BIOLOGY AND BEHAVIOR

Organization of the Nervous System

The three types of neurons in the nervous system are motor (efferent), interneurons, and sensory (afferent).

The **parasympathetic** branch of the autonomic system is focused on "rest-and-digest" responses and the **sympathetic** branch is focused on "fight-or-flight" responses.

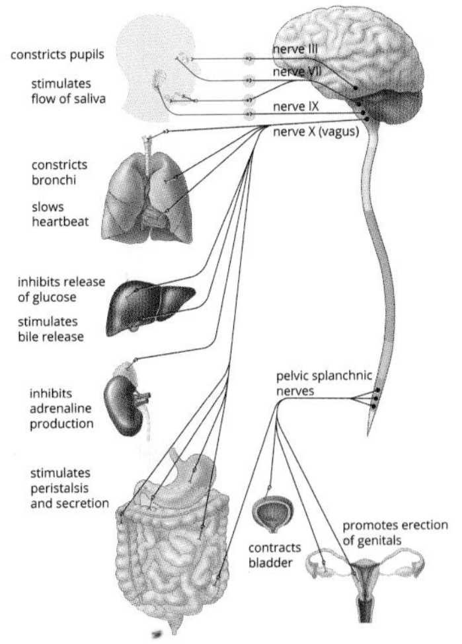

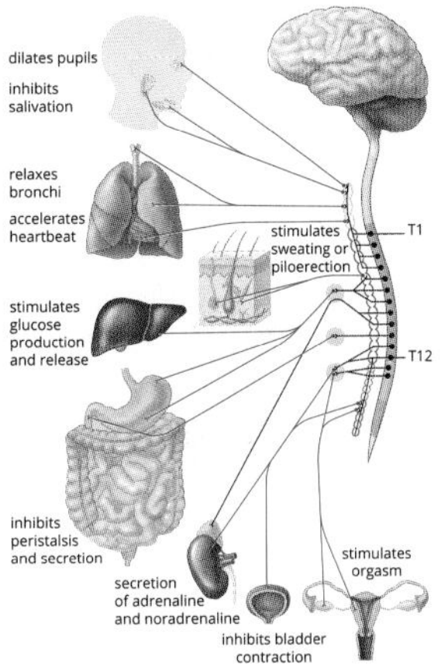

Organization of the Brain

- **Hindbrain:** contains the cerebellum, medulla oblongata, and reticular formation
- **Midbrain:** contains the inferior and superior colliculi
- **Forebrain:** contains the thalamus, hypothalamus, basal ganglia, limbic system, and cerebral cortex

Parts of the Forebrain

- **Thalamus:** relay station for sensory information
- **Hypothalamus:** maintains homeostasis and integrates with the endocrine system through the **hypophyseal portal system** that connects it to the **anterior pituitary**
- **Basal ganglia:** smoothens movements and helps maintain postural stability
- **Limbic system:** controls emotion and memory. Includes **septal nuclei** (pleasure-seeking), **amygdala** (fear and aggression), **hippocampus** (memory), and **fornix** (communication within limbic system).

The **cerebral cortex** is divided into four lobes.

Lobe	Function
Frontal	Executive function, impulse control, long-term planning (prefrontal cortex), motor function (primary motor cortex), speech production (Broca's area)
Parietal	Sensation of touch, pressure, temperature, and pain (somatosensory cortex); spatial processing, orientation, and manipulation
Occipital	Visual processing
Temporal	Sound processing (auditory cortex), speech perception (Wernicke's area), memory, and emotion (limbic system)

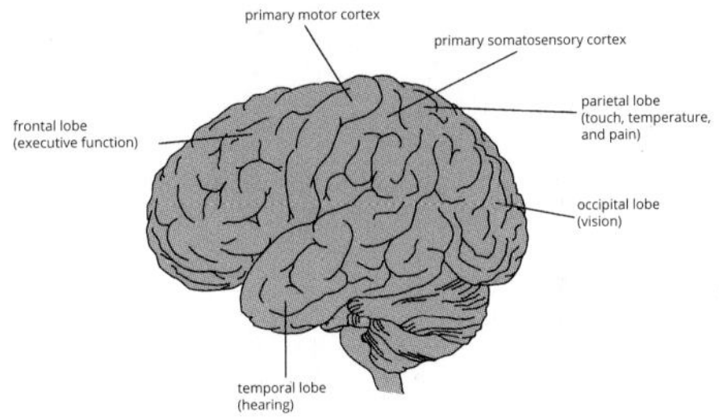

Methods of Mapping the Brain

- EEG
- rCBF
- CT
- PET
- MRI
- fMRI

Influences on Behavior

Neurotransmitter	Behavior
Acetylcholine	Voluntary muscle control, parasympathetic nervous system, attention, alertness
Epinephrine and Norepinephrine	Fight-or-flight responses, wakefulness, alertness
Dopamine	Smooth movements, postural stability
Serotonin	Mood, sleep, eating, dreaming
GABA, Glycine	Brain "stabilization"
Glutamate	Brain "excitation"
Endorphins	Natural painkillers

Nature *vs.* **nurture** is a debate regarding the contributions of genetics (nature) and environment (nurture) to an individual's traits. Family, twin, and adoption studies are used to study nature *vs.* nurture.

SENSATION AND PERCEPTION

Sensation *vs.* Perception

Sensation is the conversion of physical stimuli into neurological signals, while **perception** is the processing of sensory information to make sense of its significance.

- **Sensory receptors** respond to stimuli and trigger electrical signals.
- Sensory neurons transmit information from sensory receptors to the CNS.
- Sensory stimuli are transmitted to **projection areas** in the brain, which further analyze the sensory input.

a

perceived

Weber's law: states that the just-noticeable difference for a stimulus is proportional to the magnitude of the stimulus, and this proportion is constant over most of the range of possible stimuli

Signal detection theory: studies the effects of nonsensory factors, such as experiences, motives, and expectations, on perception of stimuli

	Subject's Response: "Yes"	Subject's Response: "No"
Signal Present	Hit	Miss
Signal Absent	False alarm	Correct negative

Response bias: examined using signal detection experiments with four possible outcomes: hits, misses, false alarms, and correct negatives

Vision

The eye is an organ specialized to detect light in the form of photons.

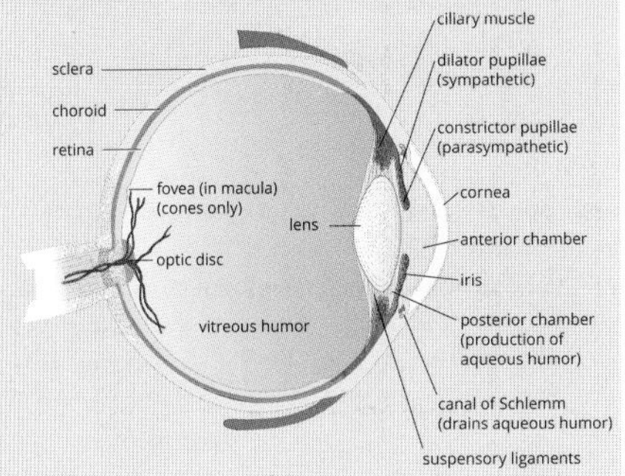

Visual pathway: retina → optic nerve → optic chiasm → optic tracts → lateral geniculate nucleus (LGN) of thalamus → visual radiations → visual cortex

Hearing and Vestibular Sense

The ear transduces sound waves into electrical signals that can be interpreted by the brain.

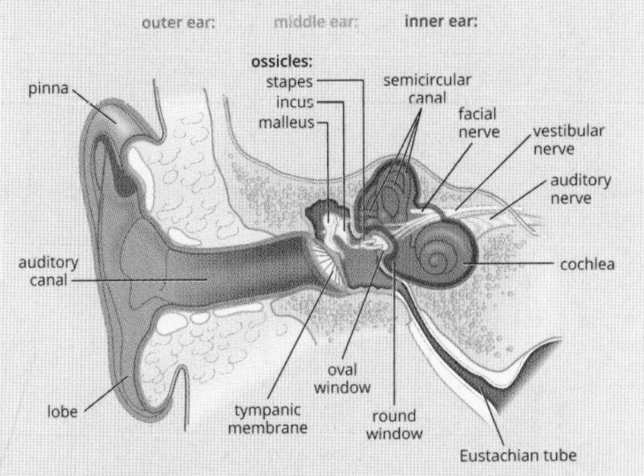

- **Cochlea:** detects sound
- **Utricle** and **saccule:** detect linear acceleration
- **Semicircular canals:** detect rotational acceleration

Auditory pathway: cochlea → vestibulocochlear nerve → medial geniculate nucleus (MGN) of thalamus → auditory cortex

Other Senses

- **Smell:** detection of volatile or aerosolized chemicals by **olfactory chemoreceptors** (**olfactory nerves**)
- **Taste:** detection of dissolved compounds by **taste buds** in **papillae**
- **Somatosensation:** four touch modalities (pressure, vibration, pain, and temperature)
- **Kinesthetic sense (proprioception):** ability to tell where one's body is in space

Object Recognition

- **Bottom-up (data-driven) processing:** recognition of objects by parallel processing and feature detection. Slower, but less prone to mistakes
- **Top-down (conceptually-driven) processing:** recognition of an object by memories and expectations, with little attention to detail. Faster, but more prone to mistakes
- **Gestalt principles:** ways that the brain can infer missing parts of an image when it is incomplete

LEARNING AND MEMORY

Learning

- **Habituation:** the process of becoming used to a stimulus
- **Dishabituation:** occurs when a second stimulus intervenes, causing a **resensitization** to the original stimulus
- **Observational learning:** the acquisition of behavior by watching others
- **Associative learning:** pairing together stimuli and responses, or behaviors and consequences
- **Classical conditioning:** a form of associative learning in which a neutral stimulus becomes associated with an **unconditioned stimulus** such that the neutral stimulus alone produces the same response as the unconditioned stimulus; the neutral stimulus thus becomes a **conditioned stimulus**

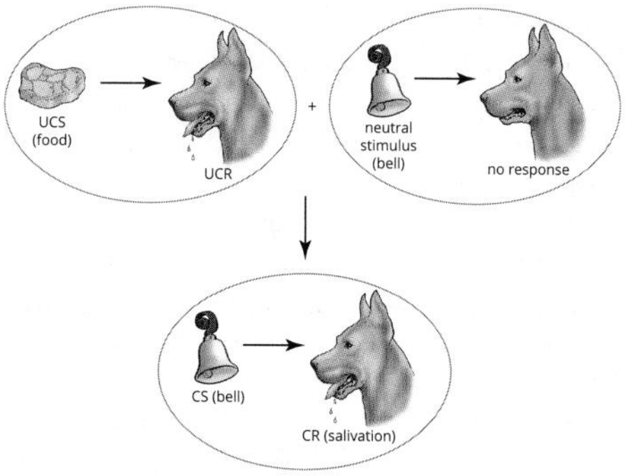

- **Operant conditioning:** a form of associative learning in which the frequency of a behavior is modified using **reinforcement** (increases behavior) or **punishment** (decreases behavior)

Behavior	Stimulus Added	Stimulus Removed
Continues	Positive reinforcement	Negative reinforcement
Stops	Positive punishment	Negative punishment

Memory

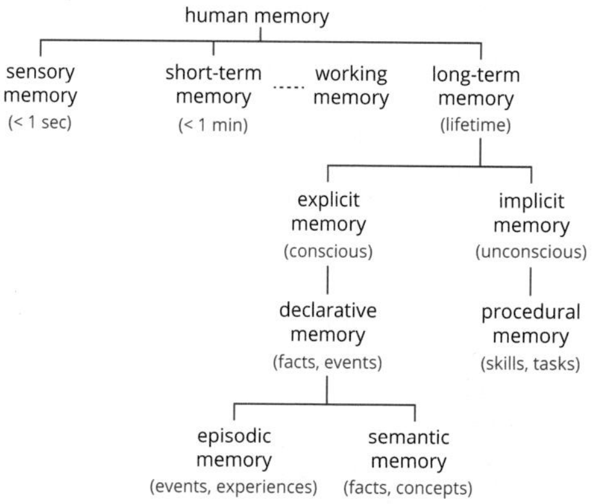

- **Encoding:** the process of putting new information into memory

Facts are stored via **semantic networks. Retrieval** of information is often based on **priming** interconnected nodes of the semantic network.

Recognition of information is stronger than **recall**.

COGNITION, CONSCIOUSNESS, AND LANGUAGE

Consciousness

Stage	EEG Waves	Features
Awake	Beta and alpha	Able to perceive, process, access, and express information
1	Theta	Light sleep
2	Theta	Sleep spindles and K complexes
3/4	Delta	Slow-wave sleep; dreams; declarative memory consolidation; some sleep disorders
REM	Mostly beta	Appears awake physiologically; dreams; paralyzed; procedural memory consolidation; some sleep disorders

Sleep disorders include **dyssomnias** (amount or timing of sleep), such as insomnia, narcolepsy, sleep apnea, and sleep deprivation; and **parasomnias** (odd behaviors during sleep), such as night terrors and sleepwalking (somnambulism).

Consciousness-Altering Drugs

Drug addiction is mediated by the **mesolimbic pathway**, which includes the **nucleus accumbens, medial forebrain bundle**, and **ventral tegmental area**. Dopamine is the main neurotransmitter.

Drug Group	Function
Depressants (alcohol, barbiturates, benzodiazepines)	Sense of relaxation and reduced anxiety
Stimulants (amphetamines, cocaine, ecstasy)	Increased arousal
Opiates/opioids (heroin, morphine, opium, pain pills)	Decreased reaction to pain; euphoria
Hallucinogens (LSD, peyote, mescaline, ketamine, psilocybin-containing mushrooms)	Distortions of reality and fantasy; introspection

Marijuana has some features of depressants, stimulants, and hallucinogens (in very high doses).

Piaget's Stages of Cognitive Development

- **Sensorimotor stage:** focuses on manipulating the environment to meet physical needs through **circular reactions; object permanence** ends this stage
- **Preoperational stage:** focuses on **symbolic thinking, egocentrism** (inability to imagine what another person thinks or feels), and **centration** (focusing on only one aspect of a phenomenon)
- **Concrete operational stage:** focuses on understanding the feelings of others and manipulating physical (concrete) objects
- **Formal operational stage:** focuses on abstract thought and problem-solving

Problem-Solving and Decision-Making

Problem-solving techniques include **trial-and-error, algorithms, deductive reasoning** (deriving conclusions from general rules) and **inductive reasoning** (deriving generalizations from evidence).

Heuristics (simplified principles used to make decisions, "rules of thumb"), biases, intuition, and emotions may assist decision-making, but may also lead to erroneous or problematic decisions.

Attention

- **Selective attention:** allows one to pay attention to a particular stimulus while determining if additional stimuli require attention in the background
- **Divided attention:** uses **automatic processing** to pay attention to multiple activities at one time

Language Areas in the Brain

- **Wernicke's area:** language comprehension; damage results in **Wernicke's aphasia** (speak fluently but have difficulty understanding language)
- **Broca's area:** motor function of speech; damage results in **Broca's aphasia** (speak comprehensibly in short sentences with great effort)
- **Arcuate fasciculus:** connects Wernicke's and Broca's areas; damage results in **conduction aphasia** (the inability to repeat words despite intact speech generation and comprehension)

MOTIVATION, EMOTION, AND STRESS

Motivation

Motivation is the purpose or driving force behind our actions.

- **Extrinsic:** based on external circumstances
- **Intrinsic:** based on internal drive or perception

Motivation theories

- **Instinct theory:** innate, fixed patterns of behavior in response to stimuli
- **Arousal theory:** the state of being awake and reactive to stimuli; aim for optimal level of arousal for a given task (Yerkes–Dodson law)

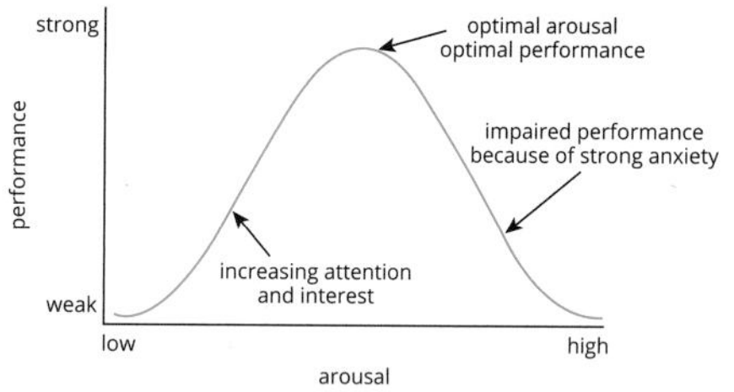

- **Drive reduction theory:** individuals act to relieve internal states of tension
- **Maslow's hierarchy of needs:** prioritizes needs into five categories: physiological needs (highest priority), safety and security, love and belonging, self-esteem, and self-actualization (lowest priority)

Emotion

Seven universal emotions: happiness, sadness, contempt, surprise, fear, disgust, anger

Theories of emotion:

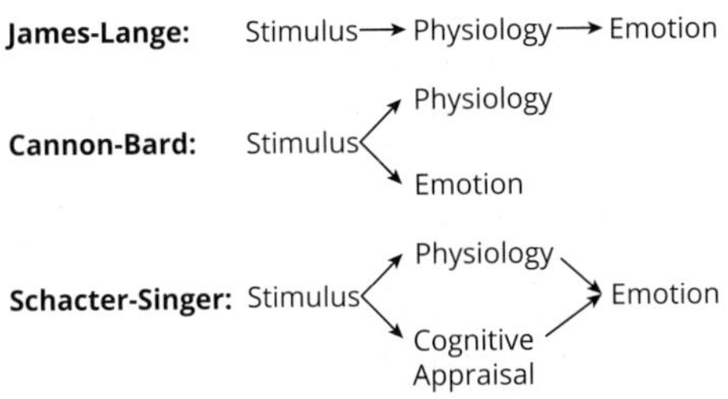

Stress

Stress: the physiological and cognitive response to challenges or life changes

- **Primary appraisal:** classifying a potential stressor as irrelevant, benign–positive, or stressful
- **Secondary appraisal:** directed at evaluating whether the organism can cope with the stress, based on harm, threat, and challenge

Stressor (distress or eustress): anything that leads to a stress response; can include environmental, social, psychological, chemical, and biological stressors

The three stages of the **general adaptation syndrome** are alarm, resistance, and exhaustion.

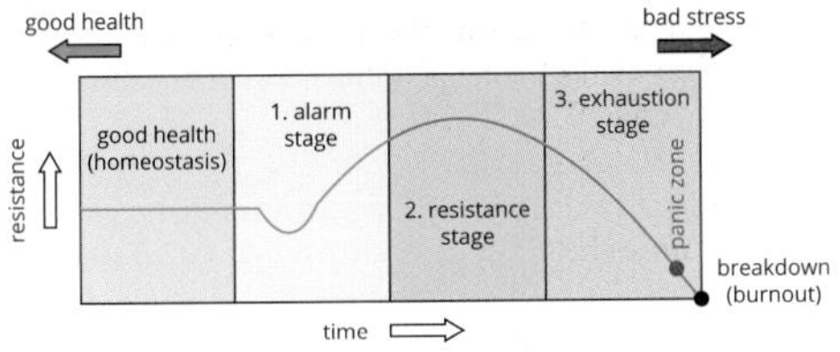

PSYCHOLOGICAL DISORDERS

***Diagnostic and Statistical Manual of Mental Disorders* (DSM):** the guide by which most psychological disorders are characterized, described, and diagnosed.

Schizophrenia and psychotic disorders

Schizophrenia: psychotic disorder characterized by distortions of reality and disturbances in content and form of thought, perception, and behavior. **Positive symptoms** include hallucinations, delusions, and disorganized thought and behavior. **Negative symptoms** include disturbance of affect and avolition.

Depressive disorders

- **Major depressive disorder:** contains at least one major depressive episode
- **Persistent depressive disorder:** a depressed mood (either **dysthymia** or major depression) for at least two years
- **Seasonal affective disorder:** the colloquial name for major depressive disorder with seasonal onset, with depression occurring during winter months

Bipolar and related disorders

- **Bipolar I disorder:** contains at least one manic episode
- **Bipolar II disorder:** contains at least one hypomanic episode and at least one major depressive episode
- **Cyclothymic disorder:** contains hypomanic episodes with dysthymia

Anxiety disorders

- **Generalized anxiety disorder:** constant disproportionate and persistent worry
- **Specific phobias:** irrational fears of specific objects
- **Social anxiety disorder:** anxiety due to social or performance situations
- **Agoraphobia:** fear of places or situations where it is hard for an individual to escape
- **Panic disorder:** recurrent attacks of intense, overwhelming fear and sympathetic nervous system activity with no clear stimulus. It may lead to **agoraphobia**.

Obsessive–compulsive disorder: obsessions (persistent, intrusive thoughts and impulses) and **compulsions** (repetitive tasks that relieve tension but cause significant impairment)

Body dysmorphic disorder: unrealistic negative evaluation of one's appearance or a specific body part

Dissociative disorders

- **Dissociative amnesia:** inability to recall past experience. May involve **dissociative fugue**, a sudden change in location that can involve the assumption of a new identity
- **Dissociative identity disorder:** two or more personalities that take control of behavior
- **Depersonalization/derealization disorder:** feelings of detachment from the mind and body, or from the environment

IDENTITY AND PERSONALITY

Self-Concept and Identity

- **Self-concept:** the sum of the ways in which we describe ourselves: in the present, who we used to be, and who we might be in the future
- **Identities:** individual components of our self-concept related to the groups to which we belong
- **Self-esteem:** our evaluation of ourselves
- **Self-efficacy:** the degree to which we see ourselves as being capable of a given skill in a given situation
- **Locus of control:** a self-evaluation that refers to the way we characterize the influences in our lives. Either **internal** (success or failure is a result of our own actions) or **external** (success or failure is a result of outside factors)

Formation of Identity

Freud's stages of psychosexual development

- Based on tensions caused by the **libido**, with failure at any given stage leading to **fixation**

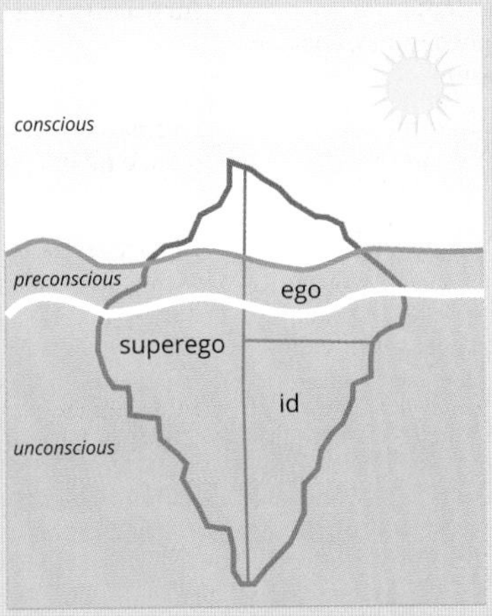

Erikson's stages of psychosocial development

- Stem from conflicts that are the result of decisions we are forced to make about ourselves and the environment around us at each phase of our lives
- Stages are trust *vs.* mistrust, autonomy *vs.* shame and doubt, initiative *vs.* guilt, industry *vs.* inferiority, identity *vs.* role confusion, intimacy *vs.* isolation, generativity *vs.* stagnation, integrity *vs.* despair

Kohlberg's theory of moral reasoning development

- Describes the approaches of individuals to resolving moral dilemmas
- Six stages are divided into three main phases: **preconventional**, **conventional**, and **postconventional**

Vygotsky's theory of cultural and biosocial development

- **Zone of proximal development:** area of learning where one cannot progress on their own, but can with assistance from a "knowledgeable other"

Personality

Psychoanalytic perspective: personality results from unconscious urges and desires

- Freud: id, superego, ego
- Jung: collective unconscious, archetypes

Humanistic perspective: emphasizes internal feelings of healthy individuals as they strive toward happiness and self-realization

- Maslow: hierarchy of needs
- Rogers: unconditional positive regard

Type and trait theory: personality can be described as a number of identifiable traits that carry characteristic behaviors

- Type theories of personality: ancient Greek humors, Sheldon's **somatotypes**, division into **Types A** and **B**, and the **Myers–Briggs Type Inventory**
- Eysenck's three major traits: psychoticism, extraversion, neuroticism
- Trait theorists' Big Five: openness, conscientiousness, extraversion, agreeableness, and neuroticism (OCEAN)
- Allport's three basic types of traits: cardinal, central, and secondary

Somatic symptom and related disorders

- **Somatic symptom disorder:** at least one somatic symptom, which may or may not be linked to an underlying medical condition, that causes disproportionate concern
- **Illness anxiety disorder:** preoccupation with having or coming down with a serious medical condition
- **Conversion disorder:** unexplained symptoms affecting motor or sensory function

Personality disorders

Patterns of inflexible, maladaptive behavior that cause distress or impaired functioning

- **Cluster A** (odd, eccentric): paranoid, schizotypal, schizoid
- **Cluster B** (dramatic, emotional, erratic, "wild"): antisocial, borderline, histrionic, narcissistic
- **Cluster C** (anxious, fearful, "worried"): avoidant, dependent, obsessive–compulsive

SOCIAL PROCESSES, ATTITUDES, AND BEHAVIOR

Group Psychology

- **Social facilitation:** tendency to perform at a different level (better or worse) when others are around
- **Deindividuation:** loss of self-awareness in large groups; can lead to drastic changes in behavior
- **Bystander effect:** in a group, individuals are less likely to respond to a person in need
- **Peer pressure:** social influence placed on an individual by other individuals they consider equals
- **Group polarization:** tendency towards making decisions in a group that are more extreme than the thoughts of the individual group members
- **Groupthink:** tendency to make decisions based on ideas and solutions that arise within the group without considering outside ideas

Culture

- **Assimilation:** one culture begins to melt into another
- **Multiculturalism:** encouragement of multiple cultures within a community to enhance diversity
- **Subculture:** a group that distinguishes itself from the primary culture to which it belongs

Socialization

- **Socialization:** the process of developing and spreading norms, customs, and beliefs
- **Norms:** boundaries of acceptable behavior within society
- **Stigma:** extreme disapproval or dislike of a person or group based on perceived differences
- **Deviance:** any violation of norms, rules, or expectations within a society
- **Conformity:** changing beliefs or behaviors in order to fit into a group or society
- **Compliance:** individuals change behavior based on the request of others; techniques for gaining compliance include **foot-in-the-door**, **door-in-the-face**, **lowball**, and **that's-not-all**
- **Obedience:** change in behavior based on a command from someone seen as an authority figure

SOCIAL INTERACTION

Elements of Social Interaction

- **Status:** a position in society used to classify individuals. Can be **ascribed** (involuntarily assigned), **achieved** (voluntarily earned), or **master** (primary identity)
- **Role:** set of beliefs, values, and norms that define the expectations of a certain status
- **Group:** two or more individuals with similar characteristics who share a sense of unity
- **Network:** observable pattern of social relationships between individuals or groups
- **Organization:** group with a structure and culture designed to achieve specific goals; exists outside of each individual's membership within the organization

Self-Presentation and Interacting with Others

- **Display rules:** unspoken rules that govern the expression of emotion
- **Impression management:** maintenance of a public image through various strategies
- **Dramaturgical approach:** individuals create images of themselves in the same way that actors perform a role in front of an audience

SOCIAL THINKING

Social Behavior

- **Interpersonal attraction:** influenced by physical, social, and psychological factors
- **Aggression:** behavior with the intention to cause harm or increase social dominance
- **Attachment:** an emotional bond to another person; usually refers to the bond between a child and a caregiver
- **Altruism:** helping behavior in which the person's intent is to benefit someone else at a personal cost

SOCIAL PERCEPTION AND BEHAVIOR

Attribution Theory

Focuses on the tendency for individuals to infer the causes of other people's behavior

- **Dispositional (internal)** causes relate to the features of the person who is being considered
- **Situational (external)** causes relate to features of the surroundings or social context
- **Correspondent inference theory:** describes attributions made by observing the intentional (especially unexpected) behaviors performed by another person
- **Fundamental attribution error:** bias toward making dispositional attributions rather than situational attributions

Stereotypes, Prejudice, and Discrimination

- **Stereotypes:** attitudes and impressions that are made based on limited and superficial information
- **Self-fulfilling prophecy:** the phenomenon of a stereotype creating an expectation of a particular group, which creates conditions that lead to confirmation of this stereotype
- **Stereotype threat:** a feeling of anxiety about confirming a negative stereotype
- **Prejudice:** an irrationally based attitude prior to actual experience
- **Ethnocentrism:** the practice of making judgments about other cultures based on the values and beliefs of one's own culture (**in-group** *vs.* **out-group**)
- **Cultural relativism:** studying social groups and cultures on their own terms
- **Discrimination:** when prejudicial attitudes cause differences in treatment of a group

SOCIAL STRUCTURE AND DEMOGRAPHICS

Sociology: Theories and Institutions

- **Functionalism:** macro-level theory focused on how parts of society work together
- **Conflict theory:** focuses on how unequal division of resources create power differentials
- **Symbolic interactionism:** the study of how individuals interact through a shared understanding of words, gestures, and other symbols
- **Social constructionism:** explores how individuals and groups make decisions to agree upon a given social reality

Culture

- **Material culture:** physical items one associates with a given group (art, clothing, foods, buildings)
- **Symbolic culture:** the ideas associated with a cultural group

Demographics

Demographics: the statistical arm of sociology

Migration: the movement of people into (immigration) or out of (emigration) a geographical location

Demographic transition: a model used to represent drops in birth and death rates as a result of industrialization

SOCIAL STRATIFICATION

Social Class

Social stratification is based on **socioeconomic status (SES)**.

- **Class:** a category of people with shared socioeconomic characteristics
- **Power:** the capacity to influence people through real or perceived rewards and punishments
- **Social capital:** the investment people make in society in return for economic or collective rewards
- **Social reproduction:** the passing on of social inequality, especially poverty, to other generations
- **Poverty:** low SES; in the US, the poverty line is the government's calculation of the minimum income requirements to acquire the minimum necessities of life

Epidemiology

Incidence: $\frac{\text{new cases}}{\text{population at risk}}$ per time

Prevalence: $\frac{\text{number of cases (new or old)}}{\text{total population}}$ per time

Morbidity: the burden or degree of illness associated with a given disease

Mortality: deaths caused by a given disease

AMINO ACIDS, PEPTIDES, AND PROTEINS

Amino Acids Found in Proteins

Amino acids have an amino group, carboxylic acid, a hydrogen atom, and an **R group** attached to a central α-carbon.

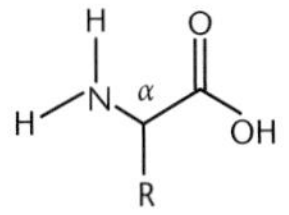

Full Name	3-Letter Code	1-Letter Code	Structure	pK_a	Group	Special Properties
Glycine	Gly	G	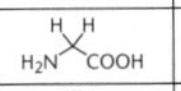	Neutral	Small	Not chiral; found in structural loops
Alanine	Ala	A	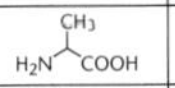	Neutral	Small, nonpolar	
Serine	Ser	S	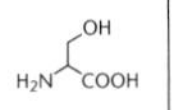	Neutral	Polar	Can form H-bonds; can be phosphorylated to introduce a negative charge
Threonine	Thr	T	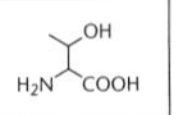	Neutral	Polar	Can form H-bonds; can be phosphorylated to introduce a negative charge
Cysteine	Cys	C	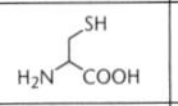	Slightly basic	Polar	Forms disulfide bridges, important for 3° and 4° structure
Valine	Val	V	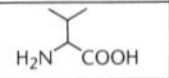	Neutral	Nonpolar	
Leucine	Leu	L	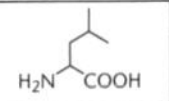	Neutral	Nonpolar	
Isoleucine	Ile	I	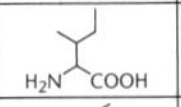	Neutral	Nonpolar	
Methionine	Met	M	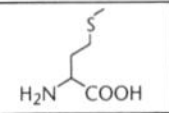	Neutral	Nonpolar	"Start" amino acid (can also be found at other positions)
Proline	Pro	P	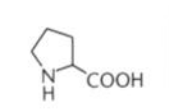	Neutral	Nonpolar	The only cis-amino acid; side chain part of peptide bond; introduces kinks in α-helices; found in loops and turns
Phenylalanine	Phe	F	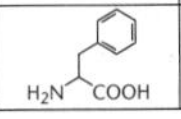	Neutral	Nonpolar	Aromatic

Acid–Base Chemistry of Amino Acids

Amino acids are amphoteric.

- At low (acidic) pH: fully protonated
- When pH = pI: zwitterion
- At high (basic) pH: fully deprotonated

pI is determined by averaging the pK_a values that refer to protonation and deprotonation of the zwitterion.

Full Name	3-Letter Code	1-Letter Code	Structure	pK_a	Group	Special Properties
Tyrosine	Tyr	Y	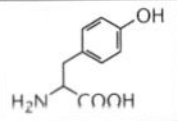	Neutral	Nonpolar	Aromatic; can be phosphorylated to introduce a negative charge
Tryptophan	Trp	W	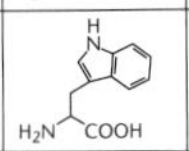	Neutral	Nonpolar	Aromatic
Aspartate	Asp	D	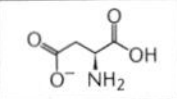	Acidic	Negatively charged at physiological pH	Side chain can form salt bridge
Glutamate	Glu	E	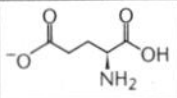	Acidic	Negatively charged at physiological pH	Side chain can form salt bridge
Asparagine	Asn	N	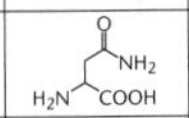	Neutral	Polar	Side chain can form H-bonds
Glutamine	Gln	Q	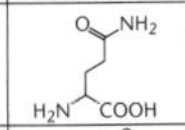	Neutral	Polar	Side chain can form H-bonds
Histidine	His	H	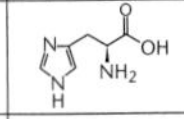	Slightly acidic	Polar	Aromatic; can be positively charged at acidic pH
Lysine	Lys	K	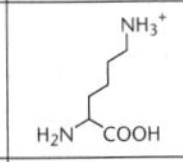	Basic	Positively charged at physiological pH	Side chain can form salt bridge; can be acetylated to mask the positive charge (important in DNA-protein interaction)
Arginine	Arg	R	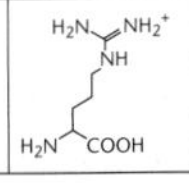	Basic	Positively charged	Side chain can form salt bridge

Peptide Bond Formation and Hydrolysis

Peptide bond formation is a **condensation (dehydration)** reaction with a nucleophilic amino group attacking an electrophilic carbonyl. Peptide bonds are broken by **hydrolysis**.

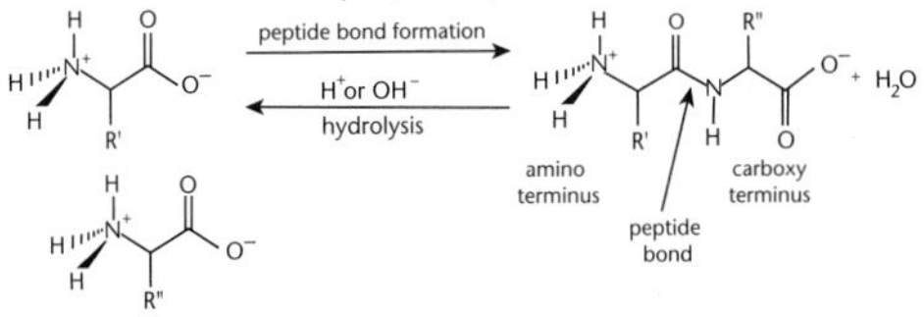

Protein Structure

Primary structure: linear sequence of amino acids

Secondary structure: local structure stabilized by noncovalent bonds; includes **α-helices** and **β-sheets**

Tertiary structure: three-dimensional structure stabilized by hydrophobic interactions, acid–base interactions (salt bridges), hydrogen bonding, and disulfide bonds

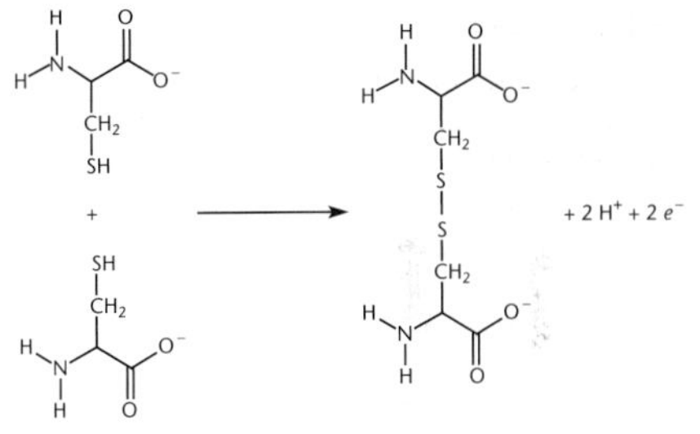

cysteine cystine

Quaternary structure: interactions between subunits
Heat and solutes can cause **denaturation.**

ENZYMES

Enzymes, like all catalysts, lower the activation energy necessary for reactions. They do not alter the free energy (ΔG) or enthalpy (ΔH) change that accompanies the reaction nor the final equilibrium position; rather, they change the rate (kinetics) at which equilibrium is reached.

- **Ligases** are responsible for joining two large biomolecules, often of the same type.
- **Isomerases** catalyze the interconversion of isomers, including both constitutional and stereoisomers.
- **Lyases** catalyze cleavage without the addition of water and without the transfer of electrons. The reverse reaction (synthesis) is usually more biologically important.
- **Hydrolases** catalyze cleavage with the addition of water.
- **Oxidoreductases** catalyze oxidation–reduction reactions that involve the transfer of electrons.
- **Transferases** move a functional group from one molecule to another molecule.

Michaelis–Menten

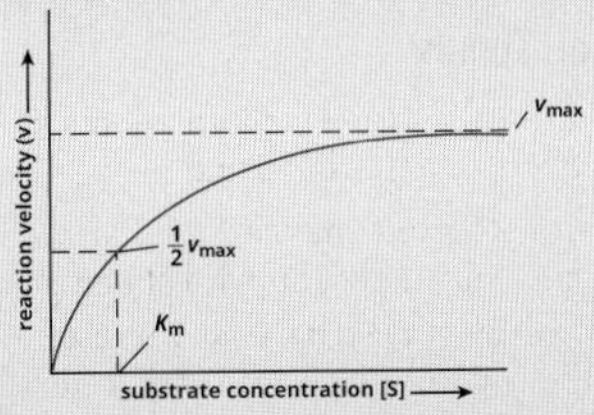

Cooperative enzymes show a **sigmoidal** curve.

Lineweaver–Burk

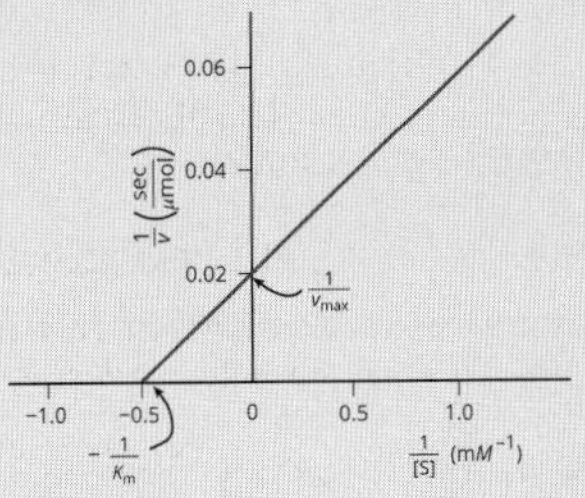

Enzyme Kinetics

Saturation kinetics: As substrate concentration increases, the reaction rate also increases until a maximum value is reached.

$$v = \frac{v_{max}[S]}{K_m + [S]}$$

At one-half v_{max}, $[S] = K_m$

$$k_{cat} = \frac{v_{max}}{[\text{enzyme}]}$$

$$\text{catalytic efficiency} = \frac{k_{cat}}{K_m}$$

Regulation of Enzyme Activity

	Competitive	Noncompetitive	Mixed	Uncompetitive
Binding Site	Active site	Allosteric site	Allosteric site	Enzyme-substrate complex
Impact on K_m	Increases	No change	Increases or decreases	Decreases
Impact on v_{max}	No change	Decreases	Decreases	Decreases

NONENZYMATIC PROTEIN FUNCTION AND PROTEIN ANALYSIS

Protein analysis

Polyacrylamide gel electrophoresis (PAGE): proteins migrate through porous matrix according to size and charge. **Native PAGE** is used to analyze the protein in folded state, whereas **SDS-PAGE** uses detergent to break all noncovalent interactions and analyzes the unfolded state. **Reducing** reagents can be used to break covalent disulfide bonds.

Cellular Functions and Biosignaling

Structural proteins: generally fibrous. Include **collagen, elastin, keratin, actin,** and **tubulin**

Motor proteins: capable of force generation through a conformational change. Include **myosin, kinesin,** and **dynein**

Cell adhesion molecules (CAM): bind cells to other cells or surfaces. Include **cadherins, integrins,** and **selectins**

Ion channels can be used for regulating ion flow into or out of a cell. There are three main types of ion channels: **ungated channels, voltage-gated channels,** and **ligand-gated channels.**

Enzyme-linked receptors participate in cell signaling through extracellular ligand binding and initiation of second messenger cascades.

G protein-coupled receptors have a membrane-bound protein associated with a trimeric **G protein.** They also initiate second messenger systems.

CARBOHYDRATE STRUCTURE AND FUNCTION

Carbohydrate Classification

Carbohydrates are organized by their number of carbon atoms and functional groups.

- 3-carbon sugars are **trioses**, 4-carbon sugars are **tetroses**, and so on.
- Sugars with aldehydes as their most oxidized group are **aldoses**; sugars with ketones as their most oxidized group are **ketoses**.

Sugars with the highest-numbered chiral carbon with the –OH group on the right (in a Fischer projection) are D-sugars; those with the –OH on the left are L-sugars. D- and L-forms of the same sugar are **enantiomers**.

Diastereomers differ at at least one—but not all—chiral carbons. Also include:

- **Epimers** differ at exactly one chiral carbon.
- **Anomers** are a subtype of epimers that differ at the anomeric carbon.

Cyclic Sugar Molecules

Cyclization describes the ring formation of carbohydrates from their straight-chain forms.

When rings form, the anomeric carbon can take on either an α- or β-conformation.

The **anomeric carbon** is the new chiral center formed in ring closure; it was the carbon containing the carbonyl in the straight-chain form.

- **α-anomers** have the –OH on the anomeric carbon *trans* to the free $-CH_2OH$ group.
- **β-anomers** have the –OH on the anomeric carbon *cis* to the free $-CH_2OH$ group.

During **mutarotation**, one anomeric form shifts to another, with the straight-chain form as an intermediate.

Monosaccharides

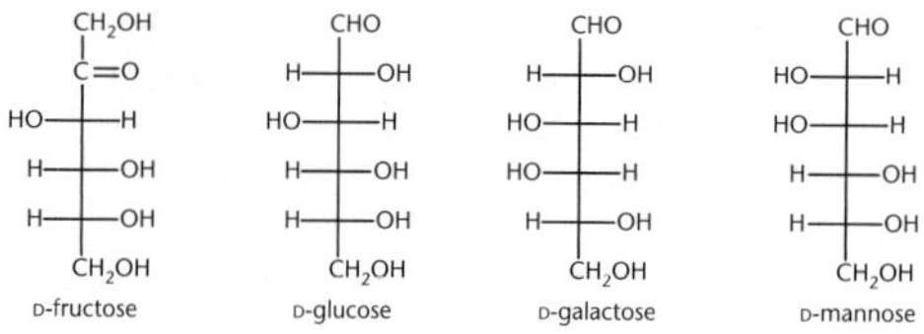

Monosaccharides are single carbohydrate units and can undergo three main reactions: **oxidation–reduction**, **esterification**, and **glycoside formation**.

Glycoside formation is the basis for building complex carbohydrates and requires the anomeric carbon to link to another sugar.

Sugars with a –H replacing an –OH group are termed **deoxy sugars**.

Disaccharides

Common **disaccharides** include **sucrose** (glucose-α-1,2-fructose), **lactose** (galactose-β-1,4-glucose), and **maltose** (glucose-α-1,4-glucose).

Polysaccharides

- **Cellulose:** main structural component of plant cell walls; main source of fiber in the human diet
- **Starches (amylose and amylopectin):** main energy storage forms for plants
- **Glycogen:** a major energy storage form for animals

Reducing sugars

Any sugar with an anomeric carbon not bound in a glycosidic bond will react with reagents like **Tollens'** and **Benedict's**.

DNA AND BIOTECHNOLOGY

DNA Structure

Nucleosides contain a five-carbon sugar bonded to a nitrogenous base; **nucleotides** are nucleosides with one to three phosphate groups added. ATP is a high-energy nucleotide with an adenosine nucleoside.

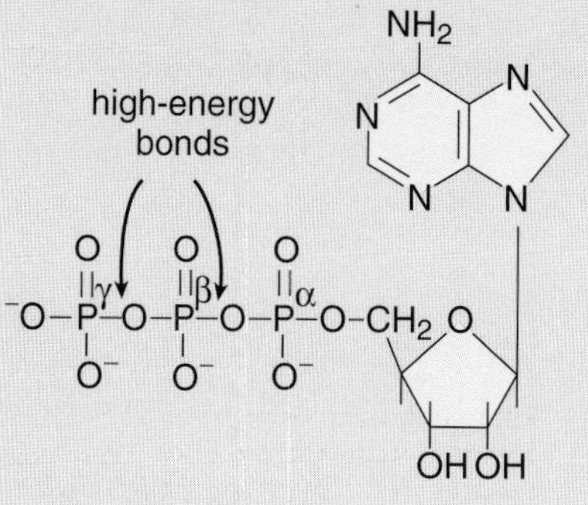

Nucleotides in DNA contain deoxyribose; in RNA, they contain ribose.

Nucleotides are abbreviated by letter: adenine (A), cytosine (C), guanine (G), thymine (T), and uracil (U).

Watson-Crick Model

- The DNA backbone is composed of alternating sugar and phosphate groups, and is always read **5' to 3'**.
- There are two strands with **antiparallel** polarity, wound into a **double helix**.
- **Purines** (A and G) always pair with **pyrimidines** (C, U, and T). In DNA, A pairs with T (via two hydrogen bonds) and C pairs with G (via three hydrogen bonds). In RNA, A pairs with U (via two hydrogen bonds).
- **Chargaff's rules:** purines and pyrimidines are equal in number in a DNA molecule. The amount of A equals the amount of T, and the amount of C equals the amount of G.

DNA strands can be pulled apart (**denatured**) and brought back together (**reannealed**).

Eukaryotic Chromosome Organization

DNA is organized into 46 chromosomes in human cells.

In eukaryotes, DNA is wound around **histone proteins** (H2A, H2B, H3, and H4) to form **nucleosomes**, which may be stabilized by another histone protein (H1). DNA and its associated histones make up **chromatin** in the nucleus.

- **Heterochromatin** is dense, transcriptionally silent DNA.
- **Euchromatin** is less dense, transcriptionally active DNA.

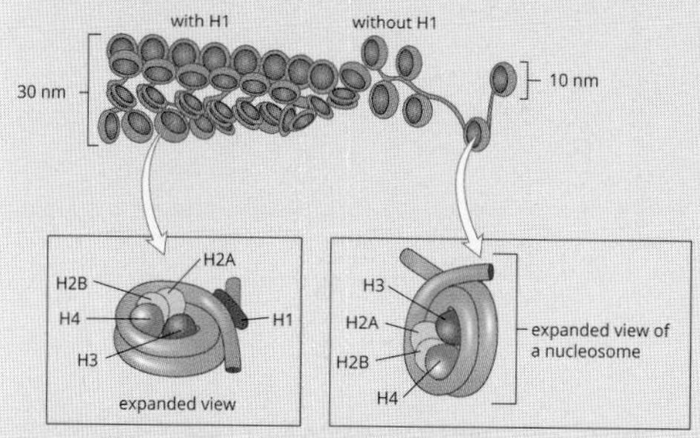

Telomeres are the ends of chromosomes. They contain high GC-content to prevent DNA unraveling.

Centromeres hold sister chromatids together until they are separated during anaphase in mitosis. They also contain a high GC-content.

DNA Replication

Step in Replication	Prokaryotic Cells	Eukaryotic Cells (Nuclei)
Origin of replication	One per chromosome	Multiple per chromosome
Unwinding of DNA double helix	Helicase	Helicase
Stabilization of unwound template strands	Single-stranded DNA-binding protein	Single-stranded DNA-binding protein
Synthesis of RNA primers	Primase	Primase
Synthesis of DNA	DNA polymerase III	DNA polymerases α, δ, and ε
Removal of RNA primers	DNA polymerase I (5′→3′ exonuclease)	RNase H (5′→3′ exonuclease)
Replacement of RNA with DNA	DNA polymerase I	DNA polymerase δ
Joining of Okazaki fragments	DNA ligase	DNA ligase
Removal of positive supercoils ahead of advancing replication forks	DNA topoisomerases (DNA gyrase)	DNA topoisomerases
Synthesis of telomeres	Not applicable	Telomerase

DNA replication is **semiconservative**: one old **parent strand** and one new **daughter strand** is incorporated into each of the two new DNA molecules.

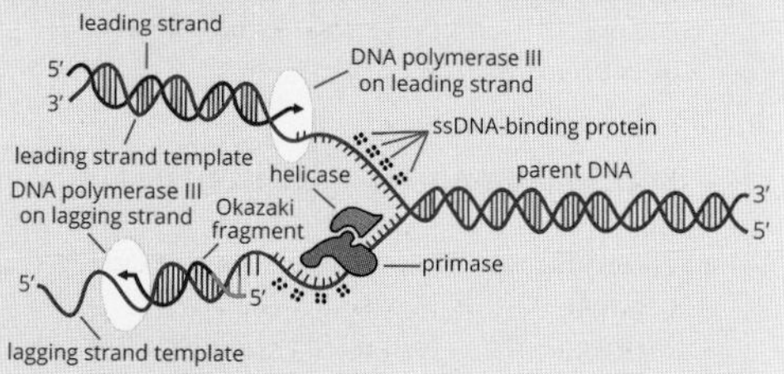

DNA polymerase synthesizes new DNA strands, reading the template DNA 3′ to 5′ and synthesizing the new strand 5′ to 3′.

- The **leading strand** requires only one primer and can then be synthesized continuously.
- The **lagging strand** requires many primers and is synthesized in discrete sections called **Okazaki fragments**.

Recombinant DNA and Biotechnology

Recombinant DNA is DNA composed of nucleotides from two different sources.

DNA cloning introduces a fragment of DNA into a **vector plasmid**. A **restriction enzyme** (**restriction endonuclease**) cuts both the plasmid and the fragment, leaving them with **sticky ends**, which can bind. Restriction enzyme sites are often palindromic.

Once replicated, the bacterial cells can be used to create a protein of interest, or can be lysed to allow for isolation of the fragment of interest from the vector.

DNA libraries are large collections of known DNA sequences.

- **Genomic libraries** contain large fragments of DNA, including both coding and noncoding regions of the genome. They cannot be used to make recombinant proteins or for gene therapy.
- **cDNA libraries (expression libraries)** are generated by reverse transcribing mRNA of sample tissue. The resulting DNA library only includes exons of expressed genes. They can be used to make recombinant proteins or for gene therapy.

Hybridization is the joining of complementary base pair sequences.

Polymerase chain reaction (PCR) is an automated process by which millions of copies of a DNA sequence can be created from a very small sample by hybridization.

DNA molecules can be separated by size using **agarose gel electrophoresis**.

Southern blotting can be used to detect the presence and quantity of various DNA strands in a sample. After electrophoresis, the sample is transferred to a membrane that can be **probed** with single-stranded DNA molecules to look for a sequence of interest.

DNA sequencing uses **dideoxyribonucleotides**, which terminate the DNA chain because they lack a 3′–OH group.

RNA AND THE GENETIC CODE

Central Dogma: DNA → RNA → proteins

The Genetic Code

Degenerate code allows multiple codons to encode for the same amino acid.

- **Initiation:** AUG (methionine)
- **Termination:** UAA, UGA, UAG
- Redundancy and **wobble** (third base in the codon) allow mutations to occur without affecting the protein.

Point mutations can cause:

- **Silent** mutations, with no effect on protein synthesis
- **Nonsense (truncation)** mutations, which produce a premature stop codon
- **Missense** mutations, which produce a codon that codes for a different amino acid
- **Frameshift mutations**, which result from nucleotide addition or deletion and change the reading frame of subsequent codons

RNA is structurally similar to DNA except:

- Substitution of a ribose sugar for deoxyribose
- Substitution of uracil for thymine
- Single-stranded instead of double-stranded

There are three major types of RNA in transcription:

- **Messenger RNA (mRNA):** carries the message from DNA in the nucleus via transcription of the gene; travels into the cytoplasm to be translated
- **Transfer RNA (tRNA):** brings in amino acids; recognizes the codon on the mRNA using its anticodon
- **Ribosomal RNA (rRNA):** makes up much of the ribosome; enzymatically active

Transcription

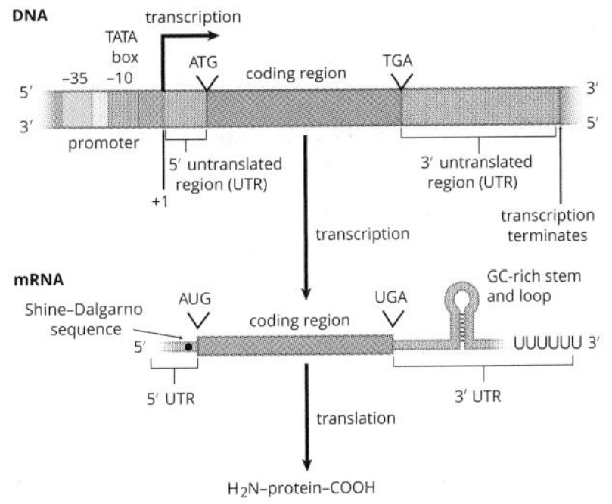

Steps:

- Helicase and topoisomerase unwind DNA double helix.
- **RNA polymerase II** binds to **TATA box** within **promoter** region of gene (25 base pairs upstream from first transcribed base).
- **hnRNA** synthesized from DNA template (antisense) strand.

Posttranscriptional modifications:

- 7-methylguanylate triphosphate cap added to 5′ end
- Polyadenosyl (poly-A) tail added to 3′ end
- Splicing done by **spliceosome**; introns removed and exons ligated together. **Alternative splicing** combines different exons to acquire different gene products.

Translation

Occurs at the ribosome.

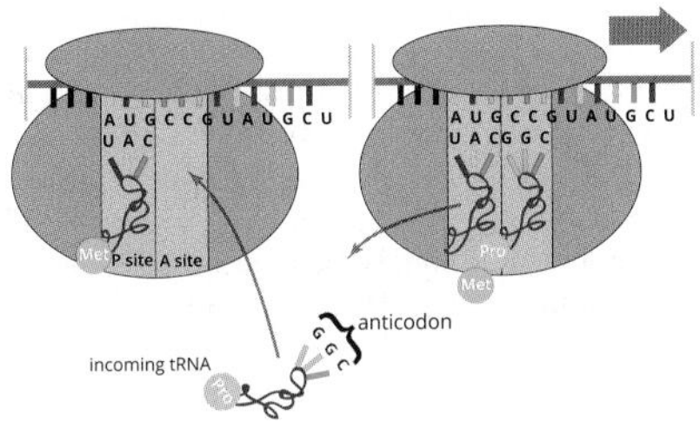

Three stages: **initiation**, **elongation**, **termination**

Posttranslational modifications:

- Folding by **chaperones**
- Formation of quaternary structure
- Cleavage of proteins or signal sequences
- Covalent addition of other biomolecules (phosphorylation, carboxylation, glycosylation, prenylation)

Control of Gene Expression in Prokaryotes

Operons (Jacob–Monod model) are inducible or repressible clusters of genes transcribed as a single mRNA.

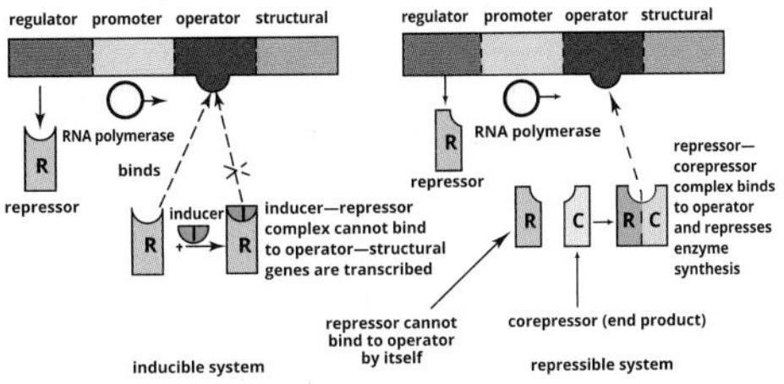

Control of Gene Expression in Eukaryotes

Transcription factors search for promoter and enhancer regions in the DNA.

- **Promoters** are within 25 base pairs of the transcription start site.
- **Enhancers** are more than 25 base pairs away from the transcription start site.

BIOLOGICAL MEMBRANES

Membrane Transport

Osmotic pressure, a **colligative property**, is the pressure applied to a pure solvent to prevent osmosis and is related to the concentration of the solution.

$$\Pi = iMRT$$

Passive transport does not require ATP because the molecule is moving down its concentration gradient or from an area of higher concentration to an area of lower concentration.

- **Simple diffusion** does not require a transporter. Small, nonpolar molecules passively move from an area of high concentration to an area of low concentration until equilibrium is achieved.
- **Osmosis** describes the diffusion of water across a selectively permeable membrane.
- **Facilitated diffusion** uses transport proteins to move impermeable solutes across the cell membrane.

Active transport requires energy in the form of ATP (**primary**) or an existing favorable ion gradient (**secondary**). Secondary active transport can be further classified as **symport** or **antiport**.

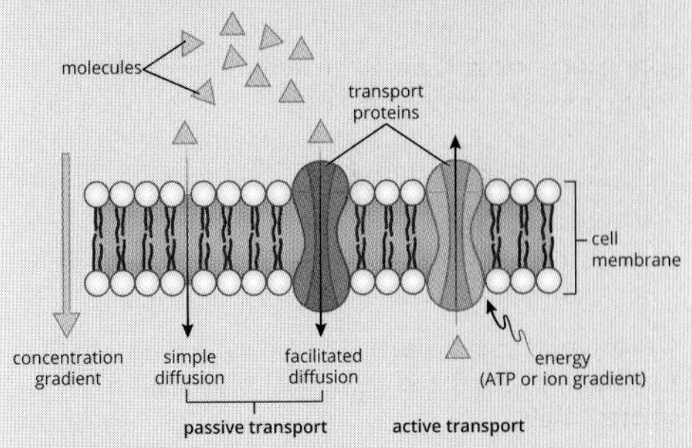

Endocytosis and **exocytosis** are methods of engulfing material into cells or releasing material to the exterior of cells, both via the cell membrane. **Pinocytosis** is the ingestion of liquid into the cell from vesicles formed from the cell membrane and **phagocytosis** is the ingestion of solid material.

CARBOHYDRATE METABOLISM

Glycolysis

Occurs in the cytoplasm of all cells, and does not require oxygen. Yields 2 ATP per glucose. Important enzymes include:

- **Glucokinase:** present in liver and pancreatic β cells, responsive to insulin; phosphorylates glucose
- **Hexokinase:** present in all tissue; phosphorylates glucose to trap it in cells
- **Phosphofructokinase-1 (PFK-1):** rate-limiting step
- **Phosphofructokinase-2 (PFK-2):** produces F2,6-BP, which activates PFK-1
- **Glyceraldehyde-3-phosphate dehydrogenase:** produces NADH
- **3-phosphoglycerate kinase** and **pyruvate kinase:** perform **substrate-level phosphorylation**

Glucokinase/hexokinase, PFK-1, and pyruvate kinase catalyze irreversible reactions.

The NADH produced in glycolysis is oxidized aerobically by the mitochondrial electron transport chain and anaerobically by cytoplasmic **lactate dehydrogenase**.

Pyruvate Dehydrogenase

- Converts pyruvate to acetyl-CoA. Stimulated by insulin and inhibited by acetyl-CoA.

The Citric Acid Cycle

Takes place in mitochondrial matrix. Main purpose is to oxidize acetyl-CoA to CO_2 and generate high-energy electron carriers (NADH and $FADH_2$) and GTP.

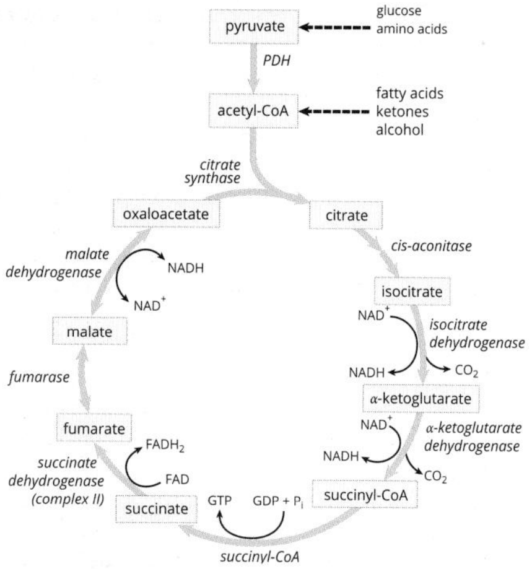

The Electron Transport Chain

Takes place on the matrix-facing surface of the inner mitochondrial membrane.

NADH donates electrons to the chain, which are passed from one complex to the next. Reduction potentials increase down the chain, until the electrons end up on oxygen, which has the highest reduction potential.

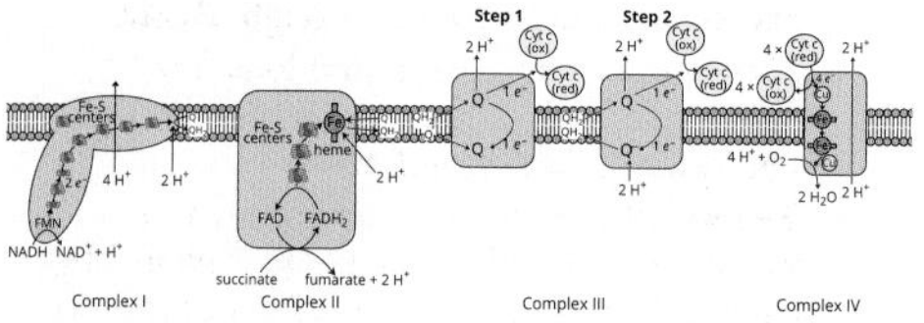

NADH cannot cross the inner mitochondrial membrane, so must use one of two shuttle mechanisms to transfer its electrons to energy carriers in the mitochondrial matrix: the **glycerol 3-phosphate shuttle** or the **malate–aspartate shuttle**.

Oxidative Phosphorylation

The **proton-motive force** is the electrochemical gradient generated by the electron transport chain across the inner mitochondrial membrane. The intermembrane space has a higher concentration of protons than the matrix; this gradient stores energy, which can be used to form ATP via **chemiosmotic coupling**.

ATP synthase is the enzyme responsible for generating ATP from ADP and an inorganic phosphate (P_i).

Summary of the energy yield of the various carbohydrate metabolism processes:

- Glycolysis: 2 NADH and 2 ATP
- Pyruvate dehydrogenase: 1 NADH (2 NADH per molecule of glucose because each glucose forms two molecules of pyruvate)
- Citric acid cycle: 3 NADH, 1 $FADH_2$, and 1 GTP (6 NADH, 2 $FADH_2$, and 2 GTP per molecule of glucose)
- Each NADH: 2.5 ATP; 10 NADH form 25 ATP
- Each $FADH_2$: 1.5 ATP; 2 $FADH_2$ form 3 ATP
- GTP are converted to ATP.
- 2 ATP from glycolysis + 2 ATP (GTP) from citric acid cycle + 25 ATP from NADH + 3 ATP from $FADH_2$ = 32 ATP per molecule of glucose (optimal). 30–32 ATP per molecule of glucose is the commonly accepted range for energy yield.

Glycogenesis and Glycogenolysis

Glycogenesis (glycogen synthesis) is the building of glycogen using two main enzymes:

- **Glycogen synthase**, which creates α-1,4 glycosidic links between glucose molecules. It is activated by insulin in the liver and muscles.
- **Branching enzyme**, which moves a block of oligoglucose from one chain and connects it as a branch using an α-1,6 glycosidic link.

Glycogenolysis is the breakdown of glycogen using two main enzymes:

- **Glycogen phosphorylase**, which removes single glucose 1-phosphate molecules by breaking α-1,4 glycosidic links. In the liver, it is activated by glucagon to prevent low blood sugar. In exercising skeletal muscle, it is activated by epinephrine and AMP to provide glucose for the muscle itself.
- **Debranching enzyme**, which moves a block of oligoglucose from one branch and connects it to the chain using an α-1,4 glycosidic link.

Gluconeogenesis

Occurs in both the cytoplasm and mitochondria, predominantly in the liver. Most of gluconeogenesis is just the reverse of glycolysis, using the same enzymes.

The three irreversible steps of glycolysis must be bypassed by different enzymes:

- Pyruvate carboxylase and PEP carboxykinase bypass pyruvate kinase
- Fructose-1,6-bisphosphatase bypasses phosphofructokinase-1
- Glucose-6-phosphatase bypasses hexokinase/glucokinase

The Pentose Phosphate Pathway

Occurs in the cytoplasm of most cells, generating **NADPH** and sugars for biosynthesis. Rate-limiting enzyme is **glucose-6-phosphate dehydrogenase**, which is activated by $NADP^+$ and insulin and inhibited by NADPH.

BIOENERGETICS AND REGULATION OF METABOLISM

Metabolic States

- In the **postprandial/well-fed (absorptive) state**, insulin secretion is high and anabolic metabolism prevails.
- In the **postabsorptive (fasting) state**, insulin secretion decreases while glucagon and catecholamine secretion increases.
- Prolonged fasting (**starvation**) dramatically increases glucagon and catecholamine secretion. Most tissues rely on fatty acids.

LIPID AND AMINO ACID METABOLISM

Lipid Transport

Lipids are transported via **chylomicrons**, **VLDL**, **IDL**, **LDL**, and **HDL**.

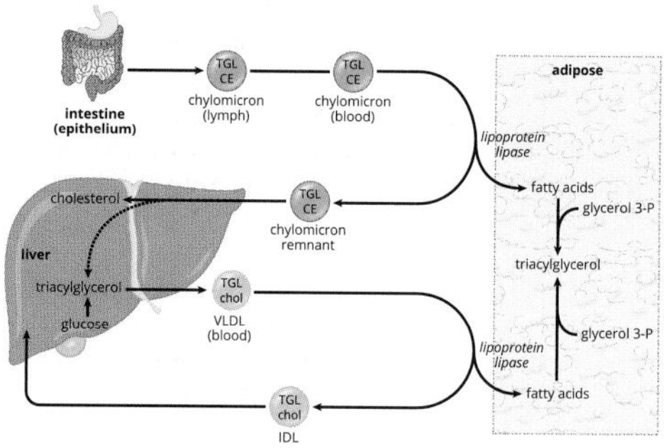

Cholesterol Metabolism

- Cholesterol may be obtained through dietary sources or through synthesis in the liver.
- The key enzyme in cholesterol biosynthesis is **HMG-CoA reductase.**

Palmitic acid, the only fatty acid that humans can synthesize, is produced in the cytoplasm from acetyl-CoA transported out of the mitochondria.

Fatty acid oxidation occurs in the mitochondria, following transport by the carnitine shuttle, via ***β*-oxidation**.

Ketone bodies form (**ketogenesis**) during a prolonged starvation state due to excess acetyl-CoA in the liver. **Ketolysis** regenerates acetyl-CoA for use as an energy source in peripheral tissues.

Protein Catabolism

Protein digestion occurs primarily in the small intestine. Carbon skeletons of amino acids are used for energy, either through gluconeogenesis or ketone body formation. Amino groups are fed into the **urea cycle** for excretion.

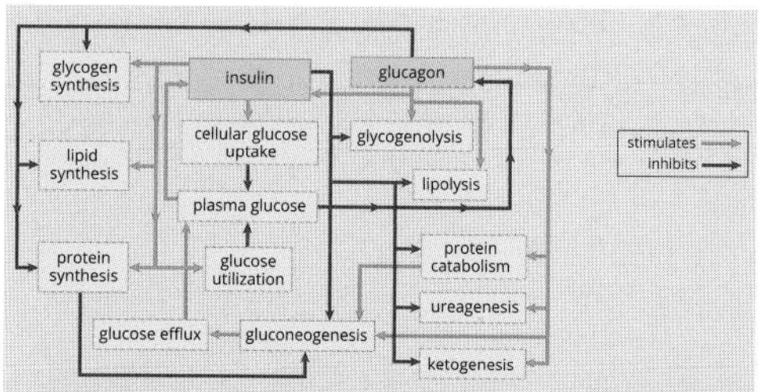

Tissue-Specific Metabolism

- Liver: maintains blood glucose through glycogenolysis and gluconeogenesis. Processes lipids, cholesterol, bile, urea, and toxins.
- Adipose: stores and releases lipids
- Resting muscle: conserves carbohydrates as glycogen and uses free fatty acids for fuel
- Active muscle: may use anaerobic metabolism, oxidative phosphorylation, direct phosphorylation (creatine phosphate), or fatty acid oxidation
- Cardiac muscle: uses fatty acid oxidation
- Brain: uses glucose except in prolonged starvation, when it can use ketolysis

THE CELL

Organelles of Eukaryotic Cells

- **Nucleus:** contains all of the genetic material necessary for replication of the cell
- **Mitochondrion:** location of many metabolic processes (pyruvate dehydrogenase, citric acid cycle, ETC, oxidative phosphorylation, β-oxidation, some of gluconeogenesis, urea cycle) and ATP production
- **Lysosomes:** membrane-bound structures containing hydrolytic enzymes capable of breaking down many different substrates
- **Rough endoplasmic reticulum:** interconnected membranous structure with ribosomes studding the outside; site of synthesis of proteins destined for insertion into a membrane or secretion
- **Smooth endoplasmic reticulum:** interconnected membranous structure where lipid synthesis and detoxification occurs
- **Golgi apparatus:** membrane-bound sacs where posttranslational modification of proteins occurs
- **Peroxisomes:** organelle containing hydrogen peroxide; site of β-oxidation of very long chain fatty acids

Fluid Mosaic Model and Membrane Traffic

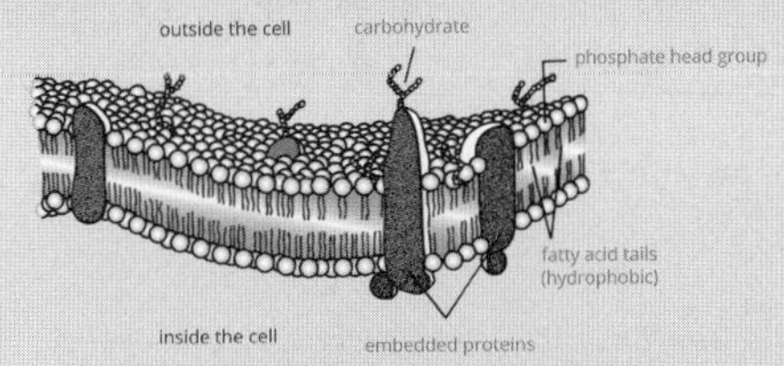

- Phospholipid bilayer with cholesterol and embedded proteins
- Exterior: hydrophilic phosphate head groups
- Interior: hydrophobic fatty acids

The original form of the **cell theory** consisted of three basic tenets:

- All living things are composed of cells.
- The cell is the basic functional unit of life.
- Cells arise only from preexisting cells.

A fourth tenet has been added as a result of advances in molecular biology: cells carry genetic information in the form of DNA. This genetic material is passed on from parent to daughter cell.

Eukaryotes contain membrane-bound organelles such as a nucleus, while prokaryotes are simpler cells without a nucleus.

Prokaryotes

- Classified by shape: Spherical bacteria are known as **cocci**, while rod-shaped bacteria are known as **bacilli**. Spiral-shaped bacteria are known as **spirilli**.
- Cell wall and cell membrane form the envelope. Composition of the cell wall further classifies bacteria into gram-positive and gram-negative. **Gram-positive** bacteria have large quantities of peptidoglycan in the cell wall, while **gram-negative** bacteria have much smaller quantities of peptidoglycan with lipopolysaccharides.
- Structure of flagella in bacteria is much different than that of eukaryotes. Eukaryotic flagella contain a basal body that serves as the engine for motion.
- All prokaryotes divide by **binary fission**. The circular chromosome replicates and attaches to the cell wall; the plasma membrane and cell wall grow along the midline, forming daughter cells.

REPRODUCTION

Cell Division

- G_1: cell increases its organelles and cytoplasm
- S: DNA replication
- G_2: same as G_1
- M: the cell divides in two
- Mitosis = PMAT
- Meiosis = PMAT × 2

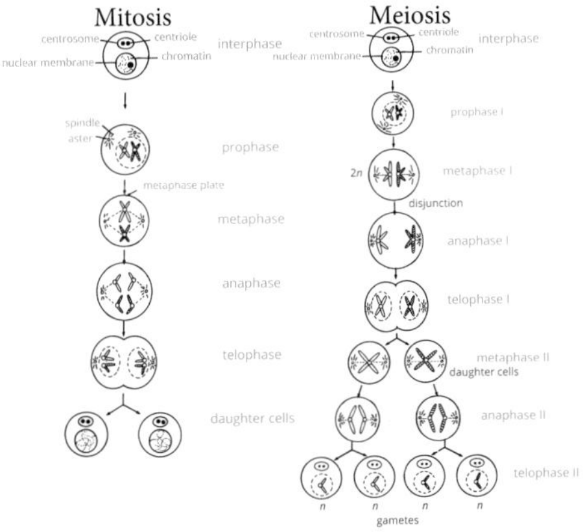

Sexual Reproduction

Meiosis I:

- Two pairs of sister chromatids form tetrads during prophase I.
- Crossing over leads to genetic recombination in prophase I.
- Homologous chromosomes separate during metaphase I.

Meiosis II:

- Essentially identical to mitosis, but no replication.
- Meiosis occurs in **spermatogenesis** (sperm formation) and **oogenesis** (egg formation).

Four Stages of Early Development

Cleavage: mitotic divisions

Implantation: embryo implants during blastula stage

Gastrulation: ectoderm, endoderm, and mesoderm form

Neurulation: germ layers develop a nervous system

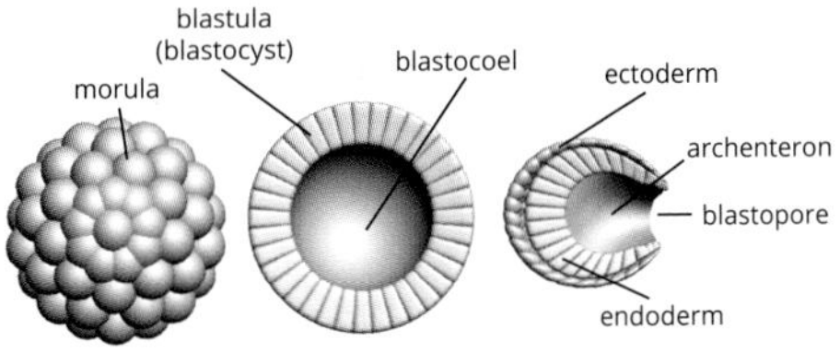

Ectoderm "Attract"oderm	Nervous system, epidermis, lens of eye, inner ear
Endoderm "Endernal" organs	Lining of digestive tract, lungs, liver and pancreas
Mesoderm "Means"oderm	Muscles, skeleton, circulatory system, gonads, kidney

The Liver's Roles in Homeostasis

1. Gluconeogenesis
2. Processing of nitrogenous wastes (urea)
3. Detoxification of wastes/chemicals/drugs
4. Storage of iron and vitamin A
5. Synthesis of bile and blood proteins
6. β-Oxidation of fatty acids to ketones
7. Interconversion of carbohydrates, fats, and amino acids

Layers of the Skin

- Stratum corneum
- Stratum lucidum
- Stratum granulosum
- Stratum spinosum
- Stratum basalis

HOMEOSTASIS

Osmoregulation

- **Filtration** at the glomerulus. Filtrate (fluid and small solutes) passes through. *Passive*
- **Secretion** of acids, bases, and ions from interstitial fluid to filtrate. Maintains pH, [K+] and [waste]. *Passive and Active*
- **Reabsorption:** essential substances and water flow from filtrate to blood. Enabled by osmolarity gradient and selective permeability of the walls. *Passive and Active*

Hormonal Regulation

Aldosterone

Stimulates Na^+ and water reabsorption

- Secreted from adrenal cortex in response to low blood pressure
- Regulated by the renin–angiotensin–aldosterone system

ADH (Vasopressin)

Increases collecting duct's permeability to water to increase water reabsorption

- Released from the posterior pituitary in response to high blood osmolarity

Kidneys regulate blood osmolarity and volume. The functional unit is the nephron.

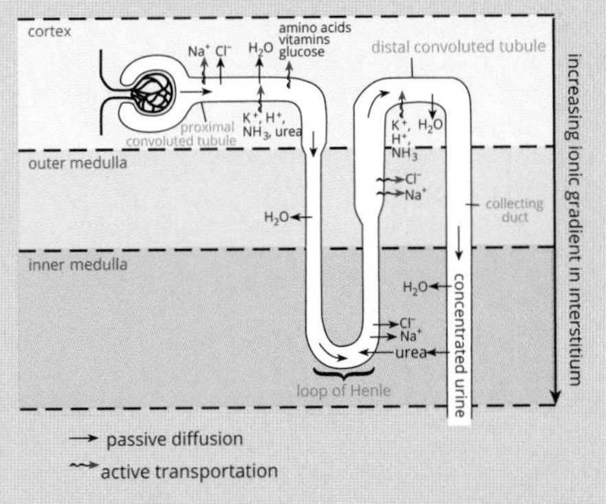

ENDOCRINE SYSTEM

Direct hormones directly stimulate organs; tropic hormones stimulate other glands.
Mechanisms of hormone action: **peptides** act via second messengers and **steroids** act via hormone/receptor binding to DNA. Amino acid-derivative hormones may do either.

Hormone	Source	Action
Follicle-stimulating (FSH)	Anterior pituitary	Stimulates follicle maturation; spermatogenesis
Luteinizing (LH)		Stimulates ovulation; testosterone synthesis
Adrenocorticotropic (ACTH)		Stimulates adrenal cortex to make and secrete glucocorticoids
Thyroid-stimulating (TSH)		Stimulates the thyroid to produce thyroid hormones
Prolactin		Stimulates milk production and secretion
Endorphins		Inhibits the perception of pain in the brain
Growth hormone		Stimulates bone and muscle growth/lipolysis
Oxytocin	Hypothalamus; stored in posterior pituitary	Stimulates uterine contractions during labor, milk secretion during lactation
Antidiuretic (ADH, vasopressin)		Stimulates water reabsorption in kidneys
Thyroid hormones (T_3, T_4)	Thyroid	Stimulates metabolic activity
Calcitonin		Decreases (tones down) blood calcium level
Parathyroid hormone	Parathyroid	Increases blood calcium level
Glucocorticoids	Adrenal cortex	Increases blood glucose level and decreases protein synthesis; anti-inflammatory
Mineralocorticoids		Increases sodium and water reabsorption in kidneys
Epinephrine, Norepinephrine	Adrenal medulla	Increases blood glucose level and heart rate
Glucagon	Pancreas	Stimulates conversion of glycogen to glucose in the liver; increases blood glucose
Insulin		Lowers blood glucose; increases glycogen stores
Somatostatin		Suppresses secretion of glucagon and insulin
Testosterone	Testes	Maintains male secondary sex characteristics
Estrogen	Ovary/Placenta	Maintains female secondary sex characteristics
Progesterone		Promotes growth/maintenance of endometrium
Melatonin	Pineal	Regulates sleep–wake cycles
Atrial natriuretic peptide	Heart	Involved in osmoregulation and vasodilation
Thymosin	Thymus	Stimulates T-cell development

Four Stages of Menstrual Cycle:

1. **Follicular:** FSH causes growth of a follicle
2. **Ovulation:** LH causes follicle to release egg
3. **Luteal:** corpus luteum forms
4. **Menstruation:** endometrial lining sheds

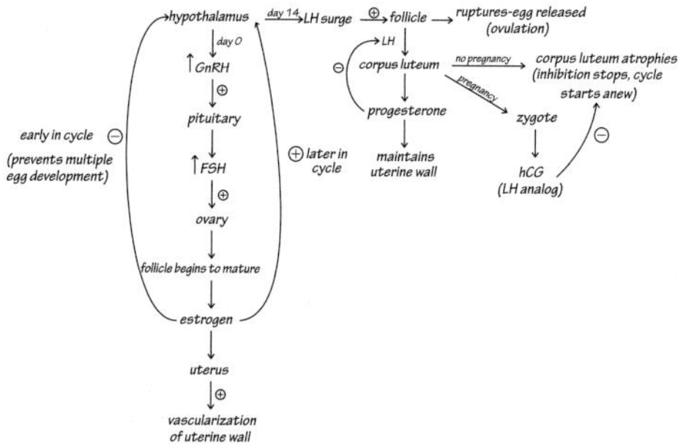

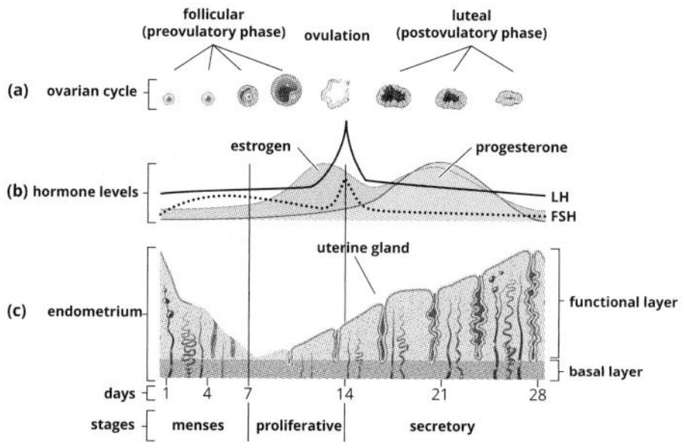

NERVOUS SYSTEM

The functional unit is the neuron:

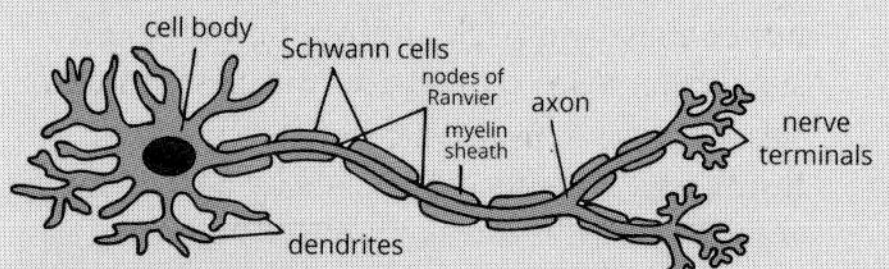

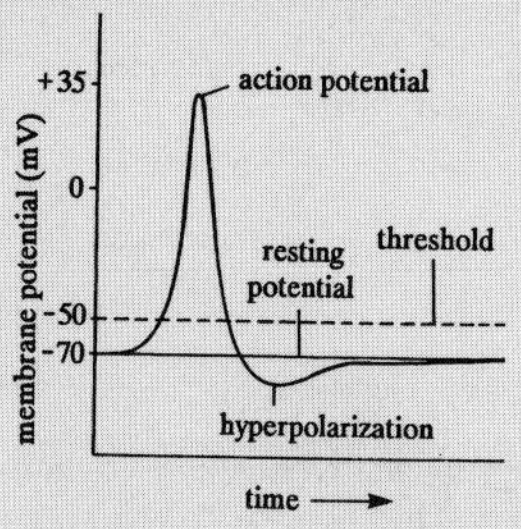

I	Rest	All gates closed
II	Depolarization	Na^+ gates open
III	Repolarization	Na^+ gates inactivate K^+ gates open
IV	Hyperpolarization	All gates closed

Resting Potential:

- Na^+/K^+ ATPase creates gradient of high $[Na^+]$ outside the cell, high $[K^+]$ inside the cell
- Movement of ions down their concentration gradient through **leak channels** establishes resting potential

Action Potential:

- Stimulus acts on the neuron, depolarizing the membrane of the cell body

Impulse Propagation:

- Depolarization (Na^+ rushing into axon) followed by repolarization (K^+ rushing out of axon) along the nerve axon

The Synapse:

- At the synaptic knob, voltage-gated Ca^{2+} channels open, sending Ca^{2+} into the cell.
- Vesicles fuse with presynaptic membrane sending the neurotransmitter across the **synaptic cleft**.
- Neurotransmitter binds to receptors on the postsynaptic membrane, triggering depolarization.

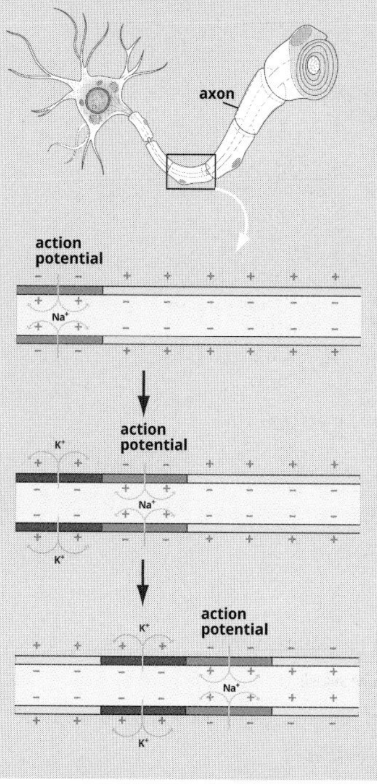

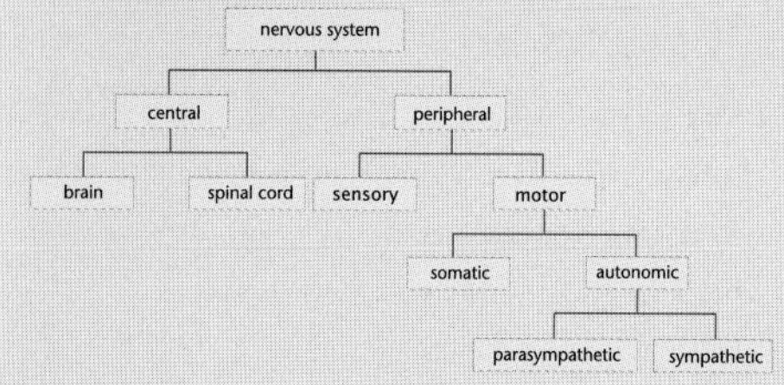

MUSCULOSKELETAL SYSTEM

Sarcomere

- Contractile unit of the fibers in skeletal muscle
- Contains thin actin and thick myosin filaments

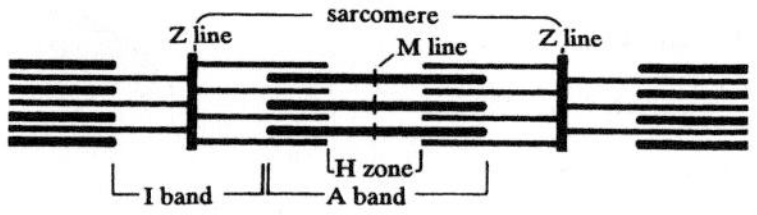

Contraction

Initiation:

- Depolarization of a neuron leads to an action potential.

Sarcomere shortening:

- Sarcoplasmic reticulum releases Ca^{2+}.
- Ca^{2+} binds to troponin on the actin filament.
- Tropomyosin shifts, exposing myosin-binding sites.
- Myosin binds, ATPase activity allows myosin to pull thin filaments towards the center of the H zone, and then ATP causes dissociation.

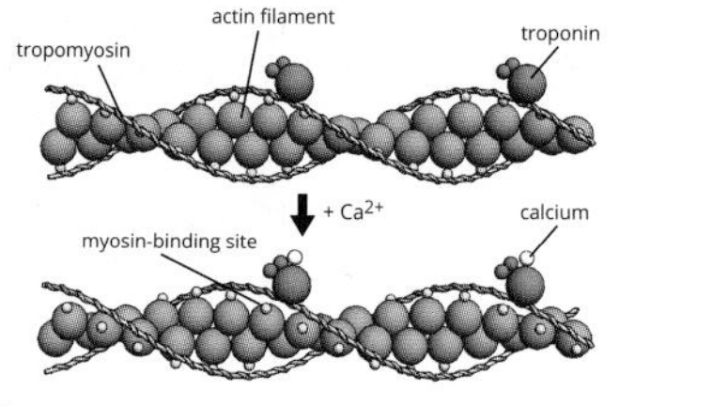

Relaxation:

- Ca^{2+} is pumped back into the sarcoplasmic reticulum.

Bone Formation and Remodeling

- **Osteoblast:** builds bone
- **Osteoclast:** breaks down bone
- **Reformation:** inorganic ions are absorbed from the blood for use in bone
- **Degradation (resorption):** inorganic ions are released into the blood

CIRCULATION

Circulatory Pathway Through Heart

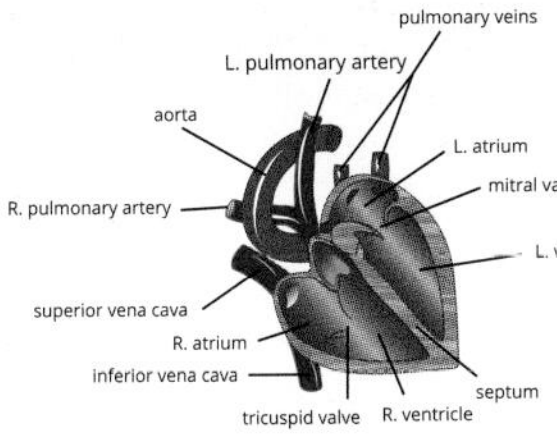

Superior and inferior vena cava → right atrium → right ventricle → pulmonary arteries → lungs→ pulmonary veins → left atrium → left ventricle → aorta → body

Three portal systems: Blood travels through an extra capillary bed before returning to the heart.

- Liver (hepatic), kidney, and brain (hypophyseal)

Fetal Circulation

- **Foramen ovale:** connects right and left atria
- **Ductus arteriosus:** connects pulmonary artery to aorta. Along with foramen ovale, shunts blood away from lungs
- **Ductus venosus:** connects umbilical vein to inferior vena cava, connecting umbilical circulation to central circulation

Blood Components

Plasma: aqueous mixture of nutrients, wastes, hormones, blood proteins, gases, and salts

Erythrocytes (red blood cells): carry oxygen

- Hemoglobin: four subunits carry O_2 and CO_2. Iron controls binding and releasing.
- Oxygen–hemoglobin dissociation:

Factors leading to right shift of curve:

- ↑ Temperature
- **Bohr Effect**

↓ pH, ↑ P_{CO_2}

- O_2 release to tissues enhanced when H^+ allosterically binds to Hb. ↑ P_{CO_2} leads to ↑ $[H^+]$:

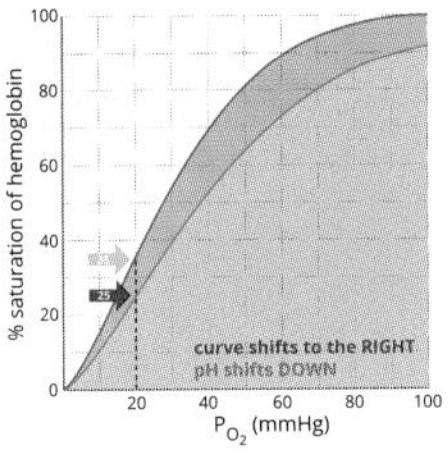

$$CO_2 + H_2O \underset{}{\overset{\text{carbonic anhydrase}}{\rightleftharpoons}} H_2CO_3 \rightleftharpoons H^+ + HCO_3^-$$

Leukocytes (white blood cells): function in immunity

Platelets: clotting

- Platelets release thromboplastin, which (along with cofactors calcium and vitamin K) converts inactive prothrombin to active thrombin.
- Thrombin converts fibrinogen into fibrin, which surrounds blood cells to form the clot.

Blood Typing

Antigens are located on the surface of red blood cells.

Blood type	RBC antigen	Antibodies	Donates to:	Receives From:
A	A	anti-B	A, AB	A, O
B	B	anti-A	B, AB	B, O
AB	A, B	None	AB only	All
O	None	anti-A, B	All	O only

Blood cells with Rh factor are Rh^+; these individuals produce no anti-Rh antibody. Rh^- blood cells lack the antigen; these individuals produce an antibody if exposed.

RESPIRATION

Gas Exchange

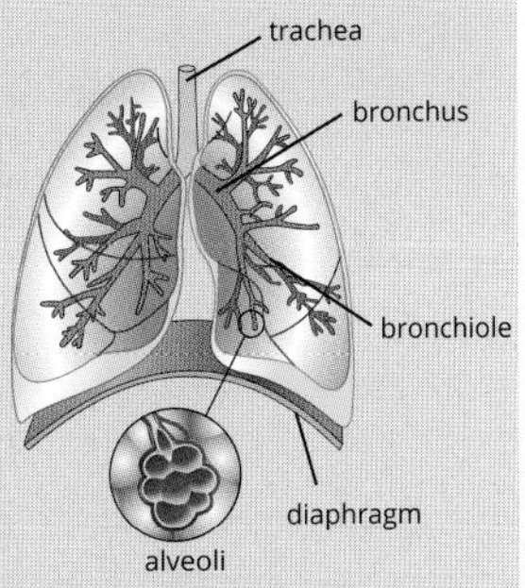

- Exchange occurs across the thin walls of **alveoli.**
- Deoxygenated blood enters the pulmonary capillaries that surround the alveoli.
- O_2 from the inhaled air diffuses down its gradient into the capillaries, where it binds with hemoglobin and returns to the heart.
- CO_2 from the tissues diffuses from the capillaries to the alveoli, and is exhaled.

Fetal Respiration

- Fetal hemoglobin has a higher affinity for oxygen than adult hemoglobin.
- Gas and nutrient exchanges occur across the placenta.

DIGESTION

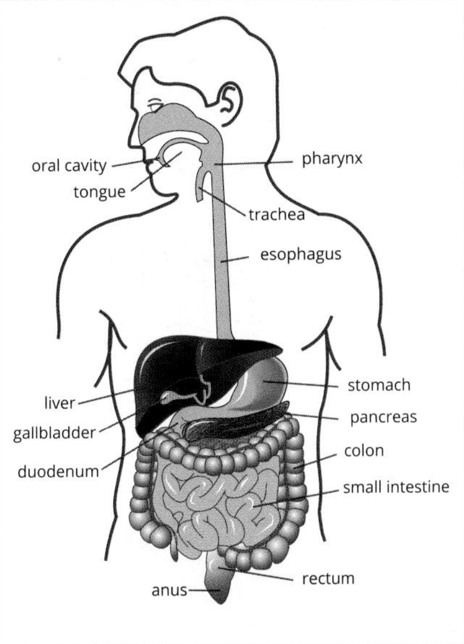

IMMUNE SYSTEM

- The body distinguishes between "self" and "nonself" (antigens).

Humoral Immunity (Specific Defense)

B-lymphocytes → **memory cells**: remember antigen, speed up secondary response

B-lymphocytes → **plasma cells** make and release antibodies (**IgG**, **IgA**, **IgM**, **IgD**, **IgE**), which induce antigen phagocytosis

- **Active imumunity:** antibodies are produced during an immune response
- **Passive immunity:** antibodies produced by one organism are transferred to another organism

Cell-Mediated Immunity (Specific Defense)

T-lymphocytes →

- **cytotoxic T-cells**: destroy cells directly
- **helper T-cells**: activate B- and T-cells and macrophages by secreting lymphokines
- **suppressor T-cells**: regulate B- and T-cells to decrease anti-antigen activity
- **memory cells**

Nonspecific Immune Response

Includes skin, passages lined with cilia, macrophages, inflammatory response, and interferons (proteins that help prevent the spread of a virus)

Lymphatic System

- Lymph vessels meet at the thoracic duct in the upper chest and neck, draining into the left subclavian vein of the cardiovascular system.
- Vessels carry **lymph** (excess interstitial fluid), and **lacteals** collect fats by absorbing chylomicrons in the small intestine.
- **Lymph nodes** are swellings along the vessels with phagocytic cells (macrophages); they remove foreign particles from lymph.

Lipid Digestion

- When chyme is present, the duodenum secretes the hormone cholecystokinin (CCK) into the blood.
- CCK stimulates the secretion of pancreatic enzymes and bile, and promotes satiety.
- Bile is made in the liver and emulsifies fat in the small intestine; it's not an enzyme.
- Lipase is an enzyme made in the pancreas that hydrolyzes lipids in the small intestine.

Carbohydrate Digestion

Enzyme	Production Site	Function Site	Hydrolysis Reaction
Salivary amylase (ptyalin)	Salivary glands	Mouth	Starch → maltose
Pancreatic amylase	Pancreas	Small intestine	Starch → maltose
Maltase	Intestinal glands	Small intestine	Maltose → 2 glucoses
Sucrase	Intestinal glands	Small intestine	Sucrose → glucose, fructose
Lactase	Intestinal glands	Small intestine	Lactose → glucose, galactose

Protein Digestion

Enzyme	Production Site	Function Site	Function
Pepsin	Gastric glands (chief cells)	Stomach	Hydrolyzes specific peptide bonds
Trypsin	Pancreas	Small Intestine	Hydrolyzes specific peptide bonds Converts chymotrypsinogen to chymotrypsin
Chymotrypsin			Hydrolyzes specific peptide bonds
Carboxypeptidases A and B			Hydrolyzes terminal peptide bond at C-terminus
Aminopeptidase	Intestinal glands		Hydrolyzes terminal peptide bond at N-terminus
Dipeptidases			Hydrolyzes part of amino acids
Enteropeptidase			Converts trypsinogen and procarboxypeptidases to active form

CLASSICAL GENETICS

Law of segregation: Homologous alleles (chromosomes) separate so that each gamete has one copy of each gene.

- If both parents are Rr, the alleles separate to give a genotypic ratio of 1:2:1 and a phenotypic ratio of 3:1.

Law of independent assortment: Alleles of unlinked genes assort independently in meiosis.

- For two traits: AaBb parents will produce AB, Ab, aB, and ab gametes.
- The phenotypic ratio for this cross is 9:3:3:1.

Statistical Calculations

- The probability of producing a genotype that requires multiple events to occur equals the *product* of the probability of each event.
- The probability of producing a genotype that can be the result of multiple different events equals the *sum* of each probability minus the probability of multiple events occurring.

Genetic Mapping

- Crossing over during meiosis I can unlink genes (prophase I).
- Genes are most likely unlinked when far apart.
- One map unit is 1% recombinant frequency (1 centimorgan).

Given recombination frequencies

X and Y: 8%

X and Z: 12%

Y and Z: 4%

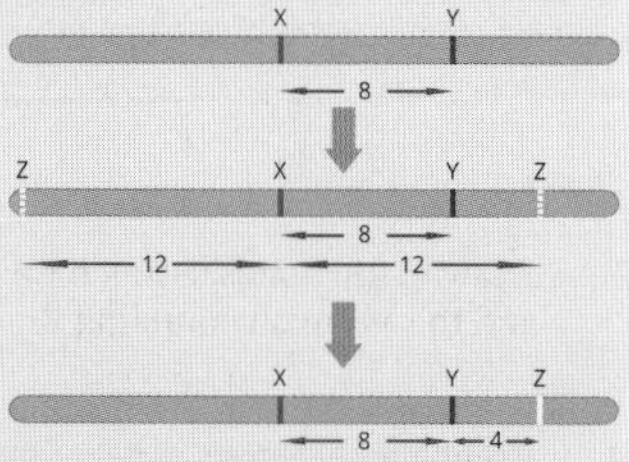

Patterns of Inheritance

- Autosomal recessive: may skip generations
- Autosomal dominant: appears in every generation
- X-linked (sex-linked): no male-to-male transmission, and more males are affected

EVOLUTION

- When frequencies are stable, the population is in **Hardy–Weinberg equilibrium:** no mutations, large population, random mating, no migration, and equal reproductive success

$$p + q = 1;\ p^2 + 2pq + q^2 = 1$$

p = frequency of dominant allele

q = frequency of recessive allele

p^2 = frequency of dominant homozygotes

$2pq$ = frequency of heterozygotes

q^2 = frequency of recessive homozygotes

MOLECULAR GENETICS

Nucleic Acids

- Basic unit: nucleotide (sugar, nitrogenous base, phosphate)
- DNA's sugar: deoxyribose; RNA's sugar: ribose
- 2 types of bases: double-ringed purines (adenine, guanine) and single-ringed pyrimidines (cytosine, uracil, thymine)
- DNA double helix: antiparallel strands joined by base pairs (A=T, G≡C)
- RNA is usually single-stranded: A pairs with U, not T

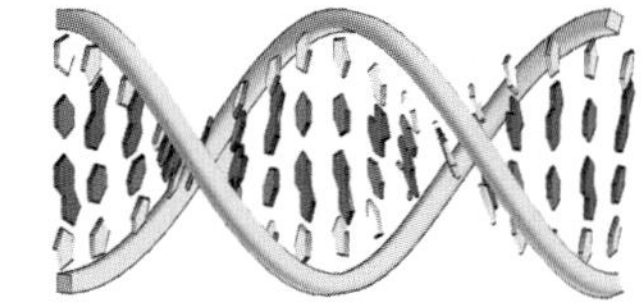

Transcriptional Regulation (Prokaryotes)

Regulated by the **operon:**

- **Structural genes:** have DNA that codes for protein
- **Operator gene:** repressor binding site
- **Promoter gene:** RNA polymerase's 1st binding site
- **Inducible systems** need an inducer for transcription to occur. **Repressible systems** need a corepressor to inhibit transcription.

Mutations

- **Point:** One nucleotide is substituted by another; they are silent if the sequence of amino acids doesn't change.
- **Frameshift:** Insertions or deletions shift reading frame. Protein doesn't form, or is nonfunctional.

Viruses

- Acellular structures of double- or single-stranded DNA or RNA in a protein coat
- **Lytic cycle:** virus kills the host cell
- **Lysogenic cycle:** virus enters host genome

GENETICS OF PROKARYOTIC CELLS

Many bacteria contain **plasmids**, or extragenomic material. Plasmids that can be integrated into the genome are known as **episomes**.

- **Transformation** occurs when a bacterium acquires a piece of genetic material from the environment and integrates that piece of genetic material into the host cell genome. This is a common method by which antibiotic resistance can be acquired.
- **Conjugation** is the bacterial form of mating (sexual reproduction). It involves two cells forming a cytoplasmic bridge between them that allows for the transfer of genetic material. The transfer is one-way, from the donor male (+) to the recipient female (–). The bridge is made from appendages called **sex pili** that are found on the donor male. To form the pilus, bacteria must contain plasmids known as **sex factors**.
- **Transduction** occurs when a bacteriophage acquires genetic information from a host cell. Sometimes, when the new virions are assembled in a host cell, some of the genetic material from the host cell is packaged along with the viral genetic material. Then, the bacteriophage infects another bacterium, resulting in transfer of bacterial genetic material.

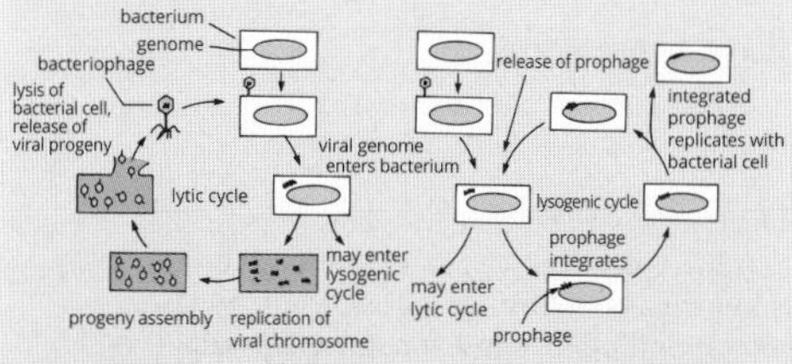

DATA ANALYSIS

A researcher performed the following experiments in order to investigate the metabolism of two different strains of bacteria, Strain 1 and Strain 2.

Experiment 1

Strains 1 and 2 were incubated in separate broth cultures for 24 hours at 37°C. A sample of each culture was streaked onto three different plates—A, B, and C—each containing a different starch–agar medium; the plates were then incubated for another 48 hours at 37°C. The plates were then examined for surface colony growth and stained with iodine solution to determine the extent of starch digestion.

Table 1

	Surface Colony Growth			Starch Digestion		
	A	B	C	A	B	C
Strain 1	+	+	+	–	–	–
Strain 2	+	+	–	+	+	–

key: + = growth/digestion; – = no growth/digestion

Experiment 2

The two strains were incubated in the same manner as in Experiment 1. Two 100 mL portions of agar were poured into two beakers, which were maintained at 43°C. Next, 0.2 mL of broth culture from Strain 1 was pipetted into the first beaker, and 0.2 mL of broth culture from Strain 2 was pipetted into the second beaker. The agar was swirled around to distribute the bacteria evenly through the media, and then poured onto plates. These plates were incubated for 48 hours at 37°C and then examined for colony growth both on the agar surface and lower down within the oxygen-poor agar layer.

Table 2

	Surface Colony Growth	Deep-Agar Colony Growth
Strain 1	+	–
Strain 2	+	+

key: + = growth; – = no growth

Once incubated, bacteria will grow if nutrients they can metabolize are available. Keep this in mind as you interpret the procedure and results.

Experiment 1 and Table 1: What are the important aspects? **Two strains** (1 and 2) undergo **identical incubation** on **3 plates with different starch agars.** Look at Table 1, one strain at a time. The researcher observes growth and starch digestion. Strain 1 grows on all plates, but doesn't digest the starch: it must be using another nutrient to grow. We don't know that Strain 1 *can't* digest starch—we just know that it's not digesting it during these 48 hours. Strain 2 uses starch to grow on plates A and B, but doesn't digest starch or grow on plate C. Again, we don't know that Strain 2 *can't* digest the starch in medium C—we just know it's not doing so during these 48 hours.

Experiment 2 and Table 2: Note the significant differences between the two experiments. This time, the strains were **separately** distributed **within the agar** instead of jointly streaked on top of multiple agars. The researcher observes growth on top and within, the assumption being that the top is oxygen-rich and within is oxygen-poor. What does it mean that Strain 1 only grows in an oxygen-rich environment? It is an obligate aerobe that requires oxygen for metabolism. What does it mean that Strain 2 can grow in oxygen-rich *and* oxygen-poor environments? It is a facultative or aerotolerant anaerobe.

ATOMIC STRUCTURE

Atomic weight: The weighted average of the masses of the naturally occurring isotopes of an element, in amu per atom

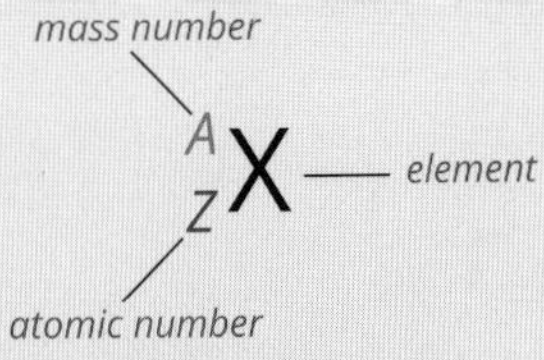

A **mole** is a unit used to count particles and is represented by **Avogadro's number**, 6.022×10^{23} particles.

$$\text{Moles} = \frac{\text{mass of a sample}}{\text{molar mass}}$$

Isotopes: For a given element, multiple species of atoms with the same number of protons (same atomic number) but different numbers of neutrons (different mass numbers)

Planck's quantum theory: Energy emitted as electromagnetic radiation from matter exists in discrete bundles called quanta.

Bohr's Model of the Hydrogen Atom

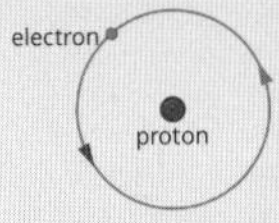

Energy of electron $= E = \frac{-R_H}{n^2}$

Electromagnetic energy of photons $= E = \frac{hc}{\lambda}$

The group of hydrogen emission lines corresponding to transitions from upper levels $n > 2$ to $n = 2$ is known as the **Balmer series**, while the group corresponding to transitions between upper levels $n > 1$ to $n = 1$ is known as the **Lyman series**.

Absorption spectrum: Characteristic energy bands where electrons absorb energy

Quantum Mechanical Model of Atoms

Heisenberg uncertainty principle: It is impossible to determine with perfect accuracy the momentum and the position of an electron simultaneously.

Quantum Numbers:

#	Character	Symbol	Value
1st	Shell	n	n
2nd	Subshell	l	From zero to $n-1$
3rd	Orbital	m_ℓ	Between l and $-l$
4th	Spin	m_s	$+\frac{1}{2}$ or $-\frac{1}{2}$

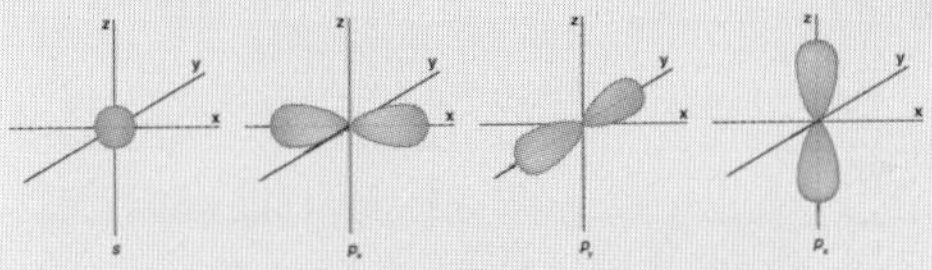

s-orbital *p*-orbitals

Principal quantum number (n): The larger the integer value of n, the higher the energy level and radius of the electron's orbit. The maximum number of electrons in energy level n is $2n^2$.

Azimuthal quantum number (l): Refers to subshells. The four subshells corresponding to $l = 0$, 1, 2, and 3 are known as *s*, *p*, *d*, and *f*, respectively. The maximum number of electrons that can exist within a subshell is given by the equation $4l + 2$.

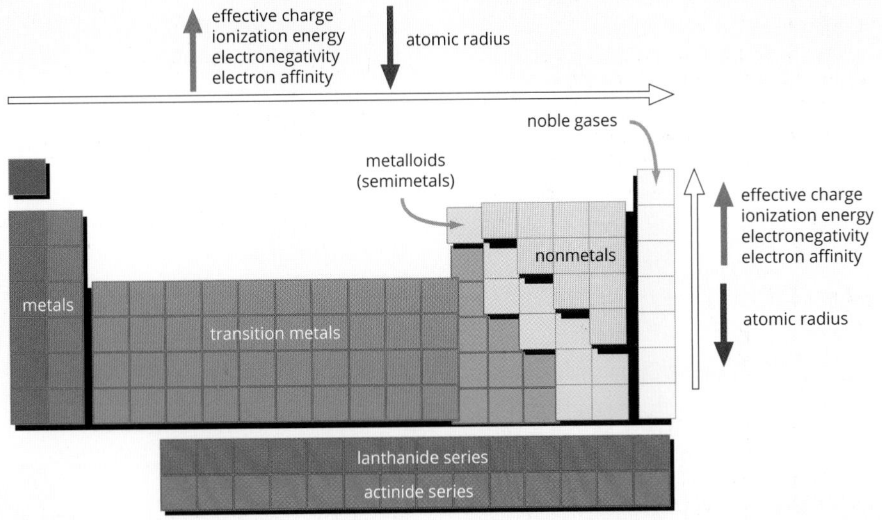

Magnetic quantum number (m_l): This specifies the particular orbital within a subshell where an electron is highly likely to be found at a given point in time.

Spin quantum number (m_s): The spin of a particle is its intrinsic angular momentum and is a characteristic of the particle, like its charge.

Electron Configuration

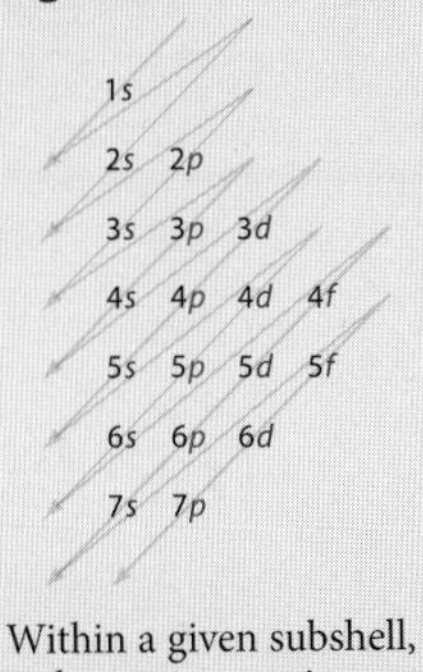

Hund's rule: Within a given subshell, orbitals are filled such that there are a maximum number of half-filled orbitals with parallel spins.

Valence electrons: Electrons of an atom that are in its outer energy shell and that are available for bonding.

BONDING & CHEMICAL INTERACTIONS

Octet Rule:

- An atom will bond until it has a full outermost shell.
- An atom wants to have a configuration similar to that of Group VIII (noble gases).

Exceptions: Some elements are stable with fewer than 8 electrons: H (2), He (2), Li (2), Be (4), B (6). Atoms found in or beyond the third period can have more than eight valence electrons because some of the valence electrons may occupy *d*-orbitals. These atoms can have more than four bonds in Lewis structures.

For instance, the sulfate ion can be drawn in at least six resonance forms, many of which have two double bonds attached to a different combination of oxygen atoms.

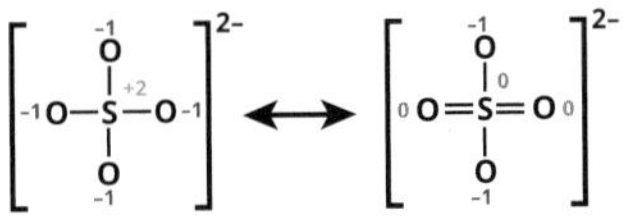

Covalent Bond Notation

Lewis structure: The chemical symbol of an element surrounded by dots, each representing one of the *s* or *p* valence electrons of the atom.

Steps for drawing Lewis structures:

1. Write the skeletal structure of the compound.
   H–C–N
2. Count all the valence electrons of the atoms.
3. Draw single bonds between the central atom and the atoms surrounding it.
   H : C : N
4. Complete the octets of all atoms bonded to the central atom, using the remaining valence electrons still to be assigned.
   H : C : N̈ :
5. Place any extra electrons on the central atom.
   H – C ≡ N̈

Formal Charges

Formal charge is the charge an atom would have if all the electrons in bonds were shared equally.

Geometry and polarity of covalent molecules

Polar covalent bond: Bonding electron pair is not shared equally, but pulled toward more electronegative atom

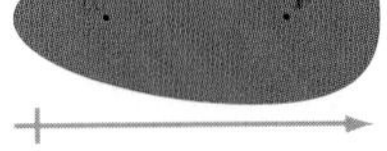

Polarity of molecules: Depends on the polarity of the constituent bonds and on the shape of the molecule. A molecule with nonpolar bonds is always nonpolar; a molecule with polar bonds may be polar or nonpolar depending on the orientation of the bond dipoles.

The overall shape of the molecule determines whether the molecule is in fact polar or not. For instance, the four bond dipoles for the CCl_4 molecule point to the vertices of the tetrahedron and cancel each other.

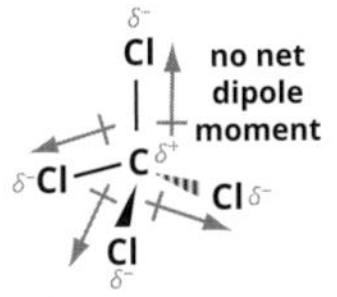

Regions of Electron Density	Example	Geometric Arrangement of Electron Pairs around the Central Atom	Shape	Angle between Electron Pairs
2	$BeCl_2$	X—A—X	linear	180°
3	BH_3	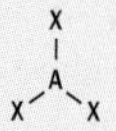	trigonal planar	120°
4	CH_4	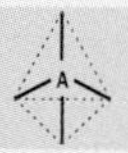	tetrahedral	109.5°
5	PCl_5	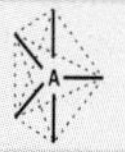	trigonal bipyramidal	90°, 120°, 180°
6	SF_6	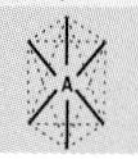	octahedral	90°, 180°

Complex Ion (Coordination Compound)

A Lewis acid–base adduct with a cation bonded to at least one electron pair donor (including water). Donor molecules are called **ligands** and use **coordinate covalent bonds**. The central cation can be bonded to the same ligand multiple times in a process called **chelation**.

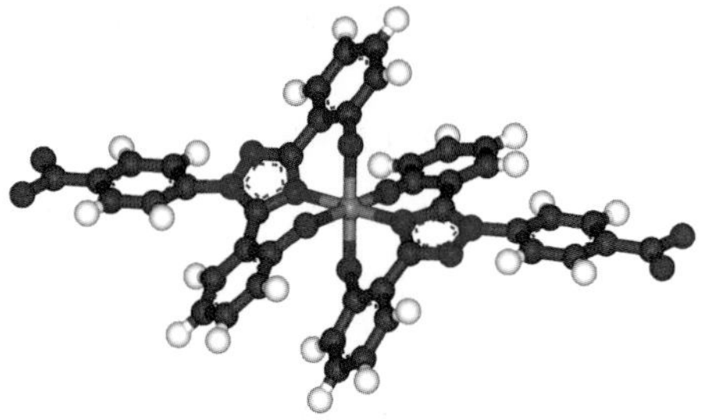

Intermolecular Forces

1. **Hydrogen bonding:** The partial positive charge of the hydrogen atom interacts with the partial negative charge located on the electronegative atoms (F, O, N) of nearby molecules.

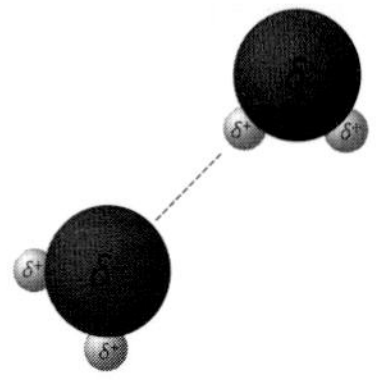

2. **Dipole–dipole interactions:** Polar molecules orient themselves such that the positive region of one molecule is close to the negative region of another molecule.

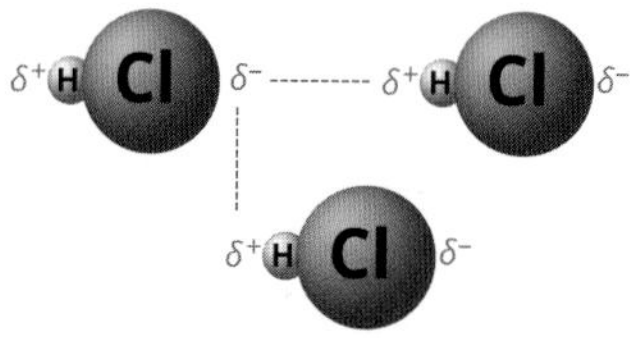

3. **Dispersion forces:** The bonding electrons in covalent bonds may appear to be equally shared between two atoms, but at any particular point in time they will be located randomly throughout the orbital. This permits unequal sharing of electrons, causing transient polarization and counterpolarization of the electron clouds of neighboring molecules, inducing the formation of more dipoles.

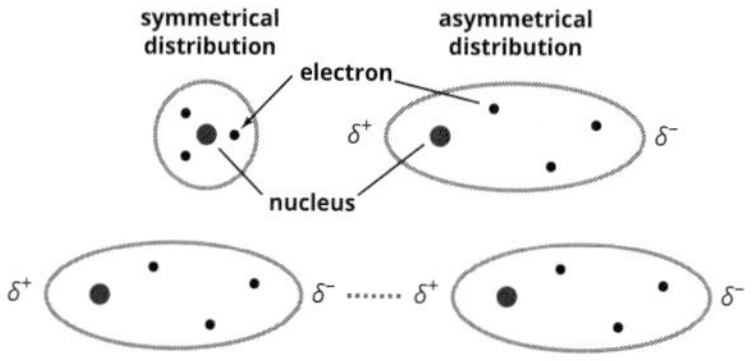

KINETICS & EQUILIBRIUM

Experimental determination of rate law: The values of k, x, and y in the rate law equation (rate = $k[A]^x[B]^y$) must be determined experimentally for a given reaction at a given temperature. The rate is usually measured as a function of the initial concentrations of the reactants, A and B.

Efficiency of Reactions

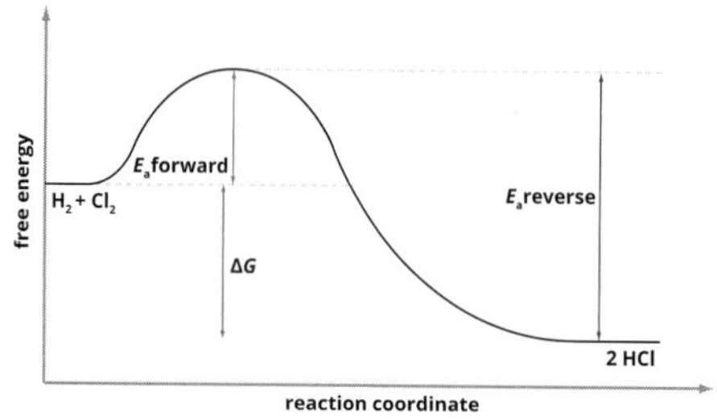

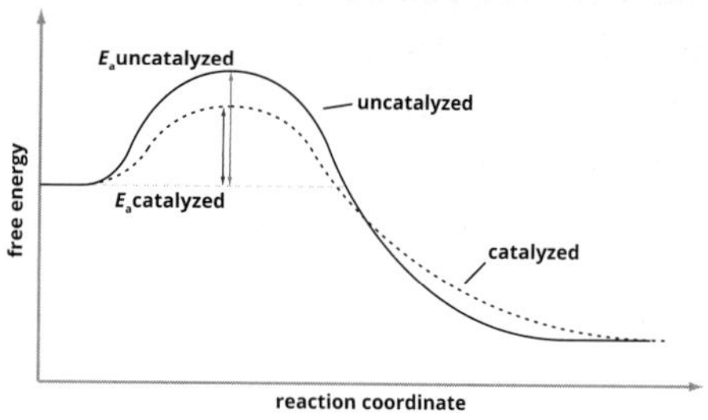

Law of Mass Action

$$aA + bB \rightleftharpoons cC + dD$$

$$K_c = \frac{[C]^c[D]^d}{[A]^a[B]^b}$$

K_c is the equilibrium constant (c stands for concentration).

Properties of the Equilibrium Constant

Pure solids and liquids don't appear in expressions.

K_{eq} is characteristic of a given system at a given temperature.

If $K_{eq} >> 1$, an equilibrium mixture of reactants and products will contain very little of the reactants compared to the products.

If $K_{eq} << 1$, an equilibrium mixture of reactants and products will contain very little of the products compared to the reactants.

If K_{eq} is close to 1, an equilibrium mixture of products and reactants will contain approximately equal amounts of the two.

Le Châtelier's principle is used to determine the direction in which a reaction at equilibrium will proceed when subjected to a stress, such as a change in concentration, pressure, volume, or temperature. The key is to remember that a system to which these kinds of stresses are applied tends to change so as to relieve the applied stress.

In a nutshell:

$A + B \rightleftharpoons C$ + heat	
Will shift to **RIGHT**	Will shift to **LEFT**
1. If more A or B added	1. If more C added
2. If C taken away	2. If A or B taken away
3. If pressure applied or volume reduced (assuming A, B, and C are gases)	3. If pressure reduced or volume increased (assuming A, B, and C are gases)
4. If temperature reduced	4. If temperature increased

COMPOUNDS & STOICHIOMETRY

A **mole** is the amount of a substance that contains the same number of particles that are found in a 12.000 g sample of carbon-12.

The **molecular** or **formula weight** is measured in amu per molecule (or formula unit). The **molar mass** is measured in grams per mole.

Combustion reactions: A fuel, such as a hydrocarbon, is reacted with an oxidant, such as oxygen, to produce an oxide and water.

$$CH_4\ (g) + 2\ O_2\ (g) \rightarrow CO_2\ (g) + 2\ H_2O\ (g)$$

Combination reactions: Two or more reactants form one product.

$$S\ (s) + O_2\ (g) \rightarrow SO_2\ (g)$$

Decomposition reactions: A compound breaks down into two or more substances, usually as a result of heating or electrolysis.

$$2\ HgO\ (s) \rightarrow 2\ Hg\ (l) + O_2\ (g)$$

Single-displacement reactions: An atom (or ion) of one compound is replaced by an atom of another element.

$$Zn\ (s) + CuSO_4\ (aq) \rightarrow Cu\ (s) + ZnSO_4\ (aq)$$

Double-displacement reactions: Also called metathesis reactions; elements from two different compounds displace each other to form two new compounds.

$$CaCl_2\ (aq) + 2\ AgNO_3\ (aq) \rightarrow Ca(NO_3)_2\ (aq) + 2\ AgCl\ (s)$$

Net ionic equations: These types of equations are written showing only the species that actually participate in the reaction. Consider the following equation:

$$Zn\ (s) + Cu^{2+}\ (aq) + SO_4^{2-}\ (aq) \rightarrow Cu\ (s) + Zn^{2+}\ (aq) + SO_4^{2-}\ (aq)$$

The spectator ion (SO_4^{2-}) does not take part in the overall reaction, but simply remains in solution throughout. The net ionic equation would be:

$$Zn\ (s) + Cu^{2+}\ (aq) \rightarrow Cu\ (s) + Zn^{2+}\ (aq)$$

Neutralization reactions: These are specific double-displacement reactions that occur when an acid reacts with a base to produce a solution of a salt (and, usually, water):

$$HCl\ (aq) + NaOH\ (aq) \rightarrow NaCl\ (aq) + H_2O\ (l)$$

Factors affecting reaction rates: reactant concentrations, temperature, medium, catalysts

Catalysts are unique substances that increase reaction rate without being consumed; they do this by lowering the activation energy.

THERMOCHEMISTRY

The law of conservation of energy dictates that energy can be neither created nor destroyed, but that all thermal, chemical, potential, and kinetic energies are interconvertible.

Systems:

Isolated: no exchange of energy/matter with the environment. Bomb calorimetry creates a nearly isolated system.

Closed: can exchange energy but not matter with the environment

Open: can exchange both energy and matter with the environment. Human beings are open systems because they can take in energy and matter (eat), release matter into the environment (respiration, urination, defecation), and release energy into the environment (heat transfer from the skin and mucous membranes).

System processes

Isothermal: temperature of system remains constant

Adiabatic: no heat exchange occurs

Isobaric: pressure of system remains constant

Isovolumetric (isochoric): volume remains constant

Heat: the transfer of thermal energy from one object to another

Endothermic: reactions that absorb thermal energy

Exothermic: reactions that release thermal energy

Endergonic: reactions that are nonspontaneous

Exergonic: reactions that are spontaneous

Constant-volume and constant-pressure calorimetry: used to indicate conditions under which the heat flow is measured

$q = mc\Delta T$, where q is the heat absorbed or released in a given process, m is the mass, c is the specific heat, and ΔT is the change in temperature

States and state functions: are described by the macroscopic properties of the system. These properties' magnitudes depend only on the initial and final states of the system, and not on the path of the change. Common state functions include pressure, density, temperature, volume, enthalpy, internal energy, free energy, and entropy.

Enthalpy (H): is used to express heat changes at constant pressure

Standard heat of formation (ΔH°_f): the enthalpy change that would occur if one mole of a compound was formed directly from its elements in their standard states

Standard heat of reaction (ΔH°_{rxn}): the hypothetical enthalpy change that would occur if the reaction were carried out under standard conditions

$$\Delta H^\circ_{rxn} = (\text{sum of } \Delta H^\circ_f \text{ of products}) - (\text{sum of } \Delta H^\circ_f \text{ of reactants})$$

Hess's law: states that enthalpies of reactions are additive

The reverse of any reaction has an enthalpy of the same magnitude as that of the forward reaction, but its sign is opposite.

Bond dissociation energy: an average of the energy required to break a particular type of bond in one mole of gaseous molecules:

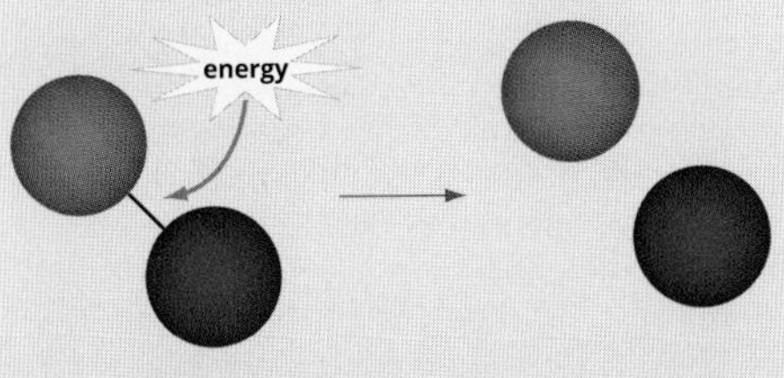

Bond enthalpy: The standard heat of reaction can be calculated using the values of bond dissociation energies of particular bonds (given in a table).

$$\Delta H^\circ_{rxn} = \sum \Delta H_{\text{bonds broken}} - \sum \Delta H_{\text{bonds formed}}$$

Entropy (S): the measure of the distribution of energy ("randomness") throughout a system

$$\Delta S_{\text{universe}} = \Delta S_{\text{system}} + \Delta S_{\text{surroundings}}$$

Gibbs free energy (G): combines the two factors that affect the spontaneity of a reaction—changes in enthalpy, ΔH, and changes in entropy, ΔS

$$\Delta G = \Delta H - T\Delta S$$

If ΔG is negative, the reaction is spontaneous.

If ΔG is positive, the reaction is nonspontaneous.

If ΔG is zero, the system is in a state of equilibrium; thus, $\Delta H = T\Delta S$.

ΔH	ΔS	Outcome
–	+	Spontaneous at all temps.
+	–	Nonspontaneous at all temps.
+	+	Spontaneous only at high temps.
–	–	Spontaneous only at low temps.

Reaction quotient (Q): Once a reaction commences, the standard state conditions no longer hold. For the reaction:

$$a\text{A} + b\text{B} \rightleftharpoons c\text{C} + d\text{D}$$

$$Q = \frac{[\text{C}]^c[\text{D}]^d}{[\text{A}]^a[\text{B}]^b}$$

THE GAS PHASE

1 atm = 760 mmHg ≡ 760 torr = 101,325 Pa

Do not confuse STP with standard conditions—the two standards involve different temperatures and are used for different purposes. STP (0˚C or 273 K, 1 atm) is generally used for gas law calculations; standard conditions (25˚C or 298 K, 1 atm, 1 M concentrations) is used when measuring standard enthalpy, entropy, Gibbs free energy, and electromotive force.

Boyle's Law

$$PV = k \text{ or } P_1V_1 = P_2V_2$$

Charles's Law

$$\frac{V}{T} = k \text{ or } \frac{V_1}{T_1} = \frac{V_2}{T_2}$$

Gay-Lussac's Law

$$\frac{P}{T} = k \text{ or } \frac{P_1}{T_1} = \frac{P_2}{T_2}$$

Avogadro's Principle

$$\frac{n}{V} = k \text{ or } \frac{n_1}{V_1} = \frac{n_2}{V_2}$$

Combined Gas Law

Integrates Boyle's Law, Charles's Law, and Gay-Lussac's Law

$$\frac{P_1V_1}{T_1} = \frac{P_2V_2}{T_2}$$

Ideal Gas Law

$$PV = nRT$$

Real Gases

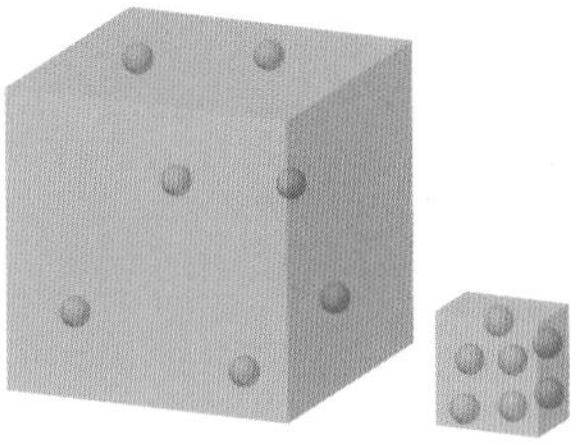

Decreasing the volume of a sample of gas makes it behave less ideally because the individual gas particles are in closer proximity in a smaller volume. (The volume of the gas particles themselves becomes appreciable, and they are more likely to engage in intermolecular interactions.)

Deviations due to pressure: As the pressure of a gas increases, the particles are pushed closer and closer together. At moderately high pressure, a gas's volume is less than would be predicted by the ideal gas law due to intermolecular attraction.

Deviations due to temperature: As the temperature of a gas decreases, the average velocity of the gas molecules decreases and the attractive intermolecular forces become increasingly significant. Increased intermolecular attraction causes the gas to have a smaller volume than would be predicted. At extremely low temperatures, the volume of the gas particles themselves causes the gas to have a larger volume than would be predicted.

1 mole of gas at STP = 22.4 L

Dalton's law of partial pressures: states that the total pressure of a gaseous mixture is equal to the sum of the partial pressures of the individual components

$$P_T = P_A + P_B + P_C + \ldots$$

$$P_A = P_TX_A$$

where $X_A = \dfrac{n_A}{n_T}\ \dfrac{\text{(moles of A)}}{\text{(total moles)}}$

Kinetic molecular theory of gases: an explanation of gaseous molecular behavior based on the motion of individual molecules

Average molecular speed: the temperature of the system dictates the speed of a gas molecule, since it is a measure of the average kinetic energy

$$K = \frac{1}{2}mv^2 = \frac{3}{2}k_BT$$

PHASES & PHASE CHANGES

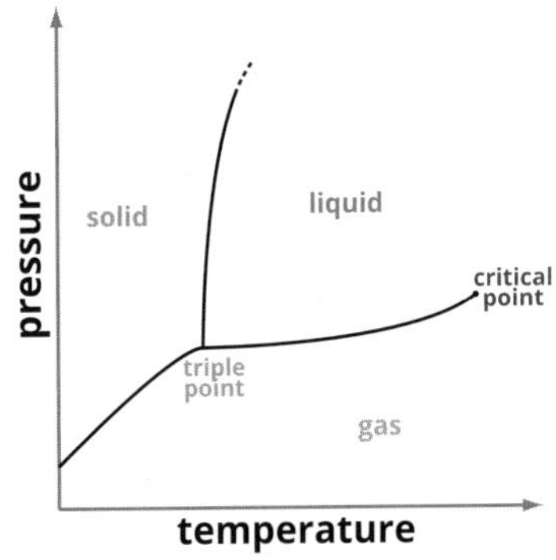

Colligative properties: These are physical properties derived solely from the number of particles present, not the nature of those particles. These properties are usually associated with dilute solutions. Molality (m) is often used, in addition to the van 't Hoff factor (i) for ionic compounds.

Freezing point depression

$$\Delta T_f = iK_fm$$

Boiling point elevation

$$\Delta T_b = iK_bm$$

Osmotic pressure

$$\Pi = MRT$$

Vapor pressure lowering (Raoult's law)

$$P_A = X_A P^\circ_A;\ P_B = X_B P^\circ_B$$

Solutions that obey Raoult's Law are called ideal solutions.

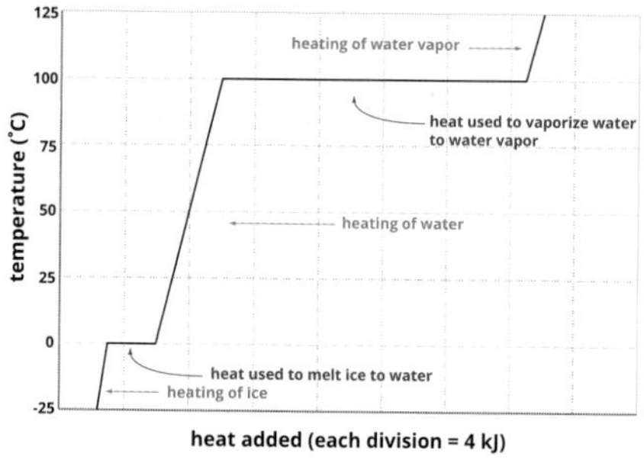

Graham's law of diffusion and effusion

Diffusion: occurs when gas molecules distribute through a volume by random motion

Effusion: the flow of gas particles under pressure from one compartment to another through a small opening:

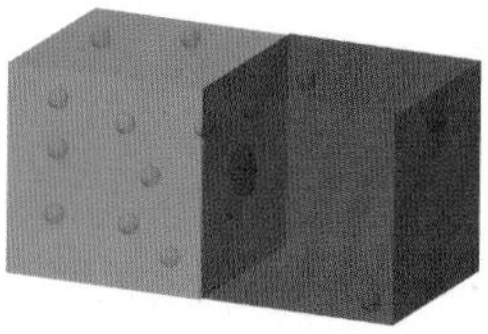

Both diffusion and effusion have the same formula:

$$\frac{r_1}{r_2} = \sqrt{\left(\frac{m_2}{m_1}\right)}$$

SOLUTIONS

Solubility rules

1. All salts containing alkali metal (Group 1) or ammonium (NH_4^+) cations are water-soluble.
2. All salts containing the nitrate (NO_3^-) or acetate (CH_3COO^-) anions are water-soluble.
3. All chlorides, bromides, and iodides are water-soluble, with the exception of Ag^+, Pb^{2+}, and Hg^{2+}.
4. All salts of the sulfate ion (SO_4^{2-}) are water-soluble, with the exception of Ca^{2+}, Sr^{2+}, Ba^{2+}, and Pb^{2+}.
5. All metal oxides are insoluble, with the exception of the alkali metals and CaO, SrO, BaO, all of which hydrolyze to form solutions of the corresponding metal hydroxides.
6. All hydroxides are insoluble, with the exception of the alkali metals and Ca^{2+}, Sr^{2+}, and Ba^{2+}.
7. All carbonates (CO_3^{2-}), phosphates (PO_4^{3-}), sulfides (S^{2-}), and sulfites (SO_3^{2-}) are insoluble, with the exception of the alkali metals and ammonium.

Units of Concentration

Percent composition by mass:

$$\frac{\text{Mass of solute}}{\text{Mass of solution}} \times 100\%$$

Mole fraction: $\frac{\text{\# of mol of compound}}{\text{total \# of moles in system}}$

Molarity: $\frac{\text{\# of mol of solute}}{\text{liter of solution}}$

Molality: $\frac{\text{\# of mol of solute}}{\text{kg of solvent}}$

Normality: $\frac{\text{\# of gram equivalent weights of solute}}{\text{liter of solution}}$

ACIDS AND BASES

Arrhenius definition: An acid is a species that produces excess H^+ (protons) in an aqueous solution, and a base is a species that produces excess OH^- (hydroxide ions).

Brønsted–Lowry definition: An acid is a species that donates protons, while a base is a species that accepts protons.

Lewis definition: An acid is an electron pair acceptor, and a base is an electron pair donor.

Properties of Acids and Bases

$$pH = -\log[H^+] = \log\left(\frac{1}{[H^+]}\right)$$

$$pOH = -\log[OH^-] = \log\left(\frac{1}{[OH^-]}\right)$$

$$H_2O\ (l) \rightleftharpoons H^+\ (aq) + OH^-\ (aq)$$

$$K_w = [H^+][OH^-] = 10^{-14}$$

$$pH + pOH = 14$$

Weak Acids and Bases

$$HA\ (aq) + H_2O\ (l) \rightleftharpoons H_3O^+\ (aq) + A^-\ (aq)$$

$$K_a = \frac{[H_3O^+][A^-]}{[HA]}$$

$$K_b = \frac{[B^+][OH^-]}{[BOH]}$$

Strong acids: HCl, HI, HBr, H_2SO_4, $HClO_3$, $HClO_4$, HNO_3

Strong bases: LiOH, NaOH, KOH, RbOH, CsOH, $Ca(OH)_2$, $Sr(OH)_2$, $Ba(OH)_2$

Any acid or base not on the above list is considered weak.

Amphoteric species: is one that can act either as an acid or a base, depending on its chemical environment

Titration and Buffers

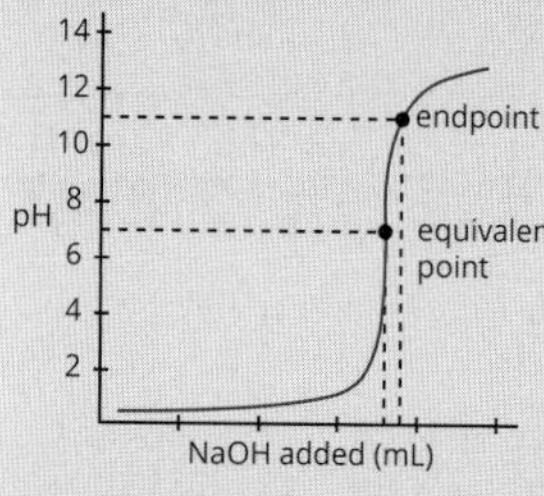

strong acid and strong base

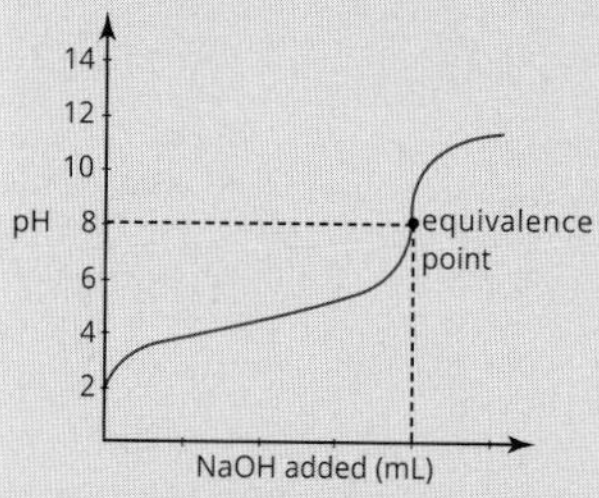

weak acid and strong base

Titration is a procedure used to determine the molarity of an acid or base by reacting a known volume of a solution of unknown concentration with a known volume of a solution of known concentration. The half-equivalence point defines $pH = pK_a$

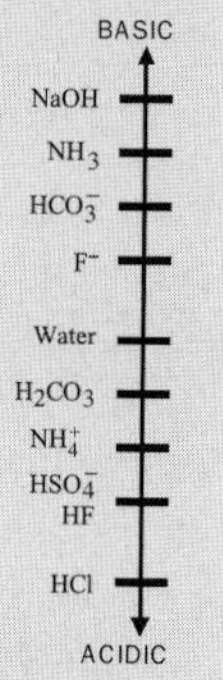

Henderson–Hasselbalch equation: is used to estimate the pH of a solution in the buffer region where the concentrations of the species and its conjugate are present in approximately equal concentrations

$$pH = pK_a + \log\frac{[\text{conjugate base}]}{[\text{weak acid}]}$$

$$pOH = pK_b + \log\frac{[\text{conjugate acid}]}{[\text{weak base}]}$$

REDOX REACTIONS & ELECTROCHEMISTRY

Oxidation: loss of electrons

Reduction: gain of electrons

Oxidizing agent: causes another atom to undergo oxidation, and is itself reduced

Reducing agent: causes another atom to be reduced, and is itself oxidized

Galvanic Cells

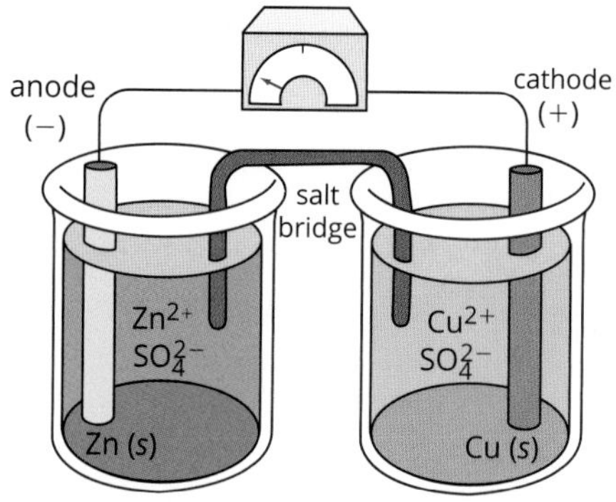

A redox reaction occurring in a galvanic cell has a negative ΔG and is therefore a spontaneous reaction. Galvanic cell reactions supply energy and are used to do work.

This energy can be harnessed by placing the oxidation–reduction half-reactions in separate containers called **half-cells**. The half-cells are then connected by an apparatus that allows for the flow of electrons.

Electrolytic Cells

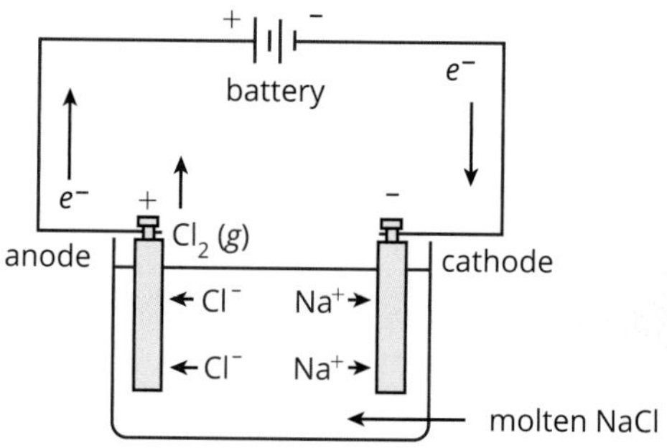

A redox reaction occurring in an electrolytic cell has a positive ΔG and is therefore nonspontaneous. In electrolysis, electrical energy is required to induce a reaction. The oxidation and reduction half-reactions are usually placed in one container.

Reduction potential of each species is defined as the tendency of a species to acquire electrons and be reduced. Standard reduction potential, E°, is measured under standard conditions: 25°C, 1 M concentration for each ion in the reaction, a partial pressure of 1 atm for each gas and metals in their pure state.

Standard reduction potentials are used to calculate the standard electromotive force (emf or E°_{cell}) of a reaction, the difference in potential between two half-cells.

$$\text{emf} = E^\circ_{\text{red, cathode}} - E^\circ_{\text{red, anode}}$$

Gibbs free energy, ΔG, is the thermodynamic criterion for determining the spontaneity of a reaction.

$$\Delta G = -nFE_{cell}$$

NOMENCLATURE

1. Find the longest carbon chain containing the principal functional group (highest-priority groups are generally the most oxidized).
2. Number the carbon chain so that the principal functional group gets lowest possible number.
3. Proceed to number the chain so that the lowest set of numbers is obtained for the substituents.
4. Name the substituents and assign each a number.
5. Complete the name by listing substituents in alphabetical order; place commas between numbers and dashes between numbers and words.

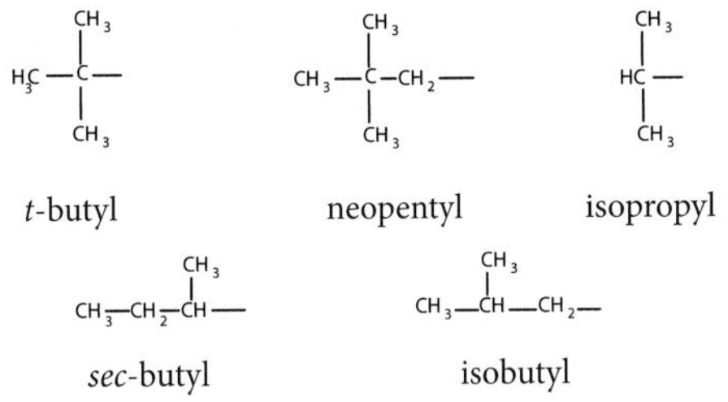

Functional Group	Prefix	Suffix
Carboxylic acid	*carboxy–*	*–oic acid*
Anhydrides	*alkanoyloxy-carbonyl–*	*anhydride*
Esters	*alkoxycarbonyl–*	*–oate*
Amides	*carbomoyl–*	*–amide*
Aldehydes	*oxo–*	*–al*
Ketones	*oxo–* or *keto–*	*–one*
Alcohols	*hydroxy–*	*–ol*

ISOMERS

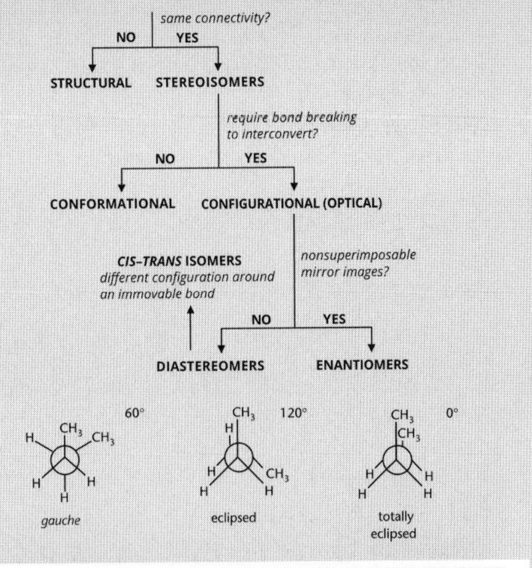

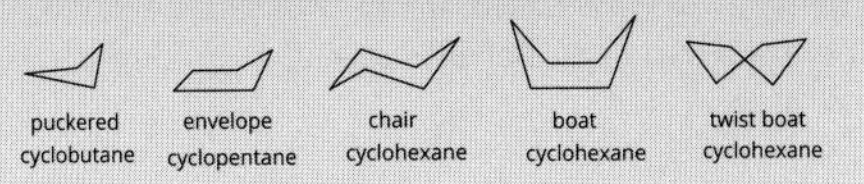

conformations of cyclic hydrocarbons

Physical properties are characteristics of processes that don't change the composition of matter, such as melting point, boiling point, solubility, odor, color, and density.

Chemical properties have to do with the reactivity of the molecule with other molecules.

Stereoisomers

Conformational isomers

Differ by rotation around a single (σ) bond

- **Staggered conformations** have groups 60° apart, as seen in a **Newman projection**. ***anti*** = largest groups are 180° apart; ***gauche*** = 60° apart.
- **Eclipsed conformations** have groups directly in front of each other. **Totally eclipsed** = largest groups are directly in front of each other; strain is maximized.

Cyclic Strain

Comes from:

- **Angle strain:** stretch or compress angles from normal size
- **Torsional strain:** from eclipsing conformations
- **Nonbonded strain:** from interactions with substituents on nonadjacent carbons. In cyclohexane, the largest substituent usually takes equatorial position to reduce nonbonded strain

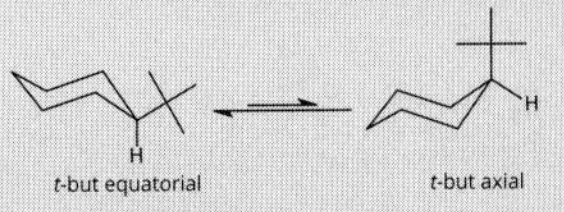

Configurational Isomers

Can only be interchanged by breaking and reforming bonds

- **Enantiomers:** nonsuperimposable mirror images; have opposite stereochemistry at every chiral carbon. Same chemical and physical properties except for rotation of plane-polarized light and reactions in a chiral environment

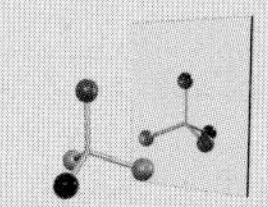

Racemic mixtures and *meso* compounds are optically inactive.

- **Diastereomers:** non-mirror-image stereoisomers. Differ at some, but not all, chiral centers. They have different chemical and physical properties.
- ***Cis–trans*:** subtype of diastereomers in which groups differ in position about an immovable bond (such as a double bond or in a cycloalkane).

Absolute Configuration

An alkene is (*Z*) if the highest-priority substituents are on the same side of the double bond, and (*E*) if on opposite sides.

A stereocenter's configuration is determined by putting the lowest-priority group in the back and drawing a circle from group 1 to 2 to 3 in descending priority. If this circle is clockwise, the stereocenter is (***R***); if it is counterclockwise, the stereocenter is (**S**).

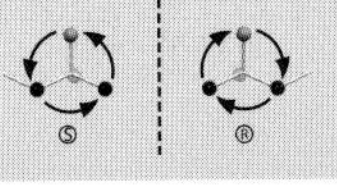

BONDING

Bond order	single	double	triple
Bond type	σ	σ π	σ 2 π
Hybridization	sp^3	sp^2	sp
Angles	109.5°	120°	180°
Example	C–C	C=C	C≡C

ALKANES

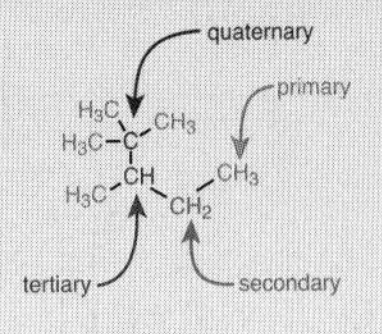

Combustion

$$C_3H_8 + 5\ O_2 \rightarrow 3\ CO_2 + 4\ H_20 + \text{heat}$$

S_N1	S_N2
2 steps	1 step
Favored in polar protic solvents	Favored in polar aprotic solvents
3° > 2° > 1° > methyl	Methyl > 1° > 2° > 3°
rate = k[RL]	rate = k[Nu][RL]
Racemic products	Optically active and inverted products
Strong nucleophile not required	Favored with strong nucleophile

S_N1

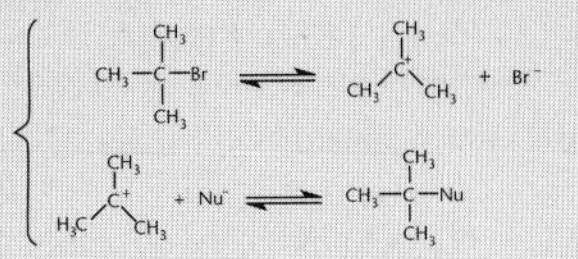

S_N2

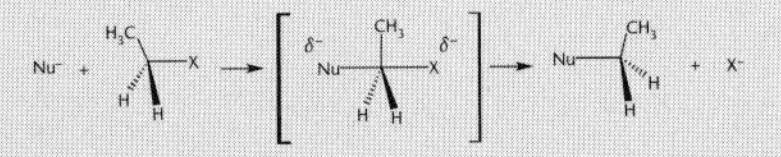

Nucleophiles

Nucleophile = "nucleus-loving"; tend to have lone pairs or π bonds that can form new bonds to electrophiles. Nucleophilicity is increased by increasing electron density.

Nucleophilicity is determined by four major factors:

- Charge: Nucleophilicity increases with increasing electron density (more negative charge).
- Electronegativity: Nucleophilicity decreases as electronegativity increases because these atoms are less likely to share electron density.
- Steric hindrance: Bulkier molecules are less nucleophilic.
- Solvent: Protic solvents can inhibit nucleophilicity by protonating the nucleophile or through hydrogen bonding.

In aprotic solvents, nucleophilicity parallels basicity:

$$F^- > Cl^- > Br^- > I^-$$

In protic solvents, good bases pick up protons and are worse nucleophiles:

$$I^- > Br^- > Cl^- > F^-$$

Electrophiles

Electrophile = "electron-loving"; tend to have a positive charge or positively polarized atom that accepts an electron pair from a nucleophile. Electrophilicity is increased by increasing the positive charge.

Most common electrophiles:

- Carbonyl carbon
- Substrate carbon in an alkane
- Carbocations

Leaving Groups

Leaving groups = molecular fragments that retain the electrons after **heterolysis** (breaking a bond, with both electrons being given to one of the two products). The best leaving groups will be able to stabilize the extra electrons.

Most common leaving groups:

- Weak bases
- Large groups with resonance
- Large groups with electron-withdrawing atoms

DETERMINING ORGANIC MECHANISMS

Step 1: Know Your Nomenclature

If given compound names in a question stem or passage, be able to draw them. If working with reaction diagrams, be able to name the compounds.

Step 2: Identify the Functional Groups

What functional groups are in the molecule? Do these functional groups act as acids or bases? How oxidized is the carbon? Are there functional groups that act as good nucleophiles, electrophiles, or leaving groups? This will help define a category of reactions that can occur with the given functional groups.

Step 3: Identify the Other Reagents

Are the other reagents acidic or basic? Are they specific to a particular reaction? Are they good nucleophiles or a specific solvent? Are they good oxidizing or reducing agents?

Step 4: Identify the Most Reactive Functional Group(s)

More oxidized carbons tend to be more reactive to both nucleophile–electrophile reactions and oxidation–reduction reactions. Note the presence of protecting groups that exist to prevent a particular functional group from reacting.

Step 5: Identify the First Step of the Reaction

- If the reaction involves an acid or a base: protonation or deprotonation
- If the reaction involves a nucleophile: nucleophile attacks electrophile, forming a bond
- If the reaction involves an oxidizing or reducing agent: most oxidized functional group is oxidized or reduced, accordingly

Step 6: Consider Stereoselectivity

If there is more than one product, the major product will generally be determined by differences in strain or stability between the two molecules. Products with **conjugation** (alternating single and multiple bonds) are significantly more stable than those without.

ALCOHOLS

- Higher boiling points than alkanes due to hydrogen bonding
- Weakly acidic hydroxyl hydrogen

Synthesis

- Addition of water to double bonds
- S_N1 and S_N2 reactions
- Reduction of carboxylic acids, aldehydes, ketones, and esters
  - Aldehydes and ketones with $NaBH_4$ or $LiAlH_4$
  - Esters and carboxylic acids with $LiAlH_4$

Reactions

Substitution reactions after protonation or leaving group conversion

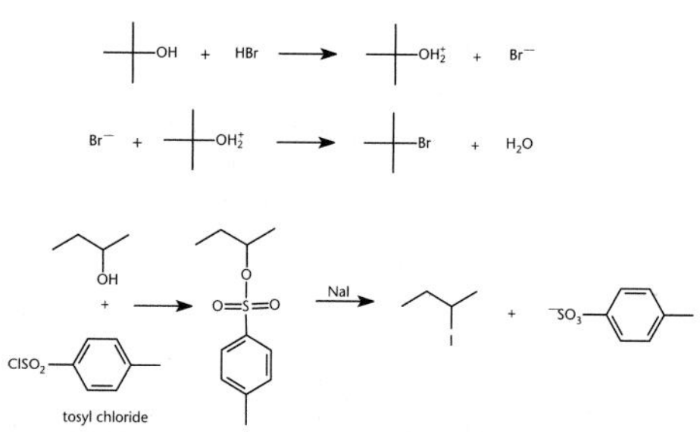

ORGANIC OXIDATION–REDUCTION

- **Level 0** (no bonds to heteroatoms): alkanes
- **Level 1**: alcohols, alkyl halides, amines
- **Level 2**: aldehydes, ketones, imines
- **Level 3**: carboxylic acids, anhydrides, esters, amides
- **Level 4** (four bonds to heteroatoms): carbon dioxide

Oxidation = loss of electrons, fewer bonds to hydrogens, more bonds to heteroatoms (O, N, halogens)

Reduction = gain of electrons, more bonds to hydrogens, fewer bonds to heteroatoms

Oxidizing Agents

Good oxidizing agents have a high affinity for electrons (such as O_2, O_3, and Cl_2) or unusually high oxidation states (like Mn^{7+} in permanganate, MnO_4^-, and Cr^{6+} in chromate, CrO_4^{2-}).

Reducing Agents

Good reducing agents include sodium, magnesium, aluminum, and zinc, which have low electronegativities and ionization energies. Metal hydrides are also good reducing agents, like NaH, CaH_2, $LiAlH_4$, and $NaBH_4$, because they contain the H^- ion.

Oxidation

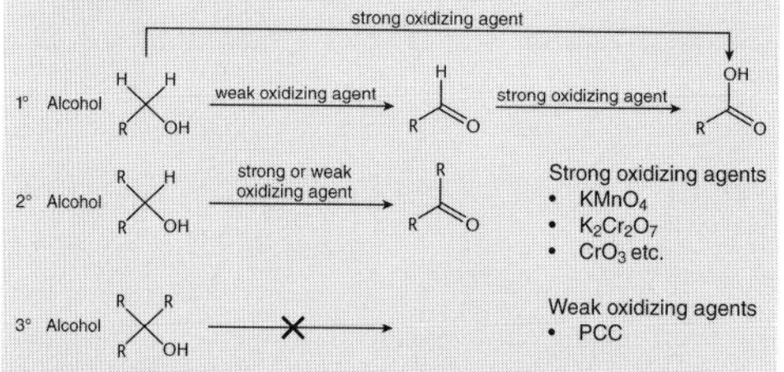

Reduction

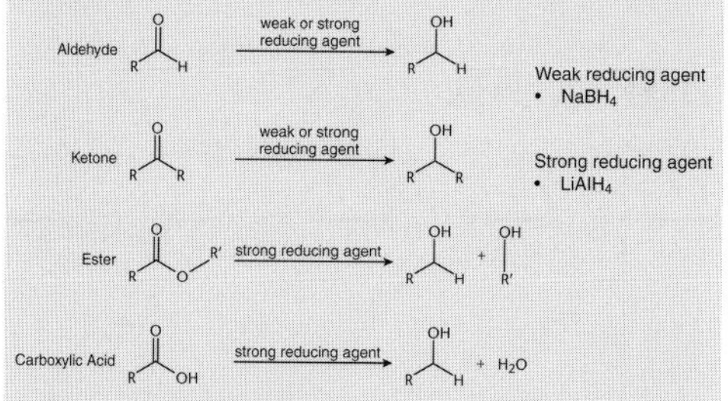

Alcohols and Reactivity

Alcohols can be converted to mesylates or tosylates to make them better leaving groups for nucleophilic substitution reactions.

- **Mesylates** ($-SO_3CH_3$) are derived from methanesulfonic acid.
- **Tosylates** ($-SO_3C_6H_4CH_3$) are derived from toluenesulfonic acid.

Alcohols can be used as **protecting groups** for carbonyls, as reaction with a dialcohol forms an unreactive acetal. After other reactions, the protecting group can be removed with aqueous acid.

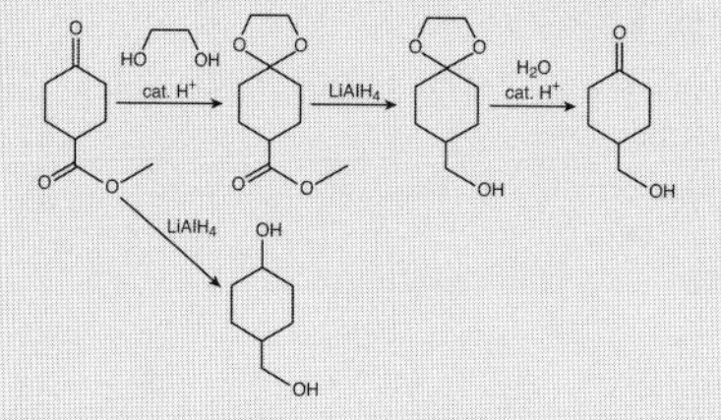

PHENOLS & QUINONE DERIVATIVES

The hydrogen of the hydroxyl group of a phenol is particularly acidic because the oxygen-containing anion is resonance-stabilized by the ring.

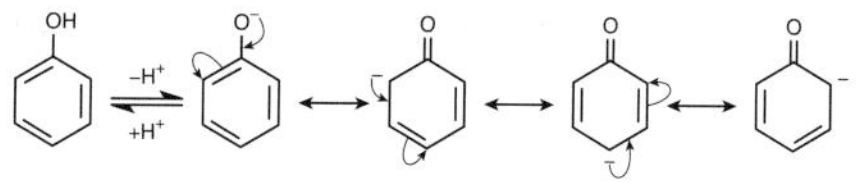

Quinones and Hydroxyquinones

Treatment of phenols with oxidizing agents produces **quinones**.

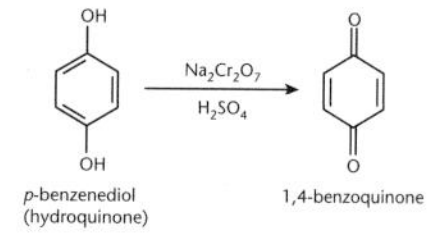

These molecules can be further oxidized to form a class of molecules called hydroxyquinones. Many hydroxyquinones have biological activity.

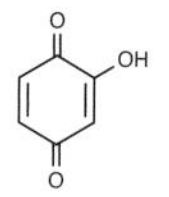

Ubiquinone

Ubiquinone is also called **coenzyme Q** and is a vital electron carrier associated with Complexes I, II, and III of the electron transport chain.

Ubiquinone can be reduced to **ubiquinol**, which can later be reoxidized to ubiquinone. This is sometimes called the **Q cycle**.

ALDEHYDES

The dipole moment of aldehydes causes an elevation of boiling point, but not as high as alcohols because there is no hydrogen bonding.

Synthesis

- Oxidation of primary alcohols
- Ozonolysis of alkenes

Reactions

Reactions of enols (Michael additions)

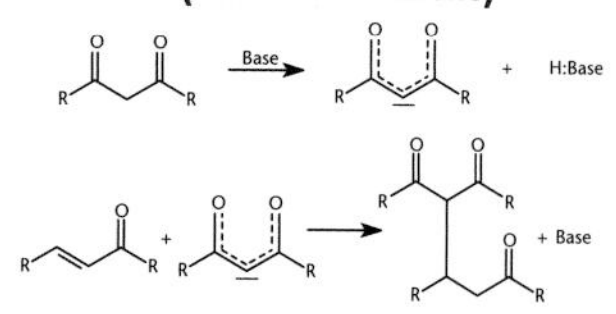

Nucleophilic addition to a carbonyl

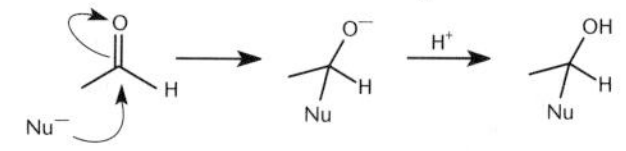

Aldol condensation

An aldehyde acts both as nucleophile (enol form) and electrophile (keto form). One carbonyl forms an enolate, which attacks the other carbonyl. After the aldol is formed, a dehydration reaction results in an α,β-unsaturated carbonyl.

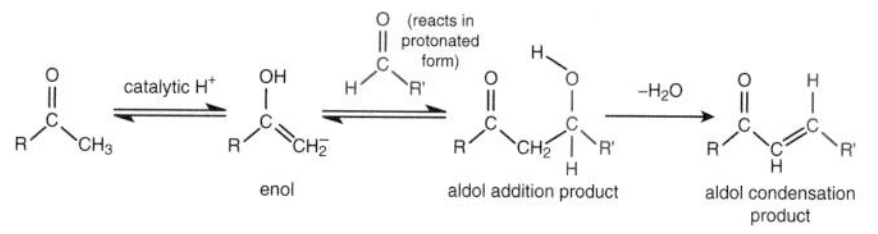

Decarboxylation

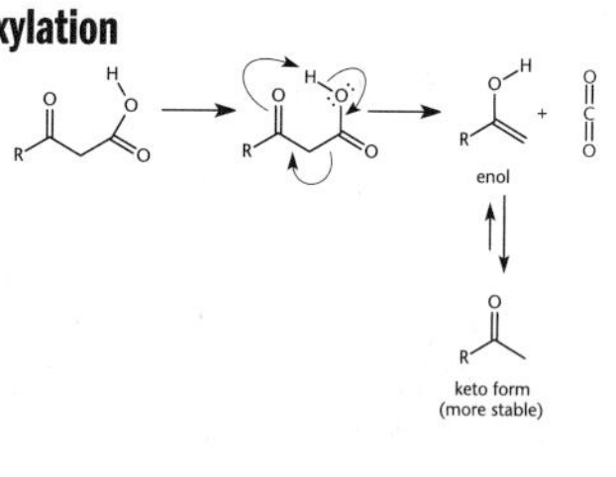

CARBOXYLIC ACIDS

Carboxylic acids have pK_a values around 4.5 due to resonance stabilization of the conjugate base. Electronegative atoms increase acidity with inductive effects. Boiling point is higher than alcohols because of the ability to form two hydrogen bonds.

Synthesis

Oxidation of primary alcohols with $KMnO_4$

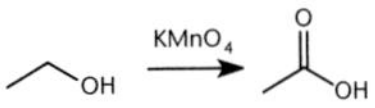

Reactions

Formation of soap by reacting carboxylic acids with NaOH; arrange in micelles

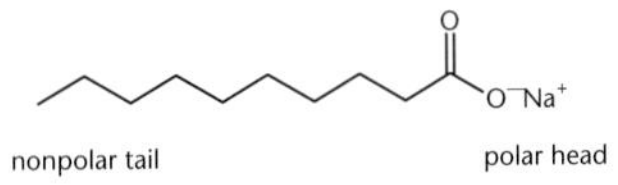

Nucleophilic acyl substitution

- General mechanism

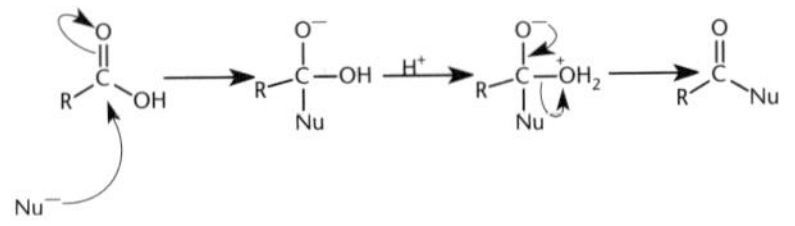

- Reduction to alcohols

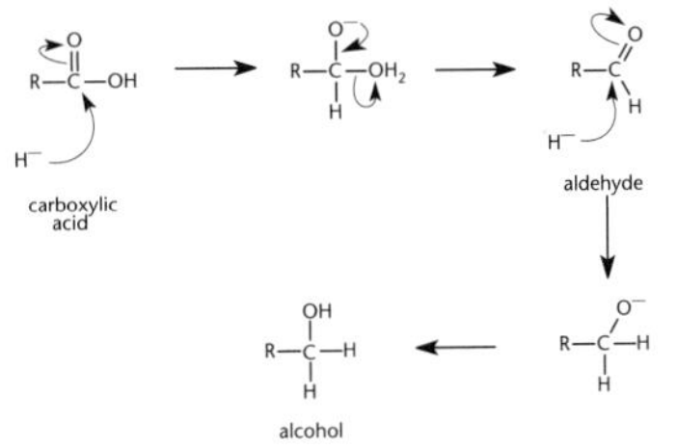

Decarboxylation

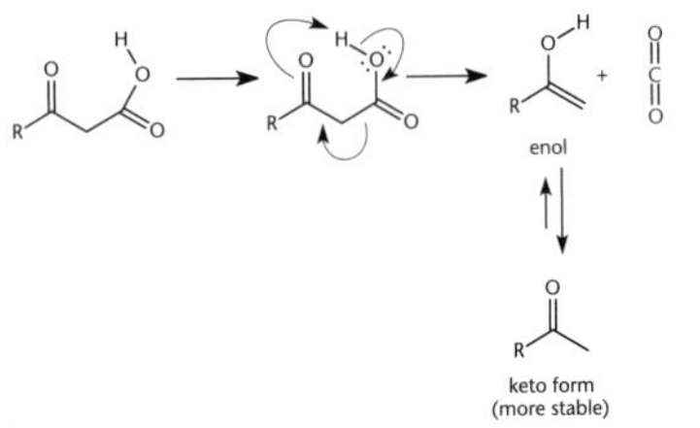

CYCLIC CARBOXYLIC ACID DERIVATIVES

Lactams

Cyclic amides are called **lactams**. These are named according to the carbon atom bonded to the nitrogen: β-lactams contain a bond between the β-carbon and the nitrogen, γ-lactams contain a bond between the γ-carbon and the nitrogen, and so forth.

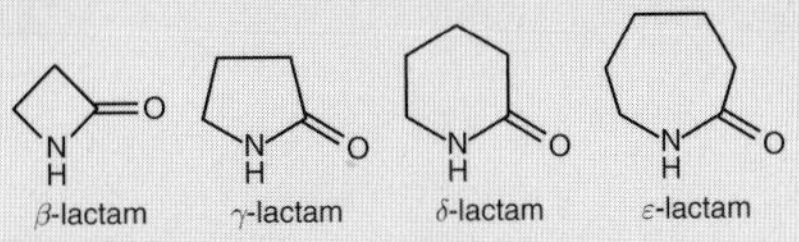

Lactones

Cyclic esters are called **lactones**. These are named not only based on the carbon bonded to the oxygen, but also the length of the carbon chain itself.

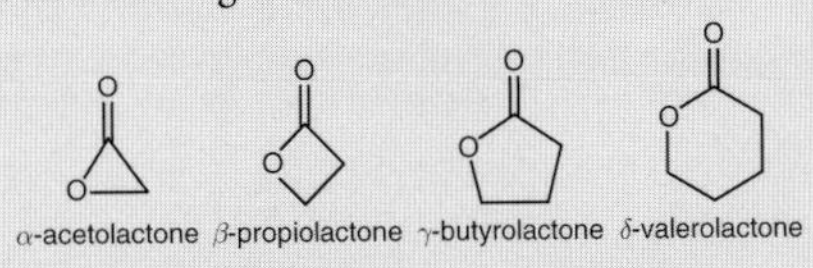

CARBOXYLIC ACID DERIVATIVES

Carboxylic acid derivatives contain three bonds to heteroatoms (O, N, halides, and so forth). As such, they can be interconverted through nucleophilic acyl substitution by swapping leaving groups.

Carboxylic acid derivatives can be ranked based on descending reactivity:

- Acyl halides are the most reactive
- Anhydrides
- Carboxylic acids and esters
- Amides are the least reactive

A reaction that proceeds down the order of reactivity can occur spontaneously by nucleophilic acyl substitution.

A reaction that proceeds up the order of reactivity requires special catalysts and specific reaction conditions.

Anhydrides

Synthesis via dehydration of two carboxylic acids

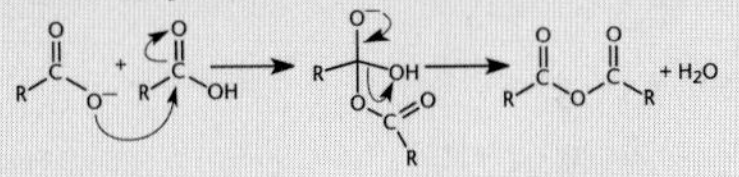

Intramolecular formation of a cyclic anhydride

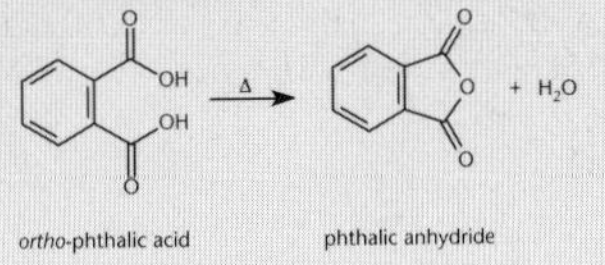

NITROGEN-CONTAINING COMPOUNDS

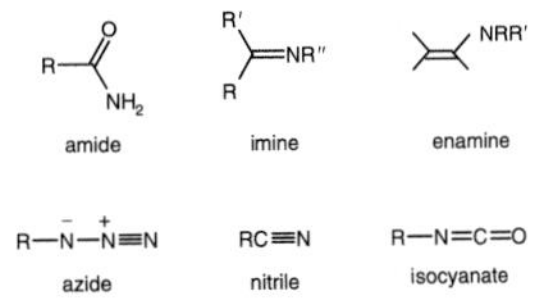

Strecker Synthesis

Reagents: aldehyde, ammonium chloride (NH_4Cl), potassium cyanide (KCN)

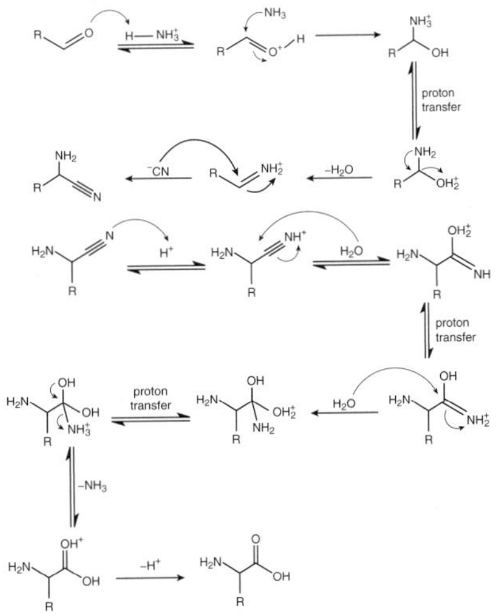

Gabriel (Malonic-Ester) Synthesis

Reagents: potassium phthalimide, diethyl bromomalonate

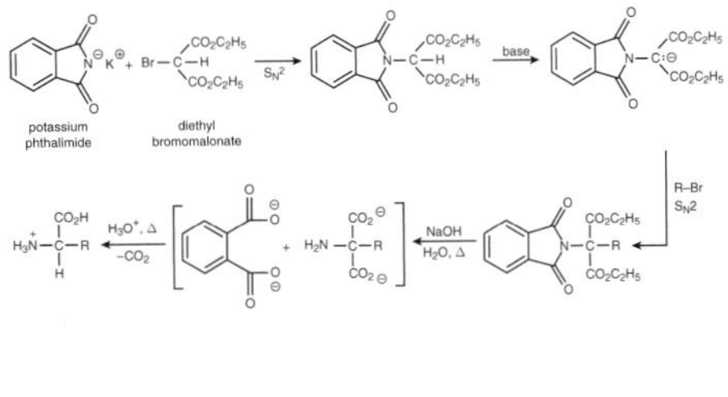

Amides

Formation from an anhydride

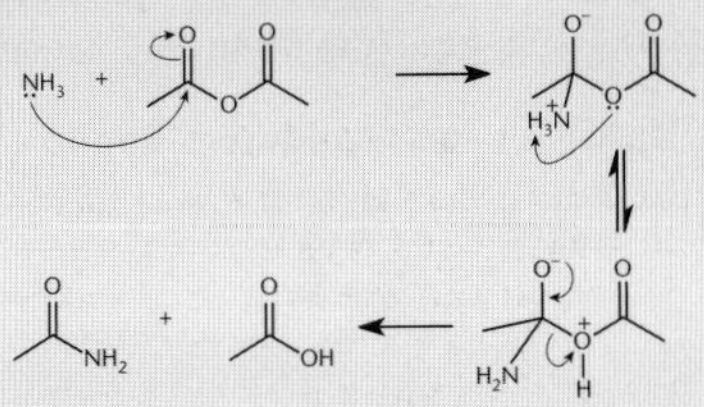

Formation from an ester

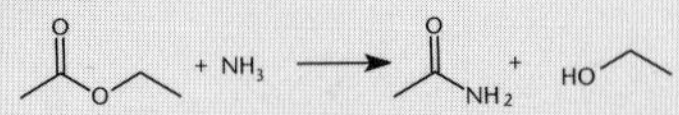

Hydrolysis (requires acid)

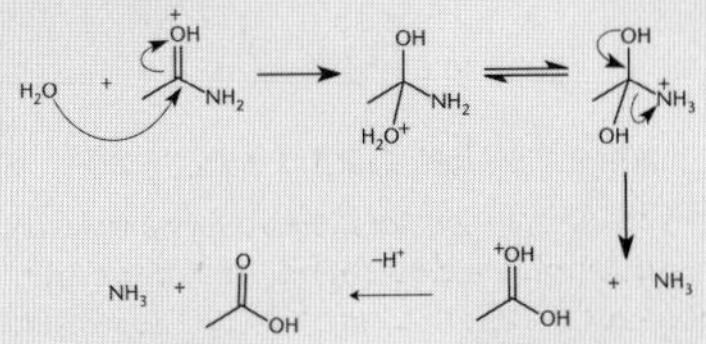

Reduction to an amine

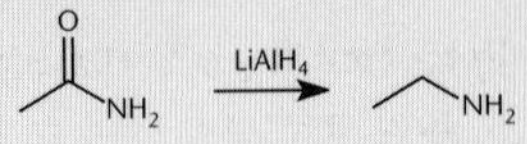

Esters

Transesterification

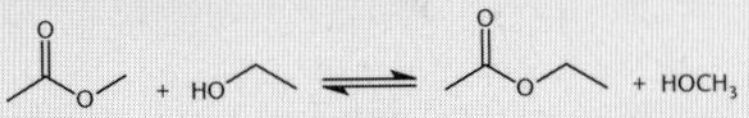

Hydrolysis

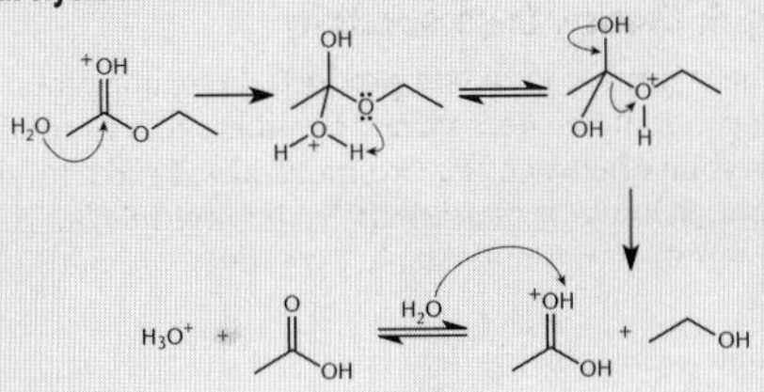

Reduction

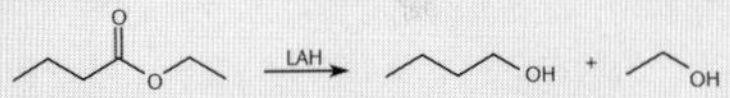

Saponification

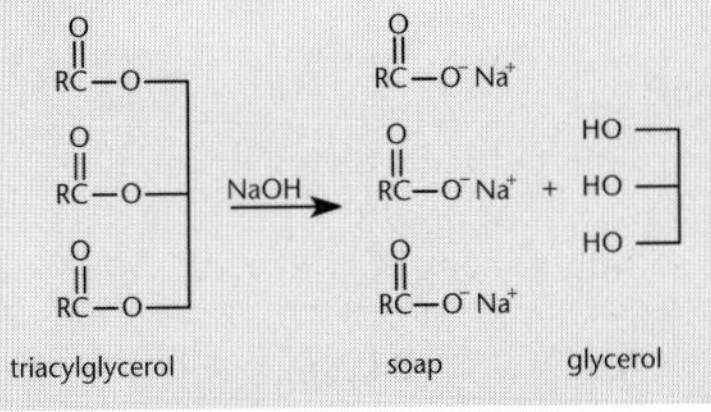

PHOSPHORUS-CONTAINING COMPOUNDS

- **Phosphoric acid** is a **phosphate group** or **inorganic phosphate** (P_i). At physiologic pH, inorganic phosphate includes both hydrogen phosphate (HPO_4^{2-}) and dihydrogen phosphate ($H_2PO_4^-$).
- **Pyrophosphate** (PP_i) is $P_2O_7^{4-}$, which is released during the formation of phosphodiester bonds in DNA. Pyrophosphate is unstable in aqueous solution, and is hydrolyzed to form two molecules of inorganic phosphate.

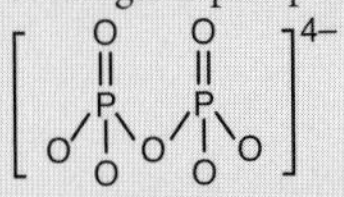

- Nucleotides with phosphate groups, such ATP, GTP, and those in DNA, are referred to as **organic phosphates**.

PURIFICATION METHODS

Extraction separates dissolved substances based on differential solubility in aqueous *vs.* organic solvents.

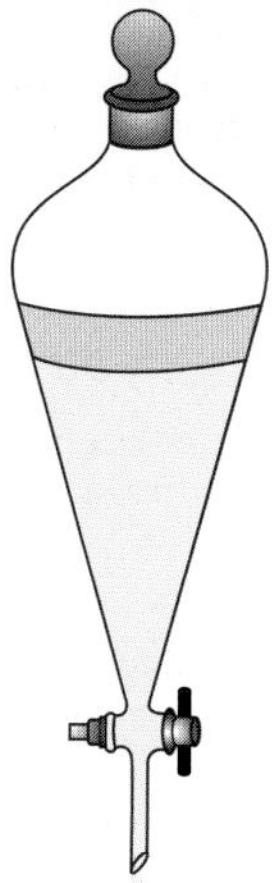

Filtration separates solids from liquids.

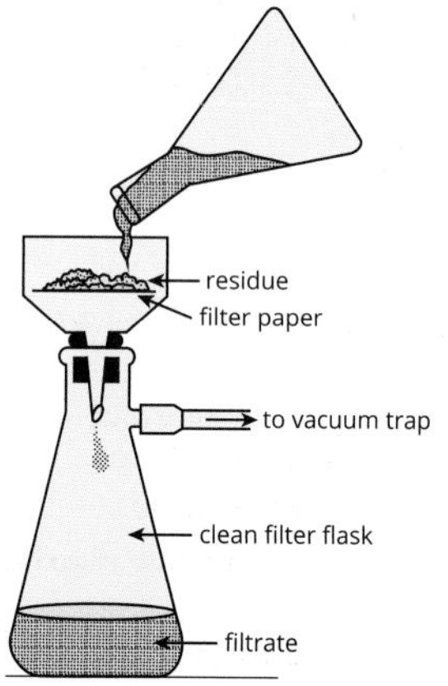

vacuum filtration

Chromatography uses a stationary phase and a mobile phase to separate compounds based on polarity and/or size.

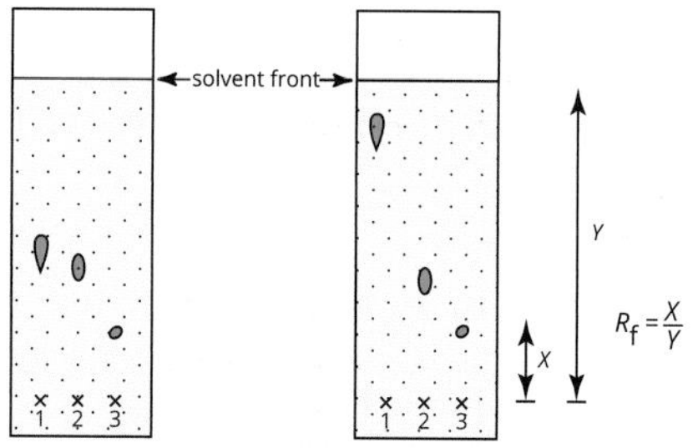

thin-layer chromatograms

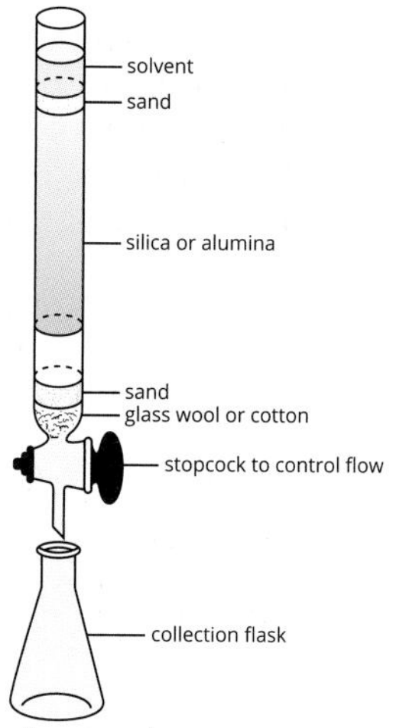

column chromatography

Distillation separates liquids based on boiling point, which depends on intermolecular forces. Types are simple, fractional, and vacuum.

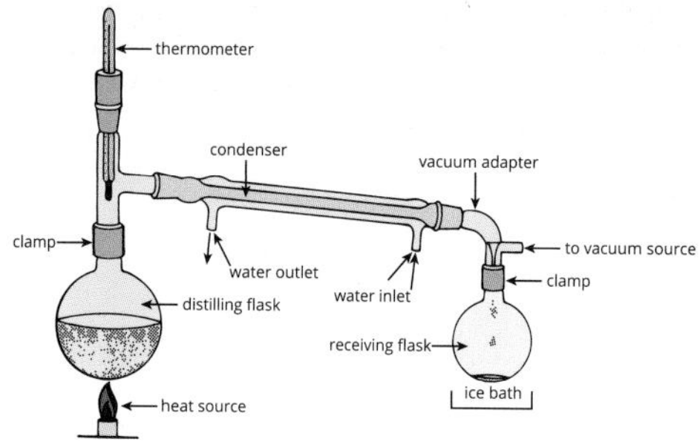

vacuum distillation

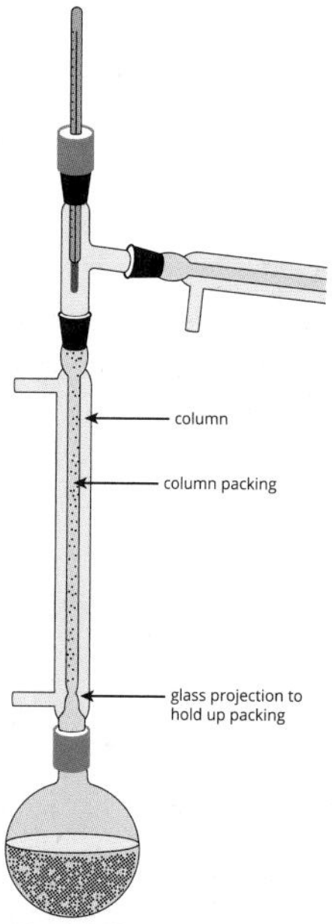

fractional distillation

Simple distillation can be used to separate two liquids with boiling points below 150°C and at least 25°C apart.

Vacuum distillation should be used when a liquid to be distilled has a boiling point above 150°C. To prevent degradation of the product, the incident pressure is lowered, thereby lowering the boiling point.

Fractional distillation should be used when two liquids have boiling points less than 25°C apart. By introducing a fractionation column, the sample boils and refluxes back down over a larger surface area, improving the purity of the distillate.

Recrystallization separates solids based on differential solubility in varying temperatures.

Electrophoresis is used to separate biological macromolecules based on size and/or charge.

SPECTROSCOPY

Infrared spectroscopy measures molecular vibrations of characteristic functional groups.

Functional Group	Wavenumber (cm^{-1})	Vibration
Alcohols	3100 — 3500	O—H (broad)
Ketones	1700 — 1750	C=O
Aldehydes	2700 — 2900	(O)C—H
	1700 — 1750	C=O
Carboxylic acids	1700 — 1750	C=O
	2800 — 3200	O—H (broad)
Amines	3100 — 3500	N—H (sharp)

UV spectroscopy involves passing ultraviolet light through a chemical sample and plotting absorbance *vs.* wavelength. It is most useful for studying compounds containing double bonds and heteroatoms with lone pairs.

^{1}H–NMR is a form of **nuclear magnetic resonance.**

Type of Proton	Approximate Chemical Shift δ (ppm) Downfield from TMS
RCH_3	0.9
RCH_2	1.25
R_3CH	1.5
–CH=CH	4.6–6
–C≡CH	2–3
Ar–H	6–8.5
–CHX	2–4.5
–CHOH/–CHOR	3.4–4
RCHO	9–10
RCHCO–	2–2.5
–CHCOOH/–CHCOOR	2–2.6
$-CHOH-CH_2OH$	1–5.5
ArOH	4–12
–COOH	10.5–12
$-NH_2$	1–5

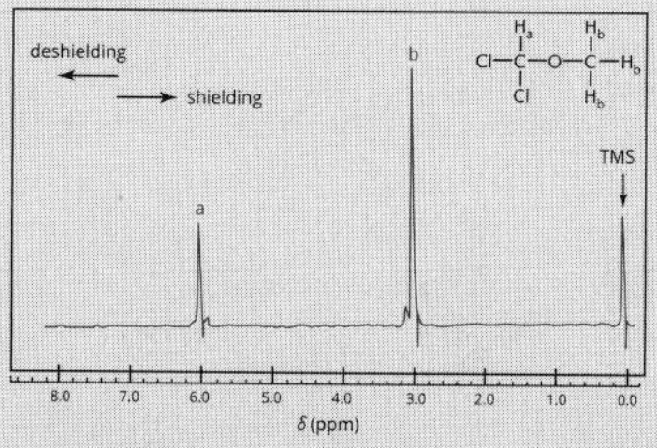

When analyzing an NMR spectrum, look for:

- **Types of protons:** corresponds to the number of peaks seen in the spectrum
- **Position of peaks:** the further left-shifted (downfield) the peak, the more deshielded the proton. Usually this corresponds to more electron-withdrawing groups
- **Integration of peaks:** the larger the integration, the more protons contained under the peak
- **Splitting:** hydrogens on adjacent carbons will split a peak into $n + 1$ subpeaks, where n is the number of hydrogens on the adjacent carbon

Type of Chromatography	Mobile Phase	Stationary Phase	Common Use
Thin-layer or Paper	Nonpolar solvent	Polar card	Identify a sample
Reverse-phase	Polar solvent	Nonpolar card	Identify a sample
Column	Nonpolar solvent	Polar gel or powder	Separate a sample into components
Ion-exchange	Nonpolar solvent	Charged beads in column	Separate components by charge
Size-exclusion	Nonpolar solvent	Polar, porous beads in column	Separate components by size
Affinity	Nonpolar solvent	Beads coated with antibody or receptor for a target molecule	Purify a molecule (usually a protein) of interest
Gas (GC)	Inert gas	Crushed metal or polymer	Separate vaporizable compounds
High-performance liquid (HPLC)	Nonpolar solvent	Small column with concentration gradient	Similar to column, but more precise

KINEMATICS

Vectors: physical quantities with both magnitude and direction

- Examples: force, velocity

Scalars: physical quantities that have magnitude, but no direction

- Examples: mass, speed

Displacement (Δx): the change in position that goes in a straight-line path from the initial position to the final position; independent of the path taken (SI unit: m)

Average velocity: $\bar{\mathbf{v}} = \frac{\Delta \mathbf{x}}{\Delta t}$ (SI units: $\frac{m}{s}$)

Acceleration: the rate of change of an object's velocity; it is a vector quantity: $\mathbf{a} = \frac{\Delta \mathbf{v}}{\Delta t}$ (SI units: $\frac{m}{s^2}$)

Linear Motion

$\mathbf{v} = \mathbf{v}_0 + \mathbf{a}t$

$\mathbf{x} = \mathbf{v}_0 t + \frac{1}{2}\mathbf{a}t^2$

$\mathbf{v}^2 = \mathbf{v}_0^2 + 2\mathbf{ax}$

$\bar{\mathbf{v}} = \frac{(\mathbf{v}_0 + \mathbf{v})}{2}$

$\mathbf{x} = \bar{\mathbf{v}}t = \left(\frac{(\mathbf{v}_0 + \mathbf{v})}{2}\right)t$

- When solving for time, there will be two values for t: when the projectile is initially launched and when it impacts the ground.
- To find max height, remember that the vertical velocity of the projectile is 0 at the highest point of the path.

Projectile Motion

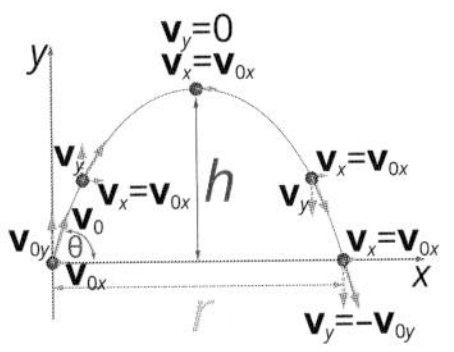

- Vertical component of velocity = $v \sin \theta$
- Horizontal component of velocity = $v \cos \theta$

Frictional forces

Static friction (f_s): is the force that must be overcome to set an object in motion. It has the formula: $0 \leq f_s \leq \mu_s N$

Kinetic friction (f_k): opposes the motion of objects moving relative to each other. It has the formula: $f_k = \mu_k N$

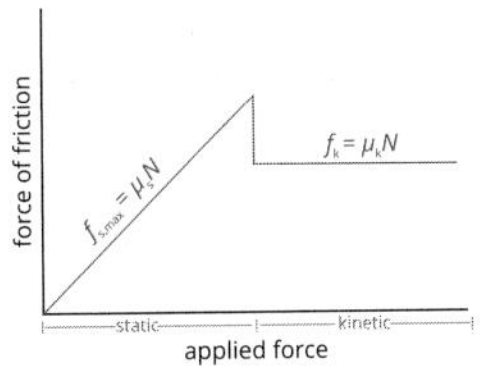

Newton's first law (law of inertia): A body in a state of motion or at rest will remain in that state unless acted upon by a net force.

Newton's second law: When a net force is applied to a body of mass m, the body will be accelerated in the same direction as the force applied to the mass. This is expressed by the formula $\mathbf{F} = m\mathbf{a}$ [SI unit: newton (N) = $\frac{kg.m}{s^2}$].

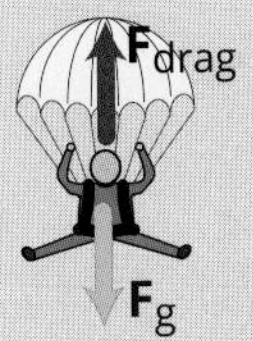

- $F_{gravity} > F_{drag}$: person accelerates downward
- $F_g = F_{drag}$: terminal velocity is reached (person travels at constant velocity)

WORK AND ENERGY

Work: For a constant force F acting on an object that moves a displacement of **d**, the work is $W = Fd \cos \theta$. (For a force perpendicular to the displacement, $W = 0$.) [SI unit: joule = N·m]

System Work

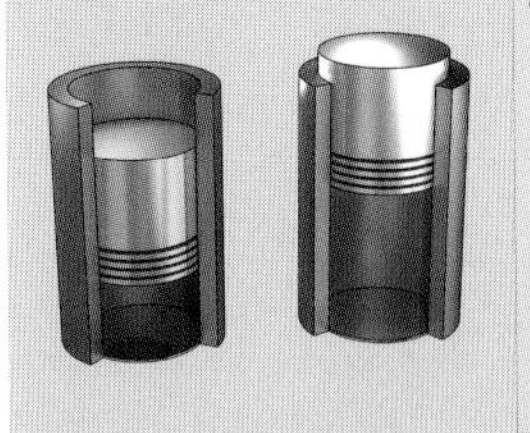

- When the piston expands, work is done *by* the system ($W > 0$).
- When the piston compresses the gas, work is done *on* the system ($W < 0$).
- The area under a P *vs.* V curve is the amount of work done in a system.

Power: the rate at which work is performed; it is given by: $P = \frac{W}{\Delta t}$ (SI unit: watt = $\frac{J}{s}$)

Mechanical Energy

Energy is a scalar quantity (SI unit: joule).

Kinetic energy: the energy associated with moving objects. It is given by:

$$K = \frac{1}{2}mv^2$$

Potential energy: the energy associated with a body's position. Gravitational potential energy of an object is due to the force of gravity acting on it and is expressed as: $U = mgh$

Total mechanical energy

$$E = U + K$$

Mechanical energy is conserved when the sum of kinetic and potential energies remains constant.

Work–Energy Theorem

Relates the work performed by all forces acting on a body in a particular time interval to the change in energy at that time:

$$W = \Delta E$$

Conservation of Energy

When there are no nonconservative forces (such as friction) acting on a system, the total mechanical energy remains constant: $\Delta E = \Delta K + \Delta U = 0$

NEWTON'S LAWS

Newton's third law: If body A exerts a force on body B, then B will exert a force back onto A that is equal in magnitude, but opposite in direction. This can be expressed as $\mathbf{F}_b = -\mathbf{F}_a$.

Newton's law of gravitation: All forms of matter experience an attractive force to other forms of matter in the universe. The magnitude of the force is represented by: $F = \frac{Gm_1m_2}{r^2}$

- **Mass (m):** a scalar quantity that measures a body's inertia
- **Weight ($\mathbf{F}_g$):** a vector quantity that measures a body's gravitational attraction to the earth ($\mathbf{F}_g = m\mathbf{g}$)

Uniform circular motion:

$a_c = \frac{v^2}{r}$

$F_c = \frac{mv^2}{r}$

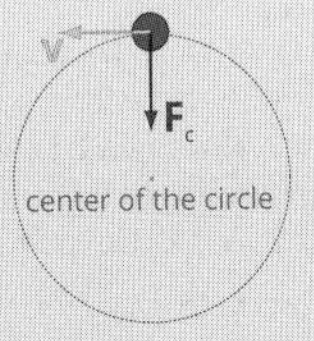

Equilibrium

First condition of equilibrium: An object is in translational equilibrium when the sum of forces pushing it one direction is counterbalanced by the sum of forces acting in the opposite direction. It can be expressed as $\Sigma\mathbf{F} = 0$.

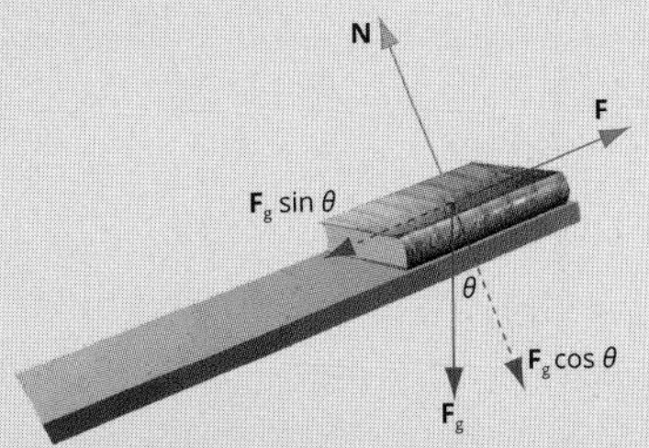

Problem-Solving Guide

- Resolve the forces into x- and y-components.
- $\Sigma\mathbf{F} = 0$ must be true for equilibrium; therefore, $\Sigma\mathbf{F}_x = 0$ and $\Sigma\mathbf{F}_y = 0$.

THERMODYNAMICS

Thermal Expansion

Linear expansion: the increase in length by most solids when heated

Mnemonic: when temperature increases, the length of a solid increases "a Lot"($\alpha L \Delta T$)

$$\Delta L = \alpha L \Delta T$$

Volume expansion: the increase in volume of fluids when heated

$$\Delta V = \beta V \Delta T$$

Heat Transfer

Conduction: the direct transfer of energy via molecular collisions

Convection: the transfer of heat by the physical motion of a fluid

Radiation: the transfer of energy by electromagnetic waves

Specific Heat

$Q = mc\Delta T$ (mnemonic: looks like MCAT)

- Can only be used to find Q when the object does not change phase
- $Q > 0$ means heat is gained; $Q < 0$ means heat is lost

[Common units: joules, calories, or Calories (kcal)]

Heat of transformation: the quantity of heat required to change the phase of 1 g of a substance.

$Q = mL$ (phase changes are isothermal processes)

First law of thermodynamics: $\Delta U = Q - W$

Process	First Law Becomes
Adiabatic ($Q = 0$)	$\Delta U = -W$
Constant volume ($W = 0$)	$\Delta U = Q$
Isothermal ($\Delta U = 0$)	$Q = W$

Second law of thermodynamics: In any thermodynamic process that moves from one state of equilibrium to another, the entropy of the system and environment together will either increase or remain unchanged.

HYDROSTATICS & FLUID DYNAMICS

Density (ρ) $= \frac{m}{V}$ [SI units: $\frac{kg}{m^3}$]

Specific gravity $= \frac{\rho_{substance}}{\rho_{water}}$ [no units]; $\rho_{water} = 10^3 \frac{kg}{m^3}$

Weight $= \rho g V$

Pressure: a scalar quantity defined as force per unit area: $P = \frac{F}{A}$ [SI units: pascal $= \frac{N}{m^2}$]

- For static fluids of uniform density in a sealed vessel, pressure: $P = \rho g z$
- **Absolute pressure** in a fluid due to gravity somewhere below the surface is given by the equation $P = P_o + \rho g z$
- **Gauge pressure:** $P_g = P - P_{atm}$

Continuity equation: $A_1 v_1 = A_2 v_2$

Bernoulli's equation: $P + \frac{1}{2}\rho v^2 + \rho g h =$ constant

Archimedes' Principle

$F_{buoy} = \rho_{fluid}\, g V_{submerged}$

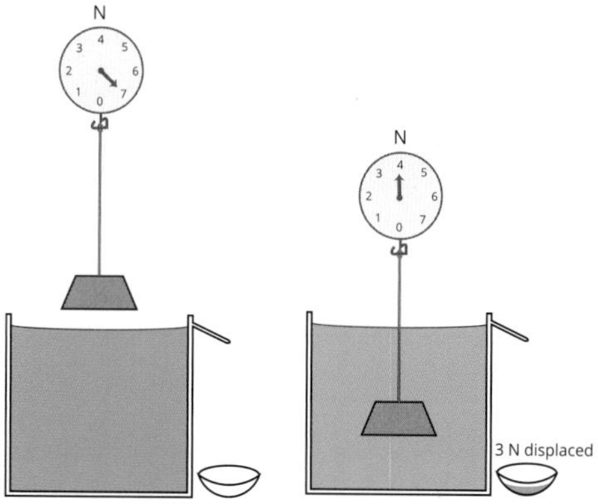

- The buoyant force is equal to the weight of the displaced fluid.
  - If the weight of the fluid displaced is less than the object's weight, the object will sink.
  - If the weight of the fluid displaced is greater than or equal to the object's weight, then it will float.

Pascal's Principle

- A change in the pressure applied to an enclosed fluid is transmitted undiminished to every portion of the fluid and to the walls of the containing vessel.

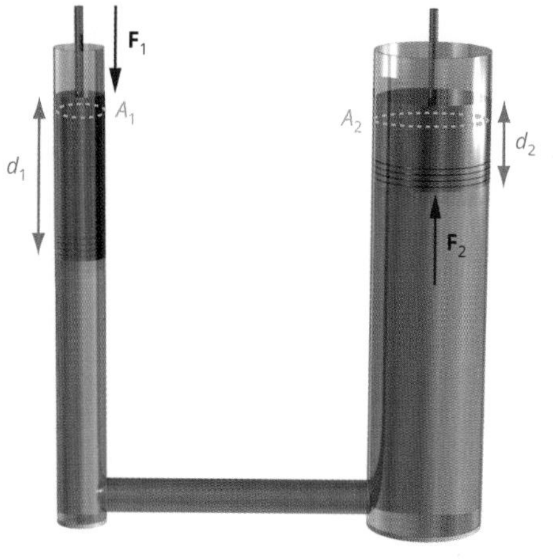

$$P = \frac{F_1}{A_1} = \frac{F_2}{A_2} \text{ and } A_1 d_1 = A_2 d_2$$

so, $W = F_1 d_1 = F_2 d_2$

ELECTROSTATICS

Coulomb's Law

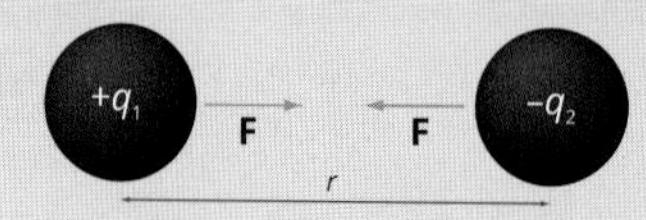

$$F = \frac{k q_1 q_2}{r^2} \text{ [SI units: newton]}$$

Electric Field

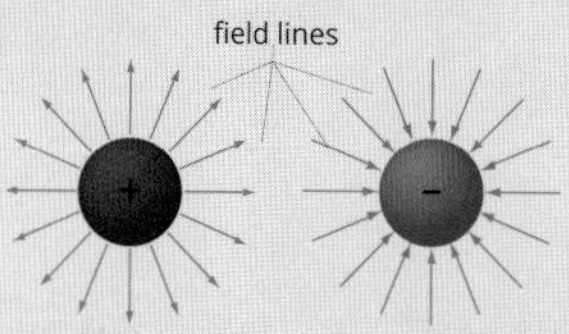

$$E = \frac{F_e}{q} = \frac{kQ}{r^2} \text{ [SI units: } \frac{N}{C} \text{ or } \frac{V}{m}\text{]}$$

- A positive point charge will move in the same direction as the electric field vector; a negative charge will move in the opposite direction.

Electrical Potential Energy (*U*)

The electrical potential energy of a charge q at a point in space is the amount of work required to move it from infinity to that point.

$$U = q\Delta V = qEd = \frac{kQq}{r} \text{ [SI units: J]}$$

Electric Dipoles

- **p** is the dipole moment ($\mathbf{p} = q\mathbf{d}$).
- The dipole feels no net translational force, but experiences a torque about the center causing it to rotate so that the dipole moment aligns with the electric field.

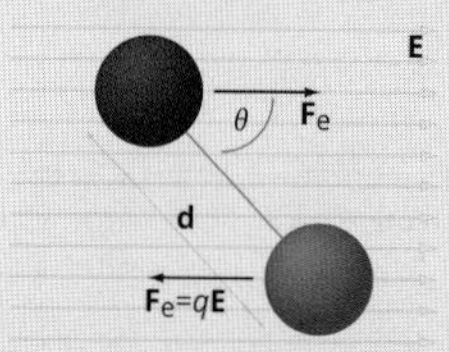

Electrical Potential

The amount of work required to move a positive test charge q from infinity to a particular point divided by the test charge: $V = \frac{U}{q}$ [SI units: volt $= \frac{J}{C}$]

Potential Difference (Voltage)

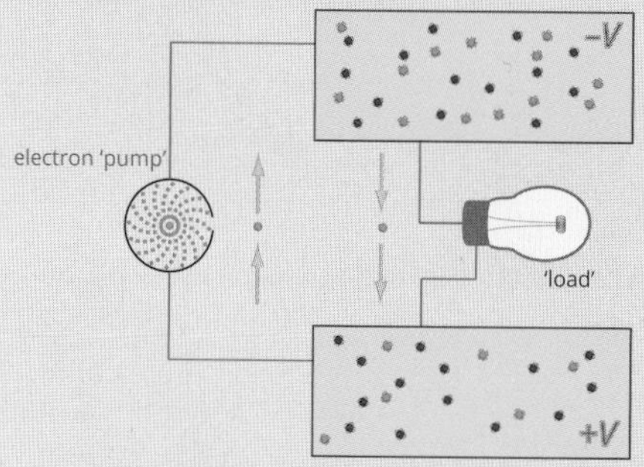

$$\text{Voltage } (\Delta V) = \frac{W}{q} = \frac{kQ}{r} \text{ [SI units: volt} = \frac{J}{C}\text{]}$$

- When two oppositely charged parallel plates are separated by a distance d, an electric field is created, and a potential difference exists between the plates, given by: $V = Ed$

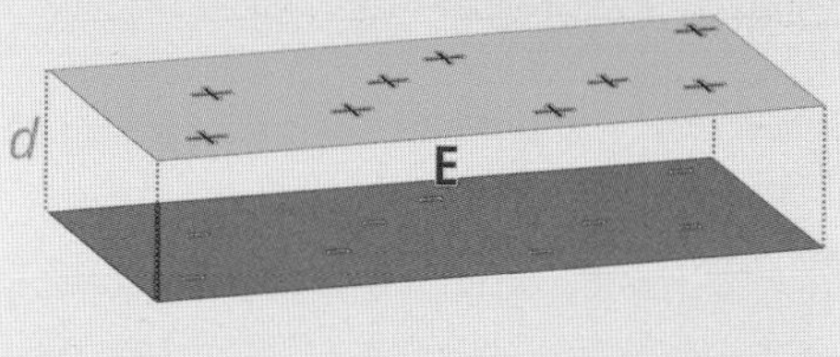

CIRCUITS

Current: the flow of electric charge. Current is given by:

$$I = \frac{Q}{\Delta t} \text{ [SI units: ampère (A)} = \frac{C}{s}\text{]}$$

(The direction of current is the direction positive charge would flow, or from high to low potential.)

Ohm's Law and Resistance

$V = IR$ (can be applied to entire circuit or individual resistors)

Resistance: opposition to the flow of charge. $R = \frac{\rho L}{A}$ (Resistance increases with increasing temperatures for most materials.)

[SI Units: ohm (Ω)]

Circuit Laws

Kirchhoff's laws:

1. At any junction within a circuit, the sum of current flowing into that point must equal the sum of current leaving.
2. The sum of voltage sources equals the sum of voltage drops around a closed-circuit loop.

Series Circuits

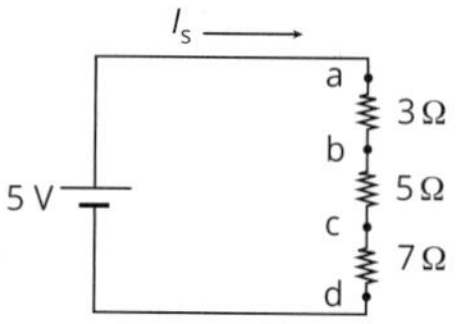

$R_{eq} = R_1 + R_2 + R_3 + \ldots$
$V_T = V_1 + V_2 + V_3 + \ldots$
$I_T = I_1 = I_2 = I_3 = \ldots$

Parallel Circuits

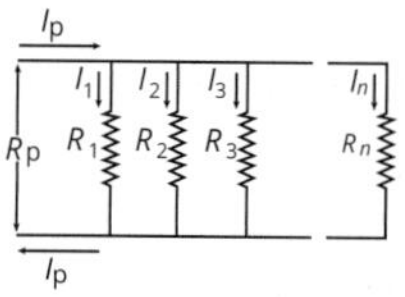

$\frac{1}{R_{eq}} = \frac{1}{R_1} + \frac{1}{R_2} + \frac{1}{R_3} + \ldots$
$V_T = V_1 = V_2 = V_3 = \ldots$
$I_T = I_1 + I_2 + I_3 + \ldots$

Power Dissipated by Resistors

$$P = IV = \frac{V^2}{R} = I^2 R$$

Capacitors

Capacitance: the ability to store charge per unit voltage. It is given by: $C = \frac{Q}{V}$

$$C' = \kappa \frac{\varepsilon_0 A}{d}$$

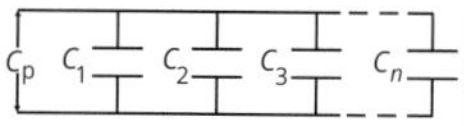

Capacitors in parallel: add
$C_{eq} = C_1 + C_2 + C_3 + \ldots$

Capacitors in series: add as reciprocals, then take reciprocal of sum
$\frac{1}{C_{eq}} = \frac{1}{C_1} + \frac{1}{C_2} + \frac{1}{C_3} + \ldots$

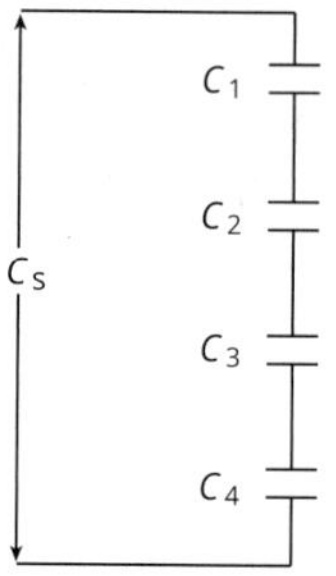

Energy Stored by Capacitors

$$U = \frac{1}{2}QV = \frac{1}{2}CV^2 = \frac{1}{2}\frac{Q^2}{C}$$

WAVES

Describing Waves

Longitudinal wave

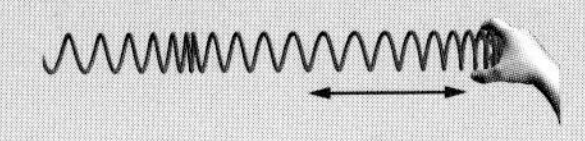

Transverse wave

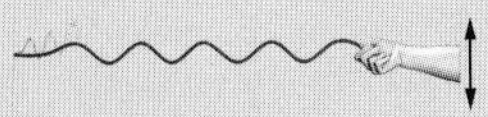

Wave formulas

$$f = \frac{1}{T}$$

$$v = f\lambda$$

Standing Waves

Strings

$\lambda = \frac{2L}{n}$ $(n = 1, 2, 3\ldots)$

$f = \frac{nv}{2L}$ $(n = 1, 2, 3\ldots)$

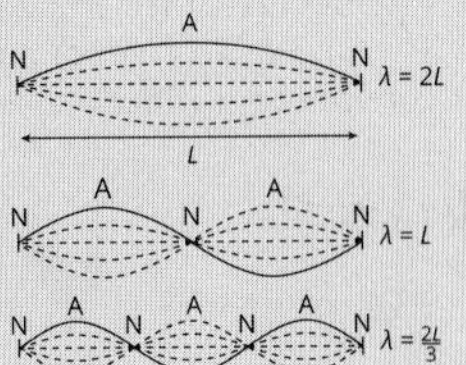

The ends of the strings are always nodes. Nodes occur where the displacement is zero.

Open pipes

$\lambda = \frac{2L}{n}$ $(n = 1, 2, 3\ldots)$

$f = \frac{nv}{2L}$ $(n = 1, 2, 3\ldots)$

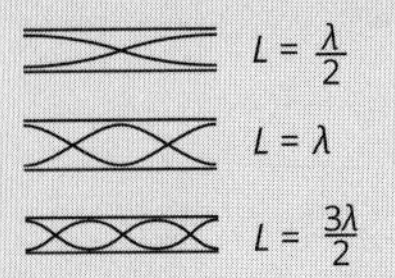

The open ends of the pipes are always antinodes (max amplitude).

Closed pipes

$\lambda = \frac{4L}{n}$ $(n = 1, 3, 5\ldots)$

$f = \frac{nv}{4L}$ $(n = 1, 3, 5\ldots)$

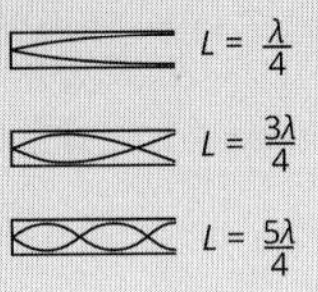

The closed end of the pipe is always a node, and the open end is always an antinode.

SOUND

Sound propagates through a deformable medium by the oscillation of particles parallel to the direction of the wave's propagation.

Intensity $(I) = \frac{P}{A}$ [SI units: $\frac{\text{W}}{\text{m}^2}$]

Sound level $(\beta) = 10 \log \left(\frac{I}{I_0}\right)$ [unit: decibel = dB]

(Note than an increase of 10 dB is an increase in intensity by a factor of 10. An increase of 20 dB is an increase in intensity by a factor of 100.)

Doppler Effect

- When a source and a detector move relative to one another, the perceived frequency of the sound received differs from the actual frequency emitted.

$$f' = f\frac{(v \pm v_D)}{(v \mp v_S)}$$

Stationary source: $v_s = 0$

Stationary detector: $v_D = 0$

Observer and detector moving closer:

- + sign in numerator
- – sign in denominator

Observer and detector moving apart:

- – sign in numerator
- + sign in denominator

OPTICS

Refraction

$n = \frac{c}{v}$ (speed of light $= 3 \times 10^8 \frac{\text{m}}{\text{s}}$)

Snell's law: $n_1 \sin \theta_1 = n_2 \sin \theta_2$. When $n_2 > n_1$, light bends toward the normal; when $n_2 < n_1$, light bends away from the normal.

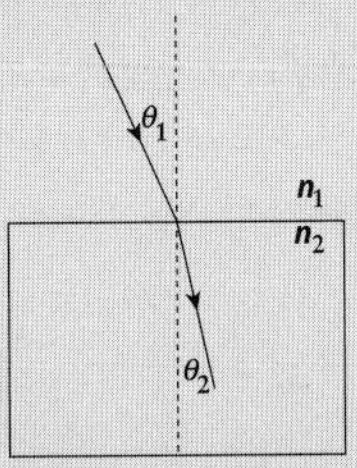

Converging system (convex lens, concave mirror)

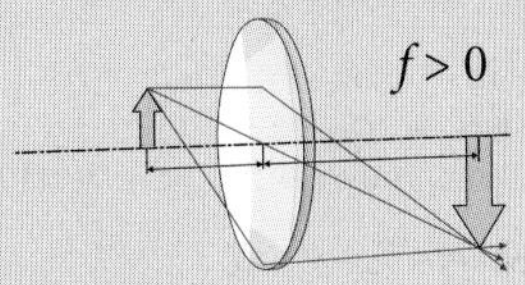

	Mirrors	Lens
Focal length (f)	(+) = concave (converging)	(+) = convex (converging)
	(–) = convex (diverging)	(–) = concave (diverging)
Object distance (o)	(+) = real object (in front of mirror)	(+) = real object (in front of lens)
	(–) = virtual object (behind mirror)	(–) = virtual object (behind lens)
Image distance (i)	(+) = real image (in front of mirror)	(+) = real image (in front of lens)
	(–) = virtual image (behind mirror)	(–) = virtual image (behind lens)
Magnification (m)	(+) = upright image	(+) = upright image
	(–) = inverted image	(–) = inverted image

	Converging systems					Diverging systems
o relative to i	$o > 2f$	$o = 2f$	$2f > o > f$	$o = f$	$o < f$	All o distances
image	real, inverted, reduced	real, inverted, same	real, inverted, magnified	no image	virtual, upright, magnified	virtual, upright, reduced

Diverging system (concave lens, convex mirror)

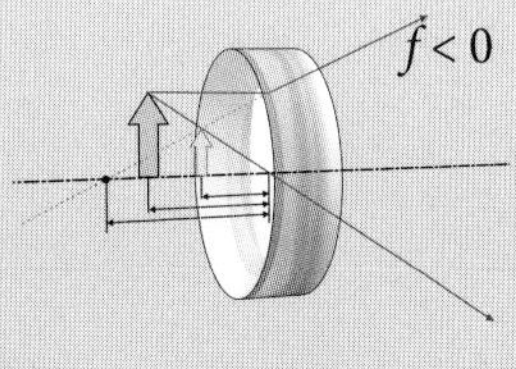

$$\frac{1}{f} = \frac{1}{o} + \frac{1}{i}$$

Magnification $(m) = \frac{-i}{o}$

- $|m| < 1$ image reduced; $|m| > 1$ image enlarged; $|m| = 1$ image same size

$$P = \frac{1}{f} (D = m^{-1})$$

ATOMIC AND NUCLEAR PHENOMENA

Photoelectric Effect

$E = hf = \frac{hc}{\lambda}$

$K = hf - W$

> K is the maximum kinetic energy of an ejected electron; W is the minimum energy required to eject an electron, called the work function.

Nuclear Binding Energy

Mass defect: the difference between the sum of the masses of nucleons in the nucleus and the mass of the nucleus. The mass defect results from the conversion of matter to energy, embodied by: $E = mc^2$. This energy is the **binding energy** that holds nucleons within the nucleus.

Exponential Decay

Half-life

$n = n_0 e^{-\lambda t}$

Alpha decay

${}^{238}_{92}\text{U} \rightarrow {}^{234}_{90}\text{Th} + {}^{4}_{2}\text{He}$

Beta-minus decay

${}^{137}_{55}\text{Cs} \rightarrow {}^{137}_{56}\text{Ba} + {}^{0}_{-1}e^- + \overline{\nu}_e$

Beta-plus decay

${}^{22}_{11}\text{Na} \rightarrow {}^{22}_{10}\text{Ne} + {}^{0}_{+1}e^+ + \nu_e$

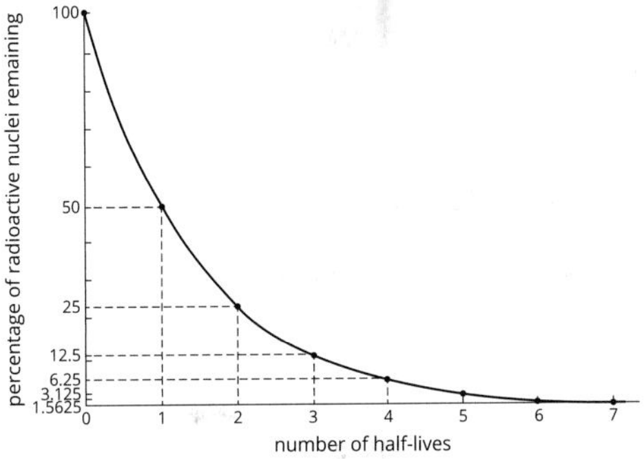

Gamma decay

${}^{12}_{6}\text{C}^* \rightarrow {}^{12}_{6}\text{C} + {}^{0}_{0}\text{Y}$

MATHEMATICS

Estimation

Scientific notation: A method of simplifying calculations by reducing numbers to a significand between one and ten and the exponent power of ten: $0.0000037 = 3.7 \times 10^{-6}$. Allows estimation by powers of ten, which is often all that is necessary on the MCAT.

Multiplication: If you round one number up, round the other down to compensate.

Division: If you round one number up, round the other up to compensate.

Roots and Logarithms

x	x^2	x	x^2	x	x^2	x	x^2
1	1	**6**	36	**11**	121	**16**	256
2	4	**7**	49	**12**	144	**17**	289
3	9	**8**	64	**13**	169	**18**	324
4	16	**9**	81	**14**	196	**19**	361
5	25	**10**	100	**15**	225	**20**	400

This table can be used to estimate even-powered roots of numbers. When taking square roots of a number raised to a power, remember not to take the square root of the exponent, but to divide it by two.

Logarithmic identities

$$\log A \times B = \log A + \log B$$

$$\log \frac{A}{B} = \log A - \log B$$

$$\log A^B = B \log A$$

$$\log \frac{1}{A} = -\log A$$

Converting common and natural logarithms

$$\log x = \frac{\ln x}{2.303}$$

$$\log (n \times 10^m) \approx m + 0.n$$

Trigonometry

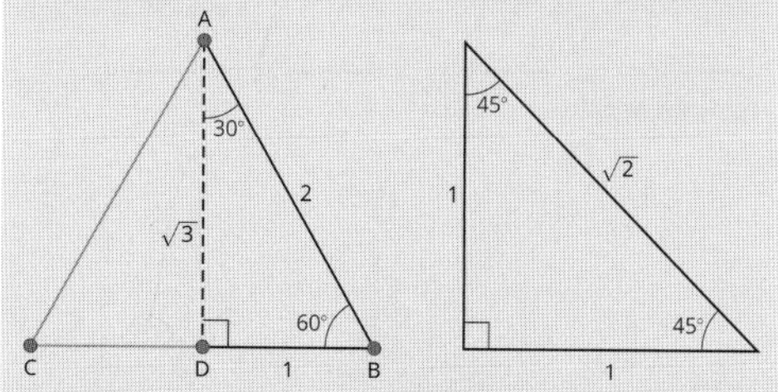

$$\sin \theta = \frac{\text{opposite}}{\text{hypotenuse}}$$

$$\cos \theta = \frac{\text{adjacent}}{\text{hypotenuse}}$$

$$\tan \theta = \frac{\text{opposite}}{\text{adjacent}}$$

Vector Addition and Subtraction

Tip-to-tail method of finding resultant of two vectors:

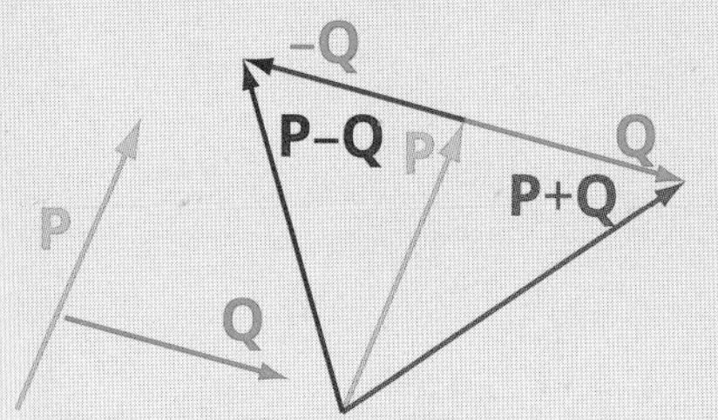

Finding the resultant using the component method:

- Resolve vectors into x- and y-components
- Sum all the vectors in the x-direction to get the resultant for the x-direction, and do the same for the y-components
- The magnitude of the resultant $R = \sqrt{R_x^2 + R_y^2}$

Right-Hand Rule for Finding Direction of Cross-Product Resultant

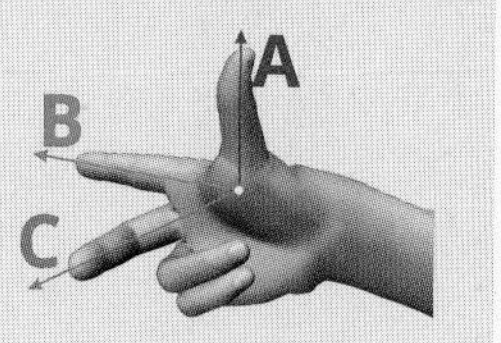

The right-hand rule is used to find the direction of a vector that is the product of two other vectors. If **C** = **A** × **B**, then **C** is represented by the palm while **A** is represented by the thumb and **B** is represented by the fingers.

RESEARCH DESIGN

Question Selection

Scientific method: determine whether sufficient background exists and whether the question is testable

FINER method: determine whether a study is **F**easible, **I**nteresting, **N**ovel, **E**thical, and **R**elevant

Causality

Controls: experimental subjects that are maintained with similar but noninterventional treatments to establish causality

Hill's criteria: help determine the strength of causal relationships. Only temporality is necessary.

Error Sources

- **Small sample size:** amplifies the effects of statistical anomalies
- **Defects in precision and accuracy:** create random or systematic variations in the data

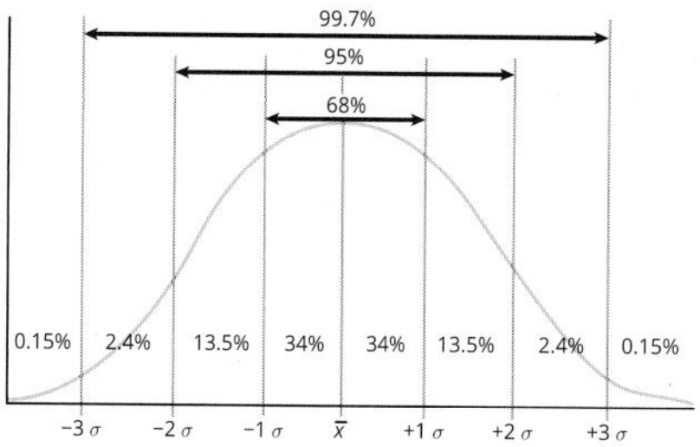

- **Bias:** systematic data error. Common types include **selection bias, detection bias,** and the **Hawthorne effect**. Minimized by proper participant selection, blinding, and randomization.
- **Confounding:** an analysis error wherein a variable that has a relationship with the other two variables is overlooked

Ethics

- **Beneficence:** the requirement to do good
- **Nonmaleficence:** "do no harm"
- **Autonomy:** the right of individuals to make decisions for themselves
- **Justice:** the need to consider only morally relevant differences between patients and to distribute healthcare resources fairly

Generalizability

Statistical significance and causality do not make something generalizable or a good intervention. **Clinical significance** and the **target population** must also be considered.

DATA ANALYSIS

Measures of Central Tendency and Distribution

- **Mean:** the average of the data points; impacted heavily by outliers
- **Median:** the central value of a data set; not affected by outliers
- **Mode:** the most common data point(s); not affected by outliers
- **Range:** the difference between the largest and smallest value in a set; impacted heavily by outliers
- **Standard deviation:** a measure of how spread out values are from the mean; affected by outliers

$$\sigma = \sqrt{\frac{\sum_{i=1}^{n} (x_i - \bar{x})^2}{n-1}}$$

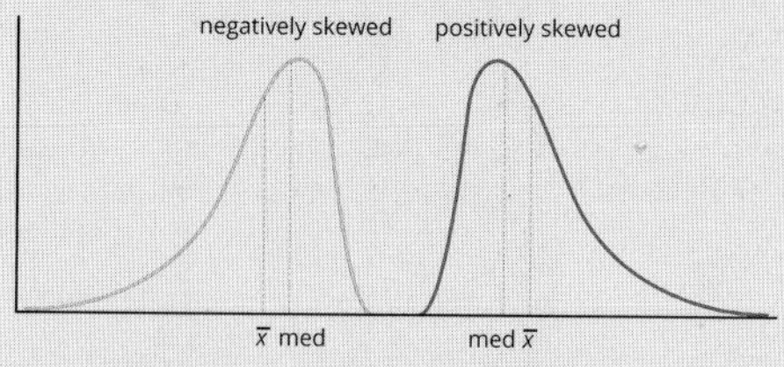

Probability

- **Mutually exclusive:** two events that cannot occur together
- **Independent:** the probability of either event is not affected by the occurrence of the other

For independent events:

$$P(\text{A and B}) = P(\text{A}) \times P(\text{B})$$

$$P(\text{A or B}) = P(\text{A}) + P(\text{B}) - P(\text{A and B})$$

Probability is usually expressed as a percent, but all math should be completed using decimals.

Statistical Testing

- **Null hypothesis:** a hypothesis of no difference; always the comparator
- ***p*-value:** the probability that results were obtained by chance given that the null hypothesis is true
- **Confidence interval:** a range of values believed to contain the true value with a given level of certainty

Visual Data Interpretation

- **Graphs:** analyze the axes first to determine whether the scale is linear, logarithmic, or semilog and what the units are. Determine whether relationships are direct or inverse.
- **Pie charts:** compare portions of data to a whole or relative responses of a group
- **Bar charts and histograms:** compare absolute or relative responses between groups
- **Box plots:** contain information about measures of central tendency and distribution; may be comparative or single

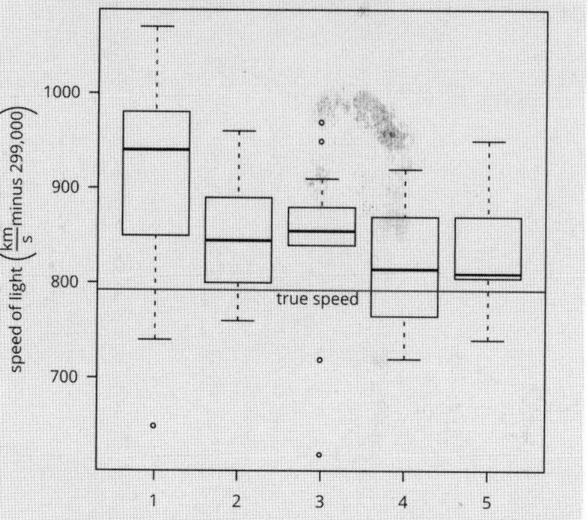

KAPLAN

MCAT® BIOCHEMISTRY REVIEW 2024–2025

ONLINE + BOOK

Edited by Alexander Stone Macnow, MD

ACKNOWLEDGMENTS

Editor-in-Chief, 2024–2025 Edition
M. Dominic Eggert

Contributing Editors, 2024–2025 Edition
Christopher Durland; Charles Pierce, MD; Jason Selzer

Prior Edition Editorial Staff: Brandon Deason, MD; Christopher Durland; M. Dominic Eggert; Tyler Fara; Elizabeth Flagge; Adam Grey; Jason Selzer; Lauren K. White

Published by Kaplan North America, LLC dba Kaplan Publishing
1515 West Cypress Creek Road
Fort Lauderdale, Florida 33309

ISBN: 978-1-5062-8681-5

10 9 8 7 6 5 4 3 2 1

TABLE OF CONTENTS

GO ONLINE
kaptest.com/booksonline

THE *KAPLAN MCAT REVIEW* TEAM

Alexander Stone Macnow, MD
Editor-in-Chief

Tyra Hall-Pogar, PhD
Editor

Bela G. Starkman, PhD
Editor

Joshua D. Brooks, PhD
Kaplan MCAT Faculty

Alisha Maureen Crowley
Kaplan MCAT Faculty

Samer T. Ismail
Kaplan MCAT Faculty

Kelly Kyker-Snowman, MS
Kaplan MCAT Faculty

Christopher Lopez
Kaplan MCAT Faculty

M. Dominic Eggert
Editor

Faculty Reviewers and Editors: Elmar R. Aliyev; James Burns; Jonathan Cornfield; Brandon Deason, MD; Nikolai Dorofeev, MD; Benjamin Downer, MS; Colin Doyle; Christopher Durland; Marilyn Engle; Eleni M. Eren; Raef Ali Fadel; Elizabeth Flagge; Adam Grey; Justine Harkness, PhD; Scott Huff; Ae-Ri Kim, PhD; Elizabeth A. Kudlaty; Ningfei Li; John P. Mahon; Matthew A. Meier; Nainika Nanda; Caroline Nkemdilim Opene; Kaitlyn E. Prenger; Uneeb Qureshi; Derek Rusnak, MA; Kristen L. Russell, ME; Michael Paul Tomani, MS; Lauren K. White; Nicholas M. White; Kerranna Williamson, MBA; Allison Ann Wilkes, MS; and Tony Yu

Thanks to Rebecca Anderson; Jeff Batzli; Eric Chiu; Tim Eich; Samantha Fallon; Tyler Fara; Owen Farcy; Dan Frey; Robin Garmise; Rita Garthaffner; Joanna Graham; Allison Gudenau; Allison Harm; Beth Hoffberg; Aaron Lemon-Strauss; Keith Lubeley; Diane McGarvey; Petros Minasi; Beena P V; John Polstein; Deeangelee Pooran-Kublall, MD, MPH; Rochelle Rothstein, MD; Larry Rudman; Srividhya Sankar; Sylvia Tidwell Scheuring; Carly Schnur; Aiswarya Sivanand; Todd Tedesco; Karin Tucker; Lee Weiss; Christina Wheeler; Kristen Workman; Amy Zarkos; and the countless others who made this project possible.

GETTING STARTED CHECKLIST

Getting Started Checklist

- [ ] Register for your free online assets—including full-length tests, Science Review Videos, and additional practice materials—at **www.kaptest.com/moreonline**.
- [ ] Create a study calendar that ensures you complete content review and sufficient practice by Test Day!
- [ ] As you finish a chapter and the online practice for that chapter, check it off on the table of contents.
- [ ] Register to take the MCAT at **www.aamc.org/mcat**.
- [ ] Set aside time during your prep to make sure the rest of your application—personal statement, recommendations, and other materials—is ready to go!
- [ ] Take a moment to admire your completed checklist, then get back to the business of prepping for this exam!

PREFACE

And now it starts: your long, yet fruitful journey toward wearing a white coat. Proudly wearing that white coat, though, is hopefully only part of your motivation. You are reading this book because you want to be a healer.

If you're serious about going to medical school, then you are likely already familiar with the importance of the MCAT in medical school admissions. While the holistic review process puts additional weight on your experiences, extracurricular activities, and personal attributes, the fact remains: along with your GPA, your MCAT score remains one of the two most important components of your application portfolio—at least early in the admissions process. Each additional point you score on the MCAT pushes you in front of thousands of other students and makes you an even more attractive applicant. But the MCAT is not simply an obstacle to overcome; it is an opportunity to show schools that you will be a strong student and a future leader in medicine.

We at Kaplan take our jobs very seriously and aim to help students see success not only on the MCAT, but as future physicians. We work with our learning science experts to ensure that we're using the most up-to-date teaching techniques in our resources. Multiple members of our team hold advanced degrees in medicine or associated biomedical sciences, and are committed to the highest level of medical education. Kaplan has been working with the MCAT for over 50 years and our commitment to premed students is unflagging; in fact, Stanley Kaplan created this company when he had difficulty being accepted to medical school due to unfair quota systems that existed at the time.

We stand now at the beginning of a new era in medical education. As citizens of this 21st-century world of healthcare, we are charged with creating a patient-oriented, culturally competent, cost-conscious, universally available, technically advanced, and research-focused healthcare system, run by compassionate providers. Suffice it to say, this is no easy task. Problem-based learning, integrated curricula, and classes in interpersonal skills are some of the responses to this demand for an excellent workforce—a workforce of which you'll soon be a part.

We're thrilled that you've chosen us to help you on this journey. Please reach out to us to share your challenges, concerns, and successes. Together, we will shape the future of medicine in the United States and abroad; we look forward to helping you become the doctor you deserve to be.

Good luck!

Alexander Stone Macnow, MD
Editor-in-Chief
Department of Pathology and Laboratory Medicine
Hospital of the University of Pennsylvania

BA, Musicology—Boston University, 2008
MD—Perelman School of Medicine at the University of Pennsylvania, 2013

ABOUT THE MCAT

Anatomy of the MCAT

Here is a general overview of the structure of Test Day:

Section	Number of Questions	Time Allotted
Test-Day Certification		4 minutes
Tutorial (optional)		10 minutes
Chemical and Physical Foundations of Biological Systems	59	95 minutes
Break (optional)		10 minutes
Critical Analysis and Reasoning Skills (CARS)	53	90 minutes
Lunch Break (optional)		30 minutes
Biological and Biochemical Foundations of Living Systems	59	95 minutes
Break (optional)		10 minutes
Psychological, Social, and Biological Foundations of Behavior	59	95 minutes
Void Question		3 minutes
Satisfaction Survey (optional)		5 minutes

The structure of the four sections of the MCAT is shown below.

Chemical and Physical Foundations of Biological Systems	
Time	95 minutes
Format	• 59 questions • 10 passages • 44 questions are passage-based, and 15 are discrete (stand-alone) questions. • Score between 118 and 132
What It Tests	• Biochemistry: 25% • Biology: 5% • General Chemistry: 30% • Organic Chemistry: 15% • Physics: 25%

Critical Analysis and Reasoning Skills (CARS)	
Time	90 minutes
Format	• 53 questions • 9 passages • All questions are passage-based. There are no discrete (stand-alone) questions. • Score between 118 and 132
What It Tests	Disciplines: • Humanities: 50% • Social Sciences: 50% Skills: • *Foundations of Comprehension*: 30% • *Reasoning Within the Text:* 30% • *Reasoning Beyond the Text*: 40%
Biological and Biochemical Foundations of Living Systems	
Time	95 minutes
Format	• 59 questions • 10 passages • 44 questions are passage-based, and 15 are discrete (stand-alone) questions. • Score between 118 and 132
What It Tests	• Biochemistry: 25% • Biology: 65% • General Chemistry: 5% • Organic Chemistry: 5%
Psychological, Social, and Biological Foundations of Behavior	
Time	95 minutes
Format	• 59 questions • 10 passages • 44 questions are passage-based, and 15 are discrete (stand-alone) questions. • Score between 118 and 132
What It Tests	• Biology: 5% • Psychology: 65% • Sociology: 30%
Total	
Testing Time	375 minutes (6 hours, 15 minutes)
Total Seat Time	447 minutes (7 hours, 27 minutes)
Questions	230
Score	472 to 528

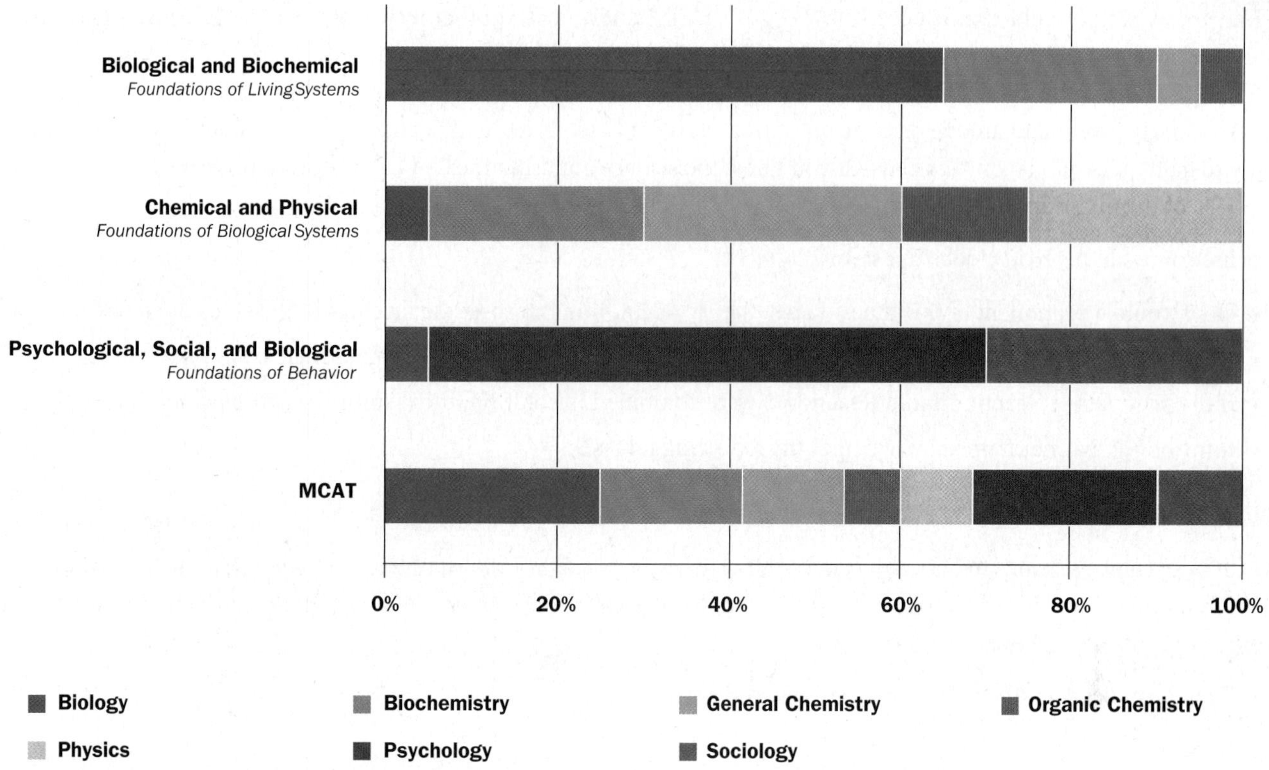

Scientific Inquiry and Reasoning Skills (SIRS)

The AAMC has defined four *Scientific Inquiry and Reasoning Skills* (SIRS) that will be tested in the three science sections of the MCAT:

1. *Knowledge of Scientific Concepts and Principles* (35% of questions)
2. *Scientific Reasoning and Problem-Solving* (45% of questions)
3. *Reasoning About the Design and Execution of Research* (10% of questions)
4. *Data-Based and Statistical Reasoning* (10% of questions)

Let's see how each one breaks down into more specific Test Day behaviors. Note that the bullet points of specific objectives for each of the SIRS are taken directly from the *Official Guide to the MCAT Exam*; the descriptions of what these behaviors mean and sample question stems, however, are written by Kaplan.

Skill 1: *Knowledge of Scientific Concepts and Principles*

This is probably the least surprising of the four SIRS; the testing of science knowledge is, after all, one of the signature qualities of the MCAT. Skill 1 questions will require you to do the following:

- Recognize correct scientific principles
- Identify the relationships among closely related concepts
- Identify the relationships between different representations of concepts (verbal, symbolic, graphic)
- Identify examples of observations that illustrate scientific principles
- Use mathematical equations to solve problems

At Kaplan, we simply call these Science Knowledge or Skill 1 questions. Another way to think of Skill 1 questions is as "one-step" problems. The single step is either to realize which scientific concept the question stem is suggesting or to take the concept stated in the question stem and identify which answer choice is an accurate application of it. Skill 1 questions are particularly prominent among discrete questions (those not associated with a passage). These questions are an opportunity to gain quick points on Test Day—if you know the science concept attached to the question, then that's it! On Test Day, 35% of the questions in each science section will be Skill 1 questions.

Here are some sample Skill 1 question stems:

- How would a proponent of the James–Lange theory of emotion interpret the findings of the study cited in the passage?
- Which of the following most accurately describes the function of FSH in the human menstrual cycle?
- If the products of Reaction 1 and Reaction 2 were combined in solution, the resulting reaction would form:
- Ionic bonds are maintained by which of the following forces?

Skill 2: *Scientific Reasoning and Problem-Solving*

The MCAT science sections do, of course, move beyond testing straightforward science knowledge; Skill 2 questions are the most common way in which it does so. At Kaplan, we also call these Critical Thinking questions. Skill 2 questions will require you to do the following:

- Reason about scientific principles, theories, and models
- Analyze and evaluate scientific explanations and predictions
- Evaluate arguments about causes and consequences
- Bring together theory, observations, and evidence to draw conclusions
- Recognize scientific findings that challenge or invalidate a scientific theory or model
- Determine and use scientific formulas to solve problems

Just as Skill 1 questions can be thought of as "one-step" problems, many Skill 2 questions are "two-step" problems, and more difficult Skill 2 questions may require three or more steps. These questions can require a wide spectrum of reasoning skills, including integration of multiple facts from a passage, combination of multiple science content areas, and prediction of an experiment's results. Skill 2 questions also tend to ask about science content without actually mentioning it by name. For example, a question might describe the results of one experiment and ask you to predict the results of a second experiment without actually telling you what underlying scientific principles are at work—part of the question's difficulty will be figuring out which principles to apply in order to get the correct answer. On Test Day, 45% of the questions in each science section will be Skill 2 questions.

Here are some sample Skill 2 question stems:

- Which of the following experimental conditions would most likely yield results similar to those in Figure 2?
- All of the following conclusions are supported by the information in the passage EXCEPT:
- The most likely cause of the anomalous results found by the experimenter is:
- An impact to a person's chest quickly reduces the volume of one of the lungs to 70% of its initial value while not allowing any air to escape from the mouth. By what percentage is the force of outward air pressure increased on a 2 cm^2 portion of the inner surface of the compressed lung?

Skill 3: *Reasoning About the Design and Execution of Research*

The MCAT is interested in your ability to critically appraise and analyze research, as this is an important day-to-day task of a physician. We call these questions Skill 3 or Experimental and Research Design questions for short. Skill 3 questions will require you to do the following:

- Identify the role of theory, past findings, and observations in scientific questioning
- Identify testable research questions and hypotheses
- Distinguish between samples and populations and distinguish results that support generalizations about populations
- Identify independent and dependent variables
- Reason about the features of research studies that suggest associations between variables or causal relationships between them (such as temporality and random assignment)
- Identify conclusions that are supported by research results
- Determine the implications of results for real-world situations
- Reason about ethical issues in scientific research

Over the years, the AAMC has received input from medical schools to require more practical research skills of MCAT test takers, and Skill 3 questions are the response to these demands. This skill is unique in that the outside knowledge you need to answer Skill 3 questions is not taught in any one undergraduate course; instead, the research design principles needed to answer these questions are learned gradually throughout your science classes and especially through any laboratory work you have completed. It should be noted that Skill 3 comprises 10% of the questions in each science section on Test Day.

Here are some sample Skill 3 question stems:

- What is the dependent variable in the study described in the passage?
- The major flaw in the method used to measure disease susceptibility in Experiment 1 is:
- Which of the following procedures is most important for the experimenters to follow in order for their study to maintain a proper, randomized sample of research subjects?
- A researcher would like to test the hypothesis that individuals who move to an urban area during adulthood are more likely to own a car than are those who have lived in an urban area since birth. Which of the following studies would best test this hypothesis?

Skill 4: *Data-Based and Statistical Reasoning*

Lastly, the science sections of the MCAT test your ability to analyze the visual and numerical results of experiments and studies. We call these Data and Statistical Analysis questions. Skill 4 questions will require you to do the following:

- Use, analyze, and interpret data in figures, graphs, and tables
- Evaluate whether representations make sense for particular scientific observations and data
- Use measures of central tendency (mean, median, and mode) and measures of dispersion (range, interquartile range, and standard deviation) to describe data
- Reason about random and systematic error

- Reason about statistical significance and uncertainty (interpreting statistical significance levels and interpreting a confidence interval)
- Use data to explain relationships between variables or make predictions
- Use data to answer research questions and draw conclusions

Skill 4 is included in the MCAT because physicians and researchers spend much of their time examining the results of their own studies and the studies of others, and it's very important for them to make legitimate conclusions and sound judgments based on that data. The MCAT tests Skill 4 on all three science sections with graphical representations of data (charts and bar graphs), as well as numerical ones (tables, lists, and results summarized in sentence or paragraph form). On Test Day, 10% of the questions in each science section will be Skill 4 questions.

Here are some sample Skill 4 question stems:

- According to the information in the passage, there is an inverse correlation between:
- What conclusion is best supported by the findings displayed in Figure 2?
- A medical test for a rare type of heavy metal poisoning returns a positive result for 98% of affected individuals and 13% of unaffected individuals. Which of the following types of error is most prevalent in this test?
- If a fourth trial of Experiment 1 was run and yielded a result of 54% compliance, which of the following would be true?

SIRS Summary

Discussing the SIRS tested on the MCAT is a daunting prospect given that the very nature of the skills tends to make the conversation rather abstract. Nevertheless, with enough practice, you'll be able to identify each of the four skills quickly, and you'll also be able to apply the proper strategies to solve those problems on Test Day. If you need a quick reference to remind you of the four SIRS, these guidelines may help:

Skill 1 (**Science Knowledge**) questions ask:

- Do you remember this science content?

Skill 2 (**Critical Thinking**) questions ask:

- Do you remember this science content? And if you do, could you please apply it to this novel situation?
- Could you answer this question that cleverly combines multiple content areas at the same time?

Skill 3 (**Experimental and Research Design**) questions ask:

- Let's forget about the science content for a while. Could you give some insight into the experimental or research methods involved in this situation?

Skill 4 (**Data and Statistical Analysis**) questions ask:

- Let's forget about the science content for a while. Could you accurately read some graphs and tables for a moment? Could you make some conclusions or extrapolations based on the information presented?

Critical Analysis and Reasoning Skills (CARS)

The *Critical Analysis and Reasoning Skills* (CARS) section of the MCAT tests three discrete families of textual reasoning skills; each of these families requires a higher level of reasoning than the last. Those three skills are as follows:

1. *Foundations of Comprehension* (30% of questions)
2. *Reasoning Within the Text* (30% of questions)
3. *Reasoning Beyond the Text* (40% of questions)

These three skills are tested through nine humanities- and social sciences–themed passages, with approximately 5 to 7 questions per passage. Let's take a more in-depth look into these three skills. Again, the bullet points of specific objectives for each of the CARS are taken directly from the *Official Guide to the MCAT Exam*; the descriptions of what these behaviors mean and sample question stems, however, are written by Kaplan.

Foundations of Comprehension

Questions in this skill will ask for basic facts and simple inferences about the passage; the questions themselves will be similar to those seen on reading comprehension sections of other standardized exams like the SAT® and ACT®. *Foundations of Comprehension* questions will require you to do the following:

- Understand the basic components of the text
- Infer meaning from rhetorical devices, word choice, and text structure

This admittedly covers a wide range of potential question types including Main Idea, Detail, Inference, and Definition-in-Context questions, but finding the correct answer to all *Foundations of Comprehension* questions will follow from a basic understanding of the passage and the point of view of its author (and occasionally that of other voices in the passage).

Here are some sample *Foundations of Comprehension* question stems:

- **Main Idea**—The author's primary purpose in this passage is:
- **Detail**—Based on the information in the second paragraph, which of the following is the most accurate summary of the opinion held by Schubert's critics?
- **(Scattered) Detail**—According to the passage, which of the following is FALSE about literary reviews in the 1920s?
- **Inference (Implication)**—Which of the following phrases, as used in the passage, is most suggestive that the author has a personal bias toward narrative records of history?
- **Inference (Assumption)**—In putting together the argument in the passage, the author most likely assumes:
- **Definition-in-Context**—The word "obscure" (paragraph 3), when used in reference to the historian's actions, most nearly means:

Reasoning Within the Text

While *Foundations of Comprehension* questions will usually depend on interpreting a single piece of information in the passage or understanding the passage as a whole, *Reasoning Within the Text* questions require more thought because they will ask you to identify the purpose of a particular piece of information in the context of the passage, or ask how one piece of information relates to another. *Reasoning Within the Text* questions will require you to:

- Integrate different components of the text to draw relevant conclusions

The CARS section will also ask you to judge certain parts of the passage or even judge the author. These questions, which fall under the *Reasoning Within the Text* skill, can ask you to identify authorial bias, evaluate the credibility of cited sources, determine the logical soundness of an argument, identify the importance of a particular fact or statement in the context of the passage, or search for relevant evidence in the passage to support a given conclusion. In all, this category includes Function and Strengthen–Weaken (Within the Passage) questions, as well as a smattering of related—but rare—question types.

Here are some sample *Reasoning Within the Text* question stems:

- **Function**—The author's discussion of the effect of socioeconomic status on social mobility primarily serves which of the following functions?
- **Strengthen–Weaken (Within the Passage)**—Which of the following facts is used in the passage as the most prominent piece of evidence in favor of the author's conclusions?
- **Strengthen–Weaken (Within the Passage)**—Based on the role it plays in the author's argument, *The Possessed* can be considered:

Reasoning Beyond the Text

The distinguishing factor of *Reasoning Beyond the Text* questions is in the title of the skill: the word *Beyond*. Questions that test this skill, which make up a larger share of the CARS section than questions from either of the other two skills, will always introduce a completely new situation that was not present in the passage itself; these questions will ask you to determine how one influences the other. *Reasoning Beyond the Text* questions will require you to:

- Apply or extrapolate ideas from the passage to new contexts
- Assess the impact of introducing new factors, information, or conditions to ideas from the passage

The *Reasoning Beyond the Text* skill is further divided into Apply and Strengthen–Weaken (Beyond the Passage) questions, and a few other rarely appearing question types.

Here are some sample *Reasoning Beyond the Text* question stems:

- **Apply**—If a document were located that demonstrated Berlioz intended to include a chorus of at least 700 in his *Grande Messe des Morts*, how would the author likely respond?
- **Apply**—Which of the following is the best example of a "virtuous rebellion," as it is defined in the passage?
- **Strengthen–Weaken (Beyond the Passage)**—Suppose Jane Austen had written in a letter to her sister, "My strongest characters were those forced by circumstance to confront basic questions about the society in which they lived." What relevance would this have to the passage?
- **Strengthen–Weaken (Beyond the Passage)**—Which of the following sentences, if added to the end of the passage, would most WEAKEN the author's conclusions in the last paragraph?

CARS Summary

Through the *Foundations of Comprehension* skill, the CARS section tests many of the reading skills you have been building on since grade school, albeit in the context of very challenging doctorate-level passages. But through the two other skills (*Reasoning Within the Text* and *Reasoning Beyond the Text*), the MCAT demands that you understand the deep structure of passages and the arguments within them at a very advanced level. And, of course, all of this is tested under very tight timing restrictions: only 102 seconds per question—and that doesn't even include the time spent reading the passages.

Here's a quick reference guide to the three CARS skills:

Foundations of Comprehension questions ask:

- Did you understand the passage and its main ideas?
- What does the passage have to say about this particular detail?
- What must be true that the author did not say?

Reasoning Within the Text questions ask:

- What's the logical relationship between these two ideas from the passage?
- How well argued is the author's thesis?

Reasoning Beyond the Text questions ask:

- How does this principle from the passage apply to this new situation?
- How does this new piece of information influence the arguments in the passage?

Scoring

Each of the four sections of the MCAT is scored between 118 and 132, with the median at approximately 125. This means the total score ranges from 472 to 528, with the median at about 500. Why such peculiar numbers? The AAMC stresses that this scale emphasizes the importance of the central portion of the score distribution, where most students score (around 125 per section, or 500 total), rather than putting undue focus on the high end of the scale.

Note that there is no wrong answer penalty on the MCAT, so you should select an answer for every question—even if it is only a guess.

The AAMC has released the 2019–2021 correlation between scaled score and percentile, as shown on the following page. It should be noted that the percentile scale is adjusted and renormalized over time and thus can shift slightly from year to year. Percentile rank updates are released by the AAMC around May 1 of each year.

Total Score	Percentile	Total Score	Percentile
528	100	499	41
527	100	498	38
526	100	497	35
525	100	496	32
524	100	495	29
523	99	494	26
522	99	493	24
521	98	492	21
520	97	491	19
519	96	490	17
518	95	489	15
517	94	488	13
516	92	487	11
515	90	486	10
514	88	485	8
513	86	484	7
512	83	483	6
511	80	482	5
510	77	481	4
509	74	480	3
508	71	479	2
507	68	478	2
506	65	477	1
505	61	476	1
504	58	475	<1
503	55	474	<1
502	51	473	<1
501	48	472	<1
500	45		

Source: AAMC. 2022. *Summary of MCAT Total and Section Scores.* Accessed October 2022. **https://students-residents.aamc.org/mcat-research-and-data/percentile-ranks-mcat-exam**

Further information on score reporting is included at the end of the next section (see *After Your Test*).

MCAT Policies and Procedures

We strongly encourage you to download the latest copy of *MCAT® Essentials*, available on the AAMC's website, to ensure that you have the latest information about registration and Test Day policies and procedures; this document is updated annually. A brief summary of some of the most important rules is provided here.

MCAT Registration

The only way to register for the MCAT is online. You can access AAMC's registration system at **www.aamc.org/mcat**.

The AAMC posts the schedule of testing, registration, and score release dates in the fall before the MCAT testing year, which runs from January into September. Registration for January through June is available earlier than registration for later dates, but see the AAMC's website for the exact dates each year. There is one standard registration fee, but the fee for changing your test date or test center increases the closer you get to your MCAT.

Fees and the Fee Assistance Program (FAP)

Payment for test registration must be made by MasterCard or VISA. As described earlier, the fee for rescheduling your exam or changing your testing center increases as one approaches Test Day. In addition, it is not uncommon for test centers to fill up well in advance of the registration deadline. For these reasons, we recommend identifying your preferred Test Day as soon as possible and registering. There are ancillary benefits to having a set Test Day, as well: when you know the date you're working toward, you'll study harder and are less likely to keep pushing back the exam. The AAMC offers a Fee Assistance Program (FAP) for students with financial hardship to help reduce the cost of taking the MCAT, as well as for the American Medical College Application Service (AMCAS®) application. Further information on the FAP can be found at **www.aamc.org/students/applying/fap**.

Testing Security

On Test Day, you will be required to present a qualifying form of ID. Generally, a current driver's license or United States passport will be sufficient (consult the AAMC website for the full list of qualifying criteria). When registering, take care to spell your first and last names (middle names, suffixes, and prefixes are not required and will not be verified on Test Day) precisely the same as they appear on this ID; failure to provide this ID at the test center or differences in spelling between your registration and ID will be considered a "no-show," and you will not receive a refund for the exam.

During Test Day registration, other identity data collected may include: a digital palm vein scan, a Test Day photo, a digitization of your valid ID, and signatures. Some testing centers may use a metal detection wand to ensure that no prohibited items are brought into the testing room. Prohibited items include all electronic devices, including watches and timers, calculators, cell phones, and any and all forms of recording equipment; food, drinks (including water), and cigarettes or other smoking paraphernalia; hats and scarves (except for religious purposes); and books, notes, or other study materials. If you require a medical device, such as an insulin pump or pacemaker, you must apply for accommodated testing. During breaks, you are allowed access to food and drink, but not to electronic devices, including cell phones.

Testing centers are under video surveillance and the AAMC does not take potential violations of testing security lightly. The bottom line: *know the rules and don't break them.*

Accommodations

Students with disabilities or medical conditions can apply for accommodated testing. Documentation of the disability or condition is required, and requests may take two months—or more—to be approved. For this reason, it is recommended that you begin the process of applying for accommodated testing as early as possible. More information on applying for accommodated testing can be found at **www.aamc.org/students/applying/mcat/accommodations**.

After Your Test

When your MCAT is all over, no matter how you feel you did, be good to yourself when you leave the test center. Celebrate! Take a nap. Watch a movie. Get some exercise. Plan a trip or outing. Call up all of your neglected friends or message them on social media. Go out for snacks or drinks with people you like. Whatever you do, make sure that it has absolutely nothing to do with thinking too hard—you deserve some rest and relaxation.

Perhaps most importantly, do not discuss specific details about the test with anyone. For one, it is important to let go of the stress of Test Day, and reliving your exam only inhibits you from being able to do so. But more significantly, the Examinee Agreement you sign at the beginning of your exam specifically prohibits you from discussing or disclosing exam content. The AAMC is known to seek out individuals who violate this agreement and retains the right to prosecute these individuals at their discretion. This means that you should not, under any circumstances, discuss the exam in person or over the phone with other individuals—including us at Kaplan—or post information or questions about exam content to Facebook, Student Doctor Network, or other online social media. You are permitted to comment on your "general exam experience," including how you felt about the exam overall or an individual section, but this is a fine line. In summary: *if you're not certain whether you can discuss an aspect of the test or not, just don't do it!* Do not let a silly Facebook post stop you from becoming the doctor you deserve to be.

Scores are typically released approximately one month after Test Day. The release is staggered during the afternoon and evening, ending at 5 p.m. Eastern. This means that not all examinees receive their scores at exactly the same time. Your score report will include a scaled score for each section between 118 and 132, as well as your total combined score between 472 and 528. These scores are given as confidence intervals. For each section, the confidence interval is approximately the given score ±1; for the total score, it is approximately the given score ±2. You will also be given the corresponding percentile rank for each of these section scores and the total score.

AAMC Contact Information

For further questions, contact the MCAT team at the Association of American Medical Colleges:

MCAT Resource Center
Association of American Medical Colleges
www.aamc.org/mcat
(202) 828-0600
www.aamc.org/contactmcat

HOW THIS BOOK WAS CREATED

The *Kaplan MCAT Review* project began shortly after the release of the *Preview Guide for the MCAT 2015 Exam*, 2nd edition. Through thorough analysis by our staff psychometricians, we were able to analyze the relative yield of the different topics on the MCAT, and we began constructing tables of contents for the books of the *Kaplan MCAT Review* series. A dedicated staff of 30 writers, 7 editors, and 32 proofreaders worked over 5,000 combined hours to produce these books. The format of the books was heavily influenced by weekly meetings with Kaplan's learning science team.

In the years since this book was created, a number of opportunities for expansion and improvement have occurred. The current edition represents the culmination of the wisdom accumulated during that time frame, and it also includes several new features designed to improve the reading and learning experience in these texts.

These books were submitted for publication in April 2023. For any updates after this date, please visit www.kaptest.com/retail-book-corrections-and-updates.

If you have any questions about the content presented here, email KaplanMCATfeedback@kaplan.com. For other questions not related to content, email booksupport@kaplan.com.

Each book has been vetted through at least ten rounds of review. To that end, the information presented in these books is true and accurate to the best of our knowledge. Still, your feedback helps us improve our prep materials. Please notify us of any inaccuracies or errors in the books by sending an email to KaplanMCATfeedback@kaplan.com.

USING THIS BOOK

Kaplan MCAT Biochemistry Review, and the other six books in the *Kaplan MCAT Review* series, bring the Kaplan classroom experience to you—right in your home, at your convenience. This book offers the same Kaplan content review, strategies, and practice that make Kaplan the #1 choice for MCAT prep.

This book is designed to help you review the biochemistry topics covered on the MCAT. Please understand that content review—no matter how thorough—is not sufficient preparation for the MCAT! The MCAT tests not only your science knowledge but also your critical reading, reasoning, and problem-solving skills. Do not assume that simply memorizing the contents of this book will earn you high scores on Test Day; to maximize your scores, you must also improve your reading and test-taking skills through MCAT-style questions and practice tests.

Learning Objectives

At the beginning of each section, you'll find a short list of objectives describing the skills covered within that section. Learning objectives for these texts were developed in conjunction with Kaplan's learning science team, and have been designed specifically to focus your attention on tasks and concepts that are likely to show up on your MCAT. These learning objectives will function as a means to guide your study, and indicate what information and relationships you should be focused on within each section. Before starting each section, read these learning objectives carefully. They will not only allow you to assess your existing familiarity with the content, but also provide a goal-oriented focus for your studying experience of the section.

MCAT Concept Checks

At the end of each section, you'll find a few open-ended questions that you can use to assess your mastery of the material. These MCAT Concept Checks were introduced after numerous conversations with Kaplan's learning science team. Research has demonstrated repeatedly that introspection and self-analysis improve mastery, retention, and recall of material. Complete these MCAT Concept Checks to ensure that you've got the key points from each section before moving on!

Science Mastery Assessments

At the beginning of each chapter, you'll find 15 MCAT-style practice questions. These are designed to help you assess your understanding of the chapter before you begin reading the chapter. Using the guidance provided with the assessment, you can determine the best way to review each chapter based on your personal strengths and weaknesses. Most of the questions in the Science Mastery Assessments focus on the first of the *Scientific Inquiry and Reasoning Skills* (*Knowledge of Scientific Concepts and Principles)*, although there are occasional questions that fall into the second or fourth SIRS (*Scientific Reasoning and Problem-Solving* and *Data-Based and Statistical Reasoning*, respectively). You can complete each chapter's assessment in a testing interface in your online resources, where you'll also find a test-like passage set covering the same content you just studied to ensure you can also apply your knowledge the way the MCAT will expect you to!

Guided Examples with Expert Thinking

Embedded in each chapter of this book is a Guided Example with Expert Thinking. Each of these guided examples will be located in the same section as the content used in that example. Each example will feature an MCAT-level scientific article, that simulates an MCAT experiment passage. Read through the passage as you would on the real MCAT, referring to the Expert Thinking material to the right of the passage to clarify the key information you should be gathering from each paragraph. Read and attempt to answer the associated question once you have worked through the passage. There is a full explanation, including the correct answer, following the given question. These passages and questions are designed to help build your critical thinking, experimental reasoning, and data interpretation skills as preparation for the challenges you will face on the MCAT.

Sidebars

The following is a guide to the five types of sidebars you'll find in *Kaplan MCAT Biochemistry Review:*

- **Bridge:** These sidebars create connections between science topics that appear in multiple chapters throughout the *Kaplan MCAT Review* series.
- **Key Concept:** These sidebars draw attention to the most important takeaways in a given topic, and they sometimes offer synopses or overviews of complex information. If you understand nothing else, make sure you grasp the Key Concepts for any given subject.
- **MCAT Expertise:** These sidebars point out how information may be tested on the MCAT or offer key strategy points and test-taking tips that you should apply on Test Day.
- **Mnemonic:** These sidebars present memory devices to help recall certain facts.
- **Real World:** These sidebars illustrate how a concept in the text relates to the practice of medicine or the world at large. While this is not information you need to know for Test Day, many of the topics in Real World sidebars are excellent examples of how a concept may appear in a passage or discrete (stand-alone) question on the MCAT.

What This Book Covers

The information presented in the *Kaplan MCAT Review* series covers everything listed on the official MCAT content lists. Every topic in these lists is covered in the same level of detail as is common to the undergraduate and postbaccalaureate classes that are considered prerequisites for the MCAT. Note that your premedical classes may include topics not discussed in these books, or they may go into more depth than these books do. Additional exposure to science content is never a bad thing, but all of the content knowledge you are expected to have walking in on Test Day is covered in these books.

Chapter profiles, on the first page of each chapter, represent a holistic look at the content within the chapter, and will include a pie chart as well as text information. The pie chart analysis is based directly on data released by the AAMC, and will give a rough estimate of the importance of the chapter in relation to the book as a whole. Further, the text portion of the Chapter Profiles includes which AAMC content categories are covered within the chapter. These are referenced directly from the AAMC MCAT exam content listing, available on the testmaker's website.

You'll also see new High-Yield badges scattered throughout the sections of this book:

In This Chapter

1.1 Amino Acids Found in Proteins

High-Yield

LEARNING OBJECTIVES

After Chapter 1.1, you will be able to:

These badges represent the top 100 topics most tested by the AAMC. In other words, according to the testmaker and all our experience with their resources, a High-Yield badge means more questions on Test Day.

This book also contains a thorough glossary and index for easy navigation of the text.

In the end, this is your book, so write in the margins, draw diagrams, highlight the key points—do whatever is necessary to help you get that higher score. We look forward to working with you as you achieve your dreams and become the doctor you deserve to be!

Studying with This Book

In addition to providing you with the best practice questions and test strategies, Kaplan's team of learning scientists are dedicated to researching and testing the best methods for getting the most out of your study time. Here are their top four tips for improving retention:

Review multiple topics in one study session. This may seem counterintuitive—we're used to practicing one skill at a time in order to improve each skill. But research shows that weaving topics together leads to increased learning. Beyond that consideration, the MCAT often includes more than one topic in a single question. Studying in an integrated manner is the most effective way to prepare for this test.

Customize the content. Drawing attention to difficult or critical content can ensure you don't overlook it as you read and re-read sections. The best way to do this is to make it more visual—highlight, make tabs, use stickies, whatever works. We recommend highlighting only the most important or difficult sections of text. Selective highlighting of up to about 10% of text in a given chapter is great for emphasizing parts of the text, but over-highlighting can have the opposite effect.

Repeat topics over time. Many people try to memorize concepts by repeating them over and over again in succession. Our research shows that retention is improved by spacing out the repeats over time and mixing up the order in which you study content. For example, try reading chapters in a different order the second (or third!) time around. Revisit practice questions that you answered incorrectly in a new sequence. Perhaps information you reviewed more recently will help you better understand those questions and solutions you struggled with in the past.

Take a moment to reflect. When you finish reading a section for the first time, stop and think about what you just read. Jot down a few thoughts in the margins or in your notes about why the content is important or what topics came to mind when you read it. Associating learning with a memory is a fantastic way to retain information! This also works when answering questions. After answering a question, take a moment to think through each step you took to arrive at a solution. What led you to the answer you chose? Understanding the steps you took will help you make good decisions when answering future questions.

Online Resources

In addition to the resources located within this text, you also have additional online resources awaiting you at **www.kaptest.com/booksonline**. Make sure to log on and take advantage of free practice and other resources!

Please note that access to the online resources is limited to the original owner of this book.

STUDYING FOR THE MCAT

The first year of medical school is a frenzied experience for most students. To meet the requirements of a rigorous work schedule, students either learn to prioritize their time or else fall hopelessly behind. It's no surprise, then, that the MCAT, the test specifically designed to predict success in medical school, is a high-speed, time-intensive test. The MCAT demands excellent time-management skills, endurance, and grace under pressure both during the test as well as while preparing for it. Having a solid plan of attack and sticking with it are key to giving you the confidence and structure you need to succeed.

Creating a Study Plan

The best time to create a study plan is at the beginning of your MCAT preparation. If you don't already use a calendar, you will want to start. You can purchase a planner, print out a free calendar from the Internet, use a built-in calendar or app on one of your smart devices, or keep track using an interactive online calendar. Pick the option that is most practical for you and that you are most likely to use consistently.

Once you have a calendar, you'll be able to start planning your study schedule with the following steps:

1. **Fill in your obligations and choose a day off.**

   Write in all your school, extracurricular, and work obligations first: class sessions, work shifts, and meetings that you must attend. Then add in your personal obligations: appointments, lunch dates, family and social time, etc. Making an appointment in your calendar for hanging out with friends or going to the movies may seem strange at first, but planning social activities in advance will help you achieve a balance between personal and professional obligations even as life gets busy. Having a happy balance allows you to be more focused and productive when it comes time to study, so stay well-rounded and don't neglect anything that is important to you.

   In addition to scheduling your personal and professional obligations, you should also plan your time off. Taking some time off is just as important as studying. Kaplan recommends taking at least one full day off per week, ideally from all your study obligations but at minimum from studying for the MCAT.

2. **Add in study blocks around your obligations.**

   Once you have established your calendar's framework, add in study blocks around your obligations, keeping your study schedule as consistent as possible across days and across weeks. Studying at the same time of day as your official test is ideal for promoting recall, but if that's not possible, then fit in study blocks wherever you can.

   To make your studying as efficient as possible, block out short, frequent periods of study time throughout the week. From a learning perspective, studying one hour per day for six days per week is much more valuable than studying for six hours all at once one day per week. Specifically, Kaplan recommends studying for no longer than three hours in one sitting. Within those three-hour blocks, also plan to take ten-minute breaks every hour. Use these breaks to get up from your seat, do some quick stretches, get a snack and drink, and clear your mind. Although ten minutes of break for every 50 minutes of studying may sound like a lot, these breaks will allow you to deal with distractions and rest your brain so that, during the 50-minute study blocks, you can remain fully engaged and completely focused.

3. **Add in your full-length practice tests.**

   Next, you'll want to add in full-length practice tests. You'll want to take one test very early in your prep and then spread your remaining full-length practice tests evenly between now and your test date. Staggering tests in this way allows you to form a baseline for comparison and to determine which areas to focus on right away, while also providing realistic feedback throughout your prep as to how you will perform on Test Day.

When planning your calendar, aim to finish your full-length practice tests and the majority of your studying by one week before Test Day, which will allow you to spend that final week completing a brief review of what you already know. In your online resources, you'll find sample study calendars for several different Test Day timelines to use as a starting point. The sample calendars may include more focus than you need in some areas, and less in others, and it may not fit your timeline to Test Day. You will need to customize your study calendar to your needs using the steps above.

The total amount of time you spend studying each week will depend on your schedule, your personal prep needs, and your time to Test Day, but it is recommended that you spend somewhere in the range of 300–350 hours preparing before taking the official MCAT. One way you could break this down is to study for three hours per day, six days per week, for four months, but this is just one approach. You might study six days per week for more than three hours per day. You might study over a longer period of time if you don't have much time to study each week. No matter what your plan is, ensure you complete enough practice to feel completely comfortable with the MCAT and its content. A good sign you're ready for Test Day is when you begin to earn your goal score consistently in practice.

How to Study

The MCAT covers a large amount of material, so studying for Test Day can initially seem daunting. To combat this we have some tips for how to take control of your studying and make the most of your time.

Goal Setting

To take control of the amount of content and practice required to do well on the MCAT, break the content down into specific goals for each week instead of attempting to approach the test as a whole. A goal of "I want to increase my overall score by 5 points" is too big, abstract, and difficult to measure on the small scale. More reasonable goals are "I will read two chapters each day this week." Goals like this are much less overwhelming and help break studying into manageable pieces.

Active Reading

As you go through this book, much of the information will be familiar to you. After all, you have probably seen most of the content before. However, be very careful: Familiarity with a subject does not necessarily translate to knowledge or mastery of that subject. Do not assume that if you recognize a concept you actually know it and can apply it quickly at an appropriate level. Don't just passively read this book. Instead, read actively: Use the free margin space to jot down important ideas, draw diagrams, and make charts as you read. Highlighting can be an excellent tool, but use it sparingly: highlighting every sentence isn't active reading, it's coloring. Frequently stop and ask yourself questions while you read (e.g., *What is the main point? How does this fit into the overall scheme of things? Could I thoroughly explain this to someone else?*). By making connections and focusing on the grander scheme, not only will you ensure you know the essential content, but you also prepare yourself for the level of critical thinking required by the MCAT.

Focus on Areas of Greatest Opportunity

If you are limited by only having a minimal amount of time to prepare before Test Day, focus on your biggest areas of opportunity first. Areas of opportunity are topic areas that are highly tested and that you have not yet mastered. You likely won't have time to take detailed notes for every page of these books; instead, use your results from practice materials to determine

which areas are your biggest opportunities and seek those out. After you've taken a full-length test, make sure you are using your performance report to best identify areas of opportunity. Skim over content matter for which you are already demonstrating proficiency, pausing to read more thoroughly when something looks unfamiliar or particularly difficult. Begin with the Science Mastery Assessment at the beginning of each chapter. If you can get all of those questions correct within a reasonable amount of time, you may be able to quickly skim through that chapter, but if the questions prove to be more difficult, then you may need to spend time reading the chapter or certain subsections of the chapter more thoroughly.

Practice, Review, and Tracking

Leave time to review your practice questions and full-length tests. You may be tempted, after practicing, to push ahead and cover new material as quickly as possible, but failing to schedule ample time for review will actually throw away your greatest opportunity to improve your performance. The brain rarely remembers anything it sees or does only once. When you carefully review the questions you've solved (and the explanations for them), the process of retrieving that information reopens and reinforces the connections you've built in your brain. This builds long-term retention and repeatable skill sets—exactly what you need to beat the MCAT!

One useful tool for making the most of your review is the How I'll Fix It (HIFI) sheet. You can create a HIFI sheet, such as the sample below, to track questions throughout your prep that you miss or have to guess on. For each such question, figure out why you missed it and supply at least one action step for how you can avoid similar mistakes in the future. As you move through your MCAT prep, adjust your study plan based on your available study time and the results of your review. Your strengths and weaknesses are likely to change over the course of your prep. Keep addressing the areas that are most important to your score, shifting your focus as those areas change. For more help with making the most of your full-length tests, including a How I'll Fix It sheet template, make sure to check out the videos and resources in your online syllabus.

Section	Q #	Type or Topic	Why I missed it	How I'll fix it
Chem/Phys	*42*	*Nuclear chem.*	*Confused electron absorption and emission*	*Reread Physics Chapter 9.2*
Chem/Phys	*47*	K_{eq}	*Didn't know right equation*	*Memorize equation for* K_{eq}
CARS	*2*	*Detail*	*Didn't read "not" in answer choice*	*Slow down when finding match*
CARS	*4*	*Inference*	*Forgot to research answer*	*Reread passage and predict first*

Where to Study

One often-overlooked aspect of studying is the environment where the learning actually occurs. Although studying at home is many students' first choice, several problems can arise in this environment, chief of which are distractions. Studying can be a mentally draining process, so as time passes, these distractions become ever more tempting as escape routes. Although you may have considerable willpower, there's no reason to make staying focused harder than it needs to be. Instead of studying at home, head to a library, quiet coffee shop, or another new location whenever possible. This will eliminate many of the usual distractions and also promote efficient studying; instead of studying off and on at home over the course of an entire day, you can stay at the library for three hours of effective studying and enjoy the rest of the day off from the MCAT.

No matter where you study, make your practice as much like Test Day as possible. Just as is required during the official test, don't have snacks or chew gum during your study blocks. Turn off your music, television, and phone. Practice on the computer with your online resources to simulate the computer-based test environment. When completing practice questions, do your work on scratch paper or noteboard sheets rather than writing directly on any printed materials since you won't have that option on Test Day. Because memory is tied to all of your senses, the more test-like you can make your studying environment, the easier it will be on Test Day to recall the information you're putting in so much work to learn.

CHAPTER 1

AMINO ACIDS, PEPTIDES, AND PROTEINS

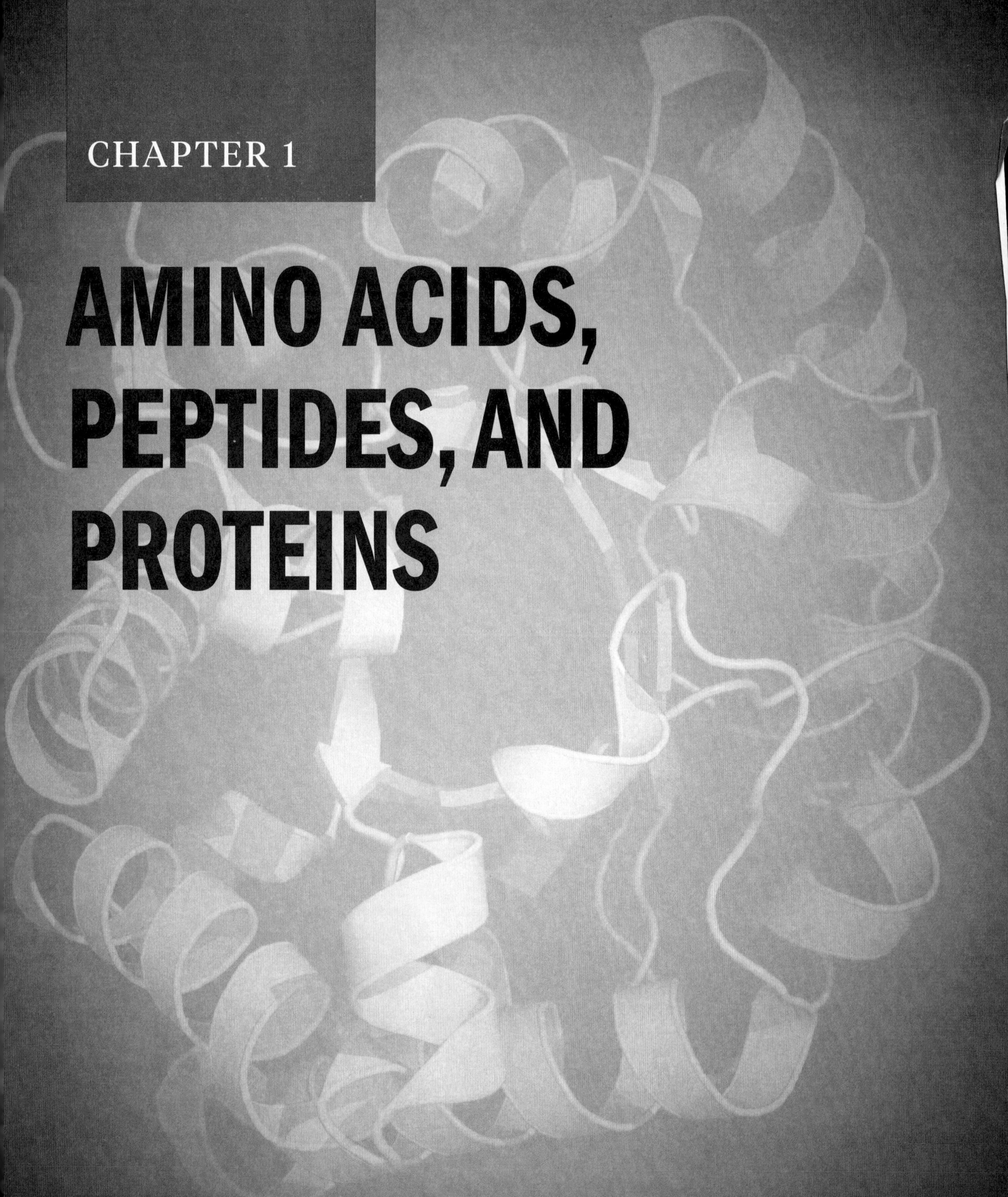

SCIENCE MASTERY ASSESSMENT

Every pre-med knows this feeling: there is so much content I have to know for the MCAT! How do I know what to do first or what's important?

While the high-yield badges throughout this book will help you identify the most important topics, this Science Mastery Assessment is another tool in your MCAT prep arsenal. This quiz (which can also be taken in your online resources) and the guidance below will help ensure that you are spending the appropriate amount of time on this chapter based on your personal strengths and weaknesses. Don't worry though—skipping something now does not mean you'll never study it. Later on in your prep, as you complete full-length tests, you'll uncover specific pieces of content that you need to review and can come back to these chapters as appropriate.

How to Use This Assessment

If you answer 0–7 questions correctly:

Spend about 1 hour to read this chapter in full and take limited notes throughout. Follow up by reviewing **all** quiz questions to ensure that you now understand how to solve each one.

If you answer 8–11 questions correctly:

Spend 20–40 minutes reviewing the quiz questions. Beginning with the questions you missed, read and take notes on the corresponding subchapters. For questions you answered correctly, ensure your thinking matches that of the explanation and you understand why each choice was correct or incorrect.

If you answer 12–15 questions correctly:

Spend less than 20 minutes reviewing all questions from the quiz. If you missed any, then include a quick read-through of the corresponding subchapters, or even just the relevant content within a subchapter, as part of your question review. For questions you got correct, ensure your thinking matches that of the explanation and review the Concept Summary at the end of the chapter.

1. In a neutral solution, most amino acids exist as:
   - A. positively charged compounds.
   - B. zwitterions.
   - C. negatively charged compounds.
   - D. hydrophobic molecules.

2. At pH 7, the charge on a glutamic acid molecule is:
   - A. −2.
   - B. −1.
   - C. 0.
   - D. +1.

3. Which of the following statements is most likely to be true of nonpolar R groups in aqueous solution?
   - A. They are hydrophilic and found buried within proteins.
   - B. They are hydrophilic and found on protein surfaces.
   - C. They are hydrophobic and found buried within proteins.
   - D. They are hydrophobic and found on protein surfaces.

4. Scientists discover a cDNA sequence for an uncharacterized protein. In their initial studies, they use a computer program designed to predict protein structure. Which of the following levels of protein structure can be most accurately predicted?
   - A. Primary structure
   - B. Secondary structure
   - C. Tertiary structure
   - D. Quaternary structure

5. How many distinct tripeptides can be formed from one valine molecule, one alanine molecule, and one leucine molecule?
   - A. 1
   - B. 3
   - C. 6
   - D. 27

6. Which of the following best describes the change in entropy that occurs during protein folding?
   - A. Entropy of both the water and the protein increase.
   - B. Entropy of the water increases; entropy of the protein decreases.
   - C. Entropy of the water decreases; entropy of the protein increases.
   - D. Entropy of both the water and the protein decrease.

7. An α-helix is most likely to be held together by:
   - A. disulfide bonds.
   - B. hydrophobic effects.
   - C. hydrogen bonds.
   - D. ionic attractions between side chains.

8. Which of the following is least likely to cause denaturation of proteins?
   - A. Heating the protein to 100°C
   - B. Adding 8 M urea
   - C. Moving it to a more hypotonic environment
   - D. Adding a detergent such as sodium dodecyl sulfate

9. A particular α-helix is known to cross the cell membrane. Which of these amino acids is most likely to be found in the transmembrane portion of the helix?
   - A. Glutamate
   - B. Lysine
   - C. Phenylalanine
   - D. Aspartate

5/15

10. Which of these amino acids has a chiral carbon in its side chain?
    I. Serine
    II. Threonine
    III. Isoleucine

    A. I only
    B. II only
    C. II and III only
    D. I, II, and III

11. Following translation and folding, many receptor tyrosine kinases exist as monomers in their inactive state on the cell membrane. Upon the binding of a ligand, these proteins dimerize and initiate a signaling cascade. During this process, their highest element of protein structure changes from:
    A. secondary to tertiary.
    B. tertiary to quaternary.
    C. primary to secondary.
    D. secondary to quaternary.

12. Which of these amino acids has a side chain that can become ionized in cells?
    A. Histidine
    B. Leucine
    C. Proline
    D. Threonine

13. In lysine, the pK_a of the side chain is about 10.5. Assuming that the pK_a of the carboxyl and amino groups are 2 and 9, respectively, the pI of lysine is closest to:
    A. 5.5.
    B. 6.2.
    C. 7.4.
    D. 9.8.

14. Which of the following is a reason for conjugating proteins?
    I. To direct their delivery to a particular organelle
    II. To direct their delivery to the cell membrane
    III. To add a cofactor needed for their activity

    A. I only
    B. II only
    C. II and III only
    D. I, II, and III

15. Collagen consists of three helices with carbon backbones that are tightly wrapped around one another in a "triple helix." Which of these amino acids is most likely to be found in the highest concentration in collagen?
    A. Proline
    B. Glycine
    C. Threonine
    D. Cysteine

V - A - I   A - I - V

V - I - A

Answer Key

1. **B**
2. **B**
3. **C**
4. **A**
5. **C**
6. **B**
7. **C**
8. **C**
9. **C**
10. **C**
11. **B**
12. **A**
13. **D**
14. **D**
15. **B**

Detailed explanations can be found at the end of the chapter.

CHAPTER 1

AMINO ACIDS, PEPTIDES, AND PROTEINS

In This Chapter

CHAPTER PROFILE

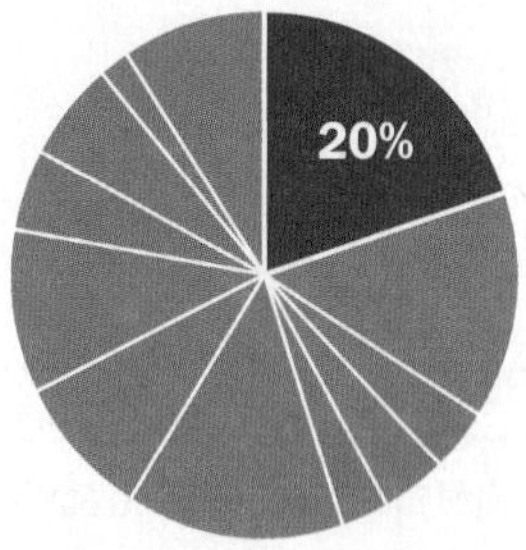

The content in this chapter should be relevant to about 20% of all questions about biochemistry on the MCAT.

This chapter covers material from the following AAMC content categories:

1A: Structure and function of proteins and their constituent amino acids

5D: Structure, function, and reactivity of biologically-relevant molecules

Normal hemoglobin: HbA
Sickle cell mutation: HBS
has 4 chains → 1 change in the surface of hemoglobin, in 2 of those chains, 6th amino acid glutamic acid to valine
causes deoxygenated form of HbS to aggregate

Introduction

How important are amino acids? Consider sickle cell disease. People with sickle cell disease have red blood cells that, under certain conditions, can become rigid and sickle-shaped. Those sickle-shaped cells can become stuck in capillaries, blocking them. In severe cases, it can block enough of the blood supply to cause damage to several organs, such as the kidneys, liver, and spleen. This happens because of a mutation in hemoglobin, the protein in red blood cells that transports oxygen. Remarkably, the difference between the normal form of hemoglobin, HbA, and the one that causes sickle cell disease, HbS, is a seemingly minor one. All it takes is a change in a single amino acid on the surface of hemoglobin: the sixth amino acid in two of its four chains is changed from glutamic acid to valine. That minor difference allows the deoxygenated form of HbS to aggregate and precipitate, which leads to the sickled shape—and all the symptoms—of sickle cell disease.

In this chapter, we'll take a look at the basics of proteins by focusing on the amino acids that compose them and how those amino acids contribute to the physical and chemical properties of proteins.

MCAT EXPERTISE

This chapter represents a whopping 20% of all biochemistry questions you will see on Test Day. That makes amino acids one of the highest yield subjects within any of the review books! Make sure to work sufficient study of these materials into your study plan.

1.1 Amino Acids Found in Proteins

High-Yield

LEARNING OBJECTIVES

After Chapter 1.1, you will be able to:

- Recognize common abbreviations for amino acids, such as Glu and Y
- Distinguish the stereochemistries, typical cellular locations, and reactivities of the 20 major amino acids
- Identify the major amino acids, such as:

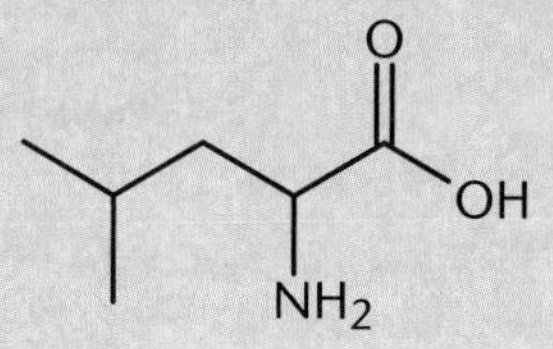

MCAT EXPERTISE

The "High-Yield" badge on this section indicates that the content is frequently tested on the MCAT.

Amino acids are molecules that contain two functional groups: an amino group ($-NH_2$) and a carboxyl group ($-COOH$). In this chapter, we'll focus specifically on the α-amino acids, in which the amino group and the carboxyl group are bonded to the same carbon, the α-carbon of the carboxylic acid. Think of the α-carbon as the central carbon of the amino acid, as shown in Figure 1.1.

BRIDGE

Remember that for carboxylic acids, the α-carbon is the carbon *adjacent* to the carboxyl carbon. The structure and nomenclature of carboxylic acids are discussed in Chapter 8 of *MCAT Organic Chemistry Review*.

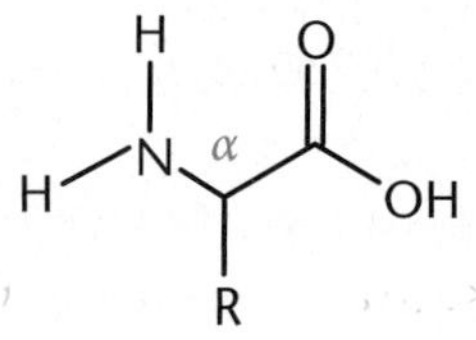

Figure 1.1 Amino Acid Structure

In addition to the amino and carboxyl groups, the α-carbon has two other groups attached to it: a hydrogen atom and a **side chain**, also called an **R group**, which is specific to each amino acid. The side chains determine the properties of amino acids, and therefore their functions.

KEY CONCEPT

The side chains (R groups) of amino acids determine their chemical properties.

A Note on Terminology

Amino acids do not *need* to have both the amino and carboxyl groups bonded to the same carbon. For example, the neurotransmitter γ-*aminobutyric acid* (GABA) has the amino group on the gamma (γ) carbon, *three* carbons away from the carboxyl group. Similarly, not every amino acid found in the human body is specified by a codon in the genetic code or incorporated into proteins. One example is *ornithine*, one of the intermediates in the urea cycle, the metabolic process by which the body excretes excess nitrogen. There are also some amino acids that are specifically modified for specialized roles in the body; for example, lysine is sometimes converted into pyrrolysine.

MCAT EXPERTISE

While the MCAT *could* include passages on GABA or other nonstandard amino acids, they are *not* part of the background information you're expected to know for Test Day.

That said, the Association of American Medical Colleges (AAMC) has specifically stated they'll focus on the 20 α-amino acids encoded by the human genetic code, also called **proteinogenic amino acids**. So, for the rest of this chapter, we'll use the term *amino acid* to refer specifically to these compounds.

Stereochemistry of Amino Acids

For most amino acids, the α-carbon is a chiral (or stereogenic) center, as it has four different groups attached to it. Thus, most amino acids are optically active. The one exception is **glycine**, which has a hydrogen atom as its R group, making it achiral, as shown in Figure 1.2.

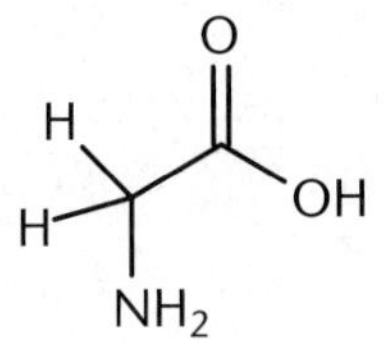

Figure 1.2 Glycine

All chiral amino acids used in eukaryotes are L-amino acids, so the amino group is drawn on the left in a Fischer projection, as demonstrated in Figure 1.3. In the Cahn–Ingold–Prelog system, this translates to an (*S*) absolute configuration for almost all chiral amino acids. The only exception is **cysteine**, which, while still being an L-amino acid, has an (*R*) absolute configuration because the $-CH_2SH$ group has priority over the $-COOH$ group.

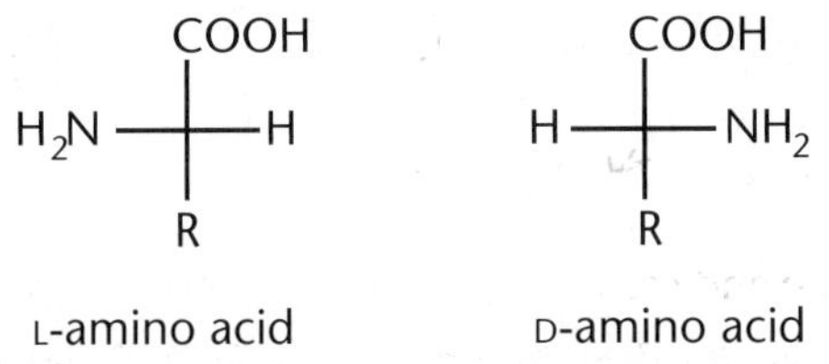

Figure 1.3 L- and D-Amino Acids

KEY CONCEPT

Except for glycine, all amino acids are chiral—and except for cysteine, all of them have an (*S*) absolute configuration.

REAL WORLD

While L-amino acids are the only ones found in eukaryotic proteins, D-amino acids do exist. One example is *gramicidin*, an antibiotic produced by a soil bacterium called *Bacillus brevis*, in which D- and L-amino acids alternate in the primary structure.

Structures of the Amino Acids

There are several ways to classify amino acids. In this section, we'll break them down by the structures of their side chains.

Nonpolar, Nonaromatic Side Chains

Seven amino acids, shown in Figure 1.4a, fall into this class. **Glycine**, discussed earlier, has a single hydrogen atom as its side chain and is therefore achiral. It is also the smallest amino acid. Four other amino acids—**alanine**, **valine**, **leucine**, and **isoleucine**—have alkyl side chains containing one to four carbons.

MCAT EXPERTISE

The AAMC's practice materials have made it clear that test takers are expected to know the structures, names, and three-letter and one-letter abbreviations for the amino acids.

Methionine is one of only two amino acids that contains a sulfur atom in its side chain. Nevertheless, because the sulfur has a methyl group attached, it is considered relatively nonpolar.

Finally, **proline** is unique in that it forms a *cyclic* amino acid. In all the other amino acids, the amino group is attached *only* to the α-carbon. In proline, however, the amino nitrogen becomes a part of the side chain, forming a five-membered ring. That ring places notable constraints on the flexibility of proline, which limits where it can appear in a protein and can have significant effects on proline's role in secondary structure.

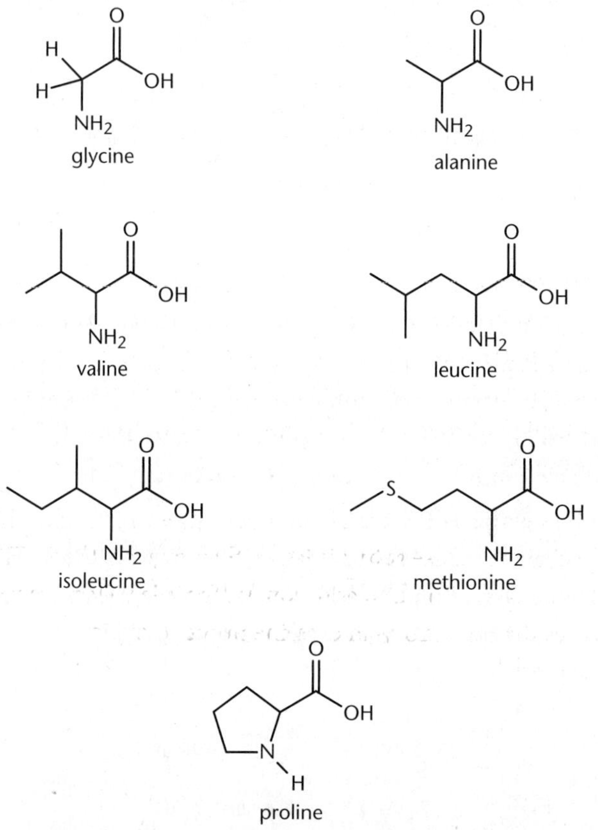

Figure 1.4a Amino Acids with Nonpolar, Nonaromatic Side Chains

MCAT EXPERTISE

The MCAT writers strive to avoid misuse of terminology. Some textbooks problematically describe proline as an *imino* acid because the amino nitrogen forms two bonds to carbon. The MCAT won't use this term because an *imine* is specifically a molecule with a carbon-nitrogen double bond.

Aromatic Side Chains

Three amino acids have uncharged aromatic side chains and are depicted in Figure 1.4b. The largest of these is **tryptophan**, which has a double-ring system that contains a nitrogen atom. The smallest is **phenylalanine**, which has a benzyl side chain (a benzene ring plus a $-CH_2-$ group). Adding an $-OH$ group to phenylalanine gives the third member, **tyrosine**. While phenylalanine is relatively nonpolar, the $-OH$ group makes tyrosine relatively polar.

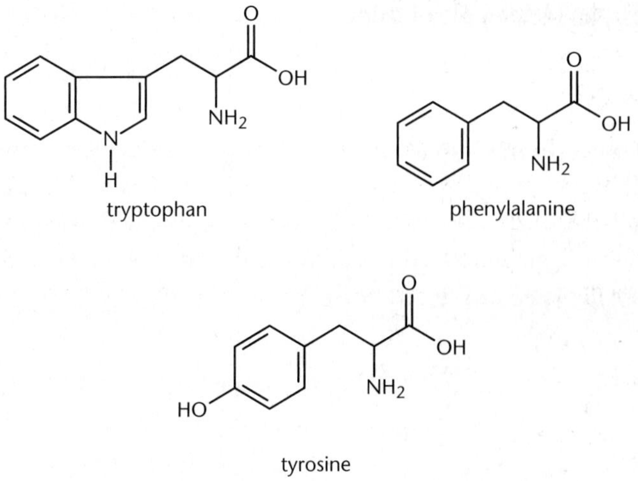

Figure 1.4b Amino Acids with Aromatic Side Chains

Polar Side Chains

Five amino acids, shown in Figure 1.4c, have side chains that are polar but not aromatic. **Serine** and **threonine** both have –OH groups in their side chains, which makes them highly polar and able to participate in hydrogen bonding. **Asparagine** and **glutamine** have amide side chains. Unlike the amino group common to all amino acids, the amide nitrogens do *not* gain or lose protons with changes in pH; they do not become charged.

BRIDGE

Make sure you know your carboxylic acid derivatives for Test Day! They are discussed in Chapter 9 of *MCAT Organic Chemistry Review.*

The last amino acid with a polar side chain is **cysteine**, which has a **thiol** (–SH) group in its side chain. Because sulfur is larger than oxygen, the S–H bond is longer and weaker than the O–H bond. In addition, sulfur is less electronegative than oxygen. This leaves the thiol group in cysteine prone to oxidation, a reaction we'll study later in this chapter.

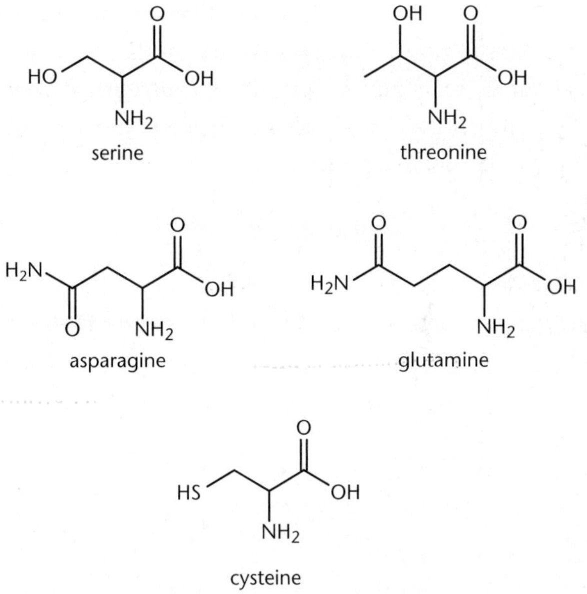

Figure 1.4c Amino Acids with Polar Side Chains

Negatively Charged (Acidic) Side Chains

Only two of the 20 amino acids have negative charges on their side chains at physiological pH (7.4). Those two are **aspartic acid** (**aspartate**), which is related to asparagine, and **glutamic acid** (**glutamate**), which is related to glutamine. Unlike asparagine and glutamine, aspartate and glutamate have carboxylate ($-COO^-$) groups in their side chains, rather than amides. Note that aspartate is simply the deprotonated form of aspartic acid, and glutamate is the deprotonated form of glutamic acid. These two amino acids are depicted in Figure 1.4d.

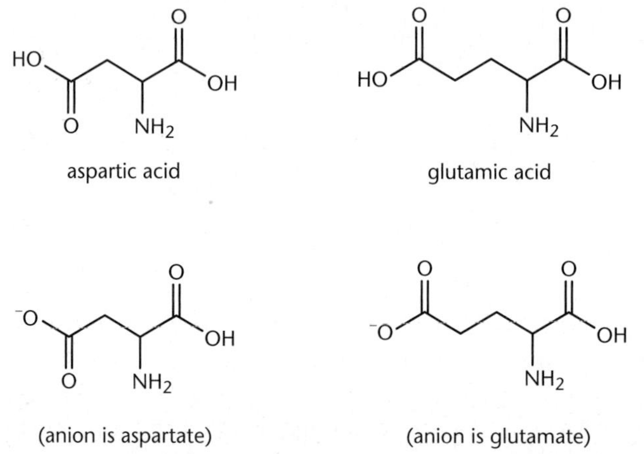

Figure 1.4d Amino Acids with Negatively Charged Side Chains

MCAT EXPERTISE

On the MCAT, you're likely to see anion names (aspartate and glutamate) instead of acid names (aspartic acid and glutamic acid) because most acids in cells exist in the deprotonated form. This also applies to molecules other than amino acids (*malate* instead of *malic acid*).

BRIDGE

The catalytic triad found in *chymotrypsin* makes use of the histidine side chain's ability to gain a proton. The histidine residue in its active site removes a proton from the —OH group of a serine residue side chain, which facilitates nucleophilic attack by the serine residue on the carbonyl carbon atom of the substrate. Chymotrypsin's role as a digestive enzyme is discussed in Chapter 9 of *MCAT Biology Review*.

Positively Charged (Basic) Side Chains

The remaining three amino acids, shown in Figure 1.4e, have side chains that have positively charged nitrogen atoms. **Lysine** has a terminal primary amino group, while **arginine** has three nitrogen atoms in its side chain; the positive charge is delocalized over all three nitrogen atoms. The final amino acid, **histidine**, has an aromatic ring with two nitrogen atoms (this ring is called an **imidazole**). You might be wondering how histidine can acquire a positive charge. The pK_a of the side chain is relatively close to 7.4—it's about 6—so, at physiologic pH, one nitrogen atom is protonated and the other isn't. Under more acidic conditions, the second nitrogen atom can become protonated, giving the side chain a positive charge.

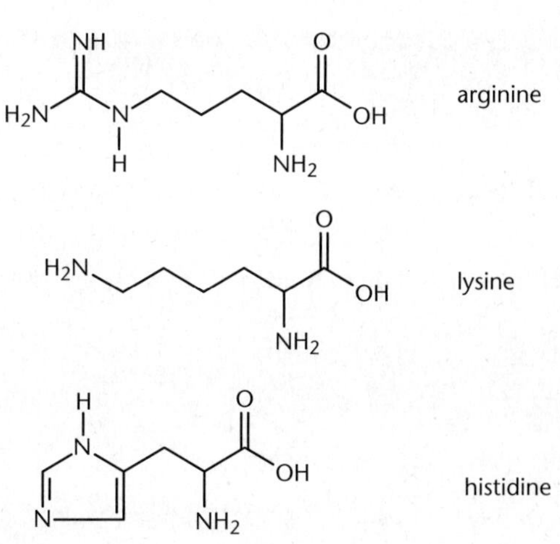

Figure 1.4e Amino Acids with Positively Charged Side Chains

Hydrophobic and Hydrophilic Amino Acids

Classifying amino acid side chains as hydrophobic or hydrophilic is actually a very complex matter. For example, tyrosine has both an –OH group and an aromatic ring—so which one "wins"?

A few clear conclusions can be drawn, though. First, the amino acids with long alkyl side chains—alanine, isoleucine, leucine, valine, and phenylalanine—are all strongly hydrophobic and thus more likely to be found in the interior of proteins, away from water on the surface of the protein. Second, all the amino acids with charged side chains—positively charged histidine, arginine, and lysine, plus negatively charged glutamate and aspartate—are hydrophilic, as are the amides asparagine and glutamine. The remaining amino acids lie somewhere in the middle and are neither particularly hydrophilic nor particularly hydrophobic.

KEY CONCEPT

The surface of a protein tends to be rich in amino acids with charged side chains. Strongly hydrophobic amino acids tend to be found in the interior of proteins.

Amino Acid Abbreviations

Now that we have explored the structures of the 20 proteinogenic amino acids, it is worth mentioning that you are expected to be able to identify an amino acid on the MCAT not only by name, but also by its three-letter and one-letter abbreviations. These abbreviations are listed in Table 1.1.

MCAT EXPERTISE

Three-letter abbreviations are used to identify amino acids in many contexts. One-letter abbreviations are primarily used when space is at a premium as with formulas of long protein sequences, the labeling of individual amino acids in figures, and mutation shorthand. While each type of mutation has its own notation, substitution is the most likely to show up on Test Day. For example, "E6V" indicates that the sixth amino acid (glutamic acid, E) has been changed to valine (V).

MCAT EXPERTISE

It bears repeating: the structures and abbreviations (both three- and one-letter) have been tested *heavily* on both natural science sections of the MCAT. Make sure you know this page by heart!

AMINO ACID	THREE-LETTER ABBREVIATION	ONE-LETTER ABBREVIATION
Alanine	Ala	A
Arginine	Arg	R
Asparagine	Asn	N
Aspartic acid	Asp	D
Cysteine	Cys	C
Glutamic acid	Glu	E
Glutamine	Gln	Q
Glycine	Gly	G
Histidine	His	H
Isoleucine	Ile	I
Leucine	Leu	L
Lysine	Lys	K
Methionine	Met	M
Phenylalanine	Phe	F
Proline	Pro	P
Serine	Ser	S
Threonine	Thr	T
Tryptophan	Trp	W
Tyrosine	Tyr	Y
Valine	Val	V

Table 1.1 Three- and One-Letter Abbreviations of Amino Acids

MCAT CONCEPT CHECK 1.1

Before you move on, assess your understanding of the material with these questions.

1. What are the four groups attached to the central (α) carbon of a proteinogenic amino acid?

____

2. What is the stereochemistry of the chiral amino acids that appear in eukaryotic proteins?
   - L or D?
   - (*R*) or (*S*)? (Exception:) _______________

3. Which amino acids fit into each of these categories? (Note: The number in parentheses indicates the number of amino acids in that category.)
   - Nonpolar, nonaromatic (7):

   ____

   - Aromatic (3):

   ____

   - Polar (5):

   ____

   - Negatively charged/acidic (2):

   ____

   - Positively charged/basic (3):

   ____

4. Where do hydrophobic amino acids tend to reside within a protein? What about hydrophilic ones?
   - Hydrophobic:

   ____

   - Hydrophilic:

   ____

5. Identify the amino acids below by their one-letter abbreviation.

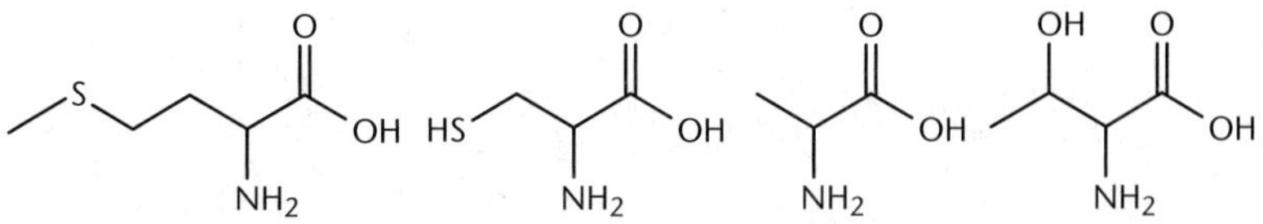

BRIDGE

Solutions to concept checks for a given chapter in *MCAT Biochemistry Review* can be found near the end of the chapter in which the concept check is located, following the Concept Summary for that chapter.

1.2 Acid-Base Chemistry of Amino Acids

LEARNING OBJECTIVES

After Chapter 1.2, you will be able to:

- Identify the predominant ion form of the generic amino acid backbone given a pH value
- Calculate pI values for an amino acid given pK_a values for backbone and side chains
- Predict the general form of the titration curve for an amino acid

The AAMC loves to use amino acids to test your understanding of acid–base chemistry because they have both an acidic carboxylic acid group and a basic amino group. That makes them **amphoteric species**, as they can either accept a proton or donate a proton; how they react depends on the pH of their environment. The key to understanding the behavior of amino acids is to remember two facts:

- Ionizable groups tend to gain protons under acidic conditions and lose them under basic conditions. So, in general, at low pH, ionizable groups tend to be protonated; at high pH, they tend to be deprotonated.
- The pK_a of a group is the pH at which, on average, half of the molecules of that species are deprotonated; that is, [protonated version of the ionizable group] = [deprotonated version of the ionizable group] or $[HA] = [A^-]$. If the pH is less than the pK_a, a majority of the species will be protonated. If the pH is higher than the pK_a, a majority of the species will be deprotonated.

MCAT EXPERTISE

You are *not* expected to know exact values for isoelectric points or side chain pK_a values. The MCAT will either provide you with numerical data to use in answering a question or test clear-cut distinctions that can be made without additional information (such as, *Which is more hydrophilic, valine or lysine?* but not *Which is more hydrophobic, valine or alanine?*).

Protonation and Deprotonation

Because all amino acids have at least two groups that can be deprotonated, they all have at least two pK_a values. The first one, pK_{a_1}, is the pK_a for the carboxyl group and is usually around 2. For most amino acids, the second pK_a value, pK_{a_2}, is the pK_a for the amino group, which is usually between 9 and 10. For amino acids with an ionizable side chain, there will be three pK_a values, but we'll come back to that later. As an example, let's take glycine, which doesn't have an ionizable side chain.

KEY CONCEPT

Like all polyprotic acids, each ionizable proton has its own pK_a at which it is "half-deprotonated."

Positively Charged under Acidic Conditions

At pH 1 (below even the pH of the stomach), there are plenty of protons in solution. Because we're far below the pK_a of the amino group, the amino group will be fully protonated ($-NH_3^+$) and thus positively charged. Because we're also below the pK_a of the carboxylic acid group, it too will be fully protonated ($-COOH$) and thus neutral. Therefore, at very acidic pH values, amino acids tend to be positively charged, as shown in Figure 1.5.

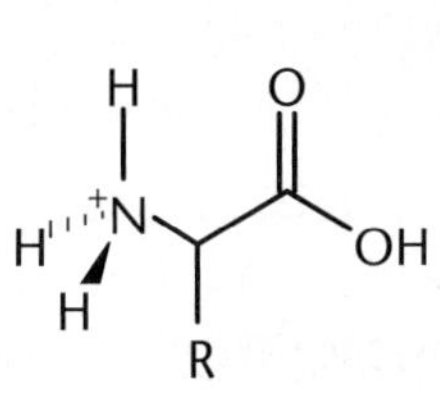

Figure 1.5 Amino Acid Structure at Acidic pH

Zwitterions at Intermediate pH

If we increase the pH of the amino acid solution from pH 1 to pH 7.4, the normal pH of human blood, we've moved far above the pK_a of the carboxylic acid group. At physiological pH, you will not find amino acids with the carboxylate group protonated (–COOH) and the amino group unprotonated ($-NH_2$). Under these conditions, the carboxyl group will be in its conjugate base form and be deprotonated, becoming $-COO^-$. Conversely, we're still well below the pK_a of the basic amino group, so it will remain fully protonated and in its conjugate acid form ($-NH_3^+$). Thus, we have a molecule that has both a positive charge and a negative charge, but overall, the molecule is electrically neutral. We call such molecules dipolar ions, or **zwitterions** (from the German *zwitter*, or "hybrid"), as depicted in Figure 1.6. The two charges neutralize one another, and zwitterions exist in water as internal salts.

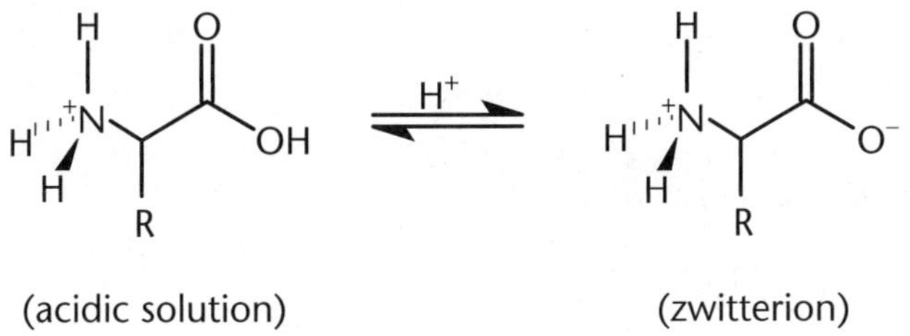

Figure 1.6 Carboxylic Acids Become Deprotonated at Neutral pH, Forming Zwitterions

Negatively Charged under Basic Conditions

Milk of magnesia, which is often used as an antacid, has a pH around 10.5. At that pH, the carboxylate group is already deprotonated and thus remains $-COO^-$. On the other hand, we are now well above the pK_a for the amino group, so it deprotonates too, becoming $-NH_2$. So, at highly basic pH, glycine is now negatively charged, as depicted in Figure 1.7.

KEY CONCEPT

At very acidic pH values, amino acids tend to be positively charged. At very alkaline pH values, amino acids tend to be negatively charged.

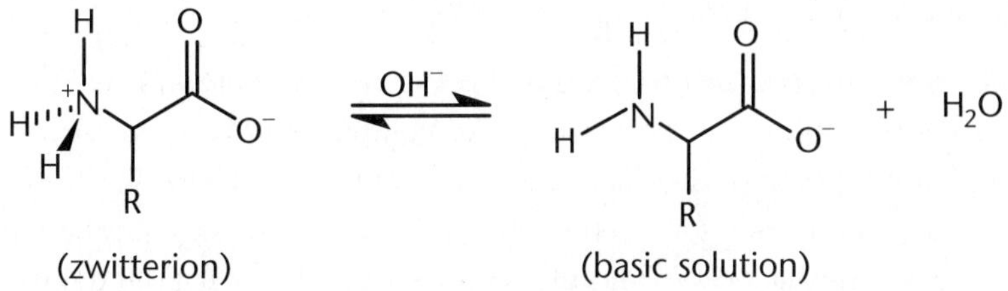

Figure 1.7 Amino Groups Become Deprotonated at Basic pH, Forming an Anion

Titration of Amino Acids

Because of these acid–base properties, amino acids are great candidates for titrations. We assume that the titration of each proton occurs as a distinct step, resembling that of a simple monoprotic acid. Thus, the titration curve looks like a combination of two monoprotic acid titration curves (or three curves, if the side chain is charged). Figure 1.8 shows the titration curve for glycine. After we inspect this curve, we'll look at the differences for the amino acids with charged side chains.

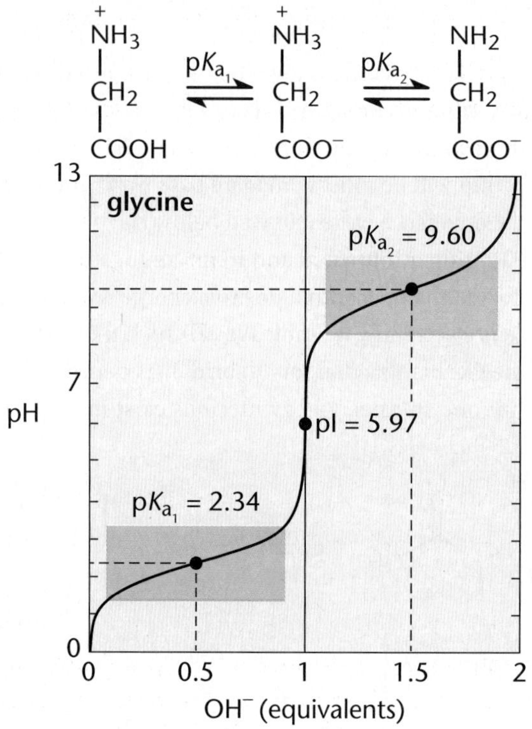

Figure 1.8 Titration Curve for Glycine

KEY CONCEPT

When the pH of a solution is approximately equal to the pK_a of the solute, the solution acts as a buffer.

Imagine an acidic 1 M glycine solution. At low pH values, glycine exists predominantly as $^+NH_3CH_2COOH$; it is fully protonated, with a positive charge. As the solution is titrated with NaOH, the carboxyl group will deprotonate first because it is more acidic than the amino group. When 0.5 equivalents of base have been added to the solution, the concentrations of the fully protonated glycine and its zwitterion, $^+NH_3CH_2COO^-$, are equal; that is, $[^+NH_3CH_2COOH] = [^+NH_3CH_2COO^-]$. At this point, the pH equals pK_{a_1}. Remember: when the pH is close to the pK_a value of a solute, the solution is acting as a buffer and the titration curve is relatively flat, as demonstrated in the blue boxes in the diagram.

As we add more base, the carboxylate group goes from half-deprotonated to fully deprotonated. The amino acid stops acting like a buffer, and pH starts to increase rapidly during this phase. When we've added 1.0 equivalent of base, glycine exists exclusively as the zwitterion form (remember, we started with 1.0 equivalent of glycine). This means that every molecule is now electrically neutral, and thus the pH equals the **isoelectric point (pI)** of glycine. This is true of all amino acids: the isoelectric point is the pH at which the molecule is electrically neutral. For neutral amino acids, it can be calculated by averaging the two pK_a values for the amino and carboxyl groups:

$$\text{pI}_{\text{neutral amino acid}} = \frac{\text{p}K_{\text{a,NH}_3^+\text{ group}} + \text{p}K_{\text{a,COOH group}}}{2}$$

Equation 1.1

For glycine, the pI value is $(2.34 + 9.60) \div 2 = 5.97$. Remember that when the molecule is neutral, it is especially sensitive to pH changes, and the titration curve is nearly vertical.

As we continue adding base, glycine passes through a second buffering phase as the amino group deprotonates; again, the pH remains relatively constant. When 1.5 equivalents of base have been added, the concentration of the zwitterion form equals the concentration of the fully deprotonated form; that is, $[^+NH_3CH_2COO^-] = [NH_2CH_2COO^-]$, and the pH equals p$K_{a_2}$. Once again, the titration curve is nearly horizontal. Finally, when we've added 2.0 equivalents of base, the amino acid has become fully deprotonated, and all that remains is $NH_2CH_2COO^-$; additional base will only increase the pH further.

KEY CONCEPT

When the pH of an amino acid solution equals the isoelectric point (pI) of the amino acid, it exists as electrically neutral molecules. The pI is calculated as the average of the two nearest pK_a values. For amino acids with non-ionizable side chains, the pI is usually around 6.

Amino Acids with Charged Side Chains

For amino acids with charged side chains, such as glutamic acid and lysine, the titration curve has an extra "step," but works along the same principles as described above.

Because glutamic acid has two carboxyl groups and one amino group, its charge in its fully protonated state is still +1. It undergoes the first deprotonation, losing the proton from its main carboxyl group, just as glycine does. At that point, it is electrically neutral. When it loses its second proton, just as with glycine, its overall charge will be −1. However, the second proton that is removed in this case comes from the side chain carboxyl group, *not* the amino group! This is a relatively acidic group, with a pK_a of around 4.2. The result is that the pI of glutamic acid is much lower than that of glycine, around 3.2. The isoelectric point for an acidic amino acid can be calculated as follows:

$$\text{pI}_{\text{acidic amino acid}} = \frac{\text{p}K_{\text{a,R group}} + \text{p}K_{\text{a,COOH group}}}{2}$$

Equation 1.2

Lysine, on the other hand, has two amino groups and one carboxyl group. Thus, its charge in its fully protonated state is +2, not +1. Losing the carboxyl proton, which still happens around pH 2, brings the charge down to +1. Lysine does not become electrically neutral until it loses the proton from its main amino group, which happens around pH 9. It gets a negative charge when it loses the proton on the amino group in its side chain, which happens around pH 10.5. Thus, the isoelectric point of lysine is the average of the pK_a values for the amino group and side chain; the pI is around 9.75. The isoelectric point for a basic amino acid can be calculated as follows:

$$\text{pI}_{\text{basic amino acid}} = \frac{\text{p}K_{\text{a,NH}_3^+\text{ group}} + \text{p}K_{\text{a,R group}}}{2}$$

Equation 1.3

The take-home message: amino acids with acidic side chains have relatively low isoelectric points, while those with basic side chains have relatively high ones.

KEY CONCEPT

Amino acids with acidic side chains have pI values well below 6; amino acids with basic side chains have pI values well above 6.

MCAT CONCEPT CHECK 1.2

Before you move on, assess your understanding of the material with these questions.

1. For a generic amino acid, $NH_2CRHCOOH$, with an uncharged side chain, what would be the predominant form at each of the following pH values?
   - pH = 1:

   ____
   - pH = 7:

   ____
   - pH = 11:

   ____

2. Given the following pK_a values, what is the value of the pI for each of the amino acids listed below?
   - Aspartic acid (pK_{a_1} = 1.88, pK_{a_2} = 3.65, pK_{a_3} = 9.60): pI = __________
   - Arginine (pK_{a_1} = 2.17, pK_{a_2} = 9.04, pK_{a_3} = 12.48): pI = __________
   - Valine (pK_{a_1} = 2.32, pK_{a_2} = 9.62): pI = __________

1.3 Peptide Bond Formation and Hydrolysis

High-Yield

LEARNING OBJECTIVES

After Chapter 1.3, you will be able to:

- Recognize the relationship of nomenclature with length, such as predicting the length of a compound called a "tripeptide"
- Apply the hydrolytic mechanisms of trypsin and chymotrypsin to novel peptide chains
- Predict the products of peptide bond formation and cleavage reactions:

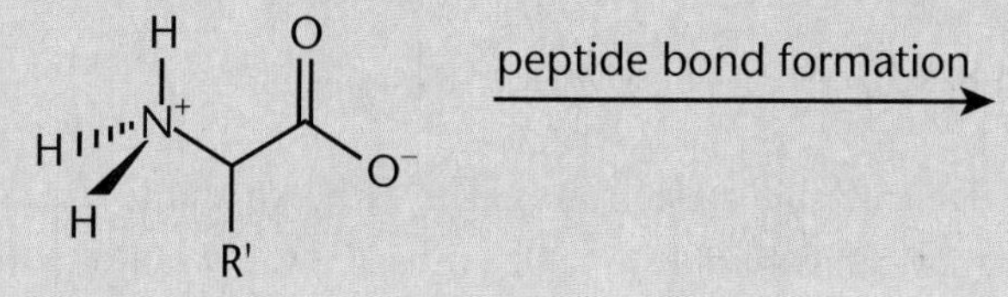

Peptides are composed of amino acid subunits, sometimes called **residues**, as shown in Figure 1.9. **Dipeptides** consist of two amino acid residues; **tripeptides** have three. The term **oligopeptide** is used for relatively small peptides, up to about 20 residues; while longer chains are called **polypeptides**.

BRIDGE

For Test Day, you also need to know how peptide bonds are formed in the context of ribosomes, which is covered in Chapter 7 of *MCAT Biochemistry Review*.

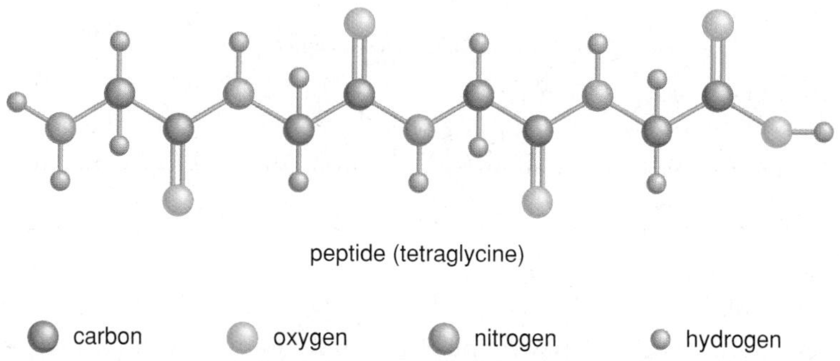

Figure 1.9 Peptide Residues

The residues in peptides are joined together through **peptide bonds**, a specialized form of an amide bond, which form between the $-COO^-$ group of one amino acid and the NH_3^+ group of another amino acid. This forms the functional group $-C(O)NH^-$. In this section, we'll look at the key reactions involved in forming and breaking peptide bonds.

Peptide Bond Formation

Peptide bond formation is an example of a **condensation** or **dehydration** reaction because it results in the removal of a water molecule (H_2O); it can also be viewed as an acyl substitution reaction, which can occur with all carboxylic acid derivatives. When a peptide bond forms, as shown in Figure 1.10, the electrophilic carbonyl carbon on the first amino acid is attacked by the nucleophilic amino group on the second amino acid. After that attack, the hydroxyl group of the carboxylic acid is kicked off. The result is the formation of a peptide (amide) bond.

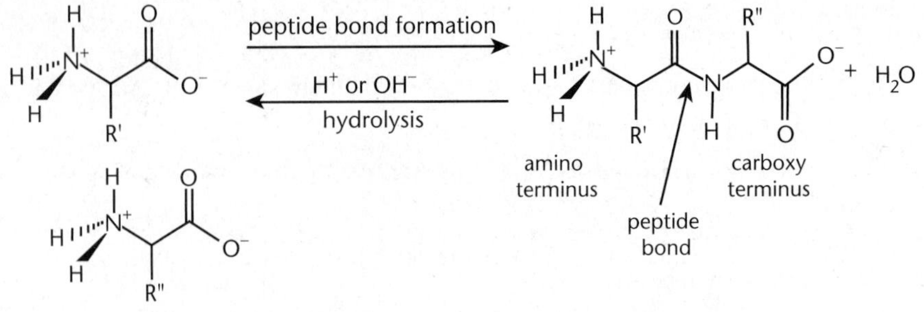

Figure 1.10 Peptide Bond Formation and Cleavage

Because amide groups have delocalizable π electrons in the carbonyl and in the lone pair on the amino nitrogen, they can exhibit resonance; thus, the C–N bond in the amide has partial double bond character, as shown in Figure 1.11.

BRIDGE

The peptide is drawn in the same order that it is synthesized by ribosomes: from the N-terminus to the C-terminus! Translation is covered in Chapter 7 of *MCAT Biochemistry Review*.

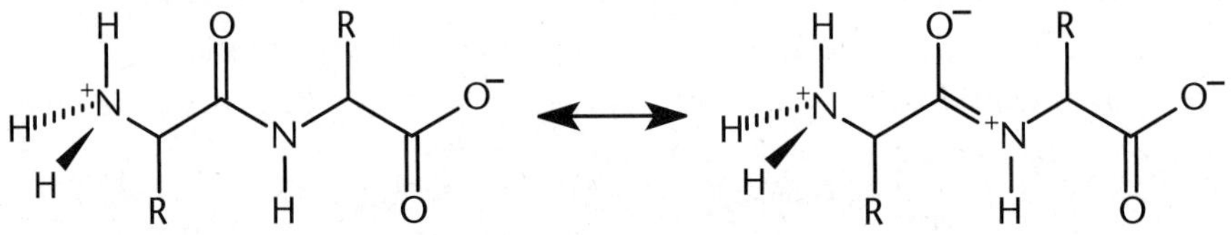

Figure 1.11 Resonance in the Peptide Bond

As a result, rotation of the protein backbone around its C–N amide bonds is restricted, which makes the protein more rigid. Rotation around the remaining bonds in the backbone, however, is not restricted, as those remain single (σ) bonds.

When a peptide bond forms, the free amino end is known as the amino terminus or **N-terminus**, while the free carboxyl end is the carboxy terminus or **C-terminus**. By convention, peptides are drawn with the N-terminus on the left and the C-terminus on the right; similarly, they are read from N-terminus to C-terminus.

Peptide Bond Hydrolysis

MCAT EXPERTISE

You do *not* need to memorize the specific amino acids that hydrolytic enzymes recognize or the exact mechanisms for those reactions. On the other hand, you could certainly encounter a passage describing them.

For enzymes to carry out their function, peptides need to be relatively stable in solution. Therefore, they don't normally fall apart on their own. On the other hand, in order to digest proteins, we need to break them down into their component amino acids. In organic chemistry, amides can be hydrolyzed using acid or base catalysis.

In living organisms, however, hydrolysis is catalyzed by hydrolytic enzymes such as *trypsin* and *chymotrypsin*. Both are specific, in that they only cleave at specific points in the peptide chain: trypsin cleaves at the carboxyl end of arginine and lysine, while chymotrypsin cleaves at the carboxyl end of phenylalanine, tryptophan, and tyrosine. While you don't need to know the exact mechanism of how these enzymes catalyze hydrolysis, you do need to understand the main idea: they break apart the amide bond by adding a hydrogen atom to the amide nitrogen and an OH group to the carbonyl carbon. This is the reverse reaction shown before in Figure 1.10.

MCAT CONCEPT CHECK 1.3

Before you move on, assess your understanding of the material with these questions.

1. What is the difference between an amino acid, a dipeptide, a tripeptide, an oligopeptide, and a polypeptide?

___

2. What molecule is released during formation of a peptide bond?

___

3. If chymotrypsin cleaves at the carboxyl end of phenylalanine, tryptophan, and tyrosine, how many oligopeptides would be formed in enzymatic cleavage of the following molecule with chymotrypsin?

   Val – Phe – Glu – Lys – Tyr – Phe – Trp – Ile – Met – Tyr – Gly – Ala

1.4 Primary and Secondary Protein Structure

High-Yield

LEARNING OBJECTIVES

After Chapter 1.4, you will be able to:

- Describe all four levels of protein structure
- Recognize the unique role of proline in secondary protein structure
- Recall the structural features of α-helices and β-pleated sheets

Proteins are polypeptides that range from just a few amino acids in length up to thousands. They serve many functions in biological systems, functioning as enzymes, hormones, membrane pores and receptors, and elements of cell structure. Proteins are the main actors in cells; the genetic code, after all, is simply a recipe for making thousands of proteins.

Proteins have four levels of structure: **primary** (1°), **secondary** (2°), **tertiary** (3°), and **quaternary** (4°). In this section, we'll examine the first two; we'll discuss tertiary and quaternary structure in the next section.

Primary Structure

The primary structure of a protein is the linear arrangement of amino acids coded in an organism's DNA. It's the sequence of amino acids, listed from the N-terminus, or amino end, to the C-terminus, or carboxyl end. So, for example, the first ten amino acids of the β-chain of hemoglobin are normally valine, histidine, leucine, threonine,

MCAT EXPERTISE

The MCAT will not expect you to memorize the exact primary sequence of any protein!

proline, glutamate, glutamate, lysine, serine, and alanine. Primary structure is stabilized by the formation of covalent peptide bonds between adjacent amino acids.

The primary structure alone encodes all the information needed for folding at all of the higher structural levels; the secondary, tertiary, and quaternary structures a protein adopts are the most energetically favorable arrangements of the primary structure in a given environment. The primary structure of a protein can be determined by a laboratory technique called **sequencing**. This is most easily done using the DNA that coded for that protein, although it can also be done from the protein itself.

Secondary Structure

KEY CONCEPT

The primary structure of a protein is the order of its amino acids. The two main secondary structures are the α-helix and β-pleated sheet, which both result from hydrogen bonding.

A protein's secondary structure is the local structure of neighboring amino acids. Secondary structures are primarily the result of hydrogen bonding between nearby amino acids. The two most common secondary structures are **α-helices** and **β-pleated sheets**. The key to the stability of both structures is the formation of intramolecular hydrogen bonds between different residues.

α-Helices

The α-helix, shown in Figure 1.12, is a rodlike structure in which the peptide chain coils clockwise around a central axis. The helix is stabilized by intramolecular hydrogen bonds between a carbonyl oxygen atom and an amide hydrogen atom four residues down the chain. The side chains of the amino acids in the α-helical conformation point away from the helix core. The α-helix is an important component in the structure of **keratin**, a fibrous structural protein found in human skin, hair, and fingernails.

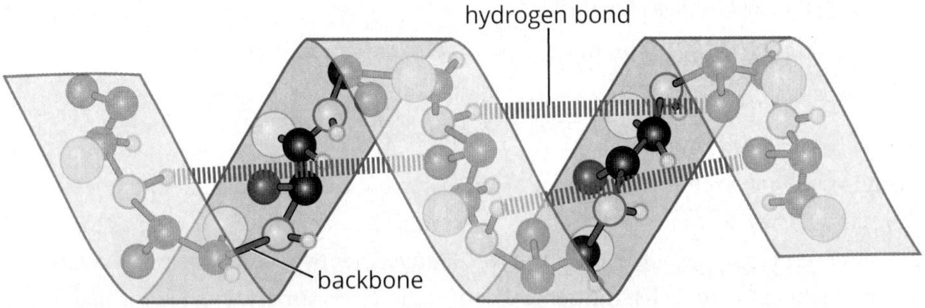

Figure 1.12 Hydrogen Bonding and Spatial Configuration of an α-Helix

β-Pleated Sheets

In β-pleated sheets, which can be parallel or antiparallel, the peptide chains lie alongside one another, forming rows or strands held together by hydrogen bonds between carbonyl oxygen atoms on one chain and amide hydrogen atoms in an adjacent chain, as shown in Figure 1.13. To accommodate as many hydrogen bonds as possible, the β-pleated sheets assume a pleated, or rippled, shape. The R groups of amino residues point above and below the plane of the β-pleated sheet. *Fibroin*, the primary protein component of silk fibers, is composed of β-pleated sheets.

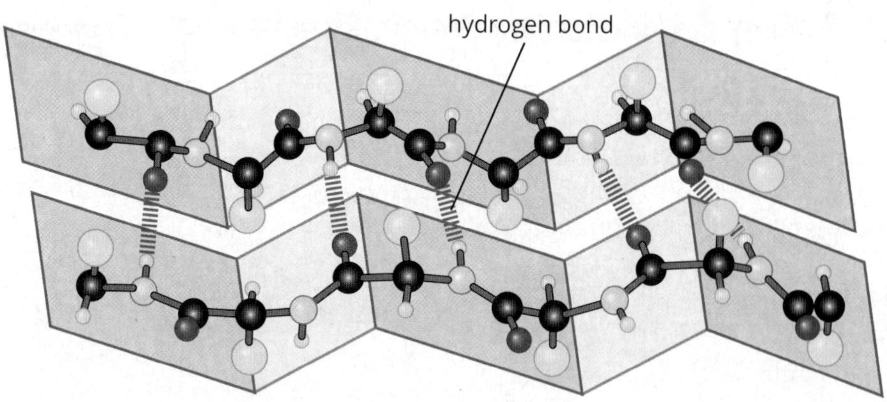

Figure 1.13 Hydrogen Bonding and Spatial Configuration of a β-Pleated Sheet

Secondary Structures and Proline

Because of its rigid cyclic structure, proline will introduce a kink in the peptide chain when it is found in the middle of an α-helix. Proline residues are thus rarely found in α-helices, except in helices that cross the cell membrane. Similarly, it is rarely found in the middle of pleated sheets. On the other hand, proline is often found in the turns between the chains of a β-pleated sheet, and it is often found as the residue at the start of an α-helix.

MCAT CONCEPT CHECK 1.4

Before you move on, assess your understanding of the material with these questions.

1. What are the definitions of primary and secondary structure, and how do they differ in subtypes and the bonds that stabilize them?

Structural Element	Definition	Subtypes	Stabilizing Bonds
Primary structure (1°)			
Secondary structure (2°)			

2. What role does proline serve in secondary structure?

____

3. Describe the key structural features of the following secondary structures.
   - α-helix:

   ____

   - β-pleated sheet:

   ____

1.5 Tertiary and Quaternary Protein Structure

High-Yield

LEARNING OBJECTIVES

After Chapter 1.5, you will be able to:

- Identify the major structural components of tertiary and quaternary protein structure
- Recognize the relationship between protein folding and the solvation layer
- Recall the nomenclature of proteins with prosthetic groups, such as nucleoproteins

Proteins can be broadly divided into **fibrous** proteins, such as **collagen**, that have structures that resemble sheets or long strands, and **globular** proteins, such as **myoglobin**, that tend to be spherical (that is, like a globe). These are caused by tertiary and quaternary protein structures, both of which are the result of protein folding.

Tertiary Structure

KEY CONCEPT

The tertiary structure of a protein is primarily the result of moving hydrophobic amino acid side chains into the interior of the protein.

A protein's tertiary structure is its three-dimensional shape. Tertiary structures are mostly determined by hydrophilic and hydrophobic interactions between R groups of amino acids. Hydrophobic residues prefer to be on the interior of proteins, which reduces their proximity to water. Hydrophilic N–H and C=O bonds found in the polypeptide chain get pulled in by these hydrophobic residues. These hydrophilic bonds can then form electrostatic interactions and hydrogen bonds that further stabilize the protein from the inside. As a result of these hydrophobic interactions, most of the amino acids on the surface of proteins have hydrophilic (polar or charged) R groups; highly hydrophobic R groups, such as phenylalanine, are almost never found on the surface of a protein.

The three-dimensional structure can also be determined by hydrogen bonding, as well as acid–base interactions between amino acids with charged R groups, creating salt bridges. A particularly important component of tertiary structure is the presence of **disulfide bonds**, the bonds that form when two **cysteine** molecules become oxidized to form **cystine**, as shown in Figure 1.14. Disulfide bonds create loops in the protein chain. In addition, disulfide bonds determine how wavy or curly human hair is: the more disulfide bonds, the curlier it is. Note that forming a disulfide bond requires the loss of two protons and two electrons (oxidation).

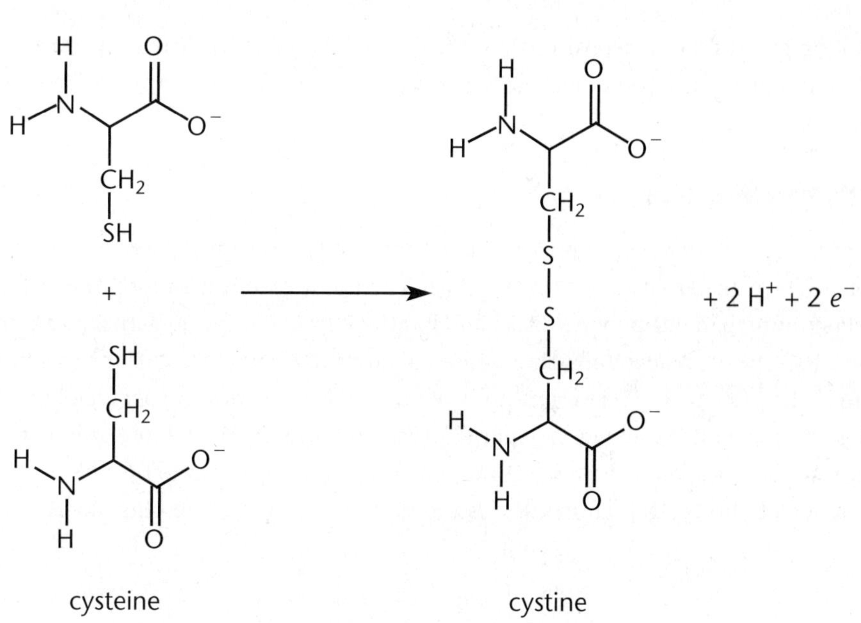

Figure 1.14 Disulfide Bond Formation

The exact details of protein folding are beyond the scope of the MCAT, but the basic idea is that the secondary structures probably form first, and then hydrophobic interactions and hydrogen bonds cause the protein to "collapse" into its proper three-dimensional structure. Along the way, it adopts intermediate states known as **molten globules**. Protein folding is an extremely rapid process: from start to finish, it typically takes much less than a second.

If a protein loses its tertiary structure, a process commonly called **denaturation**, it loses its function.

Folding and the Solvation Layer

Why do hydrophobic residues tend to occupy the interior of a protein, while hydrophilic residues tend to accumulate on the exterior portions? The answer can be summed up in one word: entropy.

Whenever a solute dissolves in a solvent, the nearby solvent molecules form a **solvation layer** around that solute. From an enthalpy standpoint, even hydrocarbons are more stable in aqueous solution than in organic ones ($\Delta H < 0$). However, when a hydrophobic side chain, such as those in phenylalanine and leucine, is placed in aqueous solution, the water molecules in the solvation layer cannot form hydrogen bonds with the side chain. This forces the nearby water molecules to rearrange themselves into specific arrangements to maximize hydrogen bonding—which means a negative change in entropy, ΔS. Remember that negative changes in entropy represent increasing order (decreasing disorder) and thus are unfavorable. This entropy change makes the overall process nonspontaneous ($\Delta G > 0$).

BRIDGE

Make sure you understand the basic thermodynamic properties of enthalpy, entropy, and Gibbs free energy, discussed in Chapter 7 of *MCAT General Chemistry Review*. On Test Day, they can be tested on both natural sciences sections!

On the other hand, putting hydrophilic residues such as serine or lysine on the exterior of the protein allows the nearby water molecules more latitude in their positioning, thus increasing their entropy ($\Delta S > 0$), and making the overall solvation process spontaneous. Thus, by moving hydrophobic residues away from water molecules and hydrophilic residues toward water molecules, a protein achieves maximum stability.

Quaternary Structure

All proteins have elements of primary, secondary, and tertiary structure; not all proteins have quaternary structure. Quaternary structures only exist for proteins that contain more than one polypeptide chain. For these proteins, the quaternary structure is an aggregate of smaller globular peptides, or **subunits**, and represents the functional form of the protein. The classic examples of quaternary structure are hemoglobin and immunoglobulins, shown in Figures 1.15a and 1.15b. Hemoglobin consists of four distinct subunits, each of which can bind one molecule of oxygen. Similarly, immunoglobulin G (IgG) antibodies also contain a total of four subunits each.

MNEMONIC

The primary structure of a protein acts like letters. The secondary structure acts like words: only certain orderings of letters make sense (CAT is a word, while CAQ is not). The tertiary structure acts like sentences: words combine to form a functioning whole. The quaternary structure acts like paragraphs: they're not always present, but subunits can combine to make a cohesive whole.

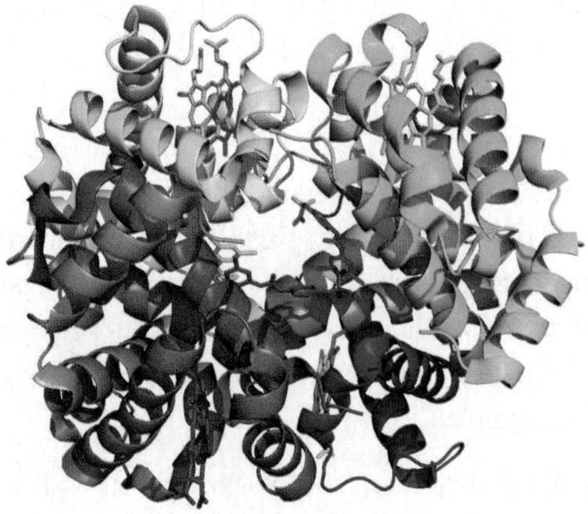

Figure 1.15a Hemoglobin
Heme molecules are visible in each chain.

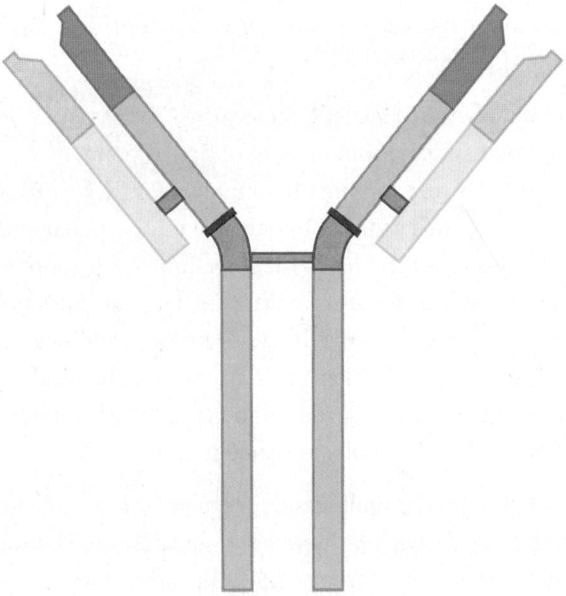

Figure 1.15b Immunoglobulin G

The formation of quaternary structures can serve several roles. First, they can be more stable, by further reducing the surface area of the protein complex. Second, they can reduce the amount of DNA needed to encode the protein complex. Third, they can bring catalytic sites close together, allowing intermediates from one reaction to be directly shuttled to a second reaction. Finally, and most important, they can induce **cooperativity**, or **allosteric effects**. We'll discuss this much further in the next chapter (especially for hemoglobin), but the basic idea is that one subunit can undergo conformational or structural changes, which either enhance or reduce the activity of the other subunits.

BRIDGE

The reduction of genetic material is crucial for viruses. The genome for most viruses is tiny. Thus, their viral coats typically consist of one small protein repeated dozens or even hundreds of times. Viral structure is discussed in Chapter 1 of *MCAT Biology Review*.

Conjugated Proteins

Conjugated proteins derive part of their function from covalently attached molecules called **prosthetic groups**. These prosthetic groups can be organic molecules, such as vitamins, or even metal ions, such as iron. Proteins with lipid, carbohydrate, and nucleic acid prosthetic groups are referred to as **lipoproteins**, **glycoproteins**, and **nucleoproteins**, respectively. These prosthetic groups have major roles in determining the function of their respective proteins. For example, each of hemoglobin's subunits (as well as myoglobin) contains a prosthetic group called **heme**. The heme group, which contains an iron atom in its core, binds to and carries oxygen; as such, hemoglobin is inactive without the heme group. These groups can also direct the protein to be delivered to a certain location, such as the cell membrane, nucleus, lysosome, or endoplasmic reticulum.

BIOCHEMISTRY GUIDED EXAMPLE WITH EXPERT THINKING

Ricin is a highly toxic ribosome-inactivating protein (RIP) that can be obtained easily from the widely available castor bean, *Ricinus communis*, making it a potential bioterrorist and biowarfare agent. There is no known antidote, but toxoid and recombinant vaccines have been shown to be effective in raising protective immunity and preventing the lethal effects of ricin.

This is just background info on ricin and vaccines

Currently, variants of ricin that do not bind to ribosomes exist, and show promising results as a human immunogen in Phase 1 clinical trials. However, the vaccines suffer from instability and aggregation, and can still cause serious effects like vascular leak syndrome (VLS). Based on previous X-ray crystal structures of RTA1-33/44-198 (an inactive variant), introduction of a disulfide bond stabilizes a disordered loop. However, it is unclear whether the mutations made to introduce the disulfide bond improve overall protein stability and how the mutant proteins interact with VLS receptors in animal models.

Problem statement: issue with current vaccines

Possible solution: introduce disulfide bonds, which may help with stability

A series of RTA1-33/44-198 mutants were created and purified. The number of free cysteines were assayed using Ellman's reagent, which reacts with free sulfhydryl groups to yield a colored product. The melting temperature (apparent T_m) of each purified protein was determined using circular dichroism measurements. Finally, each construct was assayed for its ability to induce VLS in animal models. The results are detailed in Table 1 below.

Measured: free cysteines (via assay), melting temperature, and ability to induce VLS

RTA1-33/44-198 types	Number of free Cys	Apparent T_m (°C)	Disruption of VLS?
wild-type	0.97 ± 0.03	57.9 ± 0.03	No
R48C/T77C	1.00 ± 0.08	62.9 ± 0.22	No
V49C/E99C	0.96 ± 0.05	62.9 ± 0.21	No
R48C/T77C/D75N	1.04 ± 0.02	63.2 ± 0.26	Yes
V49C/E99C/V76I	0.99 ± 0.03	62.6 ± 0.21	Yes
V49C/E99C/D75N	1.10 ± 0.06	62.2 ± 0.13	Yes
R48C/T77C/V76I	1.89 ± 0.03	59.3 ± 0.60	Yes

Table 1

Look for trends and outliers! The last construct has a different number of free Cys and a T_m similar to WT; the bottom four constructs disrupt VLS

Adapted from Janosi, L., Compton, J. R., Legler, P. M., Steele, K. E., Davis, J. M., Matyas, G. R., & Millard, C. B. (2013). Disruption of the putative vascular leak peptide sequence in the stabilized ricin vaccine candidate RTA1-33/44-198. *Toxins*, 5(2), 224-48. doi:10.3390/toxins5020224.

Is R48C/T77C/V76I a suitable candidate for further testing? Why or why not?

This question is asking us to interpret the study results, but we'll want to start with the purpose of the study to be able to go through the data efficiently. The goal is to develop a vaccine for ricin poisoning. The second paragraph starts with what has already been done, which is the creation of a possible working vaccine. Since it's based on the ricin protein, we can use our background knowledge and critical reasoning to assume that the vaccine is similar enough to the ricin protein to elicit a proper immune response, but does not inhibit ribosome function. Notice the keyword "however" in the second paragraph—this indicates that there is still a problem. In this case, the current vaccine is not stable, which would presumably affect its efficacy. Also, the vaccine seems to have a serious side effect (VLS), which is something the researchers want to eliminate. We're given a hint about a possible solution to the stability issue—creating a disulfide bond. This means that the disulfide is not native to the protein, but created by mutating select amino acids to cysteines.

Following that possible solution in paragraph 2, the researchers generated a series of protein mutations, which are outlined in the first column of Table 1. Notice the notation: letter-number-letter. We know from the passage that these are mutants and, in looking at this code, we can infer that the first letter is the original amino acid, the number is its position in the sequence, and the second letter is the mutated amino acid. This style of notation is common in scientific papers, so we'll likely want to keep this in mind even on Test Day as a possibility when we see similar notation. For instance, R48C is arginine at position 48 mutated to cysteine. Notice that in each mutation, there is a pair of amino acids mutated to cysteine to create the opportunity for a disulfide bond. The second column tells us about the success of creating a disulfide bond. Since the wild-type protein has one free cysteine, and the mutants introduce two more cysteines for the purpose of a creating a disulfide bond, a successful disulfide bond formation will eliminate two sulfhydryls, leaving the original free cysteine. R48C/T77C/V76I has approximately two (1.89 ± 0.03) free cysteines, suggesting an incomplete formation of the disulfide bond. The third column determines the effect of the disulfide bond formation on stability. Melting temperature (T_m) is a great indication for stability—the higher the temperature, the more energy it takes to break all bonds to unfold the protein. Both wild-type and R48C/T77C/V76I have markedly lower T_m compared to the other constructs, which we can conclude means they have reduced stability. Finally, the last column provides information about whether the construct induced VLS. We can see that R48C/T77C/V76I did not induce VLS, making it 'safer' from the perspective of risk for this dangerous syndrome.

Given the data from the passage, while R48C/T77C/V76I does address the issue of not inducing VLS in animal models, the construct is not stable, and therefore would not be suitable for additional testing.

MCAT CONCEPT CHECK 1.5

Before you move on, assess your understanding of the material with these questions.

1. What are the definitions of tertiary and quaternary structure, and how do they differ in subtypes and the bonds that stabilize them?

Structural Element	Definition	Subtypes	Stabilizing Bonds
Tertiary structure (3°)			
Quaternary structure (4°)			

2. What is the primary motivation for hydrophobic residues in a polypeptide to move to the interior of the protein?

____

3. List three different prosthetic groups that can be attached to a protein and name the conjugated protein.

____

1.6 Denaturation

LEARNING OBJECTIVE

After Chapter 1.6, you will be able to:

- Predict the impact of denaturation via heat or solute

BRIDGE

Heat denatures proteins for the same reason that raising a reaction's temperature increases its rate: increased average kinetic energy of molecules means increased molecular motion. The relationship between temperature and kinetic energy is discussed in Chapter 7 of *MCAT General Chemistry Review*.

In the previous section, we discussed protein folding. The reverse of this process is **denaturation**, in which a protein loses its three-dimensional structure. Although it is sometimes reversible, denaturation is often irreversible; whether its denaturation is reversible or not, unfolded proteins cannot catalyze reactions. The two main causes of denaturation are heat and solutes.

As with all molecules, when the temperature of a protein increases, its average kinetic energy increases. When the temperature gets high enough, this extra energy can be enough to overcome the hydrophobic interactions that hold a protein together, causing the protein to unfold. This is what happens when egg whites are cooked: in the uncooked egg whites, albumin is folded, which makes it transparent; cooking them causes the albumin molecules to denature and aggregate, forming a solid, rubbery white mass that will not revert to its transparent form.

On the other hand, solutes such as urea denature proteins by directly interfering with the forces that hold the protein together. They can disrupt tertiary and quaternary structures by breaking disulfide bridges, reducing cystine back to two cysteine residues. They can even overcome the hydrogen bonds and other side chain interactions that hold α-helices and β-pleated sheets intact. Similarly, detergents such as SDS (sodium dodecyl sulfate, also called sodium lauryl sulfate) can solubilize proteins, disrupting noncovalent bonds and promoting denaturation.

KEY CONCEPT

Denatured proteins lose their three-dimensional structure and are thus inactive.

MCAT CONCEPT CHECK 1.6

Before you move on, assess your understanding of the material with this question.

1. Why are proteins denatured by heat and solutes, respectively?
   - Heat:

   ___

   - Solutes:

   ___

Conclusion

Nearly every part of a cell involves proteins in some way, from the nucleus to the mitochondria to the cell membrane. The MCAT will test your understanding of key concepts regarding amino acids because the amino acids that compose a protein determine its structure. In the next chapter, we'll discuss the best-known function of proteins: their role as enzymes.

GO ONLINE

You've reviewed the content, now test your knowledge and critical thinking skills by completing a test-like passage set in your online resources!

CONCEPT SUMMARY

Amino Acids Found in Proteins

- **Amino acids** have four groups attached to a central (α) carbon: an amino group, a carboxylic acid group, a hydrogen atom, and an **R group**.
  - The R group determines chemistry and function of that amino acid.
  - Twenty amino acids appear in the proteins of eukaryotic organisms.
- The stereochemistry of the α-carbon is L for all chiral amino acids in eukaryotes.
  - D-amino acids can exist in prokaryotes.
  - All chiral amino acids except **cysteine** have an (*S*) configuration.
  - All amino acids are chiral except **glycine**, which has a hydrogen atom as its R group.
- Side chains can be polar or nonpolar, aromatic or nonaromatic, charged or uncharged.
  - **Nonpolar, nonaromatic:** glycine, alanine, valine, leucine, isoleucine, methionine, proline
  - **Aromatic:** tryptophan, phenylalanine, tyrosine
  - **Polar:** serine, threonine, asparagine, glutamine, cysteine
  - **Negatively charged (acidic):** aspartate, glutamate
  - **Positively charged (basic):** lysine, arginine, histidine
- Amino acids with long alkyl chains are hydrophobic, and those with charges are hydrophilic; many others fall somewhere in between.

Acid-Base Chemistry of Amino Acids

- Amino acids are **amphoteric**; that is, they can accept or donate protons.
- The **pK_a** of a group is the pH at which half of the species are deprotonated; $[HA] = [A^-]$.
- Amino acids exist in different forms at different pH values.
  - At low (acidic) pH, the amino acid is fully protonated.
  - At pH near the pI of the amino acid, the amino acid is a neutral **zwitterion**.
  - At high (alkaline) pH, the amino acid is fully deprotonated.
- The **isoelectric point (pI)** of an amino acid without a charged side chain can be calculated by averaging the two pK_a values.
- Amino acids can be titrated.
  - The titration curve is nearly flat at the pK_a values of the amino acid.
  - The titration curve is nearly vertical at the pI of the amino acid.

- Amino acids with charged side chains have an additional pK_a value, and their pI is calculated by averaging the two pK_a values that correspond to protonation and deprotonation of the zwitterion.
  - Amino acids without charged side chains have a pI around 6.
  - Acidic amino acids have a pI well below 6.
  - Basic amino acids have a pI well above 6.

Peptide Bond Formation and Hydrolysis

- Dipeptides have two amino acid residues; tripeptides have three. Oligopeptides have a "few" amino acid residues (<20); polypeptides have "many" (>20).
- Forming a peptide bond is a **condensation** or **dehydration** reaction (releasing one molecule of water).
  - The nucleophilic amino group of one amino acid attacks the electrophilic carbonyl group of another amino acid.
  - Amide bonds are rigid because of resonance.
- Breaking a peptide bond is a **hydrolysis** reaction.

Primary and Secondary Protein Structure

- **Primary structure** is the linear sequence of amino acids in a peptide and is stabilized by peptide bonds.
- **Secondary structure** is the local structure of neighboring amino acids, and is stabilized by hydrogen bonding between amino groups and nonadjacent carboxyl groups.
  - α-**helices** are clockwise coils around a central axis.
  - β-**pleated sheets** are rippled strands that can be parallel or antiparallel.
  - **Proline** can interrupt secondary structure because of its rigid cyclic structure.

Tertiary and Quaternary Protein Structure

- **Tertiary structure** is the three-dimensional shape of a single polypeptide chain, and is stabilized by hydrophobic interactions, acid–base interactions (salt bridges), hydrogen bonding, and disulfide bonds.
  - **Hydrophobic interactions** push hydrophobic R groups to the interior of a protein, which increases entropy of the surrounding water molecules and creates a negative Gibbs free energy.
  - **Disulfide bonds** occur when two **cysteine** molecules are oxidized and create a covalent bond to form **cystine**.
- **Quaternary structure** is the interaction between peptides in proteins that contain multiple subunits.
- Proteins with covalently attached molecules are termed **conjugated proteins**. The attached molecule is a **prosthetic group**, and may be a metal ion, vitamin, lipid, carbohydrate, or nucleic acid.

Denaturation

- Both heat and increasing solute concentration can lead to loss of three-dimensional protein structure, which is termed **denaturation**.

ANSWERS TO CONCEPT CHECKS

1.1

1. The four groups are an amino group ($-NH_2$), a carboxylic acid group ($-COOH$), a hydrogen atom, and an R group.
2. All chiral eukaryotic amino acids are L. All chiral eukaryotic amino acids are (*S*), with the exception of cysteine (because cysteine is the only amino acid with an R group that has a higher priority than a carboxylic acid according to Cahn–Ingold–Prelog rules).
3. Nonpolar, nonaromatic: glycine, alanine, valine, leucine, isoleucine, methionine, proline

   Aromatic: tryptophan, phenylalanine, tyrosine

   Polar: serine, threonine, asparagine, glutamine, cysteine

   Negatively charged/acidic: aspartate, glutamate

   Positively charged/basic: lysine, arginine, histidine
4. Hydrophobic amino acids tend to reside in the interior of a protein, away from water. Hydrophilic amino acids tend to remain on the surface of the protein, in contact with water.
5. From left to right the amino acids are methionine (M), cysteine (C), alanine (A), and threonine (T): MCAT.

1.2

1. pH = 1: $^{+}NH_3CRHCOOH$; pH = 7: $^{+}NH_3CRHCOO^-$; pH = 11: $NH_2CRHCOO^-$
2. Aspartic acid: $pI = (1.88 + 3.65) \div 2 = 2.77$

   Arginine: $pI = (9.04 + 12.48) \div 2 = 10.76$

   Valine: $pI = (2.32 + 9.62) \div 2 = 5.97$

1.3

1. These species differ by the number of amino acids that make them up: amino acid = 1, dipeptide = 2, tripeptide = 3, oligopeptide = "few" (< 20), polypeptide = "many" (> 20)
2. Water (H_2O)
3. 4: Val – Phe; Glu – Lys – Tyr; Ile – Met – Tyr; Gly–Ala. A single amino acid on its own is not considered an oligopeptide.

1.4

1.

Structural Element	Definition	Subtypes	Stabilizing Bonds
Primary structure (1°)	Linear sequence of amino acids in chain	(none)	Peptide (amide) bond
Secondary structure (2°)	Local structure determined by nearby amino acids	• α-helix • β-pleated sheet	Hydrogen bonds

2. Proline's rigid structure causes it to introduce kinks in α-helices or create turns in β-pleated sheets.
3. The α-helix is a rod-like structure in which the peptide chain coils clockwise around a central axis. In β-pleated sheets the peptide chains lie alongside one another, forming rows or strands held together by intramolecular hydrogen bonds between carbonyl oxygen atoms on one chain and amide hydrogen atoms in an adjacent chain.

1.5

1.

Structural Element	Definition	Subtypes	Stabilizing Bonds
Tertiary structure (3°)	Three-dimensional shape of protein	• Hydrophobic interactions • Acid–base/salt bridges • Disulfide links	• van der Waals forces • Hydrogen bonds • Ionic bonds • Covalent bonds
Quaternary structure (4°)	Interaction between separate subunits of a multisubunit protein	(none)	Same as tertiary structure

2. Moving hydrophobic residues to the interior of a protein increases entropy by allowing water molecules on the surface of the protein to have more possible positions and configurations. This positive ΔS makes $\Delta G < 0$, stabilizing the protein.
3. Examples of common prosthetic groups include lipids, carbohydrates, and nucleic acids; they are known as lipoproteins, glycoproteins, and nucleoproteins, respectively.

1.6

1. Heat denatures proteins by increasing their average kinetic energy, thus disrupting hydrophobic interactions. Solutes denature proteins by disrupting elements of secondary, tertiary, and quaternary structure.

SCIENCE MASTERY ASSESSMENT EXPLANATIONS

1. **B**

Most amino acids (except the acidic and basic amino acids) have two sites for protonation: the carboxylic acid and the amine. At neutral pH, the carboxylic acid will be deprotonated ($-COO^-$) and the amine will remain protonated ($-NH_3^+$). This dipolar ion is a zwitterion, so **(B)** is the correct answer.

2. **B**

Glutamic acid is an acidic amino acid because it has an extra carboxyl group. At neutral pH, both carboxyl groups are deprotonated and thus negatively charged. The amino group has a positive charge because it remains protonated at pH 7. Overall, therefore, glutamic acid has a net charge of -1, and **(B)** is correct. Notice that you do not even need to know the pI values to solve this question; as an acidic amino acid, glutamic acid must have a pI below 7.

3. **C**

Nonpolar groups are not capable of forming dipoles or hydrogen bonds; this makes them hydrophobic. Burying hydrophobic R groups inside proteins means they don't have to interact with water, which is polar. This makes **(C)** correct. **(A)** and **(B)** are incorrect because nonpolar molecules are hydrophobic, not hydrophilic; **(D)** is incorrect because they are not generally found on protein surfaces.

4. **A**

The cDNA sequence is a DNA copy of the mRNA used to generate a protein. A computer program can quickly identify the amino acid that corresponds to each codon and generate a list of these amino acids. This amino acid sequence is the primary structure of the protein. These observations support **(A)** as the correct answer. By contrast, the secondary, tertiary, and quaternary structures involve higher level interactions between the backbone and R groups and are increasingly difficult to predict.

5. **C**

There are three choices for the first amino acid, leaving two choices for the second, and one choice for the third. Multiplying those numbers gives us a total of $3 \times 2 \times 1 = 6$ distinct tripeptides. (Using the one-letter codes for valine (V), alanine (A), and leucine (L), those six tripeptides are VAL, VLA, ALV, AVL, LVA, and LAV.)

6. **B**

As the protein folds, it takes on an organized structure and thus its entropy decreases. However, the opposite trend is true for the water surrounding the protein. Prior to protein folding, hydrophobic amino acid residues are exposed and the water molecules must form structured hydration shells around these hydrophobic residues. During folding, these hydrophobic residues are generally buried in the interior of the protein so that the surrounding water molecules gain more latitude in their interactions. Thus, the entropy of the surrounding water increases, making the correct answer **(B)**.

7. **C**

The α-helix is held together primarily by hydrogen bonds between the carboxyl groups and amino groups of amino acids. Disulfide bridges, **(A)**, and hydrophobic effects, **(B)**, are primarily involved in tertiary structures, not secondary. Even if they were charged, the side chains of amino acids are too far apart to participate in strong interactions in secondary structure.

8. **C**

High salt concentrations and detergents can denature a protein, as can high temperatures. But moving a protein to a hypotonic environment—that is, a lower solute concentration—should not lead to denaturation.

9. **C**

An amino acid likely to be found in a transmembrane portion of an α-helix will be exposed to a hydrophobic environment, so we need an amino acid with a hydrophobic side chain. The only choice that has a hydrophobic side chain is **(C)**, phenylalanine. The other choices are all polar or charged.

10. **C**

Every amino acid except glycine has a chiral α-carbon, but only two of the 20 amino acids—threonine and isoleucine—also have a chiral carbon in their side chains as well. Thus, the correct answer is **(C)**. Just as only one configuration is normally seen at the α carbon, only one configuration is seen in the side chain chiral carbon.

11. **B**

In their inactive state, the receptor tyrosine kinases are fully folded single polypeptide chains and thus have tertiary structure. When these monomers dimerize, they become a protein complex and thus have elements of quaternary structure. This change from tertiary to quaternary structure justifies **(B)**.

12. **A**

Histidine has an ionizable side chain: its imidazole ring has a nitrogen atom that can be protonated. None of the remaining answers have ionizable atoms in their side chains.

13. **D**

Because lysine has a basic side chain, we ignore the pK_a of the carboxyl group, and average the pK_a of the side chain and the amino group; the average of 9 and 10.5 is 9.75, which is closest to **(D)**.

14. **D**

Conjugated proteins can have lipid or carbohydrate "tags" added to them. These tags can indicate that these proteins should be directed to the cell membrane (especially lipid tags) or to specific organelles (such as the lysosome). They can also provide the activity of the protein; for example, the heme group in hemoglobin is needed for it to bind oxygen. Thus, **(D)** is the correct answer.

15. **B**

Because collagen has a triple helix, the carbon backbones are very close together. Thus, steric hindrance is a potential problem. To reduce that hindrance, we need small side chains; glycine has the smallest side chain of all: a hydrogen atom.

Consult your online resources for additional practice. **GO ONLINE**

EQUATIONS TO REMEMBER

(1.1) **Isoelectric point of a neutral amino acid:**

$$\mathrm{pI}_{\text{neutral amino acid}} = \frac{\mathrm{p}K_{\mathrm{a,NH_3^+\ group}} + \mathrm{p}K_{\mathrm{a,COOH\ group}}}{2}$$

(1.2) **Isoelectric point of an acidic amino acid:**

$$\mathrm{pI}_{\text{acidic amino acid}} = \frac{\mathrm{p}K_{\mathrm{a,R\ group}} + \mathrm{p}K_{\mathrm{a,COOH\ group}}}{2}$$

(1.3) **Isoelectric point of a basic amino acid:**

$$\mathrm{pI}_{\text{basic amino acid}} = \frac{\mathrm{p}K_{\mathrm{a,NH_3^+\ group}} + \mathrm{p}K_{\mathrm{a,R\ group}}}{2}$$

SHARED CONCEPTS

Biochemistry Chapter 2
Enzymes

Biochemistry Chapter 3
Nonenzymatic Protein Function and Protein Analysis

Biochemistry Chapter 7
RNA and the Genetic Code

Biology Chapter 1
The Cell

Biology Chapter 9
The Digestive System

General Chemistry Chapter 7
Thermochemistry

Organic Chemistry Chapter 8
Carboxylic Acids

Organic Chemistry Chapter 9
Carboxylic Acid Derivatives

CHAPTER 2

ENZYMES

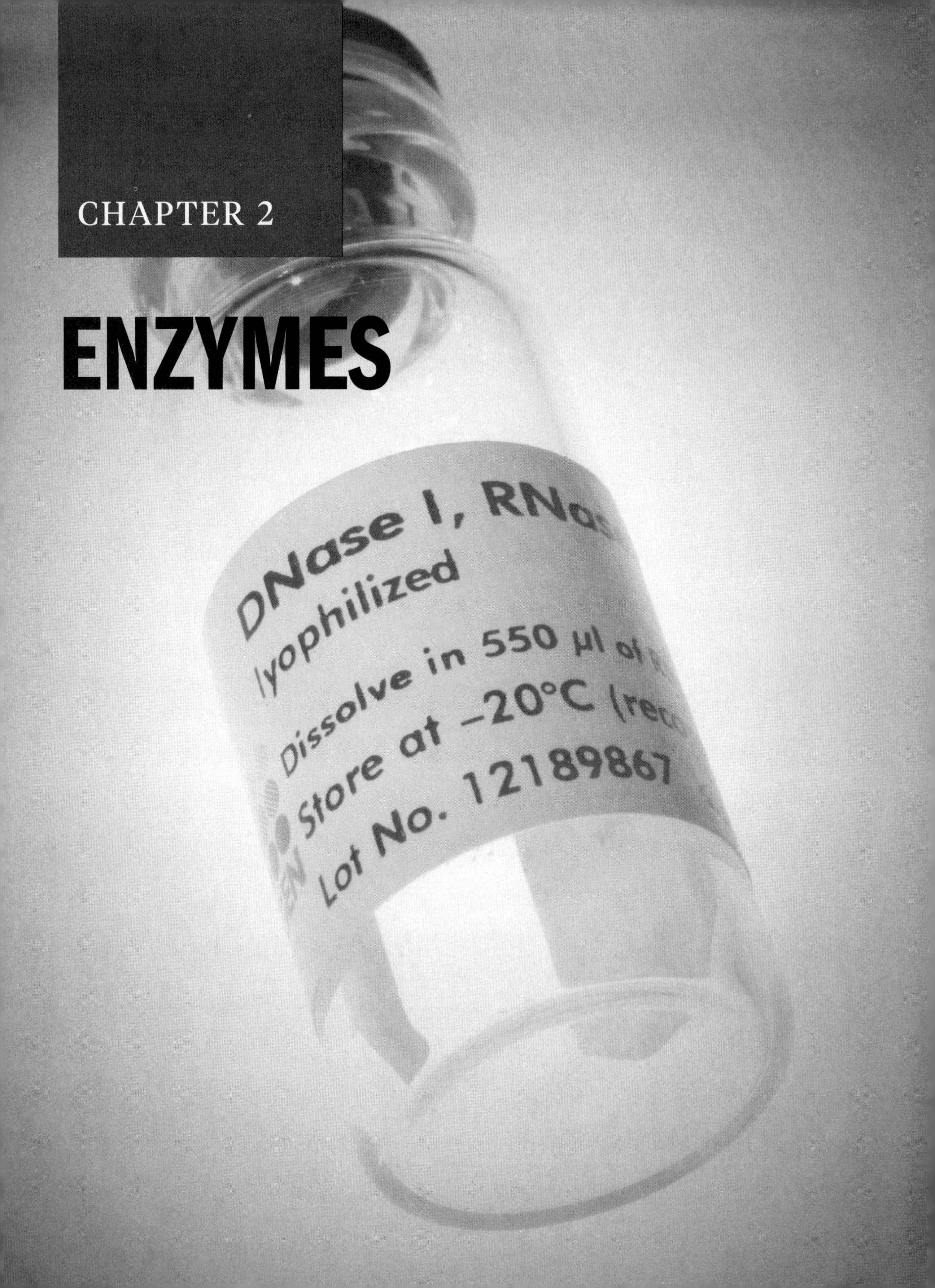

SCIENCE MASTERY ASSESSMENT

Every pre-med knows this feeling: there is so much content I have to know for the MCAT! How do I know what to do first or what's important?

While the high-yield badges throughout this book will help you identify the most important topics, this Science Mastery Assessment is another tool in your MCAT prep arsenal. This quiz (which can also be taken in your online resources) and the guidance below will help ensure that you are spending the appropriate amount of time on this chapter based on your personal strengths and weaknesses. Don't worry though—skipping something now does not mean you'll never study it. Later on in your prep, as you complete full-length tests, you'll uncover specific pieces of content that you need to review and can come back to these chapters as appropriate.

How to Use This Assessment

If you answer 0–7 questions correctly:

Spend about 1 hour to read this chapter in full and take limited notes throughout. Follow up by reviewing **all** quiz questions to ensure that you now understand how to solve each one.

If you answer 8–11 questions correctly:

Spend 20–40 minutes reviewing the quiz questions. Beginning with the questions you missed, read and take notes on the corresponding subchapters. For questions you answered correctly, ensure your thinking matches that of the explanation and you understand why each choice was correct or incorrect.

If you answer 12–15 questions correctly:

Spend less than 20 minutes reviewing all questions from the quiz. If you missed any, then include a quick read-through of the corresponding subchapters, or even just the relevant content within a subchapter, as part of your question review. For questions you got correct, ensure your thinking matches that of the explanation and review the Concept Summary at the end of the chapter.

1. Consider a biochemical reaction A → B, which is catalyzed by *A–B dehydrogenase*. Which of the following statements is true?
   - **A.** The reaction will proceed until the enzyme concentration decreases.
   - **B.** The reaction will be most favorable at 0°C.
   - **C.** A component of the enzyme is transferred from A to B.
   - **D.** The free energy change (ΔG) of the catalyzed reaction is the same as for the uncatalyzed reaction.

2. Which of the following statements about enzyme kinetics is FALSE?
   - **A.** An increase in the substrate concentration (at constant enzyme concentration) leads to proportional increases in the rate of the reaction.
   - **B.** Most enzymes operating in the human body work best at a temperature of 37°C.
   - **C.** An enzyme–substrate complex can either form a product or dissociate back into the enzyme and substrate.
   - **D.** Maximal activity of many human enzymes occurs around pH 7.4.

3. Some enzymes require the presence of a nonprotein molecule to behave catalytically. An enzyme devoid of this molecule is called a(n):
   - **A.** holoenzyme.
   - **B.** apoenzyme.
   - **C.** coenzyme.
   - **D.** zymoenzyme.

4. Which of the following factors determine an enzyme's specificity?
   - **A.** The three-dimensional shape of the active site
   - **B.** The Michaelis constant
   - **C.** The type of cofactor required for the enzyme to be active
   - **D.** The prosthetic group on the enzyme

5. Human DNA polymerase is removed from the freezer and placed in a 60°C water bath. Which of the following best describes the change in enzyme activity as the polymerase sample comes to thermal equilibrium with the water bath?
   - **A.** Increases then decreases
   - **B.** Decreases then plateaus
   - **C.** Increases then plateaus
   - **D.** Decreases then increases

6. In the equation below, substrate C is an allosteric inhibitor to enzyme 1. Which of the following is another mechanism necessarily caused by substrate C?

$$\mathrm{A} \xrightarrow[\text{enzyme 1}]{} \mathrm{B} \xrightarrow[\text{enzyme 2}]{} \mathrm{C}$$

   - **A.** Competitive inhibition
   - **B.** Irreversible inhibition
   - **C.** Feedback enhancement
   - **D.** Negative feedback

7. The activity of an enzyme is measured at several different substrate concentrations, and the data are shown in the table below.

[S] (m*M*)	$V\left(\frac{\text{mmol}}{\text{sec}}\right)$
0.01	1
0.05	9.1
0.1	17
0.5	50
1	67
5	91
10	95
50	99
100	100

K_m for this enzyme is approximately:
   - **A.** 0.5
   - **B.** 1.0
   - **C.** 10.0
   - **D.** 50.0

Questions 8 and 9 refer to the following statement:

Consider a reaction catalyzed by enzyme A with a K_m value of 5×10^{-6} M and v_{max} of $20 \frac{\text{mmol}}{\text{min}}$.

8. At a concentration of 5×10^{-6} M substrate, the rate of the reaction will be:
   - **A.** $10 \frac{\text{mmol}}{\text{min}}$.
   - **B.** $20 \frac{\text{mmol}}{\text{min}}$.
   - **C.** $30 \frac{\text{mmol}}{\text{min}}$.
   - **D.** $40 \frac{\text{mmol}}{\text{min}}$.

9. At a concentration of 5×10^{-4} M substrate, the rate of the reaction will be:
   - **A.** $10 \frac{\text{mmol}}{\text{min}}$.
   - **B.** $15 \frac{\text{mmol}}{\text{min}}$.
   - **C.** $20 \frac{\text{mmol}}{\text{min}}$.
   - **D.** $30 \frac{\text{mmol}}{\text{min}}$.

10. The graph below shows kinetic data obtained for flu virus enzyme activity as a function of substrate concentration in the presence and absence of two antiviral drugs.

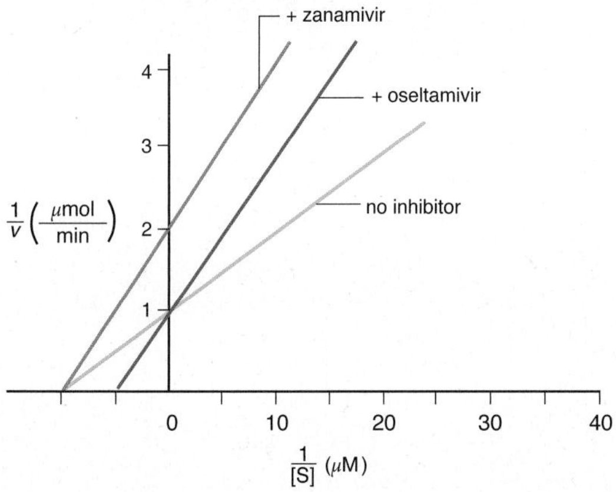

Based on the graph, which of the following statements is correct?
   - **A.** Both drugs are noncompetitive inhibitors of the viral enzyme.
   - **B.** Oseltamivir increases the K_m value for the substrate compared to Relenza.
   - **C.** Zanamivir increases the v_{max} value for the substrate compared to Tamiflu.
   - **D.** Both drugs are competitive inhibitors of the viral enzyme.

11. The conversion of ATP to cyclic AMP and inorganic phosphate is most likely catalyzed by which class of enzyme?
   - **A.** Ligase
   - **B.** Hydrolase
   - **C.** Lyase
   - **D.** Transferase

12. Which of the following is NOT a method by which enzymes decrease the activation energy for biological reactions?
   - **A.** Modifying the local charge environment
   - **B.** Forming transient covalent bonds
   - **C.** Acting as electron donors or receptors
   - **D.** Breaking bonds in the enzyme irreversibly to provide energy

13. A certain enzyme that displays positive cooperativity has four subunits, two of which are bound to substrate. Which of the following statements must be true?
   - **A.** The affinity of the enzyme for the substrate has just increased.
   - **B.** The affinity of the enzyme for the substrate has just decreased.
   - **C.** The affinity of the enzyme for the substrate is half of what it would be if four sites had substrate bound.
   - **D.** The affinity of the enzyme for the substrate is greater than with one substrate bound.

14. Which of the following is LEAST likely to be required for a series of metabolic reactions?
   - **A.** Triacylglycerol acting as a coenzyme
   - **B.** Oxidoreductase enzymes
   - **C.** Magnesium acting as a cofactor
   - **D.** Transferase enzymes

15. How does the ideal temperature for a reaction change with and without an enzyme catalyst?
   - **A.** The ideal temperature is generally higher with a catalyst than without.
   - **B.** The ideal temperature is generally lower with a catalyst than without.
   - **C.** The ideal temperature is characteristic of the reaction, not the enzyme.
   - **D.** No conclusion can be made without knowing the enzyme type.

Answer Key

1. **D**
2. **A**
3. **B**
4. **A**
5. **A**
6. **D**
7. **A**
8. **A**
9. **C**
10. **B**
11. **C**
12. **D**
13. **D**
14. **A**
15. **B**

Detailed explanations can be found at the end of the chapter.

CHAPTER 2

ENZYMES

In This Chapter

CHAPTER PROFILE

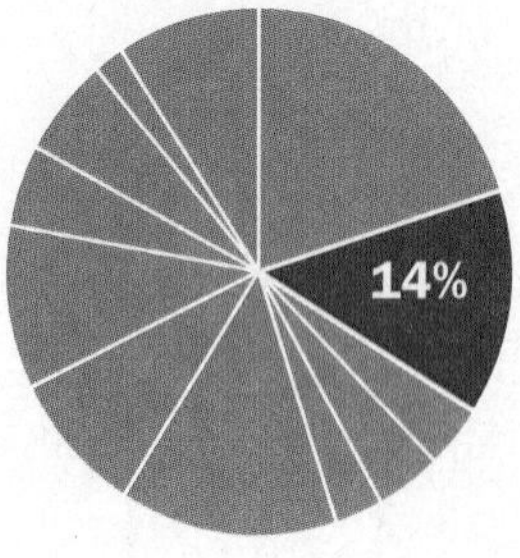

The content in this chapter should be relevant to about 14% of all questions about biochemistry on the MCAT.

This chapter covers material from the following AAMC content categories:

1A: Structure and function of proteins and their constituent amino acids

5E: Principles of chemical thermodynamics and kinetics

Introduction

Obesity is increasingly common in the United States and is paralleled by an increase in high blood pressure, or hypertension. This is extremely relevant to medical students because hypertension increases the risk of stroke, heart failure, and kidney failure.

Each year, physicians encourage millions of Americans to improve their diets, add exercise to their daily regimens, or even take prescription drugs to control their hypertension. Many of these anti-hypertensive medications are called ACE (*angiotensin-converting enzyme*) inhibitors. In healthy patients, ACE catalyzes a reaction that converts a peptide called angiotensin I to angiotensin II. The angiotensin II peptide then not only directly causes constriction of the blood vessels to raise blood pressure, but also stimulates the release of the hormone aldosterone, which activates the kidneys to reabsorb more water back into the bloodstream. The increase in blood volume also increases blood pressure. Physicians take advantage of this complicated pathway with a straightforward solution: stop the pathway early by inhibiting ACE and blood pressure will decrease.

Enzymes are crucial proteins that dramatically increase the rate of biological reactions. They're used to regulate homeostatic mechanisms in every organ system and are highly regulated themselves by environmental conditions, activators, and inhibitors. These regulators may be naturally occurring or may be given as a drug, such as the ACE inhibitors used to treat hypertension. Some enzymes are kept in an inactivated form called a zymogen and are only activated as needed. In this chapter, we'll learn about how enzymes work and how different conditions influence their activity. We'll also see how enzymes are regulated, which will help us tie together concepts about every organ system and metabolic process we learn about for the MCAT.

2.1 Enzymes as Biological Catalysts

High-Yield

LEARNING OBJECTIVES

After Chapter 2.1, you will be able to:

- Explain the major features of enzyme function, including specificity and catalysis
- Describe all six classes of enzymes: oxidoreductases, transferases, hydrolases, lyases, isomerases, and ligases
- Recognize how enzymes affect thermodynamics and kinetics of a reaction

Enzymes are incredibly important as biological catalysts. **Catalysts** do not impact the thermodynamics of a biological reaction; that is, the ΔH_{rxn} and equilibrium position do not change. Instead, they help the reaction proceed at a much faster rate. As a catalyst, the enzyme is not changed during the course of the reaction. Enzymes increase the reaction rate of a process by a factor of 100, 1000, or even 1,000,000,000,000 (10^{12}) times when compared to the uncatalyzed reaction. Without this increase, we wouldn't be alive. Table 2.1 summarizes the key points to remember about enzymes.

Lower the activation energy
Increase the rate of the reaction
Do not alter the equilibrium constant
Are not changed or consumed in the reaction (which means that they will appear in both the reactants and products)
Are pH- and temperature-sensitive, with optimal activity at specific pH ranges and temperatures
Do not affect the overall ΔG of the reaction
Are specific for a particular reaction or class of reactions

Table 2.1 Key Features of Enzymes

Enzyme Classifications

Enzymes are picky. The molecules upon which an enzyme acts are called substrates; a given enzyme will only catalyze a single reaction or class of reactions with these substrates, a property known as **enzyme specificity**. For example, *urease* only catalyzes the breakdown of urea. *Chymotrypsin*, on the other hand, can cleave peptide bonds around the amino acids phenylalanine, tryptophan, and tyrosine in a variety of polypeptides. Although those amino acids aren't identical, they all contain an aromatic ring, which makes chymotrypsin specific for a class of molecules.

Enzymes can be classified into six categories, based on their function or mechanism. We'll review each type of enzyme and give examples of those that you are most likely to see on Test Day. If you encounter an unfamiliar enzyme on the MCAT, keep in mind that most enzymes have descriptive names ending in the suffix ***–ase***: *lactase*, for example, breaks down lactose.

Oxidoreductases

Oxidoreductases catalyze oxidation–reduction reactions; that is, the transfer of electrons between biological molecules. They often have a cofactor that acts as an electron carrier, such as NAD^+ or $NADP^+$. In reactions catalyzed by oxidoreductases, the electron donor is known as the **reductant**, and the electron acceptor is known as the **oxidant**. Enzymes with *dehydrogenase* or *reductase* in their names are usually oxidoreductases. Enzymes in which oxygen is the final electron acceptor often include *oxidase* in their names.

BRIDGE

The convention for naming reductants and oxidants of oxidoreductases is the same as the convention for naming reducing agents and oxidizing agents in general and organic chemistry. This is a good time to brush up on oxidation-reduction reactions if you haven't seen them in a while—they're covered in Chapter 11 of *MCAT General Chemistry Review* and Chapter 4 of *MCAT Organic Chemistry Review.*

Transferases

Transferases catalyze the movement of a functional group from one molecule to another. For example, in protein metabolism, an *aminotransferase* can convert aspartate and α-ketoglutarate, as a pair, to glutamate and oxaloacetate by moving the amino group from aspartate to α-ketoglutarate. Most transferases will be straightforwardly named, but remember that *kinases* are also a member of this class. **Kinases** catalyze the transfer of a phosphate group, generally from ATP, to another molecule.

Hydrolases

Hydrolases catalyze the breaking of a compound into two molecules using the addition of water. In common usage, many hydrolases are named only for their substrate. For example, one of the most common hydrolases you will encounter on the MCAT is a *phosphatase*, which cleaves a phosphate group from another molecule. Other hydrolases include *peptidases*, *nucleases*, and *lipases,* which break down proteins, nucleic acids, and lipids, respectively.

Lyases

Lyases catalyze the cleavage of a single molecule into two products. They do not require water as a substrate and do not act as oxidoreductases. Because most enzymes can also catalyze the reverse of their specific reactions, the synthesis of two molecules into a single molecule may also be catalyzed by a lyase. When fulfilling this function, it is common for them to be referred to as *synthases.*

MNEMONIC

Major Enzyme Classifications: **LI'L HOT**

- **L**igase
- **I**somerase
- **L**yase
- **H**ydrolase
- **O**xidoreductase
- **T**ransferase

Isomerases

Isomerases catalyze the rearrangement of bonds within a molecule. Some isomerases can also be classified as oxidoreductases, transferases, or lyases, depending on the mechanism of the enzyme. Keep in mind that isomerases catalyze reactions between stereoisomers as well as constitutional isomers.

Ligases

Ligases catalyze addition or synthesis reactions, generally between large similar molecules, and often require ATP. Synthesis reactions with smaller molecules are generally accomplished by lyases. Ligases are most likely to be encountered in nucleic acid synthesis and repair on Test Day.

Impact on Activation Energy

BRIDGE

Gibbs free energy and endergonic/exergonic reactions are covered in Chapter 7 of *MCAT General Chemistry Review*.

Recall that thermodynamics relates the relative energy states of a reaction in terms of its products and reactants. An **endergonic** reaction is one that requires energy input ($\Delta G > 0$), whereas an **exergonic** reaction is one in which energy is given off ($\Delta G < 0$). Remember that *endo–* means "in" and *exo–* means "out," so endergonic reactions take in energy as they proceed, whereas exergonic reactions release energy as they proceed. We can look at the reaction diagram in Figure 2.1 to see this demonstrated more clearly.

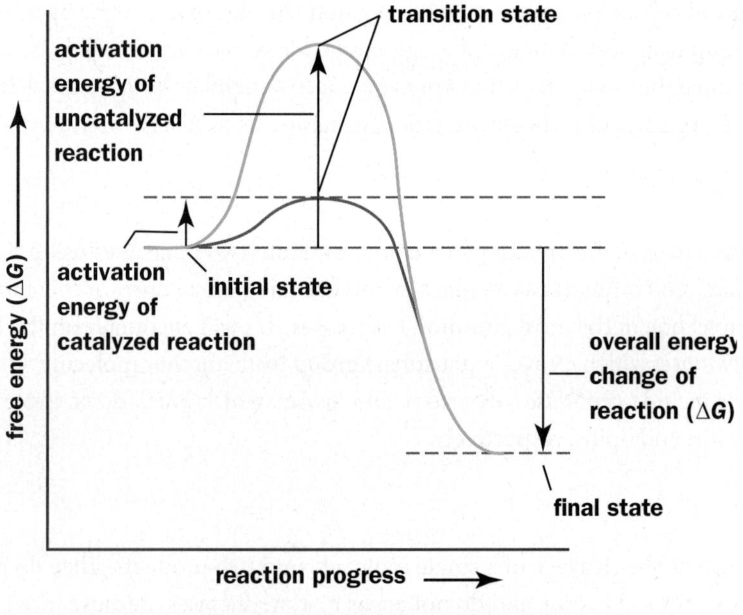

Figure 2.1 Exergonic Reaction Diagram
The activation energy required for a catalyzed reaction is lower than that of an uncatalyzed reaction while the ΔG (and ΔH) remains the same.

The reaction shown in Figure 2.1 is spontaneous. Note that the ΔG for this reaction is negative. A very important characteristic of enzymes is that they do not alter the overall free energy change for a reaction, nor do they change the equilibrium of a reaction. Rather, they affect the rate (kinetics) at which a reaction occurs; thus, they can affect how quickly a reaction gets to equilibrium but not the actual equilibrium state itself. For example, a reaction could take years to approach equilibrium without an enzyme. In comparison, with the enzyme, equilibrium might be attained within seconds. Enzymes ensure that many important reactions can occur in a reasonable amount of time in biological systems. Recall that enzymes, as catalysts, are unchanged by the reaction. What is the functional consequence of this? Far fewer copies of the enzyme are required relative to the overall amount of substrate because one enzyme can act on many, many molecules of substrate over time.

Catalysts exert their effect by lowering the **activation energy** of a reaction; in other words, they make it easier for the substrate to reach the transition state. Imagine having to walk to the other side of a tall hill. The only way to get there is to climb to the top of the hill and then walk down the other side—but wouldn't it be easier if the top of the hill was cut off so one wouldn't have to climb so high? That's exactly what catalysts do for chemical reactions when they make it easier for substrates to achieve their transition state. Most reactions catalyzed by enzymes are technically reversible, although that reversal may be extremely energetically unfavorable and therefore essentially nonexistent.

MCAT CONCEPT CHECK 2.1

Before you move on, assess your understanding of the material with these questions.

1. How do enzymes function as biological catalysts?

____

2. What is enzyme specificity?

____

3. What are the names and main functions of the six different classes of enzymes?

Name	Function

4. In what ways do enzymes affect the thermodynamics *vs.* the kinetics of a reaction?

____

2.2 Mechanisms of Enzyme Activity

High-Yield

LEARNING OBJECTIVES

After Chapter 2.2, you will be able to:

- Differentiate between coenzymes and cofactors
- Compare the induced fit and lock and key models of enzyme function

While enzyme mechanisms will vary depending on the reaction that is being catalyzed, they tend to share some common features. Enzymes may act to provide a favorable microenvironment in terms of charge or pH, stabilize the transition state, or bring reactive groups nearer to one another in the active site. The formation of the enzyme–substrate complex in the active site of an enzyme is the key catalytic activity of the enzyme, which reduces the activation energy of the reaction as described above. This interaction between a substrate and the active site of an enzyme also accounts for the selectivity and some regulatory mechanisms of enzymes.

Enzyme–Substrate Binding

The molecule upon which an enzyme acts is known as its **substrate**. The physical interaction between these two is referred to as the **enzyme–substrate complex**. The **active site** is the location within the enzyme where the substrate is held during the chemical reaction, as shown in Figure 2.2.

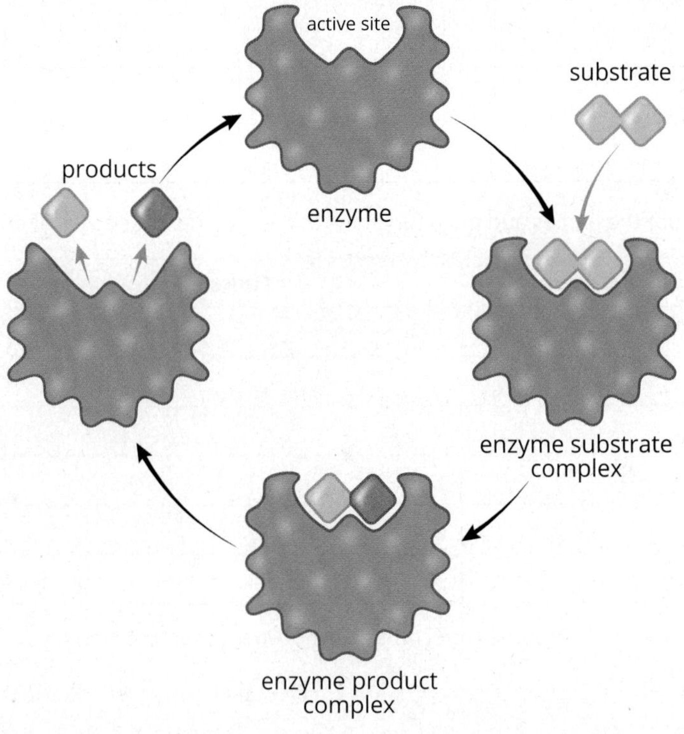

Figure 2.2 Reaction Catalysis in the Active Site of an Enzyme

The active site assumes a defined spatial arrangement in the enzyme–substrate complex, which dictates the specificity of that enzyme for a molecule or group of molecules. Hydrogen bonding, ionic interactions, and transient covalent bonds within the active site all stabilize this spatial arrangement and contribute to the efficiency of the enzyme. Two competing theories explain how enzymes and substrates interact, but one of the two is better supported than the other.

Lock and Key Theory

The **lock and key theory** is aptly named. It suggests that the enzyme's active site (lock) is already in the appropriate conformation for the substrate (key) to bind. As shown in Figure 2.3, the substrate can then easily fit into the active site, like a key into a lock or a hand into a glove. No alteration of the tertiary or quaternary structure is necessary upon binding of the substrate.

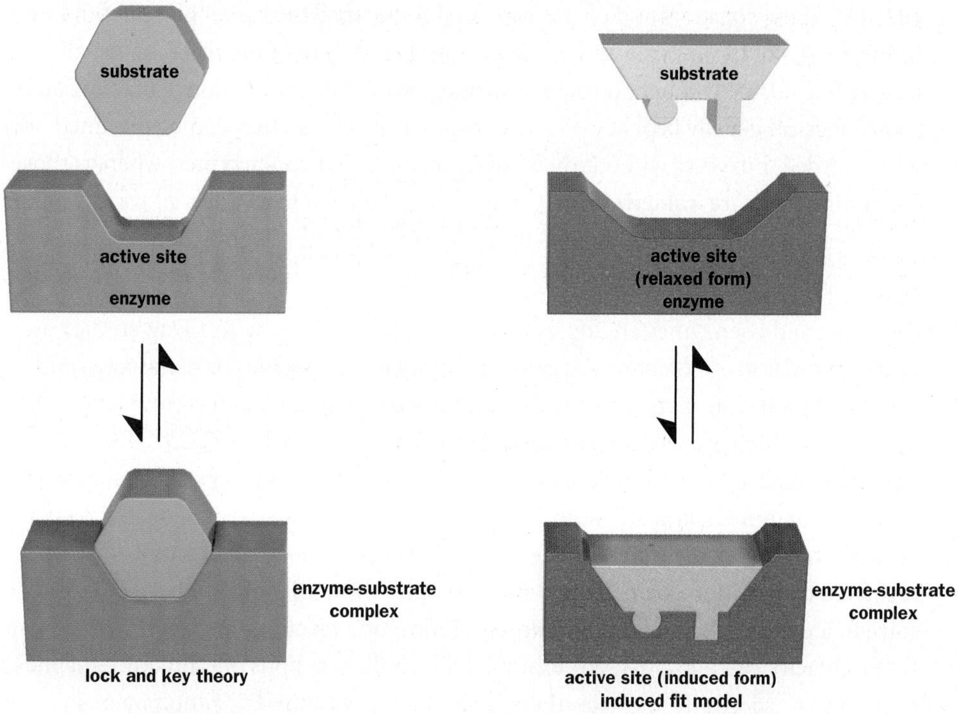

Figure 2.3 Lock and Key Theory *vs.* Induced Fit Model for Enzyme Catalysis

Induced Fit Model

The more scientifically accepted theory is the induced fit model; this is the one you are more likely to see referenced on Test Day. Imagine that the enzyme is a foam stress ball and the substrate is a frustrated MCAT student's hand. What's the desired interaction? The student wants to release some stress and relax. As the student's hand squeezes the ball, both change conformation. The ball is no longer spherical and the hand is no longer flat because they adjust to fit each other well. In this case, the substrate (the student) has induced a change in the shape of the enzyme (the stress ball). This interaction requires energy, and therefore, this part of the reaction is endergonic. Once the student lets go of the stress ball, we have our desired product: a relaxed, more confident test taker. Letting go of the stress ball is pretty easy and doesn't require extra energy; so, this part of the reaction is exergonic. Just like enzymes, foam stress balls return to their original shape once their crushers (substrates) let go of them. On a molecular level, demonstrated in Figure 2.3, the induced fit model starts with a substrate and an enzyme active site that don't seem to fit together. However, once the substrate is present and ready to interact with the active site, the molecules find that the induced form, or transition state, is more comfortable for both of them. Thus, the shape of the active site becomes truly complementary only after the substrate begins binding to the enzyme. Similarly, a substrate of the wrong type will not cause the appropriate conformational shift in the enzyme. Thus, the active site will not be adequately exposed, the transition state is not preferred, and no reaction occurs.

Cofactors and Coenzymes

REAL WORLD

Deficiencies in vitamin cofactors can result in devastating disease. Thiamine is an essential cofactor for several enzymes involved in cellular metabolism and nerve conduction. Thiamine deficiency, often a result of excess alcohol consumption and poor diet, results in diseases including Wernicke-Korsakoff syndrome. In this disorder, patients suffer from a variety of neurologic deficits, including delirium, balance problems, and, in severe cases, the inability to form new memories.

Many enzymes require nonprotein molecules called **cofactors** or **coenzymes** to be effective. These cofactors and coenzymes tend to be small in size so they can bind to the active site of the enzyme and participate in the catalysis of the reaction, usually by carrying charge through ionization, protonation, or deprotonation. Cofactors and coenzymes are usually kept at low concentrations in cells, so they can be recruited only when needed. Enzymes without their cofactors are called **apoenzymes**, whereas those containing them are **holoenzymes**. Cofactors are attached in a variety of ways, ranging from weak noncovalent interactions to strong covalent ones. Tightly bound cofactors or coenzymes that are necessary for enzyme function are known as **prosthetic groups**.

Cofactors and coenzymes are topics that we are likely to see on Test Day, so they are important to know. Cofactors are generally inorganic molecules or metal ions, and are often ingested as dietary minerals. Coenzymes are small organic groups, the vast majority of which are vitamins or derivatives of vitamins such as NAD^+, FAD, and coenzyme A. The water-soluble vitamins include the B complex vitamins and ascorbic acid (vitamin C), and are important coenzymes that must be replenished regularly because they are easily excreted. The fat-soluble vitamins—A, D, E, and K—are better regulated by partition coefficients, which quantify the ability of a molecule to dissolve in a polar *vs.* nonpolar environment. Enzymatic reactions are not restricted to a single cofactor or coenzyme. For example, metabolic reactions often require magnesium, NAD^+ (derived from vitamin B_3), and biotin (vitamin B_7) simultaneously.

BRIDGE

Vitamins come in two major classes: fat- and water-soluble. This is important to consider in digestive diseases, where different parts of the gastrointestinal tract may be affected by different disease processes. Because different parts of the gastrointestinal tract specialize in the absorption of different types of biomolecules, loss of different parts of the gastrointestinal tract or its accessory organs may result in different vitamin deficiencies. The digestive system is discussed in Chapter 9 of *MCAT Biology Review*.

The MCAT is unlikely to expect memorization of the B vitamins; however, familiarity with their names may make biochemistry passages easier on Test Day:

- B_1: thiamine
- B_2: riboflavin
- B_3: niacin
- B_5: pantothenic acid
- B_6: pyridoxal phosphate
- B_7: biotin
- B_9: folic acid
- B_{12}: cyanocobalamin

MCAT CONCEPT CHECK 2.2

Before you move on, assess your understanding of the material with these questions.

1. How do the lock and key theory and induced fit model differ?

Lock and Key	Induced Fit

2. What do cofactors and coenzymes do? How do they differ?

2.3 Enzyme Kinetics

High-Yield

LEARNING OBJECTIVES

After Chapter 2.3, you will be able to:

- Predict how changes in enzyme and solute concentration will affect enzyme kinetics
- Define enzyme cooperativity
- Compare Lineweaver–Burk and Michaelis–Menten plots
- Explain key points on a Lineweaver–Burk or Michaelis–Menten plot:

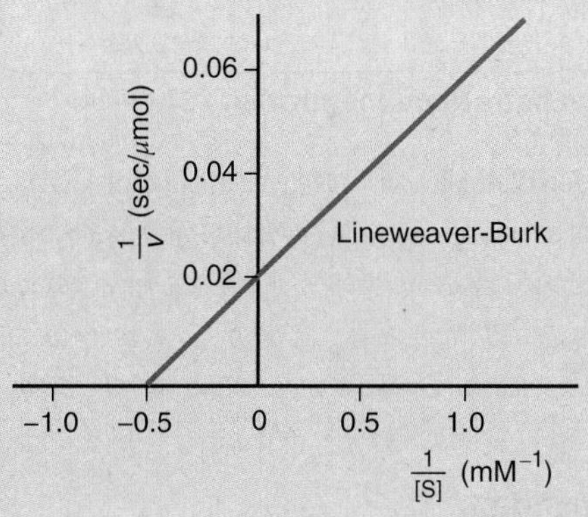

Kinetics of Monomeric Enzymes

Enzyme kinetics is a high-yield topic that can score us several points on Test Day. Just as the relief our student derives from squeezing a stress ball depends on a number of factors, such as size and shape of the ball and the student's baseline level of stress, enzyme kinetics are dependent on factors like environmental conditions and concentrations of substrate and enzyme.

The concentrations of the substrate, [S], and enzyme, [E], greatly affect how quickly a reaction will occur. Let's say that we have 100 stress balls (enzymes) and only 10 frustrated students (substrates) to derive stress relief from them. This represents a high enzyme concentration relative to substrate. Because there are many active sites available, we will quickly form products (students letting go and feeling relaxed); in a chemical sense, we would reach equilibrium quickly. As we slowly add more substrate (students), the rate of the reaction will increase; that is, more people will relax in the same amount of time because we have plenty of available stress balls for them to squeeze. However, as we add more and more people (and start approaching 100 students), we begin to level off and reach a maximal rate of relaxation. There are fewer and fewer available stress balls until finally all active sites are occupied. Unlike before, inviting more students into the room will not change the rate of the reaction. It cannot go any faster once it has reached **saturation**. At this rate, the enzyme is working at maximum velocity, denoted by $\mathbf{v_{max}}$. The only way to increase v_{max} is by increasing the enzyme concentration. In the cell, this can be accomplished by inducing the expression of the gene encoding the enzyme. These concepts are represented graphically in Figure 2.4.

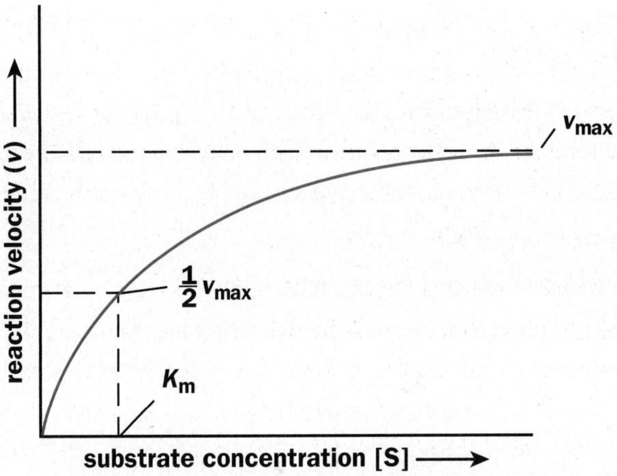

Figure 2.4 Michaelis-Menten Plot of Enzyme Kinetics
As the amount of substrate increases, the enzyme is able to increase its rate of reaction until it reaches a maximum enzymatic reaction rate (v_{max}); once v_{max} is reached, adding more substrate will not increase the rate of reaction.

Michaelis-Menten Equation

For most enzymes, the Michaelis–Menten equation describes how the rate of the reaction, v, depends on the concentration of both the enzyme, [E], and the substrate, [S], which forms product, [P]. Enzyme–substrate complexes form at a rate k_1. The ES complex can either dissociate at a rate k_{-1} or turn into E + P at a rate k_{cat}:

$$E + S \underset{k_{-1}}{\overset{k_1}{\rightleftharpoons}} ES \xrightarrow{k_{cat}} E + P$$

Equation 2.1

Note that in either case, the enzyme is again available. On Test Day, the concentration of enzyme will be kept constant. Under these conditions, we can relate the velocity of the enzyme to substrate concentration using the Michaelis–Menten equation:

$$v = \frac{v_{\text{max}}\,[\text{S}]}{K_{\text{m}} + [\text{S}]}$$

Equation 2.2

Some important and Test Day–relevant math can be derived from this equation. When the reaction rate is equal to half of v_{max}, $K_{\text{m}} = [\text{S}]$:

$$\frac{v_{\text{max}}}{2} = \frac{v_{\text{max}}[\text{S}]}{K_{\text{m}} + [\text{S}]}$$
$$v_{\text{max}}(K_{\text{m}} + [\text{S}]) = 2(v_{\text{max}}[\text{S}])$$
$$K_{\text{m}} + [\text{S}] = 2[\text{S}]$$
$$K_{\text{m}} = [\text{S}]$$

K_{m} can, therefore, be understood to be the substrate concentration at which half of the enzyme's active sites are full (half the stress balls are in use). $\mathbf{K_m}$ is the **Michaelis constant** and is often used to compare enzymes. Under certain conditions, K_{m} is a measure of the affinity of the enzyme for its substrate. When comparing two enzymes, the one with the higher K_{m} has the lower affinity for its substrate because it requires a higher substrate concentration to be half-saturated. The K_{m} value is an intrinsic property of the enzyme–substrate system and cannot be altered by changing the concentration of substrate or enzyme.

For a given concentration of enzyme, the Michaelis–Menten relationship generally graphs as a hyperbola, as seen in the Michaelis–Menten plot in Figure 2.4. When substrate concentration is less than K_{m}, changes in substrate concentration will greatly affect the reaction rate. At high substrate concentrations exceeding K_{m}, the reaction rate increases much more slowly as it approaches v_{max}, where it becomes independent of substrate concentration.

The variable v_{max} represents maximum enzyme velocity and is measured in moles of enzyme per second. Also, v_{max} can be mathematically related to $\mathbf{k_{cat}}$, which has units of s^{-1}:

$$v_{max} = [\text{E}]k_{\text{cat}}$$

Equation 2.3

Qualitatively speaking, k_{cat} measures the number of substrate molecules "turned over," or converted to product, per enzyme molecule per second. Most enzymes have k_{cat} values between 101 and 103. The Michaelis–Menton equation above can be restated using k_{cat}:

$$v = \frac{k_{\text{cat}}[\text{E}][\text{S}]}{K_{\text{m}} + [\text{S}]}$$

KEY CONCEPT

We can assess an enzyme's affinity for a substrate by noting the K_{m}. A low K_{m} reflects a high affinity for the substrate (low [S] required for 50% enzyme saturation). Conversely, a high K_{m} reflects a low affinity of the enzyme for the substrate.

At very low substrate concentrations, where $K_m >> [S]$, this derived equation can be further simplified as:

$$v = \frac{k_{cat}}{K_m}[E][S]$$

The ratio of k_{cat}/K_m is referred to as the **catalytic efficiency** of the enzyme. A large k_{cat} (high turnover) or a small K_m (high substrate affinity) will result in a higher catalytic efficiency, which indicates a more efficient enzyme.

Lineweaver–Burk Plots

The Lineweaver–Burk plot is a double reciprocal graph of the Michaelis–Menten equation. The same data graphed in this way yield a straight line as shown in Figure 2.5. The actual data are represented by the portion of the graph to the right of the y-axis, but the line is extrapolated into the upper left quadrant to determine its intercept with the x-axis. The intercept of the line with the x-axis gives the value of $-\frac{1}{K_m}$. The intercept of the line with the y-axis gives the value of $\frac{1}{v_{max}}$. The Lineweaver–Burk plot is especially useful when determining the type of inhibition that an enzyme is experiencing because v_{max} and K_m can be compared without estimation.

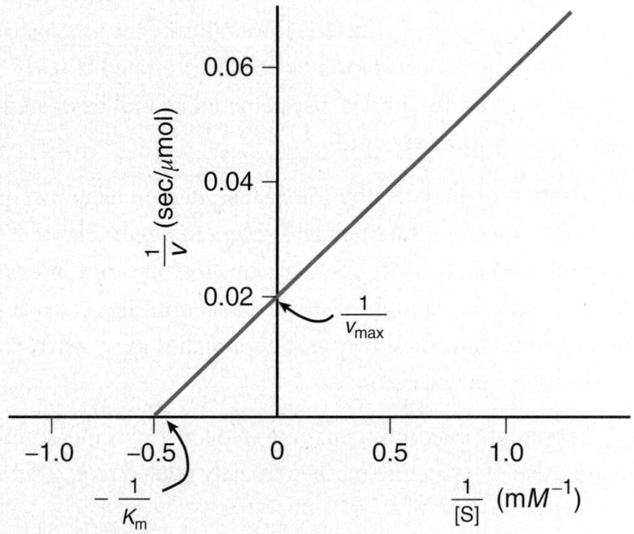

Figure 2.5 Experimentally Determined Lineweaver-Burk (Double Reciprocal) Plot Used to Calculate the Values of K_m and v_{max}

Cooperativity

MCAT EXPERTISE

The cooperative binding of hemoglobin, which acts as a transport protein rather than an enzyme, results in a characteristic sigmoidal binding curve that is an MCAT favorite.

Certain enzymes do not show the normal hyperbola when graphed on a Michaelis–Menten plot (v vs. [S]), but rather show sigmoidal (S-shaped) kinetics owing to cooperativity among substrate binding sites, as shown in Figure 2.6. Cooperative enzymes have multiple subunits and multiple active sites. Subunits and enzymes may exist in one of two states: a low-affinity tense state (T) or a high-affinity relaxed state (R). Binding of the substrate encourages the transition of other subunits from the

T state to the R state, which increases the likelihood of substrate binding by these other subunits. Conversely, loss of substrate can encourage the transition from the R state to the T state, and promote dissociation of substrate from the remaining subunits. Think of cooperative enzyme kinetics like a party. As more people start arriving, the atmosphere becomes more relaxed and the party seems more appealing, but as people start going home the party dies down and more people are encouraged to leave so the tense hosts can clean up. Enzymes showing cooperative kinetics are often regulatory enzymes in pathways, like *phosphofructokinase-1* in glycolysis. Cooperative enzymes are also subject to activation and inhibition, both competitively and through allosteric sites.

Cooperativity can also be quantified using a numerical value called **Hill's coefficient**. The value of Hill's coefficient indicates the nature of binding by the molecule:

- If Hill's coefficient > 1, positively cooperative binding is occurring, such that after one ligand is bound the affinity of the enzyme for further ligand(s) increases.
- If Hill's coefficient < 1, negatively cooperative binding is occurring, such that after one ligand is bound the affinity of the enzyme for further ligand(s) decreases.
- If Hill's coefficient $= 1$, the enzyme does not exhibit cooperative binding.

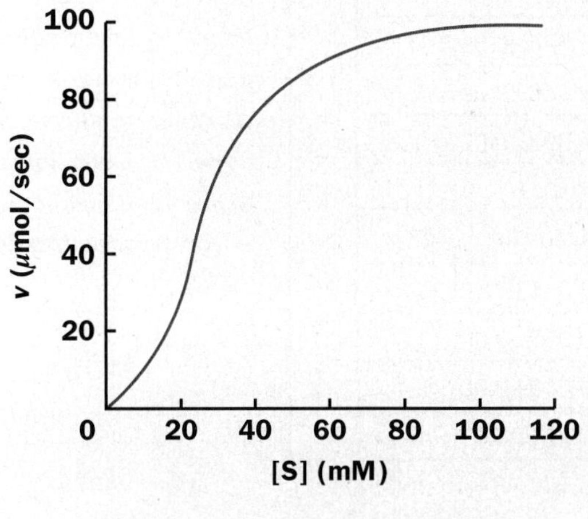

Figure 2.6 Cooperative Enzyme Kinetics

BIOCHEMISTRY GUIDED EXAMPLE WITH EXPERT THINKING

The PH1704 protease from *Pyrococcus horikoshii* OT3 is a hyperthermophilic enzyme that belongs to the DJ-1/ThiJ/PfpI superfamily. One of its members, the human protein DJ-1, has recently been reported to cause certain types of early-onset Parkinsonism. Thus, an increasing number of studies on this superfamily are being conducted. Despite this growing interest, few members of this superfamily have been biochemically characterized.

This is just a lot of context; the useful info is that PH1704 is a protease, which means it is an enzyme that cleaves peptide bonds

PH1704 has both endopeptidase (cleaves nonterminal amino acids) and aminopeptidase (cleaves amino acids from the N-terminus) activity.

2 kinds of protease activity for this enzyme

Further analysis suggests that PH1704 specifically cleaves after arginine.

Probably important—cleaves after arginine!

Two 7-amino-4-methylcoumarin (AMC)-linked substrates were used in kinetic assays: R-AMC and AAFR-AMC.

AMC sounds like a molecule attached to amino acids or peptides

Predictive substrate docking studies pinpointed Tyr-120 in the active site, possibly involved in aromatic and hydrophobic interaction with the substrate. Therefore, Tyr-120 was chosen for mutation to analyze the effects on PH1704 kinetics, and the results are shown in Table 1 below.

Y120 seems like an important residue

Enzyme	Aminopeptidase (R-AMC)		
	K_{cat} (min^{-1})	K_m (μM)	K_{cat}/K_m (min^{-1} μM^{-1})
WT	0.646±0.05	12±0.65	0.052±0.008
Y120S	0.147±0.01	9.0±0.43	0.024±0.004
Y120W	1.2±0.07	20.6±0.77	0.066±0.005
Y120P	4.37±0.12	11.3±0.59	0.398±0.025
Enzyme	**Endopeptidase (AAFR-AMC)**		
	K_{cat} (min^{-1})	K_m (μM)	K_{cat}/K_m (min^{-1} μM^{-1})
WT	0.11±0.02	10±0.2	0.018±0.004
Y120S	0.084±0.01	6.5±0.4	0.017±0.003
Y120W	0.12±0.01	16.0±1.5	0.019±0.001
Y120P	1.13±0.07	5.4±0.3	0.21±0.03

Table 1

Trends: catalytic efficiency (k_{cat}/K_m) seems much higher for Y120P, Y120S is much slower at producing product in both cases (lower k_{cat}), and, in general, efficiency is higher for aminopeptidase than for endopeptidase activity

Adapted from Zhan, D., Bai, A., Yu, L., Han, W., & Feng, Y. (2014). Characterization of the PH1704 protease from *Pyrococcus horikoshii* OT3 and the critical functions of Tyr120. *PLoS One*, 9(9), e103902. doi:10.1371/journal.pone.010390.

According to the data, does PH1704 have equivalent aminopeptidase and endopeptidase activity? Why or why not?

The question asks us for data analysis, so we know we should start by making sure we understand what the given material is telling us. A quick scan of the passage reveals unfamiliar enzymes, terminology, and a data-packed table, so a careful read of the passage for the big picture will be important in order to relate what the table is trying to prove. We are also definitely going to need to bring in some of our outside knowledge about enzymes. The passage describes an enzyme called PH1704, which has several characteristics outlined in the first half of the paragraph. We're told it's a protease, which means it breaks peptide bonds, and it's hyperthermophilic. Breaking down the term hyperthermophilic, we get *hyper-* (higher) *-thermo-* (heat) *-philic* (love), and we can thus deduce that the enzyme is from a bacterial species that lives in high temperatures. Next, we're told it's an endopeptidase (*endo-* meaning between) and an aminopeptidase with a strong preference for arginine. There are two substrates described in the study. Notice how only R-AMC can be used to discern the aminopeptidase activity, and AAFR-AMC can be used to test endopeptidase activity. Finally, we're told that Tyr-120 can be important for activity, so researchers created mutations of this residue and the kinetic information of the resulting mutants is described in Table 1.

The question asks us to determine whether PH1704 acts equally as an aminopeptidase and an endopeptidase. In order to answer this question, first note that the mutation data for Y120 is not needed since we are only being asked about the wild-type PH1704 enzyme.

All we really need is a comparison between the WT enzyme with R-AMC as a substrate, and WT enzyme with AAFR-AMC as a substrate. Also, we need to determine whether k_{cat}, k_m, or k_{cat}/k_m will be most useful. Recall that k_{cat} provides information about how much product is produced per unit time, and k_m is a measure of substrate affinity. To have an enzyme that is maximally efficient, you want both a high catalytic turnover (high k_{cat}) and a high substrate affinity (low k_m), so the best comparison would be the k_{cat}/k_m data, which is equal to the catalytic efficiency of an enzyme. The catalytic efficiency for PH1704 as an aminopeptidase is 0.052 $min^{-1}/\mu M$, and for PH1704 as an endopeptidase efficiency is 0.018 $min^{-1}/\mu M$.

Since these values of catalytic efficiency are different when measuring aminopeptidase and endopeptidase activity, we can conclude that PH1704 functions more effectively as an aminopeptidase than as an endopeptidase.

MCAT CONCEPT CHECK 2.3

Before you move on, assess your understanding of the material with these questions.

1. What are the effects of increasing [S] on enzyme kinetics? What about increasing [E]?
   - Increasing [S]:
   - Increasing [E]:
2. How are the Michaelis–Menten and Lineweaver–Burk plots similar? How are they different?
   - Similarities:
   - Differences:
3. What does K_m represent? What would an increase in K_m signify?
4. What do the *x*- and *y*-intercepts in a Lineweaver–Burk plot represent?
   - *x*-intercept:
   - *y*-intercept:
5. What is enzyme cooperativity?

2.4 Effects of Local Conditions on Enzyme Activity

High-Yield

LEARNING OBJECTIVES

After Chapter 2.4, you will be able to:

- Predict how changes to the environment will alter enzyme behavior
- Estimate the ideal pH and temperature for enzymes found in the human body

The activity of an enzyme is heavily influenced by its environment; in particular, temperature, acidity or alkalinity (pH), and high salinity have significant effects on the ability of an enzyme to carry out its function. Note that the terms **enzyme activity**, **enzyme velocity**, and **enzyme rate** are all used synonymously on the MCAT.

Temperature

Enzyme-catalyzed reactions tend to double in velocity for every 10°C increase in temperature until the optimum temperature is reached; for the human body, this is 37°C (98.6°F or 310 K). After this, activity falls off sharply, as the enzyme will denature at higher temperatures, as shown in Figure 2.7. Some enzymes that are overheated may regain their function if cooled. A real-life example of temperature dependence occurs in Siamese cats. Siamese cats are dark on their faces, ears, tails, and feet but white elsewhere. Why? The enzyme responsible for pigmentation, *tyrosinase*, is mutated in Siamese cats. It is ineffective at body temperature but at cooler temperatures becomes active. Thus, only the tail, feet, ears, and face (cooled by air passing through the nose and mouth) have an active form of the enzyme and are dark.

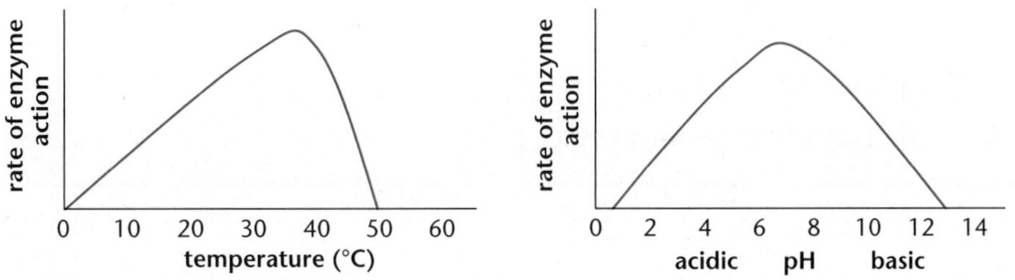

Figure 2.7 Effects of Temperature and pH on the Rate of Enzyme Action

pH

Most enzymes also depend on pH in order to function properly, not only because pH affects the ionization of the active site, but also because changes in pH can lead to denaturation of the enzyme. For enzymes that circulate and function in human blood, this optimal pH is 7.4, as shown in Figure 2.7. A pH < 7.35 in human blood is termed acidemia. Even though it's more basic than *chemically* neutral 7.0, it is more acidic than *physiologically* neutral 7.4. Where might exceptions to this pH 7.4 occur?

BRIDGE

The pH levels in the stomach and intestine, and their effects on these gastric and pancreatic enzymes, are covered in Chapter 9 of *MCAT Biology Review*.

Both are in our digestive tract. Pepsin, which works in the stomach, has maximal activity around pH 2, whereas pancreatic enzymes, which work in the small intestine, work best around pH 8.5.

Salinity

While the effect of salinity or osmolarity is not generally of physiologic significance, altering the concentration of salt can change enzyme activity *in vitro*. Increasing levels of salt can disrupt hydrogen and ionic bonds, causing a partial change in the conformation of the enzyme, and in some cases causing denaturation.

MCAT CONCEPT CHECK 2.4

Before you move on, assess your understanding of the material with these questions.

1. What are the effects of temperature, pH, and salinity on the function of enzymes?
   - Temperature:

   ____

   - pH:

   ____

   - Salinity:

   ____

2. What is the ideal temperature for most enzymes in the body? The ideal pH?
   - Ideal temperature: ______ °C = ______ °F = ______ K
   - Ideal pH (most enzymes): ______
   - Ideal pH (gastric enzymes): ______
   - Ideal pH (pancreatic enzymes): ______

2.5 Regulation of Enzyme Activity

High-Yield

LEARNING OBJECTIVES

After Chapter 2.5, you will be able to:

- Explain feedback inhibition and irreversible inhibition
- Differentiate between the four types of reversible inhibition
- Differentiate between transient and covalent enzyme modifications
- Recall the traits of zymogens

Although enzymes are useful, the body must be able to control when they work; for example, enzymes involved in mitosis should be shut off when cells are no longer dividing (in the G_0 phase). This may be accomplished in a variety of ways, as described below.

Feedback Regulation

Enzymes are often subject to regulation by products further down a given metabolic pathway, a process called **feedback regulation**. Less often, enzymes may be regulated by intermediates that precede the enzyme in the pathway, also called **feed-forward regulation**. This is clearly evident in the study of metabolism, as discussed in Chapters 9 through 12 of *MCAT Biochemistry Review*. While there are some examples of feedback activation, feedback inhibition is far more common. Feedback inhibition, or **negative feedback**, helps maintain homeostasis: once we have enough of a given product, we want to turn off the pathway that creates that product, rather than creating more. In feedback inhibition, the product may bind to the active site of an enzyme or multiple enzymes that acted earlier in its biosynthetic pathway, thereby competitively inhibiting these enzymes and making them unavailable for use. This is schematically represented in Figure 2.8, as we see product D feeding back to inhibit the first enzyme in the pathway.

BRIDGE

Negative feedback is an important topic in both enzymology and the endocrine system. Remember that most hormonal feedback loops are also inhibited by negative feedback. The endocrine system is discussed in Chapter 5 of *MCAT Biology Review*.

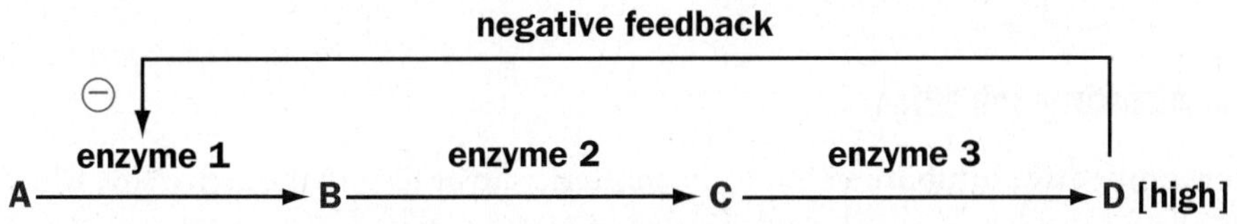

Figure 2.8 Feedback Inhibition by the Product of a Metabolic Pathway
A high concentration of the product, D, inhibits enzyme 1, slowing the entire pathway.

Reversible Inhibition

There are four types of reversible inhibition: competitive, noncompetitive, mixed, and uncompetitive. On Test Day, you will most often encounter competitive and noncompetitive inhibition, but be aware of the differences in the four types. Table 2.2 at the end of this section summarizes the features of each type of reversible inhibition.

Competitive Inhibition

REAL WORLD

The concept of competitive inhibition has relevance in the clinical setting. For example, methanol (wood alcohol), if ingested, is enzymatically converted to toxic metabolites, which can cause blindness and even death. Administration of intravenous ethanol is the treatment of choice for a patient suffering from methanol poisoning. Ethanol works by competing with methanol for the active sites of the enzymes involved.

Competitive inhibition simply involves occupancy of the active site. Substrates cannot access enzymatic binding sites if there is an inhibitor in the way. Competitive inhibition can be overcome by adding more substrate so that the substrate-to-inhibitor ratio is higher. If more molecules of substrate are available than molecules of inhibitor, then the enzyme will be more likely to bind substrate than inhibitor (assuming the enzyme has equal affinity for both molecules). Adding a competitive inhibitor does not alter the value of v_{max} because if enough substrate is added, it will outcompete the inhibitor and be able to run the reaction at maximum velocity. A competitive inhibitor does increase the measured value of K_m. This is because the substrate concentration has to be higher to reach half the maximum velocity in the presence of the inhibitor. A Lineweaver–Burk plot comparing an enzyme with and without a competitive inhibitor is shown in Figure 2.9.

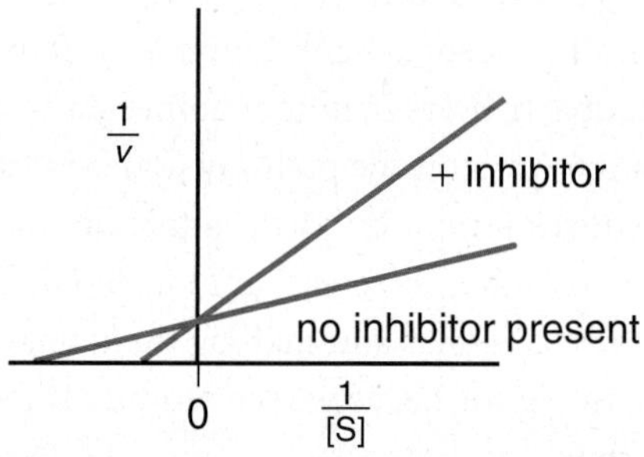

Figure 2.9 Lineweaver-Burk Plot of Competitive Inhibition

Noncompetitive Inhibition

Noncompetitive inhibitors bind to an allosteric site instead of the active site, which induces a change in enzyme conformation. Allosteric sites are non-catalytic regions of the enzyme that bind regulators. Because the two molecules do not compete for the same site, inhibition is considered noncompetitive and cannot be overcome by adding more substrate. Noncompetitive inhibitors bind equally well to the enzyme and the enzyme–substrate complex, unlike mixed inhibitors. Once the enzyme's conformation is altered, no amount of extra substrate will be conducive to forming an enzyme–substrate complex. Adding a noncompetitive inhibitor decreases the measured value of v_{max} because there is less enzyme available to react; it does not, however, alter the value of K_m because any copies of the enzyme that are still active maintain the same affinity for their substrate. A Lineweaver–Burk plot of an enzyme with and without a noncompetitive inhibitor is shown in Figure 2.10.

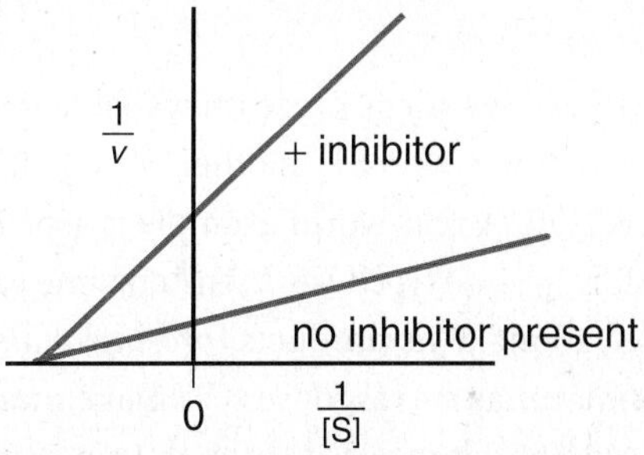

Figure 2.10 Lineweaver-Burk Plot of Noncompetitive Inhibition

Mixed Inhibition

Mixed inhibition results when an inhibitor can bind to either the enzyme or the enzyme–substrate complex, but has different affinity for each. If the inhibitor had the same affinity for both, it would be a noncompetitive inhibitor. Mixed inhibitors do not bind at the active site, but at an allosteric site. Mixed inhibition alters the experimental value of K_m depending on the preference of the inhibitor for the enzyme *vs.* the enzyme–substrate complex. If the inhibitor preferentially binds to the enzyme, it increases the K_m value (lowers affinity); if the inhibitor binds to the enzyme–substrate complex, it lowers the K_m value (increases affinity). In either case, v_{max} is decreased. On a Lineweaver–Burk plot, the curves for the activity with and without the inhibitor intersect at a point that is not on either axis.

Uncompetitive Inhibition

Uncompetitive inhibitors bind only to the enzyme–substrate complex and essentially lock the substrate in the enzyme, preventing its release. This can be interpreted as increasing affinity between the enzyme and substrate. Because the enzyme–substrate complex has already formed upon binding, uncompetitive inhibitors must bind at an allosteric site; in fact, it is the formation of the enzyme–substrate complex that creates a conformational change that allows the uncompetitive inhibitor to bind. Thus, uncompetitive inhibitors lower K_m and v_{max}. On a Lineweaver–Burk plot, the curves for activity with and without an uncompetitive inhibitor are parallel.

	COMPETITIVE	NONCOMPETITIVE	MIXED	UNCOMPETITIVE
Binding Site	Active site	Allosteric site	Allosteric site	Allosteric site
Impact on K_m	Increases	Unchanged	Increases or Decreases	Decreases
Impact on v_{max}	Unchanged	Decreases	Decreases	Decreases

Table 2.2 Comparison of Reversible Inhibitors

Irreversible Inhibition

In this type of inhibition, the active site is made unavailable for a prolonged period of time, or the enzyme is permanently altered. In other words, this type of inhibition is not easily overcome or reversed. A real-world example is aspirin. Acetylsalicylic acid (aspirin) irreversibly modifies *cyclooxygenase-1*. The enzyme can no longer bind its substrate (*arachidonic acid*) to make its products (*prostaglandins*), which are involved in modulating pain and inflammatory responses. To make more prostaglandins, new cyclooxygenase-1 will have to be synthesized through transcription and translation. Irreversible inhibition is a prime drug mechanism, and something that you will come across often in medical school.

Regulated Enzymes

Allosteric Enzymes

Enzymes that are allosteric have multiple binding sites. The active site is present, as well as at least one other site that can regulate the availability of the active site. These are known as **allosteric sites**. **Allosteric enzymes** alternate between an active and an inactive form. The inactive form cannot carry out the enzymatic reaction. Molecules that bind to the allosteric site may be either **allosteric activators** or **allosteric inhibitors**. Binding of either causes a conformational shift in the protein; however, the effect differs. An activator will result in a shift that makes the active site more available for binding to the substrate, whereas an inhibitor will make it less available. In addition to being able to alter the conformation of the protein, binding of activators or inhibitors may alter the activity of the enzyme. As shown in Figure 2.6 above, Michaelis–Menten plots of cooperative allosteric enzyme kinetics often have a sigmoidal (S-shaped) curve.

Covalently Modified Enzymes

In addition to transient interactions, enzymes are often subject to covalent modification. Enzymes can be activated or deactivated by **phosphorylation** or **dephosphorylation**. One cannot predict whether phosphorylation or dephosphorylation will activate an enzyme without experimental determination. **Glycosylation**, the covalent attachment of sugar moieties, is another covalent enzyme modification. Glycosylation can tag an enzyme for transport within the cell, or can modify protein activity and selectivity. Specific mechanisms for the modification of enzymes by glycosylation are still being studied, and are beyond the scope of the MCAT.

BRIDGE

Consider that digestive enzymes, discussed in Chapter 9 of *MCAT Biology Review*, chew up fats, proteins, and carbohydrates—the very same compounds of which our body is made. How do these enzymes know to digest your food but not your body? Simply put, they don't! So, we regulate their activity in a coordinated manner using feedback mechanisms and other substances.

Zymogens

Certain enzymes are particularly dangerous if they are not tightly controlled. These include the digestive enzymes like *trypsin*, which, if released from the pancreas in an uncontrolled manner, would digest the organ itself. To avoid this danger, these enzymes and many others are secreted as inactive **zymogens** like *trypsinogen*.

Zymogens contain a catalytic (active) domain and regulatory domain. The regulatory domain must be either removed or altered to expose the active site. Apoptotic enzymes (*caspases*) exhibit similar regulation. Most zymogens have the suffix *–**ogen***.

MCAT CONCEPT CHECK 2.5

Before you move on, assess your understanding of the material with these questions.

1. What is feedback inhibition?

____

2. Of the four types of reversible inhibitors, which could potentially increase K_m?

____

3. What is irreversible inhibition?

____

4. What are some examples of transient and covalent enzyme modifications?

   - Transient:

   ____

   - Covalent:

   ____

5. Why are some enzymes released as zymogens?

____

Conclusion

Our current chapter focused on the way in which cells are able to carry out the reactions necessary for life. We began with a discussion of the types of enzymes that you are likely to encounter on Test Day before reviewing thermodynamics and kinetics in relation to enzymes, which are biological catalysts. We went on to discuss the analysis of kinetic data with two different types of graphs, and talked about cooperativity. Because catalysts are generally most active in their native environment, we considered the impact of temperature, pH, and salinity on their activity. All of these are likely to appear on Test Day.

Enzymes need to be regulated; we analyzed the basics of feedback mechanisms. We talked about inhibitors of enzymes, which may be reversible or irreversible. The difference between the types of reversible inhibition is a key Test Day concept. Finally, we discussed changes in enzyme activity that may include allosteric activation, covalent modification, or cleavage of inactive zymogens. Let's move on now to discuss the nonenzymatic functions of proteins. You will notice many parallels between the new material and the concepts described in this chapter, like binding affinity. By the end of the next chapter, you'll be ready to face any protein question the MCAT can throw at you!

You've reviewed the content, now test your knowledge and critical thinking skills by completing a test-like passage set in your online resources!

GO ONLINE

CONCEPT SUMMARY

Enzymes as Biological Catalysts

- **Enzymes** are biological catalysts that are unchanged by the reactions they catalyze and are reusable.
- Each enzyme catalyzes a single reaction or type of reaction with high specificity.
  - **Oxidoreductases** catalyze oxidation–reduction reactions that involve the transfer of electrons.
  - **Transferases** move a functional group from one molecule to another molecule.
  - **Hydrolases** catalyze cleavage with the addition of water.
  - **Lyases** catalyze cleavage without the addition of water and without the transfer of electrons. The reverse reaction (synthesis) is often more important biologically.
  - **Isomerases** catalyze the interconversion of isomers, including both constitutional isomers and stereoisomers.
  - **Ligases** are responsible for joining two large biomolecules, often of the same type.
- **Exergonic reactions** release energy; ΔG is negative.
- Enzymes lower the activation energy necessary for biological reactions.
- Enzymes do not alter the free energy (ΔG) or enthalpy (ΔH) change that accompanies the reaction nor the final equilibrium position; rather, they change the rate (kinetics) at which equilibrium is reached.

Mechanisms of Enzyme Activity

- Enzymes act by stabilizing the transition state, providing a favorable microenvironment, or bonding with the substrate molecules.
- Enzymes have an **active site**, which is the site of catalysis.
- Binding to the active site is explained by the **lock and key theory** or the **induced fit model**.
  - The lock and key theory hypothesizes that the enzyme and substrate are exactly complementary.
  - The induced fit model hypothesizes that the enzyme and substrate undergo conformational changes to interact fully.
- Some enzymes require metal cation **cofactors** or small organic **coenzymes** to be active.

Enzyme Kinetics

- Enzymes experience **saturation kinetics**: as substrate concentration increases, the reaction rate does as well until a maximum value is reached.
- **Michaelis–Menten** and **Lineweaver–Burk** plots represent this relationship as a hyperbola and line, respectively.
- Enzymes can be compared on the basis of their K_m and v_{max} values.
- **Cooperative enzymes** display a sigmoidal curve because of the change in activity with substrate binding.

Effects of Local Conditions on Enzyme Activity

- Temperature and pH affect an enzyme's activity *in vivo*; changes in temperature and pH can result in denaturing of the enzyme and loss of activity due to loss of secondary, tertiary, or, if present, quaternary structure.
- *In vitro*, salinity can impact the action of enzymes.

Regulation of Enzyme Activity

- Enzyme pathways are highly regulated and subject to inhibition and activation.
- **Feedback inhibition** is a regulatory mechanism whereby the catalytic activity of an enzyme is inhibited by the presence of high levels of a product later in the same pathway.
- **Reversible inhibition** is characterized by the ability to replace the inhibitor with a compound of greater affinity or to remove it using mild laboratory treatment.
  - **Competitive inhibition** results when the inhibitor is similar to the substrate and binds at the active site. Competitive inhibition can be overcome by adding more substrate. v_{max} is unchanged, K_m increases.
  - **Noncompetitive inhibition** results when the inhibitor binds with equal affinity to the enzyme and the enzyme–substrate complex. v_{max} is decreased, K_m is unchanged.
  - **Mixed inhibition** results when the inhibitor binds with unequal affinity to the enzyme and the enzyme–substrate complex. v_{max} is decreased, K_m is increased or decreased depending on if the inhibitor has higher affinity for the enzyme or enzyme–substrate complex.
  - **Uncompetitive inhibition** results when the inhibitor binds only with the enzyme–substrate complex. K_m and v_{max} both decrease.

- **Irreversible inhibition** alters the enzyme in such a way that the active site is unavailable for a prolonged duration or permanently; new enzyme molecules must be synthesized for the reaction to occur again.
- Regulatory enzymes can experience activation as well as inhibition.
  - **Allosteric** sites can be occupied by activators, which increase either affinity or enzymatic turnover.
  - **Phosphorylation** (covalent modification with phosphate) or **glycosylation** (covalent modification with carbohydrate) can alter the activity or selectivity of enzymes.
  - **Zymogens** are secreted in an inactive form and are activated by cleavage.

ANSWERS TO CONCEPT CHECKS

2.1

1. Catalysts are characterized by two main properties: they reduce the activation energy of a reaction, thus speeding up the reaction, and they are not used up in the course of the reaction. Enzymes improve the environment in which a particular reaction takes place, which lowers its activation energy. They are also regenerated at the end of the reaction to their original form.
2. Enzyme specificity refers to the idea that a given enzyme will only catalyze a given reaction or type of reaction. For example, *serine/threonine-specific protein kinases* will only place a phosphate group onto the hydroxyl group of a serine or threonine residue.
3.

Name	Function
Ligase	Addition or synthesis reactions, generally between large molecules, often require ATP
Isomerase	Rearrangement of bonds within a compound
Lyase	Cleavage of a single molecule into two products, or synthesis of small organic molecules
Hydrolase	Breaking of a compound into two molecules using the addition of water
Oxidoreductase	Oxidation–reduction reactions (transferring electrons)
Transferase	Movement of a functional group from one molecule to another

4. Enzymes have no effect on the overall thermodynamics of the reaction; they have no effect on the ΔG or ΔH of the reaction, although they do lower the energy of the transition state, thus lowering the activation energy. However, enzymes have a profound effect on the kinetics of a reaction. By lowering activation energy, equilibrium can be achieved faster (although the equilibrium position does not change).

2.2

1.

Lock and Key	Induced Fit
• Active site of enzyme fits exactly around substrate • No alterations to tertiary or quaternary structure of enzyme • Less accurate model	• Active site of enzyme molds itself around substrate only when substrate is present • Tertiary and quaternary structure is modified for enzyme to function • More accurate model

2. Cofactors and coenzymes both act as activators of enzymes. Cofactors tend to be inorganic (minerals), while coenzymes tend to be small organic compounds (vitamins). In both cases, these regulators induce a conformational change in the enzyme that promotes its activity. Tightly bound cofactors or coenzymes that are necessary for enzyme function are termed prosthetic groups.

2.3

1. Increasing [S] has different effects, depending on how much substrate is present to begin with. When the substrate concentration is low, an increase in [S] causes a proportional increase in enzyme activity. At high [S], however, when the enzyme is saturated, increasing [S] has no effect on activity because v_{max} has already been attained.

   Increasing [E] will always increase v_{max}, regardless of the starting concentration of enzyme.
2. Both the Michaelis–Menten and Lineweaver–Burk relationships account for the values of K_m and v_{max} under various conditions. They both provide simple graphical interpretations of these two variables and are derived from the Michaelis–Menten equation. However, the axes of these graphs and visual representation of this information is different between the two. The Michaelis–Menten plot is *v vs.* [S], which creates a hyperbolic curve for monomeric enzymes. The Lineweaver–Burk plot, on the other hand, is $\frac{1}{v}$ *vs.* $\frac{1}{[S]}$, which creates a straight line.
3. K_m is a measure of an enzyme's affinity for its substrate, and is defined as the substrate concentration at which an enzyme is functioning at half of its maximal velocity. As K_m increases, an enzyme's affinity for its substrate decreases.
4. The *x*-intercept represents $-\frac{1}{K_m}$; the *y*-intercept represents $\frac{1}{v_{max}}$.
5. Cooperativity refers to the interactions between subunits in a multisubunit enzyme or protein. The binding of substrate to one subunit induces a change in the other subunits from the T (tense) state to the R (relaxed) state, which encourages binding of substrate to the other subunits. In the reverse direction, the unbinding of substrate from one subunit induces a change from R to T in the remaining subunits, promoting unbinding of substrate from the remaining subunits.

2.4

1. As temperature increases, enzyme activity generally increases (doubling approximately every 10°C). Above body temperature, however, enzyme activity quickly drops off as the enzyme denatures. Enzymes are maximally active within a small pH range; outside of this range, activity drops quickly with changes in pH as the ionization of the active site changes and the protein is denatured. Changes in salinity can disrupt bonds within an enzyme, causing disruption of tertiary and quaternary structure, which leads to loss of enzyme function.
2. Ideal temperature: 37°C = 98.6°F = 310 K

   Ideal pH for most enzymes is 7.4; for gastric enzymes, around 2; for pancreatic enzymes, around 8.5.

2.5

1. Feedback inhibition refers to the product of an enzymatic pathway turning off enzymes further back in that same pathway. This helps maintain homeostasis: as product levels rise, the pathway creating that product is appropriately downregulated.
2. A competitive inhibitor increases K_m because the substrate concentration has to be higher to reach half the maximum velocity in the presence of the inhibitor. A mixed inhibitor will increase K_m only if the inhibitor preferentially binds to the enzyme over the enzyme–substrate complex.
3. Irreversible inhibition refers to the prolonged or permanent inactivation of an enzyme, such that it cannot be easily renatured to gain function.
4. Examples of transient modifications include allosteric activation or inhibition. Examples of covalent modifications include phosphorylation and glycosylation.
5. Zymogens are precursors of active enzymes. It is critical that certain enzymes (like the digestive enzymes of the pancreas) remain inactive until arriving at their target site.

SCIENCE MASTERY ASSESSMENT EXPLANATIONS

1. **D**

Enzymes catalyze reactions by lowering their activation energy, and are not changed or consumed during the course of the reaction. While the activation energy is lowered, the free energy of the reaction, ΔG, remains unchanged in the presence of an enzyme. A reaction will continue to occur in the presence or absence of an enzyme; it simply runs slower without the enzyme, eliminating **(A)**. Most physiological reactions are optimized at body temperature, 37°C, eliminating **(B)**. Finally, dehydrogenases catalyze oxidation–reduction reactions, not transfer reactions, eliminating **(C)**.

2. **A**

Most enzymes in the human body operate at maximal activity around a temperature of 37°C and a pH of 7.4, which is the pH of most body fluids. In addition, as characterized by the Michaelis–Menten equation, enzymes form an enzyme–substrate complex, which can either dissociate back into the enzyme and substrate or proceed to form a product. So far, we can eliminate **(B)**, **(C)**, and **(D)**, so let's check **(A)**. An increase in the substrate concentration, while maintaining a constant enzyme concentration, leads to a proportional increase in the rate of the reaction only initially. However, once most of the active sites are occupied, the reaction rate levels off, regardless of further increases in substrate concentration. At high concentrations of substrate, the reaction rate approaches its maximal velocity and is no longer changed by further increases in substrate concentration.

3. **B**

An enzyme devoid of its necessary cofactor is called an apoenzyme and is catalytically inactive.

4. **A**

An enzyme's specificity is determined by the three-dimensional shape of its active site. Regardless of which explanation for enzyme specificity we are discussing (lock and key or induced fit), the active site determines which substrate the enzyme will react with.

5. **A**

As the temperature of the DNA polymerase sample increases from 0°C to the usual physiological temperature, i.e. 37°C, the enzyme's activity will increase. However, at temperatures above 37°C, the enzyme's activity will rapidly decline due to denaturation.

6. **D**

By limiting the activity of enzyme 1, the rest of the pathway is slowed, which is the definition of negative feedback. **(A)** is incorrect because there is no competition for the active site with allosteric interactions. While many products do indeed competitively inhibit an enzyme in the pathway that creates them, this is an example of an allosterically inhibited enzyme. There is not enough information for **(B)** to be correct because we aren't told whether the inhibition is reversible. In general, allosteric interactions are temporary. **(C)** is incorrect because it is the opposite of what occurs when enzyme 1 activity is reduced.

7. **A**

While the equations given in the text are useful, recognizing relationships is even more important. You can see that as substrate concentration increases significantly, there is only a small change in the rate. This occurs as we approach v_{max}. Because the v_{max} is near $100\ \frac{\text{mmol}}{\text{min}}$, $\frac{v_{max}}{2}$ equals $50\ \frac{\text{mmol}}{\text{min}}$. The substrate concentration giving this rate is 0.5 mM and corresponds to K_m; therefore, **(A)** is correct.

8. **A**

As with the last question, relationships are important. At a concentration of $5 \times 10^{-6}\ M$, enzyme A is working at one-half of its v_{max} because the concentration is equal to the K_m of the enzyme. Therefore, one-half of $20\ \frac{\text{mmol}}{\text{min}}$ is $10\ \frac{\text{mmol}}{\text{min}}$, which corresponds to **(A)**.

9. **C**

At a concentration of 5×10^{-4} *M*, there is 100 times more substrate than present at half maximal velocity. At high values (significantly larger than the value of K_m), the enzyme is at or near its v_{max}, which is $20\,\frac{\text{mmol}}{\text{min}}$.

10. **B**

Based on the graph, when the substrate is present, oseltamivir results in the same v_{max} and a higher K_m compared to when no inhibitor is added. These are hallmarks of competitive inhibitors. Noncompetitive inhibitors result in decreased v_{max} and the same K_m as the uninhibited reaction, which is shown by the zanamivir line in the graph. Because the question is only comparing the values between the two inhibitors, and not the enzyme without inhibitor, the mechanism of inhibition is less important to determine than the values of K_m and v_{max}. This is a great example of why previewing the answer choices works well in the sciences.

11. **C**

Lyases are responsible for the breakdown of a single molecule into two molecules without the addition of water or the transfer of electrons. Lyases often form cyclic compounds or double bonds in the products to accommodate this. Water was not a reactant, and no cofactor was mentioned; thus lyase, **(C)**, remains the best answer choice.

12. **D**

Enzymes are not altered by the process of catalysis. A molecule that breaks intramolecular bonds to provide activation energy would not be able to be reused.

13. **D**

Cooperative enzymes demonstrate a change in affinity for the substrate depending on how many substrate molecules are bound and whether the last change was accomplished because a substrate molecule was bound or left the active site of the enzyme. Because we cannot determine whether the most recent reaction was binding or dissociation, **(A)** and **(B)** are eliminated. We can make absolute comparisons though. For enzymes expressing positive cooperativity, the unbound enzyme has the lowest affinity for substrate, and the enzyme with all but one subunit bound has the highest. The increase in affinity is not necessarily linear. Furthermore, if all four sites have substrate bound, the enzyme cannot bind to any more substrate. Therefore, **(C)** is not true. An enzyme with two subunits occupied must have a higher affinity for the substrate than the same enzyme with only one subunit occupied; thus, **(D)** is correct.

14. **A**

Triglycerides are unlikely to act as coenzymes for a few reasons, including their large size, neutral charge, and ubiquity in cells. Cofactors and coenzymes tend to be small in size, such as metal ions like **(C)** or small organic molecules. They can usually carry a charge by ionization, protonation, or deprotonation. Finally, they are usually in low, tightly regulated concentrations within cells. Metabolic pathways would be expected to include both oxidation–reduction reactions and movement of functional groups, thus eliminating **(B)** and **(D)**.

15. **B**

The rate of reaction increases with temperature because of the increased kinetic energy of the reactants, but reaches a peak temperature because the enzyme denatures with the disruption of hydrogen bonds at excessively high temperatures. In the absence of enzyme, this peak temperature is generally much hotter. Heating a reaction provides molecules with an increased chance of achieving the activation energy, but the enzyme catalyst would typically reduce activation energy. Keep in mind that thermodynamics and kinetics are not interchangeable, so we are not considering the impact of heat on the equilibrium position.

Consult your online resources for additional practice. **GO ONLINE**

EQUATIONS TO REMEMBER

(2.1) **Michaelis–Menten rates:** $E + S \underset{k_{-1}}{\overset{k_1}{\rightleftharpoons}} ES \overset{k_{cat}}{\rightarrow} E + P$

(2.2) **Michaelis–Menten equation:** $v = \dfrac{v_{max}\,[S]}{K_m + [S]}$

(2.3) **Turnover number (k_{cat}):** $v_{max} = [E]k_{cat}$

SHARED CONCEPTS

Biochemistry Chapter 1
Amino Acids, Peptides, and Proteins

Biochemistry Chapter 12
Bioenergetics and Regulation of Metabolism

Biology Chapter 5
The Endocrine System

Biology Chapter 9
The Digestive System

General Chemistry Chapter 5
Chemical Kinetics

General Chemistry Chapter 7
Thermochemistry

General Chemistry Chapter 11
Oxidation–Reduction Reactions

CHAPTER 3

NONENZYMATIC PROTEIN FUNCTION AND PROTEIN ANALYSIS

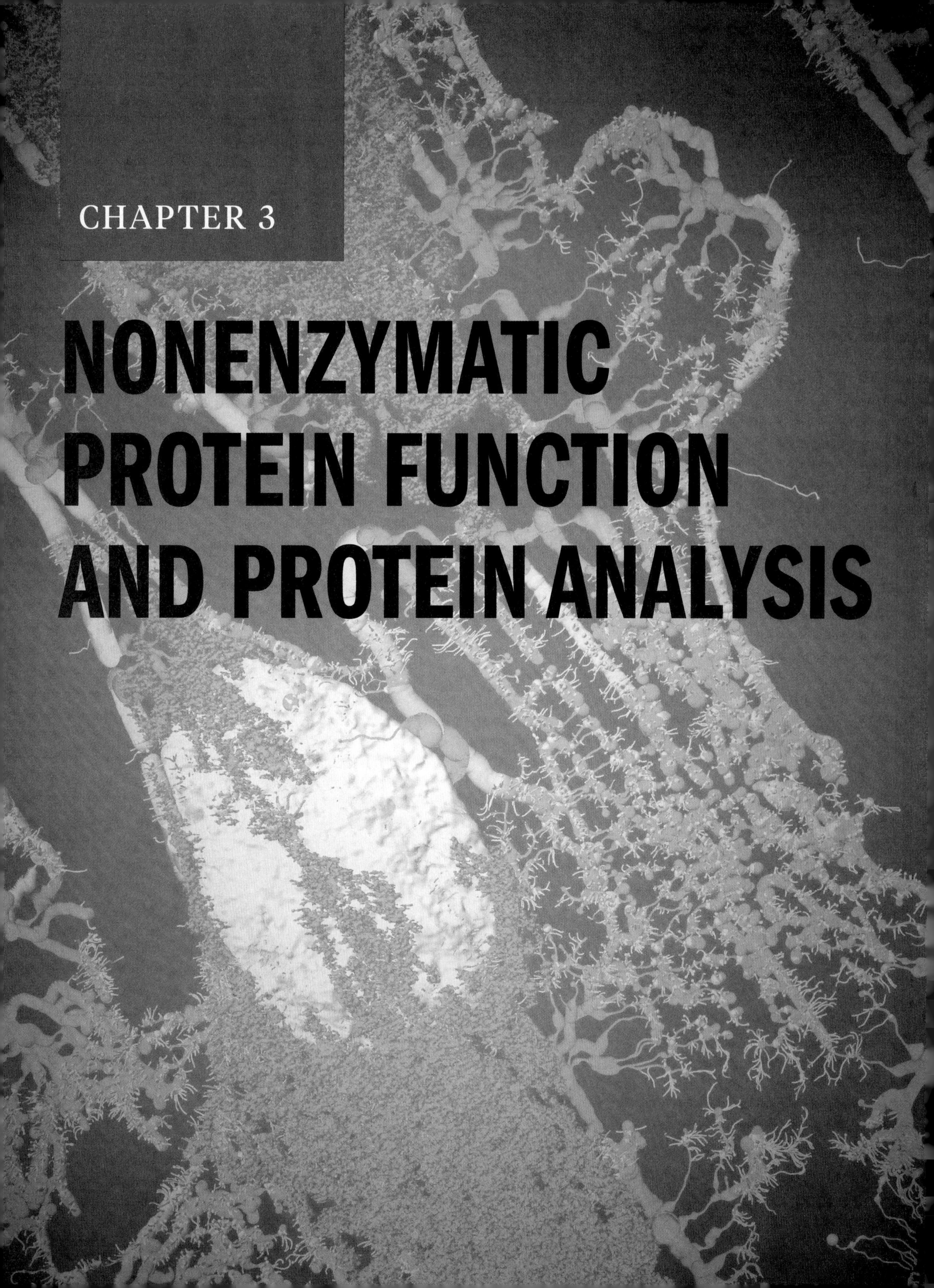

SCIENCE MASTERY ASSESSMENT

Every pre-med knows this feeling: there is so much content I have to know for the MCAT! How do I know what to do first or what's important?

While the high-yield badges throughout this book will help you identify the most important topics, this Science Mastery Assessment is another tool in your MCAT prep arsenal. This quiz (which can also be taken in your online resources) and the guidance below will help ensure that you are spending the appropriate amount of time on this chapter based on your personal strengths and weaknesses. Don't worry though—skipping something now does not mean you'll never study it. Later on in your prep, as you complete full-length tests, you'll uncover specific pieces of content that you need to review and can come back to these chapters as appropriate.

How to Use This Assessment

If you answer 0–7 questions correctly:

Spend about 1 hour to read this chapter in full and take limited notes throughout. Follow up by reviewing **all** quiz questions to ensure that you now understand how to solve each one.

If you answer 8–11 questions correctly:

Spend 20–40 minutes reviewing the quiz questions. Beginning with the questions you missed, read and take notes on the corresponding subchapters. For questions you answered correctly, ensure your thinking matches that of the explanation and you understand why each choice was correct or incorrect.

If you answer 12–15 questions correctly:

Spend less than 20 minutes reviewing all questions from the quiz. If you missed any, then include a quick read-through of the corresponding subchapters, or even just the relevant content within a subchapter, as part of your question review. For questions you got correct, ensure your thinking matches that of the explanation and review the Concept Summary at the end of the chapter.

1. At what pH can protein A best be obtained through electrophoresis? (Note: MM = molar mass)

Protein	pI	MM
Protein A	4.5	25,000
Protein B	6.0	10,000
Protein C	9.5	12,000

   A. 2.5
   B. 3.5
   C. 4.5
   D. 5.5

2. What is the function of sodium dodecyl sulfate (SDS) in SDS-PAGE?
   A. SDS stabilizes the gel matrix, improving resolution during electrophoresis.
   B. SDS solubilizes proteins to give them uniformly negative charges, so the separation is based purely on size.
   C. SDS raises the pH of the gel, separating multiunit proteins into individual subunits.
   D. SDS solubilizes proteins to give them uniformly positive charges, so separation is based purely on pH.

3. Which of the following is NOT involved in cell migration?
   A. Dynein
   B. Flagella
   C. Actin
   D. Centrioles

4. Which of the following proteins is most likely to be found extracellularly?
   A. Tubulin
   B. Myosin
   C. Collagen
   D. Actin

5. Hormones are found in the body in very low concentrations, but tend to have a strong effect. What type of receptor are hormones most likely to act on?
   I. Ligand-gated ion channels
   II. Enzyme-linked receptors
   III. G protein-coupled receptors

   A. I only
   B. III only
   C. II and III only
   D. I, II, and III

6. Which of the following is most likely to be found bound to a protein in the body?
   A. Sodium
   B. Potassium
   C. Chloride
   D. Calcium

7. Which of the following characteristics is NOT attributed to antibodies?
   A. Antibodies bind to more than one distinct antigen.
   B. Antibodies label antigens for targeting by other immune cells.
   C. Antibodies can cause agglutination by interaction with antigen.
   D. Antibodies have two heavy chains and two light chains.

8. Which ion channels are responsible for maintaining the resting membrane potential?

A. Ungated channels
B. Voltage-gated channels
C. Ligand-gated channels
D. No ion channels are involved in maintenance of the resting membrane potential.

9. Which of the following is NOT a component of all trimeric G proteins?

A. G_α
B. G_β
C. G_γ
D. G_i

10. Which of the following methods would be best to separate large quantities of the following proteins? (Note: MM = molar mass)

Protein	pI	MM
Protein A	6.5	28,000
Protein B	6.3	70,000
Protein C	6.6	200,000

A. Ion-exchange chromatography
B. Size-exclusion chromatography
C. Isoelectric focusing
D. Native PAGE

11. Which amino acids contribute most significantly to the pI of a protein?

I. Lysine
II. Glycine
III. Arginine

A. I only
B. I and II only
C. I and III only
D. II and III only

12. How does the gel for isoelectric focusing differ from the gel for traditional electrophoresis?

A. Isoelectric focusing uses a gel with much larger pore sizes to allow for complete migration.
B. Isoelectric focusing uses a gel with SDS added to encourage a uniform negative charge.
C. Isoelectric focusing uses a gel with a pH gradient that encourages a variable charge.
D. The gel is unchanged in isoelectric focusing; the protein mixture is treated before loading.

13. Which protein properties allow UV spectroscopy to be used as a method of determining concentration?

A. Proteins have partially planar characteristics in peptide bonds.
B. Globular proteins cause scattering of light.
C. Proteins contain aromatic groups in certain amino acids.
D. All organic macromolecules can be assessed with UV spectroscopy.

14. A protein collected through affinity chromatography displays no activity even though it is found to have a high concentration using the Bradford protein assay. What best explains these findings?

A. The Bradford reagent was prepared incorrectly.
B. The active site is occupied by free ligand.
C. The protein is bound to the column.
D. The protein does not catalyze the reaction of interest.

15. What property of protein-digesting enzymes allows for a sequence to be determined without fully degrading the protein?

A. Selectivity
B. Sensitivity
C. Turnover
D. Inhibition

Answer Key

1. **D**
2. **B**
3. **D**
4. **C**
5. **C**
6. **D**
7. **A**
8. **A**
9. **D**
10. **B**
11. **C**
12. **C**
13. **C**
14. **B**
15. **A**

Detailed explanations can be found at the end of the chapter.

CHAPTER 3

NONENZYMATIC PROTEIN FUNCTION AND PROTEIN ANALYSIS

In This Chapter

CHAPTER PROFILE

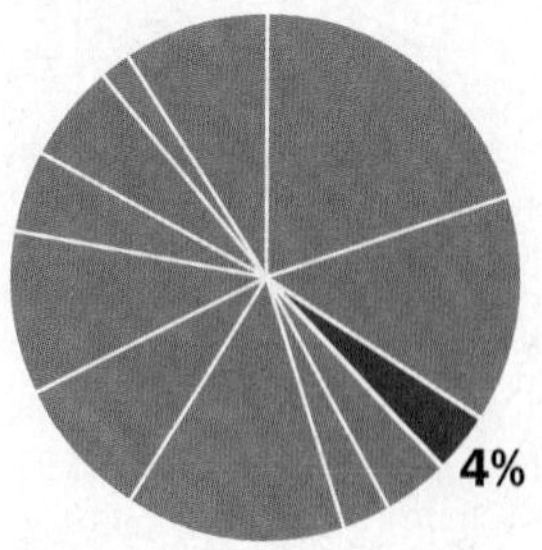

The content in this chapter should be relevant to about 4% of all questions about biochemistry on the MCAT.

This chapter covers material from the following AAMC content categories:

1A: Structure and function of proteins and their constituent amino acids

3A: Structure and functions of the nervous and endocrine systems, and ways in which these systems coordinate the organ systems

5C: Separation and purification methods

5D: Structure, function, and reactivity of biologically relevant molecules

Introduction

Did you ever wonder why some athletes eat raw eggs when training? It doesn't help with digestion or increase enzymatic activity throughout the body; rather, all that protein is used for muscle building. While muscle building does increase cytoplasm and all of the enzymes found therein, the biggest increase is seen in structural and motor proteins like actin and myosin. Valid concerns about bacteria in and on eggs have stopped most athletes from drinking raw eggs, but protein shakes and massive containers of whey protein have replaced them on the shelves of health-food stores, pharmacies, and supermarkets.

In this chapter, we will examine some of the structural and motor proteins that athletes love to build, as well as more complex protein functions in humans, including biosignaling. Finally, we'll learn how to determine which proteins—and their concentrations—are in those eggs through separation and quantitative analysis.

3.1 Cellular Functions

LEARNING OBJECTIVES

After Chapter 3.1, you will be able to:

- Compare and contrast cytoskeletal proteins and motor proteins
- Associate collagen, elastin, keratins, actin, and tubulin with their major functions
- Describe the adhesive properties of cadherins, integrins, and selectins
- Predict the possible outcomes of an antibody binding to its antigen

Typical functions provided by proteins within the cell include supporting cellular shape and organization and acting as enzymes. The enzymatic functions of proteins were detailed in Chapter 2 of *MCAT Biochemistry Review* and we are now ready to look at other protein functions. Structural and motor proteins are found in abundance within individual cells and are also found in the extracellular matrix.

Structural Proteins

The cytoskeleton can be thought of as a three-dimensional web or scaffolding system for the cell. It is comprised of proteins that are anchored to the cell membrane by embedded protein complexes. In addition to intracellular support, extracellular matrices composed of proteins also support the tissues of the body. Tendons, ligaments, cartilage, and basement membranes are all proteinaceous. The primary structural proteins in the body are collagen, elastin, keratin, actin, and tubulin. Structural proteins generally have highly repetitive secondary structure and a supersecondary structure—a repetitive organization of secondary structural elements together sometimes referred to as a **motif**. This regularity gives many structural proteins a fibrous nature.

Collagen

Collagen has a characteristic trihelical fiber (three left-handed helices woven together to form a secondary right-handed helix) and makes up most of the extracellular matrix of connective tissue. It is found throughout the body and is important in providing strength and flexibility.

REAL WORLD

The importance of the structure of collagen is highlighted in the disorder *osteogenesis imperfecta*, also referred to as brittle bone disease. Collagen—a major component of bone—forms a unique and specific secondary helical structure based on the abundance of the amino acid glycine. The replacement of glycine with other amino acids can cause improper folding of the collagen protein and cell death, leading to bone fragility.

Elastin

Elastin is another important component of the extracellular matrix of connective tissue. Its primary role is to stretch and then recoil like a spring, which restores the original shape of the tissue.

Keratins

Keratins are intermediate filament proteins found in epithelial cells. Keratins contribute to the mechanical integrity of the cell and also function as regulatory proteins. Keratin is the primary protein that makes up hair and nails.

Actin

Actin is a protein that makes up microfilaments and the thin filaments in myofibrils. It is the most abundant protein in eukaryotic cells. Actin proteins have a positive side and a negative side; this polarity allows motor proteins to travel unidirectionally along an actin filament, like a one-way street.

Tubulin

Tubulin is the protein that makes up microtubules. Microtubules are important for providing structure, chromosome separation in mitosis and meiosis, and intracellular transport with kinesin and dynein, described in the next section. Like actin, tubulin has polarity: the negative end of a microtubule is usually located adjacent to the nucleus, whereas the positive end is usually in the periphery of a cell.

Motor Proteins

Some structural proteins also have motor functions in the presence of motor proteins. The motile cilia and flagella of bacteria and sperm are prime examples, as is the contraction of the sarcomere in muscle. **Motor proteins** also display enzymatic activity, acting as **ATPases** that power the conformational change necessary for motor function. Motor proteins have transient interactions with either actin or microtubules.

Myosin is the primary motor protein that interacts with actin. In addition to its role as the thick filament in a myofibril, myosin can be involved in cellular transport. Each myosin subunit has a single head and neck; movement at the neck is responsible for the power stroke of sarcomere contraction.

Kinesins and **dyneins** are the motor proteins associated with microtubules. They have two heads, at least one of which remains attached to tubulin at all times. Kinesins play key roles in aligning chromosomes during metaphase and depolymerizing microtubules during anaphase of mitosis. Dyneins are involved in the sliding movement of cilia and flagella. Both proteins are important for vesicle transport in the cell, but have opposite polarities: kinesins bring vesicles toward the positive end of the microtubule, and dyneins bring vesicles toward the negative end. In neurons, we see a classic example of these motor proteins' polarities. Kinesins bring vesicles of neurotransmitter to the positive end of the axonal microtubules (toward the synaptic terminal). In contrast, dyneins bring vesicles of waste or recycled neurotransmitter back toward the negative end of the microtubule (toward the soma) through retrograde transport. The activity of kinesins is illustrated in Figure 3.1 below.

BRIDGE

Motor proteins are responsible for muscle contraction and cellular movement. Take a moment to review sarcomere structure in Chapter 11 of *MCAT Biology Review* as another example of the interaction between motor proteins and the cytoskeleton.

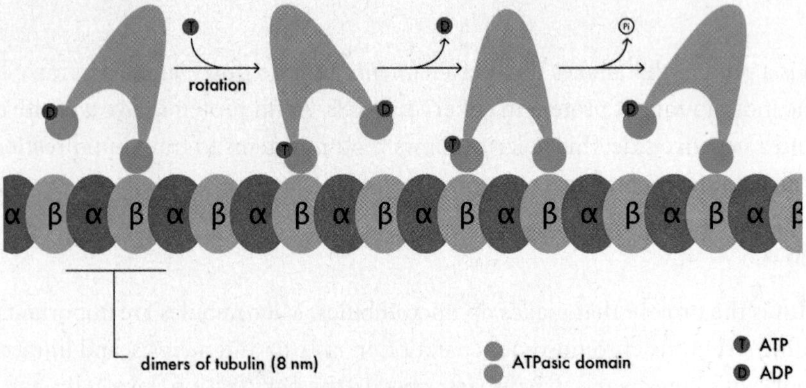

Figure 3.1 Stepwise Activity of Kinesins
Kinesins move along microtubules in a stepping motion such that one or both heads remain attached at all times.

Binding Proteins

While proteins primarily exert enzymatic or structural functions within the cell, they also can have stabilizing functions in individual cells and the body. Proteins that act in this way transport or sequester molecules by binding to them. **Binding proteins** include hemoglobin, calcium-binding proteins, DNA-binding proteins (often transcription factors), and others. Each binding protein has an affinity curve for its molecule of interest; the oxyhemoglobin dissociation curve is one well-known example. This curve differs depending on the goal of the binding protein. When sequestration of a molecule is the goal, the binding protein usually has high affinity for its target across a large range of concentrations so it can keep it bound at nearly 100 percent. A transport protein, which must be able to bind or unbind its target to maintain steady-state concentrations, is likely to have varying affinity depending on the environmental conditions.

Cell Adhesion Molecules

Cell adhesion molecules (**CAMs**) are proteins found on the surface of most cells and aid in binding the cell to the extracellular matrix or other cells. While there are a number of different types of CAMs, they are all integral membrane proteins. Adhesion molecules can be classified into three major families: cadherins, integrins, and selectins.

Cadherins

Cadherins are a group of glycoproteins that mediate calcium-dependent cell adhesion. Cadherins often hold similar cell types together, such as epithelial cells. Different cells usually have type-specific cadherins; for example, epithelial cells use E-cadherin while nerve cells use N-cadherin.

Integrins

Integrins are a group of proteins that all have two membrane-spanning chains called α and β. These chains are very important in binding to and communicating with the extracellular matrix. Integrins also play a very important role in cellular signaling and can greatly impact cellular function by promoting cell division, apoptosis, or other processes. For example, integrin $\alpha_{IIb}\beta_3$ allows platelets to stick to fibrinogen, a clotting factor, which causes activation of platelets to stabilize the clot. Other integrins are used for white blood cell migration, stabilization of epithelium on its basement membrane, and other processes.

Selectins

Selectins are unique because they bind to carbohydrate molecules that project from other cell surfaces. These bonds are the weakest formed by the CAMs discussed here. Selectins are expressed on white blood cells and the endothelial cells that line blood vessels. Like integrins, they play an important role in host defense, including inflammation and white blood cell migration, as shown in Figure 3.2.

REAL WORLD

Many medications target selectins and integrins. For example, research has shown that the ability of cancer cells to metastasize (break away from a tumor and invade other distant tissues) is associated with unique expression patterns of CAMs. By targeting these CAMs, metastasis may be avoided. To stop the clotting process during heart attacks, other medications target CAMs used by platelets.

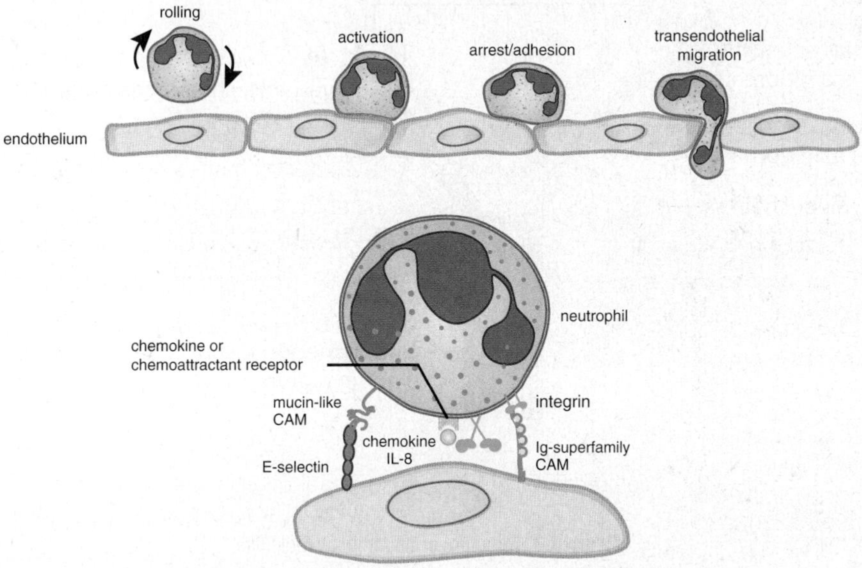

Figure 3.2 White Blood Cell Migration Using Selectins and Integrins
Many other proteins are involved in white blood cell migration, but are outside the scope of the MCAT.

Immunoglobulins

The immune system is very complex and is made up of many different types of cells and proteins. These cells and proteins have a common purpose: to rid the body of foreign invaders. The most prominent type of protein found in the immune system is the antibody. **Antibodies**, also called **immunoglobulins** (**Ig**) are proteins produced by B-cells that function to neutralize targets in the body, such as toxins and bacteria, and then recruit other cells to help eliminate the threat. Antibodies are Y-shaped proteins that are made up of two identical heavy chains and two identical light chains, as shown in Figure 3.3. Disulfide linkages and noncovalent interactions hold the heavy and light chains together. Each antibody has an **antigen-binding region** at the tips of the "Y." Within this region, there are specific polypeptide sequences that will bind one, and only one, specific antigenic sequence. The remaining part of the antibody molecule is known as the constant region, which is involved in recruitment and binding of other cells of the immune system, such as macrophages. Thus, when antibodies bind to their targets, called **antigens**, they can cause one of three outcomes:

- Neutralizing the antigen, making the pathogen or toxin unable to exert its effect on the body
- Marking the pathogen for destruction by other white blood cells immediately; this marking function is also called **opsonization**
- Clumping together (**agglutinating**) the antigen and antibody into large insoluble protein complexes that can be phagocytized and digested by macrophages

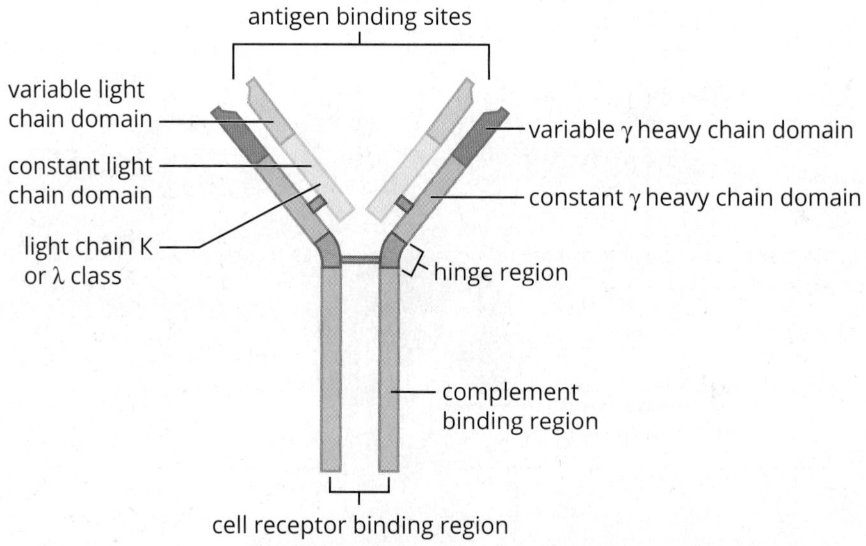

Figure 3.3 Structure of an Antibody Molecule

MCAT CONCEPT CHECK 3.1

Before you move on, assess your understanding of the material with these questions.

1. How do cytoskeletal proteins differ from motor proteins?

____

2. True or False: Motor proteins are not enzymes.

3. What could permit a binding protein involved in sequestration to have a low affinity for its substrate and still have a high percentage of substrate bound?

____

4. What are the three main classes of cell adhesion molecules? What type of adhesion does each class form?

Cell Adhesion Molecule	Type of Adhesion

5. When an antibody binds to its antigen, what are the three possible outcomes of this interaction?

1. ____
2. ____
3. ____

3.2 Biosignaling

LEARNING OBJECTIVES

After Chapter 3.2, you will be able to:

- Contrast enzyme-linked receptors with G protein-coupled receptors
- Distinguish between ungated channels, voltage-gated channels, and ligand-gated channels
- Recognize key features of transport kinetics and biosignaling processes

Biosignaling is a process in which cells receive and act on signals. Proteins participate in biosignaling in different capacities, including acting as extracellular ligands, transporters for facilitated diffusion, receptor proteins, and second messengers. The proteins involved in biosignaling can have functions in substrate binding or enzymatic activity.

Ion Channels

Ion channels are proteins that create specific pathways for charged molecules. They are classified into three main groups that have different mechanisms of opening, but that all permit facilitated diffusion of charged particles. **Facilitated diffusion**, a type of passive transport, is the diffusion of molecules down a concentration gradient through a pore in the membrane created by this transmembrane protein. It is used for molecules that are impermeable to the membrane (large, polar, or charged). Facilitated diffusion allows integral membrane proteins to serve as channels for these substrates to avoid the hydrophobic fatty acid tails of the phospholipid bilayer. The three main types of ion channels are ungated, voltage-gated, and ligand-gated.

REAL WORLD

Hundreds of ion channels have been identified that function in cell signaling and cell excitability. In addition, ion channels are drug targets in the treatment of everything from heart disease (calcium channel blockers) to seizures (sodium channel blockers) to irritable bowel syndrome (acetylcholine receptor/cation channel blockers).

Ungated Channels

As their name suggests, **ungated channels** have no gates and are therefore unregulated. For example, all cells possess ungated potassium channels. This means there will be a net efflux of potassium ions through these channels unless potassium is at equilibrium.

Voltage-Gated Channels

In **voltage-gated channels**, the gate is regulated by the membrane potential change near the channel. For example, many excitable cells such as neurons possess voltage-gated sodium channels. The channels are closed under resting conditions, but membrane depolarization causes a protein conformation change that allows them to quickly open and then quickly close as the voltage increases. Voltage-gated nonspecific sodium–potassium channels are found in cells of the sinoatrial node of the heart. Here, they serve as the pacemaker current; as the voltage drops, these channels open to bring the cell back to threshold and fire another action potential, as shown in Figure 3.4.

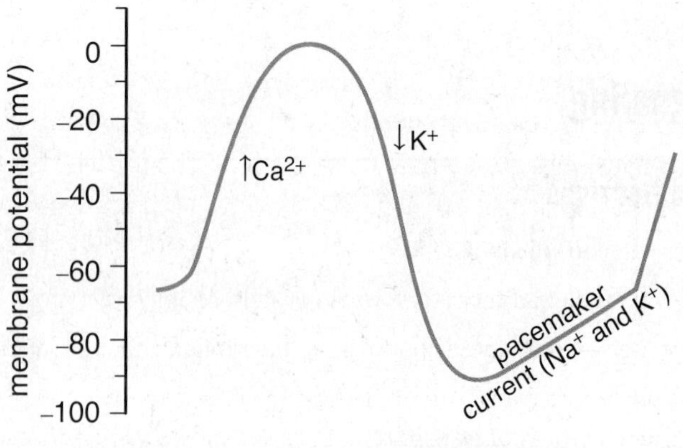

Figure 3.4 Action Potential of the Sinoatrial Node

Ligand-Gated Channels

For **ligand-gated channels**, the binding of a specific substance or ligand to the channel causes it to open or close. For example, neurotransmitters act at ligand-gated channels at the postsynaptic membrane: the inhibitory neurotransmitter γ-aminobutyric acid (GABA) binds to a chloride channel and opens it.

The K_m and v_{max} parameters that apply to enzymes are also applicable to transporters such as ion channels in membranes. The kinetics of transport can be derived from the Michaelis–Menten and Lineweaver–Burk equations, where K_m refers to the solute concentration at which the transporter is functioning at half of its maximum activity.

BRIDGE

The activity at the neuromuscular junction and most chemical synapses relies on ligand-gated ion channels. The nervous system especially makes use of this type of gating, as well as voltage-gated ion channels, as discussed in Chapter 4 of *MCAT Biology Review*.

Enzyme-Linked Receptors

Membrane receptors may also display catalytic activity in response to ligand binding. These **enzyme-linked receptors** have three primary protein domains: a membrane-spanning domain, a ligand-binding domain, and a catalytic domain. The **membrane-spanning domain** anchors the receptor in the cell membrane. The **ligand-binding domain** is stimulated by the appropriate ligand and induces a conformational change that activates the **catalytic domain.** This often results in the initiation of a **second messenger cascade.** *Receptor tyrosine kinases* (RTK) are classic examples. RTKs are composed of a monomer that dimerizes upon ligand binding. The dimer is the active form that phosphorylates additional cellular enzymes, including the receptor itself (autophosphorylation). Other classes of enzyme-linked receptors include *serine/threonine-specific protein kinases* and *receptor tyrosine phosphatases.*

KEY CONCEPT

Biosignaling can take advantage of either existing gradients (ion channels) or second messenger cascades (enzyme-linked receptors and G protein-coupled receptors).

G Protein-Coupled Receptors

G protein-coupled receptors (**GPCR**) are a large family of integral membrane proteins involved in signal transduction. They are characterized by their seven membrane-spanning α-helices. The receptors differ in specificity of the ligand-binding area found on the extracellular surface of the cell. In order for GPCRs to transmit signals to an effector in the cell, they utilize a **heterotrimeric G protein.** G proteins are named for their intracellular link to guanine nucleotides (GDP and GTP). The binding of a ligand increases the affinity of the receptor for the G protein. The binding of the G protein represents a switch to the active state and affects the intracellular signaling pathway. There are several different G proteins that can result in either stimulation or inhibition of the signaling pathway. There are three main types of G proteins:

- G_s stimulates adenylate cyclase, which increases levels of cAMP in the cell.
- G_i inhibits adenylate cyclase, which decreases levels of cAMP in the cell.
- G_q activates *phospholipase* C, which cleaves a phospholipid from the membrane to form PIP_2. PIP_2 is then cleaved into DAG and IP_3; IP_3 can open calcium channels in the endoplasmic reticulum, increasing calcium levels in the cell.

MNEMONIC

Functions of heterotrimeric G proteins:

- G_s **s**timulates.
- G_i **i**nhibits.
- "Mind your **p**'s and **q**'s": G_q activates **p**hospholipase C.

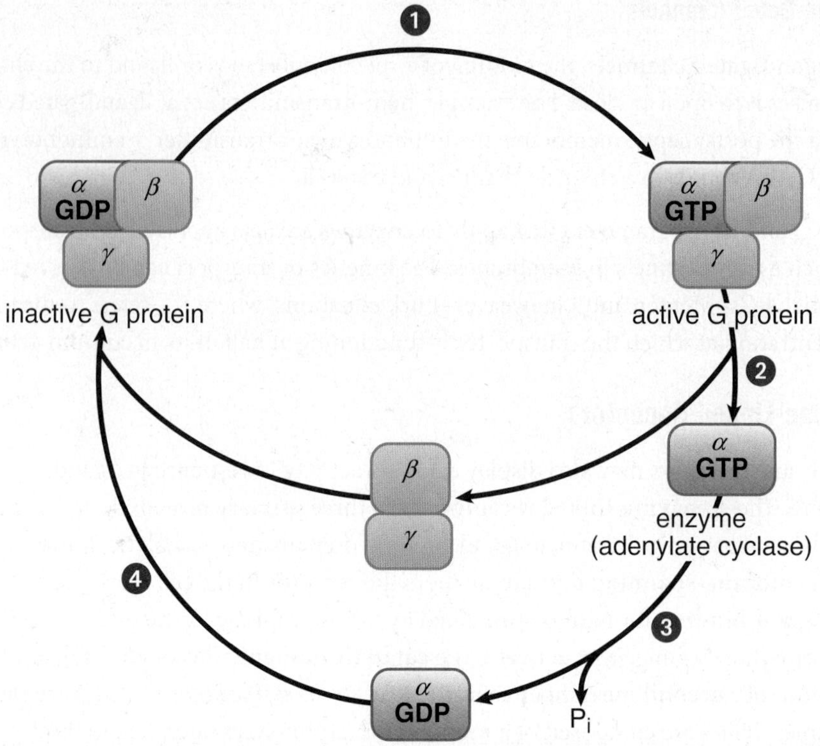

Figure 3.5 Trimeric G Protein Cycle (G_s or G_i)

The three subunits that comprise the G protein are α, β, and γ. In its inactive form, the **α subunit** binds GDP and is in a complex with the **β and γ subunits**. When a ligand binds to the GPCR, the receptor becomes activated and, in turn, engages the corresponding G protein, as shown in Step 1 of Figure 3.5. Once GDP is replaced with GTP, the α subunit is able to dissociate from the β and γ subunits (Step 2). The activated α subunit alters the activity of ***adenylate cyclase***. If the α subunit is α_s, then the enzyme is activated; if the α subunit is α_i, then the enzyme is inhibited. Once GTP on the activated α subunit is dephosphorylated to GDP (Step 3), the α subunit will rebind to the β and γ subunits (Step 4), rendering the G protein inactive.

MCAT CONCEPT CHECK 3.2

Before you move on, assess your understanding of the material with these questions.

1. Contrast enzyme-linked receptors with G protein-coupled receptors:

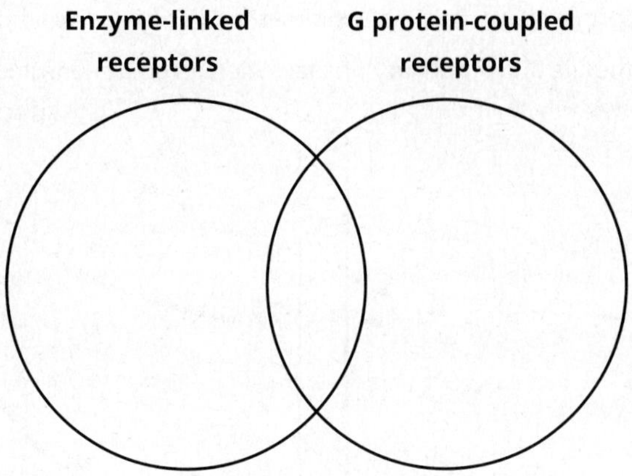

2. What type of ion channel is active at all times?

____

3. How do transport kinetics differ from enzyme kinetics?

____

3.3 Protein Isolation

High-Yield

LEARNING OBJECTIVES

After Chapter 3.3, you will be able to:

- Recall the major categories of electrophoresis and chromatography
- Select the appropriate protein isolation method in a given situation
- Identify the mobile and stationary phases when given a separatory apparatus:

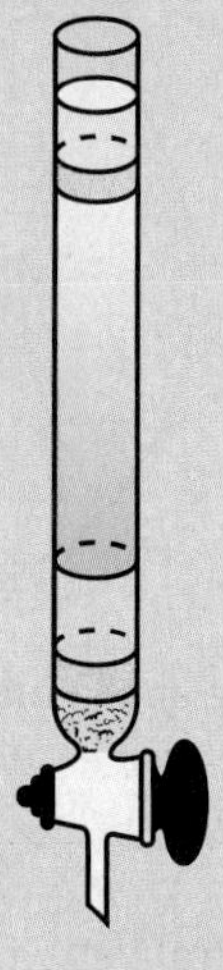

In order to better understand a specific protein, it is important to be able to isolate the protein for study. The purification of proteins can be considered an art form when one considers the difficulty of isolating just one protein from a cell containing hundreds to thousands of proteins. Luckily, as Chapter 1 of *MCAT Biochemistry Review* highlighted, there is a great amount of variation in the physical and chemical properties of proteins and these differences can be exploited in order to purify the protein of interest. Proteins and other biomolecules are isolated from body tissues or cell cultures by cell lysis and **homogenization**—crushing, grinding, or blending the tissue of interest into an evenly mixed solution. **Centrifugation** can then isolate proteins from much smaller molecules before other isolation techniques must be employed. The most common isolation techniques are electrophoresis and chromatography, either of which can be used for native or denatured proteins.

Electrophoresis

One method of separating proteins is with **electrophoresis**. In molecular biology, this is one of the most important analytical techniques. Electrophoresis works by subjecting compounds to an electric field, which moves them according to their net charge and size. Negatively charged compounds will migrate toward the positively charged anode, and positively charged compounds will migrate toward the negatively charged cathode. The velocity of this migration, known as the **migration velocity** of a molecule, **v**, is directly proportional to the electric field strength, **E**, and to the net charge on the molecule, z, and is inversely proportional to a frictional coefficient, f, which depends on the mass and shape of the migrating molecules:

$$v = \frac{Ez}{f}$$

Equation 3.1

Polyacrylamide gel is the standard medium for protein electrophoresis. The gel is a slightly porous matrix mixture, which solidifies at room temperature. Proteins travel through this matrix in relation to their size and charge. The gel acts like a sieve, allowing smaller particles to pass through easily while retaining large particles. Therefore, a molecule will move faster through the medium if it is small, highly charged, or placed in a large electric field. Conversely, molecules will migrate slower (or not at all) when they are bigger and more convoluted, electrically neutral, or placed in a small electric field. The size of a standard polyacrylamide gel allows multiple samples to be run simultaneously, as shown in Figure 3.6.

BRIDGE

Electrophoresis uses an electrolytic cell ($\Delta G > 0$, $E_{cell} < 0$), as described in Chapter 12 of *MCAT General Chemistry Review*. Remember that anions always move toward the anode and cations always move toward the cathode.

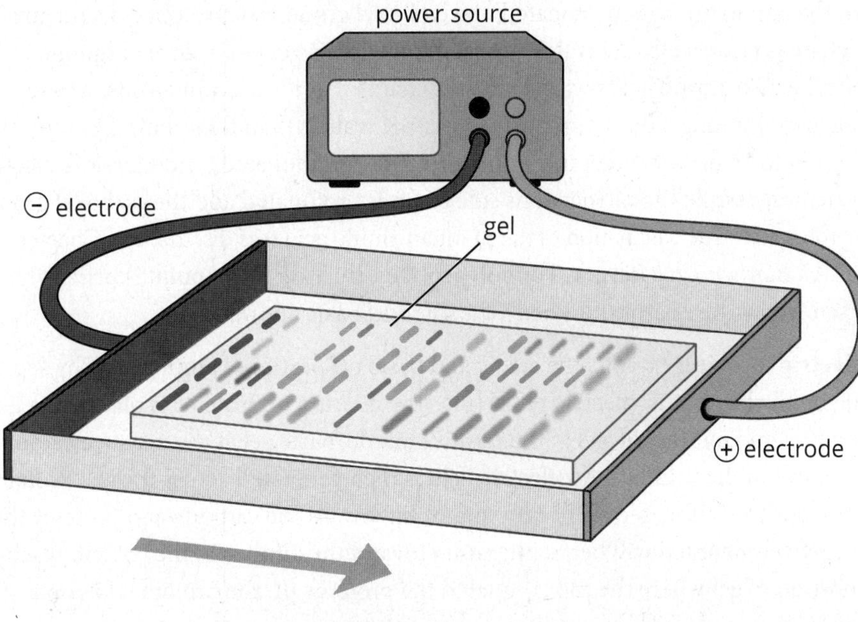

Figure 3.6 Electrophoresis
As an electrolytic (nonspontaneous) cell, electrophoresis moves charged particles toward their respective oppositely charged electrodes; the larger the particle, the more slowly it migrates.

Native PAGE

Polyacrylamide gel electrophoresis (**PAGE**) is a method for analyzing proteins in their native states. Unfortunately, PAGE is limited by the varying mass-to-charge and mass-to-size ratios of cellular proteins because multiple different proteins may experience the same level of migration. In PAGE, the functional native protein can be recovered from the gel after electrophoresis, but only if the gel has not been stained because most stains denature proteins. PAGE is most useful to compare the molecular size or the charge of proteins known to be similar in size from other analytic methods like SDS-PAGE (described below) or size-exclusion chromatography.

SDS-PAGE

MCAT EXPERTISE

For analytic purposes, protein atomic mass is typically expressed in **daltons (Da)**. A dalton is an alternative term for molar mass $\left(\frac{g}{mol}\right)$. The average molar mass of one amino acid is ~100 daltons, or 100 $\frac{g}{mol}$.

Sodium dodecyl sulfate (SDS)–polyacrylamide gel electrophoresis is a useful tool because it separates proteins on the basis of relative molecular mass alone. The SDS-PAGE technique starts with the premise of PAGE but adds SDS, a detergent that disrupts all noncovalent interactions. It binds to proteins and creates large chains with net negative charges, thereby neutralizing the protein's original charge and denaturing the protein. As the proteins move through the gel, the only variables affecting their velocity are **E**, the electric field strength, and *f*, the frictional coefficient, which depends on mass. After separation, the gel can be stained so the protein bands can be visualized and the results recorded.

Isoelectric Focusing

Proteins can be separated on the basis of their **isoelectric point (pI)**. The pI is the pH at which the protein or amino acid is electrically neutral, with an equal number of positive and negative charges. For individual amino acids this electrically neutral form is called a ***zwitterion***. For most amino acids, the zwitterion form occurs when the amino group is protonated, the carboxyl group is deprotonated, and any side chain is electrically neutral. The exceptions to this general rule are arginine and lysine, two amino acids with basic side chains. For these amino acids, whose nitrogen-containing side chains have higher pK_a values than their amino groups, the zwitterion form occurs when the amino group is deprotonated (and therefore electrically neutral), while the nitrogenous side chain is protonated and the carboxyl group is deprotonated. The calculation of the pI for an amino acid was discussed in Chapter 1 of *MCAT Biochemistry Review*. For polypeptides, the isoelectric point is primarily determined by the relative numbers of acidic and basic amino acids.

KEY CONCEPT

In isoelectric focusing, a protein stops moving when pH = pI.

Isoelectric focusing exploits the acidic and basic properties of amino acids by separating on the basis of isoelectric point (pI). The mixture of proteins is placed in a gel with a pH gradient (acidic gel at the positive anode, basic gel at the negative cathode, and neutral in the middle). An electric field is then generated across the gel. Proteins that are positively charged will begin migrating toward the cathode and proteins that are negatively charged will begin migrating toward the anode. As the protein reaches the portion of gel where the pH is equal to the protein's pI, the protein takes on a neutral charge and will stop moving.

MNEMONIC

Anode in isoelectric focusing: **A+**
Anode has **a**cidic (H^+-rich) gel and a (+) charge.

Let's take a deeper look and see how this works. We'll start with a protein that has a pI of 9. When the protein is in an environment with a pH of 9, it will carry no net charge. If we place this protein onto the gel at a pH of 7, there will be more protons around the protein. These protons will attach to the available basic sites on the protein, creating a net positive charge on the molecule. This charge will then cause the protein to be attracted to the negatively charged cathode, which is located on the basic side of the gradient. As the protein moves closer to the cathode, the pH of the gel slowly increases. Eventually, as the protein nears a pH of 9, the protons creating the positive charge will dissociate, and the protein will become neutral again. A quick way to remember the pH of each end of the gel is to recall that we associate acids with protons, which carry a positive charge, and thus the anode is positively charged. We associate bases with the negatively charged hydroxide ion, which gives us the negatively charged cathode.

Chromatography

Chromatography is another tool that uses physical and chemical properties to separate and identify compounds from a complex mixture. Chromatography refers to a variety of techniques that require the homogenized protein mixture to be fractionated through a porous matrix. One of the reasons chromatography is a valuable tool is that the isolated proteins are immediately available for identification and quantification. In all forms of chromatography discussed here, the concept is identical: the more similar the compound is to its surroundings (by polarity, charge, and so on), the more it will stick to and move slowly through its surroundings. Chromatography is preferred over electrophoresis when large amounts of protein are being separated.

BRIDGE

Chromatography and other separatory methods are also discussed in Chapter 12 of *MCAT Organic Chemistry Review*.

The process begins by placing the sample onto a solid medium called the **stationary phase** or **adsorbent**. The next step is to run the mobile phase through the stationary phase. This will allow the sample to run through the stationary phase, or **elute**. Depending on the relative affinity of the sample for the stationary and mobile phases, different substances will migrate through at different speeds. That is, components that have a high affinity for the stationary phase will barely migrate at all; components with a high affinity for the mobile phase will migrate much more quickly. The amount of time a compound spends in the stationary phase is referred to as the **retention time**. Varying retention times of each compound in the solution results in separation of the components within the stationary phase, or **partitioning**, as demonstrated in Figure 3.7. Each component can then be isolated individually for study.

KEY CONCEPT

All chromatography is about the affinity of a substance for the mobile and stationary phases, except for size-exclusion chromatography.

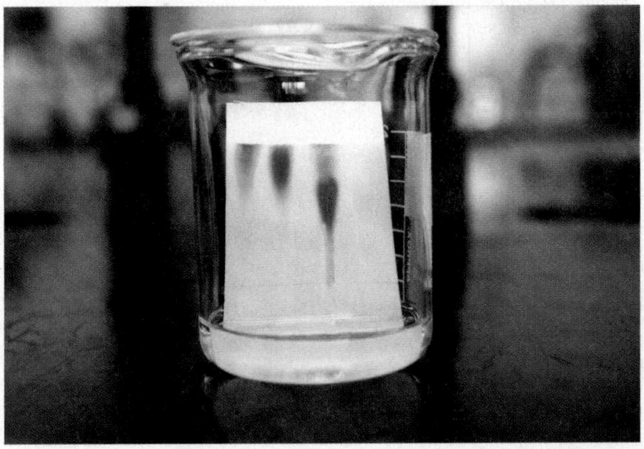

Figure 3.7 Partitioning of Black Ink
Thin-layer chromatography; original spot placed on the bottom of the card. Components with high retention times remain near the bottom of the card; components with low retention times have migrated toward the top of the card.

We can use myriad different media as our stationary phase, each one exploiting different properties that allow us to separate out our compound. In chromatography for protein separation, common properties include charge, pore size, and specific affinities.

Column Chromatography

In **column chromatography**, a column is filled with silica or alumina beads as an adsorbent, and gravity moves the solvent and compounds down the column, shown in Figure 3.8. As the solution flows through the column, both size and polarity have a role in determining how quickly a compound moves through the polar silica or alumina beads: the less polar the compound, the faster it can elute through the column (short retention time). In column chromatography, the solvent polarity, pH, or salinity can easily be changed to help elute the protein of interest.

Eventually, the solvent drips out of the end of the column, and different fractions that leave the column are collected over time. Each fraction contains bands that correspond to different compounds. After collection, the solvent can be evaporated and the compounds of interest kept. Column chromatography is particularly useful in biochemistry because it can be used to separate and collect other macromolecules besides proteins, such as nucleic acids.

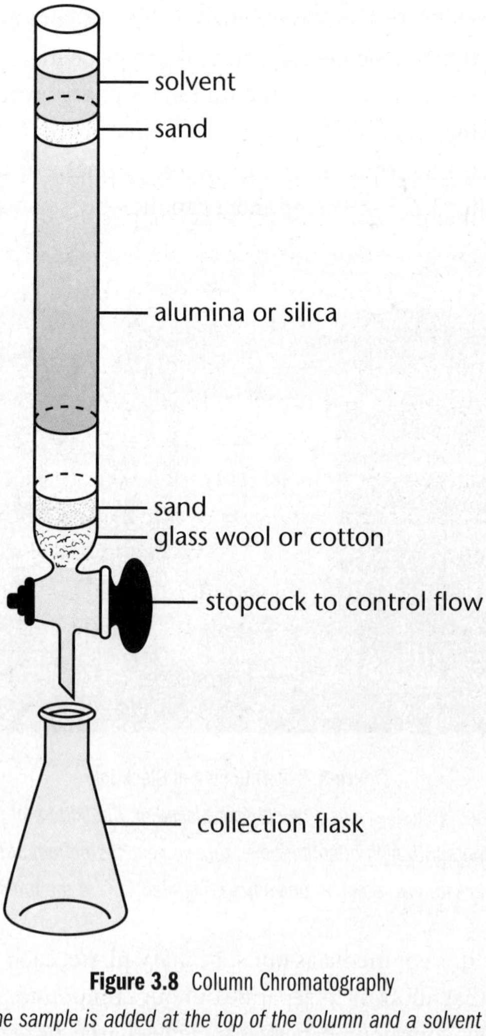

Figure 3.8 Column Chromatography

The sample is added at the top of the column and a solvent is poured over it. The more similar the sample is to the solvent (mobile phase), the more quickly it will elute; the more similar it is to the alumina or silica (stationary phase), the more slowly it will elute—if at all.

Ion-Exchange Chromatography

In this method, the beads in the column are coated with charged substances, so they attract or bind compounds that have an opposite charge. For instance, a positively charged column will attract and hold a negatively charged protein as it passes though the column, either increasing its retention time or retaining it completely. After all other compounds have moved through the column, a salt gradient is used to elute the charged molecules that have stuck to the column.

Size-Exclusion Chromatography

In this method, the beads used in the column contain tiny pores of varying sizes. These tiny pores allow small compounds to enter the beads, thus slowing them down. Large compounds can't fit into the pores, so they will move around them and travel through the column faster. It is important to remember that in this type of chromatography, the small compounds are slowed down and retained longer—which may be counterintuitive. The size of the pores may be varied so that molecules of different molecular weights can be fractionated. A common approach in protein purification is to use an ion-exchange column followed by a size-exclusion column.

Affinity Chromatography

We can also customize columns to bind any protein of interest by creating a column with high affinity for that protein. This can be accomplished by coating beads with a receptor that binds the protein or a specific antibody to the protein; in either case, the protein is retained in the column. Common stationary phase molecules include nickel, which is used in separation of genetically engineered proteins with histidine tags; antibodies or antigens; and enzyme substrate analogues, which mimic the natural substrate for an enzyme of interest. Once the protein is retained in the column, it can be eluted by washing the column with a free receptor (or target or antibody), which will compete with the bead-bound receptor and ultimately free the protein from the column. Eluents can also be created with a specific pH or salinity level that disrupts the bonds between the ligand and the protein of interest. The only drawback of the elution step is that the recovered substance can be bound to the eluent. If, for example, the eluent was an inhibitor of an enzyme, it could be difficult to remove.

BIOCHEMISTRY GUIDED EXAMPLE WITH EXPERT THINKING

Phospholipases A2 (PLA2) comprise a set of extracellular and intracellular enzymes that catalyze the hydrolysis of the sn-2 fatty acyl bond of phospholipids to yield fatty acids and lysophospholipids. The extracellular (secreted) PLA2 enzymes (sPLA2) have low molecular masses (13–18 kDa) and do not manifest significant fatty acid selectivity *in vitro*. Mammalian sPLA2 enzymes are well characterized; however, much less is known about aquatic sPLA2 enzymes and hence their study represents a great potential source for discovering new enzymes.

Lots of intro details; of most importance is that PLA2 cuts phospholipids

Characteristics of sPLA2

This passage is definitely going to focus on aquatic sPLA2

Pancreases from stingrays were harvested and subjected to multiple purification protocols, including ammonium sulfate precipitation and purification columns while monitoring sPLA2 activity. The final purification step involved a reverse phase high-performance liquid chromatography (RP-HPLC) C8 (nonpolar octylsilane) column, using a dynamic gradient composed of water and acetonitrile. As time increases, the proportion of water decreases and concentration of acetonitrile increases up to 80%. As seen below in Figure 1A, the eluate was monitored at 280 nm, and the fraction at 23 min was analyzed by 15% SDS-PAGE under reducing conditions and stained with Coomassie blue in Figure 1B.

Methods: multiple purifications

Final purification: stationary phase (nonpolar) and mobile phase (water and acetonitrile)

Figure shows two things: chromatogram and SDS-PAGE gel

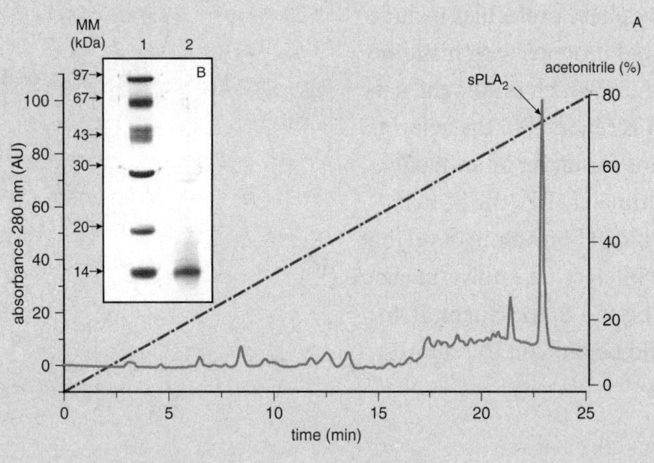

Trends: Fig 1A: big peak at ~23 min at high ACN concentration; Fig 1B: single band at ~14 kDa

Figure 1A (graph) and Figure 1B (blot)

Adapted from Bacha, A. B., Karray, A., Bouchaala, E., Gargouri, Y., & Ali, Y. B. (2011). Purification and biochemical characterization of pancreatic phospholipase A2 from the common stingray *Dasyatis pastinaca*. *Lipids in Health and Disease*, 10, 32. doi:10.1186/1476-511X-10-32

According to the data, what is the approximate monomeric molecular weight of sPLA2? Why is it biologically relevant that sPLA2 required a high acetonitrile concentration to elute off the column?

With "according to the data", this question stem is letting us know we'll need to use one or both parts of the figure to answer. So, let's start with a quick scan of the passage to see the topic and the kind of information presented to better understand the context of the data. The text is focused on a protein called phospholipase A2 (PLA2), and Figure 1 shows peaks with a gel picture inset. The bulk of the passage seems method-heavy (as indicated by the usage of column names and Figure references). We have two questions to answer: the first is asking for the size of the protein, while the second asks for a connection between the biology behind PLA2 and the way PLA2 interacts with the column.

To determine the monomeric molecular weight of sPLA2, we'll need information from the SDS-PAGE data in Figure 1B. We know from our background content knowledge that an SDS-PAGE gel under reducing conditions will denature proteins and sever any disulfide bonds. Therefore, the bands that appear should only correspond to monomers, and monomers are what this question asked about. The first lane is a series of molecular weight standards measured in kilodaltons (kDa), which are used to estimate the molecular weight of unknown proteins. We're told that the fraction at 23 minutes, which corresponds to the sPLA2 peak on the chromatogram, is analyzed in lane 2 of the gel. The band in lane 2 corresponding to sPLA2 is right next to the 14 kDa standard in lane 1, implying that the sPLA2 protein has a weight of approximately 14 kDa as well. As an extra measure of verification, paragraph 1 stated that sPLA2s have a molecular weight between 13–18 kDa.

Paragraph 2 discusses the method of the experiment, which will help us answer the second part of the question stem. For all the detail in paragraph 2, RP-HPLC is just a type of a column chromatography. Like all types of column chromatography, RP-HPLC has a stationary phase (the column) and a mobile phase (the solvent). We're told that the column is nonpolar, which means nonpolar molecules will stick inside the column. We're also told that the solvent changes composition over time—starting as mostly water, but ending as mostly acetonitrile. Why is this change in composition significant? We recall that water is a polar solvent, while acetonitrile is closer to nonpolar. Therefore, early on, when the solvent is mostly water, polar molecules will flush out of the column because like dissolves like. But near the end of the experiment, when the solvent is mostly acetonitrile, the now nonpolar solvent will dislodge nonpolar molecules. So, nonpolar molecules will elute off the column near the end of the experiment. Finally, we observe that the sPLA2 protein elutes off the column near the end, when the solvent is mostly acetonitrile. This observation implies that the sPLA2 protein is net nonpolar; the nonpolar protein had initially stuck to the nonpolar column, but the protein eventually eluted out of the column once the solvent became nonpolar enough to solvate the protein.

We can thus conclude that sPLA2 monomers have a molecular weight of around 14 kDa and, from the experimental procedure, we can conclude that sPLA2 proteins have a high affinity for nonpolar substances—first for the walls of the nonpolar column, and later for the nonpolar acetonitrile solvent. This behavior makes biological sense because the biological substrates of the sPLA2 protein are phospholipids!

MCAT CONCEPT CHECK 3.3

Before you move on, assess your understanding of the material with these questions.

1. What separation methods can be used to isolate a protein on the basis of isoelectric point?

   ____

2. What are the relative benefits of native PAGE compared to SDS-PAGE?

   ____

3. What are two potential drawbacks of affinity chromatography?

   1. ______________________________
   2. ______________________________

4. True or False: In size-exclusion chromatography, the largest molecules elute first.

3.4 Protein Analysis

LEARNING OBJECTIVES

After Chapter 3.4, you will be able to:

- Recall the traits that are typically analyzed in proteins
- Describe the Edman degradation and the Bradford assay
- Recognize the limitations of protein separation and analysis techniques

Separating proteins from one another is generally only the first step in analysis. The next step is to study the isolated protein. Protein structure, function, or quantity is often of interest for a researcher or a commercial laboratory. Even after protein identification, protein analysis tools may be used. For example, in the case of protein synthesis for commercial use, purity of the product must be periodically assessed. The protein can be studied as a whole or broken down so that its parts can be examined.

Protein Structure

BRIDGE

NMR and other forms of spectroscopy are also discussed in Chapter 11 of *MCAT Organic Chemistry Review*.

Protein structure can be determined through **X-ray crystallography** and **nuclear magnetic resonance (NMR) spectroscopy**. Before crystallographic analysis, the protein must be isolated and crystallized. X-ray crystallography is the most reliable and common method; 75 percent of the protein structures known today were analyzed through this method. Crystallography measures electron density on an extremely high-resolution scale and can also be used for nucleic acids. An X-ray diffraction pattern is generated in this method, as shown in Figure 3.9. The small dots in the diffraction pattern can then be interpreted to determine the protein's structure.

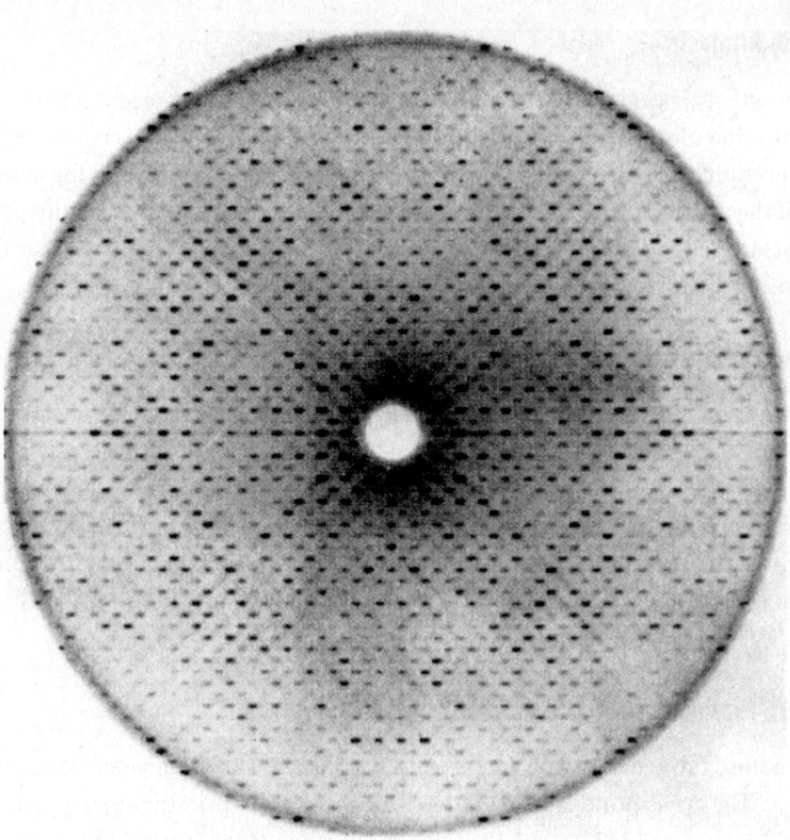

Figure 3.9 Diffraction Pattern in X-Ray Crystallography

The minority of protein structure determination (25 percent) has been accomplished through NMR, as discussed in Chapter 11 of *MCAT Organic Chemistry Review*.

Amino Acid Composition

The amino acids that compose a protein can be determined by complete protein hydrolysis and subsequent chromatographic analysis. However, the random nature of hydrolysis prevents amino acid sequencing. To determine the primary structure of a protein, sequential digestion of the protein with specific cleavage enzymes is used. Small proteins are best analyzed with the **Edman degradation**, which uses cleavage to sequence proteins of up to 50 to 70 amino acids. The Edman degradation selectively and sequentially removes the N-terminal amino acid of the protein, which can be analyzed via mass spectroscopy.

For larger proteins, digestion with *chymotrypsin*, *trypsin*, and *cyanogen bromide*, a synthetic reagent, may be used. This digestion selectively cleaves proteins at specific amino acid residues, creating smaller fragments that can then be analyzed by electrophoresis or the Edman degradation. Because disulfide links and salt bridges are broken to reduce the protein to its primary structure, their positions cannot be determined by these methods.

REAL WORLD

Like PCR gene sequencing, protein amino acid sequencing can be automated in a stepwise manner. By combining the information from both techniques, researchers can determine where on a chromosome the gene coding a particular protein resides.

Activity Analysis

Protein activity is generally determined by monitoring a known reaction with a given concentration of substrate and comparing it to a standard. Activity is correlated with concentration but is also affected by the purification methods used and the conditions of the assay. Reactions with a color change have particular applicability because microarrays can rapidly identify the samples from a chromatographic analysis that contains the compound of interest.

Concentration Determination

Concentration is determined almost exclusively through spectroscopy. Because proteins contain aromatic side chains, they can be analyzed with **UV spectroscopy** without any treatment; however, this type of analysis is particularly sensitive to sample contaminants. Proteins also cause colorimetric changes with specific reactions, particularly the **bicinchoninic acid (BCA) assay**, **Lowry reagent assay**, and **Bradford protein assay**. The Bradford method is most common because of its reliability and simplicity in basic analyses.

Bradford Protein Assay

The Bradford protein assay mixes a protein in solution with Coomassie Brilliant Blue dye. The dye is protonated and green-brown in color prior to mixing with proteins, as depicted in Figure 3.10. The dye gives up protons upon binding to amino acid groups, turning blue in the process. Ionic attractions between the dye and the protein then stabilize this blue form of the dye; thus, increased protein concentrations correspond to a larger concentration of blue dye in solution. Samples of known protein concentrations are reacted with the Bradford reagent and then absorbance is measured to create a standard curve. The unknown sample is then exposed to the same conditions, and the concentration is determined based on the standard curve. This is a very accurate method when only one type of protein is present in solution, but because of variable binding of the Coomassie dye with different amino acids, it is less accurate when more than one protein is present. The Bradford protein assay is limited by the presence of detergent in the sample or by excessive buffer.

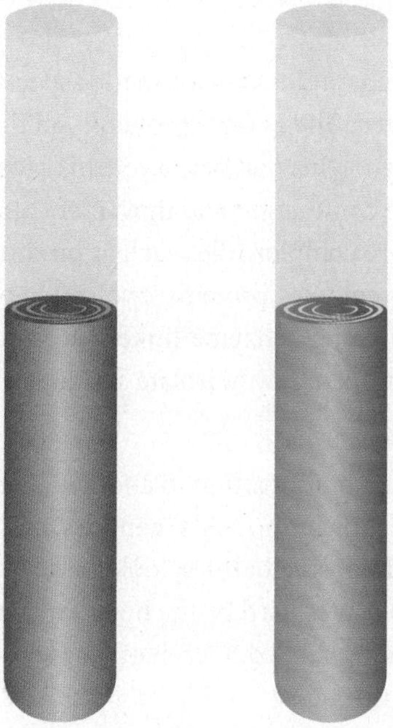

Figure 3.10 Bradford Protein Assay
The acidic form (left) has a brown-green hue; the basic form (right), which is created by interactions with proteins in solution, has a brilliant blue hue.

MCAT CONCEPT CHECK 3.4

Before you move on, assess your understanding of the material with these questions.

1. Why are proteins analyzed after isolation?

____

2. What factors would cause an activity assay to display lower activity than expected after concentration determination?

____

3. True or False: The Edman degradation proceeds from the carboxy (C-) terminus.

Conclusion

In this chapter, we have explored the nonenzymatic aspects of proteins as well as the ways proteins can be analyzed. The cellular proteins and their functions that we discussed included structural proteins that play a role in cytoskeletal architecture, motor proteins involved in muscle contraction and movement along the cytoskeleton, and other proteins that play more complex roles such as binding, immunologic function, and biosignaling. The more complex proteins involved in biosignaling highlighted in this chapter included ion channels, enzyme-linked receptors, and G protein-coupled receptors. Finally, we determined how to isolate and identify a protein and its relevant properties.

In the next chapter, we'll turn our attention to another class of biomolecules: carbohydrates. As we transition from amino acids, peptides, and proteins to monosaccharides, oligosaccharides, and polysaccharides, look for key connections between the different types of macromolecules used by the body for structure and as fuel sources. In the end, all biomolecules are related to each other through metabolism, which we'll explore in Chapters 9 through 12 of *MCAT Biochemistry Review*.

You've reviewed the content, now test your knowledge and critical thinking skills by completing a test-like passage set in your online resources!

GO ONLINE

CONCEPT SUMMARY

Cellular Functions

- **Structural proteins** compose the cytoskeleton, anchoring proteins, and much of the extracellular matrix.
  - The most common structural proteins are **collagen**, **elastin**, **keratin**, **actin**, and **tubulin**.
  - They are generally fibrous in nature.
- **Motor proteins** have one or more heads capable of force generation through a conformational change.
  - They have catalytic activity, acting as ATPases to power movement.
  - Muscle contraction, vesicle movement within cells, and cell motility are the most common applications of motor proteins.
  - Common examples include **myosin**, **kinesin**, and **dynein**.
- **Binding proteins** bind a specific substrate, either to sequester it in the body or hold its concentration at steady state.
- **Cell adhesion molecules** (**CAM**) allow cells to bind to other cells or surfaces.
  - **Cadherins** are calcium-dependent glycoproteins that hold similar cells together.
  - **Integrins** have two membrane-spanning chains and permit cells to adhere to proteins in the extracellular matrix. Some also have signaling capabilities.
  - **Selectins** allow cells to adhere to carbohydrates on the surfaces of other cells and are most commonly used in the immune system.
- **Antibodies** (or **immunoglobulins**, **Ig**) are used by the immune system to target a specific **antigen**, which may be a protein on the surface of a pathogen (invading organism) or a toxin.
  - Immunoglobulins contain a constant region and a variable region; the variable region is responsible for antigen binding.
  - Two identical heavy chains and two identical light chains form a single antibody; they are held together by disulfide linkages and noncovalent interactions.

Biosignaling

- **Ion channels** can be used for regulating ion flow into or out of a cell. There are three main types of ion channels.
  - **Ungated channels** are always open.
  - **Voltage-gated channels** are open within a range of membrane potentials.
  - **Ligand-gated channels** open in the presence of a specific binding substance, usually a hormone or neurotransmitter.

- **Enzyme-linked receptors** participate in cell signaling through extracellular ligand binding and initiation of second messenger cascades.
- **G protein-coupled receptors** have a membrane-bound protein associated with a trimeric **G protein**. They also initiate second messenger systems.
  - Ligand binding engages the G protein.
  - GDP is replaced with GTP; the α subunit dissociates from the β and γ subunits.
  - The activated α subunit alters the activity of **adenylate cyclase** or **phospholipase C**.
  - GTP is dephosphorylated to GDP; the α subunit rebinds to the β and γ subunits.

Protein Isolation

- **Electrophoresis** uses a gel matrix to observe the migration of proteins in response to an electric field.
  - **Native PAGE** maintains the protein's shape, but results are difficult to compare because the mass-to-charge ratio differs for each protein.
  - **SDS-PAGE** denatures the proteins and masks the native charge so that comparison of size is more accurate, but the functional protein cannot be recaptured from the gel.
  - **Isoelectric focusing** separates proteins by their **isoelectric point (pI)**; the protein migrates toward an electrode until it reaches a region of the gel where pH = pI of the protein.
- **Chromatography** separates protein mixtures on the basis of their affinity for a **stationary phase** or a **mobile phase**.
  - **Column chromatography** uses beads of a polar compound, like silica or alumina (stationary phase), with a nonpolar solvent (mobile phase).
  - **Ion-exchange chromatography** uses a charged column and a variably saline eluent.
  - **Size-exclusion chromatography** relies on porous beads. Larger molecules elute first because they are not trapped in the small pores.
  - **Affinity chromatography** uses a bound receptor or ligand and an eluent with free ligand or a receptor for the protein of interest.

Protein Analysis

- Protein structure is primarily determined through **X-ray crystallography** after the protein is isolated, although NMR can also be used.
- Amino acid composition can be determined by simple hydrolysis, but amino acid sequencing requires sequential degradation, such as the **Edman degradation**.
- Activity levels for enzymatic samples are determined by following the process of a known reaction, often accompanied by a color change.
- Protein concentration is also determined colorimetrically, either by UV spectroscopy or through a color change reaction.
  - **BCA assay**, **Lowry reagent assay**, and **Bradford protein assay** each test for protein and have different advantages and disadvantages.
  - The Bradford protein assay, which uses a color change from brown-green to blue, is most common.

ANSWERS TO CONCEPT CHECKS

3.1

1. Cytoskeletal proteins tend to be fibrous with repeating domains, while motor proteins tend to have ATPase activity and binding heads. Both types of protein function in cellular motility.
2. False. An enzyme is a protein or RNA molecule with catalytic activity, which motor proteins do have. Motor function is generally considered nonenzymatic, but the ATPase functionality of motor proteins indicates that these molecules do have catalytic activity.
3. If the binding protein is present in sufficiently high quantities relative to the substrate, nearly all substrate will be bound despite a low affinity.
4.

Cell Adhesion Molecule	Type of Adhesion
Cadherin	Two cells of the same or similar type using calcium
Integrin	One cell to proteins in the extracellular matrix
Selectin	One cell to carbohydrates, usually on the surface of other cells

5. Antigen–antibody interactions can result in neutralization of the pathogen or toxin, opsonization (marking) of the antigen for destruction, or creation of insoluble antigen–antibody complexes that can be phagocytized and digested by macrophages (agglutination).

3.2

1.

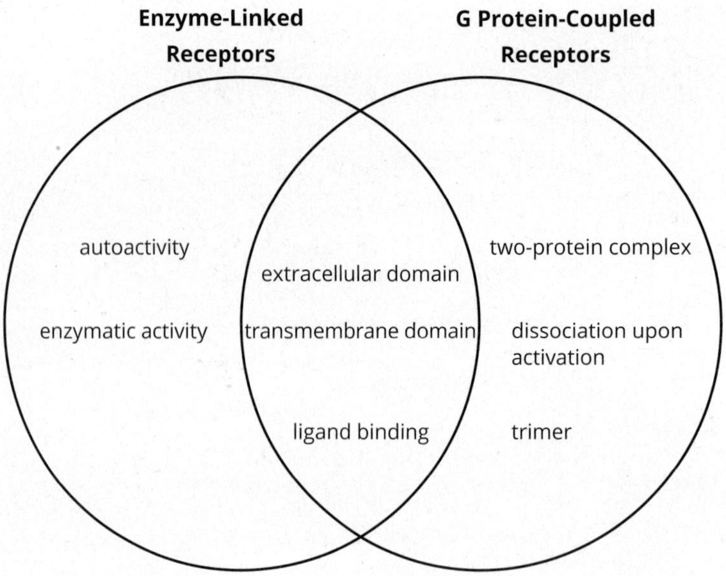

2. Ungated channels are always open.
3. Transport kinetics display both K_m and v_{max} values. They also can be cooperative, like some binding proteins. However, transporters do not have analogous K_{eq} values for reactions because there is no catalysis.

3.3

1. Isoelectric focusing and ion-exchange chromatography both separate proteins based on charge; the charge of a protein in any given environment is determined by its isoelectric point (pI).
2. Native PAGE allows a complete protein to be recovered after analysis; it also more accurately determines the relative globular size of proteins. SDS-PAGE can be used to eliminate conflation from mass-to-charge ratios.
3. The protein of interest may not elute from the column because its affinity is too high or it may be permanently bound to the free receptor in the eluent.
4. True. The small pores in size-exclusion chromatography trap smaller particles, retaining them in the column.

3.4

1. Protein isolation is generally only the first step in an analysis. The protein identity must be confirmed by amino acid analysis or activity. With unknown proteins, classification of their features is generally desired.
2. Contamination of the sample with detergent or SDS could yield an artificially increased protein level, leading to lower activity than expected (because the protein concentration was calculated as higher than its actual value). Alternatively, the enzyme could have been denatured during isolation and analysis.
3. False. The Edman degradation proceeds from the amino (N-) terminus.

SCIENCE MASTERY ASSESSMENT EXPLANATIONS

1. **D**

In most electrophoresis experiments, we attempt to separate out one component from the others. Because we are attempting to isolate protein A only, a pH that causes protein A to be negative while proteins B and C are neutral or positive will be best. pH 5.5 accomplishes this goal; proteins B and C will be positively charged. A pH of 4.5, **(C)**, would make protein A neutral, and it would thus not migrate across the gel. Any neutral impurities would also remain in the well with protein A, making this pH not the best choice.

2. **B**

Sodium dodecyl sulfate is a detergent and will digest proteins to form micelles with uniform negative charges. Because the protein is sequestered within the micelle, other factors such as charge of the protein and shape have minimal roles during separation. In essence, the protein micelles can be modeled as being spheres, dependent only on size.

3. **D**

From the given choices, all of them are involved in cell movement with the exception of **(D)**. Centrioles are composed of microtubules, but are involved in mitosis, not cell migration.

4. **C**

The most prevalent extracellular proteins are keratin, elastin, and collagen. Tubulin and actin are the primary cytoskeletal proteins, while myosin is a motor protein.

5. **C**

For a ligand present in low quantities to have a strong action, we expect it to initiate a second messenger cascade system. Second messenger systems amplify signals because enzymes can catalyze a reaction more than once while they are active, and often activate other enzymes. Both enzyme-linked receptors and G protein-coupled receptors use second messenger systems, while ion channels do not.

6. **D**

Ions that are not readily accessible in the cytoplasm or extracellular space are likely to be bound to a binding protein. Classically, calcium and magnesium are protein-bound. Without this background knowledge, the question can still be answered. Sodium, **(A)**, and potassium, **(B)**, must exist in their free states to participate in action potentials. Chloride, **(C)**, is readily excreted by the kidney, which would not be true if it were protein-bound. Calcium must be sequestered in both the bloodstream and intracellularly because calcium is used for muscle contraction, exocytosis (of neurotransmitters and other signals), and many other cellular processes that must be tightly regulated.

7. **A**

Antibodies are specific to a single antigen. Each B-cell produces a single type of antibody with a constant region that is specific to the host and a variable region that is specific to an antigen.

8. **A**

The resting membrane potential is displayed by cells that are not actively involved in signal transduction. Ungated or "leak" channels permit limited free flow of ions, while the sodium–potassium pump is also active and corrects for this leakage. Ligand-gated and voltage-gated channels are involved in cell signaling and in the pacemaker potentials of certain cells, but cause deviation from—not maintenance of—the resting membrane potential.

9. **D**

All trimeric G proteins have α, β, and γ subunits—**(A)**, **(B)**, and **(C)**, respectively. G_s, G_i, and G_q are subtypes of the G_α subunit of the trimeric G protein and differ depending on the G protein-coupled receptor's function.

10. **B**

The proteins described in the question differ primarily in their molecular weights. Their pI values are very close, so ion-exchange chromatography, **(A)**, is not a good choice. The question specifies a large quantity, which is better processed through chromatography than through electrophoresis—**(C)** and **(D)**—because the gel can only handle a small volume of protein.

11. **C**

The overall pI of a protein is determined by the relative number of acidic and basic amino acids. The basic amino acids are arginine, lysine, and histidine, and the acidic amino acids are aspartic acid and glutamic acid. Glycine's side chain is a hydrogen atom, so it will have the least contribution of all the amino acids.

12. **C**

The gel in isoelectric focusing uses a pH gradient. When a protein is in a region with a pH above its pI, it is negatively charged and moves toward the anode. When it is in a pH region below its pI, it is positively charged and moves toward the cathode. When the pH equals the pI, the migration of the protein is halted.

13. **C**

UV spectroscopy is best used with conjugated systems of double bonds. While the double bond in the peptide bond does display resonance, this is not adequate for UV absorption. However, aromatic systems are conjugated, and phenylalanine, tyrosine, and tryptophan all contain aromatic ring structures.

14. **B**

Protein activity and concentration are generally correlated. Because we have a high concentration of protein, we expect a high activity unless the protein has been damaged or inactivated in some way. The protein could have been inactivated by experimental conditions like detergents, heat, or pH; however, these are not answer choices. Rather, we must consider how the experimental procedure works. Protein elutes off of an affinity column by binding free ligand. In this situation, the binding may not have been reversed and thus the free ligand competes for the active site of the enzyme, lowering its activity.

15. **A**

The selective cleavage of proteins by digestive enzymes allows fragments of different lengths with known amino acid endpoints to be created. By cleaving the protein with several different enzymes, a basic outline of the amino acid sequence can be created.

Consult your online resources for additional practice. **GO ONLINE**

EQUATIONS TO REMEMBER

(3.1) **Migration velocity:** $\mathbf{v} = \frac{Ez}{f}$

SHARED CONCEPTS

Biochemistry Chapter 1
Amino Acids, Peptides, and Proteins

Biology Chapter 1
The Cell

Biology Chapter 8
The Immune System

Biology Chapter 11
The Musculoskeletal System

General Chemistry Chapter 12
Electrochemistry

Organic Chemistry Chapter 12
Separations and Purifications

CHAPTER 4

CARBOHYDRATE STRUCTURE AND FUNCTION

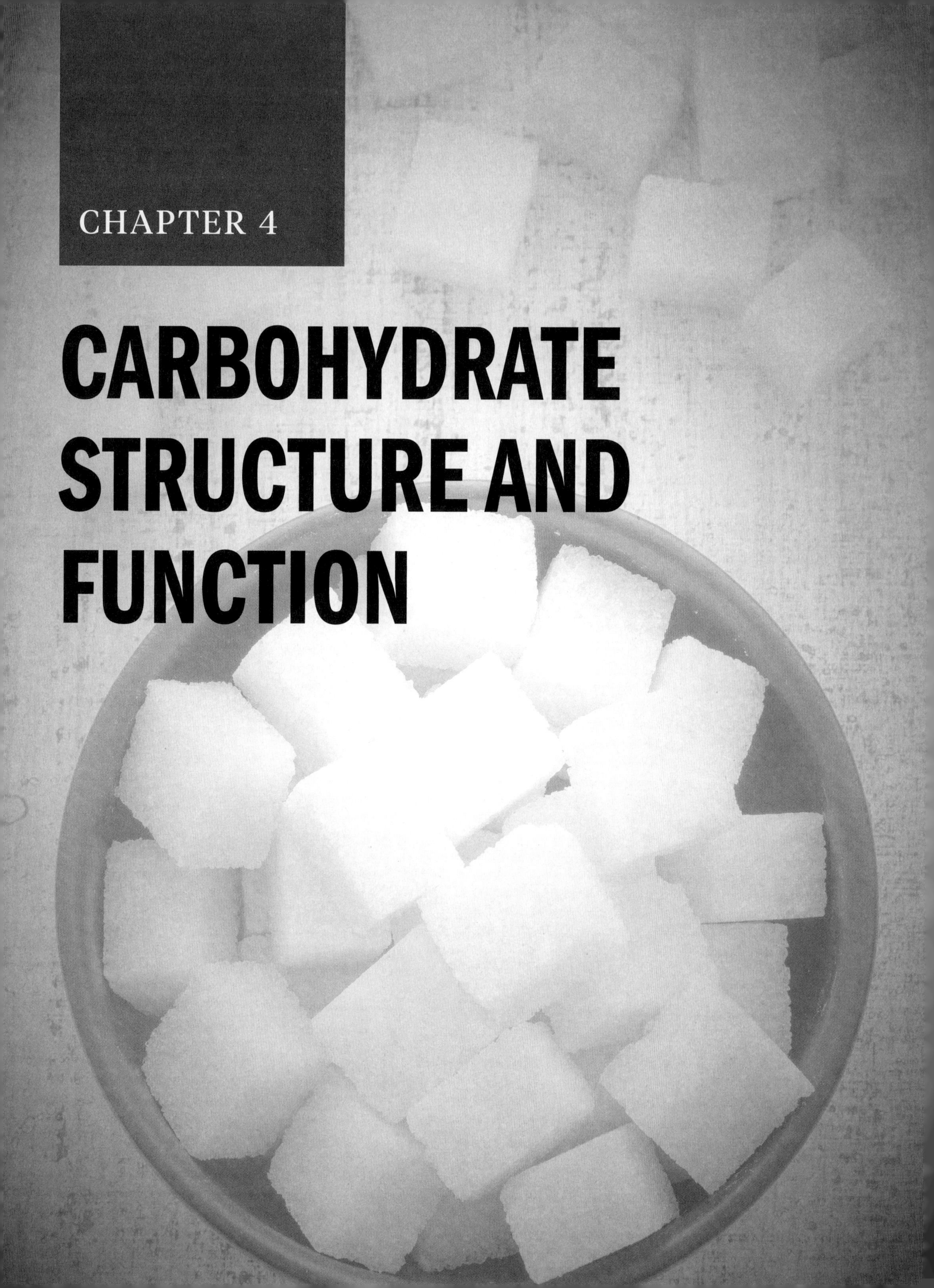

SCIENCE MASTERY ASSESSMENT

Every pre-med knows this feeling: there is so much content I have to know for the MCAT! How do I know what to do first or what's important?

While the high-yield badges throughout this book will help you identify the most important topics, this Science Mastery Assessment is another tool in your MCAT prep arsenal. This quiz (which can also be taken in your online resources) and the guidance below will help ensure that you are spending the appropriate amount of time on this chapter based on your personal strengths and weaknesses. Don't worry though—skipping something now does not mean you'll never study it. Later on in your prep, as you complete full-length tests, you'll uncover specific pieces of content that you need to review and can come back to these chapters as appropriate.

How to Use This Assessment

If you answer 0–7 questions correctly:

Spend about 1 hour to read this chapter in full and take limited notes throughout. Follow up by reviewing **all** quiz questions to ensure that you now understand how to solve each one.

If you answer 8–11 questions correctly:

Spend 20–40 minutes reviewing the quiz questions. Beginning with the questions you missed, read and take notes on the corresponding subchapters. For questions you answered correctly, ensure your thinking matches that of the explanation and you understand why each choice was correct or incorrect.

If you answer 12–15 questions correctly:

Spend less than 20 minutes reviewing all questions from the quiz. If you missed any, then include a quick read-through of the corresponding subchapters, or even just the relevant content within a subchapter, as part of your question review. For questions you got correct, ensure your thinking matches that of the explanation and review the Concept Summary at the end of the chapter.

1. When glucose is in a straight-chain formation, it:
   A. is an aldoketose.
   B. is a pentose.
   C. has five chiral carbons.
   D. is one of a group of 16 stereoisomers.

2. All of the following are true of epimers EXCEPT:
   A. they differ in configuration about only one carbon.
   B. they usually have slightly different chemical and physical properties.
   C. they are diastereomers (with the exception of glyceraldehyde).
   D. they have equal but opposite optical activities.

3. Aldonic acids are compounds that:
   A. can be oxidized, and therefore act as reducing agents.
   B. can be reduced, and therefore act as reducing agents.
   C. have been oxidized, and have acted as reducing agents.
   D. have been oxidized, and have acted as oxidizing agents.

4. The formation of α-D-glucopyranose from β-D-glucopyranose is called:
   A. glycosidation.
   B. mutarotation.
   C. enantiomerization.
   D. racemization.

5. Ketose sugars may have the ability to act as reducing sugars. Which process explains this?
   A. Ketose sugars undergo tautomerization.
   B. The ketone group is oxidized directly.
   C. Ketose sugars undergo anomerization.
   D. The ketone group is reduced directly.

6. What is the product of the following reaction?

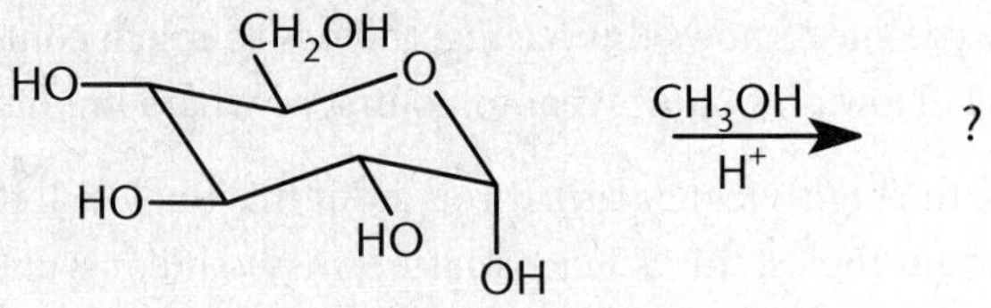

A.

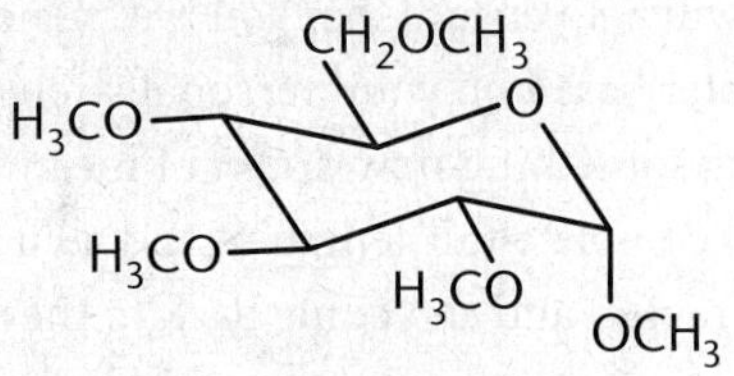

B.

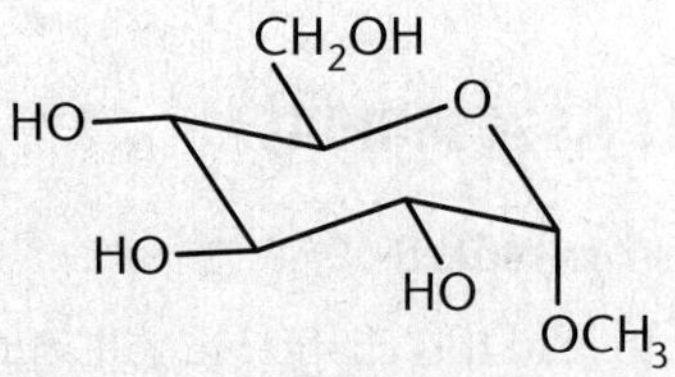

C.

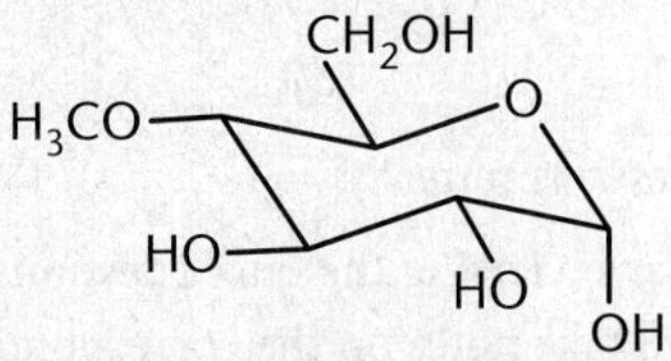

D.

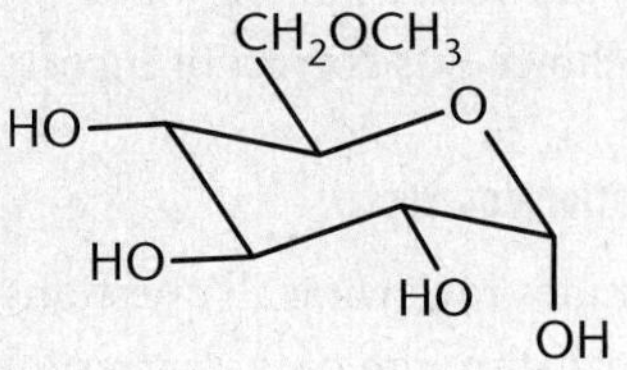

7. Which of the following enzymes cleaves polysaccharide chains and yields maltose exclusively?
   - A. α-Amylase
   - B. β-Amylase
   - C. Debranching enzyme
   - D. Glycogen phosphorylase

8. When the following straight-chain Fischer projection is converted to a chair or ring conformation, its structure will be:

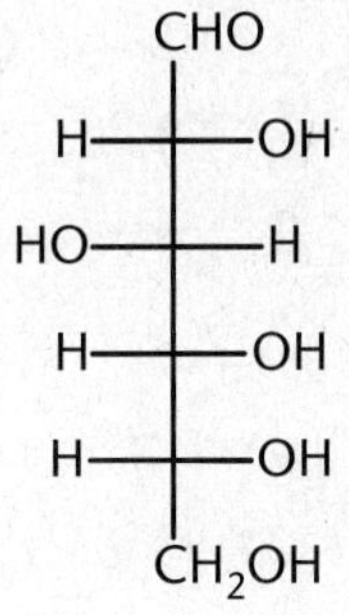

A.

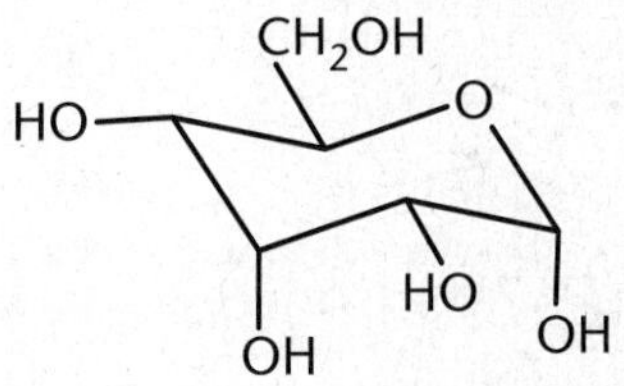

B.

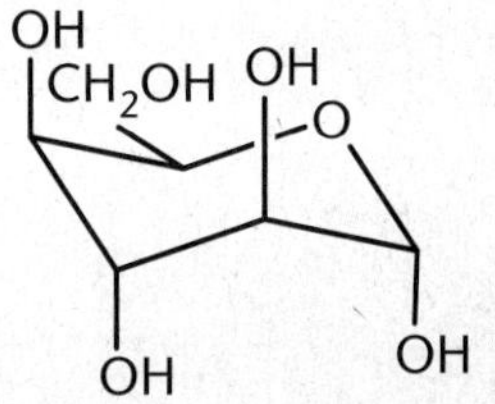

C.

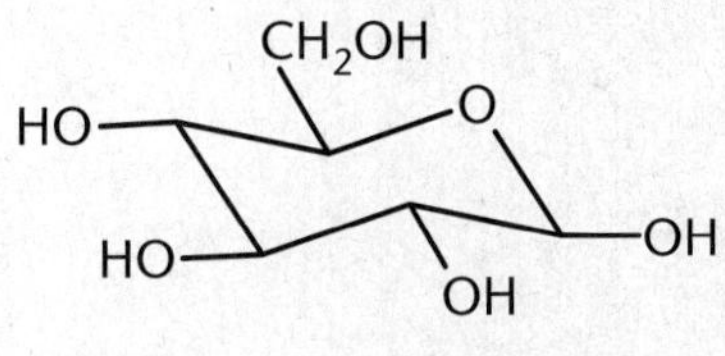

D.

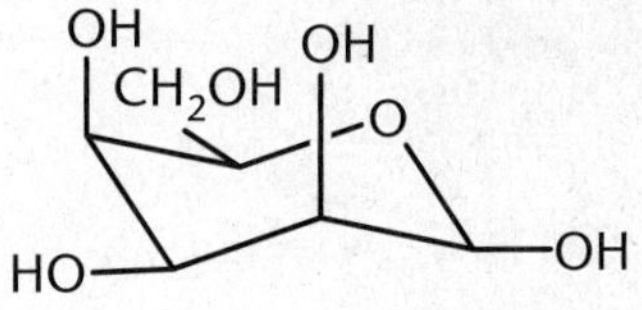

9. Why is the α-anomer of D-glucose less likely to form than the β-anomer?
   - A. The β-anomer is preferred for metabolism.
   - B. The β-anomer undergoes less electron repulsion.
   - C. The α-anomer is the more stable anomer.
   - D. The α-anomer forms more in L-glucose.

10. Which two polysaccharides share all of their glycosidic linkage types in common?
    - A. Cellulose and amylopectin
    - B. Amylose and glycogen
    - C. Amylose and cellulose
    - D. Glycogen and amylopectin

11. Which of the following is digestible by humans and is made up of only one type of monosaccharide?
    - A. Lactose
    - B. Sucrose
    - C. Maltose
    - D. Cellobiose

12. The reaction below is an example of one step in:

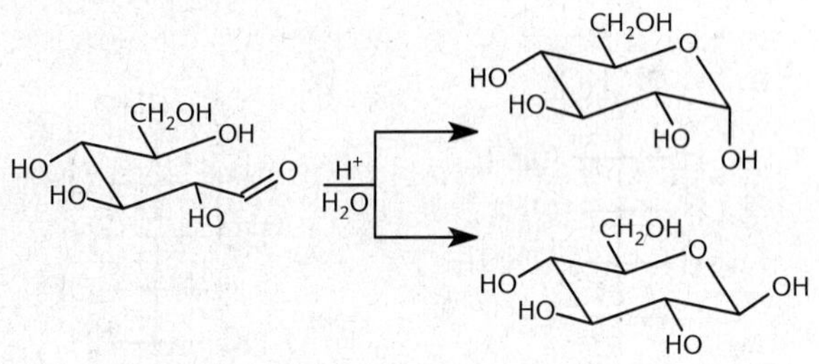

    - A. aldehyde formation.
    - B. hemiketal formation.
    - C. mutarotation.
    - D. glycosidic bond cleavage.

13. Galactose is the C-4 epimer of glucose, the structure of which is shown below. Which of the following structures is galactose?

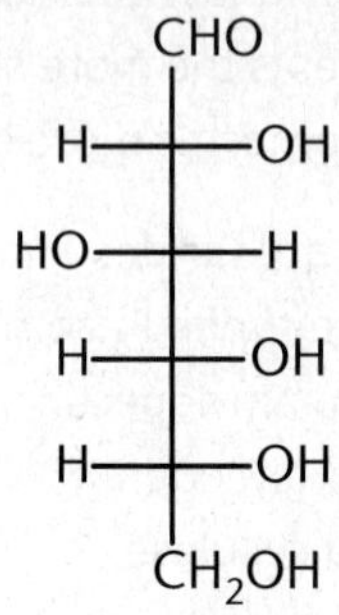

D-glucose

A.

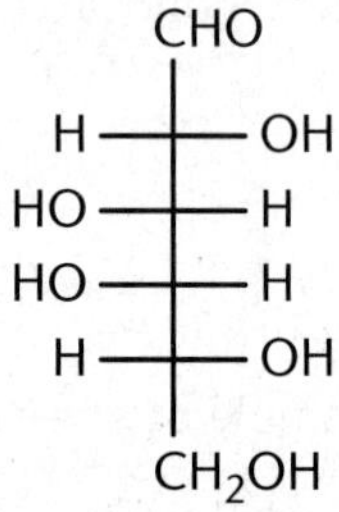

B.

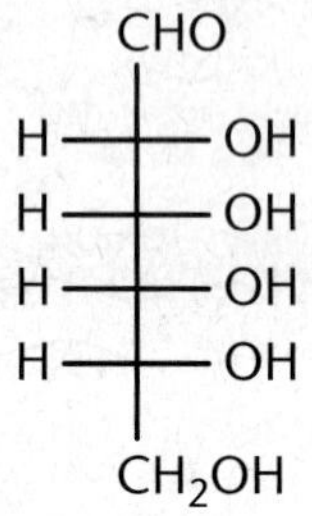

C.

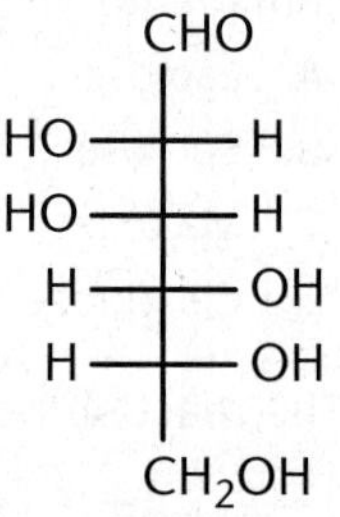

D.

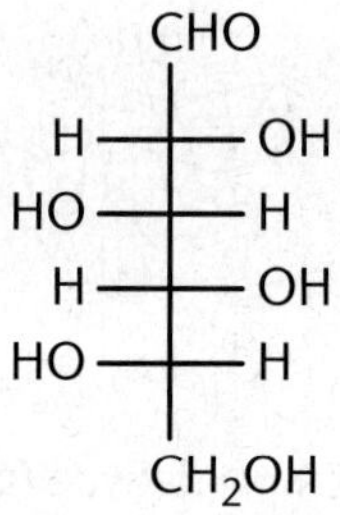

14. Andersen's disease (glycogen storage disease type IV) is a condition characterized by a deficiency in glycogen branching enzyme. Absence of this enzyme would be likely to cause all of the following effects EXCEPT:

- **A.** decreased glycogen solubility in human cells.
- **B.** slower action of glycogen phosphorylase.
- **C.** less storage of glucose in the body.
- **D.** glycogen devoid of α-1,4 linkages.

15. The cyclic forms of monosaccharides are:

- **I.** hemiacetals.
- **II.** hemiketals.
- **III.** acetals.

- **A.** I only
- **B.** III only
- **C.** I and II only
- **D.** I, II, and III

Answer Key follows on next page.

Answer Key

1. **D**
2. **D**
3. **C**
4. **B**
5. **A**
6. **B**
7. **B**
8. **C**
9. **B**
10. **D**
11. **C**
12. **C**
13. **A**
14. **D**
15. **C**

Detailed explanations can be found at the end of the chapter.

CHAPTER 4

CARBOHYDRATE STRUCTURE AND FUNCTION

In This Chapter

CHAPTER PROFILE

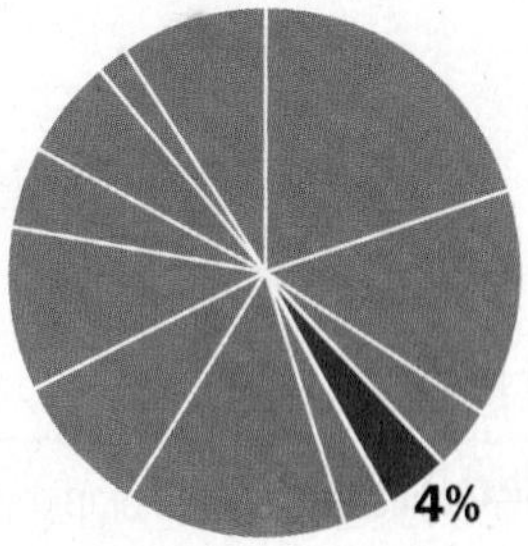

The content in this chapter should be relevant to about 4% of all questions about biochemistry on the MCAT.

This chapter covers material from the following AAMC content categories:

1D: Principles of bioenergetics and fuel molecule metabolism

5D: Structure, function, and reactivity of biologically-relevant molecules

Introduction

Carbohydrates (or, as they are known colloquially, *carbs*) have experienced a tumultuous few decades in American culinary culture. Remember the food pyramid, which advised that we consume 6 to 11 servings of carbohydrates—in the form of bread, cereal, rice, and pasta—per day? Nowadays, we're inundated with recommendations to cut down or even cut out carbs; still, carbohydrates make up most of the food and drink that continues to fill our refrigerators and cupboards. Whether or not this is healthy is debatable, as research on food choices continues. What is certain, however, is that carbohydrates are the most direct source of chemical energy for almost all organisms, ranging from single-celled protozoa to more complex organisms, such as plants and animals—including people.

From a molecular standpoint, carbohydrates used to be defined by the empirical formula $C_n(H_2O)_n$, but this definition is now considered antiquated. This formula only applies to simple monomeric sugars, which are also called monosaccharides. As simple sugars link to form complex sugars, water loss occurs, thus changing the empirical formula to $C_n(H_2O)_m$ for complex sugars.

In this chapter, we'll discuss how the various types of carbohydrates we utilize for metabolism are classified, the structures in which they exist, and the biochemical reactions they undergo.

4.1 Carbohydrate Classification

High-Yield

LEARNING OBJECTIVES

After Chapter 4.1, you will be able to:

- Recognize common features of sugar nomenclature
- Apply principles of stereoisomerism to sugar nomenclature and structure
- Distinguish enantiomers from epimers
- Classify and name a simple sugar based on its structure

Carbohydrates come in many types. They can be classified by the number of sugar moieties that make them up, the number of carbons in each sugar, the functional groups present on the molecule, and the stereochemistry of the sugar.

Nomenclature

MCAT EXPERTISE

The MCAT likes to present complex, novel molecules and then test you on the most basic information about them. Therefore, when dealing with carbohydrates on the exam, look for the functional groups we have seen before (aldehydes, ketones, and alcohols) and realize that they retain the same chemical properties that you already know.

Whenever we discuss carbohydrates (or anything else in biology), it makes sense to start with the most basic structural units, which are **monosaccharides**. The simplest monosaccharides contain three carbon atoms and are called **trioses**. Carbohydrates with four, five, and six carbon atoms are called **tetroses**, **pentoses**, and **hexoses**, respectively. Carbohydrates that contain an aldehyde group as their most oxidized functional group are called **aldoses** and those with a ketone group as their most oxidized functional group are called **ketoses**. Taken together, a six-carbon sugar with an aldehyde group would be called an *aldohexose*, while a five-carbon sugar with a ketone group would be called a *ketopentose*. The basic structure of a monosaccharide is illustrated by the simple sugar ***glyceraldehyde***, which is an aldose as shown in Figure 4.1.

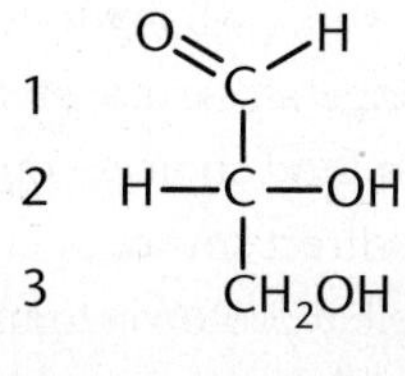

Figure 4.1 Glyceraldehyde
The simplest aldose (an aldotriose)

Glyceraldehyde is a polyhydroxylated aldehyde, or as described above, an aldose (aldehyde sugar). The numbering of carbon atoms in a monosaccharide follows the rules described in Chapter 1 of *MCAT Organic Chemistry Review*. The carbonyl carbon is the most oxidized, and therefore will always have the lowest possible number. In an aldose, the aldehyde carbon will always be carbon number one (C-1). The aldehyde carbon can participate in **glycosidic linkages**; sugars acting as substituents via this linkage are called *glycosyl* residues.

The simplest ketone sugar (ketose) is ***dihydroxyacetone***, shown in Figure 4.2. Again, the carbonyl carbon is the most oxidized; in this case, the lowest number it can be assigned is carbon number two (C-2). This is true, in fact, for most ketoses on the MCAT: the carbonyl carbon is C-2. Ketoses can also participate in glycosidic bonds at this carbon. Notice that on every monosaccharide, every carbon *other* than the carbonyl carbon will carry a hydroxyl group.

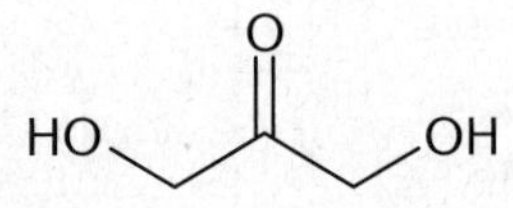

Figure 4.2 Dihydroxyacetone
The simplest ketose (a ketotriose)

Common Names

On the MCAT, a few sugars are tested by referencing their common names, or names that do not necessarily follow the nomenclature rules listed above. You should be familiar with the names of the important monosaccharides listed in Figure 4.3.

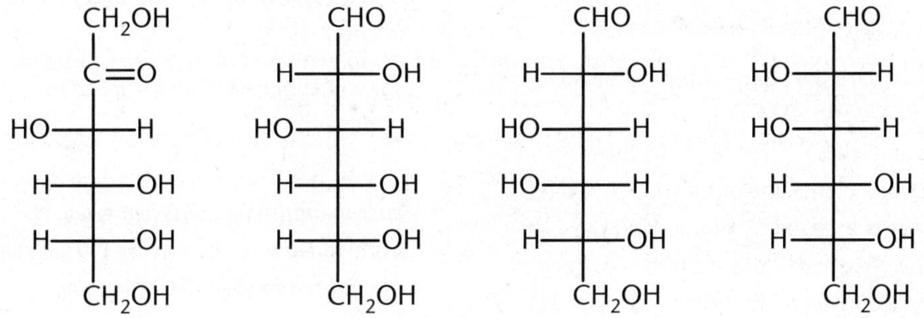

Figure 4.3 Common Names of Frequently Tested Sugars on the MCAT

BIOCHEMISTRY GUIDED EXAMPLE WITH EXPERT THINKING

Carbohydrate-based wound dressings have received increased attention in recent years for their occlusive and functionally interactive properties. They afford bacterial and odor protection, fluid balance, and elasticity. However, since all modern dressings had the same efficacy in healing as saline or paraffin gauze, there is opportunity to improve on cotton-based dressings. Proteases like human neutrophil elastase are found in high concentration in chronic wounds, which create considerable growth factor and extracellular matrix protein destruction, preventing the wound from healing. Wound dressings that selectively sequester elastase from chronic wounds are built on the concept that the properties of the protease can be used to tailor the molecular design of the wound dressing. Elastase is a glycoprotein and contains a significant carbohydrate portion shown to be glycosamine-based. There is potential for carbohydrate–carbohydrate interactions between the protein and a monosaccharide conjugated to cellulose dressing. There may be additional carbohydrate–protein interactions through the active site. In this study, researchers compared the preparation and activity of elastase in the presence of monosaccharides conjugated to citrate-cellulose.

Topic: sugar-based bandages

Details about advantages, but want to make better

Background about negative effects of elastase in wounds

We're interested in designing the sugar-based bandages to grab elastase

Reasons why the researchers think that sugar-base bandages will work to bind elastase

Purpose: which sugar works best to bind elastase?

A series of monosaccharides (Figure 1) were linked to cotton-cellulose gauze with an acid-catalyzed citric acid reaction. Varying amounts of treated gauze samples were submerged with 1 unit/mL of elastase for one hour at room temperature, after which each individual gauze sample was removed. Any unbound elastase was assayed by monitoring the spectrophotometric release of p-nitroaniline at 410 nm from the enzymatic hydrolysis of the substrate N-methoxy-succinyl-Ala-Ala-Pro-Val-p-nitroanilide. The initial activity of remaining elastase for each monosaccharide at specific amounts of treated gauze was plotted below (Figure 2).

Different sugars in Figure A linked to bandages

Experimental setup: different amounts of gauze added with set amount of elastase, then gauze removed; the remaining elastase assayed using spectrometry

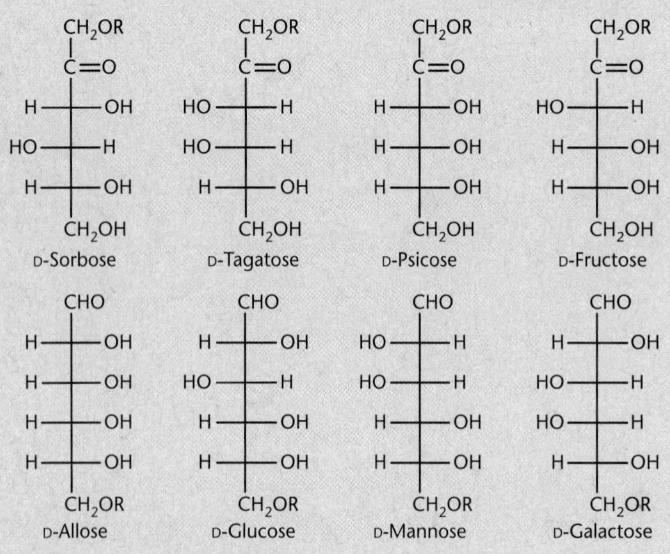

Figure 1

Sugar molecules—come back to this diagram if needed

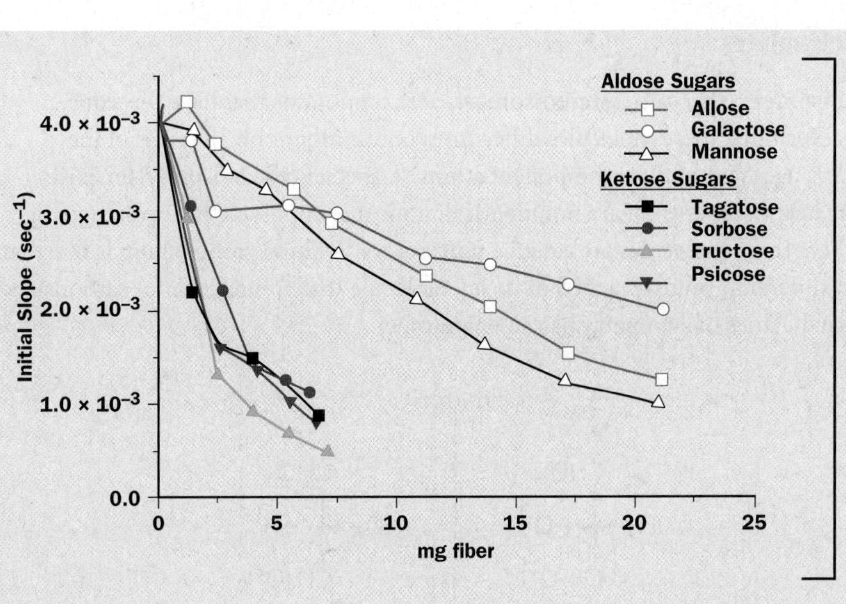

IVs: amount of gauze, type of sugar

DV: slope, which corresponds to initial elastase activity

Trend: galactose, allose, mannose have less steep lines compared to sorbose, tagalose, psicose, fructose

Figure 2

Adapted from Edwards, J. V., & Caston-Pierre, S. (2013). Citrate-linked keto- and aldo-hexose monosaccharide cellulose conjugates demonstrate selective human neutrophil elastase-lowering activity in cotton dressings. *Journal of Functional Biomaterials*, 4(2), 59-73. doi:10.3390/jfb4020059.

According to the data, which class of monosaccharide should be used in gauze to help prevent elastase-mediated wound damage?

The question asks us to select a type of monosaccharide to prevent elastase from doing damage, which means that it's important to understand the purpose of the passage and what the data tells us. The first paragraph describes how advantageous bandages currently are, but that researchers are interested in improving them by selectively binding proteases that prevent healing, like elastase.

Let's take a look at the experimental setup in paragraph 2. Since the sugar-linked bandages are soaked in a solution with elastase and then removed, the assumption is that the better the sugar binds elastase, the less elastase there is left over in the solution when the researchers assay it, after the bandage is removed. Therefore, the better the binding, the less activity there should be. The figure clearly has two sets of lines: galactose/allose/mannose have activity over a larger amount of fiber used, and, based on Figure 1, all three of these sugars are aldohexoses, which are sugars with an aldehyde at the C-1 position. Sorbose/tagatose/psicose/fructose, however, quickly drop in activity with increasing amounts of fiber, and, based on Figure 1, all four of these sugars are ketohexoses, which are sugars with a ketone at the C-2 position. To make the comparison a bit more clear, let's consider the activity for each set at 5 mg of fiber—ketohexoses have $\sim 1.5 \times 10^{-3}$ slope, and aldohexoses have $\sim 3.3 \times 10^{-3}$ slope. Since slope corresponds to activity, less activity is seen for ketohexoses with equivalent amounts of carbohydrate-bound bandage, therefore corresponding to more elastase binding.

Therefore, we can conclude that the researchers should investigate the usage of ketohexoses to help prevent elastase-mediated wound damage, since this class of sugar seems to bind elastase better than aldohexoses.

Stereochemistry

BRIDGE

Isomerism is discussed in detail in Chapter 2 of *MCAT Organic Chemistry Review*. The isomerism seen in carbohydrates is just an extension of that conversation; many sugars are related to each other as enantiomers or diastereomers.

Optical isomers, also called **stereoisomers**, are compounds that have the same chemical formula; these molecules differ from one another only in terms of the spatial arrangement of their component atoms. A special type of isomerism exists between stereoisomers that are nonidentical, nonsuperimposable mirror images of each other. These molecules are called **enantiomers**. A chiral carbon atom is one that has four different groups attached to it; any molecule that contains chiral carbons and no internal planes of symmetry has an enantiomer.

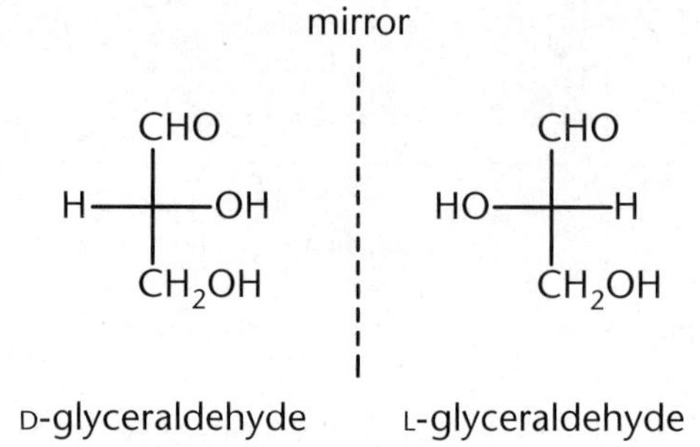

Figure 4.4 Enantiomers of Glyceraldehyde

KEY CONCEPT

The two systems for naming chiral carbons are not interchangeable! While some D-isomers are equivalent with (*R*), others are (*S*). When dealing with biomolecules like sugars, anticipate using the biochemists' method of nomenclature: D and L.

Figure 4.4 illustrates the two enantiomers of glyceraldehyde: D- and L-glyceraldehyde. The particular three-dimensional arrangement of the groups attached to the chiral carbon determines the compound's **absolute configuration**. While organic chemists use the newer (*R*) and (*S*) system when denoting absolute configuration, biochemists use the older D and L system. Notice in the figure above that D-glyceraldehyde and L-glyceraldehyde are mirror images of one another—this makes them enantiomers because they *must* have opposite absolute configurations. Because there is only one chiral carbon present, these are the only two stereoisomers that exist for glyceraldehyde. As the number of chiral carbons increases, so too does the number of possible stereoisomers because one compound may have many diastereomers. The number of possible stereoisomers of a compound can be calculated by:

KEY CONCEPT

When trying to figure out how many possible stereoisomers can exist for a multi-carbon compound, identify the number of chiral carbons (n) and plug into the formula 2^n. For example, $2^1 = 2$ stereoisomers and $2^2 = 4$ stereoisomers.

$$\text{Number of stereoisomers with common backbone} = 2^n$$

Equation 4.1

where n is the number of chiral carbons in the molecule.

KEY CONCEPT

D and L are based on the stereochemistry of glyceraldehyde. These are NOT directly related to the (+) and (−) designations denoting optical rotation.

Early in the twentieth century, scientists used glyceraldehyde to learn about the optical rotation of sugars. The results of this early study led to the **D** and **L** naming convention. D-Glyceraldehyde was later determined to exhibit a positive rotation (designated as D-(+)-glyceraldehyde), and L-glyceraldehyde a negative rotation (designated as L-(−)-glyceraldehyde). Note that the direction of rotation, (+) or (−), must be determined experimentally and cannot be determined from the D or L designation for the sugar.

On the MCAT, all monosaccharides are assigned the D or L configuration based on their relationship to glyceraldehyde. The **Fischer projection** is a simple two-dimensional drawing of stereoisomers. Recall that in a Fischer projection, the horizontal lines are wedges (out of the page), while vertical lines are dashes (into the page), as shown in Figure 4.5.

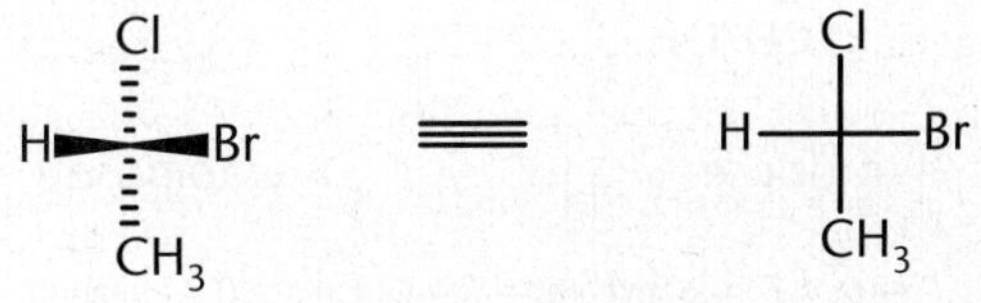

Figure 4.5 Fisher Projection
Horizontal lines are wedges (out of the page); vertical lines are dashes (into the page).

Fischer projections allow scientists to identify different enantiomers. Using this system of structural representation, all D-sugars have the hydroxide of their highest-numbered chiral center on the right, and all L-sugars have that hydroxide on the left. Because D-glucose and L-glucose are enantiomers, this means that *every* chiral center in D-glucose has the opposite configuration of L-glucose, as shown in Figure 4.6.

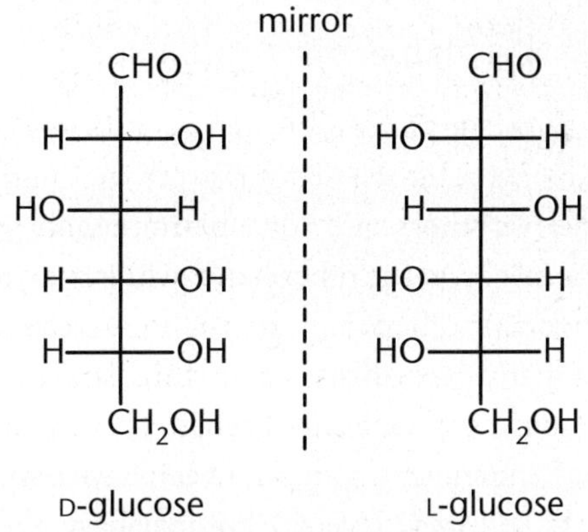

Figure 4.6 Enantiomers of Glucose

Make sure that you are familiar with these three types of stereoisomers:

1. The same sugars, in different optical families, are **enantiomers** (such as D-glucose and L-glucose).
2. Two sugars that are in the same family (both are either ketoses or aldoses, and have the same number of carbons) that are not identical and are not mirror images of each other are **diastereomers**.
3. A special subtype of diastereomers are those that differ in configuration at exactly one chiral center. These are defined as **epimers** (such as D-*ribose* and D-*arabinose*, which only differ at C-2, as shown in Figure 4.7).

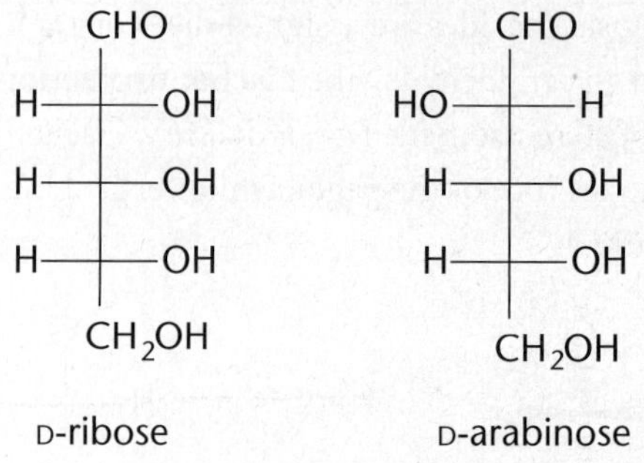

Figure 4.7 D-Ribose and D-Arabinose Are C-2 Epimers

A summary of these different types of isomers is provided in Figure 4.8, which shows four different stereoisomers of an aldotetrose, including two optical forms of *erythrose* and two optical forms of *threose*.

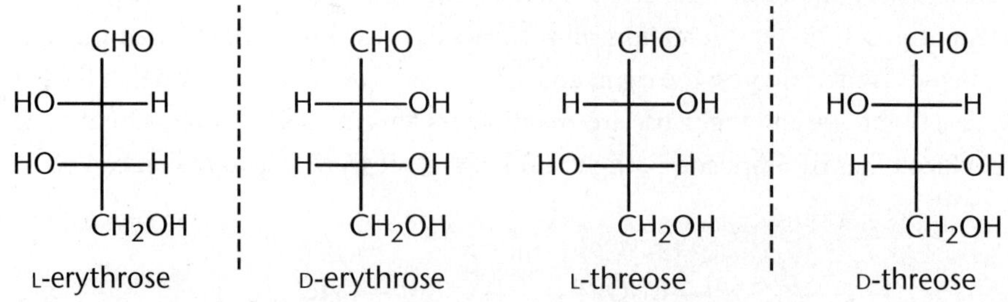

Figure 4.8 Four Stereoisomers of an Aldotetrose

Because D-erythrose and L-erythrose are nonsuperimposable mirror images of one another, they are enantiomers. On the other hand, while D-erythrose and D-threose are *not* mirror images of one another, they are still nonsuperimposable, which makes them diastereomers. Similarly, L-erythrose and D-threose are diastereomers. Because they differ in configuration at only one chiral center, they can also be defined as epimers of one another. Remember, a compound can have only one enantiomer (the left hand to its right hand, or vice versa), but may have multiple diastereomers, depending on how many (and which) chiral carbons are inverted between the two molecules.

MCAT CONCEPT CHECK 4.1

Before you move on, assess your understanding of the material with these questions.

1. What is the name for a five-carbon sugar with an aldehyde group? A six-carbon sugar with a ketone group?

___

2. Draw all of the possible D-stereoisomers of glucose in Fischer projection form.

3. Which of the diastereomers of glucose from the previous question are considered to be epimers of glucose? Enantiomers?
   - Epimers:

___

   - Enantiomers:

___

4.2 Cyclic Sugar Molecules

LEARNING OBJECTIVES

After Chapter 4.2, you will be able to:

- Convert between Haworth and Fischer projections
- Define and explain sugar-related concepts, including hemiacetal, hemiketal, pyranose, furanose, and anomeric carbon
- Predict the impact of mutarotation on conformation
- Identify the more stable anomer of a given sugar:

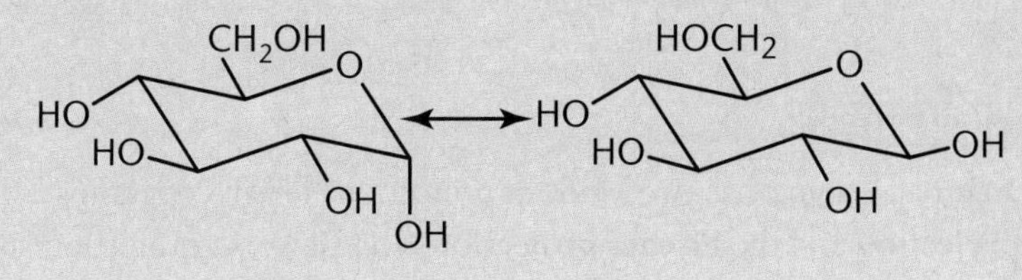

Monosaccharides contain both a hydroxyl group, which can serve as a nucleophile, and a carbonyl group, which is the most common electrophile on the MCAT. Therefore, they can undergo intramolecular reactions to form cyclic **hemiacetals** (from aldoses) and **hemiketals** (from ketoses). Due to ring strain, the only cyclic molecules that are stable in solution are six-membered **pyranose** rings or five-membered **furanose** rings. In fact, such sugars tend to exist predominantly in cyclic form. The hydroxyl group acts as the nucleophile during ring formation, so oxygen becomes a member of the ring structure. Regardless of whether hemiacetal or hemiketal is formed, the carbonyl carbon becomes chiral in this process, and is referred to as the **anomeric carbon**. Figure 4.9 demonstrates how the carbonyl containing C-1 and the hydroxyl group on C-5 of D-glucose undergo intramolecular hemiacetal formation. One of two ring forms can emerge during cyclization of a sugar molecule: α or β. Because these two molecules differ at the anomeric carbon, they are termed **anomers** of one another. In glucose, the **α-anomer** has the –OH group of C-1 *trans* to the –CH_2OH substituent (axial and down), whereas the **β-anomer** has the –OH group of C-1 *cis* to the –CH_2OH substituent (equatorial and up).

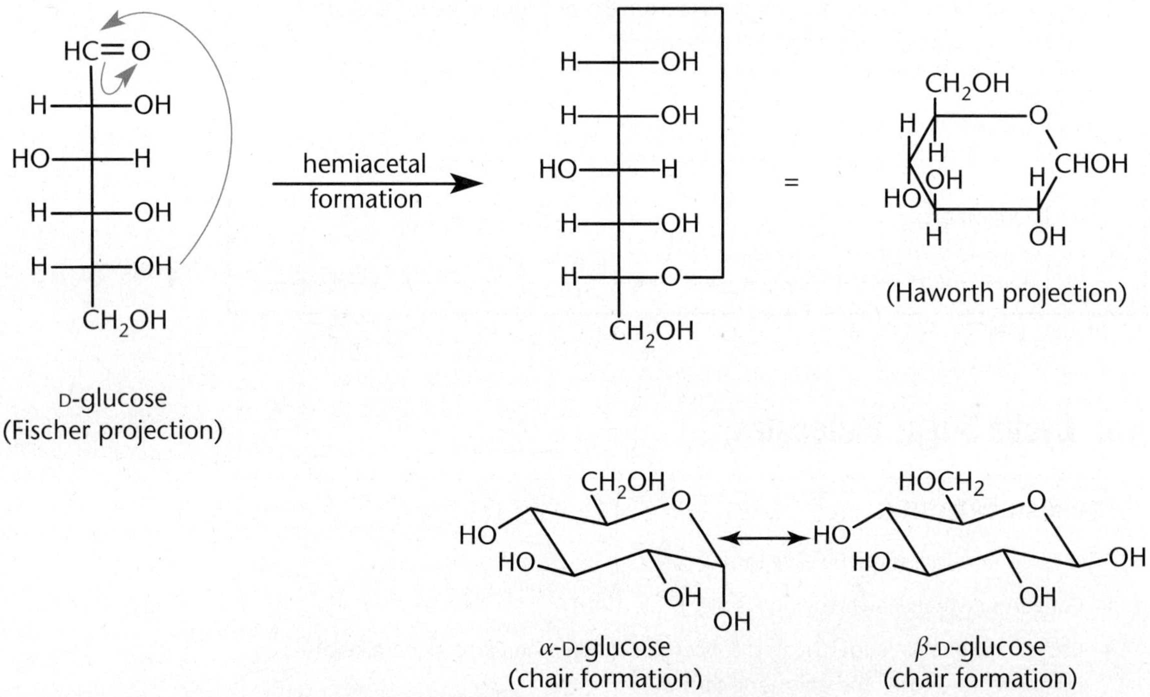

Figure 4.9 Cyclic Sugar Formation via Intramolecular Nucleophilic Addition
Glucose forms a six-membered ring with two anomeric forms: α (left) and β (right).

Hexose Conformations

Note how Figure 4.9 above has two kinds of projections for glucopyranose: the **Haworth projection** and the **Fischer projection**. The Haworth projection is a useful method for describing the three-dimensional conformations of cyclic structures. Haworth projections depict cyclic sugars as planar five- or six-membered rings with the top and bottom faces of the ring nearly perpendicular to the page. In reality the five-membered rings are very close to planar, but the pyranose rings adopt a chair-like configuration, and the substituents assume axial or equatorial positions to minimize steric hindrance. When we convert the monosaccharide from its straight-chain Fischer projection to the Haworth projection, any group on the right in the Fischer projection will point down.

Mutarotation

Exposing hemiacetal rings to water will cause them to spontaneously cycle between the open and closed form. Because the substituents on the single bond between C-1 and C-2 can rotate freely, either the α- or β-anomer can be formed, as demonstrated in Figure 4.10. This spontaneous change of configuration about C-1 is known as **mutarotation**, and occurs more rapidly when the reaction is catalyzed with an acid or base. Mutarotation results in a mixture that contains both α- and β-anomers at equilibrium concentrations (for glucose: 36% α, 64% β). In solution, the α-anomeric configuration is less favored because the hydroxyl group of the anomeric carbon is axial, adding to the steric strain of the molecule. In its solid state (not in solution), this preference can be mitigated by the anomeric effect, which helps stabilize the α-anomer, although this is outside the scope of the MCAT.

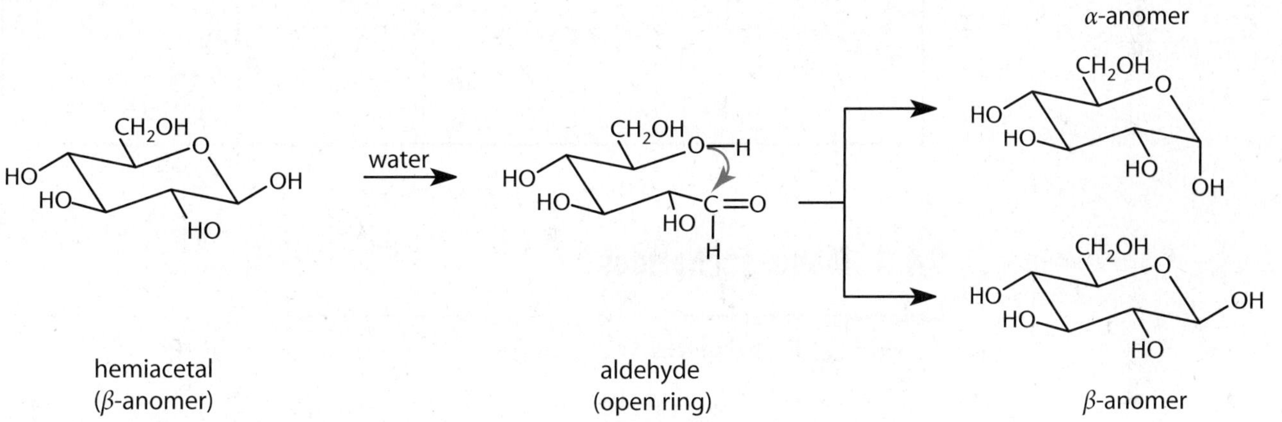

Figure 4.10 Mutarotation
Interconversion between the α- and β-anomers via ring opening and reclosing

MCAT CONCEPT CHECK 4.2

Before you move on, assess your understanding of the material with these questions.

1. Explain the relationship between the carbonyl carbon, anomeric carbon, and the alpha and beta forms of a sugar molecule.

2. Draw the less stable anomer of D-glucose in Haworth projection form.

3. Draw the less stable anomer of D-glucose in chair configuration.

4.3 Monosaccharides

LEARNING OBJECTIVES

After Chapter 4.3, you will be able to:

- Predict the products of sugar reactions, including oxidation, reduction, esterification, and glycosidic linkage formation
- Contrast Tollens' reagent and Benedict's reagent
- Apply reactions of sugars to biological contexts

Monosaccharides contain alcohols and either aldehydes or ketones. As such, these functional groups undergo the same reactions that they do when present in other compounds. These include oxidation and reduction, esterification, and nucleophilic attack (creating glycosides).

Oxidation and Reduction

One of the most important biochemical reactions in the human body is the oxidation of carbohydrates in order to yield energy. As monosaccharides switch between anomeric configurations, the hemiacetal rings spend a short period of time in the open-chain aldehyde form. Just like other aldehydes, they can be oxidized to carboxylic acids; these oxidized aldoses are called **aldonic acids**. Because aldoses can be oxidized, they are considered reducing agents. Therefore, any monosaccharide with a hemiacetal ring is considered a **reducing sugar**. When the aldose in question is in ring form, oxidation yields a **lactone** instead—a cyclic ester with a carbonyl group persisting on the anomeric carbon, as shown in Figure 4.11. Lactones, such as vitamin C, play an essential role in the human body.

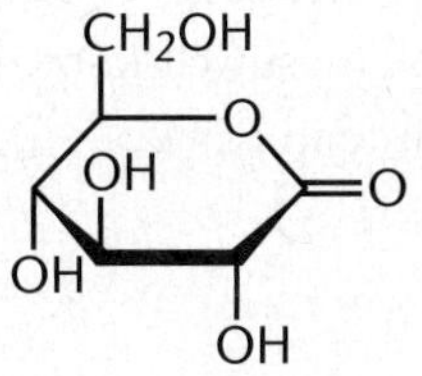

Figure 4.11 Lactone
Contains a cyclic ester

Two standard reagents are used to detect the presence of reducing sugars: Tollens' reagent and Benedict's reagent. **Tollens' reagent** must be freshly prepared, starting with silver nitrate ($AgNO_3$), which is mixed with NaOH to produce silver oxide (Ag_2O). Silver oxide is dissolved in ammonia to produce $[Ag(NH_3)_2]^+$, the actual Tollens' reagent. Tollens' reagent is reduced to produce a silvery mirror when aldehydes are present. When **Benedict's reagent** is used, the aldehyde group of an aldose is readily oxidized, indicated by a red precipitate of Cu_2O, as demonstrated in Figure 4.12. To test specifically for glucose, one may utilize the enzyme *glucose oxidase*, which does not react with other reducing sugars. A more powerful oxidizing agent, such as dilute nitric acid, will oxidize both the aldehyde and the primary alcohol (on C-6) to carboxylic acids.

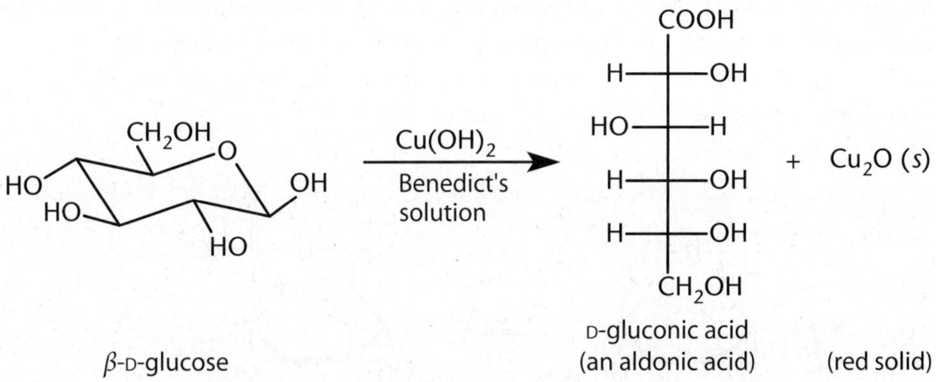

Figure 4.12 Positive Test for an Aldose Using Benedict's Reagent
Aldoses will react, forming copper(I) oxide; ketones may react more slowly.

An interesting phenomenon is that ketose sugars are also reducing sugars and give positive Tollens' and Benedict's tests. Although ketones cannot be oxidized directly to carboxylic acids, they can tautomerize to form aldoses under basic conditions, via *keto–enol* shifts. While in the aldose form, they can react with Tollens' or Benedict's reagents to form the carboxylic acid. **Tautomerization** refers to the rearrangement of bonds in a compound, usually by moving a hydrogen and forming a double bond.

In this case, the ketone group picks up a hydrogen while the double bond is moved between two adjacent carbons, resulting in an **enol**: a compound with a double bond and an alcohol group.

Reduced sugars also play an essential role in human biochemistry. When the aldehyde group of an aldose is reduced to an alcohol, the compound is considered an **alditol**. A **deoxy sugar**, on the other hand, contains a hydrogen that replaces a hydroxyl group on the sugar. The most well-known of these sugars is D-2-deoxyribose, the carbohydrate found in DNA.

Esterification

Because carbohydrates have hydroxyl groups, they are able to participate in reactions with carboxylic acids and carboxylic acid derivatives to form esters, as shown in Figure 4.13.

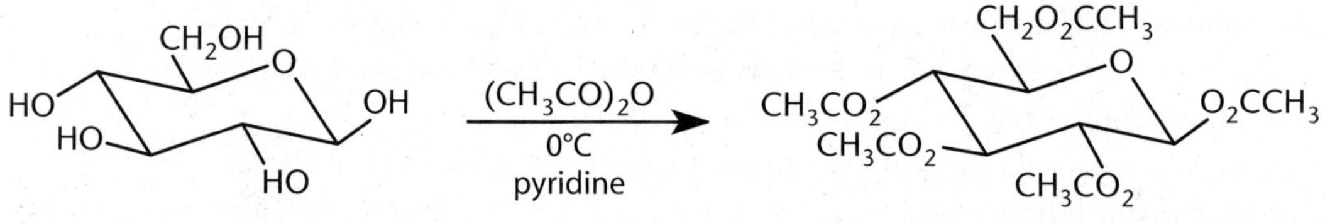

Figure 4.13 Esterification of Glucose
Acetic anhydride used as carboxylic acid derivative

BRIDGE

The action of hexokinase and glucokinase (as well as all the key glycolytic enzymes) is discussed in Chapter 9 of *MCAT Biochemistry Review*.

In the body, esterification is very similar to the phosphorylation of glucose, in which a **phosphate ester** is formed. Phosphorylation of glucose is an extremely important metabolic reaction of glycolysis in which a phosphate group is transferred from ATP to glucose, thus phosphorylating glucose while forming ADP, as shown in Figure 4.14. *Hexokinase* (or *glucokinase*, in the liver and pancreatic β-islet cells) catalyzes this reaction.

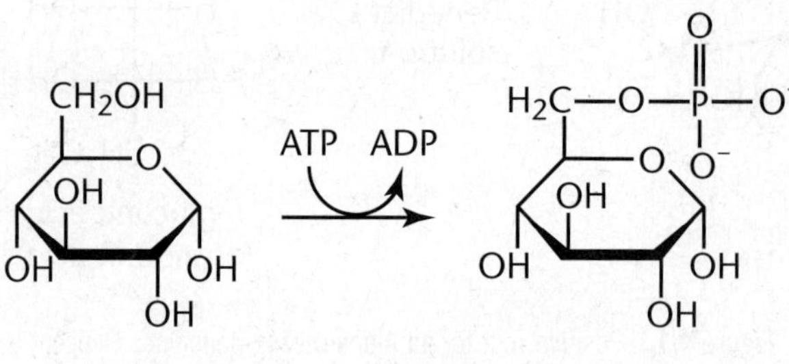

Figure 4.14 Phosphorylation of Glucose

Glycoside Formation

Hemiacetals react with alcohols to form **acetals**. The anomeric hydroxyl group is transformed into an alkoxy group, yielding a mixture of α- and β-acetals (with water as a leaving group). The resulting carbon–oxygen (C—O) bonds are called **glycosidic**

bonds, and the acetals formed are **glycosides**. An example is the reaction of glucose with ethanol shown in Figure 4.15. Equivalent reactions happen with hemiketals, forming ketals.

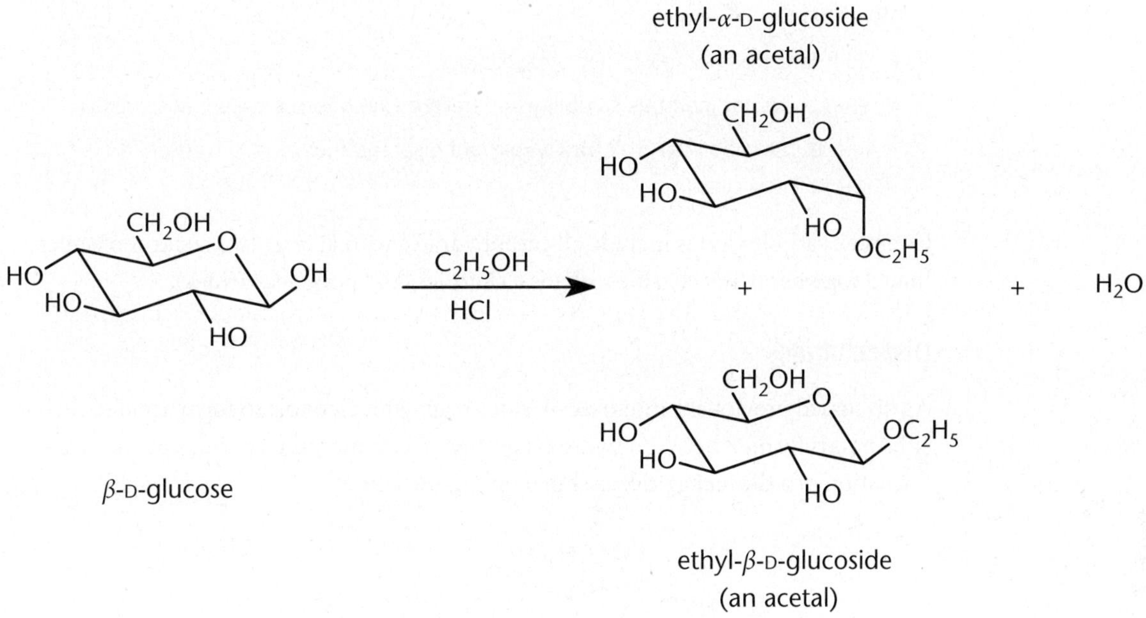

Figure 4.15 Glycosidic Linkage Formation
Hemiacetal (or hemiketal) sugars react with alcohols under acidic conditions to form acetals (or ketals).

Disaccharides and polysaccharides form as a result of glycosidic bonds between monosaccharides. Glycosides derived from furanose rings are referred to as **furanosides** and those derived from pyranose rings are called **pyranosides**. Note that glycoside formation is a dehydration reaction; thus, breaking a glycosidic bond requires hydrolysis.

MCAT CONCEPT CHECK 4.3

Before you move on, assess your understanding of the material with these questions.

1. Explain the difference between esterification and glycoside formation.

____

2. What purpose do Tollens' reagent and Benedict's reagent serve? How do they differ from each other?

____

3. From a metabolic standpoint, does it make sense for carbohydrates to get oxidized or reduced? What is the purpose of this process?

____

4.4 Complex Carbohydrates

LEARNING OBJECTIVES

After Chapter 4.4, you will be able to:

- Compare starches, glycogen, and cellulose
- Predict the comparative solubility of different starch forms based on structure
- Recognize important biologically relevant disaccharides

Complex carbohydrates include all carbohydrates with at least two sugar molecules linked together (disaccharides, oligosaccharides, and polysaccharides).

Disaccharides

As discussed previously, monosaccharides react with alcohols to form acetals. Glycosidic bonds formed between hydroxyl groups of two monosaccharides result in the formation of a **disaccharide**, as shown in Figure 4.16.

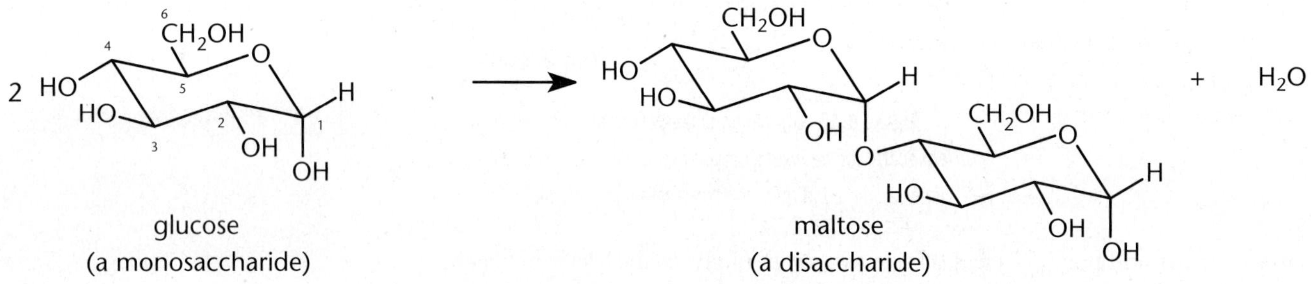

Figure 4.16 Disaccharide Formation

The hydroxyl group on the anomeric carbon reacts with the hydroxyl of another sugar to form an acetal (or ketal) with a 1,2; 1,4; or 1,6 glycosidic linkage.

Formation of an α- or β-glycosidic linkage is nonspecific in that the anomeric carbon of a cyclic sugar can react with any hydroxyl group on any other sugar molecule. The linkages are named for the configuration of the anomeric carbon and the numbers of the hydroxyl-containing carbons involved in the linkage. For example, in an α-1,6 glycosidic bond formation between two D-glucose molecules, the α-anomeric carbon of the first glucose (C-1) attaches to C-6 of the second glucose. Note that the second glucose could be either the α- or β-anomer. In the event that a glycosidic bond is formed between two anomeric carbons, this must be specified in the name. For example, a bond formed between the anomeric carbons of two α-D-glucose molecules would be termed an α,α-1,1 linkage, as demonstrated in Figure 4.17.

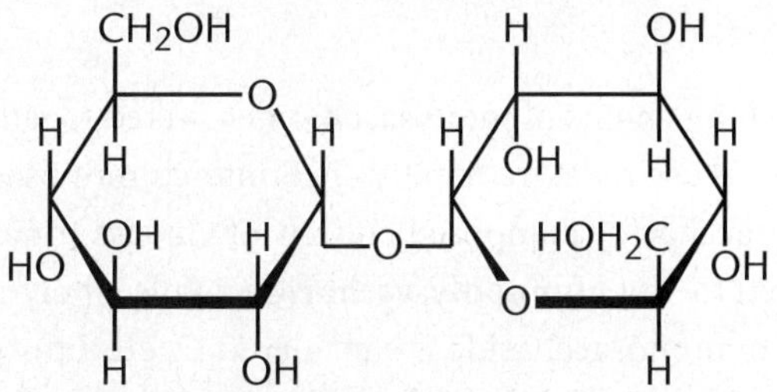

Figure 4.17 Trehalose
Example of a disaccharide with an α,α-1,1 linkage between the α-anomeric carbons of two glucose molecules

Various combinations of monosaccharides linked by glycosidic bonds result in the formation of different disaccharides. For instance, two glucose molecules linked by an α-1,4 glycosidic bond is called *maltose,* while two glucose molecules joined by a β-1,4 linkage is called *cellobiose.*

Important Disaccharides

When discussing disaccharides in a real-world context, the most important of these sugars are **sucrose, lactose,** and **maltose**. These disaccharides are commonly produced in the cell by enzymatic activity. Their molecular structures and linkages are highlighted in Figure 4.18.

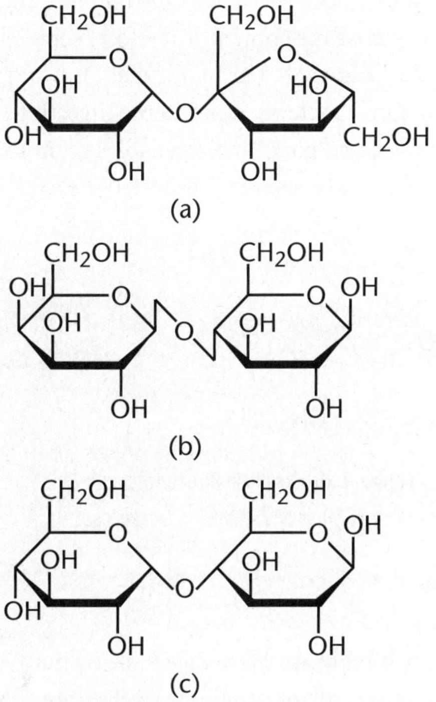

Figure 4.18 Important Disaccharides
(a) Sucrose (glucose-α-1,2-fructose), (b) Lactose (galactose-β-1,4-glucose), (c) Maltose (glucose-α-1,4-glucose)

Polysaccharides

Polysaccharides are long chains of monosaccharides linked together by glycosidic bonds. While glucose is the most frequently encountered monosaccharide, it is not the only one. A polysaccharide composed entirely of glucose (or any other monosaccharide) is referred to as a **homopolysaccharide**, while a polymer made up of more than one type of monosaccharide is considered a **heteropolysaccharide**. The three most important biological polysaccharides are cellulose, starch, and glycogen. Although these three polysaccharides have different functions, they are all composed of the same monosaccharide, D-glucose. These polysaccharides differ in configuration about the anomeric carbon and the position of glycosidic bonds, resulting in notable biological differences.

Because glycosidic bonding can occur at multiple hydroxyl groups in a monosaccharide, polymer formation can either be linear or branched. Branching happens when an internal monosaccharide in a polymer chain forms at least two glycosidic bonds, allowing branch formation. We'll take a closer look at how this is a key part of glycogen synthesis and glycogenolysis in Chapter 9 of *MCAT Biochemistry Review*.

Cellulose

Cellulose is the main structural component of plants. A homopolysaccharide, cellulose is a chain of β-D-glucose molecules linked by β-1,4 glycosidic bonds, with hydrogen bonds holding the actual polymer chains together for support. Humans are not able to digest cellulose because we lack the *cellulase* enzyme responsible for hydrolyzing cellulose to glucose monomers. Therefore, cellulose found in fruits and vegetables serves as a great source of fiber in our diet, drawing water into the gut. Cellulase is produced by some bacteria found in the digestive tract of certain animals, such as termites, cows, and goats, which enables them to digest cellulose. A portion of a cellulose chain can be seen in Figure 4.19 below.

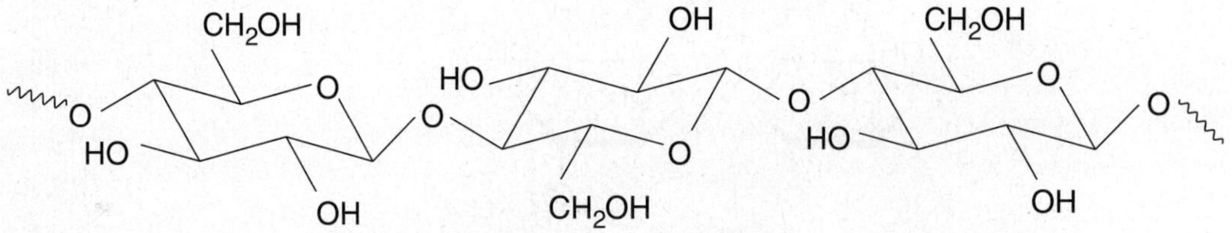

Figure 4.19 Cellulose Structure
Cellulose is a polymer of 1,4-linked β-D-glucose.

Starches

Starches are polysaccharides that are more digestible by humans because they are linked α-D-glucose monomers. Plants predominantly store starch as **amylose**, a linear glucose polymer linked via α-1,4 glycosidic bonds. Another type of starch is **amylopectin**, which starts off with the same type of linkage that amylose exhibits, but also contains branches via α-1,6 glycosidic bonds. Iodine is a well-known reagent that tests for the presence of starch and does so by fitting inside the helix conformation amylose typically makes, forming a starch–iodine complex. The structure of amylose is depicted in Figure 4.20.

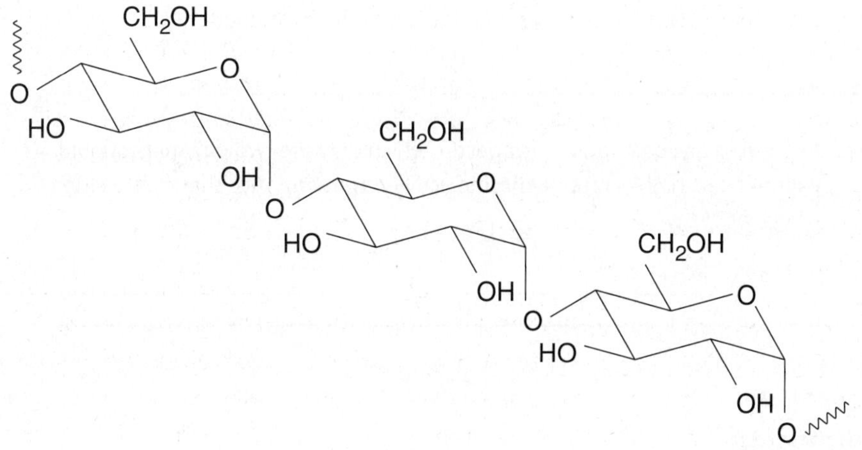

Figure 4.20 Starch Structure
Starches are polymers of 1,4-linked α-D-glucose.

Starches like amylose and amylopectin are broken down by enzymes in the body and are used as a source of energy. Amylose is degraded by *α-amylase* and *β-amylase*. **β-Amylase** cleaves amylose at the nonreducing end of the polymer (the end with acetal) to yield maltose, while **α-amylase** cleaves randomly along the chain to yield shorter polysaccharide chains, maltose, and glucose. Because amylopectin is highly branched, debranching enzymes help degrade the polysaccharide chain.

BRIDGE

The contrast between cellulose and starch digestibility exemplifies the specificity of enzymes. A slight 109.5° rotation of the anomeric carbon to form β-linkages (instead of α-linkages) is enough to make the molecule indigestible by any enzymes in humans—even though they're both D-glucose polymers! Enzyme specificity is discussed in Chapter 2 of *MCAT Biochemistry Review*.

Glycogen

Glycogen is a carbohydrate storage unit in animals. It is similar to starch, except that it has more α-1,6 glycosidic bonds (approximately one for every 10 glucose molecules, while amylopectin has approximately one for every 25), which makes it a highly branched compound. This branching optimizes the energy efficiency of glycogen and makes it more soluble in solution, thereby allowing more glucose to be stored in the body. Also, its branching pattern allows enzymes that cleave glucose from glycogen, such as *glycogen phosphorylase*, to work on many sites within the molecule simultaneously. **Glycogen phosphorylase** functions by cleaving glucose from the nonreducing end of a glycogen branch and phosphorylating it, thereby producing glucose 1-phosphate, which plays an important role in metabolism.

REAL WORLD

Hers disease, also known as glycogen storage disease (GSD) type VI, is a condition characterized by a deficiency in liver *glycogen phosphorylase*. Patients with this disease cannot break down glycogen in their livers and therefore have hepatomegaly (a swollen liver). They may also have hypoglycemia (low blood sugar) between meals because they cannot use glycogen to maintain blood glucose concentrations.

MCAT CONCEPT CHECK 4.4

Before you move on, assess your understanding of the material with these questions.

1. Which of the two forms of starch is more soluble in solution. Why?

____

2. Regarding glycogen and amylopectin, which of these two polymers should experience a higher rate of enzyme activity from enzymes that cleave side branches? Why?

____

Conclusion

This chapter examined, in depth, the unique characteristics of carbohydrates. Monosaccharides are the most basic form of carbohydrates, and in terms of human biochemistry, they typically range from three to seven carbon atoms. Classifying these monomers depends on the number of chiral centers present, which tells us the number of potential stereoisomers. Open-chain structures are most easily represented through Fischer projection diagrams; however, sugars tend to exist in ring form in biological systems, so Haworth projections are also used to depict three-dimensional structure. The most important reactions monosaccharides undergo are redox reactions, esterification, and glycoside formation—particularly when glycoside formation results in the formation of disaccharides. Polysaccharides are formed by glycosidic bonding of carbohydrates, and the polymers cellulose, starch, and glycogen are most commonly found in nature. Glycogen is the primary storage form of glucose in humans and other animals, and its unique branching structure allows for rapid access to these glucose stores.

The body has two primary energy-storage molecules: glycogen and triacylglycerols. Each has its own pros and cons—glycogen is more rapidly mobilized, but requires water of hydration, which increases its weight. Triacylglycerols serve as a long-term repository of energy, but take time to utilize. In the next chapter, we turn our attention to triacylglycerols, as well as the lipids used for structure and cell signaling.

You've reviewed the content, now test your knowledge and critical thinking skills by completing a test-like passage set in your online resources!

GO ONLINE

CONCEPT SUMMARY

Carbohydrate Classification

- Carbohydrates are organized by their number of carbon atoms and functional groups.
  - Common names are also frequently used when referring to sugars, such as glucose, fructose, and galactose.
  - Three-carbon sugars are trioses, four-carbon sugars are tetroses, and so on.
  - Sugars with aldehydes as their most oxidized group are **aldoses**; sugars with ketones as their most oxidized group are **ketoses**.
- The nomenclature of all sugars is based on the D- and L-forms of glyceraldehyde. Sugars with the highest-numbered chiral carbon with the −OH group on the right (in a Fischer projection) are D-sugars; those with the −OH on the left are L-sugars. D- and L-forms of the same sugar are **enantiomers**.
- **Diastereomers** are nonsuperimposable configurations of molecules with similar connectivity. They differ at at least one—but not all—chiral carbons. These also include epimers and anomers.
  - **Epimers** are a subtype of diastereomers that differ at exactly one chiral carbon.
  - **Anomers** are a subtype of epimers that differ at the anomeric carbon.

Cyclic Sugar Molecules

- Cyclization describes the ring formation of carbohydrates from their straight-chain forms.
- When rings form, the anomeric carbon can take on either an α- or β-conformation.
  - The **anomeric carbon** is the new chiral center formed in ring closure; it was the carbon containing the carbonyl in the straight-chain form.
  - **α-anomers** have the −OH on the anomeric carbon *trans* to the free $-CH_2OH$ group.
  - **β-anomers** have the −OH on the anomeric carbon *cis* to the free $-CH_2OH$ group.
- **Haworth projections** provide a good way to represent three-dimensional structure.
- Cyclic compounds can undergo **mutarotation**, in which they shift from one anomeric form to another with the straight-chain form as an intermediate.

Monosaccharides

- **Monosaccharides** are single carbohydrate units, with glucose as the most commonly observed monomer. They can undergo three main reactions: oxidation–reduction, esterification, and glycoside formation.
  - Aldoses can be oxidized to **aldonic acids** and reduced to **alditols**.
  - Sugars that can be oxidized are reducing agents (**reducing sugars**) themselves, and can be detected by reacting with **Tollens'** or **Benedict's reagents**.
  - Sugars with a –H replacing an –OH group are termed **deoxy sugars**.
  - Sugars can react with carboxylic acids and their derivatives, forming esters (**esterification**). **Phosphorylation** is a similar reaction in which a phosphate ester is formed by transferring a phosphate group from ATP onto a sugar.
  - **Glycoside formation** is the basis for building complex carbohydrates and requires the anomeric carbon to link to another sugar.

Complex Carbohydrates

- **Disaccharides** form as result of glycosidic bonding between two monosaccharide subunits; polysaccharides form by repeated monosaccharide or polysaccharide glycosidic bonding.
- Common disaccharides include **sucrose** (glucose-α-1,2-fructose), **lactose** (galactose-β-1,4-glucose), and **maltose** (glucose-α-1,4-glucose).
- Polysaccharides play various roles:
  - **Cellulose** is the main structural component for plant cell walls and is a main source of fiber in the human diet.
  - **Starches** (**amylose** and **amylopectin**) function as a main energy storage form for plants.
  - **Glycogen** functions as a main energy storage form for animals.

ANSWERS TO CONCEPT CHECKS

4.1

1. Aldopentose; ketohexose

2. 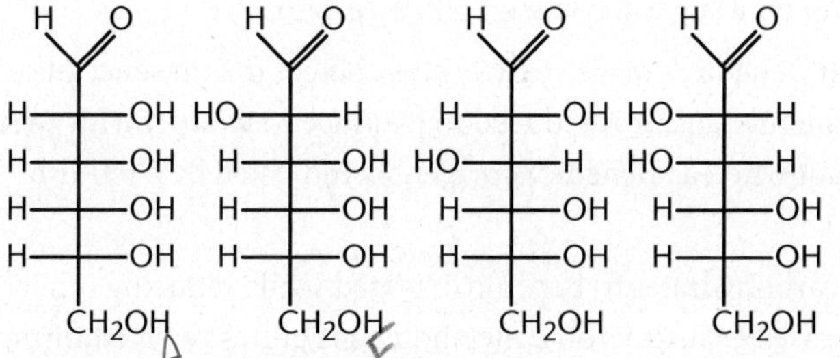

D-allose D-altrose D-glucose D-mannose

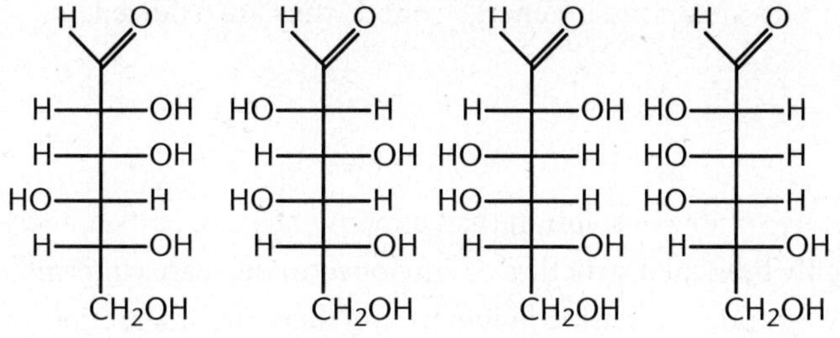

D-gulose D-idose D-galactose D-talose

3. D-Glucose's epimers are D-mannose (C-2), D-allose (C-3), and D-galactose (C-4). None of the D-stereoisomers is an enantiomer for glucose; L-glucose is the enantiomer of D-glucose.

4.2

1. During hemiacetal or hemiketal formation, the carbonyl carbon becomes chiral and is termed the anomeric carbon. The orientation of the —OH substituent on this carbon determines if the sugar molecule is the α- or β-anomer.

2. 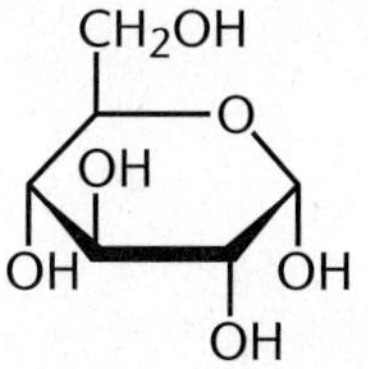

3. 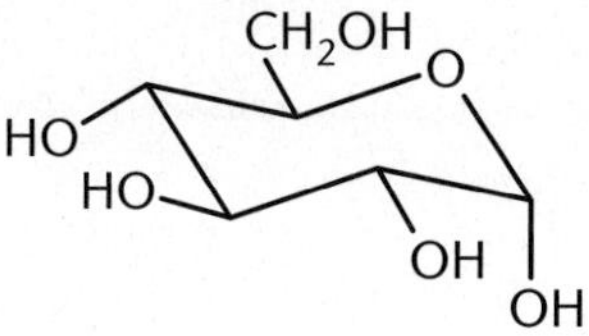

4.3

1. Esterification is the reaction by which a hydroxyl group reacts with either a carboxylic acid or a carboxylic acid derivative to form an ester. Glycoside formation refers to the reaction between an alcohol and a hemiacetal (or hemiketal) group on a sugar to yield an alkoxy group.
2. Tollens' reagent and Benedict's reagent are used to detect the presence of reducing sugars. Tollens' reagent is reduced to produce a silvery mirror when aldehydes are present whereas Benedict's reagent is indicated by a reddish precipitate of Cu_2O.
3. It makes sense for carbohydrates to become oxidized while reducing other groups. This is the case because aerobic metabolism requires reduced forms of electron carriers to facilitate processes such as oxidative phosphorylation. Because carbohydrates are a primary energy source, they are oxidized.

4.4

1. Amylopectin is more soluble in solution than amylose because of its branched structure. The highly branched structure of amylopectin decreases intermolecular bonding between polysaccharide polymers and increases interaction with the surrounding solution.
2. Glycogen has a higher rate of enzymatic branch cleavage because it contains significantly more branching than amylopectin.

SCIENCE MASTERY ASSESSMENT EXPLANATIONS

1. **D**

Glucose is an aldohexose, meaning that it has one aldehyde group and six carbons. Given this information, **(A)** and **(B)** can be eliminated. In aldose sugars, each nonterminal carbon is chiral. Therefore, glucose has four chiral centers, not five, as mentioned in **(C)**. The number of stereoisomers possible for a chiral molecule is 2^n, where n is the number of chiral carbons. Because glucose has four chiral centers, there are $2^4 = 16$ possible stereoisomers.

2. **D**

Epimers are monosaccharide diastereomers that differ in their configuration about only one carbon. As with all diastereomers, epimers have different chemical and physical properties, and their optical activities have no relation to each other. Enantiomers have equal but opposite optical activities. Therefore, **(D)** is the only statement that does not apply to epimers.

3. **C**

Aldonic acids form after the aldehyde group on a reducing sugar reduces another compound, becoming oxidized in the process.

4. **B**

Mutarotation is the interconversion between anomers of a compound. Enantiomerization and racemization, **(C)** and **(D)**, are related: enantiomerization is the formation of a mirror-image or optically inverted form of a compound, whereas racemization is moving a solution toward an equal concentration of both enantiomers. Glycosidation, **(A)**, is the addition of a sugar to another compound.

5. **A**

Ketose sugars undergo tautomerization, a rearrangement of bonds, to undergo *keto–enol* shifts. This forms an aldose, which then allows them to act as reducing sugars. A ketone group alone cannot be oxidized. Anomerization, mentioned in **(C)**, refers to ring closure of a monosaccharide, creating an anomeric carbon.

6. **B**

When glucose reacts with methanol under acid catalysis, the hemiacetal is converted to an acetal via replacement of the anomeric hydroxyl group with an alkoxy group. The result is a type of acetal known as a glycoside. This corresponds with **(B)**. The other choices all show alkoxy groups on the wrong carbon, or too many carbons.

7. **B**

β-Amylase cleaves amylose at the nonreducing end of the polymer to yield maltose exclusively, while α-amylase, **(A)**, cleaves amylose anywhere along the chain to yield short polysaccharides, maltose, and glucose. Debranching enzyme, **(C)**, removes oligosaccharides from a branch in glycogen or starches, while glycogen phosphorylase, **(D)**, yields glucose 1-phosphate.

8. **C**

Start by drawing out the Haworth projection. Recall that all the groups on the right in the Fischer projection will go on the bottom of the Haworth projection, and all the groups on the left will go on the top. Next, draw the chair structure, with the oxygen in the back right corner. Label the carbons in the ring 1 through 5, starting from the oxygen and moving clockwise around the ring. Now, draw in the lines for all the axial substituents, alternating above and below the ring. Remember to start on the anomeric C-1 carbon, where the axial substituent points down. Now start filling in the substituents. The substituent can be in either position on the anomeric carbon, so skip that one for now. The –OH groups on C-2 and C-4 should point downward while the –OH group on C-3 should point upward; **(C)**, the β-anomer of D-glucose, is the only one that matches.

9. **B**

The hydroxyl group on the anomeric carbon of the β-anomer is equatorial, thereby creating less nonbonded strain than the α-anomer, which has the hydroxyl group of the anomeric carbon in axial position.

10. **D**

Glycogen and amylopectin are the only polysaccharide forms that demonstrate branching structure, making them most similar in terms of linkage. Both glycogen and amylopectin use α-1,4 and α-1,6 linkages. Cellulose uses β-1,4 linkages and amylose does not contain α-1,6 linkages.

11. **C**

While maltose and cellobiose both have the same glucose subunits, only maltose is digestible by humans because the β-glycosidic linkages in cellobiose cannot be cleaved in the human body.

12. **C**

In solution, the hemiacetal ring of glucose will break open spontaneously and then re-form. When the ring is broken, bond rotation occurs between C-1 and C-2 to produce either the α- or the β-anomer. The reaction given in this question depicts the mutarotation of glucose. **(A)** is incorrect because the reactant is an aldehyde, not the product. **(B)** is incorrect because a hemiketal has an $-$OH group, an $-$OR group, and two $-$R groups. In addition, hemiketals are formed from ketones, and our starting reactant is an aldehyde. Finally, **(D)** is incorrect because there is no glycosidic bond in the starting reactant.

13. **A**

Galactose is a diastereomer of glucose, with the stereochemistry at C-4 (counting from the aldehyde) reversed. Being able to identify C-4 is enough to answer this question, even without looking at the glucose molecule. Because **(B)**, **(C)**, and **(D)** have identical stereochemistry at C-4, they are incorrect.

14. **D**

In Andersen's disease, glycogen is less branched than normal, thereby inducing lower solubility of glycogen. Branches reduce the interactions between adjacent chains of glycogen and encourage interactions with the aqueous environment. The smaller number of branches means that glycogen phosphorylase has fewer terminal glucose monomers on which to act, making enzyme activity slower than normal overall. Finally, without branches, the density of glucose monomers cannot be as high; therefore, the total glucose stored is lower than normal. Glycogen synthase is still functioning normally, so we would expect normal α-1,4 linkages in the glycogen of an individual with Andersen's disease but few (if any) α-1,6 linkages.

15. **C**

Monosaccharides can exist as hemiacetals or hemiketals, depending on whether they are aldoses or ketoses. When a monosaccharide is in its cyclic form, the anomeric carbon is attached to the oxygen in the ring and a hydroxyl group. Hence, it is only a hemiacetal or hemiketal because an acetal or ketal would require the $-$OH group to be converted to another $-$OR group.

Consult your online resources for additional practice. **GO ONLINE**

EQUATIONS TO REMEMBER

(4.1) **Number of stereoisomers with common backbone** $= 2^n$

SHARED CONCEPTS

Biochemistry Chapter 9
Carbohydrate Metabolism I

Biochemistry Chapter 10
Carbohydrate Metabolism II

Organic Chemistry Chapter 1
Nomenclature

Organic Chemistry Chapter 2
Isomers

Organic Chemistry Chapter 5
Alcohols

Organic Chemistry Chapter 6
Aldehydes and Ketones I

CHAPTER 5

LIPID STRUCTURE AND FUNCTION

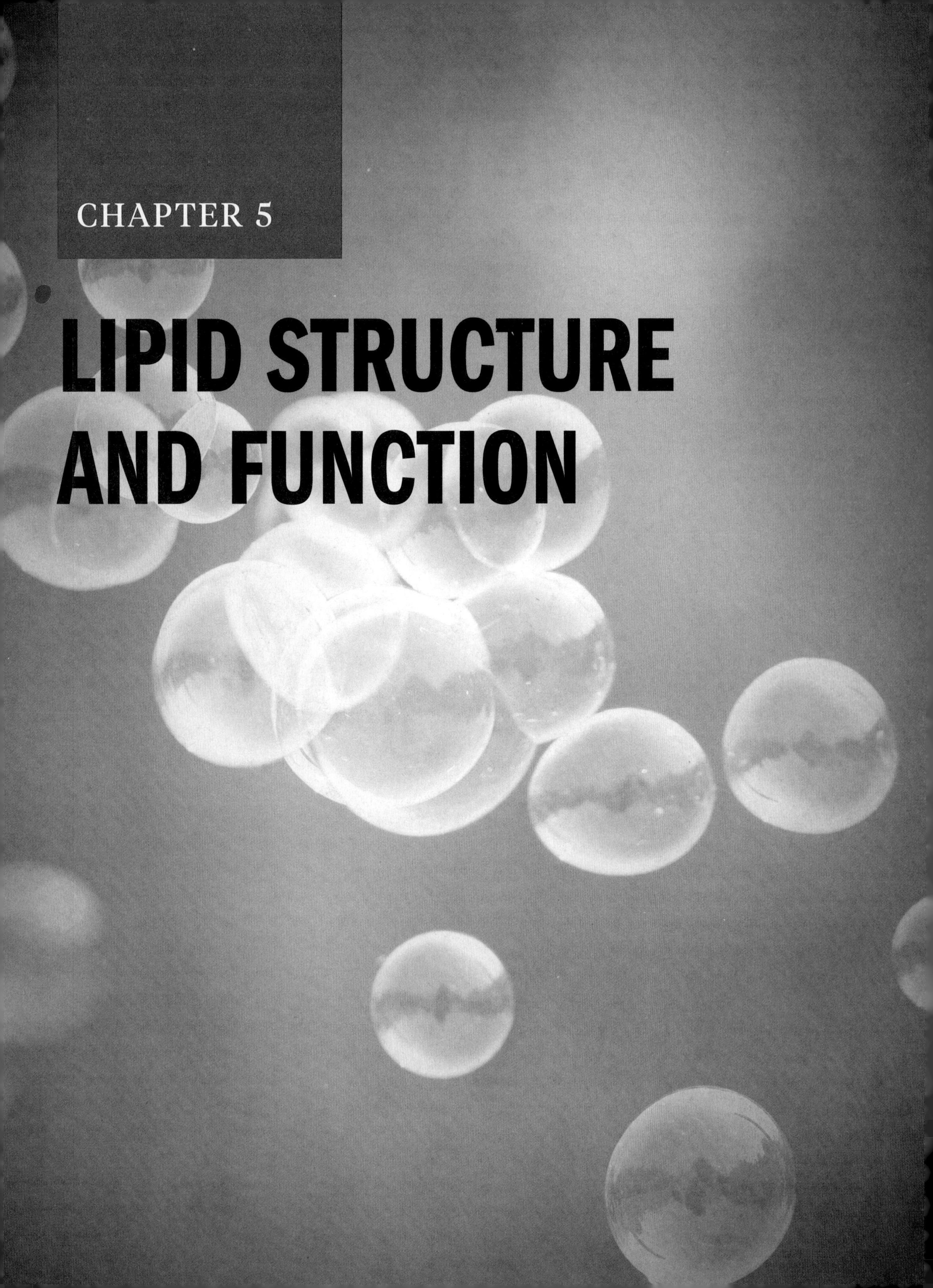

SCIENCE MASTERY ASSESSMENT

Every pre-med knows this feeling: there is so much content I have to know for the MCAT! How do I know what to do first or what's important?

While the high-yield badges throughout this book will help you identify the most important topics, this Science Mastery Assessment is another tool in your MCAT prep arsenal. This quiz (which can also be taken in your online resources) and the guidance below will help ensure that you are spending the appropriate amount of time on this chapter based on your personal strengths and weaknesses. Don't worry though—skipping something now does not mean you'll never study it. Later on in your prep, as you complete full-length tests, you'll uncover specific pieces of content that you need to review and can come back to these chapters as appropriate.

How to Use This Assessment

If you answer 0–7 questions correctly:

Spend about 1 hour to read this chapter in full and take limited notes throughout. Follow up by reviewing **all** quiz questions to ensure that you now understand how to solve each one.

If you answer 8–11 questions correctly:

Spend 20–40 minutes reviewing the quiz questions. Beginning with the questions you missed, read and take notes on the corresponding subchapters. For questions you answered correctly, ensure your thinking matches that of the explanation and you understand why each choice was correct or incorrect.

If you answer 12–15 questions correctly:

Spend less than 20 minutes reviewing all questions from the quiz. If you missed any, then include a quick read-through of the corresponding subchapters, or even just the relevant content within a subchapter, as part of your question review. For questions you got correct, ensure your thinking matches that of the explanation and review the Concept Summary at the end of the chapter.

1. Which of the following is NOT a type of glycolipid?
   A. Cerebroside
   B. Globoside
   C. Ganglioside
   D. Sphingomyelin

2. During saponification:
   A. triacylglycerols undergo a condensation reaction.
   B. triacylglycerols undergo ester hydrolysis.
   C. fatty acid salts are produced using a strong acid.
   D. fatty acid salts are bound to albumin.

3. Which of the following best describes the structure of steroids?
   A. Three cyclopentane rings, one cyclohexane ring
   B. Three cyclohexane rings, one cyclopentane ring
   C. Four carbon rings, differing in structure for each steroid
   D. Three cyclic carbon rings and a functional group

4. Soap bubbles form because fatty acid salts organize into:
   A. lysosomes.
   B. micelles.
   C. phospholipid bilayers.
   D. hydrogen bonds.

5. Steroid hormones are steroids that:
   I. have specific high-affinity receptors.
   II. travel in the bloodstream from endocrine glands to distant sites.
   III. affect gene transcription by binding directly to DNA.

   A. I only
   B. III only
   C. I and II only
   D. I and III only

6. Why are triacylglycerols used in the human body for energy storage?
   A. They are highly hydrated and therefore can store lots of energy.
   B. They always have short fatty acid chains for easy access by metabolic enzymes.
   C. The carbon atoms of the fatty acid chains are highly reduced and therefore yield more energy upon oxidation.
   D. Polysaccharides, which would actually be a better energy storage form, would dissolve in the body.

7. Which of the following is correct about fat-soluble vitamins?
   I. Vitamin E is important for calcium regulation.
   II. Vitamin D protects against cancer because it is a biological antioxidant.
   III. Vitamin K is necessary for the posttranslational introduction of calcium-binding sites.
   IV. Vitamin A is metabolized to retinal, which is important for sight.

   A. III only
   B. I and II only
   C. III and IV only
   D. II, III, and IV only

8. Which of the following is true of amphipathic molecules?
   A. They form protective spheres in any solvent, with hydrophobic molecules interior and hydrophilic molecules exterior.
   B. They have two fatty acid chains and a polar head group.
   C. They are important to the formation of the phospholipid bilayer and soap bubbles.
   D. They have a glycerol base.

9. Which of the following is/are true about sphingolipids?

- **I.** They are all phospholipids.
- **II.** They all contain a sphingosine backbone.
- **III.** They can have either phosphodiester or glycosidic linkages to their polar head groups.

- **A.** I only
- **B.** III only
- **C.** II and III only
- **D.** I, II, and III

10. Which of the following statements about saturation is FALSE?

- **A.** It can describe the number of double or triple bonds in a fatty acid tail.
- **B.** It determines at least one of the properties of membranes.
- **C.** More saturated fatty acids make for a more fluid solution.
- **D.** Fully saturated fatty acids have only single bonds.

11. Which of the following is true about glycerophospholipids?

- **A.** Glycerophospholipids can sometimes be sphingolipids, depending on the bonds in their head groups.
- **B.** Glycerophospholipids are merely a subset of phospholipids.
- **C.** Glycerophospholipids are used in the ABO blood typing system.
- **D.** Glycerophospholipids have one glycerol, one polar head group, and one fatty acid tail.

12. Which of the following statements about terpenes is FALSE?

- **A.** Terpenes are strongly scented molecules that sometimes serve protective functions.
- **B.** Terpenes are steroid precursors.
- **C.** A triterpene is made of three isoprene moieties, and therefore has 15 carbons.
- **D.** Terpenes are made by plants and insects.

13. Which of the following is true about cholesterol?

- **A.** Cholesterol always increases membrane fluidity in cells.
- **B.** Cholesterol is a steroid hormone precursor.
- **C.** Cholesterol is a precursor for vitamin A, which is produced in the skin.
- **D.** Cholesterol interacts only with the hydrophobic tails of phospholipids.

14. Which of the following statements regarding prostaglandins is FALSE?

- **A.** Prostaglandins regulate the synthesis of cAMP.
- **B.** Prostaglandin synthesis is inhibited by NSAIDs.
- **C.** Prostaglandins affect pain, inflammation, and smooth muscle function.
- **D.** Prostaglandins are endocrine hormones, like steroid hormones.

15. Which of the statements regarding waxes is FALSE?

- **A.** Waxes generally have melting points above room temperature.
- **B.** Waxes are produced only in plants and insects and therefore must be consumed by humans.
- **C.** Waxes protect against dehydration and parasites.
- **D.** Waxes are esters of long-chain fatty acids and long-chain alcohols.

Answer Key

1. **D**
2. **B**
3. **B**
4. **B**
5. **C**
6. **C**
7. **C**
8. **C**
9. **B**
10. **C**
11. **B**
12. **C**
13. **B**
14. **D**
15. **B**

Detailed explanations can be found at the end of the chapter.

CHAPTER 5

LIPID STRUCTURE AND FUNCTION

In This Chapter

CHAPTER PROFILE

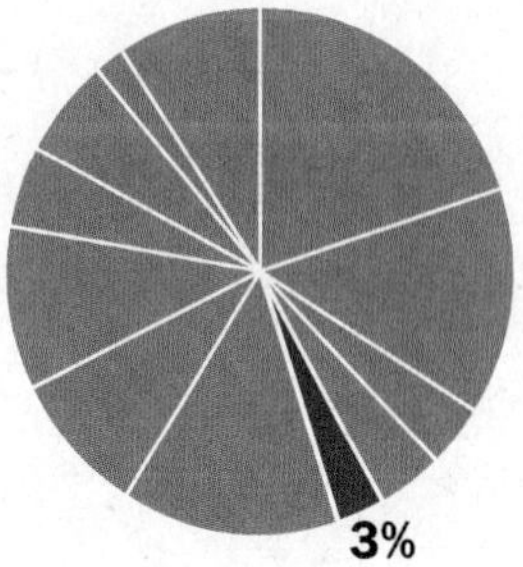

The content in this chapter should be relevant to about 3% of all questions about biochemistry on the MCAT.

This chapter covers material from the following AAMC content categories:

1D: Principles of bioenergetics and fuel molecule metabolism

3A: Structure and functions of the nervous and endocrine systems, and ways in which these systems coordinate the organ systems

5D: Structure, function, and reactivity of biologically-relevant molecules

Introduction

What do beer, human eyes, and sperm whales have in common? For all of these, lipids play a key role in some of their most interesting characteristics. The taste and smell of hops comes from lipids called *terpenes*. The ability of the human eye to respond to light (and therefore see) relies heavily on *retinal*, a lipid derived from vitamin A. Sperm whales use an enormous reservoir of *spermaceti* to dive to a depth of up to three kilometers to hunt giant squid. Spermaceti is a lipid with a density that changes dramatically with temperature—effectively allowing sperm whales to adjust their density with depth so that they can stay submerged without having to constantly fight buoyancy.

Lipids, as a class, are characterized by insolubility in water and solubility in nonpolar organic solvents. Aside from this shared feature, lipids diverge dramatically in their structural organization and biological functions, serving vital structural, signaling, and energy storage roles. In this chapter, we will explore the structural and functional characteristics of each of the major categories of lipids tested on the MCAT.

As structural building blocks, we will investigate *phospholipids* and *sterols*, which make up vesicles, liposomes, and membranes. When it comes to signaling, we will note that lipids serve multiple roles, from enzyme cofactors to light-absorbing pigments, and from intracellular messengers to hormones. Finally, we will see that lipids are the workhorse of energy storage, giving the most "bang" for the metabolic "buck" by weight.

5.1 Structural Lipids

LEARNING OBJECTIVES

After Chapter 5.1, you will be able to:

- Recall the major structural traits of phospholipids, glycerophospholipids, and sphingolipids
- Recognize how membrane lipid structure contributes to overall membrane structure and function
- Distinguish between the three types of sphingolipids
- Identify the polar and nonpolar regions of lipids:

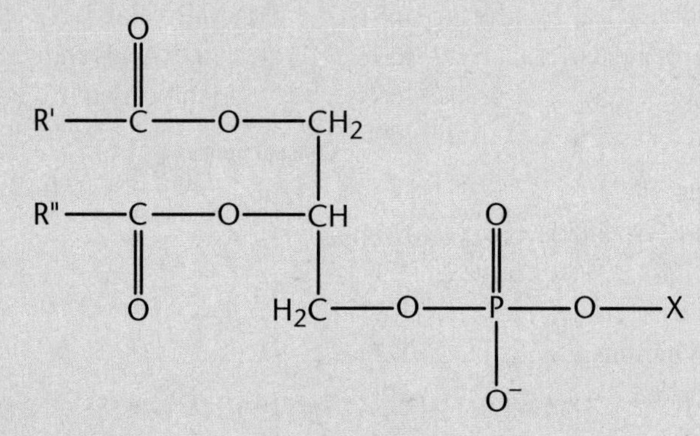

Lipids are the major component of the phospholipid bilayer, one of the most important structural parts of the cell. The unique ability of phospholipids to form a bilayer allows our cells to function as they do, separating the cell interior from the surrounding environment. We will first take a close look at the structure and role of phospholipids, glycerophospholipids, and sphingolipids. Finally, we will review the gross structural characteristics of the unique class called waxes.

Each of the membrane components is an **amphipathic** molecule, meaning that it has both hydrophilic and hydrophobic regions. For these membrane lipids, the polar head is the hydrophilic region, whereas the fatty acid tails are the hydrophobic region. When placed in aqueous solution, these molecules spontaneously form structures that allow the hydrophobic regions to group internally while the hydrophilic regions interact with water. This leads to the formation of various structures, including liposomes, micelles, and the phospholipid bilayer, shown in Figure 5.1.

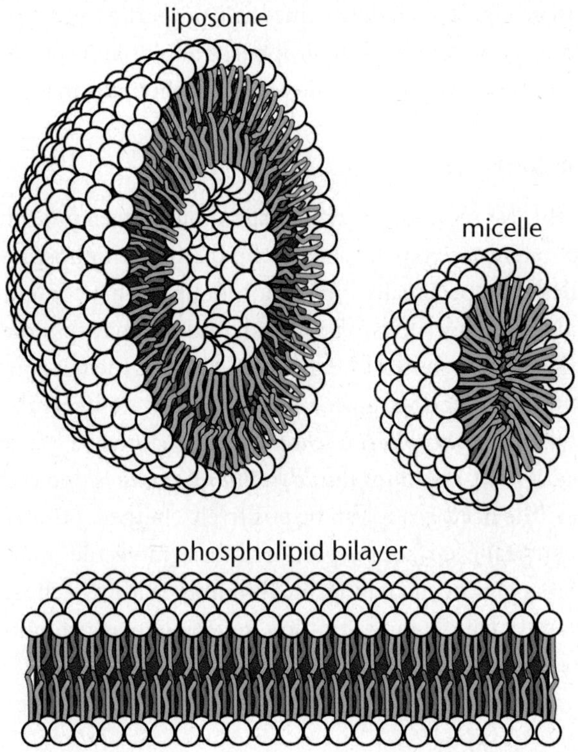

Figure 5.1 Membrane Lipids Form Various Structures in Aqueous Solutions

Phospholipids

Phospholipids contain the following elements: a phosphate and alcohol that comprise the polar head group, joined to a hydrophobic fatty acid tail by phosphodiester linkages. One or more fatty acids are attached to a backbone to form the hydrophobic tail region. Phospholipids can be further classified according to the backbone on which the molecule is built. For example, ***glycerol***, a three-carbon alcohol, forms *phosphoglycerides* or *glycerophospholipids*, and *sphingolipids* have a *sphingosine* backbone. One important thing to note, however, is that not all sphingolipids are phospholipids, as described later in this chapter.

One thing that these lipids do all share in common is a tail composed of long-chain fatty acids. These hydrocarbon chains vary by their degree of **saturation** and length. These two properties determine how the overall molecule will behave. Fully **saturated fatty acid** tails will have only single bonds; the carbon atom is considered saturated when it is bonded to four other atoms, with no π bonds. Saturated fatty acids, such as those in butter, have greater van der Waals forces and a more stable overall structure. Therefore, they form solids at room temperature. An **unsaturated fatty acid** includes one or more double bonds. Double bonds introduce kinks into the fatty acid chain, which makes it difficult for them to stack and solidify. Therefore, unsaturated fats—like olive oil—tend to be liquids at room temperature. The same rules apply in the phospholipid bilayer: phospholipids with unsaturated fatty acid tails make up more fluid regions of the phospholipid bilayer. Phospholipids, glycerophospholipids, and sphingolipids can have any of a variety of fatty acid tails and

BRIDGE

Although phospholipids are indeed the largest component of the phospholipid bilayer, nonphospholipids like glycolipids also play a role—and can be an important part of processes like cell recognition and signaling, discussed in Chapter 3 of *MCAT Biochemistry Review.*

KEY CONCEPT

Lipid properties—for all categories of lipids—are determined by the degree of saturation in fatty acid chains and the functional groups to which the fatty acid chains are bonded.

also different head groups, which determine their properties at the surface of the cell membrane. The next two sections—glycerophospholipids and sphingolipids—focus on the various polar head groups that different phospholipids may have.

Glycerophospholipids

As mentioned in the last section, glycerophospholipids are all phospholipids; yet, not all phospholipids are glycerophospholipids! **Glycerophospholipids** (or **phosphoglycerides**) are specifically those phospholipids that contain a glycerol backbone bonded by ester linkages to two fatty acids and by a phosphodiester linkage to a highly polar head group, as shown in Figure 5.2. Because the head group determines the membrane surface properties, glycerophospholipids are named according to their head group. For example, ***phosphatidylcholine*** is the name of a glycerophospholipid with a *choline* head group, and ***phosphatidylethanolamine*** is one with an *ethanolamine* head group. The head group can be positively charged, negatively charged, or neutral. The membrane surface properties of these molecules make them very important to cell recognition, signaling, and binding. Within each subtype, the fatty acid chains can vary in length and saturation, resulting in an astounding variety of functions that are the focus of active scientific research.

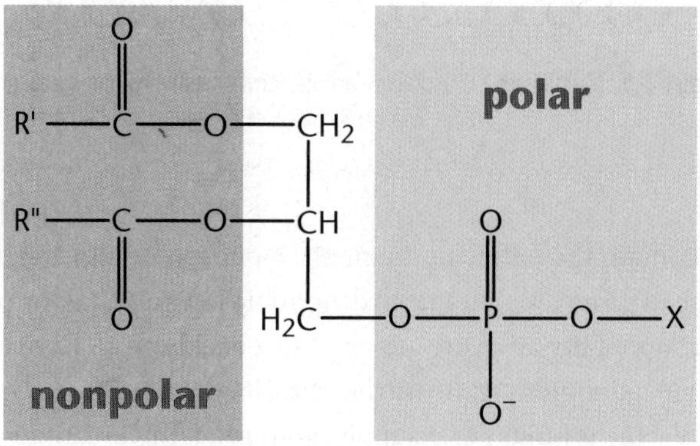

Figure 5.2 Structure of a Glycerophospholipid
X denotes the head group connected to the glycerol backbone by a phosphodiester linkage.

REAL WORLD

Although experiments in blood transfusion are recorded as early as the 17th century, blood typing wasn't developed until the 20th century. With the advent of the ABO and Rh factor blood typing systems, blood transfusions could now be successfully administered to patients with hemophilia (a clotting disorder that causes significant bleeding), during surgery, and in a number of other applications.

Sphingolipids

Blood typing makes it possible to give life-saving blood transfusions without risking potentially fatal acute hemolytic reactions. The ABO blood typing system is based on cell-surface antigens on red blood cells. These cell-surface antigens are some of the most well-known sphingolipids. Like glycerophospholipids, sphingolipids are also sites of biological recognition at the cell surface and can be bonded to various head groups and fatty acids.

Sphingolipids have a **sphingosine** or **sphingoid** (sphingosine-like) backbone, as opposed to the glycerol backbone of glycerophospholipids. These molecules also have long-chain, nonpolar fatty acid tails and polar head groups. Many sphingolipids are also phospholipids because they contain a phosphodiester linkage. However, other sphingolipids contain glycosidic linkages to sugars; any lipid linked to a sugar can be termed a ***glycolipid***. Sphingolipids are divided into four major subclasses, differing by their head group.

The simplest sphingolipid is ***ceramide***, which has a single hydrogen atom as its head group.

Sphingomyelins are the major class of sphingolipids that are also phospholipids (**sphingophospholipids**). These molecules have either phosphocholine or phosphoethanolamine as a head group, and thus contain a phosphodiester bond. Sphingomyelin head groups have no net charge. As the name implies, sphingomyelins are major components in the plasma membranes of cells producing myelin (oligodendrocytes and Schwann cells), the insulating sheath for axons.

Sphingolipids with head groups composed of sugars bonded by glycosidic linkages are considered glycolipids, as mentioned above, or, more specifically, ***glycosphingolipids***. These molecules are not phospholipids because they contain no phosphodiester linkage. Glycosphingolipids are found mainly on the outer surface of the plasma membrane and can be further classified as *cerebrosides* or *globosides*. **Cerebrosides** have a single sugar, whereas **globosides** have two or more. These molecules are also referred to as neutral glycolipids because they have no net charge at physiological pH.

The final group is composed of the most complex sphingolipids. ***Gangliosides*** are glycolipids that have polar head groups composed of oligosaccharides with one or more ***N-acetylneuraminic acid*** (**NANA**; also called **sialic acid**) molecules at the terminus and a negative charge. These molecules are also considered glycolipids because they have a glycosidic linkage and no phosphate group. Gangliosides play a major role in cell interaction, recognition, and signal transduction.

A summary of the different types of sphingolipids is provided in Figure 5.3.

REAL WORLD

Sphingolipid accumulation is associated with numerous pathological conditions. Sphingomyelins found in the myelin sheath help in signal transduction. Accumulation of sphingomyelin, resulting from lack of the enzyme *sphingomyelinase*, can result in *Niemann-Pick disease*. Symptoms can include intellectual disability and seizures. *Sulfatides* are sulfated cerebrosides associated with Alzheimer's disease.

MNEMONIC

Gangliosides are the "**gangly**" sphingolipids, with the most complex structure and functional groups (oligosaccharides and NANA) in all directions.

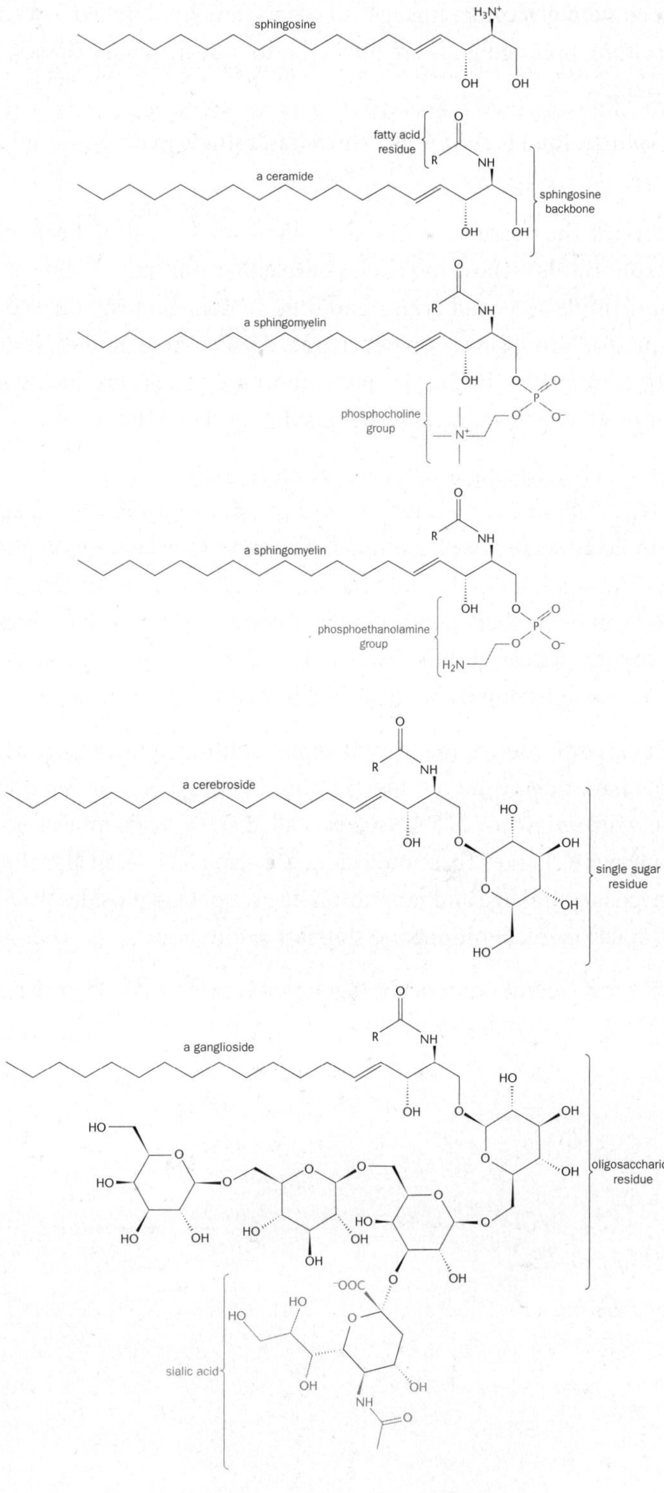

Figure 5.3 Types of Sphingolipids

Ceramide has a single hydrogen atom for a head group; sphingomyelins have phosphodiester linkages (phospholipids); cerebrosides have one sugar; globosides (not pictured) have multiple sugars; gangliosides have oligosaccharides and terminal sialic acids.

Waxes

Waxes are esters of long-chain fatty acids with long-chain alcohols. As one might expect, they form pliable solids at room temperature (what we generally think of as *wax*). Biologically, they function as protection for both plants and animals. In plants, waxes are secreted as a surface coating to prevent excessive evaporation and to protect against parasites. In animals, waxes are secreted to prevent dehydration, as a water-repellant to keep skin and feathers dry, and as lubricant. For example, *carnauba wax* is made from the leaves of the *Copernicia prunifera* palm and is used to coat candies and wax cars. Bees secrete waxes to construct shelter, as shown in Figure 5.4.

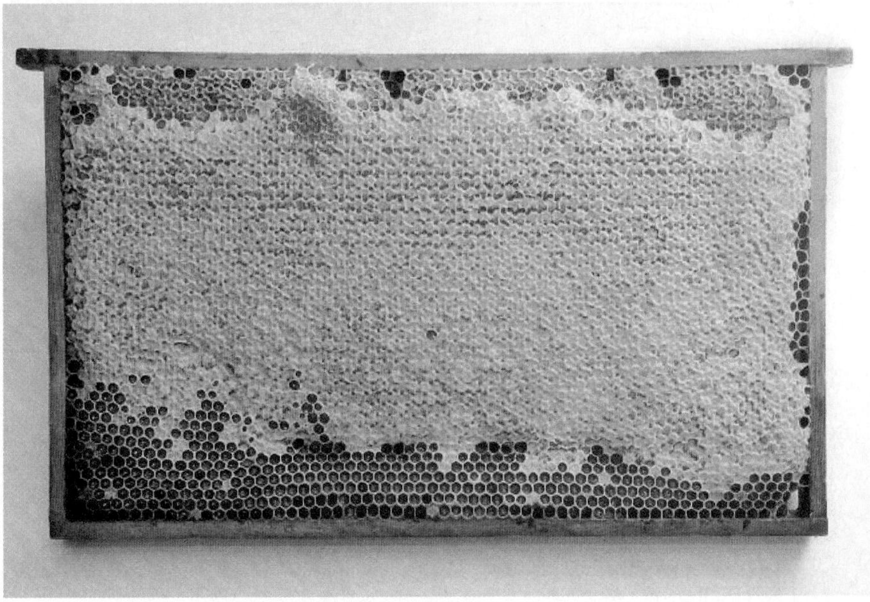

Figure 5.4 Honeycomb Structure Made from Beeswax
The solid and plastic nature of waxes, which contain esters with long alkyl chains, permits their use for structure building.

MCAT CONCEPT CHECK 5.1

Before you move on, assess your understanding of the material with these questions.

1. Which components of membrane lipids contribute to their structural role in membranes? Which components contribute to function?
   - Structure:
   - Function:

2. What is the difference between a sphingolipid that is also a phospholipid and one that is NOT?

3. Name the three main types of sphingolipids and their characteristics.

Type	Phospholipid or Glycolipid?	Functional Group(s)

4. What would happen if an amphipathic molecule were placed in a nonpolar solvent rather than an aqueous solution?

5.2 Signaling Lipids

LEARNING OBJECTIVES

After Chapter 5.2, you will be able to:

- Recall the structural features of terpenes, steroids, and prostaglandins
- Differentiate steroids from steroid hormones
- Connect prostaglandins to the symptoms associated with their presence, such as pain and inflammation
- Explain the importance of fat-soluble vitamins: A, D, E, and K

BRIDGE

Remember from Chapter 2 of *MCAT Biochemistry Review* that a coenzyme is an organic, nonprotein factor bound to an enzyme and required for its normal activity.

In addition to passive roles in structure, lipids also perform active roles in cellular signaling and as coenzymes. Lipids serve as coenzymes in the electron transport chain and in glycosylation reactions. Lipids also function as hormones that transmit signals over long distances and as intracellular messengers responding to extracellular signals. Certain special lipids with conjugated double bonds absorb light, which is extremely important for vision; others act as pigments in plants and animals. Here, we will focus on three important categories of signaling lipids: steroids, prostaglandins, and fat-soluble vitamins, as well as important precursors like terpenes.

Terpenes and Terpenoids

Before we delve into the details of downstream lipid signaling molecules, we must first turn our attention to *terpenes*. These odiferous chemicals are the metabolic precursors to steroids and other lipid signaling molecules, and have varied independent functions. **Terpenes** are a class of lipids built from ***isoprene*** (C_5H_8) moieties and share a common structural pattern with carbons grouped in multiples of five, as shown in Figure 5.5.

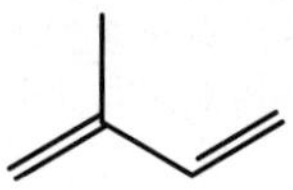

Figure 5.5 Isoprene

Terpenes are produced mainly by plants and also by some insects. They are generally strongly scented. In some cases, these pungent chemicals are part of the plant or insect's protective mechanism. The strong smell of turpentine, a derivative of resin, comes from the monoterpenes that are resin's major components; terpenes actually get their name from their original discovery in turpentine. Terpenes are also the primary components of much more pleasant-smelling essential oils extracted from plants.

Terpenes are grouped according to the number of isoprene units present; a single terpene unit contains two isoprene units. ***Monoterpenes*** ($C_{10}H_{16}$), which are abundant in both essential oils and turpentine as described above, contain two isoprene units. ***Sesquiterpenes*** (*sesqui–* meaning one-and-a-half) contain three isoprene units, and ***diterpenes*** contain four. Vitamin A, which will be discussed later in this chapter, is a diterpene from which *retinal*, a visual pigment vital for sight, is derived. ***Triterpenes***, with six isoprene units, can be converted to cholesterol and various steroids, also discussed later in this chapter. ***Carotenoids***, like *β-carotene* and *lutein*, are ***tetraterpenes*** and have eight isoprene units. Natural rubber has isoprene chains between 1000 and 5000 units long and is therefore considered a polyterpene.

Terpenoids, also sometimes referred to as isoprenoids, are derivatives of terpenes that have undergone oxygenation or rearrangement of the carbon skeleton. These compounds are further modified, as are terpenes, by the addition of an extensive variety of functional groups. Terpenoids share similar characteristics with terpenes in terms of both biological precursor function and aromatic properties, contributing to steroid biosynthesis, as well as the scents of cinnamon, eucalyptus, camphor, turmeric, and numerous other compounds. Terpenoids are named in an analogous fashion, with diterpenoids deriving from four isoprene units and so on. Terpenes and terpenoids are precursor molecules that feed into various biosynthesis pathways that produce important products, including steroids, which have widespread effects on biological function, and vitamin A, which is vital to sight.

Steroids

The term steroid probably brings to mind muscle–bound body builders or home run–hitting professional athletes. In science, and on the MCAT, steroid refers not just to the infamously abused anabolic steroids, but also to a broader class of molecules defined by their structure.

Structurally, **steroids**, shown in Figure 5.6, are metabolic derivatives of terpenes and are very different from the lipids mentioned earlier in this chapter in both structure and function. Steroids are characterized by having four cycloalkane rings fused together: three cyclohexane and one cyclopentane. Steroid functionality is determined by the oxidation status of these rings, as well as the functional groups they carry. It is important to note that the large number of carbons and hydrogens make steroids nonpolar, like the other lipids mentioned.

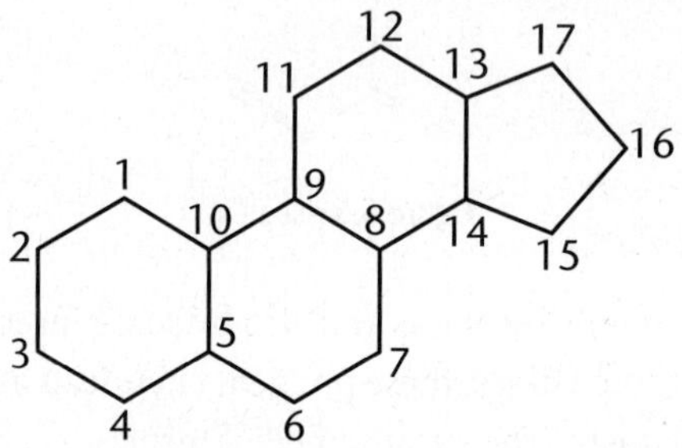

Figure 5.6 Common Steroid Structure

BRIDGE

Hormone types, including steroid hormones, are the focus of Chapter 5 of *Kaplan MCAT Biology Review*.

Keep in mind the terminology difference between steroids and steroid hormones. Steroid refers to a group defined by a particular chemical structure, demonstrated above. **Steroid hormones** are steroids that act as hormones, meaning that they are secreted by endocrine glands into the bloodstream and then travel on protein carriers to distant sites, where they can bind to specific high-affinity receptors and alter gene expression levels. Steroid hormones are potent biological signals that regulate gene expression and metabolism, affecting a wide variety of biological systems even at low concentrations. Some important steroid hormones include testosterone, various estrogens, cortisol, and aldosterone, which are discussed in Chapter 5 of *MCAT Biology Review*. Plants, like animals, also use steroids as signaling molecules.

REAL WORLD

Cholesterol can be produced *de novo* or absorbed from dietary sources. *Hypercholesterolemia*, or high cholesterol, is a condition that is strongly correlated with heart disease, in which the combination of these two cholesterol sources is excessive. Accumulation of cholesterol in arterial walls results in atherosclerosis, a hardening of the wall.

Cholesterol, shown in Figure 5.7, is a steroid of primary importance. Cholesterol is a major component of the phospholipid bilayer and is responsible for mediating membrane fluidity. Cholesterol, like a phospholipid, is an amphipathic molecule containing both hydrophilic and hydrophobic components. Interactions with both the hydrophobic tails and hydrophilic heads of phospholipids allows cholesterol to maintain relatively constant fluidity in cell membranes. At low temperatures, it keeps the cell membrane from solidifying; at high temperatures, it holds the membrane intact and prevents it from becoming too permeable. Cholesterol also serves as a precursor to many important molecules, including steroid hormones, bile acids, and vitamin D.

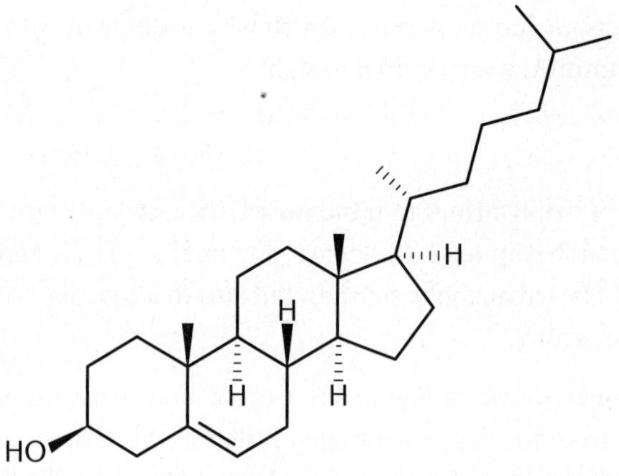

Figure 5.7 Cholesterol

Prostaglandins

Prostaglandins acquired their name because they were first thought to be produced by the prostate gland, but have since been determined to be produced by almost all cells in the body. These 20-carbon molecules are unsaturated carboxylic acids derived from ***arachidonic acid*** and contain one five-carbon ring. They act as paracrine or autocrine signaling molecules. In many tissues, the biological function of prostaglandins is to regulate the synthesis of cyclic adenosine monophosphate (cAMP), which is a ubiquitous intracellular messenger. In turn, cAMP mediates the actions of many other hormones. Downstream effects of prostaglandins include powerful effects on smooth muscle function, influence over the sleep–wake cycle, and the elevation of body temperature associated with fever and pain. Nonsteroidal anti-inflammatory drugs (NSAIDs) like aspirin inhibit the enzyme *cyclooxygenase* (COX), which aids in the production of prostaglandins.

Fat-Soluble Vitamins

A **vitamin** is an essential nutrient that cannot be adequately synthesized by the body and therefore must be consumed in the diet. Vitamins are commonly divided into water-soluble and lipid-soluble categories. Lipid-soluble vitamins can accumulate in stored fat, whereas excess water-soluble vitamins are excreted through the urine. The fat-soluble vitamins include A, D, E, and K. Each of these has important and varied functions.

Vitamin A

Vitamin A, or ***carotene***, is an unsaturated hydrocarbon that is important in vision, growth and development, and immune function. The most significant metabolite of vitamin A is the aldehyde form, ***retinal***, which is a component of the light-sensing molecular system in the human eye. ***Retinol***, the storage form of vitamin A, is also oxidized to ***retinoic acid***, a hormone that regulates gene expression during epithelial development.

MNEMONIC

One way to remember **carotene** is to remember that **carrots** are high in **vitamin A**, which is why eating carrots is colloquially suggested to improve **vision**. To remember that **vitamin D** regulates calcium, remember that it is frequently added to **milk** in order to aid in the absorption of **calcium**.

Vitamin D

Vitamin D, or ***cholecalciferol***, can be consumed or formed in a UV light–driven reaction in the skin. In the liver and kidneys, vitamin D is converted to ***calcitriol*** ($1,25\text{-}(OH)_2D_3$), the biologically active form of vitamin D. Calcitriol increases calcium and phosphate uptake in the intestines, which promotes bone production. A lack of vitamin D can result in **rickets**, a condition seen in children and characterized by underdeveloped, curved long bones as well as impeded growth.

Vitamin E

Vitamin E characterizes a group of closely related lipids called ***tocopherols*** and ***tocotrienols***. These are characterized by a substituted aromatic ring with a long isoprenoid side chain and are characteristically hydrophobic. Tocopherols are biological antioxidants. The aromatic ring reacts with free radicals, destroying them. This, in turn, prevents oxidative damage, an important contributor to the development of cancer and aging.

MNEMONIC

Vitamin **K** is for **K**oagulation.

REAL WORLD

The anticoagulant *warfarin* works by blocking the recycling of vitamin K, causing a deficiency or lowering of the active amount of vitamin K. Therefore, patients taking warfarin are recommended to stay away from food containing high amounts of vitamin K, such as green leafy vegetables.

Vitamin K

Vitamin K is actually a group of compounds, including ***phylloquinone*** (K_1) and the ***menaquinones*** (K_2). Vitamin K is vital to the posttranslational modifications required to form *prothrombin*, an important clotting factor in the blood. The aromatic ring of vitamin K undergoes a cycle of oxidation and reduction during the formation of prothrombin. Vitamin K is also required to introduce calcium-binding sites on several calcium-dependent proteins.

MCAT CONCEPT CHECK 5.2

Before you move on, assess your understanding of the material with these questions.

1. How many carbons are in a diterpene?

2. What is the difference between a steroid and a steroid hormone?

3. NSAIDs block prostaglandin production in order to reduce pain and inflammation. What do prostaglandins do to bring about these symptoms?

4. What are the names and functions of the four fat-soluble vitamins?

Name	Function

5.3 Energy Storage

LEARNING OBJECTIVES

After Chapter 5.3, you will be able to:

- Explain why energy is more optimally stored as fat than as sugar
- Recall the structure and function of triacylglycerols
- Predict the products of saponification reactions:

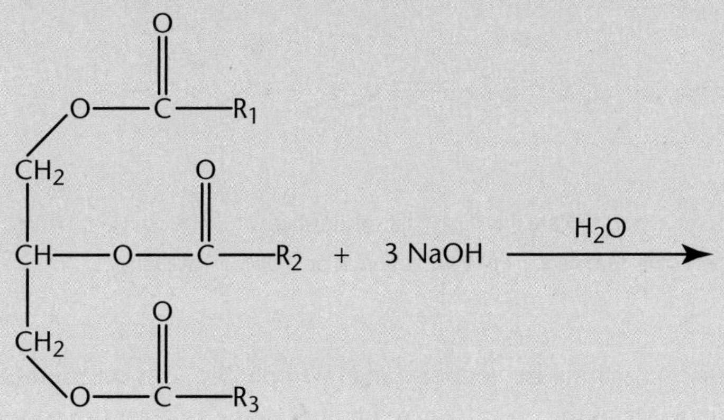

Triacylglycerols are a class of lipids specifically used for energy storage. From the body's point of view, lipids in general are a fantastic way to store energy. This is true for two major reasons. First, the carbon atoms of fatty acids are more reduced than those of sugars, which contain numerous alcohol groups. The result of this is that the oxidation of triacylglycerols yields twice the amount of energy per gram as carbohydrates, making this a far more energy-dense storage mechanism compared to polysaccharides like glycogen. Second, triacylglycerols are hydrophobic. They do not draw in water and do not require hydration for stability. This helps decrease their weight, especially in comparison to hydrophilic polysaccharides. One final perk for vertebrates surviving in colder temperatures (like penguins, polar bears, and arctic explorers) is that the layer of lipids serves a dual purpose of energy storage and insulation—it helps to retain body heat so that less energy is required to maintain a constant internal temperature.

Triacylglycerols

Triacylglycerols, also called **triglycerides**, are composed of three fatty acids bonded by ester linkages to glycerol, as shown in Figure 5.8. For most naturally occurring triacylglycerols, it is rare for all three fatty acids to be the same.

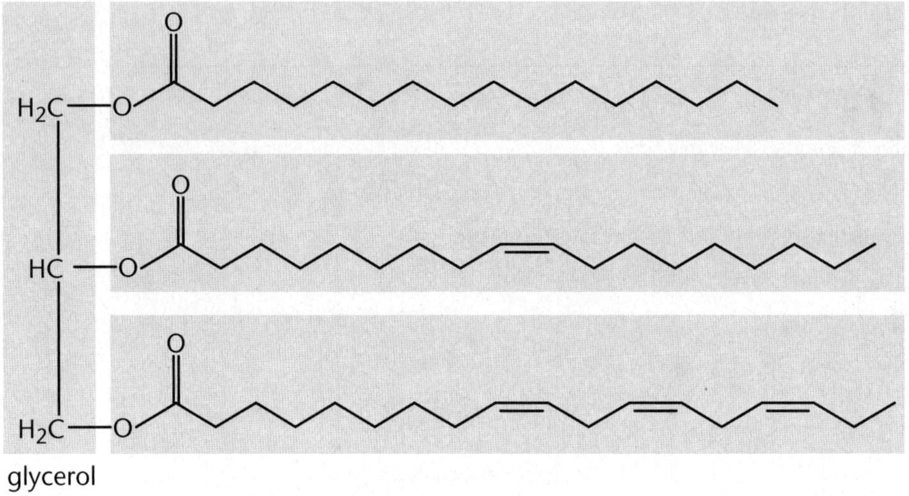

Figure 5.8 Triacylglycerol Structure
The fatty acids used here are palmitic acid, oleic acid, and α-linolenic acid.

REAL WORLD

The two main methods of energy storage in the body are as triacylglycerols in adipose tissue or as carbohydrates in glycogen. Each method has its advantages and disadvantages. For example, glycogen offers access to metabolic energy in a faster water-soluble form; however, because of its low energy density, glycogen can only provide energy for a bit less than one day. In contrast, an individual who is moderately obese with 15 to 20 kg of stored triacylglycerols in adipocytes could draw upon fat stores for months, but it takes more time to mobilize this energy.

REAL WORLD

Saponification also occurs naturally, although more slowly, in corpses and oil paintings, as the triacylglycerols are hydrolyzed by naturally occurring bases. In corpses, the result of this process is known as *adipocere*, or grave wax.

Overall, these compounds are nonpolar and hydrophobic. This contributes to their insolubility in water, as the polar hydroxyl groups of the glycerol component and the polar carboxylates of fatty acids are bonded together, decreasing their polarity.

Triacylglycerol deposits can be observed in cells as oily droplets in the cytosol. These serve as depots of metabolic fuel that can be recruited when the cell needs additional energy to divide or survive when other fuel supplies are low. Special cells in animals, known as **adipocytes**, store large amounts of fat and are found primarily under the skin, around mammary glands, and in the abdominal cavity. In plants, triacylglycerol deposits are also found in seeds as oils. Triacylglycerols travel bidirectionally in the bloodstream between the liver and adipose tissue. The physical characteristics of triacylglycerols are primarily determined by the saturation (or unsaturation) of the fatty acid chains that make them up, much like phospholipids.

Free Fatty Acids and Saponification

Free fatty acids are unesterified fatty acids with a free carboxylate group. In the body, these circulate in the blood bonded noncovalently to serum albumin. Fatty acids also make up what we know as soap, which can be produced through a process called saponification.

Saponification is the ester hydrolysis of triacylglycerols using a strong base. Traditionally, the base that is used is **lye**, the common name for sodium or potassium hydroxide. The result is the basic cleavage of the fatty acid, leaving the sodium salt of the fatty acid and glycerol, as shown in Figure 5.9. The fatty acid salt is what we know as soap.

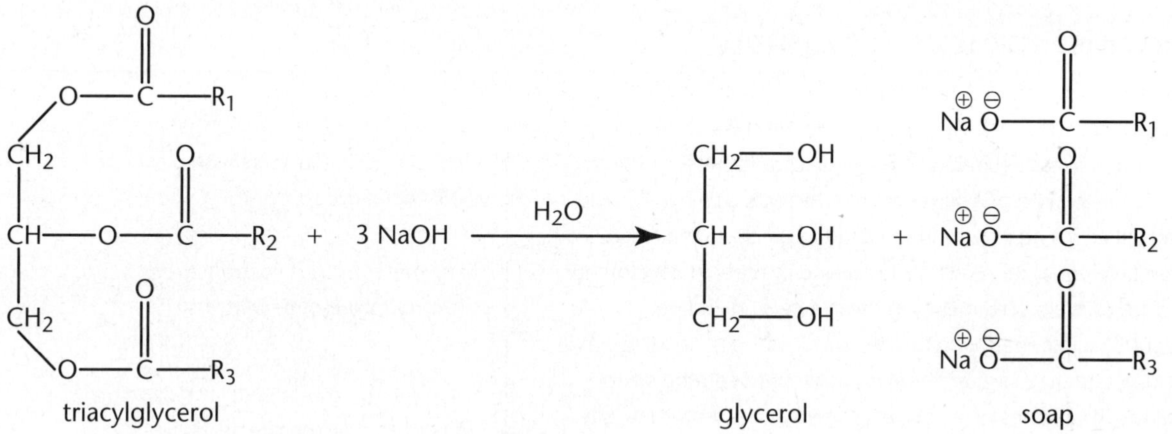

Figure 5.9 Saponification
Ester hydrolysis of a triacylglycerol using lye (NaOH)

Soaps can act as surfactants. A **surfactant** lowers the surface tension at the surface of a liquid, serving as a detergent or emulsifier. This is important to how soap works. If we try to combine an aqueous solution and oil, as with vinegar and olive oil in salad dressing, these solutions will remain in separate phases. If we were to add a soap, however, the two phases would appear to combine into a single phase, forming a **colloid**. This occurs because of the formation of **micelles**: tiny aggregates of soap with the hydrophobic tails turned inward and the hydrophilic heads turned outward, thereby shielding the hydrophobic lipid tails and allowing for overall solvation, as shown in Figure 5.10. We saw these earlier when we discussed membrane lipids.

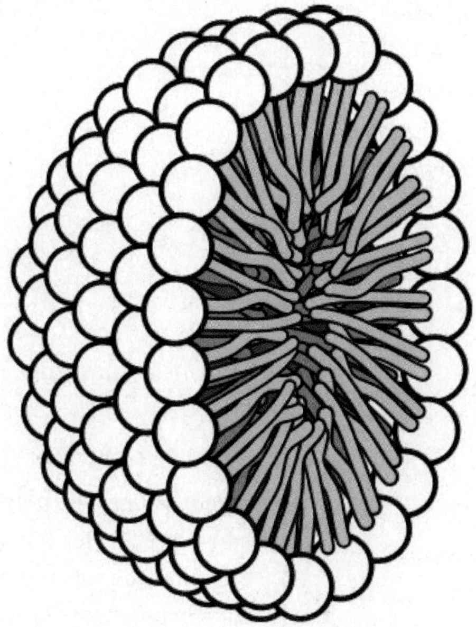

Figure 5.10 Cross-Section of a Micelle
Micelles organize in aqueous solution by forcing hydrophobic tails to the interior, allowing the hydrophilic heads to interact with water in the environment.

BIOCHEMISTRY GUIDED EXAMPLE WITH EXPERT THINKING

Sugar-based fatty acid esters usually belong to the class of non-ionic surfactants and possess desirable characteristics suitable for different applications. They consist of a sugar moiety that acts as a hydrophilic (polar) head linked via an ester bond to a fatty acid chain that acts as a hydrophobic (nonpolar) tail. There is increasing interest in developing advanced drug delivery systems using these esters, including enhancement of skin penetration and transmucosal permeability. This study aimed to investigate the relationship between the structure and activity of a series of lactose ester derivatives, enzymatically synthesized using saturated fatty acids with different chain lengths (C10–caprate; C12–laurate; C14–myristate; C16–palmitate).

Topic: a fatty acid ester with a sugar as the polar head group

Why these matter: possible usage in drug delivery through membranes

Purpose: to examine how the structure of a lactose fatty ester affects its activity

Solutions of each surfactant in water were prepared at varying concentrations and the surface tension was measured using a K100-Krüss force tensiometer with a platinum cylindrical rod probe of wetted length 1.6 mm at room temperature. The results are plotted in Figure 1 below. To examine the effect of lactose surfactants on the variation of mitochondrial membrane potential, the ratiometric dye JC-1 assay was employed. The JC-1 dye readily permeates across the cell plasma membrane where it specifically accumulates in active mitochondria, in a potential-dependent way. When present in the mitochondria, the dye forms J-aggregates, which emit fluorescence at a wavelength distinct from the wavelength the dye presents in the cytoplasm, where it remains in monomeric form. Mitochondrial depolarization, due to the dissipation of negative charges across the mitochondrial membrane because of mitochondrial disruption, is indicated by a decrease in the J-aggregate/monomer intensity ratio, thus representing an arbitrary value for mitochondrial membrane potential. The effect of different concentrations of lactose surfactants on the mitochondrial membrane potential is reported below (Figure 2).

They measured the surface tension of the different surfactants and plotted it in Fig 1

Mitochondrial membrane potential was measured in the presence of the different surfactants

A decrease in aggregate/monomer ratio indicates that the mitochondria has been disrupted

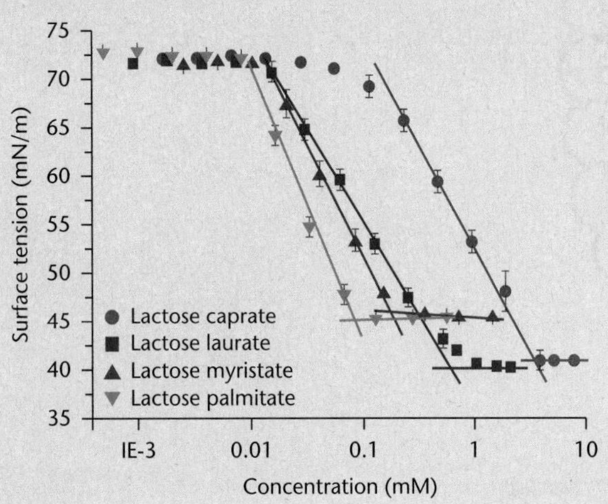

Figure 1

IVs: type of surfactant, concentration of surfactant; x-axis is a log-scale

DV: surface tension

Trend: all lines are a negative S-shaped curve; the greater the number of carbons, the lower the concentration required to decrease surface tension

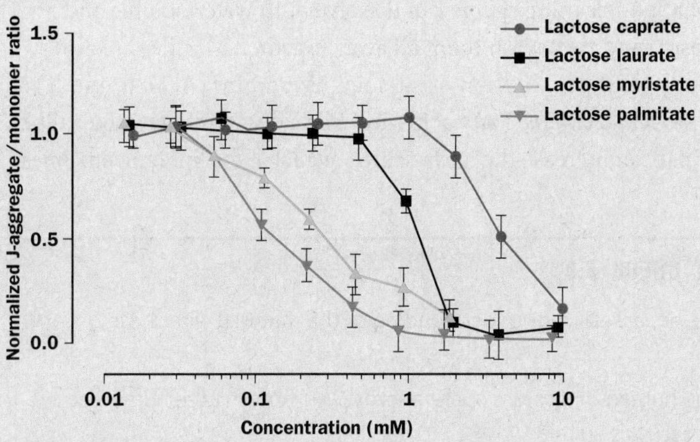

IVs: type of surfactant, concentration of surfactant; x-axis is again log-scale

DV: aggregate/monomer ratio

Trend: lines seem roughly negative S-shaped; the greater the number of carbons, the lower the concentration required to decrease the aggregate/monomer ratio

Figure 2

Adapted from Lucarini, S., Fagioli, L., Cavanagh, R., Liang, W., Perinelli, D. R., Campana, M., Stolnik, S., ... Duranti, A. (2018). Synthesis, structure-activity relationships and in vitro toxicity profile of lactose-based fatty acid monoesters as possible drug permeability enhancers. *Pharmaceutics*, 10(3), 81. doi:10.3390/pharmaceutics10030081.

If the researchers were to examine cell viability in future experiments, which of the four surfactants would be expected to be the most cytotoxic?

The question asks us to predict the outcome of a future experiment, which indicates that we need to understand the results of the current experiment in order to predict future events. In the first paragraph, we see that the purpose of the passage is to discuss how these surfactants work as a function of the number of carbons attached to the sugar head group. From our outside knowledge we want to recall that surfactants have polar head groups, fatty acid tails, and often form micelles, allowing for nonpolar compounds (like many drugs!) to dissolve in the hydrophobic interior, while the surface-exposed portion of the micelle is water-soluble. Since the question specifically asks about the cytotoxic effects of the surfactants, we can mostly ignore Figure 1, as information about surface tension would not tell us if the surfactant was cytotoxic. Quickly assessing whether or not a figure is useful is an important skill for Test Day: not all of the figures will be valuable in answering every question. The measured variable in Figure 2 is the J-aggregate/monomer ratio, and the passage tells us that a drop in this ratio indicates that the potential across the mitochondrial membrane has been disrupted. We know from our content background that a proton gradient must be built across the inner mitochondrial membrane in order for ATP to be synthesized, and without that proton gradient the cell will quickly die due to a lack of energy. It's possible that the amphiphilic nature of the surfactant is "poking" holes into the inner mitochondrial membrane, allowing for the proton gradient to dissipate without moving through ATP synthase.

Figure 2 shows that increasing carbon number in the fatty acid tail corresponds with decreasing concentration required to dissipate the mitochondrial potential. Thus, we can predict that a longer fatty acid tail will be linked with greater cytotoxic activity. Specifically, we would expect lactose palmitate to be the most cytotoxic of the four surfactants studied in the current experiment.

Nonpolar compounds can dissolve in the hydrophobic interior of the water-soluble micelle, meaning that our cleaning agents can dissolve both water-soluble and water-insoluble messes and then wash them all away together. Micelles are also important in the body for the absorption of fat-soluble vitamins (A, D, E, and K) and complicated lipids such as *lecithins*. Fatty acids and bile salts secreted by the gallbladder form micelles that can increase the surface area available for lipolytic enzymes.

MCAT CONCEPT CHECK 5.3

Before you move on, assess your understanding of the material with these questions.

1. How does the human body store spare energy? Why doesn't the human body store most energy as sugar?

   ____

2. Describe the structure and function of triacylglycerols.

   ____

3. What bonds are broken during saponification?

   ____

4. Why does soap appear to dissolve in water, and how is this fact important to cleaning?

   ____

Conclusion

In this chapter, we examined the myriad biological functions performed by lipids. We first learned the structural functions of lipids, looking at the phospholipids that are the primary component of the phospholipid bilayer and other membrane lipids. Making our way through terpenes, we looked at the structure and function of signaling lipids, examining steroid hormones in particular. We looked into the fat-soluble vitamins and their downstream functions in the body. Finally, we summarized energy storage in the form of triacylglycerols and applied our acid–base chemistry knowledge to the formation of soap. In the next chapter, we turn our attention to the final class of biomolecules: nucleic acids.

You've reviewed the content, now test your knowledge and critical thinking skills by completing a test-like passage set in your online resources!

GO ONLINE

CONCEPT SUMMARY

Structural Lipids

- Lipids are insoluble in water and soluble in nonpolar organic solvents.
- **Phospholipids** are amphipathic and form the bilayer of biological membranes.
  - They contain a hydrophilic (polar) head group and hydrophobic (nonpolar) tails.
  - The head group is attached by a **phosphodiester linkage** and, because it interacts with the environment, determines the function of the phospholipid.
  - The **saturation** of the fatty acid tails determines the fluidity of the membrane; saturated fatty acids are less fluid than unsaturated ones. Fatty acids form most of the structural thickness of the phospholipid bilayer.
  - **Glycerophospholipids** are phospholipids that contain a glycerol backbone.
- **Sphingolipids** contain a sphingosine or sphingoid backbone.
  - Many (but not all) sphingolipids are also phospholipids, containing a phosphodiester bond; these are termed **sphingophospholipids**.
  - **Sphingomyelins** are the major class of sphingophospholipids and contain a phosphatidylcholine or phosphatidylethanolamine head group. They are a major component of the myelin sheath.
  - **Glycosphingolipids** are attached to sugar moieties instead of a phosphate group. **Cerebrosides** have one sugar connected to sphingosine; **globosides** have two or more.
  - **Gangliosides** contain oligosaccharides with at least one terminal ***N*-acetylneuraminic acid** (**NANA**; also called **sialic acid**).
- **Waxes** contain long-chain fatty acids esterified to long-chain alcohols. They are used as protection against evaporation and parasites in plants and animals.

Signaling Lipids

- **Terpenes** are odiferous steroid precursors made from **isoprene**, a five-carbon molecule.
  - One terpene unit (a **monoterpene**) contains two isoprene units.
  - **Terpenoids** are derived from terpenes via oxygenation or backbone rearrangement. They have similar odorous characteristics.
- **Steroids** contain three cyclohexane rings and one cyclopentane ring. Their oxidation state and functional groups may vary.
  - **Steroid hormones** have high-affinity receptors, work at low concentrations, and affect gene expression and metabolism.
  - **Cholesterol** is a steroid important to membrane fluidity and stability; it serves as a precursor to a host of other molecules.
- **Prostaglandins** are autocrine and paracrine signaling molecules that regulate cAMP levels. They have powerful effects on smooth muscle contraction, body temperature, the sleep–wake cycle, fever, and pain.

- The fat-soluble vitamins include vitamins A, D, E, and K.
  - **Vitamin A** (**carotene**) is metabolized to **retinal** for vision and **retinoic acid** for gene expression in epithelial development.
  - **Vitamin D** (**cholecalciferol**) is metabolized to **calcitriol** in the kidneys and regulates calcium and phosphorus homeostasis in the intestines (increasing calcium and phosphate absorption), promoting bone formation. A deficiency of vitamin D causes **rickets**.
  - **Vitamin E** (**tocopherols**) act as biological antioxidants. Their aromatic rings destroy free radicals, preventing oxidative damage.
  - **Vitamin K** (**phylloquinone** and **menaquinones**) is important for formation of prothrombin, a clotting factor. It performs posttranslational modifications on a number of proteins, creating calcium-binding sites.

Energy Storage

- **Triacylglycerols** (**triglycerides**) are the preferred method of storing energy for long-term use.
  - They contain one glycerol attached to three fatty acids by ester bonds. The fatty acids usually vary within the same triacylglycerol.
  - The carbon atoms in lipids are more reduced than carbohydrates, giving twice as much energy per gram during oxidation.
  - Triacylglycerols are very hydrophobic, so they are not hydrated by body water and do not carry additional water weight.
- Animal cells specifically used for storage of large triacylglycerol deposits are called **adipocytes**.
- Free fatty acids are unesterified fatty acids that travel in the bloodstream. Salts of free fatty acids are **soaps** and can be synthesized in saponification.
  - **Saponification** is the ester hydrolysis of triacylglycerols using a strong base, like sodium or potassium hydroxide.
  - Soaps act as surfactants, forming micelles. A **micelle** can dissolve a lipid-soluble molecule in its fatty acid core, and washes away with water because of its shell of carboxylate head groups.

ANSWERS TO CONCEPT CHECKS

5.1

1. Membrane lipids are amphipathic: they have hydrophilic heads and hydrophobic tails, allowing for the formation of bilayers in aqueous solution. The fatty acid tails form the bulk of the phospholipid bilayer, and play a predominantly structural role. On the other hand, the functional differences between membrane lipids are determined by the polar head group, due to its constant exposure to the exterior environment of the phospholipid bilayer (remember, this can be either the inside or outside of the cell). The degree of unsaturation of fatty acid tails can also play a small role in function.
2. The difference is the bond between the sphingosine backbone and the head group. When this is a phosphodiester bond, it's a phospholipid (note the *phospho–* prefixes). Nonphospholipid sphingolipids include glycolipids, which contain a glycosidic linkage to a sugar.
3.

Type	Phospholipid or Glycolipid?	Functional Group(s)
Sphingomyelin	Phospholipid	Phosphatidylethanolamine/ phosphatidylcholine
Glycosphingolipid	Glycolipid	Sugars (mono- or polysaccharide)
Ganglioside	Glycolipid	Oligosaccharides and *N*-acetylneuraminic acid (NANA)

4. In a nonpolar solvent, we would see the opposite of what happens in a polar solvent like water: the hydrophilic, polar part of the molecules would be sequestered inside, while the nonpolar, hydrophobic part of the molecules would be found on the exterior and exposed to the solvent.

5.2

1. A diterpene has 20 carbon molecules in its backbone. One terpene unit is made from two isoprene units, each of which has five carbons.
2. A steroid is defined by its structure: it includes three cyclohexane rings and a cyclopentane ring. A steroid hormone is a molecule within this class that also functions as a hormone, meaning that it travels in the bloodstream, is active at low concentrations, has high-affinity receptors, and affects gene expression and metabolism.
3. Prostaglandins regulate the synthesis of cAMP, which is involved in many pathways, including those that drive pain and inflammation.

4.

Name	Function
A (carotene)	As retinal: vision; as retinoic acid: epithelial development
D (cholecalciferol)	As calcitriol: calcium and phosphate regulation
E (tocopherols)	Antioxidants, using aromatic ring
K (phylloquinone and menaquinones)	Posttranslational modification of prothrombin, addition of calcium-binding sites on many proteins

5.3

1. The human body stores energy as glycogen and triacylglycerols. Triacylglycerols are preferred because their carbons are more reduced, resulting in a larger amount of energy yield per unit weight. In addition, due to their hydrophobic nature, triacylglycerols do not need to carry extra weight from hydration.
2. Triacylglycerols, also called triglycerides, are composed of a glycerol backbone esterified to three fatty acids. They are used for energy storage.
3. The ester bonds of triacylglycerols are broken to form a glycerol molecule and the salts of fatty acids (soap).
4. Soap appears to dissolve in water because amphipathic free fatty acid salts form micelles, with hydrophobic fatty acid tails toward the center and carboxylate groups facing outward toward the water. Fat-soluble particles can then dissolve inside micelles in the soap–water solution and wash away. Water-soluble compounds can freely dissolve in the water.

SCIENCE MASTERY ASSESSMENT EXPLANATIONS

1. **D**

Glycolipids contain sugar moieties connected to their backbone. Sphingomyelin is not a glycolipid, but rather a phospholipid. This class can either have phosphatidylcholine or phosphatidylethanolamine as a head group and therefore contains a phosphodiester, not glycosidic, bond.

2. **B**

Saponification is the ester hydrolysis of triacylglycerol using a strong base like sodium or potassium hydroxide to form glycerol and fatty acid salts. This is not a condensation reaction, as in **(A)**, but a cleavage reaction. Fatty acids do travel in the body bonded to serum albumin, as in **(D)**, but that is unrelated to the process of saponification.

3. **B**

The basic backbone of steroid structure contains three cyclohexane rings and one cyclopentane ring. Although the oxidation status of these rings varies for different steroids, the overall structure does not, as in **(C)**.

4. **B**

Fatty acid salt micelles are responsible for the formation of soap bubbles. While phospholipids can form bilayers, as in **(C)**, the fatty acids in soap are free fatty acids, not phospholipids.

5. **C**

Steroid hormones are produced in endocrine glands and travel in the bloodstream to bind high-affinity receptors in the nucleus. The hormone's receptor binds to DNA as part of the hormone–receptor complex, but the hormone itself does not.

6. **C**

Triacylglycerols are highly hydrophobic and therefore not highly hydrated (which would add extra weight from the water of hydration, taking away from the energy density of these molecules), eliminating **(A)**. The fatty acid chains produce twice as much energy as polysaccharides during oxidation because they are highly reduced. The fatty acid chains vary in length and saturation.

7. **C**

Vitamin A is metabolized to retinal, which is important for sight. Vitamin D is metabolized to calcitriol, which is important for calcium regulation. Vitamin E is made up of tocopherols, which are biological antioxidants. Vitamin K is necessary for the introduction of calcium binding sites, such as during the posttranslational modification of prothrombin.

8. **C**

Phospholipids are amphipathic, as are fatty acid salts. Although amphipathic molecules take spherical forms with hydrophobic molecules interior in aqueous solution, as in **(A)**, the opposite would be true in a nonpolar solvent. **(B)** describes phospholipids and sphingolipids, and **(D)** describes triacylglycerols and phospholipids; both groups do not include fatty acid salts.

9. **B**

Sphingolipids can either have a phosphodiester bond, and therefore be phospholipids, or have a glycosidic linkage and therefore be glycolipids. Not all sphingolipids have a sphingosine backbone, as in statement II; some have related (sphingoid) compounds as backbones instead.

10. **C**

More saturated fatty acids make for a less fluid solution. This is because they can pack more tightly and form more noncovalent bonds, resulting in more energy being needed to disrupt the overall structure.

11. **B**

Glycerophospholipids are a subset of phospholipids, as are sphingomyelins. Glycerophospholipids are never sphingolipids because they contain a glycerol backbone (rather than sphingosine or a sphingoid backbone), eliminating **(A)**. Sphingolipids are used in the ABO blood typing system, eliminating **(C)**. Glycerophospholipids have a polar head group, glycerol, and two fatty acid tails, not one, as in **(D)**.

12. **C**

A triterpene is made of six isoprene moieties (remember, one terpene unit contains two isoprene units), and therefore has a 30-carbon backbone.

13. **B**

Cholesterol is a steroid hormone precursor that has variable effects on membrane fluidity depending on temperature, eliminating **(A)**. It interacts with both the hydrophobic tails and the hydrophilic heads of membrane lipids, nullifying **(D)**. It is also a precursor for vitamin D (not vitamin A), which can be produced in the skin in a UV-driven reaction, eliminating **(C)**.

14. **D**

Prostaglandins are paracrine or autocrine signaling molecules, not endocrine—they affect regions close to where they are produced, rather than affecting the entire body. Think of the swelling that happens when you bash your knee into your desk: your knee will swell, become discolored, and possibly bruise. Luckily, however, your entire body won't swell as well.

15. **B**

Waxes are also produced in animals for similar protective functions. Cerumen, or earwax, is a prime example in humans.

Consult your online resources for additional practice. GO ONLINE

SHARED CONCEPTS

Biochemistry Chapter 2
Enzymes

Biochemistry Chapter 8
Biological Membranes

Biochemistry Chapter 11
Lipid and Amino Acid Metabolism

Biology Chapter 5
The Endocrine System

Biology Chapter 9
The Digestive System

Organic Chemistry Chapter 8
Carboxylic Acids

CHAPTER 6

DNA AND BIOTECHNOLOGY

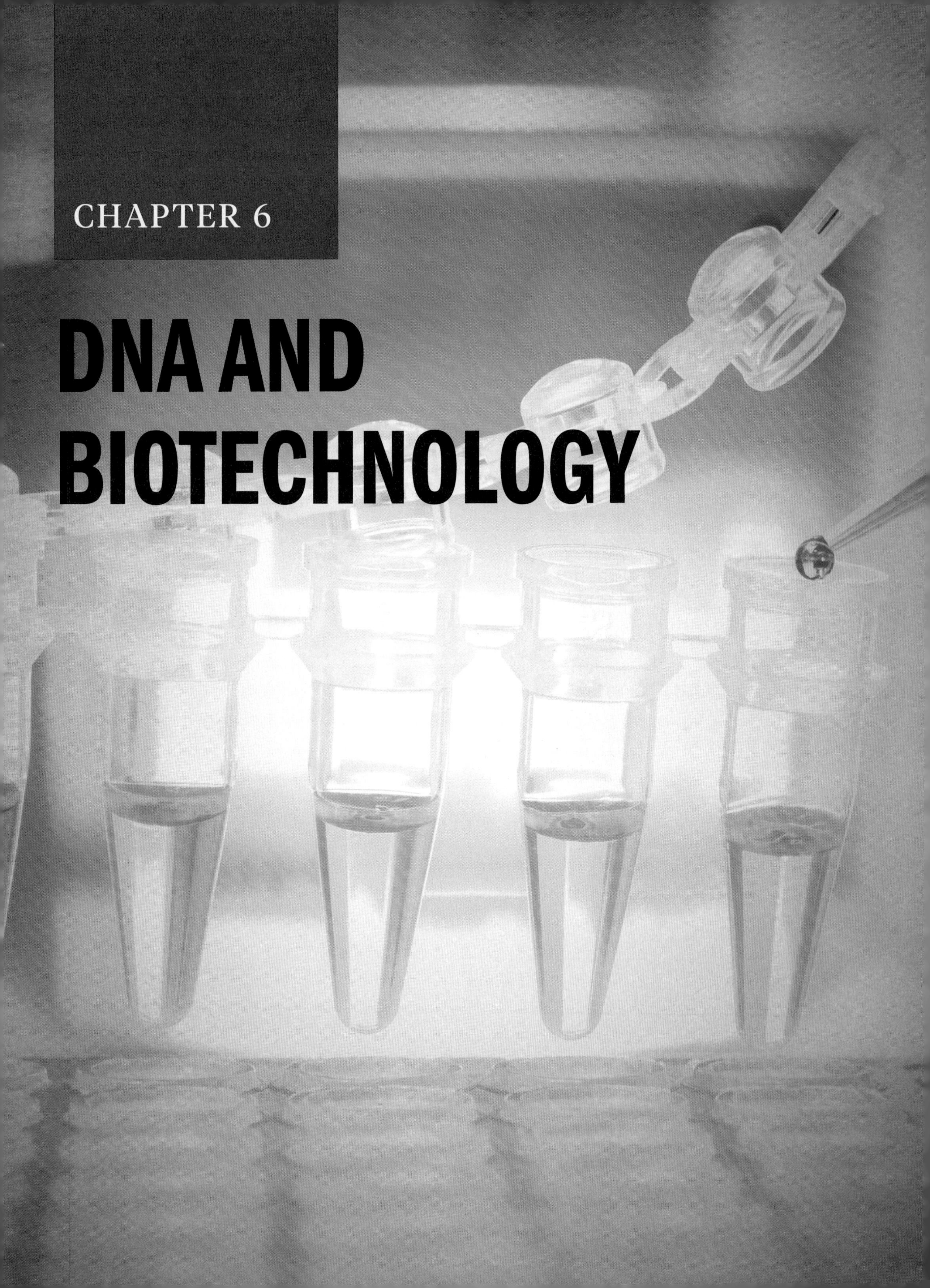

SCIENCE MASTERY ASSESSMENT

Every pre-med knows this feeling: there is so much content I have to know for the MCAT! How do I know what to do first or what's important?

While the high-yield badges throughout this book will help you identify the most important topics, this Science Mastery Assessment is another tool in your MCAT prep arsenal. This quiz (which can also be taken in your online resources) and the guidance below will help ensure that you are spending the appropriate amount of time on this chapter based on your personal strengths and weaknesses. Don't worry though—skipping something now does not mean you'll never study it. Later on in your prep, as you complete full-length tests, you'll uncover specific pieces of content that you need to review and can come back to these chapters as appropriate.

How to Use This Assessment

If you answer 0–7 questions correctly:

Spend about 1 hour to read this chapter in full and take limited notes throughout. Follow up by reviewing **all** quiz questions to ensure that you now understand how to solve each one.

If you answer 8–11 questions correctly:

Spend 20–40 minutes reviewing the quiz questions. Beginning with the questions you missed, read and take notes on the corresponding subchapters. For questions you answered correctly, ensure your thinking matches that of the explanation and you understand why each choice was correct or incorrect.

If you answer 12–15 questions correctly:

Spend less than 20 minutes reviewing all questions from the quiz. If you missed any, then include a quick read-through of the corresponding subchapters, or even just the relevant content within a subchapter, as part of your question review. For questions you got correct, ensure your thinking matches that of the explanation and review the Concept Summary at the end of the chapter.

1. In a single strand of a nucleic acid, nucleotides are linked by:
   - **A.** hydrogen bonds.
   - **B.** phosphodiester bonds.
   - **C.** ionic bonds.
   - **D.** van der Waals forces.

2. Which of the following statements regarding differences between DNA and RNA is FALSE?
   - **A.** In cells, DNA is double-stranded, whereas RNA is single-stranded.
   - **B.** DNA uses the nitrogenous base thymine; RNA uses uracil.
   - **C.** The sugar in DNA is deoxyribose; the sugar in RNA is ribose.
   - **D.** DNA strands replicate in a 5′ to 3′ direction, whereas RNA is synthesized in a 3′ to 5′ direction.

3. Which of the following DNA sequences would have the highest melting temperature?
   - **A.** CGCAACCATCCG
   - **B.** CGCAATAATACA
   - **C.** CGTAATAATACA
   - **D.** CATAACAAATCA

4. Which of the following biomolecules is LEAST likely to contain an aromatic ring?
   - **A.** Proteins
   - **B.** Purines
   - **C.** Carbohydrates
   - **D.** Pyrimidines

5. For a compound to be aromatic, all of the following must be true EXCEPT:
   - **A.** the molecule is cyclic.
   - **B.** the molecule contains $4n + 2$ π electrons.
   - **C.** the molecule contains alternating single and double bonds.
   - **D.** the molecule is planar.

6. Which of the following enzymes is NOT involved in DNA replication?
   - **A.** Primase
   - **B.** DNA ligase
   - **C.** RNA polymerase I
   - **D.** Telomerase

7. How is cDNA best characterized?
   - **A.** cDNA results from a DNA transcript with noncoding regions removed.
   - **B.** cDNA results from the reverse transcription of processed mRNA.
   - **C.** cDNA is the abbreviation for deoxycytosine.
   - **D.** cDNA is the circular DNA molecule that forms the bacterial genome.

8. Which of the following statements regarding polymerase chain reaction is FALSE?
   - **A.** Human DNA polymerase is used because it is the most accurate.
   - **B.** A primer must be prepared with a complementary sequence to part of the DNA of interest.
   - **C.** Repeated heating and cooling cycles allow the enzymes to act specifically and replaces helicase.
   - **D.** Each cycle of the polymerase chain reaction doubles the amount of DNA of interest.

9. Endonucleases are used for which of the following?
   - **I.** Gene therapy
   - **II.** Southern blotting
   - **III.** DNA repair

   - **A.** I only
   - **B.** II only
   - **C.** II and III only
   - **D.** I, II, and III

10. How does prokaryotic DNA differ from eukaryotic DNA?

- **I.** Prokaryotic DNA lacks nucleosomes.
- **II.** Eukaryotic DNA has telomeres.
- **III.** Prokaryotic DNA is replicated by a different DNA polymerase.
- **IV.** Eukaryotic DNA is circular when not restricted by centromeres.

- **A.** I only
- **B.** IV only
- **C.** II and III only
- **D.** I, II, and III only

11. Why might uracil be excluded from DNA but NOT RNA?

- **A.** Uracil is much more difficult to synthesize than thymine.
- **B.** Uracil binds adenine too strongly for replication.
- **C.** Cytosine degradation results in uracil.
- **D.** Uracil is used as a DNA synthesis activator.

12. Tumor suppressor genes are most likely to result in cancer through:

- **A.** loss of function mutations.
- **B.** gain of function mutations.
- **C.** overexpression.
- **D.** proto-oncogene formation.

13. Which of the following is an ethical concern of gene sequencing?

- **A.** Gene sequencing is invasive, thus the potential health risks must be thoroughly explained.
- **B.** Gene sequencing impacts relatives, thus privacy concerns may be raised.
- **C.** Gene sequencing is very inaccurate, which increases anxiety related to findings.
- **D.** Gene sequencing can provide false-negative results, giving a false sense of security.

14. Which of the following is NOT a difference between heterochromatin and euchromatin?

- **A.** Euchromatin has areas that can be transcribed, whereas heterochromatin is silent.
- **B.** Heterochromatin is tightly packed, whereas euchromatin is less dense.
- **C.** Heterochromatin stains darkly, whereas euchromatin stains lightly.
- **D.** Heterochromatin is found in the nucleus, whereas euchromatin is in the cytoplasm.

15. During which phase of the cell cycle are DNA repair mechanisms least active?

- **A.** G_1
- **B.** S
- **C.** G_2
- **D.** M

Answer Key

1. **B**
2. **D**
3. **A**
4. **C**
5. **C**
6. **C**
7. **B**
8. **A**
9. **D**
10. **D**
11. **C**
12. **A**
13. **B**
14. **D**
15. **D**

Detailed explanations can be found at the end of the chapter.

CHAPTER 6

DNA AND BIOTECHNOLOGY

In This Chapter

CHAPTER PROFILE

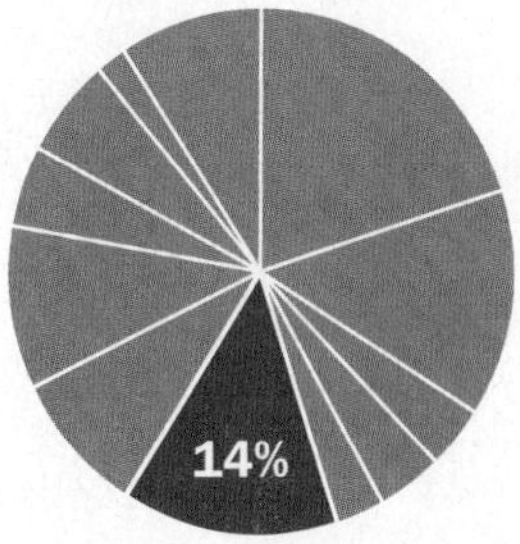

The content in this chapter should be relevant to about 14% of all questions about biochemistry on the MCAT.

This chapter covers material from the following AAMC content categories:

1B: Transmission of genetic information from the gene to the protein

5D: Structure, function, and reactivity of biologically-relevant molecules

Introduction

How do all of the cells of our body know what job to do? The cells that make up the human body have nucleic acids that instruct the cell on how to function. The nucleic acid *deoxyribonucleic acid* (DNA) stores the information in our cells and selectively shares that information when appropriate. DNA is a molecule that can be passed from generation to generation. DNA can be replicated in a carefully regulated process designed to keep the genome safe from degradation and free from errors. Seemingly small changes in the genetic code can result in life-threatening and even life-incompatible alterations to protein structure and function. In this chapter, the unique structure of DNA will be discussed, along with replication and repair processes. The primary focus will be on eukaryotic processes, but there will be some review of prokaryotic genetics to help us better understand the molecular basis of life.

Much of the advancement of medicine in the past two decades has been due to our increased understanding of molecular genetics, which has led to the creation of an entire biotechnology industry centered around genomics and the utilization of nucleic acids for various diagnostic tests and therapeutic interventions. We will also take a look at some of these important principles in this chapter.

6.1 DNA Structure

High-Yield

LEARNING OBJECTIVES

After Chapter 6.1, you will be able to:

- Identify the structures of, and distinguish the differences between, nucleotides and nucleosides
- Recognize the key features and rules of purine and pyrimidine structure and pairing
- Recall the structural differences between DNA and RNA molecules

There are two chemically distinct forms of nucleic acids within eukaryotic cells. **Deoxyribonucleic acid** (**DNA**) and **ribonucleic acid** (**RNA**) are polymers, each with distinct roles, that together create the molecules integral to life in all living organisms. DNA is the focus of this chapter and RNA will be discussed in more detail in Chapter 7 of *MCAT Biochemistry Review*. The bulk of DNA is found in chromosomes in the nucleus of eukaryotic cells, although some is also present in mitochondria and chloroplasts.

Nucleosides and Nucleotides

DNA is a macromolecule and it is essential to understand how this molecule is constructed. DNA is a *polydeoxyribonucleotide* that is composed of many *monodeoxyribonucleotides* linked together. The nomenclature of nucleic acids can be complicated, so the terms have been defined here:

- **Nucleosides** are composed of a five-carbon sugar (*pentose*) bonded to a nitrogenous base and are formed by covalently linking the base to C-1′ of the sugar, as shown in Figure 6.1. Note that the carbon atoms in the sugar are labeled with a prime symbol to distinguish them from the carbon atoms in the nitrogenous base.
- **Nucleotides** are formed when one or more phosphate groups are attached to C-5′ of a nucleoside. Often these molecules are named according to the number of phosphates present. Adenosine di- and triphosphate (ADP and ATP), for example, gain their names from the number of phosphate groups attached to the nucleoside adenosine. These are high-energy compounds because of the energy associated with the repulsion between closely associated negative charges on the phosphate groups, as shown in Figure 6.2. Nucleotides are the building blocks of DNA.

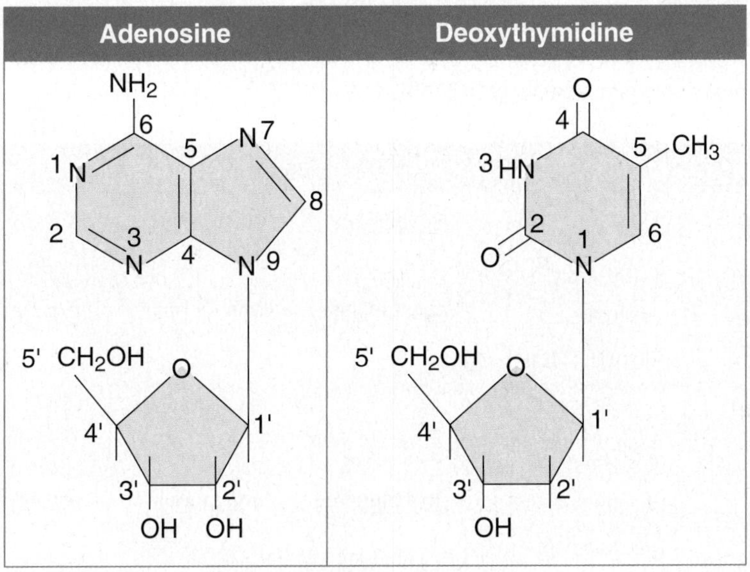

Figure 6.1 Examples of Nucleosides

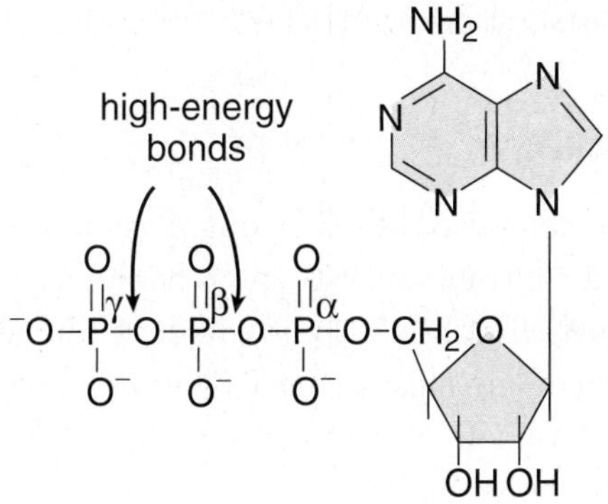

Figure 6.2 High-Energy Bonds in Adenosine Triphosphate, a Nucleotide

BRIDGE

In Chapter 3 of *MCAT General Chemistry Review*, we learned that bond breaking is usually endothermic and bond making is usually exothermic. ATP offers a biologically relevant—and MCAT tested—exception to this rule. Due to all the negative charges in close proximity, removing the terminal phosphate from ATP actually releases energy, which powers our cells.

Nucleic acids are classified according to the pentose they contain, as shown in Figure 6.3. If the pentose is **ribose**, the nucleic acid is RNA; if the pentose is **deoxyribose** (ribose with the 2′ –OH group replaced by –H), then it is DNA.

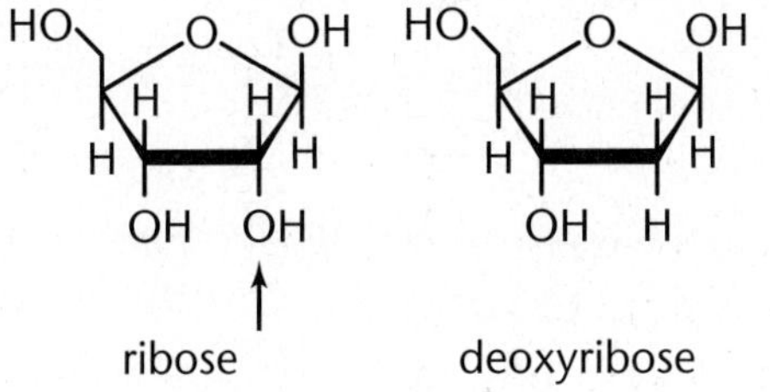

Figure 6.3 Ribose and Deoxyribose
Ribose has an –OH group at C-2; deoxyribose has an –H.

The nomenclature for the common bases, nucleosides, and nucleotides is shown in Table 6.1. Note that there is no *thymidine* listed (only *deoxythymidine*) because thymine appears almost exclusively in DNA.

BASE	NUCLEOSIDE	NUCLEOTIDES		
Adenine	Adenosine (Deoxyadenosine)	AMP (dAMP)	ADP (dADP)	ATP (dATP)
Guanine	Guanosine (Deoxyguanosine)	GMP (dGMP)	GDP (dGDP)	GTP (dGTP)
Cytosine	Cytidine (Deoxycytidine)	CMP (dCMP)	CDP (dCDP)	CTP (dCTP)
Uracil	Uridine (Deoxyuridine)	UMP (dUMP)	UDP (dUDP)	UTP (dUTP)
Thymine	(Deoxythymidine)	(dTMP)	(dTDP)	(dTTP)

Names of nucleosides and nucleotides attached to deoxyribose are shown in parentheses.

Table 6.1 Nomenclature of Important Bases, Nucleosides, and Nucleotides

Sugar–Phosphate Backbone

The backbone of DNA is composed of alternating sugar and phosphate groups; it determines the directionality of the DNA and is always read from 5′ to 3′. It is formed as nucleotides are joined by 3′–5′ phosphodiester bonds. That is, a phosphate group links the 3′ carbon of one sugar to the 5′ phosphate group of the next incoming sugar in the chain. Phosphates carry a negative charge; thus, DNA and RNA strands have an overall negative charge.

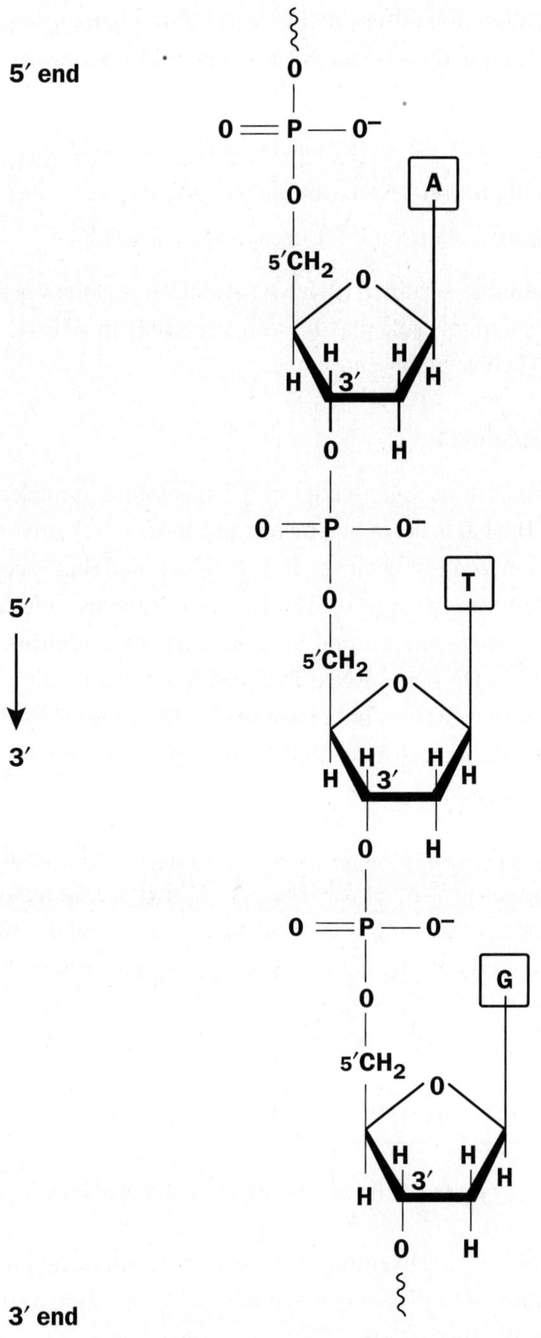

Figure 6.4 DNA Strand Polarity
DNA strands run antiparallel to one another; enzymes that replicate and transcribe DNA only work in the 5′ to 3′ direction.

Each strand of DNA has distinct 5′ and 3′ ends, creating polarity within the backbone, as shown in Figure 6.4. The 5′ end of DNA, for instance, will have an –OH or phosphate group bonded to C-5′ of the sugar, while the 3′ end has a free –OH on C-3′ of the sugar. The base sequence of a nucleic acid strand is both written and read in the 5′ to 3′ direction. Thus, the DNA strand in Figure 6.4 must be written: 5′—ATG—3′ (or simply ATG). DNA sequences can also be written in slightly different ways:

- If written backwards, the ends must be labeled: 3′—GTA—5′
- The position of phosphates may be shown: pApTpG
- "d" may be used as shorthand for deoxyribose: dAdTdG

MCAT EXPERTISE

On the MCAT, always check nucleic acids for polarity. One of the easiest ways to generate incorrect answers is to simply reverse the reading frame: 3′–GATTACA–5′ is not the same as 3′–ACATTAG–5′.

DNA is generally double-stranded (dsDNA) and RNA is generally single-stranded (ssRNA). Exceptions to this rule may be seen, especially in viruses, as described in Chapter 1 of *MCAT Biology Review*.

Purines and Pyrimidines

There are two families of nitrogen-containing bases found in nucleotides: purines and pyrimidines. The bases described below, and shown in Figure 6.5, represent the common bases in eukaryotes; however, it should be noted that exceptions may be seen in tRNA and in some prokaryotes and viruses. **Purines** contain two rings in their structure. The two purines found in nucleic acids are **adenine (A)** and **guanine (G)**; both are found in DNA and RNA. **Pyrimidines** contain only one ring in their structure. The three pyrimidines are **cytosine (C)**, **thymine (T)**, and **uracil (U)**; while cytosine is found in both DNA and RNA, thymine is only found in DNA and uracil is only found in RNA.

MNEMONIC

To remember the types and structures of these two classes of nitrogenous bases, remember to **CUT** the **PY**e (as **C**, **U**, and **T** are **py**rimidines). You can also note that pie has one ring of crust, and pyrimidines have only one ring in their structure. You can also remember **PUR**e **A**s **G**old (as **A** and **G** are **pur**ines); think of gold wedding rings. It takes two gold rings at a wedding, just like purines have two rings in their structure.

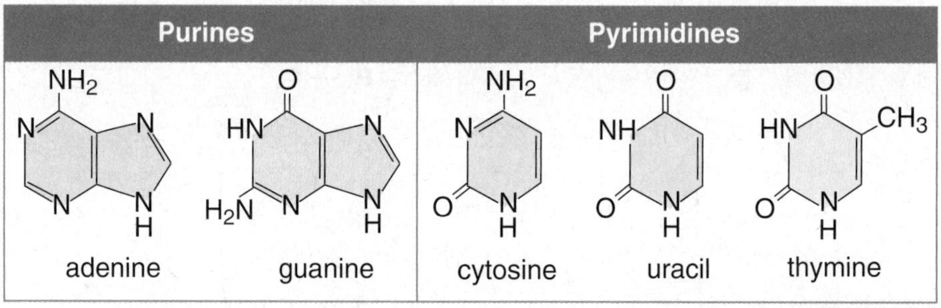

Figure 6.5 Bases Commonly Found in Nucleic Acids

Purines and pyrimidines are examples of biological aromatic heterocycles. In chemistry, the term **aromatic** describes any unusually stable ring system that adheres to the following four specific rules:

1. The compound is cyclic.
2. The compound is planar.
3. The compound is conjugated (has alternating single and multiple bonds, or lone pairs, creating at least one unhybridized *p*-orbital for each atom in the ring).
4. The compound has $4n + 2$ (where n is any integer) π electrons. This is called **Hückel's rule**.

The most common example of an aromatic compound is benzene, but many different structures obey these rules. In an aromatic compound, the extra stability is due to the delocalized π electrons, which can travel throughout the entire compound using available molecular orbitals. All six of the carbon atoms in benzene are sp^2-hybridized, and each of the six orbitals overlaps equally with its two neighbors. As a result, the delocalized electrons form two π electron clouds (one above and one below the plane of the ring), as shown in Figure 6.6. This delocalization is characteristic of all aromatic molecules, and because of this, aromatic molecules are fairly unreactive.

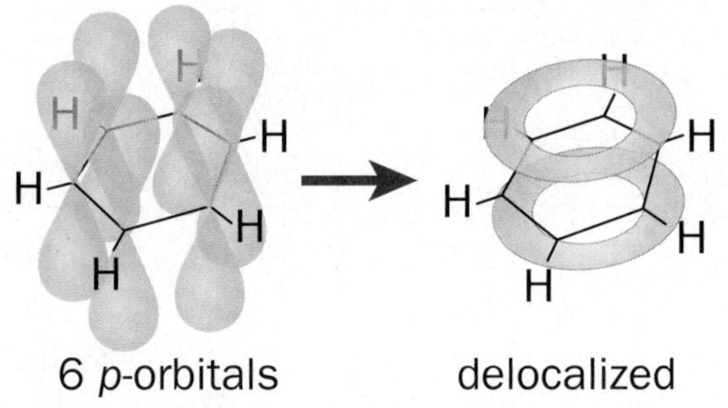

Figure 6.6 Delocalization of π Electrons in Benzene

Heterocycles are ring structures that contain at least two different elements in the ring. As shown in Figure 6.5 earlier, both purines and pyrimidines contain nitrogen in their aromatic rings. Nucleic acids are thus imbued with exceptional stability. This helps to explain the utility of nucleotides as the molecule for storing genetic information.

Watson–Crick Model

Putting this information together, we can start looking at the **Watson–Crick model** of DNA structure. In 1953, James Watson and Francis Crick presented one of the landmark findings of modern biology and medicine: the three-dimensional structure of DNA. With X-ray patterns of DNA produced by Rosalind Franklin laying the necessary foundation for their work, Watson and Crick were able to deduce the double-helical nature of DNA and propose specific base-pairing that would be the basis of a copying mechanism. In the **double helix**, two linear polynucleotide chains of DNA are wound together in a spiral orientation along a common axis. The key features of the model—some of which have already been mentioned—are:

- The two strands of DNA are antiparallel; that is, the strands are oriented in opposite directions. When one strand has polarity 5′ to 3′ *down* the page, the other strand has 5′ to 3′ polarity *up* the page.
- The sugar–phosphate backbone is on the outside of the helix with the nitrogenous bases on the inside.
- There are specific base-pairing rules, often referred to as **complementary base-pairing**, as shown in Figure 6.7. An adenine (A) is always base-paired with a thymine (T) via two hydrogen bonds. A guanine (G) always pairs with cytosine (C) via three hydrogen bonds. The three hydrogen bonds make the G–C

base pair interaction stronger. These hydrogen bonds, and the hydrophobic interactions between bases, provide stability to the double helix structure. Thus, the base sequence on one strand defines the base sequence on the other strand.

- Because of the specific base-pairing, the amount of A equals the amount of T, and the amount of G equals the amount of C. Thus, total purines will be equal to total pyrimidines overall. These properties are known as **Chargaff's rules**.

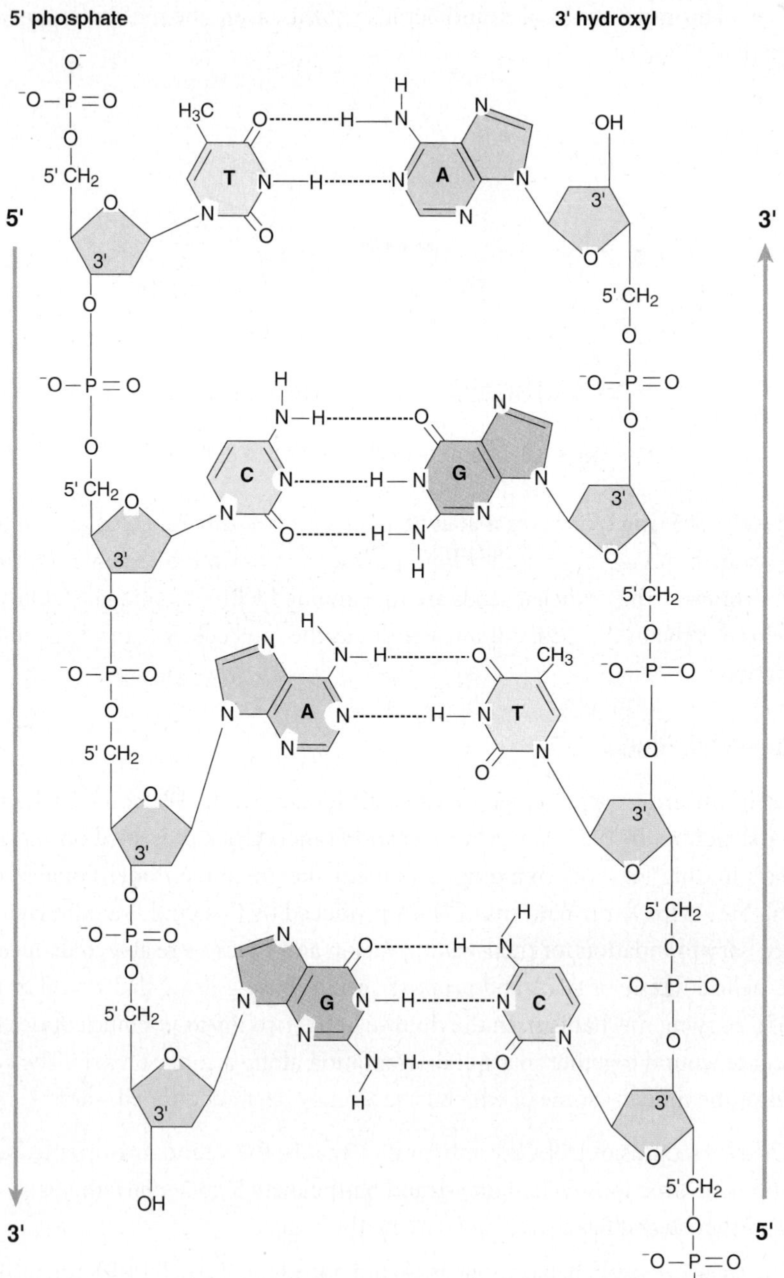

Figure 6.7 Base-Pairing in DNA

KEY CONCEPT

When writing a complementary strand of DNA, it is important to not only remember the base-pairing rules but to also keep track of the 5′ and 3′ ends. Remember that the sequences need to be both complementary and antiparallel. For example, 5′–ATCG–3′ will be complementary to 5′–CGAT–3′.

MCAT EXPERTISE

Using Chargaff's rules:

In double-stranded DNA, purines = pyrimidines:

- %A = %T
- %G = %C

If a sample of DNA has 10% G, what is the % of T?

10% G = 10% C, thus %G + %C = 20%

%A + %T = 80%, thus %T = 40%.

The double helix of most DNA is a right-handed helix, forming what is called **B-DNA**, as shown in Figure 6.8. The helix in B-DNA makes a turn every 3.4 nm and contains about 10 bases within that span. Major and minor grooves can be identified between the interlocking strands and are often the site of protein binding. Another form of DNA is called **Z-DNA** for its zigzag appearance; it is a left-handed helix that has a turn every 4.6 nm and contains 12 bases within each turn. A high GC-content or a high salt concentration may contribute to the formation of this form of DNA. No biological activity has been attributed to Z-DNA partly because it is unstable and difficult to research.

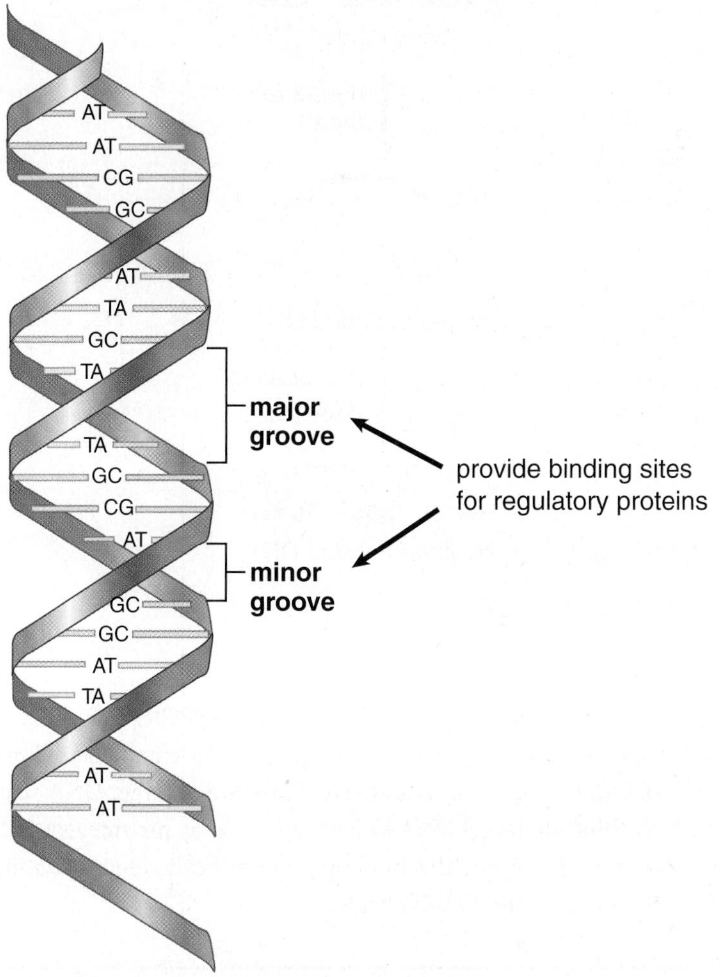

Figure 6.8 The B-DNA Double Helix

Denaturation and Reannealing

During processes such as replication and transcription, it is necessary to gain access to the DNA. The double helical nature of DNA can be **denatured** by conditions that disrupt hydrogen bonding and base-pairing, resulting in the "melting" of the double helix into two single strands that have separated from each other. Notably, none of the covalent links between the nucleotides in the backbone of the DNA break during this process. Heat, alkaline pH, and chemicals like formaldehyde and urea are commonly used to denature DNA.

Denatured, single-stranded DNA can be **reannealed** (brought back together) if the denaturing condition is slowly removed. If a solution of heat-denatured DNA is slowly cooled, for example, then the two complementary strands can become paired again, as shown in Figure 6.9.

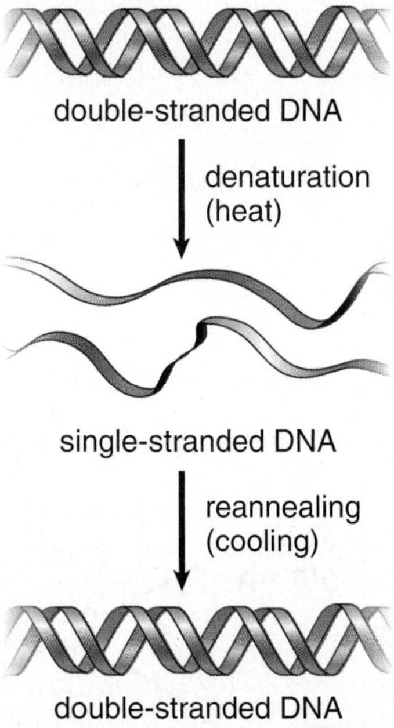

Figure 6.9 Denaturation and Reannealing of DNA

Such annealing of complementary DNA strands is also an important step in many laboratory processes, such as polymerase chain reactions (PCR) and in the detection of specific DNA sequences. In these techniques, a well-characterized **probe DNA** (DNA with known sequence) is added to a mixture of target DNA sequences. When probe DNA binds to target DNA sequences, this may provide evidence of the presence of a gene of interest. This binding process is called hybridization and is described in further detail later in this chapter.

MCAT CONCEPT CHECK 6.1

Before you move on, assess your understanding of the material with these questions.

1. What is the difference between a nucleoside and a nucleotide?

____

2. What are the base-pairing rules according to the Watson–Crick model?

____

3. What are the three major structural differences between DNA and RNA?

   1. ______________________________
   2. ______________________________
   3. ______________________________

4. How does the aromaticity of purines and pyrimidines underscore their genetic function?

____

5. If a strand of RNA contained 15% cytosine, 15% adenine, 35% guanine, and 35% uracil, would this violate Chargaff's rules? Why or why not?

____

6.2 Eukaryotic Chromosome Organization

LEARNING OBJECTIVES

After Chapter 6.2, you will be able to:

- Recall the names and the role of the five histone proteins
- Differentiate between the major characteristics of heterochromatin and euchromatin
- Describe the traits of telomeres and centromeres

There are over 6 billion bases of DNA in each human cell. It is important for the cell to organize these bases effectively. These bases must be replicated during the cell cycle and also utilized in gene expression for normal cellular functions. In humans, DNA is divided up among the 46 **chromosomes** found in the nucleus of the cell. The supercoiling of the DNA double helix does provide some compaction, but much more is necessary.

Histones

The DNA that makes up a chromosome is wound around a group of small basic proteins called **histones**, forming **chromatin**. There are five histone proteins found in eukaryotic cells. Two copies each of the histone proteins *H2A*, *H2B*, *H3*, and *H4* form a histone core and about 200 base pairs of DNA are wrapped around this protein complex, forming a **nucleosome**, as shown in Figure 6.10. Under an electron microscope, the nucleosomes look like beads on a string. The last histone, *H1*, seals off the DNA as it enters and leaves the nucleosome, adding stability to the structure. Together, the nucleosomes create a much more organized and compacted DNA.

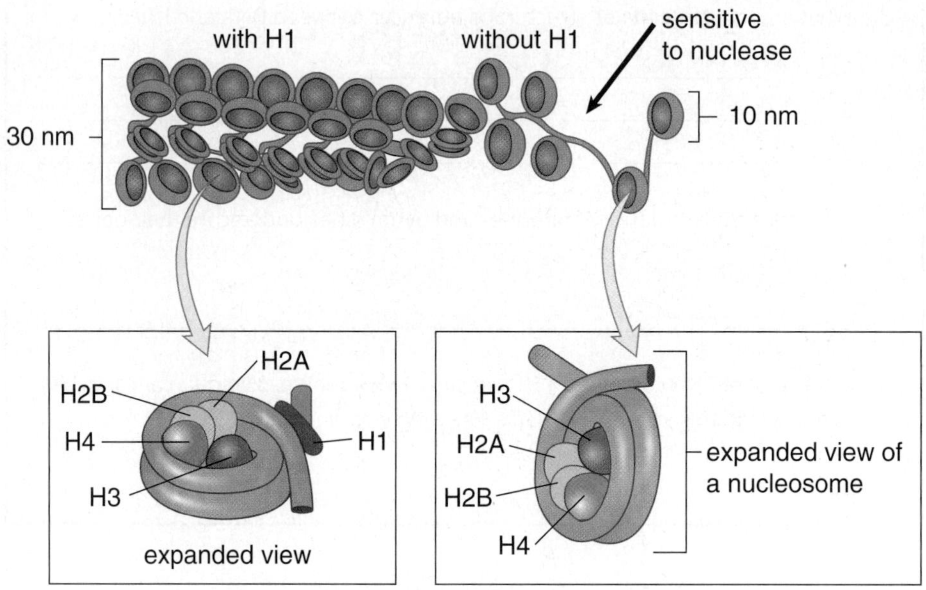

Figure 6.10 Nucleosome Structure

Nucleosomes are composed of DNA wrapped around histone proteins.

Histones are one example of **nucleoproteins** (proteins that associate with DNA). Most other nucleoproteins are acid-soluble and tend to stimulate processes such as transcription.

Heterochromatin and Euchromatin

The chromosomes have a diffuse configuration during interphase of the cell cycle. The cell will undergo DNA replication during the S phase of interphase and having the DNA uncondensed and accessible makes the process more efficient. A small percentage of the chromatin remains compacted during interphase and is referred to as **heterochromatin**. Heterochromatin appears dark under light microscopy and is transcriptionally silent. Heterochromatin often consists of DNA with highly repetitive sequences. In contrast, the dispersed chromatin is called **euchromatin**, which appears light under light microscopy. Euchromatin contains genetically active DNA. Both heterochromatin and euchromatin can be seen in the nucleus in Figure 6.11.

KEY CONCEPT

Heterochromatin is dark, dense, and silent. Euchromatin is light, uncondensed, and expressed.

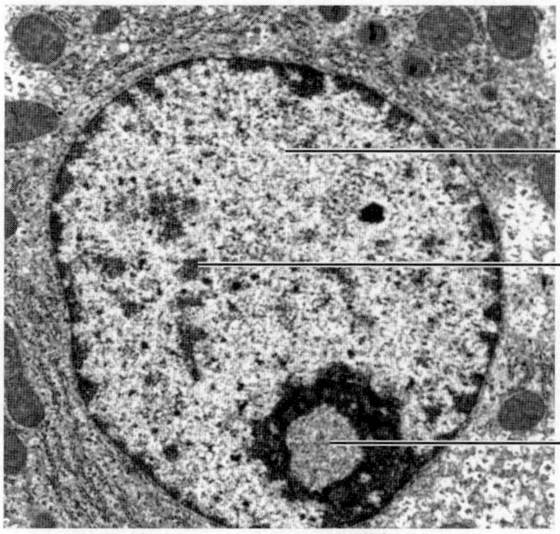

Figure 6.11 Euchromatin and Heterochromatin in an Interphase Nucleus

Telomeres and Centromeres

As described later in this chapter, DNA replication cannot extend all the way to the end of a chromosome. This will result in losing sequences and information with each round of replication. The solution for our cells is a simple repeating unit (TTAGGG) at the end of the DNA, forming a **telomere**. Some of the sequence is lost in each round of replication and can be replaced by the enzyme ***telomerase***. Telomerase is more highly expressed in rapidly dividing cells. Animal studies indicate that there are a set number of replications possible, and that the progressive shortening of telomeres contributes to aging. Telomeres also serve a second function: their high GC-content creates exceptionally strong strand attractions at the end of chromosomes to prevent unraveling; think of telomeres as "knotting off" the end of the chromosome.

Centromeres, as their name suggests, are a region of DNA found in the center of chromosomes. They are often referred to as sites of constriction because they form noticeable indentations. This part of the chromosome is composed of heterochromatin, which is in turn composed of tandem repeat sequences that also contain high GC-content. During cell division, the two sister chromatids can therefore remain connected at the centromere until microtubules separate the chromatids during anaphase.

BIOCHEMISTRY GUIDED EXAMPLE WITH EXPERT THINKING

Cisplatin is an effective chemotherapeutic agent against a number of cancers, including notoriously difficult to treat head and neck cancers. Cisplatin acts by binding DNA, which then irreversibly binds repair complexes, preventing effective repair. Cisplatin exhibits two major drawbacks that limit its application in cancer therapy—severe side effects and the rapid development of drug resistance. They are mutually connected, as adverse side effects restrict the administration of high doses, while underdosing leads to development of resistance in the cancerous cells. For this reason, drugs that sensitize cancer cells towards cisplatin could increase its therapeutic efficacy.

Topic: cisplatin is a drug used in chemotherapy; it inhibits DNA repair

Problem: cisplatin has bad side effects and cancer cells can develop resistance

Purpose: looking for a drug that makes cancer cells more susceptible to cisplatin

Four groups of mice were transfected with tumor cells by an intraperitoneal injection; 24 hours later they received 5 mg/kg cisplatin, 166 mg/kg butyrate, both cisplatin and butyrate, or a sham treatment. The life span of the mice is noted below in Table 1 along with the T/C ratio, which is the ratio between the mean life spans of the treated animals (T) and the controls (C). To further investigate the mechanism by which butyrate acts, exponentially growing HeLa cells were treated with 5 mM butyrate, 8 μM cisplatin, or both. At 4 and 24 hours after treatment, total histone fraction was isolated and equal quantities of histones were subjected to SDS-PAGE, and subsequently to western blot with anti-acetylated histone antibody. Acetylation is a post-translational modification added to lysine groups on histone proteins. The acetylation levels are expressed as a percentage of the untreated control in Figure 1 below.

First experiment: the life span of cancerous mice were measured with different treatments

Second experiment: how does butyrate act? The histone acetylation levels were measured with different treatments

Treatment	Life span (days)	T/C	*p*-value
Control	10.8 ± 2.0	1	
Butyrate	14.0 ± 4.5	1.3	0.19
Cisplatin	12.0 ± 3.5	1.1	0.53
Cisplatin + Butyrate	19.0 ± 3.4	1.8	0.0019

Table 1

IV: treatment

DV: life span

Trend: cisplatin + butyrate-treated mice had significantly longer life span

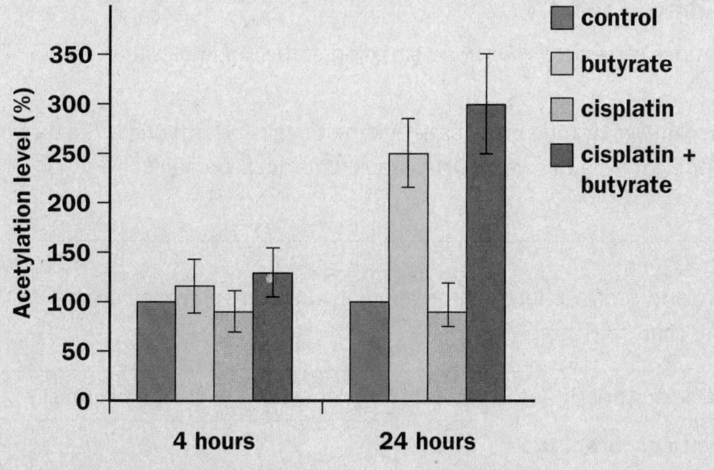

IVs: treatment, time of treatment

DV: histone acetylation

Trend: butyrate and cisplatin + butyrate had significantly higher levels of acetylation after 24 hours

Figure 1

Adapted from Koprinarova, M., Markovska, P., Iliev, I., Anachkova, B., & Russev, G. (2010). Sodium butyrate enhances the cytotoxic effect of cisplatin by abrogating the cisplatin imposed cell cycle arrest. *BMC Molecular Biology*, 11, 49. doi:10.1186/1471-2199-11-49.

Given the fact that histones are enriched with surface-exposed basic amino acids, how does butyrate enhance the cytotoxic effect of cisplatin on tumor cells?

The question stem asks us to explain the action of butyrate in conjunction with cisplatin, which means we need to dig into the experiment and results of the passage. The first paragraph tells us that cisplatin blocks DNA repair, and when targeting cancerous cells, cisplatin would likely cause cell death. Table 1 clearly shows that cisplatin alone doesn't increase the life span of mice with cancer, but coupling cisplatin with butyrate does. However, this result doesn't tell us how this paired treatment works (just that it does work), which means that we need to find this information in Figure 1. The treatments do not differ from the control after 4 hours, but butyrate and cisplatin + butyrate do increase the levels of histone acetylation. The passage tells us that histone acetylation is a post-translational addition of an acetyl group on to lysines. We know from the structure of amino acids that lysines are positively charged, so adding an acetyl group would mask the positive charge. We're also told that histones have many surface-exposed basic amino acids, and basic amino acids (like lysine and arginine) are positively charged at physiological pH. Let's also recall that when DNA is wrapped tightly around histone proteins, it is referred to as heterochromatin, which means the DNA is transcriptionally silent. Since DNA has a negative charge due to the phosphodiester backbone, acetylating the lysines on histones will remove some of the positive charge. Without that positive charge binding the negatively charged DNA, the histones will no longer be held tightly to the DNA, meaning they will dissociate from the DNA. DNA that is not tightly bound to histones forms euchromatin, which is genetically active: those genes can now be transcribed and translated. The DNA will then also be accessible to cisplatin, which will bind and stop DNA repair complexes. A build up of unrepaired DNA often causes cells to die, usually through apoptotic mechanisms.

In summary, butyrate causes DNA to separate from histones, allowing for cisplatin to bind and stop DNA repair complexes from fixing errors in the DNA, leading to eventual cell death.

MCAT CONCEPT CHECK 6.2

Before you move on, assess your understanding of the material with these questions.

1. What are the five histone proteins in eukaryotic cells? Which one is not part of the histone core around which DNA wraps to form chromatin?

____

2. Compare and contrast heterochromatin and euchromatin based on the following characteristics:

Characteristic	Heterochromatin	Euchromatin
Density of chromatin packing		
Appearance under light microscopy		
Transcriptional activity		

3. What property of telomeres and centromeres allows them to stay tightly raveled, even when the rest of DNA is uncondensed?

____

6.3 DNA Replication

LEARNING OBJECTIVES

After Chapter 6.3, you will be able to:

- List the names and functions of the major enzymes of DNA synthesis in prokaryotes and eukaryotes
- Differentiate between synthesis of the leading and lagging strands
- Explain the role of telomerase and the function of the telomere

The DNA is an organism's "blueprint" that provides not only the ability to sustain activities of life but also insight into our evolutionary past. The process of DNA replication is highly regulated to ensure as close to 100 percent perfection when making a copy of our genome as possible. DNA replication is necessary for the reproduction of a species and for any dividing cell.

Strand Separation and Origins of Replication

The human genome has about 3 billion base pairs packed into multiple chromosomes. The **replisome** or **replication complex** is a set of specialized proteins that assist the DNA polymerases. To begin the process of replication, DNA unwinds at points called **origins of replication**. The generation of new DNA proceeds in both directions, creating **replication forks** on both sides of the origin, as shown in Figure 6.12.

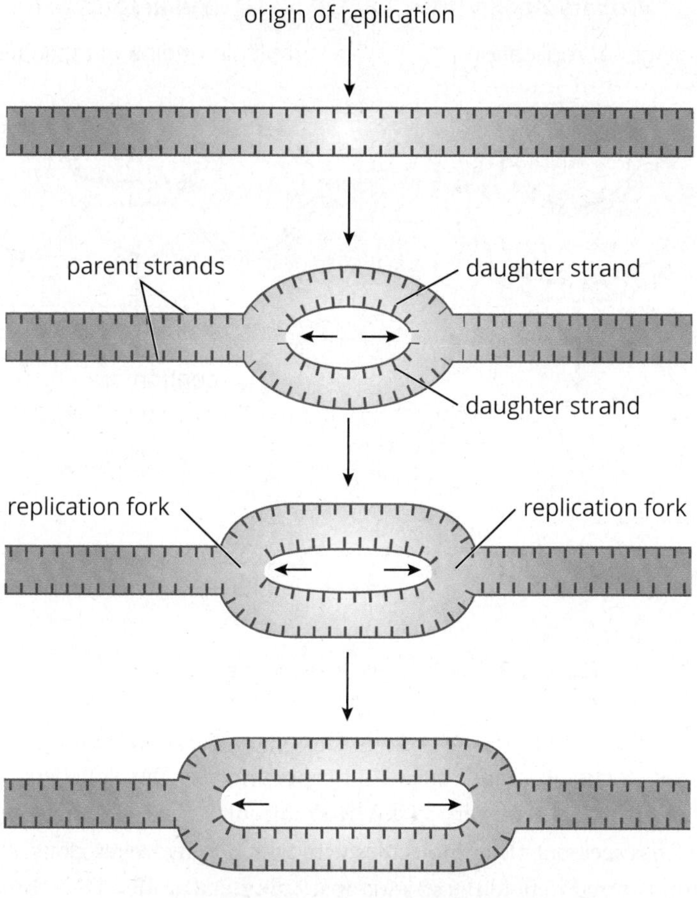

Figure 6.12 Origins of Replication
Replication forks form on both sides of the origin, increasing the efficiency of replication.

The bacterial chromosome is a closed, double-stranded circular DNA molecule with a single origin of replication. Thus, there are two replication forks that move away from each other in opposite directions around the circle. The two replication forks eventually meet, resulting in the production of two identical circular molecules of DNA.

Eukaryotic replication must copy many more bases compared to prokaryotic and is a slower process. In order to duplicate all of the chromosomes efficiently, each eukaryotic chromosome contains one linear molecule of double-stranded DNA having multiple origins of replication. As the replication forks move toward each other and **sister chromatids** are created, the chromatids will remain connected at the **centromere**. The differences between prokaryotic and eukaryotic replication patterns are shown in Figure 6.13.

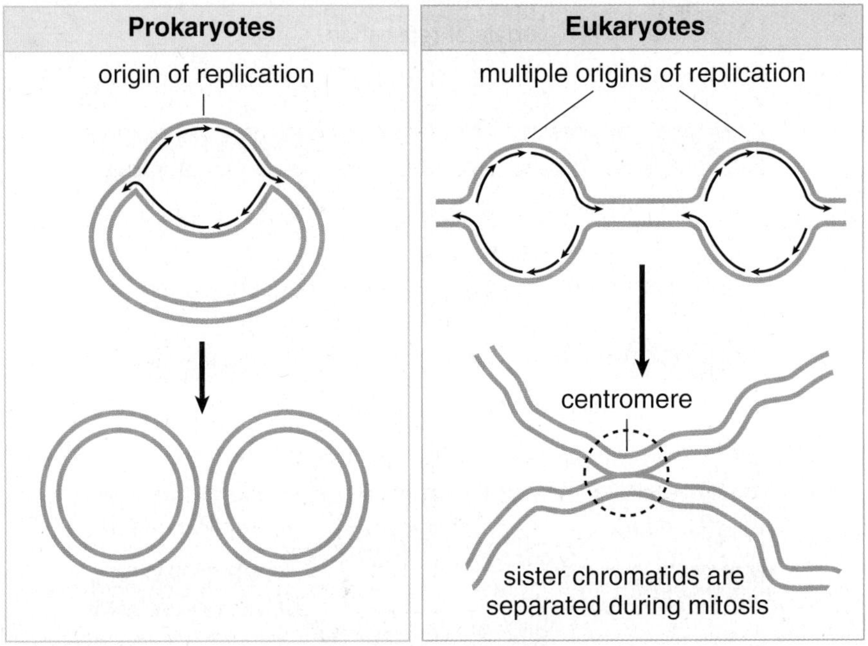

Figure 6.13 DNA Replication in Prokaryotes and Eukaryotes

REAL WORLD

Any antibiotic ending with *-floxacin* (ciprofloxacin, moxifloxacin, and so on) is called a *fluoroquinolone* and targets the prokaryotic topoisomerase *DNA gyrase*. This stops bacterial replication and slows the infection. Fluoroquinolones are routinely used for pneumonia and certain infections of the genitourinary system.

Helicase is the enzyme responsible for unwinding the DNA, generating two single-stranded template strands ahead of the polymerase. Once opened, the unpaired strands of DNA are very sticky, in a molecular sense. The free purines and pyrimidines seek out other molecules with which to hydrogen bond. Proteins are therefore required to hold the strands apart: **single-stranded DNA-binding proteins** will bind to the unraveled strand, preventing both the reassociation of the DNA strands and the degradation of DNA by ***nucleases***. As the helicase unwinds the DNA, it will cause positive supercoiling that strains the DNA helix. **Supercoiling** is a wrapping of DNA on itself as its helical structure is pushed ever further toward the telomeres during replication; picture an old-fashioned telephone cord that's become tangled on itself. To alleviate this torsional stress and reduce the risk of strand breakage, ***DNA topoisomerases*** introduce negative supercoils. They do so by working ahead of helicase, nicking one or both strands, allowing relaxation of the torsional pressure, and then resealing the cut strands.

During replication, these **parental strands** will serve as templates for the generation of new **daughter strands**. The replication process is termed **semiconservative** because one parental strand is retained in each of the two resulting identical double-stranded DNA molecules, as shown in Figure 6.14.

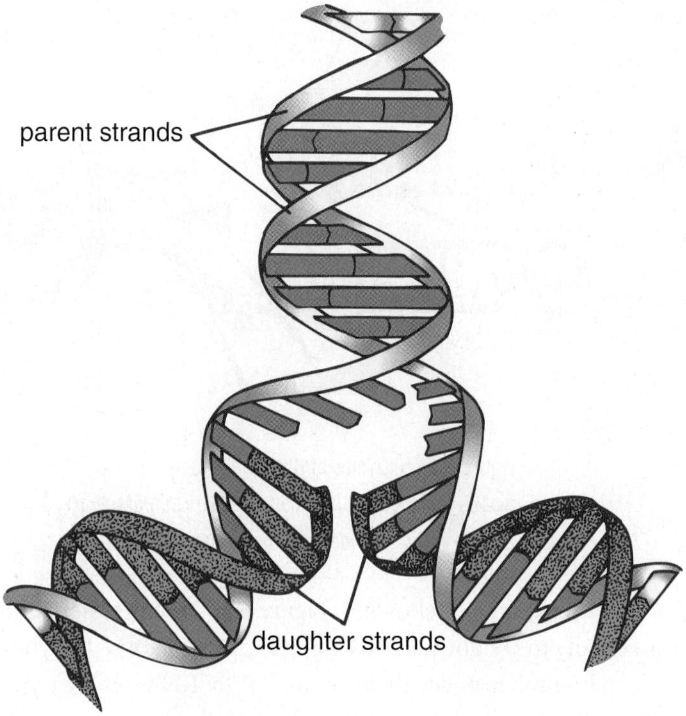

Figure 6.14 Semiconservative Replication

A new double helix is made of one old parent strand and one new daughter strand.

Synthesis of Daughter Strands

DNA polymerases are responsible for reading the DNA template, or parental strand, and synthesizing the new daughter strand. The DNA polymerase can read the template strand in a 3′ to 5′ direction while synthesizing the complementary strand in the 5′ to 3′ direction. This will result in a new double helix of DNA that has the required antiparallel orientation. Due to this directionality of the DNA polymerase, certain constraints arise. Remember that the two separated parental strands of the helix are also antiparallel to each other. Thus, at each replication fork, one strand is oriented in the correct direction for DNA polymerase; the other strand is antiparallel.

The **leading strand** in each replication fork is the strand that is copied in a continuous fashion, in the same direction as the advancing replication fork. This parental strand will be read 3′ to 5′ and its complement will be synthesized in a 5′ to 3′ manner, as discussed above.

The **lagging strand** is the strand that is copied in a direction opposite the direction of the replication fork. On this side of the replication fork, the parental strand has 5′ to 3′ polarity. DNA polymerase cannot simply read and synthesize on this strand. How does it solve this problem? Because DNA polymerase can only synthesize in the 5′ to 3′ direction from a 3′ to 5′ template, small strands called **Okazaki fragments** are produced. As the replication fork continues to move forward, it clears additional space that DNA polymerase must fill in. Each time DNA polymerase completes an Okazaki fragment, it turns around to find another gap that needs to be filled in.

KEY CONCEPT

With the exception of DNA polymerase's *reading* direction (and a few untested endonucleases), everything in molecular biology is 5′ to 3′. DNA polymerase reads 3′ to 5′, but the following processes occur 5′ to 3′:

- DNA synthesis
- DNA repair
- RNA transcription
- RNA translation (reading of codons)

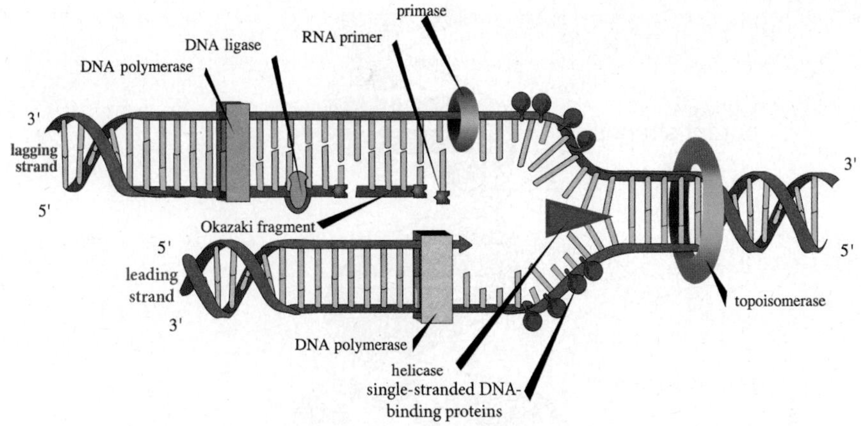

Figure 6.15 Enzymes of DNA Replication

This process involves the action of DNA helicase, gyrase, polymerase, and ligase to create two identical molecules of DNA.

The process of DNA replication is shown in Figure 6.15. The first step in the replication of DNA is actually to lay down an RNA primer. DNA cannot be synthesized *de novo*; that is, it needs another molecule to "hook on" to. RNA, on the other hand, can be directly paired with the parent strand. Thus, ***primase*** synthesizes a short primer (roughly 10 nucleotides) in the $5'$ to $3'$ direction to start replication on each strand. These short RNA sequences are constantly being added to the lagging strand because each Okazaki fragment must start with a new primer. In contrast, the leading strand requires only one, in theory (in reality, there are usually a few primers on the leading strand). ***DNA polymerase III*** (prokaryotes) or ***DNA polymerases*** $\boldsymbol{\alpha}$, $\boldsymbol{\delta}$, and ε (eukaryotes) will then begin synthesizing the daughter strands of DNA in the $5'$ to $3'$ manner. The incoming nucleotides are $5'$ deoxyribonucleotide triphosphates: dATP, dCTP, dGTP, and dTTP. As the new phosphodiester bond is made, a free *pyrophosphate* (PP_i) is released.

The RNA must eventually be removed to maintain integrity of the genome. This is accomplished by the enzyme ***DNA polymerase I*** (prokaryotes) or ***RNase H*** (eukaryotes). Then, ***DNA polymerase I*** (prokaryotes) or ***DNA polymerase*** $\boldsymbol{\delta}$ (eukaryotes) adds DNA nucleotides where the RNA primer had been. ***DNA ligase*** seals the ends of the DNA molecules together, creating one continuous strand of DNA.

While prokaryotic DNA synthesis has been worked out in great detail, and eukaryotic synthesis is considered to be very similar, there are a few differences in the enzymes involved. There are five "classic" DNA polymerases in eukaryotic cells, which are designated with the Greek letters α, β, γ, δ, and ε. Further research has revealed more polymerases named ζ through μ, but these are outside the scope of the MCAT. Table 6.2 highlights differences in the names of the enzymes associated with DNA replication in prokaryotic *vs.* eukaryotic cells; special attention should be paid to the eukaryotic DNA polymerases:

- DNA polymerases α, δ, and ε work together to synthesize both the leading and lagging strands; DNA polymerase δ also fills in the gaps left behind when RNA primers are removed

- DNA polymerase γ replicates mitochondrial DNA
- DNA polymerases β and ε are important to the process of DNA repair
- DNA polymerases δ and ε are assisted by the *PCNA* protein, which assembles into a trimer to form the **sliding clamp**. The clamp helps to strengthen the interaction between these DNA polymerases and the template strand

STEP IN REPLICATION	PROKARYOTIC CELLS	EUKARYOTIC CELLS (NUCLEI)
Origin of replication	One per chromosome	Multiple per chromosome
Unwinding of DNA double helix	Helicase	Helicase
Stabilization of unwound template strands	Single-stranded DNA-binding protein	Single-stranded DNA-binding protein
Synthesis of RNA primers	Primase	Primase
Synthesis of DNA	DNA polymerase III	DNA polymerases α, δ, and ε
Removal of RNA primers	DNA polymerase I ($5' \rightarrow 3'$ exonuclease)	RNase H ($5' \rightarrow 3'$ exonuclease)
Replacement of RNA with DNA	DNA polymerase I	DNA polymerase δ
Joining of Okazaki fragments	DNA ligase	DNA ligase
Removal of positive supercoils ahead of advancing replication forks	DNA topoisomerases (DNA gyrase)	DNA topoisomerases
Synthesis of telomeres	Not applicable	Telomerase

Table 6.2 Steps and Proteins Involved in DNA Replication

Replicating the Ends of Chromosomes

While DNA polymerase does an excellent job of synthesizing DNA, it unfortunately cannot complete synthesis of the 5′ end of the strand. Thus, each time DNA synthesis is carried out, the chromosome becomes a little shorter. To lengthen the time that cells can replicate and synthesize DNA before necessary genes are damaged, chromosomes contain **telomeres**. As described earlier, telomeres are located at the very tips of the chromosome and consist of repetitive sequences with a high GC-content. This repetition means that telomeres can be slightly degraded between replication cycles without loss of function.

MCAT CONCEPT CHECK 6.3

Before you move on, assess your understanding of the material with these questions.

1. For each of the enzymes listed below, list the function of the enzyme and if it is found in prokaryotes, eukaryotes, or both.

Enzyme	Prokaryotes/ Eukaryotes/Both	Function
Helicase		
Single-stranded DNA-binding protein		
Primase		
DNA polymerase III		
DNA polymerase α		
DNA polymerase I		
RNase H		
DNA ligase		
DNA topoisomerases		

2. Between the leading strand and lagging strand, which is more prone to mutations? Why?

____

3. What is the function of a telomere?

____

6.4 DNA Repair

LEARNING OBJECTIVES

After Chapter 6.4, you will be able to:

- Describe the major DNA repair processes, including proofreading, mismatch repair, and excision repair
- Recognize the key components and locations of each DNA repair process, including both mismatch and excision processes
- Identify major traits of oncogenes and tumor suppressor genes

The structure of DNA can be damaged in a number of ways such as exposure to chemicals or radiation. DNA is very susceptible to damage and if the damage is not corrected, it will subsequently be copied and passed on to daughter cells. Damage can include breaking of the DNA backbone, structural or spontaneous alterations of bases, or incorporation of the incorrect base during replication. Any defect in the genetic code can cause an increased risk of cancer, so the cell has multiple processes in place to catch and correct genetic errors. This helps maintain the integrity and stability of the genome from cell to cell, and from generation to generation.

Oncogenes and Tumor Suppressor Genes

Certain genes, when mutated, can lead to cancer. **Cancer** cells proliferate excessively because they are able to divide without stimulation from other cells and are no longer subject to the normal controls on cell proliferation. By definition, cancer cells are able to migrate by local invasion or **metastasis**, a migration to distant tissues by the bloodstream or lymphatic system. Over time, cancer cells tend to accumulate mutations.

Mutated genes that cause cancer are termed **oncogenes**. Oncogenes primarily encode cell cycle–related proteins. Before these genes are mutated, they are often referred to as **proto-oncogenes**. The first gene in this category to be discovered was *src* (named after *sarcoma*, a category of connective tissue cancers). The abnormal alleles encode proteins that are more active than normal proteins, promoting rapid cell cycle advancement. Typically, a mutation in only one copy is sufficient to promote tumor growth and is therefore considered dominant.

KEY CONCEPT

While the outcome of oncogenes and mutated tumor suppressor genes is the same (cancer), the actual cause is different. Oncogenes promote the cell cycle while mutated tumor suppressors can no longer slow the cell cycle. Oncogenes are like stepping on the gas pedal; mutated tumor suppressors are like cutting the brakes.

Tumor suppressor genes, like *p53* or *Rb* (*retinoblastoma*), encode proteins that inhibit the cell cycle or participate in DNA repair processes. They normally function to stop tumor progression, and are sometimes called **antioncogenes**. Mutations of these genes result in the loss of tumor suppression activity, and therefore promote cancer. Inactivation of both alleles is necessary for the loss of function because, in most cases, even one copy of the normal protein can function to inhibit tumor formation. In this example, multiple mutations or "hits" are required.

Proofreading and Mismatch Repair

DNA polymerase moves along a single strand of DNA, building the complementary strand as it goes. While DNA polymerase is almost 100 percent accurate, it does occasionally make errors.

Proofreading

During synthesis, the two double-stranded DNA molecules will pass through a part of the DNA polymerase enzyme for **proofreading**. When the complementary strands have incorrectly paired bases, the hydrogen bonds between the strands can be unstable, and this lack of stability is detected as the DNA passes through this part of the polymerase. The incorrect base is excised and can be replaced with the correct one, as shown in Figure 6.16. If both the parent and daughter strands are simply DNA, how does the enzyme discriminate which is the template strand, and which is the incorrectly paired daughter strand? It looks at the level of methylation: the template strand has existed in the cell for a longer period of time, and therefore is more heavily methylated. Methylation also plays a role in the transcriptional activity of DNA, as described in Chapter 7 of *MCAT Biochemistry Review*. This system is very efficient, correcting most of the errors put into the sequence during replication. DNA ligase, which closes the gaps between Okazaki fragments, lacks proofreading ability. Thus, the likelihood of mutations in the lagging strand is considerably higher than the leading strand.

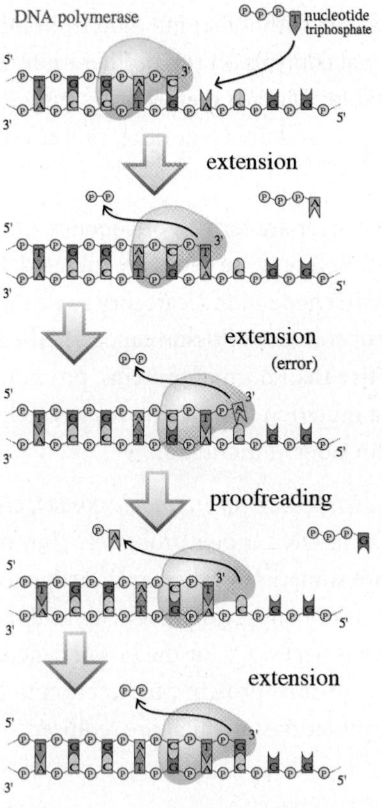

Figure 6.16 Proofreading by DNA Polymerase

Mismatch Repair

Cells also have machinery in the G_2 phase of the cell cycle for **mismatch repair**; these enzymes are encoded by genes *MSH2* and *MLH1*, which detect and remove errors introduced in replication that were missed during the S phase of the cell cycle. These enzymes are homologues of *MutS* and *MutL* in prokaryotes, which serve a similar function.

Nucleotide and Base Excision Repair

Most of the repair mechanisms involve proteins that recognize damage or a lesion, remove the damage, and then use the complementary strand as a template to fill in the gap. Our cell machinery recognizes two specific types of DNA damage in the G_1 and G_2 cell cycle phases and fixes them through nucleotide excision repair or base excision repair.

Nucleotide Excision Repair

Ultraviolet light induces the formation of dimers between adjacent thymine residues in DNA. The formation of thymine dimers interferes with DNA replication and normal gene expression, and distorts the shape of the double helix. Thymine dimers are eliminated from DNA by a **nucleotide excision repair** (**NER**) mechanism, which is a cut-and-patch process, as shown in Figure 6.17. First, specific proteins scan the DNA molecule and recognize the lesion because of a bulge in the strand. An ***excision endonuclease*** then makes nicks in the phosphodiester backbone of the damaged strand on both sides of the thymine dimer and removes the defective oligonucleotide. DNA polymerase can then fill in the gap by synthesizing DNA in the 5′ to 3′ direction, using the undamaged strand as a template. Finally, the nick in the strand is sealed by DNA ligase.

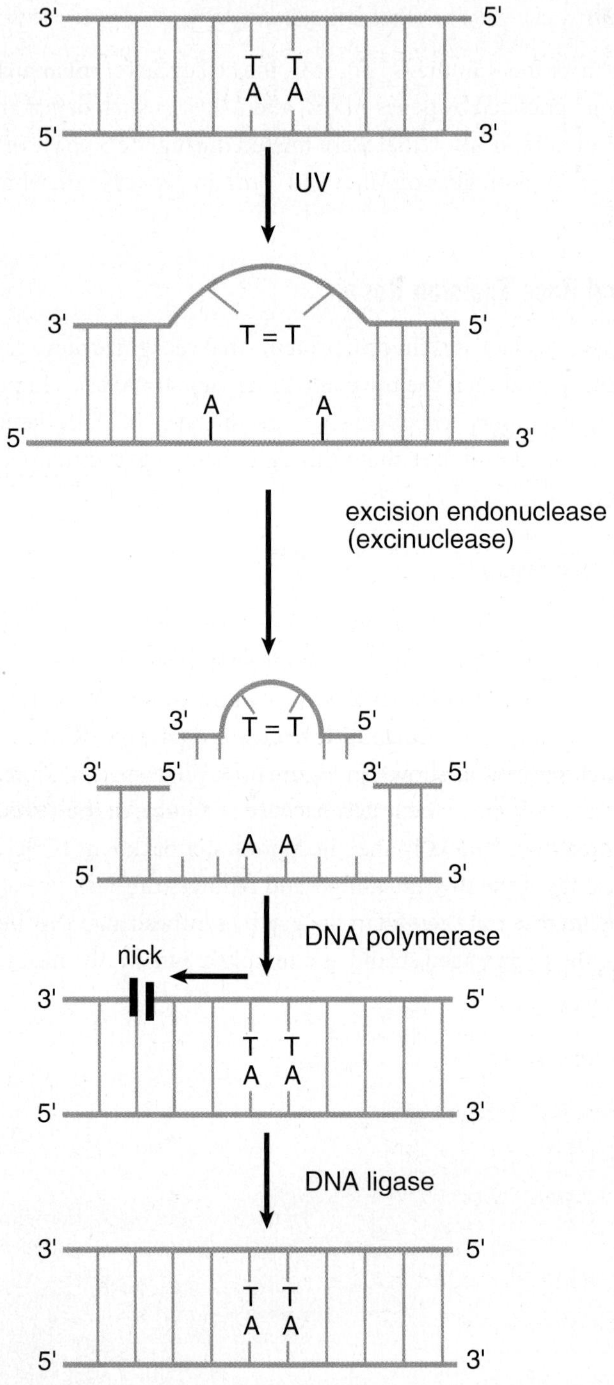

Figure 6.17 Thymine Dimer Formation and Nucleotide Excision Repair

Base Excision Repair

Alterations to bases can occur with other cellular insults. For example, thermal energy can be absorbed by DNA and may lead to cytosine deamination. This is the loss of an amino group from cytosine and results in the conversion of cytosine to uracil. Uracil should not be found in a DNA molecule and is thus easily detected as an error; however, detection systems exist for small, non-helix-distorting mutations in other bases as well. These are repaired by **base excision repair**. First, the affected base is recognized and removed by a glycosylase enzyme, leaving behind an **apurinic/apyrimidinic (AP) site**, also called an **abasic site**. The AP site is recognized by an ***AP endonuclease*** that removes the damaged sequence from the DNA. DNA polymerase and DNA ligase can then fill in the gap and seal the strand, as described above.

MCAT CONCEPT CHECK 6.4

Before you move on, assess your understanding of the material with these questions.

1. What is the difference between an oncogene and a tumor suppressor gene?

___

2. How does DNA polymerase recognize which strand is the template strand once the daughter strand is synthesized?

___

3. For each of the repair mechanisms below, in which phase of the cell cycle does the repair mechanism function? What are the key enzymes or genes specifically associated with each mechanism?

Repair Mechanism	Phase of Cell Cycle	Key Enzymes/Genes
DNA polymerase (proofreading)		
Mismatch repair		
Nucleotide excision repair		
Base excision repair		

4. What is the key structural difference in the types of lesions corrected by nucleotide excision repair *vs.* those corrected by base excision repair?

___

6.5 Recombinant DNA and Biotechnology

High-Yield

LEARNING OBJECTIVES

After Chapter 6.5, you will be able to:

- Predict the most effective DNA library technique for a given laboratory application
- Recall the inputs and outputs of biotechnology techniques, including PCR, Southern blotting, and sequencing
- Describe the differences between transgenic mice and knockout mice

Now that we have reviewed the basics of DNA structure and function, we can discuss how this knowledge has been harnessed for a variety of research and treatment innovations. **Recombinant DNA** technology allows a DNA fragment from any source to be multiplied by either gene cloning or polymerase chain reaction (PCR). This provides a means of analyzing and altering genes and proteins. It also provides the reagents necessary for genetic testing, such as carrier detection (detecting heterozygote status for a particular disease) and prenatal diagnosis of genetic diseases; it is also useful for gene therapy. Additionally, this technology can provide a source of a specific protein, such as recombinant human insulin, in almost unlimited quantities. The process of creating recombinant DNA (by gene cloning) and its benefits are shown in Figure 6.18.

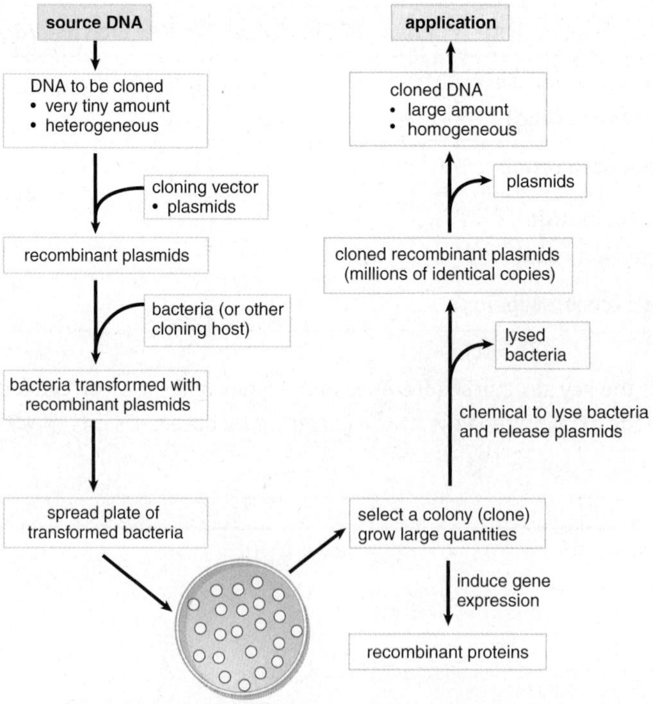

Figure 6.18 Cloning Recombinant DNA
Cloning allows production of recombinant proteins, or identification and characterization of DNA by increasing its volume and purity.

DNA Cloning and Restriction Enzymes

DNA cloning is a technique that can produce large amounts of a desired sequence. Often, the DNA to be cloned is present in a small quantity and is part of a heterogeneous mixture containing other DNA sequences. The goal is to produce a large quantity of homogeneous DNA for other applications. Cloning requires that the investigator ligate the DNA of interest into a piece of nucleic acid referred to as a **vector**, forming a **recombinant vector**. Vectors are usually bacterial or viral plasmids that can be transferred to a host bacterium after insertion of the DNA of interest. The bacteria are then grown in colonies, and a colony containing the recombinant vector is isolated. This can be accomplished by ensuring that the recombinant vector also includes a gene for antibiotic resistance; antibiotics can then kill off all of the colonies that do not contain the recombinant vector. The resulting colony can then be grown in large quantities. Depending on the investigator's goal, the bacteria can then be made to express the gene of interest (generating large quantities of recombinant protein), or can be lysed to reisolate the replicated recombinant vectors (which can be processed by restriction enzymes to release the cloned DNA from the vector).

Restriction enzymes (**restriction endonucleases**) are enzymes that recognize specific double-stranded DNA sequences. These sequences are palindromic, meaning that the 5′ to 3′ sequence of one strand is identical to the 5′ to 3′ sequence of the other strand (in antiparallel orientation). Restriction enzymes are isolated from bacteria, which are their natural source. In bacteria, they act as part of a restriction and modification system that protects the bacteria from infection by DNA viruses. Once a specific sequence has been identified, the restriction enzyme can cut through the backbones of the double helix. Thousands of restriction enzymes have been studied and many are commercially available to laboratories, allowing us to process DNA in very specific ways. Some restriction enzymes produce offset cuts, yielding sticky ends on the fragments, as shown in Figure 6.19. Sticky ends are advantageous in facilitating the recombination of a restriction fragment with the vector DNA. The vector of choice can also be cut with the same restriction enzyme, allowing the fragments to be inserted directly into the vector.

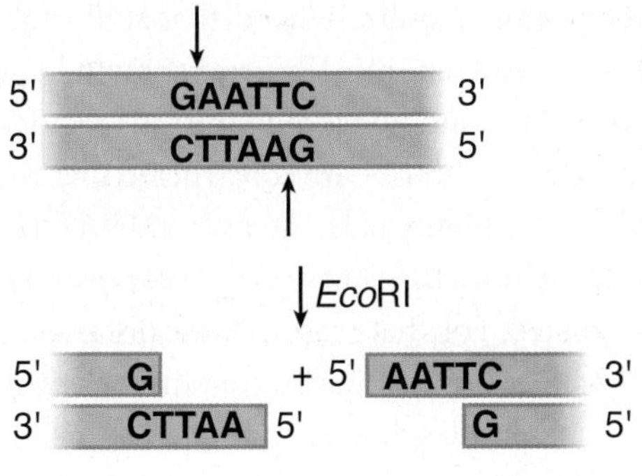

Figure 6.19 A Restriction Enzyme (*Eco*RI) Creating Sticky Ends
Restriction enzymes cut at palindromic sequences, such as GAATTC.

DNA vectors contain at least one sequence, if not many, recognized by restriction enzymes. A vector also requires an origin of replication and at least one gene for antibiotic resistance to allow for selection of colonies with recombinant plasmids, as described above. The formation of a recombinant plasmid is shown in Figure 6.20.

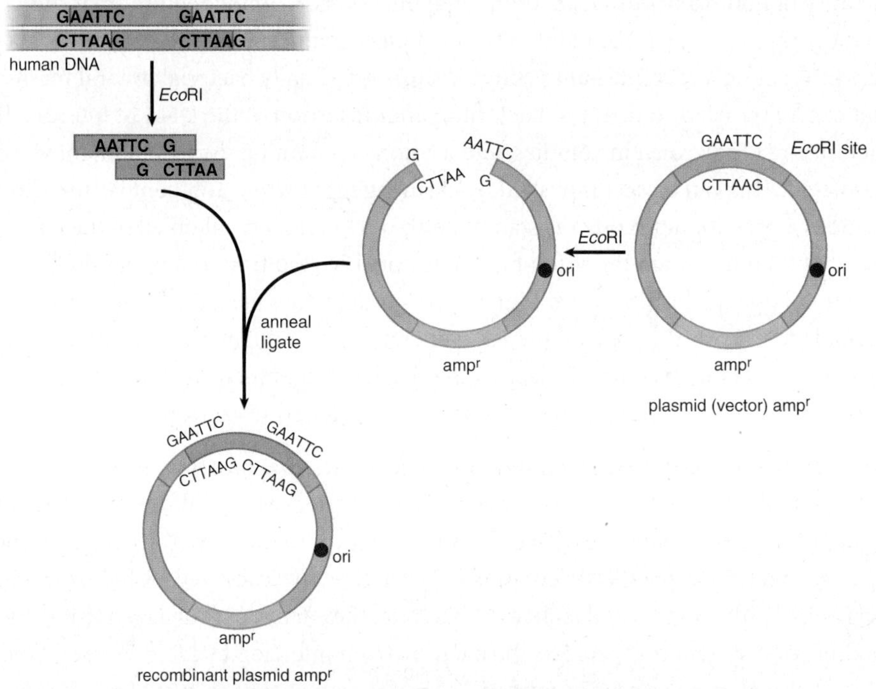

Figure 6.20 Formation of a Recombinant Plasmid Vector
ori: origin of replication; amp^r: gene for resistance to ampicillin (an antibiotic)

DNA Libraries and cDNA

DNA cloning can be used to produce DNA libraries. **DNA libraries** are large collections of known DNA sequences; in sum, these sequences could equate to the genome of an organism. To make a DNA library, DNA fragments, often digested randomly, are cloned into vectors and can be utilized for further study. Libraries can consist of either genomic DNA or cDNA. **Genomic libraries** contain large fragments of DNA, and include both coding (exon) and noncoding (intron) regions of the genome. **cDNA (complementary DNA)** libraries are constructed by reverse-transcribing processed mRNA, as shown in Figure 6.21. As such, cDNA lacks noncoding regions, such as introns, and only includes the genes that are expressed in the tissue from which the mRNA was isolated. For that reason, these libraries are sometimes called **expression libraries**. While genomic libraries contain the entire genome of an organism, genes may by chance be split into multiple vectors. Therefore, only cDNA libraries can be used to reliably sequence specific genes and identify disease-causing mutations, produce recombinant proteins (such as insulin, clotting factors, or vaccines), or produce transgenic animals. Several of these applications are discussed in more detail in subsequent sections of this chapter. Table 6.3 contrasts some of the characteristics of genomic and cDNA libraries.

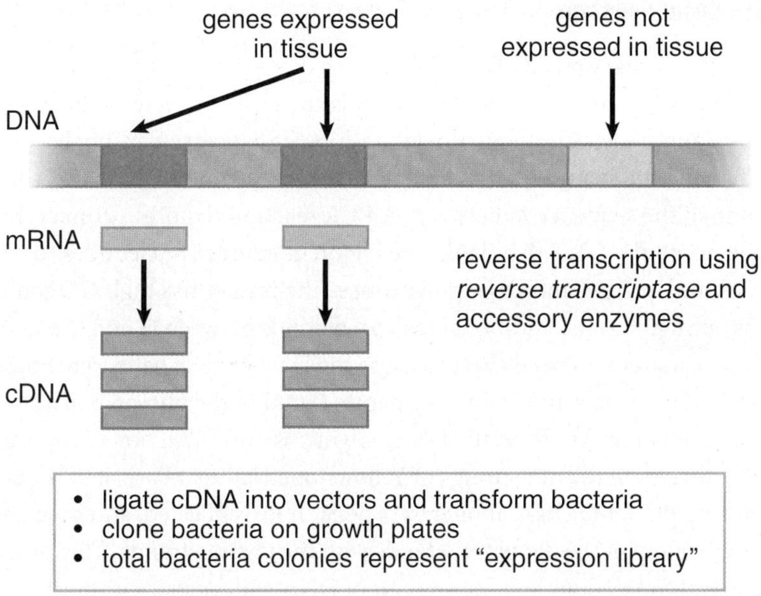

Figure 6.21 Cloning Expressed Genes by Producing cDNA

	GENOMIC LIBRARIES	cDNA (EXPRESSION) LIBRARY
Source of DNA	Chromosomal DNA	mRNA (cDNA)
Enzymes to make library	Restriction endonuclease DNA ligase	Reverse transcriptase DNA ligase
Contains nonexpressed sequences of chromosomes	Yes	No
Cloned genes are complete sequences	Not necessarily	Yes
Cloned genes contain introns	Yes	No
Promoter and enhancer sequences present	Yes, but not necessarily in same clone	No
Gene can be expressed in cloning host (recombinant proteins)	No	Yes
Can be used for gene therapy or constructing transgenic animals	No	Yes

Table 6.3 Comparison of Genomic and cDNA (Expression) Libraries

Hybridization

Another tool often used by researchers is called hybridization. **Hybridization** is the joining of complementary base pair sequences. This can be DNA–DNA recognition or DNA–RNA recognition. This technique uses two single-stranded sequences and is a vital part of polymerase chain reaction and Southern blotting.

Polymerase Chain Reaction

Polymerase chain reaction (**PCR**) is an automated process that can produce millions of copies of a DNA sequence without amplifying the DNA in bacteria. PCR is used to identify criminal suspects, familial relationships, and disease-causing bacteria and viruses. Knowing the sequences that flank the desired region of DNA allows for the amplification of the sequence in between. A PCR reaction requires **primers** that are complementary to the DNA that flanks the region of interest, nucleotides (dATP, dTTP, dCTP, and dGTP), and DNA polymerase. The primer has high GC content (40–60% is optimal), as the additional hydrogen bonds between G and C confer stability. The reaction also needs heat to cause the DNA double helix to melt apart (denature). Unfortunately, the DNA polymerase found in the human body does not work at high temperatures. Thus, the DNA polymerase from *Thermus aquaticus*, a bacteria that thrives in the hot springs of Yellowstone National Park at 70°C, is used instead. During PCR, the DNA of interest is denatured, replicated, and then cooled to allow reannealing of the daughter strands with the parent strands. This process is repeated several times, doubling the amount of DNA with each cycle, until enough copies of the DNA sequence are available for further testing.

BRIDGE

PCR provides a great example of the temperature dependence of enzymes. While human DNA polymerase denatures at the high temperatures required in PCR, the DNA polymerase from *T. aquaticus* functions optimally at these temperatures. Refer to Chapter 2 of *MCAT Biochemistry Review* for more on the link between temperature and enzyme activity.

Gel Electrophoresis and Southern Blotting

Gel electrophoresis is a technique used to separate macromolecules, such as DNA and proteins, by size and charge. Electrophoresis of proteins was discussed in detail in Chapter 3 of *MCAT Biochemistry Review*, but DNA can be separated in a similar way. All molecules of DNA are negatively charged because of the phosphate groups in the backbone of the molecule, so all DNA strands will migrate toward the anode of an electrochemical cell. The preferred gel for DNA electrophoresis is **agarose gel**, and—just like proteins in polyacrylamide gel—the longer the DNA strand, the slower it will migrate in the gel.

Gel electrophoresis is often used while performing a Southern blot. A **Southern blot** is used to detect the presence and quantity of various DNA strands in a sample. DNA is cut by restriction enzymes and then separated by gel electrophoresis. The DNA fragments are then carefully transferred to a membrane, retaining their separation. The membrane is then probed with many copies of a single-stranded DNA sequence. The **probe** will bind to its complementary sequence and form double-stranded DNA. Probes are labeled with radioisotopes or indicator proteins, both of which can be used to indicate the presence of a desired sequence.

DNA Sequencing

DNA sequencing has revolutionized the world that we live in. The applications of this technique are far-reaching, from the medical field to criminal legal system. A basic sequencing reaction contains the main players from replication, including template DNA, primers, an appropriate DNA polymerase, and all four deoxyribonucleotide triphosphates. In addition, a modified base called a ***dideoxyribonucleotide*** is added in lower concentrations. Dideoxyribonucleotides (ddATP, ddCTP, ddGTP, and ddTTP) contain a hydrogen at C-3′, rather than a hydroxyl group; thus, once one of these modified bases has been incorporated, the polymerase can no longer add to the chain. Eventually the sample will contain many fragments (as many as the number of nucleotides in the desired sequence), each one of which terminates with one of the modified bases. These fragments are then separated by size using gel electrophoresis. The last base for each fragment can be read, and because gel electrophoresis separates the strands by size, the bases can easily be read in order.

REAL WORLD

The Human Genome Project, initiated in 1991, involved the identification of all 3 billion base pairs of the human DNA sequence. The first draft of this project was completed in 2000. This project demonstrated that although humans appear to be quite different from each other, the sequence of our DNA is, in reality, highly conserved. On average, two unrelated individuals still share over 99.9% of their DNA sequences.

Applications of DNA Technology

In addition to its utility as a research tool, DNA biotechnology has led to a number of therapeutic breakthroughs, ranging from gene therapy—described in this section—to development of personalized chemotherapeutic regimens in cancer by genotyping the tumor cells. DNA technology is also used in industry, including the development of genetically modified foods that are enriched with specific nutrients and testing of the environment for risk assessment and cleanup procedures. As mentioned previously, DNA technology also plays a key role in forensic pathology and crime scene investigation. This is likely only the beginning, as biotechnology continues to be an active area of research.

Gene Therapy

Gene therapy now offers potential cures for individuals with inherited diseases. Gene therapy is intended for diseases in which a given gene is mutated or inactive, giving rise to pathology. By transferring a normal copy of the gene into the affected tissues, the pathology should be fixed, essentially curing the individual. For instance, about half of children with *severe combined immunodeficiency* (SCID) have a mutation in the gene encoding the γ chain common to several of the interleukin receptors. By placing a working copy of the gene for the γ chain into a virus, one can transmit the functional gene into human cells. The first successful case of gene therapy was for SCID (caused by a different mutation) in 1990.

For gene replacement therapy to be a realistic possibility, efficient gene delivery vectors must be used to transfer the cloned gene into the target cells' DNA. Because viruses naturally infect cells to insert their own genetic material, most gene delivery vectors in use are modified viruses. A portion of the viral genome is replaced with the cloned gene such that the virus can infect but not complete its replication cycle, as shown in Figure 6.22. Randomly integrated DNA poses a risk of integrating near and activating a host oncogene. Among the children treated for SCID, a small number have developed leukemias (cancers of white blood cells).

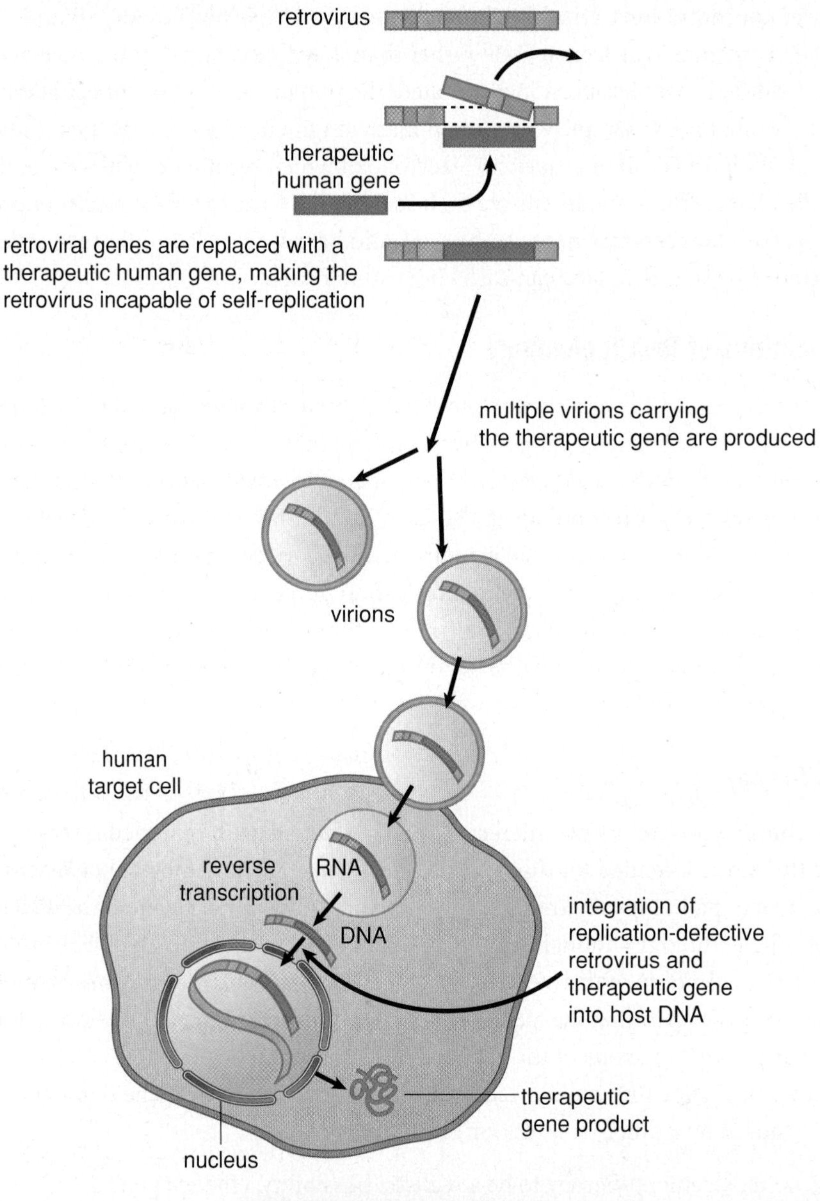

Figure 6.22 Retroviral Gene Therapy
The example given here uses a retrovirus, but other viruses may also be used for gene therapy.

Transgenic and Knockout Mice

Once DNA has been isolated, it can be introduced into eukaryotic cells. **Transgenic mice** are altered at their **germ line** by introducing a cloned gene into fertilized ova or into embryonic stem cells. The cloned gene that is introduced is referred to as a **transgene**. If the transgene is a disease-producing allele, the transgenic mice can be used to study the disease process from early embryonic development through adulthood. A similar approach can be used to produce **knockout mice**, in which a gene has been intentionally deleted (knocked out). These mice provide valuable models in which to study human diseases.

There are different approaches to developing transgenic mice. A cloned gene may be microinjected into the nucleus of a newly fertilized ovum. Rarely, the gene may subsequently incorporate into the nuclear DNA of the zygote. The ovum is implanted into a surrogate, and, if successful, the resulting offspring will contain the transgene in all of their cells, including their germ line cells (gametes). Consequently, the transgene will also be passed to *their* offspring. The transgene coexists in the animals with their own copies of the gene, which have not been deleted. This approach is useful for studying dominant gene effects but is less useful as a model for recessive disease because the number of copies of the gene that insert into the genome cannot be controlled; the transgenic mice may each contain a different number of copies of the transgene. This method is demonstrated in Figure 6.23.

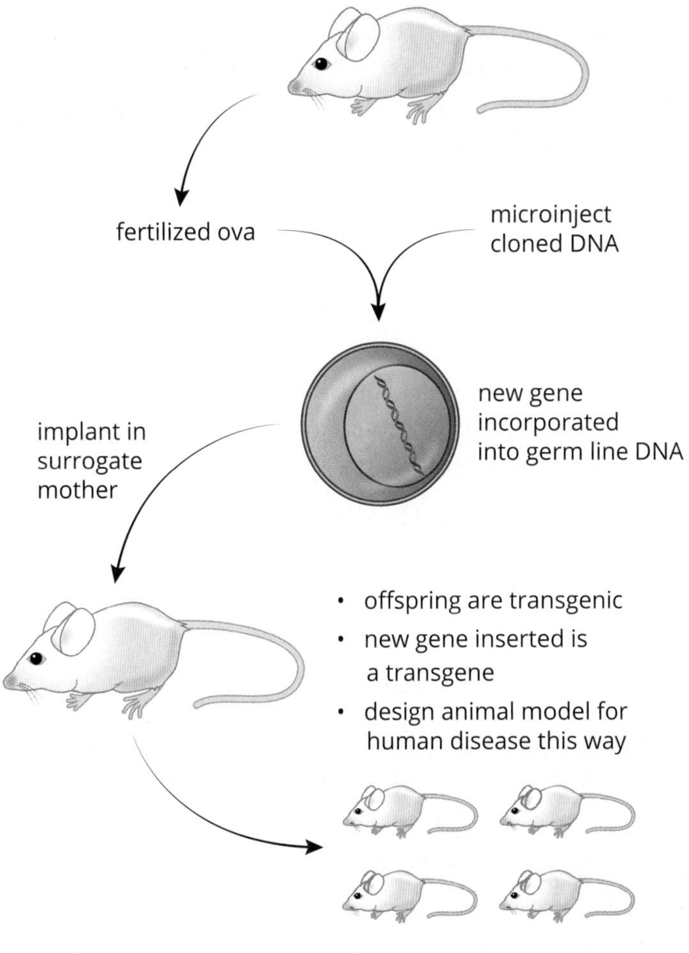

Figure 6.23 Creation of a Transgenic Mouse

Embryonic stem cell lines can also be used for developing transgenic mice. Advantages of using stem cell lines are that the cloned genes can be introduced in cultures, and that one can select for cells with the transgene successfully inserted. The altered stem cells are injected into developing blastocysts and implanted into surrogates. The blastocyst itself is thus composed of two types of stem cells: the ones containing the transgene and the original blastocyst cells that lack the transgene. The resulting offspring is a ***chimera***, meaning that it has patches of cells, including germ cells, derived from each of the two lineages. This is evident if the two cell lineages (transgenic cells and host blastocyst) come from mice with different coat colors. The chimeras will have patchy coats of two colors, allowing them to be easily identified. These chimeras can then be bred to produce mice that are heterozygous for the transgene and mice that are homozygous for the transgene.

REAL WORLD

The story of Jesse Gelsinger is one particularly harrowing example of the problems that biotechnology can create. Diagnosed with mild *ornithine transcarbamylase* (OTC) deficiency, a defect of the urea cycle, Gelsinger volunteered for a clinical trial of gene therapy. During the trial (which was also fraught with questionable consent practices), Gelsinger died from a massive immune response to the viral vector, leading to multiple organ failure and brain death. He was 18 years old.

Safety and Ethics

The different procedures and techniques that have been reviewed provide great insight for researchers in many different fields of study. However, it is also important to acknowledge the potential risks associated with these technologies. Safety concerns such as increased resistance in viruses and bacteria can impact both humans and the environment in which we live. Ethical dilemmas arise: Is it ethical to test for life-threatening genetic diseases and potentially terminate a pregnancy based on the results? What about testing for eye or hair color? What are the ethical questions around choosing human test subjects? If a disease-causing gene were found in one individual of a family, does this need to be communicated to other relatives at risk, potentially violating principles of privacy? Is it permissible to carry out potentially risky therapies in individuals whose illnesses makes them unable to communicate? The medical community and bioethicists at large continue to wrestle with this question: How much should we meddle with our own genetic makeup?

MCAT CONCEPT CHECK 6.5

Before you move on, assess your understanding of the material with these questions.

1. When creating a DNA library, what are some of the advantages of genomic libraries? What about cDNA libraries?
    - Genomic:

    ____

    - cDNA:

    ____

2. What does PCR accomplish for a researcher? What about Southern blotting?
    - PCR:

    ____

    - Southern blotting:

    ____

3. During DNA sequencing, why does the DNA polymer stop growing once a dideoxyribonucleotide is added?

    ____

4. What is the difference between a transgenic and a knockout mouse?

    ____

Conclusion

In this chapter, the DNA molecule was discussed. The importance of this molecule as an archive in the cell was highlighted. The unique structure of the DNA double helix and complementary base-pairing are integral to DNA molecules' ability to replicate and pass information from cell to cell and from generation to generation. Replication of DNA is a complex process involving many enzymes and proteins that are highly coordinated to ensure efficiency. The discoveries of DNA structure and function aid us in understanding how cellular processes take place but also provide us with many tools to exploit in the laboratory.

DNA is one of the most heavily tested concepts on the MCAT. This makes sense because not only has our understanding of the molecule increased exponentially over the last few decades, but also our ability to manipulate DNA. This has led to the creation of an entire industry of biotechnology that will assuredly grow during your career as a medical student and physician. In the next chapter, we turn to DNA's counterpart, RNA. We'll explore how the genes discussed in this chapter can actually turn into functional proteins through the key processes of transcription and translation.

GO ONLINE

You've reviewed the content, now test your knowledge and critical thinking skills by completing a test-like passage set in your online resources!

CONCEPT SUMMARY

DNA Structure

- **Deoxyribonucleic acid** (**DNA**) is a macromolecule that stores genetic information in all living organisms.
- **Nucleosides** contain a five-carbon sugar bonded to a nitrogenous base; **nucleotides** are nucleosides with one to three phosphate groups added.
    - Nucleotides in DNA contain **deoxyribose**; in RNA, they contain **ribose**.
    - Nucleotides are abbreviated by letter: **adenine** (**A**), **cytosine** (**C**), **guanine** (**G**), **thymine** (**T**), and **uracil** (**U**).
- DNA is organized according to the **Watson–Crick model**.
    - The backbone is composed of alternating sugar and phosphate groups, and is always read **5′ to 3′**.
    - There are two strands with **antiparallel** polarity, wound into a **double helix**.
    - **Purines** (A and G) always pair with **pyrimidines** (C, U, and T). In DNA, A pairs with T (via two hydrogen bonds) and C pairs with G (via three hydrogen bonds). RNA does not contain thymine, but contains uracil instead; thus, in RNA, A pairs with U (via two hydrogen bonds).
    - Purines and pyrimidines are biological aromatic heterocycles. **Aromatic** compounds are cyclic, planar, and **conjugated**, and contain $4n + 2$ π electrons (where n is any integer; **Hückel's rule**). Heterocycles are ring structures that contain at least two different elements in the ring.
    - **Chargaff's rules** state that purines and pyrimidines are equal in number in a DNA molecule, and that because of base-pairing, the amount of adenine equals the amount of thymine, and the amount of cytosine equals the amount of guanine.
    - Most DNA is B-DNA, forming a right-handed helix. Low concentrations of Z-DNA, with a zigzag shape, may be seen with high GC-content or high salt concentration.
- DNA strands can be pulled apart (**denatured**) and brought back together (**reannealed**). Heat, alkaline pH, and chemicals like formaldehyde and urea can cause denaturation of DNA; removal of these conditions may result in reannealing of the strands.

Eukaryotic Chromosome Organization

- DNA is organized into 46 chromosomes in human cells.
- In eukaryotes, DNA is wound around **histone proteins** (H2A, H2B, H3, and H4) to form **nucleosomes**, which may be stabilized by another histone protein (H1). As a whole, DNA and its associated histones make up **chromatin** in the nucleus.
  - **Heterochromatin** is dense, transcriptionally silent DNA that appears dark under light microscopy.
  - **Euchromatin** is less dense, transcriptionally active DNA that appears light under light microscopy.
- **Telomeres** are the ends of chromosomes. They contain high GC-content to prevent unraveling of the DNA. During replication, telomeres are slightly shortened, although this can be (partially) reversed by the enzyme telomerase.
- **Centromeres** are located in the middle of chromosomes and hold sister chromatids together until they are separated during anaphase in mitosis. They also contain a high GC-content to maintain a strong bond between chromatids.

DNA Replication

- The **replisome** (**replication complex**) is a set of specialized proteins that assist the DNA polymerases.
- To replicate DNA, it is first unwound at an **origin of replication** by **helicases**. This produces two **replication forks** on either side of the origin.
  - Prokaryotes have a circular chromosome that contains only one origin of replication.
  - Eukaryotes have linear chromosomes that contain many origins of replication.
- Unwound strands are kept from reannealing or being degraded by **single-stranded DNA-binding proteins**.
- **Supercoiling** causes torsional strain on the DNA molecule, which can be released by **DNA topoisomerases**, which create nicks in the DNA molecule.
- DNA replication is **semiconservative**: one old **parent strand** and one new **daughter strand** is incorporated into each of the two new DNA molecules.
- DNA cannot be synthesized without an adjacent nucleotide to hook onto, so a small RNA primer is put down by **primase**.

- **DNA polymerase III** (prokaryotes) or **DNA polymerases** α, δ, and ε (eukaryotes) can then synthesize a new strand of DNA; they read the template DNA 3′ to 5′ and synthesize the new strand 5′ to 3′.
  - The **leading strand** requires only one primer and can then be synthesized continuously in its entirety.
  - The **lagging strand** requires many primers and is synthesized in discrete sections called **Okazaki fragments**.
- RNA primers can later be removed by **DNA polymerase I** (prokaryotes) or **RNase H** (eukaryotes), and filled in with DNA by DNA polymerase I (prokaryotes) or DNA polymerase δ (eukaryotes). **DNA ligase** can then fuse the DNA strands together to create one complete molecule.

DNA Repair

- **Oncogenes** develop from mutations of **proto-oncogenes**, and promote cell cycling. They may lead to **cancer**, which is defined by unchecked cell proliferation with the ability to spread by local invasion or **metastasize** (migrate to distant sites via the bloodstream or lymphatic system).
- **Tumor suppressor genes** code for proteins that reduce cell cycling or promote DNA repair; mutations of tumor suppressor genes can also lead to cancer.
- During replication, DNA polymerase **proofreads** its work and excises incorrectly matched bases. The daughter strand is identified by its lack of methylation and corrected accordingly.
- **Mismatch repair** also occurs during the G_2 phase of the cell cycle, using the genes *MSH2* and *MLH1*.
- **Nucleotide excision repair** fixes helix-deforming lesions of DNA (such as thymine dimers) via a cut-and-patch process that requires an **excision endonuclease**.
- **Base excision repair** fixes nondeforming lesions of the DNA helix (such as cytosine deamination) by removing the base, leaving an **apurinic/apyrimidinic (AP) site**. An **AP endonuclease** then removes the damaged sequence, which can be filled in with the correct bases.

Recombinant DNA and Biotechnology

- **Recombinant DNA** is DNA composed of nucleotides from two different sources.
- **DNA cloning** introduces a fragment of DNA into a **vector plasmid**. **A restriction enzyme (restriction endonuclease)** cuts both the plasmid and the fragment, which are left with **sticky ends**. Once the fragment binds to the plasmid, it can be introduced into a bacterial cell and permitted to replicate, generating many copies of the fragment of interest.
  - Vectors contain an origin of replication, the fragment of interest, and at least one gene for antibiotic resistance (to permit for selection of that colony after replication).
  - Once replicated, the bacterial cells can be used to create a protein of interest, or can be lysed to allow for isolation of the fragment of interest from the vector.
- **DNA libraries** are large collections of known DNA sequences.
  - **Genomic libraries** contain large fragments of DNA, including both coding and noncoding regions of the genome. They cannot be used to make recombinant proteins or for gene therapy.
  - **cDNA libraries (expression libraries)** contain smaller fragments of DNA, and only include the exons of genes expressed by the sample tissue. They can be used to make recombinant proteins or for gene therapy.
- **Hybridization** is the joining of complementary base pair sequences.
  - **Polymerase chain reaction (PCR)** is an automated process by which millions of copies of a DNA sequence can be created from a very small sample by hybridization.
  - DNA molecules can be separated by size using **agarose gel electrophoresis**.
  - **Southern blotting** can be used to detect the presence and quantity of various DNA strands in a sample. After electrophoresis, the sample is transferred to a membrane that can be **probed** with single-stranded DNA molecules to look for a sequence of interest.
- **DNA sequencing** uses **dideoxyribonucleotides**, which terminate the DNA chain because they lack a $3'$ –OH group. The resulting fragments can be separated by gel electrophoresis, and the sequence can be read directly from the gel.
- **Gene therapy** is a method of curing genetic deficiencies by introducing a functional gene with a viral vector.

- **Transgenic mice** are created by integrating a gene of interest into the germ line or embryonic stem cells of a developing mouse.
  - Organisms that contain cells from two different lineages (such as mice formed by integration of transgenic embryonic stem cells into a normal mouse blastocyst) are called **chimeras**.
  - Transgenic mice can be mated to select for the transgene.
- **Knockout mice** are created by deleting a gene of interest.
- Biotechnology brings up a number of safety and ethical issues, including pathogen resistance and the ethics of choosing individuals for specific traits.

ANSWERS TO CONCEPT CHECKS

6.1

1. Nucleosides contain a five-carbon sugar (pentose) and nitrogenous base. Nucleotides are composed of a nucleoside plus one to three phosphate groups.
2. A pairs with T (in DNA) or U (in RNA), using two hydrogen bonds. C pairs with G, using three hydrogen bonds.
3. DNA contains deoxyribose, while RNA contains ribose. DNA contains thymine, while RNA contains uracil. Usually, DNA is double-stranded, while RNA is single-stranded.
4. The aromaticity of nucleic acids makes these compounds very stable and unreactive. Stability is important for storing genetic information and avoiding spontaneous mutations.
5. This does not violate Chargaff's rules. RNA is single-stranded, and thus the complementarity seen in DNA does not hold true. For single-stranded RNA, %C does not necessarily equal %G; %A does not necessarily equal %U.

6.2

1. The five histone proteins are H1, H2A, H2B, H3, and H4. H1 is the only one not in the histone core.
2.

Characteristic	Heterochromatin	Euchromatin
Density of chromatin packing	Dense	Not dense (uncondensed)
Appearance under light microscopy	Dark	Light
Transcriptional activity	Silent	Active

3. High GC-content increases hydrogen bonding, making the association between DNA strands very strong at telomeres and centromeres.

6.3

1.

Enzyme	Prokaryotes/ Eukaryotes/Both	Function
Helicase	Both	Unwinds DNA double helix
Single-stranded DNA-binding protein	Both	Prevents reannealing of DNA double helix during replication
Primase	Both	Places ~10-nucleotide RNA primer to begin DNA replication
DNA polymerase III	Prokaryotes	Adds nucleotides to growing daughter strand
DNA polymerase α	Eukaryotes	Adds nucleotides to growing daughter strand
DNA polymerase I	Prokaryotes	Fills in gaps left behind after RNA primer excision
RNase H	Eukaryotes	Excises RNA primer
DNA ligase	Both	Joins DNA strands (especially between Okazaki fragments)
DNA topoisomerases	Both	Reduces torsional strain from positive supercoils by introducing nicks in DNA strand

2. The lagging strand is more prone to mutations because it must constantly start and stop the process of DNA replication. Additionally, it contains many more RNA primers, all of which must be removed and filled in with DNA.
3. Telomeres are the ends of eukaryotic chromosomes and contain repetitive sequences of noncoding DNA. These protect the chromosome from losing important genes from the incomplete replication of the 5′ end of the DNA strand.

6.4

1. Oncogenes (or, more properly, proto-oncogenes) code for cell cycle–promoting proteins; when mutated, a proto-oncogene becomes an oncogene, promoting rapid cell cycling. Tumor suppressor genes code for repair or cell cycle–inhibiting proteins; when mutated, the cell cycle is allowed to proceed unchecked. Oncogenes are like stepping on the gas pedal, mutated tumor suppressor genes are like cutting the brakes.

2. The parent strand is more heavily methylated, whereas the daughter strand is barely methylated at all. This allows DNA polymerase to distinguish between the two strands during proofreading.

3.

Repair Mechanism	Phase of Cell Cycle	Key Enzymes/Genes
DNA polymerase (proofreading)	S	DNA polymerase
Mismatch repair	G_2	*MSH2, MLH1*(*MutS* and *MutL* in prokaryotes)
Nucleotide excision repair	G_1, G_2	Excision endonuclease
Base excision repair	G_1, G_2	Glycosylase, AP endonuclease

4. Nucleotide excision repair corrects lesions that are large enough to distort the double helix; base excision repair corrects lesions that are small enough not to distort the double helix.

6.5

1. Genomic libraries include all of the DNA in an organism's genome, including noncoding regions. This may be useful for studying DNA in introns, centromeres, or telomeres. cDNA libraries only include expressed genes from a given tissue, but can be used to express recombinant proteins or to perform gene therapy.
2. PCR increases the number of copies of a given DNA sequence and can be used for a sample containing very few copies of the DNA sequence. Southern blotting is useful when searching for a particular DNA sequence because it separates DNA fragments by length and then probes for a sequence of interest.
3. Dideoxyribonucleotides lack the 3′ –OH group that is required for DNA strand elongation. Thus, once a dideoxyribonucleotide is added to a growing DNA molecule, no more nucleotides can be added because dideoxyribonucleotides have no 3′ –OH group with which to form a bond.
4. Transgenic mice have a gene introduced into their germ line or embryonic stem cells to look at the effects of that gene; they are therefore best suited for studying the effects of dominant alleles. Knockout mice are those in which a gene of interest has been removed, rather than added.

SCIENCE MASTERY ASSESSMENT EXPLANATIONS

1. **B**

Nucleotides bond together to form polynucleotides. The 3′ hydroxyl group of one nucleotide's sugar joins the 5′ hydroxyl group of the adjacent nucleotide's sugar by a phosphodiester bond. Hydrogen bonding, **(A)**, is important for holding complementary strands together, but does not play a role in the bonds formed between adjacent nucleotides on a single strand.

2. **D**

Because we are looking for the false statement, we have to read each choice to eliminate those that are true or find one that is overtly false. Let's quickly review the main differences between DNA and RNA. In cells, DNA is double-stranded, with a deoxyribose sugar and the nitrogenous bases A, T, C, and G. RNA, on the other hand, is usually single-stranded, with a ribose sugar and the bases A, U, C, and G. **(D)** is false because both DNA replication and RNA synthesis proceed in a 5′ to 3′ direction.

3. **A**

The melting temperature of DNA is the temperature at which a DNA double helix separates into two single strands (denatures). To do this, the hydrogen bonds linking the base pairs must be broken. Cytosine binds to guanine with three hydrogen bonds, whereas adenine binds to thymine with two hydrogen bonds. The amount of heat needed to disrupt the bonding is proportional to the number of bonds. Thus, the higher the GC-content in a DNA segment, the higher the melting point.

4. **C**

Aromatic rings must contain conjugated π electrons, which require alternating single and multiple bonds, or lone pairs. In carbohydrate ring structures, only single bonds are present, thus preventing aromaticity. Nucleic acids contain aromatic heterocycles, while proteins will generally contain at least one aromatic amino acid (tryptophan, phenylalanine, or tyrosine).

5. **C**

For a compound to be aromatic, it must be cyclic, planar, conjugated, and contain $4n + 2$ π electrons, where n is any integer. Conjugation requires that every atom in the ring have at least one unhybridized p-orbital. While most examples of aromatic compounds have alternating single and double bonds, compounds can be aromatic if they contain triple bonds as well; this would still permit at least one unhybridized p-orbital.

6. **C**

During DNA replication, the strands are separated by DNA helicase. At the replication fork, primase, **(A)**, creates a primer for the initiation of replication, which is followed by DNA polymerase. On the lagging strand, Okazaki fragments form and are joined by DNA ligase, **(B)**. After the chromosome has been processed, the ends, called telomeres, are replicated with the assistance of the enzyme telomerase, **(D)**. RNA polymerase I is located in the nucleolus and synthesizes rRNA.

7. **B**

cDNA (complementary DNA) is formed from a processed mRNA strand by reverse transcription. cDNA is used in DNA libraries and contains only the exons of genes that are transcriptionally active in the sample tissue.

8. **A**

The polymerase chain reaction is used to clone a sequence of DNA using a DNA sample, a primer, free nucleotides, and enzymes. The polymerase from *Thermus aquaticus* is used because the reaction is regulated by thermal cycling, which would denature human enzymes.

9. **D**

Endonucleases are enzymes that cut DNA. They are used by the cell for DNA repair. They are also used by scientists during DNA analysis, as restriction enzymes are endonucleases. Restriction enzymes are used to cleave DNA before electrophoresis and Southern blotting, and to introduce a gene of interest into a viral vector for gene therapy.

10. **D**

Prokaryotic DNA is circular and lacks histone proteins, and thus does not form nucleosomes. Both prokaryotic and eukaryotic DNA are replicated by DNA polymerases, although these polymerases differ in identity. Eukaryotic DNA is organized into chromatin, which can condense to form linear chromosomes; only prokaryotes have circular chromosomes. Only eukaryotic DNA has telomeres.

11. **C**

One common DNA mutation is the transition from cytosine to uracil in the presence of heat. DNA repair enzymes recognize uracil and correct this error by excising the base and inserting cytosine. RNA exists only transiently in the cell, such that cytosine degradation is insignificant. Were uracil to be used in DNA under normal circumstances, it would be impossible to tell if a base *should* be uracil or if it is a damaged cytosine nucleotide.

12. **A**

Oncogenes are most likely to result in cancer through activation, **(B)**, while tumor suppressor genes are most likely to result in cancer through inactivation.

13. **B**

One of the primary ethical concerns related to gene sequencing is the issue of consent and privacy. Because genetic screening provides information on direct relatives, there are potential violations of privacy in communicating this information to family members who may be at risk. There are not significant physical risks, eliminating **(A)**, and gene sequencing is fairly accurate, eliminating **(C)** and **(D)**.

14. **D**

Euchromatin has a classic "beads on a string" appearance that stains lightly, while heterochromatin is tightly packed and stains darkly. Heterochromatin is primarily composed of inactive genes or untranslated regions, while euchromatin is able to be expressed. All chromatin is found in the nucleus, not the cytoplasm.

15. **D**

Mismatch repair mechanisms are active during S phase (proofreading) and G_2 phase (*MSH2* and *MLH1*), eliminating **(B)** and **(C)**. Nucleotide and base excision repair mechanisms are most active during the G_1 and G_2 phases, also eliminating **(A)**. These mechanisms exist during interphase because they are aimed at *preventing* propagation of the error into daughter cells during M phase (mitosis).

Consult your online resources for additional practice. GO ONLINE

SHARED CONCEPTS

Biochemistry Chapter 4
Carbohydrate Structure and Function

Biochemistry Chapter 7
RNA and the Genetic Code

Biology Chapter 1
The Cell

Biology Chapter 2
Reproduction

Biology Chapter 3
Embryogenesis and Development

Biology Chapter 12
Genetics and Evolution

CHAPTER 7

RNA AND THE GENETIC CODE

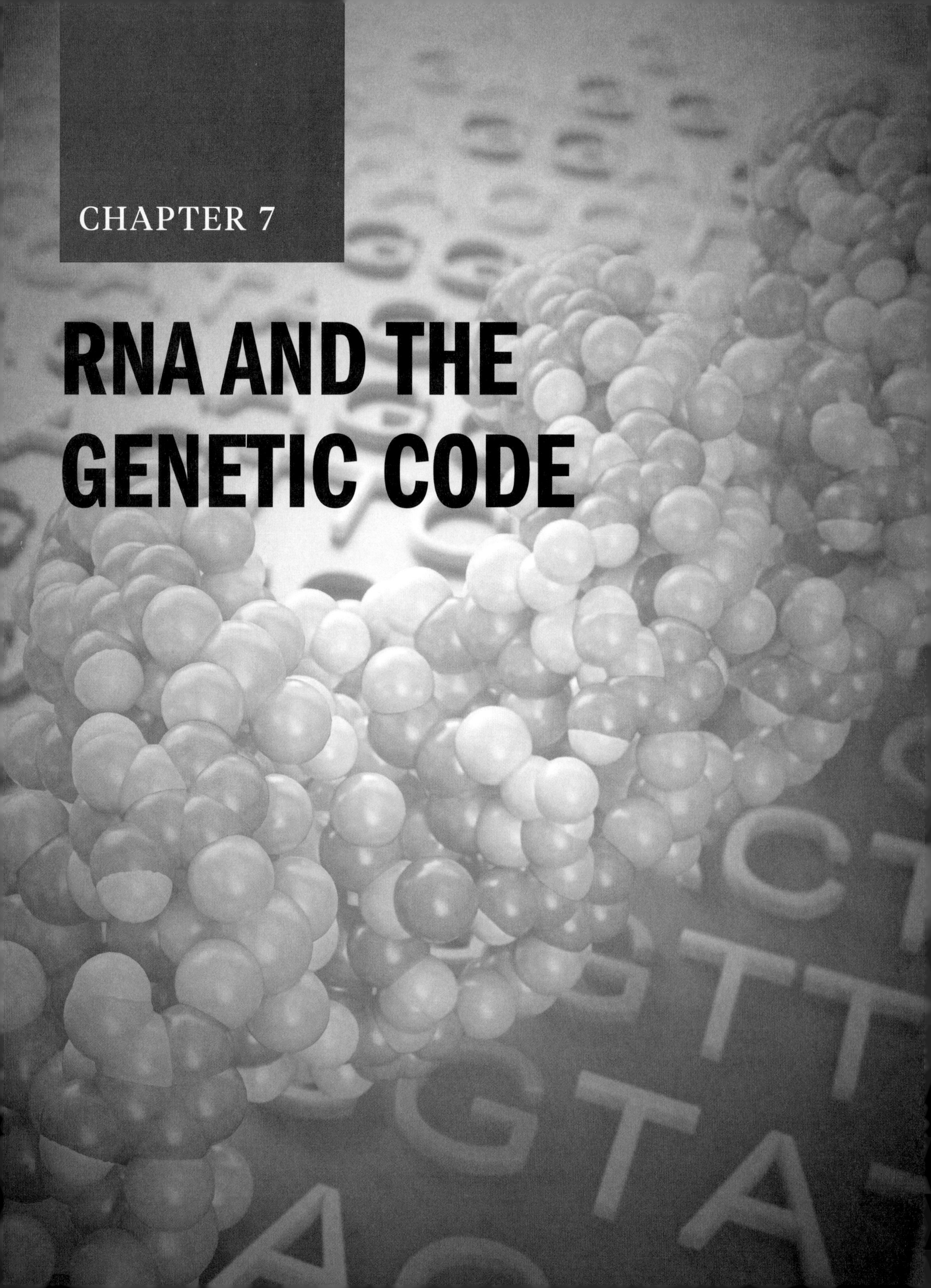

SCIENCE MASTERY ASSESSMENT

Every pre-med knows this feeling: there is so much content I have to know for the MCAT! How do I know what to do first or what's important?

While the high-yield badges throughout this book will help you identify the most important topics, this Science Mastery Assessment is another tool in your MCAT prep arsenal. This quiz (which can also be taken in your online resources) and the guidance below will help ensure that you are spending the appropriate amount of time on this chapter based on your personal strengths and weaknesses. Don't worry though—skipping something now does not mean you'll never study it. Later on in your prep, as you complete full-length tests, you'll uncover specific pieces of content that you need to review and can come back to these chapters as appropriate.

How to Use This Assessment

If you answer 0–7 questions correctly:

Spend about 1 hour to read this chapter in full and take limited notes throughout. Follow up by reviewing **all** quiz questions to ensure that you now understand how to solve each one.

If you answer 8–11 questions correctly:

Spend 20–40 minutes reviewing the quiz questions. Beginning with the questions you missed, read and take notes on the corresponding subchapters. For questions you answered correctly, ensure your thinking matches that of the explanation and you understand why each choice was correct or incorrect.

If you answer 12–15 questions correctly:

Spend less than 20 minutes reviewing all questions from the quiz. If you missed any, then include a quick read-through of the corresponding subchapters, or even just the relevant content within a subchapter, as part of your question review. For questions you got correct, ensure your thinking matches that of the explanation and review the Concept Summary at the end of the chapter.

1. What role does peptidyl transferase play in protein synthesis?
   - **A.** It transports the initiator aminoacyl-tRNA complex.
   - **B.** It helps the ribosome to advance three nucleotides along the mRNA in the 5′ to 3′ direction.
   - **C.** It holds the protein in its tertiary structure.
   - **D.** It catalyzes the formation of a peptide bond.

2. A mutation in which of the following components of the lac operon would lead to a significant reduction in the expression of lactase (one of the structural genes)?
   - **A.** Operator
   - **B.** Regulatory gene
   - **C.** Promoter
   - **D.** Structural genes

3. Topoisomerases are enzymes involved in:
   - **A.** DNA replication and transcription.
   - **B.** posttranscriptional processing.
   - **C.** RNA synthesis and translation.
   - **D.** posttranslational processing.

4. Val-tRNA^{Val} is the tRNA that carries valine to the ribosome during translation. Which of the following sequences gives an appropriate anticodon for this tRNA? (Note: Refer to Figure 7.5 for a genetic code table.)
   - **A.** CAU
   - **B.** AUC
   - **C.** UAC
   - **D.** GUG

5. Enhancers are transcriptional regulatory sequences that function by enhancing the activity of:
   - **A.** RNA polymerase at a single promoter site.
   - **B.** RNA polymerase at multiple promoter sites.
   - **C.** spliceosomes and lariat formation in the ribosome.
   - **D.** transcription factors that bind to the promoter but not to RNA polymerase.

6. In the genetic code of human nuclear DNA, one of the codons specifying the amino acid tyrosine is UAC. If one nucleotide is changed and the codon is mutated to UAG, what type of mutation will occur?
   - **A.** Silent mutation
   - **B.** Missense mutation
   - **C.** Nonsense mutation
   - **D.** Frameshift mutation

7. Which of the following is NOT used by eukaryotes to increase the transcription of a gene?
   - **A.** Gene duplication
   - **B.** Histone acetylation
   - **C.** DNA methylation
   - **D.** Enhancers

8. When trypsin converts chymotrypsinogen to chymotrypsin, some molecules of chymotrypsin bind to a repressor, which in turn binds to an operator region and prevents further transcription of trypsin. This is most similar to which of the following operons?
   - **A.** *trp* operon during lack of tryptophan
   - **B.** *trp* operon during abundance of tryptophan
   - **C.** *lac* operon during lack of lactose
   - **D.** *lac* operon during abundance of lactose

9. Which of the following RNA molecules or proteins is NOT found in the spliceosome during intron excision?
   - **A.** snRNA
   - **B.** hnRNA
   - **C.** shRNA
   - **D.** snRNPs

10. A 4-year-old toddler with cystic fibrosis (CF) is seen by his physician for an upper respiratory infection. Prior genetic testing has shown that there has been a deletion of three base pairs in exon 10 of the *CFTR* gene that affects codons 507 and 508. The nucleotide sequence in this region for normal and mutant alleles is shown below (*X* denotes the missing nucleotide):

Codon Number	506	507	508	509	510	511
Normal gene (coding strand)	ATC	ATC	TTT	GGT	GTT	TCC
Mutant gene (coding strand)	ATC	AT*X*	*XX*T	GGT	GTT	TCC

What effect will this mutation have on the amino acid sequence of the protein encoded by the *CFTR* gene? (Note: Refer to Figure 7.5 for a genetic code table.)

A. Deletion of a phenylalanine residue with no change in the C-terminus sequence
B. Deletion of a leucine residue with no change in the C-terminus sequence
C. Deletion of a phenylalanine residue with a change in the C-terminus sequence
D. Deletion of a leucine residue with a change in the C-terminus sequence

11. A gene encodes a protein with 150 amino acids. There is one intron of 1000 base pairs (bp), a 5′-untranslated region of 100 bp, and a 3′-untranslated region of 200 bp. In the final mRNA, about how many bases lie between the start AUG codon and final termination codon?

A. 150
B. 450
C. 650
D. 1750

12. Peptidyl transferase connects the carboxylate group of one amino acid to the amino group of an incoming amino acid. What type of linkage is created in this peptide bond?

A. Ester
B. Amide
C. Anhydride
D. Ether

13. A eukaryotic cell has been found to exhibit a truncation mutation that creates an inactive RNA polymerase I enzyme. Which type of RNA will be affected by this inactivation?

A. rRNA
B. tRNA
C. snRNA
D. hnRNA

14. You have just sequenced a piece of DNA that reads as follows:

5′—TCTTTGAGACATCC—3′

What would the base sequence of the mRNA transcribed from this DNA be?

A. 5′—AGAAACUCUGUAGG—3′
B. 5′—GGAUGUCUCAAAGA—3′
C. 5′—AGAAACTCTGTAGG—3′
D. 5′—GGATCTCTCAAAGA—3′

15. Double-stranded RNA cannot be translated by the ribosome and is marked for degradation in the cell. Which of the following strands of RNA would prevent mature mRNA in the cytoplasm from being translated?

A. Identical mRNA to the one produced
B. Antisense mRNA to the one produced
C. mRNA with thymine substituted for uracil
D. Sense mRNA to the one produced

Answer Key

1. **D**
2. **C**
3. **A**
4. **C**
5. **A**
6. **C**
7. **C**
8. **B**
9. **C**
10. **A**
11. **B**
12. **B**
13. **A**
14. **B**
15. **B**

Detailed explanations can be found at the end of the chapter.

CHAPTER 7

RNA AND THE GENETIC CODE

In This Chapter

CHAPTER PROFILE

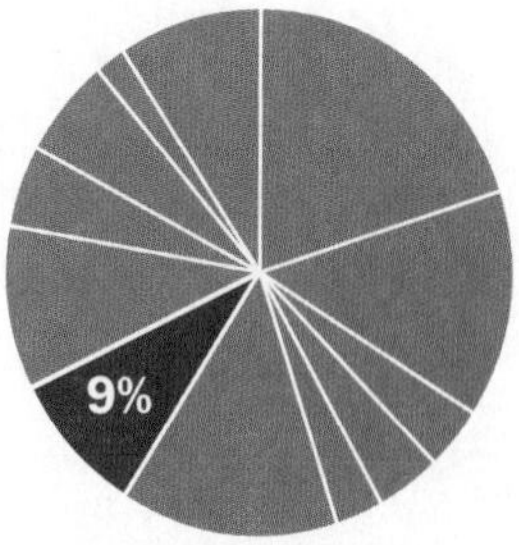

The content in this chapter should be relevant to about 9% of all questions about biochemistry on the MCAT.

This chapter covers material from the following AAMC content categories:

1B: Transmission of genetic information from the gene to the protein

5D: Structure, function, and reactivity of biologically-relevant molecules

Introduction

Hepatitis C virus (HCV) continues to be a major cause of cirrhosis and liver failure in the United States. Usually associated with intravenous drug use, hepatitis C causes ongoing damage and inflammation in the liver, leading to the formation of scar tissue that replaces the normal cells of the organ. Over time, this buildup of scar tissue makes the liver unable to keep up with the metabolic demands of the body, and liver failure ensues. To fight this virus, infected hepatocytes release interferon, a peptide signal that—as the name suggests—interferes with viral replication. Because viruses must hijack the host cell's machinery to replicate, one way the body can limit the spread of the virus is by shutting off the processes of transcription and translation. Interferon not only curtails these processes in virally infected cells, but also induces the production of *RNase L*, which cleaves RNA in cells to further reduce the ability of the virus to replicate. Coupled with other immune defenses, interferon thus serves as an efficient mechanism to protect the body from viral pathogens.

Even in normal, healthy cells, the first step in expressing genetic information is transcription of the information in the base sequence of a double-stranded DNA molecule to form a single-stranded molecule of RNA. The second step is translating that nucleotide sequence into a protein. Not every cell, though, expresses every gene product, and control of gene expression leads to the differentiation of the totipotent zygote into all of the tissues of the body. In this chapter, we will discuss the process through which proteins are produced along with the controls that modulate each step of the path.

7.1 The Genetic Code

High-Yield

LEARNING OBJECTIVES

After Chapter 7.1, you will be able to:

- Differentiate between three different types of RNA: mRNA, tRNA, and rRNA
- Transcribe a DNA sequence like "GAATTCG" into its mRNA conjugate
- Define the concepts of wobble and degeneracy
- Identify the translation outcomes of key codons, including AUG, UAG, UAA, and UGA
- Predict the likely impact of different mutation types on the resulting peptide

An organism must be able to store and preserve its genetic information, pass that information along to future generations, and express that information as it carries out all the processes of life. We know that DNA and RNA share the same language: they both code using nitrogenous bases. Proteins, however, are composed of amino acids, which constitute a different language altogether. Therefore, we use the genetic code to translate this genetic information into proteins.

While nucleotides play a crucial role in maintaining our genetic identity from generation to generation, it is the proteins they encode that help organisms develop and perform the necessary functions of life. The major steps involved in the transfer of genetic information are illustrated in the **central dogma of molecular biology**, as shown in Figure 7.1. Classically, a **gene** is a unit of DNA that encodes a specific protein or RNA molecule, and through transcription and translation, that gene can be expressed. Although this sequence is now complicated by our increased knowledge of the ways in which genes and nucleic acids may be expressed, it is still useful as a general working definition of the processes of DNA replication, transcription, and translation. We have already discussed DNA synthesis, but will continue learning more about gene expression in the rest of this chapter.

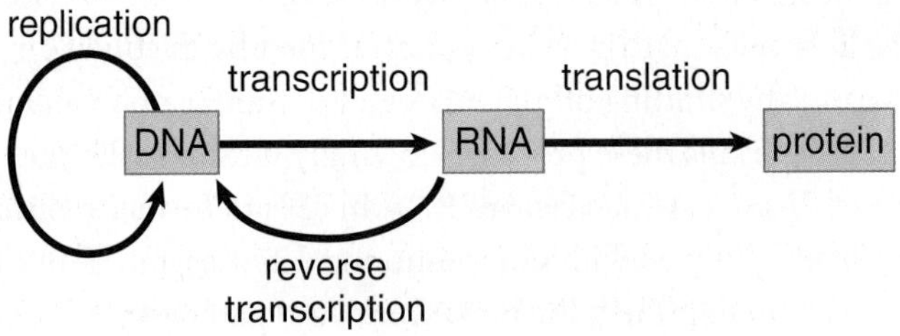

Figure 7.1 The Central Dogma of Molecular Biology

The relationship between the sequence found in double-stranded DNA, single-stranded RNA, and protein is illustrated in Figure 7.2 for a prototypical gene. Messenger RNA is synthesized in the $5' \rightarrow 3'$ direction and is complementary and antiparallel to the DNA template strand. The ribosome translates the mRNA in the $5' \rightarrow 3'$ direction, as it synthesizes the protein from the amino terminus (N-terminus) to the carboxy terminus (C-terminus).

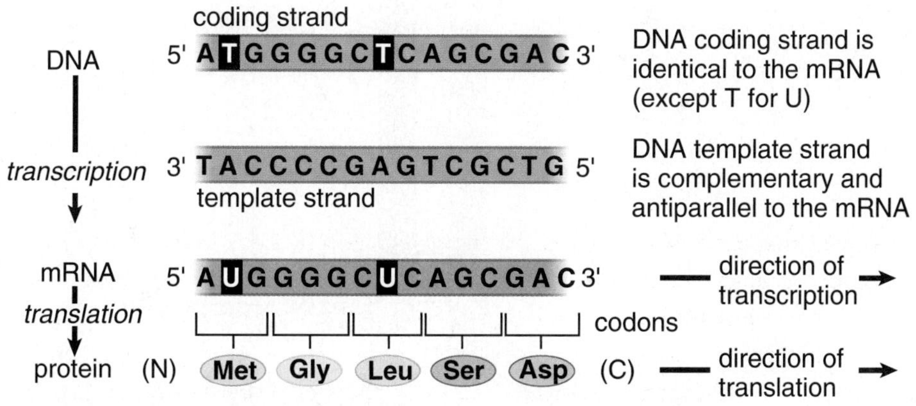

Figure 7.2 Flow of Genetic Information from DNA to Protein

Types of RNA

There are three main types of RNA found in cells: mRNA, tRNA, and rRNA. Each of the main types is described below, but regulatory and specialized forms of RNA are also described later in the chapter.

Messenger RNA (mRNA)

Messenger RNA (**mRNA**) carries the information specifying the amino acid sequence of the protein to the ribosome. mRNA is transcribed from template DNA strands by *RNA polymerase* enzymes in the nucleus of cells. Then, mRNA may undergo a host of posttranscriptional modifications prior to its release from the nucleus. mRNA is the only type of RNA that contains information that is translated into protein; to do so, it is read in three-nucleotide segments termed **codons**. In eukaryotes, mRNA is **monocistronic**, meaning that each mRNA molecule translates into only one protein product. Thus, in eukaryotes, the cell has a different mRNA molecule for each of the thousands of different proteins made by that cell. In prokaryotes, mRNA may be **polycistronic**, and starting the process of translation at different locations in the mRNA can result in different proteins. The process of creating mature mRNA will be discussed in the next section of this chapter.

KEY CONCEPT

mRNA is the messenger of genetic information. DNA codes for proteins but cannot perform any of the important enzymatic reactions that proteins are responsible for in cells. mRNA takes the information from the DNA to the ribosomes, where creation of the primary protein structure occurs.

Transfer RNA (tRNA)

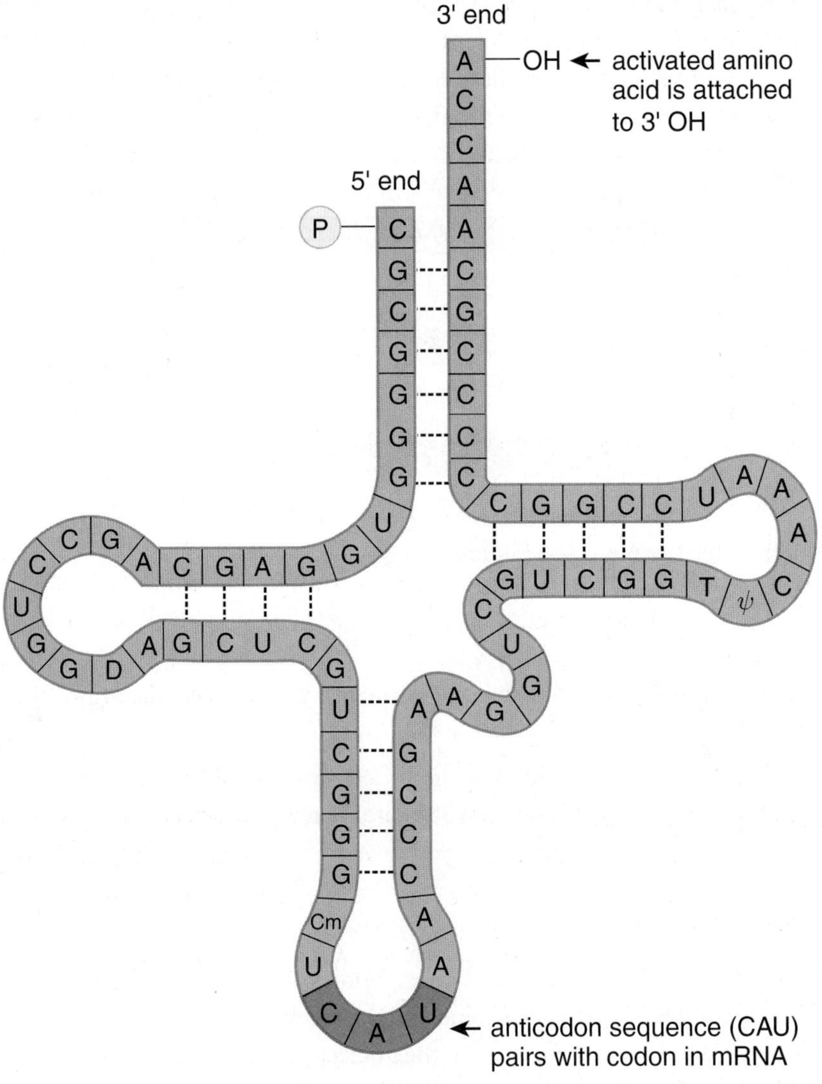

Figure 7.3 The Structure of tRNA

Transfer RNA (tRNA) is responsible for converting the language of nucleic acids to the language of amino acids and peptides. Each tRNA molecule contains a folded strand of RNA that includes a three-nucleotide anticodon, as shown in Figure 7.3. This anticodon recognizes and pairs with the appropriate codon on an mRNA molecule while in the ribosome. There are 20 amino acids in eukaryotic proteins, each of which is represented by at least one codon. To become part of a nascent polypeptide in the ribosome, amino acids are connected to a specific tRNA molecule; such tRNA molecules are said to be **charged** or **activated** with an amino acid, as shown in Figure 7.4. Mature tRNA is found in the cytoplasm.

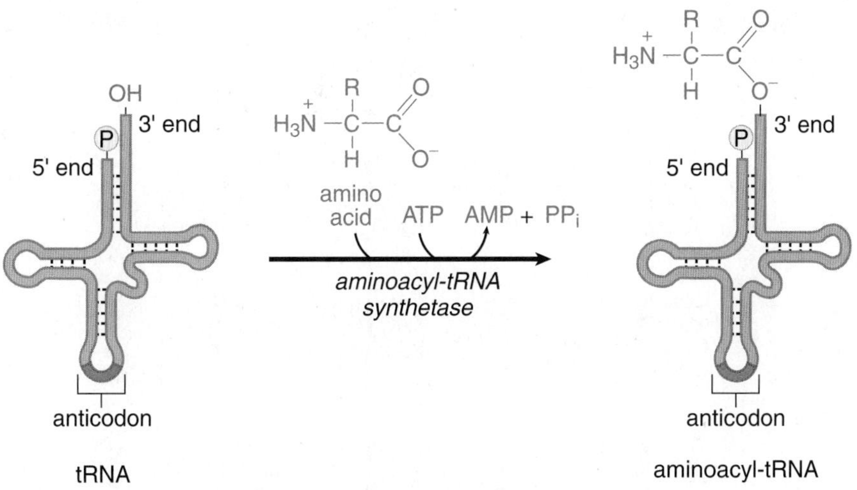

Figure 7.4 Activation of Amino Acid for Protein Synthesis

Each type of amino acid is activated by a different ***aminoacyl-tRNA synthetase*** that requires two high-energy bonds from ATP, implying that the attachment of the amino acid is an energy rich bond. The aminoacyl-tRNA synthetase transfers the activated amino acid to the 3′ end of the correct tRNA. Each tRNA has a CCA nucleotide sequence where the amino acid binds. The high-energy aminoacyl-tRNA bond will be used to supply the energy needed to create a peptide bond during translation.

Ribosomal RNA (rRNA)

Ribosomal RNA (**rRNA**) is synthesized in the nucleolus and functions as an integral part of the ribosomal machinery used during protein assembly in the cytoplasm. Many rRNA molecules function as **ribozymes**; that is, enzymes made of RNA molecules instead of peptides. rRNA helps catalyze the formation of peptide bonds and is also important in splicing out its own introns within the nucleus. The complex structure of the ribosome is described later in this chapter.

Codons

If a gene sequence is a "sentence" describing a protein, then its basic unit is a three-letter "word" known as the **codon**, which is translated into an amino acid. Genetic code tables, such as the one in Figure 7.5, serve as an easy way to determine the amino acid that is translated from each mRNA codon. Each codon consists of three bases; thus, there are 64 codons. Note how all codons are written in the 5′ → 3′ direction, and the code is unambiguous, in that each codon is specific for one and only one amino acid.

First Position (5' End)	Second Position: U	C	A	G	Third Position (3' End)
U	UUU, UUC Phe UUA, UUG Leu	UCU, UCC, UCA, UCG Ser	UAU, UAC Tyr UAA, UAG Stop	UGU, UGC Cys UGA Stop UGG Trp	U C A G
C	CUU, CUC, CUA, CUG Leu	CCU, CCC, CCA, CCG Pro	CAU, CAC His CAA, CAG Gln	CGU, CGC, CGA, CGG Arg	U C A G
A	AUU, AUC, AUA Ile AUG Met	ACU, ACC, ACA, ACG Thr	AAU, AAC Asn AAA, AAG Lys	AGU, AGC Ser AGA, AGG Arg	U C A G
G	GUU, GUC, GUA, GUG Val	GCU, GCC, GCA, GCG Ala	GAU, GAC Asp GAA, GAG Glu	GGU, GGC, GGA, GGG Gly	U C A G

Figure 7.5 The Genetic Code

KEY CONCEPT

Each codon represents only one amino acid; however, most amino acids are represented by multiple codons.

Note that 61 of the codons code for one of the 20 amino acids, while three codons encode for the termination of translation. This code is universal across species (although there are some exceptions in the mitochondria that are not necessary to know for the MCAT).

During translation, the codon of the mRNA is recognized by a complementary **anticodon** on a transfer RNA (tRNA). The anticodon sequence allows the tRNA to pair with the codon in the mRNA. Because base-pairing is involved, the orientation of this interaction will be antiparallel. For example, the aminoacyl tRNA Ile-$tRNA^{Ile}$ has an anticodon sequence 5′—GAU—3′, allowing it to pair with the isoleucine codon 5′—AUC—3′, as seen in Figure 7.6.

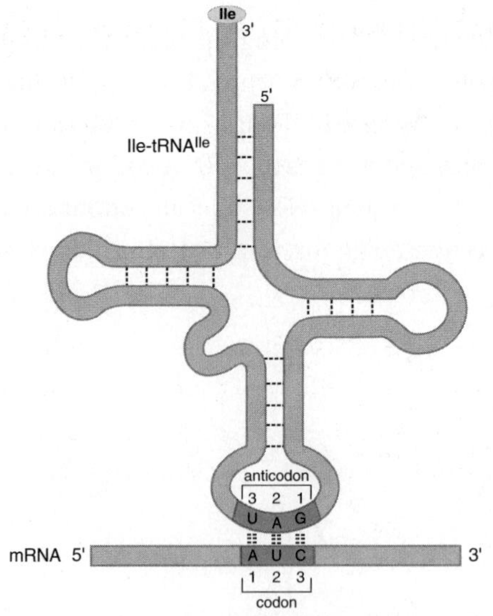

Figure 7.6 Base Pairing of an Aminoacyl-tRNA with a Codon in mRNA

Every preprocessed eukaryotic protein starts with the exact same amino acid: methionine. Because every protein begins with methionine, the codon for methionine (AUG) is considered the **start codon** for translation of the mRNA into protein. There are also three codons that encode for termination of protein translation; there are no charged tRNA molecules that recognize these codons, which leads to the release of the protein from the ribosome. The three **stop codons** are UGA, UAA, and UAG.

MNEMONIC

Stop codons:

- **UAA–U A**re **A**nnoying
- **UGA–U G**o **A**way
- **UAG–U A**re **G**one

Mutations

Degeneracy and Wobble

The genetic code is **degenerate** because more than one codon can specify a single amino acid. In fact, all amino acids, except for methionine and tryptophan, are encoded by multiple codons. Referring back to Figure 7.5, we can see that for the amino acids with multiple codons, the first two bases are usually the same, and the third base in the codon is variable. We refer to this variable third base in the codon as the **wobble position**. Wobble is an evolutionary development designed to protect against mutations in the coding regions of our DNA. Mutations in the wobble position tend to be called **silent** or **degenerate**, which means there is no effect on the expression of the amino acid and therefore no adverse effects on the polypeptide sequence. The amino acid glycine, for example, requires that only the first two nucleotides of the codon be GG. The third nucleotide could be A, C, G, or U, and the amino acid composition of the protein would remain the same.

KEY CONCEPT

The degeneracy of the genetic code allows for mutations in DNA that do not always result in altered protein structure or function. Usually, a mutation within an intron will also not change the protein sequence because introns are cleaved out of the mRNA transcript prior to translation.

Missense and Nonsense Mutations

If a mutation occurs and it affects one of the nucleotides in a codon, it is known as a **point mutation**. Although we've already discussed the silent point mutation in the wobble position, other point mutations can have a severe detrimental effect depending on where the mutation occurs in the genome. Because these point mutations can affect the primary amino acid sequence of the protein, they are called **expressed mutations**. Expressed point mutations fall into two categories: missense and nonsense.

- **Missense mutation**—a mutation where one amino acid substitutes for another
- **Nonsense mutation**—a mutation where the codon now encodes for a premature stop codon (also known as a **truncation mutation**)

Frameshift Mutations

The three nucleotides of a codon are referred to as the **reading frame**. Point mutations occur when one nucleotide is changed, but a **frameshift mutation** occurs when some number of nucleotides are added to or deleted from the mRNA sequence. Insertion or deletion of nucleotides will shift the reading frame, usually resulting in changes in the amino acid sequence or premature truncation of the protein. The effects of frameshift mutations are typically more serious than point mutations, although it is heavily dependent on where within the DNA sequence the mutation actually occurred. A synopsis of the different types of mutations can be found in Figure 7.7.

REAL WORLD

Cystic fibrosis is most commonly caused by a frameshift mutation: a deletion at codon 508 in the polypeptide chain of the *CFTR* chloride channel gene. The subsequent loss of a phenylalanine residue at this position results in a defective chloride ion channel. This altered protein never reaches the cell membrane, leading to blocked passage of salt and water into and out of cells. As a result of this blockage, cells that line the passageways of the lungs, pancreas, and other organs produce an abnormally thick, sticky mucus that traps bacteria, increasing the likelihood of infection in patients.

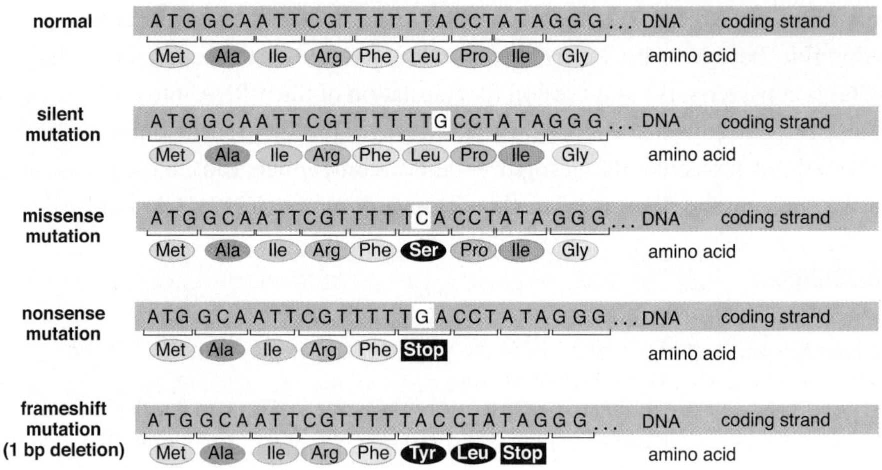

Figure 7.7 Some Common Types of Mutations in DNA

MCAT CONCEPT CHECK 7.1

Before you move on, assess your understanding of the material with these questions.

1. What are the roles of the three main types of RNA?
   - mRNA:

   - tRNA:

   - rRNA:

   ---

2. The three-base sequences listed below are DNA sequences. Using Figure 7.5, which amino acid is encoded by each of these sequences, after transcription and translation?
   - GAT:

   - ATT:

   - CGC:

   - CCA:

   ---

3. Which mRNA codon is the start codon, and what amino acid does it code for? Which mRNA codons are the stop codons?
   - Start codon: ____________; codes for: ____________
   - Stop codons: ____________

4. What is wobble, and what role does it serve?

____

5. For each of the mutations listed below, what changes in DNA sequence are observed, and what effect do they have on the encoded peptide?

Type of Mutation	Change in DNA Sequence	Effect on Encoded Protein
Silent (degenerate)		
Missense		
Nonsense		
Frameshift		

7.2 Transcription

High-Yield

LEARNING OBJECTIVES

After Chapter 7.2, you will be able to:

- Explain how each of the eukaryotic RNA polymerases (I, II, and III) impacts transcription
- Identify where RNA polymerase would bind to start transcription on a DNA strand
- Determine the mRNA that results from a given hnRNA molecule:

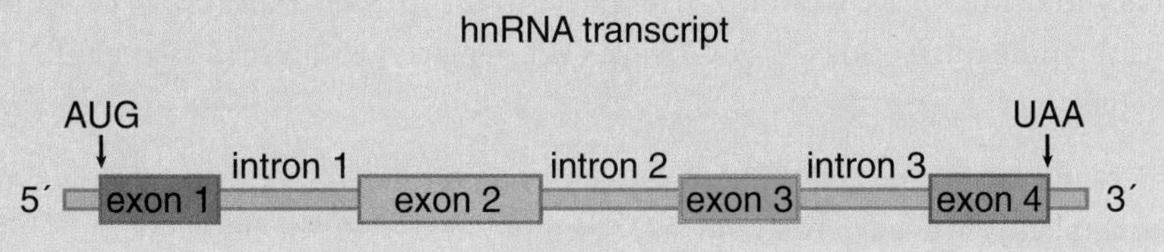

Although DNA contains the actual coding sequence for a protein, the machinery to generate that protein is located in the cytoplasm. DNA cannot leave the nucleus, as it will be quickly degraded, so it must use RNA to transmit genetic information. The creation of mRNA from a DNA template is known as **transcription**, and while mRNA is the only type of RNA that carries information from DNA directly, there are many other types of RNA that exist, two of which will play important roles during protein translation: transfer RNA (tRNA) and ribosomal RNA (rRNA).

Mechanism of Transcription

Transcription produces a copy of only one of the two strands of DNA. During initiation of transcription, several enzymes, including ***helicase*** and ***topoisomerase***, are involved in unwinding the double-stranded DNA and preventing formation of supercoils, as described in Chapter 6 of *MCAT Biochemistry Review*. This step is important in allowing the transcriptional machinery access to the DNA and the particular gene of interest. Transcription results in a single strand of mRNA, synthesized from one of the two nucleotide strands of DNA called the **template strand** (or the **antisense strand**). The newly synthesized mRNA strand is both antiparallel and complementary to the DNA template strand.

MNEMONIC

When we transcribe information, we use the same language to write it down (like in court, when the judge asks the court reporter to read back the transcript—the reporter speaks the same language as written). Translation is exactly what it says: we are changing the language. RNA translation changes the language from nucleotides to amino acids.

RNA is synthesized by a *DNA-dependent RNA polymerase*; RNA polymerase locates genes by searching for specialized DNA regions known as **promoter regions**. In eukaryotes, ***RNA polymerase II*** is the main player in transcribing mRNA, and its binding site in the promoter region is known as the **TATA box**, named for its high concentration of thymine and adenine bases. **Transcription factors** help the RNA polymerase locate and bind to this promoter region of the DNA, helping to establish where transcription will start. Unlike *DNA polymerase III*, which we reviewed during DNA replication, RNA polymerase does not require a primer to start generating a transcript.

In eukaryotes, there are three types of RNA polymerases, but only one is involved in the transcription of mRNA:

- *RNA polymerase I* is located in the nucleolus and synthesizes rRNA
- *RNA polymerase II* is located in the nucleus and synthesizes hnRNA (pre-processed mRNA) and some small nuclear RNA (snRNA)
- *RNA polymerase III* is located in the nucleus and synthesizes tRNA and some rRNA

KEY CONCEPT

Transcription is subject to the $5' \rightarrow 3'$ rule, just like DNA synthesis. Synthesis of nucleic acids always occurs in the $5' \rightarrow 3'$ direction.

RNA polymerase travels along the template strand in the $3' \rightarrow 5'$ direction, which allows for the construction of transcribed mRNA in the $5' \rightarrow 3'$ direction. Unlike DNA polymerase, RNA polymerase does not proofread its work, so the synthesized transcript will not be edited. The **coding strand** (or **sense strand**) of DNA is not used as a template during transcription. Because the coding strand is also complementary to the template strand, it is identical to the mRNA transcript except that all the thymine nucleotides in DNA have been replaced with uracil in the mRNA molecule.

In the vicinity of a gene, a numbering system is used to identify the location of important bases in the DNA strand, as shown in Figure 7.8. The first base transcribed from DNA to RNA is defined as the $+1$ base of that gene region. Bases to the left of this start point (upstream, or toward the $5'$ end) are given negative numbers:

−1, −2, −3, and so on. Bases to the right (downstream, or toward the 3′ end) are denoted with positive numbers: +2, +3, +4, and so on. Thus, no nucleotide in the gene is numbered 0. The TATA box, where RNA polymerase II binds, usually falls around −25.

Transcription will continue along the DNA coding region until the RNA polymerase reaches a termination sequence or stop signal, which results in the termination of transcription. The DNA double helix then re-forms, and the primary transcript formed is termed **heterogeneous nuclear RNA (hnRNA)**. mRNA is derived from hnRNA via posttranscriptional modifications, as described below.

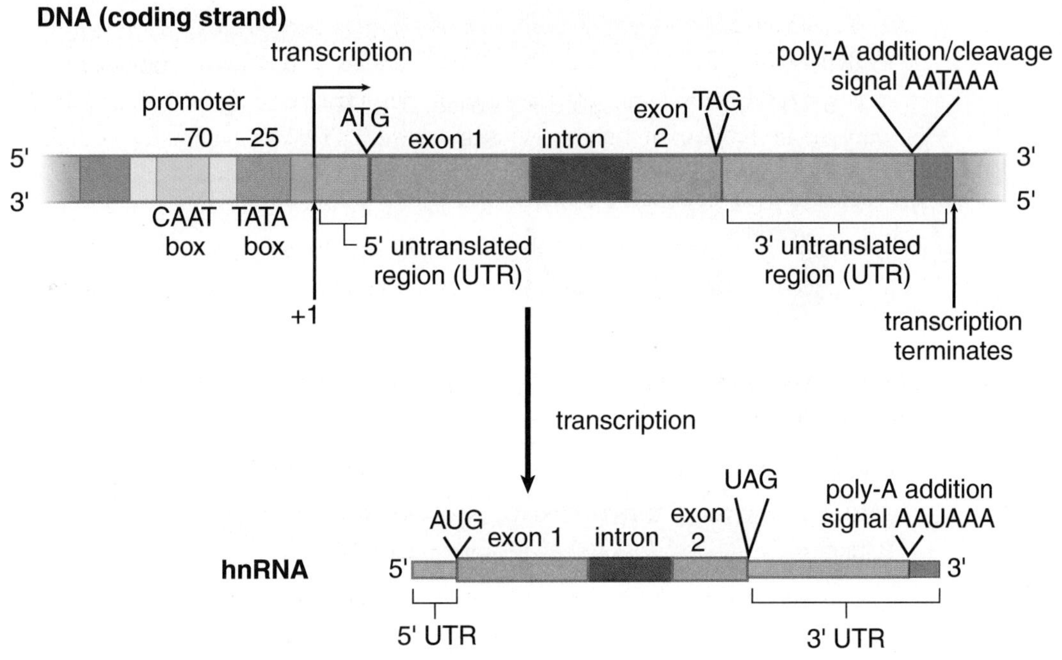

Figure 7.8 Transcription of DNA to hnRNA

Posttranscriptional Processing

Before the hnRNA can leave the nucleus and be translated to protein, it must undergo three specific processes to allow it to interact with the ribosome and survive the conditions of the cytoplasm, as demonstrated in Figure 7.9. You can think of the nucleus as the happy home of the cell; the DNA strands are the caregivers, and the hnRNA is their child. The child must mature in order to survive.

KEY CONCEPT

The MCAT commonly tests post-transcriptional processing:

- Intron/exon splicing
- 5′ cap
- 3′ poly-A tail

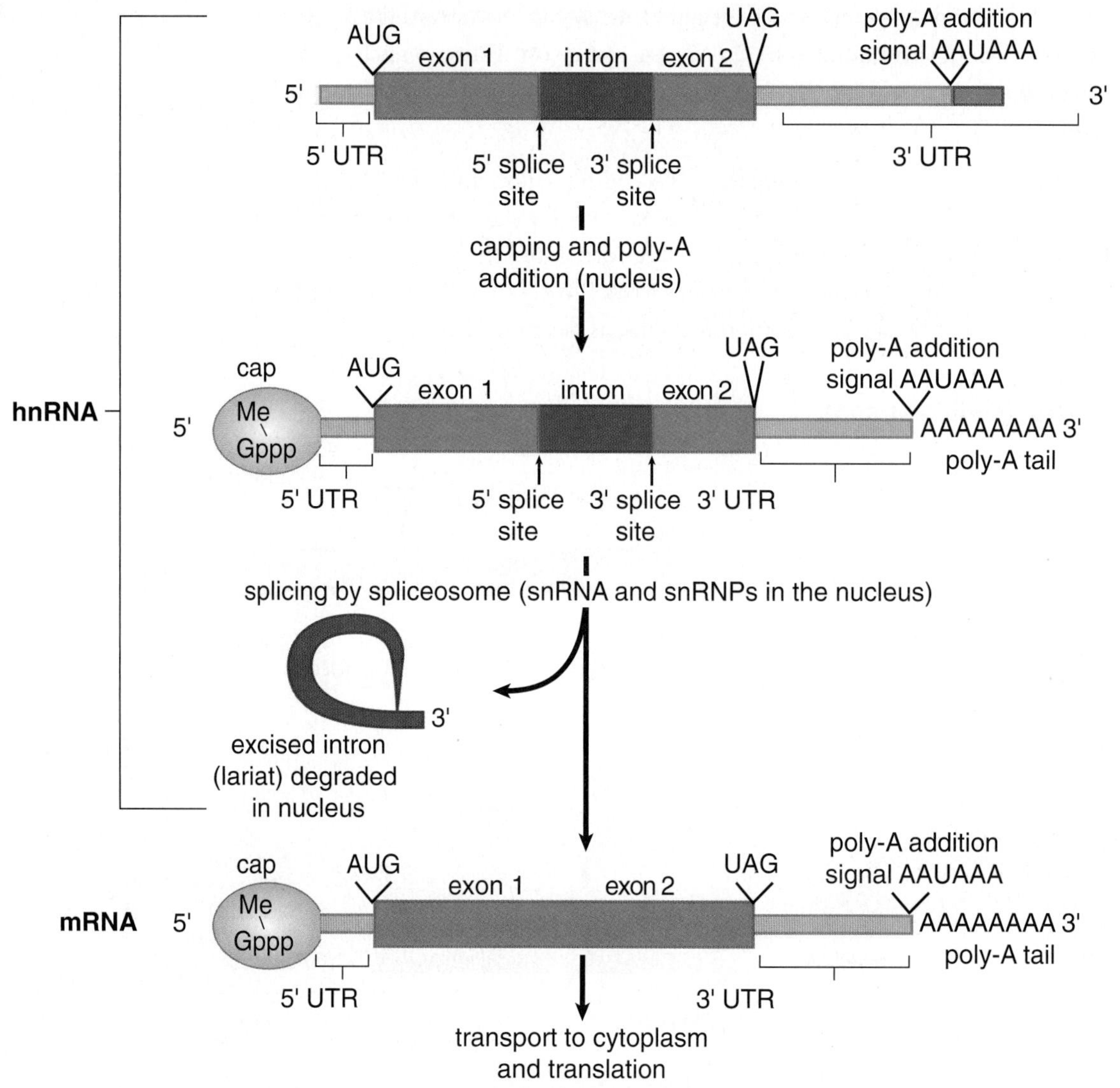

Figure 7.9 Processing Eukaryotic hnRNA to Form mRNA

MNEMONIC

Introns stay **in** the nucleus; **ex**ons will **ex**it the nucleus as part of the mRNA.

Splicing: Introns and Exons

Maturation of the hnRNA includes splicing of the transcript to remove noncoding sequences (**introns**) and ligate coding sequences (**exons**) together. Splicing is accomplished by the **spliceosome**. In the spliceosome, **small nuclear RNA** (**snRNA**) molecules couple with proteins known as **small nuclear ribonucleoproteins** (also known as **snRNPs**, or "snurps"). The snRNP/snRNA complex recognizes both the 5′ and 3′ splice sites of the introns. These noncoding sequences are excised in the form of a **lariat** (lasso-shaped structure) and then degraded.

The evolutionary function of introns in eukaryotic cells is not currently well-understood; however, scientists hypothesize that introns play an important role in the regulation of cellular gene expression levels and in maintaining the size of our genome. The existence of introns has also been hypothesized to allow for rapid protein evolution. Many eukaryotic proteins share peptide sequences in common, suggesting that the genes encoding for these particular peptides may employ a modular function; that is, they contain standard sequences that can be swapped in and out, depending on the needs of the cell.

5′ Cap

At the 5′ end of the hnRNA molecule, a **7-methylguanylate triphosphate cap** is added. The cap is actually added during the process of transcription and is recognized by the ribosome as the binding site. It also protects the mRNA from degradation in the cytoplasm.

3′ Poly-A Tail

A **polyadenosyl (poly-A) tail** is added to the 3′ end of the mRNA transcript and protects the message against rapid degradation. It is composed of adenine bases. Think of the poly-A tail as a fuse for a "time bomb" for the mRNA transcript: as soon as the mRNA leaves the nucleus, it will start to get degraded from its 3′ end. The longer the poly-A tail, the more time the mRNA will be able to survive before being digested in the cytoplasm. The poly-A tail also assists with export of the mature mRNA from the nucleus.

At this point, when only the exons remain and the cap and tail have been added, the cell has created the mature mRNA that can now be transported into the cytoplasm for protein translation. Untranslated regions of the mRNA (UTRs) will still exist at the 5′ and 3′ edges of the transcript because the ribosome initiates translation at the start codon (AUG) and will end at a stop codon (UAA, UGA, UAG).

For some genes in eukaryotic cells, however, the primary transcript of hnRNA may be spliced together in different ways to produce multiple variants of proteins encoded by the same original gene. This process is known as **alternative splicing**, and it is illustrated in Figure 7.10. By utilizing alternative splicing, an organism can make many more different proteins from a limited number of genes. For reference, humans are estimated to make at least 100,000 proteins, but the number of human genes is only about 20,000–25,000. Don't worry about memorizing these numbers, though; they are constantly changing with new research. Alternative splicing is also known to function in the regulation of gene expression, in addition to generating protein diversity.

REAL WORLD

Mutations in splice sites can lead to abnormal proteins. For example, mutations that interfere with proper splicing of β-globulin mRNA are responsible for some cases of *β-thalassemia*, a group of blood disorders that hinder the production and efficacy of hemoglobin in the blood. Splice site mutations are one of the few mutations in noncoding DNA that may still have an effect on the translated protein.

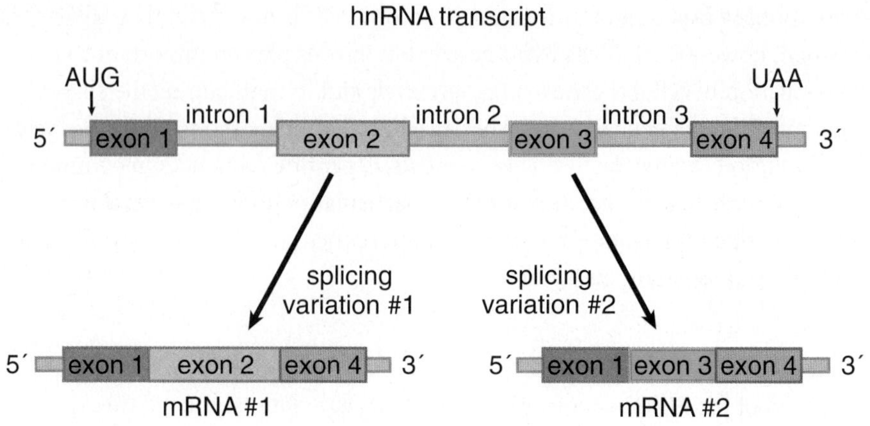

Figure 7.10 Alternative Splicing of Eukaryotic hnRNA to Produce Different Proteins

MCAT CONCEPT CHECK 7.2

Before you move on, assess your understanding of the material with these questions.

1. What is the role of each eukaryotic RNA polymerase?
   - RNA polymerase I:

   ____

   - RNA polymerase II:

   ____

   - RNA polymerase III:

   ____

2. When starting transcription, where does RNA polymerase bind?

   ____

3. What are the three major posttranscriptional modifications that turn hnRNA into mature mRNA?

   1. ______________________________
   2. ______________________________
   3. ______________________________

4. What is alternative splicing, and what does it accomplish?

   ____

7.3 Translation

High-Yield

LEARNING OBJECTIVES

After Chapter 7.3, you will be able to:

- Describe the steps of translation: initiation, elongation, and termination
- Distinguish different types of posttranslational modifications, such as phosphorylation and glycosylation
- Explain the role of the functional sites in a ribosome:

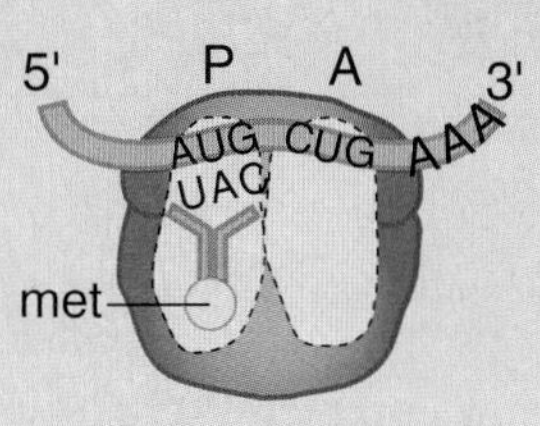

Once the mRNA transcript is created and processed, it can exit the nucleus through **nuclear pores**. Once in the cytoplasm, mRNA finds a ribosome to begin the process of **translation**—converting the mRNA transcript into a functional protein. Translation is a complex process that requires mRNA, tRNA, ribosomes, amino acids, and energy in the form of GTP.

KEY CONCEPT

Terminology and 5′ ⟶ 3′

- DNA ⟶ DNA = replication: new DNA synthesized in 5′ ⟶ 3′ direction
- DNA ⟶ RNA = transcription: new RNA synthesized in 5′ ⟶ 3′ direction (template is read 3′ ⟶ 5′)
- RNA ⟶ protein = translation: mRNA read in 5′ ⟶ 3′ direction

The Ribosome

As mentioned earlier, the anticodon of the tRNA binds to the codon on the mature mRNA in the ribosome. The **ribosome** is composed of proteins and rRNA. In both prokaryotes and eukaryotes, there are large and small subunits; the subunits only bind together during protein synthesis. The structure of the ribosome dictates its main function, which is to bring the mRNA message together with the charged aminoacyl-tRNA complex to generate the protein. There are three binding sites in the ribosome for tRNA: the A site (aminoacyl), P site (peptidyl), and E site (exit). These are described further in the section on translation below.

Eukaryotic ribosomes contain four strands of rRNA, designated the 28S, 18S, 5.8S, and the 5S rRNAs; the "S" values indicate the size of the strand. The genes for some of the rRNAs (28S, 18S, and 5.8S rRNAs) used to construct the ribosome are found in the nucleolus. RNA polymerase I transcribes the 28S, 18S, and 5.8S rRNAs as a single unit within the nucleolus, which results in a 45S ribosomal precursor RNA. This 45S pre-rRNA is processed to become the 18S rRNA of the 40S (small) ribosomal subunit and the 28S and 5.8S rRNAs of the 60S (large) ribosomal subunit. RNA polymerase III transcribes the 5S rRNA, which is also found in the 60S ribosomal subunit; this process takes place outside of the nucleolus. The ribosomal subunits created are the 60S and 40S subunits; these subunits join during protein synthesis to form the whole 80S ribosome.

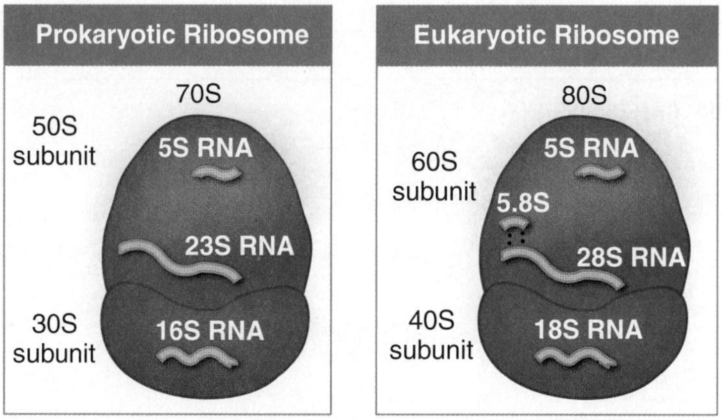

Figure 7.11 The Composition of Prokaryotic and Eukaryotic Ribosomes

REAL WORLD

The fact that prokaryotic and eukaryotic ribosomes have slightly different structures is no small fact. This difference allows us to target antibiotics, like macrolides (*azithromycin*, *erythromycin*), tetracyclines (*doxycycline*), *vancomycin*, and others to bacterial cells with fewer side effects to humans.

In comparison with eukaryotes, prokaryotes have 50S and 30S large and small subunits, which assemble to create the complete 70S ribosome. Note that the "S" value is determined experimentally by studying the behavior of particles in a ultracentrifuge; thus, the numbers of each subunit and each rRNA are not additive because they are based on size and shape, not size alone. The structure of eukaryotic and prokaryotic ribosomes are shown in Figure 7.11.

Mechanism of Translation

Translation occurs in the cytoplasm in prokaryotes and eukaryotes. In prokaryotes, the ribosomes start translating before the mRNA is complete; in eukaryotes, however, transcription and translation occur at separate times and in separate locations within the cell. The process of translation occurs in three stages, as shown in Figure 7.12: **initiation**, **elongation**, and **termination**. Specialized factors for initiation (initiation factors, IF), elongation (elongation factors, EF), and termination (release factors, RF), as well as GTP are required for each step.

Initiation

The small ribosomal subunit binds to the mRNA. In prokaryotes, the small subunit binds to the **Shine–Dalgarno sequence** in the 5′ untranslated region of the mRNA. In eukaryotes, the small subunit binds to the 5′ cap structure. The charged **initiator tRNA** binds to the AUG **start codon** through base-pairing with its anticodon within the P site of the ribosome. The initial amino acid in prokaryotes is *N-formylmethionine* (fMet); in eukaryotes, it's methionine.

The large subunit then binds to the small subunit, forming the completed initiation complex. This is assisted by **initiation factors (IF)** that are not permanently associated with the ribosome.

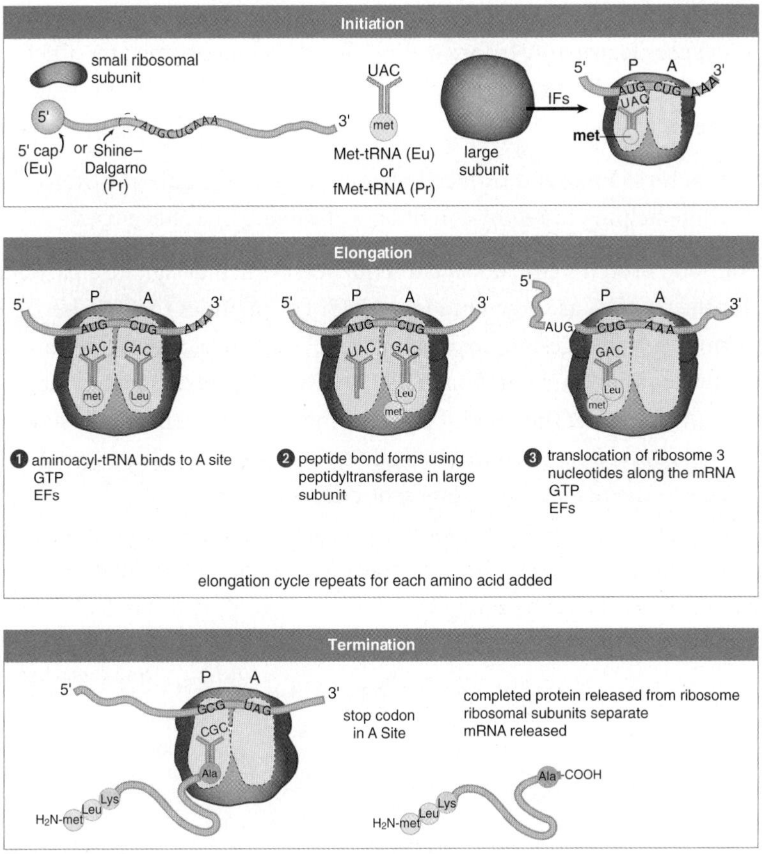

Figure 7.12 Steps in Translation

Elongation

Elongation is a three-step cycle that is repeated for each amino acid added to the protein after the initiator methionine. During elongation, the ribosome moves in the 5′ to 3′ direction along the mRNA, synthesizing the protein from its amino (N-) to carboxyl (C-) terminus. The ribosome contains three very important binding sites:

- The **A site** holds the incoming aminoacyl-tRNA complex. This is the next amino acid that is being added to the growing chain, and is determined by the mRNA codon within the A site.
- The **P site** holds the tRNA that carries the growing polypeptide chain. It is also where the first amino acid (methionine) binds because it is starting the polypeptide chain. A **peptide bond** is formed as the polypeptide is passed from the tRNA in the P site to the tRNA in the A site. This requires ***peptidyl transferase***, an enzyme that is part of the large subunit. GTP is used for energy during the formation of this bond.

MNEMONIC

Order of sites in the ribosome during translation: **APE**.

- The **E site** (not shown in Figure 7.12) is where the now inactivated (uncharged) tRNA pauses transiently before exiting the ribosome. As the now-uncharged tRNA enters the E site, it quickly unbinds from the mRNA and is ready to be recharged.

Elongation factors (**EF**) assist by locating and recruiting aminoacyl-tRNA along with GTP, while helping to remove GDP once the energy has been used.

Some eukaryotic proteins contain signal sequences, which designate a particular destination for the protein, as shown in Figure 7.13. For peptides that will be secreted, such as hormones and digestive enzymes, a signal sequence directs the ribosome to move to the endoplasmic reticulum (ER), so that the protein can be translated directly into the lumen of the rough ER. From there, the protein can be sent to the Golgi apparatus and be secreted from a vesicle via exocytosis. Other signal sequences direct proteins to the nucleus, lysosomes, or cell membrane.

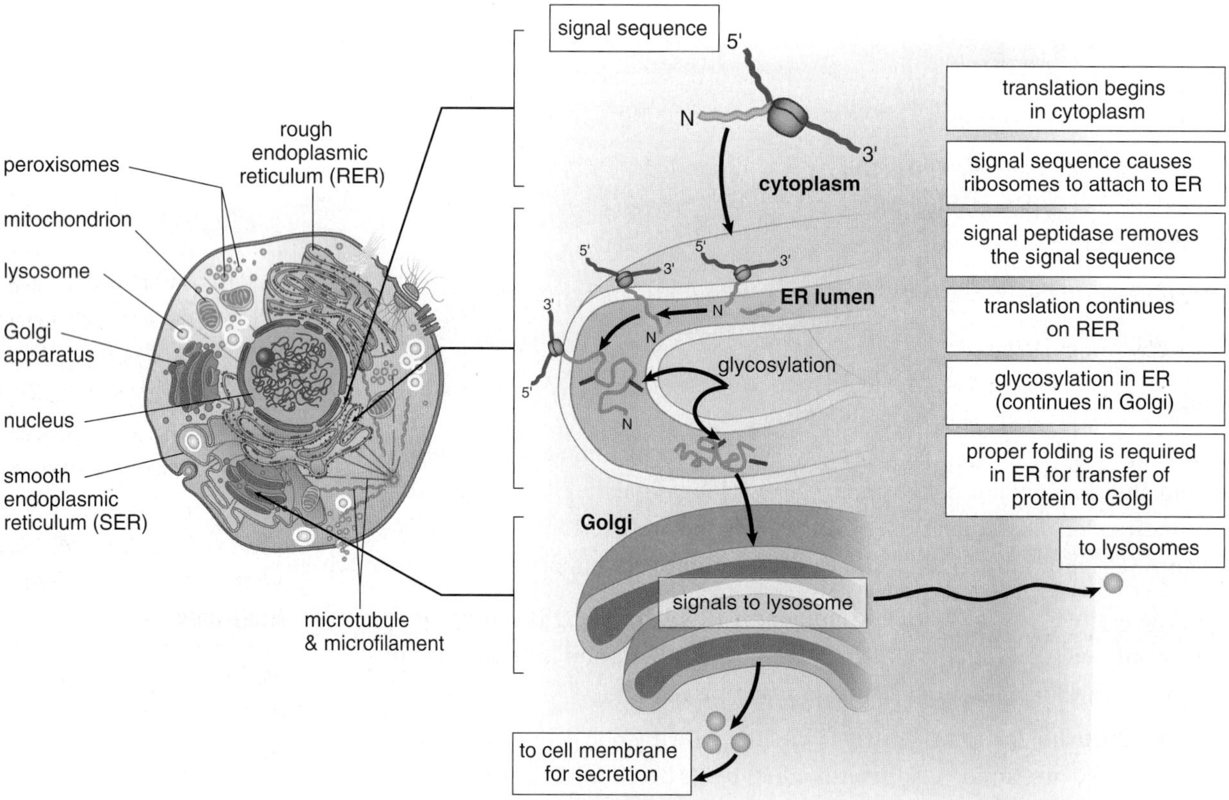

Figure 7.13 Synthesis of Secretory, Membrane, and Lysosomal Proteins

Termination

When any of the three stop codons moves into the A site, a protein called **release factor** (**RF**) binds to the termination codon, causing a water molecule to be added to the polypeptide chain. The addition of this water molecule allows peptidyl transferase and **termination factors** to hydrolyze the completed polypeptide chain from the final tRNA. The polypeptide chain will then be released from the tRNA in the P site, and the two ribosomal subunits will dissociate.

Posttranslational Processing

The nascent polypeptide chain is subject to posttranslational modifications before it will become a functioning protein, similar to how hnRNA is modified prior to being released from the nucleus. One essential step for the final synthesis of the protein is proper folding. There is a specialized class of proteins called **chaperones**, the main function of which is to assist in the protein-folding process.

Many proteins are also modified by cleavage events. A common example of this is insulin, which needs to be cleaved from a larger, inactive peptide to achieve its active form. In peptides with signal sequences, the signal sequence must be cleaved if the protein is to enter the organelle and accomplish its function.

In peptides with quaternary structure, subunits come together to form the functional protein. A classic example is hemoglobin, which is composed of two alpha chains and two beta chains.

Other biomolecules may be added to the peptide via the following processes:

- **Phosphorylation**—addition of a phosphate group (PO_4^{2-}) by protein kinases to activate or deactivate proteins; phosphorylation in eukaryotes is most commonly seen with serine, threonine, and tyrosine
- **Carboxylation**—addition of carboxylic acid groups, usually to serve as calcium-binding sites
- **Glycosylation**—addition of oligosaccharides as proteins pass through the ER and Golgi apparatus to determine cellular destination
- **Prenylation**—addition of lipid groups to certain membrane-bound enzymes

REAL WORLD

Posttranslational modifications are often important for proper protein functioning. For example, several clotting factors, including prothrombin, require posttranslational carboxylation of some of their glutamic acid residues in order to function properly. Vitamin K is required as a cofactor for these reactions; thus, vitamin K deficiency may result in a bleeding disorder.

BIOCHEMISTRY GUIDED EXAMPLE WITH EXPERT THINKING

Profilins (Pfn) are a family of actin-monomer binding proteins that strongly inhibit spontaneous elongation of pointed ends of actin filaments, but promote barbed-ended elongation through the addition of ATP-bound monomeric actin. Since actin polymerization is a fundamental component of many physiological properties, the goal of this study is to elucidate the regulation of Pfn1 (the most abundant isoform of Pfn in mammals) by phosphorylation.

Intro to topic: Pfn moderates actin through two mechanisms

Goal: better understand regulation of Pfn1 through phosphorylation

Pfn1 is known to be phosphorylated on tyrosine and serine residues. Using sequence analysis software, threonine-89 was also identified as a possible phosphorylation site by protein kinase A (PKA). To examine the role of threonine-89 in Pfn1 expression, two Pfn1 constructs were created—T89D and T89A. Human embryonic kidney cells (HEK-293) expressing indicated green fluorescent protein-fused Pfn1 (GFP Pfn1) constructs (GFP Pfn1 T89D, T89A, and wild-type) were lysed with either non-denaturing (containing 1% NP-40) or denaturing (containing 1% NP-40, 2% SDS as a mild denaturant for one buffer, and the other with 6 M urea as a strong denaturant in addition) extraction buffers. Misfolded proteins are generally insoluble unless some denaturant is present. HEK-293 lysates were subject to a western blot, where lysates were immunoblotted with anti-tubulin antibody as a loading control, anti-GFP antibody, and anti-Pfn1 antibody specific for endogenous Pfn1.

PKA possibly phosphorylates T89

T89D and T89A mutants made to analyze role of phosphorylation

Cells expressing the 3 constructs were broken apart with one of 3 types of solutions: non-, mild, and strongly denaturing

Ignore the results for tubulin; it's just a control

This will show if any of the constructs are expressed

This will show the Pfn1 that's already expressed in the cells

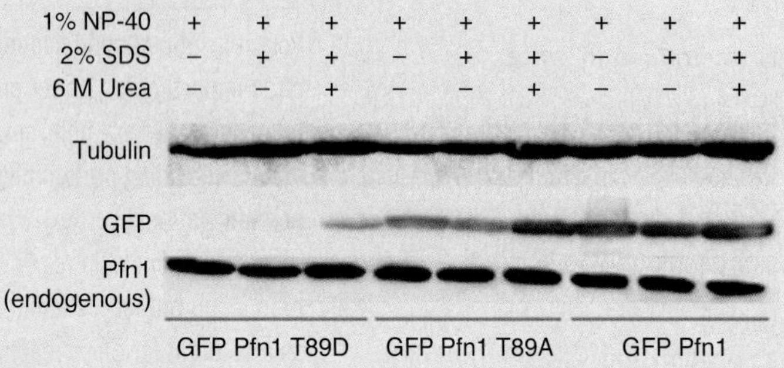

Lots of info here, so focus on what's changing: the GFP row shows the most change so it's probably the most important

Figure 1

Adapted from Gau, D., Veon, W., Zeng, X., Yates, N., Shroff, S. G., Koes, D. R., & Roy, P. (2016). Threonine 89 is an important residue of profilin-1 that is phosphorylatable by protein kinase A. *PLoS One*, 11(5), e0156313. doi:10.1371/journal.pone.0156313.

What is the purpose of mutating the potential phosphorylation site to aspartic acid and alanine, respectively? What is the implication for expression of Pfn1?

Since the question is asking for a reason behind the experimental design, our focus should be on understanding the way the experiment was designed. The passage is focused on clarifying how phosphorylation regulates Pfn1. We know from our content background that phosphorylation of an amino acid (specifically serine, threonine, and tyrosine) will turn a polar amino acid into one that is negatively charged. If we didn't remember that, we could also infer it by thinking about the charge on a phosphate group, which is highly negative. We have enough information to answer the first question. Mutating a threonine phosphorylation site to aspartic acid (which is negatively charged) would mimic the site being constantly phosphorylated, while mutating to alanine would mimic the site being constantly dephosphorylated, since alanine residues cannot be phosphorylated.

One possible phosphorylation site, T89, was identified, and three GFP constructs were made—one mimicking phosphorylation (T89D, lanes 1–3), one eliminating phosphorylation (T89A, lanes 4–6), and one unmodified (lanes 7–9). The GFP tag allows the experimenters to see whether the GFP-fused construct is being expressed (whether the protein is being made). We're told this experimental procedure is a western blot, a technique in which a specific antibody of interest will bind to proteins that were separated on a gel. In western blots, a band appears when the antibody successfully binds to protein. The rows above the gel image display experimental conditions for each of the lanes. All lanes have 1% NP-40, which we're told is non-denaturing. We should recall that the word denaturing means that a substance changes the 3-D structure of a protein. So, non-denaturing means that NP-40 won't change the shape of the protein by itself. The lanes with 2% SDS are in mild denaturing conditions, and the lanes with 2% SDS and 6 M urea are in strong denaturing conditions. Continuing by that same definition, we know that strong denaturing conditions will unfold and solubilize all proteins, greatly changing their 3-D structure. If we look at the row probing for GFP, we see that there is no band for non- and mild denaturing conditions, but there is a faint band under strong denaturing conditions for only the T89D construct. We can see that the lanes for both the wild type and T89A, regardless of condition, are mostly the same. Finally, recall that phosphorylation is a post-translational event, so a change in the phosphorylation state of the protein would occur after Pfn1 has been translated, and wouldn't work to affect its expression.

Therefore, we can conclude that mutating the threonine residue can mimic the effect of constantly phosphorylated or dephosphorylated Pfn. Second, since we only see a GFP band when T89D is in the presence of a strong denaturant, phosphorylation of Pfn1 may cause the protein to fold in a way that makes it insoluble, thereby targeting the protein for degradation. Follow-up studies are required to verify the exact mechanism of action by which this occurs. Therefore, because T89D represents the "always phosphorylated" version of Pfn1, and T89D only appears on the gel in strongly denaturing conditions, we can conclude that Pfn1, when phosphorylated, isn't available/expressed. We can thus conclude that phosphorylation of Pfn1 can potentially be used to down-regulate the availability of Pfn1 for usage with actin polymerization.

MCAT CONCEPT CHECK 7.3

Before you move on, assess your understanding of the material with these questions.

1. What are the three steps of translation?

    1. ______________________________
    2. ______________________________
    3. ______________________________

2. What are the roles of each site in the ribosome?

    - A site:

    ____

    - P site:

    ____

    - E site:

    ____

3. What are the major posttranslational modifications that occur in proteins?

    ____

7.4 Control of Gene Expression in Prokaryotes

High-Yield

LEARNING OBJECTIVES

After Chapter 7.4, you will be able to:

- Recognize the transcriptional controls on key operons such as the *lac* and *trp* operons
- Differentiate between positive and negative control systems
- Explain the role of the different sections of a standard operon

An organism's DNA encodes all of the RNA and protein molecules required to construct its cells. Yet organisms are able to differentially express their genes to make cell-specific products necessary for cellular development at specific times. In the next section, we'll look at these processes in eukaryotic cells; for now, we'll focus on the regulatory processes governing gene expression in prokaryotes—rules that are necessary in determining which subset of genes are selectively expressed or silenced in the prokaryotic cell.

Operon Structure

The simplest example of an on–off switch that regulates gene expression levels in prokaryotes was discovered in *E. coli,* which regulates the expression of many genes according to food sources that are available in the environment. For example, five genes in *E. coli* encode for enzymes that manufacture the amino acid tryptophan, and these are arranged in a cluster on the chromosome. By sharing a single common promoter region on the DNA sequence, these genes are transcribed as a group. This type of structure is called an **operon**—a cluster of genes transcribed as a single mRNA; this particular cluster in *E. coli* is known as the *trp* operon. Operons are incredibly common in the prokaryotic cell.

The **Jacob–Monod model** is used to describe the structure and function of operons. In this model, operons contain structural genes, an operator site, a promoter site, and a regulator gene, as shown in Figure 7.14. The **structural gene** codes for the protein of interest. Upstream of the structural gene is the **operator site**, a nontranscribable region of DNA that is capable of binding a repressor protein. Further upstream is the **promoter site**, which is similar in function to promoters in eukaryotes: it provides a place for RNA polymerase to bind. Furthest upstream is the **regulator gene**, which codes for a protein known as the **repressor**. There are two types of operons: inducible systems and repressible systems.

KEY CONCEPT

Operons include both inducible and repressible systems, and offer a simple on–off switch for gene control in prokaryotes.

Inducible Systems

In **inducible systems**, the repressor is bonded tightly to the operator system and thereby acts as a roadblock. RNA polymerase is unable to get from the promoter to the structural gene because the repressor is in the way. Such systems—in which the binding of a protein reduces transcriptional activity—are called **negative control** mechanisms. To remove that block, an inducer must bind the repressor protein so that RNA polymerase can move down the gene, as shown in Figure 7.14. Inducible systems operate on a principle analogous to competitive inhibition for enzyme activity: as the concentration of the inducer increases, it will pull more copies of the repressor off of the operator region, freeing up those genes for transcription. This system is useful because it allows gene products to be produced only when they are needed.

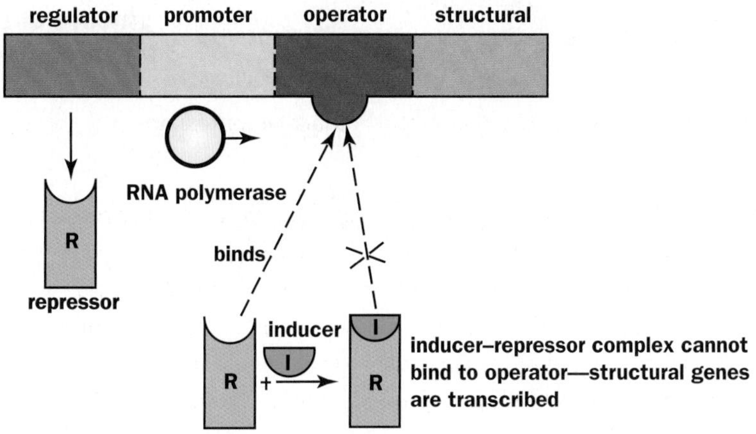

Figure 7.14 Inducible Systems
Allow for gene transcription only when an inducer is present to bind the otherwise present repressor protein

KEY CONCEPT

Negative control—The binding of a protein to DNA stops transcription.
Positive control—The binding of a protein to DNA increases transcription.
Inducible system—The system is normally "off" but can be made to turn "on," given a particular signal.
Repressible system—The system is normally "on" but can be made to turn "off," given a particular signal.

Any combination of control and system are possible; the *lac* operon is a negative inducible system whereas the *trp* operon is a negative repressible system.

A classic example of an inducible system is the *lac* operon, which contains the gene for *lactase*, as demonstrated in Figure 7.15. Bacteria can digest lactose, but it is more energetically expensive than digesting glucose. Therefore, bacteria only want to use this option if lactose is high and glucose is low. The *lac* operon is induced by the presence of lactose; thus, these genes are only transcribed when it is useful to the cell.

The *lac* operon is assisted by binding of the **catabolite activator protein** (**CAP**). CAP is a transcriptional activator used by *E. coli* when glucose levels are low to signal that alternative carbon sources should be used. Falling levels of glucose cause an increase in the signaling molecule cyclic AMP (cAMP), which binds to CAP. This induces a conformational change in CAP that allows it to bind the promoter region of the operon, further increasing transcription of the lactase gene. Such systems—in which the binding of a molecule increases transcription of a gene—are called **positive control** mechanisms.

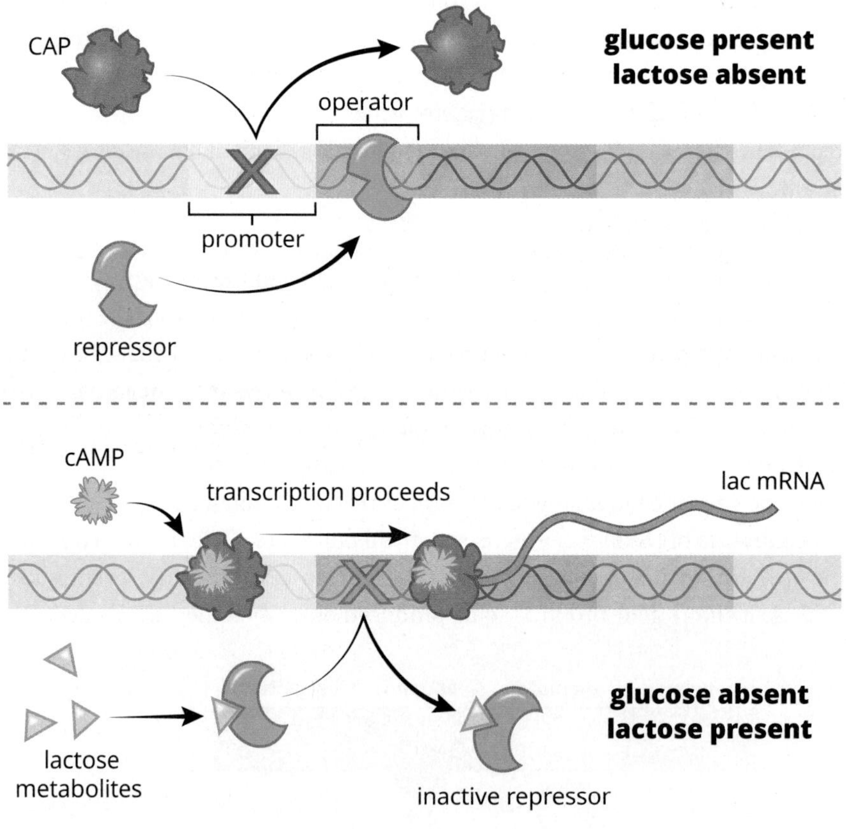

Figure 7.15 The *lac* Operon
An example of an inducible system

Repressible Systems

Repressible systems allow constant production of a protein product. In contrast to the inducible system, the repressor made by the regulator gene is inactive until it binds to a **corepressor**. This complex then binds the operator site to prevent further transcription, as shown in Figure 7.16. Repressible systems tend to serve as negative feedback; often, the final structural product can serve as a corepressor. Thus, as its levels increase, it can bind the repressor, and the complex will attach to the operator region to prevent further transcription of the same gene.

The *trp* operon, described above, operates in this way as a negative repressible system. When tryptophan is high in the local environment, it acts as a corepressor. The binding of two molecules of tryptophan to the repressor causes the repressor to bind to the operator site. Thus, the cell turns off its machinery to synthesize its own tryptophan, which is an energetically expensive process because of its easy availability in the environment.

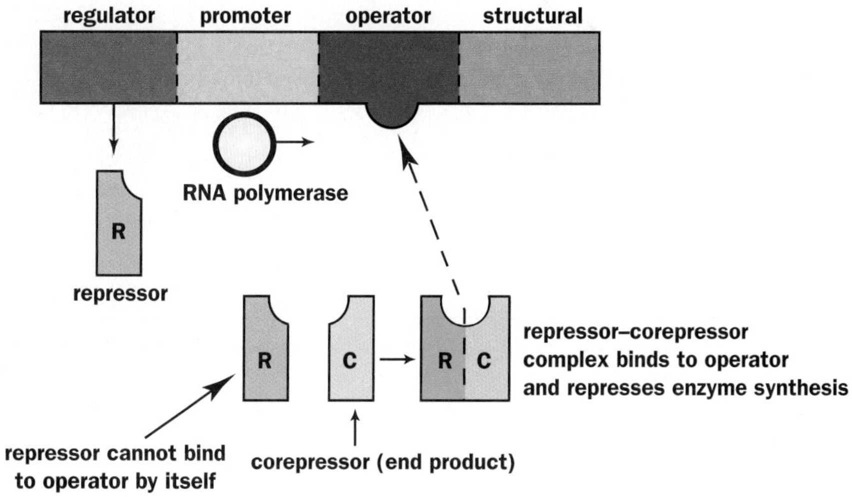

Figure 7.16 Repressible Systems
Continually allow gene transcription unless a corepressor binds to the repressor to stop transcription

MCAT CONCEPT CHECK 7.4

Before you move on, assess your understanding of the material with these questions.

1. What type of operon is the *trp* operon? The *lac* operon?
   - *trp*: ____________________________
   - *lac*: ____________________________

2. From 5′ to 3′, what are the components of the operon, and what are their roles?

Component	Role

3. What is a positive control system? What is a negative control system?
   - Positive control system:

   ____

   - Negative control system:

   ____

7.5 Control of Gene Expression in Eukaryotes

High-Yield

LEARNING OBJECTIVES

After Chapter 7.5, you will be able to:

- Identify the different mechanisms that can be used to regulate or amplify the expression of a gene
- Predict how histone and DNA modification will affect the ratio of heterochromatin to euchromatin

Genomic expression in eukaryotes is considerably more complex than in prokaryotes, and you will need to know those differences for Test Day. Regulation of gene expression is an essential feature that helps in maintaining the overall functionality of cells. In addition to basic transcriptional enzymes, however, there are a host of other regulatory proteins that play a prominent role in controlling gene expression levels in the cell.

Transcription Factors

Transcription factors are transcription-activating proteins that search the DNA looking for specific DNA-binding motifs. Transcription factors tend to have two recognizable domains: a DNA-binding domain and an activation domain. The **DNA-binding domain** binds to a specific nucleotide sequence in the promoter region or to a DNA **response element** (a sequence of DNA that binds only to specific transcription factors) to help in the recruitment of transcriptional machinery. The **activation domain** allows for the binding of several transcription factors and other important regulatory proteins, such as RNA polymerase and histone acetylases, which function in the remodeling of the chromatin structure.

Gene Amplification

Once the transcription complex is formed, basal (or low-level) transcription can begin and maintain moderate, but adequate, levels of the protein encoded by this gene in the cell. There are times, however, when the expression must be increased, or **amplified**, in response to specific signals such as hormones, growth factors, and other intracellular conditions. Eukaryotic cells accomplish this through enhancers and gene duplication.

Enhancers

Response elements outside the normal promoter regions can be recognized by specific transcription factors to enhance transcription levels. Several response elements may be grouped together to form an **enhancer**, which allows for the control of one gene's expression by multiple signals. Figure 7.17 demonstrates a eukaryotic example of an enhancer. Signal molecules, such as cyclic AMP (cAMP), cortisol, and estrogen, bind to specific receptors. For the examples given, these receptors are cyclic AMP response element-binding protein (CREB), the glucocorticoid (cortisol) receptor, and the estrogen receptor, respectively; all are transcription factors that bind to their respective response elements within the enhancer. Other proteins are involved in this process, but are outside the scope of the MCAT. Note that the large distance between the enhancer and promoter regions for a given gene means that DNA often must bend into a hairpin loop to bring these elements together spatially.

KEY CONCEPT

The DNA regulatory base sequences (such as promoters, enhancers, and response elements) are known as *cis* regulators because they are in the same vicinity as the gene they control. Transcription factors, however, have to be produced and translocated back to the nucleus; thus they are called *trans* regulators because they travel through the cell to their point of action.

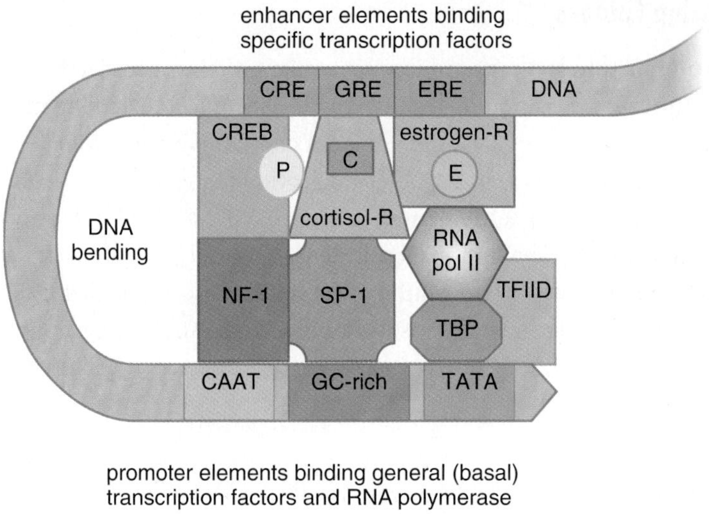

Figure 7.17 Stimulation of Transcription by an Enhancer and Its Associated Transcription Factors

Enhancer regions in the DNA can be up to 1000 base pairs away from the gene they regulate and can even be located within an intron, or noncoding region, of the gene. They differ from upstream promoter elements in their locations because upstream promoter elements must be within 25 bases of the start of a gene. By utilizing enhancer regions, genes have an increased likelihood to be amplified because of the variety of signals that can increase transcription levels.

Gene Duplication

Cells can also increase the expression of a gene product by duplicating the relevant gene. Genes can be duplicated in series on the same chromosome, yielding many copies in a row of the same genetic information. Genes can also be duplicated in parallel by opening the gene with helicases and permitting DNA replication only of that gene; cells can continue replicating the gene until hundreds of copies of the gene exist in parallel on the same chromosome.

Regulation of Chromatin Structure

In eukaryotic cells, DNA is packaged in the nucleus as chromatin, which requires chromatin remodeling to allow transcription factors and the transcriptional machinery easier access to the DNA. **Heterochromatin** is tightly coiled DNA that appears dark under the microscope; its tight coiling makes it inaccessible to the transcription machinery, so these genes are inactive. **Euchromatin**, on the other hand, is looser and appears light under the microscope; the transcription machinery can access the genes of interest, so these genes are active. Remodeling of the chromatin structures regulates gene expression levels in the cell.

Histone Acetylation

Transcription factors that bind to the DNA can recruit other coactivators such as ***histone acetylases***. These proteins are involved in chromatin remodeling, as shown in Figure 7.18, because they acetylate lysine residues found in the amino terminal tail regions of histone proteins. **Acetylation** of histone proteins decreases the positive charge on lysine residues and weakens the interaction of the histone with DNA, resulting in an open chromatin conformation that allows for easier access of the transcriptional machinery to the DNA.

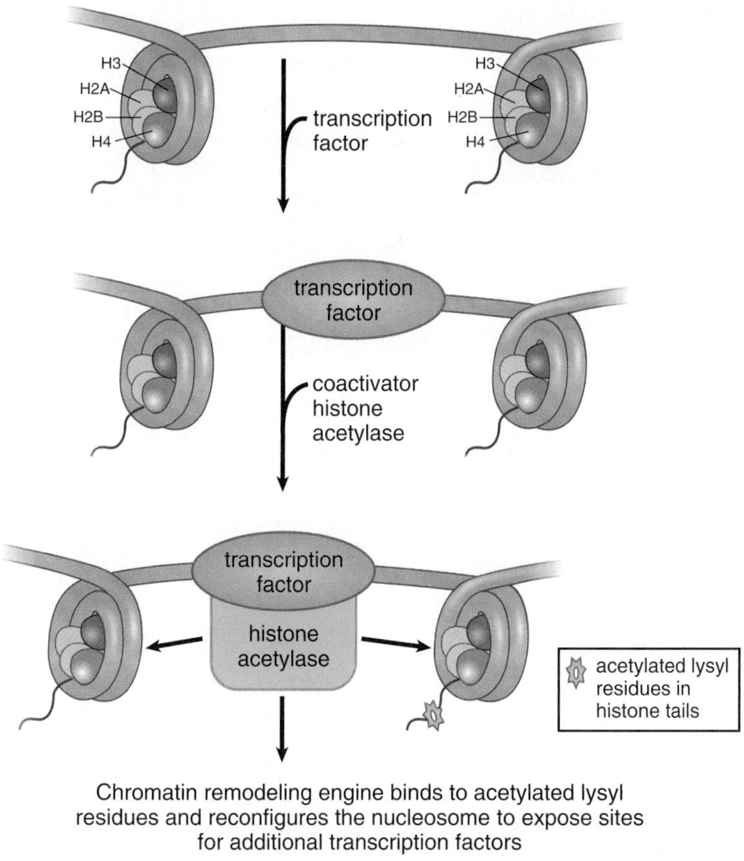

Figure 7.18 Chromatin Remodeling by Acetylation
Increases space between histones, allowing better access to DNA for transcription factors

Specific patterns of histone acetylation can lead to increased gene expression levels. On the other hand, gene silencing can occur just as easily with chromatin remodeling. ***Histone deacetylases*** are proteins that function to remove acetyl groups from histones, which results in a closed chromatin conformation and overall decrease in gene expression levels in the cell.

DNA Methylation

DNA methylation is also involved in chromatin remodeling and regulation of gene expression levels in the cell. ***DNA methylases*** add methyl groups to cytosine and adenine nucleotides; methylation of genes is often linked with the silencing of gene expression. During development, methylation plays an important role in silencing genes that no longer need to be activated. Heterochromatin regions of the DNA are much more heavily methylated, hindering access of the transcriptional machinery to the DNA.

MCAT CONCEPT CHECK 7.5

Before you move on, assess your understanding of the material with these questions.

1. In an enhancer, what are the differences between signal molecules, transcription factors, and response elements?

____

2. By what histone and DNA modifications can genes be silenced in eukaryotic cells? Would these processes increase the proportion of heterochromatin or euchromatin?

____

Conclusion

To carry out the functions of life, we must produce around 100,000 different proteins using our 20,000–25,000 available genes. Every protein in the biosphere is produced through the central dogma of molecular biology, as genes in DNA are transcribed into mRNA and then translated into a functional protein. This is a complex, highly regulated process in both prokaryotes and eukaryotes, and questions on transcription and translation, and their regulation, are frequent on the MCAT.

The last two chapters focused on the important roles played by many organelles in the cell, including the nucleus, nucleolus, ribosome, rough endoplasmic reticulum, and Golgi apparatus. After secreted proteins such as hormones and digestive enzymes are produced, they make their way to the plasma membrane for exocytosis. It is this last stop that we'll examine in the next chapter: the structure, function, and biochemistry of biological membranes.

You've reviewed the content, now test your knowledge and critical thinking skills by completing a test-like passage set in your online resources!

GO ONLINE

CONCEPT SUMMARY

The Genetic Code

- The **central dogma** states that DNA is transcribed to RNA, which is translated to protein.
- A degenerate code allows multiple codons to encode for the same amino acid.
    - Initiation (start) codon: AUG
    - Termination (stop) codons: UAA, UGA, UAG
- Redundancy and **wobble** (third base in the codon) allows mutations to occur without effects in the protein.
- Point mutations can cause:
    - **Silent** mutations with no effect on protein synthesis.
    - **Nonsense** (**truncation**) mutations that produce a premature stop codon.
    - **Missense** mutations that produce a codon that codes for a different amino acid.
- **Frameshift mutations** result from nucleotide addition or deletion, and change the reading frame of subsequent codons.
- RNA is structurally similar to DNA except:
    - Substitution of a ribose sugar for deoxyribose
    - Substitution of uracil for thymine
    - It is single-stranded instead of double-stranded
- There are three types of RNA with separate jobs in transcription:
    - **Messenger RNA** (**mRNA**) carries the message from DNA in the nucleus via transcription of the gene; it travels into the cytoplasm to be translated.
    - **Transfer RNA** (**tRNA**) brings in amino acids and recognizes the codon on the mRNA using its anticodon.
    - **Ribosomal RNA** (**rRNA**) makes up the ribosome and is enzymatically active.

Transcription

- **Helicase** unwinds the DNA double helix.
- **RNA polymerase II** binds to the **TATA box** within the **promoter** region of the gene (25 base pairs upstream from first transcribed base).
- **hnRNA** is synthesized from the DNA template (antisense) strand.

- Posttranscriptional modifications include:
  - A 7-methylguanylate triphosphate cap is added to the 5′ end.
  - A polyadenosyl (poly-A) tail is added to the 3′ end.
  - Splicing is done by snRNA and snRNPs in the **spliceosome**; introns are removed in a **lariat** structure, and exons are ligated together.
  - Prokaryotic cells can increase the variability of gene products from one transcript through **polycistronic genes** (in which starting transcription in different sites within the gene leads to different gene products).
  - Eukaryotic cells can increase variability of gene products through **alternative splicing** (combining different exons in a modular fashion to acquire different gene products).

Translation

- tRNA translates the codon into the correct amino acid.
- Ribosomes are the factories where translation (protein synthesis) occurs.
- There are three stages of **translation**.
  - **Initiation** in prokaryotes occurs when the 30S ribosome attaches to the **Shine–Dalgarno sequence** and scans for a start codon; it lays down *N*-formylmethionine in the P site of the ribosome.
  - Initiation in eukaryotes occurs when the 40S ribosome attaches to the 5′ cap and scans for a start codon; it lays down methionine in the P site of the ribosome.
  - **Elongation** involves the addition of a new aminoacyl-tRNA into the A site of the ribosome and transfer of the growing polypeptide chain from the tRNA in the P site to the tRNA in the A site. The now uncharged tRNA pauses in the E site before exiting the ribosome.
  - **Termination** occurs when the codon in the A site is a stop codon; a **release factor** places a water molecule on the polypeptide chain and thus releases the protein.
  - Initiation, elongation, and release factors help with each step in recruitment and assembly/disassembly of the ribosome.
- Posttranslational modifications include:
  - Folding by **chaperones**
  - Formation of quaternary structure
  - Cleavage of proteins or signal sequences
  - Covalent addition of other biomolecules (phosphorylation, carboxylation, glycosylation, prenylation)

Control of Gene Expression in Prokaryotes

- The **Jacob–Monod model** of repressors and activators explains how operons work.
    - **Operons** are inducible or repressible clusters of genes transcribed as a single mRNA.
- **Inducible systems** (such as the *lac* operon) are bonded to a **repressor** under normal conditions; they can be turned on by an **inducer** pulling the repressor from the **operator site**.
- **Repressible systems** (such as the *trp* operon) are transcribed under normal conditions; they can be turned off by a corepressor coupling with the repressor and the binding of this complex to the operator site.

Control of Gene Expression in Eukaryotes

- **Transcription factors** search for promoter and enhancer regions in the DNA.
    - **Promoters** are within 25 base pairs of the transcription start site.
    - **Enhancers** are more than 25 base pairs away from the transcription start site.
    - Modification of chromatin structure affects the ability of transcriptional enzymes to access the DNA through histone acetylation (increases accessibility) or DNA methylation (decreases accessibility).

ANSWERS TO CONCEPT CHECKS

7.1

1. mRNA carries information from DNA by traveling from the nucleus (where it is transcribed) to the cytoplasm (where it is translated). tRNA translates nucleic acids to amino acids by pairing its anticodon with mRNA codons; it is charged with an amino acid, which can be added to the growing peptide chain. rRNA forms much of the structural and catalytic component of the ribosome, and acts as a ribozyme to create peptide bonds between amino acids.
2. • GAT: mRNA codon = AUC; Isoleucine (Ile)
   • ATT: mRNA codon = AAU; Asparagine (Asn)
   • CGC: mRNA codon = GCG; Alanine (Ala)
   • CCA: mRNA codon = UGG; Tryptophan (Trp)
3. The start codon is AUG, which codes for methionine; the stop codons are UAA, UGA, and UAG.
4. Wobble refers to the fact that the third base in a codon often plays no role in determining which amino acid is translated from that codon. For example, any codon starting with "CC" codes for proline, regardless of which base is in the third (wobble) position. This is protective because mutations in the wobble position will not have any effect on the protein translated from that gene.
5.

Type of Mutation	Change in DNA Sequence	Effect on Encoded Protein
Silent (degenerate)	Substitution of bases in the wobble position, introns, or noncoding DNA	No change observed
Missense	Substitution of one base, creating an mRNA codon that matches a different amino acid	One amino acid is changed in the protein; variable effects on function depending on specific change
Nonsense	Substitution of one base, creating a stop codon	Early truncation of protein; variable effects on function, but usually more severe than missense mutations
Frameshift	Insertion or deletion of bases, creating a shift in the reading frame of the mRNA	Change in most amino acids after the site of insertion or deletion; usually the most severe of the types listed here

7.2

1. RNA polymerase I synthesizes most rRNA. RNA polymerase II synthesizes mRNA (hnRNA) and snRNA. RNA polymerase III synthesizes tRNA and some rRNA.
2. RNA polymerase II binds to the TATA box, which is located within the promoter region of a relevant gene, at about −25.
3. The major posttranscriptional modifications are:
   - Splicing: removal of introns, joining of exons; uses snRNA and snRNPs in the spliceosome to create a lariat, which is then degraded; exons are ligated together
   - 5′ cap: addition of a 7-methylguanylate triphosphate cap to the 5′ end of the transcript
   - 3′ poly-A tail: addition of adenosine bases to the 3′ end to protect against degradation
4. Alternative splicing is the ability of some genes to use various combinations of exons to create multiple proteins from one hnRNA transcript. This increases protein diversity and allows a species to maximize the number of proteins it can create from a limited number of genes.

7.3

1. Initiation, elongation, and termination
2. A site: binds incoming aminoacyl-tRNA using codon–anticodon pairing

   P site: holds growing polypeptide until peptidyl transferase forms peptide bond and polypeptide is handed to A site

   E site: transiently holds uncharged tRNA as it exits the ribosome
3. Posttranslational modifications include proper folding by chaperones, formation of quaternary structure, cleavage of proteins or signal sequences, and addition of other biomolecules (phosphorylation, carboxylation, glycosylation, prenylation).

7.4

1. The *trp* operon is a negative repressible system; the *lac* operon is a negative inducible system.
2.

Component	Role
Regulator gene	Transcribed to form repressor protein
Promoter site	Site of RNA polymerase binding (similar to promoters in eukaryotes)
Operator site	Binding site for repressor protein
Structural gene	The gene of interest; its transcription is dependent on the repressor being absent from the operator site

3. Positive control systems require the binding of a protein to the operator site to increase transcription. Negative control systems require the binding of a protein to the operator site to decrease transcription.

7.5

1. Signal molecules include steroid hormones and second messengers, which bind to their receptors in the nucleus. These receptors are transcription factors that use their DNA-binding domain to attach to a particular sequence in DNA called a response element. Once bonded to the response element, these transcription factors can then promote increased expression of the relevant gene.
2. Histone deacetylation and DNA methylation will both downregulate the transcription of a gene. These processes allow the relevant DNA to be clumped more tightly, increasing the proportion of heterochromatin.

SCIENCE MASTERY ASSESSMENT EXPLANATIONS

1. **D**

Peptidyl transferase is an enzyme that catalyzes the formation of a peptide bond between the incoming amino acid in the A site and the growing polypeptide chain in the P site. Initiation and elongation factors help transport charged tRNA molecules into the ribosome and advance the ribosome down the mRNA transcript, as in **(A)** and **(B)**. Chaperones maintain a protein's three-dimensional shape as it is formed, as in **(C)**.

2. **C**

The promoter functions as a recruitment site for RNA polymerase and is required for gene expression. A mutation in this region would hinder RNA polymerase recruitment, resulting in a decrease in gene expression. These observations support **(C)** as the correct answer. By contrast, mutations in the operator and regulatory genes would render the repressor less able to block transcription, leading to the opposite effect, i.e. an increase in lactase expression. This result eliminates both **(A)** and **(B)**. Finally, mutations in the structural genes could lead to the production of a nonfunctional enzyme, but are unlikely to affect gene expression, eliminating **(D)**.

3. **A**

Topoisomerases, such as prokaryotic DNA gyrase, are involved in DNA replication and mRNA synthesis (transcription). DNA gyrase is a type of topoisomerase that enhances the action of helicase enzymes by the introduction of negative supercoils into the DNA molecule. These negative supercoils facilitate DNA replication by keeping the strands separated and untangled.

4. **C**

There are four different codons for valine: GUU, GUC, GUA, and GUG. Through base-pairing, we can determine that the proper anticodon must end with "AC." Remember that the codon and anticodon are antiparallel to each other, and that nucleic acids are always written $5' \rightarrow 3'$ on the MCAT. Therefore, we are looking for an answer that ends with "AC" (rather than starting with "CA").

5. **A**

Specific transcription factors bind to a specific DNA sequence, such as an enhancer, and to RNA polymerase at a single promoter sequence. They enable the RNA polymerase to transcribe the specific gene for that enhancer more efficiently.

6. **C**

UAG is one of the three known stop codons, so changing tyrosine to a stop codon must be a nonsense (or truncation) mutation.

7. **C**

In this question, the correct answer is the answer that is *not* associated with increased transcription. DNA methylation, **(C)**, is associated with silencing of gene expression. Regions of DNA with poor gene expression, called heterochromatin, are heavily methylated. These modifications significantly decrease the ability of RNA polymerase to access DNA.

8. **B**

The example given is a sample of repression due to the abundance of a corepressor. In other words, this is a repressible system that is currently blocking transcription. For the *trp* operon, an abundance of tryptophan in the environment allows for the repressor to bind tryptophan and then to the operator site. This blocks transcription of the genes required to synthesize tryptophan within the cell. The system described is a repressible system; the *lac* operon is an inducible system, in which an inducer binds to the repressor, thus permitting transcription.

9. **C**

shRNA (short hairpin RNA) is a useful biotechnology tool used in RNA interference. It is not, however, produced in the nucleus for use in the spliceosome. It targets mRNA to be degraded in the cytoplasm; it is not utilized in splicing of the hnRNA (heterogeneous nuclear RNA). snRNA (small nuclear RNA) and snRNPs (small nuclear ribonucleoproteins), however, do bind to the hnRNA to induce splicing.

10. **A**

In this table, we are given the sequence of the sense (coding) DNA strand. This will be identical to the mRNA transcript, except all thymine nucleotides will be replaced with uracil. With the deletion of these three bases, codon 507 changes from AUC to AUU in the transcript; these both code for isoleucine due to wobble. However, codon 508 (UUU in the transcript) has been lost. UUU codes for phenylalanine. The C-terminus sequence will remain unchanged because the deletion of three bases (exactly one codon) will not throw off the reading frame. For reference, the mutant reading frames would be:

(Note: refer back to Figure 7.5 for a table of the genetic code)

AUC	AUU	GGU	GUU	UCC

11. **B**

The intron will not be a part of the final, processed mRNA, and the untranslated regions of the mRNA will not be turned into amino acids. Translation will begin with codon 1 (which would be AUG). Because there are 150 amino acids, we can surmise that there will be 151 codons. Each codon will use 3 nucleotides, so $150 \times 3 = 450$ because codon 151 will be the stop codon.

12. **B**

Peptidyl transferase connects the incoming amino terminal to the previous carboxyl terminal; the only functional group listed here with a carbonyl and amino group is the amide. Peptide bonds are thus amide linkages, and the correct answer is **(B)**.

13. **A**

RNA polymerase I in eukaryotes is found in the nucleolus and is in charge of transcribing most of the rRNA for use during ribosomal creation. RNA polymerase II is responsible for hnRNA and snRNA. RNA polymerase III is responsible for tRNA and the 5S rRNA.

14. **B**

To answer this question correctly, we must remember that mRNA will be antiparallel to DNA. Our answer should be 5′ to 3′ mRNA, with the 5′ end complementary to the 3′ end of the DNA that is being transcribed. Thus, the mRNA transcribed from this strand will be 5′—GGAUGUCUCAAAGA—3′. mRNA contains uracil, rather than thymine.

15. **B**

The mRNA produced has the same structure as the sense strand of DNA (with uracils instead of thymines). Because bonding of nucleic acids is always complementary but antiparallel, the antisense strand of mRNA would be the one that binds to the produced mRNA, creating double-stranded RNA that is then degraded once found in the cytoplasm.

Consult your online resources for additional practice. GO ONLINE

SHARED CONCEPTS

Biochemistry Chapter 1
Amino Acids, Peptides, and Proteins

Biochemistry Chapter 2
Enzymes

Biochemistry Chapter 6
DNA and Biotechnology

Biology Chapter 1
The Cell

Biology Chapter 3
Embryogenesis and Development

Biology Chapter 12
Genetics and Evolution

CHAPTER 8

BIOLOGICAL MEMBRANES

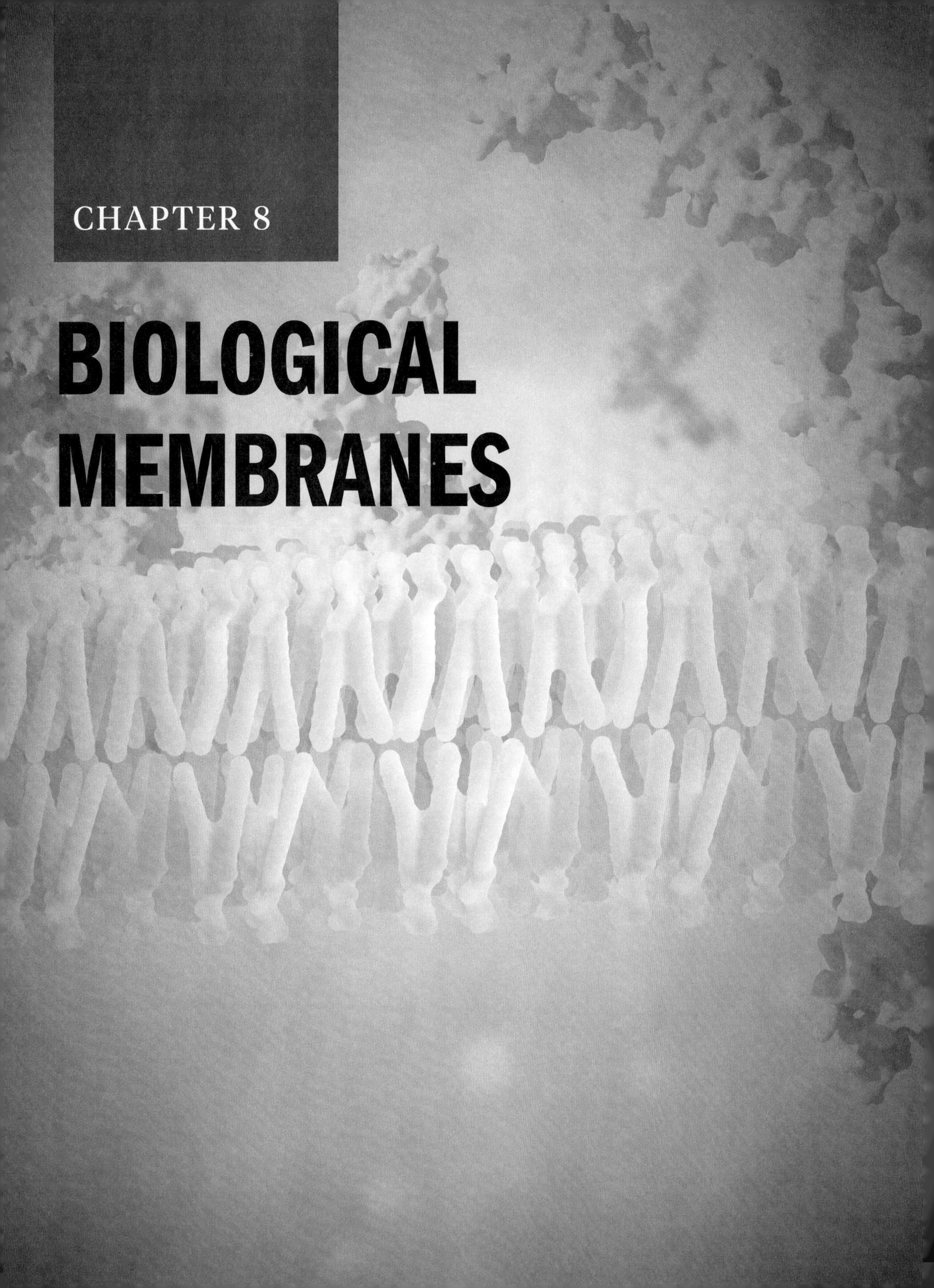

SCIENCE MASTERY ASSESSMENT

Every pre-med knows this feeling: there is so much content I have to know for the MCAT! How do I know what to do first or what's important?

While the high-yield badges throughout this book will help you identify the most important topics, this Science Mastery Assessment is another tool in your MCAT prep arsenal. This quiz (which can also be taken in your online resources) and the guidance below will help ensure that you are spending the appropriate amount of time on this chapter based on your personal strengths and weaknesses. Don't worry though—skipping something now does not mean you'll never study it. Later on in your prep, as you complete full-length tests, you'll uncover specific pieces of content that you need to review and can come back to these chapters as appropriate.

How to Use This Assessment

If you answer 0–7 questions correctly:

Spend about 1 hour to read this chapter in full and take limited notes throughout. Follow up by reviewing **all** quiz questions to ensure that you now understand how to solve each one.

If you answer 8–11 questions correctly:

Spend 20–40 minutes reviewing the quiz questions. Beginning with the questions you missed, read and take notes on the corresponding subchapters. For questions you answered correctly, ensure your thinking matches that of the explanation and you understand why each choice was correct or incorrect.

If you answer 12–15 questions correctly:

Spend less than 20 minutes reviewing all questions from the quiz. If you missed any, then include a quick read-through of the corresponding subchapters, or even just the relevant content within a subchapter, as part of your question review. For questions you got correct, ensure your thinking matches that of the explanation and review the Concept Summary at the end of the chapter.

1. A student is trying to determine the type of membrane transport occurring in a cell. The student finds that the molecule to be transported is very large and polar, and when transported across the membrane, no energy is required. Which of the following is the most likely mechanism of transport?
   - **A.** Active transport
   - **B.** Simple diffusion
   - **C.** Facilitated diffusion
   - **D.** Exocytosis

2. A researcher treats a solution containing animal cells with ouabain, a poisonous substance that interferes with the sodium–potassium ATPase embedded in the cell membrane, and the cell lyses as a result. Which of the following statements best describes ouabain's effects?
   - **A.** Treatment with ouabain results in high levels of extracellular calcium.
   - **B.** Treatment with ouabain results in high levels of extracellular potassium and sodium.
   - **C.** Treatment with ouabain increases intracellular concentrations of sodium.
   - **D.** Treatment with ouabain decreases intracellular concentrations of sodium.

3. Resting membrane potential depends on:
   - **I.** the differential distribution of ions across the membrane.
   - **II.** active transport processes.
   - **III.** selective permeability of the phospholipid bilayer.

   - **A.** I only
   - **B.** I and III only
   - **C.** II and III only
   - **D.** I, II, and III

4. Which of the following is NOT a function of the cell membrane?
   - **A.** Cytoskeletal attachment
   - **B.** Protein synthesis
   - **C.** Transport regulation
   - **D.** Second messenger reservoir

5. The dynamic properties of molecules in the cell membrane are most rapid in:
   - **A.** phospholipids moving within the plane of the membrane.
   - **B.** phospholipids moving between the layers of the membrane.
   - **C.** proteins moving within the plane of the membrane.
   - **D.** proteins exiting the cell through exocytosis.

6. Which lipid type is LEAST likely to contribute to membrane fluidity?
   - **A.** Unsaturated glycerophospholipids
   - **B.** *trans* glycerophospholipids
   - **C.** Cholesterol
   - **D.** Unsaturated sphingolipids

7. A membrane receptor is most likely to be a(n):
   - **A.** embedded protein with catalytic activity.
   - **B.** transmembrane protein with sequestration activity.
   - **C.** membrane-associated protein with sequestration activity.
   - **D.** transmembrane protein with catalytic activity.

8. Which of the following is NOT a cell–cell junction in animals?
   - **A.** Desmosomes
   - **B.** Gap junctions
   - **C.** Plasmodesmata
   - **D.** Tight junctions

9. Which of the following is true of diffusion and osmosis?

A. Diffusion and osmosis rely on the concentration gradient of only the compound of interest.
B. Diffusion and osmosis rely on the concentration gradient of all compounds in a cell.
C. Diffusion and osmosis will proceed in the same direction if there is only one solute.
D. Diffusion and osmosis cannot occur simultaneously.

10. The bulk movement of liquid into a cell through vesicular infoldings is known as:

A. phagocytosis.
B. pinocytosis.
C. exocytosis.
D. drinking.

11. Which of the following is LEAST likely to be the resting membrane potential of a cell?

A. −70 mV
B. −55 mV
C. 0 mV
D. +35 mV

12. How does the inner mitochondrial membrane differ from the outer mitochondrial membrane?

A. The inner mitochondrial membrane is more permeable and lacks cholesterol.
B. The inner mitochondrial membrane is less permeable and lacks cholesterol.
C. The inner mitochondrial membrane is more permeable and has cholesterol.
D. The inner mitochondrial membrane is less permeable and has cholesterol.

13. For most cells, the extracellular calcium concentration is around 10,000 times higher than the intracellular calcium concentration. What is the membrane potential established by this electrochemical gradient?

A. −123 mV
B. −61.5 mV
C. +61.5 mV
D. +123 mV

14. Which of the following statements conflicts with the fluid mosaic model?

A. The cell membrane is static in structure.
B. Membrane components can be derived from multiple biomolecules.
C. Hydrophobic interactions stabilize the lipid bilayer.
D. Proteins are asymmetrically distributed within the cell membrane.

15. Which of the following is a sphingolipid?

A. Lecithin
B. Phosphatidylinositol
C. Cholesterol
D. Ganglioside

Answer Key

1. **C**
2. **C**
3. **D**
4. **B**
5. **A**
6. **B**
7. **D**
8. **C**
9. **A**
10. **B**
11. **C**
12. **B**
13. **D**
14. **A**
15. **D**

Detailed explanations can be found at the end of the chapter.

CHAPTER 8

BIOLOGICAL MEMBRANES

In This Chapter

Introduction

Biological membranes are a stunning combination of opposites and contrasts. They are exceptionally thin, structurally bland, and relatively straightforward to describe. Yet, they define the borders of cells, tissues, and organelles; carry out a significant number of the biological functions within cells; and are an unending source of scientific inquiry and discovery. The most commonly tested biological membrane on the MCAT is the plasma membrane. At first, the plasma membrane seems like it's only a shell—just a barrier that defines the cell. But the plasma membrane plays roles in signaling, entry of nutrients and expulsion of waste, cell recognition, transport of materials between tissues, and even electronic functions.

Cell membranes have both a stretchy, flexible component (phospholipids) and an abundance of stabilizing molecules (cholesterol and protein) to make sure that everything remains intact. In this chapter, we will examine the general function, composition, and transport properties of biological membranes. We will conclude by taking a look at a few specialized cell membranes within the body, in addition to specific membrane properties.

CHAPTER PROFILE

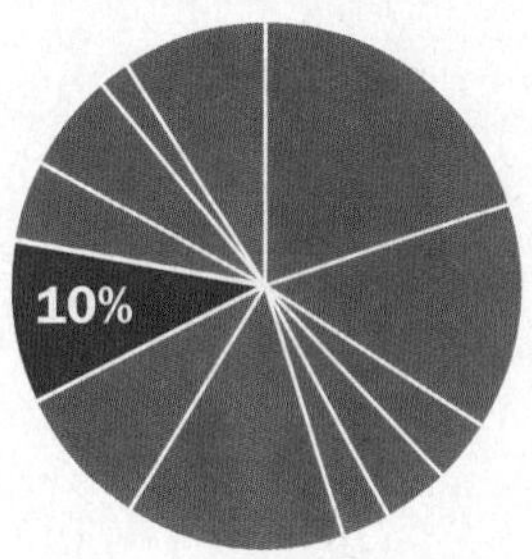

The content in this chapter should be relevant to about 10% of all questions about biochemistry on the MCAT.

This chapter covers material from the following AAMC content categories:

2A: Assemblies of molecules, cells, and groups of cells within single cellular and multicellular organisms

3A: Structure and functions of the nervous and endocrine systems, and ways in which these systems coordinate the organ systems

8.1 Fluid Mosaic Model

LEARNING OBJECTIVES

After Chapter 8.1, you will be able to:

- Describe the functions of flippases and lipid rafts
- Order a given list of membrane components from least to most abundant

The **cell (plasma) membrane** is often described as a semipermeable phospholipid bilayer. This phrase alone describes both the function and structure of the cell membrane: as a semipermeable barrier, it chooses which particles can enter and leave the cell at any point in time. This selectivity is mediated not only by the various channels and carriers that poke holes in the membrane, but also by the membrane itself. Composed primarily of two layers of phospholipids, the cell membrane permits fat-soluble compounds to cross easily, while larger and water-soluble compounds must seek alternative entry. The cell membrane is illustrated in Figure 8.1; the theory that underlies the structure and function of the cell membrane is referred to as the **fluid mosaic model**.

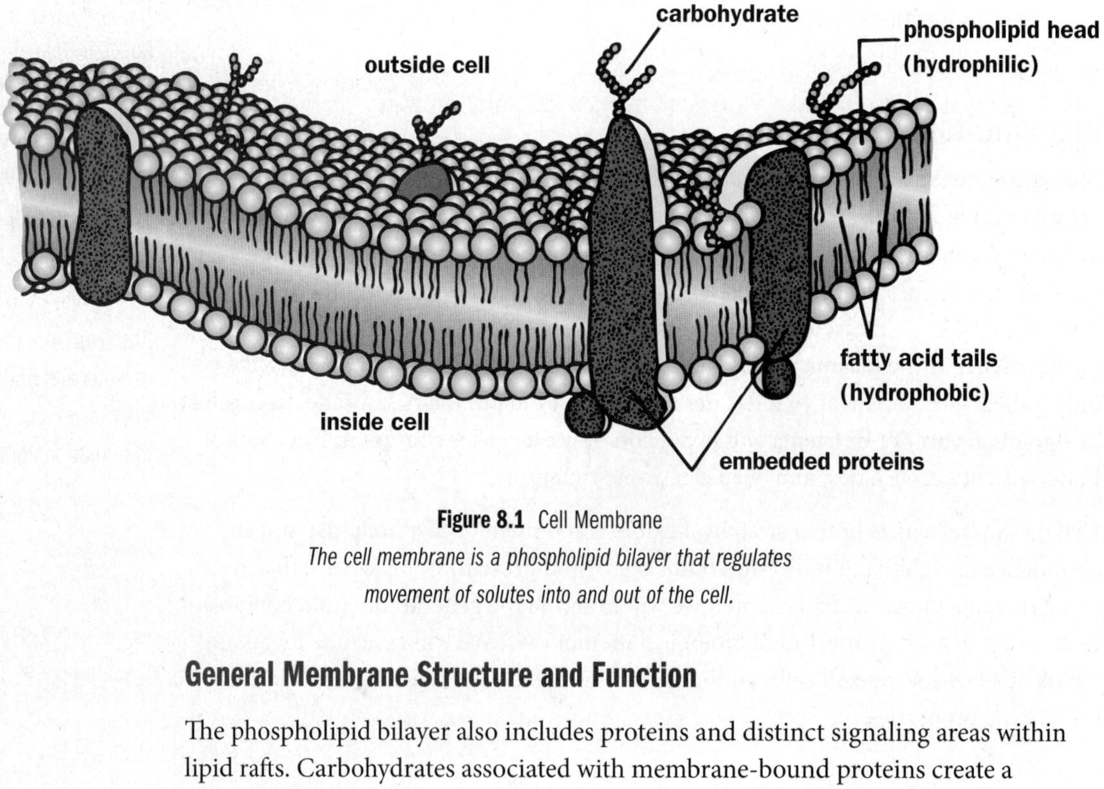

Figure 8.1 Cell Membrane
The cell membrane is a phospholipid bilayer that regulates movement of solutes into and out of the cell.

General Membrane Structure and Function

The phospholipid bilayer also includes proteins and distinct signaling areas within lipid rafts. Carbohydrates associated with membrane-bound proteins create a **glycoprotein coat**. The **cell wall** of plants, bacteria, and fungi contain higher levels of carbohydrates.

The main function of the cell membrane is to protect the interior of the cell from the external environment. Cellular membranes selectively regulate traffic into and out of the cell and are involved in both intracellular and intercellular communication and transport. Cell membranes also contain proteins embedded within the lipid bilayer that act as cellular receptors during signal transduction. These proteins play an important role in regulating and maintaining overall cellular activity.

Membrane Dynamics

The cell membrane functions as a stable semisolid barrier between the cytoplasm and the environment, but it is in a constant state of flux on the molecular level. **Phospholipids** move rapidly in the plane of the membrane through simple diffusion. This can be seen when fusing two membranes that have been tagged with different labels; the tags will migrate with their associated lipids until both types are rapidly intermixed. **Lipid rafts** are collections of similar lipids with or without associated proteins that serve as attachment points for other biomolecules; these rafts often serve roles in signaling. Both lipid rafts and proteins also travel within the plane of the membrane, but more slowly. Lipids can also move between the membrane layers, but this is energetically unfavorable because the polar head group of the phospholipid must be forced through the nonpolar tail region in the interior of the membrane. Specialized enzymes called **flippases** assist in the transition or "flip" between layers.

Dynamic changes in the concentrations of various membrane proteins are mediated by gene regulation, endocytotic activity, and protein insertion. Many cells, particularly those involved in biosignaling processes, can up- or downregulate the number of specific cellular receptors on their surface in order to meet cellular requirements.

REAL WORLD

Many antidepressants increase levels of neurotransmitters in the brain, but the effects take longer to appear than the changes in neurochemistry. The reason for this delay is that the nervous system must still upregulate its postsynaptic receptors to respond to the new levels of neurotransmitter.

MCAT CONCEPT CHECK 8.1

Before you move on, assess your understanding of the material with these questions.

1. Describe the role of flippases and lipid rafts in biological membranes.
   - Flippases:

   ____

   - Lipid rafts:

   ____

2. List the following membrane components in order from most plentiful to least plentiful: carbohydrates, lipids, proteins, nucleic acids.

   ________ > ________ > ________ > ________

8.2 Membrane Components

High-Yield

LEARNING OBJECTIVES

After Chapter 8.2, you will be able to:

- Describe the role of cholesterol in cell membranes
- Define the three classes of membrane proteins: transmembrane, embedded, and membrane-associated proteins
- Differentiate between gap junctions, tight junctions, desmosomes, and hemidesmosomes
- Identify level of saturation, as well as the hydrophilic and hydrophobic portions of a phospholipid:

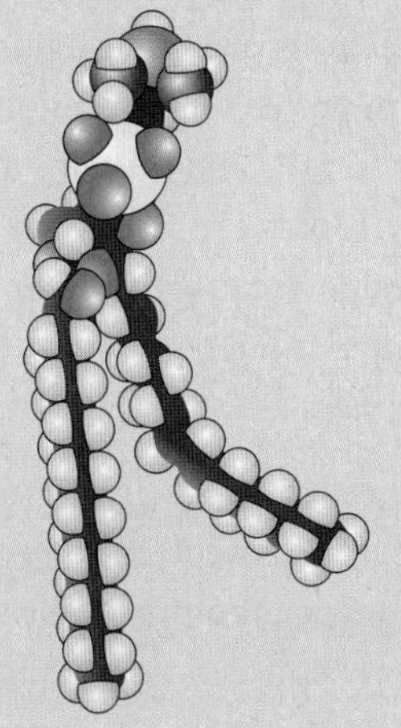

While the fluid mosaic model outlines the general composition of the membrane, the MCAT expects us to have a stronger grasp of the specifics, especially as it pertains to lipids and proteins.

Lipids

The cell membrane is composed predominantly of lipids with some associated proteins and carbohydrates. At times, the cell membrane as a whole will be referred to as a phospholipid bilayer, as it is the primary component of this barrier around the cell. Within the cell membrane, there are a large number of phospholipids with very few free fatty acids. In addition, steroid molecules and cholesterol, which lend fluidity to the membrane, and waxes, which provide membrane stability, help to maintain the structural integrity of the cell. While the structural details of these lipids were discussed in detail in Chapter 5 of *MCAT Biochemistry Review*, we will briefly describe their key points here.

Fatty Acids and Triacylglycerols

Fatty acids are carboxylic acids that contain a hydrocarbon chain and terminal carboxyl group. **Triacylglycerols**, also referred to as **triglycerides**, are storage lipids involved in human metabolic processes. They contain three fatty acid chains esterified to a glycerol molecule. Fatty acid chains can be saturated or unsaturated. **Unsaturated fatty acids** are regarded as "healthier" fats because they tend to have one or more double bonds and exist in liquid form at room temperature; in the plasma membrane, these characteristics impart fluidity to the membrane. Humans can only synthesize a few of the unsaturated fatty acids; the rest come from essential fatty acids in the diet that are transported as triacylglycerols from the intestine inside **chylomicrons**. Two important essential fatty acids for humans are *α-linolenic acid* and *linoleic acid*. **Saturated fatty acids** are the main components of animal fats and tend to exist as solids at room temperature. Saturated fats are found in processed foods and are considered less healthy. When incorporated into phospholipid membranes, saturated fatty acids decrease the overall membrane fluidity.

REAL WORLD

Trans fats, which result from the partial hydrogenation of some unsaturated fatty acids, have been banned from certain stores and cities because of their health risks. Part of the health concern is due to their ability to lower membrane fluidity, in addition to the tendency of *trans* fats to accumulate and form plaques in blood vessels.

Phospholipids

By substituting one of the fatty acid chains of triacylglycerol with a phosphate group, a polar head group joins the nonpolar tails, forming a **glycerophospholipid**, commonly called a phospholipid. Phospholipids spontaneously assemble into **micelles** (small monolayer vesicles) or **liposomes** (bilayered vesicles) due to hydrophobic interactions. Glycerophospholipids are used for membrane synthesis and can produce a hydrophilic surface layer on lipoproteins such as *very-low-density lipoprotein* (VLDL), a lipid transporter. In addition, phospholipids are the primary component of cell membranes. Phospholipids serve not only structural roles, but can also serve as second messengers in signal transduction. The phosphate group also provides an attachment point for water-soluble groups, such as *choline* (*phosphatidylcholine*, also known as *lecithin*) or *inositol* (*phosphatidylinositol*). A comparison of triacylglycerols and glycerophospholipids is shown in Figure 8.2.

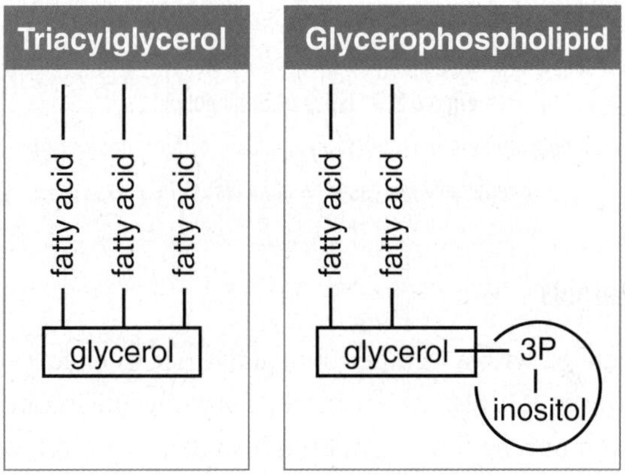

Figure 8.2 Triacylglycerol and Glycerophospholipid (Phosphatidylinositol)

MCAT EXPERTISE

The ratio of certain sphingolipids to glycerophospholipids can help to identify particular membranes within the cell, but memorizing this information is unnecessary for Test Day. Where small details like this are important, they will be provided in a passage.

Sphingolipids

Sphingolipids are also important constituents of cell membranes. Although sphingolipids do not contain glycerol, they are similar in structure to glycerophospholipids, in that they contain a hydrophilic region and two fatty acid–derived hydrophobic tails. The various classes of sphingolipids shown in Figure 8.3 differ primarily in the identity of their hydrophilic regions. Classes of sphingolipids and their hydrophilic groups include **ceramide**, **sphingomyelins**, **cerebrosides**, and **gangliosides**.

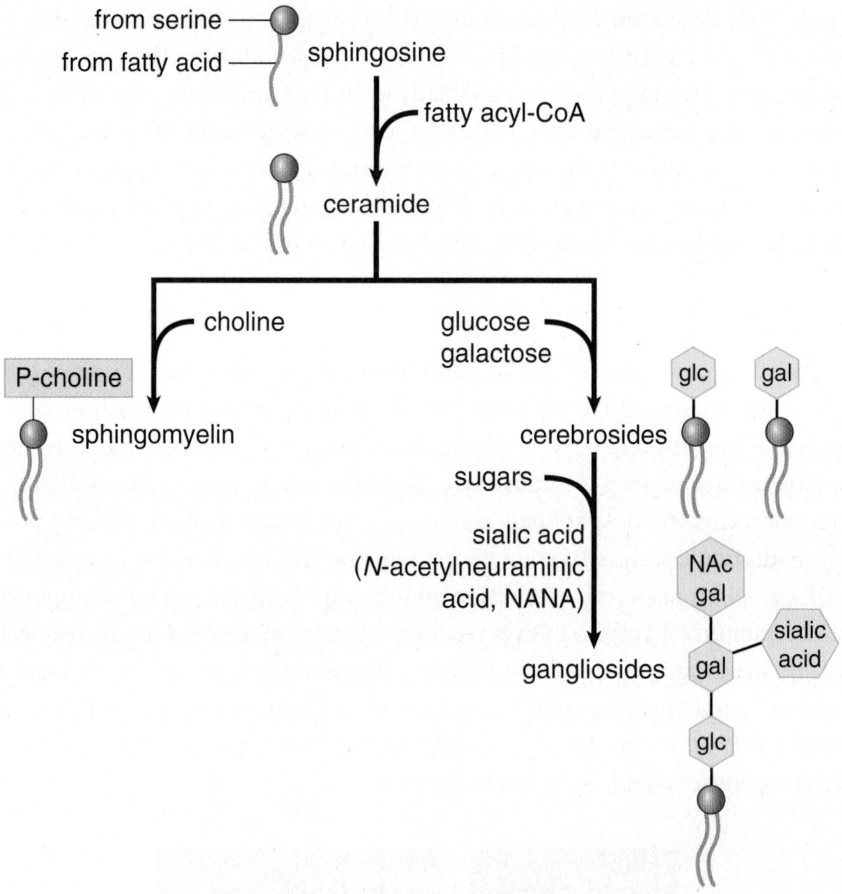

Figure 8.3 Types of Sphingolipids
Sphingolipids are sequentially modified to form each of the biologically necessary molecules in the class.

Cholesterol and Steroids

Cholesterol is associated with a number of negative health effects and receives a lot of negative press; however, it is also a very important molecule in our cells. **Cholesterol** not only regulates membrane fluidity, but it is also necessary in the synthesis of all **steroids**, which are derived from cholesterol.

The structure of cholesterol is similar to that of phospholipids in that cholesterol contains both a hydrophilic and hydrophobic region. Membrane stability is derived from interactions with both the hydrophilic and hydrophobic regions that make up the phospholipid bilayer. While cholesterol stabilizes adjacent phospholipids, it also occupies space between them. This prevents the formation of crystal structures in the membrane, increasing fluidity at lower temperatures. At high temperatures, cholesterol has the opposite effect: by limiting movement of phospholipids within the bilayer, it decreases fluidity and helps hold the membrane intact. By mass, cholesterol composes about 20 percent of the cell membrane; by mole fraction, it makes up about half. This large ratio of cholesterol to phospholipid ensures that the membrane remains fluid.

Waxes

Waxes are a class of lipids that are extremely hydrophobic and are rarely found in the cell membranes of animals, but are sometimes found in the cell membranes of plants. A wax is composed of a long-chain fatty acid and a long-chain alcohol, which contribute to the high melting point of these substances. When present within the cell membrane, waxes can provide both stability and rigidity within the nonpolar tail region only. Most waxes serve an extracellular function in protection or waterproofing.

Proteins

The **fluid mosaic model** also accounts for the presence of three types of membrane proteins, as shown in Figure 8.4. **Transmembrane proteins** pass completely through the lipid bilayer. **Embedded proteins**, on the other hand, are associated with only the interior (cytoplasmic) or exterior (extracellular) surface of the cell membrane. Together, transmembrane and embedded proteins are considered **integral proteins** because of their association with the interior of the plasma membrane, which is usually assisted by one or more membrane-associated domains that are partially hydrophobic. **Membrane-associated (peripheral) proteins** may be bound through electrostatic interactions with the lipid bilayer, especially at lipid rafts, or to other transmembrane or embedded proteins, like the G proteins found in G protein-coupled receptors. Transporters, channels, and receptors are generally transmembrane proteins.

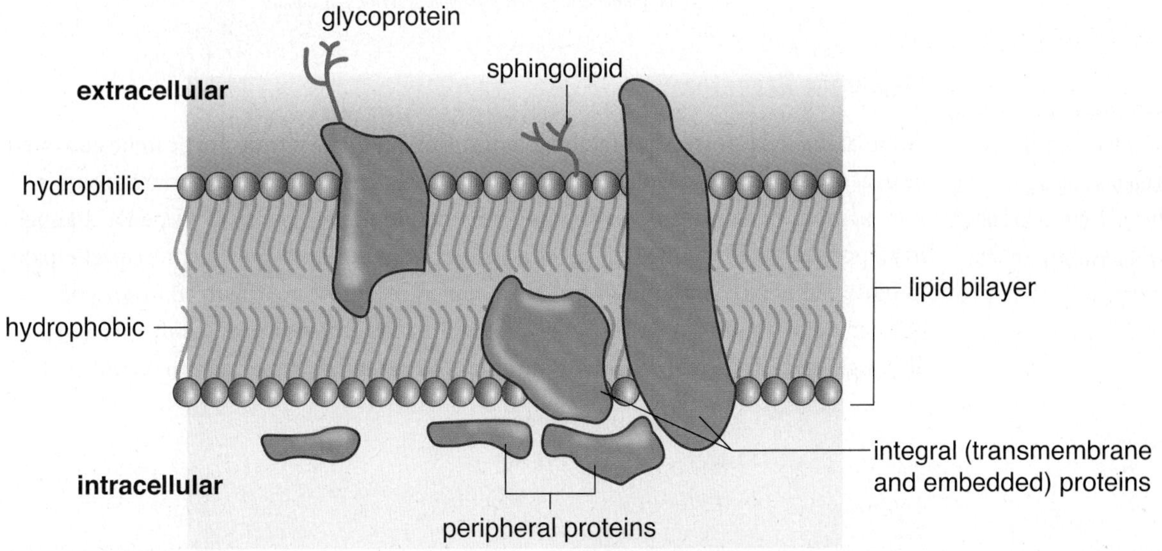

Figure 8.4 Plasma Membrane Proteins

Carbohydrates

Carbohydrates are generally attached to protein molecules on the extracellular surface of cells. Because carbohydrates are generally hydrophilic, interactions between glycoproteins and water can form a coat around the cell, as shown in Figure 8.5. In addition, carbohydrates can act as signaling and recognition molecules. For example, blood group (ABO) antigens on red blood cells are sphingolipids that differ only in their carbohydrate sequence. Our immune systems and some pathogens take advantage of these membrane carbohydrates and membrane proteins to target particular cells.

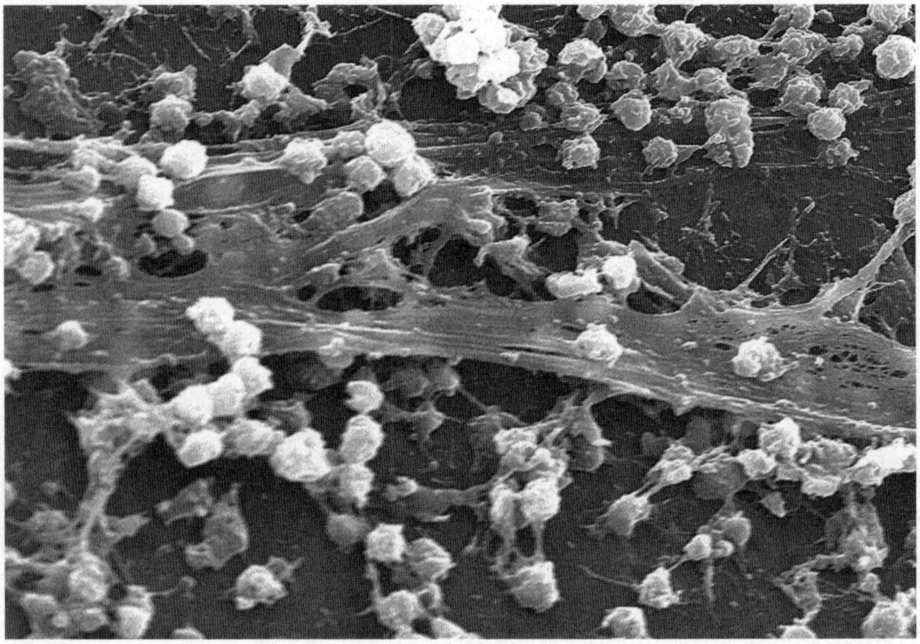

Figure 8.5 Extracellular Membrane-Associated Carbohydrates
Staphylococcus aureus bacteria embedded in bands of extracellular polysaccharides and glycolipids, forming a biofilm

BRIDGE

Biosignaling is a major function of the cell membrane. Receptors and signal cascades are covered in more detail in Chapter 3 of *MCAT Biochemistry Review*.

Membrane Receptors

Some of the transporters for facilitated diffusion and active transport can be activated or deactivated by **membrane receptors**, which tend to be transmembrane proteins. For example, ligand-gated ion channels are membrane receptors that open a channel in response to the binding of a specific ligand. Other membrane receptors participate in biosignaling; for example, G protein-coupled receptors are involved in several different signal transduction cascades. Membrane receptors are generally proteins, although there are some carbohydrate and lipid receptors, especially in viruses.

Cell–Cell Junctions

Cells within tissues can form a cohesive layer via intercellular junctions. These junctions provide direct pathways of communication between neighboring cells or between cells and the extracellular matrix. Cell–cell junctions are generally comprised of **cell adhesion molecules** (CAM), which are proteins that allow cells to recognize each other and contribute to proper cell differentiation and development.

Gap Junctions

Gap junctions allow for direct cell–cell communication and are often found in small bunches together. Gap junctions are also called **connexons** and are formed by the alignment and interaction of pores composed of six molecules of **connexin**, as shown in Figure 8.6. They permit movement of water and some solutes directly between cells. Proteins are generally not transferred through gap junctions.

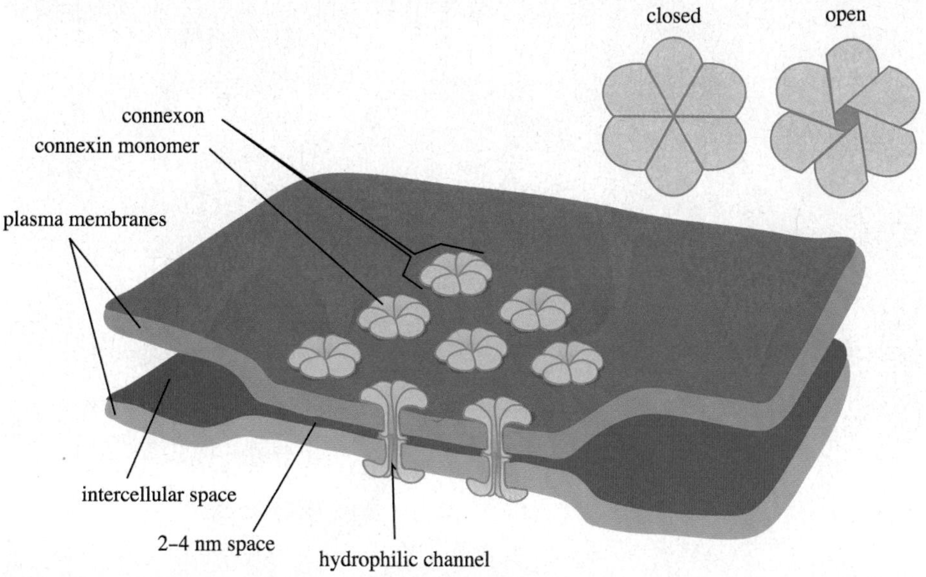

Figure 8.6 Gap Junction
A connexon (gap junction) is composed of six monomers of connexin and permits travel of solutes between cells.

Tight Junctions

Tight junctions prevent solutes from leaking into the space between cells via a **paracellular** route. Tight junctions are found in epithelial cells and function as a physical link between the cells as they form a single layer of tissue. Tight junctions can limit permeability enough to create a transepithelial voltage difference based on differing concentrations of ions on either side of the epithelium. To be effective, tight junctions must form a continuous band around the cell; otherwise, fluid could leak through spaces between tight junctions.

MNEMONIC

Tight junctions form a water**tight** seal, preventing paracellular transport of water and solutes.

BRIDGE

Tight junctions are found in the lining of renal tubules, where they restrict passage of solutes and water without cellular control. Nephrons are discussed in Chapter 10 of *MCAT Biology Review*.

Desmosomes

Desmosomes bind adjacent cells by anchoring to their cytoskeletons. Desmosomes are formed by interactions between transmembrane proteins associated with intermediate filaments inside adjacent cells, as shown in Figure 8.7. Desmosomes are primarily found at the interface between two layers of epithelial tissue. **Hemidesmosomes** have a similar function, but their main function is to attach epithelial cells to underlying structures, especially the basement membrane.

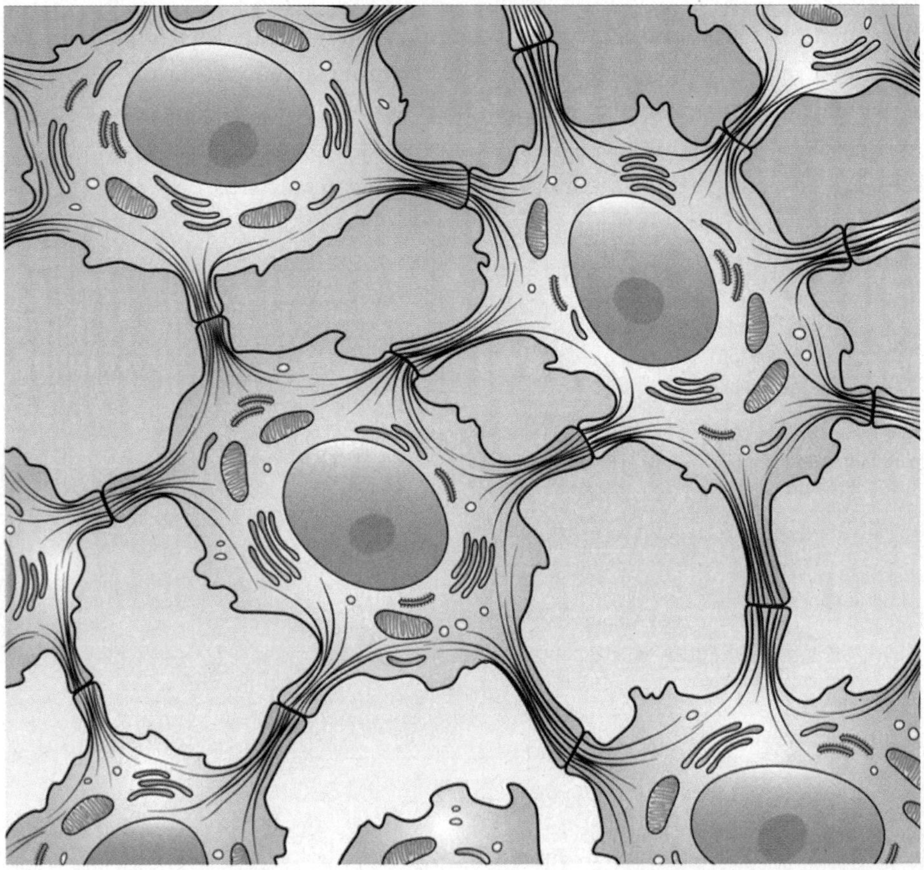

Figure 8.7 Desmosomes Between Adjacent Cells

MCAT CONCEPT CHECK 8.2

Before you move on, assess your understanding of the material with these questions.

1. In the following phospholipid, determine whether the fatty acids are saturated or unsaturated and label their hydrophobic and hydrophilic regions.

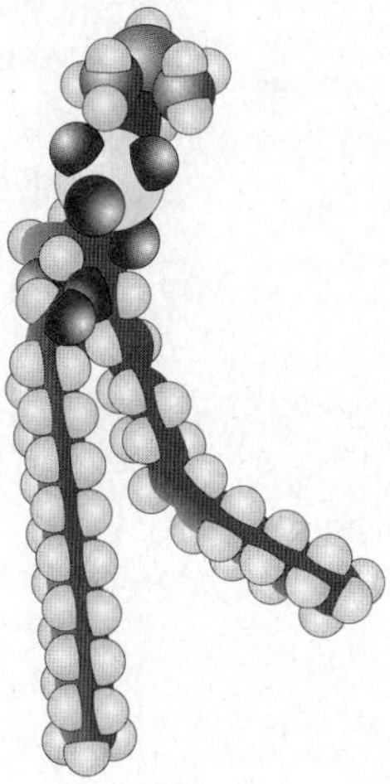

2. How does cholesterol play a role in the fluidity and stability of the plasma membrane?

____

3. What are the three classes of membrane proteins? How are they each most likely to function?

   1. ____
   2. ____
   3. ____

4. Contrast gap junctions and tight junctions.

   - Gap junctions:

____

   - Tight junctions:

____

BIOCHEMISTRY GUIDED EXAMPLE WITH EXPERT THINKING

Transplantation of pancreatic islets into patients who have Type 1 diabetes is hampered by inflammatory reactions at the transplantation site leading to dysfunction and death of insulin producing beta-cells. Recently, it was discovered that co-transplantation of neural crest stem cells (NCSCs) together with islet cells may improve transplantation outcomes. However, it could not be determined whether protection was obtained by the release of soluble factors, or whether direct cell–cell contact was required. Another investigation was conducted to describe the in vitro interaction between NCSCs and insulin-producing beta-TC6 cells that may mediate protection against cytokine-induced beta-cell death.

Problem statement: transplanting insulin producing cells causes inflammation, leading to failure of transplant

Possible solution: using NCSCs with transplant, but not sure how it works

Goal of study: figure out how NCSCs interact with pancreatic cells to protect against death

NCSCs were plated on laminin-coated plates or 0.4 micrometer cell inserts and after three days, beta-TC6 cells were added. The inserts allow for passage of soluble factors, but not direct cell-to-cell contact. After 48 hours, cytokines IL-1β and IFN-β were added. Finally, 48 hours later, cells were labeled with propidium iodide, trypsinized, and analyzed for cell death by flow cytometry. The experiment was repeated except that beta-TC6 cells were plated first, then NCSCs were added after 48 hours. Results plotted below are means for five independent experiments.
** denotes $p < 0.01$

Lots of sequential steps in the experimental setup, which may be important for understanding the figure. There's a specific order in which cells are plated, as well as whether inserts were used.

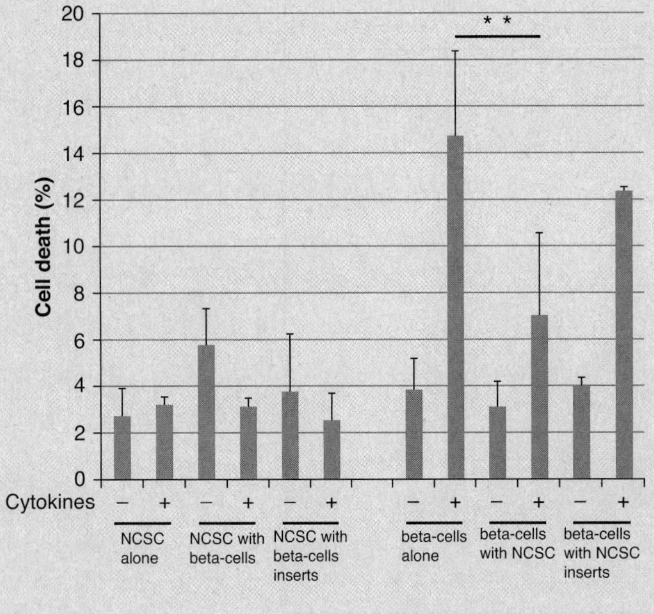

Figure 1

IV: order in which cell type plated, ECM or insert used, cytokine omitted or added

DV: cell death

Trend: significant difference between beta-cell alone and beta-cell with NCSC (no insert)

Adapted from Ngamjariyawat, A., Turpaev, K., Vasylovska, S., Kozlova, E. N., & Welsh, N. (2013). Co-culture of neural crest stem cells (NCSC) and insulin producing beta-TC6 cells results in cadherin junctions and protection against cytokine-induced beta-cell death. *PLoS One*, 8(4), e61828. doi:10.1371/journal.pone.0061828.

Based on this experiment, are NCSCs protecting beta islet cells from cytokine-induced cell death through direct contact, or through indirect contact?

Since the question requires data from the figure, we need to have a solid understanding of the results. The experimental question is asking whether beta-cells require direct contact with NCSCs, or whether the NCSCs are secreting soluble factors that are mediating protection from cytokine-mediated cell death. We'll need to refer to the passage for more information on these phenomena and how they interact. In the introduction to the experiment we can see that we are learning about co-transplantation of NCSCs and beta-cells, and that the experiments are trying to determine why co-transplantation is more effective than transplanting beta-cells alone. The way this was tested in the experimental setup is through the usage of cell inserts, which we are told in paragraph 2 will allow for the passage of factors, but not cell-cell contact.

The results on the left (first 6 bars) correspond to where NCSCs are plated first, then beta-cells are added with and without inserts. All 6 bars are roughly equal and the addition of cytokines do not seem to induce additional cell death, meaning these results cannot be used to make any conclusions since the expected control response (beta-cells inducing cell death in the presence of cytokines) is not shown. Taking a look at the next six columns in the graph, we can see that these are the experiments with the beta-cells being plated first. NCSCs were added 48 hours later, either with or without insert. The graph tells us that in the presence of cytokines, beta-cells alone show a high percentage of cell death (the expected control response), but having the NCSCs without insert shows a significant drop in cell death. This effect goes away when the insert is reintroduced: beta-cells with the NCSC insert have a higher level of cell death, though it's unclear whether that difference is significant.

Because the inserts obstruct cell-to-cell contact, we can conclude that direct contact between beta-cells and NCSCs is required for protection against cytokine-mediated cell death.

8.3 Membrane Transport

High-Yield

LEARNING OBJECTIVES

After Chapter 8.3, you will be able to:

- Explain the driving factors behind passive transport mechanisms
- Contrast symport and antiport mechanisms for active transport
- Relate osmotic pressure to the direction of osmosis:

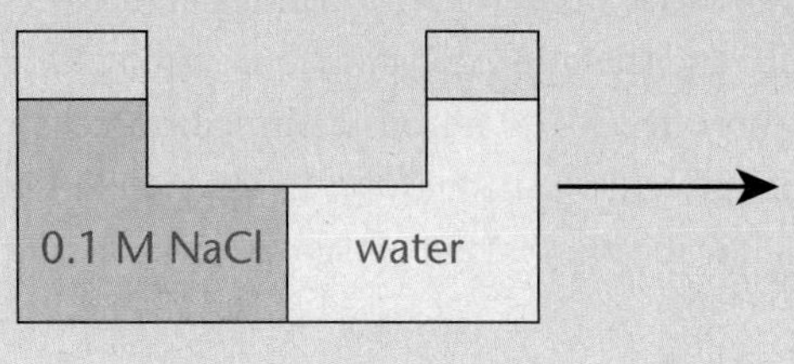

The cell membrane functions to control movement of substances into and out of the cell; however, it varies in its selectivity for different substances. Transport of small nonpolar molecules occurs rapidly through the cell membrane via diffusion, while ions and larger molecules require more specialized transport processes. The different membrane traffic processes are classified as either active or passive, and are driven by concentration gradients or intracellular energy stores.

MCAT EXPERTISE

An important point to keep in mind is that all transmembrane movement is based on concentration gradients, which are an MCAT favorite; understanding concentration gradients will net you points on Test Day. Remember that the gradient will tell us whether this process will be passive or active.

Concentration Gradients

Transport processes can be classified as active or passive depending on their thermodynamics. Spontaneous processes that do not require energy (negative ΔG) proceed through **passive transport**, while those that are nonspontaneous and require energy (positive ΔG) proceed through **active transport**. Diffusion, facilitated diffusion, and osmosis generally increase in rate as temperature increases, while active transport may or may not be affected by temperature, depending on the enthalpy (ΔH) of the process. The primary thermodynamic motivator in most passive transport is an increase in entropy (ΔS).

Passive Transport

Passive transport processes are those that do not require intracellular energy stores but rather utilize the concentration gradient to supply the energy for particles to move.

Simple Diffusion

The most basic of all membrane traffic processes is **simple diffusion**, in which substrates move down their concentration gradient directly across the membrane. Only particles that are freely permeable to the membrane are able to undergo simple diffusion. There is potential energy in a chemical gradient; some of this energy is dissipated as the gradient is utilized during simple diffusion. We can liken this process to a ball rolling down a hill: there is potential energy in the ball when it sits at the top of the hill, and as the ball spontaneously rolls down the hill, some of the energy is dissipated.

Osmosis

Osmosis is a specific kind of simple diffusion that concerns water; water will move from a region of lower solute concentration to one of higher solute concentration. That is, it will move from a region of higher water concentration (more dilute solution) down its gradient to a region of lower water concentration (more concentrated solution). Osmosis is important in several places, most notably when the solute itself is impermeable to the membrane. In such a case, water will move to try to bring solute concentrations to equimolarity, as shown in Figure 8.8. If the concentration of solutes inside the cell is higher than the surrounding solution, the solution is said to be **hypotonic**; such a solution will cause a cell to swell as water rushes in, sometimes to the point of bursting (lysing). A solution that is more concentrated than the cell is termed a **hypertonic** solution, and water will move out of the cell. If the solutions inside and outside are equimolar, they are said to be **isotonic**. A key point here is that isotonicity does not prevent movement; rather, it prevents the *net* movement of particles. Water molecules will continue to move; however, the cell will neither gain nor lose water overall.

REAL WORLD

Osmolarity explains why pure water should never be given intravenously for resuscitation. Red blood cells have an osmolarity around 300 $\frac{\text{mOsm}}{\text{L}}$, while pure water has an osmolarity of 0 $\frac{\text{mOsm}}{\text{L}}$. Water would rush into the red blood cells, causing them to burst. To avoid this, saline or dextrose-containing solutions are used.

MNEMONIC

To remember that water flows into a cell placed in hyp**O**tonic solution, imagine the cell swelling to form a giant letter **O**.

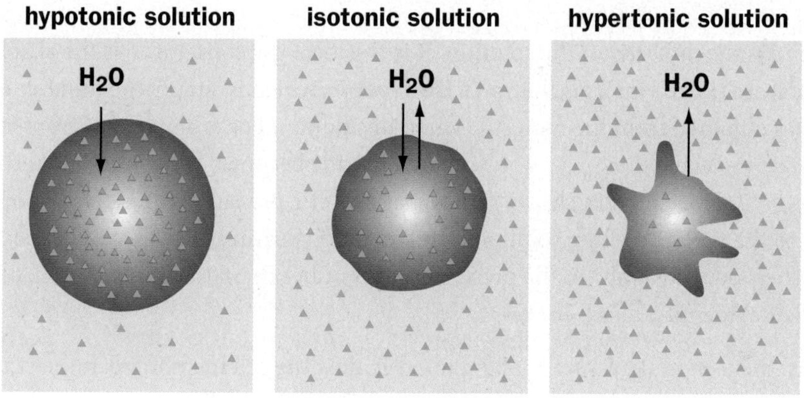

Figure 8.8 Osmosis
Water moves from areas of low solute (high water) concentration to high solute (low water) concentration.

One method of quantifying the driving force behind osmosis is osmotic pressure. **Osmotic pressure** is a **colligative property**: a physical property of solutions that is dependent on the concentration of dissolved particles but not on the chemical identity of those dissolved particles. Other examples of colligative properties include vapor pressure depression (Raoult's Law), boiling point elevation, and freezing point depression.

To illustrate osmotic pressure, consider a container separated into two compartments by a semipermeable membrane, just like the membranes in our cells. One compartment contains pure water, while the other contains water with dissolved solutes. The membrane allows water but not solutes to pass through. Because substances tend to flow, or diffuse, from higher to lower concentration (which results in an increase in entropy), water will diffuse from the compartment containing pure water into the compartment containing the water–solute mixture. This net flow will cause the water level in the compartment containing the solution to rise above the level in the compartment containing pure water, as shown in Figure 8.9.

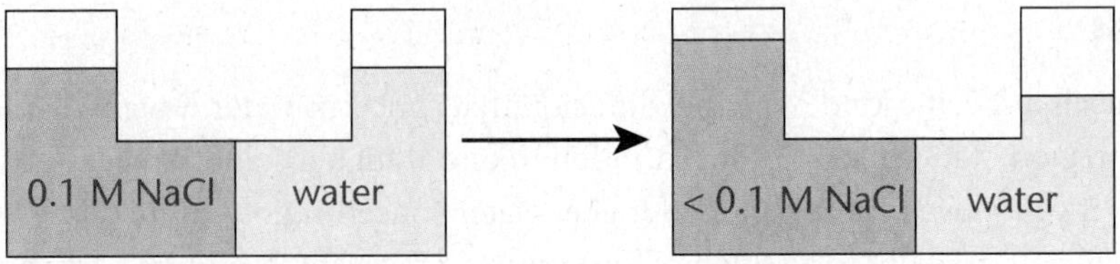

Figure 8.9 Change in Water Level Due to Osmotic Pressure

Because the solute cannot pass through the membrane, the concentrations of solute in the two compartments can never be equal. However, the hydrostatic pressure exerted by the water level in the solute-containing compartment will eventually oppose the influx of water; thus, the water level will only rise to the point at which it exerts a sufficient pressure to counterbalance the tendency of water to flow across the membrane. This pressure, defined as the **osmotic pressure** (Π) of the solution, is given by the formula:

$$\Pi = iMRT$$

Equation 8.1

where M is the molarity of the solution, R is the ideal gas constant, T is the absolute temperature (in kelvins), i is the **van't Hoff factor**, which is simply the number of particles obtained from the molecule when in solution. For example, glucose remains one intact molecule, so $i_{\text{glucose}} = 1$; sodium chloride becomes two ions (Na^+ and Cl^-), so $i_{\text{NaCl}} = 2$. The equation clearly shows that osmotic pressure is directly proportional to the molarity of the solution. Thus, osmotic pressure, like all colligative properties, depends only on the presence and number of particles in solution, but not their actual identity.

In cells, the osmotic pressure is maintained against the cell membrane, rather than the force of gravity. If the osmotic pressure created by the solutes within a cell exceeds the pressure that the cell membrane can withstand, the cell will lyse. Generally, osmotic pressure is best thought of as a "sucking" pressure, drawing water into the cell in proportion to the concentration of the solution.

Facilitated Diffusion

KEY CONCEPT

Unless otherwise specified, *semipermeable membrane* refers to a membrane governed by the same permeability rules as biological membranes: small, nonpolar, lipid-soluble particles (and water) can pass through freely, while large, polar, or charged particles cannot.

Facilitated diffusion is simple diffusion for molecules that are impermeable to the membrane (large, polar, or charged); the energy barrier is too high for these molecules to cross freely. Facilitated diffusion requires integral membrane proteins to serve as transporters or channels for these substrates.

The classic examples of facilitated diffusion involve a carrier or channel protein. **Carriers** are only open to one side of the cell membrane at any given point. This model is similar to a revolving door because the substrate binds to the transport protein (walks in), remains in the transporter during a conformational change (spins), and then finally dissociates from the substrate-binding site of the transporter (walks out). Binding of the substrate molecule to the transporter protein induces a conformational change; for a brief time, the carrier is in the **occluded state**, in which the carrier is not open to either side of the phospholipid bilayer. In addition to carriers, **channels** are also viable transporters for facilitated diffusion. Channels may be in an open or closed conformation. In their open conformation, channels are exposed to both sides of the cell membrane and act like a tunnel for the particles to diffuse through, thereby permitting much more rapid transport kinetics. The activity of the three main types of ion channels is discussed in Chapter 3 of *MCAT Biochemistry Review*.

Active Transport

Active transport results in the net movement of a solute against its concentration gradient, just like rolling a ball uphill. Active transport always requires energy, but the source of this energy can vary. **Primary active transport** uses ATP or another energy molecule to directly power the transport of molecules across a membrane. Generally, primary active transport involves the use of a *transmembrane ATPase*. **Secondary active transport**, also known as **coupled transport**, also uses energy to transport particles across the membrane; however, in contrast to primary active transport, there is no direct coupling to ATP hydrolysis. Instead, secondary active transport harnesses the energy released by one particle going *down* its electrochemical gradient to drive a different particle *up* its gradient. When both particles flow the same direction across the membrane, it is termed **symport**. When the particles flow in opposite directions, it is called **antiport**. Active transport is important in many tissues. For instance, primary active transport maintains the membrane potential of neurons in the nervous system. The kidneys use secondary active transport, usually driven by sodium, to reabsorb and secrete various solutes into and out of the filtrate.

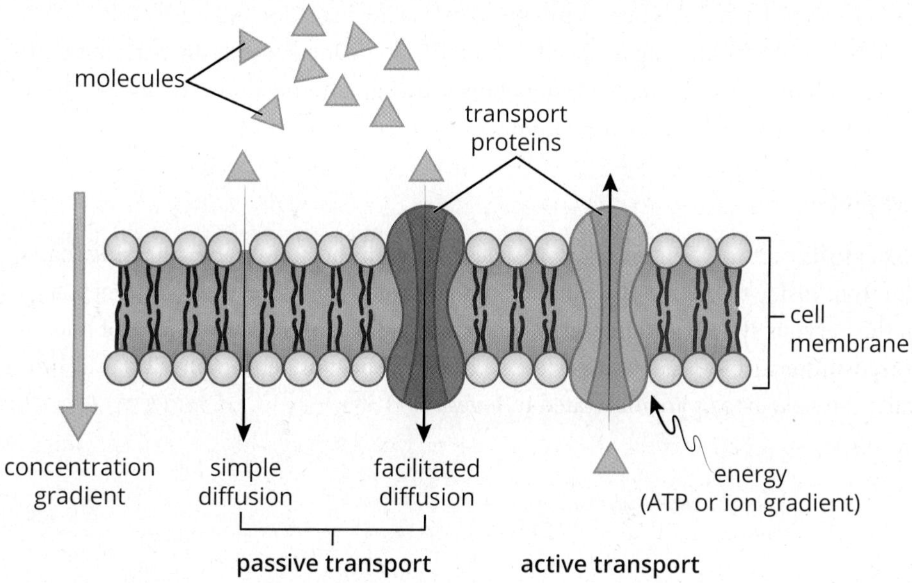

Figure 8.10 Membrane Transport Processes
The movement of solutes across the cell membrane is mediated by concentration gradients.

Figure 8.10 shows simple diffusion, facilitated diffusion, and active transport. Table 8.1 summarizes these types of movement as well as osmosis.

	SIMPLE DIFFUSION	OSMOSIS	FACILITATED DIFFUSION	ACTIVE TRANSPORT
Concentration gradient of solute	High → Low	Low → High	High → Low	Low → High
Membrane protein required	No	No	Yes	Yes
Energy required	No—this is a passive process	No—this is a passive process	No—this is a passive process	Yes—this is an active process; requires energy
Example molecule(s) transported	Small, nonpolar (O_2, CO_2)	H_2O	Polar molecules (glucose) or ions (Na^+, Cl^-)	Polar molecules or ions (Na^+, Cl^-, K^+)

Table 8.1 Membrane Transport Processes

Endocytosis and Exocytosis

Endocytosis

Endocytosis occurs when the cell membrane invaginates and engulfs material to bring it into the cell. The material is encased in a vesicle, which is important because cells will sometimes ingest toxic substances. **Pinocytosis** is the endocytosis of fluids and dissolved particles, whereas **phagocytosis** is the ingestion of large solids such as bacteria. Substrate binding to specific receptors embedded within the plasma membrane will initiate the process of endocytosis. Invagination will then be initiated and carried out by **vesicle-coating proteins**, most notably clathrin.

Exocytosis

Exocytosis occurs when secretory vesicles fuse with the membrane, releasing material from inside the cell to the extracellular environment. Exocytosis is important in the nervous system and intercellular signaling. For instance, exocytosis of neurotransmitters from synaptic vesicles is a crucial aspect of neuron physiology. Both endo- and exocytosis are illustrated in Figure 8.11.

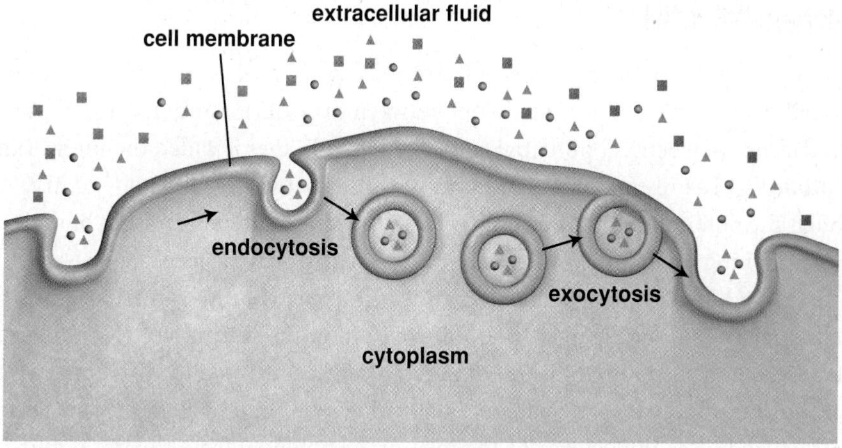

Figure 8.11 Endocytosis and Exocytosis

MCAT CONCEPT CHECK 8.3

Before you move on, assess your understanding of the material with these questions.

1. What is the primary thermodynamic factor responsible for passive transport?

____

2. What is the relationship between osmotic pressure and the direction of osmosis through a semipermeable membrane?

____

3. Compare the two types of active transport. What is the difference between symport and antiport?

____

8.4 Specialized Membranes

LEARNING OBJECTIVES

After Chapter 8.4, you will be able to:

- Identify the channels involved in maintenance of the resting membrane potential
- Calculate resting membrane potential using the Nernst equation
- Distinguish between the different regions of the mitochondrion

The membranes of most organelles are similar to the cell membrane in both composition and general characteristics; however, it is important to note that some membranes are specialized to accomplish specific functions. For instance, the sarcolemma of muscle cells must maintain a membrane potential for muscle contraction to occur. Membrane composition may also be altered slightly, especially in the case of mitochondria.

Membrane Potential

The impermeability of the cell membrane to ions and the selectivity of ion channels both lead to an electrochemical gradient between the exterior and interior of cells. The difference in electrical potential across cell membranes is called the **membrane potential,** V_m. The resting potential for most cells is between -40 and -80 mV, although the potential can rise as high as $+35$ mV during depolarization of the cell. Maintaining membrane potential requires energy because ions may passively diffuse through the cell membrane over time using **leak channels**; therefore, an ion transporter or pump such as the **sodium–potassium pump (Na^+/K^+ ATPase)** regulates the concentration of intracellular and extracellular sodium and potassium ions. Chloride ions also participate in establishing membrane potential. The **Nernst equation** can be used to determine the membrane potential from the intra- and extracellular concentrations of the various ions:

$$E = \frac{RT}{zF}\ln\frac{[\text{ion}]_{\text{outside}}}{[\text{ion}]_{\text{inside}}} = \frac{61.5}{z}\log\frac{[\text{ion}]_{\text{outside}}}{[\text{ion}]_{\text{inside}}}$$

Equation 4.2

where R is the ideal gas constant, T is the temperature in kelvins, z is the charge of the ion, and F is the Faraday constant $\left(96{,}485\ \frac{\text{C}}{\text{mol } e^-}\right)$. The simplification to 61.5 in the numerator assumes body temperature, 310 K. The **Goldman–Hodgkin–Katz voltage equation** flows from the Nernst equation, taking into account the relative contribution of each major ion to the membrane potential:

$$V_m = 61.5\log\left[\frac{P_{Na^+}\times[Na^+]_{\text{outside}} + P_{K^+}\times[K^+]_{\text{outside}} + P_{Cl^-}\times[Cl^-]_{\text{inside}}}{P_{Na^+}\times[Na^+]_{\text{inside}} + P_{K^+}\times[K^+]_{\text{inside}} + P_{Cl^-}\times[Cl^-]_{\text{outside}}}\right]$$

Equation 4.3

where P represents the permeability for the relevant ion. Note that chloride is inverted relative to the other ions because it carries a negative charge.

BRIDGE

The cell membrane is often compared to a capacitor because opposite charges are maintained on either side of the membrane. Capacitance is discussed in Chapter 6 of *MCAT Physics and Math Review.*

Sodium-Potassium Pump

There is a steady-state resting relationship between ion diffusion and the **Na^+/K^+ ATPase**. One of the main functions of the Na^+/K^+ ATPase is to maintain a low concentration of sodium ions and high concentration of potassium ions intracellularly by pumping three sodium ions out for every two potassium ions pumped in. This movement of ions removes one positive charge from the intracellular space of the cell, which maintains the negative resting potential of the cell. As mentioned before, the cell membrane also contains leak channels that allow ions, such as Na^+ and K^+, to passively diffuse into or out of the cell down their concentration gradients. Cell membranes are more permeable to K^+ ions than Na^+ ions at rest because there are more K^+ leak channels than Na^+ leak channels. The combination of Na^+/K^+ ATPase activity and leak channels together maintain a stable resting membrane potential.

Mitochondrial Membranes

Mitochondria are referred to as the "powerhouse" of the cell because of their ability to produce ATP by oxidative respiration. Mitochondria contain two membranes: the inner and outer mitochondrial membranes.

Outer Mitochondrial Membrane

The **outer mitochondrial membrane** is highly permeable due to many large pores that allow the passage of ions and small proteins. The outer membrane completely surrounds the inner mitochondrial membrane, with the presence of a small **intermembrane space** in between the two layers.

Inner Mitochondrial Membrane

The **inner mitochondrial membrane** has a much more restricted permeability compared to the outer mitochondrial membrane. Structurally, the inner mitochondrial membrane contains numerous infoldings, known as **cristae**, which increase the available surface area for the integral proteins associated with the membrane. These proteins, discussed in Chapter 10 of *MCAT Biochemistry Review*, are involved in the electron transport chain and ATP synthesis. The inner membrane also encloses the **mitochondrial matrix**, where the citric acid cycle produces high-energy electron carriers used in the electron transport chain. The inner mitochondrial membrane contains a very high level of *cardiolipin* and does not contain cholesterol.

MCAT CONCEPT CHECK 8.4

Before you move on, assess your understanding of the material with these questions.

1. How is the resting membrane potential maintained?

____

____

____

2. Given the following data, calculate the resting membrane potential of this cell:

Ion	Permeability (Relative)	Intracellular Concentration	Extracellular Concentration
Na^+	0.05	14 mM	140 mM
K^+	1	120 mM	4 mM
Cl^-	0	12 mM	120 mM

____

____

____

3. What distinguishes the inner mitochondrial membrane from other biological membranes? What is the pH gradient between the cytoplasm and the intermembrane space?

____

____

____

Conclusion

Understanding biological membranes becomes increasingly important as you progress in your medical career. At this point, you should have a strong foundation of knowledge about the fluid mosaic model and how membranes exist dynamically. We've also covered the components of cell membranes, with a special emphasis on lipids and the phospholipid bilayer. We reviewed some basic physical properties of the cell, including cell–cell junctions. We also examined membrane transport, such as passive transport (simple diffusion, facilitated diffusion, and osmosis) and active transport, before briefly touching upon endocytosis and exocytosis. Finally, we reviewed specialized membranes within cells. Up to now, you have been exposed to each of the classes of molecules and some of their applications both experimentally and within the cell. This comprehensive review should provide you with a better understanding of what will be expected of you on Test Day and briefly introduce you to topics that you will learn more about in medical school.

The first seven chapters of *MCAT Biochemistry Review* focused on various types of biomolecules, their structures, and their functions. In this chapter, we applied this knowledge of biomolecules to make sense of biological membranes. In the remaining four chapters, we'll turn our attention to the metabolic pathways by which the body builds, stores, and burns these biomolecules.

You've reviewed the content, now test your knowledge and critical thinking skills by completing a test-like passage set in your online resources!

GO ONLINE

CONCEPT SUMMARY

Fluid Mosaic Model

- The **fluid mosaic model** accounts for the presence of lipids, proteins, and carbohydrates in a dynamic, semisolid plasma membrane that surrounds cells.
- The plasma membrane contains proteins embedded within the **phospholipid bilayer**.
- The membrane is not static.
    - Lipids move freely in the plane of the membrane and can assemble into **lipid rafts**.
    - **Flippases** are specific membrane proteins that maintain the bidirectional transport of lipids between the layers of the phospholipid bilayer in cells.
    - Proteins and carbohydrates may also move within the membrane, but are slowed by their relatively large size.

Membrane Components

- Lipids are the primary membrane component, both by mass and mole fraction.
    - **Triacylglycerols** and **free fatty acids** act as phospholipid precursors and are found in low levels in the membrane.
    - **Glycerophospholipids** replace one fatty acid with a phosphate group, which is often linked to other hydrophilic groups.
    - **Cholesterol** is present in large amounts and contributes to membrane fluidity and stability.
    - **Waxes** are present in very small amounts, if at all; they are most prevalent in plants and function in waterproofing and defense.
- Proteins located within the cell membrane act as transporters, cell adhesion molecules, and enzymes.
    - **Transmembrane proteins** can have one or more hydrophobic domains and are most likely to function as receptors or channels.
    - **Embedded proteins** are most likely part of a catalytic complex or involved in cellular communication.
    - **Membrane-associated proteins** may act as recognition molecules or enzymes.
- Carbohydrates can form a protective **glycoprotein coat** and also function in cell recognition.
- Extracellular ligands can bind to membrane receptors, which function as channels or enzymes in second messenger pathways.

- Cell–cell junctions regulate transport intracellularly and intercellularly.
  - **Gap junctions** allow for the rapid exchange of ions and other small molecules between adjacent cells.
  - **Tight junctions** prevent **paracellular** transport, but do not provide intercellular transport.
  - **Desmosomes** and **hemidesmosomes** anchor layers of epithelial tissue together.

Membrane Transport

- **Concentration gradients** help to determine appropriate membrane transport mechanisms in cells.
- **Osmotic pressure**, a **colligative property**, is the pressure applied to a pure solvent to prevent osmosis and is used to express the concentration of the solution.
  - It is often better conceptualized as a "sucking" pressure in which a solution is drawing water in, proportional to its concentration.
- **Passive transport** does not require energy because the molecule is moving down its concentration gradient or from an area with higher concentration to an area with lower concentration.
  - **Simple diffusion** does not require a transporter. Small, nonpolar molecules passively move from an area of high concentration to an area of low concentration until equilibrium is achieved.
  - **Osmosis** describes the diffusion of water across a selectively permeable membrane.
  - **Facilitated diffusion** uses transport proteins to move impermeable solutes across the cell membrane.
- **Active transport** requires energy in the form of ATP or an existing favorable ion gradient.
  - Active transport may be **primary** or **secondary** depending on the energy source. Secondary active transport can be further classified as **symport** or **antiport**.
- **Endocytosis** and **exocytosis** are methods of engulfing material into cells or releasing material to the exterior of cells, both via the cell membrane. **Pinocytosis** is the ingestion of liquid into the cell in vesicles formed from the cell membrane and **phagocytosis** is the ingestion of larger, solid molecules.

Specialized Membranes

- The composition of cell membranes is fairly consistent; however, there are some cells that contain specialized membranes.
- **Membrane potential** is maintained by the sodium–potassium pump and leak channels.
  - The electrical potential created by one ion can be calculated using the **Nernst equation**.
  - The resting potential of a membrane at physiological temperature can be calculated using the **Goldman–Hodgkin–Katz voltage equation**, which is derived from the Nernst equation.
- The mitochondrial membrane differs from the cell membrane:
  - The outer mitochondrial membrane is highly permeable to metabolic molecules and small proteins.
  - The inner mitochondrial membrane surrounds the mitochondrial matrix, where the citric acid cycle produces electrons used in the electron transport chain and where many other enzymes important in cellular respiration are located. The inner mitochondrial membrane also does not contain cholesterol.

ANSWERS TO CONCEPT CHECKS

8.1

1. Flippases are responsible for the movement of phospholipids between the layers of the plasma membrane because it is otherwise energetically unfavorable. Lipid rafts are aggregates of specific lipids in the membrane that function as attachment points for other biomolecules and play roles in signaling.
2. Lipids, including phospholipids, cholesterol, and others, are most plentiful; proteins, including transmembrane proteins (channels and receptors), membrane-associated proteins, and embedded proteins, are next most plentiful; carbohydrates, including the glycoprotein coat and signaling molecules, are next; nucleic acids are essentially absent.

8.2

1. The hydrophilic region is at the top of this diagram. While you need not be able to recognize it, the head group is phosphatidylcholine in this example. The hydrophobic region is at the bottom and is composed of two fatty acid tails. The tail on the left is saturated; the tail on the right is unsaturated, as evidenced by the kink in its chain.
2. Cholesterol moderates membrane fluidity by interfering with the crystal structure of the cell membrane and occupying space between phospholipid molecules at low temperatures, and by restricting excessive movement of phospholipids at high temperatures. Cholesterol also provides stability by cross-linking adjacent phospholipids through interactions at the polar head group and hydrophobic interactions at the nearby fatty acid tail.
3. Transmembrane proteins are most likely to serve as channels or receptors. Embedded membrane proteins are most likely to have catalytic activity linked to nearby enzymes. Membrane-associated (peripheral) proteins are most likely to be involved in signaling or are recognition molecules on the extracellular surface.
4. Gap junctions allow for the intercellular transport of materials and do not prevent paracellular transport of materials. Tight junctions are not used for intercellular transport but do prevent paracellular transport. Gap junctions are in discontinuous bunches around the cell, while tight junctions form bands around the cell.

8.3

1. The primary thermodynamic factor responsible for passive transport is entropy.
2. As osmotic pressure increases, more water will tend to flow into the compartment to decrease solute concentration. Osmotic pressure is often considered a "sucking" pressure because water will move toward the compartment with the highest osmotic pressure.
3. Primary active transport uses ATP as an energy source for the movement of molecules against their concentration gradient, while secondary active transport uses an electrochemical gradient to power the transport. Symport moves both particles in secondary active transport across the membrane in the same direction, while antiport moves particles across the cell membrane in opposite directions.

8.4

1. The membrane potential, which results from a difference in the number of positive and negative charges on either side of the membrane, is maintained primarily by the sodium–potassium pump, which moves three sodium ions out of the cell for every two potassium ions pumped in, and to a minor extent by leak channels that allow the passive transport of ions.
2. $$V_m = 61.5 \log \left[\frac{P_{Na^+} \times [Na^+]_{outside} + P_{K^+} \times [K^+]_{outside} + P_{Cl^-} \times [Cl^-]_{inside}}{P_{Na^+} \times [Na^+]_{inside} + P_{K^+} \times [K^+]_{inside} + P_{Cl^-} \times [Cl^-]_{outside}}\right]$$
$$= 61.5 \log \left[\frac{0.05 \times [140] + 1 \times [4] + 0 \times [12]}{0.05 \times [14] + 1 \times [120] + 0 \times [120]}\right] = 61.5 \log \left[\frac{7 + 4}{0.7 + 120}\right]$$
$$= 61.5 \log \left[\frac{11}{120.7}\right] \approx 60 \log \frac{1}{10} = -60\ \text{mV}$$

   The exact value is -64.0 mV
3. The inner mitochondrial membrane lacks cholesterol, which differentiates it from most other biological membranes. There is no pH gradient between the cytoplasm and the intermembrane space because the outer mitochondrial membrane has such high permeability to biomolecules (the proton-motive force of the mitochondria is across the inner mitochondrial membrane, not the outer mitochondrial membrane).

SCIENCE MASTERY ASSESSMENT EXPLANATIONS

1. **C**

We are asked to identify the type of transport that would allow a large, polar molecule to cross the membrane without any energy expenditure. This scenario describes facilitated diffusion, which uses a transport protein (or channel) to facilitate the movement of large, polar molecules across the nonpolar, hydrophobic membrane. Facilitated diffusion, like simple diffusion, does not require energy.

2. **C**

This question requires an understanding of osmosis and the action of the sodium–potassium pump. When a cell is placed in a hypertonic solution (a solution having a higher solute concentration than the cell), fluid will diffuse out of the cell and result in cell shrinkage. When a cell is placed in hypotonic solution (a solution having a lower solute concentration than the cell), fluid will diffuse from the solution into the cell, causing the cell to expand and possibly lyse. The sodium–potassium pump moves three sodium ions out of the cell for every two potassium ions it lets into the cell. Therefore, inhibition of the sodium–potassium pump by ouabain will cause a net increase in the sodium concentration inside the cell and water will diffuse in, causing the cell to swell and then lyse.

3. **D**

The polarization of the membrane at rest is the result of an uneven distribution of ions between the inside and outside of the cell. This difference is achieved through active pumping of ions (predominantly sodium and potassium) into and out of the cell and the selective permeability of the membrane, which allows only certain ions to cross.

4. **B**

Ribosomes are the site of protein synthesis within a cell and are not coupled to the cell membrane. The cell membrane functions as a site for cytoskeletal attachment, **(A)**, through proteins and lipid rafts. Transport regulation, **(C)**, is accomplished through channels, transporters, and selective permeability, while the phospholipids act as a reagent for second messenger formation, **(D)**.

5. **A**

Movement of individual molecules in the cell membrane will be affected by size and polarity, just as with diffusion. Lipids are much smaller than proteins in the plasma membrane and will move more quickly. Lipids will move fastest within the plane of the cell membrane because the polar head group does not need to pass through the hydrophobic tail region in the same way that it would if it were moving between the membrane layers.

6. **B**

Compounds that contribute to membrane fluidity will lower the melting point or disrupt the crystal structure. Cholesterol, **(C)**, and unsaturated lipids, **(A)** and **(D)**, are known for these functions. *trans* glycerophospholipids tend to increase the melting point of the membrane and therefore decrease membrane fluidity.

7. **D**

Membrane receptors must have both an extracellular and intracellular domain; therefore, they are considered transmembrane proteins. In order to initiate a second messenger cascade, they typically display enzymatic activity, although some may act strictly as channels.

8. **C**

Plasmodesmata are cell–cell junctions that are found in plants, not animals. Gap junctions, tight junctions, desmosomes, and hemidesmosomes are all found in animals, particularly in epithelia.

9. **A**

The movement of any molecule is dependent on multiple factors, including electric potential, membrane solubility, and concentration gradient. While the electric potential takes into account multiple molecules, the movement of any one solute or water by diffusion or osmosis is dependent only on the concentration gradient of that molecule.

10. **B**

The endocytosis (bulk uptake through vesicle formation) of fluid is known as pinocytosis. Phagocytosis, **(A)**, is the endocytotic intake of solids, while exocytosis, **(C)**, is a method of releasing vesicular contents. Drinking, **(D)**, does not apply on a cellular level.

11. **C**

Cell membranes are most likely to have a resting membrane potential that is nonzero because the resting membrane potential creates a state that is capable of responding to stimuli. Signaling molecules and channels would not be as useful with a membrane potential of zero. The values given in the answer choices correspond to different stages of the action potential, but the key information is that a resting potential of 0 mV does not maintain gradients for later activity.

12. **B**

The outer mitochondrial membrane is very permeable while the inner membrane is highly impermeable. The inner mitochondrial membrane is unique within the cell because it lacks cholesterol.

13. **D**

The Nernst equation relates the intra- and extracellular concentrations of an ion to the potential created by that gradient. At physiological temperature, it can be simplified to $E = \frac{61.5}{z} \log \frac{[\text{ion}]_{\text{outside}}}{[\text{ion}]_{\text{inside}}}$. For calcium, $z = +2$ (Ca^{2+}) and the ratio of $[\text{ion}_{\text{outside}}]$ to $[\text{ion}_{\text{inside}}] = 10^4$. Plugging in, we get:

$$E = \frac{61.5}{+2} \log 10^4 = \frac{61.5}{+2} \times 4 = 123 \text{ mV}$$

14. **A**

The fluid mosaic model accounts for a dynamic membrane. In this model, membrane components contain both fatty and carbohydrate-derived components, eliminating **(B)**. Further, the membrane is stabilized by the hydrophobic interactions of both fatty acid tails and membrane proteins, which may be found on the cytosolic or extracellular side of the membrane, or may run directly through the membrane; thus, **(C)** and **(D)** are also eliminated.

15. **D**

Gangliosides, along with ceramide, sphingomyelin, and cerebrosides, are sphingolipids.

Consult your online resources for additional practice. GO ONLINE

EQUATIONS TO REMEMBER

(8.1) **Osmotic pressure:** $\Pi = iMRT$

(8.2) **Nernst equation:** $E = \frac{RT}{zF}\ln\frac{[\text{ion}]_{\text{outside}}}{[\text{ion}]_{\text{inside}}} = \frac{61.5}{z}\log\frac{[\text{ion}]_{\text{outside}}}{[\text{ion}]_{\text{inside}}}$

(8.3) **Goldman–Hodgkin–Katz voltage equation:**

$$V_{\text{m}} = 61.5\log\left[\frac{P_{\text{Na}^+}\times[\text{Na}^+]_{\text{outside}} + P_{\text{K}^+}\times[\text{K}^+]_{\text{outside}} + P_{\text{Cl}^-}\times[\text{Cl}^-]_{\text{inside}}}{P_{\text{Na}^+}\times[\text{Na}^+]_{\text{inside}} + P_{\text{K}^+}\times[\text{K}^+]_{\text{inside}} + P_{\text{Cl}^-}\times[\text{Cl}^-]_{\text{outside}}}\right]$$

SHARED CONCEPTS

Biochemistry Chapter 3
Nonenzymatic Protein Function and Protein Analysis

Biochemistry Chapter 5
Lipid Structure and Function

Biology Chapter 1
The Cell

Biology Chapter 10
Homeostasis

General Chemistry Chapter 9
Solutions

Physics and Math Chapter 5
Electrostatics

CHAPTER 9

CARBOHYDRATE METABOLISM I: GLYCOLYSIS, GLYCOGEN, GLUCONEOGENESIS, AND THE PENTOSE PHOSPHATE PATHWAY

SCIENCE MASTERY ASSESSMENT

Every pre-med knows this feeling: there is so much content I have to know for the MCAT! How do I know what to do first or what's important?

While the high-yield badges throughout this book will help you identify the most important topics, this Science Mastery Assessment is another tool in your MCAT prep arsenal. This quiz (which can also be taken in your online resources) and the guidance below will help ensure that you are spending the appropriate amount of time on this chapter based on your personal strengths and weaknesses. Don't worry though—skipping something now does not mean you'll never study it. Later on in your prep, as you complete full-length tests, you'll uncover specific pieces of content that you need to review and can come back to these chapters as appropriate.

How to Use This Assessment

If you answer 0–7 questions correctly:

Spend about 1 hour to read this chapter in full and take limited notes throughout. Follow up by reviewing **all** quiz questions to ensure that you now understand how to solve each one.

If you answer 8–11 questions correctly:

Spend 20–40 minutes reviewing the quiz questions. Beginning with the questions you missed, read and take notes on the corresponding subchapters. For questions you answered correctly, ensure your thinking matches that of the explanation and you understand why each choice was correct or incorrect.

If you answer 12–15 questions correctly:

Spend less than 20 minutes reviewing all questions from the quiz. If you missed any, then include a quick read-through of the corresponding subchapters, or even just the relevant content within a subchapter, as part of your question review. For questions you got correct, ensure your thinking matches that of the explanation and review the Concept Summary at the end of the chapter.

1. Which of the following transporters is used by cells in the liver to store excess glucose and by beta cells in the pancreas as a glucose sensor?
   - **A.** GLUT 1
   - **B.** GLUT 2
   - **C.** GLUT 3
   - **D.** GLUT 4

2. Which of the following organs does NOT require a constant supply of glucose from the blood for energy during a fast?
   - **A.** Red blood cells
   - **B.** Brain
   - **C.** Pancreas
   - **D.** Liver

3. When insulin is released, it acts to increase the absorption of glucose into skeletal muscle predominantly through which of the following transporters?
   - **A.** GLUT 1
   - **B.** GLUT 2
   - **C.** GLUT 3
   - **D.** GLUT 4

4. After an overnight fast, which of the following enzymes would be expected to have little, if any, physiological activity?
   - **A.** Malate dehydrogenase
   - **B.** Glucokinase
   - **C.** α-Ketoglutarate dehydrogenase
   - **D.** Phosphofructokinase-1

5. Which of the following enzymes is NOT used to trap sugar in the cell?
   - **A.** Hexokinase
   - **B.** Galactokinase
   - **C.** Phosphofructokinase
   - **D.** Fructokinase

6. When fatty acid β-oxidation predominates in the liver, mitochondrial pyruvate is most likely to be:
   - **A.** carboxylated to phosphoenolpyruvate for entry into gluconeogenesis.
   - **B.** oxidatively decarboxylated to acetyl-CoA for oxidation in the citric acid cycle.
   - **C.** carboxylated to oxaloacetate for entry into gluconeogenesis.
   - **D.** reduced to lactate in the process of fermentation.

7. A biopsy is done on a child with an enlarged liver and shows accumulation of glycogen granules with single glucose residues remaining at the branch points near the periphery of the granule. The most likely genetic defect is in the gene encoding:
   - **A.** α-1,4 phosphorylase (glycogen phosphorylase).
   - **B.** α-1,4:α-1,6 transferase (branching enzyme).
   - **C.** α-1,4:α-1,4 transferase (part of debranching enzyme complex).
   - **D.** α-1,6 glucosidase (part of debranching enzyme complex).

8. An investigator is measuring the activity of various enzymes involved in reactions of intermediary metabolism. One of the enzymes has greatly decreased activity compared to reference values. The buffer of the assay contains citrate. Which of the following enzymes will most likely be directly affected by the use of citrate?
   - **A.** Fructose-2,6-bisphosphatase
   - **B.** Isocitrate dehydrogenase
   - **C.** Phosphofructokinase-1
   - **D.** Pyruvate carboxylase

9. After a brief period of intense exercise, the activity of muscle pyruvate dehydrogenase is greatly increased. This increased activity is most likely due to:
   - **A.** decreased ADP.
   - **B.** increased acetyl-CoA.
   - **C.** increased NADH/NAD^+ ratio.
   - **D.** increased pyruvate concentration.

10. The metabolism of which of the following sugars would be LEAST affected by the inhibition of the enzyme phosphofructokinase-1?
   - **A.** Lactose
   - **B.** Fructose
   - **C.** Glucose
   - **D.** Galactose

11. A patient is given antibiotics to treat a urinary tract infection and develops an episode of red blood cell lysis. Further studies show weakness of the plasma membrane and Heinz bodies (collections of oxidized hemoglobin). Which of the following enzymes is most likely defective in this patient?
   - **A.** Fructose-1,6-bisphosphatase
   - **B.** Glucose-6-phosphate dehydrogenase
   - **C.** Hexokinase
   - **D.** Pyruvate kinase

12. The unique enzymes of gluconeogenesis are used to circumvent specific irreversible steps of glycolysis. Which of the following correctly pairs an enzyme from glycolysis with its corresponding enzyme(s) used in gluconeogenesis?
   - **A.** Phosphofructokinase-1/fructose-1,6-bisphosphatase
   - **B.** Pyruvate dehydrogenase/pyruvate carboxylase and phosphoenolpyruvate carboxykinase
   - **C.** Hexokinase/glucokinase
   - **D.** Pyruvate kinase/glucose-6-phosphatase

13. After an overnight fast, which of the following processes would be expected to occur at an elevated rate compared with the well-fed state?
   - **A.** Glycolysis
   - **B.** Glycogenolysis
   - **C.** Glycogenesis
   - **D.** Glycerol synthesis

14. Andersen disease is caused by a mutation in branching enzyme and is associated with cirrhosis. Scientists theorize the cause is likely an immune response against abnormal glycogen. Which of the following best describes the ratio of glycogen α-1,4 to α-1,6 linkages in individuals with this disorder?
   - **A.** Elevated
   - **B.** Decreased
   - **C.** No difference
   - **D.** Cannot determine

15. Each of the following catalyzes a rate-limiting step of a carbohydrate metabolism pathway EXCEPT:
   - **A.** hexokinase.
   - **B.** glycogen synthase.
   - **C.** glucose-6-phosphate dehydrogenase.
   - **D.** fructose-1,6-bisphosphatase.

Answer Key

1. **B**
2. **D**
3. **D**
4. **B**
5. **C**
6. **C**
7. **D**
8. **C**
9. **D**
10. **B**
11. **B**
12. **A**
13. **B**
14. **A**
15. **A**

Detailed explanations can be found at the end of the chapter.

CHAPTER 9

CARBOHYDRATE METABOLISM I: GLYCOLYSIS, GLYCOGEN, GLUCONEOGENESIS, AND THE PENTOSE PHOSPHATE PATHWAY

In This Chapter

CHAPTER PROFILE

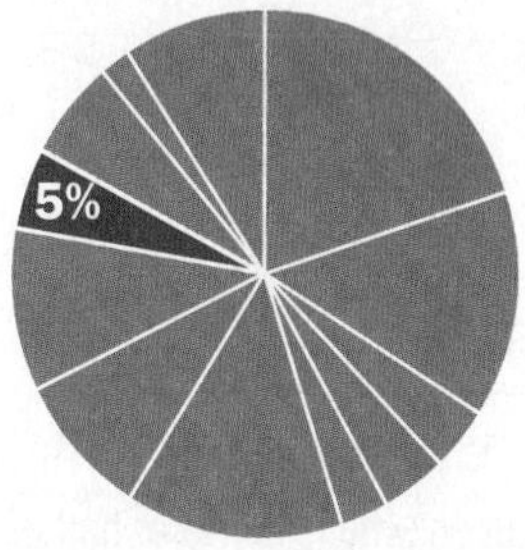

The content in this chapter should be relevant to about 5% of all questions about biochemistry on the MCAT.

This chapter covers material from the following AAMC content categories:

1D: Principles of bioenergetics and fuel molecule metabolism

5D: Structure, function, and reactivity of biologically-relevant molecules

Introduction

Maintaining a constant blood glucose concentration around $100\frac{\text{mg}}{\text{dL}}$ (5.6 mM) is of the utmost importance in the body: high blood sugar causes long-term damage to the retina, kidney, blood vessels, and nerves, while low blood sugar can cause autonomic disturbances, seizures, and even coma. Without the ability to take in glucose constantly, the body must find ways to store and release glucose as it is needed. And given the variety of food we eat on a daily basis, the body must find ways to use all of the various carbohydrates it takes in.

There's a complex interplay between the neurological, endocrine, digestive, and excretory systems to maintain this blood glucose concentration, much of which is discussed in Chapter 12 of *MCAT Biochemistry Review*. In this chapter, we'll take a look at the metabolic pathways that involve glucose: the methods by which our bodies digest glucose and other monosaccharides, store and release glucose for energy, generate glucose from other biomolecules, and use glucose to create some of the coenzymes and substrates needed for biosynthesis.

This chapter is the first of four that focus on metabolism in *MCAT Biochemistry Review*. Here, we focus on metabolic processes of glucose that do not require oxygen; in Chapter 10, we'll turn our focus to the processes that only occur under aerobic conditions. In Chapter 11, we'll explore the metabolism of lipids and amino acids. Finally, in Chapter 12, we'll bring all of metabolism together with a focus on bioenergetics and the regulation of metabolism overall.

9.1 Glucose Transport

LEARNING OBJECTIVES

After Chapter 9.1, you will be able to:

- List the locations and functions of the GLUT 2 and GLUT 4 glucose transport proteins
- Predict how increased blood glucose levels will impact GLUT 2 and GLUT 4 activity

Glucose entry into most cells is driven by concentration and is independent of sodium, unlike absorption from the digestive tract. Normal glucose concentration in peripheral blood is 5.6 mM (normal range: 4–6 mM). There are four glucose transporters, called GLUT 1 through GLUT 4. GLUT 2 and GLUT 4 are the most significant of these because they are located only in specific cells and are highly regulated.

BRIDGE

The K_m is the concentration of substrate when an enzyme is active at half of its maximum velocity (v_{max}). The lower the K_m, the higher the enzyme's affinity for the substrate. See Chapter 2 of *MCAT Biochemistry Review* for more on Michaelis-Menten enzyme kinetics.

GLUT 2 is a low-affinity transporter in hepatocytes and pancreatic cells. After a meal, blood traveling through the hepatic portal vein from the intestine is rich in glucose. GLUT 2 captures the excess glucose primarily for storage. When the glucose concentration drops below the K_m for the transporter, much of the remainder bypasses the liver and enters the peripheral circulation. The K_m of GLUT 2 is quite high (~15 mM). This means that the liver will pick up glucose in proportion to its concentration in the blood (first-order kinetics). In other words, the liver will pick up excess glucose and store it preferentially after a meal, when blood glucose levels are high. In the β-islet cells of the pancreas, GLUT 2, along with the glycolytic enzyme *glucokinase*, serves as the glucose sensor for insulin release.

REAL WORLD

Diabetes mellitus is caused by a disruption of the insulin/GLUT 4 mechanism. In type 1 diabetes, insulin is absent and cannot stimulate the insulin receptor. In type 2 diabetes, the receptor becomes insensitive to insulin and fails to bring GLUT 4 transporters to the cell surface. In both cases, blood glucose rises, leading to immediate symptoms (increased urination, increased thirst, ketoacidosis) and long-term symptoms (blindness, heart attacks, strokes, nerve damage).

GLUT 4 is in adipose tissue and muscle and responds to the glucose concentration in peripheral blood. The rate of glucose transport in these two tissues is increased by insulin, which stimulates the movement of additional GLUT 4 transporters to the membrane by a mechanism involving exocytosis, as shown in Figure 9.1. The K_m of GLUT 4 is close to the normal glucose levels in blood (~5 mM). This means that the transporter is saturated when blood glucose levels are just a bit higher than normal. When a person has high blood sugar concentrations, these transporters will still permit only a constant rate of glucose influx because they will be saturated (zero-order kinetics). Then how can cells with GLUT 4 transporters increase their intake of glucose? By increasing the number of GLUT 4 transporters on their surface.

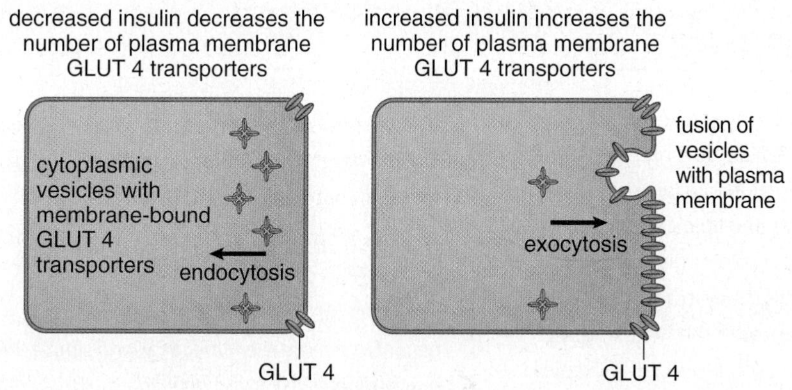

Figure 9.1 Insulin Regulation of Glucose Transport in Muscle and Adipose Cells

Although basal levels of transport occur in all cells independently of insulin, the transport rate increases in adipose tissue and muscle when insulin levels rise. Muscle stores excess glucose as glycogen, and adipose tissue requires glucose to form dihydroxyacetone phosphate (DHAP), which is converted to glycerol phosphate to store incoming fatty acids as *triacylglycerols*.

MCAT CONCEPT CHECK 9.1

Before you move on, assess your understanding of the material with these questions.

1. Compare and contrast GLUT 2 and GLUT 4:

	GLUT 2	GLUT 4
Important tissues		
K_m		
Saturated at normal glucose levels?		
Responsive to insulin?		

2. How does insulin promote glucose entry into cells?

____

BIOCHEMISTRY GUIDED EXAMPLE WITH EXPERT THINKING

Malignant cells increase their expression of glycolytic enzymes and glucose uptake to markedly enhance glycolysis (aerobic glycolysis; the Warburg effect), which leads to the production of a large amount of ATP and biomolecules such as nucleic acids and lipids essential for cell survival and division. In order to clarify the role of glycolysis in ATP production in malignant and normal cells, the intracellular levels of ATP were measured upon treatment with the hexokinase II inhibitor 3BrPA at 10, 30, and 50 μM, in malignant RPMI8226 multiple myeloma (MM) cells. Data were expressed relative to values for untreated cells (Figure 1). MM cells are known to reside in the bone marrow with normal hematopoietic cells. To compare the effects of inhibiting glycolysis on ATP production between malignant and normal cells, $CD138^+$ primary MM cells and $CD138^-$ non-MM bone marrow mononuclear cells (BMMCs) were cultured for 60 minutes with 50 μM of 3BrPA, and cellular levels of ATP were measured (Figure 2). Finally, to evaluate the effects of 3BrPA on cell viability, RPMI8226 and peripheral blood mononuclear cells (PBMCs), which are non-MM, were cultured for 24 hours with 3BrPA at the indicated concentrations. The cells were stained with propidium iodide (PI), which binds more intensely to non-viable cells, and analyzed by flow cytometry (Figure 3).

This intro is contextualizing the research, so it'll only be helpful if there are questions on the broader context of the study

Purpose statement: explain role of glycolysis to make ATP in cancerous and normal cells

With all of the acronyms in the passage it'll be helpful to replace them mentally with simpler words and add notes to your scratch board: 3BrPA with "glycolytic inhibitor" and RPMI8226 with "cancer"

Fig 2: same as Fig 1, but comparing to normal cells

Replace $CD138^+$ with "cancer", $CD138^-$ with "normal"

This indicates what "new" thing is coming in the next data set

Rephrase: glycolytic inhibitor added to cancer and normal cells

The dye will pick up dead cells!

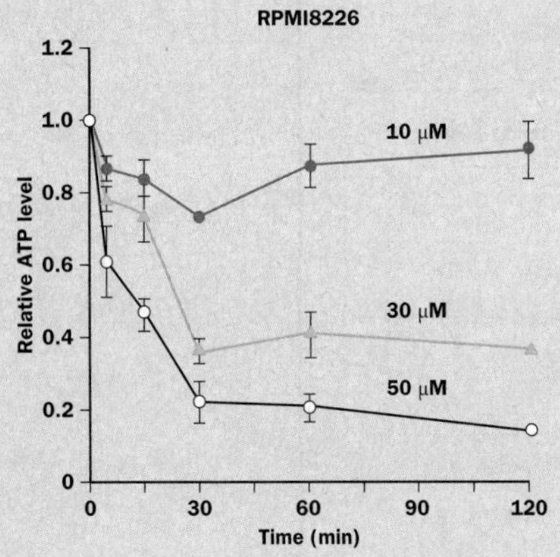

Figure 1

IVs: concentration of glycolytic inhibitor and time

DV: ATP levels

Trend: as glycolysis inhibitor conc goes up, ATP levels decrease in cancer cells

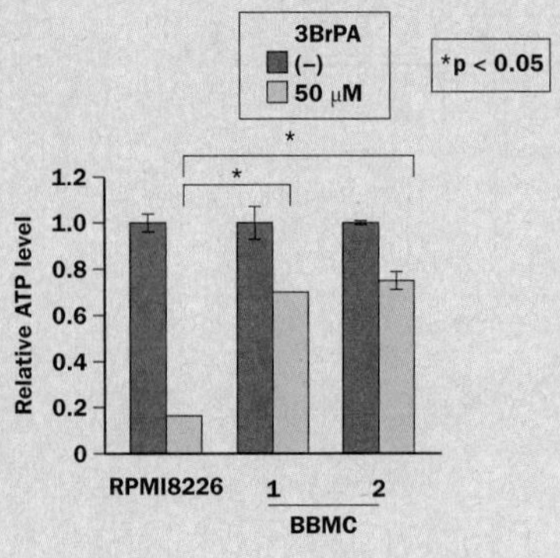

Figure 2

IVs: cancer vs. normal cell type, presence/absence of glycolytic inhibitor

DV: ATP levels

Trend: glycolytic inhibitor lowers ATP levels more in cancer cells compared to normal cells

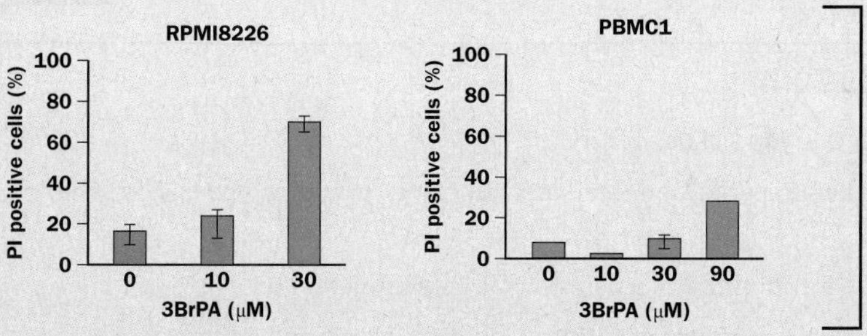

Two sets of graphs, though we can rephrase to essentially make it into one

IVs: normal vs. cancer cells, glycolytic inhibitor concentrations

DVs: levels of dead cells

Trend: the glycolytic inhibitor kills off more cancer cells compared to normal cells

Figure 3

Adapted from Nakano, A., Tsuji, D., Miki, H., Cui, Q., El Sayed, S. M., Ikegame, A., ... Abe, M. (2011). Glycolysis inhibition inactivates ABC transporters to restore drug sensitivity in malignant cells. *PLoS One*, 6(11), e27222.

According to the data, do the results support the usage of glycolytic inhibitors like 3BrPA to preferentially target malignant cells? Why or why not?

This question is going to require us to understand what this experiment is testing and how the results are gathered, so let's start by making sure we understand the passage fully. A quick scan of this passage reveals multiple challenges: lots of acronyms, unfamiliar jargon and experimental techniques, and four experimental graphs. While each piece of data will be distinct, they will all be centered around supporting the experiment's purpose. The second sentence states that the overall purpose of this passage is to explore how cancer cells primarily use glycolysis, and how this preference can be used to specifically target tumors.

In Figure 1, we can see what's happening to ATP levels over time in multiple myeloma cells treated with hexokinase inhibitor. Looking at the data, we see that over time, the bigger the dose (written above the lines) of inhibitor, the more the ATP level in the cancer cells drops. If glycolysis is the primary way cancer cells produce ATP, which is what the passage stated in the first sentence, then the results in Figure 1 can be said to support this hypothesis.

Figure 2 shows a comparison of ATP production in the presence and absence of the inhibitor to cancer cells (RPMI8226 and $CD138^{+}$) and normal cells ($CD138^{-}$). While there is a drop in ATP when treated with the inhibitor in all the cell types, there is a statistical difference in the ATP levels of cancer vs. normal cells when the inhibitor is present. The brackets at the top of this figure indicate a statistically significant difference between the cancer cell line with the inhibitor and normal cell lines with the inhibitor. These kinds of statistical significance indications in a graph often point us toward where we should be heading to solve passage-based questions on the MCAT. This is the first piece of evidence that shows how inhibiting glycolysis has a bigger effect on cancer cells compared to normal, because we saw a statistically significant difference between those groups.

However, the most impactful proof comes in Figure 3. The cells have been treated with PI, which the passage tells us will stain non-viable (dead) cells more intensely. The cancer cells have progressively more dead cells (indicated by higher bars) with increasing amounts of the glycolytic inhibitor, which we can see in the first graph of Figure 3, while the normal cells (the second graph of Figure 3) show far fewer dead cells even at the highest dose. To directly compare, one can estimate that ~70% of cancer cells are PI positive with 30 μM 3BrPA, whereas ~10% of nonmalignant cells are PI positive with the same concentration of 3BRPA.

Because the results in Figure 3 tell us that glycolytic inhibitor 3BrPA is far more effective in killing cancerous vs. noncancerous cell lines, the findings are supportive of the idea that 3BrPA could possibly be used to target and treat cancerous cells.

9.2 Glycolysis

High-Yield

LEARNING OBJECTIVES

After Chapter 9.2, you will be able to:

- Recall the key steps, key intermediates, reactants, products, and key enzymes of glycolysis
- Explain the function and mechanism of lactate fermentation
- Explain the unique effects of glycolysis on hemoglobin and erythrocytes
- Recall function and regulatory mechanisms when given an enzyme of glycolysis, such as phosphoglycerate kinase

BRIDGE

Red blood cells extrude their mitochondria during development, as discussed in Chapter 7 of *MCAT Biology Review*. This helps them carry out their function (carrying oxygen) in two ways:

- Maximizing volume available for hemoglobin, the primary oxygen-carrying protein
- Stopping the red blood cell from utilizing the oxygen it's supposed to be carrying to oxygen-depleted bodily tissues

REAL WORLD

Because glycolysis is necessary in every cell of the body, there are no known diseases caused by the complete absence of any enzyme in glycolysis; in other words, being unable to carry out glycolysis is incompatible with life. Partial enzyme defects are also rare, but include *pyruvate kinase deficiency*.

All cells can carry out glycolysis. In a few tissues, most importantly red blood cells, glycolysis represents the only energy-yielding pathway available because red blood cells lack mitochondria, which are required for the citric acid cycle, electron transport chain, oxidative phosphorylation, and fatty acid metabolism (β-oxidation). Glucose is the major monosaccharide that enters the pathway, but others such as galactose and fructose can also feed into it.

Glycolysis is a cytoplasmic pathway that converts glucose into two *pyruvate* molecules, releasing a modest amount of energy captured in two substrate-level phosphorylations and one oxidation reaction. If a cell has mitochondria and oxygen, the energy carriers produced in glycolysis (NADH) can feed into the aerobic respiration pathway to generate energy for the cell. If either mitochondria or oxygen is lacking (such as in erythrocytes or exercising skeletal muscle, respectively), glycolysis may occur anaerobically, although some of the available energy is lost.

Glycolysis also provides intermediates for other pathways. In the liver, glycolysis is part of the process by which excess glucose is converted to fatty acids for storage.

Important Enzymes of Glycolysis

While glycolysis contains many different steps, as illustrated in Figure 9.2, the MCAT predominantly tests on the enzymes that are highly regulated or that serve an important energetic function. Therefore, we'll focus our attention on five of these enzymes.

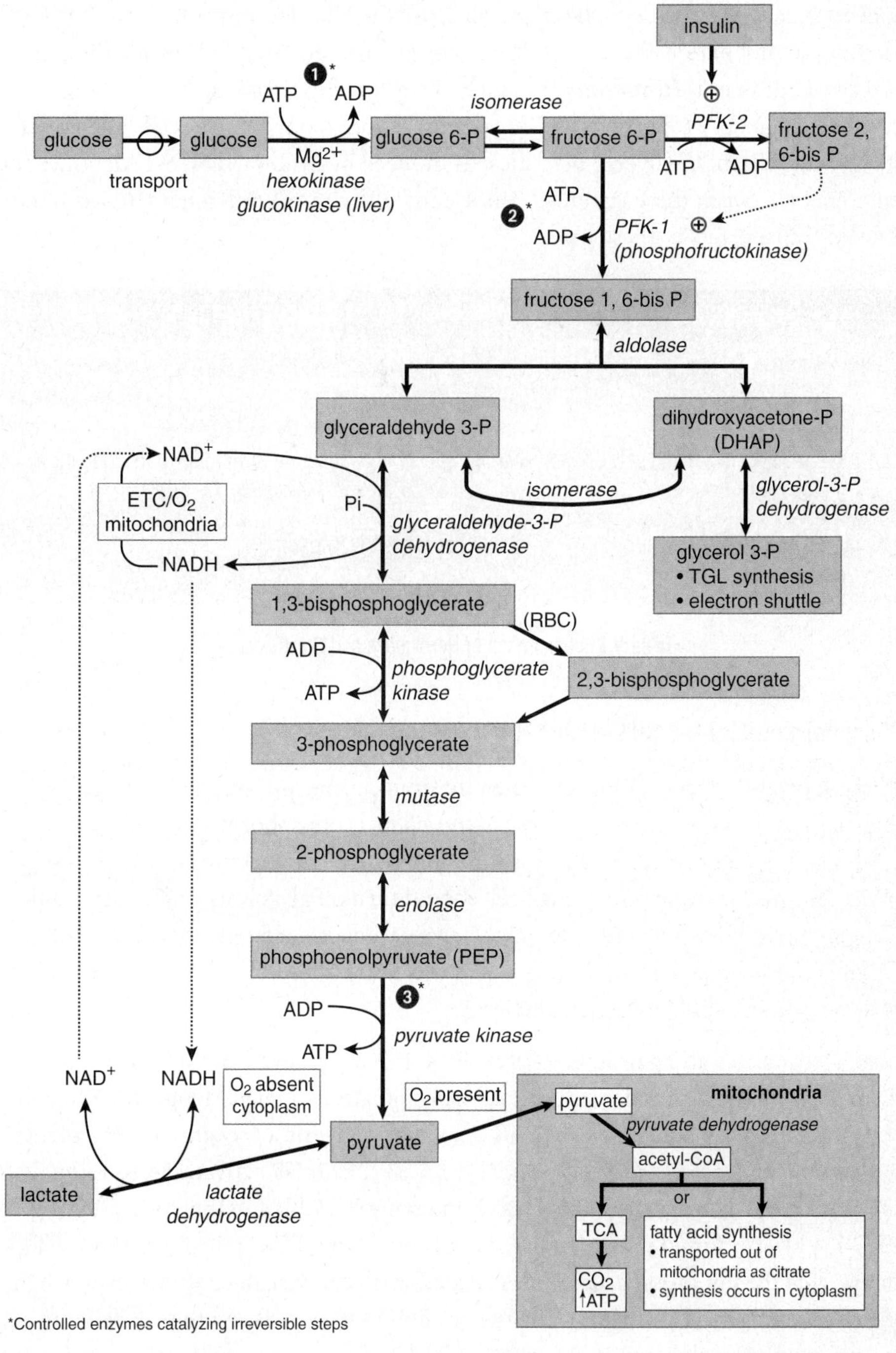

Figure 9.2 Glycolysis

Hexokinase and Glucokinase

The first steps in glucose metabolism in any cell are transport across the membrane and phosphorylation by kinase enzymes inside the cell to prevent glucose from leaving via the transporter. Remember from Chapter 2 of *MCAT Biochemistry Review* that kinases attach a phosphate group from ATP to their substrates. Glucose enters the cell by facilitated diffusion or active transport; in either case, these kinases convert glucose to *glucose 6-phosphate*. Because the GLUT transporters are specific for glucose (not *phosphorylated* glucose), the glucose gets "trapped" inside the cell and cannot leak out. ***Hexokinase*** is widely distributed in tissues and is inhibited by its product, glucose 6-phosphate. ***Glucokinase*** is found only in liver cells and pancreatic β-islet cells; in the liver, glucokinase is induced by insulin. Table 9.1 identifies the differences between these enzymes. These coincide with the differences between the glucose transporters in these tissues.

HEXOKINASE	GLUCOKINASE
Present in most tissues	Present in hepatocytes and pancreatic β-islet cells (along with GLUT 2, acts as the glucose sensor)
Low K_m (reaches maximum velocity at low [glucose])	High K_m (acts on glucose proportionally to its concentration)
Inhibited by glucose 6-phosphate	Induced by insulin in hepatocytes

Table 9.1 Comparison of Hexokinase and Glucokinase

KEY CONCEPT

Of all the enzymes the MCAT is most likely to test you on, the rate-limiting enzymes for each process are at the top of the list:

- Glycolysis: *phosphofructokinase-1*
- Fermentation: *lactate dehydrogenase*
- Glycogenesis: *glycogen synthase*
- Glycogenolysis: *glycogen phosphorylase*
- Gluconeogenesis: *fructose-1,6-bisphosphatase*
- Pentose Phosphate Pathway: *glucose-6-phosphate dehydrogenase*

Phosphofructokinases (PFK-1 and PFK-2)

Phosphofructokinase-1 (**PFK-1**) is the rate-limiting enzyme and main control point in glycolysis. In this reaction, *fructose 6-phosphate* is phosphorylated to *fructose 1,6-bisphosphate* using ATP. PFK-1 is inhibited by ATP and citrate, and activated by AMP. This makes sense because the cell should turn off glycolysis when it has sufficient energy (high ATP) and turn on glycolysis when it needs energy (high AMP). Citrate is an intermediate of the citric acid cycle, so high levels of citrate also imply that the cell is producing sufficient energy.

Insulin stimulates and glucagon inhibits PFK-1 in hepatocytes by an indirect mechanism involving PFK-2 and fructose 2,6-bisphosphate, as shown in Figure 9.2. Insulin activates ***phosphofructokinase-2*** (**PFK-2**), which converts a tiny amount of *fructose 6-phosphate* to *fructose 2,6-bisphosphate* (F2,6-BP). F2,6-BP activates PFK-1. On the other hand, glucagon inhibits PFK-2, lowering F2,6-BP and thereby inhibiting PFK-1. PFK-2 is found mostly in the liver. By activating PFK-1, it allows these cells to override the inhibition caused by ATP so that glycolysis can continue, even when the cell is energetically satisfied. The metabolites of glycolysis can thus be fed into the production of glycogen, fatty acids, and other storage molecules rather than just being burned to produce ATP.

BRIDGE

In Chapter 11 of *MCAT General Chemistry Review*, we learn that oxidation is loss of electrons and reduction is gain of electrons. While this is true with biomolecules, it may be easier to think of oxidation as increasing bonds to oxygen or other heteroatoms (atoms besides C and H) and reduction as increasing bonds to hydrogen, as discussed in Chapter 4 of *MCAT Organic Chemistry Review*. Thus, the conversion of NAD^+ to NADH is a reduction reaction.

Glyceraldehyde-3-Phosphate Dehydrogenase

Glyceraldehyde-3-phosphate dehydrogenase catalyzes an oxidation and addition of inorganic phosphate (P_i) to its substrate, *glyceraldehyde 3-phosphate*. This results in the production of a high-energy intermediate *1,3-bisphosphoglycerate* and the reduction of NAD^+ to NADH. If glycolysis is aerobic, the NADH can be oxidized by the mitochondrial electron transport chain, providing energy for ATP synthesis by oxidative phosphorylation.

3-Phosphoglycerate Kinase

3-Phosphoglycerate kinase transfers the high-energy phosphate from 1,3-bisphosphoglycerate to ADP, forming ATP and *3-phosphoglycerate*. This type of reaction, in which ADP is directly phosphorylated to ATP using a high-energy intermediate, is referred to as **substrate-level phosphorylation**. In contrast to oxidative phosphorylation in mitochondria, substrate-level phosphorylations are not dependent on oxygen, and are the only means of ATP generation in an anaerobic tissue.

Pyruvate Kinase

The last enzyme in aerobic glycolysis, pyruvate kinase catalyzes a substrate-level phosphorylation of ADP using the high-energy substrate *phosphoenolpyruvate* (PEP). ***Pyruvate kinase*** is activated by fructose 1,6-bisphosphate from the PFK-1 reaction. This is referred to as **feed-forward activation**, meaning that the product of an earlier reaction of glycolysis (fructose 1,6-bisphosphate) stimulates, or prepares, a later reaction in glycolysis (by activating pyruvate kinase).

Fermentation

In the absence of oxygen, **fermentation** will occur. The key fermentation enzyme in mammalian cells is ***lactate dehydrogenase***, which oxidizes NADH to NAD^+, replenishing the oxidized coenzyme for glyceraldehyde-3-phosphate dehydrogenase. Without mitochondria and oxygen, glycolysis would stop when all the available NAD^+ had been reduced to NADH. By reducing pyruvate to *lactate* and oxidizing NADH to NAD^+, lactate dehydrogenase prevents this potential problem from developing. There is no net loss of carbon in this process: pyruvate and lactate are both three-carbon molecules. In aerobic tissues, lactate does not normally form in significant amounts. However, when oxygenation is poor (during strenuous exercise in skeletal muscle, a heart attack, or a stroke), most cellular ATP is generated by anaerobic glycolysis, and lactate production increases.

In yeast cells, fermentation is the conversion of pyruvate (three carbons) to ethanol (two carbons) and carbon dioxide (one carbon). While the end products are different, the result of both mammalian and yeast fermentation is the same: replenishing NAD^+.

Important Intermediates of Glycolysis

Glycolysis serves as a crossroads for a number of metabolic processes; the intermediates of glycolysis are often used to link different pathways during both catabolism and anabolism. Three of these intermediates are worth highlighting:

- ***Dihydroxyacetone phosphate*** (**DHAP**) is used in hepatic and adipose tissue for triacylglycerol synthesis. DHAP is formed from fructose 1,6-bisphosphate. It can be isomerized to *glycerol 3-phosphate*, which can then be converted to *glycerol*, the backbone of triacylglycerols.
- 1,3-Bisphosphoglycerate (1,3-BPG) and phosphoenolpyruvate (PEP) are high-energy intermediates used to generate ATP by substrate-level phosphorylation. This is the only ATP gained in anaerobic respiration.

MNEMONIC

Irreversible steps of glycolysis:
How **G**lycolysis **P**ushes **F**orward the **P**rocess: **K**inases.

- **H**exokinase
- **G**lucokinase
- **PF**K-1
- **P**yruvate **K**inase

BRIDGE

Adaptation to high altitudes (low pO_2) involves:

- Increased respiration
- Increased oxygen affinity for hemoglobin (initial)
- Increased rate of glycolysis
- Increased [2,3-BPG] in RBC (over a 12–24 hour period)
- Normalized oxygen affinity for hemoglobin restored by the increased level of 2,3-BPG
- Increased hemoglobin (over days to weeks)

Gas exchange is discussed in Chapter 6 of *MCAT Biology Review*, and effects on hemoglobin are discussed in Chapter 7 of *MCAT Biology Review*.

BRIDGE

Remember the other physiological changes that promote a **right** shift of the oxygen dissociation curve (the Bohr effect), discussed in Chapter 7 of *MCAT Biology Review*:

- High 2,3-BPG
- Low pH
- High $[H^+]$
- High pCO_2

These all occur during exercise, giving the mnemonic: "Exercise is the **right** thing to do."

Irreversible Enzymes

Three enzymes in the pathway catalyze reactions that are irreversible. This keeps the pathway moving in only one direction. However, the liver must be able to generate new glucose from other biomolecules through gluconeogenesis, which is essentially the reverse of glycolysis. Because of the irreversible enzymes of glycolysis, different reactions, and therefore different enzymes, must be used at these three points:

- Glucokinase or hexokinase
- PFK-1
- Pyruvate kinase

Glycolysis in Erythrocytes

In erythrocytes (red blood cells), anaerobic glycolysis represents the only pathway for ATP production, yielding a net 2 ATP per glucose.

Red blood cells have ***bisphosphoglycerate mutase***, which produces ***2,3-bisphosphoglycerate* (2,3-BPG)** from 1,3-BPG in glycolysis. Remember that *mutases* are enzymes that move a functional group from one place in a molecule to another; in this case, the phosphate is moved from the 1-position to the 2-position. 2,3-BPG binds allosterically to the β-chains of hemoglobin A (HbA) and decreases its affinity for oxygen. This effect of 2,3-BPG is seen in the oxygen dissociation curve for HbA, shown in Figure 9.3. The rightward shift in the curve is sufficient to allow unloading of oxygen in tissues, but still allows 100 percent saturation in the lungs. An abnormal increase in erythrocyte 2,3-BPG might shift the curve far enough so that HbA is not fully saturated in the lungs.

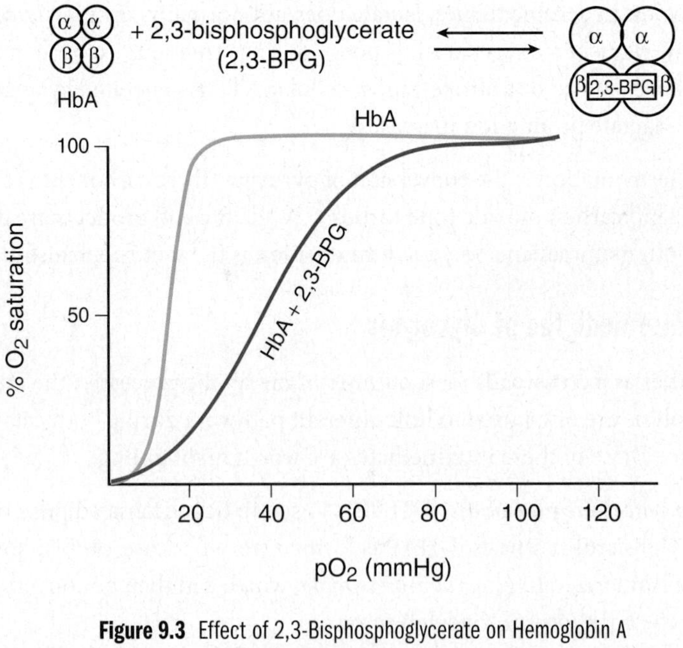

Figure 9.3 Effect of 2,3-Bisphosphoglycerate on Hemoglobin A

Although 2,3-BPG binds to HbA, it does not bind well to fetal hemoglobin (HbF), with the result that HbF has a higher affinity for oxygen than maternal HbA. This allows transplacental passage of oxygen from mother to fetus.

MCAT CONCEPT CHECK 9.2

Before you move on, assess your understanding of the material with these questions.

1. What are the function and key regulators of the following enzymes? Which ones are reversible?

Hexokinase

- Function:

___

- Regulation:

___

- Reversible?

___

Glucokinase

- Function:

___

- Regulation:

___

- Reversible?

___

Phosphofructokinase-1 (PFK-1)

- Function:

___

- Regulation:

___

- Reversible?

___

Glyceraldehyde-3-phosphate dehydrogenase

- Function:

___

- Reversible?

___

3-phosphoglycerate kinase

- Function:

- Reversible?

Pyruvate kinase

- Function:

- Regulation:

- Reversible?

2. Why must pyruvate undergo fermentation for glycolysis to continue?

3. Why is it necessary that fetal hemoglobin does not bind 2,3-BPG?

9.3 Other Monosaccharides

LEARNING OBJECTIVES

After Chapter 9.3, you will be able to:

- Explain the importance of trapping a sugar in the cell and linking its metabolism with the glycolysis pathway
- Recognize the key enzymes, reactants, and products of galactose and fructose metabolism

While glucose represents the primary monosaccharide used by cells, other monosaccharides such as *galactose* and *fructose* can also contribute to ATP production by feeding into glycolysis or other metabolic processes. These monosaccharides are tested far less frequently than glucose on the MCAT, but are included here to compare and contrast their metabolism with glycolysis. In particular, notice the similarities between Figure 9.2 (glycolysis) and Figures 9.4 (galactose metabolism) and 9.5 (fructose metabolism).

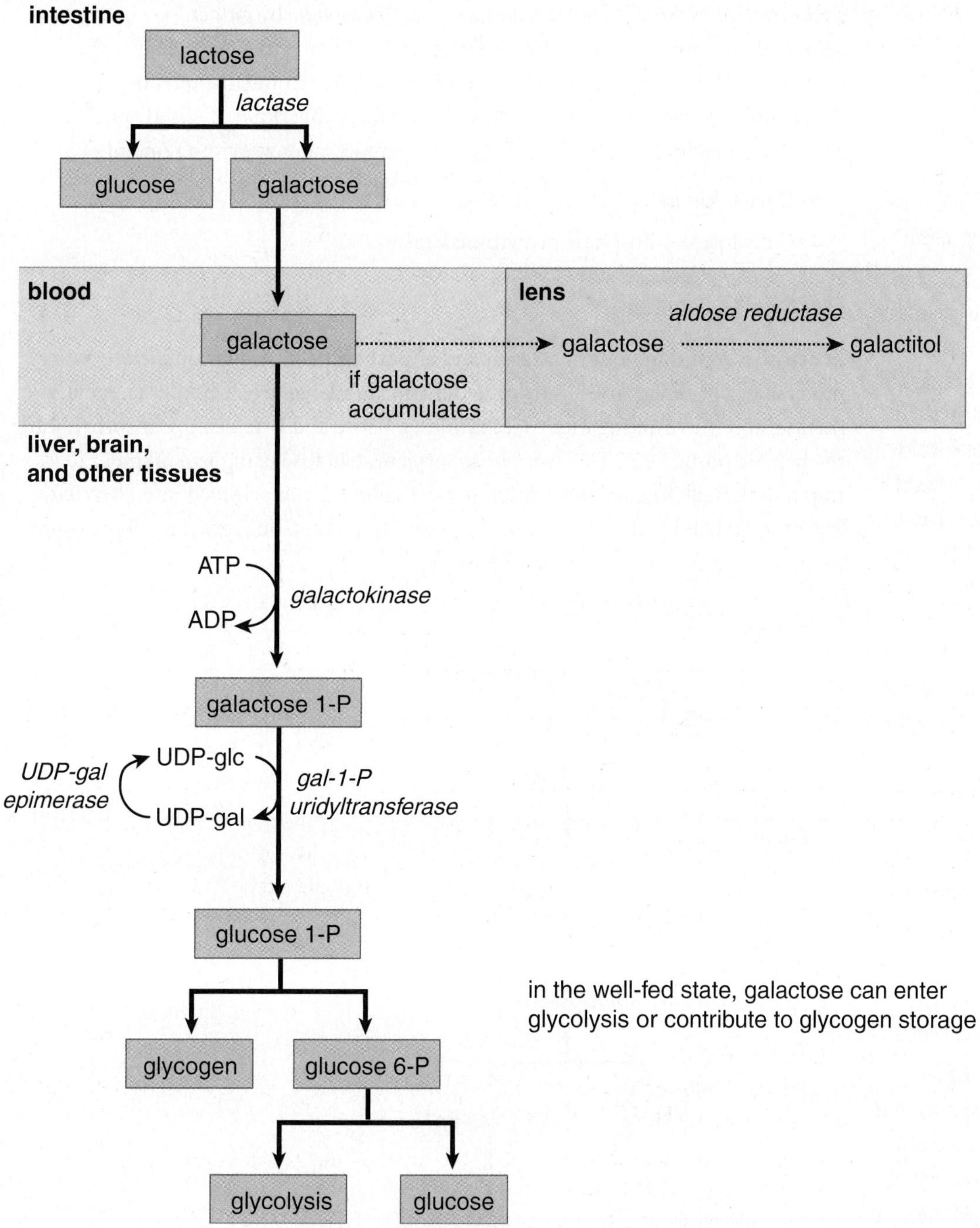

Figure 9.4 Galactose Metabolism

Galactose Metabolism

An important source of **galactose** in the diet is the disaccharide *lactose* present in milk. Lactose is hydrolyzed to galactose and glucose by *lactase,* which is a brush-border enzyme of the duodenum. Along with other monosaccharides, galactose reaches the liver through the hepatic portal vein. Once transported into tissues, galactose is phosphorylated by ***galactokinase***, trapping it in the cell. The resulting *galactose 1-phosphate* is converted to *glucose 1-phosphate* by ***galactose-1-phosphate uridyltransferase*** and an *epimerase*. **Epimerases** are enzymes that catalyze the conversion of one sugar epimer to another; remember from Chapter 4 of *MCAT Biochemistry Review* that epimers are diastereomers that differ at exactly one chiral carbon. The pathway is shown in Figure 9.4; important enzymes to remember are:

- Galactokinase
- Galactose-1-phosphate uridyltransferase

Fructose Metabolism

Fructose is found in honey and fruit and as part of the disaccharide *sucrose* (common table sugar). Sucrose is hydrolyzed by the duodenal brush-border enzyme *sucrase*, and the resulting monosaccharides, glucose and fructose, are absorbed into the hepatic portal vein. The liver phosphorylates fructose using ***fructokinase*** to trap it in the cell. The resulting *fructose 1-phosphate* is then cleaved into *glyceraldehyde* and DHAP by *aldolase B*. Smaller amounts are metabolized in renal proximal tubules. The pathway is shown in Figure 9.5.

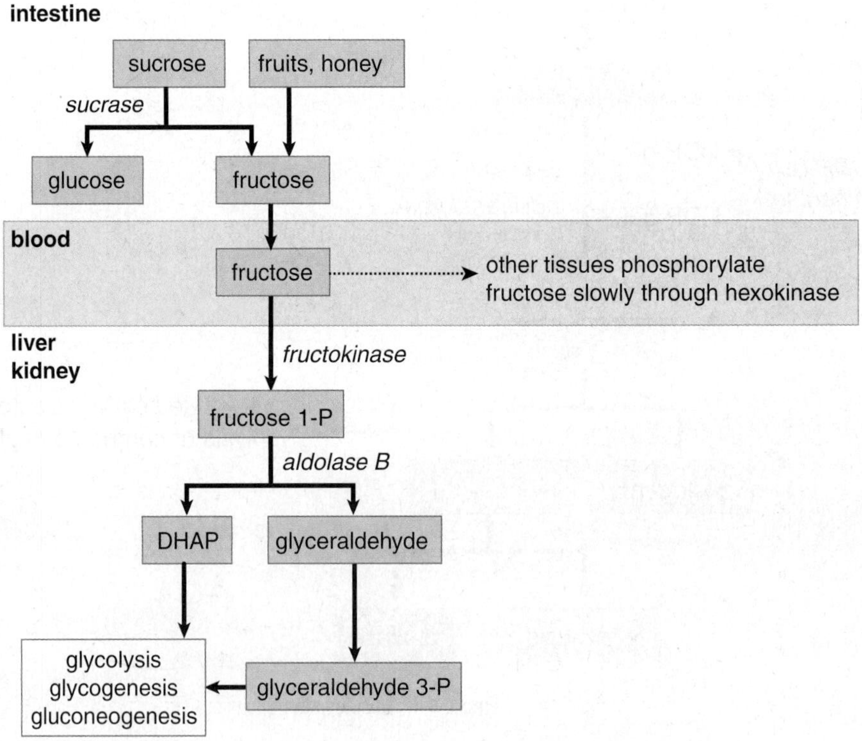

Figure 9.5 Fructose Metabolism

REAL WORLD

Primary lactose intolerance is caused by a hereditary deficiency of lactase. *Secondary lactose intolerance* can be precipitated at any age by gastrointestinal disturbances that cause damage to the intestinal lining, where lactase is found.

Common symptoms of lactose intolerance include vomiting, bloating, explosive and watery diarrhea, cramps, and dehydration. The symptoms can be attributed to bacterial fermentation of lactose, which produces a mixture of CH_4, H_2, and small organic acids. The acids are osmotically active and result in the movement of water into the intestinal lumen.

REAL WORLD

Genetic deficiencies of galactokinase or galactose-1-phosphate uridyltransferase lead to galactosemia. Cataracts are a characteristic finding, which result from the conversion of excess galactose in the blood to galactitol in the lens of the eye by aldose reductase. Galactitol is a polyol (a carbon chain with many alcohol groups) and, as such, is hydrophilic. Accumulation of galactitol in the lens causes osmotic damage and cataracts. Deficiency of galactose-1-phosphate uridyltransferase is more severe because, in addition to causing galactosemia, it leads to galactose 1-phosphate getting stuck intracellularly in the liver, brain, and other tissues and not diffusing out.

KEY CONCEPT

Because dihydroxyacetone phosphate (DHAP) and glyceraldehyde, the products of fructose metabolism, are downstream from the key regulatory and rate-limiting enzyme of glycolysis (PFK-1), a high-fructose drink supplies a quick source of energy in both aerobic and anaerobic cells.

MCAT CONCEPT CHECK 9.3

Before you move on, assess your understanding of the material with these questions.

1. Which enzyme is responsible for trapping galactose in the cell? What enzyme in galactose metabolism results in a product that can feed directly into glycolysis, linking the two pathways?
   - "Trapping" enzyme:

   - "Linking" enzyme:

   ---

2. Which enzyme is responsible for trapping fructose in the cell? What enzyme in fructose metabolism results in a product that can feed directly into glycolysis, linking the two pathways?
   - "Trapping" enzyme:

   - "Linking" enzyme:

9.4 Pyruvate Dehydrogenase

LEARNING OBJECTIVES

After Chapter 9.4, you will be able to:

- Recall the reactants and products of the pyruvate dehydrogenase complex
- Describe the relationship between acetyl-CoA levels and PDH activity

Pyruvate from aerobic glycolysis enters mitochondria, where it may be converted to ***acetyl-CoA*** for entry into the citric acid cycle if ATP is needed, or for fatty acid synthesis if sufficient ATP is present. The ***pyruvate dehydrogenase complex*** **(PDH)** reaction, shown in Figure 9.6, is irreversible and cannot be used to convert acetyl-CoA to pyruvate or to glucose. Pyruvate dehydrogenase in the liver is activated by insulin, whereas in the nervous system, the enzyme is not responsive to hormones. This makes sense because high insulin levels signal to the liver that the individual is in a well-fed state; thus, the liver should not only burn glucose for energy, but shift the fatty acid equilibrium toward production and storage, rather than oxidation (fatty acid synthesis, discussed in Chapter 11 of *MCAT Biochemistry Review*, starts from citrate produced in the citric acid cycle).

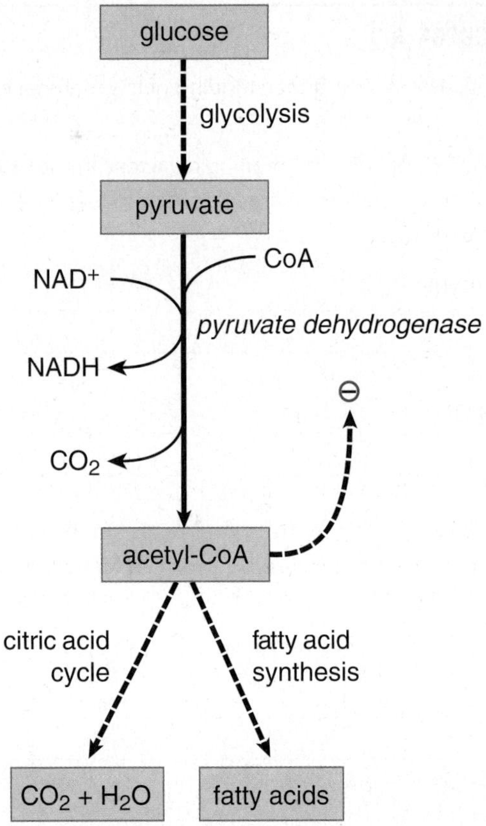

Figure 9.6 Pyruvate Dehydrogenase

Pyruvate dehydrogenase is actually a complex of enzymes carrying out multiple reactions in succession. The details of each of these reactions are covered in Chapter 10 of *MCAT Biochemistry Review*, but an overview of the enzyme is provided here because it represents one of three possible fates of pyruvate: conversion to acetyl-CoA by PDH, conversion to lactate by lactate dehydrogenase, or conversion to *oxaloacetate* by *pyruvate carboxylase.*

This large complex requires multiple cofactors and coenzymes, including *thiamine pyrophosphate*, *lipoic acid*, CoA, FAD, and NAD^+. Insufficient amounts of any of these cofactors or coenzymes can result in metabolic derangements.

Pyruvate dehydrogenase is inhibited by its product acetyl-CoA. This control is important in several contexts and should be considered along with pyruvate carboxylase, the other mitochondrial enzyme that uses pyruvate (introduced in gluconeogenesis, later in this chapter). Essentially, the buildup of acetyl-CoA (which happens during β-oxidation) causes a shift in metabolism: pyruvate is no longer converted into acetyl-CoA (to enter the citric acid cycle), but rather into oxaloacetate (to enter gluconeogenesis).

REAL WORLD

A deficiency in thiamine (vitamin B_1) can result in:

- *Beriberi*, which is characterized by congestive heart failure or nerve damage.
- *Wernicke-Korsakoff syndrome*, which is characterized by difficulty walking, uncoordinated eye movements, confusion, and memory disturbances.

Giving glucose to an individual with thiamine deficiency can lead to severe lactic acidosis and other metabolic derangements because pyruvate cannot be converted into acetyl-CoA without the vitamin. This is why thiamine must be given before an infusion of glucose in individuals suspected to have thiamine deficiency (such as alcoholics).

MCAT CONCEPT CHECK 9.4

Before you move on, assess your understanding of the material with these questions.

1. What are the reactants of the pyruvate dehydrogenase complex? What are the products?
   - Reactants:

   ___

   - Products:

   ___

2. How does acetyl-CoA affect PDH complex activity? Why?

   ___

9.5 Glycogenesis and Glycogenolysis

LEARNING OBJECTIVES

After Chapter 9.5, you will be able to:

- Recall the key enzymes, reactants, and products in glycogenesis and glycogenolysis
- Describe the features of glycogen storage diseases
- Recognize the structural features of glycogen and the major glycosidic links within a glycogen granule:

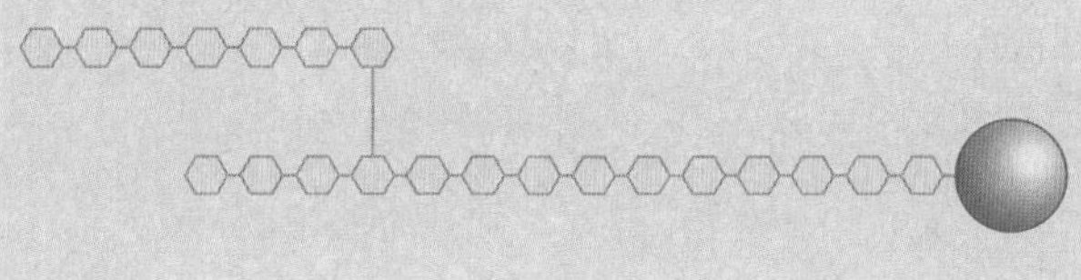

Glycogen, a branched polymer of glucose, represents a storage form of glucose. Glycogen synthesis and degradation occur primarily in liver and skeletal muscle, although other tissues store smaller quantities. Glycogen is stored in the cytoplasm as granules. Each granule has a central protein core with polyglucose chains radiating outward to form a sphere, as shown in Figure 9.7. Glycogen granules composed entirely of linear chains have the highest density of glucose near the core. If the chains are branched, the glucose density is highest at the periphery of the granule, allowing more rapid release of glucose on demand.

KEY CONCEPT

The glycogen in the liver and in skeletal muscle serve two quite different roles. Liver glycogen is broken down to maintain a constant level of glucose in the blood; muscle glycogen is broken down to provide glucose to the muscle during vigorous exercise.

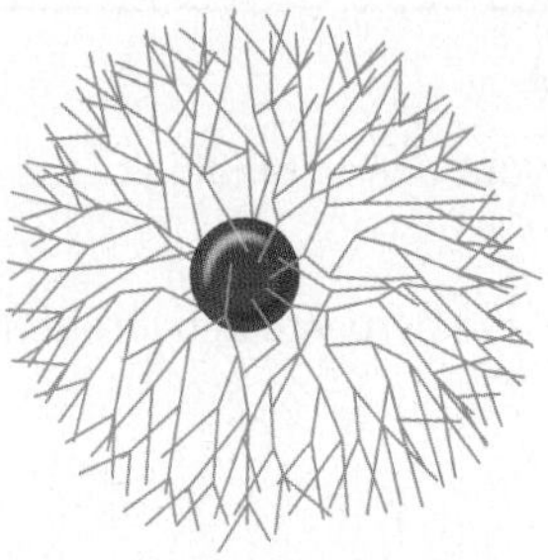

Figure 9.7 A Glycogen Granule

Glycogen stored in the liver is a source of glucose that is mobilized between meals to prevent low blood sugar, whereas muscle glycogen is stored as an energy reserve for muscle contraction.

While our focus is on human metabolism, it is worth mentioning that plants also store excess glucose in long α-linked chains of glucose called **starch**, as seen in Figure 9.8.

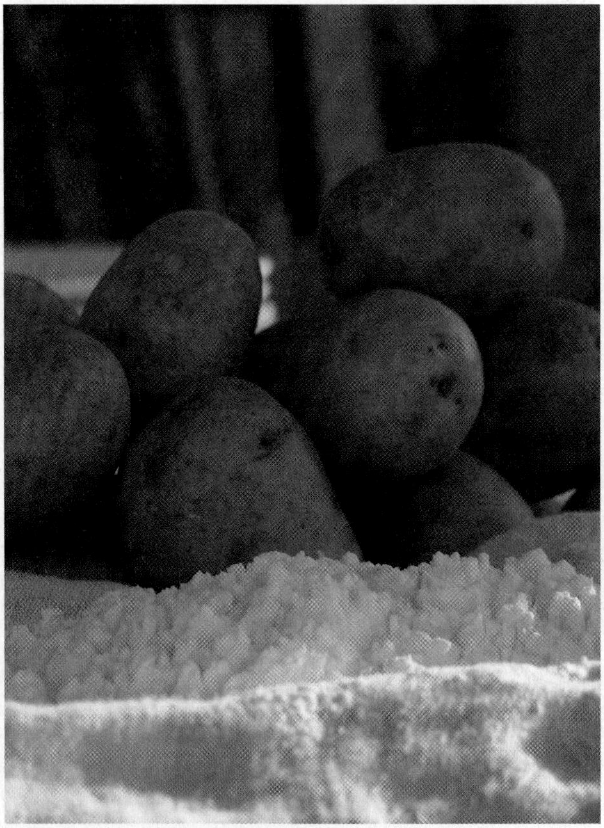

Figure 9.8 Potatoes and Potato Starch

Glycogenesis

Glycogenesis is the synthesis of glycogen granules. It begins with a core protein called *glycogenin*. As shown in Figure 9.9, glucose addition to a granule begins with glucose 6-phosphate, which is converted to glucose 1-phosphate. This glucose 1-phosphate is then activated by coupling to a molecule of *uridine diphosphate* (UDP), which permits its integration into the glycogen chain by glycogen synthase. This activation occurs when glucose 1-phosphate interacts with *uridine triphosphate* (UTP), forming UDP-glucose and a *pyrophosphate* (PP_i).

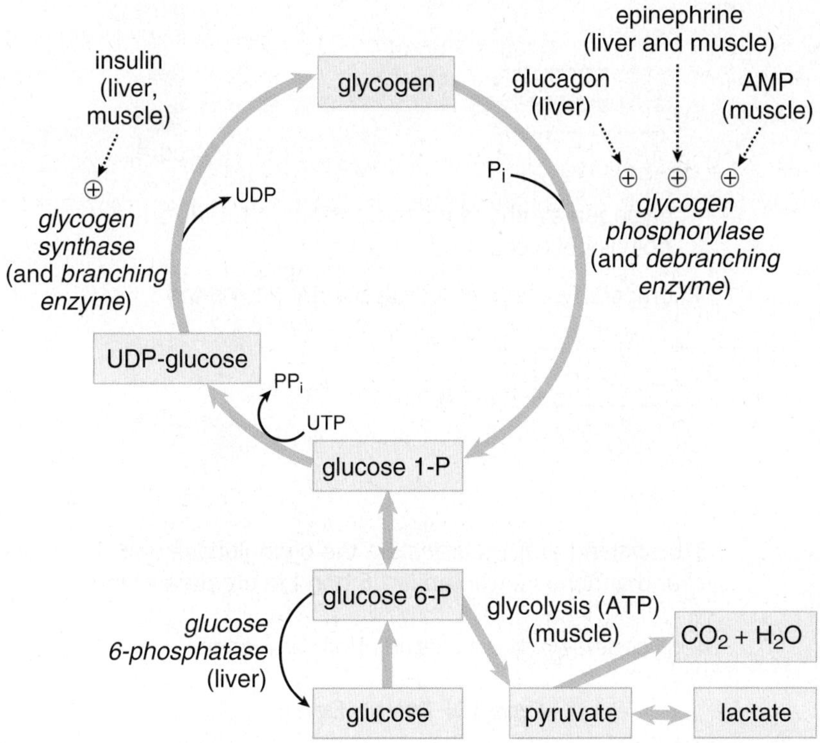

Figure 9.9 Glycogen Metabolism

Glycogen Synthase

Glycogen synthase is the rate-limiting enzyme of glycogen synthesis and forms the α-1,4 glycosidic bond found in the linear glucose chains of the granule. It is stimulated by glucose 6-phosphate and insulin. It is inhibited by epinephrine and glucagon through a protein kinase cascade that phosphorylates and inactivates the enzyme.

Branching Enzyme (Glycosyl α-1,4:α-1,6 Transferase)

Branching enzyme is responsible for introducing α-1,6-linked branches into the granule as it grows. The process by which the branch is introduced is shown schematically in Figure 9.10. Branching enzyme:

- Hydrolyzes one of the α-1,4 bonds to release a block of oligoglucose (a few glucose molecules bonded together in a chain), which is then moved and added in a slightly different location.
- Forms an α-1,6 bond to create a branch.

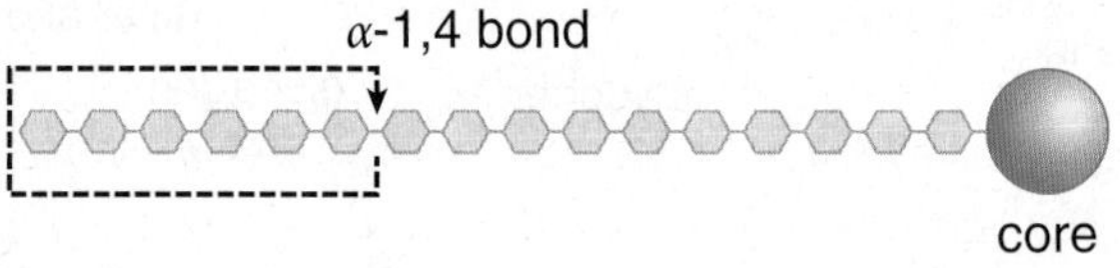

1. glycogen synthase makes a linear α-1,4-linked polyglucose chain ( )
2. branching enzyme hydrolyzes an α-1,4 bond

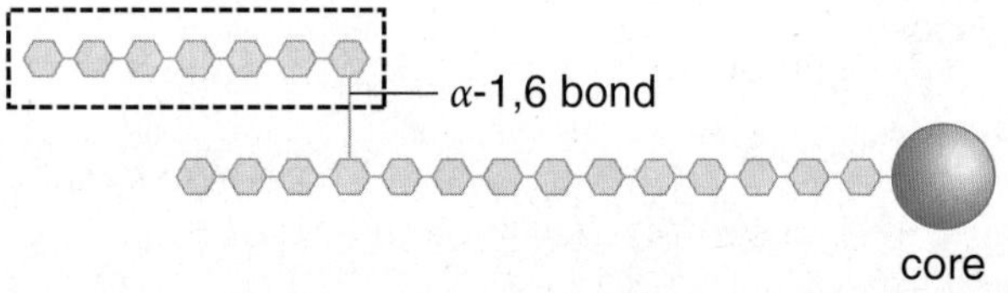

3. branching enzyme transfers the oligoglucose unit and attaches it with an α-1,6 bond to create a branch
4. glycogen synthase extends both branches

Figure 9.10 Branching Enzyme

MNEMONIC

α-1,**4** keeps the same branch moving "**4**ward"; α-1,6 (one-**six**) "puts a branch in the **mix**."

Glycogenolysis

The rate-limiting enzyme of **glycogenolysis**, the process of breaking down glycogen, is *glycogen phosphorylase*. In contrast to a *hydrolase*, a *phosphorylase* breaks bonds using an inorganic phosphate instead of water. The glucose 1-phosphate formed by glycogen phosphorylase is converted to glucose 6-phosphate by the same mutase used in glycogen synthesis, as shown in Figure 9.9.

MCAT EXPERTISE

Under the pressure of Test Day, it can be easy to misread words. When given a passage or question about carbohydrate metabolism, be sure you focus so you can distinguish between *glycolysis*, *glycogenesis*, *glycogenolysis*, and *gluconeogenesis*.

Glycogen Phosphorylase

Glycogen phosphorylase breaks α-1,4 glycosidic bonds, releasing glucose 1-phosphate from the periphery of the granule. It cannot break α-1,6 bonds and therefore stops when it nears the outermost branch points. Glycogen phosphorylase is activated by glucagon in the liver, so that glucose can be provided for the rest of the body. In skeletal muscle, it is activated by AMP and epinephrine, which signal that the muscle is active and requires more glucose. It is inhibited by ATP.

Debranching Enzyme (Glucosyl α-1,4:α-1,4 Transferase and α-1,6 Glucosidase)

Debranching enzyme is a two-enzyme complex that deconstructs the branches in glycogen that have been exposed by glycogen phosphorylase. The two-step process by which this occurs is diagrammed in Figure 9.11. Debranching enzyme:

- Breaks an α-1,4 bond adjacent to the branch point and moves the small oligoglucose chain that is released to the exposed end of the other chain.
- Forms a new α-1,4 bond.
- Hydrolyzes the α-1,6 bond, releasing the single residue at the branch point as free glucose. This represents the only free glucose produced directly in glycogenolysis (as opposed to the glucose produced from glucose 1-phosphate, which must be converted by a mutase to glucose 6-phosphate before it can be converted to glucose via the enzyme *glucose-6-phosphatase*).

KEY CONCEPT

Debranching enzyme is actually made up of two enzymes with different functions: one moves the terminal end of a glycogen chain to the branch point (α-1,4:α-1,4 transferase), and one removes the glucose monomer actually present at the branch point (α-1,6 glucosidase).

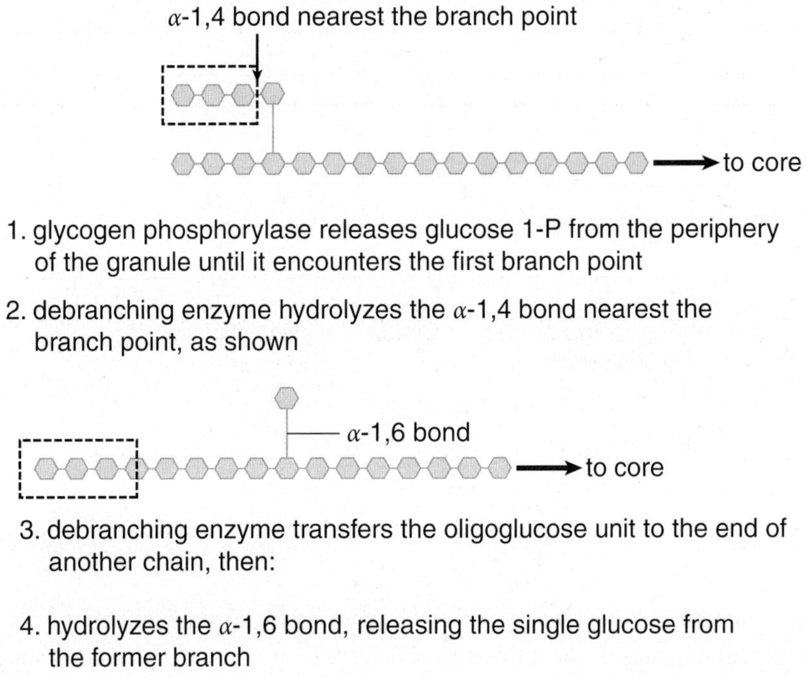

Figure 9.11 Debranching Enzyme

Glycogen Storage Diseases

There are a number of genetic deficiencies that can impact the metabolism of glycogen. The clinical features of a metabolic glycogen defect depend on a few important factors: which enzyme is affected, the degree to which that enzyme's activity is decreased, and which isoform of the enzyme is affected. **Isoforms** are slightly different versions of the same protein; in the case of glycogen enzymes, there are often different isoforms of the enzymes in the liver and muscle. These deficiencies are termed ***glycogen storage diseases*** because all are characterized by accumulation or lack of glycogen in one or more tissues.

REAL WORLD

The most common glycogen storage disease is *von Gierke's disease*, a defect in glucose-6-phosphatase. Because this enzyme is also the last step of gluconeogenesis, this process is also affected, leading to periods of extremely low blood sugar between meals. These patients therefore need continuous feeding with carbohydrates to maintain blood sugar. With the buildup of glucose 6-phosphate in liver cells, the liver enlarges and is damaged over time.

MCAT CONCEPT CHECK 9.5

Before you move on, assess your understanding of the material with these questions.

1. What is the structure of glycogen? What types of glycosidic links exist in a glycogen granule?

____

2. What are the two main enzymes of glycogenesis, and what does each accomplish?

 1. _______________
 2. _______________

3. What are the two main enzymes of glycogenolysis, and what does each accomplish?

 1. _______________
 2. _______________

9.6 Gluconeogenesis

LEARNING OBJECTIVES

After Chapter 9.6, you will be able to:

- Recognize the conditions that favor gluconeogenesis
- Recall the four enzymes unique to gluconeogenesis, and relate them to the enzymes that catalyze the opposite process in glycolysis
- Detail the regulatory role of acetyl-CoA in the metabolism of pyruvate

KEY CONCEPT

Insulin acts to lower blood sugar levels; the counterregulatory hormones, which include glucagon, epinephrine, cortisol, and growth hormone, act to raise blood sugar levels by stimulating glycogenolysis and gluconeogenesis. The regulation of metabolism is discussed in Chapter 12 of *MCAT Biochemistry Review.*

The liver maintains glucose levels in blood during fasting through either glycogenolysis or **gluconeogenesis**. The kidney can also carry out gluconeogenesis, although its contribution is much smaller. These pathways are promoted by glucagon and epinephrine, which act to raise blood sugar levels, and are inhibited by insulin, which acts to lower blood sugar levels. During fasting, glycogen reserves drop dramatically in the first 12 hours, during which time gluconeogenesis increases. After 24 hours, it represents the sole source of glucose. Important substrates for gluconeogenesis are:

- Glycerol 3-phosphate (from stored fats, or triacylglycerols, in adipose tissue)
- Lactate (from anaerobic glycolysis)
- Glucogenic amino acids (from muscle proteins)

The last item of this list merits some explaining. Amino acids can be subclassified as glucogenic, ketogenic, or both. **Glucogenic amino acids** (all except leucine and lysine) can be converted into intermediates that feed into gluconeogenesis, while **ketogenic amino acids** can be converted into ketone bodies, which can be used as an alternative fuel, particularly during periods of prolonged starvation. See Chapter 11 of *MCAT Biochemistry Review* for more information on amino acid and protein metabolism.

BRIDGE

Amino acids and proteins are extremely important topics for the MCAT. Check out Chapter 1 of *MCAT Biochemistry Review* for more information on amino acids, peptides, and proteins.

Dietary fructose and galactose can also be converted to glucose in the liver, as described earlier in this chapter.

In humans, while glucose is converted into acetyl-CoA through glycolysis and pyruvate dehydrogenase, it is not possible to convert acetyl-CoA back to glucose. Because most fatty acids are metabolized solely to acetyl-CoA, they are not a major source of glucose either. One minor exception is fatty acids with an odd number of carbon atoms (for example, fatty acid tails containing 17 carbons), which yield a small amount of *propionyl-CoA*, which is glucogenic.

The pathway of gluconeogenesis is diagrammed in Figure 9.12. Each of the important gluconeogenic intermediates—lactate, alanine, and glycerol 3-phosphate—have enzymes that convert them into glycolytic intermediates.

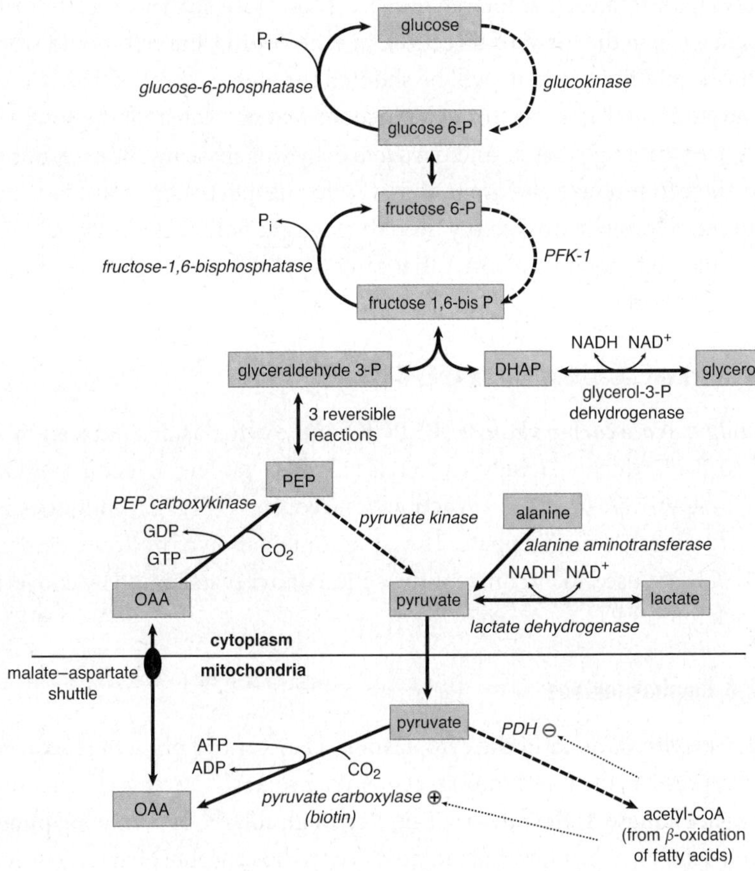

Figure 9.12 Gluconeogenesis

Lactate is converted to pyruvate by *lactate dehydrogenase*. Alanine is converted to pyruvate by *alanine aminotransferase*. Glycerol 3-phosphate is converted to dihydroxyacetone phosphate (DHAP) by *glycerol-3-phosphate dehydrogenase*.

Important Enzymes of Gluconeogenesis

Most steps in gluconeogenesis represent a reversal of glycolysis and have thus been omitted from the diagram. However, the four important enzymes to know are those required to catalyze reactions that circumvent the irreversible steps of glycolysis in the liver (those catalyzed by glucokinase, phosphofructokinase-1, and pyruvate kinase).

Pyruvate Carboxylase

KEY CONCEPT

Because glycolysis contains three irreversible steps (those catalyzed by hexokinase, phosphofructokinase-1, and pyruvate kinase), different enzymes must exist in gluconeogenesis to allow the body to revert pyruvate to glucose.

Pyruvate carboxylase is a mitochondrial enzyme that is activated by acetyl-CoA (from β-oxidation). The product, oxaloacetate (OAA), is a citric acid cycle intermediate and cannot leave the mitochondrion. Rather, it is reduced to *malate*, which can leave the mitochondrion via the malate–aspartate shuttle, which is described in Chapter 10 of *MCAT Biochemistry Review*. Once in the cytoplasm, malate is oxidized to OAA. The fact that acetyl-CoA activates pyruvate carboxylase is an important point. Acetyl-CoA inhibits pyruvate dehydrogenase because a high level of acetyl-CoA implies that the cell is energetically satisfied and need not run the citric acid cycle in the forward direction; in other words, the cell should stop burning glucose. Rather, pyruvate will be shunted through pyruvate carboxylase to help generate additional glucose through gluconeogenesis. Note that the source of acetyl-CoA is not from glycolysis and pyruvate dehydrogenase in this case, but from fatty acids. Thus, to produce glucose in the liver during gluconeogenesis, fatty acids must be burned to provide this energy, stop the forward flow of the citric acid cycle, and produce massive amounts of OAA that can eventually lead to glucose production for the rest of the body.

Phosphoenolpyruvate Carboxykinase (PEPCK)

Phosphoenolpyruvate carboxykinase **(PEPCK)** in the cytoplasm is induced by glucagon and cortisol, which generally act to raise blood sugar levels. It converts OAA to phosphoenolpyruvate (PEP) in a reaction that requires GTP. PEP continues in the pathway to fructose 1,6-bisphosphate. Thus, the combination of pyruvate carboxylase and PEPCK are used to circumvent the action of pyruvate kinase by converting pyruvate back into PEP.

Fructose-1,6-Bisphosphatase

Fructose-1,6-bisphosphatase in the cytoplasm is a key control point of gluconeogenesis and represents the rate-limiting step of the process. It reverses the action of phosphofructokinase-1, the rate-limiting step of glycolysis, by removing phosphate from fructose 1,6-bisphosphate to produce fructose 6-phosphate. A common pattern to note is that *phosphatases* oppose kinases. Fructose-1,6-bisphosphatase is activated by ATP and inhibited by AMP and fructose 2,6-bisphosphate. This should make sense: high levels of ATP imply that a cell is energetically satisfied enough to produce glucose for the rest of the body, whereas high levels of AMP imply that a cell needs energy and cannot afford to produce energy for the rest of the body before satisfying its own requirements. Fructose 2,6-bisphosphate (F2,6-BP) is sometimes thought of as a marker for satisfactory energy levels in liver cells. It helps these cells override the inhibition of phosphofructokinase-1 that occurs when high levels of acetyl-CoA are formed, signaling to the liver cell that it should shift its function from burning to storing fuel. F2,6-BP, produced by PFK-2, controls both gluconeogenesis and glycolysis (in the liver). Recall from the earlier discussion of this enzyme and Figure 9.2 that PFK-2 is activated by insulin and inhibited by glucagon. Thus, glucagon will lower F2,6-BP and stimulate gluconeogenesis, whereas insulin will increase F2,6-BP and inhibit gluconeogenesis.

Glucose-6-Phosphatase

Glucose-6-phosphatase is found only in the lumen of the endoplasmic reticulum in liver cells. Glucose 6-phosphate is transported into the ER, and free glucose is transported back into the cytoplasm, from where it can diffuse out of the cell using GLUT transporters. The absence of glucose-6-phosphatase in skeletal muscle means that muscle glycogen cannot serve as a source of blood glucose and rather is for use only within the muscle. Glucose-6-phosphatase is used to circumvent glucokinase and hexokinase, which convert glucose to glucose 6-phosphate.

Although alanine is the major glucogenic amino acid, almost all amino acids are also glucogenic. Most of these are converted by individual pathways to citric acid cycle intermediates, then to malate, following the same path from there to glucose.

It is important to note that glucose produced by hepatic (liver-based) gluconeogenesis does not represent an energy source for the liver. Gluconeogenesis requires expenditure of ATP that is provided by β-oxidation of fatty acids. Therefore, as mentioned above, hepatic gluconeogenesis is always dependent on β-oxidation of fatty acids in the liver. During periods of low blood sugar, adipose tissue releases these fatty acids by breaking down triacylglycerols to glycerol (which can also be converted to the gluconeogenic intermediate DHAP) and free fatty acids.

Although the acetyl-CoA from fatty acids cannot be converted into glucose, it can be converted into ketone bodies as an alternative fuel for cells, including the brain. Extended periods of low blood sugar are thus usually accompanied by high levels of ketones in the blood. Ketone bodies can be thought of as a transportable form of acetyl-CoA that is primarily utilized in periods of extended starvation.

KEY CONCEPT

Because gluconeogenesis requires acetyl-CoA to occur (to inhibit pyruvate dehydrogenase and stimulate pyruvate carboxylase), gluconeogenesis is inextricably linked to fatty acid oxidation. The source of acetyl-CoA cannot be glycolysis because this would just burn the glucose that is being generated in gluconeogenesis.

REAL WORLD

Because red blood cells lack mitochondria, they cannot carry out aerobic metabolism. Rather, pyruvate is converted to lactic acid to regenerate NAD^+. However, lactate is acidic; it must be removed from the bloodstream to avoid acidifying the blood. Red blood cells deliver this lactate to the liver, where it can be converted back into pyruvate and, through gluconeogenesis, become glucose for the red blood cells to use. This is known as the Cori cycle: glucose is converted to lactate in red blood cells, and lactate is converted to glucose in liver cells.

MCAT CONCEPT CHECK 9.6

Before you move on, assess your understanding of the material with these questions.

1. Under what physiological conditions should the body carry out gluconeogenesis?

____

2. What are the four enzymes unique to gluconeogenesis? Which irreversible glycolytic enzymes do they replace?

Gluconeogenic Enzyme	Replaces

3. How does acetyl-CoA shift the metabolism of pyruvate?

____

4. Given that the glycogen storage disorder von Gierke's disease affects the last enzyme of gluconeogenesis, predict the associated metabolic derangement that occurs.

____

9.7 The Pentose Phosphate Pathway

LEARNING OBJECTIVES

After Chapter 9.7, you will be able to:

- Identify the two major products of the pentose phosphate pathway
- Explain the three primary functions of NADPH in cellular respiration

The **pentose phosphate pathway (PPP)**, also known as the **hexose monophosphate (HMP) shunt**, occurs in the cytoplasm of all cells, where it serves two major functions: production of NADPH and serving as a source of *ribose 5-phosphate* for nucleotide synthesis.

An abbreviated diagram of the pathway is shown in Figure 9.13. The first part of the PPP begins with glucose 6-phosphate, ends with *ribulose 5-phosphate*, and is irreversible. This part produces NADPH and involves the important rate-limiting enzyme ***glucose-6-phosphate dehydrogenase*** **(G6PD)**. G6PD is induced by insulin because the abundance of sugar entering the cell under insulin stimulation will be shunted into both fuel utilization pathways (glycolysis and aerobic respiration), as well as fuel storage pathways (fatty acid synthesis, glycogenesis, and the PPP). The shunt is also inhibited by its product, NADPH, and is activated by one of its reactants, $NADP^+$.

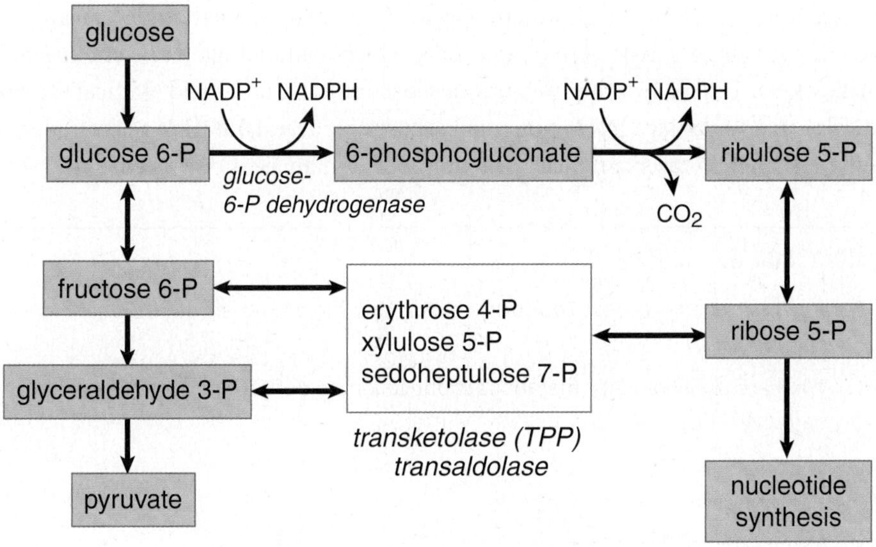

Figure 9.13 The Pentose Phosphate Pathway

The second part of the pathway, beginning with ribulose 5-phosphate, represents a series of reversible reactions that produce an equilibrated pool of sugars for biosynthesis, including ribose 5-phosphate for nucleotide synthesis. Because fructose 6-phosphate and glyceraldehyde 3-phosphate are among the sugars produced, intermediates can feed back into glycolysis; conversely, pentoses can be made from glycolytic intermediates without going through the G6PD reaction. These interconversions are primarily accomplished by the enzymes *transketolase* and *transaldolase*.

Functions of NADPH

While their names appear similar, NADPH and NADH are not the same thing. In the cell, NAD^+ acts as a high-energy electron acceptor from a number of biochemical reactions. It thus can be thought of as a potent oxidizing agent because it helps another molecule be oxidized (and thus is reduced itself during the process). The NADH produced from this reduction of NAD^+ can then feed into the electron transport chain to indirectly produce ATP.

Conversely, **NADPH** primarily acts as an electron donor in a number of biochemical reactions. It thus can be thought of as a potent reducing agent because it helps other molecules be reduced (and thus is oxidized itself during the process). Cells require NADPH for a variety of functions, including:

- Biosynthesis, mainly of fatty acids and cholesterol
- Assisting in cellular bleach production in certain white blood cells, thereby contributing to bactericidal activity
- Maintenance of a supply of reduced *glutathione* to protect against reactive oxygen species (acting as the body's natural antioxidant)

REAL WORLD

G6PD deficiency is an X-linked disorder and is the most common inherited enzyme defect in the world. Because the PPP is critically important in maintaining levels of glutathione, which helps break down peroxides, these individuals are susceptible to oxidative stress, especially in red blood cells, which carry a large concentration of oxygen. Ingestion of certain oxidizing compounds (especially particular antibiotics and antimalarial medications) or infections can lead to high concentrations of reactive oxygen species, which cause red blood cell lysis. It is hypothesized that the defect evolved because it provides some resistance to malaria infection. G6PD deficiency has also been called *favism* because fava beans are a highly oxidizing food that will also cause hemolysis in these individuals.

BRIDGE

The ribulose 5-phosphate created in the PPP is isomerized to ribose 5-phosphate, the backbone of nucleic acids. When coupled to a nitrogenous base, it forms a nucleotide that can be integrated into RNA. Make sure to review RNA synthesis (transcription; Chapter 7 of *MCAT Biochemistry Review*), as well as DNA synthesis (Chapter 6 of *MCAT Biochemistry Review*), because these are highly tested topics on the MCAT.

KEY CONCEPT

NADPH and NADH are not the same thing. NAD^+ is an energy carrier; NADPH is used in biosynthesis, in the immune system, and to help prevent oxidative damage.

This last function is important in protecting cells from free radical oxidative damage caused by peroxides. Hydrogen peroxide, H_2O_2, is produced as a byproduct in aerobic metabolism, and can break apart to form hydroxide radicals, $OH^{\bullet}$. Free radicals can attack lipids, including those in the phospholipids of the membrane. When oxidized, these lipids lose their function and can weaken the membrane, causing cell lysis. This is especially true in red blood cells, which contain high levels of oxygen, which, when oxidized by other free radicals, becomes the superoxide radical $O_2^{\bullet}$. Free radicals can also damage DNA, potentially causing cancer. **Glutathione** is a reducing agent that can help reverse radical formation before damage is done to the cell.

MCAT CONCEPT CHECK 9.7

Before you move on, assess your understanding of the material with these questions.

1. What are the two major metabolic products of the pentose phosphate pathway (PPP)?

    1. ____________________
    2. ____________________

2. What are three primary functions of NADPH?

    1. ____________________
    2. ____________________
    3. ____________________

Conclusion

This chapter is critically important in your studying for the MCAT. The processes of carbohydrate metabolism that do not require oxygen are heavily tested, as is their integration. The body has evolved in such a way that we can use, store, or create fuel 24 hours a day, depending on the demands of the internal and external environment. We can turn on pathways when we need them and turn them off when we don't. And the regulation of these pathways makes sense: for example, acetyl-CoA—a downstream product of glycolysis—can turn off the process of glycolysis and allow us to either store extra sugar as other biomolecules or generate sugar anew if we need it. Return to this chapter repeatedly during your studies to maximize points on metabolism on Test Day. In the next chapter, we'll turn our attention to the oxygen-requiring carbohydrate metabolism processes, including the citric acid cycle, the electron transport chain (ETC), and oxidative phosphorylation.

You've reviewed the content, now test your knowledge and critical thinking skills by completing a test-like passage set in your online resources!

GO ONLINE

CONCEPT SUMMARY

Glucose Transport

- **GLUT 2** is found in the liver (for glucose storage) and pancreatic β-islet cells (as part of the glucose sensor). It has a high K_m.
- **GLUT 4** is found in adipose tissue and muscle and is stimulated by insulin. It has a low K_m.

Glycolysis

- **Glycolysis** occurs in the cytoplasm of all cells and does not require oxygen. It yields 2 ATP per molecule of glucose.
- Important glycolytic enzymes include:
  - **Glucokinase**, which converts glucose to glucose 6-phosphate. It is present in the pancreatic β-islet cells as part of the glucose sensor and is responsive to insulin in the liver.
  - **Hexokinase**, which converts glucose to glucose 6-phosphate in peripheral tissues.
  - **Phosphofructokinase-1 (PFK-1)**, which phosphorylates fructose 6-phosphate to fructose 1,6-bisphosphate in the rate-limiting step of glycolysis. PFK-1 is activated by AMP and fructose 2,6-bisphosphate (F2,6-BP) and is inhibited by ATP and citrate.
  - **Phosphofructokinase-2 (PFK-2)**, which produces the F2,6-BP that activates PFK-1. It is activated by insulin and inhibited by glucagon.
  - **Glyceraldehyde-3-phosphate dehydrogenase** produces NADH, which can feed into the electron transport chain.
  - **3-phosphoglycerate kinase** and **pyruvate kinase** each perform **substrate-level phosphorylation**, placing an inorganic phosphate (P_i) onto ADP to form ATP.
- The enzymes that catalyze irreversible reactions are glucokinase/hexokinase, PFK-1, and pyruvate kinase.
- The NADH produced in glycolysis is oxidized by the mitochondrial electron transport chain when oxygen is present.
- If oxygen or mitochondria are absent, the NADH produced in glycolysis is oxidized by cytoplasmic **lactate dehydrogenase**. Examples include red blood cells, skeletal muscle (during short, intense bursts of exercise), and any cell deprived of oxygen.

Other Monosaccharides

- **Galactose** comes from lactose in milk. It is trapped in the cell by **galactokinase**, and converted to glucose 1-phosphate via **galactose-1-phosphate uridyltransferase** and an epimerase.
- **Fructose** comes from honey, fruit, and sucrose (common table sugar). It is trapped in the cell by **fructokinase**, and then cleaved by **aldolase B** to form glyceraldehyde and DHAP.

Pyruvate Dehydrogenase

- **Pyruvate dehydrogenase** refers to a complex of enzymes that convert pyruvate to acetyl-CoA.
- It is stimulated by insulin and inhibited by acetyl-CoA.

Glycogenesis and Glycogenolysis

- **Glycogenesis** (glycogen synthesis) is the production of glycogen using two main enzymes:
  - **Glycogen synthase**, which creates α-1,4 glycosidic links between glucose molecules. It is activated by insulin in liver and muscle.
  - **Branching enzyme**, which moves a block of oligoglucose from one chain and adds it to the growing glycogen as a new branch using an α-1,6 glycosidic link.
- **Glycogenolysis** is the breakdown of glycogen using two main enzymes:
  - **Glycogen phosphorylase**, which removes single glucose 1-phosphate molecules by breaking α-1,4 glycosidic links. In the liver, it is activated by glucagon to prevent low blood sugar; in exercising skeletal muscle, it is activated by epinephrine and AMP to provide glucose for the muscle itself.
  - **Debranching enzyme**, which moves a block of oligoglucose from one branch and connects it to the chain using an α-1,4 glycosidic link. It also removes the branchpoint, which is connected via an α-1,6 glycosidic link, releasing a free glucose molecule.

Gluconeogenesis

- **Gluconeogenesis** occurs in both the cytoplasm and mitochondria, predominantly in the liver. There is a small contribution from the kidneys.
- Most of gluconeogenesis is simply the reverse of glycolysis, using the same enzymes. The three irreversible steps of glycolysis must be bypassed by different enzymes:
    - **Pyruvate carboxylase** converts pyruvate into oxaloacetate, which is converted to phosphoenolpyruvate by **phosphoenolpyruvate carboxykinase** (**PEPCK**). Together, these two enzymes bypass pyruvate kinase. Pyruvate carboxylase is activated by acetyl-CoA from β-oxidation; PEPCK is activated by glucagon and cortisol.
    - **Fructose-1,6-bisphosphatase** converts fructose 1,6-bisphosphate to fructose 6-phosphate, bypassing phosphofructokinase-1. This is the rate-limiting step of gluconeogenesis. It is activated by ATP directly and glucagon indirectly (via decreased levels of fructose 2,6-bisphosphate). It is inhibited by AMP directly and insulin indirectly (via increased levels of fructose 2,6-bisphosphate).
    - **Glucose-6-phosphatase** converts glucose 6-phosphate to free glucose, bypassing glucokinase. It is found only in the endoplasmic reticulum of the liver.

The Pentose Phosphate Pathway

- The **pentose phosphate pathway** (**PPP**), also known as the **hexose monophosphate** (**HMP**) **shunt**, occurs in the cytoplasm of most cells, generating **NADPH** and sugars for biosynthesis (derived from ribulose 5-phosphate).
- The rate-limiting enzyme is **glucose-6-phosphate dehydrogenase**, which is activated by $NADP^+$ and insulin and inhibited by NADPH.

ANSWERS TO CONCEPT CHECKS

9.1

1.

	GLUT 2	GLUT 4
Important tissues	Liver, pancreas	Adipose tissue, muscle
K_m	High (~15 mM)	Low (~5 mM)
Saturated at normal glucose levels?	No—cannot be saturated under normal physiological conditions	Yes—saturated when glucose levels are only slightly above 5 mM
Responsive to insulin?	No (but serves as glucose sensor to cause release of insulin in pancreatic β-cells)	Yes

2. GLUT 4 is saturated when glucose levels are only slightly above 5 mM, so glucose entry can only be increased by increasing the number of transporters. Insulin promotes the fusion of vesicles containing preformed GLUT 4 with the cell membrane.

9.2

1.
- Hexokinase phosphorylates glucose to form glucose 6-phosphate, "trapping" glucose in the cell. It is inhibited by glucose 6-phosphate. It is irreversible.
- Glucokinase also phosphorylates and "traps" glucose in liver and pancreatic cells, and works with GLUT 2 as part of the glucose sensor in β-islet cells. In liver cells, it is induced by insulin. It is irreversible.
- PFK-1 catalyzes the rate-limiting step of glycolysis, phosphorylating fructose 6-phosphate to fructose 1,6-bisphosphate using ATP. It is inhibited by ATP, citrate, and glucagon. It is activated by AMP, fructose 2,6-bisphosphate, and insulin. It is irreversible.
- Glyceraldehyde-3-phosphate dehydrogenase generates NADH while phosphorylating glyceraldehyde 3-phosphate to 1,3-bisphosphoglycerate. It is reversible.
- 3-Phosphoglycerate kinase performs a substrate-level phosphorylation, transferring a phosphate from 1,3-bisphosphoglycerate to ADP, forming ATP and 3-phosphoglycerate. It is reversible.
- Pyruvate kinase performs another substrate-level phosphorylation, transferring a phosphate from phosphoenolpyruvate (PEP) to ADP, forming ATP and pyruvate. It is activated by fructose 1,6-bisphosphate. It is irreversible.

2. Fermentation must occur to regenerate NAD^+, which is in limited supply in cells. Fermentation generates no ATP or energy carriers; it merely regenerates the coenzymes needed in glycolysis.
3. The binding of 2,3-BPG decreases hemoglobin's affinity for oxygen. Fetal hemoglobin must be able to "steal" oxygen from maternal hemoglobin at the placental interface; therefore, it would be disadvantageous to lower its affinity for oxygen.

9.3

1. Galactose is phosphorylated by galactokinase, trapping it in the cell. Galactose-1-phosphate uridyltransferase produces glucose 1-phosphate, a glycolytic intermediate, thus linking the pathways.
2. Fructose is phosphorylated by fructokinase, trapping it in the cell (with a small contribution from hexokinase). Aldolase B produces dihydroxyacetone phosphate (DHAP) and glyceraldehyde (which can be phosphorylated to form glyceraldehyde 3-phosphate), which are glycolytic intermediates, thus linking the pathways.

9.4

1. Pyruvate, NAD^+, and CoA are the reactants of the PDH complex. Acetyl-CoA, NADH, and CO_2 are the products.
2. Acetyl-CoA inhibits the PDH complex. As a product of the enzyme complex, a buildup of acetyl-CoA from either the citric acid cycle or fatty acid oxidation signals that the cell is energetically satisfied and that the production of acetyl-CoA should be slowed or stopped. Pyruvate can then be used to form other products, such as oxaloacetate for use in gluconeogenesis.

9.5

1. Glycogen is made up of a core protein of glycogenin with linear chains of glucose emanating out from the center, connected by α-1,4 glycosidic links. Some of these chains are branched, which requires α-1,6 glycosidic links.
2. Glycogen synthase attaches the glucose molecule from UDP-glucose to the growing glycogen chain, forming an α-1,4 link in the process. Branching enzyme creates a branch by breaking an α-1,4 link in the growing chain and moving a block of oligoglucose to another location in the glycogen granule. The oligoglucose is then attached with an α-1,6 link.
3. Glycogen phosphorylase removes a glucose molecule from glycogen using a phosphate, breaking the α-1,4 link and creating glucose 1-phosphate. Debranching enzyme moves all of the glucose from a branch to a longer glycogen chain by breaking an α-1,4 link and forming a new α-1,4 link to the longer chain. The branchpoint is left behind; this is removed by breaking the α-1,6 link to form a free molecule of glucose.

9.6

1. Gluconeogenesis occurs when an individual has been fasting for >12 hours. To carry out gluconeogenesis, hepatic (and renal) cells must have enough energy to drive the process of glucose creation, which requires sufficient fat stores to undergo β-oxidation.
2.

Gluconeogenic Enzyme	Replaces
Pyruvate carboxylase	Pyruvate kinase
Phosphoenolpyruvate carboxykinase (PEPCK)	Pyruvate kinase
Fructose-1,6-bisphosphatase	Phosphofructokinase-1
Glucose-6-phosphatase	Glucokinase

3. Acetyl-CoA inhibits pyruvate dehydrogenase complex while activating pyruvate carboxylase. The net effect is to shift from burning pyruvate in the citric acid cycle to creating new glucose molecules for the rest of the body. The acetyl-CoA for this regulation comes predominantly from β-oxidation, not glycolysis.
4. The last enzyme in gluconeogenesis is glucose-6-phosphatase so patients with von Gierke's disease are unable to perform gluconeogenesis in addition to glycogenolysis. This means patients will be unable to produce glucose during periods of fasting (resulting in hypoglycemia). Furthermore, given a blocker in the gluconeogenic pathway, a buildup of intermediates (including lactate resulting in lactic acidosis) would also be expected.

9.7

1. The two major metabolic products of the pentose phosphate pathway are ribose 5-phosphate and NADPH.
2. NADPH is involved in lipid biosynthesis, bactericidal bleach formation in certain white blood cells, and maintenance of glutathione stores to protect against reactive oxygen species.

SCIENCE MASTERY ASSESSMENT EXPLANATIONS

1. **B**

The GLUT 2 receptor, **(B)**, has a high K_m and is expressed in hepatocytes of the liver. When the concentration of glucose in the blood is high, glucose is transported into the liver with first order kinetics. Also, in the pancreas, GLUT 2 and glucokinase serve as a glucose sensor. These observations together support **(B)** as the right answer.

2. **D**

The liver, like all cells, needs a constant supply of glucose; however, it is able to produce its own glucose through gluconeogenesis (cells in the kidney can also complete low levels of gluconeogenesis). The other cells listed here are absolutely dependent on a glucose source from the blood for energy, although they may also use other fuels in addition to glucose. For example, the brain can utilize ketone bodies during lengthy periods of starvation; however, it still requires at least some glucose for proper function.

3. **D**

GLUT is an abbreviation for glucose transporter and describes a family of sugar transporters with varying distributions and activities. GLUT 4 is found in adipose tissue and muscle, and mediates insulin-stimulated glucose uptake; in fact, it is the only insulin-responsive glucose transporter. Insulin acts via its receptor to translocate GLUT 4 to the plasma membrane. GLUT 4 in skeletal muscle is also stimulated by exercise through an insulin-independent pathway.

4. **B**

After an overnight fast, the liver is producing glucose and glucokinase activity would be insignificant. Glucokinase is used to trap extra glucose in liver cells as part of a storage mechanism; with low blood glucose, liver cells would be generating new glucose, not storing it. It is also in the pancreas, where it serves as a glucose sensor; if glucose levels are low, it has little activity in this tissue as well. Malate dehydrogenase, **(A)**, and α-ketoglutarate dehydrogenase, **(C)**, are citric acid cycle enzymes. Phosphofructokinase-1, **(D)**, is a glycolytic enzyme. Other enzymes used in glycolysis, the citric acid cycle, or gluconeogenesis, such as phosphofructokinase-1, would be expected to maintain normal activity after an overnight fast, using glucose derived from glycogen or gluconeogenesis, rather than orally ingested glucose.

5. **C**

This question asks for an enzyme whose role is *not* to trap sugar in the cell. Phosphofructokinase **(C)** is the rate-limiting enzyme of glycolysis. Its role is to phosphorylate fructose-6-phosphate to fructose-1,6-bisphosphate during the third step of glycolysis. Importantly, the substrate of phosphofructokinase, i.e. fructose-6-phosphate, has already been once phosphorylated before reaching phosphofructokinase. Therefore, fructose-6-phosphate is already trapped in the cell before even reaching phosphofructokinase. For this reason, it cannot be said that phosphofructokinase is used to trap sugar in the cell. By contrast, **(A)**, **(B)**, and **(D)**, can be eliminated because hexokinase phosphorylates glucose, galactokinase phosphorylates galactose, and fructokinase phosphorylates fructose, each reaction trapping the previously unphosphorylated sugar in the cell.

6. **C**

Pyruvate is converted primarily into three main intermediates: acetyl-CoA, **(B)**, for the citric acid cycle (via pyruvate dehydrogenase complex); lactate, **(D)**, during fermentation (via lactate dehydrogenase); or oxaloacetate, **(C)**, for gluconeogenesis (via pyruvate carboxylase). High levels of acetyl-CoA, which is produced during β-oxidation, will inhibit pyruvate dehydrogenase and shift the citric acid cycle to run in the reverse direction, producing oxaloacetate for gluconeogenesis. Acetyl-CoA also stimulates pyruvate carboxylase directly.

7. **D**

The pattern described for this child's glycogen demonstrates appropriate production: there are long chains of glucose monomers, implying that glycogen synthase works. There are also branch points, implying that branching enzyme, **(B)** works. During glycogenolysis, it seems that the child is able to remove individual glucose monomers and process glycogen down to the branch point itself, which requires glycogen phosphorylase, **(A)**, and α-1,4:α-1,4 transferase, **(C)**. The metabolic problem here is removing the final glucose at the branch point, which is an α-1,6 (not α-1,4) link. This requires **(D)**, α-1,6 glucosidase.

8. **C**

Citrate is produced by citrate synthase from acetyl-CoA and oxaloacetate. This reaction takes place in the mitochondria. When the citric acid cycle slows down, citrate accumulates. In the cytosol, it acts as a negative allosteric regulator of phosphofructokinase-1, the enzyme that catalyzes the rate-limiting step of glycolysis.

9. **D**

In most biochemical pathways, only a few enzymatic reactions are under regulatory control. These often occur either at the beginning of pathways or at pathway branch points. The pyruvate dehydrogenase (PDH) complex controls the link between glycolysis and the citric acid cycle, and decarboxylates pyruvate (the end product of glycolysis) with production of NADH and acetyl-CoA (the substrate for the citric acid cycle). After intense exercise, one would expect PDH to be highly active to generate ATP. ADP levels, **(A)**, should be high because ATP was just burned by the muscle. Acetyl-CoA, **(B)**, is an inhibitor of PDH, causing a shift of pyruvate into the gluconeogenic pathway. A high NADH/NAD^+ ratio, **(C)**, would imply that the cell is already energetically satisfied and not in need of energy, which would not be expected in intensely exercising muscle.

10. **B**

In this question, the right answer will be the molecule whose metabolism will be the *least* impacted by the inhibition of phosphofructokinase-1 (PFK-1). The enzyme PFK-1 catalyzes the rate-limiting step of glycolysis. So sugars that enter the glycolytic pathway after this rate-limiting step, i.e. downstream of PFK-1, would be least impacted by inhibition of PFK-1. Given this criterion, recall the metabolic pathway of fructose, choice **(B)**, which is phosphorylated and then cleaved into glyceraldehyde and DHAP, both of which enter glycolysis downstream of PFK-1. Therefore the metabolism of fructose does not depend on PFK-1, and would therefore be least impacted by the inhibition of PFK-1, making **(B)** the correct answer. By contrast, glucose, **(C)**, is metabolised using the the usual glycolytic pathway, and would therefore be impacted by inhibition of PFK-1. Similarly, galactose, **(D)**, is phosphorylated and subsequently isomerized into glucose-6-phosphate, which then follows the usual pathway and would therefore be impacted by inhibition of PFK-1. And lactose, **(A)**, is cleaved by lactase into glucose and galactose. For these reasons, **(A)**, **(B)**, and **(D)** can be eliminated.

11. **B**

Based on the question stem, we can infer that the antibiotics must have been an oxidative stress on the patient (antibiotics, antimalarial medications, infections, certain foods like fava beans, and other common exposures can induce an oxidative stress). The pentose phosphate pathway is responsible for generating NADPH, which is used to reduce glutathione, one of the natural antioxidants present in the body. In individuals with glucose-6-phosphate dehydrogenase (G6PD) deficiency, NADPH cannot be produced at sufficient levels, and oxidative stresses lead to cell membrane and protein (hemoglobin) damage. Note that you do not need to actually know the disease to answer this question; merely knowing that the enzyme must be from the pentose phosphate pathway, which is involved in mitigating oxidative stress, is sufficient.

12. **A**

The irreversible enzymes in glycolysis are hexokinase (or glucokinase in liver and pancreatic β-cells), phosphofructokinase-1, and pyruvate kinase. Pyruvate dehydrogenase is not considered a glycolytic enzyme because it requires the mitochondria to function. The list below shows the correct pairing of glycolytic enzymes with gluconeogenic enzymes:

- Hexokinase or glucokinase/glucose-6-phosphatase
- Phosphofructokinase-1/fructose-1,6-bisphosphatase
- Pyruvate kinase/pyruvate carboxylase and phosphoenolpyruvate carboxykinase (PEPCK)

13. **B**

After a fast, the liver must contribute glucose into the bloodstream through two main processes: glycogenolysis (early to intermediate fasting) and gluconeogenesis (intermediate to late fasting). The other processes would continue at normal basal levels or have decreased activity after a fast.

14. **A**

A deficiency in branching enzyme would result in chains of unbranched glycogen. Since glycogen synthase is not affected, the chain length would be normal, indicating a normal abundance of α-1,4 linkages. However, a loss of branching would correspond to a decrease in α-1,6, linkages. Thus, the ratio of α-1,4 to α-1,6 would increase as division by a smaller denominator yields a larger value, making **(A)** the correct answer.

15. **A**

Hexokinase catalyzes an important irreversible step of glycolysis, but it is not the rate-limiting step. Phosphofructokinase-1 catalyzes the rate-limiting step of glycolysis. Glycogen synthase, **(B)**, catalyzes the rate-limiting step of glycogenesis; glucose-6-phosphate dehydrogenase, **(C)**, catalyzes the rate-limiting step of the pentose phosphate pathway; and fructose-1,6-bisphosphatase, >**(D)**, catalyzes the rate-limiting step of gluconeogenesis.

Consult your online resources for additional practice.

GO ONLINE

SHARED CONCEPTS

Biochemistry Chapter 4
Carbohydrate Structure and Function

Biochemistry Chapter 10
Carbohydrate Metabolism II

Biochemistry Chapter 12
Bioenergetics and Regulation of Metabolism

Biology Chapter 7
The Cardiovascular System

General Chemistry Chapter 5
Chemical Kinetics

General Chemistry Chapter 11
Oxidation–Reduction Reactions

CHAPTER 10

CARBOHYDRATE METABOLISM II: AEROBIC RESPIRATION

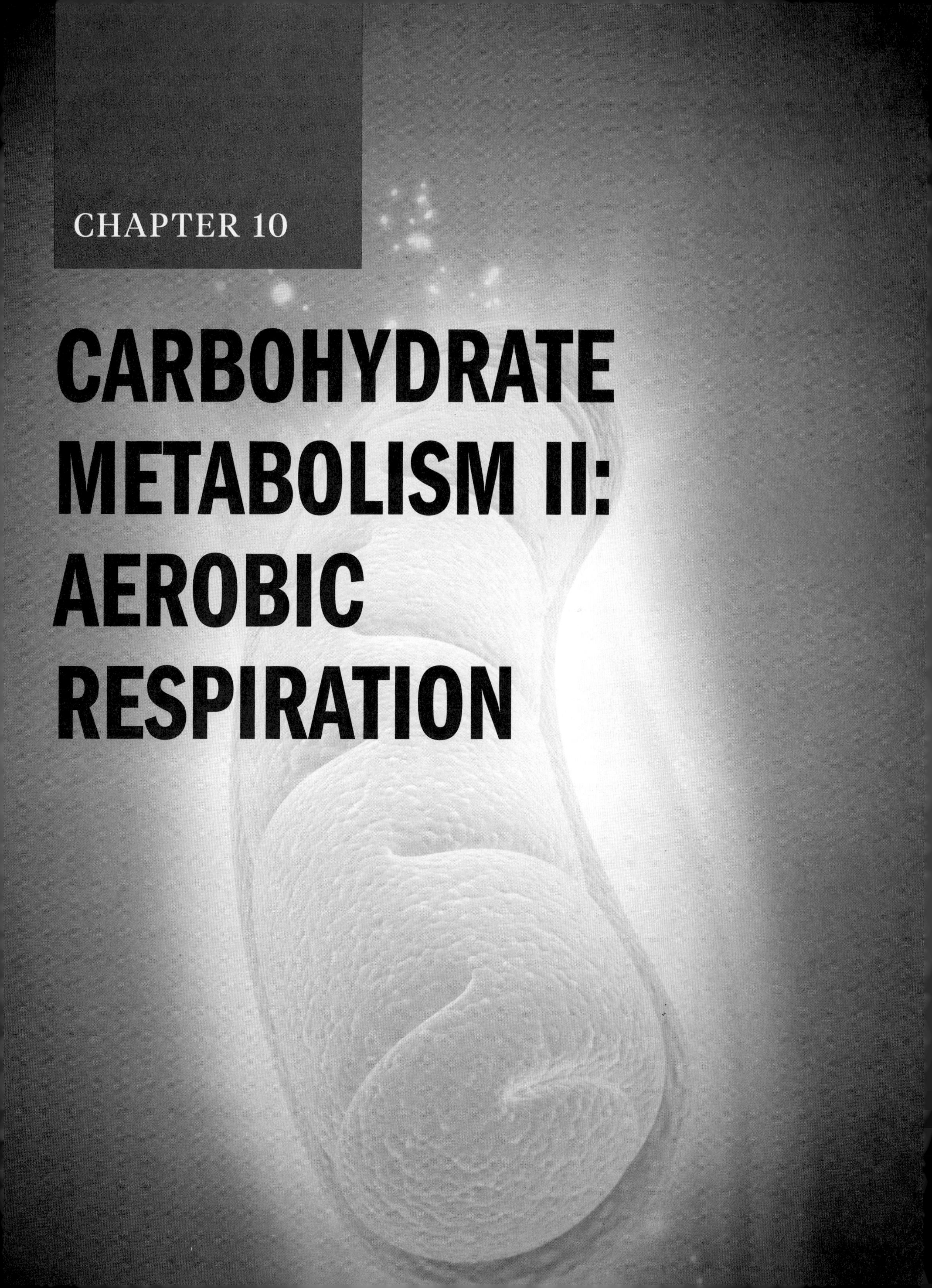

SCIENCE MASTERY ASSESSMENT

Every pre-med knows this feeling: there is so much content I have to know for the MCAT! How do I know what to do first or what's important?

While the high-yield badges throughout this book will help you identify the most important topics, this Science Mastery Assessment is another tool in your MCAT prep arsenal. This quiz (which can also be taken in your online resources) and the guidance below will help ensure that you are spending the appropriate amount of time on this chapter based on your personal strengths and weaknesses. Don't worry though—skipping something now does not mean you'll never study it. Later on in your prep, as you complete full-length tests, you'll uncover specific pieces of content that you need to review and can come back to these chapters as appropriate.

How to Use This Assessment

If you answer 0–7 questions correctly:

Spend about 1 hour to read this chapter in full and take limited notes throughout. Follow up by reviewing **all** quiz questions to ensure that you now understand how to solve each one.

If you answer 8–11 questions correctly:

Spend 20–40 minutes reviewing the quiz questions. Beginning with the questions you missed, read and take notes on the corresponding subchapters. For questions you answered correctly, ensure your thinking matches that of the explanation and you understand why each choice was correct or incorrect.

If you answer 12–15 questions correctly:

Spend less than 20 minutes reviewing all questions from the quiz. If you missed any, then include a quick read-through of the corresponding subchapters, or even just the relevant content within a subchapter, as part of your question review. For questions you got correct, ensure your thinking matches that of the explanation and review the Concept Summary at the end of the chapter.

1. During a myocardial infarction, the oxygen supply to an area of the heart is dramatically reduced, forcing the cardiac myocytes to switch to anaerobic metabolism. Under these conditions, which of the following enzymes would be activated by increased levels of intracellular AMP?
   - **A.** Succinate dehydrogenase
   - **B.** Phosphofructokinase-1
   - **C.** Isocitrate dehydrogenase
   - **D.** Pyruvate dehydrogenase

2. A patient has been exposed to a toxic compound that increases the permeability of mitochondrial membranes to protons. Which of the following metabolic changes would be expected in this patient?
   - **A.** Increased ATP levels
   - **B.** Increased oxygen utilization
   - **C.** Increased ATP synthase activity
   - **D.** Decreased pyruvate dehydrogenase activity

3. Which of the following INCORRECTLY pairs a metabolic process with its site of occurrence?
   - **A.** Glycolysis—cytosol
   - **B.** Citric acid cycle—outer mitochondrial membrane
   - **C.** ATP phosphorylation—cytosol and mitochondria
   - **D.** Electron transport chain—inner mitochondrial membrane

4. Which of the following processes has the following net reaction?

   $$2\ \text{acetyl-CoA} + 6\ NAD^+ + 2\ FAD + 2\ GDP + 2\ P_i + 6\ H_2O \rightarrow 4\ CO_2 + 6\ NADH + 2\ FADH_2 + 2\ GTP + 6\ H^+ + 2\ \text{CoA–SH}$$

   - **A.** Pyruvate decarboxylation
   - **B.** Fermentation
   - **C.** Tricarboxylic acid cycle
   - **D.** Electron transport chain

5. In glucose degradation under aerobic conditions:
   - **A.** oxygen is the final electron acceptor.
   - **B.** oxygen is necessary for all ATP synthesis.
   - **C.** net water is consumed.
   - **D.** the proton-motive force is necessary for all ATP synthesis.

6. Fatty acids enter the catabolic pathway in the form of:
   - **A.** glycerol.
   - **B.** adipose tissue.
   - **C.** acetyl-CoA.
   - **D.** ketone bodies.

7. All of the following methods are used to produce acetyl-CoA in cells EXCEPT for one. What is the exception?
   - **A.** Decarboxylation of pyruvate
   - **B.** Catabolism of ketogenic amino acids
   - **C.** Reduction of fatty acids
   - **D.** Metabolism of alcohol

8. In which part of the cell is cytochrome *c* located?
   - **A.** Mitochondrial matrix
   - **B.** Outer mitochondrial membrane
   - **C.** Inner mitochondrial membrane
   - **D.** Cytosol

9. Which of the following correctly shows the amount of ATP produced from the given high-energy carriers?
   - **A.** $FADH_2 \rightarrow 1$ ATP
   - **B.** $FADH_2 \rightarrow 1.5$ ATP
   - **C.** NADH $\rightarrow 3$ ATP
   - **D.** NADH $\rightarrow 3.5$ ATP

10. Why is it preferable to cleave thioester links rather than typical ester links in aerobic metabolism?
    - **A.** Oxygen must be conserved for the electron transport chain.
    - **B.** Thioester hydrolysis has a higher energy yield.
    - **C.** Typical ester hydrolysis cannot occur *in vivo*.
    - **D.** Thioester cleavage requires more energy.

11. Which enzyme converts GDP to GTP?
    - **A.** Nucleosidediphosphate phosphatase
    - **B.** Nucleosidediphosphate kinase
    - **C.** Isocitrate dehydrogenase
    - **D.** Pyruvate dehydrogenase

12. Which of the following best explains why cytosolic NADH can yield potentially less ATP than mitochondrial NADH?
    - **A.** Cytosolic NADH always loses energy when transferring electrons.
    - **B.** Once NADH enters the matrix from the cytosol, it becomes $FADH_2$.
    - **C.** Electron transfer from cytosol to matrix can take more than one pathway.
    - **D.** There is an energy cost for bringing cytosolic NADH into the matrix.

13. In high doses, aspirin functions as a mitochondrial uncoupler. How would this affect glycogen stores?
    - **A.** It causes depletion of glycogen stores.
    - **B.** It has no effect on glycogen stores.
    - **C.** It promotes additional storage of glucose as glycogen.
    - **D.** Its effect on glycogen stores varies from cell to cell.

14. Which complex does NOT contribute to the proton-motive force?
    - **A.** Complex I
    - **B.** Complex II
    - **C.** Complex III
    - **D.** Complex IV

15. Which of the following directly provides the energy needed to form ATP in the mitochondrion?
    - **A.** Electron transfer in the electron transport chain
    - **B.** An electrochemical proton gradient
    - **C.** Oxidation of acetyl-CoA
    - **D.** β-Oxidation of fatty acids

Answer Key

1. **B**
2. **B**
3. **B**
4. **C**
5. **A**
6. **C**
7. **C**
8. **C**
9. **B**
10. **B**
11. **B**
12. **C**
13. **A**
14. **B**
15. **B**

Detailed explanations can be found at the end of the chapter.

CHAPTER 10

CARBOHYDRATE METABOLISM II: AEROBIC RESPIRATION

In This Chapter

CHAPTER PROFILE

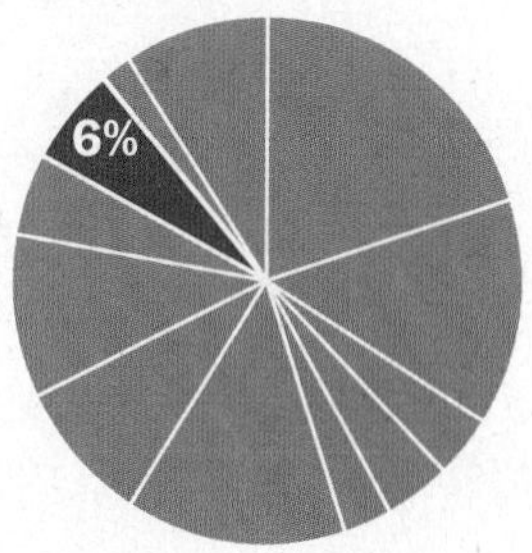

The content in this chapter should be relevant to about 6% of all questions about biochemistry on the MCAT.

This chapter covers material from the following AAMC content category:

1D: Principles of bioenergetics and fuel molecule metabolism

Introduction

Have you ever heard that eating peach pits is deadly? Before you start panicking about the snack you had during your study break, you should know that the accuracy of such a statement is debatable. While it is true that digesting peach pits can result in the formation of trace amounts of cyanide, the concentration is far too low to be clinically worrisome. Cyanide is a poison that binds irreversibly to *cytochrome* a/a_3, a protein located in the electron transport chain of the mitochondria. Why can this be deadly? Blocking the electron transport chain (ETC) inhibits aerobic respiration from yielding the ATP the body requires to function properly. Cyanide poisoning leaves cells unable to utilize oxygen for aerobic respiration because it blocks oxygen from binding to the ETC. Therefore, symptoms resemble those of tissue hypoxia: perceived difficulty breathing, general weakness, and, in higher doses, cardiac arrest followed by death within minutes.

But what about the metabolic pathways described in Chapter 9 of *MCAT Biochemistry Review*—don't they produce energy without oxygen? While glycolysis does not depend on oxygen, it only yields a net 2 ATP per molecule of glucose, which is not nearly enough to maintain the body's energy requirements. This brings us to two of the most tested topics on the MCAT: the citric acid cycle and oxidative phosphorylation.

In this chapter, we'll take a close look at what's gained when the products of glycolysis and other derivatives of metabolic pathways enter the citric acid cycle. We'll also look at how this process is regulated with regard to the substrates, products, and reactions involved. Lastly, we'll observe what happens when this cycle's products undergo oxidative phosphorylation, with particular emphasis on how the electron transport chain facilitates the process and the ATP that is yielded.

10.1 Acetyl-CoA

LEARNING OBJECTIVES

After Chapter 10.1, you will be able to:

- Detail four potential energy sources for the synthesis of acetyl-CoA
- Identify the major inputs and outputs through the pyruvate dehydrogenase complex

The **citric acid cycle**, also called the **Krebs cycle** or the **tricarboxylic acid (TCA) cycle**, occurs in the mitochondria. The main function of this cycle is the oxidation of acetyl-CoA to CO_2 and H_2O. In addition, the cycle produces the high-energy electron-carrying molecules NADH and $FADH_2$. Acetyl-CoA can be obtained from the metabolism of carbohydrates, fatty acids, and amino acids, making it a key molecule in the crossroads of many metabolic pathways and a highly testable compound.

Methods of Forming Acetyl-CoA

MCAT EXPERTISE

Similar to the *gluco-/glyco-* terminology in Chapter 9 of *MCAT Biochemistry Review*, it is critical to keep straight the various enzymes containing *pyruvate: pyruvate dehydrogenase* (PDH), its two regulators (*PDH kinase* and *PDH phosphatase*), and *pyruvate carboxylase*, an enzyme in gluconeogenesis.

Recall from Chapter 9 of *MCAT Biochemistry Review* that after glucose undergoes glycolysis, its product, *pyruvate*, enters the mitochondrion via active transport and is oxidized and decarboxylated. These reactions are catalyzed by a multienzyme complex called the ***pyruvate dehydrogenase complex***, which is located in the mitochondrial matrix. As we take a deeper look at the enzymes that make up this complex, as well as the substrates and products of their reactions, it is helpful to follow the carbons in the molecules. For example, the three-carbon pyruvate is cleaved into a two-carbon acetyl group and carbon dioxide. This reaction is irreversible, which explains why glucose cannot be formed directly from acetyl-CoA. In mammals, pyruvate dehydrogenase complex is made up of five enzymes: *pyruvate dehydrogenase* (PDH), *dihydrolipoyl transacetylase*, *dihydrolipoyl dehydrogenase*, *pyruvate dehydrogenase kinase*, and *pyruvate dehydrogenase phosphatase*. While the first three work in concert to convert pyruvate to acetyl-CoA, the latter two regulate the actions of PDH. Figure 10.1 shows the overall reaction for the conversion of pyruvate to acetyl-CoA. The reaction is exergonic $\left(\Delta G^{\circ\prime} = -33.4\,\frac{\text{kJ}}{\text{mol}}\right)$. The complex is inhibited by an accumulation of acetyl-CoA and NADH that can occur if the electron transport chain is not properly functioning or is inhibited.

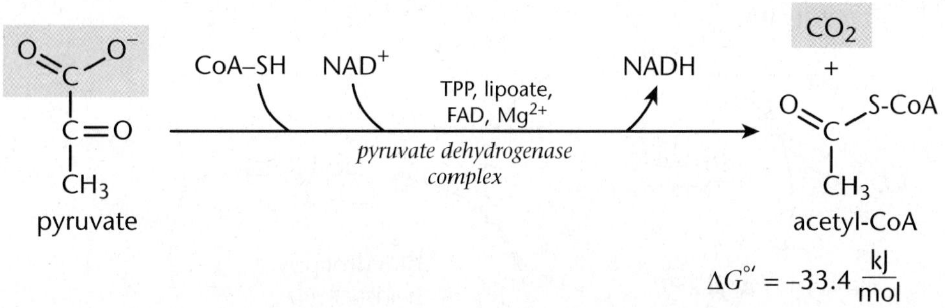

Figure 10.1 Overall Reaction of Pyruvate Dehydrogenase Complex

Note that **coenzyme A (CoA)** is written as CoA−SH in the reaction above. This is because CoA is a thiol, containing an −SH group. When acetyl-CoA forms, it does so via covalent attachment of the acetyl group to the −SH group, resulting in the formation of a thioester, which contains sulfur instead of the typical oxygen ester -OR. The formation of a thioester rather than a typical ester is worth noting because of the high-energy properties of thioesters. That is to say, when a thioester undergoes a reaction such as hydrolysis, a significant amount of energy will be released. This can be enough to drive other reactions forward, like the citric acid cycle. The pyruvate dehydrogenase complex enzymes needed to catalyze acetyl-CoA formation are listed below in sequential order, and the mechanism is shown in Figure 10.2.

- **Pyruvate dehydrogenase (PDH):** Pyruvate is oxidized, yielding CO_2, while the remaining two-carbon molecule binds covalently to *thiamine pyrophosphate* (vitamin B_1, TPP). TPP is a coenzyme held by noncovalent interactions to PDH. Mg^{2+} is also required.
- **Dihydrolipoyl transacetylase:** The two-carbon molecule bonded to TPP is oxidized and transferred to lipoic acid, a coenzyme that is covalently bonded to the enzyme. Lipoic acid's disulfide group acts as an oxidizing agent, creating the acetyl group. The acetyl group is now bonded to lipoic acid via thioester linkage. After this, dihydrolipoyl transacetylase catalyzes the CoA−SH interaction with the newly formed thioester link, causing transfer of an acetyl group to form acetyl-CoA. Lipoic acid is left in its reduced form.
- **Dihydrolipoyl dehydrogenase:** Flavin adenine dinucleotide (FAD) is used as a coenzyme in order to reoxidize lipoic acid, allowing lipoic acid to facilitate acetyl-CoA formation in future reactions. As lipoic acid is reoxidized, FAD is reduced to $FADH_2$. In subsequent reactions, this $FADH_2$ is reoxidized to FAD, while NAD^+ is reduced to NADH.

REAL WORLD

In studies of pathologies that affect the central cholinergic system such as Alzheimer's disease, Huntington's disease, and even alcoholism, a decrease in glucose metabolism and oxidative phosphorylation has been observed in the brain. Ongoing research will hopefully determine if the resulting lack of acetyl-CoA could be a cause of the disease or a result of the disease. With decreased amounts of acetyl-CoA, not only is energy production a concern, but also the production of the neurotransmitter acetylcholine.

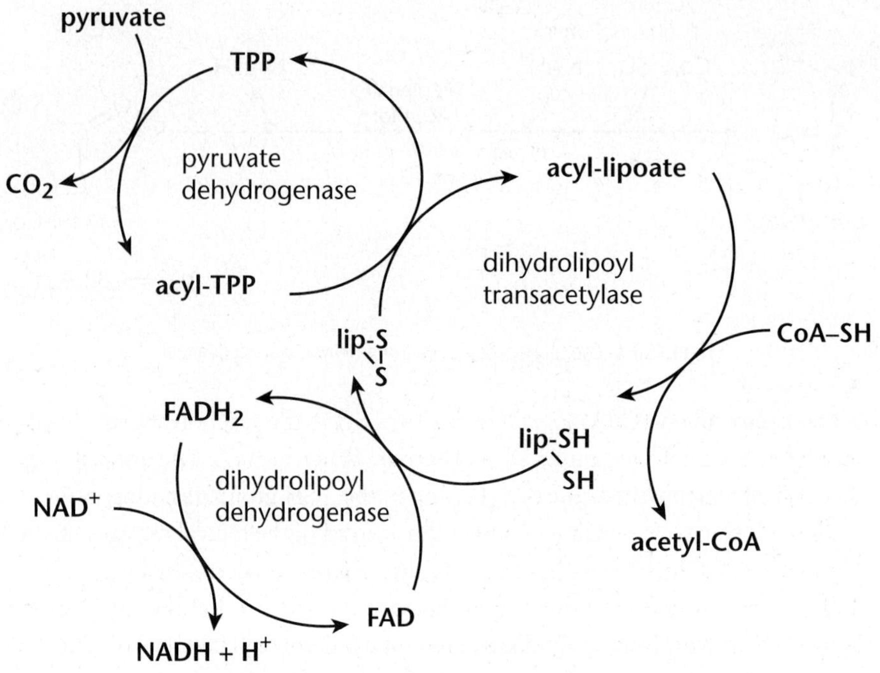

Figure 10.2 Mechanism of Pyruvate Dehydrogenase

While glycolysis is a heavily reviewed and heavily tested contributor to the production of acetyl-CoA, other pathways are capable of forming acetyl-CoA. These pathways act on fatty acids, ketogenic amino acids, ketone bodies, and alcohol. Descriptions of these pathways are provided below. The ultimate production of acetyl-CoA allows all of these pathways to culminate in the final common pathway of the citric acid cycle.

BRIDGE

Once formed, mitochondrial acyl-CoA can undergo β-oxidation. This process is discussed in Chapter 11 of *MCAT Biochemistry Review*.

- **Fatty acid oxidation (β-oxidation):** In the cytosol, a process called **activation** causes a thioester bond to form between carboxyl groups of fatty acids and CoA–SH. Because this activated *fatty acyl-CoA* cannot cross the inner mitochondrial membrane, the fatty acyl group is transferred to *carnitine* via a transesterification reaction, as shown in Figure 10.3. Carnitine is a molecule that can cross the inner membrane with a fatty acyl group in tow. Once acyl-carnitine crosses the inner membrane; it transfers the fatty acyl group to a mitochondrial CoA–SH via another transesterification reaction. In other words, carnitine's function is merely to carry the acyl group from a cytosolic CoA–SH to a mitochondrial CoA–SH. Once acyl-CoA is formed in the matrix, β-oxidation can occur, which removes two-carbon fragments from the carboxyl end.

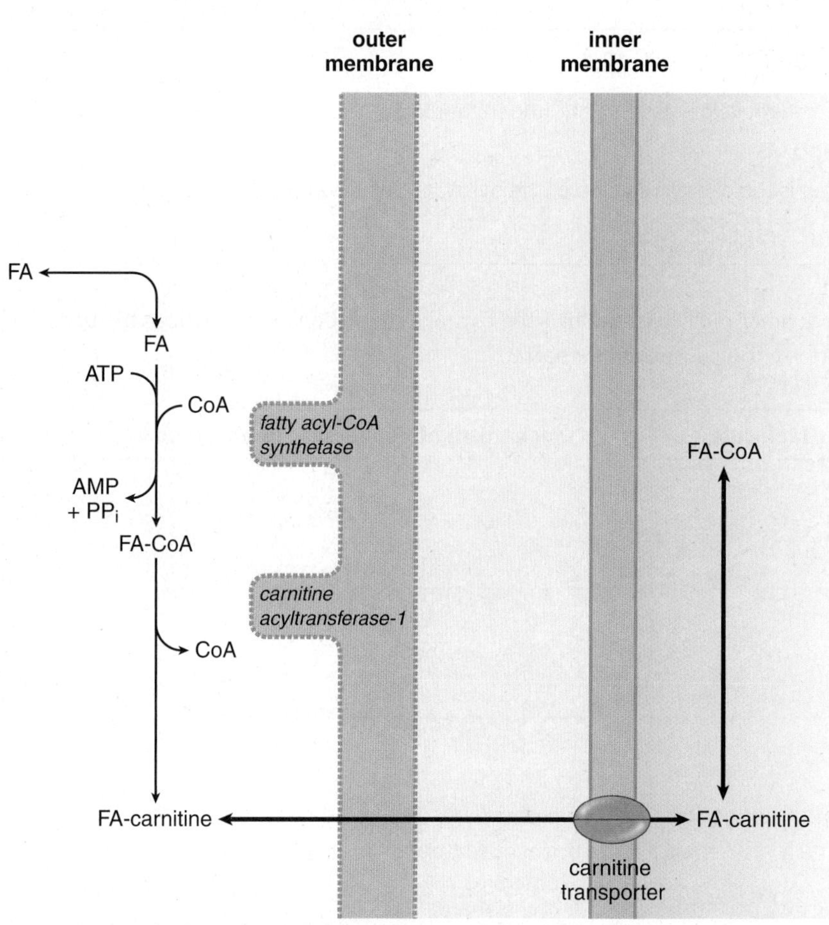

Figure 10.3 Fatty Acid Activation and Transport

- **Amino acid catabolism:** Certain amino acids can be used to form acetyl-CoA. These amino acids must lose their amino group via transamination; their carbon skeletons can then form ketone bodies. These amino acids are termed *ketogenic* for that reason. The conversion of ketone bodies to acetyl-CoA is mentioned below.
- **Ketones:** Although acetyl-CoA is typically used to produce ketones when the pyruvate dehydrogenase complex is inhibited, the reverse reaction can occur as well.
- **Alcohol:** When alcohol is consumed in moderate amounts, the enzymes ***alcohol dehydrogenase*** and ***acetaldehyde dehydrogenase*** convert it to acetyl-CoA. However, this reaction is accompanied by NADH buildup, which inhibits the Krebs cycle. Therefore, the acetyl-CoA formed through this process is used primarily to synthesize fatty acids.

REAL WORLD

While the brain normally uses glucose for energy, under conditions such as starvation, ketone bodies can become the brain's major source of energy.

MCAT CONCEPT CHECK 10.1

Before you move on, assess your understanding of the material with these questions.

1. What is the overall reaction of the pyruvate dehydrogenase complex?

 ____

2. What other molecules can be used to make acetyl-CoA, and how does the body perform this conversion for each?

Molecule	Mechanism of Conversion to Acetyl-CoA

10.2 Reactions of the Citric Acid Cycle

High-Yield

LEARNING OBJECTIVES

After Chapter 10.2, you will be able to:

- Explain the purpose of the citric acid cycle, including major inputs/outputs
- Identify the importance of key enzymes within the citric acid cycle
- Recall the inhibitors and activators of the enzymes citrate synthase, isocitrate dehydrogenase, and alpha-ketoglutarate dehydrogenase complex

The citric acid cycle takes place in the mitochondrial matrix and begins with the coupling of a molecule of acetyl-CoA to a molecule of *oxaloacetate*. While parts of this molecule are oxidized to carbon dioxide and both energy (GTP) and energy carriers (NADH and $FADH_2$) are produced, the other substrates and products of the cycle are reused over and over again. Although oxygen is not directly required in the cycle, the pathway will not occur anaerobically. This is because NADH and $FADH_2$ will accumulate if oxygen is not available for the electron transport chain and will inhibit the cycle. As we look at the individual reactions that take place during the citric acid cycle, it cannot be overemphasized that this process is exactly what it's called: a *cycle*, not just a series of reactions. An overview of the cycle is provided in Figure 10.4, and we'll take a deeper look at those steps below.

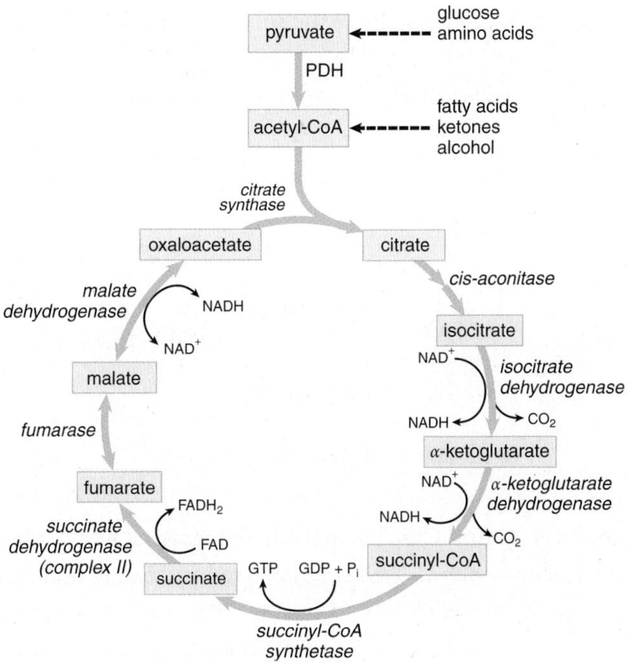

Figure 10.4 The Citric Acid Cycle

Key Reactions

Step 1—Citrate Formation: First, acetyl-CoA and *oxaloacetate* undergo a condensation reaction to form *citryl-CoA*, an intermediate. Then, the hydrolysis of citryl-CoA yields citrate and CoA–SH. This reaction is catalyzed by *citrate synthase.* As discussed in Chapter 2 of *MCAT Biochemistry Review*, *synthases* are enzymes that form new covalent bonds without needing significant energy. This second part of this step energetically favors the formation of citrate and helps the cycle revolve in the forward direction. This reaction can be seen in Figure 10.5.

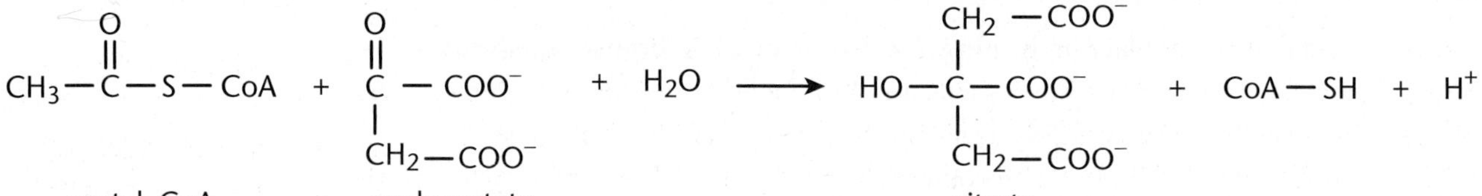

Figure 10.5 Citrate Formation

Step 2—Citrate Isomerized to Isocitrate: Achiral citrate is isomerized to one of four possible isomers of *isocitrate*. First, citrate binds at three points to the enzyme *aconitase*. Then water is lost from citrate, yielding cis-*aconitate*. Finally, water is added back to form isocitrate. The enzyme is a metalloprotein that requires Fe^{2+}. In Figure 10.6, you can see that this results in a switching of a hydrogen and a hydroxyl group. Overall, this step is necessary to facilitate the subsequent oxidative decarboxylation.

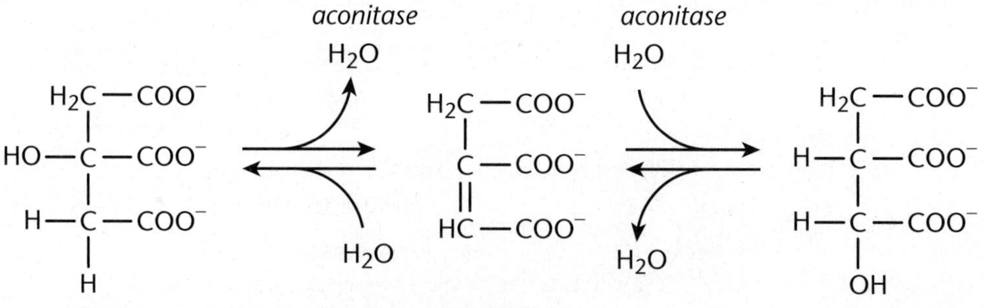

Figure 10.6 Citrate Isomerized to Isocitrate

Step 3—α-Ketoglutarate and CO_2 Formation: Isocitrate is first oxidized to *oxalosuccinate* by *isocitrate dehydrogenase*. Then oxalosuccinate is decarboxylated to produce *α-ketoglutarate* and CO_2, as shown in Figure 10.7. This is a very important step to know for Test Day because isocitrate dehydrogenase is the rate-limiting enzyme of the citric acid cycle. The first of the two carbons from the cycle is lost here. This is also the first NADH produced from intermediates in the cycle.

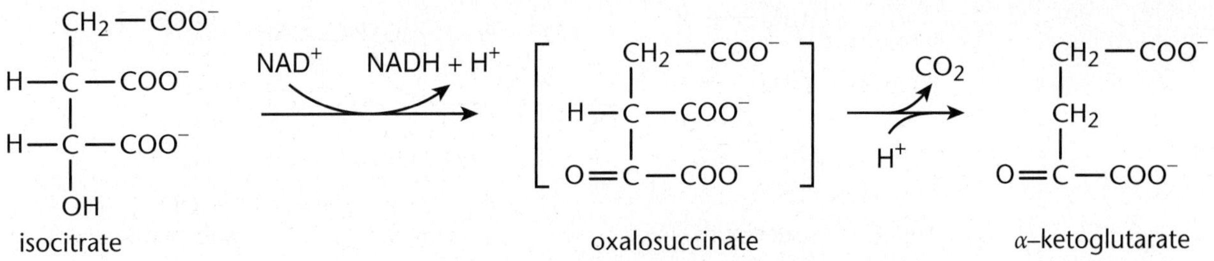

Figure 10.7 α-Ketoglutarate and CO_2 Formation

Step 4—Succinyl-CoA and CO_2 Formation: These reactions are carried out by the *α-ketoglutarate dehydrogenase complex*, which is similar in mechanism, cofactors, and coenzymes to the pyruvate dehydrogenase (PDH) complex. In the formation of succinyl-CoA, α-ketoglutarate and CoA come together and produce a molecule of carbon dioxide, as shown in Figure 10.8. This carbon dioxide represents the second and last carbon lost from the cycle. Reducing NAD^+ produces another NADH.

KEY CONCEPT

Dehydrogenases are a subtype of *oxidoreductases* (enzymes that catalyze an oxidation-reduction reaction). Dehydrogenases transfer a hydride ion (H^-) to an electron acceptor, usually NAD^+ or FAD. Therefore, whenever you see *dehydrogenase* in aerobic metabolism, be on the lookout for a high-energy electron carrier being formed!

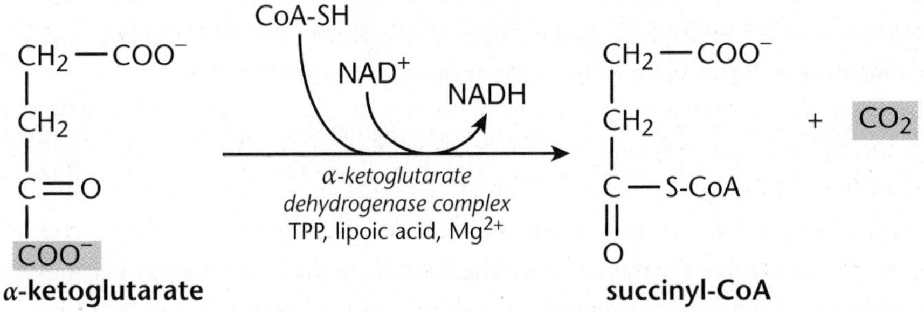

Figure 10.8 Succinyl-CoA and CO_2 Formation

Step 5—Succinate Formation: Hydrolysis of the thioester bond on succinyl-CoA yields *succinate* and CoA–SH, and is coupled to the phosphorylation of GDP to GTP. This reaction is catalyzed by *succinyl-CoA synthetase*, as shown in Figure 10.9. *Synthetases*, unlike *synthases*, create new covalent bonds *with* energy input. Recall the earlier discussion about thioester bonds with regard to acetyl-CoA: they're unique in that their hydrolysis is accompanied by a significant release of energy. Therefore, phosphorylation of GDP to GTP is driven by the energy released by thioester hydrolysis. Once GTP is formed, an enzyme called *nucleosidediphosphate kinase* catalyzes phosphate transfer from GTP to ADP, thus producing ATP. Note that this is the only time in the entire citric acid cycle that ATP is produced directly; ATP production occurs predominantly within the electron transport chain.

KEY CONCEPT

Citrate *synthase* doesn't require energy input in order to form covalent bonds, but succinyl-CoA *synthetase* certainly does. Pay careful attention to enzyme names: little things can add up to careless mistakes on Test Day otherwise!

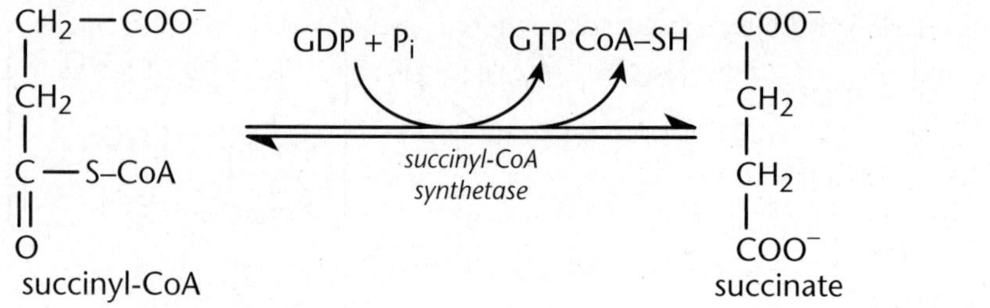

Figure 10.9 Succinate Formation

Step 6—Fumarate Formation: This is the only step of the citric acid cycle that doesn't take place in the mitochondrial matrix; instead, it occurs on the inner membrane. Let's look at why: succinate undergoes oxidation to yield *fumarate*. This reaction is catalyzed by *succinate dehydrogenase*. Succinate dehydrogenase is considered a **flavoprotein** because it is covalently bonded to FAD, the electron acceptor in this reaction. This enzyme is an integral protein on the inner mitochondrial membrane. As succinate is oxidized to fumarate, FAD is reduced to $FADH_2$. Each molecule of $FADH_2$ then passes the electrons it carries to the electron transport chain, which eventually leads to the production of 1.5 ATP (unlike NADH, which will give rise to 2.5 ATP). FAD is the electron acceptor in this reaction because the reducing power of succinate is not great enough to reduce NAD^+.

MNEMONIC

Substrates of Citric Acid Cycle: **P**lease, **C**an **I** **K**eep **S**elling **S**eashells **F**or **M**oney, **O**fficer?

- **P**yruvate
- **C**itrate
- **I**socitrate
- α-**K**etoglutarate
- **S**uccinyl-CoA
- **S**uccinate
- **F**umarate
- **M**alate
- **O**xaloacetate

Step 7—Malate Formation: The enzyme *fumarase* catalyzes the hydrolysis of the alkene bond in fumarate, thereby giving rise to *malate*. Although two enantiomeric forms are possible, only L-malate forms in this reaction.

Step 8—Oxaloacetate Formed Anew: The enzyme *malate dehydrogenase* catalyzes the oxidation of malate to *oxaloacetate*. A third and final molecule of NAD^+ is reduced to NADH. The newly formed oxaloacetate is ready to take part in another turn of the citric acid cycle, and we've gained all of the high-energy electron carriers possible from one turn of the cycle. The last steps of the citric acid cycle—from succinate to oxaloacetate—are shown in Figure 10.10.

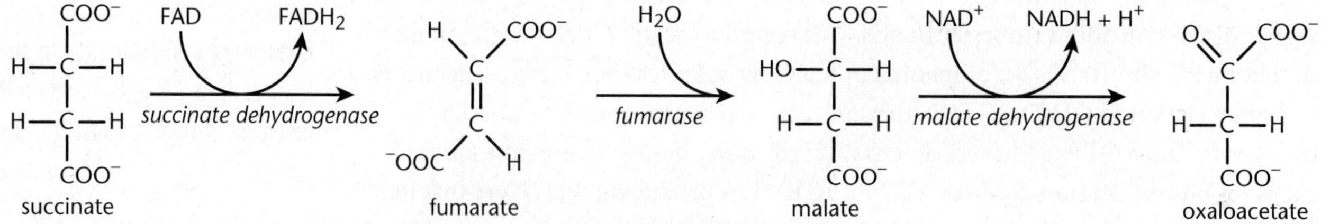

Figure 10.10 The Final Steps of the Citric Acid Cycle

Net Results and ATP Yield

Now let's take a step back and see what our net yield is from the steps we just took. Starting with the pyruvate dehydrogenase complex, recall that the products of this reaction include one acetyl-CoA and one NADH. In the citric acid cycle, steps 3, 4, and 8 each produce one NADH, while step 6 forms one $FADH_2$. Step 5 yields one GTP, which can be converted to ATP. Two carbons leave the cycle in the form of CO_2.

Each NADH can be converted to approximately 2.5 ATP, while each $FADH_2$ molecule can yield about 1.5 ATP. The total amount of chemical energy harvested per pyruvate is listed below.

Pyruvate Dehydrogenase Complex:

$$\text{pyruvate} + \text{CoA–SH} + \text{NAD}^+ \rightarrow \text{acetyl-CoA} + \textbf{NADH} + \text{CO}_2 + \text{H}^+$$

Citric Acid Cycle:

$$\text{acetyl-CoA} + 3\ \text{NAD}^+ + \text{FAD} + \text{GDP} + \text{P}_i + 2\ \text{H}_2\text{O} \rightarrow$$
$$2\ \text{CO}_2 + \text{CoA–SH} + \textbf{3 NADH} + 3\ \text{H}^+ + \textbf{FADH}_2 + \textbf{GTP}$$

ATP Production:

- 4 NADH $\rightarrow$ 10 ATP (2.5 ATP per NADH)
- 1 $FADH_2$ $\rightarrow$ 1.5 ATP (1.5 ATP per $FADH_2$)
- 1 GTP $\rightarrow$ 1 ATP
- Total: 12.5 ATP per pyruvate = 25 ATP per glucose

Glycolysis yields two ATP and two NADH, providing another seven molecules of ATP; thus, the net yield of ATP for one glucose molecule from glycolysis through oxidative phosphorylation is 30–32 ATP. Note that the efficiency of glycolysis varies slightly from cell to cell, so there is a range of ATP yield from one molecule of glucose.

Regulation

Let's say it's Test Day, and you see the following question: *Which of the following is an inhibitor of isocitrate dehydrogenase?* Before you start to panic, take a step back and use critical thinking. Where have we heard of isocitrate dehydrogenase—or merely isocitrate—before? The Krebs cycle. By knowing this, you can already make a fair attempt at such a question. Because energy (ATP) and energy carriers (NADH and $FADH_2$) are products of this process, it makes sense that these molecules would have a negative feedback effect on the citric acid cycle. Always consider the big picture when faced with questions like these. For now, we'll outline how regulation occurs throughout the citric acid cycle; look for the recurring theme that energy products inhibit energy production processes.

Pyruvate Dehydrogenase Complex Regulation

Even upstream from its actual starting point, the citric acid cycle can be regulated. The mechanism by which this happens is phosphorylation of PDH, which is facilitated by the enzyme ***pyruvate dehydrogenase kinase***. Thus, whenever levels of ATP rise, phosphorylating PDH inhibits acetyl-CoA production. Conversely, the pyruvate dehydrogenase complex is reactivated by the enzyme ***pyruvate dehydrogenase phosphatase*** in response to high levels of ADP. By removing a phosphate from PDH, pyruvate dehydrogenase phosphatase is able to reactivate acetyl-CoA production. Acetyl-CoA also has a negative feedback effect on its own production. When using alternative fuel sources such as fats, the acetyl-CoA production is sufficient to make it redundant to continue producing acetyl-CoA from carbohydrate metabolism—that's part of why eating a high-fat meal fills you up so quickly! ATP and NADH, as markers of the cell being satisfied energetically, also inhibit PDH.

Control Points of the Citric Acid Cycle

There are three essential checkpoints that regulate the citric acid cycle from within, and allosteric activators and inhibitors regulate all of them. The details of these mechanisms are outlined below and in Figure 10.11.

- **Citrate synthase:** ATP and NADH function as allosteric inhibitors of citrate synthase, which makes sense because both are products (indirect and direct, respectively) of the enzyme. Citrate also allosterically inhibits citrate synthase directly, as does succinyl-CoA.
- **Isocitrate dehydrogenase:** As we discussed in the beginning of this section, this enzyme that catalyzes the citric acid cycle is likely to be inhibited by energy products: ATP and NADH. Conversely, ADP and NAD^+ function as allosteric activators for the enzyme and enhance its affinity for substrates.
- **α-Ketoglutarate dehydrogenase complex:** Once again, the reaction products of succinyl-CoA and NADH function as inhibitors of this enzyme complex. ATP is also inhibitory and slows the rate of the cycle when the cell has high levels of ATP. The complex is stimulated by ADP and calcium ions.

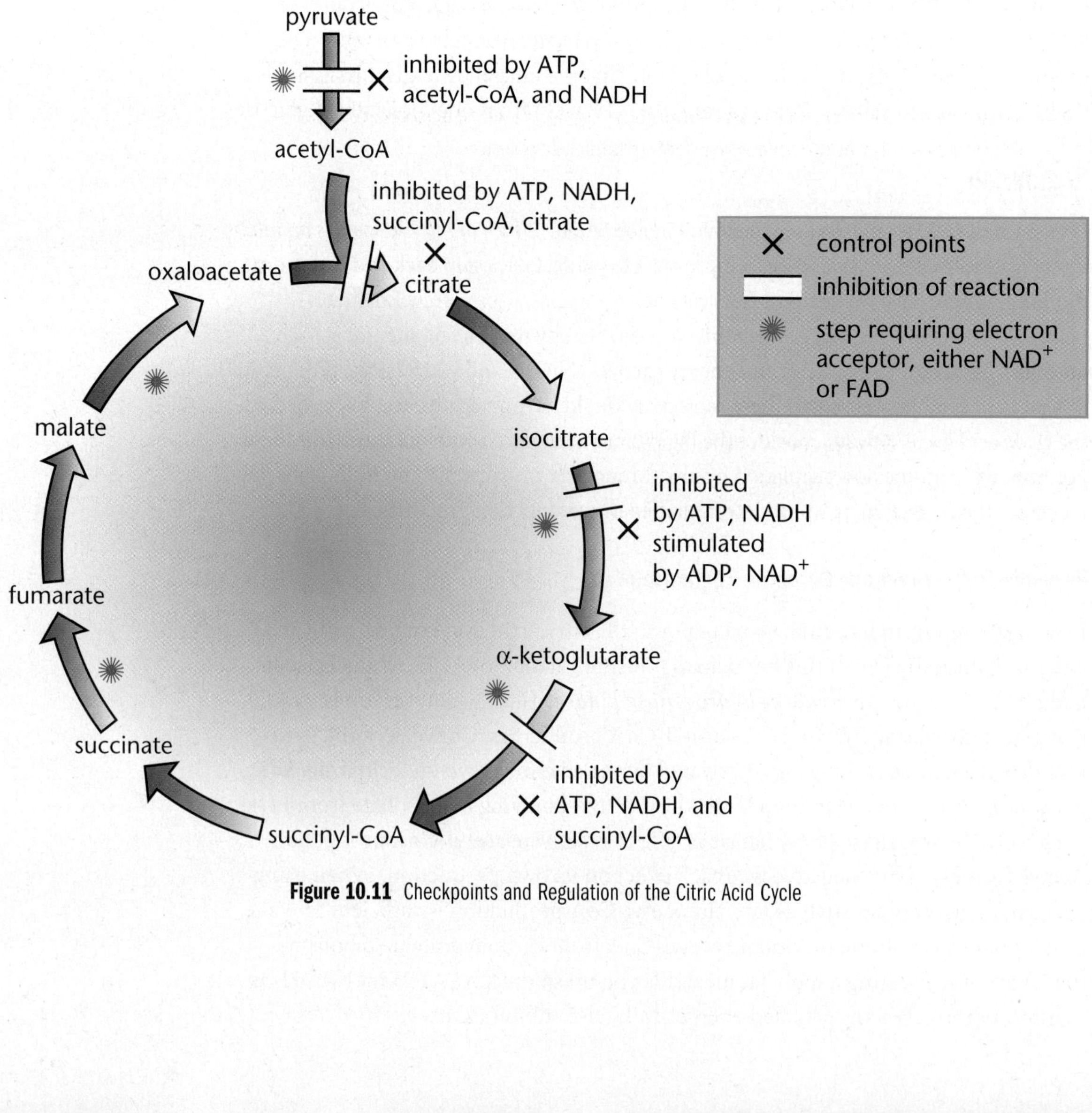

Figure 10.11 Checkpoints and Regulation of the Citric Acid Cycle

Note that high levels of ATP and NADH inhibit the citric acid cycle, while high levels of ADP and NAD^+ promote it. This isn't a coincidence! When energy is being consumed in large amounts, more and more ATP is converted to ADP and NADH is converted to NAD^+. It is therefore the ATP/ADP ratio and NADH/NAD^+ ratio that help determine whether the citric acid cycle will be inhibited or activated. During a metabolically active state, ADP and NAD^+ levels should rise as ATP and NADH levels decline, thus inducing activation at all the various checkpoints described above, replacing the energy used up by active tissues.

MCAT CONCEPT CHECK 10.2

Before you move on, assess your understanding of the material with these questions.

1. What is the purpose of all the reactions that collectively make up the citric acid cycle?

___

2. What enzyme catalyzes the rate-limiting step of the citric acid cycle?

___

3. What are the three main sites of regulation within the citric acid cycle? What molecules inhibit and activate the three main checkpoints?

Checkpoints	Inhibitors	Activators

10.3 The Electron Transport Chain

High-Yield

LEARNING OBJECTIVES

After Chapter 10.3, you will be able to:

- Connect the reactions of the electron transport chain to the generation of ATP
- Distinguish between the two shuttle mechanisms for NADH transport into the mitochondrion
- Recall the inputs, outputs, and major components of the four complexes of the electron transport chain:

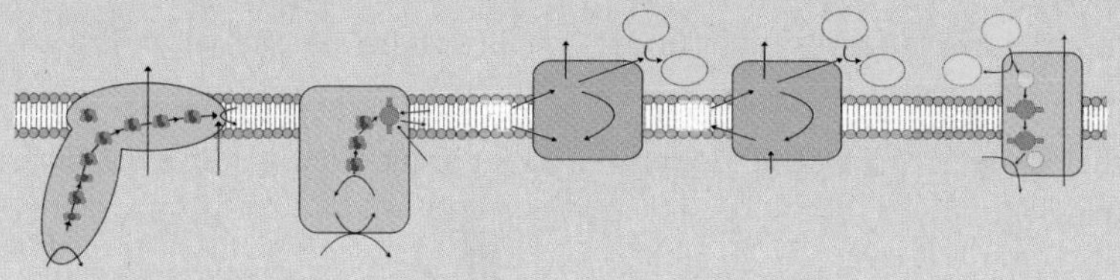

The electron transport chain is the final common pathway that utilizes the harvested electrons from different fuels in the body. It is important to make the distinction that it is not the flow of electrons but the proton gradient it generates that ultimately produces ATP. Aerobic metabolism is the most efficient way of generating energy in living systems, and the mitochondrion is the reason why. In eukaryotes, the aerobic components of respiration are executed in mitochondria, while anaerobic processes such as glycolysis and fermentation occur in the cytosol. Looking at Figure 10.12, notice how the components of the mitochondria are critical in the harvesting of energy. The citric acid cycle takes place in the mitochondrial matrix. The assemblies needed to complete oxidative phosphorylation are housed adjacent to the matrix in the inner membrane of the mitochondria. The inner mitochondrial membrane is assembled into folds called ***cristae***, which maximize surface area. It is the inner mitochondrial membrane that will be essential for generating ATP using the **proton-motive force**, an electrochemical proton gradient generated by the complexes of the electron transport chain.

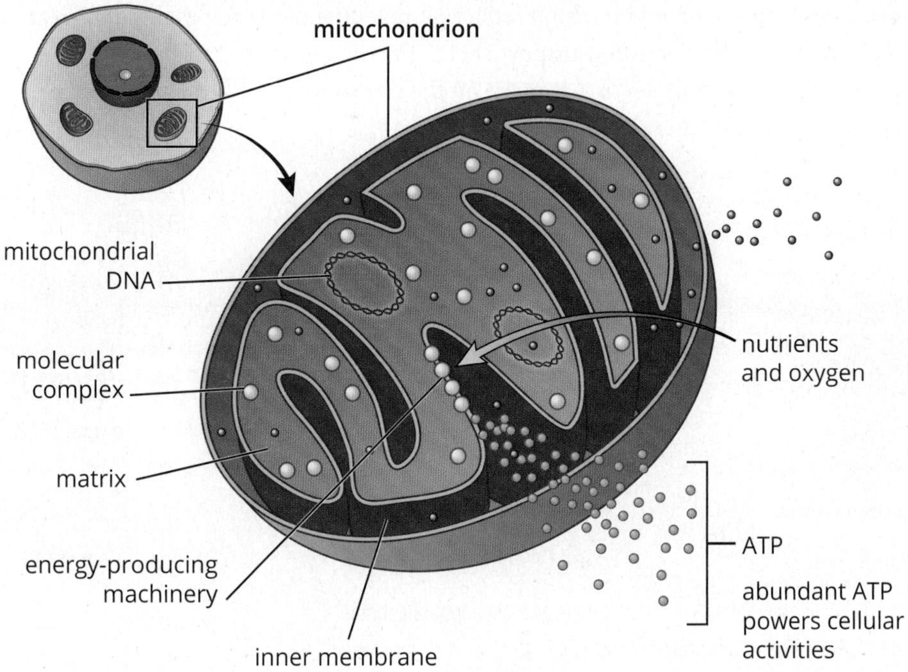

Figure 10.12 Mitochondrial Structure

The final step in aerobic respiration is actually two steps: electron transport along the inner mitochondrial membrane and the generation of ATP via ADP phosphorylation. While these two processes are actually separate entities, they are very much coupled, so explaining these steps together makes a great deal of sense. The electron-rich molecules NADH and $FADH_2$ are formed as byproducts at earlier steps in respiration. They transfer their electrons to carrier proteins located along the inner mitochondrial membrane. Finally, these electrons are given to oxygen in the form of hydride ions (H^-) and water is formed. While this is happening, energy released from transporting electrons facilitates proton transport at three specific locations in the chain. Protons are moved from the mitochondrial matrix into the intermembrane space of the mitochondria, thereby creating a greater concentration gradient of hydrogen ions that can be used to drive ATP production.

Electron Flow and Complexes

The formation of ATP is endergonic and electron transport is an exergonic pathway. By coupling these reactions, the energy yielded by one reaction can fuel the other. In order for energy to be harnessed via electron transport reactions, the proteins along the inner membrane must transfer the electrons donated by NADH and $FADH_2$ in a specific order and direction. The physical property that determines the direction of electron flow is reduction potential. Recall from Chapter 12 of *MCAT General Chemistry Review* that if you pair two molecules with different reduction potentials, the molecule with the higher potential will be reduced, while the other molecule will become oxidized. The electron transport chain is therefore nothing more than a series of oxidations and reductions that occur via the same mechanism. NADH is a good electron donor, and the high reduction potential of oxygen makes it a great final acceptor in the electron transport chain. The organizational structure of the membrane-bound complexes that make up the transport chain is diagrammed in Figure 10.13 and further detailed below.

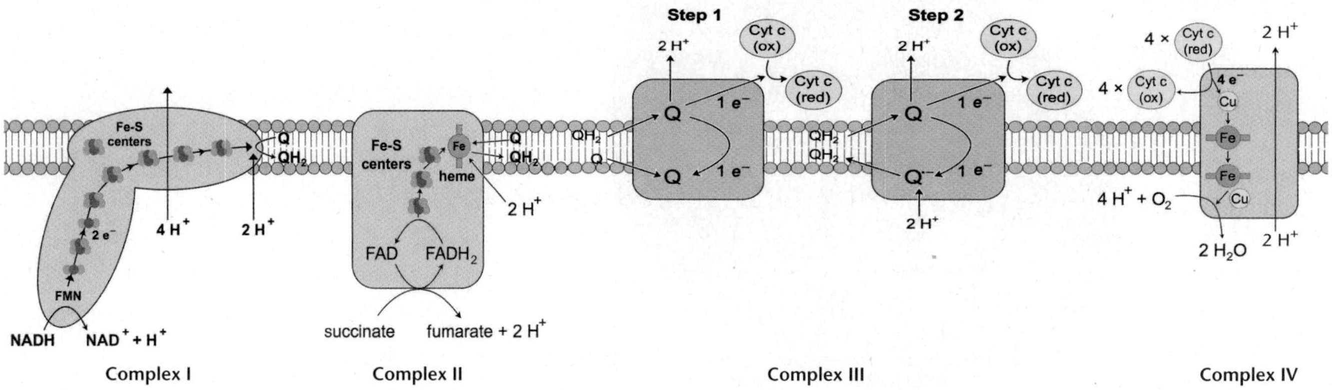

Figure 10.13 Respiratory Complexes on the Inner Mitochondrial Membrane

*Steps 1 and 2 of Complex III are drawn as two separate steps here for clarity; however, the same **$CoQH_2$-cytochrome c oxidoreductase** complex is used for both steps.*

- **Complex I (*NADH-CoQ oxidoreductase*):** The transfer of electrons from NADH to coenzyme Q (CoQ) is catalyzed in this first complex. This complex has over 20 subunits, but the two highlighted here include a protein that has an iron–sulfur cluster and a flavoprotein that oxidizes NADH. The flavoprotein has a coenzyme called *flavin mononucleotide* (FMN) covalently bonded to it. FMN is quite similar in structure to FAD, flavin adenine dinucleotide. The first step in the reaction involves NADH transferring its electrons over to FMN, thereby becoming oxidized to NAD^+ as FMN is reduced to $FMNH_2$. Next, the flavoprotein becomes reoxidized while the iron–sulfur subunit is reduced. Finally, the reduced iron–sulfur subunit donates the electrons it received from $FMNH_2$ to coenzyme Q (also called *ubiquinone*). Coenzyme Q becomes $CoQH_2$. This first complex is one of three sites where proton pumping occurs, as four protons are moved to the intermembrane space.

$$NADH + H^+ + FMN \rightarrow NAD^+ + FMNH_2$$
$$FMNH_2 + 2\ Fe{-}S_{oxidized} \rightarrow FMN + 2\ Fe{-}S_{reduced} + 2\ H^+$$
$$2\ Fe{-}S_{reduced} + CoQ + 2\ H^+ \rightarrow 2\ Fe{-}S_{oxidized} + CoQH_2$$

The net effect is passing high-energy electrons from NADH to CoQ to form $CoQH_2$:

$$NADH + H^+ + CoQ \rightarrow NAD^+ + CoQH_2$$

- **Complex II (*Succinate-CoQ oxidoreductase*):** Just like Complex I, Complex II transfers electrons to coenzyme Q. While Complex I received electrons from NADH, Complex II actually receives electrons from succinate. Remember that succinate is a citric acid cycle intermediate, and that it is oxidized to fumarate upon interacting with FAD. FAD is covalently bonded to Complex II, and once succinate is oxidized, it's converted to $FADH_2$. After this, $FADH_2$ gets reoxidized to FAD as it reduces an iron–sulfur protein. The final step reoxidizes the iron–sulfur protein as coenzyme Q is reduced. Because succinate dehydrogenase was responsible for oxidizing succinate to fumarate in the citric acid cycle, it makes sense that succinate dehydrogenase is also a part of Complex II. It should be noted that no hydrogen pumping occurs here to contribute to the proton gradient.

$$\text{succinate} + \text{FAD} \rightarrow \text{fumarate} + \text{FADH}_2$$
$$\text{FADH}_2 + \text{Fe—S}_{\text{oxidized}} \rightarrow \text{FAD} + \text{Fe—S}_{\text{reduced}}$$
$$\text{Fe—S}_{\text{reduced}} + \text{CoQ} + 2\,\text{H}^+ \rightarrow \text{Fe—S}_{\text{oxidized}} + \text{CoQH}_2$$

The net effect is passing high-energy electrons from succinate to CoQ to form $CoQH_2$:

$$\text{succinate} + \text{CoQ} + 2\,\text{H}^+ \rightarrow \text{fumarate} + \text{CoQH}_2$$

- **Complex III (*$CoQH_2$-cytochrome* c *oxidoreductase*):** Also called cytochrome reductase, this complex facilitates the transfer of electrons from coenzyme Q to cytochrome *c* in a few steps. Though Complex III is drawn as two separate complexes in Figure 10.13 to illustrate the sequential reactions that occur within the complex, both of these steps are occurring within the same complex, using the same coenzyme Q. The overall reaction is written below. The following steps involve the oxidation and reduction of ***cytochromes***: proteins with heme groups in which iron is reduced to Fe^{2+} and reoxidized to Fe^{3+}.

$$\text{CoQH}_2 + 2 \text{ cytochrome } c \text{ [with Fe}^{3+}] \rightarrow$$
$$\text{CoQ} + 2 \text{ cytochrome } c \text{ [with Fe}^{2+}] + 2\,\text{H}^+$$

In the transfer of electrons from iron, only one electron is transferred per reaction, but because coenzyme Q has two electrons to transfer, two cytochrome *c* molecules will be needed. Complex III's main contribution to the proton-motive force is via the **Q cycle**. In the Q cycle, two electrons are shuttled from a molecule of *ubiquinol* ($CoQH_2$) near the intermembrane space to a molecule of *ubiquinone* (CoQ) near the mitochondrial matrix. Another two electrons are attached to heme moieties, reducing two molecules of cytochrome *c*. A carrier containing iron and sulfur assists this process. In shuttling these electrons, four protons are also displaced to the intermembrane space; therefore, the Q cycle continues to increase the gradient of the proton-motive force across the inner mitochondrial membrane.

- **Complex IV (*cytochrome* c *oxidase*):** This complex facilitates the culminating step of the electron transport chain: transfer of electrons from cytochrome *c* to oxygen, the final electron acceptor. This complex includes subunits of cytochrome *a*, cytochrome a_3, and Cu^{2+} ions. Together, cytochromes *a* and a_3 make up *cytochrome oxidase*. Through a series of redox reactions, cytochrome oxidase gets oxidized as oxygen, becomes reduced, and forms water. This is the final location on the transport chain where proton pumping occurs, as two protons are moved across the membrane. The role proton pumping plays in ATP synthesis is an essential one that we will describe in detail next. The overall reaction is:

$$4 \text{ cytochrome } c \text{ [with Fe}^{2+}] + 4\,\text{H}^+ + \text{O}_2 \rightarrow$$
$$4 \text{ cytochrome } c \text{ [with Fe}^{3+}] + 2\,\text{H}_2\text{O}$$

BRIDGE

Ubiquinone can be created from its corresponding phenol by oxidation and represents an example of a quinone (2,5-cyclohexadiene-1,4-diones). These fascinating compounds are explored in Chapter 5 of *MCAT Organic Chemistry Review*.

KEY CONCEPT

Both coenzyme Q and cytochrome *c* aren't technically part of the complexes we're describing. However, because both are able to move freely in the inner mitochondrial membrane, this degree of mobility allows these carriers to transfer electrons by physically interacting with the next component of the transport chain.

KEY CONCEPT

Cyanide, mentioned in the introduction to this chapter, is an inhibitor of cytochrome subunits *a* and a_3. The cyanide anion is able to attach to the iron group and prevent the transfer of electrons. Tissues that rely heavily on aerobic respiration such as the heart and the central nervous system can be greatly impacted.

BIOCHEMISTRY GUIDED EXAMPLE WITH EXPERT THINKING

Mitochondrial disorders are genetically and clinically heterogeneous, mainly affecting energy-demanding organs due to impaired oxidative phosphorylation. Complex I deficiency (NADH:ubiquinone oxidoreductase) in the electron transport chain is the most prevalent oxidative phosphorylation disorder; treatment options are currently limited and successes are often anecdotal.

Focus on the big idea: there is a disease where Complex I of the ETC is broken

There have been reports of increased muscle endurance by diet modification, and, following these reports, this study seeks to examine dietary treatment options for Complex I deficiency.

Possible treatment and goal of study: see if diet helps with symptoms

A Dutch female patient with known Complex I deficiency was subjected to HPLC-based metabolite profiling on blood plasma and urine to reveal metabolic abnormalities. The patient's muscle endurance was examined by performing a bicycle test, with dietary intake for this assessment based on the patient's usual diet, in which 34.5% of the energy was derived from fat.

Assessing how long the patient biked as a measure of muscle endurance

A dietary intervention study was then performed where the patient was instructed to consume a high-carbohydrate diet for 3 weeks with 25% of the energy derived from fat, and subsequently a high-fat diet for 3 weeks with 55% of the energy derived from fat. The same bicycle endurance test was performed after each diet. Differences in muscle endurance during the bicycle test were examined with direct substrate infusion, comparing intra-lipid infusion to glucose infusion.

Five different conditions: normal diet, high-carb diet, high fat diet, glucose infused, fat infused

In each of the conditions, the mean oxygen consumption ($VO_{2\ mean}$) was also measured during the bicycle test. The results are plotted below.

Also assessed oxygen consumed during the bike test

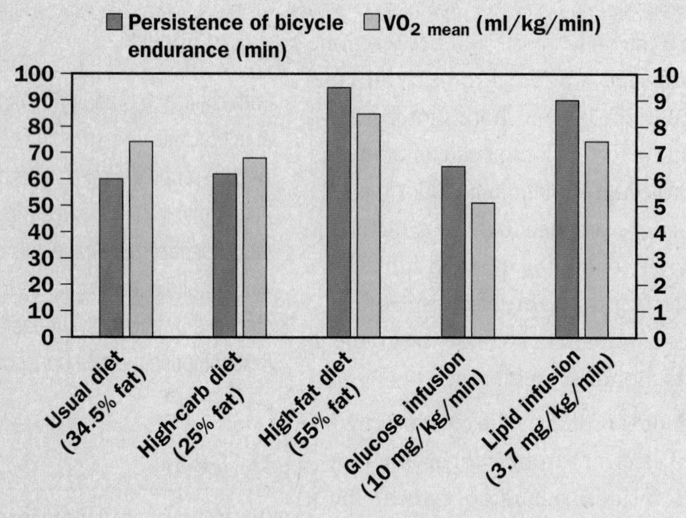

Figure 1

IVs: five diet conditions

DVs: time spent biking and how much oxygen consumed

Trend: longest bike endurance and highest oxygen consumption with high-fat diet, lowest with glucose infusion

Adapted from Theunissen, T., Gerards, M., Hellebrekers, D., van Tienen, F. H., Kamps, R., Sallevelt, S., … Smeets, H. (2017). Selection and characterization of palmitic acid responsive patients with an OXPHOS Complex I defect. *Frontiers in Molecular Neuroscience*, 10, 336. doi:10.3389/fnmol.2017.00336.

According to the data, what is the best treatment option for the patient's Complex I deficiency and why?

The question stem starts with "according to the data", so we need to ensure that we have a firm understanding of the passage presenting the context for that data. The experimental context introduced in paragraph 1 is a malfunction of Complex I in the ETC, and the hypothesis centers on dietary treatment that can help increase muscle endurance. We can recall from our content background that the ETC functions to transfer electrons from NADH and $FADH_2$ to electron acceptors, thereby creating a proton gradient to fuel the production of ATP. The coupling of the ETC to ATP synthase is termed oxidative phosphorylation and requires the availability of oxygen, as oxygen is the final electron acceptor in the ETC. Since ATP is required for muscle contraction, and oxygen is an essential component of the ETC, both high endurance and high oxygen consumption would indicate a high level of aerobic respiration.

The question asks us about the mechanism behind the best treatment option, so we must now analyze the data to see which treatment was best. According to the graph, the high-fat diet allowed the patient to endure the bicycle test the longest, and have the highest level of oxygen consumption. Therefore, the best treatment option is a diet with a high proportion of fat. This conclusion is supported by the fact that lipid infusion also gave higher values compared to glucose infusion, though not as much as the high-fat diet. The next aspect of the question to address is to examine the "why?"—why does ingesting high-fat work this way? Again, using prior knowledge, recall that metabolism of fats generates acetyl-CoA, and acetyl-CoA can then enter the citric acid cycle to produce NADH and $FADH_2$. Complex I receives electrons from NADH, and Complex II receives electrons from $FADH_2$, so in this patient with a Complex I disorder, only the production of $FADH_2$ is fueling aerobic respiration. So, why is there such a large difference between the high-fat and high-carbohydrate diets, especially considering the fact that metabolism of glucose will also eventually generate acetyl-CoA? Glycolysis (break down of glucose into pyruvate) only generates NADH, so the ratio of $FADH_2$/NADH is higher in fat metabolism vs. carbohydrate metabolism, leading to more efficient generation of energy by funneling more electron carriers to Complex II.

In summary, the best treatment for the patient's Complex I deficiency is the high-fat diet, due to increased funneling of electron carriers to Complex II.

The Proton-Motive Force

Let's take a step back and look at the proton gradient that formed as electrons were passed along the ETC. As $[H^+]$ increases in the intermembrane space, two things happen simultaneously: pH drops in the intermembrane space, and the voltage difference between the intermembrane space and matrix increases due to proton pumping. Together, these two changes contribute to what is referred to as an **electrochemical gradient**: a gradient that has both chemical and electrostatic properties. Because it is based on protons, we often refer to the electrochemical gradient across the inner mitochondrial membrane as the proton-motive force. Any electrochemical gradient stores energy, and it will be the responsibility of ***ATP synthase*** to harness this energy to form ATP from ADP and an inorganic phosphate.

NADH Shuttles

As we look at the net ATP yield per glucose, note that a range exists between 30 and 32. This is because efficiency of aerobic respiration varies between cells. This variable efficiency is caused by the fact that cytosolic NADH formed through glycolysis cannot directly cross into the mitochondrial matrix. Because it cannot contribute its electrons to the transport chain directly, it must find alternate means of transportation referred to as **shuttle mechanisms**. A shuttle mechanism transfers the high-energy electrons of NADH to a carrier that can cross the inner mitochondrial membrane. Depending on which of the two shuttle mechanisms NADH participates in, either 1.5 or 2.5 ATP will end up being produced. Let's take a look at the two mechanisms:

BRIDGE

Glycerol 3-phosphate is an important link between lipid metabolism, discussed in Chapter 11 of *MCAT Biochemistry Review*, and glycolysis, discussed in Chapter 9. Its ability to be converted to DHAP, an intermediate of glycolysis, means that the glycerol of triacylglycerols can be shunted into glycolysis for energy.

- **Glycerol 3-phosphate shuttle:** The cytosol contains one isoform of *glycerol-3-phosphate dehydrogenase*, which oxidizes cytosolic NADH to NAD^+ while forming glycerol 3-phosphate from dihydroxyacetone phosphate (DHAP). On the outer face of the inner mitochondrial membrane, there exists another isoform of glycerol-3-phosphate dehydrogenase that is FAD-dependent. This mitochondrial FAD is the oxidizing agent, and ends up being reduced to $FADH_2$. Once reduced, $FADH_2$ proceeds to transfer its electrons to the ETC via Complex II, thus generating 1.5 ATP for every molecule of cytosolic NADH that participates in this pathway, which is shown in Figure 10.14.
- **Malate–aspartate shuttle:** Cytosolic oxaloacetate, which cannot pass through the inner mitochondrial membrane, is reduced to malate, which can. This is accomplished by cytosolic *malate dehydrogenase*. Accompanying this reduction is the oxidation of cytosolic NADH to NAD^+. Once malate crosses into the matrix, mitochondrial malate dehydrogenase reverses the reaction to form mitochondrial NADH. Now that NADH is in the matrix, it can pass along its electrons to the ETC via Complex I and generate 2.5 ATP per molecule of NADH. Recycling the malate requires oxidation to oxaloacetate, which can be transaminated to form aspartate. Aspartate crosses into the cytosol, and can be reconverted to oxaloacetate to restart the cycle, as shown in Figure 10.15.

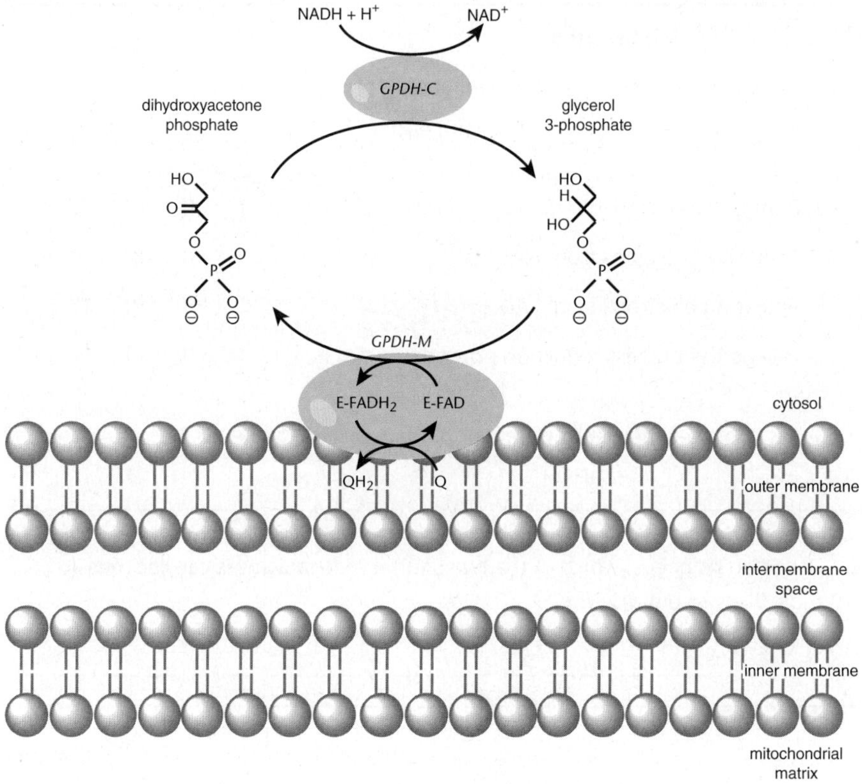

Figure 10.14 Glycerol-3-Phosphate Shuttle

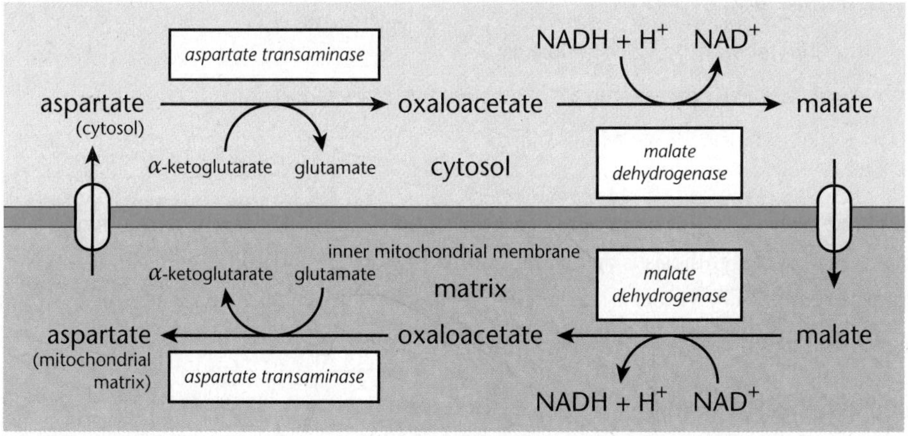

Figure 10.15 Malate-Aspartate Shuttle

MCAT CONCEPT CHECK 10.3

Before you move on, assess your understanding of the material with these questions.

1. Which complex(es) are associated with each of the following? (circle all that apply)

• Pumping a proton into the intermembrane space	I	II	III	IV
• Acquiring electrons from NADH	I	II	III	IV
• Acquiring electrons from $FADH_2$	I	II	III	IV
• Having the highest reduction potential	I	II	III	IV

2. What role does the electron transport chain play in the generation of ATP?

____

3. Based on its needs, which of the two shuttle mechanisms is cardiac muscle most likely to utilize? Why?

____

10.4 Oxidative Phosphorylation

LEARNING OBJECTIVES

After Chapter 10.4, you will be able to:

- Compare and contrast the ETC and oxidative phosphorylation
- Explain why the ETC generates more ATP than the direct reduction of oxygen by NADH

REAL WORLD

A small fraction—only 13 of approximately 100 polypeptides-that are necessary for oxidative phosphorylation are encoded by mitochondrial DNA. The significance of this fact is that mitochondrial DNA has a mutation rate nearly ten times higher than that of nuclear DNA.

We have arrived at the payout site of aerobic respiration: ATP synthesis. Knowing the nuances of ATP synthesis is an absolute must by Test Day. The link between electron transport and ATP synthesis starts with a protein complex called ATP synthase, which spans the entire inner mitochondrial membrane and protrudes into the matrix.

Chemiosmotic Coupling

The proton-motive force interacts with the portion of ATP synthase that spans the membrane, which is called the F_0 portion. $\mathbf{F_0}$ functions as an ion channel, so protons travel through F_0 along their gradient back into the matrix. As this happens, a process called **chemiosmotic coupling** allows the chemical energy of the gradient to be harnessed as a means of phosphorylating ADP, thus forming ATP. In other words, the ETC generates a high concentration of protons in the intermembrane space; the protons then flow through the F_0 ion channel of ATP synthase back into the matrix. As this happens, the other portion of ATP synthase, which is called the **$\mathbf{F_1}$ portion**, utilizes the energy released from this electrochemical gradient to phosphorylate ADP to ATP, as demonstrated in Figure 10.16. The specific mechanism by which ADP is actually phosphorylated is still a matter of debate.

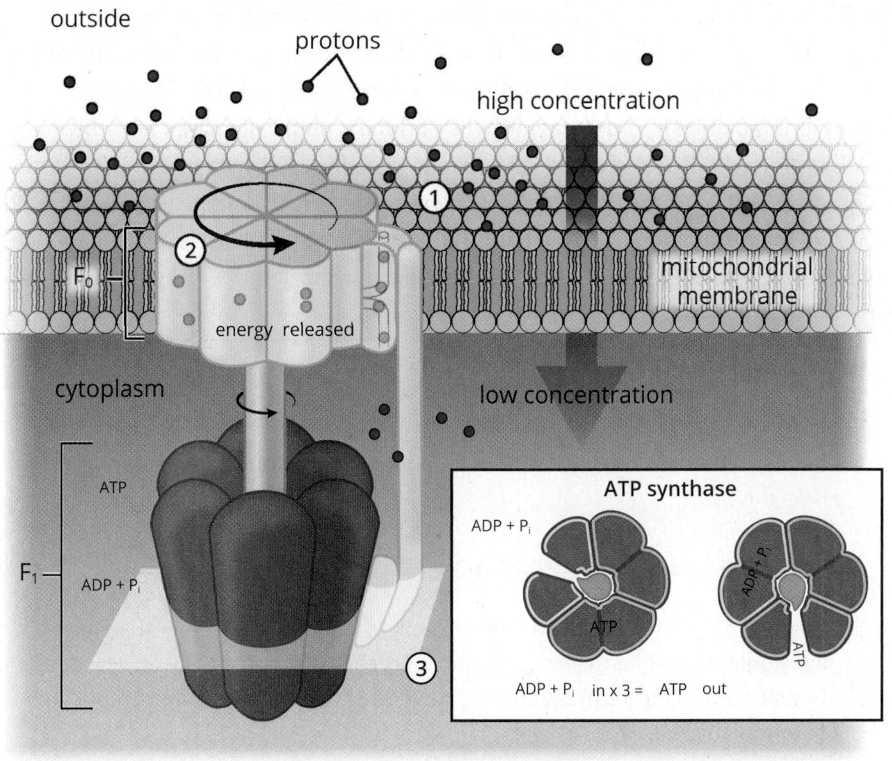

Figure 10.16 ATP Synthase Reaction

ATP synthase generates ATP from ADP and inorganic phosphate by allowing high-energy protons to move down the concentration gradient created by the electron transport chain.

Chemiosmotic coupling describes a direct relationship between the proton gradient and ATP synthesis. It is the predominant mechanism accepted in the scientific community when describing oxidative phosphorylation. However, another mechanism called **conformational coupling** suggests that the relationship between the proton gradient and ATP synthesis is indirect. Instead, ATP is released by the synthase as a result of conformational change caused by the gradient. In this mechanism, the F_1 portion of ATP synthase is reminiscent of a turbine, spinning within a stationary compartment to facilitate the harnessing of gradient energy for chemical bonding.

So we now know how we generate ATP, but how much energy was required to do so? When the proton-motive force is dissipated through the F_0 portion of ATP synthase, the free energy change of the reaction, $\Delta G^{\circ\prime}$, is $-220\,\frac{\text{kJ}}{\text{mol}}$, a highly exergonic reaction. This makes sense because phosphorylating ADP to form ATP is an endergonic process. So, by coupling these reactions, the energy harnessed from one reaction can drive another.

Regulation

Because the citric acid cycle provides the electron-rich molecules that feed into the ETC, it should come as no surprise that the rates of oxidative phosphorylation and the citric acid cycle are closely coordinated. Always think of O_2 and ADP as the key regulators of oxidative phosphorylation. If O_2 is limited, the rate of oxidative phosphorylation decreases, and the concentrations of NADH and $FADH_2$ increase. The accumulation of NADH, in turn, inhibits the citric acid cycle. The coordinated

MCAT EXPERTISE

When tackling complex mechanisms such as chemiosmotic coupling on Test Day, it's easy to make mistakes such as interpreting *a pH drop* to be *a $[H^+]$ drop* instead of a rise in proton concentration. Always read actively to avoid such mistakes.

REAL WORLD

Uncouplers are compounds that prevent ATP synthesis without affecting the ETC, thus greatly decreasing the efficiency of the ETC/oxidative phosphorylation pathway. Because ADP builds up and ATP synthesis decreases, the body responds to this perceived lack of energy by increasing O_2 consumption and NADH oxidation. The energy produced from the transport of electrons is released as heat. An example would be the fever experienced with toxic levels of salicylates, including aspirin.

regulation of these pathways is known as **respiratory control**. In the presence of adequate O_2, the rate of oxidative phosphorylation is dependent on the availability of ADP. The concentrations of ADP and ATP are reciprocally related; an accumulation of ADP is accompanied by a decrease in ATP and the amount of energy available to the cell. Therefore, ADP accumulation signals the need for ATP synthesis. ADP allosterically activates isocitrate dehydrogenase, thereby increasing the rate of the citric acid cycle and the production of NADH and $FADH_2$. The elevated levels of these reduced coenzymes, in turn, increase the rate of electron transport and ATP synthesis.

MCAT CONCEPT CHECK 10.4

Before you move on, assess your understanding of the material with these questions.

1. What is the difference between the ETC and oxidative phosphorylation? What links the two?

   ____

2. The $\Delta G°$ of NADH reducing oxygen directly is significantly greater than any individual step along the electron transport chain. If this is the case, why does transferring electrons along the ETC generate more ATP than direct reduction of oxygen by NADH?

   ____

Conclusion

Both topics discussed in this chapter—the citric acid cycle and oxidative phosphorylation—take place in the mitochondria. In the mitochondrial matrix, the citric acid cycle completely oxidizes acetyl-CoA to carbon dioxide. While this happens, energy is conserved via reduction reactions, forming high-energy electron carriers such as $FADH_2$ and NADH. ATP is also indirectly formed via GTP synthesis. These electron-rich carriers then transfer their electrons to the electron transport chain, which is located along the inner mitochondrial membrane. A series of oxidation–reduction reactions occurs in specific complexes until oxygen, the final electron acceptor, gets reduced and forms H_2O. This electrical pathway generates an electrochemical proton gradient that is harnessed by ATP synthase to generate ATP. The link between these two processes is highlighted by the fact that control of the citric acid cycle is NADH-dependent. When NADH accumulates, isocitrate dehydrogenase inhibition occurs, thus stopping both the citric acid cycle and electron transport chain.

It is worth noting that, while glycolysis is a major source of acetyl-CoA for the citric acid cycle, fatty acids also serve as an important source. In the next chapter, we turn our attention to the metabolism of two other types of biomolecules: lipids and amino acids.

You've reviewed the content, now test your knowledge and critical thinking skills by completing a test-like passage set in your online resources!

GO ONLINE

CONCEPT SUMMARY

Acetyl-CoA

- **Acetyl-CoA** contains a high-energy thioester bond that can be used to drive other reactions when hydrolysis occurs.
- It can be formed from pyruvate via **pyruvate dehydrogenase complex**, a five-enzyme complex in the mitochondrial matrix that forms—and is also inhibited by—acetyl-CoA and NADH.
  - **Pyruvate dehydrogenase** (PDH) oxidizes pyruvate, creating CO_2; it requires thiamine pyrophosphate (vitamin B_1, TPP) and Mg^{2+}.
  - **Dihydrolipoyl transacetylase** oxidizes the remaining two-carbon molecule using lipoic acid, and transfers the resulting acetyl group to CoA, forming acetyl-CoA.
  - **Dihydrolipoyl dehydrogenase** uses FAD to reoxidize lipoic acid, forming $FADH_2$. This $FADH_2$ can later transfer electrons to NAD^+, forming NADH that can feed into the electron transport chain.
  - **Pyruvate dehydrogenase kinase** phosphorylates PDH when ATP or acetyl-CoA levels are high, turning it off.
  - **Pyruvate dehydrogenase phosphatase** dephosphorylates PDH when ADP levels are high, turning it on.
- Acetyl-CoA can be formed from fatty acids, which enter the mitochondria using carriers.
  - The fatty acid couples with CoA in the cytosol to form fatty acyl-CoA, which moves to the intermembrane space.
  - The acyl (fatty acid) group is transferred to carnitine to form acyl-carnitine, which crosses the inner membrane.
  - The acyl group is transferred to a mitochondrial CoA to re-form fatty acyl-CoA, which can undergo β-oxidation to form acetyl-CoA.
- Acetyl-CoA can be formed from the carbon skeletons of ketogenic amino acids, ketone bodies, and alcohol.

Reactions of the Citric Acid Cycle

- The **citric acid cycle** takes place in the mitochondrial matrix.
- Its main purpose is to oxidize carbons in intermediates to CO_2 and generate high-energy electron carriers (NADH and $FADH_2$) and GTP.
- Key enzymes and reactions:
  - **Citrate synthase** couples acetyl-CoA to oxaloacetate and then hydrolyzes the resulting product, forming **citrate** and CoA–SH. This enzyme is regulated by negative feedback from ATP, NADH, succinyl-CoA, and citrate.
  - **Aconitase** isomerizes citrate to **isocitrate**.
  - **Isocitrate dehydrogenase** oxidizes and decarboxylates isocitrate to form **α-ketoglutarate**. This enzyme generates the first CO_2 and first NADH of the cycle. As the rate-limiting step of the citric acid cycle, it is heavily regulated: ATP and NADH are inhibitors; ADP and NAD^+ are activators.
  - **α-Ketoglutarate dehydrogenase complex** acts similarly to PDH complex, metabolizing **α-ketoglutarate** to form **succinyl-CoA**. This enzyme generates the second CO_2 and second NADH of the cycle. It is inhibited by ATP, NADH, and succinyl-CoA; it is activated by ADP and Ca^{2+}.
  - **Succinyl-CoA synthetase** hydrolyzes the thioester bond in succinyl-CoA to form **succinate** and CoA–SH. This enzyme generates the one GTP generated in the cycle.
  - **Succinate dehydrogenase** oxidizes succinate to form **fumarate**. This **flavoprotein** is anchored to the inner mitochondrial membrane because it requires FAD, which is reduced to form the one $FADH_2$ generated in the cycle.
  - **Fumarase** hydrolyzes the alkene bond of fumarate, forming **malate**.
  - **Malate dehydrogenase** oxidizes malate to **oxaloacetate**. This enzyme generates the third and final NADH of the cycle.

The Electron Transport Chain

- The **electron transport chain** takes place on the matrix-facing surface of the inner mitochondrial membrane.
- NADH donates electrons to the chain, which are passed from one complex to the next. As the ETC progresses, reduction potentials increase until oxygen, which has the highest reduction potential, receives the electrons.
  - **Complex I** (**NADH-CoQ oxidoreductase**) uses an iron–sulfur cluster to transfer electrons from NADH to flavin mononucleotide (FMN), and then to **coenzyme Q** (**CoQ**), forming $CoQH_2$. Four protons are translocated by Complex I.
  - **Complex II** (**Succinate-CoQ oxidoreductase**) uses an iron–sulfur cluster to transfer electrons from succinate to FAD, and then to CoQ, forming $CoQH_2$. No proton pumping occurs at Complex II.

- **Complex III** (**$CoQH_2$-cytochrome *c* oxidoreductase**) uses an iron–sulfur cluster to transfer electrons from $CoQH_2$ to heme, forming cytochrome *c* as part of the **Q cycle**. Four protons are translocated by Complex III.
- **Complex IV** (**cytochrome *c* oxidase**) uses cytochromes and Cu^{2+} to transfer electrons in the form of hydride ions (H^-) from cytochrome *c* to oxygen, forming water. Two protons are translocated by Complex IV.

- NADH cannot cross the inner mitochondrial membrane. Therefore, one of two available shuttle mechanisms to transfer electrons in the mitochondrial matrix must be used.
  - In the **glycerol 3-phosphate shuttle**, electrons are transferred from NADH to dihydroxyacetone phosphate (DHAP), forming glycerol 3-phosphate. These electrons can then be transferred to mitochondrial FAD, forming $FADH_2$.
  - In the **malate–aspartate shuttle**, electrons are transferred from NADH to oxaloacetate, forming malate. Malate can then cross the inner mitochondrial membrane and transfer the electrons to mitochondrial NAD^+, forming NADH.

Oxidative Phosphorylation

- The **proton-motive force** is the electrochemical gradient generated by the electron transport chain across the inner mitochondrial membrane. The intermembrane space has a higher concentration of protons than the matrix; this gradient stores energy, which can be used to form ATP via **chemiosmotic coupling**.
- **ATP synthase** is the enzyme responsible for generating ATP from ADP and an inorganic phosphate (P_i).
  - The **F_0 portion** is an ion channel, allowing protons to flow down the gradient from the intermembrane space to the matrix.
  - The **F_1 portion** uses the energy released by the gradient to phosphorylate ADP into ATP.
- The following is a summary of the energy yield of the various carbohydrate metabolism processes:
  - Glycolysis generates 2 NADH and 2 ATP.
  - Pyruvate dehydrogenase generates 1 NADH per molecule of pyruvate. Because each glucose forms two molecules of pyruvate, this complex produces a net of 2 NADH.
  - The citric acid cycle generates 3 NADH, 1 $FADH_2$, and 1 GTP (6 NADH, 2 $FADH_2$, and 2 GTP per molecule of glucose).
  - Each NADH yields 2.5 ATP; 10 NADH form 25 ATP.
  - Each $FADH_2$ yields 1.5 ATP; 2 $FADH_2$ form 3 ATP.
  - GTP are converted to ATP.
  - 2 ATP from glycolysis + 2 ATP (GTP) from the citric acid cycle + 25 ATP from NADH + 3 ATP from $FADH_2$ = 32 ATP per molecule of glucose (optimal). Inefficiencies of the system and variability between cells make 30–32 ATP/glucose the commonly accepted range for energy yield.

ANSWERS TO CONCEPT CHECKS

10.1

1. Pyruvate + CoA–SH + NAD^+ → acetyl-CoA + CO_2 + NADH + H^+
2.

Molecule	Mechanism of Conversion to Acetyl-CoA
Fatty acids	Shuttle acyl group from cytosolic CoA–SH to mitochondrial CoA–SH via carnitine; then undergo β-oxidation
Ketogenic amino acids	Transaminate to lose nitrogen; convert carbon skeleton into ketone body, which can be converted into acetyl-CoA
Ketones	Reverse of ketone body formation
Alcohol	Alcohol dehydrogenase and acetaldehyde dehydrogenase convert alcohol into acetyl-CoA

10.2

1. Complete oxidation of carbons in intermediates to CO_2 so that reduction reactions can be coupled with CO_2 formation, thus forming energy carriers such as NADH and $FADH_2$ for the electron transport chain.
2. Isocitrate dehydrogenase
3.

Checkpoints	Inhibitors	Activators
Citrate synthase	ATP, NADH, succinyl-CoA, citrate	None
Isocitrate dehydrogenase	ATP, NADH	ADP, NAD^+
α-Ketoglutarate complex	ATP, NADH, succinyl-CoA	ADP, Ca^{2+}

10.3

1. - Pumping a proton into the intermembrane space: I, III, and IV
   - Acquiring electrons from NADH: I
   - Acquiring electrons from $FADH_2$: II
   - Having the highest reduction potential: IV (reduction potentials increase along the ETC)
2. The electron transport chain generates the proton-motive force, an electrochemical gradient across the inner mitochondrial membrane, which provides the energy for ATP synthase to function.
3. The malate–aspartate shuttle. Because this mechanism is the more efficient one, it makes sense for a highly aerobic organ such as the heart to utilize it in order to maximize its ATP yield.

10.4

1. The ETC is made up of the physical set of intermembrane proteins located on the inner mitochondrial matrix, and they undergo oxidation–reduction reactions as they transfer electrons to oxygen, the final electron acceptor. As electrons are transferred, a proton-motive force is generated in the intermembrane space. Oxidative phosphorylation is the process by which ATP is generated via harnessing the proton gradient, and it utilizes ATP synthase to do so.
2. By splitting up electron transfer into several complexes, enough energy is released to facilitate the creation of a proton gradient at many locations, rather than just one. The greater the proton gradient is, the greater the ATP generation will be. Direct reduction of oxygen by NADH would release a significant amount of energy to the environment, resulting in inefficient electron transport.

SCIENCE MASTERY ASSESSMENT EXPLANATIONS

1. **B**

Phosphofructokinase-1 (PFK-1), which catalyzes the rate-limiting step of glycolysis, is the only enzyme listed here that functions under anaerobic conditions. The other enzymes are all involved in the oxygen-requiring processes discussed in this chapter. Succinate dehydrogenase, **(A)**, appears in both the citric acid cycle and as part of Complex II of the electron transport chain. Isocitrate dehydrogenase, **(C)**, catalyzes the rate-limiting step of the citric acid cycle. Pyruvate dehydrogenase, **(D)**, is one of the five enzymes that make up the pyruvate dehydrogenase complex.

2. **B**

The increased permeability of the inner mitochondrial membrane allows the proton-motive force to be dissipated through locations besides the F_0 portion of ATP synthase. Therefore, ATP synthase is less active and is forming less ATP, invalidating **(A)** and **(C)**. The body will attempt to regenerate the proton-motive force by increasing fuel catabolism, eliminating **(D)**. This increase in fuel use requires more oxygen utilization in the electron transport chain.

3. **B**

The citric acid cycle takes place in the mitochondrial matrix, not the outer mitochondrial membrane. While most citric acid cycle enzymes are located within the matrix, succinate dehydrogenase is located on the inner mitochondrial membrane.

4. **C**

It is not necessary to have all the net reactions memorized for each metabolic process to answer this question; all we need is to identify a few key reactants and products. In this case, we start with acetyl-CoA and end with CoA–SH. We also notice that in this reaction, NAD^+ and FAD are reduced to NADH and $FADH_2$, and that CO_2 is formed. The only metabolic process in which all of the above reactions would occur is the citric acid cycle, also called the tricarboxylic acid (TCA) or Krebs cycle.

5. **A**

This question is testing our general knowledge of cellular respiration. Notice that all types of cellular respiration (aerobic and anaerobic) start with the degradation of glucose by glycolysis. In aerobic respiration, oxygen is the final electron acceptor, and water is therefore produced at the end of the electron transport chain. While oxygen is needed for aerobic respiration in order to produce the optimal 32 molecules of ATP per glucose, it is not the only method by which ATP is produced. Glycolysis still provides 2 ATP per glucose without the need for oxygen, thus making **(B)** and **(D)** incorrect. Water, mentioned in **(C)**, is produced in aerobic metabolism, not consumed.

6. **C**

Fat molecules stored in adipose tissue can be hydrolyzed by lipases to fatty acids and glycerol. While glycerol can be converted into glyceraldehyde 3-phosphate, a glycolytic intermediate, a fatty acid must first be activated in the cytoplasm by coupling the fatty acid to CoA–SH, forming fatty acyl-CoA. The fatty acid is then transferred to a molecule of carnitine, which can carry it across the inner mitochondrial membrane. Once inside, the fatty acid is transferred to a mitochondrial CoA–SH, re-forming fatty acyl-CoA. Through fatty acid oxidation, this fatty acyl-CoA can become acetyl-CoA, which enters the citric acid cycle.

7. **C**

Based on the wording of this question, three choices are used to produce acetyl-CoA and one is not. As part of aerobic metabolism, decarboxylation of pyruvate by the pyruvate dehydrogenase complex yields acetyl-CoA, NADH, and CO_2. Other sources of acetyl-CoA include amino acid catabolism, beta oxidation of fatty acids, and alcohol metabolism. Fatty acids are produced via reduction of acetyl-CoA and cannot be further reduced, making **(C)** correct.

8. **C**

Cytochrome *c* carries electrons from $CoQH_2$-cytochrome *c* oxidoreductase (Complex III) to cytochrome *c* oxidase (Complex IV) as part of the electron transport chain. The ETC takes place on the inner mitochondrial membrane.

9. **B**

During oxidative phosphorylation, energy is harvested from the energy carriers $FADH_2$ and NADH in order to form ATP. One molecule of mitochondrial $FADH_2$ is oxidized to produce 1.5 molecules of ATP. Similarly, one molecule of mitochondrial NADH is oxidized to produce 2.5 molecules of ATP in the electron transport chain.

10. **B**

Thioester links release a great deal of energy when hydrolyzed, making them well-suited as respiration reaction drivers. They are particularly useful because they release more energy than typical ester cleavage. It is thioester formation, not hydrolysis, that requires a great deal of energy, making **(D)** incorrect.

11. **B**

The conversion of GDP to GTP is a phosphorylation reaction, in which a phosphate group is added to a molecule. Such reactions are catalyzed by kinases. Nomenclature is helpful here, as nucleosidediphosphate kinase is the only enzyme that contains *kinase* in its name.

12. **C**

The wording of these answer choices is critical. The electrons from cytosolic NADH can enter the mitochondrion through one of two shuttle mechanisms: the glycerol 3-phosphate shuttle, which ultimately moves these electrons to mitochondrial FAD, and the malate–aspartate shuttle, which ultimately moves these electrons to mitochondrial NAD^+. If the electrons are transferred using the malate–aspartate shuttle, then no energy is lost, making **(A)** and **(D)** incorrect. NADH cannot enter the matrix directly, making **(B)** incorrect. It is the fact that electrons can use more than one pathway—one of which loses energy that could be used for ATP synthesis—that accounts for the potentially decreased yield of ATP from cytosolic NADH.

13. **A**

Uncouplers inhibit ATP synthesis without affecting the electron transport chain. Because the body must burn more fuel to maintain the proton-motive force, glycogen stores will be mobilized to feed into glycolysis, then the TCA, and finally oxidative phosphorylation.

14. **B**

Complex II is the only complex of the ETC that does not contribute to the proton gradient. Complexes I and III each add four protons to the gradient; Complex IV adds two protons to the gradient.

15. **B**

While all of the other answers contribute to energy production, it is the electrochemical gradient (proton-motive force) that directly drives the phosphorylation of ATP by the F_1 portion of ATP synthase.

Consult your online resources for additional practice. GO ONLINE

SHARED CONCEPTS

Biochemistry Chapter 2
Enzymes

Biochemistry Chapter 4
Carbohydrate Structure and Function

Biochemistry Chapter 9
Carbohydrate Metabolism I

Biochemistry Chapter 11
Lipid and Amino Acid Metabolism

Biochemistry Chapter 12
Bioenergetics and Regulation of Metabolism

General Chemistry Chapter 12
Electrochemistry

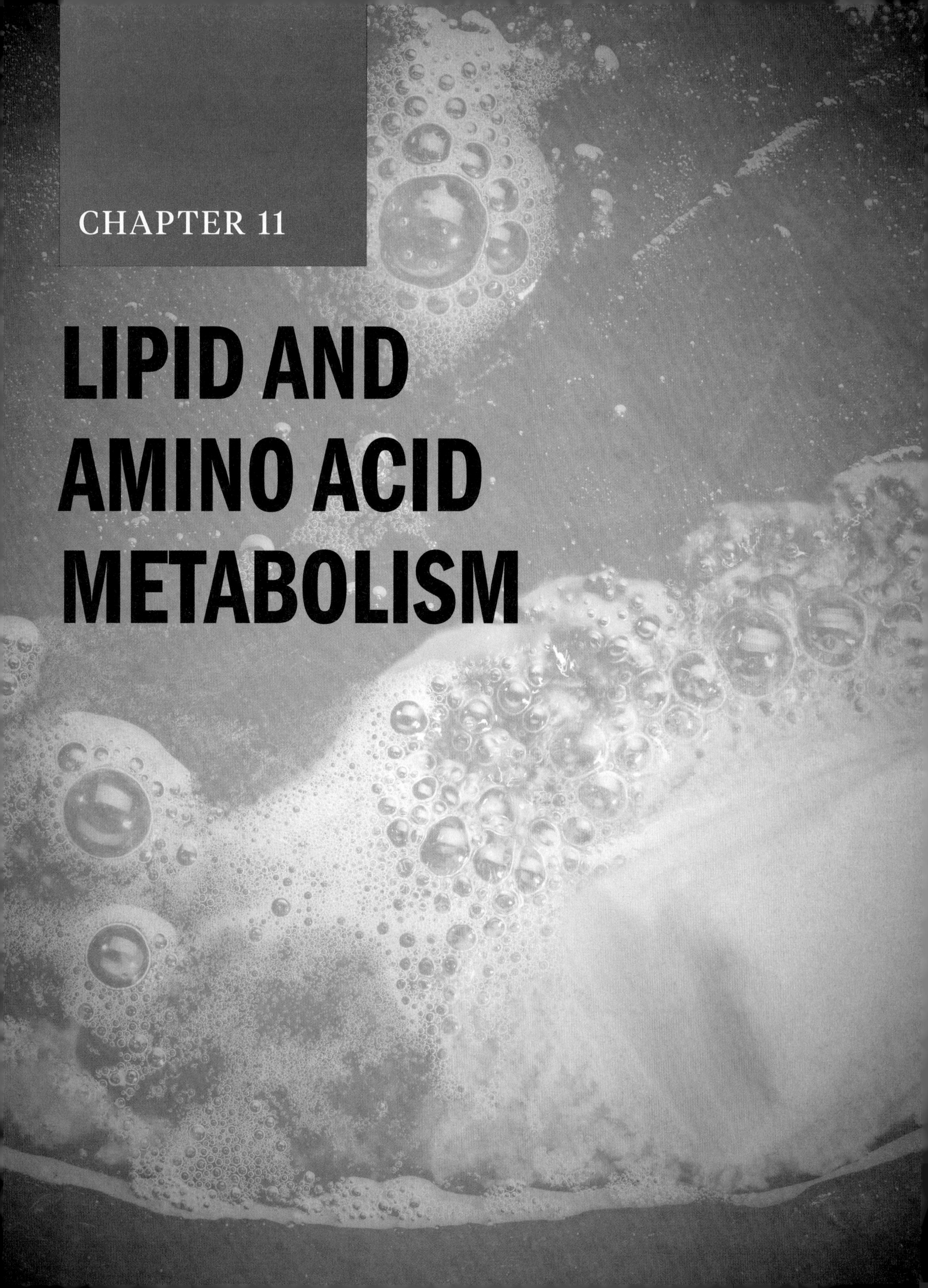

CHAPTER 11

LIPID AND AMINO ACID METABOLISM

SCIENCE MASTERY ASSESSMENT

Every pre-med knows this feeling: there is so much content I have to know for the MCAT! How do I know what to do first or what's important?

While the high-yield badges throughout this book will help you identify the most important topics, this Science Mastery Assessment is another tool in your MCAT prep arsenal. This quiz (which can also be taken in your online resources) and the guidance below will help ensure that you are spending the appropriate amount of time on this chapter based on your personal strengths and weaknesses. Don't worry though—skipping something now does not mean you'll never study it. Later on in your prep, as you complete full-length tests, you'll uncover specific pieces of content that you need to review and can come back to these chapters as appropriate.

How to Use This Assessment

If you answer 0–7 questions correctly:

Spend about 1 hour to read this chapter in full and take limited notes throughout. Follow up by reviewing **all** quiz questions to ensure that you now understand how to solve each one.

If you answer 8–11 questions correctly:

Spend 20–40 minutes reviewing the quiz questions. Beginning with the questions you missed, read and take notes on the corresponding subchapters. For questions you answered correctly, ensure your thinking matches that of the explanation and you understand why each choice was correct or incorrect.

If you answer 12–15 questions correctly:

Spend less than 20 minutes reviewing all questions from the quiz. If you missed any, then include a quick read-through of the corresponding subchapters, or even just the relevant content within a subchapter, as part of your question review. For questions you got correct, ensure your thinking matches that of the explanation and review the Concept Summary at the end of the chapter.

1. Which of the following hormones does NOT directly regulate the activity of hormone-sensitive lipase in adipose tissue?
   - **A.** Insulin
   - **B.** Glucogen
   - **C.** Epinephrine
   - **D.** Cortisol

2. What is the fate of long-chain fatty acids that are contained within micelles?
   - **A.** Transport into chylomicrons released into the lymphatic system
   - **B.** Transport into chylomicrons released into the circulatory system
   - **C.** Direct diffusion across the intestine into the lymphatic system
   - **D.** Direct diffusion across the intestine into the circulatory system

3. During fatty acid mobilization, which of the following occur(s)?
   - **I.** HSL is activated.
   - **II.** Free fatty acids are released.
   - **III.** Gluconeogenesis proceeds in adipocytes.

   - **A.** I only
   - **B.** III only
   - **C.** I and II only
   - **D.** II and III only

4. How do chylomicrons and VLDL differ?
   - **A.** Chylomicrons contain apoproteins, VLDL do not.
   - **B.** Chylomicrons are synthesized in the intestine, VLDL are synthesized in the liver.
   - **C.** Chylomicrons transport triacylglycerol, VLDL transport cholesterol.
   - **D.** VLDL are another term for chylomicron remnants; they differ in age.

5. Which of the following could result from an absence of apolipoproteins?
   - **I.** An inability to secrete lipid transport lipoproteins
   - **II.** An inability to endocytose lipoproteins
   - **III.** A decreased ability to remove excess cholesterol from blood vessels

   - **A.** I only
   - **B.** III only
   - **C.** I and II only
   - **D.** I, II, and III

6. Statin drugs inhibit HMG-CoA reductase. As such, they are likely prescribed for:
   - **A.** hypercholesterolemia (high cholesterol).
   - **B.** hypertriglyceridemia (high triacylglycerol).
   - **C.** hypocholesterolemia (low cholesterol).
   - **D.** visceral adiposity (obesity).

7. What is the function of LCAT?
   - **A.** LCAT catalyzes the production of cholesteryl esters.
   - **B.** LCAT catalyzes the production of cholesterol.
   - **C.** LCAT catalyzes the transfer of cholesteryl esters.
   - **D.** LCAT catalyzes the transfer of cholesterol.

8. Which fatty acid can be synthesized by humans?
   - **A.** 12:0
   - **B.** 16:0
   - **C.** 16:1
   - **D.** 18:3

9. Which of the following best characterizes the process of fatty acid synthesis?
   A. Two reductions followed by a dehydration and bond formation
   B. Reduction followed by activation, bond formation, dehydration, and reduction
   C. Activation followed by bond formation, reduction, dehydration, and reduction
   D. Activation followed by bond formation, oxidation, dehydration, and reduction

10. Which of the following best describes how the body creates or processes ketone bodies?
    A. Ketone bodies are produced in the peroxisomes of liver cells during periods of fasting.
    B. Acetyl-CoA is converted into acetoacetate, 3-hydroxybutyrate, or acetone, all of which are utilized for energy.
    C. Ketone bodies are produced in the mitochondria of liver cells after prolonged fasting.
    D. The brain is the first organ to use ketone bodies.

11. The majority of triacylglycerols stored in adipocytes originate from:
    A. synthesis in the adipocyte.
    B. dietary intake.
    C. ketone bodies.
    D. synthesis in the liver.

12. 2,4-Dienoyl-CoA reductase is used in the oxidation of:
    A. saturated fatty acids.
    B. monounsaturated fatty acids.
    C. polyunsaturated fatty acids.
    D. cholesterol.

13. Which of the following is true regarding ketolysis?
    A. Ketolysis occurs only in the brain.
    B. Ketolysis occurs in the liver.
    C. Ketolysis generates acetyl-CoA.
    D. Ketolysis increases glucose metabolism.

14. Which of the following amino acids will provide the most energy when degraded?
    A. Glycine
    B. Alanine
    C. Valine
    D. Isoleucine

15. Which of the following is LEAST likely to result from protein degradation and processing by the liver?
    A. Fatty acids
    B. Glucose
    C. Acetoacetate
    D. 3-Hydroxybutyrate

Answer Key

1. **B**
2. **A**
3. **C**
4. **B**
5. **D**
6. **A**
7. **A**
8. **B**
9. **C**
10. **C**
11. **D**
12. **C**
13. **C**
14. **D**
15. **A**

Detailed explanations can be found at the end of the chapter.

CHAPTER 11

LIPID AND AMINO ACID METABOLISM

In This Chapter

Introduction

For weeks before the winter season begins, bears and certain mammals increase their food intake to prepare for hibernation. During this time, they increase their weight by storing energy. Different organisms store fuel and supplies in different ways. Hamsters store extra food in pouches in their cheeks. Cacti absorb and conserve water in preparation for dry seasons. But hibernating animals store extra calories as fat. Over the course of the winter, fat stores are mobilized and metabolized for basic bodily functions, which are minimal during hibernation. Come spring and summer, these reserves will be replenished in preparation for the next winter season. Humans also store extra energy as fat. While we may not hibernate through the winter, fat stores allow us to store energy to use during prolonged periods without food.

As discussed in Chapter 8 of *MCAT Biochemistry Review*, lipids play a major role in maintaining the structure and function of cells; however, they also have important roles as storage molecules for energy and in biological signaling. In this chapter, we'll examine the metabolism of lipids, starting with ingestion of food particles and continuing through absorption, transport, and energy catabolism. We will also cover energy storage via lipid synthesis, as well as the metabolism of cholesterol and ketone bodies. In addition, we will learn about how protein degradation feeds into lipid and carbohydrate pathways and the urea cycle.

CHAPTER PROFILE

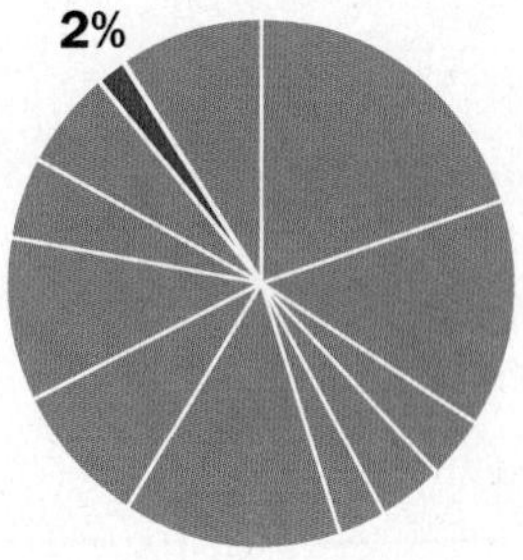

The content in this chapter should be relevant to about 2% of all questions about Biochemistry on the MCAT.

This chapter covers material from the following AAMC content category:

1D: Principles of bioenergetics and fuel molecule metabolism

MCAT EXPERTISE

Chapter 11 contains some of the most complex and difficult material in this book. However, the content within this chapter is not particularly high-yield on Test Day, as can be seen in the chapter profile above. This chapter is still worth reviewing, but its content will be most relevant to students seeking full mastery of all testable content for an extremely competitive score.

11.1 Lipid Digestion and Absorption

LEARNING OBJECTIVES

After Chapter 11.1, you will be able to:

- Differentiate between lipid digestion in the stomach and lipid digestion in the intestines
- Identify the methods by which lipids can enter circulation
- Describe the structure of a micelle

In addition to being a major source of energy in the body, lipids serve a variety of other functions in the body. For instance, some fat-soluble vitamins play roles as coenzymes; prostaglandins and steroid hormones are necessary in the control and maintenance of homeostasis. Aberrant lipid metabolism may also be associated with clinical manifestations such as atherosclerosis and obesity.

Digestion

Dietary fat consists mainly of **triacylglycerols**, with the remainder comprised of **cholesterol**, **cholesteryl esters**, **phospholipids**, and free **fatty acids**. Lipid digestion is minimal in the mouth and stomach; lipids are transported to the small intestine essentially intact. Upon entry into the duodenum, **emulsification** occurs, which is the mixing of two normally immiscible liquids (in this case, fat and water). Formation of an emulsion increases the surface area of the lipid, which permits greater enzymatic interaction and processing. Emulsification is aided by bile, which contains **bile salts**, **pigments**, and **cholesterol**; bile is secreted by the liver and stored in the gallbladder. Finally, the pancreas secretes ***pancreatic lipase***, ***colipase***, and ***cholesterol esterase*** into the small intestine; together, these enzymes hydrolyze the lipid components to *2-monoacylglycerol*, free fatty acids, and cholesterol. Figure 11.1 summarizes the digestion and absorption of dietary lipid components.

BRIDGE

Digestion is covered in Chapter 9 of *MCAT Biology Review*

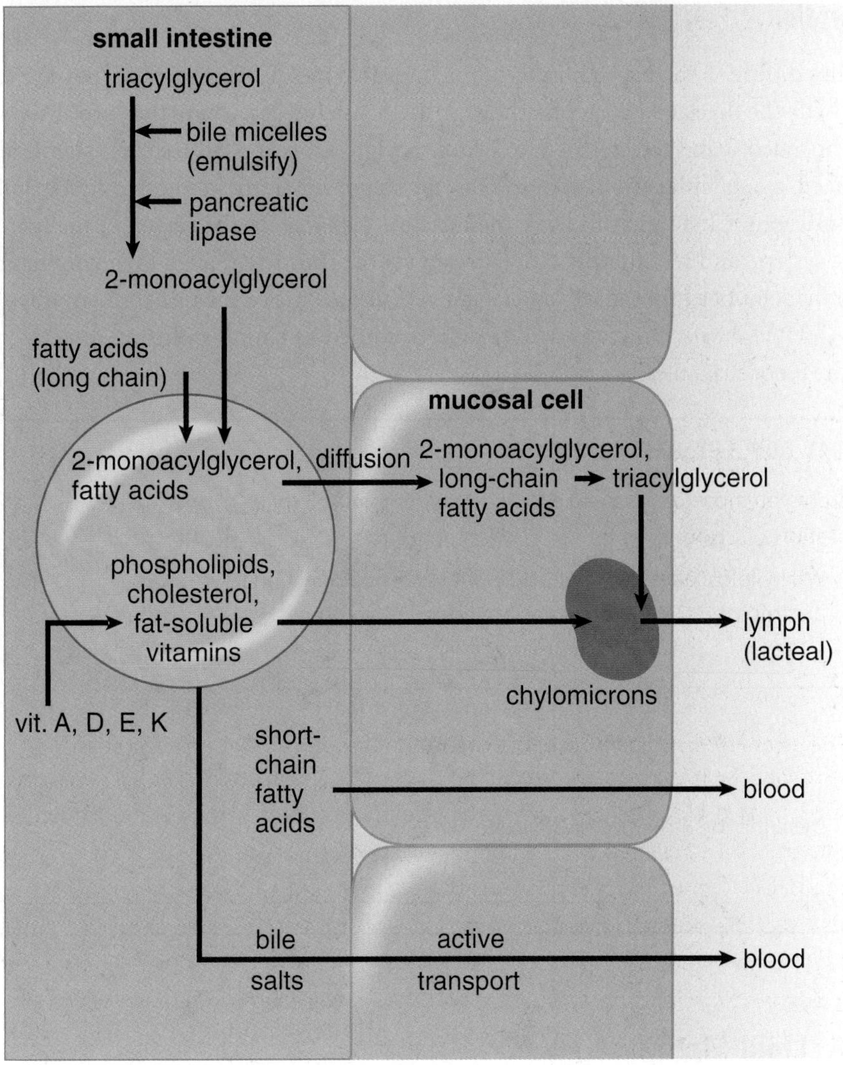

Figure 11.1 Absorption of Lipids

Micelle Formation

Emulsification is followed by absorption of fats by intestinal cells. Free fatty acids, cholesterol, 2-monoacylglycerol, and bile salts contribute to the formation of **micelles**, which are clusters of amphipathic lipids that are soluble in the aqueous environment of the intestinal lumen. Essentially, micelles are water-soluble spheres with a lipid-soluble interior. Micelles are vital in digestion, transport, and absorption of lipid-soluble substances starting from the duodenum all the way to the end of the ileum. At the end of the ileum, bile salts are actively reabsorbed and recycled; any fat that remains in the intestine will pass into the colon, and ultimately ends up in the stool.

BRIDGE

Absorption in the small intestine and colon follows a characteristic pattern. This is a good time to review digestion, discussed in Chapter 9 of *MCAT Biology Review*, to create a complete schema for the absorption and metabolism of all the macronutrients.

Absorption

Micelles diffuse to the brush border of the intestinal mucosal cells where they are absorbed. The digested lipids pass through the brush border, where they are absorbed into the mucosa and re-esterified to form triacylglycerols and cholesteryl esters and packaged, along with certain apoproteins, fat-soluble vitamins, and other lipids, into **chylomicrons**. Chylomicrons leave the intestine via **lacteals**, the vessels of the lymphatic system, and re-enter the bloodstream via the **thoracic duct**, a long lymphatic vessel that empties into the left subclavian vein at the base of the neck. The more water-soluble short-chain fatty acids can be absorbed by simple diffusion directly into the bloodstream.

MCAT CONCEPT CHECK 11.1

Before you move on, assess your understanding of the material with these questions.

1. When lipids leave the stomach, what stages of digestion have been accomplished? What enzymes are added to accomplish the next phase?

2. True or False: All lipids enter the circulation through the lymphatic system.

3. Describe the structure of a micelle.

11.2 Lipid Mobilization

LEARNING OBJECTIVES

After Chapter 11.2, you will be able to:

- Identify the conditions and hormones that promote lipid mobilization
- Predict the ratio of free fatty acids per glycerol molecule broken down via lipid mobilization

At night, the body is in the postabsorptive state, utilizing energy stores instead of food for fuel. In the postabsorptive state, fatty acids are released from adipose tissue and used for energy. Although human adipose tissue does not respond directly to glucagon, a fall in insulin levels activates a ***hormone-sensitive lipase*** (**HSL**) that hydrolyzes triacylglycerols, yielding fatty acids and glycerol. Epinephrine and cortisol can also activate HSL, as shown in Figure 11.2; we will discuss the effects of these hormones on metabolism in more detail in the next chapter. Released glycerol from fat may be transported to the liver for glycolysis or gluconeogenesis. HSL is effective within adipose cells, but ***lipoprotein lipase*** (**LPL**) is necessary for the metabolism of chylomicrons and very-low-density lipoproteins (VLDL). LPL is an enzyme that can release free fatty acids from triacylglycerols in these lipoproteins.

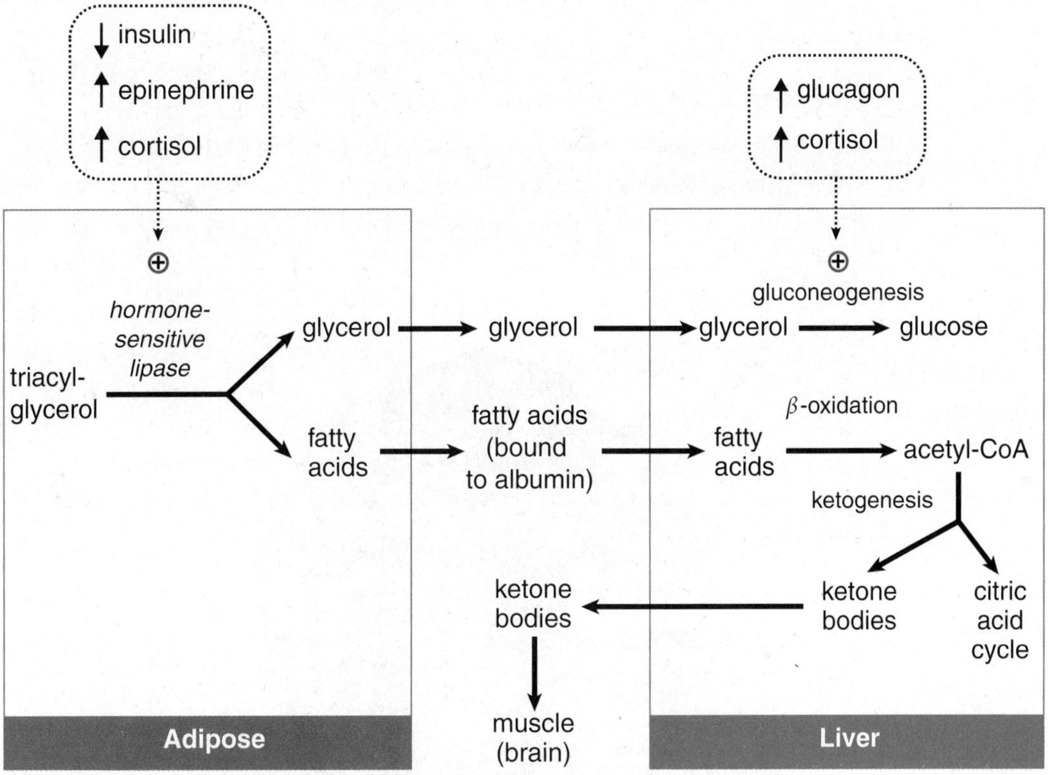

Figure 11.2 Mobilization of Triacylglycerols and Metabolism by the Liver

MCAT CONCEPT CHECK 11.2

Before you move on, assess your understanding of the material with these questions.

1. A patient who has diabetes begins insulin injections for management of blood glucose levels. What is the expected impact on the patient's weight?

____

2. What is the ratio of free fatty acids to glycerol produced through lipid mobilization?

____

11.3 Lipid Transport

LEARNING OBJECTIVES

After Chapter 11.3, you will be able to:

- Describe the means of transport for free fatty acids in the blood
- Order lipoproteins according to percentage of protein and lipid transported
- Explain the relationship between the liver and the intestinal epithelium in relation to lipoproteins
- Recall the major structural components of a lipoprotein

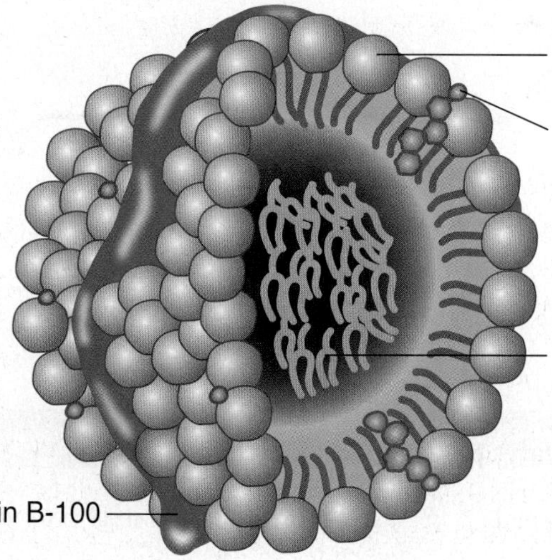

Figure 11.3 Lipoprotein Structure

While free fatty acids are transported through the blood in association with albumin, a carrier protein, triacylglycerol and cholesterol are transported in the blood as **lipoproteins**: aggregates of **apolipoproteins** and lipids, as shown in Figure 11.3. Lipoproteins are named according to their density, which increases in direct proportion to the percentage of protein in the particle. Chylomicrons are the least dense, with the highest fat-to-protein ratio. VLDL (very-low-density lipoprotein) is slightly more dense, followed by IDL (intermediate-density), LDL (low-density), and HDL (high-density). The main functions of each lipoprotein are shown in Table 11.1. Note that chylomicrons and VLDL primarily carry triacylglycerols, but also contain small quantities of cholesteryl esters. LDL and HDL are primarily cholesterol transport molecules.

LIPOPROTEIN	FUNCTIONS
Chylomicrons	Transport dietary triacylglycerols, cholesterol, and cholesteryl esters from intestine to tissues
VLDL	Transports triacylglycerols and fatty acids from liver to tissues
IDL (VLDL remnants)	Picks up cholesteryl esters from HDL to become LDL Picked up by the liver
LDL	Delivers cholesterol into cells
HDL	Picks up cholesterol accumulating in blood vessels Delivers cholesterol to liver and steroidogenic tissues Transfers apolipoproteins to other lipoproteins

Table 11.1 Classes of Lipoproteins

Chylomicrons

Chylomicrons are highly soluble in both lymphatic fluid and blood and function in the transport of dietary triacylglycerols, cholesterol, and cholesteryl esters to other tissues. Assembly of chylomicrons occurs in the intestinal lining and results in a nascent chylomicron that contains lipids and apolipoproteins.

VLDL (Very-Low-Density Lipoprotein)

VLDL metabolism is similar to that of chylomicrons; however, VLDL is produced and assembled in liver cells. Like chylomicrons, the main function of VLDL is the transport of triacylglycerols to other tissues. VLDLs also contain fatty acids that are synthesized from excess glucose or retrieved from chylomicron remnants.

KEY CONCEPT

Chylomicrons and VLDL primarily carry triacylglycerols. LDL and HDL primarily carry cholesterol. IDL is intermediate; it is a transition state between VLDL and LDL, occurring as the primary lipid within the lipoprotein changes from triacylglycerol to cholesterol.

IDL (Intermediate-Density Lipoprotein)

Once triacylglycerol is removed from VLDL, the resulting particle is referred to as either a **VLDL remnant** or **IDL**. Some IDL is reabsorbed by the liver by apolipoproteins on its exterior, and some is further processed in the bloodstream. For example, some IDL picks up cholesteryl esters from HDL to become LDL. IDL thus exists as a transition particle between triacylglycerol transport (associated with chylomicrons and VLDL) and cholesterol transport (associated with LDL and HDL). This process is shown in Figure 11.4.

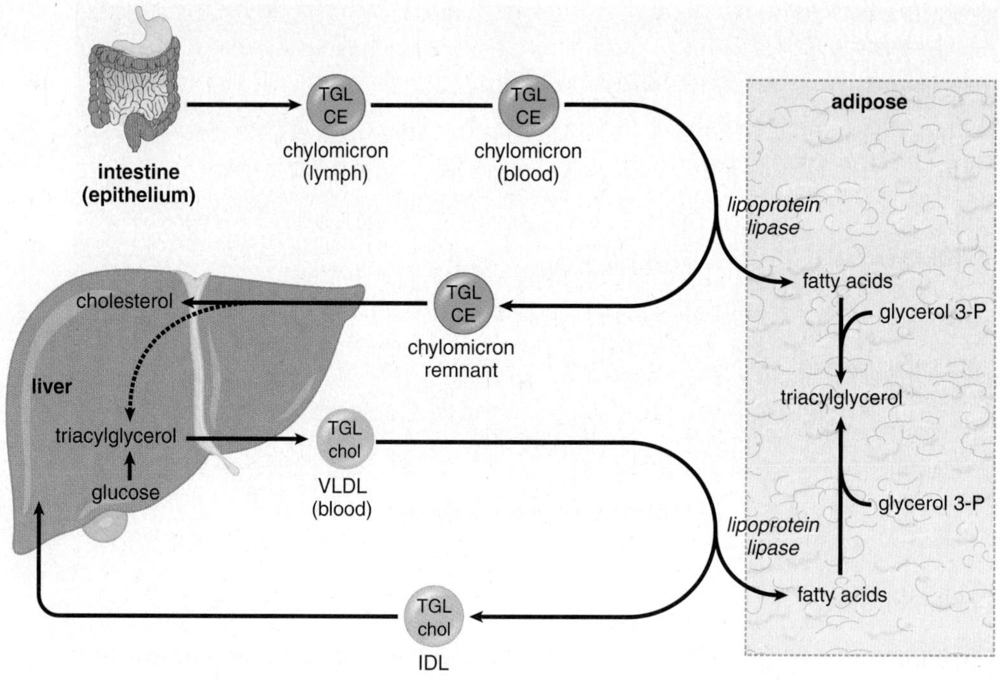

Figure 11.4 Lipid Transport in Lipoproteins
TGL = triacylglycerol; CE = cholesteryl esters; chol = cholesterol

LDL (Low-Density Lipoprotein)

Although both LDL and HDL are primarily cholesterol particles, the majority of the cholesterol measured in blood is associated with **LDL**. The normal role of LDL is to deliver cholesterol to tissues for biosynthesis. However, cholesterol also plays an important role in cell membranes. In addition, bile acids and salts are made from cholesterol in the liver, and many other tissues require cholesterol for steroid hormone synthesis (steroidogenesis).

REAL WORLD

When a physician orders a blood test for cholesterol, they are actually measuring levels of LDL and HDL in the blood. HDL is often considered "good" cholesterol because it picks up excess cholesterol from blood vessels for excretion.

HDL (High-Density Lipoprotein)

HDL is synthesized in the liver and intestines and released as dense, protein-rich particles into the blood. HDL contains apolipoproteins used for cholesterol recovery—that is, the cleaning up of excess cholesterol from blood vessels for excretion. HDL also delivers some cholesterol to steroidogenic tissues and transfers necessary apolipoproteins to some of the other lipoproteins.

Apolipoproteins

Apolipoproteins, also referred to as **apoproteins**, form the protein component of the lipoproteins described above. Apolipoproteins are receptor molecules and are involved in signaling. While it is highly unlikely that specific functions of each apolipoprotein will be tested on the MCAT, they are briefly summarized below to illustrate their diverse purposes:

- **apoA-I:** activates LCAT, an enzyme that catalyzes cholesterol esterification
- **apoB-48:** mediates chylomicron secretion
- **apoB-100:** permits uptake of LDL by the liver
- **apoC-II:** activates lipoprotein lipase
- **apoE:** permits uptake of chylomicron remnants and VLDL by the liver

MCAT CONCEPT CHECK 11.3

Before you move on, assess your understanding of the material with these questions.

1. What is the primary method of transporting free fatty acids in the blood?

____

2. Order the lipoproteins from greatest percentage of protein to least percentage of protein. Circle the molecules that are primarily involved in triacylglycerol transport.

____

3. Lipoproteins are synthesized primarily by which two organs?

____

4. When physicians order a lipid panel to evaluate a patient, which value do they prefer to see over a minimum threshold rather than below a maximum?

____

11.4 Cholesterol Metabolism

LEARNING OBJECTIVES

After Chapter 11.4, you will be able to:

- Predict optimal conditions for HMG-CoA reductase activity
- Recall the functions of the citrate shuttle, HMG-CoA reductase, LCAT, and CETP

Cholesterol is a ubiquitous component of all cells in the human body and plays a major role in the synthesis of cell membranes, steroid hormones, bile acids, and vitamin D.

Sources

Most cells derive their cholesterol from LDL or HDL, but some cholesterol may be synthesized *de novo*. *De novo* synthesis of cholesterol occurs in the liver and is driven by acetyl-CoA and ATP. The **citrate shuttle** carries mitochondrial acetyl-CoA into the cytoplasm, where synthesis occurs. NADPH (from the pentose phosphate pathway) supplies reducing equivalents. Synthesis of ***mevalonic acid*** in the smooth endoplasmic reticulum (SER) is the rate-limiting step in cholesterol biosynthesis and is catalyzed by ***3-hydroxy-3-methylglutaryl*** **(HMG)** ***CoA reductase***. Cholesterol synthesis is regulated in several ways. First, increased levels of cholesterol can inhibit further synthesis by a feedback inhibition mechanism. Next, insulin promotes cholesterol synthesis. Control over *de novo* cholesterol synthesis is also dependent on regulation of HMG-CoA reductase gene expression in the cell.

Specific Enzymes

Specialized enzymes involved in the transport of cholesterol include LCAT and CETP. ***Lecithin–cholesterol acyltransferase*** **(LCAT)** is an enzyme found in the bloodstream that is activated by HDL apoproteins. LCAT adds a fatty acid to cholesterol, which produces soluble cholesteryl esters such as those in HDL. HDL cholesteryl esters can be distributed to other lipoproteins like IDL, which becomes LDL by acquiring these cholesteryl esters. The **cholesteryl ester transfer protein** **(CETP)** facilitates this transfer process.

MCAT CONCEPT CHECK 11.4

Before you move on, assess your understanding of the material with these questions.

1. Under what conditions is HMG-CoA reductase most active? In what cellular region does it exist?

____

____

____

2. What proteins are specific to the formation and transmission of cholesteryl esters, and what are their functions?

____

____

11.5 Fatty Acids and Triacylglycerols

LEARNING OBJECTIVES

After Chapter 11.5, you will be able to:

- Recall and sequence the five steps in the addition of acetyl-CoA to a growing fatty acid chain
- Differentiate β-oxidation of unsaturated fatty acids from that of saturated fatty acids
- Identify the cellular locations involved in fatty acid synthesis and modification
- Name fatty acids and predict their structure based on their nomenclature:

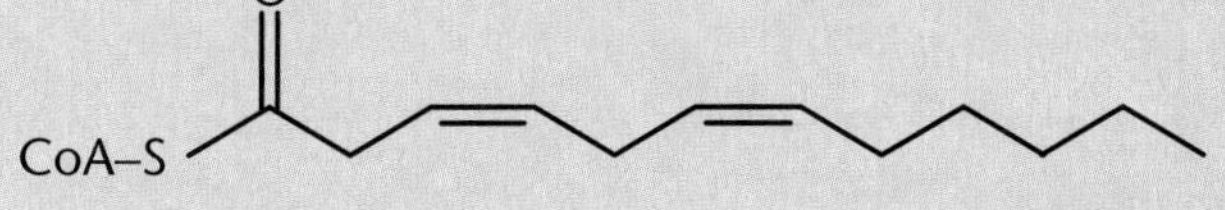

Fatty acids are long-chain carboxylic acids. The carboxyl carbon is carbon 1, and carbon 2 is referred to as the ***α-carbon***. Fatty acids found within the body occur as salts that are capable of forming micelles or are esterified to other compounds, such as the membrane lipids discussed in Chapter 8 of *MCAT Biochemistry Review*.

Nomenclature

REAL WORLD

Trans double bonds are uncommon in natural fatty acids; they predominate in fatty acids found in margarine and other foods that use partial hydrogenation of vegetable oils in their preparation. Compared with liquid oils, these partially hydrogenated fatty acids are solids at room temperature. These fatty acids contribute to arterial diseases and decreased membrane fluidity.

When describing a fatty acid, the total number of carbons is given along with the number of double bonds, written as *carbons:double bonds*. Further description can be given by indicating the position and isomerism of the double bonds in an unsaturated fatty acid. **Saturated fatty acids** have no double bonds while **unsaturated fatty acids** have one or more double bonds. Humans can synthesize only a few of the unsaturated fatty acids; the rest come from essential fatty acids found in the diet that are transported in chylomicrons as triacylglycerols from the intestine. Two important essential fatty acids are ***α-linolenic acid*** and ***linoleic acid***. These polyunsaturated fatty acids, as well as other acids formed from them, are important in maintaining cell membrane fluidity, which is critical for proper functioning of the cell. The **omega (ω) numbering system** is also used for unsaturated fatty acids. The ω designation describes the position of the last double bond relative to the end of the chain and identifies the major precursor fatty acid. For example, linoleic acid (18:2 *cis*,*cis*-9,12) is the precursor of the ω-6 family, which includes *arachidonic acid*. α-Linolenic acid (18:3 all-*cis*-9,12,15) is the primary precursor of the ω-3 family. Double bonds in natural fatty acids are generally in the *cis* configuration.

Synthesis

Fatty acids used by the body for fuel are supplied primarily by the diet. In addition, excess carbohydrate and protein acquired from the diet can be converted to fatty acids and stored as energy reserves in the form of triacylglycerols. Lipid and carbohydrate synthesis are often called **nontemplate synthesis** processes because they do not rely directly on the coding of a nucleic acid, unlike protein and nucleic acid synthesis.

Fatty Acid Biosynthesis

Fatty acid biosynthesis, shown in Figure 11.5, occurs in the liver and its products are subsequently transported to adipose tissue for storage. Adipose tissue can also synthesize smaller quantities of fatty acids. Both of the major enzymes of fatty acid synthesis, *acetyl-CoA carboxylase* and *fatty acid synthase*, are also stimulated by insulin. ***Palmitic acid*** (***palmitate***) is the primary end product of fatty acid synthesis.

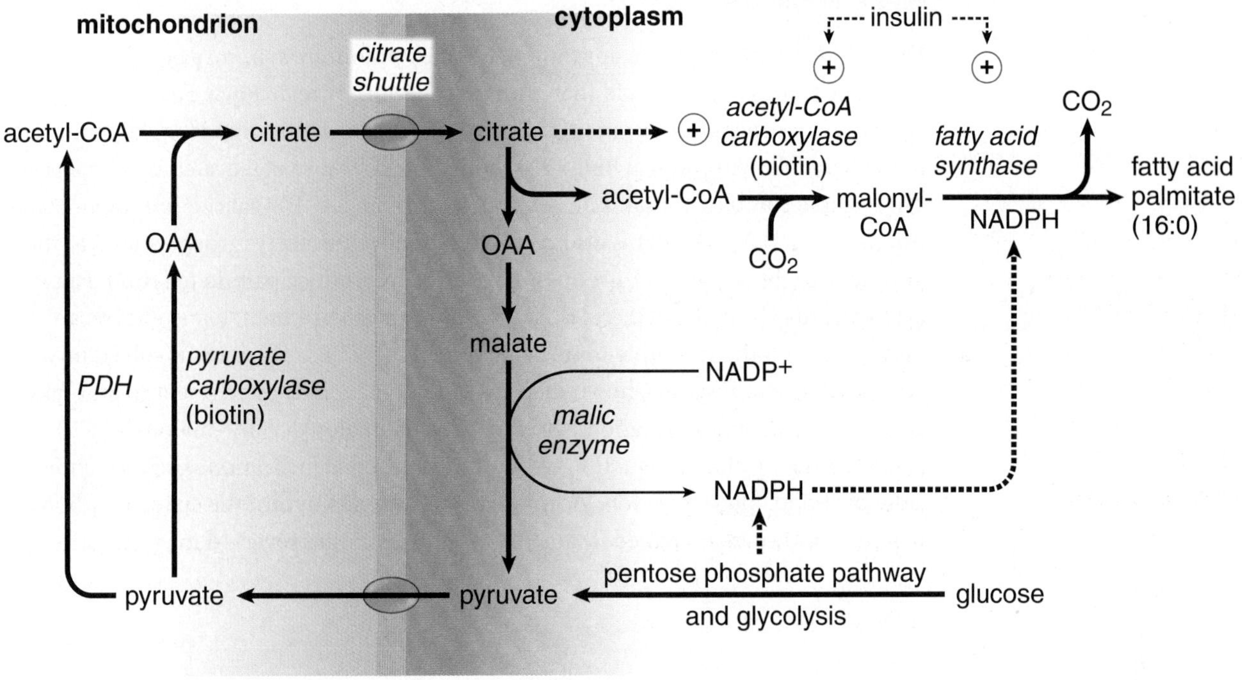

Figure 11.5 Fatty Acid Synthesis from Glucose

Acetyl-CoA Shuttling

Following a large meal, acetyl-CoA accumulates in the mitochondrial matrix and needs to be moved to the cytosol for fatty acid biosynthesis. Acetyl-CoA is the product of the ***pyruvate dehydrogenase complex***, and it couples with *oxaloacetate* to form *citrate* at the beginning of the citric acid cycle. Remember that *isocitrate dehydrogenase* is the rate-limiting enzyme of citric acid cycle; as the cell becomes energetically satisfied, it slows the citric acid cycle, which causes citrate accumulation. Citrate can then diffuse across the mitochondrial membrane. In the cytosol, ***citrate lyase*** splits citrate back into acetyl-CoA and oxaloacetate. The oxaloacetate can then return to the mitochondrion to continue moving acetyl-CoA.

Acetyl-CoA Carboxylase

Acetyl-CoA is activated in the cytoplasm for incorporation into fatty acids by acetyl-CoA carboxylase, the rate-limiting enzyme of fatty acid biosynthesis. **Acetyl-CoA carboxylase** requires biotin and ATP to function, and adds CO_2 to acetyl-CoA to form *malonyl-CoA*. The enzyme is activated by insulin and citrate. The CO_2 added to form malonyl-CoA is never actually incorporated into the fatty acid because it is removed by fatty acid synthase during addition of the activated acetyl group to the fatty acid.

Fatty Acid Synthase

Fatty acid synthase is more appropriately called ***palmitate synthase*** because palmitate is the only fatty acid that humans can synthesize *de novo*. Fatty acid synthase is a large multienzyme complex found in the cytosol that is rapidly induced in the liver following a meal high in carbohydrates because of elevated insulin levels. The enzyme complex contains an acyl carrier protein (ACP) that requires *pantothenic acid* (vitamin B_5). NADPH is also required to reduce the acetyl groups added to the fatty acid. Eight acetyl-CoA groups are required to produce palmitate (16:0). Fatty acyl-CoA may be elongated and desaturated, to a limited extent, using enzymes associated with the smooth endoplasmic reticulum (SER). The steps involved in fatty acid biosynthesis are shown in Figure 11.6 and include attachment to an acyl carrier protein, bond formation between activated malonyl-CoA (malonyl-ACP) and the growing chain, reduction of a carbonyl group, dehydration, and reduction of a double bond. These reactions occur over and over again until the sixteen-carbon palmitate molecule is created. Many of these reactions are reversed in β-oxidation.

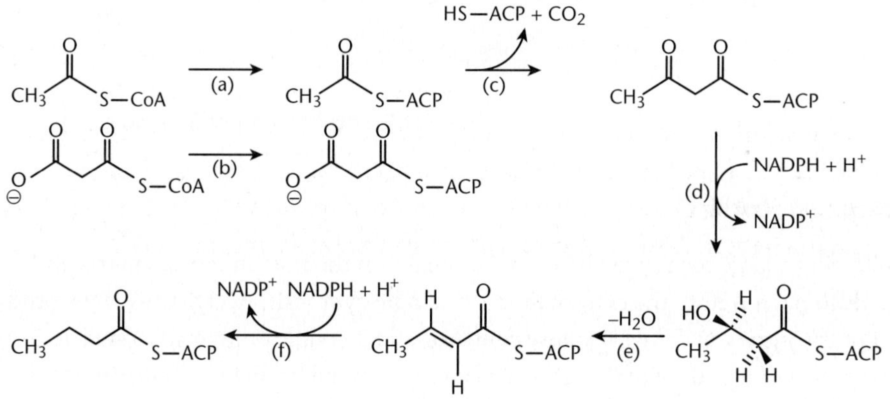

Figure 11.6 Action of Fatty Acid Synthase

Reactions include activation of the growing chain (a) and malonyl-CoA (b) with ACP, bond formation between these activated molecules (c), reduction of a carbonyl to a hydroxyl group (d), dehydration (e), and reduction to a saturated fatty acid (f).

KEY CONCEPT

Fatty acid synthesis and β-oxidation are reverse processes. Both involve transport across the mitochondrial membrane, followed by a series of redox reactions, but always in the opposite direction of one another. Understanding one process will enable you to answer questions about both pathways.

Triacylglycerol (Triglyceride) Synthesis

Triacylglycerols, the storage form of fatty acids, are formed by attaching three fatty acids (as fatty acyl-CoA) to glycerol. Triacylglycerol formation from fatty acids and *glycerol 3-phosphate* occurs primarily in the liver and somewhat in adipose tissue, with a small contribution directly from the diet, as well. In the liver, triacylglycerols are packaged and sent to adipose tissue as very-low-density lipoproteins (VLDL), leaving only a small amount of stored triacylglycerols.

Oxidation

Most fatty acid catabolism proceeds via **β-oxidation** that occurs in the mitochondria; however, peroxisomal β-oxidation also occurs. Branched-chain fatty acids may also undergo α-oxidation, depending on the branch points, while ω-oxidation in the endoplasmic reticulum produces dicarboxylic acids. You should be aware that these processes exist; however, the mechanisms are beyond the scope of the MCAT. We will take an in-depth look at β-oxidation, which will be much more heavily tested. Insulin indirectly inhibits β-oxidation while glucagon stimulates this process.

Activation

When fatty acids are metabolized, they first become activated by attachment to CoA, which is catalyzed by ***fatty-acyl-CoA synthetase***. The product is generically referred to as a fatty acyl-CoA or acyl-CoA. Specific examples would be acetyl-CoA containing a 2-carbon acyl group, or palmitoyl-CoA with a 16-carbon acyl group.

Fatty Acid Entry into Mitochondria

Short-chain fatty acids (2 to 4 carbons) and medium-chain fatty acids (6 to 12 carbons) diffuse freely into mitochondria, where they are oxidized. In contrast, while long-chain fatty acids (14 to 20 carbons) are also oxidized in the mitochondria, they require transport via a carnitine shuttle, as shown in Figure 11.7. ***Carnitine acyltransferase I*** is the rate-limiting enzyme of fatty acid oxidation. Very long chain fatty acids (over 20 carbons) are oxidized elsewhere in the cell.

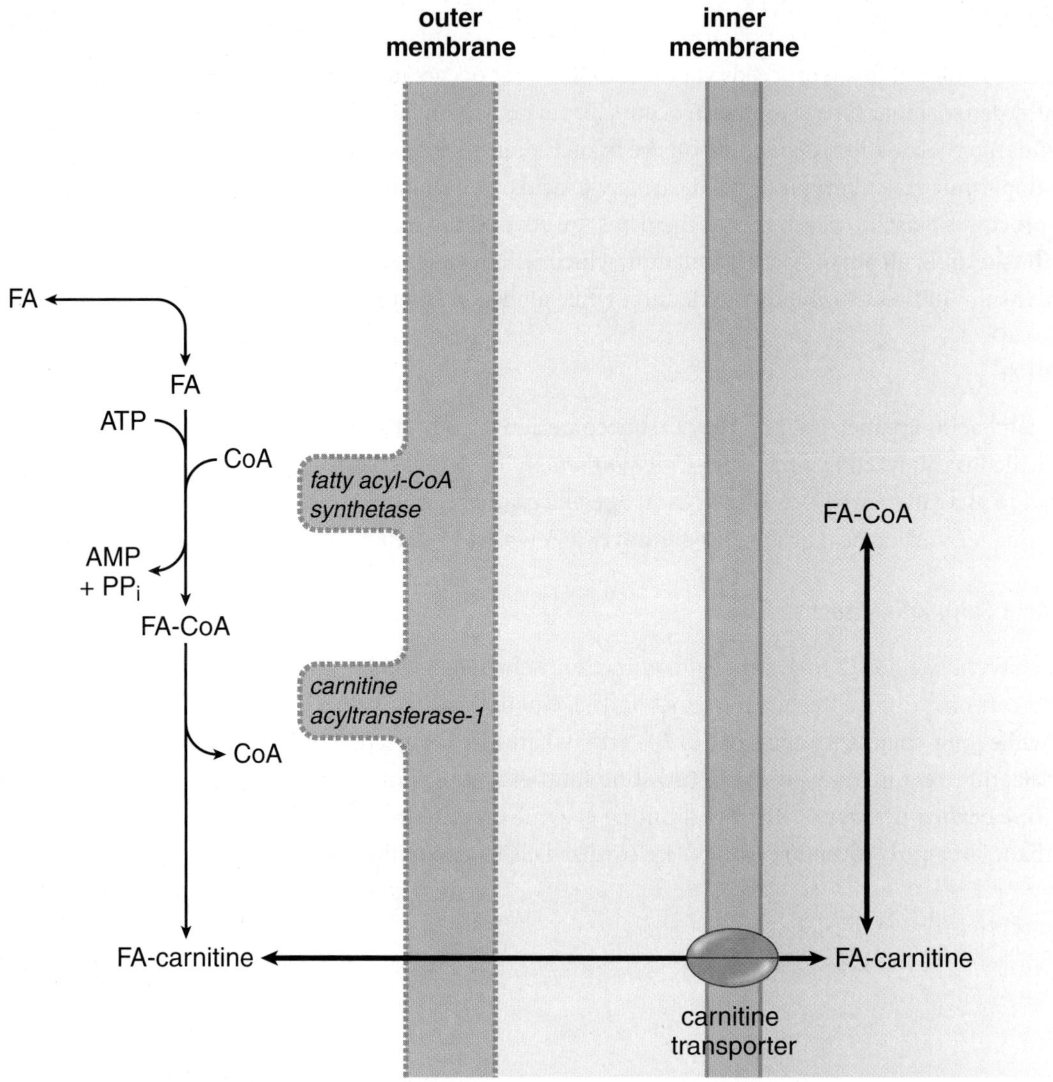

Figure 11.7 Fatty Acid Activation and Transport

β-Oxidation in Mitochondria

β-Oxidation reverses the process of fatty acid synthesis by oxidizing and releasing (rather than reducing and linking) molecules of acetyl-CoA. The pathway is a repetition of four steps; each four-step cycle releases one acetyl-CoA and reduces NAD^+ and FAD (producing NADH and $FADH_2$). The $FADH_2$ and NADH are oxidized in the electron transport chain, producing ATP. In muscle and adipose tissue, acetyl-CoA enters the citric acid cycle. In the liver, acetyl-CoA, which cannot be converted to glucose, stimulates gluconeogenesis by activating *pyruvate carboxylase*. In a fasting state, the liver produces more acetyl-CoA from β-oxidation than is used in the citric acid cycle. Much of the acetyl-CoA is used to synthesize ketone bodies (essentially two acetyl-CoA molecules linked together) that are released into the bloodstream and transported to other tissues.

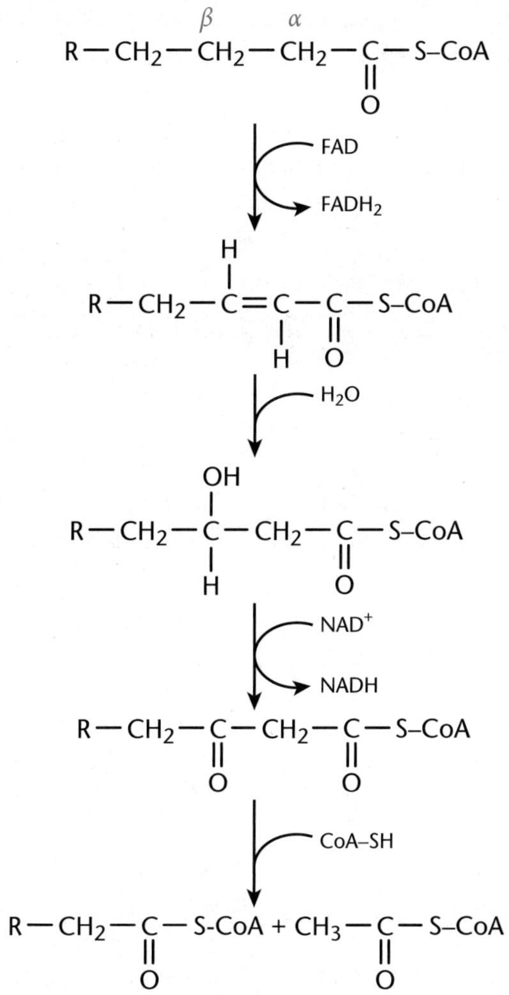

Figure 11.8 β-Oxidation

The four steps of β-oxidation, illustrated in Figure 11.8, are:

1. Oxidation of the fatty acid to form a double bond
2. Hydration of the double bond to form a hydroxyl group
3. Oxidation of the hydroxyl group to form a carbonyl (β-ketoacid)
4. Splitting of the β-ketoacid into a shorter acyl-CoA and acetyl-CoA

This process then continues until the chain has been shortened to two carbons, creating a final acetyl-CoA.

Fatty acids with an odd number of carbon atoms undergo β-oxidation in the same manner as even-numbered carbon fatty acids for the most part. The only difference is observed during the final cycle, where even-numbered fatty acids for the most part yield two acetyl-CoA molecules (from the four-carbon remaining fragment) and odd-numbered fatty acids yield one acetyl-CoA and one *propionyl-CoA* (from the five-carbon remaining fragment), as shown in Figure 11.9. Propionyl-CoA is converted to *methylmalonyl-CoA* by ***propionyl-CoA carboxylase***, which requires biotin (vitamin B_7). Methylmalonyl-CoA is then converted into *succinyl-CoA* by ***methylmalonyl-CoA mutase***, which requires cobalamin (vitamin B_{12}). Succinyl-CoA is a citric acid cycle intermediate and can also be converted to malate to enter the gluconeogenic pathway in the cytosol. Odd-carbon fatty acids thus represent an exception to the rule that fatty acids cannot be converted to glucose in humans.

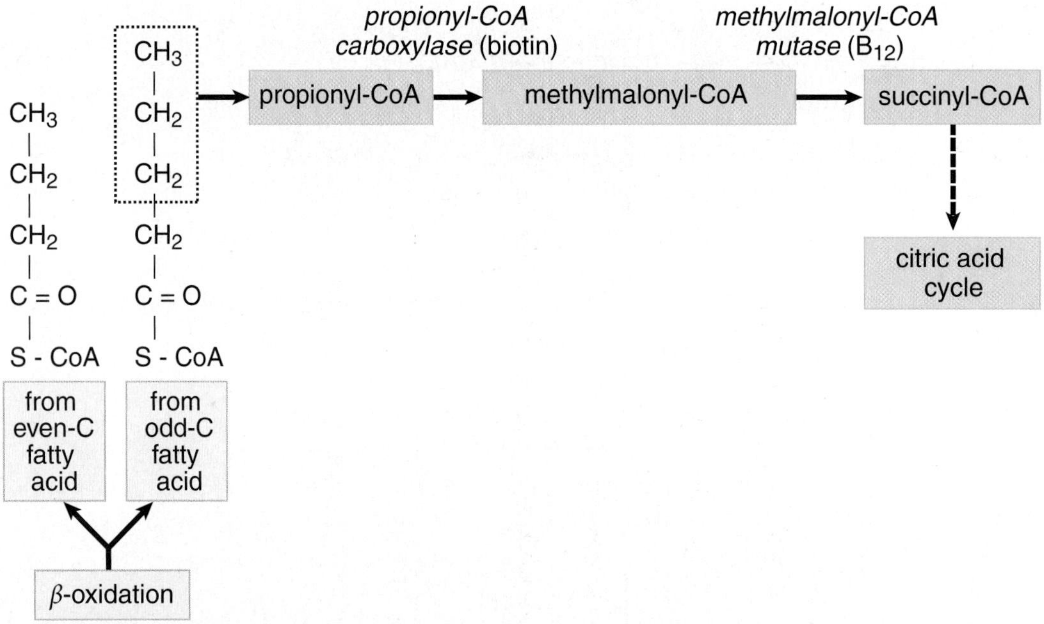

Figure 11.9 The Propionic Acid Pathway

Until now we've been discussing the oxidation of saturated fatty acids. In unsaturated fatty acids, two additional enzymes are necessary because double bonds can disturb the stereochemistry needed for oxidative enzymes to act on the fatty acid. To function, these enzymes can have at most one double bond in their active site; this bond must be located between carbons 2 and 3. ***Enoyl-CoA isomerase***, shown in Figure 11.10, rearranges *cis* double bonds at the 3,4 position to *trans* double bonds at the 2,3 position once enough acetyl-CoA has been liberated to isolate the double bond within the first three carbons. In monounsaturated fatty acids this single step permits β-oxidation to proceed.

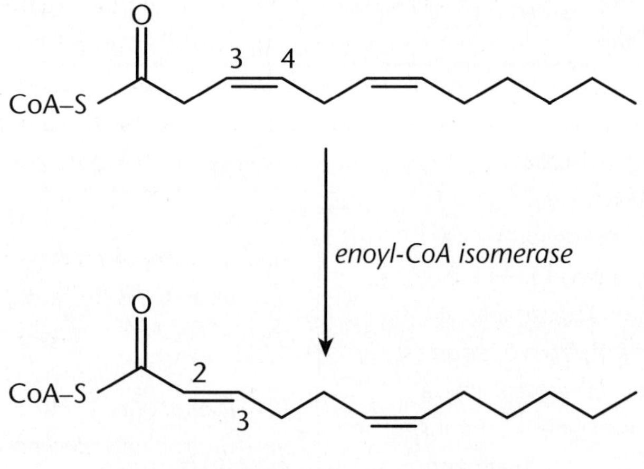

Figure 11.10 Reaction of Enoyl-CoA Isomerase

In polyunsaturated fatty acids, a further reduction is required using ***2,4-dienoyl-CoA reductase*** to convert two conjugated double bonds to just one double bond at the 3,4 position, where it will then undergo the same rearrangement as monounsaturated fatty acids (as shown in Figure 11.11) to form a *trans* 2,3 double bond.

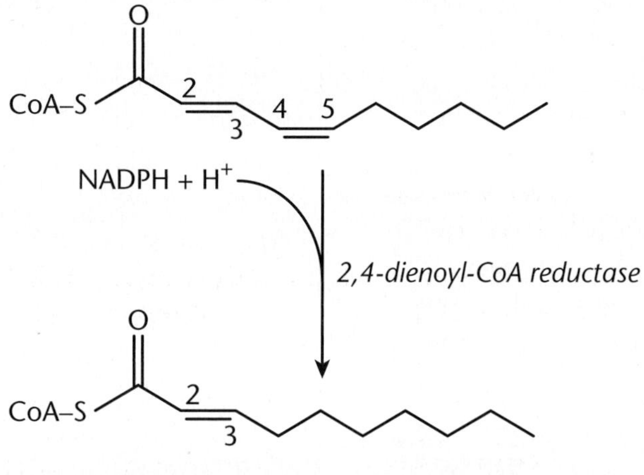

Figure 11.11 Reaction of 2,4-Dienoyl-CoA Reductase

BIOCHEMISTRY GUIDED EXAMPLE WITH EXPERT THINKING

Propionic acidemia (PA) is a life-threatening disease caused by the deficiency of a mitochondrial biotin-dependent enzyme known as propionyl coenzyme-A carboxylase (PCC). This enzyme is responsible for degrading the metabolic intermediate propionyl coenzyme-A (PP-CoA) to create methylmalonyl-CoA (MM-CoA). PP-CoA is commonly found as the end product to β-oxidation of fatty acid chains with an odd number of carbons. PP-CoA is also a metabolic intermediate arising from the normal turnover of several essential amino acids. The native PCC holoenzyme is composed of six α (PCCA) and six β (PCCB) subunits. Both types of subunits must be functional for the enzyme to be operative. Deficiency in either or both PCC subunits and the consequent accumulation of PP-CoA leads to the pathogenesis of PA.

Topic: PA is a disease caused by malfunction of enzyme PCC

Lots of details here describing how important PCC is to metabolism

Detail about PCC structure: 6 α and 6 β; need both subunits to work

Enzyme replacement therapy is an approach that aims to restore the activity of an enzyme in cases of deficiency or abnormal production. To overcome the challenge of delivery and targeting proteins to the mitochondria of living cells, two groups of peptide fusions called twin-arginine translocation (TAT) and mitochondrial targeting sequences (MTS) were employed. Purified constructs of subunit alone, TAT-MTS fusions with PCCA or PCCB, or TAT fusions with PCCA or PCCB were incubated for various time periods with PCCA- and PCCB-defective whole cell lymphocytes. The lymphocytes endogenously express the non-defective PCC subunit. Mitochondria were subsequently isolated, lysed, and the reactions were terminated by the addition of trichloroacetic acid. Levels of MM-CoA were assayed using ultra performance liquid chromatography tandem mass spectrometry (UPLC-MS/MS). Normal and PCCA- or PCCB-deficient (def) cells were included as controls. The results are plotted in Figures 1 and 2 below.

Experimental technique used in passage tries to restore activity of deficient PCC

Issue: difficult to target externally produced proteins to mitochondria

Solution: CPP and MTS are fused to protein of interest to get them into mitochondria

Constructs with different combination of PCC subunit and peptide fusions

Assayed levels of MM-CoA as a measure of PCC activity

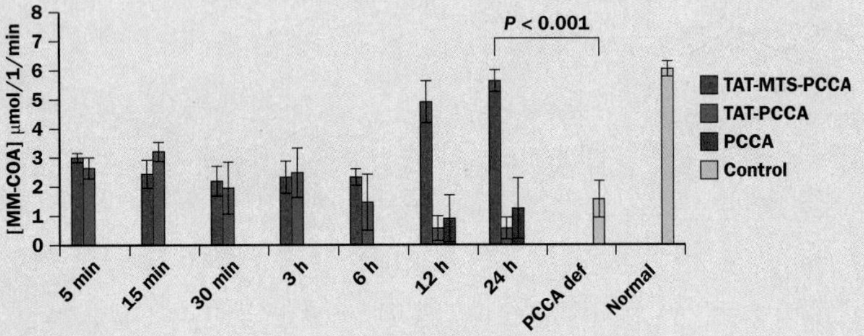

Figure 1

IVs: time assayed, type of construct

DV: levels of MM-CoA

Trend: significant difference in MM-CoA levels 24 hours after TAT-MTS-PCCA added compared to absence of PCCA

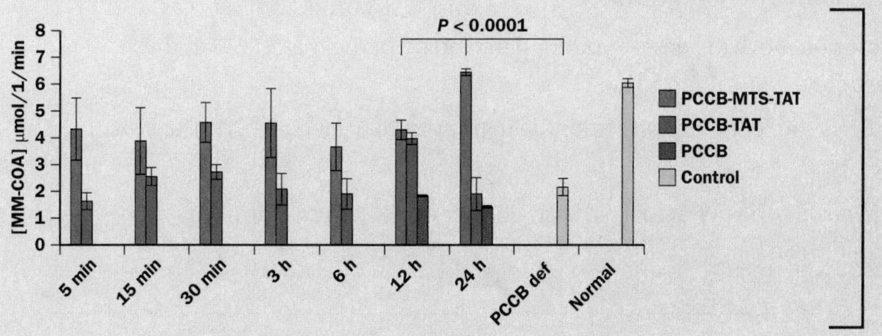

IVs: time assayed, type of construct

DV: levels of MM-CoA

Trend: significant difference in MM-CoA levels 12 and 24 hours after PCCB-MTS-TAT added compared to absence of PCCB

Figure 2

Adapted from Darvish-Damavandi, M., Ho, H.K., & Kang, T.S. (2016) Towards the development of an enzyme replacement therapy for the metabolic disorder propionic acidemia. *Molecular Genetics and Metabolism Reports*, 8, 51-60. doi:10.1016/j.ymgmr.2016.06.009.

According to the data, are MTS-TAT-PCC constructs able to successfully rescue PCC activity in deficient mitochondria?

This question begins with "according to the data", meaning it will require us to understand and analyze the data presented in the context of the experiment described in the passage. Given we have multiple, complex figures, it's important to get some context on the experiments and what the data represent first. The researchers are exploring treatment options for a disease caused by deficient PCC, which is an important metabolic enzyme in the mitochondria. We're told that PCC requires both types of subunits in order to function properly. Common methods of restoring protein activity in cells are at the transcriptional/translational level within the cell, but the method employed in this study produces the required protein outside of the cell, then adds the protein back into the cell. We should know from our content background that proteins are generally polar, so the challenge is getting the protein past the lipid bilayers of both the cellular and the mitochondrial membranes. The researcher's solution to this problem is to fuse PCC subunits to peptides that not only get PCC through the membranes, but also target the mitochondria. Also, note that the cell lines still express the non-deficient subunit: the cell lines in Figure 1 still express functional PCCB, so PCCA must be added and delivered to the mitochondria for there to be PCC activity; the opposite is true for the cell lines in Figure 2.

Diving into the data, the experimental layout and the results are similar for both PCCA and PCCB fusions. When the PCC-subunit is fused to TAT alone, or in the absence of fusion, the levels of MM-CoA are similar. However, when the PCC-subunit is fused to both MTS and TAT, we see significantly higher levels of MM-CoA. The first paragraph tells us that PCC will catalyze PP-CoA to produce MM-CoA, the product being measured in the experiment, so high levels of MM-CoA correlate to PCC activity.

Therefore, these results indicate that PCC activity can be rescued by exogenously expressing PCC-subunits and fusing them to both mitochondrial-targeting and cell-permeating proteins.

MCAT CONCEPT CHECK 11.5

Before you move on, assess your understanding of the material with these questions.

1. Draw the following fatty acids: palmitic acid, 18:3 (all-*cis*-9,12,15), an ω-6.

2. What are the five steps in the addition of acetyl-CoA to a growing fatty acid chain?

   1. ______________________________
   2. ______________________________
   3. ______________________________
   4. ______________________________
   5. ______________________________

3. How does β-oxidation of unsaturated fatty acids differ from that of saturated fatty acids?

   ____

4. True or False: Fatty acids are synthesized in the cytoplasm and modified by enzymes in the smooth endoplasmic reticulum.

11.6 Ketone Bodies

LEARNING OBJECTIVES

After Chapter 11.6, you will be able to:

- Predict when fatty acids would be used to create ketone bodies rather than glucose
- Recall the conditions that favor ketogenesis and ketolysis

KEY CONCEPT

Ketone bodies are essentially transportable forms of acetyl-CoA. They are produced by the liver and used by other tissues during prolonged starvation.

In the fasting state, the liver converts excess acetyl-CoA from β-oxidation of fatty acids into the **ketone bodies** ***acetoacetate*** and ***3-hydroxybutyrate*** (***β-hydroxybutyrate***), which can be used for energy in various tissues. Cardiac and skeletal muscle and the renal cortex can metabolize acetoacetate and 3-hydroxybutyrate to acetyl-CoA. During fasting periods, muscle will metabolize ketones as rapidly as the liver releases them, preventing accumulation in the bloodstream. After a week of fasting, ketones reach a concentration in the blood that is high enough for the brain to begin metabolizing them. The processes of ketogenesis and ketolysis are shown in Figure 11.12.

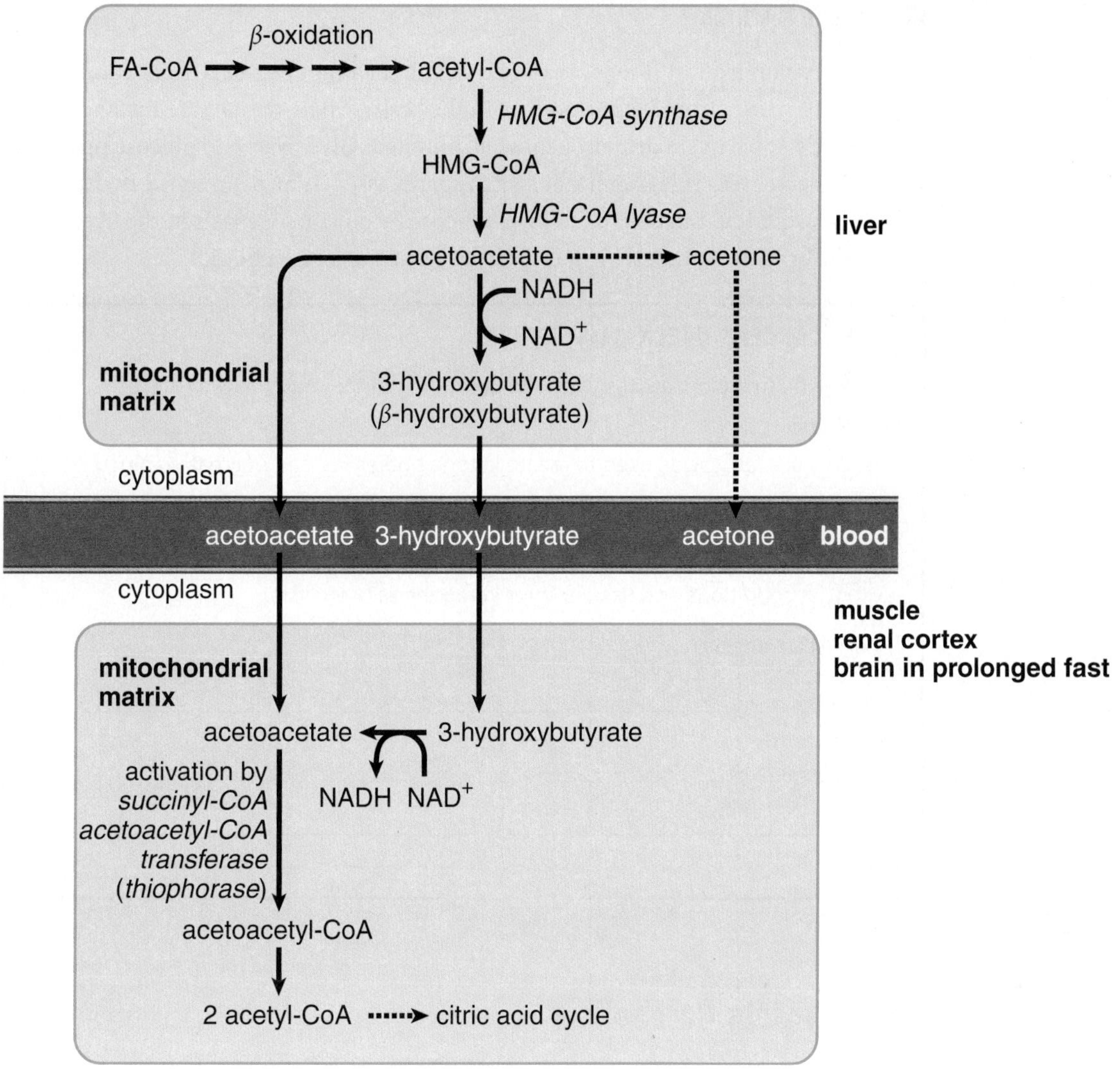

Figure 11.12 Ketogenesis and Ketolysis

Ketogenesis

Ketogenesis occurs in the mitochondria of liver cells when excess acetyl-CoA accumulates in the fasting state. ***HMG-CoA synthase*** forms HMG-CoA, and ***HMG-CoA lyase*** breaks down HMG-CoA into acetoacetate, which can subsequently be reduced to 3-hydroxybutyrate. Acetone is a minor side product that is formed but will not be used as energy for tissues.

Ketolysis

Acetoacetate picked up from the blood is activated in the mitochondria by ***succinyl-CoA acetoacetyl-CoA transferase*** (commonly called ***thiophorase***), an enzyme present only in tissues outside the liver. During this reaction, acetoacetate is oxidized to acetoacetyl-CoA. The liver lacks this enzyme, so it cannot catabolize the ketone bodies that it produces.

REAL WORLD

A significant increase in ketone levels in the blood can lead to ketoacidosis, a potentially dangerous medical condition. This occurs most often with fatty acid breakdown in type 1 (insulin-dependent) diabetes mellitus.

Ketolysis in the Brain

During a prolonged fast (longer than one week), the brain begins to derive up to two-thirds of its energy from ketone bodies. In the brain, when ketones are metabolized to acetyl-CoA, pyruvate dehydrogenase is inhibited. Glycolysis and glucose uptake in the brain decreases. This important switch spares essential protein in the body, which otherwise would be catabolized to form glucose by gluconeogenesis in the liver, and allows the brain to indirectly metabolize fatty acids as ketone bodies.

MCAT CONCEPT CHECK 11.6

Before you move on, assess your understanding of the material with these questions.

1. Why are fatty acids used to create ketone bodies instead of creating glucose?

___

2. What conditions and tissues favor ketogenesis? Ketolysis?
   - Ketogenesis:

   ___

   - Ketolysis:

   ___

11.7 Protein Catabolism

LEARNING OBJECTIVES

After Chapter 11.7, you will be able to:

- Identify common sources for acetyl-CoA used in lipid synthesis
- Recall the location(s) associated with large amounts of protein digestion
- Predict what will happen to the carbon skeleton, amino groups, and side chains of proteins that have been broken down

KEY CONCEPT

Metabolism is directed toward conserving tissues to the greatest extent possible, especially the brain and heart. Digestion of protein compromises muscle—potentially that of the heart—so it is unlikely to occur under normal conditions.

Protein is very rarely used as an energy source because it is so important for other functions; routinely breaking down protein would result in serious illness. However, under conditions of extreme energy deprivation, proteins can be used for energy. In order to provide a reservoir of amino acids for protein building by the cell, proteins must be digested and absorbed.

Proteolysis (the breakdown of proteins) begins in the stomach with ***pepsin*** and continues with the pancreatic proteases ***trypsin***, ***chymotrypsin***, and ***carboxypeptidases A*** and ***B***, all of which are secreted as zymogens. Protein digestion is completed by the small intestinal brush-border enzymes ***dipeptidase*** and ***aminopeptidase***. The main end products of protein digestion are amino acids, dipeptides, and tripeptides. Absorption of amino acids and small peptides through the luminal membrane is accomplished by secondary active transport linked to sodium. At the basal membrane, simple and facilitated diffusion transports amino acids into the bloodstream. Figure 11.13 illustrates the major transport mechanisms involved in moving amino acids across the luminal and basal membranes of intestinal cells.

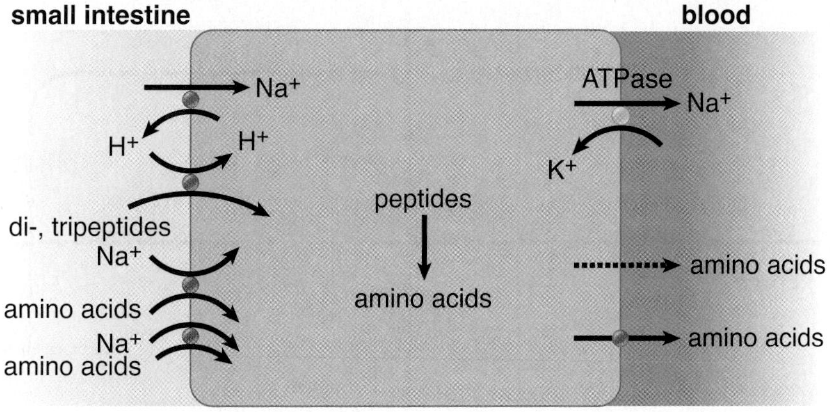

Figure 11.13 Absorption of Amino Acids and Peptides in the Intestine

Protein obtained from the diet or from the body (during prolonged fasting or starvation) may be used as an energy source. Body protein is catabolized primarily in muscle and liver. Amino acids released from proteins usually lose their amino group through **transamination** or **deamination**. The remaining carbon skeleton can be used for energy. Amino acids are classified by their ability to turn into specific metabolic intermediates: **glucogenic** amino acids (all but leucine and lysine) can be converted into glucose through gluconeogenesis; **ketogenic** amino acids (leucine and lysine, as well as isoleucine, phenylalanine, threonine, tryptophan, and tyrosine, which are also glucogenic as well) can be converted into acetyl-CoA and ketone bodies.

The amino groups removed by transamination or deamination constitute a potential toxin to the body in the form of ammonia, and must be excreted safely. The **urea cycle**, shown in Figure 11.14, occurs in the liver and is the body's primary way of removing excess nitrogen from the body. The MCAT is highly unlikely to test on the steps and intermediates of the urea cycle directly, but it is provided here as a point of reference.

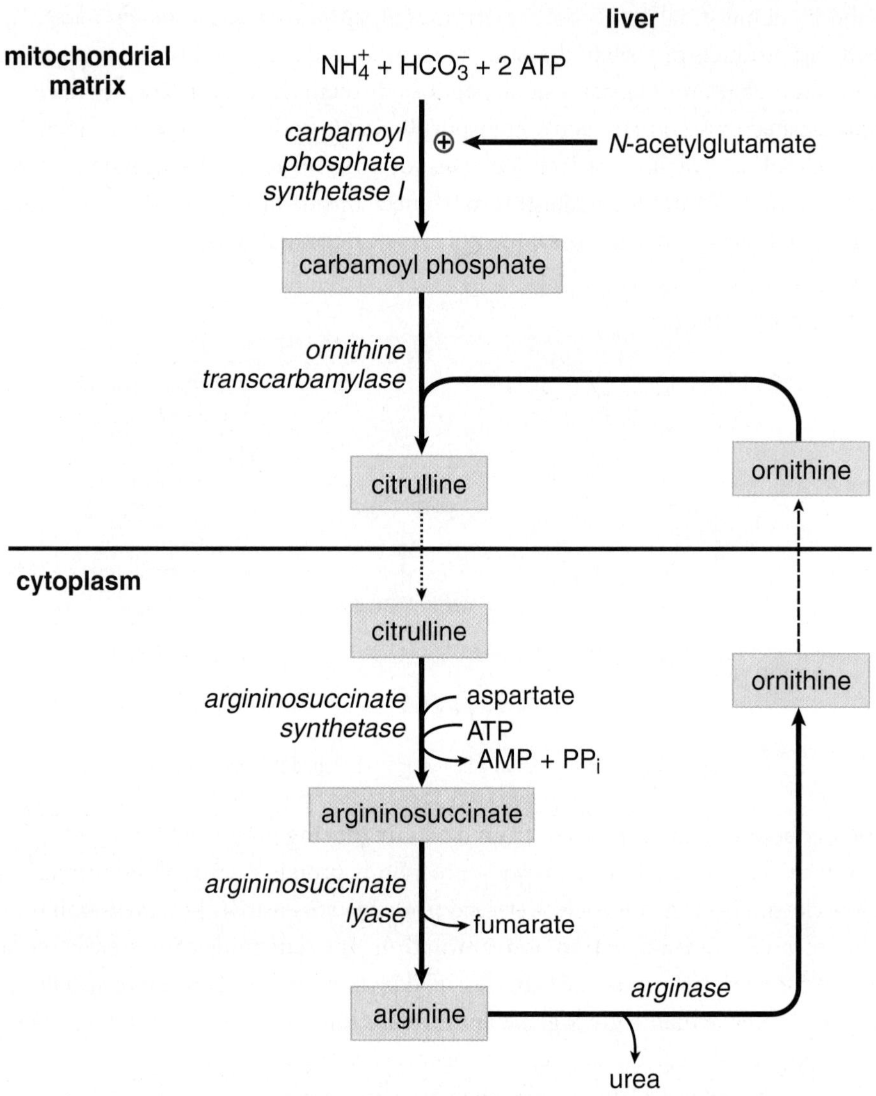

Figure 11.14 The Urea Cycle

The fate of the side chain from each amino acid depends on its chemistry. Basic amino acid side chains feed into the urea cycle, while the other side chains act like the carbon skeleton and produce energy through gluconeogenesis or ketone production.

MCAT CONCEPT CHECK 11.7

Before you move on, assess your understanding of the material with these questions.

1. True or False: Bodily proteins will commonly be broken down to provide acetyl-CoA for lipid synthesis.

2. Where does the bulk of protein digestion occur?

___

3. During protein processing, what is the eventual fate of each of the following components: carbon skeleton, amino group, and side chains?
   - Carbon skeleton:

___

   - Amino group:

___

   - Side chains:

___

Conclusion

At this point, we have examined all of the vital metabolic processes of the cell. In this chapter, we reviewed dietary lipids and different ways that lipids are metabolized in the cell. We also covered lipid transport in blood and lymphatic fluid and the mobilization of lipids from adipocytes. In addition, we went over the structure, synthesis, and breakdown of fatty acids required to address the energy needs of the cell. The importance of ketone bodies and how they are utilized by the cell during periods of starvation were also reviewed. Finally, we went over digestion and metabolism of proteins and amino acids.

Metabolism of the different macromolecules does not occur in isolation, as you've already seen: the acetyl-CoA produced in fatty acid oxidation regulates the pyruvate dehydrogenase complex and pyruvate carboxylase to create a shift in carbohydrate metabolism from glycolysis and the citric acid cycle to gluconeogenesis. In the next chapter, we'll dive into how the different pathways fit together and will integrate the metabolic knowledge that you've compiled in Chapters 9, 10, and 11 of *MCAT Biochemistry Review.*

GO ONLINE

You've reviewed the content, now test your knowledge and critical thinking skills by completing a test-like passage set in your online resources!

CONCEPT SUMMARY

Lipid Digestion and Absorption

- Mechanical digestion of lipids occurs primarily in the mouth and stomach.
- Chemical digestion of lipids occurs in the small intestine and is facilitated by **bile**, **pancreatic lipase**, **colipase**, and **cholesterol esterase**.
- Digested lipids may form **micelles** for absorption or be absorbed directly.
- Short-chain fatty acids are absorbed across the intestine into the blood.
- Long-chain fatty acids are absorbed as micelles and assembled into **chylomicrons** for release into the lymphatic system.

Lipid Mobilization

- Lipids are mobilized from adipocytes by **hormone-sensitive lipase**.
- Lipids are mobilized from lipoproteins by **lipoprotein lipase**.

Lipid Transport

- **Chylomicrons** are the transport mechanism for dietary triacylglycerol molecules and are transported via the lymphatic system.
- **VLDL** transports newly synthesized triacylglycerol molecules from the liver to peripheral tissues in the bloodstream.
- **IDL** is a **VLDL remnant** in transition between triacylglycerol and cholesterol transport; it picks up cholesteryl esters from HDL.
- **LDL** primarily transports cholesterol for use by tissues.
- **HDL** is involved in the reverse transport of cholesterol.
- **Apoproteins** control interactions between lipoproteins.

Cholesterol Metabolism

- Cholesterol may be obtained through dietary sources or through *de novo* synthesis in the liver.
- The key enzyme in cholesterol biosynthesis is **HMG-CoA reductase.**
- **LCAT** catalyzes the formation of cholesteryl esters for transport with HDL.
- **CETP** catalyzes the transition of IDL to LDL by transferring cholesteryl esters from HDL.

Fatty Acids and Triacylglycerols

- Fatty acids are carboxylic acids, typically with a single long chain, although they can be branched.
- **Saturated fatty acids** have no double bonds between carbons. **Unsaturated fatty acids** have one or more double bonds.
- Fatty acids are synthesized in the cytoplasm from acetyl-CoA transported out of the mitochondria.
  - Synthesis includes five steps: activation, bond formation, reduction, dehydration, and a second reduction.
  - These steps are repeated eight times to form **palmitic acid**, the only fatty acid that humans can synthesize.
- Fatty acid oxidation occurs in the mitochondria following transport by the carnitine shuttle.
  - **β-Oxidation** uses cycles of oxidation, hydration, oxidation, and cleavage.
  - Branched and unsaturated fatty acids require special enzymes.
  - Unsaturated fatty acids use an **isomerase** and an additional **reductase** during cleavage.

Ketone Bodies

- Ketone bodies form (**ketogenesis**) during a prolonged starvation state due to excess acetyl-CoA in the liver.
- **Ketolysis** regenerates acetyl-CoA for use as an energy source in peripheral tissues.
- The brain can derive up to two-thirds of its energy from ketone bodies during prolonged starvation.

Protein Catabolism

- Protein digestion occurs primarily in the small intestine.
- Catabolism of cellular proteins occurs only under conditions of starvation.
- Carbon skeletons of amino acids are used for energy, either through gluconeogenesis or ketone body formation. Amino groups are fed into the **urea cycle** for excretion. The fate of a side chain depends on its chemistry.

ANSWERS TO CONCEPT CHECKS

11.1

1. Physical digestion is accomplished in the mouth and the stomach, reducing the particle size. Beginning in the small intestine, pancreatic lipase, colipase, cholesterol esterase, and bile assist in the chemical digestion of lipids. In the more distal portion of the small intestine, absorption occurs.
2. False. Small free fatty acids enter the circulation directly.
3. Micelles are collections of lipids with their hydrophobic ends oriented toward the center and their charged ends oriented toward the aqueous environment. Micelles collect lipids within their hydrophobic centers.

11.2

1. An increase in insulin levels will increase lipid storage and decrease lipid mobilization from adipocytes, leading to weight gain in patients who have diabetes and begin insulin injections.
2. The ratio of free fatty acids to glycerol is 3:1. A triacylglycerol molecule is composed of glycerol and three fatty acids.

11.3

1. Free fatty acids remain in the blood, bonded to albumin and other carrier proteins. A much smaller amount will remain unbonded.
2. With respect to protein content, HDL > LDL > IDL > VLDL > chylomicrons. VLDL and chylomicrons are the primary triacylglycerol transporters. HDL and LDL are mostly involved in cholesterol transport.
3. Lipoproteins are synthesized primarily by the intestine and liver.
4. As mentioned in the chapter, HDL is often considered "good" cholesterol because it picks up excess cholesterol from blood vessels for excretion. Because of this crucial role, HDL values are checked for being over a minimum value.

11.4

1. HMG-CoA reductase is most active in the absence of cholesterol and when stimulated by insulin. Cholesterol reduces the activity of HMG-CoA reductase, which is located in the smooth endoplasmic reticulum.
2. LCAT catalyzes the esterification of cholesterol to form cholesteryl esters. CETP promotes the transfer of cholesteryl esters from HDL to IDL, forming LDL.

11.5

1. Palmitic acid (16:0):

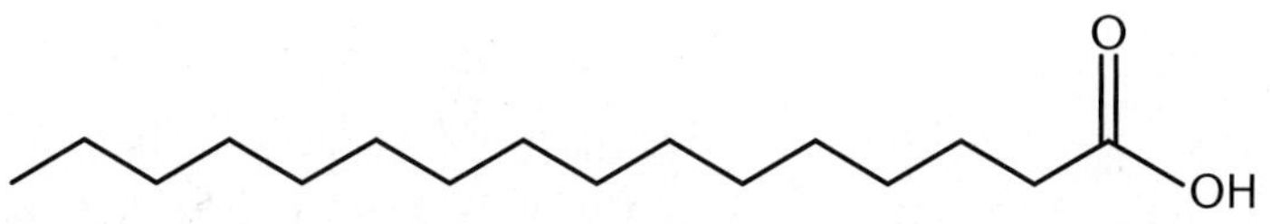

α-Linolenic acid (18:3 all-*cis*-9,12,15), an ω-3 fatty acid:

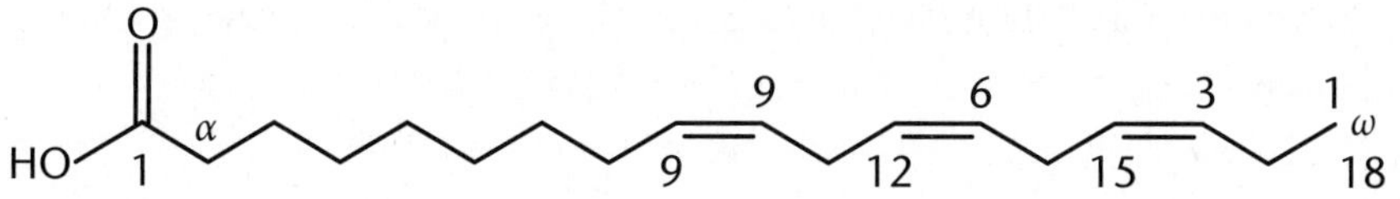

Linoleic acid (18:2 *cis*,*cis*-9,12), an ω-6 fatty acid:

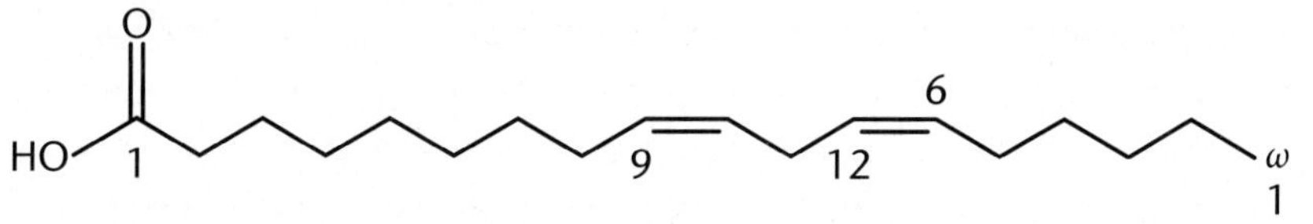

Note: As long as the last double bond is in the same position relative to the end of the chain, many answers are possible for the ω-6 fatty acid.

2. The steps in the attachment of acetyl-CoA to a fatty acid chain are attachment to acyl carrier protein, bond formation between molecules, reduction of a carbonyl group, dehydration, and reduction of a double bond. These steps are shown in Figure 11.6.
3. There is an additional isomerase and an additional reductase for the β-oxidation of unsaturated fatty acids, which provide the stereochemistry necessary for further oxidation.
4. True.

11.6

1. Fatty acid degradation results in large amounts of acetyl-CoA, which cannot enter the gluconeogenic pathway to produce glucose. Only odd-numbered fatty acids can act as a source of carbon for gluconeogenesis; even then, only the final malonyl-CoA molecule can be used. Energy is packaged into ketone bodies for consumption by the brain and muscles.
2. Ketogenesis is favored by a prolonged fast and occurs in the liver. It is stimulated by increasing concentrations of acetyl-CoA. Ketolysis is also favored during a prolonged fast, but is stimulated by a low-energy state in muscle and brain tissues and does not occur in the liver.

11.7

1. False. Proteins are more valuable to the cell than lipids, thus they will not commonly be broken down for lipid synthesis.
2. The bulk of protein digestion occurs in the small intestine.
3. The carbon skeleton is transported to the liver for processing into glucose or ketone bodies. The amino group will feed into the urea cycle for excretion. Side chains are processed depending on their composition. Basic side chains will be processed like amino groups, while other functional groups will be treated like the carbon skeleton.

SCIENCE MASTERY ASSESSMENT EXPLANATIONS

1. **B**

This question asks for the hormone that does not directly regulate the activity of hormone-sensitive lipase (HSL). Hormone sensitive lipase is an enzyme that cleaves fatty acids from their glycerol backbones, releasing these free fatty acids for use in energy production. HSL is directly activated by epinephrine and cortisol, so **(C)** and **(D)** can be eliminated. Regarding insulin vs. glucagon, observe that free fatty acid mobilization, and therefore HSL activity, is generally associated with low blood sugar, which is also associated with elevated glucagon levels. However, glucagon does not directly regulate the activity of HSL. Rather, HSL is activated by a drop in insulin levels. For this reason, insulin does directly regulate HSL activity, and therefore **(A)** can be eliminated. Only glucagon, **(B)**, does not directly influence HSL activity. Therefore **(B)** is the correct answer.

2. **A**

Short-chain fatty acids are soluble in the intestinal lumen, and thus do not interact with micelles as longer fatty acid chains do. The long-chain fatty acids are taken up by the intestinal cells and packaged into triacylglycerols for transport as chylomicrons. Chylomicrons exit the intestine through lacteals that feed into the lymphatic system, which joins with the bloodstream in the base of the neck through the thoracic duct.

3. **C**

During fatty acid mobilization, there is a breakdown of triacylglycerols in adipocytes by hormone-sensitive lipase (HSL). This breakdown results in the release of three fatty acids and a glycerol molecule. The glycerol may be used by the liver for gluconeogenesis, but adipocytes do not have the ability to carry out gluconeogenesis.

4. **B**

Chylomicrons and VLDL are very similar. Both contain apolipoproteins and primarily transport triacylglycerols, eliminating **(A)** and **(C)**. The only major difference between them is the tissue of origin. Chylomicrons transport dietary triacylglycerol and originate in the small intestine, while VLDL transport newly synthesized triacylglycerols and originate in the liver.

5. **D**

While the transport and lipid binding functions of most lipoproteins are independent of the apolipoprotein component, the interaction of these lipoproteins with the environment is controlled almost exclusively by apolipoproteins. Lipoproteins cannot exit or enter cells without apolipoproteins, and are unable to transfer lipids without specialized apolipoproteins or cholesterol-specific enzymes.

6. **A**

Statins are drugs that are prescribed to treat high cholesterol and act as competitive inhibitors of HMG-CoA reductase. HMG-CoA reductase is the rate-limiting enzyme of *de novo* cholesterol synthesis; inhibition of this enzyme lowers production of cholesterol, thus lowering overall levels of cholesterol.

7. **A**

LCAT adds a fatty acid to cholesterol, producing cholesteryl esters, which dissolve in the core of HDL, allowing HDL to transport cholesterol from the periphery to the liver.

8. **B**

Humans can only synthesize one fatty acid, palmitic acid. Palmitic acid is fully saturated and therefore does not contain any double bonds. Palmitic acid has 16 carbons, and is synthesized from eight molecules of acetyl-CoA. In shorthand notation, palmitic acid is written as 16:0 (16 carbons, no double bonds).

9. **C**

The steps in fatty acid synthesis are activation (attachment to acyl carrier protein), bond formation (between malonyl-CoA and the growing fatty acid chain), reduction (of a carboxyl group), dehydration, and reduction (of a double bond).

10. **C**

Ketone bodies are produced in the mitochondria of liver cells as acetyl-CoA accumulates during fasting, consistent with **(C)**. On the other hand, to eliminate **(B)**, observe that while acetyl-CoA is indeed converted to acetoacetate, 3-hydroxybutyrate, or acetone, the acetone that is produced is only a byproduct and is not used for energy, which conflicts with the assertion in **(B)** that "all of which are used for energy." Muscle cells will begin using ketone bodies for energy before the brain. The brain will only start using ketone bodies once they have accumulated to higher concentrations in the blood, eliminating choice **(D)**.

11. **D**

The liver is the major metabolic organ in the body and is responsible for much of the synthesis and interconversion of fuel sources. Most of the triacylglycerols that are synthesized in the liver are transported as VLDL to adipose tissue for storage. Both the adipocytes, **(A)**, and dietary intake, **(B)**, constitute a minor source of triacylglycerols.

12. **C**

In order for the enzymes of fatty acid oxidation to operate, there can be, at most, one double bond in the area of enzyme activity, and it must be oriented between carbons 2 and 3. In order to accomplish this in monounsaturated fatty acids, an isomerase is employed. When there are multiple double bonds that fall within the enzymatic binding site, both an isomerase and 2,4-dienoyl-CoA reductase are required for the oxidative enzymes to act on the fatty acid. For this question, simply recognizing that *dienoyl* refers to having multiple double bonds is sufficient to arrive at the answer.

13. **C**

Ketolysis is the breakdown of ketone bodies to acetyl-CoA for energy. This process occurs in the brain and muscle tissues, but cannot occur in the liver, which lacks an enzyme necessary for ketone body breakdown. Ketolysis is not associated with an increase in glucose metabolism because it most often occurs under conditions of starvation.

14. **D**

The energy contribution of an amino acid depends on its ability to be turned into glucose through gluconeogenesis (glucogenic amino acids), ketone bodies (ketogenic amino acids), or both. All of the amino acids listed in the answer choices are glucogenic; isoleucine is also ketogenic. The energy acquired from an amino acid will also depend on the number of carbons it can donate to these energy-creating processes, which depends on the size of its side chain. Isoleucine has the largest side chain of the answer choices, and will thus contribute the most energy per molecule.

15. **A**

The degradation of protein and processing by the liver implies a prolonged starvation state; protein will not be used for energy unless absolutely necessary. Thus, gluconeogenesis is the most likely process. When gluconeogenesis is not possible, easily metabolized molecules, such as ketone bodies, are synthesized. Fatty acid production occurs when energy is being stored; proteins would not be broken down to store energy in fatty acids.

Consult your online resources for additional practice. GO ONLINE

SHARED CONCEPTS

Biochemistry Chapter 1
Amino Acids, Peptides, and Proteins

Biochemistry Chapter 5
Lipid Structure and Function

Biochemistry Chapter 8
Biological Membranes

Biochemistry Chapter 12
Bioenergetics and Regulation of Metabolism

Biology Chapter 9
The Digestive System

Biology Chapter 10
Homeostasis

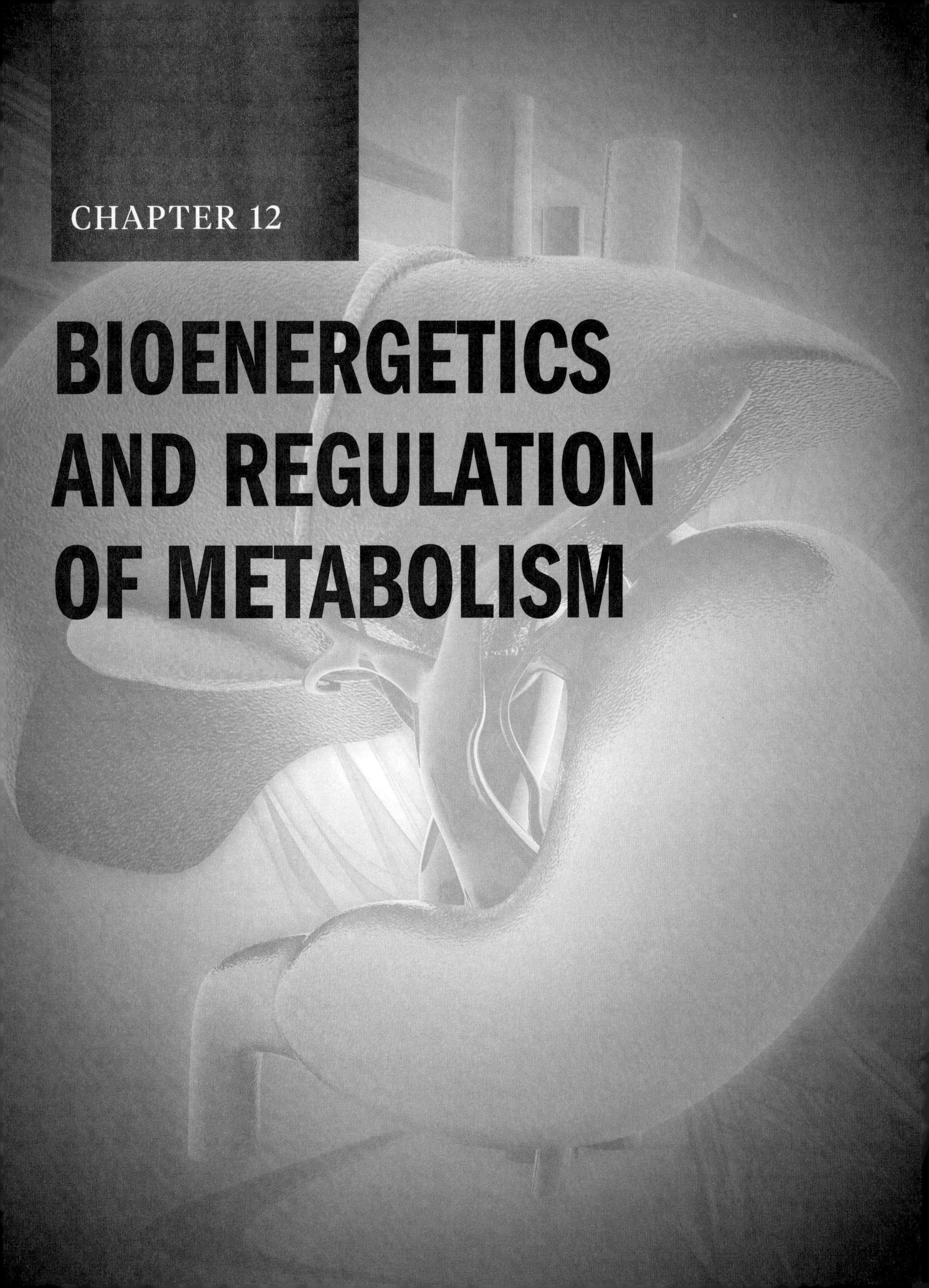

CHAPTER 12

BIOENERGETICS AND REGULATION OF METABOLISM

SCIENCE MASTERY ASSESSMENT

Every pre-med knows this feeling: there is so much content I have to know for the MCAT! How do I know what to do first or what's important?

While the high-yield badges throughout this book will help you identify the most important topics, this Science Mastery Assessment is another tool in your MCAT prep arsenal. This quiz (which can also be taken in your online resources) and the guidance below will help ensure that you are spending the appropriate amount of time on this chapter based on your personal strengths and weaknesses. Don't worry though—skipping something now does not mean you'll never study it. Later on in your prep, as you complete full-length tests, you'll uncover specific pieces of content that you need to review and can come back to these chapters as appropriate.

How to Use This Assessment

If you answer 0–7 questions correctly:

Spend about 1 hour to read this chapter in full and take limited notes throughout. Follow up by reviewing **all** quiz questions to ensure that you now understand how to solve each one.

If you answer 8–11 questions correctly:

Spend 20–40 minutes reviewing the quiz questions. Beginning with the questions you missed, read and take notes on the corresponding subchapters. For questions you answered correctly, ensure your thinking matches that of the explanation and you understand why each choice was correct or incorrect.

If you answer 12–15 questions correctly:

Spend less than 20 minutes reviewing all questions from the quiz. If you missed any, then include a quick read-through of the corresponding subchapters, or even just the relevant content within a subchapter, as part of your question review. For questions you got correct, ensure your thinking matches that of the explanation and review the Concept Summary at the end of the chapter.

1. Adding heat to a closed biological system will do all of the following EXCEPT:
   A. increase the internal energy of the system.
   B. increase the average of the vibrational, rotational, and translational energies.
   C. cause the system to do work to maintain a fixed internal energy.
   D. increase the enthalpy of the system.

2. At 25°C the $\Delta G°$ for a certain reaction $A \rightleftharpoons B + 2\,C$ is 0. If the concentration of A, B, and C in the cell at 25°C are all 10 mM, how does the ΔG compare to the measurement taken with 1 M concentrations?
   A. ΔG is greater than $\Delta G°$, thus the reaction is spontaneous.
   B. ΔG is less than $\Delta G°$, thus the reaction is spontaneous.
   C. ΔG is greater than $\Delta G°$, thus the reaction is nonspontaneous.
   D. ΔG is less than $\Delta G°$, thus the reaction is nonspontaneous.

3. Which of the following statements is true about the hydrolysis of ATP?
   A. The free energy of ATP hydrolysis is independent of pH.
   B. One mole of creatine phosphate can phosphorylate two moles of ADP.
   C. The free energy of hydrolysis of ATP is nearly the same as for ADP.
   D. ATP yields cyclic AMP after two hydrolysis reactions.

4. The reduction half-reaction in the last step of the electron transport chain is:
   A. $O_2 + 4e^- + 4\,H^+ \rightarrow 2\,H_2O$
   B. $NADPH \rightarrow NADP^+ + e^- + H^+$
   C. $NADP^+ + e^- + H^+ \rightarrow NADPH$
   D. Ubiquinone (Q) $\rightarrow$ Ubiquinol (QH_2)

5. The ability to exist in both an oxidized and a reduced state is characteristic of:
   A. adenosine triphosphate (ATP).
   B. electron carriers.
   C. regulatory enzymes.
   D. peptide hormones.

6. What energy state was described in the introduction to this chapter?
   A. Absorptive
   B. Postabsorptive
   C. Starvation
   D. Vegetative

7. Which of the following correctly pairs a tissue with its preferred energy source in the well fed state?
   A. Liver - ketone bodies
   B. Adipose tissue - fatty acids
   C. Brain - amino acids
   D. Cardiac muscle - fatty acids

8. How do hormonal controls of glycogen metabolism differ from allosteric controls?
   A. Hormonal control is systemic and covalent.
   B. Hormonal control is local and covalent.
   C. Hormonal control is systemic and noncovalent.
   D. Hormonal control is local and noncovalent.

9. Which of the following tissues is most dependent on insulin?

- **A.** Active skeletal muscle
- **B.** Resting skeletal muscle
- **C.** Cardiac muscle
- **D.** Smooth muscle

10. Glucocorticoids have been implicated in stress-related weight gain because:

- **A.** they increase appetite and decrease satiety signals.
- **B.** they increase the activity of catabolic hormones.
- **C.** they increase glucose levels, which causes insulin secretion.
- **D.** they interfere with activity of the leptin receptor.

11. In the absence of oxygen, which tissue will experience damage most rapidly?

- **A.** Skin
- **B.** Brain
- **C.** Red blood cells
- **D.** Liver

12. A respiratory quotient approaching 0.7 indicates metabolism primarily of which macromolecule?

- **A.** Carbohydrates
- **B.** Lipids
- **C.** Nucleic acids
- **D.** Amino acids

13. Which of the following side effects would be anticipated in someone taking leptin to promote weight loss?

- **A.** Drowsiness
- **B.** Increased appetite
- **C.** Irritability
- **D.** Fever

14. Which of the following statements is FALSE?

- **A.** Growth hormone participates in glucose counterregulation.
- **B.** T_4 acts more slowly than T_3.
- **C.** ATP stores are turned over more than 10,000 times daily.
- **D.** Catecholamines stimulate the sympathetic nervous system.

15. Which process is expected to begin earliest in a prolonged fast?

- **A.** Ketone bodies are used by the brain.
- **B.** Glycogen storage is halted.
- **C.** Proteins are broken down.
- **D.** Enzyme phosphorylation and dephosphorylation.

Answer Key

1. **C**
2. **B**
3. **C**
4. **A**
5. **B**
6. **B**
7. **D**
8. **A**
9. **B**
10. **C**
11. **B**
12. **B**
13. **A**
14. **C**
15. **D**

Detailed explanations can be found at the end of the chapter.

CHAPTER 12

BIOENERGETICS AND REGULATION OF METABOLISM

In This Chapter

CHAPTER PROFILE

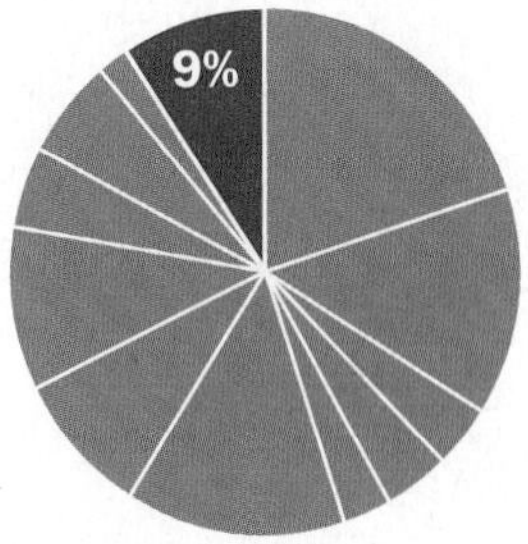

The content in this chapter should be relevant to about 9% of all questions about biochemistry on the MCAT.

This chapter covers material from the following AAMC content categories:

1D: Principles of bioenergetics and fuel molecule metabolism

5E: Principles of chemical thermodynamics and kinetics

Introduction

You got up this morning with a really ambitious plan: study for the MCAT! The day started with a big breakfast, and then you dove into *MCAT Biochemistry Review*. A few chapters in you noticed your stomach growling, but you were having so much fun that you ignored it. A little while later, your body realized it wasn't getting any more food for a while, but it still needed energy. Where does it come from?

The human body is an incredible system. When we skip lunch on a study day, we produce hormones that help raise the level of certain energy molecules in the bloodstream, mainly glucose. This is a good thing because the brain relies solely on glucose for most of its metabolism, and we always want to be thinking at our peak. Glucose in the blood comes from either our diet, such as when we eat a big breakfast, or from our fuel stores, through the processes of gluconeogenesis and glycogenolysis. These processes, just like the formation and consumption of ATP, are highly regulated.

In this chapter, we'll highlight the basic principles of bioenergetics, including thermodynamics: the sources of energy and the reactions that play a key role in moving that energy around. Then we'll examine the different energy states of the body before taking a look at the intimate relationship of hormones with metabolism. We'll spend some time examining the regulation of metabolism, regulatory enzymes for some common pathways, and how specific tissues preferentially metabolize particular macronutrients. By the end of this chapter, you'll be able to tell where and how your food is being used, and you probably won't choose to skip lunch again—no matter how much fun you're having!

12.1 Thermodynamics and Bioenergetics

High-Yield

LEARNING OBJECTIVES

After Chapter 12.1, you will be able to:

- Describe the relationship between $\Delta G°$ and $\Delta G°'$
- Explain why heat can be used as a measure of internal energy for biological systems
- Predict the spontaneity of a reaction given the signs of ΔH and ΔS

If we take a look back at what we learned about thermodynamics in Chapter 3 of *MCAT Physics and Math Review* and Chapter 7 of *MCAT General Chemistry Review*, it becomes evident that we already know quite a bit. However, most of the data that we've seen so far has been obtained under standard-state conditions (25°C, 1 atm pressure, and 1 M concentrations). These assumptions work in a chemistry lab, but must be adjusted for application in the human body.

Biological Systems

MCAT EXPERTISE

The energy of chemical reactions is described as part of general chemistry, while work is generally associated with physics. Be aware that on Test Day, you will see crossover that allows you to draw on knowledge of the other subjects and to use that background information to your advantage.

Biological systems are often considered **open systems** because they can exchange both energy and matter with the environment. Energy is exchanged in the form of mechanical work when something is moved over a distance, or as heat energy. Matter is exchanged through food consumption and elimination, as well as respiration. Most biochemical studies are performed on the cellular or subcellular level rather than in an entire organism. These systems can be considered **closed** because there is no exchange of matter with the environment. In such a system, we can make useful simplifications about the internal energy, U. **Internal energy** is the sum of all of the different interactions between and within atoms in a system; vibration, rotation, linear motion, and stored chemical energies all contribute.

Because the system is closed, the change in internal energy can come only in the form of work or heat. This can be represented mathematically through the First Law of Thermodynamics, $\Delta U = Q - W$. Work in thermodynamics refers to changes in pressure and volume. These are constant in most living systems, so the only quantity of interest in determining internal energy is heat.

Enthalpy, Entropy, and Free Energy

Bioenergetics is the term used to describe energy states in biological systems. Changes in **free energy** (ΔG) provide information about chemical reactions and can predict whether a chemical reaction is favorable and will occur. In biological systems, ATP plays a crucial role in transferring energy from energy-releasing catabolic processes to energy-requiring anabolic processes.

Whether a chemical reaction proceeds is determined by the degree to which enthalpy and entropy change during a chemical reaction. **Enthalpy** measures the overall change in heat of a system during a reaction. At constant pressure and volume, enthalpy (ΔH) and thermodynamic heat exchange (Q) are equal. Changes in **entropy** (ΔS) measure the degree of disorder or energy dispersion in a system. While the MCAT will not test on the level of statistical thermodynamics, this conceptual understanding of entropy (ΔS) will be helpful. Entropy carries the units $\frac{\text{J}}{\text{K}}$.

When combined together mathematically, along with temperature (T), these quantities can be related through the Gibbs free energy equation:

$$\Delta G = \Delta H - T\Delta S$$

Equation 12.1

which predicts the direction in which a chemical reaction proceeds spontaneously. Spontaneous reactions proceed in the forward direction, exhibit a net loss of free energy, and therefore have a negative ΔG. In contrast, nonspontaneous reactions, which would be spontaneous in the reverse direction, exhibit a net gain of energy and have a positive ΔG. Free energy approaches zero as the reaction proceeds to equilibrium and there is no net change in concentration of reactants or products.

BRIDGE

Enthalpy, entropy, and free energy are discussed more thoroughly in Chapter 7 of *MCAT General Chemistry Review*.

Physiological Conditions

The change in free energy (ΔG) that we have been discussing up to this point predicts changes occurring at any concentration of products and reactants and at any temperature. In contrast, standard free energy (ΔG°) is the energy change that occurs at standard concentrations of 1 M, pressure of 1 atm, and temperature of 25°C. These can be related by the equation:

$$\Delta G = \Delta G^\circ + \text{R}T\ln(Q)$$

Equation 12.2

where R is the universal gas constant, T is the temperature, and Q is the reaction quotient. Biochemical analysis works well under all standard conditions except one: pH. A 1 M concentration of protons would correspond to a pH of 0, which is far too acidic for most biochemical reactions. Therefore, in the **modified standard state,** $[\text{H}^+] = 10^{-7}$ M and the pH is 7. With this additional condition, ΔG° is given the special symbol $\Delta G^{\circ\prime}$, indicating that it is standardized to the neutral buffers used in biochemistry. Note that if the concentrations of other reactants and products differ from 1 M, these must still be adjusted for in the equation above.

The shift in ΔG as a result of changing concentration is not universally toward or away from spontaneity. There is a general trend that reactions with more products than reactants have a more negative ΔG, while reactions with more reactants than products have a more positive ΔG. While this trend is useful for making quick assessments, always double check with numbers on Test Day.

MCAT CONCEPT CHECK 12.1

Before you move on, assess your understanding of the material with these questions.

1. What conditions does $\Delta G^{\circ\prime}$ adjust for that are not considered with ΔG°?

   ____

2. Why can heat be used as a measure of internal energy in living systems?

   ____

   ____

3. Complete the following table relating the change in entropy and enthalpy of a reaction with whether the reaction is spontaneous.

	$+\Delta H$	$-\Delta H$
$+\Delta S$		
$-\Delta S$		

12.2 The Role of ATP

High-Yield

LEARNING OBJECTIVES

After Chapter 12.2, you will be able to:

- Predict the impact of ATP coupling on the energetics of a reaction
- Calculate free energy change for an overall reaction given energetic data for component reactions
- Relate the structure of ATP to its role as an energy carrier

The human body can make use of different energy sources with roughly the same efficiency, but all nutrient molecules are not created equally. For example, fats are much more energy-rich than carbohydrates, proteins, or ketones. Complete combustion of fat results in 9 $\frac{\text{kcal}}{\text{g}}$ of energy, compared with only 4 $\frac{\text{kcal}}{\text{g}}$ derived from carbohydrates, proteins, or ketones. Because fats are so much more energy-dense than other biomolecules, they are preferred for long-term energy storage. Think of the difference between fats and carbohydrates like the difference between a 16-GB and an 8-GB storage drive. The storage drive with a greater capacity occupies the same amount of physical space, but holds twice as much data. While different energy sources provide greater or lesser caloric values, the end goal is to have energy in a readily available form. For the cell, this is **adenosine triphosphate** (**ATP**), shown in Figure 12.1.

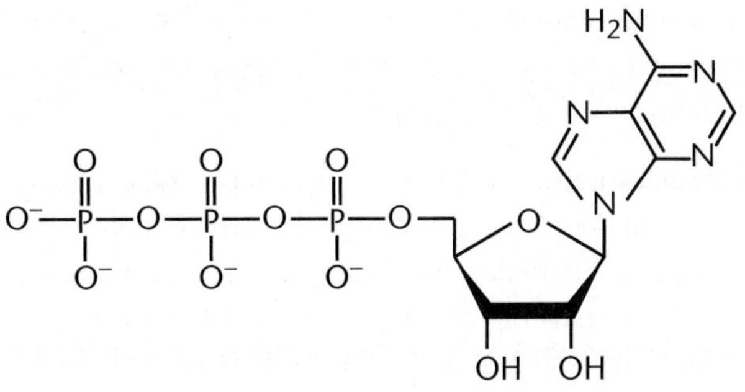

Figure 12.1 Adenosine Triphosphate (ATP)

ATP as an Energy Carrier

ATP is the major energy currency in the body. It is a mid-level energy carrier, as seen in Table 12.1, and is formed from **substrate-level phosphorylation**, as well as **oxidative phosphorylation**. Why do we want ATP to be a mid-level carrier and not a higher-level one? Think about your wallet. If you never had the ability to get change back after a purchase, what type of bill would you want in abundance? One dollar bills! Similarly, ATP cannot get back the "leftover" free energy after a reaction, so it's best to use a carrier with a smaller free energy. ATP provides about 30 $\frac{\text{kJ}}{\text{mol}}$ of energy under physiological conditions. If a reaction only requires 10 $\frac{\text{kJ}}{\text{mol}}$ to overcome a positive ΔG value, then 20 $\frac{\text{kJ}}{\text{mol}}$ have been wasted. The waste would be even higher with a higher-energy compound like creatine phosphate.

COMPOUND	$\Delta G^{\circ\prime} \frac{\text{kj}}{\text{mol}}$	FUNCTION
cAMP	−50.4	Second messenger
Creatine phosphate	−43.3	Direct phosphorylation in muscle
ATP	−30.5	Energy turnover in all cell types
Glucose 6-phosphate	−13.9	Intermediate of glycolysis and gluconeogenesis
AMP	−9.2	ATP synthesis

Table 12.1 Free Energy of Hydrolysis for Key Metabolic Phosphate Compounds

Remember that most of the ATP in a cell is produced by mitochondrial *ATP synthase*, as described in Chapter 10 of *MCAT Biochemistry Review*, but some ATP is produced during glycolysis and (indirectly from GTP) in the citric acid cycle.

ATP consists of an adenosine molecule attached to three phosphate groups, and is generated from ADP and P_i with energy input from an exergonic reaction or electrochemical gradient. ATP is consumed either through hydrolysis or the transfer of a phosphate group to another molecule. If one phosphate group is removed, **adenosine diphosphate (ADP)** is produced; if two phosphate groups are removed, **adenosine monophosphate (AMP)** is the result. In a single day, an average-sized person uses about 90 percent of body weight in ATP but only has about 50 grams of ATP available at any given time. Continuous recycling of ATP, ADP, and P_i more than 1000 times per day accounts for this discrepancy.

What makes ATP such a good energy carrier is its high-energy phosphate bonds. The negative charges on the phosphate groups experience repulsive forces with one another, and the ADP and P_i molecules that form after hydrolysis are stabilized by resonance. While ATP doesn't rapidly break down on its own in the cell, it is much more stable after hydrolysis. This accounts for the very negative value of ΔG. Under standard conditions $\Delta G°$ is about $-55\ \frac{\text{kJ}}{\text{mol}}$. At pH 7 and with excess magnesium, the standard free energy change is still $-30.5\ \frac{\text{kJ}}{\text{mol}}$. ADP, which also displays charge repulsion and resonance stabilization after hydrolysis, has similar ΔG values, but AMP has a much smaller $\Delta G°$ near $-9.2\ \frac{\text{kJ}}{\text{mol}}$.

Hydrolysis and Coupling

ATP hydrolysis is most likely to be encountered in the context of **coupled reactions**. Many coupled reactions use ATP as an energy source. For example, the movement of sodium and potassium against their electrochemical gradients requires energy, which is harnessed from the hydrolysis of ATP.

KEY CONCEPT

ATP is used to fuel energetically unfavorable reactions or to activate or inactivate other molecules.

ATP cleavage is the transfer of a high-energy phosphate group from ATP to another molecule. Generally, this activates or inactivates the target molecule. With these **phosphoryl group transfers**, the overall free energy of the reaction will be determined by taking the sum of the free energies of the individual reactions.

Phosphoryl Group Transfers

BRIDGE

Hess's law, discussed in Chapter 7 of *MCAT General Chemistry Review*, applies for all of the state functions, including pressure, density, temperature, volume, enthalpy, internal energy, free energy, and entropy.

ATP can provide a phosphate group as a reactant. For example, in the phosphorylation of glucose in the early stages of glycolysis, ATP donates a phosphate group to glucose to form glucose 6-phosphate. The information in Table 12.1 indicates the free energy of hydrolysis, which can be conceptualized as the transfer of the phosphate group to water. To determine the free energy of phosphoryl group transfer to another biological molecule, one could use Hess's law and calculate the difference in free energy between the reactants and products:

$$\begin{array}{rll} \text{creatine phosphate} + H_2O \rightarrow \text{creatine} + P_i & \Delta G°' = -43.3\ \frac{\text{kJ}}{\text{mol}} & \\ \text{ADP} + P_i \rightarrow \text{ATP} + H_2O & \Delta G°' = \ \ 30.5\ \frac{\text{kJ}}{\text{mol}} & \text{(reverse reaction from Table 12.1)} \\ \hline \text{creatine phosphate} + \text{ADP} \rightarrow \text{creatine} + \text{ATP} & \Delta G°' = -12.8\ \frac{\text{kJ}}{\text{mol}} & \end{array}$$

MCAT CONCEPT CHECK 12.2

Before you move on, assess your understanding of the material with these questions.

1. How does coupling with ATP hydrolysis alter the energetics of a reaction?

---

2. Explain why ATP is an inefficient molecule for long-term energy storage.

---

3. Using Table 12.1, calculate the free energy change for the synthesis of ATP from cAMP and inorganic phosphate. Note: cAMP is hydrolyzed to AMP, and the free energy of hydrolysis for ATP and ADP is approximately equal.

12.3 Biological Oxidation and Reduction

High-Yield

LEARNING OBJECTIVES

After Chapter 12.3, you will be able to:

- Explain the benefits of analyzing half reactions for biological oxidation–reduction reactions
- Recall soluble electron carriers, such as NADH and CoQ, and the pathways they are paired with

Many key enzymes in ATP synthesis and other biochemical pathways have oxidoreductase activity.

Half-Reactions

Just as you practiced with general chemistry, an important skill in biochemistry is to be able to divide oxidation–reduction reactions into their half-reaction components to determine the number of electrons being transferred. For example, in lactic acid fermentation, pyruvate and NADH are converted to lactate and NAD^+ by *lactate dehydrogenase*. This reaction can be broken down into half-reactions as follows:

Overall reaction	$C_3H_4O_3 + NADH + H^+$	$\rightarrow$	$C_3H_6O_3 + NAD^+$
Reduction	$C_3H_4O_3 + 2\,H^+ + 2e^-$	$\rightarrow$	$C_3H_6O_3$
Oxidation	$NADH$	$\rightarrow$	$NAD^+ + H^+ + 2e^-$

Remember that spontaneous oxidation–reduction reactions have a negative value of ΔG and a positive value of E (electromotive force).

BRIDGE

Oxidation–reduction reactions, discussed in Chapter 11 of *MCAT General Chemistry Review* and Chapter 4 of *MCAT Organic Chemistry Review*, are a staple of general chemistry and are characteristic of oxidoreductase enzymes. Take a moment to identify the oxidizing and reducing agents in the reaction catalyzed by lactate dehydrogenase.

Electron Carriers

In the cytoplasm, there are several molecules that act as **high-energy electron carriers**. These are all soluble and include NADH, NADPH, $FADH_2$, ubiquinone, cytochromes, and glutathione. Some of these electron carriers are used by the mitochondrial electron transport chain, which leads to the oxidative phosphorylation of ADP to ATP. As electrons are passed down the electron transport chain, they give up their free energy to form the proton-motive force across the inner mitochondrial membrane. In addition to soluble electron carriers, there are membrane-bound electron carriers embedded within the inner mitochondrial membrane. One such carrier is flavin mononucleotide (FMN), which is bonded to complex I of the electron transport chain and can also act as a soluble electron carrier. In general, proteins with prosthetic groups containing iron–sulfur clusters are particularly well suited for the transport of electrons.

Flavoproteins

REAL WORLD

Deficiency of riboflavin, a key component of flavoproteins, leads to a lack of growth, failure to thrive, and eventual death in experimental models. In humans, riboflavin deficiency is very rare, but may occur in severely malnourished individuals.

Flavoproteins contain a modified vitamin B_2, or ***riboflavin***. They are nucleic acid derivatives, generally either ***flavin adenine dinucleotide*** (**FAD**) or ***flavin mononucleotide*** (**FMN**). Flavoproteins are most notable for their presence in the mitochondria and chloroplasts as electron carriers. Flavoproteins are also involved in the modification of other B vitamins to active forms. Finally, flavoproteins function as coenzymes for enzymes in the oxidation of fatty acids, the decarboxylation of pyruvate, and the reduction of glutathione.

MCAT CONCEPT CHECK 12.3

Before you move on, assess your understanding of the material with these questions.

1. What is an advantage of analyzing the half-reactions in biological oxidation and reduction reactions?

 ____

2. Name three soluble electron carriers and their relevant metabolic pathways in the cell.

Electron Carrier	Metabolic Pathway(s)

12.4 Metabolic States

LEARNING OBJECTIVES

After Chapter 12.4, you will be able to:

- Identify disequilibriums that are maintained at energetic cost within the cell
- Compare the behavior of different tissues during postprandial, postabsorptive, and prolonged fasting states
- Associate the three metabolic states with related hormone activity

One of the key differences between general chemistry and biochemistry is whether or not equilibrium is seen as a desirable state. Biochemists emphatically believe that it is not! Equilibrium is a fixed state, which prevents us from storing any energy for later use or creating an excitable environment. Instead, biochemists seek a state of homeostasis. **Homeostasis** is a physiological tendency toward a relatively stable state that is maintained and adjusted, often with the expenditure of energy. Most compounds in the body are actually maintained at a homeostatic level that is different from equilibrium, which allows us to store potential energy; for example, keeping sodium concentrations much higher outside a neuron than inside it creates a gradient that stores energy. In this state, reactions can proceed such that equilibrium is put off for a long time (someone born today can delay equilibrium for about 80 years).

The pathways that are operational in fuel metabolism depend on the nutritional status of the organism. Shifts between storage and mobilization of a particular fuel, as well as shifts among the types of fuel being used, are very pronounced when going from the well-fed state to an overnight fast, and finally to a prolonged state of starvation. We'll take a look at how fuel metabolism is regulated in each state. Remember that in addition to the "big-picture view" discussed here, the specific regulatory steps of each pathway are discussed in the previous chapters of *MCAT Biochemistry Review*: Chapter 9 (glycolysis, glycogenesis, glycogenolysis, gluconeogenesis, and the pentose phosphate pathway), Chapter 10 (the citric acid cycle, electron transport chain, and oxidative phosphorylation), and Chapter 11 (fatty acid and cholesterol synthesis, β-oxidation, ketogenesis and ketolysis, and amino acid metabolism).

Postprandial (Absorptive) State

The **postprandial state**, also called the **absorptive** or **well-fed state**, occurs shortly after eating. This state is marked by greater **anabolism** (synthesis of biomolecules) and fuel storage than **catabolism** (breakdown of biomolecules for energy). Nutrients flood in from the gut and make their way via the hepatic portal vein to the liver, where they can be stored or distributed to other tissues of the body. The postprandial state generally lasts three to five hours after eating a meal.

Just after eating, blood glucose levels rise and stimulate the release of insulin. The three major target tissues for insulin are the liver, muscle, and adipose tissue, as shown in Figure 12.2. Insulin promotes glycogen synthesis in liver and muscle. After the glycogen stores are filled, the liver converts excess glucose to fatty acids and triacylglycerols. Insulin promotes triacylglycerol synthesis in adipose tissue and protein synthesis in muscle, as well as glucose entry into both tissues. After a meal, most of the energy needs of the liver are met by the oxidation of excess amino acids.

Two types of cells—nervous tissue and red blood cells—are notably insensitive to insulin. Nervous tissue derives energy from oxidizing glucose to CO_2 and water in both the well-fed and normal fasting states. Only in prolonged fasting does this situation change. Red blood cells can only use glucose anaerobically for all their energy needs, regardless of the individual's metabolic state.

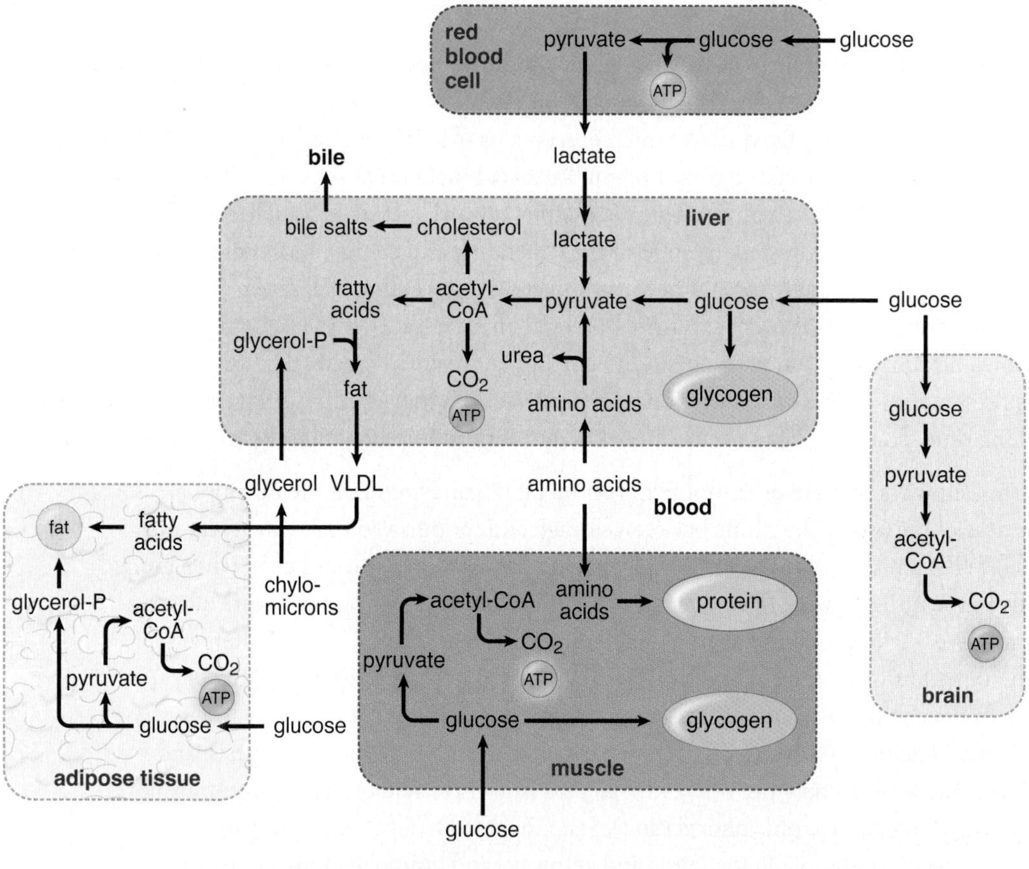

Figure 12.2 Metabolic Profile of the Postprandial (Absorptive) State

Postabsorptive (Fasting) State

Glucagon, cortisol, epinephrine, norepinephrine, and growth hormone oppose the actions of insulin. These hormones are sometimes termed **counterregulatory hormones** because of their effects on skeletal muscle, adipose tissue, and the liver, which are opposite to the actions of insulin. In the liver, glycogen degradation and the release of glucose into the blood are stimulated, as shown in Figure 12.3. Hepatic gluconeogenesis is also stimulated by glucagon, but the response is slower than that of glycogenolysis. Whereas glycogenolysis begins almost immediately at the beginning of the postabsorptive state, gluconeogenesis takes about 12 hours to hit maximum velocity.

The release of amino acids from skeletal muscle and fatty acids from adipose tissue are both stimulated by the decrease in insulin and by an increase in levels of epinephrine. Once carried into the liver, amino acids and fatty acids can provide the necessary carbon skeletons and energy required for gluconeogenesis.

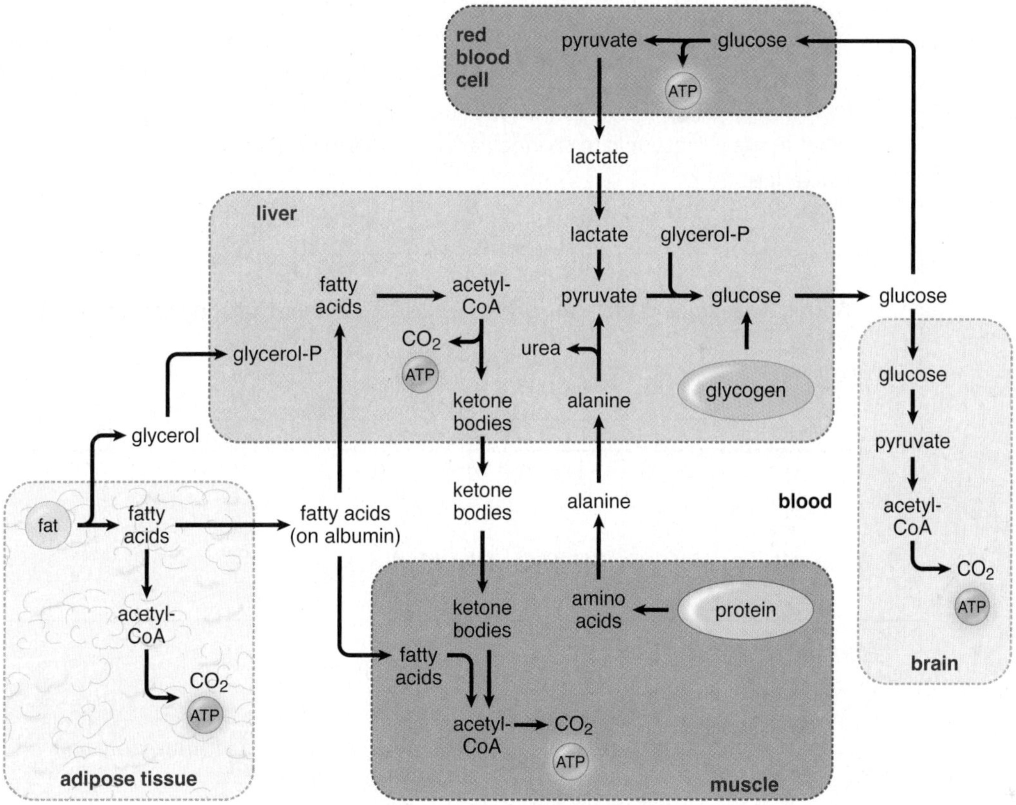

Figure 12.3 Metabolic Profile of the Postabsorptive (Fasting) State

Prolonged Fasting (Starvation)

Levels of glucagon and epinephrine are markedly elevated during starvation. Increased levels of glucagon relative to insulin result in rapid degradation of glycogen stores in the liver. As liver glycogen stores are depleted, gluconeogenic activity continues and plays an important role in maintaining blood glucose levels during prolonged fasting; after about 24 hours, gluconeogenesis is the predominant source of glucose for the body. Lipolysis is rapid, resulting in excess acetyl-CoA that is used in the synthesis of ketone bodies. Once levels of fatty acids and ketones are high enough in the blood, muscle tissue will utilize fatty acids as its major fuel source and the brain will adapt to using ketones for energy. After several weeks of fasting, the brain derives approximately two-thirds of its energy from ketones and one-third from glucose. The shift from glucose to ketones as the major fuel reduces the quantity of amino acids that must be degraded to support gluconeogenesis, which spares proteins that are vital for other functions. Cells that have few, if any, mitochondria, like red blood cells, continue to be dependent on glucose for their energy.

MCAT CONCEPT CHECK 12.4

Before you move on, assess your understanding of the material with these questions.

1. Provide an example of disequilibrium that is maintained at the expense of cellular energy.

___

2. What tissue is least able to change its fuel source in periods of prolonged starvation?

___

3. During what stage is there the greatest decrease in the circulating concentration of insulin?

___

12.5 Hormonal Regulation of Metabolism

LEARNING OBJECTIVES

After Chapter 12.5, you will be able to:

- Describe the impact of key metabolic hormones, such as insulin, glucagon, and thyroid hormones, on metabolic function
- Apply knowledge of the metabolic hormones to a given disease state
- Recall the general structures and traits of metabolic hormones:

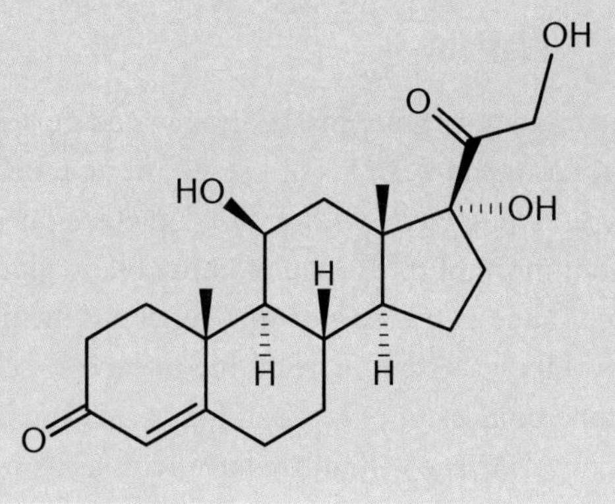

If each cell were acting independently of one another, metabolism would be a random process that could not be coordinated with outside events like meals or exertion. In order to make the most efficient use of the resources available, metabolism must be regulated across the entire organism. This regulation is accomplished best through hormonal means. Water-soluble **peptide hormones**, like insulin, are able to rapidly adjust the metabolic processes of cells via second messenger cascades, while certain fat-soluble **amino acid–derivative hormones**, like thyroid hormones, and **steroid hormones**, like cortisol, enact longer-range effects by exerting regulatory actions at the transcriptional level. Hormone levels are regulated by feedback loops with other endocrine structures, such as the hypothalamic–pituitary axis, or by the biomolecule upon which they act; for example, insulin causes a decrease in blood glucose, which removes the trigger for continued insulin release. Next, we'll examine the specific actions of several hormones involved in the regulation of metabolism and in maintaining homeostasis, including insulin and glucagon, epinephrine, glucocorticoids, and thyroid hormones.

Insulin and Glucagon

Insulin

Insulin is a peptide hormone secreted by the **β-cells** of the pancreatic islets of Langerhans, as shown in Figure 12.4. It is a key player in the uptake and storage of glucose. Glucose is absorbed by peripheral tissues via facilitated transport mechanisms that utilize glucose transporters located in the cell membrane. The tissues that require insulin for effective uptake of glucose are adipose tissue and resting skeletal muscle. Tissues in which glucose uptake is not affected by insulin include:

- Nervous tissue
- Kidney tubules
- Intestinal mucosa
- Red blood cells (erythrocytes)
- β-cells of the pancreas

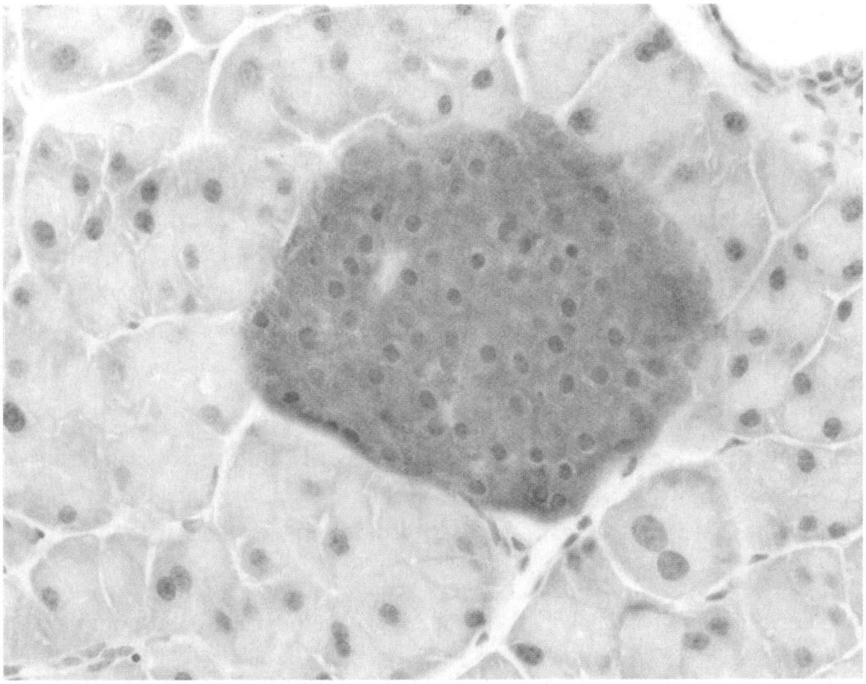

Figure 12.4 Insulin (Light Brown) in Pancreatic β-Cells

Take note of the differences between these types of tissues. Some tissues that require insulin actively store glucose when it is present in high concentrations, while other tissues that do not require insulin must still be able to absorb glucose even when the glucose concentration is low.

Insulin impacts the metabolism of the different nutrient classes in different ways. For carbohydrates, insulin increases the uptake of glucose and increases carbohydrate metabolism in muscle and fat. Increased glucose in muscle can be used as additional fuel to burn during exercise, or can be stored as glycogen. Insulin also increases glycogen synthesis in the liver by increasing the activity of *glucokinase* and *glycogen synthase*, while decreasing the activity of enzymes that promote glycogen breakdown (*glycogen phosphorylase* and *glucose-6-phosphatase*).

While the primary effects of insulin are on carbohydrate metabolism, it also changes the way that the body processes other macromolecules. For instance, insulin increases amino acid uptake by muscle cells, thereby increasing levels of protein synthesis and decreasing breakdown of essential proteins. Insulin also exhibits a significant impact on the metabolism of fats, especially in the liver and adipocytes. The effects of insulin on the metabolism of fats are described below.

Insulin increases:

- Glucose and triacylglycerol uptake by fat cells
- *Lipoprotein lipase* activity, which clears VLDL and chylomicrons from the blood
- Triacylglycerol synthesis (lipogenesis) in adipose tissue and the liver from acetyl-CoA

Insulin decreases:

- Triacylglycerol breakdown (lipolysis) in adipose tissue
- Formation of ketone bodies by the liver

The most important controller of insulin secretion is plasma glucose. Above a threshold of 100 $\frac{\text{mg}}{\text{dL}}$, or about 5.6 mM glucose, insulin secretion is directly proportional to plasma glucose. For glucose to promote insulin secretion, it must not only enter the β-cell but also be metabolized, increasing intracellular ATP concentration. Increased ATP leads to calcium release in the cell, which promotes exocytosis of preformed insulin from intracellular vesicles. Insulin secretion is also affected by signaling initiated by other hormones, such as glucagon and somatostatin.

REAL WORLD

Patients with type 1 diabetes mellitus are incapable of synthesizing insulin, but still synthesize glucagon. This combination increases blood sugar much more than if an individual were to lose all pancreatic function or to develop insulin insensitivity.

Glucagon

Glucagon is a peptide hormone secreted by the **α-cells** of the pancreatic islets of Langerhans, as shown in Figure 12.5. The primary target for glucagon action is the hepatocyte. Glucagon acts through second messengers to cause the following effects:

- Increased liver glycogenolysis. Glucagon activates glycogen phosphorylase and inactivates glycogen synthase.

- Increased liver gluconeogenesis. Glucagon promotes the conversion of pyruvate to phosphoenolpyruvate by *pyruvate carboxylase* and *phosphoenolpyruvate carboxykinase* (PEPCK). Glucagon increases the conversion of fructose 1,6-bisphosphate to fructose 6-phosphate by *fructose-1,6-bisphosphatase.*
- Increased liver ketogenesis and decreased lipogenesis.
- Increased lipolysis in the liver. Glucagon activates *hormone-sensitive lipase* in the liver. Because the action is on the liver and not the adipocyte, glucagon is not considered a major fat-mobilizing hormone.

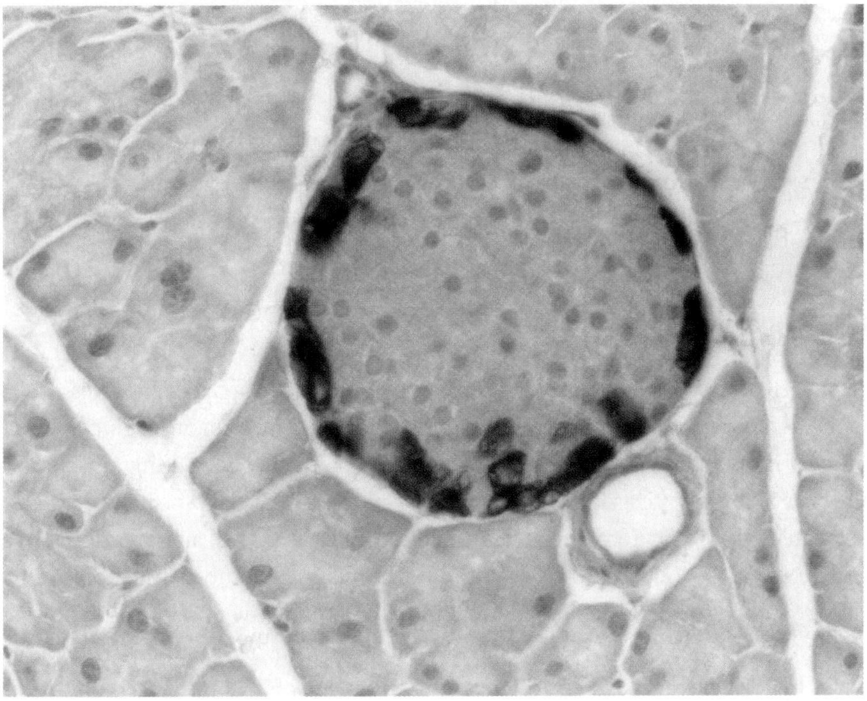

Figure 12.5 Glucagon (Dark Brown) in Pancreatic α-Cells

Low plasma glucose (hypoglycemia) is the most important physiological promoter of glucagon secretion, and elevated plasma glucose (hyperglycemia) is the most important inhibitor. Amino acids, especially basic amino acids (arginine, lysine, histidine), also promote the secretion of glucagon. Thus, glucagon is secreted in response to the ingestion of a meal rich in proteins.

Functional Relationship of Glucagon and Insulin

Insulin, associated with a well-fed, absorptive metabolic state, and glucagon, associated with a postabsorptive metabolic state, usually oppose each other with respect to pathways of energy metabolism. Enzymes that are phosphorylated by glucagon are generally dephosphorylated by insulin; enzymes that are phosphorylated by insulin are generally dephosphorylated by glucagon. Figure 12.6 displays a feedback diagram of the interaction of insulin and glucagon on plasma glucose concentration, as well as fat and protein metabolism.

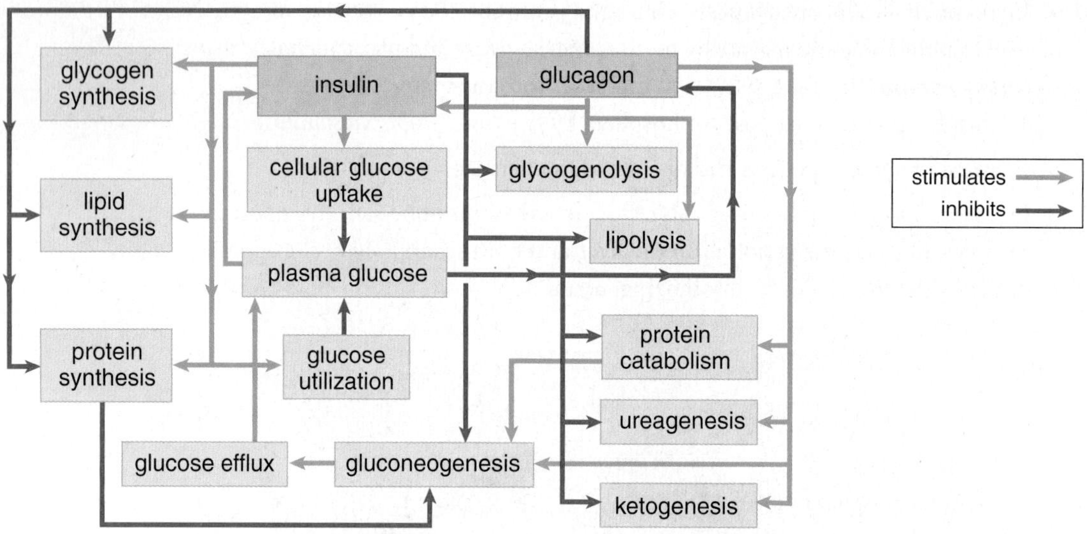

Figure 12.6 Relationship of Glucagon and Insulin in Metabolism

BRIDGE

The endocrine system, discussed in Chapter 5 of *MCAT Biology Review*, is a major regulator of homeostasis. Like the glucocorticoids and catecholamines, mineralocorticoids and sex hormones are also synthesized by the adrenal glands and play a more minor role in metabolism.

Glucocorticoids

Glucocorticoids from the adrenal cortex are responsible for part of the stress response. In order to make a getaway in the "fight-or-flight" response, glucose must be rapidly mobilized from the liver in order to fuel actively contracting muscle cells while fatty acids are released from adipocytes. Glucocorticoids, especially **cortisol**, are secreted with many forms of stress, including exercise, cold, and emotional stress. Cortisol, shown in Figure 12.7, is a steroid hormone that promotes the mobilization of energy stores through the degradation and increased delivery of amino acids and increased lipolysis. Cortisol also elevates blood glucose levels, increasing glucose availability for nervous tissue through two mechanisms. First, cortisol inhibits glucose uptake in most tissues (muscle, lymphoid, and fat) and increases hepatic output of glucose via gluconeogenesis, particularly from amino acids. Second, cortisol has a permissive function that enhances the activity of glucagon, epinephrine, and other catecholamines. Long-term exposure to glucocorticoids may be required clinically, but causes persistent hyperglycemia, which stimulates insulin. This actually promotes fat storage in the adipose tissue, rather than lipolysis.

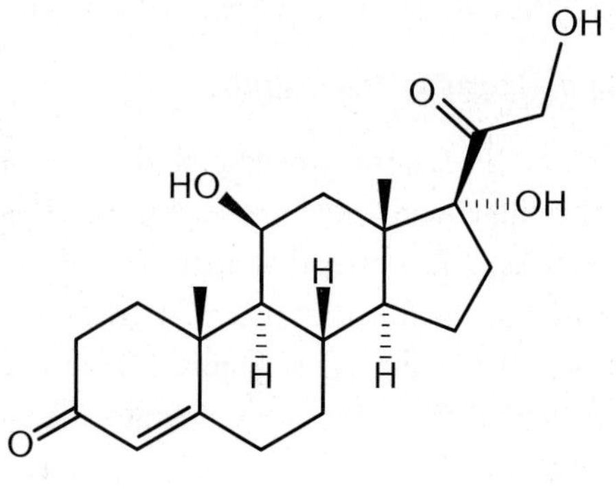

Figure 12.7 Structure of Cortisol

An enlarged adrenal gland (with a tumor of the adrenal cortex) is shown in Figure 12.8. While the adrenal cortex produces steroid hormones (glucocorticoids, mineralocorticoids, and sex hormones), the adrenal medulla produces catecholamines.

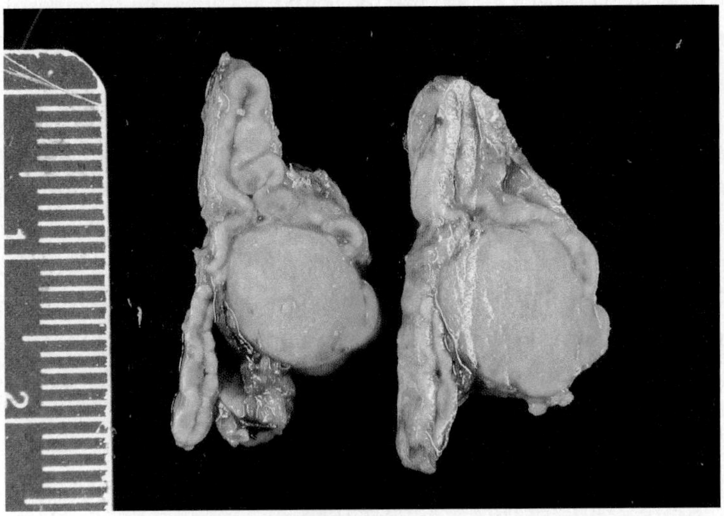

Figure 12.8 Adrenal Gland (Enlarged)
The adrenal cortex (yellow) and adrenal medulla (brown interior) are visible on both slices.

Catecholamines

Catecholamines are secreted by the adrenal medulla and include **epinephrine** and **norepinephrine**, also known as **adrenaline** and **noradrenaline**. The structures of these hormones are shown in Figure 12.9. Catecholamines increase the activity of liver and muscle glycogen phosphorylase, thus promoting glycogenolysis. This increases glucose output by the liver. Glycogenolysis also increases in skeletal muscle, but because muscle lacks glucose-6-phosphatase, glucose cannot be released by skeletal muscle into the bloodstream; instead, it is metabolized by the muscle tissue itself. Catecholamines act on adipose tissue to increase lipolysis by increasing the activity of hormone-sensitive lipase. Glycerol from triacylglycerol breakdown is a minor substrate for gluconeogenesis. Epinephrine also acts directly on target organs like the heart to increase the basal metabolic rate through the sympathetic nervous system. This increase in metabolic function is often associated with an *adrenaline rush.*

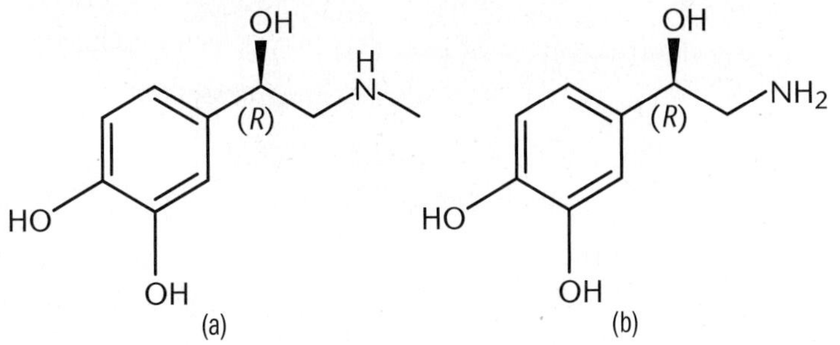

Figure 12.9 Structures of Adrenal Catecholamines
(a) Epinephrine; (b) Norepinephrine

Thyroid Hormones

REAL WORLD

While thyroid hormones are not responsible for day-to-day adjustments in metabolism, insufficient thyroid hormone levels (hypothyroidism) can cause symptoms including cold intolerance, fatigue, weight gain, and depression as metabolism suffers. Excessive thyroid hormone levels (hyperthyroidism) can cause rapid weight loss, anxiety, jitteriness, and fever.

Thyroid hormone activity is largely permissive. In other words, thyroid hormone levels are kept more or less constant, rather than undulating with changes in metabolic state. Thyroid hormones increase the basal metabolic rate, as evidenced by increased O_2 consumption and heat production when they are secreted. The increase in metabolic rate produced by a dose of ***thyroxine*** (**T_4**) occurs after a latency of several hours but may last for several days, while ***triiodothyronine*** (**T_3**) produces a more rapid increase in metabolic rate and has a shorter duration of activity. The subscript numbers refer to the number of iodine atoms in the hormone; iodine atoms are represented by purple spheres in the structures shown in Figure 12.10. T_4 can be thought of as the precursor to T_3; *deiodonases* (enzymes that remove iodine from a molecule) are located in target tissues and convert T_4 to T_3. Thyroid hormones have their primary effects in lipid and carbohydrate metabolism. They accelerate cholesterol clearance from the plasma and increase the rate of glucose absorption from the small intestine. Epinephrine requires thyroid hormones to have a significant metabolic effect.

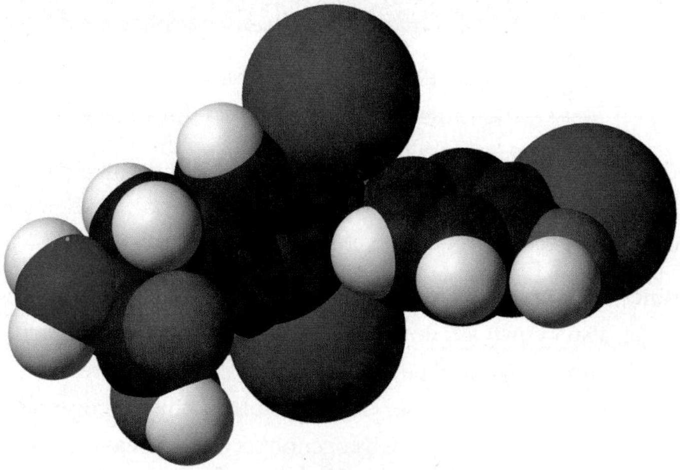

(a)

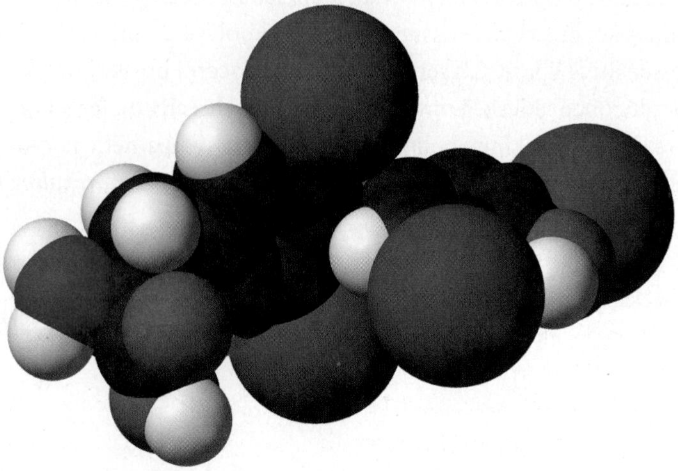

(b)

Figure 12.10 Structures of Thyroid Hormones
(a) Triiodothyronine (T_3); (b) Thyroxine (T_4)

MCAT CONCEPT CHECK 12.5

Before you move on, assess your understanding of the material with these questions.

1. Describe the primary metabolic function of each of the following hormones:
   - Insulin:

   ___

   - Glucagon:

   ___

   - Cortisol:

   ___

   - Catecholamines:

   ___

   - Thyroid hormones (T_3/T_4):

   ___

2. Thyroid storm is a potentially lethal state of extreme hyperthyroidism in which T_3 and T_4 levels are significantly above normal limits. What vital sign abnormalities might be expected in a patient with thyroid storm?

   ___

12.6 Tissue-Specific Metabolism

LEARNING OBJECTIVES

After Chapter 12.6, you will be able to:

- Identify the preferred fuel sources and fuel quantities for different tissue types, including skeletal muscle and the brain
- Recall the metabolic functions of the liver

Tissues have evolved so that their metabolic needs are met in a way corresponding to their form and function. The major sites of metabolic activity in the body are the liver, skeletal and cardiac muscles, brain, and adipocytes. Connective tissue and epithelial cells do not make major contributions to the consumption of energy. Remember though, that epithelial cells are the primary secretory cells, so they are involved in the regulation of metabolism. We have already discussed how the body operates under different nutritional conditions. The organ-specific patterns of fuel utilization in the well-fed and fasting states are summarized in Table 12.2.

ORGAN	WELL-FED	FASTING
Liver	Glucose and amino acids	Fatty acids
Resting skeletal muscle	Glucose	Fatty acids, ketones
Cardiac muscle	Fatty acids	Fatty acids, ketones
Adipose tissue	Glucose	Fatty acids
Brain	Glucose	Glucose (ketones in prolonged fast)
Red blood cells	Glucose	Glucose

Table 12.2 Preferred Fuels in the Well-Fed and Fasting States

Liver

Two major roles of the liver in fuel metabolism are to maintain a constant level of blood glucose under a wide range of conditions and to synthesize ketones when excess fatty acids are being oxidized. After a meal, glucose concentration in the portal blood is elevated. The liver extracts excess glucose and uses it to replenish its glycogen stores. Any glucose remaining in the liver is then converted to acetyl-CoA and used for fatty acid synthesis. The increase in insulin after a meal stimulates both glycogen synthesis and fatty acid synthesis in the liver. The fatty acids are converted to triacylglycerols and released into the blood as **very-low-density lipoproteins (VLDL)**. In the well-fed state, the liver derives most of its energy from the oxidation of excess amino acids. Between meals and during prolonged fasts, the liver releases glucose into the blood. The increase in glucagon during fasting promotes both glycogen degradation and gluconeogenesis. Lactate from anaerobic metabolism, glycerol from triacylglycerols, and amino acids provide carbon skeletons for glucose synthesis.

Adipose Tissue

After a meal, elevated insulin levels stimulate glucose uptake by adipose tissue. Insulin also triggers fatty acid release from VLDL and **chylomicrons** (which carry triacylglycerols absorbed from the gut). Lipoprotein lipase, an enzyme found in the capillary bed of adipose tissue, is also induced by insulin. The fatty acids that are released from lipoproteins are taken up by adipose tissue and re-esterified to triacylglycerols for storage. The glycerol phosphate required for triacylglycerol synthesis comes from glucose that is metabolized in adipocytes as an alternative product of glycolysis. Insulin can also effectively suppress the release of fatty acids from adipose tissue. During the fasting state, decreased levels of insulin and increased epinephrine activate **hormone-sensitive lipase** in fat cells, allowing fatty acids to be released into circulation.

Skeletal Muscle

Resting Muscle

The major fuels of skeletal muscle are glucose and fatty acids. Because of its enormous bulk, skeletal muscle is the body's major consumer of fuel. After a meal, insulin promotes glucose uptake in skeletal muscle, which replenishes glycogen stores and amino acids used for protein synthesis. Both excess glucose and amino acids can also be oxidized for energy. In the fasting state, resting muscle uses fatty acids derived from free fatty acids circulating in the bloodstream. Ketone bodies may also be used if the fasting state is prolonged.

Active Muscle

The primary fuel used to support muscle contraction depends on the magnitude and duration of exercise as well as the major fibers involved. A very short-lived source of energy (2–7 seconds) comes from **creatine phosphate**, which transfers a phosphate group to ADP to form ATP. Skeletal muscle has stores of both glycogen and some triacylglycerols. Blood glucose and free fatty acids may also be used. Short bursts of high-intensity exercise are also supported by anaerobic glycolysis drawing on stored muscle glycogen. During moderately high-intensity, continuous exercise, oxidation of glucose and fatty acids are both important, but after 1 to 3 hours of continuous exercise at this level, muscle glycogen stores become depleted, and the intensity of exercise declines to a rate that can be supported by oxidation of fatty acids.

BRIDGE

Fast-twitch muscle fibers have a high capacity for anaerobic glycolysis but are quick to fatigue. They are involved primarily in short-term, high-intensity exercise. Slow-twitch muscle fibers in arm and leg muscles are well vascularized and primarily oxidative. They are used during prolonged, low-to-moderate intensity exercise and resist fatigue. Slow-twitch fibers and the number of their mitochondria increase dramatically in trained endurance athletes. The musculoskeletal system is discussed in Chapter 11 of *MCAT Biology Review*.

Cardiac Muscle

Unlike other tissues of the body, cardiac myocytes prefer fatty acids as their major fuel, even in the well-fed state. When ketones are present during prolonged fasting, they can also be used. Thus, not surprisingly, cardiac myocytes most closely parallel skeletal muscle during extended periods of exercise. In patients with cardiac hypertrophy (thickening of the heart muscle), this situation reverses to some extent. In a failing heart, glucose oxidation increases and β-oxidation falls.

Brain

Although the brain represents only 2 percent of total body weight, it obtains 15 percent of the cardiac output, uses 20 percent of the total O_2, and consumes 25 percent of the total glucose, the brain's primary fuel. Blood glucose levels are tightly regulated to maintain a sufficient glucose supply for the brain (and sufficient concentration while studying). Normal function depends on a continuous glucose supply from the bloodstream. In hypoglycemic conditions $\left(< 70\ \frac{\text{mg}}{\text{dL}}\right)$, hypothalamic centers in the brain sense a fall in blood glucose level, and the release of glucagon and epinephrine is triggered. Fatty acids cannot cross the blood–brain barrier and are therefore not used at all as an energy source. Between meals, the brain relies on blood glucose supplied by either hepatic glycogenolysis or gluconeogenesis. Only during prolonged fasting does the brain gain the capacity to use ketone bodies for energy, and even then, the ketone bodies only supply approximately two-thirds of the fuel; the remainder is glucose.

BIOCHEMISTRY GUIDED EXAMPLE WITH EXPERT THINKING

A diet high in fat, low in carbohydrates, and sufficient in protein will automatically shift energy production in the body from being primarily dependent on glucose to primarily driven by ketone bodies. This dietary approach, termed a "ketogenic diet," was developed nearly 100 years ago as a metabolic therapy to mimic the metabolic changes that occur during fasting after observing that, upon halting food intake, seizures would stop in epileptic patients. Metabolic dysfunction is increasingly appreciated as a fundamental pathology across disease states, including neurodegenerative diseases, brain cancer, and treatment or reversal of type II diabetes and metabolic syndrome. Furthermore, implementing a ketogenic diet has shown improvement in these diseases. However, to date, there is no confirmation of any fundamental metabolic mechanism(s) that could explain the diverse beneficial effects seen across these numerous diseases.

Ketogenic diet (KD) = high fat, low carbs

KD known to help with epilepsy

A number of diseases are improved with KD

Researchers don't know how KD works to help so many different diseases

One possible avenue is exploring differential cellular energy production, which depends on the metabolic coenzyme nicotinamide adenine dinucleotide (NAD^+), a marker for mitochondrial and cellular health. Furthermore, NAD^+ activates downstream signaling pathways (such as the sirtuin enzymes) associated with major benefits such as longevity and reduced inflammation; thus, increasing NAD^+ is a coveted therapeutic endpoint. The Diagram 1 below outlines the usage of NAD^+ during the metabolism of glucose and ketone bodies (β-hydroxybutyrate and acetoacetate).

Possible mechanism: may depend on the role of NAD^+ in energy production

NAD^+ is a good candidate because it has overall broad health benefits

β-hydroxybutyrate and acetoacetate are both ketone bodies

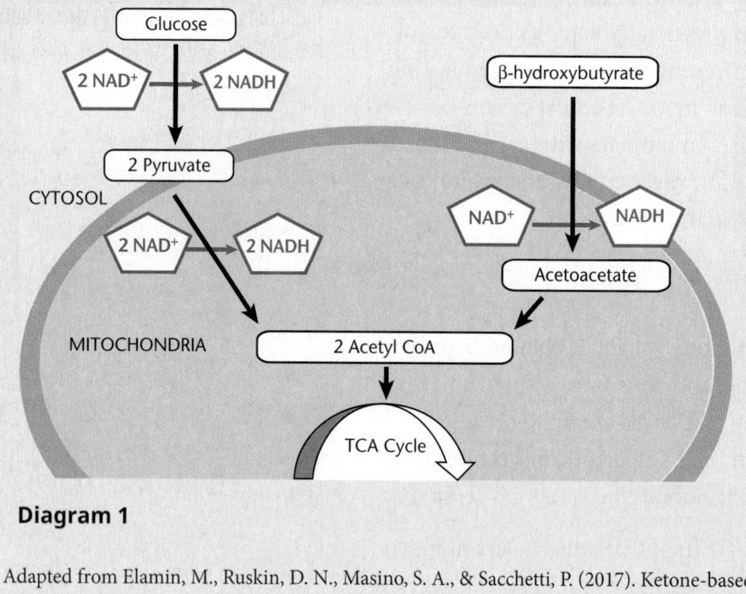

Diagram 1

Glucose uses 4 NAD^+ to get to 2 acetyl-CoA; β-hydroxybutyrate uses 1 NAD^+ to get to 2 acetyl-CoA

Adapted from Elamin, M., Ruskin, D. N., Masino, S. A., & Sacchetti, P. (2017). Ketone-based metabolic therapy: is increased NAD^+ a primary mechanism? *Frontiers in Molecular Neuroscience*, 10, 377. doi:10.3389/fnmol.2017.00377

Given the information in the passage, if the researchers were to assay mice that were fed a ketogenic diet versus normal chow, how would the NAD^+/NADH ratio in ketogenic mice compare to that of normal mice? Why would the researchers likely be more interested in measuring NAD^+/NADH ratios specifically in the brain?

The first question asks us to compare the NAD^+/NADH ratio in KD mice to that of mice that were fed a normal diet, which means we should be combining our content background with the information in the passage to generate an answer. We know normal diets tend to be high in carbohydrates, whereas a ketogenic diet will be high in ketone bodies. Diagram 1 demonstrates that the metabolism of glucose and the metabolism of β-hydroxybutyrate each produce two acetyl-CoA molecules. However, the metabolism of glucose converts four NAD^+ molecules to NADH, while the metabolism of β-hydroxybutyrate only converts one NAD^+ molecule to NADH. This difference generates a higher NAD^+/NADH ratio in those mice that are subsisting on a KD diet, as NADH levels are relatively constant (due to its production from other sources in the body) but NAD^+ availability has increased.

The answer to the second question is superficially answered in the first paragraph—many of the diseases mentioned are focused on the brain (epilepsy, neurodegenerative diseases, brain cancer). However, if we dig a little deeper into our content background, we know that the brain can use only glucose or ketone bodies as its source of energy and there are no energy storage molecules, like glycogen or adipose cells, present in the brain. So, even in the early days of a ketogenic diet, while other tissues are still using alternative energy sources such as fatty acids, the brain is already shifting to utilizing a higher proportion of ketone bodies. Thus, an increased NAD^+/NADH ratio, as well as its potential associated benefits, will occur in the brain sooner and to a greater extent than anywhere else in the body. The passage states that NAD^+ activates pathways involving sirtuin enzymes, which reduce inflammation and fight the aging process. Such physiological changes also indirectly explain why a ketogenic diet could potentially help in so many brain-based diseases.

In short, mice on ketogenic diets would likely have a higher NAD^+/NADH ratio compared to mice on a normal diet, and NAD^+ levels in the brain would likely be more susceptible to diet changes because the brain only relies on plasma glucose and ketone bodies for energy.

MCAT CONCEPT CHECK 12.6

Before you move on, assess your understanding of the material with these questions.

1. What is the preferred fuel for most cells in the well-fed state? What is the exception and its preferred fuel?
   - Preferred fuel: ______________
   - Exception: ______________ Preferred fuel: ______________

2. What organ consumes the greatest amount of glucose relative to its percentage of body mass?

   ____

3. Describe the major metabolic functions of the liver.

   ____

   ____

   ____

12.7 Integrative Metabolism

LEARNING OBJECTIVES

After Chapter 12.7, you will be able to:

- Predict changes to respiratory quotient with changes in activity
- Explain the role of leptin, ghrelin, and orexin in regulating body mass
- Apply knowledge of measurement methods for metabolism to analytical approaches in a lab setting

MCAT EXPERTISE

The MCAT does not expect you to know what levels are healthy for any of these indicators, but can easily pose data interpretation questions related to them.

Analysis of Metabolism

There are several methods of analyzing metabolic control of an organism. In humans, levels of glucose, thyroid hormones and thyroid-stimulating hormone, insulin, glucagon, oxygen, and carbon dioxide can all be measured in the blood. Because these hormones and substrates have a predictable effect on metabolism, they can be used as indicators of metabolic function. They can also be used as indicators of disorders, as in the case of blood glucose or thyroid-stimulating hormone.

Respirometry allows accurate measurement of the respiratory quotient, which differs depending on the fuels being used by the organism. The **respiratory quotient (RQ)** can be measured experimentally, and can be calculated as:

$$RQ = \frac{CO_2 \text{ produced}}{O_2 \text{ consumed}}$$

Equation 12.3

for the complete combustion of a given fuel source. The respiratory quotient for carbohydrates is around 1.0, while the respiratory quotient for lipids is around 0.7. In resting individuals, the respiratory quotient is generally around 0.8, indicating that both fat and glucose are consumed. The respiratory quotient changes under conditions of high stress, starvation, and exercise as predicted by the actions of different hormones.

Calorimeters can measure **basal metabolic rate (BMR)** based on heat exchange with the environment. Human calorimetry makes use of large insulated chambers with specialized heat sinks to determine energy expenditure. Because of the isolationist nature of testing and the expense of creating a calorimetry chamber, other measures of BMR are preferred. Because of previous experimentation, BMR can be estimated based on age, weight, height, and phenotypical sex.

Regulation of Body Mass

Until now, we've been discussing metabolism on a very small scale, but metabolic controls are also involved in maintaining body mass (weight loss or gain). Body mass is determined by several factors, including water, carbohydrates, proteins, and lipids, while nucleic acids do not contribute significantly to its maintenance. The overall mass of carbohydrates and proteins tends to be stable over time, although it can be modified slightly by periods of prolonged starvation or by significant muscle-building activities. Water is very quickly adjusted by the endocrine system and the kidneys; therefore, it does not factor into our discussion of obesity and weight regulation. Water is the primary source of frequent minor weight fluctuations because it is subject to rapid adjustment. Therefore, lipids, stored in adipocytes, are the primary factor in the gradual change of body mass over time.

An individual who is maintaining body weight consumes the same amount of energy that is spent on average each day. If energy consumed is greater than energy expenditure over a significant period of time, then fat stores begin to accumulate. The opposite is also seen. If an energy deficit exists where calories consumed are less than calories burned, then a decrease in weight is observed. As individuals increase in mass, basal metabolic rate (the amount of energy required for one sedentary day) also increases. Thus, a caloric excess will cause an increase in body mass until equilibrium is reached between the new basal metabolic rate and the existing intake. In weight loss the reverse trend is seen.

This effect does have a threshold that differs between individuals. Small adjustments in intake, even over a prolonged period of time, are partially or fully compensated by changes in energy expenditure. Similarly, a small increase or decrease in activity level will be compensated by changes in hunger. Deliberate alterations of body mass require alterations above this threshold level, which is larger in negative energy balance than in positive energy balance—in other words, larger changes must be made to lose weight than to gain it.

Diet (energy intake) and exercise (energy expenditure), genetics, socioeconomic status, and geography all play key roles in weight control. As described earlier, hormonal control by thyroid hormones, cortisol, epinephrine, glucagon, and insulin is critical to the integration of metabolism. In addition, there are hormones that control hunger and satiety, including *ghrelin*, *orexin*, and *leptin*. Have you ever wondered why, even if you don't feel hungry, when you walk into your favorite restaurant you're suddenly ravenous? This is the job of ghrelin and orexin. **Ghrelin** is secreted by the stomach in response to signals of an impending meal. Sight, sound, taste, and especially smell all act as signals for its release. Ghrelin increases appetite and also stimulates secretion of orexin. **Orexin** further increases appetite, and is also involved in alertness and the sleep–wake cycle. Hypoglycemia is also a trigger for orexin release. **Leptin** is a hormone secreted by fat cells that decreases appetite by suppressing orexin production. Genetic variations in the leptin molecule and its receptors have been implicated in obesity; a knockout mouse unable to produce leptin is shown on the left in Figure 12.11. These messengers and receptors are the target of current research; for now, questions regarding body mass modifications on the MCAT mostly come down to diet and exercise.

BRIDGE

Motivation, a psychological concept discussed in Chapter 5 of *MCAT Behavioral Sciences Review*, is often linked with physiological drives and signaling pathways. The hypothalamus, which produces orexin and responds to leptin and ghrelin, is responsible for regulating hunger, thirst, and libido.

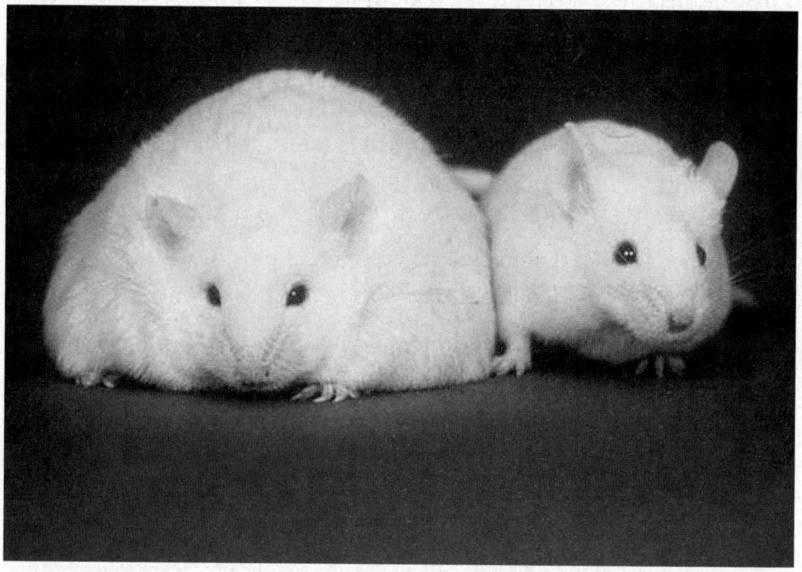

Figure 12.11 Leptin Knockout Mouse (left) Compared to Normal Mouse (right)

Body mass can be measured and tracked using the **body mass index (BMI)**, which is given by:

$$BMI = \frac{\text{mass}}{\text{height}^2}$$

Equation 12.4

where mass is measured in kilograms and height is measured in meters. A normal BMI is considered to be between 18.5 and 25; values lower than this are considered underweight. A BMI between 25 and 30 is considered overweight, whereas a BMI over 30 is considered **obese**.

MCAT CONCEPT CHECK 12.7

Before you move on, assess your understanding of the material with these questions.

1. How is the respiratory quotient expected to change when a person transitions from resting to brief exercise?

____

2. True or False: Body mass can be predicted by the leptin receptor phenotype and caloric intake alone.

3. True or False: It is easier to gain weight than to lose weight.

4. If you were designing a study to assess metabolism, which measurement method would you choose? Defend your answer.

____

Conclusion

In this chapter, we reviewed the principles of thermodynamics and thermochemistry that were introduced in general chemistry and physics and their applications to biological systems. We looked at the specific energy molecules of human metabolism, sources of energy, and key reaction types in ATP synthesis and hydrolysis. We compared different energy states and their impact on overall metabolism and tissue-specific metabolism.

At this point you should have a decent idea about how to determine what energy sources are being used from experimental data, and be able to make predictions about the changes in metabolism under varying conditions. Congratulations, because this is the last chapter of *MCAT Biochemistry Review* and you're just about ready to tackle any of the challenges that you will face on Test Day. Continue practicing, and try not to skip lunch!

GO ONLINE

You've reviewed the content, now test your knowledge and critical thinking skills by completing a test-like passage set in your online resources!

CONCEPT SUMMARY

Thermodynamics and Bioenergetics

- Biological systems are considered:
  - **Open**, wherein matter and energy can be exchanged with the environment, or
  - **Closed**, wherein only energy can be exchanged with the environment.
  - This determination is made based on the examination of the entire organism or an isolated process.
- Changes in **enthalpy** in a closed biological system are equal to changes in **internal energy**, which is equal to **heat exchange** within the environment.
- No work is performed in a closed biological system because pressure and volume remain constant.
- **Entropy** is a measure of energy dispersion in a system.
- Physiological concentrations are usually much less than standard concentrations.
- Free energy calculations must be adjusted for pH ($\boldsymbol{\Delta G^{\circ\prime}}$), temperature ($37°C = 98.6°F = 310\ K$), and concentrations.

The Role of ATP

- ATP is a mid-level energy molecule.
- ATP contains high-energy phosphate bonds that are stabilized upon hydrolysis by resonance, ionization, and loss of charge repulsion.
- ATP provides energy through **hydrolysis** and **coupling** to energetically unfavorable reactions.
- ATP can also participate in **phosphoryl group transfers** as a phosphate donor.

Biological Oxidation and Reduction

- Biological **oxidation** and **reduction** reactions can be broken down into component **half-reactions.**
- Half-reactions provide useful information about stoichiometry and thermodynamics.
- Many oxidation–reduction reactions involve an electron carrier to transport high-energy electrons.
- **Electron carriers** may be soluble or membrane-bound.
  - **Flavoproteins** are one subclass of electron carriers that are derived from riboflavin (vitamin B_2).

Metabolic States

- **Equilibrium** is an undesirable state for most biochemical reactions because organisms need to harness free energy to survive.
- In the **postprandial/well-fed (absorptive)** state, insulin secretion is high and anabolic metabolism prevails.
- In the **postabsorptive (fasting)** state, insulin secretion decreases while glucagon and catecholamine secretion increases.
  - This state is observed in short-term fasting (overnight).
  - There is a transition to catabolic metabolism.
- Prolonged fasting (**starvation**) dramatically increases glucagon and catecholamine secretion.
  - Most tissues rely on fatty acids.
  - At maximum, $\frac{2}{3}$ of the brain's energy can be derived from ketone bodies.

Hormonal Regulation of Metabolism

- **Insulin** and **glucagon** have opposing activities during most aspects of metabolism.
  - Insulin causes a decrease in blood glucose levels by increasing cellular uptake.
  - Insulin increases the rate of anabolic metabolism.
  - Insulin secretion by pancreatic β-cells is regulated by blood glucose levels.
  - Glucagon increases blood glucose levels by promoting gluconeogenesis and glycogenolysis in the liver.
  - Glucagon secretion by pancreatic α-cells is stimulated by both low glucose and high amino acid levels.
- **Glucocorticoids** increase blood glucose in response to stress by mobilizing fat stores and inhibiting glucose uptake.
  - Glucocorticoids increase the impact of glucagon and catecholamines.
- **Catecholamines** promote glycogenolysis and increase basal metabolic rate through their sympathetic nervous system activity.
- **Thyroid hormones** modulate the impact of other metabolic hormones and have a direct impact on basal metabolic rate.
  - T_3 is more potent than T_4, but has a shorter half-life and is available in lower concentrations in the blood.
  - T_4 is converted to T_3 at the tissues.

Tissue-Specific Metabolism

- The liver is the most metabolically diverse tissue.
  - Hepatocytes are responsible for the maintenance of blood glucose levels by glycogenolysis and gluconeogenesis in response to pancreatic hormone stimulation.
  - The liver also participates in the processing of lipids and cholesterol, bile, urea, and toxins.
- Adipose tissue stores lipids under the influence of insulin and releases them under the influence of epinephrine.
- Skeletal muscle metabolism differs based on the current activity level and fiber type.
  - Resting muscle conserves carbohydrates in glycogen stores and uses free fatty acids from the bloodstream.
  - Active muscle may use anaerobic metabolism, oxidative phosphorylation of glucose, direct phosphorylation from creatine phosphate, or fatty acid oxidation, depending on fiber type and exercise duration.
- Cardiac muscle uses fatty acid oxidation in both the well-fed and fasting states.
- The brain and other nervous tissues consume glucose in all metabolic states, except for prolonged fasts, where up to $\frac{2}{3}$ of the brain's fuel may come from ketone bodies.

Integrative Metabolism

- Metabolic rates can be measured using **calorimetry**, **respirometry**, consumption tracking, or measurement of blood concentrations of substrates and hormones.
- Composition of fuel that is actively consumed by the body is estimated by the **respiratory quotient (RQ)**.
- Body mass regulation is multifactorial with consumption and activity as modifiable factors.
  - The hormones **leptin**, **ghrelin**, and **orexin**, as well as their receptors, play a role in body mass.
  - Long-term changes in body mass result from changes in lipid storage.
  - Changes in consumption or activity must surpass a **threshold** to cause weight change. The threshold is lower for weight gain than for weight loss.
  - Body mass can be measured and tracked using the **body mass index (BMI)**.

ANSWERS TO CONCEPT CHECKS

12.1

1. $\Delta G^{\circ\prime}$ adjusts only for the pH of the environment by fixing it at 7. Temperature and concentrations of all other reagents are still fixed at their values from standard conditions and must be adjusted for if they are not 1 M.
2. The cellular environment has a relatively fixed volume and pressure, which eliminates work from our calculations of internal energy; if $\Delta U = Q - W$ and $W = 0$, $\Delta U = Q$.
3.

	$+\Delta H$	$-\Delta H$
$+\Delta S$	Spontaneous at high temperatures	Spontaneous
$-\Delta S$	Nonspontaneous	Spontaneous at low temperatures

12.2

1. ATP hydrolysis yields about $30\,\frac{\text{kJ}}{\text{mol}}$ of energy, which can be harnessed to drive other reactions forward. This may either allow a nonspontaneous reaction to occur or increase the rate of a spontaneous reaction.
2. ATP is an intermediate-energy storage molecule and is not energetically dense. The high-energy bonds in ATP and the presence of a significant charge make it an inefficient molecule to pack into a small space. Long-term storage molecules are characterized by energy density and stable, nonrepulsive bonds, primarily seen in lipids.
3.

$$\begin{array}{lr} \text{cAMP} + H_2O \rightarrow \text{AMP} & \Delta G^{\circ\prime} = -50.4\,\frac{\text{kJ}}{\text{mol}} \\ \text{AMP} + P_i \rightarrow \text{ADP} + H_2O & \Delta G^{\circ\prime} = 30.5\,\frac{\text{kJ}}{\text{mol}} \\ \text{ADP} + P_i \rightarrow \text{ATP} + H_2O & \Delta G^{\circ\prime} = 30.5\,\frac{\text{kJ}}{\text{mol}} \\ \hline \text{cAMP} + 2P_i \rightarrow \text{ATP} + H_2O & \Delta G^{\circ\prime} = 10.6\,\frac{\text{kJ}}{\text{mol}} \end{array}$$

12.3

1. Analyzing half-reactions can help to determine the number of electrons being transferred. This type of analysis also facilitates balancing equations and the determination of electrochemical potential if reduction potentials are provided.
2.

Electron Carrier	Metabolic Pathway(s)
NADH	Glycolysis, fermentation, citric acid cycle, electron transport chain
NADPH	Pentose phosphate pathway, lipid biosynthesis, bleach formation, oxidative stress, photosynthesis
Ubiquinone (CoQ)	Electron transport chain
Cytochromes	Electron transport chain
Glutathione	Oxidative stress

12.4

1. Any excitable cell is maintained in a state of disequilibrium. Classic examples include muscle tissue and neurons. In addition, cell volume and membrane transport are regulated by the action of the sodium–potassium pump, which can maintain a stable disequilibrium state in most tissues.
2. Cells that rely solely on anaerobic respiration are the least adaptable to different energy sources. Therefore, red blood cells are the least flexible during periods of prolonged starvation and stay reliant on glucose.
3. During the postabsorptive state, there is the greatest decrease in insulin levels. The concentrations of the counterregulatory hormones (glucagon, cortisol, epinephrine, norepinephrine, and growth hormone) begin to rise.

12.5

1. Insulin promotes glucose uptake by adipose tissue and muscle, glucose utilization in muscle cells, and macromolecule storage (glycogenesis, lipogenesis). Glucagon increases blood glucose levels by promoting glycogenolysis, gluconeogenesis, lipolysis, and ketogenesis. Cortisol increases lipolysis and amino acid mobilization, while decreasing glucose uptake in certain tissues and enhancing the activity of other counterregulatory hormones. Catecholamines increase glycogenolysis in muscle and liver and lipolysis in adipose tissue. Thyroid hormones increase basic metabolic rate and potentiate the activity of other hormones.
2. Thyroid storm presents with hyperthermia (high temperature), tachycardia (fast heart rate), hypertension (high blood pressure), and tachypnea (high respiratory rate).

12.6

1. The preferred fuel for most cells in the well-fed state is glucose; the exception is cardiac muscle, which prefers fatty acids.
2. The brain consumes the greatest amount of glucose relative to its percentage of body mass.
3. The liver is responsible for maintaining a steady-state concentration of glucose in the blood through glucose uptake and storage, glycogenolysis, and gluconeogenesis. The liver also participates in cholesterol and fat metabolism, the urea cycle, bile synthesis, and the detoxification of foreign substances.

12.7

1. As a person begins to exercise, the proportion of energy derived from glucose increases. This transition to almost exclusively carbohydrate metabolism will cause the respiratory quotient to approach 1.
2. False; energy expenditure, genetics, socioeconomic status, geography, and other hormones also play a role in body mass regulation.
3. True; the threshold is lower for uncompensated weight gain than it is for uncompensated weight loss. Therefore, it is easier to surpass this threshold and gain weight than to lose weight.
4. The methods described in the text include chemical analysis, which is objective and can quantify specific metabolic substrates, products, and enzymes; calorimetry, which is most accurate for basal metabolic rate but also most expensive; respirometry, which provides basic information about fuel sources; and caloric analysis at constant weight (food and exercise logs), which is the least invasive. Any of these answers could be defended.

SCIENCE MASTERY ASSESSMENT EXPLANATIONS

1. **C**

In a closed biological system, enthalpy, heat, and internal energy are all directly related because there is no change in pressure or volume. Because pressure and volume are fixed, work cannot be done, thus **(C)** is correct.

2. **B**

To solve this question, we can use the equation $\Delta G = \Delta G^\circ + RT \ln Q$. Q, the reaction quotient, is $\frac{[B][C]^2}{[A]}$ for this reaction. Plugging in the variables, we get:

$$\Delta G = 0 + RT \ln \frac{[10 \times 10^{-3}][10 \times 10^{-3}]^2}{[10 \times 10^{-3}]}$$
$$= RT \ln 10^{-4} = -4\,RT \ln 10.$$

Because both R and T are positive, and natural log values being greater than 0, we know that ΔG must be negative and therefore lower than the original value. A negative ΔG corresponds to a spontaneous reaction.

3. **C**

The hydrolysis of ATP is energetically favorable because there are repulsive negative charges that are relieved when hydrolyzed, and the new compounds are stabilized by resonance. This is true of both ATP and ADP. Some of the other answer choices are tempting, though. In **(A)**, ATP hydrolysis relies on pH because a protonated ATP molecule contains less negative charge and therefore experiences less repulsive force. For **(B)**, the energy released by one mole of creatine phosphate upon hydrolysis is not sufficient to phosphorylate two moles of ADP according to Table 12.1; creatine phosphate donates one phosphate group to a molecule of ADP, so one mole of creatine phosphate will phosphorylate one mole of ADP. For **(D)**, the removal of two phosphate groups from ATP yields AMP, not cyclic AMP.

4. **A**

Reduction is a gain of electrons, which eliminates **(B)** because it is an oxidation reaction. NADPH, **(C)**, is a product of the pentose phosphate pathway. Ubiquinone, **(D)**, transfers electrons during the course of the electron transport chain, but is not the final electron acceptor. This title belongs to oxygen.

5. **B**

In order to transport electrons, electron carriers like flavoproteins must be able to exist in a stable oxidized state and a stable reduced form. ATP can be dephosphorylated but is generally not oxidized or reduced. Regulatory enzymes may also be phosphorylated or dephosphorylated but are not generally oxidized or reduced.

6. **B**

Skipping a single meal is not a prolonged fast. However, the increase in hormones that promote gluconeogenesis and glycogenolysis indicates that the absorptive phase has ended.

7. **D**

In the well-fed state, the liver runs off of glucose and amino acids, the brain and adipose tissue run off of glucose, and cardiac muscle runs off of fatty acids. Only **(D)** correctly pairs the tissue with its energy source.

8. **A**

Hormonal controls are coordinated to regulate the metabolic activity of the entire organism, while allosteric controls can be local or systemic. The modification of the enzymes of glycogen metabolism by insulin and glucagon is either through phosphorylation or dephosphorylation, both of which modify covalent bonds.

9. **B**

Adipose tissue and resting skeletal muscle require insulin for glucose uptake. Active skeletal muscle, **(A)**, uses creatine phosphate and glycogen (regulated by epinephrine and AMP) to maintain its energy requirements.

10. **C**

Short-term glucocorticoid exposure causes a release of glucose and the hydrolysis of fats from adipocytes. However, if this glucose is not used for metabolism, it causes an increase in glucose level which promotes fat storage. The net result is the release of glucose from the liver to be converted into lipids in the adipose tissue under insulin stimulation.

11. **B**

The brain uses aerobic metabolism of glucose exclusively and therefore is very sensitive to oxygen levels. The extremely high oxygen requirement of the brain (20% of the body's oxygen content) relative to its size (2% of total body weight) implies that brain is the most sensitive organ to oxygen deprivation.

12. **B**

The respiratory quotient (RQ) gives an indication of the primary fuel being utilized. An RQ around 0.7 indicates lipid metabolism, 0.8–0.9 indicates amino acid metabolism, **(D)**, and 1.0 indicates carbohydrate metabolism, **(A)**. Nucleic acids do not contribute significantly to the respiratory quotient.

13. **A**

Leptin acts to decrease appetite by inhibiting the production of orexin. Orexin is also associated with alertness, so decreasing the level of orexin in the body is expected to cause drowsiness. Even without this information, the answer should be apparent because the body tends to maintain an energy balance. If consumption decreases, energy expenditures are expected to decrease as well.

14. **C**

ATP stores are turned over about 1,000 times per day, not 10,000.

15. **D**

A prolonged fast is characterized by an increase in glucagon, which accomplishes its cellular activity by phosphorylating and dephosphorylating metabolic enzymes. Glycogen storage, **(B)**, is then halted, but this requires enzyme regulation by glucagon to occur. Later in the postabsorptive state, protein breakdown, **(C)**, begins. Eventually, in starvation, ketone bodies, **(A)**, are used by the brain for its main energy source.

Consult your online resources for additional practice. **GO ONLINE**

EQUATIONS TO REMEMBER

(12.1) **Gibbs free energy:** $\Delta G = \Delta H - T\Delta S$

(12.2) **Modified standard state:** $\Delta G = \Delta G^{\circ} + RT\ln(Q)$

(12.3) **Respiratory quotient:** $\text{RQ} = \frac{CO_2 \text{ produced}}{O_2 \text{ consumed}}$

(12.4) **Body mass index:** $\text{BMI} = \frac{\text{mass}}{\text{height}^2}$

SHARED CONCEPTS

Biochemistry Chapter 9
Carbohydrate Metabolism I

Biochemistry Chapter 10
Carbohydrate Metabolism II

Biochemistry Chapter 11
Lipid and Amino Acid Metabolism

Biology Chapter 5
The Endocrine System

General Chemistry Chapter 11
Oxidation–Reduction Reactions

Physics and Math Chapter 3
Thermodynamics

GLOSSARY

Absolute configuration–The nomenclature system used for the three-dimensional arrangement of atoms in isomers; the most common systems are D/L and (*R*)/(*S*).

Acetal–A carbon atom bonded to an alkyl group, two –OR groups, and a hydrogen.

Acetyl-CoA–An important metabolic intermediate that links glycolysis and β-oxidation to the citric acid cycle; can also be converted into ketone bodies.

Activation–The conversion of a biomolecule to its active or usable form, such as activation of tRNA with an amino acid or activation of a fatty acid with CoA to form fatty acyl-CoA.

Activation energy–The energy required to change the state of a molecule or group of molecules to the transition state; the energy required for a reaction to occur.

Active site–The catalytically active portion of an enzyme.

Active transport–The movement of a molecule against its concentration gradient with energy investment; primary active transport uses ATP, whereas secondary active transport uses a favorable transport gradient of a different molecule.

Activity–The measure of the catalytic activity of an enzyme, also called the velocity or rate. It is often measured as a v_{max} and may be analyzed after protein isolation.

Activity analysis–The determination of the enzymatic activity of an isolated protein by interaction with a substrate; usually colorimetric in nature.

Adenosine triphosphate (ATP)–The primary energy molecule of the body; it releases energy by breaking the bond with the terminal phosphate to form ADP and inorganic phosphate.

Adipocyte–A cell specializing in fat storage.

Aerobic respiration–A collection of energy-producing metabolic processes that require oxygen, including the citric acid cycle, electron transport chain, and oxidative phosphorylation.

Agglutination–Clumping of particles caused by the binding of antibody to target antigen.

Aldose–A sugar in which the highest-order functional group is an aldehyde; can be categorized by number of carbons (triose, tetrose, pentose, hexose, etc.).

Allosteric enzymes–Enzymes that experience changes in their conformation as a result of interactions at sites other than the active site, called allosteric sites; conformational changes may increase or decrease enzyme activity.

α-Helix–An element of secondary structure, marked by clockwise coiling of amino acids around a central axis.

Alternative splicing–The production of multiple different but related mRNA molecules from a single primary transcript of hnRNA.

Amino acid–A dipolar compound containing an amino group ($-NH_2$) and a carboxyl group ($-COOH$).

Amphipathic–Having both hydrophilic and hydrophobic regions.

Amphoteric–The ability to act as an acid or base.

Amplification–Increased transcription (and translation) of a gene in response to hormones, growth factors, and other intracellular conditions.

Anabolism–The series of metabolic processes that result in the consumption of energy and the synthesis of molecules.

Anaerobic respiration–The series of energy-producing metabolic processes that do not require oxygen, including glycolysis and fermentation.

Anomers–A subtype of epimers in which the chiral carbon with inverted configuration was the carbonyl carbon (anomeric carbon).

Antibody–A specialized protein molecule produced by lymphocytes for interaction with antigens; antibodies consist of two heavy and two light chains that have constant and variable regions. Antibodies, also called immunoglobulins, are mediators of the immune response.

Anticodon–A three-nucleotide sequence on a tRNA molecule that pairs with a corresponding mRNA codon during translation.

Antigen–The region of a molecule that interacts with an antibody; in most cases, antigens are proteins.

Apoenzyme–An enzyme devoid of the prosthetic group, coenzyme, or cofactor necessary for normal activity.

Apolipoproteins–Protein molecules responsible for the interaction of lipoproteins with cells and the transfer of lipid molecules between lipoproteins; also called apoproteins.

Aromaticity–The ability of a molecule to delocalize π electrons around a conjugated ring, creating exceptional stability.

Basal metabolic rate–The amount of energy consumed in a given period of time by a resting organism.

β-Oxidation–The catabolism of fatty acids to acetyl-CoA.

β-Pleated sheet–An element of secondary structure, marked by peptide chains lying alongside one another, forming rows or strands.

Bile–A mixture of salts, pigments, and cholesterol that acts to emulsify lipids in the small intestine.

Binding proteins–Proteins that transport or sequester molecules by binding to them. Binding proteins have affinity curves for their molecules of interest.

Bioenergetics–Biochemistry of the energy involved in bond interactions in biological organisms.

Biosignaling–The process by which cells receive and act on messages.

Bradford protein assay–A colorimetric method of determining the concentration of protein in an isolate against a protein standard; relies on a transition of absorption between bound and unbound Coomassie Brilliant Blue dye.

Cahn–Ingold–Prelog system–The system used to name isomers ((*E*) *vs.* (*Z*); (*R*) *vs.* (*S*)), based on the atomic numbers of their substituents and their orientation in three-dimensional space.

Calorimeter–A device for measuring the heat change during the course of a reaction.

Carboxylation–The addition of carboxylic acid groups to a molecule.

Carotenoids–A group of molecules that are tetraterpenes (made of eight isoprene units).

Catabolism–The series of metabolic processes that result in the release of energy and the breakdown of molecules.

Catalyst–A substance or enzyme that increases the rate of a reaction by lowering activation energy. Catalysts are not consumed during the catalyzed reaction.

Catalytic efficiency–The ratio of k_{cat}/K_m. Catalytic efficiency is directly related to efficiency of enzyme function.

Catecholamines–Mediators of the sympathetic nervous system and adrenal gland; include epinephrine and norepinephrine.

Cell adhesion molecules–Specialized structural proteins that are involved in cell–cell junctions as well as transient cellular interactions; common cell adhesion molecules are cadherins, integrins, and selectins.

Cellulose–A homopolysaccharide of glucose, and the main structural component of plants. Cellulose is indigestible for humans.

Central dogma of molecular biology–The major steps in the transfer of genetic information, from transcription of DNA to RNA to translation of that RNA to protein.

Centrifugation–The process of separating components on the basis of their density and resistance to flow by spinning a sample at very high speeds; the highest density materials form a solid pellet and the lowest density materials remain in the supernatant (liquid portion).

Centromere–The area of a chromosome where sister chromatids are joined; it is also the point of attachment to the spindle fiber during mitosis and meiosis.

Ceramide–The simplest sphingolipid, with a single hydrogen as its head group.

Cerebroside–A sphingolipid containing a carbohydrate as a head group.

Chaperones–Proteins that assist in protein folding during posttranslational processing.

Chargaff's rule–DNA from any source should have a 1:1 ratio of pyrimidine to purine bases, with adenine equal to thymine and cytosine equal to guanine.

Chemiosmotic coupling–The utilization of the proton-motive force generated by the electron transport chain to drive ATP synthesis in oxidative phosphorylation.

Chiral–Describes a molecule with a nonsuperimposable mirror image.

Chiral center–A carbon atom bonded to four different substituents; a chiral compound must have at least one chiral center.

Cholesterol–A molecule containing four linked aromatic rings; cholesterol provides both fluidity and stability to cell membranes and is the precursor for steroid hormones.

Chromatid–Each of the two chromosomal strands formed by DNA replication in the S phase of the cell cycle, held together by the centromere. Identical pairs of chromatids are referred to as sister chromatids.

Chromatography–The process of separating molecules by their interactions with a stationary phase and a mobile phase; most chromatographic methods rely on the chemical similarity of molecules, with the exception of size-exclusion chromatography.

Chromosome–A filamentous body found within the nucleus of a eukaryotic cell or nucleoid region of a prokaryotic cell, composed of DNA.

Citric acid cycle–A metabolic pathway that produces GTP, energy carriers, and carbon dioxide as it burns acetyl-CoA; also called the Krebs cycle or tricarboxylic acid (TCA) cycle; can share intermediates with many other metabolic processes including fatty acid and cholesterol synthesis, gluconeogenesis, amino acid metabolism, and others.

Closed system–A system capable of exchanging energy, but not matter, with the environment.

Coding strand–The strand of DNA that is not used as a template during transcription; also called the sense strand.

Codon–A three-nucleotide sequence in an mRNA molecule that pairs with an appropriate tRNA anticodon during translation.

Coenzyme–An organic molecule that helps an enzyme carry out its function.

Cofactor–An inorganic molecule or ion that helps an enzyme carry out its function.

Colligative properties–Physical properties that change according to the concentration of solutes, but not their identity. Colligative properties include vapor pressure depression, boiling point elevation, freezing point depression, and osmotic pressure.

Colloid–A mixture composed of large molecules of one substance suspended within another substance.

Competitive inhibition–A decrease in enzyme activity that results from the interaction of an inhibitor with the active site of an enzyme; competitive inhibition can be overcome by addition of excess substrate.

Condensation reaction–A reaction in which the removal of a water molecule accompanies the formation of a bond; also called a dehydration reaction.

Conformational coupling–A less-accepted mechanism of ATP synthase activity in which the protons cause a conformational change that releases ATP from ATP synthase.

Conjugated protein–A protein that derives part of its function from covalently attached molecules (prosthetic groups).

Cooperativity–The interaction between subunits of a multi-subunit protein in which binding of substrate to one subunit increases the affinity of other subunits for the substrate; unbinding of substrate from one unit decreases the affinity of other subunits for the substrate.

Corepressor–A species that binds with a repressor, allowing the complex to bind to the operator region of an operon, stopping transcription of the relevant gene.

Cristae–The infoldings of the inner mitochondrial membrane that increase the surface area available for electron transport chain complexes.

C-terminus–The free carboxyl end of a polypeptide.

Dalton (Da)–Molar mass unit used for protein molecular weight. One amino acid weighs approximately 100 Da, or $100\frac{\text{g}}{\text{mol}}$.

Degeneracy–A characteristic of the genetic code, in which more than one codon can specify a single amino acid.

Denaturation–The loss of secondary, tertiary, or quaternary structure in a protein, leading to loss of function.

Deoxyribonucleic acid (DNA)–A nucleic acid found exclusively in the nucleus that codes for all of the genes necessary for life; transcribed to mRNA and always read 5′ to 3′.

Desmosomes–Cell–cell junctions that anchor layers of epithelial cells to one another.

Diastereomers–Compounds with at least one—but not all—chiral carbons in inverted configurations; differ in physical properties.

Diprotic–Containing two hydrogens (acid), or being able to pick up two hydrogens (base).

Disulfide bond–A covalent interaction between the –SH groups of two cysteine residues; an element of tertiary and quaternary structure.

Edman degradation–A stepwise process for determining the amino acid sequence in an isolated protein.

Electrochemical gradient–An uneven separation of ions across a biological membrane, resulting in potential energy.

Electrophoresis–The process of separating compounds on the basis of size and charge using a porous gel and an electric field; protein electrophoresis generally uses polyacrylamide, while nucleic acid electrophoresis generally uses agarose.

Elongation–The three-step cycle that is repeated for each amino acid being added to a protein during translation.

Emulsification–The mixing of two normally immiscible liquids.

Enantiomers–Compounds that are nonsuperimposable mirror images; have the same physical and chemical properties except for rotation of plane-polarized light and interaction with a chiral environment.

Endocytosis–The transport of molecules into a cell through the invagination of cell membrane and the formation of a vesicle; phagocytosis is the endocytosis of solid, pinocytosis is the endocytosis of liquid.

Endothermic reaction–A reaction that requires heat (positive ΔH).

Enhancer–A collection of several response elements that allow for the control of one gene's expression by multiple signals.

Enthalpy–The overall change in heat of a system during a reaction.

Entropy–The disorder of a system; systems in which entropy is increased are generally favored.

Enzyme–A biological molecule with catalytic activity; includes many proteins and some RNA molecules. Enzymes are specified for target substrate molecules.

Enzyme-linked receptor–A transmembrane protein that displays catalytic activity in response to ligand binding.

Epimers–A subtype of diastereomers that differ in absolute configuration at exactly one chiral carbon.

Euchromatin–The looser, less-dense collections of DNA that appear light colored under a microscope; transcriptionally active.

Exocytosis–The transport of molecules out of a cell by release from a transport vesicle; the vesicle fuses to the cell membrane during secretion.

Exon–A portion of hnRNA that is spliced with other exons to form mature mRNA.

Exothermic reaction–A reaction that releases heat (negative ΔH).

Facilitated diffusion–The movement of solute molecules across the cell membrane down their concentration gradients through a transport protein or channel; used for ions and large or polar molecules.

Fatty acid–A monocarboxylic acid without additional substituents; fatty acids may be saturated (all single bonds) or unsaturated (contain at least one double bond); natural fatty acids are in the *cis* conformation.

Feedback inhibition–The inhibition of an enzyme by its product (or a product further down a metabolic pathway); used to maintain homeostasis.

Feed-forward activation–The stimulation of an enzyme by an intermediate that precedes the enzyme in a metabolic pathway.

Fermentation–The conversion of pyruvate to either ethanol and carbon dioxide (yeast) or lactic acid (animal cells); does not require oxygen.

Fibrous protein–A protein composed of long sheets or strands, such as collagen.

Fischer projection–A method of drawing organic molecules in which horizontal lines are coming out of the page (wedges) and vertical lines are going into the page (dashes).

Flavin adenine dinucleotide (FAD)–An energy carrier that accepts electrons and feeds them into the electron transport chain.

Flavoprotein–A protein bonded to FAD.

Fluid mosaic model–The representation of the plasma membrane as a dynamic phospholipid bilayer with interactions of cholesterol, proteins, and carbohydrates.

Frameshift mutation–A change in DNA in which the reading frame of the codons in mRNA is shifted due to the insertion or deletion of nucleotides (other than in multiples of three).

Fructose–A monosaccharide found predominantly in fruit and honey.

Furanose–A five-membered ring sugar.

G protein-coupled receptors–A special class of membrane receptors with an associated GTP-binding protein; activation of a G protein-coupled receptor involves dissociation and GTP hydrolysis.

Galactose–A monosaccharide found predominantly in dairy.

Ganglioside–A sphingolipid with a head group containing an oligosaccharide and one or more *N*-acetylneuraminic acid (NANA) molecules.

Gap junctions–Cell–cell junctions that allow for the passage of small molecules between adjacent cells.

Gene–A unit of DNA that encodes a specific protein or RNA molecule.

Globoside–A sphingolipid with multiple carbohydrate groups attached as a head group.

Globular protein–A protein with a roughly spherical structure, such as myoglobin.

Glucagon–A mediator of glucose release that is secreted by pancreatic α-cells; rises in response to low blood glucose.

Glucogenic–Describes amino acids that can be converted into intermediates that feed into gluconeogenesis; all except leucine and lysine.

Gluconeogenesis–The production of glucose from other biomolecules; carried out by the liver and kidney.

Glucose–The primary monosaccharide used for fuel by all cells of the body, with the formula $C_6H_{12}O_6$.

Glycerol–A three-carbon alcohol that serves as the backbone for glycerophospholipids, sphingolipids, and triacylglycerols.

Glycerophospholipid–Also referred to as a phosphoglyceride; a lipid containing a glycerol backbone with a phosphate group, bonded by ester linkages to two fatty acids.

Glycogen–A branched polymer of glucose that represents a storage form of glucose.

Glycogenesis–The synthesis of glycogen granules.

Glycogenolysis–The breakdown of glycogen granules.

Glycolysis–The breakdown of glucose to two molecules of pyruvate, with the formation of energy carriers (NADH); occurs under both aerobic and anaerobic conditions.

Glycosidic linkage–The bond between the anomeric carbon of a sugar and another molecule.

Glycosphingolipid–A sphingolipid with a head group composed of sugars; includes cerebrosides and globosides.

Glycosylation–The addition of sugars to a molecule.

Haworth projection–A method for depicting cyclic sugars as planar rings with –OH groups sticking up or down from the plane of the sugar.

Hemiacetal–A carbon atom bonded to an alkyl group, an –OR group, an –OH group, and a hydrogen.

Hemiketal–A carbon atom bonded to two alkyl groups, an –OR group, and an –OH group.

Hess's law–A relationship that states that the total change in any state function is the same regardless of the path taken or the number of steps, and is equal to the difference between initial and final values of that state function.

Heterochromatin–The tightly coiled DNA that appears dark colored under a microscope; transcriptionally inactive.

Heterogeneous nuclear RNA (hnRNA)–The precursor to processed mRNA; converted to mRNA by adding a poly-A tail and 5′ cap and splicing out introns.

Hill's coefficient–A quantitative measure of cooperative binding effects in enzymes.

Histone–A structural protein about which DNA is coiled in eukaryotic cells. Histone association with DNA can be altered by acetylation of histone proteins or methylation of the DNA strand.

Holoenzyme–An enzyme that has already bound a required prosthetic group, coenzyme, or cofactor.

Homeostasis–The stable internal state of an organism; homeostasis is not synonymous with equilibrium.

Homogenization–The process of breaking cell membranes and creating a uniform mixture of cell components for further separation; may be accomplished chemically or physically.

Hormone-sensitive lipase–The enzyme responsible for the mobilization of fatty acids from adipocytes; responds to a decrease in insulin levels.

Hückel's rule–One condition for aromaticity, which states the compound must have $4n + 2$ (where n is any integer) π electrons.

Hybridization–In research techniques involving DNA, the joining of complementary base pair sequences.

Hydrolase–An enzyme that catalyzes the cleavage of a molecule with the addition of water.

Hydrolysis–Breaking a covalent bond with the assistance of a water molecule.

Hydrophilic–Being attracted to water; describes polar and charged compounds and those that can participate in hydrogen bonding.

Hydrophobic–Being repelled by water; describes nonpolar, uncharged compounds (usually lipids or certain R groups of amino acids).

Hypertonic–A solution that has a greater concentration than the one to which it is being compared.

Hypotonic–A solution that has a lower concentration than the one to which it is being compared.

Induced fit model–The best-supported of the most prominent theories of enzyme specificity; states that the enzyme and substrate experience a change in conformation during binding to increase complementarity. Usually contrasted with the lock and key theory.

Inducible system–An operon that requires an inducer to remove a repressor protein from the operator site to begin transcription of the relevant gene.

Initiation–The start of translation, in which the small subunit of the ribosome binds to the mRNA molecule, and the first tRNA (methionine or *N*-formylmethionine) is bound to the start codon (AUG).

Insulin–The primary mediator of carbohydrate metabolism that is secreted by pancreatic β-cells; rises in response to high blood glucose.

Internal energy–The sum of all of the different interactions between and within atoms in a system; vibration, rotation, linear motion, and stored chemical energies all contribute.

Intron–A portion of hnRNA that is spliced out to form mRNA; remains in the nucleus during processing.

Ion channels–Proteins that form a pore through the membrane in which they are embedded.

Irreversible inhibition–A decrease in enzyme activity that results from the interaction of an inhibitor that binds permanently at either the active site or an allosteric site; in laboratory settings, irreversible inhibitors are sometimes called suicide substrates.

Isoelectric focusing–A specialized method of separating proteins by their isoelectric point using electrophoresis; the gel is modified to possess a pH gradient.

Isoelectric point (pI)–The pH at which an amino acid is predominantly in zwitterionic form.

Isoform–A slightly different version of the same protein, often specific to a given tissue.

Isomerase–An enzyme that catalyzes the constitutional or stereochemical rearrangement of a molecule.

Isotonic–A solution that has the same concentration as the one to which it is being compared.

Jacob–Monod model–The description of the structure and function of operons in prokaryotes, in which operons have structural genes, an operator site, a promoter site, and a regulator gene.

k_{cat}–Rate of catalytic conversion of substrate. This value gives the number of substrate molecules turned over per enzyme molecule per second.

Ketal–A carbon atom bonded to two alkyl groups and two –OR groups.

Ketogenesis–The synthesis of ketone bodies from the metabolic products of β-oxidation or amino acid metabolism; occurs under conditions of starvation.

Ketogenic–Describes amino acids that can be converted into ketone bodies.

Ketolysis–The breakdown of ketone bodies for use as acetyl-CoA.

Ketose–A sugar in which the highest-order functional group is a ketone; can be categorized by number of carbons (triose, tetrose, pentose, hexose, and so on).

Kinase–A specific transferase protein that catalyzes the movement of a phosphate group, generally from ATP, to a molecule of interest.

K_m–The concentration of substrate at which an enzyme runs at half its maximal velocity; a measure of enzyme affinity (the higher the K_m, the lower the affinity).

Lactose–A disaccharide composed of glucose and galactose.

Lariat–The lasso-shaped structure formed during the removal of introns in mRNA processing.

Ligase–An enzyme that catalyzes the synthesis of large polymeric biomolecules, most commonly nucleic acids.

Lipid–A molecule that is insoluble in water and soluble in nonpolar organic solvents.

Lipoprotein–The transport mechanism for lipids within the circulatory and lymphatic systems; includes chylomicrons and VLDL, which transport triacylglycerols; and HDL, IDL, and LDL, which transport cholesterol and cholesteryl esters.

Lock and key theory–One of the two most prominent theories of enzyme specificity; states that the enzyme and the substrate have a static but complementary state. Less supported than the induced fit model.

Lyase–An enzyme that catalyzes the cleavage or synthesis of a molecule without the addition or loss of water.

Maltose–A disaccharide composed of two glucose molecules.

Matrix–The contents of the inner mitochondrial membrane; includes soluble enzymes of the electron transport chain and mitochondrial DNA.

Membrane–In cell biology, a double layer of phospholipids and proteins that forms the boundaries of cells and organelles within cells.

Membrane receptors–Transmembrane protein molecules that act enzymatically or as ion channels to participate in signal transduction.

Messenger RNA (mRNA)–The strand of RNA formed after transcription of DNA; transfers to the cytoplasm to be translated.

Micelle–A collection of fatty acid or phospholipid molecules oriented to minimize free energy through hydrophobic and hydrophilic interactions; generally a sphere with a hydrophobic core and hydrophilic exterior.

Migration velocity–the velocity at which a compound moves through a gel during electrophoresis.

Missense mutation–A mutation in which one amino acid is substituted for by a different amino acid.

Mitochondria–The organelle responsible for aerobic respiration, generating ATP from the breakdown products of other biomolecules and energy carriers reduced in various metabolic pathways; contains an inner and outer membrane.

Mixed inhibition–A decrease in enzyme activity that results from the interaction of an inhibitor with an allosteric site; mixed inhibitors bind to free enzyme and to substrate-bound enzyme with different affinities. They cannot be overcome by addition of substrate and impact both K_m and v_{max}.

Molten globules–Intermediate states in the folding of a protein.

Monocistronic–The coding pattern of eukaryotes in which one mRNA molecule codes for only one protein.

Monoprotic–Containing only one hydrogen (acid), or being able to pick up only one hydrogen (base).

Monosaccharide–A single sugar monomer; common examples are glucose, galactose, and fructose.

Motor proteins–Proteins that are involved in cell motility through interactions with structural proteins; motor proteins have ATPase activity and include myosin, kinesin, and dynein.

Mutarotation–The rapid interconversion between different anomers of a sugar.

Negative control–In prokaryotic genetics, an operon that requires the binding of a protein to decrease transcription.

Nicotinamide adenine dinucleotide (NAD^+)–An energy carrier that accepts electrons and feeds them into the electron transport chain.

Nicotinamide adenine dinucleotide phosphate ($NADP^+$)–An electron donor produced in the pentose phosphate pathway that is involved in biosynthesis, oxidative stress, and immune function.

NMR spectroscopy–A method of determining molecular structure that uses the relative position of carbons and hydrogens determined by the relative shielding and spins of electrons observed when molecule is exposed to a magnetic field.

Noncompetitive inhibition–A decrease in enzyme activity that results from the interaction of an inhibitor with an allosteric site; noncompetitive inhibitors bind equally well to free enzyme and to substrate-bound enzyme. They cannot be overcome by addition of substrate.

Nonsense mutation–A mutation in which a coding codon is changed to a stop codon. Also called a truncation mutation.

Nontemplate synthesis–The method of *de novo* synthesis of lipids and carbohydrates that relies on gene expression and enzyme specificity rather than the genetic template of DNA or RNA.

N-terminus–The free amino end of a polypeptide.

Nuclear pore–A hole in the nuclear envelope that permits the entrance and exit of substrates.

Nucleoside–Molecule composed of a pentose bound to a nitrogenous base at the C-1′ position of the sugar.

Nucleotide–Molecule composed of one or more phosphate groups bound to the C-5′ position of a nucleoside.

Nucleotide excision repair–Method for removing thymine dimers from DNA strands via a cut-and-patch process.

Okazaki fragments–Small strands formed on the lagging strand during DNA synthesis due to the unidirectional nature of DNA synthesis.

Oncogenes–Mutated genes that cause cancer.

Open system–A system capable of exchanging both matter and energy with the environment.

Operator site–A component of the operon in prokaryotes; a nontranscribable region of DNA that is capable of binding a repressor protein.

Operon–In prokaryotes, a cluster of genes transcribed as a single mRNA that can be regulated by repressors or inducers, depending on the system.

Opsonization–The marking of a pathogen by an antibody for later destruction.

Origins of replication–Sites at which DNA unwinds to allow replication of new DNA. Generation of new DNA in both directions occurs at origins of replication, resulting in replication forks.

Osmosis–The simple diffusion of water.

Osmotic pressure–The pressure necessary to counteract the effect of an osmotic gradient against pure water; one of the colligative properties.

Oxidative phosphorylation–The transfer of a phosphate group, generally to ATP that is powered by a gradient formed by oxidation–reduction reactions; occurs in the mitochondria.

Oxidoreductase–An enzyme that catalyzes an oxidation–reduction reaction, often using an electron carrier as a cofactor.

Pancreatic lipase–The primary enzyme involved in the digestion of lipids.

Pancreatic proteases–The enzymes that are primarily responsible for the digestion of proteins in the small intestine; they include trypsin, chymotrypsin, and carboxypeptidases A and B, and are secreted as zymogens.

Paracellular transport–The transport of materials through the interstitial space without interactions with the cytoplasm or cell membrane.

Passive transport–The movement of a molecule down its concentration gradient without energy investment; includes simple and facilitated diffusion and osmosis.

Pentose phosphate pathway–A metabolic process that produces NADPH and ribose 5-phosphate for nucleotide synthesis.

Peptide–A molecule composed of more than one amino acid residue; can be subdivided into dipeptides (two amino acids), tripeptides (3), oligopeptides (up to 20), and polypeptides (more than 20).

Peptide bond–An amide bond between the carboxyl group of one amino acid and the amino group of another amino acid.

Phospholipid–A lipid containing a phosphate and alcohol (glycerol or sphingosine) joined to hydrophobic fatty acid tails.

Phosphorylation–The placement of a phosphate group onto a compound.

pK_a–The pH at which half of the of the molecules of a given acid are deprotonated; $[HA] = [A^-]$.

Point mutation–The substitution of one nucleotide for another in DNA.

Polarity–An uneven sharing of electrons in a molecule, creating a slightly positive side and a slightly negative side.

Polycistronic–The coding pattern of prokaryotes, in which one mRNA may code for multiple proteins.

Polymerase chain reaction–An automated process to produce copies of a DNA sequence without use of bacteria for amplification.

Polyprotic–Containing more than one hydrogen (acid), or being able to pick up more than one hydrogen (base).

Polysaccharide–A long chain of monosaccharides linked by glycosidic bonds; can be divided into homopolysaccharides (only one type of monosaccharide is used) and heteropolysaccharides (more than one type of monosaccharide is used).

Positive control–In prokaryotic genetics, an operon that requires the binding of a protein to increase transcription.

Postprandial state–State shortly after eating characterized by increased anabolism and fuel storage. Also referred to as the absorptive or well-fed state.

Prenylation–The addition of lipid groups to a molecule.

Primary structure–The linear sequence of amino acids in a polypeptide.

Promoter region–The portion of DNA upstream from a gene; contains the TATA box, which is the site where RNA polymerase II binds to start transcription.

Prostaglandin–A group of 20-carbon molecules that are unsaturated carboxylic acids derived from arachidonic acid; act as paracrine or autocrine hormones.

Prosthetic group–A cofactor or coenzyme that is covalently bonded to a protein to permit its function. Proteins with lipid, carbohydrate, and nucleic acid prosthetic groups are referred to as lipoproteins, glycoproteins, and nuceloproteins, respectively.

Protein–A molecule made up of at least one chain of amino acids joined by peptide bonds.

Proteinogenic–The ability of certain (20) amino acids to be integrated into proteins.

Proton-motive force–The proton concentration gradient across the inner mitochondrial membrane that is created in the electron transport chain and used in oxidative phosphorylation.

Purine–Nitrogen-containing base found in nucleotides possessing a two-ring structure. The purines are adenine and guanine.

Pyranose–A six-membered ring sugar.

Pyrimidine–Nitrogen-containing base found in nucleotides possessing a one-ring structure. The three pyrimidines are cytosine, thymine, and uracil.

Pyruvate–An important metabolic intermediate that can feed into the citric acid cycle, fermentation, or gluconeogenesis.

Q cycle–The shuttling of electrons between ubiquinol and ubiquinone in the inner mitochondrial membrane as a part of Complex III's function.

Quaternary structure–The interaction between different subunits of a multi-subunit protein; stabilized by R group interactions.

Reaction coupling–The tendency of unfavorable biological reactions to occur concurrently with favorable reactions, often catalyzed by a single enzyme.

Reading frame–In translation, the three nucleotides that make up a codon.

Recombinant DNA–DNA that has been formed by combining genetic material from multiple sources in a laboratory.

Reducing sugar–A sugar that can reduce other compounds and can be detected by Tollens' or Benedict's reagent.

Regulator gene–In an operon, the gene that codes for the repressor protein.

Release factor–The protein that binds to the stop codon during termination of translation.

Renaturation–The regaining of the correct secondary, tertiary, and quaternary structure after denaturation of a protein.

Replisome–Set of specialized proteins that assist DNA polymerase during replication.

Repressible system–An operon that requires a repressor to bind to a corepressor before binding to the operator site to stop transcription of the relevant gene.

Repressor–For enzymes, an inhibitor of enzyme action; for operons, a species that binds to the operator region to stop transcription of the relevant gene.

Respiratory control–The coordinated regulation of the different aerobic metabolic processes.

Respiratory quotient–A numerical representation that can be used to determine the most prevalent type of biomolecule being used in metabolism; the ratio of carbon dioxide produced to oxygen consumed.

Respirometry–A method of measuring metabolism through the consumption of oxygen.

Resting membrane potential–The electrical potential that results from the unequal distribution of charge around the cell membrane; resting membrane potential characterizes a cell that has not been stimulated.

Restriction enzyme–Enzymes that recognize palindromic double-stranded DNA sequences and cut through the backbone of the double helix at those locations.

Ribonucleic acid (RNA)–A nucleic acid found in both the nucleus and cytoplasm and most closely linked with transcription and translation, as well as some gene regulation.

Ribosomal RNA (rRNA)–The structural and enzymatic RNA found in ribosomes that takes part in translation.

Ribosome–Organelle composed of RNA and protein; it translates mRNA during protein synthesis.

Ribozyme–An RNA molecule with enzymatic activity.

Saponification–The reaction between a fatty acid and a strong base, resulting in a negatively charged fatty acid anion bound to a metal ion; creates soap.

Saturation–The presence or absence of double bonds in a fatty acid; saturated fatty acids have only single bonds, whereas unsaturated fatty acids have at least one double bond.

Secondary structure–The local structure of neighboring amino acids; most common are α-helices and β-pleated sheets.

Sequencing–Determining the order of amino acids in a polypeptide, or of nucleotides in a nucleic acid.

Shine–Dalgarno sequence–The site of initiation of translation in prokaryotes.

Shuttle mechanism–A method of functionally transferring a compound across a membrane without the actual molecule crossing; common examples are the glycerol 3-phosphate shuttle and malate–aspartate shuttle.

Sialic acid–The common name of *N*-acetylneuraminic acid (NANA), which is the terminal portion of the head group in a ganglioside.

Side chain–The variable component of an amino acid that gives the amino acid its identity and chemical properties; also called an R group.

Silent mutation–A mutation in the wobble position of a codon or noncoding DNA that leads to no change in the protein produced during translation.

Simple diffusion–The movement of solute molecules through the cell membrane down their concentration gradients without a transport protein; used for small, nonpolar, lipophilic molecules and water.

Single-stranded DNA-binding protein–Proteins that bind to unraveled DNA strands to prevent reassociation of DNA or degradation of DNA during replication events.

Small nuclear ribonucleoproteins (snRNPs)–The protein portion of the spliceosome complex.

Small nuclear RNA (snRNA)–The RNA portion of the spliceosome complex.

Sodium-potassium pump–An ATPase that exchanges three sodium cations for two potassium cations; responsible for maintaining cell volume and the resting membrane potential.

Solvation layer–The layer of solvent particles that interacts directly with the surface of a dissolved species.

Sphingolipid–A lipid containing a sphingosine or sphingoid backbone, bonded to fatty acid tails; include ceramide, sphingomyelins, glycosphingolipids, and gangliosides.

Sphingomyelin–A sphingophospholipid containing a sphingosine backbone and a phosphate head group.

Spliceosome–The apparatus used for splicing out introns and bringing exons together during mRNA processing.

Starch–A branched polymer of glucose used for energy storage in plants; common examples are amylose and amylopectin.

Start codon–The first codon in an mRNA molecule that codes for an amino acid (AUG for methionine or *N*-formylmethionine).

Stereoisomers–Compounds that have the same chemical formula and backbone, differing only in their spatial orientation; also called optical isomers.

Steroid–A derivative of cholesterol.

Stop codon–The last codon of translation (UAA, UGA, or UAG); release factor binds here, terminating translation.

Structural gene–Within an operon, the region that codes for the protein of interest.

Structural proteins–Proteins that are involved in the cytoskeleton and extracellular matrix; they are generally fibrous in nature and include collagen, elastin, keratin, actin, and tubulin.

Substrate–The molecule upon which an enzyme acts.

Substrate-level phosphorylation–The transfer of a phosphate group from a high-energy compound to ATP or another compound; occurs in glycolysis.

Sucrose–A disaccharide composed of glucose and fructose.

Supercoiling–Wrapping of DNA on itself during replication, characterized by torsional stress and potential for strand breakage.

Surfactant–A compound that lowers the surface tension between two solutions, acting as a detergent or emulsifier.

TATA box–The site of binding for RNA polymerase II during transcription; named for its high concentration of thymine and adenine bases.

Tautomerization–The rearrangement of bonds within a compound, usually by moving a hydrogen and forming a double bond.

Telomere–Repeating unit at the end of DNA that protects against the loss of information with repeated DNA replication.

Template strand–The strand of DNA that is transcribed to form mRNA; also called the antisense strand.

Termination–The end of translation, in which the ribosome finds a stop codon and release factor binds it, allowing the peptide to be freed from the ribosome.

Terpene–A class of lipids built from isoprene moieties; have carbon groups in multiples of five.

Terpenoid–A terpene derivative that has undergone oxygenation or rearrangement of the carbon skeleton.

Tertiary structure–The three-dimensional shape of a polypeptide, stabilized by numerous interactions between R groups.

Thyroid hormones–The primary permissive metabolic hormones involved in the regulation of the basal metabolic rate.

Tight junctions–Cell–cell junctions that prevent the paracellular transport of materials; tight junctions form a collar around cells and link cells within a single layer.

Titration–A laboratory technique in which a solution of unknown concentration is mixed with a solution of known concentration to determine the unknown concentration.

Transcellular transport–The transport of materials through the cell; requires interaction with the cytoplasm and may require transport proteins.

Transcription–The production of an mRNA molecule from a strand of DNA.

Transcription factors–Proteins that help RNA polymerase II locate and bind to the promoter region of DNA.

Transfer RNA (tRNA)–A folded strand of RNA that contains a three-nucleotide anticodon that pairs with an appropriate mRNA codon during translation and is charged with the corresponding amino acid.

Transferase–An enzyme that catalyzes the transfer of a functional group.

Translation–The production of a protein from an mRNA molecule.

Triacylglycerol–A glycerol molecule esterified to three fatty acid molecules; the most common form of fat storage within the body.

Uncompetitive inhibition–A decrease in enzyme activity that results from the interaction with an inhibitor at the allosteric site; uncompetitive inhibitors bind only to the substrate-bound enzyme and cannot be overcome by addition of substrate.

UV spectroscopy–A method of determining the concentration of protein in an isolate by comparison against a protein standard; relies on the presence of aromatic amino acids. It can also be used with nucleic acids and other compounds.

van't Hoff factor–The number of particles obtained from a molecule when dissociated in solution.

Vitamin–An organic essential coenzyme that assists an enzyme in carrying out its action.

v_{max}–Maximum velocity for a given quantity of enzyme. v_{max} occurs when the enzyme is fully saturated.

Watson-Crick model–This model proposed the structure of DNA as a double stranded helix.

Wax–A high-melting point lipid composed of a very long chain alcohol and a very long chain fatty acid.

Wobble–The third nucleotide of a codon that often plays no role in specifying an amino acid; an evolutionary development designed to protect against mutations.

X-ray crystallography–A method of determining molecular structure using apparent bond angles and diffraction and refraction of X-rays.

Zwitterion–A molecule that contains charges, but is neutral overall. Most often used to describe amino acids.

Zymogen–An enzyme that is secreted in an inactive form and must be activated by cleavage; common examples are digestive enzymes.

INDEX

Note: Material in figures or tables is indicated by italic *f* or *t* after the page number.

B

C

D

H

M

ART CREDITS

Chapter 1 Cover—Image credited to Yikrazuul. From Wikimedia Commons.

Figure 1.15a—Image credited to ibreakstock. From Shutterstock.

Chapter 3 Cover—Image credited to Heiti Paves. From Shutterstock.

Figure 3.7—Image credited to ggw. From Shutterstock.

Figure 3.9—Image credited to User: Dcrjsr. From Wikimedia Commons. Copyright © 1971. Used under license: CC-BY-3.0.

Chapter 4 Cover—Image credited to Sea Wave. From Shutterstock.

Chapter 5 Cover—Image credited to Captain Yeo. From Shutterstock.

Figure 5.4—Image credited to User: Alex Hindemith. From Wikimedia Commons.

Chapter 6 Cover—Image credited to: anyaivanova. From Shutterstock.

Figure 6.16—Image credited to Madeline Price Ball. From Wikimedia Commons. Copyright © 2011.

Chapter 7 Cover—Image credited to: Mopic. From Shutterstock.

Chapter 8 Cover—Image credited to somersault1824. From Shutterstock.

Figure 8.7—Image credited to Holly Fischer. From Wikimedia Commons. Copyright © 2013. Used under license: CC-BY-3.0.

Image in Concept Check 8.2—Image credited to ellepigrafica. From Shutterstock.

Chapter 9 Cover—Image credited to Christian Bertrand. From Shutterstock.

Chapter 10 Cover—Image credited to RAJ CREATIONZS. From Shutterstock.

Chapter 11 Cover—Image credited to Bernd Juergens. From Shutterstock.

Chapter 12 Cover—Image credited to O2 creationz. From Shutterstock.

Figure 12.8—Image credited to Michael Feldman, MD, PhD. From Wikimedia Commons. Copyright © 2005. Used under license: CC-BY-2.0.

Notes

Notes

Notes

Notes

Notes

Notes

Notes

KAPLAN

MCAT® GENERAL CHEMISTRY REVIEW 2024–2025

ONLINE + BOOK

Edited by Alexander Stone Macnow, MD

ACKNOWLEDGMENTS

Editor-in-Chief, 2024–2025 Edition
M. Dominic Eggert

Contributing Editors, 2024–2025 Edition
Christopher Durland; Charles Pierce, MD; Jason Selzer

Prior Edition Editorial Staff: Brandon Deason, MD; Christopher Durland; M. Dominic Eggert; Tyler Fara; Elizabeth Flagge; Adam Grey; Jason Selzer; Lauren K. White

Published by Kaplan North America, LLC dba Kaplan Publishing
1515 West Cypress Creek Road
Fort Lauderdale, Florida 33309

ISBN: 978-1-5062-8693-8

10 9 8 7 6 5 4 3

TABLE OF CONTENTS

GO ONLINE

kaptest.com/booksonline

THE *KAPLAN MCAT REVIEW* TEAM

Alexander Stone Macnow, MD
Editor-in-Chief

Áine Lorié, PhD
Editor

Derek Rusnak, MA
Editor

Mikhail Alexeeff
Kaplan MCAT Faculty

Laura L. Ambler
Kaplan MCAT Faculty

Krista L. Buckley, MD
Kaplan MCAT Faculty

Kristen L. Russell, ME
Editor

Pamela Willingham, MSW
Editor

Melinda Contreras, MS
Kaplan MCAT Faculty

Samantha Fallon
Kaplan MCAT Faculty

Jason R. Selzer
Kaplan MCAT Faculty

M. Dominic Eggert
Editor

Faculty Reviewers and Editors: Elmar R. Aliyev; James Burns; Jonathan Cornfield; Alisha Maureen Crowley; Nikolai Dorofeev, MD; Benjamin Downer, MS; Colin Doyle; Christopher Durland; Marilyn Engle; Eleni M. Eren; Raef Ali Fadel; Elizabeth Flagge; Adam Grey; Rohit Gupta, Jonathan Habermacher; Tyra Hall-Pogar, PhD; Justine Harkness, PhD; Scott Huff; Samer T. Ismail; Ae-Ri Kim, PhD; Elizabeth A. Kudlaty; Kelly Kyker-Snowman, MS; Ningfei Li; John P. Mahon; Brandon McKenzie; Matthew A. Meier; Nainika Nanda; Caroline Nkemdilim Opene; Kaitlyn E. Prenger; Uneeb Qureshi; Jason Selzer; Allison St. Clair; Bela G. Starkman, PhD; Chris Sun; Michael Paul Tomani, MS; Bonnie Wang; Ethan Weber; Lauren K. White; Nicholas M. White; Allison Ann Wilkes, MS; Kerranna Williamson, MBA; and Tony Yu.

Thanks to Rebecca Anderson; Jeff Batzli; Eric Chiu; Tim Eich; Tyler Fara; Owen Farcy; Dan Frey; Robin Garmise; Rita Garthaffner; Joanna Graham; Allison Gudenau; Allison Harm; Beth Hoffberg; Aaron Lemon-Strauss; Keith Lubeley; Diane McGarvey; Petros Minasi; Beena P V; John Polstein; Deeangelee Pooran-Kublall, MD, MPH; Rochelle Rothstein, MD; Larry Rudman; Srividhya Sankar; Sylvia Tidwell Scheuring; Carly Schnur; Aiswarya Sivanand; Todd Tedesco; Karin Tucker; Lee Weiss; Christina Wheeler; Kristen Workman; Amy Zarkos; and the countless others who made this project possible.

GETTING STARTED CHECKLIST

Getting Started Checklist

- [ ] Register for your free online assets—including full-length tests, Science Review Videos, and additional practice materials—at **www.kaptest.com/moreonline**.
- [ ] Create a study calendar that ensures you complete content review and sufficient practice by Test Day!
- [ ] As you finish a chapter and the online practice for that chapter, check it off on the table of contents.
- [ ] Register to take the MCAT at **www.aamc.org/mcat**.
- [ ] Set aside time during your prep to make sure the rest of your application—personal statement, recommendations, and other materials—is ready to go!
- [ ] Take a moment to admire your completed checklist, then get back to the business of prepping for this exam!

PREFACE

And now it starts: your long, yet fruitful journey toward wearing a white coat. Proudly wearing that white coat, though, is hopefully only part of your motivation. You are reading this book because you want to be a healer.

If you're serious about going to medical school, then you are likely already familiar with the importance of the MCAT in medical school admissions. While the holistic review process puts additional weight on your experiences, extracurricular activities, and personal attributes, the fact remains: along with your GPA, your MCAT score remains one of the two most important components of your application portfolio—at least early in the admissions process. Each additional point you score on the MCAT pushes you in front of thousands of other students and makes you an even more attractive applicant. But the MCAT is not simply an obstacle to overcome; it is an opportunity to show schools that you will be a strong student and a future leader in medicine.

We at Kaplan take our jobs very seriously and aim to help students see success not only on the MCAT, but as future physicians. We work with our learning science experts to ensure that we're using the most up-to-date teaching techniques in our resources. Multiple members of our team hold advanced degrees in medicine or associated biomedical sciences, and are committed to the highest level of medical education. Kaplan has been working with the MCAT for over 50 years and our commitment to premed students is unflagging; in fact, Stanley Kaplan created this company when he had difficulty being accepted to medical school due to unfair quota systems that existed at the time.

We stand now at the beginning of a new era in medical education. As citizens of this 21st-century world of healthcare, we are charged with creating a patient-oriented, culturally competent, cost-conscious, universally available, technically advanced, and research-focused healthcare system, run by compassionate providers. Suffice it to say, this is no easy task. Problem-based learning, integrated curricula, and classes in interpersonal skills are some of the responses to this demand for an excellent workforce—a workforce of which you'll soon be a part.

We're thrilled that you've chosen us to help you on this journey. Please reach out to us to share your challenges, concerns, and successes. Together, we will shape the future of medicine in the United States and abroad; we look forward to helping you become the doctor you deserve to be.

Good luck!

Alexander Stone Macnow, MD
Editor-in-Chief
Department of Pathology and Laboratory Medicine
Hospital of the University of Pennsylvania

BA, Musicology—Boston University, 2008
MD—Perelman School of Medicine at the University of Pennsylvania, 2013

ABOUT THE MCAT

Anatomy of the MCAT

Here is a general overview of the structure of Test Day:

Section	Number of Questions	Time Allotted
Test-Day Certification		4 minutes
Tutorial (optional)		10 minutes
Chemical and Physical Foundations of Biological Systems	59	95 minutes
Break (optional)		10 minutes
Critical Analysis and Reasoning Skills (CARS)	53	90 minutes
Lunch Break (optional)		30 minutes
Biological and Biochemical Foundations of Living Systems	59	95 minutes
Break (optional)		10 minutes
Psychological, Social, and Biological Foundations of Behavior	59	95 minutes
Void Question		3 minutes
Satisfaction Survey (optional)		5 minutes

The structure of the four sections of the MCAT is shown below.

Chemical and Physical Foundations of Biological Systems	
Time	95 minutes
Format	• 59 questions • 10 passages • 44 questions are passage-based, and 15 are discrete (stand-alone) questions. • Score between 118 and 132
What It Tests	• Biochemistry: 25% • Biology: 5% • General Chemistry: 30% • Organic Chemistry: 15% • Physics: 25%

Critical Analysis and Reasoning Skills (CARS)	
Time	90 minutes
Format	• 53 questions • 9 passages • All questions are passage-based. There are no discrete (stand-alone) questions. • Score between 118 and 132
What It Tests	Disciplines: • Humanities: 50% • Social Sciences: 50% Skills: • *Foundations of Comprehension*: 30% • *Reasoning Within the Text*: 30% • *Reasoning Beyond the Text*: 40%
Biological and Biochemical Foundations of Living Systems	
Time	95 minutes
Format	• 59 questions • 10 passages • 44 questions are passage-based, and 15 are discrete (stand-alone) questions. • Score between 118 and 132
What It Tests	• Biochemistry: 25% • Biology: 65% • General Chemistry: 5% • Organic Chemistry: 5%
Psychological, Social, and Biological Foundations of Behavior	
Time	95 minutes
Format	• 59 questions • 10 passages • 44 questions are passage-based, and 15 are discrete (stand-alone) questions. • Score between 118 and 132
What It Tests	• Biology: 5% • Psychology: 65% • Sociology: 30%
Total	
Testing Time	375 minutes (6 hours, 15 minutes)
Total Seat Time	447 minutes (7 hours, 27 minutes)
Questions	230
Score	472 to 528

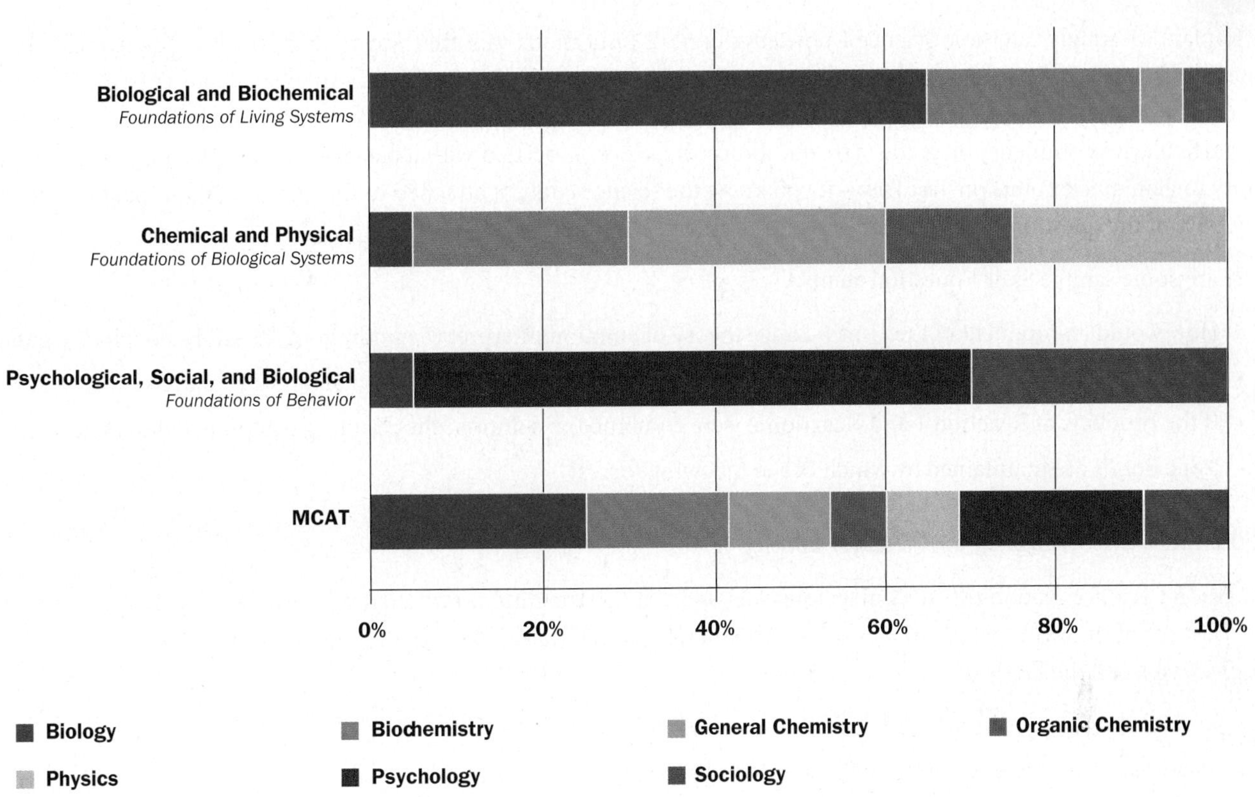

Scientific Inquiry and Reasoning Skills (SIRS)

The AAMC has defined four *Scientific Inquiry and Reasoning Skills* (SIRS) that will be tested in the three science sections of the MCAT:

1. *Knowledge of Scientific Concepts and Principles* (35% of questions)
2. *Scientific Reasoning and Problem-Solving* (45% of questions)
3. *Reasoning About the Design and Execution of Research* (10% of questions)
4. *Data-Based and Statistical Reasoning* (10% of questions)

Let's see how each one breaks down into more specific Test Day behaviors. Note that the bullet points of specific objectives for each of the SIRS are taken directly from the *Official Guide to the MCAT Exam*; the descriptions of what these behaviors mean and sample question stems, however, are written by Kaplan.

Skill 1: *Knowledge of Scientific Concepts and Principles*

This is probably the least surprising of the four SIRS; the testing of science knowledge is, after all, one of the signature qualities of the MCAT. Skill 1 questions will require you to do the following:

- Recognize correct scientific principles
- Identify the relationships among closely related concepts
- Identify the relationships between different representations of concepts (verbal, symbolic, graphic)
- Identify examples of observations that illustrate scientific principles
- Use mathematical equations to solve problems

At Kaplan, we simply call these Science Knowledge or Skill 1 questions. Another way to think of Skill 1 questions is as "one-step" problems. The single step is either to realize which scientific concept the question stem is suggesting or to take the concept stated in the question stem and identify which answer choice is an accurate application of it. Skill 1 questions are particularly prominent among discrete questions (those not associated with a passage). These questions are an opportunity to gain quick points on Test Day—if you know the science concept attached to the question, then that's it! On Test Day, 35% of the questions in each science section will be Skill 1 questions.

Here are some sample Skill 1 question stems:

- How would a proponent of the James–Lange theory of emotion interpret the findings of the study cited in the passage?
- Which of the following most accurately describes the function of FSH in the human menstrual cycle?
- If the products of Reaction 1 and Reaction 2 were combined in solution, the resulting reaction would form:
- Ionic bonds are maintained by which of the following forces?

Skill 2: *Scientific Reasoning and Problem-Solving*

The MCAT science sections do, of course, move beyond testing straightforward science knowledge; Skill 2 questions are the most common way in which it does so. At Kaplan, we also call these Critical Thinking questions. Skill 2 questions will require you to do the following:

- Reason about scientific principles, theories, and models
- Analyze and evaluate scientific explanations and predictions
- Evaluate arguments about causes and consequences
- Bring together theory, observations, and evidence to draw conclusions
- Recognize scientific findings that challenge or invalidate a scientific theory or model
- Determine and use scientific formulas to solve problems

Just as Skill 1 questions can be thought of as "one-step" problems, many Skill 2 questions are "two-step" problems, and more difficult Skill 2 questions may require three or more steps. These questions can require a wide spectrum of reasoning skills, including integration of multiple facts from a passage, combination of multiple science content areas, and prediction of an experiment's results. Skill 2 questions also tend to ask about science content without actually mentioning it by name. For example, a question might describe the results of one experiment and ask you to predict the results of a second experiment without actually telling you what underlying scientific principles are at work—part of the question's difficulty will be figuring out which principles to apply in order to get the correct answer. On Test Day, 45% of the questions in each science section will be Skill 2 questions.

Here are some sample Skill 2 question stems:

- Which of the following experimental conditions would most likely yield results similar to those in Figure 2?
- All of the following conclusions are supported by the information in the passage EXCEPT:
- The most likely cause of the anomalous results found by the experimenter is:
- An impact to a person's chest quickly reduces the volume of one of the lungs to 70% of its initial value while not allowing any air to escape from the mouth. By what percentage is the force of outward air pressure increased on a 2 cm^2 portion of the inner surface of the compressed lung?

Skill 3: *Reasoning About the Design and Execution of Research*

The MCAT is interested in your ability to critically appraise and analyze research, as this is an important day-to-day task of a physician. We call these questions Skill 3 or Experimental and Research Design questions for short. Skill 3 questions will require you to do the following:

- Identify the role of theory, past findings, and observations in scientific questioning
- Identify testable research questions and hypotheses
- Distinguish between samples and populations and distinguish results that support generalizations about populations
- Identify independent and dependent variables
- Reason about the features of research studies that suggest associations between variables or causal relationships between them (such as temporality and random assignment)
- Identify conclusions that are supported by research results
- Determine the implications of results for real-world situations
- Reason about ethical issues in scientific research

Over the years, the AAMC has received input from medical schools to require more practical research skills of MCAT test takers, and Skill 3 questions are the response to these demands. This skill is unique in that the outside knowledge you need to answer Skill 3 questions is not taught in any one undergraduate course; instead, the research design principles needed to answer these questions are learned gradually throughout your science classes and especially through any laboratory work you have completed. It should be noted that Skill 3 comprises 10% of the questions in each science section on Test Day.

Here are some sample Skill 3 question stems:

- What is the dependent variable in the study described in the passage?
- The major flaw in the method used to measure disease susceptibility in Experiment 1 is:
- Which of the following procedures is most important for the experimenters to follow in order for their study to maintain a proper, randomized sample of research subjects?
- A researcher would like to test the hypothesis that individuals who move to an urban area during adulthood are more likely to own a car than are those who have lived in an urban area since birth. Which of the following studies would best test this hypothesis?

Skill 4: *Data-Based and Statistical Reasoning*

Lastly, the science sections of the MCAT test your ability to analyze the visual and numerical results of experiments and studies. We call these Data and Statistical Analysis questions. Skill 4 questions will require you to do the following:

- Use, analyze, and interpret data in figures, graphs, and tables
- Evaluate whether representations make sense for particular scientific observations and data
- Use measures of central tendency (mean, median, and mode) and measures of dispersion (range, interquartile range, and standard deviation) to describe data
- Reason about random and systematic error

- Reason about statistical significance and uncertainty (interpreting statistical significance levels and interpreting a confidence interval)
- Use data to explain relationships between variables or make predictions
- Use data to answer research questions and draw conclusions

Skill 4 is included in the MCAT because physicians and researchers spend much of their time examining the results of their own studies and the studies of others, and it's very important for them to make legitimate conclusions and sound judgments based on that data. The MCAT tests Skill 4 on all three science sections with graphical representations of data (charts and bar graphs), as well as numerical ones (tables, lists, and results summarized in sentence or paragraph form). On Test Day, 10% of the questions in each science section will be Skill 4 questions.

Here are some sample Skill 4 question stems:

- According to the information in the passage, there is an inverse correlation between:
- What conclusion is best supported by the findings displayed in Figure 2?
- A medical test for a rare type of heavy metal poisoning returns a positive result for 98% of affected individuals and 13% of unaffected individuals. Which of the following types of error is most prevalent in this test?
- If a fourth trial of Experiment 1 was run and yielded a result of 54% compliance, which of the following would be true?

SIRS Summary

Discussing the SIRS tested on the MCAT is a daunting prospect given that the very nature of the skills tends to make the conversation rather abstract. Nevertheless, with enough practice, you'll be able to identify each of the four skills quickly, and you'll also be able to apply the proper strategies to solve those problems on Test Day. If you need a quick reference to remind you of the four SIRS, these guidelines may help:

Skill 1 (Science Knowledge) questions ask:

- Do you remember this science content?

Skill 2 (Critical Thinking) questions ask:

- Do you remember this science content? And if you do, could you please apply it to this novel situation?
- Could you answer this question that cleverly combines multiple content areas at the same time?

Skill 3 (Experimental and Research Design) questions ask:

- Let's forget about the science content for a while. Could you give some insight into the experimental or research methods involved in this situation?

Skill 4 (Data and Statistical Analysis) questions ask:

- Let's forget about the science content for a while. Could you accurately read some graphs and tables for a moment? Could you make some conclusions or extrapolations based on the information presented?

Critical Analysis and Reasoning Skills (CARS)

The *Critical Analysis and Reasoning Skills* (CARS) section of the MCAT tests three discrete families of textual reasoning skills; each of these families requires a higher level of reasoning than the last. Those three skills are as follows:

1. *Foundations of Comprehension* (30% of questions)
2. *Reasoning Within the Text* (30% of questions)
3. *Reasoning Beyond the Text* (40% of questions)

These three skills are tested through nine humanities- and social sciences-themed passages, with approximately 5 to 7 questions per passage. Let's take a more in-depth look into these three skills. Again, the bullet points of specific objectives for each of the CARS are taken directly from the *Official Guide to the MCAT Exam*; the descriptions of what these behaviors mean and sample question stems, however, are written by Kaplan.

Foundations of Comprehension

Questions in this skill will ask for basic facts and simple inferences about the passage; the questions themselves will be similar to those seen on reading comprehension sections of other standardized exams like the SAT® and ACT®. *Foundations of Comprehension* questions will require you to do the following:

- Understand the basic components of the text
- Infer meaning from rhetorical devices, word choice, and text structure

This admittedly covers a wide range of potential question types including Main Idea, Detail, Inference, and Definition-in-Context questions, but finding the correct answer to all *Foundations of Comprehension* questions will follow from a basic understanding of the passage and the point of view of its author (and occasionally that of other voices in the passage).

Here are some sample *Foundations of Comprehension* question stems:

- **Main Idea**—The author's primary purpose in this passage is:
- **Detail**—Based on the information in the second paragraph, which of the following is the most accurate summary of the opinion held by Schubert's critics?
- **(Scattered) Detail**—According to the passage, which of the following is FALSE about literary reviews in the 1920s?
- **Inference (Implication)**—Which of the following phrases, as used in the passage, is most suggestive that the author has a personal bias toward narrative records of history?
- **Inference (Assumption)**—In putting together the argument in the passage, the author most likely assumes:
- **Definition-in-Context**—The word "obscure" (paragraph 3), when used in reference to the historian's actions, most nearly means:

Reasoning Within the Text

While *Foundations of Comprehension* questions will usually depend on interpreting a single piece of information in the passage or understanding the passage as a whole, *Reasoning Within the Text* questions require more thought because they will ask you to identify the purpose of a particular piece of information in the context of the passage, or ask how one piece of information relates to another. *Reasoning Within the Text* questions will require you to:

- Integrate different components of the text to draw relevant conclusions

The CARS section will also ask you to judge certain parts of the passage or even judge the author. These questions, which fall under the *Reasoning Within the Text* skill, can ask you to identify authorial bias, evaluate the credibility of cited sources, determine the logical soundness of an argument, identify the importance of a particular fact or statement in the context of the passage, or search for relevant evidence in the passage to support a given conclusion. In all, this category includes Function and Strengthen–Weaken (Within the Passage) questions, as well as a smattering of related—but rare—question types.

Here are some sample *Reasoning Within the Text* question stems:

- **Function**—The author's discussion of the effect of socioeconomic status on social mobility primarily serves which of the following functions?
- **Strengthen–Weaken (Within the Passage)**—Which of the following facts is used in the passage as the most prominent piece of evidence in favor of the author's conclusions?
- **Strengthen–Weaken (Within the Passage)**—Based on the role it plays in the author's argument, *The Possessed* can be considered:

Reasoning Beyond the Text

The distinguishing factor of *Reasoning Beyond the Text* questions is in the title of the skill: the word *Beyond*. Questions that test this skill, which make up a larger share of the CARS section than questions from either of the other two skills, will always introduce a completely new situation that was not present in the passage itself; these questions will ask you to determine how one influences the other. *Reasoning Beyond the Text* questions will require you to:

- Apply or extrapolate ideas from the passage to new contexts
- Assess the impact of introducing new factors, information, or conditions to ideas from the passage

The *Reasoning Beyond the Text* skill is further divided into Apply and Strengthen–Weaken (Beyond the Passage) questions, and a few other rarely appearing question types.

Here are some sample *Reasoning Beyond the Text* question stems:

- **Apply**—If a document were located that demonstrated Berlioz intended to include a chorus of at least 700 in his *Grande Messe des Morts*, how would the author likely respond?
- **Apply**—Which of the following is the best example of a "virtuous rebellion," as it is defined in the passage?
- **Strengthen–Weaken (Beyond the Passage)**—Suppose Jane Austen had written in a letter to her sister, "My strongest characters were those forced by circumstance to confront basic questions about the society in which they lived." What relevance would this have to the passage?
- **Strengthen–Weaken (Beyond the Passage)**—Which of the following sentences, if added to the end of the passage, would most WEAKEN the author's conclusions in the last paragraph?

CARS Summary

Through the *Foundations of Comprehension* skill, the CARS section tests many of the reading skills you have been building on since grade school, albeit in the context of very challenging doctorate-level passages. But through the two other skills (*Reasoning Within the Text* and *Reasoning Beyond the Text*), the MCAT demands that you understand the deep structure of passages and the arguments within them at a very advanced level. And, of course, all of this is tested under very tight timing restrictions: only 102 seconds per question—and that doesn't even include the time spent reading the passages.

Here's a quick reference guide to the three CARS skills:

Foundations of Comprehension questions ask:

- Did you understand the passage and its main ideas?
- What does the passage have to say about this particular detail?
- What must be true that the author did not say?

Reasoning Within the Text questions ask:

- What's the logical relationship between these two ideas from the passage?
- How well argued is the author's thesis?

Reasoning Beyond the Text questions ask:

- How does this principle from the passage apply to this new situation?
- How does this new piece of information influence the arguments in the passage?

Scoring

Each of the four sections of the MCAT is scored between 118 and 132, with the median at approximately 125. This means the total score ranges from 472 to 528, with the median at about 500. Why such peculiar numbers? The AAMC stresses that this scale emphasizes the importance of the central portion of the score distribution, where most students score (around 125 per section, or 500 total), rather than putting undue focus on the high end of the scale.

Note that there is no wrong answer penalty on the MCAT, so you should select an answer for every question—even if it is only a guess.

The AAMC has released the 2019–2021 correlation between scaled score and percentile, as shown on the following page. It should be noted that the percentile scale is adjusted and renormalized over time and thus can shift slightly from year to year. Percentile rank updates are released by the AAMC around May 1 of each year.

Total Score	Percentile	Total Score	Percentile
528	100	499	41
527	100	498	38
526	100	497	35
525	100	496	32
524	100	495	29
523	99	494	26
522	99	493	24
521	98	492	21
520	97	491	19
519	96	490	17
518	95	489	15
517	94	488	13
516	92	487	11
515	90	486	10
514	88	485	8
513	86	484	7
512	83	483	6
511	80	482	5
510	77	481	4
509	74	480	3
508	71	479	2
507	68	478	2
506	65	477	1
505	61	476	1
504	58	475	<1
503	55	474	<1
502	51	473	<1
501	48	472	<1
500	45		

Source: AAMC. 2022. *Summary of MCAT Total and Section Scores*. Accessed October 2022.
https://students-residents.aamc.org/mcat-research-and-data/percentile-ranks-mcat-exam

Further information on score reporting is included at the end of the next section (see *After Your Test*).

MCAT Policies and Procedures

We strongly encourage you to download the latest copy of *MCAT® Essentials*, available on the AAMC's website, to ensure that you have the latest information about registration and Test Day policies and procedures; this document is updated annually. A brief summary of some of the most important rules is provided here.

MCAT Registration

The only way to register for the MCAT is online. You can access AAMC's registration system at **www.aamc.org/mcat**.

The AAMC posts the schedule of testing, registration, and score release dates in the fall before the MCAT testing year, which runs from January into September. Registration for January through June is available earlier than registration for later dates, but see the AAMC's website for the exact dates each year. There is one standard registration fee, but the fee for changing your test date or test center increases the closer you get to your MCAT.

Fees and the Fee Assistance Program (FAP)

Payment for test registration must be made by MasterCard or VISA. As described earlier, the fee for rescheduling your exam or changing your testing center increases as one approaches Test Day. In addition, it is not uncommon for test centers to fill up well in advance of the registration deadline. For these reasons, we recommend identifying your preferred Test Day as soon as possible and registering. There are ancillary benefits to having a set Test Day, as well: when you know the date you're working toward, you'll study harder and are less likely to keep pushing back the exam. The AAMC offers a Fee Assistance Program (FAP) for students with financial hardship to help reduce the cost of taking the MCAT, as well as for the American Medical College Application Service (AMCAS®) application. Further information on the FAP can be found at **www.aamc.org/students/applying/fap**.

Testing Security

On Test Day, you will be required to present a qualifying form of ID. Generally, a current driver's license or United States passport will be sufficient (consult the AAMC website for the full list of qualifying criteria). When registering, take care to spell your first and last names (middle names, suffixes, and prefixes are not required and will not be verified on Test Day) precisely the same as they appear on this ID; failure to provide this ID at the test center or differences in spelling between your registration and ID will be considered a "no-show," and you will not receive a refund for the exam.

During Test Day registration, other identity data collected may include: a digital palm vein scan, a Test Day photo, a digitization of your valid ID, and signatures. Some testing centers may use a metal detection wand to ensure that no prohibited items are brought into the testing room. Prohibited items include all electronic devices, including watches and timers, calculators, cell phones, and any and all forms of recording equipment; food, drinks (including water), and cigarettes or other smoking paraphernalia; hats and scarves (except for religious purposes); and books, notes, or other study materials. If you require a medical device, such as an insulin pump or pacemaker, you must apply for accommodated testing. During breaks, you are allowed access to food and drink, but not to electronic devices, including cell phones.

Testing centers are under video surveillance and the AAMC does not take potential violations of testing security lightly. The bottom line: *know the rules and don't break them.*

Accommodations

Students with disabilities or medical conditions can apply for accommodated testing. Documentation of the disability or condition is required, and requests may take two months—or more—to be approved. For this reason, it is recommended that you begin the process of applying for accommodated testing as early as possible. More information on applying for accommodated testing can be found at **www.aamc.org/students/applying/mcat/accommodations**.

After Your Test

When your MCAT is all over, no matter how you feel you did, be good to yourself when you leave the test center. Celebrate! Take a nap. Watch a movie. Get some exercise. Plan a trip or outing. Call up all of your neglected friends or message them on social media. Go out for snacks or drinks with people you like. Whatever you do, make sure that it has absolutely nothing to do with thinking too hard—you deserve some rest and relaxation.

Perhaps most importantly, do not discuss specific details about the test with anyone. For one, it is important to let go of the stress of Test Day, and reliving your exam only inhibits you from being able to do so. But more significantly, the Examinee Agreement you sign at the beginning of your exam specifically prohibits you from discussing or disclosing exam content. The AAMC is known to seek out individuals who violate this agreement and retains the right to prosecute these individuals at their discretion. This means that you should not, under any circumstances, discuss the exam in person or over the phone with other individuals—including us at Kaplan—or post information or questions about exam content to Facebook, Student Doctor Network, or other online social media. You are permitted to comment on your "general exam experience," including how you felt about the exam overall or an individual section, but this is a fine line. In summary: *if you're not certain whether you can discuss an aspect of the test or not, just don't do it!* Do not let a silly Facebook post stop you from becoming the doctor you deserve to be.

Scores are typically released approximately one month after Test Day. The release is staggered during the afternoon and evening, ending at 5 p.m. Eastern Standard Time. This means that not all examinees receive their scores at exactly the same time. Your score report will include a scaled score for each section between 118 and 132, as well as your total combined score between 472 and 528. These scores are given as confidence intervals. For each section, the confidence interval is approximately the given score ± 1; for the total score, it is approximately the given score ± 2. You will also be given the corresponding percentile rank for each of these section scores and the total score.

AAMC Contact Information

For further questions, contact the MCAT team at the Association of American Medical Colleges:

MCAT Resource Center
Association of American Medical Colleges
www.aamc.org/mcat
(202) 828-0600
www.aamc.org/contactmcat

HOW THIS BOOK WAS CREATED

The *Kaplan MCAT Review* project began shortly after the release of the *Preview Guide for the MCAT 2015 Exam*, 2nd edition. Through thorough analysis by our staff psychometricians, we were able to analyze the relative yield of the different topics on the MCAT, and we began constructing tables of contents for the books of the *Kaplan MCAT Review* series. A dedicated staff of 30 writers, 7 editors, and 32 proofreaders worked over 5,000 combined hours to produce these books. The format of the books was heavily influenced by weekly meetings with Kaplan's learning-science team.

In the years since this book was created, a number of opportunities for expansion and improvement have occurred. The current edition represents the culmination of the wisdom accumulated during that time frame, and it also includes several new features designed to improve the reading and learning experience in these texts.

These books were submitted for publication in April 2023. For any updates after this date, please visit www.kaptest.com/retail-book-corrections-and-updates.

If you have any questions about the content presented here, email KaplanMCATfeedback@kaplan.com. For other questions not related to content, email booksupport@kaplan.com.

Each book has been vetted through at least ten rounds of review. To that end, the information presented in these books is true and accurate to the best of our knowledge. Still, your feedback helps us improve our prep materials. Please notify us of any inaccuracies or errors in the books by sending an email to KaplanMCATfeedback@kaplan.com.

USING THIS BOOK

Kaplan MCAT General Chemistry Review, and the other six books in the *Kaplan MCAT Review* series, bring the Kaplan classroom experience to you—right in your home, at your convenience. This book offers the same Kaplan content review, strategies, and practice that make Kaplan the #1 choice for MCAT prep.

This book is designed to help you review the general chemistry topics covered on the MCAT. Please understand that content review—no matter how thorough—is not sufficient preparation for the MCAT! The MCAT tests not only your science knowledge but also your critical reading, reasoning, and problem-solving skills. Do not assume that simply memorizing the contents of this book will earn you high scores on Test Day; to maximize your scores, you must also improve your reading and test-taking skills through MCAT-style questions and practice tests.

Learning Objectives

At the beginning of each section, you'll find a short list of objectives describing the skills covered within that section. Learning objectives for these texts were developed in conjunction with Kaplan's learning science team, and have been designed specifically to focus your attention on tasks and concepts that are likely to show up on your MCAT. These learning objectives will function as a means to guide your study, and indicate what information and relationships you should be focused on within each section. Before starting each section, read these learning objectives carefully. They will not only allow you to assess your existing familiarity with the content, but also provide a goal-oriented focus for your studying experience of the section.

MCAT Concept Checks

At the end of each section, you'll find a few open-ended questions that you can use to assess your mastery of the material. These MCAT Concept Checks were introduced after numerous conversations with Kaplan's learning science team. Research has demonstrated repeatedly that introspection and self-analysis improve mastery, retention, and recall of material. Complete these MCAT Concept Checks to ensure that you've got the key points from each section before moving on!

Science Mastery Assessments

At the beginning of each chapter, you'll find 15 MCAT-style practice questions. These are designed to help you assess your understanding of the chapter before you begin reading the chapter. Using the guidance provided with the assessment, you can determine the best way to review each chapter based on your personal strengths and weaknesses. Most of the questions in the Science Mastery Assessments focus on the first of the *Scientific Inquiry and Reasoning Skills* (*Knowledge of Scientific Concepts and Principles*), although there are occasional questions that fall into the second or fourth SIRS *Scientific Reasoning and Problem-Solving* and *Data-Based and Statistical Reasoning*, respectively). You can complete each chapter's assessment in a testing interface in your online resources, where you'll also find a test-like passage set covering the same content you just studied to ensure you can also apply your knowledge the way the MCAT will expect you to!

Sidebars

The following is a guide to the five types of sidebars you'll find in *Kaplan MCAT General Chemistry Review:*

- **Bridge:** These sidebars create connections between science topics that appear in multiple chapters throughout the *Kaplan MCAT Review* series.
- **Key Concept:** These sidebars draw attention to the most important takeaways in a given topic, and they sometimes offer synopses or overviews of complex information. If you understand nothing else, make sure you grasp the Key Concepts for any given subject.
- **MCAT Expertise:** These sidebars point out how information may be tested on the MCAT or offer key strategy points and test-taking tips that you should apply on Test Day.
- **Mnemonic:** These sidebars present memory devices to help recall certain facts.
- **Real World:** These sidebars illustrate how a concept in the text relates to the practice of medicine or the world at large. While this is not information you need to know for Test Day, many of the topics in Real World sidebars are excellent examples of how a concept may appear in a passage or discrete (stand-alone) question on the MCAT.

What This Book Covers

The information presented in the *Kaplan MCAT Review* series covers everything listed on the official MCAT content lists. Every topic in these lists is covered in the same level of detail as is common to the undergraduate and postbaccalaureate classes that are considered prerequisites for the MCAT. Note that your premedical classes may include topics not discussed in these books, or they may go into more depth than these books do. Additional exposure to science content is never a bad thing, but all of the content knowledge you are expected to have walking in on Test Day is covered in these books.

Chapter profiles, on the first page of each chapter, represent a holistic look at the content within the chapter, and will include a pie chart as well as text information. The pie chart analysis is based directly on data released by the AAMC, and will give a rough estimate of the importance of the chapter in relation to the book as a whole. Further, the text portion of the Chapter Profiles includes which AAMC content categories are covered within the chapter. These are referenced directly from the AAMC MCAT exam content listing, available on the testmaker's website.

You'll also see new High-Yield badges scattered throughout the sections of this book:

In This Chapter

1.1 Amino Acids Found in Proteins

High-Yield

LEARNING OBJECTIVES

After Chapter 1.1, you will be able to:

- Recognize common abbreviations for amino acids, such as Glu and Y

These badges represent the top 100 topics most tested by the AAMC. In other words, according to the testmaker and all our experience with their resources, a High-Yield badge means more questions on Test Day.

This book also contains a thorough glossary and index for easy navigation of the text.

In the end, this is your book, so write in the margins, draw diagrams, highlight the key points—do whatever is necessary to help you get that higher score. We look forward to working with you as you achieve your dreams and become the doctor you deserve to be!

Studying with This Book

In addition to providing you with the best practice questions and test strategies, Kaplan's team of learning scientists are dedicated to researching and testing the best methods for getting the most out of your study time. Here are their top four tips for improving retention:

Review multiple topics in one study session. This may seem counterintuitive—we're used to practicing one skill at a time in order to improve each skill. But research shows that weaving topics together leads to increased learning. Beyond that consideration, the MCAT often includes more than one topic in a single question. Studying in an integrated manner is the most effective way to prepare for this test.

Customize the content. Drawing attention to difficult or critical content can ensure you don't overlook it as you read and re-read sections. The best way to do this is to make it more visual—highlight, make tabs, use stickies, whatever works. We recommend highlighting only the most important or difficult sections of text. Selective highlighting of up to about 10% of text in a given chapter is great for emphasizing parts of the text, but over-highlighting can have the opposite effect.

Repeat topics over time. Many people try to memorize concepts by repeating them over and over again in succession. Our research shows that retention is improved by spacing out the repeats over time and mixing up the order in which you study content. For example, try reading chapters in a different order the second (or third!) time around. Revisit practice questions that you answered incorrectly in a new sequence. Perhaps information you reviewed more recently will help you better understand those questions and solutions you struggled with in the past.

Take a moment to reflect. When you finish reading a section for the first time, stop and think about what you just read. Jot down a few thoughts in the margins or in your notes about why the content is important or what topics came to mind when you read it. Associating learning with a memory is a fantastic way to retain information! This also works when answering questions. After answering a question, take a moment to think through each step you took to arrive at a solution. What led you to the answer you chose? Understanding the steps you took will help you make good decisions when answering future questions.

Online Resources

In addition to the resources located within this text, you also have additional online resources awaiting you at **www.kaptest.com/booksonline**. Make sure to log on and take advantage of free practice and other resources!

Please note that access to the online resources is limited to the original owner of this book.

STUDYING FOR THE MCAT

The first year of medical school is a frenzied experience for most students. To meet the requirements of a rigorous work schedule, students either learn to prioritize their time or else fall hopelessly behind. It's no surprise, then, that the MCAT, the test specifically designed to predict success in medical school, is a high-speed, time-intensive test. The MCAT demands excellent time-management skills, endurance, and grace under pressure both during the test as well as while preparing for it. Having a solid plan of attack and sticking with it are key to giving you the confidence and structure you need to succeed.

Creating a Study Plan

The best time to create a study plan is at the beginning of your MCAT preparation. If you don't already use a calendar, you will want to start. You can purchase a planner, print out a free calendar from the Internet, use a built-in calendar or app on one of your smart devices, or keep track using an interactive online calendar. Pick the option that is most practical for you and that you are most likely to use consistently.

Once you have a calendar, you'll be able to start planning your study schedule with the following steps:

1. **Fill in your obligations and choose a day off.**

   Write in all your school, extracurricular, and work obligations first: class sessions, work shifts, and meetings that you must attend. Then add in your personal obligations: appointments, lunch dates, family and social time, etc. Making an appointment in your calendar for hanging out with friends or going to the movies may seem strange at first, but planning social activities in advance will help you achieve a balance between personal and professional obligations even as life gets busy. Having a happy balance allows you to be more focused and productive when it comes time to study, so stay well-rounded and don't neglect anything that is important to you.

   In addition to scheduling your personal and professional obligations, you should also plan your time off. Taking some time off is just as important as studying. Kaplan recommends taking at least one full day off per week, ideally from all your study obligations but at minimum from studying for the MCAT.

2. **Add in study blocks around your obligations.**

   Once you have established your calendar's framework, add in study blocks around your obligations, keeping your study schedule as consistent as possible across days and across weeks. Studying at the same time of day as your official test is ideal for promoting recall, but if that's not possible, then fit in study blocks wherever you can.

   To make your studying as efficient as possible, block out short, frequent periods of study time throughout the week. From a learning perspective, studying one hour per day for six days per week is much more valuable than studying for six hours all at once one day per week. Specifically, Kaplan recommends studying for no longer than three hours in one sitting. Within those three-hour blocks, also plan to take ten-minute breaks every hour. Use these breaks to get up from your seat, do some quick stretches, get a snack and drink, and clear your mind. Although ten minutes of break for every 50 minutes of studying may sound like a lot, these breaks will allow you to deal with distractions and rest your brain so that, during the 50-minute study blocks, you can remain fully engaged and completely focused.

3. **Add in your full-length practice tests.**

   Next, you'll want to add in full-length practice tests. You'll want to take one test very early in your prep and then spread your remaining full-length practice tests evenly between now and your test date. Staggering tests in this way allows you to form a baseline for comparison and to determine which areas to focus on right away, while also providing realistic feedback throughout your prep as to how you will perform on Test Day.

When planning your calendar, aim to finish your full-length practice tests and the majority of your studying by one week before Test Day, which will allow you to spend that final week completing a brief review of what you already know. In your online resources, you'll find sample study calendars for several different Test Day timelines to use as a starting point. The sample calendars may include more focus than you need in some areas, and less in others, and it may not fit your timeline to Test Day. You will need to customize your study calendar to your needs using the steps above.

The total amount of time you spend studying each week will depend on your schedule, your personal prep needs, and your time to Test Day, but it is recommended that you spend somewhere in the range of 300–350 hours preparing before taking the official MCAT. One way you could break this down is to study for three hours per day, six days per week, for four months, but this is just one approach. You might study six days per week for more than three hours per day. You might study over a longer period of time if you don't have much time to study each week. No matter what your plan is, ensure you complete enough practice to feel completely comfortable with the MCAT and its content. A good sign you're ready for Test Day is when you begin to earn your goal score consistently in practice.

How to Study

The MCAT covers a large amount of material, so studying for Test Day can initially seem daunting. To combat this, we have some tips for how to take control of your studying and make the most of your time.

Goal Setting

To take control of the amount of content and practice required to do well on the MCAT, break the content down into specific goals for each week instead of attempting to approach the test as a whole. A goal of "I want to increase my overall score by 5 points" is too big, abstract, and difficult to measure on the small scale. More reasonable goals are "I will read two chapters each day this week." Goals like this are much less overwhelming and help break studying into manageable pieces.

Active Reading

As you go through this book, much of the information will be familiar to you. After all, you have probably seen most of the content before. However, be very careful: Familiarity with a subject does not necessarily translate to knowledge or mastery of that subject. Do not assume that if you recognize a concept you actually know it and can apply it quickly at an appropriate level. Don't just passively read this book. Instead, read actively: Use the free margin space to jot down important ideas, draw diagrams, and make charts as you read. Highlighting can be an excellent tool, but use it sparingly: highlighting every sentence isn't active reading, it's coloring. Frequently stop and ask yourself questions while you read (e.g., *What is the main point? How does this fit into the overall scheme of things? Could I thoroughly explain this to someone else?).* By making connections and focusing on the grander scheme, not only will you ensure you know the essential content, but you also prepare yourself for the level of critical thinking required by the MCAT.

Focus on Areas of Greatest Opportunity

If you are limited by only having a minimal amount of time to prepare before Test Day, focus on your biggest areas of opportunity first. Areas of opportunity are topic areas that are highly tested and that you have not yet mastered. You likely won't have time to take detailed notes for every page of these books; instead, use your results from practice materials to determine

which areas are your biggest opportunities and seek those out. After you've taken a full-length test, make sure you are using your performance report to best identify areas of opportunity. Skim over content matter for which you are already demonstrating proficiency, pausing to read more thoroughly when something looks unfamiliar or particularly difficult. Begin with the Science Mastery Assessment at the beginning of each chapter. If you can get all of those questions correct within a reasonable amount of time, you may be able to quickly skim through that chapter, but if the questions prove to be more difficult, then you may need to spend time reading the chapter or certain subsections of the chapter more thoroughly.

Practice, Review, and Tracking

Leave time to review your practice questions and full-length tests. You may be tempted, after practicing, to push ahead and cover new material as quickly as possible, but failing to schedule ample time for review will actually throw away your greatest opportunity to improve your performance. The brain rarely remembers anything it sees or does only once. When you carefully review the questions you've solved (and the explanations for them), the process of retrieving that information reopens and reinforces the connections you've built in your brain. This builds long-term retention and repeatable skill sets—exactly what you need to beat the MCAT!

One useful tool for making the most of your review is the How I'll Fix It (HIFI) sheet. You can create a HIFI sheet, such as the sample below, to track questions throughout your prep that you miss or have to guess on. For each such question, figure out why you missed it and supply at least one action step for how you can avoid similar mistakes in the future. As you move through your MCAT prep, adjust your study plan based on your available study time and the results of your review. Your strengths and weaknesses are likely to change over the course of your prep. Keep addressing the areas that are most important to your score, shifting your focus as those areas change. For more help with making the most of your full-length tests, including a How I'll Fix It sheet template, make sure to check out the videos and resources in your online syllabus.

Section	Q #	Topic or Type	Why I missed it	How I'll fix it
Chem/Phys	*42*	*Nuclear chem.*	*Confused electron absorption and emission*	*Reread Physics Chapter 9.2*
Chem/Phys	*47*	K_{eq}	*Didn't know right equation*	*Memorize equation for* K_{eq}
CARS	*2*	*Detail*	*Didn't read "not" in answer choice*	*Slow down when finding match*
CARS	*4*	*Inference*	*Forgot to research answer*	*Reread passage and predict first*

Where to Study

One often-overlooked aspect of studying is the environment where the learning actually occurs. Although studying at home is many students' first choice, several problems can arise in this environment, chief of which are distractions. Studying can be a mentally draining process, so as time passes, these distractions become ever more tempting as escape routes. Although you may have considerable willpower, there's no reason to make staying focused harder than it needs to be. Instead of studying at home, head to a library, quiet coffee shop, or another new location whenever possible. This will eliminate many of the usual distractions and also promote efficient studying; instead of studying off and on at home over the course of an entire day, you can stay at the library for three hours of effective studying and enjoy the rest of the day off from the MCAT.

No matter where you study, make your practice as much like Test Day as possible. Just as is required during the official test, don't have snacks or chew gum during your study blocks. Turn off your music, television, and phone. Practice on the computer with your online resources to simulate the computer-based test environment. When completing practice questions, do your work on scratch paper or noteboard sheets rather than writing directly on any printed materials since you won't have that option on Test Day. Because memory is tied to all of your senses, the more test-like you can make your studying environment, the easier it will be on Test Day to recall the information you're putting in so much work to learn.

CHAPTER 1

ATOMIC STRUCTURE

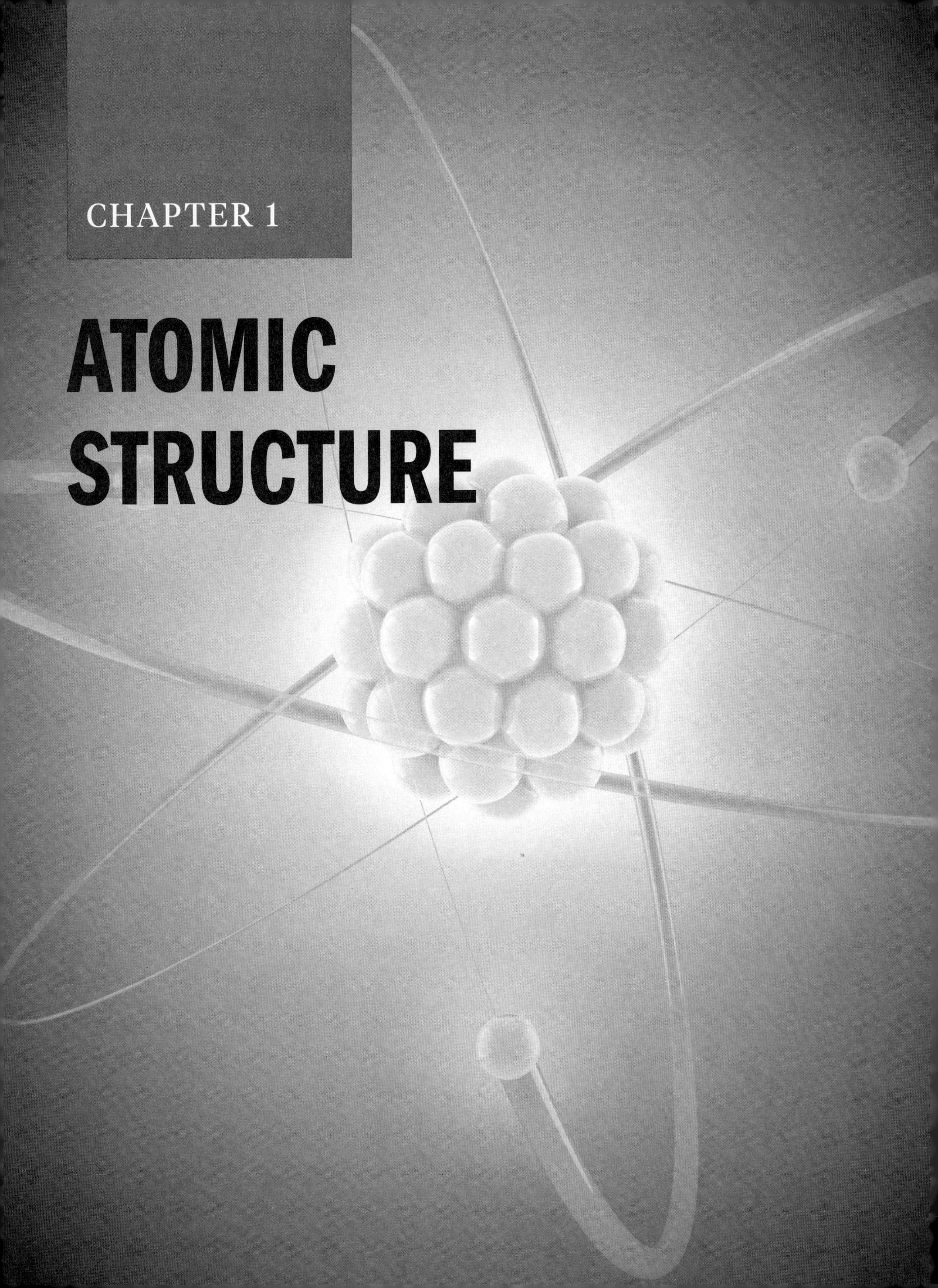

SCIENCE MASTERY ASSESSMENT

Every pre-med knows this feeling: there is so much content I have to know for the MCAT! How do I know what to do first or what's important?

While the high-yield badges throughout this book will help you identify the most important topics, this Science Mastery Assessment is another tool in your MCAT prep arsenal. This quiz (which can also be taken in your online resources) and the guidance below will help ensure that you are spending the appropriate amount of time on this chapter based on your personal strengths and weaknesses. Don't worry though—skipping something now does not mean you'll never study it. Later on in your prep, as you complete full-length tests, you'll uncover specific pieces of content that you need to review and can come back to these chapters as appropriate.

How to Use This Assessment

If you answer 0–7 questions correctly:

Spend about 1 hour to read this chapter in full and take limited notes throughout. Follow up by reviewing **all** quiz questions to ensure that you now understand how to solve each one.

If you answer 8–11 questions correctly:

Spend 20–40 minutes reviewing the quiz questions. Beginning with the questions you missed, read and take notes on the corresponding subchapters. For questions you answered correctly, ensure your thinking matches that of the explanation and you understand why each choice was correct or incorrect.

If you answer 12–15 questions correctly:

Spend less than 20 minutes reviewing all questions from the quiz. If you missed any, then include a quick read-through of the corresponding subchapters, or even just the relevant content within a subchapter, as part of your question review. For questions you answered correctly, ensure your thinking matches that of the explanation and review the Concept Summary at the end of the chapter.

1. Which of the following is the correct electron configuration for Zn^{2+}?
   A. $1s^22s^22p^63s^23p^64s^03d^{10}$
   B. $1s^22s^22p^63s^23p^64s^23d^8$
   C. $1s^22s^22p^63s^23p^64s^23d^{10}$
   D. $1s^22s^22p^63s^23p^64s^03d^8$

2. Which of the following quantum number sets is possible?
   A. $n = 2; l = 2; m_l = 1; m_s = +\frac{1}{2}$
   B. $n = 2; l = 1; m_l = -1; m_s = +\frac{1}{2}$
   C. $n = 2; l = 0; m_l = -1; m_s = -\frac{1}{2}$
   D. $n = 2; l = 0; m_l = 1; m_s = -\frac{1}{2}$

3. What is the maximum number of electrons allowed in a single atomic energy level in terms of the principal quantum number n ?
   A. $2n$
   B. $2n + 2$
   C. $2n^2$
   D. $2n^2 + 2$

4. Which of the following equations describes the maximum number of electrons that can fill a subshell?
   A. $2l + 2$
   B. $4l + 2$
   C. $2l^2$
   D. $2l^2 + 2$

5. Which of the following atoms only has paired electrons in its ground state?
   A. Sodium
   B. Iron
   C. Cobalt
   D. Helium

6. An electron returns from an excited state to its ground state, emitting a photon at $\lambda = 500$ nm. What would be the magnitude of the energy change if one mole of these photons were emitted? (Note: $h = 6.626 \times 10^{-34}$ J · s, $N_A = 6.02 \times 10^{23}$ mol^{-1})
   A. 3.98×10^{-21} J
   B. 3.98×10^{-19} J
   C. 2.39×10^{3} J
   D. 2.39×10^{5} J

7. Suppose an electron falls from $n = 4$ to its ground state, $n = 1$. Which of the following effects is most likely?
   A. A photon is absorbed.
   B. A photon is emitted.
   C. The electron moves into a *p*-orbital.
   D. The electron moves into a *d*-orbital.

8. Which of the following isotopes of carbon is LEAST likely to be found in nature?
   A. ^{6}C
   B. ^{12}C
   C. ^{13}C
   D. ^{14}C

9. Which of the following best explains the inability to measure position and momentum exactly and simultaneously according to the Heisenberg uncertainty principle?
   A. Imprecision in the definition of the meter and kilogram
   B. Limits on accuracy of existing scientific instruments
   C. Error in one variable is increased by attempts to measure the other
   D. Discrepancies between the masses of nuclei and of their component particles

10. Which of the following electronic transitions would result in the greatest gain in energy for a single hydrogen electron?

A. An electron moves from $n = 6$ to $n = 2$.
B. An electron moves from $n = 2$ to $n = 6$.
C. An electron moves from $n = 3$ to $n = 4$.
D. An electron moves from $n = 4$ to $n = 3$.

11. Suppose that an atom fills its orbitals as shown:

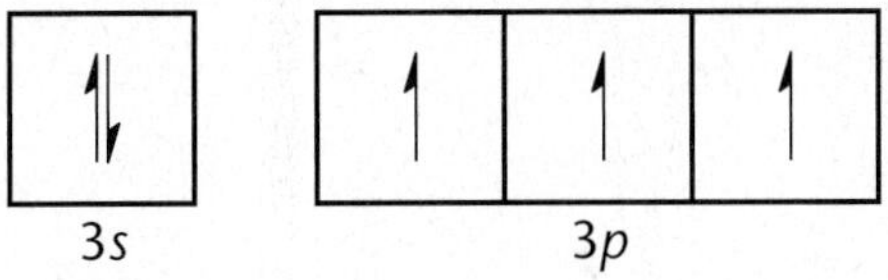

Such an electron configuration most clearly illustrates which of the following laws of atomic physics?

A. Hund's rule
B. Heisenberg uncertainty principle
C. Bohr model
D. Rutherford model

12. How many total electrons are in a ^{133}Cs cation?

A. 54
B. 55
C. 78
D. 132

13. The atomic weight of hydrogen is 1.008 amu. What is the percent composition of hydrogen by isotope, assuming that hydrogen's only isotopes are ^{1}H and ^{2}D?

A. 92% H, 8% D
B. 99.2% H, 0.8% D
C. 99.92% H, 0.08% D
D. 99.992% H, 0.008% D

14. Consider the two sets of quantum numbers shown in the table, which describe two different electrons in the same atom.

n	l	m_l	m_s
2	1	1	$+\frac{1}{2}$
3	1	−1	$+\frac{1}{2}$

Which of the following terms best describes these two electrons?

A. Parallel
B. Opposite
C. Antiparallel
D. Paired

15. Which of the following species is represented by the electron configuration $1s^22s^22p^63s^23p^64s^13d^5$?

I. Cr
II. Mn^{+}
III. Fe^{2+}

A. I only
B. I and II only
C. II and III only
D. I, II, and III

Answer Key

1. **A**
2. **B**
3. **C**
4. **B**
5. **D**
6. **D**
7. **B**
8. **A**
9. **C**
10. **B**
11. **A**
12. **A**
13. **B**
14. **A**
15. **B**

Detailed explanations can be found at the end of the chapter.

CHAPTER 1

ATOMIC STRUCTURE

In This Chapter

CHAPTER PROFILE

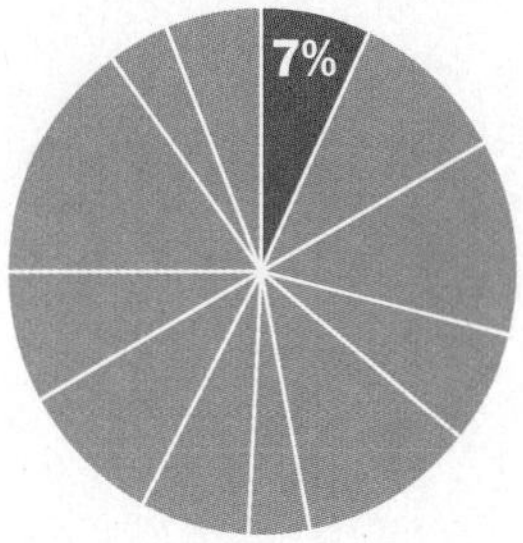

The content in this chapter should be relevant to about 7% of all questions about general chemistry on the MCAT.

This chapter covers material from the following AAMC content category:

4E: Atoms, nuclear decay, electronic structure, and atomic chemical behavior

Introduction

Chemistry is the investigation of the atoms and molecules that make up our bodies, our possessions, the food we eat, and the world around us. There are different branches of chemistry, three of which are tested directly on the MCAT: general (inorganic) chemistry, organic chemistry, and biochemistry. Ultimately, all investigations in chemistry are seeking to answer the questions that confront us in the form—the shape, structure, mode, and essence—of the physical world that surrounds us.

Many students feel similarly about general chemistry and physics: *But I'm premed,* they say. *Why do I need to know any of this? What good will this be when I'm a doctor? Do I only need to know this for the MCAT?* Recognize that to be an effective doctor, one must understand the physical building blocks that make up the human body. Pharmacologic treatment is based on chemistry; many diagnostic tests used every day detect changes in the chemistry of the body.

So, let's get down to the business of learning and remembering the principles of the physical world that help us understand what all this "stuff" is, how it works, and why it behaves the way it does—at both the molecular and macroscopic levels. In the process of reading through these chapters and applying your knowledge to practice questions, you'll prepare yourself for success not only on the *Chemical and Physical Foundations of Biological Systems* section of the MCAT but also in your future career as a physician.

MCAT EXPERTISE

The building blocks of the atom are also the building blocks of knowledge for the general chemistry concepts tested on the MCAT. By understanding these particles, we will be able to use that knowledge as the "nucleus" of understanding for all of general chemistry.

This first chapter starts our review of general chemistry with a consideration of the fundamental unit of matter—the atom. First, we focus on the subatomic particles that make it up: protons, neutrons, and electrons. We will also review the Bohr and quantum mechanical models of the atom, with a particular focus on the similarities and differences between them.

1.1 Subatomic Particles

LEARNING OBJECTIVES

After Chapter 1.1, you will be able to:

- Identify the subatomic particles most important for determining various traits of an atom, including charge, atomic number, and isotope
- Determine the number of protons, neutrons, and electrons within an isotope, such as ^{14}C

Although you may have encountered in your university-level chemistry classes such subatomic particles as *quarks*, *leptons*, and *gluons*, the MCAT's approach to atomic structure is much simpler. There are three subatomic particles that you must understand: protons, neutrons, and electrons.

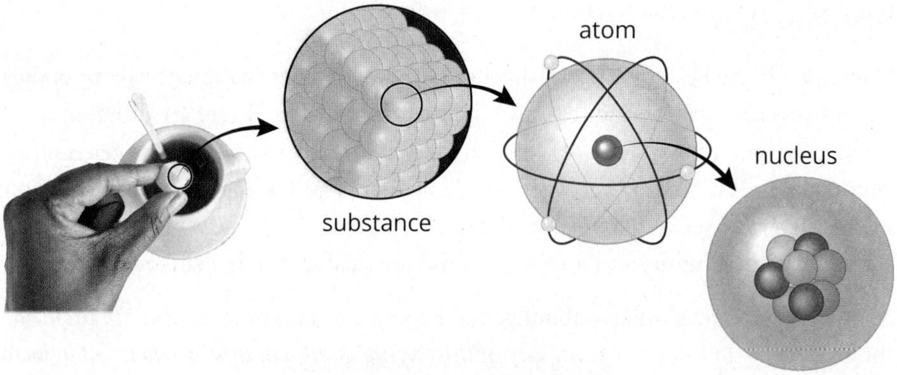

Figure 1.1 Matter: From Macroscopic to Microscopic

Protons

Protons are found in the **nucleus** of an atom, as shown in Figure 1.1. Each proton has an amount of charge equal to the fundamental unit of charge ($e = 1.6 \times 10^{-19}$ C), and we denote this fundamental unit of charge as "+1 *e*" or simply "+1" for the proton. Protons have a mass of approximately one **atomic mass unit (amu)**. The **atomic number** (*Z*) of an element, as shown in Figure 1.2, is equal to the number of protons found in an atom of that element. As such, it acts as a unique identifier for each element because elements are defined by the number of protons they contain. For example, all atoms of oxygen contain eight protons; all atoms of gadolinium contain 64 protons. While all atoms of a given element have the same atomic number, they do not necessarily have the same mass—as we will see in our discussion of isotopes.

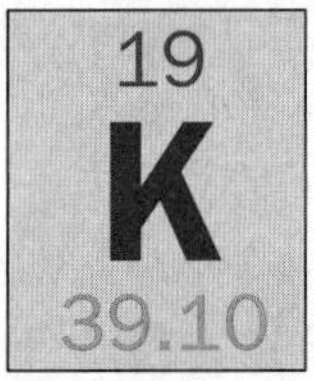

Figure 1.2 Potassium, from the Periodic Table
Potassium has the symbol K (Latin: kalium), atomic number 19, and atomic weight of approximately 39.1.

Neutrons

Neutrons, as the name implies, are neutral—they have no charge. A neutron's mass is only slightly larger than that of the proton, and together, the protons and the neutrons of the nucleus make up almost the entire mass of an atom. Every atom has a characteristic **mass number** (*A*), which is the sum of the protons and neutrons in the atom's nucleus. A given element can have a variable number of neutrons; thus, while atoms of the same element always have the same atomic number, they do not necessarily have the same mass number. Atoms that share an atomic number but have different mass numbers are known as **isotopes** of the element, as shown in Figure 1.3. For example, carbon ($Z = 6$) has three naturally occurring isotopes: ${}^{12}_{6}C$, with six protons and six neutrons; ${}^{13}_{6}C$, with six protons and seven neutrons; and ${}^{14}_{6}C$, with six protons and eight neutrons. The convention ${}^{A}_{Z}X$ is used to show both the atomic number (Z) and the mass number (A) of atom X.

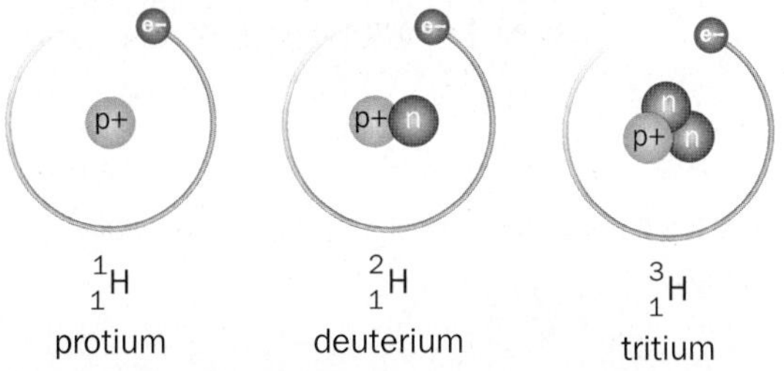

Figure 1.3 Various Isotopes of Hydrogen
Atoms of the same element have the same atomic number ($Z = 1$) but may have varying mass numbers ($A = 1, 2,$ or 3).

Electrons

Electrons move through the space surrounding the nucleus and are associated with varying levels of energy. Each electron has a charge equal in magnitude to that of a proton, but with the opposite (negative) sign, denoted by "$-1\ e$" or simply "-1." The mass of an electron is approximately $\frac{1}{2000}$ that of a proton. Because subatomic particles' masses are so small, the electrostatic force of attraction between the unlike charges of the proton and electron is far greater than the gravitational force of attraction based on their respective masses.

BRIDGE

Valence electrons will be very important to us in both general and organic chemistry. Knowing how tightly held those electrons are will allow us to understand many of an atom's properties and how it interacts with other atoms, especially in bonding. Bonding is so important that it is discussed in Chapter 3 of both *MCAT General Chemistry Review* and *MCAT Organic Chemistry Review*.

Electrons move around the nucleus at varying distances, which correspond to varying levels of electrical potential energy. The electrons closer to the nucleus are at lower energy levels, while those that are further out (in higher **electron shells**) have higher energy. The electrons that are farthest from the nucleus have the strongest interactions with the surrounding environment and the weakest interactions with the nucleus. These electrons are called **valence electrons**; they are much more likely to become involved in bonds with other atoms because they experience the least electrostatic pull from their own nucleus. Generally speaking, the valence electrons determine the reactivity of an atom. As we will discuss in Chapter 3 of *MCAT General Chemistry Review*, the sharing or transferring of these valence electrons in bonds allows elements to fill their highest energy level to increase stability. In the neutral state, there are equal numbers of protons and electrons; losing electrons results in the atom gaining a positive charge, while gaining electrons results in the atom gaining a negative charge. A positively charged atom is called a **cation**, and a negatively charged atom is called an **anion**.

Some basic features of the three subatomic particles are shown in Table 1.1.

SUBATOMIC PARTICLE	SYMBOL	RELATIVE MASS	CHARGE	LOCATION
Proton	p, p^+, or ^1_1H	1	+1	Nucleus
Neutron	n^0 or ^1_0n	1	0	Nucleus
Electron	e^- or $^0_{-1}e$	0	−1	Orbitals

Table 1.1 Subatomic Particles

BRIDGE

Solutions to concept checks for a given chapter in *MCAT General Chemistry Review* can be found near the end of the chapter in which the concept check is located, following the Concept Summary for that chapter.

Example: Determine the number of protons, neutrons, and electrons in a nickel-58 atom and in a nickel-60 +2 cation.

Solution: ^{58}Ni has an atomic number of 28 and a mass number of 58. Therefore, ^{58}Ni will have 28 protons, 28 electrons, and 58 − 28, or 30, neutrons.

$^{60}Ni^{2+}$ has the same number of protons as the neutral ^{58}Ni atom. However, $^{60}Ni^{2+}$ has a positive charge because it has lost two electrons; thus, Ni^{2+} will have 26 electrons. Also, the mass number is two units higher than for the ^{58}Ni atom, and this difference in mass must be due to two extra neutrons; thus, it has a total of 32 neutrons.

MCAT CONCEPT CHECK 1.1

Before you move on, assess your understanding of the material with these questions.

1. Which subatomic particle is the most important for determining each of the following properties of an atom?
   - Charge:

   ____

   - Atomic number:

   ____

   - Isotope:

   ____

2. In nuclear medicine, isotopes are created and used for various purposes; for instance, ^{18}O is created from ^{18}F. Determine the number of protons, neutrons, and electrons in each of these species.

Particle	Protons	Neutrons	Electrons
^{18}O			
^{18}F			

1.2 Atomic Mass *vs.* Atomic Weight

LEARNING OBJECTIVES

After Chapter 1.2, you will be able to:

- Describe atomic mass and atomic weight
- Recall the units of molar mass
- Predict the number of protons, neutrons, and electrons in a given isotope

There are a few different terms used by chemists to describe the heaviness of an element: atomic mass and mass number, which are essentially synonymous, and atomic weight. While the atomic weight is a constant for a given element and is reported in the periodic table, the atomic mass or mass number varies from one isotope to another. In this section, carefully compare and contrast the different definitions of these terms—because they are similar, they can be easy to mix up on the MCAT.

Atomic Mass

As we've seen, the mass of one proton is approximately one amu. The size of the atomic mass unit is defined as exactly $\frac{1}{12}$ the mass of the carbon-12 atom, approximately 1.66×10^{-24} g. Because the carbon-12 nucleus has six protons and six neutrons, an amu is approximately equal to the mass of a proton or a neutron. The difference in mass between protons and neutrons is extremely small; in fact, it is approximately equal to the mass of an electron.

The **atomic mass** of an atom (in amu) is nearly equal to its **mass number**, the sum of protons and neutrons (in reality, some mass is lost as binding energy, as discussed in Chapter 9 of *MCAT Physics and Math Review*). Atoms of the same element with varying mass numbers are called **isotopes** (from the Greek for "same place"). Isotopes differ in their number of neutrons and are referred to by the name of the element followed by the mass number; for example, carbon-12 or iodine-131. Only the three isotopes of hydrogen, shown in Figure 1.3, are given unique names: *protium* (Greek: "first") has one proton and an atomic mass of 1 amu; *deuterium* ("second") has one proton and one neutron and an atomic mass of 2 amu; *tritium* ("third") has one proton and two neutrons and an atomic mass of 3 amu. Because isotopes have the same number of protons and electrons, they generally exhibit similar chemical properties.

KEY CONCEPT

- Atomic number (Z) = number of protons
- Mass number (A) = number of protons + number of neutrons
- Number of protons = number of electrons (in a neutral atom)
- Electrons are not included in mass calculations because they are much smaller.

Atomic Weight

In nature, almost all elements exist as two or more isotopes, and these isotopes are usually present in the same proportions in any sample of a naturally occurring element. The weighted average of these different isotopes is referred to as the **atomic weight** and is the number reported on the periodic table. For example, chlorine has two main naturally occurring isotopes: chlorine-35 and chlorine-37. Chlorine-35 is about three times more abundant than chlorine-37; therefore, the atomic weight of chlorine is closer to 35 than 37. On the periodic table, it is listed as 35.5. Figure 1.4 illustrates the half-lives of the different isotopes of the elements; because half-life corresponds with stability, it also helps determine the relative proportions of these different isotopes.

KEY CONCEPT

When an element has two or more isotopes, no one isotope will have a mass exactly equal to the element's atomic weight. Bromine, for example, is listed in the periodic table as having a mass of 79.9 amu. This is an average of the two naturally occurring isotopes, bromine-79 and bromine-81, which occur in almost equal proportions. There are no bromine atoms with an actual mass of 79.9 amu.

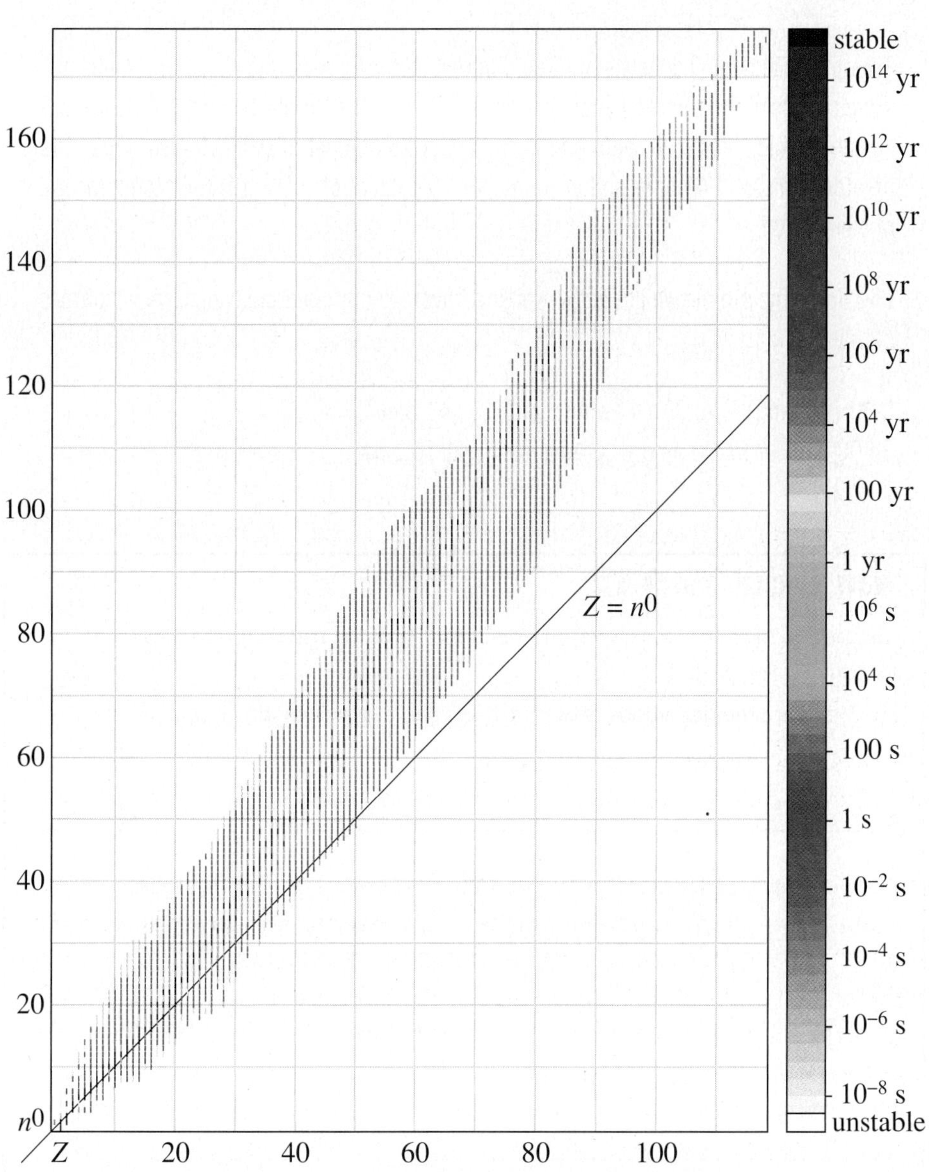

Figure 1.4 Half-Lives of the Different Isotopes of Elements
Half-life is a marker of stability; generally, longer-lasting isotopes are more abundant.

The utility of the atomic weight is that it represents both the mass of the "average" atom of that element, in amu, and the mass of one mole of the element, in grams. A mole is a number of "things" (atoms, ions, molecules) equal to **Avogadro's number**, $N_A = 6.02 \times 10^{23}$. For example, the atomic weight of carbon is 12.0 amu, which means that the average carbon atom has a mass of 12.0 amu (carbon-12 is *far* more abundant than carbon-13 or carbon-14), and 6.02×10^{23} carbon atoms have a combined mass of 12.0 grams.

MNEMONIC

Atomic **mass** is nearly synonymous with **mass** number. Atomic **weight** is a **weighted** average of naturally occurring isotopes of that element.

Example: Element Q consists of three different isotopes: A, B, and C. Isotope A has an atomic mass of 40 amu and accounts for 60 percent of naturally occurring Q. Isotope B has an atomic mass of 44 amu and accounts for 25 percent of Q. Finally, isotope C has an atomic mass of 41 amu and accounts for 15 percent of Q. What is the atomic weight of element Q?

Solution: The atomic weight is the weighted average of the naturally occurring isotopes of that element:

$$0.60\,(40\text{ amu}) + 0.25\,(44\text{ amu}) + 0.15\,(41\text{ amu}) =$$
$$24.00\text{ amu} + 11.00\text{ amu} + 6.15\text{ amu} = 41.15\text{ amu}$$

MCAT CONCEPT CHECK 1.2

Before you move on, assess your understanding of the material with these questions.

1. What are the definitions of atomic mass and atomic weight?
   - Atomic mass:

   ____

   - Atomic weight:

   ____

2. While molar mass is typically written in grams per mole $\left(\frac{\text{g}}{\text{mol}}\right)$, is the ratio moles per gram $\left(\frac{\text{mol}}{\text{g}}\right)$ also acceptable?

   ____

3. Calculate and compare the subatomic particles that make up the following atoms.

Isotope	Protons	Neutrons	Electrons
^{19}O			
^{16}O			
^{17}O			
^{19}F			
^{16}F			
^{238}U			
^{240}U			

1.3 Rutherford, Planck, and Bohr

High-Yield

LEARNING OBJECTIVES

After Chapter 1.3, you will be able to:

- Calculate the energy of transition for a valence electron that jumps energy levels
- Calculate the wavelength of an emitted photon given the energy emitted by an electron
- Calculate the energy of a photon given its wavelength

In 1910, Ernest Rutherford provided experimental evidence that an atom has a dense, positively charged nucleus that accounts for only a small portion of the atom's volume. Eleven years earlier, Max Planck developed the first quantum theory, proposing that energy emitted as electromagnetic radiation from matter comes in discrete bundles called **quanta**. The **energy** of a quantum, he determined, is given by the **Planck relation**:

$$E = hf$$

Equation 1.1

where h is a proportionality constant known as **Planck's constant**, equal to 6.626×10^{-34} J · s, and f (sometimes designated by the Greek letter nu, ν) is the frequency of the radiation.

Bohr Model

In 1913, Danish physicist Niels Bohr used the work of Rutherford and Planck to develop his model of the electronic structure of the hydrogen atom. Starting from Rutherford's findings, Bohr assumed that the hydrogen atom consisted of a central proton around which an electron traveled in a circular orbit. He postulated that the centripetal force acting on the electron as it revolved around the nucleus was created by the electrostatic force between the positively charged proton and the negatively charged electron.

Bohr used Planck's quantum theory to correct certain assumptions that classical physics made about the pathways of electrons. Classical mechanics postulates that an object revolving in a circle, such as an electron, may assume an infinite number of values for its radius and velocity. The angular momentum ($L = mvr$) and kinetic energy $\left(K = \frac{1}{2}mv^2\right)$ of the object could therefore take on any value. However, by incorporating Planck's quantum theory into his model, Bohr placed restrictions on the possible values of the angular momentum. Bohr predicted that the possible values for the **angular momentum** of an electron orbiting a hydrogen nucleus could be given by:

$$L = \frac{nh}{2\pi}$$

Equation 1.2

MCAT EXPERTISE

The "High-Yield" badge on this section indicates that the content is frequently tested on the MCAT.

BRIDGE

Recall from Chapter 8 of *MCAT Physics Review* that the speed of light (or any wave) can be calculated using $v = f\lambda$. The speed of light, c, is $3 \times 10^8 \frac{\text{m}}{\text{s}}$. This equation can be incorporated into the equation for quantum energy to provide different derivations.

MCAT EXPERTISE

When you see a formula in your review or on Test Day, focus on ratios and relationships. This simplifies our calculations to a conceptual understanding, which is usually enough to lead us to the right answer. Further, the MCAT tends to ask how changes in one variable may affect another variable, rather than a plug-and-chug application of complex equations.

where n is the principal quantum number, which can be any positive integer, and h is Planck's constant. Because the only variable is the principal quantum number, the angular momentum of an electron changes only in discrete amounts with respect to the principal quantum number. Note the similarities between quantized angular momentum and Planck's concept of quantized energy.

Bohr then related the permitted angular momentum values to the **energy of the electron** to obtain:

$$E = -\frac{R_H}{n^2}$$

Equation 1.3

where R_H is the experimentally determined **Rydberg unit of energy**, equal to $2.18 \times 10^{-18} \frac{J}{\text{electron}}$. Therefore, like angular momentum, the energy of the electron changes in discrete amounts with respect to the quantum number. A value of zero energy was assigned to the state in which the proton and electron are separated completely, meaning that there is no attractive force between them. Therefore, the electron in any of its quantized states in the atom will have an attractive force toward the proton; this is represented by the negative sign in Equation 1.3. Ultimately, the only thing the energy equation is saying is that the energy of an electron increases—becomes less negative—the farther out from the nucleus that it is located (increasing n). This is an important point: while the magnitude of the fraction is getting smaller, the actual value it represents is getting larger (becoming less negative).

KEY CONCEPT

At first glance, it may not be clear that the energy (E) is directly proportional to the principal quantum number (n) in Equation 1.3. Take notice of the negative sign, which causes the values to approach zero from a more negative value as n increases (thereby increasing the energy). Negative signs are as important as a variable's location in a fraction when it comes to determining proportionality.

Think of the concept of quantized energy as being similar to the change in gravitational potential energy that you experience when you ascend or descend a flight of stairs. Unlike a ramp, on which you could take an infinite number of steps associated with a continuum of potential energy changes, a staircase only allows you certain changes in height and, as a result, allows only certain discrete (quantized) changes of potential energy.

Bohr came to describe the structure of the hydrogen atom as a nucleus with one proton forming a dense core, around which a single electron revolved in a defined pathway (**orbit**) at a discrete energy value. If one could transfer an amount of energy exactly equal to the difference between one orbit and another, this could result in the electron "jumping" from one orbit to a higher-energy one. These orbits had increasing radii, and the orbit with the smallest, lowest-energy radius was defined as the ground state ($n = 1$). More generally, the **ground state** of an atom is the state of lowest energy, in which all electrons are in the lowest possible orbitals. In Bohr's model, the electron was promoted to an orbit with a larger radius (higher energy), the atom was said to be in the excited state. In general, an atom is in an **excited state** when at least one electron has moved to a subshell of higher than normal energy. Bohr likened his model of the hydrogen atom to the planets orbiting the sun, in which each planet traveled along a roughly circular pathway at set distances—and energy values—from the sun. Bohr's Nobel Prize-winning model was reconsidered over the next two decades but remains an important conceptualization of atomic behavior. In particular, remember that we now know that electrons are *not* restricted to specific pathways, but tend to be localized in certain regions of space.

MCAT EXPERTISE

Note that all systems tend toward minimal energy; thus on the MCAT, atoms of any element will generally exist in the ground state unless subjected to extremely high temperatures or irradiation.

Applications of the Bohr Model

The Bohr model of the hydrogen atom (and other one-electron systems, such as He^{+} and Li^{2+}) is useful for explaining the atomic emission and absorption spectra of atoms.

Atomic Emission Spectra

At room temperature, the majority of atoms in a sample are in the ground state. However, electrons can be excited to higher energy levels by heat or other energy forms to yield excited states. Because the lifetime of an excited state is brief, the electrons will return rapidly to the ground state, resulting in the emission of discrete amounts of energy in the form of photons, as shown in Figure 1.5.

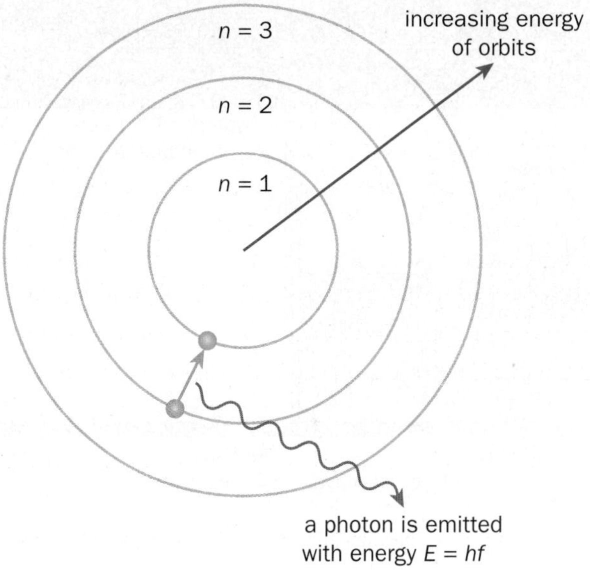

Figure 1.5 Atomic Emission of a Photon as a Result of a Ground State Transition

The electromagnetic energy of these photons can be determined using the following equation:

$$E = \frac{hc}{\lambda}$$

Equation 1.4

where h is Planck's constant, c is the speed of light in a vacuum $\left(3.00 \times 10^8 \ \frac{\text{m}}{\text{s}}\right)$, and λ is the wavelength of the radiation. Note that Equation 1.4 is just a combination of two other equations: $E = hf$ and $c = f\lambda$.

The electrons in an atom can be excited to different energy levels. When these electrons return to their ground states, each will emit a photon with a wavelength characteristic of the specific energy transition it undergoes. As described above, these energy transitions do not form a continuum, but rather are quantized to

MNEMONIC

As electrons go from a lower energy level to a higher energy level, they get **AHED**:

- **A**bsorb light
- **H**igher potential
- **E**xcited
- **D**istant (from the nucleus)

REAL WORLD

Emissions from electrons dropping from an excited state to a ground state give rise to fluorescence. What we see is the color of the emitted light.

certain values. Thus, the spectrum is composed of light at specified frequencies. It is sometimes called a **line spectrum**, where each line on the emission spectrum corresponds to a specific electron transition. Because each element can have its electrons excited to a different set of distinct energy levels, each possesses a unique **atomic emission spectrum**, which can be used as a fingerprint for the element. One particular application of atomic emission spectroscopy is in the analysis of stars and planets: while a physical sample may be impossible to procure, the light from a star can be resolved into its component wavelengths, which are then matched to the known line spectra of the elements as shown in Figure 1.6.

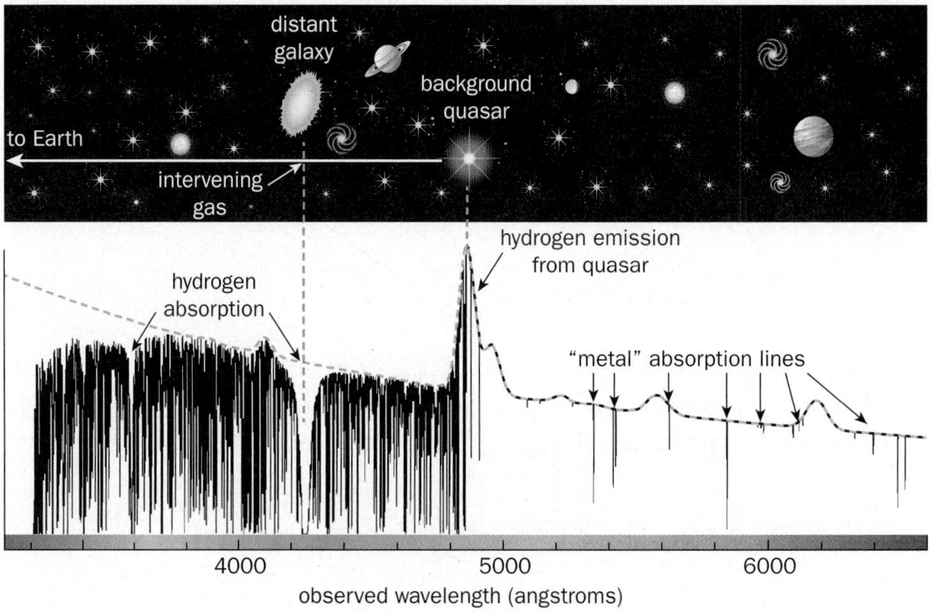

Figure 1.6 Line Spectrum with Transition Wavelengths for Various Celestial Bodies

The Bohr model of the hydrogen atom explained the atomic emission spectrum of hydrogen, which is the simplest emission spectrum among all the elements. The group of hydrogen emission lines corresponding to transitions from energy levels $n \geq 2$ to $n = 1$ is known as the **Lyman series**. The group corresponding to transitions from energy levels $n \geq 3$ to $n = 2$ is known as the **Balmer series** and includes four wavelengths in the visible region. The Lyman series includes larger energy transitions than the Balmer series; it therefore has shorter photon wavelengths in the UV region of the electromagnetic spectrum. The **Paschen series** corresponds to transitions from $n \geq 4$ to $n = 3$. These energy transition series can be seen in Figure 1.7.

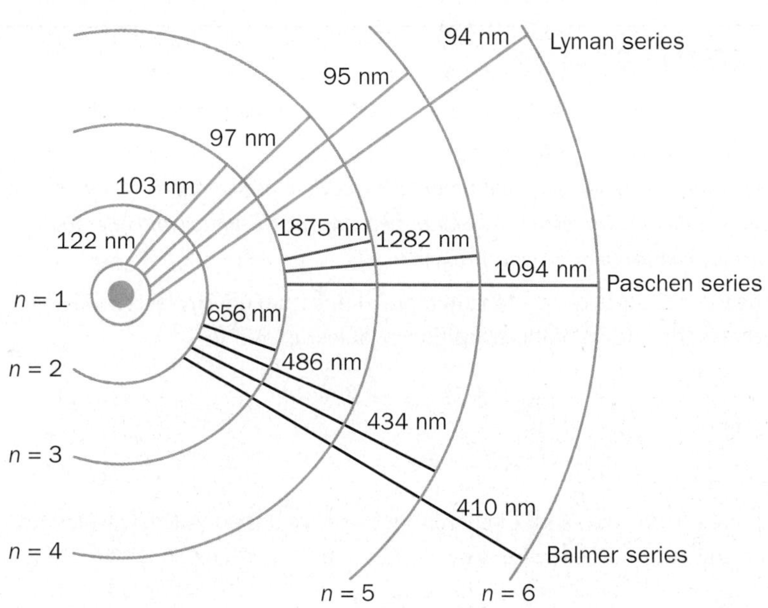

Figure 1.7 Wavelengths of Electron Orbital Transitions
Energy is inversely proportional to wavelength: $E = hf = \frac{hc}{\lambda}$.

The energy associated with a change in the principal quantum number from a higher initial value n_i to a lower final value n_f is equal to the energy of the photon predicted by Planck's quantum theory. Combining Bohr's and Planck's calculations, we can derive:

$$E = \frac{hc}{\lambda} = R_H\left[\frac{1}{n_i^2} - \frac{1}{n_f^2}\right]$$

Equation 1.5

This complex-appearing equation essentially says: *The energy of the emitted photon corresponds to the difference in energy between the higher-energy initial state and the lower-energy final state.*

KEY CONCEPT

It may seem strange to see an equation that has *initial* minus *final*, where most equations usually have final minus initial. But ultimately, this equation is designed to work just like you'd expect: If an atom emits a photon, the equation gives a negative value for energy, indicating a decrease. You can easily check this for yourself by using $n_i = 2$ and $n_f = 1$.

Atomic Absorption Spectra

When an electron is excited to a higher energy level, it must absorb exactly the right amount of energy to make that transition. This means that exciting the electrons of a particular element results in energy absorption at specific wavelengths. Thus, in addition to a unique emission spectrum, every element possesses a characteristic **absorption spectrum**. Not surprisingly, the wavelengths of absorption correspond exactly to the wavelengths of emission because the difference in energy between levels remains unchanged. Identification of elements in the gas phase requires absorption spectra.

Atomic emission and absorption spectra are complex topics, but the takeaway is that each element has a characteristic set of energy levels. For electrons to move from a lower energy level to a higher energy level, they must absorb the right amount of energy to do so. They absorb this energy in the form of light. Similarly, when electrons move from a higher energy level to a lower energy level, they emit the same amount of energy in the form of light.

BRIDGE

ΔE is the same for absorption or emission between any two energy levels according to the conservation of energy, as discussed in Chapter 2 of *MCAT Physics and Math Review*. This is also the same as the energy of the photon of light absorbed or emitted.

REAL WORLD

Absorption is the basis for the color of compounds. We see the color of the light that is *not* absorbed by the compound.

MCAT CONCEPT CHECK 1.3

Before you move on, assess your understanding of the material with these questions.

Note: *For these questions, try to estimate the calculations without a calculator to mimic Test Day conditions. Double-check your answers with a calculator and refer to the answers for confirmation of your results.*

1. The valence electron in a lithium atom jumps from energy level $n = 2$ to $n = 4$. What is the energy of this transition in joules? In eV?
   (Note: $R_H = 2.18 \times 10^{-18} \frac{J}{\text{electron}} = 13.6 \frac{eV}{\text{electron}}$)

   ____

2. If an electron emits 3 eV of energy, what is the corresponding wavelength of the emitted photon? (Note: 1 eV $= 1.60 \times 10^{-19}$ J, $h = 6.626 \times 10^{-34}$ J $\cdot$ s)

   ____

3. Calculate the energy of a photon of wavelength 662 nm. (Note: $h = 6.626 \times 10^{-34}$ J $\cdot$ s)

   ____

1.4 Quantum Mechanical Model of Atoms

LEARNING OBJECTIVES

After Chapter 1.4, you will be able to:

- Identify the four quantum numbers, the potential range of values for each, and their relationship to the electron they represent
- Compare the orbital diagram for a neutral atom, such as sulfur (S), to an ion such as S^{2-}
- Differentiate between paramagnetic and diamagnetic compounds
- Determine the number of valence electrons in a given atom

While Bohr's model marked a significant advancement in the understanding of the structure of atoms, his model ultimately proved inadequate to explain the structure and behavior of atoms containing more than one electron. The model's failure was a result of not taking into account the repulsion between multiple electrons surrounding the nucleus. Modern quantum mechanics has led to a more rigorous and generalizable study of the electronic structure of atoms. The most important difference between Bohr's model and the modern quantum mechanical model is that Bohr postulated that electrons follow a clearly defined circular pathway or orbit at a fixed distance from the nucleus, whereas modern quantum mechanics has shown that this is not the case. Rather, we now understand that electrons move rapidly and are localized within regions of space around the nucleus called **orbitals**. The confidence by which those in Bohr's time believed they could identify the location (or pathway) of the electron was now replaced by a more modest suggestion that the best we can do is describe the probability of finding an electron within a given region of space surrounding the nucleus. In the current quantum mechanical model, it is impossible to pinpoint exactly where an electron is at any given moment in time. This is expressed best by the **Heisenberg uncertainty principle**: *It is impossible to simultaneously determine, with perfect accuracy, the momentum and the position of an electron.* If we want to assess the position of an electron, the electron has to stop (thereby removing its momentum); if we want to assess its momentum, the electron has to be moving (thereby changing its position). This can be seen visually in Figure 1.8.

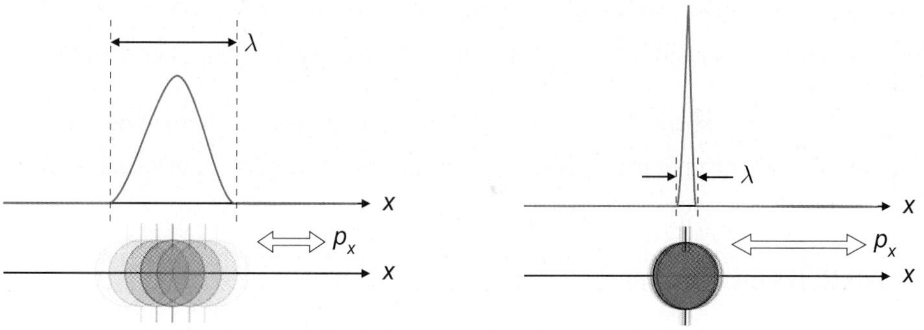

Figure 1.8 Heisenberg Uncertainty Principle
Known momentum and uncertain position (left); known position but uncertain momentum (right). λ = confidence interval of position; p_x = confidence interval of momentum.

Quantum Numbers

Modern atomic theory postulates that any electron in an atom can be completely described by four quantum numbers: n, l, m_l, and m_s. Furthermore, according to the **Pauli exclusion principle**, no two electrons in a given atom can possess the same set of four quantum numbers. The position and energy of an electron described by its quantum numbers are known as its *energy state*. The value of n limits the values of l, which in turn limit the values of m_l. In other words, for a given value of n, only particular values of l are permissible; given a value of l, only particular values of m_l are permissible. The values of the quantum numbers qualitatively give information about the size, shape, and orientation of the orbitals. As we examine the four quantum numbers more closely, pay attention especially to l and m_l because these two tend to give students the greatest difficulty.

MCAT EXPERTISE

Think of the quantum numbers as becoming more specific as one goes from n to l to m_l to m_s. This is like an address: one lives in a particular state (n), in a particular city (l), on a particular street (m_l), at a particular house number (m_s).

BRIDGE

Remember, a larger integer value for the principal quantum number indicates a larger radius and higher energy. This is similar to gravitational potential energy, as discussed in Chapter 2 of *MCAT Physics Review*, where the higher or farther the object is above the Earth, the higher its potential energy will be.

Principal Quantum Number

The first quantum number is commonly known as the **principal quantum number** and is denoted by the letter ***n***. This is the quantum number used in Bohr's model that can theoretically take on any positive integer value. The larger the integer value of n, the higher the energy level and radius of the electron's **shell**. Within each shell, there is a capacity to hold a certain number of electrons, given by:

$$\text{Maximum number of electrons within a shell} = 2n^2$$

Equation 1.6

where n is the principal quantum number. The difference in energy between two shells decreases as the distance from the nucleus increases because the energy difference is a function of $\left[\frac{1}{n_i^2} - \frac{1}{n_f^2}\right]$. For example, the energy difference between the $n = 3$ and the $n = 4$ shells $\left(\frac{1}{9} - \frac{1}{16}\right)$ is less than the energy difference between the $n = 1$ and the $n = 2$ shells $\left(\frac{1}{1} - \frac{1}{4}\right)$. This can be seen in Figure 1.7. Remember that electrons do not travel in precisely defined orbits; it just simplifies the visual representation of the electrons' motion.

Azimuthal Quantum Number

KEY CONCEPT

For any principal quantum number n, there will be n possible values for l, ranging from 0 to $(n - 1)$.

The second quantum number is called the **azimuthal (angular momentum) quantum number** and is designated by the letter ***l***. The second quantum number refers to the shape and number of **subshells** within a given principal energy level (shell). The azimuthal quantum number is very important because it has important implications for chemical bonding and bond angles. The value of n limits the value of l in the following way: for any given value of n, the range of possible values for l is 0 to $(n - 1)$. For example, within the first principal energy level, $n = 1$, the only possible value for l is 0; within the second principal energy level, $n = 2$, the possible values for l are 0 and 1. A simpler way to remember this relationship is that the n-value also tells you the number of possible subshells. Therefore, there's only one subshell $(l = 0)$ in the first principal energy level; there are two subshells ($l = 0$ and 1) within the second principal energy level; there are three subshells ($l = 0$, 1, and 2) within the third principal energy level, and so on.

Spectroscopic notation refers to the shorthand representation of the principal and azimuthal quantum numbers. The principal quantum number remains a number, but the azimuthal quantum number is designated by a letter: the $l = 0$ subshell is called s; the $l = 1$ subshell is called p; the $l = 2$ subshell is called d; and the $l = 3$ subshell is called f. Thus, an electron in the shell $n = 4$ and subshell $l = 2$ is said to be in the $4d$ subshell. The spectroscopic notation for each subshell is demonstrated in Figure 1.9.

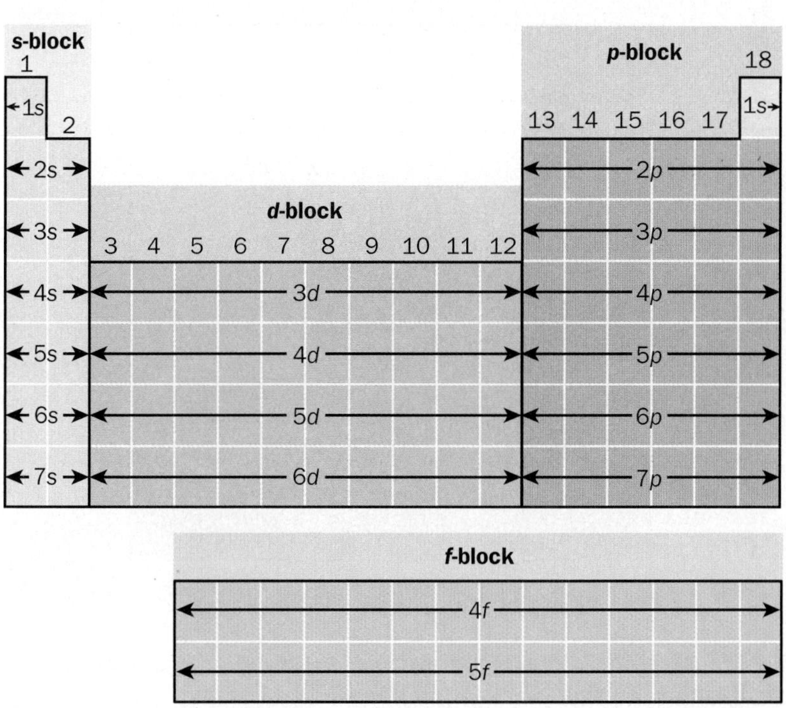

Figure 1.9 Spectroscopic Notation for Every Subshell on the Periodic Table

Within each subshell, there is a capacity to hold a certain number of electrons, given by:

$$\text{Maximum number of electrons within a subshell} = 4l + 2$$

Equation 1.7

where l is the azimuthal quantum number. The energies of the subshells increase with increasing l value; however, the energies of subshells from different principal energy levels may overlap. For example, the 4*s* subshell will have a lower energy than the 3*d* subshell.

Figure 1.10 provides an example of computer-generated probability maps of the first few electron clouds in a hydrogen atom. This provides a rough visual representation of the shapes of different subshells.

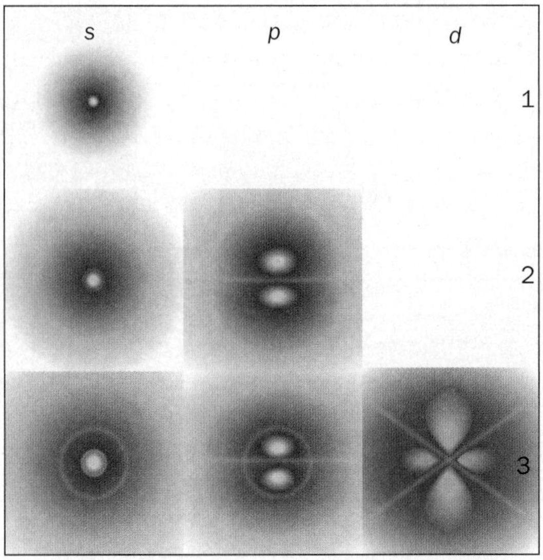

Figure 1.10 Electron Clouds of Various Subshells

Magnetic Quantum Number

The third quantum number is the **magnetic quantum number** and is designated $\boldsymbol{m_l}$. The magnetic quantum number specifies the particular **orbital** within a subshell where an electron is most likely to be found at a given moment in time. Each orbital can hold a maximum of two electrons. The possible values of m_l are the integers between $-l$ and $+l$, including 0. For example, the *s* subshell, with $l = 0$, limits the possible m_l values to 0, and because there is a single value of m_l, there is only one orbital in the *s* subshell. The *p* subshell, with $l = 1$, limits the possible m_l values to -1, 0, and $+1$, and because there are three values for m_l, there are three orbitals in the *p* subshell. The *d* subshell has five orbitals (-2 to $+2$), and the *f* subshell has seven orbitals (-3 to $+3$). The shape of the orbitals, like the number of orbitals, is dependent on the subshell in which they are found. The orbitals in the *s* subshell are spherical, while the three orbitals in the *p* subshell are each dumbbell-shaped and align along the *x*-, *y*-, and *z*-axes. In fact, the *p*-orbitals are often referred to as p_x, p_y, and p_z. The first five orbitals—1*s*, 2*s*, 2p_x, 2p_y, and 2p_z—are demonstrated in Figure 1.11. Note the similarity to the images in Figure 1.10.

KEY CONCEPT

For any value of l, there will be $2l + 1$ possible values for m_l. For any n, this produces n^2 orbitals. For any value of n, there will be a maximum of $2n^2$ electrons (two per orbital).

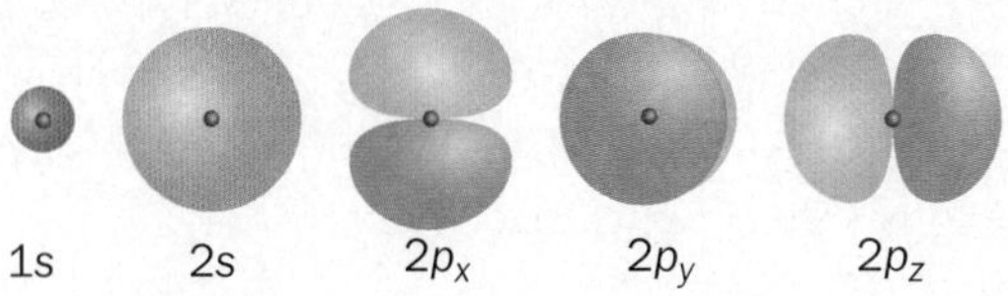

Figure 1.11 The First Five Atomic Orbitals

The shapes of the orbitals in the *d* and *f* subshells are much more complex, and the MCAT will not expect you to answer questions about their appearance. The shapes of orbitals are defined in terms of a concept called probability density, the likelihood that an electron will be found in a particular region of space.

Take a look at the 2*p* block in the periodic table. As mentioned above, 2*p* contains three orbitals. If each orbital can contain two electrons, then six electrons can be added during the course of filling the 2*p*-orbitals. As atomic number increases, so too does the number of electrons (assuming the species is neutral). Therefore, it should be no surprise that the *p* block contains six groups of elements. The *s* block contains two elements in each row of the periodic table, the *d* block contains ten elements, and the *f* block contains fourteen elements.

Spin Quantum Number

The fourth quantum number is called the **spin quantum number** and is denoted by m_s. In classical mechanics, an object spinning about its axis has an infinite number of possible values for its angular momentum. However, this does not apply to the electron, which has two spin orientations designated $+\frac{1}{2}$ and $-\frac{1}{2}$. Whenever two electrons are in the same orbital, they must have opposite spins. In this case, they are often referred to as being **paired**. Electrons in different orbitals with the same m_s values are said to have **parallel spins**.

The quantum numbers for the orbitals in the second principal energy level, with their maximum number of electrons noted in parentheses, are shown in Table 1.2.

N	2 (8)			
l	0 (2)	1 (6)		
m_l	0 (2)	+1 (2)	0 (2)	−1 (2)
m_s	$+\frac{1}{2}, -\frac{1}{2}$	$+\frac{1}{2}, -\frac{1}{2}$	$+\frac{1}{2}, -\frac{1}{2}$	$+\frac{1}{2}, -\frac{1}{2}$

Table 1.2 Quantum Numbers for the Second Principal Energy Level

Electron Configurations

For a given atom or ion, the pattern by which subshells are filled, as well as the number of electrons within each principal energy level and subshell, are designated by its **electron configuration**. Electron configurations use spectroscopic notation, wherein the first number denotes the principal energy level, the letter designates the subshell, and the superscript gives the number of electrons in that subshell. For example, $2p^4$ indicates that there are four electrons in the second (*p*) subshell of the second principal energy level. This also implies that the energy levels below 2*p* (that is, 1*s* and 2*s*) have already been filled, as shown in Figure 1.12.

MCAT EXPERTISE

Remember that the shorthand used to describe the electron configuration is derived directly from the quantum numbers.

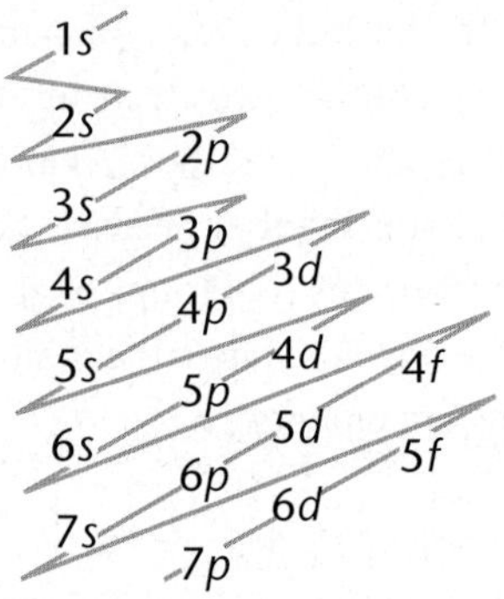

Figure 1.12 Electron Subshell Flow Diagram

To write out an atom's electron configuration, one needs to know the order in which subshells are filled. Electrons fill from lower- to higher-energy subshells, according to the **Aufbau principle** (also called the **building-up principle**), and each subshell will fill completely before electrons begin to enter the next one. The order need not be memorized because there are two very helpful ways of recalling this. The ***n* + *l* rule** can be used to rank subshells by increasing energy. This rule states that the lower the sum of the values of the first and second quantum numbers, $n + l$, the lower the energy of the subshell. This is a helpful rule to remember for Test Day. If two subshells possess the same $n + l$ value, the subshell with the lower n value has a lower energy and will fill with electrons first.

Example: Which will fill first, the 5*d* subshell or the 6*s* subshell?

Solution: For 5*d*, $n = 5$ and $l = 2$, so $n + l = 7$. For 6*s*, $n = 6$ and $l = 0$, so $n + l = 6$. Therefore, the 6*s* subshell has lower energy and will fill first.

An alternative way to approach electron configurations is through simply reading the periodic table. One must remember that the lowest *s* subshell is 1*s*, the lowest *p* subshell is 2*p*, the lowest *d* subshell is 3*d*, and the lowest *f* subshell is 4*f*. This can be seen in Figure 1.9. Then, we can simply read across the periodic table to get to the element of interest, filling subshells along the way. To do this, we must know the correct position of the lanthanide and actinide series (the *f* block), as shown in Figure 1.13. In most representations of the periodic table, the *f* block is pulled out and placed below the rest of the table. This is purely an effect of graphic design—placing the *f* block in its correct location results in a lot of excess white space on a page.

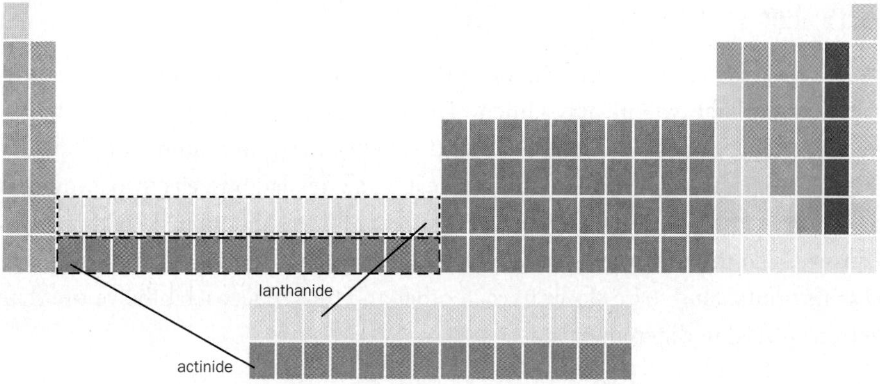

Figure 1.13 Periodic Table with Lanthanide and Actinide Series Inserted
The f block fits between the s block and d block in the periodic table.

Electron configurations can be abbreviated by placing the noble gas that precedes the element of interest in brackets. For example, the electron configuration of any element in period four (starting with potassium) can be abbreviated by starting with [Ar].

Example: What is the electron configuration of osmium ($Z = 76$)?

Solution: The noble gas that comes just before osmium is xenon ($Z = 54$). Therefore, the electron configuration can begin with [Xe]. Continuing across the periodic table, we pass through the 6*s* subshell (cesium and barium), the 4*f* subshell (the lanthanide series; remember its position on the periodic table!), and into the 5*d* subshell. Osmium is the sixth element in the 5*d* subshell, so the configuration is [Xe] $6s^2 4f^{14} 5d^6$.

This method works for neutral atoms, but how does one write the electron configuration of an ion? Negatively charged ions (**anions**) have additional electrons that fill according to the same rules as above; for example, if fluorine's electron configuration is [He] $2s^2 2p^5$, then F^- is [He] $2s^2 2p^6$. Positively charged ions (**cations**) are a bit more complicated: start with the neutral atom, and remove electrons from the subshells with the highest value for *n* first. If multiple subshells are tied for the highest *n* value, then electrons are removed from the subshell with the highest *l* value among these.

Example: What is the electron configuration of Fe^{3+}?

Solution: The electron configuration of iron is [Ar] $4s^2 3d^6$. Electrons are removed from the 4*s* subshell before the 3*d* subshell because it has a higher principal quantum number. Therefore, Fe^{3+} has a configuration of [Ar] $3d^5$, not [Ar] $4s^2 3d^3$.

MCAT EXPERTISE

Many general chemistry courses teach the flow diagram in Figure 1.12 as a method to determine the order of subshell filling in electron configurations. However, on Test Day, it can be both time-consuming and error-prone, resulting in incorrect electron configurations. Learning to read the periodic table, as described here, is the best method.

Hund's Rule

In subshells that contain more than one orbital, such as the $2p$ subshell with its three orbitals, the orbitals will fill according to **Hund's rule**, which states that, within a given subshell, orbitals are filled such that there are a maximum number of half-filled orbitals with parallel spins. Like finding a seat on a crowded bus, electrons would prefer to have their own seat (orbital) before being forced to double up with another electron. Of course, the basis for this preference is electron repulsion: electrons in the same orbital tend to be closer to each other and thus repel each other more than electrons placed in different orbitals.

Example: According to Hund's rule, what are the orbital diagrams for nitrogen and iron?

Solution: Nitrogen has an atomic number of 7. Thus, its electron configuration is $1s^2 2s^2 2p^3$. According to Hund's rule, the two *s*-orbitals will fill completely, while the three *p*-orbitals will each contain one electron, all with parallel spins.

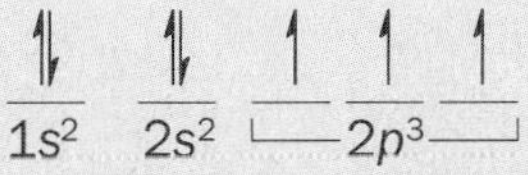

Iron has an atomic number of 26. As determined earlier, its electron configuration is [Ar] $4s^2 3d^6$. The electrons will fill all of the subshells except for the 3*d*, which will contain four orbitals with parallel (upward) spin and one orbital with electrons of both spin directions.

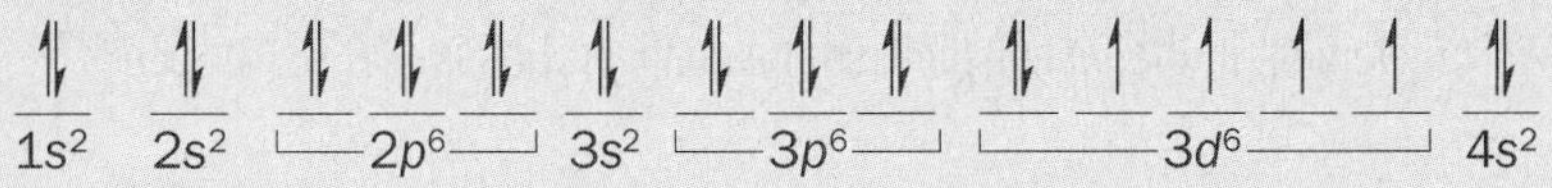

Subshells may be listed either in the order in which they fill (4*s* before 3*d*) or with subshells of the same principal quantum number grouped together, as shown here. Both methods are correct.

An important corollary from Hund's rule is that half-filled and fully filled orbitals have lower energies (higher stability) than other states. This creates two notable exceptions to electron configuration that are often tested on the MCAT: chromium (and other elements in its group) and copper (and other elements in its group). Chromium ($Z = 24$) should have the electron configuration [Ar] $4s^2 3d^4$ according to the rules established earlier. However, moving one electron from the 4*s* subshell to the 3*d* subshell allows the 3*d* subshell to be half-filled: [Ar] $4s^1 3d^5$ (remember that *s* subshells can hold two electrons and *d* subshells can hold ten). While moving the 4*s* electron up to the 3*d*-orbital is energetically unfavorable, the extra stability from making the 3*d* subshell half-filled outweighs that cost. Similarly, copper ($Z = 29$) has the electron configuration [Ar] $4s^1 3d^{10}$, rather than [Ar] $4s^2 3d^9$; a full *d* subshell outweighs the cost of moving an electron out of the 4*s* subshell. Other elements in the same group have similar behavior, moving one electron from the highest *s* subshell to the highest *d* subshell. Similar shifts can be seen with *f* subshells, but they are *never* observed for the *p* subshell; the extra stability doesn't outweigh the cost.

The presence of paired or unpaired electrons affects the chemical and magnetic properties of an atom or molecule. Materials composed of atoms with unpaired electrons will orient their spins in alignment with a magnetic field, and the material will thus be weakly attracted to the magnetic field. These materials are considered **paramagnetic**. An example is shown in Figure 1.14 where a set of iron orbs is influenced by a magnet. The metallic spheres that are close enough to be induced by the magnet are attracted to the magnet and move toward it.

MNEMONIC

Remember that **para**magnetic means that a magnetic field will cause **para**llel spins in unpaired electrons and therefore cause an attraction.

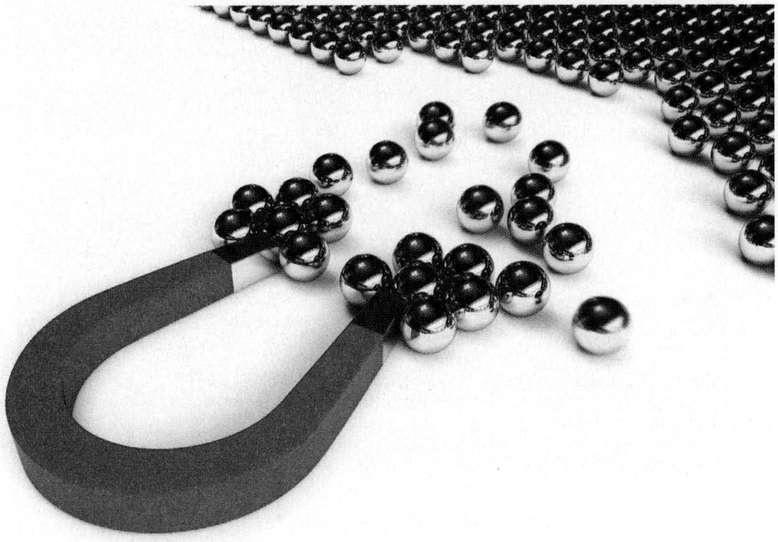

Figure 1.14 Attraction of Paramagnetic Iron Spheres to a Magnet

Materials consisting of atoms that have only paired electrons will be slightly repelled by a magnetic field and are said to be **diamagnetic**. In Figure 1.15, a piece of pyrolytic graphite is suspended in the air over strong neodymium magnets. All the electrons in this *allotrope* (configuration) of carbon are paired because of covalent bonding between layers of the material, and are thus opposed to being reoriented. Given sufficiently strong magnetic fields beneath an object, any diamagnetic substance can be made to levitate.

REAL WORLD

The concept behind "maglev" or magnetic levitation is no longer science fiction. Using powerful magnetic fields and strongly diamagnetic materials, some transportation systems have developed frictionless, high speed rail networks such as Japan's SCMaglev.

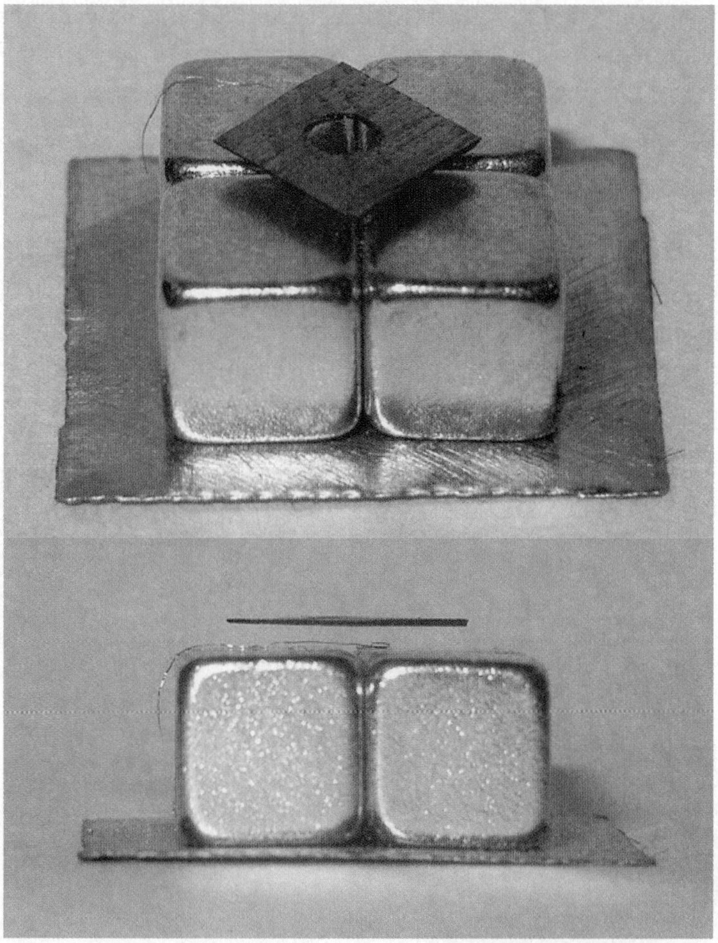

Figure 1.15 Diamagnetic Pyrolytic Graphite

Valence Electrons

MCAT EXPERTISE

The valence electron configuration of an atom helps us understand its properties and is ascertainable from the periodic table (the only "cheat sheet" available on the MCAT!). On Test Day, you will be able to access a periodic table by clicking on the button labeled "Periodic Table" on the bottom left of the screen. Use it as needed!

The valence electrons of an atom are those electrons that are in its outermost energy shell, are most easily removed, and are available for bonding. In other words, the valence electrons are the "active" electrons of an atom and to a large extent dominate the chemical behavior of the atom. For elements in Groups IA and IIA (Groups 1 and 2), only the highest *s* subshell electrons are valence electrons. For elements in Groups IIIA through VIIIA (Groups 13 through 18), the highest *s* and *p* subshell electrons are valence electrons. For transition elements, the valence electrons are those in the highest *s* and *d* subshells, even though they have different principal quantum numbers. For the lanthanide and actinide series, the valence electrons are those in the highest *s* and *f* subshells, even though they have different principal quantum numbers. All elements in period three (starting with sodium) and below may accept electrons into their *d* subshell, which allows them to hold more than eight electrons in their valence shell. This allows them to violate the octet rule, as discussed in Chapter 3 of *MCAT General Chemistry Review*.

Example: Which electrons are the valence electrons of elemental vanadium, elemental selenium, and the sulfur atom in a sulfate ion?

Solution: Vanadium has five valence electrons: two in its 4*s* subshell and three in its 3*d* subshell.

Selenium has six valence electrons: two in its 4*s* subshell and four in its 4*p* subshell. Selenium's 3*d* electrons are not part of its valence shell.

Sulfur in a sulfate ion has 12 valence electrons: its original six plus six more from the oxygens to which it is bonded. Sulfur's 3*s* and 3*p* subshells can contain only eight of these 12 electrons; the other four electrons have entered the sulfur atom's 3*d* subshell, which is normally empty in elemental sulfur.

MCAT CONCEPT CHECK 1.4

Before you move on, assess your understanding of the material with these questions.

1. If given the following quantum numbers, which element(s) do they likely refer to? (Note: Assume that these quantum numbers describe the valence electrons in the element.)

n	*l*	Possible Elements
2	1	
3	0	
5	3	
4	2	

2. Write out and compare an orbital diagram for a neutral oxygen (O) atom and an O^{2-} ion.

---

3. Magnetic resonance angiography (MRA) is a technique that can resolve defects like stenotic (narrowed) arteries. A contrast agent like gadolinium or manganese injected into the blood stream interacts with the strong magnetic fields of the MRI device to produce such images. Based on their orbital configurations, are these contrast agents paramagnetic or diamagnetic?

---

4. Determine how many valence electrons come from each subshell in the following atoms:

Atom	*s*-electrons	*p*-electrons	*d*-electrons	*f*-electrons	Total Valence Electrons
P in PO_4^{3-}					
O in PO_4^{3-}					
Ir					
Cf					

Conclusion

Congratulations! You've made it through the first chapter! Now that we have covered topics related to the most fundamental unit of matter—the atom—you're set to advance your understanding of the physical world in more complex ways. This chapter described the characteristics and behavior of the three subatomic particles: the proton, neutron, and electron. In addition, it compared and contrasted two models of the atom. The Bohr model is adequate for describing the structure of one-electron systems, such as the hydrogen atom or the helium ion, but fails to adequately describe the structure of more complex atoms. The quantum mechanical model theorizes that electrons are found not in discrete orbits, but in "clouds of probability," or orbitals, by which we can predict the likelihood of finding electrons within given regions of space surrounding the nucleus. Both theories tell us that the energy levels available to electrons are not infinite but discrete and that the energy difference between levels is a precise amount called a quantum. The four quantum numbers completely describe the location and energy of any electron within a given atom. Finally, we learned two simple recall methods for the order in which electrons fill the shells and subshells of an atom and that the valence electrons are the reactive electrons in an atom. In the next chapter, we'll take a look at how the elements are organized on the periodic table and will then turn our attention to their bonding behavior—based on valence electrons—in Chapter 3 of *MCAT General Chemistry Review*.

You've reviewed the content, now test your knowledge and critical thinking skills by completing a test-like passage set in your online resources!

GO ONLINE

CONCEPT SUMMARY

Subatomic Particles

- **A proton** has a positive charge and mass around 1 amu; a **neutron** has no charge and mass around 1 amu; an **electron** has a negative charge and negligible mass.
- The **nucleus** contains the protons and neutrons, while the electrons move around the nucleus.
- The **atomic number** is the number of protons in a given element.
- The **mass number** is the sum of an element's protons and neutrons.

Atomic Mass *vs.* Atomic Weight

- **Atomic mass** is essentially equal to the mass number, the sum of an element's protons and neutrons.
  - **Isotopes** are atoms of a given element (same atomic number) that have different mass numbers. They differ in the number of neutrons.
  - Most isotopes are identified by the element followed by the mass number (such as carbon-12, carbon-13, and carbon-14).
  - The three isotopes of hydrogen go by different names: protium, deuterium, and tritium.
- **Atomic weight** is the weighted average of the naturally occurring isotopes of an element. The periodic table lists atomic weights, not atomic masses.

Rutherford, Planck, and Bohr

- Rutherford first postulated that the atom had a dense, positively charged nucleus that made up only a small fraction of the volume of the atom.
- In the **Bohr model of the atom**, a dense, positively charged nucleus is surrounded by electrons revolving around the nucleus in orbits with distinct energy levels.
- The energy difference between energy levels is called a **quantum**, first described by Planck.
  - Quantization means that there is not an infinite range of energy levels available to an electron; electrons can exist only at certain energy levels. The energy of an electron increases the farther it is from the nucleus.
  - The **atomic absorption spectrum** of an element is unique; for an electron to jump from a lower energy level to a higher one, it must absorb an amount of energy precisely equal to the energy difference between the two levels.
  - When electrons return from the excited state to the ground state, they emit an amount of energy that is exactly equal to the energy difference between the two levels; every element has a characteristic **atomic emission spectrum**, and sometimes the electromagnetic energy emitted corresponds to a frequency in the visible light range.

Quantum Mechanical Model of Atoms

- The **quantum mechanical model** posits that electrons do not travel in defined orbits but rather are localized in orbitals; an **orbital** is a region of space around the nucleus defined by the probability of finding an electron in that region of space.
- The **Heisenberg uncertainty principle** states that it is impossible to know both an electron's position and its momentum *exactly* at the same time.
- There are four **quantum numbers**; these numbers completely describe any electron in an atom.
  - The **principal quantum number**, $\boldsymbol{n}$, describes the average energy of a **shell**.
  - The **azimuthal quantum number**, $\boldsymbol{l}$, describes the **subshells** within a given principal energy level (*s*, *p*, *d*, and *f*).
  - The **magnetic quantum number**, $\boldsymbol{m_l}$, specifies the particular **orbital** within a subshell where an electron is likely to be found at a given moment in time.
  - The **spin quantum number**, $\boldsymbol{m_s}$, indicates the spin orientation $\left(\pm\frac{1}{2}\right)$ of an electron in an orbital.
- The **electron configuration** uses **spectroscopic notation** (combining the *n* and *l* values as a number and letter, respectively) to designate the location of electrons.
  - For example, $1s^2 2s^2 2p^6 3s^2$ is the electron configuration for magnesium: a neutral magnesium atom has 12 electrons—two in the *s* subshell of the first energy level, two in the *s* subshell of the second energy level, six in the *p* subshell of the second energy level, and two in the *s* subshell of the third energy level; the two electrons in the 3*s* subshell are the valence electrons for the magnesium atom.
- Electrons fill the principal energy levels and subshells according to increasing energy, which can be determined by the **$n + l$ rule**.
- Electrons fill orbitals according to **Hund's rule**, which states that subshells with multiple orbitals (*p*, *d*, and *f*) fill electrons so that every orbital in a subshell gets one electron before any of them gets a second.
  - **Paramagnetic** materials have unpaired electrons that align with magnetic fields, attracting the material to a magnet.
  - **Diamagnetic** materials have all paired electrons, which cannot easily be realigned; they are repelled by magnets.
- **Valence electrons** are those electrons in the outermost shell available for interaction (bonding) with other atoms.
  - For the representative elements (those in Groups 1, 2, and 13–18), the valence electrons are found in *s*- and/or *p*-orbitals.
  - For the transition elements, the valence electrons are found in *s*- and either *d*- or *f*-orbitals.
  - Many atoms interact with other atoms to form bonds that complete an octet in the valence shell.

ANSWERS TO CONCEPT CHECKS

1.1

1. Charge is determined by the number of electrons present. Atomic number is determined by the number of protons. Isotope is determined by the number of neutrons (while protons make up part of the mass number, it is the number of neutrons that explains the variability between isotopes).
2. ^{18}O: 8 p^+, 10 n^0, 8 e^-. ^{18}F: 9 p^+, 9 n^0, 9 e^-.

1.2

1. Atomic mass is (just slightly less than) the sum of the masses of protons and neutrons in a given atom of an element. Atoms of the same element with different mass numbers are isotopes of each other. The atomic weight is the weighted average of the naturally occurring isotopes of an element.
2. This ratio is an equivalent concept. It is therefore acceptable, as long as units can be cancelled in dimensional analysis.
3.

Isotope	Protons	Neutrons	Electrons
^{19}O	8	11	8
^{16}O	8	8	8
^{17}O	8	9	8
^{19}F	9	10	9
^{16}F	9	7	9
^{238}U	92	146	92
^{240}U	92	148	92

1.3

1. $$E = R_H\left[\frac{1}{n_i^2} - \frac{1}{n_f^2}\right] = 2.18 \times 10^{-18}\left[\frac{1}{2^2} - \frac{1}{4^2}\right] \approx 2 \times 10^{-18}\left[\frac{3}{16}\right]$$
$$\approx 3.75 \times 10^{-19}\text{ J} \approx 4 \times 10^{-19}\text{ J} \left(\text{actual value is } 4.09 \times 10^{-19}\text{ J}\right).$$
$$E = R_H\left[\frac{1}{n_i^2} - \frac{1}{n_f^2}\right] = 13.6\left[\frac{1}{2^2} - \frac{1}{4^2}\right] \approx (14)\left[\frac{3}{16}\right]$$
$$= \left(\frac{14 \times 3}{16}\right) = \left(\frac{7}{8} \times 3\right) = \left(\frac{21}{8}\right) \approx 2.5 \text{ (actual value is 2.55 eV).}$$

2. $3\,\text{eV}\left(1.60\times10^{-19}\ \frac{\text{J}}{\text{eV}}\right) = 4.8\times10^{-19}\ \text{J}$

$$E = \frac{hc}{\lambda} \rightarrow \lambda = \frac{hc}{E} = \frac{\left(6.626\times10^{-34}\ \text{J}\cdot\text{s}\right)\left(3.00\times10^{8}\ \frac{\text{m}}{\text{s}}\right)}{\left(4.8\times10^{-19}\ \text{J}\right)}$$

$$\approx \frac{(6.6\times3)\left(10^{-34}\times10^{8}\right)}{4.8\times10^{-19}} = \frac{6.6\times10^{-26}}{1.6\times10^{-19}} \approx \frac{6.4\times10^{-26}}{1.6\times10^{-19}} = \frac{64}{16}\times10^{-26+19}$$

$$= 4\times10^{-7}\ \text{m} = 400\ \text{nm}\ \left(\text{actual value} = 4.14\times10^{-7} = 414\ \text{nm}\right)$$

3. $E = \frac{hc}{\lambda} = \frac{\left(6.626\times10^{-34}\ \text{J}\cdot\text{s}\right)\left(3.00\times10^{8}\ \frac{\text{m}}{\text{s}}\right)}{\left(6.62\times10^{-7}\ \text{m}\right)}$

$$= \frac{(6.626\times3.00)\left(10^{-34}\times10^{8}\right)}{6.62\times10^{-7}} = \frac{3.00\times10^{-26}}{10^{-7}} = 3.00\times10^{-26+7}$$

$$= 3.00\times10^{-19}\ \text{J}$$

1.4

1.

n	l	**Possible Elements**
2	1	2*p*: B, C, N, O, F, Ne
3	0	3*s*: Na, Mg
5	3	5*f*: Actinide series
4	2	4*d*: Y, Zr, Nb, Mo, Tc, Ru, Rh, Pd, Ag, Cd

2. Both O and O^{2-} have fully filled 1*s*- and 2*s*-orbitals. O has four electrons in the 2*p* subshell; two are paired, and the other two each have their own orbital. O^{2-} has six electrons in the 2*p* subshell, all of which are paired in the three *p*-orbitals.
3. Both these molecules have unfilled valence electron shells with relatively few paired electrons; therefore, they are paramagnetic.
4.

Atom	***s*-electrons**	***p*-electrons**	***d*-electrons**	***f*-electrons**	**Total Valence Electrons**
P in PO_4^{3-}	2	6	2	0	10
O in PO_4^{3-}	2	6	0	0	8
Ir	2	0	7	0	9
Cf	2	0	0	10	12

SCIENCE MASTERY ASSESSMENT EXPLANATIONS

1. **A**

Remember that when electrons are removed from an element, forming a cation, they will be removed from the subshell with the highest *n* value first. Zn^0 has 30 electrons, so it would have an electron configuration of $1s^22s^22p^63s^23p^64s^23d^{10}$. The 4*s* subshell has the highest principal quantum number, so it is emptied first, forming $1s^22s^22p^63s^23p^64s^03d^{10}$. **(B)** implies that electrons are pulled out of the *d* subshell, **(C)** presents the configuration of the uncharged zinc atom, and **(D)** shows the configuration that would exist if four electrons were removed.

2. **B**

The azimuthal quantum number *l* cannot be higher than $n - 1$, ruling out **(A)**. The m_l number, which describes the chemical's magnetic properties, can only be an integer value between $-l$ and l. It cannot be equal to ± 1 if $l = 0$; this would imply that the *s* subshell has three orbitals (-1, 0, and 1) when we know it can only have one. This rules out **(C)** and **(D)**.

3. **C**

For any value of *n*, there will be a maximum of $2n^2$ electrons; that is, two per orbital. This can also be determined from the periodic table. There are only two elements (H and He) that have valence electrons in the $n = 1$ shell. Eight elements (Li to Ne) have valence electrons in the $n = 2$ shell. This is the only equation that matches this pattern.

4. **B**

This formula describes the number of electrons in terms of the azimuthal quantum number *l*, which ranges from 0 to $n - 1$, with *n* being the principal quantum number. A table of the maximum number of electrons per subshell is provided here:

Subshell	Azimuthal Quantum Number (l)	Number of Electrons
s	0	2
p	1	6
d	2	10
f	3	14

5. **D**

The only answer choice without unpaired electrons in its ground state is helium. Recall from the chapter that a diamagnetic substance is identified by the lack of unpaired electrons in its shell. A substance without unpaired electrons, like helium, cannot be magnetized by an external magnetic field and is actually slightly repelled. Elements that come at the end of a block (Group IIA, the group containing Zn, and the noble gases, most notably) have only paired electrons.

6. **D**

The problem requires the MCAT favorite equation $E = \frac{hc}{\lambda}$, where $h = 6.626 \times 10^{-34}\ \text{J} \cdot \text{s}$ (Planck's constant), $c = 3.00 \times 10^8\ \frac{\text{m}}{\text{s}}$ is the speed of light, and λ is the wavelength of the light. This question asks for the energy of one mole of photons, so we must multiply by Avogadro's number, $N_A = 6.02 \times 10^{23}\ \text{mol}^{-1}$.

The setup is: $E = \frac{hc}{\lambda} \times N_A$

$$= \frac{\left(6.626 \times 10^{-34}\ \text{J} \cdot \text{s}\right)\left(3.00 \times 10^8\ \frac{\text{m}}{\text{s}}\right)}{\left(500 \times 10^{-9}\ \text{m}\right)} \times \left(6.02 \times 10^{23}\ \text{mol}^{-1}\right)$$

$$= \frac{(6.626 \times 3 \times 6.02)\left(10^{-34} \times 10^8 \times 10^{23}\right)}{500 \times 10^{-9}} \approx \frac{(7 \times 3 \times 6)\left(10^{-3}\right)}{500 \times 10^{-9}}$$

$$= \frac{(21 \times 6)\left(10^{-3}\right)}{500 \times 10^{-9}} \approx \frac{125}{500} \times 10^{-3+9} = \frac{1}{4} \times 10^6 = 2.5 \times 10^5\ \text{J}$$

As we rounded during calculation, we must find the answer choice that most closely matches this value. **(D)** is the closest match.

7. **B**

Because the electron is moving into the $n = 1$ shell, the only subshell available is the 1*s* subshell, which eliminates **(C)** and **(D)**. There will be some energy change, however, as the electron must lose energy to return to the minimum-energy ground state. That will require emitting radiation in the form of a photon.

8. **A**

Recall that the superscript refers to the mass number of an atom, which is equal to the number of protons plus the number of neutrons present in an element. Sometimes a text will list the atomic number, *Z*, as a subscript under the mass number, *A*. According to the periodic table, carbon contains six protons; therefore, its atomic number is 6. Isotopes all have the same number of protons, but differ in the number of neutrons. Almost all atoms with $Z > 1$ have at least one neutron. Carbon is most likely to have a mass number of 12, for six protons and six neutrons, as in **(B)**. **(C)** and **(D)** are possible isotopes that would have more neutrons than ^{12}C. The ^{6}C isotope is unlikely. It would mean that there are 6 protons and 0 neutrons. As shown in Figure 1.4, this would be a highly unstable isotope.

9. **C**

The limitations placed by the Heisenberg uncertainty principle are caused by limitations inherent in the measuring process: if a particle is moving, it has momentum, but trying to measure that momentum necessarily creates uncertainty in the position. Even if we had an exact definition of the meter, as in **(A)**, or perfect measuring devices, as in **(B)**, we still wouldn't be able to measure position *and* momentum simultaneously *and* exactly.

10. **B**

For the electron to *gain* energy, it must absorb energy from photons to jump up to a higher energy level. There is a bigger jump between $n = 2$ and $n = 6$ than there is between $n = 3$ and $n = 4$.

11. **A**

The MCAT covers the topics in this chapter qualitatively more often than quantitatively. It is critical to be able to distinguish the fundamental principles that determine electron organization, which are usually known by the names of the scientists who discovered or postulated them. The Heisenberg uncertainty principle, **(B)**, refers to the inability to know the momentum and position of a single electron simultaneously. The Bohr model, **(C)**, was an early attempt to describe the behavior of the single electron in a hydrogen atom. The Rutherford model, **(D)**, described a dense, positively charged nucleus. The element shown here, phosphorus, is often used to demonstrate Hund's rule because it contains a half-filled *p* subshell. Hund's rule explains that electrons fill empty orbitals first before doubling up electrons in the same orbital.

12. **A**

The quickest way to solve this problem is to use the periodic table and find out how many protons are in Cs atoms; there are 55. Neutral Cs atoms would also have 55 electrons. A stable Cs cation will have a single positive charge because it has one unpaired *s*-electron. This translates to one fewer electron than the number of protons or 54 electrons.

13. **B**

The easiest way to approach this problem is to set up a system of two algebraic equations, where H and D are the percentages of H (mass = 1 amu) and D (mass = 2 amu), respectively. Your setup should look like the following system:

$$\text{H} + \text{D} = 1 \text{ (percent H} + \text{percent D} = 100\%)$$

$$1\ \text{H} + 2\ \text{D} = 1.008 \text{ (atomic weight calculation)}$$

Rearranging the first equation and substituting into the second yields $(1 - D) + 2D = 1.008$, or $D = 0.008$. 0.008 is 0.8%, so there is 0.8% D.

14. **A**

The terms in the answer choices refer to the magnetic spin of the two electrons. The quantum number m_s represents this property as a measure of an electron's intrinsic spin. These electrons' spins are parallel, in that their spins are aligned in the same direction ($m_s = +\frac{1}{2}$ for both species).

15. **B**

When dealing with ions, you cannot directly approach electronic configurations based on the number of electrons they currently hold. First examine the neutral atom's configuration, and then determine which electrons are removed.

Neutral Atom's Configuration	Ion's Configuration
Cr^0: [Ar] $4s^1 3d^5$	—
Mn^0: [Ar] $4s^2 3d^5$	Mn^+: [Ar] $4s^1 3d^5$
Fe^0: [Ar] $4s^2 3d^6$	Fe^{2+}: [Ar] $4s^0 3d^6$

Due to the stability of half-filled *d*-orbitals, neutral chromium assumes the electron configuration of [Ar] $4s^1 3d^5$. Mn must lose one electron from its initial configuration to become the Mn^+ cation. That electron would come from the 4*s* subshell according to the rule that the first electron removed comes from the highest-energy shell. Fe must lose two electrons to become Fe^{2+}. They'll both be lost from the same orbital; the only way Fe^{2+} could hold the configuration in the question stem would be if one *d*-electron and one *s*-electron were lost together.

Consult your online resources for additional practice. GO ONLINE

EQUATIONS TO REMEMBER

(1.1) **Planck relation (frequency):** $E = hf$

(1.2) **Angular momentum of an electron (Bohr model):** $L = \frac{nh}{2\pi}$

(1.3) **Energy of an electron (Bohr model):** $E = -\frac{R_H}{n^2}$

(1.4) **Planck relation (wavelength):** $E = \frac{hc}{\lambda}$

(1.5) **Energy of electron transition (Bohr model):** $E = R_H\left[\frac{1}{n_i^2} - \frac{1}{n_f^2}\right]$

(1.6) **Maximum number of electrons within a shell:** $2n^2$

(1.7) **Maximum number of electrons within a subshell:** $4l + 2$

SHARED CONCEPTS

General Chemistry Chapter 2
The Periodic Table

General Chemistry Chapter 3
Bonding and Chemical Interactions

Organic Chemistry Chapter 3
Bonding

Physics and Math Chapter 2
Work and Energy

Physics and Math Chapter 8
Light and Optics

Physics and Math Chapter 9
Atomic and Nuclear Phenomena

CHAPTER 2

THE PERIODIC TABLE

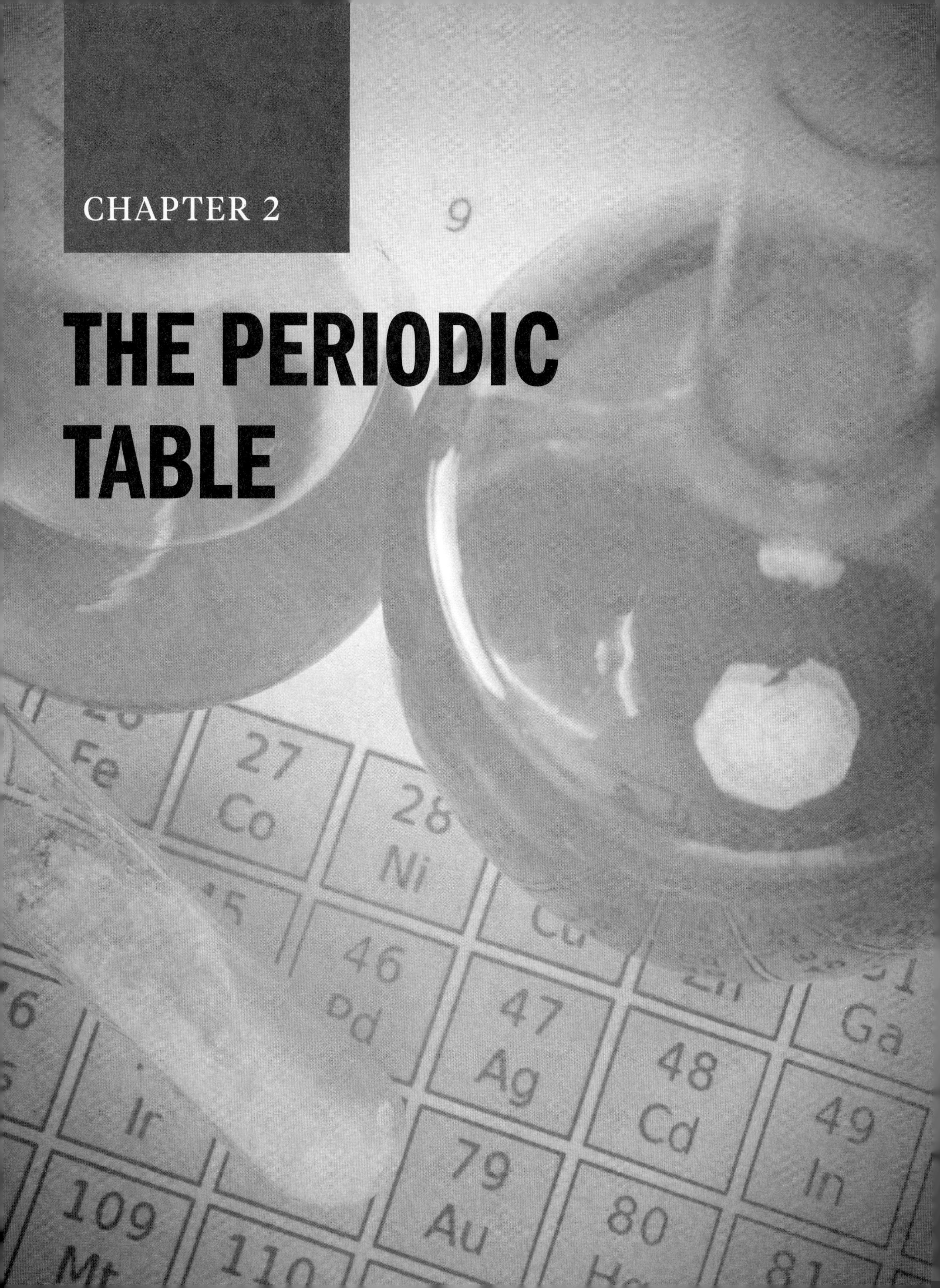

SCIENCE MASTERY ASSESSMENT

Every pre-med knows this feeling: there is so much content I have to know for the MCAT! How do I know what to do first or what's important?

While the high-yield badges throughout this book will help you identify the most important topics, this Science Mastery Assessment is another tool in your MCAT prep arsenal. This quiz (which can also be taken in your online resources) and the guidance below will help ensure that you are spending the appropriate amount of time on this chapter based on your personal strengths and weaknesses. Don't worry though—skipping something now does not mean you'll never study it. Later on in your prep, as you complete full-length tests, you'll uncover specific pieces of content that you need to review and can come back to these chapters as appropriate.

How to Use This Assessment

If you answer 0–7 questions correctly:

Spend about 1 hour to read this chapter in full and take limited notes throughout. Follow up by reviewing **all** quiz questions to ensure that you now understand how to solve each one.

If you answer 8–11 questions correctly:

Spend 20–40 minutes reviewing the quiz questions. Beginning with the questions you missed, read and take notes on the corresponding subchapters. For questions you answered correctly, ensure your thinking matches that of the explanation and you understand why each choice was correct or incorrect.

If you answer 12–15 questions correctly:

Spend less than 20 minutes reviewing all questions from the quiz. If you missed any, then include a quick read-through of the corresponding subchapters, or even just the relevant content within a subchapter, as part of your question review. For questions you answered correctly, ensure your thinking matches that of the explanation and review the Concept Summary at the end of the chapter.

1. Lithium and sodium have similar chemical properties. For example, both can form ionic bonds with chloride. Which of the following best explains this similarity?
   - **A.** Both lithium and sodium ions are positively charged.
   - **B.** Lithium and sodium are in the same group of the periodic table.
   - **C.** Lithium and sodium are in the same period of the periodic table.
   - **D.** Both lithium and sodium have low atomic weights.

2. Carbon and silicon are the basis of biological life and synthetic computing, respectively. While these elements share many chemical properties, which of the following best describes a difference between the two elements?
   - **A.** Carbon has a smaller atomic radius than silicon.
   - **B.** Silicon has a smaller atomic radius than carbon.
   - **C.** Carbon has fewer valence electrons than silicon.
   - **D.** Silicon has fewer valence electrons than carbon.

3. Which of the following elements has the highest electronegativity?
   - **A.** Mg
   - **B.** Cl
   - **C.** Zn
   - **D.** I

4. Ionization energy contributes to an atom's chemical reactivity. Which of the following shows an accurate ranking of ionization energies from lowest to highest?
   - **A.** First ionization energy of Be < second ionization energy of Be < first ionization energy of Li
   - **B.** First ionization energy of Be < first ionization energy of Li < second ionization energy of Be
   - **C.** First ionization energy of Li < first ionization energy of Be < second ionization energy of Be
   - **D.** First ionization energy of Li < second ionization energy of Be < first ionization energy of Be

5. Antimony is used in some antiparasitic medications—specifically those targeting *Leishmania donovani*. What type of element is antimony?
   - **A.** Metal
   - **B.** Metalloid
   - **C.** Halogen
   - **D.** Nonmetal

6. The properties of atoms can be predicted, to some extent, by their location within the periodic table. Which property or properties increase in the direction of the arrows shown?

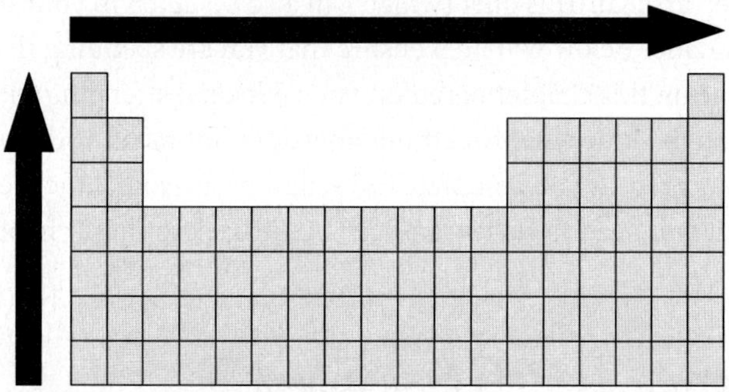

   I. Electronegativity
   II. Atomic radius
   III. First ionization energy

   - **A.** I only
   - **B.** I and II only
   - **C.** I and III only
   - **D.** II and III only

7. Metals are often used for making wires that conduct electricity. Which of the following properties of metals explains why?
   - **A.** Metals are malleable.
   - **B.** Metals have low electronegativities.
   - **C.** Metals have valence electrons that can move freely.
   - **D.** Metals have high melting points.

8. Which of the following is an important property of the group of elements shaded in the periodic table below?

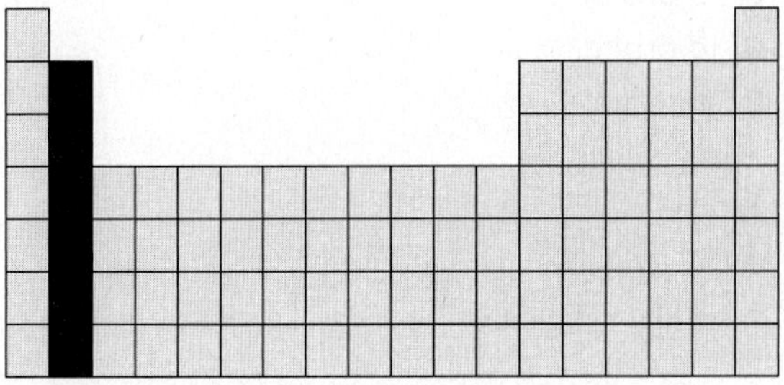

A. These elements are the best electrical conductors in the periodic table.
B. These elements form divalent cations.
C. The second ionization energy for these elements is lower than the first ionization energy.
D. The atomic radii of these elements decrease as one moves down the column.

9. When dissolved in water, which of the following ions is most likely to form a complex ion with H_2O?
A. Na^+
B. Fe^{2+}
C. Cl^-
D. S^{2-}

10. How many valence electrons are present in elements in the third period?
A. 2
B. 3
C. The number decreases as the atomic number increases.
D. The number increases as the atomic number increases.

11. Arsenic mediates some of its toxic effects via the inhibition of acetyl-CoA formation and the inhibition of the enzyme succinic dehydrogenase to decrease ATP production. In addition to its metabolic effects, arsenic can also replace phosphorus in many reactions. Which of the following best explains the similarity between these two elements?
A. Similar atomic numbers
B. Similar number of electrons
C. Similar valence configuration
D. Similar atomic radius

12. Of the four atoms depicted here, which has the highest electron affinity?

A.
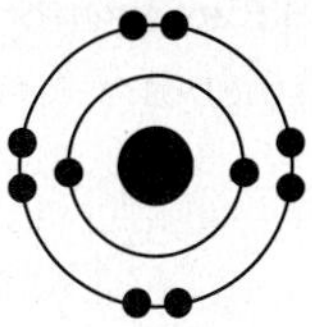

B.
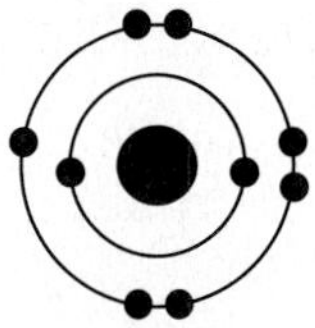

C.
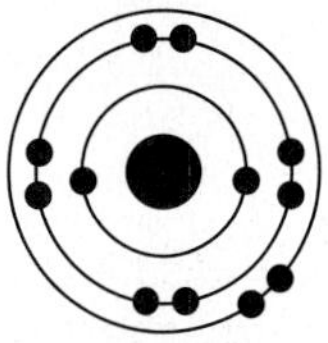

D.
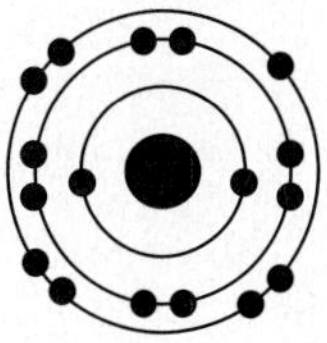

13. Which of the following atoms or ions has the largest effective nuclear charge?

A. Cl

B. Cl^-

C. K

D. K^+

14. Why do halogens often form ionic bonds with alkaline earth metals?

A. The alkaline earth metals have much higher electron affinities than the halogens.

B. By sharing electrons equally, the alkaline earth metals and halogens both form full octets.

C. Within the same row, the halogens have smaller atomic radii than the alkaline earth metals.

D. The halogens have much higher electron affinities than the alkaline earth metals.

15. What is the highest-energy orbital of elements with valence electrons in the $n = 3$ shell?

A. *s*-orbital

B. *p*-orbital

C. *d*-orbital

D. *f*-orbital

Answer Key follows on next page.

Answer Key

1. **B**
2. **A**
3. **B**
4. **C**
5. **B**
6. **C**
7. **C**
8. **B**
9. **B**
10. **D**
11. **C**
12. **D**
13. **D**
14. **D**
15. **C**

Detailed explanations can be found at the end of the chapter.

CHAPTER 2

THE PERIODIC TABLE

In This Chapter

CHAPTER PROFILE

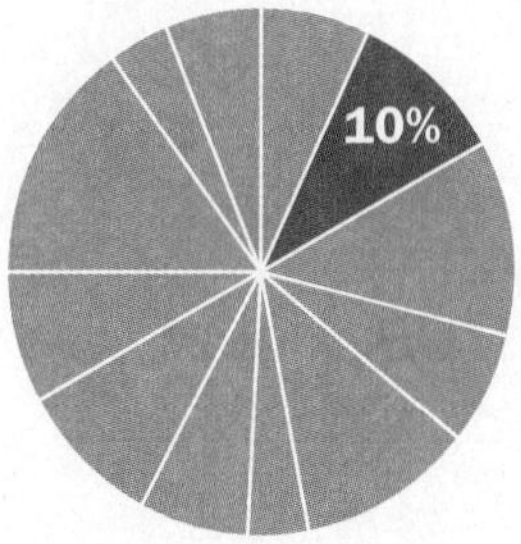

The content in this chapter should be relevant to about 10% of all questions about general chemistry on the MCAT.

This chapter covers material from the following AAMC content category:

4E: Atoms, nuclear decay, electronic structure, and atomic chemical behavior

Introduction

The pharmacological history of lithium is an interesting window into the scientific and medical communities' attempts to take advantage of the chemical and physical properties of an element for human benefit. By the mid-1800s, the medical community was showing great interest in theories that linked uric acid to a myriad of maladies. When it was discovered that solutions of lithium carbonate dissolved uric acid, therapeutic preparations containing lithium carbonate salt became popular. Even nonmedical companies tried to profit from lithium's reputation as a cure-all by adding it to their soft drinks.

Eventually, fascination with theories of uric acid wore off, and lithium's time in the spotlight seemed to be coming to an end. Then, in the 1940s, doctors began to recommend salt-restricted diets for cardiac patients. Lithium chloride was made commercially available as a sodium chloride (table salt) substitute. Unfortunately, lithium is quite toxic at fairly low concentrations, and when medical literature in the late 1940s reported several incidents of severe poisonings and multiple deaths—some associated with only minor lithium overdosing—U.S. companies voluntarily withdrew all lithium salts from the market. Right around this time, John Cade, a psychiatrist from Australia, proposed the use of lithium salts for the treatment of mania. Cade's clinical trials were quite successful. In fact, his use of lithium salts to control mania was the first instance of successful medical treatment of a mental illness, and lithium carbonate became commonly prescribed in Europe for manic behavior. Not until 1970 did the U.S. Food and Drug Administration finally approve the use of lithium carbonate for manic symptoms.

Lithium (Li) is the element with the atomic number 3. It is a very soft alkali metal, and under standard conditions, it is the least dense solid element (specific gravity = 0.53). Lithium is so reactive that it does not naturally occur on earth in its elemental form and is found only in various salt compounds.

Why would medical scientists pay attention to this particular element? What would make doctors believe that lithium chloride would be a good substitute for sodium chloride for patients on salt-restricted diets? The answers lie in the periodic table.

2.1 The Periodic Table

LEARNING OBJECTIVES

After Chapter 2.1, you will be able to:

- Explain how the modern periodic table is organized
- Differentiate between representative and nonrepresentative elements

In 1869, the Russian chemist Dmitri Mendeleev published the first version of his **Periodic Table of the Elements**, which showed that ordering the known elements according to atomic weight revealed a pattern of periodically recurring physical and chemical properties. Since then, the periodic table has been revised, using the work of English physicist Henry Moseley, to organize the elements based on increasing atomic number (the number of protons in an element) rather than atomic weight. Using this revised table, many properties of elements that had not yet been discovered could be predicted. The periodic table creates a visual representation of the **periodic law**, which states: *the chemical and physical properties of the elements are dependent, in a periodic way, upon their atomic numbers.*

BRIDGE

Recall from Chapter 1 of *MCAT General Chemistry Review* that periods (rows) graphically represent the principal quantum number, and groups (columns) help to determine the valence electron configuration.

The modern periodic table arranges the elements into **periods** (rows) and **groups** or **families** (columns), based on atomic number. There are seven periods representing the principal quantum numbers $n = 1$ through $n = 7$ for the *s*- and *p*-block elements. Each period is filled sequentially, and each element in a given period has one more proton and one more electron than the element to its left (in their neutral states). Groups contain elements that have the same electronic configuration in their **valence shell** and share similar chemical properties.

MCAT EXPERTISE

Relating valence electrons to reactivity is important. Elements with similar valence electron configurations generally behave in similar ways, as long as they are the same type (metal, nonmetal, or metalloid).

The electrons in the valence shell, known as the **valence electrons**, are the farthest from the nucleus and have the greatest amount of potential energy. Their higher potential energy and the fact that they are held less tightly by the nucleus allows them to become involved in chemical bonds with the valence electrons of other atoms; thus, the valence shell electrons largely determine the chemical reactivity and properties of the element.

The Roman numeral above each group represents the number of valence electrons elements in that group have in their neutral state. The Roman numeral is combined with the letter A or B to separate the elements into two larger classes. The **A elements** are known as the **representative elements** and include groups IA through VIIIA. The elements in these groups have their valence electrons in the orbitals of either *s* or *p* subshells. The **B elements** are known as the **nonrepresentative elements** and include both the **transition elements**, which have valence electrons in the *s* and *d* subshells, and the **lanthanide** and **actinide series**, which have valence electrons in the *s* and *f* subshells. For the representative elements, the Roman numeral and the letter designation determine the electron configuration. For example, an element in Group VA has five valence electrons with the configuration s^2p^3. As described in Chapter 1 of *MCAT General Chemistry Review*, the nonrepresentative elements may have unexpected electron configurations, such as chromium ($4s^13d^5$) and copper ($4s^13d^{10}$). In the modern IUPAC identification system, the groups are numbered 1 to 18 and are not subdivided into Group A and Group B elements.

MCAT CONCEPT CHECK 2.1

Before you move on, assess your understanding of the material with these questions.

1. Mendeleev's table was arranged by atomic weight, but the modern periodic table is arranged by:

____

2. Which of the following are representative elements (A), and which are nonrepresentative (B)?

Element	A or B	Element	A or B	Element	A or B	Element	A or B
Ag		Al		K		P	
Pb		Li		Pu		U	
Cu		Cf		Zn		B	
N		Np		O		He	

2.2 Types of Elements

LEARNING OBJECTIVES

After Chapter 2.2, you will be able to:

- Classify elements as metal, nonmetal, or metalloid
- Predict the traits of an element given its location on a periodic table:

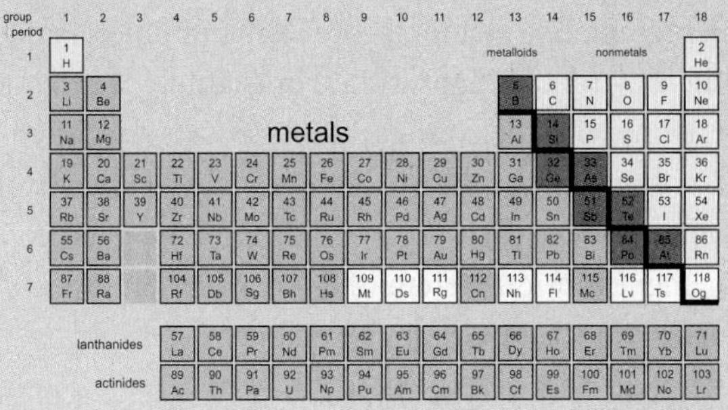

When we consider the trends of chemical reactivity and physical properties together, we can begin to identify groups of elements with similar characteristics. These larger collections are divided into three categories: metals, nonmetals, and metalloids (also called semimetals).

Metals

Metals are found on the left side and in the middle of the periodic table. They include the active metals, the transition metals, and the lanthanide and actinide series of elements. Metals are **lustrous** (shiny) solids, except for mercury, which is a liquid under standard conditions. They generally have high melting points and densities, but there are exceptions, such as lithium, which has a density about half that of water. Metals have the ability to be deformed without breaking; the ability of metal to be hammered into shapes is called **malleability**, and its ability to be pulled or drawn into wires is called **ductility**. At the atomic level, a metal is defined by a low effective nuclear charge, low electronegativity (high **electropositivity**), large atomic radius, small ionic radius, low ionization energy, and low electron affinity. All of these characteristics are manifestations of the ability of metals to easily give up electrons.

Many of the transition metals (Group B elements) have two or more **oxidation states** (charges when forming bonds with other atoms). Because the valence electrons of all metals are only loosely held to their atoms, they are free to move, which makes metals good **conductors** of heat and electricity. The valence electrons of the active metals are found in the *s* subshell; those of the transition metals are found in the *s* and *d* subshells; and those of the lanthanide and actinide series elements are in the *s* and *f* subshells. Some transition metals—copper, nickel, silver, gold, palladium, and platinum—are relatively nonreactive, a property that makes them ideal for the production of coins and jewelry.

KEY CONCEPT

Alkali and alkaline earth metals are both metallic in nature because they easily lose electrons from the *s* subshell of their valence shells.

An example of a metal is shown in Figure 2.1 with a copper wire. The wire exhibits luster, malleability, and ductility. It is used as a wire because it also exhibits good heat and electrical conductivity.

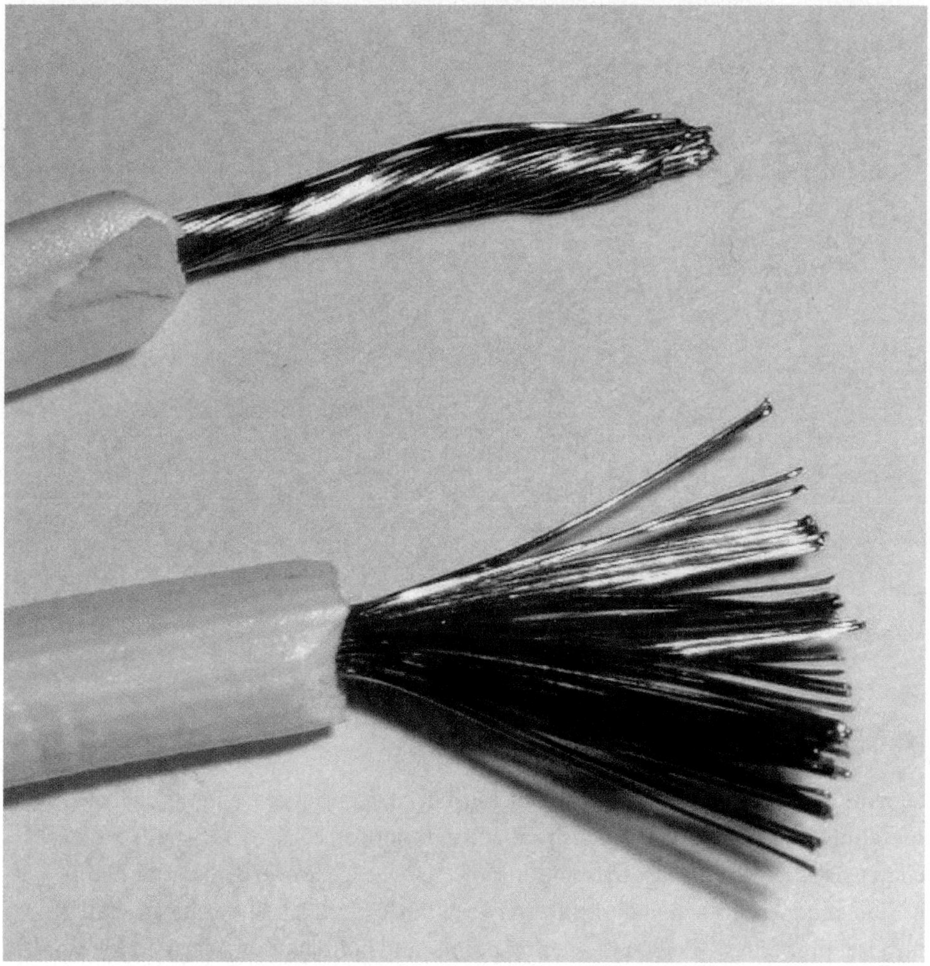

Figure 2.1 Copper (Cu) Metal Wire

Nonmetals

Nonmetals are found predominantly on the upper right side of the periodic table. Nonmetals are generally brittle in the solid state and show little or no metallic luster. They have high ionization energies, electron affinities, and electronegativities, as well as small atomic radii and large ionic radii. They are usually poor conductors of heat and electricity. All of these characteristics are manifestations of the *inability* of nonmetals to easily give up electrons. Nonmetals are less unified in their chemical and physical properties than the metals.

Carbon, shown in Figure 2.2, is a stereotypical nonmetal that retains a solid structure but is brittle, nonlustrous, and generally a poor conductor of heat and electricity.

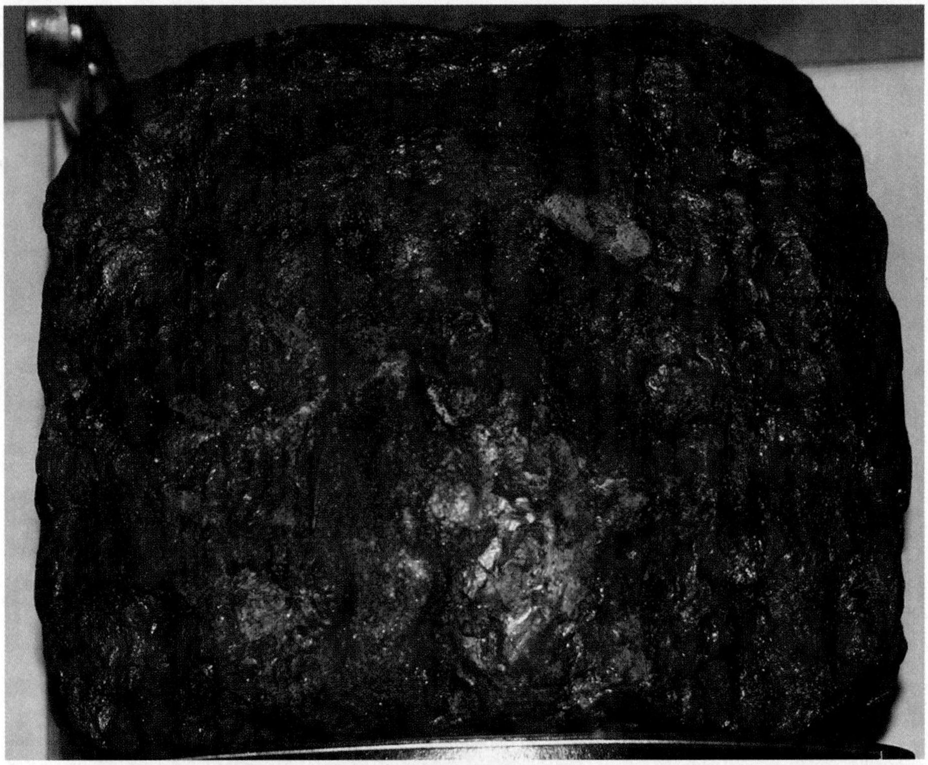

Figure 2.2 Charcoal, Composed of the Nonmetal Carbon (C)

Metalloids

Separating the metals and nonmetals are a stair-step group of elements called the **metalloids**. The metalloids are also called **semimetals** because they share some characteristics with both metals and nonmetals. The electronegativities and ionization energies of the metalloids lie between those of metals and nonmetals. Their physical properties—densities, melting points, and boiling points—vary widely and can be combinations of metallic and nonmetallic characteristics. For example, silicon (Si) has a metallic luster but is brittle and a poor conductor. The reactivities of the metalloids are dependent on the elements with which they are reacting. Boron (B), for example, behaves like a nonmetal when reacting with sodium (Na) and like a metal when reacting with fluorine (F). The elements classified as metalloids form a "staircase" on the periodic table and include boron, silicon, germanium (Ge), arsenic (As), antimony (Sb), tellurium (Te), polonium (Po), and astatine (At). While there is debate over polonium and astatine's status as metalloids, most sources label them as such. Figure 2.3 color-codes the major classifications of elements on the periodic table.

REAL WORLD

Metalloids share some properties with metals and others with nonmetals. For instance, metalloids make good semiconductors due to their partial conductivity of electricity.

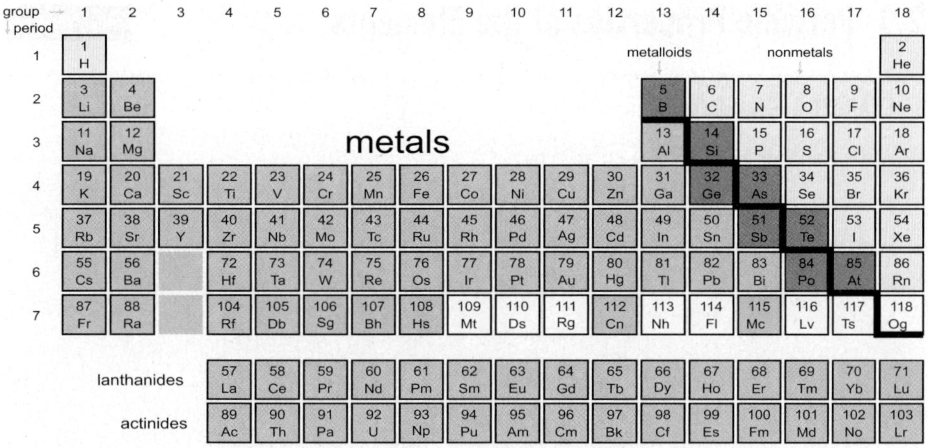

Figure 2.3 Periodic Table, Coded by Element Type

MCAT CONCEPT CHECK 2.2

Before you move on, assess your understanding of the material with these questions.

1. Based on their location in the periodic table, identify a few elements that likely possess the following properties:
   - Luster:

   ____

   - Poor conductivity of heat and electricity:

   ____

   - Good conductivity but brittle:

   ____

2. Classify the following elements as metals (M), nonmetals (NM), or metalloids (MO):

Element	Class	Element	Class	Element	Class	Element	Class
Ag		**Al**		**K**		**P**	
Pb		**Li**		**Pu**		**U**	
Cu		**As**		**Zn**		**B**	
Si		**Np**		**O**		**He**	

2.3 Periodic Properties of the Elements

High-Yield

LEARNING OBJECTIVES

After Chapter 2.3, you will be able to:

- Compare the atomic radius of neutral atoms to their ions
- Rank elements by ionization energy, electron affinity, electronegativity, or atomic radius:

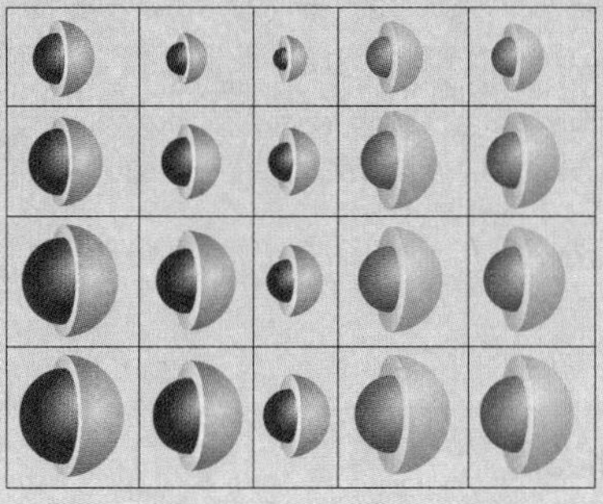

MCAT EXPERTISE

Don't try to memorize the periodic table. You will have access to it on Test Day through the test interface. *Do* understand its configuration and trends so that you can use it efficiently to get a higher score!

BRIDGE

Z_{eff} relies on the principles of electrostatic forces defined in Chapter 5 of *MCAT Physics and Math Review.* The values q_1 and q_2 can represent the net charge of the nucleus and valence electron shell, respectively. The larger each charge gets (going to the right in the periodic table), the higher the value of Z_{eff}.

The MCAT does *not* expect you to have memorized the entire periodic table. Fortunately, the periodic table is a guide unto itself, a self-referencing localization system for all of the elements. Remember, the modern table is organized in such a way to represent visually the periodicity of chemical and physical properties of the elements. The periodic table, then, can provide you with a tremendous amount of information that otherwise would have to be memorized. Note, though, that while you do not need to memorize the periodic table for the MCAT, you *do* need to understand the trends within the periodic table that help predict the chemical and physical behaviors of the elements.

Before exploring the periodic trends, let's take stock of three key rules that control how valence electrons work in an atom. First, as we've already mentioned, as one moves from left to right across a period, electrons and protons are added one at a time. As the positivity of the nucleus increases, the electrons surrounding the nucleus, including those in the valence shell, experience a stronger electrostatic pull toward the center of the atom. This causes the electron cloud, which is the outer boundary defined by the valence shell electrons, to move closer and bind more tightly to the nucleus. This electrostatic attraction between the valence shell electrons and the nucleus is known as the **effective nuclear charge (Z_{eff})**, a measure of the net positive charge experienced by the outermost electrons. This pull is somewhat mitigated by nonvalence electrons that reside closer to the nucleus. For elements in the same period, Z_{eff} increases from left to right. The parts of an atom responsible for Z_{eff} are illustrated in Figure 2.4.

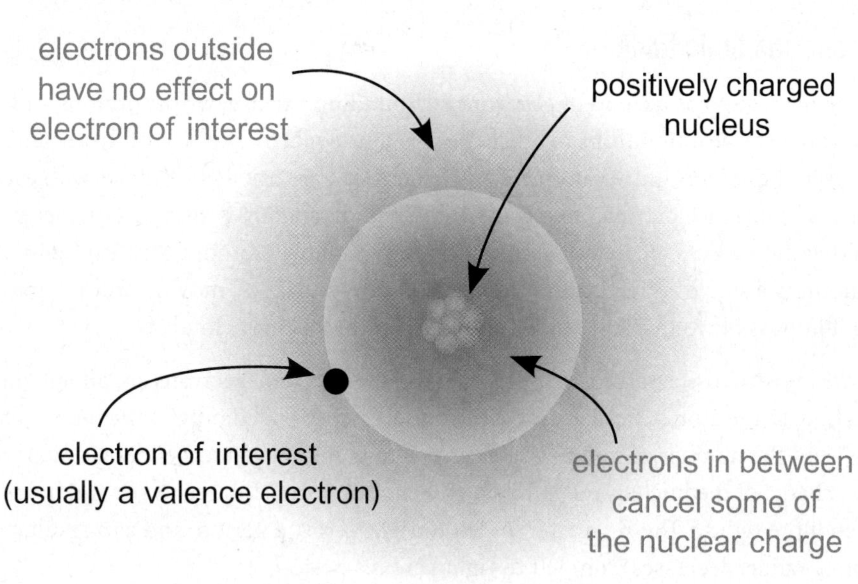

Figure 2.4 Factors that Determine Effective Nuclear Charge (Z_{eff})

Second, as one moves down the elements of a given group, the **principal quantum number** increases by one each time. This means that the valence electrons are increasingly separated from the nucleus by a greater number of filled principal energy levels, which can also be called inner shells. The result of this increased separation is a reduction in the electrostatic attraction between the valence electrons and the positively charged nucleus. These outermost electrons are held less tightly as the principal quantum number increases. As one goes down in a group, the increased shielding created by the inner shell electrons cancels the increased positivity of the nucleus. Thus, the Z_{eff} is more or less constant among the elements within a given group. Despite this fact, the valence electrons are held less tightly to the nucleus as one moves down a group due to the increased separation between valence electrons and the nucleus.

Third, elements can also gain or lose electrons in order to achieve a stable octet formation representative of the **noble (inert) gases** (Group VIIIA or Group 18). In Chapter 3 of *MCAT General Chemistry Review*, we will discuss how the **octet rule** is hardly a rule at all because there are many exceptions. For now, keep in mind that elements, especially the ones that have biological roles, tend to be most stable with eight electrons in their valence shell.

These three facts are guiding principles as we work toward an understanding of the trends demonstrated in the periodic table. In fact, the trend for effective nuclear charge across a period and the impact of increasing the number of inner shells down a group will help derive all the trends we discuss below.

KEY CONCEPT

Atomic radius refers to the size of a neutral element, while an ionic radius is dependent on *how* the element ionizes based on its element type and group number.

MCAT EXPERTISE

Atomic radius is essentially opposite that of all other periodic trends. While others increase going up and to the right, atomic radius increases going down and to the left.

Atomic and Ionic Radii

Think of an atom as a cloud of electrons surrounding a dense core of protons and neutrons. The **atomic radius** of an element is thus equal to one-half of the distance between the centers of two atoms of an element that are briefly in contact with each other. The distance between two centers of circles in contact is akin to a diameter, making this radius calculation simple. The atomic radius cannot be measured by examining a single atom because the electrons are constantly moving around, making it impossible to mark the outer boundary of the electron cloud.

As we move across a period from left to right, protons and electrons are added one at a time to the atoms. Because the electrons are being added only to the outermost shell and the number of inner-shell electrons remains constant, the increasing positive charge of the nucleus pulls the outer electrons more closely inward and holds them more tightly. The Z_{eff} increases left to right across a period, and as a result, atomic radius decreases from left to right across a period.

As we move down a group, the increasing principal quantum number implies that the valence electrons will be found farther away from the nucleus because the number of inner shells is increasing, separating the valence shell from the nucleus. Although the Z_{eff} remains essentially constant, the atomic radius increases down a group. Within each group, the largest atom will be at the bottom, and within each period, the largest atom will be in Group IA (Group 1). For reference, the largest atomic radius in the periodic table belongs to cesium (Cs, 260 pm), and the smallest belongs to helium (He, 25 pm). Francium is typically not considered because it is exceptionally rare in nature. Figure 2.5 displays a graph of atomic radius *vs.* atomic number, with Group IA elements possessing the largest atomic radius in each row.

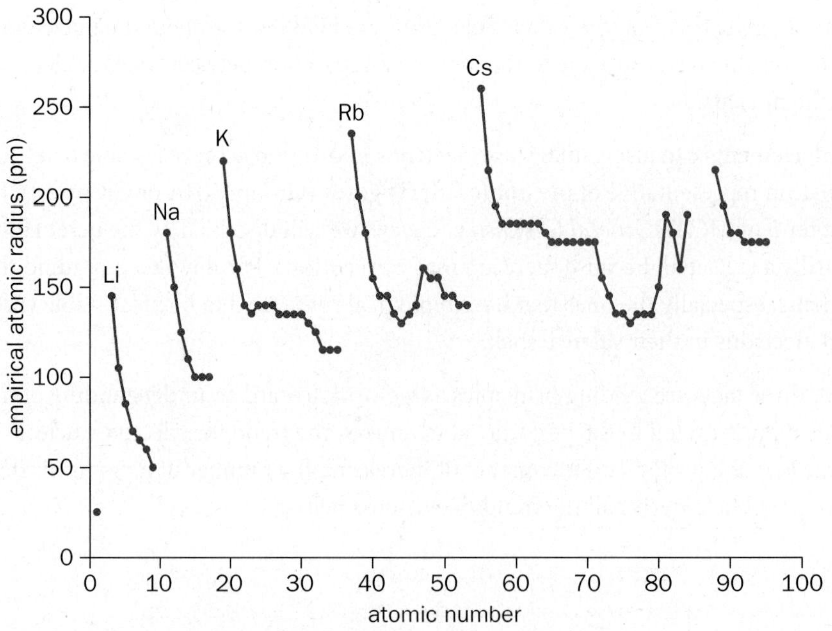

Figure 2.5 Atomic Radius (in pm) *vs.* Atomic Number

Unlike atomic radii, **ionic radii** will require some critical thinking and periodic table geography to determine. In order to understand ionic radii, we must make two generalizations. One is that metals lose electrons and become positive, while nonmetals gain electrons and become negative. The other is that metalloids can go in either direction, but tend to follow the trend based on which side of the metalloid line they fall on. Thus, silicon (Si) behaves more like a nonmetal, while germanium (Ge) tends to act more like a metal. On the MCAT, these generalizations can also be inferred from information found in passages and questions, such as oxidation states in compounds.

For nonmetals close to the metalloid line, their group number dictates that they require more electrons than other nonmetals to achieve the electronic configuration seen in Group VIIIA (Group 18). These nonmetals gain electrons while their nuclei maintain the same charge. Therefore, these nonmetals close to the metalloid line possess a larger ionic radius than their counterparts closer to Group VIIIA.

For metals, the trend is similar but opposite. Metals closer to the metalloid line have more electrons to lose to achieve the electronic configuration seen in Group VIIIA. Because of this, the ionic radius of metals near the metalloid line is dramatically smaller than that of other metals. Metals closer to Group IA have fewer electrons to lose and therefore experience a less drastic reduction in radius during ionization. These changes are illustrated in Figure 2.6. Note that tellurium (Te) behaves as a nonmetal and boron (B) behaves as a metal; under varying conditions, these metalloids can have opposite behavior.

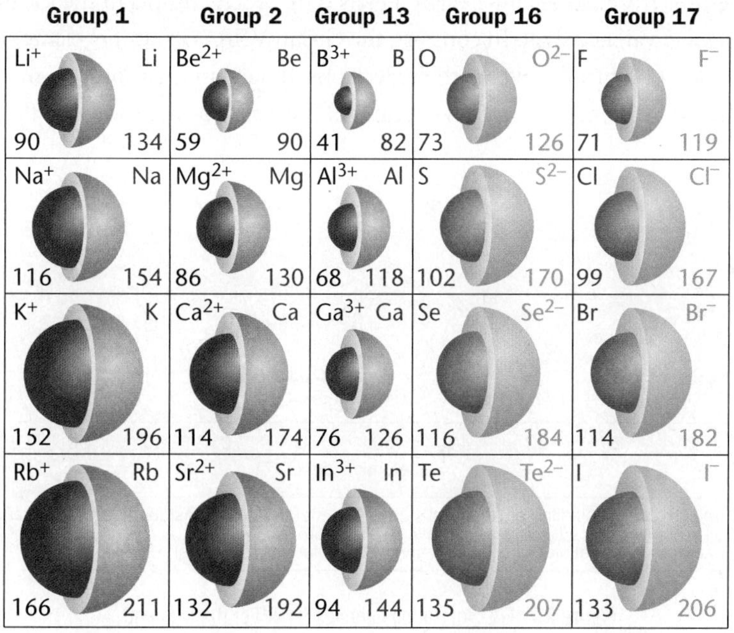

Figure 2.6 Ionic Radii (in pm) for Various Metals and Nonmetals
Neutral atoms are shown in purple; cations in black; anions in green.

Ionization Energy

Ionization energy (IE), also known as **ionization potential**, is the energy required to remove an electron from a gaseous species. Removing an electron from an atom always requires an input of heat, which makes it an **endothermic process**. The greater the atom's Z_{eff} or the closer the valence electrons are to the nucleus, the more tightly bound they are. This makes it more difficult to remove one or more electrons, increasing the ionization energy. Thus, ionization energy increases from left to right across a period and from bottom to top in a group. The subsequent removal of a second or third electron requires increasing amounts of energy because the removal of more than one electron means that the electrons are being removed from an increasingly cationic (positive) species. The energy necessary to remove the first electron is called the **first ionization energy**; the energy necessary to remove the second electron from the univalent cation (X^+) to form the divalent cation (X^{2+}) is called the **second ionization energy**, and so on. For example:

$$Mg(g) \rightarrow Mg^+(g) + e^- \qquad \text{first ionization energy} = 738\ \frac{kJ}{mol}$$

$$Mg^+(g) \rightarrow Mg^{2+}(g) + e^- \qquad \text{second ionization energy} = 1450\ \frac{kJ}{mol}$$

Elements in Groups IA and IIA (Groups 1 and 2), such as lithium and beryllium, have such low ionization energies that they are called the **active metals**. The active metals do not exist naturally in their neutral forms; they are always found in ionic compounds, minerals, or ores. The loss of one electron from the alkali metals (Group IA) or the loss of two electrons from the alkaline earth metals (Group IIA) results in the formation of a stable, filled valence shell. In contrast, the Group VIIA (Group 17) elements—the halogens—do not typically give up their electrons. In fact, in their ionic form, they are generally anions. The first ionization energies of the elements are shown in Figure 2.7.

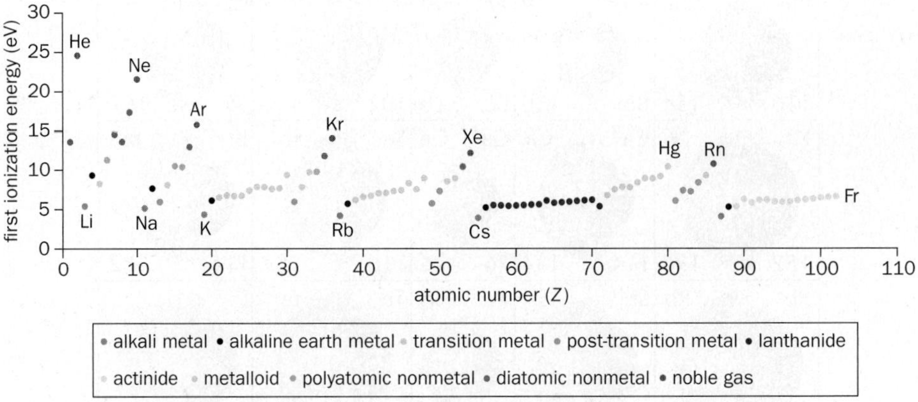

Figure 2.7 First Ionization Energies (in eV) of the Elements

The values for second ionization energies are disproportionally larger for Group IA monovalent cations (like Na^+) but generally not that much larger for Group IIA or subsequent monovalent cations (like Mg^+). This is because removing one electron from a Group IA metal results in a noble gas-like electron configuration.

MCAT EXPERTISE

First ionization energy (IE) will always be smaller than second IE, which will always be smaller than third IE. However, the degree to which the IE increases provides clues about the identity of the atom. If losing a certain number of electrons gives an element a noble gas-like electron configuration, then removing a subsequent electron will cost much more energy. For example:

$$Mg^{2+}(g) \rightarrow Mg^{3+}(g) + e^-$$

$$\text{third ionization energy} = 7730\ \frac{kJ}{mol}$$

Group VIIIA (Group 18) elements, or noble or inert gases, are the least likely to give up electrons. They already have a stable electron configuration and are unwilling to disrupt that stability by giving up an electron. Therefore, noble gases are among the elements with the highest ionization energies.

Electron Affinity

Halogens are the most "greedy" group of elements on the periodic table when it comes to electrons. By acquiring one additional electron, a halogen is able to complete its octet and achieve a noble gas configuration. This **exothermic** process expels energy in the form of heat. **Electron affinity** refers to the energy dissipated by a gaseous species when it gains an electron. Note the electron affinity is essentially the opposite concept from ionization energy. Because this is an exothermic process, ΔH_{rxn} has a negative sign; however, the electron affinity is reported as a positive number. This is because electron affinity refers to the energy dissipated: if 200 $\frac{kJ}{mol}$ of energy is released, $\Delta H_{rxn} = -200\ \frac{kJ}{mol}$, and the electron affinity is 200 $\frac{kJ}{mol}$. The stronger the electrostatic pull (the higher the Z_{eff}) between the nucleus and the valence shell electrons, the greater the energy release will be when the atom gains the electron. Thus, electron affinity increases across a period from left to right. Because the valence shell is farther away from the nucleus as the principal quantum number increases, electron affinity decreases in a group from top to bottom. Groups IA and IIA (Groups 1 and 2) have very low electron affinities, preferring to give up electrons to achieve the octet configuration of the noble gas in the previous period. Conversely, Group VIIA (Group 17) elements have very high electron affinities because they need to gain only one electron to achieve the octet configuration of the noble gases (Group VIIIA or Group 18) in the same period. Although the noble gases would be predicted to have the highest electron affinities according to the trend, they actually have electron affinities on the order of zero because they already possess a stable octet and cannot readily accept an electron. Most metals also have low electron affinity values, as can be seen in Figure 2.8.

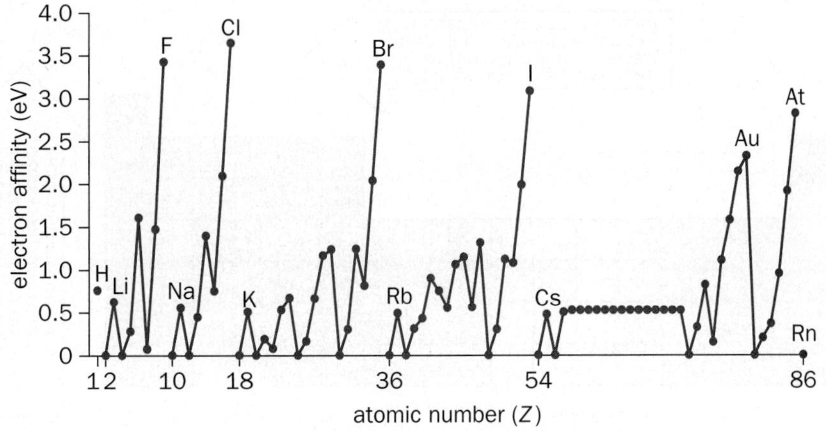

Figure 2.8 Electron Affinities (in eV) of the Elements

Electronegativity

Electronegativity is a measure of the attractive force that an atom will exert on an electron in a chemical bond. The greater the electronegativity of an atom, the more it attracts electrons within a bond. Electronegativity values are related to ionization energies: the lower the ionization energy, the lower the electronegativity; the higher the ionization energy, the higher the electronegativity. The first three noble gases are exceptions: despite their high ionization energies, these elements have negligible electronegativity because they do not often form bonds.

The electronegativity value is a relative measure, and there are different scales used to express it. The most common scale is the **Pauling electronegativity scale**, which ranges from 0.7 for cesium, the least electronegative (most electropositive) element, to 4.0 for fluorine, the most electronegative element. Electronegativity increases across a period from left to right and decreases in a group from top to bottom. Figure 2.9 shows the electronegativity values of the elements.

KEY CONCEPT

- Cs = largest, least electronegative
- F = smallest, most electronegative

H 2.1																	He
Li 1.0	Be 1.5											B 2.0	C 2.5	N 3.0	O 3.5	F 4.0	Ne
Na 0.9	Mg 1.2											Al 1.5	Si 1.8	P 2.1	S 2.5	Cl 3.0	Ar
K 0.8	Ca 1.0	Sc 1.3	Ti 1.5	V 1.6	Cr 1.6	Mn 1.5	Fe 1.8	Co 1.9	Ni 1.8	Cu 1.9	Zn 1.6	Ga 1.6	Ge 1.8	As 2.0	Se 2.4	Br 2.8	Kr
Rb 0.8	Sr 1.0	Y 1.2	Zr 1.4	Nb 1.6	Mo 1.8	Tc 1.9	Ru 2.2	Rh 2.2	Pd 2.2	Ag 1.9	Cd 1.7	In 1.7	Sn 1.8	Sb 1.9	Te 2.1	I 2.5	Xe
Cs 0.7	Ba 0.9	Lu	Hf 1.3	Ta 1.5	W 1.7	Re 1.9	Os 2.2	Ir 2.2	Pt 2.2	Au 2.4	Hg 1.9	Tl 1.8	Pb 1.9	Bi 1.9	Po 2.0	At 2.2	Rn
Fr 0.7	Ra 0.9	Lr	Rf	Db	Sg	Bh	Hs	Mt	Ds	Rg	Cn	Uut	Fl	Uup	Lv	Uus	Uuo

Figure 2.9 Pauling Electronegativity Values of the Elements

The periodic trends are summarized together in Figure 2.10.

KEY CONCEPT

Periodic Trends

Left ⟶ Right

- Atomic radius ↓
- Ionization energy ↑
- Electron affinity ↑
- Electronegativity ↑

Top ⟶ Bottom

- Atomic radius ↑
- Ionization energy ↓
- Electron affinity ↓
- Electronegativity ↓

Note: Atomic radius is always opposite the other trends. Ionic radius is variable.

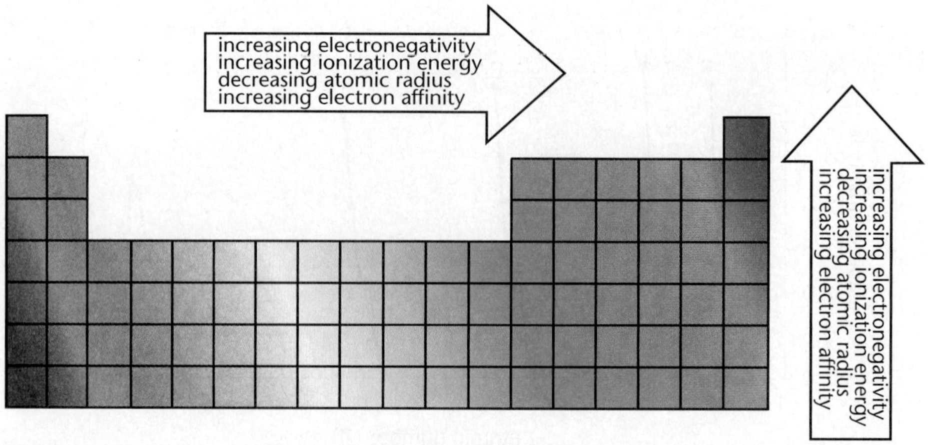

Figure 2.10 Periodic Trends

MCAT CONCEPT CHECK 2.3

Before you move on, assess your understanding of the material with these questions.

1. In each of the following pairs, which has the larger radius?
   - F or F^- ______________
   - K or K^+ ______________

2. Rank the following elements by decreasing first ionization energy: calcium (Ca), carbon (C), germanium (Ge), potassium (K)
   1. ______________
   2. ______________
   3. ______________
   4. ______________

3. Rank the following elements by increasing electron affinity: barium (Ba), copper (Cu), sulfur (S), yttrium (Y)
   1. ______________
   2. ______________
   3. ______________
   4. ______________

4. Rank the following elements by decreasing electronegativity: antimony (Sb), neon (Ne), oxygen (O), thallium (Tl)
   1. ______________
   2. ______________
   3. ______________
   4. ______________

5. Rank the following elements by increasing atomic radius: niobium (Nb), praseodymium (Pr), tantalum (Ta), xenon (Xe)
   1. ______________
   2. ______________
   3. ______________
   4. ______________

2.4 The Chemistry of Groups

LEARNING OBJECTIVES

After Chapter 2.4, you will be able to:

- Identify the groups on the periodic table by the properties they exhibit
- Connect periodic table groups 1, 2, 16, 17, 18, and 3–12 to their common names

What follows is a discussion of the major groups you are likely to encounter on the MCAT. While it is rare to be tested on every group, it is important to understand the overarching trends we have already discussed and how they relate across different groups.

Alkali Metals (IA)

The **alkali metals** (Group IA or Group 1) possess most of the classic physical properties of metals, except that their densities are lower than those of other metals (as described for lithium earlier in this chapter). The alkali metals have only one loosely bound electron in their outermost shells. Their Z_{eff} values are very low, giving them the largest atomic radii of all the elements in their respective periods. This low Z_{eff} value also explains the other trends: low ionization energies, low electron affinities, and low electronegativities. Alkali metals easily lose one electron to form univalent cations, and they react readily with nonmetals—especially the halogens—as in NaCl. Figure 2.11 illustrates the reaction of an alkali metal with water, a stereotypically violent reaction.

REAL WORLD

Due to their high reactivity with water and air, most alkali metals are stored in mineral oil.

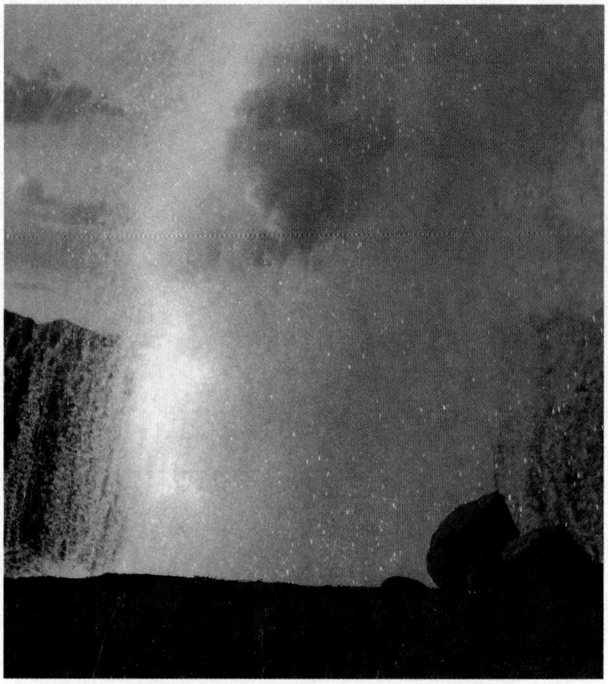

Figure 2.11 Reaction of Sodium with Water
Group IA metals react violently with water, forming strong bases.

Alkaline Earth Metals (IIA)

The **alkaline earth metals** (Group IIA or Group 2) also possess many properties characteristic of metals. They share most of the characteristics of the alkali metals, except that they have slightly higher effective nuclear charges and thus slightly smaller atomic radii. They have two electrons in their valence shell, both of which are easily removed to form divalent cations. Together, the alkali and alkaline earth metals are called the active metals because they are so reactive that they are not naturally found in their elemental (neutral) state.

Chalcogens (VIA)

The **chalcogens** (Group VIA or Group 16) are an eclectic group of nonmetals and metalloids. While not as reactive as the halogens, they are crucial for normal biological functions. They each have six electrons in their valence electron shell and, due to their proximity to the metalloids, generally have small atomic radii and large ionic radii. Oxygen is the most important element in this group for many reasons; it is one of the primary constituents of water, carbohydrates, and other biological molecules. Sulfur is also an important component of certain amino acids and vitamins. Selenium also is an important nutrient for microorganisms and has a role in protection from oxidative stress. The remainder of this group is primarily metallic and generally toxic to living organisms. It is important to note that, at high concentrations, many of these elements—no matter how biologically useful—can be toxic or damaging.

BRIDGE

Many of the molecules discussed in metabolism, covered in Chapters 9 through 12 of *MCAT Biochemistry Review,* utilize lighter nontoxic elements from the chalcogen group (oxygen and sulfur). Many of the heavier chalcogens are toxic metals.

Halogens (VIIA)

The **halogens** (Group VIIA or Group 17) are highly reactive nonmetals with seven valence electrons. These elements are desperate to complete their octets by gaining one additional electron. The physical properties of this group are variable. At standard conditions, the halogens range from gaseous (F_2 and Cl_2) to liquid (Br_2) to solid (I_2) forms. Their chemical reactivity is more uniform, and, due to their very high electronegativities and electron affinities, they are especially reactive toward the alkali and alkaline earth metals. Fluorine (F) has the highest electronegativity of all the elements. The halogens are so reactive that they are not naturally found in their elemental state but rather as ions (called **halides**) or diatomic molecules. Diatomic iodine at standard conditions can be seen in Figure 2.12.

MCAT EXPERTISE

Halogens are frequently tested on the MCAT. Remember that they only need one more electron to have a noble gas-like electron configuration (full valence shell).

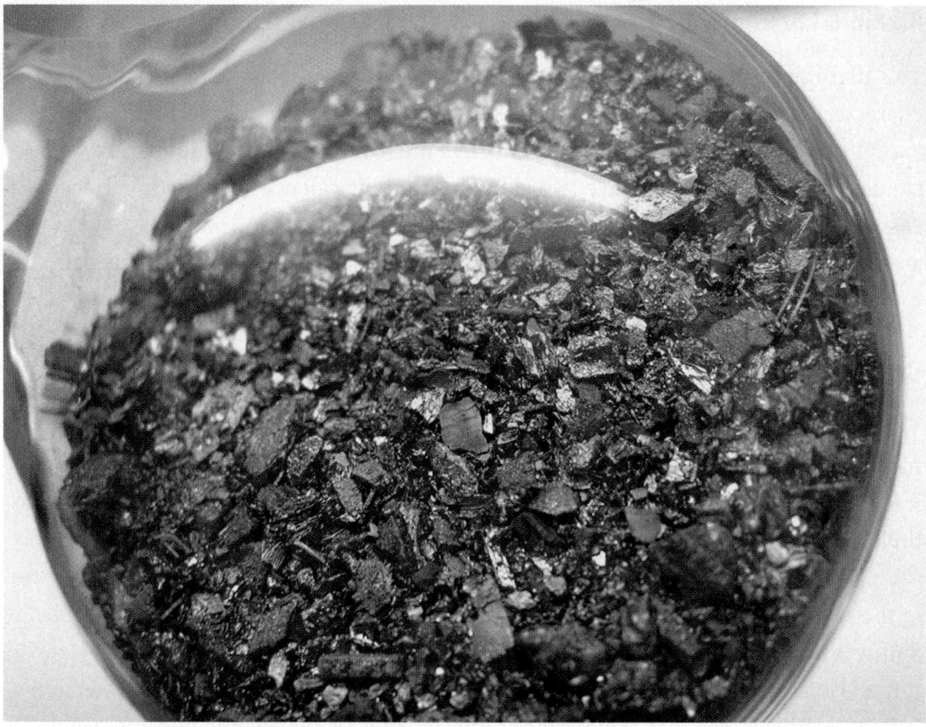

Figure 2.12 Iodine in Standard State (Diatomic Iodine)

Noble Gases (VIIIA)

The **noble gases** (Group VIIIA or Group 18) are also known as **inert gases** because they have minimal chemical reactivity due to their filled valence shells. They have high ionization energies, little or no tendency to gain or lose electrons, and (for He, Ne, and Ar, at least), no measurable electronegativities. The noble gases have extremely low boiling points and exist as gases at room temperature. Noble gases have found a commercial niche as lighting sources, as seen in Figure 2.13, due to their lack of reactivity.

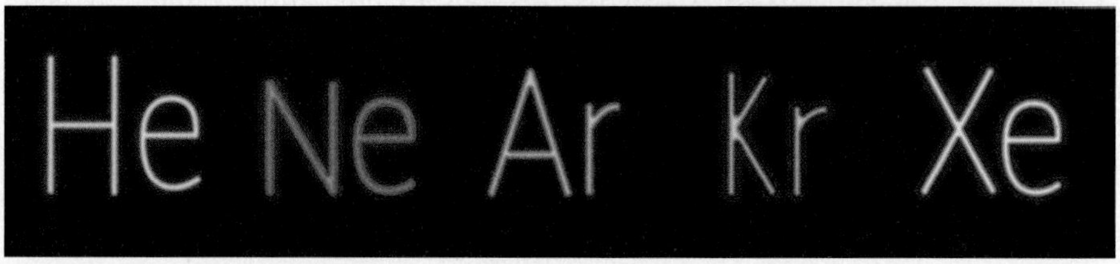

Figure 2.13 Noble Gases Used in "Neon" Signs

Transition Metals (B)

The **transition elements** (Groups IB to VIIIB or Groups 3 to 12) are considered to be metals and as such have low electron affinities, low ionization energies, and low electronegativities. These metals are very hard and have high melting and boiling points. They tend to be quite malleable and are good conductors due to the loosely held electrons that progressively fill the *d*-orbitals in their valence shells. One of the unique properties of the transition metals is that many of them can have different possible charged forms or **oxidation states** because they are capable of losing different numbers of electrons from the *s*- and *d*-orbitals in their valence shells. For instance, copper (Cu) can exist in either the +1 or the +2 oxidation state, and manganese (Mn) can exist in the +2, +3, +4, +6, or +7 oxidation state. Because of this ability to attain different positive oxidation states, transition metals form many different ionic compounds. These different oxidation states often correspond to different colors; solutions with transition metal-containing complexes are often vibrant, as shown in Figure 2.14.

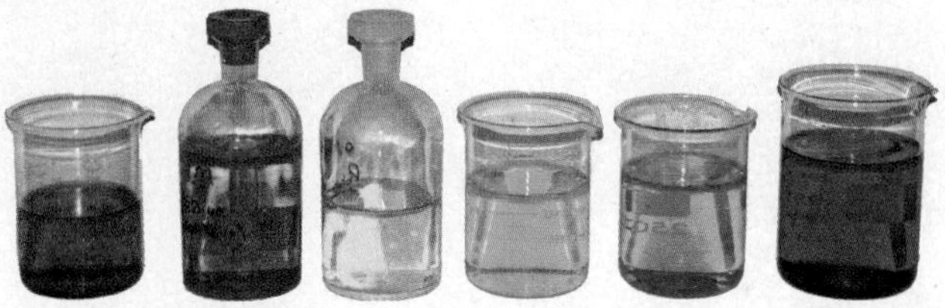

Figure 2.14 Solutions of Transition Metal-Containing Compounds

From left to right: cobalt(II) nitrate, $Co(NO_3)_2$ (red); potassium dichromate, $K_2Cr_2O_7$ (orange); potassium chromate, K_2CrO_4 (yellow); nickel(II) chloride, $NiCl_2$ (green); copper(II) sulfate, $CuSO_4$ (blue); potassium permanganate, $KMnO_4$ (violet)

These complex ions tend to associate in solution either with molecules of water (**hydration complexes**, such as $CuSO_4 \cdot 5\ H_2O$) or with nonmetals (such as $[Co(NH_3)_6]Cl_3$). This ability to form complexes contributes to the variable solubility of certain transition metal-containing compounds. For example, AgCl is insoluble in water but quite soluble in aqueous ammonia due to the formation of the complex ion $[Ag(NH_3)_2]^+$. The formation of complexes causes the *d*-orbitals to split into two energy sublevels. This enables many of the complexes to absorb certain frequencies of light—those containing the precise amount of energy required to raise electrons from the lower- to the higher-energy *d*-orbitals. The frequencies not absorbed (known as the subtraction frequencies) give the complexes their characteristic colors.

BRIDGE

Many transition metals act as cofactors for enzymes, including vanadium, chromium, manganese, iron, cobalt, nickel, copper, and zinc. Cofactors and coenzymes are discussed in Chapter 2 of *MCAT Biochemistry Review*.

This brings up an important point about the perception of color: when we perceive an object as a particular color, it is because that color is *not* absorbed—but rather reflected—by the object. If an object absorbs a given color of light and reflects all others, our brain mixes these **subtraction frequencies** and we perceive the **complementary color** of the frequency that was absorbed. This is best illustrated with an example. *Carotene* is a photosynthetic pigment that strongly absorbs blue light but reflects other colors. Thus, our brains interpret the color of carotene as the result of white light *minus* blue light, which is yellow light. The complementary colors are shown in Figure 2.15; while the MCAT is unlikely to ask you to name the complement of a given color, the relationship between complementary colors, as explained here, is fair game. It should also be noted that the manner in which colors mix in this scheme is distinctly different from mixing, say, paint colors. The differences between these two schemes, termed additive and subtractive color mixing, respectively, are outside the scope of the MCAT.

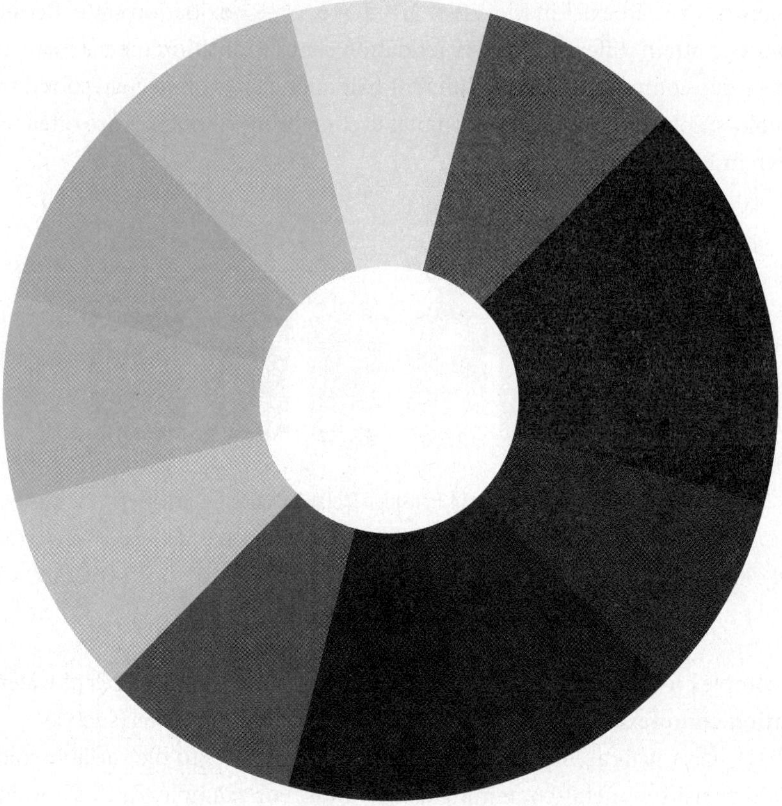

Figure 2.15 Red-Green-Blue (Additive) Color Wheel
Each color is directly across the circle from its complementary color; commonly referenced complementary pairs include red/cyan, green/magenta, and blue/yellow.

MCAT CONCEPT CHECK 2.4

Before you move on, assess your understanding of the material with this question.

1. For each of the properties listed below, write down the groups of the periodic table that exhibit those properties.
   - High reactivity to water:
   ____
   - Six valence electrons:
   ____
   - Contain at least one metal:
   ____
   - Multiple oxidation states:
   ____
   - Negative oxidation states:
   ____
   - Possess a full octet in the neutral state:
   ____

Conclusion

Now that we have completed our review of the Periodic Table of the Elements, commit to understanding (not just memorizing) the trends of physical and chemical properties of the elements. They will help you quickly answer many questions on the MCAT. As you progress through the chapters of this book, a foundational understanding of the elements will help you develop a richer, more nuanced understanding of their general and particular behaviors. Topics in general chemistry that may have given you trouble in the past will be understandable from the perspective of the behaviors and characteristics that you have reviewed here.

More broadly, you will see a diverse array of elements from the groups we have discussed here that are critical or detrimental to biological function. In addition, you may begin to see why the human body utilizes certain elements for specific purposes, taking advantage of the periodic trends discussed here.

GO ONLINE

You've reviewed the content, now test your knowledge and critical thinking skills by completing a test-like passage set in your online resources!

CONCEPT SUMMARY

The Periodic Table

- The **Periodic Table of the Elements** organizes the elements according to their atomic numbers and reveals a pattern of similar chemical and physical properties among elements.
  - Rows are called **periods** and are based on the same principal energy level, *n*.
  - Columns are called **groups**. Elements in the same group have the same valence shell electron configuration.

Types of Elements

- The elements on the periodic table belong to one of three types.
  - **Metals** are shiny (**lustrous**), conduct electricity well, and are **malleable** and **ductile**. Metals are found on left side and middle of the periodic table.
  - **Nonmetals** are dull, poor conductors of electricity, and are brittle. Nonmetals are found on right side of the periodic table.
  - **Metalloids** possess characteristics of both metals and nonmetals and are found in a stair-step pattern starting with boron (B).

Periodic Properties of the Elements

- **Effective nuclear charge** (**Z_{eff}**) is the net positive charge experienced by electrons in the valence shell and forms the foundation for all periodic trends.
  - Z_{eff} increases from left to right across a period, with little change in value from top to bottom in a group.
  - Valence electrons become increasingly separated from the nucleus as the principal energy level, *n*, increases from top to bottom in a group.
- **Atomic radius** decreases from left to right across a period and increases from top to bottom in a group.
- **Ionic radius** is the size of a charged species. The largest nonmetallic ionic radii and the smallest metallic ionic radii exist at the metalloid boundary.
  - Cations are generally smaller than their corresponding neutral atom.
  - Anions are generally larger than their corresponding neutral atom.
- **Ionization energy** is the amount of energy necessary to remove an electron from the valence shell of a gaseous species; it increases from left to right across a period and decreases from top to bottom in a group.
- **Electron affinity** is the amount of energy released when a gaseous species gains an electron in its valence shell; it increases from left to right across a period and decreases from top to bottom in a group.
- **Electronegativity** is a measure of the attractive force of the nucleus for electrons within a bond; it increases from left to right across a period and decreases from top to bottom in a group.

The Chemistry of Groups

- **Alkali metals** typically take on an oxidation state of +1 and prefer to lose an electron to achieve a noble gas-like configuration; they and the alkaline earth metals are the most reactive of all metals.
- **Alkaline earth metals** take on an oxidation state of +2 and can lose two electrons to achieve noble gas-like configurations.
- **Chalcogens** take on oxidation states of −2 or +6 (depending on whether they are nonmetals or metals, respectively) in order to achieve noble gas configuration. They are very biologically important.
- **Halogens** typically take on an oxidation state of −1 and prefer to gain an electron to achieve noble gas-like configurations; these nonmetals have the highest electronegativities.
- **Noble gases** have a fully filled valence shell in their standard state and prefer not to give up or take on additional electrons; they have very high ionization energies and (for He, Ne, and Ar), virtually nonexistent electronegativities and electron affinities.
- **Transition metals** are unique because they take on multiple oxidation states, which explains their ability to form colorful complexes with nonmetals in solution and their utility in certain biological systems.

ANSWERS TO CONCEPT CHECKS

2.1

1. The modern periodic table is arranged in order by atomic number.
2.

Element	A or B	Element	A or B	Element	A or B	Element	A or B
Ag	B	**Al**	A	**K**	A	**P**	A
Pb	A	**Li**	A	**Pu**	B	**U**	B
Cu	B	**Cf**	B	**Zn**	B	**B**	A
N	A	**Np**	B	**O**	A	**He**	A

2.2

1. Metals have luster. Nonmetals have poor conductivity. Metalloids exhibit brittleness but good conductivity. Any answers within each of these categories are acceptable.
2.

Element	Class	Element	Class	Element	Class	Element	Class
Ag	M	**Al**	M	**K**	M	**P**	NM
Pb	M	**Li**	M	**Pu**	M	**U**	M
Cu	M	**As**	MO	**Zn**	M	**B**	MO
Si	MO	**Np**	M	**O**	NM	**He**	NM

2.3

1. $F^- > F$; $K > K^+$. The ionic radii of anions are larger than the associated atomic radii, while the ionic radii of cations are smaller.
2. Ionization energy: carbon > germanium > calcium > potassium
3. Elcctron affinity: barium < yttrium < copper < sulfur
4. Electronegativity: oxygen > antimony > thallium > neon
5. Atomic radius: xenon < niobium < tantalum < praseodymium

2.4

1.
   - High reactivity to water: Groups 1 and 2
   - Six valence electrons: Groups 6 and 16
   - Contain at least one metal: Groups 1 through 15
   - Multiple oxidation states: All groups; most notably Groups 3 through 12 (transition metals)
   - Negative oxidation states: Almost all groups; most notably Groups 14 through 17 (nonmetals)
   - Possess a full octet in the neutral state: Group 18

SCIENCE MASTERY ASSESSMENT EXPLANATIONS

1. **B**

The periodic table is organized into periods (rows) and groups (columns). Groups (columns) are particularly significant because they represent sets of elements with the same valence electron configuration, which in turn will dictate many of the chemical properties of those elements. Although **(A)** is true, the fact that both ions are positively charged does not explain the similarity in chemical properties; most metals produce positively charged ions. **(C)** is not true because lithium and sodium are in the same group, not period. Finally, although lithium and sodium do have relatively low atomic weights, so do several other elements that do not share the same properties, eliminating **(D)**.

2. **A**

As one moves from top to bottom in a group (column), extra electron shells accumulate, despite the fact that the valence configurations remain identical. These extra electron shells provide shielding between the positive nucleus and the outermost electrons, decreasing the electrostatic attraction and increasing the atomic radius. Because carbon and silicon are in the same group, and silicon is farther down in the group, silicon will have a larger atomic radius because of its extra electron shell.

3. **B**

This question requires knowledge of the trends of electronegativity within the Periodic Table. Electronegativity increases as one moves from left to right for the same reasons that effective nuclear charge increases. Electronegativity decreases as one moves down the Periodic Table because there are more electron shells separating the nucleus from the outermost electrons. In this question, chlorine is the furthest toward the top-right corner of the Periodic Table, making **(B)** the correct answer.

4. **C**

Ionization energy increases from left to right, so the first ionization energy of lithium is lower than that of beryllium. Second ionization energy is always larger than first ionization energy, so beryllium's second ionization energy should be the highest value. This is because removing an additional electron from Be^{+} requires one to overcome a significantly larger electrostatic force.

5. **B**

Antimony (Sb) is on the right side of the periodic table, but not far right enough to be a nonmetal, **(D)**. It certainly does not lie far enough to the right to fall in Group VIIA (Group 17), which would classify it as a halogen, **(C)**. While sources have rarely classified antimony as a metal, **(A)**, it is usually classified as a metalloid, **(B)**.

6. **C**

Electronegativity describes how strong an attraction an element will have for electrons in a bond. A nucleus with a larger effective nuclear charge will have a higher electronegativity; Z_{eff} increases toward the right side of a period. A stronger nuclear pull will also lead to increased first ionization energy, as the forces make it more difficult to remove an electron. The vertical arrow can be explained by the size of the atoms. As size decreases, the positive charge becomes more effective at attracting electrons in a chemical bond (higher electronegativity), and the energy required to remove an electron (ionization energy) increases.

7. **C**

All four descriptions of metals are true, but the most significant property that contributes to the ability of metals to conduct electricity is the fact that they have valence electrons that can move freely. Malleability, **(A)**, is the ability to shape a material with a hammer, which does not play a role in conducting electricity. The low electronegativity and high melting points of metals, **(B)** and **(D)**, also do not play a major role in the conduction of electricity.

8. **B**

This block represents the alkaline earth metals, which form divalent cations, or ions with a +2 charge. All of the elements in Group IIA have two electrons in their outermost *s* subshell. Because loss of these two electrons would leave a full octet as the outermost shell, becoming a divalent cation is a stable configuration for all of the alkaline earth metals. Although some of these elements might be great conductors, they are not as effective as the alkali metals, eliminating **(A)**. **(C)** is also incorrect because, although forming a divalent cation is a stable configuration for the alkaline earth metals, the second ionization energy is still always higher than the first. Finally, **(D)** is incorrect because atomic radii increase when moving down a group of elements because the number of electron shells increases.

9. **B**

Iron is a transition metal. Transition metals can often form more than one ion. Iron, for example, can be Fe^{2+} or Fe^{3+}. The transition metals, in these various oxidation states, can often form hydration complexes with water. Part of the significance of these complexes is that, when a transition metal can form a complex, its solubility within the related solvent will increase. The other ions given might dissolve readily in water, but because none of them are transition metals, they will not likely form complexes.

10. **D**

This question is simple if one recalls that periods refer to the rows in the periodic table, while groups or families refer to the columns. Within the same period, an additional valence electron is added with each step toward the right side of the table.

11. **C**

Phosphorous and arsenic are both found in group 5A, indicating that they have a similar number of valence electrons. Since the valence electron configuration is one of the main determinants of bonding, elements with similar valence states react similarly, supporting **(C)**.

12. **D**

The correct answer to this question may be surprising because this question illustrates an important exception to a trend. Electron affinity generally increases as one moves up and to the right on the periodic table. Based on this trend alone, one might expect that the atom fluorine, depicted in **(B)**, would be correct. However, the correct answer is chlorine, **(D)**, even despite the fact that chlorine is below fluorine on the periodic table. The diagrams in the answer choices help make sense of this apparent exception: Fluorine and chlorine have the same valence electron configuration and have a similar amount of effective nuclear charge. However, when an electron is added to fluorine's valence shell, that negative charge is added to the second energy shell, which is quite small in physical size, meaning that the new electron is crowded into a small energy shell with seven other electrons. As a result, energy is still released when an electron is added to fluorine, but not as much energy as might be predicted by the general trend alone. By contrast, when an additional electron is added to a chlorine atom, that new electron adds to the third energy shell, so there is less repulsion among the valence electrons, leading to a slightly greater electron affinity for chlorine. Thus, chlorine, **(D)**, has the highest electron affinity and is the right answer.

13. **D**

The effective nuclear charge refers to the strength with which the protons in the nucleus can pull on electrons. This phenomenon helps to explain electron affinity, electronegativity, and ionization energy. The effective nuclear charge can be calculated by subtracting the number of non-valence electrons from the number of protons. In **(A)** and **(B)**, chlorine has 17 protons and 10 non-valence electrons, giving it a Z_{eff} of 7. Next, elemental potassium, **(C)**, has the lowest effective nuclear charge because it contains additional inner shells that shield its valence electron from the nucleus. With 19 protons and 18 non-valence electrons, it has a Z_{eff} of 1. **(D)**, ionic potassium, has a higher effective nuclear charge than any of the other options. It has the same electron configuration as Cl^- (10 non-valence electrons) but contains two extra protons in its nucleus, and thus has a Z_{eff} of 9.

14. **D**

Ionic bonds are formed through unequal sharing of electrons. These bonds typically occur because the electron affinities of the two bonded atoms differ greatly. For example, the halogens have high electron affinities because adding a single electron to their valence shells would create full valence shells. In contrast, the alkaline earth metals have very low electron affinities and are more likely to be electron donors because the loss of two electrons would leave them with full valence shells. **(A)** states the opposite and is incorrect because the halogens have high electron affinity and the alkaline earth metals have low electron affinity. **(B)** is incorrect because equal sharing of electrons is a classic description of covalent bonding, not ionic. **(C)** is a true statement, but is not relevant to why ionic bonds form.

15. **C**

When $n = 3$, $l = 0$, 1, or 2. The highest value for l in this case is 2, which corresponds to the *d* subshell. Although the 3*d* block appears to be part of the fourth period, it still has the principal quantum number $n = 3$. In general, the subshells within an energy shell increase in energy as follows: $s < p < d < f$ (although there is no 3*f* subshell).

Consult your online resources for additional practice. GO ONLINE

SHARED CONCEPTS

General Chemistry Chapter 1
Atomic Structure

General Chemistry Chapter 3
Bonding and Chemical Interactions

General Chemistry Chapter 4
Compounds and Stoichiometry

Organic Chemistry Chapter 3
Bonding

Physics and Math Chapter 5
Electrostatics and Magnetism

Physics and Math Chapter 9
Atomic and Nuclear Phenomena

CHAPTER 3

BONDING AND CHEMICAL INTERACTIONS

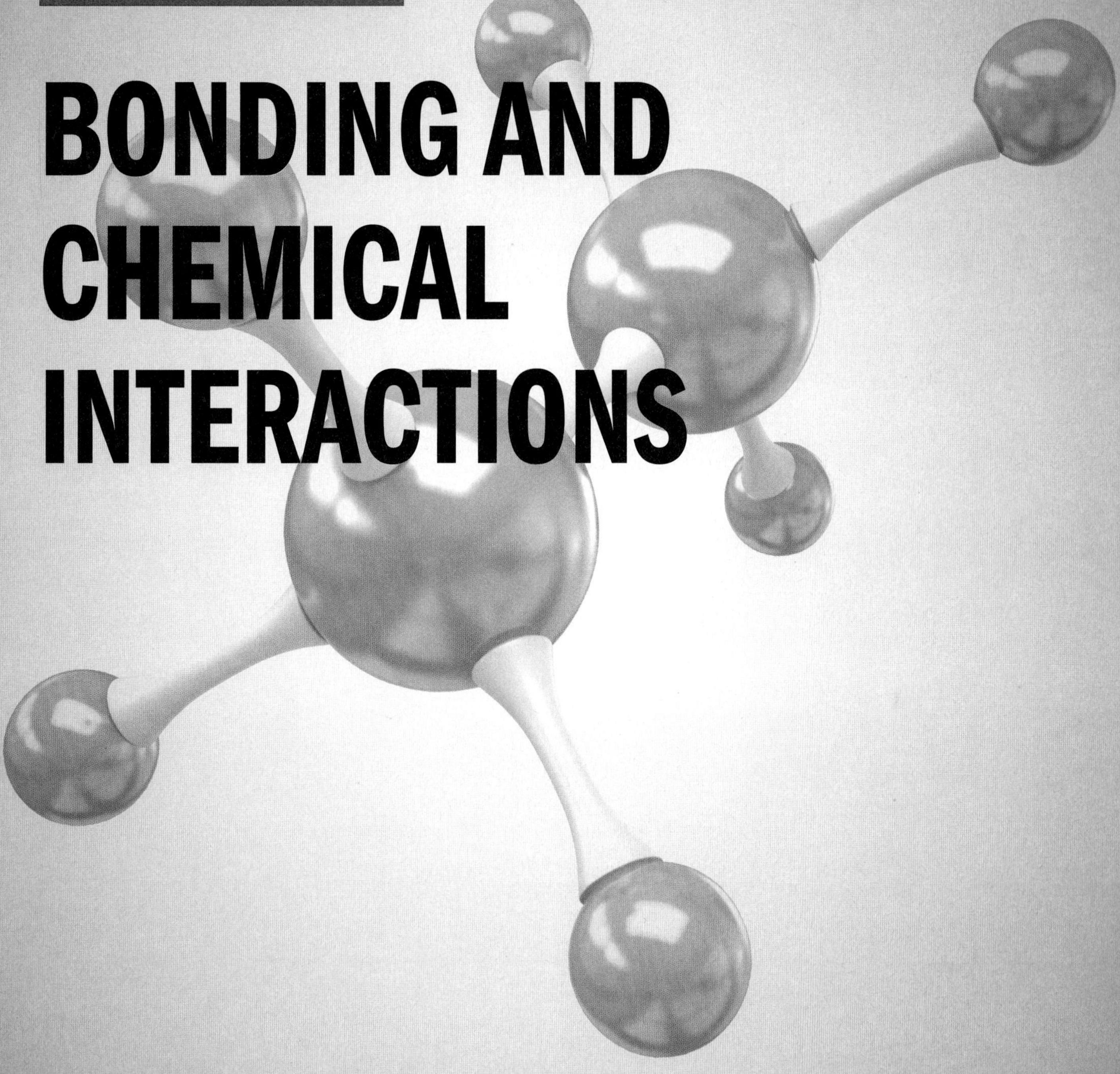

SCIENCE MASTERY ASSESSMENT

Every pre-med knows this feeling: there is so much content I have to know for the MCAT! How do I know what to do first or what's important?

While the high-yield badges throughout this book will help you identify the most important topics, this Science Mastery Assessment is another tool in your MCAT prep arsenal. This quiz (which can also be taken in your online resources) and the guidance below will help ensure that you are spending the appropriate amount of time on this chapter based on your personal strengths and weaknesses. Don't worry though—skipping something now does not mean you'll never study it. Later on in your prep, as you complete full-length tests, you'll uncover specific pieces of content that you need to review and can come back to these chapters as appropriate.

How to Use This Assessment

If you answer 0–7 questions correctly:

Spend about 1 hour to read this chapter in full and take limited notes throughout. Follow up by reviewing **all** quiz questions to ensure that you now understand how to solve each one.

If you answer 8–11 questions correctly:

Spend 20–40 minutes reviewing the quiz questions. Beginning with the questions you missed, read and take notes on the corresponding subchapters. For questions you answered correctly, ensure your thinking matches that of the explanation and you understand why each choice was correct or incorrect.

If you answer 12–15 questions correctly:

Spend less than 20 minutes reviewing all questions from the quiz. If you missed any, then include a quick read-through of the corresponding subchapters, or even just the relevant content within a subchapter, as part of your question review. For questions you answered correctly, ensure your thinking matches that of the explanation and review the Concept Summary at the end of the chapter.

1. What is the character of the bonds in carbon dioxide?
   A. Ionic
   B. Polar covalent
   C. Nonpolar covalent
   D. Coordinate covalent

2. Which of the following molecules contains the oxygen atoms with the most negative average formal charge?
   A. H_2O
   B. CO_3^{2-}
   C. O_3
   D. CH_2O

3. Which of the following elements does NOT break the octet rule?
   A. Be
   B. S
   C. Na
   D. P

4. Which of the following correctly ranks the compounds below by ascending boiling point?
   I. Acetone
   II. KCl
   III. Kr
   IV. Isopropyl alcohol

   A. I < II < IV < III
   B. III < IV < I < II
   C. II < IV < I < III
   D. III < I < IV < II

5. Both CO_3^{2-} and ClF_3 have three atoms bonded to a central atom. What is the best explanation for why CO_3^{2-} has trigonal planar electronic geometry, while ClF_3 has trigonal bipyramidal electronic geometry?
   A. CO_3^{2-} has multiple resonance structures, while ClF_3 does not.
   B. CO_3^{2-} has a charge of −2, while ClF_3 has no charge.
   C. ClF_3 has lone pairs on its central atom, while CO_3^{2-} has none.
   D. CO_3^{2-} has lone pairs on its central atom, while ClF_3 has none.

6. Which of the following elements, when paired together, would form ionic bonds?
   I. Mg
   II. Cl
   III. O
   IV. H

   A. II and IV
   B. I and II
   C. II and III
   D. III and IV

7. Despite the fact that both C_2H_2 and HCN contain triple bonds, the lengths of these triple bonds are not equal. Which of the following is the best explanation for this finding?
   A. In C_2H_2, the bond is shorter because it is between atoms of the same element.
   B. The two molecules have different resonance structures.
   C. Carbon is more electronegative than hydrogen.
   D. Nitrogen is more electronegative than carbon.

8. Which of the following is the best explanation of the phenomenon of hydrogen bonding?
- **A.** Hydrogen has a strong affinity for holding onto valence electrons.
- **B.** Hydrogen can only hold two valence electrons.
- **C.** Electronegative atoms disproportionately carry shared electron pairs when bonded to hydrogen.
- **D.** Hydrogen bonds have ionic character.

9. Which of the following best describes the number and character of the bonds in an ammonium cation?
- **A.** Three polar covalent bonds
- **B.** Four polar covalent bonds, of which none are coordinate covalent bonds
- **C.** Four polar covalent bonds, of which one is a coordinate covalent bond
- **D.** Four polar covalent bonds, of which two are coordinate covalent bonds

10. Although the octet rule dictates much of molecular structure, some atoms can violate the octet rule by being surrounded by more than eight electrons. Which of the following is the best explanation for why some atoms can exceed the octet?
- **A.** Atoms that exceed the octet already have eight electrons in their outermost electron shell.
- **B.** Atoms that exceed the octet only do so when bonding with transition metals.
- **C.** Atoms that exceed the octet can do so because they have *d*-orbitals in which extra electrons can reside.
- **D.** Some atoms can exceed the octet because they are highly electronegative.

11. Which of the following types of intermolecular forces provides the most accurate explanation for why noble gases can liquefy?
- **A.** Hydrogen bonding
- **B.** Ion–dipole interactions
- **C.** Dispersion forces
- **D.** Dipole–dipole interactions

12. In the structure shown, which atom(s) have the most positive charge?

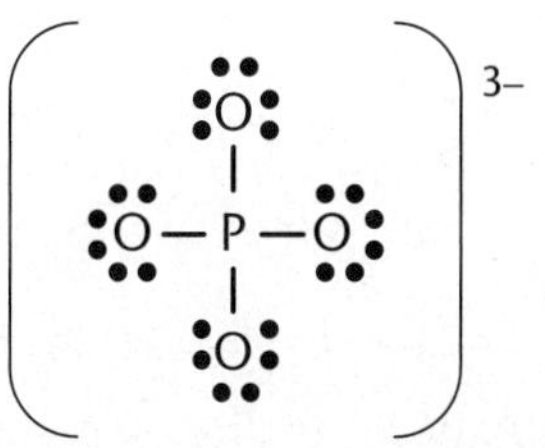

- **A.** The phosphorus atom has the most positive charge.
- **B.** All atoms share the charge equally.
- **C.** The four oxygen atoms share the highest charge.
- **D.** The oxygen atom at the peak of the trigonal pyramidal geometry has the most positive charge.

13. Which of the following is the best name for the new bond formed in the reaction shown?

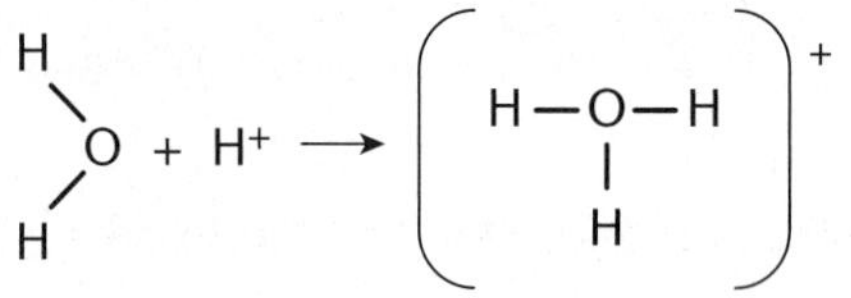

- **A.** Nonpolar covalent bond
- **B.** Ionic bond
- **C.** Coordinate covalent bond
- **D.** Hydrogen bond

14. Both BF_3 and NH_3 have three atoms bonded to the central atom. Which of the following is the best explanation for why the geometry of these two molecules is different?
- **A.** BF_3 has three bonded atoms and no lone pairs, which makes its geometry trigonal pyramidal.
- **B.** NH_3 is nonpolar, while BF_3 is polar.
- **C.** NH_3 has three bonded atoms and one lone pair, which makes its geometry trigonal pyramidal.
- **D.** BF_3 is nonpolar, while NH_3 is polar.

15. Which of the following compounds has the highest melting point?
- **A.** Sucrose
- **B.** NaCl
- **C.** Glycerol
- **D.** H_2O

Answer Key

1. **B**
2. **B**
3. **C**
4. **D**
5. **C**
6. **B**
7. **D**
8. **C**
9. **C**
10. **C**
11. **C**
12. **A**
13. **C**
14. **C**
15. **B**

Detailed explanations can be found at the end of the chapter.

CHAPTER 3

BONDING AND CHEMICAL INTERACTIONS

In This Chapter

CHAPTER PROFILE

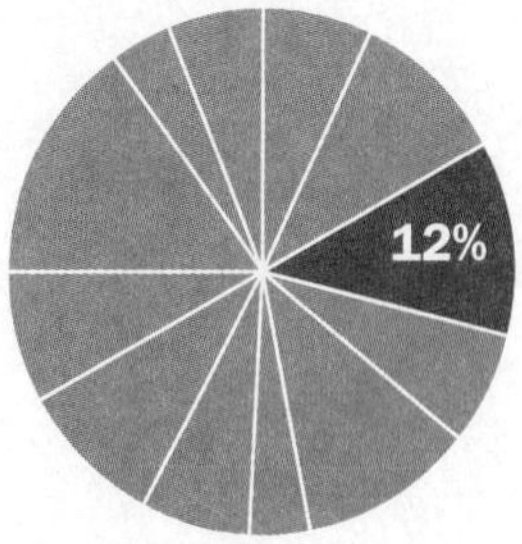

The content in this chapter should be relevant to about 12% of all questions about general chemistry on the MCAT.

This chapter covers material from the following AAMC content categories:

4C: Electrochemistry and electrical circuits and their elements

5B: Nature of molecules and intermolecular interactions

Introduction

The Maillard reaction is one of the most important chemical processes that occurs while cooking. The reaction mechanism itself is one with which you are closely familiar from your studies of organic chemistry: a nucleophilic reaction between the amino terminus of the peptide chain of a protein and the carbonyl functionality of a sugar to form an *N*-substituted glycosylamine. This compound undergoes a complex series of rearrangements and other reactions to produce a set of compounds that gives cooked food its pleasing color and delectable flavor. This reaction is especially important for browning meat.

When the surface of the meat comes into contact with the hot surface of a pan or grill, the proteins and sugars on the meat's exterior begin interacting via the Maillard reaction. The pan must be sufficiently hot to bring the exterior of the meat to a temperature of 155°C (310°F), the optimal temperature for the reaction to occur. So how does a grill master achieve the impossible: generating very high heat for the exterior but not overcooking the interior? The answer lies, in part, in drying the meat. When meat that has a lot of water on its exterior surface hits the hot pan, the first process that takes place is the boiling of the water. Boiling is a phase change from liquid to gas and occurs at a constant temperature; water's boiling point is 100°C (212°F). Because this temperature is considerably lower than that necessary for the Maillard reaction, no browning will occur and the flavor compounds will not form. The lesson here is: if you want a tasty steak, always dry the surface of your meat!

Of course, the real lesson is the topic of discussion for this chapter: bonding and chemical interactions. We will not address complex chemical bonding, such as that which takes place in the Maillard reaction, in this chapter. Rather, this chapter will address the basics of chemical bonding and interactions. Here, we will investigate the nature and behavior of covalent and ionic bonds. We will also review a system—Lewis structures—by which bonding electrons are accounted for, and we will address the main principles of valence shell electron pair repulsion (VSEPR) theory. Finally, we will recount the various modes of interaction between molecules: intermolecular forces.

3.1 Bonding

LEARNING OBJECTIVES

After Chapter 3.1, you will be able to:

- Compare and contrast ionic and covalent compounds
- Identify elements that do not obey the octet rule
- Apply periodic trends to determine whether a covalent bond is polar or nonpolar:

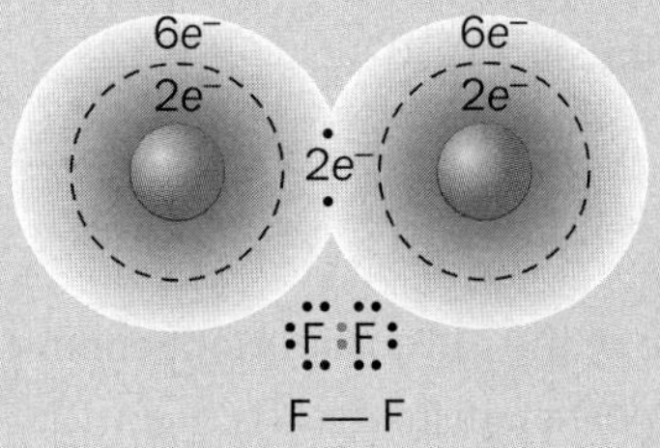

The atoms of most elements, except for a few noble gases, can combine to form **molecules**. The atoms within these molecules are held together by strong attractive forces called **chemical bonds**, which are formed via the interaction of the valence electrons of the combining atoms. The chemical and physical properties of the resulting compound are usually very different from those of the constituent elements. For example, elemental sodium, an alkali metal, is so reactive that it can actually produce fire when reacting with water because the reaction is highly exothermic. Diatomic chlorine gas is so toxic that it was used for chemical warfare during World War I. However, when sodium and chlorine react, the biologically important compound NaCl (table salt) is produced.

The Octet Rule

How do atoms join together to form compounds? In the example above, how do the sodium and the chlorine atoms form sodium chloride? For many molecules, the constituent atoms bond according to the **octet rule**, which states that an atom tends to bond with other atoms so that it has eight electrons in its outermost shell, thereby forming a stable electron configuration similar to that of the noble gases. An example of an octet configuration is shown for the noble gas argon (Ar) in Figure 3.1.

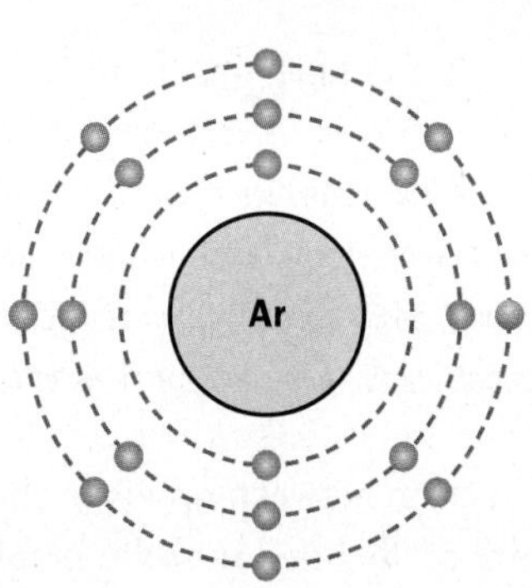

Figure 3.1 Electron Configuration of Argon
As a noble gas, argon has a complete octet in its valence shell.

However, this is more of a "rule of thumb," because there are more elements that can be exceptions to the rule than those that follow the rule. These "exceptional" elements include hydrogen, which can only have two valence electrons (achieving the configuration of helium); lithium and beryllium, which bond to attain two and four valence electrons, respectively; boron, which bonds to attain six valence electrons; and all elements in period 3 and greater, which can expand the valence shell to include more than eight electrons by incorporating *d*-orbitals. For example, in certain compounds, chlorine can form seven covalent bonds, thereby holding 14 electrons in its valence shell.

KEY CONCEPT

The octet rule is the desire of all atoms to achieve noble gas configuration. However, keep in mind that there are many exceptions to this rule.

A simple way to remember all the exceptions is as follows:

- **Incomplete octet:** These elements are stable with fewer than 8 electrons in their valence shell and include hydrogen (stable with 2 electrons), helium (2), lithium (2), beryllium (4), and boron (6).
- **Expanded octet:** Any element in period 3 and greater can hold more than 8 electrons, including phosphorus (10), sulfur (12), chlorine (14), and many others.
- **Odd numbers of electrons:** Any molecule with an odd number of valence electrons cannot distribute those electrons to give eight to each atom; for example, nitric oxide (NO) has eleven valence electrons.

Another way to remember the exceptions is to remember the common elements that almost always abide by the octet rule: carbon, nitrogen, oxygen, fluorine, sodium, and magnesium. Note that nonmetals gain electrons and metals lose electrons to achieve their respective complete octets.

Types of Bonds

We classify chemical bonds into two distinct types: ionic and covalent.

In **ionic bonding**, one or more electrons from an atom with a low ionization energy, typically a metal, are transferred to an atom with a high electron affinity, typically a nonmetal. An illustration of such a process is shown for our initial example, sodium chloride, in Figure 3.2.

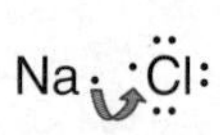

Figure 3.2 Formation of an Ionic Bond
Sodium (Na) has a low ionization energy, easily releasing an electron; chlorine (Cl) has a high electron affinity, easily absorbing that electron into its valence shell. In this example, both atoms achieve an octet formation.

The resulting electrostatic attraction between opposite charges is what holds the ions together. This is the nature of the bond in sodium chloride, where the positively charged sodium cation is electrostatically attracted to the negatively charged chloride anion. It is important to note that this type of electrostatic attraction creates lattice structures consisting of repeating rows of cations and anions, rather than individual molecular bonds, as shown in Figure 3.3.

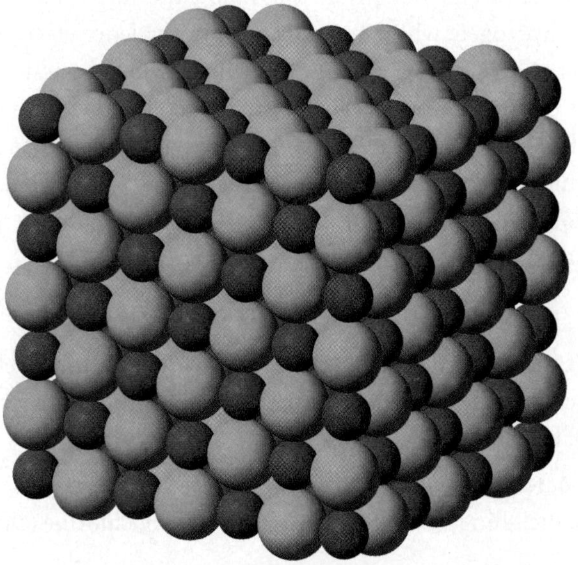

Figure 3.3 Crystal Lattice Structure of Sodium Chloride
Sodium = purple; chloride = green

BRIDGE

Electronegativity, discussed in Chapter 2 of *MCAT General Chemistry Review,* is a property that addresses how an individual atom acts within a bond and will help us understand the formation of molecules from atoms with different electronegativities.

In **covalent bonding**, an electron pair is shared between two atoms, typically nonmetals, that have relatively similar values of electronegativity. The degree to which the pair of electrons is shared equally or unequally between the two atoms determines the degree of polarity in the covalent bond. For example, if the electron pair is shared equally, the covalent bond is nonpolar; and if the pair is shared unequally, the bond is polar. If both of the shared electrons are contributed by only one of the two atoms, the bond is called **coordinate covalent**.

An example of nonpolar covalent bonding is shown for diatomic fluorine in Figure 3.4. Each atom has seven electrons in its valence shell, and by sharing one of these electrons from each atom, they can each form an octet. Unlike ionic crystal lattices, covalent compounds consist of individually bonded molecules.

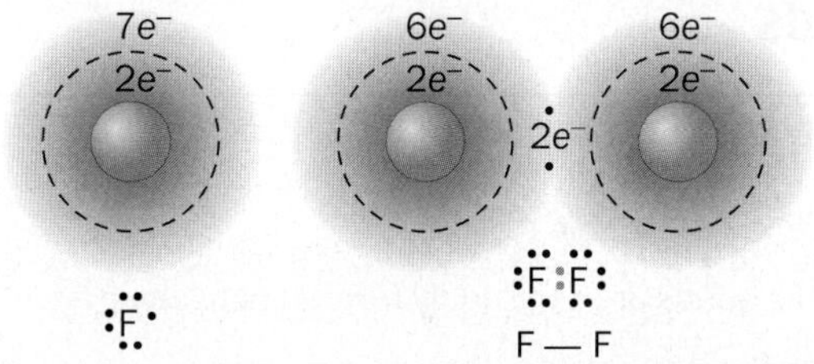

Figure 3.4 Formation of a Covalent Bond

Fluorine (F) has seven valence electrons; by sharing one electron from each atom, both fluorine atoms achieve an octet formation.

MCAT CONCEPT CHECK 3.1

Before you move on, assess your understanding of the material with these questions.

1. Describe the atomic differences between ionic and covalent compounds:
   - Ionic:

   - Covalent:

   ---

2. List three elements that do not follow the octet rule and explain why:

Element	Why It Violates the Octet Rule

3. Which periodic trend determines whether a covalent bond is polar or nonpolar?

3.2 Ionic Bonds

LEARNING OBJECTIVES

After Chapter 3.2, you will be able to:

- Explain why ionic bonds are commonly formed between metals and nonmetals
- Recall the major characteristics of ionic compounds

MNEMONIC

Me**T**als lose electrons to become ca**T**ions = posi**T**ive (+) ions

Nonmetals gain electrons to become a**N**ions = **N**egative (−) ions

Ionic bonds form between atoms that have significantly different electronegativities. The atom that loses the electrons becomes a **cation**, and the atom that gains electrons becomes an **anion**. The ionic bond is the result of an electrostatic force of attraction between the opposite charges of these ions. Electrons are not shared in an ionic bond. For this electron transfer to occur, the difference in electronegativity must be greater than 1.7 on the Pauling scale.

The MCAT won't expect you to memorize the Pauling scale, but recognize that ionic bonds are generally formed between a metal and a nonmetal. For example, alkali and alkaline earth metals of Groups IA and IIA (Groups 1 and 2, respectively) readily form ionic bonds with the halogens of Group VIIA (Group 17). The atoms of the active metals loosely hold onto their electrons, whereas the halogens are more likely to gain an electron to complete their valence shell. The differences in bonding behavior for these classes of elements, and their differences in electronegativity values (ΔEN), explain the formation of ionic compounds such as cesium chloride ($\Delta EN = 2.3$), potassium iodide ($\Delta EN = 1.7$), and sodium fluoride ($\Delta EN = 3.1$).

Ionic compounds have characteristic physical properties that you should recognize for Test Day. Because of the strength of the electrostatic force between the ionic constituents of the compound, ionic compounds have very high melting and boiling points. For example, the melting point of sodium chloride is 801°C. Many ionic compounds dissolve readily in water and other polar solvents and, in the molten or aqueous state, are good conductors of electricity. In the solid state, the ionic constituents of the compound form a **crystalline lattice** consisting of repeating positive and negative ions, as shown earlier in Figure 3.3. With this arrangement, the attractive forces between oppositely charged ions are maximized, and the repulsive forces between ions of like charge are minimized.

MCAT CONCEPT CHECK 3.2

Before you move on, assess your understanding of the material with these questions.

1. Why do ionic bonds tend to form between metals and nonmetals?

2. Describe five characteristics of ionic compounds.

 •

 •

 •

 •

 •

3.3 Covalent Bonds

High-Yield

LEARNING OBJECTIVES

After Chapter 3.3, you will be able to:

- Explain the relationship between bond strength, bond length, and bond energy
- Identify the values of ΔEN for which polar covalent, nonpolar covalent, and ionic bonds will form
- Predict the molecular geometry of a molecule given its formula
- Draw Lewis dot structures for simple molecules, including resonance structures, such as:

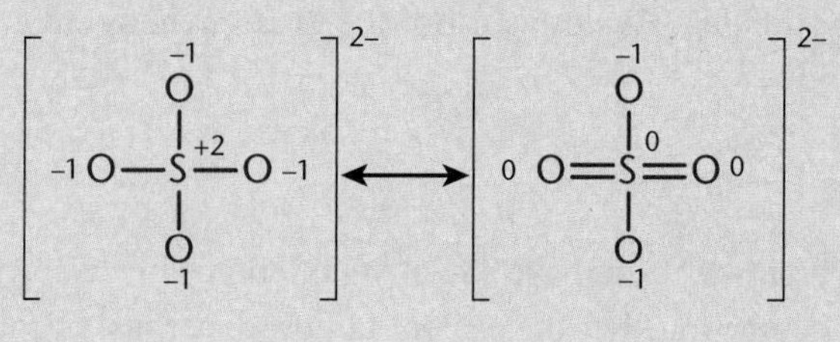

When two or more atoms with similar electronegativities interact, the energy required to form ions through the complete transfer of one or more electrons is greater than the energy that would be released upon the formation of an ionic bond. That is, when two atoms of similar tendency to attract electrons form a compound, it is energetically unfavorable to create ions. Rather than transferring electrons to form octets, the atoms share electrons. The bonding force between the atoms is not ionic; instead, there is an attraction that each electron in the shared pair has for the two positive nuclei of the bonded atoms.

MCAT EXPERTISE

Think of bonds as a tug-of-war between two atoms. When the difference in electronegativity is great (more than 1.7), then the "stronger" atom wins all of the electrons and becomes the anion. When the electronegativity values are relatively similar, then we have a stalemate, or a covalent bond with mostly equal sharing of electrons.

Covalent compounds contain discrete molecular units with relatively weak intermolecular interactions. As a result, compounds like carbon dioxide (CO_2) tend to have lower melting and boiling points. In addition, because they do not break down into constituent ions, they are poor conductors of electricity in the liquid state or in aqueous solutions.

Properties of Covalent Compounds

The formation of one covalent bond may not be sufficient to fill the valence shell for a given atom. Thus, many atoms can form bonds with more than one other atom, and most atoms can form multiple bonds with other atoms. Two atoms sharing one, two, or three pairs of electrons are said to be joined by a **single**, **double**, or **triple covalent bond**, respectively. The number of shared electron pairs between two atoms is called the **bond order**; hence, a single bond has a bond order of one, a double bond has a bond order of two, and a triple bond has a bond order of three. There are three important characteristics of a covalent bond to explain: bond length, bond energy, and polarity.

Bond Length

Bond length is the average distance between the two nuclei of atoms in a bond. As the number of shared electron pairs increases, the two atoms are pulled closer together, resulting in a decrease in bond length. Thus, for a given pair of atoms, a triple bond is shorter than a double bond, which is shorter than a single bond.

KEY CONCEPT

You will see this inverse relationship between bond length and strength in both organic and general chemistry.

	Bond Length	Bond Strength
C—C	longest	weakest
C=C	medium	medium
C≡C	shortest	strongest

Know this relationship on Test Day and you'll earn quick points!

Bond Energy

Bond energy is the energy required to break a bond by separating its components into their isolated, gaseous atomic states. The greater the number of pairs of electrons shared between the atomic nuclei, the more energy is required to break the bonds holding the atoms together. Thus, triple bonds have the greatest bond energy, and single bonds have the lowest bond energy. We will discuss bond energy and calculations involving bond enthalpy in Chapter 7 of *MCAT General Chemistry Review*. By convention, the greater the bond energy is, the stronger the bond.

Polarity

Polarity occurs when two atoms have a relative difference in electronegativities. When these atoms come together in covalent bonds, they must negotiate the degree to which the electron pairs will be shared. The atom with the higher electronegativity gets the larger share of the electron density. A polar bond creates a dipole, with the positive end of the dipole at the less electronegative atom and the negative end at the more electronegative atom, as shown in Figure 3.5.

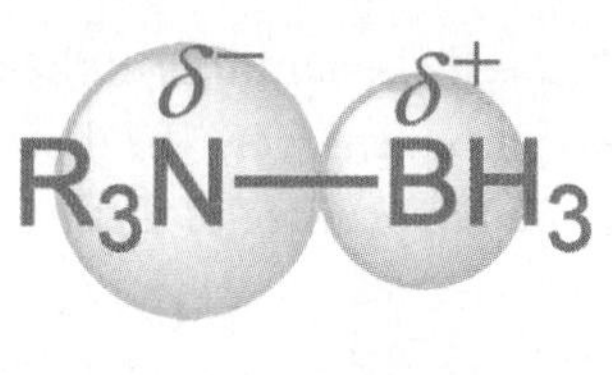

Figure 3.5 Polar Covalent Bond in an Amine Borane
Nitrogen takes on a partial negative charge (δ^-), boron takes on a partial positive charge (δ^+).

When atoms that have identical or nearly identical electronegativities share electron pairs, they do so with equal distribution of the electrons. This is called a **nonpolar covalent bond**, and there is no separation of charge across the bond. Note that only bonds between atoms of the same element will have exactly the same electronegativity and therefore exhibit a purely equal distribution of electrons. The seven common diatomic molecules are H_2, N_2, O_2, F_2, Cl_2, Br_2, and I_2. At the same time, many bonds are close to nonpolar. Any bond between atoms with a difference in electronegativity less than 0.5 is generally considered nonpolar.

MNEMONIC

Here's a quick way to remember the naturally occurring diatomic elements on the periodic table: they form the number **7** on the periodic table (except for H), there are **7** of them, and most of them are in Group **VIIA**: H_2, N_2, O_2, F_2, Cl_2, Br_2, I_2.

Polar Covalent Bond

Atoms that differ moderately in their electronegativities will share electrons unevenly, resulting in **polar covalent bonds**. While the difference in their electronegativities (between 0.5 and 1.7) is not enough to result in the formation of an ionic bond, it is sufficient to cause a separation of charge across the bond. This results in the more electronegative element acquiring a greater portion of the electron density, taking on a **partial negative charge** (δ^-), and the less electronegative element acquiring a smaller portion of the electron density, taking on a **partial positive charge** (δ^+). For instance, the covalent bond in HCl is polar because the two atoms have a moderate difference in electronegativity ($\Delta EN = 0.9$). In this bond, the chlorine atom gains a partial negative charge, and the hydrogen atom gains a partial positive charge. The difference in charge between the atoms is indicated by an arrow crossed at its tail end (giving the appearance of a "plus" sign) and pointing toward the negative end, as shown in Figure 3.6.

MCAT EXPERTISE

The range of electronegativities for nonpolar bonds is roughly 0 to 0.5. Polar bonds are found from 0.5 to 1.7, and ionic bonds are at 1.7 and above. Some chemistry courses allude to a grey area from 1.7 to 2.0. For the MCAT, if a molecule in this range has a metal and nonmetal, then it is effectively ionic; otherwise, it is polar covalent.

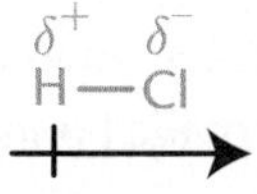

Figure 3.6 Dipole Moment of HCl

A molecule that has such a separation of positive and negative charges is called a polar molecule. The **dipole moment** of the polar bond or polar molecule is a vector quantity given by the equation:

$$\mathbf{p} = q\mathbf{d}$$

Equation 3.1

where **p** is the dipole moment, q is the magnitude of the charge, and **d** is the displacement vector separating the two partial charges. The dipole moment vector, represented by an arrow pointing from the positive to the negative charge, is measured in **Debye units** (coulomb–meters).

BRIDGE

The chemistry that creates coordinate covalent bonds appears in many forms. These reactions can be called nucleophile-electrophile reactions, described in Chapter 4 of *MCAT Organic Chemistry Review*; Lewis acid–base reactions, described in Chapter 10 of *MCAT General Chemistry Review*, or complexation reactions, described in Chapter 9 of *MCAT General Chemistry Review.*

Coordinate Covalent Bonds

In a **coordinate covalent bond**, both of the shared electrons originated on the same atom. Generally, this means that a lone pair of one atom attacked another atom with an unhybridized *p*-orbital to form a bond, as shown in Figure 3.7. Once such a bond forms, however, it is indistinguishable from any other covalent bond. The distinction is only helpful for keeping track of the valence electrons and formal charges. Coordinate covalent bonds are typically found in Lewis acid–base reactions, described in Chapter 10 of *MCAT General Chemistry Review.* A Lewis acid is any compound that will accept a lone pair of electrons, while a Lewis base is any compound that will donate a pair of electrons to form a covalent bond.

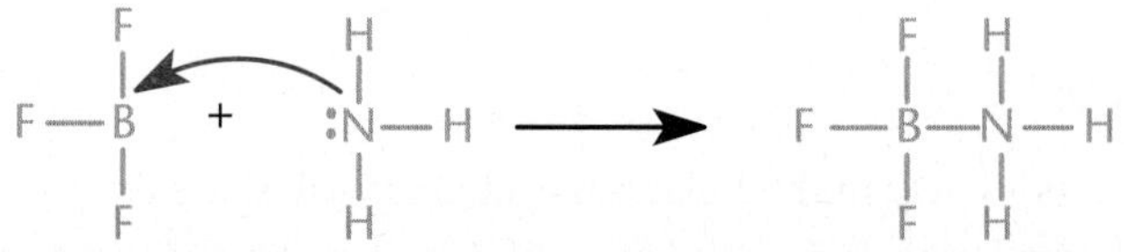

Figure 3.7 Coordinate Covalent Bond

Here, NH_3 donates a pair of electrons to form a coordinate covalent bond; thus, it acts as a Lewis base. At the same time, BF_3 accepts this pair of electrons to form the coordinate covalent bond; thus, it acts as a Lewis acid.

Covalent Bond Notation

The electrons involved in a covalent bond are in the valence shell and are **bonding electrons**, while those electrons in the valence shell that are not involved in covalent bonds are **nonbonding electrons**. The unshared electron pairs are also known as lone pairs because they are associated only with one atomic nucleus. Because atoms can bond with other atoms in many different combinations, the **Lewis structure** system of notation was developed to keep track of the bonded and nonbonded electron pairs.

Think of Lewis structures as a bookkeeping method for electrons. The number of valence electrons attributed to a particular atom in the Lewis structure of a molecule is not necessarily the same as the number of valence electrons in the neutral atom. This difference accounts for the **formal charge** of an atom in a Lewis structure. Often, more than one Lewis structure can be drawn for a molecule. If the possible Lewis structures differ in their bond connectivity or arrangement, then the Lewis structures represent different possible compounds. However, if the Lewis structures show the same bond connectivity and differ only in the arrangement of the electron pairs, then these structures represent different resonance forms of a single compound. Note that Lewis structures do not represent the actual or even theoretical geometry of a real compound. Their usefulness lies in showing the different possible ways in which atoms may be combined to form different compounds or resonance forms of a single compound.

When more than one arrangement can be made, one can assess the likelihood of each arrangement by checking the formal charges on the atoms in each arrangement. The arrangement that minimizes the number and magnitude of formal charges is usually the most stable arrangement of the compound.

Lewis Structures

A Lewis structure, or **Lewis dot diagram**, is the chemical symbol of an element surrounded by dots, each representing one of the *s* or *p* valence electrons of the atom. The Lewis symbols of the elements in the second period of the periodic table are shown in Table 3.1.

·Li	Lithium	·N̈· (with one dot below)	Nitrogen
·Be·	Beryllium	·Ö:	Oxygen
·Ḃ·	Boron	·F̤̈:	Fluorine
·Ċ· (with one dot below)	Carbon	:N̤̈e:	Neon

Table 3.1 Lewis Symbols for Period 2 Elements

KEY CONCEPT

In drawing Lewis dot structures, remember that some atoms can expand their octets by utilizing the *d*-orbitals in their outer shell. This will only take place with atoms in period 3 or greater.

Just as a Lewis symbol is used to represent the distribution of valence electrons in an atom, it can also be used to represent the distribution of valence electrons in a molecule. For example, the Lewis symbol for a fluoride ion, F^-, is $:\ddot{\underset{..}{F}}:^-$ the Lewis structure of the diatomic molecule F_2 is $:\ddot{\underset{..}{F}}-\ddot{\underset{..}{F}}:$. Certain rules must be followed in assigning a Lewis structure to a molecule. The steps for drawing a Lewis structure are outlined here, using HCN as an example.

MCAT EXPERTISE

The number of dots in Lewis Structure notation comes from group numbers. Lithium is in Group IA and therefore has one electron (dot). Carbon is in Group IVA and has four dots.

- Draw out the backbone of the compound—that is, the arrangement of atoms. In general, the least electronegative atom is the central atom. Hydrogen (always) and the halogens F, Cl, Br, and I (usually) occupy a terminal position.

  In HCN, H must occupy an end position. Of the remaining two atoms, C is the least electronegative and, therefore, occupies the central position. Therefore, the skeletal structure is as follows:

  $$H—C—N$$

- Count all the valence electrons of the atoms. The number of valence electrons of the molecule is the sum of the valence electrons of all atoms present:

  H has 1 valence electron
  C has 4 valence electrons
  N has 5 valence electrons; therefore,
  HCN has a total of 10 valence electrons.

- Draw single bonds between the central atom and the atoms surrounding it. Each single bond corresponds to a pair of electrons:

$$H:C:N$$

- Complete the octets of all atoms bonded to the central atom, using the remaining valence electrons left to be assigned. Recall that H is an exception to the octet rule because it can only have two valence electrons. In this example, H already has two valence electrons from its bond with C.

$$H:C:\ddot{\underset{..}{N}}:$$

- Place any extra electrons on the central atom. If the central atom has less than an octet, try to write double or triple bonds between the central and surrounding atoms using the lone pairs on the surrounding atoms.

The HCN structure above does not satisfy the octet rule for C because C only has four valence electrons. Therefore, two lone electron pairs from the N atom must be moved to form two more bonds with C, creating a triple bond between C and N. To make it easier to visualize, bonding electron pairs are represented as lines. You should be familiar with both dot and line notation for bonds.

$$H-C\equiv N:$$

Now, the octet rule is satisfied for all three atoms; C and N have eight valence electrons, and H has two valence electrons.

Formal Charge

To determine if a Lewis structure is representative of the actual arrangement of atoms in a compound, one must calculate the formal charge of each atom. In doing so, assume a perfectly equal sharing of all bonded electron pairs, regardless of actual differences in electronegativity. In other words, assume that each electron pair is split evenly between the two nuclei in the bond. The difference between the number of electrons assigned to an atom in a Lewis structure and the number of electrons normally found in that atom's valence shell is the **formal charge**. A simple equation you can use to calculate formal charge is:

$$\text{formal charge} = V - N_{\text{nonbonding}} - \frac{1}{2} N_{\text{bonding}}$$

Equation 3.2

where V is the normal number of electrons in the atom's valence shell, $N_{\text{nonbonding}}$ is the number of nonbonding electrons, and N_{bonding} is the number of bonding electrons (double the number of bonds because each bond has two electrons). The charge of an ion or compound is equal to the sum of the formal charges of the individual atoms comprising the ion or compound.

MNEMONIC

A less formal way to calculate formal charge is with the formula:

Formal charge = valence electrons − dots − sticks

Where a "dot" refers to a lone electron and a "stick" refers to a bond.

Example: Calculate the formal charge on the central N atom of $[NH_4]^+$.

Solution: The Lewis structure of $[NH_4]^+$ is:

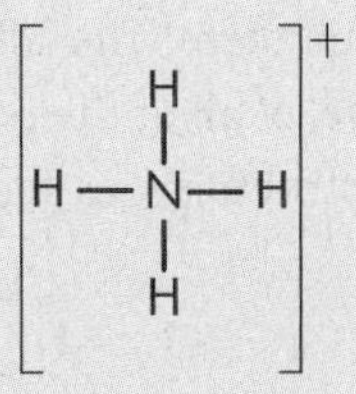

Nitrogen is in Group VA; thus, it has five valence electrons. In $[NH_4]^+$, N has four bonds (eight bonding electrons and zero nonbonding electrons).

Thus, $V = 5$; $N_{bonding} = 8$; $N_{nonbonding} = 0$

$$\text{Formal charge} = 5 - 0 - \frac{1}{2}(8) = +1$$

Thus, the formal charge on the N atom in $[NH_4]^+$ is $+1$.

One can also use logic to determine formal charge. As drawn, N has four bonds. Assuming equal sharing of the electrons in the bonds, this means N has four valence electrons. In its normal state, N has five valence electrons. Thus, nitrogen has one fewer electron than its normal state, and has a $+1$ charge.

Let us offer a brief note of explanation on the difference between formal charge and oxidation number: formal charge underestimates the effect of electronegativity differences, whereas oxidation numbers overestimate the effect of electronegativity differences, assuming that the more electronegative atom has a 100 percent share of the bonding electron pair. For example, in a molecule of CO_2 (carbon dioxide), the formal charge on each of the atoms is 0, but the oxidation number of each of the oxygen atoms is –2 and of the carbon is +4. In reality, the distribution of electron density between the carbon and oxygen atoms lies somewhere between the extremes predicted by the formal charges and the oxidation states.

BRIDGE

Resonance is an important topic in both general and organic chemistry. It allows for greater stability, delocalizing electrons and charges over what is known as a π (pi) system. Resonance in organic molecules is discussed in Chapter 3 of *MCAT Organic Chemistry Review.*

Resonance

As suggested earlier, it may be possible to draw two or more Lewis structures that demonstrate the same arrangement of atoms but that differ in the specific placement of the electrons. These are called **resonance structures** and are represented with a double-headed arrow between them. The actual electronic distribution in the compound is a hybrid, or composite, of all of the possible resonance structures. For example, SO_2 has three resonance structures, as shown in Figure 3.8.

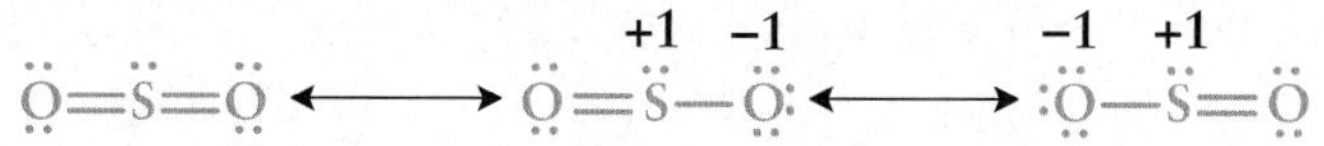

Figure 3.8 Resonance Structures for SO_2
The double-headed arrows indicate that these molecules are involved in a resonance hybrid.

The nature of the bonds within the actual compound is a hybrid of these three structures. If one were to evaluate the spectral data, it would indicate that the two S—O bonds are identical and equivalent. This phenomenon is known as resonance, and the actual structure of the compound is called the **resonance hybrid**.

The first resonance structure in Figure 3.8 is significantly more stable than the other two structures. Consequently, it is the major contributor to the resonance hybrid. In general, the more stable the structure, the more it contributes to the character of the resonance hybrid. In Figure 3.8, the minor contributors contain formal charges, indicating decreased stability. One can use formal charge to assess the stability of resonance structures according to the following guidelines:

- A Lewis structure with small or no formal charges is preferred over a Lewis structure with large formal charges.
- A Lewis structure with less separation between opposite charges is preferred over a Lewis structure with a large separation of opposite charges.
- A Lewis structure in which negative formal charges are placed on more electronegative atoms is more stable than one in which the negative formal charges are placed on less electronegative atoms.

Example: Write the resonance structures for $[NCO]^-$.

Solution:

1. C is the least electronegative of the three given atoms. Therefore, the C atom occupies the central position in the skeletal structure of $[NCO]^-$:

$$N - C - O$$

2. N has 5 valence electrons;
C has 4 valence electrons;
O has 6 valence electrons;
and the species has one negative charge.
Total valence electrons $= 5 + 4 + 6 + 1 = 16$

3. Draw single bonds between the central C atom and the surrounding atoms, N and O. Draw a pair of electrons to represent each bond.

$$N:C:O$$

4. Complete the octets of N and O with the remaining 12 electrons.

$$:\underset{..}{\ddot{N}}:C:\underset{..}{\ddot{O}}:$$

5. The C octet is incomplete. There are three ways in which double and triple bonds can be formed to complete the C octet: two lone pairs from the O atom can be used to form a triple bond between the C and O atoms:

$$:\overset{-2}{\underset{..}{\ddot{N}}} - \overset{0}{C} \equiv \overset{+1}{\ddot{O}}$$

Or one lone electron pair can be taken from both O and N to form two double bonds, one between N and C, the other between O and C:

$$:\overset{-1}{\underset{..}{N}} = \overset{0}{C} = \overset{0}{\underset{..}{O}}:$$

Or two lone electron pairs can be taken from the N atom to form a triple bond between the C and N atoms:

$$:\overset{0}{N} \equiv \overset{0}{C} - \overset{-1}{\underset{..}{\ddot{O}}}:$$

All three are resonance structures of $[NCO]^-$

6. Assign formal charges to each atom of each resonance structure.
The most stable structure is this:

$$:\overset{0}{N} \equiv \overset{0}{C} - \overset{-1}{\underset{..}{\ddot{O}}}:$$

because the charges are minimized, and the negative formal charge is on the most electronegative atom, O.

Exceptions to the Octet Rule

As stated previously, the octet rule has many exceptions. In addition to hydrogen, helium, lithium, beryllium, and boron, which are exceptions because they cannot or do not usually reach the octet, all elements in or beyond the third period may be exceptions because they can take on more than eight electrons in their valence shells. These electrons can be placed into orbitals of the *d* subshell, and as a result, atoms of these elements can form more than four bonds. On Test Day, don't automatically discount a Lewis structure with a central atom that has more than four bonds—the testmakers may be testing your ability to recognize that many atoms can expand their valence shells beyond the octet.

MCAT EXPERTISE

Don't be surprised if you can draw more than two resonance structures for a molecule or ion. Becoming proficient at drawing and, more importantly, recognizing resonance structures will save you time on Test Day.

Consider the sulfate ion, SO_4^{2-}. In the Lewis structure for the sulfate ion, giving the sulfur 12 valence electrons permits three of the five atoms to be assigned a formal charge of zero. The sulfate ion can be drawn in at least six resonance forms, many of which have two double bonds attached to a different combination of oxygen atoms. Figure 3.9 shows two of the possible forms.

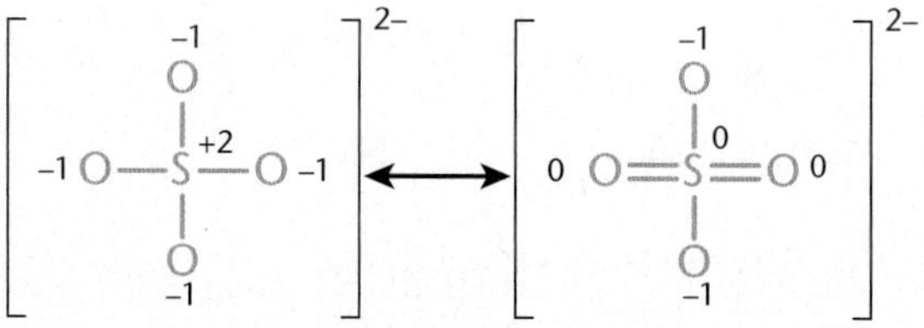

Figure 3.9 Two Different Resonance Forms of the Sulfate Ion

Geometry and Polarity

Because Lewis dot structures do not suggest or reflect the actual geometric arrangement of atoms in a compound, we need another system to provide this information. One such system is known as the **valence shell electron pair repulsion** (**VSEPR**) **theory**.

Valence Shell Electron Pair Repulsion (VSEPR) Theory

VSEPR theory uses Lewis dot structures to predict the molecular geometry of covalently bonded molecules. It states that the three-dimensional arrangement of atoms surrounding a central atom is determined by the repulsions between bonding and nonbonding electron pairs in the valence shell of the central atom. These electron pairs arrange themselves as far apart as possible, thereby minimizing repulsive forces. The following steps are used to predict the geometrical structure of a molecule using the VSEPR theory:

- Draw the Lewis dot structure of the molecule.
- Count the total number of bonding and nonbonding electron pairs in the valence shell of the central atom.

- Arrange the electron pairs around the central atom so that they are as far apart as possible. For example, the compound AX_2 has the Lewis structure X:A:X. The A atom has two bonding electron pairs in its valence shell. To position these electron pairs as far apart as possible, their geometric structure should be linear:

$$X - A - X$$

A summary of electronic geometries as predicted by VSEPR theory is shown in Table 3.2.

REGIONS OF ELECTRON DENSITY	EXAMPLE	GEOMETRIC ARRANGEMENT OF ELECTRON PAIRS AROUND THE CENTRAL ATOM	SHAPE	ANGLE BETWEEN ELECTRON PAIRS
2	$BeCl_2$	X - A - X	linear	180°
3	BH_3	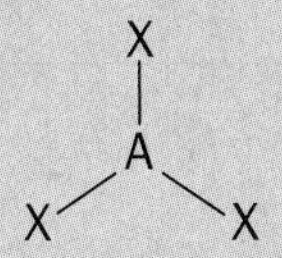	trigonal planar	120°
4	CH_4	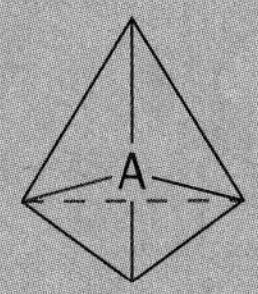	tetrahedral	109.5°
5	PCl_5	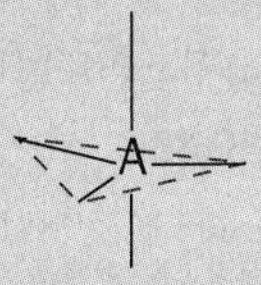	trigonal bipyramidal	90°, 120°, 180°
6	SF_6	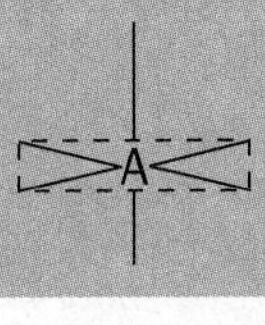	octahedral	90°, 180°

Table 3.2 VSEPR Theory
This table lists the five most common electronic configurations of molecules.

MCAT EXPERTISE

According to the AAMC's official content lists, you need to be prepared to draw and identify structural formulas for molecules involving H, C, N, O, F, S, P, Si, and Cl. Rather than memorizing these elements, however, just be familiar with the process of creating a Lewis diagram for any element and predicting its three-dimensional shape from VSEPR theory.

Example: Predict the molecular geometry of NH_3.

Solution:

1. The Lewis structure of NH_3 is:

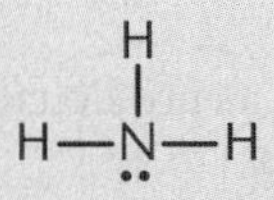

2. The central atom, N, has three bonding electron pairs and one nonbonding electron pair, for a total of four electron pairs.

3. The four electron pairs will be farthest apart when they occupy the corners of a tetrahedron. Because one of the four electron pairs is a lone pair, the observed molecular geometry is trigonal pyramidal, shown below.

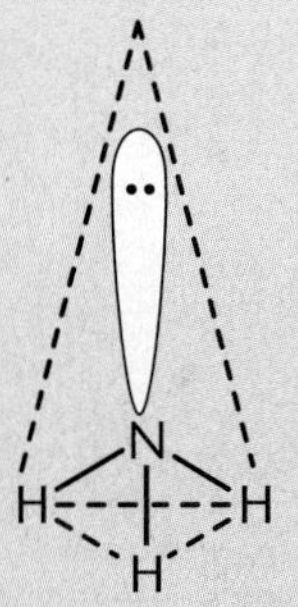

In describing the shape of a molecule, only the arrangement of atoms (not electrons) is considered. Even though the electron pairs are arranged tetrahedrally, the shape of NH_3 is pyramidal. It is not trigonal planar because the lone pair repels the three bonding electron pairs, causing them to move as far apart as possible.

KEY CONCEPT

The shapes from Table 3.2 refer to *electronic geometry*, which is different from *molecular geometry.* In the worked example, notice that the ammonia molecule has a tetrahedral *electronic* structure, but is considered to have a *molecular* structure that is trigonal pyramidal.

Example: Predict the geometry of CO_2.

Solution: The Lewis structure of CO_2 is $\ddot{\underset{..}{O}}::C::\ddot{\underset{..}{O}}$

The double bond behaves just like a single bond for the purposes of predicting molecular shape. This compound has two groups of electrons around the carbon. According to the VSEPR theory, the two sets of electrons will orient themselves 180° apart, on opposite sides of the carbon atom, minimizing electron repulsion. Therefore, the molecular structure of CO_2 is linear: $\ddot{\underset{..}{O}}=C=\ddot{\underset{..}{O}}$

One subtlety that the MCAT loves to test is the difference between electronic geometry and molecular geometry. **Electronic geometry** describes the spatial arrangement of all pairs of electrons around the central atom, including both the bonding and the lone pairs. In contrast, the **molecular geometry** describes the spatial arrangement of only the bonding pairs of electrons. The **coordination number**, which is the number of atoms that surround and are bonded to a central atom, is the relevant factor when determining molecular geometry. For example, consider that CH_4 (methane), NH_3 (ammonia), and H_2O all have the same electronic geometry: in each compound, four pairs of electrons surround the central atom. This is tetrahedral electronic geometry. However, because each molecule has a different coordination number, they have different molecular geometries. In molecular geometry, methane has tetrahedral geometry, ammonia has trigonal pyramidal geometry, and water is identified as angular or bent.

MCAT EXPERTISE

CH_4, NH_3, and H_2O all have a tetrahedral electronic geometry, but differ in their molecular shapes:

CH_4 is tetrahedral, NH_3 is pyramidal, and H_2O is bent or angular.

The distinction is important, and the MCAT will primarily focus on molecular geometry. However, there is one important implication of electronic geometry: the determination of the **ideal bond angle**. Tetrahedral electronic geometry, for example, is associated with an ideal bond angle of 109.5°; however, nonbonding pairs are able to exert more repulsion than bonding pairs because these electrons reside closer to the nucleus. Thus, the angle in ammonia is closer to 107°, and the angle in water is 104.5°.

Polarity of Molecules

When two atoms of different electronegativities bond covalently, sharing one or more pairs of electrons, the resulting bond is polar, with the more electronegative atom possessing the greater share of the electron density. However, the presence of bond dipoles does not necessarily result in a molecular dipole; that is, an overall separation of charge across the molecule. We must first consider the molecular geometry and the vector addition of the bond dipoles based upon that molecular geometry. A compound with nonpolar bonds is always nonpolar. However, a compound with polar bonds may be polar or nonpolar, depending upon the spatial orientation of the polar bonds in the molecule. If the compound has a molecular geometry such that the bond dipole moments cancel each other out (that is, if the vector sum is zero), then the result is a nonpolar compound. For example, CCl_4 (carbon tetrachloride) has four polar C–Cl bonds, but because the molecular geometry of carbon tetrachloride is tetrahedral, the four bond dipoles point to the vertices of the tetrahedron and, therefore, cancel each other out, resulting in a nonpolar compound, as shown in Figure 3.10.

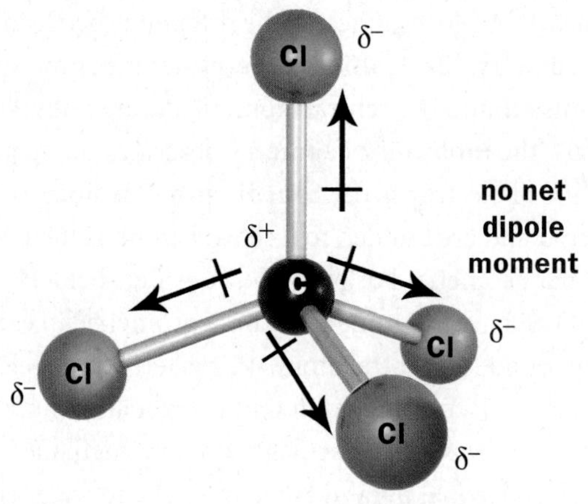

Figure 3.10 CCl_4 is a Nonpolar Compound with Four Polar Bonds

MCAT EXPERTISE

Be careful! If you spot a polar bond in a molecule, the molecule can be either polar or nonpolar. On the contrary, when you see only nonpolar bonds in a molecule, the structure *must* be nonpolar. When in doubt, draw out relevant structures on your scratch paper on Test Day.

However, when the molecular geometry is arranged such that the bond dipoles do not cancel each other out, the molecule will have a net dipole moment and will therefore be polar. For instance, the O–H bonds in H_2O are polar, with each hydrogen atom assuming a partial positive charge and the oxygen assuming a partial negative charge. Recall that the molecular geometry of water is angular (bent). Therefore, the vector summation of the bond dipoles results in a molecular dipole moment from the partially positive hydrogen end to the partially negative oxygen end, as illustrated in Figure 3.11.

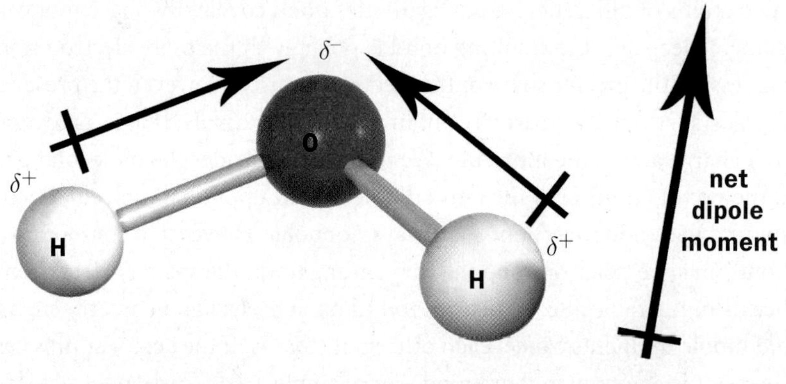

Figure 3.11 H_2O is a Polar Molecule with Two Polar Bonds

BRIDGE

Quantum Numbers (Chapter 1 of *MCAT General Chemistry Review*) revisited:

For any value of *n*, there are *n* values of *l* $(0 \rightarrow n - 1)$.

- $l = 0 \rightarrow s$
- $l = 1 \rightarrow p$
- $l = 2 \rightarrow d$
- $l = 3 \rightarrow f$

For any value of *l*, there are $2l + 1$ values of *ml* (number of orbitals); values range from $-l$ to l.

Atomic and Molecular Orbitals

To finish the discussion of covalent bonds, we need to address the concept of atomic and molecular orbitals. Recall the model of the atom as a dense, positively charged nucleus surrounded by a cloud of electrons organized into orbitals (regions in space surrounding the nucleus within which there are certain probabilities of finding an electron). The four quantum numbers describe the energy and position of an electron in an atom. While the principal quantum number, *n*, indicates the average energy level of the shell, the azimuthal quantum number, *l*, describes the subshells within each principal energy level. When $l = 0$, this indicates the *s* subshell, which has one orbital that is spherical in shape. The 1*s*-orbital $(n = 1, l = 0, m_l = 0)$ is plotted in Figure 3.12.

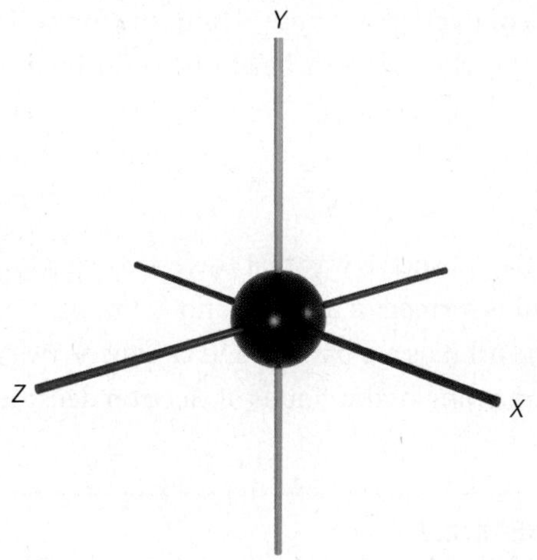

Figure 3.12 1*s*-Orbital

When $l = 1$, this indicates the *p* subshell, which has three orbitals shaped like barbells along the *x*-, *y*-, and *z*-axes at right angles to each other. The 2*p*-orbitals ($n = 2, l = 1, m_l = -1, 0,$ and $+1$) are plotted in Figure 3.13.

Although well beyond the scope of the MCAT, mathematical analysis of the wave functions of the orbitals is used to determine and assign plus and minus signs to each lobe of the *p*-orbitals. The shapes of the five *d*-orbitals and the seven *f*-orbitals are more complex and do not need to be memorized for the MCAT.

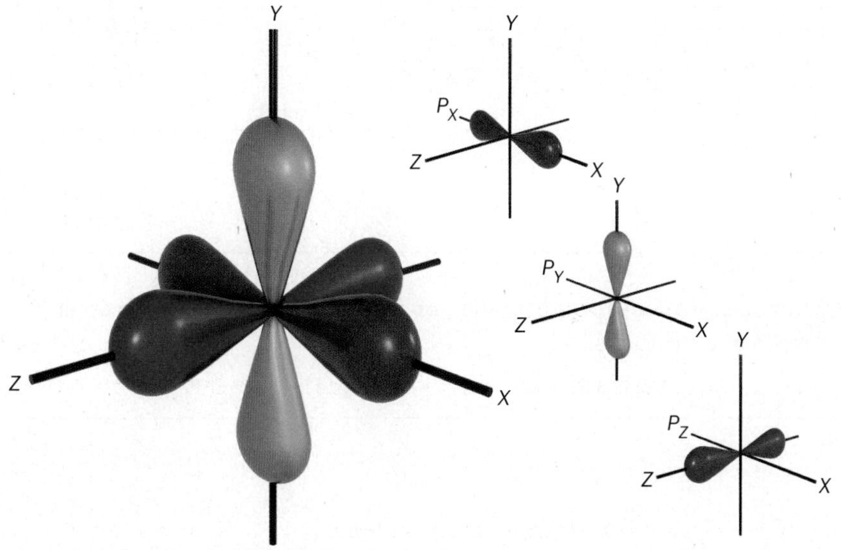

Figure 3.13 *p*-Orbitals on the *x*-, *y*-, and *z*-Axes

When two atoms bond to form a compound, the atomic orbitals interact to form a **molecular orbital** that describes the probability of finding the bonding electrons in a given space. Molecular orbitals are obtained by combining the wave functions of the atomic orbitals. Qualitatively, the overlap of two atomic orbitals describes this molecular orbital. If the signs of the two atomic orbitals are the same, a **bonding orbital** forms. If the signs are different, an **antibonding orbital** forms.

Two different patterns of overlap are observed in the formation of molecular bonds. When orbitals overlap head-to-head, the resulting bond is a **sigma (σ) bond.** σ bonds allow for free rotation about their axes because the electron density of the bonding orbital is a single linear accumulation between the atomic nuclei.

When the orbitals overlap in such a way that there are two parallel electron cloud densities, a **pi (π) bond** is formed. π bonds do not allow for free rotation because the electron densities of the orbitals are parallel and cannot be twisted in such a way that allows continuous overlapping of the clouds of electron densities.

MCAT CONCEPT CHECK 3.3

Before you move on, assess your understanding of the material with these questions.

1. Describe the relationship between bond strength, bond length, and bond energy.

   ---

2. For what values of ΔEN will a nonpolar covalent bond form? Polar covalent? Ionic?

   - Nonpolar covalent:

   - Polar covalent:

   - Ionic:

   ---

3. Draw a Lewis dot structure for the carbonate ion (CO_3^{2-}) and its two other resonance structures.

   ---

4. Predict the molecular geometries of the following molecules:
   - PCl_5:
   - MgF_2:
   - AlF_3:
   - UBr_6:
   - SiH_4:

3.4 Intermolecular Forces

LEARNING OBJECTIVES

After Chapter 3.4, you will be able to:

- Order the intermolecular forces from strongest to weakest
- Describe what occurs during dipole-dipole, hydrogen bonding, and London dispersion force interactions
- Predict what intermolecular forces are possible for given interacting molecules:

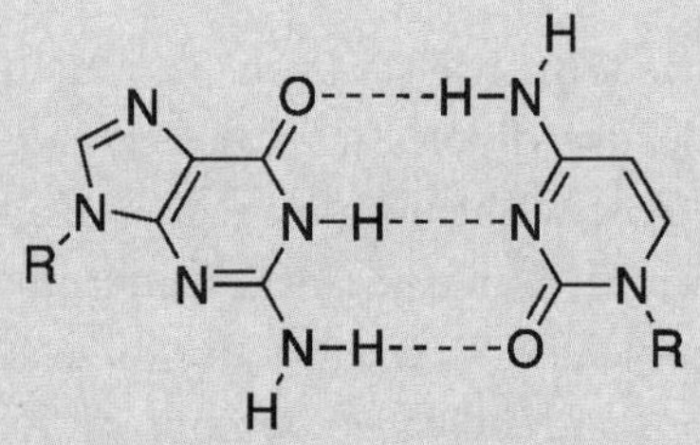

Atoms and compounds participate in weak electrostatic interactions. The strength of these **intermolecular forces** can impact certain physical properties, such as melting and boiling points. The weakest of the intermolecular interactions are the dispersion forces, also known as London forces. Next are the dipole–dipole interactions, which are of intermediate strength. Finally, we have the strongest type of interaction, the hydrogen bond, which is a misnomer because there is no actual sharing or transfer of electrons. We must keep in mind, however, that even hydrogen bonds, the strongest of these interactions, only have about 10 percent of the strength of a covalent bond. Therefore, these electrostatic interactions can be overcome with small or moderate amounts of energy.

BRIDGE

These intermolecular forces are the bonding forces that keep a substance together in its solid or liquid state and determine whether two substances are miscible or immiscible in solution. Solutions and solubility are discussed in Chapter 9 of *MCAT General Chemistry Review.*

London Dispersion Forces

The bonding electrons in nonpolar covalent bonds may appear to be shared equally between two atoms, but at any point in time, they will be located randomly throughout the orbital. In a given moment, the electron density may be unequally distributed between the two atoms. This results in a rapid polarization and counterpolarization of the electron cloud and the formation of short-lived dipole moments. Subsequently, these dipoles interact with the electron clouds of neighboring compounds, inducing the formation of more dipoles. The momentarily negative end of one molecule will cause the closest region in any neighboring molecule to become temporarily positive itself. This causes the other end of the neighboring molecule to become temporarily negative, which in turn induces other molecules to become temporarily polarized, and the cycle begins again. The attractive or repulsive interactions of these short-lived and rapidly shifting dipoles are known as **London dispersion forces**, a type of **van der Waals force**.

REAL WORLD

While dispersion forces (a type of van der Waals force) are the weakest of the intermolecular attractions, when there are millions of these interactions there is an amazing power of adhesion. This is demonstrated by geckos' feet; the animal's ability to climb smooth, vertical, and even inverted surfaces is due to dispersion forces.

Dispersion forces are the weakest of all of the intermolecular interactions because they are the result of induced dipoles that change and shift moment to moment. They do not extend over long distances and are, therefore, significant only when molecules are in close proximity. The strength of the London force also depends on the degree and ease by which the molecules can be polarized—that is, how easily the electrons can be shifted around. Large molecules are more easily polarizable than comparable smaller molecules and thus possess greater dispersion forces.

Despite their weak nature, don't underestimate the importance of dispersion forces. If it weren't for them, the noble gases would not liquefy at any temperature because no other intermolecular forces exist between the noble gas atoms. The low temperatures at which noble gases liquefy are indicative of the very small magnitude of the dispersion forces between the atoms.

Dipole–Dipole Interactions

Polar molecules tend to orient themselves in such a way that the oppositely charged ends of the respective molecular dipoles are closest to each other: the positive region of onc molecule is close to the negative region of another molecule. This arrangement is energetically favorable because an attractive electrostatic force is formed between the two molecules. This attractive force is denoted by dashed lines in most molecular notations and indicates a temporary bonding interaction, as shown in Figure 3.14.

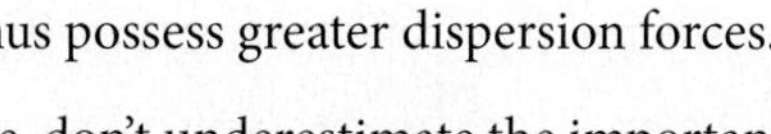

Figure 3.14 Dipole–Dipole Interactions in HCl

BRIDGE

In organic chemistry, carbonyl groups possess distinct dipoles that facilitate nucleophilic attacks. This is the focus of almost all of the reactions in Chapters 6 to 9 of *MCAT Organic Chemistry Review.*

Dipole–dipole interactions are present in the solid and liquid phases but become negligible in the gas phase because of the significantly increased distance between gas particles. Polar species tend to have higher melting and boiling points than nonpolar species of comparable molecular weight due to these interactions. Realize that London forces and dipole–dipole interactions are different not in kind but in duration. Both are electrostatic forces between opposite partial charges; the difference is only in the transience or permanence of the molecular dipole.

Hydrogen Bonds

Hydrogen bonds are a favorite topic on the MCAT. A hydrogen bond is a specific, unusually strong form of dipole–dipole interaction that may be intra- or intermolecular. Hydrogen bonds are not actually bonds—there is no sharing or transferring of electrons between two atoms. When hydrogen is bonded to one of three highly electronegative atoms—nitrogen, oxygen, or fluorine—the hydrogen atom carries only a small amount of the electron density in the covalent bond.

MNEMONIC

Hydrogen bonds: Pick up the **FON** (phone):

Hydrogen bonds exist in molecules containing a hydrogen bonded to **F**luorine, **O**xygen, or **N**itrogen.

The hydrogen atom essentially acts as a naked proton. The positively charged hydrogen atom interacts with the partial negative charge of fluorine, oxygen, or nitrogen on nearby molecules. Substances that display hydrogen bonding tend to have unusually high boiling points compared to compounds of similar molecular weights that do not exhibit hydrogen bonding. The difference derives from the energy required to break the hydrogen bonds. Hydrogen bonding, shown in Figure 3.15, is particularly important in the behavior of water, alcohols, amines, and carboxylic acids.

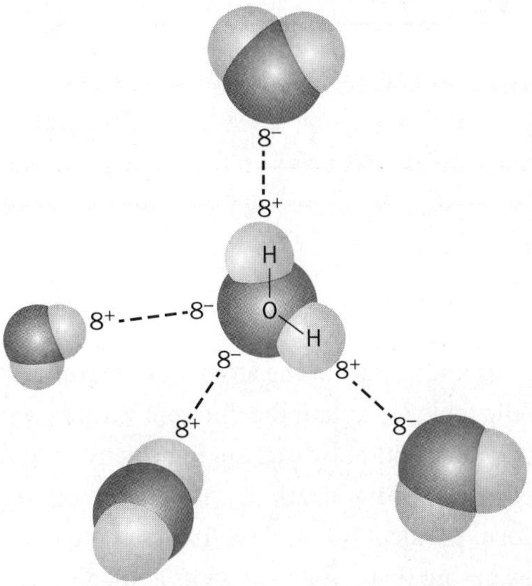

Figure 3.15 Hydrogen Bonding in Water

Many biochemical molecules, such as nucleotides, have different regions that are stabilized by hydrogen bonding, as shown in Figure 3.16. It is not an overstatement to say that, were it not for water's ability to form hydrogen bonds and exist in the liquid state at room temperature, we would not exist (at least not in the form we recognize as "human").

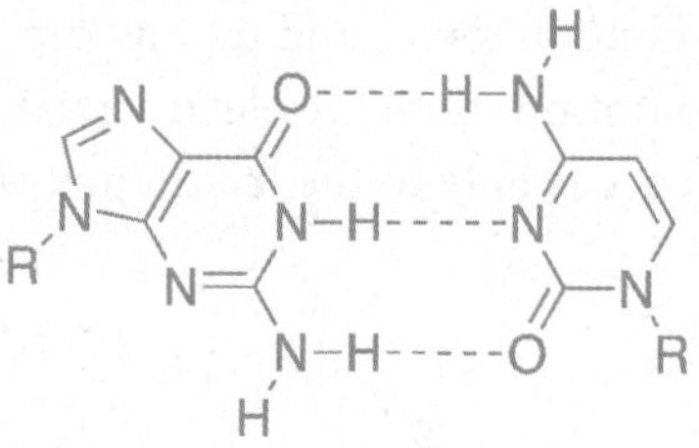

Figure 3.16 Hydrogen Bonding between Guanine and Cytosine

MCAT CONCEPT CHECK 3.4

Before you move on, assess your understanding of the material with these questions.

1. Rank the major intermolecular forces from strongest to weakest:

    1. ____________________
    2. ____________________
    3. ____________________

2. Describe what occurs during dipole–dipole interactions.

    ____

3. In order to exhibit hydrogen bonding, what must be true of a given molecule?

    ____

Conclusion

This chapter built on our knowledge of the atom and the trends demonstrated by the elements in the periodic table to explain the different ways by which atoms partner together to form compounds, either by exchanging electrons to form ions, which are then held together by electrostatic attractions between opposite charges; or by sharing electrons to form covalent bonds. We discussed the nature and characteristics of covalent bonds, noting their relative lengths and energies, as well as polarities. A review of Lewis dot structures and VSEPR theory will prepare you for predicting likely bond arrangements, resonance structures, and molecular geometries. Finally, we compared the relative strengths of the most important intermolecular electrostatic interactions, noting that even the strongest of these—hydrogen bonding—is still much weaker than an actual covalent bond. The next time you're "browning" some of your food in a pan or the oven, take a moment to consider what's happening at the atomic and molecular level. It's not just cooking; it's science!

You've reviewed the content, now test your knowledge and critical thinking skills by completing a test-like passage set in your online resources!

GO ONLINE

CONCEPT SUMMARY

Bonding

- Chemical bonds can be ionic or covalent.
- Elements will form bonds to attain a noble gas-like electron configuration.
- The **octet rule** states that elements will be most stable with eight valence electrons. However, there are many exceptions to this rule:
  - Elements with an incomplete octet are stable with fewer than eight electrons and include H, He, Li, Be, and B.
  - Elements with an expanded octet are stable with more than eight electrons and include all elements in period 3 or greater.
  - Compounds with an odd number of electrons cannot have eight electrons on each element.

Ionic Bonds

- An **ionic bond** is formed via the transfer of one or more electrons from an element with a relatively low ionization energy to an element with a relatively high electron affinity.
  - Ionic bonds occur between elements with large differences in electronegativity ($\Delta EN > 1.7$), usually between metals and nonmetals.
  - A positively charged ion is called a **cation**. A negatively charged ion is called an **anion**.
  - The resulting electrostatic attraction between the ions causes them to remain in close proximity, forming the bond.
  - Ionic compounds form **crystalline lattices**—large, organized arrays of ions.
- Ionic compounds have unique physical and chemical properties.
  - Ionic compounds tend to dissociate in water and other polar solvents.
  - Ionic solids tend to have high melting points.

Covalent Bonds

- A **covalent bond** is formed via the sharing of electrons between two elements of similar electronegativities.
- **Bond order** refers to whether a covalent bond is a single bond, double bond, or triple bond. As bond order increases, **bond strength** increases, **bond energy** increases, and **bond length** decreases.

- Covalent bonds can be categorized as nonpolar or polar based on the nature of the elements involved.
  - **Nonpolar bonds** result in molecules in which both atoms have exactly the same electronegativity; some bonds are considered nonpolar when there is a very small difference in electronegativity between the atoms ($\Delta EN < 0.5$), even though they are technically slightly polar.
  - **Polar bonds** form when there is a significant difference in electronegativities ($\Delta EN = 0.5$ to 1.7), but not enough to transfer electrons and form an ionic bond. In a polar bond, the more electronegative element takes on a partial negative charge, and the less electronegative element takes on a partial positive charge.
- **Coordinate covalent bonds** result when a single atom provides both bonding electrons while the other atom does not contribute any; coordinate covalent bonds are most often found in Lewis acid–base chemistry.
- **Lewis dot symbols** are a chemical representation of an atom's valence electrons.
- Drawing a complete Lewis dot structure requires a balance of valence, bonding, and nonbonding electrons in a molecule or ion.
- **Formal charges** exist when an atom is surrounded by more or fewer valence electrons than it has in its neutral state (assuming equal sharing of electrons in a bond).
- For any molecule with a π (pi) system of electrons, **resonance structures** exist; these represent all of the possible configurations of electrons—stable and unstable—that contribute to the overall structure.
- The **valence shell electron pair repulsion (VSEPR) theory** predicts the three-dimensional molecular geometry of covalently bonded molecules. In this theory, electrons—whether bonding or nonbonding—arrange themselves to be as far apart as possible from each other in three-dimensional space, leading to characteristic geometries.
  - Nonbonding electrons exert more repulsion than bonding electrons because they reside closer to the nucleus.
  - **Electronic geometry** refers to the position of all electrons in a molecule, whether bonding or nonbonding. **Molecular geometry** refers to the position of only the bonding pairs of electrons in a molecule.
- The **polarity of molecules** is dependent on the dipole moment of each bond and the sum of the dipole moments in a molecular structure.
  - All polar molecules contain polar bonds.
  - Nonpolar molecules may contain nonpolar bonds, or polar bonds with dipole moments that cancel each other.
- σ and π bonds describe the patterns of overlap observed when molecular bonds are formed.
  - **Sigma (σ) bonds** are the result of head-to-head overlap.
  - **Pi (π) bonds** are the result of the overlap of two parallel electron cloud densities.

Intermolecular Forces

- **Intermolecular forces** are electrostatic attractions between molecules. They are significantly weaker than covalent bonds (which are weaker than ionic bonds).
  - **London dispersion forces** are the weakest interactions, but are present in all atoms and molecules. As the size of the atom or structure increases, so does the corresponding London dispersion force.
  - **Dipole–dipole interactions**, which occur between the oppositely charged ends of polar molecules, are stronger than London forces; these interactions are evident in the solid and liquid phases but negligible in the gas phase due to the distance between particles.
  - **Hydrogen bonds** are a specialized subset of dipole–dipole interactions involved in intra- and intermolecular attraction; hydrogen bonding occurs when hydrogen is bonded to one of three very electronegative atoms—fluorine, oxygen, or nitrogen.

ANSWERS TO CONCEPT CHECKS

3.1

1. Ionic bonds form between ions and involve gain or loss of electrons. Covalent bonds occur when electrons are shared between atoms.
2. Any three examples that form incomplete octets (H, He, Li, Be, B) or expanded octets (Period 3 and greater) are acceptable.
3. The polarity in a covalent bond is determined by differences in electronegativity between the two atoms involved.

3.2

1. Metals lose electrons because they have low ionization energies, while nonmetals gain electrons because they have high electron affinities. These processes are complementary, leading to the formation of an ionic bond.
2. Some characteristics of ionic compounds include high melting and boiling points due to electrostatic attractions, solubility of ions in water due to interactions with polar solvents, good conductors of heat and electricity, crystal lattice arrangement to minimize repulsive forces, and large electronegativity differences between ions, among other possible answers.

3.3

1. Bond strength is defined by the electrostatic attraction between nuclei and electrons; multiple bonds (higher bond order) increases strength. Bond length is a consequence of these attractions. The stronger the bond, the shorter it is. Bond energy is the minimum amount of energy needed to break a bond. The stronger the bond, the higher the bond energy.
2. Nonpolar covalent bonds form with $\Delta EN = 0$ to 0.5. Polar covalent bonds form with $\Delta EN = 0.5$ to 1.7. Ionic bonds form with $\Delta EN = 1.7$ or higher.
3. 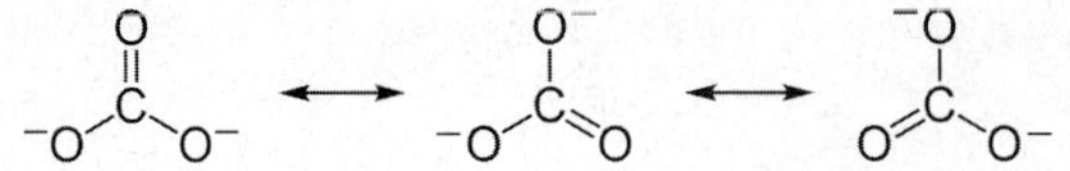
4. PCl_5: trigonal bipyramidal, MgF_2: linear, AlF_3: trigonal planar, UBr_6: octahedral, SiH_4: tetrahedral

3.4

1. Hydrogen bonding > dipole–dipole interactions > dispersion (London) forces
2. A dipole consists of a segment of a molecule with partial positive and partial negative regions. The positive end of one molecule is attracted to the negative end of another molecule, and vice-versa.
3. To experience hydrogen bonding, a molecule must contain a hydrogen bonded to a very electronegative atom (nitrogen, oxygen, or fluorine).

SCIENCE MASTERY ASSESSMENT EXPLANATIONS

1. **B**

Carbon dioxide, CO_2, has a double bond between carbon and each of its oxygen atoms. In polar covalent bonds, the difference in electronegativity between the bonded atoms is great enough to cause electrons to move disproportionately toward the more electronegative atom; hence the bonds are polar. But the electronegativity difference is not great enough to completely transfer electrons to the more electronegative atom; hence the bonds are covalent. Because oxygen has somewhat greater electronegativity compared to carbon, the bonds of carbon dioxide are polar covalent.

2. **B**

To answer this question, one must understand the contribution of resonance structures to average formal charge. In **(B)**, there are three possible resonance structures. Each of the three oxygen atoms carries a formal charge of -1 in two out of the three structures. This averages to approximately $-\frac{2}{3}$ charge on each oxygen atom, which is more negative than in the other answer choices. Both water and formaldehyde, **(A)** and **(D)**, have no formal charge on the oxygen. Ozone, **(C)**, has a $-\frac{1}{2}$ on two of the three oxygens and a $+1$ charge on the central oxygen.

3. **C**

This question is asking for an element that reliably follows the octet rule. There are only a few elements that do not break the octet rule, including carbon, nitrogen, oxygen, fluorine, sodium, and magnesium. Thus, **(C)** is correct. To eliminate **(A)**, **(B)**, and **(D)**, observe that the remaining elements can have other valences; Be is stable with a valence of four electrons, while both S and P can expand their octets.

4. **D**

The key to answering this question is to understand the types of intermolecular forces that exist in each of these molecules because larger intermolecular forces correspond to higher boiling points. Kr is a noble gas with a full octet, so the only intermolecular forces present are London dispersion forces, the weakest type of intermolecular forces. Acetone and isopropyl alcohol are both polar, so both have dipole–dipole interactions, which are stronger than dispersion forces. However, isopropyl alcohol can also form hydrogen bonds, increasing its boiling point. Finally, the strongest interactions are ionic bonds, which exist in potassium chloride.

5. **C**

The central carbon in carbonate has no lone pairs. It has three resonance structures, each of which involves a double bond between carbon and one of the three oxygens. Having made four bonds, carbon has no further orbitals for bonding or to carry lone pairs. This makes carbonate's geometry trigonal planar. Alternatively, ClF_3 also has three bonds; however, chloride still maintains two extra lone pairs. These lone pairs each inhabit one orbital, meaning that the central chloride must organize five items about itself: three bonds to fluorides and two lone pairs. The best configuration for maximizing the distance between all of these groups is trigonal bipyramidal. **(A)** and **(B)** are true statements but do not account for the difference in geometry.

6. **B**

Ionic bonds are formed between elements with large differences in electronegativity, i.e. between metals and nonmetals. Mg is a metal, whereas Cl, O, and H are all nonmetals. Since **(B)** contains a metal and nonmetal, it is correct. **(A)**, **(C)**, and **(D)** all describe covalent bonds. While HCl does ionize in aqueous solution, it exists as a polar covalent compound in the gaseous state.

7. **D**

Bond lengths decrease as the bond order increases, and they also decrease with larger differences in electronegativity. In this case, because both C_2H_2 and HCN have triple bonds, we cannot compare the bond lengths based on bond order. We must then rely on other periodic trends. The bond length decreases when moving to the right along the periodic table's rows because more electronegative atoms have shorter atomic radii. The nitrogen in HCN is likely to hold its electrons closer, or in a shorter radius, than the carbons in C_2H_2.

8. **C**

Electronegative atoms bonded to hydrogen disproportionately pull covalently bonded electrons toward themselves, which leaves hydrogen with a partial positive character. That partial positive charge is attracted to nearby negative or partial negative charges, such as those on other electronegative atoms.

9. **C**

First recall that ammonium is NH_4^+, while ammonia is NH_3. Ammonium is formed by the association of NH_3, an uncharged molecule with a lone pair on the nitrogen, with a positively charged hydrogen cation. In other words, NH_3 is a Lewis base, while H^+ is a Lewis acid. This type of bonding between a Lewis acid and base is a coordinate covalent bond.

10. **C**

All atoms in the third period or greater have *d*-orbitals, which can hold an additional 10 electrons. The typical "octet" electrons reside in *s*- and *p*-orbitals, but elements in period 3 or higher can place electrons into these *d*-orbitals.

11. **C**

All of the listed types of forces describe interactions between different types of molecules. However, noble gases are entirely uncharged and do not have polar covalent bonds, ionic bonds, or dipole moments. Therefore, the only intermolecular forces experienced by noble gases are London dispersion forces. Although these interactions are small in magnitude, they are necessary for condensation into a liquid.

12. **A**

In this Lewis diagram, the phosphate molecule has an overall formal charge of -3. The four oxygen atoms would each be assigned a formal charge of -1. Given the overall charge of -3 and the -1 charge on each oxygen, the phosphorus must have a formal charge of $+1$.

13. **C**

The reaction in this question shows a water molecule, which has two lone pairs of electrons on the central oxygen, combining with a free hydrogen cation. The resulting molecule, H_3O^+ has formed a new bond between H^+ and H_2O. This bond is created via the sharing of one of oxygen's lone pairs with the free H^+ ion. This represents the donation of a shared pair of electrons from a Lewis base (H_2O) to a Lewis acid (H^+, electron acceptor). This type of bond is called a coordinate covalent bond.

14. **C**

NH_3 has three hydrogen atoms bonded to the central nitrogen, which also has a lone pair. These four groups—three atoms, one lone pair—lead NH_3 to assume tetrahedral electronic geometry yet trigonal pyramidal molecular geometry. The nitrogen in ammonia is sp^3-hybridized. By hybridizing all three *p*-orbitals and the one *s*-orbital, four groups are arranged about the central atom, maximizing the distances between the groups to minimize the energy of the molecule with a tetrahedral configuration. In contrast, BF_3 has three atoms and no lone pairs, resulting in sp^2-hybridization. Its shape is called trigonal planar.

15. **B**

When a compound melts, the interactions between molecules must be broken to a sufficient extent to enable movement. In NaCl, these interactions are ionic. On the other hand, solids made of molecules of sucrose, glycerol, or water are held together by hydrogen bonds. Due to the greater electrostatic attraction between the full charges of ionic bonds, the ionic bonds of NaCl are significantly stronger than hydrogen bonds of other molecules. Thus, NaCl has the highest melting point, consistent with **(B)**.

Consult your online resources for additional practice. GO ONLINE

EQUATIONS TO REMEMBER

(3.1) **Dipole moment:** $\mathbf{p} = q\mathbf{d}$

(3.2) **Formal charge:** $V - N_{\text{nonbonding}} - \frac{1}{2} N_{\text{bonding}}$

SHARED CONCEPTS

General Chemistry Chapter 1
Atomic Structure

General Chemistry Chapter 2
The Periodic Table

General Chemistry Chapter 4
Compounds and Stoichiometry

Organic Chemistry Chapter 3
Bonding

Organic Chemistry Chapter 4
Analyzing Organic Reactions

Physics and Math Chapter 5
Electrostatics and Magnetism

CHAPTER 4

COMPOUNDS AND STOICHIOMETRY

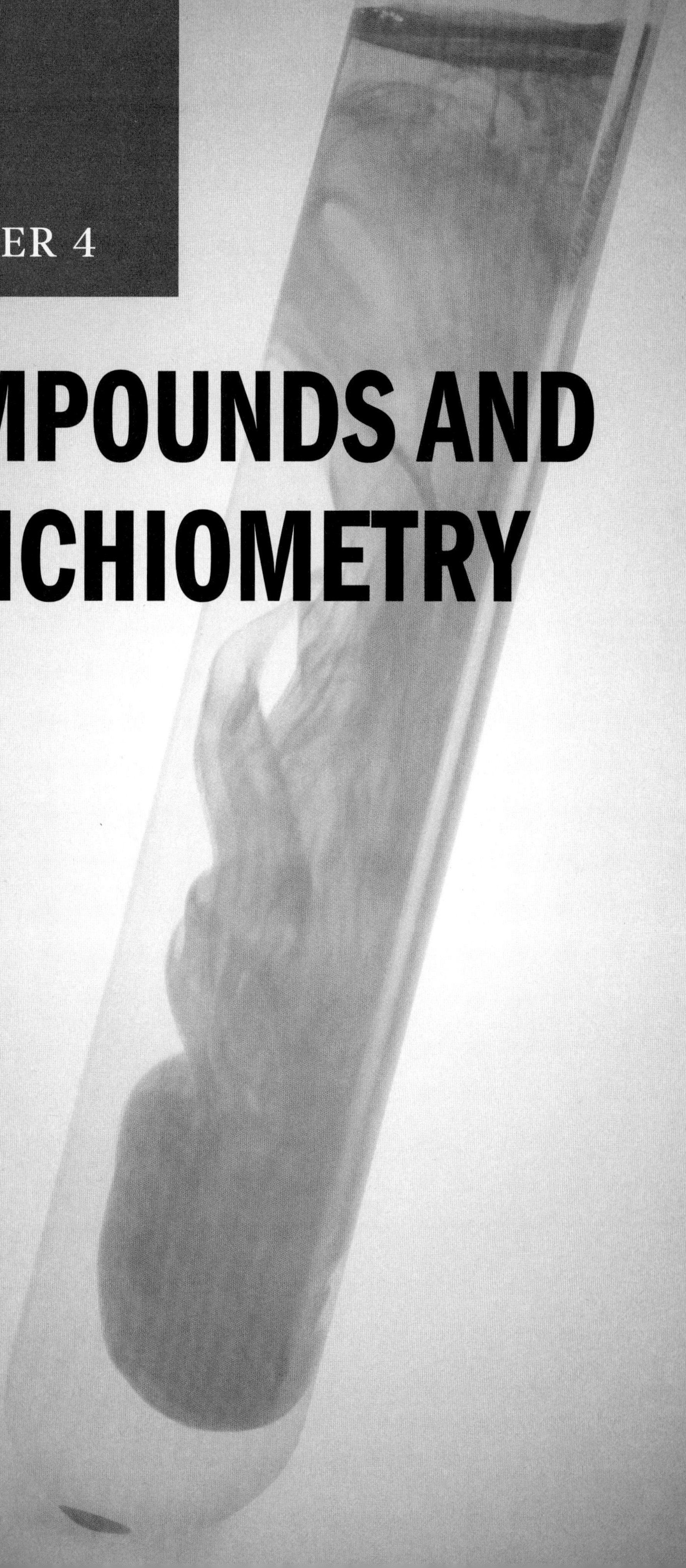

SCIENCE MASTERY ASSESSMENT

Every pre-med knows this feeling: there is so much content I have to know for the MCAT! How do I know what to do first or what's important?

While the high-yield badges throughout this book will help you identify the most important topics, this Science Mastery Assessment is another tool in your MCAT prep arsenal. This quiz (which can also be taken in your online resources) and the guidance below will help ensure that you are spending the appropriate amount of time on this chapter based on your personal strengths and weaknesses. Don't worry though—skipping something now does not mean you'll never study it. Later on in your prep, as you complete full-length tests, you'll uncover specific pieces of content that you need to review and can come back to these chapters as appropriate.

How to Use This Assessment

If you answer 0–7 questions correctly:

Spend about 1 hour to read this chapter in full and take limited notes throughout. Follow up by reviewing **all** quiz questions to ensure that you now understand how to solve each one.

If you answer 8–11 questions correctly:

Spend 20–40 minutes reviewing the quiz questions. Beginning with the questions you missed, read and take notes on the corresponding subchapters. For questions you answered correctly, ensure your thinking matches that of the explanation and you understand why each choice was correct or incorrect.

If you answer 12–15 questions correctly:

Spend less than 20 minutes reviewing all questions from the quiz. If you missed any, then include a quick read-through of the corresponding subchapters, or even just the relevant content within a subchapter, as part of your question review. For questions you answered correctly, ensure your thinking matches that of the explanation and review the Concept Summary at the end of the chapter.

1. Which of the following best describes ionic compounds?
   - **A.** Ionic compounds are formed from molecules containing two or more atoms.
   - **B.** Ionic compounds are formed of charged particles and are measured by molecular weight.
   - **C.** Ionic compounds are formed of charged particles that share electrons equally.
   - **D.** Ionic compounds are three-dimensional arrays of charged particles.

2. Which of the following compounds has a formula weight between 74 and 75 grams per mole?
   - **A.** KCl
   - **B.** $C_4H_{10}O$
   - **C.** $MgCl_2$
   - **D.** BF_3

3. Which of the following is the gram equivalent weight of H_2SO_4 with respect to protons?
   - **A.** 49.1 g
   - **B.** 98.1 g
   - **C.** 147.1 g
   - **D.** 196.2 g

4. Which of the following molecules CANNOT be expressed by the empirical formula CH?
   - **A.** Benzene
   - **B.** Ethyne
   - **C.** 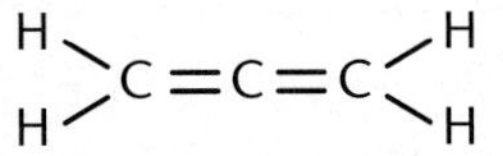
   - **D.** 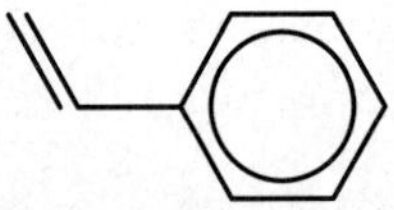

5. In which of the following compounds is the percent composition of carbon by mass closest to 62 percent?
   - **A.** Acetone
   - **B.** Ethanol
   - **C.** Propane
   - **D.** Methanol

6. What is the most specific characterization of the reaction shown?

$$Ca(OH)_2\ (aq) + H_2SO_4\ (aq) \rightarrow CaSO_4\ (aq) + H_2O\ (l)$$

   - **A.** Single-displacement
   - **B.** Neutralization
   - **C.** Double-displacement
   - **D.** Oxidation–reduction

7. In the reaction shown, if 39.05 g of Na_2S are reacted with 85.5 g of $AgNO_3$, how much of the excess reagent will be left over once the reaction has gone to completion?

$$Na_2S + 2\ AgNO_3 \rightarrow Ag_2S + 2\ NaNO_3$$

   - **A.** 19.5 g Na_2S
   - **B.** 26.0 g Na_2S
   - **C.** 41.4 g $AgNO_3$
   - **D.** 74.3 g $AgNO_3$

8. Using a given mass of $KClO_3$, how would one calculate the mass of oxygen produced in the following reaction, assuming it goes to completion?

$$2\ KClO_3 \rightarrow 2\ KCl + 3\ O_2$$

   - **A.** $\dfrac{(\text{grams } KClO_3 \text{ consumed})(3 \text{ moles } O_2)(\text{molar mass } O_2)}{(\text{molar mass } KClO_3)(2 \text{ moles } KClO_3)}$
   - **B.** $\dfrac{(\text{grams } KClO_3 \text{ consumed})(\text{molar mass } O_2)}{(\text{molar mass } KClO_3)(2 \text{ moles } KClO_3)}$
   - **C.** $\dfrac{(\text{molar mass } KClO_3)(2 \text{ moles } KClO_3)}{(\text{grams } KClO_3 \text{ consumed})(\text{molar mass } O_2)}$
   - **D.** $\dfrac{(\text{grams } KClO_3 \text{ consumed})(3 \text{ moles } O_2)}{(\text{molar mass } KClO_3)(2 \text{ moles } KClO_3)(\text{molar mass } O_2)}$

9. Aluminum metal can be used to remove tarnish from silver when the two solid metals are placed in water, according to the following reaction:

$$3\ AgO + 2\ Al \rightarrow 3\ Ag + Al_2O_3$$

This reaction is a:

I. double-displacement reaction.
II. single-displacement reaction.
III. oxidation–reduction reaction.
IV. combination reaction.

A. II only
B. IV only
C. I and III only
D. II and III only

10. Which of the following types of reactions generally have the same number of reactants and products?

I. Double-displacement reactions
II. Single-displacement reactions
III. Combination reactions

A. I only
B. II only
C. I and II only
D. II and III only

11. Diethyl zinc is a very unstable compound. When exposed to air, it reacts with oxygen to produce zinc oxide, carbon dioxide, and water. The unbalanced reaction is shown below.

$$Zn(C_2H_5)_2 + O_2 \rightarrow ZnO + CO_2 + H_2O$$

What is the coefficient for carbon dioxide in the balanced reaction?

A. 4
B. 5
C. 6
D. 7

12. In the process of photosynthesis, carbon dioxide and water combine with energy to form glucose and oxygen, according to the following equation:

$$CO_2 + H_2O \xrightarrow{h\nu} C_6H_{12}O_6 + O_2$$

What is the theoretical yield of glucose if 30 grams of water are reacted with excess carbon dioxide and energy, according to the equation above?

A. 30.0 g
B. 50.0 g
C. 300.1 g
D. 1801 g

13. In the following reaction:

$$Au_2S_3\ (s) + H_2\ (g) \rightarrow Au\ (s) + H_2S\ (g)$$

If 2 moles of Au_2S_3 (*s*) is reacted with 5 moles of hydrogen gas, what is the limiting reagent?

A. Au_2S_3 (*s*)
B. H_2 (*g*)
C. Au (*s*)
D. H_2S (*g*)

14. Which of the following would make the strongest electrolytic solution?

A. A nonpolar covalent compound with significant solubility.
B. An ionic compound composed of one cation with +3 charge and three anions with −1 charge.
C. A polar covalent compound with a small dissociation constant.
D. An ionic compound composed of two cations with +1 charge and one anion with −2 charge.

15. Carbon disulfide and nitrous oxide, when ignited, react exothermically to produce elemental sulfur, nitrogen, and carbon dioxide. Since this reaction produces a "woof" sound, it is sometimes referred to as the Barking Dog reaction. Which of the following represents the balanced chemical reaction?

A. $8\ N_2O + 4\ CS_2 \rightarrow S_8 + 4\ CO_2 + 8\ N_2$
B. $6\ N_2O + 4\ CS_2 \rightarrow S_8 + 4\ CO_2 + 6\ N_2$
C. $8\ N_2O + 2\ CS_2 \rightarrow S_8 + 2\ CO_2 + 8\ N_2$
D. $7\ N_2O + 5\ CS_2 \rightarrow S_8 + 4\ CO_2 + 7\ N_2$

Answer Key

1. **D**
2. **A**
3. **A**
4. **C**
5. **A**
6. **B**
7. **A**
8. **A**
9. **D**
10. **C**
11. **A**
12. **B**
13. **B**
14. **B**
15. **A**

Detailed explanations can be found at the end of the chapter.

CHAPTER 4

COMPOUNDS AND STOICHIOMETRY

In This Chapter

CHAPTER PROFILE

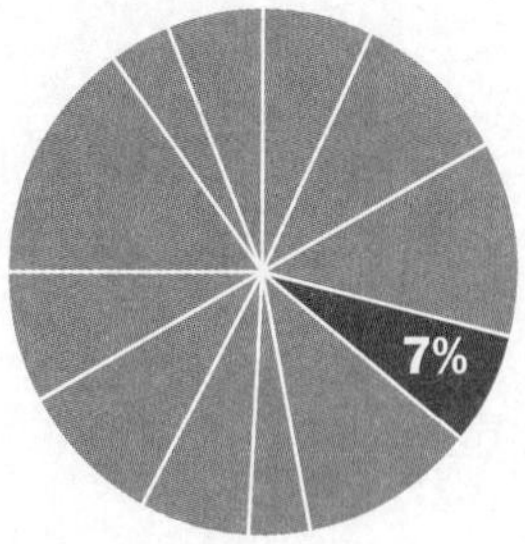

The content in this chapter should be relevant to about 7% of all questions about general chemistry on the MCAT.

This chapter covers material from the following AAMC content categories:

4C: Electrochemistry and electrical circuits and their elements

4E: Atoms, nuclear decay, electronic structure, and atomic chemical behavior

5A: Unique nature of water and its solutions

Introduction

Oh—what is that smell? It smells like rancid almonds. Then you notice a few green bugs whose backs give the impression of a shield. *Stink bugs!* A stink bug "stinks" because it produces a highly concentrated solution of volatile compounds that we perceive as malodorous, noxious, and irritating. Interestingly enough, the primary compounds in the stink bug's stink bomb are hydrogen cyanide—a highly toxic compound that inhibits *cytochrome* c *oxidase*, thereby blocking aerobic respiration—and benzaldehyde. Like many other aromatic compounds, benzaldehyde vaporizes at room temperature and reaches the olfactory system as gas particles. Benzaldehyde is also the key ingredient in artificial almond extract. At low concentrations, it produces a pleasant aroma of toasted almonds. However, at high concentrations, its odor is that of rotten almonds, and it is a noxious irritant to the skin, eyes, and respiratory tract.

Benzaldehyde is a compound composed of seven carbon atoms, six hydrogen atoms, and one oxygen atom. One mole of benzaldehyde has a mass of approximately 106 grams. It can react with other atoms or compounds to form new **compounds**—pure substances composed of two or more elements in a fixed proportion. Compounds can be broken down by chemical means to produce their constituent elements or other compounds. They are characterized by describing their physical and chemical properties.

This chapter focuses on compounds and their reactions. It reviews the various ways in which compounds are represented, using empirical and molecular formulas and percent composition. There is a brief overview of the major classes of chemical reactions, which we will examine more closely in subsequent chapters, and finally, there is a recap of the steps involved in balancing chemical equations with a particular focus on identifying limiting reagents and calculating reaction yields.

4.1 Molecules and Moles

LEARNING OBJECTIVES

After Chapter 4.1, you will be able to:

- Calculate the molar mass of a given substance, such as AgCN
- Calculate the number of moles of a molecule given its mass in grams
- Compare the number of molecules in two different compounds given their gram weights and molecular formulas
- Determine the normality of a solution

A **molecule** is a combination of two or more atoms held together by covalent bonds. Molecules are the smallest units of compounds that display their identifying properties. Molecules can be composed of two or more atoms of the same element (such as N_2 and O_2) or may be composed of atoms of different elements, as in CO_2 (carbon dioxide), $SOCl_2$ (thionyl chloride), and C_6H_5CHO (benzaldehyde). Because reactions usually involve a very large number of molecules—far too many to count individually—we usually measure amounts of compounds in terms of moles or grams, using molar mass to interconvert between these units.

BRIDGE

Ionic compounds form from combinations of elements with large electronegativity differences, such as sodium and chlorine. Molecular compounds form from elements of similar electronegativity, such as carbon with oxygen. The difference between ionic and covalent bonds is discussed in Chapter 3 of *MCAT General Chemistry Review*.

Ionic compounds do not form true molecules because of the way in which the oppositely charged ions arrange themselves in the solid state. As solids, they can be considered as nearly infinite three-dimensional arrays of the charged particles that comprise the compound. As described in Chapter 3 of *MCAT General Chemistry Review*, solid NaCl is a coordinated lattice in which each of the Na^+ ions is surrounded by Cl^- ions and each of the Cl^- ions is surrounded by Na^+ ions. This makes it rather difficult to clearly define a sodium chloride molecule, and the term **formula unit**, representing the empirical formula of the compound, is used instead. Because no molecule actually exists, molecular weight becomes meaningless, and the term **formula weight** is used instead.

Molecular Weight

Remember that the term **atomic weight** is a misnomer because it is actually a weighted average of the masses of the naturally occurring isotopes of an element, not their weights. The same applies here to our discussion of **molecular weight**. Molecular weight, then, is simply the sum of the atomic weights of all the atoms in a molecule, and its units are atomic mass units (amu) per molecule. Similarly, the **formula weight** of an ionic compound is found by adding up the atomic weights of the constituent ions according to its empirical formula, and its units are also amu per molecule.

Example: What is the molecular weight of $SOCl_2$?

Solution: To find the molecular weight of $SOCl_2$, add together the atomic weights of each of the atoms.

1 S: 1×32.1 amu	=	32.1 amu
1 O: 1×16.0 amu	=	16.0 amu
2 Cl: 2×35.5 amu	=	71.0 amu
Total molecular weight	=	119.1 amu per molecule

Mole

A **mole** is a quantity of any substance (atoms, molecules, dollar bills, kittens—anything) equal to the number of particles that are found in 12 grams of carbon-12 $\left({}^{12}_{6}\text{C}\right)$. This number of particles is defined as **Avogadro's number** (N_A), $6.022 \times 10^{23}\ \text{mol}^{-1}$. One mole of a compound has a mass in grams equal to the molecular or formula weight of the compound in amu. For example, one molecule of H_2CO_3 (carbonic acid) has a mass of 62 amu; one mole of the compound has a mass of 62 grams. The mass of one mole of a compound is called its **molar mass** and is usually expressed in $\frac{\text{g}}{\text{mol}}$. The term *molecular weight* is sometimes used incorrectly to imply molar mass; remember, molecular weight is measured in $\frac{\text{amu}}{\text{molecule}}$, not $\frac{\text{g}}{\text{mol}}$.

KEY CONCEPT

Remember that Avogadro's number (and the mole) are just units of convenience, like the dozen is a convenient unit for eggs.

The formula for determining the number of moles of a sample substance is:

$$\text{Moles} = \frac{\text{Mass of sample (g)}}{\text{Molar mass}\left(\frac{\text{g}}{\text{mol}}\right)}$$

Equation 4.1

This equation is often used in stoichiometry and titration problems.

Example: How many moles are in 9.53 g of $MgCl_2$?

Solution: First, find the molar mass of $MgCl_2$.

$$\left(1 \times 24.3\ \frac{\text{g}}{\text{mol}}\right) + \left(2 \times 35.5\ \frac{\text{g}}{\text{mol}}\right) = 95.3\ \frac{\text{g}}{\text{mol}}$$

Now, solve for the number of moles.

$$\frac{9.53\ \text{g}}{95.3\ \frac{\text{g}}{\text{mol}}} = 0.10\ \text{mol MgCl}_2$$

Equivalent Weight

Equivalent weight and the related concept of **equivalents** are a source of confusion for many students. Part of the problem may be the context in which equivalents and equivalent weights are usually discussed: acid–base reactions, oxidation–reduction reactions, and precipitation reactions, all three of which can be sources of confusion and anxiety on their own. Therefore, let's start with a more basic discussion of equivalents.

Often, certain elements or compounds can act more potently than others in performing certain reactions. For example, one mole of HCl has the ability to donate one mole of hydrogen ions (H^+) in solution, but one mole of H_2SO_4 has the ability to donate two moles of hydrogen ions, and one mole of H_3PO_4 has the ability to donate three moles of hydrogen ions. To gather one mole of hydrogen ions for a particular acid–base reaction, we could use one mole of HCl, a half-mole of H_2SO_4, or one-third of a mole of H_3PO_4. Or, consider the difference between Na and Mg: one mole of sodium has the ability to donate one mole of electrons, while one mole of magnesium has the ability to donate two moles of electrons. This provides context for the concept of **equivalents**: How many moles of the *thing we are interested in* (protons, hydroxide ions, electrons, or ions) will one mole of a given compound produce? Sodium will donate one mole of electrons (one equivalent), but magnesium will donate two moles of electrons (two equivalents).

BRIDGE

The idea of *equivalents* is related to the concept of normality, which is explained in the discussion of acids and bases in Chapter 10 of *MCAT General Chemistry Review*.

So far, this discussion has been focused on the mole-to-mole relationship between, say, an acid compound and the hydrogen ions it donates. However, sometimes we need to work in units of mass rather than moles. Just as one mole of HCl will donate one mole of hydrogen ions, a certain mass of HCl (about 36.5 g) will also donate one equivalent of hydrogen ions. This amount of a compound, measured in grams, that produces one equivalent of the particle of interest is called the **gram equivalent weight** and can be calculated from:

MCAT EXPERTISE

Whenever confronting a stoichiometry problem, always look for normality by identifying an equivalent unit (protons, hydroxide ions, electrons, ions) and then multiplying it by the number of moles or molar concentration to find the normal concentration.

$$\text{Gram equivalent weight} = \frac{\text{Molar mass}}{n}$$

Equation 4.2

where n is the number of particles of interest produced or consumed per molecule of the compound in the reaction. For example, one would need 31 grams of H_2CO_3 $\left(\text{molar mass} = 62\ \frac{\text{g}}{\text{mol}}\right)$ to produce one equivalent of hydrogen ions because each molecule of H_2CO_3 can donate two hydrogen ions ($n = 2$). Simply put, the equivalent weight of a compound is the mass that provides one mole of the particle of interest.

If the amount of a compound in a reaction is known and we need to determine how many equivalents are present, use the equation:

$$\text{Equivalents} = \frac{\text{Mass of compound (g)}}{\text{Gram equivalent weight (g)}}$$

Equation 4.3

Finally, we can now introduce the measurement of normality. **Normality (*N*)** is a measure of concentration, given in the units $\frac{\text{equivalents}}{\text{L}}$. On the MCAT, it is most commonly used for hydrogen ion concentration. Thus, a 1 *N* solution of acid contains a concentration of hydrogen ions equal to 1 mole per liter; a 2 *N* solution of acid contains a concentration of hydrogen ions equal to 2 moles per liter. The actual concentration of the acidic compound may be the same or different from the normality because different compounds are able to donate different numbers of hydrogen ions. In a 1 *N* HCl solution, the molarity of HCl is 1 *M* because HCl is a monoprotic acid; in a 1 *N* H_2CO_3 solution, the molarity of H_2CO_3 is 0.5 *M* because H_2CO_3 is a diprotic acid. Note that normality calculations always assume that a reaction will proceed to completion; while carbonic acid does not fully dissociate in solution, it can be reacted with enough base for each molecule to give up both of its protons. The conversion from normality to molarity of a given solute is:

$$\text{Molarity} = \frac{\text{Normality}}{n}$$

Equation 4.4

where *n* is the number of protons, hydroxide ions, electrons, or ions produced or consumed by the solute.

Figure 4.1 shows the titration of the diprotic acid H_2CO_3 with a base. The *x*-axis indicates that two equivalents of base are needed to neutralize both protons of this acid.

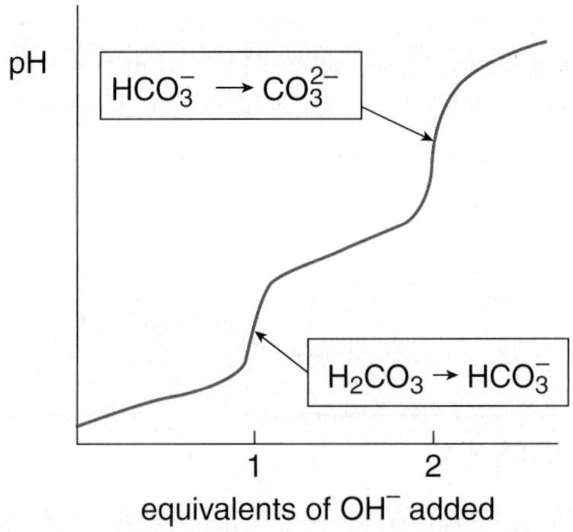

Figure 4.1 Titration of Carbonic Acid with a Base
Carbonic acid is diprotic, so two equivalents of base are required to neutralize both protons of the acid.

There is a real benefit to working with equivalents and normality because it allows a direct comparison of the quantities of the entity we are most interested in. In an acid–base reaction, we care about the hydrogen or hydroxide ions; where the ions come from is not really the primary concern. It is convenient to be able to say that one equivalent of acid (hydrogen ions) will neutralize one equivalent of base (hydroxide ions), but the same could not necessarily be said if we were dealing with moles of acidic compounds and moles of basic compounds. For example, one mole of HCl will not completely neutralize one mole of $Ca(OH)_2$ because one mole of HCl will donate one equivalent of acid, but $Ca(OH)_2$ will donate two equivalents of base.

KEY CONCEPT

In acid–base chemistry, the gram equivalent weight represents the mass of acid that yields one mole of protons, or the mass of base that yields one mole of hydroxide ions.

Example: What is the gram equivalent weight (GEW) of sulfuric acid?

Solution: First, find the molar mass of H_2SO_4.

$$\left(2 \times 1.0 \frac{\text{g}}{\text{mol H}}\right) + \left(1 \times 32.1 \frac{\text{g}}{\text{mol S}}\right) + \left(4 \times 16.0 \frac{\text{g}}{\text{mol O}}\right) = 98.1 \frac{\text{g}}{\text{mol H}_2\text{SO}_4}$$

Next, identify the equivalents: protons (H^+), because these are transferred in acid-base reactions. The number of protons in sulfuric acid (n) is 2.

Now, calculate the gram equivalent weight.

$$\text{Gram equivalent weight} = \frac{\text{Molar mass}}{n}$$

$$\text{GEW} = \frac{98.1 \frac{\text{g}}{\text{mol H}_2\text{SO}_4}}{2 \frac{\text{mol H}^+}{\text{mol H}_2\text{SO}_4}} = 49.05 \frac{\text{g}}{\text{mol H}^+}$$

Example: What is the normality of a 2 M $Mg(OH)_2$ solution?

Solution: First, identify the number of equivalents (n). There are two hydroxide ions (OH^-) for each molecule of $Mg(OH)_2$, which is the equivalent of interest because magnesium hydroxide is a base.

Then, calculate the normality.

$$\text{Normality} = \text{molarity} \times n = 2\ M \times 2 \frac{\text{equiv OH}^-}{\text{mol Mg(OH)}_2} = 4\ N\ \text{Mg(OH)}_2$$

MCAT CONCEPT CHECK 4.1

Before you move on, assess your understanding of the material with these questions.

1. Calculate the molar masses of the following substances:
   - NaBr:

   - $SrCl_2$:

   - $C_6H_{12}O_6$:

     ---

2. Calculate the number of moles in 100 g of each of the following substances:
   - NaBr:
   - $SrCl_2$:
   - $C_6H_{12}O_6$:
3. How do the number of molecules in 18 g of H_2O compare to the number of formula units in 58.5 g of NaCl?
4. Determine the normality of the following solutions: (Note: The species of interest is H^+.)
   - 0.25 *M* H_3PO_4:
   - 95 g PO_4^{3-} in 100 mL solution:

4.2 Representation of Compounds

LEARNING OBJECTIVES

After Chapter 4.2, you will be able to:

- Recall the similarities and differences between molecular and empirical formulas
- Calculate the percent composition by mass of a compound, such as $C_6H_{12}O_6$
- Determine the empirical formula of a compound given its percent composition by mass

There are different ways of representing compounds and their constituent atoms. We've already reviewed a couple of these systems in Chapter 3 of *MCAT General Chemistry Review*: Lewis dot structures and VSEPR theory. In organic chemistry, it is common to encounter skeletal representations of compounds, called **structural formulas**, that show the various bonds between the constituent atoms of a compound. Inorganic (general) chemistry typically represents compounds by showing the constituent atoms without representing the actual bond connectivity or atomic arrangement. For example, the formula $C_6H_{12}O_6$ (glucose) tells us that this particular

BRIDGE

Many of these representations are discussed in more detail in Chapter 2 of *MCAT Organic Chemistry Review.* Understanding the theory behind such representations will help convert between different projections and representations with ease.

compound consists of six atoms of carbon, twelve atoms of hydrogen, and six atoms of oxygen, but there is no indication of how the different atoms are arranged or how many bonds exist between each of the atoms.

Law of Constant Composition

The **law of constant composition** states that any pure sample of a given compound will contain the same elements in an identical mass ratio. For example, every sample of water will contain two hydrogen atoms for every one oxygen atom, or—in terms of mass—for every one gram of hydrogen, there will be eight grams of oxygen.

REAL WORLD

Even biologically important molecules, such as water and amino acids on Earth are, by composition, the same anywhere else in the universe, even though densities and other physical properties may differ.

Empirical and Molecular Formulas

There are two ways to express the formula of a compound. The **empirical formula** gives the simplest whole-number ratio of the elements in the compound. The **molecular formula** gives the exact number of atoms of each element in the compound and is a multiple of the empirical formula. For example, the empirical formula for benzene is CH, while the molecular formula is C_6H_6. For some compounds, the empirical and molecular formulas are identical, as is the case for H_2O. As previously discussed, ionic compounds, such as NaCl or $CaCO_3$, will only have empirical formulas.

BRIDGE

An empirical formula of CH_2O is indicative of a monosaccharide. Common monosaccharides include glucose, fructose, and galactose. The structures of these monosaccharides—and of carbohydrates in general—are discussed in Chapter 4 of *MCAT Biochemistry Review*.

Percent Composition

The **percent composition** of an element (by mass) is the percent of a specific compound that is made up of a given element. To determine the percent composition of an element in a compound, the following formula is used:

$$\text{Percent composition} = \frac{\text{Mass of element in formula}}{\text{Molar mass}} \times 100\%$$

Equation 4.5

MCAT EXPERTISE

Percent composition is a common way for stoichiometry to be tested on the MCAT. Practice these problems to build up speed and efficiency for Test Day.

One can calculate the percent composition of an element by using either the empirical or the molecular formula. It is also possible to determine the molecular formula given both the percent compositions and molar mass of a compound. The following examples demonstrate such calculations.

Example: What is the percent composition of chromium in $K_2Cr_2O_7$?

Solution: The molar mass of $K_2Cr_2O_7$ is:

$$\left(2 \times 39.1 \frac{\text{g}}{\text{mol}}\right) + \left(2 \times 52.0 \frac{\text{g}}{\text{mol}}\right) + \left(7 \times 16.0 \frac{\text{g}}{\text{mol}}\right)$$

$$\approx (2 \times 40) + (2 \times 50) + (7 \times 16)$$

$$= 292 \frac{\text{g}}{\text{mol}} \left(\text{actual value} = 294.2 \frac{\text{g}}{\text{mol}}\right)$$

Calculate the percent composition of Cr:

$$\text{Percent composition} = \frac{2 \times 52.0 \frac{\text{g}}{\text{mol}}}{294.2 \frac{\text{g}}{\text{mol}}} \times 100\%$$

$$\approx \frac{2 \times 50}{300} \times 100\% = \frac{100}{300} \times 100\%$$

$$= 33\% \text{ (actual value} = 35.4\%)$$

Example: What are the empirical and molecular formulas of a carbohydrate that contains 40.9% carbon, 4.58% hydrogen, and 54.52% oxygen and has a molar mass of $264 \frac{\text{g}}{\text{mol}}$?

Method One: First, determine the number of moles of each element in the compound by assuming a 100-gram sample; this converts the percentage of each element present directly into grams of that element. Then convert grams to moles:

$$\text{moles C} = \frac{40.9 \text{ g}}{12 \frac{\text{g}}{\text{mol}}} \approx 3.4 \text{ mol}$$

$$\text{moles H} = \frac{4.58 \text{ g}}{1 \frac{\text{g}}{\text{mol}}} \approx 4.6 \text{ mol}$$

$$\text{moles O} = \frac{54.52 \text{ g}}{16 \frac{\text{g}}{\text{mol}}} \approx 3.4 \text{ mol}$$

Next, find the simplest whole number ratio of the elements by dividing the number of moles for each compound by the smallest number out of all obtained in the previous step.

$$\text{C: } \frac{3.4}{3.4} = 1.00; \text{ H: } \frac{4.6}{3.4} \approx 1.33; \text{ O: } \frac{3.4}{3.4} = 1.00$$

Finally, the empirical formula is obtained by converting the numbers obtained into whole numbers by multiplying them by an integer value.

$$\text{Empirical formula} = C_1H_{1.33}O_1 \times 3 = C_3H_4O_3$$

To determine the molecular formula, divide the molar mass (264 g/mol, given in the question stem) by the empirical formula weight. The resulting value gives the number of empirical formula units in the molecular formula.

The formula weight of the empirical formula $C_3H_4O_3$ is:

$$\left(3 \times 12.0 \frac{\text{g}}{\text{mol C}}\right) + \left(4 \times 1.0 \frac{\text{g}}{\text{mol H}}\right) + \left(3 \times 16.0 \frac{\text{g}}{\text{mol O}}\right) = 88 \frac{\text{g}}{\text{mol total}}$$

$$\text{ratio of } \frac{\text{molecular formula}}{\text{empirical formula}} = \frac{264 \frac{\text{g}}{\text{mol}}}{88 \frac{\text{g}}{\text{mol}}} = 3$$

Finally, find the molecular formula by multiplying by this ratio:

$C_3H_4O_3 \times 3 = C_9H_{12}O_9$. The molecular formula is $C_9H_{12}O_9$.

MCAT EXPERTISE

When there are two methods for approaching a problem, be well-versed in both. Knowing multiple ways to solve a problem will help you tackle questions efficiently.

Method Two: When the molar mass is given, it is generally easier to find the molecular formula first. This is accomplished by multiplying the molar mass by the given percentages to find the mass of each element present in one mole of compound, then dividing by the respective atomic weights to find the mole ratio of the elements:

$$\text{moles C} = \frac{(0.409)(264 \text{ g})}{12 \frac{\text{g}}{\text{mol}}} \approx \frac{(0.4)(270)}{12} \approx \frac{270}{30} = 9 \text{ mol}$$

$$\text{moles H} = \frac{(0.0458)(264 \text{ g})}{1 \frac{\text{g}}{\text{mol}}} \approx \frac{(0.05)(270)}{1} \approx 13 \text{ mol}$$

$$\text{moles O} = \frac{(0.5452)(264 \text{ g})}{16 \frac{\text{g}}{\text{mol}}} \approx \frac{(0.5)(270)}{16} \approx \frac{270}{30} = 9 \text{ mol}$$

KEY CONCEPT

The molecular formula is either the same as the empirical formula or a multiple of it. To calculate the molecular formula, you need to know the mole ratio (this will give you the empirical formula) and the molar mass (molar mass divided by empirical formula weight will give the multiplier for the empirical formula-to-molecular formula conversion).

At first glance, this gives a molecular formula of $C_9H_{13}O_9$. However, familiarity with carbohydrates indicates that a molecular formula of $C_9H_{12}O_9$ fits the ratio CH_2O, and takes rounding error into account. The empirical formula can now be found by reducing the subscript ratio to the simplest integer values ($C_3H_4O_3$).

MCAT CONCEPT CHECK 4.2

Before you move on, assess your understanding of the material with these questions.

1. What are some similarities and differences between molecular and empirical formulas?
   - Similarities:

   ____

   - Differences:

   ____

2. Find the percent composition (by mass) of sodium, carbon, and oxygen in sodium carbonate (Na_2CO_3):
   - Sodium:
   - Carbon:
   - Oxygen:

3. Experimental data from the combustion of an unknown compound indicates that it is 28.5% iron, 24.0% sulfur, and 49.7% oxygen by mass. What is its empirical formula?

4.3 Types of Chemical Reactions

LEARNING OBJECTIVES

After Chapter 4.3, you will be able to:

- Describe the series of events in a single displacement, double displacement, neutralization, or combustion reaction
- Classify a reaction and predict its products given the reactants:

$$CH_4 + 2O_2 \rightarrow$$

BRIDGE

Many of the reactions we will discuss here have analogs in *MCAT Organic Chemistry Review* and *MCAT Biochemistry Review*. Be sure to understand the relationships between the products and reactants because it will help simplify more advanced reactions.

This section reviews the major classes of chemical reactions. We will begin with a classification of major types of reactions seen on the MCAT and then discuss methods to recognize their products. It is important to understand the conventions of reaction mechanisms. In the following section, we will discuss how to properly balance chemical equations.

Combination Reactions

A **combination reaction** has two or more reactants forming one product. The formation of water by burning hydrogen gas in air is an example of a combination reaction. This reaction is highlighted in Figure 4.2.

KEY CONCEPT

Combination reactions have more reactants than products: **A + B → C**

$$2\,H_2\,(g) + O_2\,(g) \rightarrow 2\,H_2O\,(g)$$

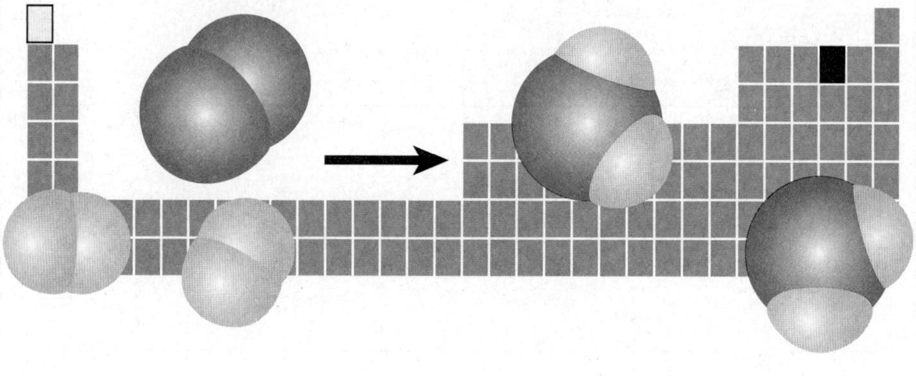

Figure 4.2 Formation of Water from Hydrogen and Oxygen

KEY CONCEPT

Decomposition reactions generally have more products than reactants. **A** $\longrightarrow$ **B** + **C**

Decomposition Reactions

A **decomposition** reaction is the opposite of a combination reaction: a single reactant breaks down into two or more products, usually as a result of heating, high-frequency radiation, or electrolysis. An example of decomposition is the breakdown of mercury(II) oxide. (The Δ [delta] sign over a reaction arrow represents the addition of heat.)

$$2\,HgO\,(s) \xrightarrow{\Delta} 2\,Hg\,(l) + O_2\,(g)$$

An example of a reaction that utilizes high-frequency light is the decomposition of silver chloride crystals, shown in Figure 4.3, in the presence of sunlight. The ultraviolet component of sunlight has sufficient energy to catalyze certain chemical reactions. For silver chloride, exposure to sunlight results in a decomposition reaction that yields a rust-colored product that consists of separated silver and chlorine.

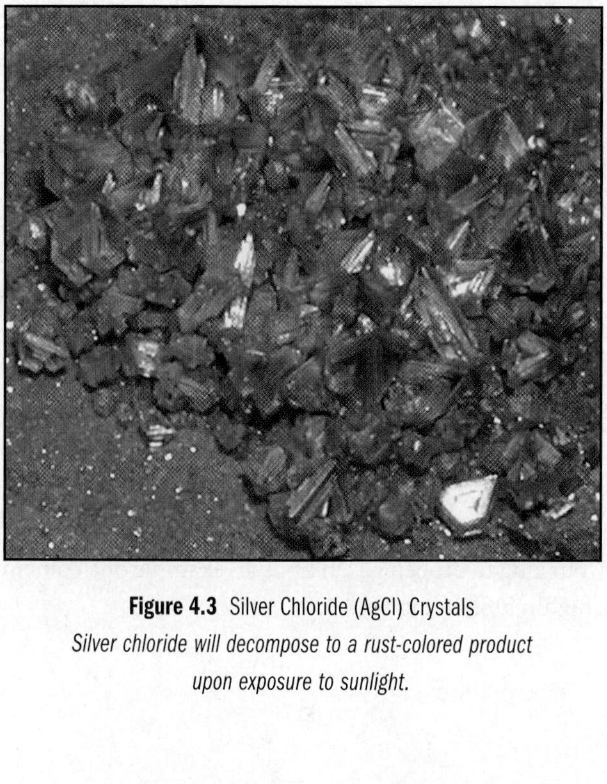

Figure 4.3 Silver Chloride (AgCl) Crystals
Silver chloride will decompose to a rust-colored product upon exposure to sunlight.

Combustion Reactions

A **combustion reaction** is a special type of reaction that involves a fuel—usually a hydrocarbon—and an oxidant (normally oxygen). In its most common form, these reactants form the two products of carbon dioxide and water. For example, the balanced equation expressing the combustion of methane is shown in Figure 4.4.

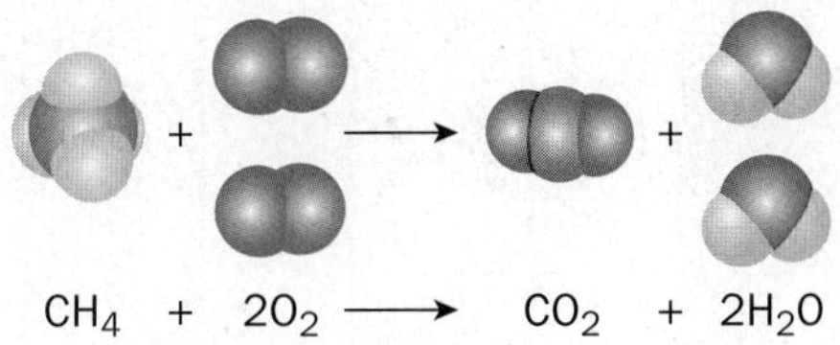

Figure 4.4 Combustion of Methane

Single-Displacement Reactions

A **single-displacement reaction** occurs when an atom or ion in a compound is replaced by an atom or ion of another element. For example, solid copper metal will displace silver ions in a clear solution of silver nitrate to form a blue copper nitrate solution and solid silver metal.

$$Cu\ (s) + AgNO_3\ (aq) \rightarrow Ag\ (s) + CuNO_3\ (aq)$$

Single-displacement reactions are often further classified as oxidation–reduction reactions, which will be discussed in greater detail in Chapter 11 of *MCAT General Chemistry Review*. For example, Ag in $AgNO_3$ has an oxidation state of $+1$, but when it leaves the compound, it gains one electron (the Ag^+ is reduced to Ag). On the other hand, copper loses an electron (oxidation) when it joins the nitrate ion.

Double-Displacement Reactions

In **double-displacement reactions**, also called **metathesis reactions**, elements from two different compounds swap places with each other to form two new compounds. This type of reaction occurs when one of the products is removed from the solution as a precipitate or gas or when two of the original species combine to form a weak electrolyte that remains undissociated in solution. For example, when solutions of calcium chloride and silver nitrate are combined, insoluble silver chloride forms in a solution of calcium nitrate.

$$CaCl_2\ (aq) + 2\ AgNO_3\ (aq) \rightarrow Ca(NO_3)_2\ (aq) + 2\ AgCl\ (s)$$

A series of double-displacement reactions is depicted in Figure 4.5. Shown are illustrations of test tubes in which $Zn(NO_3)_2$ is dissolved in solutions to precipitate solid zinc salts. From left to right, the solutions are $(NH_4)_2S$, NaOH, and Na_2CO_3.

KEY CONCEPT

Combustion involves oxidation (using O_2 or similar) of a fuel (typically a hydrocarbon).

MCAT EXPERTISE

Combustion reactions are usually conducted with hydrocarbon fuels, but they can also use elements such as sulfur or other compounds such as sugars. The products can differ, but carbon dioxide and water are almost always present. Therefore, it is important to recognize the reactants and products of this reaction type because you may see it in various contexts.

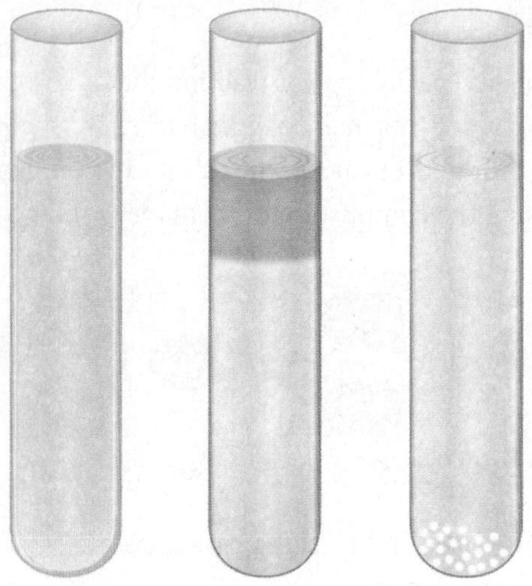

Figure 4.5 Illustration of Double-Displacement Reactions Forming Zinc Salts
Left: $(NH_4)_2S$ solution, producing ZnS (s). Middle: $NaOH$ solution, producing $Zn(OH)_2$ (s). Right: Na_2CO_3 solution, producing $ZnCO_3$ (s).

Neutralization Reactions

Neutralization reactions are a specific type of double-displacement reaction in which an acid reacts with a base to produce a salt (and, usually, water). For example, hydrochloric acid and sodium hydroxide will react to form sodium chloride and water:

$$HCl\ (aq) + NaOH\ (aq) \rightarrow NaCl\ (aq) + H_2O\ (l)$$

Reactions between acids and bases are not always visible. The addition of an indicator or use of indicator strips, as shown in Figure 4.6, can determine when the reaction has occurred.

BRIDGE

Acids and bases combine in neutralization reactions to produce salts (and, usually, water). Acid-base chemistry is discussed in Chapter 10 of *MCAT General Chemistry Review.*

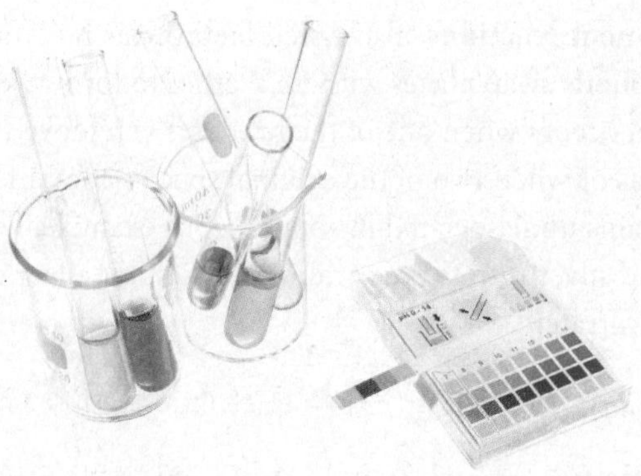

Figure 4.6 Indicator Strip Tested in Solutions of Varying pH
After an indicator strip is placed in a solution, the indicator strip (right) can be read using the indicator key.

MCAT CONCEPT CHECK 4.3

Before you move on, assess your understanding of the material with these questions.

1. Describe in words what occurs when $Zn(NO_3)_2$ is dissolved in $(NH_4)_2S$:

____

2. Complete and classify the most likely reactions in the table below:

Reactants	Conditions	Products	Reaction Type
$2\ H_2 + O_2$	$\rightarrow$		
$Al(OH)_3 + H_3PO_4$	$\rightarrow$		
$2\ H_2O$	$\xrightarrow{\text{electricity}}$		
$NaNO_3 + CuOH$	$\rightarrow$		
$Zn + AgCl$	$\rightarrow$		

4.4 Balancing Chemical Equations

High-Yield

LEARNING OBJECTIVES

After Chapter 4.4, you will be able to:

- Balance a chemical equation

Because chemical equations express how much and what types of reactants must be used to obtain a given quantity of product, it is of utmost importance that the reaction be balanced so as to reflect the **laws of conservation of mass** and **charge**. The mass of the reactants consumed must equal the mass of products generated. More specifically, one must ensure that the number of atoms of each element on the reactant side equals the number of atoms of that element on the product side. **Stoichiometric coefficients**, which are the numbers placed in front of each compound, are used to indicate the relative number of moles of a given species involved in the reaction. For example, the balanced equation expressing the combustion of nonane is:

$$C_9H_{20}\ (g) + 14\ O_2\ (g) \rightarrow 9\ CO_2\ (g) + 10\ H_2O\ (l)$$

The coefficients indicate that one mole of C_9H_{20} gas must be reacted with fourteen moles of O_2 gas to produce nine moles of carbon dioxide and ten moles of water. In general, stoichiometric coefficients are given as whole numbers.

The steps taken to balance a chemical reaction are necessary to ensure that calculations regarding the reaction are performed correctly. Let's review the steps involved in balancing a chemical equation, using an example.

MCAT EXPERTISE

It is unlikely that you will come across a question that explicitly asks you to balance an equation. However, you will need to recognize unbalanced reactions and quickly add the necessary coefficients. To balance a reaction, look at the number of atoms of each element and the charge on both sides (especially for oxidation-reduction reactions).

Example: Balance the following reaction:

$$C_4H_{10}\ (l) + O_2\ (g) \rightarrow CO_2\ (g) + H_2O\ (l)$$

Method One: First, balance the carbons (4 on reactant side) in the products. Carbons are a good choice to start with because they appear only once on both sides of the reaction:

$$C_4H_{10}\ (l) + O_2\ (g) \rightarrow \mathbf{4}\ CO_2\ (g) + H_2O\ (l)$$

Then, balance the hydrogens (10 on reactant side) in the products. Again, hydrogens appear only once on each side, making them a good choice to work on next:

$$C_4H_{10}\ (l) + O_2\ (g) \rightarrow 4\ CO_2\ (g) + \mathbf{5}\ H_2O\ (l)$$

Next, balance the oxygens (now 13 on product side) in the reactants. Note that oxygens appear in multiple reactants and products, making them the most complex atom to balance and therefore the best to leave until the end:

$$C_4H_{10}\ (l) + \frac{13}{2}\ O_2\ (g) \rightarrow 4\ CO_2\ (g) + 5\ H_2O\ (l)$$

Next, produce a whole number ratio. In this case, double each coefficient.

$$2\ C_4H_{10}\ (l) + 13\ O_2\ (g) \rightarrow 8\ CO_2\ (g) + 10\ H_2O\ (l)$$

Finally, check that all of the elements and the total charges are balanced correctly. If there is a difference in total charge between the reactants and products, then the charge will also have to be balanced. (Instructions for balancing charge in oxidation–reduction reactions are found in Chapter 11 of *MCAT General Chemistry Review*.)

Method Two: First, if in doubt, take a guess. Assume there are 4 of the first reactant and balance the carbons appropriately.

$$\mathbf{4}\ C_4H_{10}\ (l) + O_2\ (g) \rightarrow \mathbf{16}\ CO_2\ (g) + H_2O\ (l)$$

Second, balance the hydrogens (40 on reactant side) in the products.

$$4\ C_4H_{10}\ (l) + O_2\ (g) \rightarrow 16\ CO_2\ (g) + \mathbf{20}\ H_2O\ (l)$$

Third, balance the oxygens (now 52 on product side) in the reactants.

$$4\ C_4H_{10}\ (l) + \mathbf{26}\ O_2\ (g) \rightarrow 16\ CO_2\ (g) + 20\ H_2O\ (l)$$

Fourth, produce the simplest whole number ratio through the greatest common factor. In this case, divide each side by 2.

$$2\ C_4H_{10}\ (l) + 13\ O_2\ (g) \rightarrow 8\ CO_2\ (g) + 10\ H_2O\ (l)$$

Finally, check that all of the elements and the total charges are balanced correctly. Notice that both methods produce a multiple of our final answer. These ratios are both correct, but in terms of the stoichiometry one performs on the MCAT, the simpler the numbers are, the easier calculations will become.

KEY CONCEPT

When balancing equations, focus on the least represented elements first and work your way to the most represented element of the reaction (usually oxygen or hydrogen). If you're stuck, take a guess for the coefficient of the first reactant and balance the remainder appropriately.

MCAT CONCEPT CHECK 4.4

Before you move on, assess your understanding of the material with this question.

1. Balance the following reactions:
   - __ Fe + __ $Cl_2 \rightarrow$ __ $FeCl_3$
   - __ Zn + __ $HCl \rightarrow$ __ $ZnCl_2$ + __ H_2
   - __ C_5H_{12} + __ $O_2 \rightarrow$ __ CO_2 + __ H_2O
   - __ $Pb(NO_3)_2$ + __ $AlCl_3 \rightarrow$ __ $PbCl_2$ + __ $Al(NO_3)_3$

4.5 Applications of Stoichiometry

LEARNING OBJECTIVES

After Chapter 4.5, you will be able to:

- Calculate the grams of product produced given the quantities of reactant
- Identify the limiting reagent within a reaction
- Calculate the mass of excess reagent in a reaction with a limiting reagent
- Calculate the percent yield of a reaction

Perhaps the most useful information to glean from a balanced reaction is the mole ratio of reactants consumed-to-products generated. One can also generate the mole ratio of one reactant to another or one product to another. All of these ratios can be generated using the stoichiometric coefficients. In the formation of water ($2\ H_2 + O_2 \rightarrow 2\ H_2O$), for example, one can determine that, for every one mole of hydrogen gas consumed, one mole of water can be produced; for every one mole of oxygen gas consumed, two moles of water can be produced. Furthermore, mole-to-mole, hydrogen gas is being consumed at a rate twice that of oxygen gas.

Stoichiometry problems usually involve at least a few unit conversions, so take care when working through these types of problems to ensure that units cancel out appropriately to lead to the desired units of the answer choices.

KEY CONCEPT

Stoichiometry, an application of dimensional analysis, is often simplified to a series of three fractions. These fractions demonstrate an underlying three-step process:

- Convert from the given units to moles
- Use the mole ratio
- Convert from moles to the desired units

Pay close attention to the following problem, which demonstrates a clear and easy-to-follow method for keeping track of the numbers, calculations, and unit conversions.

Example: How many grams of calcium chloride are needed to prepare 71.7 g of silver chloride according to the following equation?

$$CaCl_2\ (aq) + 2\,AgNO_3\ (aq) \rightarrow Ca(NO_3)_2\ (aq) + 2\,AgCl\ (s)$$

Solution: Noting first that the equation is balanced, 1 mole of $CaCl_2$ is reacted with 2 moles of $AgNO_3$ to yield 2 moles of AgCl. The molar mass of $CaCl_2$ is 111.1 g, and the molar mass of AgCl is 143.4 g. The given quantity is 71.7 g AgCl.

$$71.7\text{ g AgCl} \times \left[\frac{1\text{ mol AgCl}}{143.4\text{ g AgCl}}\right]\left[\frac{1\text{ mol CaCl}_2}{2\text{ mol AgCl}}\right]\left[\frac{111.1\text{ g CaCl}_2}{1\text{ mol CaCl}_2}\right]$$

$$\approx \frac{72}{144} \times \frac{1}{2} \times \frac{110}{1} = \frac{1}{2} \times \frac{1}{2} \times \frac{110}{1} = \frac{110}{4}$$

$$= 27.5\text{ g CaCl}_2\ (\text{actual value} = 27.775\text{ g})$$

Thus, about 27.8 g $CaCl_2$ are needed to produce 71.7 g AgCl.

MCAT EXPERTISE

Common conversions used in stoichiometry include:

- 1 mole of any ideal gas at STP = 22.4 L
- 1 mole of any substance = 6.022×10^{23} particles (Avogadro's number)
- 1 mole of any substance = its molar mass in grams (from the periodic table)

Limiting Reagent

Rarely are reactants added in the exact stoichiometric proportions shown in the balanced equation of a reaction. As a result, in most reactions, one reactant will be used up or consumed first. This reactant is known as the **limiting reagent** (or reactant) because it limits the amount of product that can be formed in the reaction. The reactants that remain after all the limiting reagent is used up are called **excess reagents** (or reactants).

MCAT EXPERTISE

When the quantities of two reactants are given on the MCAT, expect to have to figure out which is the limiting reagent.

Figure 4.7 shows a reaction vessel that has significant amounts of reactants A and B, which react in equal amounts to produce product C. On the left, before the reaction, there is more reactant A than B. After the reaction is over, there is more product C but there is reactant A left over. Thus, reactant A is considered in excess, and reactant B is considered limiting.

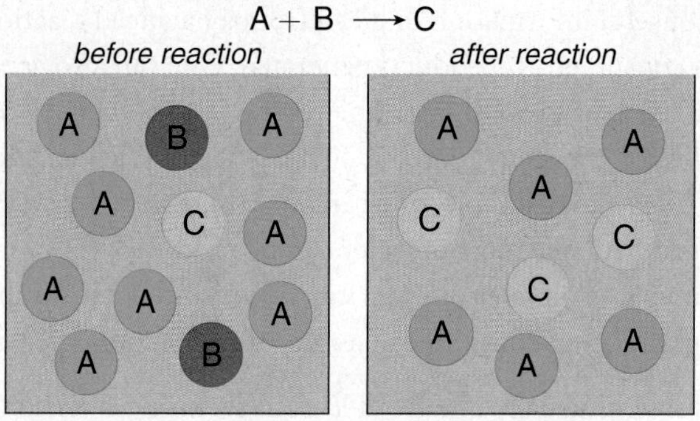

Figure 4.7 Reaction with a Limiting Reagent
A is considered an excess reagent; B is the limiting reagent.

For problems involving the determination of the limiting reagent, keep in mind two principles:

1. All comparisons of reactants must be done in units of moles. Gram-to-gram comparisons will be useless and may even be misleading.
2. It is not the absolute mole quantities of the reactants that determine which reactant is the limiting reagent. Rather, the rate at which the reactants are consumed (the stoichiometric ratios of the reactants), combined with the absolute mole quantities determines which reactant is the limiting reagent.

Example: If 27.9 g of Fe react with 24.1 g of S to produce FeS, what would be the limiting reagent? How many grams of excess reagent would be present in the vessel at the end of the reaction?

The balanced equation is $Fe + S \longrightarrow FeS$.

Solution: First, determine the number of moles for each reactant.

$$27.9 \text{ g Fe} \times \frac{1 \text{ mol Fe}}{55.8 \text{ g Fe}} \approx 28 \times \frac{1}{56} = 0.5 \text{ mol Fe}$$

$$24.1 \text{ g S} \times \frac{1 \text{ mol S}}{32.1 \text{ g S}} \approx 24 \times \frac{1}{32} = 0.75 \text{ mol S}$$

Because 1 mole of Fe is needed to react with 1 mole of S and there are 0.5 moles Fe for the given 0.75 moles S, the limiting reagent is Fe. Thus, 0.5 moles of Fe will react with 0.5 moles of S, leaving an excess of 0.25 moles of S in the vessel. The mass of the excess reagent will be:

$$0.25 \text{ mol} \times \frac{32.1 \text{ g S}}{1 \text{ mol S}} \approx 8 \text{ g S}$$

Yield

The **yield** of a reaction can refer to either the amount of product predicted (theoretical yield) or actually obtained (raw or actual yield) when a reaction is carried out. **Theoretical yield** is the maximum amount of product that can be generated as predicted from the balanced equation, assuming that all of the limiting reactant is consumed, no side reactions have occurred, and the entire product has been collected. Theoretical yield is rarely ever attained through the actual chemical reaction. **Actual yield** is the amount of product one actually obtains during the reaction. The ratio of the actual yield to the theoretical yield, multiplied by 100 percent, gives the **percent yield**:

$$\text{Percent yield} = \frac{\text{Actual yield}}{\text{Theoretical yield}} \times 100\%$$

Equation 4.6

MCAT EXPERTISE

An experimentally based passage that involves a chemical reaction may include a pseudo-discrete question that involves finding the percent yield.

Example: What is the percent yield for a reaction in which 28 g of Cu is produced by reacting 32.7 g of Zn in excess $CuSO_4$ solution?

Solution: The balanced equation is as follows:

$$\text{Zn}\ (s) + \text{CuSO}_4\ (aq) \rightarrow \text{Cu}\ (s) + \text{ZnSO}_4\ (aq)$$

Calculate the theoretical yield for Cu.

$$32.7\ \text{g Zn} \times \left[\frac{1\ \text{mol Zn}}{65.4\ \text{g Zn}}\right]\left[\frac{1\ \text{mol Cu}}{1\ \text{mol Zn}}\right]\left[\frac{63.5\ \text{g Cu}}{1\ \text{mol Cu}}\right]$$
$$\approx 33 \times \frac{1}{66} \times \frac{1}{1} \times \frac{64}{1} = \frac{1}{2} \times \frac{64}{1} = 32\ (\text{actual value} = 31.8\ \text{g Cu})$$

This 31.8 g represents the theoretical yield. Finally, determine the percent yield.

$$\frac{28\ \text{g}}{31.8\ \text{g}} \times 100\% \approx \frac{28}{32} \times 100\% = \frac{7}{8} \times 100\% = 87.5\%$$

MCAT CONCEPT CHECK 4.5

Before you move on, assess your understanding of the material with these questions.

Questions 1–3 refer to the following unbalanced equation:

$$\text{Na}\ (s) + \text{O}_2\ (g) \rightarrow \text{Na}_2\text{O}\ (s)$$

1. Balance the chemical equation:

$$\_\_\ \text{Na}\ (s) + \_\_\ \text{O}_2\ (g) \rightarrow \_\_\ \text{Na}_2\text{O}\ (s)$$

2. If 46 g Na and 32 g O_2 are provided, find the maximum number of moles of sodium oxide produced.

____

3. Identify the limiting reagent, and find the mass of the excess reagent left over once the reaction has run to completion.

____

4. $Be(OH)_2$ is produced when water reacts with BeO. Starting with 2.5 kg BeO in excess water, and producing 1.1 kg $Be(OH)_2$, what is the percent yield of this reaction?

____

4.6 Ions

LEARNING OBJECTIVES

After Chapter 4.6, you will be able to:

- Determine whether a molecule will act as an electrolyte in solution
- Recall the common polyatomic ions, including their names and charges

Ionic compounds are of particular interest to chemists because certain important types of chemical reactions—acid–base and oxidation–reduction reactions, for instance—commonly take place in ionic solutions. For stoichiometry problems, the goal with ions is to identify oxidation states. This will allow us to determine electron equivalents, balance equations, and deduce chemical formulas from nomenclature.

Cations and Anions

In Chapter 3 of *MCAT General Chemistry Review*, we discussed how ionic compounds are made up of positively charged **cations**, usually metals, and negatively charged **anions**, usually nonmetals. This rule does not always hold true for elements like hydrogen, which can act like an anion or cation but is still classified as a nonmetal, as shown in Figure 4.8. Ionic compounds are held together by **ionic bonds**, which rely on the force of electrostatic attraction between oppositely charged particles.

BRIDGE

The magnitude of the electrostatic force in an ionic bond follows the same conventions described for Coulomb's law in Chapter 5 of *MCAT Physics and Math Review*. The distance between nuclei in ionic bonds is inversely proportional to the force. Therefore, ionic compounds with long bond distances are much more weakly held together.

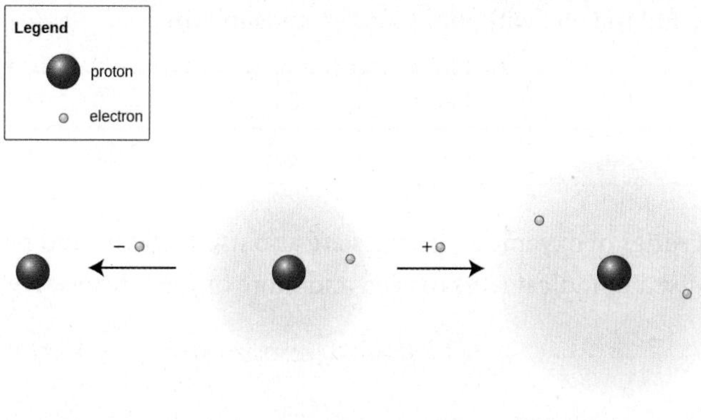

No. of protons	1	1	1
No. of electrons	0	1	2
Charge	+1	0	−1
Notation	H^+	H	H^-
Classification	cation	neutral (not an ion)	anion

Figure 4.8 Oxidation States of Hydrogen

The nomenclature of ionic compounds is based on the names of the component ions:

1. For elements (usually metals) that can form more than one positive ion, the charge is indicated by a Roman numeral in parentheses following the name of the element.

Fe^{2+}	Iron(II)	Cu^{+}	Copper(I)
Fe^{3+}	Iron(III)	Cu^{2+}	Copper(II)

MCAT EXPERTISE

It is unlikely that *-ous* or *-ic* endings will be required for most problem-solving. Passages tend to provide reaction schemes that allow you to deduce any unfamiliar compound's formulas. However, it is still important to understand the nomenclature for discrete questions.

2. An older, less commonly used method is to add the endings ***–ous*** or ***–ic*** to the root of the Latin name of the element to represent the ions with lesser and greater charge, respectively.

Fe^{2+}	Ferrous	Cu^{+}	Cuprous
Fe^{3+}	Ferric	Cu^{2+}	Cupric

3. Monatomic anions are named by dropping the ending of the name of the element and adding ***–ide***.

H^{-}	Hydride	S^{2-}	Sulfide
F^{-}	Fluoride	N^{3-}	Nitride
O^{2-}	Oxide	P^{3-}	Phosphide

MNEMONIC

The "**lite**st" anions have the fewest oxygens; the heaviest anions **ate** the most oxygens.

4. Many polyatomic anions contain oxygen and are therefore called **oxyanions.** When an element forms two oxyanions, the name of the one with less oxygen ends in ***–ite***, and the one with more oxygen ends in ***–ate***.

NO_2^-	Nitrite	SO_3^{2-}	Sulfite
NO_3^-	Nitrate	SO_4^{2-}	Sulfate

5. In extended series of oxyanions, prefixes are also used. ***Hypo–*** and hyper, written as ***per–***, are used to indicate less oxygen and more oxygen, respectively.

ClO^-	Hypochlorite
ClO_2^-	Chlorite
ClO_3^-	Chlorate
ClO_4^-	Perchlorate

6. Polyatomic anions often gain one or more H^+ ions to form anions of lower charge. The resulting ions are named by adding the word **hydrogen** or **dihydrogen** to the front of the anion's name. An older method uses the prefix ***bi–*** to indicate the addition of a single hydrogen ion.

HCO_3^-	Hydrogen carbonate or bicarbonate
HSO_4^-	Hydrogen sulfate or bisulfate
$H_2PO_4^-$	Dihydrogen phosphate

7. Other common polyatomic ions that may be useful to know are in Table 4.1.

CHARGE	FORMULA	NAME
+1	NH_4^+	Ammonium
−1	$C_2H_3O_2^-$	Acetate
	CN^-	Cyanide
	MnO_4^-	Permanganate
	SCN^-	Thiocyanate
−2	CrO_4^{2-}	Chromate
	$Cr_2O_7^{2-}$	Dichromate
−3	BO_3^{3-}	Borate

Table 4.1 Other Common Polyatomic Ions

Ion Charges

Ionic species, by definition, have charge. Cations have positive charge, and anions have negative charge. Some elements are only found naturally in their charged forms, while others may exist naturally in the charged or uncharged state. Some elements can even have several different charges or **oxidation states**, depending on the other atoms in a compound.

Some of the charged atoms or molecules that are on the MCAT include the active metals—the alkali metals (Group IA or Group 1) and the alkaline earth metals (Group IIA or Group 2), which have charges of +1 and +2, respectively, in the natural state.

Nonmetals, which are found on the right side of the periodic table, generally form anions. For example, all the halogens (Group VIIA or Group 17) form monatomic anions with a charge of −1 because they already have 7 electrons and aim to fill an octet.

In summary, all elements in a given group tend to form monatomic ions with the same charge (for example, all Group IA elements have a charge of +1 in their ionic state). Note that there are anionic species that contain metallic elements (for example, MnO_4^- [permanganate] and CrO_4^{2-} [chromate]); even so, the metals have positive oxidation states. Also note that in the oxyanions of the halogens, such as ClO^- and ClO_2^-, the halogen is assigned a positive oxidation state.

For nonrepresentative elements like many of the transition metals, such as copper, iron, and chromium, there are numerous positively charged states. These states need not be memorized. Qualitatively, the color of a solution can be indicative of the oxidation state of a given element in the solution. The same element in different oxidation states can undergo different electron transitions and therefore absorb different frequencies of light. In Figure 4.9, this phenomenon is shown for various plutonium salts with different oxidation states for plutonium indicated in Roman numerals.

BRIDGE

Remember that alkali metals are not typically found in nature in their uncharged state because they are highly reactive with moisture. Instead, they are found as cations in salts (like NaCl).

BRIDGE

Oxyanions of transition metals like the MnO_4^- and CrO_4^{2-} ions have an inordinately high oxidation number on the metal. As such, they tend to gain electrons in order to reduce this oxidation number and thus make good oxidizing agents. Good oxidizing and reducing agents are discussed in Chapter 4 of *MCAT Organic Chemistry Review*.

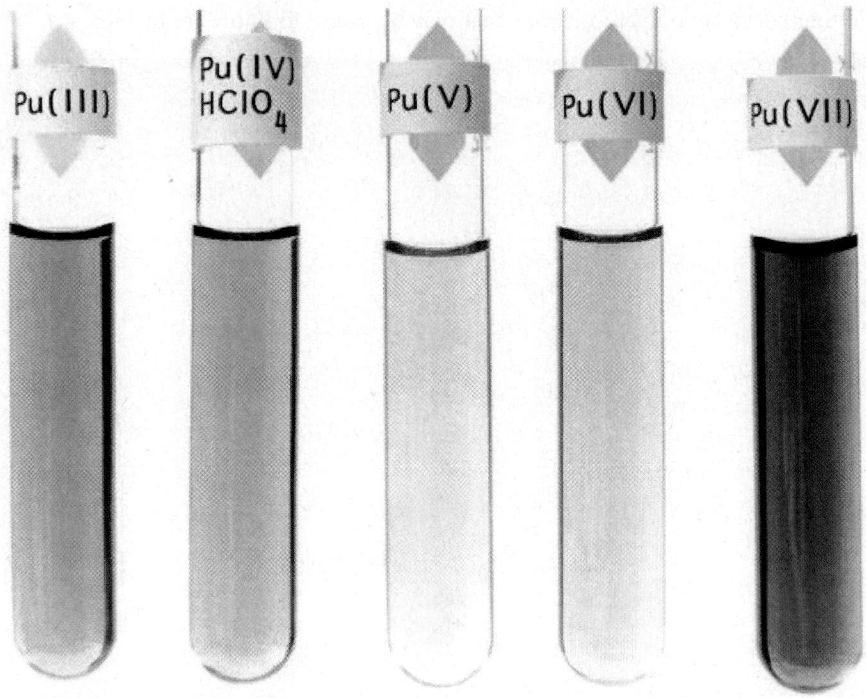

Figure 4.9 Solutions with Various Plutonium Oxidation States

The trends of **ionicity**, as we've described here, are helpful but are complicated by the fact that many elements have intermediate electronegativity and are consequently less likely to form ionic compounds, and by the left-to-right transition from metallic to nonmetallic character on the periodic table.

Electrolytes

In spite of the fact that ionic compounds are composed of ions, solid ionic compounds tend to be poor conductors of electricity because the charged particles are rigidly set in place by the lattice arrangement of the crystalline solid. In aqueous solutions, however, the lattice arrangement is disrupted by the ion–dipole interactions between the ionic components and the water molecules. The cations and anions are now free to move, and as a result, the solution of ions is able to conduct electricity.

MCAT EXPERTISE

Ionic compounds make good electrolytes because they dissolve most readily. Nonpolar covalent compounds are the weakest because they do not form current-carrying ions.

Solutes that enable solutions to carry currents are called **electrolytes**. The electrical conductivity of aqueous solutions is governed by the presence and concentration of ions in the solution. Subsequently, the number of electron equivalents being transferred in such a system, such as in electrochemical cells, varies. Pure water, which has no ions other than the very few hydrogen ions and hydroxide ions that result from water's low-level autodissociation, is a very poor conductor.

The tendency of an ionic solute to dissolve, or **solvate**, into its constituent ions in water may be high or low. A solute is considered a strong electrolyte if it dissociates completely into its constituent ions. Examples of strong electrolytes include certain ionic compounds, such as NaCl and KI, and molecular compounds with highly polar covalent bonds that dissociate into ions when dissolved, such as HCl in water. An example of solvation of such compounds is shown in Figure 4.10.

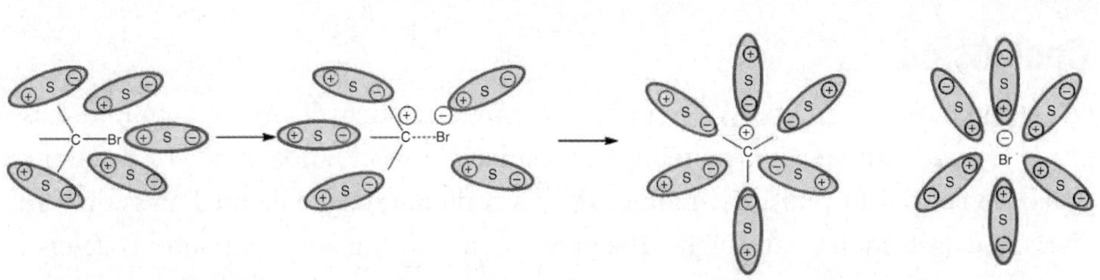

Figure 4.10 Solvation of a Polar Covalent Compound
S indicates a solvent particle.

A weak electrolyte, on the other hand, ionizes or hydrolyzes incompletely in aqueous solution, and only some of the solute is dissolved into its ionic constituents. Examples include Hg_2I_2 ($K_{sp} = 4.5 \times 10^{-29}$), acetic acid and other weak acids, and ammonia and other weak bases. Many compounds do not ionize at all in water, retaining their molecular structure in solution, which may also limit their solubility. These compounds are called nonelectrolytes and include many nonpolar gases and organic compounds, such as O_2 (*g*), CO_2 (*g*), and glucose.

BRIDGE

Because electrolytes ionize in solution, they will produce a larger effect on colligative properties, described in Chapter 9 of *MCAT General Chemistry Review*, than one would expect from the given concentration.

MCAT CONCEPT CHECK 4.6

Before you move on, assess your understanding of the material with these questions.

1. Label the following solutions as electrolytes or nonelectrolytes: (Note: Assume these compounds are all in aqueous solution.)

• HCl	Electrolyte	Nonelectrolyte
• Sucrose	Electrolyte	Nonelectrolyte
• $MgBr_2$	Electrolyte	Nonelectrolyte
• CH_4	Electrolyte	Nonelectrolyte

2. Identify the following ions as cations or anions, and then provide the formula or chemical symbol:

Ion	Cation or Anion	Formula
Phosphate		
Hypochlorite		
Ammonium		
Phosphide		
Bicarbonate		
Nitrite		
Chromium(II)		

Conclusion

We began our consideration of compounds with benzaldehyde. As a compound, it is made from constituent atoms of different elements in a set ratio defined by its empirical or molecular formula. Each molecule of a compound has a defined mass that is measured as its molecular weight. The mass of one mole of any compound is determined from its molar mass in the units of grams per mole. We reviewed the basic classifications of reactions commonly tested on the MCAT: combination, decomposition, combustion, single-displacement, double-displacement, and neutralization reactions. Furthermore, we are now confident in our understanding of the steps necessary to balance any chemical reaction; we are ready to tackle more stoichiometric problems in preparation for Test Day.

Before moving to the next chapters discussing chemical kinetics and thermodynamics, let us offer our congratulations to you. By completing these first four chapters, you have been introduced to the fundamental concepts of chemistry—everything from the structure of the atom and trends of the elements to bonding and the formation of compounds. The understanding you have gained so far will be the foundation for your comprehension of even the most difficult general chemistry concepts tested on the MCAT. Keep moving forward with your review of general chemistry; don't get stuck in the details. Those details will be learned best through the application of the basic principles to MCAT practice passages and questions.

You've reviewed the content, now test your knowledge and critical thinking skills by completing a test-like passage set in your online resources!

GO ONLINE

CONCEPT SUMMARY

Molecules and Moles

- **Compounds** are substances composed of two or more elements in a fixed proportion.
- **Molecular weight** is the mass (in amu) of the constituent atoms in a compound as indicated by the molecular formula.
- **Molar mass** is the mass of one mole (**Avogadro's number** or 6.022×10^{23} particles) of a compound; usually measured in grams per mole.
- **Gram equivalent weight** is a measure of the mass of a substance that can donate one equivalent of the species of interest.
- **Normality** is the ratio of equivalents per liter; it is related to **molarity** by multiplying the molarity by the number of equivalents present per mole of compound.
- **Equivalents** are moles of the species of interest; equivalents are most often seen in acid–base chemistry (hydrogen ions or hydroxide ions) and oxidation–reduction reactions (moles of electrons or other ions).

Representation of Compounds

- The **law of constant composition** states that any pure sample of a compound will contain the same elements in the same mass ratio.
- The **empirical formula** is the smallest whole-number ratio of the elements in a compound.
- The **molecular formula** is either the same as or a multiple of the empirical formula; it gives the exact number of atoms of each element in a compound.
- To calculate **percent composition** by mass, determine the mass of the individual element and divide by the molar mass of the compound.

Types of Chemical Reactions

- **Combination reactions** occur when two or more reactants combine to form one product.
- **Decomposition reactions** occur when one reactant is chemically broken down into two or more products.
- **Combustion reactions** occur when a fuel and an oxidant (typically oxygen) react, forming the products water and carbon dioxide (if the fuel is a hydrocarbon).

- **Displacement reactions** occur when one or more atoms or ions of one compound are replaced with one or more atoms or ions of another compound.
  - **Single-displacement reactions** occur when an ion of one compound is replaced with another element.
  - **Double-displacement reactions** occur when elements from two different compounds trade places with each other to form two new compounds.
- **Neutralization reactions** are those in which an acid reacts with a base to form a salt (and, usually, water).

Balancing Chemical Equations

- Chemical equations must be balanced to perform stoichiometric calculations.
- **Balanced equations** are determined using the following steps in order:
  - Balancing the least common atoms
  - Balancing the more common atoms (usually hydrogen and oxygen)
  - Balancing charge, if necessary

Applications of Stoichiometry

- Balanced equations can be used to determine the **limiting reagent**, which is the reactant that will be consumed first in a chemical reaction.
- The other reactants present are termed **excess reagents.**
- **Theoretical yield** is the amount of product generated if all of the limiting reactant is consumed with no side reactions.
- **Actual yield** is typically lower than theoretical yield.
- **Percent yield** is calculated by dividing actual yield by theoretical yield and converting to a percentage.

Ions

- Like organic chemistry, ions in general chemistry have a system of nomenclature:
  - Roman numerals are used for nonrepresentative elements to denote ionic charge.
  - ***–ous*** endings can also be used to indicate lesser charge, while ***–ic*** endings indicate greater charge.
  - All monatomic anions end in ***–ide***.
  - Oxyanions are given a suffix indicating how oxidized the central atom is. Those that contain a lesser amount of oxygen are given the suffix ***–ite***, and those with a greater amount are given the suffix ***–ate***.

    - Oxyanion series with more than two members are given an additional level of nomenclature. The species with the fewest oxygens is given the prefix ***hypo–***, and the species with the most oxygens is given the prefix ***per–***.
    - Polyatomic ions containing hydrogen denote the number of hydrogens using ***hydrogen*** or ***bi–*** to denote one, or ***dihydrogen*** to denote two.
- **Ionic charges** are predictable by group number and type of element (metal or nonmetal) for representative elements, but are generally unpredictable for non-representative elements.
    - Metals form positively charged cations based on group number.
    - Nonmetals form negatively charged anions based on the number of electrons needed to achieve an octet.
- **Electrolytes** contain equivalents of ions from molecules that dissociate in solution. The strength of an electrolyte depends on its degree of dissociation or **solvation**.

ANSWERS TO CONCEPT CHECKS

4.1

1. NaBr: $23 + 79.9 \approx 23 + 80 = 103\,\frac{\text{g}}{\text{mol}}$

   $SrCl_2$: $87.6 + (2 \times 35.5) = 87.6 + 71 = 158.6\,\frac{\text{g}}{\text{mol}}$

   $C_6H_{12}O_6$: $(6 \times 12) + (12 \times 1) + (6 \times 16) = 180\,\frac{\text{g}}{\text{mol}}$

2. NaBr: $\frac{100\text{ g}}{103\,\frac{\text{g}}{\text{mol}}} = 0.97\text{ moles}$

   Note that the denominator is greater than the numerator by approximately 3 percent, and the actual value is less than 1 by approximately 3 percent. This approximation can be used to quickly estimate answers that are close to one.

   $SrCl_2$: $\frac{100\text{ g}}{158.6\,\frac{\text{g}}{\text{mol}}} \approx \frac{100}{160} = \frac{10}{16} = \frac{5}{8} = 0.625\text{ moles}$

   Note that the answer is a fraction based on eighths. As these are commonly used on the MCAT, knowing the values for 1/8 through 7/8 can be useful for many problems.

   $C_6H_{12}O_6$: $\frac{100\text{ g}}{180\,\frac{\text{g}}{\text{mol}}} = \frac{10}{18} = \frac{5}{9} = 0.555\text{ moles}$

   Note that the final fraction is in ninths. Dividing by nine follows a standard pattern that is useful to know for the MCAT: 1/9 = 0.111, 2/9 = 0.222, 3/9 = 0.333, etc.

3. Both values equal one mole of the given substance. The number of entities in a mole is always the same (Avogadro's number, $6.022 \times 10^{23}\text{ mol}^{-1}$).

4. Normality is calculated as $N = M \times \frac{\text{equivalents}}{\text{mole}}$.

   For H_3PO_4 : $0.25\ M\ H_3PO_4 \times \frac{3\text{ equiv }H^+}{\text{mol }H_3PO_4} = 0.75\ N\ H_3PO_4$.

   For PO_4^{3-} the grams must first be converted to moles, then to normality. PO_4^{3-} has a molecular mass of 95, giving

   $$\frac{95\text{ g}}{100\text{ mL}} = \frac{950\text{ g}}{1\text{ L}} = \frac{10\text{ mol}}{1\text{ L}} = 10\ M\ PO_4^{3-}$$

   $$10\ M\ PO_4^{3-} \times \frac{3\text{ equiv }H^+}{\text{mol }PO_4^{3-}} = 30\ N\ PO_4^{3-}.$$

4.2

1. Both molecular and empirical formulas contain the same elements in the same ratios. They differ in that molecular formulas give the actual number of atoms of each element in the compound; empirical formulas give only the ratio and therefore may or may not give the actual number of atoms.
2. The molar mass of sodium carbonate is given by $(2 \times 23) + (1 \times 12) + (3 \times 16) = 106 \ \frac{\text{g}}{\text{mol}}$. The percent compositions are:

$$\text{Na: } \frac{2 \times \left(23 \ \frac{\text{g}}{\text{mol}}\right)}{106 \ \frac{\text{g}}{\text{mol}}} \times 100\% \approx \frac{46}{100} \times 100\% = 46\% \text{ (actual value} = 43.4\%)$$

$$\text{O: } \frac{3 \times \left(16 \ \frac{\text{g}}{\text{mol}}\right)}{106 \ \frac{\text{g}}{\text{mol}}} \times 100\% \approx \frac{48}{100} \times 100\% = 48\% \text{ (actual value} = 45.3\%)$$

$$\text{C: } \frac{1 \times \left(12 \ \frac{\text{g}}{\text{mol}}\right)}{106 \ \frac{\text{g}}{\text{mol}}} \times 100\% \approx \frac{12}{100} \times 100\% = 12\% \text{ (actual value} = 11.3\%)$$

   Note that in all three cases, the estimation reduces the value of the denominator, thus making the calculated value larger than the actual value.

3. Start by assuming a 100 g sample, which represents 28.5 g Fe, 24.0 g S, and 49.7 g O. Next, divide each number of grams by the atomic weight to determine the number of moles:

$$\text{Fe: } \frac{28.5 \text{ g}}{55.8 \ \frac{\text{g}}{\text{mol}}} \approx \frac{28}{56} = 0.5 \text{ moles}$$

$$\text{S: } \frac{24 \text{ g}}{32.1 \ \frac{\text{g}}{\text{mol}}} \approx \frac{24}{32} = \frac{3}{4} = 0.75 \text{ moles}$$

$$\text{O: } \frac{49.7 \text{ g}}{16 \ \frac{\text{g}}{\text{mol}}} \approx \frac{48}{16} = 3 \text{ moles}$$

   Next, find the multiplier that gives all three compounds integer values of moles. Using sulfur, multiplying 0.75 moles $\times$ 4 = 3 moles. Using 4 as a multiplier for all three compounds gives the ratio 2 Fe : 3 S : 12 O. This gives an empirical formula of $Fe_2S_3O_{12}$.

4.3

1. Ammonium cations swap places with (or displace) zinc cations yielding ammonium nitrate and zinc(II) sulfide. Zinc(II) sulfide then precipitates out of solution as a solid salt.

2.

Reactants	Conditions	Products	Reaction Type
$2\ H_2 + O_2$	$\longrightarrow$	$2\ H_2O$	Combination
$Al(OH)_3 + H_3PO_4$	$\longrightarrow$	$3\ H_2O + AlPO_4$	Neutralization (a type of double-displacement)
$2\ H_2O$	$\xrightarrow{\text{electricity}}$	$2\ H_2 + O_2$	Decomposition
$NaNO_3 + CuOH$	$\longrightarrow$	$NaOH + CuNO_3$	Double-displacement (metathesis)
$Zn + AgCl$	$\longrightarrow$	$ZnCl + Ag$	Single-displacement

4.4

1.
- $2\ Fe + 3\ Cl_2 \rightarrow 2\ FeCl_3$
- $Zn + 2\ HCl \rightarrow ZnCl_2 + H_2$
- $C_5H_{12} + 8\ O_2 \rightarrow 5\ CO_2 + 6\ H_2O$
- $3\ Pb(NO_3)_2 + 2\ AlCl_3 \rightarrow 3\ PbCl_2 + 2\ Al(NO_3)_3$

4.5

1. $4\ Na\ (s) + O_2\ (g) \rightarrow 2\ Na_2O\ (s)$

2. $46\text{ g Na} \times \left[\frac{1\text{ mol Na}}{23\text{ g Na}}\right] = 2\text{ mol Na};\ 32\text{ g }O_2 \times \left[\frac{1\text{ mol }O_2}{32\text{ g }O_2}\right] = 1\text{ mol }O_2$

   Because 4 sodium atoms are needed for every oxygen molecule, sodium will run out first. To determine the amount of Na_2O formed:

$$2\text{mol Na} \times \left[\frac{2\text{ mol }Na_2O}{4\text{ mol Na}}\right] = 1\text{ mol }Na_2O$$

3. The limiting reagent is Na because 4 sodium atoms are needed for every oxygen molecule.

$$2\text{ mol Na} \times \left[\frac{1\text{ mol }O_2}{4\text{ mol Na}}\right] = 0.5\text{ mol }O_2$$

   will be used, so $1.0 - 0.5\text{ mol }O_2 = 0.5\text{ mol }O_2$ will remain. In grams, this is:

$$0.5\text{ mol }O_2 \times \left[\frac{32\text{ g }O_2}{1\text{ mol }O_2}\right] = 16\text{ g excess }O_2$$

4. Reaction: $BeO + H_2O \rightarrow Be(OH)_2$

   Theoretical yield:

$$2500 \text{ g BeO} \times \left[\frac{1 \text{ mol BeO}}{25 \text{ g BeO}}\right]\left[\frac{1 \text{ mol Be(OH)}_2}{1 \text{ mol BeO}}\right]\left[\frac{43 \text{ g Be(OH)}_2}{1 \text{ mol Be(OH)}_2}\right] = 4300 \text{ g Be(OH)}_2$$

$$\text{Percent yield} = \frac{\text{Actual yield}}{\text{Theoretical yield}} \times 100\% = \frac{1100 \text{ g}}{4300 \text{ g}} \times 100\% \approx \frac{11}{44} \times 100\%$$

$$= 25\% \text{ yield (actual value} = 25.6\%)$$

4.6

1. Electrolytes: HCl, $MgBr_2$; Nonelectrolytes: sucrose, CH_4
2.

Ion	Cation or Anion	Formula
Phosphate	Anion	PO_4^{3-}
Hypochlorite	Anion	ClO^-
Ammonium	Cation	NH_4^+
Phosphide	Anion	P^{3-}
Bicarbonate	Anion	HCO_3^-
Nitrite	Anion	NO_2^-
Chromium(II)	Cation	Cr^{2+}

SCIENCE MASTERY ASSESSMENT EXPLANATIONS

1. **D**

Ionic compounds are composed of atoms held together by ionic bonds. Ionic bonds associate charged particles with large differences in electronegativity. Rather than forming molecules or being measured by molecular weight, as in **(A)** and **(B)**, ionic compounds form large arrays of ions in crystalline solids and are measured with formula weights. In ionic bonds, electrons are not really shared but rather are donated from the less electronegative atom to the more electronegative atom, eliminating **(C)**.

2. **A**

Of the compounds listed, both **(B)** and **(D)** are covalent compounds and thus are measured in molecular weights, not formula weights. The formula weight of $MgCl_2$ is much too high (24.3 amu + 2 × 35.5 amu = 95.3 amu per formula unit), eliminating **(C)**. Only KCl fits the criteria (39.1 amu + 35.5 amu = 74.6 amu).

3. **A**

First, it is helpful to know the molar mass of one mole of H_2SO_4, which is found by adding the atomic weights of the atoms that constitute the molecule:

$$\left(2 \times 1.0 \ \frac{\text{g}}{\text{mol H}}\right) + \left(1 \times 32.1 \ \frac{\text{g}}{\text{mol S}}\right) + \left(4 \times 16.0 \ \frac{\text{g}}{\text{mol O}}\right) = 98.1 \ \frac{\text{g}}{\text{mol H}_2\text{SO}_4}.$$

Gram equivalent weight is the mass (in grams) that would release one mole of protons. Because sulfuric acid has two hydrogens per molecule, the gram equivalent weight is 98.1 g divided by 2, or 49.1 g.

4. **C**

The definition of an empirical formula is a formula that represents a molecule with the simplest ratio, in whole numbers, of the elements comprising the compound. In this case, given the empirical formula CH, any molecule with carbon and hydrogen atoms in a 1:1 ratio would be accurately represented by this empirical formula. **(C)** has three carbon atoms and four hydrogen atoms. Both its molecular and empirical formulas would be C_3H_4 because this formula represents the smallest whole-number ratio of its constituent elements.

5. **A**

The percent composition by mass of any given element within a molecule is equal to the mass of that element in the molecule divided by the molar mass of the compound, times 100%. In this case, acetone, C_3H_6O, has

$$\frac{3 \times 12 \ \frac{\text{g}}{\text{mol C}}}{\left(3 \times 12 \ \frac{\text{g}}{\text{mol C}}\right) + \left(6 \times 1 \ \frac{\text{g}}{\text{mol H}}\right) + \left(16 \ \frac{\text{g}}{\text{mol O}}\right)}$$

$$= \frac{36 \ \frac{\text{g}}{\text{mol}}}{58 \ \frac{\text{g}}{\text{mol}}} = \frac{18}{29} \approx \frac{2}{3} \approx 66.7\%.$$

This is an overestimation, and the actual value will be lower; it is closest to 62% out of the four choices available. **(B)**, ethanol, is $\frac{24 \ \frac{\text{g}}{\text{mol C}}}{46 \ \frac{\text{g}}{\text{mol total}}} \approx 50\%$. This is an underestimation, and the actual value will be higher but nowhere near 62%. **(C)**, propane, is C_3H_8, and calculates to be $\frac{36 \ \frac{\text{g}}{\text{mol c}}}{44 \ \frac{\text{g}}{\text{mol total}}} \approx \frac{9}{11} \approx 80\%$ carbon. This is an underestimation, and therefore the actual value cannot be 62%. Finally, **(D)**, methanol, is $\frac{12 \ \frac{\text{g}}{\text{mol C}}}{32 \ \frac{\text{g}}{\text{mol total}}} = \frac{3}{8} = 37.5\%$ carbon.

Note that all four of these compounds are commonly encountered on the MCAT, and you should be familiar with the structure and composition of each, including their common names.

6. **B**

This reaction is a classic example of a neutralization reaction, in which an acid and a base react to form a salt and, usually, water. Although this reaction also fits the criteria for a double-displacement reaction, **(C)**, in which two molecules essentially exchange ions with each other, neutralization is a more specific description of the process.

7. **A**

In this question, you are first given the masses of both reactants used to start the reaction. To figure out what will be left over, we must first determine which species is the limiting reagent. The formula weight of Na_2S is

$$\left(2\times\frac{23\text{ g}}{\text{mol Na}}\right)+\left(1\times\frac{32.1\text{ g}}{\text{mol S}}\right)=78.1\ \frac{\text{g}}{\text{mol}}\ \text{Na}_2\text{S}.$$

The formula weight of $AgNO_3$ is

$$\left(1\times\frac{107.9\text{ g}}{\text{mol Ag}}\right)+\left(1\times\frac{14\text{ g}}{\text{mol N}}\right)+\left(3\times\frac{16\text{ g}}{\text{mol O}}\right)=169.9\ \frac{\text{g}}{\text{mol}}\ \text{AgNO}_3.$$

From this, we can determine that we are given:

$$\frac{39.05\text{ g Na}_2\text{S}}{78.1\ \frac{\text{g}}{\text{mol}}}=0.5\text{ mol Na}_2\text{S}$$

$$\text{and}\quad\frac{85.5\text{ g AgNO}_3}{169.9\ \frac{\text{g}}{\text{mol}}}=0.5\text{ mol AgNO}_3.$$

Because we need two moles of $AgNO_3$ for every mole of Na_2S, $AgNO_3$ is the limiting reagent, and the correct answer choice will be in grams of Na_2S. If 0.5 mol of $AgNO_3$ are used up, and Na_2S will be consumed at half the rate of $AgNO_3$ (based on their mole ratio), then 0.25 mol Na_2S will be used up. We then have 0.25 mol excess Na_2S, which has a mass of

$$0.25\text{ mol}\times\left(\frac{78.1\text{ g}}{\text{mol}}\right)\approx\frac{1}{4}\times\frac{80}{1}=20\text{ g}\ (\text{actual value}=19.5\text{ g}).$$

8. **A**

This is a question best answered by dimensional analysis. Keeping in mind that molar mass is measured in grams of a substance per moles of that substance, only **(A)** comes out with the units of grams of oxygen. **(B)** has the units of grams per mole of oxygen, not grams of oxygen. **(C)** has the units of moles per gram of oxygen. **(D)** has the units of mol^2 per gram of oxygen.

9. **D**

In the reaction, there is a single displacement, with the silver in silver oxide being replaced by the aluminum to form aluminum oxide. This single-displacement reaction also necessitates a transfer of electrons in an oxidation–reduction reaction; silver, for example, changes from the +2 oxidation state to neutral. Aluminum changes from neutral to the +3 oxidation state.

10. **C**

Typically, both single-displacement and double-displacement reactions have two reactants that swap either one or two components between the two species. Combination reactions, on the other hand, have more reactants than products because the reactants combine together to form the product.

11. **A**

In the unbalanced reaction given in the question stem, zinc is already balanced. Next check carbon. There are 4 carbon atoms in the reactants and 1 in the product, so add a coefficient of 4 to carbon dioxide on the product side. Next, check hydrogen. There are 10 hydrogen atoms in the reactants and 2 in the products, so add a coefficient of 5 to water on the product side. Finally, check oxygen. There are 2 oxygen atoms in the reactants and 14 in the products, so add a coefficient of 7 to molecular oxygen on the reactant side. These alterations yield the balanced reaction

$$\text{Zn}(\text{C}_2\text{H}_5)_2+7\ \text{O}_2\rightarrow\text{ZnO}+4\ \text{CO}_2+5\ \text{H}_2\text{O}$$

Because of the coefficient of 4 in front of the CO_2 molecule on the product side, the answer is **(A)**.

12. **B**

The equation given is unbalanced, so the first step must be to balance it:

$$6\ CO_2 + 6\ H_2O \xrightarrow{h\nu} C_6H_{12}O_6 + 6\ O_2$$

The theoretical yield is the amount of product synthesized if the limiting reagent is completely used up. This question therefore asks how much glucose is produced if the limiting reagent is 30 grams of water. Using the three-fraction method discussed in this chapter to solve for the mass of glucose produced gives:

$$30.0\ g\ H_2O \times \left[\frac{1\ mol\ H_2O}{18\ g\ H_2O}\right]\left[\frac{1\ mol\ C_6H_{12}O_6}{6\ mol\ H_2O}\right]\left[\frac{180\ g\ C_6H_{12}O_6}{1\ mol\ C_6H_{12}O_6}\right]$$
$$= 50\ g\ C_6H_{12}O_6$$

Thus, 50 grams of glucose are produced.

13. **B**

A limiting reagent is by definition a reactant. Because Au and H_2S are products, they cannot act as limiting reagents, eliminating **(C)** and **(D)**. Next, note that the given equation is unbalanced and the first step is to balance it:

$$Au_2S_3\ (s) + 3\ H_2\ (g) \rightarrow 2\ Au\ (s) + 3\ H_2S\ (g)$$

The problem states that 2 moles of gold(III) sulfide and 5 moles of hydrogen gas are available. To use up both moles of gold(III) sulfide, 6 moles of hydrogen gas are needed because there is a 1:3 ratio between these reactants. Since only 5 moles of hydrogen gas are present, that will have to be the limiting reagent.

14. **B**

The best electrolytes dissociate readily (have a high dissociation constant) and are ionic compounds with large amounts of cations and anions. This rules out **(A)** and **(C)**. **(D)** has fewer total ions with a smaller total magnitude of charge and therefore is not as strong an electrolyte as **(B)**.

15. **A**

One approach to answering this question might be to write out an unbalanced equation using the description in the question stem, and then balance that equation. But a faster method is elimination. Three of the given chemical equations are not properly balanced, while one is. Check one element at a time. Observe that in this question, the oxygen atoms in equation **(A)** are balanced, but oxygen is not balanced in **(B)**, **(C)**, and **(D)**. Thus **(A)** must be the correct answer.

Consult your online resources for additional practice. GO ONLINE

EQUATIONS TO REMEMBER

(4.1) **Moles from mass:** $\text{Moles} = \frac{\text{Mass of a sample}}{\text{Molar mass}}$

(4.2) **Gram equivalent weight:** $\text{GEW} = \frac{\text{Molar mass}}{n}$

(4.3) **Equivalents from mass:** $\text{Equivalents} = \frac{\text{Mass of compound}}{\text{Gram equivalent weight}}$

(4.4) **Molarity from normality:** $\text{Molarity} = \frac{\text{Normality}}{n}$

(4.5) **Percent composition:** $\%\ \text{composition} = \frac{\text{Mass of element in formula}}{\text{Molar mass}} \times 100\%$

(4.6) **Percent yield:** $\%\ \text{yield} = \frac{\text{Actual yield}}{\text{Theoretical yield}} \times 100\%$

SHARED CONCEPTS

General Chemistry Chapter 2
The Periodic Table

General Chemistry Chapter 3
Bonding and Chemical Interactions

General Chemistry Chapter 9
Solutions

General Chemistry Chapter 10
Acids and Bases

General Chemistry Chapter 11
Oxidation–Reduction Reactions

Physics and Math Chapter 5
Electrostatics and Magnetism

CHAPTER 5

CHEMICAL KINETICS

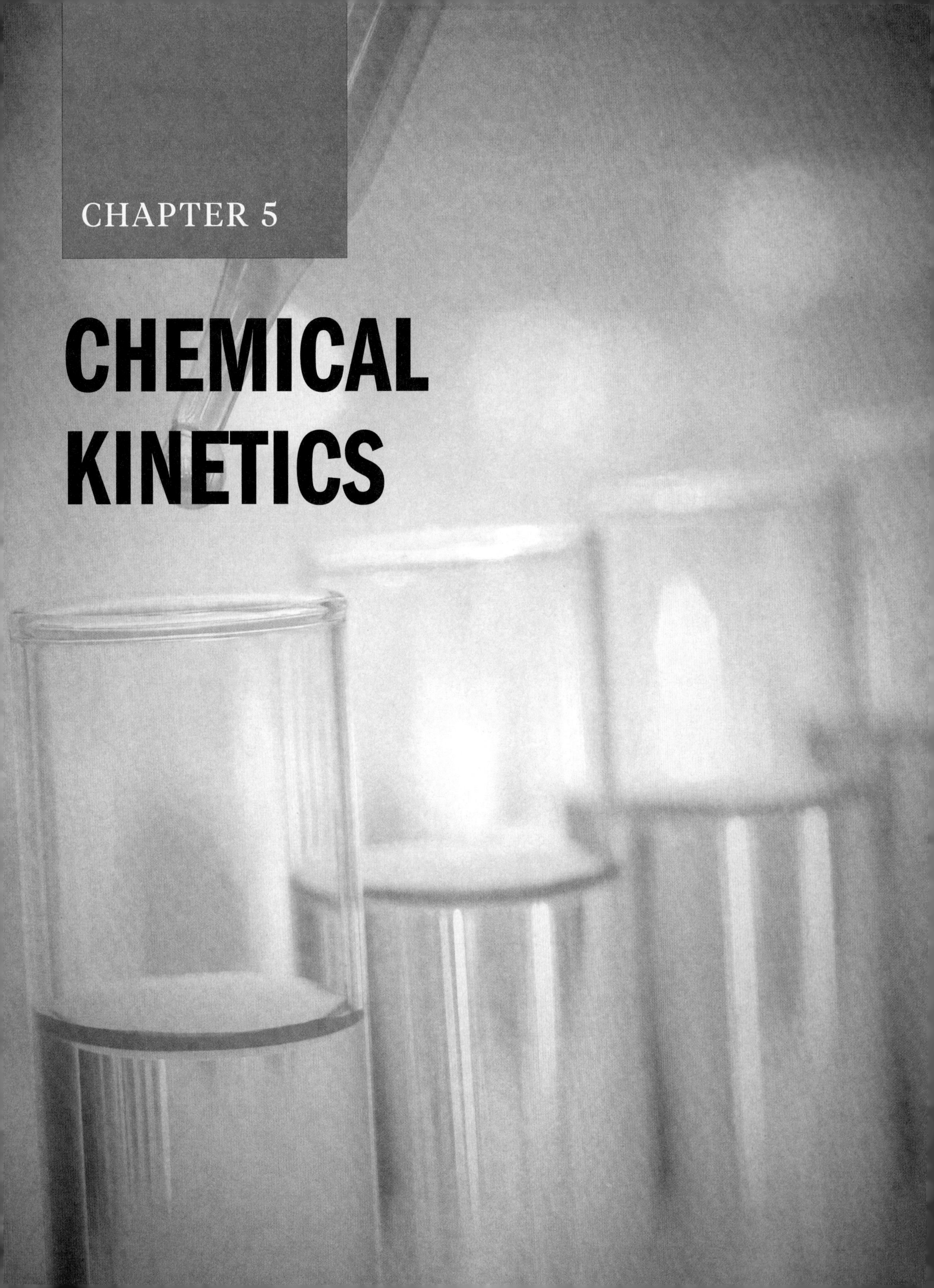

SCIENCE MASTERY ASSESSMENT

Every pre-med knows this feeling: there is so much content I have to know for the MCAT! How do I know what to do first or what's important?

While the high-yield badges throughout this book will help you identify the most important topics, this Science Mastery Assessment is another tool in your MCAT prep arsenal. This quiz (which can also be taken in your online resources) and the guidance below will help ensure that you are spending the appropriate amount of time on this chapter based on your personal strengths and weaknesses. Don't worry though—skipping something now does not mean you'll never study it. Later on in your prep, as you complete full-length tests, you'll uncover specific pieces of content that you need to review and can come back to these chapters as appropriate.

How to Use This Assessment

If you answer 0–7 questions correctly:

Spend about 1 hour to read this chapter in full and take limited notes throughout. Follow up by reviewing **all** quiz questions to ensure that you now understand how to solve each one.

If you answer 8–11 questions correctly:

Spend 20–40 minutes reviewing the quiz questions. Beginning with the questions you missed, read and take notes on the corresponding subchapters. For questions you answered correctly, ensure your thinking matches that of the explanation and you understand why each choice was correct or incorrect.

If you answer 12–15 questions correctly:

Spend less than 20 minutes reviewing all questions from the quiz. If you missed any, then include a quick read-through of the corresponding subchapters, or even just the relevant content within a subchapter, as part of your question review. For questions you answered correctly, ensure your thinking matches that of the explanation and review the Concept Summary at the end of the chapter.

1. In a third-order reaction involving two reactants and two products, doubling the concentration of the first reactant causes the rate to increase by a factor of 2. What will happen to the rate of this reaction if the concentration of the second reactant is cut in half?
   - **A.** It will increase by a factor of 2.
   - **B.** It will increase by a factor of 4.
   - **C.** It will decrease by a factor of 2.
   - **D.** It will decrease by a factor of 4.

2. In a certain equilibrium process, the activation energy of the forward reaction ($\Delta G_f^{\ddagger}$) is greater than the activation energy of the reverse reaction ($\Delta G_r^{\ddagger}$). This reaction is:
   - **A.** endothermic.
   - **B.** exothermic.
   - **C.** spontaneous.
   - **D.** nonspontaneous.

3. A reactant in a second-order reaction at a certain temperature is increased by a factor of 4. By how much is the rate of the reaction altered?
   - **A.** It is unchanged.
   - **B.** It is increased by a factor of 4.
   - **C.** It is increased by a factor of 16.
   - **D.** It cannot be determined from the information given.

4. The concentrations of all reactants in a zero-order reaction are increased two-fold. What is the new rate of the reaction?
   - **A.** It is unchanged.
   - **B.** It is decreased by a factor of 2.
   - **C.** It is increased by a factor of 2.
   - **D.** It cannot be determined from the information given.

5. Which of the following experimental methods should NEVER affect the rate of a reaction?
   - **A.** Placing an exothermic reaction in an ice bath.
   - **B.** Increasing the pressure of a reactant in a closed container.
   - **C.** Putting the reactants into an aqueous solution.
   - **D.** Removing the product of an irreversible reaction.

6. What would increasing the concentration of reactants accomplish in a solution containing a saturated catalyst?
   - **A.** It would increase the rate constant but not the reaction rate.
   - **B.** It would decrease the rate constant but increase the reaction rate.
   - **C.** It would increase the rate constant and increase the reaction rate.
   - **D.** The reaction rate would be unaffected.

7. A certain chemical reaction has the following rate law:

$$\text{rate} = k[NO_2][Br_2]$$

Which of the following statements necessarily describe(s) the kinetics of this reaction?

   - **I.** The reaction is second-order.
   - **II.** The amount of NO_2 consumed is equal to the amount of Br_2 consumed.
   - **III.** The rate will not be affected by the addition of a compound other than NO_2 and Br_2.

   - **A.** I only
   - **B.** I and II only
   - **C.** II and III only
   - **D.** I, II, and III

8. The following data shown in the table were collected for the combustion of the theoretical compound XH_4:

$$XH_4 + 2\ O_2 \rightarrow XO_2 + 2\ H_2O$$

Trial	$[XH_4]_{initial}$ (M)	$[O_2]_{initial}$ (M)	$\text{Rate}_{initial}$ $\left(\frac{M}{\text{min}}\right)$
1	0.6	0.6	12.4
2	0.6	2.4	49.9
3	1.2	2.4	198.3

What is the rate law for the reaction described here?
   - **A.** rate $= k[XH_4][O_2]$
   - **B.** rate $= k[XH_4][O_2]^2$
   - **C.** rate $= k[XH_4]^2[O_2]$
   - **D.** rate $= k[XH_4]^2[O_2]^2$

9. Which of the following best describes the purpose of a catalyst?
   A. Catalysts are used up in the reaction, increasing reaction efficiency.
   B. Catalysts increase the rate of the reaction by lowering the activation energy.
   C. Catalysts alter the thermodynamics of the reaction to facilitate the formation of products or reactants.
   D. Catalysts stabilize the transition state by bringing it to a higher energy.

10. If the rate law for a reaction is:

$$\text{rate} = k[A]^0[B]^2[C]^1$$

What is the overall order of the reaction?
   A. 0
   B. 2
   C. 3
   D. 4

For questions 11–13, consider the following energy diagram shown below:

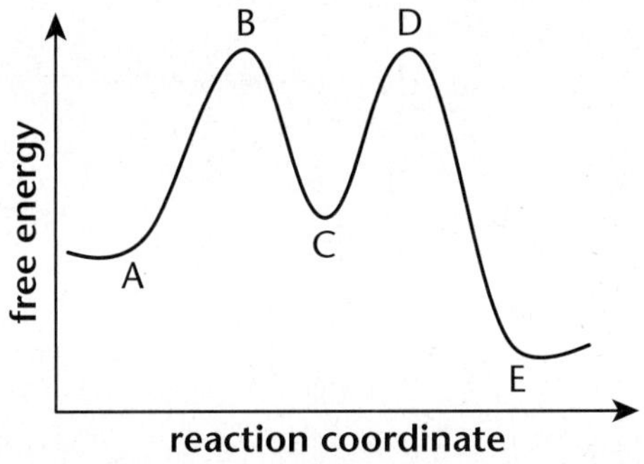

11. The overall reaction depicted by this energy diagram is:
   A. endergonic, because point B is higher than point A.
   B. endergonic, because point C is higher than point A.
   C. exergonic, because point D is higher than point E.
   D. exergonic, because point A is higher than point E.

12. Which process has the highest activation energy?
   A. The first step of the forward reaction
   B. The first step of the reverse reaction
   C. The second step of the forward reaction
   D. The second step of the reverse reaction

13. Point C in this reaction profile refers to the:
   A. reactants.
   B. products.
   C. transition state.
   D. intermediates.

14. The following system obeys second-order kinetics.

$$2\,NO_2 \rightarrow NO_3 + NO \quad \text{(slow)}$$

$$NO_3 + CO \rightarrow NO_2 + CO_2 \quad \text{(fast)}$$

What is the rate law for this reaction?
   A. rate $= k[NO_2][CO]$
   B. rate $= k[NO_2]^2[CO]$
   C. rate $= k[NO_2][NO_3]$
   D. rate $= k[NO_2]^2$

15. The potential energy diagram shown represents four different reactions.

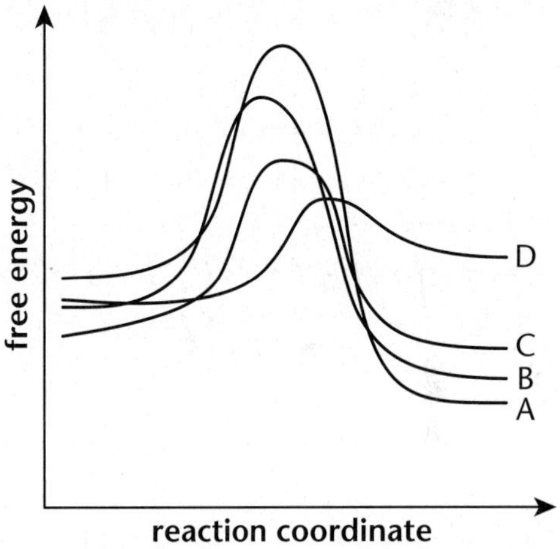

Assuming identical conditions, which of the reactions displayed on the energy diagram proceeds the fastest?
   A. A
   B. B
   C. C
   D. D

Answer Key

1. **D**
2. **D**
3. **D**
4. **A**
5. **D**
6. **D**
7. **A**
8. **C**
9. **B**
10. **C**
11. **D**
12. **B**
13. **D**
14. **D**
15. **D**

Detailed explanations can be found at the end of the chapter.

CHAPTER 5

CHEMICAL KINETICS

In This Chapter

CHAPTER PROFILE

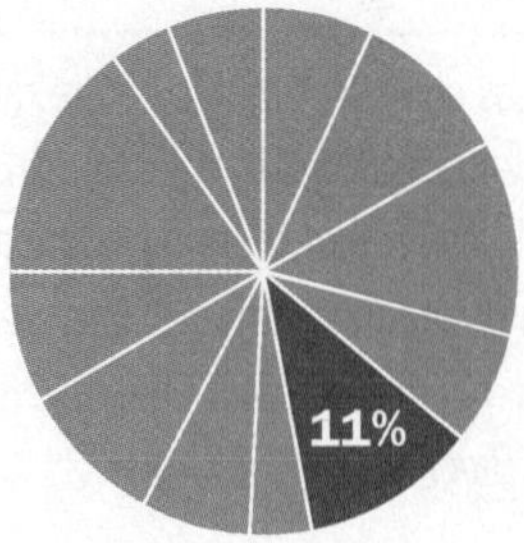

The content in this chapter should be relevant to about 11% of all questions about general chemistry on the MCAT.

This chapter covers material from the following AAMC content categories:

1A: Structure and function of proteins and their constituent amino acids

5E: Principles of chemical thermodynamics and kinetics

Introduction

The following chapters focus on two primary topics: chemical kinetics and chemical equilibrium. As the term suggests, chemical kinetics is the study of reaction rates, the effects of reaction conditions on these rates, and the mechanisms implied by such observations. We start with kinetics because the molecular basis of reactions provides us with a framework of reaction chemistry. Following this, we will explore the equilibria of these reactions, which are related to—but distinct from—the kinetics of the reactions.

You may already have a fairly good understanding of equilibrium and the differences between spontaneous and nonspontaneous reactions. For instance, the utilization of ATP in the body is a spontaneous reaction that can be used to provide thermochemical energy for other reactions. While the equilibrium tells us that ATP will favor dissociation, it tells us nothing about its rate of dissociation. And, in fact, various conditions in the body can alter the rate at which ATP is synthesized and utilized for energy—primarily temperature. Some of the symptoms of hyper- and hypothermia are related to changes in metabolism caused by changes in temperature and reaction kinetics.

More broadly, we will see how multistep reactions, such as those seen in substrate-level and oxidative phosphorylation in biochemistry, have intermediate steps that have crucial kinetic limitations.

5.1 Chemical Kinetics

High-Yield

LEARNING OBJECTIVES

After Chapter 5.1, you will be able to:

- Describe the series of events within a multistep mechanism
- Explain the meaning and importance of a rate-determining step
- Describe activation energy
- Compare and contrast transition state theory and collision theory

BRIDGE

Enzymes selectively enhance the rate of certain reactions by a factor of 10^2 to 10^{12} over other thermodynamically feasible reaction pathways. Enzyme function is discussed in Chapter 2 of *MCAT Biochemistry Review*.

Reactions can be spontaneous or nonspontaneous; the change in **Gibbs free energy** (**ΔG**) determines whether or not a reaction will occur by itself without outside assistance. However, even if a reaction is spontaneous, this does not necessarily mean that it will run quickly. In fact, nearly every biochemical reaction that enables life to exist, while perhaps spontaneous, proceeds so slowly that, without the aid of enzymes and other catalysts, measurable reaction progress might not actually occur over the course of an average human lifetime. And enzymes, like many other catalyzed reactions, can be saturated and experience a maximal turnover rate, as shown in Figure 5.1. For now, however, let us review reaction mechanisms, rates, rate laws, and the factors that pertain to simple chemical systems.

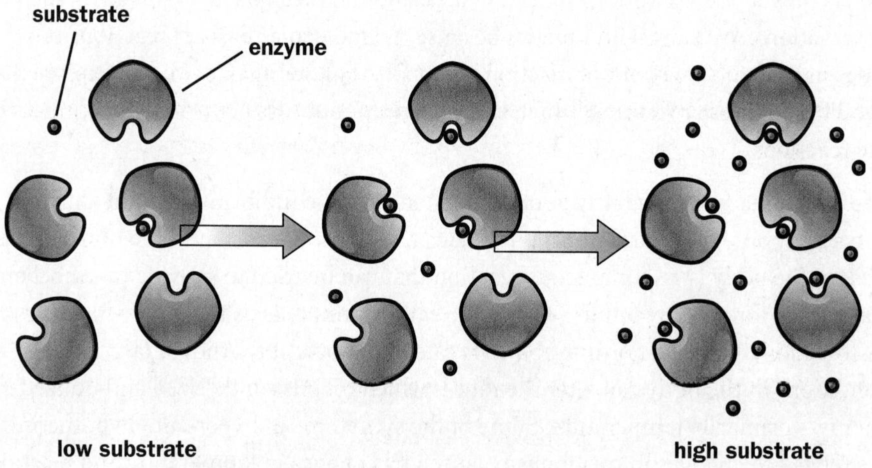

Figure 5.1 Enzymes, as Biological Catalysts, Can Be Saturated
High substrate conditions saturate the active sites of the enzyme, leading to maximal turnover.

Reaction Mechanisms

Very rarely is the balanced reaction equation, used for determining limiting reactants and yields, an accurate representation of the actual steps involved in the chemical process from reactants to products. Many reactions proceed by more than one step, the series of which is known as the **mechanism** of a reaction, and the sum of which gives the overall reaction. Knowing the accepted mechanism of a reaction may help explain the reaction's rate, position of equilibrium, and thermodynamic characteristics. Consider this generic reaction:

$$A_2 + 2\ B \rightarrow 2\ AB$$

On its own, this equation seems to imply a mechanism in which two molecules of B collide with one molecule of A_2 to form two molecules of AB. Suppose instead, however, that the reaction actually takes place in two steps:

$$\text{Step 1: } A_2 + B \rightarrow A_2B \qquad \text{(slow)}$$

$$\text{Step 2: } A_2B + B \rightarrow 2\ AB \qquad \text{(fast)}$$

Note that the two steps, taken together, give the overall net reaction. The molecule A_2B, which does not appear in the overall reaction, is called an **intermediate**. Reaction intermediates are often difficult to detect because they may be consumed almost immediately after they are formed, but a proposed mechanism that includes intermediates can be supported through kinetic experiments. One of the most important points to remember is that the slowest step in any proposed mechanism is called the **rate-determining step** because it acts like a kinetic bottleneck, preventing the overall reaction from proceeding any faster than that slowest step.

BRIDGE

Mechanisms are proposed pathways for a reaction that must coincide with rate data information from experimental observation. Reaction mechanisms are a major topic in organic chemistry and metabolism; Chapters 5 through 10 of *MCAT Organic Chemistry Review* and Chapters 9 through 11 of *MCAT Biochemistry Review* focus almost exclusively on reaction mechanisms in specific contexts.

KEY CONCEPT

The rate of the whole reaction is only as fast as the rate-determining step.

Molecular Basis of Chemical Reactions

It's one thing to say A_2 *reacts with 2 B to form 2 AB*; it's quite another to be able to describe, as precisely as possible, the actual interactions that occur between A_2 and B to produce AB at some rate. Various theories have been proposed to explain the events that are taking place at the atomic level through the process of a reaction.

Collision Theory of Chemical Kinetics

For a reaction to occur, molecules must collide with each other. The **collision theory of chemical kinetics** states that the rate of a reaction is proportional to the number of collisions per second between the reacting molecules.

The theory suggests, however, that not all collisions result in a chemical reaction. An effective collision (one that leads to the formation of products) occurs only if the molecules collide with each other in the correct orientation and with sufficient energy to break their existing bonds and form new ones. The minimum energy of collision necessary for a reaction to take place is called the **activation energy**, E_a, or the **energy barrier**. Only a fraction of colliding particles have enough kinetic energy to exceed the activation energy. This means that only a fraction of all collisions are effective. The rate of a reaction can therefore be expressed as follows:

$$\text{rate} = Z \times f$$

Equation 5.1

where Z is the total number of collisions occurring per second and f is the fraction of collisions that are effective. A much more quantitatively rigorous analysis of the collision theory can be accomplished through the **Arrhenius equation**, which is normally given as:

$$k = Ae^{\frac{-E_a}{RT}}$$

Equation 5.2

where k is the rate constant of a reaction, A is the frequency factor, E_a is the activation energy of the reaction, R is the ideal gas constant, and T is the temperature in kelvin. The **frequency factor**, also known as the **attempt frequency** of the reaction, is a measure of how often molecules in a certain reaction collide, with the unit s^{-1}. Activation energy is a subject that will be touched upon briefly in the following subsection and more qualitatively in future chapters.

Overall, what is important here in studying the Arrhenius equation is not the actual calculation (because those involving Euler's number, *e*, and natural logs, ln, are not commonly found on the MCAT), but rather the relationships between the variables and the exponent rules that govern the equation.

MCAT EXPERTISE

Low activation energy and high temperatures make the negative exponent of the Arrhenius equation smaller in magnitude and thus increase the rate constant k.

For example, a simple relationship between A and k is evident in the equation. As the frequency factor of the reaction increases, the rate constant of the reaction also increases in a direct relationship. More complex relationships can also be seen in this equation. For example, if the temperature (T) of a chemical system were to increase to infinity, while all other variables are held constant, the value of the exponent would have a magnitude less than 1. However, before assuming that the rate constant is going to decrease as a result, note the presence of the negative sign. As the magnitude of the exponent gets smaller, it actually moves from a more negative value toward zero. The exponent thus becomes less negative (or more positive), which means that the rate constant actually increases. This should make sense conceptually because the rate of a reaction increases with temperature.

The frequency factor can be increased by increasing the number of molecules in a vessel. When there are more molecules, the opportunities for collision are increased, as shown in Figure 5.2.

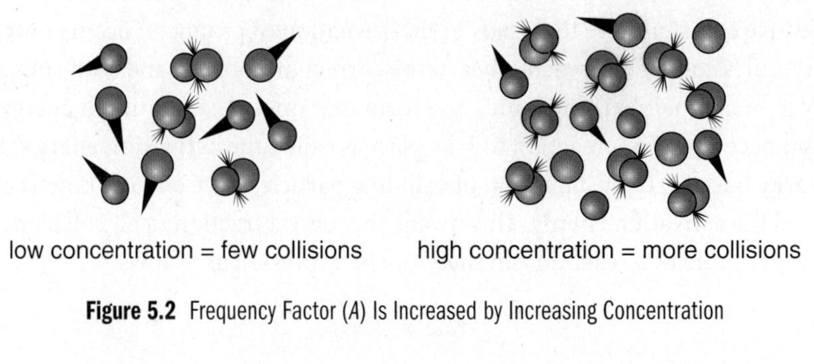

Figure 5.2 Frequency Factor (A) Is Increased by Increasing Concentration

Transition State Theory

When molecules collide with energy equal to or greater than the activation energy, they form a transition state in which the old bonds are weakened and the new bonds begin to form. The transition state then dissociates into products, fully forming the new bonds. For the reaction $A_2 + 2\ B \rightarrow 2\ AB$, the progress along the **reaction coordinate**, which traces the reaction from reactants to products, can be represented as shown in Figure 5.3.

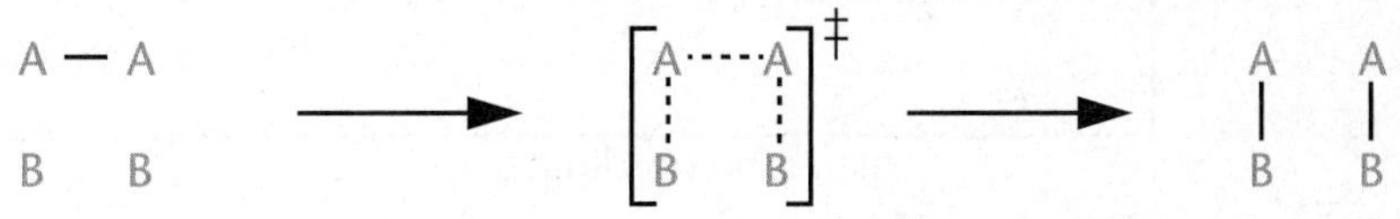

Figure 5.3 The Transition State

KEY CONCEPT

Relative to reactants and products, transition states have the highest energy. They are only theoretical structures and cannot be isolated. Nevertheless, we can still use the proposed structures to better understand the reactions in which they are involved.

The **transition state**, also called the **activated complex**, has greater energy than both the reactants and the products and is denoted by the symbol ‡. The energy required to reach this transition state is the activation energy. Once an activated complex is formed, it can either dissociate into the products or revert to reactants without any additional energy input. Transition states are distinguished from reaction intermediates in that transition states are theoretical constructs that exist at the point of maximum energy, rather than distinct identities with finite lifetimes.

A free energy diagram illustrates the relationship between the activation energy, the free energy of the reaction, and the free energy of the system. The most important features to recognize in such diagrams are the relative energies of all of the products and reactants. The **free energy change of the reaction (ΔG_{rxn})** is the difference between the free energy of the products and the free energy of the reactants. A negative free energy change indicates an **exergonic reaction** (energy is given off), and a positive free energy change indicates an **endergonic reaction** (energy is absorbed). The transition state exists at the peak of the energy diagram. The difference in free energy between the transition state and the reactants is the activation energy of the forward reaction; the difference in free energy between the transition state and the products is the activation energy of the reverse reaction.

KEY CONCEPT

$+\Delta G$ = endergonic = energy absorbed

$-\Delta G$ = exergonic = energy given off

For example, consider the formation of HCl from H_2 and Cl_2. The overall reaction is:

$$H_2\ (g) + Cl_2\ (g) \rightleftharpoons 2\ HCl\ (g)$$

Figure 5.4 shows that the reaction is exergonic. The free energy of the products is less than the free energy of the reactants; energy is released, and the free energy change of the reaction is negative.

MCAT EXPERTISE

Kinetics and thermodynamics should be considered separately. Note that the activation energy can be lowered without affecting the ΔG. In fact, this is how catalysts increase the rate of a reaction.

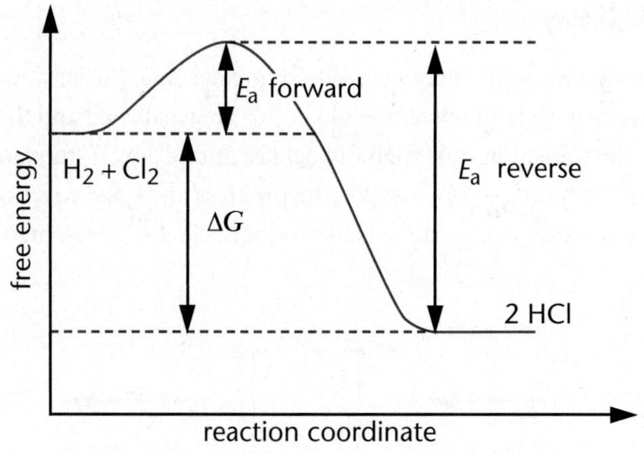

Figure 5.4 Reaction Diagram for the Formation of HCl
On the left are the reactants (H_2 and Cl_2) and on the right are the products (2 HCl); this reaction is exergonic, and forward and reverse activation energies are shown.

Factors Affecting Reaction Rate

Before we delve into the specifics of rate calculations, it is helpful to understand the conditions that can alter experimental rates.

Reaction Concentrations

The greater the concentrations of the reactants, the greater the number of effective collisions per unit time. Recall that this leads to an increase in the frequency factor (A) of the Arrhenius equation. Therefore, the reaction rate will increase for all but zero-order reactions, which will be discussed shortly. For reactions occurring in the gaseous state, the partial pressures of the gas reactants serve as a measure of concentration, as discussed in Chapter 8 of *MCAT General Chemistry Review*.

Temperature

For nearly all reactions, the reaction rate will increase as the temperature increases. Because the temperature of a substance is a measure of the particles' average kinetic energy, increasing the temperature increases the average kinetic energy of the molecules. Consequently, the proportion of reactants gaining enough energy to surpass E_a (and thus capable of undergoing reaction) increases with higher temperature. All reactions—even the nuclear reactions shown in Figure 5.5—are temperature-dependent and experience an optimal temperature for activity.

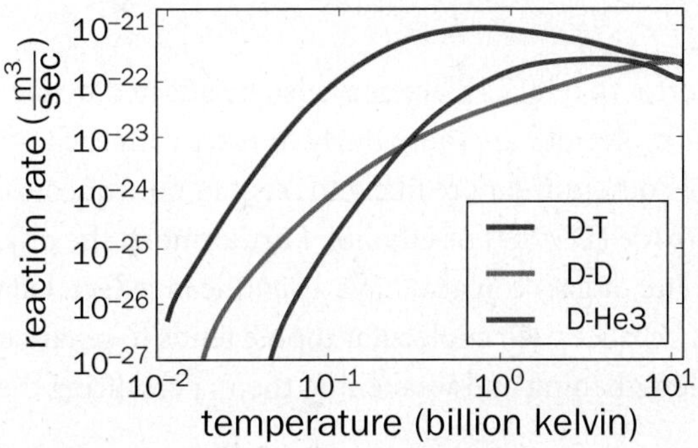

Figure 5.5 All Reactions Are Temperature-Dependent
Examples shown are nuclear fusion reactions; at extreme temperatures, the nucleus itself begins to break down.

You'll often hear that raising the temperature of a system by 10°C will result in an approximate doubling of the reaction rate. Be careful with this approximation because it is *generally* true for biological systems but not so for many other systems. Further, even in biological systems, if the temperature gets too high, a catalyst may denature—and then the reaction rate plummets. Figure 5.6 shows a general curve for an enzymatic reaction that is optimal between 35°C and 40°C (body temperature). Notice that the curve falls sharply after 40°C, at which point denaturation has occurred.

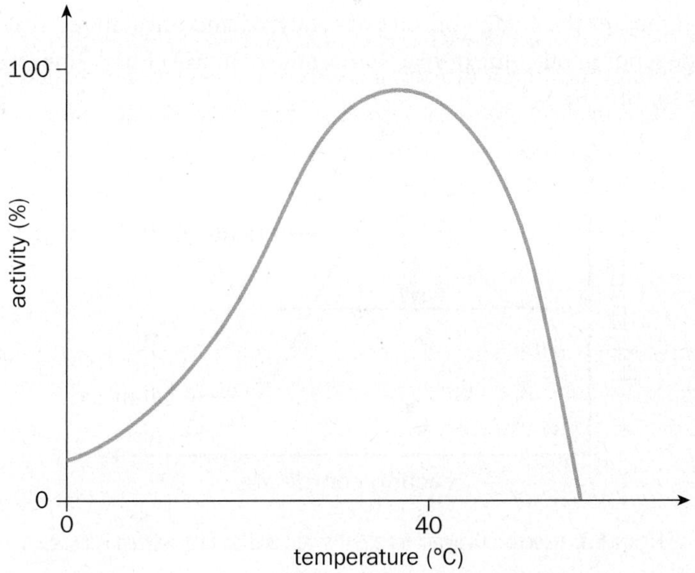

Figure 5.6 An Activity *vs.* Temperature Curve for a Generic Human Enzyme

Medium

The rate at which a reaction takes place may also be affected by the medium in which it takes place. Some molecules are more likely to react with each other in aqueous environments, while others are more likely to react in nonaqueous solvents, such as in dimethyl sulfoxide (DMSO) or ethanol. Furthermore, the physical state of the medium (liquid, solid, or gas) can also have a significant effect. Generally, polar solvents are preferred because their molecular dipole tends to polarize the bonds of the reactants, thereby lengthening and weakening them, permitting the reaction to occur faster.

Catalysts

Catalysts are substances that increase reaction rate without themselves being consumed in the reaction. Catalysts interact with the reactants, either by adsorption or through the formation of intermediates, and stabilize them so as to reduce the activation energy necessary for the reaction to proceed. While many catalysts, including all enzymes, chemically interact with the reactants, they return to their original chemical state upon formation of the products. They may increase the frequency of collisions between the reactants; change the relative orientation of the reactants, making a higher percentage of the collisions effective; donate electron density to the reactants; or reduce intramolecular bonding within reactant molecules. In **homogeneous catalysis**, the catalyst is in the same phase (solid, liquid, gas) as the reactants. In **heterogeneous catalysis**, the catalyst is in a distinct phase. Figure 5.7 compares the energy profiles of catalyzed and uncatalyzed reactions. Note that, depending on context, reaction profiles can use either Gibbs free energy or enthalpy for the *y*-axis.

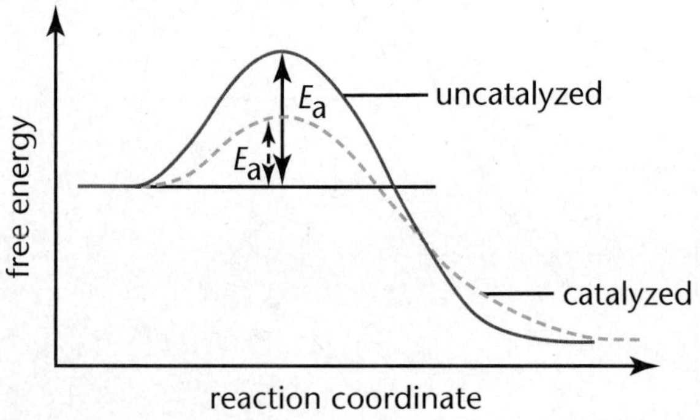

Figure 5.7 Reaction Diagram for a Catalyzed and an Uncatalyzed Reaction

Notice that the only effect of the catalyst is the decrease in the energies of activation, E_a, for both the forward and reverse reactions. The presence of the catalyst has no impact on the free energies of the reactants or the products or the difference between them. This means that catalysts change only the rates of reactions, and in fact, change the forward rate and the reverse rate by the same factor. Consequently, they have no impact whatsoever on the equilibrium position or the measurement of K_{eq}. Remember that, as useful as catalysts are in biological and nonbiological systems, catalysts

BRIDGE

Equilibrium, like biological homeostasis, is a dynamic process that seeks to find balance in all systems. We can use this concept to our advantage on the MCAT in all seven of the basic sciences. Equilibria are dynamic, meaning that they *do* undergo change but their *net* change will be zero.

are not miracle workers: they will not transform a nonspontaneous reaction into a spontaneous one; they only make spontaneous reactions move more quickly toward equilibrium.

MCAT CONCEPT CHECK 5.1

Before you move on, assess your understanding of the material with these questions.

1. Describe in words what is occurring in the following two-step mechanism:

$$\text{Step 1: } A_2B + A_2B \rightarrow A_4B_2$$
$$\text{Step 2: } A_4B_2 \rightarrow 2A_2 + B_2$$

____

2. What does it mean for a step in a mechanism to be the rate-determining step?

____

3. What is activation energy?

____

4. How does the transition state theory compare with the collision theory of chemical kinetics?

    - Transition state theory:

____

    - Collision theory:

____

5.2 Reaction Rates

LEARNING OBJECTIVES

After Chapter 5.2, you will be able to:

- Predict the impact of changing temperature, concentration, and catalyst presence on rate of reaction for a zero, first, or second-order reaction
- Determine the rate law and rate order for a reaction, given experimental reaction rate data:

Trial	$[A]_{initial}$ (M)	$[B]_{initial}$ (M)	rate $_{initial}$ $\left(\frac{M}{s}\right)$
1	1.00	1.00	2.0
2	1.00	2.00	8.1
3	2.00	2.00	15.9

Reactions, unfortunately, do not come with handy built-in speedometers. To determine the rate at which a reaction proceeds, we must take measurements of the concentrations of reactants and products and note their change over time.

Definition of Rate

If we consider a generic reaction, $2\,A + B \rightarrow C$, in which one mole of C can be produced from two moles of A and one mole of B, we can describe the rate of this reaction in terms of either the disappearance of reactants over time or the appearance of products over time. Because the reactants, by definition, are being consumed in the process of formation of the products, we place a negative sign in front of the rate expression for the reactants. For the above reaction, the rate of the reaction with respect to A is $-\frac{\Delta[A]}{\Delta t}$, with respect to B is $-\frac{\Delta[B]}{\Delta t}$, and with respect to C is $+\frac{\Delta[C]}{\Delta t}$. Notice that the stoichiometric coefficients for the reaction are not equal, which means that the rates of change of concentrations are not equal. Because two moles of A are consumed for every mole of B consumed, the rate of consumption of A is twice the rate of consumption of B. Furthermore, for every two moles of A consumed, only one mole of C is produced; thus, we can say that the rate of consumption of A is twice the rate of production of C. Based on the stoichiometry, we can see that the rate of consumption of B is equal to the rate of production of C. To show a standard rate of reaction in which the rates with respect to all reaction species are equal, the rate of concentration change of each species should be divided by the species' stoichiometric coefficients. Thus, for the general reaction $aA + bB \rightarrow cC + dD$:

$$\text{rate} = -\frac{\Delta[A]}{a\Delta t} = -\frac{\Delta[B]}{b\Delta t} = \frac{\Delta[C]}{c\Delta t} = \frac{\Delta[D]}{d\Delta t}$$

Equation 5.3

Rate is expressed in the units of moles per liter per second $\left(\frac{\text{mol}}{\text{L}\cdot\text{s}}\right)$ or molarity per second $\left(\frac{M}{\text{s}}\right)$.

Determination of Rate Law

In the *Chemical and Physical Foundations of Biological Systems* section of the MCAT, it is unlikely that the testmakers will provide a reaction equation that one can merely look at and write the correct rate law. Therefore, on the MCAT, whenever a question asks to determine the rate law for a reaction, the first thing to look for is experimental data.

For nearly all forward, irreversible reactions, the rate is proportional to the concentrations of the reactants, with each concentration raised to some experimentally determined exponent. For the general reaction

$$aA + bB \rightarrow cC + dD$$

the rate is proportional to $[A]^x[B]^y$. By including a proportionality constant, k, we can say that rate is determined according to the following equation:

$$\text{rate} = k[A]^x[B]^y$$

Equation 5.4

where k is the reaction rate coefficient or rate constant and the exponents x and y are the orders of the reaction. This expression is called the **rate law**. Remember that rate is always measured in units of concentration over time; that is, molarity per second. The exponents x and y (or x, y, and z, if there are three reactants) can be used to state the order of the reaction with respect to each reactant or overall: x is the order with respect to reactant A, and y is the order with respect to reactant B. The overall order of the reaction is the sum of x and y. These exponents may be integers or fractions and must be determined experimentally. The MCAT will focus almost exclusively on zero-, first-, second-, and third-order reactions. In most cases, the exponents will be integers.

Before we go any further in our consideration of rate laws, we must offer a few warnings about common traps in chemical kinetics. The first—and most common—is the assumption that the orders of a reaction are the same as the stoichiometric coefficients in the balanced overall equation. Pay close attention: *On the MCAT, the values of* x *and* y *are almost never the same as the stoichiometric coefficients*. The orders of a reaction must be determined experimentally. There are only two cases in which the stoichiometric coefficients match the orders of the reaction. The first is when the reaction mechanism is a single step and the balanced overall reaction is reflective of the entire chemical process. The second is when the complete reaction mechanism is given and the rate-determining step is indicated. The stoichiometric coefficients on the reactant side of the rate-determining step are equal to the orders of the reaction. Occasionally, even this can get a little complicated when the rate-determining step involves an intermediate as a reactant, in which case one must derive the intermediate molecule's concentration by the **law of mass action** (that is, the equilibrium constant expression) for the step that produced the intermediate.

MCAT EXPERTISE

Remember that the stoichiometric coefficients for the overall reaction are often different from those for the rate law and will, therefore, not be the same as the order of the reaction.

MCAT EXPERTISE

Note that the exponents in the rate law are *not* equal to the stoichiometric coefficients, unless the reaction occurs via a single-step mechanism. Note that product concentrations *never* appear in a rate law. Don't fall into the exceedingly common trap of confusing the rate law with an equilibrium expression!

The second common trap is mistaking the equilibrium constant expression (law of mass action) for the rate law. The expressions for both look similar; if you're not alert on Test Day, you may mistake one for the other or use one when you should be using the other. The expression for equilibrium includes the concentrations of all the species in the reaction, both reactants and products. The expression for chemical kinetics—the rate law expression—includes only the reactants. K_{eq} indicates where the reaction's equilibrium position lies. The rate indicates how quickly the reaction will get there.

The third trap regards the rate constant, k. Technically speaking, k is not a constant because its particular value for any specific chemical reaction will depend on the activation energy for that reaction and the temperature at which the reaction takes place. However, for a specific reaction, at a specific temperature, the rate constant is indeed a constant. For a reversible reaction, the K_{eq} is equal to the ratio of the rate constant for the forward reaction, k, divided by the rate constant for the reverse reaction, k_{-1}.

The fourth and final trap is that the notion and principles of equilibrium apply to the system only at the end of the reaction; that is, after the system has already reached equilibrium. On the other hand, while the reaction rate can theoretically be measured at any time, it is usually measured at or near the beginning of the reaction to minimize the effects of the reverse reaction.

Experimental Determination of Rate Law

This has already been stated a few times, but it bears repeating: The values of k, x, and y in the rate law equation (rate $= k[A]^x[B]^y$) must be determined experimentally for a given reaction at a given temperature. Although rate laws can be quite complex and the orders of the reaction difficult to discern, the MCAT limits its coverage of this topic to fairly straightforward reaction mechanisms, experimental data, and rate laws.

On the MCAT, experimental data for determining rate order is usually provided as a chart that includes the initial concentrations of the reactants and the initial rates of product formation as a function of the reactant concentrations. Often, the data for three or four trials are included in this chart.

To use this data, identify a pair of trials in which the concentration of one of the reactants is changed while the concentrations of all other reactants remain constant. Under these conditions, any change in the rate of product formation from one trial to the other (*if* there is any change) is fully attributable to the change in concentration of that one reactant. Consider a reaction with two reactants, A and B, forming product C. Imagine two trials in which the concentration of A is constant, while the concentration of B doubles. If the rate of the formation of product C has subsequently quadrupled, then the exponent on [B] must be two. Why? Looking at the generic rate law (rate $= k[A]^x[B]^y$), the logic should look something like this: *Doubling [B] has resulted in a quadrupling of the rate, so to determine the order of the reaction, y, with respect to B, I need to calculate the exponent to which the number 2 must be raised to equal 4. Because* $2^y = 4$, $y = 2$.

The next step is to repeat this process for the other reactant, using data from a different pair of trials, making sure that the concentration of only the reactant we are trying to analyze is changed from one trial to the other while the concentrations of all other reactants remain the same. Once the orders of the reaction have been determined with respect to each reactant, we can write the complete rate law, replacing the exponents x and y with actual numbers. To determine the value of the rate constant k, plug in actual values from any one of the trials; pick whichever trial has the most arithmetically convenient numbers.

MCAT EXPERTISE

The testmakers love rate problems. Why? Because solving these questions requires a real understanding of proportionality and variable relationships. With practice, you'll be able to do these quickly in your head with minimal paper-and-pencil calculations. Remember to look for pairs of reaction trials in which the concentration of only one species changes while the others remain constant.

Example: Given the data below, find the rate law for the following reaction at 300 K:

$$A + B \rightarrow C + D$$

Trial	$[A]_{initial}$ (M)	$[B]_{initial}$ (M)	$rate_{initial}$ $\left(\frac{M}{s}\right)$
1	1.00	1.00	2.0
2	1.00	2.00	8.1
3	2.00	2.00	15.9

Solution: First, look for two trials in which the concentrations of all but one of the substances are held constant.

In Trials 1 and 2, the concentration of A is kept constant, while the concentration of B is doubled. The rate increases by a factor of approximately 4. Since k and [A] are constant between the two trials, the rate is proportional to [B] raised to some power (the symbol $\propto$ means "is proportional to"):

$$\text{rate} = k[A]^x[B]^y \xrightarrow{k \text{ and } [A] \text{ are constant}} \text{rate} \propto [B]^y$$

Specifically, the relationship between the change in rate and the change in concentration of B can be written as: $\Delta \text{ rate} = \Delta[B]^y$. For this specific set of data, the proportionality becomes: $4 = [2]^y$.

In other words, since the rate was multiplied by 4, and [B] was multiplied by 2, y must be equal to 2. Based on what is known so far, the rate law becomes $\text{rate} = k[A]^x[B]^2$.

In Trials 2 and 3, the concentration of B is kept constant, while the concentration of A is doubled. The rate increases by a factor of approximately 2. Since k and [B] are constant between the two trials, rate is proportional to [A] raised to some power:

$$\text{rate} = k[A]^x[B]^2 \xrightarrow{k \text{ and } [B] \text{ are constant}} \text{rate} \propto [A]^x$$

The relationship between the change in rate and the change in concentration of B can be written as: $\Delta\text{rate} = \Delta[\text{A}]^x$. For this specific set of data, the proportionality becomes: $2 = [2]^x$.

In other words, since the rate was multiplied by 2, and [A] was multiplied by 2, x must be equal to 1.

Therefore, rate $= k[\text{A}]^1[\text{B}]^2$, more typically written as rate $= k[\text{A}][\text{B}]^2$ as raising a value to the first power is equivalent to the value (e.g., $2^1 = 2$). The order of the reaction is 1 with respect to A and 2 with respect to B; the overall reaction order is thus $1 + 2 = 3$.

To calculate k, substitute the values from any one of the trials into the rate law. In this case, trial 1 is chosen because the numbers are straightforward to manipulate:

$$\text{rate} = k[\text{A}][\text{B}]^2$$
$$2.0\,\frac{M}{\text{s}} = k[1.00\,M][1.00\,M]^2$$
$$k = 2.0\,M^{-2}\,\text{s}^{-1}$$

Therefore, the final rate law is rate $= 2.0\,M^{-2}\,\text{s}^{-1}\,[\text{A}][\text{B}]^2$.

Reaction Orders

We classify chemical reactions as zero-order, first-order, second-order, higher-order, or mixed-order on the basis of kinetics. We will continue to consider the generic reaction $a\text{A} + b\text{B} \rightarrow c\text{C} + d\text{D}$ for this discussion.

Zero-Order Reaction

A **zero-order reaction** is one in which the rate of formation of product C is independent of changes in concentrations of any of the reactants, A and B. These reactions have a constant reaction rate equal to the rate constant (rate coefficient), k. The rate law for a zero-order reaction is:

$$\text{rate} = k[\text{A}]^0[\text{B}]^0 = k$$

where k has units of $\frac{M}{\text{s}}$. Remember that the rate constant itself is dependent on temperature; thus, it is possible to change the rate for a zero-order reaction by changing the temperature. The only other way to change the rate of a zero-order reaction is by the addition of a catalyst, which lowers the activation energy, thereby increasing the value of k.

Plotting a zero-order reaction on a concentration *vs.* time curve results in a linear graph, as shown in Figure 5.8. This line shows that the rate of formation of product is independent of the concentration of reactant. The slope of such a line is the opposite of the rate constant, k.

MCAT EXPERTISE

Temperature and the addition of a catalyst are the only factors that can change the rate of a zero-order reaction.

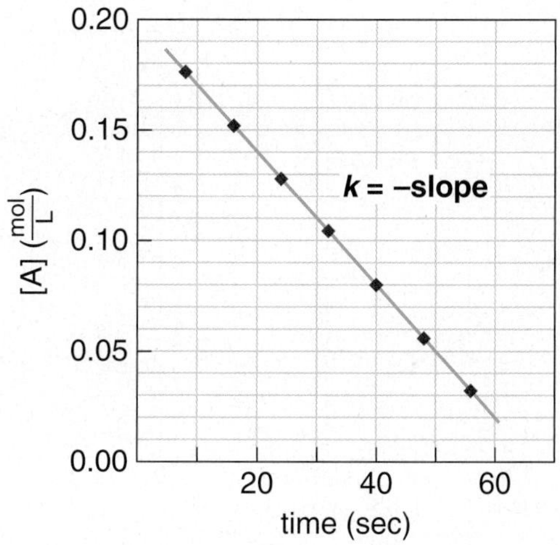

Figure 5.8 Kinetics of a Zero-Order Reaction
Note that the rate of reaction, k, is the opposite of the slope.

First-Order Reaction

A **first-order reaction** has a rate that is directly proportional to only one reactant, such that doubling the concentration of that reactant results in a doubling of the rate of formation of the product. The rate law for a first-order reaction is

$$\text{rate} = k[\text{A}]^1 \text{ or rate} = k[\text{B}]^1$$

where k has units of s^{-1}. A classic example of a first-order reaction is the process of radioactive decay. From the rate law, in which the rate of decrease of the amount of a radioactive isotope A is proportional to the amount of A:

$$\text{rate} = -\frac{\Delta[\text{A}]}{\Delta t} = k[\text{A}]$$

The concentration of radioactive substance A at any time t can be expressed mathematically as:

$$[\text{A}]_t = [\text{A}]_0 e^{-kt}$$

Equation 5.5

where $[\text{A}]_t$ is the concentration of A at time t, $[\text{A}]_0$ is the initial concentration of A, k is the rate constant, and t is time. It is important to recognize that a first-order rate law with a single reactant suggests that the reaction begins when the molecule undergoes a chemical change all by itself, without a chemical interaction, and usually without a physical interaction with any other molecule.

Plotting a first-order reaction on a concentration *vs.* time curve results in a nonlinear graph, as shown in Figure 5.9. This curve shows that the rate of formation of product is dependent on the concentration of reactant. Plotting ln [A] *vs.* time reveals a straight line; the slope of such a line is the opposite of the rate constant, *k*.

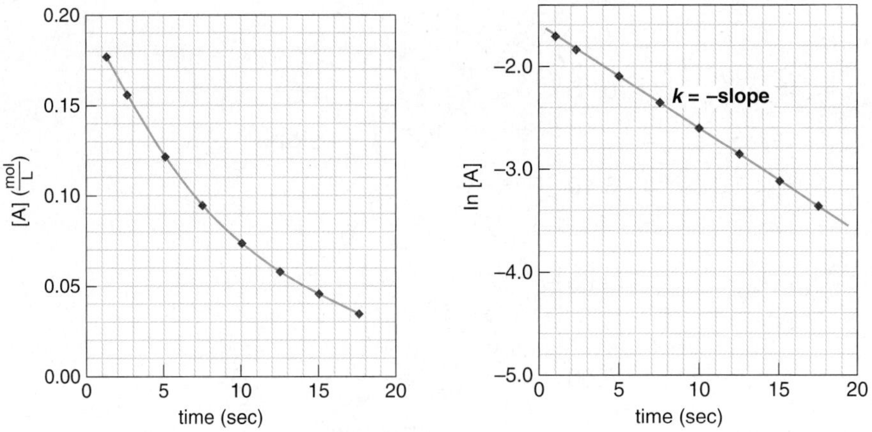

Figure 5.9 Kinetics of a First-Order Reaction
On the left, note that the rate of reaction is dependent on reactant concentration; on the right, note that the rate constant is the opposite of the slope of a graph of ln [A] vs. time.

Second-Order Reaction

A **second-order reaction** has a rate that is proportional to either the concentrations of two reactants or to the square of the concentration of a single reactant. The following rate laws all reflect second-order reactions:

$$\text{rate} = k[\text{A}]^1[\text{B}]^1 \text{ or rate} = k[\text{A}]^2 \text{ or rate} = k[\text{B}]^2$$

where *k* has units of $M^{-1}\text{ s}^{-1}$. It is important to recognize that a second-order rate law often suggests a physical collision between two reactant molecules, especially if the rate law is first-order with respect to each of the two reactants.

Plotting a reaction that is second-order with respect to a single reactant on a concentration *vs.* time curve results in a nonlinear graph, as shown in Figure 5.10. This curve shows that the rate of formation of product is dependent on the concentration of reactant. Plotting $\frac{1}{[\text{A}]}$ *vs.* time reveals a linear curve; the slope of such a curve is equal to the rate constant, *k*.

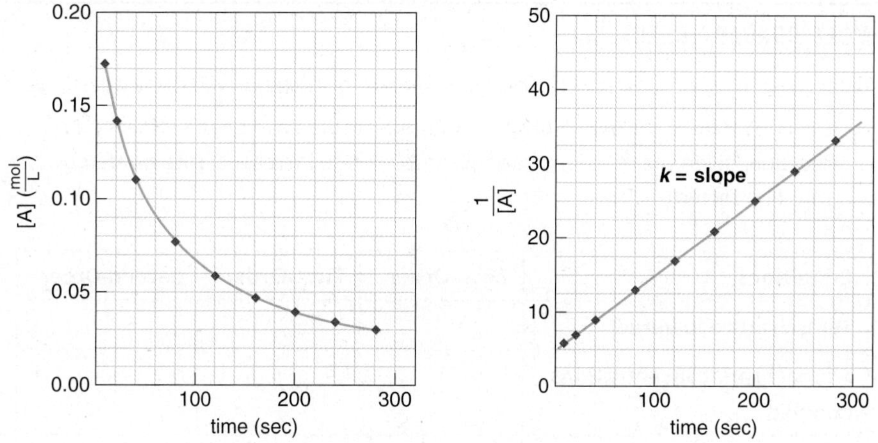

Figure 5.10 Kinetics of a Second-Order Reaction
On the left, note that the rate of reaction is dependent on reactant concentration; on the right, note that the rate constant is equal to the slope of a graph of $\frac{1}{[A]}$ vs. time.

Higher-Order Reactions

Fortunately, there are very few noteworthy reactions in which a single reaction step involves a termolecular process; in other words, there are few processes with third-order rates. This is because it is far more rare for three particles to collide simultaneously with the correct orientation and sufficient energy to undergo a reaction.

Mixed-Order Reactions

Mixed-order reactions sometimes refer to non-integer orders (fractions) and in other cases to reactions with rate orders that vary over the course of the reaction. Fractions are more specifically described as **broken-order**. In recent times, the term mixed-order has come to refer solely to reactions that change order over time. Knowing those two definitions will be sufficient for Test Day.

An example of a mixed-order rate law is given by:

$$\text{rate} = \frac{k_1[\text{C}][\text{A}]^2}{k_2 + k_3[\text{A}]}$$

where A represents a single reactant and C, a catalyst. The overall reaction and its mechanism are beyond the relevance and scope of the MCAT, and the derivation of this rate law is even more unnecessary for Test Day; however, understanding what is implied by this equation is important. The result of the large value for [A] at the beginning of the reaction is that $k_3[\text{A}] \gg k_2$, and the reaction will appear to be first-order with respect to A. (Note: The symbol "$\gg$" means "much-greater-than", implying, in this context, that the contribution of k_2 to the denominator "$k_2 + [\text{A}]k_3$" is negligible.) At the end of the reaction, when [A] is low, $k_2 \gg k_3[\text{A}]$, making the reaction appear second-order with respect to A. While the MCAT will not ask you to derive a rate expression for a mixed-order reaction, you are responsible for being able to recognize how the rate order changes as the reactant concentration changes.

MCAT CONCEPT CHECK 5.2

Before you move on, assess your understanding of the material with these questions.

1. Describe the effects the following conditions would have on the initial rate of reaction, given the reaction order: (Examples: rate increased, rate divided by 2, rate unaffected)

Conditions	Zero-Order	First-Order	Second-Order
Temperature lowered			
All reactants' concentrations doubled			
Catalyst added			

2. Determine the rate law and rate order for the following reaction:

$$A + B + C \rightarrow D$$

Trial	$[A]_{initial}$ (M)	$[B]_{initial}$ (M)	$[C]_{initial}$ (M)	$rate_{initial}$ $\left(\frac{M}{s}\right)$
1	1.00	1.00	1.00	2.0
2	1.00	2.00	1.00	2.1
3	2.00	1.00	1.00	15.9
4	2.00	1.00	2.00	32.2

Conclusion

We began with a consideration of chemical reactions and the mechanisms that illustrate the individual steps necessary to transform reactants into products. We demonstrated the way to derive a reaction's rate law through the analysis of experimental data, and we looked at the factors that can affect the rates of chemical reactions.

After such an overview, you should begin to appreciate that many chemical principles in the human body rely on the principles of chemical kinetics. Why does the body maintain a certain temperature? Primarily to stabilize the enzymes that catalyze the metabolic reactions necessary for life. Why does the body maintain a pH buffer? Altering the concentration of protons affects not only the ability of an enzyme to maintain its secondary, tertiary, and quaternary structure, but can also directly affect the collisions between reactants. You will begin to appreciate these and many other questions from a clinical perspective throughout your medical career. In the next chapter, we will investigate chemical equilibria, which—although related to kinetics—are distinct (and commonly confused!) topics.

You've reviewed the content, now test your knowledge and critical thinking skills by completing a test-like passage set in your online resources!

GO ONLINE

CONCEPT SUMMARY

Chemical Kinetics

- The change in **Gibbs free energy** (ΔG) determines whether or not a reaction is spontaneous.
- **Chemical mechanisms** propose a series of steps that make up the overall reaction.
  - **Intermediates** are molecules that exist within the course of a reaction but are neither reactants nor products overall.
  - The slowest step, also known as the **rate-determining step**, limits the maximum rate at which the reaction can proceed.
- The **collision theory** states that a reaction rate is proportional to the number of effective collisions between the reacting molecules.
  - For a collision to be effective, molecules must be in the proper orientation and have sufficient kinetic energy to exceed the **activation energy**.
  - The **Arrhenius equation** is a mathematical way of representing collision theory.
- The **transition state theory** states that molecules form a **transition state** or **activated complex** during a reaction in which the old bonds are partially dissociated and the new bonds are partially formed.
  - From the transition state, the reaction can proceed toward products or revert back to reactants.
  - The transition state is the highest point on a free energy reaction diagram.
- Reaction rates can be affected by a number of factors.
  - Increasing the concentration of reactant will increase reaction rate (except for zero-order reactions) because there are more effective collisions per time.
  - Increasing the temperature will increase reaction rate because the particles' kinetic energy is increased.
  - Changing the medium can increase or decrease reaction rate, depending on how the reactants interact with the medium.
  - Adding a catalyst increases reaction rate because it lowers the activation energy. **Homogeneous catalysts** are the same phase as the reactants; **heterogeneous catalysts** are a different phase.

Reaction Rates

- Reaction rates are measured in terms of the rate of disappearance of a reactant or appearance of a product.
- **Rate laws** take the form of rate $= k[A]^x[B]^y$.
  - The **rate orders** usually do not match the stoichiometric coefficients.
  - Rate laws must be determined from experimental data.

- The rate order of a reaction is the sum of all individual rate orders in the rate law.
- **Zero-order reactions** have a constant rate that does not depend on the concentration of reactant.
  - The rate of a zero-order reaction can only be affected by changing the temperature or adding a catalyst.
  - A concentration *vs.* time curve of a zero-order reaction is a straight line; the slope of such a line is equal to $-k$.
- **First-order reactions** have a nonconstant rate that depends on the concentration of reactant.
  - A concentration *vs.* time curve of a first-order reaction is nonlinear.
  - The slope of a ln [A] *vs.* time plot is $-k$ for a first-order reaction.
- **Second-order reactions** have a nonconstant rate that depends on the concentration of reactant.
  - A concentration *vs.* time curve of a second-order reaction is nonlinear.
  - The slope of a $\frac{1}{[A]}$ *vs.* time plot is k for a second-order reaction.
- **Broken-order reactions** are those with noninteger orders.
- **Mixed-order reactions** are those that have a rate order that changes over time.

ANSWERS TO CONCEPT CHECKS

5.1

1. Two molecules of A_2B come together in a combination reaction to form an intermediate, A_4B_2, which subsequently decomposes to produce the final products, two molecules of A_2 and one molecule of B_2.
2. The rate-determining step is the slowest step of a reaction. It determines the overall rate of the reaction because the reaction can only proceed as fast as the rate at which this step occurs.
3. The activation energy is the minimum energy needed for a chemical reaction to occur.
4. Both theories require a certain activation energy to be overcome in order for a reaction to occur (therefore not all reactions will occur). The transition state theory focuses on forming a high-energy activated complex that can then proceed forward or backward, forming the products or reverting to the reactants, respectively. The collision theory focuses on the energy and orientation of reactants, and considers each potential reaction to be "all-or-nothing" (either there is enough energy to form the products, or there is not).

5.2

1.

Conditions	Zero-Order	First-Order	Second-Order
Temperature lowered	rate decreased	rate decreased	rate decreased
All reactants' concentrations doubled	rate unaffected	rate doubled	rate multiplied by 4
Catalyst added	rate increased	rate increased	rate increased

2. This question asks for the rate law and rate order for the following reaction:

$$A + B + C \rightarrow D$$

Trial	$[A]_{initial}$ (M)	$[B]_{initial}$ (M)	$[C]_{initial}$ (M)	$rate_{initial}$ $\left(\frac{M}{s}\right)$
1	1.00	1.00	1.00	2.0
2	1.00	2.00	1.00	2.1
3	2.00	1.00	1.00	15.9
4	2.00	1.00	2.00	32.2

Start by writing the generic rate law for the reaction: rate $= k[A]^x[B]^y[C]^z$.

In a complex rate law problem, always check for the possibility of a reagent that has no impact on the rate law. Looking at Trials 1 and 2, the concentration of B is doubled with no change in the rate. Thus, reagent B has no impact on the rate law, and its exponent is zero. The rate law can be updated to rate $= k[A]^x[B]^0[C]^z$.

Next, compare Trials 1 and 3. The concentration of A doubles, the concentrations of B and C remain constant, and the rate increases by a factor of approximately 8. This results in the proportionality $\Delta\text{rate} = \Delta[A]^x$, so $8 = 2^x$, giving $x = 3$. The rate law can now be updated to rate $= k[A]^3[B]^0[C]^z$.

Finally, compare Trials 3 and 4. The concentration of C doubles, the concentrations of A and B remain constant, and the rate approximately doubles. This results in the proportionality $\Delta\text{rate} = \Delta\,[C]^z$, so $2 = 2^z$, giving $z = 1$. The rate law can now be updated to rate $= k[A]^3[B]^0[C]^1$.

Thus, the final rate law is: rate $= k[A]^3[B]^0[C]^1 = k[A]^3[C]$. The rate order is $3 + 0 + 1 = 4$.

SCIENCE MASTERY ASSESSMENT EXPLANATIONS

1. **D**

Based on the information given in the question, the rate is first-order with respect to the concentration of the first reactant; when the concentration of that reactant doubles, the rate also doubles. Because the reaction is third-order, the sum of the exponents in the rate law must be equal to 3. Therefore, the reaction order with respect to the other reactant must be $3 - 1 = 2$. If the concentration of this second reactant is multiplied by $\frac{1}{2}$, the rate will be multiplied by $\left(\frac{1}{2}\right)^2 = \frac{1}{4}$.

2. **D**

Before you try to answer this question, you should draw a free energy diagram for the system.

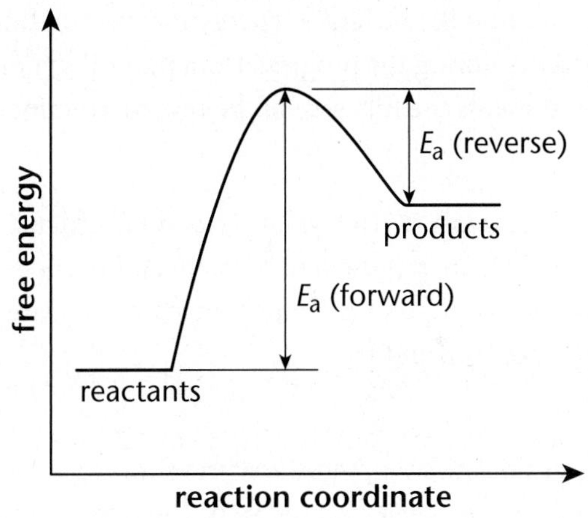

If the activation energy of the forward reaction is greater than the activation energy of the reverse reaction, then the products must have a higher free energy than the reactants. The overall energy of the system is higher at the end than it was in the beginning. The net free energy change is positive, indicating an endergonic (nonspontaneous) reaction. The terms endothermic, **(A)**, and exothermic, **(B)**, are associated with enthalpy. While free energy does depend on enthalpy, it also depends on entropy; there is not enough information in the question stem to reliably determine the sign of the entropy change of the reaction.

3. **D**

A second-order reaction can be second-order with respect to one reactant, or first-order with respect to two different reactants. In this case, one reactant was increased by a factor of 4. If the reaction is second-order with respect to this reactant, the rate law will be rate $= k[A]^2[B]^0$ and the rate will increase by a factor of 16. If it is first-order with respect to this reactant and first-order with respect to another reactant, the rate law will be rate $= k[A]^1[B]^1$, and the rate will increase by a factor of 4. We do not know which of these is the correct rate law and, thus, cannot determine the effect on the rate.

4. **A**

By definition, zero-order reactions are unaffected by the concentrations of any reactants in the reaction. Thus, changing the concentrations of these reactants will not affect the rate.

5. **D**

The question asks which alteration does NOT affect the rate of the reaction. Temperature directly affects the rate constant (k), making **(A)** incorrect. Changing the partial pressure of a gas will affect the number of effective collisions per time. This makes **(B)** incorrect—but note that concentration changes will not affect the rate of zero-order reactions. Solvents affect the rate of reactions depending on how the reactants interact with the solvent, making **(C)** incorrect. Removing the product of an irreversible reaction, **(D)**, should not affect the rate of the reaction because the rate law does not depend on the concentrations of products.

6. **D**

While increasing the concentration of reactants can alter the reaction rate in first- or higher-order reactions, saturated solutions containing a catalyst have a maximum turnover rate and cannot increase the rate constant or the reaction rate any higher by adding more reactant molecules.

7. **A**

If the sum of the exponents (orders) of the concentrations of each species in the rate law is equal to 2, then the reaction is second-order. The exponents in the rate law are unrelated to stoichiometric coefficients, so NO_2 and Br_2 could have any stoichiometric coefficients in the original reaction and still be a second-order reaction, invalidating statement II. Statement III is incorrect because the rate can be affected by a wide variety of compounds. A catalyst, for example, could increase the rate.

8. **C**

Start with the generic rate law: rate $= k[XH_4]^x[O_2]^y$. In the first two trials, the concentration of XH_4 is held constant while the concentration of O_2 is multiplied by 4, and the rate of the reaction also increases by a factor of approximately 4. This gives the proportion $\Delta\text{rate} = [O_2]^y$, or $4 = 4^y$, meaning $y = 1$. The rate law can be updated to: rate $= k[XH_4]^x[O_2]^1$.

In the last two trials, the concentration of O_2 is held constant while the concentration of XH_4 is doubled, and the rate of the reaction is increased by a factor of approximately 4. This gives $\Delta\text{rate} = [XH_4]^x$, or $4 = 2^x$, and $x = 2$. The rate law can be updated to: rate $= k[XH_4]^2[O_2]^1$. The final version of the rate law is: rate $= k[XH_4]^2[O_2]$.

9. **B**

By definition, a catalyst increases the rate of a reaction by lowering the activation energy, making it easier for both the forward and reverse reactions to overcome this energy barrier. Catalysts are neither used up in the reaction, nor do they alter the equilibrium of a reaction, eliminating **(A)** and **(C)**. Finally, catalysts stabilize the transition state by lowering its energy, not raising it, eliminating **(D)**.

10. **C**

The overall order of a reaction is the sum of the individual orders in the reaction. Therefore, the rate order is $0 + 2 + 1 = 3$.

11. **D**

A system is exergonic if energy is released by the reaction. For exergonic reactions, the net energy change is negative, and the free energy of the final products is lower than the free energy of the initial reactants. Point E, which represents the energy of the final products, is lower on the energy diagram than point A, which represents the energy of initial reactants. Thus, energy must have been given off, and the reaction is exergonic.

12. **B**

The activation energy of a reaction is represented by the distance on the *y*-axis from the energy of the reactants to the peak energy prior to formation of products. The activation energy of the first step of the forward reaction, for example, is equal to the distance along the *y*-axis from point A to point B. The largest energy increase on this graph occurs during the progress from point E to point D, which represents the first step of the reverse reaction.

13. **D**

Intermediates exist at "valleys" in reaction diagrams. Reactants, **(A)**, are represented by point A. Products, **(B)**, are represented by point E. Transition states, **(C)**, are represented by points B and D.

14. **D**

To answer this question, recall that the slow step of a reaction is the rate-determining step. The rate is always related to the concentrations of the reactants in the rate-determining step (*not* the overall reaction), so NO_2 is the only compound that should be included in the correct answer. The concentration of NO_2 is squared in the rate law because the question stem tells us that the system obeys second-order kinetics.

15. **D**

The faster a reaction can reach its activation energy, the faster it will proceed to completion. Because this question states that all conditions are equal, the reaction with the lowest activation energy will have the fastest rate. In the diagram, **(D)** has the lowest activation energy.

Consult your online resources for additional practice. GO ONLINE

EQUATIONS TO REMEMBER

(5.1) **Collision theory:** rate $= Z \times f$

(5.2) **Arrhenius equation:** $k = Ae^{\frac{-E_a}{RT}}$

(5.3) **Definition of rate:** rate $= -\frac{\Delta[A]}{a\Delta t} = -\frac{\Delta[B]}{b\Delta t} = \frac{\Delta[C]}{c\Delta t} = \frac{\Delta[D]}{d\Delta t}$

for the general reaction $aA + bB \rightarrow cC + dD$

(5.4) **Rate law:** rate $= k[A]^x[B]^y$

(5.5) **Radioactive decay:** $[A]_t = [A]_0e^{-kt}$

SHARED CONCEPTS

Biochemistry Chapter 2
Enzymes

General Chemistry Chapter 3
Bonding and Chemical Interactions

General Chemistry Chapter 6
Equilibrium

General Chemistry Chapter 7
Thermochemistry

Organic Chemistry Chapter 4
Analyzing Organic Reactions

Physics and Math Chapter 3
Thermodynamics

CHAPTER 6

EQUILIBRIUM

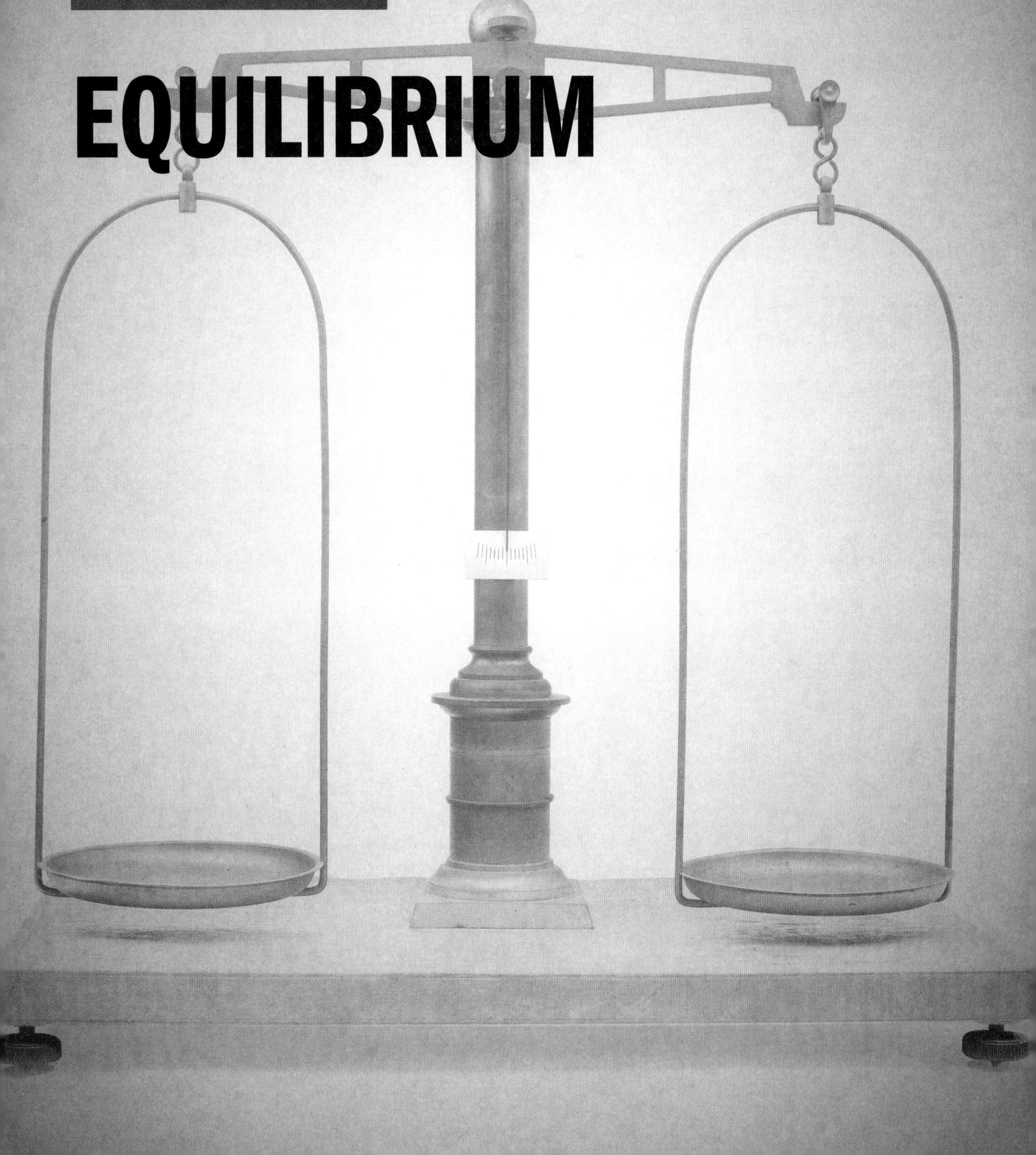

SCIENCE MASTERY ASSESSMENT

Every pre-med knows this feeling: there is so much content I have to know for the MCAT! How do I know what to do first or what's important?

While the high-yield badges throughout this book will help you identify the most important topics, this Science Mastery Assessment is another tool in your MCAT prep arsenal. This quiz (which can also be taken in your online resources) and the guidance below will help ensure that you are spending the appropriate amount of time on this chapter based on your personal strengths and weaknesses. Don't worry though—skipping something now does not mean you'll never study it. Later on in your prep, as you complete full-length tests, you'll uncover specific pieces of content that you need to review and can come back to these chapters as appropriate.

How to Use This Assessment

If you answer 0–7 questions correctly:

Spend about 1 hour to read this chapter in full and take limited notes throughout. Follow up by reviewing **all** quiz questions to ensure that you now understand how to solve each one.

If you answer 8–11 questions correctly:

Spend 20–40 minutes reviewing the quiz questions. Beginning with the questions you missed, read and take notes on the corresponding subchapters. For questions you answered correctly, ensure your thinking matches that of the explanation and you understand why each choice was correct or incorrect.

If you answer 12–15 questions correctly:

Spend less than 20 minutes reviewing all questions from the quiz. If you missed any, then include a quick read-through of the corresponding subchapters, or even just the relevant content within a subchapter, as part of your question review. For questions you answered correctly, ensure your thinking matches that of the explanation and review the Concept Summary at the end of the chapter.

1. A reaction is found to stop just before all reactants are converted to products. Which of the following could be true about this reaction?
   - **A.** The reaction is irreversible, and the forward rate is greater than the reverse rate.
   - **B.** The reaction is irreversible, and the reverse rate is too large for products to form.
   - **C.** The reaction is reversible, and the forward rate is equal to the reverse rate.
   - **D.** The reaction is reversible, and the reverse rate is greater than the forward rate.

2. What is the equilibrium expression for the reaction $Cu_2SO_4\ (s) \rightleftharpoons 2\ Cu^+\ (aq) + SO_4^{2-}\ (aq)$?
   - **A.** $\frac{[Cu^+]^2[SO_4^{2-}]}{[Cu_2SO_4]}$
   - **B.** $\frac{2 \times [Cu^+][SO_4^{2-}]}{[Cu_2SO_4]}$
   - **C.** $[Cu^+][SO_4^{2-}]$
   - **D.** $[Cu^+]^2[SO_4^{2-}]$

3. Carbonated beverages are produced by dissolving carbon dioxide in water to produce carbonic acid:

   $$CO_2\ (g) + H_2O\ (l) \rightleftharpoons H_2CO_3\ (aq)$$

   When a bottle containing carbonated water is opened, the taste of the beverage gradually changes as the carbonation is lost. Which of the following statements best explains this phenomenon?
   - **A.** The change in pressure and volume causes the reaction to shift to the left, thereby decreasing the amount of aqueous carbonic acid.
   - **B.** The change in pressure and volume causes the reaction to shift to the right, thereby decreasing the amount of gaseous carbon dioxide.
   - **C.** Carbonic acid reacts with environmental oxygen and nitrogen.
   - **D.** Carbon dioxide reacts with environmental oxygen and nitrogen.

4. Which of the following best describes how to favor the production of the kinetic product over the thermodynamic product?
   - **A.** High temperature and short reaction time
   - **B.** Low temperature and short reaction time
   - **C.** High temperature and long reaction time
   - **D.** Low temperature and long reaction time

5. If $K_c \gg 1$:
   - **A.** the equilibrium mixture will favor products over reactants.
   - **B.** the equilibrium mixture will favor reactants over products.
   - **C.** the equilibrium concentrations of reactants and products are equal.
   - **D.** the reaction is essentially irreversible.

6. Acetic acid dissociates in solution according to the following equation:

   $$CH_3COOH \rightleftharpoons CH_3COO^- + H^+$$

   If sodium acetate is added to a solution of acetic acid in excess water, which of the following effects would be observed in the solution?
   - **A.** Decreased pH
   - **B.** Increased pH
   - **C.** Decreased pK_{eq} (pK_a)
   - **D.** Increased pK_{eq} (pK_a)

Questions 7 and 8 refer to the reaction below:

$$FeI\ (aq) + I_2\ (g) \rightarrow FeI_3\ (aq)$$

7. Which of the following would increase the formation of product?
   - **A.** Decreasing the volume of the container
   - **B.** Decreasing the pressure of the container
   - **C.** Increasing the volume of the container
   - **D.** Decreasing the volume of the container while maintaining a constant pressure

8. If this reaction were exothermic, what effect would decreasing the temperature have on the equilibrium?
   A. The forward reaction rate and the reverse reaction rate both increase.
   B. The forward reaction rate decreases while the reverse reaction rate increases.
   C. The forward reaction rate increases while the reverse reaction rate decreases.
   D. The forward reaction rate and the reverse reaction rate both decrease.

9. Which of the following actions does NOT affect the equilibrium position of a reaction?
   A. Adding or removing heat.
   B. Adding or removing a catalyst.
   C. Increasing or decreasing concentrations of reactants.
   D. Increasing or decreasing volumes of reactants.

10. In a sealed 1 L container, 1 mole of nitrogen gas reacts with 3 moles of hydrogen gas to form 0.05 moles of NH_3 at equilibrium. Which of the following is closest to the K_c of the reaction?
   A. 0.0001
   B. 0.001
   C. 0.01
   D. 0.1

11. Increasing temperature can alter the K_{eq} of a reaction. Why might increasing temperature indefinitely be unfavorable for changing reaction conditions?
   A. The equilibrium constant has a definite limit that cannot be surpassed.
   B. The products or reactants can decompose at high temperatures.
   C. Increasing temperature would decrease pressure, which may or may not alter reaction conditions.
   D. If a reaction is irreversible, its K_{eq} will resist changes in temperature.

12. How does the change in free energy compare between the kinetic and thermodynamic product?
   A. The free energy change for the kinetic product is greater since it is less stable.
   B. The free energy change for the kinetic product is greater since it is more stable.
   C. The free energy change for the thermodynamic product is greater since it is less stable.
   D. The free energy change for the thermodynamic product is greater since it is more stable.

13. Compound A has a K_a (equilibrium constant of acid dissociation) of approximately 10^{-4}. Which of the following compounds is most likely to react with a solution of compound A?
   A. HNO_3
   B. NO_2
   C. NH_3
   D. N_2O_5

14. Consider the following two reactions:

$$3\text{ A} + 2\text{ B} \rightleftharpoons 3\text{ C} + 4\text{ D (Reaction 1)}$$

$$4\text{ D} + 3\text{ C} \rightleftharpoons 3\text{ A} + 2\text{ B (Reaction 2)}$$

If K_{eq} for reaction 1 is equal to 0.1, what is K_{eq} for reaction 2?
   A. 0.1
   B. 1
   C. 10
   D. 100

15. Which of the following statements best describes the effect of lowering the temperature of the following reaction?

$$\text{A} + \text{B} \rightleftharpoons \text{C} + \text{D} \qquad \Delta H = -1.12\,\frac{\text{kJ}}{\text{mol}}$$

   A. [C] and [D] would increase.
   B. [A] and [B] would increase.
   C. ΔH would increase.
   D. ΔH would decrease.

Answer Key

1. **C**
2. **D**
3. **A**
4. **B**
5. **A**
6. **B**
7. **A**
8. **C**
9. **B**
10. **A**
11. **B**
12. **D**
13. **C**
14. **C**
15. **A**

Detailed explanations can be found at the end of the chapter.

CHAPTER 6

EQUILIBRIUM

In This Chapter

CHAPTER PROFILE

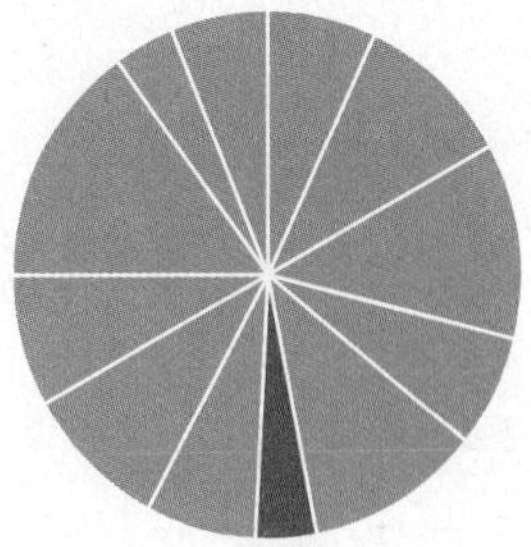

The content in this chapter should be relevant to about 4% of all questions about general chemistry on the MCAT.

This chapter covers material from the following AAMC content categories:

1D: Principles of bioenergetics and fuel molecule metabolism

5A: Unique nature of water and its solutions

5E: Principles of chemical thermodynamics and kinetics

Introduction

You're on the first call of your pediatrics rotation. You get a page: *Come to the emergency room, now*, the resident says. *They just brought in a kid with DKA*. DKA, as you know, stands for diabetic ketoacidosis and is a fairly common way for undiagnosed type I diabetes mellitus to present. You remember from your second-year classes about endocrine pathophysiology that ketoacidosis can arise as a result of the body's metabolism of fatty acids when insulin production shuts down. Fatty acids are metabolized into ketone bodies as an alternative energy source to glucose. Some of the ketones produced are ketoacids, and as the diabetic crisis continues and worsens, the concentration of these ketoacids increases (termed metabolic acidosis), resulting in a plasma pH below 7.35.

As you enter the child's room, the examination is already under way; the child is young, about ten years old, conscious but agitated, and the most obvious sign—which you notice immediately—is rapid, shallow breathing. You ask why the child is hyperventilating, and the resident takes a piece of paper and writes the following:

$$CO_2\ (g) + H_2O\ (l) \rightleftharpoons H_2CO_3\ (aq) \rightleftharpoons H^+\ (aq) + HCO_3^-\ (aq)$$

The child's breathing begins to slow and realization dawns on you. *It's Le Châtelier's principle! The respiratory system is trying to compensate for the metabolic acidosis; the increased breathing rate allows the child to blow off more CO_2, which causes the equilibrium to shift to the left. Hydrogen ions combine with bicarbonate ions to produce carbonic acid, which decomposes into CO_2 gas that's expelled from the lungs. The result*

MCAT EXPERTISE

The AAMC has shown that it will only rarely directly test the details of equilibrium in this chapter. However, you'll need an excellent conceptual understanding of equilibrium to master many other high-yield topics, such as acid-base chemistry (Chapter 10 of *MCAT General Chemistry Review*) and enzymes (Chapter 2 of *MCAT Biochemistry Review*).

is a decrease in the plasma hydrogen ion concentration, which stabilizes the pH and keeps it from getting too low. Wow, chemistry really is essential for medical school!

Chemical equilibrium is the dynamic state of a chemical reaction in which the concentrations of reactants and products stabilize over time in a low-energy configuration. Pay particular attention to the concepts of chemical equilibrium because we will return to these topics during our review of solutions, acid–base chemistry, and oxidation–reduction reactions.

6.1 Equilibrium

LEARNING OBJECTIVES

After Chapter 6.1, you will be able to:

- Determine the sign of ΔG and the direction of a reaction given its K_{eq} constant
- Calculate K_{eq} for a reaction
- Write the equilibrium constant expression for a reaction:
  $$3\,H_2\,(g) + N_2\,(g) \rightleftharpoons 2\,NH_3\,(g)$$

In the previous chapter, we danced around the term *equilibrium*. We warned you not to confuse the chemical equilibrium expression for the rate expression. We stressed that catalysts make reactions go faster toward their equilibrium position, but that they can't actually change the equilibrium position or alter the value of K_{eq}. The principles and concepts that are the focus of this chapter will direct our discussion in the upcoming chapters about some of the most important general chemistry topics for the MCAT: solutions, acids and bases, and oxidation–reduction reactions.

Dynamic Equilibria and Reversibility

So far, most of the reactions we've covered are **irreversible**; that is, the reaction proceeds in one direction only, the reaction goes to completion, and the maximum amount of product formed is determined by the amount of limiting reagent initially present. **Reversible** reactions are those in which the reaction can proceed in one of two ways: forward (toward the products or "to the right") and reverse (toward the reactants or "to the left"). Reversible reactions usually do not proceed to completion because the products can react together to reform the reactants. When the reaction system is closed and no reactants or products are added or removed, the system will eventually settle into a state in which the rate of the forward reaction equals the rate of the reverse reaction and the concentrations of the products and reactants remain constant. In this **dynamic equilibrium**, the forward and reverse reactions are still occurring—they haven't stopped, as they do in a **static equilibrium**—but they are going at the same rate; thus, there is no net change in the concentrations of the products or reactants, as shown in Figure 6.1.

BRIDGE

Many biochemical reactions can be classified as reversible, and their activation energies are lowered by enzymes. Irreversible biochemical steps are sometimes termed "committed" because they cannot be reversed in their pathways. These steps also tend to be the rate-limiting steps of metabolic pathways, which are discussed in Chapters 9 through 11 of *MCAT Biochemistry Review.*

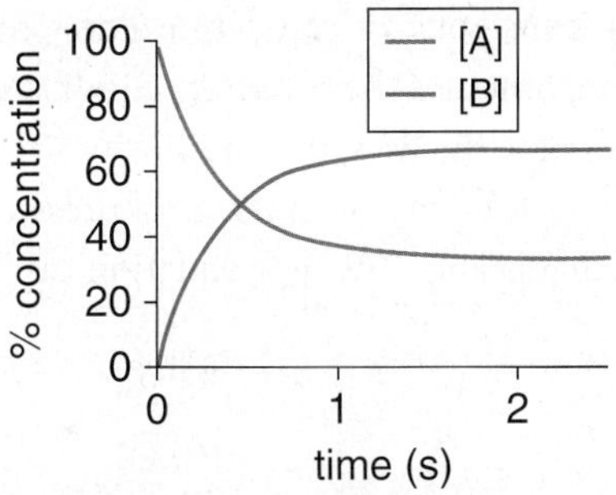

Figure 6.1 Dynamic Equilibrium Occurs when Forward and Reverse Rates Are Equal

Consider the generic reversible reaction illustrated in Figure 6.1:

$$A \rightleftharpoons B$$

At equilibrium, the concentrations of A and B are constant (although not necessarily equal), and the reactions A → B and B → A continue to occur at equal rates.

Equilibrium can be thought of as a balance between the forward and reverse reactions. Better still, equilibrium should be understood on the basis of **entropy**, which is the measure of the distribution of energy throughout a system or between a system and its environment. For a reversible reaction at a given temperature, the reaction will reach equilibrium when the system's entropy—or energy distribution—is at a maximum and the Gibbs free energy of the system is at a minimum.

BRIDGE

In Chapter 7 of *MCAT General Chemistry Review*, we will explore the more "classic" MCAT definition of entropy—a measure of the disorder of a system. It is important to realize, though, that the units of entropy $\left(\frac{J}{K \cdot mol}\right)$ imply a distribution of energy in a system.

Law of Mass Action

For a generic reversible reaction $aA + bB \rightleftharpoons cC + dD$, the **law of mass action** states that, if the system is at equilibrium at a constant temperature, then the following ratio is constant:

$$K_{eq} = \frac{[C]^c[D]^d}{[A]^a[B]^b}$$

Equation 6.1

KEY CONCEPT

At equilibrium, the rate of the forward reaction equals the rate of the reverse reaction, entropy is at a maximum, and Gibbs free energy is at a minimum. This links the concepts of thermodynamics and kinetics.

The law of mass action is actually related to the expressions for the rates of the forward and reverse reactions. Consider the following one-step reversible reaction:

$$2\,A \rightleftharpoons B + C$$

Because the reaction occurs in one step, the rates of the forward and reverse reactions are given by:

$$\text{rate}_f = k_f[A]^2 \text{ and } \text{rate}_r = k_r[B][C]$$

When $\text{rate}_f = \text{rate}_r$, the system is in equilibrium. Because the rates are equal, we can set the rate expressions for the forward and reverse reactions equal to each other:

$$k_f[A]^2 = k_r[B][C] \rightarrow \frac{k_f}{k_r} = \frac{[B][C]}{[A]^2}$$

Because k_f and k_r are both constants, we can define a new constant K_c, where K_c is called the **equilibrium constant** and the subscript c indicates that it is in terms of concentration. When dealing with gases, the equilibrium constant is referred to as K_p, and the subscript p indicates that it is in terms of pressure. For dilute solutions, K_c and K_{eq} are used interchangeably. The new equation can thus be written:

KEY CONCEPT

For most purposes, you will not need to distinguish between different *K* values. For dilute solutions, $K_{eq} = K_c$ and both are calculated in units of concentration.

$$K_c = K_{eq} = \frac{[B][C]}{[A]^2}$$

While the forward and the reverse reaction rates are equal at equilibrium, the concentrations of the reactants and products are not usually equal. This means that the forward and reverse reaction rate constants, k_f and k_r, respectively, are not usually equal to each other. The ratio of k_f to k_r is K_c:

$$K_c = K_{eq} = \frac{k_f}{k_r}$$

KEY CONCEPT

Remember the warning in Chapter 5 of *MCAT General Chemistry Review* about confusing equilibrium expressions and rate laws? In equilibrium expressions, the exponents are equal to the coefficients in the balanced equation. In rate laws, the exponents must be determined experimentally and often do not equal the stoichiometric coefficients.

When a reaction occurs in more than one step, the equilibrium constant for the overall reaction is found by multiplying together the equilibrium constants for each step of the reaction. When this is done, the equilibrium constant for the overall reaction is equal to the concentrations of the products divided by the concentrations of the reactants in the overall reaction, with each concentration term raised to the stoichiometric coefficient for the respective species. The forward and reverse rate constants for the *n*th step are designated k_n and k_{-n}, respectively. For example, if the reaction $aA + bB \rightleftharpoons cC + dD$ occurs in three steps, each with a forward and reverse rate, then:

$$K_c = \frac{k_1 k_2 k_3}{k_{-1} k_{-2} k_{-3}} = \frac{[C]^c [D]^d}{[A]^a [B]^b}$$

Example: What is the expression for the equilibrium constant for the following reaction?

$$3\ H_2\ (g) + N_2\ (g) \rightleftharpoons 2\ NH_3\ (g)$$

Solution:

$K_c = K_{eq} = \frac{[NH_3]^2}{[H_2]^3[N_2]}$. The K_p of this reaction would be: $\frac{(P_{NH_3})^2}{(P_{H_2})^3 \times P_{N_2}}$

Reaction Quotient

The law of mass action defines the position of equilibrium; however, equilibrium is a state that is only achieved through time. Depending on the actual rates of the forward and reverse reactions, equilibrium might be achieved in microseconds or millennia. What can serve as a "timer" to indicate how far the reaction has proceeded toward equilibrium? This role is served by the **reaction quotient, *Q***. At any point in time during a reaction, we can measure the concentrations of all of the reactants and products and calculate the reaction quotient according to the following equation:

$$Q_c = \frac{[C]^c[D]^d}{[A]^a[B]^b}$$

Equation 6.2

This equation looks identical to the equation for K_{eq}. It is the same form, but the information it provides is quite different. While the concentrations used for the law of mass action are equilibrium (constant) concentrations, the concentrations of the reactants and products are not constant when calculating a value for Q of a reaction. Thus, the utility of Q is not the value itself but rather the comparison that can be made between Q at any given moment in the reaction to the known K_{eq} for the reaction at a particular temperature. Le Châtelier's principle, which will be elaborated upon shortly, will then guide the reaction. For any reaction, if:

- $Q < K_{eq}$, then the forward reaction has not yet reached equilibrium.
  - There is a greater concentration of reactants (and smaller concentration of products) than at equilibrium.
  - The forward rate of reaction is increased to restore equilibrium.
- $Q = K_{eq}$, then the reaction is in dynamic equilibrium.
  - The reactants and products are present in equilibrium proportions.
  - The forward and reverse rates of reaction are equal.
- $Q > K_{eq}$, then the forward reaction has exceeded equilibrium.
  - There is a greater concentration of products (and smaller concentration of reactants) than at equilibrium.
  - The reverse rate of reaction is increased to restore equilibrium.

Any reaction that has not yet reached the equilibrium state, as indicated by $Q < K_{eq}$, will continue spontaneously in the forward direction (consuming reactants to form products) until the equilibrium ratio of reactants and products is reached. Any reaction in the equilibrium state will continue to react in the forward and reverse directions, but the reaction rates for the forward and reverse reactions will be equal, and the concentrations of the reactants and products will be constant, such that $Q = K_{eq}$. A reaction that is beyond the equilibrium state, as indicated by $Q > K_{eq}$, will proceed in the reverse direction (consuming products to form reactants) until the equilibrium ratio of reactants and products is reached again. Once a reaction is at equilibrium, any further movement in either the forward direction (resulting in an increase in products) or in the reverse direction (resulting in the reformation of reactants) will be nonspontaneous. This trend is illustrated in Figure 6.2.

KEY CONCEPT

- $Q < K_{eq}$: $\Delta G < 0$, reaction proceeds in forward direction
- $Q = K_{eq}$: $\Delta G = 0$, reaction is in dynamic equilibrium
- $Q > K_{eq}$, $\Delta G > 0$: reaction proceeds in reverse direction

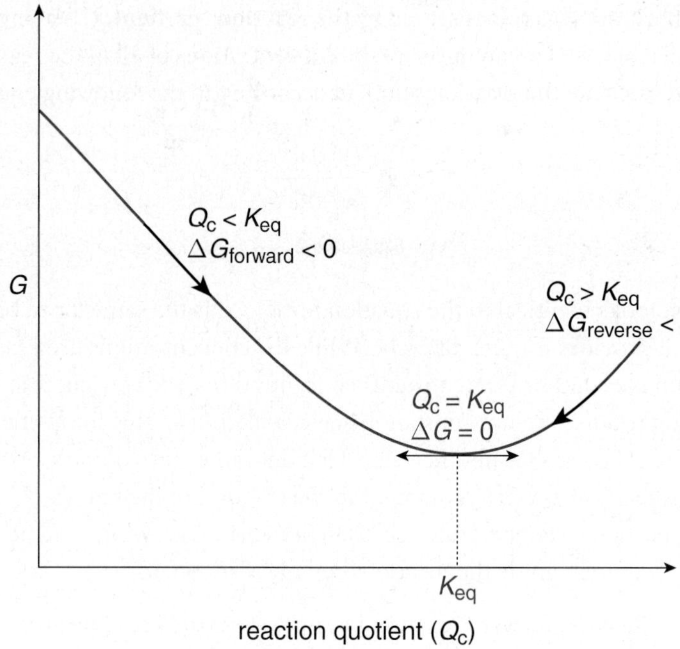

Figure 6.2 Gibbs Free Energy *vs.* Reaction Quotient

In Chapter 7 of *MCAT General Chemistry Review*, we'll further discuss how the spontaneity of these systems is related to enthalpy and entropy.

Properties of the Law of Mass Action

Make sure to remember the following characteristics of the law of mass action and equilibrium constant expressions:

- The concentrations of pure solids and pure liquids do not appear in the equilibrium constant expression. This is because the equilibrium expression is technically based on the activities of compounds, not concentrations; the activities of pure solids and liquids are defined to be 1. For the purposes of the MCAT, there is a negligible difference between concentration and activity.
- K_{eq} is characteristic of a particular reaction at a given temperature; the equilibrium constant is temperature-dependent.
- The larger the value of K_{eq}, the farther to the right the equilibrium position.
- If the equilibrium constant for a reaction written in one direction is K_{eq}, the equilibrium constant for the reverse reaction is $\frac{1}{K_{eq}}$.

Equilibrium Calculations

Calculations involving the equilibrium constant can take several forms but are also highly repetitive. Although we have discussed K_{eq} in this chapter, equilibrium constants and related calculations appear in solutions (K_{sp}), acids and bases (K_w, K_a, and K_b), and enzyme kinetics (K_d, K_b, and K_a). Thus, learning the "ins and outs" of equilibrium calculations has a large payoff on the MCAT.

One of the first concepts to grasp is the scale of the equilibrium constant. In an ideal situation, the concentrations of products and reactants would all be the same, and regardless of their actual concentrations would reduce to 1:1 ratios. In this case, K_{eq} would equal 1. In the real world, this situation doesn't exist, as it is unlikely that any reaction would have exactly equal concentrations of products and reactants at equilibrium. However, a K_{eq} of 1 can be a valuable reference point, given that $K_{eq} = \frac{[\text{products}]}{[\text{reactants}]}$.

If the concentration of products is greater than the concentration of reactants, K_{eq} becomes a "top heavy" fraction and must be greater than 1. On the other hand, if the concentration of reactants is greater than that of products, K_{eq} becomes a "bottom heavy" fraction and must be less than 1. Keep in mind, however, that K_{eq} is often expressed as a single value using exponents, and the sign and scale of these exponents gives even more information about the relative quantities of reactants and products. A reaction that strongly favors products will have a large, positive exponent, and the larger the exponent, the less reactant that will be present at equilibrium. In other words, a large positive exponent indicates a reaction that goes almost to completion.

On the other hand, a large negative exponent indicates a reaction that strongly favors reactants at equilibrium. In this case, only a small amount of reactant is converted to product. When performing equilibrium calculations, a K_{eq} with a large negative exponent allows a very convenient and very necessary shortcut to be used: the amount that has reacted can be considered negligible compared to the amount of reactant that remains.

Consider the reaction $A \leftrightarrow B + C$, with $K_{eq} = 10^{-12}$ and a starting concentration of $[A] = 1\ M$. The K_{eq} expression can be written as:

$$K_{eq} = \frac{[C][B]}{[A]}$$

If x amount of A has reacted, x amount of C and x amount of B have been produced at equilibrium, and the equilibrium concentration of A will be $[1 - x]\ M$. Substituting these values into the K_{eq} expression gives:

$$K_{eq} = 10^{-12} = \frac{(x)(x)}{(1-x)} = \frac{x^2}{1-x}$$

Unfortunately, performing the calculations required by this equation would give us a polynomial function that would be extremely burdensome to solve. However, the value of K_{eq} has a large negative exponent, allowing us to use the "x is negligible" shortcut. Relative to the 1 M starting concentration, the amount that has reacted is so small, based on $K_{eq} = 10^{-12}$, that we can assume x is negligible and round the denominator to the starting concentration:

$$10^{-12} = \frac{x^2}{1}$$

The problem is much more readily solved, and the value for x is found to be 10^{-6}. This confirms our estimate that x is negligible compared to 1, since $x = 0.000001$, and $[1 - (0.00001)] \approx 1$.

MCAT EXPERTISE

You may have been previously taught to solve these types of equilibrium problems using a technique referred to as an ICEbox. On Test Day, generating an entire ICEbox table takes valuable time and effort, and this technique can be shortcut using logic alone. Practice solving equilibrium problems without the ICEbox technique, using the methods described in this chapter, for a faster solution on Test Day.

BRIDGE

Equilibrium constants are calculated for many types of reactions, and go by many different names. For solubility problems (*MCAT General Chemistry Review* Chapter 9), K_{eq} is known as K_{sp}. For acids and bases (*MCAT General Chemistry Review* Chapter 10), K_{eq} is known as K_a, K_b, or K_w. For enzyme kinetics (*MCAT Biochemistry Review* Chapter 2), K_{eq} is known as K_d, K_b, or K_a.

If the value for K_{eq} is within one to two orders of magnitude of one, or if the concentration of reactant that goes to product is within two orders of magnitude of the initial concentration of reactant, this estimation will not be valid. Likewise, if the value of K_{eq} is significantly larger than one, this estimation cannot be used. In both cases, the amount that reacts will be significant compared to the starting concentration of reactant. However, these situations are unlikely to be tested on the MCAT.

Example: 3 moles of N_2O_4 is placed in a 0.5 L container and allowed to reach equilibrium according to the following reaction:

$$N_2O_4\ (g) \leftrightarrow 2\,NO_2\ (g)$$

What is the equilibrium concentration of NO_2, given K_{eq} for the reaction is 6×10^{-6}?

Solution: Start by writing the expression for K_{eq}: $K_{eq} = \frac{[NO_2]^2}{[N_2O_4]}$

Note that the concentration of NO_2 is squared due to its coefficient of 2 in the balanced reaction. Next, determine the starting concentration of N_2O_4, taking into account that the initial volume is 500 mL = 0.5 L: $\frac{3\ M}{0.5\ L} = \frac{[N_2O_4]}{1\ L}$

$$[N_2O_4] = \frac{(3)(1)}{(0.5)} = 6\ M$$

Thus, the starting concentration of $N_2O_4 = 6\ M$. Next, using x to represent the amount of N_2O_4 that reacts, $2x$ to represent the amount of NO_2 that is produced, and 10^{-6} for the value of K_{eq}, plug into the expression for the equilibrium constant:

$$K_{eq} = 6 \times 10^{-6} = \frac{[2x]^2}{[6 - x]} \approx \frac{[2x]^2}{[6]}$$

Note that the small negative exponent in the value of K_{eq} indicates that x will be negligible in comparison to 6 M, allowing the K_{eq} expression to be simplified, and x to be determined as follows:

$$6 \times 10^{-6} = \frac{4x^2}{6}$$

$$36 \times 10^{-6} = 4x^2$$

$$x^2 = \frac{36 \times 10^{-6}}{4} = 9 \times 10^{-6}$$

$$x = 3 \times 10^{-3}\ M$$

However, be careful to note that this is the value of x, which represents the amount of N_2O_4 that reacts. The final answer must represent the amount of NO_2 produced, which is twice the amount of N_2O_4 that reacts, or $2x$. Thus the final answer is the concentration of NO_2, which is $6 \times 10^{-3}\ M$.

MCAT CONCEPT CHECK 6.1

Before you move on, assess your understanding of the material with these questions.

1. Given that [product] = 0.075 *M* and [reactant] = 1.5 *M*, determine the direction of reaction and the sign of the free energy change for reactions with the following K_{eq} values: (Note: Assume that the reaction has only one product and one reactant, and that the stoichiometric coefficient for each is 1.)

K_{eq}	Direction of Reaction	ΔG
5.0×10^{-2}		
5.0×10^{-3}		
5.0×10^{-1}		

2. Write the equilibrium constant expression for the following reactions:

- $CO\ (g) + 2\ H_2\ (g) \rightleftharpoons CH_3OH\ (g)$:

____

- $H_3PO_4\ (aq) + H_2O\ (l) \rightleftharpoons H_2PO_4^-\ (aq) + H_3O^+\ (aq)$:

____

3. Consider the hypothetical reaction A $\leftrightarrow$ B + C.

   For each of the following, determine if the amount of reactant A that has converted to product at equilibrium will be negligible compared to the starting concentration of A.

K_{eq}	Initial Concentration of A (*M*)	Is the amount reacted negligible?
1.0×10^{-12}	1	
1.0×10^{-2}	0.1	
1.0×10^{-3}	0.001	
1.0×10^{-15}	0.001	

4. The following reaction has a K_{eq} of 2.1×10^{-7}. Given an initial concentration for A equal to 0.1 *M* and an initial concentration of B equal to 0.2 *M*, what is the equilibrium concentration of C? Is the approximation that *x* is negligible valid for this calculation?

$$A\ (aq) + B\ (aq) \leftrightarrow C\ (g) + D\ (s)$$

6.2 Le Châtelier's Principle

LEARNING OBJECTIVES

After Chapter 6.2, you will be able to:

- Use Le Châtelier's principle to determine how changing conditions, including pH, temperature, pressure, and concentration changes, will affect a reaction previously in equilibrium

MCAT EXPERTISE

Le Châtelier's principle applies to a wide variety of systems and, therefore, appears as a fundamental concept in all three MCAT science sections.

Le Châtelier's principle states that if a stress is applied to a system, the system shifts to relieve that applied stress. Regardless of the form the stress takes, the reaction is temporarily moved out of its equilibrium state. This is either because the concentrations or partial pressures of the system are no longer in the equilibrium ratio or because the equilibrium ratio itself has changed as a result of a change in the temperature of the system. The reaction then responds by reacting in whichever direction—either forward or reverse—will result in a reestablishment of the equilibrium state.

Changes in Concentration

BRIDGE

The bicarbonate buffer system is a classic example of Le Châtelier's principle applied to physiology:

$CO_2\ (g) + H_2O\ (l) \rightleftharpoons H_2CO_3\ (aq) \rightleftharpoons H^+\ (aq) + HCO_3^-\ (aq)$

In the tissues, there is a relatively high concentration of CO_2, and the reaction shifts to the right. In the lungs, CO_2 is lost, and the reaction shifts to the left. Note that blowing off CO_2 (hyperventilation) is used as a mechanism for dealing with acidemia (excess H^+ in the blood). This buffer system plays a key role in the respiratory, circulatory, and excretory systems, discussed in Chapters 6, 7, and 10 of *MCAT Biology Review*, respectively.

When reactants or products are added or removed from a reaction in equilibrium, the reaction is moved from its minimum energy state. With the change in concentration of one or more of the chemical species, the system now has a ratio of products to reactants that is not equal to the equilibrium ratio. In other words, changing the concentration of either a reactant or a product results in $Q_c \neq K_{eq}$. If reactants are added (or products are removed), $Q_c < K_{eq}$, and the reaction will spontaneously react in the forward direction, increasing the value of Q_c until $Q_c = K_{eq}$. If reactants are removed (or products are added), $Q_c > K_{eq}$, and the reaction will spontaneously react in the reverse direction, thereby decreasing the value of Q_c until once again $Q_c = K_{eq}$. Put simply, the system will always react in the direction away from the added species or toward the removed species.

We often take advantage of Le Châtelier's principle to improve the yield of chemical reactions. For example, in the industrial production of chemicals, products of reversible reactions are removed as they are formed to prevent the reactions from reaching their equilibrium states. The reaction will continue to react in the forward direction, producing more and more products—assuming reactants are continually replaced as they are consumed. One could also drive a reaction forward by starting with high concentrations of reactants. This will lead to an increase in the absolute quantities of products formed, although the reaction will still eventually reach its equilibrium state unless products are removed as they are formed.

Changes in Pressure (and Volume)

Because liquids and solids are essentially incompressible, only chemical reactions that involve at least one gaseous species will be affected by changes in the system's pressure and volume. When a system is compressed, its volume decreases and its total pressure increases. This increase in the total pressure is associated with an increase in the partial pressures of each gas in the system, and this results in the system no longer being in the equilibrium state, such that Q_p does not equal K_{eq}. The system will move forward or in reverse, always toward whichever side has the lower total number of moles of gas. This is a consequence of the ideal gas law, which tells us that there is a direct relationship between the number of moles of gas and the pressure of the gas. If one increases the pressure of a system, it will respond by decreasing the total number of gas moles, thereby decreasing the pressure. Note that this scenario assumes that the volume of the system was decreased and then held constant while the system returned to its equilibrium state. When one expands the volume of a system, the total pressure and the partial pressures decrease. The system is no longer in its equilibrium state and will react in the direction of the side with the greater number of moles of gas in order to restore the pressure.

Consider the following reaction:

$$N_2\ (g) + 3\ H_2\ (g) \rightleftharpoons 2\ NH_3\ (g)$$

The left side of the reaction has a total of four moles of gas molecules, while the right side has only two moles. When the pressure of this system is increased, the system will react in the direction that produces fewer moles of gas. In this case, that direction is to the right, and more ammonia will form. However, if the pressure is decreased, the system will react in the direction that produces more moles of gas; thus, the reverse reaction will be favored, and more nitrogen and hydrogen gas will reform.

Changes in Temperature

Le Châtelier's principle tells us that changing the temperature of a system will also cause the system to react in a particular way to return to its equilibrium state. However, unlike the effect of changing concentrations or pressures, the result of changing temperature is not a change in the reaction quotient, Q_c or Q_p, but a change in K_{eq}. The change in temperature does not cause the concentrations or partial pressures of the reactants and products to change immediately, so Q immediately after the temperature change is the same as before the temperature change. Thus, because K_{eq} is now a different value, Q no longer equals K_{eq}. The system has to move in whichever direction allows it to reach its new equilibrium state at the new temperature. That direction is determined by the enthalpy of the reaction. If a reaction is endothermic ($\Delta H > 0$), heat functions as a reactant; if a reaction is exothermic ($\Delta H < 0$), heat functions as a product. Thinking about heat as a reactant or product allows us to apply the same principles we used with concentration changes to temperature changes.

For example, consider the following endothermic reaction, shown in Figure 6.3:

$$N_2O_4\ (g) \overset{\Delta}{\rightleftharpoons} 2\ NO_2\ (g)$$

KEY CONCEPT

The reaction

A (*aq*) + 2 B (*g*) ⇌ C (*g*) + heat

Will shift to the right if...	Will shift to the left if...
A or B is added	C is added
C is removed	A or B is removed
the pressure is increased or the volume is reduced	the pressure is reduced or the volume is increased
the temperature is reduced	the temperature is increased

The equilibrium position can be shifted by changing the temperature. When heat is added and the temperature increases, the reaction shifts to the right, and the flask turns reddish-brown due to an increase in $[NO_2]$. When heat is removed and the temperature decreases, the reaction shifts to the left, and the flask turns more transparent due to an increase in N_2O_4. This demonstrates Le Châtelier's principle because the equilibrium shifts in the direction that consumes energy.

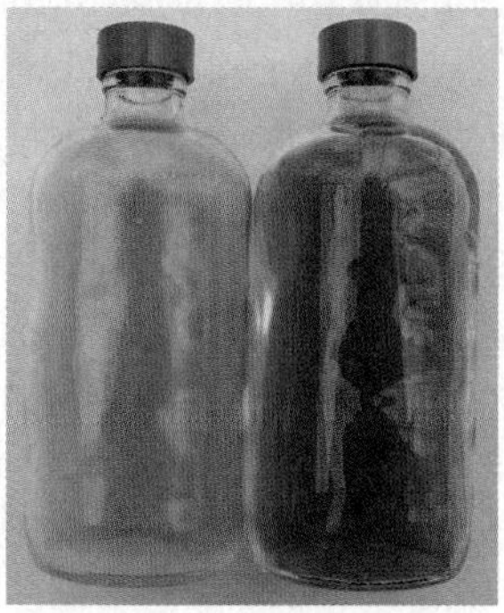

Figure 6.3 Example of a Reversible Endothermic Reaction, $N_2O_4\ (g) \rightleftharpoons 2\ NO_2\ (g)$
Left: As temperature decreases, the equilibrium favors N_2O_4 production, turning the reaction vessel more transparent. Right: As temperature increases, the equilibrium favors NO_2 production, turning the reaction vessel reddish-brown.

MCAT CONCEPT CHECK 6.2

Before you move on, assess your understanding of the material with this question.

1. Describe what would happen in the following situations:
   - In the reaction $H_2SO_4\ (aq) \rightleftharpoons H^+\ (aq) + HSO_4^-\ (aq)$, the pH has been increased:

   ____

   - In the reaction $2\ C\ (s) + O_2\ (g) \rightleftharpoons 2\ CO\ (g)$, the pressure of the reaction vessel is decreased:

   ____

   - In the reaction $CH_4\ (g) + 2\ O_2\ (g) \rightleftharpoons CO_2\ (g) + 2\ H_2O\ (l)$ + heat, the reaction vessel is warmed:

   ____

   - In the reaction $H_3PO_4\ (aq) + H_2O\ (l) \rightleftharpoons H_3O^+\ (aq) + H_2PO_4^-\ (aq)$, water is removed (without changing temperature):

   ____

6.3 Kinetic and Thermodynamic Control

LEARNING OBJECTIVES

After Chapter 6.3, you will be able to:

- Identify the conditions that will cause a reaction to favor the kinetic or the thermodynamic product
- Distinguish between a kinetic and thermodynamic pathway on a reaction coordinate diagram

Having covered the fundamentals of kinetics and thermodynamics, we come upon a topic that bridges all chemical systems: control of a reaction. In particular, biochemical reactions often require regulation in a precise manner to be useful to an organism. The applications of kinetic and thermodynamic control are common on the MCAT and range from metabolic reactions requiring high-energy phosphate molecules, such as ATP to the effects of temperature and solvents on enzyme activity.

The examples below consider unimolecular systems through the lens of the transition state theory. Figure 6.4 shows starting materials (reactants) at a certain energy level. These reactants can undergo two different sets of reactions. At lower temperatures (with smaller heat transfer), a **kinetic product** is formed. At higher temperatures (with larger heat transfer), a **thermodynamic product** is formed.

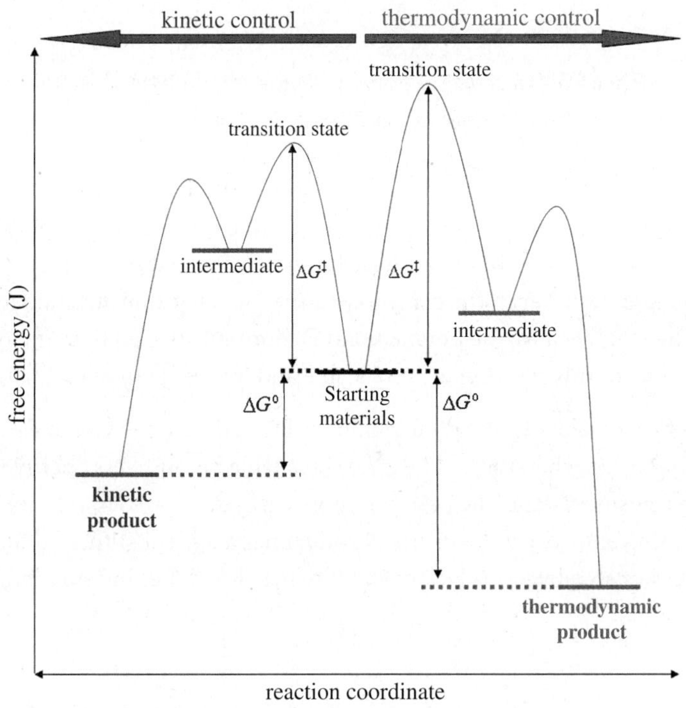

Figure 6.4 Kinetic and Thermodynamic Control of a Reaction
The kinetic pathway requires less free energy to reach the transition state, but results in a higher-energy (less stable) product.

Note that the free energy that must be added for the kinetic pathway is lower than that of the thermodynamic pathway. Therefore, the kinetic products often form faster than the thermodynamic products and are sometimes called "fast" products. On the other hand, the free energy of the thermodynamic product is significantly lower than that of the kinetic product. Thermodynamic products are therefore associated with greater stability, and with a more negative ΔG than kinetic products.

The stability of organic molecules is covered in Chapter 2 of *MCAT Organic Chemistry Review* and is dependent on torsional strain, angle strain, and nonbonded strain. In this example, we consider the conversion of 2-methylcyclohexanone to its thermodynamic product and its kinetic product, as shown in Figure 6.5. Both reactions require a base (B^-) in order to catalyze the conversion, yet two different products are produced.

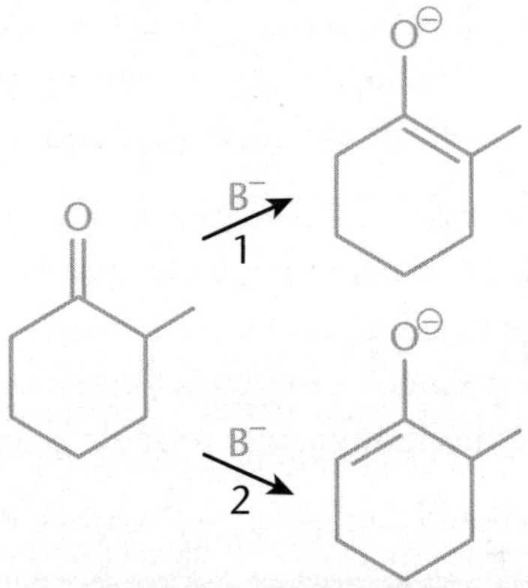

Figure 6.5 Conversion of 2-methylcyclohexanone to (1) Thermodynamic Product and (2) Kinetic Product

For the thermodynamic pathway **(1)**, the double bond is located between C-1 and the methyl group. It requires more energy to form the transition state of this reaction because the base must overcome the steric hindrance created by the methyl group. The base squeezes in to reach the carbon with the methyl group attached to abstract a proton. However, because the double bond is more substituted than the other pathway, the product of this reaction is more stable and less likely to react further.

For the kinetic pathway **(2)**, the double bond is located between C-1 and C-6. This pathway is preferred when there is little heat available because less energy is needed to reach the transition state. The base can more easily reach C-6 to remove a proton, and the resulting enolate can form. This product has a less substituted double bond, which reduces its stability. This lack of stability may leave the ring susceptible to further attack.

MCAT CONCEPT CHECK 6.3

Before you move on, assess your understanding of the material with these questions.

1. What conditions favor formation of a kinetic product? A thermodynamic product?
   - Kinetic product:

   ____

   - Thermodynamic product:

   ____

2. On a reaction coordinate diagram, how would the kinetic pathway appear as compared to the thermodynamic pathway?

   ____

Conclusion

We've discussed some very important concepts and principles in the past two chapters related to the studies of reaction rates and chemical equilibria. In this chapter, we began with the law of mass action and the significance of the equilibrium state of a chemical reaction. With our understanding of the significance of K_{eq} and Q, we are able to predict the direction that a reaction will go in response to various stresses—concentration, pressure, or temperature changes—that might be applied to a system.

The concept of homeostasis in biology is a direct result of the energy associated with disturbing equilibria in the body. Reactions are often held slightly out of the equilibrium state to generate energy. Many pathologies you will encounter in your future career in medicine will have a fundamental basis in disturbed chemical equilibria—just wait until you start ordering metabolic panels on your patients!

GO ONLINE

You've reviewed the content, now test your knowledge and critical thinking skills by completing a test-like passage set in your online resources!

CONCEPT SUMMARY

Equilibrium

- **Reversible** reactions eventually reach a state in which energy is minimized and entropy is maximized.
  - Chemical equilibria are **dynamic**—the reactions are still occurring, just at a constant rate.
  - The concentrations of reactants and products remain constant because the rate of the forward reaction equals the rate of the reverse reaction.
- The **law of mass action** gives the expression for the equilibrium constant, K_{eq}. The reaction quotient, Q, has the same form but can be calculated at any concentrations of reactants and products.
  - Q is a calculated value that relates the reactant and product concentrations at any given time during a reaction.
  - K_{eq} is the ratio of products to reactants at equilibrium, with each species raised to its stoichiometric coefficient. K_{eq} for a reaction is constant at a constant temperature.
  - Pure solids and liquids do not appear in the law of mass action; only gases and aqueous species do.
- Comparison of Q to K_{eq} provides information about where the reaction is with respect to its equilibrium state.
  - If $Q < K_{eq}$, $\Delta G < 0$, and the reaction proceeds in the forward direction.
  - If $Q = K_{eq}$, $\Delta G = 0$, and the reaction is in dynamic equilibrium.
  - If $Q > K_{eq}$, $\Delta G > 0$, and the reaction proceeds in the reverse direction.
- Equilibrium calculations are broadly applicable to many areas of chemistry but are often formulaic in their application. The magnitude of K_{eq} determines the balance of a reaction and whether the amount that has reacted can be treated as negligible when compared to other concentrations.
  - If $K_{eq} > 1$, the products are present in greater concentration at equilibrium.
  - If $K_{eq} \approx 1$, products and reactants are both present at equilibrium at reasonably similar levels.
  - If $K_{eq} < 1$, the reactants are present in greater concentration at equilibrium.
  - If $K_{eq} \lll 1$, the amount of reactants that have been converted to products can be considered negligible in comparison to the initial concentration of reactants.

Le Châtelier's Principle

- **Le Châtelier's principle** states that when a chemical system experiences a stress, it will react so as to restore equilibrium.
- There are three main types of stresses applied to a system: changes in concentration, pressure and volume, and temperature.
  - Increasing the concentration of reactants or decreasing the concentration of products will shift the reaction to the right. Increasing the concentration of products or decreasing the concentration of reactants will shift the reaction to the left.
  - Increasing pressure on a gaseous system (decreasing its volume) will shift the reaction toward the side with fewer moles of gas. Decreasing pressure on a gaseous system (increasing its volume) will shift the reaction toward the side with more moles of gas.
  - Increasing the temperature of an endothermic reaction or decreasing the temperature of an exothermic reaction will shift the reaction to the right. Decreasing the temperature of an endothermic reaction or increasing the temperature of an exothermic reaction will shift the reaction to the left.

Kinetic and Thermodynamic Control

- Reactions may have both kinetic and thermodynamic products that can be regulated by temperature and the presence of a catalyst.
  - **Kinetic products** are higher in free energy than thermodynamic products and can form at lower temperatures. These are sometimes termed "fast" products because they can form more quickly under such conditions.
  - **Thermodynamic products** are lower in free energy than kinetic products and are therefore more stable. Despite proceeding more slowly than the kinetic pathway, the thermodynamic pathway is more spontaneous (more negative ΔG).

ANSWERS TO CONCEPT CHECKS

6.1

1. First calculate the value of Q from the given concentrations:

$$Q = \frac{[\text{products}]}{[\text{reactants}]} = \frac{0.075}{1.5} = \frac{7.5 \times 10^{-2}}{1.5} = 5 \times 10^{-2}.$$

Q can now be compared to each value of K_{eq} to predict the direction of the reaction.

K_{eq}	Direction of Reaction	ΔG
5.0×10^{-2}	At equilibrium: no net reaction	0
5.0×10^{-3}	$Q_c > K_{eq}$: proceeds toward reactants (left)	Positive
5.0×10^{-1}	$Q_c < K_{eq}$: proceeds toward products (right)	Negative

2. $K_p = \dfrac{P_{CH_3OH}}{P_{CO} \times \left(P_{H_2}\right)^2}$

$$K_c = K_a = \frac{[H_2PO_4^-][H_3O^+]}{[H_3PO_4]}$$

3. The concentration of a reactant that converts to product can be considered negligible if it is two or more orders of magnitude less than the initial concentration of the reactant.

K_{eq}	Initial Concentration of A (M)	Is the amount reacted negligible?
1×10^{-12}	1	Yes
1×10^{-2}	0.1	No
1×10^{-3}	0.001	No
1×10^{-15}	0.001	Yes

4. The first step in solving is to write the equation for K_{eq} for the reaction: $A(aq) + B(aq) \leftrightarrow C(g) + D(s)$.

$$K_{eq} = \frac{[C]}{[A][B]} = 2.1 \times 10^{-7}$$

Note that the equation for K_{eq} does not include product D because D is a solid.

Next, using the initial concentrations for A and B and x for the amount that has reacted, plug into the equation for K_{eq}:

$$K_{eq} = \frac{[C]}{[A][B]} = \frac{[x]}{[0.1 - x][0.2 - x]}$$

Given that $K_{eq} = 2.1 \times 10^{-7}$, the concentrations of A and B are sufficiently large that x can be considered negligible in comparison to both. This allows the equation for K_{eq} to be simplified and solved:

$$K_{eq} = 2.1 \times 10^{-7} \approx \frac{x}{[0.1][0.2]}$$

$$x = \left(2.1 \times 10^{-7}\right)(0.1)(0.2) = 4.2 \times 10^{-9}$$

The value of $x = 4.2 \times 10^{-9}$ is equal to both the equilibrium concentration of C and the amount of A and B that have reacted. The approximation that x is negligible compared to the initial concentrations of A and B is valid.

6.2

1. - Increasing pH of $H_2SO_4\ (aq) \rightleftharpoons H^+\ (aq) + HSO_4^-\ (aq)$: $[H^+]$ decreases, shifting reaction to the right.
   - Decreasing pressure of $2\ C\ (s) + O_2\ (g) \rightleftharpoons 2\ CO\ (g)$: Reaction shifts right, favoring the side with more moles of gas.
   - Warming $CH_4\ (g) + 2O_2\ (g) \rightleftharpoons CO_2\ (g) + 2\ H_2O\ (l)$ + heat: Reaction shifts left, using the additional heat energy to produce more reactants.
   - Removing water from $H_3PO_4\ (aq) + H_2O\ (l) \rightleftharpoons H_3O^+\ (aq) + H_2PO_4^-\ (aq)$: Reaction shifts left. All concentrations would increase proportionately; because there are more products than reactants (and the stoichiometric coefficient is 1 for each reactant and product), the value of Q will increase.

6.3

1. Kinetic products are favored at low temperatures with low heat transfer. Thermodynamic products are favored at high temperatures with high heat transfer.
2. Kinetic pathways require a smaller gain in free energy to reach the transition state. They also have a higher free energy of the products, with a smaller difference in free energy between the transition state and the products.

SCIENCE MASTERY ASSESSMENT EXPLANATIONS

1. **C**

This scenario likely describes a situation in which a reaction has reached equilibrium very far to the right (with high product concentration and low reactant concentration). This reaction must be reversible because the reaction did not proceed all the way to the right. Any reaction in equilibrium has equal forward and reverse rates of reaction.

2. **D**

Recall that pure solids and liquids do not appear in the equilibrium expression; thus, this K_{eq} has no denominator because the only reactant is a solid, cuprous sulfate. This could also be called K_{sp} because a solid is dissociating into ions in solution. The correct K_{eq} should have $[Cu^+]$ squared because its stoichiometric coefficient is 2.

3. **A**

Carbon dioxide gas evolves and leaves the bottle, which decreases the total pressure of the reactants. Le Châtelier's principle explains that a decrease in pressure shifts the equilibrium to increase the number of moles of gas present. This particular reaction will shift to the left, which in turn will decrease the amount of carbonic acid and increase the amount of carbon dioxide and water. Oxygen and nitrogen are not highly reactive and are unlikely to combine spontaneously with carbon dioxide or carbonic acid, as in **(C)** and **(D)**.

4. **B**

Recall that when multiple products are possible and an equilibrium exists between these multiple products, one product will be called the kinetic product and the other the thermodynamic product. The transition state leading to the kinetic product is lower in energy, so that the kinetic product is formed more rapidly in solution. However, the kinetic product is less stable than the thermodynamic product. The end result is that the equilibrium of products initially favors the kinetic product, but eventually favors the more stable thermodynamic product. Taking these factors together, to favor the kinetic product, conduct the reaction for a short duration, so that the thermodynamic product does not have much chance to form. Also, the reaction should be conducted at a lower temperature to help stabilize the otherwise less stable kinetic product. These factors—low temperature and short reaction time—justify choice **(B)**.

5. **A**

The larger the value of K_{eq} (whether K_c or K_p), the larger the ratio of products to reactants. Therefore, if $K_c \gg 1$, there are significantly larger concentrations of products than reactants at equilibrium. Even with a large K_{eq}, the reaction will ultimately reach equilibrium far toward the products side and is therefore reversible, eliminating **(D)**.

6. **B**

Adding sodium acetate increases the number of acetate ions present. According to Le Châtelier's principle, this change will push this reaction to the left, resulting in a decrease in the number of free H^+ ions. Because pH is determined by the hydrogen ion concentration, a decrease in the number of free protons will increase the pH. An acid's K_a (which is simply the K_{eq} for acid dissociation) will remain constant under a given temperature and pressure, eliminating **(C)** and **(D)**.

7. **A**

Both increasing the pressure of the container and decreasing the volume would favor the side with fewer moles of gas, which is the product side. This makes **(B)** and **(C)** incorrect. **(D)** would not disturb the equilibrium—the significance of decreasing the volume of the container in most equilibria is that there is an increase in pressure; in this case, however, the pressure remains constant despite the change in volume.

8. **C**

An exothermic reaction produces heat. Decreasing the temperature favors product formation, resulting in an increase in the forward reaction rate with a concomitant decrease in the reverse reaction rate.

9. **B**

The equilibrium of a reaction can be changed by several factors. Adding or subtracting heat, **(A)**, would shift the equilibrium based on the enthalpy change of the reaction. Increasing reactant concentrations would shift the equilibrium in the direction of the product, and the opposite would occur if reactant concentrations were decreased, eliminating **(C)**. Changing the volume of a reactant would affect any reaction with gaseous reactants or products, eliminating **(D)**. While adding or removing a catalyst would change the reaction rates, it would not change where the equilibrium lies.

10. **A**

Start with the balanced equation for the reaction of H_2 and N_2 to produce NH_3: $N_2 + 3\ H_2 \rightleftharpoons 2\ NH_3$.

Next, write out $K_c = K_{eq} = \frac{[NH_3]^2}{[N_2][H_2]^3}$. Because the volume is 1 L, the amount of each gas in moles is equal to the value of the concentration of each gas in moles per liter (M). The relatively small amount of NH_3 produced indicates that it will be possible to consider the amount of N_2 and H_2 that reacts to be negligible compared to their starting concentrations. Putting the amounts of each reactant and product into the K_{eq} expression gives:

$$K_{eq} = \frac{[NH_3]^2}{[N_2][H_2]^3} = \frac{[0.05]^2}{[1-x][3-x]^3} \approx \frac{[0.05]^2}{[1][3]^3} = \frac{\left[5\times10^{-2}\right]^2}{27}$$

$$K_{eq} = \frac{25\times10^{-4}}{27} \approx \frac{25\times10^{-4}}{25} = 1\times10^{-4} = 0.0001$$

11. **B**

At extremely high temperatures, reactants or products may decompose, which will affect the equilibrium and potentially destroy the desired products. **(A)** implies that reactions have limits, which is true; however, this does not make increasing temperature unfavorable. **(C)** is false because increasing temperature would also increase pressure, assuming constant volume. **(D)** is incorrect because it refers to properties of irreversible reactions, which would not be involved in an equilibrium between products and reactants.

12. **D**

The thermodynamic product is more stable than the kinetic product, making the thermodynamic product lower in energy. Because the energy of the product is lower, the *change* in free energy is greater for the thermodynamic product compared to the kinetic product. Thus, **(D)** is correct.

13. **C**

K_a is equal to the ratio of products to reactants, with each species raised to its stoichiometric coefficient. A compound with a K_a greater than 10^{-7} contains more H^+ cations than HA^- anions at equilibrium, which makes it an acid. This means that the compound in question is likely to react with a compound that is basic. Of the four answer choices, NH_3 is the only base.

14. **C**

Reaction 2 is the reverse of reaction 1. This means that K_{eq} for reaction 2 is the inverse of K_{eq} of reaction 1, so the answer is $\frac{1}{0.1} = \frac{1}{\frac{1}{10}} = 10$.

15. **A**

A negative ΔH value indicates an exothermic reaction, meaning that the forward reaction produces heat. Visualize this as follows:

$$A + B \rightleftharpoons C + D + \text{heat}$$

This means that removing heat by decreasing the temperature is similar to removing any other product of the reaction. To compensate for this loss, the reaction will shift to the right, causing an increase in the concentrations of C and D, as well as a decrease in the concentrations of A and B.

Consult your online resources for additional practice. **GO ONLINE**

EQUATIONS TO REMEMBER

(6.1) **Equilibrium constant:** $K_{eq} = \frac{[C]^c[D]^d}{[A]^a[B]^b}$

(6.2) **Reaction quotient:** $Q_c = \frac{[C]^c[D]^d}{[A]^a[B]^b}$

SHARED CONCEPTS

Biochemistry Chapter 2
Enzymes

General Chemistry Chapter 5
Chemical Kinetics

General Chemistry Chapter 7
Thermochemistry

General Chemistry Chapter 9
Solutions

General Chemistry Chapter 10
Acids and Bases

Organic Chemistry Chapter 2
Isomers

CHAPTER 7

THERMOCHEMISTRY

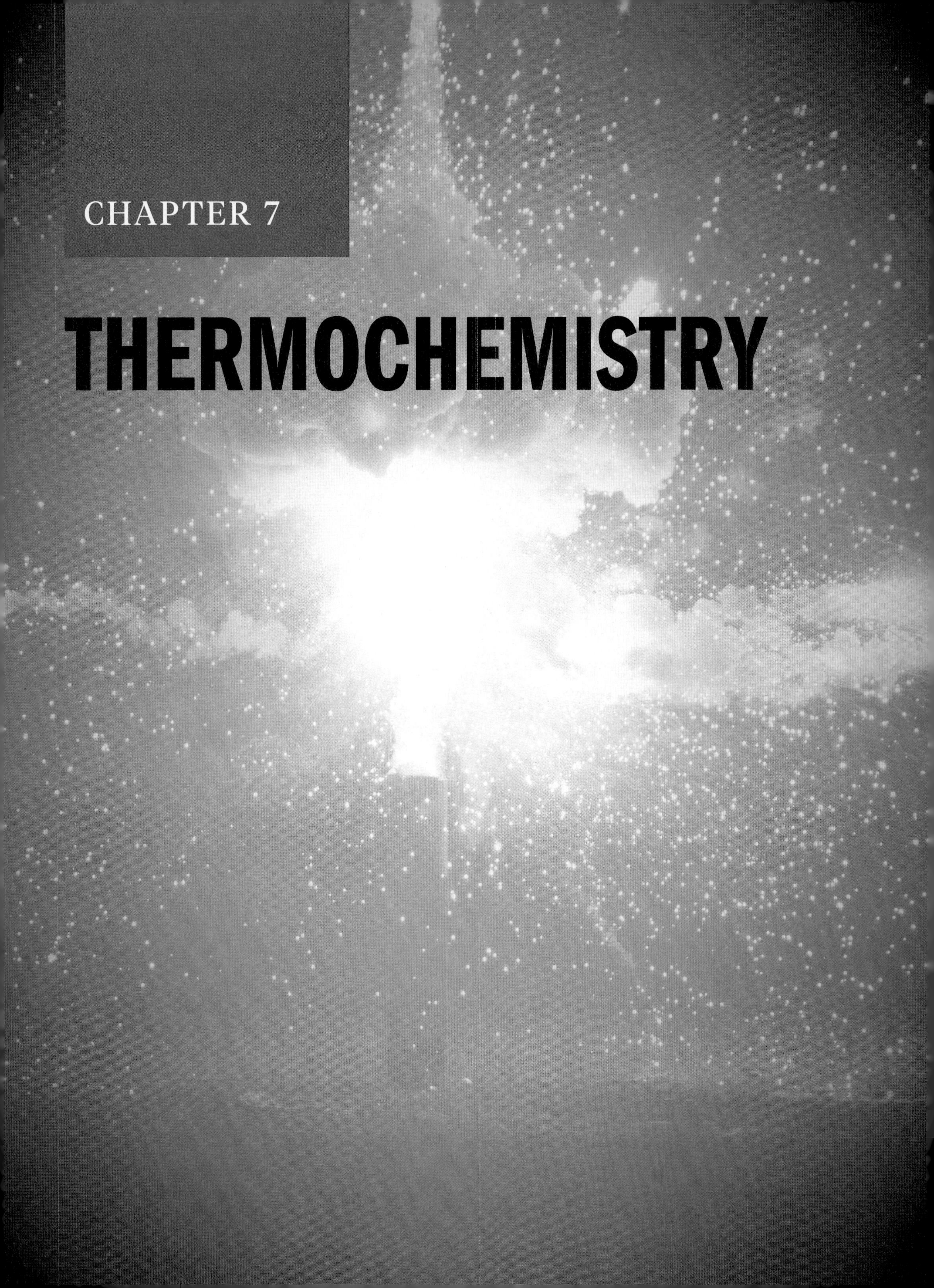

SCIENCE MASTERY ASSESSMENT

Every pre-med knows this feeling: there is so much content I have to know for the MCAT! How do I know what to do first or what's important?

While the high-yield badges throughout this book will help you identify the most important topics, this Science Mastery Assessment is another tool in your MCAT prep arsenal. This quiz (which can also be taken in your online resources) and the guidance below will help ensure that you are spending the appropriate amount of time on this chapter based on your personal strengths and weaknesses. Don't worry though—skipping something now does not mean you'll never study it. Later on in your prep, as you complete full-length tests, you'll uncover specific pieces of content that you need to review and can come back to these chapters as appropriate.

How to Use This Assessment

If you answer 0–7 questions correctly:

Spend about 1 hour to read this chapter in full and take limited notes throughout. Follow up by reviewing **all** quiz questions to ensure that you now understand how to solve each one.

If you answer 8–11 questions correctly:

Spend 20–40 minutes reviewing the quiz questions. Beginning with the questions you missed, read and take notes on the corresponding subchapters. For questions you answered correctly, ensure your thinking matches that of the explanation and you understand why each choice was correct or incorrect.

If you answer 12–15 questions correctly:

Spend less than 20 minutes reviewing all questions from the quiz. If you missed any, then include a quick read-through of the corresponding subchapters, or even just the relevant content within a subchapter, as part of your question review. For questions you answered correctly, ensure your thinking matches that of the explanation and review the Concept Summary at the end of the chapter.

1. Consider the cooling of an ideal gas in a closed system. This process is illustrated in the pressure–volume graph shown in the following figure.

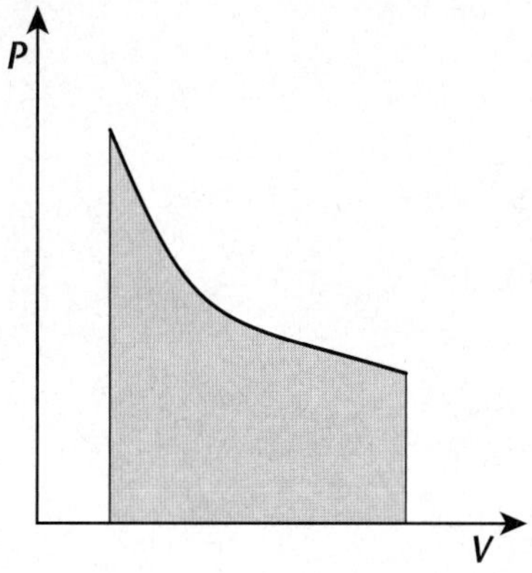

Based on this information, the process may be:
   A. adiabatic.
   B. isobaric.
   C. isothermal.
   D. isochoric.

2. A pot of water at 100°C sits on a heating element and boils. Which of the following best characterizes this phase change process?
   A. Isothermal expansion
   B. Adiabatic expansion
   C. Isovolumetric heating
   D. Adiabatic compression

3. Pure sodium metal spontaneously combusts upon contact with room temperature water. What is true about the equilibrium constant of this combustion reaction at 25°C?
   A. $K_{eq} < 0$
   B. $0 < K_{eq} < 1$
   C. $K_{eq} = 1$
   D. $K_{eq} > 1$

4. Which of the following processes has the most exothermic standard heat of combustion?
   A. Combustion of ethane
   B. Combustion of propane
   C. Combustion of *n*-butane
   D. Combustion of *n*-pentane

5. Methanol reacts with acetic acid to form methyl acetate and water.

Type of Bond	Bond Dissociation Energy $\left(\frac{kJ}{mol}\right)$
C–C	348
C–H	415
C=O	805
O–H	463
C–O	360

Based on the values in the table above, what is the heat of reaction in $\frac{kJ}{mol}$?
   A. 0
   B. 464
   C. 824
   D. 1288

6. Which of the following refers to the temperature and pressure at which all three phases exist in equilibrium?
   A. Critical point
   B. Triple point
   C. Deposition
   D. State function

7. A 10 g sample of water is brought from 40°C to boiling and is completely boiled to the gas phase. Which of the following expressions represents the total amount of energy required if the final temperature of the vapor is 100°C? (The heat of vaporization of water is 2,260 J/g.)
   A. (10 g)(40°C)(4.2 J/g°C) + (2,260 J/g)(10 g)
   B. (10 g)(40°C)(4.2 J/g°C) + (2,260 J/°C)(60°C)
   C. (10 g)(60°C)(4.2 J/g°C) + (2,260 J/g)(10 g)
   D. (10 g)(60°C)(4.2 J/g°C) + (2,260 J/°C)(60°C)

8. Consider the chemical reaction in the vessel depicted in the following diagram.

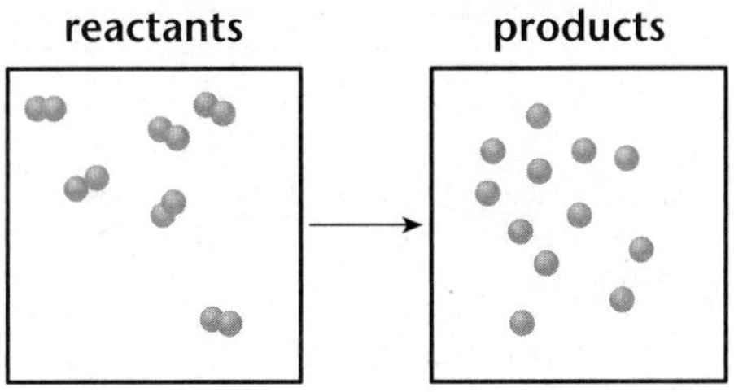

   A. The reaction is spontaneous.
   B. The reaction is nonspontaneous.
   C. The reaction is at equilibrium.
   D. There is not enough information to determine if the reaction is spontaneous.

9. Suppose $\Delta G^\circ_{rxn} = -2000 \frac{J}{mol}$ for a chemical reaction. At 300 K, what is the change in Gibbs free energy in $\frac{J}{mol}$?
   A. $\Delta G = -2000 + (300\text{ K})(8.314)(\ln Q)$
   B. $\Delta G = -2000 - (300\text{ K})(8.314)(\ln Q)$
   C. $\Delta G = -2000 + (300\text{ K})(8.314)(\log Q)$
   D. $\Delta G = -2000 - (300\text{ K})(8.314)(\log Q)$

10. A chemical reaction has a negative enthalpy and a negative entropy. Which of the following terms necessarily describes this reaction?
   A. Exothermic
   B. Endothermic
   C. Exergonic
   D. Endergonic

11. Which of the following statements is true of a process that is spontaneous in the forward direction?
   A. $\Delta G > 0$ and $K_{eq} > Q$
   B. $\Delta G > 0$ and $K_{eq} < Q$
   C. $\Delta G < 0$ and $K_{eq} > Q$
   D. $\Delta G < 0$ and $K_{eq} < Q$

12. Which of the following reactions has the greatest decrease in entropy?
   A. $2\ NH_3\ (g) \rightarrow 3\ H_2\ (g) + N_2\ (g)$
   B. $2\ Na\ (s) + Cl_2\ (g) \rightarrow 2\ NaCl\ (s)$
   C. $2\ H_2O_2\ (l) \rightarrow 2\ H_2O\ (l) + O_2\ (g)$
   D. $Zn\ (s) + CuSO_4\ (aq) \rightarrow ZnSO_4\ (aq) + Cu\ (s)$

13. A reaction coordinate for a chemical reaction is displayed in the graph below.

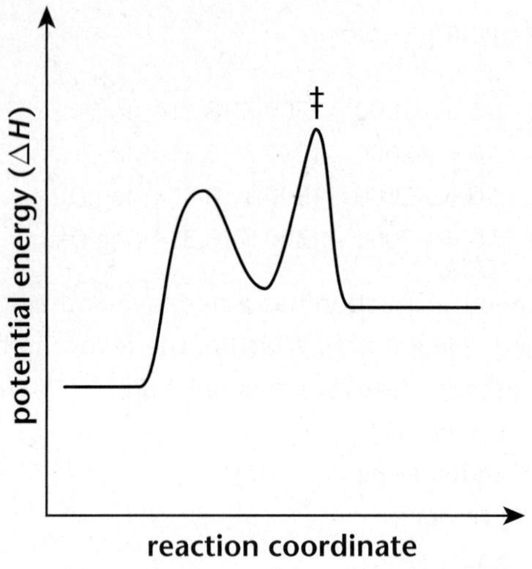

Which of the following terms describes the energy of this reaction?

A. Endothermic
B. Exothermic
C. Endergonic
D. Exergonic

14. The process of melting NaCl requires a large amount of energy due to the strong attraction between ions. A researcher finds that 58 g of salt melts at 1060 K and requires a heat input of 30,000 J. What is the change in entropy?

A. 28 J/K
B. 1,580 J/K
C. 61,000 J/K
D. Not enough information is provided

15. Explosions are necessarily characterized by:

A. $\Delta G < 0$.
B. $\Delta H > 0$.
C. $\Delta S < 0$.
D. $T < 0$.

Answer Key follows on next page.

Answer Key

1. **A**
2. **A**
3. **D**
4. **D**
5. **A**
6. **B**
7. **C**
8. **D**
9. **A**
10. **A**
11. **C**
12. **B**
13. **A**
14. **A**
15. **A**

Detailed explanations can be found at the end of the chapter.

CHAPTER 7

THERMOCHEMISTRY

In This Chapter

CHAPTER PROFILE

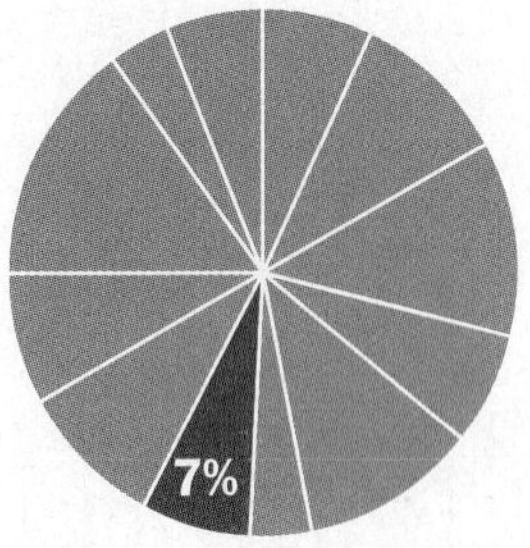

The content in this chapter should be relevant to about 7% of all questions about general chemistry on the MCAT.

This chapter covers material from the following AAMC content categories:

1D: Principles of bioenergetics and fuel molecule metabolism

5E: Principles of chemical thermodynamics and kinetics

Introduction

Styrofoam cups are such good insulators that they can be used as holding containers for certain calorimetry experiments. Coffee-cup calorimetry, which uses Styrofoam cups to measure heats of solution and specific heats of metals and other materials, is low-tech, yet it can produce remarkably accurate results as long as care has been taken to calibrate the calorimeter and to minimize heat loss through the top of the container. The next time you are at your favorite coffee chain, think about what occurs when cold cream is added to hot coffee. If we took the time to measure the masses and temperatures of the hot coffee and the cold cream before mixing them, measured the drink's temperature after it had been stirred, and looked up the specific heats of water and cream, we would have enough information to calculate the amount of heat exchanged between the hot coffee and the cold cream.

This chapter will review the basic principles of thermochemistry, which is the study of the energy changes that accompany chemical and physical processes. Starting with the first law of thermodynamics, which states that energy is never created nor destroyed but—at most—simply changed from one form to another, we will quantify the various exchanges in energy as a system moves from some initial state to a final state. As we go along, we will define what is meant by system and surroundings, state functions, heat, enthalpy, entropy, and Gibbs free energy.

7.1 Systems and Processes

LEARNING OBJECTIVES

After Chapter 7.1, you will be able to:

- Identify the system and its surroundings given a situation involving transfer of heat
- Recall the features of isothermal, adiabatic, isobaric, and isovolumetric processes

Students often have some anxiety over what constitutes a *system* and what—by exclusion from the system—constitutes the *surroundings* or *environment*. Perhaps the problem isn't so much the definitions themselves but the way in which the boundary between the two can be shifted to suit the needs of the experimenter or observer. Simply put, the **system** is the matter that is being observed—the total amount of reactants and products in a chemical reaction. It could be the amount of solute and solvent used to create a solution. It could be the gas inside a balloon. Then, the **surroundings**, or **environment**, are everything outside of that system. However, the boundary between system and surroundings is not permanently fixed and can be moved. For example, one might consider the mass of coffee in a coffee cup to be the system and the cup containing it to be part of the environment. This setup would likely be used if someone was interested in determining the amount of heat transferred from the hot coffee to the cooler coffee cup. Alternatively, one might define the system as the hot coffee and the cup together, and the environment as the air surrounding the coffee cup. This setup would likely be used if someone was interested in calculating the heat exchange between the hot coffee and cup system and the cooler surrounding air. The boundary can be extended out farther and farther, until the entire mass of the universe is ultimately included in the system. At this point, there are no surroundings. Again, where the boundary is placed is a decision based on what phenomenon one is interested in studying.

Thermodynamic Terminology

Systems can be characterized by whether or not they can exchange heat or matter with the surroundings. A system may be characterized as follows:

- **Isolated:** The system cannot exchange energy (heat and work) or matter with the surroundings; for example, an insulated bomb calorimeter.
- **Closed:** The system can exchange energy (heat and work) but not matter with the surroundings; for example, a steam radiator.
- **Open:** The system can exchange both energy (heat and work) and matter with the surroundings; for example, a pot of boiling water.

When a system experiences a change in one or more of its properties (such as concentrations of reactants or products, temperature, or pressure), it undergoes a **process**.

While processes, by definition, are associated with a change of the state of a system, some processes are uniquely identified by some property that is constant throughout the process. Many of these processes create special conditions because they allow us to simplify the **first law of thermodynamics**:

$$\Delta U = Q - W$$

Equation 7.1

where ΔU is the change in internal energy of the system, Q is the heat added to the system, and W is the work done by the system.

For example, **isothermal processes** occur when the system's temperature is constant. Constant temperature implies that the total internal energy of the system (U) is constant throughout the process. This is because temperature and internal energy are directly proportional. When U is constant, $\Delta U = 0$ and the first law simplifies to $Q = W$ (the heat added to the system equals the work done by the system). An isothermal process appears as a hyperbolic curve on a pressure–volume graph (P–V graph). Work is represented by the area under such a curve, as shown in Figure 7.1.

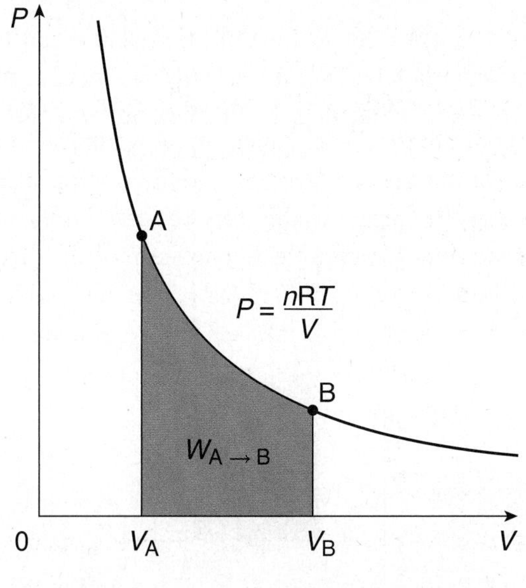

Figure 7.1 Graph of an Isothermal Expansion
Temperature is constant in an isothermal process; thus, the area under the curve represents not only the work performed by the gas, but also the heat that entered the system.

Adiabatic processes occur when no heat is exchanged between the system and the environment; thus, the thermal energy of the system is constant throughout the process. When $Q = 0$, the first law simplifies to $\Delta U = -W$ (the change in internal energy of the system is equal to work done *on* the system [the opposite of work done *by* the system]). An adiabatic process also appears hyperbolic on a P–V graph, as shown in Figure 7.2.

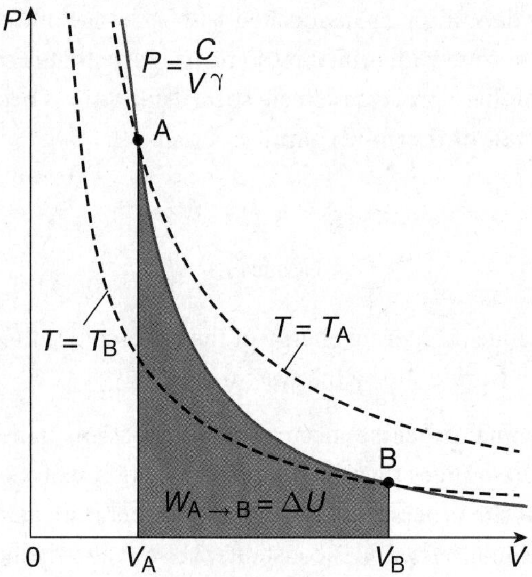

Figure 7.2 Graph of an Adiabatic Expansion
Heat exchange is zero in an adiabatic process; temperature is not constant (as shown by the dotted lines).

Isobaric processes occur when the pressure of the system is constant. Isothermal and isobaric processes are common because it is usually easy to control temperature and pressure. Isobaric processes do not alter the first law, but note that an isobaric process appears as a flat line on a P–V graph, as shown in Figure 7.3.

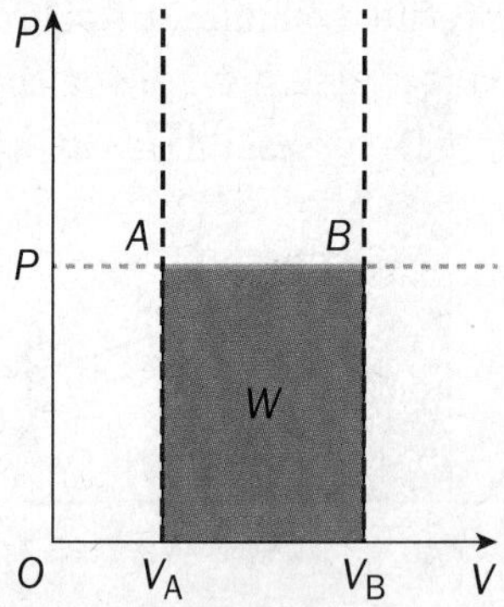

Figure 7.3 Graph of an Isobaric Expansion
Pressure is constant in an isobaric process; the slope of the line is therefore zero.

BRIDGE

The terms isothermal, adiabatic, isobaric, and isovolumetric (isochoric) may seem familiar because they are also discussed in Chapter 3 of MCAT *Physics and Math Review*.

Finally, **isovolumetric (isochoric) processes** experience no change in volume. Because the gas neither expands nor compresses, no work is performed in such a process. Thus, the first law simplifies to $\Delta U = Q$ (the change in internal energy is equal to the heat added to the system). An isovolumetric process is a vertical line on a P–V graph; the area under the curve, which represents the work done by the gas, is zero.

Processes themselves can also be classified as spontaneous or nonspontaneous. A **spontaneous process** is one that can occur by itself without having to be driven by energy from an outside source. Calculating the change in the Gibbs free energy (ΔG) for a process, such as a chemical reaction, allows us to predict whether the process will be spontaneous or nonspontaneous. As discussed later in the chapter, the same quantities that are used to calculate the change in the Gibbs free energy, ΔH and ΔS, can also tell us whether the process will be temperature dependent; that is, spontaneous at some temperatures and nonspontaneous at others.

Spontaneous reactions, as mentioned in Chapters 5 and 6 of *MCAT General Chemistry Review*, will not necessarily happen quickly and may not go to completion. Many spontaneous reactions have very high activation energies and, therefore, rarely take place. For example, when was the last time you saw a match ignite itself? However, providing a quantity of thermal energy (generated by the friction associated with striking the match) that equals or exceeds the activation energy will allow the match to light and burn spontaneously. At this point, the combustion of the chemical components of the match using molecular oxygen in the air will not need any additional external energy once the activation energy has been supplied.

Some spontaneous reactions proceed very slowly. The role of enzymes—biological catalysts—is to selectively enhance the rate of certain spontaneous (but slow) chemical reactions so that the biologically necessary products can be formed at a rate sufficient for sustaining life. As we discussed in Chapter 6 of *MCAT General Chemistry Review*, some reactions do not go to completion but settle into a low-energy state called equilibrium. Spontaneous reactions may go to completion, but many simply reach equilibrium with dynamically stable concentrations of reactants and products. A common method for supplying energy for nonspontaneous reactions is by **coupling** nonspontaneous reactions to spontaneous ones, as shown in Figure 7.4.

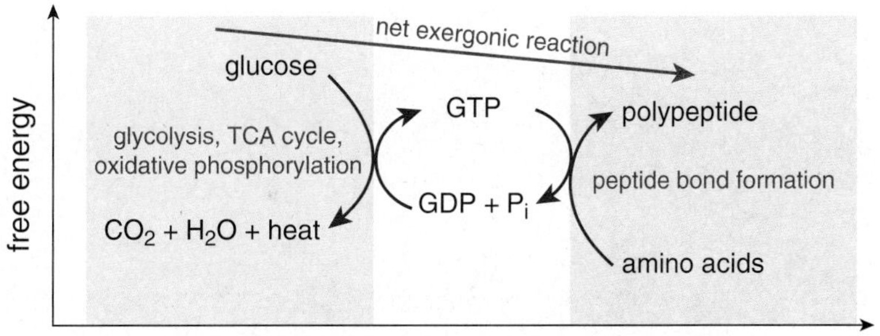

Figure 7.4 Coupling of Reactions
The combustion of glucose is exergonic; the formation of peptide bonds is endergonic. Energy from the combustion of glucose can be stored in the bonds in GTP, which are then lysed to provide the energy for forming peptide bonds.

MCAT CONCEPT CHECK 7.1

Before you move on, assess your understanding of the material with these questions.

1. A person snaps an ice pack and places it on one leg. In terms of energy transfer, what would be considered the system and what would be the surroundings in this scenario?
   - System:
   - Surroundings:
2. What is unique about each of the following types of processes?
   - Isothermal:
   - Adiabatic:
   - Isobaric:
   - Isovolumetric (isochoric):

7.2 States and State Functions

LEARNING OBJECTIVES

After Chapter 7.2, you will be able to:

- Recall standard conditions and the calculations they are used for
- Distinguish between a state function and a process function
- List the common state functions
- Identify the triple point and critical point on a phase diagram:

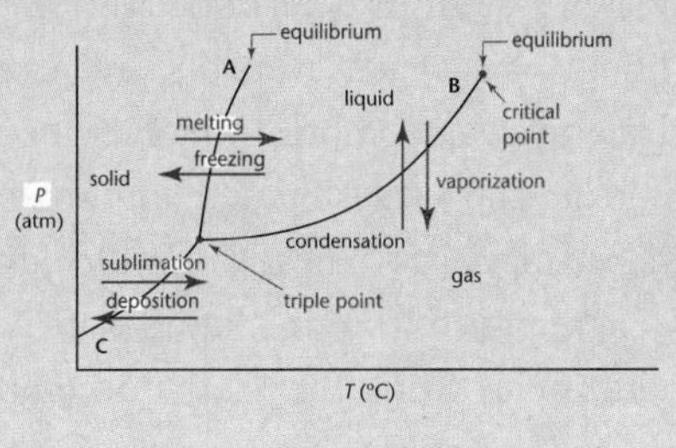

The state of a system can be described by certain macroscopic properties. These properties, or **state functions**, describe the system in an equilibrium state. They cannot describe the process of the system; that is, how the system got to its current equilibrium. They are useful only for comparing one equilibrium state to another. The pathway taken from one equilibrium state to another is described quantitatively by the **process functions**, the most important of which are work (W) and heat (Q).

Overview

The state functions include pressure (P), density (ρ), temperature (T), volume (V), enthalpy (H), internal energy (U), Gibbs free energy (G), and entropy (S). When the state of a system changes from one equilibrium to another, one or more of these state functions will change. In addition, while state functions are independent of the path (process) taken, they are not necessarily independent of one another. For example, Gibbs free energy is related to enthalpy, temperature, and entropy.

Because systems can be in different equilibrium states at different temperatures and pressures, a set of **standard conditions** has been defined for measuring the enthalpy, entropy, and Gibbs free energy changes of a reaction. The standard conditions are defined as 25°C (298 K), 1 atm pressure, and 1 M concentrations. Don't confuse standard conditions with **standard temperature and pressure (STP)**, for which the temperature is 0°C (273 K) and pressure is 1 atm. Standard conditions are used for kinetics, equilibrium, and thermodynamics problems; STP is used for ideal gas calculations.

Under standard conditions, the most stable form of a substance is called the **standard state** of that substance. You should recognize the standard states for some elements and compounds commonly encountered on the MCAT. For example, H_2 (g), H_2O (l), NaCl (s), O_2 (g), and C (s, graphite) are the most stable forms of these substances under standard conditions. Recognizing whether or not a substance is in its standard

MNEMONIC

State functions: When I'm under **pressure** and feeling **dense**, all I want to do is watch **TV** and get **HUGS**.

Pressure (P), density (ρ), temperature (T), volume (V), enthalpy (H), internal energy (U), Gibbs free energy (G), and entropy (S).

MCAT EXPERTISE

On the MCAT, be sure that you do not confuse standard conditions in thermodynamics with standard temperature and pressure (STP), which is used in gas law calculations:

- Standard conditions: 25°C (298 K), 1 atm pressure, 1 M concentrations
- STP: 0°C (273 K), 1 atm pressure

state is important for thermochemical calculations, such as heats of reactions and—in particular—heats of formation. The changes in enthalpy, entropy, and free energy that occur when a reaction takes place under standard conditions are called the **standard enthalpy**, **standard entropy**, and **standard free energy changes**, respectively, and are symbolized by ΔH°, ΔS°, and ΔG°. The degree sign in these variables represents zero, as the standard state is used as the "zero point" for all thermodynamic calculations.

Phase Changes

KEY CONCEPT

As with all equilibria, the rates of the forward and reverse processes will be the same when considering phase changes.

Phase diagrams are graphs that show the standard and nonstandard states of matter for a given substance in an isolated system, as determined by temperatures and pressures. **Phase changes** (solid $\rightleftharpoons$ liquid $\rightleftharpoons$ gas) are reversible, and an equilibrium of phases will eventually be reached at any given combination of temperature and pressure. For example, at 0°C and 1 atm in an isolated system, ice and water exist in an equilibrium. In other words, some of the ice may absorb heat (from the liquid water) and melt, but because that heat is being removed from the liquid water, an equal amount of the liquid water will freeze and form ice. Thus, the relative amounts of ice and water remain constant. Equilibrium between the liquid and gas states of water will be established in a closed container at room temperature and atmospheric pressure, such as a plastic water bottle with the cap screwed on tightly. Most of the water in the bottle will be in the liquid phase, but a small number of molecules at the surface will gain enough kinetic energy to escape into the gas phase; likewise, a small number of gas molecules will lose sufficient kinetic energy to reenter the liquid phase. After a while, equilibrium is established, and the relative amounts of water in the liquid and gas phases become constant—at standard conditions, equilibrium occurs when the air above the water has about 3 percent water vapor by mass. Phase equilibria are analogous to the dynamic equilibria of reversible chemical reactions: the concentrations of reactants and products are constant because the rates of the forward and reverse reactions are equal.

Gas–Liquid Equilibrium

The temperature of any substance in any phase is related to the average kinetic energy of the molecules that make up the substance. However, not all of the molecules have exactly the same instantaneous speeds. Therefore, the molecules possess a range of instantaneous kinetic energy values. In the liquid phase, the molecules are relatively free to move around one another. Some of the molecules near the surface of the liquid may have enough kinetic energy to leave the liquid phase and escape into the gaseous phase. This process is known as **evaporation** or **vaporization**. Each time the liquid loses a high-energy particle, the temperature of the remaining liquid decreases. Evaporation is an endothermic process for which the heat source is the liquid water. Of course, the liquid water itself may be receiving thermal energy from some other source, as in the case of a puddle of water drying up under the hot summer sun or a pot of water on the stovetop. Given enough energy, the liquid will completely evaporate.

Boiling is a specific type of vaporization that occurs only under certain conditions. Any liquid will lose some particles to the vapor phase over time; however, boiling is the rapid bubbling of the entire liquid with rapid release of the liquid as gas particles.

While evaporation happens in all liquids at all temperatures, boiling can only occur above the boiling point of a liquid and involves vaporization through the entire volume of the liquid.

In a covered or closed container, the escaping molecules are trapped above the solution. These molecules exert a countering pressure, which forces some of the gas back into the liquid phase; this process is called **condensation**. Condensation is facilitated by lower temperature or higher pressure. Atmospheric pressure acts on a liquid in a manner similar to that of an actual physical lid. As evaporation and condensation proceed, the respective rates of the two processes become equal, and equilibrium is reached. The pressure that the gas exerts over the liquid at equilibrium is the vapor pressure of the liquid. Vapor pressure increases as temperature increases because more molecules have sufficient kinetic energy to escape into the gas phase. The temperature at which the vapor pressure of the liquid equals the ambient (also known as external, applied, or incident) pressure is called the **boiling point**.

Liquid–Solid Equilibrium

We've already illustrated the equilibrium that can exist between the liquid and the solid phases of water at 0°C. Even though the atoms or molecules of a solid are confined to specific locations, each atom or molecule can undergo motions about some equilibrium position. These vibrational motions increase when heat is applied. From our understanding of entropy, we can say that the availability of energy **microstates** increases as the temperature of the solid increases. In basic terms, this means that the molecules have greater freedom of movement, and energy disperses. If atoms or molecules in the solid phase absorb enough energy, the three-dimensional structure of the solid will break down, and the atoms or molecules will escape into the liquid phase. The transition from solid to liquid is called **fusion** or **melting**. The reverse process, from liquid to solid, is called **solidification**, **crystallization**, or **freezing**. The temperature at which these processes occur is called the **melting point** or **freezing point**, depending on the direction of the transition. Whereas pure crystalline solids have distinct, very precise melting points, amorphous solids, such as glass, plastic, chocolate, and candle wax, tend to melt (or solidify) over a larger range of temperatures due to their less-ordered molecular structure.

Gas–Solid Equilibrium

The final phase equilibrium is that which exists between the gaseous and solid phases. When a solid goes directly into the gas phase, the process is called **sublimation**. Dry ice (solid CO_2) sublimes at room temperature and atmospheric pressure; the absence of the liquid phase makes it a convenient dry refrigerant. The reverse transition, from the gaseous to the solid phase, is called **deposition**. In organic chemistry laboratories, a device known as a **cold finger** may be used to purify a product that is heated under reduced pressure, causing it to sublime. The desired product is usually more volatile than the impurities, so the gas is purer than the original product and the impurities are left in the solid state. The gas then deposits onto the cold finger, which has cold water flowing through it, yielding a purified solid product that can be collected.

Phase Diagrams

Phase diagrams are graphs that show the temperatures and pressures at which a substance will be thermodynamically stable in a particular phase. They also show the temperatures and pressures at which phases will be in equilibrium.

The lines on a phase diagram are called the **lines of equilibrium** or the **phase boundaries** and indicate the temperature and pressure values for the equilibria between phases. The lines of equilibrium divide the diagram into three regions corresponding to the three phases—solid, liquid, and gas—and they themselves represent the phase transformations. The phase diagram for a single compound is shown in Figure 7.5.

MCAT EXPERTISE

On the MCAT, you should be able to identify and understand each area and every line of a phase diagram.

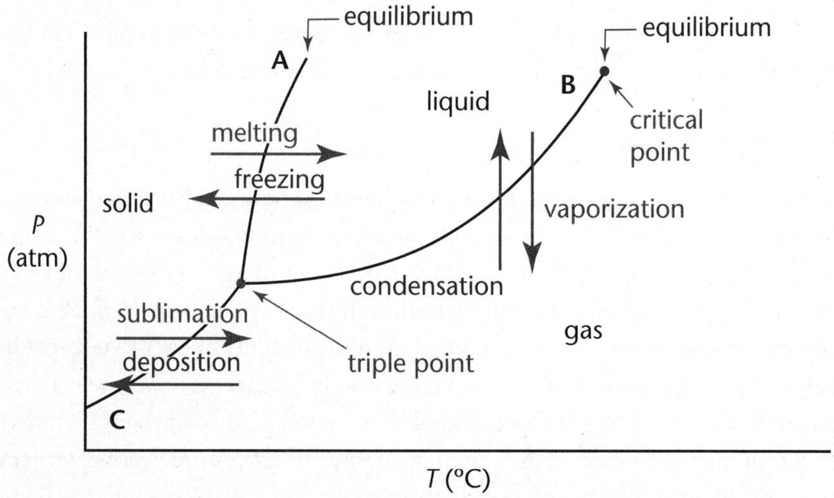

Figure 7.5 Phase Diagram for a Single Compound

REAL WORLD

Because of water's unique properties, ice floats and skates flow smoothly over ice rinks. This all "boils" down to the negative slope of the solid–liquid equilibrium line in its phase diagram. Because the density of ice is less than that of liquid water, an increase in pressure (at a constant temperature) will actually melt ice (the opposite of what is seen for the substance in Figure 7.5).

Line **A** represents the solid–liquid interface, line **B** the liquid–gas interface, and line **C** the solid–gas interface. In general, the gas phase is found at high temperatures and low pressures, the solid phase is found at low temperatures and high pressures, and the liquid phase is found at moderate temperatures and moderate pressures. The point at which the three phase boundaries meet is called the **triple point**. This is the temperature and pressure at which the three phases exist in equilibrium. The phase boundary that separates the solid and the liquid phases extends indefinitely from the triple point. The phase boundary between the liquid and gas phases, however, terminates at a point called the **critical point**. This is the temperature and pressure above which there is no distinction between the phases. Although this may seem to be an impossibility—after all, it's always possible to distinguish between the liquid and the solid phase—such **supercritical fluids** are perfectly logical. As a liquid is heated in a closed system its density decreases and the density of the vapor sitting above it increases. The critical point is the temperature and pressure at which the two densities become equal and there is no distinction between the two phases. The heat of vaporization at this point and for all temperatures and pressures above the critical point values is zero.

MCAT CONCEPT CHECK 7.2

Before you move on, assess your understanding of the material with these questions.

1. What are standard conditions? When are standard conditions used for calculations?

____

2. What is the definition of a state function? A process function?

- State function:

____

- Process function:

____

3. List at least five common state functions:

- ____________________
- ____________________
- ____________________
- ____________________
- ____________________

4. Identify the triple point and critical point on the diagram below. What is the definition of the triple point? The critical point?

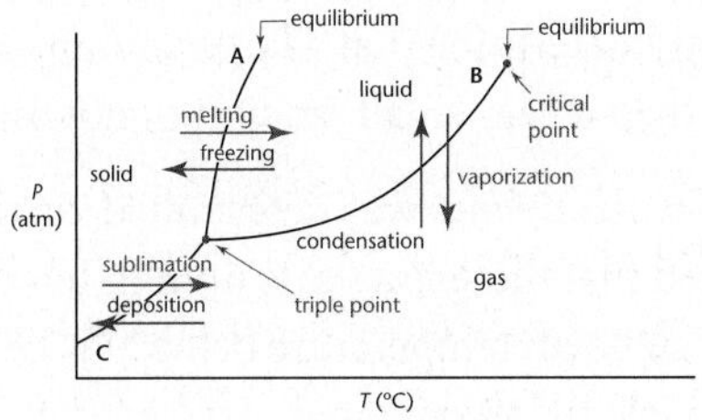

- Triple point:

____

- Critical point:

____

7.3 Heat

LEARNING OBJECTIVES

After Chapter 7.3, you will be able to:

- Differentiate between temperature and heat
- Compare specific heat and heat capacity
- Recall the specific heat of water
- Describe the processes for constant-volume and constant-pressure calorimetry:

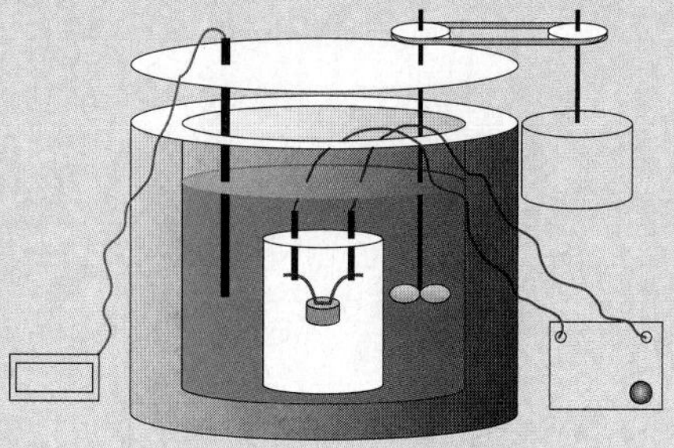

KEY CONCEPT

Remember that heat and temperature are different. Heat is a specific form of energy that can enter or leave a system, while temperature is a measure of the average kinetic energy of the particles in a system.

Before we can examine the first of the four state functions that are the focus of this chapter, we must address the topic of heat, which is a source of confusion for many students. Perhaps the greatest barrier to a proper understanding of heat is the semantic conflation of the terms *heat* and *temperature*. Many people use these terms interchangeably in everyday conversation, but this obscures the lexicon of thermodynamics. **Temperature (*T*)** is related to the average kinetic energy of the particles of a substance. Temperature is the way that we scale how hot or cold something is. We are familiar with a few temperature scales: Fahrenheit, Celsius, and Kelvin. The average kinetic energy of the particles in a substance is related to the **thermal energy (enthalpy)** of the substance, but because we must also include consideration of how much substance is present to calculate total thermal energy content, the most we can say about temperature is that when a substance's thermal energy increases, its temperature also increases. Nevertheless, we cannot say that something that is hot necessarily has greater thermal energy (in absolute terms) than a substance that is cold. For example, we might determine that a large amount of lukewarm water has a greater *total* heat content than a very small amount of hot water.

The absolute temperature scale, Kelvin, was determined via the third law of thermodynamics, which elucidated that there is a finite limit to temperature below which nothing can exist. There can be no temperature below 0 K because, by definition, the system is said to be unable to lose any more heat energy. Quantum mechanics describes a state of molecular motions possible below absolute zero, but this is beyond the scope of the MCAT.

Overview

Heat (Q) is the transfer of energy from one substance to another as a result of their differences in temperature. In fact, the **zeroth law of thermodynamics** implies that objects are in thermal equilibrium only when their temperatures are equal. Heat is therefore a process function, not a state function: we can quantify how much thermal energy is transferred between two or more objects as a result of their difference in temperatures by measuring the heat transferred.

Remember that the first law of thermodynamics states that the change in the total internal energy (ΔU) of a system is equal to the amount of heat (Q) transferred to the system minus the amount of work (W) done by the system: $\Delta U = Q - W$.

Because heat and work are measured independently, we can assess the transfer of energy in the form of heat through any process regardless of the amount of work done. Processes in which the system absorbs heat are called **endothermic** ($\Delta Q > 0$), while those processes in which the system releases heat are called **exothermic** ($\Delta Q < 0$). The unit of heat is the unit of energy: joule (J) or calorie (cal), for which 1 cal = 4.184 J. **Enthalpy (ΔH)** is equivalent to heat (Q) under constant pressure, which is an assumption the MCAT usually makes for thermodynamics problems.

When substances of different temperatures are brought into thermal contact with each other—that is, some physical arrangement that allows heat transfer—energy will move from the warmer substance to the cooler substance. When a substance undergoes an endothermic or exothermic reaction, heat energy will be exchanged between the system and the environment.

The process of measuring transferred heat is called **calorimetry**. Two basic types of calorimetry include constant-pressure calorimetry and constant-volume calorimetry. The coffee-cup calorimeter, introduced at the beginning of this chapter, is a low-tech example of a constant-pressure calorimeter, while a bomb calorimeter is an example of a constant-volume calorimeter.

The heat (q) absorbed or released in a given process is calculated via the equation:

$$q = mc\Delta T$$

Equation 7.2

where m is the mass, c is the specific heat of the substance, and ΔT is the change in temperature (in kelvin or degrees Celsius). **Specific heat** is defined as the amount of energy required to raise the temperature of one gram of a substance by one degree Celsius (or one kelvin). Specific heat values will generally be provided on Test Day, but one constant to remember is the specific heat of $H_2O\,(l)$: $c_{H_2O} = 1\ \frac{\text{cal}}{\text{g} \cdot \text{K}}$.

It requires less heat to raise the temperature of a glass of water the same amount as a swimming pool. While these two items have the same specific heat, c, they have different **heat capacities**—the product mc (mass times specific heat).

REAL WORLD

One of the most important ways that the body works to prevent overheating is through the production of sweat—an exocrine secretion of water, electrolytes, and urea. However, it is not the *production* of sweat that is the cooling mechanism. It's the *evaporation* of the sweat that helps cool the body. Evaporation (vaporization) from the liquid to gas phase is an endothermic process: energy must be absorbed from the body for the particles of the liquid to gain enough kinetic energy to escape into the gas phase. Hot, arid desert air has a lower partial pressure of water vapor than humid, tropical air, so sweat vaporizes more readily in the dry air than it does in the humid air. Accordingly, most people will feel more comfortable in dry heat than in humid heat.

MNEMONIC

The equation for heat transfer, given a specific heat, is the same as the test you're studying for! $q = mc\Delta T$ looks a lot like "q equals MCAT."

REAL WORLD

When walking barefoot, a blacktop *feels* much hotter than a wooden walkway even when they are the same temperature. This is because they have different specific heats.

Constant-Pressure and Constant-Volume Calorimetry

To picture the setup of a **constant-pressure calorimeter**, just think of the coffee-cup calorimeter: an insulated container covered with a lid and filled with a solution in which a reaction or some physical process, such as dissolution, is occurring. The incident pressure, which is atmospheric pressure, remains constant throughout the process, and the temperature can be measured as the reaction progresses. There should be sufficient thermal insulation (such as Styrofoam) to ensure that the heat being measured is an accurate representation of the reaction, without gain or loss of heat to the environment. Other commercial applications of these same principles include home insulation, padded clothing, and certain food containers such as thermoses.

The term **bomb calorimeter** may sound rather ominous, but a more accurate descriptive term is **decomposition vessel**. This better reflects what is actually taking place in **constant-volume calorimetry**. As shown in Figure 7.6, a sample of matter, typically a hydrocarbon, is placed in the steel decomposition vessel, which is then filled with almost pure oxygen gas. The decomposition vessel is then placed in an insulated container holding a known mass of water. The contents of the decomposition vessel are ignited by an electric ignition mechanism. The material combusts (burns) in the presence of the oxygen, and the heat that evolves is the heat of the combustion reaction. Because $W = P\Delta V$, no work is done in an isovolumetric process ($\Delta V = 0$), so $W_{calorimeter} = 0$. Furthermore, because of the insulation, the whole calorimeter can be considered isolated from the rest of the universe, so we can identify the system as the sample plus the oxygen and steel vessel, and the surroundings as the water.

REAL WORLD

Tests looking at plasma proteins or cancer diagnostics in medicine have utilized differential scanning calorimetry (DSC), which is a constant-pressure device, to identify blood components. Such results have shown that thermal properties of major plasma proteins are altered from early- to late-stage tumors.

REAL WORLD

Bomb calorimeters have helped elucidate the thermodynamic properties of various chemical compounds, including food additives, to determine nutritional value (the caloric content of the additive).

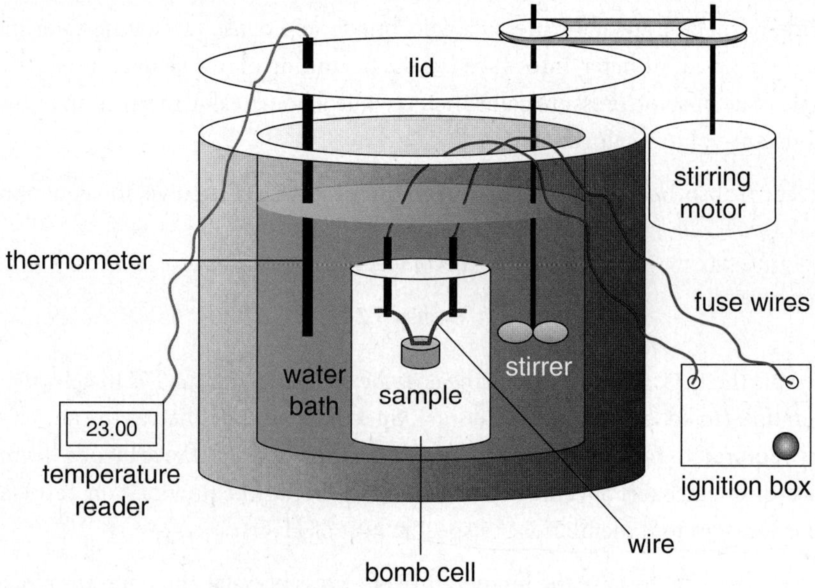

Figure 7.6 Diagram of a Bomb Calorimeter

Because no heat is exchanged between the calorimeter and the rest of the universe, $Q_{calorimeter}$ is 0. So,

$$\Delta U_{system} + \Delta U_{surroundings} = \Delta U_{calorimeter} = Q_{calorimeter} - W_{calorimeter} = 0$$

Therefore,

$$\Delta U_{system} = -\Delta U_{surroundings}$$

and because no work is done,

$$q_{system} = -q_{surroundings}$$
$$m_{steel}c_{steel}\Delta T + m_{oxygen}c_{oxygen}\Delta T = -m_{water}c_{water}\Delta T$$

Note that by using the layer of insulation to isolate the entire calorimeter from the rest of the universe, we've created an adiabatic process. This means that no heat is exchanged between the calorimeter and the rest of the universe, but it *is* exchanged between the steel decomposition vessel and the surrounding water. As the previous derivation shows, heat exchange between the system and its surroundings makes it possible for us to calculate the heat of combustion.

Example: One cup containing 100 grams of water at 300 K is mixed into another cup containing 200 g of water at 450 K. What is the equilibrium temperature of the system? (Note: Assume that the pressure is sufficiently high to avoid boiling.)

Solution: The two liquids undergo thermal exchange; thus, the heat given off by one liquid will be equal to the heat absorbed by the other.

$$q_{cold} = -q_{hot}$$
$$m_{cold}c_{H_2O}\Delta T_{cold} = m_{hot}c_{H_2O}(-\Delta T_{hot})$$

Now plug in the values from the question. Because we are solving for final (equilibrium) temperature of a mixture, we can use any value of *c* so long as we are consistent for both liquids (in this case we have two quantities of water and will use $c_{H_2O} = 1\frac{\text{cal}}{\text{g}\cdot\text{K}}$).

$$m_{cold}c_{H_2O}\Delta T_{cold} = m_{hot}c_{H_2O}(-\Delta T_{hot})$$
$$(100\text{ g})\left(1\frac{\text{cal}}{\text{g}\cdot\text{K}}\right)(T_f - 300\text{ K}) = (200\text{ g})\left(1\frac{\text{cal}}{\text{g}\cdot\text{K}}\right)(450\text{ K} - T_f)$$
$$100\,T_f - 30{,}000\text{ cal} = 90{,}000\text{ cal} - 200\,T_f$$
$$300\,T_f = 120{,}000$$
$$T_f = \frac{120{,}000}{300} = 400\text{ K}$$

MCAT EXPERTISE

Knowing that heat can transfer energy from a system to the surroundings is a key concept tested on calorimetry questions. Whenever you are asked about equilibrium questions regarding the final temperature of a two-liquid (or liquid–solid) system, remember that the colder object gains thermal energy and the hotter object loses it. You should instinctively realize that a metal bar at 1000 K is hotter than a bath of water at 298 K even though water has a high specific heat. Thus, set up the equation as $q_{cold} = -q_{hot}$. This form of the equation avoids the pesky sign notation issues in the ΔT equation encountered in most general chemistry texts.

Heating Curves

When a compound is heated, the temperature rises until the melting or boiling point is reached. Then, the temperature remains constant as the compound is converted to the next phase (liquid or gas, respectively). Once the entire sample is converted, then the temperature begins to rise again. This is depicted in the heating curves in Figure 7.7.

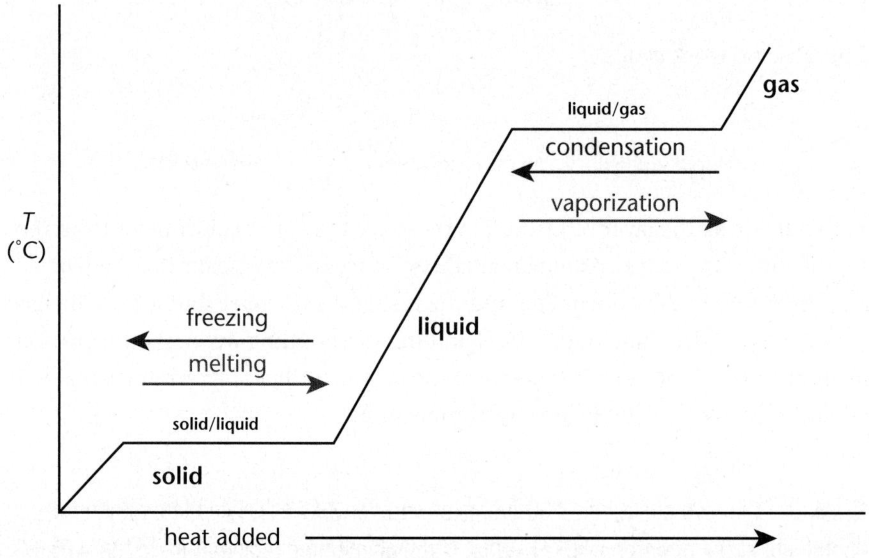

Figure 7.7 Heating Curve for a Single Compound

Heating curves show that phase change reactions do not undergo changes in temperature. For this reason, we cannot use $q = mc\Delta T$ during this interval because $\Delta T = 0$. We know intuitively that heat must continue to be added in order for the whole solid to melt, so where does this heat go? The solid absorbs energy, which allows particles to overcome the attractive forces that hold them in a rigid, three-dimensional arrangement. When melting an ice cube, all of the heat added during the process is used to overcome the intermolecular forces between water molecules in ice, forming liquid water. Once all of the ice has been turned into liquid water, the temperature of the liquid water can then increase again. The converse is also true: removing heat from a liquid at the solid–liquid phase transition temperature will cause the formation of a rigid lattice of water molecules.

During phase changes, we must use values based on enthalpy. When transitioning at the solid–liquid boundary, the **enthalpy** (or **heat**) **of fusion** (**ΔH_{fus}**) must be used to determine the heat transferred during the phase change. When transitioning from solid to liquid, the change in enthalpy will be positive because heat must be added; when transitioning from a liquid to a solid, the change in enthalpy will be negative because heat must be removed. At the liquid–gas boundary, the **enthalpy** (or **heat**) **of vaporization** (**ΔH_{vap}**) must be used, and its sign convention also follows a similar pattern. These are utilized in the equation

$$q = mL$$

Equation 7.3

where m is the mass and L is the **latent heat**, a general term for the enthalpy of an isothermal process, given in the units $\frac{\text{cal}}{\text{g}}$.

The total amount of heat needed to cross multiple phase boundaries is simply a summation of the heats for changing the temperature of each of the respective phases and the heats associated with phase changes.

KEY CONCEPT

We need a different formula to calculate q during phase changes when $\Delta T = 0$. If we used $q = mc\Delta T$, we'd erroneously think $q = 0$.

Example: What amount of energy is required to change a 90 gram ice cube at $-10°\text{C}$ to vapor at $110°\text{C}$? (Note: $c_{\text{H}_2\text{O}\,(l)} = 4.18 \frac{\text{J}}{\text{g}\cdot\text{K}}$, $c_{\text{H}_2\text{O}\,(s)} = 2.18 \frac{\text{J}}{\text{g}\cdot\text{K}}$, $c_{\text{H}_2\text{O}\,(g)} = 2.00 \frac{\text{J}}{\text{g}\cdot\text{K}}$, $\Delta H_{\text{fus}} = 6.02 \frac{\text{kJ}}{\text{mol}}$, $\Delta H_{\text{vap}} = 40.67 \frac{\text{kJ}}{\text{mol}}$)

Solution: Some of the constants given are in terms of mass (g), and some are in terms of moles, so we should convert the mass (90 g) to moles:

$$n = \frac{90\ \text{g H}_2\text{O}}{18 \frac{\text{g}}{\text{mol}}} = \frac{10}{2} = 5 \text{ moles H}_2\text{O}$$

Because we are beginning in the ice phase, we must heat the ice cube to the solid-liquid phase transition, which occurs at $0°\text{C}$. This first step involves a change in temperature, so we must use the heat formula that contains ΔT and all the pertinent variables for ice (solid water). Also, it is important to match all results in terms of J and kJ for the different steps of the calculation.

$$q_1 = m_{\text{ice}} c_{\text{ice}} \Delta T_1$$

$$q_1 = (90\ \text{g})\left(2.18 \frac{\text{J}}{\text{g}\cdot\text{K}}\right)(10\ \text{K}) \approx 90 \times 2 \times 10 = 1800\ \text{J} = 1.8\ \text{kJ}$$

In step 2, we must convert the ice into liquid form. During this phase change, there will be no temperature change.

$$q_2 = mL = n_{\text{H}_2\text{O}} \Delta H_{\text{fus}}$$

$$q_2 = (5\ \text{mol})\left(6.02 \frac{\text{kJ}}{\text{mol}}\right) \approx 5 \times 6 = 30\ \text{kJ}$$

In step 3, we heat the water to its liquid-gas phase transition temperature at $100°\text{C}$.

$$q_3 = m_{\text{water}} c_{\text{water}} \Delta T_3$$

$$q_3 = (90\ \text{g})\left(4.18 \frac{\text{J}}{\text{g}\cdot\text{K}}\right)(100\ \text{K}) \approx 90 \times 4 \times 100 = 36{,}000\ \text{J} = 36\ \text{kJ}$$

In step 4, we vaporize the water. Again, no temperature change will occur during this phase change.

$$q_4 = mL = n_{\text{H}_2\text{O}} \Delta H_{\text{vap}}$$

$$q_4 = (5\ \text{mol})\left(40.67 \frac{\text{kJ}}{\text{mol}}\right) \approx 5 \times 40 = 200\ \text{kJ}$$

In step 5, we must finally heat the water to the target temperature of 110°C.

$$q_5 = m_{steam}c_{steam}\Delta T_5$$

$$q_5 = (90\text{ g})\left(2.00\frac{\text{J}}{\text{g}\cdot\text{K}}\right)(10\text{ K}) = 90 \times 2 \times 10 = 1800\text{ J} = 1.8\text{ kJ}$$

The total heat required for this whole phase change from beginning to end is:

$$q_{tot} = q_1 + q_2 + q_3 + q_4 + q_5$$

$$q_{tot} = 1.8 + 30 + 36 + 200 + 1.8$$

$$q_{tot} \approx 2 + 30 + 36 + 200 + 2 = 270\text{ kJ (actual value} = 274.8\text{ kJ)}$$

A question *this* involved is unlikely to be seen on the MCAT because so many steps must be calculated. However, understanding the significance and rationale of this calculation is definitely within the scope of the test.

MCAT EXPERTISE

It is not in your best interest to memorize all the possible values for c and ΔH for Test Day. The MCAT will provide constants as needed, especially if the system is not water. That being said, practicing with heat calculations for water solutions and gaining familiarity with the heat capacities of water will help on Test Day.

MCAT CONCEPT CHECK 7.3

Before you move on, assess your understanding of the material with these questions.

1. Contrast temperature and heat.
   - Temperature:

   ____

   - Heat:

   ____

2. Contrast specific heat and heat capacity.
   - Specific heat:

   ____

   - Heat capacity:

   ____

3. Contrast constant-volume and constant-pressure calorimetry.
   - Constant-volume:

   ____

   - Constant-pressure:

   ____

4. What is the specific heat of liquid water (in calories)?

7.4 Enthalpy

LEARNING OBJECTIVES

After Chapter 7.4, you will be able to:

- Distinguish between endothermic and exothermic reactions
- Determine the enthalpy of a molecule or atom given reaction data:

$$C\ (s,\ \text{graphite}) + 2\ H_2\ (g) \rightarrow CH_4\ (g)$$

$$CH_4\ (g) + 2\ O_2\ (g) \rightarrow CO_2\ (g) + 2\ H_2O\ (l) \qquad \Delta H_a = -890.4\ \frac{\text{kJ}}{\text{mol}}$$

$$C\ (s,\ \text{graphite}) + O_2\ (g) \rightarrow CO_2\ (g) \qquad \Delta H_b = -393.5\ \frac{\text{kJ}}{\text{mol}}$$

$$2 \times \left[H_2\ (g) + \tfrac{1}{2}\ O_2\ (g) \rightarrow H_2O\ (l)\right] \qquad \Delta H_g = 2 \times -285.8\ \frac{\text{kJ}}{\text{mol}}$$

Most reactions in the laboratory occur under constant pressure (at 1 atm) in closed thermodynamic systems. To express heat changes at constant pressure, chemists use the term **enthalpy (*H*)**. Enthalpy is a state function, so we can calculate the change in enthalpy (ΔH) for a system that has undergone a process—for example, a chemical reaction—by comparing the enthalpy of the final state to the enthalpy of the initial state, irrespective of the path taken. The change in enthalpy is equal to the heat transferred into or out of the system at constant pressure. To find the enthalpy change of a reaction, ΔH_{rxn}, one must subtract the enthalpy of the reactants from the enthalpy of the products:

$$\Delta H_{rxn} = H_{products} - H_{reactants}$$

Equation 7.4

A positive ΔH_{rxn} corresponds to an endothermic process, and a negative ΔH_{rxn} corresponds to an exothermic process. It is not possible to measure enthalpy directly; only ΔH can be measured, and only for certain fast and spontaneous processes. Thus, several methods have been developed to calculate ΔH for any process.

Standard Heat of Formation

The **standard enthalpy of formation** of a compound, ΔH°_f, is the enthalpy required to produce one mole of a compound from its elements in their standard states. Remember that *standard state* refers to the most stable physical state of an element or compound at 298 K and 1 atm. Note that ΔH°_f of an element in its standard state, by definition, is zero. The ΔH°_f values of most known substances are tabulated. You do not need to memorize these values because they will be provided for you.

Standard Heat of Reaction

The **standard enthalpy of a reaction**, ΔH°_{rxn}, is the enthalpy change accompanying a reaction being carried out under standard conditions. This can be calculated by taking the difference between the sum of the standard heats of formation for the products and the sum of the standard heats of formation of the reactants:

$$\Delta H^\circ_{rxn} = \Sigma\, \Delta H^\circ_{f,products} - \Sigma\, \Delta H^\circ_{f,reactants}$$

Equation 7.5

Hess's Law

KEY CONCEPT

State functions are always path independent.

Enthalpy is a state function and is a property of the equilibrium state, so the pathway taken for a process is irrelevant to the change in enthalpy from one equilibrium state to another. As a consequence of this, **Hess's law** states that enthalpy changes of reactions are additive. When thermochemical equations (chemical equations for which energy changes are known) are added to give the net equation for a reaction, the corresponding heats of reaction are also added to give the net heat of reaction, as shown in Figure 7.8.

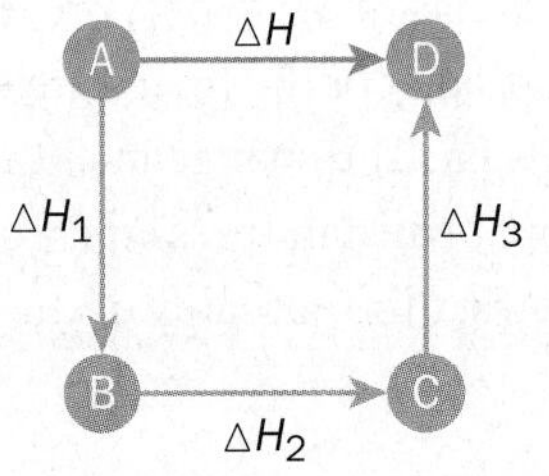

Figure 7.8 Illustration of Hess's Law: Forming Product (D) from Reactant (A)
Because enthalpy is a state function, $\Delta H = \Delta H_1 + \Delta H_2 + \Delta H_3$

Hess's law is embodied in the enthalpy equations we've already introduced. For example, we can describe any reaction as the result of breaking down the reactants into their component elements, then forming the products from these elements. The enthalpy change for the reverse of any reaction has the same magnitude, but the opposite sign, as the enthalpy change for the forward reaction. Therefore,

$$\Delta H_{reactants \rightarrow elements} = -\Delta H_{elements \rightarrow reactants}$$

The ΔH_{rxn} can be written as:

$$\Delta H_{rxn} = \Delta H_{reactants \rightarrow elements} + \Delta H_{elements \rightarrow products}$$

which is another way of writing

$$\Delta H^\circ_{rxn} = \Sigma\, \Delta H^\circ_{f,products} - \Sigma\, \Delta H^\circ_{f,reactants}$$

Consider the following phase change:

$$Br_2(l) \rightarrow Br_2(g) \qquad \Delta H^\circ_{rxn} = 31\ \frac{kJ}{mol}$$

The enthalpy change for the phase change is called the heat of vaporization (ΔH°_{vap}). As long as the initial and final states exist at standard conditions, the ΔH°_{rxn} will always equal the ΔH°_{vap}, irrespective of the particular pathway that the process takes. For example, it's possible that Br_2 (*l*) could first decompose to Br atoms, which then recombine to form Br_2 (*g*), rather than simply boiling from the liquid to gaseous state. However, because the net reaction is the same, the change in enthalpy will be the same.

Example: Given the following thermochemical equations:

(a) $CH_4\,(g) + 2\,O_2\,(g) \rightarrow CO_2\,(g) + 2\,H_2O\,(l)$ $\quad \Delta H_a = -890.4\,\frac{kJ}{mol}$

(b) $C\,(s,\text{graphite}) + O_2\,(g) \rightarrow CO_2\,(g)$ $\quad \Delta H_b = -393.5\,\frac{kJ}{mol}$

(c) $H_2\,(g) + \frac{1}{2}\,O_2\,(g) \rightarrow H_2O\,(l)$ $\quad \Delta H_c = -285.8\,\frac{kJ}{mol}$

Calculate ΔH for this reaction:

(d) $C\,(s,\text{graphite}) + 2\,H_2\,(g) \rightarrow CH_4\,(g)$

Solution: Equations (a), (b), and (c) must be combined to obtain equation (d). Because equation (d) contains only C, H_2, and CH_4, we must eliminate O_2, CO_2, and H_2O from the first three equations. Equation (a) is reversed to move CH_4 to the product side (equation (e) below). Next, equation (b) is left as is (we will call this equation (f) for consistency below) and (c) is multiplied by 2 (equation (g) below). Then, (d) can be calculated from (e) + (f) + (g):

(e) $CO_2\,(g) + 2\,H_2O\,(l) \rightarrow CH_4\,(g) + 2\,O_2\,(g)$ $\quad \Delta H_e = 890.4\,\frac{kJ}{mol}$

(f) $C\,(s,\text{graphite}) + O_2\,(g) \rightarrow CO_2\,(g)$ $\quad \Delta H_f = -393.5\,\frac{kJ}{mol}$

(g) $2 \times \left[H_2\,(g) + \frac{1}{2}\,O_2\,(g) \rightarrow H_2O\,(l)\right]$ $\quad \Delta H_g = 2 \times -285.8\,\frac{kJ}{mol}$

$C\,(s,\text{graphite}) + 2\,H_2\,(g) \rightarrow CH_4\,(g)$ $\quad \Delta H_d = \Delta H_e + \Delta H_f + \Delta H_g$

$$\Delta H_d = 890.4 + (-393.5) + [2 \times (-285.8)] \approx 900 + (-400) - (2 \times 285)$$

$$\Delta H_d = 900 - 400 - 570 = -70\,\frac{kJ}{mol}\ \left(\text{actual value} = -74.7\,\frac{kJ}{mol}\right)$$

It is important to realize that Hess's law applies to *any* state function, including entropy and Gibbs free energy.

MCAT EXPERTISE

When doing a problem like this on the MCAT, make sure to switch signs when you reverse the equation. Also, make sure to multiply by the correct stoichiometric coefficients when performing your calculations.

Bond Dissociation Energy

Hess's law can also be expressed in terms of **bond enthalpies**, also called **bond dissociation energies**. Bond dissociation energy is the average energy that is required to break a particular type of bond between atoms in the gas phase—remember, bond dissociation is an endothermic process. Bond dissociation energy is given in the units $\frac{\text{kJ}}{\text{mol of bonds broken}}$ and is often given in tables on the MCAT in a format similar to Table 7.1.

BOND	ENTHALPY $\left(\Delta H, \frac{\text{kJ}}{\text{mol}}\right)$
O=O	498
C—H	415
H—H	436

Table 7.1 Sample Bond Enthalpies

KEY CONCEPT

Because it takes energy to pull two atoms apart, bond breakage is generally endothermic. The reverse process, bond formation, is generally exothermic.

Bond enthalpies are the averages of the bond energies for the same bond in many different compounds. For example, the C—H bond enthalpy $\left(415\ \frac{\text{kJ}}{\text{mol}}\right)$ is averaged from measurements of the individual C—H bond enthalpies of thousands of different organic compounds. Note that bond formation, the opposite of bond breaking, has the same magnitude of energy but is negative rather than positive; that is, energy is released when bonds are formed. Remember that atoms generally form bonds to become more stable (often by completing an octet). Thus, it makes sense that bond formation is exothermic and bond dissociation is endothermic. The enthalpy change associated with a reaction is given by

$$\Delta H^\circ_{\text{rxn}} = \Sigma\,\Delta H_{\text{bonds broken}} - \Sigma\,\Delta H_{\text{bonds formed}} = \text{total energy absorbed} - \text{total energy released}$$

Equation 7.6

Example: Calculate the enthalpy change for the following reaction:

$$C\,(s) + 2\,H_2\,(g) \rightarrow CH_4\,(g) \qquad \Delta H = ?$$

Bond dissociation energies of H—H and C—H bonds are $436\,\frac{kJ}{mol}$ and $415\,\frac{kJ}{mol}$, respectively. The ΔH_f of C (g) is $715\,\frac{kJ}{mol}$.

Solution: CH_4 is formed from free elements in their standard states (C in solid state and H_2 in gaseous state). Thus, here $\Delta H_{rxn} = \Delta H_f$. The reaction can be written in three steps:

$$\begin{array}{ll} \text{(a) } C\,(s) \rightarrow C\,(g) & \Delta H_1 \\ \text{(b) } 2\,[H_2\,(g) \rightarrow 2\,H\,(g)] & 2 \times \Delta H_2 \\ \text{(c) } C\,(g) + 4\,H\,(g) \rightarrow CH_4\,(g) & \Delta H_3 \end{array}$$

with $\Delta H_f = \Delta H_1 + (2 \times \Delta H_2) + \Delta H_3$.

$$\Delta H_1 = \Delta H_f \text{ of } C(g) = 715\,\frac{kJ}{mol}$$

ΔH_2 is the energy required to break the H—H bond of one mole of H_2, so $\Delta H_2 =$ bond enthalpy of $H_2 = 436\,\frac{kJ}{mol}$. Note that reaction (b) is doubled in order to produce 4 atoms of H from two molecules of H_2.

ΔH_3 is the energy released when 4 C—H bonds are formed. Because energy is released when bonds are formed, ΔH_3 is negative.

$$\Delta H_3 = -(4 \times \text{bond energy of C—H}) = -\left(4 \times 415\,\frac{kJ}{mol}\right) = -1660\,\frac{kJ}{mol}$$

Therefore, for the entire reaction,

$$\Delta H_{rxn} = \Delta H_f = 715\,\frac{kJ}{mol} + \left(2 \times 436\,\frac{kJ}{mol}\right) - 1660\,\frac{kJ}{mol}$$

$$\Delta H_{rxn} \approx 700 + (2 \times 450) - 1660 = 700 + 900 - 1660 = -60\,\frac{kJ}{mol}$$

$$\left(\text{actual value} = -73\,\frac{kJ}{mol}\right)$$

Standard Heat of Combustion

As the name implies, the **standard heat of combustion,** ΔH°_{comb}, is the enthalpy change associated with the combustion of a fuel. Because measurements of enthalpy change require a reaction to be spontaneous and fast, combustion reactions are the ideal processes for such measurements. Most combustion reactions presented on the MCAT occur in the presence of atmospheric oxygen, but keep in mind that there are other combustion reactions in which oxygen is not the oxidant. Diatomic fluorine, for example, can be used as an oxidant. In addition, hydrogen gas will combust with chlorine gas to form gaseous hydrochloric acid and, in the process, will evolve a large amount of heat and light as is characteristic of combustion reactions. The reactions listed in the CH_4 (*g*) example shown earlier are combustion reactions with O_2 (*g*) as the oxidant. Therefore, the enthalpy change listed for each of the three reactions is the ΔH_{comb} for each of the reactions.

The glycolytic pathway, described in Chapter 9 of *MCAT Biochemistry Review*, is also a combustion reaction that utilizes a fuel (glucose) mixed with an oxidant (oxygen) to produce carbon dioxide and water.

$$C_6H_{12}O_6 + 6\,O_2 \rightarrow 6\,CO_2 + 6\,H_2O$$

KEY CONCEPT

The larger the alkane reactant, the more numerous the combustion products.

The heat of combustion for this reaction is found in a similar fashion to that of Hess's Law. Given the numerous reactions and pathways involved, we can determine the overall enthalpy of the reaction, as shown in Figure 7.9.

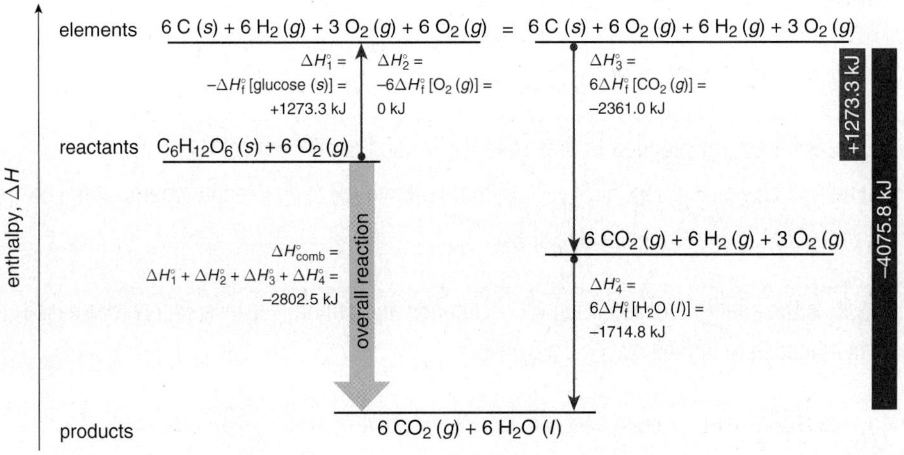

Figure 7.9 Determining the Enthalpy of Glycolysis

MCAT CONCEPT CHECK 7.4

Before you move on, assess your understanding of the material with these questions.

1. Define endothermic and exothermic processes.
   - Endothermic:

   ____

   - Exothermic:

   ____

2. Given the following reactions, determine the enthalpy of:

$C\ (s, \text{graphite}) + \frac{1}{2}\ O_2 \rightarrow CO.$

$C\ (s, \text{graphite}) + O_2 \rightarrow CO_2 \quad \Delta H = -393.5\ \frac{\text{kJ}}{\text{mol}}$

$CO + \frac{1}{2}\ O_2 \rightarrow CO_2 \quad \Delta H = -283\ \frac{\text{kJ}}{\text{mol}}$

---

3. What is the enthalpy of reaction for the reaction: $2\ H_2O\ (g) \rightarrow 2\ H_2\ (g) + O_2\ (g)$, given the following and bond enthalpies: $H{-}H = 436\ \frac{\text{kJ}}{\text{mol}}$, $O{=}O = 498\ \frac{\text{kJ}}{\text{mol}}$, $O{-}O = 146\ \frac{\text{kJ}}{\text{mol}}$, and $O{-}H = 463\ \frac{\text{kJ}}{\text{mol}}$

7.5 Entropy

LEARNING OBJECTIVES

After Chapter 7.5, you will be able to:

- Order the phases of matter from lowest to highest entropy
- Define entropy in terms of its relation to energy distribution and disorder
- Predict the direction of change in entropy within a given reaction

Many students are perplexed by the concept of entropy. Enthalpy makes intuitive sense, especially when the energy change from reactants to products is large, fast, and dramatic (as in combustion reactions involving explosions). Entropy seems to be less intuitive—except that it isn't. Consider, for example, how "normal" each of the following seems: hot tea cools down, frozen drinks melt, iron rusts, buildings crumble, balloons deflate, living things die and decay, and so on.

These examples have a common denominator: in each of them, energy of some form is going from being localized or concentrated to being spread out or dispersed. The thermal energy in the hot tea is spreading out to the cooler air that surrounds it. The thermal energy in the warmer air is spreading out to the cooler frozen drink. The chemical energy in the bonds of elemental iron and oxygen is released and dispersed as a result of the formation of the more stable, lower-energy bonds of iron oxide (rust). The potential energy of the building is released and dispersed in the form of light, sound, and heat as the building crumbles and falls. The energy of the pressurized air is released to the surrounding atmosphere as the balloon deflates. The chemical energy of all the molecules and atoms in living flesh is released into the environment during the process of death and decay.

The **second law of thermodynamics** states that energy spontaneously disperses from being localized to becoming spread out if it is not hindered from doing so. Pay attention to this: *the usual way of thinking about entropy as "disorder" must not be taken too literally, a trap that many students fall into. Be very careful in thinking about entropy as disorder*. The old analogy between a messy (disordered) room and entropy is deficient and may not only hinder understanding but actually increase confusion.

KEY CONCEPT

Entropy changes that accompany phase changes can be easily estimated, at least qualitatively. For example, freezing is accompanied by a decrease in entropy, as the relatively disordered liquid becomes a well-ordered solid. Meanwhile, boiling is accompanied by a large increase in entropy, as the liquid becomes a much more disordered gas. For any substance, sublimation will be the phase transition with the greatest increase in entropy.

Entropy is the measure of the spontaneous dispersal of energy at a specific temperature: *how much* energy is spread out, or *how widely* spread out energy becomes, in a process. The equation for calculating the change in entropy is:

$$\Delta S = \frac{Q_{\text{rev}}}{T}$$

Equation 7.7

where ΔS is the change in entropy, Q_{rev} is the heat that is gained or lost in a reversible process, and T is the temperature in kelvin. The units of entropy are usually $\frac{\text{J}}{\text{mol}\cdot\text{K}}$. When energy is distributed into a system at a given temperature, its entropy increases. When energy is distributed out of a system at a given temperature, its entropy decreases.

Notice that the second law states that energy will spontaneously disperse; it does not say that energy can never be localized or concentrated. However, the concentration of energy will rarely happen spontaneously in a closed system. Work usually must be done to concentrate energy. For example, refrigerators work against the direction of spontaneous heat flow (that is, they counteract the flow of heat from the "warm" exterior of the refrigerator to the "cool" interior), thereby "concentrating" energy outside of the system in the surroundings. As a result, refrigerators consume a lot of energy to accomplish this movement of energy against the temperature gradient.

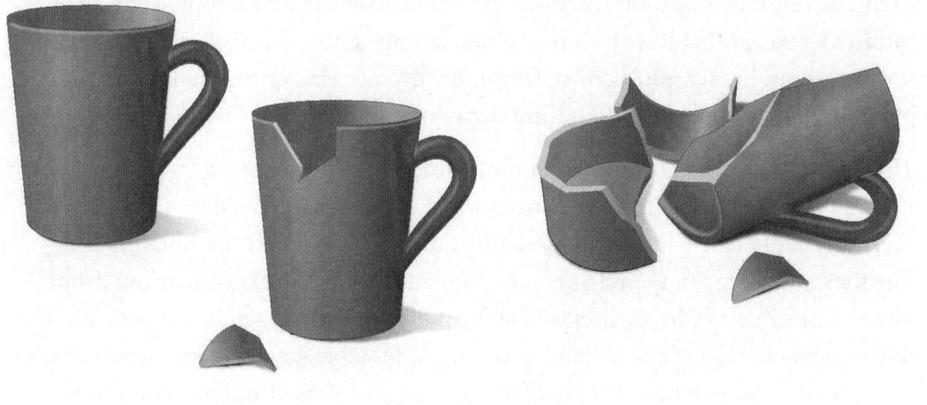

Figure 7.10 Entropy in the Kitchen
A new coffee mug can break if dropped, but a broken mug cannot put itself back together, one example of the asymmetry of time. The broken mug's entropy is higher than the new mug's.

The second law has been described as *time's arrow* because there is a unidirectional limitation on the movement of energy by which we recognize *before and after* or *new and old*, as shown in Figure 7.10. For example, you would instantly recognize whether a video recording of an explosion was running forward or backward. Another way of understanding this is to say that energy in a closed system will spontaneously spread out, and entropy will increase if it is not hindered from doing so. Remember that a system can be variably defined to include the entire universe; in fact, the second law ultimately claims that the entropy of the universe is increasing.

$$\Delta S_{\text{universe}} = \Delta S_{\text{system}} + \Delta S_{\text{surroundings}} > 0$$

Equation 7.8

Entropy is a state function, so a change in entropy from one equilibrium state to another is pathway independent and only depends upon the difference in entropies of the final and initial states. Further, the standard entropy change for a reaction, $\Delta S^\circ_{\text{rxn}}$, can be calculated using the standard entropies of the reactants and products—much like enthalpy:

$$\Delta S^\circ_{\text{rxn}} = \Sigma\, \Delta S^\circ_{\text{f,products}} - \Sigma\, \Delta S^\circ_{\text{f,reactants}}$$

Equation 7.9

MCAT CONCEPT CHECK 7.5

Before you move on, assess your understanding of the material with these questions.

1. Rank the phases of matter from lowest to highest entropy.

____

2. Describe entropy in terms of energy dispersal and disorder.

____

3. Do the following situations result in an increase or decrease in entropy?

Reaction	ΔS
$H_2O\ (l) \rightarrow H_2O\ (s)$	
Dry ice sublimates into carbon dioxide	
$NaCl\ (s) \rightarrow NaCl\ (aq)$	
$N_2\ (g) + 3\ H_2\ (g) \rightarrow 2\ NH_3\ (g)$	
An ice pack is placed on a wound	

7.6 Gibbs Free Energy

LEARNING OBJECTIVES

After Chapter 7.6, you will be able to:

- Determine the Gibbs free energy for a reaction at varying temperatures
- Predict the temperature necessary for a temperature-dependent reaction to be at equilibrium
- Identify how changing concentrations of reactant or product will alter the progress of a reaction

The final state function that we will examine in this chapter is **Gibbs free energy, *G***. This state function is a combination of the three that we've just examined: temperature, enthalpy, and entropy. The change in Gibbs free energy, ΔG, is a measure of the change in the enthalpy and the change in entropy as a system undergoes a process, and it indicates whether a reaction is spontaneous or nonspontaneous. The change in the free energy is the maximum amount of energy released by a process—occurring at constant temperature and pressure—that is available to perform useful work. The change in Gibbs free energy is defined as follows:

MNEMONIC

Gibbs free energy: $\Delta G = \Delta H - T\Delta S$
Goldfish are (equals sign) Horrible without (minus sign) Tartar Sauce.

$$\Delta G = \Delta H - T\Delta S$$

Equation 7.10

where T is the temperature in kelvin and $T\Delta S$ represents the total amount of energy that is absorbed by a system when its entropy increases reversibly.

Overview

A helpful visual aid for conceptualizing Gibbs free energy is to think of it as a valley between two hills. Just as a ball would tend to roll down the hill into the valley and eventually come to rest at the lowest point in the valley, any system—including chemical reactions—will move in whichever direction results in a reduction of the free energy of the system. The bottom of the valley represents equilibrium, and the sides of the hill represent the various points in the pathway toward or away from equilibrium. This is shown graphically in Figure 7.11, which was also discussed in the previous chapter.

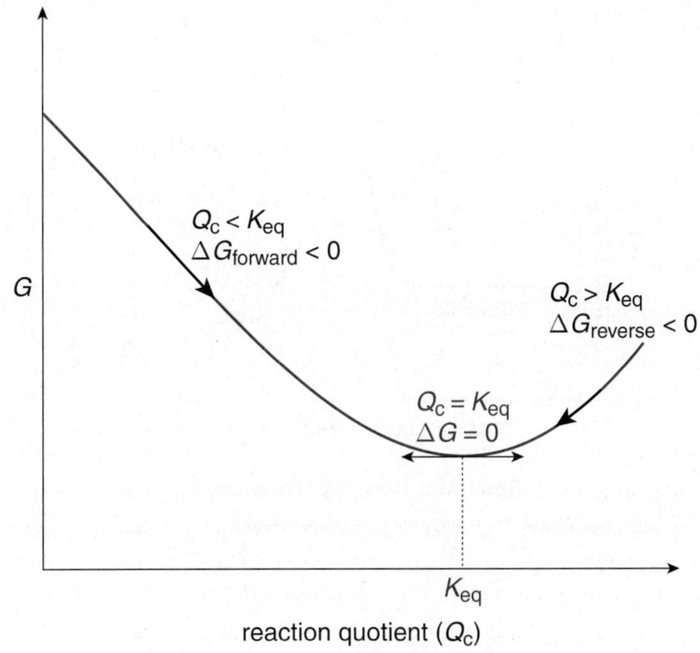

Figure 7.11 Gibbs Free Energy and Spontaneity
A decrease in Gibbs free energy indicates that a reaction is spontaneous. When an equilibrated system is disturbed, it will spontaneously act to restore equilibrium.

Movement toward the equilibrium position is associated with a decrease in Gibbs free energy ($\Delta G < 0$) and is spontaneous. When a system releases energy, it is said to be **exergonic**, as shown in Figure 7.12.

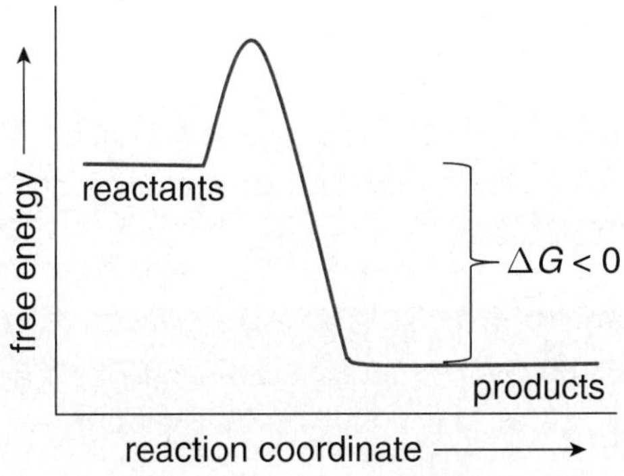

Figure 7.12 Exergonic Reaction Profile
Exergonic reactions release energy and are spontaneous ($\Delta G_{rxn} < 0$).

On the other hand, movement away from the equilibrium position is associated with an increase in Gibbs free energy ($\Delta G > 0$) and is nonspontaneous. Such a reaction is said to be **endergonic**, as shown in Figure 7.13.

MCAT EXPERTISE

Be careful not to confuse endergonic/exergonic (describing Gibbs free energy) with endothermic/exothermic (describing enthalpy).

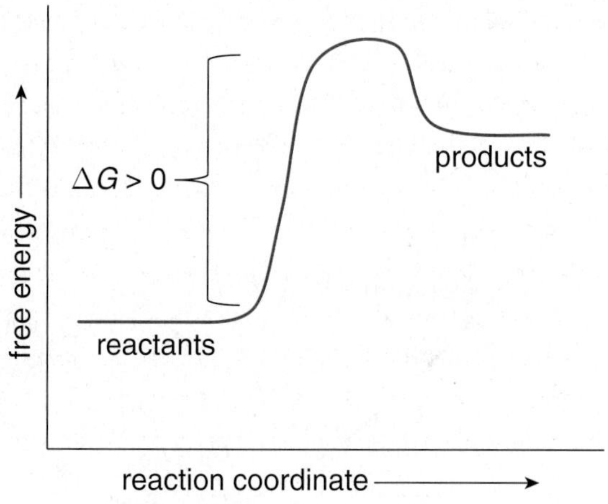

Figure 7.13 Endergonic Reaction Profile
Endergonic reactions absorb energy and are nonspontaneous ($\Delta G_{rxn} > 0$).

Once at the energy minimum state—equilibrium—the system will resist any changes to its state, and the change in free energy is zero. To summarize:

1. If ΔG is negative, the reaction is spontaneous.
2. If ΔG is positive, the reaction is nonspontaneous.
3. If ΔG is zero, the system is in a state of equilibrium; $\Delta H = T\Delta S$.

KEY CONCEPT

Recall that thermodynamics and kinetics are separate topics. When a reaction is thermodynamically spontaneous, it has no bearing on how fast it goes. It only means that it will proceed *eventually* without external energy input.

You should recall that phase equilibria are states in which more than one phase exists. As with all equilibria, the change in Gibbs free energy must be equal to zero ($\Delta G = 0$). For an equilibrium between a gas and a solid,

$$\Delta G = G\,(g) - G\,(s) = 0$$

Therefore,

$$G\,(g) = G\,(s)$$

Because the temperature in Gibbs free energy is in kelvin, it is always positive. Therefore, the effects of the signs of ΔH and ΔS on the spontaneity of a process can be summarized as in Table 7.2.

ΔH	ΔS	OUTCOME
+	+	Spontaneous at high *T*
+	−	Nonspontaneous at all *T*
−	+	Spontaneous at all *T*
−	−	Spontaneous at low *T*

Table 7.2 Effects of ΔH, ΔS, and *T* on Spontaneity

KEY CONCEPT

ΔG is temperature dependent when ΔH and ΔS have the same sign.

Phase changes are examples of temperature-dependent processes. The phase changes of water should be familiar to you; have you ever wondered why water doesn't boil at, say, 20°C instead of 100°C? When water boils, hydrogen bonds are broken, and the water molecules gain sufficient energy to escape into the gas phase. Thus, boiling is an endothermic process, and ΔH is positive. As thermal energy is transferred to the water molecules, energy is distributed through the molecules entering the gas phase. Thus, entropy is positive and the term $T\Delta S$ is positive. If both ΔH and $T\Delta S$ are positive, the reaction will only be spontaneous if $T\Delta S$ is greater than ΔH, resulting in a negative ΔG. These conditions are met only when the temperature of the system is greater than 373 K (100°C). Below 100°C, the free energy change is positive, and boiling is nonspontaneous; the water remains a liquid. At 100°C, $\Delta H - T\Delta S = 0$, and an equilibrium is established between the liquid and gas phases in such a way that the water's vapor pressure equals the ambient pressure. This is the definition of the boiling point: the temperature at which the vapor pressure equals the ambient pressure.

It is important to remember that the rate of a reaction depends on the activation energy E_a, not ΔG. Spontaneous reactions may be fast or slow. Sometimes a reversible reaction may produce two products that differ both in their stability (as measured by the change in the free energy associated with their production) and in their kinetics (as measured by their respective activation energies). Sometimes, the thermodynamically more stable product will have the slower kinetics due to higher activation energy. In this situation, we talk about kinetic *vs.* thermodynamic reaction control, which is discussed in Chapter 6 of *MCAT General Chemistry Review*. For a period of time after the reaction begins, the major product will be the one that is produced more quickly as a result of its lower activation energy. The reaction can be said to be under kinetic control at this time. Given enough time, however, and assuming a reversible reaction, the dominant product will be the thermodynamically more stable product as a result of its lower free energy value. The reaction can then be said to be under thermodynamic control. Eventually, the reaction will reach equilibrium, as defined by its K_{eq}.

Standard Gibbs Free Energy

The free energy change of reactions can be measured under standard state conditions to yield the **standard free energy, ΔG°_{rxn}**. For standard free energy determinations, the concentrations of any solutions in the reaction are 1 *M*. The standard free energy of formation of a compound, ΔG°_f, is the free energy change that occurs when 1 mole of a compound in its standard state is produced from its respective elements in their standard states under standard state conditions. The standard free energy of formation for any element under standard state conditions is, by definition, zero. The standard free energy of a reaction, ΔG°_{rxn}, is the free energy change that occurs when that reaction is carried out under standard state conditions; that is, when the reactants are converted to the products at standard conditions of temperature (298 K) and pressure (1 atm). Like enthalpy and entropy, the free energy of the reaction can be calculated from the free energies of formation of the reactants and products:

$$\Delta G^\circ_{rxn} = \sum \Delta G^\circ_{f,products} - \sum \Delta G^\circ_{f,reactants}$$

Equation 7.11

Free Energy, K_{eq}, and Q

We can derive the standard free energy change for a reaction from the equilibrium constant K_{eq} for the reaction using the equation:

$$\Delta G^{\circ}_{rxn} = -RT \ln K_{eq}$$

Equation 7.12

where R is the ideal gas constant, T is the temperature in kelvin, and K_{eq} is the equilibrium constant. This equation allows us to make not only quantitative evaluations of the free energy change of a reaction, but also qualitative assessments of the spontaneity of the reaction. The greater the value of K_{eq}, the more positive the value of its natural logarithm. The more positive the natural logarithm, the more negative the standard free energy change. The more negative the standard free energy change, the more spontaneous the reaction.

Once a reaction begins, however, the standard state conditions (specifically 1 M solutions) no longer apply. The value of the equilibrium constant must be replaced with another number that is reflective of where the reaction is in its path toward equilibrium. To determine the free energy change for a reaction that is in progress, we relate ΔG_{rxn} (not ΔG°_{rxn}) to the reaction quotient, Q:

KEY CONCEPT

Note that the right side of this equation is similar to Equation 7.12. The use of the Q indicates that the system is not at equilibrium.

$$\Delta G_{rxn} = \Delta G^{\circ}_{rxn} + RT \ln Q = RT \ln \frac{Q}{K_{eq}}$$

Equation 7.13

As described in Chapter 6 of *MCAT General Chemistry Review*, if the ratio of $\frac{Q}{K_{eq}}$ is less than one ($Q < K_{eq}$), then the natural logarithm will be negative, and the free energy change will be negative, so the reaction will spontaneously proceed forward until equilibrium is reached. If the ratio of $\frac{Q}{K_{eq}}$ is greater than one ($Q > K_{eq}$), then the natural logarithm will be positive, and the free energy change will be positive. In that case, the reaction will spontaneously move in the reverse direction until equilibrium is reached. Of course, if the ratio is equal to one, the reaction quotient is equal to the equilibrium constant; the reaction is at equilibrium, and the free energy change is zero ($\ln 1 = 0$).

Reaction profiles of free energy can be altered by the presence of catalysts. While the overall free energy change of the reaction is not altered, the activation energy required to accomplish the reaction is reduced significantly in the presence of a catalyst, as shown in Figure 7.14.

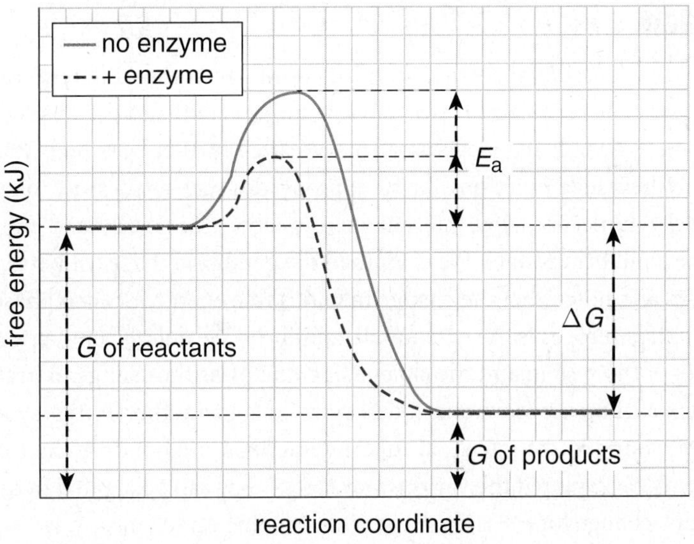

Figure 7.14 Catalysts Alter Kinetics but Not Equilibrium or Free Energy Change

MCAT CONCEPT CHECK 7.6

Before you move on, assess your understanding of the material with these questions.

1. The Haber–Bosch process creates ammonia through several reactions, the final step of which is

$$N_2 + 3\,H_2 \rightarrow 2\,NH_3 \left(\Delta H_{rxn} = -93\,\frac{kJ}{mol},\ \Delta S_{rxn} = -198\,\frac{J}{mol \cdot K}\right)$$

Determine what the Gibbs free energy of this reaction is at standard conditions and at 500 K:

- At standard conditions:

____

- At 500 K:

____

2. At what temperature would the reaction described above be at equilibrium?

____

3. If you were to suddenly flood the reaction vessel with significant amounts of ammonia, what would occur?

____

Conclusion

We began our discussion of thermochemistry with a review of different ways in which we characterize systems (open, closed, and isolated) and processes (isothermal, adiabatic, isobaric, and isovolumetric). We then further classified systems according to their state functions—system properties such as pressure, density, temperature, volume, enthalpy, internal energy, Gibbs free energy, and entropy that describe the equilibrium state. We examined the equilibria that exist between the different phases and noted that the change in Gibbs free energy for each phase change in equilibrium is zero, as is the case for all equilibria. We defined enthalpy as the heat content of the system and the change in enthalpy as the change in heat content of the system as it moves from one equilibrium state to another. Enthalpy is defined as the energy found in the intermolecular interactions and bonds of the compounds in the system. We explored the various ways Hess's law can be applied to calculate the total enthalpy change for a series of reactions. Moving on to entropy, we described this property as a measure of the degree to which energy in a system becomes spread out through a process. There is danger in thinking too literally about entropy as "disorder" because a system's entropy may be increasing even if there is no observable change in the system's macroscopic disorder (such as ice warming from $-10°C$ to $-5°C$). Gibbs free energy combines the effects of temperature, enthalpy, and entropy, and the change in Gibbs free energy determines whether a process will be spontaneous or nonspontaneous. When the change in Gibbs free energy is negative, the process is spontaneous, but when the change in Gibbs free energy is positive, the process is nonspontaneous.

Many reactions in the body must be spontaneous in order for cells to function. While there are some nonspontaneous reactions in our body, we are able to couple them to thermodynamically favorable (exergonic) reactions that allow the cell to perform even more complex functions.

You've reviewed the content, now test your knowledge and critical thinking skills by completing a test-like passage set in your online resources!

GO ONLINE

CONCEPT SUMMARY

Systems and Processes

- Systems are classified based on what is or is not exchanged with the surroundings.
  - **Isolated systems** exchange neither matter nor energy with the environment.
  - **Closed systems** can exchange energy but not matter with the environment.
  - **Open systems** can exchange both energy and matter with the environment.
- Processes can be characterized based on a single constant property.
  - **Isothermal** processes occur at a constant temperature.
  - **Adiabatic** processes exchange no heat with the environment.
  - **Isobaric** processes occur at a constant pressure.
  - **Isovolumetric** (**isochoric**) processes occur at a constant volume.

States and State Functions

- **State functions** describe the physical properties of an equilibrium state; they are pathway independent and include pressure, density, temperature, volume, enthalpy, internal energy, Gibbs free energy, and entropy.
- **Standard conditions** are defined as 298 K, 1 atm, and 1 *M* concentrations.
- The **standard state** of an element is its most prevalent form under standard conditions; **standard enthalpy**, **standard entropy**, and **standard free energy** are all calculated under standard conditions.
- **Phase changes** exist at characteristic temperatures and pressures.
  - **Fusion** (**melting**) and **freezing** (**crystallization** or **solidification**) occur at the boundary between the solid and the liquid phases.
  - **Vaporization** (**evaporation** or **boiling**) and **condensation** occur at the boundary between the liquid and the gas phases.
  - **Sublimation** and **deposition** occur at the boundary between the solid and gas phases.
  - At temperatures above the **critical point**, the liquid and gas phases are indistinguishable.
  - At the **triple point**, all three phases of matter exist in equilibrium.
- The **phase diagram** for a system graphs the phases and phase equilibria as a function of temperature and pressure.

Heat

- Temperature and heat are not the same thing.
  - **Temperature** is a scaled measure of the average kinetic energy of a substance.
  - **Heat** is the transfer of energy that results from differences of temperature between two substances.
- The heat content of a system undergoing heating, cooling, or phase changes is the sum of all the respective energy changes.

Enthalpy

- **Enthalpy** is a measure of the potential energy of a system found in intermolecular attractions and chemical bonds.
- **Hess's law** states that the total change in potential energy of a system is equal to the changes of potential energies of the individual steps of the process.
- Enthalpy can also be calculated using heats of formation, heats of combustion, or bond dissociation energies.

Entropy

- **Entropy**, while often thought of as disorder, is a measure of the degree to which energy has been spread throughout a system or between a system and its surroundings.
  - Entropy is a ratio of heat transferred per mole per unit kelvin.
  - Entropy is maximized at equilibrium.

Gibbs Free Energy

- **Gibbs free energy** is derived from both enthalpy and entropy values for a given system.
- The change in Gibbs free energy determines whether a process is spontaneous or nonspontaneous.
  - $\Delta G < 0$: reaction proceeds in forward direction (spontaneous)
  - $\Delta G = 0$: reaction is in dynamic equilibrium
  - $\Delta G > 0$: reaction proceeds in reverse direction (nonspontaneous)
- Gibbs free energy depends on temperature; temperature-dependent processes change between spontaneous and nonspontaneous, depending on the temperature.

ANSWERS TO CONCEPT CHECKS

7.1

1. The boundary between system and surroundings could be placed anywhere. Most commonly, the ice pack would be considered the chemical system using up energy, and the person (and the remainder of the universe) constitutes the surroundings that are providing the heat for the ice pack to function.
2. - Isothermal: no change in temperature; $\Delta U = 0$, $Q = W$
   - Adiabatic: no heat exchange; $Q = 0$, $\Delta U = -W$
   - Isobaric: no change in pressure; line appears flat in a P–V graph
   - Isovolumetric (isochoric): no change in volume; $W = 0$, $\Delta U = Q$

7.2

1. Kinetics, equilibrium, and thermodynamics calculations use standard conditions, which are 25°C (298 K), 1 atm pressure, and 1 *M* concentrations.
2. State functions are properties of a system at equilibrium and are independent of the path taken to achieve the equilibrium; they may be dependent on one another. Process functions define the path between equilibrium states and include *Q* (heat) and *W* (work).
3. State functions include pressure (*P*), density (ρ), temperature (*T*), volume (*V*), enthalpy (*H*), internal energy (*U*), Gibbs free energy (*G*), and entropy (*S*).
4. The triple point is the specific combination of temperature and pressure at which all three phases are in equilibrium. The critical point is the temperature and pressure above which the liquid and gas phases are indistinguishable and the heat of vaporization is zero.

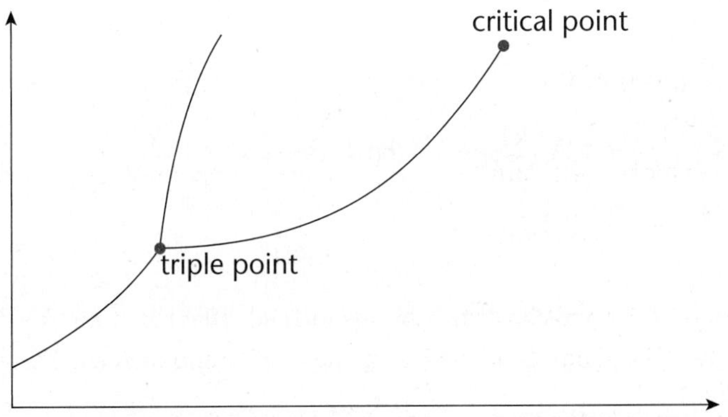

7.3

1. Temperature is an indirect measure of the thermal content of a system that looks at average kinetic energy of particles in a sample. Heat is the thermal energy transferred between objects as a result of differences in their temperatures.
2. Specific heat (*c*) is the energy required to raise the temperature of one gram of a substance by one degree Celsius. Heat capacity (*mc*) is the product of mass and specific heat and is the energy required to raise any given amount of a substance one degree Celsius.
3. A constant-pressure calorimeter (coffee cup calorimeter) is exposed to constant (atmospheric) pressure. As the reaction proceeds, the temperature of the contents is measured to determine the heat of the reaction. A constant-volume calorimeter (bomb calorimeter) is one in which heats of certain reactions (like combustion) can be measured indirectly by assessing temperature change in a water bath around the reaction vessel.
4. $c_{H_2O\,(l)} = 1\ \frac{\text{cal}}{\text{g}\cdot\text{K}}$

7.4

1. Endothermic reactions involve an increase in heat content of a system from the surroundings ($\Delta H > 0$), while exothermic reactions involve a release of heat content from a system ($\Delta H < 0$).
2. To reach the net equation $C(s, \text{graphite}) + \frac{1}{2} O_2 \rightarrow CO$, the second reaction must be reversed along with the sign of its enthalpy of reaction.

$$C(s, \text{graphite}) + O_2 \rightarrow CO_2 \qquad \Delta H = -393.5\ \frac{\text{kJ}}{\text{mol}}$$

$$CO_2 \rightarrow CO + \frac{1}{2} O_2 \qquad \Delta H = +283\ \frac{\text{kJ}}{\text{mol}}$$

Adding the enthalpies gives:

$$-393.5\ \frac{\text{kJ}}{\text{mol}} + 283\ \frac{\text{kJ}}{\text{mol}} \approx -400 + 285 = -115\ \frac{\text{kJ}}{\text{mol}}$$

$$\left(\text{actual value} = -110.5\ \frac{\text{kJ}}{\text{mol}}\right)$$

3. Enthalpy of reaction = bonds broken – bonds formed. There are four O–H bonds broken, two H–H bonds formed, and one O=O bond formed. Therefore,

$$\Delta H_{\text{rxn}} = \text{bonds broken} - \text{bonds formed}$$

$$\Delta H_{\text{rxn}} = (4 \times \text{O–H}) - [(2 \times \text{H–H}) + (1 \times \text{O=O})]$$

$$\Delta H_{\text{rxn}} = \left(4 \times 463\ \frac{\text{kJ}}{\text{mol}}\right) - \left[\left(2 \times 436\ \frac{\text{kJ}}{\text{mol}}\right) + \left(1 \times 498\ \frac{\text{kJ}}{\text{mol}}\right)\right]$$

$$\Delta H_{\text{rxn}} \approx (4 \times 450) - [(2 \times 435) + (500)] = 1800 - (870 + 500)$$

$$\Delta H_{\text{rxn}} = 1800 - 1370 = 430\ \frac{\text{kJ}}{\text{mol}} \left(\text{actual value} = 482\ \frac{\text{kJ}}{\text{mol}}\right)$$

7.5

1. Solids have the lowest entropy, followed by liquids, with gases having the highest entropy.
2. Entropy increases as a system has more disorder or freedom of movement, and energy is dispersed in a spontaneous system. Entropy of the universe can never be decreased spontaneously.
3.

Reaction	ΔS
H_2O (*l*) → H_2O (*s*)	Decrease (freezing)
Dry ice sublimates into carbon dioxide	Increase (sublimation)
NaCl (*s*) → NaCl (*aq*)	Increase (dissolution)
N_2 (*g*) + 3 H_2 (*g*) → 2 NH_3 (*g*)	Decrease (fewer moles of gas)
An ice pack is placed on a wound	Increase (heat is transferred)

7.6

1. At standard conditions:

$$\Delta G = \Delta H - T\Delta S = -93{,}000\ \frac{\text{J}}{\text{mol}} - (298\ \text{K})\left(-198\ \frac{\text{J}}{\text{mol}\cdot\text{K}}\right) \approx$$

$$-93{,}000 - (300 \times -200) = -93{,}000 + 60{,}000 = -33{,}000\ \frac{\text{J}}{\text{mol}} = -33\ \frac{\text{kJ}}{\text{mol}}$$

$$\left(\text{actual} = -34.0\ \frac{\text{kJ}}{\text{mol}}\right)$$

At 500 K:

$$\Delta G = \Delta H - T\Delta S = -93{,}000\ \frac{\text{J}}{\text{mol}} - (500\ \text{K})\left(-198\ \frac{\text{J}}{\text{mol}\cdot\text{K}}\right) \approx$$

$$-93{,}000 - (500 \times -200) = -93{,}000 + 100{,}000 = 7{,}000\ \frac{\text{J}}{\text{mol}} = 7\ \frac{\text{kJ}}{\text{mol}}$$

$$\left(\text{actual} = 6\ \frac{\text{kJ}}{\text{mol}}\right)$$

2. The system is at equilibrium when $\Delta G = 0$:

$$\Delta G = \Delta H - T\Delta S$$

$$0 = -93{,}000\ \frac{\text{J}}{\text{mol}} - \left[(T)\left(-198\ \frac{\text{J}}{\text{mol}\cdot\text{K}}\right)\right] 93{,}000 \approx 200\ T$$

$$T = \frac{93{,}000}{200} = \frac{930}{2} = 465\ \text{K}\ (\text{actual} = 470\ \text{K}).$$

3. The value of Q would increase significantly, causing the system to shift left, forming more reactants until the system again reached equilibrium.

SCIENCE MASTERY ASSESSMENT EXPLANATIONS

1. **A**

This process may be adiabatic. Given that the gas was cooled, it did not maintain constant temperature, eliminating **(C)**. Isobaric and isovolumetric processes appear as horizontal and vertical lines in pressure–volume graphs, respectively, eliminating **(B)** and **(D)**. Adiabatic processes appear hyperbolic on pressure–volume graphs, as illustrated here.

2. **A**

Since the temperature during a phase change is constant, all phase changes are isothermal processes. During boiling, heat is added to the system to break the intermolecular attractions between the water molecules. As the water molecules vaporize, they expand outward, occupying a larger volume. Thus, boiling is an isothermal expansion, consistent with **(A)**.

3. **D**

Solve this question using the equation $\Delta G^\circ_{rxn} = -RT \ln K_{eq}$. ΔG°_{rxn} is negative (as it must be for a spontaneous reaction), and R and T are always positive. Therefore, $\ln K_{eq}$ must also be positive for the sign convention to work out correctly. Since $\ln(1) = 0$, the natural logarithm of any number greater than 1 will be positive, and the natural logarithm of any number less than 1 will be negative. In order for $\ln K_{eq}$ to be a positive number, K_{eq} must be greater than 1.

4. **D**

Combustion often involves the reaction of a hydrocarbon with oxygen to produce carbon dioxide and water. Longer hydrocarbon chains yield greater amounts of combustion products and release more heat in the process—that is, the reaction is more exothermic. Of the hydrocarbons listed here, *n*-pentane is the longest chain.

5. **A**

At first glance, this might seem like a math-heavy problem, but it really doesn't require any calculations at all. We just have to keep track of which bonds are broken and which bonds are formed. Remember, breaking bonds requires energy, while forming bonds releases energy. Two bonds are broken: a C–O bond between the carbonyl carbon and oxygen of acetic acid 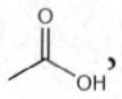, and an O–H bond between the hydroxyl oxygen and hydrogen of methanol 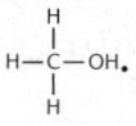. Two bonds are also formed: a C–O bond between the carbonyl carbon and the oxygen of methyl acetate 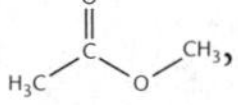, and an O–H bond between a hydroxyl group and a hydrogen to form water 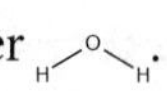. Given that the same two bonds are broken and formed in this reaction, the energy change must be 0 $\frac{\text{kJ}}{\text{mol}}$.

6. **B**

At the triple point (triple for three phases), the solid, liquid, and gas phases exist in equilibrium, consistent with **(B)**. On the other hand, the critical point refers to the temperature and pressure above which gases and liquids are indistinguishable, so **(A)** can be eliminated.

7. **C**

There are two parts to this computation. First, the water must be heated from 40°C to 100°C, then it must be vaporized. To calculate the energy required to heat the water, use the formula $q = mc\Delta T$. Plugging in values yields (10 g)(60°C)(4.2 J/g°C). Next, calculate the energy required to vaporize using the equation $q = mL$. Plugging in values yields (2,260 J/g)(10 g). Finally combine the two energies together: (10 g)(60°C)(4.2 J/g°C) + (2,260 J/g)(10 g), matching **(C)**.

8. **D**

There is not enough information available to determine the free energy of this reaction. While the entropy is clearly increasing (there are more particles in the system), it is unclear what the enthalpy change is. Because bonds are breaking, the reaction should be endothermic, meaning that both ΔS and ΔH are positive. In this case, it is a temperature-dependent process, and—without a temperature given—we cannot determine the sign on ΔG.

9. **A**

This problem asks for the free energy of a reaction at nonstandard conditions, which can be determined with the equation $\Delta G = \Delta G^\circ + RT \ln Q$.

10. **A**

A reaction with a negative enthalpy is, by definition, exothermic. Because both enthalpy and entropy are negative, this is a temperature-dependent process, and the reaction will be both endergonic and exergonic—but only at particular temperatures, eliminating **(C)** and **(D)**.

11. **C**

For a process to progress forward spontaneously, Q must be less than K_{eq} and will therefore have a tendency to move in the direction toward equilibrium. A spontaneous reaction's free energy is negative by convention.

12. **B**

This question is asking for a reaction with the greatest decrease in entropy, so the phases of the reactants and products must be evaluated. In general, the entropy of gases is the highest, while the entropy of solids is the lowest. Thus, a reaction in which gases react to produce solids will have a significant entropy decrease. In reaction **(B)**, a gaseous reactant forms a solid product, so the entropy decreases, making **(B)** correct. By contrast, the other reactions have either a minimal change or increase in entropy. In reaction **(A)**, two moles of gaseous reactants become four moles of gaseous product, so the entropy increases. In **(C)**, a liquid reactant forms a gaseous product, so entropy likewise increases. In reaction **(D)**, each side of the equation has a solid and an aqueous component, so there is approximately no change in entropy.

13. **A**

Eliminate **(C)** and **(D)**, which describe the free energy of reaction and cannot be determined from this graph. While most reaction coordinate graphs we've explored in this book use free energy for the *y*-axis, this one uses potential energy (enthalpy). If the heat of formation of the products is greater than that of the reactants, the reaction is endothermic. We can determine this information from their relative positions on the graph: because the products are higher than the reactants, this is an endothermic reaction.

14. **A**

The entropy change can be calculated using the formula $\Delta S = q/T$. Note that more information is given in the question than is necessary, so ignore the mass. Plugging in values yields: $\Delta S = 30{,}000\ \text{J} / 1{,}060\ \text{K} = 28\ \text{J/K}$. Thus, **(A)** is correct.

15. **A**

In an explosion, a significant amount of heat energy is released, meaning that the reaction is exothermic ($\Delta H < 0$), eliminating **(B)**. The entropy change associated with an explosion is positive because energy is dispersed over a much larger area, eliminating **(C)**. If this is true, the expression $\Delta H - T\Delta S$ must be negative, indicating that this is an exergonic process ($\Delta G < 0$). Absolute temperature can never be negative, eliminating **(D)**.

Consult your online resources for additional practice. **GO ONLINE**

EQUATIONS TO REMEMBER

(7.1) **First law of thermodynamics:** $\Delta U = Q - W$

(7.2) **Heat transfer (no phase change):** $q = mc\Delta T$

(7.3) **Heat transfer (during phase change):** $q = mL$

(7.4) **Generalized enthalpy of reaction:** $\Delta H_{rxn} = H_{products} - H_{reactants}$

(7.5) **Standard enthalpy of reaction:** $\Delta H^{\circ}_{rxn} = \Sigma\, \Delta H^{\circ}_{f,products} - \Sigma\, \Delta H^{\circ}_{f,reactants}$

(7.6) **Bond enthalpy:** $\Delta H^{\circ}_{rxn} = \Sigma\, \Delta H_{bonds\ broken} - \Sigma\, \Delta H_{bonds\ formed} =$ total energy absorbed − total energy released

(7.7) **Entropy:** $\Delta S = \frac{Q_{rev}}{T}$

(7.8) **Second law of thermodynamics:** $\Delta S_{universe} = \Delta S_{system} + \Delta S_{surroundings} > 0$

(7.9) **Standard entropy of reaction:** $\Delta S^{\circ}_{rxn} = \Sigma\, \Delta S^{\circ}_{f,products} - \Sigma\, \Delta S^{\circ}_{f,reactants}$

(7.10) **Gibbs free energy:** $\Delta G = \Delta H - T\Delta S$

(7.11) **Standard Gibbs free energy of reaction:**

$$\Delta G^{\circ}_{rxn} = \Sigma\, \Delta G^{\circ}_{f,products} - \Sigma\, \Delta G^{\circ}_{f,reactants}$$

(7.12) **Standard Gibbs free energy from equilibrium constant:**

$$\Delta G^{\circ}_{rxn} = -RT \ln K_{eq}$$

(7.13) **Gibbs free energy from reaction quotient:**

$$\Delta G_{rxn} = \Delta G^{\circ}_{rxn} + RT \ln Q = RT \ln \frac{Q}{K_{eq}}$$

SHARED CONCEPTS

General Chemistry Chapter 3
Bonding and Chemical Interactions

General Chemistry Chapter 4
Compounds and Stoichiometry

General Chemistry Chapter 5
Chemical Kinetics

General Chemistry Chapter 6
Equilibrium

Physics and Math Chapter 2
Work and Energy

Physics and Math Chapter 3
Thermodynamics

CHAPTER 8

THE GAS PHASE

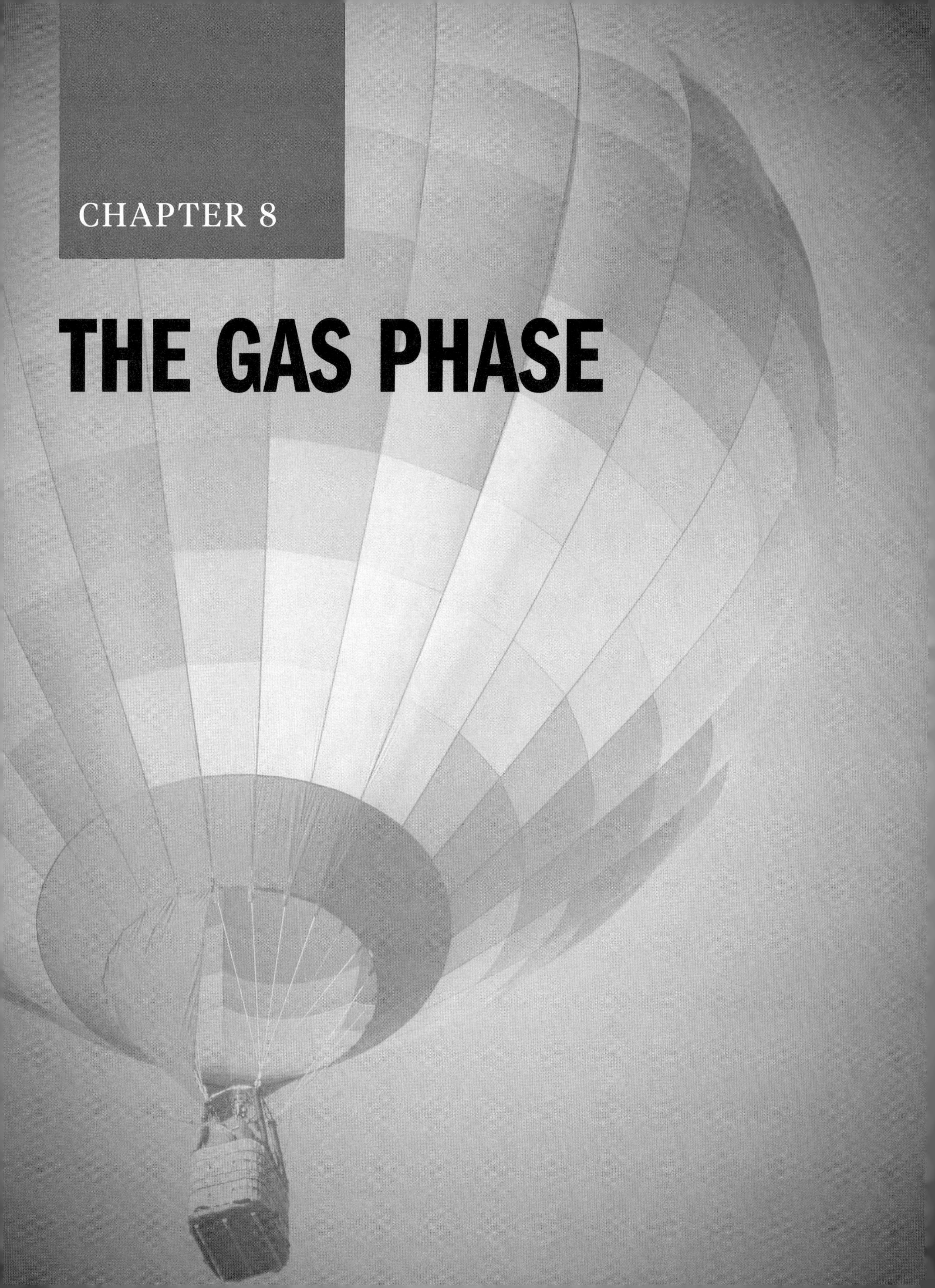

SCIENCE MASTERY ASSESSMENT

Every pre-med knows this feeling: there is so much content I have to know for the MCAT! How do I know what to do first or what's important?

While the high-yield badges throughout this book will help you identify the most important topics, this Science Mastery Assessment is another tool in your MCAT prep arsenal. This quiz (which can also be taken in your online resources) and the guidance below will help ensure that you are spending the appropriate amount of time on this chapter based on your personal strengths and weaknesses. Don't worry though—skipping something now does not mean you'll never study it. Later on in your prep, as you complete full-length tests, you'll uncover specific pieces of content that you need to review and can come back to these chapters as appropriate.

How to Use This Assessment

If you answer 0–7 questions correctly:

Spend about 1 hour to read this chapter in full and take limited notes throughout. Follow up by reviewing **all** quiz questions to ensure that you now understand how to solve each one.

If you answer 8–11 questions correctly:

Spend 20–40 minutes reviewing the quiz questions. Beginning with the questions you missed, read and take notes on the corresponding subchapters. For questions you answered correctly, ensure your thinking matches that of the explanation and you understand why each choice was correct or incorrect.

If you answer 12–15 questions correctly:

Spend less than 20 minutes reviewing all questions from the quiz. If you missed any, then include a quick read-through of the corresponding subchapters, or even just the relevant content within a subchapter, as part of your question review. For questions you answered correctly, ensure your thinking matches that of the explanation and review the Concept Summary at the end of the chapter.

1. Which of the following sets of conditions would be LEAST likely to result in ideal gas behavior?
   A. High pressure and low temperature
   B. Low temperature and large volume
   C. High pressure and large volume
   D. Low pressure and high temperature

2. What is the density of neon gas in $\frac{g}{L}$ at STP?
   A. 452.3
   B. 226.0
   C. 1.802
   D. 0.9018

3. A leak of helium gas through a small hole occurs at a rate of $3.22 \times 10^{-5}\ \frac{mol}{s}$. How will the leakage rates of neon and oxygen gases compare to helium at the same temperature and pressure?
   A. Neon will leak faster than helium; oxygen will leak faster than helium.
   B. Neon will leak faster than helium; oxygen will leak slower than helium.
   C. Neon will leak slower than helium; oxygen will leak faster than helium.
   D. Neon will leak slower than helium; oxygen will leak slower than helium.

4. A 0.10 g piece of magnesium is placed in a beaker of hydrochloric acid. Hydrogen gas is generated according to the following equation:

$$Mg\ (s) + 2\ HCl\ (aq) \rightarrow MgCl_2\ (aq) + H_2\ (g)$$

The gas is collected over water at 25°C, and the gauge pressure during the experiment reads 784 mmHg.

The gas displaces a volume of 100 mL. The vapor pressure of water at 25°C is approximately 24.0 mmHg. Based on this data, how many moles of hydrogen are produced in this reaction?
(Note: $R = 0.0821\ \frac{L \cdot atm}{mol \cdot K} = 8.314\ \frac{J}{K \cdot mol}$.)
   A. 4.04×10^{-5} moles hydrogen
   B. 4.09×10^{-3} moles hydrogen
   C. 3.07×10^{-2} moles hydrogen
   D. 3.11 moles hydrogen

5. Ideal gases:
   I. have no volume.
   II. have particles with no attractive forces between them.
   III. have no mass.

   A. I only
   B. II only
   C. I and II only
   D. I, II, and III

6. Which of the following best explains the difference in ideal behavior between nitrogen and fluoromethane gas?
   A. Nitrogen gas is more ideal because it is smaller and forms stronger intermolecular interactions.
   B. Nitrogen gas is more ideal because it is smaller and forms weaker intermolecular interactions.
   C. Fluoromethane is more ideal because it is larger and forms stronger intermolecular interactions.
   D. Fluoromethane is more ideal because it is smaller and forms weaker intermolecular interactions.

7. The kinetic molecular theory states that:
   A. the average kinetic energy of a molecule of gas is directly proportional to the temperature of the gas in kelvin.
   B. collisions between gas molecules are inelastic.
   C. gas particles occupy discrete areas of space.
   D. all gas molecules have the same kinetic energy at the same temperature.

8. The plots of two gases at STP are shown below. One of the gases is 1.0 L of helium, and the other is 1.0 L of bromine. Which plot corresponds to each gas and why?

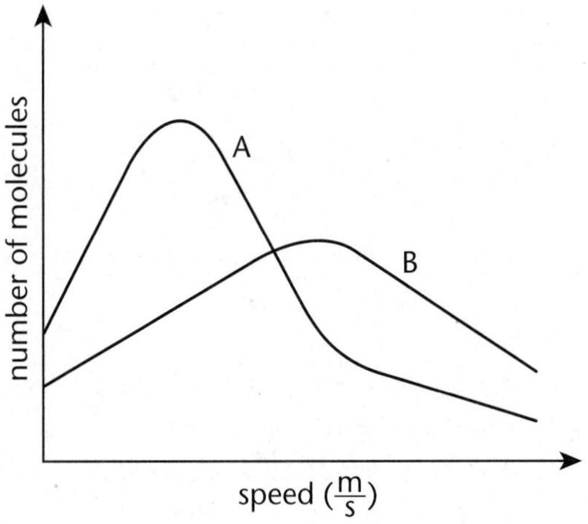

A. Curve A is helium and curve B is bromine because helium has a smaller molar mass than bromine.
B. Curve A is helium and curve B is bromine because the average kinetic energy of bromine is greater than the average kinetic energy of helium.
C. Curve A is bromine and curve B is helium because helium has a smaller molar mass than bromine.
D. Curve A is bromine and curve B is helium because the average kinetic energy of bromine is greater than the average kinetic energy of helium.

9. At sea level and 25°C, the solubility of oxygen gas in water is 1.25×10^{-3} *M*. In Denver, a city in the United States that lies high above sea level, the atmospheric pressure is 0.800 atm. What is the solubility of oxygen in water in Denver?
A. 1.00×10^{-3} *M*
B. 1.05×10^{-3} *M*
C. 1.50×10^{-3} *M*
D. 2.56×10^{-3} *M*

10. Given that the gases at the center of the sun have an average molar mass of 2.00 $\frac{g}{mol}$, compressed to a density of 1.20 $\frac{g}{cm^3}$ under 1.30×10^9 atm of pressure, what is the temperature at the center of the sun?
A. 2.6×10^4 K
B. 2.6×10^6 K
C. 2.6×10^7 K
D. 2.6×10^{10} K

11. The gaseous state of matter is characterized by which of the following properties?
I. Gases are compressible.
II. Gases assume the volume of their containers.
III. Gas particles exist as diatomic molecules.

A. I only
B. I and II only
C. II and III only
D. I, II, and III

12. A gas at a temperature of 27°C has a volume of 60.0 mL. What temperature change is needed to increase this gas to a volume of 90.0 mL?
A. A reduction of 150°C
B. An increase of 150°C
C. A reduction of 13.5°C
D. An increase of 13.5°C

13. How do a significant decrease in temperature and volume affect ideal gas behavior, respectively?
A. Both lead to more ideal behavior.
B. A lower temperature leads to deviations from ideal behavior, while lower volume causes more ideal behavior.
C. A lower temperature leads to more ideal behavior, while lower volume causes more ideal behavior.
D. Both lead to deviations in ideal behavior.

14. In which of the following situations is it impossible to predict how the pressure will change for a gas sample?
A. The gas is cooled at a constant volume.
B. The gas is heated at a constant volume.
C. The gas is heated, and the volume is simultaneously increased.
D. The gas is cooled, and the volume is simultaneously increased.

15. Experimenters notice that the molar concentration of dissolved oxygen in an enclosed water tank has decreased to one-half its original value. In an attempt to counter this decrease, they quadruple the partial pressure of oxygen in the container. What is the final concentration of the gas?
A. Half of the original concentration
B. The same as the original concentration
C. Double the original concentration
D. Quadruple the original concentration

Answer Key

1. **A**
2. **D**
3. **D**
4. **B**
5. **B**
6. **B**
7. **A**
8. **C**
9. **A**
10. **C**
11. **B**
12. **B**
13. **D**
14. **C**
15. **C**

Detailed explanations can be found at the end of the chapter.

CHAPTER 8

THE GAS PHASE

In This Chapter

CHAPTER PROFILE

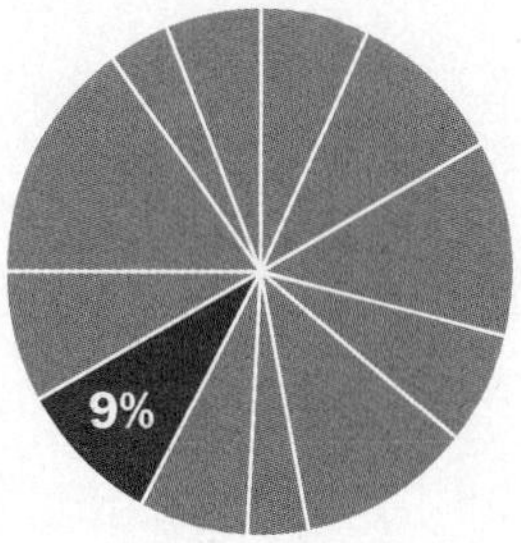

The content in this chapter should be relevant to about 9% of all questions about general chemistry on the MCAT.

This chapter covers material from the following AAMC content categories:

3B: Structure and integrative functions of the main organ systems

4B: Importance of fluids for the circulation of blood, gas movement, and gas exchange

Introduction

Let's start this chapter with a thought experiment. Imagine a helium balloon tied to the gearshift lever between the seats of a car and allowed to float freely. What do you think will happen to the balloon as the car accelerates forward? You might think, based on how you feel when you are in an accelerating vehicle, that the balloon will be pushed backwards due to its inertia. However, the balloon's movement isn't what we might predict: the balloon shifts forward as the car accelerates!

The molar mass of helium is 4 $\frac{\text{g}}{\text{mol}}$, while that of air, which is mostly nitrogen and oxygen, is about 29 $\frac{\text{g}}{\text{mol}}$. This means that air is about seven times denser than helium. Because the air in which the balloon is floating is more dense than the balloon itself, the air has greater inertia. Therefore, as the car accelerates forward, everything that has significant mass, including the air in the car, resists the forward motion (has inertia) and shifts toward the back of the car (even though, of course, everything in the car is accelerating forward, just not as quickly as the car itself). As the air shifts toward the back, a pressure gradient builds up such that there is greater air pressure in the back of the car than in the front, and this pressure difference results in a pushing force against the balloon that is directed from the back toward the front. Responding to this force, the balloon shifts forward in the direction of the car's acceleration. Who would have thought that general chemistry and physics could be so much fun?

In this chapter, we will discuss some MCAT favorites—the gas phase and the ideal gas laws. We will begin our discussion with ideal gases and the laws that govern their behavior. We will then examine the kinetic molecular theory that describes ideal gases and conclude with an evaluation of the ways in which the behavior of real gases deviates from that predicted by the ideal gas law.

8.1 The Gas Phase

LEARNING OBJECTIVES

After Chapter 8.1, you will be able to:

- Identify the unique characteristics of the gas phase
- Predict how pressure will change in different positions and locations, including underwater
- Recall the conditions at STP and standard conditions

Matter can exist in three different physical forms, called **phases** or **states**: gas, liquid, and solid. We have discussed liquids in the context of intermolecular forces and solids in the context of organized crystals in Chapter 3 of *MCAT General Chemistry Review*. The gaseous phase may be the simplest to understand because all gases display similar behavior and follow similar laws regardless of their particular chemical identities. Like liquids, gases are classified as fluids because they can flow and take on the shapes of their containers. However, the atoms or molecules in a gaseous sample move rapidly and are far apart from each other. In addition, only very weak intermolecular forces exist between gas particles; this results in certain characteristic physical properties, such as the ability to expand to fill any volume. Gases are also easily—although not infinitely—compressible, which distinguishes them from liquids.

Variables

We can define the state of a gaseous sample by four variables: **pressure (*P*)**, **volume (*V*)**, **temperature (*T*)**, and number of **moles (*n*)**.

Gas pressures are usually expressed in units of **atmospheres (atm)** or in **millimeters of mercury (mmHg)**, which are equivalent to **torr**. The SI unit for pressure, however, is the **pascal (Pa)**. The mathematical relationships among all of these units are as follows:

$$1 \text{ atm} = 760 \text{ mmHg} \equiv 760 \text{ torr} = 101.325 \text{ kPa}$$

Medical devices that measure blood pressure are termed **sphygmomanometers**, and the most clinically relevant unit of measurement for them is mmHg. In fact many medical devices utilize the same conceptual design of a **barometer**, shown in Figure 8.1, to continuously monitor blood pressure.

REAL WORLD

Blood pressure is measured by a sphygmomanometer, which uses units of mmHg. A normal adult blood pressure is considered less than 120 mmHg systolic and 80 mmHg diastolic ($<$120/80). Hypertension (high blood pressure) is defined as having at least two blood pressure readings $>$140 mmHg systolic or $>$90 mmHg diastolic.

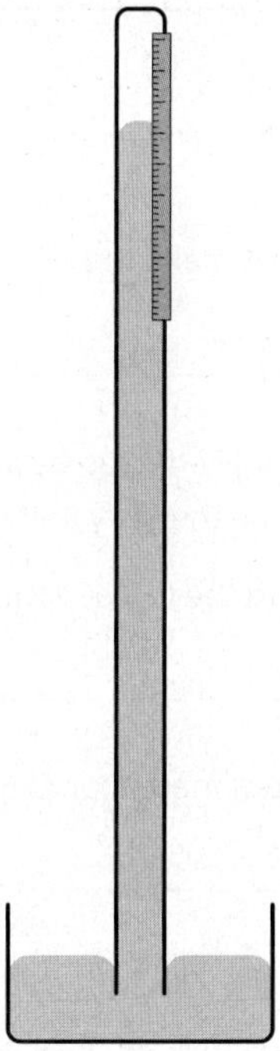

Figure 8.1 Schematic of a Simple Mercury Barometer

In order to explain why the mercury rises in a barometer, we must summarize the forces at play here. **Atmospheric pressure** creates a downward force on the pool of mercury at the base of the barometer while the mercury in the column exerts an opposing force (its weight) based on its density. The weight of the mercury creates a vacuum in the top of the tube. When the external air exerts a higher force than the weight of the mercury in the column, the column rises. When the external air exerts a lower force than the weight of the mercury, the column falls. Thus, a reading can be obtained by measuring the height of the mercury column (in mm), which will be directly proportional to the atmospheric pressure being applied.

BRIDGE

Fluid dynamics is an important concept discussed in Chapter 4 of *MCAT Physics and Math Review* that applies to multiple aspects of the gas laws covered here, including the functionality of a mercury barometer.

It is important to mention here that atmospheric pressure is not the only external pressure that can exert this force. For instance, a clinical blood pressure cuff creates a force that is opposed by the person's systolic and diastolic arterial blood pressure.

The volume of a gas is generally expressed in liters (L) or milliliters (mL). Temperature is usually given in kelvin (K), although degrees Celsius (°C) may be used instead. Many processes involving gases take place under **standard temperature and pressure (STP)**, which refers to conditions of 273 K (0°C) and 1 atm.

A note of caution: **STP conditions** are not identical to **standard state conditions**. The two standards involve different temperatures and are used for different purposes. STP (273 K and 1 atm) is generally used for gas law calculations; standard state conditions (298 K, 1 atm, 1 *M* concentrations) are used when measuring standard enthalpy, entropy, free energy changes, and electrochemical cell voltage.

MCAT EXPERTISE

On the MCAT, remember that STP is different from standard state. Temperature at STP is 0°C (273 K). Temperature at standard state is 25°C (298 K).

MCAT CONCEPT CHECK 8.1

Before you move on, assess your understanding of the material with these questions.

1. Name some characteristics that make the gas phase unique:

____

2. A mercury barometer is primarily affected by atmospheric pressure. What would happen to the level of the mercury in the column if:
   - the barometer was moved to the top of a mountain?

   ____

   - the barometer was placed ten meters under water?

   ____

3. What are the conditions for STP?

____

4. What are the standard conditions?

____

8.2 Ideal Gases

High-Yield

LEARNING OBJECTIVES

After Chapter 8.2, you will be able to:

- Apply the ideal gas equation to calculations of pressure, temperature, volume, or number of moles
- Calculate the density of a substance given its molecular formula, current pressure, and current temperature
- Apply Avogadro's principle, Boyle's law, Charles's law, Gay–Lussac's law, and the combined ideal gas law to given scenarios
- Solve problems using Dalton's law of partial pressures and Henry's law

KEY CONCEPT

An ideal gas follows the gas laws we will discuss at all pressures and temperatures. A real gas deviates from these laws at high pressures (low volumes) and low temperatures because of intermolecular forces or volume effects.

When we examine the behavior of gases under varying conditions of temperature and pressure, we assume that the gases are ideal. An **ideal gas** represents a hypothetical gas with molecules that have no **intermolecular forces** and occupy no volume. Although **real gases** deviate from this ideal behavior at high pressures (low volumes) and low temperatures, many compressed real gases demonstrate behavior that is close to ideal.

Ideal Gas Law

The ideal gas law was first stated in 1834 by Benoît Paul Émile Clapeyron, more than 170 years after Sir Robert Boyle performed his experimental studies on the relationship between pressure and volume in the gas state. In fact, by the time the ideal gas law found its expression, Boyle's law, Charles's law, and Dalton's law had already been well-established. Historical considerations aside, it will benefit us to examine the ideal gas law first so that we can then understand the other laws, which had been identified earlier, to be only special cases of the ideal gas law.

The ideal gas law shows the relationship among four variables that define a sample of gas:

$$PV = n\mathrm{R}T$$

Equation 8.1

where P is the pressure, V is the volume, n is the number of moles, and T is the temperature. R represents the **ideal gas constant**, which has a value of $8.21 \times 10^{-2}\ \frac{\mathrm{L \cdot atm}}{\mathrm{mol \cdot K}}$. Be aware that the gas constant can be expressed in other units. On the MCAT, you may also encounter R given as $8.314\ \frac{\mathrm{J}}{\mathrm{K \cdot mol}}$, which is derived when SI units of pascal (for pressure) and cubic meters (for volume) are substituted into the ideal gas law. Although the relevant values for R will be provided on Test Day if needed, it is important to recognize the appropriate value for R based on the units of the variables given in a passage or question stem.

The ideal gas law is used to determine the missing term when given all of the others. It can also be used to calculate the change in a term while holding two of the others constant. It is most commonly used to solve for volume or pressure at any given temperature and number of moles; Figure 8.2 shows graphs of P-V relationships at increasing temperatures.

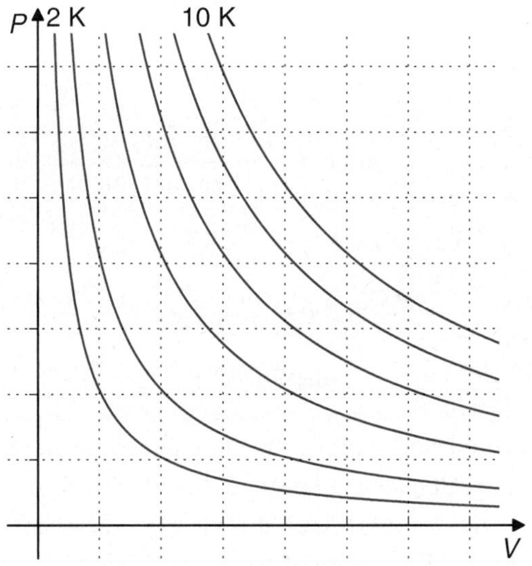

Figure 8.2 Ideal Gas Isothermal Curves

When n, R, and T are held constant, one can easily analyze the relationship between pressure and volume.

Example: What volume would 12 g of helium occupy at 27°C and a pressure of 380 mmHg?

Solution: The ideal gas law can be used, but first, all of the variables must be converted to units that will correspond to the expression of the gas constant as $8.21 \times 10^{-2}\ \frac{\text{L} \cdot \text{atm}}{\text{mol} \cdot \text{K}}$.

$$P = 380\ \text{mmHg}\left[\frac{1\ \text{atm}}{760\ \text{mmHg}}\right] = 0.5\ \text{atm}$$

$$T = 27^\circ\text{C} + 273 = 300\ \text{K}$$

$$n = 12\ \text{g He}\left[\frac{1\ \text{mol}}{4.0\ \text{g}}\right] = 3\ \text{mol He}$$

$$PV = nRT$$

$$(0.5\ \text{atm})(V) = (3\ \text{mol He})\left(0.0821\ \frac{\text{L} \cdot \text{atm}}{\text{mol} \cdot \text{K}}\right)(300\ \text{K})$$

$$0.5\ V \approx 3 \times 8 \times 3$$

$$V = 144\ \text{L}\ (\text{actual} = 148\ \text{L})$$

BRIDGE

Round numbers to speed up your arithmetic on Test Day. For instance, constants such as 0.0821 can be rounded to 0.08. Choices will be sufficiently different so that your estimated answer will be nearly identical to the true answer choice. Arithmetic and math strategies are discussed in Chapter 10 of *MCAT Physics and Math Review.*

The ideal gas law is useful not only for standard calculations of pressure, volume, or temperature of a gas under a given set of conditions, but also for determinations of gas density and molar mass.

Density

We define **density** (ρ) as the ratio of the mass per unit volume of a substance. The densities of gases are usually expressed in units of grams per liter. The ideal gas law contains variables for volume and number of moles, so we can rearrange the law to calculate the density of any gas:

$$PV = nRT$$

$$\text{where } n = \frac{m\ (\text{mass})}{M\ (\text{molar mass})}$$

$$\text{Therefore, } PV = \frac{m}{M}RT$$

$$\text{and } \rho = \frac{m}{V} = \frac{PM}{RT}$$

Equation 8.2

A different approach could start with the fact that a mole of an ideal gas at STP occupies 22.4 L. We can then calculate the effect of changes in pressure and temperature when they differ from STP conditions, predicting the volume of the gas. Finally, we'll calculate the density by dividing the mass by the predicted volume. The following equation, the **combined gas law**, is an amalgam of some of the special cases we will discuss in the following section. It can be used to relate changes in temperature, volume, and pressure of a gas:

$$\frac{P_1V_1}{T_1} = \frac{P_2V_2}{T_2}$$

Equation 8.3

where the subscripts 1 and 2 refer to the two states of the gas (at STP and at the conditions of actual temperature and pressure, for example). This equation assumes the number of moles stays constant.

To calculate a change in volume, the equation is rearranged as follows:

$$V_2 = V_1\left[\frac{P_1}{P_2}\right]\left[\frac{T_2}{T_1}\right]$$

V_2 is then used to find the density of the gas under nonstandard conditions:

$$\rho = \frac{m}{V_2}$$

On Test Day, it may be helpful to visualize how the changes in pressure and temperature affect the volume of the gas, and this can serve as a check to avoid accidentally switching the values of pressure and temperature in the numerator and denominator. For example, one could predict that doubling the temperature of a gas would result in doubling its volume, and doubling the pressure of a gas would result in halving the volume, so doubling both the temperature and pressure at the same time results in a final volume that is equal to the original volume.

Example: What is the density of CO_2 gas at 2 atm and 273°C?

Solution: At STP, a mole of gas occupies 22.4 L. Because the increase in pressure to 2 atm decreases volume proportionally, 22.4 L must be multiplied by $\frac{1\text{ atm}}{2\text{ atm}} = 0.5$. Because the increase in temperature increases volume proportionally, the temperature factor will be $\frac{546\text{ K}}{273\text{ K}} = 2$.

$$V_2 = \left[\frac{22.4\text{ L}}{\text{mol}}\right]\left[\frac{1\text{ atm}}{2\text{ atm}}\right]\left[\frac{546\text{ K}}{273\text{ K}}\right] = 22.4\,\frac{\text{L}}{\text{mol}}$$

$$\rho = \frac{44\,\frac{\text{g}}{\text{mol}}}{22.4\,\frac{\text{L}}{\text{mol}}} \approx 2\,\frac{\text{g}}{\text{L}}\left(\text{actual} = 1.96\,\frac{\text{g}}{\text{L}}\right).$$

Molar Mass

Sometimes the identity of a gas is unknown, and the molar mass, discussed in Chapter 4 of *MCAT General Chemistry Review*, can be determined in order to identify it. Using the equation for density derived from the ideal gas law, we can calculate the molar mass of a gas experimentally in the following way:

The pressure and temperature of a gas contained in a bulb of a given volume are measured, and the mass of the bulb with the sample is measured. Then, the bulb is evacuated—the gas is removed—and the mass of the empty bulb is determined. The mass of the bulb with the sample minus the mass of the evacuated bulb gives the mass of the sample. Finally, the density of the sample is determined by dividing the mass of the sample by the volume of the bulb. This gives the density at the given temperature and pressure.

Using $V_2 = V_1\left[\frac{P_1}{P_2}\right]\left[\frac{T_2}{T_1}\right]$, we then calculate the volume of the gas at STP, substituting 273 K for T_2 and 1 atm for P_2. The ratio of the sample mass divided by V_2 gives the density of the gas at STP. The molar mass can then be calculated as the product of the gas's density at STP and the STP volume of one mole of gas, 22.4 $\frac{\text{L}}{\text{mol}}$:

$$M = (\rho_{\text{STP}})\left(22.4\ \frac{\text{L}}{\text{mol}}\right)$$

Example: What is the molar mass of a 22.4 L sample of gas that has a mass of 225 g at a temperature of 273°C and a pressure of 10 atm?

Solution: Determine how the current conditions compare to STP, and use this to set up a proportional relationship. Be careful to note the differences between degrees C and K, and current versus STP conditions.

$$\frac{P_1V_1}{T_1} = \frac{P_2V_2}{T_2} \text{ giving } V_2 = V_1\left[\frac{P_1}{P_2}\right]\left[\frac{T_2}{T_1}\right]$$

$$V_{\text{STP}} = V_1\left[\frac{P_1}{P_{\text{STP}}}\right]\left[\frac{T_{\text{STP}}}{T_1}\right] = 22.4\ \text{L}\left[\frac{10\ \text{atm}}{1\ \text{atm}}\right]\left[\frac{273\ \text{K}}{546\ \text{K}}\right] = 22.4 \times 10 \times \frac{1}{2} = 112\ \text{L}$$

$$\frac{225\ \text{g}}{112\ \text{L}} \approx 2\ \frac{\text{g}}{\text{L}} \text{ at STP}$$

$$M = 2\ \frac{\text{g}}{\text{L}}\left[\frac{22.4\ \text{L}}{\text{mol}}\right] \approx 44.8\ \frac{\text{g}}{\text{mol}}$$

Special Cases

Now that we have considered the ideal gas law as the mathematical relationship between four variables that define the state of a gas (pressure, volume, temperature, and moles of gas), we can examine the other laws that preceded its discovery. Even though the following laws were developed before the ideal gas law, it is conceptually helpful to think of them as special cases of the more general ideal gas law.

Avogadro's Principle

One important discovery that preceded Clapeyron's formulation of the ideal gas law was **Avogadro's principle**, which states that all gases at a constant temperature and pressure occupy volumes that are directly proportional to the number of moles of gas present. Equal amounts of all gases at the same temperature and pressure will occupy equal volumes. As discussed above, one mole of any gas, irrespective of its chemical identity, will occupy 22.4 liters at STP.

$$\frac{n}{V} = k \text{ or } \frac{n_1}{V_1} = \frac{n_2}{V_2}$$

Equation 8.4

where k is a constant, n_1 and n_2 are the number of moles of gas 1 and gas 2, respectively, and V_1 and V_2 are the volumes of the gases, respectively. This can be summarized in the following statement: *as the number of moles of gas increases, the volume increases in direct proportion.*

Example: A 2.0 L sample at 100°C and 20 atm contains 5 moles of a gas. If an additional 25 moles of gas at the same pressure and temperature are added, what is the final volume of the gas?

Solution: If pressure and temperature are held constant, the ideal gas law reduces to Avogadro's principle:

$$\frac{n_1}{V_1} = \frac{n_2}{V_2}$$

$$\frac{5\text{ mol}}{2.0\text{ L}} = \frac{5\text{ mol} + 25\text{ mol}}{V_2}$$

$$V_2 = \frac{30\text{ mol} \times 2.0\text{ L}}{5\text{ mol}} = 12.0\text{ L}$$

Boyle's Law

Robert Boyle conducted a series of experimental studies in 1660 that led to his formulation of a law that now bears his name: **Boyle's law**. His work showed that, for a given gaseous sample held at constant temperature (isothermal conditions), the volume of the gas is inversely proportional to its pressure:

$$PV = k \text{ or } P_1V_1 = P_2V_2$$

Equation 8.5

where k is a constant, and the subscripts 1 and 2 represent two different sets of pressure and volume conditions. Careful examination of Boyle's law shows that it is, indeed, simply the special case of the ideal gas law in which n and T are constant.

KEY CONCEPT

Boyle's law is a derivation of the ideal gas law and states that pressure and volume are inversely related: when one increases, the other decreases.

A plot of volume *vs.* pressure for a gas—the inverse of the curves in Figure 8.2—is shown in Figure 8.3.

MCAT EXPERTISE

Sometimes it is easier to remember the shape of the graph to help you recall the variables' relationship on Test Day. Here we can see that, as pressure increases, the volume decreases, and vice-versa. These ratios and relationships will often allow you to answer questions on the MCAT without having to do much math.

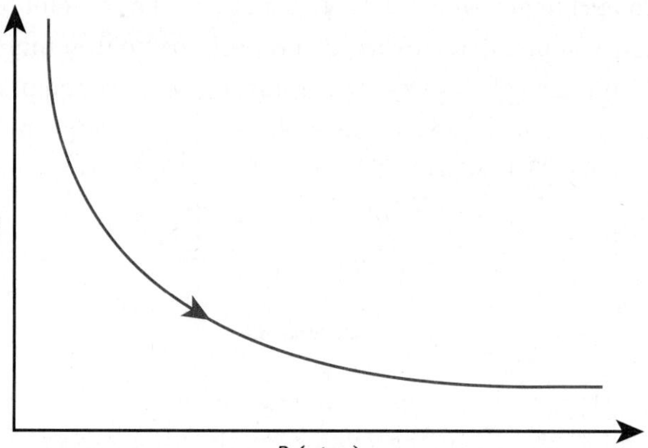

Figure 8.3 Boyle's Law (Isothermal Compression)
As pressure increases, volume decreases.

Example: What would be the volume of a 1 L sample of helium if its pressure is changed from 12 atm to 4 atm under isothermal conditions?

Solution: If the number of moles of gas and temperature are held constant, the ideal gas law reduces to Boyle's law:

$$P_1V_1 = P_2V_2$$

$$(12\text{ atm})(1\text{ L}) = (4\text{ atm})(V_2)$$

$$V_2 = \frac{12\text{ atm} \times 1\text{ L}}{4\text{ atm}} = 3\text{ L}$$

Charles's Law

KEY CONCEPT

Charles's law is also a derivation of the ideal gas law and states that volume and temperature are directly proportional: when one increases, the other increases in direct proportion.

In the early 19th century, Joseph Louis Gay-Lussac published findings based, in part, on earlier unpublished work by Jacques Charles; hence, the law of Charles and Gay-Lussac is more commonly known simply as **Charles's law**. The law states that, at constant pressure, the volume of a gas is proportional to its absolute temperature, expressed in kelvin. Expressed mathematically, Charles's law is

$$\frac{V}{T} = k \text{ or } \frac{V_1}{T_1} = \frac{V_2}{T_2}$$

Equation 8.6

where, again, k is a proportionality constant and the subscripts 1 and 2 represent two different sets of temperature and volume conditions. Careful examination of Charles's law shows that it is another special case of the ideal gas law in which n and P are constant.

A plot of temperature *vs.* volume is shown in Figure 8.4. Note that if one extrapolates the V *vs.* T plot for a gas back to where $T = 0$ (absolute zero), we find that $V = 0$!

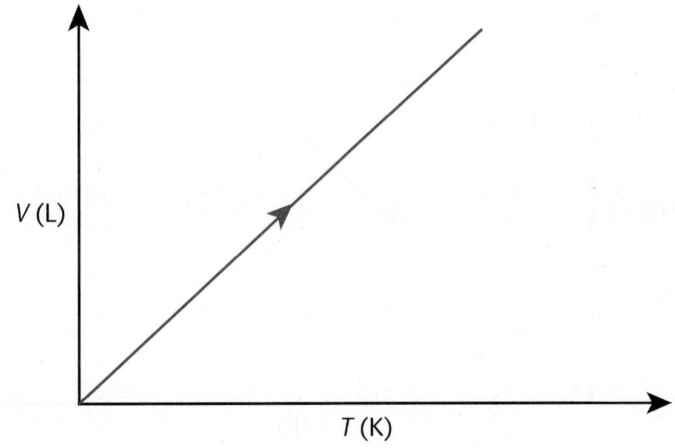

Figure 8.4 Charles's Law (Isobaric Expansion)
As temperature increases, volume increases.

REAL WORLD

While the temperature of 0K cannot be physically attained, curves such as Charles's law were originally used to figure out its value.

Example: If the temperature of 2 L of gas at constant pressure is changed from 290 K to 580 K, what would be its final volume?

Solution: If the number of moles of gas and pressure are held constant, the ideal gas law reduces to Charles's law:

$$\frac{V_1}{T_1} = \frac{V_2}{T_2}$$

$$\frac{2\text{ L}}{290\text{ K}} = \frac{V_2}{580\text{ K}}$$

$$V_2 = \frac{2\text{ L} \times 580\text{ K}}{290\text{ K}} = 4\text{ L}$$

Gay-Lussac's Law

Gay-Lussac's law is complementary to Charles's Law. It utilizes the same derivation from the ideal gas law, but it relates pressure to temperature instead. Expressed mathematically, Gay-Lussac's law is

$$\frac{P}{T} = k \text{ or } \frac{P_1}{T_1} = \frac{P_2}{T_2}$$

Equation 8.7

where, again, k is a proportionality constant, and the subscripts 1 and 2 represent two different sets of temperature and pressure conditions. Careful examination of Gay-Lussac's law shows that it is another special case of the ideal gas law in which n and V are constant.

Figure 8.5 graphs this concept, which is nearly identical to Charles's law. Again, an increase in temperature will increase the pressure in direct proportion.

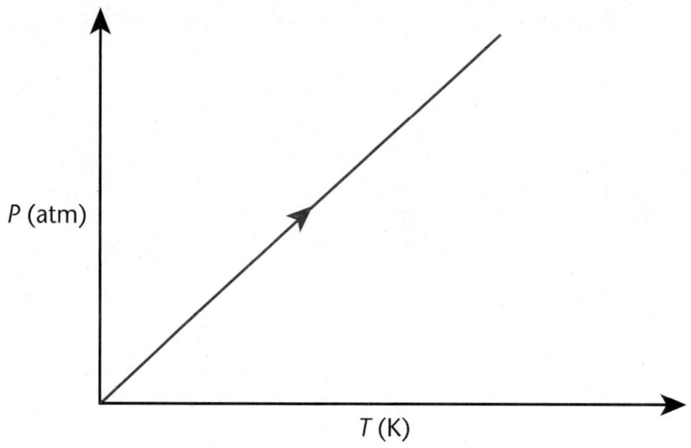

Figure 8.5 Gay-Lussac's Law (Isovolumetric Heating)
As temperature increases, pressure increases.

Example: If the pressure of a sample of gas with a temperature of 300 K changes from 2 atm to 5 atm during heating, what would be the final temperature if volume is held constant?

Solution: If the number of moles of gas and volume are held constant, the ideal gas law reduces to Gay-Lussac's law:

$$\frac{P_1}{T_1} = \frac{P_2}{T_2}$$

$$\frac{2\text{ atm}}{300\text{ K}} = \frac{5\text{ atm}}{T_2}$$

$$T_2 = \frac{5\text{ atm} \times 300\text{ K}}{2\text{ atm}} = 750\text{ K}$$

MCAT EXPERTISE

Understanding how the combined gas law functions helps avoid the need to memorize every other special case of the ideal gas law. Read the question stem or passage with an eye toward the quantities that remain constant to know when assumptions can be made.

Combined Gas Law

As discussed earlier, the **combined gas law** (Equation 8.3) was a combination of many of the preceding laws. This law relates pressure and volume (Boyle's law) in the numerator, and relates the variations in temperature to both volume (Charles's law) and pressure (Gay-Lussac's law) simultaneously. When using this equation, take care to place all of the variables in the right place.

Dalton's Law of Partial Pressures

When two or more gases that do not chemically interact are found in one vessel, each gas will behave independently of the others. That is, each gas will behave as if it were the only gas in the container. Therefore, the pressure exerted by each gas in the mixture will be equal to the pressure that the gas would exert if it were the only one in the container. The pressure exerted by each individual gas is called the **partial pressure** of that gas. In 1801, John Dalton derived an expression, now known as **Dalton's law of partial pressures**, which states that the total pressure of a gaseous mixture is equal to the sum of the partial pressures of the individual components. The equation for Dalton's law is

$$P_T = P_A + P_B + P_C + \cdots$$

Equation 8.8

where P_T is the total pressure in the container, and P_A, P_B, and P_C are the partial pressures of gases A, B, and C, respectively.

KEY CONCEPT

When more than one gas is in a container, each contributes to the whole as if it were the only gas present. Add up all of the pressures of the individual gases and you get the whole pressure of the system.

The partial pressure of a gas is related to its mole fraction and can be determined using the following equation:

$$P_A = X_A P_T$$

$$\text{where } X_A = \frac{\text{moles of gas A}}{\text{total moles of gas}}$$

Equation 8.9

Example: A vessel contains 0.75 mol of nitrogen, 0.20 mol of hydrogen, and 0.05 mol of fluorine at a total pressure of 2.5 atm. What is the partial pressure of each gas?

Solution: First calculate the mole fraction of each gas.

$$X_{N_2} = \frac{0.75 \text{ mol}}{1.00 \text{ mol}} = 0.75 \quad X_{H_2} = \frac{0.20 \text{ mol}}{1.00 \text{ mol}} = 0.20 \quad X_{F_2} = \frac{0.05 \text{ mol}}{1.00 \text{ mol}} = 0.05$$

Then calculate the partial pressure.

$$P_A = X_A P_T$$

$$P_{N_2} = (0.75)(2.5 \text{ atm}) = 1.875 \text{ atm}$$

$$P_{H_2} = (0.20)(2.5 \text{ atm}) = 0.5 \text{ atm}$$

$$P_{F_2} = (0.05)(2.5 \text{ atm}) = 0.125 \text{ atm}$$

Henry's Law

The difference in gas solubility between fluids was explained by William Henry in 1803. What Henry noticed was that, at various applied pressures, the concentration of a gas in a liquid increased or decreased. This was a characteristic of a gas's vapor pressure. **Vapor pressure** is the pressure exerted by evaporated particles above the surface of a liquid. Evaporation, as discussed in Chapter 7 of *MCAT General Chemistry Review*, is a dynamic process that requires the molecules at the surface of a liquid to gain enough energy to escape into the gas phase.

Vapor pressure from the evaporated molecules forces some of the gas back into the liquid phase, and equilibrium is reached between evaporation and condensation. Mathematically, this is expressed as:

$$[A] = k_H \times P_A \text{ or } \frac{[A]_1}{P_1} = \frac{[A]_2}{P_2} = k_H$$

Equation 8.10

KEY CONCEPT

The solubility of a gas will increase with increasing partial pressure of the gas.

where [A] is the concentration of A in solution, k_H is Henry's constant, and P_A is the partial pressure of A. The value of Henry's constant depends on the identity of the gas.

According to this relationship, solubility (concentration) and pressure are directly related. In biology, this is a critically important relationship for gas and nutrient exchange. As discussed in Chapter 6 of *MCAT Biology Review*, lung tissue—at the microscopic level—is organized into grapelike clusters of sacs called alveoli. These sacs are perfused by capillaries that allow for the exchange of carbon dioxide and oxygen, as shown in Figure 8.6. If the atmospheric pressure changes, as it does from sea level to high altitude, then the partial pressure of oxygen in the atmosphere also changes (as explained by Dalton's law), and the amount of gas exchanged is altered accordingly; if the partial pressure of a particular gas is elevated, such as when giving hyperbaric oxygen, the amount of that gas dissolved in the blood is also elevated.

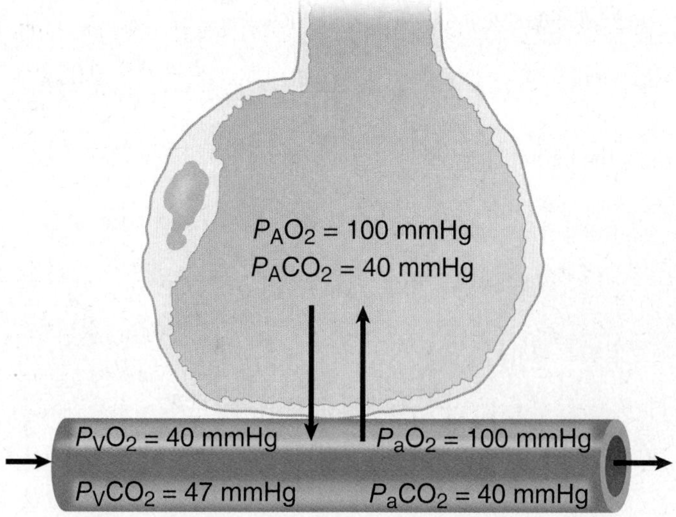

Figure 8.6 Alveolar Capillary Gas Exchange
In medicine, A represents alveolar concentrations, V represents venous concentrations, and a represents arterial concentrations.

Example: If 4×10^{-4} moles of gas are dissolved in 2 L of solution under an ambient pressure of 2 atm, what will be the molar concentration of the gas under 10 atm?

Solution: Start by determining the initial concentration of the gas in solution.

$$[A]_1 = \frac{4 \times 10^{-4} \text{ mol}}{2 \text{ L}} = 2 \times 10^{-4}\ M$$

Next, utilize the direct relationship between solubility and pressure according to Henry's law.

$$\frac{[A]_1}{P_1} = \frac{[A]_2}{P_2}$$

$$\frac{2 \times 10^{-4}\ M}{2 \text{ atm}} = \frac{[A]_2}{10 \text{ atm}}$$

$$[A]_2 = \frac{(2 \times 10^{-4}\ M)(10 \text{ atm})}{2 \text{ atm}} = 10^{-3}\ M$$

MCAT CONCEPT CHECK 8.2

Before you move on, assess your understanding of the material with these questions.

1. A container with 4 moles of a gas at a pressure of 8 atm has a volume of 12 liters. What is its temperature? (Note: $R = 8.21 \times 10^{-2} \frac{\text{L} \cdot \text{atm}}{\text{mol} \cdot \text{K}}$)

2. What is the density of argon gas at 4 atm and 127°C?

3. A 20 L sample at 300°C and 5 atm of pressure contains 2 moles of a gas. If an additional 3 moles of gas at the same pressure and temperature are added, what is the final total volume of the gas?

4. What would be the volume of a 2 L sample of neon if its pressure is changed from 1 atm to 40 atm under isothermal conditions?

5. If the temperature of 6 L of gas at constant pressure is changed from 27°C to 127°C, what would be its final volume?

6. If the pressure of a sample of gas with a temperature of 227°C is changed from 5 atm to 2 atm during cooling, what would be the final temperature?

7. A vessel contains 8 mol O_2, 3 mol CH_4, and 1 mol CO_2 at a total pressure of 240 atm. What is the partial pressure of each gas?

8. How can the concentration of carbon dioxide in sodas or other carbonated beverages be so much higher than that of atmospheric carbon dioxide?

8.3 Kinetic Molecular Theory

LEARNING OBJECTIVES

After Chapter 8.3, you will be able to:

- Recall the assumptions made by kinetic molecular theory
- Calculate the average speed of a gas, given its temperature
- Compare the relative speeds of two different gases at the same temperature
- Apply Graham's law to situations involving gas effusion:

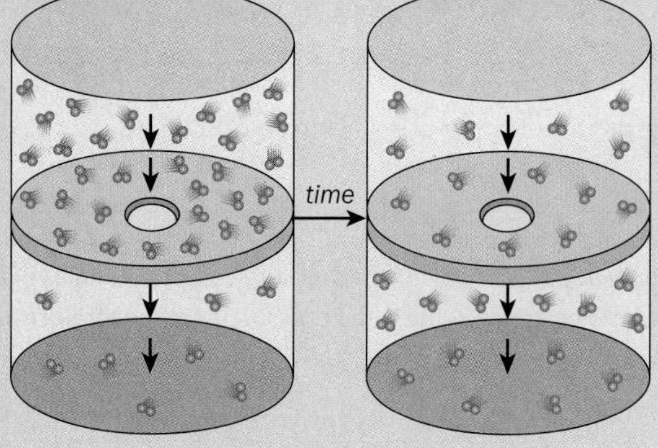

The **kinetic molecular theory** was developed in the second half of the 19th century, well after the laws describing gas behavior had been developed. The kinetic molecular theory was used to *explain* the behavior of gases, which the other laws merely *described.* The gas laws demonstrate that all gases show similar physical characteristics and behavior irrespective of their particular chemical identity. The behavior of real gases deviates from the ideal behavior predicted under the assumptions of this theory, but these deviations can be corrected for in calculations. The combined efforts of James Maxwell, Ludwig Boltzmann, and others led to a simple explanation of gaseous molecular behavior based on the motion of individual molecules. Like the gas laws, the kinetic molecular theory was developed in reference to ideal gases, although it can be applied with reasonable accuracy to real gases as well.

Assumptions

To simplify the model proposed by the kinetic molecular theory, certain assumptions are made:

1. Gases are made up of particles with volumes that are negligible compared to the container volume.
2. Gas atoms or molecules exhibit no intermolecular attractions or repulsions.
3. Gas particles are in continuous, random motion, undergoing collisions with other particles and the container walls.
4. Collisions between any two gas particles (or between particles and the container walls) are elastic, meaning that there is conservation of both momentum and kinetic energy.
5. The average kinetic energy of gas particles is proportional to the absolute temperature of the gas (in kelvin), and it is the same for all gases at a given temperature, irrespective of chemical identity or atomic mass.

Applications

It is fairly straightforward to imagine gas particles as little rubber balls bouncing off each other and off the walls of the container. Of course, rubber balls, like real gas particles, have measurable mass and volume, and not even the bounciest rubber balls will collide in a completely elastic manner. Still, this provides an apt visualization of the behaviors described by the kinetic molecular theory.

Average Molecular Speeds

According to the kinetic molecular theory of gases, the average kinetic energy of a gas particle is proportional to the absolute temperature of the gas:

$$KE = \frac{1}{2} mv^2 = \frac{3}{2} k_B T$$

Equation 8.11

where k_B is the **Boltzmann constant** $\left(1.38 \times 10^{-23} \frac{J}{K}\right)$, which serves as a bridge between the macroscopic and microscopic behaviors of gases (that is, as a bridge between the behavior of the gas as a whole and the individual gas molecules). This equation shows that the speed of a gas particle is related to its absolute temperature. However, because of the large number of rapidly and randomly moving gas particles, which may travel only nanometers before colliding with another particle or the container wall, the speed of an individual gas molecule is nearly impossible to define. Therefore, the speeds of gases are defined in terms of their average molecular speed. One way to define an average speed is to determine the average kinetic energy

MCAT EXPERTISE

Understanding concepts will be much more fruitful on Test Day than memorizing all of the facts. The higher the temperature, the faster the molecules move. The larger the molecules, the slower they move.

per particle and then calculate the speed to which this corresponds. The resultant quantity, known as the **root-mean-square speed** (**u_{rms}**), is given by the following equation:

$$u_{rms} = \sqrt{\frac{3RT}{M}}$$

Equation 8.12

where R is the ideal gas constant, T is the temperature, and M is the molar mass.

A **Maxwell–Boltzmann distribution curve** shows the distribution of gas particle speeds at a given temperature. Figure 8.7 shows a distribution curve of molecular speeds at two temperatures, T_1 and T_2, where T_2 is greater than T_1. Notice that the bell-shaped curve flattens and shifts to the right as the temperature increases, indicating that at higher temperatures, more molecules are moving at higher speeds.

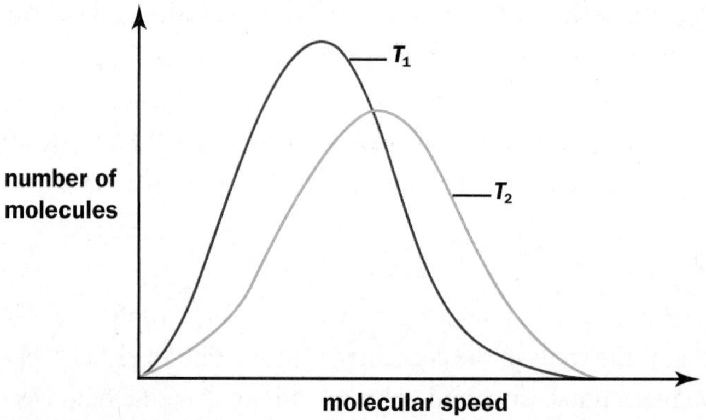

Figure 8.7 Maxwell-Boltzmann Distribution Curves of Molecular Speeds at Two Different Temperatures

Example: What is the average speed of xenon difluoride molecules at 20°C?

Solution: The ideal gas constant $R = 8.314 \frac{J}{K \cdot mol}$ should be used, and the molar mass of xenon difluoride is $169.3 \frac{g}{mol}$. M must be expressed in $\frac{kg}{mol}$ because joules are also derived from kilograms.

$$u_{rms} = \sqrt{\frac{3RT}{M}}$$

$$u_{rms} = \sqrt{\frac{(3)\left(8.314 \frac{J}{K \cdot mol}\right)(293\ K)}{0.17 \frac{kg}{mol}}}$$

$$u_{rms} \approx \sqrt{\frac{(3)(8)(300)}{0.18}} = \sqrt{\frac{(8)(300)}{0.06}} = \sqrt{(8)(5{,}000)} = \sqrt{40{,}000}$$

$$u_{rms} \approx 200\ \frac{m}{s}\ \left(\text{actual} = 208\ \frac{m}{s}\right)$$

Graham's Law of Diffusion and Effusion

The movement of molecules from high concentration to low concentration through a medium (such as air or water) is called **diffusion**, as shown in Figure 8.8.

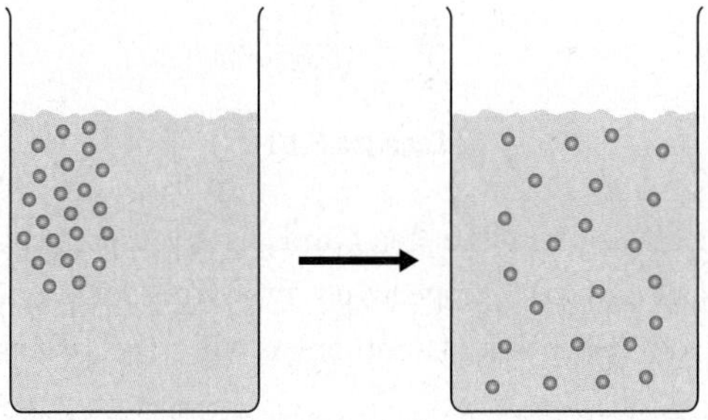

Figure 8.8 Diffusion of Solutes in a Solvent

The kinetic molecular theory of gases predicts that heavier gases diffuse more slowly than lighter ones because of their differing average speeds, as shown in Figure 8.9. Because all gas particles have the same average kinetic energy at the same temperature, it must be true that particles with greater mass travel at a slower average speed.

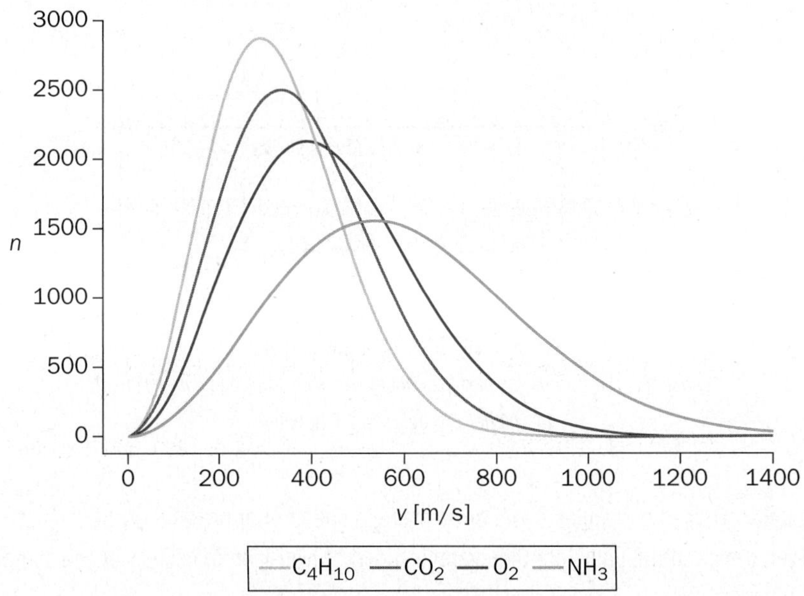

Figure 8.9 Maxwell-Boltzmann Distribution Curves of Molecular Speeds for Gases with Different Molar Masses

The more massive the gas particles, the slower their average speed.

In 1832, Thomas Graham showed mathematically that, under isothermal and isobaric conditions, the rates at which two gases diffuse are inversely proportional to the square roots of their molar masses. This is called **Graham's law**, which is written mathematically as:

$$\frac{r_1}{r_2} = \sqrt{\frac{M_2}{M_1}}$$

Equation 8.13

where r_1 and r_2 are the diffusion rates of gas 1 and gas 2, respectively, and M_1 and M_2 are the molar masses of gas 1 and gas 2, respectively. From this equation, we can see that a gas that has a molar mass four times that of another gas will travel half as fast as the lighter gas.

Effusion is the flow of gas particles under pressure from one compartment to another through a small opening, as shown in Figure 8.10. Graham used the kinetic molecular theory of gases to show that, for two gases at the same temperature, the rates of effusion are proportional to the average speeds. He then expressed the rates of effusion in terms of molar mass and found that the relationship is the same as that for diffusion.

REAL WORLD

Clinically, a pleural effusion is a condition in which fluid enters the intrapleural space through small openings in the capillaries or lymphatic vessels. This causes a pressure buildup around the lungs that hinders breathing.

KEY CONCEPT

Diffusion—When gases mix with one another.

Effusion—When a gas moves through a small hole under pressure.

Both will be slower for larger molecules.

Both conditions use the same equation.

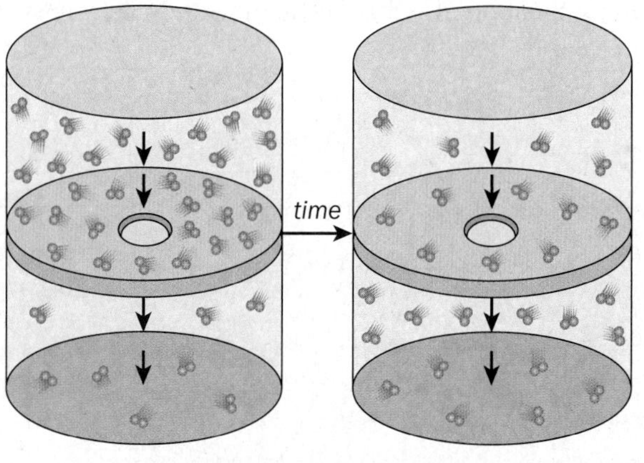

Figure 8.10 Effusion of Gas Particles

Effusion is the flow of gas particles under pressure from one compartment to another through a small opening.

Example: Oxygen molecules travel at an average speed of approximately 500 $\frac{m}{s}$ at a given temperature. Calculate the average speed of hydrogen molecules at the same temperature.

Solution: Oxygen's molar mass is 32 $\frac{g}{mol}$. Hydrogen's molar mass is 2 $\frac{g}{mol}$. Plugging into Graham's law, we get:

$$\frac{r_1}{r_2} = \sqrt{\frac{M_2}{M_1}} \rightarrow r_2 = r_1\sqrt{\frac{M_1}{M_2}}$$

$$r_2 = 500\ \frac{m}{s}\sqrt{\frac{32\ \frac{g}{mol}}{2\ \frac{g}{mol}}} = 500\ \frac{m}{s} \times 4 = 2000\ \frac{m}{s}$$

MCAT CONCEPT CHECK 8.3

Before you move on, assess your understanding of the material with these questions.

1. What are the assumptions made by the kinetic molecular theory?

   ____

2. What is the average speed of helium atoms at −173°C?

   ____

3. If neon gas travels at 400 $\frac{m}{s}$ at a given temperature, calculate the average speed of krypton at the same temperature.

   ____

4. Hydrogen sulfide (H_2S) has a very strong rotten egg odor. Methyl salicylate (C_8H_8O) has a wintergreen odor, and benzaldehyde (C_7H_6O) has a pleasant almond odor. If the vapors for these three substances were released at the same time from across a room, in which order would one smell the odors? Explain your answer.

   ____

8.4 Real Gases

LEARNING OBJECTIVES

After Chapter 8.4, you will be able to:

- Distinguish between real gases and ideal gases
- Predict how differences in attractive forces or volumes will affect real gas behavior

Throughout our discussions of the laws and theory that describe and explain the behaviors of gases, we have stressed that the fundamental assumption is a gas that behaves ideally. However, our world is not one of ideal gases but rather real ones. Real gases have particles that occupy nonnegligible volumes and that interact with each other in measurable ways. In general, the ideal gas law is a good approximation of the behavior of real gases, but all real gases deviate from ideal gas behavior to some extent, particularly when the gas atoms or molecules are forced into close proximity under high pressure (at low volume) or at low temperature. These effects are implied by Figure 8.11, which shows isothermal lines on a pressure–volume graph for a real gas. Compare these lines to the ideal isotherms in Figure 8.2. Under these nonideal conditions, the intermolecular forces and the particles' volumes become significant.

MCAT EXPERTISE

At high temperature and low pressure (high volume), deviations from ideality are usually small; good approximations can still be made from the ideal gas law.

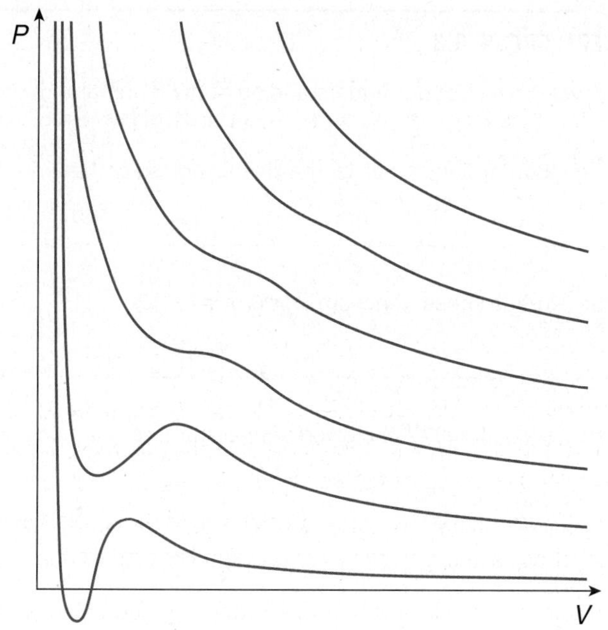

Figure 8.11 Real Gas Isothermal Curves
Compare these lines to the ideal gas isotherms in Figure 8.2.

MCAT EXPERTISE

On the MCAT, an understanding of nonideal conditions will help with determining how gases' behaviors may deviate.

Deviations Due to Pressure

As the pressure of a gas increases, the particles are pushed closer and closer together. As the condensation pressure for a given temperature is approached, intermolecular attraction forces become more and more significant, until the gas condenses into a liquid.

At moderately high pressure (a few hundred atmospheres), a gas's volume is less than would be predicted by the ideal gas law due to intermolecular attraction. At extremely high pressures, however, the size of the particles becomes relatively large compared to the distance between them, and this causes the gas to take up a larger volume than would be predicted by the ideal gas law. That is, while the ideal gas law assumes that a gas can be compressed to take up zero volume, this is not actually physically possible—the gas particles themselves will take up space.

Deviations Due to Temperature

As the temperature of a gas is decreased, the average speed of the gas molecules decreases and the attractive intermolecular forces become increasingly significant. As the condensation temperature is approached for a given pressure, intermolecular attractions eventually cause the gas to condense to a liquid state.

Like deviations due to pressure, as the temperature of a gas is reduced toward its condensation point (which is the same as its boiling point), intermolecular attraction causes the gas to have a smaller volume than that which would be predicted by the ideal gas law. The closer a gas is to its boiling point, the less ideally it acts. At extremely low temperatures, gases will again occupy more space than predicted by the ideal gas law because the particles cannot be compressed to zero volume.

van der Waals Equation of State

There are several gas equations that attempt to correct for the deviations from ideality that occur when a gas does not closely follow the ideal gas law. The van der Waals equation of state is one such equation:

$$\left(P + \frac{n^2 a}{V^2}\right)(V - nb) = nRT$$

Equation 8.14

where a and b are physical constants experimentally determined for each gas. The a term corrects for the attractive forces between molecules and, as such, will be smaller for gases that are small and less polarizable (such as helium), larger for gases that are larger and more polarizable (such as Xe or N_2), and largest for polar molecules such as HCl and NH_3. The b term corrects for the volume of the molecules themselves. Larger molecules thus have larger values of b. Numerical values for a are generally much larger than those for b.

Example: By what percentage does the real pressure of 1 mole of ammonia in a 1 liter flask at 227°C deviate from its ideal pressure? (Note: $R = 0.0821 \frac{L \cdot atm}{mol \cdot K}$; for NH_3, $a = 4.2$, $b = 0.037$)

Solution: According to the ideal gas law,

$$P = \frac{nRT}{V} = \frac{(1\text{ mol})\left(0.0821 \frac{L \cdot atm}{mol \cdot K}\right)(500\text{ K})}{1\text{ L}} = \frac{(0.0821)(1000)}{2}$$

$$= \frac{82.1}{2} = 41.5\text{ atm}$$

According to the van der Waals equation of state,

$$P = \frac{nRT}{V - nb} - \frac{n^2 a}{V^2} = \left[\frac{(1\text{ mol})\left(0.0821 \frac{L \cdot atm}{mol \cdot K}\right)(500\text{ K})}{1\text{ L} - (1\text{ mol})(0.037)}\right] - \left[\frac{(1\text{ mol})^2(4.2)}{(1\text{ L})^2}\right]$$

$$P = \frac{41.5}{0.963} - 4.2 \approx [41.5 + 4\%(41.5)] \approx 43 - 4 \approx 39\text{ atm (actual} = 38.8\text{ atm)}$$

The pressure is thus approximately $41.5 - 38.8 = 2.7$ atm less than would be predicted from the ideal gas law, representing an error of

$$\frac{2.7\text{ atm}}{41.5\text{ atm}} \times 100\% \approx \frac{3}{40} \times 100\% = 7.5\text{ percent.}$$

KEY CONCEPT

Note that if a and b are both zero, the van der Waals equation of state reduces to the ideal gas law.

MNEMONIC

a is the van der Waals term for the **a**ttractive forces.

b is the van der Waals term for **b**ig particles.

MCAT EXPERTISE

Be familiar with the concepts embodied by this equation but do not bother memorizing it; if the testmakers want you to apply the equation, it will be provided in a passage or question stem.

MCAT CONCEPT CHECK 8.4

Before you move on, assess your understanding of the material with these questions.

1. In what ways do real gases differ from ideal gases?

____

2. Which gas will exert a higher pressure under the same, nonideal conditions: methane or chloromethane?

____

3. If methane and isobutane are placed in the same size container under the same conditions, which will exert the higher pressure (consider both as having negligible attractive forces)?

____

Conclusion

In this chapter, we reviewed the basic characteristics and behaviors of gases. The ideal gas law shows the mathematical relationship among four variables associated with gases: pressure, volume, temperature, and number of moles. We examined special cases of the ideal gas law in which temperature (Boyle's law), pressure (Charles's law), or volume (Gay-Lussac's law) is held constant. Henry's law helped explain the principles behind dissolution of gases in liquids and gas exchange in biological systems. We also examined Dalton's law, which relates the partial pressure of a gas to its mole fraction and the sum of the partial pressures of all the gases in a system to the total pressure of the system. The kinetic molecular theory of gases provided the explanation for the behaviors of ideal gases as described by the ideal gas law. Finally, we examined the ways in which real gases deviate from the predicted behaviors of ideal gases. The van der Waals equation of state is a useful equation for correcting deviations caused by molecular interactions and volumes.

From helium-filled balloons to the bubbles of carbon dioxide in a glass of soda, from the pressurized gases used for scuba diving to the air we breathe on land, gases are all around us. And yet, all the different gases that bubble, flow, and settle in and through our daily living experiences behave in remarkably similar ways. Human life is dependent on the exchange of two gases: oxygen and carbon dioxide—to that end, expect that the MCAT will frequently test gases because of their importance in our everyday lives.

You've reviewed the content, now test your knowledge and critical thinking skills by completing a test-like passage set in your online resources!

GO ONLINE

CONCEPT SUMMARY

The Gas Phase

- Gases are the least dense phase of matter.
- Gases are fluids and therefore conform to the shapes of their containers.
- Gases are easily compressible.
- Gas systems are described by the variables **temperature (*T*)**, **pressure (*P*)**, **volume (*V*)**, and **number of moles (*n*)**.
- Important pressure equivalencies include
  $1\ \text{atm} = 760\ \text{mmHg} \equiv 760\ \text{torr} = 101.325\ \text{kPa}$.
- A **simple mercury barometer** measures incident (usually atmospheric) pressure. As pressure increases, more mercury is forced into the column, increasing its height. As pressure decreases, mercury flows out of the column under its own weight, decreasing its height.

Ideal Gases

- **Standard temperature and pressure (STP)** is 273 K (0°C) and 1 atm.
- Equations for ideal gases assume negligible mass and volume of gas molecules.
- Regardless of the identity of the gas, equimolar amounts of two gases will occupy the same volume at the same temperature and pressure. At STP, one mole of an ideal gas occupies 22.4 L.
- The **ideal gas law** describes the relationship between the four variables of the gas state for an ideal gas.
- **Avogadro's principle** is a special case of the ideal gas law for which the pressure and temperature are held constant; it shows a direct relationship between the number of moles of gas and volume.
- **Boyle's law** is a special case of the ideal gas law for which temperature and number of moles are held constant; it shows an inverse relationship between pressure and volume.
- **Charles's law** is a special case of the ideal gas law for which pressure and number of moles are held constant; it shows a direct relationship between temperature and volume.
- **Gay-Lussac's law** is a special case of the ideal gas law for which volume and number of moles are held constant; it shows a direct relationship between temperature and pressure.
- The **combined gas law** is a combination of Boyle's, Charles's, and Gay-Lussac's laws; it shows an inverse relationship between pressure and volume along with direct relationships between pressure and volume with temperature.

- **Dalton's law of partial pressures** states that individual gas components of a mixture of gases will exert individual pressures in proportion to their **mole fractions**. The total pressure of a mixture of gases is equal to the sum of the partial pressures of the component gases.
- **Henry's law** states that the amount of gas dissolved in solution is directly proportional to the partial pressure of that gas at the surface of a solution.

Kinetic Molecular Theory

- The **kinetic molecular theory** attempts to explain the behavior of gas particles. It makes a number of assumptions about the gas particles:
  - Gas particles have negligible volume.
  - Gas particles do not have intermolecular attractions or repulsions.
  - Gas particles undergo random collisions with each other and the walls of the container.
  - Collisions between gas particles (and with the walls of the container) are elastic.
  - The average kinetic energy of the gas particles is directly proportional to temperature.
- **Graham's law** describes the behavior of gas diffusion or effusion, stating that gases with lower molar masses will diffuse or effuse faster than gases with higher molar masses at the same temperature.
  - **Diffusion** is the spreading out of particles from high to low concentration.
  - **Effusion** is the movement of gas from one compartment to another through a small opening under pressure.

Real Gases

- **Real gases** deviate from ideal behavior under high pressure (low volume) and low temperature conditions.
  - At moderately high pressures, low volumes, or low temperatures, real gases will occupy less volume than predicted by the ideal gas law because the particles have intermolecular attractions.
  - At extremely high pressures, low volumes, or low temperatures, real gases will occupy more volume than predicted by the ideal gas law because the particles occupy physical space.
  - The **van der Waals equation of state** is used to correct the ideal gas law for intermolecular attractions (a) and molecular volume (b).

ANSWERS TO CONCEPT CHECKS

8.1

1. Gases are compressible fluids with rapid molecular motion, large intermolecular distances, and weak intermolecular forces.
2. At the top of the mountain, atmospheric pressure is lower, causing the column to fall. Under water, hydrostatic pressure is exerted on the barometer in addition to atmospheric pressure, causing the column to rise.
3. STP: $T = 273$ K (0°C), $P = 1$ atm
4. Standard conditions: $T = 298$ K (25°C), $P = 1$ atm, concentrations = 1 M

8.2

1. $PV = nRT \rightarrow T = \frac{PV}{nR} = \frac{(8\text{ atm})(12\text{ L})}{(4\text{ mol})\left(0.0821\ \frac{\text{L}\cdot\text{atm}}{\text{mol}\cdot\text{K}}\right)} \approx \frac{8\times 3}{0.08} = \frac{3}{0.01} = 300\text{ K}$

   $(\text{actual} = 292.3\text{K})$

2. $\rho = \frac{m}{V} = \frac{PM}{RT} = \frac{(4\text{ atm})\left(39.9\ \frac{\text{g}}{\text{mol}}\right)}{\left(0.0821\ \frac{\text{L}\cdot\text{atm}}{\text{mol}\cdot\text{K}}\right)(400\text{ K})} \approx 5\ \frac{\text{g}}{\text{L}}$

   $\left(\text{actual} = 4.85\ \frac{\text{g}}{\text{L}}\right)$

3. $\frac{n_1}{V_1} = \frac{n_2}{V_2} \rightarrow V_2 = \frac{n_2 \times V_1}{n_1} = \frac{(2+3\text{ mol})(20\text{ L})}{2\text{ mol}} = 50\text{ L}$
4. $P_1V_1 = P_2V_2 \rightarrow V_2 = \frac{P_1V_1}{P_2} = \frac{(1\text{ atm})(2\text{ L})}{40\text{ atm}} = 0.05\text{ L}$
5. $\frac{V_1}{T_1} = \frac{V_2}{T_2} \rightarrow V_2 = \frac{V_1 \times T_2}{T_1} = \frac{(6\text{ L})(400\text{ K})}{300\text{ K}} = 8\text{ L}$
6. $\frac{P_1}{T_1} = \frac{P_2}{T_2} \rightarrow T_2 = \frac{P_2 \times T_1}{P_1} = \frac{(2\text{ atm})(500\text{ K})}{5\text{ atm}} = 200\text{ K}$
7. There are twelve total moles of gas, so the mole fractions of each gas are:

   $X_{O_2} = \frac{8\text{ mol } O_2}{12\text{ mol}} = \frac{2}{3} = 0.67;\ X_{CH_4} = \frac{3\text{ mol } CH_4}{12\text{ mol}} = \frac{1}{4} = 0.25;$

   $X_{CO_2} = \frac{1\text{ mol } CO_2}{12\text{ mol}} = 0.083$

   Then multiply each mole fraction by the total pressure to get the partial pressures (this is typically simpler with fractions than with decimals):

   $P_{O_2} = \frac{2}{3}(240\text{ atm}) = 160\text{ atm};\ P_{CH_4} = \frac{1}{4}(240\text{ atm}) = 60\text{ atm};$

   $P_{CO_2} = \frac{1}{12}(240\text{ atm}) = 20\text{ atm}$

8. High pressures of carbon dioxide gas are forced on top of the liquid in sodas, increasing its concentration in the liquid.

8.3

1. Assumptions in the kinetic molecular theory include: negligible volume of gas particles, no intermolecular forces, random motion, elastic collisions, and proportionality between absolute temperature and energy.

2. $$u_{rms} = \sqrt{\frac{3\,RT}{M}} = \sqrt{\frac{3\left(8.314\ \frac{\text{J}}{\text{mol}\cdot\text{K}}\right)(100\ \text{K})}{0.004\ \frac{\text{kg}}{\text{mol}}}} \approx \sqrt{\frac{(3)(8)(100)}{4\times10^{-3}}}$$
$$= \sqrt{(3)(8)(25)\left(10^{3}\right)}$$
$$u_{rms} = \sqrt{(3)(200)\left(10^{3}\right)} = \sqrt{600\times10^{3}} = \sqrt{60\times10^{4}}$$
$$\approx \sqrt{64}\times\sqrt{10^{4}}$$
$$u_{rms} = 8\times10^{2} = 800\ \frac{\text{m}}{\text{s}}\ \left(\text{actual} = 790\ \frac{\text{m}}{\text{s}}\right)$$

3. $$\frac{r_1}{r_2} = \sqrt{\frac{M_2}{M_1}} \rightarrow r_2 = r_1\sqrt{\frac{M_1}{M_2}} = 400\ \frac{\text{m}}{\text{s}}\sqrt{\frac{20.2\ \frac{\text{g}}{\text{mol}}}{83.8\ \frac{\text{g}}{\text{mol}}}} \approx 400\times\frac{1}{2} = 200\ \frac{\text{m}}{\text{s}}$$
$$\left(\text{actual} = 196.4\ \frac{\text{m}}{\text{s}}\right)$$

4. The rotten egg odor (hydrogen sulfide) first, almond (benzaldehyde) next, and wintergreen (methyl salicylate) last. Because all of the gases have the same temperature, they have the same kinetic energy; thus, the lightest molecules travel the fastest.

8.4

1. Real gas molecules have nonnegligible volume and attractive forces. Real gases deviate from ideal gases at high pressure (low volume) and low temperature.
2. According to the van der Waals equation, if a is increased while b remains negligible, the correction term $\left(\frac{n^2a}{V^2}\right)$ gets larger, and the pressure drops to compensate. Therefore, methane will behave more ideally than chloromethane because a is smaller for methane. The real pressure of methane will thus be higher (closer to ideal).
3. Isobutane is larger and will thus have a larger correction term for the size of the molecule, b. This makes the term $V - nb$ smaller. The pressure or volume must rise to compensate. Because the two gases are in the same size container, isobutane must exert a higher pressure.

SCIENCE MASTERY ASSESSMENT EXPLANATIONS

1. **A**

Gases deviate from ideal behavior at higher pressures and lower volumes and temperatures, all of which force molecules closer together. The closer they are, the more they can participate in intermolecular forces, which violates the definition of an ideal gas. At low temperatures, the kinetic energy of the particles is reduced, so collisions with other particles or the walls of the container are more likely to result in significant changes in kinetic energy.

2. **D**

Density equals mass divided by volume. The mass of 1 mole of neon gas equals 20.2 grams. At STP, 1 mole of neon occupies 22.4 L.

$$\text{density} = \rho = \frac{\text{mass}}{\text{volume}} = \frac{20.2\ \text{g}}{22.4\ \text{L}} \approx \frac{10}{11} < 1\ \frac{\text{g}}{\text{L}}$$

$$\left(\text{actual} = 0.902\ \frac{\text{g}}{\text{L}}\right)$$

3. **D**

Graham's law of effusion states that the relative rates of effusion of two gases at the same temperature and pressure are given by the inverse ratio of the square roots of the masses of the gas particles. In other words, a gas with a higher molar mass will leak more slowly than a gas with a lower molar mass. Both neon and oxygen gases will leak at slower rates than helium because they both have more mass than helium.

4. **B**

The pressure of the gas is calculated by subtracting the vapor pressure of water from the measured pressure during the experiment: 784 mmHg − 24 mmHg = 760 mmHg, or 1 atm. This is because the reaction is carried out in an aqueous environment; the water present will contribute to the partial pressures of the gas over the liquid. The ideal gas law can be used to calculate the moles of hydrogen gas. The volume of the gas is 0.100 L, the temperature is 298 K, and $R = 0.0821\ \frac{\text{L}\cdot\text{atm}}{\text{mol}\cdot\text{K}}$. Plugging in gives:

$$n = \frac{PV}{RT} = \frac{(1\ \text{atm})(0.1\ \text{L})}{\left(0.0821\ \frac{\text{L}\cdot\text{atm}}{\text{mol}\cdot\text{K}}\right)(298\ \text{K})} \approx \frac{1}{0.8 \times 300}$$

$$= \frac{1}{240} \approx \frac{1}{250} = 0.004$$

(A) incorrectly substitutes 8.314 into the gas law, rather than 0.0821. Remember that the value of R depends on the other variables in the equation; using 1 atm in the numerator necessitates using 0.0821. **(C)** incorrectly substitutes the wrong R and keeps the pressure in mmHg. **(D)** also keeps the pressure in mmHg.

5. **B**

Ideal gases are said to have no attractive forces between molecules. While each particle within the gas is considered to have negligible volume, ideal gases as a whole certainly do have a measurable volume, thus option I is eliminated. Gases have molar masses, thus option III is eliminated.

6. **B**

Deviations from ideal behavior are due either to large particle size and/or strong intermolecular forces between molecules. Nitrogen gas consists of two nitrogen atoms triple bonded. This molecule is therefore relatively small and its nonpolar triple bond leads to very weak intermolecular forces. Together, these observations support **(B)** as the correct answer. By contrast, fluoromethane consists of all single bonds, making this molecule somewhat larger. Furthermore, due to the polarity of the carbon-fluorine bond, this molecule can participate in dipole-dipole interactions. Fluoromethane would therefore exhibit greater deviations from ideal behavior.

7. **A**

The average kinetic energy is directly proportional to the temperature of a gas in kelvin. The kinetic molecular theory states that collisions between molecules are elastic and thus do not result in a loss of energy, eliminating **(B)**. Gas particles are assumed to take up negligible space in kinetic molecular theory, eliminating **(C)**. While the average kinetic energy of any gas as a whole is the same at a given temperature, the particles themselves have a distribution of speeds (as seen in the Maxwell–Boltzmann distribution curve), eliminating **(D)**.

8. **C**

At STP, the difference between the distribution of speeds for helium and bromine gas is due to the difference in molar mass. Helium has a smaller molar mass than bromine. Particles with small masses travel faster than those with large masses, so the helium gas corresponds to curve B, which has a higher average speed. Because the gases are at the same temperature (273 K), they have the same average kinetic energy, eliminating **(B)** and **(D)**.

9. **A**

The solubility of gases in liquids is directly proportional to the atmospheric pressure, as shown by Henry's law.

$$\frac{[O_2]_1}{P_1} = \frac{[O_2]_2}{P_2}$$

$$\frac{1.25\times10^{-3}\,M}{1.000\text{ atm}} = \frac{[O_2]_2}{0.8000\text{ atm}}$$

$$[O_2]_2 = \frac{0.8\times1.25\times10^{-3}}{1} = \frac{8}{10}\times\frac{5}{4}\times10^{-3} = 1\times10^{-3}\,M$$

Note that the use of fractions allows this problem to be simplified more readily than it would be with decimals.

10. **C**

The ideal gas law can be modified to include density (ρ) because the number of moles of gas, n, is equal to the mass divided by the molar mass. Thus, $PV = nRT = \frac{m}{M}RT \rightarrow P = \frac{m}{V}\times\frac{RT}{M} = \frac{\rho RT}{M}$. Isolating for temperature gives:

$$T = \frac{PM}{\rho R}$$

$$T = \frac{\left(1.3\times10^{9}\text{ atm}\right)\left(2.00\ \frac{\text{g}}{\text{mol}}\right)}{\left(1.2\ \frac{\text{g}}{\text{cm}^3}\right)\left(1000\ \frac{\text{cm}^3}{\text{L}}\right)\left(0.0821\ \frac{\text{L}\cdot\text{atm}}{\text{mol}\cdot\text{K}}\right)}$$

$$\approx \frac{\left(1.3\times2\times10^{9}\right)}{(1)(1000)(0.1)} \approx \frac{2.6\times10^{9}}{100}$$

$$\approx 2.6\times10^{7}\text{ K}$$

11. **B**

Gases are easily compressible because they travel freely with large amounts of space between molecules. Because gas particles are far apart from each other and in rapid motion, they tend to take up the volume of their container. Many gases exist as diatomic molecules, but this is not a property that characterizes all gases, eliminating option III.

12. **B**

We will use Charles's law. First, we must convert the temperature to kelvin by adding 273 to get 300 K as the initial temperature. Think of this as a proportionality: If the volume is multiplied by $\frac{3}{2}$, the temperature will also have to be multiplied by $\frac{3}{2}$. Thus the final temperature is 450 K, which represents a 150 K increase (which is equivalent to an increase of 150°C).

13. **D**

A decrease in temperature leads to a decrease in the kinetic energy of the particles so intermolecular interactions become more significant. This change leads to deviations from ideal behavior. Similarly, decreases in volume cause the volume of the particles themselves to become significant. This change also leads to deviations from ideal behavior. Thus, **(D)** is correct.

14. **C**

Both a change in temperature and a change in volume can affect a gas's pressure. So if one of those two variables is kept constant, as in **(A)** and **(B)**, we'll definitely be able to predict which way the pressure will change. At a constant volume, heating the gas will increase its pressure, and cooling the gas will decrease it. What about when both temperature and volume are changing? If both changes have the same effect on pressure, then we can still predict which way it will change. This is the case in **(D)**. Cooling the gas and increasing its volume both decrease pressure. **(C)**, on the other hand, presents too vague a scenario for us to predict definitively the change in pressure. Heating the gas would amplify the pressure, while increasing the volume would decrease it. Without knowing the magnitude of each influence, it's impossible to say whether the pressure would increase, decrease, or stay the same.

15. **C**

Initially the concentration of the gas is decreased to one-half its original value. Recall that concentration (solubility) and partial pressure are directly related—as one increases, the other increases. If the experimenters then quadruple the partial pressure of oxygen in the vessel, the solubility is also increased by a factor of four. One-half times four gives twice the original concentration value. Misreading the answer choices as being related to the concentration before the experimenters increased the partial pressure leads to **(D)**.

Consult your online resources for additional practice. GO ONLINE

EQUATIONS TO REMEMBER

(8.1) **Ideal gas law:** $PV = n\text{R}T$

(8.2) **Density of a gas:** $\rho = \frac{m}{V} = \frac{PM}{\text{R}T}$

(8.3) **Combined gas law:** $\frac{P_1V_1}{T_1} = \frac{P_2V_2}{T_2}$

(8.4) **Avogadro's principle:** $\frac{n}{V} = k$ or $\frac{n_1}{V_1} = \frac{n_2}{V_2}$

(8.5) **Boyle's law:** $PV = k$ or $P_1V_1 = P_2V_2$

(8.6) **Charles's law:** $\frac{V}{T} = k$ or $\frac{V_1}{T_1} = \frac{V_2}{T_2}$

(8.7) **Gay-Lussac's law:** $\frac{P}{T} = k$ or $\frac{P_1}{T_1} = \frac{P_2}{T_2}$

(8.8) **Dalton's law (total pressure from partial pressures):** $P_\text{T} = P_\text{A} + P_\text{B} + P_\text{C} + \cdots$

(8.9) **Dalton's law (partial pressure from total pressure):** $P_\text{A} = X_\text{A}P_\text{T}$

(8.10) **Henry's law:** $[\text{A}] = k_\text{H} \times P_\text{A}$ or $\frac{[\text{A}]_1}{P_1} = \frac{[\text{A}]_2}{P_2} = k_\text{H}$

(8.11) **Average kinetic energy of a gas:** $KE = \frac{1}{2}mv^2 = \frac{3}{2}k_\text{B}T$

(8.12) **Root-mean-square speed:** $u_\text{rms} = \sqrt{\frac{3\text{R}T}{M}}$

(8.13) **Graham's law:** $\frac{r_1}{r_2} = \sqrt{\frac{M_2}{M_1}}$

(8.14) **van der Waals equation of state:** $\left(P + \frac{n^2a}{V^2}\right)(V - nb) = n\text{R}T$

SHARED CONCEPTS

Biology Chapter 6
The Respiratory System

General Chemistry Chapter 3
Bonding and Chemical Interactions

General Chemistry Chapter 6
Equilibrium

Physics and Math Chapter 2
Work and Energy

Physics and Math Chapter 3
Thermodynamics

Physics and Math Chapter 4
Fluids

CHAPTER 9

SOLUTIONS

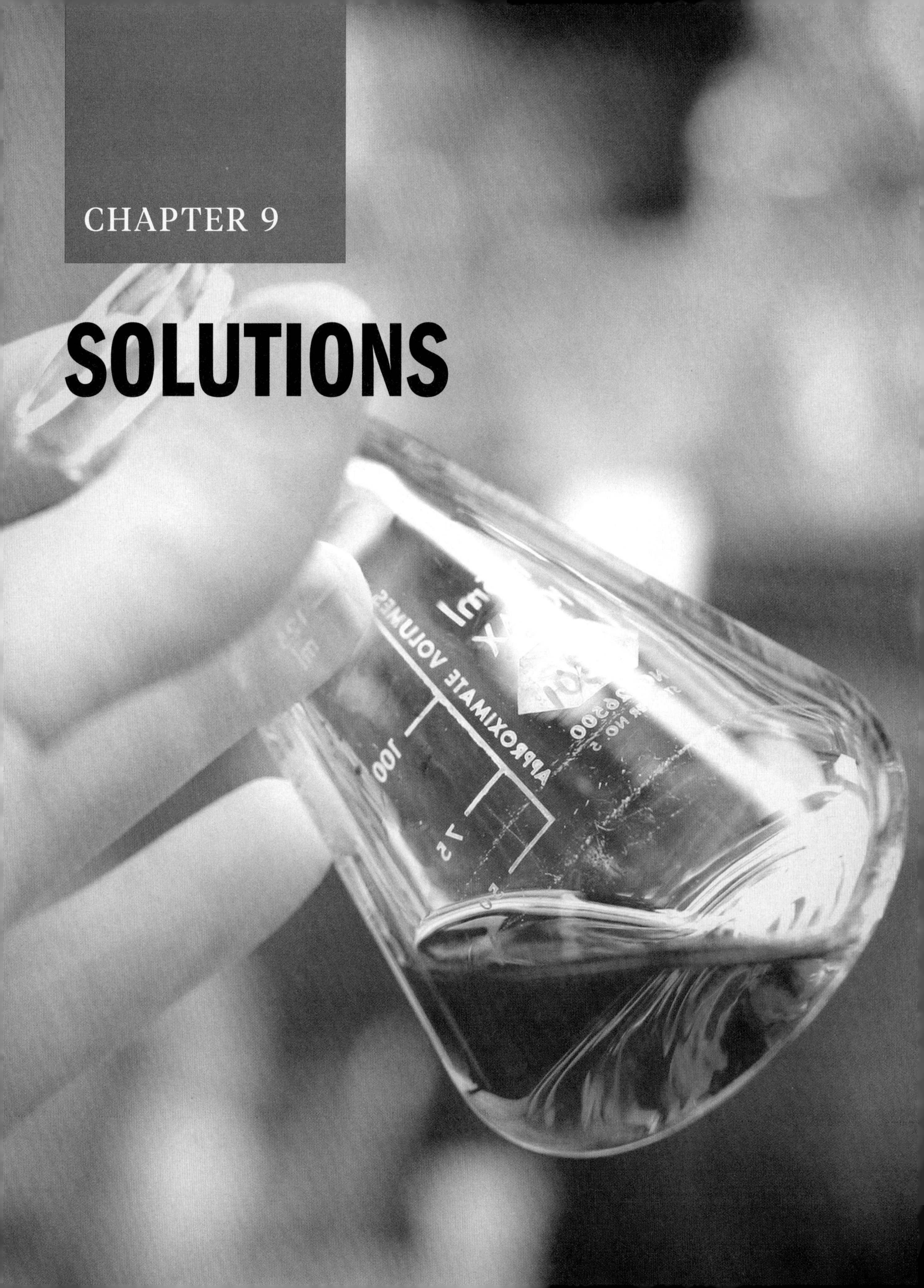

SCIENCE MASTERY ASSESSMENT

Every pre-med knows this feeling: there is so much content I have to know for the MCAT! How do I know what to do first or what's important?

While the high-yield badges throughout this book will help you identify the most important topics, this Science Mastery Assessment is another tool in your MCAT prep arsenal. This quiz (which can also be taken in your online resources) and the guidance below will help ensure that you are spending the appropriate amount of time on this chapter based on your personal strengths and weaknesses. Don't worry though—skipping something now does not mean you'll never study it. Later on in your prep, as you complete full-length tests, you'll uncover specific pieces of content that you need to review and can come back to these chapters as appropriate.

How to Use This Assessment

If you answer 0–7 questions correctly:

Spend about 1 hour to read this chapter in full and take limited notes throughout. Follow up by reviewing **all** quiz questions to ensure that you now understand how to solve each one.

If you answer 8–11 questions correctly:

Spend 20–40 minutes reviewing the quiz questions. Beginning with the questions you missed, read and take notes on the corresponding subchapters. For questions you answered correctly, ensure your thinking matches that of the explanation and you understand why each choice was correct or incorrect.

If you answer 12–15 questions correctly:

Spend less than 20 minutes reviewing all questions from the quiz. If you missed any, then include a quick read-through of the corresponding subchapters, or even just the relevant content within a subchapter, as part of your question review. For questions you answered correctly, ensure your thinking matches that of the explanation and review the Concept Summary at the end of the chapter.

1. An aqueous solution was prepared by mixing 70 g of an unknown nondissociating solute into 100 g of water. The solution has a boiling point of 101.0°C. What is the molar mass of the solute?

(Note: $K_b = 0.512 \frac{K \cdot kg}{mol}$)

A. $358.4 \frac{g}{mol}$

B. $32.3 \frac{g}{mol}$

C. $123.2 \frac{g}{mol}$

D. $233.6 \frac{g}{mol}$

2. Which phases of solvent and solute can form a solution?

I. Solid solvent, gaseous solute
II. Solid solvent, solid solute
III. Gaseous solvent, gaseous solute

A. I and II only
B. I and III only
C. II and III only
D. I, II, and III

3. Two organic liquids, pictured in the figure below, are combined to form a solution. Based on their structures, will the solution closely obey Raoult's law?

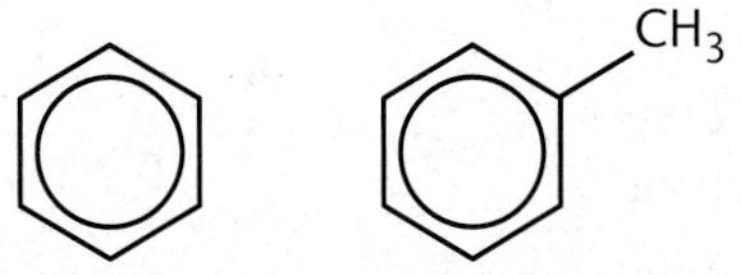

A. Yes; the liquids differ due to the additional methyl group on toluene and, therefore, will not deviate from Raoult's law.
B. Yes; the liquids are very similar and, therefore, will not deviate from Raoult's law.
C. No; the liquids differ due to the additional methyl group on toluene and, therefore, will deviate from Raoult's law.
D. No; the liquids both contain benzene rings, which will interact with each other and cause deviation from Raoult's law.

4. Which of the following explanations best describes the mechanism by which solute particles affect the melting point of ice?

A. Melting point is elevated because the kinetic energy of the substance increases.
B. Melting point is elevated because the kinetic energy of the substance decreases.
C. Melting point is depressed because solute particles interfere with lattice formation.
D. Melting point is depressed because solute particles enhance lattice formation.

5. The process of formation of a salt solution can be better understood by breaking the process into three steps:

1. Breaking the solute into its individual components
2. Making room for the solute in the solvent by overcoming intermolecular forces in the solvent
3. Allowing solute–solvent interactions to occur to form the solution

Which of the following correctly lists the enthalpy changes for these three steps, respectively?

A. Endothermic, exothermic, endothermic
B. Exothermic, endothermic, endothermic
C. Exothermic, exothermic, endothermic
D. Endothermic, endothermic, exothermic

6. The entropy change when a solution forms can be expressed by the term ΔS°_{soln}. When water molecules become ordered around an ion as it dissolves, the ordering would be expected to make a negative contribution to ΔS°_{soln}. An ion that has more charge density will have a greater hydration effect, or ordering of water molecules. In an experiment, an equimolar amount of each of the following aqueous soluble compounds is dissolved in its own test tube containing 100 mL of water. Which will have the most negative contribution to ΔS°_{soln}? (Assume that the charge density of each ion is equal to its actual charge.)

A. KCl
B. CsI
C. BeF_2
D. NaCl

7. When ammonia, NH_3, is used as a solvent, it can form complex ions. For example, dissolving AgCl in NH_3 will result in the complex ion $[Ag(NH_3)]^{2+}$. What effect would the formation of complex ions have on the solubility of a compound like AgCl in NH_3?
   - **A.** The solubility of AgCl will increase because complex ion formation will cause more ions to exist in solution, which interact with AgCl to cause it to dissociate.
   - **B.** The solubility of AgCl will increase because complex ion formation will consume Ag^+ ions and cause the equilibrium to shift away from solid AgCl.
   - **C.** The solubility of AgCl will decrease because Ag^+ ions are in complexes, and the Ag^+ ions that are not complexed will associate with Cl^- to form solid AgCl.
   - **D.** The solubility of AgCl will decrease because complex ion formation will consume Ag^+ ions and cause the equilibrium to shift toward the solid AgCl.

8. One hundred grams of sucrose are dissolved in a cup of hot water at 80°C. The cup of water contains 300.00 mL of water. What is the percent composition by mass of sugar in the resulting solution? (Note: Sucrose = $C_{12}H_{22}O_{11}$, density of water at 80°C = $0.975\ \frac{g}{mL}$)
   - **A.** 25.0%
   - **B.** 25.5%
   - **C.** 33.3%
   - **D.** 34.2%

9. Which of the following combinations of liquids would be expected to have a vapor pressure higher than the vapor pressure that would be predicted by Raoult's law?
   - **A.** Ethanol and hexane
   - **B.** Acetone and water
   - **C.** Isopropanol and methanol
   - **D.** Nitric acid and water

10. The salt KCl is dissolved in a beaker. To an observer holding the beaker, the solution begins to feel colder as the KCl dissolves. From this observation, one could conclude that:
   - **A.** ΔS°_{soln} is large enough to overcome the unfavorable ΔH°_{soln}.
   - **B.** KCl is mostly insoluble in water.
   - **C.** ΔS°_{soln} must be negative when KCl dissolves.
   - **D.** boiling point depression will occur in this solution.

11. Which of the following will cause the greatest increase in the boiling point of water when it is dissolved in 1.00 kg H_2O?
   - **A.** 0.4 mol calcium sulfate
   - **B.** 0.5 mol iron(III) nitrate
   - **C.** 1.0 mol acetic acid
   - **D.** 1.0 mol sucrose

12. Reverse osmosis is a process that allows fresh water to be obtained by using pressure to force an impure water source through a semi-permeable membrane that only allows water molecules to pass. What is the minimum pressure that would be required to purify seawater at 25°C that has a total osmolarity of 1,000 mOsm/L?
   - **A.** 23.5 atm
   - **B.** 24.5 atm
   - **C.** 24,000 atm
   - **D.** 24,500 atm

13. Lead is a toxic element that can cause many symptoms, including intellectual disabilities in children. If a body of water is polluted with lead ions at 200 ppb (parts per billion), what is the concentration of lead expressed as molarity? (Note: The density of water is $1\ \frac{g}{mL}$, and ppb = grams per 10^9 grams of solution)
   - **A.** $9.7 \times 10^{-10}\ M\ Pb^{2+}$
   - **B.** $9.7 \times 10^{-7}\ M\ Pb^{2+}$
   - **C.** $6.2 \times 10^{-7}\ M\ Pb^{2+}$
   - **D.** $6.2 \times 10^{-6}\ M\ Pb^{2+}$

14. A saturated solution of aqueous cobalt(III) hydroxide ($K_{sp} = 1.6 \times 10^{-44}$) is added to a saturated solution of aqueous thallium(III) hydroxide ($K_{sp} = 6.3 \times 10^{-46}$). What is likely to occur?

A. Both cobalt(III) hydroxide and thallium(III) hydroxide remain stable in solution.

B. Thallium(III) hydroxide precipitates and cobalt(III) hydroxide remains stable in solution.

C. Cobalt(III) hydroxide precipitates and thallium(III) hydroxide remains stable in solution.

D. Both thallium(III) hydroxide and cobalt(III) hydroxide precipitate.

15. The following equilibrium exists when AgBr ($K_{sp} = 5.35 \times 10^{-13}$) is in solution:

$$\text{AgBr}\ (s) \rightleftharpoons \text{Ag}^{+}\ (aq) + \text{Br}^{-}\ (aq)$$

What is the solubility of AgBr in a solution of 0.0010 *M* NaBr?

A. $5.35 \times 10^{-13}\ \frac{\text{g}}{\text{L}}$

B. $1.04 \times 10^{-12}\ \frac{\text{g}}{\text{L}}$

C. $5.35 \times 10^{-10}\ \frac{\text{g}}{\text{L}}$

D. $1.04 \times 10^{-7}\ \frac{\text{g}}{\text{L}}$

Answer Key follows on next page.

Answer Key

1. **A**
2. **D**
3. **B**
4. **C**
5. **D**
6. **C**
7. **B**
8. **B**
9. **A**
10. **A**
11. **B**
12. **B**
13. **B**
14. **A**
15. **D**

Detailed explanations can be found at the end of the chapter.

CHAPTER 9

SOLUTIONS

In This Chapter

CHAPTER PROFILE

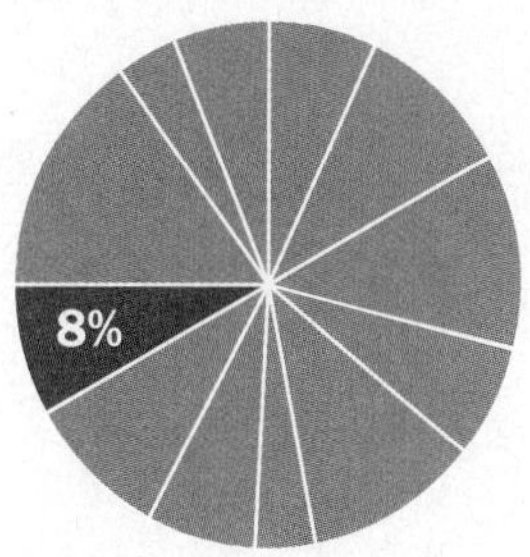

The content in this chapter should be relevant to about 8% of all questions about general chemistry on the MCAT.

This chapter covers material from the following AAMC content categories:

2A: Assemblies of molecules, cells, and groups of cells within single cellular and multicellular organisms

5A: Unique nature of water and its solutions

Introduction

What do first aid instant cold packs and sweet tea have in common? Not much, you might think—but both, in fact, demonstrate the same principles of solution chemistry. Instant cold packs contain two compartments, one holding water and the other ammonium nitrate. When the barrier between the two compartments is broken, it allows the ammonium nitrate to dissolve into the water. Sweet tea is made by dissolving a large amount of sugar into strongly brewed tea.

The creation of both the ammonium nitrate and sugar solutions is an endothermic process. However, the formation of the ammonium nitrate solution is much more endothermic than the formation of the sugar solution. This is why ammonium nitrate is useful in instant cold packs. When it dissolves in water, the system must absorb an amount of energy equal to $6.14 \frac{\text{kcal}}{\text{mol}}$ of ammonium nitrate. The heat is absorbed from the surrounding environment, so the pack feels cool to the touch.

Although the dissolution of sugar into water is not as strongly endothermic, we nevertheless have an intuitive understanding that the process is endothermic because we all know that the easiest way to dissolve lots of sugar into water (such as in tea or coffee) is to heat up the water and then add the sugar. Because heating the water increases the solubility of sugar, it must be that the dissolution of sugar into water is an endothermic process—think of Le Châtelier's principle and changes in temperature from Chapter 6.

In this chapter, our focus will be on the characteristics and behaviors of solutions, the nature of solutions, the formation of aqueous solutions, the measurements of solution concentration, and finally the qualitative and quantitative evaluation of solution equilibria.

9.1 Nature of Solutions

High-Yield

LEARNING OBJECTIVES

After Chapter 9.1, you will be able to:

- Describe the process of solvation
- Define key terms involved in solutions, such as complex, solubility, and saturation
- Explain how to increase solubility of a compound
- Recall the solubility rules and apply them to predict solubility of a compound

Many important chemical reactions, both in the laboratory and in nature, take place in solutions, including almost all reactions in living organisms. **Solutions** are homogeneous (the same throughout) mixtures of two or more substances that combine to form a single phase, usually the liquid phase. The MCAT will focus almost exclusively on solids dissolved into aqueous solutions, but it's important to remember that solutions can be formed from different combinations of the three phases of matter. For example, gases can be dissolved in liquids (carbonating soda); liquids can be dissolved in other liquids (ethanol in water); solids can even be dissolved in other solids (metal alloys). Incidentally, gases "dissolved" into other gases can be thought of as solutions, but are more properly defined only as **mixtures** because gas molecules do not interact all that much chemically, as described by the kinetic molecular theory of gases. As a point of clarification: all solutions are considered mixtures, but not all mixtures are considered solutions.

A solution consists of a **solute** (such as NaCl, NH_3, $C_6H_{12}O_6$, or CO_2) dissolved (dispersed) in a solvent (such as H_2O, benzene, or ethanol). The **solvent** is the component of the solution that remains in the same phase after mixing. If the two substances are already in the same phase (for example, a solution of two liquids), the solvent is the component present in greater quantity. If the two same-phase components are in equal proportions in the solution, then the component that is more commonly used as a solvent in other contexts is considered the solvent. Solute molecules move about freely in the solvent and interact with it by way of intermolecular forces such as ion–dipole, dipole–dipole, or hydrogen bonding. Dissolved solute molecules are also relatively free to interact with other dissolved molecules of different chemical identities; consequently, chemical reactions occur easily in solution.

Solvation

Solvation is the electrostatic interaction between solute and solvent molecules. This is also known as **dissolution**, and when water is the solvent, it can be called **hydration**. Solvation involves breaking intermolecular interactions between solute molecules and between solvent molecules and forming new intermolecular interactions between solute and solvent molecules together, as shown in Figure 9.1 (which was also shown in Chapter 4 of *MCAT General Chemistry Review* in the context of ions).

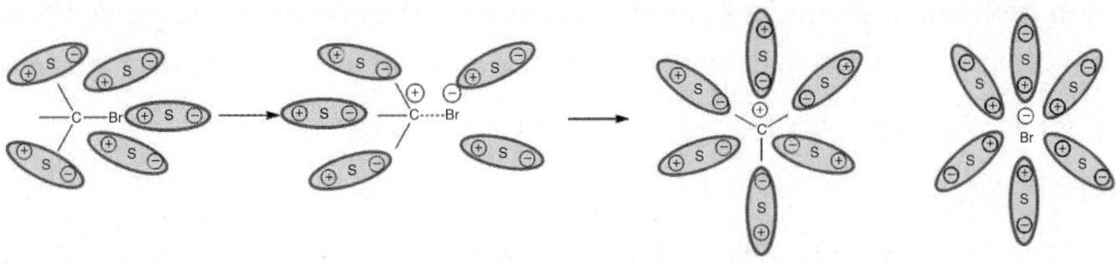

Figure 9.1 Solvation of a Polar Covalent Compound
S indicates a solvent particle.

When the new interactions are stronger than the original ones, solvation is exothermic, and the process is favored at low temperatures. The dissolution of gases into liquids, such as CO_2 into water, is an exothermic process because the only significant interactions that must be broken are those between water molecules—CO_2, as a gas, demonstrates minimal intermolecular interaction. Le Châtelier's principle tells us this is the reason that lowering the temperature of a liquid favors solubility of a gas in the liquid.

When the new interactions are weaker than the original ones, solvation is endothermic and the process is favored at high temperatures. Most dissolutions are of this type. Two such examples have already been given: dissolving ammonium nitrate or sugar into water. Because the new interactions between the solute and solvent are weaker than the original interactions between the solute molecules and between the solvent molecules, energy (heat) must be supplied to facilitate the formation of these weaker, less stable interactions. Sometimes the overall strength of the new interactions is approximately equal to the overall strength of the original interactions. In this case, the overall enthalpy change for the dissolution is close to zero. These types of solutions approximate the formation of an **ideal solution**, for which the enthalpy of dissolution is equal to zero.

The spontaneity of dissolution is dependent not only on the enthalpy change; solutions may form spontaneously for both endothermic and exothermic dissolutions. The second property that contributes to the spontaneity of dissolution is the entropy change that occurs in the process. At constant temperature and pressure, entropy always increases upon dissolution. As with any process, the spontaneity of dissolution depends on the change in Gibbs free energy: spontaneous processes are associated with a decrease in free energy, while nonspontaneous processes are associated with an increase in free energy. Thus, whether or not dissolution will happen spontaneously depends on both the change in enthalpy and the change in entropy for the solute and solvent of the system.

Consider, for example, the formation of another common solution: sodium chloride dissolved in water. When NaCl dissolves in water, its component ions dissociate from each other and become surrounded by water molecules. For this new interaction to occur, ionic bonds between Na^+ and Cl^- must be broken, and hydrogen bonds between water molecules must also be broken. This step requires energy and is therefore endothermic. Because water is polar, it can interact with each of the component ions through ion–dipole interactions: the partially positive hydrogen end of the water molecules will surround the Cl^- ions, and the partially negative oxygen end of the water molecules will surround the Na^+ ions, as shown in Figure 9.2. The formation of these ion–dipole

BRIDGE

Proteins dissolve in solution with their most hydrophilic amino acids on the outside and hydrophobic amino acids on the inside because this maximizes the increase in entropy during dissolution. As described in Chapter 1 of *MCAT Biochemistry Review*, a protein dissolves by forming a solvation layer.

bonds is exothermic, but the magnitude is slightly less than the energy required to break the ionic bonds and hydrogen bonds. As a result, the overall dissolution of table salt into water is endothermic $\left(+3.87\ \frac{\text{kJ}}{\text{mol}}\right)$ and favored at high temperatures.

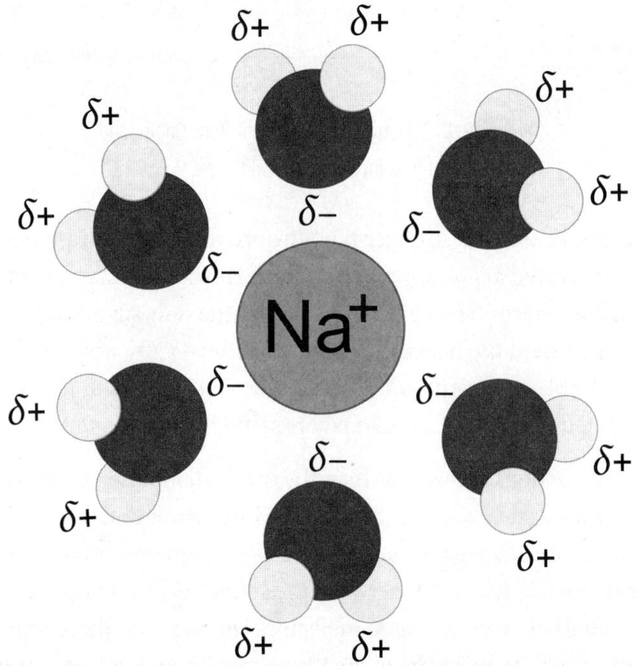

Figure 9.2 Solvation of Na^+ Ions in Aqueous Solutions

We've considered the enthalpy change for the formation of a sodium chloride solution, and now we need to examine the entropy change. Remember that entropy can be thought of as the degree to which energy is dispersed throughout a system or the amount of energy distributed from the system to the surroundings at a given temperature. Another way to understand entropy is the measure of molecular disorder, or the number of energy **microstates** available to a system at a given temperature. When solid sodium chloride dissolves into water, the rigidly ordered arrangement of the sodium and chloride ions is broken up as the ion–ion interactions are disrupted and new ion–dipole interactions with the water molecules are formed. The ions, freed from their lattice arrangement, have a greater number of energy microstates available to them (in simpler terms, they are freer to move around in different ways), and consequently, their energy is more distributed and their entropy increases. The water, however, becomes more restricted in its movement because it is now interacting with the ions. The number of energy microstates available to it (that is, the water molecules' ability to move around in different ways) is reduced, so the entropy of the water decreases. In the end, the increase in the entropy experienced by the dissolved sodium chloride is greater than the decrease in the entropy experienced by the water, so the overall entropy change is positive—energy is, overall, dispersed by the dissolution of sodium chloride in water. Because of the relatively low endothermicity and relatively large positive change in entropy, sodium chloride will spontaneously dissolve in liquid water ($\Delta G = \Delta H - T\Delta S$).

Solubility

We often want to know more than just whether or not dissolution of a solute into a solvent will be spontaneous or nonspontaneous—we also want to know how much solute will dissolve into a given solvent. The **solubility** of a substance is the maximum amount of that substance that can be dissolved in a particular solvent at a given temperature. When this maximum amount of solute has been added, the dissolved solute is in equilibrium with its undissolved state, and we say that the solution is **saturated.** If more solute is added, it will not dissolve. For example, at 25°C, a maximum of 90.9 g glucose will dissolve in 100 mL H_2O. Thus, the solubility of glucose is 909 $\frac{g}{L}$. If more glucose is added to an already saturated glucose solution, it will not dissolve but rather will remain in solid form, **precipitating** to the bottom of the container. A solution in which the proportion of solute to solvent is small is said to be **dilute,** and one in which the proportion is large is said to be **concentrated.** Note that both dilute and concentrated solutions are still considered unsaturated if the maximum equilibrium concentration (saturation) has not yet been reached.

The solubility of substances in different solvents is ultimately a function of thermodynamics. When the change in Gibbs free energy for the dissolution reaction is negative at a given temperature, the process will be spontaneous, and the solute is said to be soluble. When the change in Gibbs free energy is positive, the process will be nonspontaneous, and the solute is said to be insoluble. Some solute–solvent systems have negative changes in free energy with very large magnitudes, so the equilibrium reaction strongly favors the dissolution of the solute. In general, solutes are considered soluble if they have a molar solubility above 0.1 *M* in solution. Others have only slightly negative changes in free energy, so the equilibrium position lies closer to the undissociated (reactants) side of the reaction. Those solutes that dissolve minimally in the solvent (molar solubility under 0.1 *M*) are called **sparingly soluble salts.**

Aqueous Solutions

The most common type of solution is the **aqueous solution,** in which the solvent is water. The aqueous state is denoted by the symbol (*aq*). Aqueous solutions rely on the interactions between water molecules and solutes in solutions. We have mentioned previously that hydration is often the process through which dissolution occurs. It is also important to note that in some solutions, such as acids, the formation of a complex called the **hydronium ion (H_3O^+)** can occur. This is facilitated by the transfer of a hydrogen ion (H^+) from a molecule in solution to a water molecule (H_2O). The reaction of acetic acid (H^+ donor) with water is shown in Figure 9.3.

$$CH_3COOH\ (aq) + H_2O\ (l) \rightleftharpoons CH_3COO^-\ (aq) + H_3O^+\ (aq)$$

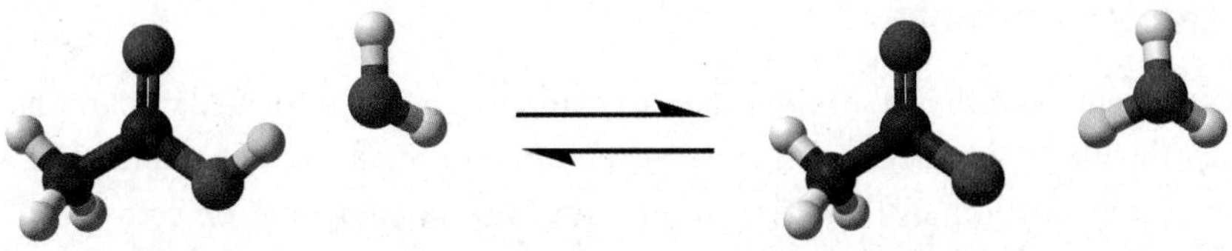

Figure 9.3 Transfer of a Proton in Solution, Forming the Hydronium Ion
The transferred proton is highlighted in green.

It is important to realize that H^+ is never found alone in solution because a free proton is difficult to isolate; rather, it is found bonded to an electron pair donor (carrier) molecule such as a water molecule. This is an example of a coordinate covalent bond. The hydronium ion and its effects on the solubilities of other compounds using Le Châtelier's principle will be described further in Chapter 10 of *MCAT General Chemistry Review*.

Because aqueous solutions are so common and so important to biological systems, the MCAT focuses on them above all others. In aqueous solutions, there are seven general solubility rules:

1. All salts containing ammonium (NH_4^+) and alkali metal (Group 1) cations are water-soluble.
2. All salts containing nitrate (NO_3^-) and acetate (CH_3COO^-) anions are water-soluble.
3. Halides (Cl^-, Br^-, I^-), excluding fluorides, are water-soluble, with the exceptions of those formed with Ag^+, Pb^{2+}, and Hg_2^{2+}.
4. All salts of the sulfate ion (SO_4^{2-}) are water-soluble, with the exceptions of those formed with Ca^{2+}, Sr^{2+}, Ba^{2+}, and Pb^{2+}.
5. All metal oxides are insoluble, with the exception of those formed with the alkali metals, ammonium, and CaO, SrO, and BaO, all of which hydrolyze to form solutions of the corresponding metal hydroxides.
6. All hydroxides are insoluble, with the exception of those formed with the alkali metals, ammonium, and Ca^{2+}, Sr^{2+}, and Ba^{2+}.
7. All carbonates (CO_3^{2-}), phosphates (PO_4^{3-}), sulfides (S^{2-}), and sulfites (SO_3^{2-}) are insoluble, with the exception of those formed with the alkali metals and ammonium.

MCAT EXPERTISE

Because most solutions in the real world involve water as the solvent, it is not a surprise that solutions are common on the MCAT. These solubility rules are not bad to know, but memorizing them all may be a little excessive. It is never a bad thing to know facts, but being able to apply them is more important. Know rules 1 and 2 for sure, and be aware of some of the more common insoluble exceptions, like Pb^{2+} and Ag^+.

The MCAT will not expect memorization of all of the solubility rules, but it is worth knowing two absolutes: all salts of Group 1 metals, and all nitrate salts are soluble. Otherwise, *familiarity* with rules listed above will suffice—the MCAT generally supplies solubility information for most compounds. Sodium and nitrate ions are generally used as counterions to what is actually chemically important; for example, if a pH problem gives a sodium formate concentration of 0.10 *M*, it is *really* indicating that the concentration of the formate ion is 0.10 *M* because the sodium ion concentration does not affect pH. The only time one needs to worry about the nitrate ion concentration is in an oxidation–reduction reaction, for the nitrate ion can function—although only weakly—as an oxidizing agent. In all other cases with nitrate ions, only focus on the cation as the chemically reacting species.

Complex Ion Formation

We have mentioned the hydronium ion as a complex that forms in acidic solutions, but it is worthwhile to mention that there are even more varied forms of complex ions that can appear in solution. By definition, a **complex ion**—or **coordination compound**—refers to a molecule in which a cation is bonded to at least one electron pair donor (which could include the water molecule). The electron pair donor molecules are called **ligands**. An example of such a **complexation reaction** is shown for the *tetraaquadioxouranyl* cation, which has water (*aqua–*) and oxygen (*oxo–*) ligands, in Figure 9.4.

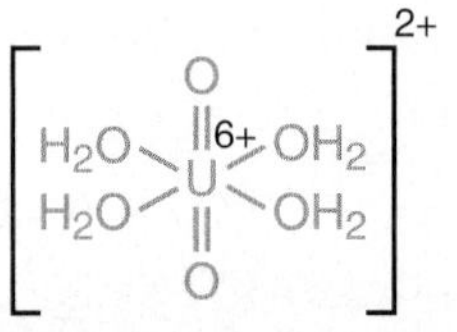

Figure 9.4 Structure of the Tetraaquadioxouranyl Complex Cation
Water and oxygen act as ligands with a U^{6+} cation.

Complexes are held together with **coordinate covalent bonds**, in which an electron pair donor (a Lewis base) and an electron pair acceptor (a Lewis acid) form very stable Lewis acid–base adducts. Most general chemistry courses do not stress the biological importance of coordination compounds. However, complex ions have profound biological applications in macromolecules such as proteins. For instance, many active sites of proteins utilize complex ion binding and transition metal complexes to carry out their function. One classic example is the iron cation in hemoglobin, which can carry oxygen, carbon dioxide, and carbon monoxide as ligands, as shown in Figure 9.5.

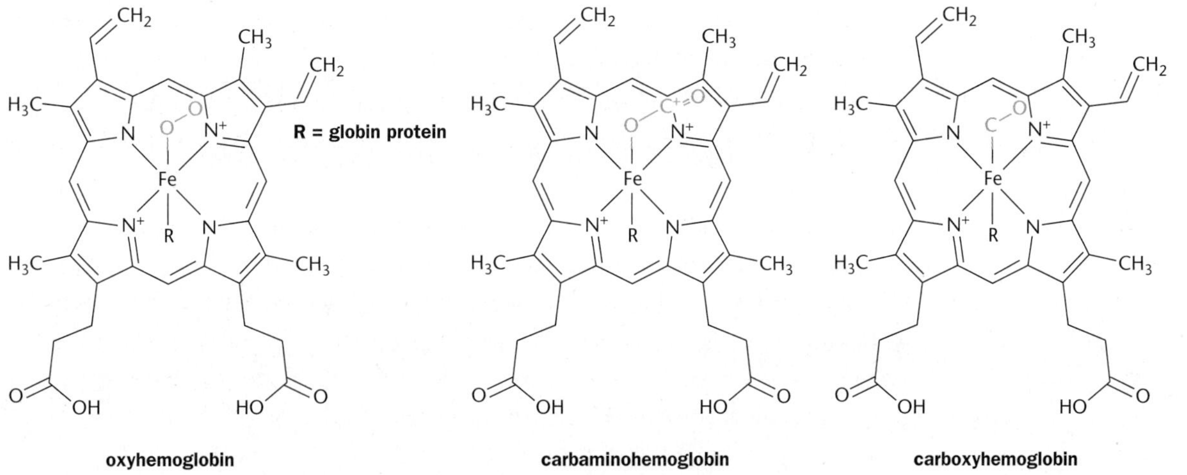

Figure 9.5 Hemoglobin Is a Classic Example of Biochemical Complex Formation
The iron in hemoglobin can bind various gases, leading to the formation of oxyhemoglobin (O_2), carbaminohemoglobin (CO_2), and carboxyhemoglobin (CO).

Many coenzymes (vitamins) and cofactors also contain complexes of transition metals, such as cobalamin (vitamin B_{12}), shown in Figure 9.6. The presence of a transition metal allows coenzymes and cofactors to bind other ligands or assist with electron transfer.

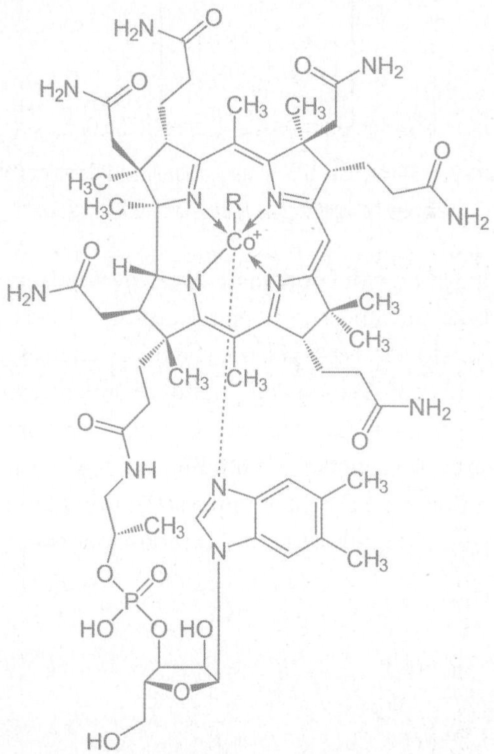

Figure 9.6 Cobalamin (Vitamin B_{12}) Contains a Cobalt Complex

Physical and chemical properties of complex ions are diverse, including a wide range of solubilities and varied chemical reactions. Inorganic complex ions are often fun to characterize because they tend to have vibrant, distinctive colors, as illustrated in Figure 9.7.

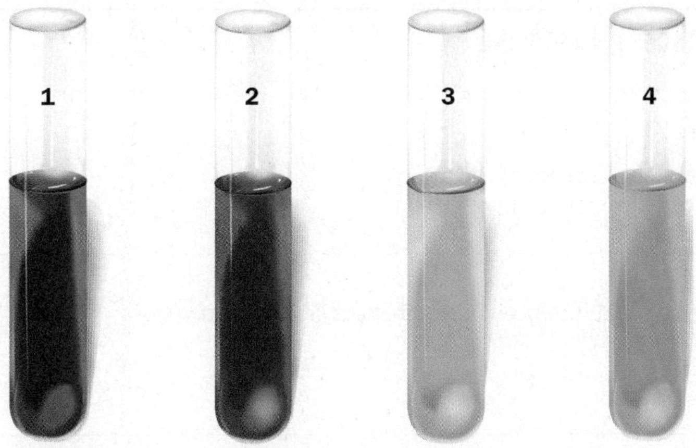

Figure 9.7 Nickel(II) Ion Complexes Display Distinctive Colors
The characteristic colors of Nickel (II) Ion complexes are, from left to right: 1) hexaamminenickel(II), 2) tris(ethylenediamine)nickel(II), 3) tetrachloronickelate(II), and 4) hexaaquanickel(II)

In some complexes, the central cation can be bonded to the same ligand in multiple places. This is called **chelation**, and it generally requires large organic ligands that can double back to form a second (or even third) bond with the central cation. Chelation therapy is often used to sequester toxic metals (lead, arsenic, mercury, and so on). Even biologically necessary metals, such as iron, can be toxic in overload states; an example of iron being chelated is shown in Figure 9.8.

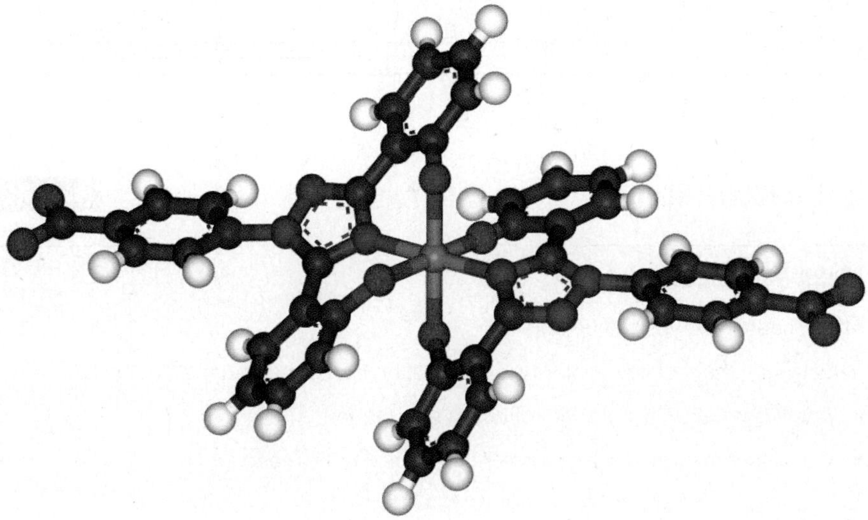

Figure 9.8 Chelation of Iron with Two Molecules of Deferasirox

MCAT CONCEPT CHECK 9.1

Before you move on, assess your understanding of the material with these questions.

1. Describe the process of solvation.

____

2. Describe the differences between solubility and saturation:

   •

____

   •

____

3. What is one way in which solubility of a compound can be increased?

____

4. Name two ions that form salts that are always soluble:

   •

____

   •

____

9.2 Concentration

High-Yield

LEARNING OBJECTIVES

After Chapter 9.2, you will be able to:

- Calculate the molality, molarity, or normality of a compound in solution
- Apply $M_iV_i = M_fV_f$ to calculate dilution of a solution
- Calculate mole fraction and percent composition by mass

Concentration denotes the amount of solute dissolved in a solvent. There are many different ways of expressing concentration, and different units have been standardized for specific everyday situations. For example, alcohol content in liquors like vodka, gin, or rum is expressed in volume percent (volume of solute divided by volume of solution times 100 percent). Alcoholic proof is twice the volume percent. The sugar content of orange juice and other fruit juices is measured in units of degrees Brix (°Bx), which is a mass percent: mass of glucose divided by mass of solution times 100 percent.

Units of Concentration

On the MCAT, concentrations are commonly expressed as percent composition by mass, mole fraction, molarity, molality, and normality.

MCAT EXPERTISE

It is important to have a good idea of how to work with all of these ways of expressing concentration because more than one may show up on Test Day.

Percent Composition by Mass

The **percent composition by mass** is given by the equation

$$\frac{\text{mass of solute}}{\text{mass of solution}} \times 100\%$$

Equation 9.1

Percent composition is used not only for aqueous solutions, but also for metal alloys and other solid-in-solid solutions.

Example: What is the percent composition by mass of a salt water solution if 100 g of the solution contains 20 g of NaCl?

Solution: $\frac{\text{mass of solute}}{\text{mass of solution}} \times 100\% = \frac{20\text{ g}}{100\text{ g}} \times 100\%$

$= 20\%$ NaCl solution

Mole Fraction

The **mole fraction** (X) of a compound is given by the equation

$$X_A = \frac{\text{moles of A}}{\text{total moles of all species}}$$

Equation 9.2

The sum of the mole fractions in a system will always equal 1. The mole fraction is used to calculate the vapor pressure depression of a solution, described later in this chapter, as well as the partial pressures of gases in a system, described in Chapter 8 of *MCAT General Chemistry Review*.

Example: If 184 g glycerol ($C_3H_8O_3$) is mixed with 180 g water, what will be the mole fractions of the two components? (Note: Molar mass of $H_2O = 18\ \frac{g}{mol}$; molar mass of $C_3H_8O_3 = 92\ \frac{g}{mol}$)

Solution: First, determine the number of moles of each compound:

$$180\text{ g water} \times \left[\frac{1\text{ mol}}{18\text{ g}}\right] = 10\text{ moles water}$$

$$184\text{ g glycerol} \times \left[\frac{1\text{ mol}}{92\text{ g}}\right] = 2\text{ moles glycerol}$$

$$\text{Total number of moles} = 10 + 2 = 12\text{ moles}$$

Then, determine the mole fractions:

$$X_{\text{water}} = \frac{10\text{ mol water}}{12\text{ mol total}} = \frac{5}{6} = 0.83$$

$$X_{\text{glycerol}} = \frac{2\text{ mol glycerol}}{12\text{ mol total}} = \frac{1}{6} = 0.17$$

Molarity

The **molarity** (*M*) of a solution is defined as

$$M = \frac{\text{moles of solute}}{\text{liters of solution}}$$

Equation 9.3

Solution concentrations are usually expressed in terms of molarity, and this is the most common unit for concentration on the MCAT. Unless otherwise specified, representations of concentration using brackets—such as $[Na^+]$—indicate molarity. Note that the volume term in the denominator of molarity refers to the solution volume, *not* the volume of solvent used to prepare the solution—although the two values are often close enough to approximate the solution volume using the solvent volume. Molarity is used for rate laws, the law of mass action, osmotic pressure, pH and pOH, and the Nernst equation.

MCAT EXPERTISE

Note that for dilute solutions, the volume of the solution is approximately equal to the volume of solvent used, which simplifies our calculations on Test Day. However, technical questions could ask you to distinguish between these two. For example, when you add two kilograms of sucrose (table sugar) to a liter of water at room temperature (achieving saturation), the volume of solution is certainly larger than 1 L!

Example: If enough water is added to 11 g of $CaCl_2$ to make 100 mL of solution, what is the molarity of the solution?

Solution: First, calculate the number of moles of $CaCl_2$:

$$11\text{ g CaCl}_2\left[\frac{1\text{ mol}}{111.1\text{ g}}\right]=0.1\text{ mol CaCl}_2$$

Then determine the molarity:

$$M=\frac{\text{moles of solute}}{\text{liters of solution}}$$

$$M=\frac{0.1\text{ mol}}{100\text{ mL}\times\frac{1\text{ L}}{1000\text{ mL}}}=\frac{0.1}{0.1}=1\ M$$

Molality

The **molality (*m*)** of a solution is defined as

$$m=\frac{\text{moles of solute}}{\text{kilograms of solvent}}$$

Equation 9.4

For dilute aqueous solutions at 25°C, the molality is approximately equal to molarity because the density of water at this temperature is 1 kilogram per liter. However, note that this is an approximation and true only for dilute aqueous solutions. As aqueous solutions become more concentrated with solute, their densities become significantly different from that of pure water; most water-soluble solutes have molar masses significantly greater than that of water, so the density of the solution increases as the concentration increases. You won't use molality very often, so be mindful of the special situations when it is required: boiling point elevation and freezing point depression.

Example: If 10 g NaOH are dissolved in 500 g of water, what is the molality of the solution?

Solution: First, calculate the number of moles of NaOH:

$$10\text{ g NaOH}\left[\frac{1\text{ mol}}{40\text{ g}}\right]=0.25\text{ mol NaOH}$$

Then determine the molality:

$$m=\frac{\text{moles of solute}}{\text{kilograms of solvent}}$$

$$m=\frac{0.25\text{ mol}}{500\text{ g}\times\frac{1\text{ kg}}{1000\text{ g}}}=\frac{0.25}{0.5}=0.5\ m$$

Normality

We discussed the related concepts of gram equivalent weight, equivalents, and normality in Chapter 4 of *MCAT General Chemistry Review*. The **normality** (***N***) of a solution is equal to the number of equivalents of interest per liter of solution. An equivalent is a measure of the reactive capacity of a molecule. Most simply, an equivalent is equal to a mole of the species of interest—protons, hydroxide ions, electrons, or ions.

MCAT EXPERTISE

Simple ideas on Test Day will make things easier. So, when you come across normality, think of it as *molarity of the stuff of interest* in the reaction.

To calculate the normality of a solution, we need to know what purpose the solution serves because it is the concentration of the reactive species with which we are concerned. For example, in acid–base reactions, we are most concerned with the concentration of hydrogen ions; in oxidation–reduction reactions, we are most concerned with the concentration of electrons. Normality is unique among concentration units in that it is reaction dependent. For example, in acidic solution, 1 mole of the permanganate ion (MnO_4^-) will readily accept 5 moles of electrons, so a 1 *M* solution would be 5 *N*. However, in alkaline solution, 1 mole of permanganate will accept only 1 mole of electrons, so in alkaline solution, a 1 *M* permanganate solution would be 1 *N*.

MCAT EXPERTISE

This equation is worthy of memorization. Note that a similar equation is used for the equivalence point in acid-base chemistry, as discussed in Chapter 10 of *MCAT General Chemistry Review*.

Dilution

A solution is diluted when solvent is added to a solution of higher concentration to produce a solution of lower concentration. The concentration of a solution after dilution can be determined using the equation

$$M_iV_i = M_fV_f$$

Equation 9.5

where *M* is molarity, *V* is volume, and the subscripts i and f refer to the initial and final values, respectively.

MCAT EXPERTISE

Though not a unique means of measuring concentration or dilution, the term "parts-per" can be used to indicate concentration of a dissolved substance in a solution (most commonly water). Parts-per-million (ppm, 10^{-6}) is the most common usage. If a problem states there is one ppm of substance X in water, that would indicate there is 1 mg/L of water, as there would be 1 millionth of a gram per gram of water, and the density of water is 1 g/mL. On Test Day, prior to converting from ppm, make sure to assess whether conversion to a different unit of measure is actually required, as this conversion can typically be avoided on the MCAT.

Example: A chemist wishes to prepare 300 mL of a 1.1 *M* NaOH solution from a 5.5 *M* NaOH stock solution. What volume of stock solution should be diluted with pure water to obtain the desired solution?

Solution:

$$M_iV_i = M_fV_f \rightarrow V_i = \frac{M_fV_f}{M_i}$$

$$V_i = \frac{(1.1\ M)(300\ \text{mL})}{(5.5\ M)} = \frac{300}{5} = 60\ \text{mL}$$

Note that one can use mL or L in the equation, as long as the units are consistent.

MCAT CONCEPT CHECK 9.2

Before you move on, assess your understanding of the material with these questions.

1. If you mix 180 g of the following compounds in 250 L of water $\left(\text{density} = 1\,\frac{\text{kg}}{\text{L}}\right)$, what are their concentrations in molality, molarity, and normality (for acid–base chemistry)?

Compound	Molality	Molarity	Normality
Glucose $\left(180\,\frac{\text{g}}{\text{mol}}\right)$			
Carbonate $\left(60\,\frac{\text{g}}{\text{mol}}\right)$			

2. You are working in a sewage treatment facility and are assaying chlorine in a water sample. You need to dilute the water sample from 100 ppm stock to 25 ppm and create 100 mL of solution. Calculate the amount of stock solution needed and determine how you would create your final solution:

____

____

____

3. A stock solution for making typical IV saline bags contains 90.0 g of NaCl per 10 liters of water $\left(\text{density} = 1\,\frac{\text{g}}{\text{mL}}\right)$. What is the mole fraction and the percent composition by mass of NaCl in the saline solutions?
   - Mole fraction:

____

   - Percent composition by mass:

____

9.3 Solution Equilibria

High-Yield

LEARNING OBJECTIVES

After Chapter 9.3, you will be able to:

- Calculate molar solubility for a compound given its K_{sp} and vice versa
- Calculate ion product for a solution
- Given K_{sp}, predict when a solute may dissociate or precipitate in order to reach equilibrium
- Predict the impact of a common ion on the dissolution of a compound

The process of solvation, like other reversible chemical and physical processes, tends toward an equilibrium position, defined as the lowest energy state of a system under a given set of temperature and pressure conditions. Systems move spontaneously toward the equilibrium position, and any movement away from equilibrium is nonspontaneous. In the process of creating a solution, the equilibrium is defined as the **saturation point**, where the solute concentration is at its maximum value for the given temperature and pressure. Immediately after solute has been introduced into a solvent, most of the change taking place is dissociation because no dissolved solute is initially present. However, once solute is dissolved, the reverse process—precipitation of the solute—will begin to occur.

When the solution is dilute (unsaturated), the thermodynamically favored process is dissolution, and initially, the rate of dissolution will be greater than the rate of precipitation. As the solution becomes more concentrated and approaches saturation, the rate of dissolution lessens, while the rate of precipitation increases. Eventually, the saturation point of the solution is reached. The solution now exists in a state of dynamic equilibrium for which the rates of dissolution and precipitation are equal, and the concentration of dissolved solute reaches a steady-state (constant) value. Neither dissolution nor precipitation is more thermodynamically favored at equilibrium because favoring either would necessarily result in the solution no longer being in a state of equilibrium. At this point, the change in free energy is zero, as is the case for all systems at equilibrium.

An ionic solid introduced into a polar solvent dissociates into its component ions, and the dissociation of such a solute in solution may be represented by

$$\mathrm{A}_m\mathrm{B}_n\,(s) \rightleftharpoons m\,\mathrm{A}^{n+}\,(aq) + n\,\mathrm{B}^{m-}\,(aq)$$

On Test Day, the first step for any solution stoichiometry or solution equilibrium question is to write out the balanced dissociation reaction for the ionic compound in question. This first step is essential for correctly calculating the solubility product constant, ion product, molar solubility, or for determining the outcome of the common ion effect. In other words, it is the essential first step for nearly every solution chemistry problem on the MCAT.

Solubility Product Constants

Most solubility problems on the MCAT deal with solutions of sparingly soluble salts, which are ionic compounds that have very low solubility in aqueous solutions. You may wonder why any ionic compound would not be highly soluble in water. The degree of solubility is determined by the relative changes in enthalpy and entropy associated with the dissolution of the ionic solute at a given temperature and pressure. One common sparingly soluble salt is silver chloride, AgCl, which dissociates in water according to the following equation:

$$AgCl\ (s) \rightleftharpoons Ag^{+}\ (aq) + Cl^{-}\ (aq)$$

The law of mass action can be applied to a solution at equilibrium; that is to say, when the solution is saturated and the solute concentration is at a maximum and is dynamically stable. For a saturated solution of an ionic compound with the formula A_mB_n, the equilibrium constant for its solubility in aqueous solution, called the **solubility product constant (K_{sp})**, can be expressed by:

$$K_{sp} = [A^{n+}]^m[B^{m-}]^n$$

Equation 9.6

where the concentrations of the ionic constituents are equilibrium (saturation) concentrations. For example, we can express the K_{sp} of silver chloride as:

$$K_{sp} = [Ag^{+}][Cl^{-}]$$

You'll notice that, for the law of mass action of solutions, there is no denominator. Remember that pure solids and liquids do not appear in the equilibrium constant. Because the silver chloride solution was formed by adding pure solid silver chloride to pure water, neither the solid silver chloride nor the water is included. Indeed, dissociation reactions—by definition—have a solid salt as a reactant; thus, K_{sp} expressions should never have denominators.

Solubility product constants, like all other equilibrium constants (K_{eq}, K_a, K_b, and K_w) are temperature dependent. When the solution consists of a gas dissolved into a liquid, the value of the equilibrium constant, and hence the position of equilibrium (saturation), will also depend on pressure. Generally speaking, the solubility product constant increases with increasing temperature for non-gas solutes and decreases for gas solutes. Higher pressures favor dissolution of gas solutes, and therefore the K_{sp} will be larger for gases at higher pressures than at lower ones.

As solute dissolves into the solvent, the system approaches saturation, at which point no more solute can be dissolved and any excess will precipitate to the bottom of the container. We may not know whether the solution has reached saturation, and so to determine where the system is with respect to the equilibrium position, we can calculate a value called the **ion product (*IP*)**, which is analogous to the reaction quotient, Q, for other chemical reactions. The ion product equation has the same form as the equation for the solubility product constant:

$$IP = [A^{n+}]^m[B^{m-}]^n$$

Equation 9.7

MCAT EXPERTISE

On the MCAT, if you remember that K_{sp} is just a specialized form of K_{eq}, then you can simplify a lot of problems by using the same concepts that you do for all equilibria, including Le Châtelier's principle.

REAL WORLD

Because gases become more soluble in solution as pressure increases, divers who have spent time at significant depths under water will have more nitrogen gas dissolved in their blood because nitrogen gas is the main inert gas in the air we breathe. If divers rise to the surface too quickly, the abrupt decompression will lead to an abrupt decrease in gas solubility in the plasma, resulting in the formation of nitrogen gas bubbles in the bloodstream. The gas bubbles can get lodged in the small vasculature of the peripheral tissue, mostly around the large joints of the body, causing pain and tissue damage (hence the name, the *bends*). The condition is painful and dangerous and can be fatal if not properly treated.

KEY CONCEPT

$IP < K_{sp}$: unsaturated, solute will continue to dissolve

$IP = K_{sp}$: saturated, solution is at equilibrium

$IP > K_{sp}$: supersaturated, precipitation will occur

The difference is that the concentrations used in the ion product equation are the concentrations of the ionic constituents at that given moment in time, which may differ from equilibrium concentrations. As with the reaction quotient *Q*, the utility of the ion product lies in comparing its value to that attained at equilibrium, K_{sp}. Each salt has its own distinct K_{sp} at a given temperature. If, at a given set of conditions, a salt's *IP* is less than the salt's K_{sp}, then the solution is not yet at equilibrium and is considered **unsaturated**. For unsaturated solutions, dissolution is thermodynamically favored over precipitation. If the *IP* is greater than the K_{sp}, then the solution is beyond equilibrium, and the solution is considered **supersaturated**. It is possible to create a supersaturated solution by dissolving solute into a hot solvent and then slowly cooling the solution. A supersaturated solution is thermodynamically unstable, and any disturbance to the solution, such as the addition of more solid solute or other solid particles, or further cooling of the solution, will cause spontaneous precipitation of the excess dissolved solute. If the calculated *IP* is equal to the known K_{sp}, then the solution is at equilibrium—the rates of dissolution and precipitation are equal—and the solution is considered **saturated**. The molarity of a solute in a saturated solution is called the **molar solubility** of that substance.

Example: The molar solubility of $Fe(OH)_3$ in an aqueous solution was determined to be $4 \times 10^{-10}\ \frac{mol}{L}$. What is the value of the K_{sp} for $Fe(OH)_3$ at the same temperature and pressure?

Solution: The molar solubility is given as 4×10^{-10} *M*. The equilibrium concentration of each ion can be determined from the molar solubility and the balanced dissociation reaction of $Fe(OH)_3$. The dissociation reaction is:

$$Fe(OH)_3\ (s) \rightleftharpoons Fe^{3+}\ (aq) + 3\ OH^-\ (aq)$$

$$K_{sp} = [Fe^{3+}][OH^-]^3$$

The molar solubility can be expressed as *x*, the amount of $Fe(OH)_3$ that dissolves to make a saturated solution at equilibrium. As it dissolves, $Fe(OH)_3$ dissociates to create *x* of Fe^{2+} and 3*x* of OH^-. This can be entered into the K_{sp} equation to give:

$$K_{sp} = [x][3x]^3$$

If the molar solubility *x* is 4×10^{-10} *M*, then $x = 4 \times 10^{-10}$ *M* $Fe(OH)_3$ has dissolved, yielding $x = 4 \times 10^{-10}$ *M* Fe^{3+} and $3x = 3 \times 4 \times 10^{-10}$ *M* OH^- (because there are three OH^- ions released per $Fe(OH)_3$ molecule dissolved). Thus,

$$K_{sp} = [Fe^{3+}][OH^-]^3$$

$$K_{sp} = (4 \times 10^{-10}\ M)(3 \times 4 \times 10^{-10}\ M)^3 = (4 \times 10^{-10}) \times \left[3^3 \times (4 \times 10^{-10})^3\right]$$

$$K_{sp} = 3^3 \times (4 \times 10^{-10})^4 = 27(4 \times 10^{-10})^4 = 27 \times 256 \times 10^{-40} \approx 30 \times 250 \times 10^{-40}$$

$$K_{sp} \approx 7500 \times 10^{-40} = 7.5 \times 10^{-37}\ (\text{actual} = 6.9 \times 10^{-37})$$

Example: What are the concentrations of each of the ions in a saturated solution of CuBr, given that the K_{sp} of CuBr is 6.27×10^{-9} at 25°C? If 3 g CuBr are dissolved in water to make 1 L of solution at 25°C, would the solution be saturated, unsaturated, or supersaturated?

Solution: The first step is to write out the dissociation reaction:

$$CuBr\ (s) \longrightarrow Cu^{+}\ (aq) + Br^{-}\ (aq)$$

$$K_{sp} = [Cu^{+}][Br^{-}]$$

Let x equal the molar solubility of CuBr, which is the amount of CuBr that dissolves at equilibrium. The concentration of Cu^{+} and Br^{-} will each equal x.

$$K_{sp} = x \cdot x = x^2$$

$$6.27 \times 10^{-9} = x^2$$

$$6.3 \times 10^{-9} \approx x^2$$

$$63 \times 10^{-10} \approx x^2 \approx 64 \times 10^{-10}$$

$$8 \times 10^{-5} \approx x \text{ (actual value} = 7.9 \times 10^{-5})$$

Therefore, $[Cu^{+}]$ is about 8×10^{-5} *M*, and $[Br^{-}]$ is also about 8×10^{-5} *M*. Note that 8×10^{-5} *M* also represents the molar solubility of copper(I) bromide.

Next, we convert 3 g of CuBr into moles:

$$3\text{ g} \times \frac{1\text{mol CuBr}}{143.5\text{ g}} \approx \frac{3}{150} \approx \frac{3}{1.5 \times 10^2} \approx 2 \times 10^{-2}\text{ mol}$$

2×10^{-2} mol CuBr in 1 L of solution represents a molarity of 2×10^{-2} *M*, which is more than 100 times higher than the molar solubility of CuBr. Therefore, this is a supersaturated solution.

KEY CONCEPT

Every sparingly soluble salt of general formula *MX* will have $K_{sp} = x^2$, where x is the molar solubility (assuming no common ion effect).

KEY CONCEPT

Every sparingly soluble salt of general formula MX_2 will have $K_{sp} = 4x^3$, where x is the molar solubility (assuming no common ion effect).

KEY CONCEPT

Every sparingly soluble salt of general formula MX_3 will have $K_{sp} = 27x^4$, where x is the molar solubility (assuming no common ion effect).

Finally, let's return to our discussion of complex ions and their solubility factors. Much like the examples we have seen previously, the solubility of complex ion solutions is determined by the K_{sp}. The formation of complex ions increases the solubility of a salt in solution.

For instance, consider free iron(III) (Fe^{3+}) in a solution of water. If a cyanide solution were added, an exceptionally stable iron and cyanide metal complex would form as the water molecules solvating the iron are replaced by excess cyanide ions:

$$Fe^{3+}(aq) + 6CN^{-}(aq) \rightleftharpoons [Fe(CN)_6]^{3-}(aq) \qquad K_f = 1.0 \times 10^{31}$$

Knowing the intricacies of why complexes are more stable in solution than isolated ions is beyond the scope of the MCAT; however, it should make sense that, if a complex ion contains multiple polar bonds between the ligands and the central metal ion, it should be able to engage in a very large amount of dipole–dipole interactions. This stabilizes the dissolution of the complex ion. The end result is that such complexes tend to have very high K_{sp} values.

When forming a complex ion, one must often use a mixture of solutions. For this reason, a distinction must be made between the K_{sp} of the solution and that of the complex ion itself. The dissolution of the original solution is termed K_{sp}, and the subsequent formation of the complex ion in solution is termed $\mathbf{K_f}$ (the **formation** or **stability constant** of the complex in solution). An example is shown below in which the diamminesilver(I) complex is formed in a silver chloride solution:

$$AgCl(s) \rightleftharpoons Ag^+(aq) + Cl^-(aq) \quad K_{sp} = 1.8 \times 10^{-10} = [Ag^+][Cl^-]$$

$$Ag^+(aq) + 2NH_3(aq) \rightleftharpoons [Ag(NH_3)_2]^+ \quad K_f = 1.6 \times 10^7 = \frac{[[Ag(NH_3)_2]^+]}{[Ag^+][NH_3]^2}$$

Notice that the formation constant (K_f) of the complex ion is significantly larger than the K_{sp} of the compound providing the metal ion. This is part of the explanation for why the initial dissolution of the metal ion is the rate-limiting step of complex ion formation. However, Le Châtelier's principle is at play in these reactions as well. Ultimately, complex ions form to become more soluble in solution. And as an amount of silver ion is being used up to form the complex ion itself, the dissociation reaction of AgCl shifts to the right, providing more silver for complex ion formation.

Example: A 0.1 mol sample of CuS is added to 1.00 L of 1.00 *M* NH_3. What is the final concentration of the complex ion, tetraamminecopper(II)?

$$CuS\ (s) \rightleftharpoons Cu^{2+}(aq) + S^{2-}\ (aq) \quad K_{sp} = 8 \times 10^{-37}$$

$$Cu^{2+}(aq) + 4\,NH_3\ (aq) \rightleftharpoons [Cu\,(NH_3)_4]^{2+}(aq) \quad K_f = 1.1 \times 10^{13}$$

Solution: First determine the amount of copper ion produced from copper sulfide (CuS) in solution. Comparison of the two equilibrium constants shows that the CuS dissociation has a K_{sp} of 8×10^{-37}, indicating that this reaction is unlikely to proceed as the forward reaction is not favorable. However, if the formation of the complex ion occurs simultaneously, the large K_f of 1.1×10^{13} for this process will drive the dissociation of CuS forward as the Cu^{2+} ions are consumed in the second reaction due to Le Châtlier's principle. Note that, even without quantitative analysis, the large value of K_f is a sign that the formation of the product of the second reaction will be highly favorable. In fact, if these two reactions are simultaneous, the CuS will ultimately be completely consumed due to this effect.

Thus, the amount of Cu^{2+} available to react is given by $[Cu^{2+}] = \frac{0.1\text{ mol}}{1.00\text{ L}} = 0.1\ M$. The reactions given show a 1:1 relationship between the Cu^{2+} available and the $[Cu(NH_3)_4]^{2+}$ that is generated. In other words, almost all of the Cu^{2+} ions will be used up to form the complex. Therefore, the concentration of the $[Cu(NH_3)_4]^{2+}$ complex ion is 0.1 *M*.

Common Ion Effect

The solubility of a substance varies depending on the temperature of the solution, the solvent, and in the case of a gas-phase solute, the pressure. Solubility is also affected by the addition of other substances to the solution. The effect of a complex ion increasing the solubility of a substance is not typical and is—in fact—opposite to the effect seen in many mixtures of solutions.

One of the more challenging solution chemistry problems on the MCAT is calculation of the equilibrium concentration of a salt in a solution that already contains one of the ions in that salt. The solubility of a salt is considerably reduced when it is dissolved in a solution that already contains one of its constituent ions as compared to its solubility in a pure solvent. This reduction in molar solubility is called the **common ion effect**. As described above, the molar solubility of a compound is its concentration (in moles per liter) at equilibrium at a given temperature. If X moles of A_mB_n (*s*) can be dissolved in one liter of solution to reach saturation, then the molar solubility of A_mB_n (*s*) is X molar.

Pay attention to the effect of the common ion: its presence results in a reduction in the molar solubility of the salt. Note, however, that the presence of the common ion has no effect on the value of the solubility product constant itself. For example, if a salt such as CaF_2 is dissolved into water already containing Ca^{2+} ions (from some other salt, perhaps $CaCl_2$), the solution will dissolve less CaF_2 than would an equal amount of pure water.

The common ion effect is really Le Châtelier's principle in action. Because the solution already contains one of the constituent ions from the products side of the dissociation equilibrium, the system will shift toward the left side, reforming the solid salt. As a result, molar solubility for the solid is reduced, and less of the solid dissolves in the solution—although the K_{sp} remains constant.

One can take advantage of the common ion effect to separate out specific compounds in a solution mixture. For example, in a solution of silver salts, one could add sodium or potassium chloride to preferentially precipitate silver(I) chloride. By adding an appropriate counterion in excess, the dissociation reaction shifts to the left, forming the solid salt.

Example: The K_{sp} of AgI in aqueous solution is 8.5×10^{-17}. If a 1×10^{-5} *M* solution of $AgNO_3$ is saturated with AgI, what will be the final concentration of the iodide ion?

Solution: The concentration of Ag^+ in the original $AgNO_3$ solution will be 1×10^{-5} *M* because $AgNO_3$ will fully dissociate (review the solubility rules from earlier in this chapter). Some small amount of AgI will dissociate into the solution, which is the molar solubility *x* of AgI under these conditions. The net silver concentration from both $AgNO_3$ and AgI will become $1 \times 10^{-5}\ M + x$. Because no iodide was present in solution until the AgI began dissociating, the concentration of iodide will be *x*. Thus, the K_{sp} expression for the dissociation of AgI can be written as:

$$K_{sp} = [Ag^+][I^-]$$
$$8.5 \times 10^{-17} = [1 \times 10^{-5}\ M + x][x]$$

Given that the value of K_{sp} for this reaction is 10^{-16}, only a minuscule amount of AgI will be dissociated. Thus, the value of *x* is sufficiently small to be negligible when added to 10^{-5}. The math simplifies to:

$$8.5 \times 10^{-17} = [1 \times 10^{-5}\ M][x]$$
$$8.5 \times 10^{-12} = x$$

This question asks for the concentration of iodide, which—based on the equilibrium expression—is represented by *x*. Thus, $[I^-] = 8.5 \times 10^{-12}\ M$.

MCAT CONCEPT CHECK 9.3

Before you move on, assess your understanding of the material with these questions.

1. Calculate the K_{sp} of $Ni(OH)_2$ in water, given that its molar solubility is $5.2 \times 10^{-6}\ M$.

2. The K_{sp} of $Ba(OH)_2$ is 5.0×10^{-3}. Assuming that barium hydroxide is the only salt added to form a solution, calculate the ion product of the following solutions based on the concentration of Ba^{2+}. Then, predict the behavior of the given solutions (dissolution, equilibrium, or precipitation):

$[Ba^{2+}]$	Ion Product	Behavior of Solution
0.5 *M*		
0.1 *M*		
0.05 *M*		

3. What is the molar solubility of $Zn(OH)_2$ ($K_{sp} = 4.1 \times 10^{-17}$) in a 0.1 *M* solution of NaOH?

9.4 Colligative Properties

LEARNING OBJECTIVES

After Chapter 9.4, you will be able to:

- Recall the names, equations, and applications of the common colligative properties
- Describe the relationship between molality and molarity for a compound
- Calculate the boiling point, freezing point, vapor pressure, or osmotic pressure of a solution

The **colligative properties** are physical properties of solutions that are dependent on the concentration of dissolved particles but not on the chemical identity of the dissolved particles. These properties—vapor pressure depression, boiling point elevation, freezing point depression, and osmotic pressure—are usually associated with dilute solutions.

Raoult's Law

Raoult's law accounts for **vapor pressure depression** caused by solutes in solution. As solute is added to a solvent, the vapor pressure of the solvent decreases proportionately. For example, consider compound A in Figure 9.9. Compound A in its pure form (mole fraction = 1.0) has a particular vapor pressure, indicated by P_A°. At the same temperature, compound B has a lower vapor pressure, indicated by P_B°. Note that, as the concentration of B increases, the vapor pressure of A decreases. Indeed, as more solute is dissolved into solvent (as more B is dissolved into A), the vapor pressure of the solvent decreases.

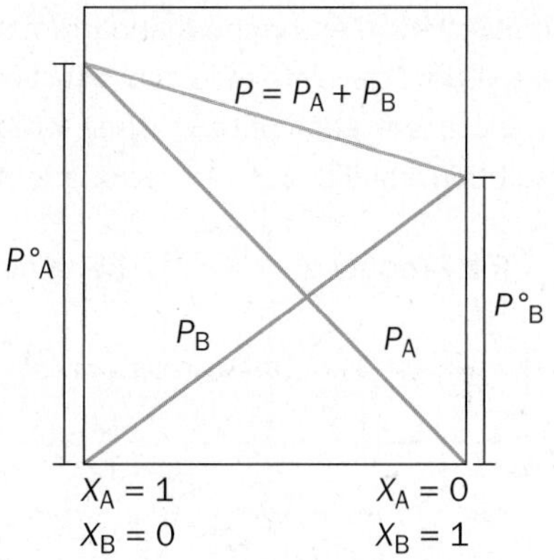

Figure 9.9 Raoult's Law

As more of solute B is dissolved in solvent A, the vapor pressure of solvent A decreases.

On a molecular level, the presence of the solute molecules can block the evaporation of solvent molecules but not their condensation. This reduces the vapor pressure of the solution compared to the pure solvent, as seen in Figure 9.10.

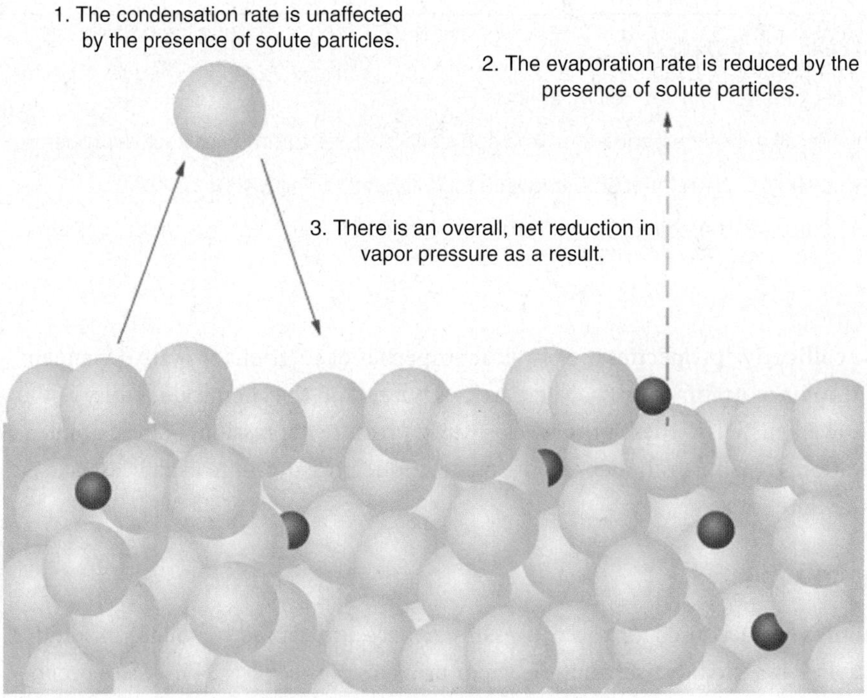

Figure 9.10 Molecular Basis of Raoult's Law

Raoult's law is expressed mathematically as:

$$P_A = X_A P_A^{\circ}$$

Equation 9.8

where P_A is the vapor pressure of solvent A when solutes are present, X_A is the mole fraction of the solvent A in the solution, and P_A° is the vapor pressure of solvent A in its pure state.

Raoult's law holds only when the attraction between the molecules of the different components of the mixture is equal to the attraction between the molecules of any one component in its pure state. When this condition does not hold, the relationship between mole fraction and vapor pressure will deviate from Raoult's law. Solutions that obey Raoult's law are called ideal solutions.

KEY CONCEPT

Vapor pressure depression goes hand in hand with boiling point elevation. The lowering of a solution's vapor pressure would mean that a higher temperature is required to match atmospheric pressure, thereby raising the boiling point.

Example: What is the change in vapor pressure when 180 grams of glyceraldehyde ($C_3H_6O_3$) are added to 0.18 L of water at 100°C?

Solution: The density of water at 100°C is close to $1\,\frac{\text{g}}{\text{mL}}$, and the vapor pressure of water at the same temperature is 1 atm because this is the boiling point of water.

In order to find the mole fraction of the solvent, first find the molar mass of the solute (glyceraldehyde) and solvent (water). 180 g glyceraldehyde represents 2 moles of glyceraldehyde. 0.18 L of water has a mass around 180 g, which represents 10 moles of water. The mole fraction of water is therefore $\frac{10\text{ mol water}}{12\text{ mol total}}=\frac{5}{6}=0.83$.

To find the vapor pressure change, we want to find the difference in the old pressure and the new pressure. The new pressure can be calculated from Raoult's law:

$$P_A = X_A P_A^\circ = (0.83)(1\text{ atm}) = 0.83\text{ atm.}$$

The change in vapor pressure is therefore 1 atm − 0.83 atm = 0.17 atm.

Example: What is the vapor pressure at room temperature of a mixture containing 58 g butane (C_4H_{10}) and 172 g hexane (C_6H_{14})? (Note: The vapor pressures of pure butane and pure hexane are 172 kPa and 17.6 kPa, respectively, at 25°C.)

Solution: First, determine the number of moles of each substance. 58 g butane represents 1 mole of butane. 172 g hexane represents 2 moles of hexane. Then, determine the mole fractions of each component of the mixture.

$$X_{\text{butane}} = \frac{\text{moles of butane}}{\text{total moles}} = \frac{1}{3}$$
$$X_{\text{hexane}} = \frac{\text{moles of hexane}}{\text{total moles}} = \frac{2}{3}$$

Then, calculate the vapor pressure of each component:

$$P^{\circ}_{\text{butane}} = X_{\text{butane}} P_{\text{butane}} = \frac{1}{3}(172\text{ kPa}) \approx \frac{1}{3}(180\text{ kPa}) = 60\text{ kPa}$$
$$P^{\circ}_{\text{hexane}} = X_{\text{hexane}} P_{\text{hexane}} = \frac{2}{3}(17.6\text{ kPa}) \approx \frac{2}{3}(18\text{ kPa}) = 12\text{ kPa}$$

The total vapor pressure is the sum of the two vapor pressures. Thus, the total vapor pressure is $60 + 12 = 72$ kPa (actual = 69.1 kPa).

Boiling Point Elevation

When a nonvolatile solute is dissolved into a solvent to create a solution, the boiling point of the solution will be greater than that of the pure solvent. The boiling point is the temperature at which the vapor pressure of the liquid equals the ambient (incident) pressure. We've just seen that adding solute to a solvent results in a decrease in the vapor pressure of the solvent in the solution. If the vapor pressure of a solution is lower than that of the pure solvent, then more energy (and consequently a higher temperature) will be required before its vapor pressure equals the ambient pressure. The extent to which the boiling point of a solution is raised relative to that of the pure solvent is given by the formula

$$\Delta T_{\text{b}} = iK_{\text{b}}m$$

Equation 9.9

where ΔT_{b} is the increase in boiling point, i is the van't Hoff factor, K_{b} is a proportionality constant characteristic of a particular solvent (which will be provided on Test Day), and m is the molality of the solution. The **van't Hoff factor** corresponds to the number of particles into which a compound dissociates in solution. For example, $i = 2$ for NaCl because each formula unit of sodium chloride dissociates into two particles—a sodium ion and a chloride ion—when it dissolves. Covalent molecules such as glucose do not readily dissociate in water and thus have i values of 1.

MCAT EXPERTISE

The boiling point elevation formula calculates the amount that the normal boiling point is raised. The value calculated is not the boiling point itself.

Example: 400 g $AlCl_3$ is dissolved in 1.5 L of water at room temperature $\left(K_b = 0.512\ \frac{K \cdot kg}{mol}\right)$. How much does the boiling point increase after adding the aluminum chloride?

Solution: Water at room temperature has a density of $1\ \frac{g}{mL}$. Therefore, 1.5 L is the same as 1.5 kg. The van't Hoff factor for aluminum chloride is 4 because it breaks down to form 1 aluminum cation and 3 chloride anions. To determine the molality, we will also need to know how many moles 400 g $AlCl_3$ represents.

$$400\ g\ AlCl_3 \times \frac{1\ mol}{133.5\ g} \approx 3\ mol\ AlCl_3$$

The molality is therefore $\frac{3\ mol\ AlCl_3}{1.5\ kg} = 2\ m$.

Then, plug into the boiling point elevation equation.

$$\Delta T_b = iK_b m = (4)\left(0.512\ \frac{K \cdot kg}{mol}\right)(2\ m) \approx 4\ K\ (\text{actual} = 4.1\ K)$$

Freezing Point Depression

The presence of solute particles in a solution interferes with the formation of the lattice arrangement of solvent molecules associated with the solid state. Thus, a greater amount of energy must be removed from the solution (resulting in a lower temperature) in order for the solution to solidify. For example, pure water freezes at 0°C, but for every mole of solute dissolved in 1 kg of water, the freezing point is lowered by 1.86°C. Therefore, the K_f for water is $1.86\ \frac{K \cdot kg}{mol}$. As is the case for K_b, the values for K_f are unique to each solvent and will be provided on Test Day. The formula for calculating the freezing point depression for a solution is

$$\Delta T_f = iK_f m$$

Equation 9.10

where ΔT_f is the freezing point depression, i is the van't Hoff factor, K_f is the proportionality constant characteristic of a particular solvent, and m is the molality of the solution. Freezing point depression is a colligative property and depends only on the concentration of particles, not on their identities.

Example: 400 g of $AlCl_3$ is dissolved in 1.5 L of water at room temperature $\left(K_f = 1.86\ \frac{K \cdot kg}{mol}\right)$. What is the new freezing point of this solution?

Solution: Using the same variables for i and m from the previous example,

$$\Delta T_f = iK_f m = (4)\left(1.86\ \frac{K \cdot kg}{mol}\right)(2\ m) \approx 15\ K(\text{actual} = 14.9\ K)$$

The normal freezing point of water is 273 K. The freezing point is going to be depressed (or decreased) by 15 K. The new freezing point is therefore $273 - 15 = 258\ K = -15°C$.

MCAT EXPERTISE

As with boiling point elevation, there is a distinction between the calculated value and a final answer. The freezing point depression calculates the amount that the normal freezing point is lowered. As always, read the question to determine if it is asking for the change in temperature (ΔT) or the new (altered) boiling or freezing point.

This effect is the explanation for why many people in colder climates salt icy roads in the winter. Salt mixes with the snow and ice and initially dissolves into the small amount of liquid water that is in equilibrium with the solid phase (the snow and ice). The solute in solution causes a disturbance to the equilibrium such that the rate of melting is unchanged (because the salt can't interact with the solid water that is stabilized in a rigid lattice arrangement), but the rate of freezing is decreased (the solute displaces some of the water molecules from the solid–liquid interface and prevents liquid water from entering into the solid phase).

This imbalance causes more ice to melt than water to freeze. Melting is an endothermic process, so heat is initially absorbed from the liquid solution, causing the solution temperature to fall below the ambient temperature. Now, there is a temperature gradient, and heat flows from the warmer air to the cooler aqueous solution; this additional heat facilitates more melting—even though the temperature of the solution is actually colder than it was before the solute was added! The more the ice melts into liquid water, the more the solute is dispersed through the liquid. The resulting salt solution, by virtue of the presence of the solute particles, has a lower freezing point than the pure water and remains in the liquid state even at temperatures that would normally cause pure water to freeze.

Osmotic Pressure

Osmotic pressure is covered primarily in Chapter 8 of *MCAT Biochemistry Review*, but a brief recap is provided here. **Osmotic pressure** refers to a "sucking" pressure generated by solutions in which water is drawn into a solution. Formally, the osmotic pressure is the amount of pressure that must be applied to counteract this attraction of water molecules for the solution. The equation for osmotic pressure is:

$$\Pi = iMRT$$

Equation 9.11

where Π is the osmotic pressure, i is the van't Hoff factor, M is the molarity of the solution, R is the ideal gas constant, and T is the temperature.

Water moves in the direction of higher solute concentration. For instance, pure water (no solute concentration) will traverse a semipermeable membrane to a solution containing solute particles (such as NaCl) and increase the level of the water as a result, as shown in Figure 9.11.

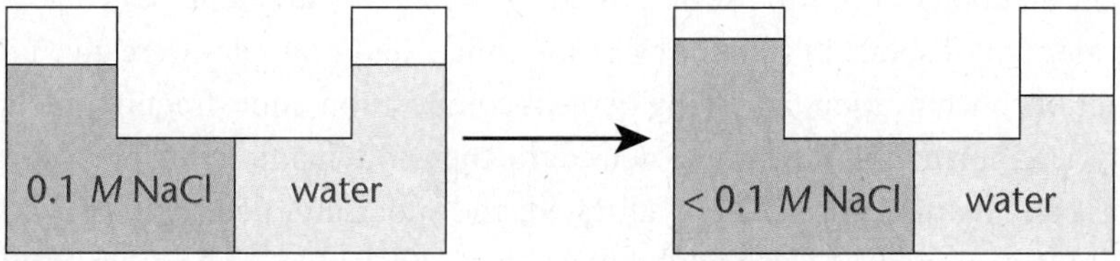

Figure 9.11 Change in Water Level Due to Osmotic Pressure

MCAT CONCEPT CHECK 9.4

Before you move on, assess your understanding of the material with these questions.

1. What is a colligative property?

____

2. How are molality and molarity related for water? How are they related for other solvents?
   - Water:

   ____

   - Other solvents:

   ____

3. Determine the vapor pressure of a solution containing 190 g $MgCl_2$ in 540 g water at room temperature: (Note: The vapor pressure of pure water at 25°C is 3.2 kPa.)

____

4. Determine the new boiling point of a solution containing 190 g $MgCl_2$ in 1500 g water at room temperature: $\left(K_b = 0.512\ \frac{K \cdot kg}{mol}\right)$

____

5. Determine the freezing point depression of a solution containing 58.5 g of NaCl in 1800 g of water at room temperature: $\left(K_f = 1.86\ \frac{K \cdot kg}{mol}\right)$

____

Conclusion

Our review of solution chemistry has provided an opportunity for us to consider the nature of solutions, solutes, and solvents, and the interactions between solutes and solvents in the formation of solutions. We reviewed solubility and the rules that reflect the solubility of common compounds in water. The different ways of expressing the amount of solute in solution were identified, and examples were given for each unit of concentration, including percent composition, mole fraction, molarity, molality, and normality. Next, we reviewed the thermodynamic principles of solution equilibria and defined unsaturated, saturated, and supersaturated solutions with respect to ion product (*IP*) and solubility product constant (K_{sp}). Subsequently, we discussed the common ion effect from the perspective of Le Châtelier's principle for a solution at equilibrium. And finally, we examined the colligative properties of solutions and the mathematics that govern them. The colligative properties—vapor pressure depression, boiling point elevation, freezing point depression, and osmotic pressure—are physical properties of solutions that depend on the concentration of dissolved particles but not on their chemical identities.

You've reviewed the content, now test your knowledge and critical thinking skills by completing a test-like passage set in your online resources!

GO ONLINE

CONCEPT SUMMARY

Nature of Solutions

- **Solutions** are homogeneous **mixtures** composed of two or more substances.
  - They combine to form a single phase, generally the liquid phase.
  - **Solvent** particles surround **solute** particles via electrostatic interactions in a process called **solvation** or **dissolution**.
  - **Aqueous solutions** are most important for the MCAT; solvation in water can also be called **hydration**.
  - Most dissolutions are endothermic, although the dissolution of gas into liquid is exothermic.
- **Solubility** is the maximum amount of a solute that can be dissolved in a given solvent at a given temperature; it is often expressed as **molar solubility**—the molarity of the solute at saturation.
- **Complex ions** or **coordination compounds** are composed of metallic ions bonded to various neutral compounds and anions, referred to as **ligands**.
  - Formation of **complex ions** increases the solubility of otherwise insoluble ions (the opposite of the common ion effect).
  - The process of forming a complex ion involves electron pair donors and electron pair acceptors such as those seen in **coordinate covalent bonding**.

Concentration

- There are many ways of expressing concentration.
  - **Percent composition by mass** (mass of solute per mass of solution times 100%) is used for aqueous solutions and solid-in-solid solutions.
  - The **mole fraction** (moles of solute per total moles) is used for calculating vapor pressure depression and partial pressures of gases in a system.
  - **Molarity** (moles of solute per liters of solution) is the most common unit for concentration and is used for rate laws, the law of mass action, osmotic pressure, pH and pOH, and the Nernst equation.
  - **Molality** (moles of solute per kilograms of solvent) is used for boiling point elevation and freezing point depression.
  - **Normality** (number of equivalents per liters of solution) is the molarity of the species of interest and is used for acid–base and oxidation–reduction reactions.

Solution Equilibria

- Saturated solutions are in equilibrium at that particular temperature.
- The **solubility product constant** (K_{sp}) is simply the equilibrium constant for a dissociation reaction.
- Comparison of the **ion product** (*IP*) to K_{sp} determines the level of saturation and behavior of the solution:
  - $IP < K_{sp}$: the solution is unsaturated, and if more solute is added, it will dissolve
  - $IP = K_{sp}$: the solution is saturated (at equilibrium), and there will be no change in concentrations
  - $IP > K_{sp}$: the solution is supersaturated, and a precipitate will form
- Formation of a complex ion in solution greatly increases solubility.
  - The **formation** or **stability constant** (K_f) is the equilibrium constant for complex formation. Its value is usually much greater than K_{sp}.
  - The formation of a complex increases the solubility of other salts containing the same ions because it uses up the products of those dissolution reactions, shifting the equilibrium to the right (the opposite of the common ion effect).
  - The **common ion effect** decreases the solubility of a compound in a solution that already contains one of the ions in the compound. The presence of that ion in solution shifts the dissolution reaction to the left, decreasing its dissociation.

Colligative Properties

- **Colligative properties** are physical properties of solutions that depend on the concentration of dissolved particles but not on their chemical identity.
- **Vapor pressure depression** follows **Raoult's law**.
  - The presence of other solutes decreases the evaporation rate of a solvent without affecting its condensation rate, thus decreasing its vapor pressure.
  - Vapor pressure depression also explains boiling point elevation—as the vapor pressure decreases, the temperature (energy) required to boil the liquid must be raised.
- **Freezing point depression** and **boiling point elevation** are shifts in the phase equilibria dependent on the molality of the solution.
- **Osmotic pressure** is primarily dependent on the molarity of the solution.
- For solutes that dissociate, the **van't Hoff factor** (*i*) is used in freezing point depression, boiling point elevation, and osmotic pressure calculations.

ANSWERS TO CONCEPT CHECKS

9.1

1. Solvation refers to the breaking of intermolecular forces between solute particles and between solvent particles, with formation of intermolecular forces between solute and solvent particles. In an aqueous solution, water is the solvent.
2. Solubility is the amount of solute contained in a solvent. Saturation refers to the maximum solubility of a compound at a given temperature; one cannot dissolve any more of the solute just by adding more at this temperature.
3. Solubility of solids can be increased by increasing temperature. Solubility of gases can be increased by decreasing temperature or increasing the partial pressure of the gas above the solvent (Henry's law).
4. Group I metals, ammonium, nitrate, and acetate salts are always soluble.

9.2

1.

Compound	Molality	Molarity	Normality
Glucose $\left(180\ \frac{\text{g}}{\text{mol}}\right)$	$\frac{1\text{ mol}}{250\text{ kg solvent}} = 0.004\ m$	$\frac{1\text{ mol}}{250\text{ L solution}} = 0.004\ m$	0.004 *N* (glucose does not dissociate)
Carbonate $\left(60\ \frac{\text{g}}{\text{mol}}\right)$	$\frac{3\text{ mol}}{250\text{ kg solvent}} = 0.012\ m$	$\frac{3\text{ mol}}{250\text{ L solution}} = 0.012\ m$	Approximately 0.024 *N* (twice the molarity)

Please note that the denominator for molality uses kilograms of *solvent*, whereas the denominator for molarity uses liters of *total solution*. These quantities are not necessarily the same and so you must be careful!

An example will help clarify the difference: Suppose 1 mol of solute were added to 1 L of water. 1 L of water has mass 1 kg, so you would simply use 1 kg solvent in the denominator of the molality computation, because molality's denominator is the mass of the solvent itself. However, when adding 1 mol solute to 1 L water, the volume of the final solution will likely be significantly larger than 1 L, because the solute itself takes up space. Therefore, you could not simply plug 1 L into the molarity equation, because molarity's denominator depends on the total volume of the final, mixed solution. Instead, you would need to remeasure the total, final volume, and use that number when computing molarity.

All that said, in the problem in the concept check, the initial volume of solvent is so large (250 L) that the added solute will not appreciably change the volume of final solution. Therefore, in this case, we were able to add 250 L directly into the molarity computation.

2. $M_iV_i = M_fV_f \rightarrow V_i = \frac{M_fV_f}{M_i} = \frac{(25\text{ ppm})(100\text{ mL})}{(100\text{ ppm})} = 25\text{ mL}$.

Thus, start with 25 mL of the stock solution and add 75 mL pure water to get 100 mL of solution with 25 ppm Cl_2.

3. $X_{NaCl} = \frac{\text{moles of NaCl}}{\text{total moles}} = \frac{90\text{ g}\left[\frac{1\text{ mol}}{58.5\text{ g}}\right]}{90\text{ g}\left[\frac{1\text{ mol}}{58.5\text{ g}}\right] + 10^4\text{ g}\left[\frac{1\text{ mol}}{18\text{ g}}\right]} \approx \frac{90\left(\frac{1}{60}\right)}{90\left(\frac{1}{60}\right) + 10^4\left(\frac{1}{20}\right)}$

$\approx \frac{1.5}{1.5 + 500} \approx \frac{1.5}{500} \approx \frac{1.5}{5 \times 10^2} \approx \frac{1}{3} \times 10^{-2} \approx 3 \times 10^{-3}\ (\text{actual} = 2.8 \times 10^{-3})$

Percent composition $= \frac{\text{mass of solute}}{\text{mass of solution}} \times 100\% = \frac{90\text{ g}}{90\text{ g} + 10^4\text{ g}} \times 100\% \approx$

$\frac{90}{10^4} \times 100\% = 0.9\%\ (\text{actual} = 0.89\%)$

9.3

1. First, write out the balanced equation: $Ni(OH)_2 \rightarrow Ni^{2+} + 2OH^-$

Next, identify that the molar solubility x represents the amount of $Ni(OH)_2$ that dissociates, creating x of Ni^{2+} and $2x$ of OH^-. Write out the K_{sp} equation, and plug in the values of x to solve for K_{sp}:

$K_{sp} = [Ni^{2+}][OH^-]^2 = x(2x)^2$

$K_{sp} = (5.2 \times 10^{-6})(2 \times 5.2 \times 10^{-6})^2$

$K_{sp} = (5 \times 10^{-6})(10 \times 10^{-6})^2 \approx (5 \times 10^{-6})(10^{-5})^2$

$K_{sp} \approx 5 \times 10^{-6} \times 10^{-10} = 5 \times 10^{-16}\ (\text{actual value} = 5.6 \times 10^{-16})$

2. Start with the balanced reaction and calculation for K_{sp}, which can also be used to calculate Q. Keep in mind that for every x of $Ba(OH)_2$ that dissolves, x of Ba^{2+} will be produced, and $2x$ of OH^-.

$Ba(OH)_2 \rightarrow Ba^{2+} + 2OH^-$

$K_{sp} = [Ba^{2+}][OH^-]^2$

$[Ba^{2+}]$	Ion Product	Behavior of Solution
0.5 M	$(0.5\ M)(1\ M)^2 = 0.5$	$0.5 > 5.0 \times 10^{-3} \rightarrow$ precipitation
0.1 M	$(0.1\ M)(0.2\ M)^2 = 4.0 \times 10^{-3}$	$4.0 \times 10^{-3} < 5.0 \times 10^{-3} \rightarrow$ dissolution
0.05 M	$(0.05\ M)(0.1\ M)^2 = 5.0 \times 10^{-4}$	$5.0 \times 10^{-4} < 5.0 \times 10^{-3} \rightarrow$ dissolution

Note that the concentration of hydroxide is double that of barium. While there will be a very small contribution of hydroxide from the autoionization of water, this amount is negligible compared to the values given in the question.

3. Start by writing the balanced reaction for the least soluble salt in the problem: $Zn(OH)_2 \rightarrow Zn^{2+} + 2\ OH^-$. Next, write out the K_{sp} equation and enter the variables for the concentrations. The Zn^{2+} concentration will equal x, the molar solubility under these conditions, but the OH^- concentration will come from two contributors: the dissociated $Zn(OH)_2$, and the 0.1 *M* NaOH solution. This results in the following K_{sp} expression: $K_{sp} = [Zn^{2+}][OH^-]^2 = (x)(0.1 + 2x)^2$. Since the K_{sp} for $Zn(OH)_2$ is 4.1×10^{-17}, x will be negligible compared to the 0.1 *M* from NaOH. The K_{sp} expression simplifies to: $K_{sp} = (x)(0.1)^2$. Thus, $4.1 \times 10^{-17} = 0.01x$. $x =$ molar solubility of $Zn(OH)_2 = 4.1 \times 10^{-15}$.

9.4

1. Colligative properties are those that depend on the amount of solute present, but not the actual identity of the solute particles. Examples include vapor pressure depression, boiling point elevation, freezing point depression, and osmotic pressure.
2. Molarity (*M*) and molality (*m*) are nearly equal at room temperature. This is only because 1 L solution is approximately equal to 1 kg solvent for dilute solutions (the denominators of the molarity and molality equations, respectively). For other solvents, molarity and molality differ significantly because their densities are not 1 $\frac{g}{mL}$ like water.
3. $190\ g\ MgCl_2 \times \frac{1\ mol}{95.3\ g} = 2\ mol\ MgCl_2$. $540\ g\ H_2O \times \frac{1\ mol}{18\ g} = 30\ mol\ H_2O$

$$X_{water} = \frac{30\ \text{moles water}}{32\ \text{total moles}}$$

$$P_{water} = X_{water} P^{\circ}_{water} = \frac{30\ \text{moles water}}{32\ \text{total moles}} \times (3.2\ kPa) = 3.0\ kPa$$

4. $T_b = iK_b m = (3)\left(0.512\ \frac{K \cdot kg}{mol}\right)\left(\frac{2\ mol\ MgCl_2}{1.5\ kg\ water}\right) \approx 2\ K\ (\text{actual} = 2.04\ K)$

The new boiling point will be $373 + 2 = 375$ K.

5. $\Delta T_f = iK_f m = (2)\left(1.86\ \frac{K \cdot kg}{mol}\right)\left(\frac{1\ mol\ NaCl}{1.8\ kg\ water}\right) \approx 2\ K\ (\text{actual} = 2.06\ K)$

SCIENCE MASTERY ASSESSMENT EXPLANATIONS

1. **A**

The equation $\Delta T_b = iK_b m$ can be used to solve this problem. The change in boiling point is 101.0 – 100 = 1.0°C. Then, plug that into:

$$\Delta T_b = iK_b m \rightarrow m = \frac{\Delta T_b}{iK_b} = \frac{1.0\text{ K}}{(1)\left(0.512\ \frac{\text{K}\cdot\text{kg}}{\text{mol}}\right)} \approx 2\ m$$

The van't Hoff factor for this solute is 1 because the molecule does not dissociate into smaller components. Then, convert to grams of solute using the definition of molality:

$$\text{molality} = \frac{\text{moles of solute}}{\text{kg of solvent}} \rightarrow \text{moles of solute}$$
$$= (2\,m)(0.1\text{ kg}) = 0.2\text{ mol.}$$

The mass used in this equation is 0.1 kg because 100 mL of water has a mass of 0.1 kg. Then, determine the molar mass:

$\text{molar mass} = \frac{70\text{ g}}{0.2\text{ mol}} = 350\ \frac{\text{g}}{\text{mol}}$, which is closest to **(A)**.

2. **D**

All three choices can make a solution as long as the two components create a mixture that is of uniform appearance (homogeneous). Hydrogen in platinum is an example of a gas in a solid. Brass and steel are examples of homogeneous mixtures of solids. The air we breathe is an example of a homogeneous mixture of gases; while these are more commonly referred to as mixtures, they still fit the criteria of a solution.

3. **B**

Benzene and toluene are both organic liquids and have very similar properties. They are both nonpolar and are almost exactly the same size. Raoult's law states that ideal solution behavior is observed when solute–solute, solvent–solvent, and solute–solvent interactions are all very similar. Therefore, benzene and toluene in solution will be predicted to behave as a nearly ideal solution.

4. **C**

Melting point depresses upon solute addition, making **(A)** and **(B)** incorrect. Solute particles interfere with lattice formation, the highly organized state in which solid molecules align themselves. Colder-than-normal conditions are necessary to create the solid structure.

5. **D**

The first step will most likely be endothermic because energy is required to break molecules apart. The second step is also endothermic because the intermolecular forces in the solvent must be overcome to allow incorporation of solute particles. The third step will most likely be exothermic because polar water molecules will interact with the dissolved ions, creating a stable solution and releasing energy.

6. **C**

BeF_2 will cause the most negative contribution to ΔS°_{soln} through the hydration effect because Be^{2+} cation has the highest charge density compared to the other ions. All of the other ions have a charge density of +1 or −1, whereas Be^{2+} has a charge density of magnitude two.

7. **B**

Formation of complex ions between silver ions and ammonia will cause more molecules of solid AgCl to dissociate. The equilibrium is driven toward dissociation because the Ag^+ ions are essentially being removed from solution when they complex with ammonia. This rationale is based upon Le Châtelier's principle, stating that when a chemical equilibrium experiences a change in concentration, the system will shift to counteract that change.

8. **B**

The mass percent of a solute equals the mass of the solute divided by the mass of the total solution times 100%. $\text{mass }\% = \frac{\text{mass of solute}}{\text{total mass of solution}} \times 100\%$. Plug in the values given for sucrose, the volume of water and the density of water to determine the % mass of sucrose:

$$\frac{(100\text{ g sucrose})}{(300\text{ mL }H_2O)(0.975\text{ g/mL}) + 100\text{ g sucrose}} \times 100\%$$
$$\approx \frac{100}{300+100} \times 100\% = \frac{100}{400} \times 100\% = 25\%$$

Keep in mind that in rounding while calculating, the denominator was estimated to be larger than the actual value, thus giving an answer that is slightly lower than the actual value. Thus, the correct answer is **(B)**, 25.5%. **(A)** results if rounding error is not taken into account. While these answers are very close, the mass of the water must be slightly *less* than 300 g, given the density value, so the percent composition of sucrose must be slightly *higher* than 25%. If the solute's mass is not added to the solvent's, the calculated value is 34.2%, which is **(D)**. **(C)** neglects both the addition step and the rounding error.

9. **A**

Mixtures that have a higher vapor pressure than predicted by Raoult's law have stronger solvent–solvent and solute–solute interactions than solvent–solute interactions. Therefore, particles do not want to stay in solution and more readily evaporate, creating a higher vapor pressure than an ideal solution. Two liquids that have different properties, like hexane (hydrophobic) and ethanol (hydrophilic, small) in **(A)**, would not have many interactions with each other and would cause positive deviation (i.e. higher vapor pressure). **(B)** and **(C)** are composed of liquids that are similar to one another and would not show significant deviation from Raoult's law. **(D)** contains two liquids that would interact very well with each other, which would actually cause a negative deviation from Raoult's law—when attracted to one other, solutes and solvents prefer to stay in liquid form and have a lower vapor pressure than predicted by Raoult's law.

10. **A**

Dissolution is governed by enthalpy and entropy, which are related by the equation $\Delta G^\circ_{soln} = \Delta H^\circ_{soln} - T\Delta S^\circ_{soln}$. The cooling of the solution indicates that heat is used up in this bond-breaking reaction. In other words, dissolution is endothermic, and ΔH is positive. The reaction is occurring spontaneously, so ΔG must be negative. The only way that a positive ΔH can result in a negative ΔG is if entropy, ΔS, is a large, positive value as in **(A)**. Conceptually, that means that the only way the solid can dissolve is if the increase in entropy is great enough to overcome the increase in enthalpy. **(B)** is incorrect because it is clearly stated in the question stem that KCl dissolves; further, all salts of Group 1 metals are soluble. **(C)** is incorrect because ΔS°_{soln} must be positive in order for KCl to dissolve. Finally, **(D)** is incorrect because solute dissolution would cause the boiling point to elevate, not depress. It is also not a piece of evidence that could be found simply by observing the beaker's temperature change.

11. **B**

The equation to determine the change in boiling point of a solution is as follows: $\Delta T_b = iK_b m$. m is the molality of the solution, and K_b is the boiling point elevation constant. In this case, the solvent is always water, so K_b will be the same for each solution. What is needed is the number of dissociated particles from each of the original species. This is referred to as the van't Hoff factor (i) and is multiplied by molality to give a normality (the concentration of the species of interest—in this case, all particles). The normality values determine which species causes the greatest change in boiling point.

Species	Number of Moles	Number of Dissolved Particles	$i \times m$ (Normality)
$CaSO_4$	0.4	2	0.8
$Fe(NO_3)_3$	0.5	4	2.0
CH_3COOH	1.0	Between 1 and 2 (acetic acid is a weak acid and a low percentage of the molecules will dissociate into 2 particles)	Between 1.0 and 2.0
$C_{12}H_{22}O_{11}$	1.0	1	1.0

The choice is between iron(III) nitrate and acetic acid. The fact that acetic acid is a weak acid indicates that only a few particles will dissociate into H^+ and acetate. Therefore, the normality of the acetic acid will be much closer to 1.0 than 2.0.

12. **B**

Osmotic pressure is given by the formula $\Pi = iMRT$. Entering the values from the question stem gives:

$$\Pi = \left(1000 \times 10^{-3}\,\text{mOsm/L}\right)(0.0812\ \text{L}\cdot\text{atm/mol}\cdot\text{K})(298\ \text{K})$$
$$\approx 1 \times 0.08 \times 300 = 24\ \text{atm}\ (\text{actual value} = 24.2\ \text{atm})$$

Notice that the concentration of seawater is given for all solutes, which represents $i \times M$. It is also given in mOsm/L, which is converted to moles per liter by multiplying by 10^{-3}. Also, the question asks for the minimum pressure required, which means that the correct answer choice must be slightly above the calculated pressure in order for reverse osmosis to proceed.

13. **B**

200 ppb of Pb^{2+} is equivalent to 200 grams of Pb^{2+} in 10^9 grams of solution; given the extremely low concentration of lead, the mass of the water can be assumed to be approximately 10^9 grams, as well. To solve, set up a dimensional analysis question. The units needed at the end are moles per liter (molarity), so convert from grams of lead to moles of lead and grams of water to liters of water:

$$\left[\frac{200 \text{ g Pb}^{2+}}{10^9 \text{ g H}_2\text{O}}\right]\left[\frac{10^3 \text{ g H}_2\text{O}}{1 \text{ L}}\right]\left[\frac{1 \text{ mol Pb}^{2+}}{207.2 \text{ g Pb}^{2+}}\right] \approx \frac{200\times10^3}{200\times10^9}$$

$$= 1\times10^{-6}\ M = 10\times10^{-7}\ M$$

$$\left(\text{actual value} = 9.67\times10^{-7}\ M\right)$$

Note that the denominator was rounded to a smaller number, meaning the estimated answer is slightly larger than the actual value.

14. **A**

This question is actually more complicated than it seems since hydroxide is involved. In aqueous solution, the concentration of hydroxide from the autoionization of water is 10^{-7} M. This concentration is significantly greater (approximately 10,000× greater) than the amount of hydroxide that would be produced by the dissociation of either salt. Thus, the concentration of hydroxide is set by water, not by the dissociation of cobalt(III) hydroxide and thallium(III) hydroxide. When the two solutions are mixed, the concentration of hydroxide does not change. However, in mixing the two solutions, the concentration of the metal ions decreases as a consequence of dilution. As a result, both solutions would be below saturation, justifying **(A)** as the correct answer.

15. **D**

The solubility of AgBr can be determined using the K_{sp} value given in the equation. Some amount of AgBr will dissolve; this is the molar solubility x for these conditions. When AgBr dissociates, there will be x amount of silver(I) formed and x amount of bromide—which is added to the 0.0010 M Br^- already present from NaBr.

$$\text{AgBr} \rightleftharpoons \text{Ag}^+ + \text{Br}^-$$

$$K_{sp} = \left[\text{Ag}^+\right]\left[\text{Br}^-\right]$$

$$5.35\times10^{-13} = (x)(0.0010\ M + x)$$

Given the K_{sp} of 5.4 × 10^{-13}, x will be negligible compared to 0.0010 M. Thus, the math can be simplified to:

$$5.35\times10^{-13} = (x)(0.0010)$$

$$x = \frac{5.35\times10^{-13}}{10^{-3}} = 5.35\times10^{-10}$$

Therefore, x, the molar solubility, is 5.35 × 10^{-10}, which looks like **(C)**. However, the units of the answer choices are grams per liter, not molarity, and the result must be multiplied by the molar mass $\left(187.8\ \frac{\text{g}}{\text{mol}}\right)$:

$$5.35\times10^{-10}\ \frac{\text{mol}}{\text{L}}\times187.8\ \frac{\text{g}}{\text{mol}} \approx 5\times10^{-10}\times200$$

$$= 1{,}000\times10^{-10} = 1\times10^{-7}$$

which is close to **(D)**. Note that a very accurate approximation was reached by rounding down the first number and rounding up the second, balancing the error.

Consult your online resources for additional practice. **GO ONLINE**

EQUATIONS TO REMEMBER

(9.1) **Percent composition by mass:** $\frac{\text{mass of solute}}{\text{mass of solution}} \times 100\%$

(9.2) **Mole fraction:** $X_A = \frac{\text{moles of A}}{\text{total moles of all species}}$

(9.3) **Molarity:** $M = \frac{\text{moles of solute}}{\text{liters of solution}}$

(9.4) **Molality:** $m = \frac{\text{moles of solute}}{\text{kilograms of solvent}}$

(9.5) **Dilution formula:** $M_iV_i = M_fV_f$

(9.6) **Solubility product constant:** $K_{sp} = [A^{n+}]^m[B^{m-}]^n$

(9.7) **Ion product:** $IP = [A^{n+}]^m[B^{m-}]^n$

(9.8) **Raoult's law (vapor pressure depression):** $P_A = X_AP_A^\circ$

(9.9) **Boiling point elevation:** $\Delta T_b = iK_bm$

(9.10) **Freezing point depression:** $\Delta T_f = iK_fm$

(9.11) **Osmotic pressure:** $\Pi = iMRT$

SHARED CONCEPTS

Biology Chapter 10
Homeostasis

General Chemistry Chapter 3
Bonding and Chemical Interactions

General Chemistry Chapter 6
Equilibrium

General Chemistry Chapter 7
Thermochemistry

General Chemistry Chapter 10
Acids and Bases

General Chemistry Chapter 12
Electrochemistry

CHAPTER 10

ACIDS AND BASES

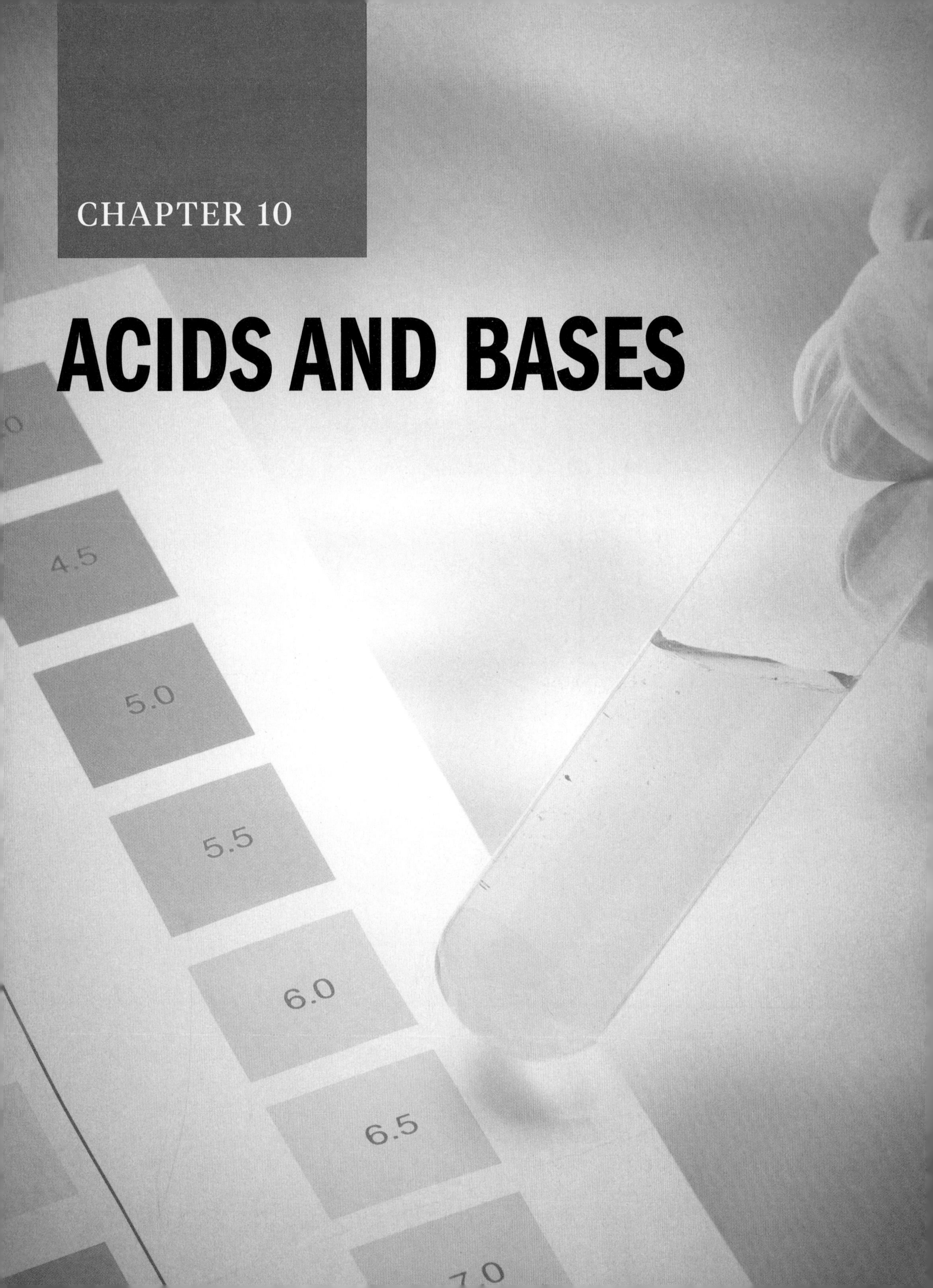

SCIENCE MASTERY ASSESSMENT

Every pre-med knows this feeling: there is so much content I have to know for the MCAT! How do I know what to do first or what's important?

While the high-yield badges throughout this book will help you identify the most important topics, this Science Mastery Assessment is another tool in your MCAT prep arsenal. This quiz (which can also be taken in your online resources) and the guidance below will help ensure that you are spending the appropriate amount of time on this chapter based on your personal strengths and weaknesses. Don't worry though—skipping something now does not mean you'll never study it. Later on in your prep, as you complete full-length tests, you'll uncover specific pieces of content that you need to review and can come back to these chapters as appropriate.

How to Use This Assessment

If you answer 0–7 questions correctly:

Spend about 1 hour to read this chapter in full and take limited notes throughout. Follow up by reviewing **all** quiz questions to ensure that you now understand how to solve each one.

If you answer 8–11 questions correctly:

Spend 20–40 minutes reviewing the quiz questions. Beginning with the questions you missed, read and take notes on the corresponding subchapters. For questions you answered correctly, ensure your thinking matches that of the explanation and you understand why each choice was correct or incorrect.

If you answer 12–15 questions correctly:

Spend less than 20 minutes reviewing all questions from the quiz. If you missed any, then include a quick read-through of the corresponding subchapters, or even just the relevant content within a subchapter, as part of your question review. For questions you answered correctly, ensure your thinking matches that of the explanation and review the Concept Summary at the end of the chapter.

1. Which of the following is not a Brønsted–Lowry base?
   - A. 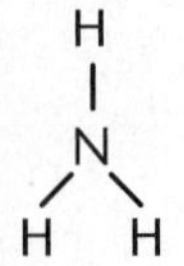
   - B. F^-
   - C. 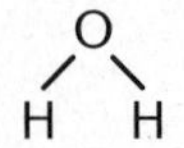
   - D. H—O—N=O

2. Which of the following is closest to the pH of a solution containing 5 m*M* H_2SO_4?
   - A. 1
   - B. 2
   - C. 3
   - D. 4

3. Which of the following represents chloric acid?
   - A. $HClO_3$
   - B. ClO_3^-
   - C. $HClO_2$
   - D. HClO

4. Which of the following bases is the weakest?
   - A. KOH
   - B. NH_3
   - C. CH_3NH_2
   - D. $Ca(OH)_2$

5. What is the gram equivalent weight of phosphoric acid?
   - A. 32 g
   - B. 49 g
   - C. 98 g
   - D. 294 g

6. What is the pH of a solution with an ammonium concentration of 70 m*M* and an ammonia concentration of 712 m*M*? (Note: The pK_b of ammonia is 3.45.)
   - A. 2.45
   - B. 4.45
   - C. 9.55
   - D. 11.55

Questions 7–9 refer to the titration curve of acid X shown below:

Titration Curve of Weak Acid X

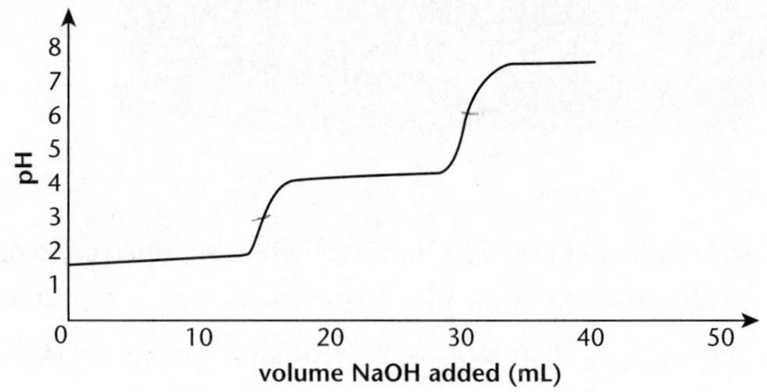

7. What is the approximate value of pK_{a1}?
   - A. 1.9
   - B. 2.9
   - C. 3.8
   - D. 4.1

8. At what pH is the second equivalence point?
   - A. pH = 3.0
   - B. pH = 4.1
   - C. pH = 5.9
   - D. pH = 7.2

9. What is the approximate value of pK_{a2}?
   - A. 3.6
   - B. 4.1
   - C. 5.5
   - D. 7.2

10. What is the gram equivalent weight of phosphoric acid?
    - A. 24.5 g
    - B. 32.7 g
    - C. 49.0 g
    - D. 98.0 g

11. What is the $[H_3O^+]$ of a 2 *M* aqueous solution of a weak acid HXO_2 with $K_a = 3.2 \times 10^{-5}$?
    - A. 6.4×10^{-5} *M*
    - B. 1.3×10^{-4} *M*
    - C. 4.0×10^{-3} *M*
    - D. 8.0×10^{-3} *M*

12. A solution is prepared with an unknown concentration of a theoretical compound with a K_a of exactly 1.0. What is the pH of this solution?
    - A. Higher than 7
    - B. Exactly 7
    - C. Less than 7
    - D. There is not enough information to answer the question.

13. Which of the following is NOT a characteristic of an amphoteric species?
    - A. Amphoteric species can act as an acid or a base, depending on its environment.
    - B. Amphoteric species can act as an oxidizing or reducing agent, depending on its environment.
    - C. Amphoteric species are sometimes amphiprotic.
    - D. Amphoteric species are always nonpolar.

14. What is the approximate pH of a 1.2×10^{-5} *M* aqueous solution of NaOH?
    - A. 4.92
    - B. 7.50
    - C. 9.08
    - D. 12.45

15. How many liters of 2 *M* $Ba(OH)_2$ are needed to titrate a 4 L solution of 6 *M* H_3PO_4?
    - A. 1.33 L
    - B. 12 L
    - C. 18 L
    - D. 56 L

Answer Key

1. **D**
2. **B**
3. **A**
4. **B**
5. **A**
6. **D**
7. **A**
8. **C**
9. **B**
10. **B**
11. **D**
12. **C**
13. **D**
14. **C**
15. **C**

Detailed explanations can be found at the end of the chapter.

CHAPTER 10

ACIDS AND BASES

In This Chapter

CHAPTER PROFILE

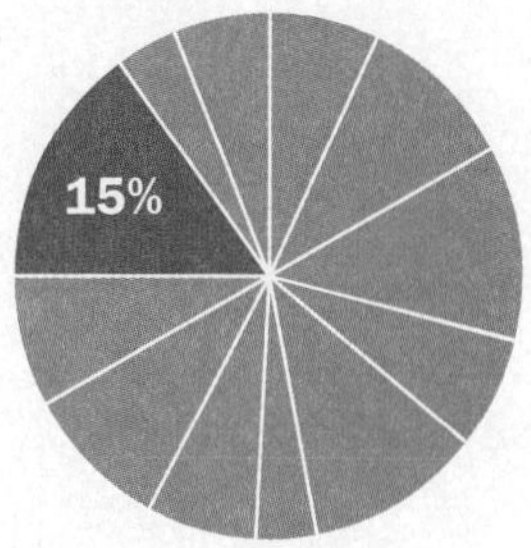

The content in this chapter should be relevant to about 15% of all questions about general chemistry on the MCAT.

This chapter covers material from the following AAMC content categories:

4D: How light and sound interact with matter

5A: Unique nature of water and its solutions

Introduction

Some medications can be applied as drops, salves, or creams to mucous membranes. Others are injected. Some employ a transdermal patch, while others are swallowed or inhaled. The route of administration of a drug compound is related to both the location of its target tissue (local or systemic), as well as the chemical and physical properties of the compound. For example, compounds that are water-soluble can be administered intravenously (an aqueous solution dripped directly into the bloodstream), while those that are lipid-soluble can be administered transcutaneously (via a patch or a cream) or orally (in a pill or liquid suspension). The polarity, size, and charge of the drug compound will determine its solubility in polar or nonpolar environments and will be major contributing factors in determining the most effective and efficient route of administration.

Whether a drug compound has an ionic charge is usually a function of the acidic or basic nature of the compound. For example, a basic organic compound that is insoluble in water when neutral can be reacted with an acid to form a salt; because this salt is ionic, it is water-soluble. Correspondingly, an acidic organic compound that is insoluble in water when neutral can be reacted with a base to form a water-soluble salt. On the other hand, the protonated (acidic cationic) form of an organic compound can be reacted with a base to neutralize the compound and release it from its salt, changing (and usually reversing) its solubility in water.

Medical professionals aren't the only ones concerned about drug solubilities and routes of administration—there's a science to illicit drugs, too. One of the clearest examples of this is the difference between the two major forms of cocaine, a large alkaloid compound derived from the coca plant. Most commonly, the alkaloid compound is reacted with hydrochloric acid (which protonates its tertiary amine functional group), extracted with water, and dried to a water-soluble powder (cocaine hydrochloride); this powder either is snorted (insufflated) into the nasal cavity, where it is absorbed into the capillary beds, or is injected directly into the venous circulation. The second form of cocaine, the salt form, has a very high boiling point, which is close to the temperature at which cocaine degrades, and cannot be smoked. To produce a vaporizable form of cocaine that can be inhaled from a pipe, the cocaine hydrochloride must be reacted with a base, typically either ammonia (to produce pure freebase cocaine) or sodium bicarbonate (to produce crack cocaine, which is less pure). The base reacts with the protonated tertiary amine, removing the hydrogen ion to reform the neutral alkaloid compound. The freebase cocaine is water-insoluble and usually extracted with ether, or it is left in the aqueous solution, which is heated and evaporated. The freebase and crack forms of cocaine have much lower boiling points; consequently, they can be smoked without risk of degradation.

In this chapter, our focus will be on those two classes of compounds—acids and bases—which are involved in so many important reactions. Acid–base reactions are an important topic for the MCAT; in fact, neutralization reactions are some of the most commonly tested reaction types on Test Day. We will begin with a review of the different definitions of acids and bases and their properties, including their characterization as either strong or weak. Focusing on weak acids and bases, we will discuss the significance of the equilibrium constants K_a and K_b for acids and bases, respectively. Finally, we will review acid–base titrations and buffer systems.

10.1 Definitions

LEARNING OBJECTIVES

After Chapter 10.1, you will be able to:

- Compare and contrast the Arrhenius, Brønsted–Lowry, and Lewis definitions for acids and bases
- Predict the acid formula and name for an anion using Arrhenius acid naming trends
- Identify amphoteric species, and determine whether they are amphiprotic as well

Over the last century, chemists have used different definitions to identify compounds as acids or bases. Three definitions emerged, with each more inclusive than the former one.

Arrhenius

The first and most specific definition of an acid or base is the Arrhenius definition. An **Arrhenius acid** will dissociate to form an excess of H^+ in solution, and an **Arrhenius base** will dissociate to form an excess of OH^- in solution. These behaviors are generally limited to aqueous acids and bases. Arrhenius acids and bases are easily identified; acids contain H at the beginning of their formula (HCl, HNO_3, H_2SO_4, and so on) and bases contain OH at the end of their formula (NaOH, $Ca(OH)_2$, $Fe(OH)_3$, and so on).

MCAT EXPERTISE

Any mention of the Arrhenius definition on Test Day will likely be in comparison to other definitions of acids. The Arrhenius definition is by far the most restrictive; the Brønsted-Lowry and Lewis definitions predominate on the MCAT.

Brønsted-Lowry

A more inclusive definition of acids and bases was proposed independently by Johannes Brønsted and Thomas Lowry in 1923. A **Brønsted–Lowry acid** is a species that donates hydrogen ions (H^+), while a **Brønsted–Lowry base** is a species that accepts them.

The advantage of this definition over Arrhenius's is that it is not limited to aqueous solutions. For example, OH^-, NH_3, and F^- are all Brønsted–Lowry bases because each has the ability to accept a hydrogen ion. However, neither NH_3 nor F^- can be classified as Arrhenius bases because they do not dissociate to produce an excess of OH^- ions in aqueous solutions. According to both of these definitions, there is only one way for a species to be an acid: producing hydrogen ions. The only differences between the two definitions for acids are the requirement of an aqueous medium in the Arrhenius definition and the acidity of water. In the Arrhenius definition, water is not considered an acid—it does not produce an excess of H^+ in solution. Water is, on the other hand, a Brønsted–Lowry acid because it is able to donate a proton to other species. Most acid–base chemistry reactions on the MCAT will involve the transfer of hydrogen ions in accordance with the Brønsted–Lowry definitions.

MCAT EXPERTISE

Every Arrhenius acid (or base) can also be classified as a Brønsted-Lowry acid (or base). Every Brønsted-Lowry acid (or base) can also be classified as a Lewis acid (or base). This logic does not always work the other way (for example, NH_3 is a Brønsted-Lowry base, but not an Arrhenius base).

Brønsted–Lowry acids and bases always occur in pairs because the definitions require the transfer of a proton from the acid to the base. These are **conjugate acid–base pairs**, as described in the next section. For example, in the autoionization of water, H_3O^+ is the conjugate acid and OH^- is the conjugate base, as shown in Figure 10.1.

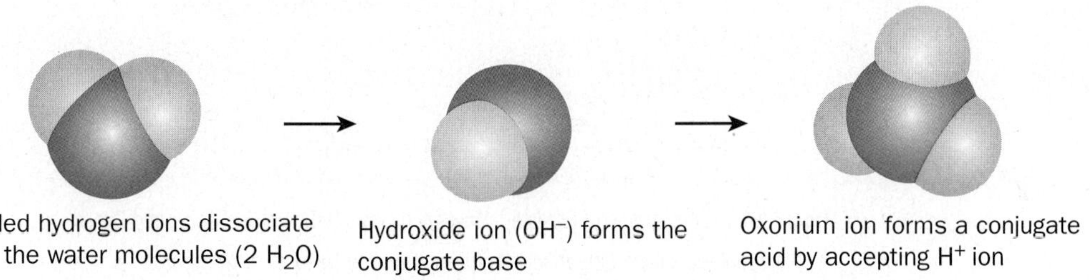

Figure 10.1 Autoionization of Water into Its Conjugate Acid and Conjugate Base
The hydroxide ion is the conjugate base; the oxonium (hydronium) ion is the conjugate acid.

$$H_2O\ (l) + H_2O\ (l) \leftrightharpoons H_3O^+\ (aq) + OH^-\ (aq)$$

Lewis

At approximately the same time as Brønsted and Lowry's publications, Gilbert Lewis also proposed a definition for acids and bases. A **Lewis acid** is defined as an electron pair acceptor, and a **Lewis base** is defined as an electron pair donor, as shown in Figure 10.2. The electron pair being donated is a lone pair and is not involved in any other bonds.

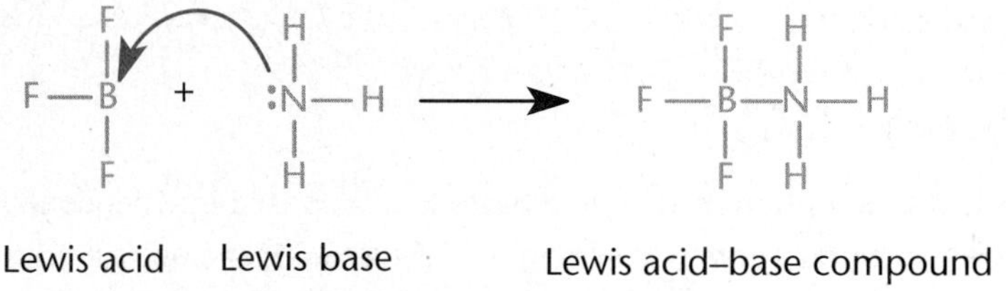

Figure 10.2 Lewis Acid-Base Chemistry
Boron trifluoride serves as the Lewis acid, accepting a lone pair. Ammonia serves as a Lewis base, donating a lone pair.

MNEMONIC

The Br**ø**nsted-L**o**wry definition revolves around pr**o**t**o**ns; the **L**ewis definition around **e**lectrons.

On the MCAT, Lewis acid–base chemistry appears with many names. The underlying idea is that one species pushes a lone pair to form a bond with another. This same chemistry can be called coordinate covalent bond formation (discussed in Chapter 3 of *MCAT General Chemistry Review*), complex ion formation (discussed in Chapter 9 of *MCAT General Chemistry Review*), or nucleophile–electrophile interactions (discussed in Chapter 4 of *MCAT Organic Chemistry Review*).

There is an intuitive approach to understanding the differences in the definitions we have discussed so far. The Lewis definition relies on a behavior that is not vastly different from the Brønsted–Lowry interactions—the only difference is the focus. For Brønsted–Lowry acids and bases, we follow the exchange of the hydrogen ion (H^+), which is essentially a naked proton. In the Lewis definition, the focus of the reaction is no longer on the proton, but instead the electrons forming the coordinate covalent bond. This difference can be seen using curved arrows, as shown in Figure 10.3.

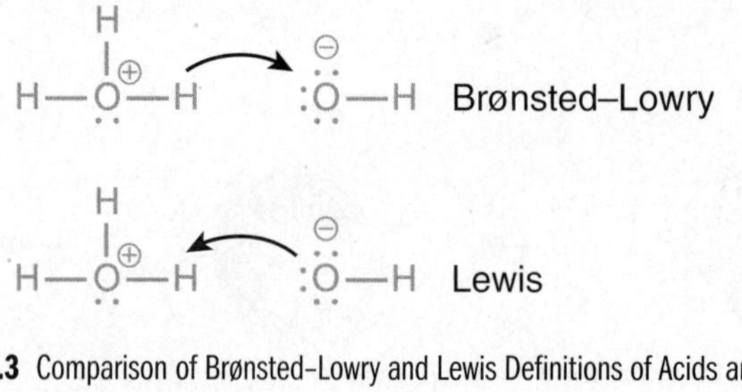

Figure 10.3 Comparison of Brønsted-Lowry and Lewis Definitions of Acids and Bases
In the Brønsted-Lowry definition, the focus is on the transfer of the proton. In the Lewis definition, the focus is on the attack of the Lewis acid (electrophile) by the lone pair of the Lewis base (nucleophile).

Note that the Lewis definition is the most inclusive: every Arrhenius acid is also a Brønsted–Lowry acid, and every Brønsted–Lowry acid is also a Lewis acid (and likewise for bases). However, the converse is not necessarily true. The Lewis definition encompasses some species not included within the Brønsted–Lowry definition; for example, BF_3 and $AlCl_3$ are species that can each accept an electron pair, which qualifies them as Lewis acids, but they lack a hydrogen ion to donate, disqualifying them as both Arrhenius and Brønsted–Lowry acids.

On the MCAT, you may encounter Lewis acids in the context of organic chemistry reactions because Lewis acids are often used as catalysts.

Amphoteric Species

An **amphoteric** species is one that reacts like an acid in a basic environment and like a base in an acidic environment. In the Brønsted–Lowry sense, an amphoteric species can either gain or lose a proton, making it **amphiprotic** as well. On the MCAT, water is the most common example. When water reacts with a base, it behaves as an acid:

$$H_2O + B^- \rightleftharpoons HB + OH^-$$

When water reacts with an acid, it behaves as a base:

$$HA + H_2O \rightleftharpoons H_3O^+ + A^-$$

The partially dissociated conjugate base of a polyvalent acid is usually amphoteric. For example, HSO_4^- can either gain a proton to form H_2SO_4 or lose a proton to form SO_4^{2-}. The hydroxides of certain metals (such as Al, Zn, Pb, and Cr) are also amphoteric. Furthermore, species that can act as both oxidizing and reducing agents are often considered to be amphoteric as well because by accepting or donating electron pairs, they act as Lewis acids or bases, respectively.

Complex amphoteric molecules include amino acids that have a *zwitterion* intermediate with both cationic and anionic character, as shown in Figure 10.4. Such species are discussed in great detail in Chapter 1 of *MCAT Biochemistry Review*.

KEY CONCEPT

Water, amino acids, and partially deprotonated polyprotic acids such as bicarbonate and bisulfate are common examples of amphoteric and amphiprotic substances. Metal oxides and hydroxides are also considered amphoteric but not necessarily amphiprotic because they do not give off protons.

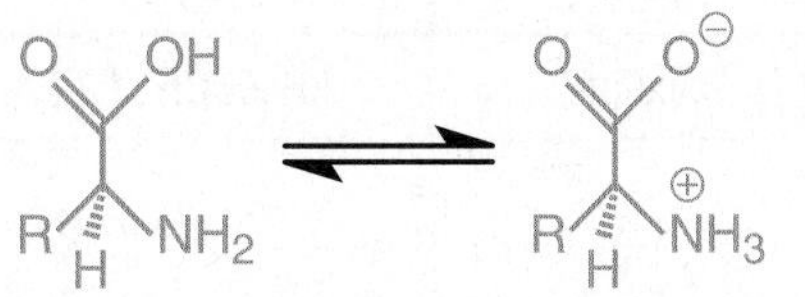

Figure 10.4 Amino Acid Zwitterions Are Complex Amphoteric Species
The amino group can release a proton (acid) and the carboxylate group can accept a proton (base).

Acid-Base Nomenclature

The names of most acids are related to the names of their parent anions (the anion that combines with H^+ to form the acid). Acids formed from anions with names that end in *–ide* have the prefix ***hydro*–** and the ending ***–ic***.

F^-	Fluoride	HF	Hydrofluoric acid
Cl^-	Chloride	HCl	Hydrochloric acid
Br^-	Bromide	HBr	Hydrobromic acid

Acids formed from oxyanions are called oxyacids. If the anion ends in *–ite* (less oxygen), then the acid will end with ***–ous acid***. If the anion ends in *–ate* (more oxygen), then the acid will end with ***–ic acid***. Prefixes in the names of the anions are retained. Some common examples include the following:

ClO^-	Hypochlorite	HClO	Hypochlorous acid
ClO_2^-	Chlorite	$HClO_2$	Chlorous acid
ClO_3^-	Chlorate	$HClO_3$	Chloric acid
ClO_4^-	Perchlorate	$HClO_4$	Perchloric acid
NO_2^-	Nitrite	HNO_2	Nitrous acid
NO_3^-	Nitrate	HNO_3	Nitric acid
CO_3^{2-}	Carbonate	H_2CO_3	Carbonic acid
SO_4^{2-}	Sulfate	H_2SO_4	Sulfuric acid
PO_4^{3-}	Phosphate	H_3PO_4	Phosphoric acid
BO_3^{3-}	Borate	H_3BO_3	Boric acid
CrO_4^{2-}	Chromate	H_2CrO_4	Chromic acid
CH_3COO^-	Acetate	CH_3COOH	Acetic acid

MCAT EXPERTISE

There are some exceptions to the nomenclature rules. For instance, MnO_4^- is called permanganate even though there are no MnO_3^- or MnO_2^- ions.

MCAT CONCEPT CHECK 10.1

Before you move on, assess your understanding of the material with these questions.

1. Compare and contrast the three definitions for acids and bases:

Definition	Acid	Base
Arrhenius		
Brønsted-Lowry		
Lewis		

2. Utilizing Arrhenius acid naming trends, predict the acid formula and name for the following anions:

Anion	Acid Formula	Acid Name
MnO_4^-		
Titanate (TiO_3^{2-})		
I^-		
IO_4^-		

3. Identify which reactants are amphoteric species in the following reactions. For those species, determine if the compound is also amphiprotic.

Reaction	Amphoteric Reactant	Amphiprotic? (Y or N)
$HCO_3^- + HBr \rightleftharpoons H_2CO_3 + Br^-$		
$3\ HCl + Al(OH)_3 \rightleftharpoons AlCl_3 + 3\ H_2O$		
$2\ HBr + ZnO \rightleftharpoons ZnBr_2 + H_2O$		

10.2 Properties

High-Yield

LEARNING OBJECTIVES

After Chapter 10.2, you will be able to:

- Predict the behavior of an acid or base in water given its K_a or K_b value, respectively
- Apply the mathematical relationships between pH, pOH, and ion concentration
- Recall the mathematical relationship between K_a, K_b, and K_w
- Determine concentration of hydrogen ions given molarity and K_a or K_b of a solution
- Identify acids, bases, conjugate acids, and conjugate bases in a reaction: $H_2O\ (l) + H_2O\ (l) \rightleftharpoons H_3O^+\ (aq) + OH^-\ (aq)$

Acids and bases are usually characterized according to their relative tendencies to either donate or accept hydrogen ions. Furthermore, aqueous acid and base solutions can be characterized according to their concentrations of hydrogen and hydroxide ions.

Autoionization of Water and Hydrogen Ion Equilibria

Because many acid–base reactions take place in water—especially on the MCAT—it is very important to understand the behavior of acidic and basic compounds in water. Only then can one fully appreciate the meaning and significance of such terms as *strong acid*, *weak base*, or measurements of pH and pOH.

The Acid–Base Behavior of Water

As described above, water is an **amphoteric** species: in the presence of a base it reacts as an acid, and in the presence of an acid, it reacts as a base. As an amphoteric compound, water can react with itself in a process called **autoionization**, seen previously in Figure 10.1. The autoionization of water is represented by the equation:

$$H_2O\ (l) + H_2O\ (l) \rightleftharpoons H_3O^+\ (aq) + OH^-\ (aq)$$

One water molecule donates a hydrogen ion to another water molecule to produce the **hydronium ion** (H_3O^+) and the **hydroxide ion** (OH^-). Many general chemistry courses depict the hydrogen ion simply as H^+, rather than as H_3O^+.

This is acceptable for representing the chemistry, but it is important to remember that the proton is never isolated in the solution; it is always attached to water or some other species that has the ability to accept it. Autoionization of water is a reversible reaction; therefore, the expression above is in equilibrium. For pure water at 298 K, the **water dissociation constant, K_w**, has been experimentally determined:

$$K_w = [H_3O^+][OH^-] = 10^{-14} \text{ at } 25^\circ\text{C (298 K)}$$

Equation 10.1

Each mole of water that autoionizes produces one mole each of hydrogen (or hydronium) ions and hydroxide ions, so the concentrations of the hydrogen ions and hydroxide ions are always equal in pure water at equilibrium. Thus, the concentration of each of the ions in pure water at equilibrium at 298 K is 10^{-7} *M*.

However, the concentrations of the two ions will not always be equal. In fact, they will only be equal when the solution is neutral. Nevertheless, the product of their respective concentrations will always equal 10^{-14} when the temperature of the solution is 298 K. For example, if a species donates hydrogen ions to pure water, the hydrogen ion concentration will increase, causing the system to shift toward the reactants in the autoionization process. The result is a decrease in the hydroxide ion concentration and a return to the equilibrium state. This is Le Châtelier's principle in action: the addition of product to a system at equilibrium causes the system to shift away from the products and toward the reactants. The shift away from the products necessarily decreases the hydroxide ion concentration such that the product of the concentrations of the dissolved ions equals K_w. The addition of a species that accepts hydrogen ions results in a decrease in the hydrogen ion concentration and causes the system to shift toward the products, thereby replacing hydrogen ions. This shift necessarily increases the hydroxide ion concentration and returns the system to equilibrium.

Before we introduce the scales used in measuring concentrations of hydrogen ions and hydroxide ions in different acid–base solutions, it is worthwhile to emphasize an important thermodynamic principle regarding the water dissociation constant (K_w) expression. K_w is an equilibrium constant; unless the temperature of the water is changed, the value for K_w cannot be changed. Thus, the product of the concentrations of the hydrogen ions and the hydroxide ions in an aqueous solution at 298 K must always equal 10^{-14}. However, at different temperatures, the value for K_w changes. At temperatures above 298 K, K_w will increase; this is a direct result of the endothermic nature of the autoionization reaction.

MCAT EXPERTISE

The MCAT loves to test this concept: the value of K_w, like any other equilibrium constant, is dependent only on temperature. Therefore, isolated changes in concentration, pressure, or volume will not affect K_w.

pH and pOH Scales

The concentrations of hydrogen ions and hydroxide ions in aqueous solutions can vary significantly, making the range of measurements on a linear scale unmanageable. The concentration scales for acidic and basic solutions are condensed into something more manageable through expression in logarithmic terms. These logarithmic scales are the **pH** and the **pOH** scales for the concentrations of hydrogen and hydroxide ions, respectively.

BRIDGE

Logarithmic scales are used to condense very large absolute differences into small scale differences. Remember that sound level (dB) also uses a logarithmic scale, as discussed in Chapter 7 of *MCAT Physics and Math Review.*

Using a logarithmic scale is not only mathematically convenient, but also useful for calculations. For instance, the reactivity of an acidic solution is not a function of hydrogen ion concentration but instead of the *logarithm* of the hydrogen ion concentration. pH and pOH are prototypical examples of p scales. A **p scale** is defined as the negative logarithm of the number of items.

The pH and pOH of a solution are given by:

$$\text{pH} = -\log\left[\text{H}^+\right] = \log\frac{1}{\left[\text{H}^+\right]}$$

$$\text{pOH} = -\log\left[\text{OH}^-\right] = \log\frac{1}{\left[\text{OH}^-\right]}$$

Equation 10.2

For pure water at equilibrium and 298 K, the concentration of hydrogen ions equals the concentration of hydroxide ions (10^{-7} *M*). Therefore, pure water at 298 K has a pH of 7 and a pOH of 7 ($-\log 10^{-7} = 7$). If we take the negative logarithm of the entire water dissociation constant expression ($[H_3O^+][OH^-] = 10^{-14}$), we find:

$$\text{pH} + \text{pOH} = 14$$

Equation 10.3

Equation 10.3 holds true for all aqueous solutions at 298 K. As pH increases, pOH decreases by the same amount. This relationship can be seen in Figure 10.5 below.

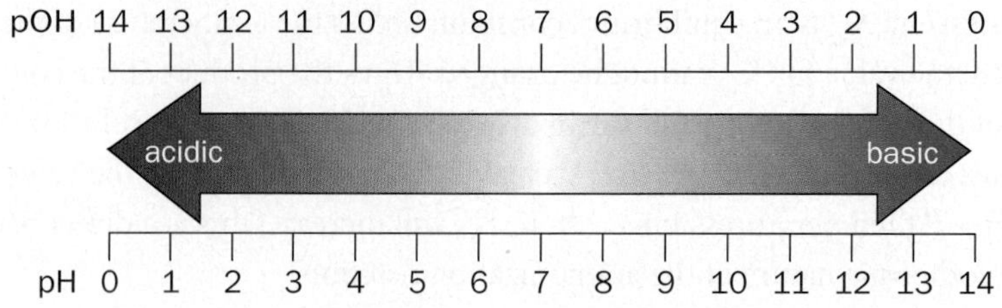

Figure 10.5 pH and pOH Scales
pH + pOH = 14 for aqueous solutions at 298 K.

For an aqueous solution at 298 K, a pH less than 7 (or pOH greater than 7) indicates a relative excess of hydrogen ions, and the solution is acidic; a pH greater than 7 (or pOH less than 7) indicates a relative excess of hydroxide ions, and the solution is basic. A pH (and pOH) equal to 7 indicates equal concentrations of hydrogen and hydroxide ions, resulting in a neutral solution.

MCAT EXPERTISE

The K_w (like all equilibrium constants) will change if the temperature changes and, in turn, will change the significance of the pH scale. Be careful and read the system conditions given on the MCAT: pH = 7 = neutral is only valid at 25°C.

Estimating Scale Values

An essential skill to hone for Test Day is the ability to quickly convert pH, pOH, pK_a, and pK_b values into nonlogarithmic form and vice-versa.

When the original value is a power of ten, the operation is relatively straightforward: changing the sign on the exponent gives the corresponding p scale value directly. For example, if $[H^+] = 0.001$ or 10^{-3}, then the pH = 3 and pOH = 11. Or, if $K_b = 1.0 \times 10^{-12}$, then p$K_b$ = 12.

More difficulty arises when the value is not an exact power of ten. Rest assured that the MCAT is not a math test and is not interested in determining your ability to perform complex logarithmic calculations; an exact logarithmic calculation of a number that is not an integer power of ten is unnecessary on the MCAT. The testmakers are interested, however, in testing the ability to apply mathematical concepts appropriately in solving certain problems.

One can obtain a relatively close approximation of a p scale value using the following shortcut: if the nonlogarithmic value is written in proper scientific notation, it will be in the form $n \times 10^{-m}$, where n is a number between 1 and 10. Taking the negative logarithm and simplifying, the p value will be:

$$-\log\left(n \times 10^{-m}\right) = -\log(n) - \log\left(10^{-m}\right)$$
$$= m - \log(n)$$

BRIDGE

In general, math using logarithms frequently appears on the MCAT; make sure to review how these mathematical concepts work in Chapter 10 of *MCAT Physics and Math Review*. Specifically, the equation pH + pOH = 14 comes from the fact that the log of a product is equal to the sum of logs; that is, $\log(xy) = \log x + \log y$.

Because n is a number between 1 and 10, its logarithm will be a decimal between 0 and 1 ($\log 1 = 0$ and $\log 10 = 1$). The closer n is to 1, the closer $\log n$ will be to 0; the closer n is to 10, the closer $\log n$ will be to 1. As a reasonable approximation, one can say that:

$$\text{p value} \approx m - 0.n$$

Equation 10.4

where $0.n$ represents sliding the decimal point of n one position to the left (dividing n by ten).

Example: If the K_a of an acid is 1.8×10^{-5}, then what is its pK_a?

Solution: $pK_a = -\log(1.8 \times 10^{-5}) = 5 - \log 1.8 \approx 5 - 0.18$
$= 4.82$ (actual $= 4.74$)

MCAT EXPERTISE

Learning how to estimate when using logarithms is an important skill that can save a lot of time on Test Day.

Strong Acids and Bases

Strong acids and bases completely dissociate into their component ions in aqueous solutions. For example, when sodium hydroxide is added to water, the ionic compound dissociates according to the net ionic equation:

$$NaOH\ (s) \rightarrow Na^+\ (aq) + OH^-\ (aq)$$

Hence, in a 1 M NaOH solution, complete dissociation yields 1 M Na^+ and 1 M OH^-. The pH and pOH for this solution can be calculated as follows:

$$pH = 14 - pOH = 14 - (-\log[OH^-]) = 14 + \log(1\ M) = 14 + 0 = 14$$

Virtually no undissociated strong acid or base, such as NaOH, will remain in solution. This is why the dissociation of strong acids and bases is said to go to completion. In the NaOH example above, we assume that the concentration of OH^- from the autoionization of water is negligible due to addition of a strong base. The contribution of OH^- and H^+ ions from the autoionization of water is negligible if the concentration of the acid or base is significantly greater than 10^{-7} M. On the other hand, if the concentration of acid or base is close to 10^{-7} M, then the contribution from the autoionization of water is important.

MCAT EXPERTISE

Acid–base reactions that consist of a single-headed arrow generally indicate strong acids or bases (complete dissociation with no reversibility).

Example: Calculate the pH of a 1×10^{-8} M solution of HCl.

Solution: At first, one may calculate the pH as $-\log[H^+] = -\log 10^{-8}\ M = 8$. However, this answer is not feasible: a pH of 8 cannot describe an acidic solution at 298 K because the presence of the acid will increase the hydrogen ion concentration to above 10^{-7} M, resulting in an acidic pH below 7.

Recognize that the acid concentration in this question is actually ten times less than the equilibrium concentration of hydrogen ions in pure water generated by the autoionization of water. Consequently, the hydrogen ion concentration from the water itself is significant and cannot be ignored. This can be represented in the equilibrium expression in which *x* represents the concentration of H_3O^+ and OH^- resulting from the autoionization of water:

$$K_w = [H_3O^+][OH^-] = [x + 10^{-8}][x] = 10^{-14}$$

Solving for *x* (which would require a quadratic equation—math that is beyond the scope of the MCAT) gives $x = 9.5 \times 10^{-8}$ *M*. The total concentration of hydrogen ions is $[H^+]_{total} = (9.5 \times 10^{-8}) + (1.0 \times 10^{-8}) = 1.05 \times 10^{-7}$ *M*. Notice that this is extremely close to the concentration of H^+ in pure water. The pH of this acidic solution can now be calculated as $pH = -\log(1.05 \times 10^{-7}) \approx 7$ (actual $= 6.98$). This pH is slightly lower than 7, as expected for a very dilute acidic solution. The point of all of this is: *stay alert and keep thinking critically, no matter how familiar the problem setups might seem to you!*

Strong acids commonly encountered on the MCAT include HCl (hydrochloric acid), HBr (hydrobromic acid), HI (hydroiodic acid), H_2SO_4 (sulfuric acid), HNO_3 (nitric acid), and $HClO_4$ (perchloric acid). Strong bases commonly encountered include NaOH (sodium hydroxide), KOH (potassium hydroxide), and other soluble hydroxides of Group IA metals. Calculation of the pH and pOH of strong acids and bases assumes complete dissociation of the acid or base in solution.

Example: What is the pH of a solution with $[HClO_4] = 10$ *M*?

Solution: Because perchloric acid is a strong acid, it will fully dissociate in solution. Therefore, $[H^+] = 10$ *M* (note that the contribution from the autoionization of water is negligible). $pH = -\log [H^+] = -\log 10$ *M* $= -1$.

This question points out that the pH scale does not "end" at 0 and 14. There can be negative pH values and pH values greater than 14—but this implies a very high concentration of a strong acid or base.

Weak Acids and Bases

Before going any further in our discussion of acids and bases as *strong* or *weak*, verify that you are making the distinction between the chemical behavior of an acid or base with respect to its tendency to dissociate (that is, strong bases completely dissociate in aqueous solutions) and the concentrations of acid and base solutions. Although we may casually describe a solution's concentration as *strong* or *weak*, it is preferable to use the terms *concentrated* and *dilute*, respectively, because they are unambiguously associated with concentrations, rather than chemical behavior.

Continuing our focus on the chemical behavior of acids and bases, we will now consider those acids and bases that only partially dissociate in aqueous solutions. These are called **weak acids and bases**. A weak monoprotic acid, HA, will dissociate partially in water to achieve an equilibrium state:

$$HA\ (aq) + H_2O\ (l) \rightleftharpoons H_3O^+\ (aq) + A^-\ (aq)$$

Because the system exists in an equilibrium state, we can write the dissociation equation to determine the **acid dissociation constant (K_a)** as:

$$K_a = \frac{[H_3O^+][A^-]}{[HA]}$$

Equation 10.5

The smaller the K_a, the weaker the acid, and consequently, the less it will dissociate. Note that water, as a pure liquid, is not incorporated into the equilibrium expression.

A weak monovalent Arrhenius base, BOH, undergoes dissociation to yield B^+ and OH^- in solution:

$$BOH\ (aq) \rightleftharpoons B^+\ (aq) + OH^-\ (aq)$$

The **base dissociation constant (K_b)** can be calculated as:

$$K_b = \frac{[B^+][OH^-]}{[BOH]}$$

Equation 10.6

The smaller the K_b, the weaker the base, and consequently, the less it will dissociate. As with the acid dissociation expression, water is not included because it is a pure liquid.

Generally speaking, we can characterize a species as a weak acid if its K_a is less than 1.0 and as a weak base if its K_b is less than 1.0. On the MCAT, molecular (nonionic) weak bases are almost exclusively amines.

Conjugate Acid–Base Pairs

Because the Brønsted–Lowry definition of an acid–base reaction is one in which a hydrogen ion (proton) is transferred from an acid to a base, the two always occur in pairs called conjugates. A **conjugate acid** is the acid formed when a base gains a proton, and a **conjugate base** is the base formed when an acid loses a proton. For example,

$$HCO_3^-\ (aq) + H_2O\ (l) \rightleftharpoons CO_3^{2-}\ (aq) + H_3O^+\ (aq)$$

CO_3^{2-} is the conjugate base of HCO_3^-, a weak acid, and H_3O^+ is the conjugate acid of H_2O, a weak base. To find the K_a, we consider the equilibrium concentrations of the dissolved species:

$$K_a = \frac{[CO_3^{2-}][H_3O^+]}{[HCO_3^-]}$$

The reaction between bicarbonate and water is reversible. The reverse reaction would be:

$$CO_3^{2-}\ (aq) + H_2O\ (l) \rightleftharpoons HCO_3^-\ (aq) + OH^-\ (aq)$$

We can write the K_b for CO_3^{2-} as:

$$K_b = \frac{[HCO_3^-][OH^-]}{[CO_3^{2-}]}$$

If one adds the previous two reversible reactions, the net reaction is simply the dissociation of water:

$$\begin{array}{c} \cancel{HCO_3^-} + H_2O \rightleftharpoons \cancel{CO_3^{2-}} + H_3O^+ \\ \cancel{CO_3^{2-}} + H_2O \rightleftharpoons \cancel{HCO_3^-} + OH^- \\ \hline 2\,H_2O \rightleftharpoons H_3O^+ + OH^- \end{array}$$

Because the net reaction is the autoionization of water, the equilibrium constant for the reaction is $K_w = [H_3O^+][OH^-] = 10^{-14}$, which is the product of K_a and K_b. Remember: the product of the concentrations of the hydrogen ion and the hydroxide ion must always equal 10^{-14} for acidic or basic aqueous solutions. Because water is an amphoteric species (both a weak acid and a weak base), all acid–base reactivity in water ultimately reduces to the acid–base behavior of water, and all acidic or basic aqueous solutions are governed by the dissociation constant for water. Thus, if the dissociation constant for one species or its conjugate is known, then the dissociation constant for the other can be determined using the following equations:

KEY CONCEPT

Be aware of the relationship between conjugate acids and bases because you will need to recognize these entities on the MCAT. Removing a proton from a molecule produces the conjugate base, and adding a proton produces the conjugate acid.

$$K_{a,\text{acid}} \times K_{b,\text{conjugate base}} = K_w = 10^{-14}$$

$$K_{b,\text{base}} \times K_{a,\text{conjugate acid}} = K_w = 10^{-14}$$

Equation 10.7

As is evident from these equations, K_a and K_b are inversely related. In other words, if K_a is large, then K_b is small, and vice-versa. By this logic, a strong acid (K_a approaching ∞) will produce a very weak conjugate base (for example, HCl is a strong acid and Cl^- is a very weak base), and a strong base will produce a very weak conjugate acid (for example, NaOH is a strong base and H_2O is a very weak acid). The conjugate of a strong acid or base is sometimes termed **inert** because it is almost completely unreactive.

BRIDGE

This thermodynamic preference for the bicarbonate ion intermediate is a major reason why the bicarbonate buffer system in the body is ideal for maintaining a stable pH. The homeostatic mechanisms involved are discussed in Chapter 6 of *MCAT Biology Review*.

On the other hand, weak acids and bases tend to have conjugates that are also weak. As seen above, CO_3^{2-} is a weak base; its conjugate acid, HCO_3^- is a weak acid. As it turns out, for this specific example, the reaction of CO_3^{2-} with water to produce HCO_3^- and OH^- occurs to a greater extent—is more thermodynamically favorable—than the reaction of HCO_3^- and water to produce CO_3^{2-} and H_3O^+. This fact makes this equilibrium ideal for buffering solutions as part of the bicarbonate buffer system, discussed in Chapter 6 of *MCAT Biology Review*.

One important theme for acid strength is the effect of induction. Electronegative elements positioned near an acidic proton increase acid strength by pulling electron density out of the bond holding the acidic proton. This weakens proton bonding and facilitates dissociation. Thus, acids that have electronegative elements nearer to acidic hydrogens are stronger than those that do not, as shown in Figure 10.6.

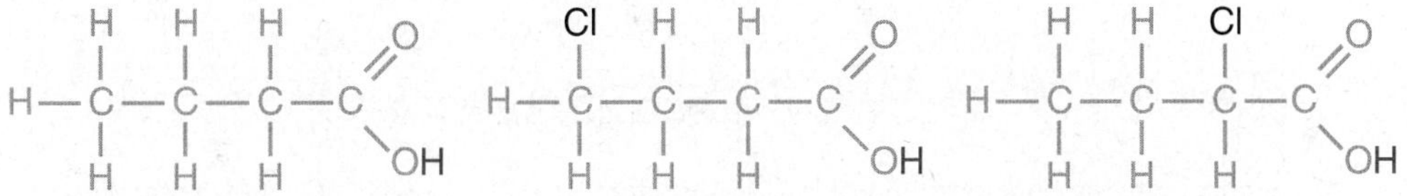

Figure 10.6 Inductive Effects from Electronegative Elements Increase Acidity

Applications of K_a and K_b

The most common use of acid and base dissociation constants is to determine the concentration of one of the species in solution at equilibrium. On Test Day, you may be asked to calculate the concentration of the hydrogen ion (or pH), the concentration of the hydroxide ion (or pOH), or the concentration of either the original acid or base.

Example: Calculate the concentration of H_3O^+ in a 2.0 *M* aqueous solution of acetic acid, CH_3COOH. (Note: $K_a = 1.8 \times 10^{-5}$)

Solution: First, write the equilibrium reaction:

$$CH_3COOH\ (aq) + H_2O\ (l) \rightleftharpoons H_3O^+\ (aq) + CH_3COO^-\ (aq)$$

Next, write the expression for the acid dissociation constant:

$$K_a = \frac{[H_3O^+][CH_3COO^-]}{[CH_3COOH]} = 1.8 \times 10^{-5}$$

Then, recognize that acetic acid is a weak acid, so the concentration of CH_3COOH at equilibrium is equal to its initial concentration, 2.0 *M*, minus the amount dissociated, *x*. Likewise, $[H_3O^+] = [CH_3COO^-] = x$ because each molecule of CH_3COOH dissociates into one H^+ ion and one CH_3COO^- ion. Note that the contribution of H_3O^+ from water is negligible. Thus, the equation can be rewritten as follows:

$$K_a = \frac{[x][x]}{[2.0\ M - x]} = 1.8 \times 10^{-5}$$

Remember that the value of x is generally very small. Therefore, we can approximate that $2.0\ M - x \approx 2.0\ M$. This is further supported because acetic acid is a weak acid and only slightly dissociates in water. This simplifies the calculations:

$$K_a = \frac{[x][x]}{2.0\ M} = 1.8 \times 10^{-5}$$

$$x^2 = 3.6 \times 10^{-5} = 36 \times 10^{-6}$$

$$x = 6 \times 10^{-3}\ M$$

x represents the concentration of H_3O^+; therefore, $[H_3O^+] = 6 \times 10^{-3}\ M$. Note: When required to take the square root, adjust the coefficient as needed to make the power of 10 an even number. This way the square root only requires cutting the power of 10 in half.

In this example, note that x is significantly lower than the initial concentration of acetic acid ($2.0\ M$), which validates the approximation; otherwise, it would have been necessary to solve for x using the quadratic formula. Fortunately, the value of x on Test Day is almost always sufficiently small to make this approximation. A rule of thumb is that the approximation is valid as long as x is less than 5 percent of the initial concentration. This typically occurs when K_a is at least 100 times smaller than the concentration of the starting solution. For example, if K_a is 10^{-4} and the concentration of the starting solution is $0.01\ M$ ($10^{-2}\ M$), then the ratio between the values is 10^2 or 100. The error in this calculation should be no more than $\frac{1}{100} = 1\%$. On the other hand, if the K_a is 10^{-3} and the concentration is still $0.01\ M$, then the ratio between the values becomes 10, which could lead to $\frac{1}{10} = 10\%$ error. This degree of error may not be useful when identifying an answer choice on the MCAT.

Students often feel nervous making the assumption that x is negligible because they want to see precise answer choices. However, keep in mind that the MCAT quite deliberately tests students' ability to make reasonable assumptions under timed conditions to arrive at a feasible answer choice. Part of the skill of taking the MCAT is rounding appropriately to simplify math.

BRIDGE

Remember the reaction types discussed in Chapter 4 of *MCAT General Chemistry Review*? Go back and review the section on neutralization reactions if this equation doesn't look familiar to you.

Salt Formation

Acids and bases may react with each other to form a salt and often (but not always) water, in what is termed a **neutralization reaction**. For example,

$$HA\ (aq) + BOH\ (aq) \rightarrow BA\ (s) + H_2O\ (l)$$

The salt may precipitate out or remain ionized in solution, depending on its solubility and the amount produced. In general, neutralization reactions go to completion. The reverse reaction, in which the salt ions react with water to give back the acid or base, is known as **hydrolysis**.

Four combinations of strong and weak acids and bases are possible:

- Strong acid + strong base: $HCl + NaOH \rightarrow NaCl + H_2O$
- Strong acid + weak base: $HCl + NH_3 \rightarrow NH_4Cl$
- Weak acid + strong base: $HClO + NaOH \rightarrow NaClO + H_2O$
- Weak acid + weak base: $HClO + NH_3 \rightarrow NH_4ClO$

The products of a reaction between equal concentrations of a strong acid and a strong base are equimolar amounts of salt and water. The acid and base neutralize each other, so the resulting solution is neutral (pH = 7), and the ions formed in the reaction will not react with water because they are inert conjugates.

The product of a reaction between a strong acid and a weak base is also a salt, but often no water will be formed because weak bases are often not hydroxides. In this case, the cation of the salt is a weak acid and will react with the water solvent, re-forming some of the weak base through hydrolysis. For example:

- Reaction I: $HCl\ (aq) + NH_3\ (aq) \rightarrow NH_4^+\ (aq) + Cl^-\ (aq)$
- Reaction II: $NH_4^+\ (aq) + H_2O\ (l) \rightarrow NH_3\ (aq) + H_3O^+\ (aq)$

NH_4^+ is the conjugate acid of a weak base (NH_3) and is stronger than the conjugate base (Cl^-) of the strong acid, HCl. NH_4^+ will then transfer a proton to H_2O to form the hydronium ion. The increase in the concentration of the hydronium ion causes the system to shift away from autoionization, thereby reducing the concentration of hydroxide ion. Consequently, the concentration of the hydronium ion will be greater than that of the hydroxide ion at equilibrium, and as a result, the pH of the solution will fall below 7. This should make sense: a strong acid and a weak base produce a slightly acidic solution.

On the other hand, when a weak acid reacts with a strong base, the pH of the solution at equilibrium will be within the basic range because the salt hydrolyzes, with concurrent formation of hydroxide ions. The increase in hydroxide ion concentration will cause the system to shift away from autoionization, thereby reducing the concentration of the hydronium ion. Consequently, the concentration of the hydroxide ion will be greater than that of the hydronium ion at equilibrium, and as a result, the pH of the solution will rise above 7. Consider the reaction of acetic acid, CH_3COOH (weak acid) with sodium hydroxide, NaOH (strong base):

- Reaction I: $CH_3COOH\ (aq) + NaOH\ (aq) \rightarrow Na^+\ (aq) + CH_3COO^-\ (aq) + H_2O\ (l)$
- Reaction II: $CH_3COO^-\ (aq) + H_2O\ (l) \rightarrow CH_3COOH\ (aq) + OH^-\ (aq)$

The pH of a solution containing a weak acid and a weak base depends on the relative strengths of the reactants. For example, the weak acid HClO has a K_a of 3.2×10^{-8}, and the weak base NH_3 has a $K_b = 1.8 \times 10^{-5}$. Thus, an aqueous solution of HClO and NH_3 is basic because the K_a for HClO is less than the K_b for NH_3. That is, HClO is weaker as an acid than NH_3 is as a base. At equilibrium, therefore, the concentration of hydroxide ions will be greater than the concentration of hydronium ions in the aqueous solution.

In biology and biochemistry, neutralization reactions are often condensation reactions because they form bonds with a small molecule as a byproduct (usually water). The peptide bonds in proteins, for example, are created from the reaction of a carboxyl group (acid) and an amino group (base), while forming a water molecule, as shown in Figure 10.7. The salt in this reaction is the polypeptide itself; breaking it apart requires hydrolysis.

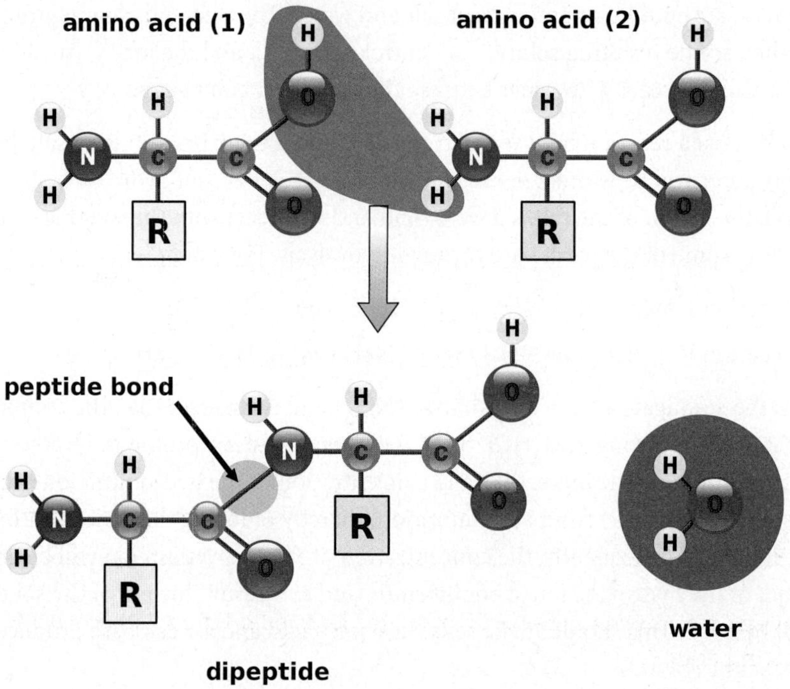

Figure 10.7 Peptide Bond Formation
An acidic carboxyl group reacts with a basic amino group.

MCAT CONCEPT CHECK 10.2

Before you move on, assess your understanding of the material with these questions.

1. What is an amphoteric species?

___

2. If a compound has a K_a value ≫ water, what does it mean about its behavior in solution? How does this compare with a solution that has only a slightly higher K_a than water?

___

3. If a compound has a K_b value ≫ water, what does it mean about its behavior in solution? How does this compare with a solution that has only a slightly higher K_b than water?

___

4. Complete the blank cells in the table by utilizing the mathematical relationships between pH, pOH, and ion concentrations. (Note: Round the numbers given and use logarithmic approximations to determine p values, without a calculator, to simulate Test Day math.)

pH	$[H_3O^+]$	pOH	$[OH^-]$	Acid or Base?
4				
	8.89×10^{-4} *M*			
		5.19		
			1.88×10^{-6} *M*	

5. What is the mathematical relationship between K_a, K_b, and K_w?

____

6. Identify the conjugate acid–base pairings in the reactions below:

Reaction	Acid	Base	Conjugate Acid	Conjugate Base
$H_2CO_3 + H_2O \rightleftharpoons HCO_3^- + H_3O^+$				
$H_2PO_4^- + H_2O \rightleftharpoons H_3PO_4 + OH^-$				

7. Determine the concentration of hydrogen ions and pH of a solution of 0.2 *M* acetic acid ($K_a = 1.8 \times 10^{-5}$).

____

10.3 Polyvalence and Normality

LEARNING OBJECTIVES

After Chapter 10.3, you will be able to:

- Describe how equivalents of acid or base are calculated
- Calculate the normality of a solution given its formula and molarity

The relative acidity or basicity of an aqueous solution is determined by the relative concentrations of acid and base equivalents. An **acid equivalent** is equal to one mole of H^+ (or, more properly, H_3O^+) ions; a **base equivalent** is equal to one mole of OH^- ions. Some acids and bases are **polyvalent**; that is, each mole of the acid or base liberates more than one acid or base equivalent. Under the

Brønsted–Lowry definition, such acids or bases could also be termed **polyprotic**. For example, the divalent diprotic acid H_2SO_4 undergoes the following dissociation in water:

$$H_2SO_4\,(aq) + H_2O\,(l) \rightarrow H_3O^+\,(aq) + HSO_4^-\,(aq)$$
$$HSO_4^-\,(aq) + H_2O\,(l) \rightleftharpoons H_3O^+\,(aq) + SO_4^{2-}\,(aq)$$

One mole of H_2SO_4 produces two acid equivalents (2 moles of H_3O^+). Notice that the first dissociation goes to completion, but the second dissociation reaches an equilibrium state. The acidity or basicity of a solution depends on the concentration of acidic or basic equivalents that can be liberated. The quantity of acidic or basic capacity is directly indicated by the solution's **normality**, described in Chapter 9 of *MCAT General Chemistry Review*. For example, each mole of H_3PO_4 yields three moles (equivalents) of H_3O^+. Therefore, a 2 M H_3PO_4 solution would be 6 N.

BRIDGE

To review normality in more detail, revisit the calculations performed in Chapter 4 of *MCAT General Chemistry Review*. These are critical calculations for polyvalent acids and bases.

Another measurement useful for acid–base chemistry is **gram equivalent weight**. Chapter 4 of *MCAT General Chemistry Review* defined and discussed this term extensively. The gram equivalent weight is the mass of a compound that produces one equivalent (one mole of charge). For example, H_2SO_4 (molar mass: 98 $\frac{g}{mol}$) is a divalent acid, so each mole of the acid compound yields two acid equivalents. The gram equivalent weight is $98 \div 2 = 49$ grams. That is, the complete dissociation of 49 grams of H_2SO_4 will yield one acid equivalent (one mole of H_3O^+). Common polyvalent acids include H_2SO_4, H_3PO_4, and H_2CO_3. Common polyvalent bases include $Al(OH)_3$, $Ca(OH)_2$, and $Mg(OH)_2$.

MCAT CONCEPT CHECK 10.3

Before you move on, assess your understanding of the material with these questions.

1. What species are considered the equivalents for acids and bases, respectively?
   - Acids:

   ____

   - Bases:

   ____

2. Calculate the normality of the following solutions:
   - 2 M $Al(OH)_3$:

   ____

   - 16 M H_2SO_4:

   ____

10.4 Titration and Buffers

High-Yield

LEARNING OBJECTIVES

After Chapter 10.4, you will be able to:

- Select an appropriate indicator for a given acid–base reaction
- Explain the purpose of a buffer solution
- Identify the pH range of the equivalence point for different combinations of acids and bases, for example, weak acid + weak base
- Calculate the pH or pOH of a known solution
- Identify the buffering region, half-equivalence point, equivalence point, and endpoint of a titration reaction:

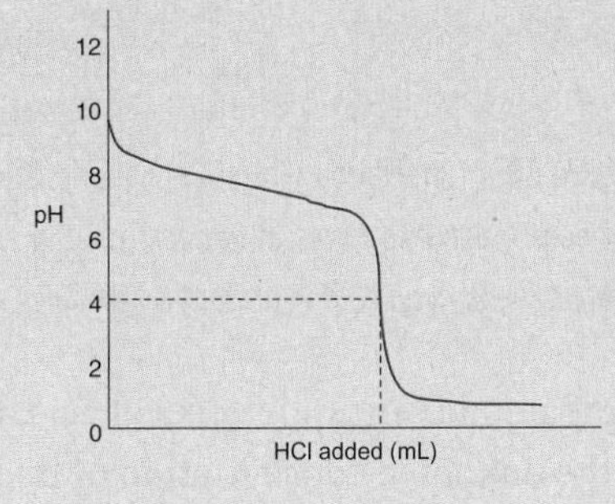

Titration is a procedure used to determine the concentration of a known reactant in a solution. There are different types of titrations, including acid–base, oxidation–reduction, and complexometric (metal ion). The MCAT frequently tests the first two types. Complexometric (metal ion) titrations are outside the scope of the MCAT but focus on formation of complex ions, as described in Chapter 9 of *MCAT General Chemistry Review*.

General Principles

Titrations are performed by adding small volumes of a solution of known concentration (the **titrant**) to a known volume of a solution of unknown concentration (the **titrand**) until completion of the reaction is achieved at the **equivalence point**.

Acid–Base Equivalence Points

In acid–base titrations, the equivalence point is reached when the number of acid equivalents present in the original solution equals the number of base equivalents added, or vice-versa. It is important to emphasize that, while a strong acid/strong base titration will have its equivalence point at a pH of 7, the equivalence point does *not* always occur at pH 7. When titrating polyprotic acids or bases (discussed later in this chapter), there are multiple equivalence points, as each acidic or basic conjugate species is titrated separately. This is shown in the speciation plot in Figure 10.8.

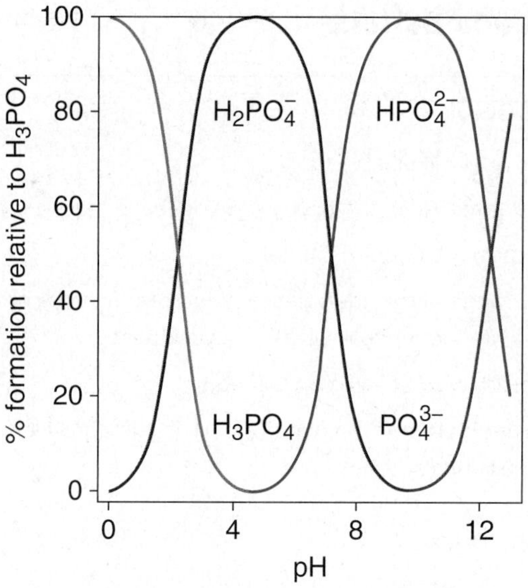

Figure 10.8 Speciation Plot of Phosphoric Acid
At any given pH, only two forms of the acid exist in solution; thus, each conjugate is titrated separately.

At the equivalence point, the number of equivalents of acid and base are equal. This fact allows us to calculate the unknown concentration of the titrand through the equation:

$$N_a V_a = N_b V_b$$

Equation 10.8

where N_a and N_b are the acid and base normalities, respectively, and V_a and V_b are the volumes of acid and base solutions, respectively. Note that, as long as both volumes use the same units, the units used do not have to be liters.

The equivalence point in an acid–base titration is determined in two common ways: evaluated by using a graphical method, plotting the pH of the unknown solution as a function of added titrant by using a **pH meter**, or estimated by watching for a color change of an added **indicator**.

KEY CONCEPT

Indicators change color as they shift between their conjugate acid and base forms:

$$\underset{\text{(color 1)}}{\text{H} - \text{Indicator}} \rightleftharpoons \text{H}^+ + \underset{\text{(color 2)}}{\text{Indicator}^-}$$

Because this is an equilibrium process, we can apply Le Châtelier's principle. Adding H^+ shifts the equilibrium to the left. Adding OH^- removes H^+ and therefore shifts the equilibrium to the right.

Indicators

Indicators are weak organic acids or bases that have different colors in their protonated and deprotonated states. This small structural change—the binding or release of a proton—leads to a change in the absorption spectrum of the molecule, which we perceive as a color change. Indicators are generally vibrant and can be used in low concentrations without significantly altering the equivalence point. The indicator must always be a weaker acid or base than the acid or base being titrated; otherwise, the indicator would be titrated first! The point at which the indicator changes to its final color is not the equivalence point but rather the **endpoint**. If the indicator is chosen correctly and the titration is performed well, the volume difference between the endpoint and the equivalence point is negligible and may be corrected for or simply ignored.

Acid–base titrations can be performed for different combinations of strong and weak acids and bases. The most useful combinations involve at least one strong species. Weak acid/weak base titrations can be done but are not very accurate and therefore are rarely performed. The pH curve for the titration of a weak acid and weak base lacks the sharp change that normally indicates the equivalence point. Furthermore, indicators are less useful because the pH change is far more gradual.

Strong Acid and Strong Base

Let's consider the titration of 10 mL of a 0.1 *N* solution of HCl with a 0.1 *N* solution of NaOH. Plotting the pH of the solution *vs.* the quantity of NaOH added gives the curve shown in Figure 10.9.

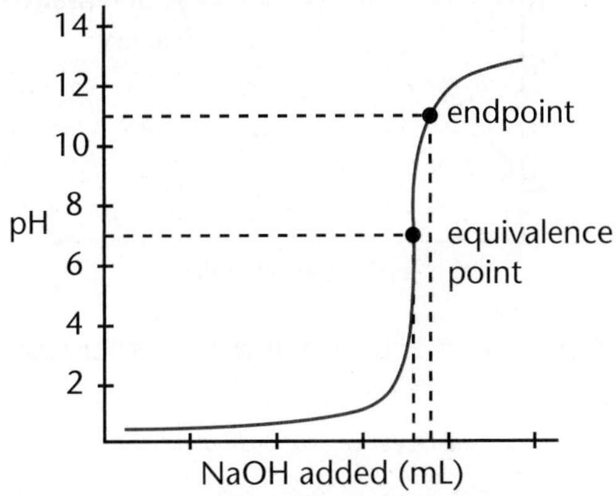

Figure 10.9 Monoprotic Strong Acid and Strong Base Titration Curve
A strong base, NaOH, is titrated into a solution of strong acid, HCl, to yield an equivalence point of pH = 7.

Because HCl is a strong acid and NaOH is a strong base, the equivalence point of the titration will be at pH 7, and the solution will be neutral. Note that the endpoint shown is close to, but not exactly equal to, the equivalence point; selection of a better indicator, one that changes colors at, say, pH 8, would have given a better approximation. Still, the amount of error introduced by the use of an indicator that changes color around pH 11 rather than pH 8 is not especially significant; it represents a mere fraction of a milliliter of excess NaOH solution.

In the early part of the curve when little base has been added, the acidic species predominates, so the addition of small amounts of base will not appreciably change either the $[OH^-]$ or the pH. Similarly, in the last part of the titration curve when an excess of base has been added, the addition of small amounts of base will not change the $[OH^-]$ significantly, and the pH will remain relatively constant. The addition of base will alter the concentrations of H^+ and OH^- near the equivalence point, and will elicit the most substantial changes in pH in that region. Remember: the equivalence point for strong acid/strong base titrations is always at pH 7 (for monovalent species).

MCAT EXPERTISE

Any question involving the selection of an ideal indicator will require you to know what the pH of the reaction at the equivalence point will be, whether graphically or mathematically. Once you have determined where the equivalence point is, select the indicator that has the closest pK_a value to it.

KEY CONCEPT

Compare the relative strength of the two solutions in a titration to determine if the pH of the equivalence point is less than, equal to, or greater than 7:

- Strong acid + weak base: equivalence point pH < 7
- Strong acid + strong base: equivalence point pH $= 7$
- Weak acid + strong base: equivalence point pH > 7

If one uses a pH meter to chart the change in pH as a function of volume of titrant added, a good approximation can be made of the equivalence point by locating the midpoint of the region of the curve with the steepest slope.

Weak Acid and Strong Base

Titration of a weak acid, such as CH_3COOH, with a strong base, such as NaOH, produces the titration curve shown in Figure 10.10.

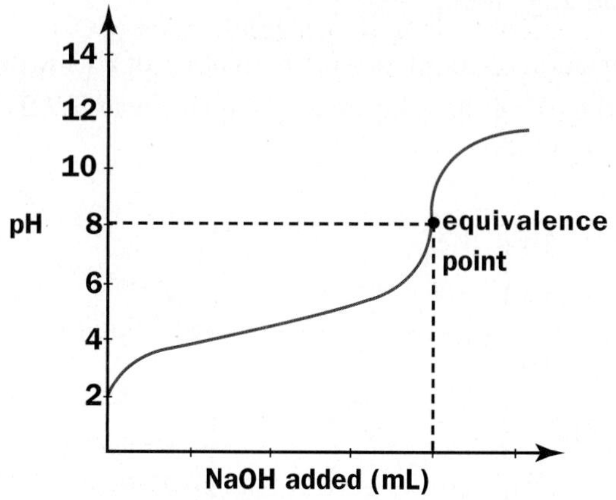

Figure 10.10 Weak Acid and Strong Base Titration Curve
A strong base, NaOH, is titrated into a solution of weak acid, CH_3COOH, to yield an equivalence point of pH > 7.

Compare Figure 10.10 with the curve in Figure 10.9. The first difference is that the initial pH of the weak acid solution is greater than the initial pH of the strong acid solution. Weak acids do not dissociate to the same degree that strong acids do; therefore, the concentration of H_3O^+ will generally be lower (and pH will be higher) in an equimolar solution of weak acid. The second difference is the shapes of the curves. The pH curve for the strong acid/strong base titration shows a steeper, more sudden rise in pH at the equivalence point. In the weak acid/strong base titration, the pH changes gradually early on in the titration and has a less sudden rise at the equivalence point. The third difference is the position of the equivalence point. While the equivalence point for a strong acid/strong base titration is pH 7, the equivalence point for a weak acid/strong base titration is above 7. This is because the reaction between the weak acid (HA) and strong base (OH^-) produces a weak conjugate base (A^-) and even weaker conjugate acid (H_2O). This produces a greater concentration of hydroxide ions than hydrogen ions at equilibrium (due to the common ion effect on the autoionization of water). Therefore, the equivalence point for weak acid/strong base titration is always in the basic range of the pH scale.

Strong Acid and Weak Base

The appearance of the titration curve for a weak base titrand and strong acid titrant will look like an inversion of the curve for a weak acid titrand and strong base titrant. The initial pH will be in the basic range (typical range: pH 10–12) and will demonstrate a gradual drop in pH with the addition of strong acid. The equivalence point will be in the acidic pH range because the reaction between the weak base and strong acid will produce a weak conjugate acid and even weaker conjugate base, as shown in Figure 10.11. The stronger conjugate acid will result in an equilibrium state with a concentration of hydrogen ions greater than that of the hydroxide ions. Therefore, the equivalence point for a weak base/strong acid titration is always in the acidic range of the pH scale.

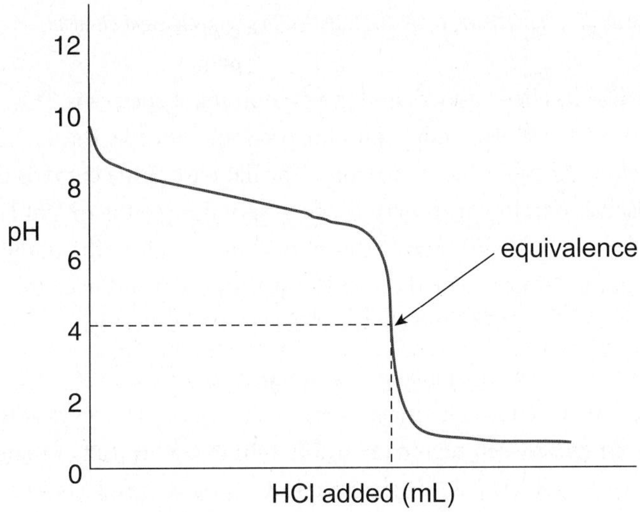

Figure 10.11 Strong Acid and Weak Base Titration Curve
A strong acid, HCl, is titrated into a solution of weak base, NH_3*, to yield an equivalence point of pH* < 7*.*

Weak Acid and Weak Base

The appearance of the titration curve for a weak base titrand and weak acid titrant will look like an intermediate of the previous types discussed. Because both the titrant and the titrand are weak, the initial pH is generally in the 3–11 range and will demonstrate a very shallow drop at the equivalence point. The equivalence point will be near neutral pH because the reaction is partially dissociative for both species.

Polyvalent Acids and Bases

The titration curve for a polyvalent acid or base looks different from that for a monovalent acid or base. Figure 10.12 shows the titration of Na_2CO_3 with HCl, in which the divalent (diprotic) acid H_2CO_3 is the ultimate product.

MCAT EXPERTISE

To identify which type of titration is being shown in a graph, identify the starting position in the graph (pH $\gg 7 =$ titrand is a strong base, > 7 (slightly) $=$ weak base, < 7 (slightly) $=$ weak acid, and $\ll 7$ pH $=$ strong acid), and determine where the equivalence point is. Think of titrations like tug-of-war: the stronger the acid or base, the more it pulls the equivalence point into its pH territory.

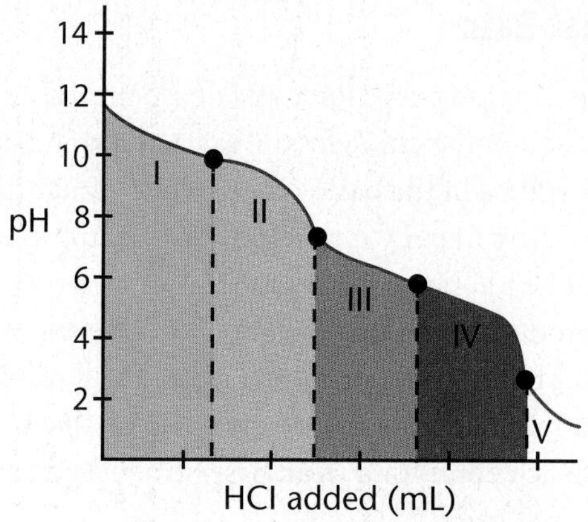

Figure 10.12 Polyvalent Titration
The multiple equivalence points indicate that this is a polyvalent titration.

In region I, little acid has been added, and the predominant species is CO_3^{2-}. In region II, more acid has been added, and the predominant species are CO_3^{2-} and HCO_3^-, in relatively equal concentrations. The flat part of the curve is the first buffer region (discussed in the next section), corresponding to the pK_a of HCO_3^- ($K_a = 5.6 \times 10^{-11}$; p$K_a = 10.25$). The center of the buffer region (the point between regions I and II) is sometimes termed the **half-equivalence point** because it occurs when half of a given species has been protonated (or deprotonated).

Region III begins with the equivalence point, at which all of the CO_3^{2-} is finally titrated to HCO_3^-. As the curve illustrates, a rapid change in pH occurs at the equivalence point (the point between regions II and III). In the latter part of region III, the predominant species is HCO_3^-, although some H_2CO_3 has formed as well.

At the beginning of region IV, the acid has neutralized approximately half of the HCO_3^-, and now H_2CO_3 and HCO_3^- are in roughly equal concentrations. This flat region is the second buffer region (and second half-equivalence point, between regions III and IV) of the titration curve, corresponding to the pK_a of H_2CO_3 ($K_a = 4.3 \times 10^{-7}$; p$K_a = 6.37$). Region V starts with the second equivalence point, as all of the HCO_3^- is finally converted to H_2CO_3. Again, a rapid change in pH is observed near the equivalence point (the point between regions IV and V) as acid is added.

The titrations of the acidic and basic amino acids (which have acidic or basic side chains, respectively) will show curves similar to the one shown in Figure 10.12. But rather than two equivalence points, there will in fact be three: one corresponding to the titration of the carboxyl group and a second corresponding to the titration of the amino group, both of which are attached to the central carbon, as well as a third corresponding to either the acidic or basic side chain.

Buffers

A **buffer solution** consists of a mixture of a weak acid and its salt (which is composed of its conjugate base and a cation) or a mixture of a weak base and its salt (which is composed of its conjugate acid and an anion). Two examples of buffers that are common in the laboratory—and commonly tested on the MCAT—are a solution of acetic acid (CH_3COOH) and its salt, sodium acetate ($CH_3COO^-Na^+$), and a solution of ammonia (NH_3) and its salt, ammonium chloride ($NH_4^+Cl^-$). The acetic acid/sodium acetate solution is considered an acid buffer, and the ammonium chloride/ammonia solution is a base buffer. Buffer solutions have the useful property of resisting changes in pH when small amounts of acid or base are added. Consider a buffer solution of acetic acid and sodium acetate: (Note: The sodium ion has not been included because it is not involved in the acid–base reaction.)

$$CH_3COOH\ (aq) + H_2O\ (l) \rightleftharpoons H_3O^+\ (aq) + CH_3COO^-\ (aq)$$

When a small amount of strong base, such as NaOH, is added to the buffer, the OH^- ions from the NaOH react with the H_3O^+ ions present in the solution; subsequently, more acetic acid dissociates (the system shifts to the right), restoring the $[H_3O^+]$. The weak acid component of the buffer thereby serves to neutralize the strong base that has been added. The resulting increase in the concentration of the acetate ion (the conjugate base) does not create nearly as large an increase in hydroxide ions as the unbuffered NaOH would. Thus, the addition of the strong base does not result in a significant increase in $[OH^-]$ and does not appreciably change the pH.

Likewise, when a small amount of HCl is added to the buffer, H^+ ions from the HCl react with the acetate ions to form acetic acid. Acetic acid is weaker than the added hydrochloric acid (which has been neutralized by the acetate ions), so the increased concentration of acetic acid does not significantly contribute to the hydrogen ion concentration in the solution. Because the buffer maintains $[H^+]$ at approximately constant values, the pH of the solution is relatively unchanged.

The Bicarbonate Buffer System

In the human body, one of the most important buffers is the H_2CO_3/HCO_3^- conjugate pair in the plasma component of the blood, called the **bicarbonate buffer system**. Specifically, carbonic acid (H_2CO_3) and its conjugate base, bicarbonate (HCO_3^-), form a weak acid buffer for maintaining the pH of the blood within a fairly narrow physiological range. CO_2 (*g*), one of the waste products of cellular respiration, also has low solubility in aqueous solutions. The majority of the CO_2 transported from peripheral tissues to the lungs (where it will be exhaled out) is dissolved in the plasma in a "disguised" form through the bicarbonate buffer system. CO_2 (*g*) and water react in the following manner:

$$CO_2\ (g) + H_2O\ (l) \rightleftharpoons H_2CO_3\ (aq) \rightleftharpoons H^+\ (aq) + HCO_3^-\ (aq)$$

The bicarbonate buffer system is tied to the respiratory system. In conditions of metabolic acidosis (production of excess plasma H^+ not caused by the respiratory system itself), the breathing rate will increase to compensate and blow off a greater amount of carbon dioxide gas; this causes the system to shift to the left, thereby reducing $[H^+]$ and buffering against dramatic and dangerous changes to the blood pH. It is interesting to note that the bicarbonate buffer system ($pK_a = 6.37$) maintains a pH around 7.4, which is actually slightly outside the optimal buffering capacity of

REAL WORLD

A number of conditions can affect the delicate pH balance of tissues in the body, including chronic obstructive pulmonary disease (COPD), renal tubular acidosis (RTA), diabetic ketoacidosis (DKA), lactic acidosis, metabolic diseases, poisonings and ingestions, and hyperventilation. The buffer system must be well maintained to mitigate these changes.

the system. Buffers have a narrow range of optimal activity ($pK_a \pm 1$). This actually makes sense—it is far more common for acidemia (too much acid in the blood) to occur than alkalemia (too much base in the blood). As acidemia becomes more severe, the buffer system actually becomes more effective and more resistant to further lowering of the pH.

The Henderson–Hasselbalch Equation

The **Henderson–Hasselbalch equation** is used to estimate the pH or pOH of a buffer solution. For a weak acid buffer solution:

$$\text{pH} = \text{p}K_a + \log \frac{[\text{A}^-]}{[\text{HA}]}$$

Equation 10.9

where $[\text{A}^-]$ is the concentration of the conjugate base and [HA] is the concentration of the weak acid. Note that when [conjugate base] = [weak acid], the pH = pK_a because log (1) = 0. This occurs at the half-equivalence points in a titration, and buffering capacity is optimal at this pH.

Likewise, for a weak base buffer solution:

$$\text{pOH} = \text{p}K_b + \log \frac{[\text{B}^+]}{[\text{BOH}]}$$

Equation 10.10

where $[\text{B}^+]$ is the concentration of conjugate acid and [BOH] is the concentration of the weak base. Similar to acid buffers, pOH = pK_b when [conjugate acid] = [weak base]. Buffering capacity is optimal at this pOH.

The Henderson–Hasselbalch equation is, in reality, just a rearrangement of the acid (or base) dissociation constant:

$$K_a = \frac{[\text{H}_3\text{O}^+][\text{A}^-]}{[\text{HA}]}$$

$$-\log K_a = -\log \frac{[\text{H}_3\text{O}^+][\text{A}^-]}{[\text{HA}]}$$

$$-\log K_a = -\log [\text{H}_3\text{O}^+] - \log \frac{[\text{A}^-]}{[\text{HA}]}$$

$$\text{p}K_a = \text{pH} - \log \frac{[\text{A}^-]}{[\text{HA}]}$$

$$\text{pH} = \text{p}K_a + \log \frac{[\text{A}^-]}{[\text{HA}]}$$

One subtlety of buffer systems and Henderson–Hasselbalch calculations that usually goes unnoticed or is misunderstood by students is the effect of changing the concentrations of the conjugate pair but not changing the ratio of their concentrations. Clearly, changing the ratio of the conjugate base to the acid will lead to a change in the pH of the buffer solution. But what about changing the concentrations while maintaining a constant ratio? What would happen if the concentrations of both the acid and its conjugate base were doubled? While the pH would not change, the **buffering capacity**—the ability to which the system can resist changes in pH—has doubled. In other words, addition of a small amount of acid or base to this system will now cause even less deviation in the pH. As mentioned earlier, the buffering capacity is generally maintained within 1 pH unit of the pK_a value.

Example: What is the pH of a solution made from 1 L of 0.05 *M* acetic acid (CH_3COOH, $K_a = 1.8 \times 10^{-5}$) mixed with 500 mL of 1 *M* acetate (CH_3COO^-)?

Solution: First, determine the concentrations of acetic acid and acetate in the final solution. Because two solutions were mixed, there will be some dilution of both the acetic acid and acetate.

$$N_{i,CH_3COOH}V_{i,CH_3COOH} = N_{f,CH_3COOH}V_{f,CH_3COOH} \rightarrow N_{f,CH_3COOH} = \frac{N_{i,CH_3COOH}V_{i,CH_3COOH}}{V_{f,CH_3COOH}}$$

$$N_{f,CH_3COOH} = \frac{(0.05\ N)(1\ L)}{(1.5\ L)} = 0.033\ N$$

$$N_{i,CH_3COO^-}V_{i,CH_3COO^-} = N_{f,CH_3COO^-}V_{f,CH_3COO^-} \rightarrow N_{f,CH_3COO^-} = \frac{N_{i,CH_3COO^-}V_{i,CH_3COO^-}}{V_{f,CH_3COO^-}}$$

$$N_{f,CH_3COO^-} = \frac{(1\ N)(0.5\ L)}{(1.5\ L)} = 0.33\ N$$

Then, use the Henderson-Hasselbalch equation.

$$pH = pK_a + \log\frac{[A^-]}{[HA]} = -\log(1.8 \times 10^{-5}) + \log\frac{0.33\ N}{0.033\ N}$$

$$pH \approx 4.82 + 1 = 5.82\ (\text{actual} = 5.74)$$

MCAT CONCEPT CHECK 10.4

Before you move on, assess your understanding of the material with these questions.

1. Describe each of the following parts of a titration curve:
   - Buffering region:

   ____

   - Half-equivalence point:

   ____

   - Equivalence point:

   ____

   - Endpoint:

   ____

2. For a reaction involving a strong base and a weak acid, which of the following indicators would be best to indicate the endpoint of the titration? (Circle the correct answer.)
   - Phenolphthalein ($pK_a = 9.7$)
   - Bromothymol blue ($pK_a = 7.1$)
   - Bromocresol green ($pK_a = 4.7$)
   - Methyl yellow ($pK_a = 3.3$)

3. In which part of the pH range (acidic, basic, or neutral) will the equivalence points fall for each of the following titrations?
   - Strong acid + weak base:

   ____

   - Strong base + weak acid:

   ____

   - Strong acid + strong base:

   ____

   - Weak acid + weak base:

   ____

4. What is the purpose of a buffer solution?

   ____

5. What are the pH and pOH of a solution containing 5 mL of 5 *M* benzoic acid ($K_a = 6.3 \times 10^{-5}$) and 100 mL of 0.005 *M* benzoate solution?

   ____

Conclusion

In this chapter, we have reviewed the important principles of acid–base chemistry. We clarified the differences among the three definitions of acids and bases, including the nomenclature of some common Arrhenius acids. We investigated important properties of acids and bases, including the important acid–base behavior of water (autoionization) and hydrogen ion equilibria. We explained the mathematics of the pH and pOH logarithmic scales and demonstrated a useful Test Day shortcut for approximating the logarithmic value of hydrogen ion or hydroxide ion concentrations. Strong acids and bases are defined as compounds that completely dissociate in aqueous solutions, and weak acids and bases are compounds that only partially dissociate (to an equilibrium state). We discussed neutralization and salt formation upon reaction of acids and bases, and finally, we applied our fundamental understanding of acid–base reactivity to titrations and buffer systems. Titrations are useful for determining the concentration of a known acid or base solution. Weak acid and weak base buffers are useful for minimizing changes in pH upon addition of a strong acid or base.

You've just accomplished a major task in the overall effort to earn points on Test Day. It's okay if you didn't understand everything on this first pass. Go back and review the concepts that were challenging for you and then complete the questions at the end of the chapter and MCAT practice passages to test your knowledge. Don't be alarmed if you find yourself reviewing parts or all of a chapter a second or third time—repetition is the key to success.

You are now two chapters away from completing this review of general chemistry. While we don't want to offer our congratulations prematurely, we want to acknowledge all the hard work you've invested in this process. Keep it up: success on Test Day is within your reach!

GO ONLINE

You've reviewed the content, now test your knowledge and critical thinking skills by completing a test-like passage set in your online resources!

CONCEPT SUMMARY

Definitions

- **Arrhenius acids** dissociate to produce an excess of hydrogen ions in solution. **Arrhenius bases** dissociate to produce an excess of hydroxide ions in solution.
- **Brønsted–Lowry acids** are species that can donate hydrogen ions. **Brønsted–Lowry bases** are species that can accept hydrogen ions.
- **Lewis acids** are electron-pair acceptors. **Lewis bases** are electron-pair donors.
- All Arrhenius acids and bases are Brønsted–Lowry acids and bases, and all Brønsted–Lowry acids and bases are Lewis acids and bases; however, the converse of these statements is not necessarily true (that is, not all Lewis acids and bases are Brønsted–Lowry acids and bases, and not all Brønsted–Lowry acids and bases are Arrhenius acids and bases).
- **Amphoteric** species are those that can behave as an acid or base. **Amphiprotic** species are amphoteric species that specifically can behave as a Brønsted–Lowry acid or Brønsted–Lowry base.
  - Water is a classic example of an amphoteric, amphiprotic species—it can accept a hydrogen ion to become a hydronium ion, or it can donate a hydrogen ion to become a hydroxide ion.
  - Conjugate species of polyvalent acids and bases can also behave as amphoteric and amphiprotic species.

Properties

- The **water dissociation constant,** K_w, is 10^{-14} at 298 K. Like other equilibrium constants, K_w is only affected by changes in temperature.
- **pH** and **pOH** can be calculated given the concentrations of H_3O^+ and OH^- ions, respectively. In aqueous solutions, pH + pOH = 14 at 298 K.
- **Strong acids and bases** completely dissociate in solution.
- **Weak acids and bases** do not completely dissociate in solution and have corresponding **dissociation constants** (K_a and K_b, respectively).
- In the Brønsted–Lowry definition, acids have conjugate bases that are formed when the acid is deprotonated. Bases have conjugate acids that are formed when the base is protonated.
  - Strong acids and bases have very weak (**inert**) conjugates.
  - Weak acids and bases have weak conjugates.
- **Neutralization reactions** form salts and (sometimes) water.

Polyvalence and Normality

- An **equivalent** is defined as one mole of the species of interest.
- In acid–base chemistry, **normality** is the concentration of acid or base equivalents in solution.
- **Polyvalent** acids and bases are those that can donate or accept multiple electrons. The normality of a solution containing a polyvalent species is the molarity of the acid or base times the number of protons it can donate or accept.

Titration and Buffers

- **Titrations** are used to determine the concentration of a known reactant in a solution.
  - The **titrant** has a known concentration and is added slowly to the titrand to reach the equivalence point.
  - The **titrand** has an unknown concentration but a known volume.
- The **half-equivalence point** is the midpoint of the **buffering region**, in which half of the titrant has been protonated (or deprotonated); thus, $[HA] = [A^-]$ and a buffer is formed.
- The **equivalence point** is indicated by the steepest slope in a titration curve; it is reached when the number of acid equivalents in the original solution equals the number of base equivalents added, or vice-versa.
  - Strong acid and strong base titrations have equivalence points at $pH = 7$.
  - Weak acid and strong base titrations have equivalence points at $pH > 7$.
  - Weak base and strong acid titrations have equivalence points at $pH < 7$.
  - Weak acid and weak base titrations can have equivalence points above or below 7, depending on the relative strength of the acid and base.
- **Indicators** are weak acids or bases that display different colors in their protonated and deprotonated forms.
  - The indicator chosen for a titration should have a pK_a close to the pH of the expected equivalence point.
  - The **endpoint** of a titration is when the indicator reaches its final color.
- Multiple buffering regions and equivalence points are observed in polyvalent acid and base titrations.
- **Buffer solutions** consist of a mixture of a weak acid and its conjugate salt or a weak base and its conjugate salt; they resist large fluctuations in pH.
- **Buffering capacity** refers to the ability of a buffer to resist changes in pH; maximal buffering capacity is seen within 1 pH point of the pK_a of the acid in the buffer solution.
- The **Henderson–Hasselbalch equation** quantifies the relationship between pH and pK_a for weak acids and between pOH and pK_b for weak bases; when a solution is optimally buffered, $pH = pK_a$ and $pOH = pK_b$.

ANSWERS TO CONCEPT CHECKS

10.1

1.

Definition	Acid	Base
Arrhenius	Dissociates to form excess H^+ in solution	Dissociates to form excess OH^- in solution
Brønsted–Lowry	H^+ donor	H^+ acceptor
Lewis	Electron pair acceptor	Electron pair donor

2.

Anion	Acid Formula	Acid Name
$\mathbf{MnO_4^-}$	$HMnO_4$	Permanganic acid
Titanate ($\mathbf{TiO_2^{2-}}$)	H_2TiO_3	Titanic acid
$\mathbf{I^-}$	HI	Hydroiodic acid
$\mathbf{IO_4^-}$	HIO_4	Periodic acid

3.

Reaction	Amphoteric Reactant	Amphiprotic? (Y or N)
$HCO_3^- + HBr \rightarrow H_2CO_3 + Br^-$	HCO_3^-	Yes
$3\ HCl + Al(OH)_3 \rightarrow AlCl_3 + 3\ H_2O$	$Al(OH)_3$	No
$2\ HBr + ZnO \rightarrow ZnBr_2 + H_2O$	ZnO	No

10.2

1. An amphoteric species can act as an acid or a base.
2. High K_a indicates a strong acid, which will dissociate completely in solution. Having a K_a slightly greater than water means the acid is a weak acid with minimal dissociation.
3. High K_b indicates a strong base, which will dissociate completely in solution. Having a K_b slightly greater than water means the base is a weak base with minimal dissociation.

4.

pH	$[H_3O^+]$	pOH	$[OH^-]$	Acid or Base?
4	10^{-4} *M*	10	10^{-10} *M*	Acid
3.05	8.89×10^{-4} *M*	10.95	1.12×10^{-11} *M*	Acid
8.81	1.55×10^{-9} *M*	5.19	6.46×10^{-6} *M*	Base
8.27	5.32×10^{-9} *M*	5.73	1.88×10^{-6} *M*	Base

(Note: Exact answers are provided; your rounded answers should be relatively close to those listed here.)

5. $K_a \times K_b = K_w$

6.

Reaction	Acid	Base	Conjugate Acid	Conjugate Base
$H_2CO_3 + H_2O \rightleftharpoons HCO_3^- + H_3O^+$	H_2CO_3	H_2O	H_3O^+	HCO_3^-
$H_2PO_4^- + H_2O \rightleftharpoons H_3PO_4 + OH^-$	H_2O	$H_2PO_4^-$	H_3PO_4	OH^-

7. $K_a = \dfrac{[CH_3COO^-][H_3O^+]}{[CH_3COOH]} = \dfrac{[x][x]}{[0.2\,M - x]} \approx \dfrac{x^2}{0.2}$. Therefore, $x^2 = 3.6 \times 10^{-6}$ $\rightarrow x \approx 2 \times 10^{-3}$ *M* (actual $= 1.9 \times 10^{-3}$ *M*). Then, pH $= -\log H_3O^+ \approx$ $3 - 0.2 = 2.8$ (actual $= 2.72$)

10.3

1. Acids use moles of H^+ (H_3O^+) as an equivalent. Bases use moles of OH^- as an equivalent.
2. 6 N $Al(OH)_3$; 32 N H_2SO_4

10.4

1. The buffering region occurs when [HA] $\approx$ [A^-] and is the flattest portion of the titration curve (resistant to changes in pH). The half-equivalence point is the center of the buffering region, where [HA] = [A^-]. The equivalence point is the steepest point of the titration curve, and occurs when the equivalents of acid present equal the equivalents of base added (or vice-versa). The endpoint is the pH at which an indicator turns its final color.
2. Phenolphthalein would be the preferred indicator for this titration.
3. A strong acid and weak base have an equivalence point in the acidic range. A strong base and weak acid have an equivalence point in the basic range. A strong acid and strong base have an equivalence point at pH = 7 (neutral). A weak acid and weak base can have an equivalence point in the acidic, neutral, or basic range, depending on the relative strengths of the acid and base.
4. A buffer solution is designed to resist changes in pH and has optimal buffering capacity within 1 pH point from its pK_a.

5. Recall from section 10.2 on Properties that the concentrations of the conjugate acid and conjugate base in the final solution must first be calculated due to the dilution from mixing the two solutions together. The calculation below follows that step, but leaves the values unsolved for so that some of their components can be cancelled and simplified:

$$\text{pH} = \text{p}K_a + \log\frac{[\text{A}^-]}{[\text{HA}]} = -\log\left(6.3\times10^{-5}\right) + \log\frac{\left[\frac{(0.005\text{ N})(100\text{ mL})}{(105\text{ mL})}\right]}{\left[\frac{(5\ N)(5\text{ mL})}{(105\text{ mL})}\right]}$$

$$\text{pH} \approx 4.37 + \log\frac{(0.005\text{ N})(100\text{ mL})}{(5\text{ N})(5\text{ mL})} = 4.37 + \log\frac{0.5}{25} = 4.37 + \log\left(2\times10^{-2}\right)$$

$$\approx 4.37 - 1.8 = 2.57\ (\text{actual} = 2.50)$$

$$\text{pOH} \approx 14 - 2.57 = 11.43\ (\text{actual} = 11.5)$$

SCIENCE MASTERY ASSESSMENT EXPLANATIONS

1. **D**

A Brønsted–Lowry base is defined as a proton acceptor. Ammonia, fluoride, and water—**(A)**, **(B)**, and **(C)**, respectively—each accept a proton. **(D)**, HNO_2, is a far better Brønsted–Lowry acid, donating a proton to a solution.

2. **B**

First, convert the concentration to $5 \times 10^{-3}\ M$. Next, because sulfuric acid is a strong acid, we can assume that, for the majority of sulfuric acid molecules (although not all), both protons will dissociate. The concentration of hydrogen ions is therefore $2 \times 5 \times 10^{-3}$, or 10^{-2}. The equation for pH is $\text{pH} = -\log\,[\text{H}^+]$. If $[\text{H}^+] = 10^{-2}\ M$, then $\text{pH} = 2$.

3. **A**

Answering this question is simply a matter of knowing nomenclature. Acids ending in *–ic* are derivatives of anions ending in *–ate,* while acids ending in *–ous* are derivatives of anions ending in *–ite*. ClO_3^-, **(B)**, is chlorate because it has more oxygen than the other commonly occurring ion, ClO_2^-, which is named chlorite. Therefore, $HClO_3$ is chloric acid. $HClO_2$, **(C)**, represents chlorous acid. HClO, **(D)**, represents hypochlorous acid.

4. **B**

Soluble hydroxides of Group IA and IIA metals are strong bases, eliminating **(A)** and **(D)**. **(B)** and **(C)** are both weak bases; however, methylamine contains an alkyl group, which is electron-donating. This increases the electron density on the nitrogen in methylamine, making it a stronger (Lewis) base. Therefore, ammonia is the weakest base.

5. **A**

The gram equivalent weight of an acid is equal to its molecular weight divided by the equivalents of H^+ that the acid can produce. Phosphoric acid, H_3PO_4, has three dissociable hydrogen atoms and can thus produce 3 equivalents of protons. Its molecular weight is 98 g/mol. Thus, the gram equivalent weight is (98 g/mol)/(3 equivalents/mol) = 32.6 grams/equivalent, matching **(A)**.

6. **D**

The question is asking for pH, but because of the information given, we must first find the pOH and then subtract it from 14 to get the pH. Use the Henderson–Hasselbalch equation:

$$\text{pOH} = \text{p}K_\text{b} + \log\frac{[\text{conjugate acid}]}{[\text{base}]} = 3.45 + \log\frac{70\ \text{m}M}{712\ \text{m}M}$$

$$\approx 3.45 + \log\frac{1}{10} = 3.45 - 1 = 2.45$$

If the pOH = 2.45, the pH = 14 − 2.45 = 11.55.

7. **A**

The first $\text{p}K_\text{a}$ in this curve can be estimated by eye. It is located halfway between the starting point (when no base had yet been added) and the first equivalence point (the first steep portion of the graph, around 15 mL). This point is at approximately 7–8 mL on the *x*-axis, which corresponds to a pH of approximately 1.9. Notice that this region experiences very little change in pH, which is the defining characteristic of a buffer region.

8. **C**

The second equivalence point is the midpoint of the second steep increase in slope. This corresponds to approximately pH = 5.9.

9. **B**

The value of the second pK_a is found at the midpoint between the first and second equivalence points. In this curve, that corresponds to pH = 4.1. Just like the first pK_a, it is in the center of a flat buffering region.

10. **B**

Gram equivalent weight is the weight (in grams) that releases 1 acid or base equivalent from a compound. Because H_3PO_4 contains 3 protons, we find the gram equivalent weight by dividing the mass of one mole of the species by 3. The molar mass of phosphoric acid is 98 $\frac{g}{mol}$, so the gram equivalent weight is 32.7 g.

11. **D**

This question requires the application of the acid dissociation constant. Weak acids do not dissociate completely; therefore, all three species that appear in the balanced equation will be present in solution. Hydrogen ions and conjugate base anions dissociate in equal amounts, so $[H^+] = [XO_2^-]$. If the initial concentration of HXO_2 was 2 M and some amount x dissociates, we will have x amount of H_3O^+ and XO_2^- at equilibrium, with 2 $M - x$ amount of HXO_2 at equilibrium.

$$K_a = \frac{[H_3O^+][XO_2^-]}{[HXO_2]} = \frac{(x)(x)}{2\,M - x} \approx \frac{x^2}{2}$$

Note that x was considered negligible when added or subtracted, per usual. Solving for x, we get:

$$\frac{x^2}{2} = 3.2\times10^{-5} \rightarrow x^2 = 6.4\times10^{-5} = 64\times10^{-6}$$

$$\rightarrow x = 8\times10^{-3}\ M$$

12. **C**

A higher K_a implies a stronger acid. Weak acids usually have a K_a that is several orders of magnitude below 1. The pK_a of a compound is the pH at which there are equal concentrations of acid and conjugate base; the pK_a of this compound would be $-\log 1 = 0$. With such a low pK_a, this compound must be an acid. Therefore, the pH of any concentration of this compound must be below 7.

13. **D**

An amphoteric species is one that can act either as an acid or a base, depending on its environment. Proton transfers are classic oxidation–reduction reactions, so **(A)** and **(B)** are true. **(C)** is true because many amphoteric species, such as water and bicarbonate, can either donate or accept a proton. **(D)** is false, and thus the correct answer because amphoteric species can be either polar or nonpolar in nature.

14. **C**

NaOH is a strong base; as such, there will be $1.2 \times 10^{-5}\ M\ OH^-$ in solution. Based on this information alone, the pOH must be between 4 and 5, and the pH must be between 9 and 10. Using the shortcut, pOH $\approx 5 - 0.12 = 4.88$. pH $= 14 -$ pOH $= 9.12$ (actual $= 9.08$).

15. **C**

Use the equivalence point equation: $N_aV_a = N_bV_b$. $Ba(OH)_2$ can dissociate to give two hydroxide ions, so its normality is 2 $M \times 2 = 4$ N. H_3PO_4 can dissociate to give three hydronium ions, so its normality is 6 $M \times 3 = 18$ N. Plugging into the equation, we get $(18\text{ N})(4\text{ L}) = (4\text{ N})(V_b)$. Therefore, V_b is 18 L.

Consult your online resources for additional practice. GO ONLINE

EQUATIONS TO REMEMBER

(10.1) **Autoionization constant for water:** $K_w = [H_3O^+][OH^-] = 10^{-14}$ at 25°C (298 K)

(10.2) **Definitions of pH and pOH:** $\text{pH} = -\log[H^+] = \log \frac{1}{[H^+]}$

$$\text{pOH} = -\log[OH^-] = \log \frac{1}{[OH^-]}$$

(10.3) **Relationship of pH and pOH at 298 K:** $\text{pH} + \text{pOH} = 14$

(10.4) **p scale value approximation:** p value $\approx m - 0.n$

(10.5) **Acid dissociation constant:** $K_a = \frac{[H_3O^+][A^-]}{[HA]}$

(10.6) **Base dissociation constant:** $K_b = \frac{[B^+][OH^-]}{[BOH]}$

(10.7) **Relationship of K_a and K_b at 298 K:** $K_{a,\text{acid}} \times K_{b,\text{conjugate base}} = K_w = 10^{-14}$;

$$K_{b,\text{base}} \times K_{a,\text{conjugate acid}} = K_w = 10^{-14}$$

(10.8) **Equivalence point:** $N_a V_a = N_b V_b$

(10.9) **Henderson–Hasselbalch equation (acid buffer):** $\text{pH} = \text{p}K_a + \log \frac{[A^-]}{[HA]}$

(10.10) **Henderson–Hasselbalch equation (base buffer):** $\text{pOH} = \text{p}K_b + \log \frac{[B^+]}{[BOH]}$

SHARED CONCEPTS

Biology Chapter 6
The Respiratory System

Biology Chapter 10
Homeostasis

General Chemistry Chapter 3
Bonding and Chemical Interactions

General Chemistry Chapter 9
Solutions

Organic Chemistry Chapter 4
Analyzing Organic Reactions

Physics and Math Chapter 10
Mathematics

CHAPTER 11

OXIDATION–REDUCTION REACTIONS

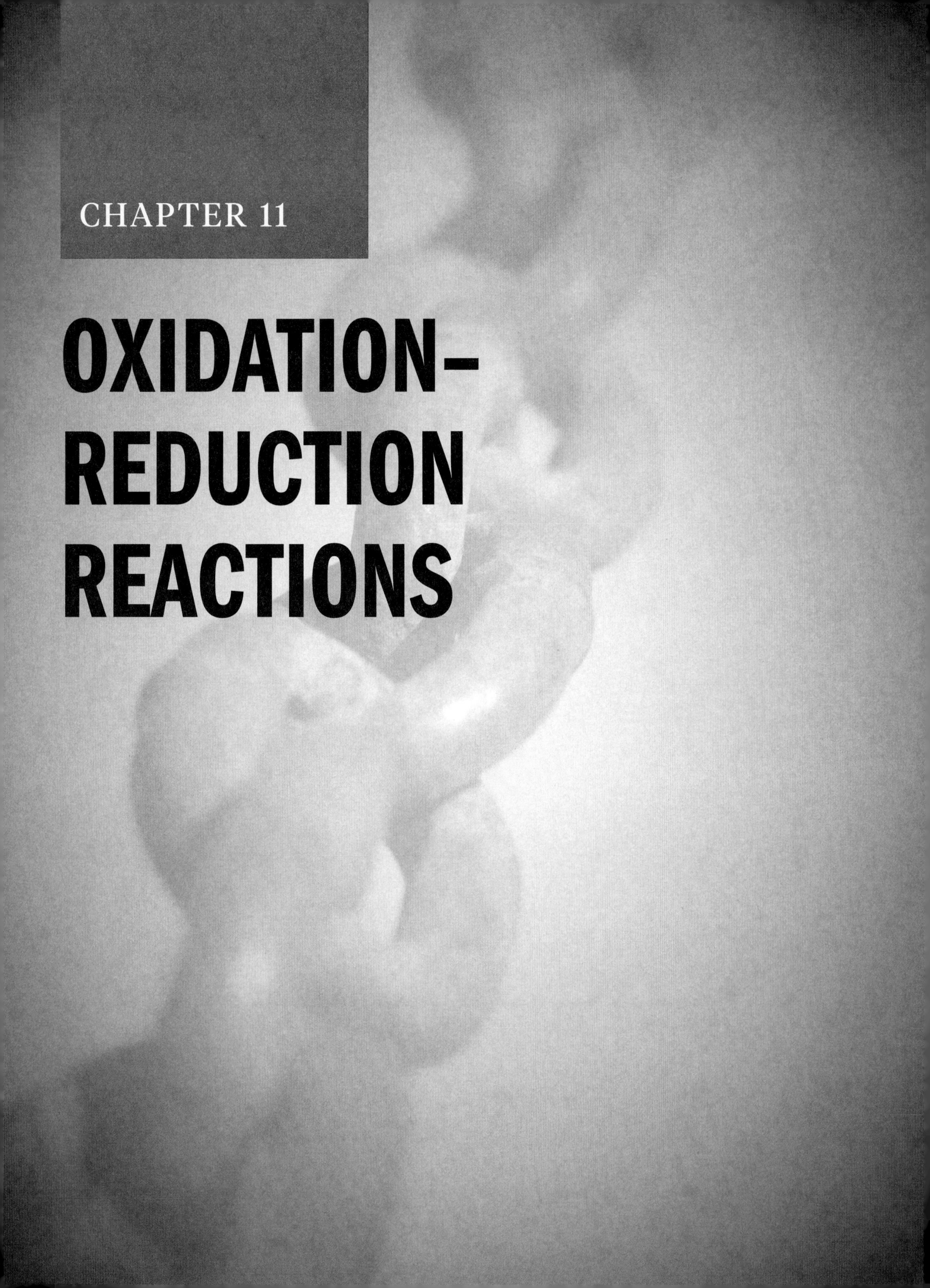

SCIENCE MASTERY ASSESSMENT

Every pre-med knows this feeling: there is so much content I have to know for the MCAT! How do I know what to do first or what's important?

While the high-yield badges throughout this book will help you identify the most important topics, this Science Mastery Assessment is another tool in your MCAT prep arsenal. This quiz (which can also be taken in your online resources) and the guidance below will help ensure that you are spending the appropriate amount of time on this chapter based on your personal strengths and weaknesses. Don't worry though—skipping something now does not mean you'll never study it. Later on in your prep, as you complete full-length tests, you'll uncover specific pieces of content that you need to review and can come back to these chapters as appropriate.

How to Use This Assessment

If you answer 0–7 questions correctly:

Spend about 1 hour to read this chapter in full and take limited notes throughout. Follow up by reviewing **all** quiz questions to ensure that you now understand how to solve each one.

If you answer 8–11 questions correctly:

Spend 20–40 minutes reviewing the quiz questions. Beginning with the questions you missed, read and take notes on the corresponding subchapters. For questions you answered correctly, ensure your thinking matches that of the explanation and you understand why each choice was correct or incorrect.

If you answer 12–15 questions correctly:

Spend less than 20 minutes reviewing all questions from the quiz. If you missed any, then include a quick read-through of the corresponding subchapters, or even just the relevant content within a subchapter, as part of your question review. For questions you answered correctly, ensure your thinking matches that of the explanation and review the Concept Summary at the end of the chapter.

1. Consider the following equation:

$$6\ Na\ (s) + 2\ NH_3\ (aq) \rightarrow 2\ Na_3N\ (s) + 3\ H_2\ (g)$$

Which species acts as an oxidizing agent?

A. Na
B. N in NH_3
C. H in NH_3
D. H_2

2. How many electrons are involved in the following half-reaction after it is balanced?

$$Cr_2O_7^{2-} + H^+ + e^- \rightarrow Cr^{2+} + H_2O$$

A. 2
B. 8
C. 12
D. 16

3. Lithium aluminum hydride ($LiAlH_4$) is often used in laboratories because of its tendency to donate a hydride ion. Which of the following roles would lithium aluminum hydride likely play in a reaction?

A. Strong reducing agent only
B. Strong oxidizing agent only
C. Both a strong reducing agent and strong oxidizing agent
D. Neither a strong reducing agent nor a strong oxidizing agent

4. What is the oxidation number of chlorine in NaClO?

A. −1
B. 0
C. +1
D. +2

5. The following electronic configurations represent elements in their neutral form. Which element is the strongest oxidizing agent?

A. $1s^22s^22p^63s^23p^64s^2$
B. $1s^22s^22p^63s^23p^64s^23d^5$
C. $1s^22s^22p^63s^23p^64s^23d^{10}4p^1$
D. $1s^22s^22p^63s^23p^64s^23d^{10}4p^5$

6. Which of the following is the correct net ionic reaction for the reaction of copper with silver(I) nitrate?

A. $Cu + AgNO_3 \rightarrow Cu(NO_3)_2 + Ag$
B. $Cu + 2\ Ag^+ + 2\ NO_3^- \rightarrow Cu^{2+} + 2\ NO_3^- + 2\ Ag$
C. $2\ Ag^+ + 2\ NO_3^- \rightarrow 2\ NO_3^- + 2\ Ag^+$
D. $Cu + 2\ Ag^+ \rightarrow Cu^{2+} + 2\ Ag$

7. One way to test for the presence of iron in solution is by adding potassium thiocyanate to the solution. The product when this reagent reacts with iron is $FeSCN^{2+}$, which creates a dark red color in solution via the following net ionic equation:

$$Fe^{3+} + SCN^- \rightarrow FeSCN^{2+}$$

How many grams of iron sulfate would be needed to produce 2 moles of $FeSCN^{2+}$?

A. 110 g
B. 220 g
C. 400 g
D. 500 g

8. During the assigning of oxidation numbers, which of the following elements would most likely be determined last?

A. Ar
B. F
C. Sr
D. Ir

9. As methanol is converted to methanal, and then methanoic acid, the oxidation number of the carbon:

A. increases.
B. decreases.
C. increases, then decreases.
D. decreases, then increases.

10. In the compound KH_2PO_4, which element has the highest oxidation number?

A. K
B. H
C. P
D. O

11. If a certain metal has multiple oxidation states, its acidity as an oxide generally increases as the oxidation state increases. Therefore, which of the following tungsten compounds is likely to be the strongest acid?

A. WO_2
B. WO_3
C. W_2O_3
D. W_2O_5

12. Consider the following steps in the reaction between oxalic acid and chlorine:

I. $Cl_2 + H_2O \rightarrow HOCl + Cl^- + H^+$
II. $H_2C_2O_4 \rightarrow H^+ + HC_2O_4^-$
III. $HOCl + HC_2O_4^- \rightarrow H_2O + Cl^- + 2\ CO_2$

Which of these steps, occurring in aqueous solution, is an example of a disproportionation reaction?

A. I only
B. III only
C. I and III only
D. I, II, and III

13. Potentiometry in an oxidation–reduction titration is analogous to performing an acid–base titration with a(n):

A. acidic indicator.
B. basic indicator.
C. pH meter.
D. oxidizing agent.

14. After balancing the following oxidation–reduction reaction, what is the sum of the stoichiometric coefficients of all of the reactants and products?

$$S_8\ (s) + NO_3^-\ (aq) \rightarrow SO_3^{2-}\ (aq) + NO\ (g)$$

A. 4
B. 50
C. 91
D. 115

15. An assay is performed to determine the gold content in a supply of crushed ore. One method for pulling gold out of ore is to react it in a concentrated cyanide (CN^-) solution. The equation is provided below:

$$Au + NaCN + O_2 + H_2O \rightarrow Na[Au(CN)_2] + NaOH$$

An indicator is used during this reaction, and approximately 100 mL of a 2 *M* NaCN solution is used to reach the endpoint. How many moles of Au are present in the crushed ore?

A. 0.01 mol
B. 0.02 mol
C. 0.10 mol
D. 0.20 mol

Answer Key

1. **C**
2. **B**
3. **A**
4. **C**
5. **D**
6. **D**
7. **C**
8. **D**
9. **A**
10. **C**
11. **B**
12. **A**
13. **C**
14. **D**
15. **C**

Detailed explanations can be found at the end of the chapter.

CHAPTER 11

OXIDATION–REDUCTION REACTIONS

In This Chapter

CHAPTER PROFILE

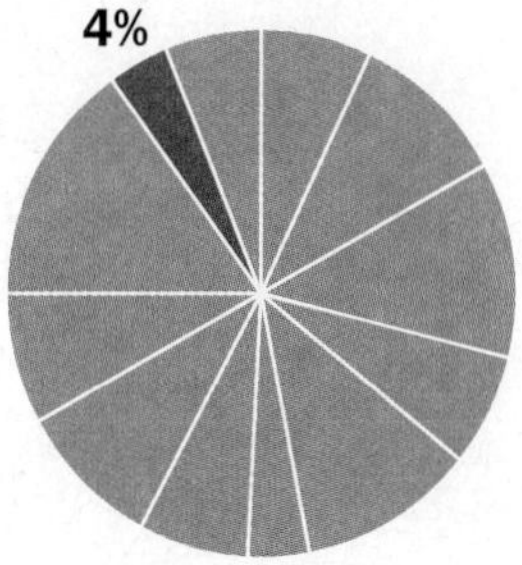

The content in this chapter should be relevant to about 4% of all questions about general chemistry on the MCAT.

This chapter covers material from the following AAMC content categories:

4E: Atoms, nuclear decay, electronic structure, and atomic chemical behavior

5A: Unique nature of water and its solutions

Introduction

You're on a night call in the emergency department (ED) when a 5-month-old infant patient's chart appears on your screen. You click through the triage notes and read what the caregiver reports: *poor sucking ability and loss of head control and motor skills*. You're puzzled by the findings and the previous ED admissions of lactic acidosis. You suspect diabetic ketoacidosis (DKA), liver, or kidney diseases—and possibly even poisoning—but nothing seems to fit. Minutes later, the child is brought into the examination room and does not stop crying. Over the course of an hour, another episode of lactic acidosis develops. The child is eventually admitted to the neonatal intensive care unit for long-term care.

Later, you ask the neonatologist about the patient. They point you to the charts and a genetic test performed shortly after birth. The child was diagnosed with Leigh disease, an extremely rare mitochondrial disorder. In Leigh disease, a number of key mitochondrial enzymes are disrupted and the process of oxidative phosphorylation is never achieved. Specifically, some of the most important enzymes that catalyze oxidation–reduction reactions, such as the *pyruvate dehydrogenase complex* and *succinate dehydrogenase complex*, are affected. When pyruvate cannot be oxidized to acetyl-CoA, it is instead fermented to lactic acid.

In biological systems, oxidation is coincident with the loss of electrons, sometimes in the form of hydrogen (dehydrogenation). The enzymes that catalyze these oxidations are called *dehydrogenases*. Many other macromolecules besides enzymes, such as vitamins, also carry out their functions by oxidizing or reducing other compounds. Iron in hemoglobin likewise undergoes rounds of oxidation and reduction as it carries oxygen from the lungs to tissues.

In this chapter, we focus our attention on the movement of electrons in chemical reactions. Such reactions are called oxidation–reduction (redox) reactions because they always occur in pairs. Oxidation–reduction reactions are particularly important because they tie into a number of topics in organic chemistry and biochemistry. In fact, Chapters 5 through 10 of *MCAT Organic Chemistry Review* and Chapters 9 through 11 of *MCAT Biochemistry Review* all touch on oxidation–reduction reactions in different sets of molecules.

11.1 Oxidation-Reduction Reactions

LEARNING OBJECTIVES

After Chapter 11.1, you will be able to:

- Separate a redox reaction into oxidation and reduction half-reactions
- Balance a redox reaction
- Identify the oxidizing agent, reducing agent, and relevant oxidation states for a given reaction: $SnCl_2 + PbCl_4 \rightarrow SnCl_4 + PbCl_2$

Reactions that involve the transfer of electrons from one chemical species to another can be classified as **oxidation–reduction (redox) reactions**.

Oxidation and Reduction

MNEMONIC

Redox reactions: choose one of the mnemonics and stick with it!

- **OIL RIG**: **O**xidation **I**s **L**oss of electrons, **R**eduction **I**s **G**ain of electrons.
- **LEO** the lion says **GER**: **L**oss of **E**lectrons is **O**xidation, **G**ain of **E**lectrons is **R**eduction.
- **LEORA** says **GEROA**: **L**oss of **E**lectrons is **O**xidation (**R**educing **A**gent), **G**ain of **E**lectrons is **R**eduction (**O**xidizing **A**gent).

The law of conservation of charge states that electrical charge can be neither created nor destroyed. Thus, an isolated loss or gain of electrons cannot occur; **oxidation** (loss of electrons) and **reduction** (gain of electrons) must occur simultaneously, resulting in an electron transfer called a **redox reaction**. An **oxidizing agent** causes another atom in a redox reaction to undergo oxidation and is itself reduced. A **reducing agent** causes the other atom to be reduced and is itself oxidized. There are various mnemonics to remember these terms, as highlighted in the sidebar.

Being familiar with some common oxidizing and reducing agents can save significant time on Test Day, especially in organic chemistry reactions. Some of the commonly used agents on the MCAT are listed in Table 11.1. Note that almost all oxidizing agents contain oxygen or another strongly electronegative element (such as a halogen). Reducing agents often contain metal ions or hydrides (H^-).

OXIDIZING AGENTS	REDUCING AGENTS
O_2	CO
H_2O_2	C
F_2, Cl_2, Br_2, I_2 (halogens)	B_2H_6
H_2SO_4	Sn^{2+} and other pure metals
HNO_3	Hydrazine*
NaClO	Zn(Hg)*
$KMnO_4$*	Lindlar's catalyst*
CrO_3, $Na_2Cr_2O_7$*	$NaBH_4$*
Pyridinium chlorochromate (PCC)*	$LiAlH_4$*
NAD^+, FADH**	NADH, $FADH_2$**

* These oxidizing agents and reducing agents are commonly seen in organic chemistry reactions.

** These and other biochemical redox reagents often act as energy carriers in biochemistry reactions.

Table 11.1 Common Oxidizing and Reducing Agents

Note that biochemical redox reagents such as NAD^+ tend to act as both oxidizing and reducing agents at different times during metabolic pathways. As such, they act as mediators of energy transfer during many metabolic processes, as shown in Figure 11.1.

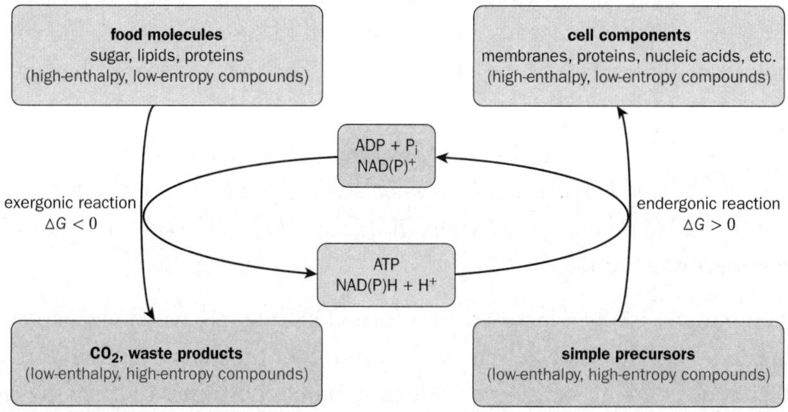

Figure 11.1 Oxidation and Reduction of Biochemical Compounds Serves as a Method of Energy Transfer

On a technical level, the term oxidizing agent or reducing agent is applied specifically to the atom that gains or loses electrons, respectively. However, many science texts will describe the compound as a whole (CrO_3, rather than Cr^{6+}) as the oxidizing or reducing agent.

Assigning Oxidation Numbers

It is important, of course, to know which atom is oxidized and which is reduced. **Oxidation numbers** are assigned to atoms in order to keep track of the redistribution of electrons during chemical reactions. Based on the oxidation numbers of the reactants and products, it is possible to determine how many electrons are gained or lost by each atom.

The oxidation number of an atom in a compound is assigned according to the following rules:

1. *The oxidation number of a free element is zero.* For example, the atoms in N_2, P_4, S_8, and He all have oxidation numbers of zero.
2. *The oxidation number for a monatomic ion is equal to the charge of the ion.* For example, the oxidation numbers for Na^+, Cu^{2+}, Fe^{3+}, Cl^-, and N^{3-} are +1, +2, +3, −1, and −3, respectively.
3. *The oxidation number of each Group IA element in a compound is +1.*
4. *The oxidation number of each Group IIA element in a compound is +2.*
5. *The oxidation number of each Group VIIA element in a compound is −1, except when combined with an element of higher electronegativity.* For example, in HCl, the oxidation number of Cl is −1; in HOCl, however, the oxidation number of Cl is +1.
6. *The oxidation number of hydrogen is usually +1; however, its oxidation number is −1 in compounds with less electronegative elements (Groups IA and IIA).* Hydrogen is +1 in HCl, but −1 in NaH.
7. *In most compounds, the oxidation number of oxygen is −2.* The two exceptions are peroxides (O_2^{2-}), for which the charge on each oxygen is −1, and compounds with more electronegative elements, such as OF_2, in which oxygen has a +2 charge.
8. *The sum of the oxidation numbers of all the atoms present in a neutral compound is zero. The sum of the oxidation numbers of the atoms present in a polyatomic ion is equal to the charge of the ion.* Thus, for (SO_4^{2-}), the sum of the oxidation numbers must be −2.

Oxidation number is often confused with **formal charge**, discussed in Chapter 3 of *MCAT General Chemistry Review*. Both account for the perceived charge on an element, but do so in different ways. Oxidation number assumes unequal division of electrons in bonds, "awarding" the electrons to the more electronegative element. Formal charge, on the other hand, assumes equal division of electrons in bonds, "awarding" one electron to each atom in the bond. In reality, the distribution of electron density lies somewhere between these two extremes. The assigning of oxidation numbers can be seen in Figure 11.2.

BRIDGE

In Chapter 3 of *MCAT General Chemistry Review,* we illustrated that metals form cations and nonmetals form anions. To form a cation, a metal must lose electrons. Therefore, metals like to get oxidized (lose electrons) and act as good reducing agents. Nonmetals, on the other hand, like to get reduced (gain electrons) and act as good oxidizing agents.

MCAT EXPERTISE

Think of the oxidation number as the typical charge of an element based on its group number, metallicity, and general location in the periodic table.

KEY CONCEPT

The conventions of formula writing put cation first and anion second. Thus HCl implies H^+, and NaH implies H^-. Use the way the compound is written on the MCAT along with the periodic table to determine oxidation states.

MCAT EXPERTISE

Don't forget that you can click on "Periodic table" to pull it up on Test Day. Note the trends for assigning oxidation numbers; these general rules will help reduce the need to memorize individual oxidation numbers. Be aware that the transition metals can take on multiple oxidation states and therefore multiple oxidation numbers.

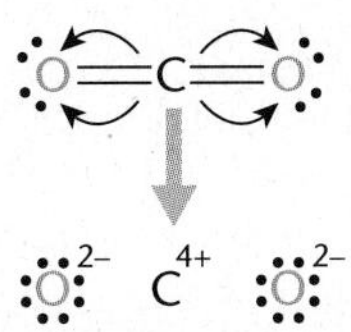

Figure 11.2 Assigning Oxidation Numbers to Carbon Dioxide

When assigning oxidation numbers, start with the known atoms (usually Groups I and II, halides, and oxygen) and use this information to determine the oxidation states of the other atoms. Keep in mind that most transition metals can take on multiple oxidation states. When transition metals are oxidized or reduced, the absorption and emission of light from a metal is altered such that different frequencies are absorbed. For this reason, changes of oxidation state in transition metals usually correspond to a color change.

Example: Assign oxidation numbers to the atoms in the following reaction to determine the oxidizing and reducing agents.

$$SnCl_2 + PbCl_4 \rightarrow SnCl_4 + PbCl_2$$

Solution: All of these species are neutral, so the oxidation numbers of each compound must add up to zero. In $SnCl_2$, tin must have an oxidation number of +2 because there are two chlorines present and each chlorine has an oxidation number of −1. Similarly, the oxidation number of Sn in $SnCl_4$ is +4; the oxidation number of Pb is +4 in $PbCl_4$ and +2 in $PbCl_2$.

The oxidation number of Sn goes from +2 to +4; it loses electrons and thus is oxidized, making it the reducing agent. Because the oxidation number of Pb has decreased from +4 to +2, it gains electrons and is reduced, making it the oxidizing agent. The sum of the charges on both sides of the reaction is equal to zero, so charge has been conserved. Keep in mind that oxidation state also plays a role in nomenclature; the reactants in this reaction would be called tin(II) chloride and lead(IV) chloride.

Balancing Oxidation-Reduction Reactions

By assigning oxidation numbers to the reactants and products, one can determine how many moles of each species are required for conservation of charge and mass, which is necessary to balance the equation. To balance a redox reaction, both the net charge and the number of atoms must be equal on both sides of the equation. The most common method for balancing redox equations is the **half-reaction method**, also known as the **ion–electron method**, in which the equation is separated into two half-reactions—the oxidation part and the reduction part. Each half-reaction is balanced separately, and they are then added to give a balanced overall reaction.

KEY CONCEPT

Oxidizing agents oxidize *other* molecules, but are themselves *reduced*. Reducing agents reduce *other* molecules, but are themselves *oxidized*. If you determine one ion to be an oxidizing agent then the other must be a reducing agent.

MCAT EXPERTISE

Methodical, step-by-step approaches like the half-reaction method are great for the MCAT. Usually, you will not have to go through *all* of these steps before you can narrow down your answer choices and may be able to find the correct answer partway through the problem with a little critical thinking.

Example: Balance this redox reaction using the half-reaction method:

$$MnO_4^- + I^- \rightarrow I_2 + Mn^{2+}$$

Step 1: Separate the two half-reactions.

$$I^- \rightarrow I_2$$
$$MnO_4^- \rightarrow Mn^{2+}$$

Step 2: Balance the atoms of each half-reaction. First, balance all atoms except H and O. Next, in an acidic solution, add H_2O to balance the O atoms and then add H^+ to balance the H atoms. In a basic solution, use OH^- and H_2O to balance the O and H atoms.

$$2\,I^- \rightarrow I_2$$
$$MnO_4^- + 8\,H^+ \rightarrow Mn^{2+} + 4\,H_2O$$

Step 3: Balance the charges of each half-reaction. Add electrons as necessary to one side of the reaction so that the charges are equal on both sides.

$$2\,I^- \rightarrow I_2 + 2\,e^-$$
$$MnO_4^- + 8\,H^+ + 5\,e^- \rightarrow Mn^{2+} + 4\,H_2O$$

Step 4: Both half-reactions must have the same number of electrons so that they cancel each other out in the next step. In this example, you need to multiply the oxidation half-reaction by 5 and the reduction half-reaction by 2.

$$10\,I^- \rightarrow 5\,I_2 + 10\,e^-$$
$$2\,MnO_4^- + 16\,H^+ + 10\,e^- \rightarrow 2\,Mn^{2+} + 8\,H_2O$$

Step 5: Add the half-reactions, canceling out terms that appear on both sides of the reaction arrow.

$$2\,MnO_4^- + 16\,H^+ + 10\,I^- \rightarrow 2\,Mn^{2+} + 5\,I_2 + 8\,H_2O$$

Step 6: Confirm that mass and charge are balanced. There is a +4 net charge on each side of the reaction equation, and the atoms are stoichiometrically balanced.

MCAT CONCEPT CHECK 11.1

Before you move on, assess your understanding of the material with these questions.

1. For each of the reactions below, identify the oxidation states of the relevant atoms, the oxidizing agent, and the reducing agent:

Reaction	Oxidation Numbers	Oxidizing Agent	Reducing Agent
$2\ KI + H_2 \rightarrow 2\ K + 2\ HI$			
$Al + BPO_4 \rightarrow B + AlPO_4$			

2. Identify the oxidation and reduction half-reactions in the following redox reaction:

$$Zn + Cu^{2+} \rightarrow Zn^{2+} + Cu$$

- Oxidation:

- Reduction:

3. Balance the following redox reaction using the half-reaction method:

$$Mg\ (s) + HNO_3\ (aq) \rightarrow Mg^{2+}\ (aq) + NO\ (g)$$

11.2 Net Ionic Equations

LEARNING OBJECTIVES

After Chapter 11.2, you will be able to:

- Identify the element undergoing disproportionation and the oxidation state of the products for a given reaction
- Apply redox reaction principles to balance and solve application-style problems, such as ones that involve redox titrations
- Determine the net ionic equation for a reaction:
$$Zn\ (s) + CuSO_4\ (aq) \rightarrow Cu\ (s) + ZnSO_4\ (aq)$$

When we discussed reaction types in Chapter 4 of *MCAT General Chemistry Review*, we left out the rationale for why certain elements come together and others do not. Now that we have discussed oxidation–reduction reactions, it should be clearer that the gain and loss of electrons drives the formation of many compounds, especially ionic ones. Below, we will revisit many important reaction types and understand their basis in oxidation–reduction reactions.

Overview

In our discussion of acids and bases, we focused only on the presence of protons and hydroxide ions, with little concern for which species actually provided those ions. Similarly, in redox reactions, our focus is on the shifting of electrons more so than the identities of the ions themselves. Consider the following single-displacement reaction:

$$Zn\ (s) + CuSO_4\ (aq) \rightarrow Cu\ (s) + ZnSO_4\ (aq)$$

If we split the various species into all of the ions present, we get the **complete ionic equation**:

$$Zn\ (s) + Cu^{2+}\ (aq) + SO_4^{2-}\ (aq) \rightarrow Cu\ (s) + Zn^{2+}\ (aq) + SO_4^{2-}\ (aq)$$

Note that the sulfate ion is present on both sides of the equation in the same form; this ion is chemically inert during this reaction. In other words, the sulfate is not taking part in the overall reaction but simply remaining in the solution unchanged. We call such species **spectator ions**. Because the sulfate ion is not involved in the oxidation–reduction reaction, we can simplify the reaction to its **net ionic equation**, showing only the species that actually participate in the reaction:

$$Zn\ (s) + Cu^{2+}\ (aq) \rightarrow Cu\ (s) + Zn^{2+}\ (aq)$$

MCAT EXPERTISE

Look for compounds such as polyatomic anions that retain their charge before and after reactions; these are usually spectator ions and will *not* be found in the net ionic equation.

When writing net ionic equations, all aqueous compounds should be split into their constituent ions. Solid salts, on the other hand, should be kept together as a single entity. Let's return to some of the other reactions we have seen previously, including combination, decomposition, combustion, and double-displacement (metathesis) reactions.

Combination Reactions

In **combination reactions**, two or more species come together to form a product. For example:

$$\overset{0}{H_2}\ (g) + \overset{0}{F_2}\ (g) \rightarrow 2\ \overset{+1}{H}\overset{-1}{F}\ (aq)$$

The relevant half-reactions would be:

$$H_2 \rightarrow 2\ H^+ + 2\ e^-$$

$$F_2 + 2\ e^- \rightarrow 2\ F^-$$

The net ionic equation is:

$$H_2 + F_2 \rightarrow 2\ H^+ + 2\ F^-$$

In this reaction, molecular hydrogen acts as a reducing agent as it is oxidized from 0 to +1. Molecular fluorine is the oxidizing agent as it is reduced from 0 to −1. In this reaction, there is no spectator ion.

Decomposition Reactions

In **decomposition reactions**, one product breaks down into two or more species. For example:

$$(\overset{-3}{N}\overset{+1}{H}_4)_2\overset{+6}{Cr}_2\overset{-2}{O}_7\,(aq) \rightarrow \overset{0}{N}_2\,(g) + \overset{+3}{Cr}_2\overset{-2}{O}_3\,(s) + 4\,\overset{+1}{H}_2\overset{-2}{O}\,(g)$$

The relevant half-reactions would be:

$$2\,NH_4^+ \rightarrow N_2 + 8\,H^+$$
$$Cr_2O_7 + 8\,H^+ \rightarrow Cr_2O_3 + 4\,H_2O$$

The net ionic equation is:

$$2\,NH_4^+ + Cr_2O_7^{2-} \rightarrow N_2 + Cr_2O_3 + 4\,H_2O$$

In this reaction, the nitrogen atom in the ammonium cation acts as a reducing agent as it is oxidized from -3 to 0. The chromium in the dichromate anion acts as the oxidizing agent as it is reduced from $+6$ to $+3$. In this reaction, there is no spectator ion. Note that the net ionic equation is not significantly different from the original balanced equation.

Combustion Reactions

In **combustion reactions**, a fuel (usually a hydrocarbon) is mixed with an oxidant (usually oxygen), forming carbon dioxide and water. For example:

$$\overset{-4}{C}\overset{+1}{H}_4\,(g) + 2\,\overset{0}{O}_2\,(g) \rightarrow \overset{+4}{C}\overset{-2}{O}_2\,(g) + 2\,\overset{+1}{H}_2\overset{-2}{O}\,(l)$$

The relevant half-reactions would be:

$$CH_4 + 2\,H_2O \rightarrow CO_2 + 8\,H^+ + 8\,e^-$$
$$2\,O_2 + 8\,H^+ + 8\,e^- \rightarrow 4\,H_2O$$

The net ionic equation is identical to the overall balanced equation because there are no spectator ions and no aqueous species:

$$CH_4 + 2\,O_2 \rightarrow CO_2 + 2\,H_2O$$

Combustion reactions can have complex half-reactions, depending on the type of fuel used. In this instance, carbon in methane is the reducing agent as it is oxidized from -4 to $+4$. Molecular oxygen is the oxidizing agent as it is reduced from 0 to -2.

Double-Displacement (Metathesis) Reactions

Double-displacement or **metathesis reactions** involve the switching of counterions. Because all ions generally retain their oxidation state, these are not usually oxidation–reduction reactions. For example:

$$\overset{+1}{Ag}\overset{-1}{\overbrace{NO_3}}\,(aq) + \overset{+1}{H}\overset{-1}{Cl}\,(aq) \rightarrow \overset{+1}{H}\overset{-1}{\overbrace{NO_3}}\,(aq) + \overset{+1}{Ag}\overset{-1}{Cl}\,(s)$$

Because all species retain the same oxidation numbers, this is not considered oxidation–reduction. The net ionic reaction would be:

$$Ag^{+} + Cl^{-} \rightarrow AgCl$$

The nitrate anion and hydrogen cation both act as spectator ions in this reaction.

In double-displacement reactions where both reactants and both products are aqueous, there is no net ionic reaction. For example:

$$\overset{+1}{Na}\overbrace{NO_3}^{-1}(aq) + \overset{+1}{H}\overset{-1}{Cl}(aq) \rightarrow \overset{+1}{H}\overbrace{NO_3}^{-1}(aq) + \overset{+1}{Na}\overset{-1}{Cl}(aq)$$

This reaction is not an oxidation–reduction reaction because no species change their oxidation states. Further, because all species are aqueous, the complete ionic reaction is:

$$Na^{+} + NO_3^{-} + H^{+} + Cl^{-} \rightarrow H^{+} + NO_3^{-} + Na^{+} + Cl^{-}$$

Because all of the ions appear on both sides of the reaction, there is no net ionic reaction.

Disproportionation Reactions

Disproportionation (or **dismutation**) is a specific type of redox reaction in which an element undergoes both oxidation and reduction in producing its products. Many biological enzymes utilize a disproportionation mechanism. An example of such a reaction is the catalysis of peroxides by *catalase*, an enzyme found in peroxisomes. Catalase is a critical biological enzyme used to protect cells from excessive oxidation by free radicals or reactive oxygen species. The activity of catalase can be seen when disinfecting a wound with hydrogen peroxide:

$$2\ \overset{+1}{H_2}\overset{-1}{O_2}\ (aq) \xrightarrow[\text{catalase}]{} 2\ \overset{+1}{H_2}\overset{-2}{O}\ (l) + \overset{0}{O_2}\ (g)$$

As can be seen from this reaction, oxygen is disproportioned between water and molecular oxygen. In hydrogen peroxide, each oxygen has an oxidation state of -1 (the peroxide ion has a charge of -2 overall). In water, oxygen has an oxidation state of -2, and in molecular oxygen, it has an oxidation state of 0. Therefore, the oxygen is both reduced and oxidized in this reaction.

Another related biological disproportionation mechanism is that of the enzyme *superoxide dismutase*. As the name implies, a *dismutase* catalyzes dismutation. This enzyme disproportions oxygen free radicals in the reaction

$$2\,\overset{-\frac{1}{2}}{O_2^{\bullet -}} + 2\overset{+1}{H^{+}} \rightarrow \overset{+1}{H_2}\overset{-1}{O_2} + \overset{0}{O_2}$$

where peroxide and oxygen are the disproportioned products. The oxidation state of oxygen in the free radical is $-\frac{1}{2}$ (a negative charge divided over two oxygen atoms), and it is reduced to -1 in the peroxide and oxidized to 0 in molecular oxygen.

Biochemical disproportionation reactions—and oxidation–reduction reactions in biological systems in general—are usually accomplished by enzymes. Structurally, these enzymes often have metals such as Cu and Zn in their active sites that act as reducing agents, as shown in Figure 11.3.

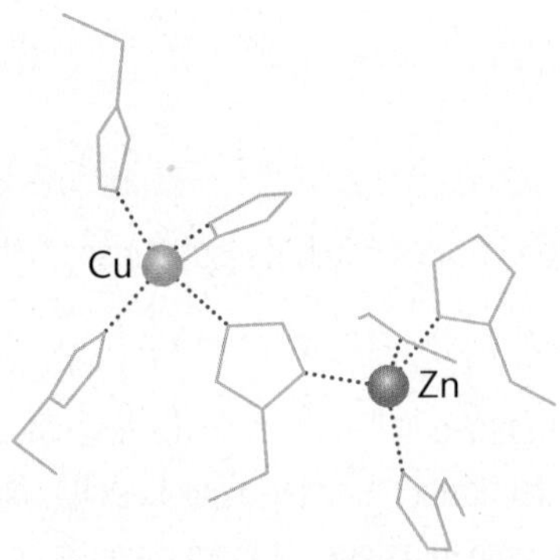

Figure 11.3 Active Site of Superoxide Dismutase
Cu and Zn atoms act as reducing agents, losing electrons during catalysis. The atoms are stabilized in position by histidine residues.

Oxidation–Reduction Titrations

Oxidation–reduction titrations are similar in setup to acid–base titrations, but the focus is different. Whereas acid–base titrations follow the movement of protons, as discussed in Chapter 10 of *MCAT General Chemistry Review*, redox titrations follow the transfer of charge (as electrons) to reach the equivalence point. Redox titrations can utilize indicators that change color at a particular voltage (emf) value. Some common indicators are listed in Table 11.2. As for acid–base titrations, it is not necessary to memorize these indicators, but rather to understand their utility.

INDICATOR	VOLTAGE OF COLOR CHANGE	OXIDIZED FORM	REDUCED FORM
Bipyridine metal complexes	About +1 V	Colorless (Ru), Cyan (Fe)	Yellow (Ru), Red (Fe)
Diphenylamine	+0.76 V	Violet	Colorless
Safranin	+0.24/−0.29 V*	Red-Violet	Colorless

* Safranin is unique in that its color change is not only voltage dependent, but also pH dependent.

Table 11.2 Common Indicators for Oxidation–Reduction (Redox) Titrations

One prototypical redox titration involves the use of starch indicators to identify iodine complexes. This specific redox titration is called an iodimetric titration because it relies on the titration of free iodine radicals. The presence of iodine is initially determined by a dark solution in the presence of starch, and at the endpoint of the titration, a colorless solution develops. A common general chemistry laboratory experiment involves the standardization of a thiosulfate solution using iodimetry, as described in the example below.

Example: A group of students prepares to standardize a $Na_2S_2O_3$ solution. 32 mL of the $Na_2S_2O_3$ solution is titrated into 50 mL of a 0.01 *M* KIO_3 solution to reach the equivalence point. They first titrate the KIO_3 solution until it loses color, then add a starch indicator until the reaction is complete. The reaction proceeds in these two steps:

$$IO_3^- + I^- + H^+ \rightarrow I_3^- + H_2O$$
$$I_3^- + S_2O_3^{2-} \rightarrow I^- + S_4O_6^{2-}$$

Determine the concentration of the sodium thiosulfate solution at the beginning of the experiment.

Solution: The titration is performed in two steps. In the first step, the iodate is converted into triiodide anions. The initial titration creates a colorless I_3^- solution in water, which then requires a starch indicator for the remainder of the titration.

In the second step, the triiodide ions are then reduced in the presence of thiosulfate to determine its concentration. Note that the reactions are unbalanced. It would be tempting to balance the first equation as:

$$IO_3^- + 2\,I^- + 6\,H^+ \rightarrow I_3^- + 3\,H_2O$$

However, this reaction has a charge of $+3$ on the reactants side and -1 on the products side. In oxidation-reduction chemistry, we must balance not only for stoichiometry but also for charge. The correct balanced equations are:

$$IO_3^- + 8\,I^- + 6\,H^+ \rightarrow 3\,I_3^- + 3\,H_2O$$
$$I_3^- + 2\,S_2O_3^{2-} \rightarrow 3\,I^- + S_4O_6^{2-}$$

Keeping in mind that each iodate is used to make three triiodide anions, and each triiodide anion interacts with two thiosulfate anions, the mole ratio of thiosulfate to iodate is six to one:

$$IO_3^- + 8\,I^- + 6\,H^+ \rightarrow 3\,I_3^- + 3\,H_2O$$
$$3\,I_3^- + 6\,S_2O_3^{2-} \rightarrow 9\,I^- + 3\,S_4O_6^{2-}$$

Then, use stoichiometry to determine the molarity of the thiosulfate solution from the 50 mL potassium iodate solution.

$$0.01\,M\,IO_3^-\,[0.05\text{ L}]\left[\frac{6\text{ mol }S_2O_3^{2-}}{1\text{ mol }IO_3^-}\right] = 3 \times 10^{-3}\text{ mol}$$

Now, we can use the volume to find the molarity.

$$M_{S_2O_3^{2-}} = \frac{3 \times 10^{-3}\text{ mol}}{32\text{ mL}\left[\frac{1\text{ L}}{1000\text{ mL}}\right]} = \frac{3 \times 10^{-3}}{32 \times 10^{-3}} \approx \frac{3}{30} = 0.1\ M\ (\text{actual} = 0.094\ M)$$

Potentiometric titration is a form of redox titration where no indicator is used. Instead, the electrical potential difference (voltage) is measured using a voltmeter. As a redox titration progresses, its voltage changes; this is analogous to following an acid–base titration with a pH meter instead of a color indicator.

MCAT CONCEPT CHECK 11.2

Before you move on, assess your understanding of the material with these questions.

1. Write the net ionic equations for the reactions below:
   - $CuNO_3\ (aq) + NaCl\ (aq) \rightarrow CuCl\ (s) + NaNO_3\ (aq)$

   ____

   - $Mg\ (s) + AlCl_3\ (aq) \rightarrow Al\ (s) + MgCl_2\ (aq)$

   ____

2. In each of the reactions below, which element undergoes disproportionation? What are that element's oxidation states in the products?

$$3\ Cl_2\ (g) + 6\ NaOH\ (aq) \rightarrow 5\ NaCl\ (aq) + NaClO_3\ (aq) + 3\ H_2O\ (l)$$

$$S_2O_3^{2-}\ (aq) + 2\ H^+\ (aq) \rightarrow S\ (s) + SO_2\ (g) + H_2O\ (l)$$

   - Element undergoing disproportionation:

   ____

   - Oxidation states in products:

   ____

   - Element undergoing disproportionation:

   ____

   - Oxidation states in products:

   ____

3. A sample is assayed for lead by a redox titration with $I_3^-\ (aq)$. A 10.00 g sample is crushed, dissolved in sulfuric acid, and passed over a reducing agent so that all the lead is in the form Pb^{2+}. The $Pb^{2+}\ (aq)$ is completely oxidized to Pb^{4+} by 32.60 mL of a 0.7 *M* solution of NaI_3. The balanced equation for the reaction is:

$$I_3^- + (aq) + Pb^{2+}\ (aq) \rightarrow Pb^{4+}\ (aq) + 3\ I^-\ (aq)$$

   Calculate the mass of lead in the sample.

   ____

Conclusion

In this chapter, we covered the essential MCAT topic of oxidation–reduction reactions. We reviewed the rules for assigning oxidation numbers to help us keep track of the movement of electrons from the species that are oxidized (reducing agents) to the species that are reduced (oxidizing agents). We also covered the sequence of steps involved in balancing half-reactions, redox titrations, and disproportionation reactions.

In addition to understanding the fundamental chemical principles behind these reactions, you will begin to see these concepts resurface in *MCAT Organic Chemistry Review* and *MCAT Biochemistry Review*. Oxidation–reduction reactions are often used for energy transfer in biological systems, and any deficiencies in such systems are profoundly deleterious (such as metabolic, mitochondrial, and immunologic diseases). Our next chapter—the last of *MCAT General Chemistry Review*—brings the principles of oxidation–reduction reactions to their application in electrochemical cells. By the end of the next chapter, you will have reviewed all of the general chemistry knowledge required for Test Day!

You've reviewed the content, now test your knowledge and critical thinking skills by completing a test-like passage set in your online resources!

GO ONLINE

CONCEPT SUMMARY

Oxidation–Reduction Reactions

- **Oxidation** is a loss of electrons, and **reduction** is a gain of electrons; the two are paired together in what is known as an **oxidation–reduction** (**redox**) reaction.
- An **oxidizing agent** facilitates the oxidation of another compound and is reduced itself in the process; a **reducing agent** facilitates the reduction of another compound and is itself oxidized in the process.
  - Common oxidizing agents almost all contain oxygen or a similarly electronegative element.
  - Common reducing agents often contain metal ions or hydrides (H^-).
- To assign oxidation numbers, one must know the common oxidation states of the representative elements.
  - Any free element or diatomic species has an oxidation number of zero.
  - The oxidation number of a monatomic ion is equal to the charge of the ion.
  - When in compounds, Group IA metals have an oxidation number of $+1$; Group IIA metals have an oxidation number of $+2$.
  - When in compounds, Group VIIA elements have an oxidation number of -1 (unless combined with an element with higher electronegativity).
  - The oxidation state of hydrogen is $+1$ unless it is paired with a less electronegative element, in which case it is -1.
  - The oxidation state of oxygen is usually -2, except in peroxides (when its charge is -1) or in compounds with more electronegative elements.
  - The sum of the oxidation numbers of all the atoms present in a compound is equal to the overall charge of that compound.
- When balancing redox reactions, the **half-reaction method**, also called the **ion–electron method**, is the most common.
  - Separate the two half-reactions.
  - Balance the atoms of each half-reaction. Start with all the elements besides H and O. In acidic solution, balance H and O using water and H^+. In basic solution, balance H and O using water and OH^-.
  - Balance the charges of each half-reaction by adding electrons as necessary to one side of the reaction.
  - Multiply the half-reactions as necessary to obtain the same number of electrons in both half-reactions.
  - Add the half-reactions, canceling out terms on both sides of the reaction arrow.
  - Confirm that the mass and charge are balanced.

Net Ionic Equations

- A **complete ionic equation** accounts for all of the ions present in a reaction. To write a complete ionic reaction, split all aqueous compounds into their relevant ions. Keep solid salts intact.
- **Net ionic equations** ignore spectator ions to focus only on the species that actually participate in the reaction. To obtain a net ionic reaction, subtract the ions appearing on both sides of the reaction, which are called **spectator ions**.
  - For reactions that contain no aqueous salts, the net ionic equation is generally the same as the overall balanced reaction.
  - For double displacement (metathesis) reactions that do not form a solid salt, there is no net ionic reaction because all ions remain in solution and do not change oxidation number.
- **Disproportionation (dismutation) reactions** are a type of redox reaction in which one element is both oxidized and reduced, forming at least two molecules containing the element with different oxidation states.
- **Oxidation–reduction titrations** are similar in methodology to acid–base titrations. These titrations follow transfer of charge.
  - Indicators used in such titrations change color when certain voltages of solutions are achieved.
  - **Potentiometric titration** is a form of redox titration in which a voltmeter or external cell measures the electromotive force (emf) of a solution. No indicator is used, and the equivalence point is determined by a sharp change in voltage.

ANSWERS TO CONCEPT CHECKS

11.1

1.

Reaction	Oxidation Numbers	Oxidizing Agent	Reducing Agent
$2\ KI + H_2 \rightarrow 2\ K + 2\ HI$	$2\ \overset{+1}{K}\overset{-1}{I} + \overset{0}{H_2} \rightarrow 2\overset{0}{K} + 2\ \overset{+1}{H}\overset{-1}{I}$	K^+ (charge goes from +1 to 0)	H_2 (charge goes from 0 to +1)
$Al + BPO_4 \rightarrow B + AlPO^4$	$\overset{0}{Al} + \overset{+3}{B}\overbrace{PO_4}^{-3} \rightarrow \overset{0}{B} + \overset{+3}{Al}\overbrace{PO_4}^{-3}$	B^{3+} (charge goes from +3 to 0)	Al (charge goes from 0 to +3)

2. Oxidation: $Zn \rightarrow Zn^{2+} + 2\ e^-$

   Reduction: $Cu^{2+} + 2\ e^- \rightarrow Cu$

3. 1. $\begin{cases} Mg \rightarrow Mg^{2+} \\ HNO_3 \rightarrow NO \end{cases}$

   2. $\begin{cases} Mg \rightarrow Mg^{2+} \\ HNO_3 + 3H^+ \rightarrow NO + 2H_2O \end{cases}$

   3. $\begin{cases} Mg \rightarrow Mg^{2+} + 2e^- \\ HNO_3 + 3H^+ + 3e^- \rightarrow NO + 2H_2O \end{cases}$

   4. $\begin{cases} 3Mg \rightarrow 3Mg^{2+} + 6e^- \\ 2HNO_3 + 6H^+ + 6e^- \rightarrow 2NO + 4H_2O \end{cases}$

   5. $2HNO_3 + 3Mg + 6H^+ \rightarrow 2NO + 3Mg^{2+} + 4H_2O$

11.2

1. $Cu^+ + Cl^- \rightarrow CuCl$
   $3\ Mg + 2\ Al^{3+} \rightarrow 3\ Mg^{2+} + 2\ Al$ (don't forget to balance the reaction!)
2. In the first reaction, chlorine undergoes disproportionation to have a −1 oxidation state in NaCl and a +5 oxidation state in $NaClO_3$.
   In the second reaction, sulfur undergoes disproportionation to have a 0 oxidation state in elemental sulfur and +4 oxidation state in SO_2.
3. $0.7\ M\ I_3^-\left[32.60 \times 10^{-3}\ L\right]\left[\frac{1\ mol\ Pb^{2+}}{1\ mol\ I_3^-}\right]\left[\frac{207.2\ g\ Pb^{2+}}{1\ mol\ Pb^{2+}}\right] \approx 0.7 \times 3 \times 2 = 4.2\ g$

   (actual = 4.73 g)

   Note that question 3 also included the extraneous value 10.0 g, which is not needed to calculate the mass of lead produced.

SCIENCE MASTERY ASSESSMENT EXPLANATIONS

1. **C**

The oxidizing agent is the species that is reduced in any given equation. In this problem, six hydrogen atoms with +1 oxidation states in NH_3 are reduced to three neutral H_2 molecules.

2. **B**

First, balance the atoms in the equation:

$$Cr_2O_7^{2-} + 14\,H^+ \rightarrow 2\,Cr^{2+} + 7\,H_2O$$

Now, adjust the number of electrons to balance the charge. Currently, the left side has a charge of +12 (−2 from dichromate and +14 from protons). The right side has a charge of +4 (+2 from each chromium cation). To decrease the charge on the left side from +12 to +4, we should add 8 electrons:

$$Cr_2O_7^{2-} + 14\,H^+ + 8\,e^- \rightarrow 2\,Cr^{2+} + 7\,H_2O$$

3. **A**

Hydride ions are composed of a hydrogen nucleus with two electrons, thereby giving it a negative charge and a considerable tendency to donate electrons. $LiAlH_4$ is therefore a strong reducing agent. Strong reducing agents tend to have metals or hydrides; strong oxidizing agents tend to have oxygen or a similarly electronegative element.

4. **C**

In NaClO (sodium hypochlorite), sodium carries its typical +1 charge, and oxygen carries its typical −2 charge. This means that the chlorine atom must carry a +1 charge in order to balance the overall charge of zero.

5. **D**

A strong oxidizing agent will be easily reduced, meaning that it will have a tendency to gain electrons. Atoms usually gain electrons if they are one or two electrons away from filling up their valence shell. **(A)** has a full 4*s*-orbital, meaning that it can only gain an electron if it gains an entire subshell. **(B)** has a stable, half-full 3*d*-orbital, so it is unlikely to pick up electrons unless it can gain five. **(C)** has only a single electron in the outer shell, which is more likely lost upon ionization. **(D)** would fill up its 4*p*-orbital by gaining one electron, so it is easily reduced.

6. **D**

A net ionic equation represents each of the aqueous ions comprising the reactants and products as individual ions, instead of combining them as formula units. Thus, **(A)** is not a net ionic reaction. The term *net* means that the correct answer does not include any spectator ions (ions that do not participate in the reaction). In this reaction, nitrate (NO_3^-) remains unchanged. Therefore, **(B)** and **(C)** are eliminated.

7. **C**

What you are shown is a net ionic equation. If two moles of FeSCN are created, two moles of Fe^{3+} must be used because the mole ratio is 1:1. Iron sulfate has the formula $Fe_2(SO_4)_3$ because sulfate has a charge of −2 and iron has a charge of +3 (based on the net ionic equation). Therefore, one mole of iron sulfate is needed to make two moles of iron for the reaction. The molar mass of iron sulfate is

$$2 \times 55.8\,\frac{g}{mol} + 3 \times 32.1\,\frac{g}{mol} + 12 \times 16.0\,\frac{g}{mol} = 399.9\,\frac{g}{mol}$$

This most closely matches answer **(C)**. The most common error would be to calculate the amount of iron, which would be 111.6 g, **(A)**.

8. **D**

When assigning oxidation numbers, one starts with elements of known oxidation state first, and determines the oxidation state of the other elements by deduction. As a noble gas, argon, **(A)**, will always have an oxidation state of 0. As a Group VIIA element, fluorine, **(B)**, will have an oxidation state of 0 (by itself) or −1 (in a compound). As a Group IIA element, strontium, **(C)**, will have an oxidation state of 0 (by itself) or +2 (in a compound). Like most transition metals, iridium, **(D)**, can have various oxidation states, ranging from −3 to +8. Therefore, one would have to determine the oxidation states of other atoms in an iridium-containing compound to determine iridium's oxidation number.

9. **A**

The formula for methanol is H_3COH, for methanal is HCHO, and for methanoic acid is HCOOH. If we assign oxidation numbers to carbon in each molecule, it starts at -2, then becomes 0, then becomes $+2$:

$$\overset{+1}{H_3}\overset{-2}{C}\overset{-2}{O}\overset{+1}{H} \rightarrow \overset{+1}{H}\overset{0}{C}\overset{+1}{H}\overset{-2}{O} \rightarrow \overset{+1}{H}\overset{+2}{C}\overset{-2}{O}\overset{-2}{O}\overset{+1}{H}$$

In general, it is often easier to think of oxidation as a gain of bonds to oxygen (or a similarly electronegative element) or loss of bonds to hydrogen for organic compounds. Therefore, because the carbon is oxidized as one converts from an alcohol to an aldehyde to a carboxylic acid, the oxidation number must increase.

10. **C**

Start with the atoms that have oxidation states of which you are certain. Potassium is a Group IA metal, and therefore must have an oxidation state of $+1$. Hydrogen is almost always $+1$, unless it is paired with a less electronegative element (which is not the case here). Oxygen is generally -2. Because there are four oxygens, they create a total negative charge of -8 which is partially balanced by two hydrogens $(+2)$ and potassium $(+1)$. Therefore, phosphorus has a $+5$ charge, making it the highest oxidation state.

11. **B**

Recall that oxygen has an oxidation state of -2. Therefore, in tungsten(IV) oxide, **(A)**, tungsten has an oxidation state of $+4$. In tungsten(VI) oxide, **(B)**, it has an oxidation state of $+6$. In tungsten(III) oxide, **(C)**, it is $+3$. In tungsten pentoxide, **(D)**, it is $+5$.

12. **A**

Step I is a disproportionation reaction because chlorine starts with an oxidation state of 0 in the reactants and ends up with an oxidation state of $+1$ in HOCl and -1 as Cl^-. In the other reactions, no element appears with different oxidation states in two different products. Therefore, only step I is a disproportionation reaction.

13. **C**

Potentiometry refers to carrying out an oxidation–reduction titration with a voltmeter present to get precise readings of the reaction's electromotive force (emf) to determine the endpoint. This is analogous to using a pH meter in an acid–base titration because it uses technology to get precise readings for plotting a titration curve. Indicators, as in **(A)** and **(B)**, can be used in both acid–base and redox titrations, but provide a qualitative (rather than quantitative) analysis of the titration. Oxidizing and reducing agents are used in redox titrations, not acid–base titrations, eliminating **(D)**.

14. **D**

Utilize the method described earlier to balance this redox reaction. The balanced half-reactions are:

$$S_8 + 24\ H_2O \rightarrow 8\ SO_3^{2-} + 48\ H^+ + 32\ e^-$$

$$NO_3^- + 4\ H^+ + 3\ e^- \rightarrow NO + 2\ H_2O$$

To get equal numbers of electrons in each half-reaction, the oxidation half-reaction will have to be multiplied by 3, and the reduction half-reaction will have to be multiplied by 32:

$$3\ S_8 + 72\ H_2O \rightarrow 24\ SO_3^{2-} + 144\ H^+ + 96\ e^-$$

$$32\ NO_3^- + 128\ H^+ + 96\ e^- \rightarrow 32\ NO + 64\ H_2O$$

This makes the overall reaction:

$$3\ S_8 + 32\ NO_3^- + 8\ H_2O \rightarrow 24\ SO_3^{2-} + 32\ NO + 16\ H^+$$

The sum of the stoichiometric coefficients is therefore: $3 + 32 + 8 + 24 + 32 + 16 = 115$.

15. **C**

First, balance the chemical equation:

$$4\ Au + 8\ NaCN + O_2 + 2\ H_2O \rightarrow 4\ Na[Au(CN)_2] + 4\ NaOH$$

Now, determine the number of moles of NaCN used in the reaction:

$$0.1\ L \times 2\ \frac{mol}{L} = 0.2\ mol\ NaCN$$

If 0.2 mol NaCN are used in the reaction, then 0.2 mol NaCN $\times \dfrac{4\ mol\ Au}{8\ mol\ NaCN} = 0.1$ mol Au is oxidized.

Consult your online resources for additional practice. GO ONLINE

SHARED CONCEPTS

Biochemistry Chapter 2
Enzymes

Biochemistry Chapter 10
Carbohydrate Metabolism II

Biology Chapter 7
The Cardiovascular System

General Chemistry Chapter 10
Acids and Bases

General Chemistry Chapter 12
Electrochemistry

Organic Chemistry Chapter 4
Analyzing Organic Reactions

CHAPTER 12

ELECTROCHEMISTRY

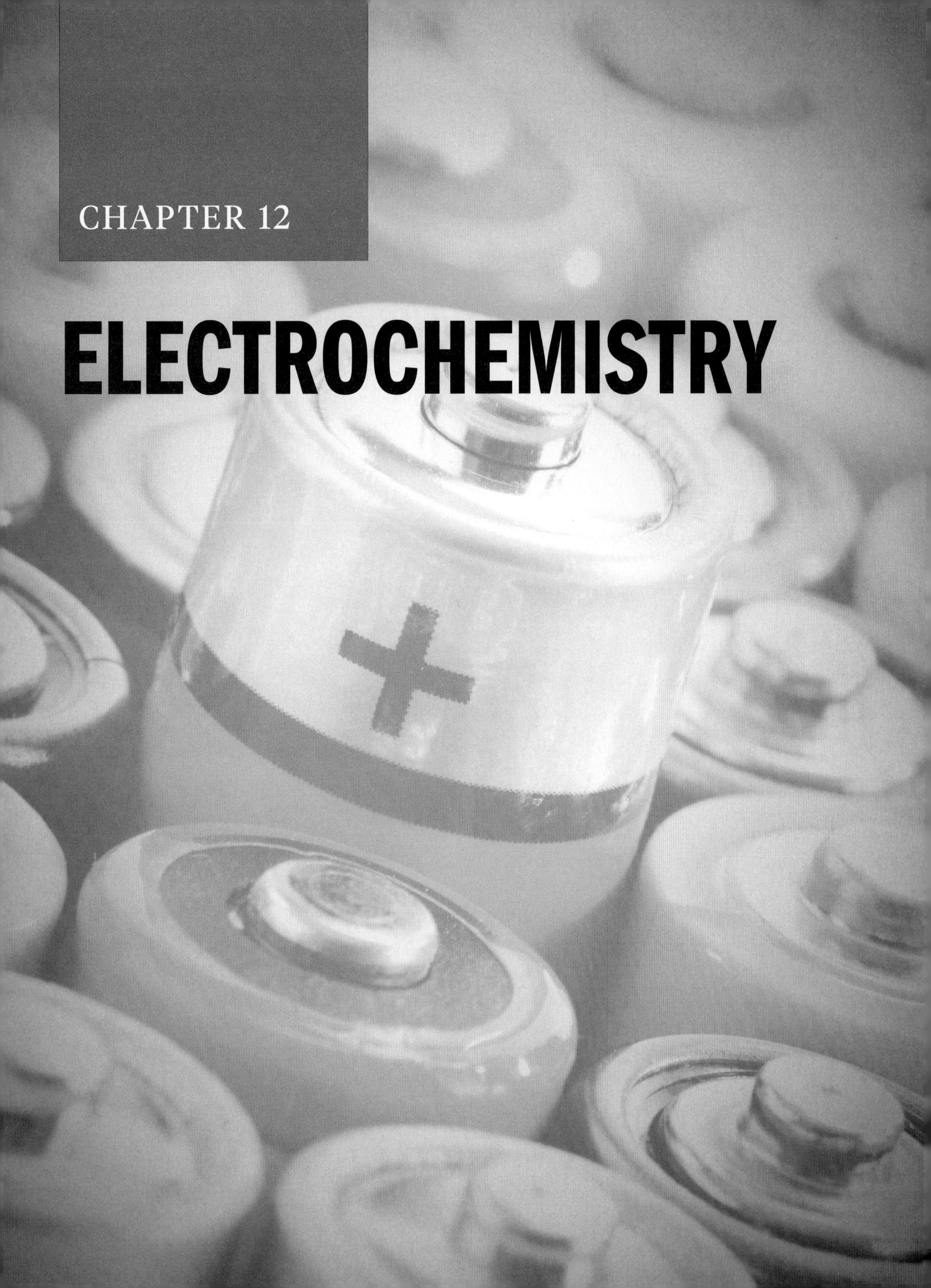

SCIENCE MASTERY ASSESSMENT

Every pre-med knows this feeling: there is so much content I have to know for the MCAT! How do I know what to do first or what's important?

While the high-yield badges throughout this book will help you identify the most important topics, this Science Mastery Assessment is another tool in your MCAT prep arsenal. This quiz (which can also be taken in your online resources) and the guidance below will help ensure that you are spending the appropriate amount of time on this chapter based on your personal strengths and weaknesses. Don't worry though—skipping something now does not mean you'll never study it. Later on in your prep, as you complete full-length tests, you'll uncover specific pieces of content that you need to review and can come back to these chapters as appropriate.

How to Use This Assessment

If you answer 0–7 questions correctly:

Spend about 1 hour to read this chapter in full and take limited notes throughout. Follow up by reviewing **all** quiz questions to ensure that you now understand how to solve each one.

If you answer 8–11 questions correctly:

Spend 20–40 minutes reviewing the quiz questions. Beginning with the questions you missed, read and take notes on the corresponding subchapters. For questions you answered correctly, ensure your thinking matches that of the explanation and you understand why each choice was correct or incorrect.

If you answer 12–15 questions correctly:

Spend less than 20 minutes reviewing all questions from the quiz. If you missed any, then include a quick read-through of the corresponding subchapters, or even just the relevant content within a subchapter, as part of your question review. For questions you answered correctly, ensure your thinking matches that of the explanation and review the Concept Summary at the end of the chapter.

1. Rusting occurs due to the oxidation–reduction reaction of iron with environmental oxygen:

$$4\ Fe\ (s) + 3\ O_2\ (g) \rightarrow 2\ Fe_2O_3\ (s)$$

Some metals cannot react with oxygen in this fashion.

Which of the following best explains why iron can?

A. Iron has a more positive reduction potential than those metals, making it more likely to donate electrons to oxygen.
B. Iron has a more positive reduction potential than those metals, making it more likely to accept electrons from oxygen.
C. Iron has a less positive reduction potential than those metals, making it more likely to donate electrons to oxygen.
D. Iron has a less positive reduction potential than those metals, making it more likely to accept electrons from oxygen.

2. Given the following standard reduction potentials:

$$Zn^{2+} + 2\ e^- \rightarrow Zn \qquad E^\circ_{red} = -0.763\ V$$

$$Ag^+ + e^- \rightarrow Ag \qquad E^\circ_{red} = +0.337\ V$$

What is the standard electromotive force of the following reaction?

$$Zn^{2+} + 2\ Ag \rightarrow 2\ Ag^+ + Zn$$

A. -2.2 V
B. -1.1 V
C. $+1.1$ V
D. $+2.2$ V

3. Consider the following data:

$$Hg^{2+} + 2\ e^- \rightarrow Hg \qquad E^\circ_{red} = +0.85\ V$$

$$Cu^+ + e^- \rightarrow Cu \qquad E^\circ_{red} = +0.52\ V$$

$$Zn^{2+} + 2\ e^- \rightarrow Zn \qquad E^\circ_{red} = -0.76\ V$$

$$Al^{3+} + 3\ e^- \rightarrow Al \qquad E^\circ_{red} = -1.66\ V$$

The anode of a certain galvanic cell is composed of copper. Which of the metals from the data table can be used at the cathode, assuming equal concentrations of the two electrolyte solutions?

A. Hg
B. Cu
C. Zn
D. Al

4. An electrolytic cell is filled with water. Which of the following will move toward the cathode of such a cell?

I. H^+ ions
II. O^{2-} ions
III. Electrons

A. I only
B. II only
C. I and III only
D. II and III only

5. If the value of E°_{cell} is known, what other data is needed to calculate ΔG°?

A. Equilibrium constant
B. Reaction quotient
C. Temperature of the system
D. Half-reactions of the cells

6. Which of the following compounds is LEAST likely to be found in the salt bridge of a galvanic cell?
   A. NaCl
   B. SO_3
   C. $MgSO_3$
   D. NH_4NO_3

7. If the surface area of electrode material in an electrochemical cell is tripled, what else is necessarily tripled?
   I. E°_{cell}
   II. Current
   III. K_{eq}

   A. I only
   B. II only
   C. I and II only
   D. II and III only

8. Which of the following can alter the emf of an electrochemical cell?
   A. The mass of the electrodes
   B. The length of the wire connecting the half-cells
   C. The overall size of the battery
   D. The temperature of the solutions in the half-cells

9. Which of the following statements could be true about a Na–Cd cell, based on the information below?

$$Na^+ + e^- \rightarrow Na \qquad E^\circ_{red} = -2.71 \text{ V}$$

$$Cd^{2+} + 2e^- \rightarrow Cd \qquad E^\circ_{red} = -0.40 \text{ V}$$

   A. It is a galvanic cell, and sodium is the cathode.
   B. It is an electrolytic cell, and cadmium is the anode.
   C. It is a galvanic cell, with $E^\circ_{cell} = 3.11$ V.
   D. It is an electrolytic cell, with $E^\circ_{cell} = -3.11$ V.

10. Which of the following expressions correctly describes the relationship between standard electromotive force and standard change in free energy?
   A. $\Delta G^\circ = -nF(E^\circ_{red,anode} - E^\circ_{red,cathode})$
   B. $E^\circ_{cell} = \frac{nF}{RT} \ln K_{eq}$
   C. $E^\circ_{cell} = -\frac{RT}{nF} \ln K_{eq}$
   D. $\Delta G^\circ = nF(E^\circ_{red,anode} - E^\circ_{red,cathode})$

11. Which of the following choices is indicative of a spontaneous reaction, assuming standard conditions?
   A. E°_{cell} is negative.
   B. $Q = K_{eq}$
   C. The cell is a concentration cell.
   D. $K_{eq} > 1$

12. For a cell with the following half-reactions:

Anode: $SO_2 + 2\ H_2O \rightarrow SO_4^{2-} + 4\ H^+ + 2\ e^-$

Cathode: $Pd^{2+} + 2\ e^- \rightarrow Pd$

How would decreasing the pH of the solution inside the cell affect the electromotive force (emf)?
   A. The emf would decrease.
   B. The emf would remain the same.
   C. The emf would increase.
   D. The emf would become zero.

13. An electrolytic cell necessarily has:
   A. $\Delta S^\circ > 0$
   B. $\Delta G^\circ < 0$
   C. $K_{eq} < 1$
   D. $E^\circ_{cell} > 0$

14. Which of the following is the best explanation for the fact that a larger mass of electrodes are required for lead–acid batteries, as compared to other batteries, to produce a certain current?

A. The lead–acid electrolyte, sulfuric acid, is diprotic and incompletely dissociates in solution.
B. The energy density of lead–acid electrodes is higher than that of other batteries.
C. The electrolytes in other batteries less readily dissociate than those of lead–acid batteries.
D. The energy density of lead–acid electrodes is lower than that of other batteries.

15. Which of the following best describes why overcharging a Ni–Cd battery is not detrimental?

A. The energy density of a Ni–Cd battery is high, so it can store more charge than other batteries per its mass.
B. The electrodes of a Ni–Cd battery can discharge through the circuit when they are fully charged.
C. The Ni–Cd battery will stop accepting electrons from an outside source when its electrodes are recharged.
D. Ni–Cd batteries have a high surge current and can dissipate the overcharge before damage can occur to electrodes.

Answer Key follows on next page.

Answer Key

1. **C**
2. **B**
3. **A**
4. **C**
5. **D**
6. **B**
7. **B**
8. **D**
9. **B**
10. **D**
11. **D**
12. **A**
13. **C**
14. **D**
15. **C**

Detailed explanations can be found at the end of the chapter.

CHAPTER 12

ELECTROCHEMISTRY

In This Chapter

CHAPTER PROFILE

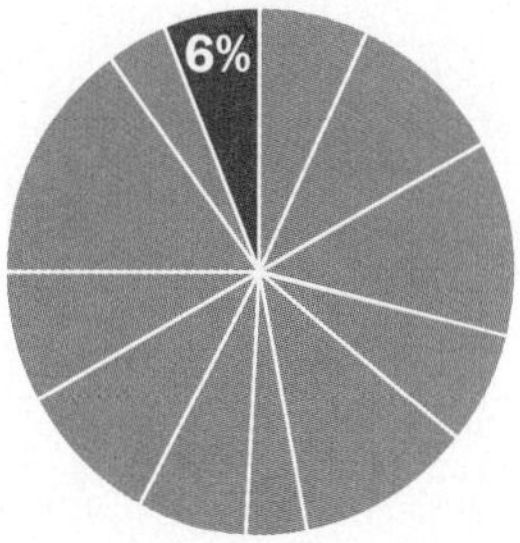

The content in this chapter should be relevant to about 6% of all questions about general chemistry on the MCAT.

This chapter covers material from the following AAMC content categories:

1D: Principles of bioenergetics and fuel molecule metabolism

3A: Structure and functions of the nervous and endocrine systems and ways in which these systems coordinate the organ systems

4C: Electrochemistry and electrical circuits and their elements

5E: Principles of chemical thermodynamics and kinetics

Introduction

The mitochondria are powerhouses of energy. Their primary purpose is to manufacture a deliverable and usable form of energy. By now, you are well aware of the complex processes by which the potential energy in the chemical bonds of carbohydrates, amino acids, and lipids is converted into the potential energy of the phosphate bond in adenosine triphosphate (ATP). ATP is then delivered to different parts of the cell, where it is used to energize most of the processes essential to the maintenance of life.

The mitochondria generate tremendous amounts of ATP—in humans, the average daily turnover of ATP is more than 50 kilograms! Without a continuous supply and replenishment of ATP, we wouldn't survive. ATP powers the contraction of our heart muscle and maintains the membrane potential essential for neurological function, among thousands of other essential roles. How do the mitochondria manufacture these packets of life-sustaining energy? Remember that mitochondria rely on their double-membrane structure to carry out the electron transport chain and oxidative phosphorylation. As such, mitochondria truly act as batteries of the cell. In fact, note the similarity between the proton-motive force of the mitochondria and the electromotive force of electrochemistry. Are these two terms the same thing or—at the very least—similar in nature?

Indeed, mitochondria and batteries do function in similar ways. Specifically, mitochondria function most similarly to concentration cells. In both concentration cells and mitochondria, a concentration gradient of ions between two separated compartments—connected to each other by some means of charge conduction—establishes an electrical potential difference (voltage). This voltage, called electromotive force in concentration cells and proton-motive force in the mitochondria, provides the drive to move charge from one compartment to the other, creating current. In the concentration cell, an oxidation–reduction reaction takes place, and electrons move in the direction that causes the concentration gradient to be dissipated. In the mitochondria, the charge buildup is in the form of a hydrogen ion (proton) gradient between the intermembrane space and the matrix. Embedded in the inner membrane is *ATP synthase*, which serves a dual role as a proton channel and a catalyst for the formation of the high-energy phosphate bond in ATP. As the hydrogen ions flow down their electrochemical gradient, energy is dissipated, and this energy is harnessed by ATP synthase to form ATP.

In this final chapter of *MCAT General Chemistry Review*, we will focus our attention on the study of various electrochemical cells. Utilizing our knowledge of oxidation–reduction reactions from Chapter 11, we will study how these principles can be applied to create different types of electrochemical cells, including galvanic (voltaic), electrolytic, and concentration cells. Regarding the thermodynamics of electrochemistry, we will focus on the significance of reduction potentials and examine the relationship between electromotive force, the equilibrium constant, and Gibbs free energy.

12.1 Electrochemical Cells

High-Yield

LEARNING OBJECTIVES

After Chapter 12.1, you will be able to:

- Distinguish between electrolytic and galvanic cells
- Describe electrolytic and galvanic cells
- Predict which electrode will act as the cathode or anode in an electrolytic or a galvanic cell
- Calculate ΔG and emf values for a given galvanic or electrolytic cell
- Apply the Nernst equation to electrochemical cell questions

Electrochemical cells are contained systems in which oxidation–reduction reactions occur. There are three fundamental types of electrochemical cells: galvanic cells (also known as voltaic cells), electrolytic cells, and concentration cells. In addition, there are specific commercial cells such as Ni–Cd batteries through which we can understand these fundamental models.

Galvanic cells and concentration cells house spontaneous reactions, whereas electrolytic cells contain nonspontaneous reactions. Remember that spontaneity is indicated by the change in Gibbs free energy, ΔG. All three types contain **electrodes** where oxidation and reduction take place. For all electrochemical cells, the electrode where oxidation occurs is called the **anode**, and the electrode where reduction occurs is called the **cathode**. Other descriptors of electrochemical cells include the

MNEMONIC

Electrodes in an electrochemical cell: **AN OX** and a **RED CAT**

The **an**ode is the site of **ox**idation; **red**uction occurs at the **cat**hode.

electromotive force (**emf**), which corresponds to the voltage or electrical potential difference of the cell. If the emf is positive, the cell is able to release energy ($\Delta G < 0$), which means it is spontaneous. If the emf is negative, the cell must absorb energy ($\Delta G > 0$), which means it is nonspontaneous.

Furthermore, we can also state that, for all electrochemical cells, the movement of electrons is from anode to cathode, and the current (I) runs from cathode to anode. This point can be a point of confusion among students. In physics, it is typical to state that current is the direction of flow of a positive charge through a circuit; this model was first proposed by Ben Franklin and continues to be used among physicists. Modern chemists are interested in the flow of electrons, but may discuss the current (a theoretical flow of positive charge) as a proxy for the flow of electrons; the current and the flow of electrons are always of equal magnitude but in opposite directions.

KEY CONCEPT

Electrons move through an electrochemical cell opposite to the flow of current (I).

Last, it is important to note that all batteries are influenced by temperature changes. For instance, lead–acid batteries in cars, like most galvanic cells, tend to fail most in cold weather. The thermodynamic reasons behind this will be discussed later in this chapter.

Galvanic (Voltaic) Cells

REAL WORLD

Galvanic cells are commonly used as batteries; to be worthwhile (that is, producing energy to power some device or appliance), these batteries must be spontaneous!

All of the nonrechargeable batteries you own are **galvanic cells**, also called **voltaic cells**. Accordingly, because household batteries are used to supply energy to a flashlight or remote control, the reactions in these cells must be spontaneous. This means that the reaction's free energy is decreasing ($\Delta G < 0$) as the cell releases energy to the environment. By extension, if the free energy change is negative for these cells, their electromotive force (E_{cell}) must be positive; the free energy change and electromotive force always have opposite signs.

Let's examine the inner workings of a galvanic (voltaic) cell. Two electrodes of distinct chemical identity are placed in separate compartments, which are called **half-cells**. The two electrodes are connected to each other by a conductive material, such as a copper wire. Along the wire, there may be other various components of a circuit, such as resistors or capacitors, but for now, we'll focus on the battery itself.

Surrounding each of the electrodes is an aqueous **electrolyte** solution composed of cations and anions. As shown in the **Daniell cell** illustrated in Figure 12.1, the cations in the two half-cell solutions can be of the same element as the respective metal electrode. Connecting the two solutions is a structure called a **salt bridge**, which consists of an inert salt. When the electrodes are connected to each other by a conductive material, charge will begin to flow as the result of an oxidation–reduction reaction that is taking place between the two half-cells. The redox reaction in a galvanic cell is spontaneous, and therefore the change in Gibbs free energy for the reaction is negative ($\Delta G < 0$). As the spontaneous reaction proceeds toward equilibrium, the movement of electrons results in a conversion of electrical potential energy into kinetic energy. By separating the reduction and oxidation half-reactions into two compartments, we are able to harness this energy and use it to do work by connecting various electrical devices into the circuit between the two electrodes.

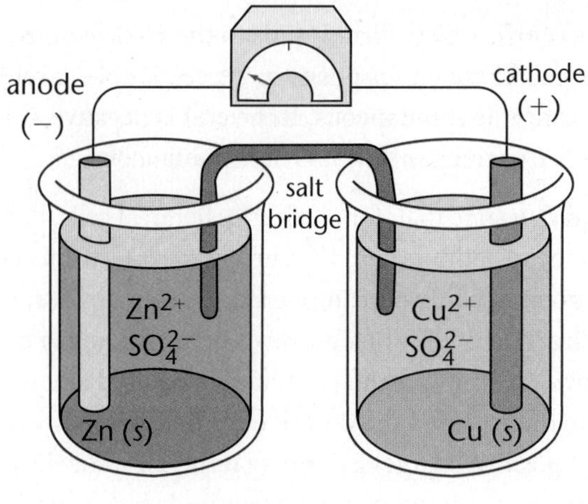

Figure 12.1 Daniell Cell

In this galvanic cell, zinc is the anode and copper is the cathode; each electrode is bathed in an electrolyte solution containing its cation and sulfate.

In the Daniell cell, a zinc electrode is placed in an aqueous $ZnSO_4$ solution, and a copper electrode is placed in an aqueous $CuSO_4$ solution. The anode of this cell is the zinc bar where Zn (*s*) is oxidized to Zn^{2+} (*aq*). The cathode is the copper bar, and it is the site of the reduction of Cu^{2+} (*aq*) to Cu (*s*). The half-cell reactions are written as follows:

$$\mathrm{Zn}\ (s) \rightarrow \mathrm{Zn}^{2+}\ (aq) + 2\ e^- \quad E_{\mathrm{red}} = -0.762\ \mathrm{V\ (anode)}$$

$$\mathrm{Cu}^{2+}\ (aq) + 2\ e^- \rightarrow \mathrm{Cu}\ (s) \quad E_{\mathrm{red}} = +0.340\ \mathrm{V\ (cathode)}$$

The net reaction is

$$\mathrm{Zn}\ (s) + \mathrm{Cu}^{2+}\ (aq) \rightarrow \mathrm{Zn}^{2+}\ (aq) + \mathrm{Cu}\ (s) \quad E_{\mathrm{cell}} = +1.102\ \mathrm{V}$$

We will discuss the calculation of cell potential in the next section. For now, appreciate that the calculation can be accomplished by knowing each half-reaction. If the two half-cells were not separated, the Cu^{2+} ions would react directly with the zinc bar, and no useful electrical work would be done. Because the solutions and electrodes are physically separated, they must be connected by a conductive material to complete the circuit.

However, if only a wire were provided for this electron flow, the reaction would soon stop because an excess positive charge would build up on the anode, and an excess negative charge would build up on the cathode. Eventually, the excessive charge accumulation would provide a countervoltage large enough to prevent the oxidation–reduction reaction from taking place, and the current would cease. This charge gradient is dissipated by the presence of a **salt bridge**, which permits the exchange of cations and anions. The salt bridge contains an inert electrolyte, usually KCl or NH_4NO_3, which contains ions that will not react with the electrodes or with the ions in solution. While the anions from the salt bridge (Cl^-) diffuse into the solution on the anode side ($ZnSO_4$) to balance out the charge of the newly created Zn^{2+} ions, the cations of the salt bridge (K^+) flow into the solution on the cathode side ($CuSO_4$) to balance out the charge of the sulfate ions left in solution when the Cu^{2+} ions are reduced to Cu and precipitate onto the electrode. This precipitation process onto the cathode itself can also be called **plating** or **galvanization**.

KEY CONCEPT

The purpose of the salt bridge is to exchange anions and cations to balance, or dissipate, newly generated charges.

During the course of the reaction, electrons flow from the zinc anode through the wire and to the copper cathode. A voltmeter can be connected to measure this electromotive force. As mentioned earlier, the anions (Cl^-) flow externally from the salt bridge into the $ZnSO_4$, and the cations (K^+) flow externally from the salt bridge into the $CuSO_4$. This flow depletes the salt bridge and, along with the finite quantity of Cu^{2+} in the solution, accounts for the relatively short lifespan of the cell.

A **cell diagram** is a shorthand notation representing the reactions in an electrochemical cell. A cell diagram for the Daniell cell is as follows:

$$Zn\ (s)\ |\ Zn^{2+}\ (1\ M)\ ||\ Cu^{2+}\ (1\ M)\ |\ Cu\ (s)$$

The following rules are used in constructing a cell diagram:

1. The reactants and products are always listed from left to right in this form:
   anode | anode solution (concentration) || cathode solution (concentration) | cathode
2. A single vertical line indicates a phase boundary.
3. A double vertical line indicates the presence of a salt bridge or some other type of barrier.

Electrolytic Cells

When comparing and contrasting galvanic and electrolytic cells, it is important to keep straight what remains consistent between the two types of cells and what differs. All types of electrochemical cells have a reduction reaction occurring at the cathode, an oxidation reaction occurring at the anode, a current flowing from cathode to anode, and electron flow from anode to cathode. However, **electrolytic cells**, in almost all of their characteristics and behavior, are otherwise the opposite of galvanic cells. Whereas galvanic cells house spontaneous oxidation–reduction reactions that generate electrical energy, electrolytic cells house nonspontaneous reactions that require the input of energy to proceed. Therefore, the change in free energy for an electrolytic cell is positive. This type of oxidation–reduction reaction driven by an external voltage source is called **electrolysis**, in which chemical compounds are decomposed. For example, electrolytic cells can be used to drive the nonspontaneous decomposition of water into oxygen and hydrogen gas. Another example, the electrolysis of molten NaCl, is illustrated in Figure 12.2.

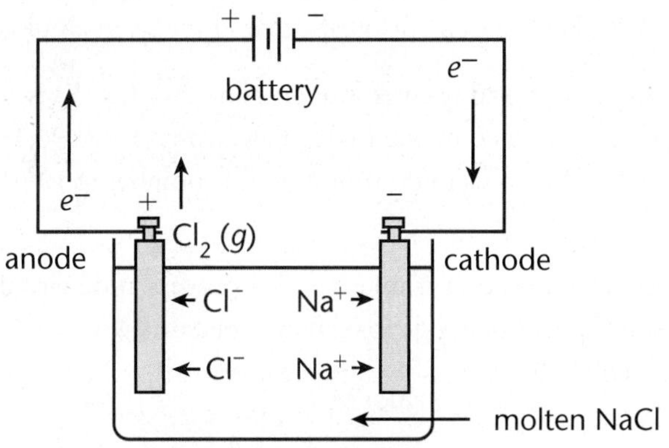

Figure 12.2 Electrolysis of Molten NaCl

MNEMONIC

Electron flow in an electrochemical cell:
A ⟶ **C** (order in the alphabet)

Electrons flow from **a**node to **c**athode in all types of electrochemical cells.

MCAT EXPERTISE

Recognize and understand the shorthand cell notation for electrochemical cells on Test Day. Passages frequently use this format rather than spelling out which reactions take place at the anode and cathode.

KEY CONCEPT

Because electrolysis is nonspontaneous, the electrode (anode or cathode) can consist of any material so long as it can resist the high temperatures and corrosion of the process.

In this electrolytic cell, molten NaCl is decomposed into Cl_2 (*g*) and Na (*l*). The external voltage source—a battery—supplies energy sufficient to drive the oxidation–reduction reaction in the direction that is thermodynamically unfavorable (nonspontaneous).

In this example, Na^+ ions migrate toward the cathode, where they are reduced to Na (*l*). At the same time, Cl^- ions migrate toward the anode, where they are oxidized to Cl_2 (*g*). Notice that the half-reactions do not need to be separated into different compartments; this is because the desired reaction is nonspontaneous. Note that sodium is a liquid at the temperature of molten NaCl; it is also less dense than the molten salt and, thus, is easily removed as it floats to the top of the reaction vessel.

This cell is used in industry as the major means of sodium and chlorine production. You may wonder why one would do so much work to obtain pure sodium and chlorine. Remember that these elements are never found naturally in their elemental form because they are so reactive. Thus, to use elemental sodium or chlorine gas in a reaction, it must be manufactured through processes such as these.

Michael Faraday was the first to define certain quantitative principles governing the behavior of electrolytic cells. He theorized that the amount of chemical change induced in an electrolytic cell is directly proportional to the number of moles of electrons that are exchanged during the oxidation–reduction reaction. The number of moles exchanged can be determined from the balanced half-reaction. In general, for a reaction that involves the transfer of *n* electrons per atom M:

$$M^{n+} + n\,e^- \rightarrow M\ (s)$$

Equation 12.1

KEY CONCEPT

Faraday's laws state that the liberation of gas and deposition of elements on electrodes is directly proportional to the number of electrons being transferred during the oxidation-reduction reaction. Here, normality or gram equivalent weight is used. These observations are proxy measurements of the amount of current flowing in a circuit.

According to this equation, one mole of metal M (*s*) will logically be produced if *n* moles of electrons are supplied to one mole of M^{n+}. Additionally, the number of moles of electrons needed to produce a certain amount of M (*s*) can now be related to the measurable electrical property of charge. One electron carries a charge of 1.6×10^{-19} coulombs (C). The charge carried by one mole of electrons can be calculated by multiplying this number by Avogadro's number, as follows:

$$\left[\frac{1.6\times10^{-19}\ \text{C}}{\text{electron}}\right]\left[\frac{6.02\times10^{23}\ \text{electrons}}{1\ \text{mol}\ e^-}\right] = 96{,}485\ \frac{\text{C}}{\text{mol}\ e^-}$$

This number is called the **Faraday constant**, and one **faraday** (**F**) is equivalent to the amount of charge contained in one mole of electrons (1 F = 96,485 C) or one equivalent. On the MCAT, you should round up this number to $10^5\ \frac{\text{C}}{\text{mol}\ e^-}$ to make calculations more manageable.

KEY CONCEPT

One faraday (F) is equivalent to the amount of charge contained in one mole of electrons (1 F = 96,485 C).

The **electrodeposition equation** summarizes this process and helps determine the number of moles of element being deposited on a plate:

$$\text{mol M} = \frac{It}{n\text{F}}$$

Equation 12.2

where mol M is the amount of metal ion being deposited at a specific electrode, I is current, t is time, n is the number of electron equivalents for a specific metal ion, and F is the Faraday constant. This equation can also be used to determine the amount of gas liberated during electrolysis.

MNEMONIC

Electrodeposition equation: Calculating **Moles of M**etal, **It** is **N**ot **F**un.
$\text{mol M} = \frac{It}{n\text{F}}$

Example: What mass of copper will be deposited in a Daniell cell if a current of 2 A flows through the cell for 3 hours?

Solution: We will use the equation $\text{mol M} = \frac{It}{n\text{F}}$

A Daniell cell uses a copper electrode in copper sulfate ($CuSO_4$) solution. Because the oxidation state of copper in solution is +2, $n = 2$. Now we can plug into the equation.

$$\text{mol M} = \frac{It}{n\text{F}} = \frac{(2\text{ A})(3\text{ hr})\left(3600\ \frac{\text{s}}{\text{hr}}\right)}{(2\text{ mol } e^-)\left(96{,}485\ \frac{\text{C}}{\text{mol } e^-}\right)} \approx \frac{3 \times 3600}{10^5}$$
$$= 0.1 \text{ mol Cu (actual} = 0.11 \text{ mol Cu)}$$

Then, we must determine the actual mass of copper being deposited.
0.1 mol Cu should have a mass of 6.35 g because the molar mass of copper is $63.5\ \frac{\text{g}}{\text{mol}}$ (actual = 7.11 g).

Concentration Cells

A **concentration cell** is a special type of galvanic cell. Like all galvanic cells, it contains two half-cells connected by a conductive material, allowing a spontaneous oxidation–reduction reaction to proceed, which generates a current and delivers energy. The distinguishing characteristic of a concentration cell is in its design: the electrodes are chemically identical. For example, if both electrodes are copper metal, they have the same reduction potential. Therefore, current is generated as a function of a concentration gradient established between the two solutions surrounding the electrodes. The concentration gradient results in a potential difference between the two compartments and drives the movement of electrons in the direction that results in equilibration of the ion gradient. The current will stop when the concentrations of ionic species in the half-cells are equal. This implies that the voltage (V) or electromotive force of a concentration cell is zero when the concentrations are equal; the voltage, as a function of concentrations, can be calculated using the **Nernst equation**.

In a biological system, a concentration cell is best represented by the cell membrane of a neuron, as shown in Figure 12.3. Sodium and potassium cations, and chlorine anions, are exchanged as needed to produce an electrical potential. The actual value depends on both the concentrations and charges of the ions. In this way, a **resting membrane potential** (V_m) can be maintained. Disturbances of the resting membrane potential, if sufficiently large, may stimulate the firing of an action potential.

BRIDGE

The maintenance of a resting membrane potential is discussed in Chapter 8 of *MCAT Biochemistry Review.* The conduction of an action potential is discussed in Chapter 4 of *MCAT Biology Review.* The transfer of ions and electrons during an action potential produces biochemical work.

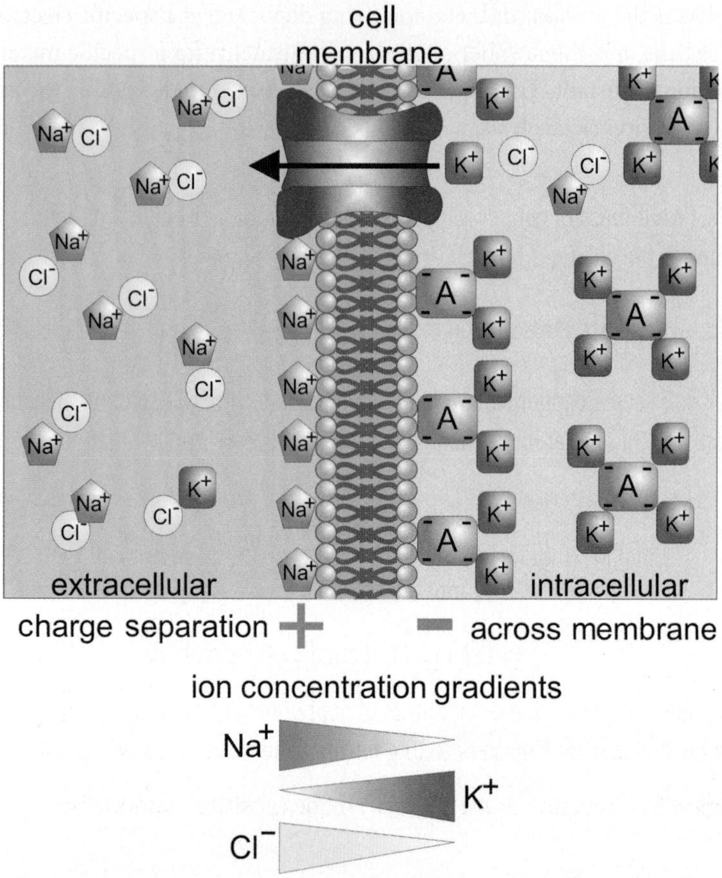

Figure 12.3 The Cell Membrane as an Example of a Concentration Cell
The electrochemical gradient created by separation of ions across the cell membrane is analogous to a cell with two electrodes composed of the same material.

Rechargeable Cells

A **rechargeable cell** or **rechargeable battery** is one that can function as both a galvanic and electrolytic cell.

Lead-Acid Batteries

A **lead-acid battery**, also known as a **lead storage battery**, is a specific type of rechargeable battery. As a voltaic cell, when fully charged, it consists of two half-cells—a Pb anode and a porous PbO_2 cathode, connected by a conductive material (concentrated 4 *M* H_2SO_4). When fully discharged, it consists of two $PbSO_4$ electroplated lead electrodes with a dilute concentration of H_2SO_4, as shown in Figure 12.4.

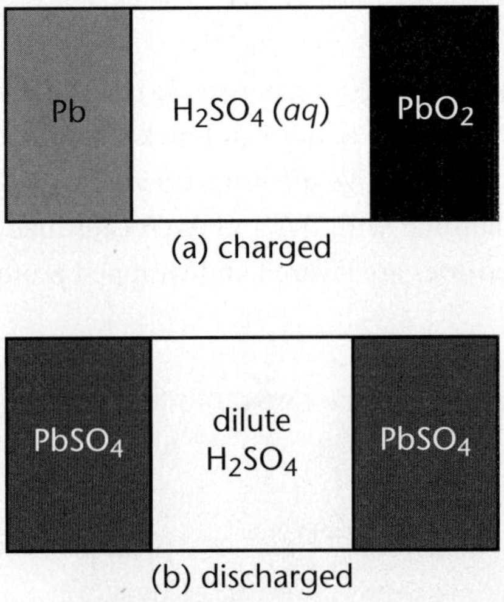

Figure 12.4 Lead-Acid Battery
When charged (a), the cell contains a Pb anode and PbO2 cathode; when discharged (b), both electrodes are coated with lead sulfate.

The oxidation half-reaction at the lead (negative) anode is:

$$Pb\ (s) + HSO_4^-\ (aq) \rightarrow PbSO_4\ (s) + H^+\ (aq) + 2\ e^- \qquad E^\circ_{red} = -0.356\ V$$

The reduction half-reaction at the lead(IV) oxide (positive) cathode is:

$$PbO_2\ (s) + SO_4^{2-}\ (aq) + 4H^+ + 2\ e^- \rightarrow PbSO_4\ (s) + 2\ H_2O \qquad E^\circ_{red} = 1.685\ V$$

Both half-reactions cause the electrodes to plate with lead sulfate ($PbSO_4$) and dilute the acid electrolyte when **discharging**. The lead anode is negatively charged and attracts the anionic bisulfate. The lead(IV) oxide cathode is a bit more complicated. This electrode is porous, which allows the electrolyte (sulfuric acid) to solvate the cathode into lead and oxide ions. Then, the hydrogen ions in solution react with the oxide ions to produce water, and the remaining sulfate ions react with the lead to produce the electroplated lead sulfate.

Overall, the net equation for a discharging lead–acid battery is:

$$Pb\ (s) + PbO_2\ (s) + 2\ H_2SO_4\ (aq) \rightarrow 2\ PbSO_4\ (s) + 2\ H_2O$$

$$E^\circ_{cell} = 1.685 - (-0.356) = 2.041\ V$$

When **charging**, the lead–acid cell is part of an electrolytic circuit. These equations and electrode charge designations are the opposite because an external source reverses the electroplating process and concentrates the acid solution—this external source is very evident when one uses jumper cables to restart a car.

Lead–acid batteries, as compared to other cells, have some of the lowest energy-to-weight ratios (otherwise known as energy density). **Energy density** is a measure of a battery's ability to produce power as a function of its weight. Lead–acid batteries, therefore, require a heavier amount of battery material to produce a certain output as compared to other batteries.

Nickel-Cadmium Batteries

Nickel–cadmium batteries are also rechargeable cells. They consist of two half-cells made of solid cadmium (the anode) and nickel(III) oxide-hydroxide (the cathode) connected by a conductive material, typically potassium hydroxide (KOH). Most of us are familiar with AA and AAA cells made of Ni–Cd materials, inside of which the electrodes are layered and wrapped around in a cylinder, as shown in Figure 12.5.

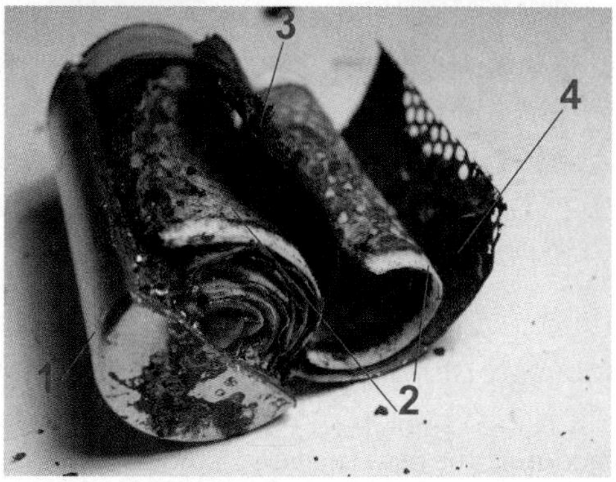

Figure 12.5 A Nickel-Cadmium Battery
(1) Metal casing, (2) salt bridge, (3) NiO(OH) cathode, (4) Cd anode

The oxidation half-reaction at the cadmium (negative) anode is:

$$\text{Cd}\,(s) + 2\,\text{OH}^-\,(aq) \rightarrow \text{Cd(OH)}_2\,(s) + 2\,e^- \qquad E^\circ_{\text{red}} = -0.86\text{ V}$$

The reduction half-reaction at the nickel oxide–hydroxide (positive) cathode is:

$$2\,\text{NiO(OH)}\,(s) + 2\,\text{H}_2\text{O} + 2\,e^- \rightarrow 2\,\text{Ni(OH)}_2\,(s) + 2\,\text{OH}^- \qquad E^\circ_{\text{red}} = 0.49\text{ V}$$

Both half-reactions cause the electrodes to plate with their respective products. Overall, the net equation for a Ni–Cd battery is:

$$2\,\text{NiO(OH)}\,(s) + \text{Cd} + 2\,\text{H}_2\text{O} \rightarrow 2\,\text{Ni(OH)}_2\,(s) + \text{Cd(OH)}_2\,(s)$$
$$E^\circ_{\text{cell}} = 0.49\ -(-0.86) = 1.35\text{ V}$$

As in our previous example, charging reverses the electrolytic cell potentials. Some Ni–Cd designs are vented for this reason to allow for the release of built-up hydrogen and oxygen gas during electrolysis.

Ni–Cd batteries have a higher energy density than lead–acid batteries. The electrochemistry of the Ni–Cd half-reactions also tends to provide higher surge current. **Surge currents** are periods of large current (amperage) early in the discharge cycle. This is preferable in appliances such as remote controls that demand rapid responses. It is important to note that modern Ni–Cd batteries have largely been replaced by more efficient **nickel–metal hydride (NiMH) batteries**. These newer batteries have more energy density, are more cost effective, and are significantly less toxic. As the name suggests, in lieu of a pure metal anode, a metal hydride is used instead.

Electrode Charge Designations

In a galvanic cell, current is spontaneously generated as electrons are released by the oxidized species at the anode and travel through the conductive material to the cathode, where reduction takes place. Because the anode of a galvanic cell is the source of electrons, it is considered the negative electrode; the cathode is considered the positive electrode, as shown in Figure 12.1 previously. Electrons, therefore, move from negative (low electrical potential) to positive (high electrical potential), while the current—the flow of positive charge—is from positive (high electrical potential) to negative (low electrical potential).

Conversely, the anode of an electrolytic cell is considered positive because it is attached to the positive pole of the external voltage source and attracts anions from the solution. The cathode of an electrolytic cell is considered negative because it is attached to the negative pole of the external voltage source and attracts cations from the solution.

In spite of this difference in designating charge (sign), oxidation always takes place at the anode and reduction always takes place at the cathode in both types of cells; electrons always flow through the wire from the anode to the cathode and current flows from cathode to anode. Finally, note that—regardless of its charge designation—the cathode always attracts cations and the anode always attracts anions. In the Daniell cell, for example, the electrons created at the anode by the oxidation of elemental zinc travel through the wire to the copper half-cell. There, they attract copper(II) cations to the cathode, resulting in the reduction of the copper ions to elemental copper, and drawing cations out of the salt bridge into the compartment. The anode, having lost electrons, attracts anions from the salt bridge at the same time that zinc(II) ions formed by the oxidation process dissolve away from the anode.

This is an important rule to understand not only for electrochemistry in the *Chemical and Physical Foundations of Biological Systems* section on Test Day, but also for electrophoresis in both this section and *Biological and Biochemical Foundations of Living Systems*. **Isoelectric focusing** is a technique used to separate amino acids or polypeptides based on their **isoelectric points (pI)**. The positively charged amino acids (protonated at the solution's pH) will migrate toward the cathode; negatively charged amino acids (deprotonated at the solution's pH) will migrate toward the anode. The technique of isoelectric focusing is discussed in detail in Chapter 3 of *MCAT Biochemistry Review*.

MNEMONIC

In a galva**n**ic cell, the a**n**ode is **n**egative.

KEY CONCEPT

In a galvanic cell, the anode is negative and the cathode is positive. In an electrolytic cell, the anode is positive and the cathode is negative. This is because an external source is used to reverse the charge of an electrolytic cell. However, in both types of cells, reduction occurs at the cathode, and oxidation occurs at the anode; cations are attracted to the cathode, and anions are attracted to the anode.

REAL WORLD

Recognize that in any system in which batteries are placed, it is important to line up cathodes and anodes. Electronics tend to have (+) and (−) designations to line up the electrodes–think jumper cables, television remotes, and button batteries in watches.

MNEMONIC

Anions are attracted to the **an**ode. **Cat**ions are attracted to the **cat**hode. This is true regardless of the type of cell (galvanic, electrolytic, or concentration cells).

MCAT CONCEPT CHECK 12.1

Before you move on, assess your understanding of the material with these questions.

1. Circle which electrode each of the following statements describes in a galvanic (voltaic) cell:

• Site of oxidation:	Anode	Cathode
• Electrons flow toward it:	Anode	Cathode
• Current flows toward it:	Anode	Cathode
• Has (–) designation:	Anode	Cathode
• Attracts cations:	Anode	Cathode

2. Circle which electrode each of the following statements describes in an electrolytic cell:

• Site of oxidation:	Anode	Cathode
• Electrons flow toward it:	Anode	Cathode
• Current flows toward it:	Anode	Cathode
• Has (–) designation:	Anode	Cathode
• Attracts cations:	Anode	Cathode

3. Write the cell diagram for the discharging state of a lead–acid battery:

____

4. Which type of cell has a positive ΔG? A positive E_{cell}?

• Positive ΔG:

____

• Positive E_{cell}:

____

5. How much current is required to produce 0.23 kg Na from a molten NaCl electrolytic cell that runs for 30 hours? Assume the cell is 100% efficient.

____

6. Fill in the following chart to summarize electrode charge designations of batteries we have analyzed:

Battery	State of Use	Galvanic or Electrolytic	Anode Material	Anode Charge	Cathode Material	Cathode Charge
Ni—Cd	Discharging					
Ni—Cd	Charging					
Molten NaCl	Discharging					
Daniell cell	Discharging					
Lead-acid	Charging					
Lead-acid	Discharging					

12.2 Cell Potentials

LEARNING OBJECTIVES

After Chapter 12.2, you will be able to:

- Describe how standard reduction potentials are measured
- Explain the importance of the sign for electromotive force
- Determine whether a cell using a given reaction is galvanic or electrolytic
- Calculate the net *E* value for a redox reaction between two species:

$$Ag^{+} + e^{-} \rightarrow Ag\ (s) \qquad E^{\circ}_{red} = +0.80\ V$$

$$Tl^{+} + e^{-} \rightarrow Tl\ (s) \qquad E^{\circ}_{red} = -0.34\ V$$

For galvanic cells, the direction of spontaneous movement of charge is from the anode, the site of oxidation, to the cathode, the site of reduction. This is simple enough to remember, but it begs the question: how do we determine which electrode species will be oxidized and which will be reduced? The relative tendencies of different chemical species to be reduced have been determined experimentally, using the tendency of the hydrogen ion (H^{+}) to be reduced as an arbitrary zero reference point.

Reduction Potentials

A reduction potential is measured in volts (V) and defined relative to the **standard hydrogen electrode** (**SHE**), which is given a potential of 0 V by convention. The species in a reaction that will be oxidized or reduced can be determined from the **reduction potential** of each species, defined as the tendency of a species to gain electrons and to be reduced. Each species has its own intrinsic reduction potential; the more positive the potential, the greater the tendency to be reduced.

KEY CONCEPT

A reduction potential is exactly what it sounds like. It tells us how likely a compound is to be reduced. The more positive the value, the more likely it is to be reduced—the more it *wants* to be reduced.

Standard reduction potential (E°_{red}) is measured under **standard conditions**: 25°C (298 K), 1 atm pressure, and 1 *M* concentrations. The relative reactivities of different half-cells can be compared to predict the direction of electron flow. A more positive E°_{red} means a greater relative tendency for reduction to occur, while a less positive E°_{red} means a greater relative tendency for oxidation to occur.

For galvanic cells, the electrode with the more positive reduction potential is the cathode, and the electrode with the less positive reduction potential is the anode. Because the species with a stronger tendency to gain electrons (that *wants* to gain electrons more) is actually doing so, the reaction is spontaneous and ΔG is negative. For electrolytic cells, the electrode with the more positive reduction potential is forced by the external voltage source to be oxidized and is, therefore, the anode. The electrode with the less positive reduction potential is forced to be reduced and is, therefore, the cathode. Because the movement of electrons is in the direction against the tendency or desires of the respective electrochemical species, the reaction is non-spontaneous and ΔG is positive.

Example: Given the following half-reactions and E°_{red} values, determine which species would be oxidized and which would be reduced in a galvanic cell.

$$Ag^+ + e^- \rightarrow Ag\ (s) \quad E^\circ_{red} = +0.80\ V$$

$$Tl^+ + e^- \rightarrow Tl\ (s) \quad E^\circ_{red} = -0.34\ V$$

Solution: E°_{red} indicates the reduction potential, or the likelihood of a compound to be reduced via a given reaction. A positive E°_{red} value indicates a spontaneous reduction, and a negative value indicates a non-spontaneous reduction. In a galvanic cell, Ag^+ will be spontaneously reduced to Ag (*s*) and Tl (*s*) will be spontaneously oxidized to Tl^+ because Ag^+ has the more positive E°_{red} and thus the more favorable reduction reaction. Therefore, the net ionic equation would be:

$$Ag^+ + Tl\ (s) \rightarrow Tl^+ + Ag\ (s)$$

which is the sum of the two spontaneous half-reactions.

It should be noted that reduction and oxidation are opposite processes. Therefore, to obtain the oxidation potential of a given half-reaction, both the reduction half-reaction and the sign of the reduction potential are reversed. For instance, from the example above, the oxidation half-reaction and oxidation potential of Tl (*s*) are:

$$Tl\ (s) \rightarrow Tl^+ + e^- \qquad E^\circ_{ox} = +0.34\ V$$

Note that, in the examples of batteries given above (lead–acid storage batteries and nickel–cadmium batteries), the oxidation half-reaction was given with the reduction potential of the reverse reaction. These two quantities have equal magnitudes but opposite signs. On the MCAT, reduction potentials are generally given rather than oxidation potentials. Therefore, all references in this book (with exception of the thallium example immediately above) are given using reduction potentials—not oxidation potentials.

The Electromotive Force

Standard reduction potentials are also used to calculate the **standard electromotive force (emf or E°_{cell})** of a reaction, which is the difference in potential (voltage) between two half-cells under standard conditions. The emf of a reaction is determined by calculating the difference in reduction potentials between the two half-cells:

$$E^\circ_{cell} = E^\circ_{red,cathode} - E^\circ_{red,anode}$$

Equation 12.3

When subtracting standard potentials, do not multiply them by the number of moles oxidized or reduced. This is because the potential of each electrode does not depend on the size of the electrode (the amount of material), but rather the identity of the material. The standard reduction potential of an electrode will not change unless the chemical identity of that electrode is changed.

KEY CONCEPT

If you need to multiply each half-reaction by a common denominator to cancel out electrons when coming up with the net ionic equation, do *not* multiply the reduction potential, E°_{red}, by that number. That would indicate a change in the chemical identity of the electrode, which is not occurring.

Example: Given that the standard reduction potentials for Sm^{3+} and $[RhCl_6]^{3-}$ are -2.41 V and $+0.44$ V, respectively, calculate the electromotive force of the following reaction:

$$Sm^{3+} + Rh + 6\,Cl^- \rightarrow [RhCl_6]^{3-} + Sm$$

Solution: First, determine the oxidation and reduction half-reactions. As written, the Rh is oxidized, and the Sm^{3+} is reduced:

$$Sm^{3+} + 3\,e^- \rightarrow Sm$$

$$Rh + 6\,Cl^- \rightarrow [RhCl_6]^{3-} + 3\,e^-$$

Now, we simply take the difference between the samarium(III) reduction potential and the hexachlororhodate(III) reduction potential. We need not change the sign on the hexachlororhodate(III) reduction potential because we are *subtracting* it from that of samarium(III).

Using the equation provided, the emf can be calculated as:
$-2.41\text{ V} - (+0.44\text{ V}) = -2.85\text{ V}$. The cell is thus electrolytic. If this were instead a galvanic cell the reaction would proceed spontaneously to the left, toward reactants, in which case the Sm would be oxidized while $[RhCl_6]^{3-}$ would be reduced with an emf of $+2.85$ V.

MCAT CONCEPT CHECK 12.2

Before you move on, assess your understanding of the material with these questions.

1. How are standard reduction potentials measured?

2. If a cell's electromotive force (emf) is denoted as a positive value, what does that mean? What if it is negative?
   - Positive emf:
   - Negative emf:

3. Given the following reactions, determine whether the cell is galvanic or electrolytic:
   - $2\ Fe^{3+}\ (aq) + 2\ Cl^-\ (aq) \rightarrow 2\ Fe^{2+}\ (aq) + Cl_2\ (g)$ ($E^\circ_{cell} = -0.59$ V):
   - $2\ Fe^{3+}\ (aq) + 2\ I^-\ (aq) \rightarrow 2\ Fe^{2+}\ (aq) + I_2\ (aq)$ ($E^\circ_{cell} = +0.25$ V):

4. Given the two half-reactions below, what would be the spontaneous oxidation-reduction reaction between these two species?

$$Fe^{3+} + 3\,e^- \rightarrow Fe \qquad E^\circ_{red} = -0.036\text{ V}$$

$$I_3^- + 2\,e^- \rightarrow 3\,I^- \qquad E^\circ_{red} = +0.534\text{ V}$$

12.3 Electromotive Force and Thermodynamics

LEARNING OBJECTIVES

After Chapter 12.3, you will be able to:

- Apply the formula $\Delta G^\circ = -RT \ln K_{eq}$ to calculations of Gibbs free energy or electromotive force
- Predict E_{cell} given reaction quotients and equilibrium constants

Throughout our discussion of electrochemistry and the different types of electrochemical cells, we have been making references to the spontaneity or nonspontaneity of the redox reactions housed in each of the different cell types. Let's now look more formally at this topic by relating free energy to electromotive force (emf) and the concentrations of the oxidation–reduction reactants and products to the voltage of a cell at a given point in time.

Gibbs Free Energy

By now, you should be familiar with the thermodynamic criterion for determining the spontaneity of a reaction: the change in Gibbs free energy, ΔG. This is the change in the amount of energy available in a chemical system to do work. In an electrochemical cell, the work done is dependent on the number of coulombs of charge transferred and the energy available. Thus, ΔG° and emf are related as follows:

$$\Delta G^\circ = -nFE^\circ_{\text{cell}}$$

Equation 12.4

where ΔG° is the standard change in free energy, n is the number of moles of electrons exchanged, F is the Faraday constant, and E°_{cell} is the standard emf of the cell. Keep in mind that, if the Faraday constant is expressed in coulombs $\left(\frac{\text{J}}{\text{V}}\right)$, then ΔG° must be expressed in J, not kJ. Notice the similarity of this relationship to that expressed in the physics formula $W = q\Delta V$ for the amount of work available or needed in the transport of a charge q across a potential difference ΔV: $n \times \text{F}$ is a charge, and E°_{cell} is a voltage. This application in electrostatics is discussed in Chapter 5 of *MCAT Physics and Math Review.*

BRIDGE

Recall from Chapter 6 of *MCAT General Chemistry Review* that, if ΔG is positive, the reaction is nonspontaneous; if ΔG is negative, the reaction is spontaneous.

Note the significance of the negative sign on the right side of the equation. ΔG° and E°_{cell} will always have opposite signs. Therefore, galvanic cells have negative ΔG° and positive E°_{cell} values; electrolytic cells have positive ΔG° and negative E°_{cell} values.

Example: Determine the standard change in free energy of a cell with the following net reaction. (Note: The standard reduction potential of iron(III) is +0.77 V; the standard reduction potential of molecular chlorine is +1.36 V.)

$$2\ Fe^{3+}\ (aq) + 2\ Cl^-\ (aq) \rightarrow 2\ Fe^{2+}\ (aq) + Cl_2\ (g)$$

Solution: First, separate the reaction into the half-reactions:

$$2\ Fe^{3+} + 2\ e^- \rightarrow 2\ Fe^{2+}$$

$$2\ Cl^- \rightarrow Cl_2 + 2\ e^-$$

In this reaction, iron(III) is reduced and is the cathode, whereas Cl^- is oxidized and is the anode. The reduction potential of chlorine is actually higher than that of iron(III); this means that the electrodes are serving the *opposite* role from their natural tendency, and the reaction is nonspontaneous. This is an electrolytic cell, and should have a negative emf value.

Now, determine the emf:

$$E^\circ_{cell} = E^\circ_{red,cathode} - E^\circ_{red,anode} = 0.77\text{ V} - 1.36\text{ V} = -0.59\text{ V}$$

Use the emf to determine the free energy change (note that as 2 electrons are transferred, $n = 2$):

$$\Delta G^\circ = -nFE^\circ_{cell} = -(2\text{ mol }e^-)\left(96{,}485\,\frac{\text{C}}{\text{mol }e^-}\right)(-0.59\text{ V})$$
$$\approx 2 \times 10^5 \times (0.6) = 1.2 \times 10^5\text{ J (actual} = 1.14 \times 10^5\text{ J)}$$

The free energy change is about +120 kJ, which represents a non-spontaneous reaction.

Reaction Quotients

So far, we have considered the calculation of a cell's emf only under standard conditions. However, electrochemical cells may have ionic concentrations that deviate from 1 *M*. Also, for the concentration cell, the concentrations of the ions in the two compartments *must* be different for there to be a measurable voltage and current. Concentration and the emf of a cell are related: emf varies with the changing concentrations of the species in the cell. When conditions deviate from standard conditions, one can use the **Nernst equation**:

$$E_{cell} = E^\circ_{cell} - \frac{RT}{nF}\ln Q$$

Equation 12.5

where E_{cell} is the emf of the cell under nonstandard conditions, E°_{cell} is the emf of the cell under standard conditions, R is the ideal gas constant, *T* is the temperature in kelvin, *n* is the number of moles of electrons, F is the Faraday constant, and Q is the reaction quotient for the reaction at a given point in time. The following simplified version of the equation can be used, assuming $T = 298$ K:

$$E_{cell} = E^\circ_{cell} - \frac{0.0592}{n}\log Q$$

Equation 12.6

This simplified version of the equation brings together R, *T* (298 K), and F, and converts the natural logarithm to the base-ten logarithm to make calculations easier.

Remember that the reaction quotient, Q, for a general reaction $a\text{A} + b\text{B} \rightarrow c\text{C} + d\text{D}$ has the form:

$$Q = \frac{[\text{C}]^c[\text{D}]^d}{[\text{A}]^a[\text{B}]^b}$$

Equation 12.7

MCAT EXPERTISE

If the Nernst equation is needed on Test Day, stick with the $\log_{10}$ version because natural logarithm calculations get very tedious.

Although the expression for the reaction quotient Q has two terms for the concentrations of reactants and two terms for the concentrations of products, remember that only the species in solution are included. When considering the case of the Daniell cell, for example, only the concentrations of zinc and copper ions are considered:

$$\mathrm{Zn}\ (s) + \mathrm{Cu}^{2+}(aq) \rightarrow \mathrm{Zn}^{2+}(aq) + \mathrm{Cu}\ (s)$$

$$Q = \frac{[\mathrm{Zn}^{2+}]}{[\mathrm{Cu}^{2+}]}$$

The emf of a cell can be measured with a **voltmeter**. A **potentiometer** is a kind of voltmeter that draws no current and gives a more accurate reading of the difference in potential between two electrodes.

Example: Find the emf of a galvanic cell at 25°C based on the following standard reduction potentials:

$$\mathrm{Fe}^{2+} + 2\,e^- \rightarrow \mathrm{Fe} \qquad E^\circ_{\mathrm{red}} = -0.44\ \mathrm{V}$$

$$\mathrm{Cl}_2 + 2\ e^- \rightarrow 2\ \mathrm{Cl}^- \qquad E^\circ_{\mathrm{red}} = +1.36\ \mathrm{V}$$

In this cell, $[\mathrm{Fe}^{2+}] = 0.01\ M$ and $[\mathrm{Cl}^-] = 0.1\ M$.

Solution: First, determine the standard cell potential. Because the chlorine half-reaction has a higher reduction potential, it will be the cathode. Iron will act as the anode. The standard cell potential is:

$$E^\circ_{\mathrm{cell}} = E^\circ_{\mathrm{red,cathode}} - E^\circ_{\mathrm{red,anode}} = 1.36\ \mathrm{V} - (-0.44\ \mathrm{V}) = +1.80\ \mathrm{V}$$

Now, determine the net ionic equation. Remember that iron is being oxidized, so its reduction half-reaction in the question stem will have to be reversed. The net ionic equation is:

$$\mathrm{Fe} + \mathrm{Cl}_2 \rightarrow \mathrm{Fe}^{2+} + 2\ \mathrm{Cl}^-$$

From this equation, we can determine the value of the reaction quotient:

$$Q = [\mathrm{Fe}^{2+}][\mathrm{Cl}^-]^2 = (0.01\ M)(0.1\ M)^2 = 10^{-4}$$

Now, plug into the Nernst equation, keeping in mind that two electrons are transferred ($n = 2$):

$$E_{\mathrm{cell}} = E^\circ_{\mathrm{cell}} - \frac{0.0592}{n}\log Q = 1.8 - \frac{0.0592}{2}\log 10^{-4}$$

$$= 1.8 + \frac{4 \times 0.0592}{2} \approx 1.8 + (2 \times 0.06) = 1.92\ \mathrm{V}$$

In this case, the cell actually has a higher voltage than it normally would due to the concentrations of ions present.

BRIDGE

While a mathematically rigorous equation, the Nernst equation has a powerful use in biochemistry for calculating resting and depolarized membrane potentials based on concentrations of ions. Its more extended version, the Goldman–Hodgkin–Katz equation, is discussed in Chapter 8 of *MCAT Biochemistry Review.* Equation 8.2 in that chapter looks slightly different than Equation 12.6 here. This is because the temperature is different (310 K rather than 298 K) and the units are different (mV instead of V).

Equilibria

As discussed in Chapter 7 of *MCAT General Chemistry Review*, $\Delta G°$ can also be determined in another manner:

$$\Delta G° = -RT \ln K_{eq}$$

Equation 12.8

where R is the ideal gas constant, T is the absolute temperature, and K_{eq} is the equilibrium constant for the reaction.

Combining the two expressions that solve for standard free energy change, we see that

$$\Delta G° = -nFE°_{cell} = -RT \ln K_{eq}$$

or

$$nFE°_{cell} = RT \ln K_{eq}$$

By extension, if the values for n, T, and K_{eq} are known, then $E°_{cell}$ for the reaction is easily calculated. On the MCAT, you will not be expected to calculate natural logarithm values in your head. That being said, these equations can still be tested but in a conceptual way.

MCAT EXPERTISE

Whether it is log or ln, remember that a logarithm will be positive when equilibrium constants are greater than 1, negative when equilibrium constants are less than 1, and 0 when equilibrium constants are equal to 1.

Analysis of the equations shows us that, for redox reactions with equilibrium constants less than 1 (equilibrium state favors the reactants), the $E°_{cell}$ will be negative because the natural logarithm of any number between 0 and 1 is negative. These properties are characteristic of electrolytic cells, which house nonspontaneous oxidation–reduction reactions. Instead, if the equilibrium constant for the reaction is greater than 1 (equilibrium state favors the products), the $E°_{cell}$ will be positive because the natural logarithm of any number greater than 1 is positive. These properties are characteristic of galvanic cells, which house spontaneous oxidation–reduction reactions. If the equilibrium constant is equal to 1 (concentrations of the reactants and products are equal at equilibrium), the $E°_{cell}$ will be equal to zero. An easy way to remember this is that $E°_{cell} = 0$ V for any concentration cell with equimolar concentrations in both half-cells because there is no net ionic equation (both half-cells contain the same ions).

KEY CONCEPT

If $E°_{cell}$ is positive, ln K_{eq} is positive. This means that K_{eq} must be greater than one and that the equilibrium lies to the right (products are favored).

Knowing the effects of concentration on equilibria, we can now derive the change in Gibbs free energy of an electrochemical cell with varying concentrations using the equation:

$$\Delta G = \Delta G° + RT \ln Q$$

Equation 12.9

where ΔG is the free energy change under nonstandard conditions, $\Delta G°$ is the free energy change under standard conditions (which can be determined from Equation 12.4 or Equation 12.8 above), R is the ideal gas constant, T is the temperature, and Q is the reaction quotient.

MCAT CONCEPT CHECK 12.3

Before you move on, assess your understanding of the material with these questions.

1. Fill in the table to show the relationships between the equilibrium constant, Gibbs free energy, and electromotive force (emf), assuming standard conditions:

K_{eq}	$\Delta G°$: (+) or (−)?	Reaction: Spontaneous or Nonspontaneous?	$E°_{cell}$: (+) or (−)?
1.2×10^{-2}			
2×10^{2}			
1			

2. Given the following reaction quotients and equilibrium constants, determine the direction of the reaction and the sign of E_{cell}:

Q	K_{eq}	Reaction Direction (Forward, Backward, or Equilibrium)	Sign of E_{cell}
10^{-3}	10^{-2}		
10^{2}	1.1		
1	1		

Conclusion

In this chapter, we covered the essential MCAT topic of electrochemistry. We reviewed the behavior of many different types of electrochemical cells. Galvanic cells rely on spontaneous oxidation–reduction reactions to produce current and supply energy. The concentration cell is a special type of galvanic cell for which the current is dependent on an ion concentration gradient rather than a difference in reduction potential between two chemically distinct electrodes. Electrolytic cells rely on external voltage sources to drive a nonspontaneous oxidation–reduction reaction called electrolysis. Finally, we considered the thermodynamics of the different cell types. Galvanic and concentration cells have positive electromotive forces (emf) and negative free energy changes, whereas electrolytic cells have negative electromotive forces and positive free energy changes.

In retrospect, the content you have learned in *MCAT General Chemistry Review* has numerous organic (biological) and inorganic applications. And as you prepare to be a physician, you must begin to understand and treat the individual as a sum of many intertwining systems and parts. Many body systems and parts rely on electrochemical cells: the heart is a self-paced electrochemical cell, the neurons of the brain and spinal cord are rechargeable concentration cells, and every cell that contains mitochondria (all cells except erythrocytes) rely on the proton-motive force across the inner mitochondrial membrane to function. Our discussion here of inorganic systems has value through analogy to many biological systems.

Without further delay, we want to offer you our heartiest congratulations for completing this final chapter of *MCAT General Chemistry Review*. The hard work, time, and energy you have invested in a careful and thorough review of the topics covered within the pages of this book will pay off on Test Day. We hope that we have been successful in meeting our goals in writing this *Kaplan MCAT Review* series: to assess the general concepts and principles essential to correctly and efficiently answer the general chemistry questions on the MCAT; to guide you in the development of critical thinking skills necessary for analyzing passages, question stems, and answer choices; and to provide holistic preparation for your Test Day experience. In addition to all of these, we aimed to relate the science to everyday life experiences and future experiences as a physician, demystify the concepts, and have some fun in the process. We are grateful for the opportunity to have been a part of your journey to success on the MCAT, and—beyond that—success in your medical education and future practice as the great physician you deserve to be!

You've reviewed the content, now test your knowledge and critical thinking skills by completing a test-like passage set in your online resources!

GO ONLINE

CONCEPT SUMMARY

Electrochemical Cells

- An **electrochemical cell** describes any cell in which oxidation–reduction reactions take place. Certain characteristics are shared between all types of electrochemical cells.
  - **Electrodes** are strips of metal or other conductive materials placed in an **electrolyte** solution.
  - The **anode** is always the site of oxidation. It attracts anions.
  - The **cathode** is always the site of reduction. It attracts cations.
  - Electrons flow from the anode to the cathode.
  - Current flows from the cathode to the anode.
- **Cell diagrams** are shorthand notation that represent the reactions taking place in an electrochemical cell.
  - Cell diagrams are written from anode to cathode with electrolytes (the solution) in between.
  - A vertical line represents a phase boundary, and a double vertical line represents a salt bridge or other physical boundary.
- **Galvanic (voltaic) cells** house spontaneous reactions ($\Delta G < 0$) with a positive electromotive force.
- **Electrolytic cells** house nonspontaneous reactions ($\Delta G > 0$) with a negative electromotive force. These nonspontaneous cells can be used to create useful products through electrolysis.
- **Concentration cells** are a specialized form of a galvanic cell in which both electrodes are made of the same material. Rather than a potential difference causing the movement of charge, it is the concentration gradient between the two solutions.
- The charge on an electrode is dependent on the type of electrochemical cell one is studying.
  - For galvanic cells, the anode is negatively charged and the cathode is positively charged.
  - For electrolytic cells, the anode is positively charged and the cathode is negatively charged.
- **Rechargeable batteries** are electrochemical cells that can experience **charging** (electrolytic) and **discharging** (galvanic) states. Rechargeable batteries are often ranked by **energy density**—the amount of energy a cell can produce relative to the mass of battery material.
  - **Lead–acid batteries**, when discharging, consist of a Pb anode and a PbO_2 cathode in a concentrated sulfuric acid solution. When charging, the $PbSO_4$-plated electrodes are dissociated to restore the original Pb and PbO_2 electrodes and concentrate the electrolyte. These cells have a low energy density.

- **Nickel–cadmium batteries (Ni–Cd)**, when discharging, consist of a Cd anode and a NiO(OH) cathode in a concentrated KOH solution. When charging, the $Ni(OH)_2$ and $Cd(OH)_2$ plated electrodes are dissociated to restore the original Cd and NiO(OH) electrodes and concentrate the electrolyte. These cells have a higher energy density than lead–acid batteries.
- **Nickel–metal hydride (NiMH)** batteries have more or less replaced Ni–Cd batteries because they have higher energy density, are more cost effective, and are significantly less toxic.

- **Surge current** is an above-average current transiently released at the beginning of the discharge phase; it wanes rapidly until a stable current is achieved.

Cell Potentials

- A **reduction potential** quantifies the tendency for a species to gain electrons and be reduced. The higher the reduction potential, the more a given species wants to be reduced.
  - **Standard reduction potentials (E°_{red})** are calculated by comparison to the **standard hydrogen electrode (SHE)** under the standard conditions of 298 K, 1 atm pressure, and 1 *M* concentrations.
  - The standard hydrogen electrode has a standard reduction potential of 0 V.
- **Standard electromotive force (E°_{cell})** is the difference in standard reduction potential between the two half-cells.
- For galvanic cells, the difference of the reduction potentials of the two half-reactions is positive; for electrolytic cells, the difference of the reduction potentials of the two half-reactions is negative.

Electromotive Force and Thermodynamics

- Electromotive force and change in free energy always have opposite signs.
  - When E°_{cell} is positive, ΔG° is negative. This is the case in galvanic cells.
  - When E°_{cell} is negative, ΔG° is positive. This is the case in electrolytic cells.
  - When E°_{cell} is 0, ΔG° is 0. This is the case in concentration cells.
- The **Nernst equation** describes the relationship between the concentration of species in a solution under nonstandard conditions and the electromotive force.
- There exists a relationship between the equilibrium constant (K_{eq}) and E°_{cell}.
  - When K_{eq} (the ratio of products' concentrations at equilibrium over reactants', raised to their stoichiometric coefficients) is greater than 1, E°_{cell} is positive.
  - When K_{eq} is less than 1, E°_{cell} is negative.
  - When K_{eq} is equal to 1, E°_{cell} is 0.

ANSWERS TO CONCEPT CHECKS

12.1

1. In a galvanic cell, the anode is the site of oxidation, has current flowing toward it, and has a (−) designation. The cathode has electrons flowing toward it and attracts cations.
2. In an electrolytic cell, the anode is the site of oxidation and has current flowing toward it. The cathode has electrons flowing toward it, has a (−) designation, and attracts cations.
3. $\text{Pb}\ (s)\ |\ \text{H}_2\text{SO}_4\ (4\ M)\ ||\ \text{H}_2\text{SO}_4\ (4\ M)\ |\ \text{PbO}_2\ (s)$
4. Electrolytic cells are nonspontaneous and have a positive ΔG. Galvanic cells are spontaneous and have a negative ΔG; therefore, they have a positive E_{cell}.
5. $$\text{mol M} = \frac{It}{n\text{F}} \rightarrow I = \frac{(\text{mol M})n\text{F}}{t} = \frac{\left(\dfrac{230\ \text{g}}{23\ \dfrac{\text{g}}{\text{mol}}}\right)\left(1\ \text{mol}\ e^-\right)\left(96{,}485\ \dfrac{\text{C}}{\text{mol}\ e^-}\right)}{30\ \text{hr}\left(\dfrac{3600\ \text{s}}{1\ \text{hr}}\right)} \approx \frac{10 \times 10^5}{10^5}$$
$$= 10\ \text{A}\ (\text{actual} = 8.93\ \text{A})$$
6.

Battery	State of Use	Galvanic or Electrolytic	Anode Material	Anode Charge	Cathode Material	Cathode Charge
Ni—Cd	Discharging	Galvanic	Cd	Negative	NiO(OH)	Positive
Ni—Cd	Charging	Electrolytic	Cd(OH)_2	Positive	Ni(OH)_2	Negative
Molten NaCl	Discharging	Electrolytic	Any	Positive	Any	Negative
Daniell cell	Discharging	Galvanic	Zn	Negative	Cu	Positive
Lead–acid	Charging	Electrolytic	PbSO_4	Positive	PbSO_4	Negative
Lead–acid	Discharging	Galvanic	Pb	Negative	PbO_2	Positive

12.2

1. A sample is measured by setting up a cell relative to a standard hydrogen electrode, which is given a reduction potential of 0 V by convention.
2. A positive emf means the cell is spontaneous (galvanic); a negative emf means the cell is nonspontaneous (electrolytic).
3. The first cell is electrolytic because it has a negative emf. The second cell is galvanic because it has a positive emf.
4. The reduction potential of triiodide is higher than iron(III), so triiodide will be reduced and iron will be oxidized: $2\ Fe + 3\ I_3^- \rightarrow 2\ Fe^{3+} + 9\ I^-$ ($E^\circ_{cell} = +0.57$ V).

12.3

1.

K_{eq}	ΔG°: (+) or (−)?	Reaction: Spontaneous or Nonspontaneous?	E°_{cell}: (+) or (−)?
1.2×10^{-2}	+	Nonspontaneous	−
2×10^{2}	−	Spontaneous	+
1	0	Not applicable—applies to any cell at equilibrium	0

Remember that $\Delta G^\circ = -RT \ln K_{eq}$; if $K_{eq} < 1$, $\ln K_{eq} < 0$, and $\Delta G^\circ > 0$. If $K_{eq} > 1$, $\ln K_{eq} > 0$, and $\Delta G^\circ < 0$. If $K_{eq} = 1$, $\ln K_{eq} = 0$, and $\Delta G^\circ = 0$.

2.

Q	K_{eq}	Reaction Direction (Forward, Backward, or Equilibrium)	Sign of E_{cell}
10^{-3}	10^{-2}	Forward	+
10^{2}	1.1	Backward	−
1	1	Equilibrium	0

Note that these calculations do not assume standard conditions, unlike question 1.

SCIENCE MASTERY ASSESSMENT EXPLANATIONS

1. **C**

In the oxidation–reduction reaction of a metal with oxygen, the metal will be oxidized (donate electrons) and oxygen will be reduced (accept electrons). This fact allows us to immediately eliminate **(B)** and **(D)**. A species with a higher reduction potential is more likely to be reduced, and a species with a lower reduction potential is more likely to be oxidized. Based on the information in the question, iron is oxidized more readily than those metals; this means that iron has a lower reduction potential.

2. **B**

To determine the standard electromotive force of a cell, simply subtract the standard reduction potentials of the two electrodes. In this case, the cathode is zinc because it is being reduced; the anode is silver because it is being oxidized. Thus,

$$E^\circ_{\text{cell}} = E^\circ_{\text{red,cathode}} - E^\circ_{\text{red,anode}} = -0.763 - 0.337 = -1.10 \text{ V}$$

While we must multiply the silver half-reaction by two to balance electrons, the actual value for the reduction potential does not change. Remember that the standard reduction potential is determined by the identity of the electrode, not the amount of it present.

3. **A**

Oxidation occurs at the anode, and reduction occurs at the cathode. Because Cu is the anode, it must be oxidized. The reduction potential of the cathode cannot be less than that of the anode for a galvanic cell. Therefore, mercury, **(A)**, must be the cathode. In a concentration cell, the same material is used as both the cathode and anode; however, this question assumes equal concentrations. If both electrolyte solutions have the same concentration, there will be no oxidation–reduction reaction and, therefore, no anode or cathode. This eliminates **(B)**.

4. **C**

In an electrolytic cell, ionic compounds are broken up into their constituents; the cations (positively charged ions) migrate toward the cathode, and the anions (negatively charged ions) migrate toward the anode. In this case, the cations are H^+ ions (protons), so option I is correct. Electrons flow from anode to cathode in all types of cells, meaning that option III is also correct. Option II is incorrect for two reasons. First, it is unlikely that the anions in any cell would be O^{2-} rather than OH^-. Second, and more significantly, these anions would flow to the anode, not the cathode.

5. **D**

This answer comes directly from the equation relating Gibbs free energy and E°_{cell}. $\Delta G^\circ = -nFE^\circ_{\text{cell}}$, where n is the number of moles of electrons transferred and F is the Faraday constant, 96,485 $\frac{\text{C}}{\text{mol } e^-}$. To determine n, one must look at the balanced half-reactions occurring in the oxidation–reduction reaction.

6. **B**

Salt bridges contain inert electrolytes. Ionic compounds, such as **(A)**, **(C)**, and **(D)**, are known to be strong electrolytes because they completely dissociate in solution. **(B)** cannot be considered an electrolyte because its atoms are covalently bonded and will not dissociate in aqueous solution. **(B)** and **(C)** may appear similar, but there is an important distinction to be made. **(C)** implies that Mg^{2+} and SO_3^{2-} are the final, dissociated ionic constituents, while **(B)** implies that neutral SO_3 would have to be dissolved in solution.

7. **B**

Potential, as measured by E°_{cell}, is dependent only on the identity of the electrodes and not the amount present. Similarly, the equilibrium constant depends only on the identity of the electrolyte solutions and the temperature. However, as the electrode material is increased, the surface area participating in oxidation–reduction reactions is increased and more electrons are released, making statement II correct.

8. **D**

E°_{cell} is dependent upon the change in free energy of the system through the equation $RT \ln K_{\text{eq}} = nFE^\circ_{\text{cell}}$. The temperature, T, appears in this equation; thus, a change in temperature will impact the E°_{cell}.

9. **B**

If this were a galvanic cell, the species with the more positive reduction potential (cadmium) would be reduced. The cathode is always reduced in an electrochemical cell, so sodium could not be the cathode in such a galvanic cell, eliminating **(A)**. Sodium would be the cathode in an electrolytic cell, however, which would make cadmium the anode. Thus, the answer is **(B)**. Note that we do not have to determine E°_{cell} because we already know the answer. However, the E°_{cell} would be $-2.71 - (-0.40) = -2.31$ V for an electrolytic cell, and $+2.31$ V for a galvanic cell, eliminating **(C)** and **(D)**.

10. **D**

There are only two equations involving standard change in free energy in electrochemical cells: $\Delta G^\circ = -nFE^\circ_{\text{cell}}$ and $\Delta G^\circ = -RT \ln K_{\text{eq}}$. Substituting $E^\circ_{\text{cell}} = E^\circ_{\text{red,cathode}} - E^\circ_{\text{red,anode}}$ into the first equation and distributing the negative sign gives **(D)**. **(A)** would be the opposite of ΔG°. Setting the two equations equal to each other, we get $RT \ln K_{\text{eq}} = nFE^\circ_{\text{cell}}$. Solving for E°_{cell}, we get $E^\circ_{\text{cell}} = \frac{RT}{nF} \ln K_{\text{eq}}$, which is the opposite of **(B)**. **(C)** incorrectly solves the algebra.

11. **D**

A spontaneous electrochemical reaction has a negative ΔG. Using the equation $\Delta G^\circ = -RT \ln K_{\text{eq}}$, $K_{\text{eq}} > 1$ would result in $\ln K_{\text{eq}} > 0$, which means $\Delta G^\circ < 0$. A negative electromotive force, **(A)**, or equilibrium state, **(B)**, would not correspond to a spontaneous reaction. Concentration cells can be spontaneous; however, if the concentration cell had reached equilibrium, it would cease to be a spontaneous reaction, eliminating **(C)**. When an answer choice *may* be true, but does not *have to* be—it is the wrong answer on Test Day.

12. **A**

A change in pH has a direct correlation to the hydrogen ion (H^+) concentration. Decreasing the pH increases the H^+ concentration, which means the concentration of products has increased in the oxidation of sulfur dioxide. This means it would be harder to liberate electrons, thus decreasing the emf. One could also view this decrease in oxidation potential as an increase in reduction potential. If $E^\circ_{\text{red,anode}}$ increases, then E°_{cell} must decrease according to $E^\circ_{\text{cell}} = E^\circ_{\text{red,cathode}} - E^\circ_{\text{red,anode}}$.

13. **C**

An electrolytic cell is nonspontaneous. Therefore, the ΔG° must be positive and E°_{cell} must be negative, eliminating **(B)** and **(D)**. The change in entropy may be positive or negative, depending on the species involved, eliminating **(A)**. According to the equation $\Delta G^\circ = -RT \ln K_{\text{eq}}$, $K_{\text{eq}} < 1$ would result in $\ln K_{\text{eq}} < 0$, which means $\Delta G^\circ > 0$.

14. **D**

Compared to other cell types, lead–acid batteries have a characteristically low energy density, **(D)**. While **(A)** is a true statement, the incomplete dissociation of sulfuric acid does not fully explain the low energy density of lead–acid batteries. **(C)** is likely to be an opposite; the more easily the electrodes dissociate, the easier it is to carry out oxidation–reduction reactions with them.

15. **C**

During the recharge cycle, Ni–Cd cells will accept current from an outside source until the Cd and NiO(OH) electrodes are pure; at this point, the reaction will stop because $Cd(OH)_2$ runs out and no more electrons can be accepted. **(A)** and **(B)** are both true statements, but they fail to explain why overcharging the battery (continuing to try to run current into the battery even when the electrodes are reverted to their original state) is not a problem with Ni–Cd batteries. Finally, surge current refers to the initial burst of current seen in some batteries; once charged, the surge current will not increase even if the power source continues to be run because no additional charge will be stored on the electrodes, eliminating **(D)**.

Consult your online resources for additional practice. **GO ONLINE**

EQUATIONS TO REMEMBER

(12.1) **Moles of electrons transferred during reduction:** $M^{n+} + n\,e^- \rightarrow M\,(s)$

(12.2) **Electrodeposition equation:** $\text{mol M} = \frac{It}{n\text{F}}$

(12.3) **Standard electromotive force of a cell:** $E^\circ_{\text{cell}} = E^\circ_{\text{red,cathode}} - E^\circ_{\text{red,anode}}$

(12.4) **Standard change in free energy from standard emf:** $\Delta G^\circ = -n\text{F}E^\circ_{\text{cell}}$

(12.5) **Nernst equation (full):** $E_{\text{cell}} = E^\circ_{\text{cell}} - \frac{\text{R}T}{n\text{F}} \ln Q$

(12.6) **Nernst equation (simplified):** $E_{\text{cell}} = E^\circ_{\text{cell}} - \frac{0.0592}{n} \log Q$

(12.7) **Reaction quotient:** $Q = \frac{[\text{C}]^c[\text{D}]^d}{[\text{A}]^a[\text{B}]^b}$

(12.8) **Standard change in free energy from equilibrium constant:**
$\Delta G^\circ = -\text{R}T \ln K_{\text{eq}}$

(12.9) **Free energy change (nonstandard conditions):** $\Delta G = \Delta G^\circ + \text{R}T \ln Q$

SHARED CONCEPTS

Biochemistry Chapter 3
Nonenzymatic Protein Function and Protein Analysis

Biochemistry Chapter 8
Biological Membranes

General Chemistry Chapter 7
Thermochemistry

General Chemistry Chapter 11
Oxidation–Reduction Reactions

Physics and Math Chapter 5
Electrostatics and Magnetism

Physics and Math Chapter 6
Circuits

GLOSSARY

Absolute zero–The temperature at which all substances have no thermal energy; 0 K or −273.15°C.

Absorption spectrum–The series of discrete lines at characteristic frequencies representing the energy required to excite an electron from the ground state.

Acid–A species that donates hydrogen ions or accepts electrons.

Acid dissociation constant (K_a)–The equilibrium constant that measures the degree of dissociation of an acid under specific conditions.

Acidic solution–An aqueous solution that contains more H^+ ions than OH^- ions; pH <7 under standard conditions.

Actinide series–The series of chemical elements atomic numbered 89–103 and falling between the *s* and *d* blocks on the periodic table.

Activation energy (E_a)–The minimum amount of energy required for a reaction to reach the transition state; also called energy barrier.

Actual yield–The experimental quantity of a substance obtained at the end of a reaction.

Adiabatic process–A process that occurs without the transfer of heat into or out of the system.

Alkali metals–Elements found in Group IA of the periodic table; highly reactive, readily losing one valence electron to form ionic compounds with nonmetals.

Alkaline earth metals–Elements found in Group IIA of the periodic table; chemistry is similar to that of the alkali metals, except that they have two valence electrons and, thus, form +2 cations.

Amphiprotic species–A species that may either gain or lose a proton.

Amphoteric species–A species capable of reacting as either an acid or base, depending on the nature of the reactants.

Angular momentum–The rotational analog of linear momentum.

Anion–An ionic species with a negative charge.

Anode–The electrode at which oxidation occurs.

Antibonding orbital–A molecular orbital formed by the overlap of two or more atomic orbitals; energy is greater than the energy of the combining atomic orbitals.

Aqueous solution–A solution in which water is the solvent.

Arrhenius acid–A species that donates protons (H^+) in aqueous solution.

Arrhenius base–A species that donates hydroxide ions (OH^-) in aqueous solution.

Arrhenius equation–A chemical kinetics equation that relates the rate constant (*k*) of a reaction with the frequency factor (*A*), the activation energy (E_a), the ideal gas constant (R), and temperature (*T*) in kelvin.

Atom–The smallest unit of an element that retains the properties of the element; it cannot be further broken down by chemical means.

Atomic mass–The mass of a given isotope of an element; closely related to the mass number.

Atomic mass unit (amu)–A unit of mass defined as $\frac{1}{12}$ the mass of a carbon-12 atom; approximately equal to the mass of one proton or one neutron.

Atomic number–The number of protons in a given element.

Atomic orbital–Describes the region of space where there is a high probability of finding an electron.

Atomic radius–The average distance between a nucleus and its outermost electron; usually measured as one-half the distance between two nuclei of an element in its elemental form.

Atomic weight–The weighted average mass of the atoms of an element, taking into account the relative abundance of all naturally occurring isotopes.

Aufbau principle–The concept that electrons fill energy levels in order of increasing energy, completely filling one sublevel before beginning to fill the next.

Autoionization–The process by which a molecule (usually water) spontaneously dissociates into cations and anions.

Avogadro's number–The number of atoms or molecules in one mole of a substance: 6.02×10^{23} mol^{-1}.

Avogadro's principle–The law stating that under the same conditions of temperature and pressure, equal volumes of different gases will have the same number of molecules.

Azimuthal quantum number (*l*)–The quantum number denoting the sublevel or subshell in which an electron can be found; reveals the shape of the orbital.

Balanced equation–An equation for a chemical reaction in which the number of atoms for each element in the reaction and the total charge are the same for the reactants and the products.

Balmer series–Part of the emission spectrum for hydrogen, representing transitions of an electron from energy levels $n > 2$ to $n = 2$.

Barometer–A tool for measuring pressure.

Base–A species that donates hydroxide ions or electron pairs or that accepts protons.

Base dissociation constant (K_b)–The equilibrium constant that measures the degree of dissociation for a base under specific conditions.

Basic solution–An aqueous solution that contains more OH^- ions than H^+ ion; $pH > 7$ under standard conditions.

Bohr model–The model of the hydrogen atom in which electrons assume certain circular orbits around a positive nucleus.

Boiling point–The temperature at which the vapor pressure of a liquid is equal to the incident pressure; the normal boiling point of any liquid is defined as its boiling point at a pressure of 1 atmosphere.

Boiling point elevation–The amount by which a given quantity of solute raises the boiling point of a liquid; a colligative property.

Bond energy–The energy (enthalpy change) required to break a particular bond under given conditions.

Bond enthalpy–The average energy that is required to break a particular type of bond between atoms in the gas phase.

Bonding electrons–Electrons located in the valence shell of an atom and involved in a covalent bond.

Bonding orbital–A molecular orbital formed by the overlap of two or more atomic orbitals; energy is less than that of the combining orbitals.

Bond length–The average distance between two nuclei in a bond; as the number of shared electron pairs increases, the bond length decreases.

Bond order–The number of shared electron pairs between two atoms; a single bond has a bond order of 1, a double bond has a bond order of 2, a triple bond has a bond order of 3.

Boyle's law–The law stating that at constant temperature, the volume of a gaseous sample is inversely proportional to its pressure.

Broken-order reaction–A reaction with noninteger orders in its rate law.

Brønsted–Lowry acid–A proton donor.

Brønsted–Lowry base–A proton acceptor.

Buffer–A solution containing a weak acid and its salt (or a weak base and its salt) that tends to resist changes in pH.

Buffer region–The portion of a titration curve in which the concentration of an acid is approximately equal to that of its conjugate base; pH remains relatively constant through this region.

Buffering capacity–The degree to which a system can resist changes in pH.

Calorie (cal)–A unit of thermal energy.

Calorimeter–An apparatus used to measure the heat absorbed or released by a reaction.

Catalyst–A substance that increases the rates of the forward and reverse directions of a specific reaction by lowering activation energy, but is itself left unchanged.

Cathode–The electrode at which reduction takes place.

Cation–An ionic species with a positive charge.

Celsius (°C)–A temperature scale defined by having 0°C equal to the freezing point of water and 100°C equal to the boiling point of water; otherwise known as the centigrade temperature scale.

Chalcogens–Elements found in Group VIA of the periodic table with diverse chemistry; the group contains metals, nonmetals (like oxygen), and metalloids; typically form –2 anions.

Charging–A state of an electrochemical cell in which an external electromotive force is being used to return a cell to its original state; during this process, electrons are transferred nonspontaneously from cathode to anode.

Charles's law–The law stating that the volume of a gas at constant pressure is directly proportional to its absolute (kelvin) temperature.

Chelation–The process of binding metal ions to the same ligand at multiple points.

Chemical bond–The interaction between two atoms resulting from the sharing or transfer of electrons.

Chemical equation–An expression used to describe the quantity and identity of the reactants and products of a reaction.

Chemical properties–Those properties of a substance related to the chemical changes that it undergoes, such as ionization energy and electronegativity.

Closed system–A system that can exchange energy but not matter with its surroundings.

Colligative properties–Those properties of solutions that depend only on the number of solute particles present but not on the nature of those particles.

Collision theory of chemical kinetics–A theory that states that the rate of a reaction is proportional to the number of collisions per second between reacting molecules that have sufficient energy to overcome the activation energy barrier; implies that only a fraction of collisions are sufficient.

Combination reaction–A reaction in which two or more reactants form a single product.

Combined gas law–A gas law that combines Boyle's law, Charles's law, and Gay-Lussac's law to state that pressure and volume are inversely proportional to each other, and each is directly proportional to temperature.

Combustion reaction–A reaction in which an oxidant (typically oxygen) reacts with a fuel (typically a hydrocarbon) to yield water and an oxide (such as carbon dioxide if between a hydrocarbon and oxygen).

Common ion effect–A shift in the equilibrium of a solution due to the addition of ions of a species already present in the reaction mixture.

Complexation reaction–A reaction in which a central cation is bound to one or more ligands.

Complex ion–A polyatomic molecule in which a central cation is bonded to electron pair donors called ligands.

Compound–A pure substance that can be decomposed to produce elements, other compounds, or both.

Compression–Reduction in the volume of a gas.

Concentrated solution–A solution with a high concentration value; the cutoff for the term "concentrated" depends on the purpose and identity of the solution.

Concentration–The amount of solute per unit of solvent or the relative amount of one component in a mixture.

Concentration cell–A cell that creates an electromotive force (emf or voltage) using a single chemical species in half-cells of varying concentration.

Condensation–The process in which a gas transitions to the liquid state.

Conductor–A material in which electrons are able to transfer energy in the form of heat or electricity.

Conjugate acid–base pair–The relationship between a Brønsted–Lowry acid and its deprotonated form, or a Brønsted–Lowry base and its protonated form.

Coordinate covalent bond–A covalent bond in which both electrons of the bonding pair are donated by one of the bonded atoms.

Coordination number–The number of atoms that are bound to a central atom.

Covalent bond–A chemical bond formed by the sharing of an electron pair between two atoms; can be in the form of single bonds, double bonds, or triple bonds.

Critical point–The point in a phase diagram beyond which the phase boundary between liquid and gas no longer exists.

Critical pressure–The vapor pressure at the critical temperature of a given substance.

Critical temperature–Also known as the critical point. The highest temperature at which the liquid and gas phases of a substance can coexist; above this temperature, the liquid and gas phases are indistinguishable.

Crystal–A solid in which atoms, ions, or molecules are arranged in a regular, three-dimensional lattice structure.

***d* subshell**–Subshell corresponding to the angular momentum quantum number $l = 2$; contains five orbitals and is found in the third and higher principal energy levels.

Dalton's law of partial pressures–The law stating that the sum of the partial pressures of the components of a gaseous mixture must equal the total pressure of the sample.

Daniell cell–An electrochemical cell in which the anode is the site of Zn metal oxidation and the cathode is the site of Cu^{2+} ion reduction.

Decomposition reaction–A reaction in which a single compound breaks down into two or more products.

Delocalized orbitals–Molecular orbitals in which electron density is spread over an entire molecule, or a portion thereof, rather than being localized between two atoms.

Density (ρ)–A physical property of a substance, defined as the mass contained in a unit of volume.

Deposition–In most chemical processes, the direct transition of a substance from the gaseous state to the solid state; in electrochemical reactions, the build-up of a solid precipitate onto an electrode.

Diamagnetism–A condition that arises when a substance has no unpaired electrons and is slightly repelled by a magnetic field.

Diffusion–The random motion of gas or solute particles across a concentration gradient, leading to uniform distribution of the gas or solute throughout the container.

Dilute solution–A solution with a low concentration of a given solute.

Dipole–A species containing bonds between elements of different electronegativities, resulting in an unequal distribution of charge.

Dipole–dipole interactions–The attractive forces between two dipoles; magnitude is dependent on both the dipole moments and the distance between the two species.

Dipole moment–A vector quantity with a magnitude that is dependent on the product of the charges and the distance between them; oriented from the positive to the negative pole.

Discharging–The state of a rechargeable electrochemical cell that is providing an electromotive force by allowing electrons to flow spontaneously from anode to cathode.

Disproportionation–An oxidation–reduction reaction in which the same species acts as the oxidizing agent and as the reducing agent; also called dismutation.

Dissociation–The separation of a single species into two separate species; usually used in reference to salts or weak acids or bases.

Double-displacement reaction–A reaction in which ions from two different compounds swap their associated counterions; typically, one of the products of this type of reaction is insoluble in solution and will precipitate.

Ductility–The property of metals that allows a material to be drawn into thinly stretched wires.

Effective nuclear charge (Z_{eff})–The charge perceived by an electron from the nucleus; applies most often to valence electrons and influences periodic trends such as atomic radius and ionization energy.

Effusion–The movement of gas from one compartment to another under pressure through a small opening; follows Graham's law.

Electrochemical cell–A cell within which an oxidation–reduction reaction takes place, containing two electrodes between which there is an electrical potential difference.

Electrode–An electrical conductor through which an electrical current enters or leaves a medium.

Electrolysis–The process in which an electrical current is used to power an otherwise nonspontaneous decomposition reaction.

Electrolyte–A compound that ionizes in water and increases the conductance of the solution.

Electrolytic cell–An electrochemical cell that uses an external voltage source to drive a nonspontaneous oxidation–reduction reaction.

Electromagnetic radiation–A wave composed of electric and magnetic fields oscillating perpendicular to each other and to the direction of propagation.

Electromagnetic spectrum–The range of all possible frequencies or wavelengths of electromagnetic radiation.

Electromotive force (emf)–The potential difference developed between the cathode and the anode of an electrochemical cell; also called voltage.

Electron (e^-)–A subatomic particle that remains outside the nucleus and carries a single negative charge; in most cases, its mass is considered to be negligible.

Electron affinity–The energy dissipated by a gaseous species when it gains an electron.

Electron configuration–The symbolic representation used to describe the electron arrangement within the energy sublevels in a given atom.

Electron spin–The intrinsic angular momentum of an electron, represented by *ms*; has arbitrary values of $+\frac{1}{2}$ and $-\frac{1}{2}$.

Electronegativity–A measure of the ability of an atom to attract the electrons in a bond; commonly measured with the Pauling scale.

Electronic geometry–The spatial arrangement of all pairs of electrons around a central atom, including both the bonding and lone pairs.

Electron shell–The space occupied by/path followed by an electron around an atom's nucleus. Electron shell (also called principal energy level) for a given electron is indicated by its principal quantum number.

Element–A substance that cannot be further broken down by chemical means; defined by its number of protons (atomic number).

Emission spectrum–A series of discrete lines at characteristic frequencies, each representing the energy emitted when electrons in an atom return from an excited state to their ground state.

Empirical formula–The simplest whole-number ratio of the different elements in a compound.

Endothermic reaction–A reaction that absorbs heat from the surroundings as the reaction proceeds (positive ΔH).

Endpoint–The point in a titration at which the indicator changes to its final color.

Energy density–An equivalence unit regarding the amount of electrochemical energy capable of being stored per unit weight; a battery with a large energy density can produce a large amount of energy with a small amount of material.

Enthalpy (H)–The heat content of a system at constant pressure; the change in enthalpy (ΔH) in the course of a reaction is the difference between the enthalpies of the products and the reactants.

Entropy (S)–A property related to dispersion of energy through a system or the degree of disorder in that system; the change in entropy (ΔS) in the course of a reaction is the difference between the entropies of the products and the reactants.

Equilibrium–The state of balance in which the forward and reverse reaction rates of a reversible reaction are equal; the concentrations of all species will remain constant over time unless there is a change in the reaction conditions.

Equilibrium constant (K_{eq})–The ratio of the concentrations of the products to the concentrations of the reactants for a certain reaction at equilibrium, all raised to their stoichiometric coefficients.

Equivalence point–The point in a titration at which the moles of acid present equal the moles of base added, or vice-versa.

Equivalent–A mole of charge in the form of electrons, protons, ions, or other measurable quantities that are produced by a substance.

Evaporation–The transition from a liquid to a gaseous state.

Excess reagent–In a chemical reaction, any reagent that does not limit the amount of product that can be formed.

Excitation–The promotion of an electron to a higher energy level by absorption of an energy quantum.

Excited state–An electronic state having a higher energy than the ground state; typically attained by the absorption of a photon of a certain energy.

Exothermic reaction–A reaction that gives off heat to the surroundings (negative ΔH) as the reaction proceeds.

***f* subshell**–The subshell corresponding to the angular momentum quantum number $l = 3$; contains seven orbitals and is found in the fourth and higher principal energy levels.

Faraday constant (F)–The total charge on 1 mole of electrons $\left(F = 96{,}485 \ \frac{C}{mol\,e^-}\right)$; not to be confused with the farad (also denoted F), a unit of capacitance.

First law of thermodynamics–The law stating that the total energy of a system and its surroundings remains constant.

First-order reaction–A reaction in which the rate is directly proportional to the concentration of only one reactant.

Fluid–A substance that flows due to weak intermolecular attractions between molecules and that takes the shape of its container; liquids and gases are considered fluids.

Formal charge–The conventional assignment of charges to individual atoms of a Lewis structure for a molecule; the total number of valence electrons in the free atom minus the total number of electrons when the atom is bonded (assuming equal splitting of the electrons in bonds).

Formula weight–The sum of the atomic weights of constituent ions according to an ionic compound's empirical formula.

Freezing–The process in which a liquid transitions to the solid state; also known as solidification or crystallization.

Freezing point–At a given pressure, the temperature at which the solid and liquid phases of a substance coexist in equilibrium; identical to the melting point.

Freezing point depression–Amount by which a given quantity of solute lowers the freezing point of a liquid; a colligative property.

Galvanic cell–An electrochemical cell that uses a spontaneous oxidation–reduction reaction to generate an electromotive force; also called a voltaic cell.

Galvanization–In electrochemical cells, the precipitation process onto the cathode itself; also called plating.

Gas–The physical state of matter possessing the most disorder, in which molecules interact through very weak attractions; found at relatively low pressure and high temperatures.

Gas constant (R)–A proportionality constant that appears in the ideal gas law equation, $PV = nRT$. Its value depends on the units of pressure, temperature, and volume used in a given situation.

Gay-Lussac's law–The law stating that the pressure of a gaseous sample at constant volume is directly proportional to its absolute temperature.

Gibbs free energy (*G*)–The energy of a system available to do work. The change in Gibbs free energy, ΔG, can be determined for a given reaction equation from the enthalpy change, temperature, and entropy change; a negative ΔG denotes a spontaneous reaction, while a positive ΔG denotes a nonspontaneous reaction.

Graham's law–The law stating that the rate of effusion or diffusion for a gas is inversely proportional to the square root of the gas's molar mass.

Gram equivalent weight (GEW)–The amount of a compound that contains 1 mole of reacting capacity when fully dissociated; one GEW equals the molar mass divided by the reactive capacity (how many of the species of interest is obtained) per formula unit.

Ground state–The unexcited state of an electron.

Group–A vertical column of the periodic table containing elements that are similar in their chemical properties; also called a family.

Half-cell–The separated compartments housing the electrodes and solutions in an electrochemical reaction.

Half-equivalence point–The point at which half a given species within a titration has been protonated or deprotonated.

Half-reaction–Either the reduction half or oxidation half of an oxidation–reduction reaction; in an electrochemical cell, each half-reaction occurs at one of the electrodes.

Halogens–The active nonmetals in Group VIIA of the periodic table, which have high electronegativities and high electron affinities.

Heat–The energy transferred spontaneously from a warmer sample to a cooler sample.

Heat of formation (ΔH_f)–The heat absorbed or released during the formation of a pure substance from its elements at a constant pressure.

Heat of fusion (ΔH_{fus})–The enthalpy change for the conversion of 1 gram or 1 mole of a solid to a liquid at constant temperature and pressure.

Heat of sublimation (ΔH_{sub})–The enthalpy change for the conversion of 1 gram or 1 mole of a solid to a gas at constant temperature and pressure.

Heat of vaporization (ΔH_{vap})–The enthalpy change for the conversion of 1 gram or 1 mole of a liquid to a gas at constant temperature and pressure.

Heisenberg uncertainty principle–The concept that states that it is impossible to determine both the momentum and position of an electron simultaneously with perfect accuracy.

Henderson–Hasselbalch equation–Equation showing the relationship of the pH or pOH of a solution to the pK_a or pK_b and the ratio of the concentrations of the dissociated species.

Henry's law–The law stating that the mass of a gas that dissolves in a solution is directly proportional to the partial pressure of the gas above the solution.

Hess's law–The law stating that the energy change in an overall reaction is equal to the sum of the energy changes in the individual reactions that comprise it.

Heterogeneous–Nonuniform in composition.

Heterogeneous catalyst–A catalyst that is not in the same phase of matter as the reactants (for example, a solid platinum catalyst reacting with hydrogen gas).

Homogeneous–Uniform in composition.

Homogeneous catalyst–A catalyst that is in the same phase of matter as the reactants (for example, an aqueous enzyme in the cytoplasm of a cell).

Hund's rule–The rule that electrons will fill into separate orbitals with parallel spins before pairing within an orbital.

Hybridization–The combination of two or more atomic orbitals to form new orbitals with properties that are intermediate between those of the original orbitals.

Hydrogen bonding–The strong attraction between a hydrogen atom bonded to a highly electronegative atom (such as nitrogen, oxygen, or fluorine) in one molecule and a highly electronegative atom in another molecule.

Hydrolysis–A reaction in which water is consumed during the breakdown of another molecule.

Hydronium ion–The H_3O^+ ion.

Hydroxide ion–The OH^- ion.

Ideal bond angle–An angle between nonbonding or bonding electron pairs that minimizes the repulsion between them.

Ideal gas–A hypothetical gas with behavior that is described by the ideal gas law under all conditions; assumes that its particles have zero volume and do not exhibit interactive forces.

Ideal gas law–The equation stating $PV = nRT$, where R is the gas constant; can be used to describe the behavior of many real gases at moderate pressures and temperatures significantly above absolute zero.

Ideal solution–A solution with an enthalpy of dissolution that is equal to zero.

Indicator–A substance used in low concentrations during a titration that changes color over a certain pH range (acid–base titrations) or at a particular electromotive force (oxidation–reduction titrations); the final color change of an indicator occurs at the endpoint of a titration.

Inert–Unreactive.

Inert gases–The elements in Group VIIIA, which contain a full octet of valence electrons in their outermost shells and are therefore very unreactive; also called noble gases.

Intermediate–A molecule that transiently exists in a multistep reaction; does not appear in the overall balanced equation.

Intermolecular forces–The attractive and repulsive forces between molecules.

Intramolecular forces–The attractive forces between atoms within a single molecule (ionic and covalent bonds).

Ion–A charged atom or molecule that results from the loss or gain of electrons.

Ion product (*IP*)–The general term for the reaction quotient of a dissolving ionic compound; compared to K_{sp} to determine the saturation status of a solution.

Ionic bond–A chemical bond formed through electrostatic interaction between positive and negative ions.

Ionic radius–The average distance from the center of the nucleus to the edge of its electron cloud; cationic radii are generally smaller than their parent metal, whereas anionic radii are generally larger than their parent nonmetal.

Ionic solid–A solid consisting of positive and negative ions arranged into crystals that are made up of regularly repeated units held together by ionic bonds.

Ionization energy–The energy required to remove an electron from the valence shell of a gaseous atom.

Irreversible reaction–A reaction that proceeds in one direction only and goes to completion.

Isobaric process–A process that occurs at constant pressure.

Isoelectric focusing–A technique used to separate amino acids or polypeptides based on their isoelectric points.

Isolated system–A system that can exchange neither matter nor energy with its surroundings.

Isothermal process–A process that occurs at constant temperature.

Isotopes–Atoms containing the same number of protons but different numbers of neutrons.

Isovolumetric process–A process that occurs at constant volume in which the system performs no work; also called an isochoric process.

Joule (J)–The unit of energy; $1\ \text{J} = 1\ \frac{\text{Kg} \cdot \text{m}^2}{\text{s}^2}$.

Kelvin (K)–A temperature scale with units equal to the units of the Celsius scale and absolute zero defined as 0 K; also called the absolute temperature scale.

Kinetic molecular theory–The theory proposed to account for the observed behavior of gases; considers gas molecules to be pointlike, volumeless particles exhibiting no intermolecular forces that are in constant random motion and undergo only completely elastic collisions with the container or other gas particles.

Kinetic product–The product of a reaction that is formed favorably at a lower temperature because thermal energy is not available to form the transition state required to create a more stable thermodynamic product; has a smaller overall difference in free energy between the products and reactants than the thermodynamic product.

Lanthanide series–The series of chemical elements atomic numbered 57–71 and falling between the S and D blocks on the periodic table.

Latent heat–The enthalpy of an isothermal process.

Law of conservation of charge–The law stating that, in a given reaction, the charge of ions in the products is equal to the charge of ions in the reactants.

Law of conservation of mass–The law stating that, in a given reaction, the mass of the products is equal to the mass of the reactants.

Law of constant composition–The law stating that the elements in a pure compound are found in specific mass ratios.

Law of mass action–The form of the equilibrium constant; has the concentrations of products over concentrations of reactants, each raised to their stoichiometric coefficients.

Le Châtelier's principle–The observation that when a system at equilibrium is disturbed or stressed, the system will react in such a way as to relieve the stress and restore equilibrium.

Lead–acid battery–An electrochemical cell in which the anode is the site of Pb metal oxidation and the cathode is the site of Pb^{4+} ion reduction. The electrolyte is a strong acid, usually sulfuric acid.

Lewis acid–A species capable of accepting an electron pair.

Lewis base–A species capable of donating an electron pair.

Lewis structure–A method of representing the shared and unshared electrons of an atom, molecule, or ion; also called a Lewis dot diagram.

Ligand–A molecule bonded to a metal ion in a coordination compound; ligands are Lewis bases that form coordinate covalent bonds with the central metal ion.

Limiting reagent–In a chemical reaction, the reactant present in such quantity as to limit the amount of product that can be formed.

Liquid–The state of matter in which intermolecular attractions are intermediate between those in gases and in solids, distinguished from the gas phase by having a definite volume and from the solid phase because molecules may mix freely.

London dispersion forces–Intermolecular forces arising from interactions between temporary dipoles in molecules.

Lyman series–A portion of the emission spectrum for hydrogen representing electronic transitions from energy levels $n > 1$ to $n = 1$.

Magnetic quantum number (m_l)–The third quantum number, defining the particular orbital of a subshell in which an electron resides; conveys information about the orientation of the orbital in space.

Malleability–A physical property of metals that defines how well an element can be shaped using a hammer.

Mass–A physical property representing the amount of matter in a given sample.

Mass number–The sum of protons and neutrons in an atom's nucleus. Can also be called atomic mass number.

Maxwell–Boltzmann distribution curve–The distribution of the molecular speeds of gas particles at a given temperature; as temperature increases, average speed increases and the distribution becomes wider and flatter.

Mechanism–The series of steps involved in a given reaction.

Melting point–The temperature at which the solid and liquid phases of a substance coexist in equilibrium; identical to the freezing point.

Metal–One of a class of elements on the left side of the periodic table possessing low ionization energies and electronegativities; readily give up electrons to form cations and possess relatively high electrical conductivity.

Metalloid–An element possessing properties intermediate between those of a metal and those of a nonmetal; also called a semimetal.

Microstate–In thermodynamics, a specific way in which energy of a system is organized.

Millimeters of mercury (mmHg)–A unit of pressure defined as the number of millimeters that mercury in a barometer is raised above its surface in a capillary tube by an external pressure; 1 torr is equal to 1 mmHg by definition, and 1 atmosphere is equal to 760 mmHg.

Mixed-order reaction–A reaction in which the reaction order changes over time in the rate law.

Mixture–A system containing multiple substances (2+) that have been physically combined but are not chemically combined.

Molality (*m*)–A concentration unit equal to the number of moles of solute per kilogram of solvent.

Molarity (*M*)–A concentration unit equal to the number of moles of solute per liter of solution.

Molar mass–The mass in grams of one mole of an element or compound.

Molar solubility–The molarity of a solute in a saturated solution.

Mole–An amount of substance equal to Avogadro's number of molecules or atoms; the mass of 1 mole of substance in grams is the same as the mass of one molecule or atom in atomic mass units.

Mole fraction (X)–A unit of concentration equal to the ratio of the number of moles of a particular component to the total number of moles for all species in the system.

Molecular formula–A formula showing the actual number and identity of all atoms in each molecule of a compound; always a whole-number multiple of the empirical formula.

Molecular geometry–The spatial arrangement of only the bonding pairs of electrons around a central atom.

Molecular orbital–The region of electron density in chemical bonding that results from the overlap of two or more atomic orbitals.

Molecular weight–The sum of the atomic weights of all the atoms in a molecule.

Molecule–The smallest polyatomic unit of an element or compound that exists with distinct chemical and physical properties.

Nernst equation–An equation that relates the voltage of an electrochemical cell to the concentrations of the reactants and products within that cell.

Net ionic equation–A reaction equation showing only the species actually participating in the reaction.

Neutral solution–An aqueous solution in which the concentration of H^+ and OH^- ions are equal (pH = 7 at 298 K).

Neutralization reaction–A reaction between an acid and base in which a salt is formed (and sometimes water).

Neutron–A subatomic particle contained within the nucleus of an atom; carries no charge and has a mass slightly larger than that of a proton.

Nickel-cadmium battery–A rechargeable electrochemical cell in which the anode is the site of Cd metal oxidation and the cathode is the site of Ni^{2+} ion reduction.

Nickel-metal hydride battery–A rechargeable electrochemical cell in which the anode is the site of metal hydride oxidation and the cathode is the site of nickel ion reduction; the nickel may be in one of many oxidation states.

Nonbonding electrons–Electrons located in the valence shell of an atom but not involved in covalent bonds.

Nonelectrolyte–A compound that does not ionize in water.

Nonmetal–One of a class of elements with high ionization energies and electron affinities that generally gain electrons to form anions; located in the upper right corner of the periodic table.

Nonpolar covalent bond–A covalent bond between elements of similar electronegativity; contains no charge separation.

Nonpolar molecule–A molecule that exhibits no net separation of charge and, therefore, no net dipole moment.

Nonrepresentative element–Elements with an expanded valence shell that includes *d*- and *f*-block electrons; also called Group B or transition elements.

Nonspontaneous process–A process that will not occur on its own without energy input from the surroundings; has a positive change in free energy.

Normality (N)–A concentration unit equal to the number of equivalents per liter of solution.

Nucleus–The small central region of an atom; a dense, positively charged area containing protons and neutrons.

Octet–Eight valence electrons in a subshell around a nucleus; imparts great stability to an atom.

Octet rule–A rule stating that bonded atoms tend to undergo reactions that will produce a complete octet of valence electrons; applies without exception only to C, N, O, and F.

Open system–A system that can exchange both energy and matter with its surroundings.

Orbital–A region of electron density around an atom or molecule containing no more than two electrons of opposite spin.

Osmosis–The movement of water through a semipermeable membrane down its concentration gradient, from low solute concentration to high solute concentration.

Osmotic pressure–The pressure that must be applied to a solution to prevent the passage of water through a semipermeable membrane down its concentration gradient; best thought of as a "sucking" pressure drawing water into solution.

Oxidation–A reaction involving the net loss of electrons, increasing oxidation number.

Oxidation number–Also called oxidation state, the number assigned to an atom in an ion or molecule that denotes its real or hypothetical charge, assuming that the most electronegative element in a bond is awarded all of the electrons in that bond.

Oxidation potential–The ability of a substance to be spontaneously oxidized; a more positive oxidation potential (measured in volts) is indicative of a substance that is easier to oxidize and will therefore more likely act as an anode in an electrochemical cell.

Oxidation-reduction (redox) reaction–A reaction that involves the transfer of electrons from one chemical species to another.

Oxidizing agent–In an oxidation–reduction reaction, the atom that facilitates the oxidation of another species; the oxidizing agent gains electrons and is thereby reduced.

***p* subshell**–The subshell corresponding to the angular momentum quantum number $l = 1$; contains three dumbbell-shaped orbitals oriented perpendicular to each other (p_x, p_y, and p_z) and is found in the second and higher principal energy levels.

Paired electrons–Two electrons in the same orbital with assigned spins of $+\frac{1}{2}$ and $-\frac{1}{2}$.

Parallel spin–In quantum mechanics, electrons in different orbitals of an atom with the same m_s values.

Paramagnetism–A condition that arises when a substance has unpaired electrons and is slightly attracted to a magnetic field.

Partial pressure–The pressure that one component of a gaseous mixture would exert if it were alone in the container.

Pascal (Pa)–The SI unit for pressure, equivalent to $\frac{N}{m^2}$; 1 atm = 101,325 Pa.

Paschen series–Part of the emission spectrum for hydrogen, representing transitions of an electron from energy levels $n \geq 4$ to $n = 3$.

Pauli exclusion principle–The principle stating that no two electrons within an atom may have an identical set of quantum numbers.

Pauling electronegativity scale–The most common scale used to express electronegativity of the elements.

Percent composition–The percentage of the total formula weight of a compound attributable to a given element.

Percent yield–The percentage of the theoretical product yield that is actually recovered when a chemical reaction occurs; obtained by dividing the actual yield by the theoretical yield and multiplying by 100%.

Period–A horizontal row of the periodic table containing elements with the same number of electron shells.

Periodic law–The law stating that the chemical properties of elements depend on the atomic number of the elements and change in a periodic fashion.

Periodic table–The visual display of all known chemical elements arranged in rows (periods) and columns (groups) according to their atomic number and electron structure.

pH–A measure of the hydrogen ion content of an aqueous solution, defined as the negative log of the H^+ (H_3O^+) concentration.

pH meter–A device used to measure the concentration of hydrogen ions in solution and report it as a pH value.

Phase–One of the three forms of matter: solid, liquid, or gas; also called state.

Phase change–Reversible transition between solid, liquid, and/or gas phase caused by shifts in temperature or pressure.

Phase diagram–A plot, usually of pressure *vs.* temperature, showing which phases of a compound will exist under any set of conditions.

Photon–The form of light which displays particulate and quantal behavior.

Physical property–A property of a substance unrelated to its chemical behavior, such as melting point, boiling point, density, or odor.

Pi (π) bond–A bond with two parallel electron cloud densities formed between two *p*-orbitals that limits the possibility of free rotation; π bonds are the second bond in a double bond and both the second and third bonds in a triple bond.

pOH–A measure of the hydroxide (OH^-) ion content of an aqueous solution, defined as the negative log of the OH^- concentration.

Polar covalent bond–A covalent bond between atoms with different electronegativities in which electron density is unevenly distributed, giving the bond positive and negative ends.

Polar molecule–A molecule possessing one or more polar covalent bonds and a geometry that allows the bond dipole moments to sum to a net dipole moment.

Polyprotic–A molecule capable of donating more than one proton.

Polyvalent acid–An acid capable of donating more than one acid equivalent.

Polyvalent base–A base capable of donating more than one hydroxide or accepting more than one proton.

Potential energy diagram–A graph that shows the potential energies of the reactants and products of a reaction during the course of the reaction; by convention, the *x*-axis shows the progress of the reaction and the *y*-axis shows potential energy.

Potentiometer–A device used to measure electromotive force (voltage). Potentiometers can be used in potentiometric titrations: redox titrations with no indicator.

Precipitate–An insoluble solid that separates from a solution; generally the result of mixing two or more solutions or of a temperature change.

Pressure–Average force per unit area measured in atmospheres (atm), torr or mmHg, or pascals (Pa); 1 atm = 760 torr ≡ 760 mmHg = 101.325 kPa.

Principal quantum number (n)–The first quantum number, which defines the energy level or shell occupied by an electron.

Process–In a system, when a change in one or more of the properties of the system occurs.

Proton (p^+)–A subatomic particle that carries a single positive charge and has a mass slightly less than 1 amu.

Quanta–In Planck's theory, discrete bundles of energy that are emitted as electromagnetic radiation from matter.

Quantum number–A number used to describe the energy levels in which electrons reside; all electrons in an element are described by a unique set of four quantum numbers.

Radioactivity–A phenomenon exhibited by certain unstable isotopes in which they undergo spontaneous nuclear transformation via emission of one or more particles.

Raoult's law–A law stating that the partial pressure of a component in a solution is proportional to the mole fraction of that component in the solution; provides an explanation for vapor pressure depression seen in solutions.

Rate constant–The proportionality constant in the rate law of a reaction; specific to a particular reaction at a given temperature.

Rate-determining step–The slowest step of a reaction mechanism; this step serves as a bottleneck on the progress of the reaction.

Rate law–A mathematical expression giving the rate of a reaction as a function of the concentrations of the reactants; must be determined experimentally.

Rate order–The exponential effect of a change in concentration of a reactant on the change of rate in a reaction; the overall rate order is the sum of all the individual reactant rate orders.

Reaction mechanism–The series of steps that occurs in the course of a chemical reaction, often including the formation and destruction of reaction intermediates.

Reaction order–In a calculation of the rate law for a reaction, the sum of the exponents to which the concentrations of reactants must be raised.

Reaction quotient (Q)–Has the same form as the equilibrium constant, but the concentrations of products and reactants may not be at equilibrium; when compared to K_{eq}, it dictates the direction a reaction will proceed spontaneously.

Reaction rate–The speed at which a substance is produced or consumed by a reaction.

Real gas–A gas that exhibits deviations from the ideal gas law due to molecular attractions and the actual volume of the gas molecules themselves.

Rechargeable battery–An electrochemical cell that can undergo a reversible oxidation–reduction process;

when discharging, it functions as a galvanic (voltaic) cell, and when charging, it functions as an electrolytic cell.

Redox titration–A specific method used to determine the concentration of an unknown solution using reducible titrants or titrands, typically by measuring voltage changes.

Reducing agent–In an oxidation–reduction reaction, the atom that facilitates the reduction of another species; the reducing agent loses electrons and is thereby oxidized.

Reduction–A reaction involving the net gain of electrons, decreasing the oxidation number.

Reduction potential–The ability of a substance to be spontaneously reduced; a more positive reduction potential (measured in volts) is indicative of a substance that is easier to reduce and will therefore more likely act as a cathode in an electrochemical cell.

Representative elements–Elements in Groups 1, 2, and 13 through 18 in the modern IUPAC table (the *s*- and *p*-blocks of the table, also called A group elements); these elements tend to have valence shells that follow the octet rule.

Resonance–A difference in the arrangement of electron pairs but not the bond connectivity or overall charge within a Lewis structure.

Resonance hybrid–A Lewis structure that represents the weighted average (by stability) of all possible resonance structures.

Reversible reaction–A reaction that can proceed in either the forward or reverse direction, and typically does not go to completion.

Root-mean-square speed (u_{rms})–The average speed of a gas molecule at a given temperature; as a scalar, it does not take direction into account.

***s* subshell**–Subshell corresponding to the angular momentum quantum number $l = 0$ and containing one spherical orbital; found in all energy levels.

Salt–An ionic substance consisting of cations and anions.

Salt bridge–A component of an electrochemical cell composed of an inert electrolyte that allows the charge gradient that builds up in the half-cells to be dissipated as a reaction occurs; contains ions that will not react with electrodes or ions in solution and that can move to balance charge.

Saturated solution–A solution containing the maximum amount of solute that can be dissolved in a particular solvent at a given temperature.

Second law of thermodynamics–The law stating that all spontaneous processes lead to an increase in the entropy of the universe.

Second-order reaction–A reaction in which the rate is directly proportional to the concentration of two reactants, or to the square of one single reactant.

Semipermeable–A quality of a membrane allowing only some components of a solution to pass through, usually including the solvent, while limiting the passage of other species.

Sigma (σ) bond–A head-to-head bond between two orbitals of different atoms that allows free rotation about its axis.

Single-displacement reaction–A reaction in which an ion of one compound is replaced with another ion; also known as a single-replacement reaction.

Solid–The phase of matter possessing the greatest order; molecules are fixed in a rigid structure.

Solubility–A measure of the amount of solute that can be dissolved in a solvent at a certain temperature.

Solubility product (K_{sp})–The equilibrium constant for the ionization reaction of a sparingly soluble salt.

Solute–The component of a solution that is present in a lesser concentration than the solvent.

Solution–A homogeneous mixture of two or more substances. It may be solid (brass), liquid (HCl (*aq*)), or gas (air).

Solvation–The electrostatic interaction between solute and solvent molecules; also called dissolution. The term hydration can be used when water is the solvent.

Solvent–The component of a solution present in the greatest amount; the substance in which the solute is dissolved.

Sparingly soluble salt–An ionic compound that has a low solubility at a given temperature.

Specific heat–The amount of heat required to raise the temperature of one gram of a substance by 1°C.

Spectator ions–Ions involved in a reaction that do not change formula, charge, or phase; normally omitted from the net ionic equation.

Spectrum–The characteristic wavelengths of electromagnetic radiation emitted or absorbed by an object, atom, or molecule.

Spectroscopic notation–The shorthand representation of the principal and azimuthal quantum numbers, in which the azimuthal number is designated by a letter rather than a number.

Sphygmomanometer–A tool for measuring blood pressure.

Spin quantum number (m_s)–The fourth quantum number, which indicates the orientation of the intrinsic spin of an electron in an atom; can only assume values of $+\frac{1}{2}$ and $-\frac{1}{2}$.

Spontaneous process–A process that will occur on its own without energy input from the surroundings; defined by a negative change in free energy.

Standard conditions–Conditions defined as 25°C, 1 atm pressure, and 1 *M* concentrations; used for measuring the standard Gibbs free energy, enthalpy, entropy, and cell electromotive force.

Standard free energy ($G°$)–The Gibbs free energy for a reaction under standard conditions.

Standard heat of combustion ($\Delta H^{\circ}_{\text{comb}}$)–The enthalpy change associated with the combustion of a fuel.

Standard hydrogen electrode (SHE)–The electrode defined as having a potential of zero under standard conditions; all oxidation and reduction potentials are measured relative to the standard hydrogen electrode at 25°C and with 1 *M* concentrations of each ion in solution.

Standard potential–The voltage associated with a half-reaction of a specific oxidation–reduction reaction; generally tabulated as reduction potentials, compared to the standard hydrogen electrode.

Standard state–The phase of matter for a certain element under standard conditions.

Standard temperature and pressure (STP)–Defined as 0°C (273 K) and 1 atm; used for measuring characteristics of an ideal gas.

State function–A function that depends on the state of a system but not on the path used to arrive at that state; includes pressure, density, temperature, volume, enthalpy, internal energy, Gibbs free energy, and entropy.

Stoichiometric coefficient–In a reaction, the number placed in front of each compound to indicate relative number of moles of that species involved in the reaction.

Stoichiometry–A form of dimensional analysis focusing on the relationships between amounts of reactants and products in a reaction.

Strong acid–An acid that undergoes complete dissociation in an aqueous solution.

Strong base–A base that undergoes complete dissociation in an aqueous solution.

Structural formula–The graphic representation of a molecule depicting how its atoms are arranged.

Sublimation–A change of phase from solid to gas without passing through the liquid phase.

Subshell–The division of electron shells or energy levels into different values of the azimuthal quantum number (*s*, *p*, *d*, and *f*); composed of orbitals.

Supercritical fluid–A substance whose current state is simultaneously a liquid and a gas—there is no distinction between the two phases.

Supersaturated–A solution which is beyond equilibrium, where ion product is greater than the solubility product constant. Supersaturated solutions are thermodynamically unstable.

Surge current–An above-average current transiently released at the beginning of the discharge phase of a battery.

Surroundings–All matter and energy in the universe not included in the particular system under consideration.

System–The matter and energy under consideration.

Temperature–A measure of the average kinetic energy of the particles in a system.

Theoretical yield–The maximal amount of product that can be obtained in a reaction; determined by stoichiometric analysis of the limiting reagent.

Thermodynamic product–The product of a reaction that is formed favorably at a higher temperature because thermal energy is available to form the transition state of the more stable product; has a larger overall difference in free energy between the products and reactants than the kinetic product.

Titrand–A solution of unknown concentration to which a solution of known concentration is added to determine its concentration.

Titrant–A solution of known concentration that is slowly added to a solution of unknown concentration to determine its concentration.

Titration–A method used to determine the concentration of an unknown solution by gradual reaction with a solution of known concentration.

Titration curve–A plot of the pH of a solution *vs.* the volume of acid or base added in an acid–base titration, or a plot of the electromotive force of a solution *vs.* the volume of oxidizing or reducing agent added in an oxidation–reduction titration.

Transition metal–Any of the elements in the B groups of the periodic table, all of which have partially filled *d* subshells.

Transition state–The point during a reaction in which old bonds are partially broken and new bonds are partially formed; has a higher energy than the reactants or products of the reaction and is also called the activated complex.

Triple point–The pressure and temperature at which the solid, liquid, and gas phases of a particular substance coexist in equilibrium.

Unsaturated solution–A solution into which more solute may be dissolved before reaching saturation.

Valence electron–An electron in the highest occupied energy level of an atom; the tendency of a given valence electron to be retained or lost determines the chemical properties of an element.

Valence shell–The outermost shell of an atom.

Valence shell electron pair repulsion (VSEPR) theory–A system that reflects the geometric arrangement of a molecule based on its Lewis dot structure; the three-dimensional structure is determined by the repulsions between bonding and nonbonding electron pairs in the valence shells of atoms.

van der Waals equation of state–One of several real gas laws, which corrects for attractive forces and the volumes of gas particles, which are assumed to be negligible in the ideal gas law.

van der Waals forces–Attractive or repulsive forces between molecules that don't arise from covalent or ionic bonds.

van't Hoff factor–The number of particles into which a compound dissociates in solution.

Vapor pressure–The partial pressure of a gaseous substance in the atmosphere above the liquid or solid with which it is in equilibrium.

Vapor pressure depression–The decrease in the vapor pressure of a liquid caused by the presence of dissolved solute; a colligative property.

Vaporization–The transformation of a liquid into a gas.

Water dissociation constant (K_w)–The equilibrium constant of the water dissociation reaction at a given temperature; equal to 10^{-14} at 25°C (298 K).

Weak acid–An acid that undergoes partial dissociation in an aqueous solution.

Weak base–A base that undergoes partial dissociation in an aqueous solution.

Yield–The amount of product obtained from a reaction.

Zero-order reaction–A reaction in which the concentrations of reactants have no effect on the overall rate.

INDEX

Note: Material in figures or tables is indicated by italic *f* or *t* after the page number.

B

C

N

Q

R

S

U

V

W

ART CREDITS

Chapter 1 Cover—Image credited to koya979. From Shutterstock.

Figure 1.1—Image credited to Grace Cary. From Getty Images. Modified from source.

Figure 1.14—Image credited to User: alphaspirit. From Shutterstock.

Chapter 2 Cover—Image credited to RTimages. From Shutterstock.

Figure 2.1—Image credited to User: Scott Ehardt. From Wikimedia Commons.

Figure 2.2—Image credited to User: Karelj. From Wikimedia Commons.

Figure 2.12—Image credited to User: Dnn87. From Wikimedia Commons. Copyright © 2008. Used under license: CC-BY-3.0.

Chapter 3 Cover—Image credited to Wire_man. From Shutterstock.

Chapter 4 Cover—Image credited to imagedb.com. From Shutterstock.

Figure 4.3—Image credited to User: Igor M Olekhnovitch. From Wikimedia Commons. Copyright © 2009. Used under license: CC-BY-3.0.

Figure 4.6—Image credited to User: butaiump. From Shutterstock.

Figure 4.9—Unless otherwise indicated, this information has been authored by an employee or employees of the University of California, operator of the Los Alamos National Laboratory under Contract No. W-7405-ENG-36 with the U.S. Department of Energy. The U.S. Government has rights to use, reproduce, and distribute this information. The public may copy and use this information without charge, provided that this Notice and any statement of authorship are reproduced on all copies. Neither the Government nor the University makes any warranty, express or implied, or assumes any liability or responsibility for the use of this information.

Figure 5.5—Image credited to User: DStrozzi. From Wikimedia Commons. Copyright © 2009. Used under license: CC-BY-2.5.

Chapter 6 Cover—Image credited to Kletr. From Shutterstock.

Chapter 7 Cover—Image credited to Michal Zduniak. From Shutterstock.

Chapter 10 Cover—Image credited to Shawn Hempel. From Shutterstock.

Chapter 12 Cover—Image credited to monticello. From Shutterstock.

Figure 12.3—Image credited to User: Synaptidude. From Wikimedia Commons. Copyright © 2011. Used under license: CC-BY-3.0.

Figure 12.4—Images credited to User: Riventree. From Wikimedia Commons. Copyright © 2011. Used under license: CC-BY-3.0.

Notes

Notes

Notes

KAPLAN

MCAT® CRITICAL ANALYSIS AND REASONING SKILLS REVIEW 2024–2025

ONLINE + BOOK

Edited by Alexander Stone Macnow, MD

ACKNOWLEDGMENTS

Editor-in-Chief, 2024–2025 Edition
M. Dominic Eggert

Contributing Editors, 2024–2025 Edition
Christopher Durland; Charles Pierce, MD; Jason Selzer

Prior Edition Editorial Staff: Brandon Deason, MD; Christopher Durland; M. Dominic Eggert; Tyler Fara; Elizabeth Flagge; Adam Grey; Jason Selzer; Lauren K. White

Published by Kaplan North America, LLC dba Kaplan Publishing
1515 West Cypress Creek Road
Fort Lauderdale, Florida 33309

ISBN: 978-1-5062-8689-1

10 9 8 7 6 5 4 3

Kaplan Publishing print books are available at special quantity discounts to use for sales promotions, employee premiums, or educational purposes. For more information or to purchase books, please call the Simon & Schuster special sales department at 866-506-1949.

TABLE OF CONTENTS

THE *KAPLAN MCAT REVIEW* TEAM

Alexander Stone Macnow, MD
Editor-in-Chief

Áine Lorié, PhD
Editor

Derek Rusnak, MA
Editor

Mikhail Alexeeff
Kaplan MCAT Faculty

Laura L. Ambler
Kaplan MCAT Faculty

Krista L. Buckley, MD
Kaplan MCAT Faculty

Kristen L. Russell, ME
Editor

Pamela Willingham, MSW
Editor

Melinda Contreras, MS
Kaplan MCAT Faculty

Samantha Fallon
Kaplan MCAT Faculty

Jason R. Selzer
Kaplan MCAT Faculty

M. Dominic Eggert
Editor

Faculty Reviewers and Editors: Elmar R. Aliyev; James Burns; Jonathan Cornfield; Alisha Maureen Crowley; Nikolai Dorofeev, MD; Benjamin Downer, MS; Colin Doyle; Christopher Durland; Marilyn Engle; Eleni M. Eren; Raef Ali Fadel; Elizabeth Flagge; Paul Forn; Adam Grey; Tyra Hall-Pogar, PhD; Mary Halton; Scott Huff; Samer T. Ismail; Ae-Ri Kim, PhD; Elizabeth A. Kudlaty; Kelly Kyker-Snowman, MS; Ningfei Li; John P. Mahon; Brandon McKenzie; Matthew A. Meier; Nainika Nanda; Caroline Nkemdilim Opene; Aishwarya Pillai; Kaitlyn E. Prenger; Uneeb Qureshi; Kristen Russell; Bela G. Starkman, PhD; Michael Paul Tomani, MS; Lauren K. White; Nicholas M. White; Allison Ann Wilkes, MS; Kerranna Williamson, MBA; MJ Wu; and Tony Yu.

Thanks to Rebecca Anderson; Jeff Batzli; Eric Chiu; Tim Eich; Tyler Fara; Owen Farcy; Dan Frey; Robin Garmise; Rita Garthaffner; Joanna Graham; Allison Gudenau; Allison Harm; Beth Hoffberg; Aaron Lemon-Strauss; Keith Lubeley; Diane McGarvey; Petros Minasi; Beena P V; John Polstein; Deeangelee Pooran-Kublall, MD, MPH; Rochelle Rothstein, MD; Larry Rudman; Srividhya Sankar; Sylvia Tidwell Scheuring; Carly Schnur; Aiswarya Sivanand; Todd Tedesco; Karin Tucker; Lee Weiss; Christina Wheeler; Kristen Workman; Amy Zarkos; and the countless others who made this project possible.

GETTING STARTED CHECKLIST

Getting Started Checklist ☑

- ☐ Register for your free online assets—including full-length tests, Science Review Videos, and additional practice materials—at **www.kaptest.com/moreonline**.
- ☐ Create a study calendar that ensures you complete content review and sufficient practice by Test Day!
- ☐ As you finish a chapter and the online practice for that chapter, check it off on the table of contents.
- ☐ Register to take the MCAT at **www.aamc.org/mcat**.
- ☐ Set aside time during your prep to make sure the rest of your application—personal statement, recommendations, and other materials—is ready to go!
- ☐ Take a moment to admire your completed checklist, then get back to the business of prepping for this exam!

PREFACE

And now it starts: your long, yet fruitful journey toward wearing a white coat. Proudly wearing that white coat, though, is hopefully only part of your motivation. You are reading this book because you want to be a healer.

If you're serious about going to medical school, then you are likely already familiar with the importance of the MCAT in medical school admissions. While the holistic review process puts additional weight on your experiences, extracurricular activities, and personal attributes, the fact remains: along with your GPA, your MCAT score remains one of the two most important components of your application portfolio—at least early in the admissions process. Each additional point you score on the MCAT pushes you in front of thousands of other students and makes you an even more attractive applicant. But the MCAT is not simply an obstacle to overcome; it is an opportunity to show schools that you will be a strong student and a future leader in medicine.

We at Kaplan take our jobs very seriously and aim to help students see success not only on the MCAT, but as future physicians. We work with our learning science experts to ensure that we're using the most up-to-date teaching techniques in our resources. Multiple members of our team hold advanced degrees in medicine or associated biomedical sciences, and are committed to the highest level of medical education. Kaplan has been working with the MCAT for over 50 years and our commitment to premed students is unflagging; in fact, Stanley Kaplan created this company when he had difficulty being accepted to medical school due to unfair quota systems that existed at the time.

We stand now at the beginning of a new era in medical education. As citizens of this 21st-century world of healthcare, we are charged with creating a patient-oriented, culturally competent, cost-conscious, universally available, technically advanced, and research-focused healthcare system, run by compassionate providers. Suffice it to say, this is no easy task. Problem-based learning, integrated curricula, and classes in interpersonal skills are some of the responses to this demand for an excellent workforce—a workforce of which you'll soon be a part.

We're thrilled that you've chosen us to help you on this journey. Please reach out to us to share your challenges, concerns, and successes. Together, we will shape the future of medicine in the United States and abroad; we look forward to helping you become the doctor you deserve to be.

Good luck!

Alexander Stone Macnow, MD
Editor-in-Chief
Department of Pathology and Laboratory Medicine
Hospital of the University of Pennsylvania

BA, Musicology—Boston University, 2008
MD—Perelman School of Medicine at the University of Pennsylvania, 2013

ABOUT THE MCAT

Anatomy of the MCAT

Here is a general overview of the structure of Test Day:

Section	Number of Questions	Time Allotted
Test-Day Certification		4 minutes
Tutorial (optional)		10 minutes
Chemical and Physical Foundations of Biological Systems	59	95 minutes
Break (optional)		10 minutes
Critical Analysis and Reasoning Skills (CARS)	53	90 minutes
Lunch Break (optional)		30 minutes
Biological and Biochemical Foundations of Living Systems	59	95 minutes
Break (optional)		10 minutes
Psychological, Social, and Biological Foundations of Behavior	59	95 minutes
Void Question		3 minutes
Satisfaction Survey (optional)		5 minutes

The structure of the four sections of the MCAT is shown below.

Chemical and Physical Foundations of Biological Systems	
Time	95 minutes
Format	• 59 questions • 10 passages • 44 questions are passage-based, and 15 are discrete (stand-alone) questions. • Score between 118 and 132
What It Tests	• Biochemistry: 25% • Biology: 5% • General Chemistry: 30% • Organic Chemistry: 15% • Physics: 25%

Critical Analysis and Reasoning Skills (CARS)	
Time	90 minutes
Format	• 53 questions • 9 passages • All questions are passage-based. There are no discrete (stand-alone) questions. • Score between 118 and 132
What It Tests	Disciplines: • Humanities: 50% • Social Sciences: 50% Skills: • *Foundations of Comprehension:* 30% • *Reasoning Within the Text:* 30% • *Reasoning Beyond the Text:* 40%
Biological and Biochemical Foundations of Living Systems	
Time	95 minutes
Format	• 59 questions • 10 passages • 44 questions are passage-based, and 15 are discrete (stand-alone) questions. • Score between 118 and 132
What It Tests	• Biochemistry: 25% • Biology: 65% • General Chemistry: 5% • Organic Chemistry: 5%
Psychological, Social, and Biological Foundations of Behavior	
Time	95 minutes
Format	• 59 questions • 10 passages • 44 questions are passage-based, and 15 are discrete (stand-alone) questions. • Score between 118 and 132
What It Tests	• Biology: 5% • Psychology: 65% • Sociology: 30%
Total	
Testing Time	375 minutes (6 hours, 15 minutes)
Total Seat Time	447 minutes (7 hours, 27 minutes)
Questions	230
Score	472 to 528

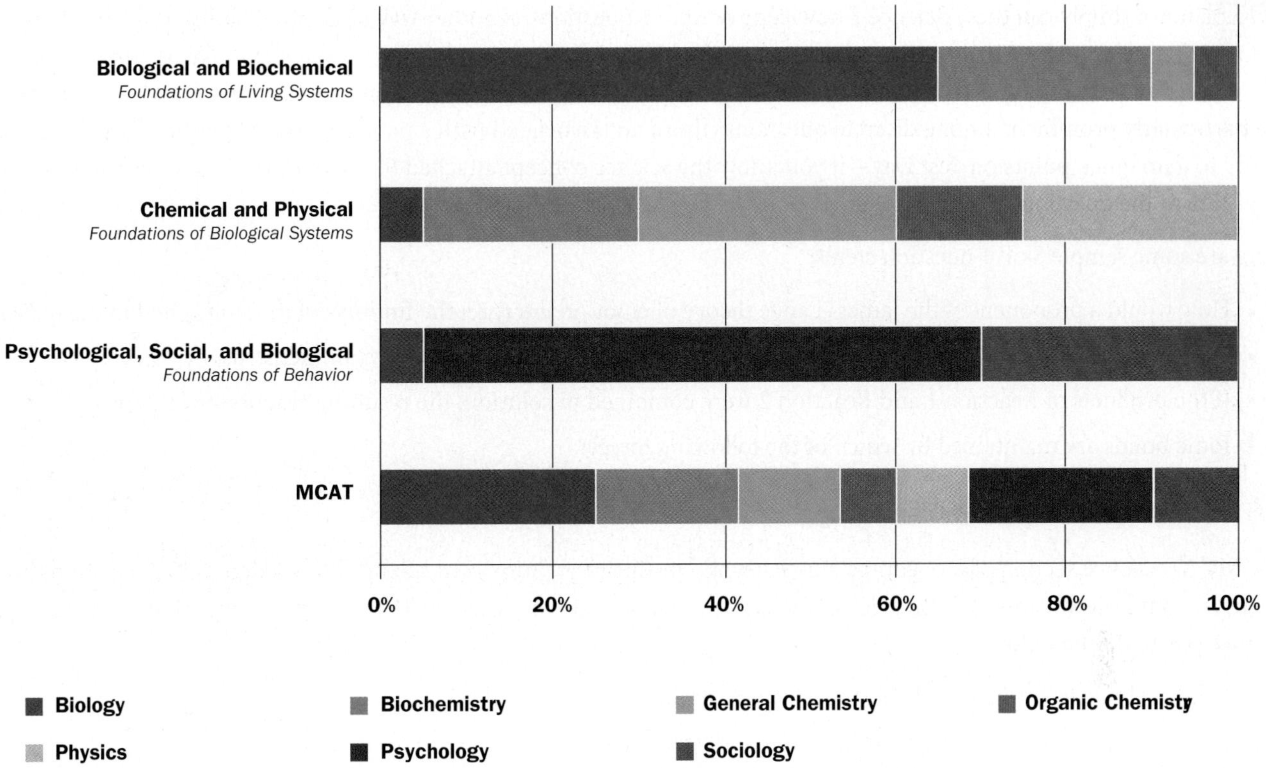

Scientific Inquiry and Reasoning Skills (SIRS)

The AAMC has defined four *Scientific Inquiry and Reasoning Skills* (SIRS) that will be tested in the three science sections of the MCAT:

1. *Knowledge of Scientific Concepts and Principles* (35% of questions)
2. *Scientific Reasoning and Problem-Solving* (45% of questions)
3. *Reasoning About the Design and Execution of Research* (10% of questions)
4. *Data-Based and Statistical Reasoning* (10% of questions)

Let's see how each one breaks down into more specific Test Day behaviors. Note that the bullet points of specific objectives for each of the SIRS are taken directly from the *Official Guide to the MCAT Exam*; the descriptions of what these behaviors mean and sample question stems, however, are written by Kaplan.

Skill 1: *Knowledge of Scientific Concepts and Principles*

This is probably the least surprising of the four SIRS; the testing of science knowledge is, after all, one of the signature qualities of the MCAT. Skill 1 questions will require you to do the following:

- Recognize correct scientific principles
- Identify the relationships among closely related concepts
- Identify the relationships between different representations of concepts (verbal, symbolic, graphic)
- Identify examples of observations that illustrate scientific principles
- Use mathematical equations to solve problems

At Kaplan, we simply call these Science Knowledge or Skill 1 questions. Another way to think of Skill 1 questions is as "one-step" problems. The single step is either to realize which scientific concept the question stem is suggesting or to take the concept stated in the question stem and identify which answer choice is an accurate application of it. Skill 1 questions are particularly prominent among discrete questions (those not associated with a passage). These questions are an opportunity to gain quick points on Test Day—if you know the science concept attached to the question, then that's it! On Test Day, 35% of the questions in each science section will be Skill 1 questions.

Here are some sample Skill 1 question stems:

- How would a proponent of the James–Lange theory of emotion interpret the findings of the study cited in the passage?
- Which of the following most accurately describes the function of FSH in the human menstrual cycle?
- If the products of Reaction 1 and Reaction 2 were combined in solution, the resulting reaction would form:
- Ionic bonds are maintained by which of the following forces?

Skill 2: *Scientific Reasoning and Problem-Solving*

The MCAT science sections do, of course, move beyond testing straightforward science knowledge; Skill 2 questions are the most common way in which they do so. At Kaplan, we also call these Critical Thinking questions. Skill 2 questions will require you to do the following:

- Reason about scientific principles, theories, and models
- Analyze and evaluate scientific explanations and predictions
- Evaluate arguments about causes and consequences
- Bring together theory, observations, and evidence to draw conclusions
- Recognize scientific findings that challenge or invalidate a scientific theory or model
- Determine and use scientific formulas to solve problems

Just as Skill 1 questions can be thought of as "one-step" problems, many Skill 2 questions are "two-step" problems, and more difficult Skill 2 questions may require three or more steps. These questions can require a wide spectrum of reasoning skills, including integration of multiple facts from a passage, combination of multiple science content areas, and prediction of an experiment's results. Skill 2 questions also tend to ask about science content without actually mentioning it by name. For example, a question might describe the results of one experiment and ask you to predict the results of a second experiment without actually telling you what underlying scientific principles are at work—part of the question's difficulty will be figuring out which principles to apply in order to get the correct answer. On Test Day, 45 percent of the questions in each science section will be Skill 2 questions.

Here are some sample Skill 2 question stems:

- Which of the following experimental conditions would most likely yield results similar to those in Figure 2?
- All of the following conclusions are supported by the information in the passage EXCEPT:
- The most likely cause of the anomalous results found by the experimenter is:
- An impact to a person's chest quickly reduces the volume of one of the lungs to 70% of its initial value while not allowing any air to escape from the mouth. By what percentage is the force of outward air pressure increased on a 2 cm^2 portion of the inner surface of the compressed lung?

Skill 3: *Reasoning About the Design and Execution of Research*

The MCAT is interested in your ability to critically appraise and analyze research, as this is an important day-to-day task of a physician. We call these questions Skill 3 or Experimental and Research Design questions for short. Skill 3 questions will require you to do the following:

- Identify the role of theory, past findings, and observations in scientific questioning
- Identify testable research questions and hypotheses
- Distinguish between samples and populations and distinguish results that support generalizations about populations
- Identify independent and dependent variables
- Reason about the features of research studies that suggest associations between variables or causal relationships between them (such as temporality and random assignment)
- Identify conclusions that are supported by research results
- Determine the implications of results for real-world situations
- Reason about ethical issues in scientific research

Over the years, the AAMC has received input from medical schools to require more practical research skills of MCAT test takers, and Skill 3 questions are the response to these demands. This skill is unique in that the outside knowledge you need to answer Skill 3 questions is not taught in any one undergraduate course; instead, the research design principles needed to answer these questions are learned gradually throughout your science classes and especially through any laboratory work you have completed. It should be noted that Skill 3 comprises 10 percent of the questions in each science section on Test Day.

Here are some sample Skill 3 question stems:

- What is the dependent variable in the study described in the passage?
- The major flaw in the method used to measure disease susceptibility in Experiment 1 is:
- Which of the following procedures is most important for the experimenters to follow in order for their study to maintain a proper randomized sample of research subjects?
- A researcher would like to test the hypothesis that individuals who move to an urban area during adulthood are more likely to own a car than are those who have lived in an urban area since birth. Which of the following studies would best test this hypothesis?

Skill 4: *Data-Based and Statistical Reasoning*

Lastly, the science sections of the MCAT test your ability to analyze the visual and numerical results of experiments and studies. We call these Data and Statistical Analysis questions. Skill 4 questions will require you to do the following:

- Use, analyze, and interpret data in figures, graphs, and tables
- Evaluate whether representations make sense for particular scientific observations and data
- Use measures of central tendency (mean, median, and mode) and measures of dispersion (range, interquartile range, and standard deviation) to describe data
- Reason about random and systematic error

- Reason about statistical significance and uncertainty (interpreting statistical significance levels and interpreting a confidence interval)
- Use data to explain relationships between variables or make predictions
- Use data to answer research questions and draw conclusions

Skill 4 is included in the MCAT because physicians and researchers spend much of their time examining the results of their own studies and the studies of others, and it's very important for them to make legitimate conclusions and sound judgments based on that data. The MCAT tests Skill 4 on all three science sections with graphical representations of data (charts and bar graphs), as well as numerical ones (tables, lists, and results summarized in sentence or paragraph form). On Test Day, 10 percent of the questions in each science section will be Skill 4 questions.

Here are some sample Skill 4 question stems:

- According to the information in the passage, there is an inverse correlation between:
- What conclusion is best supported by the findings displayed in Figure 2?
- A medical test for a rare type of heavy metal poisoning returns a positive result for 98% of affected individuals and 13% of unaffected individuals. Which of the following types of error is most prevalent in this test?
- If a fourth trial of Experiment 1 was run and yielded a result of 54% compliance, which of the following would be true?

SIRS Summary

Discussing the SIRS tested on the MCAT is a daunting prospect given that the very nature of the skills tends to make the conversation rather abstract. Nevertheless, with enough practice you'll be able to identify each of the four skills quickly, and you'll also be able to apply the proper strategies to solve those problems on Test Day. If you need a quick reference to remind you of the four SIRS, these guidelines may help:

Skill 1 (**Science Knowledge**) questions ask:

- Do you remember this science content?

Skill 2 (**Critical Thinking**) questions ask:

- Do you remember this science content? And if you do, could you please apply it to this novel situation?
- Could you answer this question that cleverly combines multiple content areas at the same time?

Skill 3 (**Experimental and Research Design**) questions ask:

- Let's forget about the science content for a while. Could you give some insight into the experimental or research methods involved in this situation?

Skill 4 (**Data and Statistical Analysis**) questions ask:

- Let's forget about the science content for a while. Could you accurately read some graphs and tables for a moment? Could you make some conclusions or extrapolations based on the information presented?

Critical Analysis and Reasoning Skills (CARS)

The *Critical Analysis and Reasoning Skills* (CARS) section of the MCAT tests three discrete families of textual reasoning skills; each of these families requires a higher level of reasoning than the last. Those three skills are as follows:

1. *Foundations of Comprehension* (30 percent of questions)
2. *Reasoning Within the Text* (30 percent of questions)
3. *Reasoning Beyond the Text* (40 percent of questions)

These three skills are tested through nine humanities- and social sciences–themed passages, with approximately 5 to 7 questions per passage. Let's take a more in-depth look into these three skills. Again, the bullet points of specific objectives for each of the CARS are taken directly from the *Official Guide to the MCAT Exam*; the descriptions of what these behaviors mean and sample question stems, however, are written by Kaplan.

Foundations of Comprehension

Questions in this skill will ask for basic facts and simple inferences about the passage; the questions themselves will be similar to those seen on reading comprehension sections of other standardized exams like the SAT® and ACT®. *Foundations of Comprehension* questions will require you to do the following:

- Understand the basic components of the text
- Infer meaning from rhetorical devices, word choice, and text structure

This admittedly covers a wide range of potential question types including Main Idea, Detail, Inference, and Definition-in-Context questions, but finding the correct answer to all *Foundations of Comprehension* questions will follow from a basic understanding of the passage and the point of view of its author (and occasionally that of other voices in the passage).

Here are some sample *Foundations of Comprehension* question stems:

- **Main Idea**—The author's primary purpose in this passage is:
- **Detail**—Based on the information in the second paragraph, which of the following is the most accurate summary of the opinion held by Schubert's critics?
- **(Scattered) Detail**—According to the passage, which of the following is FALSE about literary reviews in the 1920s?
- **Inference (Implication)**—Which of the following phrases, as used in the passage, is most suggestive that the author has a personal bias toward narrative records of history?
- **Inference (Assumption)**—In putting together the argument in the passage, the author most likely assumes:
- **Definition-in-Context**—The word "obscure" (paragraph 3), when used in reference to the historian's actions, most nearly means:

Reasoning Within the Text

While *Foundations of Comprehension* questions will usually depend on interpreting a single piece of information in the passage or understanding the passage as a whole, *Reasoning Within the Text* questions require more thought because they will ask you to identify the purpose of a particular piece of information in the context of the passage, or ask how one piece of information relates to another. *Reasoning Within the Text* questions will require you to:

- Integrate different components of the text to draw relevant conclusions

In other words, questions in this skill often ask either *How do these two details relate to one another?* or *What else must be true that the author didn't say?* The CARS section will also ask you to judge certain parts of the passage or even judge the author. These questions, which fall under the *Reasoning Within the Text* skill, can ask you to identify authorial bias, evaluate the credibility of cited sources, determine the logical soundness of an argument, identify the importance of a particular fact or statement in the context of the passage, or search for relevant evidence in the passage to support a given conclusion. In all, this category includes Function and Strengthen–Weaken (Within the Passage) questions, as well as a smattering of related—but rare—question types.

Here are some sample *Reasoning Within the Text* question stems:

- **Function**—The author's discussion of the effect of socioeconomic status on social mobility primarily serves which of the following functions?
- **Strengthen–Weaken (Within the Passage)**—Which of the following facts is used in the passage as the most prominent piece of evidence in favor of the author's conclusions?
- **Strengthen–Weaken (Within the Passage)**—Based on the role it plays in the author's argument, *The Possessed* can be considered:

Reasoning Beyond the Text

The distinguishing factor of *Reasoning Beyond the Text* questions is in the title of the skill: the word *Beyond*. Questions that test this skill, which make up a larger share of the CARS section than questions from either of the other two skills, will always introduce a completely new situation that was not present in the passage itself; these questions will ask you to determine how one influences the other. *Reasoning Beyond the Text* questions will require you to:

- Apply or extrapolate ideas from the passage to new contexts
- Assess the impact of introducing new factors, information, or conditions to ideas from the passage

The *Reasoning Beyond the Text* skill is further divided into Apply and Strengthen–Weaken (Beyond the Passage) questions, and a few other rarely appearing question types.

Here are some sample *Reasoning Beyond the Text* question stems:

- **Apply**—If a document were located that demonstrated Berlioz intended to include a chorus of at least 700 in his *Grande Messe des Morts*, how would the author likely respond?
- **Apply**—Which of the following is the best example of a "virtuous rebellion," as it is defined in the passage?
- **Strengthen–Weaken (Beyond the Passage)**—Suppose Jane Austen had written in a letter to her sister, "My strongest characters were those forced by circumstance to confront basic questions about the society in which they lived." What relevance would this have to the passage?
- **Strengthen–Weaken (Beyond the Passage)**—Which of the following sentences, if added to the end of the passage, would most WEAKEN the author's conclusions in the last paragraph?

CARS Summary

Through the *Foundations of Comprehension* skill, the CARS section tests many of the reading skills you have been building on since grade school, albeit in the context of very challenging doctorate-level passages. But through the two other skills (*Reasoning Within the Text* and *Reasoning Beyond the Text*), the MCAT demands that you understand the deep structure of passages and the arguments within them at a very advanced level. And, of course, all of this is tested under very tight timing restrictions: only 102 seconds per question—and that doesn't even include the time spent reading the passages.

Here's a quick reference guide to the three CARS skills:

Foundations of Comprehension questions ask:

- Did you understand the passage and its main ideas?
- What does the passage have to say about this particular detail?
- What must be true that the author did not say?

Reasoning Within the Text questions ask:

- What's the logical relationship between these two ideas from the passage?
- How well argued is the author's thesis?

Reasoning Beyond the Text questions ask:

- How does this principle from the passage apply to this new situation?
- How does this new piece of information influence the arguments in the passage?

Scoring

Each of the four sections of the MCAT is scored between 118 and 132, with the median at approximately 125. This means the total score ranges from 472 to 528, with the median at about 500. Why such peculiar numbers? The AAMC stresses that this scale emphasizes the importance of the central portion of the score distribution, where most students score (around 125 per section, or 500 total), rather than putting undue focus on the high end of the scale.

Note that there is no wrong answer penalty on the MCAT, so you should select an answer for every question—even if it is only a guess.

The AAMC has released the 2019–2021 correlation between scaled score and percentile, as shown on the following page. It should be noted that the percentile scale is adjusted and renormalized over time and thus can shift slightly from year to year. Percentile rank updates are released by the AAMC around May 1 of each year.

Total Score	Percentile	Total Score	Percentile
528	100	499	41
527	100	498	38
526	100	497	35
525	100	496	32
524	100	495	29
523	99	494	26
522	99	493	24
521	98	492	21
520	97	491	19
519	96	490	17
518	95	489	15
517	94	488	13
516	92	487	11
515	90	486	10
514	88	485	8
513	86	484	7
512	83	483	6
511	80	482	5
510	77	481	4
509	74	480	3
508	71	479	2
507	68	478	2
506	65	477	1
505	61	476	1
504	58	475	<1
503	55	474	<1
502	51	473	<1
501	48	472	<1
500	45		

Source: AAMC. 2022. *Summary of MCAT Total and Section Scores.* Accessed October 2022.
https://students-residents.aamc.org/mcat-research-and-data/percentile-ranks-mcat-exam

Further information on score reporting is included at the end of the next section (see *After Your Test*).

MCAT Policies and Procedures

We strongly encourage you to download the latest copy of *MCAT® Essentials*, available on the AAMC's website, to ensure that you have the latest information about registration and Test Day policies and procedures; this document is updated annually. A brief summary of some of the most important rules is provided here.

MCAT Registration

The only way to register for the MCAT is online. You can access AAMC's registration system at **www.aamc.org/mcat**.

The AAMC posts the schedule of testing, registration, and score release dates in the fall before the MCAT testing year, which runs from January into September. Registration for January through June is available earlier than registration for later dates, but see the AAMC's website for the exact dates each year. There is one standard registration fee, but the fee for changing your test date or test center increases the closer you get to your MCAT.

Fees and the Fee Assistance Program (FAP)

Payment for test registration must be made by MasterCard or VISA. As described earlier, the fee for rescheduling your exam or changing your testing center increases as one approaches Test Day. In addition, it is not uncommon for test centers to fill up well in advance of the registration deadline. For these reasons, we recommend identifying your preferred Test Day as soon as possible and registering. There are ancillary benefits to having a set Test Day, as well: when you know the date you're working toward, you'll study harder and are less likely to keep pushing back the exam. The AAMC offers a Fee Assistance Program (FAP) for students with financial hardship to help reduce the cost of taking the MCAT, as well as for the American Medical College Application Service (AMCAS®) application. Further information on the FAP can be found at **www.aamc.org/students/applying/fap**.

Testing Security

On Test Day, you will be required to present a qualifying form of ID. Generally, a current driver's license or United States passport will be sufficient (consult the AAMC website for the full list of qualifying criteria). When registering, take care to spell your first and last names (middle names, suffixes, and prefixes are not required and will not be verified on Test Day) precisely the same as they appear on this ID; failure to provide this ID at the test center or differences in spelling between your registration and ID will be considered a "no-show," and you will not receive a refund for the exam.

During Test Day registration, other identity data collected may include: a digital palm vein scan, a Test Day photo, a digitization of your valid ID, and signatures. Some testing centers may use a metal detection wand to ensure that no prohibited items are brought into the testing room. Prohibited items include all electronic devices, including watches and timers, calculators, cell phones, and any and all forms of recording equipment; food, drinks (including water), and cigarettes or other smoking paraphernalia; hats and scarves (except for religious purposes); and books, notes, or other study materials. If you require a medical device, such as an insulin pump or pacemaker, you must apply for accommodated testing. During breaks, you are allowed access to food and drink, but not to electronic devices, including cell phones.

Testing centers are under video surveillance and the AAMC does not take potential violations of testing security lightly. The bottom line: *know the rules and don't break them.*

Accommodations

Students with disabilities or medical conditions can apply for accommodated testing. Documentation of the disability or condition is required, and requests may take two months—or more—to be approved. For this reason, it is recommended that you begin the process of applying for accommodated testing as early as possible. More information on applying for accommodated testing can be found at **www.aamc.org/students/applying/mcat/accommodations**.

After Your Test

When your MCAT is all over, no matter how you feel you did, be good to yourself when you leave the test center. Celebrate! Take a nap. Watch a movie. Get some exercise. Plan a trip or outing. Call up all of your neglected friends or message them on social media. Go out for snacks or drinks with people you like. Whatever you do, make sure that it has absolutely nothing to do with thinking too hard—you deserve some rest and relaxation.

Perhaps most importantly, do not discuss specific details about the test with anyone. For one, it is important to let go of the stress of Test Day, and reliving your exam only inhibits you from being able to do so. But more significantly, the Examinee Agreement you sign at the beginning of your exam specifically prohibits you from discussing or disclosing exam content. The AAMC is known to seek out individuals who violate this agreement and retains the right to prosecute these individuals at their discretion. This means that you should not, under any circumstances, discuss the exam in person or over the phone with other individuals—including us at Kaplan—or post information or questions about exam content to Facebook, Student Doctor Network, or other online social media. You are permitted to comment on your "general exam experience," including how you felt about the exam overall or an individual section, but this is a fine line. In summary: *if you're not certain whether you can discuss an aspect of the test or not, just don't do it!* Do not let a silly Facebook post stop you from becoming the doctor you deserve to be.

Scores are typically released approximately one month after Test Day. The release is staggered during the afternoon and evening, ending at 5 p.m. Eastern Standard Time. This means that not all examinees receive their scores at exactly the same time. Your score report will include a scaled score for each section between 118 and 132, as well as your total combined score between 472 and 528. These scores are given as confidence intervals. For each section, the confidence interval is approximately the given score ± 1; for the total score, it is approximately the given score ± 2. You will also be given the corresponding percentile rank for each of these section scores and the total score.

AAMC Contact Information

For further questions, contact the MCAT team at the Association of American Medical Colleges:

MCAT Resource Center
Association of American Medical Colleges
www.aamc.org/mcat
(202) 828-0600
www.aamc.org/contactmcat

HOW THIS BOOK WAS CREATED

The *Kaplan MCAT Review* project began shortly after the release of the *Preview Guide for the MCAT 2015 Exam*, 2nd edition. Through thorough analysis by our staff psychometricians, we were able to analyze the relative yield of the different topics on the MCAT, and we began constructing tables of contents for the books of the *Kaplan MCAT Review* series. A dedicated staff of 30 writers, 7 editors, and 32 proofreaders worked over 5,000 combined hours to produce these books. The format of the books was heavily influenced by weekly meetings with Kaplan's learning-science team.

In the years since this book was created, a number of opportunities for expansion and improvement have occurred. The current edition represents the culmination of the wisdom accumulated during that time frame, and it also includes several new features designed to improve the reading and learning experience in these texts.

These books were submitted for publication in April 2023. For any updates after this date, please visit www.kaptest.com/pages/retail-book-corrections-and-updates.

If you have any questions about the content presented here, email KaplanMCATfeedback@kaplan.com. For other questions not related to content, email booksupport@kaplan.com.

Each book has been vetted through at least ten rounds of review. To that end, the information presented in these books is true and accurate to the best of our knowledge. Still, your feedback helps us improve our prep materials. Please notify us of any inaccuracies or errors in the books by sending an email to KaplanMCATfeedback@kaplan.com.

USING THIS BOOK

Kaplan MCAT Critical Analysis and Reasoning Skills Review, and the other six books in the *Kaplan MCAT Review* series, bring the Kaplan classroom experience to you—right in your home, at your convenience. This book offers the same Kaplan strategies and practice that make Kaplan the #1 choice for MCAT prep.

This book is designed to help you review the *Critical Analysis and Reasoning Skills* section of the MCAT. Unlike other books in this MCAT series, there is no content to review for the *Critical Analysis and Reasoning Skills* section. The questions are written in such a way that they do not presume any prior fund of knowledge. In other words, all the support that is needed to answer the questions correctly is found in the corresponding passages.

Learning Objectives

At the beginning of each chapter, you'll find a short list of objectives describing the skills covered within that chapter. Learning objectives for these texts were developed in conjunction with Kaplan's learning science team. They have been designed specifically to focus your attention on tasks and concepts that are likely to be relevant to your MCAT testing experience. These learning objectives will function as a means to guide your review of the chapter and indicate what information and relationships you should be focused on within each chapter. Before starting each chapter, read these learning objectives carefully. They will not only allow you to assess your existing familiarity with the content of the chapter, but also provide a goal-oriented focus for your studying experience.

Sidebars

The following is a guide to the five types of sidebars you'll find in *Kaplan MCAT Critical Analysis and Reasoning Skills Review*:

- **Bridge:** These sidebars create connections between science topics that appear in multiple chapters throughout the *Kaplan MCAT Review* series.
- **Key Concept:** These sidebars draw attention to the most important takeaways in a given topic, and they sometimes offer synopses or overviews of complex information. If you understand nothing else, make sure you grasp the Key Concepts for any given subject.
- **MCAT Expertise:** These sidebars point out how information may be tested on the MCAT or offer key strategy points and test-taking tips that you should apply on Test Day.
- **Mnemonic:** These sidebars present memory devices to help recall certain facts.
- **Real World:** These sidebars illustrate how a concept in the text relates to the practice of medicine or the world at large. While this is not information you need to know for Test Day, many of the topics in Real World sidebars are excellent examples of how a concept may appear in a passage or discrete (stand-alone) question on the MCAT.

In the end, this is your book, so write in the margins, draw diagrams, highlight the key points—do whatever is necessary to help you get that higher score. We look forward to working with you as you achieve your dreams and become the doctor you deserve to be!

Online Resources

In addition to the resources located within this text, you also have additional online resources awaiting you at **www.kaptest.com/booksonline**. Make sure to log on and take advantage of free practice and access other resources!

Please note that access to the online resources is limited to the original owner of this book.

STUDYING FOR THE MCAT

The first year of medical school is a frenzied experience for most students. To meet the requirements of a rigorous work schedule, students either learn to prioritize their time or else fall hopelessly behind. It's no surprise, then, that the MCAT, the test specifically designed to predict success in medical school, is a high-speed, time-intensive test. The MCAT demands excellent time-management skills, endurance, and grace under pressure both during the test as well as while preparing for it. Having a solid plan of attack and sticking with it are key to giving you the confidence and structure you need to succeed.

Creating a Study Plan

The best time to create a study plan is at the beginning of your MCAT preparation. If you don't already use a calendar, you will want to start. You can purchase a planner, print out a free calendar from the Internet, use a built-in calendar or app on one of your smart devices, or keep track using an interactive online calendar. Pick the option that is most practical for you and that you are most likely to use consistently.

Once you have a calendar, you'll be able to start planning your study schedule with the following steps:

1. Fill in your obligations and choose a day off.

   Write in all your school, extracurricular, and work obligations first: class sessions, work shifts, and meetings that you must attend. Then add in your personal obligations: appointments, lunch dates, family and social time, etc. Making an appointment in your calendar for hanging out with friends or going to the movies may seem strange at first, but planning social activities in advance will help you achieve a balance between personal and professional obligations even as life gets busy. Having a happy balance allows you to be more focused and productive when it comes time to study, so stay well-rounded and don't neglect anything that is important to you.

   In addition to scheduling your personal and professional obligations, you should also plan your time off. Taking some time off is just as important as studying. Kaplan recommends taking at least one full day off per week, ideally from all your study obligations but at minimum from studying for the MCAT.

2. Add in study blocks around your obligations.

   Once you have established your calendar's framework, add in study blocks around your obligations, keeping your study schedule as consistent as possible across days and across weeks. Studying at the same time of day as your official test is ideal for promoting recall, but if that's not possible, then fit in study blocks wherever you can.

   To make your studying as efficient as possible, block out short, frequent periods of study time throughout the week. From a learning perspective, studying one hour per day for six days per week is much more valuable than studying for six hours all at once one day per week. Specifically, Kaplan recommends studying for no longer than three hours in one sitting. Within those three-hour blocks, also plan to take ten-minute breaks every hour. Use these breaks to get up from your seat, do some quick stretches, get a snack and drink, and clear your mind. Although ten minutes of break for every 50 minutes of studying may sound like a lot, these breaks will allow you to deal with distractions and rest your brain so that, during the 50-minute study blocks, you can remain fully engaged and completely focused.

3. Add in your full-length practice tests.

   Next, you'll want to add in full-length practice tests. You'll want to take one test very early in your prep and then spread your remaining full-length practice tests evenly between now and your test date. Staggering tests in this way allows you to form a baseline for comparison and to determine which areas to focus on right away, while also providing realistic feedback throughout your prep as to how you will perform on Test Day.

When planning your calendar, aim to finish your full-length practice tests and the majority of your studying by one week before Test Day, which will allow you to spend that final week completing a final review of what you already know. In your online resources, you'll find sample study calendars for several different Test Day timelines to use as a starting point. The sample calendars may include more focus than you need in some areas, and less in others, and it may not fit your timeline to Test Day. You will need to customize your study calendar to your needs using the steps above.

The total amount of time you spend studying each week will depend on your schedule, your personal prep needs, and your time to Test Day, but it is recommended that you spend somewhere in the range of 300–350 hours preparing before taking the official MCAT. One way you could break this down is to study for three hours per day, six days per week, for four months, but this is just one approach. You might study six days per week for more than three hours per day. You might study over a longer period of time if you don't have much time to study each week. No matter what your plan is, ensure you complete enough practice to feel completely comfortable with the MCAT and its content. A good sign you're ready for Test Day is when you begin to earn your goal score consistently in practice.

How to Study

The MCAT covers a large amount of material and studying for Test Day can initially seem daunting. To combat this, we have some tips for how to take control of your studying and make the most of your time.

Goal Setting

To take control of the amount of content and practice required to do well on the MCAT, break the content down into specific goals for each week instead of attempting to approach the test as a whole. A goal of "I want to increase my overall score by 5 points" is too big, abstract, and difficult to measure on the small scale. More reasonable goals are "I will read two chapters each day this week." Goals like this are much less overwhelming and help break studying into manageable pieces.

Active Reading

As you go through this book, much of the information will be familiar to you. After all, you have probably seen most of the content before. However, be very careful: Familiarity with a subject does not necessarily translate to knowledge or mastery of that subject. Do not assume that if you recognize a concept you actually know it and can apply it quickly at an appropriate level. Don't just passively read this book. Instead, read actively: Use the free margin space to jot down important ideas, draw diagrams, and make charts as you read. Highlighting can be an excellent tool, but use it sparingly: highlighting every sentence isn't active reading, it's coloring. Frequently stop and ask yourself questions while you read (e.g., *What is the main point? How does this fit into the overall scheme of things? Could I thoroughly explain this to someone else?*). By making connections and focusing on the grander scheme, not only will you ensure you know the essential content, but you also prepare yourself for the level of critical thinking required by the MCAT.

Focus on Areas of Greatest Opportunity

If you are limited by only having a minimal amount of time to prepare before Test Day, focus on your biggest areas of opportunity first. Areas of opportunity are topic areas that are highly tested and that you have not yet mastered. You likely won't have time to take detailed notes for every page of these books; instead, use your results from practice materials to determine which areas are your biggest opportunities and seek those out. After you've taken a full-length test, make sure you are using your performance report to best identify areas of opportunity. Skim over content matter for which you are already demonstrating proficiency, pausing to read more thoroughly when something looks unfamiliar or particularly difficult. Consider starting with the Practice Questions at the end of each chapter. If you can get all of those questions correct within a reasonable amount of time, you may be able to quickly skim through that chapter, but if the questions prove to be more difficult, then you may need to spend time reading the chapter or certain subsections of the chapter more thoroughly.

Practice, Review, and Tracking

Leave time to review your practice questions and full-length tests. You may be tempted, after practicing, to push ahead and cover new material as quickly as possible, but failing to schedule ample time for review will actually throw away your greatest opportunity to improve your performance. The brain rarely remembers anything it sees or does only once. When you carefully review the questions you've solved (and the explanations for them), the process of retrieving that information reopens and reinforces the connections you've built in your brain. This builds long-term retention and repeatable skill sets—exactly what you need to beat the MCAT!

One useful tool for making the most of your review is the How I'll Fix It (HIFI) sheet. You can create a HIFI sheet, such as the sample below, to track questions throughout your prep that you miss or have to guess on. For each such question, figure out why you missed it and supply at least one action step for how you can avoid similar mistakes in the future. As you move through your MCAT prep, adjust your study plan based on your available study time and the results of your review. Your strengths and weaknesses are likely to change over the course of your prep. Keep addressing the areas that are most important to your score, shifting your focus as those areas change. For more help with making the most of your full-length tests, including a How I'll Fix It sheet template, make sure to check out the videos and resources in your online syllabus.

Section	Q #	Topic or Type	Why I missed it	How I'll fix it
Chem/Phys	*42*	*Nuclear chem.*	*Confused electron absorption and emission*	*Reread Physics Chapter 9.2*
Chem/Phys	*47*	K_{eq}	*Didn't know right equation*	*Memorize equation for* K_{eq}
CARS	*2*	*Detail*	*Didn't read "not" in answer choice*	*Slow down when finding match*
CARS	*4*	*Inference*	*Forgot to research answer*	*Reread passage and predict first*

Where to Study

One often-overlooked aspect of studying is the environment where the learning actually occurs. Although studying at home is many students' first choice, several problems can arise in this environment, chief of which are distractions. Studying can be a mentally draining process, so as time passes, these distractions become ever more tempting as escape routes. Although you may have considerable willpower, there's no reason to make staying focused harder than it needs to be. Instead of studying at home, head to a library, quiet coffee shop, or another new location whenever possible. This will eliminate many of the usual distractions and also promote efficient studying; instead of studying off and on at home over the course of an entire day, you can stay at the library for three hours of effective studying and enjoy the rest of the day off from the MCAT.

No matter where you study, make your practice as much like Test Day as possible. Just as is required during the official test, don't have snacks or chew gum during your study blocks. Turn off your music, television, and phone. Practice on the computer with your online resources to simulate the computer-based test environment. When completing practice questions, do your work on scratch paper or noteboard sheets rather than writing directly on any printed materials since you won't have that option on Test Day. Because memory is tied to all of your senses, the more test-like you can make your studying environment, the easier it will be on Test Day to recall the information you're putting in so much work to learn.

CHAPTER 1

ABOUT CARS

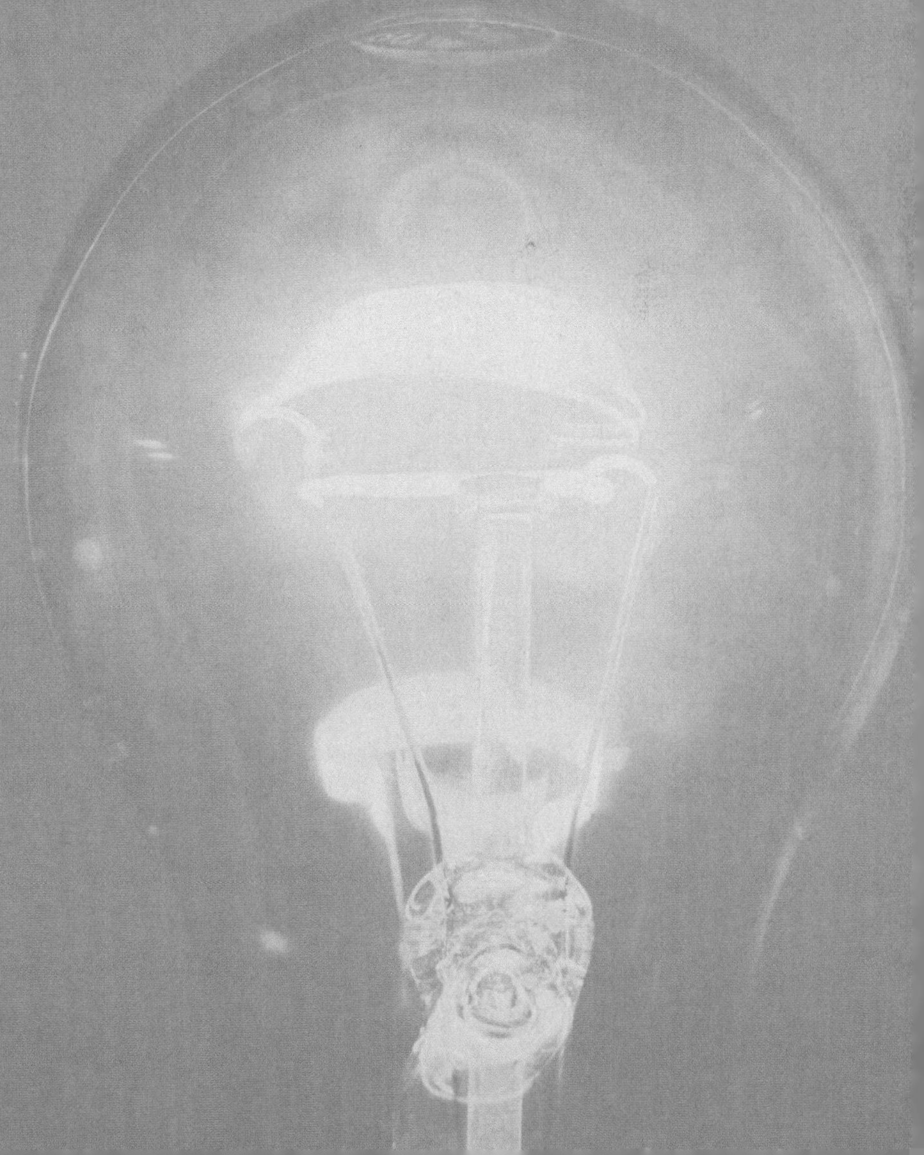

CHAPTER 1

ABOUT CARS

In This Chapter

Introduction

LEARNING OBJECTIVES

After Chapter 1, you will be able to:

- Recite the major structural features of the CARS section of the MCAT
- Recall the two major passage topic categories
- Explain the major differences between *Foundations of Comprehension*, *Reasoning Within the Text*, and *Reasoning Beyond the Text* question categories

Congratulations! You are about to embark upon an exciting journey down the path to medical school to achieve your goal of becoming a doctor. As you might expect, this particular journey will require thorough preparation. Fortunately, you don't have to prepare on your own: we are here to help!

As a pre-medical student, you have already seen at least some of the wide variety of science topics that will be tested in the three science sections of the exam. In contrast, the *Critical Analysis and Reasoning Skills* (CARS) section will present you with a variety of passages from myriad disciplines to which you may have never been exposed. You could see a musicological analysis of Johannes Brahms's 1868 masterpiece *Ein Deutsches Requiem*, a philosophical diatribe criticizing Immanuel Kant's *Metaphysics*, or a dissection of the political underpinnings of the development of the US Medicare system. For the CARS section, you will be expected to read, understand, and apply the knowledge you gain from these passages. Students often feel ill-equipped for the CARS section of the test, but Kaplan is here to help! This book will help you understand what is expected of you in CARS and will teach you the Kaplan strategies that have paved the way for many thousands of students to become the doctors they deserve to be.

In this chapter, we will go over the structure of the CARS section of the MCAT, as well as the diverse disciplines encountered in CARS passages. We'll provide a brief overview of the question categories identified by the Association of American Medical Colleges (AAMC). Finally, we'll discuss how to use this book and how it can guide you in preparing for your MCAT and the journey beyond. The journey to becoming a physician may be long, but it is extremely rewarding. Someday in the future, you'll find yourself putting on your white coat and changing patients' lives, and having the right plan for success is what will make that future possible.

1.1 The CARS Section

In some ways, the *Critical Analysis and Reasoning Skills* (CARS) section of the MCAT will be nothing new to you; it is similar to many of the standardized tests you may have taken throughout your academic career, presenting you with passages to read and multiple-choice questions to gauge your understanding. In 90 minutes, you will be presented with 9 passages, each of which will be followed by approximately 5 to 7 questions, for a total of 53 questions. The passages you encounter will be relatively short (but lengthier than the science passages on the test), typically ranging from 500 to 600 words.

Unlike reading comprehension sections you have come across previously, such as those in the SAT® or ACT®, the CARS section of the MCAT has been designed to assess analytical and reasoning skills that are required in medical school. The passages you will face in CARS will be multifaceted, incorporating advanced vocabulary, presenting varied writing styles, and requiring higher-level thought. To answer the accompanying questions, you will have to go beyond merely comprehending the content of a CARS passage: you will need to analyze its rhetorical and logical structure and assess how it impacts (or is impacted by) outside information.

1.2 Passages

The types of passages chosen for CARS consist of multiple paragraphs that require active, critical reading to answer the questions that follow. The passages included in the section are from an array of disciplines in the social sciences and humanities, as listed in Table 1.1. Approximately half of the passages (and questions) that you encounter on Test Day will fall in the realm of the humanities, while the other half will be in the social sciences. All of the passages that appear in CARS are selected from books, journals, and other publications similar to those you have come across in academic settings.

Humanities	Social Sciences
Architecture	Anthropology
Art	Archaeology
Dance	Economics
Ethics	Education
Literature	Geography
Music	History
Philosophy	Linguistics
Popular Culture	Political Science
Religion	Population Health
Studies of Diverse Cultures*	Psychology
Theater	Sociology
	Studies of Diverse Cultures*

* Note: Studies of Diverse Cultures can be tested in both humanities and social sciences passages.

Table 1.1 Humanities and Social Sciences Disciplines in the CARS Section[1]

For students who have exclusively focused on the sciences, information for the fields used in the CARS section may be presented in a strikingly different way that can sometimes seem overwhelming. This book will review the writing styles used for the passages in CARS and explain how to read these passages with purpose, which will ultimately make them much less intimidating and significantly more manageable.

1.3 Question Categories

The AAMC has identified three categories of questions in CARS that will assess your critical thinking skills: *Foundations of Comprehension*, *Reasoning Within the Text*, and *Reasoning Beyond the Text.*

Foundations of Comprehension

These questions tend to be straightforward. They will ask about the main idea of a passage, specific details from within the passage, inferences that can be drawn from the passage, or the likely meaning of a word or phrase based on context. These questions are the most similar to those you have seen in previous standardized tests because they ask only for reading comprehension (understanding what you have read). Questions in *Foundations of Comprehension* will make up approximately 30 percent of the questions in CARS, or about 16 questions.

[1] Adapted from AAMC, *The Official Guide to the MCAT 2015 Exam* (Washington, D.C.: Association of American Medical Colleges, 2014), 311–322.

In Chapter 9 of *MCAT CARS Review*, we will further dissect the four question types within *Foundations of Comprehension*:

- Main Idea
- Detail
- Inference
- Definition-in-Context

Reasoning Within the Text

Reasoning Within the Text questions require greater thought than *Foundations of Comprehension* questions because they will ask you to identify the purpose of a particular piece of information in the context of the passage, or ask how one piece of information relates to another (as a piece of evidence that supports a conclusion, for example). Questions in *Reasoning Within the Text* will also make up approximately 30 percent of the questions in CARS, or 16 questions.

In Chapter 10 of *MCAT CARS Review*, we will further dissect the two main question types within *Reasoning Within the Text* and a few other, rare questions that fit into this category:

- Function
- Strengthen–Weaken (Within the Passage)

Reasoning Beyond the Text

Reasoning Beyond the Text questions focus on two specific skills: the capacity to extrapolate information from the passage and place it within new contexts, and the ability to ascertain how new information would relate to and affect the concepts in the passage. Questions in *Reasoning Beyond the Text* will make up approximately 40 percent of the questions in CARS, or 21 questions.

In Chapter 11 of *MCAT CARS Review*, we will further dissect the two main question types within *Reasoning Beyond the Text* and a few other, rare questions that fit into this category:

- Apply
- Strengthen–Weaken (Beyond the Passage)

Conclusion

This chapter is only the beginning. Now that we have covered the structure of the CARS section, we will dive into the tools and strategies that will help you score points on Test Day. In Chapter 2, we will begin with a thorough explanation of the tools (both physical and within the testing interface) that will be available to you on Test Day.

In Chapter 3, we begin with an examination of rhetoric and its application in the CARS section, then move into analysis of arguments. Chapter 4 explains the Kaplan CARS Passage Strategy, with guidance and tips on previewing CARS passages. Chapter 5 continues the strategy with a discussion of the use of keywords to extract valuable information as you read the passage. Chapter 6 describes the three ways in which you can choose to Distill information from the passage in order to best tackle questions. Chapter 7 integrates the contents of Chapters 4, 5, and 6 into a cohesive passage strategy you can use to approach any passage presented in the CARS section. Chapter 8 introduces the Kaplan Method for CARS Questions, and this method is then applied in the three following chapters to each of the different AAMC categories. Finally, we end with a look at how to review your practice tests to find your personal test-taking pathologies and keep improving that score.

CONCEPT AND STRATEGY SUMMARY

The CARS Section

- The *Critical Analysis and Reasoning Skills* (CARS) section lasts 90 minutes and contains 53 questions, divided among 9 passages.
  - Passages range from 500 to 600 words.
  - Each passage has approximately 5 to 7 questions.
- CARS requires going beyond merely comprehending the content: you must analyze a passage's rhetorical and logical structure, and even be able to assess relationships between information given in the passage and new outside information.

Passages

- Half of the passages will be in the humanities (architecture, art, dance, ethics, literature, music, philosophy, popular culture, religion, studies of diverse cultures, and theater).
- Half of the passages will be in the social sciences (anthropology, archaeology, economics, education, geography, history, linguistics, political science, population health, psychology, sociology, and studies of diverse cultures).

Question Categories

- *Foundations of Comprehension* questions ask about the main idea of a passage, specific details from within the passage, inferences that must be true based on the passage content, or the likely meaning of a word or phrase based on context.
- *Reasoning Within the Text* questions ask you to identify the function of a particular piece of information within the context of the passage or ask how one piece of information relates to another (as a piece of evidence that supports a conclusion, for example).
- *Reasoning Beyond the Text* questions ask you to extrapolate information from the passage and place it within a new context or to ascertain how new information would relate to and affect the concepts in the passage.

CHAPTER 2

USING YOUR TEST DAY TOOLS

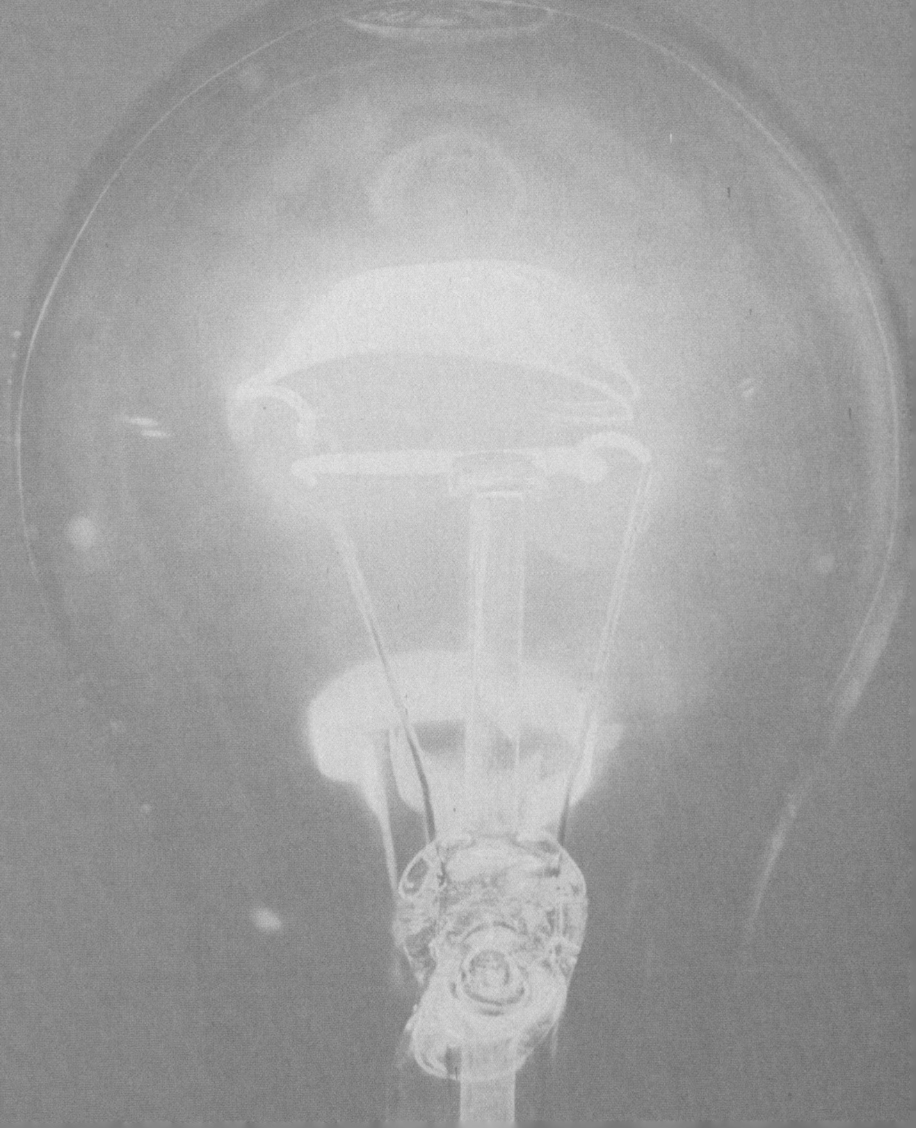

CHAPTER 2

USING YOUR TEST DAY TOOLS

In This Chapter

Introduction

LEARNING OBJECTIVES

After Chapter 2, you will be able to:

- Describe the computer-based nature of the MCAT and the writing tools available on Test Day
- Apply Test Day tools to expertly navigate and review an MCAT section
- Leverage Test Day tools while approaching MCAT passages and questions

"10 blade," "forceps," "suction"—if you've ever had the opportunity to observe a surgery or just marathon your favorite medical drama, you've likely heard these tools called for by a surgeon or an actor playing a surgeon. Even if Hollywood's portrayal of these events can be exaggerated, the truth remains that the tools of a surgeon are vital for a successful surgery. To this end, surgeons must not only be experts in their anatomical and procedural knowledge, but also experts on the tools at their disposal and their capabilities. In this way, the MCAT is much like surgery. Not only does the MCAT require science knowledge and critical reasoning, but also a thorough understanding of the tools provided on Test Day. In this chapter, we will explain the tools available to you on Test Day and explore best practices for their usage.

2.1 Test Day Tools

The MCAT has been administered as a computer-based test (CBT) since 2007. In the years since, many adjustments have been made to the CBT interface, with the latest changes (as of the writing of this textbook) occurring in January 2018. For many students beginning their MCAT studies, learning that the MCAT is administered via computer can come with feelings of uncertainty or even anxiety. But there is good news: like all aspects of the MCAT, once the nature of the challenge is understood it can be prepared for and ultimately leveraged in your favor. In fact, compared to a standardized pencil-and-paper test, the tools offered on the CBT MCAT will allow your Test Day experience to go far more smoothly! All that's needed on your end is a little knowledge and some practice with the testing interface. Before jumping into the specifics, let's discuss a few key factors to keep in mind.

Interface Controls

Inputting commands on the MCAT can be done two ways. One input method is via on-screen buttons using the mouse, and the second is via keyboard-based commands, also known as **hotkeys** Table 2.1. The MCAT aims to be as versatile as possible, so while all functions on Test Day can be accomplished with the mouse and on-screen buttons, those functions have associated hotkeys as well. As a general rule, the use of hotkeys is more efficient than on-screen controls, thus, it is recommended that test takers become comfortable with the hotkey system for the MCAT prior to Test Day. If you find yourself using a function only once or twice per section, then the keyboard shortcut may not be worth incorporating into your Test Day habits.

Shortcut	Function	Shortcut (Section Review)	Function (Section Review)
Alt + N	Advance to Next; Answer No	Alt + E	End Review of Section/ Exam
Alt + P	Return to Previous	Alt + W	Return to Section Review
Alt + V	Open Navigation	Alt + A	Review All Questions
Alt + H	Highlight/Remove Highlight	Alt + I	Review Incomplete
Alt + S	Strikethrough/Remove Strikethrough	Alt + R	Review Flagged
Alt + T	Open Periodic Table	Alt + Y	Answer Yes
Alt + C	Close Navigation/Close Periodic Table	Alt + O	Answer OK
Alt + F	Flag for Review		

Table 2.1 Keyboard Shortcuts

Selecting an Answer

The most important feature on Test Day is the ability to select an answer. This can be done in two ways. First, you can select an answer by clicking on the answer choice (either the letter or the answer). Alternatively, pressing the A, B, C, or D key on the keyboard selects the corresponding answer choice. Upon selecting an answer, the circle beside the answer choice will fill in. To deselect an answer choice, select the same answer choice again or select a different answer choice.

Noteboard Booklet

Despite being a computer-based test, on Test Day you will have the opportunity to use a test-center provided **noteboard booklet**. The noteboard booklet will be 8″ by 14″ in size, contain 9 white laminated pages, and come with a black fine point marker. The pages themselves are made of wet-erase material preventing any written work from being accidentally erased. If additional scratch-work space is needed, raise your hand and the proctor will exchange your booklet for a clean one. Strategically, it is best to exchange your noteboard booklet during the breaks in order to avoid losing your previously done scratch work and valuable test time.

The marker and noteboard booklet should be used just like a pen and paper booklet. Use of a similar noteboard booklet during practice, particularly a full-length simulation, will prevent any unforeseen frustrations on Test Day. As a general note, it is good practice to keep your written work relatively neat and organized in case you find yourself needing to revisit a question. In later chapters, we will go into greater detail about the types of information that are most useful to write down when navigating MCAT passages and questions.

2.2 Navigation Tools

Compared to a standard pencil-and-paper exam, where you can glance at upcoming questions or even flip pages back and forth, the computer-based MCAT may seem like an unnecessary nuisance. In reality, the navigation tools available on the MCAT provide time-saving opportunities not possible with a standard pencil-and-paper exam. Let's discuss the tools that will allow you to expertly navigate each section of the MCAT.

Section Interface

The section interface is the main interface you will use on Test Day (Figure 2.1), displaying both a passage and one associated question. On Test Day you will use this interface both to analyze passages and to answer questions. The features of this interface allow efficient navigation between questions and passages as you work through the section.

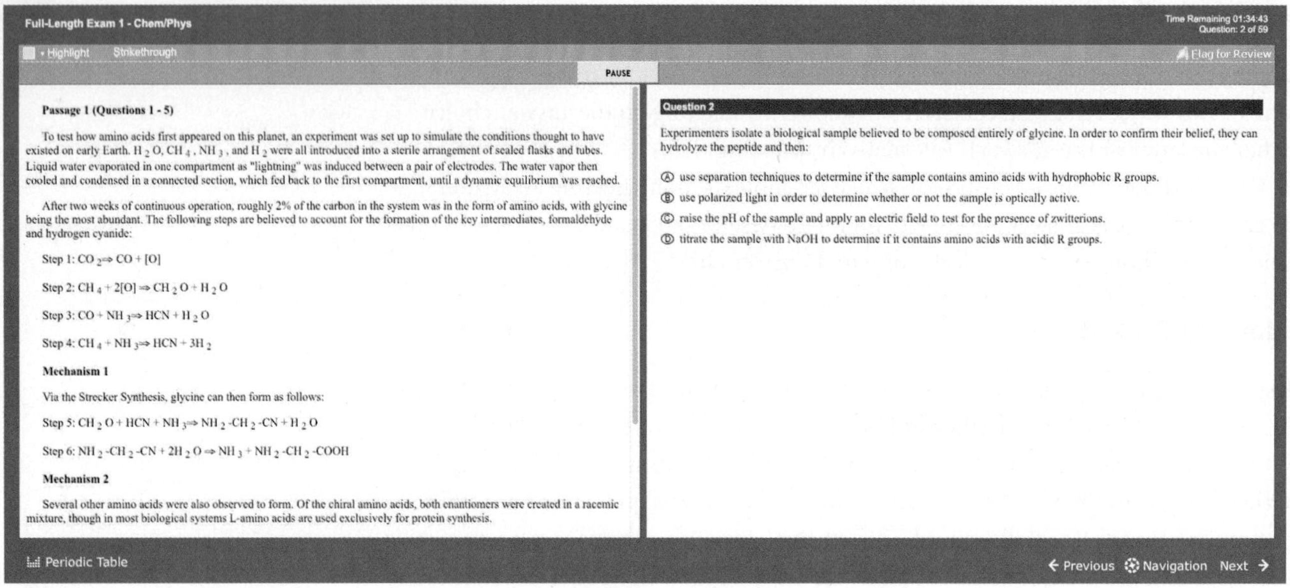

Figure 2.1 Section Interface

To navigate the section, use the three on-screen buttons at the bottom right of the screen, or their associated hotkeys:

- **Next** (Alt + N) brings up the next question.
- **Previous** (Alt + P) brings up the previous question.
- **Navigation** (Alt + V) brings up the Navigator window.

Navigator Window

The **Navigator window** lists the questions, displays question status, and displays flagged status (Figure 2.2). Understanding how to use this tool is vital for the passage strategies discussed in later chapters!

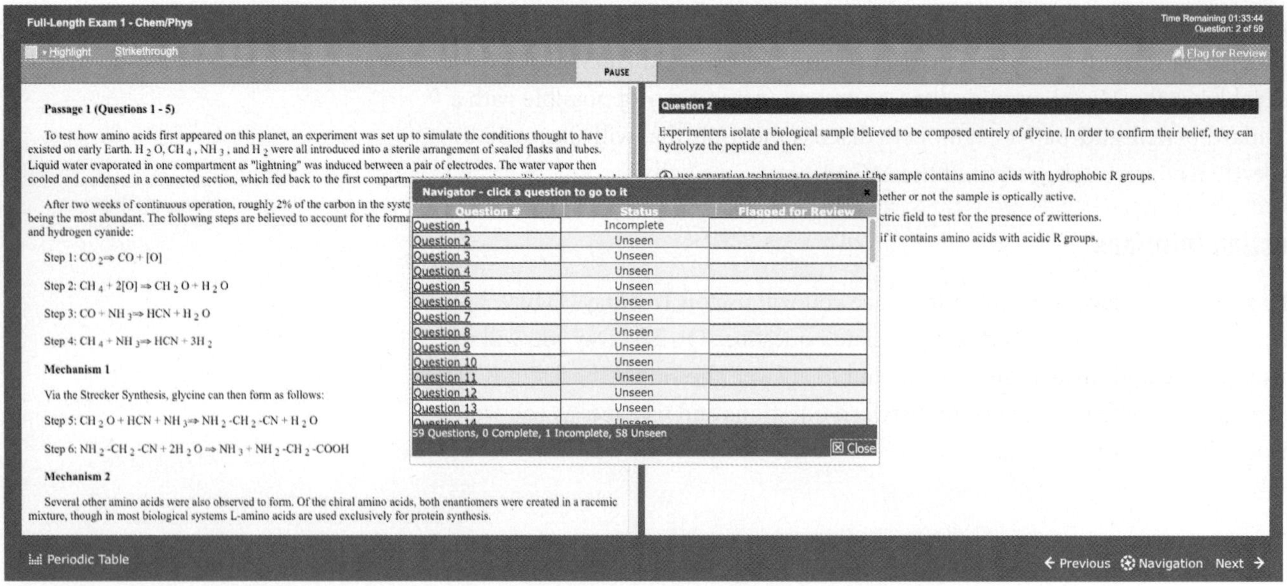

Figure 2.2 Navigator Window

The left column lists question numbers and can be used to navigate to specific questions. To do so, left-click on the question number. The center column displays question status, which updates automatically as you progress through the test:

- **Completed**—The question has an answer selected.
- **Incomplete**—The question has been seen but no answer has been selected.
- **Unseen**—The question has not been seen.

In the right column, the question's flagged status is shown. As you take the exam, you can flag a question to remind you to return to it at the end of the section. We'll expand upon this strategy later in the chapter.

The Navigator window itself can be moved by clicking and dragging the top bar and resized by clicking and dragging the borders. To close the navigation window without jumping to a different question, click **Close** or press Alt + C.

With the ability to jump to any question in the section, the Navigator window can allow a savvy MCAT tester to skip difficult passages (saving them for last) and quickly return to them near the end of the section. To skip a passage, note the title of a passage, such as "Passage 1 (Questions 1–5)," then use the Navigator window to bring up the first question of the next passage (e.g., Question 6). Returning to any previously seen passage, including passages skipped due to their difficulty, requires a bit of foresight. Reserve a space in your noteboard booklet for passage navigation, a place where you can jot down each passage number and the number of the first question associated with each passage (e.g., "P6: Q31"). When you wish to return to a skipped passage, simply bring up the Navigator window and click on the first question of the passage (e.g., Question 31). We will discuss these strategies further in Chapter 4: Previewing the Passage.

Section Review Tool

Transition from the general section interface (seen above) to the **Section Review** interface (Figure 2.3) occurs when the section is finished (more specifically, when the **Next** button is clicked on the last question of the section). The purpose of the Section Review interface is to allow the tester to return to any lingering questions and to ensure no questions remain unanswered. Toward this end, the Section Review provides three ways to review the section.

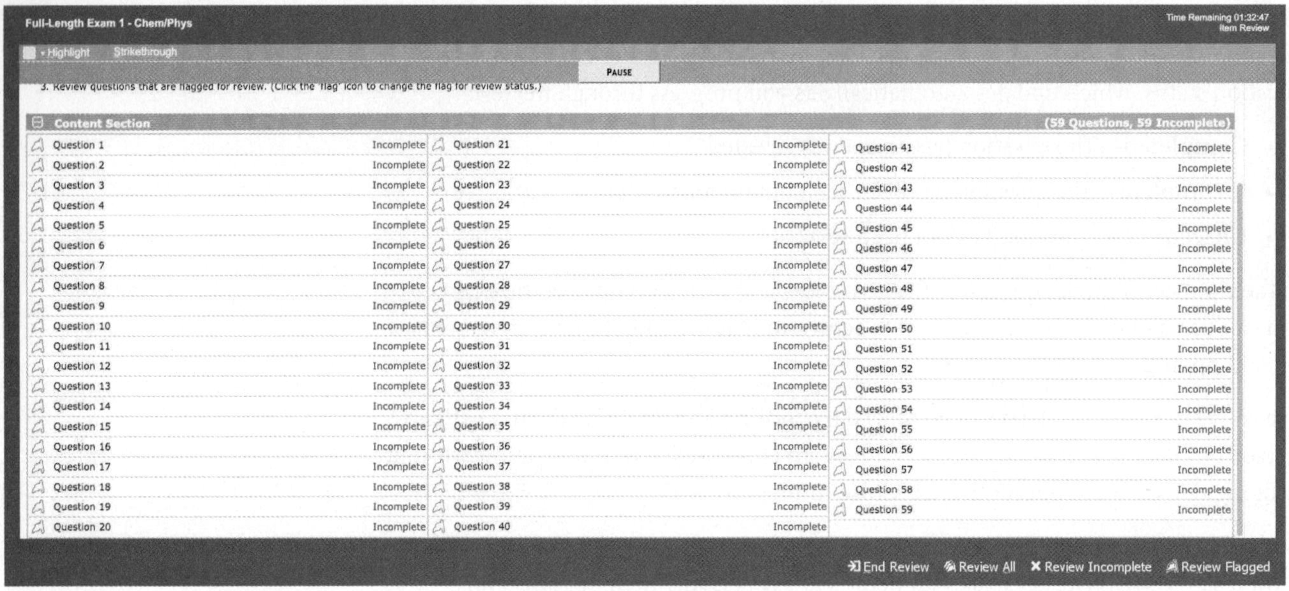

Figure 2.3 Section Review

1. **Review All (Alt + A)**—brings up Question 1 and allows for navigation to every question with the next/previous buttons.
2. **Review Incomplete (Alt + I)**—allows for review of incomplete questions only. The next and previous button only navigate to incomplete questions, skipping completed questions.
3. **Review Flagged (Alt + R)**—allows for review of flagged questions only. The next/previous buttons will only navigate to flagged questions, skipping non-flagged questions.

Similar to the Navigator window, Section Review allows you to review individual questions by clicking the question number on the screen. When viewing questions through the Section Review interface, the **Navigation** button is replaced with the **Review Section** button (Alt + V), which returns to the Section Review screen.

Most testers will have limited time remaining when they enter the Section Review interface, so it's important to use its functions strategically. We recommend using the **Review Incomplete** function to ensure no questions remain unanswered and then **Review Flagged** to return to those questions you've marked for further review. To end the section, click the **End Review** (Alt + E) button at the bottom right of the screen.

Timer and Question Progress

The time remaining and question progress are displayed at the top right of all interfaces within a section of the MCAT. Although these items can be hidden by left-clicking on them, it is highly recommended to keep both visible—they are important tools for managing your section pacing, as discussed in Chapter 4: Previewing the Passage.

2.3 Interface Tools

In addition to the tools available to navigate throughout the sections of the MCAT, the testmaker has made several other tools available via the CBT interface (Figure 2.4). Just as it takes practice to become comfortable adapting from reading books and articles on paper to reading text on a screen, so too do these interface tools require a bit of practice. But with a little dedication, using these tools will become second nature by Test Day. When you master these tools, you can efficiently highlight text, strike out text, flag questions, and call up the periodic table in the science sections.

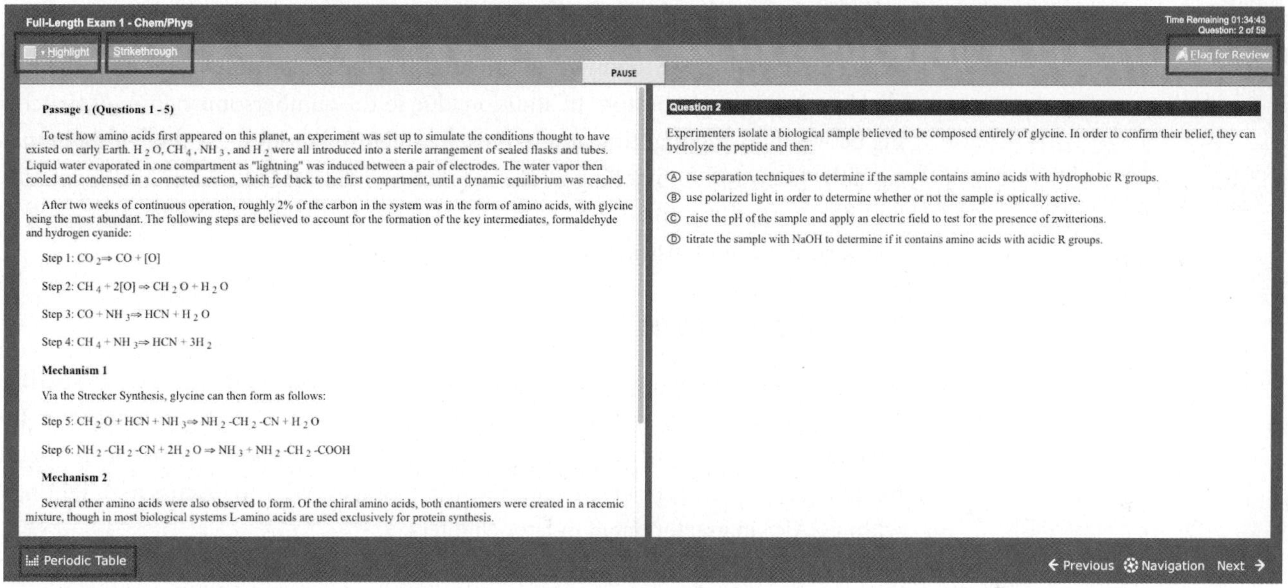

Figure 2.4 Interface Tools

Highlight Function

Much like its everyday counterpart, the highlight function highlights text in yellow. Strategically, highlighting text should stress the text's importance. To highlight text:

1. Ensure the **Highlight** option is selected in the top left corner, indicated by a yellow box (this is the default setting).
2. Use the cursor to left-click and hold while dragging over the desired text.
3. Press Alt + H or alternatively left-click the **Highlight** button in the top left of the screen.

MCAT highlighting also allows a feature that ordinary highlighting does not: erasing. Unfortunately, this process is somewhat cumbersome. To remove highlighting from text:

1. Select the **Remove Highlight** option by left-clicking the box beside the word "Highlight" in the top left corner. Alternatively, pressing Alt + H (with no text selected), then pressing the down arrow key twice, and then the space bar will also select the remove highlight option.
2. Left-click and hold while dragging over the highlighted text using the cursor.
3. Press Alt + H or left-click the **Highlight** button, ensuring that the remove highlight option is selected.

When highlighting, we highly recommend using the hotkey, Alt + H, rather than clicking the highlight button. In addition, due to the cumbersome nature of switching between the highlighting and remove highlighting modes, use the highlight tool carefully to avoid ever needing to use the remove highlight function. And if you do highlight something you didn't intend to, consider just leaving it on screen unless you're sure it would distract you.

Highlighting in Passages

If you choose to highlight within the passage, we recommend that you do so sparingly to avoid creating more work for yourself when referring back to the passage later. In general, "less is more" when it comes to highlighting. In the sciences, it can be useful to highlight key terms or given values within passages. We will discuss highlighting within CARS in greater detail in later chapters.

Highlighting in Questions

Highlighting in question stems should be used as needed. To clarify, many students will find highlighting question stems unnecessary, while others may find highlighting helps them avoid careless mistakes. For example, if you find yourself often overlooking phrases such as "is not to be expected" in question stems, spending a moment highlighting the phrase can help ensure it stays in your mind while you are answering the question. Highlighting in the answer choices, although possible, is not recommended.

Strikethrough Function

The **strikethrough** function crosses out selected text, ~~as seen here~~. Typically, this is used to indicate that the crossed out text is not important. To strikethrough text:

1. Left-click and hold while dragging over the desired text using the cursor.
2. Press Alt + S or alternatively left-click the **Strikethrough** button in the top left of the screen.

To remove strikethrough from text, click and drag to select *only* the strikethrough text, then press Alt + S. If non-strikethrough text is accidentally selected along with the strikethrough text, then the Alt + S function will strikethrough *all* selected text.

Strikethrough in Passages

Generally speaking, a limited use of the Strikethrough tool during passage reading is best. Although it is no secret that each passage on the MCAT has its own amount of "fluff" (irrelevant) text, the Strikethrough tool should be used sparingly, since it's often more efficient to simply read past the fluff than to stop and strikethrough the text. It can be difficult to determine when text is actually irrelevant in CARS passages, so we recommend using the Strikethrough tool more on passages in the science sections (where it is easier to determine when material won't be targeted by questions) than in CARS.

Strikethrough in Questions

Like highlighting, the Strikethrough tool should be used as needed in questions. Most testers find little value using the Strikethrough tool in the question stem, but find it useful to eliminate answer choices. The key here is to keep use of the tool purpose driven; do not strikethrough answer choices simply because they are wrong, as these extra seconds add up over a section! Rather, aim to use the Strikethrough tool in a way that reduces your chance of error. For instance, let's say you begin working on a question, then ultimately choose to triage it. Before moving on to the next question, first use Strikethrough on any choices you managed to eliminate. When you return to the triaged question later, those eliminated choices will remain crossed out, even if you don't remember why!

Question Flagging

The **Flag** (Alt + F) function allows testers to flag a specific question, usually to remind them to return to it at the end of the section. Flagged questions can be seen at a glance in the Navigator window and the Section Review screen. To flag a specific question, click the flag icon at the top right corner or use the hotkey Alt + F. Once flagged, the flag icon will turn yellow. In order to make the most of this function, it's important to use it sparingly. Remember, the MCAT is a timed test: if there is extra time at the end of a section, it is best spent reviewing questions you could feasibly answer. In other words, do not flag every difficult question or every question that you guess on; rather, flag only those questions that you know you could answer correctly if you just devoted some extra time to them.

It is worth pointing out that the Flag function loses much of its usefulness in the CARS section. CARS questions are completely passage based and therefore best answered shortly after analyzing the passage. Thus, you should aim to answer every question in a CARS passage before moving on to the next one, and save the Flag function for the science sections.

The Periodic Table

The periodic table of elements is made available in both the Chem/Phys and Bio/Biochem sections of the MCAT and provides for each element its symbol, atomic number, and atomic weight. To bring up the periodic table, left-click the **Periodic Table** (Alt + T) button at the bottom left. This will bring up a centered window displaying the periodic table (Figure 2.5). Similar to the Navigator window discussed previously, the Periodic Table window can be manipulated by clicking and dragging the top bar and window borders. To close the periodic table left-click Close (Alt + C).

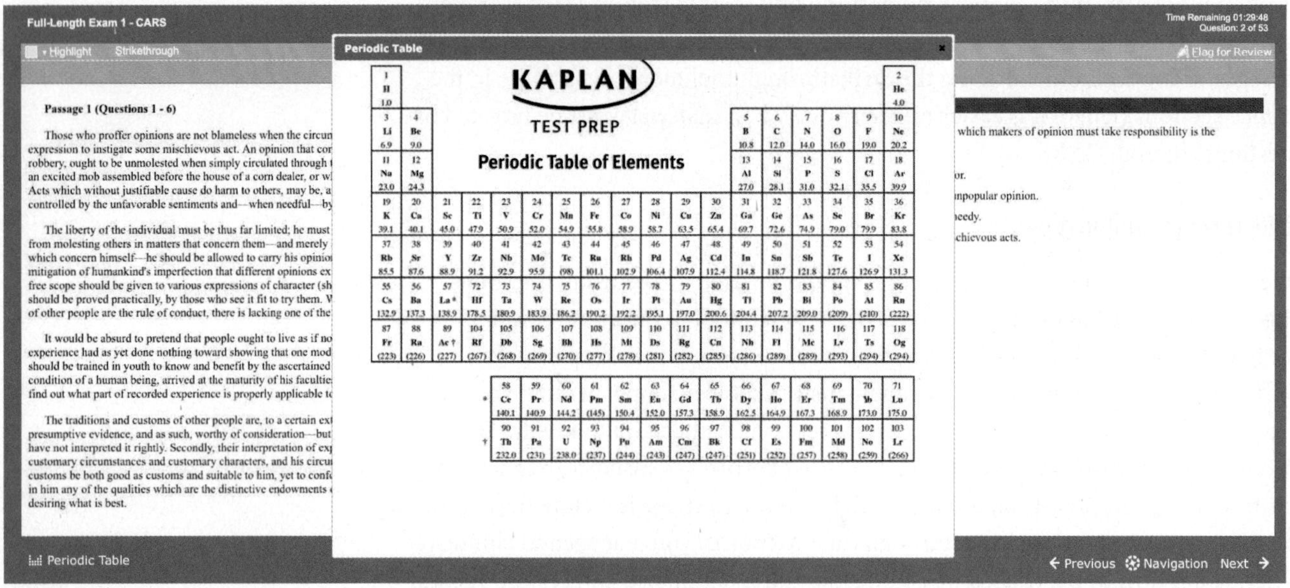

Figure 2.5 Periodic Table

Strategically, the periodic table should be used only when needed. Keep in mind that the periodic table always displays the same information and that bringing it up obscures the view of the question and passage. Thus, you should use the periodic table only when seeking a specific piece of information, e.g., an element's group or an element's atomic weight. In other words, do not bring up the periodic table simply to check if there is anything useful for a particular question. Instead, when opening up the periodic table, you should know exactly what you are looking for.

Conclusion

Well done! You've taken your first step toward mastering the computerized tools, that allow for smooth navigation of the interface on Test Day. Now you're ready to practice with them! If you're learning how to swim, it's not enough to read a book about different swim strokes; you're better off finding a shallow body of water where you can practice those strokes safely. So too with these CBT tools: to truly master them, practice using them whenever you use a test-like MCAT interface.

During your practice, you will likely find some tools are more useful to you than others, and you might even find yourself disregarding some of the recommendations in this chapter. This is perfectly acceptable: the tools are yours to make use of (or not) based on your preferences. The key is to ask yourself, before your test-taking habits become too entrenched, "Is my usage of the tools helping or hurting?" As long as it helps you, you're using the tools in the right way for you.

CONCEPT AND STRATEGY SUMMARY

Test Day Tools

- The MCAT is a **computer-based test (CBT)** with unique tools to master.
- Interacting with the CBT MCAT can be done via on-screen buttons or keyboard shortcuts, listed in Table 2.2.

Shortcut	Function	Shortcut (Section Review)	Function (Section Review)
Alt + N	Advance to Next; Answer No	Alt + E	End Review of Section/ Exam
Alt + P	Return to Previous	Alt + W	Return to Section Review
Alt + V	Open Navigation	Alt + A	Review All Questions
Alt + H	Highlight/Remove Highlight	Alt + I	Review Incomplete
Alt + S	Strikethrough/Remove Strike-through	Alt + R	Review Flagged
Alt + T	Open Periodic Table	Alt + Y	Answer Yes
Alt + C	Close Navigation/Close Periodic Table	Alt + O	Answer OK
Alt + F	Flag for Review		

Table 2.2 Keyboard Shortcuts

- On Test Day, you will be provided with a 9-page **noteboard booklet** and fine-point marker to use for scratchwork. If you need additional space, you may exchange your booklet for a clean one with the test administrator.

Navigation Tools

- **Section Interface** displays the passage and associated questions one at a time. Use the buttons listed below to navigate the section.
  - **Next** brings up next question.
  - **Previous** brings up previous question.
  - **Navigation** brings up the Navigator window, which displays the status of all questions at a glance and allows the tester to jump to any specific question.

- Use the **Navigator window** like an expert.
  - Jot down in your noteboard booklet the passage number and first question number for each passage (e.g., "P6: Q31").
  - When you wish to return to a skipped passage, simply bring up the Navigator window and click on the first question of the passage (e.g., Question 31).
- The **Section Review** interface shares most of the functions of the Navigator interface, but allows for targeted review of questions, including:
  - **Review Incomplete** allows for review of incomplete questions only.
  - **Review Flagged** allows for review of flagged questions only.
  - Use the Review Incomplete function first, then the Review Flagged before ending your section (Alt + E).
- **Timer and Question Progression** functions are located at the top right of the screen and should be kept visible to assist in your pacing strategy.

Interface Tools

- **Highlight** keywords or phrases, as needed.
  - Use the cursor to select text and the keyboard shortcut, Alt + H, to highlight text.
  - Reserve highlighting for important terms or phrases, while avoiding the need to remove highlighting.
  - Highlight key phrases in question stems that have been missed on previous questions.
  - The less text that is highlighted, the more effective it is.
- **Strikethrough** irrelevant text, as needed.
  - Use the cursor to select text and then the keyboard shortcut, Alt + S, to strikethrough text.
  - Strikethrough should be used for wrong answer choices, in particular when a question may be returned to later.
  - Strikethrough with purpose! Do not simply strikethrough wrong answers because they are wrong; this will use too much time.
- **Flag** questions that you want to return to at the end of the section.
  - Be conservative in your question flagging because there will be limited time at the end of the section.
  - You can navigate through only flagged items from the Section Review interface.
- The **periodic table** is available in the Chem/Phys and Bio/Biochem sections.
  - The periodic table contains an element symbol, atomic number, and atomic weight for each element.
  - When using the periodic table, you should know what you are looking for. Do not use the periodic table for inspiration.

CHAPTER 3

RHETORIC AND ARGUMENTS

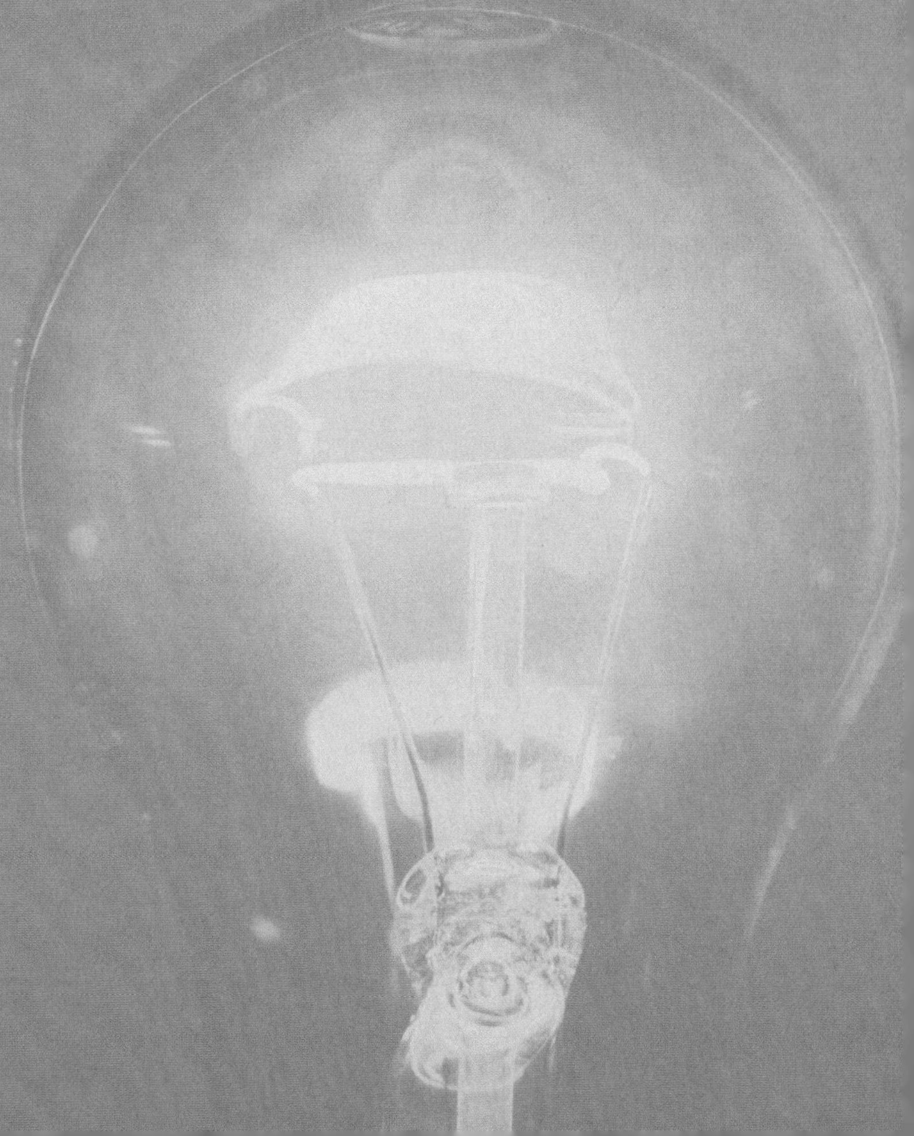

CHAPTER 3

RHETORIC AND ARGUMENTS

In This Chapter

Introduction

LEARNING OBJECTIVES

After Chapter 3, you will be able to:

- Describe the key components of rhetoric and their impact on passage reading on Test Day
- Describe the key components of an argument and their impact on passage reading on Test Day
- Use rhetorical and argument analysis to understand the central ideas of CARS passages

By now you've learned about the CARS section in outline and about the CBT tools at your disposal on Test Day, and perhaps you've even attempted a couple CARS passages yourself. During all this, you've seen that CARS passages can explore almost any topic, which may have led to the question, *"How can the CARS section be standardized if each passage discusses something unique? Isn't that the opposite of standardized?"* Well, not quite. The standardization of the CARS section is achieved not through a shared set of content topics, but rather by means of *how* the passages are written (as well as through the common types of questions accompanying each passage). Thus, rather than trying to familiarize yourself with all the topics that could show up in CARS passages on Test Day, your aim should be to recognize the common patterns authors use to construct their passages. By Test Day, whether you see passages discussing the workings of ancient Greek currency, the appeal of a mystery novel, or even the ramifications of an obscure philosophical theory, you will be comfortable analyzing these passages by identifying their basic rhetorical and argumentative components.

Toward that end, this chapter will focus on two nearly universal aspects of CARS passages, **rhetoric** and **arguments**, with the ultimate goal of introducing you to their most common (and most testable) patterns. A strong command of rhetoric and argumentation will allow you to navigate any passage on Test Day.

3.1 Key Components of Rhetoric

It is safe to assume that the authors of CARS passages are competent writers. In fact, we could even go so far as to say they are effective writers. Therefore, it makes sense to begin our discussion of *how* CARS authors construct their passages by examining rhetoric, the art of effective communication. The theory of rhetoric is a wide-ranging topic that can literally fill a university-level writing course but, fortunately, only a couple of key components of rhetoric are necessary to gain proficiency in CARS.

Rhetoric

Most of us are familiar with the device known as a **rhetorical question**. Although it ends in a question mark, a rhetorical question tends to have only one plausible and obvious answer. What makes it rhetorically effective is that it forces readers to reach the conclusion themselves, so that readers are more convinced of the intended conclusion than if the author had simply stated it. However, effective use of rhetoric is much more nuanced than simply asking questions that aren't really questions. Considered broadly, **rhetoric** is the art of effective communication, both in speech and in text. Because the MCAT is a written exam (as opposed to oral), we will discuss only the textual side of rhetoric throughout this chapter. While language may serve many purposes, the study of rhetoric tends to focus on persuasion—the attempt to influence others to adopt particular beliefs or to engage in certain behaviors. **Rhetorical analysis**, then, is an examination of speech or writing that goes beyond *what* the author is saying (the content) to consider *how* and *why* the author is saying it.

REAL WORLD

Discussion of the art of rhetoric often begins by describing the **rhetorical situation**: an interplay between author, audience, message, purpose, genre, exigence, and context. However, discussion of the rhetorical situation as a whole is not needed for the MCAT.

Many other standardized tests focus predominantly on understanding the details of what the author has said. However, the MCAT takes it a step further, sometimes asking you to use the text to infer characteristics about the author, the audience, and the goal of the passage. To that end, we will define these fundamental aspects of rhetoric (author, audience, and goal) and demonstrate how Distilling them will translate to points on Test Day.

Author and Tone

The **author**, in the most basic sense, is the individual or group that wrote the text. Authors can be distinguished by how much expertise they have on the topic at hand and by how passionate or vested in the topic they are.

Authors who are experts in a topic—and who know that their intended audience is also knowledgeable in the topic—tend to use a lot of jargon in their writing. **Jargon** refers to technical words and phrases that belong to a particular field. For example, *transcriptional repression*, *zwitterion*, and *anabolism* are all biochemical jargon; *homunculus*, *Gesellschaften*, and *negative symptoms* are all behavioral sciences jargon. Authors who are less expert, or who are writing to a less-informed audience, tend to use more common terminology and provide more explicitly detailed descriptions of their ideas. Authors who consider themselves less expert than their audiences may use an abundance of Moderating keywords, described in Chapter 5 of *MCAT CARS Review*.

MCAT EXPERTISE

The more knowledgeable authors are in a topic, the more jargon may appear in their writing. This may make for a challenging passage to read, but recognize that the MCAT does not expect you to know any field-specific terminology in CARS. Any important jargon will be defined in the passage—or the definition will be strongly implied.

Tone reflects the author's attitude toward the subject matter. When an author is passionate about a topic, this emotion often manifests as strong language. Extreme keywords, also described in Chapter 5 of *MCAT CARS Review*, may suggest that an author is emotionally invested in the piece. Less-invested authors may use more emotionally neutral words to describe the same ideas. In addition to an author's word choice, what the author chooses to discuss about a subject matter can also reveal the author's tone. For instance, an author may use neutral language, but use that neutral language to describe disadvantages of a particular activity and to list suitable alternatives. Despite the lack of Negative keywords (also discussed in Chapter 5), the author would still have a negative attitude toward the subject matter. On Test Day, aim to identify whether, and to what extent, the author's attitude toward the subject matter is positive or negative.

Determining Author Tone

MCAT EXPERTISE

On Test Day, be on the lookout for descriptive words, such as adjectives and adverbs. These words were specifically chosen by the author and can convey tone.

Identifying the author's tone can help you keep track of the author's opinions while reading the passage, but more importantly it will pay off when answering questions. Not only will you be asked questions directly focused on the attitudes and opinions of the author, but you will also see questions where simply knowing the author's tone will allow you to narrow down the answer choices. To determine the author's tone in a passage, examine the words that are used while considering the question: What imagery or feelings do these words convey? Let's try an example!

Consider this passage excerpt:

> One of the first examples of the ascendance of abstraction in 20th-century art is the Dada movement, which Lowenthal dubbed "the groundwork to abstract art and sound poetry, a starting point for performance art, a prelude to postmodernism, an influence on pop art . . . and the movement that laid the foundation for surrealism." Dadaism was ultimately premised on a philosophical rejection of the dominant culture, which is to say the dominating culture of colonialist Europe. Not content with the violent exploitation of other peoples, Europe's ruling factions once again turned inward, reigniting provincial disputes into the conflagration that came to be known by the Eurocentric epithet "World War I"—the European subcontinent apparently being the only part of the world that mattered.

It's clear that the author is discussing the Dada movement, but what is the author's view of the Dada movement? Notice how the author's chosen quotation describes the Dada movement: "...groundwork...starting point...prelude...foundation..." The quotation makes it clear that the Dada movement is one of the first instances of artistic abstraction, but why did the author choose a quotation that seems to be saying the same thing in four different ways? The answer is because the author wants to stress the influential nature of the Dada movement, implying that the author's opinion of Dadism is positive! In contrast, notice the author's word choice to describe the "dominating culture" of Europe: "violent exploitation." This is clearly negative. Furthermore, if you read the last sentence of the excerpt and thought it sounded sarcastic, you're right. This echoes the author's negative view of early twentieth-century European culture. All this provides further evidence of the author's would again support the positive view of Dadaism because the author claims Dadaism is based on a "philosophical rejection of the dominant culture."

In short, there are two opinions being put forward in this excerpt: the author's positive view of the Dada movement and his negative view of the European culture of the time. Using the author's tone, let's tackle this Inference question (Inference questions will be further discussed in Chapter 9):

1. It is reasonable to infer that the author believes that:
   - (A) the rejection of Dadaism in Europe was a cause of World War I.
   - (B) the Dada movement was an insignificant blip in art history.
   - (C) the Dada movement was a step forward for artistic abstraction.
   - (D) Dadaism should not have gained popularity in Europe.

When answering an Inference question on Test Day, you can use the author's tone to set expectations before reviewing the answer choices. Keeping in mind the author's opinions toward Dadaism and European culture of the time, let's evaluate each of the answer choices. Choice (A) suggests something negative about European culture, that its rejection of Dadaism led to World War I. We know that this author has a negative opinion about European culture, so you can't immediately eliminate this answer. But, there's more we need to unpack with this choice to determine whether it's what we're looking for. So let's see if we can eliminate any of the other choices. Choice (B) portrays Dadaism negatively with the word "insignificant" and is thus wrong. Choice (C), however, paints Dadaism in a positive light with the phrase "a step forward." This is consistent with the author's expressed opinions. On the other hand, Choice (D), like (B), represents Dadaism negatively, making (D) incorrect as well.

Using the author's tone alone, we were able to get this Inference question down to a 50/50 choice between (A) and (C)! To decide between them, simply return to the passage and verify whether the facts match up as well as the opinions do. The author never suggests that rejecting Dadaism was a cause of World War I—rather, he blames the "inward" turn of "Europe's ruling factions." However, he does describe Dadaism as an important early example of abstract art. That means (A) can be ruled out and (C) is correct.

Audience and Genre

The **audience** is the person, or persons, for whom the text is intended. In daily life, the audience could be a single person with whom you have a dialogue, but publications typically have considerably larger audiences. Many CARS passages address an academic audience—perhaps other specialists in the author's field. Even when writing for the "general public," authors may draw upon idioms, clichés, symbols, and references that may have been recognizable to people of a particular time and place, but are less commonly used today.

In CARS, you will rarely be a member of the passage's intended audience, but you can still develop the ability to recognize the audience for whom a passage was originally written. One potential source of information about the author's intended audience is the genre of the passage. The **genre** is the particular category to which the written work belongs—for example, fiction, nonfiction, drama, poetry, and so on. Genre can also represent the more tangible form of the work: book, scholarly journal article, case study, essay, letter, email, and so forth.

Determining Audience and Genre

A passage's audience and genre are tested less frequently in the CARS section than are the author's opinions and tone. Nevertheless, being able to recognize audience and genre can sometimes yield points on Test Day. To determine the audience, begin by identifying the topic of the passage, then consider *how* the author presents the major ideas in the passage. Does the author explicitly define key concepts and use simple terms that most readers would recognize? Or does the author use jargon and assume readers will already understand the intended meaning? Generally speaking, an author who writes more accessibly aims for a general audience, while an author who assumes reader knowledge is writing for an expert or specialized audience.

In terms of genre, most of the passages you'll encounter on Test Day will be nonfiction prose, excerpted from books or articles. A piece intended for a general audience is likely to be taken from a popular magazine or book, while journal articles and other scholarly publications are more often associated with specialized audiences. Let's try an example!

Consider this excerpt:

> The most prevalent argument against doctor-assisted suicide relies upon a distinction between *passive* and *active* euthanasia—in essence, the difference between killing someone and letting that person die. On this account, physicians are restricted by the Hippocratic oath to do no harm and thus cannot act in ways that would inflict the ultimate harm, death. In contrast, failing to resuscitate an individual who is dying is permitted because this would be only an instance of refraining from help and not a willful cause of harm. The common objection to this distinction, that it is vague and therefore difficult to apply, does not carry much weight. After all, applying ethical principles of *any sort* to the complexities of the world is an enterprise fraught with imprecision.

REAL WORLD

Why does the testmaker care so much about your ability to think beyond just understanding the content of an author's writing? This is a skill you'll use every day when talking with patients (to discern what they are really thinking from their body language and tone of voice) and when critically appraising research (to look for potential biases or conflicts of interest on the part of the researcher). To make good choices for your patients, you must be able to move beyond simply reading words on a page and consider the bigger picture, such as the author's goal.

The MCAT might test your ability to recognize the passage's intended audience or genre with a question like the one below.

1. Which of the following titles would best be suited for this passage?
   (A) A Medical Student Handbook: Euthanasia
   (B) Exploring the Ethics of Doctor-Assisted Suicide
   (C) A Case Study on Euthanasia
   (D) Euthanasia, Society's Next Plight

To answer this question, consider the author's tone as well as the passage's intended audience. Unlike the previous example, the author's tone is fairly neutral, with few words suggesting strong authorial opinions. Despite this, she does share one opinion in the next-to-last sentence: the common objection to the active *vs.* passive distinction is weak. This excerpt describes subject matter that might appeal to medical professionals, professors of ethics, or the general public. In this case, considering subject matter alone, it may be difficult to determine the intended audience. But by considering *how* the author constructs this passage, you can arrive at a more precise answer. The author explicitly defines concepts like active euthanasia, passive euthanasia, and the Hippocratic oath—terms that specialists such as doctors and ethics scholars would already know. Overall, the language is accessible and the amount of jargon minimal, which suggests that this article's audience is the segment of the general public that may have an interest in ethics. Choice (B), "Exploring the Ethics of Doctor-Assisted Suicide," matches the tone of the author, the topic of the passage, and the intended audience. In terms of genre, that title suggests an excerpt from a popular book or magazine, and this makes more sense than (A)'s "handbook" or (C)'s "case study," which are more specialized publications that don't fit the language of the passage.

Goal

BRIDGE

Impression management, discussed in Chapter 9 of *MCAT Behavioral Sciences Review*, focuses on how we present ourselves to accomplish specific goals. Some of the impression management strategies can be employed in writing as well, such as self-disclosure, ingratiation, and alter-casting.

The **goal** of a passage, sometimes called the purpose, is why the author wrote the passage. In other words, what was the author hoping to accomplish? In some cases, the author's goal may be simply to inform the audience. Passages with an informative goal tend to read like textbooks or encyclopedia entries, providing detailed descriptions nearly devoid of the author's opinion. In the CARS section, however, more often the goal is persuasion, in which the author aims to influence the audience to adopt new beliefs. Persuasive passages are the most common on the MCAT; most passages on Test Day will contain at least one opinion the author tries to get the reader to endorse (with varying degrees of forcefulness). Besides altering beliefs, persuasion can also motivate individuals to take action. Such persuasion is often encountered in speeches, but it could appear on the MCAT as a set of recommendations for solving a particular problem.

On Test Day, you will encounter Main Idea questions, covered in Chapter 9: Foundations of Comprehension, which will directly test your ability to distill the author's goal.

Distilling the Goal of a Passage

To distill the goal of the passage, consider the major ideas of the passage while keeping the author's tone in mind. Ask yourself, *Why did the author write this passage?* We recommend beginning your answer an infinitive verb ("to X"), such as "to explain," "to argue," or "to compare." Let's try an example!

Consider this excerpt, which includes and continues the previous excerpt:

> The most prevalent argument against doctor-assisted suicide relies upon a distinction between *passive* and *active* euthanasia—in essence, the difference between killing someone and letting that person die. On this account, physicians are restricted by the Hippocratic oath to do no harm and thus cannot act in ways that would inflict the ultimate harm, death. In contrast, failing to resuscitate an individual who is dying is permitted because this would be only an instance of refraining from help and not a willful cause of harm. The common objection to this distinction, that it is vague and therefore difficult to apply, does not carry much weight. After all, applying ethical principles of *any sort* to the complexities of the world is an enterprise fraught with imprecision.
>
> Rather, the fundamental problem with the distinction is that it is not an ethically relevant one, readily apparent in the following thought experiment. Imagine a patient who is terminally ill and hooked up to an unusual sort of life support device, one that only functioned to prevent a separate "suicide machine" from administering a lethal injection so long as the doctor pressed a button on it once per day. Would there be any relevant difference between using the suicide machine directly and not using the prevention device? The intention of the doctor would be the same (fulfilling the patient's wish to die), and the effect would be the same (an injection causing the patient's death). The only variance here is the means by which the effect comes about, and this is not an ethical difference but merely a technical one.

Consider the ideas discussed in both paragraphs and determine how they connect to serve the purpose of the passage. In the first paragraph, the author describes the distinction between active and passive euthanasia, providing examples. She then offers the "common objection" to this distinction, but immediately shoots this common objection down. In paragraph 2, the author provides *her own* objection ("fundamental problem") with the active and passive distinction: that the distinction is ethically irrelevant. The author then supports her objection with a thought experiment.

With the passage's structure laid out, the goal should be more visible. The author clearly disagrees with those who distinguish between active and passive euthanasia. After describing these terms in paragraph 1, she dedicates the entire second paragraph to debunking this distinction. But more specifically, what reason does this author give for disagreeing with this distinction? In paragraph 1, the author describes one reason why some people object to the distinction between passive and active euthanasia, which is that the distinction is vague. However, notice that the author distances herself from this point of view: she calls this "the common objection" and says it "does not carry much weight." The author's own objection comes in paragraph 2, where she claims that the distinction between passive and active euthanasia is not "ethically relevant." Thus, the author's goal is broadly persuasive and could be phrased more precisely as: *to argue that the distinction between passive and active euthanasia is not ethically relevant.* Recognizing with the goal of the passage, let's consider the following Main Idea question.

1. Which of the following best reflects the central purpose of the passage?
   - (A) To explain how euthanasia is ethically unjustified in all circumstances
   - (B) To suggest there is no distinction between active and passive euthanasia
   - (C) To contend that active and passive are not morally significant categories for euthanasia
   - (D) To argue that euthanasia is ethical only if it is neither active nor passive

Choice (C)'s phrase "morally significant" is just another way of saying "ethically relevant," so (C) best reflects the goal we distilled previously.

3.2 Key Components of Arguments

You may have noticed that we used the verb "to argue" in our formulation of the last passage's purpose. But contrary to popular usage, an "argument" in the CARS section is not a heated verbal dispute between people, but a specific kind of logical structure that authors use for persuasive purposes. In this section of the chapter, we will investigate the structure of arguments and prepare you to recognize their components in CARS passages.

Argument Structure

In the study of logic, an argument is the combination of one claim, known as the **conclusion**, and one or more other assertions, known as the **evidence**, explicitly used to support the conclusion. In this way, a mere claim becomes a supported conclusion as long as it's accompanied by supporting evidence. Evidence is like the friend who vouches for you to get into the VIP area at a nightclub (*conclusions only!*): it offers a reason to "trust" that the conclusion is what it claims to be. In other words, the evidence is an answer to the question, *"Why should I believe that conclusion?"* Together, the evidence, the conclusion, and the one-way connection between them constitute the simplest form of an **argument**. Consider the following statements:

- **Statement A:** Cats are great pets.
- **Statement B:** Cats are cute.

These two statements can create a plausible argument, but only if arranged the proper way. Specifically, you must correctly identify which of the statements is the conclusion and which is the evidence. To determine the relationship between two statements in an argument, we recommend using the One Sentence Test. Phrase a sentence in the following form: "<conclusion> because <evidence>." The order that makes more sense will reveal which statement is the evidence and which is the conclusion.

Let's try out the One Sentence Test on Statements A and B:

- Cats are great pets *because* cats are cute.
- Cats are cute *because* cats are great pets.

The first arrangement makes sense; it's logical to think that at least one reason why cats make great pets is their cuteness. That doesn't have to be the full explanation of why they're great pets, as long as it gives us some reason to believe that they are. The second arrangement, however, seems confused. An animal's appearance is based on genetics and environmental conditions, not on their relationships with humans (as pets). Notice that arguments have a one-way connection: evidence supports conclusion and not vice versa.

We can summarize the argument and its components as follows:

- **Evidence:** Cats are cute.
- **Conclusion:** Cats are great pets.
- **Argument:** Cats are great pets because they are cute. (Or, equivalently: Cats are cute and, therefore, make great pets.)

KEY CONCEPT

An argument is the combination of one claim, known as the conclusion, and one or more other assertions, known as the evidence, explicitly used to support it.

While one piece of evidence is the minimum required to support a conclusion, authors typically rely upon multiple sources of support. In fact, authors will often build layers of support for their arguments by providing additional reasons to believe the evidence. In other words, providing evidence for their evidence! So, with respect to our cat example, perhaps you're a dog person, someone who's skeptical that cats are so cute, especially compared to that new puppy your friend just adopted. You might ask, why should I believe that cats are cute? After all, that claim seems like a matter of opinion, one that you might not share. The cat advocate could attempt to address your concern by providing evidence for the original evidence, perhaps by stating that cats are cute because they have large eyes and small mouths. More formally, this argument appears as follows:

- **Evidence:** Cats have large eyes and small mouths.
- **Conclusion:** Cats are cute.
- **Argument:** Cats are cute because they have large eyes and small mouths.

This may seem peculiar because what was before called the evidence is now the conclusion. Can the exact same statement be both evidence and conclusion? Yes, but only in relation to two different claims. This is nothing special: the same woman can be both a mother and a daughter, but only to two different individuals. Anytime a claim is used to *support* something else, the claim is acting as evidence; but whenever the claim in turn is *supported by* something else, the claim is acting as a conclusion. If we treated the second argument as a "subargument" within the first, we could represent it like this:

- **Subevidence:** Cats have large eyes and small mouths.
- **Subconclusion/evidence:** Cats are cute.
- **Conclusion:** Cats are great pets.

We can also use arrows to represent the relevant support relationships, simplifying the depiction of the argument further:

MCAT EXPERTISE

When authors employ especially difficult arguments, you may find it useful to sketch a diagram on your noteboard, using arrows to denote the support connections. Place the author's main conclusion, or thesis, either at the top with arrows pointing up toward it or, as we model here, at the bottom with arrows pointing down to it. Multiple pieces of evidence for the same conclusion would appear as branches extending from a common stem; thus, we sometimes call these drawings "argument trees."

Cats have large eyes and small mouths.

↓

Cats are cute.

↓

Cats are great pets.

When determining relationships such as these, you can use the textual clues discussed in Chapter 5 of *MCAT CARS Review*, especially Evidence and Conclusion keywords (the two most important subtypes of Logic keywords). However, as noted there, these keywords are less common than the other two types, and some authors use them quite sparingly. Be alert for hidden support relationships!

With an understanding of the basic components of an argument, let's take a moment to consider how this will affect your CARS reading on Test Day. As previously stated, most passages on Test Day will contain at least one argument, but is it necessary to identify its components clearly when you first analyze it? After all, we were able to analyze the euthanasia passage from earlier without applying knowledge of arguments. But even in that analysis, we identified the author's conclusion (that the active/passive distinction is morally irrelevant) and recognized that the purpose of the passage was to argue for that conclusion. In addition, we noticed that the author supported that conclusion with a thought experiment—in other words, the thought experiment was the evidence in that argument. Thus, just as a little rhetorical analysis can aid us in better understanding the passage (and in answering more questions correctly), so too can attention to argumentation. On Test Day, you'll typically find it most worthwhile to identify conclusions because they are more often featured in questions. Often, it's enough just to note the location of evidence without spelling out exactly what it says (until prompted by a question).

KEY CONCEPT

Unstated claims in arguments are known as inferences. Inferences are either assumptions (unstated evidence) or implications (unstated conclusions).

Inferences

While an argument could contain as little as one stated conclusion and one piece of stated evidence, most arguments contain unstated, or implicit, parts as well. The most commonly appearing terms for these are *implications*, *assumptions*, and *inferences*. For the sake of precision, whenever we use the word **implication**, we specifically will refer to an unstated conclusion, and **assumption** will be used only for unstated evidence. **Inference** will be used generally to cover any unstated part of an argument, whether an implication or an assumption.

It's important to note that inferences (whether assumptions or implications) are not simply claims that are *possibly* or *probably* true given what is said. Rather, inferences *must* be true or—at the very least—must be highly probable, the most likely option among the alternatives. One way to recognize an inference is by the negative effect it would have on the argument if the inference were denied. An example will help clarify what this means.

In our previous argument about the cuteness of cats, *cats are cute because they have large eyes and small mouths,* the connection between the evidence and the conclusion might seem unclear. For that argument to be valid, we need another piece of information that connects those features (big eyes and tiny mouths) to that trait (cuteness). This additional claim is an assumption. In short, an assumption is an unstated piece of evidence that must be true in order for the conclusion to follow from the stated evidence. In this case, we can identify the assumption as follows:

- **Conclusion:** Cats are cute.
- **Evidence:** Cats have large eyes and small mouths.
- **Assumption:** Animals with large eyes and small mouths are cute.

We can be sure that we have correctly identified an assumption by considering what would happen to the conclusion if we negated that suspected assumption. So, for example, if we were to say instead that *animals with large eyes and small mouths are NOT cute,* then it would make no sense to conclude that cats are cute—because we've already stated as our evidence that they have those very features. This procedure for identifying inferences by negating them is called the Denial Test, and is explained further in Chapter 9.

So where do inferences fit into your Test Day experience? Well, it's worth mentioning that a common question type in the CARS section is the Inference question type, which will be discussed in detail in Chapter 9. So, you should have the ability to identify an argument's assumptions and implications as necessary. However, spelling out the inferences of every argument that appears in the passage is generally not a good use of your time. Instead, only consider the inferences of an argument if and when a question demands it of you.

Strengthening and Weakening Arguments

Although claims or statements can be called true or false, it is a misnomer to say that an argument is true or false. Rather, the **validity** or **strength** of arguments varies along a continuum with certain proof at one end and complete refutation at the other. Most arguments (virtually all of the ones you see on the MCAT) fall somewhere short of either extreme, with evidence making conclusions more probable and refutations making them less probable.

CARS questions, particularly Strengthen–Weaken questions (discussed in Chapters 10 and 11), will often require you to imagine how an argument's validity might be modified. More supporting evidence will *strengthen*, *bolster*, or *further* an argument. This evidence can come in many forms, and often what counts as compelling evidence will depend on the topic of the CARS passage. For instance, quotations from the novel *Moby Dick* are excellent evidence when an author is advocating for a particular interpretation of *Moby Dick*. But those same quotes—coming from a work of fiction—would not be great evidence in a passage about the history of whaling in the Atlantic ocean.

On the other hand, a claim is said to *weaken*, *challenge*, or *undermine* an argument whenever the claim's truth would make the conclusion more likely to be false. Such claims serve as refutations or counterarguments (discussed more below). Note that most refutations do not come in the form of outright contradictions of the original conclusion

KEY CONCEPT

Arguments are evaluated on the basis of their strength or validity, which varies along a spectrum. An argument is strengthened whenever the truth of its conclusion is made more probable and weakened whenever it is made less probable.

or evidence. In other words, while directly attacking a conclusion will definitely weaken an argument, there are many ways to challenge an argument other than to simply state the opposite conclusion. For example, if an author draws a general conclusion about US citizens on the basis of results from a psychological survey, then evidence that the survey used a demographically unrepresentative sample would undermine the author's argument. In this way, it is not the author's conclusion that is directly undermined, but rather the evidence (that psychological survey) the conclusion stands on.

With an understanding of how claims can strengthen or weaken an argument, let's revisit our argument on cats as great pets.

- **Subevidence:** Cats have large eyes and small mouths.
- **Subconclusion/evidence:** Cats are cute.
- **Conclusion:** Cats are great pets.

This argument could be *weakened* by a claim that many of the cutest animals of the world make terrible pets, which would undermine the assumption that cute animals make for great pets. Similarly, we might challenge the assumption that large eyes and small mouths indicate cuteness by pointing to a study that identified other features (say, floppy ears or wagging tails) as being more salient indicators of cuteness. In contrast, this argument could be *strengthened* by a study that found that most people choose pets based on their apparent cuteness or by a survey showing that a majority of people describe cats as "adorable." Any argument can be strengthened *or* weakened with the appropriate evidence!

On Test Day, strengthening and weakening arguments should be treated just like making inferences. Don't bother trying to figure out all the ways an argument could be bolstered or hindered as you read through a passage—the number of possibilities is enormous, but your time is limited. Instead, you should only make such judgments when a particular Strengthen–Weaken question (see Chapters 10 and 11) requires it.

Counterarguments

A related concept is the counterargument. **Counterarguments**, also known as refutations, objections, or challenges, are simply claims that weaken a particular conclusion. Counterarguments are often worth noting when they appear in passages, because they're high yield for questions. Counterarguments are sometimes indicated through the use of Refutation keywords, discussed in Chapter 5 of *MCAT CARS Review*.

A counterargument can take aim at any component of an argument. Consider the original version of our cats as great pets argument:

- **Evidence:** Cats are cute.
- **Conclusion:** Cats are great pets.

Each of the following are possible counterarguments:

- **Refute Evidence:** Cats are not cute.
- **Refute Conclusion:** Cats are bad pets.
- **Refute Assumption:** Cute animals make for poor pets.

When you encounter a counterargument in a passage on Test Day, consider its relative strength compared to the original argument and the author's tone when presenting it, then ask yourself, *Why did the author include this?* In most cases, authors include counterarguments for one of two reasons: either they're constructing a counterargument in order to shoot down an argument they oppose, or they're describing someone else's counterargument (and probably then refuting it!) as an indirect way of supporting their own point of view.

3.3 Analyzing Passages with Rhetoric and Arguments

Now that you've seen the basic elements of rhetorical and argumentative structure, let's consider in more detail how to apply this knowledge when reading and analyzing CARS passages.

Using Rhetoric to Analyze Passages

While analyzing passages, always be on the lookout for clues that reveal the author's tone and attitudes toward the subject matter. Pay attention to opinions suggested by the author's use of adjectives and adverbs. At the start of your CARS journey, this might mean consciously stopping and asking yourself, *What is the author's feeling about this?* With practice, you will likely begin to identify author attitudes automatically, without the need for conscious effort. In addition to tone and author opinion, the author's goal is also prime material for questions. When you finish reading a CARS passage, you should always mentally answer the question, *Why did the author write this?* Other rhetorical elements like the intended audience and the genre are really only useful to the extent that they help you to identify the author's goal or to answer a particular question.

Using Arguments to Analyze Passages

As with rhetorical analysis, logical analysis is most effective on Test Day if you focus on only some of the elements of arguments. Conclusions, in particular, should be explicitly identified because they most often appear in questions. And whenever you identify a conclusion, you should also be able to locate the evidence that supports that conclusion, but you will typically not need to unpack that evidence further unless a question demands it. Counterarguments are less common but are likely to show up in questions when they do appear, so these are also worth locating. Be particularly careful when arguments are complex, with multiple layers of evidence or counterargument; try to keep clear which particular conclusion is being supported or challenged by a specific claim. As a general rule, inferences, as well as strengthening and weakening conditions, should only be considered when directly featured in questions. See the discussion in Chapter 5 of Logic keywords for more on how to recognize arguments in passages.

Now, let's apply these skills of rhetorical and logical analysis to a sample passage. As you read the passage below, try to identify the elements of rhetoric and argument discussed in this chapter. Then compare your thoughts to the expert analysis that follows.

Sample Passage

Can we truly know anything with certainty? Since the dawn of the so-called "Early Modern" era in Western philosophy, this question has preoccupied both skeptics and their critics. Perhaps the most noteworthy challenger of the certainty-rejecting skeptics is René Descartes, who constructs in his seminal *Meditations* an elaborate argument that purports to ground all human knowledge on the indubitability of one's own existence. However, in his attempts, Descartes actually bolsters the case for skepticism. Indeed, later thinkers even cast doubt on the supposed surety of self-existence.

Dissatisfied with the dogmatism of his scholastic forebears, Descartes sought to clear away all the questionable but typically unquestioned "truths" handed down to him and his contemporaries, expecting that anything that remained after an onslaught of radical doubt would have to be known with certainty. Demolishing accepted opinions one by one would require volumes, so instead Descartes examines the basic categories of belief, rejecting any kind for which he can find plausible reasons for doubt.

The first *Meditation* begins the process by considering empirical knowledge, what is learned from experience by means of our senses. Descartes's most powerful argument relies upon the impossibility of distinguishing waking consciousness from sleeping. Who has not dreamt of "waking up" while still asleep? When I awaken, how do I know the "reality" around me is not just another layer of illusion, a dream-within-a-dream-within-a-dream? Thus, Descartes concludes that all knowledge that derives from sensation cannot be certain.

With the certainty of the *a posteriori* now eradicated, the *Meditations* turn to the *a priori*, knowledge that is independent of experience, such as mathematics and logic. This proves a more difficult task, so Descartes must introduce the possibility of a Great Deceiver, a malevolent being with godlike powers who deludes us at every turn. If I cannot prove that such an entity does not exist, then "how do I know that I am not deceived every time that I add two and three, or count the sides of a square, or judge of things yet simpler, if anything simpler can be imagined?" Readers of Orwell's *1984* might have an easier time of imagining this, recalling that Winston Smith under torture genuinely comes to believe that $2 + 2 = 5$.

If even arithmetic can be cast into doubt, then how could anything be known for sure? Descartes provides an answer in the second *Meditation*. Even if the Deceiver tricks me about everything else, he cannot delude me about my own existence: "Let him deceive me as much as he will, he can never cause me to be nothing so long as I think that I am something." Of course, this "I" that exists for certain does not include the physical body, which may just be an illusion, but is simply the thinking self or mind. Even so, Descartes builds on this proposition in the remainder of the *Meditations*, arguing first for the existence of a benevolent God who would not deceive us about anything perceived "clearly and distinctly," subsequently enabling him to claim certainty for all knowledge that results from clear perception and careful reasoning.

But is Descartes's foundation really so certain? Is it not possible to doubt the existence of one's own mind? In the *Genealogy of Morals*, Friedrich Nietzsche raises the possibility of an even more radical skepticism. Though Nietzsche uses the example of lightning, the same point might be clearer to English speakers with the statement "it is raining." Although "it" seems to suggest some agent independent of the action, the phrase simply means that raining is happening. Rather than saying with certainty that "I think," perhaps Descartes should have merely concluded that "thinking happens."

Passage Analysis

Paragraph 1

In this example we can see that not all paragraphs are created equal! Here, paragraph 1 lays out three different arguments—that of the so-called "skeptics", that of René Descartes, and that of the author. Most of the rest of the passage is simply supporting evidence for the author's argument in particular. With such a rich first paragraph, let's make sure to spend some serious brain power teasing apart the beliefs of the skeptics, Descartes, and the author herself.

The passage opens with a question intended to introduce the reader to the author's central concern: "Can we truly know anything with certainty?" The goal of this passage, as is the case with many passages that open with a single question, will be to answer this question—but at this point it is too early to tell *how* the author will answer it. As might be suspected, this question could be answered *yes* or *no*, and the author presents in the second sentence a contrast between the skeptics (who would say, *no, we can be certain about nothing*) and their critics (who would say, *yes, we can know some things for sure*). At this point, the author then introduces the figure who will soon be the star of this passage, René Descartes, and his book, the *Meditations*. In this third sentence, Descartes is clearly identified as a critic ("challenger") of the skeptics, and the author spells out clearly (in case you were unsure) that the skeptics reject the possibility of certainty, while critics accept it.

This explicit identification of the sides of the debate is our first clue that the author is targeting a more generalized audience, though the relatively high difficulty of some of the language suggests the author expects this general audience to be well educated.

After reading this chapter, you probably paused when you saw the mention of Descartes's "elaborate argument" in the third sentence. We're not told yet precisely what that argument is, but we can get some sense of his conclusion (namely, that human knowledge can be certain) based on the fact that Descartes is described as a critic of skepticism. Remember that an argument is conclusion plus evidence, and all we're told about Descartes's evidence is that it has something to do with "the indubitability of one's own existence," whatever that means.

The next-to-last sentence is a crucial one. The use of the transition "However" is a clue; Contrast keywords like this one are discussed in Chapter 5. Despite the relatively neutral tone of this sentence, it reveals an important author opinion: that Descartes's argument doesn't actually do what Descartes wants it to do! Instead, according to this author, Descartes's argument actually strengthens the case of those skeptics he was supposedly criticizing! The final sentence of this paragraph acts as a first piece of evidence for the author's conclusion, suggesting there are even more reasons to doubt Descartes's argument, though they're not yet spelled out. Because the author is challenging Descartes's argument in these last two sentences, we can see that she is making what we have identified as a counterargument.

A well-constructed opening paragraph like this one can actually reveal a lot about the passage that follows, allowing you to set expectations that make the remainder of the passage more manageable to read. Not all CARS passages contain such a helpful introduction, but when they do you should try to make the most of them. This paragraph allowed us to get a sense of the topic (the certainty of knowledge), the author's tone (largely neutral, with some notable opinions), the intended audience (educated general public), and even a sense of the author's goal (answering the question about certainty of knowledge in some way that involves Descartes). We were also able to determine the conclusion in Descartes's argument (that some knowledge can be known with certainty), as well as the conclusion in the author's counterargument (that Descartes's argument actually backfires and supports the anti-certainty position, rather than the pro-certainty position he intended). As we'll see, with so much vital information already extracted, subsequent paragraphs can be analyzed more briefly.

Paragraph 2

Paragraph 2 presents us with some background on Descartes and his argument. The author suggests that Descartes was dissatisfied with the dogmatism that passed for knowledge because he would only be happy with what can be "known with certainty." The upshot of these two dense sentences is that Descartes uses a method that might seem counterintuitive: "radical doubt," which is more or less what "skepticism" is, the view that Descartes is supposedly against! When reading this, we might begin to get the sense of how the author is going to suggest that Descartes helps the anti-certainty position more than the pro-certainty one.

Paragraph 3

Paragraph 3 gives us some details about how Descartes uses his method of doubt, so this paragraph as a whole serves as evidence for Descartes's larger conclusion. Within the paragraph, though, there is a distinctive argument attributed to Descartes (this is a case of a piece of evidence serving as a kind of subconclusion with its own subevidence). The conclusion is that "empirical knowledge," which the author defines as knowledge that comes from sensory experience, can't be known with certainty. To support this, Descartes uses as evidence the claim that we can't really tell whether we're asleep or awake. This evidence, which might seem pretty controversial by itself, is in turn supported by its own subevidence, namely, the common experience of false awakenings in dreams. The author (channeling Descartes) poses this last evidence in the form of a rhetorical question: "Who has not dreamt of 'waking up' while still asleep?" This allows the author to be more persuasive than if she simply asserted that all people have had this experience, because a claim about all human beings will often seem controversial, while a rhetorical question will look like it has one obvious and simple answer.

MCAT EXPERTISE

On Test Day, you do not have to understand every component of an argument. If pressed for time, focus on identifying the conclusion and simply knowing the location of the supporting evidence.

We can sketch out the argument presented as follows (although it does not appear in this order in the paragraph):

We have all dreamt of "waking up" while still asleep.

↓

It is impossible to distinguish waking consciousness from dreaming.

↓

All knowledge that derives from sensory experience cannot be certain.

Paragraph 4

Paragraph 4 begins with some potentially frightening Latin terms—*a posteriori* and *a priori*. But the author helpfully defines the second one as experience-independent knowledge, and implies that the first term refers to the experience-dependent knowledge discussed in the previous paragraph. From that first sentence, we can expect to see something similar in paragraph 4 as we saw in paragraph 3: a subargument that concludes that experience-independent knowledge is uncertain. If you didn't follow all of the evidence presented in this paragraph, that's okay and not as important as recognizing the conclusion. But if a question required you to delve into it, you'd want to note that the central piece of evidence for paragraph 4's argument is "the possibility of a Great Deceiver," some kind of demon that tricks us whenever we try to do mental math. The author references a much later literary work (*1984*) to try to make this strange idea more plausible (in other words, to provide subevidence for the Great Deceiver subconclusion).

Paragraph 5

Paragraph 5 opens with a question that also helpfully rehashes the major point of paragraph 4 (that mathematics and other experience-independent knowledge are uncertain). Remembering paragraph 3 too, we've seen Descartes argue that both experience-dependent and experience-independent knowledge are uncertain. So what's left? The author (quoting Descartes) answers: self-knowledge, specifically the knowledge that I, a thinking being, exist. After all, how could some hypothetical Great Deceiver fool me, unless I existed in the first place? So again we have another argument, though presented quite briefly. The conclusion is that knowledge of self-existence is certain, and the evidence is that you can't be fooled about your own existence.

The remainder of the paragraph gives us more broad details about Descartes's big argument in favor of certain knowledge (as you can see, real-life arguments can contain many, many pieces of evidence; the passage here only points to a small fraction of the evidence Descartes uses in his book). The author tells us that he argues for the existence of God (without her telling us what evidence Descartes uses) and then asserts that this subconclusion is used to provide certainty for a lot more knowledge (the references to "perception" and "reasoning" suggest both the categories of knowledge discussed in paragraphs 3 and 4). So, at the end of Descartes's argument, we see that there is reason to believe that some experience-dependent and some experience-independent knowledge can be known with certainty, despite what earlier steps in his argument seemed to suggest.

Paragraph 6

The questions at the beginning of the final paragraph are truly rhetorical questions (unlike many of the open-ended questions that appear in this passage, all of which the author tries to answer explicitly)—the author's use of "really" and "not" should be dead giveaways that she wants you to answer by saying *no, Descartes's foundation is not really so certain, and yes, it is possible to doubt the existence of your mind.* Unlike paragraphs 2–5, all of which presented Descartes's argument as he made it (with the author generally trying to make a good case for it, so it's clear that she's not being unfair to him), paragraph 6 at last tells us what the author thinks herself. And, in fact, the conclusion she reveals with these rhetorical questions is very much the one we saw at the end of paragraph 1: that Descartes's argument actually undermines the possibility of certain knowledge. To support this conclusion, the author presents a counterargument against the certainty of self-knowledge, which was the key piece of evidence at the very foundation of Descartes's argument. To support this counterargument, she draws on a point inspired by Nietzsche: just as there is no "it" that does the raining when you recognize "it is raining," there may be no "I" that does the thinking when you recognize "I am thinking." The author finishes the passage with the suggestion that Descartes could only really be sure about the existence of thinking, not about the existence of a self that thinks, a conclusion that follows from the evidence she just presented.

We can summarize the author's counterargument as follows:

There is no "it" that rains.

↓

There may be no "I" that thinks.

↓

Knowledge of even your own existence is uncertain.

↓

Descartes's argument fails to show that certain knowledge is possible.

Goal

Now that we've examined every paragraph and extracted their key rhetorical and argumentative features, we can reflect on the passage as a whole. As we expected, the author maintained a relatively neutral tone but was willing to be critical of Descartes, especially in the first and last paragraphs. The language was often high level, but the author continued to define abstract terms and break down complex arguments where she could, confirming an intended audience of educated non-experts. And now, we can more exactly formulate the author's goal and understand how she would answer the question that she opens the passage with. Her main purpose seems to be to make a counterargument against Descartes' argument, which was in favor of the possibility of certain knowledge. So she might answer that first question by saying, *no, knowledge cannot be certain, because Descartes' argument for certainty fails.* In short, we might summarize her goal as: to challenge Descartes' argument that knowledge can be certain.

Conclusion

As we saw in this chapter, rhetoric and logic can enhance our understanding of MCAT CARS passages. While CARS questions will seldom explicitly ask you to identify, say, the genre of a given passage, recognizing common rhetorical structures and features can aid your answering of other questions. Arguments, on the other hand, are often explicitly referenced in questions, so there's no debate that recognizing conclusions and their evidence is a vital Test Day skill.

Rhetoric and logic are not just ancient disciplines passed down from scholars in classical Greece, nor are they only useful when taking a standardized test like the MCAT. With the expansion of evidence-based medicine, you may find yourself answering clinical questions through a meticulous analysis of the research on the topic. For example, you may find yourself asking, *Which breast cancer screening guidelines should I follow? Do I opt for the United States Preventive Services Task Force (USPSTF), which tends to be more conservative with screening, or the American Cancer Society (ACS), which is more rigorous? Or what about the American Congress of Obstetricians and Gynecologists (ACOG), which is somewhere in between?* An effective physician would read each group's recommendations with an eye toward the identity of each group (the authors), their arguments, and each group's goals. In short, understanding logic and rhetoric is indispensable to success on the MCAT, in medical school, and beyond.

CONCEPT AND STRATEGY SUMMARY

Key Components of Rhetoric

- **Rhetoric** is the art of effective communication through writing and speaking.
- **Rhetorical analysis** is the examination of a particular work for the sake of identifying its rhetorical elements (the components of rhetorical knowledge).
- The **author** is the individual or group writing the piece.
  - Authors who are experts in a topic and are writing for knowledgeable audiences may use **jargon**, which is vocabulary specific to a particular field.
  - Authors may use more opinionated words if they are passionate about the topic at hand. Authors may use more neutral words if they are less invested or knowledgeable.
  - Tone is a reflection of how the author feels about the subject matter. Identifying the tone can be done by noticing the author's word choice and phrasing.
- The **audience** refers to the person or persons the author intended to read or hear the work and is closely related to the genre.
  - The **genre** is the category to which the written work belongs, such as a book, article, essay, letter, and so on.
- The **goal** is the reason why the author wrote the work.
  - The goal of many passages on the MCAT is to be persuasive, that is, to convince the reader to adopt new beliefs or to take action.
  - Other passages may have a goal of evoking an emotional response.
  - Authors may write with more than one goal in mind.

Key Components of Arguments

- At a minimum, arguments contain three parts: a **conclusion**, its **evidence**, and the one-way path of **support** between them.
- **Inferences** are unstated parts of arguments. They are claims that must be true given what else is said in the argument.
  - **Assumptions** are unstated pieces of evidence.
  - **Implications** are unstated conclusions.
- There are three main ways of **strengthening** an argument:
  - Provide a new piece of evidence that supports the conclusion.
  - Further support evidence that already exists to support the conclusion.
  - Challenge refutations against the conclusion.

- There are three main ways of **weakening** an argument:
    - Provide a new refutation that challenges the conclusion.
    - Further support (find new evidence for) an existing counterargument.
    - Directly challenge evidence for the conclusion.
- **Counterarguments**, also called refutations, objections, or challenges, are the opposite of evidence because they go against the conclusion.

Analyzing Passages with Rhetoric and Arguments

- Author, tone, and goal should be considered consistently while reading the passages; the intended audience should be considered only when demanded by a question.
- Rhetorical clues can be used to anticipate what is coming up in a passage.
- Conclusions and counterarguments should always be explicitly identified because they are highest yield for questions, while evidence should be located and connected to particular conclusions. Inferences and strengthening and weakening should only be considered as prompted by questions.

CHAPTER 4

PREVIEWING THE PASSAGE

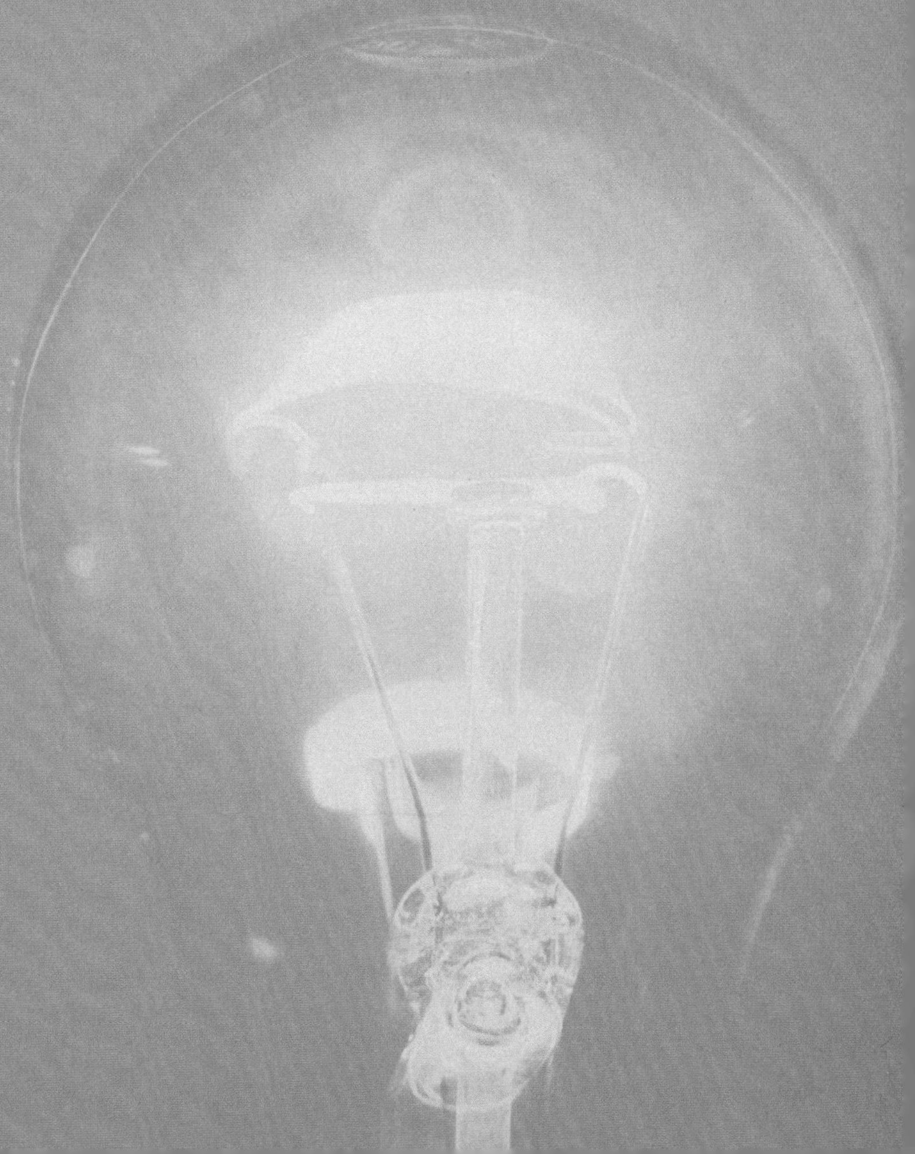

CHAPTER 4

PREVIEWING THE PASSAGE

In This Chapter

Introduction

LEARNING OBJECTIVES

After Chapter 4, you will be able to:

- Describe the timing in the CARS section
- Predict the difficulty of a CARS passage
- Determine the order in which to work the passages in a given CARS section

Great writers work with a plan, and so do great test takers. If you've ever had to make a plan to finish a project, you've already utilized this skill. Great doctors make a plan for the best way to approach a problem, be it large or small: whether in a trauma scenario or deciding on a long-term treatment plan for a patient, doing things in the proper order is a critical skill for any physician. Finding the proper order is equally important for the CARS section of the MCAT. In this chapter, we'll discuss how to take control of the section as a whole, passage by passage, so that you're driving the CARS section rather than letting it drive you.

This chapter begins by discussing the timing in the CARS section, common pitfalls in CARS, and how to overcome getting behind on time. Then we discuss how to assess a passage and techniques for knowing how difficult a passage will be for *you*. Finally, we discuss the order in which you can tackle the passages in the CARS section to maximize your score.

4.1 Timing in the CARS Section

As mentioned in the introduction to this chapter, great test takers work with a plan! In particular, CARS requires that the test taker work against both a heavy cognitive challenge and a time challenge. This chapter will discuss the best ways to meet those challenges head on, starting with the time challenge.

The CARS section is the second section that you will encounter on Test Day. In the CARS section, you have 90 minutes to read nine passages and answer 53 questions. The number of questions per passage is variable, but the goal is generally to spend about one minute per question, just like in the science sections.

As you've probably already discovered, there are several important differences between passages from the three science sections and those found in CARS. The most apparent difference is that CARS passages contain considerably more words, as well as having no images to break up the monotony of the text. Under the surface, CARS passages are much more variable, both in their range of topics and their diversity of writing styles. Moreover, unlike the science passages, which are nearly always impartial, CARS passages are often written by authors who take sides and express their opinions, although not always in a straightforward manner.

To account for these essential differences, the Kaplan Method for CARS Passages can be refined, and is shown in Figure 4.1. This chapter will focus on the very first step in this method. The remaining steps will be addressed in subsequent chapters of this book.

PREVIEW FOR DIFFICULTY

- Look for the big picture
- Assess the relative difficulty
- Decide to read *now* or *later*

CHOOSE YOUR APPROACH

- Highlighting: Best for high-difficulty passages or if low on time
- Outlining: Gives a moderate understanding of the passage and allows for more time to work on the questions
- Interrogating: Gives a strong understanding of passage but allows for less time to work on the questions

READ AND **DISTILL** THE MEANING OF EACH PARAGRAPH

- Recognize keywords to identify the most important and testable content in each paragraph
- Use your approach from the choose step to extract your major takeaways from each paragraph:
  - Highlighting—highlight 1–3 key terms and phrases per paragraph you can use to quickly locate information later
  - Outlining—create a brief label for each paragraph that summarizes the main idea of that paragraph
  - Interrogating—thoroughly examine each major idea presented in the paragraph and determine why and how the author is using the information to build an argument
- Identify the reason the passage was written before moving into the questions

Figure 4.1 The Kaplan Method for CARS Passages

Note: The Kaplan Method for CARS Passages—as well as the Kaplan Method for CARS Questions, CARS Question Types, and Wrong Answer Pathologies—are included as tear-out sheets in the back of this book.

Passage Timing

The CARS section is conveniently timed to take 90 minutes to complete nine passages and their associated questions, which means that, on average, each CARS passage should take 10 minutes to complete. This is not necessarily the case in practice, as some passages will take more than 10 minutes and some will take considerably less. That is why it must be emphasized that 10 minutes per passage is merely an average. The best test takers will organize their approach to the CARS section to deliberately take advantage of those time differences, prioritizing passages with care. Most careful test takers opt to complete passages that will take less time up front and leave the more involved passages for the end of the section, though some may vary this approach slightly based on their individual strengths.

Your time spent within each passage will not be divided evenly, either. As you'll see in Chapter 6, there are three strategies to choose from that you can deploy to Distill information from the passage. The three methods—Highlighting, Outlining, and Interrogating—take different amounts of time to complete and produce distinct outputs. Nevertheless, each method has been designed to minimize the amount of time and effort you must expend overall in approaching the passage and questions, while maximizing the number of questions you can answer correctly. Based upon which passage method you choose, you'll divide your time a bit differently between distilling passage information and answering questions. Distilling information from the passage using these methods will be discussed in Chapter 6 of *MCAT Critical Analysis and Reasoning Skills Review.*

Timing Strategy

So why should you care about timing? Why not just take your time, start from the beginning of the section, go at your own pace, and just focus on getting the questions you encounter correct? Well, consider a common pitfall that occurs before many test takers master timing: you come across a hard passage early and you find yourself spending 15 or 20 minutes on it, but by the time you're done, you're not sure you got many questions right or even understood what you read. Now you have to scramble to finish the section on time, which adds to your stress, detracts from your focus, and leaves you susceptible to mistakes you otherwise wouldn't make. It's far better to avoid such unnecessary stresses by exercising a little foresight.

Getting a high MCAT score is a numbers game: your sole objective is to get as many questions correct as possible in the time allotted. If you had to choose between an easy passage where you'll probably get all six questions correct and a difficult passage where you're more likely to get four out of seven, your best bet is to tackle the easy passage early and get those points before running out of time. Moreover, having those quick points in the bag from tackling easy passages first gives you more confidence and extra time as you work on the harder passages that remain. The MCAT scoring model specifically rewards this type of strategic thinking.

MCAT EXPERTISE

Your time on Test Day is valuable, so make sure you're using it as efficiently as you can. It is not "against the rules" to change your plan if you realize midway that it isn't working.

4.2 Previewing CARS Passages

As we discussed in the previous section, using your time effectively means prioritizing easy and quick passages over difficult and time-consuming ones. But how do you know in the first place what's hard and what's easy? And how can you make this assessment quickly enough that it doesn't create its own timing problems? This is what the Preview step of the Kaplan Method for CARS Passages is all about! When you Preview a passage, you'll be looking out for a few specific factors that you can assess quickly, enabling you to make a swift, sound judgment about the passage's difficulty. Let's consider each of these factors in turn.

Passage Topic

The first indication of the difficulty of a passage on the MCAT will be the topic. As shown in Table 1.1 in Chapter 1, passages on the CARS section come in two basic types: social sciences and humanities. Many students find that identifying the broad category for a given passage is a good first filter to determine roughly when in the 90 minute section they should approach the passage.

Social sciences passages are more likely to rely upon empirical research and data, even if they don't share the heavy focus on controlled experimentation seen in the natural science sections of the MCAT. Also, social sciences passages are more likely to focus on cause and effect relationships and are often (but not always) more logically rigorous than their humanities counterparts. In contrast, humanities passages tend to rely on different types of evidence, such as quotations from famous writers and speakers, thought experiments, or interpretations of historical events. While both types contain jargon, the jargon in the humanities can seem more daunting to many pre-med students, with references to obscure thinkers, terms borrowed from other languages, and boatloads of "ism"s with similar-sounding names.

In addition to the broad humanities *vs.* social sciences distinction, the specific discipline (from among those listed in Table 1.1) of a passage can also be useful information. As you practice with more CARS passages, you might discover some disciplines come more easily for you, perhaps because of your educational background or interests, while other disciplines are more of an ordeal. For example, if you find yourself always struggling with philosophy passages but breezing through literature passages, then your default should be to assume a philosophy passage is hard and a literature passage is easy, at least as a first guess. We recommend compiling and refining your own list of strong and weak topics as you do more CARS practice.

MCAT EXPERTISE

Use caution when approaching a CARS passage on a topic with which you are familiar. Relying upon outside information that may be true, but is not in the passage, is a surefire way to pick an Out of Scope wrong answer.

Sentence Structure

A second important influence on passage difficulty is sentence structure. Some sentences are short. Others are very long and often seem needlessly wordy with the author repeating information over and over seemingly for no reason at all! Most sentences are somewhere in between these two extremes. Unlike passage topic, which affects difficulty in a way that depends mostly on your personal interests and strengths, sentence structure tends to have a consistent influence: passages with more complex sentence structure are harder for just about everyone.

While the distance between periods (the average sentence length) is one good measure of sentence complexity, rare punctuation marks can also be helpful indicators. A passage strewn with semicolons, dashes, parentheses, or simply an excessive number of commas may suggest an author who is prone to go off on tangents, making the main points harder to follow. Remember on Test Day that you're trying to Preview passages quickly: it should only take you a few seconds to get a gut feeling of complexity based on sentence length and amount of punctuation. Any more effort than that is overthinking it.

Writing Style

While most CARS passages are standard academic prose, some authors (perhaps most notably those from earlier in history) adopt distinctive writing styles that can make the passage easier or harder to read. The exact effect usually depends on what you personally like to read, but a particularly archaic writing style can be a challenge even for a history buff. Style is not as easy to gauge as sentence structure, but you should nevertheless limit yourself to a gut-level check: take just a few seconds when assessing writing style.

MCAT EXPERTISE

Just because a style is one you don't enjoy reading doesn't mean that you won't be successful reading it on Test Day. Don't avoid passages with simpler structures just because you find their topics or styles boring.

Length

The length of the passage is perhaps the most obvious clue that you should use to identify difficulty: longer passages take more time to read. MCAT CARS passages are typically 500–600 words in length, though apparent length can be distorted based on paragraphing: a passage with a greater number of shorter paragraphs will seem longer than one with the same word count but with fewer, longer paragraphs. Paragraph length, as well, has its own impact on difficulty; it's easier to get lost when in the middle of a long paragraph that never seems to end. Both overall passage length and average paragraph length are quick and easy to assess, but be careful not to let them be the only factors shaping your judgment of difficulty.

Questions

The last noteworthy influence on passage difficulty is the number of questions associated with the passage. Remember that questions appear only one at a time in the Test Day interface. However, you can easily determine the number of questions associated with a given passage because each passage will list the range of associated question numbers, for example, "Question 32–37." You may be tempted to think more questions necessarily means a harder, more time consuming passage. But remember: passages with more questions are also worth more points!

MCAT EXPERTISE

At the top of every passage on Test Day there will be a label that tells you the range of questions associated with that passage. Using that detail makes it easy to flip between passages using the test's navigation tools. It's a good idea to make a note of the question that starts each passage on your noteboard booklet to hop easily between passages in the order that suits you.

4.3 Determining Passage Order

Whether you've worked in a hospital, volunteered in a clinic, served as a medic in the military, or just watched episodes of any medical television show, you have probably heard the word *triage*. The idea behind triaging patients is that the sickest patients get to "skip the line" so that the physician can address the most urgent needs first, minimizing further damage and fatalities among patients waiting for treatment.

The same idea can be applied to the MCAT and the CARS section. But instead of triaging to save lives, you'll be triaging to gain points, prioritizing passages to let you correctly answer as many questions as possible in the time you have. We will examine a few different ways to approach this triaging—and we recommend you experiment with each approach until you find the one that works best for you.

Section Order Strategy

One proven technique is to order the entire section by difficulty at the start of the section. Every passage on the MCAT will have a label at the top indicating the passage number and range of questions (e.g., *Passage 1 [Questions 1–7]*). This label can help you to navigate the section efficiently by jumping between the first question of each passage using the Navigator tool, discussed in Chapter 2 of *Kaplan MCAT CARS Review*. You'll need to be able to navigate between passages quickly to use the section order strategy effectively.

To use this strategy, you'll need to find a place in your noteboard booklet to list a few pieces of information, as can be seen in Figure 4.2. For each passage, write down the passage number, the number of its first question, and your triaging decision. For your triaging decision, you have a few options for how much information you want to include. You will certainly want to record your perception of the passage's difficulty. Most students prefer to record difficulty as either Easy, Medium, or Hard. However, some students prefer to simplify the decision by recording only Easy or Hard. After recording the passage's difficulty, some students also prefer to execute the Choose step by deciding whether to Highlight, Outline, or Interrogate the passage. Because the Choose step often depends heavily on passage difficulty, pairing Choose with Preview is one potential way to increase your efficiency. However, other students prefer to save the Choose decision until they have committed to a passage. Regardless of how much or how little information you prefer to record with your triaging decision, give yourself just a few seconds to decide and jot down your decision. Then use the Navigator tool to jump to the next passage (see Chapter 2), and take a few seconds to record similar information for that passage. Triaging the section in this way should take around two minutes and not more than three.

Once you've made your decisions for every passage (and have recorded something on your noteboard booklet that looks like one of the examples in Figure 4.2), then move in order of increasing difficulty: Easy passages first, then Medium (if any), and finally Hard. This approach lets you complete all of the easiest (and fastest) passages first and maximize the number of questions you answer. Further, starting with the easiest passages and slowly increasing difficulty can help you to manage stress within the section, and ensure you reach the hardest passages still full of energy. You can scratch out each passage as you complete it to have a visual representation of how much is left to do in the section.

The section order strategy is a time investment. You'll need to spend a couple minutes upfront, but the payoff will come when you move more quickly between passages as you complete them. The hard decisions primarily come at the start of the section, and then you can just focus on getting things done.

MCAT EXPERTISE

There will be stressful points during your exam; but try not to let these moments of stress "get in your head" and ruin the section as a whole. If a passage was more difficult than you expected, take a moment after you finish it to close your eyes, breathe deeply, and refocus before attacking the next passage.

MCAT EXPERTISE

In addition to your triaging decision, you can also write down a one-word clue about the passage's topic if you'd like a way to help keep the passages distinct in your mind. This can make it easier, for example, to decide which of those Hard passages to tackle first.

MCAT EXPERTISE

When reviewing a practice CARS section that you've completed, don't just consider how many points you got, but take some time to evaluate your triaging decisions. Did a passage you thought would be easy turn out to be hard for reasons you didn't originally anticipate? Adjust future triaging decisions in light of your analysis.

1	2	3	4	5	6	7	8	9
Q1	Q7	Q13	Q19	Q25	Q31	Q36	Q43	Q49
H	M	E	M	E	E	H	M	E
Econ	Lit	Psych	Ethics	Music	Art	Phil	Hist	Theat

1	2	3	4	5	6	7	8	9
Q1	Q7	Q13	Q19	Q25	Q31	Q36	Q43	Q49
H	H	E	H	E	E	H	E	E

1	7	13	19	25	31	36	43	49
H-H	M-I	E-O	H-O	E-I	E-O	H-H	M-I	E-I

E	M	H
Q13	Q7	Q1
Q25	Q19	Q36
Q31	Q43	
Q49		

Figure 4.2 Section Order Strategy Scratch Work

From the top: example scratch work with 3 levels of difficulty, passage type, passage, and question number; example scratch-work with 2 levels of difficulty, passage, and question number; example scratch work with 3 levels of difficulty, question number, and Choose step approach; and example scratchwork with 3 levels of difficulty and question number

Now *vs.* Later Strategy

An alternative to the section order strategy is the Now *vs.* Later strategy. This strategy amounts to triaging as you work through the section, instead of doing all of your triaging upfront. If you use the Now *vs.* Later strategy, you'll still perform the Preview step (perhaps combined with the Choose step) when you first encounter a passage. You'll still assign a difficulty rating to the passage. And you'll still record the passage number, difficulty, first question number, and other important details in your scratch work. The difference is, with the Now *vs.* Later strategy, you'll immediately complete any passage you decide is Easy before moving on to the next passage. Those you triage as Hard (or Medium, if you use that label too) you will save for Later. See Figure 4.3 for examples of how your noteboard booklet should look with this strategy.

For students who are particularly concerned about timing, an alternate version of Now *vs.* Later involves working both the Easy and Medium difficulty passages "now", and saving only the Hard passages for a second pass. In this version, your scratch work will be minimal, because you will only need to make note of those Hard passages that you're saving for the end. While this variant of the strategy is a great fit for many students, be warned that it may not be the best fit for everyone; some students might find that they become less efficient and more stressed when they force themselves to work through passages of moderate difficulty too early in the section.

In short, experiment with each version of the triaging strategy. You'll quickly find the version that best suits your own personality. If you like having a detailed plan for the section clearly laid out at the start, you might prefer doing all your triaging up front with the Section Order version. On the other hand, if you suffer from decision fatigue trying to assign difficulty ratings to each and every passage, you might prefer to triage as you go with the Now *vs.* Later version of the strategy. The key is optimizing the triaging strategy to work for you.

MCAT EXPERTISE

While our default recommendation is to work in order of increasing difficulty, some students find they prefer to structure the section like a hill, starting and ending with Easy passages and working the Hard passages in the middle. But regardless of which approach you adopt, you should always start with an Easy passage: data indicates that starting with a Hard passage first can negatively affect your performance across the entire section.

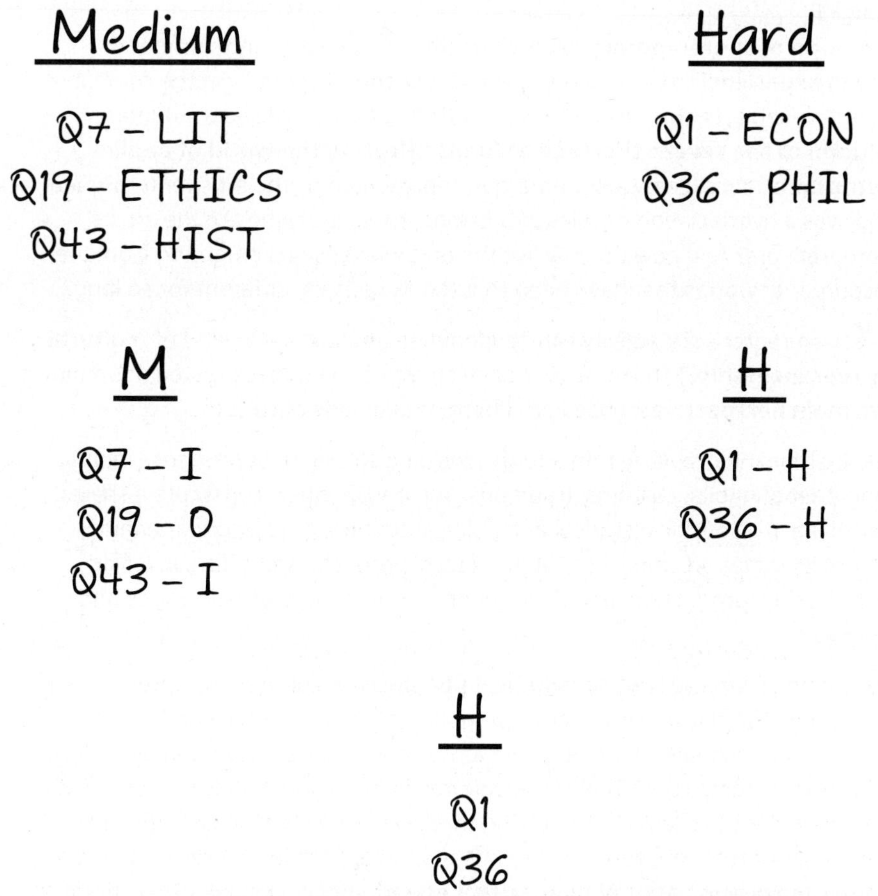

Figure 4.3 Now *vs.* Later Strategy Scratch Work

From the top: example scratch work with 2 levels of difficulty, question number, and topic; example scratch work with 2 levels of difficulty, question number, and Choose method; and example scratch work with 1 level of difficulty and question number

Applied Examples

Now let's practice some of these triaging strategies with some applied examples. The following pages feature two test-like CARS passages. We've already set in bold important lines from each passage (ones that should stand out when completing the Preview step) to help aid your decisions. Remember that your goal is only to evaluate the difficulty of the passage for you; don't bother reading the whole thing!

Passage 1

The **world of contemporary art** is characterized by a growing number of **artists experiencing an entrepreneurial venture.** Especially in the context of performing arts, this has been lived both as a necessary and a voluntary **solution to the severe shortage of funds affecting the world of public institutions.** Thus a new actor emerges, represented by the artist-entrepreneur who lives a hybridization of roles and competences. But who are the artists-entrepreneurs? And how do they live the possible tensions emerging from the encounter of worlds that have been reputed as radically different for so long?

Artists-entrepreneurs' activity can be identified as a particular kind of **"cultural entrepreneurship."** This practice has been traditionally investigated adopting **two main perspectives**, based on different meanings of culture.

As a first meaning, *culture* refers to the sociological frame of reference identifying a set of habits, customs, traditions, and beliefs which constitute a shared way of life in a specific historical and political context. As a second meaning, culture identifies a complex set of processes, products, and actors involved in the design, production, and distribution of cultural and artistic goods and services.

Descending from the **first sociological perspective**, cultural entrepreneurship represents "the skill of certain entrepreneurs to use culture as a toolkit for constructing resonant identities and motivating resource-holding audiences to allocate their resources." Therefore, cultural entrepreneurship is instrumentally identified in the process of storytelling that gives shape and legitimates new ventures. Not referring to a specific industry, the adjective *cultural* is used to identify the process of legitimization that entrepreneurs sustain, giving shape to the story of their personal and professional life.

In a second perspective, cultural entrepreneurship identifies a set of processes through which a growing number of artists and cultural professionals assume an entrepreneurial role. Cultural entrepreneurship thus identifies the activity of conceiving, producing and marketing "cultural goods and services, generating economic, cultural and social opportunities for creators while adding cultural value for consumers." The artists-entrepreneurs combine their artistic attitudes with a deep sense of business, economically sustaining the cultural enterprise in coherence with their cultural vision.

Upon investigation, what emerges with more emphasis is the tough and complex relationship between the artistic and the entrepreneurial dimensions faced by the artists-entrepreneurs. The interdependence between the two spheres emerges as a matter of fact, emphasizing the dual nature of the cultural enterprise. But duality means adopting an integral perspective that results from an intense dialogue between the two languages.

Adapted from Clacagno, M., Balzarin, L. 2016. The Artist-Entrepreneur Acting as a Gatekeeper in the Realm of Art. Venezia Arti, 25. http://doi.org/10.14277/2385-2720/VA-25-16-3

As discussed earlier, the Preview step should take just a few seconds and should really be a "gut-check" decision. As we Preview this passage, we can see that it's a humanities passage, specifically one about art. Sentence structure is moderately complex, without tons of unusual punctuation and with an average sentence length of about two lines. The writing style is a bit unusual and the author uses some humanities jargon, but there seems to be a recognizable structure to some of the paragraphs (e.g., paragraphs 4 and 5 each deal with one of a pair of "perspectives"). The passage isn't extensively long, nor are its paragraphs, so the length is manageable. This is probably a Medium passage for most students, but students who struggle with art passages would likely triage this as Hard.

Now try the Preview step with a second passage, also featuring selective use of bold to help focus your assessment.

Passage 2

Bauls are a religious group living primarily in the rural areas of West Bengal (India) and Bangladesh. They come from a variety of backgrounds, including Hindu and Muslim, and span the castes, though most are low caste. Although their roots extend more deeply, Bauls have been around at least a century. In practice and belief, they have been influenced by local traditions of the more orthodox Gauriya (Bengali) Vaishnavism, the Tantric-influenced Buddhist and Hindu Sahajiyas, and Sufism. **However, unlike many other religious groups, Bauls intentionally reverse a number of orthodox practices.** They argue that the Divine is within all humans and thus people should respect and worship humans instead of going to the temple, mosque, or church to worship something that cannot be seen. Bauls sing and compose songs that critique societal divisions and allude to their philosophy and practice. They spread their messages door to door, on trains, and in performances at large public venues.

I sought the lived experiences and perspectives of Baul women.

In [the] first 18 months of work, I carefully framed how I presented my research to my interlocutors in order to avoid the usual pitfalls of my predecessors, such as having to exchange money or prestige for information, taking initiation, or losing integrity in my research methods in other ways.

[My interaction with the Baul] brings to the forefront the postcolonial predicament concerning the relationship between ethnographers and "informants," in which the ethnographer collects "data," which is then analyzed and presented for academic scrutiny.

I have argued elsewhere that as they traverse a Baul path, those who take the teachings seriously gradually adopt cognitive and spiritual models that shift their own understanding of the world around them. Thus, they learn (or aim to learn) to recognize the ways in which society creates divisions that lead to discrimination, and to recognize the divine in all human beings, regardless of caste, gender, or religion. By listening to their explanations about the micro- and macrocosmos, by hearing their songs, and by traveling with them, they expected that I, too, would experience these shifts in understanding. The cultural specifics of their experiences may not carry home, but elements of hierarchy, discrimination, and the inherent value of all human beings are as real and important in my American communities as they are in their Bengali ones. For Bauls, issues of hierarchy and domination are religiously meaningful, and knowledge of these realities constitutes important aspects of their religious experiences.

In these and other ways, the Baul women I worked with expected me to participate in their world, particularly when they knew I shared their views. Although moments of connection have shifted my own perspectives, [a specific Baul woman's] critiques ring loudest. In demanding that I (and the many Bengalis and foreigners who enjoy her singing) support her, she refuses to let me be a complacent ethnographer. She demands dignity, and she is right to do so. Several years later, her proclamations are forcing me to rethink my ethnographic work and to reveal, as a tentative step, that I have been moved, that I have taken their words and lifeworlds seriously.

Maybe language is inadequate to explain religious experience. Bauls would certainly say so, since they insist that one can only trust and know what is personally experienced. Perhaps, then, I should acknowledge moments of connection, for instance, when [the Baul] and I discussed our views of the world, its beauty and faults, and our struggle to make sense of suffering and find ways to improve the lives of those discriminated against. Maybe it's enough for me and my interlocutors to share meaningful experiences and conversations, to be open to being inspired and transformed in the field and also back home, and to be willing to put some of those ideas into action.

Knight, L. I. (2016). "I Will Not Keep Her Book in My Home": Representing Religious Meaning among Bauls. Asianetwork Exchange: A Journal for Asian Studies in the Liberal Arts, 23(1), 30–46. DOI: http://doi.org/10.16995/ane.159

This is a social sciences passage on studies of diverse cultures, or perhaps anthropology. The topic specifically concerns religion (which is a humanities topic) but references to social sciences jargon like "ethnographers" and "informants" indicate that the passage is not exactly a humanities passage. Sentence structure is again moderately complex, without tons of unusual punctuation and with an average sentence length of about 2 or 3 lines. However, unlike the art passage, the writing style is more conversational, being more of a narrative account of the author's experiences with this culture. Regarding length: both the paragraphs (with a few exceptions) and the passage itself are longer than we saw in Passage 1, but the conversational writing style might make this an Easy passage for many students. If you struggle with studies of diverse cultures, though, you might label this one Medium or even Hard.

Previewing and triaging are skills that require practice—to establish mastery, you'll need to repeat this process over and over, any time you work on a CARS passage. Break the habit (if you have it) of doing the passages in order. Try variations of both the section order strategy and the Now *vs.* Later strategy, and reflect on their effectiveness until you find the approach that works best for you. On Test Day, the higher score you're able to earn will be worth the effort!

Conclusion

Managing your timing, Previewing effectively, and triaging efficiently are all vital skills for Test Day that can help you improve your performance and get more points on the CARS section. Practice these skills, along with those covered in the remaining chapters of this book, and you'll be well on your way to Test Day success!

The next three chapters continue the discussion of the Kaplan Method for CARS Passages with a more thorough examination of the Read and Distill steps.

CONCEPT AND STRATEGY SUMMARY

Timing in the CARS Section

- You have, on average, 10 minutes per passage on the CARS Section of the MCAT.
- The AAMC rewards students who think strategically and approach the passages out of order.

Previewing CARS Passages

- The Preview step is a quick determination of the difficulty of the passage; it should be a gut-level check that takes only a few seconds.
- Several factors influence a passage's difficulty:
  - Passage Topic
  - Sentence Structure
  - Writing Style
  - Length
  - Questions

Determining Passage Order

- There is no single correct way to order a section. The most successful students will experiment with the different strategies and choose the option that is most effective for them.
- Practice is essential to learn how to triage effectively and efficiently.
- There are two basic triaging strategies:
  - Section Order Strategy: Go through the entire section, determining the difficulty of each passage. Then, work the passages from easiest to hardest or in the order most optimal for you.
  - Now *vs.* Later Strategy: Go through the section, stopping and working any Easy passages you encounter. Write down the difficulty of other passages and return to them later, working the Hard passages last.

CHAPTER 5

READING THE PASSAGE

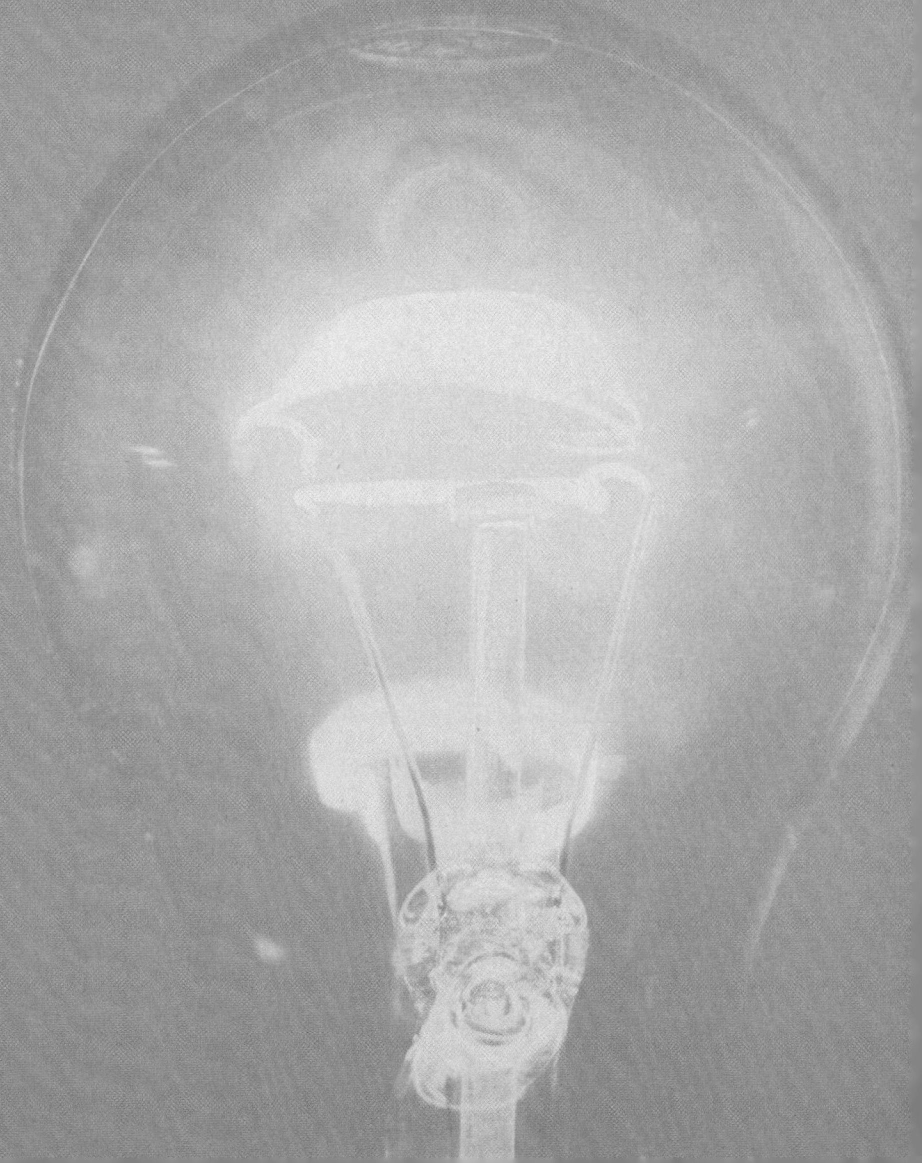

CHAPTER 5

READING THE PASSAGE

In This Chapter

Introduction

LEARNING OBJECTIVES

After Chapter 5, you will be able to:

- Apply keyword strategies within a passage to locate important themes and elements
- Identify the relationship of a sentence to its surrounding context using Relation keywords
- Connect evidence and conclusions within a passage by identifying Logic keywords
- Use Author keywords to associate author tone and opinion with text

One of the biggest mistakes you can make as a student is to think that learning how to read is a one-time occurrence, like a switch that, once flipped, fully illuminates the darkened recesses of illiteracy. It is always possible to improve your ability to read, both by refining your current approach and by broadening your comfort with a range of texts in a variety of settings. Would you read a novel for pleasure the same way you would read a textbook for homework? Once you recognize that there are many ways to analyze the written word, you can learn to customize your reading approach to fit your purpose, whether it be relaxing with a piece of fiction or reaching for that higher score on the MCAT!

KEY CONCEPT

Keywords are words and phrases commonly employed in CARS passages that serve as valuable clues for answering the accompanying questions. They fall into three broad categories: Relation, Logic, and Author.

In Chapter 3, we explored the nature of CARS passages by discussing the key components of rhetoric and argument. In Chapter 5, we'll explore strategies that will leverage keywords as a mechanism for better understanding passage structure and will build toward your ability to complete the Read and Distill step of the Kaplan Method for CARS passages. First, we will discuss the different modes of reading (reading for content, reading for purpose, and reading for reasoning) and their utility when analyzing a passage. We will then discuss keywords and their ability to clarify complex passages as part of your Read and Distill steps.

KEY CONCEPT

Any CARS passage can be understood in three different ways, which we call the modes of reading. Each mode answers at least one vital question:

- Content–*What does the text say?*
- Purpose–*What does a particular sentence do? Why does the author write?*
- Reasoning–*How are claims supported? How are claims challenged?*

5.1 Reading Strategically with Keywords

When it comes to reading dense academic prose—and this describes just about every passage in the CARS section—there are at least three ways to approach the text; that is, there are three distinct levels on which it might be appreciated. The first of these modes, **content**, is what you're most likely accustomed to looking for, whether reading for work or pleasure. On Test Day, you will want to pay attention to informational content, but you'll also want to broaden your approach to encompass the two other modes of reading: **purpose** and **reasoning**. Building on the concepts discussed in Chapter 3: Rhetoric and Arguments, reading for purpose involves identifying rhetorical components, while reading for reasoning involves identifying components of arguments.

Reading for Content

Before jumping into new ways to read CARS passages, let's briefly discuss what you are likely already familiar with, reading for content. Reading for content is focused on extracting the information from the text, discovering precisely *what* is being said. It is important to note that you will never be expected to have preexisting familiarity with the content of a passage in the CARS section; all information necessary to answer the questions is contained within the passage itself. This situation is in stark contrast to passages in the three science sections, in which you are expected to integrate outside knowledge with any new information provided in the passage.

When reading for the content, the question you should be trying to answer is *What is the author saying?* With that said, reading for content has its limitations for CARS passages, as it is unlikely that you will be a member of the passage's intended audience. Meaning, it's likely that you will not have the content background to fully understand the concepts presented in some of the harder CARS passages on Test Day. When this happens, don't panic! Instead, turn your attention toward rhetoric and arguments by reading for purpose and reasoning.

Reading for Purpose

Although there are many ways to talk about "purpose," we are specifically answering the question, *why did the author do that?* This general question can be applied to various portions of the passage and consequently reveal different aspects of the passage and author, such as:

- Why did the author use a particular word or phrase?
- Why did the author include this sentence? What does this sentence do?

- Why did the author include this paragraph? What does this paragraph do?
- Why did the author write this passage?

As you can see, we can get very specific when reading for purpose (possibly evaluating every word!), and although reading for purpose provides great insight, exploring each of these questions at every opportunity requires substantial amounts of time. Thus, it's vital to build efficient habits to ensure that reading for purpose will serve you on Test Day. As a general rule, determining the purpose of specific terms and sentences should be done when those components are major parts of the argument being built. Keywords will help you to establish when and where identifying the purpose of a portion of the passage is something you should spend time on. In contrast, determining the purpose of paragraphs and the passage as a whole should be done consistently, and is the focus of each of the Distill options in the Kaplan Method for CARS passages.

Purpose of a Particular Word or Phrase

Each CARS passage contains hundreds of words, so it is not worth your time to consider the author's intentions with every single word. Instead, you should only focus a particular term when the questions require it. **Definition-in-Context** questions (covered in Chapter 9) require you to focus on particular words and phrases, but they ask you for the meanings of terms (their content), not their purposes. In contrast, **Function** questions (covered in Chapter 10) focus exclusively on the author's intentions and will sometimes point to a brief phrase or even a single word. When assessing the purpose of a term, move outward, first thinking about how the specific sentence that contains the term functions in the larger paragraph, and then about how that paragraph functions in the passage as whole. If the term is consistent with these larger purposes, you need only look for the answer choice that best reflects the main themes of the passage. However, if something unexpected is introduced with the term, ask yourself why the author seems to be going in a different direction. Pay special attention to language that conveys feeling, whether in the term itself or in the surrounding context. If nothing else, awareness of emotionally-laden language can help you to eliminate answer choices that contain the wrong sentiments.

Purpose of a Particular Sentence

Some question types, such as Function questions, will sometimes ask about specific sentences instead. Again, if you know the larger purpose of the paragraph that contains the sentence, as well as how that paragraph functions to accomplish the author's larger purpose in the passage, then such questions will be more straightforward. When you're confused about the author's larger purposes, though, you can still use context to infer the author's intentions. Consider the following example:

> The notion of realism in literature is based largely on the implicit belief that writers can accurately transform common objects or ideas from life into words on a page while maintaining an accurate representation of the object or idea. If an author writes a novel which seems believable, meaning that a reader can imagine events in the novel actually happening, then that book is often considered a "realistic" work of literature.

BRIDGE

The amount of time you spend reading for purpose when focused on a CARS passage will depend on the Distill method you've selected for that passage as part of your Choose step. If you're Distilling by Highlighting, you will likely do very little reading for purpose, and largely rely on keywords to identify components to highlight. If you are Distilling by Outlining, you will determine the purpose of each paragraph and write it down as part of your outline. If you are Distilling by Interrogating, you will focus on the purpose of separate chunks throughout the passage on a more granular level than once per paragraph. You will always consider the purpose of the passage overall, no matter the method you have chosen. The Distill methods, and their application in the Kaplan CARS Passage Strategy, are discussed in Chapters 6 and 7.

This is a dense paragraph, consisting of two convoluted sentences. But even if you had difficulty unpacking the meaning, you can still look at the general structure of each sentence to gather information about the author's intentions. The first sentence begins with the phrase, *The notion of realism in literature is based largely on . . .*, with a long string of words following. While it may be difficult to unpack the last two-thirds of the sentence, the first third tells us that the author is explaining the basis of literary realism or, in other words, giving us the definition of that concept. Thus, the first sentence functions as an introduction and definition of a particular concept.

The second sentence, in contrast, is structured as a big if-then statement. You may have noticed the author's use of quotation marks with "*realistic*" in the then portion of the statement. This sentence is effectively saying, "if a book's author does X, then that book is realistic." In other words, this sentence is again aiming to explain what it means to have realism in literature. Since the author already gave a definition in the first sentence, the second sentence functions as an elaboration upon, or perhaps a clarification of, that definition. While the second sentence doesn't include any "transition words" (a term you may have learned about in high school or college English), the author could easily have started with a phrase like "to clarify" or "in other words" without changing the meaning or purpose of the sentence.

Often authors will include **Relation keywords**, covered later in this chapter, to emphasize these relationships between sentences. You may have learned about these in high school English or first year composition courses as "transition words" because they facilitate the movement (or transition) between sentences. In the previous example, phrases like *To clarify* or *For example* could have been used to start the second sentence. Determining the purpose of a sentence assists with reading strategically, and it also helps provide a clear prediction for Function questions (covered in Chapter 10).

Purpose of a Paragraph

Reading for purpose is particularly high yield at the level of paragraphs. While Function questions commonly ask you about the purpose of specific paragraphs, you will generally find it worthwhile to investigate each paragraph's purpose as you read, irrespective of the questions. Knowledge of how each paragraph fits into the larger whole can better enable you to eliminate answer choices for a wide variety of question types, which means more points. In Chapter 6, we will explore Kaplan's three distillation approaches to CARS passages: Highlighting, Outlining, and Interrogating. Each of these approaches includes examination of paragraph purposes, but with varying levels of specificity.

When determining a paragraph's purpose, try to get a sense of it from the opening sentence. While CARS authors are less likely than many writers to open with a topic sentence, they are occasionally straightforward, and when they aren't, you can still often pick up a few clues from that first sentence. Watch out for keywords (discussed later in this chapter) that suggest a particular transition from the previous paragraph (if there is one). Look out for changes in direction in the sentences that follow, paying particular attention again to the concluding sentence, which may contain its own transition to a following paragraph. If the paragraph goes as expected, then your initial guess at its purpose is likely accurate. But if anything surprises you, take a moment to figure out why the author would include that unexpected element. In the end, find a good answer to one of these questions: *Why did the author include this paragraph? What does this paragraph do for the passage?*

Purpose of the Passage

Chapter 3 on Rhetoric and Arguments first introduced the concept of a passage's overall purpose or goal. Indeed, a major focus of rhetoric is the study of author intentions, of what authors hope to accomplish with their writing. Regardless of which approach you choose when reading a CARS passage, it will always be worth your time to seek out the passage's goal. Make a guess about this goal as early in the passage as you can, modifying this guess if you encounter anything you didn't expect. When you finish the passage, be sure to take a moment and reflect on what you read. Ask yourself: *Did the passage accomplish what I expected it to? If not, what was the author actually trying to do?* Your answers to these questions will enable you to articulate the passage's goal in your own words, which, in turn, will translate to points on Main Idea questions and other CARS question types.

Reading for Reasoning

The final mode of reading is reading for reasoning, which focuses on the structure of arguments. Chapter 3 introduced the topic of arguments, so return there if you need a more thorough review of the topic. For present purposes, recall that an argument, at its most basic level, consists of evidence (one or more supporting statements) and a conclusion (a supported statement). When you read for reasoning, you're on the lookout for these support relationships, as well as for refutations (also discussed in Chapter 3) that challenge particular claims.

When you read for reasoning, you should ask yourself questions like the following: *What is the author trying to convince the audience to believe? Does the author give any reasons to believe this sentence is true? Does this new claim make a previous one more plausible, or does it perhaps challenge an earlier one? What evidence or refutations does the author provide for this opinion? Which claims in the passage are given the most support?* Logic keywords, discussed later this chapter, can assist you in identifying the structure of arguments in a passage.

In addition to looking out for conclusions, evidence, and refutations within paragraphs, you should also consider whether the author uses a larger argument to structure the entire passage. For example, an author might introduce a controversial claim in the first paragraph, and then provide a few different types of evidence for that claim in each of the paragraphs that follows. Alternatively, an author may introduce a claim in one paragraph, support it in the next with some evidence, and then offer additional support (sub-evidence) for that evidence in a third paragraph. At other times, an author will present a claim, perhaps even give a little evidence for it, and then go on to refute the claim in subsequent paragraphs. Being mindful of these and similar argument structures can help you better understand a wide variety of passages.

Reading and Keywords

Keywords are words and short phrases that reveal a passage's structure and its author's intentions. Keywords are the connective tissue of a text, holding ideas together in a particular way that allows the passage to do what its author wants. Keywords do not refer to a passage's major ideas (its content), but are instead common words that many readers pay little attention to: conjunctions and other transition words, prepositions, adjectives, and adverbs. Paying attention to these often-overlooked words can give you an advantage on Test Day by enhancing your understanding of even the most difficult passages.

The following sections of this chapter will introduce Relation, Logic, and Author keywords, as well as advice on using them to read strategically. At the surface level, keywords can tell you what is important in a passage, letting you know where in a passage you should be focusing your attention. Toward this end, one useful approach is to assign colors to different categories of keywords: green, yellow, and red. In this traffic light system, *green* keywords indicate that you should keep moving (expecting to see more of the same), *yellow* keywords indicate that you should slow down and look out for author opinions or shifts in the direction of the passage, and *red* keywords suggest "*Stop!* There is something important to be found."

KEY CONCEPT

The way the traffic light system should be applied to different types of keywords is discussed throughout the rest of Chapter 5. Generally speaking, Continuation keywords will be green lights, Contrast and Author keywords will be yellow lights, and Logic keywords will be red lights. However, there are exceptions to these rules, so review the following material carefully.

5.2 Relation Keywords

When tackling a CARS passage, it is essential to recognize how what you're reading now fits into the text as a whole. **Relation keywords** are words and phrases that reveal specific kinds of relationships between ideas. While there are many ways in which ideas can be related, the vast majority of Relation keywords will fall into one of two subcategories: Continuation or Contrast.

Continuation

Continuation keywords indicate that the coming material is an extension of a previous statement and include *and, also, moreover, furthermore*, and so on. In addition, phrases that indicate examples (*such as, for instance*, and *take the case of*) fall into this category, as do demonstrative pronouns (*this, that, these*, and *those*). Generally speaking, when a sentence or clause begins with a **Continuation keyword**, it will be continuing in the same vein as what came before. In other words, it won't be saying anything particularly new. As a consequence, if you understood the preceding material, you can generally read a clause that follows a Continuation keyword quickly, briskly moving through the text until a new keyword signals something different. On the other hand, if you struggled to understand a particular sentence, but see a Continuation keyword at the beginning of the next sentence, keep moving forward—the author is likely to continue with the same idea but may rephrase it in easier words. Thus, in our traffic light analogy, Continuation keywords would be *green lights*, signaling you to keep going!

Even though they are not technically *keywords*, certain punctuation marks can also indicate that a similar idea is coming up. Most notably, colons (:) and semicolons (;) are commonly employed to function as the verbal equivalent of the equals sign (=). The use of dashes—such as the ones surrounding this clause—and parentheses (the marks enclosing this phrase) also tend to indicate elaboration upon the same general theme. Finally, keep an eye out for quotation marks (""): while quotes can serve a variety of functions, one of the most common is to use another person's voice to restate the point the author just made.

Contrast

On the other hand, **Contrast keywords** will usually merit additional attention when you encounter them, as they tend to suggest more interesting (and therefore testable) relationships than Continuity keywords. Common Contrast keywords such as *but*, *yet*, *however*, *although*, and *otherwise* signal a change in the direction of the text. Like Continuation keywords, Contrast keywords serve as transitions between sentences, but they can also indicate deeper conceptual relations—the contrast between two solutions to a political problem, a point of disagreement between various critics of a literary work, or a rapid change in opinion from one time period to another, to give just a few examples. The connections between ideas are among the most commonly tested aspects of CARS passages, so strive to understand these relationships with as much specificity as the given clues allow. To this end, view Contrast keywords as *yellow lights* in our traffic light analogy. When you come across a Contrast keyword, be prepared to slow down and read carefully to ensure you follow the author's transition of thought.

MCAT EXPERTISE

When you encounter a Contrast keyword, slow down your reading or (if needed) even stop! These keywords signify a change in the author's focus or a direct contrast between two things; either way, we need to know how the trajectory of the passage is changing to keep a step ahead of the author.

While punctuation symbols often indicate continuation, this is not always true. If a punctuation symbol is accompanied by another type of keyword, the actual word or phrase generally takes precedence in determining the relationship (for example, a semicolon followed by *yet* usually suggests a point of contrast rather than continuation). This points out the greater importance of anticipating while you read; a great score in CARS depends on your ability to be a critical reader rather than a passive reader. When we passively read for pleasure, we tend to glide over text and often only understand the superficial message of the written work. In critical reading, we are continuously questioning the text and setting expectations for where the author will go with an idea. Even if they are not met, it is still worthwhile to set these expectations. In fact, when an author takes a starkly different route in a part of the passage than we expect, the testmaker is more likely to ask about the sudden contrast in the text. That which is rhetorically unusual in the passage and frustrates expectations becomes excellent material for MCAT questions.

More Complex Relationships

While the keywords considered under this heading might broadly count as Contrast keywords, they designate special types of difference and are especially ripe for CARS questions. While by no means exhaustive of the types of relations you might see on Test Day, **Oppositions**, **Sequences**, and **Comparisons** are three of the most common.

Oppositions

Words and phrases like *not*, *never*, *on the contrary*, and *as opposed to* indicate not merely a contrast but an outright **Opposition** or conflict between ideas.

Many authors of passages used in CARS like to create **dichotomies**, which are divisions of entities into two categories. These categories are considered **mutually exclusive**, meaning that they don't overlap. The use of *either ... or*, *on the one hand ... on the other hand*, and similar parallel phrase constructions are good indications of this phenomenon. Often, but not always, these dichotomies will be depicted as **exhaustive**, meaning that everything falls into one of the two categories. For example, an author writing about human behavior might claim that *all actions are either free choices or involuntary reflexes*, leaving no space for shades of gray. Because these dichotomies are frequently tested on the MCAT, treat Opposition keywords as *yellow lights*. Slow down to determine why the author is presenting this opposition and how it affects their overall argument.

Sequences

Some Relation keywords suggest a series of events advancing in time: *initially*, *first*, *second*, *third*, *next*, *subsequently*, *before*, *after*, *last*, and *finally*. These words will usually be spaced relatively evenly throughout the passage, or at least throughout a paragraph or two, so note how they organize the text into chunks. **Sequences** are something of a hybrid between Continuation and Contrast, with each word suggesting not only a connection to a larger process but also a departure from the other steps in the series. Generally, you're better off taking your time with these, at least until you have a good idea of how the sequence will unfold. However, you will often find Sequence keywords require less of a "slow down" than other yellow light keywords.

Some sequences can set up a clear contrast between time periods. *Historically*, *traditionally*, *used to*, *originally*, and—when used in comparison to a later time—*initially* and *before* can be used as time-based Contrast keywords when contrasted with words like *now*, *currently*, *modern*, *later*, and *after*. Such a setup often implies that new information was learned or discovered in the intervening time: *the traditional interpretation* vs. *a more modern understanding* or *historically, we thought* vs. *but now, we know*.

Comparisons

Sometimes, authors will evaluate ideas and rank them relative to other ideas. More often than not, authors will consider only two concepts at a time, contrasting them through the use of **Comparison keywords** like *more*, *less*, *better*, and *worse*. That said, occasionally authors will compare three or more items, or offer vague judgments of superiority (or inferiority) of one item over all others, reflected by superlatives such as *most*, *least*, *best*, and *worst*. When revealing attitudes, Comparison keywords function more like Author keywords, further explained later in the chapter.

In our traffic light analogy, Comparison keywords require more attention than most Contrast keywords and should be viewed as *yellow lights.* You should slow down and notice what entities are being compared and the author's opinion on them. A common wrong answer trap in CARS is to suggest that the author makes a comparison between two entities from the passage that were not actually directly compared. By taking special note of the comparisons the author does make, you can avoid such traps.

Table 5.1 lists examples of Relation keywords in each category. Note that some words can fit into more than one category; for example, *not* reveals a contrast, but it can also indicate a direct opposition.

Continuation	Contrast	Opposition
and	but	not/never/none
also	yet	either ... or
moreover	however	as opposed to
furthermore	although	on the contrary
like	(even) though	versus (*vs.*)
same/similar	rather (than)	on the one hand ... on the other hand
that is	in contrast	otherwise
in other words	on the other hand	**Sequence**
for example	otherwise	before/after
take the case of	nevertheless	earlier/later
for instance	whereas	previous/next
including	while	initially/subsequently/finally
such as	different	first/second/third/last
in addition	unlike	historically/traditionally/used to
plus	notwithstanding	now/currently/modern
at the same time	another	**Comparison**
as well as	instead	better/best
equally	still	worse/worst
this/that/these/those	despite	less/least
: [colon]	alternatively	more/most
; [semicolon]	unless	*-er/-est*
– [dash]	not	primarily
( ) [parentheses]	conversely	especially
" " [quotes]	contrarily	above all

Table 5.1 Common Relation Keywords

MCAT EXPERTISE

Simply memorizing lists of keywords is not sufficient to extract all of the information from a passage. A Contrast keyword can serve slightly different functions depending on the context in which the word is found. Recognize that MCAT CARS success is not about memorizing the fact that *but*, *yet*, and *however* are Contrast keywords, but is instead about understanding how Contrast keywords reveal changes in direction in a passage.

5.3 Logic Keywords

Reading for reasoning is perhaps the most difficult of the reading modes because the one-way support relationship between a conclusion and its evidence is among the most complex you'll encounter on Test Day. **Logic keywords** are words and phrases that signal these support (and refutation) relationships. Unfortunately, they tend to be relatively rare, occurring less frequently than either Relation or Author keywords in most passages. Notwithstanding these difficulties, Logic keywords are a powerful tool: once you gain proficiency in recognizing them and understanding what they entail, you'll find the many CARS questions on reasoning much less daunting.

Evidence and Conclusion

In Chapter 3: Rhetoric and Arguments, we defined an argument as a relationship between two claims, a conclusion and its evidence. To review, a **conclusion** is a claim that the author (or whomever the author is speaking for) is trying to convince the audience to believe, while pieces of **evidence** are the reasons that are given for believing it. Determine whether the conclusion is one that the author would endorse or whether it is intended to represent some other viewpoint by paying attention to nearby Author keywords (discussed later) and other clues.

Typical examples of **Evidence keywords** are *because*, *since*, *if*, *why*, *the reason is*, *for example*, *on account of*, *due to*, *as a result of*, *is justified by*, and *after all*. There is a bit less variety in **Conclusion keywords**, which also tend to occur less frequently than Evidence keywords. The most important conclusion words to know are *therefore*, *thus*, *then*, *so*, *consequently*, *leading to*, *resulting in*, *argue*, and *conclude*.

In our traffic light analogy, both Conclusion and Evidence keywords should be viewed as *red lights*. When you encounter Evidence keywords, stop and ask yourself, *What is this supporting? Where is the conclusion?* When you encounter Conclusion keywords, take note of whose conclusion it is (the author's or some other view's) and be on the lookout for its evidence (if any is provided).

MCAT EXPERTISE

Having trouble figuring out what part of the argument a Logic keyword is indicating? Try this simple substitution test: If you can replace the word or phrase with *because* or *because of*, then whatever follows is a piece of evidence. If, instead, *therefore* would preserve the meaning, the subsequent claim is a conclusion.

MCAT EXPERTISE

Sometimes Evidence and Conclusion keywords are used to signal cause-and-effect relationships, rather than arguments. This most commonly occurs in scientific and historical explanations of phenomena. Fortunately, while causation differs from argumentation in important ways, they share a consistent relationship to the Logic keyword subcategories. When used for causation, Evidence keywords will always indicate a cause and Conclusion keywords will always indicate an effect.

Refutation

Refutation keywords will not always be included in the presentation of an argument, but they are effectively the opposite of evidence—countervailing reasons for rejecting a conclusion. They include words such as *despite*, *notwithstanding*, *challenge*, *object*, *counter*, *critique*, *conflict*, and *problem*. Given the opinionated nature of Refutation keywords, you should consider *why* the author included the refutation. Was it is to attack an idea that the author has a negative view on? Or perhaps the author intentionally put forward a weak refutation only to later refute the refutation, thus supporting the original contention. No matter the purpose of the refutation, it is important that you notice it and consider its purpose—refutations are relatively rare, so if a passage features one or more of them, expect to see questions on them. For this reason, Refutation keywords should be viewed as *red lights,* as with the other Logic keywords.

Table 5.2 lists examples of Logic keywords in each category.

Evidence	Conclusion	Refutation
because (of)	therefore	despite
since	thus	notwithstanding
if	then	challenge
for example	so	undermined by
why	consequently	object/objection
the reason is	leading to	counter(argument)
as a result of	resulting in	critique/criticize
due to	argue	conflict
as evident in	conclude	doubt
justified by	imply	problem
assuming	infer	weakness
after all	suggest	called into question by

Table 5.2 Common Logic Keywords

5.4 Author Keywords

Author keywords can be among the most subtle clues that you'll encounter on Test Day, but they are crucial for answering the many questions you'll face that ask about the author's attitudes, whether directly or indirectly. Authors of passages used in CARS rarely say *I believe* or *it seems to me* (and if you do find this language, it's more often in the humanities than the social sciences). Instead, they are more likely to hint at their opinions by selecting verbs, nouns, adjectives, and adverbs that carry a particular emotional valence—a connotation of either approval or disapproval. Moreover, authors will use characteristic words and short phrases to make their claims more extreme (indicating emphasis and strengthening ideas), as well as others that moderate their claims (qualifying or limiting what they are saying and weakening ideas).

Given the importance of establishing the author's tone and opinions, it may seem appropriate to make them red lights in our traffic light analogy. However, because Author keywords are so common, they are typically best viewed as *yellow lights*: slow down and take notice, particularly noting the context of the keyword so you know *who* feels a certain way and about *what topic*. In passages with multiple arguments or viewpoints, you may have to treat some Author keywords as red lights, simply because their context is complicated enough to require you to stop and clarify which perspective holds what opinion.

Positive *vs.* Negative

Understanding the author's attitude becomes a much simpler matter if we employ a metaphor taken from the sciences. Just as an atom or molecule might possess an electrostatic charge, so too can a word or phrase contain a kind of emotional charge that may be positive or negative. Because most of the language in CARS passages tends to be "uncharged" or neutral, you'll predominantly pay attention to the exceptions—those cases in which terms have clear positive or negative connotations.

Positive keywords include nouns such as *masterpiece*, *genius*, and *triumph*; verbs such as *excel*, *succeed*, and *know*; adjectives such as *compelling*, *impressive*, and *elegant*; and adverbs such as *correctly*, *reasonably*, and *fortunately*. Among **Negative keywords** would be nouns such as *disaster*, *farce*, and *limitation*; verbs such as *miss*, *fail*, and *confuse*; adjectives such as *problematic*, *so-called*, and *deceptive*; and adverbs such as *questionably*, *merely*, and *purportedly*.

MCAT EXPERTISE

Most CARS passages contain strong, but not necessarily extreme, opinions. For example, a typical CARS passage might provide several refutations to challenge a particular theory, but its author likely wouldn't claim that the theory is "utter nonsense." Passages with neutral authors, such as might be found in a typical textbook, are not usually selected for the CARS section because they feature less testable material.

Keep in mind that, just as there is a difference between a cation with a +1 charge and one with a +3 charge, so too is there a difference between a moderately positive opinion and an extremely positive one. For instance, an author probably approves more strongly of a novelist described as *a masterful artist* than one portrayed merely as *a quality writer*. Consequently, it may be helpful to think of the author's attitude as varying along a spectrum or continuum, with extremely positive opinions on the one end and extremely negative on the other, as in Figure 5.1. Note that most authors' attitudes in CARS fall in a comfortable middle ground between being too extreme and being too moderate, as implied by the relative widths of the sections in the diagram.

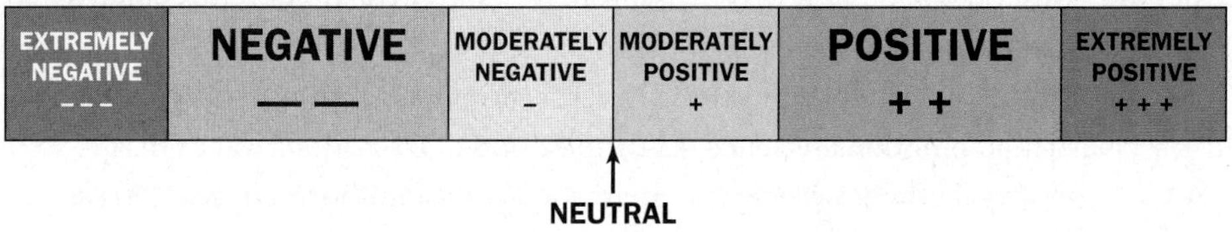

Figure 5.1 The Spectrum of Author Attitudes (Linear)

KEY CONCEPT

While they are both neutral overall, these two attitudes are very different:

- Ambivalent = having both a positive and negative opinion
- Impartial = having neither a positive nor negative opinion

Note that in addition to positive, negative, or neutral, an author can also be **ambivalent**. Ambivalence literally means *feeling both ways*, and it is as different from **impartiality**—having no strong opinion one way or another—as the set of 1 and −1 is from the number 0. Continuing the analogy with an electrostatic charge, an ambivalent attitude is like an amino acid in its *zwitterionic* form, with both a positively charged and a negatively charged end, and an impartial attitude is like an uncharged, unpolarized atom. Describing the net zero charge of a zwitterion as merely "neutral" would mean neglecting its distinctive properties. The MCAT won't let you get away with such oversimplifications!

Extreme

Placing a particular idea on the author-attitude spectrum above becomes easier by paying attention to **Extreme keywords**, a type of Author keyword that you can imagine as enhancing the charge of what the author is saying, forcing the author into one or the other extreme. These words and short phrases are functionally equivalent to exclamation points (!), offering insight into what the author feels passionately about and regards as important.

Examples of Extreme keywords include *indeed*, *very*, *really*, *quite*, *primarily*, *especially*, *obviously*, *foremost*, *always*, *in fact*, *above all*, and *it is clear that*. Note that words that indicate necessity, like *need* and *must*, also serve as Extreme keywords, as do words that indicate value judgments like *should* and *ought*—these tend to be rare in CARS passages, so they deserve special consideration when they do appear.

Moderating

Authors will sometimes modify the strength of their claims in the other direction by using qualifying language, also known as *hedging*. **Moderating keywords** are those words that set limits on claims in order to make them easier to support (because a stronger statement is always more difficult to prove than a weaker one). For example, it would be an extreme claim to say that *human beings are motivated only by greed*. Though some might agree with this formulation, the bulk of MCAT authors would sooner water it down by saying something like *in many aspects of life, humans are predominantly motivated by greed*, or even further limit it to a subset of human beings, such as *investment bankers are often motivated by greed*. Such modifications transform a controversial claim into one that is much more plausible.

Among the most important Moderating keywords are those that use the language of possibility, such as *can*, *could*, *may*, and *might*. Claims about what is possible are always weaker than claims about what is definitely true. Other Moderating keywords include limits on time or place, whether stated specifically or in vague phrases such as *now*, *here*, *at times*, *in some cases*, and *in this instance*. Still others will impose general constraints on meaning; examples include *in this sense*, *according to this interpretation*, and *in a manner of speaking*.

Accounting for Opposition

One final consideration when working with Author keywords is contradiction or opposition, a special type of Contrast keyword mentioned above. It can be particularly tricky to figure out the authors' attitudes in CARS when they use double negatives (or worse!). The key is to remember that the opposite of an extreme statement will typically be a moderate statement of the reverse charge. In the diagram below, which is just a slight rearrangement of the author attitude spectrum presented in Figure 5.2, a word of opposition will typically serve to flip the author's view 180 degrees.

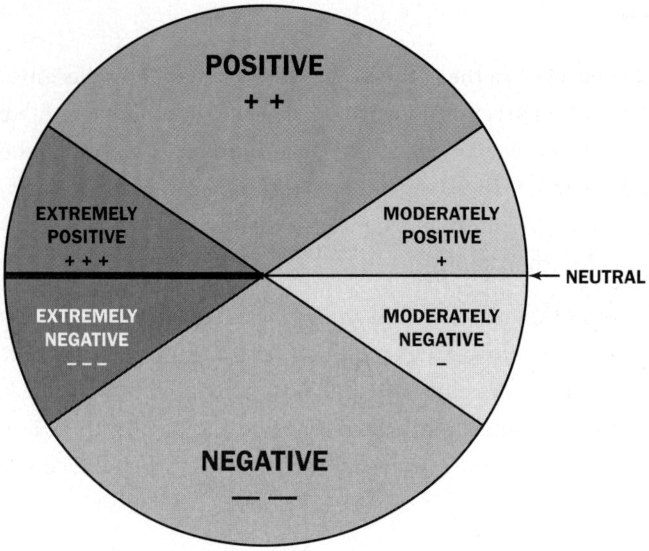

Figure 5.2 The Spectrum of Author Attitudes (Circular)

So, if an author were to claim that a particular event is *impossible*, this statement would fall somewhere in the extremely negative range. On the other hand, suggesting the situation was *not impossible* would be making a moderately positive claim, effectively saying that it was *possible*. Be aware, however, that some words retain their strength even when accompanied with *not* or some other word of opposition—for instance, *must* is extremely positive in charge, while *must not* is extremely negative in charge.

Table 5.3 lists examples of Author keywords in each category.

Positive	Negative	Extreme	Moderating
masterpiece	disaster	must	can/could
genius	farce	need/necessary	may/might
triumph	limitation	always	possibly
excel	miss	every	probably
succeed	fail	any	sometimes
know	confuse	only	on occasion
compelling	problematic	should/ought	often
impressive	so-called	indeed	tends to
elegant	deceptive	very	here
correctly	questionably	especially	now
reasonably	merely	obviously	in this case
fortunately	purportedly	above all	in some sense

Table 5.3 Common Author Keywords

Conclusion

We began this chapter with a discussion of the modes of reading and finished with a discussion of keywords, but these two topics are closely interrelated. Reading for purpose is aided by close attention to Relation and Author keywords, while reading for reasoning is made simpler when authors use Logic keywords. As you continue your CARS practice, try the reading strategies discussed in this chapter (the modes of reading, the keyword categories, and the traffic light system) until you have a solid grasp of them. In conjunction with the other Kaplan strategies, they'll help you get that higher score in CARS. The next chapter focuses on another CARS strategy: distilling passage information.

CONCEPT AND STRATEGY SUMMARY

Reading Strategically with Keywords

- **Keywords** are words and short phrases that reveal passage structure and author intentions.
- When we read for **content**, we ask, *What does the text say?*
  - You are never expected to have prior familiarity with the content of a passage in CARS.
  - When reading for content is a struggle, reading for purpose and for reasoning can help you make sense of the passage.
- When we read for **purpose**, we ask, *Why does the author include this?* and *Why does the author write?*
  - Reading for purpose is guided by **Relation keywords** and **Author keywords**.
- When we read for reasoning, we ask, *What is the conclusion? How are claims supported?* and *How are claims challenged?*
  - Reading for reasoning is guided by **Logic keywords**.
  - Differentiating between conclusions, evidence, and refutations can help you make sense of the author's larger argument in the passage.
- Keywords serve as signs that indicate where you should focus your attention. As an analogy, you can consider different categories of keywords to be different colors of a traffic light (green, yellow, and red).

Relation Keywords

- **Relation keywords** are words and phrases that reveal specific kinds of relationships between ideas.
- **Continuation keywords** indicate that the following material continues in the same vein as the preceding material (*green light*).
- **Contrast keywords** signal a change in the trajectory of the passage (*yellow light*).
- **Opposition keywords** are particularly strong Contrast keywords that create a dichotomy, or divisions of entities into two categories (*yellow light*).
  - **Mutually exclusive** categories do not overlap.
  - When dichotomies are **exhaustive**, all relevant entities fit into one or the other category.
- **Sequence keywords** suggest a series of events advancing in time. They may also be used to set up a contrast between two time periods (*yellow light*).
- **Comparison keywords** rank ideas relative to each other (*yellow light*).

Logic Keywords

- **Logic keywords** indicate relationships of support and refutation (all types are *red lights*).
- **Conclusion keywords** signal what the author is trying to convince the audience to believe.
- **Evidence keywords** indicate reasons why the audience should believe the author's claim.
- **Refutation keywords** signal reasons for rejecting a conclusion.

Author Keywords

- **Author keywords** indicate the author's feelings or opinions about a topic (*yellow light*).
- **Positive** and **Negative keywords** indicate whether an author likes, agrees with, or supports a topic, or dislikes, disagrees with, or opposes a topic. An absence of either type suggests an author is neutral with respect to a topic.
  - An author with an **ambivalent** attitude has both positive and negative opinions on a topic.
  - An author with an **impartial** attitude has neither positive nor negative opinions on a topic.
- **Extreme keywords** enhance the charge of what the author is saying.
- **Moderating keywords** permit the author to qualify a claim, or hedge.
- The opposite of an extreme statement tends to be a moderate statement with the opposite charge.

CHAPTER 6

DISTILLING PASSAGE INFORMATION

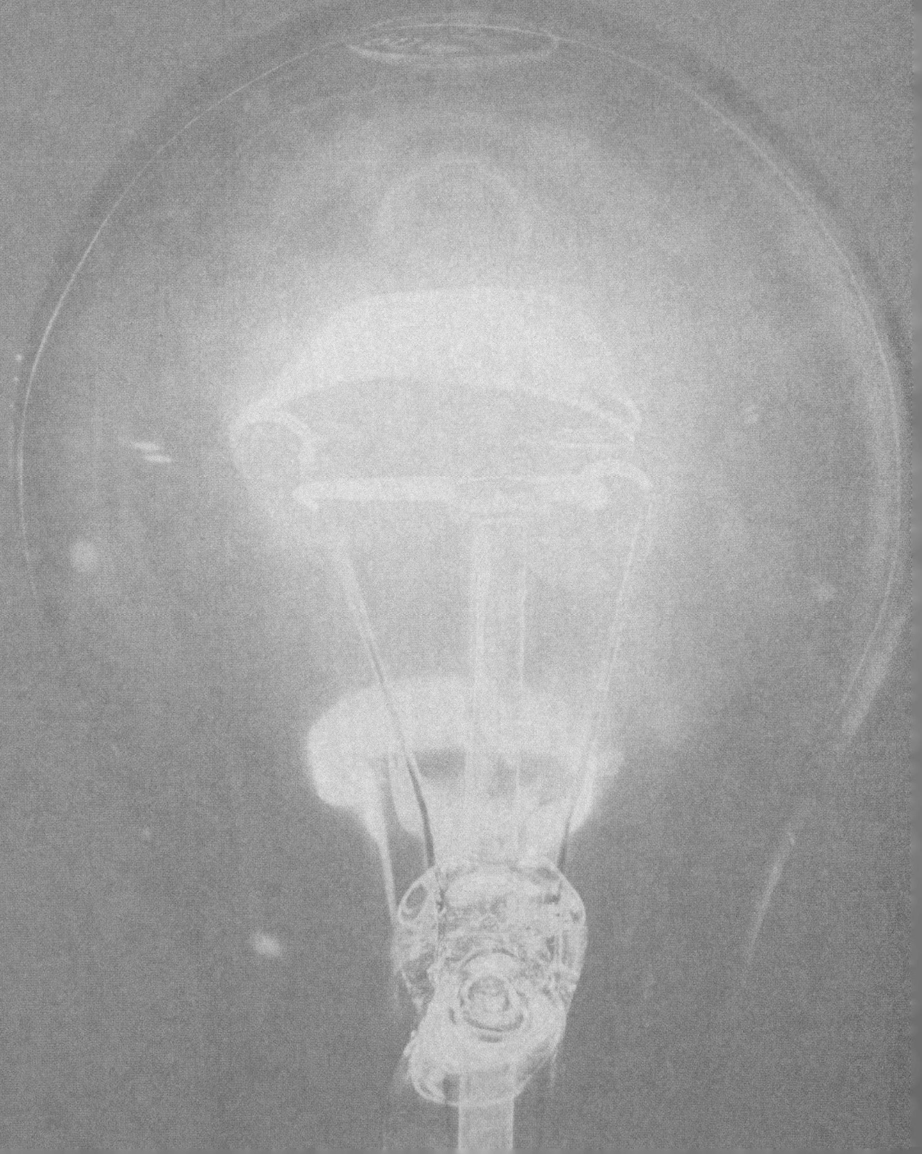

CHAPTER 6

DISTILLING PASSAGE INFORMATION

In This Chapter

Introduction

LEARNING OBJECTIVES

After Chapter 6, you will be able to:

- Differentiate between the *Highlighting*, *Outlining*, and *Interrogating* approaches to CARS passages
- Identify the types of passages best suited for each method
- Apply each of the three methods to sample MCAT passages
- Step beyond the text to analyze the underlying themes of the passage

Not all passages on the MCAT are created equal. As we discussed in Chapter 4 of *MCAT CARS Review*, you will use things like passage topic, sentence structure, writing style, and passage length to triage each passage on the test and decide which ones you want to save for later. Once you decide to attempt a passage, you must have an action plan. Just like you wouldn't treat a five year old with a cold the same way you would treat an eighty-five year old with chronic heart failure and asthma, you are not necessarily going to approach a long, complex humanities passage the same way you might approach a more concise, clear social sciences passage. Remember, one of our main tasks when working through a CARS passage is to truly understand the big picture of the passage. So, it is essential to read actively and methodically so you do not miss key details or insights. During this chapter, we'll explore different ways to approach passages so that, come Test Day, you will be equipped with both the ability to gauge the best way to handle a passage and the skill to use your chosen method on that passage effectively.

This chapter will begin by introducing three different approaches to completing MCAT CARS passages and discussing their respective pros and cons. We will then carry out a more in-depth discussion of each approach, and we will end by seeing how each approach can be applied to a sample MCAT passage.

6.1 Choosing Your Approach

Interviewing a new patient can feel like an uphill battle against an onslaught of information, and so can reading through a CARS passage. Having a solid plan for how to Distill and organize the most important information from a CARS passage allows you to gather the context you need without getting overwhelmed by extraneous material. In this section, we will introduce the three different methods for distilling a passage (each of these will be covered in depth later in this chapter as well). Note that you should plan to practice all three of these methods throughout your prep so that you can easily choose the best method for each passage on Test Day.

Triaging the Passage

Remember, we're not reading CARS passages for pleasure, the way we might read a novel or a magazine. In CARS, certain parts of the passage will inevitably contain more testable information than others. So, given the tight time constraints, you need to develop strategies to navigate through passages effectively and to identify the most important pieces of information as you read.

BRIDGE

Chapter 4 focused heavily on Previewing the passage, the process by which you will quickly gain information about the passage and determine difficulty. This allows you to triage each passage (decide whether to work it now or later), but that same information gathered in the Preview step is also used for Choosing your passage approach. Refer to Chapter 4 for more information on the Preview step.

In Chapter 4, we discussed how to determine the order in which you will work the passages. Once you have decided to commit to and read a passage, use the conclusions you made while triaging to influence the approach you use to work through that passage. For example, you will probably not approach a long, complex philosophy passage the same way you would approach a more straightforward literature passage. While a long, complex passage is often best met with a quick reading focused on identifying big picture concepts, a straightforward passage is often better handled with a more detailed read and with a greater focus on identifying the rationale behind the author's arguments. One of the best things about having multiple strategies in your toolbox is that you can pick and choose the best approach for each passage rather than sticking to a "one-size-fits-all" approach for every passage in the section; so don't be afraid to change it up as you go. As was referenced in Chapter 4, you can either wait and Choose your approach when you are actually working the passage, or you can preemptively Choose as you triage each passage. In either case, you will want to make an active decision about how you are going to Read and Distill the passage.

Keywords

A key strategy for identifying where to read thoroughly, as opposed to skimming quickly, is noting the use of keywords and punctuation. For example, since Continuation keywords indicate that more of the same is coming, if you understand what has already been stated, then save yourself time by reading quickly through that portion. Conversely, Contrast keywords indicate that a shift in focus, a new piece of information, an alternative viewpoint, or some other kind of change is up ahead, essentially telling you to slow down and to ensure that you don't miss something important. Furthermore, Conclusion keywords indicate that the major point of an argument is ahead, so it is worth stopping and ensuring that you completely understand the point before moving forward in the passage.

BRIDGE

Keywords are discussed in depth in Chapter Five.

Approaching the Passage

The ultimate goal of the Distill step of the CARS passage method is to help you identify what is most critical in each paragraph of the passage. You want to have some concept of the main idea and overall argument of each paragraph. This will save you time on questions, because you will already have a solid idea of what is contained in each paragraph and how that information fits together. As a result, you will be able to find specific details or supporting evidence in the passage more easily. We can compare this process to the scientific process of distilling a liquid: you are removing the impurities (the extraneous information) from the passage. And you are left with a purified product consisting of only the information relevant to answering the questions associated with the passage. This step can be done using one of three approaches. We'll describe each approach in broad strokes over the next couple pages. Then we'll drill down into each approach and examine how and when to implement that approach, the pros and cons of that approach, and Worked Examples.

Highlighting the Passage

For some situations, and especially in a time crunch, a thorough read of the passage that revolves around taking notes or questioning the purpose of every sentence is going to be too much to accomplish in the limited time allotted. If you are short on time, if you are unable to completely understand the content of a paragraph and you know you won't understand even with more time, or if the passage is simply too long to accomplish with the other methods, then Highlighting can be a great choice. Focus on highlighting a phrase that points to the main idea or purpose of each paragraph, so that when you return to the passage while working through a question, you can easily identify the high-yield information. Highlighting doesn't allow you to create a true paraphrase of the main idea, so you'll need to rely on finding the most helpful phrase or word already located in the paragraph. Note that if you're using the Highlighting method, you should not be highlighting random words that you don't know, or highlighting details. Instead, highlight words that will allow you to quickly relocate where main ideas were found throughout the passage. Finally, when you reach the end of the passage, take a moment to consider why the author wrote the passage. Some examples include: to argue a point, to discuss a topic, to contrast two different ideas.

From a timing perspective, the Highlighting approach is the quickest of the three methods we'll discuss. Highlighting allows you to work through the passage in 2–3 minutes. Furthermore, the highlighting you did should allow you to find main themes and search the passage more efficiently. However, you should be aware that the Highlighting method is going to require that you spend more time on the questions, as compared to the other two methods. This time will be spent returning to the passage for further research. With the Highlighting approach in particular, it is imperative that you work all passage questions immediately following the passage, with no intention of coming back to any questions after looking at other passages. Your highlighting will make the most sense immediately after you've done it, and if you look at other materials in the interim, it's unlikely that you'll be able to return to the passage and decipher your highlighting.

Outlining the Passage

When composing a paper for your high school or college English classes, you likely were asked to first create an outline. In this outline, you recorded the purpose of each paragraph you intended to write, and then you used that outline as a template for the full paper. The Outlining strategy for CARS passages is essentially the reverse of that: you will take a full passage and reverse engineer the outline that captures each paragraph's purpose. Like with the Highlighting approach, the goal of Outlining is to identify the main idea and the purpose of each paragraph. However, the Outlining approach goes a step further, asking you to use your own words to summarize the main points and to record these main points on your scratch paper. To Outline, simply jot down a summary of the purpose of each paragraph as you read. You may find a paragraph's purpose toward the beginning, middle, or end of the paragraph. But in any case, read all the way to the end of each paragraph, and only then pause to record your outline of that paragraph—this is, after all, the Outlining method, not the "note-taking" method! Finally, as with the Highlighting method, when you reach the end of the passage, take a moment to consider why the author wrote the passage. Compared to the fast, lightweight Highlighting method, the Outlining method adds two large pieces of value: first, Outlining allows you to use your own words to clearly and concisely summarize main ideas and themes, meaning you are not relying on the sometimes obtuse language used in the passage. Second, your Outline creates a "table of contents" for the passage, which should make it easier to go back and find information necessary to answer questions. Perhaps surprisingly, you can often find important information more rapidly and more precisely using your outline than you could using highlights. From a timing perspective, the Outlining approach will take you 3–4 minutes per passage.

Interrogating the Passage

The Interrogating method is based on this principle: if you take the time to fully understand why an author has written a passage, and if you reframe the passage content in a context that makes sense to you, then you will be well prepared to answer questions about that passage. In the Interrogating method, you will approach the passage by questioning why portions of the text were included and how they connect to the rest of the author's argument. Interrogating is active reading. To interrogate the passage is to continually ask "why" and "how" questions as you read. This strategy amounts to a deeper read even than Outlining. When Outlining, you are attempting to capture the main purpose at the paragraph level. But when Interrogating, your goal is to capture the purpose of each individual conclusion, piece of evidence, example, counterexample, and so on. And, as with the other methods, when you reach the end of a passage while Interrogating, you'll stop to consider why the author wrote the passage overall, in light of everything you have read. The Interrogating method sounds time consuming, and it is. But there are two major ways you'll gain time back when you Interrogate a passage. First, unlike the Outlining method, you won't write anything down while Interrogating. You won't need to. The goal of Interrogating is to generate enough comfort with the author's argument that you rarely need to refer back to the passage at all. You just won't need the reference points that Highlighting or Outlining provide. This leads to the second way that Interrogating saves time. When you have developed the skill of Interrogating, you'll be able to answer most questions confidently and immediately, usually without referring back to the passage at all. Expect that Interrogating a passage will take 4–6 minutes per passage, or peharps longer for the toughest/longest passages you could see on Test Day.

6.2 Highlighting the Passage

Each of these three approaches comes with its own strengths and weaknesses. It is up to you to determine which approach will best fit each passage. The first of these approaches is the Highlighting method, which should enable you to work through the passage in as little as 2–3 minutes.

What Is Highlighting?

The goal of the Highlighting approach is to make it easier for you to locate main ideas and high-yield information as you return to the passage to answer questions. As you read the passage, keep an eye out for main themes of each paragraph, as these themes are likely to be the focus of multiple questions. Rather than highlighting as you go, aim to read a few sentences, process the information from them, and then highlight the key phrase or phrases, if there are any. It is important to note that highlighting is for your eyes, not for your brain. You need to fight the impulse to highlight full sentences, long phrases, or every other word, and instead use your highlighting tool sparingly. By highlighting less, your focus will be drawn to keywords and main ideas, making it easier to track down correct answers. Do your best to be stringent with your highlighting, and always remember the mantra "Highlighting everything is like highlighting nothing." One more benefit to targeted and thoughtful highlighting is that it forces you to actively analyze what passage information is worth highlighting, giving you a deeper understanding of the passage as a result.

Finally, that although the Highlighting method requires the least amount of time to perform on Test Day, Highlighting does require a good deal of practice beforehand in order to learn how to highlight well.

How to Highlight as a Method

The words and phrases discussed below will be used in passages to depict major changes or unique aspects, which are highly likely to be tested. Remember, in order to easily locate important ideas when you return to the passage, only highlight the first few words of a phrase of interest.

As you work through the passage, the following are MUST highlights:

- **A term that captures the essence of the sentences around it.** For example, *generosity* to stand in for details about the numerous charitable donations made by a famous philanthropist.
- **A detail that departs from the central idea of the paragraph.** For example, a complete change in subject.
- **A word that captures or indicates a position shift.** For example, the introduction of a counterargument.
- **A word that indicates the start of a new major perspective.** For example, the introduction of a new school of thought.

In contrast with the MUST highlights, the following types of words have the potential to be tested, but it is up to you to determine the likelihood and highlight or not highlight accordingly.

The following are MAYBE highlights:

- **Specific, new terms that are defined within the passage.** For example, the word *troika* to mean a group of three people working together.
- **Names and Dates.** Often, names and dates are simply included as supplemental details. Names and dates should only be highlighted if they are a key part of an argument in the passage.

Finally, the following are things you absolutely do NOT want to highlight in the passage. While these suggestions may depart from what you might typically find yourself highlighting as you work through a textbook or academic paper, remember that the goal of Highlighting on the MCAT is to understand the main idea and to make the passage more searchable once you get to the questions.

The following are do NOT highlights:

- **Background information in the first paragraph** if it seems likely that this information will be discussed in greater detail through the rest of the passage. This situation occurs most commonly when the first paragraph is short, serving to merely introduce the topic at hand without providing significant analysis.
- **Anything in the first or last line of a paragraph.** By nature of its location, information in the first or last line of a paragraph is already easy to find, should you need to return to it.
- **Words that have the same meaning or represent the same concept as a previously highlighted word.**
- **Full sentences or more than one highlight per sentence.**

Note that while keywords like "because," "therefore," "argue," etc. indicate that a transition to new information is imminent, the words that come directly after such transition words tend to be most important to the passage. So when you identify these transition keywords in the text, consider highlighting the words that follow in order to capture the unique, highly testable passage details.

There may be instances where you are unable to identify main ideas as you read, or you simply may not understand what you are reading. In these instances, the best plan of action is to highlight words that will help you locate information quickly when questions ask about it.

As you become a more effective highlighter, you will find yourself able to skim portions of the text and feel confident that your highlighting will allow you to find relevant information without having to reread large parts of the passage.

KEY CONCEPT

Remember, you can still highlight in the other two approaches, when applicable, but the rules you use to determine what should be highlighted will differ from those listed above. With the Highlighting approach, your highlights are meant to draw your eye to main ideas and major shifts. In the other two approaches, highlights can be used to help you isolate specific ideas or details that support the information in your outline or analysis.

When to Choose Highlighting

Advantages

Though the Highlighting method can technically be used for any passage, there are certain passages where Highlighting is the preferred approach. For example, this method is particularly suitable for passages that would otherwise take a large amount of time.

Thus, Highlighting is a good choice for passages that are very long. It is often the best strategy to use if a passage appears to be particularly dense, when an in-depth analysis would take far too much time to carry out. And because Highlighting does not require paraphrasing, it is the perfect choice for passages where you struggle to understand what you are reading.

Highlighting also effectively counters passages with unusual formatting. Some passages feature long paragraphs lacking natural breaks or transitions. Because highlights draw your eye back to the information that is worth re-reading, Highlighting can help you navigate such passages. At the other end of the formatting spectrum, Highlighting is also surprisingly effective on passages that feature a large number of unusually short paragraphs. Attempting to Outline every paragraph of a passage that consists of a dozen short paragraphs would be way too time consuming, but Highlighting just the main ideas from the most important of those paragraphs is much quicker.

In summary, Highlighting allows you to utilize the computer-based testing tools to quickly parse long, dense, or unusually formatted passages. This method does not require in-depth comprehension or extensive note-taking.

Disadvantages

However, this approach is not without potential pitfalls. If you do opt to use the Highlighting method on a passage, be aware that Highlighting's rapid pace and lack of paraphrasing can lead to limited understanding of the text. So, for passages that require in-depth analysis (more common among humanities passages), a different approach might be more suitable.

BRIDGE

Faulty Use of Detail answer choices, as well as other wrong answer pathologies, are discussed in Chapter 8: Question and Answer Strategy.

Additionally, because Highlighting relies on the exact wording from the text, this method can make Faulty Use of Detail answer choices seem exceedingly tempting. Therefore, when you use this method, take the time as you work through the questions to investigate the passage and rephrase passage text, before matching to an answer choice. Keep in mind that this method requires you to frequently refer back to the text when answering questions, so choosing to Highlight a passage does not mean you're totally off the hook for in-depth passage analysis. You will just do the majority of your analysis as part of your investigation, of the questions.

Highlighting Method Example

The passage below has long paragraphs with deep discussions of abstract ideas and is relatively complex in its presentation; as such, the Highlighting method is ideal for this passage. Highlighting will help you to locate major high-yield concepts and to keep track of multiple perspectives. Your aim is to work through the passage as quickly as possible while still capturing some idea of the author's purpose. This way, you will have time to perform the deep analysis of important sections of the passage that some questions require. Remember that Highlighting goes hand-in-hand with active reading. Do not get lazy and just highlight keywords. Instead, read a couple of sentences and then challenge yourself to highlight the word or phrase that accurately describes the main idea of what you just read.

Notice that not every detail is highlighted in the passage below. Rather, only the high-yield, likely-to-be-tested ideas are targeted.

HIGHLIGHTING METHOD

Passage	Expert Thinking
Alienation is a fundamental concept in present-day thought about the human being and his/her spatial and social environment. Alienation depends on transformation; without change-for-the-better, alienation cannot exist, and therefore the concept of transformation—and not mere change—must be understood before alienation can be understood. The concepts of transformation and alienation have only been current since the nineteenth century. The theories that form the original concept of alienation are those of Hegel, Marx, and Brecht.	What did the first paragraph reveal about the passage? What are the key terms that we need to know? *Alienation is the theme of this paragraph and possibly this entire passage. However, since it is the first word of the passage, there is no need to highlight it. I need to highlight more important details, like "transformation," which according to the paragraph is critical for "alienation."* *More importantly, the end of the paragraph reveals that the passage will discuss three names. This is a cue that I should be prepared to compare and contrast the three ideas. No need to highlight the names, as the future paragraphs will soon talk about them.*
To Georg Wilhelm Friedrich Hegel, a German philosopher who lived through the French Revolution, alienation was a value-adding process of self-creativity and self-discovery, which is the origin of Hegel's idea of *entfremdung* (alienation and estrangement) as an action to become other than oneself, to enter into what is other than the spirit or to become an alien to oneself. Hegel saw alienation as an experience with positive or value-adding, long-term consequences.	What can you highlight that can portray the most information about Hegel's definition of alienation? *While I wanted to highlight* "entfremdung" *as that is a new term, I know that would not benefit me as much because that term is isolated. The better highlight is the definition: "become other than oneself." I also highlighted "positive" because I know it is important to note the author's perspective.*
To be invited into a desired social or cultural space, which is not the individual's local culture, requires extreme discipline in courtesy, education, and achievement. Hegel calls the self-sacrifice and strenuous effort it requires alienation. Hegel's alienation is the extra effort needed to raise an individual to another and desired level of culture—like the newly acquired social mobility of the social groupings he observed after the French Revolution. Only a few individuals attain alienation consciousness, because appreciating a foreign culture seems remote and unreachable, and even humiliating for the average individual. However, alienation consciousness bridges the gap(s) between cultures. Hegel's alienation is a conscious and intrinsic choice of an individual with a positive outcome for the individual and his/her society and culture over the long term. It is alienation from fellow human beings, which is different from Marx's iconic response to Hegel's theory of alienation.	This paragraph is complicated. How can the details of this paragraph be related to the previous paragraph? *This paragraph shows one application of Hegel's alienation principle. For Hegel, alienation is necessary to move from one culture to another. The phrase "bridges the gap(s)" best captures this main idea, which is why I chose to highlight it. Though other relevant phrases exist, they are too long to concisely capture the same idea. I need the highlights to be efficient so I don't highlight everything and I can quickly locate the information later on.*

HIGHLIGHTING METHOD	
Passage	**Expert Thinking**
To Karl Heinrich Marx, philosopher, economist, and sociologist, alienation was a forced separation of things—not other people—that naturally belong together, or antagonism between those who should be in harmony, with damaging long-term consequences. Marx's well-known illustration describes the production-line worker who is alienated—and deprived—from the products of his labour: profit, satisfaction, feedback, and creativity. Marx attributes alienation to the capitalistic economic system where the worker is a puppet in the hand of the capitalists. The individual workers do not have any choice in what to produce and how to produce and are therefore alienated from the product they produce. Marx's alienation is a negative experience of perpetual deficit.	What is Marx's definition of *alienation*? *I highlighted phrases and words that parallel the highlights in the Hegel paragraph. Unlike Hegel, Marx does not view alienation as positive, and sees it as "forced separation," not a way to evolve as Hegel had suggested.* *Since I am unfamiliar with Marx's philosophy, I also highlighted the detail "alienated from the product," to identify a practical example of Marx's alienation, similar to my previous paragraph's highlights.* *While this may be a lot of highlighting in such a short paragraph, I know these highlights will be impactful because it will allow me to quickly compare the three theories directly.*
Hegel's and Marx's alienation refers to unintentional and gradual processes, whereas Brecht's alienation refers to a deliberate and immediate process. Whether alienation is the result of a gradual or an immediate and deliberate process, the experience is the same: an experience of dissonance and a desire to move toward the old or a new space of comfort. To the playwright, Eugen Berthold Friedrich Brecht, alienation is the distancing and estrangement effect or *Verfremdungseffekt*, when the audience was hindered from simply identifying itself with the actions and utterances of the performers when techniques designed to distance the audience are used or when using innovative theatrical techniques to de-familiarize the familiar in order to provoke a social-critical audience.	Here we are introduced to the last opinion holder. Highlight his definition of alienation as compared to the previous two definitions. *To follow the pattern of the previous highlights, I quickly found the key characteristic of Brecht's definition of alienation. "Deliberate and immediate" is a characteristic distinct from the previous two philosophers' definitions.*

HIGHLIGHTING METHOD

Passage	Expert Thinking
The Brechtian approach identifies acceptance or reception as the opposite of rejection or alienation. To alienate is, therefore, the deliberate choice of an artist on the reaction of the audience: to receive or to not-receive. He describes it as playing in such a way that the audience was hindered from simply identifying itself with the characters in the play. Acceptance or rejection of their actions and utterances was meant to take place on a conscious plane, instead of in the audience's subconscious. The artist challenges the audience-member therefore to venture into an unfamiliar space and to experience alienation in order to encounter the unknown. Brecht's alienation might be an instantaneous distancing experience, which might have a slow-developing positive or negative long-term effect. To Hegel, Marx, and Brecht, alienation is the process whereby people become foreign to the world they are living in.	What new idea is introduced here? *This paragraph talked about abstract and complicated topics. To stay focused, I stuck with concrete details. I first highlighted "reception as the opposite" to capture Brecht's view of the relationship between acceptance and alienation. The paragraph seems to suggest that the playwright wants the audience to experience alienation, and I highlighted "venture into a unfamiliar space" to capture that idea.* *The last sentence of the passage provides a nice summary of what is shared by the three authors in their distinctive definitions of alienation. I did not need to highlight it because it is at the end and therefore easy to find.*

Adapted from Smit, E., & Nel, V. (2016). Alienation, reception and participative spatial planning on marginalised campuses during transformational processes. *Cogent Arts & Humanities*, 3(1), 1154715. https://doi.org/10.1080/23311983.2016.1154715

Choosing what to highlight and what not to highlight is a learned skill that improves with time and experience. The way to master this skill is to practice frequently, constantly asking yourself, *Was this actually worth highlighting?* Over time, this habit will fine-tune your ability to gauge what is likely to be tested and what can be written off as "fluff." And this skill will carry over even when you choose a different method for Distilling a passage.

6.3 Outlining the Passage

As we saw in the last section, Highlighting is optimal for particularly long or dense passages, or for when you are low on time. Fortunately, most CARS passages do not present these challenges, and for many of these Outlining will be a better choice. The Outlining approach focuses on identifying the main idea of each paragraph, and of the passage as a whole, before moving on to the questions. This approach lets you see how each paragraph contributes to the author's overall purpose, which enables you to predict answers to many questions more accurately, as well as eliminate wrong answer choices more efficiently. Using the Outlining method, you should take about 3–4 minutes to work through a passage.

What Is Outlining?

The goal of the Outlining approach is to the most important information from the passage and to summarize that information on your noteboard booklet. Doing so enables you to better understand the relationships among the many ideas in a passage, as well as how those ideas interlock to form the bigger picture of the passage. Consequently, before you even get to the questions, you will already have done some of the work required to answer them!

A second asset of the Outlining approach is the end result of the process: your outline. The outline you construct for a passage is a vital tool that empowers you to locate specific details necessary to answer the accompanying questions. You can think of the outline as a map for the questions. Your outline helps guide you to the information you need.

How to Build an Outline

As you read, focus on determining the main idea of each paragraph. Once you reach the end of the paragraph, paraphrase the main idea in your own words and write your paraphrase on your noteboard booklet. Optionally, you can add key features within the paragraph—major details or examples, key shifts in scope or tone, and so on. Just keep these additional notes short, if you add any at all. Also, keep in mind that your outline is for your use only. As long as you can understand it, shorthand and symbols are fair game. And feel free to throw grammar and spelling to the wind, as long as it still makes sense to you!

As you Outline, mentally note the existence of details, evidence, and examples, but don't spend too much time trying to understand these features of the passage. Use the red/yellow/green light keyword system (Chapter 5) to guide you quickly through the passage. Should a question ask about one of the passage's details or examples, a quick glance at your passage outline will tell you which paragraph to return to for further research. As you read and outline, look out for information that is more commonly tested, such as author opinions and the conclusions of arguments. Spotting testable passage content is a skill that requires practice to master. As you complete more passages, you'll have an easier time determining what material is likely to return in the questions and what can be categorized as "fluff." One potential pitfall of Outlining is wasting time by including too much in your outline. Remember that information beyond a paragraph's main idea should only be added if it helps you locate testable content more easily.

MCAT EXPERTISE

Since you won't be writing down minor details, evidence, and examples on your noteboard booklet, consider taking advantage of the highlighting tool to make it easier to find them when you return to the passage.

When to Choose Outlining

Advantages

The Outlining approach forces you to identify main ideas in your own words, which helps you predict answers quickly. As you develop the ability to make your outlines concise yet specific, you will find that you can answer many questions using your outline alone, and this will save you time. Additionally, rephrasing the key points while you construct your outline will make you less likely to select Faulty Use of Detail answer choices.

Pausing after each paragraph to construct your outline may sound time consuming, but building an outline actually saves time and lowers stress. Outlining helps you move through the passage quickly, enabling you to skim details and examples, rather than spending time deciphering parts of the passage that may not even be referenced in the questions. The Outlining strategy asks you to return to the passage as needed, so you don't have to get stressed if you don't understand every detail in every paragraph, provided you write something in your outline (even just a name or theory) that indicates where to go if a question references it.

Outlining is especially useful for highly detailed or list-driven passages that require you to return to the passage frequently to identify details in order to answer questions. It can also help you keep different points of view organized, especially in passages that describe, compare, and contrast multiple groups' opinions. Organizing details and opinions in this way is particularly effective in passages with a straightforward structure, where one main theme is covered per paragraph. In short, Outlining is usually quite effective for the typical CARS passage.

Finally, if you consider yourself to be a visual person, then having a physical map of the passage can help you organize what you read and keep you from getting lost in the minutiae.

Disadvantages

There are certain instances where Outlining may not be the best strategy to use. For example, some authors do not make their main points obvious. Time spent trying to paraphrase a rambling author is often time wasted, which can lead to stress. Likewise, if a rambling author causes you to ramble in your own outline, that's more wasted time! For these reasons, passages with wordy, dense paragraphs often lead to outlines that are wordy and dense. And getting lost in your own outline is certainly even worse than getting lost in the passage! At the other extreme, Outlining a passage with unusually short paragraphs could result in many trips to your noteboard booklet, just to paraphase a small amount of information per paragraph. As we saw in the Highlighting section, for passages with irregular formatting—very large paragraphs or unusually short paragraphs—both are better handled using Highlighting.

Additionally, though some questions can be answered directly from the outline, the Outlining method still requires you to refer back to the text when answering many question types. So, take care to limit the time you spend Outlining and save yourself enough time to investigate those questions that require it.

Building an outline, if done carelessly, can eat up a significant amount of time. Before choosing to Outline, ask yourself, "Would this passage be considerably easier to navigate with a table of contents?" Outlining is only appropriate if the answer is yes; otherwise your outline is doing you little good. Practice this and the other two strategies during your prep, and before long you'll learn when Outlining works best for you.

Outlining Method Example

The passage in this section is an excellent fit for the Outlining method because it features a simple structure with a relatively straightforward purpose. Each paragraph is organized around a single goal, and we can identify each paragraph's goal from just the first few sentences. A number of paragraphs also contain Conclusion keywords, helping us identify these paragraphs' main ideas. In addition, the author of the passage is relatively light with jargon, which makes it easier to grasp the author's claims. All of these structural clues allow us to read with a focus on the big ideas, which we'll capture directly in our outline.

OUTLINING METHOD

Passage	Expert Thinking
The world of contemporary art is characterized by a growing number of artists experiencing an entrepreneurial venture. Especially in the context of performing arts, this has been lived both as a necessary and a voluntary solution to the severe shortage of funds affecting the world of public institutions. Thus, a new actor emerges, represented by the artist–entrepreneur who lives a hybridization of roles and competences. But who are these artists–entrepreneurs? And how do they live the possible tensions emerging from the encounter of worlds that have been reputed as radically different for so long?	With a lot of passages, the first paragraph is where we want to start looking for the author's main idea. What is being introduced to us here? *The author introduces the idea of artists-entrepreneurs.* Does the author give us a direction of where we will be going with this main idea? If so, how? *This comes in the form of two rhetorical questions at the end of the paragraph. We are asked about who these artists-entrepreneurs are and how they manage to fulfill such radically different roles at the same time.* P1: art. - entrep -> who and how?
Artists–entrepreneurs' activity can be identified as a particular kind of "cultural entrepreneurship." This practice has been traditionally investigated adopting two main perspectives, based on different meanings of culture.	Paragraphs of this length will typically serve as either a quick transition or a continuation of the previous paragraph. What is the author accomplishing here? *The author introduces a new term: "cultural entrepreneurship." The author also mentions two interpretations of this idea coming from different definitions of* culture. P2: Cult. Entrep.: -> 2 persp., based on diff defns of culture
As a first meaning, *culture* refers to the sociological frame of reference identifying a set of habits, customs, traditions, and beliefs, which constitute a shared way of life in a specific historical and political context. As a second meaning, *culture* identifies a complex set of processes, products and actors involved in the design, production and distribution of cultural and artistic goods and services.	This paragraph has a pretty clear structure, as indicated by keywords. What is the author doing in this paragraph? *The author provides two definitions of* culture. *The first refers to a broad sociological phenomenon, and the second refers to specific factors involved in artistic production.* P3: 2 defns of culture
Descending from the first sociological perspective, cultural entrepreneurship represents "the skill of certain entrepreneurs to use culture as a toolkit for constructing resonant identities and motivating resource-holding audiences to allocate their resources." Therefore, cultural entrepreneurship is instrumentally identified in the process of storytelling that gives shape and legitimizes new ventures. Not referring to a specific industry, the adjective *cultural* is used to identify the process of legitimization that entrepreneurs sustain, giving shape to the story of their personal and professional life.	Using the first sentence of this paragraph as a clue, what is the author introducing to us here? *The author discusses how cultural entrepreneurship can be viewed using the first perspective, as a kind of storytelling.* P4: 1st perspec. on cult. entrep. -> storytelling

OUTLINING METHOD

Passage	Expert Thinking
In a second perspective, cultural entrepreneurship identifies a set of processes through which a growing number of artists and cultural professionals assume an entrepreneurial role. Cultural entrepreneurship thus identifies the activity of conceiving, producing and marketing "cultural goods and services, generating economic, cultural, and social opportunities for creators while adding cultural value for consumers." The artists–entrepreneurs combine their artistic attitudes with a deep sense of business, economically sustaining the cultural enterprise in coherence with their cultural vision.	Continuing from the last paragraph and using the first sentence again as a guide, what new information is provided here? *The author now looks at cultural entrepreneurship through the second perspective, as a kind of business or economic activity.* How can we outline this without making our statement too long? P5: 2nd perspec. on cult. entrep. -> business
Upon investigation, what emerges with more emphasis is the tough and complex relationship between the artistic and the entrepreneurial dimensions faced by the artists–entrepreneurs. The interdependence between the two spheres emerges as a matter of fact, emphasizing the dual nature of the cultural enterprise. But duality means adopting an integral perspective that results from an intense dialogue between the two languages.	As we come to the last paragraph, we are typically expecting the author to provide some sort of conclusion to the main idea of the passage. What is the author's conclusion? *Cultural entrepreneurship is best understood by considering both perspectives, the artistic and the entrepreneurial.* Is there any additional information provided by the author? *Yes! Seeing both dimensions requires a new perspective that can integrate both.* P6: Author: cult. entrep. has 2 sides, new perspec. integrates both

Adapted from Clacagno, M., Balzarin, L. 2016. The Artist-Entrepreneur Acting as a Gatekeeper in the Realm of Art. *Venezia Arti*, 25. http://doi.org/10.14277/2385-2720/VA-25-16-3

Effectively outlining passages on the MCAT is not a skill you master overnight. Learning to move through the passage and summarize each paragraph is challenging, so you'll need to practice this method. Many passages in this book will have a sample passage outline so that you can compare your work to that of an expert. Another good drill to improve your outlining skills is to review and re-outline each passage after you have completed and reviewed the questions. In this drill, when you re-outline the passage, you are doing so knowing what ends up actually being tested. Each time you practice this exercise, you will naturally identify important information that you should have included in your original outline, which trains you to spot that type of information the next time you outline a passage.

6.4 Interrogating the Passage

The last of the three Distill methods is the Interrogating approach. With this approach, you consider whether each new piece of information is important as you read and, if it is, you ask why that information was included by the author. This Interrogating process will help you to understand the passage in greater depth, including the elements of the text most likely to be tested. Consequently, when you get to the accompanying questions, you'll be in a better position to answer them with much less rereading of the passage. Interrogating a passage should take you about 4–6 minutes.

What Is Interrogating?

The goal of Interrogating, also referred to as **Elaborative Interrogation**, is to understand not only what each important piece of information in the passage means, but also how that piece of information fits in with the rest of the passage. This method is valuable not only for CARS, but as a method validated by learning science for strengthening working memory with any content presented in a similar, text-heavy format. In other words, not only is Interrogating valuable for CARS on the MCAT, but it's also useful for any content that you must read and understand, including textbooks, science content, and even MCAT science passages. Interrogating is a step beyond the other two methods. Highlighting and Outlining focus more on *what* the author said rather than *why* the author said it. By contrast, while Interrogating a passage, you will constantly ask yourself, *Why is this information here?* and *How does this information connect to what came before?*

How to Interrogate a Passage

The biggest thing to remember as you Interrogate a passage is that you have the leeway to spend a lot of time working through the passage, provided that the majority of that time is spent reflecting about the passage, rather than just reading it. Remember: Interrogation will put you in a position where you are preemptively generating predictions for many of the upcoming questions, so it's okay to take some serious time to Interrogate!

There are two steps involved in the Interrogation approach. In the first step, you identify a "chunk" of information as you read. Ask yourself, *Can the sentence I am currently reading be grouped together with the sentence that I just read?* Use Continuation keywords to identify chunks of the current paragraph that essentially say the same thing or build on the same concept. When you hit a yellow or red light keyword, it's time to assess whether or not you've just reached the end of a chunk. Be careful though! Sometimes these keywords are false alarms. Many keywords are commonly employed words and phrases that serve a variety of functions, and not every use signals an important transition. Even more dangerous: sometimes an author will transition to a new topic with no warning at all! Traps like these are why you must consistently be asking yourself if it makes sense to group the current sentence with what preceded it, or if you have transitioned to a new chunk. These dangers aside however, a yellow or red light keyword often means you have reached the end of a chunk.

BRIDGE

Keywords, and the keyword stoplight system, are described in Chapter 5 of *MCAT CARS Review.*

Once you have identified a meaningful chunk, the second step when Interrogating is to ask yourself what role that chunk plays in the passage. The reasoning behind this step is two-fold. First, asking and answering questions as you go makes you an active reader, which makes it easier for you to remember the information in the passage. Second, forming an answer to a *Why?* question helps you contextualize and mentally organize the information in the passage, rather than treating each sentence as isolated from the ones around it.

MCAT EXPERTISE

When answering questions in the CARS section, you should always avoid relying on outside knowledge. However, when Interrogating a passage, outside knowledge can help you to connect what you are reading to what you already understand, enabling you to comprehend and remember passage content more effectively. Just be careful when answering questions to stick with only what is in the passage; otherwise you might be lured by an Out of Scope incorrect answer!

Listed below are some examples of the types of questions you should ask yourself as you Interrogate:

- Why is this piece of information being used in this way in the argument?
- Why is this piece of information important?
- How does this relate to other information the author has shared?
- How does this chunk differ from the previous chunk?
- Why did the author choose to reference this example?
- How does this support or refute a claim made previously?
- How can I relate this content to other related content, or even to the outside world?

When to Choose Interrogating

Advantages

Once you master this approach, you will no longer need to return to the passage to answer most questions. So, even though this strategy consistently requires the most amount of time to work through the passage, it empowers you to answer questions more rapidly as you draw on the critical thinking and analysis you already performed while reading. Questions that may have seemed daunting without this method often become more approachable because Interrogating leaves you with a better understanding of the structure and purpose of every part of the passage. When you understand what the author was trying to accomplish and how each part of the passage contributes to that, you can more readily generate predictions to questions as you encounter them, and skip the time-consuming research you would otherwise be doing after Highlighting or Outlining.

By asking and answering questions as you Interrogate the passage, you also build a far stronger memory of the passage. To borrow a familiar example from the sciences, the difference between Interrogating and Outlining is similar to the difference between knowing *why* a nucleophile attacks an electrophile and only memorizing *that* it occurs. When you understand *why* phenomena occur, you are much more likely to remember them. And so it goes with CARS. When you understand *why* the author felt a certain example was needed, you are much more likely to remember that example. As you improve your elaborative interrogation skills, you'll find that you can easily recall major ideas, destructive counterarguments, important examples, and often even small, random details... at least for a long enough time to answer the passage's questions!

Finally, this approach is most ideal for tackling shorter passages, and passages that you triage as Easy or Medium difficulty. Even if they appear more difficult, passages with a single, sustained argument or a collection of several abstract arguments, which is often the case for those on law or philosophy, are typically good candidates for this approach. Interrogating can help you to better understand how all the pieces of a large argument fit together, as well as how several distinct arguments work together to accomplish the author's larger goal.

Disadvantages

Some students pick up the Interrogating technique rapidly, or find that it is already similar to their natural style of reading. For most, however, learning to use this approach can be frustrating, especially at first. Undoubtedly, even for experienced test takers, this method takes the longest out of the three Distill approaches, and it also requires the most substantial amount of analysis and critical thinking. So for those first learning this approach, there are many potential pitfalls early on. You may find that the passage is harder to understand than you expected, and now you're trapped in an over-long interrogation. Or, you might get to the questions and realize that you spent too much time focusing on parts of the passage that are not tested.

It should come as no surprise, then, that becoming a good interrogator is not a short journey. But remember, the more you practice, the more natural it will feel to constantly ask *How?* and *Why?* as you read. And as you practice more with the method, you will develop a better sense for timing and for what is testable. Even an expert interrogator will likely not decide to Interrogate every passage they see. So be sure to practice the Choose step and select the Interrogating approach only when it is your best option.

Avoid using this approach on passages that seem especially complex or long, and on passages that appear to be long lists of details or unconnected information. In particular, if you are struggling just to make sense of the sentences you are reading, let alone how they connect or why the author wrote them, then an approach like Highlighting, which relies more upon the questions to guide you to what is important in the passage, is a better bet.

Interrogating Method Example

A quick glance at this passage reveals that it is a social sciences passage. Unlike most CARS passages, it uses first-person pronouns like "I," which suggests a description of the author's personal experiences. The language is also relatively straightforward with only a little jargon, so we can expect this passage to be Easy or Medium in difficulty, which makes it a great candidate for Interrogating.

INTERROGATING METHOD

Passage	Expert Thinking
Bauls are a religious group living primarily in the rural areas of West Bengal (India) and Bangladesh. They come from a variety of backgrounds, including Hindu and Muslim, and span the castes, though most are low caste. Although their roots extend more deeply, Bauls have been around at least a century. In practice and belief, they have been influenced by local traditions of the more orthodox Gauriya (Bengali) Vaishnavism, the Tantric-influenced Buddhist and Hindu Sahajiyas, and Sufism. However, unlike many other religious groups, Bauls intentionally reverse a number of orthodox practices. They argue that the Divine is within all humans and thus people should respect and worship humans instead of going to the temple, mosque, or church to worship something that cannot be seen. Bauls sing and compose songs that critique societal divisions and allude to their philosophy and practice. They spread their messages door to door, on trains, and in performances at large public venues.	S1–8. Why has the author decided to write about and focus on the Bauls? *The author is focusing on the unique aspects of the Baul religious group, and we can infer that she finds the Bauls to be particularly interesting because of those differences. Specifically, this group is unique because, despite significant influences from other religious and ethnic groups, they have opted to reverse a number of traditional practices. The heavy use of detail suggests that the author's purpose is to describe what is distinctive about the Bauls, at least in this first paragraph, but also potentially in the rest of the passage.*
I sought the lived experiences and perspectives of Baul women. In [the] first 18 months of work, I carefully framed how I presented my research to my interlocutors in order to avoid the usual pitfalls of my predecessors, such as having to exchange money or prestige for information, taking initiation, or losing integrity in my research methods in other ways. [My interactions with the Baul] bring to the forefront the postcolonial predicament concerning the relationship between ethnographers and "informants," in which the ethnographer collects "data," which is then analyzed and presented for academic scrutiny.	S1. Why is the author using "I" and "my"? *This author is describing her personal experience with people of the Baul religion, so first-person pronouns are appropriate. Within this context, we can infer that the passage will likely contain more tone and opinion than the average CARS passage, and should stay vigilant in looking for Author keywords, as there are likely to be questions about opinion or tone.* S2. Why does the author talk about "avoid[ing] the usual pitfalls"? *The phrase suggests that ethnography (the author's field) suffers from some common problems. By making efforts to avoid these problems, the author can enhance the credibility of her research.* S3. Why does the author bring up the "postcolonial predicament," and how does it relate to her purpose? *The word "predicament" suggests this is connected to the "pitfalls" described in the preceding sentence. The use of scare quotes in the remainder of the sentence suggests that the author wants to distance herself from treating the people she lived with as "informants" presenting her with "data." In other words, she thinks there are issues with treating ethnographers like natural scientists who are dispassionately observing the world around them. This is an elaboration on how she's trying to avoid the common problems of ethnography, so it's a further attempt to increase the credibility of her description of the Baul.*

INTERROGATING METHOD

Passage	Expert Thinking
I have argued elsewhere that as they traverse a Baul path, those who take the teachings seriously gradually adopt cognitive and spiritual models that shift their own understanding of the world around them. Thus, they learn (or aim to learn) to recognize the ways in which society creates divisions that lead to discrimination, and to recognize the divine in all human beings, regardless of caste, gender, or religion. By listening to their explanations about the micro- and macrocosmos, by hearing their songs, and by traveling with them, they expected that I too would experience these shifts in understanding. The cultural specifics of their experiences may not carry home, but elements of hierarchy, discrimination, and the inherent value of all human beings are as real and important in my American communities as they are in their Bengali ones. For Bauls, issues of hierarchy and domination are religiously meaningful, and knowledge of these realities constitutes important aspects of their religious experiences.	S1–5. How did the Baul expect the author to respond to their religion? How did the author actually respond? *The Baul expected the author to adopt the same beliefs and values that they explained and demonstrated to her. She suggests that she had trouble relating to the "cultural specifics of their experiences," but was able to appreciate shared values that overlapped with her experience as an American.*
In these and other ways, the Baul women I worked with expected me to participate in their world, particularly when they knew I shared their views. Although moments of connection have shifted my own perspectives, [a specific Baul woman's] critiques ring loudest. In demanding that I (and the many Bengalis and foreigners who enjoy her singing) support her, she refuses to let me be a complacent ethnographer. She demands dignity, and she is right to do so. Several years later, her proclamations are forcing me to rethink my ethnographic work and to reveal, as a tentative step, that I have been moved, that I have taken their words and lifeworlds seriously.	S1–4. Why does the author mention the specific Baul woman's critique? *This is a continuation of the discussion of Baul expectations and the author's reaction to them. The Baul woman expected the author to change from a passive observer to an active supporter and participant. This pertains directly to the second paragraph, where the author described the problematic role of traditional ethnographers, and her efforts to avoid some of the typical problems. She concludes the paragraph by saying that her critic was right and that she's been moved to change, which suggests that she's further questioning the role of the ethnographer as a dispassionate observer.*

INTERROGATING METHOD

Passage	Expert Thinking
Maybe language is inadequate to explain religious experience. Bauls would certainly say so, since they insist that one can only trust and know what is personally experienced. Perhaps, then, I should acknowledge moments of connection. For instance, when [the Baul] and I discussed our views of the world, its beauty and faults, and our struggle to make sense of suffering and find ways to improve the lives of those discriminated against. Maybe it's enough for me and my interlocutors to share meaningful experiences and conversations, to be open to being inspired and transformed in the field and also back home, and to be willing to put some of those ideas into action.	S1–4. Why does the author conclude with a discussion of religious experiences? *The author discusses religious experience both because it's important to the Baul and because it's a further challenge to the view of the ethnographer as a detached observer. Thus, it's an appropriate conclusion since it connects the two major themes of this passage (characteristics of the Baul religion and the role of the ethnographer). Her closing sentence suggests that she has developed an alternative vision for what it means to be an ethnographer ("to share meaningful experiences, to be open to being inspired and transformed"), one that was directly shaped by her experiences with the Baul.*

Adapted from Knight, L. I. (2016). "I Will Not Keep Her Book in My Home": Representing Religious Meaning among Bauls. Asianetwork Exchange: A *Journal for Asian Studies in the Liberal Arts*, 23(1), 30–46. DOI: http://doi.org/10.16995/ane.159

Now that you've seen all three methods, remember that there is no "one-size-fits-all" when it comes to MCAT passages. As you Preview and Choose, think about which method will allow you to work through the passage and its questions most efficiently and effectively. But don't be afraid of choosing the wrong method as you start out. All things are hard before they are easy. And as you practice choosing a Distill method for each passage, you'll find you often learn as much or more from your wrong strategic decisions as you do from your right ones! The key is to make many mistakes now, while it's safe to make them, so that you have mastered all three approaches, as well as the ability to choose between them, by Test Day. And finally, know that what someone else may consider the best approach for a passage may be different from your judgement. Ultimately, the best choice for you is the one that earns you the most points. So, practice, learn from your mistakes, and watch your CARS mastery gradually improve.

Conclusion

Each of the three Distill methods discussed in this chapter provides you with a way to effectively navigate each passage while reading strategically. Perhaps as you read the description of each method, you observed that each trains you in its own way to become a better CARS test-taker overall. Highlighting trains you to rapidly identify testable information, even when you're not Highlighting. Outlining trains you to quickly summarize the main point of each paragraph, even when you're not Outlining. And Interrogating trains you to analyze the author's arguments and rhetorical choices, even when you're not Interrogating. So it is imperative that you do not utilize a "one-size-fits-all" approach. Learning the three different methods will expand your playbook on Test Day, and it will make you a much stronger test-taker along the way. The following chapter will help you further develop your ability to choose the right method for each passage and show you how each strategy can ultimately be leveraged to help you effectively answer the questions.

GO ONLINE

You've reviewed the strategy, now test your knowledge and critical thinking skills by completing a test-like passage set in your online resources!

CONCEPT AND STRATEGY SUMMARY

Choosing Your Approach

- As you triage, use things like passage length, topic complexity, and sentence structure to choose your Distill approach.
- As you work through the passage, aim to identify main ideas and key points using either the **Highlighting**, **Outlining**, or **Interrogating** approach.
- Use Contrast and Logic keywords to help you identify regions of the passage that contain high-yield, testable information and note them down accordingly, based on your approach.

Highlighting the Passage

- Highlight the main ideas in each paragraph so they are easier to find as you work through questions.
- Use your highlight tool sparingly. Avoid highlighting full sentences or wordy phrases.
- Keep an eye out for keywords that indicate structural shifts or the author's opinion and highlight a word or phrase that sums up the ideas that follow.
- Use this method on:
  - dense or complex passages that you will want to work through quickly (2–3 minutes)
  - passages that you have triaged until the end of the test
  - passages without natural transition points
- Avoid using this method on passages that require in-depth analysis (usually humanities passages).

Outlining the Passage

- Determine the main idea of each paragraph, rephrase it, and note it down on your scratch paper.
- Avoid getting caught up in details, evidence, and examples as you read.
- The act of rephrasing main ideas helps you better internalize them and read more quickly (3–4 minutes).
- Use this method for:
  - passages for which having a table of contents would be highly useful
  - highly detailed or list-driven passages
  - passages where multiple opinions are expressed and discussed
  - passages that you do not completely understand (simply jot down a relevant name or theme on your scratch paper and move on)

- Avoid Outlining when the time investment for creating the outline would not pay off, such as when you're low on time, or dealing with a rambling or unusually structured passage.

Interrogating the Passage

- Identify a "chunk" of information within the text that essentially says the same thing or builds on the same idea.
- Then ask yourself questions about the role that the chunk plays in the passage. Example questions include:
    - How does this connect to what I have read so far?
    - Why was this detail included here?
- Answering these questions as you go makes you a more active reader and helps you mentally organize the information in the passage.
- Use this method for:
    - shorter passages
    - passages you triage as Easy or Medium difficulty
    - passages with overarching arguments or collections of several arguments
- Since this method takes 4–6 minutes, avoid using it on long or complex passages, and on passages that consist of lists of details.

Worked Example

Use the Worked Example below, in tandem with the subsequent practice passages located in Chapters 7-11, to internalize and apply the strategies described in this chapter. The Worked Example matches the specifications and style of a typical MCAT *Critical Analysis and Reasoning Skills* (CARS) passage.

Start by Previewing the following passage (located on the left side of the page in this and in subsequent Worked Examples). Note its overall structure and difficulty, and consider what approach you might Choose if you were working this passage alone. Note that this is the first Worked Example in the book, and for this chapter alone, all three methods have been demonstrated on the same passage to better display how each method could be applied. This is also a reminder that passages on Test Day can be successfully navigated with whichever Distill approach, or combination of approaches, that works best for you. In future chapters, Worked Examples will only apply one of the methods, with an explanation of why that approach was chosen.

HIGHLIGHTING METHOD

Passage	Expert Thinking
One of the more well-known female writers to adopt a pen name was George Sand, born Aurore Dupin, who became one of the most prolific and admired French authors during the nineteenth century. The true identity of George Sand did not remain a secret for long, for the author used this name in her everyday life, and close friends commonly referred to her as "George."	From the first paragraph, what can you tell about what the rest of the passage will focus on? What should you highlight to capture that? *This paragraph is just a short introduction to the subject and doesn't contain any terms that jump out at me. However, I highlighted "not remain a secret" to capture the essence of having an obvious pseudonym.*
Most portraits of the author as an adult are simply George Sand and make no reference to her given name. Her son, too, adopted this new last name, even though his association with his famous author–mother did not bring him any obvious benefits. Given the name "George Sand" is radically different from Aurore Dupin's birth name, many readers have wondered how the author formulated her masculine pen name.	What is the purpose of this paragraph? What should you highlight to show that? *This paragraph includes several details in the beginning, but I did not see any as particularly high yield. These details are included to emphasize how strong the association is between this female author and her masculine pseudonym. I highlighted "wondered" because the question of why she chose this name will likely be explored in the rest of this passage.*
At least two possible answers spring to mind. The first, as indicated in Curtis Cate's biography *George Sand*, is that the pseudonym arose from a collaboration with her first lover, Jules Sandeau, with whom she co-authored several articles as well as a full-length novel entitled *Rose et Blanche*. On the advice of their publisher, the authors signed this latter work under the name "J. Sand." Once Aurore's writing began to overshadow that of Jules, she decided to sign her solo works as "Georges Sand," which eventually became simply "George Sand." Because her own literary output was a great success, she quickly became known by this name and began to use her pen name on a daily basis.	Here, the author mentions two theories. What should you highlight to efficiently capture these theories? *The first theory revolves around collaboration, so I chose to highlight that term. In addition, I highlighted "overshadow" because it better describes how the collaboration was eclipsed as Dupin started to shine. Also, I know while words like "first" are critical indicators for important ideas, highlighting that word won't actually provide me with useful information. Finally, while the author mentions "two possible answers," there's no indication here of what the second answer might be, so I'll look out for it to be introduced in a later paragraph."*
By continuing to use the name initially assigned to collaborative writings with her lover, perhaps Aurore hoped to maintain their connection. Perhaps she fondly remembered their time together and wished to have a permanent reminder. Or perhaps she simply realized that it would be much more expedient to continue to write under a name which was already familiar to her audience thanks to their joint works.	What should you highlight in this paragraph? *In this paragraph, the author continues the discussion of the first theory of Dupin's pseudonym, speculating on why she would keep this name after becoming independently successful. The author offers two potential motivations, one based on the relationship she had with her lover (remembering their "connection"), the other based on the relationship she was cultivating with her readers (using a name they would find "familiar").*

HIGHLIGHTING METHOD

Passage	Expert Thinking
Given that George Sand began writing under this masculine name around the same time as she began to roam around Paris in pants and a jacket—typically male clothing—it is not hard to understand why she chose a masculine pseudonym because, like her clothes, this male identity gave her more freedom of expression, both literally and figuratively. And once she became known as a successful author under this name, there was no reason to change. Writing under a false name allowed her to distance parts of her character—her roles as wife, mother, and lover—from the creative and literary parts that formed her role as an author. Using a male name set her apart and added to her persona as an unusual and fascinating woman. In the end, the reason why she chose this particular pen name is not nearly as important as the vast quantity of writing—articles, letters, novels, and plays—that forms her legacy to the field of French literature.	What is this paragraph about? *This paragraph continues the discussion of why it would be advantageous for Dupin to use a masculine pseudonym. The major reasons the author provides are the additional freedom that the name (as well as the male identity she affected in her clothing choices) afforded her, and the distancing it allowed her from traditional feminine roles. The author concludes the paragraph by expressing a favorable opinion of Dupin, as captured by the word "legacy." Because author opinions are frequently tested, this justifies making a third highlight in this long paragraph.*
The name could have a more symbolic meaning as well, which would give more deserved credit to the author herself. Taking each letter of "SAND" as an allusion to names, places, or people from Aurore's life, this name can be seen as a representation of Aurore's childhood and early married life. Even if George created the name, however, she was well aware of the similarity to her lover's name, and was equally aware that many readers would make this connection. As an intelligent and perceptive woman, she recognized that such an association with a male author would help to validate her early writing career before she had succeeded in establishing her own reputation as a talented and publishable author.	What's new in the last paragraph of the passage? What should you highlight? *In the final paragraph, we finally come to the second of the "two possible answers" that the author alluded to in the third paragraph. The first answer suggested that she took the name from her lover/collaborator and adapted it, while this answer suggests she had a more active role in its creation, with each letter in "SAND" representing something important from her early life. The author notes, though, that even if she made up the name, she used its masculine associations to enhance her value to potential readers before having established herself.*

OUTLINING METHOD

Passage	Expert Thinking
One of the more well-known female writers to adopt a pen name was George Sand, born Aurore Dupin, who became one of the most prolific and admired French authors during the nineteenth century. The true identity of George Sand did not remain a secret for long, for the author used this name in her everyday life, and close friends commonly referred to her as "George."	The first paragraph will often give you a hint about the author's main idea. What seems to be the author's focus? *The author introduces a writer with the pen name "George Sand" who was born Aurore Dupin.* Are there any keywords to tell you how author feels about Aurore Dupin? *Yes! ". . . one of the most prolific and admired French authors . . ."* How can we express all this information in a concise format? P1: George Sand = Aurore Dupin → + tone
Most portraits of the author as an adult are simply George Sand and make no reference to her given name. Her son, too, adopted this new last name, even though his association with his famous author-mother did not bring him any obvious benefits. Given the name "George Sand" is radically different from Aurore Dupin's birth name, many readers have wondered how the author formulated her masculine pen name.	While this is another short paragraph, make sure not to glaze over it. How does the author further narrow the main point of the passage? *The author is wondering how the pen name "George Sand" came to be, as well as why it was more popular than the writer's real name.* What would be the best way to briefly express this? Note we can abbreviate names by their initials! P2: G.S. > A.D. → question: How was G.S. created?
At least two possible answers spring to mind. The first, as indicated in Curtis Cate's biography *George Sand*, is that the pseudonym arose from a collaboration with her first lover, Jules Sandeau, with whom she co-authored several articles as well as a full-length novel entitled *Rose et Blanche*. On the advice of their publisher, the authors signed this latter work under the name "J. Sand." Once Aurore's writing began to overshadow that of Jules, she decided to sign her solo works as "Georges Sand," which eventually became simply "George Sand." Because her own literary output was a great success, she quickly became known by this name and began to use her pen name on a daily basis.	Following the logic of previous paragraphs, what are you expecting to find in this one? *The answer to the question of how G.S. name came to be. The author actually suggests there are "at least two possible answers," and provides one of them here: it was inspired by a collaboration with her first lover, Jules Sandeau.* While there is a lot of detail in this paragraph, you still want to come up with a short statement to outline it. P3: 1st answer: G.S. inspired by first love

OUTLINING METHOD	
Passage	**Expert Thinking**
By continuing to use the name initially assigned to collaborative writings with her lover, perhaps Aurore hoped to maintain their connection. Perhaps she fondly remembered their time together and wished to have a permanent reminder. Or perhaps she simply realized that it would be much more expedient to continue to write under a name which was already familiar to her audience thanks to their joint works.	Based on the first line of the paragraph, what can you expect to see in the rest of it? *Since there is a Continuation keyword present, I am expecting further development of the idea in the previous paragraph about why the writer kept using the name G.S.* P4: G.S. kept name → familiar
Given that George Sand began writing under this masculine name around the same time as she began to roam around Paris in pants and a jacket—typically male clothing—it is not hard to understand why she chose a masculine pseudonym because, like her clothes, this male identity gave her more freedom of expression, both literally and figuratively. And once she became known as a successful author under this name, there was no reason to change. Writing under a false name allowed her to distance parts of her character—her roles as wife, mother, and lover—from the creative and literary parts that formed her role as an author. Using a male name set her apart and added to her persona as an unusual and fascinating woman. In the end, the reason why she chose this particular pen name is not nearly as important as the vast quantity of writing—articles, letters, novels, plays—that forms her legacy to the field of French literature.	This is another long paragraph, but focus on what new idea is being introduced. *The author provides further justification for why the writer chose a more masculine pen name. There are multiple reasons stated and I do not want to try and write them all down in the outline. Just specifying where I can find them is enough.* P5: Further reasons to keep G.S.
The name could have a more symbolic meaning as well, which would give more deserved credit to the author herself. Taking each letter of "SAND" as an allusion to names, places, or people from Aurore's life, this name can be seen as a representation of Aurore's childhood and early married life. Even if George created the name, however, she was well aware of the similarity to her lover's name, and was equally aware that many readers would make this connection. As an intelligent and perceptive woman, she recognized that such an association with a male author would help to validate her early writing career before she had succeeded in establishing her own reputation as a talented and publishable author.	Thinking back to paragraph 3, you are still waiting for a second possibility for where the name George Sand came from. And this is exactly what this last paragraph provides. What is the second possibility? *The writer perhaps picked the name as an homage to people and places from her life.* How can you concisely outline this paragraph? P6: 2nd answer: SAND = impt ppl. & places

INTERROGATING METHOD

Passage	Expert Thinking
One of the more well-known female writers to adopt a pen name was George Sand, born Aurore Dupin, who became one of the most prolific and admired French authors during the nineteenth century. The true identity of George Sand did not remain a secret for long, for the author used this name in her everyday life, and close friends commonly referred to her as "George."	S1–2. Why is the author discussing the different names of the writer George Sand? *The writer, born Aurore Dupin, is female, but used a male pen name (George Sand) in the 19th century. I know it was common for women writers to use male pen names at this time because it was unusual for women to be published writers.* S2. Why is it important to note that her true identity wasn't a secret? *If her true identity was no secret, then she must not have been using it to mask her gender. I expect the author will go on to explain why she used this pen name.*
Most portraits of the author as an adult are simply George Sand and make no reference to her given name. Her son, too, adopted this new last name, even though his association with his famous author–mother did not bring him any obvious benefits. Given the name "George Sand" is radically different from Aurore Dupin's birth name, many readers have wondered how the author formulated her masculine pen name.	S1–2. Why does the author use the example of Sand's son taking her pen name? *The passage says that the son gained no benefit from taking her name and that the author is almost never referred to by her birth name, so it seems that this pen name was more of an identity to the writer than an attempt to disguise her gender. This makes sense based on the last paragraph.* S3. Why does the author mention that many readers wonder about the origin of Sand's pen name? *The last two paragraphs discuss how this pen name was part of the writer's identity and was clearly important to her. I expect that in the next few paragraphs, the author will discuss possible explanations of how Sand came up with her pen name that might explain why the name was so important to her.*
At least two possible answers spring to mind. The first, as indicated in Curtis Cate's biography *George Sand*, is that the pseudonym arose from a collaboration with her first lover, Jules Sandeau, with whom she co-authored several articles as well as a full-length novel entitled *Rose et Blanche*. On the advice of their publisher, the authors signed this latter work under the name "J. Sand." Once Aurore's writing began to overshadow that of Jules, she decided to sign her solo works as "Georges Sand," which eventually became simply "George Sand." Because her own literary output was a great success, she quickly became known by this name and began to use her pen name on a daily basis.	S1. Why is it important to pay attention to the fact that there are two possible answers? *This indicates that I can anticipate the structure of the remainder of this passage as it will likely be based around providing these two answers as to why she adopted a male pseudonym.* S2–5. Why does the author discuss Jules Sandeau? *Jules Sandeau was Dupin's former lover, with whom she coauthored some works. The author explains how the pseudonym they used together evolved into her own personal pen name.*

INTERROGATING METHOD

Passage	Expert Thinking
By continuing to use the name initially assigned to collaborative writings with her lover, perhaps Aurore hoped to maintain their connection. Perhaps she fondly remembered their time together and wished to have a permanent reminder. Or perhaps she simply realized that it would be much more expedient to continue to write under a name which was already familiar to her audience thanks to their joint works.	S1-3. How do the claims in this paragraph link to the previous paragraph? Why is the author not sure about the reasons? *There are three possible reasons (each signaled by a "perhaps") for why Dupin kept using that specific name. It's clear that Dupin did not state the reasons for maintaining the pen name, so the author is using historical and contextual clues to come up with reasons.*
Given that George Sand began writing under this masculine name around the same time as she began to roam around Paris in pants and a jacket—typically male clothing—it is not hard to understand why she chose a masculine pseudonym because, like her clothes, this male identity gave her more freedom of expression, both literally and figuratively. And once she became known as a successful author under this name, there was no reason to change. Writing under a false name allowed her to distance parts of her character—her roles as wife, mother, and lover—from the creative and literary parts that formed her role as an author. Using a male name set her apart and added to her persona as an unusual and fascinating woman. In the end, the reason why she chose this particular pen name is not nearly as important as the vast quantity of writing—articles, letters, novels, plays—that forms her legacy to the field of French literature.	S1–5. Why would having a male identity allow for more freedom? *After Dupin adopted the pen name, she also wore male clothing, further adopting a male persona. Given that this is the 19th century, women typically had less freedom of expression and movement. Additionally, the male name allowed her to separate her creative life from her other roles.*
The name could have a more symbolic meaning as well, which would give more deserved credit to the author herself. Taking each letter of "SAND" as an allusion to names, places, or people from Aurore's life, this name can be seen as a representation of Aurore's childhood and early married life. Even if George created the name, however, she was well aware of the similarity to her lover's name, and was equally aware that many readers would make this connection. As an intelligent and perceptive woman, she recognized that such an association with a male author would help to validate her early writing career before she had succeeded in establishing her own reputation as a talented and publishable author.	S1–4. How does this information structurally fit with the earlier paragraphs? Why does the author spend so little time on this alternative explanation? *This is the second of the "two possible answers" (P3) for how Dupin came to use George Sand for her pen name. The author speculates that SAND might be an acronym, but doesn't discuss what the letters stand for. The author grants that, even if the name was an acronym, it still had the connections to a masculine identity, which afforded Dupin a number of advantages (discussed in earlier paragraphs too). The lack of detail here suggests that the first possible answer may have better support.*

PRACTICE QUESTIONS

Passage 1 (Questions 1–6)

Peter Gay's book, *The Education of the Senses*, reexamines Victorian bourgeois attitudes about sensuality and sexuality in an attempt to discredit the pervasive and negative view of the Victorian bourgeois as repressed and repressive people whose outward prim public appearances often hypocritically masked inner lascivious thoughts and private behaviors. One of the most interesting facets of Gay's study is his discussion of the necessary, yet taboo, issue of birth control during the latter part of the nineteenth century.

Gay points out that the very process of giving birth was dangerous to both the newborn and the mother—that most women suffered greatly during the birth, that many children and new mothers died within five years of a birth, and that many women approached the child-bearing process with trepidation even though they believed that producing offspring was a woman's ultimate fulfillment. Advice or assistance from the medical profession—whether licensed doctors or self-trained midwives—was sorely lacking and inconsistent, hardly capable of reassuring the expectant mother and father about the safety of woman and baby.

In fact, the medical profession itself was largely responsible for promulgating myths and rumors about the dangers of attempting to limit family size through use of some forms of birth control, regardless of the fact that so many women and children died each year due to complications of pregnancy or birth. Some medical, religious, and social experts did acknowledge that the continual cycle of birth was not only detrimental to the health of the mother, but also could take a toll on the quality of life of the family because multiple children increased the financial burden and responsibility of the father. Furthermore, women were often caught in this cycle of pregnancy and childbirth well into their late 40s, greatly increasing the health risks and mortality rate of mother and child alike. It seemed appropriate and even necessary, then, to make efforts to limit the number of offspring in order to benefit the family unit and thus the greater good of society itself.

Nonetheless, open discussion of birth control methods, both natural and device-assisted, was rare, even between doctor and patient. Most information was passed along by word-of-mouth, which inevitably led to a great deal of unchecked misinformation that was, at times, deadly. Gay maintains that a primary motivation for this reticence was deeply ingrained in the Victorian bourgeois mindset that emphasized the value of family and traditional roles and thus encouraged women to be productive—in the very literal, procreative sense. Though concerned husbands certainly did take steps to assure that their wives and families were not jeopardized by an overabundance of offspring, a widespread effort to limit family size was not firmly rooted in society until the advent of a strong women's movement, which did not make many real and meaningful strides toward changing public attitudes and behaviors until the early twentieth century. Thus, Victorian bourgeois women were obliged to fulfill their societal role as child bearers despite very real fears about the toll this could take on their health and on the well being of their family.

1. Which of the following is NOT, according to the author, a reason that most Victorian women did not use any form of birth control?
   A. The medical profession did not offer any methods of birth control, but only vague suggestions for limiting the number of pregnancies a woman had during her lifetime.
   B. Although the risks to women were widely recognized, women were still held responsible for continuing the family line.
   C. Accurate information about safe forms of birth control was difficult to ascertain, even from doctors or midwives.
   D. Many medical experts were reluctant to discuss birth control with their patients because they themselves were not well informed about the options and consequences.

2. Which of the following, if true, would most seriously WEAKEN Gay's argument that deeply ingrained social attitudes were responsible for the lack of open discussion about birth control?
   A. The majority of Victorian women were satisfied with their role as wives and mothers.
   B. Limiting family size was inconsistent with bourgeois perceptions about social status.
   C. Bourgeois Victorians believed the ideal family consisted of fewer than five children.
   D. Many Victorian physicians actually knew that family planning would improve women's overall health.

3. The passage suggests that which of the following was commonly associated with childbirth during the Victorian era?
   I. Death of the child
   II. The need for additional family income
   III. Appreciation of the mother's suffering

   A. I only
   B. I and II only
   C. I and III only
   D. II and III only

4. Which of the following general theories would be most consistent with Gay's arguments as presented in the passage?
   A. Examination of sociohistorical context offers the modern historian little useful information about prevailing attitudes and behaviors of a certain time period.
   B. Understanding the psychological basis for social actions can help to explain apparently contradictory behavioral patterns.
   C. Social historians can best analyze past cultures by applying modern theories to the work of earlier critics.
   D. Critics should not attempt to rework prior studies of social classes because they cannot properly understand the historical context of their predecessors.

5. The passage suggests that Peter Gay is LEAST likely to agree with which of the following statements?
   A. Social critics should occasionally reexamine existing beliefs to make sure that they are appropriate.
   B. The prevailing views of Victorian bourgeois society were based on accurate sociocultural perceptions.
   C. The women's movement of the early twentieth century helped to bring the issue of birth control into the public consciousness.
   D. Sometimes, common mindsets must be altered before real social change can be accomplished.

6. Based on the passage, which of the following does the author consider was the most important factor that contributed to the high danger associated with Victorian childbirth?
   A. False and misleading information about the risks of childbirth
   B. Unsanitary conditions in the birthing rooms
   C. Successive cycles of pregnancy and childbirth
   D. Oppressive social attitudes that forced women to procreate

ANSWERS AND EXPLANATIONS

For this and all following sets of Practice Questions, examples of the text you should be Highlighting or writing down in your Outline will be included in the explanation for each passage.

Passage 1 (Questions 1–6)

Sample Highlighting

P1. "discredit"; **P2.** "trepidation"; **P3.** "responsible" and "efforts to limit"; **P4.** "unchecked misinformation" and "obliged."

Sample Outline

P1. Introduces Gay's reexamination of Victorian bourgeois attitudes; will focus on birth control

P2. Describes dangers to women and their babies; Victorian women: childbirth = "ultimate fulfillment"

P3. Doctors exacerbated the misinformation that women received, but recognized some issues with constant cycle of birth

P4. Discussion of birth control remained hidden in Victorian society—women had to fulfill their roles (until women's movement)

1. **A**

This is a Scattered Detail question asking for what is *not* stated as a reason women did not use birth control. We will need to use the process of elimination to eliminate the answers discussed in the passage. Starting with **(A)**, the medical profession's attitude about birth control is mentioned in paragraph 3. Doctors did not provide even vague advice for limiting family size, but rather "promulgat[ed] myths and rumors about the dangers of attempting to limit family size." Thus, **(A)** is the correct answer. **(B)** is mentioned at the end of paragraph 4. **(C)** is mentioned in detail in paragraph 2 and briefly mentioned again in paragraph 4. **(D)** is discussed in paragraph 3 and again at the beginning of paragraph 4.

2. **C**

This is a Strengthen–Weaken (Beyond the Passage) question focusing on what would *weaken* the author's argument. The author argues that deeply ingrained social attitudes were responsible for the lack of open discussion of birth control. We will need to consider what the social attitudes were at the time, as the right answer will contradict them. The author stated that women "believed that producing offspring was a woman's ultimate fulfillment" and that "a widespread effort to limit family size was not firmly rooted in society." A prediction for the answer would likely be something that implies that women felt that they had a different role or wanted to limit the size of the family. **(C)** best matches this prediction. **(A)** is consistent with Gay, reflecting on the idea that Victorian women "believed that producing offspring was a woman's ultimate fulfillment," and does not significantly weaken Gay's argument. **(B)** would strengthen the author's argument, as it gives an additional reason why women would not aim to limit family size—and would likely not discuss birth control openly, by extension. Finally, **(D)** would also strengthen the author's argument because it removes one of the alternative explanations why birth control was not discussed—if doctors actually knew that limiting family size was beneficial, and yet still did not discuss it openly, then it increases the likelihood that prevailing social attitudes limited discussions of birth control.

3. **B**

Because the question asks what the passage *suggests*, this is an Inference question; the Roman numeral answer choices make it a Scattered Inference question. We will need to evaluate the Roman numerals one by one to arrive at the answer. Starting with Statement I, the process of childbirth and the consequences of it were mentioned in paragraph 2. The author stated that many "children ... died within five years," so Statement I is true, and we can eliminate **(D)**. For Statement II, the author mentioned in paragraph 3 that additional children "increased the financial burden and responsibility of the father." This suggests that the family would need a larger income to support a larger family, so Statement II is also true. When we look at the answer choices, there is only one answer that has both Statements I and II, so **(B)** is the correct answer. For reference, Statement III is false because while some husbands were concerned about their wives during childbirth, it was not widespread.

4. **B**

This is an Apply question in which we need to use our understanding of the author's argument to determine which statement would be most consistent with it. The author mentioned the problems associated with childbirth in the second paragraph and the lack of action by medical professionals in paragraph 3. The author then explained that the reason birth control was not discussed was due to the current social mindset in which women were expected to be productive. This argument structure is most consistent with **(B)**. **(A)** and **(D)** are Opposites; Gay uses sociohistorical context and reworks prior studies about Victorian bourgeois attitudes—so these statements would be inconsistent with Gay's argument in the passage. **(C)** is Out of Scope as Gay does not apply modern theories to earlier critics, but rather reevaluates information and research on the Victorian bourgeoisie themselves.

5. **B**

This is an Apply question (specifically of the Response subtype) asking us what Gay would be least likely to agree with. Gay's study was a reexamination of the stereotypical beliefs about Victorian bourgeois attitudes and behaviors with regard to sexuality. We can predict that if Gay found it necessary to reevaluate attitudes toward the Victorian bourgeoisie, he must have found the existing studies and opinions to be inaccurate. **(B)** best matches this prediction. **(A)** is an Opposite because this is exactly what Gay did—so he would definitely agree with reexamining existing beliefs. **(C)** and **(D)** both pertain to the end of the passage, where the author states that widespread attempts to limit family size did not occur until a strong women's movement made meaningful strides in changing public attitudes and behaviors.

6. **A**

This is another Inference question asking what the author thought was the most important factor contributing to the danger of childbirth in the Victorian era. Without an explicit statement of which factor the author thought most important, we can look at how the argument was structured for insight. The predominant focus of the passage, which plays a role in paragraphs 2, 3, and 4, is the misinformation from the medical field. This matches closely with **(A)**. **(B)** is Out of Scope because sanitation was never discussed. **(C)** is indeed mentioned in the passage but merely as an example of one of the few things doctors recognized was problematic—it is too narrow and restricted of an answer when compared to the author's overall argument in the passage. Finally, **(D)** is Extreme; social attitudes certainly encouraged women to procreate, but the word *forced* is simply too strong.

CHAPTER 7

APPLYING THE KAPLAN PASSAGE STRATEGY

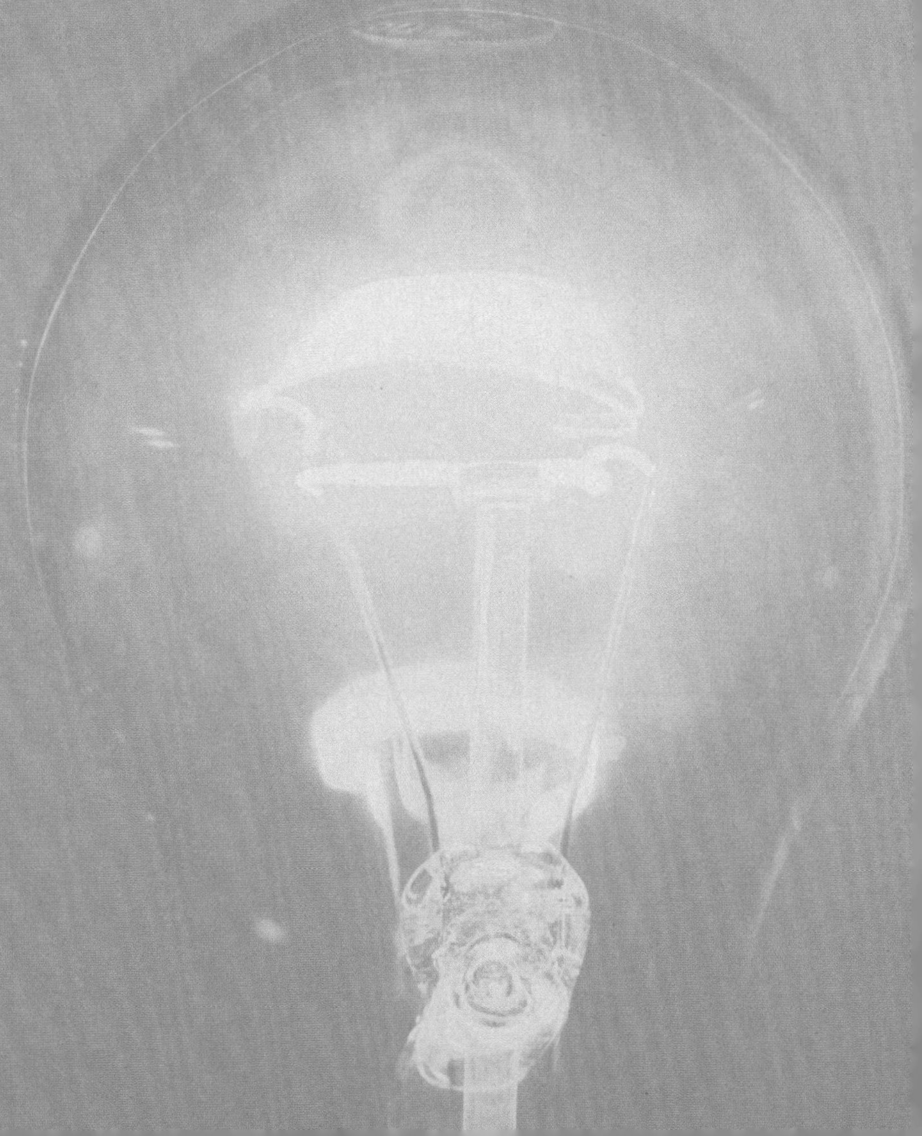

CHAPTER 7

APPLYING THE KAPLAN PASSAGE STRATEGY

In This Chapter

Introduction

LEARNING OBJECTIVES

After Chapter 7, you will be able to:

- Categorize MCAT passages by type and difficulty
- Choose the best Distill approach based on passage features
- Predict questions that are likely to be asked about a given passage

Now that we have examined how to Preview, Choose, and Read and Distill passages in the CARS section, it's time to put these strategies into action. All of the strategies will come together in this chapter. We'll start with a summary of the Kaplan Method for CARS Passages. Then we'll work through the Method with examples from the two categories of passages. The chapter concludes with a Worked Example and two practice passages.

This chapter is broken down as follows. First, we'll revisit the method in combination, and discuss how it will be applied to passages. We'll also revisit the major categories of passage type, and review their major features. Then, we will apply the Method to passages of both major types, walking through all steps of the Method and providing guided examples of applying the Method to three example passages.

7.1 The Kaplan Passage Method

The Kaplan Passage Method is a set of passage strategies that you will apply to every passage you encounter on Test Day. It begins with a scan of the passage and a determination of the order in which the passages will be handled. As you dive into a passage you'll pick an approach from the three Distill options. Then, using keywords, you will read the passage and extract the most question-relevant information.

As discussed in previous chapters, there are a variety of passage topics you will encounter on the MCAT. In fact, the AAMC lists eleven different fields in the humanities and a dozen in the social sciences (as shown in Table 7.1) that most CARS passages can be classified into. Preview, Choose, and Read and Distill (PCRD for short) is designed to address the variety of passages you will see on Test Day: Previewing enables you to work the passages in an efficient manner, Choosing ensures you match your approach to the demands of the passage, and Reading and Distilling will focus your attention on the information most likely to show up in the questions.

MCAT EXPERTISE

According to the AAMC, 50 percent of the questions in the CARS section will come from the humanities, and 50 percent will come from social sciences.

Humanities	Social Sciences
Architecture	Anthropology
Art	Archaeology
Dance	Economics
Ethics	Education
Literature	Geography
Music	History
Philosophy	Linguistics
Popular Culture	Political Science
Religion	Population Health
Studies of Diverse Cultures*	Psychology
Theater	Sociology
	Studies of Diverse Cultures*

* Note: Studies of Diverse Cultures can be tested in both humanities and social sciences passages.

Table 7.1 Humanities and Social Sciences Disciplines in the CARS Section

The goal of determining the passage subtype is to help you set your expectations appropriately, just as you would in the science section. For example, you would expect a science passage on rate kinetics to discuss rate laws, rate-of-formation tables, and reaction mechanisms. You would likely also anticipate that the associated questions will ask you to calculate a rate law using the tables and to consider topics like rate-limiting steps and catalysis. Similarly, you can set expectations about the trajectory of a CARS passage and predict what topics are more likely to be tested than others. In the following two sections, we will work through three different CARS passages together, breaking down our approach as we go, in order to give you a more comprehensive understanding of how to apply the Kaplan CARS Passage Method.

KEY CONCEPT

Think about trends you notice in passages that discuss similar topics or fall into similar disciplines. Applying these trends to future passages will give you insight into both their structure and the questions you will likely be asked, allowing you to become more efficient in navigating and distilling the passage and helping you predict and answer questions more rapidly and accurately.

Steps of the Method

As stated previously, this method can be applied to every CARS passage you encounter, so it is important to make a habit of automatically executing it as you begin each passage. Figure 7.1 shows the steps of the method.

BRIDGE

The steps of the Kaplan Method for CARS Passages are covered in greater detail in Chapters 4, 5, and 6.

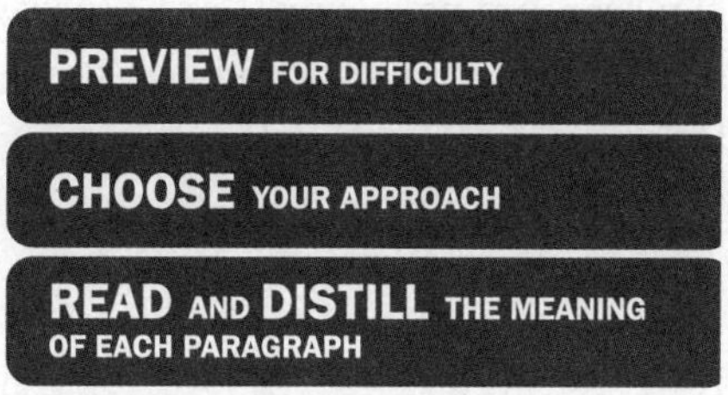

Figure 7.1 The Kaplan CARS Passage Method

Preview

The first step of the Kaplan Passage Method is to Preview the passage. As described in Chapter 4, you will look at the topic, sentence structure, writing style, length, and the first question to determine whether you want to attack the passage now or save it for later. Remember, there is a lot of variety among test takers in how they make those triage decisions and how they track those decisions on their noteboard. A topic that may be interesting to you may be kryptonite for the person sitting next to you, and as such, your preview is always going to be a very personal assessment.

Triaging and saving harder passages for the end provides two key benefits. First, it ensures that you are spending your time on the questions that you are more likely to answer correctly. It's unwise to spend excessive amounts of time on harder passages only to run out of time while working on an easier one. Second, it allows you to build confidence and a time buffer, both of which are key for when you do finally work on the harder passages.

Choose

Once you have decided to move forward with a passage, it's time to choose your approach to Distilling that passage. As discussed in Chapter 6, you can choose to Highlight, Outline, or Interrogate the passage. Each method has its own advantages and disadvantages. Rely on the analysis from your Preview step to help make this decision. In fact, many students will make their decision *as they preview* and note their choice on their noteboard. Should you choose to save a passage for later, you can either determine the approach you want to use before moving on to the next passage, or make that call when you return to the passage. Choosing the first option removes one of the steps you will have to perform when you return to the passage; however, you should remain open to changing your decision based on the time you have left.

Highlighting

The **Highlighting** approach is the quickest method for Distilling. When using this method, you should take about 2–3 minutes to work through a passage. As you read, plan to highlight important pieces of information, major shifts, and central ideas. This approach tends to work best for passages that appear to be overly dense and confusing or otherwise time consuming during your Preview step. You will typically use this strategy on passages you save until the end, because it enables you to move through the passage quickly. It is also a good option for passages that don't follow a clear structure, that is, those that lack distinctive transition points and breaks.

Outlining

The **Outlining** approach is best used to summarize the central ideas of each paragraph, while also noting the location of important pieces of information. You should be able to work through a passage in 3–4 minutes using this method. Your outline will be especially helpful in forming predictions for questions that test your understanding of the main ideas discussed in the passage, but you will need to return to the passage to answer questions asking about specific details. This is a useful approach for passages that appear to contain a large number of examples or details.

Interrogating

The **Interrogating** approach takes the most time but allows you to carry out a deep analysis of the passage as you read, enabling you to answer most questions with little rereading of the passage. However, at 4–6 minutes per passage, this is the most time consuming approach. In general, it is best used on passages you have triaged as *Now* and on shorter passages, to avoid timing becoming an issue. Passages that have complex central arguments or several distinct lines of argument are also well-suited for this approach because their questions will often ask about the logical relationships established in the passage.

Read and Distill

After deciding which approach to use, it is finally time to begin reading the passage. Note that the Read and Distill steps are grouped together because, functionally, they happen at the same time: you read with keywords, and use those keywords to guide your distillation of passage information. This is an active process of thinking and analyzing as you read. By staying engaged with the text, you help prevent a loss of focus and the need for rereading.

In Chapter 5, we discussed the importance of identifying and evaluating keywords in the passage. As you work your way through the passage, use keywords to help you identify notable shifts or key points in the text, along with author intentions and parts of arguments.

The goal of this step is to combine your knowledge of the passage types (and the questions commonly associated with them) with the most applicable passage approach in order to efficiently extract the major takeaways of each paragraph.

Highlighting

As you read, aim to highlight 1–3 key terms and phrases per paragraph that you think are likely to show up in the questions. Since the goal is to read quickly while still capturing the main points, your Distill step will primarily be limited to highlighting the main idea (or, in some cases, ideas) of each paragraph, and highlighting words that describe, support, or refute that idea. The keywords discussed in Chapter 5 will help guide you toward words worth highlighting, but remember that keywords typically indicate connections between ideas, rather than the content of the ideas themselves. So instead of highlighting keywords, focus on the concepts surrounding the keywords and note the progression of ideas through the passage.

Outlining

As you read, actively predict (and adjust your prediction as you encounter new ideas) the main idea of each paragraph. When you reach the end of a paragraph, take a moment to rephrase this main idea in your own words and write it on your noteboard. By identifying and rewording the main idea of each paragraph, you are already performing some of the analysis required to answer the questions. Thus, Outlining increases the accuracy of your predictions and saves you time on the questions. Because you are writing these main ideas on your noteboard with the Outlining method, you can use the highlighting tool to emphasize Relation, Logic, and Author keywords that you'd typically ignore when using the Highlighting method, making it easier to see important relationships and author intentions in the text. Remember that a major benefit of this method is that it allows you to read without having to memorize details. Once your paragraph label is on your noteboard, you can move on to the next paragraph without being concerned about forgetting the main idea of the previous one. It is important to remember that as you outline, you don't necessarily want to rephrase the entire paragraph. Rather, you want to select the information that answers questions like *What new information was added here?* and *What is the most testable information in this paragraph?* to include in your passage label.

Interrogating

As you read, actively examine the major idea presented in each paragraph to determine why and how the information was used by the author. Remember, this step goes beyond the Outlining method because instead of simply asking, *What information is new?*, you also want to understand the reasons for its inclusion. Use keywords to help you identify the information most likely to be tested. Also be sure to take advantage of the "Chunking" method. Don't only work through this method sentence by sentence. Rather, group similar ideas, often linked by Continuation keywords, into a chunk, before asking yourself questions about each chunk and why it was included.

This method has the most involved Distill step, as your goal is to do the majority of the work analyzing and understanding the passage before you even get to the questions. Once you've done this deep analysis, though, you won't have to spend a lot of time referring back to the passage.

In all three of the methods, the underlying goal is to help you identify the most important and testable content in each paragraph. As part of that, regardless of the method you choose to use, by the time you reach the end of the passage, you should be able to identify the reason the passage was written (the overall purpose or goal of the passage, as was discussed in the rhetoric portion of Chapter 3). If it is not clear, take a moment to consider it before jumping into the questions.

In the next section, you will get to see the Kaplan Passage Strategy applied to several examples. Use them as guides for understanding the advantages and disadvantages of each method.

7.2 Humanities Passages

Now that we have discussed the components of the Kaplan CARS Passage Method, let's apply it to a passage similar to the ones you will see on Test Day. As previously mentioned, the two broadest passage categories are humanities and social sciences. The next section will discuss the unique challenges of humanities passages and will demonstrate how the Kaplan Passage Method can be applied to these passage types.

Humanities Passages

Passages in the humanities tend to fall into two broad categories. The first category, which includes most of the passages from architecture, art, dance, literature, music, popular culture, and theater, can broadly be considered **arts passages**.

Many arts passages are characterized by the heavy use of quotations from other artists, writers, or critics, in addition to strong Author opinions and the use of descriptive language when discussing artistic examples. Often, each paragraph is structured with a claim, followed by evidentiary support. While not every Arts passage will contain these elements—literature passages, in particular, tend to have a lot of variation—the majority do, making them easy to identify and triage.

Most of the other passages in the humanities fall into the second category, which includes ethics, philosophy, religion, and studies of diverse cultures. These are broadly categorized as **philosophical passages**.

MCAT EXPERTISE

Passages with a lack of support or argumentation are likely to include *Reasoning Beyond the Text* questions, which bring in a new element of information and ask you to apply the information in the passage to a new scenario (Apply questions) or ask how the new information would impact the passage (Strengthen-Weaken [Beyond the Passage] questions). These question types are discussed in Chapter 11.

Philosophical passages tend to be very abstract, with an emphasis placed on logic. They focus on concepts and the relationships between them, and they often appeal to the reader's memory or imagination, drawing on common experiences or thought experiments (asking a question with no definite answer to help you delve deeper into the nature of things).

Keep in mind that there will be plenty of humanities passages that mix characteristics of arts and philosophical passages, as well as some passages that don't properly fit in either category. Nevertheless, this distinction is useful for setting expectations about the kind of support that a passage will use as well as the types of questions that will accompany it.

Applying the Method to Humanities Passages

Passage 1

Now, let's take a look at how to apply the Kaplan CARS Passage Method to a humanities passage, keeping the unique challenges of this passage type in mind.

Preview

Preview the passage below (do not read through it completely; there will be an opportunity for that later in the chapter), then read the analysis that follows to assess what you are already noticing and what other factors you could have considered.

> *The Monkey Kid*, written and directed by Xiao-Yen Wang, is probably one of the best Chinese feature films ever made but few Americans have seen it. Released in 1995 by the Beijing-San Francisco Film Group, the film "was an Official Selection at the 1995 Cannes International Film Festival and received the Grand Prize at the 1996 Aubervilliers International Children's Film Festival, awards for Best Film and Best Director at the 1995 Danube Film Festival, Best Foreign Film at the 1995 Fort Lauderdale International Film Festival, the Young Jury Award at the 1996 International Women's Film Festival at Créteil, and the Critic's Prize at the Cinestival 97 at Marseille."
>
> The film is the autobiographical account of director Xiao-Yen Wang's childhood in China during the Cultural Revolution, the great political upheaval that gripped Chinese society and politics from 1966–1976. Ms. Wang is not just a casual observer of the times. She is an accomplished writer and director who graduated from the Beijing Film Academy in 1982. That same class of directors came to be called the famed Fifth Generation of Chinese filmmakers and included Chen Kaige (*Farewell My Concubine*, *The Emperor and the Assassin*) and Zhang Yimou (*Curse of the Golden Flower*, *Hero*, *House of Flying Daggers*, *Ju Dou*, *Raise the Red Lantern*, *Red Sorghum*, *The Story of Qiu Ju*, and *To Live*). Ms. Wang has also written and directed two other films, *The Blank Point* (1991) and *I'm Seducible* (2006).
>
> At first glance, *The Monkey Kid* may seem like a simple slice-of-life story about one family during the Cultural Revolution, but it is much more than that. This feature film shows just how much Maoist ideology affected everyone in China, especially mothers, fathers, and children. Every family felt the turmoil in some way. What makes this film about the Cultural Revolution different from all others is that it offers a way to understand revolutionary society from a child's perspective.
>
> The main character of the film is Shi-Wei. For much of the film, Shi-Wei and her sister, Shao-Qiong, are alone in the family's apartment. Her parents live apart in two different locations in rural China as part of the campaign to have intellectuals learn from the peasants. During the film, both the father and the mother return home for short periods of time. Otherwise, Shi-Wei and Shao-Qiong must take care of themselves. They do their homework, keep the apartment tidy, shop for vegetables from street vendors, and even cook the way their parents have taught them, without any adult supervision.

The film depicts Shi-Wei as a model child. She takes on a lot of the responsibility at home while her parents are away. She also does well in school and serves as a class leader. Yet even Shi-Wei is not perfect. In one of the first scenes of the film, Shi-Wei arrives at school late because she and her friends were playing in the snow. Other students would have been punished, but Shi-Wei counts on the fact that she is a "teacher's pet." Shi-Wei just whispers some excuse to the teacher and all is forgiven.

The Monkey Kid is not a new film, but educators should not be afraid to use it in the classroom. It is especially helpful for illustrating the many ways in which Mao's cult of personality dominated this era. It offers a view of the Cultural Revolution that is both compelling and entertaining. I have used the film with great success in both undergraduate and graduate classes on modern China. Students report that more than any other film about the Cultural Revolution, *The Monkey Kid* stays with them long after its showing in class because of the story line, the acting of the children, and the effective direction. The film always generates much discussion about class divisions, ideological education, and mass mobilization.

Adapted from Andrew, A.M., 2011. The Monkey Kid: A Personal Glimpse into the Cultural Revolution. ASIANetwork Exchange: A Journal for Asian Studies in the Liberal Arts, 18(2), pp.108–111. DOI: http://doi.org/10.16995/ane.190

A quick peek at the first sentence indicates that this is likely an arts passage, since it begins by discussing a movie. The second sentence is easily identifiable as a list of the movie's accolades. Glancing at the first sentence of the next two paragraphs further supports the idea that we will be spending the passage learning more about the movie and its origins. Looking down the passage, the sentence structure appears to be generally simple.

Since this passage appears relatively straightforward and does not contain long, complex sentences, advanced vocabulary, or highly abstract ideas, this is an excellent passage to do now, rather than later, and should rank as Easy or Medium for most readers.

Choose

None of the paragraphs are extremely long, and many appear to focus on examples and specific details. Therefore, the Outlining method is ideal for this passage, as it will allow us to boil down to the simple main idea of each paragraph in a way that will facilitate answering questions with ease. Furthermore, the language and the structure are not overly complex, so an in-depth reading is not required to determine the author's goal.

Read and Distill

Given the simplicity of the wording and sentence structure, you should be able to create a well-structured outline while reading through the details more quickly. Expect to work quickly through the passage, labeling the key points and returning back to it as needed to revisit specific details and examples if asked about them in a question.

OUTLINING METHOD

Passage	Expert Thinking
The Monkey Kid, written and directed by Xiao-Yen Wang, is probably one of the best Chinese feature films ever made but few Americans have seen it. Released in 1995 by the Beijing-San Francisco Film Group, the film "was an Official Selection at the 1995 Cannes International Film Festival and received the Grand Prize at the 1996 Aubervilliers International Children's Film Festival, awards for Best Film and Best Director at the 1995 Danube Film Festival, Best Foreign Film at the 1995 Fort Lauderdale International Film Festival, the Young Jury Award at the 1996 International Women's Film Festival at Créteil, and the Critic's Prize at the Cinestival 97 at Marseille."	Ideally, the first paragraph will let us know the general direction for the rest of the passage. What is being introduced to us here? *The author introduced a Chinese film* The Monkey Kid. Does the author have an opinion on this film? *Absolutely! The phrase "one of the best" clearly indicates the author's high opinion of the film.* Notice also that the bulk of the paragraph is dedicated to describing why the author considers this one of the best films. But we don't need to outline that because it's just evidence for the conclusion we already identified. P1: The Monkey Kid = one of the best films
The film is the autobiographical account of director Xiao-Yen Wang's childhood in China during the Cultural Revolution, the great political upheaval that gripped Chinese society and politics from 1966–1976. Ms. Wang is not just a casual observer of the times. She is an accomplished writer and director who graduated from the Beijing Film Academy in 1982. That same class of directors came to be called the famed Fifth Generation of Chinese filmmakers and included Chen Kaige (*Farewell My Concubine*, *The Emperor and the Assassin*) and Zhang Yimou (*Curse of the Golden Flower*, *Hero*, *House of Flying Daggers*, *Ju Dou*, *Raise the Red Lantern*, *Red Sorghum*, *The Story of Qiu Ju*, *To Live*). Ms. Wang has also written and directed two other films, The *Blank Point* (1991) and *I'm Seducible* (2006).	Based on the previous paragraph, we can expect further description of the film to come next. What information are we given? *The author states that the film is an autobiography of the director. We are also told further information about the director.* Does the author express an opinion about the director? *Yes! Words like "accomplished" show that the author feels positive.* This paragraph contains a lot of details that simply support the author's opinion and shouldn't be included in the outline. P2: Author: Director = accomplished
At first glance, *The Monkey Kid* may seem like a simple slice-of-life story about one family during the Cultural Revolution, but it is much more than that. This feature film shows just how much Maoist ideology affected everyone in China, especially mothers, fathers, and children. Every family felt the turmoil in some way. What makes this film about the Cultural Revolution different from all others is that it offers a way to understand revolutionary society from a child's perspective.	The first sentence provides us with a contrast. What is being contrasted? *The author states that the film may seem simple at first but shows how Moaist ideology affected families. In addition, it is done from a child's perspective.* P3: Film = Maoist ideol. from child eyes

OUTLINING METHOD

Passage	Expert Thinking
The main character of the film is Shi-Wei. For much of the film, Shi-Wei and her sister, Shao-Qiong, are alone in the family's apartment. Her parents live apart in two different locations in rural China as part of the campaign to have intellectuals learn from the peasants. During the film, both the father and the mother return home for short periods of time. Otherwise, Shi-Wei and Shao-Qiong must take care of themselves. They do their homework, keep the apartment tidy, shop for vegetables from street vendors, and even cook the way their parents have taught them, without any adult supervision.	The beginning of this paragraph quickly tells us that the author is about to provide more information on what the film is about. Look out for contrasts or anything else unexpected, but otherwise don't spend too much time on this paragraph. P4: Main char description
The film depicts Shi-Wei as a model child. She takes on a lot of the responsibility at home while her parents are away. She also does well in school and serves as a class leader. Yet, even Shi-Wei is not perfect. In one of the first scenes of the film, Shi-Wei arrives at school late because she and her friends were playing in the snow. Other students would have been punished, but Shi-Wei counts on the fact that she is a "teacher's pet." Shi-Wei just whispers some excuse to the teacher and all is forgiven.	At first glance, this paragraph may seem like a continuation of the previous one. However, we do see a contrast made in the middle of it. What has changed? *The author states that even though main character is depicted as a model child, she is not perfect.* P5: Main char = model child but not perfect
The Monkey Kid is not a new film, but educators should not be afraid to use it in the classroom. It is especially helpful for illustrating the many ways in which Mao's cult of personality dominated this era. It offers a view of the Cultural Revolution that is both compelling and entertaining. I have used the film with great success in both undergraduate and graduate classes on modern China. Students report that more than any other film about the Cultural Revolution, *The Monkey Kid* stays with them long after its showing in class because of the story line, the acting of the children, and the effective direction. The film always generates much discussion about class divisions, ideological education, and mass mobilization.	Since this is the last paragraph, we expect the author to come up a with a conclusion and perhaps a reason why this film was discussed. What is the author's conclusion? *The author is advocating for this film as a great educational tool on Maoist ideology. In addition, there is evidence provided to back up the conclusion. We do not need to outline the evidence but we can make note of it.* P6: Film = great educ tool on Maoist ideol

This passage has a lot of details about the movie and its accolades, but our outline allows us to stay focused on the big ideas while being confident that we can find those details if a question requires it. Overall, the author wrote this passage to argue that this excellent movie can be used to teach students about the Maoist era in China. Given all of the details, we should certainly expect to see some Detail questions, but the CARS section is usually more interested in your understanding of the author's reasons for writing. Thus, we should also expect to see Function questions about particular details, such as why the author describes the main characters in such depth.

Passage 2

Now, let's apply the Kaplan method to another humanities passage. Pay particular attention to how we might vary our approach to this passage from that of the previous passage.

Preview

Preview (don't read) the passage below, then read the following analysis to assess what you are already noticing and what other factors you could have considered.

> The poet lives by words as the musician by sounds. One or other of the threads with which both build, investigate, decipher and seek to express wonderment refers back to the order of the originary. In the beginning was what? The network of ancient cosmogonies and the imbricate lexical and semantic web of documents and sources that give shape to our concepts bear witness to the universal operative power of both sound and syllables. The word is the purest symbol of the manifestation of being, of the being that thinks himself and expresses himself or the being that is known of, and communicated by another. Expressing the person, the word is part of its dynamism. Even if by analogy, does the same claim not apply to music?
>
> Nothing authorises us to say that Guerra Junqueiro (1850–1923) knew music or was able to read music beyond the most elementary level—even though, from a certain point he lived in a house inhabited by music. Both his daughters played piano and the youngest, Julia, excelled at the violin, to the point that, for example, in a public concert in 1898, she played the allegro from Mozart's 3rd Quintet with Gilhermina Suggia on cello; and even if he openly, to write some poetry, sought inspiration in certain pieces by Beethoven, which reminded him of those "immortal melodic souls of great epic tales that have died. . . ."
>
> Guerra Junqueiro has been a unique case in Portuguese literary history. No other poet, whatever the period being analyzed, attained such popularity. The effectiveness of the poetry-reader communication meant a mighty power of persuasion, able to seduce, charm, convince of its truth. This happened in a society marked by a high level of illiteracy in which music was the fundamental language and collective means of communicating feelings and meanings. Many, not knowing how to read, learned by ear and recited by rote extensive compositions of Guerra Junqueiro (such as "O Melro" from *A Lágrima*) or even entire books. And if knowing by heart implies an appropriation and has something of possession, it is also knowledge of the heart. It would, therefore, be useless and demeaning to ascribe his seduction to specific audiences. The

work of the poet served audiences differentiated by taste, social status, culture and political persuasion.

Words, like music, are liable to various modulations; they are, or can be, singing material. Guerra Junqueiro knew it and demanded that it was so: what "doesn't have music . . . is useless!" or what "doesn't sing, doesn't vibrate, is no good!" Based on this evaluation criterion, the verse of Junqueiro's work is stretched, loiters, stops, dances or sets off running like giddily rolling waves. Rich rhymes, vocal strata, ostensive use of metaphor, visually and aurally expressive images, pauses that are eloquent silences, sequences, reiterative structures, synaesthetic and onomatopoeic processes, a vast range of nuances, of technical-compositional, rhetorical-stylistic, ideothematic aspects, interwoven in a harmonious, seamless music, concur both for the modulation of what is the music of Junqueiro, and for direct communication with the reader or listener, easily consigning the verses to memory.

It is not, however, about reestablishing the prestige of Guerra Junqueiro, since this task would be impossible and an improbable anachronism, so intimate is the relation between text and society in the work of the poet and so disproportionately resounding was his reception. The academic project, Revisiting/Discovering Guerra Junqueiro, is rather an attempt to rescue him from the fog of oblivion and from the cultural ambiguity in which troubled circumstances, orthodoxies and conflicting powers bound him, freezing the reading and interpretation of his work and action.

Adapted from Pereira, H. (2010). From Singing Material to Intangible Poetry: The Music of Junqueiro. Journal of Science and Technology of the Arts, 2(1), 58-60. doi:http://dx.doi.org/10.7559/citarj.v2i1.195

A quick look at the first sentence indicates that this is likely an arts passage, since it begins by discussing poetry and music. The second sentence contains flowery language and abstract concepts and is followed by a question. The first sentences of the next two paragraphs discuss a poet named Guerra Junqueiro. As a result, we can assume that this passage will discuss music and poetry, specifically the work of Guerra Junqueiro. The first paragraph may seem intimidating, but it also looks like it's just an introduction to a more straightforward piece, so this passage is likely not as challenging as the first paragraph appears.

Since this passage contains advanced vocabulary and abstract ideas, this is certainly a passage that many would triage for later, likely assigning a difficulty of Hard or Medium.

Choose

This is a difficult passage to Choose an approach for, and the passage is likely to wind up being time consuming regardless of method chosen. The first paragraph is exceptionally verbose, with unnecessarily convoluted language. Subsequent paragraphs indicate that the passage is primarily focused on a single individual and his poetic work. Main ideas, for the purposes of outlining or highlighting, will be difficult to determine and require additional time regardless of method chosen. Furthermore, the passage is filled with strongly-worded, abstract claims. This abstraction and complexity suggest that the Interrogation method will be challenging to apply to this passage, but, if done correctly, will hugely facilitate answering questions. As a further benefit, Interrogating will likely allow a reader to connect the abstractions of the first paragraph with the rest of the passage, promoting deeper understanding.

If insufficient time existed to approach this passage with Interrogating, Highlighting or Outlining could be used. Specifically, the difficulty and length of the passage point to Highlighting as a way to save time. The lack of clear focus and main idea in each paragraph mean that it may be difficult to find terms to highlight as main ideas, and may even be hard to find words to write in an outline without doing a deep passage analysis.

Read and Distill

As you read, locate sentences that discuss or elaborate on a single theme. Ask yourself why the author chose to include that information and how it contributes to the author's overall purpose before moving to the next "chunk" of information. It's normal to take longer to work through a passage when you use this approach as compared to the other two, but be mindful of time and don't get lost in the minutiae. Remember, the goal is to think about the big picture, so avoid interrogating sentence by sentence. If you're struggling to generate questions in order to interrogate passages, consider going through this example by reading the questions on the right, then trying to answer them yourself. Follow up by reading the expert response and evaluating how well you did. Interrogating is a challenging method to learn and master, so if you're just starting out with it, focus on building one skill at a time!

MCAT EXPERTISE

If you encounter a tough passage like this on Test Day, don't lose your cool! The majority of passages you encounter will not be this challenging. A passage like this one should be saved for later as part of your Preview step, and when you do come back to it at the end of the section, after completing other passages, you will have a clear idea of how much time you have available to devote to the passage. Remember, when in a time crunch, Highlighting is a great approach for challenging passages. If you have sufficient time, Interrogating is the best way to clearly identify all major themes and ideas in a passage and prepare yourself for the questions to come. Choose the approach that's right for you based on the time left on the clock when you tackle difficult passages at the end of your CARS section!

INTERROGATING METHOD

Passage	Expert Thinking
The poet lives by words as the musician by sounds. One or other of the threads with which both build, investigate, decipher and seek to express wonderment refers back to the order of the originary. In the beginning was what? The network of ancient cosmogonies and the imbricate lexical and semantic web of documents and sources that give shape to our concepts bear witness to the universal operative power of both sound and syllables. The word is the purest symbol of the manifestation of being, of the being that thinks himself and expresses himself or the being that is known of, and communicated by another. Expressing the person, the word is part of its dynamism. Even if by analogy, does the same claim not apply to music?	S1–7. Why does the author build an analogy between words and music? *The author uses a lot of obtuse language here, but the first sentence makes a comparison between words and music that is reiterated with the rhetorical question at the end of the paragraph. It's tough to pin down exactly what the author is saying, but there's a general theme about words and music both having a "universal operative power," a suggestion that both are means for people to express themselves and communicate with each other. Thus, the author draws this analogy between words and music in order to highlight their similarities, specifically the way that both are used for self-expression and communication.*
Nothing authorizes us to say that Guerra Junqueiro (1850–1923) knew music or was able to read music beyond the most elementary level—even though, from a certain point he lived in a house inhabited by music. Both his daughters played piano and the youngest, Julia, excelled at the violin, to the point that, for example, in a public concert in 1898, she played the allegro from Mozart's 3rd Quintet with Gilhermina Suggia on cello; and even if he openly, to write some poetry, sought inspiration in certain pieces by Beethoven, which reminded him of those "immortal melodic souls of great epic tales that have died . . . ."	S1–2. Why does the author shift to talking about one man's experience with music and poetry? *The first paragraph drew parallels between music and words, and now the author is describing an example of a poet who is familiar with, but untrained in, music. She also mentions specific pieces of music that inspired the poet. Thus, the author uses Junqueiro as an example to reinforce her analogy between music and language from paragraph 1. In addition, as you may recall from previewing the passage, the remaining paragraphs focus on Junqueiro, so we can see that this paragraph serves to introduce us to the main topic of the passage: Junqueiro's musically inspired poetry.*

INTERROGATING METHOD

Passage	Expert Thinking
Guerra Junqueiro has been a unique case in Portuguese literary history. No other poet, whatever the period being analyzed, attained such popularity. The effectiveness of the poetry-reader communication meant a mighty power of persuasion, able to seduce, charm, convince of its truth. This happened in a society marked by a high level of illiteracy in which music was the fundamental language and collective means of communicating feelings and meanings. Many, not knowing how to read, learned by ear and recited by rote extensive compositions of Guerra Junqueiro (such as "O Melro" from *A Lágrima*) or even entire books. And if knowing by heart implies an appropriation and has something of possession, it is also knowledge of the heart. It would, therefore, be useless and demeaning to ascribe his seduction to specific audiences. The work of the poet served audiences differentiated by taste, social status, culture and political persuasion.	S1–2. Why does the author emphasize Junqueiro's popularity? *So far, there have been a lot of words in this passage, but only a few key ideas: the analogy between music and words/poetry as modes of expression, and the fact that Junqueiro's poetry was inspired by music (despite no formal musical training). We also know from our preview that the passage primarily focuses on Junqueiro's work. From this, it is reasonable to conclude that the author emphasizes Junqueiro's popularity both to justify why she decided to write about him in particular and to give her claims about the connection between music and poetry more force. After all, if she spoke about some obscure poet that nobody read anymore, then her audience would be less likely to take what she has to say seriously.* S3–8. Why does the author talk about the audience of Junqueiro? *The author presents a few key facts about Junqueiro's audience: they came from a society with limited education and literacy, they primarily communicated with music, and they learned to recite Junqueiro's poetry by listening to it (instead of reading it). Based on these facts, we can conclude that the author is suggesting that a Junqueiro poem functions exactly like a piece of music (at least for his audience), providing more support for the analogy between words and music as forms of expression.*

INTERROGATING METHOD

Passage	Expert Thinking
Words, like music, are liable to various modulations; they are, or can be, singing material. Guerra Junqueiro knew it and demanded that it was so: what "doesn't have music . . . is useless!" or what "doesn't sing, doesn't vibrate, is no good!" Based on this evaluation criterion, the verse of Junqueiro's work is stretched, loiters, stops, dances or sets off running like giddily rolling waves. Rich rhymes, vocal strata, ostensive use of metaphor, visually and aurally expressive images, pauses that are eloquent silences, sequences, reiterative structures, synaesthetic and onomatopoeic processes, a vast range of nuances, of technical-compositional, rhetorical-stylistic, ideothematic aspects, interwoven in a harmonious, seamless music, concur both for the modulation of what is the music of Junqueiro, and for direct communication with the reader or listener, easily consigning the verses to memory.	S1–4. Why does the author use such long strings of descriptive terms for Junqueiro's poetry? *This paragraph begins with a few shorter sentences, but its lengthy concluding sentence spans more than half of the paragraph and contains more than a dozen commas. Rather than attempting to make sense of every single descriptor, you should focus on the general theme: most of the descriptors use language associated with music or sound (as opposed to the written word). Thus, this long list is really just evidence for the claim that Junqueiro's poetry is musical by nature, which in turn supports the author's contention that words and music are closely related as means of expression.*
It is not, however, about reestablishing the prestige of Guerra Junqueiro, since this task would be impossible and an improbable anachronism, so intimate is the relation between text and society in the work of the poet and so disproportionately resounding was his reception. The academic project, Revisiting/Discovering Guerra Junqueiro, is rather an attempt to rescue him from the fog of oblivion and from the cultural ambiguity in which troubled circumstances, orthodoxies and conflicting powers bound him, freezing the reading and interpretation of his work and action.	S1–2. Why is the academic project NOT about reestablishing the prestige of Junqueiro? Why is the author writing about this project? *The author focused in previous paragraphs on the appeal of Junqueiro's work among those who primarily used music and spoken word to express themselves. However, contemporary audiences tend to inhabit different historical circumstances (e.g., they are more likely to be literate), so the author suggests that his work would not be received in the same way today. This serves to anticipate a potential criticism of the project, namely, that more literate and less musically-inclined audiences would not appreciate Junqueiro's poetry. Rather than restoring the former popularity of his work, the project instead aims to introduce this forgotten poet to contemporary audiences ("rescue him from the fog of oblivion") and help those audiences better interpret his work (namely, as a type of expression analogous to music, as established in previous paragraphs).*

Despite difficult language and complicated sentence structure, a deep interrogation of this passage shows us that the author actually has a fairly simple goal—one we honestly might have missed had we used a less in-depth passage method. The author uses the relationship between music and words to illustrate why Junqueiro was such a popular poet in his time and to suggest that his works deserve more attention today. Based on our analysis of the passage, we might expect to see Function questions asking why the author discussed the relationship between music and words, or an Inference question asking you why the author feels that Junqueiro's work is so important. The most challenging questions you might see with a passage of this type would ask you to expand on ideas from the passage: extending the analogy from the first paragraph or applying it to new examples.

7.3 Social Sciences Passages

Now that we have seen how the Kaplan Passage Method can be used to work through humanities passages, let's look at how it can also be applied to social sciences. The next section will discuss the unique challenges of these passages and walk you through how the Kaplan Passage Method can be applied to a social sciences passage.

Social Sciences Passages

As in the humanities, passages in the social sciences tend to fall into two broad categories. The first category, which includes most of the passages in anthropology, education, linguistics, population health, psychology, and sociology, has a **scientific** form.

Many scientific passages are characterized by the presence of numbers and reference to empirical studies as evidence. The author's opinion tends to be less obvious than in arts passages, but the presence of Author keywords can still be used to guide you to it. In some cases, a scientific passage may even look like a passage you might find in the *Psychological, Social, and Biological Foundations of Behavior* section, so it is especially important than you not bring any outside knowledge into your analysis of these types of passages.

The remaining passages tend to fall into the second category, which includes archaeology, economics, geography, history, political science, and studies of diverse cultures. These types of passages are best categorized as **historical passages**. Note that these types of passages are far more variable than the clear-cut scientific passages and may even resemble humanities passages at first glance.

Historical passages tend to draw on historical events and quotations from sources alive at the time of the events discussed. They are rarely heavily opinionated, but the nature of the subject matter itself allows authors to express strong viewpoints if they so desire. Passages dealing with history, economics, and political science often contain empirical studies, bringing in some elements of scientific passages, or heavy theoretical discussions, making them more like philosophical humanities passages.

Nevertheless, though some social sciences may appear to cross categorical boundaries, distinguishing them broadly as social science and more specifically as scientific or historical is useful for making judgments about what approach is best and what questions will likely be asked.

MCAT EXPERTISE

While psychology and sociology can be tested in both the *Critical Analysis and Reasoning Skills* section and the *Psychological, Social, and Biological Foundations of Behavior* section, the former will not require outside knowledge. In fact, bringing in outside knowledge to answer any question in the CARS section can lead you astray, drawing you toward Out of Scope answer choices.

Applying the Method to Social Sciences Passages

Now, let's take a look at how to apply the Kaplan method to a social sciences passage, keeping the unique challenges of this passage type in mind.

Preview

Preview the passage below, then read the following analysis to assess what you are already noticing and what other factors you could have considered.

The issue of climate change is undoubtedly one of the most important that humankind has faced. Yet as important as it is, it is merely one of hundreds of news items that may or may not be regularly reported in the news media. How the issue is treated in the press is a relevant inquiry to make, as research clearly indicates that an issue's salience in the media can translate directly into relevance in people's minds. We also know that media coverage is also linked to more than just awareness of a topic; it can also have an effect on policy debates and attitudes among audiences, for example.

We know that climate change is difficult for one person to openly observe, and specific weather events are not always directly linked to the larger issue of climate change. The ways that media stories on climate change are written or produced vary considerably and depend largely on media workers making explicit connections and reporting such through their outlets. However, the business of mediated news tends to favor certain kinds of coverage over others in the media. News producers look for specific crises, or spectacular events, often utilizing an episodic lens through which stories may be relayed to audiences. If there is no specific event, then the topic will be less likely to receive coverage. The issue of climate change may be important in the long term, but it may not receive ample coverage in the immediate short term. As a result, regardless of Al Gore's and Leonardo DiCaprio's efforts, the salience of global climate change may be reduced for the public, who are likely dealing with more pressing issues or things that are more immediately impactful on their lives; even the shift of presidential attention to issues such as jobs and the economy over climate change highlights this situation.

The media's attention to the problem of climate change varies considerably. One study found that coverage was events-based in France, whereas in the United States, "conflicts between scientists and politicians" received more emphasis. Coinciding with this, other studies have suggested that over the years, scientists were quoted less, and politicians more, as the topic became politicized. Another suggested that the issue of climate change was too abstract, that journalists did not have the proper background to assess the details, that there was a false sense of balance in the reports, and that scientists were not providing jargon-free language so that journalists and the public might easily understand the issue.

The topic may become relevant to news outfits when addressed in some way by government or supranational body officials, who may be dealing with incidences or policies that are linked to climate change. Besides having actual events occurring naturally in the environment, which is likely to be covered, we may see elites or organizations raising the issue and thus drawing news attention (e.g., by commissioning and issuing an environmental impact report). Research indicated that international climate summits and efforts of NGOs had a stronger impact on issue attention than weather events. This is likely also the case in the Gulf region where newspapers engage in a type of protocol journalism practicing "non-adversarial forms of journalism common in Gulf states, relying heavily on protocol news and content supplied by government and corporations," which emphasizes the importance of covering official activities and government-driven pronouncements. At the same time, the public relations literature indicates that actors are recognizing that getting out in front of an issue allows potentially for greater control of the narrative surrounding any story. That is to say, if an official of the Gulf Cooperation Council issues a press release, they are able to address the issue, while at the same time encourage a specific kind of coverage on the subject.

While a given country may not see a need to address or take immediate action on climate change, another country may be suffering the consequences of inaction. As a result of the potential for one country's policies to impact another, supranational organizations are becoming increasingly relevant in dealing with matters of regional and international dealings, including climate change.

Adapted from Freeman, B. C. (2016). Protecting the Gulf: Climate change coverage in GCC print media. Cogent Arts & Humanities, 3(1), 1212690. https://doi.org/10.1080/23311983.2016.1212690

The reference to climate change and its representation in the media indicates that this is likely a social sciences passage. Since the first sentences of the next three paragraphs build on the idea of how climate change is portrayed in the media, we can further categorize this as a historical passage, perhaps political science.

Since this passage appears straightforward, with simple sentence structure and vocabulary, this would be an Easy passage for many readers.

Choose

The passage has a straightforward topic and doesn't appear to contain significant changes in trajectory, meaning it is only of about medium difficulty. However, the length of the passage, and the fact that most of its paragraphs are long and cover multiple ideas, makes Highlighting an excellent method to use. Remember, generally Highlighting is best applied to difficult passages, but can also be a way to save time on Reading and Distilling long passages, so long as you are prepared to spend additional time answering questions!

Read and Distill

As you read, try to identify big picture topics in each paragraph. Then, use your highlighting tool to highlight one or two words that summarize those main ideas or will help you remember key points when you refer back to them. Aim to work through the passage as quickly as possible so that you have more time to come back and perform a deep analysis of part of the passage if a question specifically requires you to. If used efficiently, highlights will help you quickly locate the details needed to answer these future questions.

HIGHLIGHTING METHOD	
Passage	**Expert Thinking**
The issue of climate change is undoubtedly one of the most important that humankind has faced. Yet as important as it is, it is merely one of the hundreds of news items that may or may not be regularly reported in the news media. How the issue is treated in the press is a relevant inquiry to make, as research clearly indicates that an issue's salience in the media can translate directly into relevance in people's minds. We also know that media coverage is also linked to more than just awareness of a topic; it can also have an effect on policy debates and attitudes among audiences, for example.	What did the first paragraph reveal about the theme and the purpose of this passage? *The passage will likely talk about climate change and its relationship with the media. More specifically, the passage will investigate how the media treats, and perhaps should treat, climate change. We can highlight "treated in the press" to capture the main idea of this paragraph.*
We know that climate change is difficult for one person to openly observe, and specific weather events are not always directly linked to the larger issue of climate change. The ways that media stories on climate change are written or produced vary considerably and depend largely on media workers making explicit connections and reporting it through their outlets. However, the business of mediated news tends to favor certain kinds of coverage over others in the media. News producers look for specific crises, or spectacular events, often utilizing an episodic lens through which stories may be relayed to audiences. If there is no specific event, then the topic will be less likely to receive coverage. The issue of climate change may be important in the long term, but it may not receive ample coverage in the immediate short term. As a result, regardless of Al Gore's and Leonardo DiCaprio's efforts, the salience of global climate change may be reduced for the public, who are likely dealing with more pressing issues or things that are more immediately impactful on their lives; even the shift of presidential attention to issues such as jobs and the economy over climate change highlights this situation.	How can we use highlighting to tackle long paragraphs? What types of detail should we focus on? *We need our highlighting to break down this long paragraph. The first part of the paragraph seems to focus on how reports on climate change are heavily dependent on the media producing it. We can highlight "depend" to remind us of this, and to draw attention to the sentence surrounding it. We would not want to highlight the full phrase as it is wordy and would lower the efficiency of the highlight. The next idea is about how the media has a bias for immediate, singular events rather than focusing on the big picture. We should highlight "look for specific crises" to represent this idea. The last important idea is how this short-term focus lowers the salience of climate change significantly for the public. Here, we can highlight "reduced for the public" rather than "salience of global climate change" because the former better captures the action of the idea. The key is that the salience is reduced, and simply highlighting the word "salience" will not convey that information as well as "reduced for the public."*

HIGHLIGHTING METHOD

Passage	Expert Thinking
The media's attention to the problem of climate change varies considerably. One study found that coverage was events-based in France, whereas in the United States, "conflicts between scientists and politicians" received more emphasis. Coinciding with this, other studies have suggested that over the years, scientists were quoted less, and politicians more, as the topic became politicized. Another suggested that the issue of climate change was too abstract, that journalists did not have the proper background to assess the details, that there was a false sense of balance in the reports, and that scientists were not providing jargon-free language so that journalists and the public might easily understand the issue.	In a paragraph with a lot of details and examples, what should we highlight? *Since we know highlighting every detail will result in over-highlighting, which is not very productive, we need to focus on the main theme of these details. The first line already captures the "variability" aspect, so we won't highlight terms like "many factors." It seems that this is due to the "conflicts between scientists and politicians," which can be quickly summarized by the word "politicized."*
The topic may become relevant to news outfits when addressed in some way by government or supranational body officials, who may be dealing with incidences or policies that are linked to climate change. Besides having actual events occurring naturally in the environment, which is likely to be covered, we may see elites or organizations raising the issue and thus drawing news attention (e.g., by commissioning and issuing an environmental impact report). Research indicated that international climate summits and efforts of NGOs had a stronger impact on issue attention than weather events. This is likely also the case in the Gulf region where newspapers engage in a type of protocol journalism practicing "non-adversarial forms of journalism common in Gulf states, relying heavily on protocol news and content supplied by government and corporations," which emphasizes the importance of covering official activities and government-driven pronouncements. At the same time, the public relations literature indicates that actors are recognizing that getting out in front of an issue allows potentially for greater control of the narrative surrounding any story. That is to say, if an official of the Gulf Cooperation Council issues a press release, they are able to address the issue, while at the same time encourage a specific kind of coverage on the subject.	Another long paragraph with a lot of detail and examples. How do we use good highlighting to quickly digest this paragraph? *This paragraph introduces new actors in the climate change conversation: government and supranational bodies. We need to highlight a phrase that shows how this new idea elaborates on previous ones. Since the paragraph seems to focus on how governments and other groups can create additional media attention on the topic of climate change, we can highlight "organizations raising the issue."* *The next part introduced the Gulf region's journalism habits, which certainly stands apart from the rest of the passage. However, the general message is the same: government actions impact media activity on climate change and therefore awareness. We can also highlight "protocol journalism" to capture the idea that the key nature of the Gulf states' media is more government driven. Finally, the end of the paragraph introduces a new idea—that specific actors can not only increase media exposure but also "control the narrative" about the action as well.*

HIGHLIGHTING METHOD	
Passage	**Expert Thinking**
While a given country may not see a need to address or take immediate action on climate change, another country may be suffering the consequences of inaction. As a result of the potentials for one country's policies to impact another, supranational organizations are becoming increasingly relevant in dealing with matters of regional and international dealings, including climate change.	What does this last paragraph have to conclude? What is the final message? *This paragraph shows how one country's actions can impact others. So, we can highlight "supranational organizations" to capture the idea that institutions that go beyond nation states (what "supranational" really means) will be necessary to adequately address climate change.*

The goal of the Highlighting method is to make it easy to locate the key points of the passage, while not becoming distracted by superfluous details, examples, and digressions. In this case, our highlighting allows us to easily identify the author's main points, the structure of the passage, and key details. If a question requires it, we should feel confident that we could quickly locate where in the passage to research an answer. As a final step before moving on to the questions, always stop to consider the author's overall goal in writing the passage. In this case, the author uses the passage to discuss media attention to climate change and how that attention can be manipulated by various actors.

Conclusion

And so our discussion of how to approach passages draws to a close. The skills we've covered—understanding rhetorical elements, using keywords, reading critically, using the Kaplan Method for CARS Passages, analyzing argumentation and logic, recognizing varieties of passages, and anticipating questions—will serve you well not only on the MCAT but also in medical school and as a physician.

When you read a CARS passage, you use keywords to guide your reading and determine how information is put together. You then draw inferences and set expectations for where the author is likely to go with a given argument in order to anticipate the questions you'll be asked. Similarly, in medicine, you will listen actively to your patients, assessing whether various aspects of their chief complaint and background information are likely to help guide you to a diagnosis. By forming predictions about their diagnosis as you take their history, you can then set expectations for some of the other signs and symptoms the patient may exhibit, which then informs your physical exam. You can also anticipate the questions the patient will ask you—*What does this mean for me? Do I have to take medication for this? Does this put me at risk for anything else?*—and answer them in advance, to paint as comprehensive a picture as possible. Thus, it should come as no surprise that the *Critical Analysis and Reasoning Skills* section gets its name because it tests your ability not to comprehend dance theory, musicology, archaeology, or linguistics, but to understand how to analyze and reason through complex information.

Passages are only a part of the picture, though. While we need to read the passage to gain information, the real points come from the questions. In the next four chapters, we will shift our focus to these questions, starting with the Kaplan Method for CARS Questions and then focusing on the three major question type categories, as identified by the AAMC: *Foundations of Comprehension*, *Reasoning Within the Text*, and *Reasoning Beyond the Text.*

GO ONLINE

You've reviewed the strategy, now test your knowledge and critical thinking skills by completing a test-like passage set in your online resources!

CONCEPT AND STRATEGY SUMMARY

The Kaplan Passage Method

PREVIEW FOR DIFFICULTY

- Look for the big picture
- Assess the relative difficulty
- Decide to read *now* or *later*

CHOOSE YOUR APPROACH

- Highlighting: Best for high-difficulty passages or if low on time
- Outlining: Gives a moderate understanding of the passage and allows for more time to work on the questions
- Interrogating: Gives a strong understanding of passage but allows for less time to work on the questions

READ AND DISTILL THE MEANING OF EACH PARAGRAPH

- Recognize keywords to identify the most important and testable content in each paragraph
- Use your approach from the choose step to extract your major takeaways from each paragraph:
    - Highlighting—highlight 1–3 key terms and phrases per paragraph you can use to quickly locate information later
    - Outlining—create a brief label for each paragraph that summarizes the main idea of that paragraph
    - Interrogating—thoroughly examine each major idea presented in the paragraph and determine why and how the author is using the information to build an argument
- Identify the reason the passage was written before moving into the questions

Figure 7.2 The Kaplan Method for Passages in CARS

Humanities Passages

- **Humanities passages** include topics from architecture, art, dance, ethics, literature, music, philosophy, popular culture, religion, studies of diverse cultures, and theater. Many passages in the humanities can be considered arts passages or philosophical passages.
    - **Arts passages** tend to include strong opinions, quotations, and descriptive language to illustrate examples.
    - **Philosophical passages** tend to be abstract and heavy on logic, focusing heavily on concepts and relations between them; they often appeal to the reader's memory or imagination.

Social Sciences Passages

- **Social sciences passages** include topics from anthropology, archaeology, economics, education, geography, history, linguistics, political science, population health, psychology, sociology, and studies of diverse cultures. Many passages in the social sciences can be considered scientific passages or historical passages.
  - **Scientific passages** tend to include empirical studies and more subtle author opinions. Remember not to use any outside knowledge when working through these passages in the CARS section.
  - **Historical passages** tend to draw on historical events and quotations from sources alive at the time; they may include empirical studies or theoretical evidence, which can make them similar to the other passage varieties.

Worked Example

Use the following Worked Example, in tandem with the following practice passages, to internalize and apply the strategies described in this chapter. The Worked Example matches the specifications and style of a typical MCAT *Critical Analysis and Reasoning Skills* (CARS) passage.

Take a few moments to quickly glance over the passage in order to Preview and Choose your approach. The Outlining approach is a strong method for use with this passage. There are only two arguments to keep track of, and both are clearly laid out in terms of paragraph structure. In addition, paragraph length, sentence, and language complexity make it possible to create a short outline and still capture the main idea of the passage. As with all passages, any approach could be chosen and work for this passage, so, remember to practice all approaches as you start your CARS prep in order to determine which work best for you and in what situations!

OUTLINING METHOD

Passage	Expert Thinking
In *Prisoners of Men's Dreams*, published in 1992, Suzanne Gordon argues that American feminism has lost sight of its original goal of transforming the world into a kinder, gentler place. Gordon deplores the sort of feminism that has triumphed instead: a cold, ruthless, "equal-opportunity" feminism, which aims for women's entrance into the masculine public world and their achievement by male standards of excellence.	As with most passages, the first paragraph is where the author will give us at least a hint of the main idea. What is being introduced here? *The author mentions Suzanne Gordon, who we can abbreviate as S.G., and her argument on how American feminism has changed from kind and gentle to cold and ruthless.* Are there indications of opinions here? *Yes. The words used to describe S.G.'s position clearly indicate that she favors the "kind" form of feminism over the "cold" form. However, it's not yet clear whether the author endorses S.G.'s view.* P1: S.G.: Amer femin change = bad, kind → ruthless
The heart of the book consists of excerpts from a hundred interviews with career women, who do a lot of complaining about fatigue and disillusion. Gordon's subjects comprise an unsurprising lot, given her presupposition of modern feminism's focus on successful women as products of overcoming male-centric and male-infused social and business structures. At the end, Gordon calls for a National Care Agenda that would make "caregiving" rather than competition the ultimate American value.	Based on the previous paragraph, what are we expecting to logically follow? *Since we were introduced to a conclusion without any support, we would expect some evidence for that conclusion to come next. And this is exactly what this paragraph contains.* Is there any change in S.G.'s point of view or any indication of the author's opinion? *No. S.G. continues to emphasize the "caregiving" or kind idea of feminism, and the author's opinion remains unclear.* P2: Support for S.G.'s femin, Nat Care Agenda
Suzanne Gordon is obviously an intelligent, sympathetic, and well-meaning person, but *Prisoners of Men's Dreams* is a good example of the kind of sentimental, unlearned effusion that has become a staple of some types of contemporary feminism and that most people rightly ignore. And who could blame them? Rallying for the propulsion of women in the public and private spheres through carefully played attempts at the pity point are bound to be met with stolid expression and silenced ears.	The last two paragraphs discussed S.G.'s conclusion and the supporting evidence for it, but we still have not seen where the author stands on the issue. What is the author's opinion on the issue and what can help us determine this? *The author starts out the paragraph with a positive tone toward S.G. However, the Contrast keyword "but" precedes a change in tone: the author harshly criticizes S.G.'s idea of feminism.* Does the author provide any evidence to reinforce this point of view? *The sentence following the question provides an answer to it, a justification for why S.G.'s feminism should be ignored. The language is dense, but the author suggests some kind of problem with appealing to "pity." However, this is a detail we don't need to include in our outline.* P3: Auth: S.G. = well-meaning but unlearned

OUTLINING METHOD

Passage	Expert Thinking
Like a number of other American feminists, Gordon is completely out of her depth as a social analyst. Awkward, unintegrated quotes from Adam Smith and Woodrow Wilson are waved around to disguise her lack of familiarity with economics, history, and political science. Gordon's quote appropriations smack of the same short-sighted social phenomena that lead to "Keep Calm and Carry On" paraphernalia being plastered on the walls with complete disregard of manifest intent of the message.	The first sentence of this paragraph continues along the same line that the previous one did. This means that we are expecting more support for the author's stance unless we see a Contrast keyword. Does the author change the stance at any point? *No. The entire paragraph is dedicated to explaining why S.G. is a poor social analyst.* P4: Auth: S.G. = bad social analyst
Well, let me tell you: as a child of Italian immigrants, I happen to think that America is the most open, dynamic, creative nation on earth. As a scholar, I also know that it is capitalist America that produced the modern, independent woman. Never in history have women had more freedom of choice in regard to dress, behavior, career, and sexual orientation.	In the first sentence, we see a colon (:), which indicates that we have an example coming up and a continuation of the discussion. We only need to be on the lookout for a Contrast keyword if there is one. Does the author shift direction here? *No, the author continues to refute a view that is ascribed to S.G. by arguing for American capitalism.* P5: Auth: America = best for women now
And yet, Gordon's insistence on defining women as nurturant and compassionate drove me up the wall. My entire rebellion as a child in the Fifties was against this unctuous, preachy stuff coming from teachers, clergy, and Girl Scout leaders. This drivel was not the path to supporting and empowering this woman.	In this paragraph, we actually see the author showing strong emotion, which is uncommon in MCAT passages. Even though we see a Contrast keyword in the first line, it is there to signify the difference between S.G.'s and the author's opinions, which is not new info. P6: Auth = upset with S.G.'s feminism
This "transformative feminism" is just as repressive and reactionary as the "patriarchy" it claims to attack. Minerva save us from the cloying syrup of coercive compassion! What feminism does not need, it seems to me, is an endless recycling of Doris Day Fifties clichés about noble womanhood.	In the last paragraph, we see further strong opinion from the author. Did that opinion change compared to previous paragraphs? *No, it did not.* P7: Auth: S.G.'s "transform fem" = bad

Here's a sample outline for this passage:

P1. S.G.: Amer femin change = bad, kind → ruthless

P2. Support for S.G.'s femin, Nat Care Agenda

P3. Auth: S.G. = well-meaning but unlearned

P4. Auth: S.G. = bad social analyst

P5. Auth: America = best for women now

P6. Auth = upset with S.G.'s feminism

P7. Auth: S.G.'s "transform fem" = bad

PRACTICE QUESTIONS

Passage 1 (Questions 1–5)

In recent years, extensive media attention has been given to enormous damages awarded in the US civil litigation tort system. In 1996, 79-year-old Stella Liebeck was awarded $2.7 million in punitive damages from McDonald's after sustaining third-degree burns from spilled coffee. The system awarded Michael Gore nearly $4 million in 1994 after BMW sold him a car that had been repainted and sold as new.

Awards such as these spurred businesses, insurance companies, and lobbyists to claim an "explosion" of legal liability. In response, many legislators called for tort system reform that included limiting the amount of damages, controlling legal fees, and redefining the concept of "fault" administered by the judges. Jury verdicts that appear, on superficial inquiry, to be blatantly excessive seem to challenge our system of compensation. Some claim that juries find negligence in order to provide compensation for victims who have large medical bills and lost wages, at the expense of "deep pocket" defendants.

In his seminal article in the *Maryland Law Journal*, "Real World Torts: An Antidote to Anecdote," Marc Galanter examines the issue. As the title suggests, in order to investigate the tort system, Galanter used empirical data to examine whether, on the whole, these "anecdotes" truly represented how the system compensates injured parties.

Galanter found that all tort claims form a dispute pyramid charting the progress from an injury to a jury verdict. Injuries form the broad base of the pyramid. On the next level, approximately 8 percent of injuries become grievances (events for which an injury was noticed). Of these grievances, 85 percent become claims (where the injured brings the problem to the alleged wrongdoer), and 23.5 percent of claims become disputes (having failed to reach an informal agreement). Next, 58 percent of plaintiffs with claims contact a lawyer, and 32.8 percent of these result in a court filing. Of all court filings, only 7 percent result in a verdict, and only 34.7 percent of these are decided in favor of the plaintiff. This means that injured people gets a jury verdict in their favor only 0.007 percent of the time.

For example, medical malpractice results in approximately 100,000 deaths a year. At the tip of Galanter's pyramid, only 21 of the 100,000 deaths will result in a verdict. Finally, only 7 people will receive damage awards from a jury.

Galanter concludes that the system is hardly unbalanced in favor of plaintiffs. The proposed tort reform would actually increase insurance company profitability and reduce payments to the most seriously injured tort victims. Punitive damage awards are extremely rare, only applied in the most egregious cases, and always subject to judicial review. The awards discourage businesses from releasing harmful products into the stream of commerce.

Moreover, according to Galanter, court filings in the law division of the circuit court of Cook County have actually declined during the period from 1980 to 1994. His observations are consistent with a 1999 study by the National Center for State Courts, which found that tort filings have decreased by 9 percent since 1986. By looking at existing empirical data instead of isolated, inflammatory cases, legislators will be able to do a better job of deciding if the system is in need of reform and, if so, what type of reform is appropriate.

1. The author primarily mentions Liebeck's award (paragraph 1) in order to:
   - **A.** give an example to support the author's overall claim.
   - **B.** give an example of a verdict that is blatantly excessive.
   - **C.** give an example of a verdict that has caused legislators to call for tort reform.
   - **D.** introduce evidence for a conclusion made later in the passage.

2. Which of the following situations would be most analogous to the situation faced by a potential tort plaintiff, based on the information in paragraph 4?
   - **A.** A young basketball prospect trying to make it to the NBA
   - **B.** A group of children picking sides for a baseball game
   - **C.** A young, qualified woman looking for a job
   - **D.** An injured person trying to reach an emergency room

3. Based on the information in the passage, the author believes that Galanter's pyramid:
   - **I.** is applicable to medical claims.
   - **II.** should compel legislators to change their views.
   - **III.** is biased against "deep pocket" companies.

   - **A.** I only
   - **B.** II only
   - **C.** I and II only
   - **D.** I, II, and III

4. Which of the following, if true, would most WEAKEN the conclusion implied in paragraph 4?
   - **A.** Galanter's article was published in 1995.
   - **B.** A study showed that filings for divorce followed a much different pattern.
   - **C.** Galanter's study dealt with only product liability cases.
   - **D.** Most doctors carry medical malpractice insurance.

5. Based on the information in the passage, the author would argue for all of the following EXCEPT:
   - **A.** juries should not be so compassionate toward victims at the expense of wealthy businesses.
   - **B.** legislators should examine all data.
   - **C.** the media spotlight does not necessarily clarify problems.
   - **D.** courts might award damages as a way to ensure that businesses practice in the public's best interest.

Passage 2 (Question 6–12)

. . . [post-World-War-II Director of Policy Planning George F.] Kennan's strategy had been to try to bring about changes, over time, in the Soviet concept of international relations: to convince Russian leaders that their interests could be better served by learning to live with a diverse world rather than trying to remake it in their own image. Kennan had rejected both war and appeasement to accomplish this; it could only be done, he thought, through a long-term process of "behavior modification"—responding positively to whatever conciliatory initiatives emanated from the Kremlin, while firmly countering those that were not . . .

Kennan took the position that it was as important to reward the Kremlin for conciliatory gestures as it was to resist aggressive ones. This meant being prepared to engage in such negotiations that would produce mutually acceptable results. The [Truman] administration conveyed the appearance of being willing to discuss outstanding issues with Moscow, but Kennan regarded several of its major actions between 1948 and 1950 . . . [among them] the formation of the North Atlantic Treaty Organization (NATO) . . . would reinforce Soviet feelings of suspicion and insecurity, and hence, to narrow opportunities for negotiations . . .

The initiatives for the North Atlantic Treaty came from the Western Europeans themselves, and reflected the uneasiness they felt over the disparity in military power in Europe: the Russians had thirty divisions in Eastern and Central Europe alone; comparable combined US, British, and French forces came to fewer than ten divisions. Thus, the Western Union countries (Great Britain, France, and Benelux), together with the United States and Canada, agreed on the outlines of a treaty providing that an attack on any one of them would be regarded as an attack upon all.

Kennan had not been involved in the initial discussions, but he made clear his reservations about the course the administration chose to follow. These boiled down to three points: (1) that the Europeans had mistaken what was essentially a political threat for a military one, and that they consequently risked "a general preoccupation with military affairs, to the detriment of economic recovery"; (2) that outside the immediate North Atlantic, "which embraces a real community of defense interest firmly rooted in geography and tradition," any alliance extended to only some countries would render the rest more vulnerable . . .; (3) that an alliance made up of [Western European] nations would amount to "a final militarization of the present dividing-line through Europe," and that "no alteration, or obliteration, of that line could take place without having an accentuated military significance." Such a development might be unavoidable, "but our present policy is still directed . . . toward the eventual peaceful withdrawal of both the United States and the U.S.S.R. from the heart of Europe . . ."

These were not isolated concerns. There was worry in Washington that emphasis on rearmament would delay recovery; indeed, one condition attached to the administration's military assistance program for Western Europe was that economic revival would continue to have first priority. The question of how to include some countries without appearing to write off others also caused a great deal of agonizing: in the end, the administration stretched the concept of "North Atlantic" to encompass Italy, but refused to extend it to Greece, Turkey, Iran, or to form a comparable pact with non-communist countries of the Western Pacific. There was less concern about Kennan's third point simply because most observers already regarded division, by mid-1948, as an accomplished fact . . . Despite its reservations, the administration went on to conclude a North Atlantic Treaty and initiate a program of military assistance to its members. Kennan came to see, regretfully, that [because of military insecurity of Europeans] there were few alternatives . . .

6. The passage suggests that Kennan's "behavior modification" approach to changing the Soviet concept of international relations was:
   - A. unlikely to be successful if the Kremlin always made conciliatory gestures.
   - B. moderate in comparison with the approaches he decided to reject.
   - C. a logical outgrowth of his extensive background in behavioral psychology.
   - D. an extension of American strategy during World War II.

7. The passage suggests that the impetus for the formation of NATO was:
   - A. information that a Russian attack on Western Europe was impending.
   - B. the understanding that no nation could withstand a Russian attack without assistance.
   - C. the desire to aid the Western European economic recovery as well as to guarantee military assistance.
   - D. the fear that the Soviets would try to capitalize on their military advantage.

8. Kennan assumed which of the following in making his first counterpoint against NATO?
   - A. The formation of the military alliance would spur economic growth.
   - B. The presence of the thirty Soviet divisions did not mean they were going to attack.
   - C. The economic recovery in Europe had been progressing slowly.
   - D. It's always a mistake to make military affairs a higher priority than economic affairs.

9. Kennan's reaction to the administration's refusal to extend NATO membership to Greece, Turkey, or Iran was most likely one of:
   - A. understanding, because these countries did not have the same geographic defense interests as the Europeans.
   - B. approval of the fact that the concept of "North Atlantic" was not overextended.
   - C. disappointment that those countries could not now be employed in anti-Soviet strategy.
   - D. trepidation that these countries were now more open to potential enemy aggression.

10. Which of the following explains why the Truman administration was not worried about Kennan's objection that NATO would amount to "a final militarization of the present dividing-line through Europe"?
    - A. They believed that it would be possible to alter the line through negotiations of peaceful withdrawal.
    - B. They wanted to maintain a strong American military presence in Europe.
    - C. They felt it was too late to prevent the solidification of the dividing line.
    - D. Neither of Kennan's other two objections to NATO had given them cause for concern.

11. The passage suggests that, with regard to the reservations expressed by Kennan about NATO, the administration was:
    - A. often in agreement but ultimately undeterred.
    - B. unresponsive to his proposals for improvement.
    - C. able to counter each of his criticisms.
    - D. forced to carefully reexamine its objectives.

12. Which of the following conclusions would be most in accord with the theme of the passage?
    - A. Military alliances invariably have drawbacks that render them ineffective.
    - B. Behavioral modification is the only way to change a government's concept of international relations.
    - C. Coherent international strategy can flounder because of the military situation.
    - D. Negotiations should be conducted between two powers once military equilibrium has been established.

Answers follow on next page.

ANSWERS AND EXPLANATIONS

Passage 1 (Questions 1–5)

Sample Highlighting

P1. "litigation tort system"; **P2.** "call for tort system reform"; **P3.** "truly represent"; **P4.** "dispute pyramid" and "only 7 percent"; **P5.** "Medical malpractice"; **P6.** "damage awards"; **P7.** "declined" and "empirical data."

Sample Outline

P1. Introduction to tort system; examples of extreme damages awarded

P2. Insurance/lobbyists: tort awards too excessive

P3. Galanter examines empirical evidence

P4. Galanter pyramid findings: tiny amount of successful tort claims

P5. Malpractice ex: 7 of 100,000 win damages

P6. Galanter: system not in favor of plaintiffs; awards = good: keeps businesses in line

P7. Overall, tort filings declining without legislation, Auth: legislators should use empirical data

1. **C**

This Function question directs us back to Paragraph 1 which mentions extreme examples the tort system awards. Even without rereading, predict that Liebeck must be one of those very high monetary awards that caused lobbyists to be so aggressive in fighting against the tort system in general and call for reform. This matches **(C)**. **(A)** is not possible simply because the author does not overtly make any claims. The author is largely neutral and simply sets the facts in front of us to make our own decisions. **(B)** distorts the author's mention of "jury verdicts that appear, on superficial inquiry, to be blatantly excessive"—the use of the phrase *on superficial inquiry* implies that the author may not agree that these damages actually are excessive. Finally, **(D)** is vague enough that it could sound plausible, but there is no later argument or conclusion that requires Liebeck's award specifically. Generally, there isn't any conclusion about coffee, McDonald's, burns, or the elderly, that would depend on this example either.

2. **A**

The best description of "the situation faced by a potential tort plaintiff" in paragraph 4 is as follows: Galanter's pyramid findings demonstrated that only a tiny number of tort claims actually result in decisions in favor of the plaintiff. The main point is that there must be a tiny number of success stories from a much larger pool of individuals. This matches **(A)**. In each of the other cases, close to 100 percent success would be expected (or at least a much higher percentage than the number of young basketball prospects who make it to the NBA).

3. **C**

The combination of *Based on the information in the passage* and Roman numerals in the question stem tells us that this is a Scattered Detail question. In paragraphs 4 and 5, the author brings in the medical example to illustrate the extremely low rate of success that actually is seen in tort cases. This is not a blatant endorsement of Galanter, but coincides with Galanter's pyramid findings. Statement I is exactly the example that is being used, so eliminate **(B)**. Statement II is true because it is the recommended course of action given at the end of the passage, which is primarily supported by Galanter's pyramid argument. With **(A)** eliminated, we can investigate Statement III. This claim is actually made by lobbyists and insurance companies in paragraph 2—and is part of the larger claim that Galanter ultimately refutes. Thus, Statement III is untrue, making **(C)** the correct answer.

4. **C**

This is a Strengthen–Weaken (Beyond the Passage) question, so let's start by determining the conclusion implied by paragraph 4. The main point of Galanter's argument stems from the assumption that analyzing all of the empirical data will give the fullest picture and not allow anecdotal bias. If it were possible that the data Galanter used was false or incomplete for some reason, this would seriously weaken his argument overall. **(C)** reflects that prediction; if Galanter's study was only specific to product liability, then it can't be generalized to other similar cases or other tort suits. **(A)** reflects on the dates given in the passage—Galanter's study seems to investigate data until 1994. As long as Galanter's study was published after this point, there is no negative effect on his argument, eliminating this answer. The pattern of divorce cases, as described in **(B)**, has no effect on the argument because there is no reason to believe that divorce would (or wouldn't) follow the same patterns as tort cases. Finally, whether or not physicians have malpractice insurance does not appear to be related to the number of cases brought to court or decided in favor of the plaintiff, so **(D)** would also have no effect on Galanter's argument.

5. **A**

We are asked for arguments the author would make *based on the . . . passage*; with the word *EXCEPT* included, this must be a Scattered Inference question. While the author does not overtly state an opinion, it can be inferred that the author sides overall with Galanter's thesis. With that as a general prediction, we can eliminate any answer choice that fits with Galanter (and, by extension, the author)—and the one answer that does not fit is correct. This means that **(A)** is immediately correct. The author would not openly support being more lax to wealthy businesses at the potential detriment to victims. This position is exactly Opposite Galanter's, making it the correct answer. The other claims are all made in the passage: **(B)** is supported by the claim "By looking at existing empirical data, . . . legislators will be able to do a better job of deciding if the system is in need of reform." **(C)** is supported by the "extensive media attention" described in paragraph 1. **(D)** is supported in paragraph 6, where the author states that "awards discourage businesses from releasing harmful products into the stream of commerce."

Sample Highlighting

P1. "learning to live with" and "behavior modification"; **P2.** "willing to discuss" and "feelings of suspicion"; **P3.** "disparity in military"; **P4.** "mistaken," "vulnerable," "dividing-line," and "peaceful withdrawal"; **P5.** "economic revival," "stretched," and "less concern."

Sample Outline

P1. Kennan: use behavior modification to improve Soviet international relations

P2. Behavior modification requires positive and negative reinforcement, ex: Truman administration

P3. NATO = Western nations uneasy, think Soviet military too big: attack on 1 = attack on all

P4. Kennan's reservations about NATO: (1) political vs. military threat, (2) other countries vulnerable, (3) solidifies military line in Europe

P5. Administration agrees with Kennan's 1 and 2, assumes 3 is already fact; NATO still goes through

6. **B**

Because this question is asking about a conclusion the author implies, this is an Inference question of the Implication subtype. According to paragraph 1, behavior modifications were Kennan's advocated method to improve international relations with Soviets. It relied on consistent positive and negative responses, and not on military or extreme actions. This method is in contrast to the military strategy presented later in the passage, NATO—which Kennan opposed. Predict that Kennan's approach is more subtle and less aggressive than the other option. This matches closely with **(B)**. **(A)** isn't well-supported by the passage, and it comes across as an Opposite. *Conciliatory gestures* would mean that the Soviets are taking actions that the Western nations approve of, so this would theoretically mean that great progress (success) was underway. **(C)** ascribes an extensive background to Kennan that was never mentioned (or even hinted at) in the passage. Finally, **(D)** has two issues: first, American World-War-II strategy was not explicitly described in detail (to determine if this could be an offshoot from that), and second, it appears that Kennan's "*behavior modification*" strategy wasn't actually used by America—against Kennan's reservations.

7. **D**

This is another Inference question, so we start by identifying the relevant text in the passage. The most sensible place to go is the paragraph where NATO is first mentioned, paragraph 3. Here, we learned that Western nations were uneasy and felt that the Soviet military was too big. Specifically, Russia had more divisions than combined Western forces, and the West feared a possible (but entirely theoretical) attack. This matches closely with **(D)**. **(A)** intones a similar idea, but is Extreme and distorts the information. The attack was possible, but there was no evidence that *information* was available that showed the attack was *impending* (about to happen). **(B)** is similarly Extreme; even though certain Western European countries feared an invasion (and the passage hints at the dire fate of even smaller countries), the idea that *no nation could withstand a Russian attack* is simply too broad. Finally, **(C)** contradicts both Kennan and the administration, who say in the passage that *emphasis on rearmament would delay recovery*. Thus, while NATO did guarantee military assistance, it went directly against the principle of *aid[ing] Western European economic recovery*.

8. **B**

The word *assumed* tells us that this is an Inference question of the Assumption subtype. Our task is to find a missing piece of evidence for Kennan's first conclusion in paragraph 4. Kennan accused "the Europeans [of] mistak[ing] what was essentially a political threat for a military one." One way to attack an Assumption question is the Denial Test, described further in Chapter 9. In the Denial Test, one takes the opposite of each answer choice—whichever answer choice, when turned into its opposite, undermines Kennan's argument will be the correct answer. The opposite of **(A)** would be: *The formation of the military alliance would not spur economic growth*. This is a statement Kennan is likely to agree with, given the statement that "emphasis on rearmament would delay recovery" in paragraph 5, so it can be eliminated. The opposite of **(B)** would be: *The presence of the thirty Soviet divisions meant they were going to attack*. This undermines Kennan's argument because it means that the Europeans were not just responding to a political threat—there was a very real military threat as well. Because this negated statement ruins Kennan's argument, this must be the correct answer. Negating **(C)** would yield: *The economic recovery in Europe had been progressing quickly*. This assumption does not impact Kennan's argument and can be eliminated. Finally, **(D)** if negated would suggest that it is not always a mistake to favor military over economic affairs, but this doesn't negatively impact Kennan's argument: Kennan never suggests such an extreme position.

9. **D**

This is yet another Inference question, asking for Kennan's likely response. Kennan's second point of contention was that other countries are vulnerable. Kennan is worried that "any alliance extended to only some countries would render the rest more vulnerable." **(D)** paraphrases that prediction. Both **(A)** and **(B)** express a neutral to positive reaction, which does not match Kennan's actual response. **(C)** might sound reasonable in a real-world scenario, but Kennan was generally against uniting formally against Russia. It's doubtful, then, that he would *be disappoint[ed] that those countries could not now be employed in anti-Soviet strategy*.

10. **C**

This is a Detail question, asking for the Truman administration's thoughts on Kennan's final point of contention in paragraph 4. Paragraph 5 is where we learn what the administration's feelings actually are. The end of that paragraph serves as an excellent prediction: "most observers already regarded division, by mid-1948, as an accomplished fact." This matches **(C)**. **(A)** is a Faulty Use of Detail because it ascribes one of Kennan's opinions from the end of paragraph 4 to the Truman administration. **(B)** distorts the description of the troops in Europe. The passage discusses the Western European troops that are present, but doesn't mention how many—or whether there even are—American ones there. Further, there is no evidence in the passage that the Truman administration desired *a strong American military presence* in Europe at all. **(D)** is an Opposite: the administration agreed with Kennan on the first two points (mostly), giving them *cause for concern*.

11. **A**

This Inference question is quite similar to the Detail question that preceded it. We know from paragraph 5 that the Truman administration agreed with Kennan on two of his three points, but that they still decided to go ahead with the treaty "despite [his and their] reservations." This prediction matches nicely with answer **(A)**: the administration was *often in agreement* with Kennan but *ultimately undeterred* by the reservations that he had. **(B)** indicates that Kennan had specific *proposals*, but they were never mentioned or implied in the passage. Kennan had general strategies like "*behavior modification,*" but not specific proposals. **(C)** is patently untrue because the administration actually agreed with the majority (two out of three) of Kennan's points. Finally, **(D)** was also never directly discussed, and—if anything—the administration went ahead with actions to further *military assistance* and *economic revival* (the only two objectives that we're told about in the passage).

12. **C**

This is an excellent chance to turn the main idea of the passage into a prediction. Kennan begins by providing general suggestions on how to improve relations with Russia, before moving on to a more focused discussion on his reservations about NATO and his expectations that it would negatively impact Soviet relations. Kennan's "*behavior modification*" strategy, first introduced in paragraph 1, was hampered by the formation of NATO, and NATO was formed in response to the military imbalance in Europe. Thus, overall, Kennan clearly believed that the development of NATO was not beneficial to international relations with Russia. This matches closely with **(C)**. **(A)** and **(B)** are Extreme: NATO had *drawbacks*, sure, but was not *render[ed]...ineffective* by them. And behavioral modification is one way—but not the *only way—to change a government's concept of international relations*. **(D)** is what the members of NATO clearly thought, but it is neither a main theme of the passage nor what Kennan—the primary voice in the passage—thought.

CHAPTER 8

QUESTION AND ANSWER STRATEGY

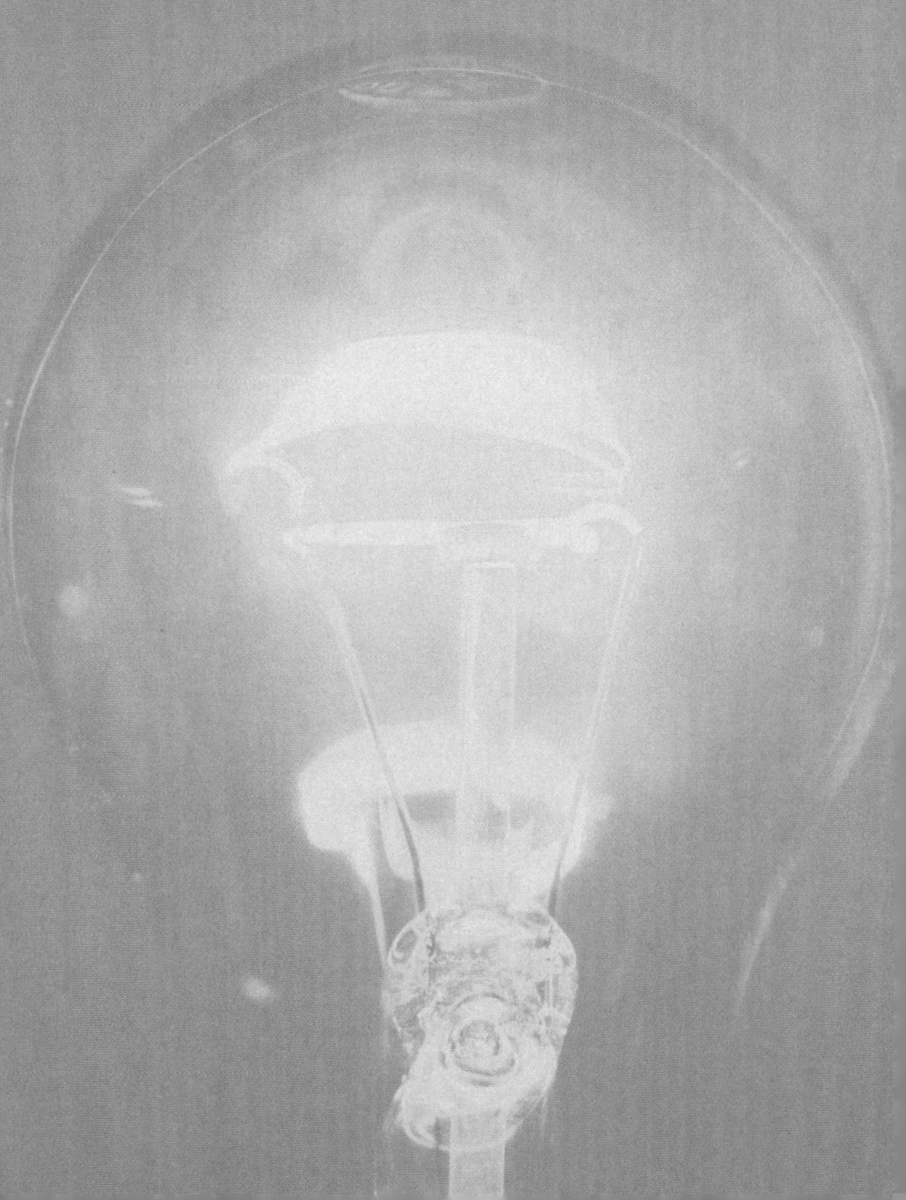

CHAPTER 8

QUESTION AND ANSWER STRATEGY

In This Chapter

Introduction

LEARNING OBJECTIVES

After Chapter 8, you will be able to:

- Solve questions by applying the Kaplan Method for CARS Questions: Type, Rephrase, Investigate, and Match
- Recognize and avoid common wrong answer pathologies
- Identify correct answers by focusing on scope, author agreement, and tone

Thus far, this book has examined the multifarious aspects of *Critical Analysis and Reasoning Skills* (CARS) passages. You've learned about their rhetorical and logical characteristics in Chapter 3. You've seen how to approach them with thoughtful Previewing in Chapter 4 and Reading in Chapter 5. Chapter 6 built on these foundations and focused on Distilling the meaning of the passage. Finally in Chapter 7, these threads were brought together as we discussed the Kaplan CARS Passage Strategy.

Now, we turn to question stems and answer choices. We'll start by outlining the Kaplan Method for CARS Questions. Subsequently, we'll look at the recurring traps that the testmaker sets for the unwary student, which we call Wrong Answer Pathologies. In the final portion, we'll consider the counterpart to pathologies: patterns common in correct answers.

8.1 The Kaplan Method for CARS Questions

In Chapter 7 of *MCAT CARS Review*, we introduced the Kaplan Method for CARS Passages and explored the ways in which it can be applied to a variety of passage types. In this section, we'll introduce the Kaplan CARS question method, which takes the basic form shown in Figure 8.1.

TYPE THE QUESTION

- Read the question, **NOT** the answers
- Identify the question type and difficulty
- Decide to attack *now* or *later* in the same passage

REPHRASE THE STEM

- Determine the task to be accomplished based on the question type
- Simplify the phrasing of the original question stem
- Translate the question into a specific piece of information you can either locate or infer

INVESTIGATE POTENTIAL SOLUTIONS

- Search for the answer in your interrogation, your outline, or the passage
- Predict what you can about the answer
- Be flexible if your initial approach fails: when in doubt, refer back to the passage itself

MATCH YOUR PREDICTION TO AN ANSWER CHOICE

- Search the answer choices for a response that is synonymous with your prediction
- Eliminate answer choices that diverge from the passage
- Select an answer and move on

Figure 8.1 The Kaplan Method for CARS Questions

Note: The Kaplan Method for CARS Questions, as well as the Kaplan Method for CARS Passages, CARS Question Types, and Wrong Answer Pathologies, are included as tear-out sheets in the back of this book.

Type

You might notice that the first step of the question method is similar to the Preview step of the Kaplan Method for CARS Passages. This is not a coincidence, but rather a consequence of the timing constraints posed by the MCAT. Every question is worth the same number of points, which means you want to avoid being derailed by any given question. It is important to approach the MCAT by being realistic about the nature of the exam: at least one or two questions within each section are so difficult that you're likely to get them wrong no matter how many minutes you spend on them. Though it may be tempting to spend a long time on a challenging question, it is better to recognize which questions those are right away, so you can instead use that time to gain more points by answering a larger number of more straightforward questions.

To that end, your first task with any question will be to read the stem, and *only* the stem, for the sake of deciding either to work on it *now* or to triage (to use an apt medical metaphor) and save it for *later in the passage*. In Chapter 4, we discussed the variety of factors used to assess the difficulty of passages during the Preview step of the Kaplan CARS Passage Method. For questions, however, difficulty is best assessed by identifying the **question type**. Because question type is the main variable to be focused on, this step of the Question Method is referred to as the Type step. The three broad categories of question that the AAMC presents in CARS were introduced in Chapter 1, and these categories can be further separated into more granular question types. Almost all *Foundations of Comprehension* questions fall into one of four types, while *Reasoning Within the Text* and *Reasoning Beyond the Text* categories can each be split into two predominant types, along with a handful of other types that only appear rarely. All of these question types are discussed in greater depth in Chapters 9–11. Starting each question with the Type step not only allows for proper assessment of difficulty but also makes Rephrasing and Investigating a question much easier. We will discuss how question type indicates difficulty and how to apply the Type step most effectively to each question type in Chapters 9–11.

Why avoid looking at the answer choices when determining question difficulty? The primary reason is that most of them are wrong. If you glance at just one of them, for instance, it's three times more likely to be incorrect than correct and could seriously mislead you about the question. Inexperienced test takers immediately jump to the answers, and the AAMC punishes them for it by wording wrong options attractively. Selecting the first answer that looks good without first thinking through the question itself is a recipe for failure. Thus, in the next steps, Rephrase and Investigate, we will cover how to think through the question before jumping to the answer choices in the Match step.

Rephrase

Once you have decided to work on a question, it's time to rephrase it. The **Rephrase** step goes beyond simply restating the question stem. The purpose of the Rephrase step is to provide you with a clear **task** and direction that you can use to approach the question. To this end, rephrase the question stem, focusing on the task itself and any relevant context given in the stem, to clearly identify what the question is demanding of you. Simpler question types like Main Idea and Definition-in-Context always involve one specific task (recognizing the big picture and explaining the meaning of part of the text as used in the passage, respectively). Even the most complex question types will have one major task to accomplish, though it may involve multiple steps. For example, almost all questions of the Apply type involve one of three tasks: gauging the author's response, predicting a likely outcome, or finding a good example (as described in Chapter 11 of *MCAT CARS Review*). Even if you feel you understand the task as phrased in the original question stem, the Rephrase step is an important check to ensure that you have fully read the question and know what you have to do to answer it. One of the most common causes of missed questions in the CARS section is misreading of question stems; taking the additional time to Rephrase will earn you valuable points on Test Day.

REAL WORLD

Think of question typing as equivalent to diagnosing a question. In medical school, you will learn the appropriate steps to undertake if a patient presents with chest pain, abdominal pain, a severe headache, confusion, and so on. The ten question types should be thought of as the "presentation" of the question, which determines the appropriate steps to take through the rest of the Kaplan Method for CARS Questions.

MCAT EXPERTISE

To avoid being enticed by wrong answer choices, cover all answer choices with your hand or your noteboard without touching the screen; leave them out of your field of view until you're ready for them in the Match step. Reading the answer choices can lead to the misinformation effect, discussed in Chapter 3 of *MCAT Behavioral Sciences Review.*

MCAT EXPERTISE

Rephrasing is a purely mental exercise. You won't want to waste time writing down a fresh question stem for each question. If a question stem is too distracting in its current form, consider using the strikethrough or highlight tools in the stem to focus on the most pertinent information.

Sometimes rephrasing is more difficult to accomplish, such as when the task is obscured by unclear language or by extraneous information in the stem. In either of these cases, try working your way backwards, starting with the part of the question directly before the question mark or colon (in a question that requires completing a sentence). Try to simplify the phrasing of that part first, and then connect it to any other relevant information in the stem. If you still struggle to identify the task of the question, consider the question type you found in the Type step, because different instances of the same question type often have similar tasks. Finally, don't waste time on Test Day writing out the rephrased question; simplifying the question in your head is usually sufficient.

It's worth pointing out that Rephrasing the stem into a task can be done even without any passage knowledge due to the standardization of CARS questions. Taking notice of common patterns will allow you to devise a plan of action even if you had difficulty with the passage itself. This skill of Rephrasing will require practice to master, but it's worth it. To help you master this step, here are some example question stems from the passage at the end of the chapter, along with sample rephrasing and identification of the task:

The author mentions Knorozov in the third paragraph in order to:

- Simplify: Why was Knorozov mentioned (P3)?
- Task: Identify how Knorozov was used to build the author's argument.

Which of the following would most call into question the author's argument about the complexity of Mayan writing?

- Simplify: What would weaken the author's argument about the complexity of Mayan writing?
- Task: Recall or refer to the author's argument on Mayan writing complexity and consider how each answer would affect that argument.

The author of the passage would be LEAST likely to agree with which of the following?

- Simplify: What would the author disagree with?
- Task: Recall or refer to the author's central ideas and arguments and identify which answer choice the author would disagree with.

MCAT EXPERTISE

If you are unable to Rephrase a question and arrive at a series of actionable steps, review the question types and their tasks in Chapters 9, 10, and 11.

Notice that the rephrased question stems are fairly similar to the original wordings. This is often the case, particularly for more straightforward questions. The simplest question stems may not even require a Rephrase: if the task is clearly stated in the stem without extraneous information, you can move on to the Investigate step. You should not need to simplify the phrasing of each question as part of your Rephrase step, but it is an option if you need to. Notice that the third question stem is simplified by converting the clunky "LEAST likely to agree" to *disagree*. Other troublesome phrases, such as double negatives, should also be simplified to avoid making careless misreading errors.

After the Rephrase step you should have a clear understanding of the task(s) to be completed in order to reach the correct answer. *How* you go about accomplishing those objectives is the focus of the Investigate step.

Investigate

The next step in the question and answer strategy is to **Investigate** potential solutions using your rephrasing of the question. Specifically, you will follow the directives in your Rephrase to **predict** what the correct answer should look like. How you use the passage to make this prediction depends on your passage approach (**Highlight**, **Outline**, or **Interrogate**).

Highlighting

A **Highlighting** approach to the passage should provide the location of important pieces of information and central ideas, but will typically lack details. Thus, the corresponding Investigate step should include rereading specific portions of the passage, as directed by the Rephrase step and the ideas highlighted. Ensure that you are not scanning the entirety of the passage during this step; instead consider the task of the question and your highlighting to determine where you should look. For example, consider the following rephrasing of the second question from above:

BRIDGE

Highlighting, Outlining, and Interrogating as approaches to CARS passages are covered in Chapters 6 and 7.

Rephrase: Understand the author's argument on the complexity of Mayan writing and consider how the answer choices affect that argument.

Investigate: Review what you've highlighted to locate where in the passage the complexity of Mayan writing was mentioned, and reread it for deeper understanding in order to form a prediction about what would weaken it.

Outlining

An **Outlining** approach to the passage should not only note the location of important pieces of information, but also summarize the central ideas of each paragraph. Thus, you should expect your written outline to be sufficient to form predictions for questions that require understanding of the main ideas. However, questions that ask about a specific detail or require inferences from passage information will often require returning to the passage. Again, ensure you are not scanning the entirety of the passage to make your prediction—use your outline to determine where to look. Now, consider the same example from before with outlining:

Rephrase: Understand the author's argument on the complexity of Mayan writing and consider how the answer choices affect that argument.

Investigate: Review your outline to find the relevant paragraph(s), as well as the conclusion of the argument if you've included it. Use that to predict what would weaken the argument or, if that's insufficient, return to the relevant paragraph(s) and review the argument's evidence to aid you.

Interrogating

An **Interrogating** approach to the passage will usually be in-depth enough to leave you with a solid understanding of the central ideas of the passage and their interconnections. As a result, you'll find you can answer many questions without even referring back to the passage. Of course, a quick double check of the passage is always allowed, but keep in mind that with an Interrogating approach there will not be much time left for passage research during the questions. Let's look at the same example one more time, now with a mind toward interrogating:

Rephrase: Understand the author's argument on the complexity of Mayan writing and consider how the answer choices affect that argument.

Investigate: Recall from your interrogation the conclusion of the argument and the type of evidence the author used to support it, and then consider how that argument might be weakened. Use that to make a prediction and only return to the passage if you get stuck.

MCAT EXPERTISE

If you ever find yourself searching the entirety of the passage during your Investigate step, you could be in trouble! When returning to the passage, you should know what you are looking for and its general location in the passage. If you don't know where in the passage to look, stop and save the question for later in the passage. It's likely that while answering the other questions in the passage, you will become more familiar with the passage and may even stumble upon the information you needed. This problem is most likely to occur when using the Highlighting method for the passage, but fortunately this quick approach should leave you with some extra time to investigate the questions.

While investigating your predictions, it's important to be mindful of how specific or in-depth your prediction should be. Predictions lay along a spectrum from focused to general. Focused predictions should be specific enough to allow you to directly match your prediction to an answer choice. In contrast, general predictions just set broad expectations about what the correct answer should include or exclude. Where your prediction falls on this spectrum primarily depends on the question type and question task. Your mantra for predicting should be *predict what you can*. Here are some examples:

The author mentions Knorozov in the third paragraph in order to:

- Focused prediction: This prediction should refer specifically to the role Knorozov plays in paragraph three.
- The correct answer choice will likely be a paraphrase of your prediction.

Which of the following would most call into question the author's argument about the complexity of Mayan writing?

- General prediction: This prediction begins with a summary of the author's conclusion about the complexity of Mayan writing and the kind of evidence used to support it. You'll be looking for something that weakens this argument.
- The correct answer will be a statement that weakens the argument by attacking its conclusion, its evidence, or an unstated assumption.

The author of the passage would be LEAST likely to agree with which of the following?

- General prediction: This prediction should consist of a brief recounting of the major ideas of the passage. You'll be looking for something inconsistent with one or more of these ideas.
- The correct answer will often be a statement that conflicts with one of the major ideas. However, in some cases, the disagreement may be with one of the more specific details of the passage, so you may need to use process of elimination, ruling out answer choices that are consistent with your summary of the major ideas.

Primed with these predictions, you will be better prepared to evaluate the array of misleading answer choices. But perhaps you're wondering: why bother with this Investigation step and with making predictions at all? After all, you've taken multiple choice tests before that included reading comprehension sections, and perhaps you've never needed much strategy to do well on them. Why change when it comes to CARS? There are several reasons why Investigating is key to success in CARS. For one, the CARS section is quite different from postsecondary reading comprehension exams. CARS passages are more likely to be on topics that you lack familiarity with, so you're less likely to have an intuitive sense of what the answers to questions will be. In addition, the answer choices in the CARS section are designed to lure testers who do not use the passage to answer the question. They often sound like something you read in the passage, or they appeal to outside information that seems right but is irrelevant. Without a thoughtful prediction you are more likely to fall for these alluring yet incorrect answer choices.

An apt analogy would be going to the grocery store hungry and without a shopping list. As many of us have experienced in this very situation, you are more likely to succumb to the influence of professional marketers, which may be peddling unhealthy food choices. If you had a grocery list, you'd be more likely to leave with healthier options and the items you actually require. Plus, you'd likely finish your grocery shopping faster, as you'll avoid aimlessly walking down the aisles trying to figure out what it was you were intending to bring home.

Finally, what should you do if you can't locate relevant information in the passage or don't know where to look? Typically such questions are best to try later, at the very end of a passage set, after you've researched the other questions and already reread some of the text. You may find that by the time you return to it, the effort you put into other questions ended up revealing an unhelpful question stem's correct answer. When you do attempt these questions, a general prediction and process of elimination will usually end up being the best plan. As a final note here, you will always want to return to these questions and at least guess before you leave the passage, since it is more effective in CARS to complete all questions when you work their relevant passages, rather than returning at the very end of the section.

Match

The final step of the question method is to **Match** your prediction to the correct answer. First evaluate the choices, and if you see an item that closely resembles what you expected, reread every word of that answer choice carefully to make sure it says precisely what you think it does. On the MCAT, correct answers are often vague and use synonyms to phrasings from the passage, rather than quoting the passage phrasing verbatim. This can make finding a match challenging. In addition, rarely will you find a word-for-word match for your prediction. Instead, your best bet is to look for a correspondence between ideas, by searching for a choice that shares a similar meaning with your prediction but uses different words. Once you have found such an answer, select it and move on to the next question. At that point, *reading the other choices will not be worth your time*—be confident that you've answered the question when you find that conceptual match.

If you aren't able to find a choice that is synonymous with your prediction, don't feel that you immediately need to resort to process of elimination (although that is a valid strategy). Part of being flexible is being able to revise your initial prediction; to set new expectations if the answer choices point you in that direction. The answer choices could technically be considered an additional source of information for arriving at the correct answer, but keep in mind that they include a lot of misinformation and so should be treated with caution.

MCAT EXPERTISE

If you read a question stem and it doesn't give you very much to work with, don't just say *I don't know* and jump straight to the answer choices. Take a moment to remember the main themes of the passage and then use those themes to help with the process of elimination. This will help you avoid being distracted by answer choices that are tempting but that do not fit with the passage.

Sometimes the question stem just doesn't give you very much to work with, and on other occasions you'll search through the answers for your prediction but find no likely match. In these cases, you will have to use the process of elimination, which may require multiple returns to the text as you research each choice individually. If you were able to set expectations during the Investigate step for wrong choices, however, less additional research will be required. Keep in mind that an answer requires only one major flaw for elimination, so the Wrong Answer Pathologies described in the next section can greatly expedite the process.

When all else fails, you can fall back on educated guessing. Eliminate whatever you can and then go with your gut among the remaining options. Never make a blind guess unless you're completely out of time and need to fill in an answer choice. Even crossing off just one wrong answer will increase your chances of randomly choosing the correct one by 33 percent, while crossing off two doubles your chances. If time allows, try working on any unanswered questions for the passage and see if that effort allows you to return to rule out additional incorrect options.

MCAT EXPERTISE

Should I compare answer choices?
Your default assumption should be that only one answer choice is flawless and that the others contain at least one flaw each, sufficient for ruling them out. However, you may occasionally find questions containing superlatives (*strongest challenge, most supported, best example,* and so on) in which you need to compare two or more answers that have the same effect but to different degrees. When making such comparisons, don't assume that an Extreme answer is necessarily wrong, especially if the question stem includes the words *if true* or similar language. A stronger answer that nevertheless produces the desired outcome would be the correct choice. Thankfully, questions that actually require distinctions of this type are rare.

8.2 Wrong Answer Pathologies

The AAMC has designed the CARS section to be a fair test of critical thinking skills. The focus on fairness is great news for test takers because it means that the questions are not designed to unfairly mislead you. There will never be a question with two correct answer choices or one in which all of the options are wrong. Each question you encounter on Test Day will have one right answer and three that are incorrect for at least one reason. Even better, there are only so many ways an answer can be incorrect; in fact, a few of them are found so frequently that you can treat them like recurring signs and symptoms of answer choice "illness." Naturally, we call them **Wrong Answer Pathologies**.

KEY CONCEPT

Wrong Answer Pathologies are the most frequent patterns found in incorrect answer choices. They are so common that you'll find at least one in just about every CARS question and even in many of the questions in the three science sections!

A choice only needs one fatal flaw to be worth eliminating, but often wrong answer options have many issues, so don't necessarily be alarmed if you ruled out a wrong answer for a different reason than the one mentioned in a practice question's explanation. In addition to having some occasional overlap, the following list of pathologies is not meant to be exhaustive; it includes only the four patterns we've identified as the most common through researching all of the released MCAT material. In the Kaplan Method for CARS Questions just detailed, pathologies function as recurring expectations for wrong answers, which you can assume fit for most of the questions you encounter (with a few significant departures noted below).

Note: The Wrong Answer Pathologies, as well as the Kaplan Method for CARS Passages, Kaplan Method for CARS Questions, and CARS Question Types, are included as tear-out sheets in the back of this book.

Faulty Use of Detail (FUD)

The testmaker will often include accurate reflections of passage details in wrong answers, primarily to appeal to those students who jump at the familiar language. What makes the use of a detail "faulty" is that it simply doesn't answer the question posed. It may be too specific for a question that requires a general answer, or it may be that the detail comes from the wrong part of the passage. Even if a choice comes from the right paragraph, the detail cited might not be relevant to the question posed, which is often the case in Strengthen–Weaken (Within the Passage) questions. A thorough prediction made in your Investigate step makes catching these FUDs much easier. Remember, the correct answer must be true to the passage and must answer the question!

Out of Scope (OS)

With the noteworthy exception of *Reasoning Beyond the Text* questions (for which this pathology does not usually apply), an answer choice that is outside the scope of the passage will inevitably be wrong. Typically, such answers will be on topic but will bring in some element that the text does not discuss. For instance, if an author never makes comparisons when discussing different ideas, an Out of Scope answer choice might involve the author ranking two or more concepts. Another common OS pattern is the suggestion that an entity or idea was the first of its kind or the most influential, when the author entirely avoids discussing its historical origins or impact. Remember that information that is unstated but strongly suggested (such as assumptions and implications) does not count as Out of Scope as will be the case with the correct answers to many *Reasoning Within the Text* questions, so don't be too quick to reject a choice as OS just because the author does not explicitly say it.

Opposite (OPP)

Whenever an answer choice contains information that directly conflicts with the passage, we call it an Opposite. Often the difference is due simply to the presence (or absence) of a single word like *not* or *except*, a prefix like *un–* or *a–*, or even a suffix like *–less* or *–free*. Be especially careful when stems or choices involve double (or triple) negatives; they're much less difficult to understand if you Rephrase them with fewer negations. Moreover, don't assume that just because two answer choices contradict each other that one of them has to be correct. For example, suppose an author argues that it is impossible to prove whether or not a divine being exists, a variant of the religious view known as *agnosticism*. If a question accompanying the passage were to ask for a claim the author agreed with, *God exists* and *There is no God* would both be Opposites of the correct answer.

REAL WORLD

A Faulty Use of Detail answer choice is like a politician who dodges a question during a debate:

- **Moderator:** *Candidate X, what will you do to improve the economy?*
- **Candidate X:** *You know, that's a wonderful question. My platform is to stand for all Americans' rights and to represent them fairly. If elected, I will help lead our country with integrity.*

Even if the candidate is being honest, the response just doesn't answer the question posed!

BRIDGE

The answers to many *Reasoning Within the Text* questions will be claims unstated by the passage that can nonetheless be inferred. Remember that inferences include assumptions (unstated evidence) and implications (unstated conclusions). Inferences are discussed in Chapter 3 of *MCAT CARS Review*.

Distortion (DIST)

Extreme answers and other answers that "twist" the ideas in the passage further than the author would prefer are what we call Distortions. Although they do not automatically make a choice incorrect, the following are common signals of distorted claims:

- Strong words like *all*, *always*, *none*, *never*, *impossible*, or *only*
- A prefix like *any*– or *every*–
- A suffix like –*est* or –*less*

MCAT authors typically do not take radical positions on issues, so it's worth noting whenever they do. In those rare cases, extreme choices would not actually be Distortions of the author's view and might be correct. The other major case in which extreme answer choices should not be immediately ruled out is when the question stem tells you that you can treat the answer choices as true and your task is only to gauge which would have the greatest impact on a particular argument. This is often the case with Strengthen–Weaken (Beyond the Passage) questions.

8.3 Signs of a Healthy Answer

If you're like most students prepping for the CARS section, you've had a dispute with at least one question explanation. *Hey, what about what the author says in the first paragraph?* you may have wondered, or perhaps you've said to yourself (or aloud!), *But couldn't you think of it like* this *instead?* While you may be in the habit of arguing for points with college professors, it does you no good to try to argue with the MCAT. The AAMC is extremely deliberate about how they word correct answers, always taking care to include exactly one per question.

Correct answer choices can vary widely in appearance, but there are patterns in how they are written as well. If the traps that can lead you astray on Test Day are appropriately called Wrong Answer Pathologies, then these corresponding traits can be thought of as indicators of good health. While the following signs are not enough by themselves to make an answer right, you can generally expect them to correspond to the correct choices in most types of questions.

MCAT EXPERTISE

The scope of a text refers to the particular aspects of a topic that the author addresses. Every paragraph in a CARS passage has its own scope, and together you can think of them as constituting the scope of the whole passage. Similarly, each answer choice will have its own scope, which could mimic any part of the author's discussion or depart from the passage entirely. It is essential to note that having the same scope doesn't necessarily mean having identical content. For instance, unstated assumptions in an argument are definitely within the scope of the passage, even though the information they contain is left unsaid by the author.

Appropriate Scope

You might say correct answers follow the "Goldilocks principle" when it comes to scope: not too broad, not too specific, but just right. The **scope** defines the limits of the discussion, or the particular aspects of the larger topic that the author really cares about. Consideration of the purpose of the passage as you Read and Distill should give you an idea of the scope of the passage overall. As a general rule (with an important exception), correct answers to MCAT questions will remain within the scope of the passage, but you can formulate a more precise expectation of what scope the correct answer needs to have by identifying the question's type and task.

Main Idea questions will always have correct answers that match the scope of the entire passage. They will typically include at least one wrong answer that is too focused (Faulty Use of Detail) and at least one that goes outside the passage entirely (Out of Scope). In contrast, Detail and Definition-in-Context questions usually require more refined scopes to identify their correct answer choices. If a clue directs you to a particular portion of the passage, the correct answer, more often than not, will have the same scope as the referenced text (or what immediately surrounds it).

The important exception to the rule that answers must remain within the scope of the author's discussion applies to the category of *Reasoning Beyond the Text* questions, addressed in Chapter 11. As their name suggests, these broaden the scope to new contexts, sometimes appearing to have no connection to the passage whatsoever. Note, however, that some *Reasoning Beyond the Text* questions will present new information in the stem but have answers that stick to the scope of the passage anyway. So be savvy with the answer choices in *Reasoning Beyond the Text* questions: while the correct answer choice will tend to lie slightly outside the scope of the passage, don't automatically rule out an answer choice just because it *happens* to be in scope.

Author Agreement

Unless a question stem explicitly asks about an alternative viewpoint or a challenge to the information presented in the passage, a correct answer choice will be consistent with what the author says. This is one reason why considerations of **tone** (most clearly reflected by Author keywords) are usually important enough to be worth including as you Read and Distill the passage (Highlight, Outline, Interrogate), as was recommended in Chapter 5. Generally, a correct answer should not contradict anything that the author says elsewhere in the passage, with the possible exception of sentences that speak in a different voice than the author's (such as quotes or references to others' opinions). In short, if it doesn't sound like something the author would say, you'll most likely want to rule it out.

Synonymous Phrasing

The correct answer should match your prediction made in your Investigate step, be it a focused or general prediction. When evaluating answer choices using your prediction, keep in mind that the AAMC often phrases their correct answers with different terms than those presented in the passage. This can lead students to mistakenly rule out correct answers as Out of Scope, simply because they contain unfamiliar language. Thus, when evaluating answer choices, it is key to remember that consistency of meaning is more important than consistency of phrasing.

Weaker Is Usually Better

One final consideration is a consequence of the fact that the AAMC tends to select passages by authors who do not take extreme views. You may find one or two passages on Test Day with more radical writers; for them, a stronger claim in the answer choices may actually be a good sign. However, for most of the passages you'll encounter, authors tend to use numerous Moderating keywords to limit the strength of their claims. Because a stronger claim has a higher burden of proof (that is, stronger evidence must be provided to support the claim), most authors avoid them to make what they write seem more plausible. Thus, you should generally give preference to answer choices that use weaker language such as *can*, *could*, *may*, *might*, *is possible*, *sometimes*, *often*, *likely*, *probably*, and *in some sense*. Exceptions to this tendency are questions that instruct you to consider the answer choices as true and gauge their effect on an argument. These were addressed earlier in the discussion of the Distortion Wrong Answer Pathology.

Conclusion

This chapter is only an introduction to the question method; the three chapters that follow are a necessary supplement for seeing how the method functions in practice. Specific strategy suggestions and Worked Examples are included for each of the most common question types and tasks, together constituting well more than 90 percent of what you'll encounter on Test Day. The explanations accompanying these sample questions will also identify their Wrong Answer Pathologies, giving you some concrete examples to go with the explanations provided here.

You've reviewed the strategy, now test your knowledge and critical thinking skills by completing a test-like passage set in your online resources!

GO ONLINE

CONCEPT AND STRATEGY SUMMARY

The Kaplan Method for CARS Questions

- **Type** the question
  - Read the question, **NOT** the answers
  - Identify the question type and difficulty
  - Decide to attack *now* or *later in the same passage*
- **Rephrase** the stem
  - Determine the task to be accomplished based on the question type
  - Simplify the phrasing of the original question stem
  - Translate the question into a specific piece of information you can either locate or infer
- **Investigate** potential solutions
  - Search for the answer in your interrogation, your outline, or the passage
  - Predict what you can about the answer
  - Be flexible if your initial approach fails: when in doubt, refer back to the passage itself
- **Match** your prediction to an answer choice
  - Search the answer choices for a response that is synonymous with your prediction
  - Eliminate answer choices that diverge from the passage
  - Select an answer and move on

Wrong Answer Pathologies

- **Faulty Use of Detail** (**FUD**) answer choices may be accurate statements, but they fail to answer the question posed.
  - The answer choice may be too specific for a question that requires a general answer.
  - The answer choice may use a detail from the wrong part of the passage.
  - The answer choice may be from the right paragraph but still not be relevant to the question posed.
- **Out of Scope** (**OS**) answer choices usually bring in some element that the passage does not discuss (and that cannot be inferred from the passage).
  - The answer choice may make connections or comparisons that the author did not discuss.
  - The answer choice may make a statement about the significance or history of an idea that the author did not.
  - The answer choice may otherwise bring in information that does not fall within the constraints of the passage.

- **Opposite** answer choices contain information that directly conflicts with the passage.
    - The answer choice may contain (or omit) a single word like *not* or *except*.
    - The answer choice may contain a prefix like *un–* or *a–* or a suffix like *–less* or *–free*.
    - The answer choice may say that a given claim is true, when the author is ambivalent.
- **Distortion** answer choices are extreme or twist the ideas in the passage further than the author would prefer.
    - The answer choice may use a strong word like *all*, *always*, *none*, *never*, *impossible*, or *only*.
    - The answer choice may contain a prefix like *any–* or *every–* or a suffix like *–est* or *–less*.
    - The answer choice is usually more radical than the author because radical positions are hard to support and are rare in MCAT passages.

Signs of a Healthy Answer

- Correct answers tend to have the right **scope**—not too broad, not too specific, but just right.
- Correct answers tend to be consistent with the author's statements and opinions.
- Correct answers use language that differs from the passage but is still consistent with the ideas discussed.
- Correct answers tend to use Moderating keywords, such as *can*, *could*, *may*, *might*, *is possible*, *sometimes*, *often*, *likely*, *probably*, and *in some sense*.

Worked Example

Use the Worked Example on the next page in tandem with the subsequent practice passages, to internalize and apply the strategies described in this chapter. The Worked Example matches the specifications and style of a typical MCAT *Critical Analysis and Reasoning Skills* (CARS) passage.

Take a few moments to quickly glance over the passage in order to Preview and Choose your approach. The following passage is well suited for the Interrogating method. With a simple structure and four medium-length paragraphs, you will be able to spend more time thinking about the connection between paragraphs and why the author includes specific details. The passage is informative and relatively straightforward, and while there are a lot of details, they are strongly tied to the central argument of the passage, making Interrogating useful for identifying the unique contribution of each major new argument component added. As with all passages, any approach could be chosen and work for this passage. So, remember to practice all approaches as you start your CARS prep in order to determine the approach that works best for you in different passage types!

INTERROGATING METHOD

Passage	Expert Thinking
Mayan signs are by nature highly pictorial, often representing in considerable detail animals, people, body parts, and objects of daily life. The pictorial principle is taken to the extreme in inscriptions composed of "full-figure" glyphs, in which individual signs and numbers become animated and are shown interacting with one another. None of this should be taken to mean that the Mayans had simple picture writing. The Mayans wrote both logographically and phonetically, and within its phonetic system alone, the Mayans had multiple options. All English words are formed from various combinations of only 26 phonetic signs. By contrast, all Mayan words can be formed from various combinations of nearly 800 consonant–vowel glyphs, each representing a full syllable. Sounds are formed by combining a particular consonant with one of the five vowels (hence a syllabary, rather than alphabet).	S1–2. Why did the author emphasize that Mayan signs are highly detailed? *The details in the images provide a lot of information, in contrast to the reader's possible preconception that signs are often simple and straightforward.* S3–7. Why is it important to note that the Mayans had two writing systems? Why does the author bring up the English language? *The author distinguishes between logographic (or pictorial) signs and phonetic (or syllabic) ones, explaining that the Mayans used both. The author uses the English language as a contrast, demonstrating that its phonetic alphabet is simpler than the Mayan phonetic syllabary, just one of their two writings systems. This is consistent with the first two sentences, providing further evidence that the Mayans had a complex system of writing.*
The combination of consonant–vowel syllabic glyphs and logographs enabled the scribes a variety of choices to write the words of their texts in detail. For example, one very common honorific title in Mayan texts is *ahaw*, meaning "lord" or "noble." *Ahaw* may be written in logographic form as a head in profile, with the distinctive headband or scarf that marked the highest nobility in Mayan society. But it is also possible to write the word as a combination of three phonetic, syllabic signs: *a–ha–wa*. Likewise, the word *pakal* ("shield") can be indicated by a depiction of a shield or by the combination of syllabic elements *pa–ka–la*.	S1–5. Why does the author describe how specific words like *ahaw* work in the Mayan language? *These words are used as examples of how logographs and phonetic language can describe the same word. This provides further evidence for the argument the author introduced in the first paragraph: having a variety of ways to depict the same concept adds to the overall complexity and utility of the Mayan writing system.*

INTERROGATING METHOD

Passage	Expert Thinking
Because many Mayan signs remain undeciphered, it's not possible to state precisely the relative proportions of logographic and syllabic signs. But a significant number of the logograms have been deciphered, and the number of deciphered syllabic signs keeps growing. Epigraphers have filled more than half of the syllabic grid (which plots the consonants of the spoken Mayan language against its vowels and thus represents the totality of signs needed to write the language). Half of the grid may seem a meager proportion, but it must be remembered that the discovery of the structure of the syllabic elements—Knorozov's main contribution—was made only a little more than 30 years ago. Furthermore, the consonant-vowel syllables that are already understood are the common ones. Many of the empty spaces in the syllabic grid remain so because they are linguistically rare; rare signs are more difficult to translate than common ones.	S1–5. Why has the author turned to discussing undeciphered Mayan signs? Why is it reasonable that approximately half of the possible Mayan signs have not been deciphered? *Keep in mind that the author is trying to build an argument that the Mayans had a particularly complex system of writing. The fact that the system is not completely understood could serve as a potential objection to this conclusion, so the author tries to set the record straight here. While a lot of the syllabary is unknown, researchers can at least identify what pieces are missing based on their knowledge of the Mayan language. It makes sense that only half have been deciphered because most of the missing pieces are uncommonly used syllables anyway and because the process of deciphering has only been going on for about 30 years (as the reference to Knorozov serves to highlight).*
Nonetheless, the pace of phonetic decipherment is bound to increase in the coming years as more resources are trained on it. One aspect of Mayan writing that may complicate this progress is the fact that different signs can have the same value. Two signs that share a value are known as allographs. Such equivalences are common in Mayan texts (there are at least five different signs that could be chosen to represent the Mayan syllable *ba*). Each scribe chose from several different signs to convey the sounds. In evaluating a particular phonetic interpretation of a syllable, it's helpful to identify as many of the variant forms as possible; the process of recognizing allographs depends on the slow work of comparing many texts in order to find variant spellings of the same word.	S1–5. Why do allographs possibly hinder deciphering Mayan writing? How does this relate to the bigger idea introduced in P1? *Allographs are two signs that share the same value, and the researchers need to compare many texts to find the different variants, slowing down the process. Ultimately, allographs relate to the central argument introduced in P1 because they indicate the complexity of Mayan writing.* *After reading the whole passage, the goal should be evident: the author writes in order to argue that the Mayan system of writing is distinctively complex and to explain some of this complexity.*

Question	Analysis
1. The author mentions Knorozov in the third paragraph in order to:	This is a Function question, which is a *Foundations of Comprehension* question. Because we read the passage noticing its rhetoric, this is a question that we can do right away. The question stem even tells us to go to paragraph 3, which deals with progress in completing the syllabic grid. Knorozov was used to justify why only about half of the syllabic grid has been filled in—he discovered the syllable structure only "a little more than 30 years ago."
A. prove that the recent discovery of Mayan signs has led to its lack of decipherment.	**(A)** is a Distortion on two counts: first, the recent discovery is of the syllable structure of the language, not the *Mayan signs* themselves; second, *prove* is far too strong a word—the author is not nearly so extreme.
B. offer an explanation for what may appear to be a relative paucity in the completion of the Mayan syllabic grid.	**(B)** fits and is the correct answer. Knorozov and his recent discovery is part of the justification for why there is so little filled in on the syllabic grid. This also fits with our interrogation of paragraph 3.
C. argue that expert linguists have been unsuccessful in their attempts to decipher and understand allographic Mayan signs.	**(C)** is a Faulty Use of Detail; the challenge presented by allographs is described in paragraph 4 and is not associated with Knorozov.
D. show how the understanding of other linguistic structures may improve the comprehension of Mayan syllabic signs.	**(D)** is a classic Out of Scope answer choice as *other linguistic structures* are never discussed in paragraph 3.

Question	Analysis
2. As used in the passage, the term "logographic" most closely refers to:	This is a Definition-in-Context question. As another *Foundations of Comprehension* question, we can do this right away. We saw "logographic" in paragraphs 1 and 2. When introduced in paragraph 1, the gist of the word was that it was a picture. Paragraph 2 then describes the writing of the word *Ahaw*: "Ahaw may be written in logographic form as a head in profile." Because a picture is used to represent the word in *logographic* form, they must be pictorial symbols.
A. a written phonetic representation of a word.	**(A)** and **(B)** are both Opposites that describe the other form of Mayan writing presented in the passage.
B. syllabic division of an individual word.	
C. representation of an idea as an image.	**(C)** simply paraphrases the idea of pictorial representation, so it's the correct answer.
D. a visual picture of an idiomatic phrase.	**(D)** is a Distortion; although logographs are visual representations, the author suggests that they represent single words, not entire *idiomatic phrase*[s].

Question	Analysis
3. The author of the passage would be LEAST likely to agree with which of the following?	This is an Apply question. Because this is a *Reasoning Beyond the Text* question type, this is one that we should save for later. The question asks what *the author . . . would be LEAST likely to agree with*, so the answer should be inconsistent with the author's beliefs. The author believes that Mayan writing is complex for several reasons but is steadily being deciphered. The correct answer will contradict this or some other point from the passage.
A. Languages with writing composed of pictorial signs can demonstrate a remarkable degree of complexity and detail.	**(A)** is an Opposite; the author would certainly agree with this statement, having expressed the belief that the language is more than just "simple picture writing"; the description of the "800 . . . glyphs," multiple ways of writ-ing the same word, and allographs support this idea.
B. Linguistic signs based on syllabic or phonetic coding may be easier to decipher than those based on visual images.	**(B)** is Out of Scope; this comparison is never made, so it's impossible to say whether the author would agree with this statement or not.
C. Pictorial languages are restricted to the expression of simple ideas because of their emphasis on images.	The author would certainly disagree with **(C)**, making it the correct answer. Mayan writing doesn't convey only *simple ideas*, the author would argue, because it's more than just "simple picture writing."
D. The existence of allographs in Mayan signs indicates the complexity of this linguistic system.	**(D)** is an Opposite; this summarizes the point of paragraph 4: allographs are a complication that makes deciphering Mayan writing more difficult.

Question	Analysis
4. The author discusses the words *ahaw* and *pakal* in order to:	This is another Function question, so we should do it right away. Where did we see the words *ahaw* and *pakal*? The words were in paragraph 2. The purpose of paragraph 2 is to explain that a logograph (picture) and a combination of syllables can both be used to represent the same word.
A. estimate the number of meanings that some common Mayan words may possess.	**(A)** Distorts the author's point: the same word can have multiple ways of being represented, not multiple *meanings*.
B. compare the flexibility of Mayan logographs to that of consonant–vowel syllables.	**(B)** is Out of Scope, as the author does not suggest a comparison between the *flexibility* of phonetic and logographic writing—just that they can both be used to write certain words.
C. illustrate the difficulty of filling in the syllabic grid due to words being linguistically rare.	**(C)** is a Faulty Use of Detail; even though *the syllabic grid* has been slow to fill due to *linguistically rare* words, this is a point from paragraph 3 rather than paragraph 2, where *ahaw* and *pakal* are introduced.
D. demonstrate that Mayan words may appear in both logographic and syllabic form.	**(D)** matches cleanly with the prediction and is the correct answer.

Question	Analysis
5. According to the author, which of the following would best address some of the decipherment problems associated with Mayan signs?	This is an Inference question, asking for a conclusion the author did not explicitly state, or an implication. Because the example is not explicitly stated in the passage, we should save this question until later. Problems with *decipherment* are mentioned in paragraphs 3 and 4. In paragraph 3, the author noted that the remaining unknown syllables are rarely used and thus harder to translate. Paragraph 4 continued the idea by talking about allographs. The author does say in the last lines of the passage that deciphering allographs depends on *comparing many texts*. Look for an answer that sounds like the points in either of these two paragraphs.
A. Additional financial and scholarly resources should be directed toward this linguistic effort.	**(A)** is a Distortion; the author argues at the beginning of paragraph 4 that the "pace of phonetic decipherment is bound to increase" as more resources are trained on it, but stops short of saying that more resources *should* be trained on it, or suggesting what *form* those resources might take. This answer choice changes a statement of fact to a recommendation, as well as interpreting *resources* far more specifically than can be justified by the passage.
B. More attention should be focused on identifying logographic signs than on categorizing syllabic signs.	**(B)** is an Opposite; because allographs are phonetic representations, the author would argue that if anything, there should be more attention given to syllabic signs than logographic signs—many of which have already been deciphered.
C. Scholars should prioritize the completion of the syllabic grid.	**(C)** Distorts the author and is extreme; the author actually seems content with the current, incomplete state of the grid and its slow but steady progress toward being filled in.
D. Careful study of comparative texts should continue in order to evaluate phonetic interpretation of each syllable.	**(D)** closely reflects statements at the end of paragraph 4 that "the process of recognizing allographs depends on the slow work of comparing many texts in order to find variant spellings of the same word." That makes it correct.

Question	Analysis
6. The author implies which of the following about the ratio of logographic to syllabic signs in Mayan writing?	This is an Inference question and best saved for later. The question stem references the ratio between two types of signs. Refer back to paragraph 3 where this is discussed. The author says that "it's not possible to state precisely the relative proportions of logographic and syllabic signs" because many of the signs are undeciphered. The clear implication is that as these signs are deciphered, the ratio will become clearer.
A. Researchers disagree about the correct way to determine it.	**(A)** is Out of Scope; the author suggests that the lack of a ratio is due to a lack of information, not because of *disagree*[ment].
B. Its practical value has failed to attract serious attention.	**(B)** is also Out of Scope, as the author doesn't indicate anything about the *practical value* of knowing this ratio.
C. A meaningful ratio will likely never be established.	**(C)** is a Distortion; the author mentions that the number of deciphered signs is growing. So, if anything, the author would argue that a ratio may be established some day in the future.
D. More work must be done before the ratio can be determined.	**(D)** matches perfectly. Once all logographs and syllables are translated, we would know the ratio—but that will require *more work*.

Question	Analysis
7. Which of the following would most call into question the author's argument about the complexity of Mayan writing?	This is a Strengthen–Weaken (Beyond the Passage) question, so we should save it until last. We need to *call* the *complexity of Mayan writing into question*; this means we need to find that answer that would make the author's conclusion less likely. Where do we see the author's argument about the complexity of Mayan writing? In paragraph 3, the author states that Mayan writing is complex due to the fact that it includes both logographic and syllabic systems. In paragraph 4, the author goes on to state that part of the problem in deciphering Mayan writing is the presence of so many allographs that scribes had to choose from when writing. To make the conclusion about complexity less likely, we need to find a statement that challenges the conclusion, a piece of evidence used to support it, or an unstated assumption.
A. It has recently been discovered that allographs are actually just stylistic differences between scribes.	**(A)** is exactly what we are looking for: if allographs are actually just stylistic differences—and not "different signs that could be chosen to represent" the same syllable, then one key piece of evidence for the author's conclusion is refuted. While this isn't a particularly strong challenge to the argument (because there's a lot more evidence provided for it in the passage), it's stronger than any of the other choices, which makes it correct.
B. The syllabic grid is only partially complete.	**(B)** is a statement made by the author in paragraph 3. The author explains in that paragraph why this lack of completion is reasonable, so this choice doesn't challenge the author's argument.
C. Other pictorial languages, such as Egyptian, have been deciphered.	**(C)** is incorrect because the relative extent of decipherment was shown in paragraph 3 not to be relevant to the author's conclusion.
D. Languages based on logographs are less complicated than modern syllabic languages.	**(D)** is incorrect because Mayan is not a purely logographic language, but uses both logographs and a phonetic syllabary. The comparison here is irrelevant to the author's argument.

PRACTICE QUESTIONS

Passage 1 (Questions 1–7)

The rich analysis of Fernand Braudel and his fellow *Annales* historians have made significant contributions to historical theory and research, not the least of which is a broad expansion of potential routes of scholastic analysis. In a departure from traditional approaches, the *Annales* historians assume that history cannot be limited to a simple recounting of conscious human actions, but must be understood in the context of forces and material conditions that underlie human behavior. Braudel was the first *Annales* historian to gain widespread support for the idea that history should synthesize data from various social sciences, especially economics, in order to provide a broader view of human societies over time (although Febvre and Bloch, founders of the *Annales* school, originated this approach).

Braudel conceived of history as the dynamic interaction of three temporalities. The first of these, the *evenementielle*, involved short-lived dramatic "events," such as battles, revolutions, and the actions of great individuals, which had preoccupied traditional historians like Carlyle. *Conjonctures* was Braudel's term for larger cyclical processes that might last up to half a century. The *longue durée*, a historical wave of great length, was for Braudel the most fascinating of the three temporalities. Here he focused on those aspects of everyday life that might remain relatively unchanged for centuries. What people ate, what they wore, their means and routes of travel—for Braudel, these things create "structures" that define the limits of potential social change for hundreds of years at a time.

Braudel's concept of the *longue durée* extended the perspective of historical physical space as well as time. Until the *Annales* school, historians had generally taken the juridical political unit—the nation-state, duchy, or whatever—as their starting point. Yet, when such enormous timespans are considered, geographical features may well have more significance for human populations than national borders. In his doctoral thesis, a seminal work on the Mediterranean during the reign of Philip II, Braudel treated the geohistory of the entire region as a "structure" that had exerted myriad influences on human lifeways since the first settlements on the shores of the Mediterranean Sea. So, the reader is given such esoteric information as the list of products that came to Spanish shores from North Africa, the seasonal routes followed by Mediterranean sheep and their shepherds, and the cities where the best ship timber could be bought.

Braudel has been faulted for the impression of his approach. With his Rabelaisian delight in concrete detail, Braudel vastly extended the realm of relevant phenomena; but this very achievement made it difficult to delimit the boundaries of observation, a task necessary to beginning any social analysis. Indeed, to identify an appropriate scope of work when all options and directions for academic inquiry are available before one's eyes is a nearly impossible task. Further, Braudel and other *Annales* historians minimize the differences among the social sciences. Nevertheless, the many similarly designed studies aimed at both professional and popular audiences indicate that Braudel asked significant questions that traditional historians had overlooked.

1. The author refers to the work of Febvre and Bloch in order to:

- **A.** illustrate the need to delimit the boundaries of observation.
- **B.** suggest the relevance of economics to historical investigation.
- **C.** debate the need for combining various social science approaches.
- **D.** show that previous *Annales* historians anticipated Braudel's focus on economics.

2. In the third paragraph, the author is primarily concerned with discussing:
   - **A.** Braudel's fascination with obscure facts.
   - **B.** Braudel's depiction of the role of geography in human history.
   - **C.** the geography of the Mediterranean region.
   - **D.** the irrelevance of national borders.

3. The passage suggests that, compared with traditional historians, *Annales* historians are:
   - **A.** more interested in other social sciences than in history.
   - **B.** critical of the achievements of famous historical figures.
   - **C.** skeptical of the validity of most economic research.
   - **D.** more interested in the underlying context of human behavior.

4. Which of the following statements would be most likely to follow the last sentence of the passage?
   - **A.** Few such studies, however, have been written by trained economists.
   - **B.** It is time, perhaps, for a revival of the Carlylean emphasis on personalities.
   - **C.** Many historians believe that Braudel's conception of three distinct "temporalities" is an oversimplification.
   - **D.** Such diverse works as Gascon's study of the Lyon and Barbara Tuchman's *A Distant Mirror* testify to his relevance.

5. According to the passage, some historians are critical of Braudel's perspective for which of the following reasons?
   - **A.** It seeks structures that underlie all forms of social activity.
   - **B.** It assumes a greater similarity among the social sciences than actually exists.
   - **C.** It fails to consider the relationship between short-term events and long-term social activity.
   - **D.** It rigidly defines boundaries for social analysis.

6. Which of the following historical phenomena would the author most likely consider an example of the *longue durée*?
   - **A.** Julius Caesar's crossing of the Rubicon, which led to a four-year civil war in Rome
   - **B.** The occurrence in ancient Rome of devastating malaria outbreaks roughly every half-century
   - **C.** A gradual shift toward a drier Mediterranean climate that lasted from 250 to 600 c.e. and impacted food availability and daily life
   - **D.** The battle of Carrhae in 53 b.c.e., in which the Parthians exterminated a large Roman army

7. Suppose Braudel was once quoted as saying, "For me, the most interesting aspects of history are those in which one person's decisions turned the tides of history." What relevance would this new information have for the passage?
   - **A.** It would weaken the author's claim that Braudel was most interested in the *longue durée* temporality.
   - **B.** It would weaken the author's claim that Braudel was not interested in the actions of great individuals.
   - **C.** It would strengthen the author's claim that Braudel was most interested in the *evenementielle* temporality.
   - **D.** It would strengthen the author's claim that Braudel considered the best historical analysis to focus on the actions of great individuals.

ANSWERS AND EXPLANATIONS

Passage 1 (Questions 1–7)

Sample Highlighting

P1. "synthesize data"; **P2.** "dramatic event," "cyclical processes," and "aspects of everyday life"; **P3.** "geographical features"; **P4.** "delimit the boundaries" and "minimizes difference."

Sample Outline

P1. *Annales vs.* traditional historians; Braudel popularized

P2. Braudel's three temporalities

P3. Expansion on *longue durée* as geohistory

P4. Braudel critics: "scope too broad, differences of social sciences blurred"; Author: "but asked new questions"

1. **D**

A classic Function question: Why did the author refer to Febvre and Bloch? Go back to the end of paragraph 1 where Febvre and Bloch are mentioned and read the surrounding text: "Braudel was the first *Annales* historian to gain widespread support of the idea that history should synthesize data from various social sciences . . . (although Febvre and Bloch, founders of the *Annales* school, originated this approach)." In other words, while Braudel popularized this approach, it was actually Febvre and Bloch who came up with it in the first place. This prediction matches closely with **(D)**, which has Febvre and Bloch *anticipat*[ing] Braudel's approach. **(A)** and **(C)** both suggest that Febvre and Bloch could be used to argue against the *Annales* approach, which is inconsistent with their roles as originators of this same approach. **(B)** tries to Distort the author's use of Febvre and Bloch: economics is clearly relevant for the *Annales* approach to historical investigation, but Febvre and Bloch are not used in the context of supporting the relevance of economics—they are mentioned only because they used economics before Braudel.

2. **B**

This is another Function question that essentially asks, *What is the role of the third paragraph*? Refer back to paragraph 3 and summarize its purpose: *Expansion on* longue durée *as geohistory*. This prediction matches closely with **(B)**, which reflects on *the role of geography in human history*. **(A)** is a Faulty Use of Detail wrong answer; the author does mention Braudel's attention to *esoteric information*, but this is a minor detail from the paragraph that misses the full purpose of expanding on the *longue durée*. **(C)** is also a Faulty Use of Detail; the *geography of the Mediterranean region* is used to support the use of geography in Braudel's approach, but the primary concern is not to discuss *the geography of the Mediterranean* specifically—rather, it is to show how geography can influence human history. **(D)** Distorts the author's words. Braudel does shy away from national borders to focus on geographic borders, but that does not mean that all national borders are *irrelevan*[t].

3. **D**

This is an Inference question. Based on the evidence presented in the passage, we should be able to infer a difference between traditional and *Annales* historians. From our initial analysis, we know that the two are contrasted in paragraph 1, so this is where we will look for clues. The key to the answer is given in the second sentence: "In a departure from traditional approaches, the *Annales* historians assume that history . . . must be understood in the context of forces and material conditions that underlie human behavior." In other words, the *Annales* historians are *more interested in the underlying context of human behavior* than traditional historians, as **(D)** states. **(A)** Distorts the author's words: the *Annales* are interested in incorporating social sciences into historical analysis, but that does not mean that they are more interested in other social sciences than in history—they are historians, after all! **(B)** is also a Distortion. The *Annales* historians propose that history is more than just the actions of famous figures, but this doesn't mean that they are *critical of* those figure's *achievements*. Finally, **(C)** is an Opposite. *Annales* historians want to incorporate economic research findings into historical analysis and so should not be *skeptical of the validity* of such approaches.

4. **D**

We want to predict what direction the author would go in if the passage were continued in this *Reasoning Beyond the Text* question. The purpose of the last paragraph was to mention criticisms of Braudel's approach and respond to those criticisms. The paragraph ends by responding to criticism by citing the contribution of Braudel's work: "studies . . . indicate that Braudel asked significant questions that traditional historians had overlooked." If another sentence were added, it should continue along the same lines of highlighting the influence or merits of Braudel. This prediction matches perfectly with **(D)**. **(A)** would backtrack on the author's support by questioning the professionalism of the authors of such studies. **(B)** is both Out of Scope and Opposite. Incorporation of the *Carlylean approach* mentioned in paragraph 2 would come out of nowhere at the end of paragraph 4, and it also represents the traditional approach to historical analysis; the author is unlikely to support a revival of this approach. Finally, **(C)** is a criticism of Braudel, and because the author is defending Braudel in the last part of the paragraph, this answer choice is an Opposite.

5. **B**

This is a Detail question, so we simply need to find the appropriate information in the passage. From our initial analysis, we know that the beginning of paragraph 4 is where the criticisms of Braudel are brought up. In fact, Braudel's critics believed his *scope* was *too broad*, and that the *differences* among *social sciences* were *blurred*. This prediction matches **(B)**. **(A)** is a Faulty Use of Detail. Braudel seeks structures like geohistory that underlie social activity in history; however, this is not in paragraph 4 and is not a criticism of Braudel. **(C)** is Out of Scope; while Braudel's "three temporalities" are discussed, the *relationship between them* is never addressed. Finally, **(D)** is an Opposite answer choice. According to paragraph 4, critics thought Braudel's approach "made it difficult to delimit the boundaries of observation." This statement is at odds with *rigidly define*[d] *boundaries* in this answer choice.

6. **C**

This is an Apply question of the Example subtype. We must use the author's description of the *longue durée* to identify a similar example. Paragraph 2 defines the three temporalities and defines the *longue durée* as being an "historical wave of great length" on the order of hundreds of years. Only **(C)** has even remotely that long of a duration, making it the correct answer. **(A)** and **(D)** are short-lived events in history just as the *evenementielle* temporality is defined in the passage. **(B)** describes a cyclical event that *occur[s] . . . roughly every half-century*, which would fit the definition of the *conjonctures* temporality described in the passage.

7. **A**

The question asks us to *suppose* new information. Thus, this is a *Reasoning Beyond the Text* question. If we glance at the answer choices, we can see that this is a Strengthen–Weaken question. The question stem introduces a hypothetical quote from Braudel that emphasizes his interest in the influence of *one person's decisions* in history. The focus on one person's influence is most similar to the *evenementielle* temporality discussed in paragraph 2. We also see in this paragraph that Braudel considered the *longue durée* the "most fascinating of the three temporalities." The quote given in the question stem would go against the information in the passage, so we can immediately cross off **(C)** and **(D)**, which claim that this quote would *strengthen* the author's claim. The logic presented here matches with **(A)**. **(B)** is a Distortion because the author claims that Braudel is most fascinated by the *longue durée* temporality, but that is not the same thing as saying Braudel is *not interested* at all in other aspects of history. In fact, Braudel gives the actions of great individuals their own temporality, the *evenementielle*, so Braudel must be at least somewhat interested in these actions.

CHAPTER 9

QUESTION TYPES I: *FOUNDATIONS OF COMPREHENSION* QUESTIONS

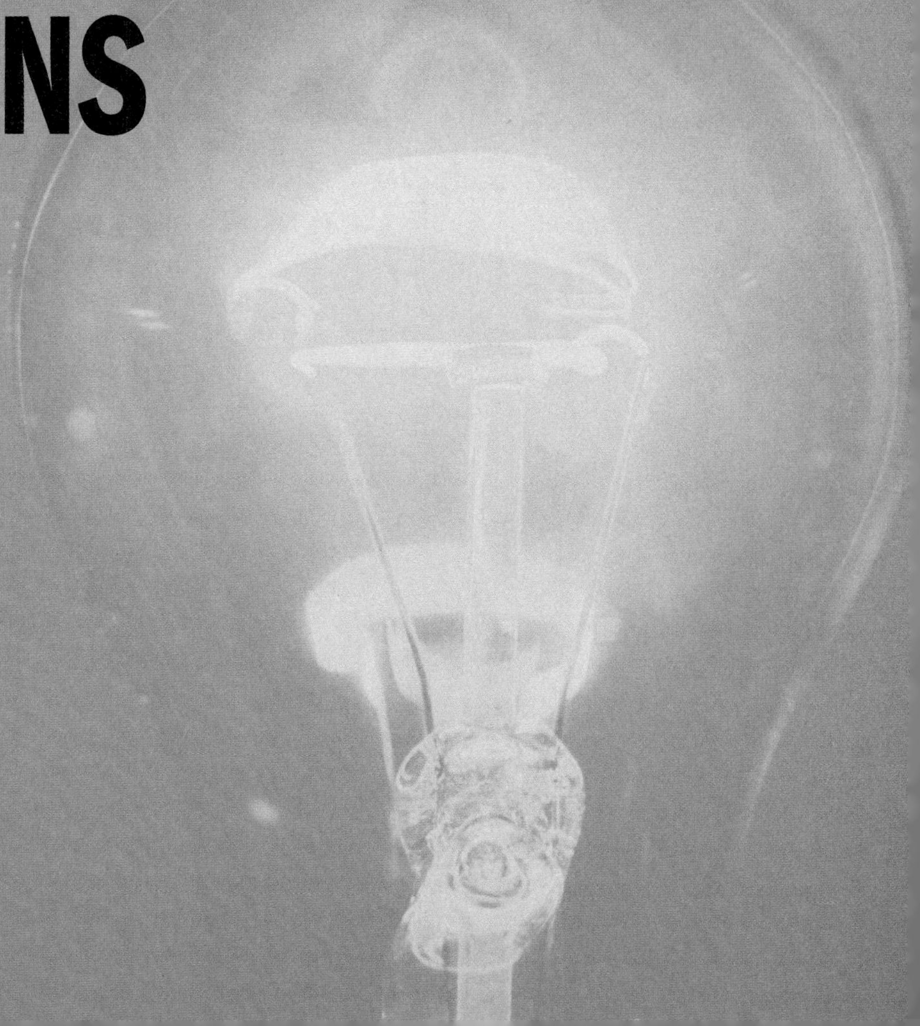

CHAPTER 9

QUESTION TYPES I: *FOUNDATIONS OF COMPREHENSION* QUESTIONS

In This Chapter

Introduction

LEARNING OBJECTIVES

After Chapter 9, you will be able to:

- Identify Main Idea, Detail, Inference, and Definition-in-Context questions
- Solve *Foundations of Comprehension* questions with strategies based on question type
- Recognize common features of *Foundations of Comprehension* questions

In order to get into college, you likely had to take an exam like the SAT® or ACT®, both of which feature sections that test reading comprehension. Most of the questions in those sections were straightforward, requiring you merely to search the text for a key fact, to define the meaning of a term used in a passage, or to identify the author's thesis. Some of the more challenging questions may have required you to imagine things from the writer's perspective or to explain why a certain word or phrase was used. Such questions can also be found in the *Critical Analysis and Reasoning Skills* (CARS) section of the MCAT, though you will find that they are generally more difficult than the analogous questions found on your precollege exams.

Chapters 9, 10, and 11 of this textbook will follow the same general pattern. For each question type, we will briefly describe distinguishing features before examining some sample question stems. Then, after discussing strategic approaches to the question type, we'll attack an example passage excerpt, providing at least one sample question of each type. The question types in this chapter all fall under the *Foundations of Comprehension* category and will be examined in the following order: Main Idea, Detail, Inference, and Definition-in-Context.

Note: The Question Types, as well as the Kaplan Method for CARS Passages, Kaplan Method for CARS Questions, and Wrong Answer Pathologies, are all included as tear-out sheets in the back of this book.

9.1 Main Idea Questions

Questions that ask about the big picture or major themes of the passage are what we call **Main Idea questions**. Only a small number of the questions in the CARS section fall into this type, but they are easy to recognize. The Kaplan Method for CARS Passages will arm you with everything you need to attack Main Idea questions, typically without referring back to the passage.

Sample Question Stems

- The author's central thesis is that:
- Which of the following best characterizes the main idea of the passage?
- The primary purpose of the passage is to:
- The author of the passage is primarily interested in:
- Which of the following titles best captures the main theme of the passage?
- The author can best be viewed as a proponent of:
- The language used in the passage makes it clear that the intended audience is:
- What is the author's central concern?

BRIDGE

Main Idea questions that ask about the audience or the medium are checking your rhetorical analysis skills. Analysis of the likely author, including the author's tone and voice, can reveal the intended audience and most likely medium. Rhetoric was discussed in Chapter 3 of *MCAT CARS Review.*

Main Idea questions will often use some variant of the phrase *central thesis*, *primary purpose*, or—of course—*main idea*, or they might make some kind of general reference to the *author*. On rare occasions, Main Idea questions will bring in a more challenging aspect of the rhetorical situation, such as the *audience* or the *medium*.

Strategy

You should decide to work on a Main Idea question as soon as you encounter it, because these questions can get you some quick points. Your best bet for your Investigate step is simply to *Go for the goal!* As discussed in Chapter 6, no matter which Distill approach you take, you will consider the overarching purpose or goal of the passage before moving on to the questions. If you encounter a Main Idea question, the purpose that you considered during your passage distillation will usually echo the correct answer. When searching for a Match in the answer choices, both the verb and the content of each answer choice should be carefully considered. For Main Idea answer choices, the verb used to describe the author's purpose in writing the passage is just as important as the content of the answer.

In the event that none of the choices come close to matching what you thought the author's purpose was, you should use a systematic process of elimination to remove Faulty Use of Detail answers that are too narrow, Out of Scope options that go too far afield, and any answer choice that has the wrong tone (positive, negative, ambivalent, or impartial) or degree (extreme *vs.* moderate) as discussed in Chapter 8 *of Critical Analysis and Reasoning Skills Review.*

MCAT EXPERTISE

The wrong answer choices in Main Idea questions are very predictable. One or more tend to be too narrow, reflecting the ideas from only one paragraph. One or more tend to be too broad, becoming Out of Scope. One or more tend to embody the wrong tone (positive, negative, ambivalent, or impartial) or degree (extreme *vs.* moderate).

Main Idea Questions—Applied Example

There is no shortage of evidence for the existence of systemic biases in ordinary human reasoning. For instance, Kahneman and Tversky in their groundbreaking 1974 work proposed the existence of a heuristic—an error-prone shortcut in reasoning—known as "anchoring." In one of their most notable experiments, participants were exposed to the spin of a roulette wheel (specially rigged to land randomly on one of only two possible results) before being asked to guess what percentage of United Nations member states were African. The half of the sample who had the roulette wheel stop at 65 guessed, on average, that 45 percent of the UN was African, while those with a result of 10 guessed only 25 percent, demonstrating that prior presentation of a random number otherwise unconnected to a quantitative judgment can still influence that judgment.

The anchoring effect has been observed on repeated other occasions, such as in Dan Ariely's experiment that used digits in Social Security numbers as an anchor for bids at an auction, and in the 1996 study by Wilson et al. that showed even awareness of the existence of anchoring bias is insufficient to mitigate its effects. The advertising industry has long been aware of this bias, the rationale for its frequent practice of featuring an "original" price before showing a "sale" price that is invariably reduced. Of course, anchoring is hardly alone among the defective tendencies in human reasoning; other systemic biases have also been experimentally identified, including loss aversion, the availability heuristic, and optimism bias.

Example:

1. The author's primary task in the passage is to:

   A. search for evidence of systemic biases in normal human thinking.
   B. discuss empirical findings on anchoring and other reasoning biases.
   C. show that anchoring is the most commonly occurring error in reasoning.
   D. demonstrate that knowledge of anchoring bias is insufficient to prevent it.

Solution: Utilizing the Kaplan Question Strategy discussed in Chapter 8, start *with the Type step.* This question asks you to identify the *primary task* of the author, which is indicative of a Main Idea question. During your Read and Distill of the passage, you should consider the overall goal of the passage, meaning that these questions can be answered quickly. Attempt and answer questions like this one as soon as you encounter them to earn quick points on Test Day.

The second step is to Rephrase the question. A simplification in this case might be *Why did the author write this passage?,* or *What was the author trying to convey to the reader?* The task in Main Idea questions is usually well defined by the question stem, so the Rephrase step should be minimal, and you may not need to generate alternate phrasing at all.

The Investigate step will remain the same for Main Idea questions no matter which method you selected in your Choose step for the passage. Main Idea questions ask you to synthesize all of the information presented into an overall purpose. To solve, you should recall your reasoning about the purpose of the passage from the end of your Distill step, then find a Match in the answer choices. In this case, the author was attempting to present evidence for systemic biases in reasoning, especially anchoring.

That prediction from your Investigate step should immediately lead you to Match **(B)**. The phrase *discuss empirical findings* is roughly equivalent in meaning to our *present evidence*. Also, the scope is right, with the answer focusing on anchoring but mentioning other biases because the author does introduce anchoring as an example with the phrase "For instance."

On Test Day, whenever you find a match for a prediction or a choice that fulfills your expectation for correctness, go with that answer and move on to the next question. For these examples, though, it's worth discussing what's wrong with the other options. **(A)** comes close and has the appropriate scope, but the verb is wrong: in the very first sentence, the author says that "There is no shortage of evidence," so why would the author's task be to *search for* something so readily available? Moving on to **(C)**, we find an Out of Scope choice: while the author says that systemic biases are common to thinking, there is never any comparison among the types mentioned. Just because the author focuses on anchoring does *not* mean that anchoring is necessarily the most frequently occurring–the author could choose to discuss it for any number of reasons other than its commonness. Finally, **(D)** is a Faulty Use of Detail because it is too specific. The referenced claim is made in the second paragraph, but it applies only to the study conducted by Wilson and others. This answer does not encompass the focus of the whole passage.

9.2 Detail Questions

Detail questions ask about what is stated explicitly in the passage. These are probably what you typically think of when you imagine a "reading comprehension" question, as they tend to require searching the text to find the missing piece. While Main Idea questions focus on the big picture, Detail questions zoom in on some of the finer points of the passage. They are by far the most common question type in the *Foundations of Comprehension* category, constituting at least half of the questions that fall under this heading.

Sample Question Stems

- According to the author's account of [topic], [concept] is:
- The author states that [person] holds the view that:
- Which of the following, according to the passage, does the author associate with the idea of [concept]?
- The author's apparent attitude toward [alternative position] is:
- Based on the discussion in [paragraph reference], the work of [artist/writer] was widely regarded as:
- The passage suggests which of the following about [topic]? [list of Roman numerals]
- The author asserts all of the following EXCEPT:
- Which of the following claims does NOT appear in the passage?

Detail questions tend to contain simple, declarative language (*is* and *are*) rather than the subjunctive mood (*would* and *could*), often include phrases like *the author states* and *according to the passage*, and can take the form of incomplete sentences ending with a colon.

The last three examples listed above fall into what is known as the Scattered subtype. A **Scattered** question is one that either employs a set of Roman numeral options or uses a word like EXCEPT, NOT, or LEAST. While just about any type of question can be Scattered—from Scattered Function to Scattered Inference—Scattered Detail is perhaps the most common example of the Scattered subtype.

Strategy

The only trick to working with Detail questions is that sometimes a seemingly straightforward question can actually require making an inference (which is, notably, another type of question in the *Foundations of Comprehension* category). If you are dealing with a true Detail question, though, you should follow the clues in the question stem, especially the content **buzzwords**, and keep these terms as a focus during your Rephrase of the question stem. You should then Investigate by using your Distill step to help you home in on the relevant portion of the passage. If you Highlighted or Outlined, the main idea of each paragraph should help you find the relevant detail. If you Interrogated, you should return to the chunk that contained the detail being asked about in the question stem. Once you find the precise sentence referenced, remember

MCAT EXPERTISE

It is easy to forget that you are working on a LEAST/NOT/EXCEPT question when you're analyzing the answer choices. Highlighting those words in the question stem can provide a visual clue that you are looking for a false statement as opposed to the three true wrong answers.

BRIDGE

Sometimes, what appears to be a Detail question will actually require you to make an inference. Inference questions include both Assumption and Implication questions, the strategies for which are discussed later in this chapter.

to read at least the sentence before and the sentence after (unless, of course, you're looking at the first or last sentence of the entire passage!) to get a bit more context. Once you've read the relevant text, complete your investigation by putting the sentence into your own words, and then look for the best match to answer the question.

MCAT EXPERTISE

For Detail questions, make sure to paraphrase the relevant text in a "short and sweet" format that will be easy to repeat to yourself while reading the answer choices. Much of the challenge of this type of question can be trying to figure out which answer choice actually matches your prediction—so make your prediction something that's easy to remember!

You will likely want to save the Scattered Detail questions you encounter for later because these will often require researching three or four different parts of the text, rather than just one. When working with these questions, your approach will vary quite a bit depending on which passage strategy you've chosen. Process of elimination is almost inevitable with questions of the Scattered subtype, but that doesn't mean you should immediately jump blindly into the answer choices. As with any question, take what you can from the stem to set some basic expectations.

Detail Questions—Applied Example

One of the first examples of the ascendance of abstraction in 20th-century art is the Dada movement, which Lowenthal dubbed "the groundwork to abstract art and sound poetry, a starting point for performance art, a prelude to postmodernism, an influence on pop art . . . and the movement that laid the foundation for surrealism." Dadaism was ultimately premised on a philosophical rejection of the dominant culture, which is to say the dominating culture of colonialist Europe. Not content with the violent exploitation of other peoples, Europe's ruling factions once again turned inward, reigniting provincial disputes into the conflagration that came to be known by the Eurocentric epithet "World War I"—the European subcontinent apparently being the only part of the world that mattered.

The absurd destructiveness of the Great War was a natural prelude to the creative absurdity of Dada. Is it any wonder that the rejection of reason made manifest by senseless atrocities should lead to the embrace of irrationality and disorder among the West's subaltern artistic communities? Marcel Janco, one of the first Dadaists, cited this rationale: "We had lost confidence in our culture. Everything had to be demolished. We would begin again after the *tabula rasa*." Thus, we find the overturning of what was once considered art: a urinal becomes the *Fountain* after Marcel Duchamp signs it "R. Mutt" in 1917, the nonsense syllables of Hugo Ball and Kurt Schwitters transform into "sound poems," and dancers in cardboard cubist costumes accompanied by foghorns and typewriters metamorphosize into the ballet *Parade*. Unsurprisingly, many commentators, including founding members, have described Dada as an "anti-art" movement. Notwithstanding such a designation, Dadaism has left a lasting imprint on modern Western art.

Example:

2. As stated in the passage, prior to the Great War, the leaders of Europe were primarily focused on:

   A. fighting one another in World War I.
   B. colonizing other parts of the globe.
   C. gazing inward at local problems.
   D. rejecting the dominant culture.

Solution: The first step to the Kaplan Method for CARS Questions is the Type step, and when the stem says *as stated in the passage*, it usually signifies a Detail question (with some exceptions). You'll most likely want to work on Detail questions right away, rather than saving them for later.

The Rephrase step is next, and this question could be rephrased into a specific task: *Find in the passage what the leaders of Europe were focused on prior to the war.* There are two buzzwords in the question stem: *the Great War* and *the leaders of Europe*. The first comes directly from the start of paragraph 2, where you can judge from the context that it must be another name for what we now call World War I. (They of course didn't know there was going to be a second one at the time!) The second buzzword does not appear verbatim, but it shows up in the synonymous phrase "Europe's ruling factions" in the last sentence of paragraph 1. In addition to reading these two sentences to refresh yourself if necessary as part of your investigation, it may be worth reading one before and one after.

When we Investigate, the preceding sentence offers a key bit of context, illustrating that the author regards European culture quite negatively, with the phrase "the dominating culture of colonialist Europe." More of the same follows with the phrase "violent exploitation of other peoples," as this author highlights Europe's past as a global colonizer. The phrase "once again turned inward" is noteworthy for mirroring the language of *focused on* featured in the question stem. Putting this all together sets a thorough expectation for the correct answer: if the turning inward happened with the Great War, then prior to that, Europe's leaders must have been looking outward, focusing on their colonial acquisitions. This prediction finds a match in **(B)**.

Among the wrong options, **(A)** is based on a misunderstanding of the terminology. Though World War I is mentioned in the prior sentence, the author calls attention to the fact that it only later came to be known by that "epithet" (name) and then in the following sentence uses another name for it. Because the two terms refer to the same event, European leaders could not be focused on it before it happened. In contrast, **(C)** is an Opposite because Europeans were actually turning outward at their colonies. Finally, **(D)** is a Faulty Use of Detail: that phrase appears almost exactly, but it actually describes the founders of the Dada movement, not the European leaders.

MCAT EXPERTISE

One of the unique critical thinking challenges on the MCAT is based on the use of synonym. Test questions and answer choices are likely to use synonymous terms, rather than directly quoting the associated passage. Keep this in mind and remain flexible in your thinking when you Investigate a question stem or search for a Match in the answer choices to a particular question.

Example:

3. Based on the passage, which of the following is not a characteristic associated with Dadaism?

   A. A renunciation of European culture
   B. A reputation as an "anti-art" movement
   C. Importance for later 20th-century art
   D. The embrace of irrational atrocities

Solution: Although the testmaker will often put the word *not* in italics or all caps, sometimes it will appear plainly in a question stem, as seen here. Don't be fooled as you Type the question: this is still a Scattered Detail question. Because Scattered Detail questions are often time-consuming, you'd likely want to make it the last question you work on in the question set. When you do commit to working through a Scattered Detail question, don't forget to Rephrase the stem and set some basic expectations. The phrasing *a characteristic associated with* is vague enough that it could mean something the author says, or it could potentially reflect another view identified in the passage. That means you can't rule out an answer choice just because it doesn't sound like something the author would say, so long as it sounds like something someone else in the passage would. Because both paragraphs are chock-full of claims about Dadaism, there's no point in searching the text to set additional expectations—you'll have to go with a more minimal prediction as the output of your Investigate step.

(A) comes directly from the author's second sentence: "Dadaism was ultimately premised on a philosophical rejection of the ... culture of colonialist Europe." The word *renunciation* is a synonym of *rejection*—so cross off this option. Moving on to the next choice, while the author explicitly rejected the idea that Dadaism is "anti-art," that view is still reflected in the passage in the next-to-last sentence, where the author writes "many commentators, including founding members, have described Dada as an 'anti-art' movement." Another way of saying that many commentators describe it that way is to say that it has a reputation. Hence, **(B)** should also be eliminated. The next characteristic is found at both the beginning of the passage, with the quotation from Lowenthal, and at the end, with the author's statement that "Dadaism has left a lasting imprint on modern Western art." With **(C)** now off the table, we know that **(D)** must be the answer—but let's check it anyway.

This choice is very close to being a characteristic; however, the word *atrocities* prevents it from being associated with Dadaism and makes it the correct choice. The key sentence is worth repeating in full in order to untangle it: "Is it any wonder that the rejection of reason made manifest by senseless atrocities should lead to the embrace of irrationality and disorder among the West's subaltern artistic communities?" The author is saying that Dadaism embraces irrationality, although not in the same way that irrationality (*rejection of reason*) manifests itself in warfare (*senseless atrocities*). The preceding sentence offers some useful clarification: "The absurd destructiveness of the Great War was a natural prelude to the creative absurdity of Dada." Notice how the word *absurd* is used to join two concepts that are typically viewed as opposites: creation and destruction. The author is suggesting that, even though both the Great War and Dadaism defied reason, they did so in dramatically different ways. This irrationality or absurdness in Dadaism stood in opposition to the atrocities of World War I; the word *embrace* in the answer choice makes this statement *not* a characteristic of Dadaism. That's why **(D)** is correct.

9.3 Inference Questions

What makes **Inference questions** distinctive is that they deal with unstated parts of arguments: information that is not explicitly written by the author but that *must* be true given what is claimed in the passage. It is crucial to understand that the correct answers to Inference questions are not simply assertions that are *possibly* true or that *could* be accurate; rather, they are necessary assumptions or at least highly probable implications. This is why Inference questions are considered *Foundations of Comprehension* rather than *Reasoning Within the Text* questions: the answers are directly implied and must be true based on the written text. We call these Inference questions because, as first noted in Chapter 3 of *MCAT CARS Review*, it is the common name of the process used to arrive at both **assumptions** (unstated evidence) and **implications** (unstated conclusions), collectively known as inferences.

Sample Question Stems

- In [paragraph reference], it is reasonable to believe that the author assumes:
- Implicit in the discussion of [topic] is the underlying assumption that:
- The passage suggests [claim] because:
- On the basis of the author's account of [topic], which of the following might reasonably be inferred?
- The author implies that [concept] is NOT:
- It is reasonable to conclude that the author regards [person or position] as:
- The author says [quotation], but also [paraphrase of different claim]. These beliefs imply:
- Which of the following inferences is most justified by information provided in the passage? [list of Roman numerals]

As these examples indicate, during the first step of the Kaplan Method for CARS Questions—in which you Type the question —you can recognize that you might be dealing with an Inference question if you see one or more of the following words (or variations of them): *assume, because, conclude, imply, infer, justify, reasonable*, or *suggest.* However, if a question stem contains any of these words and new information of some kind, then it will fall into the *Reasoning Beyond the Text* category instead (which we will discuss in Chapter 11). If there are no new elements, you are likely dealing with an Inference question.

As previously alluded to, there is actually something of a continuum between Detail and Inference questions; the position of questions on that continuum varies based on the complexity of the reasoning used to solve them. A question that tells you to make an inference might require one relatively simple step, such as canceling out a double negative or identifying a paraphrase of lines from the passage. Sometimes you'll even find you were told to look for an item that the *passage suggests* or the *author implies* but, as you Investigate, you may discover that the answer was in the text virtually word for word. In cases such as these, consider yourself fortunate, because you've uncovered a Detail question in disguise! The predictions you make for these questions will likely be more than adequate to match to the correct answer.

The downside to this ambiguity is that sometimes a question that uses simple declarative language will require a lot more critical thinking than you expected. Just because a stem includes a phrase like *the author asserts* or *as stated in the passage* (common question stems for Detail questions) does not necessarily mean that the answer is stated in a straightforward manner. Notwithstanding such trickery on the part of the AAMC, as long as you recognize the possibility that apparent Detail questions can be disguised as Inference questions and are prepared to apply the Denial Test strategy to those questions, you can avoid being fooled!

Strategy

There are only two basic tasks with the Inference question type. When you recognize that you need to make an inference, first ask yourself whether you are looking for a missing but essential piece of *evidence* (an **assumption**) or for a *conclusion* that is unstated but highly probable given what is said (an **implication**).

Assumptions

If you Rephrase the stem and your task is to identify an assumption, your Investigation should begin by determining what claim the assumption is supposed to underlie. Sometimes the question stem will say this explicitly, or it may use quoted text or paragraph numbers to refer to a particular claim. If not, depending on which passage strategy you used, you may need to go back and do research in the passage. If you need to go back to the passage as you investigate, you should reread the relevant passage sentences and isolate the specific statement, taking care to see whether there's any existing evidence in the surrounding text that's used to support the statement. Logic keywords are your best friends here, but keep in mind that a lot of authors use them sparsely, so they won't always be there to help. The Match to assumption questions might include words or ideas that are similar to a piece of evidence actually stated, so you can use any that you locate for your prediction, or just go with whatever links the evidence provided to the conclusion when you reread the text—*now I see what the author is taking for granted!*

KEY CONCEPT

Inferences are unstated parts of arguments that must be true based on what the passage says. Assumptions are unstated pieces of evidence, while implications are unstated conclusions.

Implications

If you Rephrase the stem and your task is to identify an implication, center your Investigation on any particular sentences referenced in the question stem. Watch out for Logic keywords, just as with assumptions. Now, however, you'll be looking to see whether the particular statements referenced are used to support anything else. If so, use those explicitly supported conclusions to set your expectations for the correct answer. Alternatively, if another implication occurs to you when you reread, you can use that as a prediction.

Whenever you can't find a Match for your prediction—if you thought it was a Detail question, if you didn't know where to look because the stem had no paragraph reference clues, or if the answer choices just turned out very differently than you expected—plan B is to use a special version of process of elimination known as the **Denial Test**. Let's take a look at how it works in practice.

The Denial Test

For each answer choice, negate (take the opposite of) what is being said. In question stems that end with a colon (:), you may need to take part of the text from the end of the stem and combine it with the answer choice to create a sentence that can then be denied. Be careful with sentences that already contain negative words, prefixes, and suffixes, because sometimes just removing that text is not enough to change the meaning in the proper way. If nothing else, any claim can be denied by adding *It is not the case that* to the beginning of the sentence. Once you've denied the claim, think about the effect the denied claim has on the passage. If you're not sure what effect it has, look for clues in the question stem or the answer choice itself to see if it refers to a particular part of the passage that you could reread. If it's clear that the negated claim has no significant impact, then eliminate that answer.

MCAT EXPERTISE

While the Denial Test will always reveal the correct answer in an Inference question, it's very time-consuming. If you cannot set good expectations for the right answer during the Execute step, triage the question and return to it later with the Denial Test.

When you come across an answer choice that logically conflicts with the text once you've negated it, you've likely found the correct answer. However, sometimes multiple answer choices will have denials that cause problems for the text, so when executing the Denial Test you should *always test every answer choice* and pick the one for which negation has the most detrimental impact on arguments or assertions from the passage. Keep in mind that this can be time-consuming, which is why it's generally a good idea to save a question for later if you believe the Denial test will be necessary to answer it.

It is hard to understand how the Denial Test works simply by reading about it. Check out the Worked Example below and make sure to practice the Denial Test on Inference questions to get used to using it.

Inference Questions—Applied Example

In 1941, an exuberant nationalist wrote: "We must accept wholeheartedly our duty and our opportunity as the most powerful and vital nation . . . to exert upon the world the full impact of our influence, for such purposes as we see fit and by such means as we see fit." If forced to guess the identity of the writer, many US citizens would likely suspect a German jingoist advocating for *Lebensraum*. In actuality, the sentiment was expressed by one of America's own: Henry Luce, the highly influential publisher of the magazines *Life*, *Time*, and *Fortune*. Luce sought to dub the 1900s the "American Century," calling upon the nation to pursue global hegemony as it slipped from the grasp of warring Old World empires. As a forecast of world history, Luce's pronouncement seems prescient—but is it justifiable as a normative stance?

Not all of Luce's contemporaries bought into his exceptionalist creed. Only a year later, Henry Wallace, vice president under FDR, insisted that no country had the "right to exploit other nations" and that "military [and] economic imperialism" were invariably immoral. It is a foundational assumption in ethics that the wrongness of an act is independent of the particular identity of the actor—individuals who pay no heed to moral consistency are justly condemned as hypocrites. So why should it be any different for nation-states? In accord with this principle, Wallace proselytized for "the century of the common man," for the furtherance of a "great revolution of the people," and for bringing justice and prosperity to all persons irrespective of accidents of birth. Sadly, Wallace never had the chance to lead the United States in this cosmopolitan direction; prior to Roosevelt's demise at the beginning of his fourth term, the vice presidency was handed to Harry Truman, a man whose narrow provincialism ensconced him firmly in Luce's camp. And with Truman came the ghastly atomic eradication of two Japanese cities, the dangerous precedent set by military action without congressional approval in Korea, and a Cold War with the Soviet Union that brought the world to the brink of nuclear destruction.

Example:

4. One can most justifiably conclude on the basis of the author's discussion that Henry Luce assumed that:

   A. the United States did not have the right to create a military or economic empire.
   B. nation-states are never bound by the same ethical principles that persons are.
   C. the same normative standards should apply to both Americans and Germans.
   D. moral rules that govern individual behavior do not necessarily apply to countries.

Solution: The *assumed* at the end of the question stem makes the Type step for this question straightforward: it must be an Inference question. Rephrasing the question stem should give you something along the lines of "Based on the passage, what did Henry Luce assume?" Using this rephrase, we know we're looking for an assumption from a portion of the passage relevant to Luce's argument, and we'll want to rely on our Distill technique, possibly in combination with referring back to the passage itself, in order to Investigate. Luce advocated for what the author calls the *exceptionalist* stance that the United States, as the most powerful country at the time, was free to do as it pleased. This is in contrast to Henry Wallace, who explicitly rebuffed Luce's view, so watch out for Faulty Uses of Detail answer choices that would actually describe Wallace.

Denying **(A)** yields *the United States did have the right to create a military or economic empire*, which is completely consistent with Luce's view. Eliminate it. As written, **(A)** is actually a view attributed to Wallace by the author, so it's both a FUD and an Opposite as this was the major point of disagreement between the two.

(B) contains *never*, which is an Extreme keyword, but because Luce seems to have a fairly strong position, don't jump to dismissing the answer as a Distortion quite yet. It's a bit trickier to negate: to say that it is *not* the case that some event *never* happens is the same as saying the event *sometimes* occurs. Thus, the proper negation of **(B)** is *nation-states are sometimes bound by the same ethical principles that persons are*, which is completely consistent with Luce, who presumably believes that ethical principles do apply to nations sometimes, say on those occasions when the nation in question is not the United States. Eliminate it.

For **(C)**, the contradiction would be *the same normative standards should not apply to both Americans and Germans*, which is again consistent with Luce's *"American Century"* idea. Hence, we can definitely cross off **(C)**, which, as written, is actually another one of Wallace's beliefs—a second Opposite/FUD combo.

All that remains is **(D)**, which does indeed destroy the argument if rejected. Countering it by saying *moral rules that govern individual behavior do necessarily apply to countries* would mean that they *always* apply. But this supports the anti-hypocrisy argument that the author makes in favor of Wallace and against Luce at the beginning of paragraph 2. Thus, denying **(D)** would make Henry Luce's argument fall apart, and so it is an assumption Luce has made. **(B)** was simply a more extreme version of this claim, rightly rejected as a Distortion because an author is more likely to assume a weak form of a statement than a strong one.

BRIDGE

Remember that the opposite of an Extreme Negative keyword (like *never*) is a Moderating Positive keyword (like *sometimes*). The circular view of Author keywords presented in Chapter 5 of *MCAT CARS Review* is a great way to visualize this change.

Example:

5. It is reasonable to infer that the author believes that:

   A. Harry Truman was the worst US president of the 20th century.
   B. Franklin Roosevelt did not endorse the idea of the "American Century."
   C. Henry Wallace would not have approved of the use of atomic weapons.
   D. Henry Luce did not provide an accurate historical assessment of the 1900s.

Solution: We can Type this question as an Inference question given the phrase *reasonable to infer*. With a stem like this, which has no specific clues or references, you may find Rephrasing barely changes anything, and thus choose to dive straight into the Investigate step. With a stem that gives almost no information, we have little choice but to proceed with the Denial Test. It's not entirely clear what kind of inference this is, because an author "believes" both assumptions and implications. While you can guess based on the descriptive language used that the author does not approve of Harry Truman, you do not know the writer's feelings toward any of the other American presidents in the 1900s, so denying that Truman was the worst president would not have too much of an impact. Therefore **(A)** is a Distortion, too extreme to attribute to the author.

For **(B)**, you do not really know what the author believes about Franklin Delano Roosevelt (FDR). We only know that he was the US president serving over both Wallace and Truman. Therefore, we can make no safe inferences about FDR's attitude toward Luce's point of view: this Out of Scope option should be discarded.

Negate **(C)** and you arrive at *Henry Wallace would have approved of the use of atomic weapons*. If this were so, had he become president, he would have been guilty of the very misdeeds for which the author blames Truman—and the author would be utterly inconsistent in praising the one and condemning the other. In fact, because the passage rails against hypocrisy, it is clear that the author would have to hold the two men to the same ethical standards. Thus, denying **(C)** would considerably undermine the author's argument in paragraph 2, and this is almost certainly the answer.

To make sure, finish executing the Denial Test: rejecting **(D)** would have no negative impact—in fact, it would support the author's claim that Luce's view "seem[ed] prescient" as an historical prediction. This assumption suggests that the author indeed views Luce's view as historically accurate, even if ethically questionable. You can now be confident that **(C)** is the answer.

9.4 Definition-in-Context Questions

Definition-in-Context questions are the final question type to fall into the *Foundations of Comprehension* category. The task generated from the Rephrase of these questions is always the same: define the word or phrase as it is used in the passage. These questions are infrequent on Test Day, but are straightforward and make for easy points when they do occur.

Sample Question Stems

- As used by the author, the word [term] most nearly means:
- In [paragraph reference], what is the author's most likely meaning when stating [quotation]?
- The author's choice of the phrase [term] is probably intended to suggest:
- As used in the passage, [term] refers to:
- In [paragraph reference], the author asserts that [claim]. What the author most likely means by this is:
- Which of the following is most synonymous with [concept] as discussed in the text?

This list of stems makes it clear that Definition-in-Context questions always feature a reference to a word, phrase, or an entire claim from the passage, the meaning of which you are tasked with identifying. Quotation marks and italics are common features used to call attention to the terms, but on occasion a Definition-in-Context question stem may lack these.

Strategy

Although these questions ask about the meanings of words, a dictionary will not help you here, and in some cases it could even lead you astray. Trap answers in these questions are often the common definitions of the word, which are tempting Out of Scope choices that fail to match the use of the term in the context of the passage. These questions tend to be relatively fast to solve because they refer only to small portions of the text. Thus, you should generally decide to work on these questions as soon as you see them.

Your Investigation with a Definition-in-Context question will be to go to the text and surrounding context, if necessary, to see how the word or phrase is used in the passage. With this question type, the question stems will usually contain a paragraph reference, but use your recall of your Interrogation, your Outlining, or your Highlighting if this reference is not given to locate the relevant sentence. For this question type in particular, even if you interrogated the passage, it's likely you will need to go back into the passage and reread the surrounding materials. If reading that sentence doesn't give you enough to work with, look at the sentences before and after the target term or phrase. Wrap up your Investigation with a clear prediction: define the term or phrase in your own words based on how it was used in the passage. Author keywords may be especially helpful, because answer choices with the wrong tone can immediately be ruled out.

MCAT EXPERTISE

An author may imbue common words with a special meaning in the passage. Therefore, be sure to check how the author actually uses the word in a Definition-in-Context question, rather than looking for a dictionary definition of the term. Wrong answers in these questions are often accurate definitions of the term that do not match how the term was used in the passage.

Definition-in-Context Questions—Applied Example

In 1941, an exuberant nationalist wrote: "We must accept wholeheartedly our duty and our opportunity as the most powerful and vital nation . . . to exert upon the world the full impact of our influence, for such purposes as we see fit and by such means as we see fit." If forced to guess the identity of the writer, many US citizens would likely suspect a German jingoist advocating for *Lebensraum*. In actuality, the sentiment was expressed by one of America's own: Henry Luce, the highly influential publisher of the magazines *Life*, *Time*, and *Fortune*. Luce sought to dub the 1900s the "American Century," calling upon the nation to pursue global hegemony as it slipped from the grasp of warring Old World empires. As a forecast of world history, Luce's pronouncement seems prescient—but is it justifiable as a normative stance?

Not all of Luce's contemporaries bought into his exceptionalist creed. Only a year later, Henry Wallace, vice president under FDR, insisted that no country had the "right to exploit other nations" and that "military [and] economic imperialism" were invariably immoral. It is a foundational assumption in ethics that the wrongness of an act is independent of the particular identity of the actor—individuals who pay no heed to moral consistency are justly condemned as hypocrites. So why should it be any different for nation-states? In accord with this principle, Wallace proselytized for "the century of the common man," for the furtherance of a "great revolution of the people," and for bringing justice and prosperity to all persons irrespective of accidents of birth. Sadly, Wallace never had the chance to lead the United States in this cosmopolitan direction; prior to Roosevelt's demise at the beginning of his fourth term, the vice presidency was handed to Harry Truman, a man whose narrow provincialism ensconced him firmly in Luce's camp. And with Truman came the ghastly atomic eradication of two Japanese cities, the dangerous precedent set by military action without congressional approval in Korea, and a Cold War with the Soviet Union that brought the world to the brink of nuclear destruction.

Example:

6. The author's use of the term "provincialism" in paragraph 2 comes closest in meaning to:

   A. German jingoism.
   B. economic imperialism.
   C. nationalistic exceptionalism.
   D. exuberant cosmopolitanism.

Solution: With the stereotypical Definition-in-Context question structure, Typing this question as Definition-in-Context should be a quick and easy step, with little to no Rephrase needed prior to proceeding with the Investigate step. The clue in the question stem points to the second paragraph, but the reference might still be difficult to find in a paragraph full of *-isms*. The key sentence is: "Sadly, Wallace never had the chance to lead the United States in this cosmopolitan direction; prior to Roosevelt's demise at the beginning of his fourth term, the vice presidency was handed to Harry Truman, a man whose narrow provincialism ensconced him firmly in Luce's camp." This sentence gives you a lot to work with. You can see that *provincialism* is a view attributed to Truman and Luce, who are contraposed to the "cosmopolitan" Wallace. In a passage that features a few different perspectives, it's not surprising to see a question like this that requires keeping straight who holds which view. This passage presents two major sides, and it's clear that *provincialism* represents a view that belongs to Truman, whose views align with those of Luce.

With these expectations established, look for a match in the answers. Because both nationalism (at the start of paragraph 1) and exceptionalism (at the start of paragraph 2) are views attributed to Luce, it is evident that **(C)** must be correct. **(A)** is a Faulty Use of Detail; *a German jingoist* was mentioned in the first paragraph, but this phrase is no good because Luce and Truman are both Americans. **(B)** echoes the quotation from Wallace as he criticizes Luce—"military [and] economic imperialism"—but all of the examples given for Truman show evidence of military action, not economic: "the ghastly atomic eradication of two Japanese cities, the dangerous precedent set by military action without congressional approval in Korea, and a Cold War with the Soviet Union that brought the world to the brink of nuclear destruction." The emphasis in **(B)** is therefore misplaced. Lastly, **(D)** uses a variant of *cosmopolitan*, a characteristic that was attributed to Wallace, so it's an Opposite.

Conclusion

Reading comprehension is a skill you've been honing your whole life—most exams you've had in literature and English classes have most likely centered on your ability to understand the text you read. On the MCAT, reading comprehension is important not only for answering *Foundations of Comprehension* questions, but also for understanding the passage itself. While they take many forms, including Main Idea, Detail, Inference, and Definition-in-Context, all *Foundations of Comprehension* questions share a few common features. Answering all of these question types is facilitated by a solid understanding of the structure of the passage, which can be used to locate the relevant text for the answer. The answers to all of these questions must be stated, paraphrased, or implied directly in the passage. That said, not all of these questions are asking for the same thing: these question types differ in significant ways. For example, Main Idea and Definition-in-Context questions should usually be answered as soon as you see them, whereas Detail (especially Scattered Detail) and some of the more challenging Inference questions may be more time-consuming and should, therefore, be saved until the end of the question set. Each of these questions can be Typed, Rephrased, and Investigated in predictable ways. We'll continue discussing question types in the next two chapters as we explore *Reasoning Within the Text* and *Reasoning Beyond the Text* questions.

You've reviewed the strategy, now test your knowledge and critical thinking skills by completing a test-like passage set in your online resources!

GO ONLINE

CONCEPT AND STRATEGY SUMMARY

Main Idea Questions

- **Type: Main Idea questions** ask for the author's primary goal or purpose in writing the passage.
  - These questions often contain words like *central thesis, primary purpose,* or *main idea.*
  - Less commonly, these questions may ask about a different aspect of the rhetorical situation, such as the *audience* or the *medium.*
- **Rephrase:** Phrase the question in such a way that you have a task for your Investigate step, such as *Why did the author write this passage* or *What clues in the passage tell me who the author's audience is?*
- **Investigate:** Recall the purpose that you constructed during the Distillation step of the Kaplan Passage Strategy, and predict that the correct answer will be synonymous with that purpose.
- **Match:** Your prediction should closely correlate to the right answer. If there is no clear match, or if you cannot perform any of the earlier steps of the *Kaplan Method for CARS Questions*, use the process of elimination.
  - Wrong answer choices may be too narrow (Faulty Use of Detail) or too broad (Out of Scope).
  - Wrong answer choices may have the wrong tone (positive, negative, ambivalent, or impartial) or degree (extreme *vs.* moderate).

Detail Questions

- **Type: Detail questions** ask about what is stated explicitly in the passage.
  - Unstated parts of arguments *must* be true given what is claimed in the passage.
  - Detail questions are the most likely to use the **scattered** format, which uses Roman numeral options or words like *EXCEPT, NOT,* or *LEAST.*
- **Rephrase:** Phrase the question in a way that maintains any **buzzwords** from the stem that will guide you to where in the passage you need to Investigate.
- **Investigate:** If you do not recall enough information to make a prediction, reread the relevant sentence, as well as the sentences before and after.
  - Make a concise prediction so you can repeat it to yourself between answer choices.
  - For Scattered Detail questions, locate all three of the wrong answers in the passage so you can eliminate them as options.
- **Match:** Your prediction should match the right answer. If there is no clear match, or if you cannot perform any of the earlier steps of the Kaplan Method for CARS Questions, use the process of elimination.

Inference Questions

- **Type: Inference questions** look for unstated parts of arguments.
  - These questions stems are similar to Main Idea questions, although they focus on the purpose of only one portion of the passage (usually one sentence or one paragraph).
  - **Assumptions** are unstated evidence.
  - **Implications** are unstated conclusions.
  - These question stems often contain words like *assume*, *because*, *conclude*, *imply*, *infer*, *justify*, *reasonable*, or *suggest*.
- **Rephrase:** Determine whether you are looking for an assumption (evidence) or implication (conclusion). Then, rephrase the claim the answer is supposed to support (assumptions) or be supported by (implications). It is helpful to build the directionality of the support into your Rephrase step.
- **Investigate:** Reread the relevant sentence if necessary, noting the explicit evidence and conclusions given.
  - For assumption questions, the answer is either similar to the evidence given or links the evidence to the conclusions.
  - For implication questions, the answer is either similar to the conclusions given or is another logical conclusion one could draw from the evidence.
- **Match:** Your prediction to an answer choice. If there is no clear match, or if you cannot perform any of the earlier steps of the Kaplan Method for CARS Questions, use the process of elimination, removing any answer that conflicts with the author's main argument or the paragraph's purpose.
  - Apply the Denial Test: negate each answer choice.
  - Whichever answer choice—when negated—has the most detrimental effect on the argument made in the passage is the correct answer choice.

Definition-in-Context Questions

- **Type: Definition-in-Context questions** ask you to define a word or phrase as it is used in the passage.
  - These questions often call attention to the term to be defined using quotation marks or italics, but not always.
  - Definition-in-Context questions always reference a word, phrase, or an entire claim from the passage.

- **Rephrase:** For Definition-in-Context questions, the rephrase will always look the same: *What does this word mean in this passage?*
- **Investigate:** Reread the sentence with the word or phrase, and perhaps the surrounding context, as necessary. Reword the author's definition of the term in your own voice as your prediction.
- **Match:** Your expectations should match the right answer. If there is no clear match, or if you cannot perform any of the earlier steps of the Kaplan Method for CARS Questions, use the process of elimination.

Worked Example

Use the Worked Example below, in tandem with the subsequent practice passages, to internalize and apply the strategies described in this chapter. The Worked Example matches the specifications and style of a typical MCAT *Critical Analysis and Reasoning Skills* (CARS) passage.

Take a few moments to quickly glance over the passage in order to Preview and Choose your approach. Highlighting can be beneficial when a passage is complex and the author jumps and pivots from one perspective to the next. The following passage has those qualities, and it also has unusual structural features that don't lend themselves well to Outlining or Interrogating. Thus, the Highlighting method is a strong way to approach this passage, specifically because it can be used to clearly visually indicate the points where major ideas are introduced and the points where the author shifts her focus. This will speed up efforts to find relevant information while answering questions later. As with all passages, any approach could be chosen and work for this passage, so, remember to practice all approaches as you start your CARS prep in order to determine which work best for you and in what situations!

HIGHLIGHTING METHOD

Passage	Expert Thinking
. . . Until last year, many people—but not most economists—thought that economic data told a simple tale. On one side, productivity—the average output of an average worker—was rising. And although the rate of productivity increase was very slow during the 1970s and early 1980s, the official numbers said that it had accelerated significantly in the 1990s. By 1994, an average worker was producing about 20 percent more than 1978.	What is the main theme of the passage? What words could be highlighted to demonstrate what this passage and paragraph are about? *The first sentence hints that the author is about to dispute conventional wisdom. However, this isn't the best phrase to highlight, as it's not the focus of the paragraph. A more informative highlight would be "productivity increase," as it captures what this paragraph is about.*
On the other hand, other statistics said that real, inflation-adjusted wages had not been rising at the same rate. Some commonly cited numbers showed real wages actually falling over the last 25 years. Those who did their homework knew that the gloomiest numbers overstated the case . . . Still, even the most optimistic measure, the total hourly compensation of the average worker, rose only 3 percent between 1978 and 1994 . . .	What parallel structure did you notice in this paragraph? What phrase can be highlighted to indicate the new concept introduced in this paragraph? *This paragraph's first line is similar to the "On one side" sentence in the previous paragraph. More accurately, this paragraph is a continuation of the first paragraph and completes the thought. Highlight the phrase "real wages actually falling" because it represents the conclusion of the author's first point. That is, the simple tale is how productivity went up, but real wages went down.*
. . . But now, experts tell us it may have been a figment of our statistical imaginations . . . a blue-ribbon panel of economists headed by Michael Boskin of Stanford declared that the Consumer Price Index [C.P.I.] had been systematically overstating inflation, probably by more than 1 percent per year for the last two decades, mainly failing to take account of changes in consumption patterns and product quality improvements . . .	What pivot point did you notice in this paragraph? What phrase should you highlight to capture this shift? *The first word of this paragraph indicates that the author is about to pivot into his second point. However, highlighting the "But now" phrase in the first sentence won't actually indicate what the author's point is when referring back to the passage. Instead, highlight "overstating inflation" to capture the new focus of this paragraph.* *When using the Highlighting method, do not highlight terms like C.P.I.: although it is a new term, the term is isolated and doesn't match the theme of this passage up to this point. This is the kind of term you might highlight if you were Outlining or Interrogating, as something a Definition-in-Context or Detail question might ask about.*

HIGHLIGHTING METHOD

Passage	Expert Thinking
. . . The Boskin Report, in particular, is not an official document—it will be quite a while before the government actually issues a revised C.P.I., and the eventual revision may be smaller than Boskin proposed. Still, the general outline of the resolution is pretty clear. When revisions are taken into account, productivity growth will probably look somewhat higher than before because some of the revisions will also affect how we calculate growth. But the rate of growth of real wages will look much higher—roughly in line with productivity. In other words, the whole story about workers not sharing in productivity gains will turn out to have been based on a statistical illusion . . .	How is this paragraph linked to the previous paragraph? What is the most important information in this paragraph? *A new term, "Boskin Report," is introduced, which relates to the mention of Michael Boskin in the previous paragraph. The first half of this paragraph mostly speaks about the technical aspect of the Boskin Report, but the actual main idea is about disproving that real wages are falling while productivity is climbing. Highlight "in line with productivity" or a related phrase to capture this idea. With this theme identified, this paragraph can be identified as a conceptual extension of the previous paragraph.*
It is important not to go overboard on this point. There are real problems in America, and our previous concerns were not pure hypochondriasis. For one, economic progress over the past 25 years has been much slower than in the previous 25. Even if Boskin's numbers are right, median family income—which officially has experienced virtually no gain since 1973—has risen by only about 35 percent over the past 25 years, compared with 100 percent over the previous 25. Furthermore, it is likely that if we "Boskinized" the old data—that is, if we tried to adjust the C.P.I. for the 50s and 60s to take account of changing consumption patterns and rising product quality—we would find that official numbers understated the rate of progress just as much if not more than they did in recent decades . . .	What pivots are in this paragraph? What phrases should you highlight to track the author's perspective? *In this paragraph, the author emphasizes that the claims discussed in the first two paragraphs about the "simple tale" are not totally unfounded. This can be represented by highlighting "not pure hypochondriasis". The following sentences dive into the details surrounding concerns about the economy. You could additionally highlight "understated the rate" because it parallels with the previous notion that the Boskin report is used to adjust the old data.*
. . . Moreover, while workers as a group have shared fully in national productivity gains, they have not done so equally. The overwhelming evidence of a huge increase in income inequality in America has nothing to do with price indices and is therefore unaffected by recent statistical revelations. Families in the bottom fifth, who had 5.4 percent of total income in 1970, had only 4.2 percent in 1994; over the same period, the top 5 percent went from 15.6 to 20.1. Corporate CEOs, who used to make about 35 times as much as their employees, now make 120 times as much or more . . .	What is the main idea for this paragraph? What are some low-yield details not worth highlighting? *The main idea in this paragraph is "income inequality," extending the previous paragraph's idea that the "simple tale" has some merit to it. The second half of this paragraph talks about the details of income inequality in American society. These details do not offer anything remarkably new.*

HIGHLIGHTING METHOD

Passage	Expert Thinking
. . . While these are real and serious problems, however, one thing is now clear: the truth about what is happening in America is more subtle than the simplistic morality play about greedy capitalists and oppressed workers that so many would-be sophisticates accepted only a few months ago.	What final conclusion is drawn in the last paragraph? *The last paragraph brings the passage full circle by restating a conclusion found in the first paragraph. The author is arguing against the "simple tale" that real wages are falling, and claims that the actual picture is more complicated. "More subtle" captures that idea. For details and to answer most questions, we will have to refer back to previous paragraphs.*

Question	Analysis
1. According to the passage, "Boskinization" adjusts the C.P.I. by:	The words *according to the passage* tell us this is a Detail question, which should be quick points. The term "Boskinized" appears in paragraph 5, where we find that it means that *Boskin adjusted the C.P.I. to take account of changing consumption patterns and rising product quality.*
A. increasing wages and decreasing productivity to reconcile the present disparity.	**(A)** may be tempting because Boskin's model did, in the end, increase apparent wages, but the passage makes no mention of *decreasing productivity* measures, making this choice Out of Scope. This choice also does not match with how the term "Boskinized" is used in the passage.
B. taking into account technology's role in an improved efficiency.	**(B)** is also Out of Scope because there is no mention of *technology's role* in the passage.
C. reassessing patterns of consumption and quality of product.	This choice is a spot-on match with the passage, making **(C)** the correct answer.
D. evaluating the inequalities in various levels of incomes.	**(D)** gives us an option that discusses wage inequality. However, this idea was a facet of the author's argument, not of Boskin's revisions. This is a Faulty Use of Detail answer choice.

Question	Analysis
2. The Boskin Report does all of the following EXCEPT:	The word *EXCEPT* shows us that this is a Scattered Detail question—one that might be worth skipping on Test Day until more time is available. To investigate, we must find relevant details and eliminate them systematically, keeping in mind that the correct answer is the one NOT included in the passage.
A. reveals that the C.P.I. was inaccurate.	Paragraph 3 tells us that the Boskin Report demonstrated that the C.P.I. "had been systematically overstating inflation," eliminating **(A)**.
B. reconciles the present disparity between productivity and wage levels.	Paragraph 4 shows us that Boskin did reconcile wages and productivity, eliminating **(B)**.
C. reveals the reasons for the increasing disparity between the highest and lowest income earners.	**(C)** is not present in the passage. While the income disparity was discussed, no mention was made of its causes—making this the correct answer.
D. provides possible clarification for economic progress in the 1950s and 1960s.	In paragraph 5, we see that Boskin's work, if applied to the 1950s and 1960s, "could find that official numbers understated the rate of progress," eliminating **(D)**.

Question	Analysis
3. In the first paragraph the author assumes:	The word *assumes* shows us that this is an Inference question, meaning our first Investigate action is to look back at paragraph one and its themes.
A. the total productivity of America has not seen a significant increase since the 1970s.	**(A)** can be eliminated because this is discussed in paragraph 6, rather than paragraph 1.
B. productivity is a measure of economic growth.	**(B)** The unstated evidence in paragraph 1 is that productivity is a measure of economic growth—making this the correct answer.
C. each American worker's productivity is directly proportional to overall national productivity gains.	**(C)** is Opposite, because the author states that "while workers . . . have shared . . . in national productivity gains, they have not done so equally." It is also Out of Scope because it comes from paragraph 2.
D. Boskin's report is unable to explain the discrepancy between productivity growth and wage increases.	**(D)** This paragraph focuses on *income inequality*, not *the discrepancy between productivity growth and wage increases*. Faulty Use of Detail.

Question	Analysis
4. The author's primary purpose in presenting this passage is to:	The words *primary purpose* identify this as a Main Idea question, which usually can be answered quickly. The goal in this passage that we identified when highlighting is *to argue that the C.P.I., with or without Boskin's work, understated real wages; and that the productivity/wage disparity is more complicated than it first appears.*
A. argue that overreliance on the C.P.I. is insufficient for explaining the current state of the American worker.	**(A)** is correct; the passage primarily addresses the idea that the "C.P.I. . . . understated real wages" (and therefore does not fully explain the current state of the American worker).
B. argue that wages actually increased from 1978 to 1994.	In **(B)**, the answer is far too specific as it applies only to paragraph 2 and not the entire passage.
C. argue that a capitalistic oppression of the worker is the primary cause of the current economic climate.	The *capitalist oppression of the worker* is part of the *simplistic* model dismissed in paragraph 7. Because the author does not agree with this model, **(C)** can be eliminated.
D. suggest that partisan division in Congress would be more adequate for explaining the current economic climate.	Congressional divide, while perhaps present in real life, was never mentioned in the passage, making **(D)** Out of Scope.

Question	Analysis
5. The author's use of the term "statistical imagination" in paragraph 3 most nearly indicates:	This is a Definition-in-Context question. A quick scan of paragraph 3 shows us that "statistical imagination" refers to a shortcoming of the traditional C.P.I. model, due to failure to "take account of changes in consumption patterns and product quality improvements." Be on the lookout for any wrong answers that sound like a standard definition for *imagination*.
A. wage data for the last 25 years has been falsified.	**(A)** is Out of Scope because we're never told that data was *falsified*.
B. the pessimistic view of the economy indicated by the C.P.I. is overstated due to underestimation of the significance of key variables.	**(B)** matches closely with the prediction and is the correct answer.
C. mathematical models of the economy are less accurate than anecdotal reports.	**(C)** is Out of Scope because this passage never compares *mathematical models* to *anecdotal reports* in terms of validity.
D. the C.P.I. is a completely unreliable tool for explaining the economic climate.	The C.P.I. certainly has some issues but is not the *completely unreliable tool* mentioned in **(D)**—this is Extreme.

PRACTICE QUESTIONS

Passage 1 (Questions 1–6)

The United States has less than half of the 215 million acres of wetlands that existed at the time of European settlement. Wetland conversion began upon the arrival of Europeans with their traditional antipathy to wetlands and with the will and technology to dry them out. In the mid-19th century, the federal government awarded nearly 65 million acres of wetlands to 15 states in a series of Swamp Land Acts. But the most rapid conversion occurred between the mid-1950s and mid-1970s, when an estimated 450,000 acres per year were lost, primarily to agriculture.

This conversion has meant the loss of a wide range of important wetland functions. Wetlands inhibit downstream flooding, prevent erosion along coasts and rivers, and help remove or assimilate pollutants. They support scores of endangered birds, mammals, amphibians, plants, and fishes. Wetlands provide aesthetic and open-space benefits, and some are critical groundwater exchange areas. These and other public benefits have been lost to agricultural forestry and development enterprises of all kinds, despite the fact that most of the conversion goals might have been obtained with far less wetland loss through regional planning, stronger regulation, and greater public understanding of wetland values.

At best, existing wetland laws and programs only slow the rate of loss. Despite the growing willingness of government to respond, wetland protection faces significant obstacles. Acquisition as a remedy will always be limited by severe budget constraints. The Emergency Wetlands Resources Act allocates only $40 million per year in federal funds, supplemented by relatively modest state funds, for wetland purchase. Ultimately, the wetlands that are protected will be a small percentage of the approximately 95 million acres remaining today. Wetland acquisition by private environmental groups and land trusts adds qualitatively important, but quantitatively limited, protection. Government incentives to induce wetland conservation through private initiatives are limited and poorly funded. Some private developers have recognized that business can protect selected wetlands and still profit. Recreational developments in Florida have benefited from wetland and habitat protection that preserves visual amenities. It is doubtful, however, that these business decisions to save wetlands would have occurred without strong government regulation; the marketplace does not generally recognize the public benefits of wetlands for flood control, fish and wildlife, and other long-term values.

One possible strategy (and the one presently being implemented) is to protect each and every wetland in threatened areas according to stringent permit guidelines that do not distinguish by wetland types or values. This approach may be environmentally desirable, but it has not worked. About 300,000 acres of wetlands are lost each year. An alternative strategy is to develop a regional management approach focused on valuable wetlands in selected areas that are under intense pressure. Broad regional wetland evaluations could identify critical wetland systems that meet particular local and national needs and avoid abandonment of any wetlands without careful review of the trade-offs. Cooperating federal, state, and local interests can then anticipate and seek ways to prevent wetland losses and can guide future development in areas where alternative options exist. There is no general federal authority to conduct such planning for wetland system protection. But there are several authorities under which a program to anticipate and prevent wetland losses on an area-wide basis can be developed.

1. In paragraph 1, it is reasonable to believe that the author assumes:
   - **A.** wetland conservation efforts are cost prohibitive.
   - **B.** wetland conservation began with the arrival of Europeans to the United States.
   - **C.** wetlands are a source of tourism income for many areas in the United States.
   - **D.** wetlands can be converted to agricultural purposes through currently available means.

2. According to the passage, all of the following contributed to the rapid loss of wetlands in the United States EXCEPT:
   - **A.** technological innovations implemented by European settlers.
   - **B.** development of commercial and residential real estate complexes.
   - **C.** increased rezoning for the purposes of agricultural and industrial operations.
   - **D.** conversion of wetlands for agricultural uses.

3. As used by the author, the word "authority" (paragraph 4) most nearly means:
   - **A.** a person with extensive or specialized knowledge of a subject.
   - **B.** having ascertained something from a reliable source.
   - **C.** the power to influence others due to one's knowledge about a topic.
   - **D.** a person or organization having power or control in particular.

4. Implicit in the discussion in this passage is the underlying assumption that the author believes:
   - **A.** Wetlands under intense pressure should be focused on first.
   - **B.** Using current policies, wetland losses cannot be fully combated, only minimized.
   - **C.** The loss of wildlife due to wetland losses is the only reason the government should be concerned.
   - **D.** Advocating for increased governmental spending in wetlands conservation will solve the problem of wetland losses.

5. Which of the following does the author state as beneficial functions of the wetlands?
   - **I.** Supporting communities of endangered amphibians
   - **II.** Providing renewable forestry options
   - **III.** Erosion and flood control

   - **A.** III only
   - **B.** I and II only
   - **C.** I and III only
   - **D.** I, II, and III

6. The author can best be viewed as a proponent of:
   - **A.** developing new strategies and improving current efforts to prevent wetland losses.
   - **B.** maintaining the current stringent permit guidelines to protect conservation areas.
   - **C.** promoting development of wetlands for visual amenities and aesthetic benefits.
   - **D.** current government incentives to induce wetland conservation through private business funding.

ANSWERS AND EXPLANATIONS

Passage 1 (Questions 1–6)

Sample Highlighting

P1. "wetland conversion"; **P2.** "wetland function" and "lost to"; **P3.** "obstacles" and "private initiatives"; **P4.** "alternative strategy" and "no general federal authority."

Sample Outline

P1. History of wetlands conversion

P2. Benefits of wetlands, ways loss could have been minimized

P3. Current problems with conservation efforts and ways of minimizing further loss

P4. Current solution (save all threatened wetlands) hasn't worked; proposes new regional management strategy

1. **D**

The word *assumes* signifies to us that we are approaching an Inference question type. Inference questions ask us to find the necessary connecting information. With a paragraph reference, there is clear direction on where to begin the Investigate step. In paragraph 1 we're told "Wetland conversion began upon the arrival of Europeans with their traditional antipathy to wetlands and with the will and technology to dry them out... when an estimated 450,000 acres per year were lost, primarily to agriculture." For answer choice **(A)**, costs were discussed in paragraph 3 but not paragraph 1. In answer choice **(B)** Wetland *conversion* began with the arrival of Europeans, not wetland *conservation*. Answer choice **(C)** is an Out Of Scope answer choice. While the passage is about the wetlands and they may be a source of tourism income, that topic is never discussed within the passage. This leaves answer choice **(D)** as the correct answer, and further, this is a reasonable inference, as we are told that wetlands were converted to agricultural property.

2. **C**

For this Scattered Detail question type, we will have to find three answer choices that are mentioned in the passage and eliminate them. For **(A)**, the "technological innovations" of European settlers are mentioned in paragraph 1. "Development enterprises" are listed at the end of paragraph 2, which eliminates **(B)**. **(C)**, however, cannot be found in the passage. No mention is made of *increased rezoning* of wetlands, so this must be the correct answer. Finally, "conversion of wetlands for agricultur[e]" is listed at the end of the first paragraph, which removes **(D)**.

3. **D**

Typing this question is pretty straightforward, as you are given a word from the last paragraph and asked what it means in the passage, making this a Definition-in-Context question. The best thing to do with a question like this is to reread the targeted sentence in the passage, as well as the surrounding sentences. The sentence the word appears in is "There is no general federal authority to conduct such planning for wetland system protection." This sentence alone doesn't give a full answer, but the sentence before gives the necessary context by mentioning "federal, state, and local interests," or the organizations that are in power to conduct planning which matches **(D)**. Answer choices **(A)**, **(B)**, and **(C)** are all definitions for authority, but are not the definition that the author was referencing in this passage, which makes them all Out of Scope answers.

4. **B**

This Inference question is asking for an inference the author made without a passage reference. This would be a good question to leave for your second pass through the questions. Answer choice **(A)** is a Faulty Use of Detail choice from paragraph 4 that does not answer the question being asked. In paragraph 3, the passage tells us "At best, existing wetland laws and programs only slow the rate of loss," which Matches answer choice **(B)**. Answer choice **(C)** is an Extreme answer choice; unless an author is extreme, which this author is not, an Extreme answer choice will not be correct. The author thinks that the best way to fix this problem is to apply a new regional management strategy, making **(D)** Out of Scope.

5. **C**

The Roman numeral format and the verb *state* tell us that this is a Scattered Detail question. "Beneficial functions of the wetlands" are mentioned in the first part of paragraph 2. Relevant to this question are the details that "wetlands inhibit downstream flooding, prevent erosion along coasts and rivers, . . . and support scores of endangered birds, mammals, amphibians, plants, and fishes." Statements I and III are listed in this paragraph, whereas *renewable forestry options*, Statement II, are never mentioned.

6. **A**

This is a masked Main Idea question; asking what the author is a *proponent of* is another way of asking what the author likes. The author's goal in the passage is to *describe problems with current wetland conservation efforts and to propose a new strategy*. This prediction matches well with **(A)**. In the final paragraph, the author discusses the flaws of the current permit system, so **(B)** can be eliminated as an Opposite. **(C)** can also be eliminated for similar reasons because the author is a proponent of the preservation of—not *development of*—the wetlands. Finally, the author states in the third paragraph that "government incentives to induce wetland conservation through private initiatives are limited and poorly funded," so **(D)** can also be eliminated.

CHAPTER 10

QUESTION TYPES II: *REASONING WITHIN THE TEXT* QUESTIONS

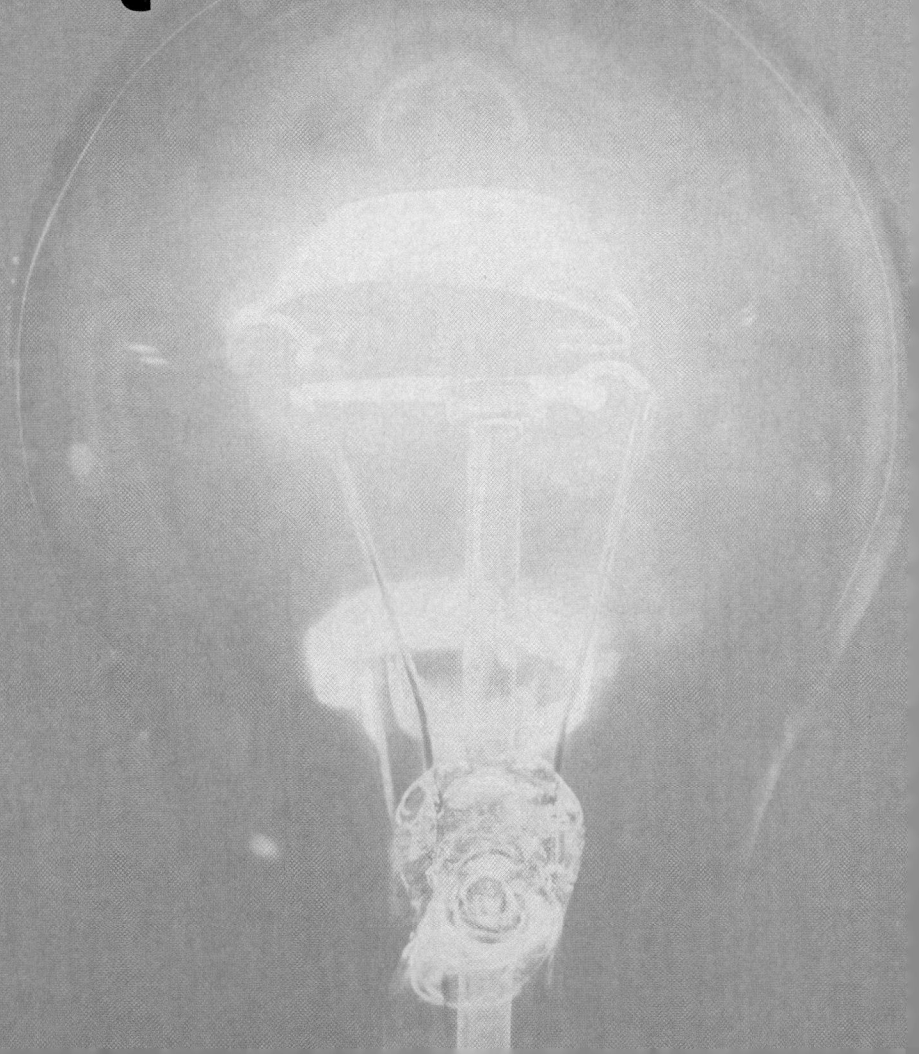

CHAPTER 10

QUESTION TYPES II: *REASONING WITHIN THE TEXT* QUESTIONS

In This Chapter

Introduction

LEARNING OBJECTIVES

After Chapter 10, you will be able to:

- Identify Function, Strengthen–Weaken, and Other *Reasoning Within the Text* questions
- Solve *Reasoning Within the Text* questions with focused strategies
- Apply the major principles of argument and logical structure to MCAT questions

In this chapter, we'll continue the treatment of question types first employed with *Foundations of Comprehension*, now examining the two types of *Reasoning Within the Text* questions that Kaplan has identified: Function questions, which ask about why the author included a piece of information or argument in the passage, and Strengthen–Weaken (Within the Passage) questions, which predominantly concern the ways in which arguments are backed by evidence and undermined by refutations. This chapter adopts the same general approach as Chapter 9: after identifying what makes the questions distinctive and offering several common question stems, we discuss strategies for each question type, illustrating them with a few Applied Examples.

Reasoning Within the Text questions account for approximately 30 percent of what you'll encounter on Test Day, according to both the AAMC's official statements and Kaplan's own extensive research of released AAMC material. In general, Function questions are roughly as common as Detail and Strengthen–Weaken (Beyond the Passage) questions, but they are less common than Apply questions. Strengthen–Weaken (Within the Passage) questions are more rare than Function questions.

Note: The question types, as well as the Kaplan Method for CARS Passages, Kaplan Method for CARS Questions, and Wrong Answer Pathologies, are included as tear-out sheets in the back of this book.

10.1 Function Questions

One of the reasons that the Kaplan Method for CARS Passages emphasizes reading for perspective (trying to understand the author's attitude and intentions) rather than just for detail is that the **Function question** type specifically asks about what the author is trying to *do* in the passage. Unlike a Main Idea question, which might ask about the overall goal of the passage, a Function question will ask about the purpose of only a portion of the passage, often in the context of the author's larger argument. Further, these questions will require some level of critical thinking about why a piece of information was included, meaning they involve an additional level of complexity beyond the *Foundations of Comprehension* question types seen in Chapter 9.

Sample Question Stems

- What is the author's apparent purpose in stating [quotation]?
- The author mentions [topic] in [paragraph reference] in order to:
- Which of the following is the most probable reason for the author's inclusion of a quotation from [person]?
- The author's reference to [concept] in [paragraph reference] is most likely supposed to show:
- When the author says [claim], she is emphasizing that:
- Which of the following is the example from [paragraph reference] most likely intended to suggest?
- The author compares [one concept] to [another concept] because:
- The author's principal motive for discussing [alternative position] is to explain that:

What should be readily apparent in the phrasing of Function questions is frequent mention of the author and the use of direct references to the text—especially through paragraph references. Language like *purpose, motive*, and *intention* indicate a Function question, as do phrases that end with *in order to* and *because*. Use these key phrases and traits to Type the question quickly. For Function questions, the Rephrase step tends to be fairly straightforward, as these questions usually state the task to be accomplished.

Strategy

Function questions are usually specific to a certain portion of the passage that can be directly referenced, making them a good option to solve now rather than later. Referring back to your Distill step will be key when working with a Function question. If you were reading for perspective by looking for Author keywords (which give a glimpse from the author's point of view), you may have already considered the information you need to answer such a question in your Distill step; it might even be highlighted or in your outline, if you chose either of those approaches. Keep in mind that, generally speaking, Function questions work in a nested way. In other words, the passage as a whole has a purpose, and each paragraph within it has a subordinate function that is distinct but that contributes to the larger whole. Each paragraph can in turn be broken down into sentences, each of which has its own particular role to play in the paragraph—and even sentences can be broken down into particular words or phrases.

Because a Function question will generally ask for the purpose of no more than a paragraph, to Investigate this question type you should recall or refer back to your Distill step for the specific paragraph (and perhaps also consider the author's overall goal in the passage). Then, if buzzwords in the question stem direct you to specific sentences, reread those portions of the paragraph if needed and think about how they fit into the purpose of the paragraph and the passage's general purpose. If you chose to Distill by Interrogating, you may find you don't even have to return to the passage, and can instead directly predict an answer. Formulate a statement of the function, and then start to look for an answer that matches.

Remember, if you can't find a perfect match, you can eliminate choices that are inconsistent with the passage at a higher level. For example, the purpose of a paragraph will not be at odds with the author's goal for the passage as a whole unless that paragraph represents a counterargument. Even when authors bring up information that conflicts with their main arguments, they commonly do so for the sake of shooting it down—answering or countering a refutation they introduced in a prior portion of the passage.

Function Questions—Applied Example

The most prevalent argument against doctor-assisted suicide relies upon a distinction between *passive* and *active* euthanasia—in essence, the difference between killing someone and letting that person die. On this account, physicians are restricted by the Hippocratic oath to do no harm and thus cannot act in ways that would inflict the ultimate harm, death. In contrast, failing to resuscitate an individual who is dying is permitted because this would be only an instance of refraining from help and not a willful cause of harm. The common objection to this distinction, that it is vague and therefore difficult to apply, does not carry much weight. After all, applying ethical principles of *any sort* to the complexities of the world is an enterprise fraught with imprecision.

Rather, the fundamental problem with the distinction is that it is not an ethically relevant one, readily apparent in the following thought experiment. Imagine a patient who is terminally ill and hooked up to an unusual sort of life support device, one that only functioned to prevent a separate "suicide machine" from administering a lethal injection so long as the doctor pressed a button on it once per day. Would there be any relevant difference between using the suicide machine directly and not using the prevention device? The intention of the doctor would be the same (fulfilling the patient's wish to die), and the effect would be the same (an injection causing the patient's death). The only variance here is the means by which the effect comes about, and this is not an ethical difference but merely a technical one.

Example:

1. The author's apparent intention in discussing the "suicide machine" in paragraph 2 is to:

    A. support his thesis using an imaginative exercise.
    B. question the idea that vagueness is ethically relevant.
    C. explain the operation of a piece of medical equipment.
    D. propose a new method for performing euthanasia.

Solution: The first step in the method is to Type this question as a Function question. This can be done by recognizing the "intention ... is to" portion of the question stem as asking why a specific piece of information was included. Your approach to Function questions will differ depending on which approach you took to the passage. However, they will all rely on one thing: knowing why the author mentioned the fact from the question stem. As this question stem has a direct task already listed, the Rephrase step is likely not necessary.

The question stem directly states a location and quoted term, meaning that whether you outlined, highlighted, or interrogated, the location of the relevant information in the passage is readily available. However, we don't actually need to dive back into the passage to answer this question. To investigate, recall the purpose of paragraph two or refer back to your outline or highlighting to find that purpose. We know that the author used the "suicide machine" thought experiment to support her argument, so this will suffice as a prediction. Going back to the text itself shouldn't be necessary unless the answer choices take us somewhere unexpected. Fortunately, that is not the case with this question, and we can see that **(A)** gives us precisely what we need. The time spent distilling the passage has been more than paid back with a quick correct response.

Among the wrong answers, **(B)** is wrong for bringing in *vagueness*, when the point of the thought experiment is to question whether the *passive/active distinction* is ethically relevant—not vagueness. **(C)** might be considered a Faulty Use of Detail because the operation of this machine is explained. However, the machine is being described not for its own sake—it's imaginary, after all—but simply to illustrate a point. The final incorrect option, **(D)**, would be a product of taking the thought experiment too literally.

10.2 Strengthen–Weaken (Within the Passage) Questions

Strengthen–Weaken questions span two of AAMC's delineated categories, but both types generally concern the logical relationships between conclusions and the evidence that *strengthens* them or the refutations that *weaken* them. Note that the only substantial difference between Strengthen–Weaken (Within the Passage) questions and Strengthen–Weaken (Beyond the Passage) questions is that the former stick to the passage as written while the latter will bring in some new element, usually appearing in the question stem, though on occasion only in the answer choices.

Sample Question Stems

- The author's suggestion that [claim] is supported in the passage by:
- For which of the following statements from the passage does the author provide the most support?
- The author states in [paragraph reference] that [claim]. This most strengthens the author's contention that:
- Which of the following objections considered in the passage most WEAKENS the author's thesis?
- Which of the following is a claim that the author makes without providing evidence?
- The view of [person] is challenged in the passage by:
- How does other information from the passage relate to the claim that [quotation]?
- What significance does the assertion that [claim] have for the author's argument?

As this list suggests, these types of questions often contain references indicating that the answers will be taken directly from the text and are heavy on words indicating connections between claims like *relate*, *support*, and *challenge*. Some question stems may be ambiguous about whether the support or challenge you're looking for will be coming from within the text or outside of it, in which case you'll also want to bear in mind the strategy for Strengthen–Weaken (Beyond the Passage) questions, detailed in Chapter 11.

Strategy

Every Strengthen–Weaken question has three pieces: **two claims** and the **connection** between them. You will always be given at least one of these elements, and your task will be to find the other(s), so begin your Investigate step by identifying where each piece can be found: either directly in the stem itself, somewhere in the passage, or in the answer choices.

If the *connection* is revealed in the question stem, it will typically be some variation of strengthen (support) or weaken (challenge), as the name of these questions suggests. However, when the connection does not occur until the answer choices, such as when a stem uses vague words like *relevance*, *significance*, or *impact*, the claims occasionally have some other relationship, such as identity (meaning the same thing) or even irrelevance. Once you know whether your task is to Strengthen, Weaken, or find some yet-to-be-discovered relevance, the next step of your investigation will be to research the status of any *claims* quoted or otherwise referenced in the question stem. The number of steps you must go through as you investigate will vary based on the number of claims in the stem.

If no other claims are mentioned, such as in a question like *Which of the following passage assertions is the LEAST supported?*, you should probably save the question for later and then use the process of elimination in your Investigate step.

KEY CONCEPT

Evidence is used to support a conclusion through a one-way relationship. A refutation is used as a counterargument against a conclusion through a one-way relationship.

If the question stem refers to two claims, then the task must be to find the nature of the relationship they share, so think about whether one claim supports the other, remembering that evidence makes a conclusion more likely to be true and refutations make conclusions less probable.

In most cases, though, you'll be presented with only one claim in the question stem, so plan to investigate the given statement as a conclusion, piece of evidence, or a refutation. Start your research with the relevant sentence, but check the surrounding text for language suggestive of a relationship. When you are researching the passage, Logic keywords are just about as important for Strengthen–Weaken questions as they are for Inference questions. If the question stem specified the relationship, pay special attention to that one; otherwise, keep an eye out for any logical connections made to the claim, using those to set expectations.

If your initial plan of attack proves unsuccessful, try process of elimination, crossing out any answer choice that does not establish the correct kind of relationship. Do not forget that support is unidirectional: if the "arrow" points the wrong way, it cannot be the right choice. So, for instance, if you are asked to find a claim that *supports* the author's thesis, a potential wrong answer is an implication that could be drawn if you assumed the thesis was true—in other words, a conclusion that the thesis itself *supported.*

Strengthen–Weaken (Within the Passage) Questions—Applied Example

The most prevalent argument against doctor-assisted suicide relies upon a distinction between *passive* and *active* euthanasia—in essence, the difference between killing someone and letting that person die. On this account, physicians are restricted by the Hippocratic oath to do no harm and thus cannot act in ways that would inflict the ultimate harm, death. In contrast, failing to resuscitate an individual who is dying is permitted because this would be only an instance of refraining from help and not a willful cause of harm. The common objection to this distinction, that it is vague and therefore difficult to apply, does not carry much weight. After all, applying ethical principles of *any sort* to the complexities of the world is an enterprise fraught with imprecision.

Rather, the fundamental problem with the distinction is that it is not an ethically relevant one, readily apparent in the following thought experiment. Imagine a terminally ill patient hooked up to an unusual sort of life support device, one that only functioned to prevent a separate "suicide machine" from administering a lethal injection so long as the doctor pressed a button on it once per day. Would there be any relevant difference between using the suicide machine directly and not using the prevention device? The intention of the doctor would be the same (fulfilling the patient's wish to die), and the effect would be the same (an injection causing the patient's death). The only variance here is the means by which the effect comes about, and this is not an ethical difference but merely a technical one.

Example:

2. Which of the following roles is played in the passage by the claim that the difference between killing and letting die is ethically relevant?

   I. It is contradicted by the assertion that the distinction between active and passive euthanasia is only technical.
   II. It bolsters the contention that applying ethical principles precisely is difficult.
   III. It underlies the most common argument against physician-assisted suicide.

   A. III only
   B. I and II only
   C. I and III only
   D. I, II, and III

Solution: The first thing to notice in your Type step is that this question is a Roman numeral question. A glance at the answer choices also tells you that this is a Strengthen–Weaken question based on the use of the words *contradicted, bolstered,* and *underlies*. The question asks about *roles* that are *played in the passage* by a statement given in the stem, so you can identify this as a Strengthen–Weaken (Within the Passage) question. However, it's a Roman numeral question, and these are usually more time-consuming. Your best bet is to save this for the end of the question set.

When you do solve this question, rephrase the base stem of the question first and leave the Roman numerals aside for the time being. Then, Investigate to find the claim referenced in the question stem. As is often the case in more complex Strengthen–Weaken (Within the Passage) questions, there is no single sentence that contains all the words in the assertion; rather, parts of it are spread throughout the text. The two lines that are most important are the opening sentences of each paragraph, the first of which refers to "the difference between killing someone and letting that person die" and the second of which maintains that "the distinction . . . is not an ethically relevant one." To Rephrase, we could ask ourselves *What is the connection between the two paragraphs?*

As you investigate, you can see that the claim that the distinction is ethically relevant must be what is "relie[d] upon" (Evidence keyword) by the so-called "most prevalent argument against doctor-assisted suicide." In other words, the claim that the distinction is ethically relevant plays a supporting role in that argument. Second, it is clear that the second paragraph is denying this claim. These initial observations already offer a sense of two roles that the distinction plays, a fairly thorough prediction.

MCAT EXPERTISE

CARS authors often use multiple *terms* (words or phrases) to describe the same *concept*, or underlying idea. On Test Day, pay special attention to the ways in which authors use terms, especially when you see Opposition keywords. When you come across dualisms, you can draw a set of columns adjacent to your map on your note board and jot down what words the author uses for each side of the contrast. This can serve as a handy reference for any synonymous language you might encounter in the questions and answer choices. So, for the ethics passage, you would put *killing* and *active euthanasia* in one column and *letting die* and *passive euthanasia* in the other.

At this point, you can start the Match step by looking at the answer choices to see how the Roman numerals are distributed. We generally recommend starting with the most common numeral or, alternatively, whichever seems easiest for you. Statements I and III both appear three times, so start with the shorter of them. Statement III suggests the claim *underlies* the most common argument, which is precisely as predicted. Therefore, Statement III must be true and **(B)** can be crossed off.

Turning to Statement I, you'll note the mention of "the distinction between active and passive euthanasia," which you were told in the first sentence was "in essence, the difference between killing someone and letting that person die." This is consistent with the expectation set earlier that the second paragraph challenges the assertion that the claim is ethically relevant. The final sentence confirms it: "this is not an ethical difference but merely a technical one." The "not" tells you that this is the contradiction that Statement I suggests, so it must also be true, eliminating **(A)**.

There are still two answer choices remaining, so you will have to deal with Statement II. The contention that it mentions did not figure into our prediction, so check the text to find the reference, which is located at the end of the first paragraph. How does this assertion relate to the original claim that the distinction is ethically relevant? The clue is the keyword that precedes the assertion: *After all*. Even though it may sound like a Conclusion keyword on the surface, it's actually an Evidence keyword, which means that this assertion about *applying ethical principles* is in truth used to support something else. Specifically, this statement bolsters the author's belief that the "common objection" to the distinction carries little weight. This is not the relationship suggested by Statement II, which says that the claim that the distinction is ethically relevant supports how hard it is to apply ethical principles precisely. Thus, Statement II is false. Only Statements I and III are true, making **(C)** the only match, and thus the correct answer.

Example:

3. On the basis of the author's discussion, which of the following items from the passage LEAST challenges the argument for the prohibition of active euthanasia?

    A. The thought experiment involving two suicide machines from the second paragraph
    B. The assertion that the distinction between passive and active euthanasia is too difficult to apply
    C. The argument that the distinction between passive and active euthanasia is only technical
    D. The claim that the effect and the intention are the same regardless of the type of euthanasia

Solution: Question 3 is somewhat tricky to untangle, with its multiple negative terms, but you can use the phrases *challenges* and *from the passage* to Type this question as a Strengthen-Weaken (Within the Passage) question—specifically, Weaken. However, the *LEAST* means a **Scattered** format, one in which you'll probably have to test all of the answer choices. Save this for later if possible.

When Rephrasing, begin by clarifying the *argument for the prohibition of active euthanasia*. Although the order after the dash in the first sentence is switched, it should be clear from the subsequent sentence that *active euthanasia* refers to the act of *killing*, which is supposedly forbidden because of the Hippocratic oath that the physician takes. This argument prohibiting active euthanasia is, in fact, the *most prevalent argument* from the first line. The correct answer, then, will be the one that challenges this argument the least.

The Scattered form suggests process of elimination as the best Investigate and Match method, but before resorting to that, it doesn't hurt to see whether the author actually talks about a challenge that she regards poorly because that could be the very answer you're seeking. Indeed, the author does say in paragraph 1 that "the common objection ... does not carry much weight." The objection referenced is that it's difficult to apply the distinction between killing and letting someone die, so this can serve as your prediction.

Looking at the answers, you can see that this prediction matches **(B)**. However, you should be cautious with this sort of question. While the passage says that the objection carries little weight, it does not say that it carries no weight at all, meaning that if there were an answer choice that had no effect or even supported the argument, that would be *even less* of a challenge. As it turns out, the remaining answer choices are all aspects of the counterargument made in the second paragraph, and all do indeed challenge the original argument. Now you can be confident that **(B)** is the correct answer.

10.3 Other *Reasoning Within the Text* Questions

There are a few rarer types of questions that do not neatly fall into either the Inference or Strengthen–Weaken (Within the Passage) categories, but that definitely concern passage reasoning and that do show up in some CARS sections. These can take many different forms and all are rare, so we'll just focus our discussion on three typical tasks.

Clarification

Questions that ask about **clarification** concern a relationship that is very similar to support, as it is also a one-way relationship. One assertion clarifies another if the two share roughly the same meaning, but the "clarifying" part is typically more specific or exact. Because the clarifying language tends to be more precise, its truth value is easier to assess, and thus you should think of "clarifying" statements as supporting evidence for "clarified" conclusions. Approach them more or less as you would a Strengthen–Weaken (Within the Passage) question, except keep in mind that the meanings should be roughly synonymous.

With the ethics passage, for instance, you could see a Clarification question like *Which of the following clarifies the author's statement that the common argument against physician-assisted suicide rests upon the distinction between passive and active euthanasia?* The answer would most likely come from one of the sentences that followed, which explained the difference between the two more concretely, including the reasons why one is supposedly permitted and the other is not. In addition to words like *clarify*, words like *explain* and *reflect* are used in questions to indicate this kind of relationship.

KEY CONCEPT

In a Clarification question, look for an answer choice that is nearly synonymous with the given claim, only that is more specific or exact.

Weakness

KEY CONCEPT

Answering a Weakness question is just like using the Denial Test, discussed in Chapter 9 for Inference questions. The difference is that the correct answer choice will be detrimental to the arguments in the passage *without* being negated.

Weakness questions are somewhat related to Inference questions, but they concern *implicit weaknesses* and *reasonable objections* to arguments discussed in the passage. Instead of the Denial Test, the best way to investigate is often via the process of elimination by directly examining the effect that answer choices have on the argument in question. The correct answer will have the most significant negative impact on the argument, perhaps even contradicting it altogether.

One example of a Weakness question for a passage we've seen would be *Which of the following is the greatest inherent weakness in the author's use of a thought experiment to support the main argument?* This is a more complex type of *Reasoning Within the Text*, and it is one among a number of rarer questions that require you to appraise the strength of the author's reasoning. The answer to this example might be the fact that thought experiments force the author to rely upon readers' imagination and intuition, which may not always result in the same conclusion as the author intended.

Paradox

KEY CONCEPT

A paradox is a set of two claims that appear to be inconsistent on the surface. The correct answer in a Paradox question will be consistent with both of the claims, and it will usually attempt to explain the surface inconsistencies between the two claims.

Finally, by a **paradox**, we mean an *apparent* logical contradiction, a set typically consisting of two assertions that seem inconsistent, but only at first glance. These will usually include two distinct claims from the text, phrased in a way to make them sound conflicting, followed by a question like *How would the author resolve this dilemma?* or *How might the passage account for this discrepancy?* Sometimes one of the claims will be a new element, which would technically make such questions *Reasoning Beyond the Text*, although they should still be approached with the same strategy in this case.

The correct answer to a Paradox question must be *consistent* with both of the claims given in the question stem. If possible, it should also not conflict with anything that the author says elsewhere in the passage. Thus, to resolve paradoxes, you should use process of elimination, marking out any answer choice that is inconsistent with one or both of the claims (or with the passage as a whole).

Conclusion

Although often variable in appearance, *Reasoning Within the Text* questions test only a few essential skills: identifying inherent weaknesses in arguments; identifying the function of parts of the argument; understanding relationships of consistency and conflict; and recognizing the connections in passages between conclusions, evidence, and refutations. Regardless of how challenging these questions may seem to you now, you have the ability to improve your reasoning skills! The solution is to practice using Logic keywords to identify support relationships, and applying the other strategies discussed in this chapter as you Type, Rephrase, and Investigate questions. These tactics will also be useful when working on the final class of questions, *Reasoning Beyond the Text*, the subject of the upcoming chapter.

GO ONLINE

You've reviewed the strategy, now test your knowledge and critical thinking skills by completing a test-like passage set in your online resources!

CONCEPT AND STRATEGY SUMMARY

Function Questions

- **Type: Function questions** ask about what the author is trying to *do* with a piece of information in the passage.
  - These questions are similar to Main Idea questions, although they focus on the purpose of only one portion of the passage (usually one sentence or one paragraph).
  - Function questions tend to use words like *purpose, motive,* or *intention,* or phrases like *in order to* or *because*
- **Rephrase:** Function questions will always have a similar Rephrase task, which will result in something similar to *What purpose does [this detail] serve in the passage?*
- **Investigate:** If buzzwords in the question stem direct you to specific sentences, recall or reread those portions, thinking about how they fit into the purpose of the paragraph and the overall passage.
- **Match:** Your expectations should match the right answer. If there is no clear match, or if you cannot perform any of the earlier steps of the Kaplan Method for CARS Questions, use the process of elimination, removing any answer that conflicts with the author's main argument or the paragraph's purpose.

Strengthen–Weaken (Within the Passage) Questions

- **Type: Strengthen–Weaken (Within the Passage) questions** concern the logical relationship between conclusions and the evidence that strengthens them or the refutations that weaken them.
  - These questions often contain words like *relate*, *support*, *challenge*, *relevance*, *significance*, or *impact*.
  - These questions are closely related to Strengthen–Weaken (Beyond the Passage) questions, which simply bring in a new piece of information rather than using information directly from the passage.
- **Rephrase:** Your Rephrase should center around the task of identifying the two pieces of information and the connection between them; you will usually be given at least one of these elements and will have to find the other(s).
  - Identify where each piece of the argument can be found: in the question stem, in the passage, or in the answer choices.
  - If no claims are given in the question stem, triage the question and answer it by process of elimination later.
  - If one claim is given in the question stem, determine if it is a conclusion, a piece of evidence, or a refutation.
  - If two claims are given in the question stem, identify the relationship between them.

- **Investigate:** Research the relevant text to determine the missing claim or the connection between the claims. Use Logic keywords to help assemble the argument.
- **Match:** Your expectations should match the right answer. If there is no clear match, or if you cannot perform any of the earlier steps of the Kaplan Method for CARS Questions, use the process of elimination.

Other Reasoning Within the Text Questions

- **Clarification questions** ask for statements that are roughly synonymous, but the clarifying statement tends to be supporting evidence for the conclusion because it is more specific or exact.
  - These questions often contain words like *clarify*, *explain*, or *reflect*.
  - Approach these questions as you would Strengthen–Weaken (Within the Passage) questions, except that the meanings of the two claims should be roughly synonymous.
- **Weakness questions** ask for implicit refutations to arguments discussed in the passage.
  - These questions often contain words like *implicit weaknesses* or *reasonable objections*.
  - Approach these questions using the Denial Test as you would for Inference questions, except that the correct answer will be the most detrimental to the argument made in the passage *without* being negated.
- **Paradox questions** ask for the resolution of an apparent logical contradiction.
  - These questions often contain words like *paradox*, *dilemma*, or *discrepancy*.
  - Approach these questions through the process of elimination, crossing out any answer choice that is inconsistent with one or both of the claims of the paradox or with the passage as a whole.

Worked Example

Use the Worked Example below, in tandem with the subsequent practice passages, to internalize and apply the strategies described in this chapter. The Worked Example matches the specifications and style of a typical MCAT *Critical Analysis and Reasoning Skills* (CARS) passage.

Take a few moments to quickly glance over the passage in order to Preview and Choose your approach. The paragraphs of this passage may seem lengthy, but most of that volume is dedicated to examples to support the conclusions that are provided at the start of each paragraph. As each paragraph appears to center around one theme with examples, Outlining should be extremely effective. To work this passage efficiently, just make sure not to fall into the trap of trying to note all the supporting details. The language and wording are not overly complex, making it relatively easy to spot those arguments and extract a short summary for the outline. As with all passages, any approach could be chosen and work for this passage, so, remember to practice and hone all approaches as you start your CARS prep!

OUTLINING METHOD

Passage	Expert Thinking
Certain contemporary forms of literary criticism draw on modern sociology and political science to understand literary works. There has been a conservative reaction to these schools of criticism, accusing them of imposing modern ideas on old texts. For example, some would consider it an implausible claim that Shakespeare's *The Tempest* can be interpreted as a play about "colonialism" and "imperialism"; after all, these terms were not even in use when Shakespeare wrote the play. These concepts must therefore be modern ones, and it is anachronistic to suppose that Shakespeare had them in mind. Besides, as Ben Jonson wrote, Shakespeare "was not of an age, but for all time," and it trivializes his genius to suppose that he had in mind the fashionable concerns of any one period. The conservative reading of *The Tempest* sees it as a play about "universal" themes like estrangement and reconciliation.	What argument does the author introduce in the first paragraph? *The author states that modern literary criticism uses modern ideas on old texts, and that there has been an accusatory reaction to this from the conservative side.* Is there evidence to back up this argument? *Yes. The author provides* The Tempest *as an example. However, we do not need to write down any details on that in our outline.* Does the author take a stance on the issue? *No keywords point to tone at this point in the passage.* P1: Conserv: modern crit uses modern bias, evidence
But writers do live in specific societies and are affected by the cultures of the times and places in which they live. The establishment of colonies—the building of empires—was an issue of keen concern in England in the early 17th century. It was a matter of national prestige and also a potential source of private wealth. All the great powers of Europe were competing for the wealth of the East and West Indies. The rich hoped to add to their fortunes; the poor hoped to begin their lives anew in the "New World." Richard Hakluyt's *Voyages*, a series of published accounts of European voyages to Asia, Africa, and the Americas, was one of the most successful publishing ventures of Elizabethan England. Moreover, although the words *colonialism* and *imperialism* had not been coined yet, the ideas they connote already existed, in the sense that some Europeans perceived ethical problems relating to empire-building. The Spanish priest Bartolomé de las Casas had already condemned the cruelty of the Spanish regime in Mexico and the Caribbean, and the French essayist Michel de Montaigne had already compared some indigenous peoples favorably with decadent Europeans.	This paragraph starts with a contrast keyword ("But"). What does that indicate is coming next? *This paragraph will center around the author disagreeing with the view from the previous paragraph.* What is the author's argument? *The author argues that while certain modern words were not used in the time of older literary texts, the ideas behind those texts already existed.* Is there support for the author's claims? *Yes. Multiple examples are provided. We do not need to try to analyze or remember all the details, as our outline will send us back to this paragraph if needed.* P2: Auth ≠ conserv, mod ideas already existed, evidence

OUTLINING METHOD

Passage	Expert Thinking
Now let us look again at *The Tempest*. Here is a play about a European family ruling a remote island by superior European technology (magic, learned from books) and the forced labor of the native population. When another group of Europeans arrives on the island, one of them imagines an ideal commonwealth in terms derived, as scholars have long recognized, from Montaigne's essay about the native people of Brazil. The prostrate Caliban reminds Trinculo of a deceased native who might be exhibited in England for crowds willing to pay to see an exotic "monster." And scholars have long recognized that the story of *The Tempest* is suggested in part by accounts of the *Sea Venture*, shipwrecked in Bermuda in 1609 on the way to the Virginia colonies.	What new ideas or themes are introduced in this paragraph? *The first sentence of this paragraph tells us that the author is coming back to* The Tempest *example. Since we do not have any Contrast keywords, it is safe to assume that the author will try to apply the argument from the previous paragraph to* The Tempest, *which conservatives used as an example in the opening paragraph. There is no need to write down specific details here.* P3: Auth: mod ideas in The Tempest
With all this in mind, are we really to believe that neither Shakespeare nor anyone who saw the play in London in 1611 was reminded of the colonial enterprise that England was then undertaking in America? Who is making the implausible claim?	How can we identify the author's conclusion? *The author used rhetorical questions to indicate a concluding thought.* What is the author's conclusion? *Those who saw the play in London were reminded of England's actions in America.* P4: Auth: conserv making implaus claim

Question	Analysis
1. The author mentions "Richard Hakluyt" primarily in order to:	This is a Function question that is asking how the author uses a particular detail in the structure of the passage. "Richard Hakluyt" was mentioned in paragraph 2, which should be the focus of our Investigate step.
A. serve as an example of authors who wrote about topics while lacking specific language to describe them.	Much of this paragraph consisted of examples of authors who were writing about topics that didn't have words for them yet. Answer choice **(A)** is correct.
B. serve as an example of a popular contemporary of Shakespeare.	While Shakespeare does appear in paragraph 1, the author doesn't suggest that Hakluyt and Shakespeare are contemporaries, making **(B)** a Faulty Use of Detail answer choice.
C. serve as an example of authors who invented new ideologies.	**(C)** is an Extreme answer choice; Hakluyt didn't invent colonialism, he just described it in his writing.
D. serve as a counter point to Bartolomé de las Casas.	**(D)** is an Opposite answer choice: Bartolomé de las Casas and Hakluyt were used in the same paragraph as examples of people who condemned colonialism and imperialism.

Question	Analysis
2. Which of the following is used in the passage to support the conservative interpretation of Shakespeare?	This is a Strengthen–Weaken (Within the Passage) question because it asks for the evidence used for a given conclusion. We know the conservative critics see Shakespeare as a timeless, "universal" playwright and not one whose themes are about only a specific time. The conservative argument in paragraph 1 hinges on the claim that the terms "colonialism" and "imperialism" did not exist yet, and therefore it would be "anachronistic to suppose that Shakespeare had them in mind."
A. Imperialism and colonialism are anachronistic terms for the 17th century.	**(A)** fits perfectly with the prediction and is the correct answer.
B. *The Tempest* has its roots in a story regarding English ships headed for America. **C.** The specific society a writer lives in is essential to understanding the writer's themes. **D.** European technology in the 17th century was far superior to other technology.	**(B)**, **(C)**, and **(D)** can be eliminated quickly because they do not come from paragraph 1, the only place where the conservatives' view is given any support. These answer choices come from paragraphs 2 and 3, which are not used to support the conservative view.

Question	Analysis
3. How would the author of this passage resolve the apparent paradox that it is an implausible claim that Shakespeare's *The Tempest* can be interpreted as a play about "colonialism" and "imperialism"?	This is an Other *Reasoning Within the Text* question. The "implausible claim" is discussed in Paragraph 1, but the author's response to that claim is discussed in the rest of the passage. By looking at our outline, we can see that the author thought those modern ideas already existed and gave examples to support that theory. In fact, the author focuses most of the passage on critiquing the argument from the first paragraph, centering around his assertion that the ideas already existed even if the words did not.
A. Ideas can only occur when they are able to be described by specific language.	**(A)** sounds like the conservative critics and is inconsistent with the author's central argument. This choice should be eliminated.
B. All ideologies are present in all stories and are ubiquitous regardless of time period.	The words *all* and *ubiquitous* indicate that **(B)** is an Extreme answer choice and should be approached with caution. For an Extreme answer choice to be correct, the author must hold an extreme viewpoint, which this author does not.
C. Even though the words had not been invented, the ideas behind them existed in the time when Shakespeare wrote *The Tempest.*	This answer choice is very close to our prediction from the Investigate step and uses moderate language. Therefore, **(C)** is the correct answer choice.
D. Thematic ideas are not present in older stories in which the author was living in a different time period.	**(D)** implies that older stories do not have thematic elements at all. This idea is inconsistent with the author's argument that "colonialism" and "imperialism" are present in *The Tempest.*

Question	Analysis
4. The author mentions the East and West Indies for what purpose (paragraph 2)?	While this question uses the word *purpose* and it may feel like a Main Idea question at first blush, it's actually asking about the function of the East and West Indies in building the author's argument. Approach this question by locating the reference in the passage and either recalling or reading the sentence before and after it. It's stated in the passage that "all the great powers of Europe were competing for the[ir] wealth" and "the building of empires—was an issue of keen concern in England in the early 17th century."
A. As an example of one of the most successful publishing ventures of Elizabethan England	**(A)** is a Faulty Use of Detail answer choice. The most successful publishing venture of Elizabethan England mentioned in the passage was "Hakluyt's *Voyages*, a series of published accounts of European voyages to Asia, Africa, and the Americas."
B. As an example of empire building that Shakespeare participated in as part of his research for *The Tempest*	There is no reference to Shakespeare witnessing firsthand the colonialism that is referenced in *The Tempest*; **(B)** is an Out Of Scope answer choice.
C. As an example of empire building that existed in when Shakespeare was writing *The Tempest*	**(C)** is closest to our investigation of the paragraph surrounding the mention of the East and West Indies and is the correct choice.
D. To show that everywhere visited by Europeans was colonized	**(D)** This is an Extreme answer choice; while the Europeans were involved in colonialism and imperialism, it is never implied that everywhere the Europeans traveled was a place they colonized.

Question	Analysis
5. The fact that the terms "colonialism" and "imperialism" were not coined yet in Shakespeare's time has what effect on the author's argument?	This is another Strengthen–Weaken (Within the Passage) question. The author's idea throughout the passage is that even though the words *colonialism* and *imperialism* did not exist, these themes were still present in *The Tempest*. Therefore, the fact that these words "were not coined yet" is consistent with—but does not strengthen or weaken—the author's argument.
A. It strengthens the author's argument about Shakespeare's works. **B.** It weakens the author's argument about *The Tempest*. **C.** It strengthens the author's argument about *Voyages*.	**(A)**, **(B)**, and **(C)** can be eliminated immediately because they state that the author's argument would be *strengthen[ed]* or *weaken[ed]*.
D. It doesn't affect the author's argument.	The prediction—that the author's argument is neither strengthened nor weakened—matches **(D)**.

PRACTICE QUESTIONS

Passage 1 (Questions 1–6)

It would be difficult to overstate the complexity of the Japanese language. The system of writing (or more properly, systems) represents a fusion of almost entirely non-native characters and a spoken language so linguistically isolated that philologists have yet to discover a precursor. Not unlike many other ancient languages, Japan lacked any system of writing at all for much of its history. Making up for lost time, though, no fewer than three different systems of writing are now employed.

The first Japanese system of writing was not Japanese. The *kanji*, a group of logographic Chinese characters, each representing a word or idea, were adopted with minimal change around the seventh century. Few languages are so geographically close yet linguistically dissimilar. As a result, the people of Japan adopted a modified Chinese pronunciation for each kanji (the *on-yomi*), while retaining the native Japanese spoken word that most closely fit each kanji's meaning (the *kun-yomi*). In modern Japanese, the *on-yomi* is used for certain kanji and the *kun-yomi* for others, with compound words often involving both. Further adding complication, the Chinese language contains many words in which variations in tone alone indicate drastically different meanings. The adaptation of these words to Japanese pronunciation led to a number of homophones that has, without hyperbole, been called "embarrassing" and "alarming" by scholars of the language.

The *hiragana* syllabary was developed in the eighth century by court women, who were not permitted to study *kanji* because they were deemed unfit to master its complexities. In response, they developed a simplified, flowing form of the kanji that represented all the sounds in spoken Japanese. Hiragana is phonetic rather than logographic and is therefore far more accessible to a foreign learner than the kanji. Because Japanese is an open language, most consonants cannot be expressed by themselves. Hiragana is therefore not strictly an alphabet. *Katakana* came about around the same time as hiragana, also as an attempt to simplify the kanji. The sparse, angular characters correspond fairly closely to the hiragana and, as befitting their origin among Buddhist monks, have a look generally considered more masculine than hiragana, which was originally called *onnade*, or "women's hand." The katakana have essentially become the print counterparts of the "cursive" hiragana.

With so many systems jostling for position, each used more or less independently of the other, it would not be unreasonable to anticipate that a national movement toward systematization of the language would settle on a single one. A national movement was in fact started after World War II: a radical idea encouraging the use of all three systems together. A glance at any Tokyo newspaper will reveal kanji used to represent most standard actions and ideas, hiragana to indicate grammatical inflections and tenses, and katakana to represent adopted non-native and technical words, as well as to indicate emphasis. The use of the three systems has become sufficiently standardized in this way that deviations often lend a piece of writing strong connotations. A piece written entirely in katakana, for example, may be disconcerting to a modern reader and may have a vaguely pre–World War II military air to it, much as a piece written all in capital letters with telegraph punctuation might in English. While such a complex system has made the language's learning curve high for native and non-native speakers alike, it has also contributed to a stunning richness of expression such that any list of world's great works of art a hundred years from now will have to be written partially in kanji, hiragana, and katakana.

1. The author mentions Chinese *kanji* (paragraph 2) for what purpose?
   - **A.** To show the large number of homophones in the language is due to the closeness of Japanese and Chinese pronunciation.
   - **B.** To illustrate that the presence of homophones in a language can be considered embarrassing.
   - **C.** To show it as a precursor to the Japanese method of writing that caused some linguistic quirks.
   - **D.** To show that homophones are dependent on variations in tone.

2. The author's primary purpose in the passage is to:
   - **A.** argue that the Japanese language is overly complex.
   - **B.** describe the origins of the Japanese language's complexity.
   - **C.** propose a simplification in how Japanese is written.
   - **D.** trace the origins of logographic writing systems.

3. According to the passage, which of the following pieces of Japanese literature would NOT likely be written entirely in katakana?
   - **A.** a modern Japanese novel
   - **B.** a list of adopted foreign words
   - **C.** a 9th-century Buddhist text
   - **D.** an early 20th-century general's log

4. Based on the author's description, open languages generally contain:
   - **A.** borrowed systems of writing and speaking from many different sources.
   - **B.** intrinsic acceptance of change and reform.
   - **C.** syllables that end in vowels.
   - **D.** few consonant sounds.

5. As can be inferred from the passage, the group of Buddhist monks who developed katakana:
   - **A.** was predominantly or entirely male.
   - **B.** used hiragana as a model.
   - **C.** was considered unfit to master the complexities of kanji.
   - **D.** was closely involved with the military of the time.

6. Which of the following is a claim the author makes without providing evidence?
   - **A.** The first Japanese system of writing was not Japanese.
   - **B.** The use of the three systems has become sufficiently standardized in a way that deviations often lend a piece of writing strong connotations.
   - **C.** Japanese lacked any system of writing at all for much of its history.
   - **D.** The katakana have essentially become the print counterparts of the "cursive" hiragana.

Answers follow on next page.

ANSWERS AND EXPLANATIONS

Passage 1 (Questions 1–6)

Sample Highlighting

P1. "linguistically isolated"; **P2.** "Chinese character"; **P3.** "Hiragana is phonetic" and "simplify the kanji"; **P4.** "sufficiently standardized" and "richness."

Sample Outline

P1. Japanese language and writing complex: at least 3 systems

P2. Chinese (logographic) introduced = kanji; on-yomi *vs.* kun-yomi

P3. Syllabic/phonetic: hiragana (feminine, script) *vs.* katakana (masculine, print)

P4. Post-WWII: All three combined and systematized, different uses for each

1. **C**

For this Function question, start with where *kanji* are mentioned. Kanji appears in paragraph 2, where the author says that the adaptation of Chinese words with variations in tone to Japanese resulted in lots of homophones. The function of including kanji is to introduce the idea that Japanese came from Chinese and doesn't have as many variations in tone as Chinese does. **(C)** fits this prediction. While **(B)** may be a true statement, it is not related to kanji and is a Faulty Use of Detail answer choice. **(D)** is an Opposite; it is the loss of "variations in tone" as words moved from Japanese to Chinese that led to the formation of homophones. As for **(A)**, the author specifically stated that "Few languages are so geographically close yet linguistically dissimilar," so we know that pronunciations must be very different.

2. **B**

This is a Main Idea question, so predict using the author's overall goal established during your Distill step: *to examine the origins and complexity of three Japanese writing systems.* Only **(B)** involves both the *origins* and *complexity* of the language. Notice that we can use a vertical scan of the first words of the answers to eliminate **(A)** and **(C)** because the author is neutral and does not make any strong *argu[ments]* or *propos[als]*. As for **(D)**, the author discussed the origins of Japanese only—not multiple *logographic writing systems*—and, even then, this answer choice is too narrow as it addresses the author's purpose only in paragraph 2.

3. **A**

This is an Apply question asking for an example of a text that would *NOT likely be written entirely in katakana.* Where does the author discuss the uses of writing in katakana? Referring back to the passage (or recalling if you used the Interrogate method for distilling the passage), we find that it is introduced in paragraph 3 and that the modern approach of using all three systems together—including katakana—is described in paragraph 4. There, the author writes that katakana is used to "represent adopted non-native and technical words, as well as to indicate emphasis" and that a piece written entirely in katakana "may be disconcerting to a modern reader and would have a pre–World War II military air" to it. Based on this information, **(B)** and **(D)** can immediately be eliminated. **(C)** can also be eliminated based on the description of the origins of *katakana* in paragraph 3: both hiragana and katakana appear around the *eighth century*, and katakana specifically "origin[ated] among Buddhist monks." The answer must, therefore, be **(A)**, which makes sense: a modern piece of literature would be expected to combine all three writing systems.

4. **C**

For this Inference question of the Implication subtype, start with where *open languages* are mentioned. Paragraph 2 states that "because Japanese is an open language, most consonants cannot be expressed by themselves." It also points out that hiragana (and, by extension, katakana) is "not strictly an alphabet," but rather a "syllabary." Taking these pieces of information together, we can determine that open languages must express consonants together with vowels and that the language is built on these consonant–vowel combinations (syllables). **(C)** reflects this idea, highlighting the syllabic nature of the language. While the author does not specifically state that vowels end syllables in Japanese, the two Japanese terms given in the paragraph—hiragana and katakana—both demonstrate this pattern. **(D)** is a Distortion because although the author does say that consonants are not often used by themselves, there is no mention that they are few in number overall. While **(A)** describes the Japanese language, it does not reflect the author's use of the more general term "open languages." Finally, **(B)** is a literal use of the word *open* and does not fit the context described by the author.

5. **A**

The word *inferred* shows that this is an Inference question. The Buddhist monks who developed katakana are highlighted in paragraph 3. Let's review the main points: katakana was created by "Buddhist monks" and looks "more masculine than hiragana." The author also notes that hiragana was developed by women and was known as "women's hand." Given the contrast between katakana and hiragana on the basis of gender, we can infer that katakana looks masculine because it was developed by men. **(A)** must therefore accurately describe this group of Buddhist monks. While **(C)** might look tempting, we know only that the women who developed hiragana were "considered unfit to master the complexities of kanji." The author never stated anything similar about the monks who developed katakana, so we cannot make that inference. In the last paragraph, the author points out that katakana now has a "vague... military air" to it for the modern reader, but that does not mean that the monks who created katakana were *closely involved with the military of the time.*

6. **C**

This is a Strengthen–Weaken question asking for a claim in the passage that lacks evidence. Note that all four answer choices are sentences taken verbatim from the passage. For this question, we will have to address each answer choice as we look for evidence that supports the claim. The "first Japanese system of writing," **(A)**, was addressed in paragraph 2. Immediately following this sentence, the description of "kanji" is given—which is that "first... system of writing." Therefore, this answer choice can be eliminated. The use of "three systems" and the effects of "deviations" from the standardized approach are detailed in paragraph 4; the subsequent "piece written entirely in katakana" is evidence to support this claim, eliminating **(B)**. **(C)** is mentioned at the end of paragraph 1, but that's all the information we get about the Japanese language before writing systems were developed. This answer is therefore correct. Finally, **(D)** is supported by the sentence that immediately precedes it, which describes the "sparse, angular characters" of katakana as counterparts to the hiragana.

CHAPTER 11

QUESTION TYPES III: *REASONING BEYOND THE TEXT* QUESTIONS

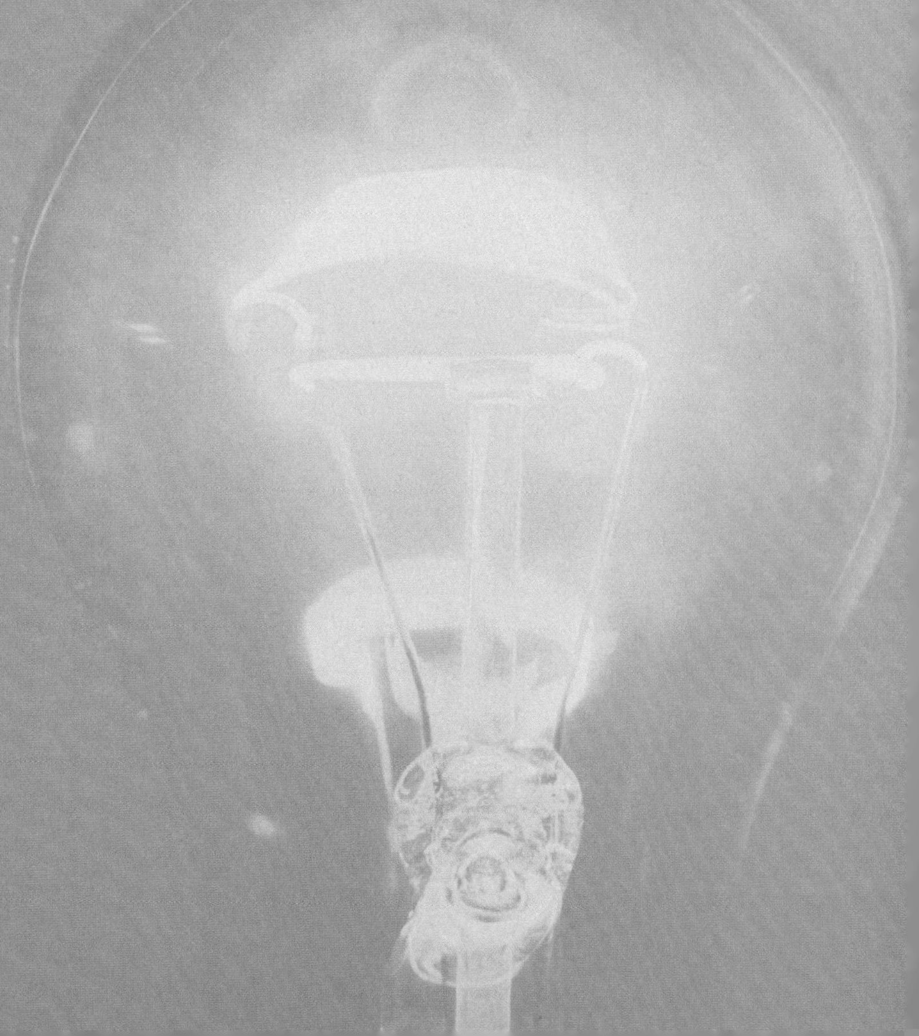

CHAPTER 11

QUESTION TYPES III: *REASONING BEYOND THE TEXT* QUESTIONS

In This Chapter

Introduction

LEARNING OBJECTIVES

After Chapter 11, you will be able to:

- Identify Apply, Strengthen–Weaken, and other *Reasoning Beyond the Text* questions
- Solve *Reasoning Beyond the Text* questions with strategies specific to each question type
- Differentiate between Probable Hypothesis, Alternative Explanation, and Passage Alteration questions

As a physician, you'll quickly realize that patients rarely present with the exact mix of signs and symptoms you may have spent countless hours memorizing in medical school. Additionally, when patients describe their symptoms, the language they use rarely coincides with the sophisticated terminology found in textbooks and journals. As a result, a large part of medical training involves interacting directly with patients in order to better understand how to assimilate the knowledge learned in class with the practicalities of real life. Medical schools are interested in students who can take information they have elicited from a patient and go a step further with it, not just matching symptoms to a diagnosis, but rather, identifying future diagnostic steps and applying information learned from prior patients to new ones. This is why this skill is so heavily tested in the *Critical Analysis and Reasoning Skills* (CARS) section. Like an ICU, the MCAT tests whether you are able to take what you have learned and apply it to a novel situation with speed and precision.

In this chapter, we'll examine the Apply and Strengthen–Weaken (Beyond the Passage) question types. As in the previous question types chapters, we'll look at some common question stems, specific strategies, and a few worked examples for each question type. We will conclude with a brief discussion of the rarer kinds of *Reasoning Beyond the Text* questions.

The AAMC reports that 40 percent of the questions in the CARS section should be classified as *Reasoning Beyond the Text.* It further divides this categorization into questions that require you to apply or extrapolate ideas from the passage to a new context (Apply questions) and those that require you to evaluate the effect new information would have if it were incorporated into the passage (Strengthen–Weaken [Beyond the Passage]). The fundamental difference between the two question types is one of direction: Apply questions ask you to determine how the passage relates to a new situation, while Strengthen–Weaken (Beyond the Passage) questions ask you to determine how the new information might affect the passage. While the AAMC suggests that the *Reasoning Beyond the Text* category is split evenly between these question types, our intensive study of released AAMC materials has shown that Apply questions tend to be slightly more common than Strengthen–Weaken (Beyond the Passage) questions. Note that it is possible, though rare, to get a question that doesn't fall into either question type but still qualifies as *Reasoning Beyond the Text.*

KEY CONCEPT

Apply and Strengthen-Weaken (Beyond the Passage) test your deductive reasoning. In both cases, a new situation is provided. Apply questions focus on how the passage relates to the new information (through a Response, Outcome, or Example). Strengthen-Weaken (Beyond the Passage) questions focus on how the new information impacts the passage.

Note: The Question Types, as well as the Kaplan Method for CARS Passages, Kaplan Method for CARS Questions, and Wrong Answer Pathologies, are included as tear-out sheets in the back of this book.

11.1 Apply Questions

Reasoning Beyond the Text questions always contain information in the question or answer choices (or both) that is not stated or suggested by the passage. *Reasoning Beyond* questions commonly begin with words like *suppose, assume,* and *imagine,* followed by an elaborate scenario, ending with a question connecting the new content to the author or passage. Apply questions will ask you to take information from the passage and apply it to a new situation. Strengthen–Weaken (Beyond the Passage) questions will test the opposite relationship, providing you with new information and then asking you to determine how it impacts the passage.

Apply questions are one of the most common of the CARS question types covered on the MCAT. In Apply questions, the text is used as a starting point that you must then apply to a new context. There are three common tasks, each constituting roughly one-third of the Apply question pool, that you will be asked to carry out. We categorize them as *Response, Outcome,* and *Example* Apply questions based on the words commonly seen in their respective question stems.

Sample Question Stems

- Consider the following: [new info]. The author would most likely respond to this by claiming:
- With which of the following claims would [the author or an alternative viewpoint from the passage] be LEAST likely to agree?
- Suppose that [details of new scenario]. Based on the passage, what would the author most likely advise in this case?
- Imagine [new info]. Which of the following, according to information presented in the passage, is the most reasonable outcome?
- If the passage's author is correct, the most likely consequence of [new situation] would be:
- Assume that [new info]. One could reasonably expect, on the basis of the passage, that:
- Which of the following best exemplifies the author's notion of [quotation from the passage]?
- Which of the following phenomena would the author most likely characterize as a [concept]?
- [New info]. The author would most likely classify this as:

At least a third of Apply question stems are similar to the first three samples above, concerning how the author (or, less frequently, another individual discussed in the passage) would respond to a particular situation. These questions commonly ask for the author's likely *response* or *reply*, a claim that the author would be *most likely to agree with*, or the statement *least consistent with* one of the views discussed.

Other Apply question stems take the form of the next three samples, investigating the most probable *outcome*, *result*, *expectation*, or *consequence* in a situation that is in some way analogous to one discussed in the passage. In other words, these questions provide you with a cause and ask about the likeliest effect, based on the passage.

Most of the remaining third of Apply question stems resemble the final three cases, asking for *examples* or *instances* of ideas discussed in the passage. Usually, the concept or term will be given, and your task is to find an item from a specified context (or from the "real world") that best exemplifies it as it was used in the passage. Question stems like the last one are rarer and more difficult, starting with an outside case and asking you how the author would categorize it: *What is this an example of?*

MCAT EXPERTISE

A lengthy question stem preceded by words like *suppose*, *imagine*, or *assume* is often a good indication of a *Reasoning Beyond the Text* question. From there, jump ahead to the last line before the question mark or colon at the end of the question stem to Type the question as either Apply or Strengthen–Weaken (Beyond) and identify the specific task being asked of you. Then, read through the new information and Rephrase carefully, always watching out for analogies to and similarities with the passage text.

Strategy

Once you've identified that new information is being provided in the question stem, you may find it helpful to jump to the end of the question stem to see what the question is really asking. This particular technique can be very helpful in your Rephrase step. Once you've picked up on the key language needed to determine the task, analyze the new information in the question stem closely for hints that connect it back to the passage. Then, go back and reread the relevant portions of the passage to make your prediction. When rephrasing the stem, keep in mind the question type and the task associated with it.

Response

For example, if the stem asks *How would the author respond to . . . ?* or *Which of the following claims would the author be most likely to endorse?*, your task is to get inside the author's head. The correct answer to a Response question should be consistent with the author's beliefs, which are typically reflected in the passage through the use of Author keywords, originally discussed in Chapter 5 of *MCAT CARS Review*. If you find yourself with a prediction that does not match directly with an answer choice, begin by eliminating any answers that are logically inconsistent with the author's assertions. If you are asked about a viewpoint other than the author's, utilize a similar strategy by putting yourself in the mind-set of the alternative perspective and recognizing what that person believes.

Outcome

If a question asks you about the probable outcomes of a scenario, look for words in the passage that indicate cause-and-effect relationships (Logic keywords). Identify any causes in the passage that are analogous to what is presented in the question stem and use their corresponding effects as the basis for your prediction.

Example

When you are called upon to identify examples, begin by finding the relevant text from the passage. Specifically focus on text that provides definitions, explanations, or the author's own examples of the concept in question. Take note of necessary conditions (which MUST occur in all instances of the concept) and sufficient conditions (which are enough on their own to make an instance qualify as that concept). Sufficient conditions are easier to match to, prediction-wise, but necessary conditions are useful when using an elimination strategy as they can be easily ruled out.

Apply Questions—Applied Example

There is no shortage of evidence for the existence of systemic biases in ordinary human reasoning. For instance, Kahneman and Tversky in their groundbreaking 1974 work proposed the existence of a heuristic—an error-prone shortcut in reasoning—known as "anchoring." In one of their most notable experiments, participants were exposed to the spin of a roulette wheel (specially rigged to land randomly on one of only two possible results) before being asked to guess what percentage of United Nations member states were African. The half of the sample who had the roulette wheel stop at 65 guessed, on average, that 45 percent of the UN was comprised of African states, while those with a result of 10 guessed only 25 percent, demonstrating that prior presentation of a random number otherwise unconnected to a quantitative judgment can still influence that judgment.

The anchoring effect has been observed on repeated other occasions, such as in Dan Ariely's experiment that used digits in Social Security numbers as an anchor for bids at an auction, and in the 1996 study by Wilson et al. that showed even awareness of the existence of anchoring bias is insufficient to mitigate its effects. The advertising industry has long been aware of this bias, the rationale for its frequent practice of featuring an "original" price before showing a "sale" price that is invariably reduced. Of course, anchoring is hardly alone among the defective tendencies in human reasoning; other systemic biases have also been experimentally identified, including loss aversion, the availability heuristic, and optimism bias.

Example:

1. Suppose a consumer who is looking for an inexpensive replacement for an outmoded refrigerator is enticed by a local retailer's ads for a discount sale promising savings of 50 percent or greater on all appliances. The author would probably warn the consumer that:

   A. sales are scams designed to exploit the consuming public.
   B. the pre-markdown prices are most likely set artificially high.
   C. heavily discounted merchandise is likely damaged or stolen.
   D. making a rational decision about what to buy is impossible.

Solution: The question starts with "suppose" so we are likely dealing with a *Reasoning Beyond* question. For your Type step, this should lead you to identify Apply as the question type, and given the relative level of difficulty of Apply questions, you may want to consider saving this question for later. Given the long question stem, you might consider skipping the new information in the stem on first read, in order to prioritize determining the task required. Your Rephrase step should result in needing to determine what the author would warn the consumer, which is a type of response. As a result, as you work through the question, you want to be thinking about views that the author holds. The ads for the sale should draw you to paragraph 2, in which the author states: "The advertising industry has long been aware of this bias, the rationale for its frequent practice of featuring an 'original' price before showing a 'sale' price that is invariably reduced." Although the author is not explicit, the use of quotation marks here is a case of "scare quotes," suggesting that the so-called "original" price is just there to make the "sale" price seem lower. Thus, it's reasonable to infer that the author would warn the consumer about the anchoring effect intended with pre-sale prices.

The closest match to this prediction is **(B)**. **(A)** can be ruled out as a Distortion because the language is too strong. Advice or admonitions that an author would provide should both be consistent with what the author says in the passage and also similar in tone. **(D)** is also a Distortion because of the word *impossible*. Finally, **(C)** is Out of Scope. The author suggests that discounts are offered to manipulate buyers into believing they have found a better deal, not to trick them into buying products that turn out to be faulty.

MCAT EXPERTISE

Although forming a prediction prior to looking at the answer choices is generally recommended, since *Reasoning Beyond the Text* questions contain new elements in the answers, sometimes looking at the first one or two answer choices can give you a better idea of the form that the correct answer will take. If the options diverge significantly from what you expected, go back and modify your original expectations before moving on to any remaining choices. Matching to the correct answer is generally less time-consuming than crossing out all three incorrect choices, so revising your prediction is usually a more optimal strategy than process of elimination.

Example:

2. Imagine that a psychologist specialized in the study of systemic reasoning biases. On the basis of the information presented, this psychologist could most reasonably be expected to:

   A. have a higher likelihood of misjudging numerical quantities when not given an anchor.
   B. make significantly fewer mistakes in reasoning than those ignorant of anchoring bias.
   C. be equally as susceptible to errors resulting from the anchoring effect as anyone else.
   D. avoid entirely the logical fallacies that ordinary human beings commit systematically.

Solution: The question stem is relatively short, so there's no need to jump to the end before reading the part after *Imagine*. Because we're searching for something *this psychologist could most reasonably be expected to do*, you can Type this as an Outcome question. Ask yourself whether the passage suggests anything about what happens to psychologists with greater knowledge of these biases in reasoning. Since there is no explicit reference, and the question stem is not heavy on other clues, expect to briefly look through the answer choices for additional clues on what to search for in the passage as the first part of your Investigate step.

The very first possibility suggests a consequence that would occur without the presentation of an anchor; however, the passage is only concerned about what happens when an anchor is present. It does not tell us anything about how accurate people's judgments of quantities are without the anchoring effect. We therefore have no basis to determine what effect having no anchor would have. Eliminate **(A)** as Out of Scope.

(B) suggests that such a psychologist would make fewer mistakes because of knowledge of the anchoring effect. Is there anything in the passage that would warrant this conclusion? The second paragraph states that Wilson and his colleagues "showed even awareness of the existence of anchoring bias is insufficient to mitigate its effects." Not only does this rule out **(B)** as an Opposite, but it also gives you an idea of what you can expect in a correct answer—that a psychologist is just as likely as anybody else to fall into these errors due to anchoring.

This revision to your Investigation pays off when you read **(C)**, which is almost an exact match for the new prediction. On Test Day, you would select this choice and move on to the next question without paying much attention to **(D)**—which could be ruled out for being a Distortion or an Opposite, constituting an even more extreme version of **(B)**.

Example:

3. Which of the following would the author be LEAST likely to consider a case of anchoring bias?

   A. An unusually high opening bid at an annual charity auction leads to a sizable increase over previous years in total proceeds collected.
   B. The sequel to a popular film is deemed a failure because it could not quite beat the record-smashing box office receipts of the original.
   C. A shipping website receives reports of greater levels of customer satisfaction after starting deliberately to overestimate delivery times.
   D. Poor initial sales figures for a new video game console motivate its manufacturer to reduce significantly the system's suggested retail price.

Solution: Despite asking for the *LEAST likely* case, we should still be able to Type this as an Example Apply question. It is hard to know what to predict based on the limited information in the question stem, but you can still set expectations about the correct answer by investigating the concept mentioned. The anchoring effect is the primary subject of this short passage, but the author only provides examples of the phenomenon without giving it an explicit definition. It's difficult to say precisely what would be sufficient to constitute anchoring bias, but we can isolate some necessary conditions. In each of the passage examples, a baseline numerical expectation, or "anchor," is set (either at random, as in the case of the experiments mentioned, or deliberately high in order to manipulate purchasers), which then skews the judgments people make about quantities. Any answer choice that satisfies these prerequisites should be eliminated because you are asked to find the *LEAST likely* example. Your Match will be found by process of elimination.

(A) is clearly a case of the anchoring effect; the passage even made mention of an experiment that used bids at an auction as the dependent variable. You can reason that the lofty opening bid must have caused other participants to heighten their appraisals of the items for sale, which in turn led to larger final sale prices and increased total proceeds.

Even though **(B)** is unlike anything found directly in the passage, it follows the model we anticipated for wrong answers. In this case, the original film is serving as the anchor that biases judgments of its sequel. Stating that the new movie *could not quite beat the record-smashing box office receipts of the original* suggests that it still generated a lot of revenue, meaning that the assessment of failure was probably in error. Because the anchoring effect is said to be a systemic bias, this implication of error should quell any remaining doubts about eliminating **(B)**.

Turning to **(C)**, we find another case that departs from the passage. Here, the anchor would be the estimated time of arrival for a particular shipment. If the site deliberately overestimates shipping times, its customers will consistently have to wait less time than they are told to expect, which will lead many to think that they are receiving excellent service. This situation is precisely analogous to the example of the original price marked down for sale, and hence it should also be eliminated.

Thus, **(D)** must be correct. While similar to one of the examples discussed on a superficial level, the monetary value of the sales (which would undoubtedly be orders of magnitude *higher* than the original price of one individual console) does not *bias* the manufacturer to lower the cost per system. Rather, this is a case of a rational response to an economic problem: when demand is too low, reduce the price.

Now, to be clear, this reduction in price could *lead to* a case of anchoring bias if, say, consumers started to purchase the console in greater quantities, believing it now to be a better deal. But the answer choice does not focus on that effect nor on any of the effects of cutting the cost, rather only mentioning its cause. And so, **(D)** is indubitably the one *LEAST likely* to count as anchoring bias for the author.

11.2 Strengthen–Weaken (Beyond the Passage) Questions

Like Strengthen–Weaken (Within the Passage) questions, **Strengthen–Weaken (Beyond the Passage) questions** explore evidence–conclusion relationships. Two notable distinctions between the two question types are that Strengthen–Weaken (Beyond the Passage) questions (1) contain at least one claim not from the passage that is unique to the question stem or answer choices and (2) treat the passage as flexible, in that they can be modified by outside forces.

Sample Question Stems

- Suppose [new info]. This new information:
- Which of the following statements, if true, would most bolster the author's argument about [topic]?
- Assume that [new info]. This assumption weakens the author's claim that:
- [New info] would most strongly support the view of:
- Recent research on [topic] suggests [new info]. Which of the following assertions from the passage is most logically consistent with these results?
- Some theorists have argued that [new info]. Based on the discussion in the passage, which of the following would present the greatest CHALLENGE to their argument?
- [New info]. In conjunction with information presented in the passage, it would be most reasonable to conclude that:
- Imagine that [new info]. What impact would this have on the arguments made in the passage?
- Which of the following study findings would most seriously undermine the author's thesis?

If the question includes new information and asks about logical relationships using words like *support*, *challenge*, and *consistency*, you can safely Type the question as a Strengthen–Weaken (Beyond the Passage) question. In some cases, the new information may be hidden in the answer choices, so watch out for clues that suggest the correct answer will come from outside the passage, such as words like *would* and *could*.

Strategy

As with Strengthen–Weaken (Within the Passage) questions, your primary task is to identify the three relevant parts: the conclusion, the evidence or refutation, and the nature of the connection (strengthen, weaken, or some unspecified relevance). Begin by determining which component (or, rarely, which two components) you are looking for, which you can target by rephrasing the question stem. Rather than reading all the new details during your first pass, jump to what immediately precedes the question mark or colon in order to figure out what the question is asking. Then, reread the question stem, keeping an eye out for any hints of analogy. Then, return back to the passage to confirm the relationship as the last step of your Investigation. Remember that Logic keywords from the passage can help you identify relevant evidence–conclusion relationships. For example, if a new experimental finding described in the question stem is similar to a study in the passage that was used to support the author's thesis, a good prediction is that this new finding will *strengthen* the author's thesis.

Note that the correct answers to Strengthen–Weaken (Beyond the Passage) questions rarely match predictions exactly the way they did for Strengthen–Weaken (Within the Passage) questions. As a result, it is more important to focus on relationships in your predictions, rather than specific wording, especially since answer choices are usually only incidentally related to the text.

BRIDGE

Strengthen-Weaken (Beyond the Passage) questions are extremely similar to Strengthen-Weaken (Within the Passage) questions, except that the former bring in new information, while the latter ask about arguments contained in the passage. Thus, a similar strategic approach can be used for both question types. Make sure to review Strengthen-Weaken (Within the Passage) questions, discussed in Chapter 10 of *MCAT CARS Review*, in tandem with this discussion of Strengthen-Weaken (Beyond the Passage) questions.

Strengthen–Weaken (Beyond the Passage) Questions—Applied Example

One of the first examples of the ascendance of abstraction in 20th-century art is the Dada movement, which Lowenthal dubbed "the groundwork to abstract art and sound poetry, a starting point for performance art, a prelude to postmodernism, an influence on pop art . . . and the movement that laid the foundation for surrealism." Dadaism was ultimately premised on a philosophical rejection of the dominant culture, which is to say the dominating culture of colonialist Europe. Not content with the violent exploitation of other peoples, Europe's ruling factions once again turned inward, reigniting provincial disputes into the conflagration that came to be known by the Eurocentric epithet "World War I"—the European subcontinent apparently being the only part of the world that mattered.

The absurd destructiveness of the Great War was a natural prelude to the creative absurdity of Dada. Is it any wonder that the rejection of reason made manifest by senseless atrocities should lead to the embrace of irrationality and disorder among the West's subaltern artistic communities? Marcel Janco, one of the first Dadaists, cited this rationale: "We had lost confidence in our culture. Everything had to be demolished. We would begin again after the *tabula rasa*." Thus, we find the overturning of what was once considered art: a urinal becomes the *Fountain* after Marcel Duchamp signs it "R. Mutt" in 1917, the nonsense syllables of Hugo Ball and Kurt Schwitters transform into "sound poems," and dancers in cardboard cubist costumes accompanied by foghorns and typewriters metamorphosize into the ballet *Parade*. Unsurprisingly, many commentators, including founding members, have described Dada as an "anti-art" movement. Notwithstanding such a designation, Dadaism has left a lasting imprint on modern Western art.

Example:

4. According to some estimates, prior to the beginning of World War I in 1914, more than four-fifths of the world's landmass was controlled by European nations or former colonies such as the United States. If this figure is accurate, what effect does it have on the passage?

   A. It bolsters the author's suggestion that European colonialism was an overbearing force.
   B. It weakens the author's assertion that World War I was instigated by provincial disputes.
   C. It strengthens the author's claim that Europe is the only place in the world that mattered.
   D. It challenges the author's insinuation that European rulers ignored the rest of the globe.

Solution: With such a long question stem, you'll want to skip right to the question itself, which asks for the *effect* on the passage. Type this as a Strengthen-Weaken (Beyond the Passage) question, and therefore, your task will be to determine the relevance of this new data. As you Rephrase the question stem, think about how the information presented either supports or challenges statements from the passage. The evidence provided has nothing to do directly with the Dada movement, which doesn't start until after the commencement of the war, but it does pertain to the author's discussion of Europe and World War I at the end of the first paragraph. So, your Investigate step will require rereading that portion of the text to see whether anything there would be impacted. The figure cited supports the author's opinionated characterization of *the dominating culture of colonialist Europe*.

(A) matches this prediction perfectly. *Overbearing* and *dominating* are synonyms, so even the language in the answer choice closely matches that in the passage. On Test Day, select this answer and then move on to the next question without reading the wrong answers.

For our purposes, however, it's worth reviewing where the others go wrong. While **(B)** may point to a claim that the author actually makes, the new information provided in the question stem does not pose a threat to it, making it a Faulty Use of Detail. The catalyst for World War I could still have been provincial disputes, regardless of how much land each country controlled. **(C)** is wrong for two reasons: first, it's Out of Scope because this is not something the author endorses; the author sarcastically states "the European subcontinent apparently being the only part of the world that mattered" when pointing out that "World" War I actually took place exclusively in Europe. Also, even if the author did have this view, the statement is a value judgment—a matter of opinion—which cannot be directly affected by geographic facts. Finally, **(D)** is also Out of Scope. Though it does contain a factual claim that would be challenged by the question stem, the author never insinuated that *European rulers ignored the rest of the globe*. Rather, the author refers to rulers "turn[ing] inward" after "violent exploitation of other peoples," suggesting they were actually gazing outward before the start of the war, the time period noted in the question stem.

Example:

5. Which of the following, if true, would most threaten what the author says in the final sentence of the second paragraph?
   A. A large majority of members of the general public, when asked to identify the most important work of art of the 1900s, fail to mention an example from the Dada movement.
   B. Other prominent 20th-century artistic movements, such as Surrealism and Pop Art, were also commonly described as "anti-art" by their most influential participants.
   C. The consensus among art historians today is that Dada was merely a brief departure from the principal themes in European art that evolved during the 20th century.
   D. Some of the founding members of the Dada movement were sympathetic to the radical view that, far from being anti-art, Dada was the purest form of art imaginable.

Solution: The hypothetical *if true* is strong evidence that the answer choices will be new elements and that this should be Typed as a Strengthen-Weaken (Beyond the Passage) question. The word *threaten* further implies that the task is to Weaken the author's claim.

After the Rephrase step, the first part of your Investigate step should involve returning to paragraph 2 and reading the last line, as referenced in the question stem, in addition to reading the preceding one for context. Though second to last sentence suggests that some people think of Dada as "anti-art," the last one contests this by pointing out Dada's "lasting imprint on modern Western art." Thus, we are most likely looking for a refutation of the author's idea that Dada was influential.

It's also possible that the correct answer challenges the author's rejection of the term *anti-art*. So, if we cancel out the confusing double negatives, the correct answer could also support the idea that Dada is anti-art.

Our first prediction matches **(C)** since the scholars' idea of a "brief departure" clashes directly with the "lasting imprint" from the text. An appeal to expert opinion is an acceptable form of evidence for most arts and literary passages. Also, since the author name drops and cites quotations frequently in the passage, consensus among experts should carry even more weight in this case.

While **(A)** does not support what the author says, it also does not pose a large challenge. Popular opinion does not necessarily reflect whether a work of art is influential or not. Additionally, leaving a "lasting imprint" is not identical to being the singularly most important movement of the century. Thus, the threat presented by **(A)** is weak at best. **(B)** is consistent with the passage, strengthening the point that simply calling a movement "anti-art" does not necessarily make it so. **(D)** has no impact on the last sentence of paragraph two. Even if some of the "founding members" of Dadaism did not think of the movement as being "anti-art," this answer choice targets the penultimate sentence—not the last one.

MCAT EXPERTISE

Appeals to authority or expert opinion are common in CARS passages, particularly those involving disciplines like the arts or literature, in which value judgments and other opinions play a prominent role. As you read, take note of the field you are reading about and the types of argumentation the author chooses to use. Quoting experts may provide decent support for a passage on an artistic movement, but such testimony will carry far less weight in more empirical social sciences like psychology or economics. Nonexpert opinions tend to carry even less weight: while authors may occasionally draw on popular opinion to support arguments, actual surveys of public opinion are seldom seen outside of a small number of cases, confined primarily to political science.

MCAT EXPERTISE

According to our research of released AAMC material, *Reasoning Beyond the Text* questions that are neither Apply nor Strengthen–Weaken (Beyond the Passage) questions are rare, numbering only one to two, on average, per CARS section.

11.3 Other *Reasoning Beyond the Text* Questions

Some questions that require you to think beyond the passage won't necessarily fall under the categories of Strengthen–Weaken (Beyond the Passage) or Apply question. Since these types of questions do not occur frequently, we will limit our discussion to three examples that have appeared on past MCAT exams.

Probable Hypothesis

In many ways, **Probable Hypothesis questions** are similar to Apply questions, but instead of asking about the outcomes of new situations, they ask about the likely causes. After presenting the new details, these stems will ask for *a probable hypothesis, the likely cause*, or *the most reasonable explanation based on the passage*. Though working backward from a given effect to its probable cause may seem more challenging, you will still use Logic keywords that reveal analogous cause–effect relationships in the passage to form your predictions. If no match to your prediction can be found, eliminate any answers that contradict claims the author states or suggests elsewhere in the passage.

Alternative Explanation

Alternative Explanation questions are also interested in potential causes. They begin by providing a phenomenon that may be pulled directly from the passage but then ask you to provide a cause that is not provided in the passage and may be dissimilar from anything previously discussed. Since it is almost impossible to form a focused prediction, expect to evaluate each answer choice and eliminate those that would not produce the result in the question stem. If you get stuck between multiple answers that seem equally likely to serve as the cause, eliminate those that would most conflict with other parts of the passage. While a correct alternative explanation won't be one the author has already provided, it should also not significantly contradict what the author has already stated.

Passage Alteration

One other less common *Reasoning Beyond the Text* question type will ask about changes that the author could make to the passage to make it consistent with new information. These are appropriately called **Passage Alteration questions**. In many ways, these are like the rare instances of *Reasoning Within the Text* questions that require resolving paradoxes, except that they will include some new information that contradicts what the author says or implies. The correct answer to these questions will typically be the one that produces the desired effect with the *least* amount of modification to ideas originally presented in the passage.

Conclusion

And so, this brings us to the end of our discussion of question types. If you are still confused about which name corresponds to which type, don't worry! The common stems, tailored strategies, and Worked Examples you have seen thus far are designed to serve only as your first exposure to the intricacies of the Kaplan Method for CARS questions, the question types and tasks, and the Wrong Answer Pathologies. Continue practicing until the Method becomes second nature for you. In the end, it will be less important to be able to name the question type than to know how to approach it. The best way to improve your performance with CARS questions is practice accompanied by effective review—the subject of our final chapter.

GO ONLINE

You've reviewed the strategy, now test your knowledge and critical thinking skills by completing a test-like passage set in your online resources!

CONCEPT AND STRATEGY SUMMARY

Apply Questions

- **Type: Apply questions** require you to take the information given in the passage and extrapolate it to a new context. These questions often begin with words like *suppose*, *consider*, or *imagine*. Apply questions typically ask for one of three tasks:
  - They may ask for the author's **Response** to a situation, using words like *response*, *reply*, *most likely to agree with*, or *least consistent with*.
  - They may ask for the most probable **Outcome** in a situation, using words like *outcome*, *result*, *expectation*, or *consequence*.
  - They may ask for an **Example** of an idea discussed in the passage, using words like *example* or *instance*.
- **Rephrase:** If the question stem is long, jump to the end to determine what it's asking. Read any information given in the question stem closely, looking for hints that connect it to the passage.
- **Investigate:** Reread the relevant text if needed, keeping in mind the specific type of Apply question involved.
  - For Response questions, determine the author's key beliefs, which are generally indicated in the passage by Author keywords.
  - For Outcome questions, pay attention to cause–effect relationships in the passage, which are generally indicated in the passage by Logic keywords.
  - For Example questions, look for passage excerpts that provide definitions, explanations, or the author's own example and note any necessary or sufficient conditions.
- **Match:** Match your expectations with the right answer. If there is no clear match, or if you cannot perform any of the earlier steps of the Kaplan Method for CARS Questions, use process of elimination.
  - Eliminate any answer choices that are inconsistent with the author's views, especially for Response questions.
  - Eliminate any answer choice that does not contain necessary conditions (which must occur in all instances of a concept), especially for Example questions.

Strengthen–Weaken (Beyond the Passage) Questions

- **Type: Strengthen–Weaken (Beyond the Passage) questions** focus on the logical relationship between conclusions and the evidence or refutations that strengthens or weaken them, respectively.
  - These questions are closely related to Strengthen–Weaken (Within the Passage) questions, which use information directly from the passage, rather than bringing in new information.
  - These questions often contain words like *relate*, *support*, *challenge*, *relevance*, *significance*, or *impact*. Words like *could* or *would* often help differentiate them from Strengthen–Weaken (Within the Passage) questions.
- **Rephrase:** Determine the two claims and the connection between them; you will usually be given at least one of these elements and be tasked with finding the other(s).
  - Identify where each piece of the argument can be found: in the question stem, in the passage, or in the answer choices.
  - If no claims are given in the question stem, plan to triage it for later and answer it using process of elimination.
  - If one claim is given in the question stem, determine if it is a conclusion, a piece of evidence, or a refutation.
  - If two claims are given in the question stem, identify the relationship between them.
- **Investigate:** Research the relevant text to determine the missing claim or the connection between them. Use Logic keywords to help assemble the argument.
- **Match:** Match your expectations with the right answer. If there is no clear match, or if you cannot perform any of the earlier steps of the Kaplan Method for CARS Questions, use process of elimination.

Other *Reasoning Beyond the Text* Questions

- **Probable Hypothesis questions** ask for causes of new situations presented in the question stem.
  - These questions often contain words like *probable hypothesis, likely cause*, or *most reasonable explanation.*
  - Approach these questions like you would Apply questions, but look specifically for analogous cause–effect relationships in the passage.
- **Alternative Explanation questions** ask for causes that differ from the ones given in the passage while still providing an explanation for a phenomenon.
  - These questions often contain words like *alternative explanation, other cause*, or *different reason.*
  - Approach these questions by eliminating answer choices that would not lead to the effect in the question stem. If you get stuck between multiple answers, eliminate those that conflict most significantly with the passage.
- **Passage Alteration questions** ask for changes the author could make to the passage to make it consistent with new information.
  - These questions often contain words like *alter, change*, or *update.*
  - Approach these questions by looking for the answer that produces the desired effect with the least amount of modification to the ideas in the passage.

Worked Example

Use the Worked Example below, in tandem with the subsequent practice passages, to internalize and apply the strategies described in this chapter. The Worked Example matches the specifications and style of a typical MCAT *Critical Analysis and Reasoning Skills* (CARS) passage.

Take a few moments to quickly glance over the passage in order to Preview and Choose your approach. An initial glance at this passage reveals that there are multiple types of art described in the body paragraphs. Interrogating this passage is a strong choice, as drawing connections between each of the mentioned art types and their underlying purpose in building the author's argument will be key to answering test questions. Further, this passage is not too long and has a structure that appears to lend itself well to chunking. Outlining would also be a strong choice, given that there are multiple terms with descriptive detail for each, and an outline is a simple way of keeping track of the location of a large number of details. In any case, we can predict during our passage Preview that the structure and high detail content of this passage will necessitate some referral back into the passage for questions regardless of Distill method chosen. As with all passages, any approach could be chosen and work for this passage, so, remember to practice all approaches as you start your CARS prep in order to determine which work best for you and in what situations!

INTERROGATING METHOD

Passage	Expert Thinking
Summer to winter to summer yet again, morning to night and then dawn once more. All things in life seem to cycle, and so, too, do trends in art. Styles, of course, do coexist and always have. Life is rarely as neatly divided between night and day as we might wish. But throughout history, art has followed one main avenue and then reversed direction time and time again, thus producing the Classicism *vs.* Romanticism (or Expressionism) dichotomy.	S1–4. Why does the author talk about such different concepts as life and art? *The author is drawing a parallel between life and art, as both life and art are apparently cyclical (in art, this refers to "style"). The author then brings up life being not neatly divided; we can predict from the start of the next sentence ("But") that art IS evenly divided, and the author is going to talk about that.* S5. Why does the author bring up Classicism and Romanticism? What do you think the author will discuss next? *These are the two main streams that art follows according to the author. Art following one path, then reversing direction seems to be a connection to the cyclical art trend noted in earlier sentences. We can anticipate that the author is going to elaborate more on the dichotomy.*
Classicism in art primarily refers to clean, cool imagery. In the High Classical period in ancient Greece, idealized sculpted figures of young men and women were perfect in proportion, the picture of health and vitality. The subsequent ancient Greek Hellenistic art swept in a more expressive era in which figures depicted actual people, with an emphasis on their individuality. Eschewing the sleek lines of the Classical period, sculptors lent their images a sense of weight so that clothing and hair looked a bit waterlogged. However, this additional substance often produced a sense of expressive motion: the goddess Nike (Victory) of Samothrace races forward as her windswept drapery creates wet wings behind her. The rational distance of the earlier Classical sculptures has given way to expressions that convey a more passionate, romantic essence.	S1–7. Why is High Classical art contrasted with Greek Hellenistic art? *High Classical art is defined by ideal sculptures with perfect proportions, whereas Greek Hellenistic art is subsequent to High Classical art, and is more expressive and weighted. The two are presented in this paragraph as examples of the two bigger art types in paragraph1: High Classical art is the first type (Classicism), and Greek Hellenistic art is the second type (Romanticism).*

INTERROGATING METHOD	
Passage	**Expert Thinking**
Not surprisingly, the French Neoclassicists, from about 1750 to 1850, looked to the Classical age for inspiration. Painting and sculpture contained the same refined, dignified qualities as the earlier work, although employing contemporary subjects. Portraits of both aristocrats and commoners reveal the late 18th- to early 19th-century "re-vision" of Classical times in everything from fashion to furniture and architecture. It was the Romanticists, though, who put the soul back into art. Their technique was looser, emitting the sense that the artist's hand had just lifted off the canvas or finished chiseling the stone. Brooding compositions described exotic locales in the Middle and Far East. Heroic stories detailed contemporary shipwrecks, battles, and civilian revolutions. Neoclassical works tasted of buttered toast where romantic pieces tasted of hot spice.	S1–8. Why is Neoclassical art contrasted with the Romanticists? *The refined Neoclassical art, which is similar to the Classical art in paragraph 2, is contrasted with the looser but exotic Romantic art. The contrast serves to highlight the dichotomy brought up in paragraph 1, were art starts in one direction (Classical) then reverses (Romanticism). We can now see a clear trend: the author is trying to provide recurring examples of the cyclic nature of art.*
Classicism evolved into two camps during the 20th century. A realism trend continued, in which artists depicted the world along the lines of human perception. The Regionalists in the early part of the century reflected life in America's backcountry. Grant Wood's 1930 painting "American Gothic" presents a no-nonsense farm couple staring the viewer straight in the eye. They exude the basic goodness and solidity of their nature. They stand together for eternity, more as emblems of an age and ideal than true individuals. Interestingly, the same cool distance resulted later on in the abstraction of Minimalism, beginning around the early 1960s. Minimalist artists created no figures or references to the outside world. Instead, the sharp edges of their geometric shapes, unmixed colors, and lack of visible brush or carving stroke embodied the same distilled, classical calm.	S1–9. How does this paragraph differ from paragraphs 2 and 3? Why does the author bring up Regionalists and Minimalists? *Paragraphs 2 and 3 focused on the Classical* vs. *Romanticism dichotomy, but in paragraph 4, the author is only talking about two streams of Classicism in the 20th century. Regionalist, focusing on ideal goodness, and Minimalists, focusing on abstract geometric shapes, are both Classical streams that embody the same cool distance. This diverges from the cyclic trend that has been emphasized since P1.*

INTERROGATING METHOD

Passage	Expert Thinking
Between these two periods, America birthed Abstract Expressionism, its most fervent art form. Painters abandoned realistic, figurative images and thrust their inner emotions or the invisible vibrations of the universe onto canvas. Virtuoso brushwork and color flash across flat surfaces with a magnetism and energy unknown before. These huge compositions take your breath away. Abstract Expressionism, the nation's first unique art movement, exudes all the brashness of a young upstart, even as the more classically oriented works that bracket this movement recall an esteemed, stately heritage.	S1–5. Why does the author bring up Abstract Expressionism as occurring between the two styles from P4? *Abstract Expressionism is not Classicism, and it is stated to be unique. However, from its description, we can see links to Romanticism, and given that this new style arises between the two Classical trends in P4, we are again returning to the theme of the cyclic nature of art.*
The time between the cycle from cool to expressive and ideal to romantic has shortened of late. The current art scene hosts art from both sides now. Perhaps the future will bring us more artists who freely sew the two ends of the continuum together.	S1–3. Why does the author see the future art movement possibly combining both dichotomies? *The time between cycles of Classicism and Romanticism seems progressively shorter and shorter until the present movement has a mix of both, and the author hopes for more mixes of the two dichotomies in the future.* *Overall, the author has built an argument that the nature of art styling is cyclical and alternates between versions of Classicism and Romanticism.*

Question	Analysis
1. Assume that most people at the time said the work of the Regionalists was emotionally overwhelming. What effect would this have on the author's arguments?	Because this question brings in new information and asks about its *effect*, this is a Strengthen–Weaken (Beyond the Passage) question. Regionalism supposedly evolved from Classicism, but *emotionally overwhelming* is a much better descriptor for Abstract Expressionism, as described in paragraph 5: these artists "thrust their inner emotions ... onto canvas, creating huge compositions [that] take your breath away." Because the new information in the question stem seems to go against the author, investigate the answer choices that include the word *weaken*.
A. It would strengthen the assertion that the time period between styles is currently shortening.	**(A)** and **(B)** can be eliminated immediately because they say *strengthen*.
B. It would strengthen the claim that Classicism primarily refers to clean, cool imagery.	
C. It would weaken the claim that art styles can coexist.	Because the new information implies that Regionalists have some expressive attributes, the claim that Classicism and Romanticism can coexist is *strengthened*, not weakened—making **(C)** an Opposite answer.
D. It would weaken the claim that Regionalism was a type of classicism.	The new evidence suggests that Regionalism could have been misclassified as Classicism when it has expressive aspects, confirming **(D)** as the correct answer.

Question	Analysis
2. In 1801, a French Neoclassicist announced that "I seek to infuse the modern era with the historical weight of a great past." On the evidence of the passage, he could have best achieved his goal by producing:	This is an Apply question of the Example subtype. Given the Roman numerals, it is a Scattered Apply question. As a French Neoclassicist, this artist would aim to have the "refined, dignified qualities" of classicism, "although employing contemporary subjects." The quote in the stem also indicates that a reference to something *historical* or the *past* should also appear in the answer choice.
I. a statue of Napoleon Bonaparte in which he is costumed plainly as an ancient Greek emperor.	In Statement I, we see Napoleon is the contemporary subject matter, but the artist is inspired by ancient times and uses a plain costume, reminiscent of Classical style. This fits the criteria, so Statement I must appear in the correct answer.
II. a full-length portrait of Romantic novelist Victor Hugo resembling one of his heroic characters.	In Statement II, representing Hugo as a hero makes no connection to the past—"refined" and "dignified" or otherwise. This falls short of what we need, so Statement II must not appear in the correct answer.
III. a painting of Queen Marie Antoinette in which she is indistinguishable from the courtiers who surround her.	Statement III similarly does not make a connection to the past, and therefore must not appear in the correct answer. Further, to make the Queen blend in with her court would be the opposite of making her appear "refined" and "dignified."
A. I only	**(A)** contains the correct statement and is the right answer.
B. III only	**(B)**, **(C)**, and **(D)** contain incorrect statements.
C. I and II only	
D. II and III only	

Question	Analysis
3. According to the passage, which of the following musical experiences is most analogous to Minimalism?	This is an Apply question asking for a musical example that is similar to Minimalism in art. Minimalism is described at the end of paragraph 4, and all of the characteristics of this style are said to "embody . . . distilled, classical calm" and is a form of Classicism that involves abstraction and ideals like calm.
A. Agitated classical music in a large concert hall	**(A)** intentionally uses the word *classical* as a Faulty Use of Detail, but the word *agitated* indicates that this music is anything but calm. Eliminate this answer choice.
B. Electronic elevator music playing quietly	Elevators are typically calm places—the phrase *elevator music* even tends to have the connotation of innocuous or boring, implying that this music is quite calm. This makes **(B)** the correct answer.
C. Hard rock music blasting through speakers	We can rule out **(C)** because *hard rock* and *blasting* indicate that this music anything but calm.
D. A repetitive tape loop of country music	A repetitive tape loop would likely be irksome and not particularly calm, making **(D)** incorrect as well. This answer choice is a good trap if you are familiar with music history, as many Minimalist composers did indeed employ tape loops in their music; however, this answer is not supported by the passage and is therefore incorrect.

Question	Analysis
4. With which statement would the author most likely DISAGREE?	This is an Inference question of the Implication subtype; we are looking for something that the author would not agree with. It is hard to form a solid prediction for this question, so analyze each answer choice and eliminate the ones that are consistent with the author's opinions or that are Out of Scope.
A. Late 18th- to early 19th-century French Romantic art had a sense of personality that Neoclassicism lacked.	**(A)** clearly addresses the dichotomy we are getting comfortable with: classical = cool, romantic = expressive. The author would agree that *Romantic art* has more personality than a Classical movement, so eliminate this answer choice.
B. At any given time, it can be difficult to pinpoint a strong dichotomy between prevailing styles and previous ones.	**(B)** reflects what the author tells us in the first paragraph: that "styles, of course, do coexist" and that "life is rarely as neatly divided ... as we might wish." This answer can be eliminated as well.
C. French Romanticism lacked an immediacy that was apparent in Neoclassical painting.	**(C)** goes against the author's description of Classicism as having a coolness and distance to it, whereas Romanticism has more expressive, emotional impact. Romanticism should have the immediacy that Classicism lacks—this answer choice is an Opposite, meaning the author would *DISAGREE* with the statement, making **(C)** the correct choice.
D. French Romanticism was the polar opposite of Neoclassicism.	This passage repeatedly draws a polar contrast between Classicism and Romanticism. **(D)** is a valid inference based on the passage and therefore can be eliminated.

Question	Analysis
5. Suppose that most late 18th-century French drawings are exotic and exciting. Which passage assertion would be most WEAKENED by this conclusion?	This is another Strengthen–Weaken (Beyond the Passage) question that provides new evidence and asks us to identify the conclusion that is most *WEAKENED* by it. The *late 18th-century* is a reference to the time period given at the beginning of the third paragraph, "1750 to 1850." This is the French Neoclassicist era—a Classical period—but *exotic* and *exciting* are descriptors of Romanticism. This implies that many artists were not actually using Classical themes at the time.
A. Classicism was more popular than Romanticism in late 18th-century France.	**(A)** uses comparative language, but how *popular* one style is in comparison to another is not addressed at all in the passage and so this choice can be eliminated.
B. The Neoclassicists' inspiration had pervasive effects.	This claim is made in paragraph 3: according to the author, Neoclassicism impacted "everything from fashion to furniture and architecture." However, because we were surprised to hear about Romanticism in a Classical period, it no longer seems that the Neoclassicists were as "pervasive" as the author described. Therefore, **(B)** is the correct answer.
C. Inner emotions can be imbued into artwork.	**(C)** is certainly a valid inference, but it is not affected in any way by the question stem's information.
D. Neoclassical works are less dramatic than works of the Classical age.	**(D)** also makes a comparison that was never mentioned explicitly in the passage—the author never addresses how *dramatic* one Classical style is compared to another Classical style.

Question	Analysis
6. Suppose that romantic artists and Classically oriented artists began borrowing heavily from one another. This finding would support the view that:	This is a Strengthen–Weaken (Beyond the Passage) question, based on the words *Suppose* and *would support the view*. The new evidence in the question stem is consistent with the final point the author makes—that these two styles may eventually be "sew[n] ... together." To carry out your Investigation, scan for an answer choice that is consistent with the passage goal.
A. Romanticism and Classicism are independent movements.	**(A)** contradicts the author's point in the last paragraph. Further, the question stem shows a case where the two movements are converging—not that they are *independent* of each other. Eliminate this answer choice.
B. the past inevitably influences the future.	**(B)** uses extreme language and was never overtly claimed by the author. While the author provides some examples of the "past ... influenc[ing] the future," such as French Neoclassicism, the word *inevitably* is far too strong, as many movements that are not strongly influenced by the past, such as Abstract Expressionism, are also described.
C. the cycle from cool to expressive art styles is shortening.	**(C)** might be tempting because it is a claim the author makes. However, "borrowing heavily" from each other at one point in time would mean there wouldn't be two distinct styles that are cycling.
D. artists might be beginning to make less of a distinction between these two schools of art.	**(D)** uses the Moderating keyword *might* and correctly states the author's main point at the end of the last paragraph. That's our match.

Question	Analysis
7. Which of the following, if true, would constitute a reason Neoclassicists looked to Classical Greece for inspiration?	For this Strengthen–Weaken (Beyond the Passage) question, we are looking for a reason Neoclassicists would look to the High Classicism style in ancient Greece for inspiration. It is challenging to make a prediction, but we should look at the answers with an eye toward the themes the author has identified as part of the Classical mode.
A. Nineteenth-century French nobility admired the ancient period because it was one in which even ordinary citizens acquired important art.	**(A)** does not address the idea of Classicism at all; further, there is no obvious reason why *nobility* would like an art style that *even ordinary citizens* could acquire. Eliminate this answer choice.
B. Neoclassical painters and architects were impressed by the wide range of human feelings that Classical Greek sculptors captured in their marble works.	**(B)** discusses *feelings*, which the passage indicates are actually the hallmark of the opposite art style: Expressionism. Eliminate this Opposite answer choice.
C. Nineteenth-century French elite idealized the cultural expressions of the ancient past as conveying regal grandeur, devoid of intense emotions.	**(C)** references the absence of emotions, which matches our understanding of Classical values. In addition, it makes sense that the *French elite* would be attracted to art that *convey[ed] regal grandeur*. This is the correct answer choice.
D. Neoclassicists found that appealing to patrons' interest in antiquity allowed them to move their style toward the Expressionist ideal.	**(D)** implies that Neoclassicists desired to move their style out of the Classical mode and into the Expressionist mode, but there is no evidence in the passage that these artists desired to do so.

PRACTICE QUESTIONS

Passage 1 (Questions 1–5)

Post-structuralist literary criticism was developed largely in reaction to Saussurian linguistic theory, which first expressed the relationship between words and the concepts they denote. In Saussurian linguistics, an actual word is referred to as a "signifier"—the "sound image" made by the word "train," for instance, constitutes a signifier. At the same time, the idea evoked by the signifier is termed a "signified." Saussure argued that the structural relationship between a signifier and a signified constituted a "linguistic sign." He saw language as made up entirely of such signs, or structural relationships, and argued that the relationship that constituted these signs was actually arbitrary and based on common usage rather than on some necessary link. He did believe, however, that certain "signifiers" (words) could be permanently linked to specific "signifieds" (concepts) in order to create stable, predictable relationships that evoked constant meanings.

In contrast to Saussurian linguistics, the post-structuralist view contends that there exists no system of describing ourselves, or of communicating with one another, which does not somehow use our indigenous language systems. To post-structuralists, language defines our identities and is required if we are to maintain those identities. In this view of language, any signifier always signifies another signifier. Definitions and meanings always take the form of metaphors: one term can only be defined as being another term. To change the meaning of a term, one must only change the metaphor through which that term is defined. Meaning shifts from one signifier to another, and because of this, no act of signification is ever fully closed or fully complete.

Because the post-structuralists do not view necessary connections as composing permanent linguistic sign relationships, they reject the idea of absolute meaning. Because language constantly shifts along a chain of meaning, "absolute" meanings cannot exist. Language in this view can never be viewed as entirely stable. Whereas Saussure believed that linguistic sign relationships could create stable, consistent meanings between terms and the images they evoke, post-structuralists argue that meaning can be established only through discourse. Thus, meaning is never absolute, immutable, or concrete because it is always dependent on the differing and constantly shifting discourse in which language terms operate.

It is here that the divergence of these two schools of thought becomes readily apparent, insofar as they concern themselves with fields beyond linguistics. The implications of the nearly irrefutable, albeit bleak, reasoning that is so fundamental to post-structural thought reach far beyond the confines of linguistics. The idea of conceptual instability is a manifestation of the existential phenomenology that heavily influenced the work of innumerable scholars in disparate fields through the 20th century. Where structuralism was grounded in linguistics and made inroads into the human sciences, the very ideas that presuppose post-structuralism are rooted more ambitiously in the central discussion of human nature. It is for this reason that existentialism and post-structuralism continue to flourish and have inserted themselves into our enduring understanding of what it is to be human while structuralism and Saussurian linguistics hold a devoted place in scarcely few discussions beyond linguistic relativism.

1. Which of the following best adheres to the post-structuralist view of meaning as presented in the passage?
   A. The words "signifier" and "signified" are expressed in different ways across several languages.
   B. All members of a literary club puts forth unique interpretations of a fairy tale based on their academic backgrounds.
   C. The relationship between a parent and child shifts dramatically during the course of a novel.
   D. All ten members of a focus group derive the same meaning from the preview of a new situation comedy.

2. In addressing a class, a professor describes the mind first as a blank slate to be written on and later as a garden to be cultivated. In light of the information in the passage, the professor's method best represents:
   A. the immutable nature of meaning.
   B. a Saussurian relationship between words and the concepts they denote.
   C. the arbitrary use of language in academia.
   D. a post-structuralist change in the meaning of a term.

3. "Broad, open-ended study is frivolous and indulgent. It is through deliberate, focused study that knowledge advances." How does this statement affect the author's argument in paragraph 4?
   A. It weakens the author's argument.
   B. It strengthens the author's argument.
   C. It neither strengthens nor weakens the author's argument.
   D. It could both strengthen and weaken different parts of the author's argument.

4. A study finds that humans taught a fabricated word and its definition immediately form an association between that word and its definition. After repeated exposure to the word in different contexts, the same people consistently offered different definitions for the word than the one they were initially given. This strengthens:
   A. post-structural theory because the initial signifier did not maintain its association with the initial signified.
   B. post-structural theory because the initial signifier was most likely understood through a metaphor that changed.
   C. Saussurian linguistic theory because of the initial association of signifier and signified.
   D. neither theory, either theory, or both theories; more information on the underlying mechanism that precipitated the change is needed.

5. Which of the following examples is LEAST analogous to the Saussurian understanding of linguistic relativism?
   A. A dog's response to the "sit" command could not be changed upon retraining, though its response to the "stop" command could be changed.
   B. A study reveals that words learned in any language stimulate the same neurons regardless of attempts to retrain the meaning of these words over several years.
   C. The definition of the word "cool" has evolved drastically over the years depending upon social context and common usage.
   D. A study revealed that the presentation of a word to a listener immediately resulted in a localized brain region becoming activated before the listener could offer the word's definition.

Answers follow on next page.

ANSWERS AND EXPLANATIONS

Passage 1 (Questions 1–5)

Sample Highlighting

P1. "linguistic signs" and "permanently linked"; **P2.** "define our identity" and "metaphors"; **P3.** "reject" and "only through discourse"; **P4.** "far beyond" and "scarcely few."

Sample Outline

P1. Saussure: arbitrary signifier (word) relation with signified (concept) = linguistic sign, can become concrete

P2. Post-structuralist: signifier defined only by other signifiers; understand through metaphors that can change

P3. Saussure = language can be stable, post-structuralist = language never stable, depends on discourse

P4. Post-structuralism endures because of broader ties to human nature; Saussurian theory restricted to linguistics

1. **B**

This question challenges us to apply our understanding of the post-structuralist theory to the answer choices in order to find an example. Paragraph 3 makes clear that the post-structuralists believe that "meaning is never absolute, immutable, or concrete." Looking for the choice that best fits with this notion brings us to **(B)**. The fact that the "unique interpretations" are due to differences in "academic backgrounds" supports the notion that exposure to different fields of discourse leads to the differences in interpretation, which is consistent with the language of paragraph 3. **(A)** cleverly uses words from the passage in a new context. The fact that words are expressed differently in different languages does not affect the absolute meaning of these words; they're expressed in various ways, as one would expect in different languages, but that doesn't mean they are defined differently. In **(C)**, the relationship between parent and child may shift, but we'd have to see some variation in interpreting the *meaning* of this shift to get us into post-structuralist territory. As for **(D)**, a lack of consensus would seem more consistent with the post-structuralist view, although it's conceivable that the ten focus-groupers arrived at their opinions through discourse with each other. However, because such a state of affairs isn't indicated, we can't assume it.

2. **D**

In Application questions like this one, we must determine how the new example relates to what's in the passage. In passages where the goal is *to explain the differences between* two things, that usually means figuring out what camp the new situation falls into. The major task here is figuring out what the professor is doing, and how it relates to the theories in the passage. When the "professor describes the mind ... as a blank slate, or as a garden," the professor is using metaphors, which brings us into the post-structuralist camp. Moreover, the metaphor is being shifted, which relates precisely to the penultimate sentence of paragraph 2: "To change the meaning of a term, one must only change the metaphor through which that term is defined." Therefore, the answer is **(D)**. **(A)** and **(B)** are Opposites because they presuppose constant meaning, whether it is described as immutable or Saussurian—Saussure posits "stable, predictable relationships that evoke constant meanings," according to the end of the first paragraph. **(C)** is Out of Scope as there is no mention of the use of language in academia in the passage.

3. **C**

This question provides new information and asks how it impacts the passage, making this a Strengthen–Weaken (Beyond the Passage) question. The new quotation suggests that widely applicable fields of study, such as post-structuralism as described in this paragraph, are frivolous and that narrowly focused fields, such as Saussurian linguistics, advance knowledge. However, let's consider the author's argument in this paragraph. The author focuses on the differences in scope between the two camps and why post-structuralism is more enduring. The author makes no mention of the advancement of knowledge or frivolity. The author may imply some partiality to post-structuralism, but there is no argument made regarding the focus of the new quotation. Thus, **(C)** is correct as this statement has no bearing on the author's argument.

4. **D**

This Strengthen–Weaken (Beyond the Passage) question challenges us to identify not only whether the new information *strengthens* post-structuralism or Saussurian theory, but also why. The first thing to recognize is that the study's results could support either theory. Even though Saussurian theory suggests that words "could be permanently linked" to concepts, it also recognizes that the relationship between a word and the concept it represents is "actually arbitrary and based on common usage rather than on some necessary link." We also know that post-structuralism definitely supports changing definitions. Thus, we have to look at the reasoning in the answer choices to determine the correct answer. **(A)** may sound tempting because the reasoning sounds as if it's disproving Saussurian theory, but remember that Saussurian theory does account for "signified" changing depending on "common usage." Also, Saussurian theory being proven incorrect wouldn't necessarily prove post-structuralism correct. **(B)** requires assumptions we just can't make because there is not enough support in the passage for it being a "metaphor that changed" that caused the change in meaning. **(C)** is also tempting because it mentions Saussurian theory and one of its tenets, although *the initial association of signifier and signified* does not really add any new information to strengthen the author's description. More importantly, this answer choice doesn't explain the all-important second half of the new information: why the association changed. Therefore, the answer must be **(D)**. This answer choice identifies the real problem with the other choices: we don't know the mechanism behind the change in association. Both theories account for a change in associations, so the mechanism by which the association changed needs to be described before we can draw any conclusions about which theory the study supports.

5. **B**

The challenge in this Application question is to transfer our knowledge of Saussurian linguistics to find three appropriate analogies or one choice that does not fit. This description appears in paragraph 1 of the passage, where the author makes it clear that "signifiers" are tied to "signifieds" in order to produce a sign, or linguistic understanding. This relationship can be, but is not necessarily, permanent. **(A)** adheres to this description well. The meaning can be permanently linked or changed, depending on the circumstances. **(B)** is Extreme in its categorization of semantic links as permanent. The passage said that links are "arbitrary and based on common usage rather than on some necessary link," so the categorization in this answer choice of all links being concrete is Extreme, and thus correct. **(C)** fits in perfectly with the previous quotation that links are "based on common usage." Finally, **(D)** is also a perfect explanation of Saussurian theory. The signifier is presented, it triggers brain activity, and the definition (signified) is provided.

CHAPTER 12

EFFECTIVE REVIEW OF CARS

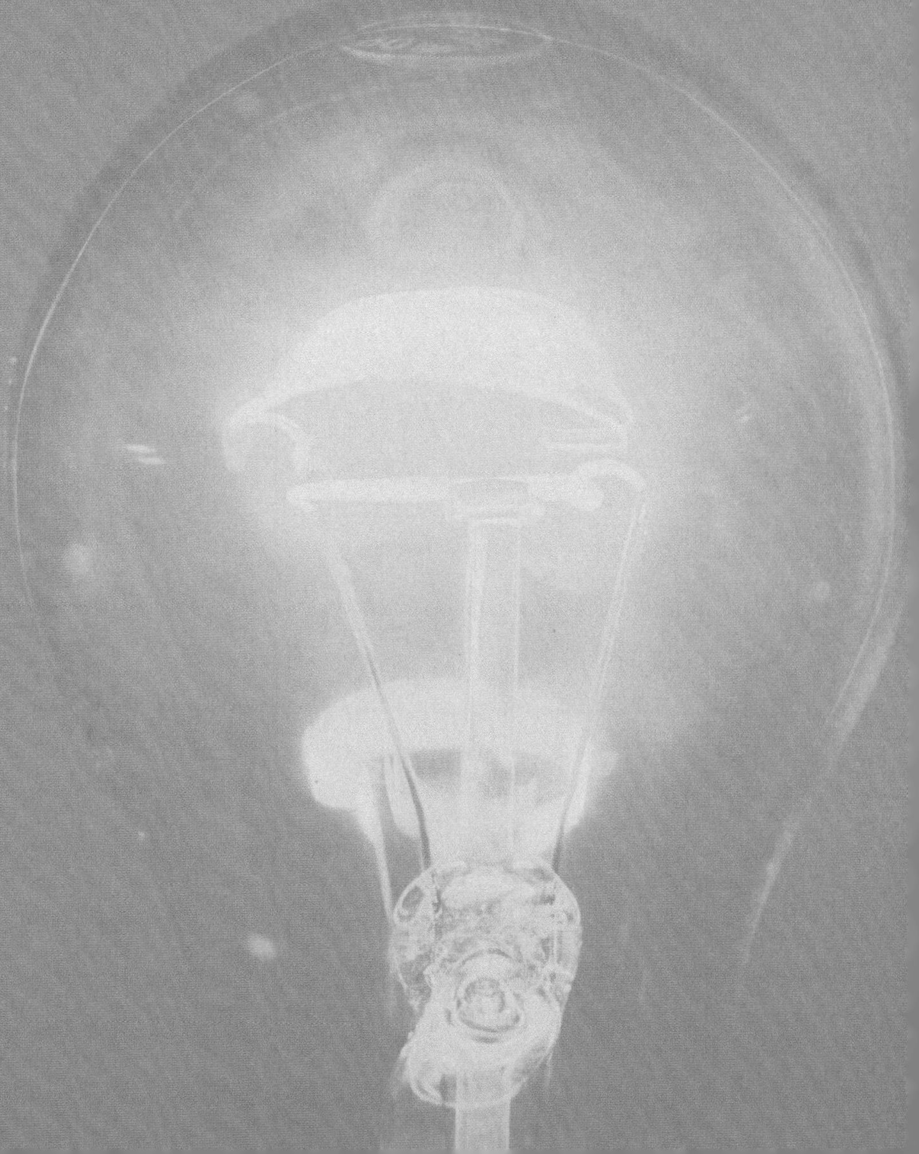

CHAPTER 12

EFFECTIVE REVIEW OF CARS

In This Chapter

Introduction

LEARNING OBJECTIVES

After Chapter 12, you will be able to:

- Troubleshoot common errors on missed questions with How I'll Fix It Sheets
- Apply post-phrasing analysis to difficult passages
- Manage and adjust your pacing within the CARS section to meet the 90-minute deadline
- Build endurance and vocabulary through targeted practice

This final chapter is a troubleshooting guide for raising your score. Experience with the CARS section is a prerequisite for the material in this chapter. So, before studying this chapter in detail, you must practice the strategies discussed throughout this book, especially the Kaplan Method for CARS Passages from Chapter 7 and the Kaplan Method for CARS Questions from Chapter 8. For the material in this chapter to be most effective, it's best if you have also taken a few timed and scored CARS sections, possibly on one or two Full-Length practice exams. Once you've built this familiarity with the CARS section—and with your personal pitfalls in the CARS section—you'll be ready for troubleshooting! We'll look at five proven ways to increase your *Critical Analysis and Reasoning Skills* (CARS) section score—including some methods you'll find useful for the science sections as well.

Hands down, the best way to improve is to learn from the mistakes you make on practice tests, which is why we begin our discussion with Kaplan's How I'll Fix It Sheets (HIFIS). The post-phrasing strategy discussed in the following section builds on the HIFIS, helping you think more like the writers of the MCAT. After we discuss post-phrasing, we'll talk about a simple approach for managing your pacing on Test Day, and we'll discuss what you can do to build your test-taking stamina. We'll close with a discussion of one final advantage you can give yourself for CARS: a stronger vocabulary.

12.1 Learning from Your Mistakes

At this juncture, you have read quite a bit about how to approach CARS, you have had the opportunity to practice, and you may even have completed one or more Full-Length Exams. Now is the time to reflect on your performance and adjust your study plan based on your personal test-taking pathologies, which are identifiable patterns in your past errors that can help to guide your future CARS studying.

How I'll Fix It Sheets

It can be overwhelming to try to discern what your strengths and areas of opportunity are by looking at an entire CARS section at once. Rather, take time to analyze each question you answered incorrectly. One way to help manage this process—and to keep a clear record of your performance over time—is to set up **How I'll Fix It Sheets** (**HIFIS**). Create a document with at least four columns: question number, question type/topic, wrong answer type chosen, and "How I'll Fix It." In the first column, make a list compiling all of the items you answered incorrectly on the test. In the second column, identify the passage topic and question type based on the Kaplan classifications we reviewed in the previous three chapters (or, if you're making a HIFIS for one of the sciences, include the question topic). The third column should include the wrong answer type you chose (Opposite, Faulty Use of Detail, Distortion, Out of Scope, content error) for the question. Lastly, in column four, take time to review your incorrect response and identify the specific reason why you got the question wrong and what steps you'll take to "fix it" (i.e. avoid this mistake in the future). Table 12.1 demonstrates what HIFIS should look like.

MCAT EXPERTISE

HIFIS are a way to create and maintain a pool of data on your own performance on the MCAT. Because they're structured as tables, spreadsheet tools can be very helpful for analyzing your HIFIS. Consider using a spreadsheet-creating program to build your HIFIS so you can add to them from multiple devices, sort them by different columns to more easily see trends, and organize them in different ways that best suit your current needs.

Question Number	Question Type/ Topic	Wrong Answer Chosen	How I'll Fix It
Full-Length 1, #12	Detail (Music)	Faulty Use of Detail	Misinterpreted the question stem. Next time, stop after reading the question ask myself "what is this question asking me to find?"
Full-Length 1, #21	Strengthen–Weaken (Within the Passage) (Art)	Faulty Use of Detail	Didn't understand question stem. Next time, stop after reading the question to ask myself whose opinion the question is asking about and whether strengthen or weaken is needed.
Full-Length 1, #38	Inference (Population Health)	Distortion	Chose an answer choice that *may* be true. Next time focus my answer choice elimination on which choices *must be true*.
Full-Length 1, #53	Main Idea (Psychology)	Distortion	Answer choice was too narrow. Next time, use my Read & Distill steps to predict an overall goal of the passage before reading the choices.

Table 12.1 Sample How I'll Fix It Sheet (HIFIS)

BRIDGE

Need some help identifying the question type for your How I'll Fix It Sheets? Don't forget to review Chapters 9, 10, and 11 of *MCAT CARS Review* for thorough coverage of each question type.

The most important element of this table is the *How I'll Fix It* column. Do not just categorize your test-taking mistakes with a generic *I didn't understand* or *careless mistake*. Such comments will not give you insight into why you missed the question nor how you can avoid that problem in the future. At the other extreme, you are never going to see this specific question again, so a hyper-specific description of exactly how you would answer this question isn't going to help you in the future either. Responses that are either too vague or too specific both result in the same problem: you're spending this time reviewing your performance, but you're not learning what to do better on the next test! The goal of HIFIS is to learn to identify questions in the future that are similar to questions you've missed in the past, and then to avoid the mistakes you made on such questions in the past. Your response in the *How I'll Fix It* column should always keep this goal in mind.

To write good *How I'll Fix It* responses, start by identifying exactly what you did wrong on the specific question you're reviewing and what behavior or thought process you would change to get the question correct, then generalize that behavior just a bit by recording only the steps of how to get the right answer without the details of that specific question. The responses in the above table illustrate this technique. Take the first response as an example. This student identifies the specific mistake and what steps to take to avoid this error, "Misinterpreted the question stem ... asking me to find?." But this student doesn't provide unnecessary details about the question or passage. In the *How I'll Fix It* column, this student also labels this mistake with the general label, "Misinterpreted question stem." In fact every one of this student's *How I'll Fix It* entries follow this formula: general label, then specific details on how to fix the problem, all with little or no information unique to the passage or question. You don't have to follow this format exactly on every question, but it is a good default.

HIFIS make it easier to identify flaws that are becoming trends, which helps you better address these trends earlier in your prep. Consider the following pairs of "bad" and "good" examples:

> **Bad:** *I missed this because the answer choice declares that Beowulf was written by an aristocrat, but the passage said that the author was only "probably" a member of the royal court. Next time, I need to read more carefully.*
> **Good:** *Misread question stem. Next time, I'll rephrase the question stem so I know exactly what is being asked.*

> **Bad:** *I missed this because I recognized "unmoved mover" from the question stem, which is in paragraph 3, but the answer they were looking for actually comes from the description of the "Central Headquarters" sentence in paragraph 4. Next time, I'll go to the right paragraph.*
> **Good:** *Referred to passage incorrectly. Next time, I'll identify which paragraph the question is asking about and use the passage to make a prediction.*

When reviewing your HIFIS, in addition to looking for trends in the *How I'll Fix It* column, compare the question type/topic column to the wrong answer chosen column to narrow the scope of your future study plan. Is there a recognizable pattern you can utilize to optimize your performance? For instance, maybe looking at the question type column, you observe that you are repeatedly missing *Reasoning Within the Text* questions. That's good information. But maybe by also comparing with the topic, you observe that you most often miss this question type on anthropology passages specifically. Now, not only have you identified a question type for further practice, but also you know to be on guard next time you're facing a *Reasoning Within the Text* question on an anthropology passage. Further, by also comparing the wrong answer chosen column, you may identify that you frequently choose Faulty Use of Detail answer choices for this question type. Use your HIFIS to plan which passage varieties you'll focus on in the future, what strategies you need to work on to ensure you understand the passage and questions, or to determine which chapters you need to reread in *MCAT CARS Review*. You want to make sure that you are moving forward with a plan that specifically supports your areas of opportunity.

REAL WORLD

In medical school, you'll attend morbidity and mortality (M&M) conferences, in which physicians review clinical and medical errors, patient complications, and other healthcare quality measures to investigate the root causes of problems in order to fix them directly. These conferences are not dissimilar to creating How I'll Fix It Sheets—you can only improve if you know what you're doing wrong!

In addition to the basic data we've discussed so far, you can optionally collect several additional pieces of data to further flesh out your HIFIS and make them even more valuable tools. You can add a column to record the time you spent on each passage and question, which can be valuable for discovering passage types, question types, or content or topic areas where you tend to fall behind. Note that when reviewing the Kaplan Review Page, the time associated with the first question in a question set will typically represent the time you spent Distilling the passage plus the time you spent answering that question. Some students also find it helpful to actually split out the one *How I'll Fix It* column into two columns: one column to capture a general label for the error and a second column to record how they'll address that error. Make your HIFIS your own by customizing them to capture data points that are most relevant to the most problematic parts of your prep.

Troubleshooting Common Wrong Answer Trends

HIFIS are a great tool for uncovering trends among your wrong answers. But of course, diagnosing and treating your errors in this way may not be something you've done before. So, let's discuss three of the most common trends among wrong answers, and what to do about them.

If you repeatedly read questions incorrectly, you are not alone—MCAT students often misread or misinterpret questions in CARS. So, if misreading questions comes up as a trend in your HIFIS, you'll know to practice the CARS question strategy. Remember, establishing the question type is a critical component of the CARS question strategy. You might be less familiar with CARS-style content, but the tradeoff is that all CARS questions are subdivided into just a few predictable question types, each with its own predictable (and practiceable!) strategy. Rephrasing the question stem to ensure you fully understand the question is also essential. As you review your practice tests, reexamine the questions and the answers you selected that were incorrect. In hindsight, when looking at the question a second time, do you find yourself shaking your head because you simply misinterpreted what was being asked? This could indicate that you are reading the question stems too hastily and moving on to the answer choices before you even know *what* you're supposed to be answering. If this is the case, force yourself to take the extra time to paraphrase a difficult question stem so that you know precisely what the question is asking. Time spent paraphrasing is not wasted time. The added clarity will allow you to Investigate more quickly, which will help you Match an answer choice rapidly and accurately. In the next section, we will discuss a review technique called post-phrasing, which is a particularly helpful exercise for any student who commonly misreads the question.

If your HIFIS demonstrates a pattern in which you keep missing the same question types, then there is an easy way to gain time and confidence on this test: start to triage those questions. First, go back and reread the appropriate chapter in *MCAT CARS Review* so you can recognize these question types with greater ease. Chapters 9, 10, and 11 introduced the major question types and highlighted the common question stems that fall into each type. Remember that triaging a question to the end of the set is the opposite of admitting defeat. Very often, as you answer the other questions in the set, you learn more about the author's argument, which maximizes your chances on the triaged question. Here's a good way to think about it: triaging a question is less like running from your foe, and more warming up before going into battle. Remember also that each question type has an associated strategy that you can practice. Many students find that their least favorite question types early on becomes among their most reliable question types by Test Day. And this turnaround starts by identifying a problematic question type using HIFIS.

Finally, don't neglect identifying the Wrong Answer Pathologies of the incorrect answers that you chose. Simply knowing the Wrong Answer Pathologies that most often sway you from choosing the correct answer may be enough to help you avoid falling for the same traps in future tests. For example, if you know that you frequently choose Out of Scope answer choices in Main Idea questions, then you'll know to ask yourself *Is this answer truly within the confines of the passage, or does it bring in something else?* before finalizing your answer for Main Idea questions in the future.

BRIDGE

Knowing your personal test-taking pathologies is essential to improving your score. In addition to looking at the question types, topics or disciplines, and how you read question stems, don't forget to look at Kaplan's classifications of Wrong Answer Pathologies (Faulty Use of Detail, Out of Scope, Opposite, and Distortion), discussed in Chapter 8 of *MCAT CARS Review.*

12.2 Thinking Like the Testmaker: Post-Phrasing

Does this scenario sound familiar? You skim through the explanation for a question that you missed, shrug, and think, "I guess I get it." When you miss a practice question, you've actually made two mistakes. Not only were you tempted by a trap answer, but also you looked right at the right answer and thought, "Nah! Not that one!" To turn today's wrong answers into tomorrow's right answers, you need a proactive technique for reviewing questions. Post-phrasing is that technique. With **post-phrasing**, you go over both why incorrect answers are wrong and why correct answers are right. This strategy is especially helpful if you frequently experience the classic test-taking dilemma: *I can usually narrow it down to two answer choices, and then I always go for the wrong one.*

To post-phrase, open a question you answered incorrectly, and make a note of the correct answer. Now, you'll carefully dissect the question. Begin by identifying the Type of the question. Recall that each question Type is associated with a general strategy so, if necessary, briefly review the general strategy for that question Type. Next, paraphrase the question stem. To make it very concrete, say your paraphrase out loud, write it down, or type it out. By doing this, you are essentially practicing a formal version of the Rephrase step from the question method. Your focus in this step should be to carefully decode what the question stem is asking you to do.

Once you've Typed the question, reviewed the best strategies for addressing that question type, and Rephrased the question, Investigate the solution. When post-phrasing, write or type out your prediction for the correct response. While you wouldn't write down a prediction on Test Day, the post-phrasing exercise is designed to ensure you are making concrete predictions as part of your Investigation. It's essential to take the time to write the prediction down: many students find that a poorly focused prediction keeps them from finding a Match on MCAT questions. The more you practice writing out your predictions during the post-phrasing process, the more routine making predictions will become.

You may notice that the description of post-phrasing, thus far, basically describes a regimented and very deliberate use of the Kaplan Method for MCAT Questions. But at the end, the focus will not be on matching your prediction anymore; after all, you already know the correct answer because you're reviewing a question you answered incorrectly. Instead, turn your attention to the incorrect answers. Determine why each incorrect answer is unsuitable. Does it fail to match your prediction? Does it have a common Wrong Answer Pathology? Are there other subtle flaws in logic or reasoning that misrepresent the author's arguments? Pay special attention to the wrong answer you actually chose. Why was this answer tempting? Why is it ultimately wrong? By taking the time to write or type out an explanation of the flaw for each incorrect answer, you'll become better at identifying flaws in future wrong answers. Finally, after all this, *now* take a look at Kaplan's explanation and check how well your reasoning matches up.

To summarize, remember this saying: *Practice alone doesn't make perfect. Perfect practice makes perfect.* Post-phrasing is that perfect practice. You are taking a question that you did not answer correctly, and you are modeling the steps, actions, and strategies that you *should have used* to get that question right, which reinforces those behaviors for next time. And lastly, after such a thorough review of a question, what's the best next step? Summarize the results of this detailed, post-phrasing investigation in your HIFIS of course. You don't have to post-phrase every question you missed on every practice exam. Instead, save post-phrasing for the questions that really deserve a thorough examination: the ones where you were stumped, where you were stuck between two answers, and the ones where you made a silly mistake that you want to forever avoid in the future.

Alternatively, a variant of post-phrasing can be used as an exercise to improve your recognition of Wrong Answer Pathologies in passages you haven't seen yet. Consider practicing with a few passages following the steps below:

1. Find a fresh CARS passage from your Kaplan resources, as well as its explanations.
2. Go through and select the correct answers for the passage. Don't read the explanations, just record the correct answers and set them aside for now.
3. Outline the passage as you normally would.
4. When you work on the questions, do so in a fundamentally different way: as above, the goal here is not to find the right answers (as you have already identified them) but to reason why each incorrect answer is wrong. Read the right

answer to be sure you understand it, but spend more time identifying the types of wrong answers presented by the other choices.

5. Look at the explanations for each incorrect answer choice and compare them with your notes. If there are any major omissions or other discrepancies in your explanations, be sure to note them prominently. The more you practice, though, the closer you should find the correspondence between your post-phrasing notes and Kaplan's explanations.

Remember, on the MCAT the right answer is not just the "most correct" answer. Each question has one right answer and three answers with objective flaws, meaning that the right answer is objectively correct because it is the only answer without flaws. Through regular post-phrasing practice, you will begin to see the patterns emerge. What seem now like very subtle flaws will soon start to seem very pronounced. As a result, you will find yourself recognizing the correct answer, the one that doesn't suffer from any flaws, and thinking *this one just feels right*. Furthermore, taking the time to post-phrase will expand your awareness of how the test is written and what the expectations are for MCAT questions. Through post-phrasing practice, you will refine your thought process and your approach to passages and questions, making you better prepared for Test Day.

BRIDGE

In addition to Wrong Answer Pathologies, take time to review the Signs of a Healthy Answer presented in Chapter 8 of *MCAT CARS Review*. These include appropriate scope, agreement with the author, and "hedging" language that creates weaker claims.

12.3 Improving Your Timing

Proper management of the clock can make a significant difference to your score in any section, but the timing constraints in the CARS section differ from those of the other sections. Consider a few basic facts about the CARS section:

- It lasts 90 minutes.
- There are 9 passages.
- There are 53 questions.

It's a simple matter of arithmetic to see that 9 passages in 90 minutes allows you 10 minutes for each passage. Because all of the points actually come from answering the questions, though, you'll want to ensure that you allot enough time for the questions. Passages vary in difficulty, meaning that some will certainly take longer to read than others, but as a rule of thumb you should aim to complete the Preview, Read, and Distill steps for the passage in about 4–5 minutes. Your timing will vary based on the Distill approach you Choose, but even the most intense Interrogation of a very challenging passage should take no longer than 6 minutes. Subtracting those combined ~40 minutes for reading leaves you with 50 minutes for the 53 questions, which works out to almost exactly one minute per question. Keep in mind that the number of questions associated with a passage can vary from 5 to 7, meaning that a more precise expectation for completing a passage and its questions is somewhere between 9–11 minutes.

MCAT EXPERTISE

While it is most common to have five to seven questions associated with a given passage, there have been instances of passages with only four or as many as eight questions. This should not significantly impact how you approach these passages, although—all else being equal—a passage with eight questions will give you more points for the same amount of reading.

Pacing Guidelines

Now, trying to ensure that each passage takes 4–5 minutes and each question a little less than one minute would actually be counterproductive: not only would you lose a substantial amount of time checking the clock, you'd likely heighten your anxiety each time you came across a question that takes a little extra time to get through. A better approach to managing your time is to check your timing only at a limited number of predetermined points during the section. We recommend checking the clock after every other passage. Assuming that you take 10 minutes to read a passage and answer its questions, you should ideally be no more than 20 minutes further into the section each time you check the clock. We recommend jotting down how much time remains when you start the third, fifth, seventh, and ninth passages (it should be at least 70, 50, 30, and 10 minutes, respectively). If your timing appears to go off-course, then during your review of the test, note which passages (and potentially Distill approaches) seem to have caused this trouble. Could you have triaged these time-consuming passages or distilled them differently, and answered more questions correctly in the limited time you had left?

Hitting these recommended time points does not leave you much of a cushion for going back to previous passages and questions, but this approach is by far the best way to maximize your score. Given that each CARS passage contains between 500 and 600 words, jumping between passages is far less realistic in CARS than in any of the science sections, where passages can be less than half that length. While it is recommended that you skip passages that you decide will be too time-consuming in your Preview step, we do not recommend that you leave a passage unfinished with the intention of returning later. Once you decide to work on a passage, commit to finishing it.

Managing Question Timing

The timing guidelines given so far are useful for managing the CARS section. But mastering the split between reading each passage and answering its questions can still be tricky. In your online resources, we record the time spent working on each question so you can get a sense of which questions take you longer than others. (Note that this mechanism requires you to click on the question when you begin working on it to accurately record this information.) Keep in mind that the time we record for the first question of each passage will include the time you spend critically Reading and Distilling the passage in the beginning. Thus, you should strive to have the first question of each set answered within around 5 minutes (or 300 seconds), and every subsequent question should be close to the one-minute mark, calculated as an average. If you've chosen to Distill primarily by Highlighting, you should expect to see that you answered your first question more quickly, and then spent more time on each question. Alternately, if you mostly choose to Distill by Interrogating, you should expect to see a time of 6 or even 7 minutes for the first question, with much shorter times for the subsequent questions in each set. If you use a mix of methods, or if you primarily use the Outlining method, 5 minutes average for the passage and first question should be your target.

MCAT EXPERTISE

If the seconds ticking down causes you too much anxiety, an alternative way of working on your timing is to use the timer on your phone or some other timepiece to "time up"—that is, to count upwards from zero to see how much time it's taking you to read the passage and to complete each question. Timers with "lap" functions can be especially useful because these can record how long each question takes. Generally, this method works best with only one or two passages at a time. Keep in mind, however, that an alternate timer cannot be used on Test Day!

Once you have a better sense of which types of passages and questions take you longer to complete, you should use this information in conjunction with what you've learned from each HIFIS to guide your *now* or *later* decisions in the first step of each method (Preview for passages and Type for questions). Beginning the section with the passages that are easiest for you will allow you to get ahead on the timing curve. Similarly, once you've committed to a passage, saving the toughest questions for the end of that set will give you an opportunity to gain additional familiarity with the passage as you work on its more manageable questions. Because questions can repeat the same theme, you may even find the answer to a challenging question while working on an easier question.

12.4 Building Endurance

Preparing for the MCAT is like preparing for a marathon. You cannot run 1 or 2 miles a day for two months and then expect to be successful in a 26.2-mile marathon. Runners ramp up to the 26.2 miles, routinely running long distances in preparation for marathon day.

How often are you studying and for how long? If you are only studying in 30- or 60-minute increments, you might find when you sit down to complete a Full-Length Exam that you have not built up your endurance for that type of test. Not only do you need to study and practice regularly, but you also need to simulate the Test Day experience, which requires concentrating for 6 hours and 15 minutes of testing time. Gear up for practice tests—and Test Day itself—by periodically holding long study and practice sessions. When working on CARS, try studying in 90-minute increments to mimic the amount of time you'll have for this section. Long study periods can also be helpful for the sciences, as you will have 95 minutes for each science section on Test Day.

12.5 Enhancing Your Vocabulary

The AAMC claims that there's no outside content required for the CARS section of the MCAT, but in truth this is not 100 percent accurate—you may come across a question that has an element of common knowledge (the number of days in a week, for example). Furthermore, while very few questions hinge on knowing the definition of a piece of jargon from outside knowledge, a strong vocabulary on Test Day can be a tremendous asset. If nothing else, you can become more comfortable with academic writing in the various disciplines that the AAMC includes in the CARS section. Do this by familiarizing yourself with plenty of examples.

BRIDGE

While you will not be expected to know the definition of a piece of jargon from outside knowledge, Definition-in-Context questions hinge on your ability to determine the meaning of a word or phrase from the rest of the passage. These questions are discussed in Chapter 9 of *MCAT CARS Review*.

The Kaplan and AAMC Full-Length Exams are, of course, the best place to go to get samples of CARS-style passages and questions. But students who want to go the extra mile also have the option of practicing with outside reading.

Reading Plan

The more often you read, the stronger your reading comprehension skills become, and the faster you evolve into a more efficient reader. This practice will help you build up a wider array of words that you recognize by sight, meaning that you'll spend less time deciphering the text. Believe it or not, reading is a skill that you can practice and improve, just like any skill. So, to prepare for CARS, read on a consistent basis. This practice this will increase your reading speed so that you can maneuver swiftly through passages.

Set up a regimented reading schedule for at least 20 minutes a day, which is just enough time to get through two passages according to the the timing guidelines for the CARS section. Also, keep an array of reading materials handy for when you have time available. This mini-library could consist of a list of links kept on a smartphone or other wireless-enabled device. It is surprising how much time we spend waiting—for a friend at a coffee shop, for a group to go out in the evening, for a professor to arrive to class, or for a meeting. These are all examples of times that could be used productively to sharpen reading skills to prepare for CARS.

When selecting materials, try to simulate the variety of passages you'll encounter on Test Day with a blend of texts from both the humanities and the social sciences. Use your HIFIS to determine which types of passages cause you the greatest confusion or frustration, the ones that slow you down the most on your Full-Length Exams. Focus on reading those problematic types of passages in particular; the more you read these difficult texts, the more familiar you will become with their jargon and with other conventions, and the less intimidating these passages will start to seem. Consider using one of the following online services to find academic journal articles in the disciplines that give you the most trouble:

- JSTOR (jstor.org)
- Oxford Journals (academic.oup.com/journals)
- Google Scholar (scholar.google.com)
- Project MUSE (muse.jhu.edu)
- The Directory of Open Access Journals (doaj.org)
- Sage Journals (journals.sagepub.com)

Whenever you come across a word that you don't recognize, stop and take a moment to look that word up and write down its definition *in your own words*. Keeping a list of these new terms and looking over them periodically will go a long way toward building your vocabulary. As your vocabulary expands, you will be able to either recognize words or swiftly infer their meaning, which will increase your efficiency both while Reading and Distilling the passage and while tackling question stems and answer choices.

In addition to learning the meanings of new words, reading humanities and social sciences articles will help you become acquainted with the major themes and concepts that frequently appear on the CARS section. Familiarity with a concept can allow you to glean more from a passage when that concept is mentioned, enabling you to read more quickly if the text simply repeats what you already know. Be careful, however, not to bring in any ideas that the passage does not include when answering its questions—there's a reason Out of Scope is a common Wrong Answer Pathology!

Because there are only nine passages in CARS, the likelihood that you will have read about the exact scenario presented in a CARS passage is not high, but it is very likely that you will have read about similar topics.

Finally, any form of academic reading forces you to think critically about the ideas the author is presenting. Just as when you practice with passages in CARS, try distilling a few paragraphs of an academic article. Focus on how the author structures the argument: what conclusion does the author want the audience to reach? What evidence is used to support that conclusion? Are there any flaws in the author's logic? Focused, regular reading will help prepare you for CARS by bolstering your reading comprehension and reasoning skills, as well as your comfort with academic texts and the challenges they bring.

Conclusion

Medical schools want to admit students with strong reasoning skills because higher-order thinking is necessary for both appropriately diagnosing patients and conducting groundbreaking research. When given a constellation of symptoms and concerns, a physician needs to generate a differential diagnosis—a list of the potential ailments described by the symptoms. From this list, the medical team must rule out unlikely diagnoses and provide evidence for the most likely diagnosis. What starts as a list of a hundred possible causes of headache—from migraines and tension-type headaches to intracranial bleeds and brain tumors—is reduced to the one most likely cause by asking appropriate questions (*When did the headache start? Where do you feel the headache? Have you ever had anything similar before?*), by performing a thorough physical exam (cranial nerve function, eye exam, looking for evidence of trauma), and by running appropriate laboratory and imaging tests (head CT, MRI, inflammatory markers).

Patients want to trust the expertise of their doctors, and you want to ensure that you are able to deliver the best treatment to your patients. The skills in CARS that enable you to determine the author's perspective, to distinguish the author's voice from others in the passage, to predict a response to a question, and to match your predictions (while eliminating incorrect answers) are the same skills that will serve you well as a physician. In the future, you may not be expected to think critically about dance theory, musicology, archaeology, and linguistics, but you will have to synthesize disparate pieces of information, consider assumptions about patient care, and respond appropriately to all parts of your patients' questions—both what they say and what they leave for you to infer. As pointed out in this chapter, the skills tested in the *Critical Analysis and Reasoning Skills* section can always be improved through pointed and actionable review of your past performance. Congratulations on reaching the end of *MCAT Critical Analysis and Reasoning Skills Review.* Though this book now comes to an end, for you this is merely a beginning—good luck on the MCAT, and in all your endeavors in medicine!

CONCEPT AND STRATEGY SUMMARY

Learning from Your Mistakes

- Create How I'll Fix It Sheets (HIFIS) to look for your test-taking pathology patterns.
    - Make a table with at least 4 columns: question number, question type, topic/discipline, and "How I'll Fix It."
    - In the How I'll Fix It column, describe the error you made in the question and what specific steps you should take to avoid this error in the future.
    - Look for patterns in your HIFIS.
- If you misread questions, be sure to slow down and rephrase the question stem to make sure you know what question you are actually trying to answer.
- Reread the relevant chapters in *MCAT Critical Analysis and Reasoning Skills Review* as needed.

Thinking Like the Testmaker: Post-Phrasing

- Find a CARS passage from your Kaplan resources, as well as its explanations. This could be a passage you have already read or a new one.
- Go through and indicate all the correct answers for the passage. Don't read the explanations—just indicate the correct answers and set aside for now.
- Distill the passage as you normally would.
- When you work on the questions, do so in a fundamentally different way: the goal is not to find the right answers (as you have already identified them). Rather, the goal is to reason why each incorrect answer is wrong. Read the right answer to be sure you understand it, but spend more time identifying the types of wrong answers presented by the other choices.
- Look at the explanations for each incorrect answer choice and compare them with your notes. If there are any major omissions or other discrepancies in your explanations, be sure to note them prominently.

Improving Your Timing

- Aim to read a passage in about 4 minutes; aim to answer each question in about one minute.
- Each passage and its questions together should take somewhere between 9 and 11 minutes.
- Check the clock after every other passage and its questions. Each passage pair should take about 20 minutes.
    - At the beginning of the section, you have 90 minutes left.
    - After two passages, you have about 70 minutes left.

- After four passages, you have about 50 minutes left.
- After six passages, you have about 30 minutes left.
- After eight passages, you have about 10 minutes left.
- After nine passages, you have 0 minutes left and are finished with the section.

Building Endurance

- Increase stamina by studying in 90-minute increments when possible (equal to the amount of time for the CARS section).
- Periodically, simulate the Test Day experience with study and practice for 6 hours and 15 minutes (equal to the amount of testing time).

Enhancing Your Vocabulary

- Read academic texts for at least 20 minutes a day to sharpen reading skills in preparation for CARS.
- Choose articles on topics that cause you trouble on Full-Length Exams (as revealed by your HIFIS).
- Practice Distilling (Highlighting, Outlining, and Interrogating) using these articles.

Notes

Notes

Notes

Notes

Notes

Notes

Notes

The Kaplan Method for CARS Passages

PREVIEW FOR DIFFICULTY

- Look for the big picture
- Assess the relative difficulty
- Decide to read *now* or *later*

CHOOSE YOUR APPROACH

- Highlighting: Best for high-difficulty passages or if low on time
- Outlining: Gives a moderate understanding of the passage and allows for more time to work on the questions
- Interrogating: Gives a strong understanding of the passage but allows for less time to work on the questions

READ AND DISTILL THE MEANING OF EACH PARAGRAPH

- Recognize keywords to identify the most important and testable content in each paragraph
- Use your approach from the Choose step to extract your major takeaways from each paragraph:
  - Highlighting—highlight 1–3 key terms and phrases per paragraph you can use to quickly locate information later
  - Outlining—create a brief label for each paragraph that summarizes the main idea of that paragraph
  - Interrogating—thoroughly examine each major idea presented in the paragraph and determine why and how the author is using the information to build an argument
- Identify the reason the passage was written before moving on to the questions

The Kaplan Method for CARS Questions

TYPE THE QUESTION

- Read the question, **NOT** the answers
- Identify the question type and difficulty
- Decide to attack *now* or *later* in the same passage

REPHRASE THE STEM

- Determine the task to be accomplished based on the question type
- Simplify the phrasing of the original question stem
- Translate the question into a specific piece of information you can either locate or infer

INVESTIGATE POTENTIAL SOLUTIONS

- Search for the answer in your interrogation, your outline, or the passage
- Predict what you can about the answer
- Be flexible if your initial approach fails: when in doubt, refer back to the passage

MATCH YOUR PREDICTION TO AN ANSWER CHOICE

- Search the answer choices for a response that is synonymous with your prediction
- Eliminate answer choices that diverge from the passage
- Select an answer and move on

CARS Question Types

	Foundations of Comprehension				Reasoning Within the Text*		Reasoning Beyond the Text*	
Question Type	**Main Idea**	**Detail**	**Inference**	**Definition-in-Context**	**Function**	**Strengthen–Weaken (Within the Passage)**	**Apply**	**Strengthen–Weaken (Beyond the Passage)**
Type	• Asks for the author's primary goal • Look for: *central thesis*, *primary purpose*, *main idea*	• Asks about what is stated explicitly in the passage • Look for: *the author states*, *according to the passage*, declarative language (*is* or *are*)	• Asks for unstated parts of arguments • Look for: *assume*, *because*, *conclude*, *imply*, *infer*, *justify*, *reasonable*, *suggest*	• Asks to define a word or phrase as it is used in the passage • Look for: a word, phrase, or claim from the passage (usually in quotes or italics)	• Asks about what the author is trying to do during the passage • Look for: *purpose*, *motive*, *intention*, *in order to*, *because*	• Asks about the logical relationship between conclusions and the evidence that strengthens them or the refutations that weaken them • Look for: *relate*, *support*, *challenge*, *relevance*, *significant*, *impact*	• Asks to take the information given in the passage and extrapolate it to a new context (author's response, probable outcome, or example) • Look for: *response*, *reply*, *most likely to agree with*, *least consistent with*, *outcome*, *result*, *expectation*, *consequence*, *example*, *instance*	• Asks about the logical relationship between conclusions and the evidence that strengthens them or the refutations that weaken them • Look for: *relate*, *support*, *challenge*, *relevance*, *significant*, *impact*, *could*, *would*
Rephrase	• Rephrase the question in such a way that you have a task for your Investigate step; this will often resemble *Why did the author write this passage?* or *What clues in the passage tell me who the author's audience is?*	• Rephrase the question in a way that maintains any buzzwords from the stem that will guide you to where in the passage you need to Investigate	• Determine whether you are looking for an assumption (evidence) or implication (conclusion) • Determine which claim the answer is supposed to support or be supported by	• Often *How is this phrase used in the passage?*	• *Why/how has the author used this [word, phrase, etc.]?*	• Determine the two claims and the connection between them; you will usually be given at least one of these elements and will have to find the other(s) • Identify where each piece of the argument can be found: in the question stem, in the passage, or in the answer choices	• If the question stem is long, jump to the end to determine what it's asking • Read any information given in the question stem closely, looking for hints that connect it to the passage	• Determine the two claims and the connection between them; you will usually be given at least one of these elements and will have to find the other(s) • Identify where each piece of the argument can be found: in the question stem, in the passage, or in the answer choices
Investigate	• Reread the goal in your outline, taking note of the charge and degree of the verb (positive *vs.* negative, extreme *vs.* moderate)	• Reread the relevant sentence, as well as the sentences before and after • Create your prediction by putting the answer in your own words • Make the prediction brief so you can repeat it to yourself between answer choices	• Reread the relevant sentence, noting explicit evidence and conclusions given • For Assumption questions, the answer is either similar to the evidence given or links the evidence to the conclusions • For Implication questions, the answer is either similar to the conclusions given or is another logical conclusion one could draw from the evidence	• Reread the sentence with the word or phrase, and perhaps the surrounding context • Rephrase the author's definition of the term in your own words	• Look at your label for the relevant paragraph and the goal at the bottom of your outline • If buzzwords in the question stem direct you to specific sentences, reread those portions, thinking about how they fit into the purpose of the paragraph and the overall passage	• Research the relevant text to determine the missing claim or the connection between the claims • Use Logic keywords to help assemble the argument	• Reread the relevant text • For Response questions, determine the author's key beliefs (Author keywords) • For Outcome questions, pay attention to cause–effect relationships (Logic keywords) • For Example questions, look for text that provides definitions, explanations, or the author's own example, noting any necessary or sufficient conditions	• Research the relevant text to determine the missing claim or the connection between the claims • Use Logic keywords to help assemble the argument
Match	• Match your expectations to the right answer • If there is no clear match, use process of elimination • Wrong answers are often too narrow or too broad • Wrong answers may have the wrong tone (positive, negative, ambivalent, or impartial) or degree (too extreme or too moderate)	• Match your expectations to the right answer • If there is no clear match, use process of elimination	• Match your expectations to the right answer • If there is no clear match, use the Denial Test (negate each answer choice; whichever answer choice—when negated—has the most detrimental effect on the argument made in the passage is the correct answer choice)	• Match your expectations to the right answer • If there is no clear match, use process of elimination	• Match your expectations to the right answer • If there is no clear match, use process of elimination • Remove any answer that conflicts with the author's main argument or the paragraph's purpose	• Match your expectations to the right answer • If there is no clear match, use process of elimination	• Match your expectations to the right answer • If there is no clear match, use process of elimination • Eliminate any answer choices that are inconsistent with the author's views • Eliminate any answer choice that does not contain necessary conditions	• Match your expectations to the right answer • If there is no clear match, use process of elimination

*Note: The *Reasoning Within the Text* and *Reasoning Beyond the Text* categories also contain a few other rare question types (described in Chapters 10 and 11 of *MCAT CARS Review*).

Wrong Answer Pathologies

Wrong Answer Pathology	What Is It?	Common Findings
Faulty Use of Detail (FUD)	Potentially an accurate statement, but one that fails to answer the question posed	• Stays too specific for a question that requires a general answer • Uses a detail from the wrong part of the passage • Comes from the right paragraph but still is not relevant
Out of Scope (OS)	A statement that brings in some element that the passage does not discuss (and that cannot be inferred from the passage)	• Makes connections or comparisons that the author did not discuss • Makes a statement about the significance or history of an idea that the author did not • Brings in other information that does not fit within the constraints of the passage
Opposite (OPP)	A statement that contains information that directly conflicts with the passage	• Contains (or omits) a single word like *not* or *except* • Contains a prefix like *un–* or *a–* or a suffix like *–less* or *–free* • Says that a given claim is true, when the author is ambivalent
Distortion (DIST)	A statement that is extreme or twists the ideas in the passage further than the author would prefer	• Uses a strong word like *all*, *always*, *none*, *never*, *impossible*, or *only* • Contains a prefix like *any–* or *every–* or a suffix like *–est* or *–less* • Is more radical than the author (radical positions are rare in MCAT passages)

KAPLAN

MCAT® ORGANIC CHEMISTRY REVIEW 2024–2025

ONLINE + BOOK

Edited by Alexander Stone Macnow, MD

ACKNOWLEDGMENTS

Editor-in-Chief, 2024–2025 Edition
M. Dominic Eggert

Contributing Editors, 2024–2025 Edition
Christopher Durland; Charles Pierce, MD; Jason Selzer

Prior Edition Editorial Staff: Brandon Deason, MD; Christopher Durland; M. Dominic Eggert; Tyler Fara; Elizabeth Flagge; Adam Grey; Lauren K. White

Published by Kaplan North America, LLC dba Kaplan Publishing
1515 West Cypress Creek Road
Fort Lauderdale, Florida 33309

ISBN: 978-1-5062-8697-6

10 9 8 7 6 5 4 3 2 1

Kaplan Publishing print books are available at special quantity discounts to use for sales promotions, employee premiums, or educational purposes. For more information or to purchase books, please call the Simon & Schuster special sales department at 866-506-1949.

TABLE OF CONTENTS

GO ONLINE

kaptest.com/booksonline

THE *KAPLAN MCAT REVIEW* TEAM

Alexander Stone Macnow, MD
Editor-in-Chief

Kelly Kyker-Snowman, MS
Kaplan MCAT Faculty

M. Dominic Eggert
Editor

Reviewers and Editors: Elmar R. Aliyev; James Burns; Jonathan Cornfield; Alisha Maureen Crowley; Brandon Deason, MD; Nikolai Dorofeev, MD; Benjamin Downer, MS; Colin Doyle; Christopher Durland; Marilyn Engle; Eleni M. Eren; Raef Ali Fadel; Elizabeth Flagge; Adam Grey; Tyra Hall-Pogar, PhD; Scott Huff; Samer T. Ismail; Elizabeth A. Kudlaty; Ningfei Li; John P. Mahon; Matthew A. Meier; Nainika Nanda; Caroline Nkemdilim Opene; Kaitlyn E. Prenger; Uneeb Qureshi; Derek Rusnak, MA; Kristen L. Russell, ME; Bela G. Starkman, PhD; Michael Paul Tomani, MS; Lauren K. White; Nicholas M. White; Allison Ann Wilkes, MS; Kerranna Williamson, MBA; and Tony Yu

Thanks to Rebecca Anderson; Jeff Batzli; Tim Eich; Samantha Fallon; Owen Farcy; Dan Frey; Robin Garmise; Rita Garthaffner; Joanna Graham; Adam Grey; Allison Gudenau; Allison Harm; Beth Hoffberg; Aaron Lemon-Strauss; Keith Lubeley; Diane McGarvey; Petros Minasi; Beena P V; John Polstein; Deeangelee Pooran-Kublall, MD, MPH; Rochelle Rothstein, MD; Larry Rudman; Srividhya Sankar; Sylvia Tidwell Scheuring; Carly Schnur; Aiswarya Sivanand; Todd Tedesco; Karin Tucker; Lee Weiss; Christina Wheeler; Kristen Workman; Amy Zarkos; and the countless others who made this project possible.

GETTING STARTED CHECKLIST

Getting Started Checklist

- [ ] Register for your free online assets—including full-length tests, Science Review Videos, and additional practice materials—at **www.kaptest.com/moreonline**.
- [ ] Create a study calendar that ensures you complete content review and sufficient practice by Test Day!
- [ ] As you finish a chapter and the online practice for that chapter, check it off on the table of contents.
- [ ] Register to take the MCAT at **www.aamc.org/mcat**.
- [ ] Set aside time during your prep to make sure the rest of your application—personal statement, recommendations, and other materials—is ready to go!
- [ ] Take a moment to admire your completed checklist, then get back to the business of prepping for this exam!

PREFACE

And now it starts: your long, yet fruitful journey toward wearing a white coat. Proudly wearing that white coat, though, is hopefully only part of your motivation. You are reading this book because you want to be a healer.

If you're serious about going to medical school, then you are likely already familiar with the importance of the MCAT in medical school admissions. While the holistic review process puts additional weight on your experiences, extracurricular activities, and personal attributes, the fact remains: along with your GPA, your MCAT score remains one of the two most important components of your application portfolio—at least early in the admissions process. Each additional point you score on the MCAT pushes you in front of thousands of other students and makes you an even more attractive applicant. But the MCAT is not simply an obstacle to overcome; it is an opportunity to show schools that you will be a strong student and a future leader in medicine.

We at Kaplan take our jobs very seriously and aim to help students see success not only on the MCAT, but as future physicians. We work with our learning science experts to ensure that we're using the most up-to-date teaching techniques in our resources. Multiple members of our team hold advanced degrees in medicine or associated biomedical sciences, and are committed to the highest level of medical education. Kaplan has been working with the MCAT for over 50 years and our commitment to premed students is unflagging; in fact, Stanley Kaplan created this company when he had difficulty being accepted to medical school due to unfair quota systems that existed at the time.

We stand now at the beginning of a new era in medical education. As citizens of this 21st-century world of healthcare, we are charged with creating a patient-oriented, culturally competent, cost-conscious, universally available, technically advanced, and research-focused healthcare system, run by compassionate providers. Suffice it to say, this is no easy task. Problem-based learning, integrated curricula, and classes in interpersonal skills are some of the responses to this demand for an excellent workforce—a workforce of which you'll soon be a part.

We're thrilled that you've chosen us to help you on this journey. Please reach out to us to share your challenges, concerns, and successes. Together, we will shape the future of medicine in the United States and abroad; we look forward to helping you become the doctor you deserve to be.

Good luck!

Alexander Stone Macnow, MD
Editor-in-Chief
Department of Pathology and Laboratory Medicine
Hospital of the University of Pennsylvania

BA, Musicology—Boston University, 2008
MD—Perelman School of Medicine at the University of Pennsylvania, 2013

ABOUT THE MCAT

Anatomy of the MCAT

Here is a general overview of the structure of Test Day:

Section	Number of Questions	Time Allotted
Test-Day Certification		4 minutes
Tutorial (optional)		10 minutes
Chemical and Physical Foundations of Biological Systems	59	95 minutes
Break (optional)		10 minutes
Critical Analysis and Reasoning Skills (CARS)	53	90 minutes
Lunch Break (optional)		30 minutes
Biological and Biochemical Foundations of Living Systems	59	95 minutes
Break (optional)		10 minutes
Psychological, Social, and Biological Foundations of Behavior	59	95 minutes
Void Question		3 minutes
Satisfaction Survey (optional)		5 minutes

The structure of the four sections of the MCAT is shown below.

Chemical and Physical Foundations of Biological Systems	
Time	95 minutes
Format	• 59 questions • 10 passages • 44 questions are passage-based, and 15 are discrete (stand-alone) questions. • Score between 118 and 132
What It Tests	• Biochemistry: 25% • Biology: 5% • General Chemistry: 30% • Organic Chemistry: 15% • Physics: 25%

Critical Analysis and Reasoning Skills (CARS)	
Time	90 minutes
Format	• 53 questions • 9 passages • All questions are passage-based. There are no discrete (stand-alone) questions. • Score between 118 and 132
What It Tests	Disciplines: • Humanities: 50% • Social Sciences: 50% Skills: • *Foundations of Comprehension*: 30% • *Reasoning Within the Text*: 30% • *Reasoning Beyond the Text*: 40%
Biological and Biochemical Foundations of Living Systems	
Time	95 minutes
Format	• 59 questions • 10 passages • 44 questions are passage-based, and 15 are discrete (stand-alone) questions. • Score between 118 and 132
What It Tests	• Biochemistry: 25% • Biology: 65% • General Chemistry: 5% • Organic Chemistry: 5%
Psychological, Social, and Biological Foundations of Behavior	
Time	95 minutes
Format	• 59 questions • 10 passages • 44 questions are passage-based, and 15 are discrete (stand-alone) questions. • Score between 118 and 132
What It Tests	• Biology: 5% • Psychology: 65% • Sociology: 30%
Total	
Testing Time	375 minutes (6 hours, 15 minutes)
Total Seat Time	447 minutes (7 hours, 27 minutes)
Questions	230
Score	472 to 528

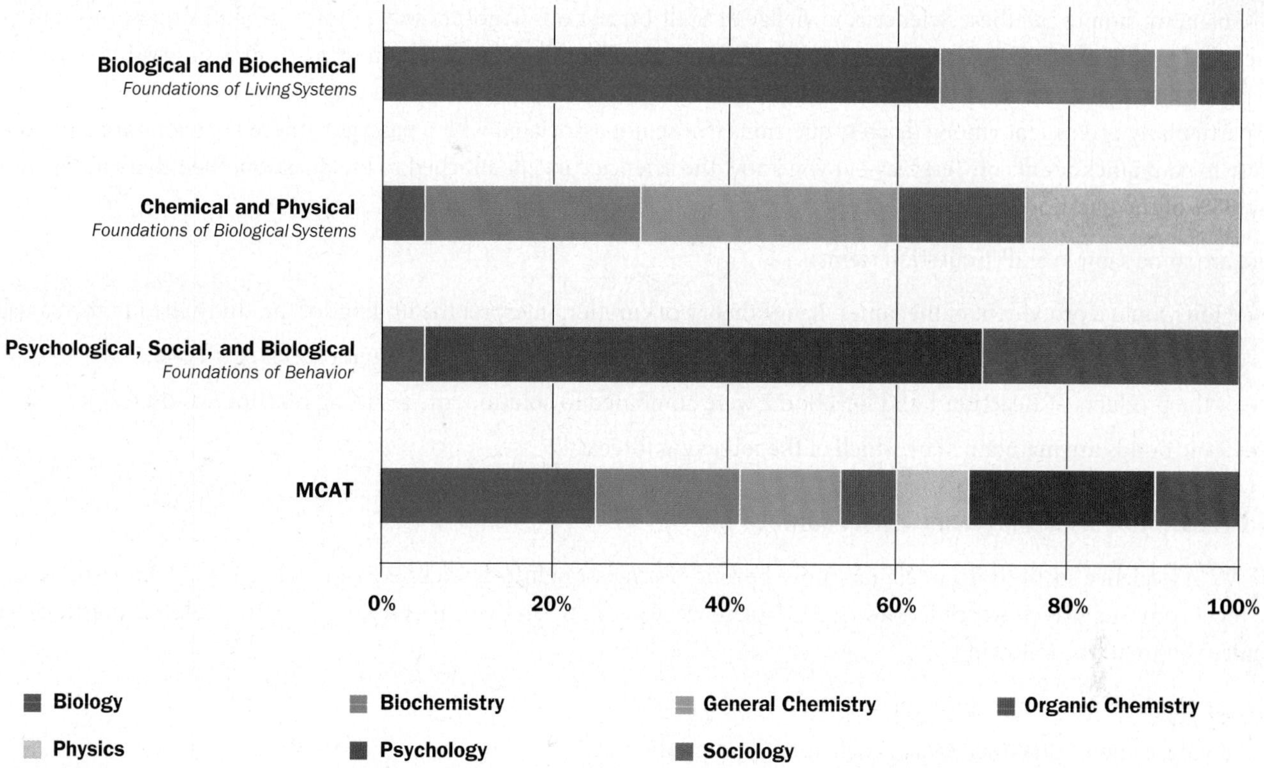

Scientific Inquiry and Reasoning Skills (SIRS)

The AAMC has defined four *Scientific Inquiry and Reasoning Skills* (SIRS) that will be tested in the three science sections of the MCAT:

1. *Knowledge of Scientific Concepts and Principles* (35% of questions)
2. *Scientific Reasoning and Problem-Solving* (45% of questions)
3. *Reasoning About the Design and Execution of Research* (10% of questions)
4. *Data-Based and Statistical Reasoning* (10% of questions)

Let's see how each one breaks down into more specific Test Day behaviors. Note that the bullet points of specific objectives for each of the SIRS are taken directly from the *Official Guide to the MCAT Exam*; the descriptions of what these behaviors mean and sample question stems, however, are written by Kaplan.

Skill 1: *Knowledge of Scientific Concepts and Principles*

This is probably the least surprising of the four SIRS; the testing of science knowledge is, after all, one of the signature qualities of the MCAT. Skill 1 questions will require you to do the following:

- Recognize correct scientific principles
- Identify the relationships among closely related concepts
- Identify the relationships between different representations of concepts (verbal, symbolic, graphic)
- Identify examples of observations that illustrate scientific principles
- Use mathematical equations to solve problems

At Kaplan, we simply call these Science Knowledge or Skill 1 questions. Another way to think of Skill 1 questions is as "one-step" problems. The single step is either to realize which scientific concept the question stem is suggesting or to take the concept stated in the question stem and identify which answer choice is an accurate application of it. Skill 1 questions are particularly prominent among discrete questions (those not associated with a passage). These questions are an opportunity to gain quick points on Test Day—if you know the science concept attached to the question, then that's it! On Test Day, 35% of the questions in each science section will be Skill 1 questions.

Here are some sample Skill 1 question stems:

- How would a proponent of the James–Lange theory of emotion interpret the findings of the study cited in the passage?
- Which of the following most accurately describes the function of FSH in the human menstrual cycle?
- If the products of Reaction 1 and Reaction 2 were combined in solution, the resulting reaction would form:
- Ionic bonds are maintained by which of the following forces?

Skill 2: *Scientific Reasoning and Problem-Solving*

The MCAT science sections do, of course, move beyond testing straightforward science knowledge; Skill 2 questions are the most common way in which it does so. At Kaplan, we also call these Critical Thinking questions. Skill 2 questions will require you to do the following:

- Reason about scientific principles, theories, and models
- Analyze and evaluate scientific explanations and predictions
- Evaluate arguments about causes and consequences
- Bring together theory, observations, and evidence to draw conclusions
- Recognize scientific findings that challenge or invalidate a scientific theory or model
- Determine and use scientific formulas to solve problems

Just as Skill 1 questions can be thought of as "one-step" problems, many Skill 2 questions are "two-step" problems, and more difficult Skill 2 questions may require three or more steps. These questions can require a wide spectrum of reasoning skills, including integration of multiple facts from a passage, combination of multiple science content areas, and prediction of an experiment's results. Skill 2 questions also tend to ask about science content without actually mentioning it by name. For example, a question might describe the results of one experiment and ask you to predict the results of a second experiment without actually telling you what underlying scientific principles are at work—part of the question's difficulty will be figuring out which principles to apply in order to get the correct answer. On Test Day, 45% of the questions in each science section will be Skill 2 questions.

Here are some sample Skill 2 question stems:

- Which of the following experimental conditions would most likely yield results similar to those in Figure 2?
- All of the following conclusions are supported by the information in the passage EXCEPT:
- The most likely cause of the anomalous results found by the experimenter is:
- An impact to a person's chest quickly reduces the volume of one of the lungs to 70% of its initial value while not allowing any air to escape from the mouth. By what percentage is the force of outward air pressure increased on a 2 cm^2 portion of the inner surface of the compressed lung?

Skill 3: *Reasoning About the Design and Execution of Research*

The MCAT is interested in your ability to critically appraise and analyze research, as this is an important day-to-day task of a physician. We call these questions Experimental and Research Design questions or Skill 3 for short. Skill 3 questions will require you to do the following:

- Identify the role of theory, past findings, and observations in scientific questioning
- Identify testable research questions and hypotheses
- Distinguish between samples and populations and distinguish results that support generalizations about populations
- Identify independent and dependent variables
- Reason about the features of research studies that suggest associations between variables or causal relationships between them (such as temporality and random assignment)
- Identify conclusions that are supported by research results
- Determine the implications of results for real-world situations
- Reason about ethical issues in scientific research

Over the years, the AAMC has received input from medical schools to require more practical research skills of MCAT test takers, and Skill 3 questions are the response to these demands. This skill is unique in that the outside knowledge you need to answer Skill 3 questions is not taught in any one undergraduate course; instead, the research design principles needed to answer these questions are learned gradually throughout your science classes and especially through any laboratory work you have completed. It should be noted that Skill 3 comprises 10% of the questions in each science section on Test Day.

Here are some sample Skill 3 question stems:

- What is the dependent variable in the study described in the passage?
- The major flaw in the method used to measure disease susceptibility in Experiment 1 is:
- Which of the following procedures is most important for the experimenters to follow in order for their study to maintain a proper, randomized sample of research subjects?
- A researcher would like to test the hypothesis that individuals who move to an urban area during adulthood are more likely to own a car than are those who have lived in an urban area since birth. Which of the following studies would best test this hypothesis?

Skill 4: *Data-Based and Statistical Reasoning*

Lastly, the science sections of the MCAT test your ability to analyze the visual and numerical results of experiments and studies. We call these Data and Statistical Analysis questions. Skill 4 questions will require you to do the following:

- Use, analyze, and interpret data in figures, graphs, and tables
- Evaluate whether representations make sense for particular scientific observations and data
- Use measures of central tendency (mean, median, and mode) and measures of dispersion (range, interquartile range, and standard deviation) to describe data
- Reason about random and systematic error

- Reason about statistical significance and uncertainty (interpreting statistical significance levels and interpreting a confidence interval)
- Use data to explain relationships between variables or make predictions
- Use data to answer research questions and draw conclusions

Skill 4 is included in the MCAT because physicians and researchers spend much of their time examining the results of their own studies and the studies of others, and it's very important for them to make legitimate conclusions and sound judgments based on that data. The MCAT tests Skill 4 on all three science sections with graphical representations of data (charts and bar graphs), as well as numerical ones (tables, lists, and results summarized in sentence or paragraph form). On Test Day, 10% of the questions in each science section will be Skill 4 questions.

Here are some sample Skill 4 question stems:

- According to the information in the passage, there is an inverse correlation between:
- What conclusion is best supported by the findings displayed in Figure 2?
- A medical test for a rare type of heavy metal poisoning returns a positive result for 98% of affected individuals and 13% of unaffected individuals. Which of the following types of error is most prevalent in this test?
- If a fourth trial of Experiment 1 was run and yielded a result of 54% compliance, which of the following would be true?

SIRS Summary

Discussing the SIRS tested on the MCAT is a daunting prospect given that the very nature of the skills tends to make the conversation rather abstract. Nevertheless, with enough practice, you'll be able to identify each of the four skills quickly, and you'll also be able to apply the proper strategies to solve those problems on Test Day. If you need a quick reference to remind you of the four SIRS, these guidelines may help:

Skill 1 (Science Knowledge) questions ask:

- Do you remember this science content?

Skill 2 (Critical Thinking) questions ask:

- Do you remember this science content? And if you do, could you please apply it to this novel situation?
- Could you answer this question that cleverly combines multiple content areas at the same time?

Skill 3 (Experimental and Research Design) questions ask:

- Let's forget about the science content for a while. Could you give some insight into the experimental or research methods involved in this situation?

Skill 4 (Data and Statistical Analysis) questions ask:

- Let's forget about the science content for a while. Could you accurately read some graphs and tables for a moment? Could you make some conclusions or extrapolations based on the information presented?

Critical Analysis and Reasoning Skills (CARS)

The *Critical Analysis and Reasoning Skills* (CARS) section of the MCAT tests three discrete families of textual reasoning skills; each of these families requires a higher level of reasoning than the last. Those three skills are as follows:

1. *Foundations of Comprehension* (30% of questions)
2. *Reasoning Within the Text* (30% of questions)
3. *Reasoning Beyond the Text* (40% of questions)

These three skills are tested through nine humanities- and social sciences-themed passages, with approximately 5 to 7 questions per passage. Let's take a more in-depth look into these three skills. Again, the bullet points of specific objectives for each of the CARS are taken directly from the *Official Guide to the MCAT Exam*; the descriptions of what these behaviors mean and sample question stems, however, are written by Kaplan.

Foundations of Comprehension

Questions in this skill will ask for basic facts and simple inferences about the passage; the questions themselves will be similar to those seen on reading comprehension sections of other standardized exams like the SAT® and ACT®. *Foundations of Comprehension* questions will require you to do the following:

- Understand the basic components of the text
- Infer meaning from rhetorical devices, word choice, and text structure

This admittedly covers a wide range of potential question types including Main Idea, Detail, Inference, and Definition-in-Context questions, but finding the correct answer to all *Foundations of Comprehension* questions will follow from a basic understanding of the passage and the point of view of its author (and occasionally that of other voices in the passage).

Here are some sample *Foundations of Comprehension* question stems:

- **Main Idea**—The author's primary purpose in this passage is:
- **Detail**—Based on the information in the second paragraph, which of the following is the most accurate summary of the opinion held by Schubert's critics?
- **(Scattered) Detail**—According to the passage, which of the following is FALSE about literary reviews in the 1920s?
- **Inference (Implication)**—Which of the following phrases, as used in the passage, is most suggestive that the author has a personal bias toward narrative records of history?
- **Inference (Assumption)**—In putting together the argument in the passage, the author most likely assumes:
- **Definition-in-Context**—The word "obscure" (paragraph 3), when used in reference to the historian's actions, most nearly means:

Reasoning Within the Text

While *Foundations of Comprehension* questions will usually depend on interpreting a single piece of information in the passage or understanding the passage as a whole, *Reasoning Within the Text* questions require more thought because they will ask you to identify the purpose of a particular piece of information in the context of the passage, or ask how one piece of information relates to another. *Reasoning Within the Text* questions will require you to:

- Integrate different components of the text to draw relevant conclusions

In other words, questions in this skill often ask either *How do these two details relate to one another?* or *What else must be true that the author didn't say?* The CARS section will also ask you to judge certain parts of the passage or even judge the author. These questions, which fall under the *Reasoning Within the Text* skill, can ask you to identify authorial bias, evaluate the credibility of cited sources, determine the logical soundness of an argument, identify the importance of a particular fact or statement in the context of the passage, or search for relevant evidence in the passage to support a given conclusion. In all, this category includes Function and Strengthen–Weaken (Within the Passage) questions, as well as a smattering of related—but rare—question types.

Here are some sample *Reasoning Within the Text* question stems:

- **Function**—The author's discussion of the effect of socioeconomic status on social mobility primarily serves which of the following functions?
- **Strengthen–Weaken (Within the Passage)**—Which of the following facts is used in the passage as the most prominent piece of evidence in favor of the author's conclusions?
- **Strengthen–Weaken (Within the Passage)**—Based on the role it plays in the author's argument, *The Possessed* can be considered:

Reasoning Beyond the Text

The distinguishing factor of *Reasoning Beyond the Text* questions is in the title of the skill: the word *Beyond*. Questions that test this skill, which make up a larger share of the CARS section than questions from either of the other two skills, will always introduce a completely new situation that was not present in the passage itself; these questions will ask you to determine how one influences the other. *Reasoning Beyond the Text* questions will require you to:

- Apply or extrapolate ideas from the passage to new contexts
- Assess the impact of introducing new factors, information, or conditions to ideas from the passage

The *Reasoning Beyond the Text* skill is further divided into Apply and Strengthen–Weaken (Beyond the Passage) questions, and a few other rarely appearing question types.

Here are some sample *Reasoning Beyond the Text* question stems:

- **Apply**—If a document were located that demonstrated Berlioz intended to include a chorus of at least 700 in his *Grande Messe des Morts*, how would the author likely respond?
- **Apply**—Which of the following is the best example of a "virtuous rebellion," as it is defined in the passage?
- **Strengthen–Weaken (Beyond the Passage)**—Suppose Jane Austen had written in a letter to her sister, "My strongest characters were those forced by circumstance to confront basic questions about the society in which they lived." What relevance would this have to the passage?
- **Strengthen–Weaken (Beyond the Passage)**—Which of the following sentences, if added to the end of the passage, would most WEAKEN the author's conclusions in the last paragraph?

CARS Summary

Through the *Foundations of Comprehension* skill, the CARS section tests many of the reading skills you have been building on since grade school, albeit in the context of very challenging doctorate-level passages. But through the two other skills (*Reasoning Within the Text* and *Reasoning Beyond the Text*), the MCAT demands that you understand the deep structure of passages and the arguments within them at a very advanced level. And, of course, all of this is tested under very tight timing restrictions: only 102 seconds per question—and that doesn't even include the time spent reading the passages.

Here's a quick reference guide to the three CARS skills:

Foundations of Comprehension questions ask:

- Did you understand the passage and its main ideas?
- What does the passage have to say about this particular detail?
- What must be true that the author did not say?

Reasoning Within the Text questions ask:

- What's the logical relationship between these two ideas from the passage?
- How well argued is the author's thesis?

Reasoning Beyond the Text questions ask:

- How does this principle from the passage apply to this new situation?
- How does this new piece of information influence the arguments in the passage?

Scoring

Each of the four sections of the MCAT is scored between 118 and 132, with the median at approximately 125. This means the total score ranges from 472 to 528, with the median at about 500. Why such peculiar numbers? The AAMC stresses that this scale emphasizes the importance of the central portion of the score distribution, where most students score (around 125 per section, or 500 total), rather than putting undue focus on the high end of the scale.

Note that there is no wrong answer penalty on the MCAT, so you should select an answer for every question—even if it is only a guess.

The AAMC has released the 2019–2021 correlation between scaled score and percentile, as shown on the following page. It should be noted that the percentile scale is adjusted and renormalized over time and thus can shift slightly from year to year. Percentile rank updates are released by the AAMC around May 1 of each year.

Total Score	Percentile	Total Score	Percentile
528	100	499	41
527	100	498	38
526	100	497	35
525	100	496	32
524	100	495	29
523	99	494	26
522	99	493	24
521	98	492	21
520	97	491	19
519	96	490	17
518	95	489	15
517	94	488	13
516	92	487	11
515	90	486	10
514	88	485	8
513	86	484	7
512	83	483	6
511	80	482	5
510	77	481	4
509	74	480	3
508	71	479	2
507	68	478	2
506	65	477	1
505	61	476	1
504	58	475	<1
503	55	474	<1
502	51	473	<1
501	48	472	<1
500	45		

Source: AAMC. 2022. *Summary of MCAT Total and Section Scores.* Accessed October 2022.
https://students-residents.aamc.org/mcat-research-and-data/percentile-ranks-mcat-exam

Further information on score reporting is included at the end of the next section (see *After Your Test*).

MCAT Policies and Procedures

We strongly encourage you to download the latest copy of *MCAT® Essentials*, available on the AAMC's website, to ensure that you have the latest information about registration and Test Day policies and procedures; this document is updated annually. A brief summary of some of the most important rules is provided here.

MCAT Registration

The only way to register for the MCAT is online. You can access AAMC's registration system at **www.aamc.org/mcat**.

The AAMC posts the schedule of testing, registration, and score release dates in the fall before the MCAT testing year, which runs from January into September. Registration for January through June is available earlier than registration for later dates, but see the AAMC's website for the exact dates each year. There is one standard registration fee, but the fee for changing your test date or test center increases the closer you get to your MCAT.

Fees and the Fee Assistance Program (FAP)

Payment for test registration must be made by MasterCard or VISA. As described earlier, the fee for rescheduling your exam or changing your testing center increases as one approaches Test Day. In addition, it is not uncommon for test centers to fill up well in advance of the registration deadline. For these reasons, we recommend identifying your preferred Test Day as soon as possible and registering. There are ancillary benefits to having a set Test Day, as well: when you know the date you're working toward, you'll study harder and are less likely to keep pushing back the exam. The AAMC offers a Fee Assistance Program (FAP) for students with financial hardship to help reduce the cost of taking the MCAT, as well as for the American Medical College Application Service (AMCAS®) application. Further information on the FAP can be found at **www.aamc.org/students/applying/fap**.

Testing Security

On Test Day, you will be required to present a qualifying form of ID. Generally, a current driver's license or United States passport will be sufficient (consult the AAMC website for the full list of qualifying criteria). When registering, take care to spell your first and last names (middle names, suffixes, and prefixes are not required and will not be verified on Test Day) precisely the same as they appear on this ID; failure to provide this ID at the test center or differences in spelling between your registration and ID will be considered a "no-show," and you will not receive a refund for the exam.

During Test Day registration, other identity data collected may include: a digital palm vein scan, a Test Day photo, a digitization of your valid ID, and signatures. Some testing centers may use a metal detection wand to ensure that no prohibited items are brought into the testing room. Prohibited items include all electronic devices, including watches and timers, calculators, cell phones, and any and all forms of recording equipment; food, drinks (including water), and cigarettes or other smoking paraphernalia; hats and scarves (except for religious purposes); and books, notes, or other study materials. If you require a medical device, such as an insulin pump or pacemaker, you must apply for accommodated testing. During breaks, you are allowed access to food and drink, but not to electronic devices, including cell phones.

Testing centers are under video surveillance and the AAMC does not take potential violations of testing security lightly. The bottom line: *know the rules and don't break them.*

Accommodations

Students with disabilities or medical conditions can apply for accommodated testing. Documentation of the disability or condition is required, and requests may take two months—or more—to be approved. For this reason, it is recommended that you begin the process of applying for accommodated testing as early as possible. More information on applying for accommodated testing can be found at **www.aamc.org/students/applying/mcat/accommodations**.

After Your Test

When your MCAT is all over, no matter how you feel you did, be good to yourself when you leave the test center. Celebrate! Take a nap. Watch a movie. Get some exercise. Plan a trip or outing. Call up all of your neglected friends or message them on social media. Go out for snacks or drinks with people you like. Whatever you do, make sure that it has absolutely nothing to do with thinking too hard—you deserve some rest and relaxation.

Perhaps most importantly, do not discuss specific details about the test with anyone. For one, it is important to let go of the stress of Test Day, and reliving your exam only inhibits you from being able to do so. But more significantly, the Examinee Agreement you sign at the beginning of your exam specifically prohibits you from discussing or disclosing exam content. The AAMC is known to seek out individuals who violate this agreement and retains the right to prosecute these individuals at their discretion. This means that you should not, under any circumstances, discuss the exam in person or over the phone with other individuals—including us at Kaplan—or post information or questions about exam content to Facebook, Student Doctor Network, or other online social media. You are permitted to comment on your "general exam experience," including how you felt about the exam overall or an individual section, but this is a fine line. In summary: *if you're not certain whether you can discuss an aspect of the test or not, just don't do it!* Do not let a silly Facebook post stop you from becoming the doctor you deserve to be.

Scores are typically released approximately one month after Test Day. The release is staggered during the afternoon and evening, ending at 5 p.m. Eastern Standard Time. This means that not all examinees receive their scores at exactly the same time. Your score report will include a scaled score for each section between 118 and 132, as well as your total combined score between 472 and 528. These scores are given as confidence intervals. For each section, the confidence interval is approximately the given score ± 1; for the total score, it is approximately the given score ± 2. You will also be given the corresponding percentile rank for each of these section scores and the total score.

AAMC Contact Information

For further questions, contact the MCAT team at the Association of American Medical Colleges:

MCAT Resource Center
Association of American Medical Colleges
www.aamc.org/mcat
(202) 828-0600
www.aamc.org/contactmcat

HOW THIS BOOK WAS CREATED

The *Kaplan MCAT Review* project began shortly after the release of the *Preview Guide for the MCAT 2015 Exam*, 2nd edition. Through thorough analysis by our staff psychometricians, we were able to analyze the relative yield of the different topics on the MCAT, and we began constructing tables of contents for the books of the *Kaplan MCAT Review* series. A dedicated staff of 30 writers, 7 editors, and 32 proofreaders worked over 5,000 combined hours to produce these books. The format of the books was heavily influenced by weekly meetings with Kaplan's learning science team.

In the years since this book was created, a number of opportunities for expansion and improvement have occurred. The current edition represents the culmination of the wisdom accumulated during that time frame, and it also includes several new features designed to improve the reading and learning experience in these texts.

These books were submitted for publication in April 2023. For any updates after this date, please visit www.kaptest.com/retail-book-corrections-and-updates.

If you have any questions about the content presented here, email KaplanMCATfeedback@kaplan.com. For other questions not related to content, email booksupport@kaplan.com.

Each book has been vetted through at least ten rounds of review. To that end, the information presented in these books is true and accurate to the best of our knowledge. Still, your feedback helps us improve our prep materials. Please notify us of any inaccuracies or errors in the books by sending an email to KaplanMCATfeedback@kaplan.com.

USING THIS BOOK

Kaplan MCAT Organic Chemistry Review, and the other six books in the *Kaplan MCAT Review* series, bring the Kaplan classroom experience to you—right in your home, at your convenience. This book offers the same Kaplan content review, strategies, and practice that make Kaplan the #1 choice for MCAT prep.

This book is designed to help you review the organic chemistry topics covered on the MCAT. Please understand that content review—no matter how thorough—is not sufficient preparation for the MCAT! The MCAT tests not only your science knowledge but also your critical reading, reasoning, and problem-solving skills. Do not assume that simply memorizing the contents of this book will earn you high scores on Test Day; to maximize your scores, you must also improve your reading and test-taking skills through MCAT-style questions and practice tests.

Learning Objectives

At the beginning of each section, you'll find a short list of objectives describing the skills covered within that section. Learning objectives for these texts were developed in conjunction with Kaplan's learning science team, and have been designed specifically to focus your attention on tasks and concepts that are likely to show up on your MCAT. These learning objectives will function as a means to guide your study, and indicate what information and relationships you should be focused on within each section. Before starting each section, read these learning objectives carefully. They will not only allow you to assess your existing familiarity with the content, but also provide a goal-oriented focus for your studying experience of the section.

MCAT Concept Checks

At the end of each section, you'll find a few open-ended questions that you can use to assess your mastery of the material. These MCAT Concept Checks were introduced after numerous conversations with Kaplan's learning science team. Research has demonstrated repeatedly that introspection and self-analysis improve mastery, retention, and recall of material. Complete these MCAT Concept Checks to ensure that you've got the key points from each section before moving on!

Science Mastery Assessments

At the beginning of each chapter, you'll find 15 MCAT-style practice questions. These are designed to help you assess your understanding of the chapter before you begin reading the chapter. Using the guidance provided with the assessment, you can determine the best way to review each chapter based on your personal strengths and weaknesses. Most of the questions in the Science Mastery Assessments focus on the first of the *Scientific Inquiry and Reasoning Skills* (*Knowledge of Scientific Concepts and Principles*), although there are occasional questions that fall into the second or fourth SIRS (*Scientific Reasoning and Problem-Solving* and *Data-Based and Statistical Reasoning*, respectively). You can complete each chapter's assessment in a testing interface in your online resources, where you'll also find a test-like passage set covering the same content you just studied to ensure you can also apply your knowledge the way the MCAT will expect you to!

Sidebars

The following is a guide to the five types of sidebars you'll find in *Kaplan MCAT Organic Chemistry Review:*

- **Bridge:** These sidebars create connections between science topics that appear in multiple chapters throughout the *Kaplan MCAT Review* series.
- **Key Concept:** These sidebars draw attention to the most important takeaways in a given topic, and they sometimes offer synopses or overviews of complex information. If you understand nothing else, make sure you grasp the Key Concepts for any given subject.
- **MCAT Expertise:** These sidebars point out how information may be tested on the MCAT or offer key strategy points and test-taking tips that you should apply on Test Day.
- **Mnemonic:** These sidebars present memory devices to help recall certain facts.
- **Real World:** These sidebars illustrate how a concept in the text relates to the practice of medicine or the world at large. While this is not information you need to know for Test Day, many of the topics in Real World sidebars are excellent examples of how a concept may appear in a passage or discrete (stand-alone) question on the MCAT.

What This Book Covers

The information presented in the *Kaplan MCAT Review* series covers everything listed on the official MCAT content lists. Every topic in these lists is covered in the same level of detail as is common to the undergraduate and postbaccalaureate classes that are considered prerequisites for the MCAT. Note that your premedical classes may include topics not discussed in these books, or they may go into more depth than these books do. Additional exposure to science content is never a bad thing, but all of the content knowledge you are expected to have walking in on Test Day is covered in these books.

Chapter profiles, on the first page of each chapter, represent a holistic look at the content within the chapter, and will include a pie chart as well as text information. The pie chart analysis is based directly on data released by the AAMC, and will give a rough estimate of the importance of the chapter in relation to the book as a whole. Further, the text portion of the Chapter Profiles includes which AAMC content categories are covered within the chapter. These are referenced directly from the AAMC MCAT exam content listing, available on the testmaker's website.

You'll also see new High-Yield badges scattered throughout the sections of this book:

In This Chapter

1.1 Amino Acids Found in Proteins

High-Yield

LEARNING OBJECTIVES

After Chapter 1.1, you will be able to:

- Recognize common abbreviations for amino acids, such as Glu and Y

These badges represent the top 100 topics most tested by the AAMC. In other words, according to the testmaker and all our experience with their resources, a High-Yield badge means more questions on Test Day.

This book also contains a thorough glossary and index for easy navigation of the text.

In the end, this is your book, so write in the margins, draw diagrams, highlight the key points—do whatever is necessary to help you get that higher score. We look forward to working with you as you achieve your dreams and become the doctor you deserve to be!

Studying with This Book

In addition to providing you with the best practice questions and test strategies, Kaplan's team of learning scientists are dedicated to researching and testing the best methods for getting the most out of your study time. Here are their top four tips for improving retention:

Review multiple topics in one study session. This may seem counterintuitive—we're used to practicing one skill at a time in order to improve each skill. But research shows that weaving topics together leads to increased learning. Beyond that consideration, the MCAT often includes more than one topic in a single question. Studying in an integrated manner is the most effective way to prepare for this test.

Customize the content. Drawing attention to difficult or critical content can ensure you don't overlook it as you read and re-read sections. The best way to do this is to make it more visual—highlight, make tabs, use stickies, whatever works. We recommend highlighting only the most important or difficult sections of text. Selective highlighting of up to about 10 percent of text in a given chapter is great for emphasizing parts of the text, but over-highlighting can have the opposite effect.

Repeat topics over time. Many people try to memorize concepts by repeating them over and over again in succession. Our research shows that retention is improved by spacing out the repeats over time and mixing up the order in which you study content. For example, try reading chapters in a different order the second (or third!) time around. Revisit practice questions that you answered incorrectly in a new sequence. Perhaps information you reviewed more recently will help you better understand those questions and solutions you struggled with in the past.

Take a moment to reflect. When you finish reading a section for the first time, stop and think about what you just read. Jot down a few thoughts in the margins or in your notes about why the content is important or what topics came to mind when you read it. Associating learning with a memory is a fantastic way to retain information! This also works when answering questions. After answering a question, take a moment to think through each step you took to arrive at a solution. What led you to the answer you chose? Understanding the steps you took will help you make good decisions when answering future questions.

Online Resources

In addition to the resources located within this text, you also have additional online resources awaiting you at **www.kaptest.com/booksonline**. Make sure to log on and take advantage of free practice and additional resources!

Please note that access to the online resources is limited to the original owner of this book.

STUDYING FOR THE MCAT

The first year of medical school is a frenzied experience for most students. To meet the requirements of a rigorous work schedule, students either learn to prioritize their time or else fall hopelessly behind. It's no surprise, then, that the MCAT, the test specifically designed to predict success in medical school, is a high-speed, time-intensive test. The MCAT demands excellent time-management skills, endurance, and grace under pressure both during the test as well as while preparing for it. Having a solid plan of attack and sticking with it are key to giving you the confidence and structure you need to succeed.

Creating a Study Plan

The best time to create a study plan is at the beginning of your MCAT preparation. If you don't already use a calendar, you will want to start. You can purchase a planner, print out a free calendar from the Internet, use a built-in calendar or app on one of your smart devices, or keep track using an interactive online calendar. Pick the option that is most practical for you and that you are most likely to use consistently.

Once you have a calendar, you'll be able to start planning your study schedule with the following steps:

1. **Fill in your obligations and choose a day off.**

   Write in all your school, extracurricular, and work obligations first: class sessions, work shifts, and meetings that you must attend. Then add in your personal obligations: appointments, lunch dates, family and social time, etc. Making an appointment in your calendar for hanging out with friends or going to the movies may seem strange at first, but planning social activities in advance will help you achieve a balance between personal and professional obligations even as life gets busy. Having a happy balance allows you to be more focused and productive when it comes time to study, so stay well-rounded and don't neglect anything that is important to you.

   In addition to scheduling your personal and professional obligations, you should also plan your time off. Taking some time off is just as important as studying. Kaplan recommends taking at least one full day off per week, ideally from all your study obligations but at minimum from studying for the MCAT.

2. **Add in study blocks around your obligations.**

   Once you have established your calendar's framework, add in study blocks around your obligations, keeping your study schedule as consistent as possible across days and across weeks. Studying at the same time of day as your official test is ideal for promoting recall, but if that's not possible, then fit in study blocks wherever you can.

   To make your studying as efficient as possible, block out short, frequent periods of study time throughout the week. From a learning perspective, studying one hour per day for six days per week is much more valuable than studying for six hours all at once one day per week. Specifically, Kaplan recommends studying for no longer than three hours in one sitting. Within those three-hour blocks, also plan to take ten-minute breaks every hour. Use these breaks to get up from your seat, do some quick stretches, get a snack and drink, and clear your mind. Although ten minutes of break for every 50 minutes of studying may sound like a lot, these breaks will allow you to deal with distractions and rest your brain so that, during the 50-minute study blocks, you can remain fully engaged and completely focused.

3. **Add in your full-length practice tests.**

   Next, you'll want to add in full-length practice tests. You'll want to take one test very early in your prep and then spread your remaining full-length practice tests evenly between now and your test date. Staggering tests in this way allows you to form a baseline for comparison and to determine which areas to focus on right away, while also providing realistic feedback throughout your prep as to how you will perform on Test Day.

When planning your calendar, aim to finish your full-length practice tests and the majority of your studying by one week before Test Day, which will allow you to spend that final week completing a brief review of what you already know. In your online resources, you'll find sample study calendars for several different Test Day timelines to use as a starting point. The sample calendars may include more focus than you need in some areas, and less in others, and it may not fit your timeline to Test Day. You will need to customize your study calendar to your needs using the steps above.

The total amount of time you spend studying each week will depend on your schedule, your personal prep needs, and your time to Test Day, but it is recommended that you spend somewhere in the range of 300–350 hours preparing before taking the official MCAT. One way you could break this down is to study for three hours per day, six days per week, for four months, but this is just one approach. You might study six days per week for more than three hours per day. You might study over a longer period of time if you don't have much time to study each week. No matter what your plan is, ensure you complete enough practice to feel completely comfortable with the MCAT and its content. A good sign you're ready for Test Day is when you begin to earn your goal score consistently in practice.

How to Study

The MCAT covers a large amount of material, so studying for Test Day can initially seem daunting. To combat this, we have some tips for how to take control of your studying and make the most of your time.

Goal Setting

To take control of the amount of content and practice required to do well on the MCAT, break the content down into specific goals for each week instead of attempting to approach the test as a whole. A goal of "I want to increase my overall score by 5 points" is too big, abstract, and difficult to measure on the small scale. More reasonable goals are "I will read two chapters each day this week." Goals like this are much less overwhelming and help break studying into manageable pieces.

Active Reading

As you go through this book, much of the information will be familiar to you. After all, you have probably seen most of the content before. However, be very careful: Familiarity with a subject does not necessarily translate to knowledge or mastery of that subject. Do not assume that if you recognize a concept you actually know it and can apply it quickly at an appropriate level. Don't just passively read this book. Instead, read actively: Use the free margin space to jot down important ideas, draw diagrams, and make charts as you read. Highlighting can be an excellent tool, but use it sparingly: highlighting every sentence isn't active reading, it's coloring. Frequently stop and ask yourself questions while you read (e.g., *What is the main point? How does this fit into the overall scheme of things? Could I thoroughly explain this to someone else?*). By making connections and focusing on the grander scheme, not only will you ensure you know the essential content, but you also prepare yourself for the level of critical thinking required by the MCAT.

Focus on Areas of Greatest Opportunity

If you are limited by only having a minimal amount of time to prepare before Test Day, focus on your biggest areas of opportunity first. Areas of opportunity are topic areas that are highly tested and that you have not yet mastered. You likely won't have time to take detailed notes for every page of these books; instead, use your results from practice materials to determine which areas are your biggest opportunities and seek those out. After you've taken a full-length test, make sure you are using your performance report to best identify areas of opportunity. Skim over content matter for which you are already demonstrating proficiency, pausing to read more thoroughly when something looks unfamiliar or particularly difficult. Begin with the Science Mastery Assessment at the beginning of each chapter. If you can get all of those questions correct within a reasonable amount of time, you may be able to quickly skim through that chapter, but if the questions prove to be more difficult, then you may need to spend time reading the chapter or certain subsections of the chapter more thoroughly.

Practice, Review, and Tracking

Leave time to review your practice questions and full-length tests. You may be tempted, after practicing, to push ahead and cover new material as quickly as possible, but failing to schedule ample time for review will actually throw away your greatest opportunity to improve your performance. The brain rarely remembers anything it sees or does only once. When you carefully review the questions you've solved (and the explanations for them), the process of retrieving that information reopens and reinforces the connections you've built in your brain. This builds long-term retention and repeatable skill sets—exactly what you need to beat the MCAT!

One useful tool for making the most of your review is the How I'll Fix It (HIFI) sheet. You can create a HIFI sheet, such as the sample below, to track questions throughout your prep that you miss or have to guess on. For each such question, figure out why you missed it and supply at least one action step for how you can avoid similar mistakes in the future. As you move through your MCAT prep, adjust your study plan based on your available study time and the results of your review. Your strengths and weaknesses are likely to change over the course of your prep. Keep addressing the areas that are most important to your score, shifting your focus as those areas change. For more help with making the most of your full-length tests, including a How I'll Fix It sheet template, make sure to check out the videos and resources in your online syllabus.

Section	Q #	Topic or Type	Why I missed it	How I'll fix it
Chem/Phys	*42*	*Nuclear chem.*	*Confused electron absorption and emission*	*Reread Physics Chapter 9.2*
Chem/Phys	*47*	K_{eq}	*Didn't know right equation*	*Memorize equation for* K_{eq}
CARS	*2*	*Detail*	*Didn't read "not" in answer choice*	*Slow down when finding match*
CARS	*4*	*Inference*	*Forgot to research answer*	*Reread passage and predict first*

Where to Study

One often-overlooked aspect of studying is the environment where the learning actually occurs. Although studying at home is many students' first choice, several problems can arise in this environment, chief of which are distractions. Studying can be a mentally draining process, so as time passes, these distractions become ever more tempting as escape routes. Although you may have considerable willpower, there's no reason to make staying focused harder than it needs to be. Instead of studying at home, head to a library, quiet coffee shop, or another new location whenever possible. This will eliminate many of the usual distractions and also promote efficient studying; instead of studying off and on at home over the course of an entire day, you can stay at the library for three hours of effective studying and enjoy the rest of the day off from the MCAT.

No matter where you study, make your practice as much like Test Day as possible. Just as is required during the official test, don't have snacks or chew gum during your study blocks. Turn off your music, television, and phone. Practice on the computer with your online resources to simulate the computer-based test environment. When completing practice questions, do your work on scratch paper or noteboard sheets rather than writing directly on any printed materials since you won't have that option on Test Day. Because memory is tied to all of your senses, the more test-like you can make your studying environment, the easier it will be on Test Day to recall the information you're putting in so much work to learn.

CHAPTER 1

NOMENCLATURE

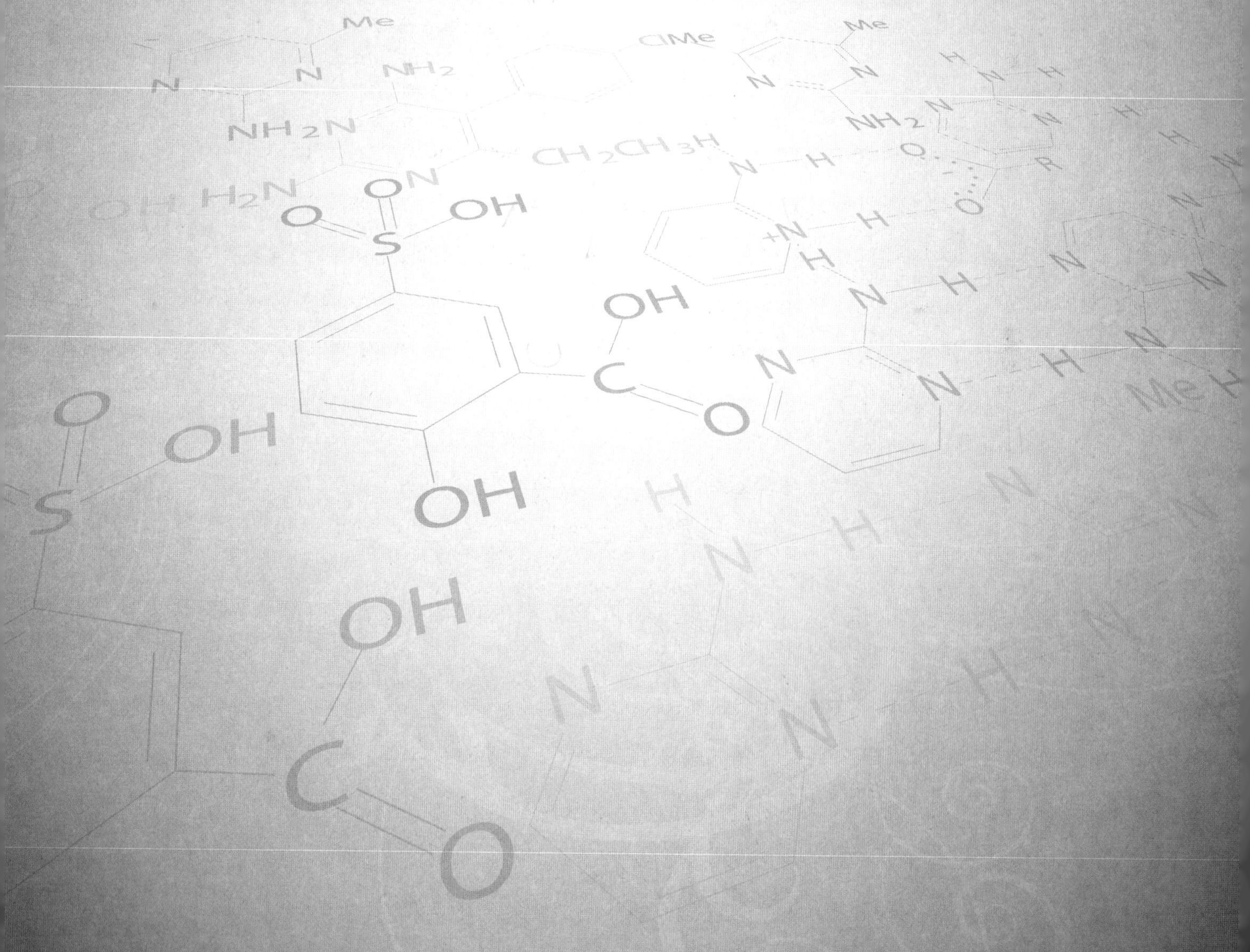

SCIENCE MASTERY ASSESSMENT

Every pre-med knows this feeling: there is so much content I have to know for the MCAT! How do I know what to do first or what's important?

While the high-yield badges throughout this book will help you identify the most important topics, this Science Mastery Assessment is another tool in your MCAT prep arsenal. This quiz (which can also be taken in your online resources) and the guidance below will help ensure that you are spending the appropriate amount of time on this chapter based on your personal strengths and weaknesses. Don't worry though—skipping something now does not mean you'll never study it. Later on in your prep, as you complete full-length tests, you'll uncover specific pieces of content that you need to review and can come back to these chapters as appropriate.

How to Use This Assessment

If you answer 0–7 questions correctly:

Spend about 1 hour to read this chapter in full and take limited notes throughout. Follow up by reviewing **all** quiz questions to ensure that you now understand how to solve each one.

If you answer 8–11 questions correctly:

Spend 20–40 minutes reviewing the quiz questions. Beginning with the questions you missed, read and take notes on the corresponding subchapters. For questions you answered correctly, ensure your thinking matches that of the explanation and you understand why each choice was correct or incorrect.

If you answer 12–15 questions correctly:

Spend less than 20 minutes reviewing all questions from the quiz. If you missed any, then include a quick read-through of the corresponding subchapters, or even just the relevant content within a subchapter, as part of your question review. For questions you got correct, ensure your thinking matches that of the explanation and review the Concept Summary at the end of the chapter.

1. Which of the following lists the correct common names for ethanal, methanal, and ethanol, respectively?
   - **A.** Acetaldehyde, formaldehyde, ethyl alcohol
   - **B.** Ethyl alcohol, propionaldehyde, isopropyl alcohol
   - **C.** Ethyl alcohol, formaldehyde, acetaldehyde
   - **D.** Isopropyl alcohol, ethyl alcohol, formaldehyde

2. Which of the following are considered terminal functional groups?
   - **I.** Aldehydes
   - **II.** Ketones
   - **III.** Carboxylic acids

   - **A.** I only
   - **B.** III only
   - **C.** I and III only
   - **D.** I, II, and III

3. If all prefixes were dropped, what would be the name of the parent root of this molecule?

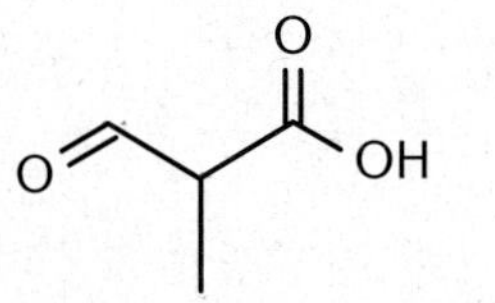

   - **A.** Propanoate
   - **B.** Propanol
   - **C.** Propanoic acid
   - **D.** Propanoic anhydride

4. What is the highest-priority functional group in this molecule?

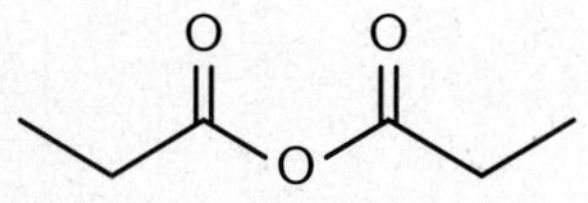

   - **A.** Anhydride
   - **B.** Carbonyl
   - **C.** Ketone
   - **D.** Alkyl chain

5. The IUPAC name for the following structure ends in what suffix?

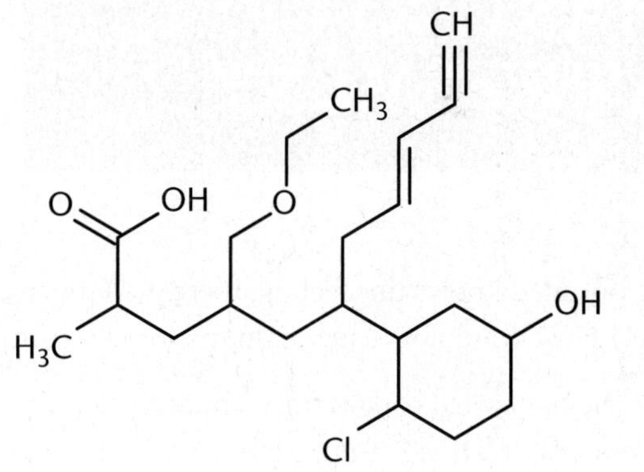

   - **A.** -ol
   - **B.** -one
   - **C.** -oic acid
   - **D.** -yne

6. Which of the two possibilities below correctly numbers the carbon backbone of this molecule?

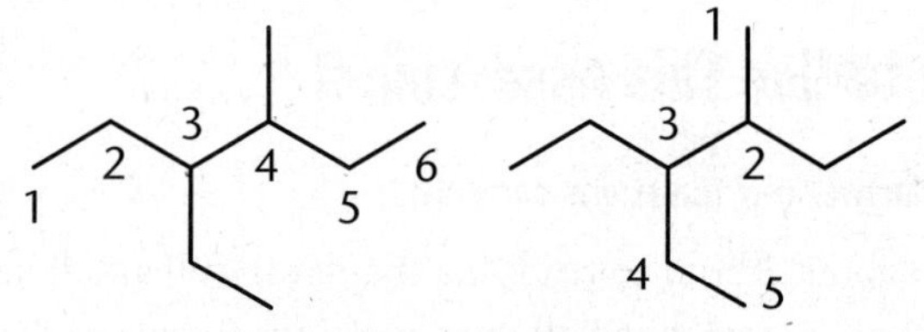

numbering scheme 1   numbering scheme 2

   - **A.** Numbering scheme 1
   - **B.** Numbering scheme 2
   - **C.** Numbering schemes 1 and 2 are equivalent and correct.
   - **D.** Numbering schemes 1 and 2 are equivalent and incorrect.

7. What is the proper structure for 2,3-dihydroxybutanedioic acid (tartaric acid)?

A.

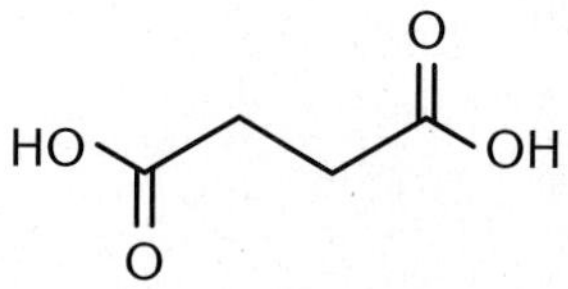

B.

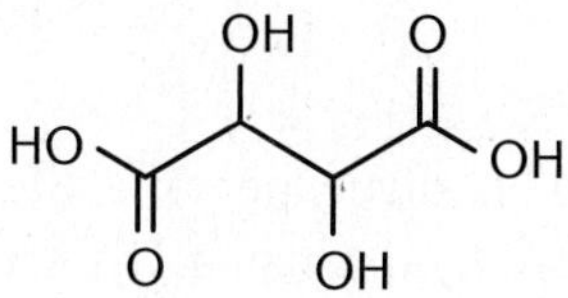

C.

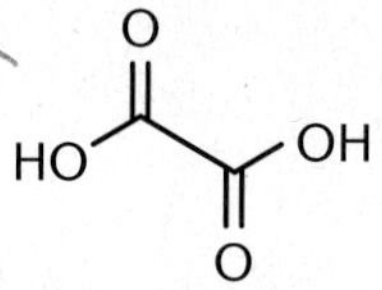

D.

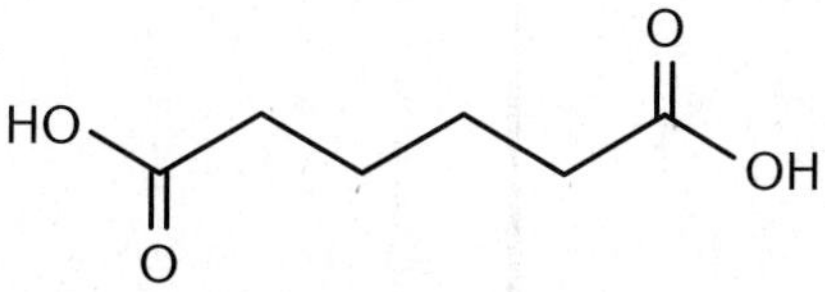

8. The common names for the aldehydes and carboxylic acids that contain only one carbon start with which prefix?

A. Para–
B. Form–
C. Meth–
D. Acet–

9. What is the IUPAC name for the following structure?

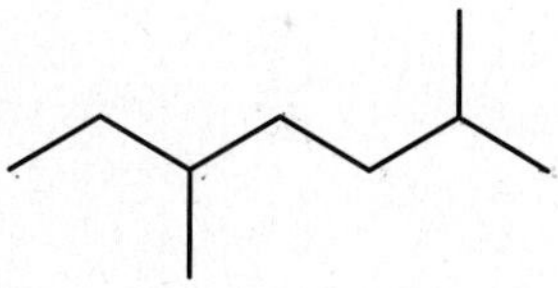

A. 2,5-dimethylheptane
B. 2-ethyl-5-methylhexane
C. 3,6-dimethylheptane
D. 5-ethyl-2-methylhexane

10. What is the IUPAC name for the following structure?

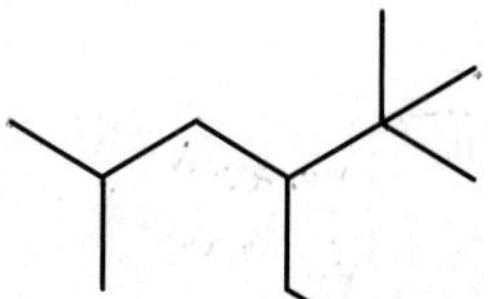

A. 4-isopropyl-2-methylhexane
B. 3-isopropyl-5-methylhexane
C. 2,2,5-trimethyl-3-ethylhexane
D. 3-ethyl-2,2,5-trimethylhexane

11. The IUPAC name for the following structure starts with what prefix?

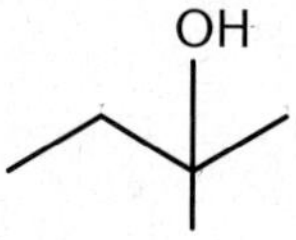

A. 3-methyl-
B. 2-methyl-
C. 2-hydroxy-
D. 3-hydroxy-

12. NADH is a coenzyme that releases high-energy electrons into the electron transport chain. It is known as nicotinamide adenine dinucleotide or diphosphopyridine nucleotide. What functional groups exist in this molecule?

I. Phosphate
II. Amide
III. Anhydride

A. I only
B. II only
C. I and II only
D. I, II, and III

13. Pyruvic acid, one of the end products of glycolysis, is commonly called acetylformic acid. Based on its common name, the structure of pyruvic acid must be:

A. 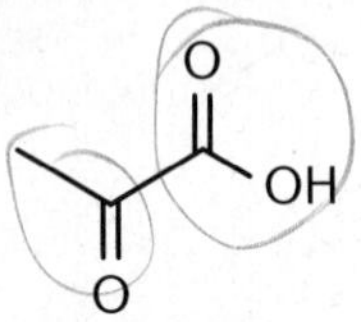

B. 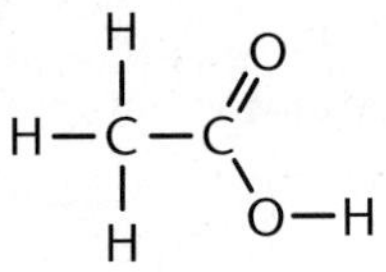

C. 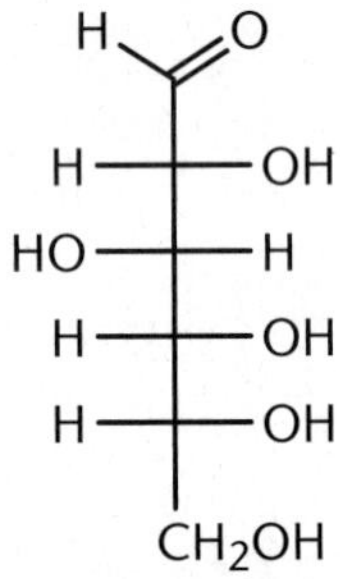

D. 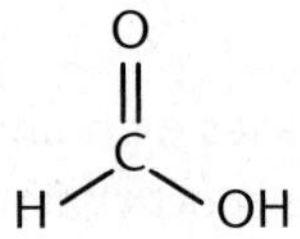

14. Which of the following are common names for carboxylic acid derivatives?

I. Acetic anhydride
II. Formic acid
III. Methyl formate

A. I and II only
B. I and III only
C. II and III only
D. I, II, and III

15. Consider the name 2,3-diethylpentane. Based on the structure implied by this name, the correct IUPAC name for this molecule is:

A. 2,3-diethylpentane.
B. 1,2-diethylbutane.
C. 3-ethyl-4-methylhexane.
D. 3-methyl-4-ethylhexane.

Answer Key follows on next page.

Answer Key

1. **A**
2. **C**
3. **C**
4. **A**
5. **C**
6. **A**
7. **B**
8. **B**
9. **A**
10. **D**
11. **B**
12. **C**
13. **A**
14. **B**
15. **C**

Detailed explanations can be found at the end of the chapter.

CHAPTER 1

NOMENCLATURE

In This Chapter

CHAPTER PROFILE

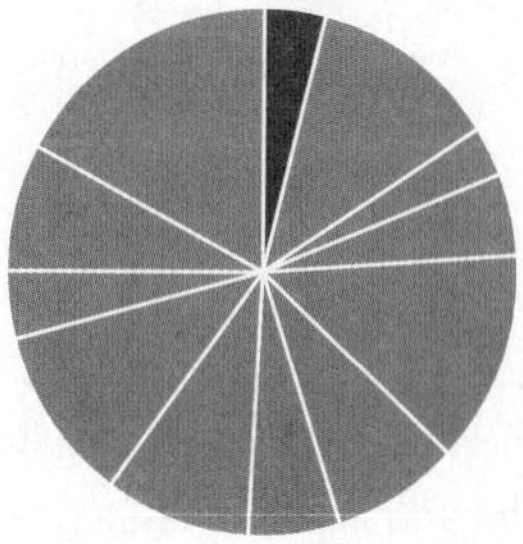

The content in this chapter should be relevant to about 4% of all questions about organic chemistry on the MCAT.

This chapter covers material from the following AAMC content category:

5D: Structure, function, and reactivity of biologically-relevant molecules

Introduction

You walk into the pharmacy looking for something to take for a headache and find an entire aisle of drugs just for that purpose: Advil, Aleve, Motrin, Tylenol, ibuprofen, naproxen, acetaminophen, and aspirin. In this list, however, there are only four distinct drugs. In the United States, it is not uncommon for drugs to be known by both generic and brand names—and sometimes, multiple brands market the same medications. As a medical student, you'll have to know both: while a doctor may order *atorvastatin 40 mg qd*, patients will tell you they're taking *Lipitor daily*.

For doctors, a generic name is sufficiently unambiguous to specify a given compound, but this is not true within the pharmaceutical industry. Medications are usually large organic compounds with many functional groups and numerous chiral centers. Chemists needed to be able to describe such compounds, as well as innumerable others. Thus, within chemistry, a specific set of rules for naming and describing compounds was designed. In this chapter, we'll examine the steps for naming a compound and then practice applying them to example compounds. By the end of the chapter, we'll have discussed the most common functional groups for Test Day and how they relate to each other in the nomenclature hierarchy. Note that you may have learned nomenclature for a number of other compounds, including ethers, epoxides, amines, imines, sulfonic acids, and others in your organic chemistry courses; we have restricted the content of this chapter to only the functional groups you are expected to identify on Test Day.

MCAT EXPERTISE

According to the AAMC, the MCAT will not include standalone, nomenclature-only organic chemistry questions (such as "name this compound" questions). But as you probably remember from your own classes, nomenclature is the very foundation of the entire subject of organic chemistry, and you will lose points on Test Day if you don't have nomenclature down cold.

1.1 IUPAC Naming Conventions

LEARNING OBJECTIVES

After Chapter 1.1, you will be able to:

- Identify the parent carbon chain in a complex molecule
- Describe how numbers are integrated into chemical nomenclature
- Apply the five steps of IUPAC nomenclature and name a molecule:

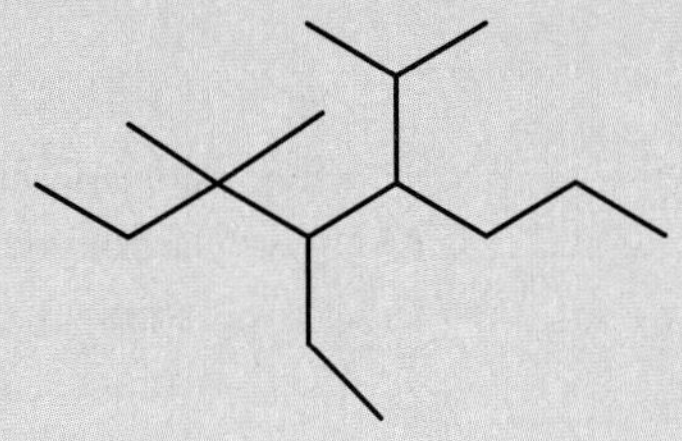

MCAT EXPERTISE

Nomenclature is often tested on the MCAT by providing the question stem and the answer choices in different formats. For example, the question stem may give you the IUPAC name of the reactant, and the answer choices may show product structures—leaving you to figure out both the structure of the reactant and the reaction taking place.

Nomenclature is one of the most important prerequisites for answering organic chemistry questions on Test Day; if you don't know which chemical compound the question is asking about, it's hard to get the answer right! That's why it's so important to understand both IUPAC and common nomenclature. Once you have a handle on these naming systems, you can easily translate question stems and focus on finding the correct answer. Let's begin by examining IUPAC naming conventions before we highlight specific compounds and functional groups.

Naming Steps

The primary goal of the **International Union of Pure and Applied Chemistry (IUPAC)** naming system is to create an unambiguous relationship between the name and structure of a compound. With the conventions established by IUPAC, no two distinct compounds have the same name. The IUPAC naming system greatly simplifies chemical naming. Once we understand the rules, we can match names to structures with ease.

1. Identify the Longest Carbon Chain Containing the Highest-Order Functional Group

This will be called the **parent chain** and will be used to determine the root of the name. Keep in mind that if there are double or triple bonds between carbons, they must be considered when identifying the highest-order functional group. We'll examine priorities of functional groups throughout this chapter, but keep in mind that the highest-priority functional group (with the most oxidized carbon) will provide the suffix. This step may sound easy, but be careful! The molecule may be drawn in such a way that the longest carbon chain is not immediately obvious. If there are two or more chains of equal length, then the more substituted chain gets priority as the parent chain. Figure 1.1 shows a hydrocarbon with the longest chain labeled.

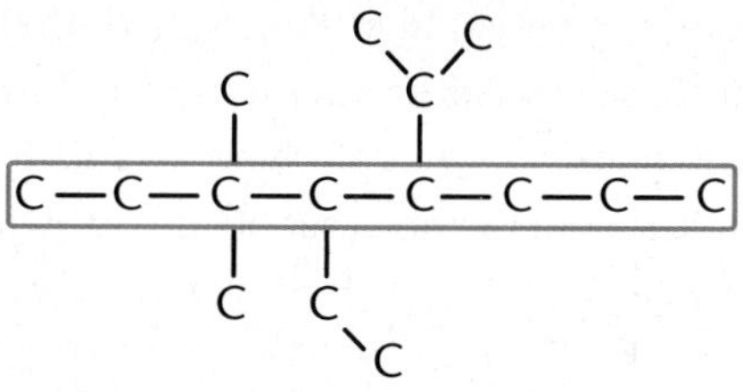

Figure 1.1 Finding the Longest Carbon Chain

2. Number the Chain

In order to appropriately name a compound, we need to number the carbon chain, as shown in Figure 1.2. As a convention, the carbon numbered 1 will be the one closest to the highest-priority functional group. If the functional groups all have the same priority, numbering the chain should make the numbers of the substituted carbons as low as possible.

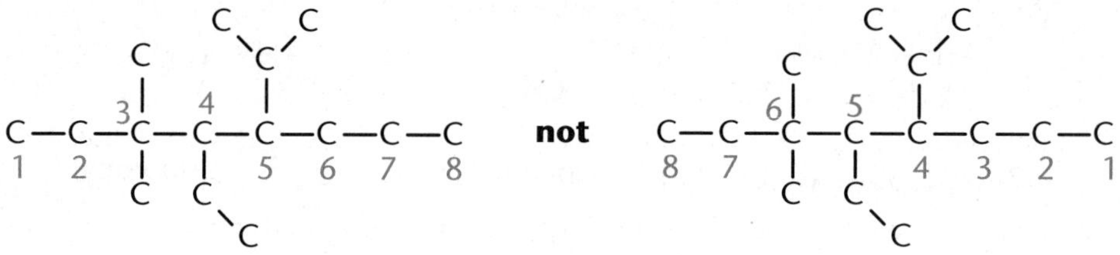

Figure 1.2 Numbering the Longest Carbon Chain
The highest-priority functional group should have the lowest possible number; if all substituents have the same priority, as in this figure, make their numbers as low as possible.

After we have discussed the functional groups most commonly tested on the MCAT, we'll review a table of those functional groups in order of priority. For now, keep in mind that the more oxidized the carbon is, the higher priority it has in the molecule. Oxidation state increases with more bonds to **heteroatoms** (atoms besides carbon and hydrogen, like oxygen, nitrogen, phosphorus, or halogens) and decreases with more bonds to hydrogen.

Just like straight chains, rings are numbered starting at the point of greatest substitution, continuing in the direction that gives the lowest numbers to the highest-priority functional groups. Somewhat counterintuitively, if there is a tie between assigning priority in a molecule with double and triple bonds, the double bond takes precedence.

3. Name the Substituents

Substituents are functional groups that are not part of the parent chain. A substituent's name will be placed at the beginning of the compound name as a prefix, followed by the name of the longest chain. Remember that only the highest-priority functional group will determine the suffix for the compound and must be part of the parent chain.

Carbon chain substituents are named like alkanes, with the suffix ***–yl*** replacing ***–ane***. The prefix ***n–*** that we see in Figure 1.3 on *n*-propyl simply indicates that this is "normal"—in other words, a straight-chain alkane. Because this prefix will not always be present, it is safe to assume that alkane substituents will be normal unless otherwise specified.

CH_3–	CH_3CH_2–	$CH_3CH_2CH_2$–
methyl	ethyl	*n*-propyl

Figure 1.3 Common Normal Alkyl Substituents
The bond on the right side of each substituent connects to the parent molecule.

In Figure 1.4, we see some examples of what alternative alkyl substituents may look like.

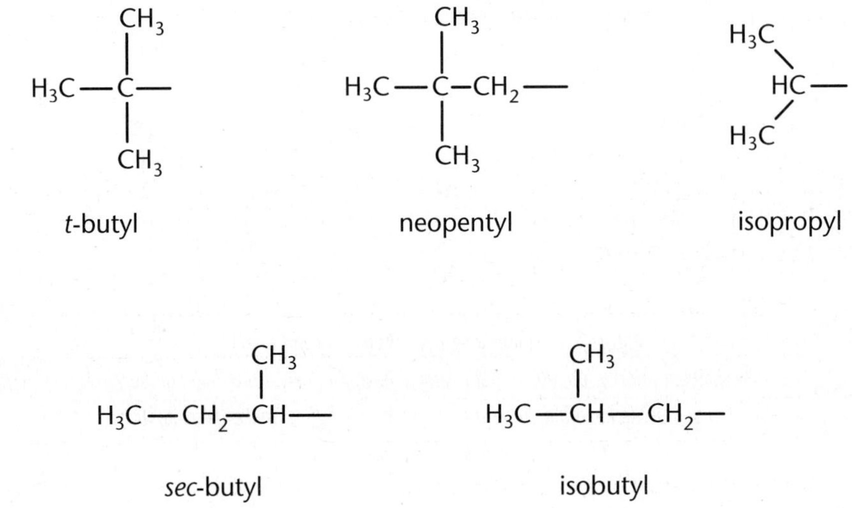

Figure 1.4 Common Alternative Alkyl Substituents
The bond on the right side of each substituent connects to the parent molecule.

If there are multiple substituents of the same type, we use the prefixes ***di–***, ***tri–***, ***tetra–***, and so on to indicate this fact. These prefixes are included directly before the substituent's name.

4. Assign a Number to Each Substituent

Pair the substituents that you have named to the corresponding numbers in the parent chain. Multiple substituents of the same type will get both the *di–*, *tri–*, and *tetra–* prefixes that we have previously noted and also a carbon number designation—even if they are on the same carbon.

5. Complete the Name

Names always begin with the names of the substituents in alphabetical order, with each substituent preceded by its number. Note, however, that prefixes like *di–*, *tri–*, and *tetra–*, as well as the hyphenated prefixes like ***n–*** and ***tert–*** (or ***t–***), are ignored while alphabetizing. Nonhyphenated roots that *are* part of the name, however, are included; these are modifiers like ***iso–***, ***neo–***, or ***cyclo–***. Then the numbers are separated from each other with commas, and from words with hyphens. Finally, we finish the name with the name of the backbone chain, including the suffix for the functional group of highest priority. Figure 1.5 shows an example of an entire hydrocarbon named with IUPAC nomenclature.

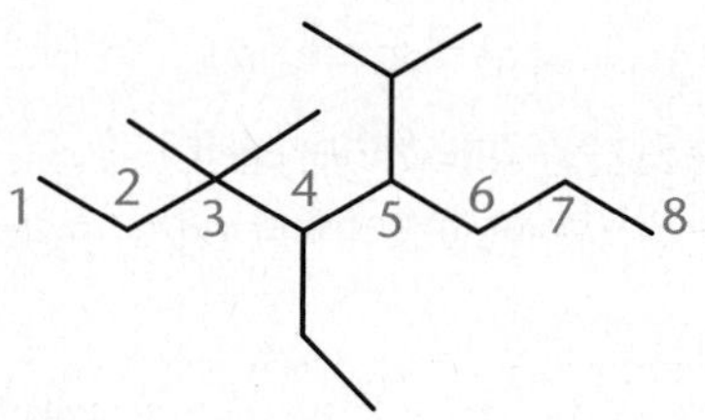

4-ethyl-5-isopropyl-3,3-dimethyloctane

Figure 1.5 An Example of a Complete IUPAC Name

MCAT CONCEPT CHECK 1.1

Before you move on, assess your understanding of the material with these questions.

1. List the steps of IUPAC nomenclature:
   1. ______________________________
   2. ______________________________
   3. ______________________________
   4. ______________________________
   5. ______________________________

2. Circle or highlight the parent chain in each of the following compounds:

$$\begin{array}{l} \quad CH_2CH_3 \\ \quad\ | \\ CH_3CH{-}CH_2{-}COOH \end{array}$$

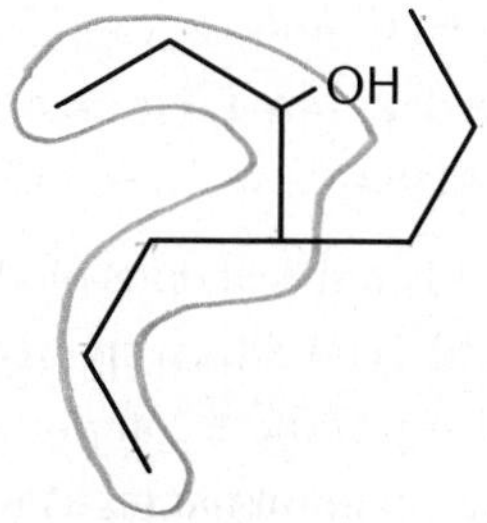

$H_3C{-}CH_3$

3. Circle and name the substituents in the following molecule, then name the molecule.

4-ethyl-2,3-dimethylheptane

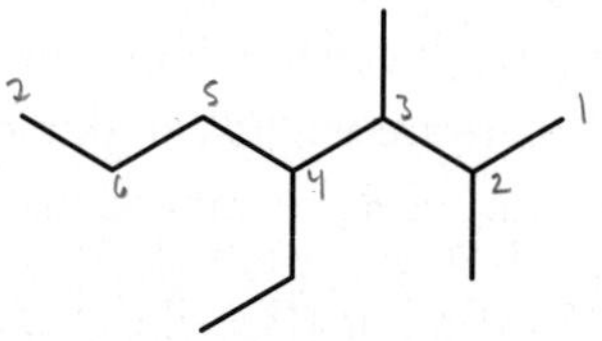

BRIDGE

Solutions to concept checks for a given chapter in *MCAT Organic Chemistry Review* can be found near the end of the chapter in which the concept check is located, following the Concept Summary for that chapter.

1.2 Hydrocarbons and Alcohols

LEARNING OBJECTIVES

After Chapter 1.2, you will be able to:

- Predict the structure of a hydrocarbon or alcohol molecule when given a simple molecular formula, such as C_9H_{20}
- Differentiate between geminal and vicinal diols
- Recall common names of key compounds, such as 2-propanol
- Apply priority rules when naming molecules with multiple functional groups, such as:

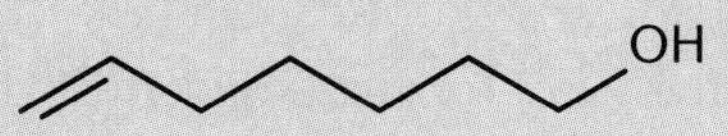

Hydrocarbons are compounds that contain only carbon and hydrogen atoms. Alcohols, on the other hand, contain at least one –OH group, which lends them additional reactivity. In this section, we'll explore the naming of hydrocarbons and alcohols.

Alkanes

Alkanes are simple hydrocarbon molecules with the formula $C_nH_{(2n+2)}$. The names for the first four of these compounds are methane (one carbon), ethane (two carbons), propane (three carbons), and butane (four carbons). Alkanes with more than four carbons have a simpler naming pattern in which the name is the Greek root describing the number of carbons followed by ***–ane***. From 5 to 12, these Greek roots are: ***pent–***, ***hex–***, ***hept–***, ***oct–***, ***non–***, ***dec–***, ***undec–***, and ***dodec–***. Some examples of alkanes are shown in Table 1.1.

Halogens are common substituents on alkanes. Alkyl halides are indicated by a prefix: ***fluoro–***, ***chloro–***, ***bromo–***, or ***iodo–***.

Alkenes and Alkynes

The MCAT does not explicitly test reactions of **alkenes** or **alkynes**, but you may still see the suffixes ***–ene*** and ***–yne***, which signify double and triple bonds, respectively. Keep in mind that many of these compounds will also have common names, and it is vital to know these common names as well. On Test Day, you are most likely to encounter double bonds in the context of unsaturated fatty acids or other biochemical compounds. The double or triple bond is named like a substituent and is indicated by the lower-numbered carbon involved in the bond. The number may precede the molecule name, as in 2-butene, or it may be placed near the suffix, as in but-2-ene; both are correct. If there are *multiple* multiple bonds, the numbering is generally separated from the suffix, as in 1,3-butadiene.

Number of Carbons	Name	Structure
1	methane	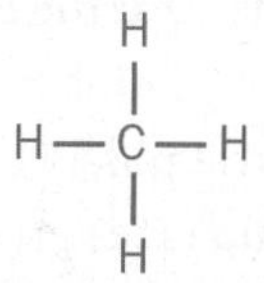
2	ethane	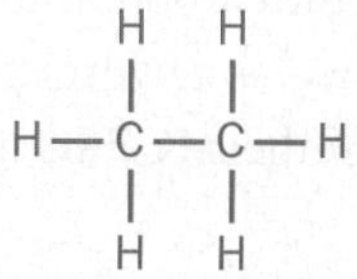
3	propane	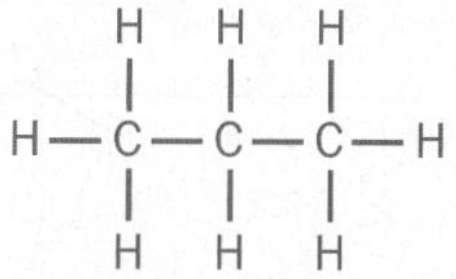
4	butane	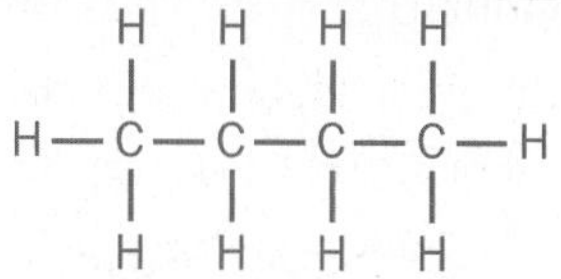
5	pentane	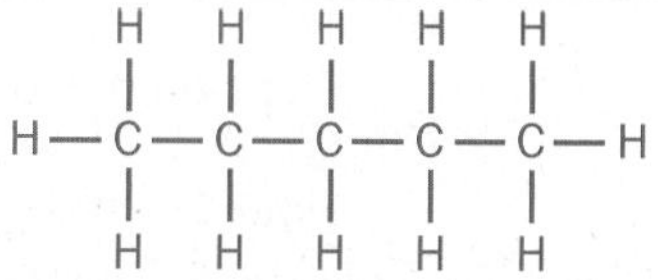
6	hexane	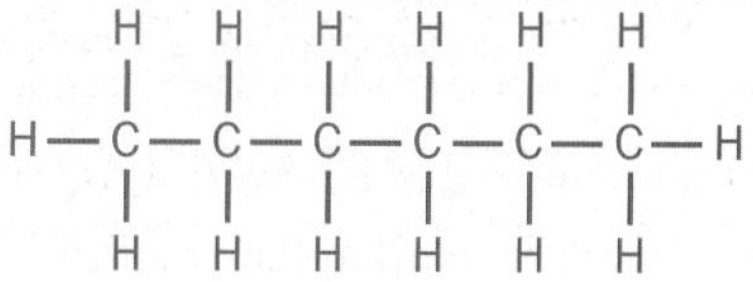
7	heptane	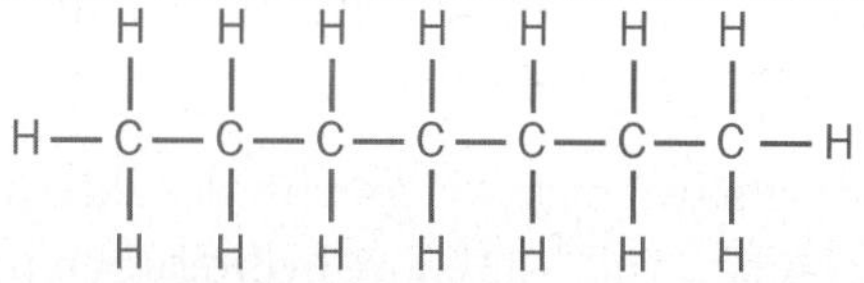
8	octane	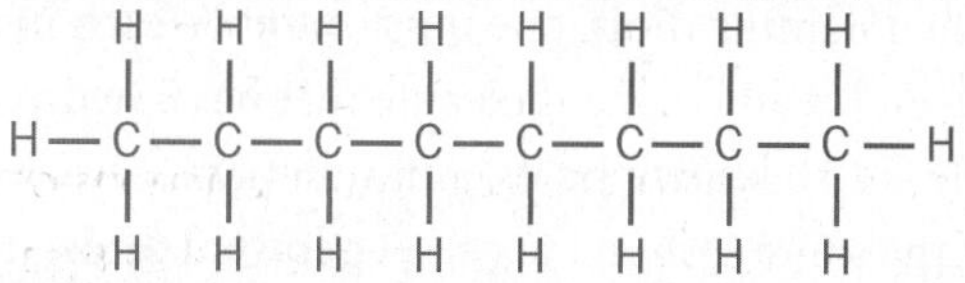

Table 1.1 Examples of Alkanes

Alcohols

Alcohols are named by replacing the *–e* at the end of the name of the corresponding alkane with the suffix ***–ol***. The chain is numbered so that the carbon attached to the hydroxyl group (–OH) gets the lowest possible number—even when there is a multiple bond present. The hydroxyl group takes precedence over multiple bonds because of the higher oxidation state of the carbon. If the alcohol is not the highest-priority functional group, then it is named as a hydroxyl substituent (***hydroxy–***). Figure 1.6 demonstrates a few alcohols and their IUPAC names.

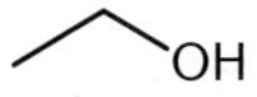

ethanol

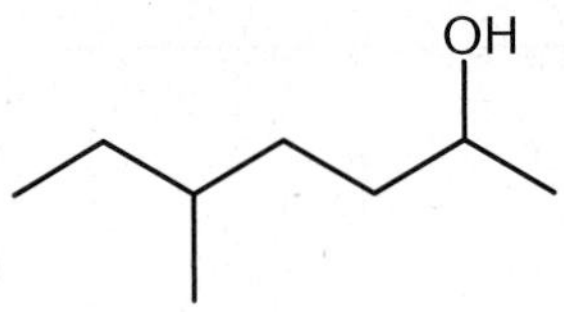

5-methyl-2-heptanol

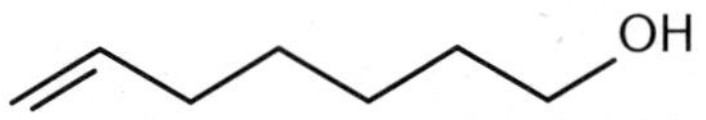

hept-6-en-1-ol

Figure 1.6 Naming Alcohols
Alcohols are more oxidized than multiple bonds, so they take priority in nomenclature and are indicated with the suffix -ol.

Alcohols are often referred to by their common names, rather than their IUPAC names. In this version of naming, the name of the alkyl group is followed by the word *alcohol*. Examples include *ethyl alcohol* (rather than ethanol) and *isopropyl alcohol* (rather than 2-propanol.)

Alcohols with two hydroxyl groups are called **diols** or **glycols** and are indicated with the suffix ***–diol***. The entire hydrocarbon name is preserved, and ***–diol*** is added. When naming diols, one must number each hydroxyl group. For example, ethane-1,2-diol is an ethane molecule that has a hydroxyl group on each carbon. This molecule is also known by its common name, ethylene glycol. Diols with hydroxyl groups on the same carbon are called **geminal diols**; diols with hydroxyl groups on adjacent carbons are called **vicinal diols**. Geminal diols, or **hydrates**, are not commonly seen because they spontaneously dehydrate (lose a water molecule) to produce carbonyl compounds with the functional group C=O.

MCAT EXPERTISE

The MCAT may use the common names for some alcohols, as well as some of the molecules we will see later. For alcohols, these include ethyl alcohol and isopropyl alcohol—know what these common names refer to!

MNEMONIC

Vicinal diols are in the **vicin**ity of each other, on adjacent carbons. **Gemin**al diols—like the **Gemin**i twins—are paired on the same carbon.

MCAT CONCEPT CHECK 1.2

Before you move on, assess your understanding of the material with these questions.

1. Fill in the correct names for the alkanes listed below. If more than one compound can be described with a given molecular formula, name the straight-chain alkane to which the formula refers and draw one alternative.

Molecular Formula	IUPAC Name (Straight-Chain Alkane)	Alternative Structure
CH_4	methyl	
C_2H_6	ethyl	
C_3H_8	butane	
C_4H_{10}	propane	
C_5H_{12}	pentane	
C_6H_{14}	hexane	
C_7H_{16}	heptane	
C_8H_{18}	octane	
C_9H_{20}	nonane	
$C_{10}H_{22}$	decane	

2. In a molecule with two double bonds adjacent to each other and an alcohol, which functional group would take precedence in naming?

alcohol

3. Is the following compound a geminal diol or a vicinal diol?

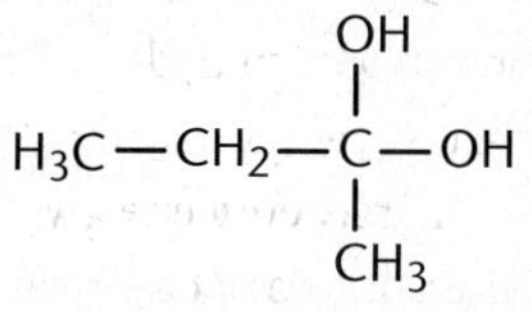

4. What are the common names for 2-propanol and ethanol?

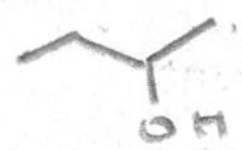

- 2-Propanol:

~~propyl butalconol~~ isopropyl alcohol

- Ethanol:

ethyl alcohol

1.3 Aldehydes and Ketones

LEARNING OBJECTIVES

After Chapter 1.3, you will be able to:

- Distinguish aldehydes from ketones
- Recall common names for methanal, ethanal, propanal, and propanone
- Determine the highest priority functional group in a complex molecule
- Apply appropriate prefixes and suffixes when naming molecules containing aldehyde and ketone groups

Aldehydes and ketones are two classes of molecules that contain a **carbonyl group**, which is a carbon double-bonded to an oxygen. Aldehydes and ketones differ in the placement of the carbonyl group: aldehydes are **chain-terminating**, meaning that they appear at the end of a parent chain, while ketones are found in the middle of carbon chains. Aldehydes and ketones do not have any leaving groups connected to the carbonyl carbon; they are only connected to alkyl chains or, in the case of aldehydes, hydrogen atoms. As we'll examine later, carboxylic acids and their derivatives do contain leaving groups connected to the carbonyl carbon.

Aldehydes

Aldehydes have a carbonyl group found at the end of the carbon chain. Because this is a terminal functional group that takes precedence over many others, it is generally attached to carbon number 1. Aldehydes are named by replacing the *–e* of the parent alkane with the suffix *–al*. When the aldehyde is at position 1, as is usually the case, we do not need to include this number in the chemical name. Figure 1.7 shows the IUPAC nomenclature for two aldehydes.

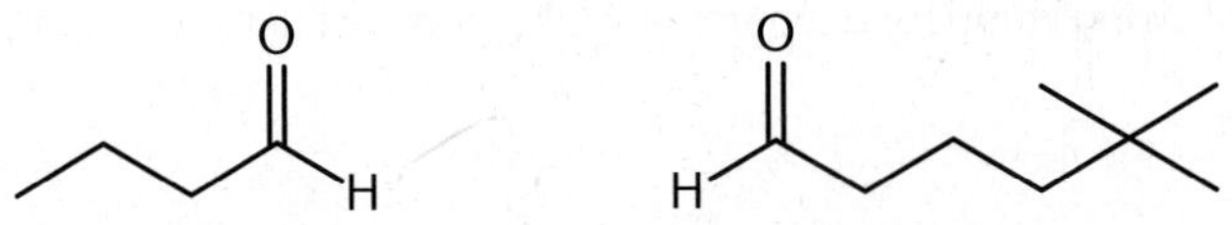

butanal   5,5-dimethylhexanal

Figure 1.7 Naming Aldehydes
The carbonyl group of the aldehyde usually does not receive a number in the name because it is a terminal functional group.

MCAT EXPERTISE

As is the case for alcohols, it is important to know both the common names and IUPAC names for common aldehydes and ketones. Make sure that you know what formaldehyde, acetaldehyde, and acetone are!

Methanal, ethanal, and propanal are referred to almost exclusively by their common names, *formaldehyde*, *acetaldehyde*, and *propionaldehyde*, rather than their IUPAC names. These molecules are shown in Figure 1.8.

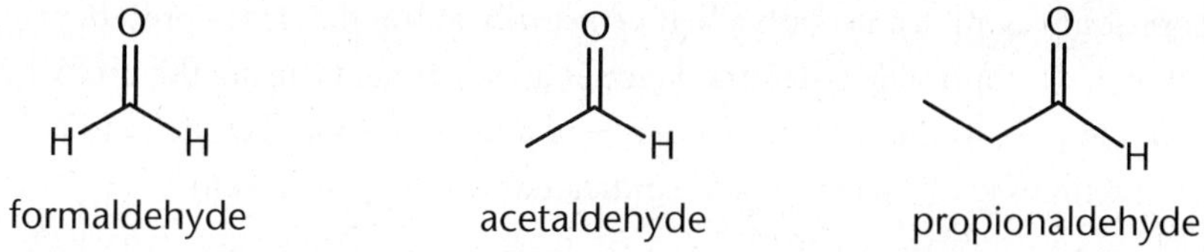

Figure 1.8 Common Names of Aldehydes

Ketones

Ketones contain a carbonyl group somewhere in the middle of the carbon chain. Because this is the case, we will always have to assign a number to the carbonyl carbon when naming ketones (except propanone, which must have the ketone on carbon 2 by default). Ketones are named by replacing the *–e* in the name of the parent alkane with the suffix ***–one***. Just as when naming other compounds, be sure to give the carbonyl the lowest possible number if it is the highest-priority group.

Ketones are commonly named by listing the alkyl groups in alphabetical order, followed by *ketone*, such as *ethylmethylketone*. *Acetone* is the smallest possible ketone molecule. Figure 1.9 includes IUPAC and common names for a number of ketones.

BRIDGE

Sugars are classified as either aldoses (aldehyde sugars) or ketoses (ketone sugars). Understanding nomenclature can help you to identify the structure of a sugar, as well as some of its physical properties. Carbohydrate structure is discussed in Chapter 4 of *MCAT Biochemistry Review*.

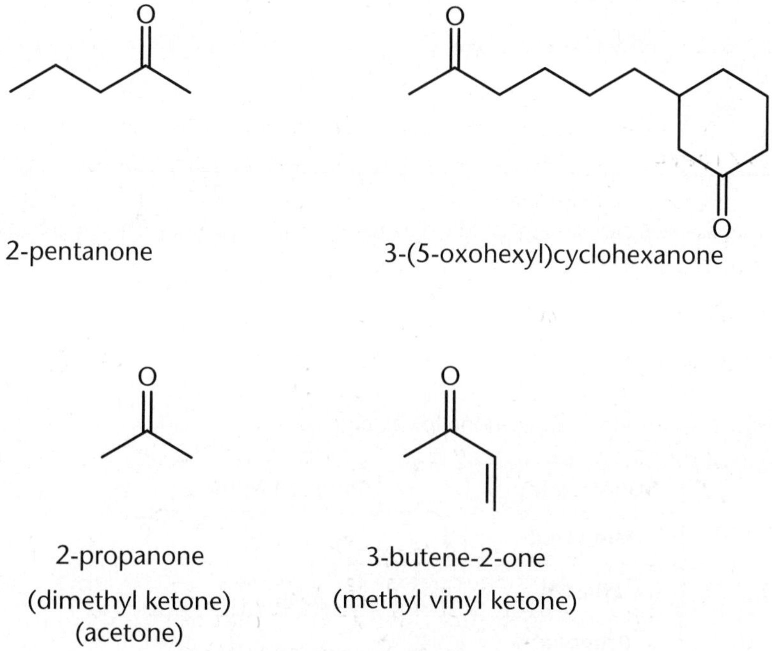

Figure 1.9 Naming Ketones
Common names are included in parentheses.

In a more complex molecule with a higher-priority group that takes precedence over the carbonyl, we name aldehydes and ketones as substituents, using the prefix ***oxo–***. This is in reference to the carbonyl oxygen and applies for both ketones and aldehydes. Sometimes ketones may also be indicated with the prefix ***keto–***.

Another convention that you may see on the MCAT is naming carbons relative to the carbonyl group. By this convention, the carbon *adjacent* to the carbonyl carbon is indicated by alpha (α). Moving away from the carbonyl, the successive carbons are referred to as beta (β), gamma (γ), and delta (δ) carbons. This applies on both sides of the carbonyl in the same fashion, so the carbons on both sides of a ketone are considered alpha carbons. This will become important when we discuss α-hydrogen acidity in Chapter 7 of *MCAT Organic Chemistry Review.*

MCAT CONCEPT CHECK 1.3

Before you move on, assess your understanding of the material with these questions.

1. What is the difference between an aldehyde and a ketone?
   - Aldehyde:

     chain terminating
   - Ketone:

     middle
2. What suffixes are used for aldehydes and ketones; how are carbonyl groups named as a substituent?
   - Aldehyde suffix: al; substituent prefix: oxo
   - Ketone suffix: one; substituent prefix: keto
3. Fill in the common names in the following chart.

IUPAC Name	Common Name
Methanal	formaldehyde
Ethanal	acetalaldehyde
Propanal	propionaldehyde
Propanone	acetone

4. For a molecule with a double bond, an aldehyde, and an alcohol, which functional group would determine the suffix when naming?

   aldehyde

1.4 Carboxylic Acids and Derivatives

LEARNING OBJECTIVES

After Chapter 1.4, you will be able to:

- Name common carboxylic acid derivatives, including esters, amides, and anhydrides
- Differentiate between common carboxylic acid derivatives

Carboxylic Acids

Carboxylic acids contain both a carbonyl group (C=O) and a hydroxyl group (–OH) on a terminal carbon. Carboxylic acids, like aldehydes, are terminal functional groups; therefore, their associated carbon is usually numbered 1. This is the most oxidized functional group that appears on the MCAT, with three bonds to oxygen; only carbon dioxide, with four bonds to oxygen, contains a more oxidized carbon. Carboxylic acids are thus the highest-priority functional group in MCAT-tested nomenclature, and all other groups are named as substituents using prefixes. Carboxylic acids are named by replacing the *–e* at the end of the name of the parent alkane with the suffix ***–oic acid***.

Once again, the common names for carboxylic acids show up fairly often on the MCAT. *Formic acid* is the common name for methanoic acid; *acetic acid* is ethanoic acid; and *propionic acid* is propanoic acid. These compounds are shown in Figure 1.10. Be sure that you know both these common names and IUPAC names for Test Day.

MCAT EXPERTISE

Did you notice that some of the common names are similar between aldehydes and carboxylic acids? Remembering that formaldehyde and formic acid both refer to molecules with methane as a parent alkane—and that acetaldehyde and acetic acid contain ethane as a parent alkane—will help consolidate this information.

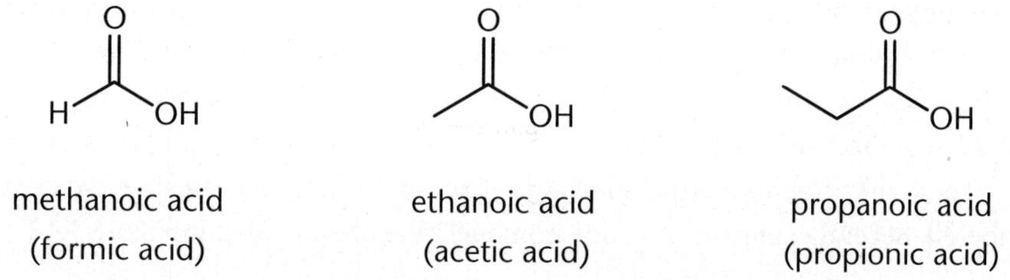

Figure 1.10 Naming Carboxylic Acids
The carboxylic acid group does not receive a number in the name because it is a terminal functional group; common names are included in parentheses.

The carboxylic acid derivatives are the final category of functional groups. These include esters, amides, and anhydrides.

Esters

Esters are common carboxylic acid derivatives. In these compounds, the hydroxyl group (–OH) is replaced with an **alkoxy group** (–OR, where R is a hydrocarbon chain). Ester nomenclature is based on the naming conventions for carboxylic acids. The first term is the alkyl name of the esterifying group. Think of this first term as an adjective describing the ester, based on the identity of the alkyl (R) group. The second term is the name of the parent acid, with *-oate* replacing the *-oic acid* suffix. For example, methanoic acid (formic acid) would form butyl methanoate with exposure to butanol under appropriate reaction conditions. Examples of ester nomenclature are shown in Figure 1.11.

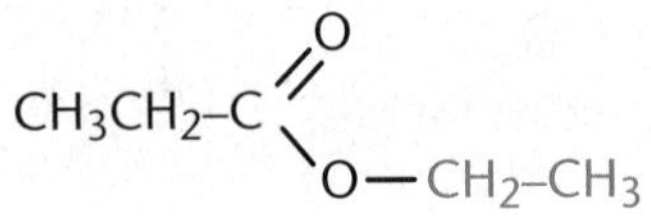

ethyl propanoate

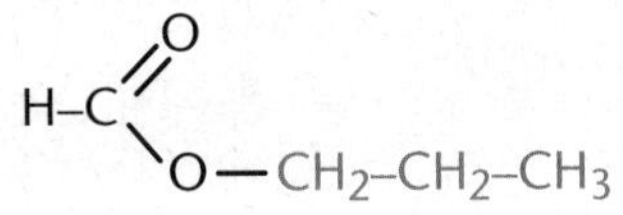

propyl methanoate

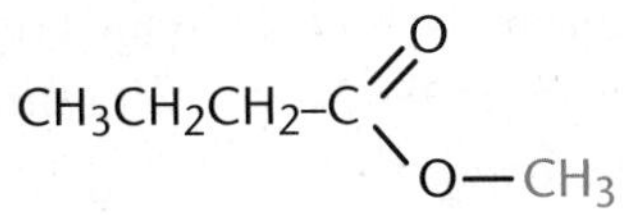

methyl butanoate

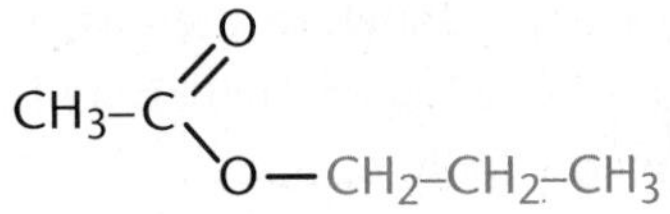

propyl ethanoate

Figure 1.11 Naming Esters
Groups bonded directly to the ester oxygen are named as substituents and are not numbered.

Amides

Another group of carboxylic acid derivatives includes **amides**. In an amide, the hydroxyl group is replaced by an **amino group** (nitrogen-containing group). These compounds can be more complex—the amino nitrogen can be bonded to zero, one, or two alkyl groups. Amides are named similarly to esters, except that the suffix becomes ***-amide***. Substituents attached to the nitrogen atom are labeled with a capital **N-**, indicating that this group is bonded to the parent molecule via a nitrogen atom. These substituents are included as prefixes in the compound name and are not numbered. Several examples of amide nomenclature are included in Figure 1.12.

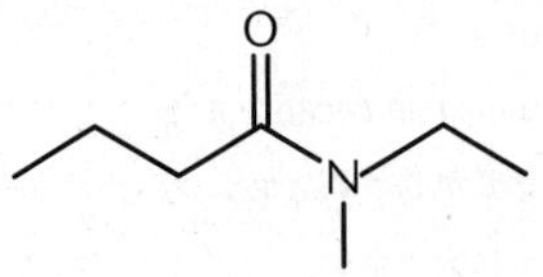

N-ethyl-*N*-methylbutanamide

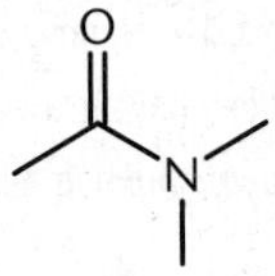

N,N-dimethylethanamide

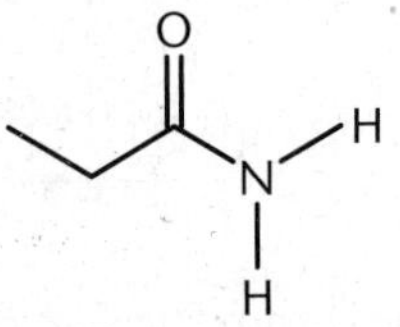

propanamide

Figure 1.12 Naming Amides
Groups bonded directly to the amide nitrogen are named as substituents with the prefix N-, *and are not numbered.*

Anhydrides

One final group of carboxylic acid derivatives is the **anhydrides.** In the formation of an anhydride from two carboxylic acid molecules, one water molecule is removed. Many anhydrides are cyclic, which may result from the intramolecular dehydration of a dicarboxylic acid. Anhydrides are named by replacing ***acid*** with ***anhydride*** in the name of the corresponding carboxylic acid if the anhydride is formed from only one type of carboxylic acid. If the anhydride is not symmetrical, both carboxylic acids are named (without the suffix *acid*) before *anhydride* is added to the name. Some examples of anhydrides are shown in Figure 1.13.

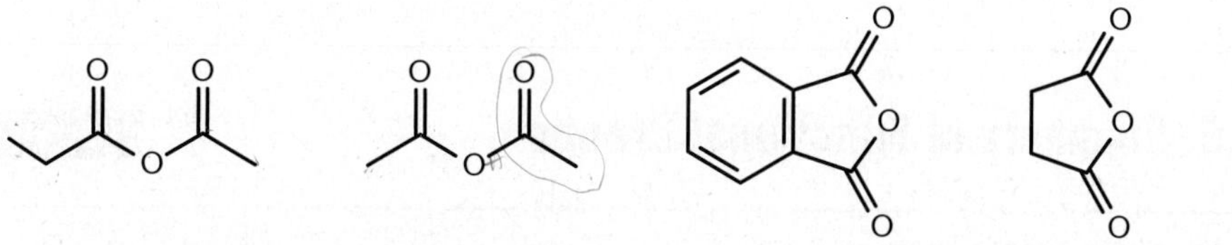

ethanoic propanoic anhydride | ethanoic anhydride (acetic anhydride) | phthalic anhydride | succinic anhydride

Figure 1.13 Naming Anhydrides
Phthalic anhydride and succinic anhydride are given as examples of cyclic anhydrides; their names need not be memorized.

MNEMONIC

Because *hydro-* is a prefix meaning *water*, and *an-* is a prefix meaning *not* or *without*, we can remember that anhydrides have had water molecules removed during formation.

MCAT CONCEPT CHECK 1.4

Before you move on, assess your understanding of the material with these questions.

1. What would be the names of the ester, amide, and anhydride derivatives of pentanoic acid? Assume that the R group on the ester is $-CH_3$ and that the amide is unsubstituted.
   - Ester:
     methyl propanoate
   - Amide:
     pentamide
   - Anhydride:
     pentanoic anhydride

2. Name the following compound:

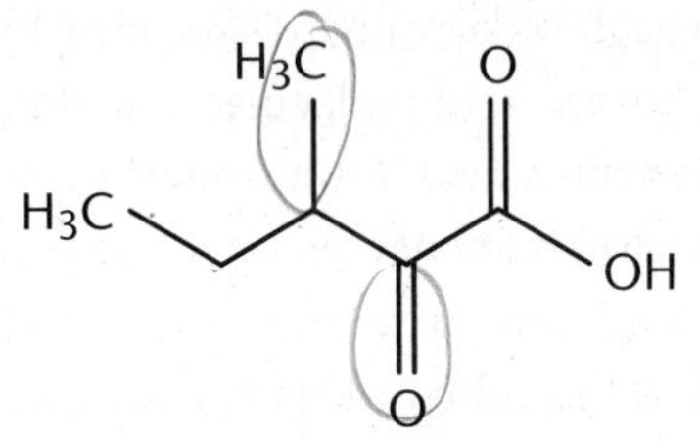

2-keto-3-methylpentanoic acid

1.5 Summary of Functional Groups

High-Yield

MCAT EXPERTISE

The "High-Yield" badge on this section indicates that the content is frequently tested on the MCAT.

LEARNING OBJECTIVES

After Chapter 1.5, you will be able to:

- Apply appropriate prefixes and suffixes for common organic functional groups

Table 1.2 lists the functional groups that you will need to know for the MCAT in order of priority, with prefixes and suffixes. Carboxylic acids are the highest-priority functional group on the MCAT. In nomenclature, use the suffix if the functional group is the highest-priority group in the molecule; otherwise, name the group as a substituent using its prefix.

KEY CONCEPT

Functional group priority is correlated with oxidation state. Carboxylic acids have the highest priority while alkanes have the lowest.

FUNCTIONAL GROUP	PREFIX	SUFFIX
Carboxylic acid	carboxy-	-oic acid
Anhydride	alkanoyloxycarbonyl-	anhydride
Ester	alkoxycarbonyl-	-oate
Amide	carbamoyl- or amido-	-amide
Aldehyde	oxo-	-al
Ketone	oxo- or keto-	-one
Alcohol	hydroxy-	-ol
Alkene*	alkenyl-	-ene
Alkyne*	alkynyl-	-yne
Alkane	alkyl-	-ane

*Note: Alkenes and alkynes are considered to be tied for priority except in cyclic compounds, where alkenes have higher priority.

Table 1.2 Major Functional Groups

Conclusion

Now that we've worked through nomenclature, we should be able to navigate MCAT organic chemistry questions with ease and confidence. Remember that even if an MCAT question is asking about a reaction or laboratory technique, translating the name of a compound in the question stem may be a necessary step to get to the answer. We have also covered the important functional groups that will show up and have taken note of the order of priority for these groups when it comes to naming compounds. Remember, the common names can be just as important on the MCAT as the IUPAC names—so knowing both is key. Now that we know the language of organic chemistry, we will learn more about the properties of molecules in the next two chapters, and then will focus on reactions of functional groups and laboratory techniques in subsequent chapters of *MCAT Organic Chemistry Review*.

GO ONLINE

You've reviewed the content, now test your knowledge and critical thinking skills by completing a test-like passage set in your online resources!

CONCEPT SUMMARY

IUPAC Naming Conventions

- The **International Union of Pure and Applied Chemistry** (**IUPAC**) has designated standards for naming chemical compounds. There are five steps in the process:
  - First, find the longest carbon chain in the compound that contains the highest-priority functional group. This is called the **parent chain**.
  - Second, number the chain in such a way that the highest-priority functional group receives the lowest possible number. This group will determine the **suffix** of the molecule.
  - Third, name the **substituents** with a **prefix**. Multiple substituents of a single type receive another prefix denoting how many are present (***di–***, ***tri–***, ***tetra–***, and so on).
  - Fourth, assign a number to each of the substituents depending on the carbon to which it is bonded.
  - Finally, complete the name by alphabetizing the substituents and separating numbers from each other by commas and from words by hyphens.

Hydrocarbons and Alcohols

- **Alkanes** are **hydrocarbons** without any double or triple bonds. They have the general formula $C_nH_{(2n+2)}$.
- Alkanes are named according to the number of carbons present followed by the suffix ***–ane***.
  - The first four alkanes are methane (CH_4), ethane (C_2H_6), propane (C_3H_8), and butane (C_4H_{10}).
  - Larger alkanes use the Greek root for the number (pentane, hexane, heptane, octane, and so on).
- **Alkenes** and **alkynes** contain double and triple bonds, respectively.
  - Alkenes are named by substituting ***–ene*** for the suffix and numbering the double bond by its lower-numbered carbon. Alkynes substitute ***–yne*** with the same numbering.
- **Alcohols** contain a hydroxyl (–OH) group, which substitutes for one or more of the hydrogens in the hydrocarbon chain.
  - Alcohols are named by substituting the suffix ***–ol*** or by using the prefix ***hydroxy–*** if a higher-priority group is present.
  - Alcohols have higher priority than double or triple bonds and alkanes.
  - Common names of alcohols include the name of the carbon chain followed by the word *alcohol*. For example, ethyl alcohol is the same compound as ethanol.
  - **Diols** contain two hydroxyl groups. They are termed **geminal** if on the same carbon or **vicinal** if on adjacent carbons.

Aldehydes and Ketones

- Aldehydes and ketones contain a **carbonyl group**—a carbon double-bonded to an oxygen.
- **Aldehydes** have the carbonyl group on a terminal carbon that is also attached to a hydrogen atom.
    - Aldehydes are named with the suffix ***–al***, or by using the prefix ***oxo–*** if a higher-priority group is present.
    - Common names of aldehydes include formaldehyde for methanal, acetaldehyde for ethanal, and propionaldehyde for propanal.
- **Ketones** have the carbonyl group on a nonterminal carbon.
    - Ketones are named with the suffix ***–one*** and share the prefix ***oxo–*** if a higher-priority group is present. Ketones can also be indicated by the prefix ***keto–***.
    - The common names of ketones are constructed by naming the alkyl groups on either side alphabetically and adding ketone. For example, 2-butanone is called ethylmethylketone.
    - Acetone is significant as the smallest ketone. Its IUPAC name is propanone.
- Carbonyl-containing compounds (aldehydes, ketones, carboxylic acids, and derivatives) also create a lettering scheme for carbons. The carbon adjacent to the carbonyl carbon is the **α-carbon**.

Carboxylic Acids and Derivatives

- **Carboxylic acids** are the highest-priority functional group because they contain three bonds to oxygen: one from a hydroxyl group and two from a carbonyl group.
- Carboxylic acids are always terminal, although their **derivatives** may occur within a molecule.
    - Carboxylic acids are named with the suffix ***–oic acid***. They are very rarely named as a prefix.
    - Common names for carboxylic acids follow the trend for aldehydes. Formic acid is methanoic acid, acetic acid is ethanoic acid, and propionic acid is propanoic acid.
- **Esters** are carboxylic acid derivatives where –OH is replaced with –OR, an **alkoxy group**.
    - Esters use the suffix ***–oate*** or the prefix ***alkoxycarbonyl–***.
    - Common names for esters are derived from the alcohol and the carboxylic acid used during synthesis.
- **Amides** replace the hydroxyl group of a carboxylic acid with an amino group that may or may not be substituted.
    - Amides use the suffix ***–amide*** or the prefix ***carbamoyl–*** or ***amido–***. Substituents attached to the amide nitrogen are designated with a capital ***N–***.

- **Anhydrides** are formed from two carboxylic acids by dehydration. They may be symmetric (two of the same acid), asymmetric (two different acids), or cyclic (intramolecular reaction of a dicarboxylic acid).
  - Anhydrides are named using the suffix ***anhydride*** in place of *acid*. If the anhydride is formed from more than one carboxylic acid, both are named in alphabetical order in the name before the word *anhydride*.

Summary of Functional Groups

- Functional groups are arranged in order of priority as follows: Carboxylic acid > anhydride > ester > amide > aldehyde > ketone > alcohol > alkene or alkyne > alkane.

ANSWERS TO CONCEPT CHECKS

1.1

1. 1. Find the longest carbon chain in the compound with the highest-order functional group; 2. Number the chain; 3. Name the substituents; 4. Assign a number to each substituent; 5. Complete the name

2.

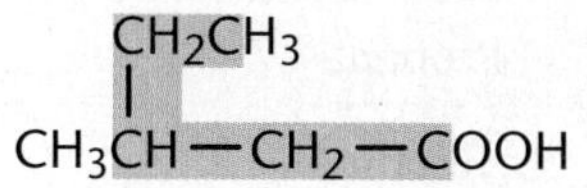

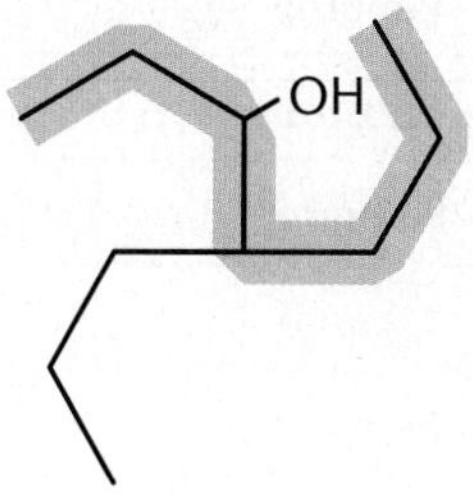

Note: There are two possible answers; however, the longest chain must include the hydroxyl group.

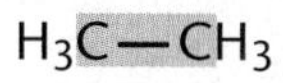

3.

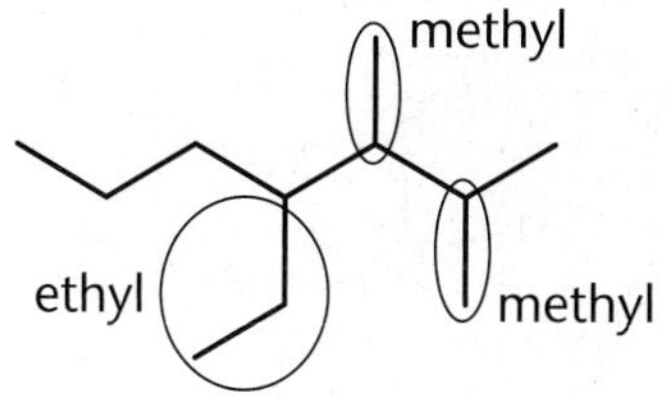

The question asks us to circle and name the substituents, but in order to determine the substituents it is necessary to identify the parent chain. So, begin by identifying the longest carbon chain that contains the highest-priority functional group. The molecule contains only alkyl functional groups, and the alkyl functional groups have the same priority, so the parent chain will be the longest continuous carbon chain (seven carbons). Once the parent chain is identified, the substituents can be circled and named as shown above.

Numbering the chain from right to left ensures that the substituents have the smallest possible locants (numbers). The substituents have already been named and numbered, so to complete the name, alphabetize the substituents (remembering that *di–* is ignored): 4-ethyl-2,3-dimethylheptane.

1.2

1.

Molecular Formula	IUPAC Name (Straight-Chain Alkane)	Alternative Structure
CH_4	Methane	No alternative structures
C_2H_6	Ethane	No alternative structures
C_3H_8	Propane	No alternative structures
C_4H_{10}	Butane	See below
C_5H_{12}	Pentane	See below
C_6H_{14}	Hexane	See below
C_7H_{16}	Heptane	See below
C_8H_{18}	Octane	See below
C_9H_{20}	Nonane	See below
$C_{10}H_{22}$	Decane	See below

Butane and all hydrocarbons that are larger than butane may have a branched appearance, which shortens the parent chain. An example is *isobutane*, properly named *methylpropane*, shown here. Any branched hydrocarbon with the correct number of carbons and no multiple bonds or rings is correct.

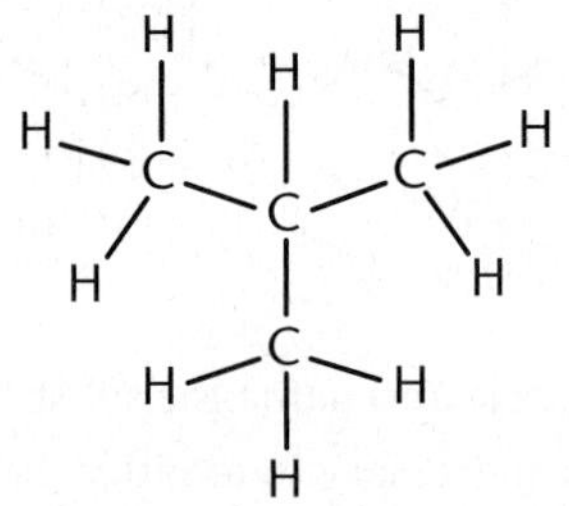

2. The alcohol would take precedence because the carbon to which it is attached has a higher oxidation state.
3. Diols are alcohols with two hydroxyl groups. In a geminal diol, these hydroxyl groups are on the same carbon (*gemini* derives from the Latin for "paired, twins"). In a *vici*nal diol, the hydroxyls are in the *vicinity* of each other—on adjacent carbons (*vicinus* derives from the Latin for "neighbor"). Thus, the compound shown is a geminal diol.
4. Isopropyl alcohol and ethyl alcohol, respectively.

1.3

1. An aldehyde has a carbonyl group at the end of the chain. A ketone has a carbonyl group somewhere in the middle of the carbon chain. Another way to think of this is that the carbonyl carbon of an aldehyde has at least one bond to a hydrogen atom, whereas the carbonyl carbon of a ketone is always bonded to two other carbons.
2. Aldehydes are referred to with the suffix *–al*, while ketones are given the suffix *–one*. Carbonyl groups of both aldehydes and ketones are labeled as *oxo–* substituents (ketones may also be called *keto–* substituents).
3.

IUPAC Name	Common Name
Methanal	Formaldehyde
Ethanal	Acetaldehyde
Propanal	Propionaldehyde
Propanone	Acetone

4. Ketones and aldehydes both take precedence over both alcohols and hydrocarbon chains, and the functional group that is the highest priority determines the suffix. Because the aldehyde is chain-terminating and therefore on carbon number 1, the aldehyde would determine the suffix when naming this compound.

1.4

1. The ester derivative would be methyl pentanoate. The amide would be pentanamide. The anhydride would be pentanoic anhydride.
2. 3-methyl-2-oxopentanoic acid

SCIENCE MASTERY ASSESSMENT EXPLANATIONS

1. **A**

The common name of ethanal is acetaldehyde, the common name of methanal is formaldehyde, and the common name of ethanol is ethyl alcohol. Isopropyl alcohol is the common name of 2-propanol. Propionaldehyde is the common name of propanal.

2. **C**

Aldehydes and carboxylic acids are characterized by their positions at the ends of carbon backbones and are thus considered terminal groups. As a result, the carbons to which they are attached are usually designated carbon 1. Ketones are internal by definition because there must be a carbon on either side of the carbonyl.

3. **C**

The highest-priority functional group in this molecule is the carboxyl group, so this will be a component of the backbone and provides the suffix of the molecule. This molecule is 2-methyl-3-oxopropanoic acid.

4. **A**

This molecule features an anhydride. The only other groups are hydrocarbon chains, which will provide part of the name of the parent root. Keep in mind that when a carbonyl group is present with a leaving group, the larger functional group (carboxylic acid, anhydride, ester, amide) takes priority over the carbonyl group alone. This molecule is propanoic anhydride.

5. **C**

Among the functional groups presented, carboxylic acids have the highest priority, and their compounds end with an *–oic acid* suffix. **(A)** denotes an alcohol, **(B)** a ketone, and **(D)** an alkyne, all of which have lower priorities than carboxylic acids. The MCAT does not test nomenclature of halides or ethers, but note that these must have lower priority than a carboxylic acid because they are less oxidized groups.

6. **A**

This molecule is 3-ethyl-4-methylhexane, not 2,3-diethylpentane. When naming alkanes, one must locate the longest carbon chain (6 carbons rather than 5 carbons), and the numbering system should give the alkyl groups the lowest possible numbers.

7. **B**

We know from the IUPAC name that we have a butanedioic acid backbone—in other words, a four-carbon backbone with carboxylic acids at either end. Adding the hydroxyl groups at carbons 2 and 3 then yields the correct structure.

8. **B**

Form– is a prefix shared by the common names of methanoic acid (formic acid) and methanal (formaldehyde).

9. **A**

The first task in naming a compound is identifying the longest carbon chain. In this case, the longest chain has seven carbons, so the parent alkane ends in *–heptane.* **(B)** and **(D)** can therefore be eliminated. Then, we must make sure that the carbons are numbered so that the substituents' position numbers are as small as possible. This compound has two methyl groups; minimizing their position numbers requires us to number the chain from right to left. These methyl groups are attached to carbons 2 and 5, so the correct IUPAC name is 2,5-dimethylheptane. **(C)** is incorrect because the position numbers of the substituents are not minimized.

10. **D**

We begin by finding the longest carbon chain; because there are no non-alkyl groups, we don't need to worry about any other groups' priorities. We then number our carbons such that the lowest possible combination of numbers is given to the various substituents. Then substituents are organized alphabetically, not numerically—eliminating **(C)**.

11. **B**

We know right away that **(C)** and **(D)** will be incorrect because a hydroxyl group is of higher priority than a methyl group. We also know that we will number the carbon chain so that the hydroxyl group receives the lowest possible position. Therefore, this molecule is 2-methyl-2-butanol, which starts with the prefix 2-methyl.

12. **C**

The suffix *–amide* in nicotinamide indicates that this compound contains an amide functional group. The prefix *diphospho–* indicates that there are two phosphate groups as well. Even if we did not know the prefix *phospho–* from this chapter, we should recognize that nucleotides, mentioned in the name of the compound, contain a sugar, a phosphate group, and a nitrogenous base. The structure of NAD^+, the oxidized form of NADH, is shown below.

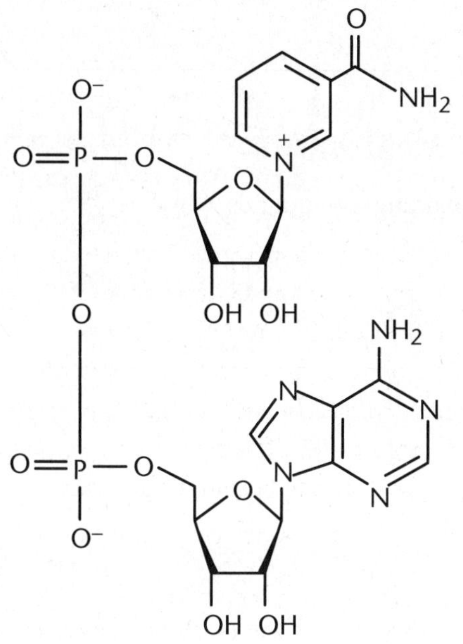

13. **A**

We can use the name acetylformic acid to figure out what our functional groups are. The prefix *acet–* refers to a two-carbon unit with one carbon in a carbonyl group—think of acetic acid, acetic anhydride, or acetaldehyde. The carbonyl carbon is the point of attachment to another functional group. Formic acid is a single-carbon carboxylic acid. Therefore, acetylformic acid is an acetyl group directly attached to formic acid, as shown in **(A)**. **(B)** shows acetic acid, or vinegar; **(C)** shows glucose; and **(D)** shows formic acid.

14. **B**

Acetic anhydride is the common name for ethanoic anhydride. Methyl formate is the common name for methyl methanoate; we can infer this from the common root *form–* and the ester suffix *–oate* (which is sometimes shortened to *–ate* for pronunciation purposes). Formic acid is the common name for methanoic acid, but this is a carboxylic acid—not a derivative.

15. **C**

Draw out the molecule, and you will see that the longest carbon chain with the substituents at the lowest possible carbon numbers is actually different from the one chosen in the original name. The correct IUPAC name for this molecule is 3-ethyl-4-methylhexane.

Consult your online resources for additional practice. **GO ONLINE**

SHARED CONCEPTS

Organic Chemistry Chapter 4
Analyzing Organic Reactions

Organic Chemistry Chapter 5
Alcohols

Organic Chemistry Chapter 6
Aldehydes and Ketones I

Organic Chemistry Chapter 8
Carboxylic Acids

Organic Chemistry Chapter 9
Carboxylic Acid Derivatives

Organic Chemistry Chapter 10
Nitrogen- and Phosphorus-Containing Compounds

CHAPTER 2

ISOMERS

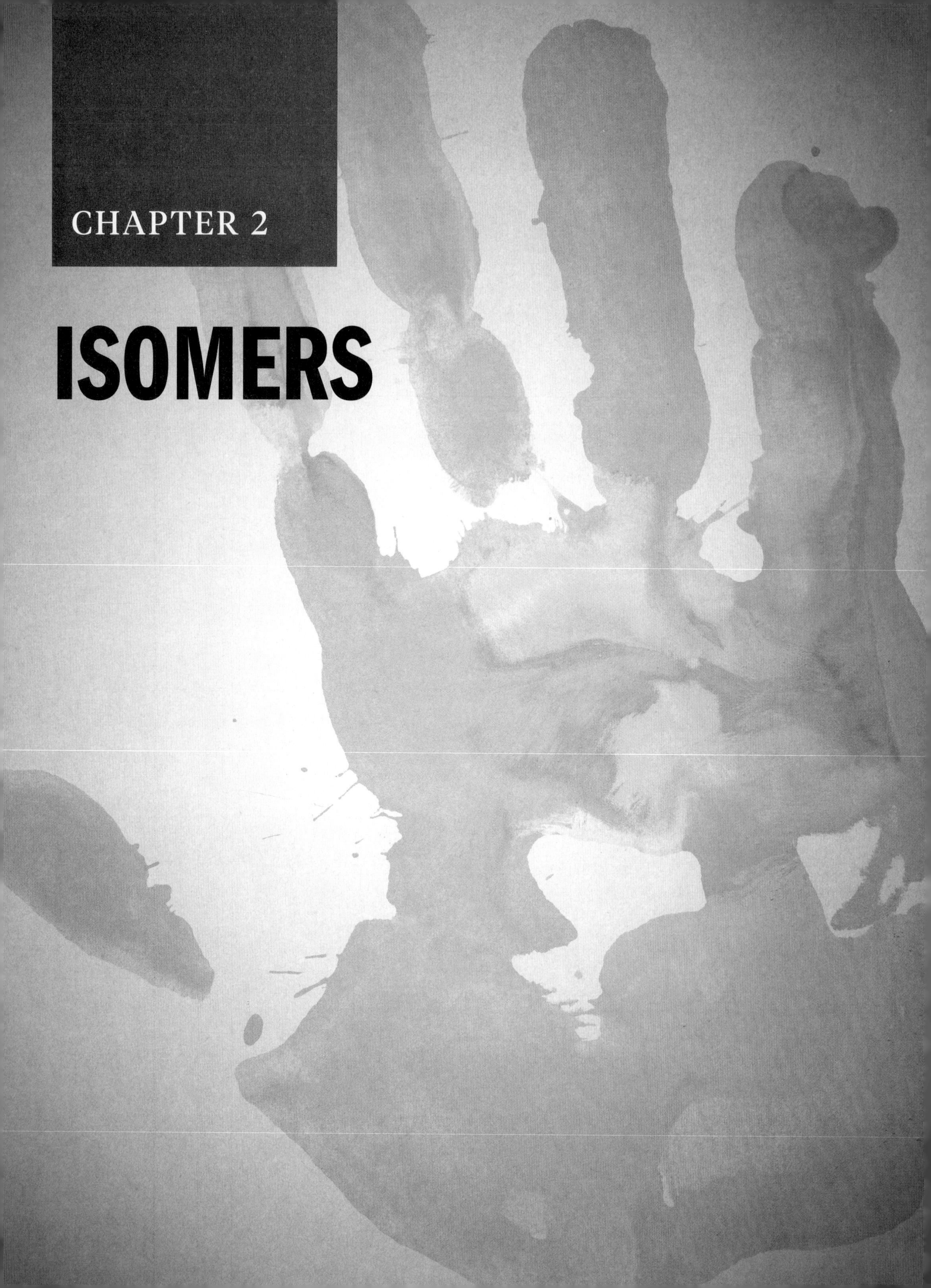

SCIENCE MASTERY ASSESSMENT

Every pre-med knows this feeling: there is so much content I have to know for the MCAT! How do I know what to do first or what's important?

While the high-yield badges throughout this book will help you identify the most important topics, this Science Mastery Assessment is another tool in your MCAT prep arsenal. This quiz (which can also be taken in your online resources) and the guidance below will help ensure that you are spending the appropriate amount of time on this chapter based on your personal strengths and weaknesses. Don't worry though—skipping something now does not mean you'll never study it. Later on in your prep, as you complete full-length tests, you'll uncover specific pieces of content that you need to review and can come back to these chapters as appropriate.

How to Use This Assessment

If you answer 0–7 questions correctly:

Spend about 1 hour to read this chapter in full and take limited notes throughout. Follow up by reviewing **all** quiz questions to ensure that you now understand how to solve each one.

If you answer 8–11 questions correctly:

Spend 20–40 minutes reviewing the quiz questions. Beginning with the questions you missed, read and take notes on the corresponding subchapters. For questions you answered correctly, ensure your thinking matches that of the explanation and you understand why each choice was correct or incorrect.

If you answer 12–15 questions correctly:

Spend less than 20 minutes reviewing all questions from the quiz. If you missed any, then include a quick read-through of the corresponding subchapters, or even just the relevant content within a subchapter, as part of your question review. For questions you got correct, ensure your thinking matches that of the explanation and review the Concept Summary at the end of the chapter.

1. Which of the following does NOT show optical activity?
   A. (*R*)-2-butanol
   B. (*S*)-2-butanol
   C. A solution containing 1 *M* (*R*)-2-butanol and 2 *M* (*S*)-2-butanol
   D. A solution containing 2 *M* (*R*)-2-butanol and 2 *M* (*S*)-2-butanol

2. How many stereoisomers exist for the following aldehyde?

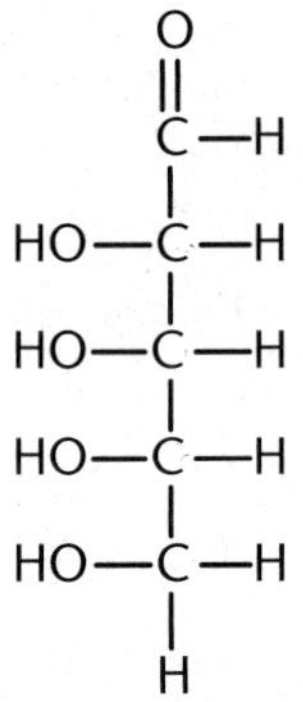

   A. 2
   B. 8
   C. 9
   D. 16

3. Which of the following compounds is optically inactive?

A. 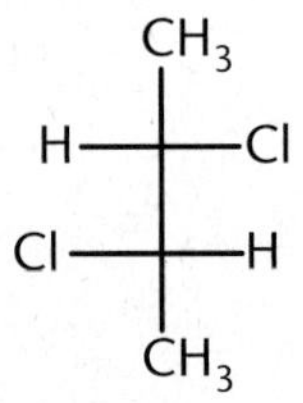

B. 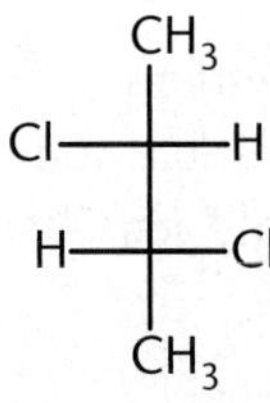

C. 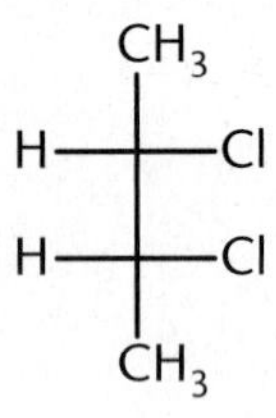

D. 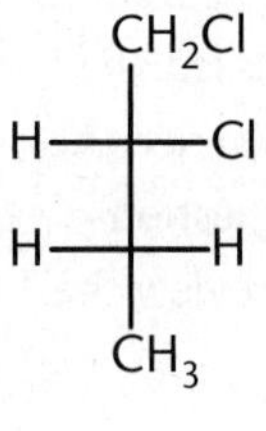

4. Cholesterol, shown below, contains how many chiral centers?

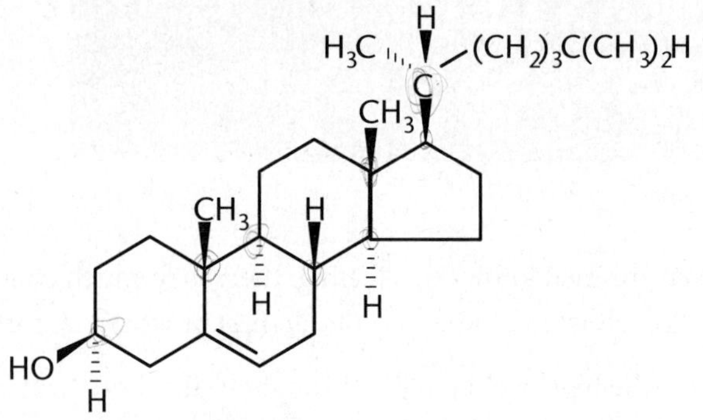

cholesterol

   A. 5
   B. 7
   C. 8
   D. 9

5. Which isomer of the following compound is the most stable?

A. 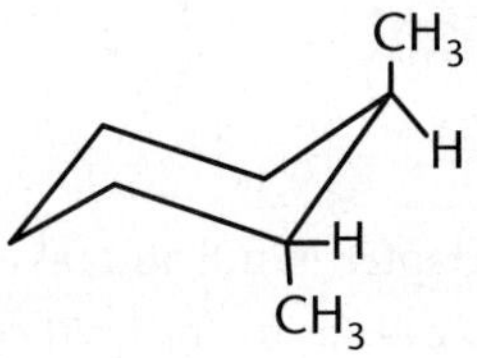

B. 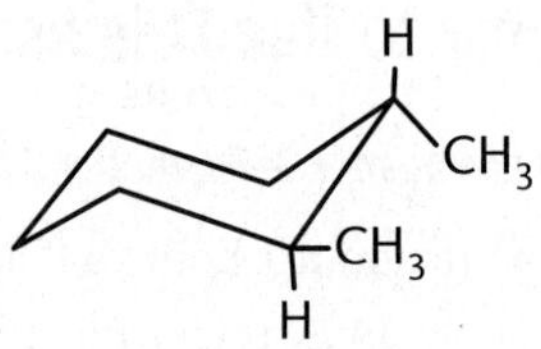

C. 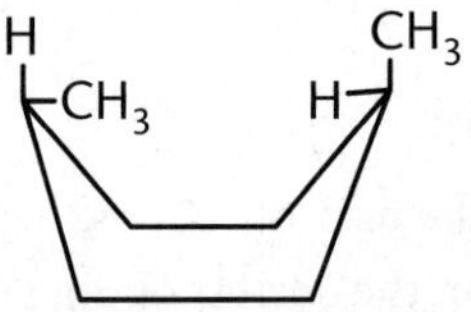

D. They are all equally stable.

6. The following reaction results in:

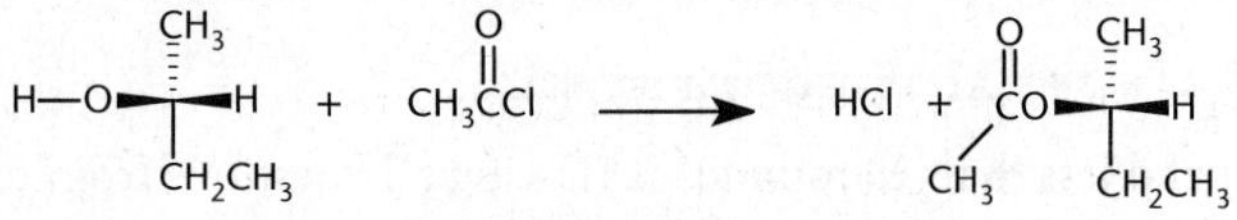

   A. retention of relative configuration and a change in the absolute configuration.
   B. a change in the relative and absolute configurations.
   C. retention of the relative and absolute configurations.
   D. retention of the absolute configuration and a change in the relative configuration.

7. The following molecules are considered to be:

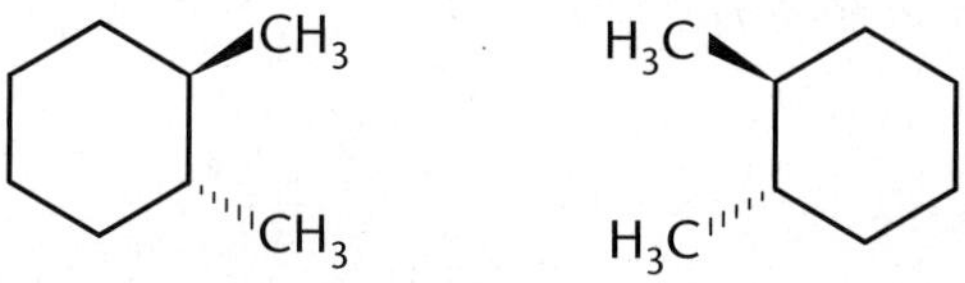

A. enantiomers.
B. diastereomers.
C. *meso* compounds.
D. structural isomers.

8. (+)-Glyceraldehyde and (−)-glyceraldehyde refer to the (*R*) and (*S*) forms of 2,3-dihydroxypropanal, respectively. These molecules are considered:
A. enantiomers.
B. diastereomers.
C. *meso* compounds.
D. structural isomers.

9. Consider (*E*)-2-butene and (*Z*)-2-butene. This is a pair of what type(s) of isomers?
I. *Cis–trans* isomers
II. Diastereomers
III. Enantiomers

A. I only
B. II only
C. I and II only
D. I and III only

10. 3-methylpentane and hexane are related in that they are:
A. enantiomers.
B. diastereomers.
C. constitutional isomers.
D. conformational isomers.

11. (*R*)-2-chloro-(*S*)-3-bromobutane and (*S*)-2-chloro-(*S*)-3-bromobutane are:
A. enantiomers.
B. diastereomers.
C. *meso* compounds.
D. the same molecule.

12. A scientist takes a 0.5 $\frac{g}{ml}$ solution of an unknown pure dextrorotatory organic molecule and places it in a test tube with a diameter of 1 cm. He observes that a plane of polarized light is rotated 12° under these conditions. What is the specific rotation of this molecule?
A. −240°
B. −24°
C. +24°
D. +240°

13. Omeprazole is a proton pump inhibitor commonly used in gastroesophageal reflux disease. When omeprazole, a racemic mixture, went off-patent, pharmaceutical companies began to manufacture esomeprazole, the (*S*)-enantiomer of omeprazole, by itself. Given 1 *M* solutions of omeprazole and esomeprazole, which solution(s) would likely exhibit optical activity?
A. Omeprazole only
B. Esomeprazole only
C. Both omeprazole and esomeprazole
D. Neither omeprazole nor esomeprazole

14. (2*R*,3*S*)-2,3-dihydroxybutanedioic acid and (2*S*,3*R*)-2,3-dihydroxybutanedioic acid are:
I. *meso* compounds.
II. the same molecule.
III. enantiomers.

A. I only
B. III only
C. I and II only
D. I and III only

15. If the methyl groups of butane are 120° apart, as seen in a Newman projection, this molecule is in its:
A. highest-energy *gauche* form.
B. lowest-energy staggered form.
C. middle-energy eclipsed form.
D. highest-energy eclipsed form.

Answer Key

1. **D**
2. **B**
3. **C**
4. **C**
5. **B**
6. **C**
7. **A**
8. **A**
9. **C**
10. **C**
11. **B**
12. **D**
13. **B**
14. **C**
15. **C**

Detailed explanations can be found at the end of the chapter.

CHAPTER 2

ISOMERS

In This Chapter

Introduction

An important way that we distinguish between molecules is by identifying **isomers** of the same compound—those that have the same molecular formula but different structures. Keep in mind that isomerism describes a relationship; just as there must be at least two children to have siblings, two molecules can be isomers to each other, but no molecule can be an isomer by itself. Throughout this chapter, we will learn how to identify these relationships and describe the similarities and differences between isomers. Figure 2.1 shows the isomer classes that we will learn more about and how they are related—feel free to come back to this figure as a reference after you have read through the more detailed explanations.

CHAPTER PROFILE

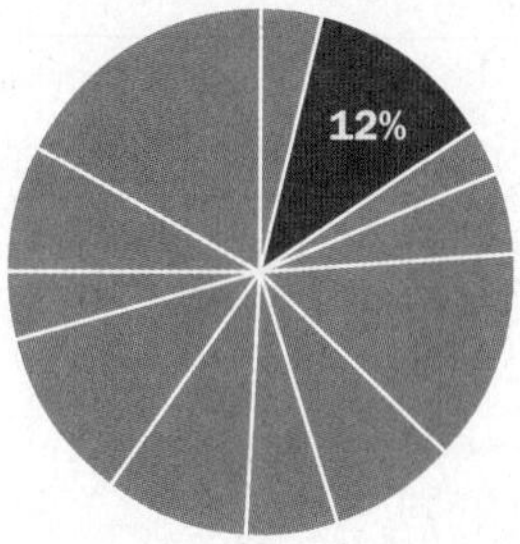

The content in this chapter should be relevant to about 12% of all questions about organic chemistry on the MCAT.

This chapter covers material from the following AAMC content categories:

1D: Principles of bioenergetics and fuel molecule metabolism

5B: Nature of molecules and intermolecular interactions

5C: Separation and purification methods

5D: Structure, function, and reactivity of biologically-relevant molecules

KEY CONCEPT

Isomers have the same molecular formula, but different structures.

2.1 Structural Isomers

LEARNING OBJECTIVES

After Chapter 2.1, you will be able to:

- Describe the shared and unique properties of structural isomers
- Explain what physical and chemical properties are
- Identify structural isomers

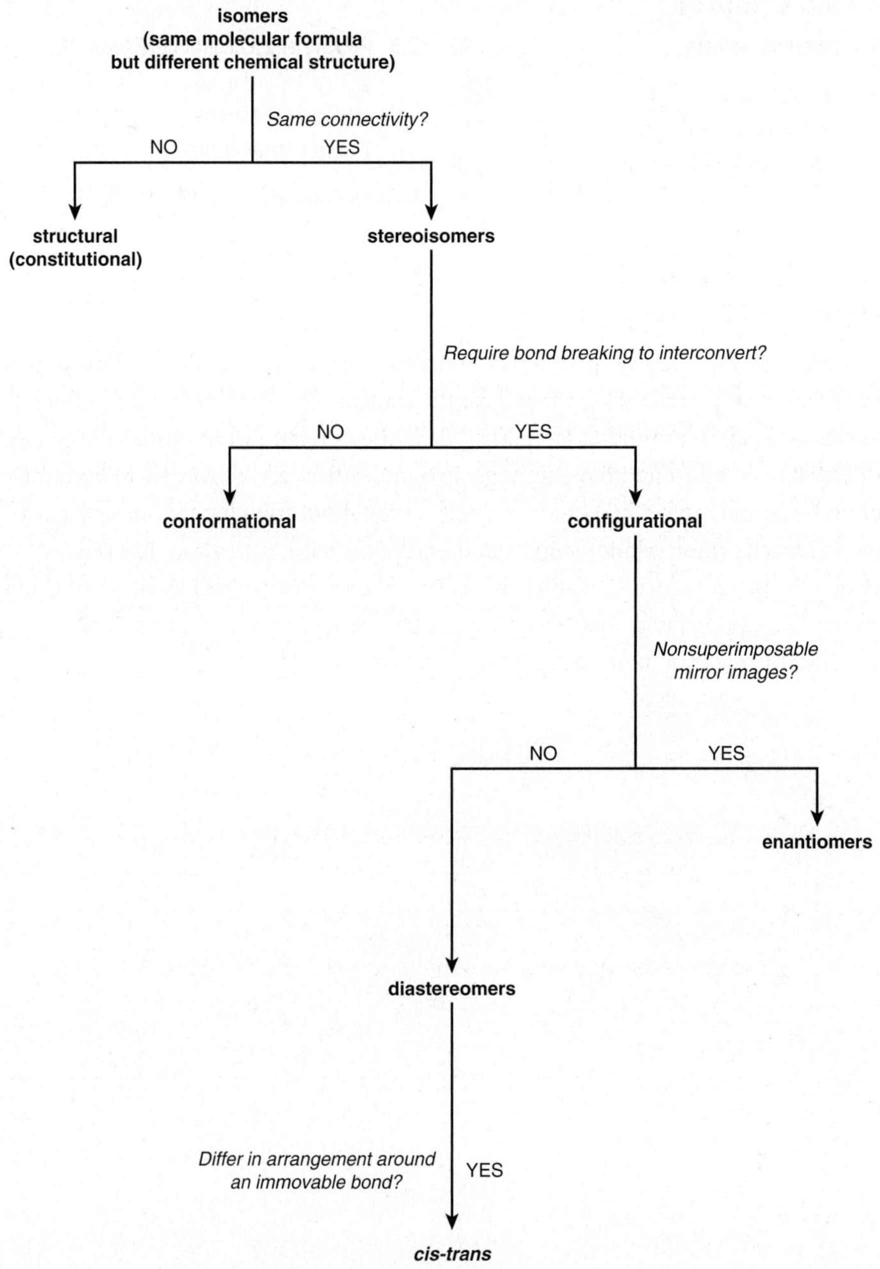

Figure 2.1 Flowchart of Isomer Relationships

Structural isomers are the least similar of all isomers. In fact, the only thing that **structural isomers** (also called **constitutional isomers**) share is their molecular formula, meaning that their molecular weights must be the same. Aside from this similarity, structural isomers are widely varied, with different chemical and physical properties. For example, five different structural isomers of C_6H_{14} are shown in Figure 2.2. Each of these molecules looks completely different but has the same number of carbon and hydrogen atoms.

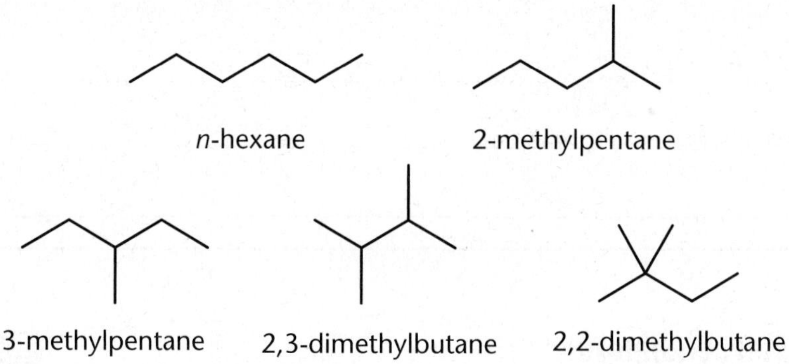

Figure 2.2 Structural (Constitutional) Isomers of C_6H_{14}

Physical and chemical properties are prime MCAT material and are often tested in the context of isomerism. **Physical properties** are characteristics of processes that don't change the composition of matter, such as melting point, boiling point, solubility, odor, color, and density. **Chemical properties** have to do with the reactivity of the molecule with other molecules and result in changes in chemical composition. In organic chemistry, the chemical properties of a compound are generally dictated by the functional groups in the molecule.

KEY CONCEPT

Physical properties: no change in composition of matter; examples include melting point, boiling point, solubility, odor, color, density.

Chemical properties: reactivity of molecule, resulting in change in composition; generally attributable to functional groups in the molecule.

MCAT CONCEPT CHECK 2.1

Before you move on, assess your understanding of the material with these questions.

1. What property or properties do structural isomers have in common?

____

2. Of the compounds cyclopropanol, 2-propanol, acetone, and prop-2-ene-1-ol, which are structural isomers of each other?

____

3. What are physical properties? Give three examples of physical properties.
   -
   -
   -

4. What are chemical properties?

2.2 Stereoisomers

High-Yield

LEARNING OBJECTIVES

After Chapter 2.2, you will be able to:

- Differentiate between conformational and configurational isomers
- Distinguish enantiomers from diastereomers
- Identify enantiomers, diastereomers, and *meso* compounds
- Convert between Newman and 3D molecular projections

Like structural isomers—and all isomers, for that matter—stereoisomers have the same chemical formula. Unlike structural isomers, however, **stereoisomers** also share the same atomic connectivity. In other words, they have the same structural backbone. Stereoisomers differ in how these atoms are arranged in space (their wedge-and-dash pattern), and all isomers that are not structural isomers fall under this category. The largest distinction within this class is between conformational and configurational isomers. **Conformational isomers** or **conformers** differ in rotation around single (σ) bonds; **configurational isomers** can be interconverted only by breaking bonds.

Conformational Isomers

Of all of the isomers, conformational isomers are the most similar. Conformational isomers are, in fact, the same molecule, only at different points in their natural rotation around single (σ) bonds.

While double bonds hold molecules in a specific position (as explained with *cis–trans* isomers later), single bonds are free to rotate. Conformational isomers arise from the fact that varying degrees of rotation around single bonds can create different levels of strain. These conformations are easy to see when the molecule is depicted in a **Newman projection**, in which the molecule is visualized along a line extending through a carbon–carbon bond axis. The classic example for demonstrating conformational isomerism in a straight chain is butane, which is shown in Figure 2.3.

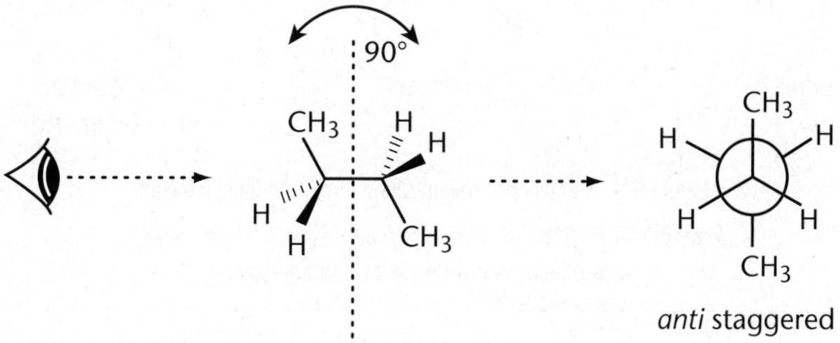

Figure 2.3 Newman Projection of Butane
Depiction of different atoms' positions from the point of view of the C-2 to C-3 bond axis.

Straight-Chain Conformations

For butane, the most stable conformation occurs when the two methyl groups (containing C-1 and C-4) are oriented 180° away from each other. In this position, there is minimal steric repulsion between the atoms' electron clouds because they are as far apart as they can possibly be. Thus, the atoms are "happiest" and in their lowest-energy state. Because there is no overlap of atoms along the line of sight (besides C-2 and C-3), the molecule is said to be in a **staggered** conformation. Specifically, it is called the ***anti*** conformation because the two largest groups are antiperiplanar (in the same plane, but on opposite sides) to each other. This is the most energetically favorable type of staggered conformation. The other type of staggered conformation, called ***gauche***, occurs when the two largest groups are 60° apart.

To convert from the *anti* to the *gauche* conformation, the molecule must pass through an **eclipsed** conformation in which the two methyl groups are 120° apart and overlap with the hydrogen atoms on the adjacent carbon. When the two methyl groups directly overlap each other with 0° separation, the molecule is said to be **totally eclipsed** and is in its highest-energy state. Totally eclipsed conformations are the least favorable energetically because the two largest groups are synperiplanar (in the same plane, on the same side). The different staggered and eclipsed conformations are demonstrated in Figures 2.3 and 2.4. For compounds larger than butane, the name of the conformation is decided by the relative positions of the two largest substituents about a given carbon–carbon bond.

MNEMONIC

It's ***gauche*** (unsophisticated or awkward) for one methyl group to stand too close to another group. Groups are **eclipsed** when they are completely in line with one another—just like a solar or lunar eclipse.

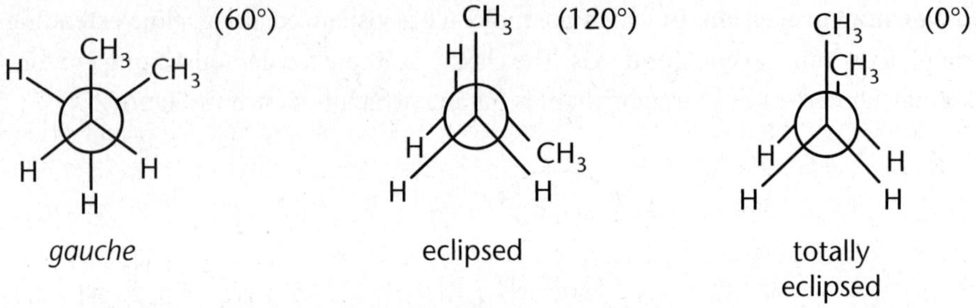

Figure 2.4 Stability of Straight-Chain Conformational Isomers
Degree measurements indicate the angle between the two largest substituents about the carbon-carbon bond.

Figure 2.5 shows the plot of potential energy *vs.* degree of rotation about the bond between C-2 and C-3 in butane. It shows the relative minima and maxima of potential energy of the molecule throughout its various conformations. Remember that every molecule wants to be in the lowest energy state possible, so the higher the energy, the less time the molecule will spend in that energetically unfavorable state.

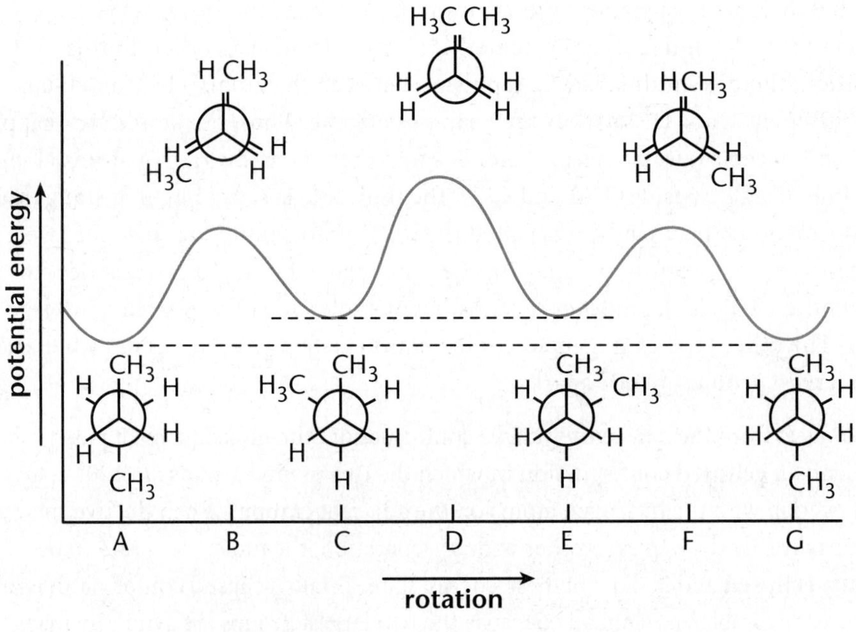

Figure 2.5 Potential Energy *vs.* Degree of Rotation about the C-2 to C-3 Bond in Butane

KEY CONCEPT

Notice that the *anti* staggered isomer (A and G) has the lowest energy, whereas the totally eclipsed isomer (D) has the highest energy.

These conformational interconversion barriers are small (19 $\frac{\text{kcal}}{\text{mol}}$ between *anti* staggered butane and totally eclipsed butane) and are easily overcome at room temperature. Nevertheless, at very low temperatures, conformational interconversions are dramatically slow. If the molecules do not possess sufficient energy to cross the energy barrier, they may not rotate at all (as happens to all molecules at absolute zero).

Cyclic Conformations

Cycloalkanes can be either fairly stable compounds or fairly unstable—depending on **ring strain**. Ring strain arises from three factors: angle strain, torsional strain, and nonbonded strain (sometimes referred to as steric strain). **Angle strain** results when bond angles deviate from their ideal values by being stretched or compressed. **Torsional strain** results when cyclic molecules must assume conformations that have eclipsed or *gauche* interactions. **Nonbonded strain (van der Waals repulsion)** results when *nonadjacent* atoms or groups compete for the same space. Nonbonded strain is the dominant source of steric strain in the **flagpole interactions** of the cyclohexane boat conformation. To alleviate the strain, cycloalkanes attempt to adopt various nonplanar conformations. Cyclobutane puckers into a slight "V" shape; cyclopentane adopts what is called an envelope conformation; and cyclohexane (the one you will undoubtedly see the most on the MCAT) exists mainly in three conformations called the **chair**, **boat**, and **twist**- or **skew-boat** forms. These cycloalkanes are shown in Figure 2.6.

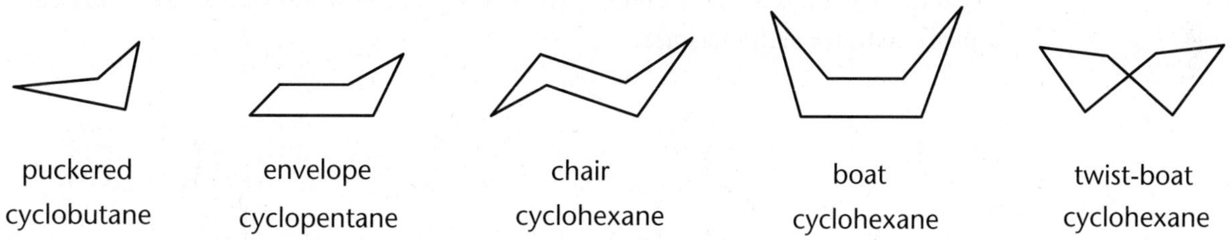

Figure 2.6 Conformations of Cycloalkanes

The most stable conformation of cyclohexane is the chair conformation, which minimizes all three types of strain. The hydrogen atoms that are perpendicular to the plane of the ring (sticking up or down) are called **axial**, and those parallel (sticking out) are called **equatorial**. The axial–equatorial orientations alternate around the ring; that is, if the wedge on C-1 is an axial group, the dash on C-2 will also be axial, the wedge on C-3 will be axial, and so on.

Cyclohexane can undergo a **chair flip** in which one chair form is converted to the other. In this process, the cyclohexane molecule briefly passes through a fourth conformation called the **half-chair** conformation. After the chair flip, all axial groups become equatorial and all equatorial groups become axial. All dashes remain dashes, and all wedges remain wedges. This interconversion can be slowed if a bulky group is attached to the ring; *tert*-butyl groups are classic examples of bulky groups on the MCAT. For substituted rings, the bulkiest group will favor the equatorial position to reduce nonbonded strain (flagpole interactions) with axial groups in the molecule, as shown in Figure 2.7.

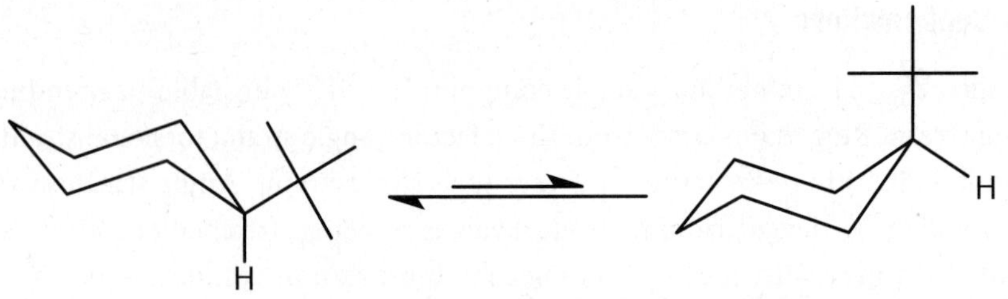

Figure 2.7 Axial and Equatorial Positions in Cyclohexane

During a chair flip, axial components become equatorial and vice versa. However, components pointing "up" (wedge) remain up and components pointing "down" (dash) remain down.

In rings with more than one substituent, the preferred chair form is determined by the larger group, which will prefer the equatorial position. These rings also have associated nomenclature. If both groups are located on the same side of the ring, the molecule is called *cis*; if they are on opposite sides of the ring, it is called *trans*, as shown in Figure 2.8. These same terms are used for molecules with double bonds, as explained later in this chapter.

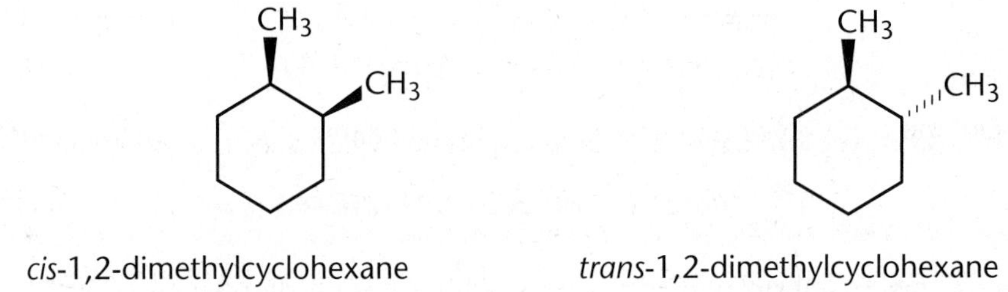

Figure 2.8 Nomenclature of Rings with Multiple Substituents

Configurational Isomers

Unlike conformational isomers that interconvert by simple bond rotation, **configurational isomers** can only change from one form to another by breaking and reforming covalent bonds. The two categories of configurational isomers are enantiomers and diastereomers. Both enantiomers and diastereomers can also be considered **optical isomers** because the different spatial arrangement of groups in these molecules affects the rotation of plane-polarized light.

Chirality

KEY CONCEPT

Chirality = handedness

An object is considered **chiral** if its mirror image cannot be superimposed on the original object; this implies that the molecule lacks an internal plane of symmetry. Chirality can also be thought of as handedness. In fact, one of the easiest visualizations of chirality is to think of a pair of hands, as shown in Figure 2.9. Although essentially identical, the left hand will not be able to fit into a right-handed glove. **Achiral** objects have mirror images that *can* be superimposed; for example, a fork is identical to its mirror image and is therefore achiral.

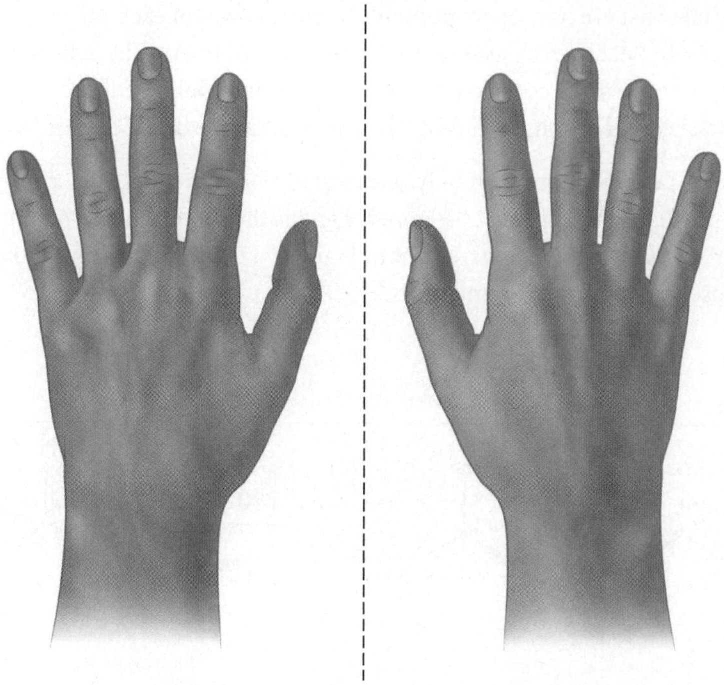

Figure 2.9 Hands as Examples of Chiral Structures
Each hand has a nonsuperimposable mirror image.

On the MCAT, you will often see this concept tested when there is a carbon atom with four different substituents. This carbon will be an asymmetrical core of optical activity and is known as a **chiral center**. As mentioned earlier, chiral centers lack a plane of symmetry. For example, the C-1 carbon atom in 1-bromo-1-chloroethane has four different substituents. As shown in Figure 2.10, this molecule is chiral because it is not superimposable on its mirror image.

MCAT EXPERTISE

Whenever you see a carbon with four different substituents, think chirality.

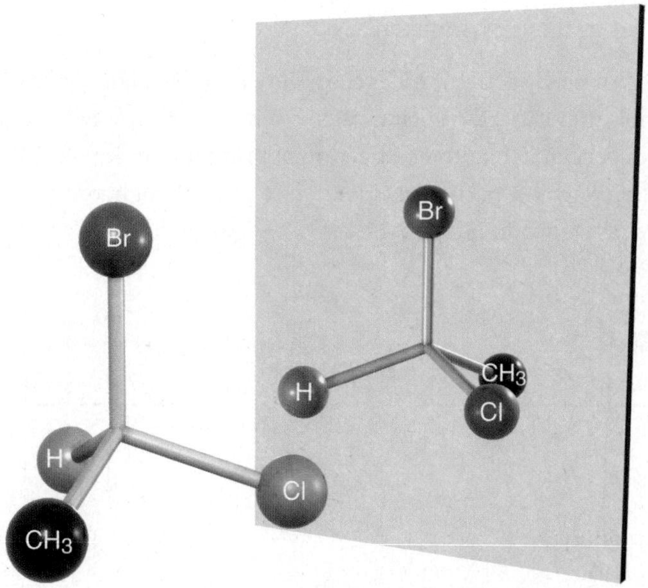

Figure 2.10 Enantiomers of 1-Bromo-1-Chloroethane

Two molecules that are nonsuperimposable mirror images of each other are called **enantiomers**. Molecules may also be related as **diastereomers**. These molecules are chiral and share the same connectivity but are not mirror images of each other. This is because they differ at some (but not all) of their multiple chiral centers.

Alternatively, a carbon atom with only *three different* substituents, such as 1,1-dibromoethane, has a plane of symmetry and is therefore **achiral**. A simple 180° rotation around a vertical axis, as shown in Figure 2.11, allows the compound to be superimposed upon its mirror image.

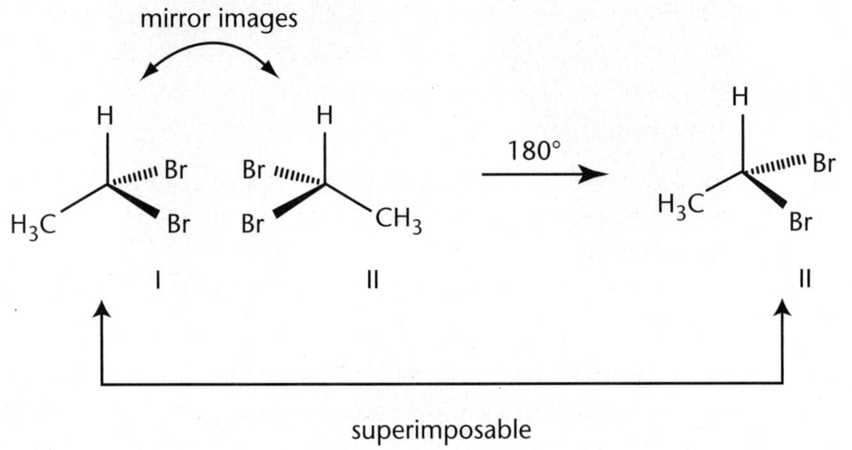

Figure 2.11 Rotation of an Achiral Molecule

Enantiomers

Enantiomers (nonsuperimposable mirror images) have the same connectivity but opposite configurations at every chiral center in the molecule. Enantiomers have identical physical and chemical properties with two notable exceptions: optical activity and reactions in chiral environments.

A compound is optically active if it has the ability to rotate plane-polarized light. Ordinary light is unpolarized, which means that it consists of waves vibrating in all possible planes perpendicular to its direction of propagation. A polarizer allows light waves oscillating only in a particular direction to pass through, producing plane-polarized light, as shown in Figure 2.12.

KEY CONCEPT

Enantiomers have nearly identical physical properties and chemical properties, but they rotate plane-polarized light in opposite directions and react differently in chiral environments.

BRIDGE

While rotation of plane-polarized light can be tested in organic chemistry questions, the polarization of light *itself* is fair game as a physics question. Be sure to review light polarization, discussed in Chapter 8 of *MCAT Physics and Math Review.*

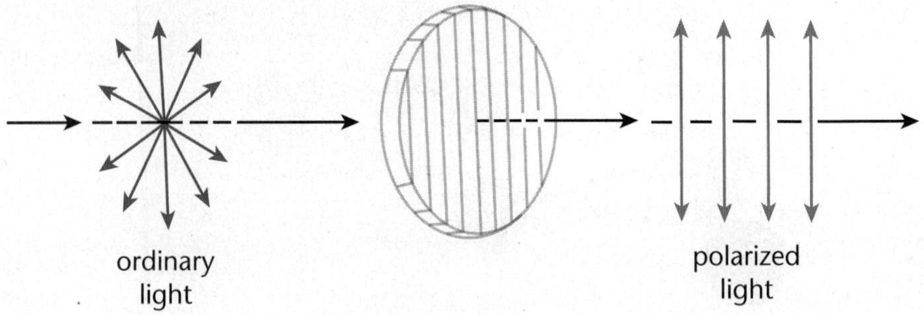

Figure 2.12 Polarizer

Optical activity refers to the rotation of this plane-polarized light by a chiral molecule. At the molecular level, one enantiomer will rotate plane-polarized light to the same magnitude but in the opposite direction of its mirror image (assuming concentration and path lengths are equal). A compound that rotates the plane of polarized light to the right, or clockwise, is dextrorotatory (d-) and is labeled (+). A compound that rotates light toward the left, or counterclockwise, is levorotatory (l-) and is labeled (−). The direction of rotation cannot be determined from the structure of a molecule and must be determined experimentally. That is, it is not related to the absolute configuration of the molecule.

The amount of rotation depends on the number of molecules that a light wave encounters. This depends on two factors: the concentration of the optically active compound and the length of the tube through which the light passes. Chemists have set standard conditions of 1 $\frac{\text{g}}{\text{mL}}$ for concentration and 1 dm (10 cm) for length to compare the optical activities of different compounds. Rotations measured at different concentrations and tube lengths can be converted to a standardized **specific rotation** using the following equation:

$$[\alpha] = \frac{\alpha_{\text{obs}}}{c \times l}$$

Equation 2.1

where $[\alpha]$ is specific rotation in degrees, α_{obs} is the observed rotation in degrees, c is the concentration in $\frac{\text{g}}{\text{mL}}$, and l is the path length in dm.

When both (+) and (−) enantiomers are present in equal concentrations, they form a **racemic mixture**. In these solutions, the rotations cancel each other out, and no optical activity is observed. If enantiomerism is analogous to handedness, racemic mixtures are the equivalent of ambidexterity. These solutions possess no handedness overall and will not rotate plane-polarized light.

The fact that enantiomers have identical physical and chemical properties prompts a question about racemic mixtures: How can one separate the mixture into its two constituent isomers? The answer lies in the relationship between enantiomers and diastereomers. Reacting two enantiomers with a single enantiomer of another compound will, by definition, lead to two diastereomers. Imagine, for example, two enantiomers that contain only one chiral carbon; these compounds could be labeled (+) and (−). If each is reacted with only the (+) enantiomer of another compound, two products would result: (+,+) and (−,+). Because these two products differ at some—but not all—chiral centers, they are necessarily diastereomers. Diastereomers have different physical properties, as we will explore momentarily. These differences enable one to separate these products by common laboratory techniques such as crystallization, filtration, distillation, and others. Once separated, these diastereomers can be reacted to regenerate the original enantiomers.

KEY CONCEPT

The system for labeling optical activity always uses d- or (+) to refer to clockwise rotation of plane-polarized light, while l- and (−) always go together and refer to counterclockwise rotation of plane-polarized light. Do not confuse this with D- or L- labels on carbohydrates or amino acids, which are based on the absolute configuration of glyceraldehyde. (*R*) and (*S*) also refer to absolute configuration, which is determined by structure. Optical activity does not consistently align with the other systems.

KEY CONCEPT

A racemic mixture displays no optical activity.

Diastereomers

Diastereomers are non-mirror-image configurational isomers. Diastereomers occur when a molecule has two or more stereogenic centers and differs at some, but not all, of these centers. The term diastereomer encompasses any stereoisomer that is not an enantiomer. For any molecule with *n* chiral centers, there are 2^n possible stereoisomers. Thus, if a compound has two chiral carbon atoms, it has a maximum of four possible stereoisomers, as shown in Figure 2.13.

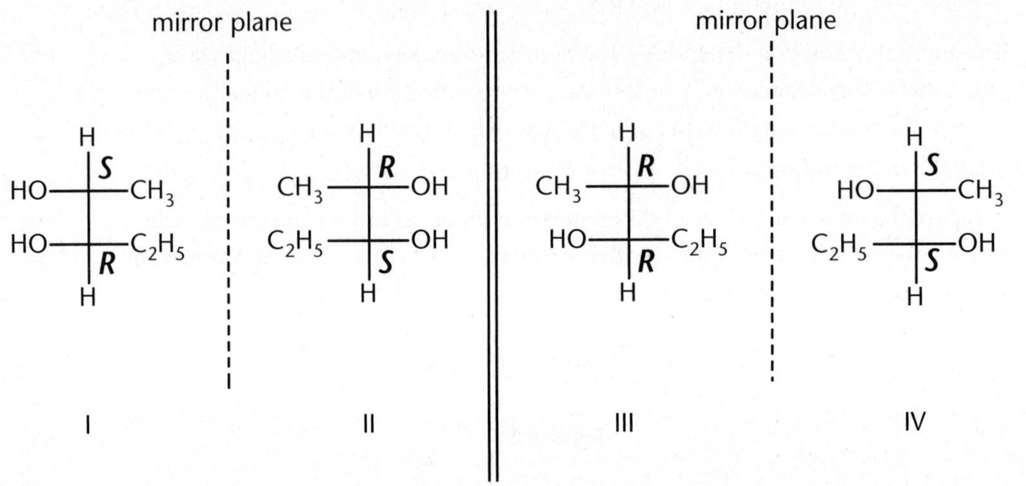

Figure 2.13 2^n Possible Stereoisomers (n = chiral centers)
Four stereoisomers with two chiral centers; enantiomers = I/II and III/IV pairs, and all other combinations are diastereomers.

In this image, one can see that I and II are mirror images of each other and are therefore enantiomers of each other. Similarly, III and IV are enantiomers. However, I and III are not. These are stereoisomers that are not mirror images and are thus diastereomers. Notice that other combinations of non-mirror-image stereoisomers are also diastereomers: I and IV, II and III, and II and IV.

Diastereomers have different chemical properties. However, they might behave similarly in particular reactions because they have the same functional groups. Because they have different arrangements in space, they will consistently have different physical properties. Diastereomers will also rotate plane-polarized light; however, knowing the specific rotation of one diastereomer gives no indication of the specific rotation of another diastereomer. This is a stark contrast from enantiomers, which will always have equal-magnitude rotations in opposite directions.

Cis–Trans Isomers

Cis–trans **isomers** (formerly called **geometric isomers**) are a specific subtype of diastereomers in which substituents differ in their position around an immovable bond, such as a double bond, or around a ring structure, such as a cycloalkane in which the rotation of bonds is greatly restricted. In simple compounds with only one substituent on either side of the immovable bond, we use the terms ***cis*** and ***trans***.

If two substituents are on the same side of the immovable bond, the molecule is considered *cis*. If they are on opposite sides, it is considered *trans*, as shown in Figure 2.8 earlier. For more complicated compounds with polysubstituted double bonds, (*E*)/(*Z*) nomenclature is used instead, as described in the next section.

MCAT EXPERTISE

While the MCAT is up-to-date with science, it is still possible to see older terms for some concepts on Test Day. Thus, it's important to know not only the current name, *cis-trans* isomers, but also the older name, geometric isomers.

Meso Compounds

For a molecule to have optical activity, it must not only have chiral centers within it, but must also lack a plane of symmetry. Thus, if a plane of symmetry exists, the molecule is not optically active even if it possesses chiral centers. This plane of symmetry can occur either through the chiral center or between chiral centers. A molecule with chiral centers that has an internal plane of symmetry is called a ***meso* compound**, an example of which is shown in Figure 2.14.

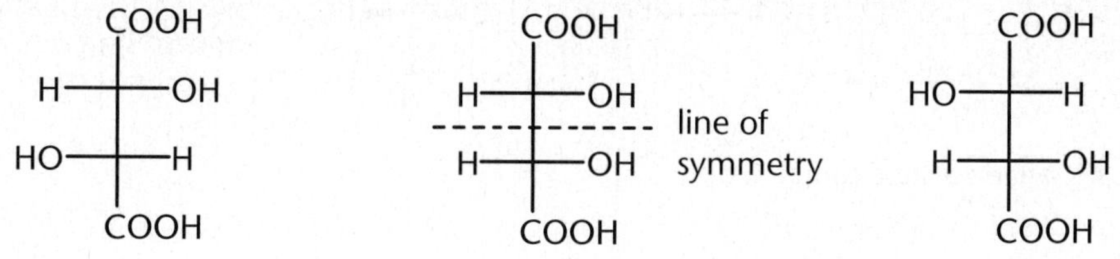

L-tartaric acid   *meso*-tartaric acid   D-tartaric acid

Figure 2.14 Example of a *Meso* Compound

As shown in this image, D- and L-tartaric acid are both optically active, but *meso*-tartaric acid has a plane of symmetry and is not optically active. This means that even though *meso*-tartaric acid has two chiral carbon atoms, the molecule as a whole does not display optical activity. *Meso* compounds are essentially the molecular equivalent of a racemic mixture.

KEY CONCEPT

Meso compounds are made up of two halves that are mirror images. Thus, as a whole they are not optically active.

MCAT CONCEPT CHECK 2.2

Before you move on, assess your understanding of the material with these questions.

1. What is the difference between a conformational and a configurational isomer?
   - Conformational:

     ____

   - Configurational:

     ____

2. Consider the six pairs that the following four molecules can make. Which pairs are enantiomers? Diastereomers?

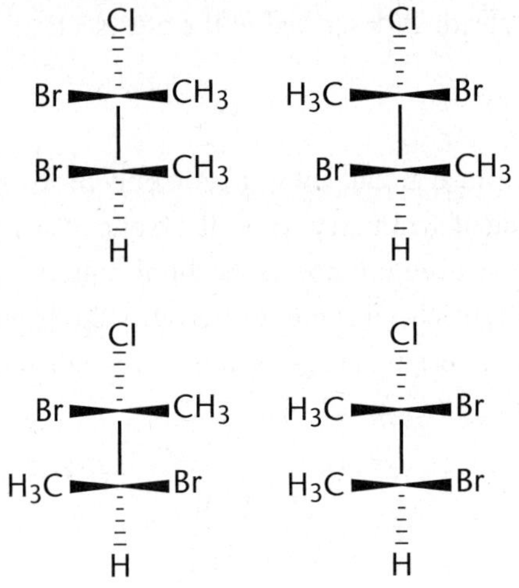

3. What is a *meso* compound?

4. Complete the Newman projection for the following compound:

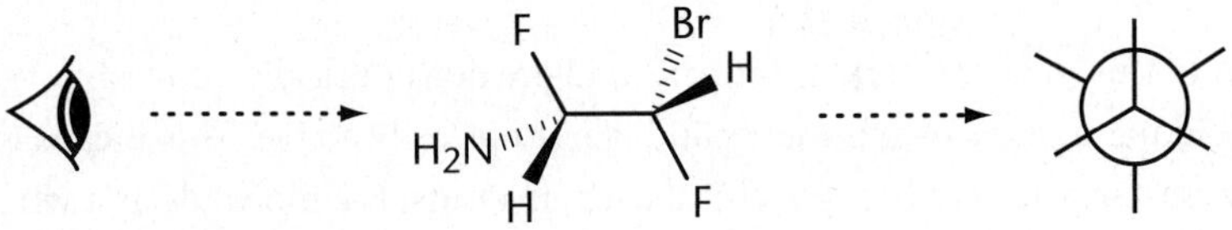

2.3 Relative and Absolute Configurations

LEARNING OBJECTIVES

After Chapter 2.3, you will be able to:

- Name *cis*, *trans*, *E*, and *Z* molecules using appropriate nomenclature
- Apply Cahn–Ingold–Prelog priority rules to molecules with up to four substituents

The **configuration** of a stereoisomer refers to the spatial arrangement of the atoms or groups in the molecule. The **relative configuration** of a chiral molecule is its configuration in relation to another chiral molecule (often through chemical interconversion). We can use the relative configuration to determine whether molecules are enantiomers, diastereomers, or the same molecule. On the other hand, the **absolute conformation** of a chiral molecule describes the exact spatial arrangement of these atoms or groups, independent of other molecules.

(*E*) and (*Z*) Forms

(*E*) and (*Z*) nomenclature is used for compounds with polysubstituted double bonds. Recall that simpler double-bond-containing compounds can use the *cis–trans* system. To determine the (*E*)/(*Z*) designation, one starts by identifying the highest-priority substituent attached to each double-bonded carbon. Using the **Cahn–Ingold–Prelog priority rules**, priority is assigned based on the atom bonded to the double-bonded carbons: the higher the atomic number, the higher the priority. If the atomic numbers are equal, priority is determined by the next atoms outward; again, whichever group contains the atom with the highest atomic number is given top priority. If a tie remains, the atoms in this group are compared one-by-one in descending atomic number order until the tie is broken. The alkene is named (***Z***) (German: *zusammen*, "together") if the two highest-priority substituents on each carbon are on the same side of the double bond and (***E***) (*entgegen*, "opposite") if they are on opposite sides, as shown in Figure 2.15.

MNEMONIC

Z = "**z**"ame side; ***E*** = "**e**"pposite side

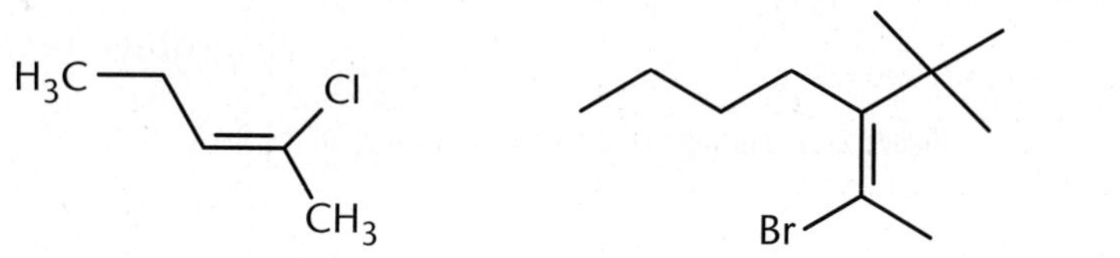

(*Z*)-2-chloro-2-pentene (*E*)-2-bromo-3-*t*-butyl-2-heptene

Figure 2.15 (*E*) and (*Z*) Designations of Alkenes

(*R*) and (*S*) Forms

(*R*) and (*S*) nomenclature is used for chiral (stereogenic) centers in molecules. We go through a set sequence to determine this absolute configuration:

Step 1: Assign Priority

Using the Cahn–Ingold–Prelog priority rules described earlier, assign priority to the four substituents, looking only at the atoms directly attached to the chiral center. Once again, higher atomic number takes priority over lower atomic number. If the atomic numbers are equal, priority is determined by the combination of the atoms attached to these atoms; if there is a double bond, it is counted as two individual bonds to that atom. If a tie is encountered, work outward from the stereocenter until the tie is broken. An example is shown in Figure 2.16.

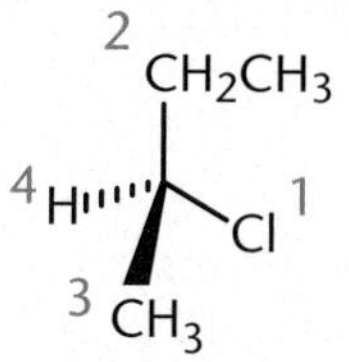

Figure 2.16 Applying the Cahn-Ingold-Prelog Priority Rules to Determine Absolute Configuration

Assign priority by the highest atomic number.

KEY CONCEPT

When assigning priority, look only at the first atom attached to the chiral carbon, not at the group as a whole. The higher the atomic number of this first atom, the higher the priority—this same system is used to determine priority for both (*E*) and (*Z*) forms, as well as (*R*) and (*S*) forms.

Step 2 (Classic Version): Arrange in Space

Orient the molecule in three-dimensional space so that the atom with the lowest priority (usually a hydrogen atom) is at the back of the molecule. Another way to think of this is to arrange the point of view so that the line of sight proceeds down the bond from the asymmetrical carbon atom (the chiral center) to the substituent with lowest priority. The three substituents with higher priority should then radiate out from the central carbon, coming out of the page, as shown in Figure 2.17.

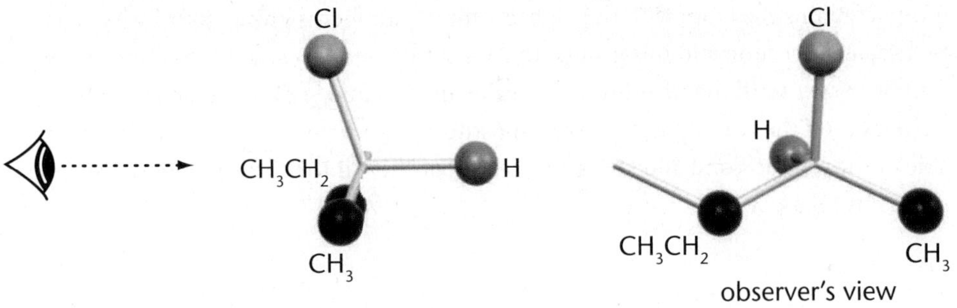

Figure 2.17 Placing the Lowest-Priority Group in the Back

Step 2 (Modified Version): Invert the Stereochemistry

If it is difficult to visualize rotating three-dimensional structures, one can simplify this process by remembering one simple rule: *any time two groups are switched on a chiral carbon, the stereochemistry is inverted.* By this logic, we can simply switch the lowest-priority group with the group at the back of the molecule (the substituent projecting into the page). We can then proceed to Step 3, keeping in mind that we have now changed the molecule to the opposite configuration. Therefore, if we use this modified step, we need to remember to switch our final answer (either (*R*) to (*S*), or (*S*) to (*R*)). This is a strategy we'll commonly use on Fischer diagrams, as described below.

Step 3: Draw a Circle

Now, imagine drawing a circle connecting the substituents from number 1 to 2 to 3. Pay no attention to the lowest-priority group; it can be skipped because it projects directly into the page. If the circle is drawn counterclockwise, the asymmetric atom is called (***S***) (Latin: *sinister*, "left"). If it is clockwise, it is called (***R***) (*rectus*, "right"), as shown in Figure 2.18. Remember to correct the stereochemistry if the modified version of Step 2 was used.

MNEMONIC

A clockwise arrangement is like turning a steering wheel clockwise, which makes a car turn **R**ight—so the chirality at that center is (***R***).

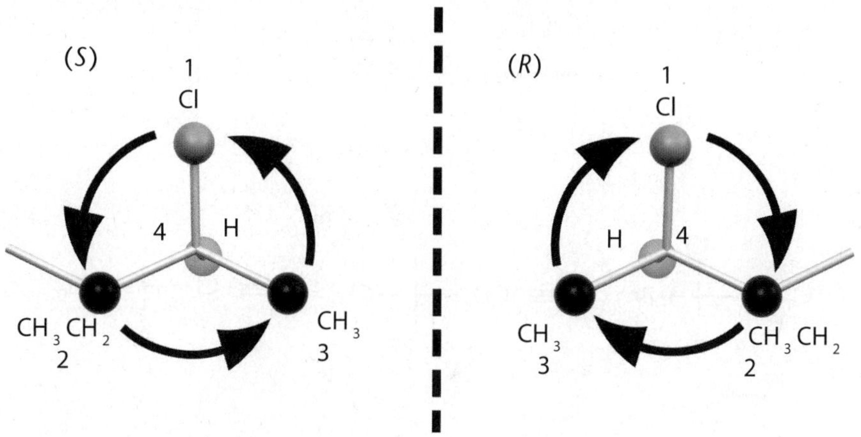

Figure 2.18 Drawing a Circle to Determine Absolute Configuration
Counterclockwise = (S); clockwise = (R)

Step 4: Write the Name

Once the (*R*)/(*S*) designation has been determined, the name can be written out. (*R*) and (*S*) are put in parentheses and separated from the rest of the name by a hyphen. If we have a compound with more than one chiral center, location is specified by a number preceding the *R* or *S* within the parentheses and without a hyphen.

Fischer Projections

On the MCAT, one way to represent three-dimensional molecules is by a **Fischer projection**. In this system, horizontal lines indicate bonds that project out from the plane of the page (wedges), whereas vertical lines indicate bonds going into the plane of the page (dashes). The point of intersection of the lines represents a carbon atom.

To determine configurations using Fischer projections, we follow the same rules listed above. Once again, we have to make sure that the lowest-priority group projects into the page. A benefit of Fischer projections is that the lowest-priority group can be on the top or bottom of the molecule and still project into the page.

Another advantage is that we can manipulate Fischer projections without changing the compound. As mentioned before, switching two substituents around a chiral carbon will invert the stereochemistry ((*R*) to (*S*), or (*S*) to (*R*)). Rotating a Fischer projection in the plane of the page by 90° will also invert the stereochemistry of the molecule. By extension, interchanging any *two* pairs of substituents will revert the compound back to its original stereochemistry, and rotating a Fischer projection in the plane of the page by 180° will also retain the stereochemistry of the molecule. These manipulations are shown in Figure 2.19.

KEY CONCEPT

To determine the absolute configuration at a chiral center:

1. Assign priority by atomic number
2. Arrange the molecule with the lowest-priority substituent in the back (or invert the stereochemistry by switching two substituents)
3. Draw a circle around the molecule from highest to lowest priority (1 to 2 to 3)
4. Clockwise = (*R*); counterclockwise = (*S*)

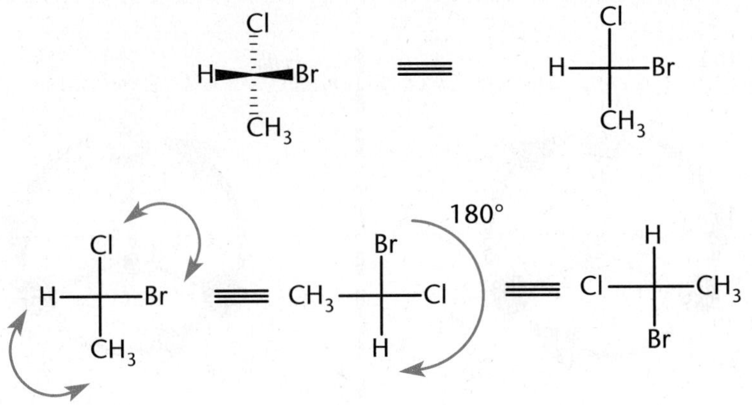

Figure 2.19 Manipulations of Fischer Projections

Again, determining the (*R*)/(*S*) designation of a Fischer projection of a compound follows the same rules as described previously. But what if our lowest-priority group is pointing to the side and, as such, pointing out of the page? Just as before, we've got a couple of different tricks to help determine the right stereochemistry.

MCAT EXPERTISE

Determine which option you prefer for Fischer projection (*R*)/(*S*) designation and stick with it. It's more efficient to have a consistent method than to use all three interchangeably.

Option 1: Make 0 Switches

Go ahead and determine the order of substituents as normal, drawing a circle from 1 to 2 to 3. Remember, number 4 doesn't count, so just skip right over it when determining the order. Then, obtain the (*R*)/(*S*) designation. The *true* designation will be the opposite of what you just obtained.

Option 2: Make 1 Switch

Swap the lowest-priority group with one of the groups on the vertical axis. Obtain the (*R*)/(*S*) designation and, once again, the *true* designation will be the opposite of what you just found.

Option 3: Make 2 Switches

In this method, start with option 2, moving the lowest-priority group into the correct position. Then, switch the other two groups as well. Because we made two switches, this molecule will have the *same* designation as the initial molecule. This is the same as holding one substituent in place and rotating the other three in order.

MCAT CONCEPT CHECK 2.3

Before you move on, assess your understanding of the material with these questions.

1. How is priority assigned under the Cahn–Ingold–Prelog priority rules?

   ____

2. Name the following compound using *E*/*Z* nomenclature:

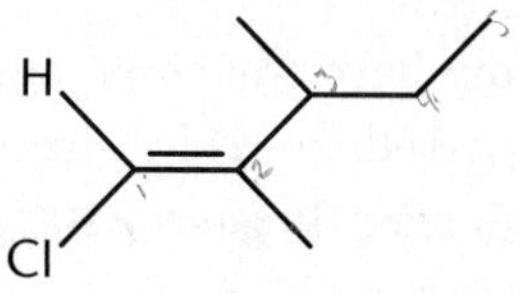

   ____

3. For each of the Fischer projection manipulations listed below, is stereochemistry retained or inverted?
   - Switching a pair of substituents: ______________
   - Switching two pairs of substituents: ______________
   - Rotating the molecule 90°: ______________
   - Rotating the molecule 180°: ______________

Conclusion

Throughout this chapter, we've seen just how many different molecules can be derived from the same molecular formula. This information is going to be essential on the MCAT—not only for questions on isomerism itself but on every single organic chemistry question you encounter. Most of the compounds we come across will have different possible isomers, and you need to be prepared to differentiate among them to find the one and only correct answer. In the next chapter, we'll explore how organic molecules are held together through discussions of hybridized orbitals and resonance.

GO ONLINE

You've reviewed the content, now test your knowledge and critical thinking skills by completing a test-like passage set in your online resources!

CONCEPT SUMMARY

Structural Isomers

- **Structural isomers** share only a molecular formula.
- They have different physical and chemical properties.

Stereoisomers

- **Conformational isomers** differ by rotation around a single (σ) bond.
  - **Staggered conformations** have groups 60° apart, as seen in a **Newman projection**. In ***anti*** **staggered** molecules, the two largest groups are 180° apart, and strain is minimized. In ***gauche*** **staggered** molecules, the two largest groups are 60° apart.
  - **Eclipsed conformations** have groups directly in front of each other as seen in a Newman projection. In **totally eclipsed conformations**, the two largest groups are directly in front of each other and strain is maximized.
  - The strain in cyclic molecules comes from **angle strain** (created by stretching or compressing angles from their normal size), **torsional strain** (from eclipsing conformations), and **nonbonded strain** (from interactions between substituents attached to nonadjacent carbons). Cyclic molecules will usually adopt nonplanar shapes to minimize this strain.
  - Substituents attached to cyclohexane can be classified as **axial** (sticking up or down from the plane of the molecule) or **equatorial** (in the plane of the molecule). Axial substituents create more nonbonded strain.
  - In cyclohexane molecules with multiple substituents, the largest substituent will usually take the equatorial position to minimize strain.
- **Configurational isomers** can only be interchanged by breaking and reforming bonds.
  - **Enantiomers** are nonsuperimposable mirror images and thus have opposite stereochemistry at every chiral carbon. They have the same chemical and physical properties except for rotation of plane-polarized light and reactions in a chiral environment.
  - **Optical activity** refers to the ability of a molecule to rotate plane-polarized light: d- or (+) molecules rotate light to the right; l- or (−) molecules rotate light to the left.
  - **Racemic mixtures**, with equal concentrations of two enantiomers, will not be optically active because the two enantiomers' rotations cancel each other out.
  - ***Meso*** **compounds**, with an internal plane of symmetry, will also be optically inactive because the two sides of the molecule cancel each other out.
  - **Diastereomers** are non-mirror-image stereoisomers. They differ at some, but not all, chiral centers. They have different chemical and physical properties.

- ***Cis–trans*** isomers are a subtype of diastereomers in which groups differ in position about an immovable bond (such as a double bond or in a cycloalkane).
- **Chiral centers** have four different groups attached to the central carbon.

Relative and Absolute Configurations

- **Relative configuration** gives the stereochemistry of a compound in comparison to another molecule.
- **Absolute configuration** gives the stereochemistry of a compound without having to compare to other molecules.
  - Absolute configuration uses the **Cahn–Ingold–Prelog priority rules**, in which priority is given by looking at the atoms connected to the chiral carbon or double-bonded carbons; whichever has the highest atomic number gets highest priority. If there is a tie, one moves outward from the chiral carbon or double-bonded carbon until the tie is broken.
- An alkene is (***Z***) if the highest-priority substituents are on the same side of the double bond and (***E***) if on opposite sides.
- A stereocenter's configuration is determined by putting the lowest priority group in the back and drawing a circle from group 1 to 2 to 3 in descending priority. If this circle is clockwise, the stereocenter is (***R***); if it is counterclockwise, the stereocenter is (***S***).
- Vertical lines in **Fischer diagrams** go into the plane of the page (dashes); horizontal lines come out of the plane of the page (wedges).
  - Switching one pair of substituents in a Fischer diagram inverts the stereochemistry of the chiral center. Switching two pairs retains the stereochemistry.
  - Rotating a Fischer diagram 90° inverts the stereochemistry of the chiral center. Rotating 180° retains the stereochemistry.

ANSWERS TO CONCEPT CHECKS

2.1

1. Structural isomers share a molecular formula, and not necessarily anything else.
2. Cyclopropanol, acetone, and prop-2-ene-1-ol are all structural isomers of each other with the chemical formula C_3H_6O. 2-Propanol has the chemical formula C_3H_8O.
3. Physical properties are aspects of a compound that do not play a role in changing chemical composition. Examples include melting point, boiling point, solubility, odor, color, and density.
4. Chemical properties are aspects of a compound that change chemical composition; in organic chemistry, chemical properties are usually dictated by the reactivity of various functional groups.

2.2

1. Conformational isomers are stereoisomers with the same molecular connectivity at different points of rotation around a single bond. Configurational isomers are stereoisomers with differing molecular connectivity.
2. Enantiomers are nonsuperimposable mirror images. That means the molecules must be mirror images that are different from one another (superimposable mirror images represent the same object). The molecules on the top-left and bottom-right are nonsuperimposable mirror images and therefore enantiomers. The same is true for the top-right and bottom-left. All other combinations are diastereomeric because the pairs differ at some, but not all, stereocenters.
3. A *meso* compound contains chiral centers but also has an internal plane of symmetry. This means that the molecule is overall achiral and will not rotate plane-polarized light.
4.

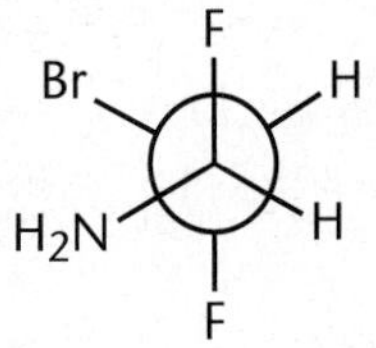

2.3

1. Priority is assigned by atomic number: the atom connected to the stereocenter or double-bonded carbon with the highest atomic number gets highest priority. If there is a tie, one works outward from the stereocenter or double-bonded carbon until the tie is broken.
2. The highest-priority functional group is an alkene, and the longest carbon chain that contains the double bond is five carbons long. So, the root will be *pent–* and the suffix will be *–ene*. There are three substituents: a chlorine and two methyls. Number the chain to give the double bond the lowest possible number, in this case from left to right. Bringing it all together gives 1-chloro-2,3-dimethyl-1-pentene. However, there are two possible configurations around the double bond. To determine (*E*)/(*Z*) designation, start by identifying the highest-priority substituents attached to each double-bonded carbon. The chlorine and butyl groups are the highest-priority substituents and are on opposite sides of the double bond (in addition to being on opposite ends of the double bond), so this molecule is (*E*)-1-chloro-2,3-dimethyl-1-pentene.
3. Switching a pair of substituents inverts stereochemistry; switching two pairs retains it. Rotating the molecule 90° inverts stereochemistry; rotating 180° retains it.

SCIENCE MASTERY ASSESSMENT EXPLANATIONS

1. **D**

This is a racemic mixture of 2-butanol because it consists of equimolar amounts of (*R*)-2-butanol and (*S*)-2-butanol. The (*R*)-2-butanol molecule rotates the plane of polarized light in one direction, and the (*S*)-2-butanol rotates it by the same angle but in the opposite direction; as a result, no net rotation of polarized light is observed.

2. **B**

The maximum number of stereoisomers of a compound equals 2^n, where n is the number of chiral carbons in the compound. In this molecule, C-1 (the aldehydic carbon) is not chiral, nor is C-5 (because it is attached to two hydrogen atoms). Therefore, with three chiral centers, there are $2^3 = 8$ stereoisomers.

3. **C**

This answer choice is an example of a *meso* compound—a compound that contains chiral centers but has an internal plane of symmetry:

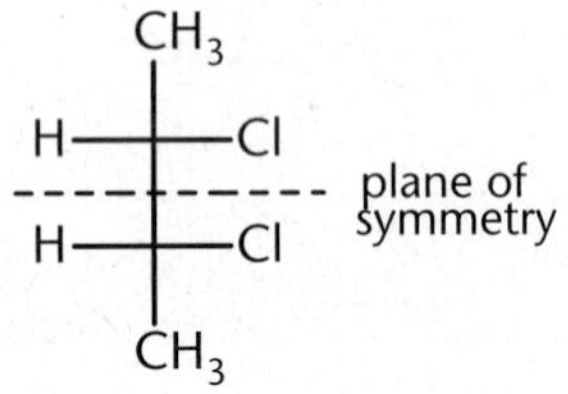

Owing to this internal plane of symmetry, the molecule is achiral and, hence, optically inactive. **(A)** and **(B)** are enantiomers of each other and will certainly show optical activity on their own. **(D)**, because it contains a chiral carbon and no internal plane of symmetry, is optically active as well.

4. **C**

To be considered a chiral center, a carbon must have four different substituents. There are eight stereocenters in this molecule, which are marked below with asterisks.

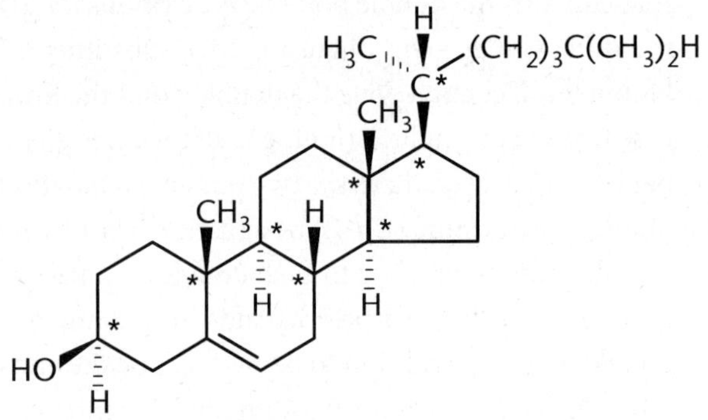

cholesterol

The other carbons are not chiral for various reasons. Many are bonded to two hydrogens; others participate in double bonds, which count as two bonds to the same atom.

5. **B**

This molecule is a chair conformation in which the two equatorial methyl groups are *trans* to each other. Because the axial methyl hydrogens do not compete for the same space as the hydrogens attached to the ring, this conformation ensures the least amount of steric strain. **(A)** would be less stable because the diaxial methyl group hydrogens are closer to the hydrogens on the ring, causing greater steric strain. **(C)** is incorrect because it is in the more unstable boat conformation.

6. **C**

The relative configuration is retained because the bonds of the stereocenter are not broken; thus, the positions of groups around the chiral carbon are maintained. The absolute configuration is also retained because both the reactant and product are (*R*).

7. **A**

These compounds are nonsuperimposable mirror images. To make analysis a bit easier, we can rotate structure II 180° to look like structure III. Structures I and III more clearly have opposite stereochemistry at every chiral center, meaning that they are enantiomers.

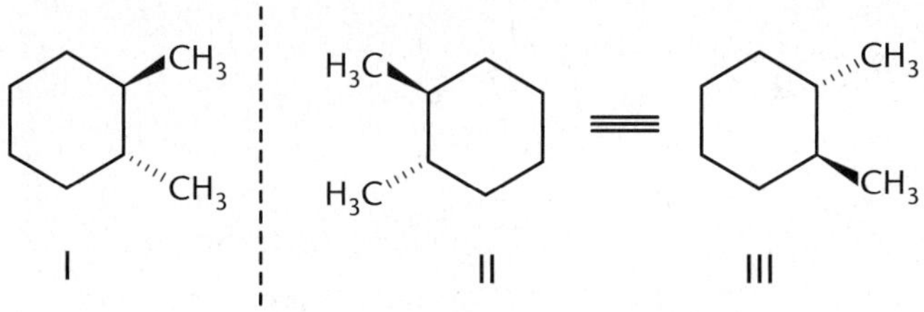

(B) is incorrect because diastereomers are stereoisomers that are not mirror images of each other. **(C)** is incorrect because *meso* compounds must contain a plane of symmetry, which neither of these molecules has. **(D)** is incorrect because structural isomers are compounds with the same molecular formula but different atomic connections. The connectivity in these two molecules is the same, which means that they are stereoisomers, not structural isomers.

8. **A**

(+)-Glyceraldehyde and (−)-glyceraldehyde, or (*R*)- and (*S*)-2,3-dihydroxypropanal, are enantiomers. Enantiomers are nonsuperimposable mirror images. Each has only one chiral center (C-2), which has opposite absolute configuration in these two molecules.

9. **C**

(*E*)-2-butene can also be called *trans*-2-butene; (*Z*)-2-butene can also be called *cis*-2-butene. As such, they are *cis–trans* isomers. Remember that *cis–trans* isomers are a subtype of diastereomers in which the position of substituents differs about an immovable bond. Diastereomers are molecules that are non-mirror-image stereoisomers (molecules with the same atomic connectivity). These are not enantiomers because they are not mirror images of each other.

10. **C**

Because they have the same molecular formula but different atomic connectivity, 3-methylpentane and hexane are constitutional isomers.

11. **B**

These two molecules are stereoisomers of one another, but are *not* nonsuperimposable mirror images. Therefore, they are diastereomers. Note that these molecules differ by at least one, but not all, chiral carbons.

12. **D**

Remember that the equation for specific rotation is $[\alpha] = \frac{\alpha_{obs}}{c \times l}$. In this example, α_{obs} is +12° (remember that dextrorotatory, or clockwise, rotation is considered positive), $c = 0.5\ \frac{g}{mL}$, $l = 1$ cm = 0.1 dm. Remember that path length is always measured in decimeters when calculating specific rotation. Therefore, the specific rotation can be calculated as:

$$[\alpha] = \frac{\alpha_{obs}}{c \times l} = \frac{+12}{\left(0.5\ \frac{g}{mL}\right) \times (0.1\ dm)} = +240°$$

13. **B**

Racemic mixtures like omeprazole contain equimolar amounts of two enantiomers and thus have no observed optical activity. Each of the two enantiomers causes rotation in opposite directions, so their effects cancel out. Esomeprazole only contains one of the two enantiomers and thus should cause rotation of plane-polarized light.

14. **C**

Draw out these structures. The two names describe the same molecule, which also happens to be a *meso* compound because it contains a plane of symmetry. These compounds are not enantiomers because they are superimposable mirror images of one another, *not* nonsuperimposable mirror images. These compounds are better termed *meso*-2,3-dihydroxybutanedioic acid:

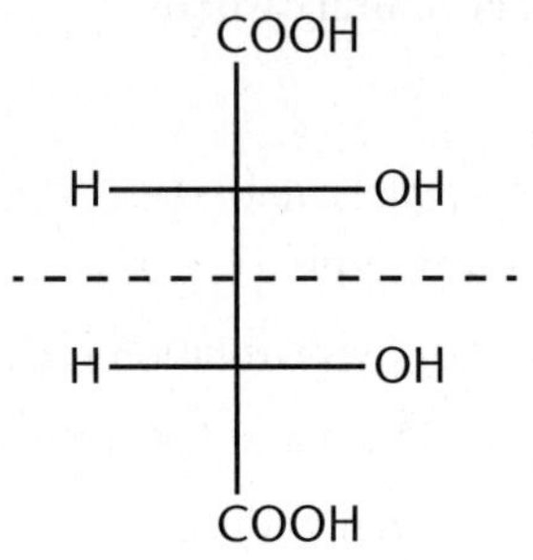

15. **C**

In butane, the position at which the two methyl groups are 120° apart is an eclipsed conformation. This has a moderate amount of energy, although not as high as a totally eclipsed conformation in which the two methyl groups are 0° apart.

Consult your online resources for additional practice. GO ONLINE

EQUATIONS TO REMEMBER

(2.1) **Specific rotation:** $[\alpha] = \frac{\alpha_{\text{obs}}}{c \times l}$

SHARED CONCEPTS

Biochemistry Chapter 1
Amino Acids, Peptides, and Proteins

Biochemistry Chapter 4
Carbohydrate Structure and Function

General Chemistry Chapter 3
Bonding and Chemical Interactions

Organic Chemistry Chapter 3
Bonding

Organic Chemistry Chapter 4
Analyzing Organic Reactions

Physics and Math Chapter 8
Light and Optics

CHAPTER 3

BONDING

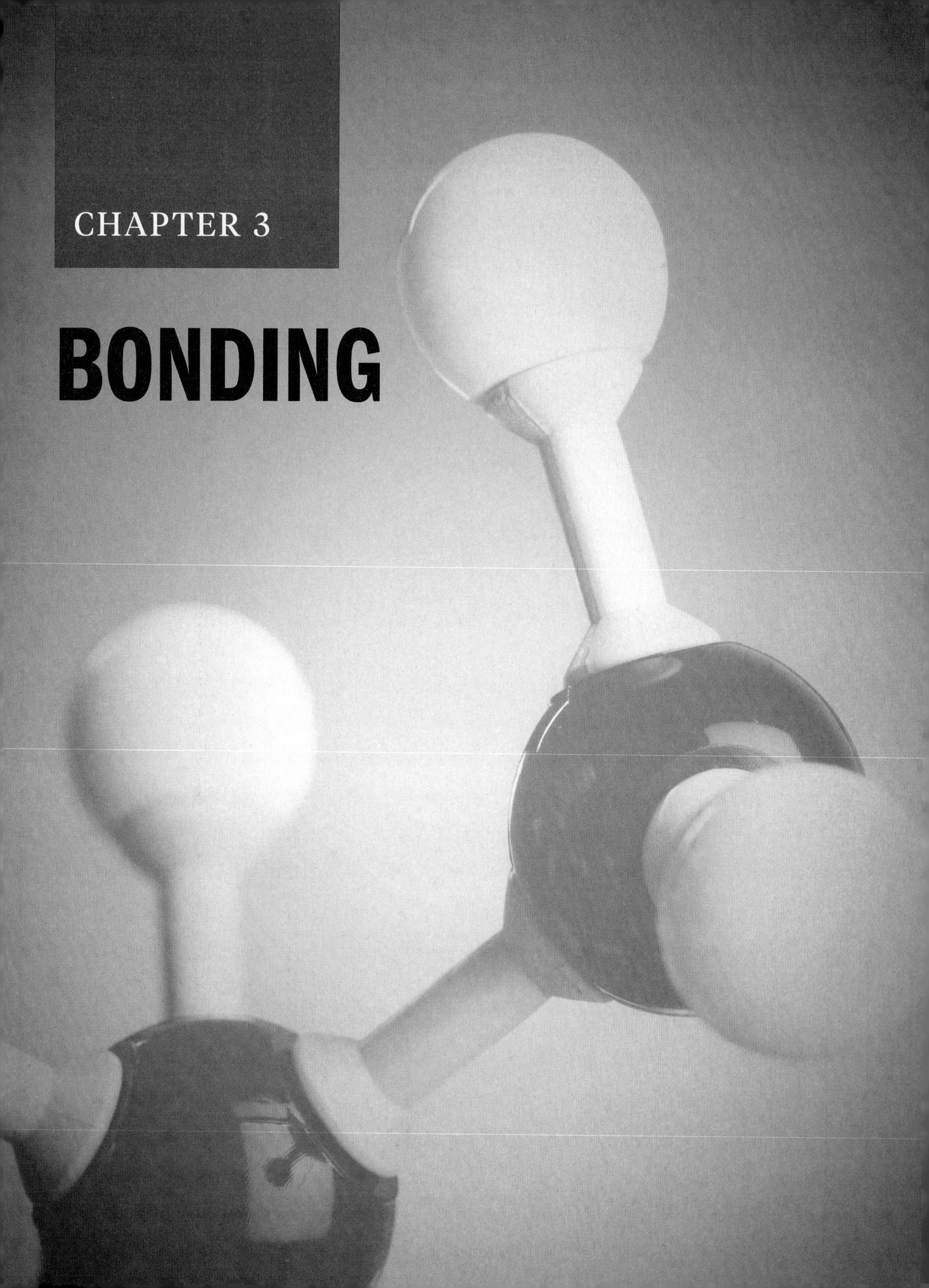

SCIENCE MASTERY ASSESSMENT

Every pre-med knows this feeling: there is so much content I have to know for the MCAT! How do I know what to do first or what's important?

While the high-yield badges throughout this book will help you identify the most important topics, this Science Mastery Assessment is another tool in your MCAT prep arsenal. This quiz (which can also be taken in your online resources) and the guidance below will help ensure that you are spending the appropriate amount of time on this chapter based on your personal strengths and weaknesses. Don't worry though—skipping something now does not mean you'll never study it. Later on in your prep, as you complete full-length tests, you'll uncover specific pieces of content that you need to review and can come back to these chapters as appropriate.

How to Use This Assessment

If you answer 0–7 questions correctly:

Spend about 1 hour to read this chapter in full and take limited notes throughout. Follow up by reviewing **all** quiz questions to ensure that you now understand how to solve each one.

If you answer 8–11 questions correctly:

Spend 20–40 minutes reviewing the quiz questions. Beginning with the questions you missed, read and take notes on the corresponding subchapters. For questions you answered correctly, ensure your thinking matches that of the explanation and you understand why each choice was correct or incorrect.

If you answer 12–15 questions correctly:

Spend less than 20 minutes reviewing all questions from the quiz. If you missed any, then include a quick read-through of the corresponding subchapters, or even just the relevant content within a subchapter, as part of your question review. For questions you got correct, ensure your thinking matches that of the explanation and review the Concept Summary at the end of the chapter.

1. Within one principal energy level, which subshell has the least energy?
   - **A.** *s*
   - **B.** *p*
   - **C.** *d*
   - **D.** *f*

2. Which of the following compounds possesses at least one σ bond?
   - **A.** CH_4
   - **B.** C_2H_2
   - **C.** C_2H_4
   - **D.** All of the above contain at least one σ bond.

3. A carbon atom participates in one double bond. As such, this carbon contains orbitals with:
   - **A.** hybridization between the *s*-orbital and one *p*-orbital.
   - **B.** hybridization between the *s*-orbital and two *p*-orbitals.
   - **C.** hybridization between the *s*-orbital and three *p*-orbitals.
   - **D.** unhybridized *s* character.

4. The hybridizations of the carbon and nitrogen atoms in CN^- are:
   - **A.** sp^3 and sp^3, respectively.
   - **B.** sp^3 and sp, respectively.
   - **C.** sp and sp^3, respectively.
   - **D.** sp and sp, respectively.

5. Which of the following hybridizations does the Be atom in BeH_2 assume?
   - **A.** sp
   - **B.** sp^2
   - **C.** sp^3
   - **D.** sp^3d

6. Two atomic orbitals may combine to form:
   - **I.** a bonding molecular orbital.
   - **II.** an antibonding molecular orbital.
   - **III.** hybridized orbitals.

   - **A.** I only
   - **B.** III only
   - **C.** I and II only
   - **D.** I, II, and III

7. Molecular orbitals can contain a maximum of:
   - **A.** one electron.
   - **B.** two electrons.
   - **C.** four electrons.
   - **D.** $2n^2$ electrons, where *n* is the principal quantum number of the combining atomic orbitals.

8. π bonds are formed by which of the following orbitals?
   - **A.** Two *s*-orbitals
   - **B.** Two *p*-orbitals
   - **C.** One *s*- and one *p*-orbital
   - **D.** Two sp^2-hybridized orbitals

9. How many σ bonds and π bonds are present in the following compound?

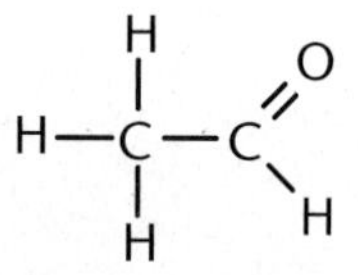

A. Six σ bonds and one π bond
B. Six σ bonds and two π bonds
C. Five σ bonds and one π bond
D. Five σ bonds and two π bonds

10. The four C–H bonds of CH_4 point toward the vertices of a tetrahedron. This indicates that the hybridization of the carbon atom in methane is:
A. *sp*.
B. sp^2.
C. sp^3.
D. sp^3d.

11. Why is a single bond stronger than a π bond?
I. π bonds have greater orbital overlap.
II. *s*-orbitals have more overlap than *p*-orbitals.
III. sp^3 hybridization is always unstable.

A. I only
B. II only
C. I and III only
D. II and III only

12. The *p* character of the bonds formed by the carbon atom in HCN is:
A. 25%.
B. 50%.
C. 67%.
D. 75%.

13. A resonance structure describes:
I. the hybrid of all possible structures that contribute to electron distribution.
II. a potential arrangement of electrons in a molecule.
III. the single form that the molecule most often takes.

A. I only
B. II only
C. I and II only
D. I, II, and III

14. An electron is known to be in the $n = 4$ shell and the $l = 2$ subshell. How many possible combinations of quantum numbers could this electron have?
A. 1
B. 2
C. 5
D. 10

15. Compared to single bonds, triple bonds are:
A. weaker.
B. longer.
C. made up of fewer σ bonds.
D. more rigid.

Answer Key

1. **A**
2. **D**
3. **B**
4. **D**
5. **A**
6. **D**
7. **B**
8. **B**
9. **A**
10. **C**
11. **B**
12. **B**
13. **B**
14. **D**
15. **D**

Detailed explanations can be found at the end of the chapter.

CHAPTER 3

BONDING

In This Chapter

CHAPTER PROFILE

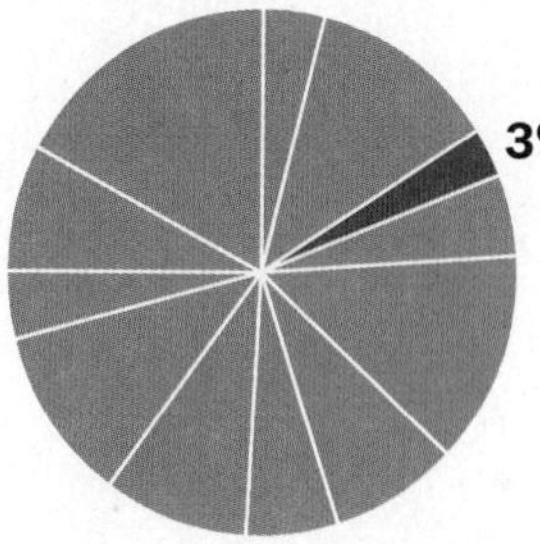

The content in this chapter should be relevant to about 3% of all questions about organic chemistry on the MCAT.

This chapter covers material from the following AAMC content categories:

4E: Atoms, nuclear decay, electronic structure, and atomic chemical behavior

5B: Nature of molecules and intermolecular interactions

Introduction

Now that we have an understanding of nomenclature and how compounds are related, we are ready to start examining the real nature of chemical bonding. Bonding determines how atoms come together to form molecules. It also governs the ways those molecules interact with the other molecules in their environment.

Organic chemistry is the study of carbon and carbon-containing compounds. What makes carbon so special? The simple answer is that carbon has unique bonding properties. Carbon is tetravalent, which means that it can form bonds with up to four other atoms, allowing for the massive versatility required to form the foundation of biomolecules and life itself. This versatility is compounded by the fact that carbon, located near the center of the periodic table, can form bonds with many different elements because of its moderate electronegativity. In addition, because carbon atoms are fairly small, the bonds that they form are strong and stable.

Remember that there are two types of chemical bonds. The first is **ionic**, in which electrons are transferred from one atom to another and the resulting ions are held together by electrostatic interactions; the second is **covalent**, in which electrons are shared between atoms. Organic chemistry is deeply rooted in covalent bonding.

3.1 Atomic Orbitals and Quantum Numbers

LEARNING OBJECTIVES

After Chapter 3.1, you will be able to:

- Describe the four quantum numbers, n, l, m_l, and m_s
- Provide ranges of possible values for each quantum number

Bonding occurs in the outermost electron shell of atoms, so an understanding of bonding is contingent on understanding the organization of electrons in an atom. Quantum numbers are discussed in detail in Chapter 1 of *MCAT General Chemistry Review*, and are briefly summarized here.

The first three quantum numbers, n, l, and m_l, describe the size, shape, number, and orientation of atomic orbitals an element possesses. The **principal quantum number, *n***, corresponds to the energy level of a given electron in an atom and is essentially a measure of size. The smaller the number, the closer the shell is to the nucleus, and the lower its energy. The possible values of n range from 1 to ∞, although the MCAT only tests on n-values up to 7.

BRIDGE

Recall from Chapter 1 of *MCAT General Chemistry Review* that quantum numbers describe the location of an electron within an atom and that each electron has a unique combination of quantum numbers according to the Pauli exclusion principle.

Within each electron shell, there can be several subshells. Subshells are described by the **azimuthal quantum number, *l***, which ranges from 0 to $n - 1$ for a given energy shell. The l-values 0, 1, 2, and 3 correspond to the *s*, *p*, *d*, and *f* subshells, respectively. Just as with the principal quantum number, energy increases as the azimuthal quantum number increases.

Within each subshell, there may be several orbitals. Orbitals are described by the **magnetic quantum number, m_l**, which ranges from $-l$ to $+l$ for a given subshell. Each type of atomic orbital has a specific shape, which describes the probability of finding an electron in a given region of space. An **s-orbital** is spherical and symmetrical, centered around the nucleus. A ***p*-orbital** is composed of two lobes located symmetrically about the nucleus and contains a **node**—an area where the probability of finding an electron is zero—at the nucleus. Picture the *p*-orbital as a dumbbell that can be positioned in three different orientations, along the *x*-, *y*-, or *z*-axis. It should make sense that there are three *p*-orbitals; the *p* subshell has the l-value of 1, so there are three possible values for m_l: -1, 0, and 1. The shapes of the first five *s*- and *p*-orbitals are shown in Figure 3.1. A ***d*-orbital** is composed of four symmetrical lobes and contains two nodes. Four of the *d*-orbitals are clover-shaped, and the fifth looks like a donut wrapped around the center of a *p*-orbital. Thankfully, the multiple complex shapes of *d*- and *f*-orbitals are rarely encountered in organic chemistry. Each orbital can hold two electrons, which are distinguished by the **spin quantum number, m_s**. The only values of m_s are $\pm\frac{1}{2}$.

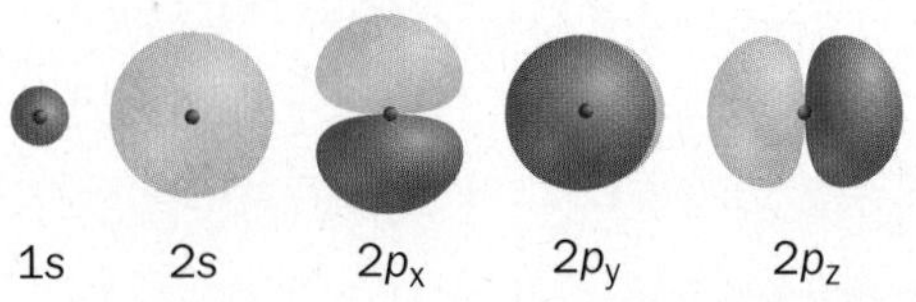

Figure 3.1 The First Five Atomic Orbitals

MCAT CONCEPT CHECK 3.1

Before you move on, assess your understanding of the material with this question.

1. Summarize the quantum numbers below. The first entry has been completed for clarification.

Symbol	Name	Describes...	Organizational Level	Possible Values
n	Principal QN	Size	Shell	1 to ∞
l				
m_l				
m_s				

3.2 Molecular Orbitals

LEARNING OBJECTIVES

After Chapter 3.2, you will be able to:

- Describe the stability and energy of bonding and antibonding orbitals
- Explain how the addition of a double or triple bond affects the electron density and molecular orbitals within a molecule
- Order the different orbital types based on strength

When two atomic orbitals combine, they form **molecular orbitals**. Molecular orbitals are obtained mathematically by adding or subtracting the wave functions of the atomic orbitals. While the mathematics of combining wave functions is outside the scope of the MCAT, some questions may ask for the visualization of molecular orbitals, as shown in Figure 3.2. If the signs of the wave functions are the same, a lower-energy (more stable) **bonding orbital** is produced. If the signs are different, a higher-energy (less stable) **antibonding orbital** is produced.

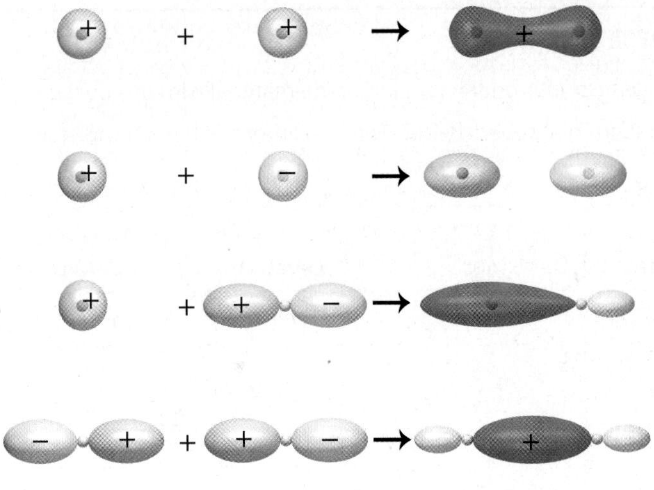

Figure 3.2 Molecular Orbitals

Molecular orbitals can be bonding or antibonding, depending on the signs of the atomic orbitals used to form them; head-to-head or tail-to-tail overlap of atomic orbitals results in a σ bond.

KEY CONCEPT

Sigma (σ) bonds are formed by head-to-head or tail-to-tail overlap of atomic orbitals. These bonds are by far the most common in organic compounds and on the MCAT.

σ and π Bonds

When a molecular orbital is formed by head-to-head or tail-to-tail overlap, as in Figure 3.2, the resulting bond is called a **sigma (σ) bond**. All **single bonds** are σ bonds, accommodating two electrons.

When two *p*-orbitals line up in a parallel (side-by-side) fashion, their electron clouds overlap, and a bonding molecular orbital, called a **pi (π) bond**, is formed. This is demonstrated in Figure 3.3. One π bond on top of an existing σ bond is a **double bond**. A σ bond and two π bonds form a **triple bond**. Unlike single bonds, which allow free rotation of atoms around the bond axis, double and triple bonds hinder rotation and, in effect, lock the atoms into position.

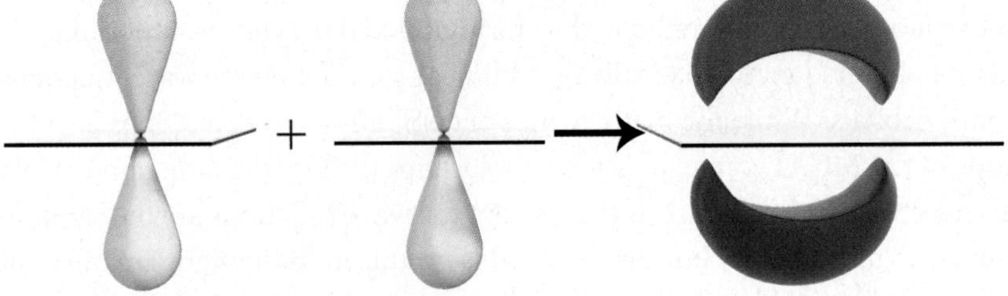

Figure 3.3 Pi (π) Bond

Electron density exists above and below the plane of the molecule, restricting rotation about a double bond.

It is important to remember that a π bond cannot exist independently of a σ bond. Only after the formation of a σ bond will the *p*-orbitals of adjacent carbons be parallel and in position to form the π bond. The more bonds that are formed between atoms, the shorter the overall bond length. Therefore, a double bond is shorter than a single bond, and a triple bond is shorter than a double bond. Shorter bonds hold atoms more closely together and are stronger than longer bonds; shorter bonds require more energy to break.

While double bonds are stronger than single bonds overall, individual π bonds are weaker than σ bonds. Therefore, it is possible to break only one of the bonds in a double bond, leaving a single bond intact. This happens often in organic chemistry, such as when *cis–trans* isomers are interconverted between conformations. Breaking a single bond requires far more energy.

As discussed previously, double and triple bonds do not freely rotate like single bonds. As such, double bonds in compounds make for stiffer molecules. Partial double-bond character in structures with resonance also restricts free rotation, resulting in more rigid structures. Proteins exhibit this kind of limited rotation because there is resonance in the amide linkages between adjacent amino acids.

KEY CONCEPT

A double bond consists of both a σ bond and a π bond; a triple bond consists of a σ bond and two π bonds. π bonds are weaker than σ bonds, but the strength is additive, making double and triple bonds stronger overall than single bonds.

MCAT CONCEPT CHECK 3.2

Before you move on, assess your understanding of the material with these questions.

1. Which is more stable: a bonding orbital or an antibonding orbital? Which has higher energy?
   - More stable:

   ____

   - Higher energy:

   ____

2. What differences would be observed in a molecule containing a double bond compared to the same molecule containing only single bonds?

   ____

3. Rank the following orbitals in decreasing order of strength: σ bond, π bond, double bond, triple bond.

   __________ > __________ > __________ > __________.

3.3 Hybridization

LEARNING OBJECTIVES

After Chapter 3.3, you will be able to:

- Recall the percentage of *s* character present in a given hybridization level, such as sp^2
- Describe the relationship between electron density and resonance structures
- Identify the hybridization of an atom within a complex molecule:

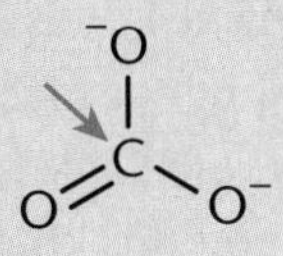

Carbon has the electron configuration $1s^22s^22p^2$ and therefore needs four electrons to complete its octet ($2s^22p^6$). A typical molecule formed by carbon is methane, CH_4. Experimentation shows that the four σ bonds in methane are equivalent. This may seem inconsistent with what we know about the asymmetrical distribution of carbon's valence electrons: two electrons in the 2*s*-orbital, one in the p_x-orbital, one in the p_y-orbital, and none in the p_z-orbital. This apparent discrepancy is accounted for by the theory of orbital **hybridization**.

sp^3

Hybrid orbitals are formed by mixing different types of orbitals. Just as with molecular orbitals, we can use advanced mathematics to merge three *p*-orbitals and one *s*-orbital. The result? As shown in Figure 3.4, this forms four identical sp^3 orbitals with new, hybridized shapes.

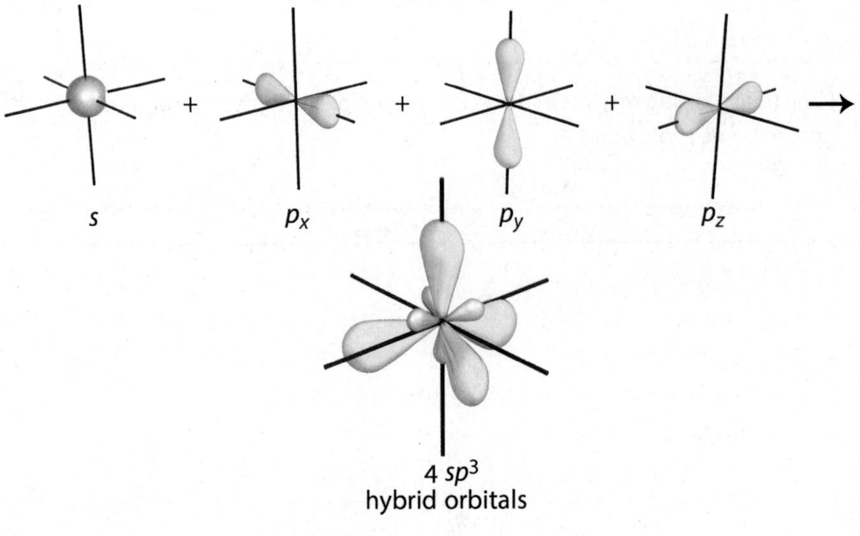

Figure 3.4 sp^3-Hybridized Orbitals
An atom with these orbitals has tetrahedral geometry, and there are no unhybridized p-orbitals to form π bonds.

All four of these orbitals point toward the vertices of a tetrahedron to minimize repulsion, which explains why carbon prefers tetrahedral geometry. The hybridization is accomplished by promoting one of the 2*s* electrons into the $2p_z$-orbital, as shown in Figure 3.5. This produces four valence orbitals, each with one electron, which can be mathematically mixed to model the hybrid orbitals.

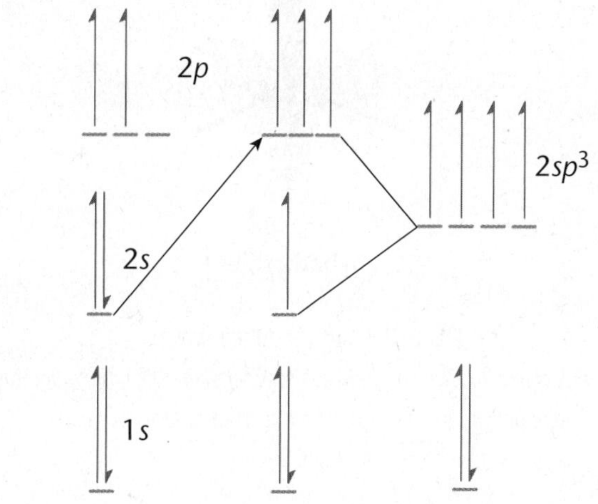

Figure 3.5 Hybridization of Carbon Orbitals

KEY CONCEPT

Hybridization is a way of making all of the bonds to a central atom equivalent to each other. The sp^3 orbitals are the reason for the tetrahedral shape that is a hallmark of carbon-containing compounds.

The MCAT sometimes tests how much "*s* character" a certain hybrid orbital has. To answer such questions, we simply need to determine what type of hybridization exists and use the name to solve the problem. For example, in sp^3 orbitals, we have one *s*- and three *p*-orbitals, so the bond has 25% *s* character and 75% *p* character.

sp^2

Although carbon is most often bonded with sp^3 hybridization, there are two other possibilities. When one *s*-orbital is mixed with two *p*-orbitals, three sp^2-hybridized orbitals are formed, as shown in Figure 3.6. These orbitals have 33% *s* character and 67% *p* character.

This is the hybridization seen in alkenes. The third *p*-orbital of each carbon is left unhybridized. This is the orbital that participates in the π bond. The three sp^2 orbitals are oriented 120° apart, which allows for maximum separation. We know that the unhybridized *p*-orbital is involved in the π component of the double bond, but what about the hybrid orbitals? In ethene, two of the sp^2 hybridized orbitals will participate in C—H bonds, and the other hybrid orbital will line up with the π bond and form the σ component of the C=C double bond.

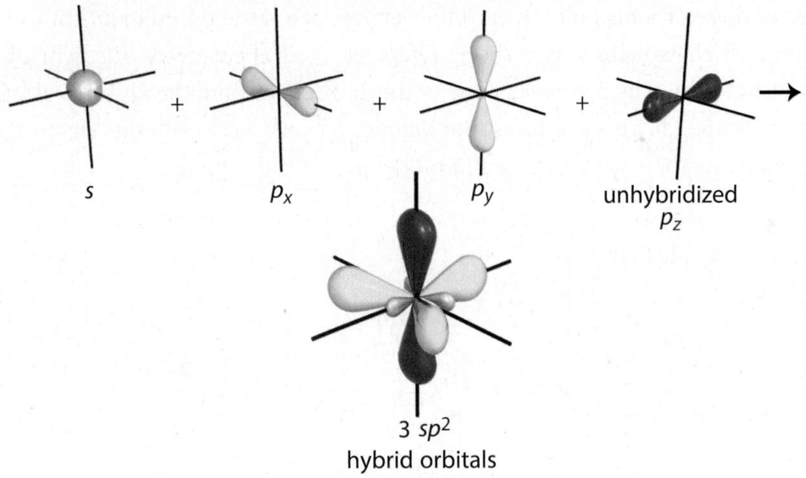

Figure 3.6 sp^2-Hybridized Orbitals
A molecule with these orbitals has trigonal planar geometry, and the one unhybridized p-orbital can be used to form a π bond.

sp

To form a triple bond, we need two of the *p*-orbitals to form π bonds, and the third *p*-orbital will combine with the *s*-orbital to form two *sp*-orbitals, as shown in Figure 3.7. These orbitals have 50% *s* character and 50% *p* character. These orbitals are oriented 180° apart, which explains the linear structure of molecules containing *sp*-hybridized carbons. The two π bonds can be between the carbon and one other atom (forming a triple bond, like ethyne), or between the carbon and two different atoms (forming two double bonds in a row, like carbon dioxide). In both cases, the molecule is linear about the *sp*-hybridized carbon.

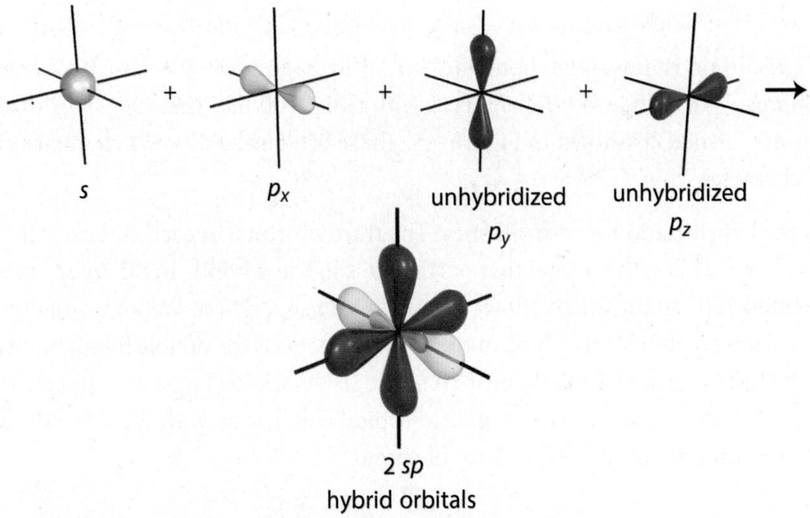

Figure 3.7 *sp*-Hybridized Orbitals
A molecule with these orbitals has linear geometry, and the two unhybridized p-orbitals can be used to form π bonds.

Resonance

Resonance delocalization of electrons occurs in molecules that have conjugated bonds. **Conjugation** requires alternating single and multiple bonds because this pattern aligns a number of unhybridized *p*-orbitals down the backbone of the molecule. π electrons can then delocalize through this *p*-orbital system, adding stability to the molecule. Resonance structures are drawn as the various transient forms the molecule takes, as shown in Figure 3.8.

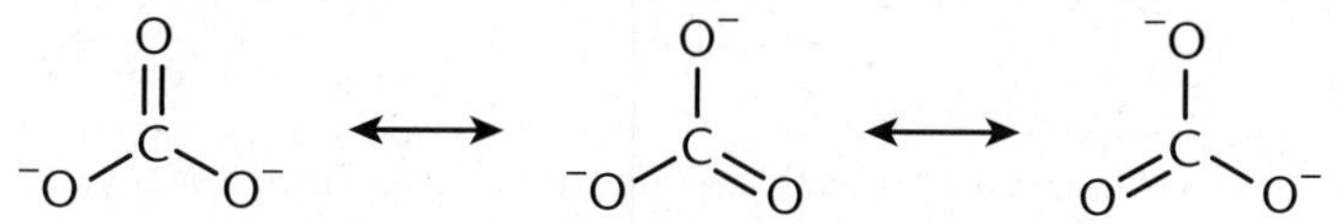

Figure 3.8 Resonance Forms of Carbonate
These forms have equal stability and therefore contribute equally to the true electron density of the molecule.

However, these forms aren't in any sort of equilibrium—the electron density is distributed throughout, making the true form a hybrid of the resonance structures, as shown with ozone in Figure 3.9.

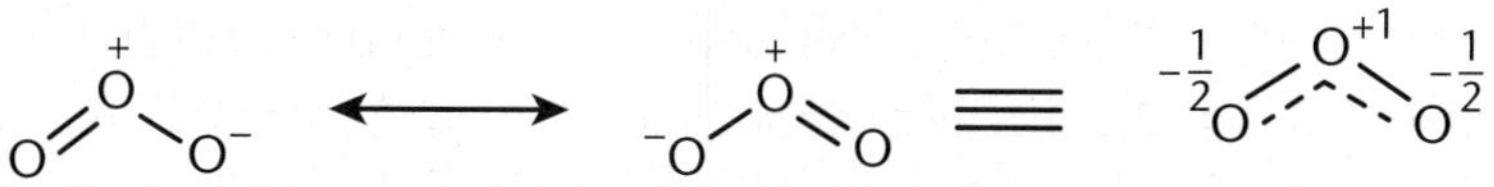

Figure 3.9 Structure of Ozone
The true electron density of ozone is somewhere between the two resonance forms, creating 1.5 bonds between each oxygen, and leaving each oxygen with a $-\frac{1}{2}$ *charge.*

If the stability of the various resonance forms differs, then the true electron density will favor the most stable form. Particular resonance structures can be favored because they lack formal charges or form full octets on highly electronegative atoms, like oxygen and nitrogen. Stabilization of positive and negative charges through induction and aromaticity can also favor certain resonance structures.

MCAT CONCEPT CHECK 3.3

Before you move on, assess your understanding of the material with these questions.

1. What is the *s* character of *sp*-, sp^2-, and sp^3-hybridized orbitals?
    - *sp*: ______________________
    - sp^2: ______________________
    - sp^3: ______________________
2. What are resonance structures? How does the true electron density of a compound relate to its resonance structures?

    ____

Conclusion

The ability of carbon to form single, double, and triple bonds (or to form σ and multiple π bonds) and to form hybrid orbitals gives rise to an entire branch of chemistry—as well as life on Earth. You may have thought this chapter was a bit brief; that's because the specifics of bonding fall mostly under the domain of general chemistry. However, without a solid grasp of orbitals and bonding, it would be difficult to explain the organic reactions that are tested on the MCAT, which will be the focus of the next seven chapters. Avoid compartmentalizing the information you learn throughout the course of your studies, as bonding plays a role in general chemistry, organic chemistry, and biochemistry, and can therefore be tested in either the *Chemical and Physical Foundations of Biological Systems* section or the *Biological and Biochemical Foundations of Living Systems* section. All of the subjects within science blend together into a seemingly complicated, yet beautifully simple, picture of the universe. The sooner you integrate the knowledge you're accumulating, the more manageable and rewarding your studying will become.

You've reviewed the content, now test your knowledge and critical thinking skills by completing a test-like passage set in your online resources!

GO ONLINE

CONCEPT SUMMARY

Atomic Orbitals and Quantum Numbers

- **Quantum numbers** describe the size, shape, orientation, and number of **atomic orbitals** an element possesses.
- The **principal quantum number, *n***, describes the energy level (shell) in which an electron resides and indicates the distance from the nucleus to the electron. Its possible values range from 1 to ∞.
- The **azimuthal quantum number, *l***, determines the subshell in which an electron resides. Its possible values range from 0 to $n - 1$. The subshell is often indicated with a letter: $l = 0$ corresponds to *s*, 1 is *p*, 2 is *d*, and 3 is *f*.
- The **magnetic quantum number, m_l**, determines the orbital in which an electron resides. Its possible values range from $-l$ to $+l$. Different orbitals have different shapes: *s*-orbitals are spherical, while *p*-orbitals are dumbbell-shaped and located on the *x*-, *y*-, or *z*-axis.
- The **spin quantum number, m_s**, describes the spin of an electron. Its possible values are $\pm\frac{1}{2}$.

Molecular Orbitals

- **Bonding orbitals** are created by head-to-head or tail-to-tail overlap of atomic orbitals of the same sign and are energetically favorable.
- **Antibonding orbitals** are created by head-to-head or tail-to-tail overlap of atomic orbitals that have opposite signs and are energetically unfavorable.
- **Single bonds** are **sigma (σ) bonds**, which contain two electrons.
- **Double bonds** contain one σ bond and one **pi (π) bond**. π bonds are created by sharing of electrons between two unhybridized *p*-orbitals that align side-by-side.
- **Triple bonds** contain one σ bond and two π bonds.
- Multiple bonds are less flexible than single bonds because rotation is not permitted in the presence of a π bond. Multiple bonds are shorter and stronger than single bonds, although individual π bonds are weaker than σ bonds.

Hybridization

- ***sp^3***-hybridized orbitals have 25% *s* character and 75% *p* character. They form tetrahedral geometry with 109.5° bond angles. Carbons with all single bonds are sp^3-hybridized.
- ***sp^2***-hybridized orbitals have 33% *s* character and 67% *p* character. They form trigonal planar geometry with 120° bond angles. Carbons with one double bond are sp^2-hybridized.
- ***sp***-hybridized orbitals have 50% *s* character and 50% *p* character. They form linear geometry with 180° bond angles. Carbons with a triple bond, or with two double bonds, are *sp*-hybridized.

- **Resonance** describes the delocalization of electrons in molecules that have conjugated bonds.
  - **Conjugation** occurs when single and multiple bonds alternate, creating a system of unhybridized *p*-orbitals down the backbone of the molecule through which π electrons can delocalize.
  - Resonance increases the stability of a molecule.
  - The various resonance forms all contribute to the true electron density of the molecule; the more stable the resonance form, the more it contributes. Resonance forms are favored if they lack formal charge, form full octets on electronegative atoms, or stabilize charges through induction and aromaticity.

ANSWERS TO CONCEPT CHECKS

3.1

1.

Symbol	Name	Describes...	Organizational Level	Possible Values
n	Principal QN	Size	Shell	1 to ∞
l	Azimuthal QN	Shape	Subshell	0 to $n - 1$
m_l	Magnetic QN	Orientation	Orbital	$-l$ to $+l$
m_s	Spin QN	Spin	—	$\pm\frac{1}{2}$

3.2

1. Bonding orbitals are more stable than antibonding orbitals. Therefore, antibonding orbitals have higher energy than bonding orbitals.
2. The differences would be in bond length (shorter in double bond than single), bond energy (higher in double bond than single), and molecular rigidity (higher in double bond than single).
3. Triple bond > double bond > σ bond > π bond. Remember that while an individual π bond is weaker than a σ bond, bond strength is additive. Therefore, double bonds are stronger than single, and triple bonds are stronger still.

3.3

1. *sp* orbitals have 50% *s* character and 50% *p* character, sp^2 orbitals have 33% *s* character and 67% *p* character, and sp^3 orbitals have 25% *s* character and 75% *p* character.
2. Resonance structures differ in their placement of electrons in hybridized *p*-orbitals and require bond conjugation to delocalize electrons in a molecule. The true electron density is a weighted average of the resonance structures of a given compound, favoring the most stable structures.

SCIENCE MASTERY ASSESSMENT EXPLANATIONS

1. **A**

The energies of the subshells within a principal quantum number are as follows: $s < p < d < f$

2. **D**

All single bonds are σ bonds; double and triple bonds each contain one σ bond and one or two π bonds, respectively. The compounds CH_4, C_2H_2, and C_2H_4 all contain at least one single bond and therefore contain at least one σ bond.

3. **B**

In a carbon with one double bond, sp^2 hybridization occurs—that is, one *s*-orbital hybridizes with two *p*-orbitals to form three sp^2-hybridized orbitals. The third *p*-orbital of the carbon atom remains unhybridized and takes part in the formation of the π bond of the double bond. Although there is an unhybridized *p*-orbital, there are no unhybridized *s*-orbitals, eliminating **(D)**.

4. **D**

The carbon and nitrogen atoms are connected by a triple bond in CN^- ($:C{\equiv}N:^-$). A triple-bonded atom is *sp* hybridized; one *s*-orbital hybridizes with one *p*-orbital to form two *sp*-hybridized orbitals. The two remaining unhybridized *p*-orbitals take part in the formation of two π bonds.

5. **A**

Beryllium has only two electrons in its valence shell. When it bonds to two hydrogens, it requires two hybridized orbitals, meaning that its hybridization must be *sp*. Note that the presence of only single bonds does not mean that the hybridization must be sp^3; this is a useful assumption for carbon, but does not apply to beryllium because of its smaller number of valence electrons. The two unhybridized *p*-orbitals around beryllium are empty in BeH_2, which takes on the linear geometry characteristic of *sp*-hybridized orbitals.

6. **D**

When atomic orbitals combine, they form molecular orbitals. When two atomic orbitals with the same sign are added head-to-head or tail-to-tail, they form bonding molecular orbitals. When two atomic orbitals with opposite signs are added head-to-head or tail-to-tail, they form antibonding molecular orbitals. Atomic orbitals can also hybridize, forming sp^3, sp^2, or *sp* orbitals.

7. **B**

Like atomic orbitals, molecular orbitals each can contain a maximum of two electrons with opposite spins. The $2n^2$ rule in **(D)** refers to the total number of electrons that can exist in a given energy shell, not in a molecular orbital.

8. **B**

π bonds are formed by the parallel overlap of unhybridized *p*-orbitals. The electron density is concentrated above and below the bonding axis. A σ bond, on the other hand, can be formed by the head-to-head overlap of two *s*-orbitals or hybridized orbitals. In a σ bond, the density of the electrons is concentrated between the two nuclei of the bonding atoms.

9. **A**

Each single bond has one σ bond, and each double bond has one σ and one π bond. In this question, there are five single bonds (five σ bonds) and one double bond (one σ bond and one π bond), which gives a total of six σ bonds and one π bond. Thus, the correct answer is **(A)**.

10. **C**

The four bonds point to the vertices of a tetrahedron, which means that the angle between two bonds is 109.5°, a characteristic of sp^3 orbitals. Hence, the carbon atom of CH_4 is sp^3-hybridized.

11. **B**

Bond strength is determined by the degree of orbital overlap; the greater the overlap, the greater the bond strength. A π bond is weaker than a single bond because there is significantly less overlap between the unhybridized *p*-orbitals of a π bond (due to their parallel orientation) than between the *s*-orbitals or hybrid orbitals of a σ bond. sp^3-hybridized orbitals can be quite stable, as evidenced by the number of carbon atoms with this hybridization forming stable compounds.

12. **B**

The carbon bond in hydrogen cyanide (H–C≡N:) is triple-bonded, and because triple bonds require two unhybridized *p*-orbitals, the carbon must be *sp*-hybridized; *sp*-hybridized orbitals have 50% *s* character and 50% *p* character.

13. **B**

A resonance structure describes an arrangement of electrons in a molecule. Different resonance structures can be derived by moving electrons in unhybridized *p*-orbitals throughout a molecule containing conjugated bonds. In molecules that contain multiple resonance structures, some are usually more stable than others; however, each resonance structure is not necessarily the most common form a molecule takes, eliminating statement III. Statement I has reversed the terminology for resonance structures: the electron density in a molecule is the weighted average of all possible resonance structures, not the other way around.

14. **D**

An electron in the $n = 4$ shell and the $l = 2$ subshell can have five different values for m_l: $-2, -1, 0, 1$, or 2. In each of these orbitals, electrons can have positive or negative spin. Thus, there are $5 \times 2 = 10$ possible combinations of quantum numbers for this electron.

15. **D**

π bonds do not permit free rotation, unlike σ bonds; this makes triple bonds more rigid than single bonds. Triple bonds are stronger and shorter bonds than single bonds, eliminating **(A)** and **(B)**. Both single and triple bonds contain one σ bond, eliminating **(C)**.

Consult your online resources for additional practice. **GO ONLINE**

SHARED CONCEPTS

Biochemistry Chapter 1
Amino Acids, Peptides, and Proteins

General Chemistry Chapter 1
Atomic Structure

General Chemistry Chapter 3
Bonding and Chemical Interactions

General Chemistry Chapter 4
Compounds and Stoichiometry

Organic Chemistry Chapter 2
Isomers

Organic Chemistry Chapter 11
Spectroscopy

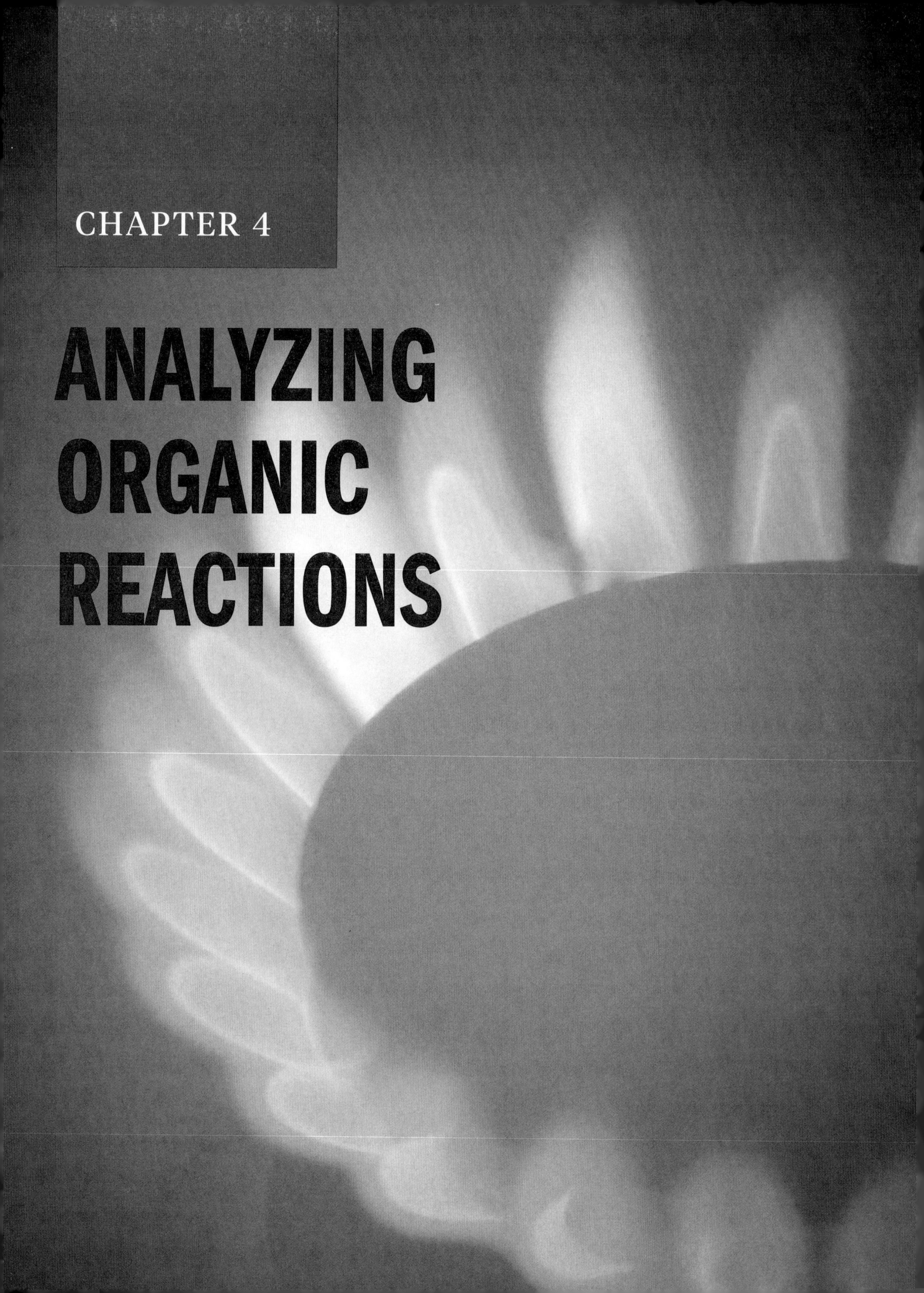

CHAPTER 4

ANALYZING ORGANIC REACTIONS

SCIENCE MASTERY ASSESSMENT

Every pre-med knows this feeling: there is so much content I have to know for the MCAT! How do I know what to do first or what's important?

While the high-yield badges throughout this book will help you identify the most important topics, this Science Mastery Assessment is another tool in your MCAT prep arsenal. This quiz (which can also be taken in your online resources) and the guidance below will help ensure that you are spending the appropriate amount of time on this chapter based on your personal strengths and weaknesses. Don't worry though—skipping something now does not mean you'll never study it. Later on in your prep, as you complete full-length tests, you'll uncover specific pieces of content that you need to review and can come back to these chapters as appropriate.

How to Use This Assessment

If you answer 0–7 questions correctly:

Spend about 1 hour to read this chapter in full and take limited notes throughout. Follow up by reviewing **all** quiz questions to ensure that you now understand how to solve each one.

If you answer 8–11 questions correctly:

Spend 20–40 minutes reviewing the quiz questions. Beginning with the questions you missed, read and take notes on the corresponding subchapters. For questions you answered correctly, ensure your thinking matches that of the explanation and you understand why each choice was correct or incorrect.

If you answer 12–15 questions correctly:

Spend less than 20 minutes reviewing all questions from the quiz. If you missed any, then include a quick read-through of the corresponding subchapters, or even just the relevant content within a subchapter, as part of your question review. For questions you got correct, ensure your thinking matches that of the explanation and review the Concept Summary at the end of the chapter.

1. Which of the following are Lewis bases?
   I. Ag^+
   II. H_2O
   III. NH_3

   A. I only
   B. I and II only
   C. II and III only
   D. I, II, and III

2. Rank the following in order of decreasing nucleophilicity in an aprotic solvent: RO^-, RCOOH, ROH, HO^-
   A. RCOOH > ROH > RO^- > HO^-
   B. HO^- > ROH > RO^- > RCOOH
   C. RO^- > HO^- > ROH > RCOOH
   D. RCOOH > RO^- > HO^- > ROH

3. Rank the following in order of decreasing electrophilicity: CR_3^+, CH_3OH, CH_3OCH_3, CH_3Cl
   A. $CH_3OCH_3 > CR_3^+ > CH_3OH > CH_3Cl$
   B. $CR_3^+ > CH_3OH > CH_3OCH_3 > CH_3Cl$
   C. $CH_3OCH_3 > CH_3Cl > CR_3^+ > CH_3OH$
   D. $CR_3^+ > CH_3Cl > CH_3OH > CH_3OCH_3$

4. Rank the following in order of decreasing leaving group ability: H_2O, HO^-, Br^-, H^-
   A. $H_2O > Br^- > HO^- > H^-$
   B. $H_2O > HO^- > Br^- > H^-$
   C. $HO^- > Br^- > H_2O > H^-$
   D. $HO^- > H^- > H_2O > Br^-$

5. Rank the following in order of decreasing oxidation state: amine, carboxylic acid, aldehyde, alkane
   A. Aldehyde, amine, alkane, carboxylic acid
   B. Carboxylic acid, aldehyde, amine, alkane
   C. Carboxylic acid, amine, aldehyde, alkane
   D. Alkane, amine, aldehyde, carboxylic acid

6. The last step in the Grignard reaction is acidification, in which the alkoxide ion is protonated to form the final alcohol product. During this reaction, the alkoxide ion acts as a:
   A. Lewis base only
   B. Brønsted–Lowry base and Lewis base
   C. Brønsted–Lowry base and Lewis acid
   D. Brønsted–Lowry base only

7. If 2-butanol was treated with dichromate, what reaction would occur?
   A. Reduction, resulting in the formation of butene
   B. Oxidation, resulting in the formation of butanoic acid
   C. Oxidation, resulting in the formation of butanone
   D. No reaction would occur.

8. If 1-hexanol was treated with pyridinium chlorochromate, what would the end product be?
   A. 2-Hexanol
   B. 2-Hexanone
   C. Hexanal
   D. Hexanoic acid

9. S_N1 reactions show first-order kinetics because:
   A. the rate-limiting step is the first step to occur in the reaction.
   B. the rate-limiting step involves only one molecule.
   C. there is only one rate-limiting step.
   D. the reaction involves only one molecule.

10. In a protic solvent, which of the following halogens would be the best nucleophile?
    A. Br^-
    B. Cl^-
    C. F^-
    D. I^-

11. Which of the compounds below can undergo oxidation by PCC?

    A. 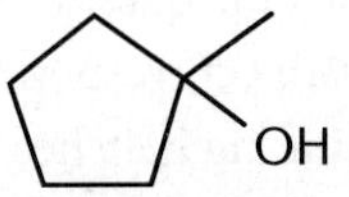

    B. 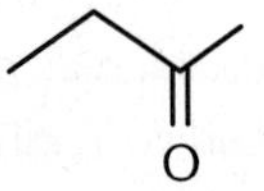

    C. 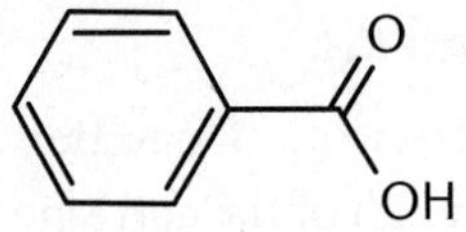

    D. 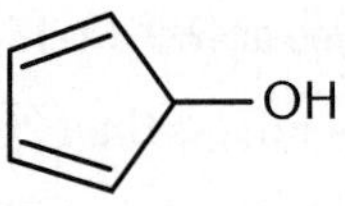

12. Which of the following substrates would most rapidly undergo an S_N2 reaction when paired with an appropriate nucleophile?

A. 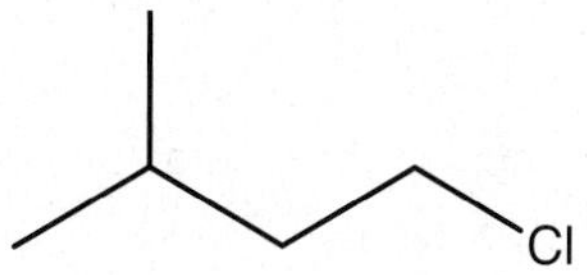

B. 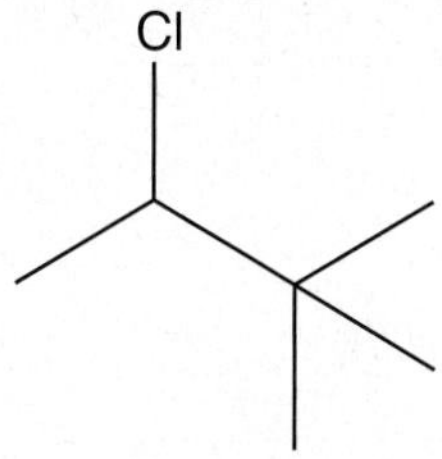

C. 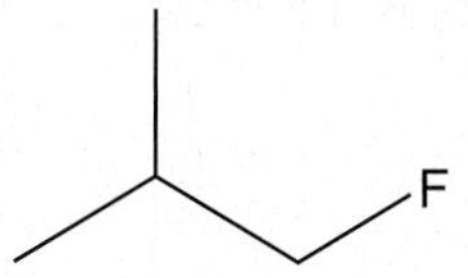

D. 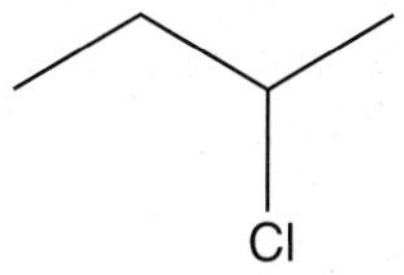

13. Which of the following solvents would be LEAST useful for a nucleophile–electrophile reaction?
   - **A.** H_2O
   - **B.** CH_3CH_2OH
   - **C.** CH_3SOCH_3
   - **D.** $CH_3CH_2CH_2CH_2CH_2CH_3$

14. Aldehydes are generally more reactive than equivalent ketones to nucleophiles. This is likely due to differences in:
   - **A.** steric hindrance.
   - **B.** leaving group ability.
   - **C.** resonance stabilization.
   - **D.** electron-withdrawing character.

15. Which conversion between carboxylic acid derivatives is NOT possible by a nucleophilic reaction?
   - **A.** Carboxylic acid to ester
   - **B.** Ester to carboxylic acid
   - **C.** Anhydride to amide
   - **D.** Ester to anhydride

Answer Key

1. **C**
2. **C**
3. **D**
4. **A**
5. **B**
6. **B**
7. **C**
8. **C**
9. **B**
10. **D**
11. **D**
12. **A**
13. **D**
14. **A**
15. **D**

Detailed explanations can be found at the end of the chapter.

CHAPTER 4

ANALYZING ORGANIC REACTIONS

In This Chapter

CHAPTER PROFILE

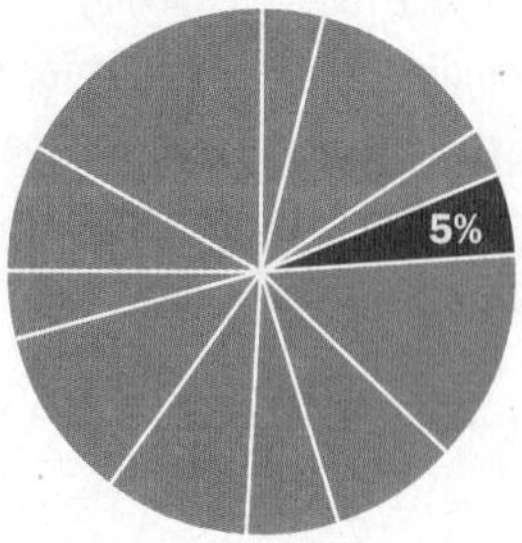

The content in this chapter should be relevant to about 5% of all questions about organic chemistry on the MCAT.

This chapter covers material from the following AAMC content categories:

1A: Structure and function of proteins and their constituent amino acids

4E: Atoms, nuclear decay, electronic structure, and atomic chemical behavior

5A: Unique nature of water and its solutions

5D: Structure, function, and reactivity of biologically-relevant molecules

Introduction

Sitting down to solve MCAT organic chemistry problems can be overwhelming at first, particularly if the reactants or reagents are new to you. The reactions on the page may seem like stage magic—fun to watch, but controlled by forces outside of our knowledge. The good news, however, is that organic chemistry isn't magic—and it is governed by sets of rules that make understanding what will happen much simpler. In this chapter, we will go over several of the aspects that determine how a complex reaction proceeds and take a brief look at functional group reactivity. Then, armed with this knowledge, we lay out the simple, sequential steps that we can use to determine which reactions will take place. Chapters 5 through 10 of *MCAT Organic Chemistry Review* focus on applications of these principles with different functional groups, so look for patterns between these reactions as you continue preparing for Test Day. With these tools in hand, you can show the MCAT that you know how the trick is done—it isn't magic.

MCAT EXPERTISE

This chapter is vital for understanding all the reactions you'll see in the next six chapters of this book (Chapters 5-10). On top of that, this material is directly tested on the MCAT as often as any other topic in organic chemistry. Make sure you know all of it!

4.1 Acids and Bases

LEARNING OBJECTIVES

After Chapter 4.1, you will be able to:

- Recall the importance of amphoteric species and common amphoteric molecules
- Describe the meaning of pK_a and pK_b values in relation to acid and base strength
- Recall common functional groups that act as acids or bases

KEY CONCEPT

An acid-base reaction will only proceed if the products that will be formed (the conjugate base of the acid and the conjugate acid of the base) are weaker than the original reactants.

In an acid–base reaction, an acid and a base react, resulting in the formation of the conjugate base of the acid and the conjugate acid of the base. This reaction proceeds so long as the reactants are more reactive, or stronger, than the products that they form. We will discuss acid and base definitions and strength in the following section. For the MCAT, we will concern ourselves with the broader Lewis and Brønsted–Lowry definitions of acids and bases. The Lewis definition concerns itself with the transfer of electrons in the formation of coordinate covalent bonds; the Brønsted–Lowry definition focuses on proton transfer.

Definitions

BRIDGE

Acids and bases are critically important material in organic chemistry, biochemistry, and general chemistry. The most extensive coverage of acids and bases is in Chapter 10 of *MCAT General Chemistry Review*.

A **Lewis acid** is defined as an **electron acceptor** in the formation of a covalent bond. Lewis acids also tend to be electrophiles, which wc will touch on in the next section. Lewis acids have vacant *p*-orbitals into which they can accept an electron pair, or are positively polarized atoms.

A **Lewis base** is defined as an **electron donor** in the formation of a covalent bond. Lewis bases also tend to be nucleophiles, which we will touch on in the next section. Lewis bases have a lone pair of electrons that can be donated, and are often anions, carrying a negative charge.

When Lewis acids and bases interact, they form **coordinate covalent bonds**—covalent bonds in which both electrons in the bond came from the same starting atom (the Lewis base), as shown in Figure 4.1.

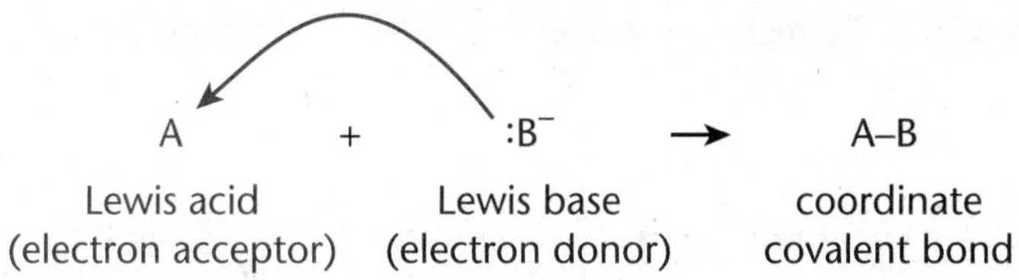

Figure 4.1 Lewis Acid-Base Reactions

In the **Brønsted–Lowry** definition, an acid is a species that can donate a proton (H^+); a base is a species that can accept a proton. Some molecules, like water, have the ability to act as either Brønsted–Lowry acids or bases, making them **amphoteric**. Water can act as an acid by donating its proton to a base, and thus becoming its conjugate base, OH^-. However, water can also act as a base by accepting a proton from an acid to become its conjugate acid, H_3O^+. The degree to which a molecule acts as an acid or a base is dependent upon the properties of the solution—water can only act as a base in an acidic solution, and only as an acid in a basic solution. Other examples of amphoteric molecules include $Al(OH)_3$, HCO_3^-, and HSO_4^-.

Acid and Base Strength

The **acid dissociation constant**, or K_a, measures the strength of an acid in solution. In the dissociation of an acid HA ($HA \rightleftharpoons H^+ + A^-$), the equilibrium constant is given by:

$$K_a = \frac{[H^+][A^-]}{[HA]}$$

Equation 4.1

and the pK_a can be calculated as:

$$pK_a = -\log K_a$$

Equation 4.2

Thus, more acidic molecules will have a smaller (or even negative) pK_a; more basic molecules will have a larger pK_a. Acids with a pK_a below −2 are considered strong acids, which almost always dissociate completely in aqueous solution. Weak organic acids often have p*K*a values between −2 and 20. pK_a values for common functional groups are shown in Table 4.1.

Functional group	Example	pK_a	Conjugate base
Alkane	$H_3CCH_2CH_2CH_3$	~50	$H_3CCH_2CH_2CH_2^{\ominus}$
Alkene	$H_2C{=}CH{-}CH_3$	~43	$H_2C{=}C^{\ominus}{-}CH_3$
Hydrogen	H– H	42	$H^{\ominus}$
Amine	NH_3	~35	$NH_2^{\ominus}$
Alkyne	R—≡—H	25	R—≡$^{\ominus}$
Ester	$H_3CO{-}C({=}O){-}CH_3$	25	$H_3CO{-}C({=}O){-}CH_2^{\ominus}$
Ketone/ Aldehyde	$H_3C{-}C({=}O){-}CH_3$	17–20 (ald.) 20–24 (ket.)	$H_3C{-}C({=}O){-}CH_2^{\ominus}$
Alcohol	$H_3C{-}OH$	17	$H_3C{-}O^{\ominus}$
Water	HO— H	16	$HO^{\ominus}$
Carboxylic acid	$H_3C{-}C({=}O){-}OH$	4	$H_3C{-}C({=}O){-}O^{\ominus}$
Hydronium ion	$H_3O^{\oplus}$	–1.7	H_2O

Weaker acid ↓ Stronger acid (top to bottom); Weaker base ↑ Stronger base (bottom to top)

Table 4.1 pK_a Values for Common Functional Groups

Generally, bond strength decreases down the periodic table, and acidity therefore increases. Also, the more electronegative an atom, the higher the acidity. When these two trends oppose each other, low bond strength takes precedence.

For the common functional groups on the MCAT, the α-hydrogens of carbonyl compounds deserve special note. **α-hydrogens** are connected to the **α-carbon**, which is a carbon adjacent to the carbonyl. Because the *enol* form of carbonyl-containing carbanions is stabilized by resonance, these are acidic hydrogens that are easily lost. We will go into greater depth about enolate chemistry in Chapters 7 through 9 of *MCAT Organic Chemistry Review*.

Common Functional Groups

We can also apply these acid and base rules directly to the functional groups that appear on the MCAT. Functional groups that act as acids include alcohols, aldehydes and ketones (at the α-carbon), carboxylic acids, and most carboxylic acid derivatives. These compounds are therefore easier to target with basic (or nucleophilic) reactants because they readily accept a lone pair.

Amines and amides are the main functional groups that act as bases—keep an eye out for these compounds in the formation of peptide bonds. The nitrogen atom of an amine can form coordinate covalent bonds by donating a lone pair to a Lewis acid.

MCAT CONCEPT CHECK 4.1

Before you move on, assess your understanding of the material with these questions.

1. When will an acid–base reaction proceed, based on the strength of the reactants and products?

____

2. What does it mean for a molecule to be amphoteric? What biologically relevant molecules are also characteristically amphoteric?

____

3. How is pK_a defined, and what does a low pK_a indicate?

____

4. What are some functional groups that classically act as acids? As bases?

   - Acids:

____

   - Bases:

____

4.2 Nucleophiles, Electrophiles, and Leaving Groups

LEARNING OBJECTIVES

After Chapter 4.2, you will be able to:

- Distinguish nucleophiles and electrophiles from Lewis acids and bases
- Compare nucleophilicity using the four main trends
- Describe the relationship between electrophile and leaving group in a substitution reaction
- Identify the traits that increase electrophilicity
- Recall the traits of a good leaving group

Almost all reactions in organic chemistry can be divided into one of two groups: oxidation–reduction reactions or nucleophile–electrophile reactions. Nucleophiles, electrophiles, and leaving groups are particularly important to the reactions of alcohols and carbonyl-containing compounds, which we will look at in depth in later chapters. Let's take a look at how each of these terms is defined.

Nucleophiles

Nucleophiles are defined as "nucleus-loving" species with either lone pairs or π bonds that can form new bonds to electrophiles. You may have noted that nucleophilicity and basicity appear to have similar definitions—and this is true! Good nucleophiles tend to be good bases. There is, however, a distinction between the two. Nucleophile strength is based on relative rates of reaction with a common electrophile—and is therefore a kinetic property. Base strength is related to the equilibrium position of a reaction—and is therefore a thermodynamic property. Some common examples of nucleophiles are shown in Figure 4.2.

KEY CONCEPT

Nucleophiles tend to have lone pairs or π bonds that can be used to form covalent bonds to electrophiles. On Test Day, look for carbon, hydrogen, oxygen, or nitrogen (CHON) with a minus sign or lone pair to identify most nucleophiles.

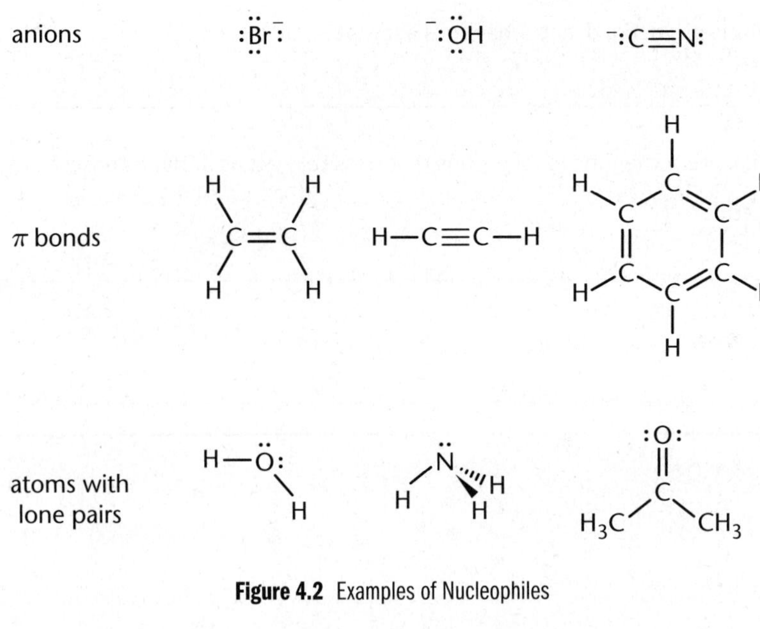

Figure 4.2 Examples of Nucleophiles

As long as the nucleophilic atom is the same, the more basic the nucleophile, the more reactive it is. This also holds when comparing atoms in the same row of the periodic table, but *not* when proceeding down a column in the periodic table. Nucleophilicity is determined by four major factors:

- **Charge:** Nucleophilicity increases with increasing electron density (more negative charge)
- **Electronegativity:** Nucleophilicity decreases as electronegativity increases because these atoms are less likely to share electron density
- **Steric hindrance:** Bulkier molecules are less nucleophilic
- **Solvent:** Protic solvents can hinder nucleophilicity by protonating the nucleophile or through hydrogen bonding

Solvent Effects

The solvent consideration is worth spending a bit more time on. In polar protic solvents, nucleophilicity increases *down* the periodic table. In polar aprotic solvents, nucleophilicity increases *up* the periodic table. Examples of both types of solvents are shown in Figure 4.3.

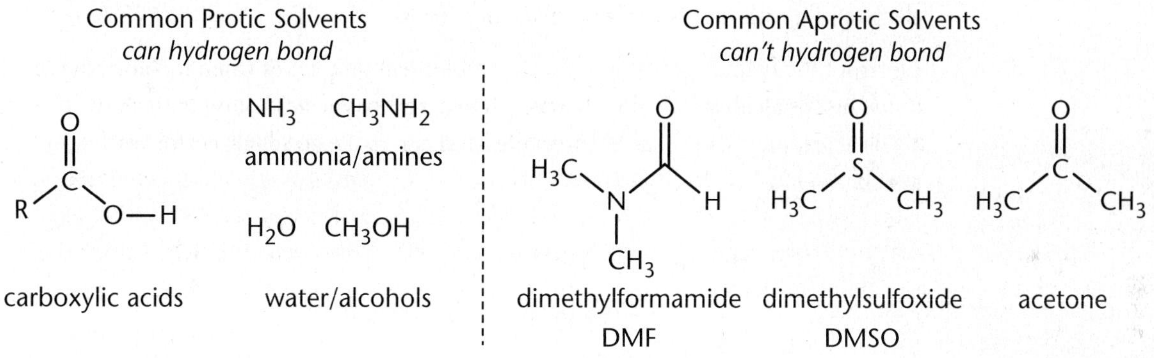

Figure 4.3 Examples of Polar Protic and Polar Aprotic Solvents

The halogens are good examples of the effects of the solvent on nucleophilicity. In protic solvents, nucleophilicity decreases in the order:

$$I^- > Br^- > Cl^- > F^-$$

This is because the protons in solution will be attracted to the nucleophile. F^- is the conjugate base of HF, a weak acid. As such, it will form bonds with the protons in solution and be less able to access the electrophile to react. I^-, on the other hand, is the conjugate base of HI, a strong acid. As such, it is less affected by the protons in solution and can react with the electrophile.

In aprotic solvents, on the other hand, nucleophilicity decreases in the order:

$$F^- > Cl^- > Br^- > I^-$$

This is because there are no protons to get in the way of the attacking nucleophile. In aprotic solvents, nucleophilicity relates directly to basicity.

MCAT EXPERTISE

If a solvent is not given on Test Day, assume that the reaction occurs in a polar solvent. Polar solvents—whether protic or aprotic—can dissolve nucleophiles and assist in any reaction in which electrons are moved. Organic chemistry is all about moving electrons, so it's less common for these reactions to be performed in nonpolar solvents.

KEY CONCEPT

We can't use nonpolar solvents in these nucleophile-electrophile reactions because our reactants are polar—they wouldn't dissolve!

We won't use nonpolar solvents with this type of reaction because we need our nucleophile to dissolve. Because charged molecules are polar by nature, a polar solvent is required to dissolve the nucleophile as well because *like dissolves like.* Examples of strong nucleophiles include HO^-, RO^-, CN^-, and N_3^-. NH_3 and RCO_2^- are fair nucleophiles, and H_2O, ROH, and RCOOH are weak or very weak nucleophiles. As far as functional groups go, amine groups tend to make good nucleophiles.

Electrophiles

Electrophiles are defined as "electron-loving" species with a positive charge or positively polarized atom that accepts an electron pair when forming new bonds with a nucleophile. Again, this definition brings to mind Lewis acids. The distinction, as with nucleophiles and bases above, is that electrophilicity is a kinetic property, whereas acidity is a thermodynamic property. Practically, however, electrophiles will almost always act as Lewis acids in reactions. A greater degree of positive charge increases electrophilicity, so a carbocation is more electrophilic than a carbonyl carbon. Some comparisons between electrophiles are drawn in Figure 4.4. Additionally, the nature of the leaving group influences electrophilicity in species without empty orbitals; better leaving groups make it more likely that a reaction will happen. If empty orbitals are present, an incoming nucleophile can make a bond with the electrophile without displacing the leaving group.

Electrophilicity and acidity are effectively identical properties when it comes to reactivity. Just as alcohols, aldehydes and ketones, carboxylic acids, and their derivatives act as acids, they also act as electrophiles and can make good targets for nucleophilic attack.

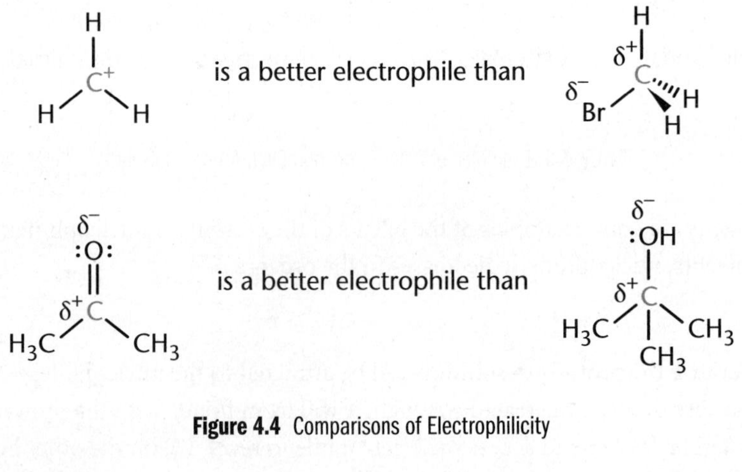

Figure 4.4 Comparisons of Electrophilicity

The carboxylic acid derivatives are often ranked by electrophilicity. Anhydrides are the most reactive, followed by carboxylic acids and esters, and then amides. In practical terms, this means that derivatives of higher reactivity can form derivatives of lower reactivity but not vice versa, similar to the acid–base reactions described previously.

Leaving Groups

Leaving groups are the molecular fragments that retain the electrons after heterolysis. **Heterolytic reactions** are essentially the opposite of coordinate covalent bond formation: a bond is broken and both electrons are given to one of the two products. The best leaving groups will be able to stabilize the extra electrons. Weak bases are more stable with an extra set of electrons and therefore make good leaving groups. By this logic, the conjugate bases of strong acids (like I^-, Br^-, and Cl^-) tend to make good leaving groups. Leaving group ability can be augmented by resonance and by inductive effects from electron-withdrawing groups: these help delocalize and stabilize negative charge.

Alkanes and hydrogen ions will almost never serve as leaving groups because they form very reactive, strongly basic anions. We can think of leaving groups and nucleophiles as serving opposite functions. In substitution reactions, the weaker base (the leaving group) is replaced by the stronger base (the nucleophile).

Nucleophilic Substitution Reactions

Nucleophilic substitution reactions are perfect examples for demonstrating nucleophile–electrophile reactions. In both S_N1 and S_N2 reactions, a nucleophile forms a bond with a substrate carbon and a leaving group leaves.

KEY CONCEPT

Just like acid-base reactions, nucleophilic attack will only occur if the reactants are more reactive than the products. Thus, the nucleophile must be more reactive than the leaving group.

S_N1 Reactions

Unimolecular nucleophilic substitution (S_N1) reactions contain two steps. The first step is the rate-limiting step in which the leaving group leaves, generating a positively charged **carbocation**. The nucleophile then attacks the carbocation, resulting in the substitution product. This mechanism is shown in Figure 4.5 below.

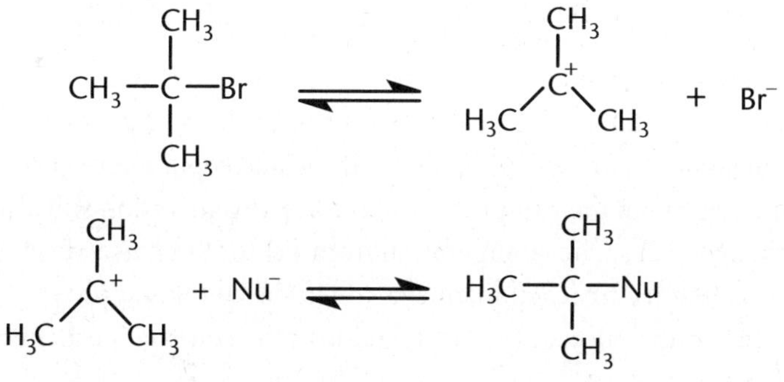

Figure 4.5 Mechanism of S_N1 Reaction
Step 1: Formation of the carbocation (rate-limiting);
Step 2: Nucleophilic attack.

The more substituted the carbocation, the more stable it is because the alkyl groups act as electron donors, stabilizing the positive charge. Because the formation of the carbocation is the rate-limiting step, the rate of the reaction depends only on the concentration of the substrate: rate $= k[R{-}L]$, where R–L is an alkyl group containing a leaving group. This is a first-order reaction; anything that accelerates the formation of the carbocation will increase the rate of an S_N1 reaction.

Because S_N1 reactions pass through a planar intermediate before the nucleophile attacks, the product will usually be a racemic mixture. The incoming nucleophile can attack the carbocation from either side, resulting in varied stereochemistry.

S_N2 Reactions

Bimolecular nucleophilic substitution (S_N2) reactions contain only one step, in which the nucleophile attacks the compound at the same time as the leaving group leaves. Because this reaction has only one step, we call it a **concerted** reaction. The reaction is called bimolecular because this single rate-limiting step involves two molecules.

In S_N2 reactions, the nucleophile actively displaces the leaving group in a **backside attack**. For this to occur, the nucleophile must be strong, and the substrate cannot be sterically hindered. Therefore, the less substituted the carbon, the more reactive it is in S_N2 reactions. Note that this is the opposite of the trend for S_N1 reactions. The one-step mechanism is shown in Figure 4.6.

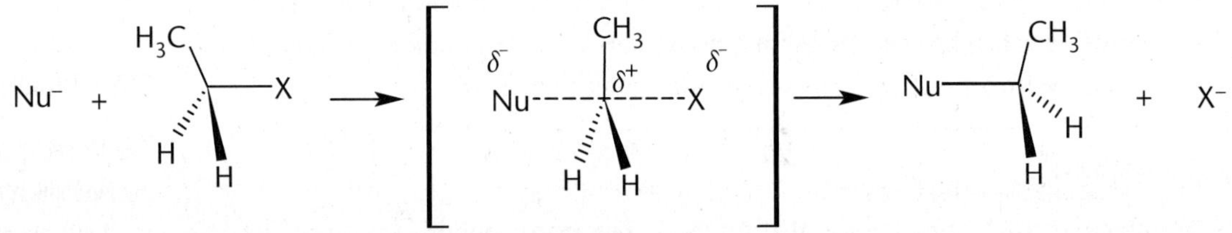

Figure 4.6 Mechanism of S_N2 Reaction

The single step of an S_N2 reaction involves two reacting species: the substrate (often an alkyl halide, tosylate, or mesylate) and the nucleophile. Therefore, the concentrations of both have a role in determining the rate: rate $= k[\text{Nu:}][\text{R–L}]$

S_N2 reactions are accompanied by an inversion of relative configuration. Much like an umbrella being turned inside out on a blustery day, the position of substituents around the substrate carbon will be inverted. If the nucleophile and leaving group have the same priority in their respective molecules, this inversion will also correspond to a change in absolute configuration from (*R*) to (*S*) or vice-versa. This is an example of a **stereospecific** reaction, one in which the configuration of the reactant determines the configuration of the product due to the reaction mechanism.

MCAT CONCEPT CHECK 4.2

Before you move on, assess your understanding of the material with these questions.

1. How do the definitions of nucleophile and electrophile differ from those of Lewis base and acid?

____

2. Rank the following molecules in order of increasing nucleophilicity: methoxide, *t*-butoxide, isopropanolate, ethoxide.

______ < ______ < ______ < ______.

3. How must the nucleophile and leaving group be related in order for a substitution reaction to proceed?

____

4. What trends increase electrophilicity?

____

5. What are some features of good leaving groups?

____

4.3 Oxidation–Reduction Reactions

LEARNING OBJECTIVES

After Chapter 4.3, you will be able to:

- Recall common oxidizing agents and the characteristics of a good oxidizing agent
- Recall common reducing agents and the characteristics of a good reducing agent
- Order a given list of molecules from most oxidized to least oxidized:

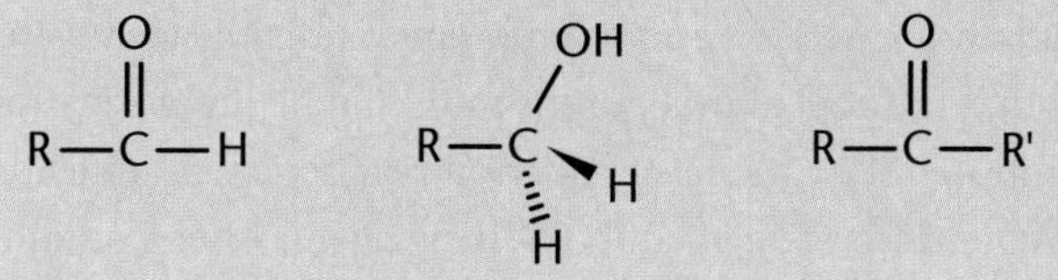

Another important class of reactions are **oxidation–reduction (redox) reactions**, in which the oxidation states of the reactants change. **Oxidation state** is an indicator of the hypothetical charge that an atom would have if all bonds were completely ionic. Oxidation state can be calculated from the molecular formula for a molecule. For example, the carbon in methane (CH_4) has an oxidation state of −4 because the hydrogens each have an oxidation state of +1. This is the most reduced form of carbon. In carbon dioxide (CO_2), each of the oxygen atoms has an oxidation state of −2, and the carbon has an oxidation state of +4. This is the most oxidized form of carbon. For an ion, the oxidation state is simply the charge—so Na^+ and S^{2-} would have oxidation states of +1 and −2, respectively. Carboxylic acids are more oxidized than aldehydes, ketones, and imines, which in turn are more oxidized than alcohols, alkyl halides, and amines.

We won't need to know too much about how to assign oxidation states in organic chemistry, but should know the definitions of oxidation and reduction. **Oxidation** refers to an increase in oxidation state, which means a loss of electrons. In organic chemistry, it is often easier to view oxidation as increasing the number of bonds to oxygen or other heteroatoms (atoms besides carbon and hydrogen). **Reduction** refers to a decrease in oxidation state, or a gain in electrons. In organic chemistry, it is often easier to view reduction as increasing the number of bonds to hydrogen.

Oxidizing Agents and Reactions

As we mentioned above, oxidation refers to an increase in oxidation state. Oxidation of a carbon atom occurs when a bond between a carbon atom and an atom that is less electronegative than carbon is replaced by a bond to an atom that is more electronegative than carbon. In practice, this usually means decreasing the number of bonds to hydrogen and increasing the number of bonds to other carbons, nitrogen, oxygen, or halides.

KEY CONCEPT

One can organize the different functional groups by "levels" of oxidation:

- Level 0 (no bonds to heteroatoms): alkanes
- Level 1: alcohols, alkyl halides, amines
- Level 2: aldehydes, ketones, imines
- Level 3: carboxylic acids, anhydrides, esters, amides
- Level 4 (four bonds to heteroatoms): carbon dioxide

The **oxidizing agent** is the element or compound in an oxidation–reduction reaction that accepts an electron from another species. Because the oxidizing agent is gaining electrons, it is said to be reduced. Good oxidizing agents have a high affinity for electrons (such as O_2, O_3, and Cl_2) or unusually high oxidation states (like Mn^{7+} in permanganate, MnO_4^-, and Cr^{6+} in chromate, CrO_4^{2-}).

Primary alcohols can be oxidized by one level to become aldehydes, or can be further oxidized to form carboxylic acids. This reaction commonly proceeds all the way to the carboxylic acid when using strong oxidizing agents such as chromium trioxide (CrO_3) or sodium or potassium dichromate ($Na_2Cr_2O_7$ or $K_2Cr_2O_7$), but can be made to stop at the aldehyde level using specific reagents such as pyridinium chlorochromate (PCC). Secondary alcohols can be oxidized to ketones.

A number of oxidation reactions and the relevant oxidizing agents are shown in Figure 4.7. Note that the goal at this point should not be memorization of these reactions, but recognition of two themes: oxidation reactions tend to feature an increase in the number of bonds to oxygen, and oxidizing agents often contain metals bonded to a large number of oxygen atoms.

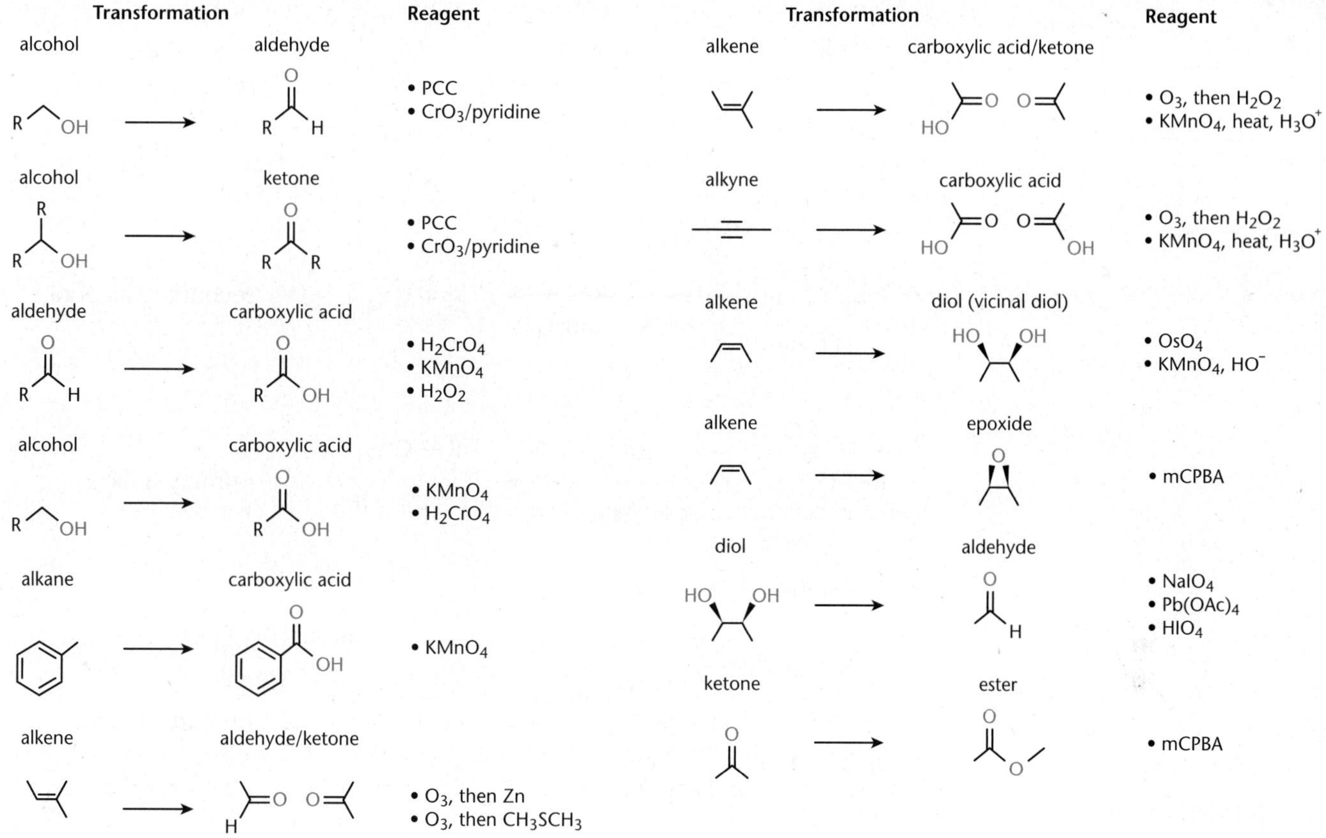

Figure 4.7 Oxidation Reactions and Common Oxidizing Agents

Reducing Agents and Reactions

Conversely, reduction refers to a decrease in oxidation state. Reduction of a carbon occurs when a bond between a carbon atom and an atom that is more electronegative than carbon is replaced by a bond to an atom that is less electronegative than carbon. In practice, this usually means increasing the number of bonds to hydrogen and decreasing the number of bonds to other carbons, nitrogen, oxygen, or halides.

Good reducing agents include sodium, magnesium, aluminum, and zinc, which have low electronegativities and ionization energies. Metal hydrides, such as NaH, CaH_2, $LiAlH_4$, and $NaBH_4$, are also good reducing agents because they contain the H^- ion.

Aldehydes and ketones will be reduced to primary and secondary alcohols, respectively. This reaction is exergonic, but exceedingly slow without a catalyst. Amides can be reduced to amines using $LiAlH_4$. This same reducing agent will reduce carboxylic acids to primary alcohols and esters to a pair of alcohols. Examples of reduction reactions are shown in Figure 4.8. Again, the focus is not on memorization, but on recognizing that reduction reactions tend to feature an increase in the number of bonds to hydrogen, and reducing agents often contain metals bonded to a large number of hydrides.

BRIDGE

Note that many of the common oxidizing and reducing agents include transition metals. This is because transition metals can often take on many different oxidation states. Their low ionization energies and presence of *d*-orbitals allow them to give up and accept electrons easily. Transition metals and periodic trends are discussed in Chapter 2 of *MCAT General Chemistry Review*.

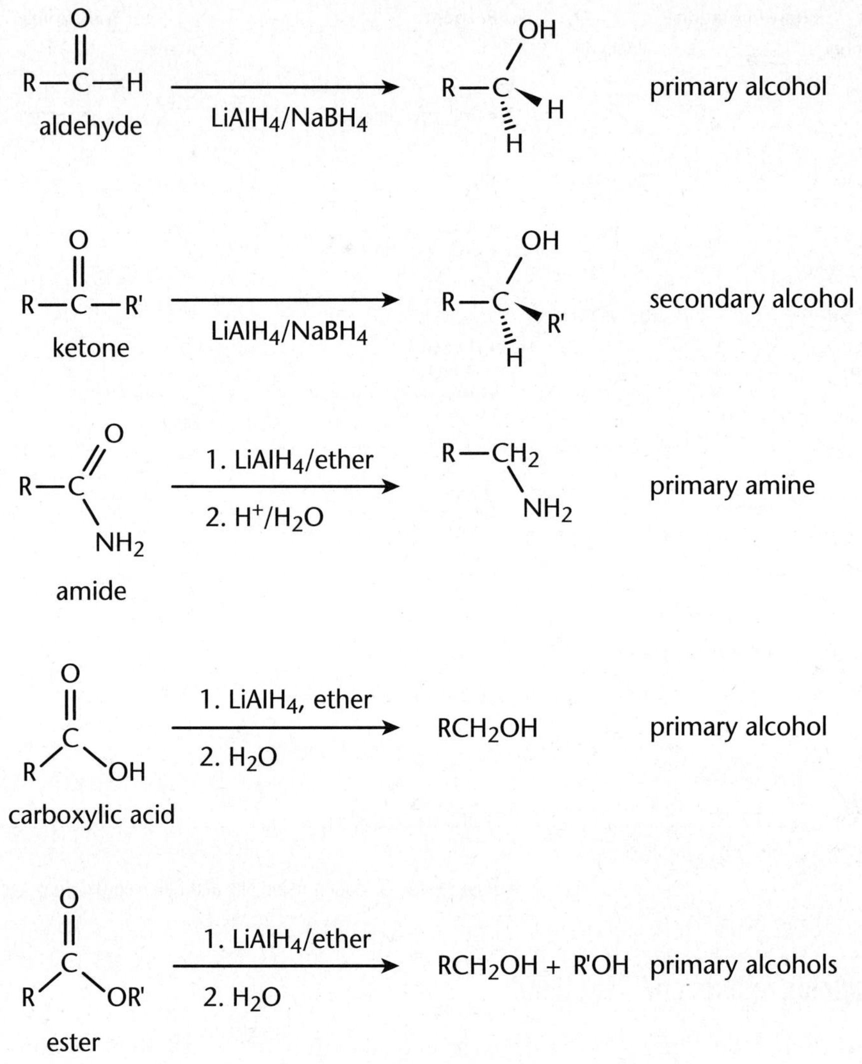

Figure 4.8 Reduction Reactions and Common Reducing Agents

MCAT CONCEPT CHECK 4.3

Before you move on, assess your understanding of the material with these questions.

1. What are some characteristics of good oxidizing agents? List some examples of common oxidizing agents.
   - Characteristics:

   ____

   - Examples:

   ____

2. What are some characteristics of good reducing agents? List some examples of common reducing agents.
   - Characteristics:

   ____

   - Examples:

   ____

3. List the following carbon-containing compounds from most oxidized carbon to most reduced: methane, carbon dioxide, ketone, alcohol, carboxylic acid
   - Most oxidized: ____________________
   - ____________________
   - ____________________
   - ____________________
   - Most reduced: ____________________

4.4 Chemoselectivity

LEARNING OBJECTIVES

After Chapter 4.4, you will be able to:

- Describe the types of compounds that are most likely to undergo S_N1 and S_N2 reactions
- Identify the two reactive centers of a carbonyl-containing compound:

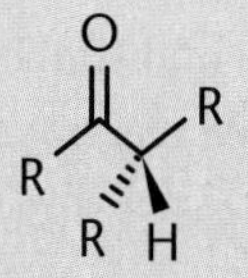

A key skill in recognizing which reactions will occur is recognizing the reactive regions within a molecule. The preferential reaction of one functional group in the presence of other functional groups is termed **chemoselectivity**.

Reactive Locations

Which site is the reactive site of a molecule depends on the type of chemistry that's occurring. A redox reagent, as described earlier, will tend to act on the highest-priority functional group. Thus, in a molecule with an alcohol and a carboxylic acid, a reducing agent is more likely to act on the carboxylic acid than on the alcohol. For a reaction involving nucleophiles and electrophiles, reactions also tend to occur at the highest-priority functional group because it contains the most oxidized carbon. A nucleophile is looking for a good electrophile; the more oxidized the carbon, the

KEY CONCEPT

The more oxidized the functional group, the more reactive it is in both nucleophile–electrophile and oxidation–reduction reactions.

more electronegative groups around it, and the larger partial positive charge it will experience. Thus, carboxylic acids and their derivatives are the first to be targeted by a nucleophile, followed by an aldehyde or ketone, followed by an alcohol or amine. Aldehydes are generally more reactive toward nucleophiles than ketones because they have less steric hindrance.

One common reactive site on the MCAT is the carbon of a carbonyl, which can be found in carboxylic acids and their derivatives, aldehydes, and ketones. Within a carbonyl-containing compound, the carbon of the carbonyl acquires a positive polarity due to the electronegativity of the oxygen. Thus, the carbonyl carbon becomes electrophilic and can be a target for nucleophiles. Further, the α-hydrogens are much more acidic than in a regular C—H bond due to the resonance stabilization of the enol form. These can be deprotonated easily with a strong base, forming an enolate, as shown in Figure 4.9. The enolate then becomes a strong nucleophile, and alkylation can result if good electrophiles are available.

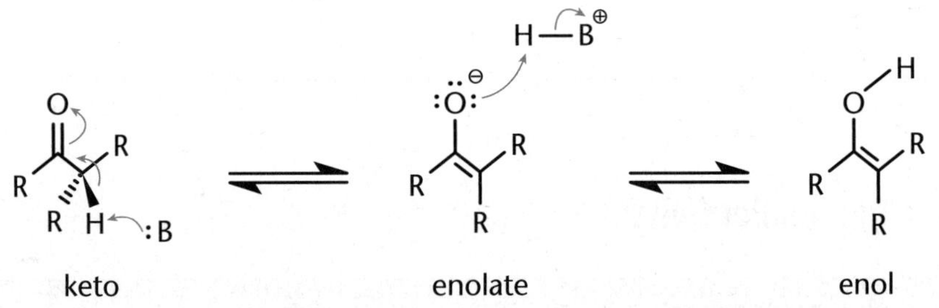

Figure 4.9 Enol and Enolate Forms of a Ketone

A second reactive site for consideration is the substrate carbon in substitution reactions. S_N1 reactions, which have to overcome the barrier of carbocation stability, prefer tertiary to secondary carbons as reactive sites, and secondary to primary. For S_N2 reactions, which have a bigger barrier in steric hindrance, methyl and primary carbons are preferred over secondary, and tertiary carbons won't react. This is all because of the mechanism of these two reactions.

Steric Protection

Steric hindrance describes the prevention of reactions at a particular location within a molecule due to the size of substituent groups. For example, S_N2 reactions won't occur with tertiary substrates. This characteristic of **steric protection** can be a useful tool in the synthesis of desired molecules and the prevention of the formation of alternative products. Effectively, bulky groups make it impossible for the nucleophile to reach the most reactive electrophile, making the nucleophile more likely to attack another region.

Another way that sterics come into play is in the protection of leaving groups. One can temporarily mask a reactive leaving group with a sterically bulky group during synthesis. For example, reduction of a molecule containing both carboxylic acids and aldehydes or ketones can result in reduction of all of the functional groups. To prevent this, the aldehyde or ketone is first converted to a nonreactive acetal or ketal, which serves as the **protecting group**, and the reaction can proceed. This reaction is shown in Figure 4.10. Another protective reaction is the reversible reduction of alcohols to *tert*-butyl ethers.

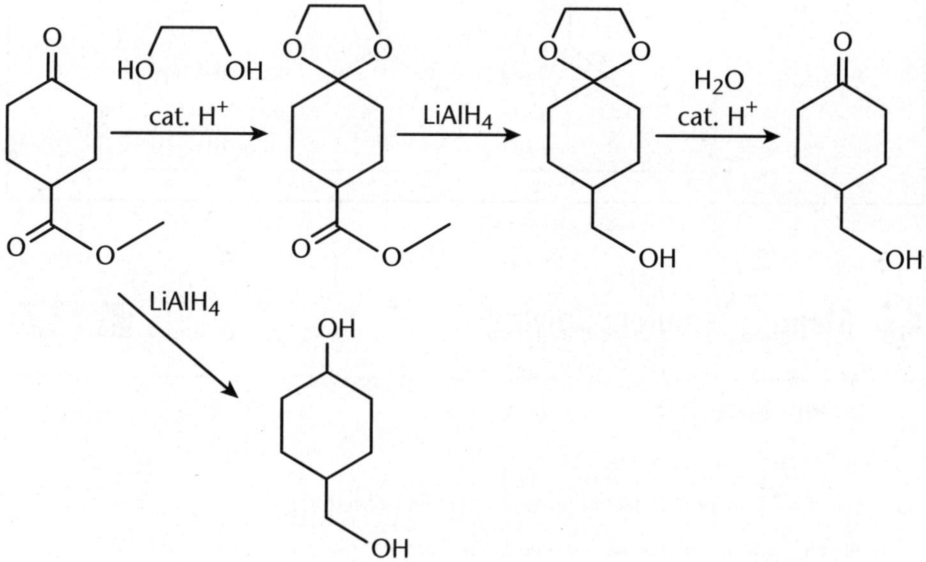

Figure 4.10 Protection of a Ketone by Conversion to an Acetal

BRIDGE

When an aldehyde is mixed with a diol (or two equivalents of alcohol), it forms an acetal. When a ketone is mixed with a diol (or two equivalents of alcohol), it forms a ketal. Acetal and ketal chemistry is discussed in Chapter 6 of *MCAT Organic Chemistry Review*.

Don't worry if this seems overwhelming—this is just a preview of what we will see in later chapters, along with a set of rules that will make it easier to understand how chemical reactions will proceed! Feel free to come back to this chapter later to remind yourself of the rules that apply across the board after reading further chapters.

MCAT CONCEPT CHECK 4.4

Before you move on, assess your understanding of the material with these questions.

1. What are the two reactive centers of carbonyl-containing compounds?
   - ________________________
   - ________________________
2. Which pair of reactants will undergo S_N1 more quickly? Why?

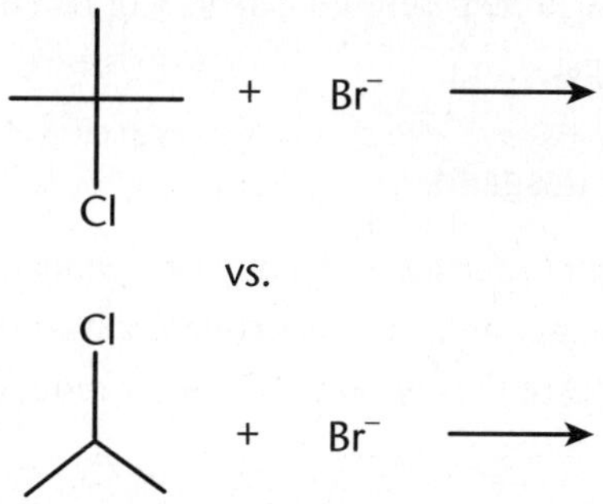

____

3. Which of the following electrophiles will be more favorable to an S_N2 reaction? Why?

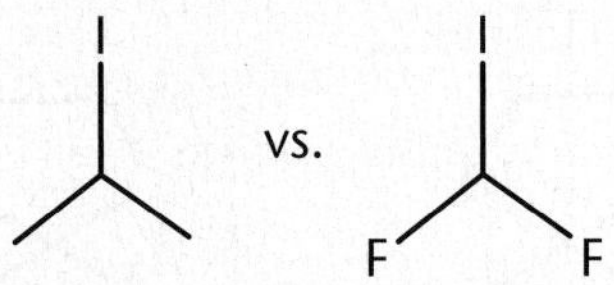

4.5 Steps to Problem Solving

High-Yield

LEARNING OBJECTIVES

After Chapter 4.5, you will be able to:

- List the six steps for solving organic chemistry reactions
- Predict how a reaction will proceed if you are not given reaction conditions

MCAT EXPERTISE

While studying organic chemistry for the MCAT, don't permit yourself to simply nod along with the reaction mechanisms—get involved! During each step of a mechanism, ask yourself how the trends and problem-solving steps in this chapter play out.

With all of these rules in hand, we can now apply our knowledge in a systematic way to simplify organic chemistry reactions that appear on the MCAT. These steps are described below.

Step 1: Know Your Nomenclature

Before you can even start to understand what reactions will occur and what products will form, it is vital to know which compounds IUPAC and common names refer to! If you're still having trouble with nomenclature, be sure to review Chapter 1 of *MCAT Organic Chemistry Review.*

Step 2: Identify the Functional Groups

Look at the organic molecules in the reaction. What functional groups are in the molecules? Do these functional groups act as acids or bases? How oxidized is the carbon? Are there functional groups that act as good nucleophiles, electrophiles, or leaving groups? This step will help define a category of reactions that can occur with the given functional groups.

Step 3: Identify the Other Reagents

In this step, determine the properties of the other reagents in the reaction. Are they acidic or basic? Are they suggestive of a particular reaction? Are they good nucleophiles or a specific solvent? Are they good oxidizing or reducing agents?

Step 4: Identify the Most Reactive Functional Group(s)

Once you've identified the functional groups in the compound and the other reagents present, this step should be relatively quick. Remember that more oxidized carbons tend to be more reactive to both nucleophile–electrophile reactions and oxidation–reduction reactions. Note the presence of protecting groups that exist to prevent a particular functional group from reacting.

Step 5: Identify the First Step of the Reaction

If the reaction involves an acid or a base, the first step will usually be protonation or deprotonation. If the reaction involves a nucleophile, the first step is generally for the nucleophile to attack the electrophile, forming a bond with it. If the reaction involves an oxidizing or reducing agent, the most oxidized functional group will be oxidized or reduced, accordingly.

Once you know what will react, think through how the reaction will go. Did the protonation or deprotonation of a functional group increase its reactivity? When the nucleophile attacks, how does the carbon respond to avoid having five bonds? Does a leaving group leave, or does a double bond get reduced to a single bond (like the opening of a carbonyl)?

Step 6: Consider Stereospecificity/Stereoselectivity

Though not all reactions are stereospecific or stereoselective, these possibilities should be considered when predicting products. For stereospecificity, consider whether the configuration of the reactant necessarily leads to a specific configuration in the product, as seen in S_N2 reactions. Stereoselectivity, on the other hand, occurs in reactions where one configuration of product is more readily formed due to product characteristics. Stereoselectivity is seen in many reactions, as different products often possess different traits which affect their relative stability. If there is more than one product, the major product will generally be determined by differences in strain or stability between the two molecules. More strained molecules (with significant angle, torsional, or nonbonded strain) are less likely to form than molecules without significant sources of strain. Products with conjugation (alternating single and multiple bonds) are significantly more stable than those without.

Example Reactions

Now, we'll apply these rules to three novel reactions. Focus on the decision-making element of this process so that you will be able to apply the same logic to reactions that appear on Test Day.

Reaction 1

We'll start with a series of reactions involving ethyl 5-oxohexanoate. First, it is reacted with 1,2-ethanediol and *p*-toluenesulfonic acid in benzene; second, with lithium aluminum hydride in tetrahydrofuran, followed by a heated acidic workup. What are the intermediates and final product?

Let's go through the steps:

1. First, let's draw out the reactants and reaction conditions.

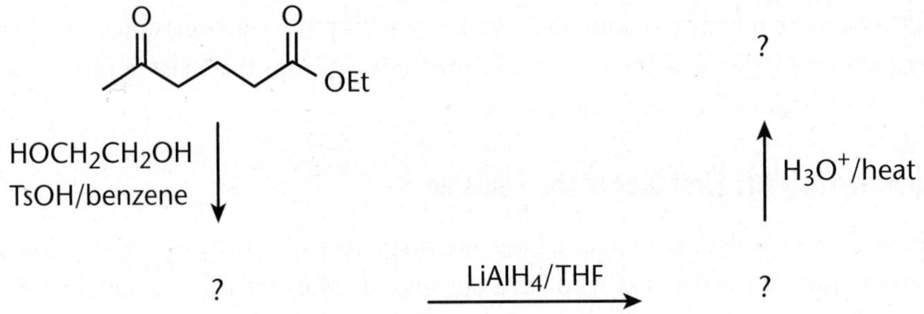

2. This molecule has an alkane backbone, a ketone, and an ester. Both of the carbonyl carbons are electrophilic targets for nucleophiles. The carbonyl oxygens can also be reduced. Acidic α-hydrogens are also present.
3. For the first part of the reaction, we have a diol, which is commonly used as a protecting group for aldehydes or ketones. Diols are nucleophiles because of lone pairs on the oxygens in the hydroxyl groups. For the second reaction, we have a reducing agent in an organic solvent. Finally, we have an acidic workup—which is often used to remove protecting groups. We're starting to get hints as to what is happening here.
4. In the first reaction, both the ketone and ester carbonyls are highly reactive. One or both of these functional groups will react in the first step.
5. The diol is a good nucleophile because it contains lone pairs on the oxygen atoms in the hydroxyl groups. Further, the presence of a diol hints at protecting the ketone carbonyl because diols are commonly used for this function. This gives our first intermediate—the ketone carbonyl will be replaced by a protected diether. The second reaction, then, will only be able to proceed on the ester. $LiAlH_4$ is a strong reducing agent, so the next reaction will be reduction of the carbonyl all the way to an alcohol. In the final reaction, the protecting group will be removed by acidic workup, leaving us with our original ketone group.
6. The product and intermediate have no stereoselectivity, so this won't be a consideration.

Let's see what we came up with. The first intermediate will have a protective diether at the ketone carbonyl. The second will show the reduction of the ester to an alcohol, with the protecting group still present. The third will be our final product.

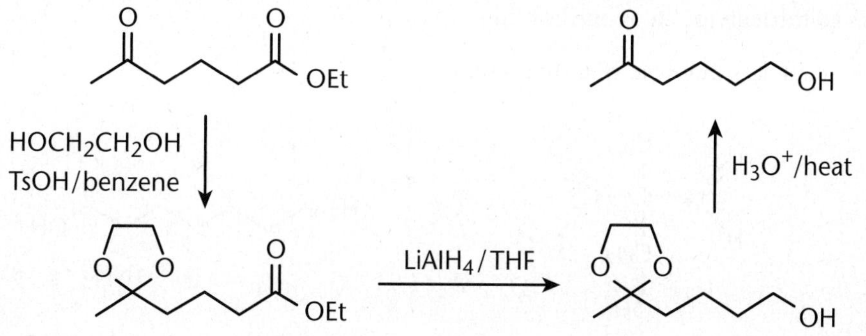

Reaction 2

If ethanol is reacted in acidic solution with potassium dichromate, what will the end product be?

Let's go through the steps again.

1. First, let's draw out our molecules.

$$CH_3CH_2OH \xrightarrow[H_2SO_4]{K_2Cr_2O_7}$$

2. This molecule has an alkane backbone and a primary alcohol. Alcohols make good nucleophiles and can also be oxidized. The hydroxyl group can also act as a leaving group, especially if it gets protonated.
3. Next, the reagents. Dichromate is a good oxidizing agent.
4. The alcohol carbon is most likely to react because it is the most oxidized.
5. The primary product of a primary alcohol with a strong oxidant like dichromate will be a carboxylic acid. One other possible product could have been an aldehyde, so this could trip us up! Remember, however, that primary alcohols can only be oxidized to aldehydes by reagents specifically designated for this purpose, like pyridinium chlorochromate (PCC). If we start with ethanol, we'll obtain ethanoic acid (acetic acid) after reaction with dichromate.
6. Stereospecificity again isn't a consideration and won't change the outcome in this reaction.

Therefore, the primary product of this reaction will be ethanoic acid.

Reaction 3

Determine the product of a reaction between 2-amino-3-hydroxypropanoic acid and 2,6-diaminohexanoic acid in aqueous solution.

Let's go through the steps one last time.

1. First, let's draw out both molecules.

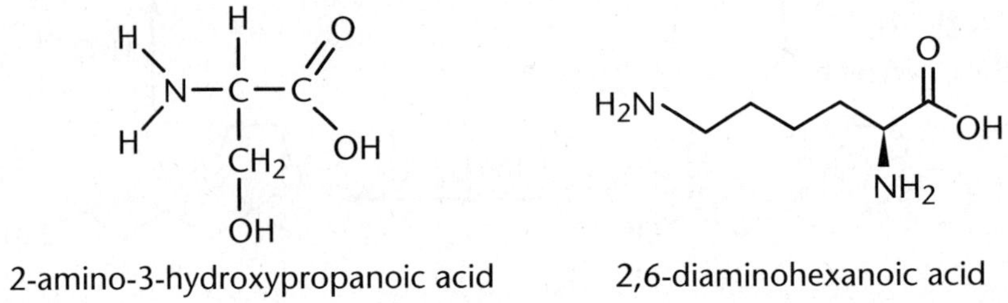

2. Both of these molecules have a carboxylic acid (which has an acidic hydrogen and an electrophilic carbonyl carbon) and an amino group (which is nucleophilic). The first molecule also has a hydroxyl group; the second has an additional amino group and a long alkane chain.
3. There are no additional reagents listed. Therefore, it will be the properties of the two reactants alone that determine how the reaction will proceed.
4. Either of the two molecules could act as the nucleophile in this reaction, and either could be the electrophile. The most reactive species are likely the nucleophilic amino groups attacking the electrophilic carbonyl carbon.
5. The first step of this reaction will be nucleophilic attack by the amino group on the electrophilic carbonyl carbon. Carbon cannot have five bonds, so the carbonyl group will have to open up. The hydroxyl group on the carboxylic acid is a poor leaving group, but proton rearrangements in the molecule turn the hydroxyl group into water, improving its leaving group ability. Then, the carbonyl will reform, kicking off the water molecule as a leaving group.
6. We might ask why the hydroxyl group on 2-amino-3-hydroxypropanoic acid doesn't react. Remember that more oxidized groups tend to be more reactive, and the carboxylic acid is significantly more oxidized than the hydroxyl group. Another question to consider is which of the amino groups of 2,6-diaminohexanoic acid will react. This is a question that is perhaps best answered retrospectively; in this case, the amino group closer to the carbonyl will react because the resulting product will be stabilized by resonance.

Does this reaction look familiar? It should! 2-amino-3-hydroxypropanoic acid and 2,6-diaminohexanoic acid are serine and lysine, respectively—in this reaction, we are forming a peptide bond. If we treat them as generic amino acids, this is the reaction:

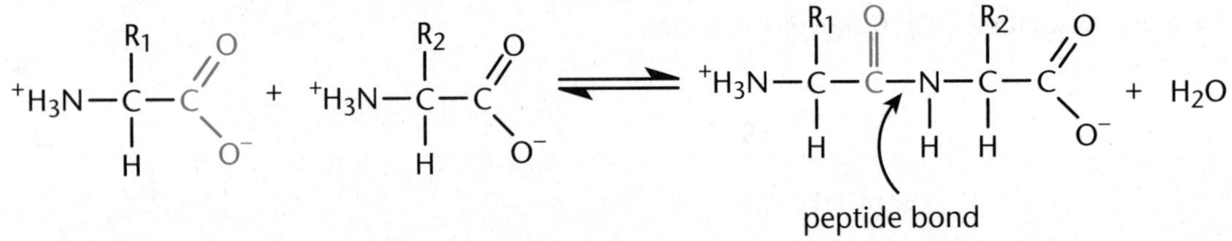

We've worked through a few problems here to get a handle on how to use this method. Once you have read further chapters and learned specific mechanisms that we did not touch on here, be sure to come back and see how these rules apply to novel reactions.

MCAT CONCEPT CHECK 4.5

Before you move on, assess your understanding of the material with these questions.

1. What are the six steps for solving organic chemistry reactions?
   1. ______________________________
   2. ______________________________
   3. ______________________________
   4. ______________________________
   5. ______________________________
   6. ______________________________
2. If there are no reaction conditions listed, what determines how the reaction will proceed?

   ____

Conclusion

In this chapter, we've outlined a framework for thinking through organic chemistry questions on the MCAT. We have discussed the various types of reactions that we may see, the properties that make them more or less likely to occur, and a few selective rules that can help us work through reactions, even if they are unfamiliar. Finally, we put this framework to the test on example problems in order to cement its application. With this framework in mind, there's nothing you can't tackle—revisit these rules and methods as you continue working through the different functional groups and their reactions in the next six chapters!

GO ONLINE

You've reviewed the content, now test your knowledge and critical thinking skills by completing a test-like passage set in your online resources!

CONCEPT SUMMARY

Acids and Bases

- **Lewis acids** are electron acceptors; they have vacant orbitals or positively polarized atoms.
- **Lewis bases** are electron donors; they have a lone pair of electrons and are often anions.
- **Brønsted–Lowry acids** are proton donors; **Brønsted–Lowry bases** are proton acceptors.
- **Amphoteric molecules** can act as either acids or bases, depending on reaction conditions. Water is a common example of an amphoteric molecule.
- The **acid dissociation constant, K_a**, is a measure of acidity. It is the equilibrium constant corresponding to the dissociation of an acid, HA, into a proton (H^+) and its conjugate base (A^-).
    - **pK_a** is the negative logarithm of K_a. A lower (or even negative) pK_a indicates a stronger acid.
    - pK_a decreases down the periodic table and as electronegativity increases.
- Alcohols, aldehydes, ketones, carboxylic acids, and carboxylic acid derivatives are common acidic functional groups. **α-hydrogens** (hydrogens connected to an **α-carbon**, a carbon adjacent to a carbonyl) are acidic.
- Amines and amides are common basic functional groups.

Nucleophiles, Electrophiles, and Leaving Groups

- **Nucleophiles** are "nucleus-loving" and contain lone pairs or π bonds. They have increased electron density and often carry a negative charge.
    - Nucleophilicity is similar to basicity; however, nucleophilicity is a kinetic property, while basicity is thermodynamic.
    - Charge, electronegativity, steric hindrance, and the solvent can all affect nucleophilicity.
    - Amino groups are common organic nucleophiles.
- **Electrophiles** are "electron-loving" and contain a positive charge or are positively polarized.
    - More positive compounds are more electrophilic.
    - Alcohols, aldehydes, ketones, carboxylic acids, and their derivatives can act as electrophiles.
- **Leaving groups** are the molecular fragments that retain the electrons after **heterolysis**.
    - The best leaving groups can stabilize additional charge through resonance or induction.
    - Weak bases (the conjugate bases of strong acids) make good leaving groups.
    - Alkanes and hydrogen ions are almost never leaving groups because they form reactive anions.

- **Unimolecular nucleophilic substitution (S_N1) reactions** proceed in two steps.
  - In the first step, the leaving group leaves, forming a **carbocation**, an ion with a positively charged carbon atom.
  - In the second step, the nucleophile attacks the planar carbocation from either side, leading to a racemic mixture of products.
  - S_N1 reactions prefer more substituted carbons because the alkyl groups can donate electron density and stabilize the positive charge of the carbocation.
  - The rate of an S_N1 reaction is dependent only on the concentration of the substrate: rate = k[R–L].
- **Bimolecular nucleophilic substitution (S_N2) reactions** proceed in one **concerted** step.
  - The nucleophile attacks at the same time as the leaving group leaves.
  - The nucleophile must perform a **backside attack**, which leads to an inversion of stereochemistry.
  - The absolute configuration is changed—(*R*) to (*S*) and vice versa—if the incoming nucleophile and the leaving group have the same priority in the molecule.
  - S_N2 reactions prefer less-substituted carbons because the alkyl groups create steric hindrance and inhibit the nucleophile from accessing the electrophilic substrate carbon.
  - The rate of an S_N2 reaction is dependent on the concentrations of both the substrate and the nucleophile: rate = k[Nu:][R–L].

Oxidation—Reduction Reactions

- The **oxidation state** of an atom is the charge it would have if all its bonds were completely ionic.
  - CH_4 is the lowest oxidation state of carbon (most reduced); CO_2 is the highest (most oxidized).
  - Carboxylic acids and carboxylic acid derivatives are the most oxidized functional groups, followed by aldehydes, ketones, and imines, followed by alcohols, alkyl halides, and amines.
- **Oxidation** is an increase in oxidation state and is assisted by oxidizing agents.
  - **Oxidizing agents** accept electrons and are reduced in the process. They have a high affinity for electrons or an unusually high oxidation state. They often contain a metal and a large number of oxygens.

- Primary alcohols can be oxidized to aldehydes by pyridinium chlorochromate (PCC) or to carboxylic acids by stronger oxidizing agents, like chromium trioxide (CrO_3) or sodium or potassium dichromate ($Na_2Cr_2O_7$ or $K_2Cr_2O_7$).
- Secondary alcohols can be oxidized to ketones by most oxidizing agents.
- Aldehydes can be oxidized to carboxylic acids by most oxidizing agents.

- **Reduction** is a decrease in oxidation state and is assisted by reducing agents.
  - **Reducing agents** donate electrons and are oxidized in the process. They have low electronegativity and ionization energy. They often contain a metal and a large number of hydrides.
  - Aldehydes, ketones, and carboxylic acids can be reduced to alcohols by lithium aluminum hydride ($LiAlH_4$).
  - Amides can be reduced to amines by $LiAlH_4$.
  - Esters can be reduced to a pair of alcohols by $LiAlH_4$.

Chemoselectivity

- Both nucleophile–electrophile and oxidation–reduction reactions tend to act at the highest-priority (most oxidized) functional group.
- One can make use of steric hindrance properties to selectively target functional groups that might not primarily react, or to protect functional groups.
  - Diols are often used as protecting groups for aldehyde or ketone carbonyls.
  - Alcohols may be protected by conversion to *tert*-butyl ethers.

Steps to Problem Solving

1. Know your nomenclature
2. Identify the functional groups
3. Identify the other reagents
4. Identify the most reactive functional group(s)
5. Identify the first step of the reaction
6. Consider stereoselectivity

ANSWERS TO CONCEPT CHECKS

4.1

1. An acid–base reaction will proceed when the acid and base react to form conjugate products that are weaker than the reactants.
2. Amphoteric species can act as either an acid or a base. Water, bicarbonate, and dihydrogen phosphate are common amphoteric species in biological systems.
3. $pK_a = -\log K_a$, where K_a is the equilibrium constant for the dissociation of an acid. pK_a indicates acid strength: a stronger acid has a lower (or even negative) pK_a.
4. Alcohols, aldehydes and ketones, carboxylic acids, and most carboxylic acid derivatives act as acids. Amines and amides act as bases.

4.2

1. Nucleophilicity and electrophilicity are based on relative rates of reactions and are therefore kinetic properties. Acidity and basicity are measured by the position of equilibrium in a protonation or deprotonation reaction and are therefore thermodynamic properties.
2. *t*-Butoxide < isopropanolate < ethoxide < methoxide. The four main determinants of nucleophilicity are charge (more negative = better nucleophile), electronegativity (more electronegative = worse nucleophile), steric hindrance (larger = worse nucleophile), and the solvent (protic solvents can protonate or hydrogen bond with the nucleophile, decreasing its reactivity). Each of these nucleophiles has the same attacking atom (oxygen), but differ in their bulkiness. The molecules with the least steric hindrance will be the more effective nucleophiles.
3. A substitution reaction will proceed when the nucleophile is a stronger base (more reactive) than the leaving group.
4. Greater positive charge increases electrophilicity, and better leaving groups increase electrophilicity by making the reaction more likely to proceed.
5. Good leaving groups can stabilize the extra electrons that result from heterolysis. Weak bases (the conjugate bases of strong acids) are good leaving groups. Resonance stabilization and inductive effects from electron-withdrawing groups also improve leaving group ability.

4.3

1. Good oxidizing agents have a high affinity for electrons or have very high oxidation states. Examples include O_2, O_3, Cl_2, permanganate (MnO_4^-), chromate (CrO_4^-), dichromate (CrO_4^{2-}), and pyridinium chlorochromate. These compounds often contain a metal and a large number of oxygen atoms.
2. Good reducing agents have low electronegativities and ionization energies or contain a hydride ion (H^-). Examples include sodium, magnesium, aluminum, zinc, sodium hydride (NaH), calcium dihydride (CaH_2), lithium aluminum hydride ($LiAlH_4$), and sodium borohydride ($NaBH_4$). These compounds often contain a metal and a large number of hydrides.
3. Carbon dioxide, carboxylic acid, ketone, alcohol, methane

4.4

1. The two reactive centers are the carbonyl carbon, which is electrophilic, and the α-hydrogens, which are acidic.
2. S_N1 reactions are most likely to occur on tertiary carbons where a carbocation can be most easily stabilized. The first reaction has a tertiary carbon containing a good leaving group while the second reaction has a secondary carbon containing a good leaving group. The first reaction will proceed more quickly.
3. S_N2 reactions are easily inhibited by steric hindrance. The fluorides are smaller than the methyls and so the difluoride molecule will be more suitable for an S_N2.

4.5

1. 1. Know your nomenclature
   2. Identify the functional groups
   3. Identify the other reagents
   4. Identify the most reactive functional group(s)
   5. Identify the first step of the reaction
   6. Consider stereoselectivity
2. If there are no reagents other than the reactants, then the properties of the functional groups on the reactants themselves (acid–base; nucleophile–electrophile) will determine the outcome.

SCIENCE MASTERY ASSESSMENT EXPLANATIONS

1. **C**

NH_3 and H_2O are Lewis bases because nitrogen and oxygen can donate lone pairs. Ag^+ is a Lewis acid because it can accept a lone pair into an unoccupied orbital.

2. **C**

Remember, good nucleophiles tend to have lone pairs or π bonds and are negatively charged or polarized. Alkoxide (OR^-) and hydroxide (OH^-) anions are strong nucleophiles. Alcohols (ROH) and carboxylic acids (RCOOH) are weak nucleophiles. The alkyl group of an alkoxide anion donates additional electron density, making it more reactive than the hydroxide ion. The carboxylic acid contains more electron-withdrawing oxygen atoms than the alcohol, making it less nucleophilic.

3. **D**

Good electrophiles are positively charged or polarized. CR_3^+ is a tertiary carbocation; it has a positive charge, which makes it very electrophilic. CH_3Cl and CH_3OH are both polarized; however, the leaving groups differ between these two. Cl^- is a weaker base than OH^- (HCl is a stronger acid than H_2O). As such, Cl^- will be more stable in solution than OH^-, which increases the electrophilic reactivity of CH_3Cl above CH_3OH. CH_3OCH_3 has a much less stable leaving group, CH_3O^-, and is therefore significantly less electrophilic.

4. **A**

Good leaving groups are weak bases, which are the conjugates of strong acids. Leaving groups must also be stable once they leave the molecule. H_2O is, by far, the most stable leaving group and will be extremely unreactive once it leaves the molecule through heterolysis. Br^- is the conjugate base of HBr; HO^- is the conjugate base of water. HBr is a much stronger acid than water, so Br^- is a better leaving group than HO^-. Finally, hydride (H^-) is a very poor leaving group because it is extremely unstable in solution.

5. **B**

Carboxylic acids are the second most oxidized form of carbon (only carbon dioxide is more oxidized). In carboxylic acids, the carbon atom has three bonds to oxygen. In aldehydes, the carbon atom has two bonds to oxygen. In amines, the carbon atom has one bond to nitrogen. In an alkane, the carbon only has bonds to other carbons and hydrogens.

6. **B**

During this reaction, the alkoxide anion accepts a proton, meaning this molecule acts as a Brønsted-Lowry base. Also, in accepting the proton, the alkoxide anion donates a lone pair of electrons to form a coordinate covalent bond with the incoming hydrogen ion. In this way, the alkoxide anion is also acting as a Lewis base. Together, these observations support **(B)**.

7. **C**

Because 2-butanol is a secondary alcohol, oxidation by a strong oxidizing agent like dichromate will result in a ketone, butanone.

8. **C**

Pyridinium chlorochromate is a weak oxidizing agent, and will oxidize an alcohol to an aldehyde. Stronger oxidizing agents are required to convert a primary alcohol to a carboxylic acid.

9. **B**

An S_N1 reaction is a first-order nucleophilic substitution reaction. It is called first-order because the rate-limiting step involves only one molecule. **(A)** is true, but does not explain why S_N1 reactions have first-order kinetics; the rate-limiting step of an S_N2 reaction is also the first (and only) step of that reaction, but S_N2 reactions have second-order kinetics, not first-order. **(C)** is a true statement as well, but again does not explain why the reaction is first-order. Finally, **(D)** is incorrect because it is the rate-limiting step, not the reaction overall, that involves only one molecule.

10. **D**

In a protic solvent, the protons in solution can attach to the nucleophile, decreasing its nucleophilicity. The larger the nucleophile, and the stronger its conjugate acid, the stronger the nucleophile will be. Of the options given, I^- will therefore be the strongest nucleophile because it is least likely to associate with the protons in solution.

11. **D**

Primary and secondary alcohols can be oxidized by PCC because the central carbon atom can form additional bonds with oxygen while losing bonds to hydrogen, justifying **(D)** as the right answer. Choices **(A)**, a tertiary alcohol; **(B)**, a ketone; and **(C)**, a carboxylic acid, cannot be oxidized by PCC because the central carbon in these molecules is already making four bonds to other carbon or oxygen atoms, and therefore cannot readily form more bonds to oxygen.

12. **A**

Steric hindrance slows S_N2 pathways, so the molecule that is fastest to react will be the one that is least sterically hindered. The reactivity trend based on steric hindrance is methyl > primary > secondary (note that tertiary substrates are too hindered to react via S_N2 at all). The molecule in **(A)** is a primary substrate, that is, the least sterically hindered, and will therefore react rapidly by an S_N2 pathway. Additionally, the molecule in **(A)** has a good leaving group. Together, these trends make **(A)** the best substrate for rapid S_N2. Note that while **(C)** also depicts a primary substrate, this molecule does not have a good leaving group, so **(C)** can be eliminated. Choices **(B)** and **(D)** can be eliminated because these molecules are secondary substrates.

13. **D**

To carry out a nucleophile–electrophile reaction, the nucleophile must be able to dissolve in the solvent. Nucleophiles are nearly always polar, and often carry a charge. Polar solvents are therefore preferred for these reactions. Hexane is a nonpolar solvent and will not be useful for a nucleophile–electrophile reaction.

14. **A**

Aldehydes have one alkyl group connected to the carbonyl carbon, whereas ketones have two. This creates more steric hindrance in ketones, which lowers their reactivity to nucleophiles. Ketones are also less reactive because their carbonyl carbon has less positive charge character; the additional alkyl group can donate electron density—the opposite of **(D)**—which decreases the electrophilicity of the compound.

15. **D**

Remember, there is a hierarchy to the reactivity of carboxylic acid derivatives that dictates how reactive they are toward nucleophilic attack. In order from highest to lowest, this is anhydrides > carboxylic acids and esters > amides. In practical terms, this means that derivatives of higher reactivity can form derivatives of lower reactivity but not vice versa. Nucleophilic attack of an ester cannot result in the corresponding anhydride because anhydrides are more reactive than esters.

Consult your online resources for additional practice. **GO ONLINE**

EQUATIONS TO REMEMBER

(4.1) **Acid dissociation constant:** $K_a = \frac{[H^+][A^-]}{[HA]}$

(4.2) **Definition of pK_a:** $pK_a = -\log K_a$

SHARED CONCEPTS

General Chemistry Chapter 5
Chemical Kinetics

General Chemistry Chapter 10
Acids and Bases

General Chemistry Chapter 11
Oxidation–Reduction Reactions

Organic Chemistry Chapter 1
Nomenclature

Organic Chemistry Chapter 5
Alcohols

Organic Chemistry Chapter 7
Aldehydes and Ketones II

CHAPTER 5

ALCOHOLS

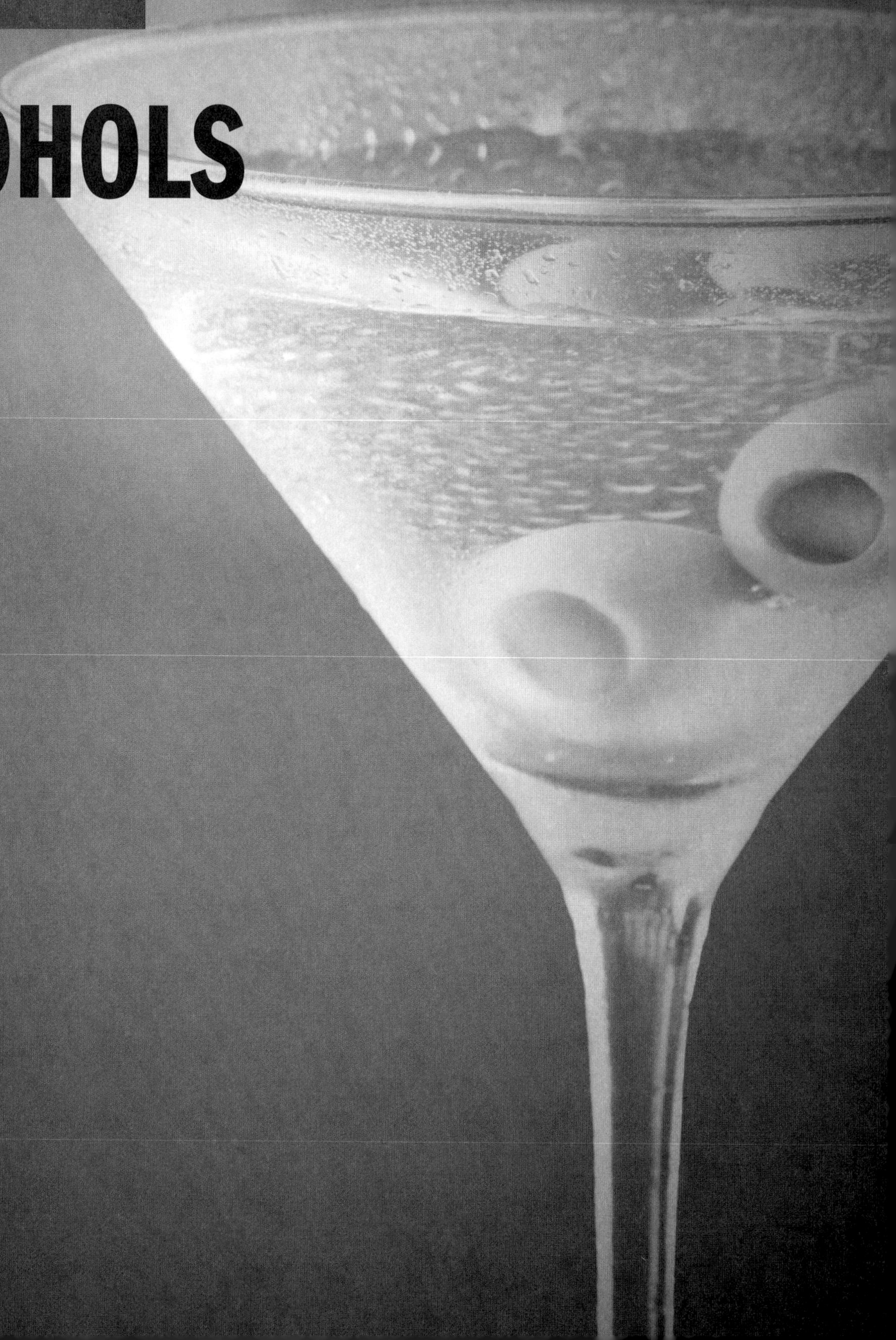

SCIENCE MASTERY ASSESSMENT

Every pre-med knows this feeling: there is so much content I have to know for the MCAT! How do I know what to do first or what's important?

While the high-yield badges throughout this book will help you identify the most important topics, this Science Mastery Assessment is another tool in your MCAT prep arsenal. This quiz (which can also be taken in your online resources) and the guidance below will help ensure that you are spending the appropriate amount of time on this chapter based on your personal strengths and weaknesses. Don't worry though—skipping something now does not mean you'll never study it. Later on in your prep, as you complete full-length tests, you'll uncover specific pieces of content that you need to review and can come back to these chapters as appropriate.

How to Use This Assessment

If you answer 0–7 questions correctly:

Spend about 1 hour to read this chapter in full and take limited notes throughout. Follow up by reviewing **all** quiz questions to ensure that you now understand how to solve each one.

If you answer 8–11 questions correctly:

Spend 20–40 minutes reviewing the quiz questions. Beginning with the questions you missed, read and take notes on the corresponding subchapters. For questions you answered correctly, ensure your thinking matches that of the explanation and you understand why each choice was correct or incorrect.

If you answer 12–15 questions correctly:

Spend less than 20 minutes reviewing all questions from the quiz. If you missed any, then include a quick read-through of the corresponding subchapters, or even just the relevant content within a subchapter, as part of your question review. For questions you got correct, ensure your thinking matches that of the explanation and review the Concept Summary at the end of the chapter.

1. Alcohols have higher boiling points than their analogous hydrocarbons because:

A. the oxygen atoms in alcohols have shorter bond lengths.
B. hydrogen bonding is present in alcohols.
C. alcohols are more acidic than their analogous hydrocarbons.
D. alcohols can be oxidized to ketones.

2. Tertiary alcohols are oxidized with difficulty because:

A. there is no hydrogen attached to the carbon with the hydroxyl group.
B. there is no hydrogen attached to the α-carbon of the carbonyl.
C. tertiary alcohols contain hydroxyl groups with no polarization.
D. they are relatively inert.

3. The IUPAC name of this molecule is:

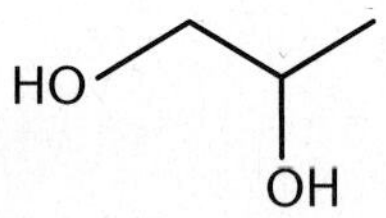

A. ethane-1,2-diol.
B. propane-1,2-diol.
C. dimethanol.
D. dipropanol.

4. The IUPAC name of this molecule is:

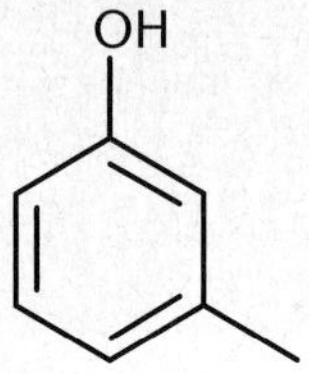

A. 2-methylcyclohexanol.
B. *m*-methylphenol.
C. *p*-methylphenol.
D. 3-methylcyclohexanol.

5. Which of the following correctly lists methanol, isobutyl alcohol, and propanol by decreasing boiling point?

A. Methanol > isobutyl alcohol > propanol
B. Isobutyl alcohol > methanol > propanol
C. Isobutyl alcohol > propanol > methanol
D. Methanol > propanol > isobutyl alcohol

6. Which of the following correctly lists hexanol, phenol, and cyclohexanol by increasing acidity of the hydroxyl hydrogen?

A. Phenol < hexanol < cyclohexanol
B. Cyclohexanol < hexanol < phenol
C. Cyclohexanol < phenol < hexanol
D. Phenol < cyclohexanol < hexanol

7. Which of the following will convert $CH_3CH_2CH_2OH$ to CH_3CH_2CHO?
   I. CrO_3
   II. PCC
   III. $K_2Cr_2O_7$

   A. I only
   B. II only
   C. I and III only
   D. I, II, and III

8. Which of the following will convert cyclohexanol to cyclohexanone?
   I. Chromium trioxide
   II. Pyridinium chlorochromate
   III. Sodium dichromate

   A. I only
   B. II only
   C. I and III only
   D. I, II, and III

9. Successfully converting 3-phenylpropanol to 3-phenylpropanoic acid by the Jones oxidation requires the oxidizing agent, the solvent, and:
   A. dilute sulfuric acid.
   B. dilute sodium hydroxide.
   C. anhydrous conditions.
   D. high temperature.

10. Treating 2-methyl-1-propanol with methylsulfonyl chloride in base, followed by reaction with pyridinium chlorochromate, and a final step in strong acid, will give an end product of:
   A. 2-methyl-1-propanol.
   B. 2-methylpropanal.
   C. 2-methylpropanoic acid.
   D. 2-methyl-1-propane.

11. Reaction of 1-phenylethanone with ethylene glycol, also known as ethane-1,2-diol, in aqueous H_2SO_4 will result in the formation of:
   A. a ketal.
   B. a carboxylic acid.
   C. an aldehyde.
   D. a hemiacetal.

12. Treatment of this molecule with CrO_3 under appropriate reaction conditions will yield which of the following molecules?

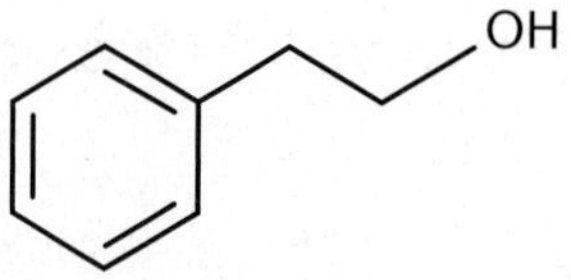

   A. 2-Phenylethanol
   B. Phenylacetaldehyde
   C. Phenylacetone
   D. 2-Phenylethanoic acid

13. In order to convert phenols into hydroxyquinones, how many steps of oxidation or reduction are required?
   A. 1 oxidation step
   B. 2 oxidation steps
   C. 1 reduction step
   D. 2 reduction steps

14. The conversion of ubiquinone to ubiquinol requires what type of reaction?
   A. Condensation
   B. Oxidation
   C. Reduction
   D. Hydrolysis

15. Which of the following will convert a cyclic acetal to a carbonyl and a dialcohol?
   A. Aqueous acid
   B. $LiAlH_4$
   C. CrO_3
   D. Acetone

Answer Key

1. **B**
2. **A**
3. **B**
4. **B**
5. **C**
6. **B**
7. **B**
8. **D**
9. **A**
10. **A**
11. **A**
12. **D**
13. **B**
14. **C**
15. **A**

Detailed explanations can be found at the end of the chapter.

CHAPTER 5

ALCOHOLS

In This Chapter

CHAPTER PROFILE

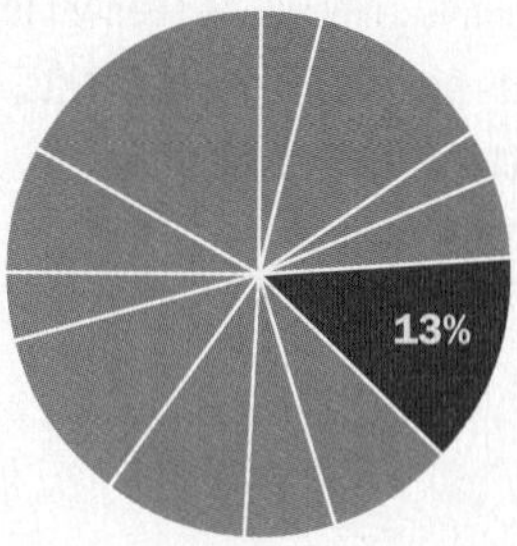

The content in this chapter should be relevant to about 13% of all questions about organic chemistry on the MCAT.

This chapter covers material from the following AAMC content category:

5D: Structure, function, and reactivity of biologically-relevant molecules

Introduction

Alcohols are probably the most popular chemicals you'll encounter in organic chemistry. Ethanol has been popular with humans for more than 10,000 years. It's not just humans, either: many animals are known to seek out rotten fruits that have fermented enough to contain moderate levels of ethanol. Note that when we talk about consuming "alcohol," we are referring exclusively to ethanol (grain alcohol). In fact, consuming other alcohols can have drastically negative effects. Methanol (wood alcohol), for example, is oxidized by the body to formic acid, which is extremely toxic to the optic nerve and retina and can cause blindness when ingested. Isopropyl alcohol, commonly used as an antiseptic, can cause severe central nervous system depression. For organic chemistry purposes, of course, we do not restrict ourselves to only one type of alcohol—many are used synthetically and in analytic techniques.

5.1 Description and Properties

LEARNING OBJECTIVES

After Chapter 5.1, you will be able to:

- Predict the relative pK_a values of two given alcohols
- Order alcohols based on boiling point

MCAT EXPERTISE

Alcohols are an important group of compounds. They will be seen on the MCAT as protic solvents, reactants, products, and prime examples of hydrogen bonding.

Alcohols have the general formula ROH, with the functional group –OH referred to as a **hydroxyl** group.

Nomenclature

Alcohols are named in the IUPAC system by replacing the ***-e*** ending of the root alkane with the ending ***-ol***. If the alcohol is the highest-priority functional group, the carbon atom attached to it receives the lowest possible number. Some examples are shown in Figure 5.1.

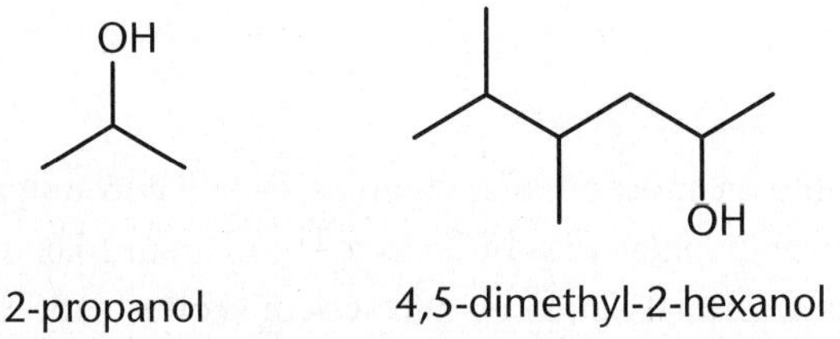

Figure 5.1 IUPAC Names of Alcohols

Alternatively, the common naming practice is to name the alkyl group as a derivative, followed by ***alcohol***, as shown in Figure 5.2.

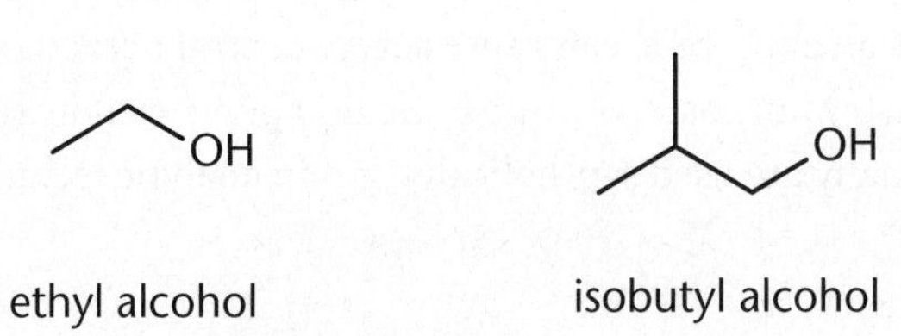

Figure 5.2 Common Names of Alcohols

When the alcohol is not the highest-priority group, it is named as a substituent, with the prefix ***hydroxy–***.

KEY CONCEPT

Aromatic alcohols are called phenols. The possible resonance between the ring and the lone pairs of the oxygen atom in the hydroxyl group make the hydrogen of the alcohol more acidic than other alcohols.

Finally, we will also see that hydroxyl groups can be attached to aromatic rings, as shown in Figure 5.3. These compounds are called **phenols**. The hydroxyl hydrogens of phenols are particularly acidic due to resonance within the phenol ring. When benzene rings contain two substituents, their relative positions must be indicated. Two groups on adjacent carbons are called ***ortho***–, or simply ***o***–. Two groups separated by a carbon are called ***meta***–, or ***m***–. Two groups on opposite sides of the ring are called ***para***–, or ***p***–.

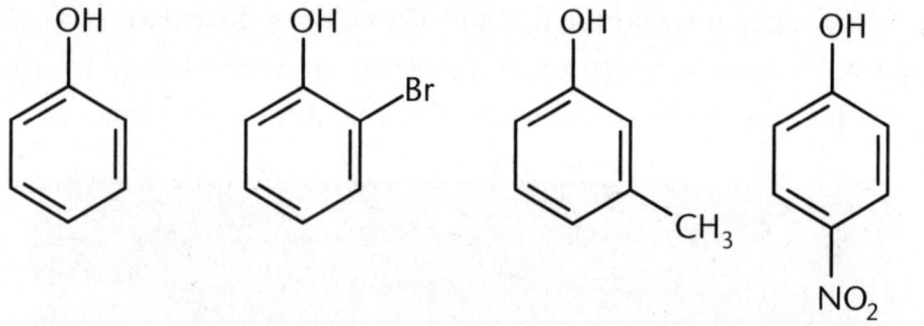

phenol   *o*-bromophenol   *m*-cresol (*m*-methylphenol)   *p*-nitrophenol

Figure 5.3 Phenols: Aromatic Alcohols

Physical Properties

One of the prominent properties of alcohols is that they are capable of intermolecular hydrogen bonding, which results in significantly higher melting and boiling points than those of analogous hydrocarbons, as shown in Figure 5.4.

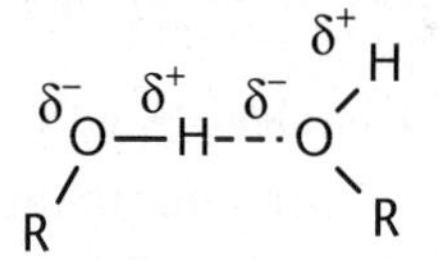

Figure 5.4 Intermolecular Hydrogen Bonding in Alcohols

Molecules with more than one hydroxyl group show greater degrees of hydrogen bonding. This is evident from the boiling points shown in Figure 5.5.

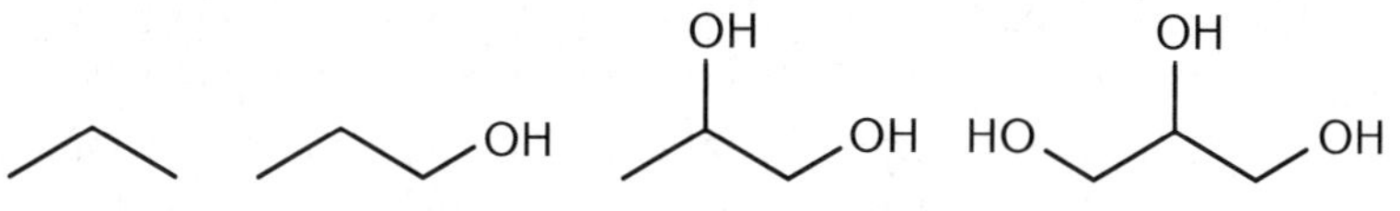

boiling point (°C)   −42.1   97.4   188.2   290.0

Figure 5.5 Boiling Points for Various Alcohols
Boiling point increases significantly with additional hydroxyl groups, which permit more hydrogen bonding.

Hydrogen bonding occurs when hydrogen atoms are attached to highly electronegative atoms like nitrogen, oxygen, or fluorine. Hydrogen bonding is the result of the extreme polarity of these bonds. In the case of a hydroxyl group, the electronegative oxygen atom pulls electron density away from the less electronegative hydrogen atom. This generates a slightly positive charge on the hydrogen and slightly negative charge on the oxygen. Then, the partially positive hydrogen of one molecule electrostatically attracts the partially negative oxygen of another molecule, generating a noncovalent bonding force known as a **hydrogen bond**.

MCAT EXPERTISE

Hydrogen bonding causes increased melting points, boiling points, and solubility in water.

The hydroxyl hydrogen is weakly acidic, and alcohols can dissociate into protons and alkoxide ions in the same way that water dissociates into protons and hydroxide ions. Table 5.1 gives pK_a values of several hydroxyl-containing compounds.

BRIDGE

Remember from Chapter 10 of *MCAT General Chemistry Review* that p$K_a = -\log K_a$. Strong acids have high K_a values and low pK_a values. Thus, phenol, which has the smallest pK_a, is the most acidic of the alcohols listed in Table 5.1.

DISSOCIATION			pK_a
H_2O	$\rightleftharpoons$	$HO^- + H^+$	14.0
CH_3OH	$\rightleftharpoons$	$CH_3O^- + H^+$	15.5
C_2H_5OH	$\rightleftharpoons$	$C_2H_5O^- + H^+$	15.9
i-PrOH	$\rightleftharpoons$	*i*-PrO$^-$ + H^+	16.5
t-BuOH	$\rightleftharpoons$	*t*-BuO$^-$ + H^+	17.0
CF_3CH_2OH	$\rightleftharpoons$	$CF_3CH_2O^- + H^+$	12.5
PhOH	$\rightleftharpoons$	PhO$^-$ + H^+	~10.0

Table 5.1 pK_a Values of Hydroxyl-Containing Compounds

Looking at Table 5.1, we can see that the hydroxyl hydrogens of phenols are more acidic than those of other alcohols. This is due to the aromatic nature of the ring, which allows for the resonance stabilization of the negative charge on oxygen, stabilizing the anion. Like other alcohols, phenols form intermolecular hydrogen bonds and have relatively high melting and boiling points. Phenols are slightly soluble in water, owing to hydrogen bonding, as are some phenol derivatives. Because phenols are much more acidic than nonaromatic alcohols, they can form salts with inorganic bases such as NaOH.

KEY CONCEPT

Charges like to be spread out as much as possible. Acidity decreases as more alkyl groups are attached because they are electron-donating, which destabilizes the alkoxide anion. Resonance or electron-withdrawing groups stabilize the alkoxide anion, making the alcohol more acidic.

The presence of other substituents on the ring has significant effects on the acidity, boiling points, and melting points of phenols. As with other compounds, electron-withdrawing substituents increase acidity, and electron-donating groups decrease acidity.

Another trend seen in Table 5.1 is that the presence of more alkyl groups in nonaromatic alcohols produces less acidic molecules. Because alkyl groups donate electron density, they destabilize a negative charge. Additionally, alkyl groups help stabilize positive charges, explaining why more substituted carbocations have higher stability than less substituted carbocations.

MCAT CONCEPT CHECK 5.1

Before you move on, assess your understanding of the material with these questions.

1. Which has a lower pK_a: ethanol or *p*-ethylphenol? Why?

____

____

____

2. Rank the following by decreasing boiling point: 1-pentanol, 1-hexanol, 1,6-hexanediol

1. ______________________________

2. ______________________________

3. ______________________________

5.2 Reactions of Alcohols

LEARNING OBJECTIVES

After Chapter 5.2, you will be able to:

- Predict the reaction of primary and secondary alcohols with strong oxidizing agents
- Recall the reagent(s) used to oxidize primary alcohols to aldehydes
- Explain the purpose of a mesylate or tosylate group
- Describe the process for protecting an aldehyde or ketone

The main reactions that we will see on the MCAT for alcohols include oxidation, preparation of mesylates and tosylates, and protection of carbonyls by alcohols.

Oxidation Reactions

Oxidation of alcohols can produce several products. Primary alcohols can be oxidized to aldehydes, but only by **pyridinium chlorochromate (PCC)**, a mild anhydrous oxidant, as shown in Figure 5.6. This reactant stops after the primary alcohol has been converted to an aldehyde because PCC lacks the water necessary to hydrate the otherwise easily hydrated aldehyde. With other oxidizing agents, aldehydes are rapidly hydrated to form **geminal diols** (1,1-diols), which can be easily oxidized to carboxylic acids.

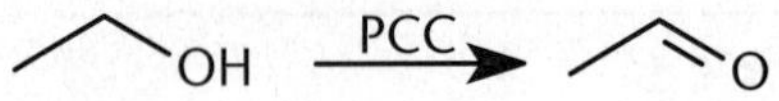

Figure 5.6 Oxidation of a Primary Alcohol to an Aldehyde by Pyridinium Chlorochromate (PCC)

Secondary alcohols can be oxidized to ketones by PCC or any stronger oxidizing agent. Tertiary alcohols cannot be oxidized because they are already as oxidized as they can be without breaking a carbon–carbon bond.

KEY CONCEPT

Alcohols are readily oxidized to carboxylic acids by any oxidizing agent other than PCC (which will only oxidize primary alcohols to aldehydes).

The oxidation of primary alcohols with a strong oxidizing agent like chromium(VI) will produce a carboxylic acid. In the process, chromium(VI) is reduced to chromium(III). Common examples of chromium-containing oxidizing agents include sodium and potassium dichromate salts ($Na_2Cr_2O_7$ and $K_2Cr_2O_7$). As with other strong oxidizing agents, these will fully oxidize primary alcohols to carboxylic acids, and secondary alcohols to ketones. An example is shown in Figure 5.7.

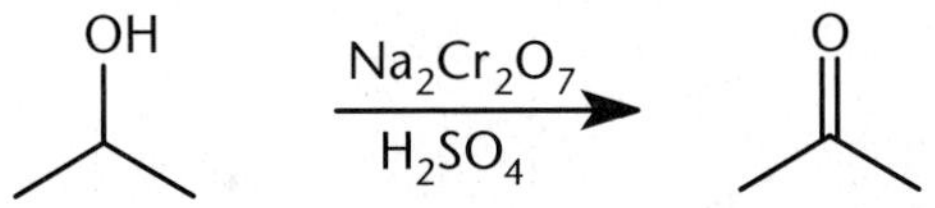

Figure 5.7 Oxidation of a Secondary Alcohol to a Ketone by a Dichromate Salt

Finally, an even stronger chromium-containing oxidizing agent is chromium trioxide, CrO_3. When dissolved with dilute sulfuric acid in acetone, this is called the **Jones oxidation**, as shown in Figure 5.8. As expected, this reaction oxidizes primary alcohols to carboxylic acids and secondary alcohols to ketones.

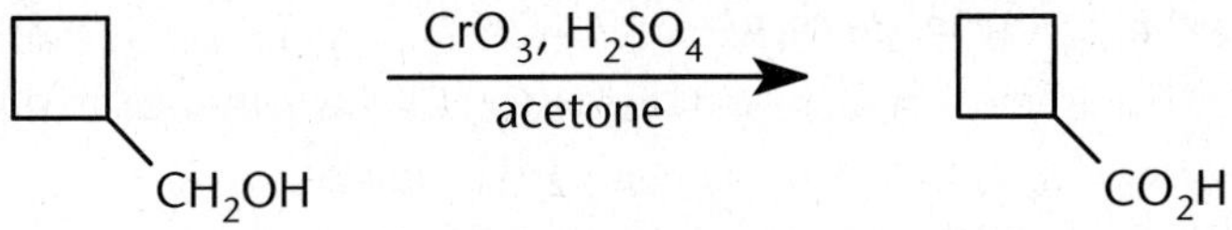

Figure 5.8 Jones Oxidation
A primary alcohol is oxidized to a carboxylic acid by CrO_3.

Mesylates and Tosylates

The hydroxyl groups of alcohols are fairly poor leaving groups for nucleophilic substitution reactions. However, they can be protonated, or reacted to form much better leaving groups called mesylates and tosylates. A **mesylate** is a compound containing the functional group $-SO_3CH_3$, derived from **methanesulfonic acid**; its anionic form is shown in Figure 5.9.

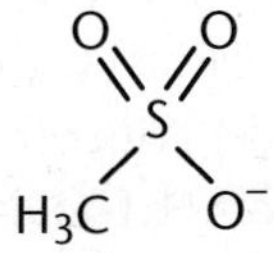

Figure 5.9 Structure of the Mesylate Anion

Mesylates are prepared using methylsulfonyl chloride and an alcohol in the presence of a base.

Tosylates contain the functional group $-SO_3C_6H_4CH_3$, derived from **toluenesulfonic acid**. These compounds are produced by the reaction of alcohols with *p*-toluenesulfonyl chloride, forming esters of toluenesulfonic acid. A tosylate is shown in Figure 5.10.

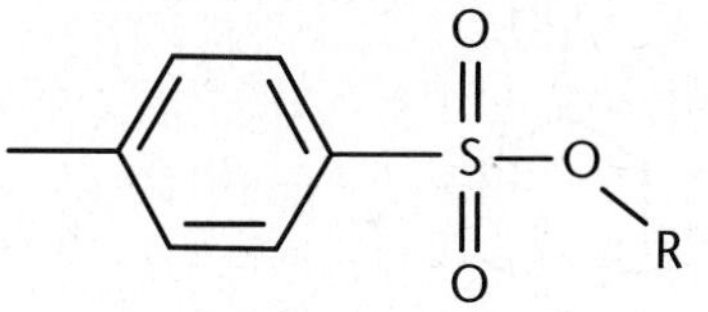

Figure 5.10 Structure of a Tosylate

In addition to making hydroxyl groups of alcohols into better leaving groups for nucleophilic substitution reactions, mesyl and tosyl groups can also serve as protecting groups when we do not want alcohols to react. These groups are protective in that they will not react with many of the other reagents that would attack alcohols, especially oxidizing agents. Thus, reacting an alcohol to form a mesylate or tosylate is sometimes performed before multistep reactions in which the desired products do not derive from the alcohol.

Protecting Groups

Alcohols can also be used as protecting groups for other functional groups themselves. For example, aldehydes and ketones can be reacted with two equivalents of an alcohol or a diol (dialcohol), forming **acetals** (primary carbons with two $-OR$ groups and a hydrogen atom) or **ketals** (secondary carbons with two $-OR$ groups). Carbonyls are very reactive with strong reducing agents like lithium aluminum hydride ($LiAlH_4$). Acetals and ketals, on the other hand, do not react with $LiAlH_4$. The acetal or ketal functionality thereby protects the aldehyde or ketone from reaction. After reducing other functionalities in the molecule, the acetal or ketal can be reverted back to a carbonyl with aqueous acid, a step called **deprotection**. These reactions are shown in Figure 5.11.

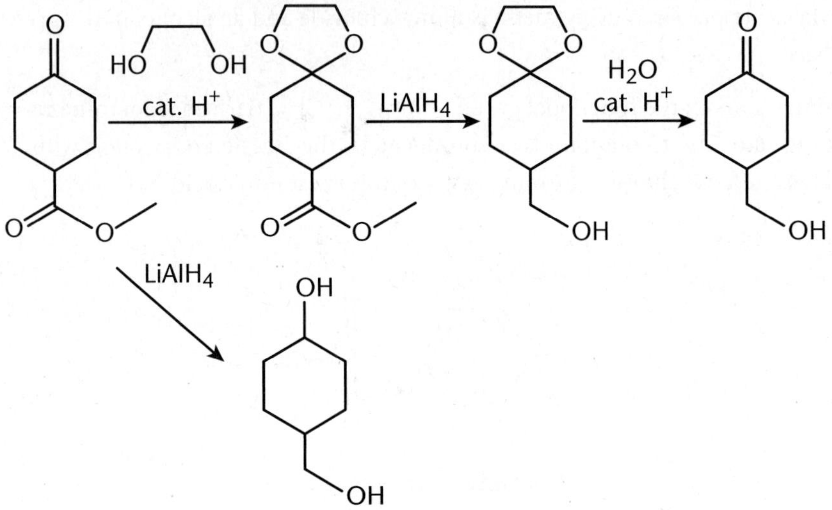

Figure 5.11 Protection of a Ketone by Ketal Formation Using a Dialcohol

MCAT CONCEPT CHECK 5.2

Before you move on, assess your understanding of the material with these questions.

1. What will happen to primary and secondary alcohols, respectively, in the presence of strong oxidizing agents?
   - Primary alcohols:

   ____

   - Secondary alcohols:

   ____

2. What is the product when 1-butanol is treated with PCC? With chromium trioxide?
   - PCC:

   ____

   - Chromium trioxide:

   ____

3. What is the purpose of a mesylate or tosylate?

   ____

4. How can aldehydes or ketones be protected using alcohols?

   ____

5.3 Reactions of Phenols

High-Yield

LEARNING OBJECTIVES

After Chapter 5.3, you will be able to:

- Recall the process for production of quinones and hydroxyquinones
- Identify the properties of ubiquinone that allow it to function as an electron carrier:

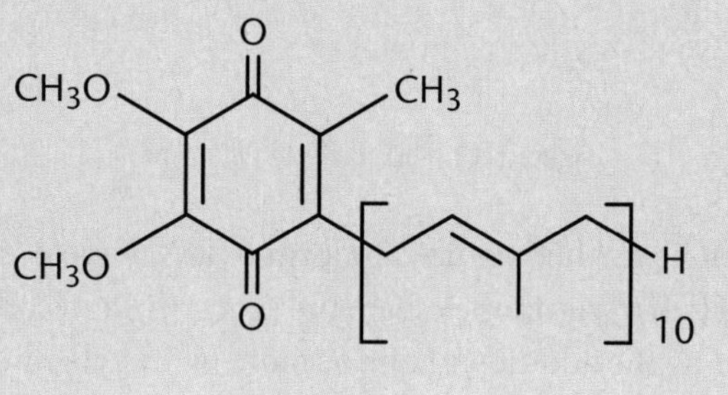

ubiquinone

Reactions of phenols proceed in similar fashion to reactions of alcohols. However, as discussed previously, the hydrogen in the hydroxyl group of phenols is particularly acidic because the oxygen-containing anion is resonance-stabilized by the ring.

Quinones and Hydroxyquinones

Treatment of phenols with oxidizing agents produces compounds called **quinones** (2,5-cyclohexadiene-1,4-diones), as shown in Figure 5.12.

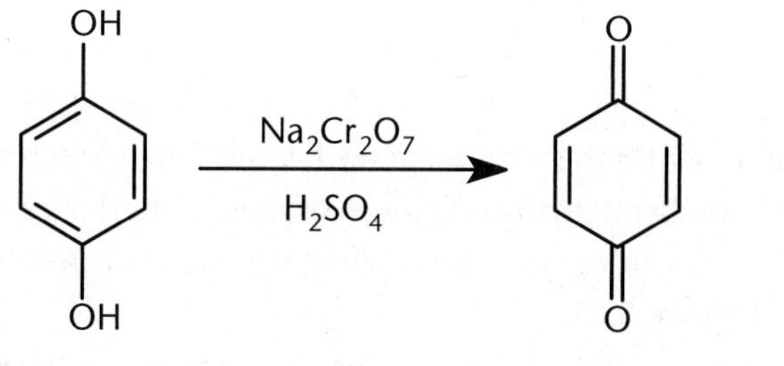

Figure 5.12 Oxidation of *p*-Benzenediol (a Hydroquinone) to a Quinone

Quinones are named by indicating the position of the carbonyls numerically and adding ***quinone*** to the name of the parent phenol. Due to the conjugated ring system, these molecules are resonance-stabilized electrophiles. Remember, however, that these are not necessarily aromatic because they lack the classic aromatic conjugated ring structure. Some quinones do have an aromatic ring, but this is not always the case. Quinones serve as electron acceptors biochemically, specifically in the electron transport chain in both photosynthesis and aerobic respiration. Vitamin K_1 is the common name of the quinone 2-methyl-3-[(2*E*)-3,7,11,15-tetramethylhexadec-2-en-1-yl]naphthoquinone, shown in Figure 5.13. This molecule is also called

phylloquinone and is important for photosynthesis and the carboxylation of some of the clotting factors in blood. Vitamin K_2, similarly, corresponds to a class of molecules called **menaquinones.**

BRIDGE

Phylloquinone and menaquinone are the common names of Vitamin K_1 and Vitamin K_2, respectively. These molecules are fat-soluble vitamins that play a role in carboxylation of clotting factors II, VII, IX, and X, and proteins C and S in blood. The functions of fat-soluble vitamins are explored in Chapter 5 of *MCAT Biochemistry Review.*

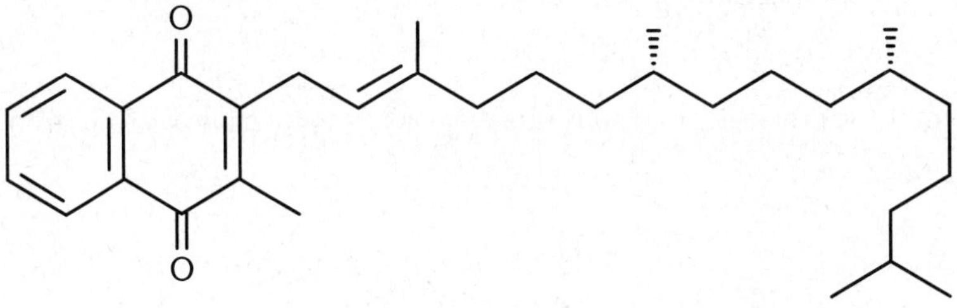

Figure 5.13 Phylloquinone (Vitamin K_1)

These molecules can be further oxidized to form a class of molecules called hydroxyquinones. **Hydroxyquinones** share the same ring and carbonyl backbone as quinones, but differ by the addition of one or more hydroxyl groups. Many hydroxyquinones have biological activity, and some are used in the synthesis of medications. One classic example is shown in Figure 5.14.

MCAT EXPERTISE

Note the subtle difference in terminology between Figure 5.12 and Figure 5.14. A *hydroquinone* is a benzene ring with two hydroxyl groups. A *hydroxyquinone* contains two carbonyls and a variable number of hydroxyl groups.

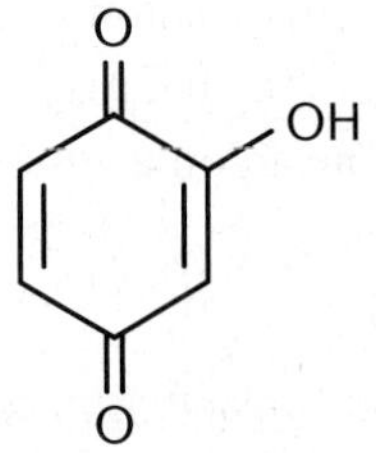

Figure 5.14 2-Hydroxy-1,4-Benzoquinone, a Hydroxyquinone

Because of resonance, hydroxyquinones behave like quinones with electron-donating groups, making these slightly less electrophilic (although still quite reactive). When naming these compounds, the position of the hydroxyl groups is indicated by a number, and the total number of hydroxyl groups (if there is more than one) is indicated by a prefix (such as *di–*, or *tri–*) with the substituent name ***hydroxy–***. Several examples are shown in Figure 5.15.

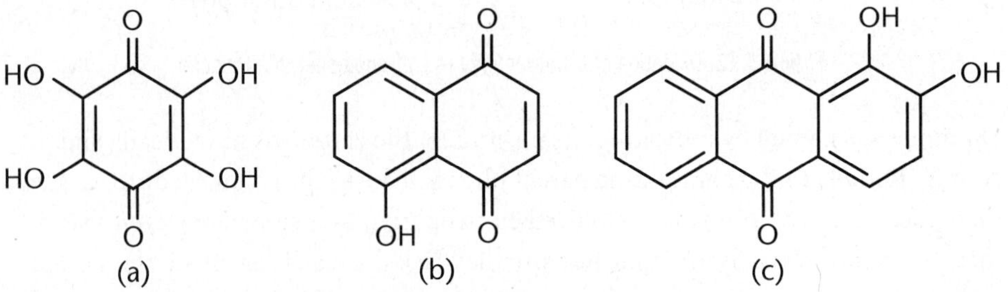

Figure 5.15 Three Examples of Hydroxyquinones
(a) Tetrahydroxybenzoquinone; (b) 5-hydroxynaphthoquinone; (c) 1,2-dihydroxyanthraquinone.

Ubiquinone

Ubiquinone is one example of a biologically active quinone. Ubiquinone is also called **coenzyme Q** and is a vital electron carrier associated with Complexes I, II, and III of the electron transport chain. Ubiquinone is the most oxidized form that this molecule takes physiologically: it can also be reduced to **ubiquinol** upon the acceptance of electrons, as shown in Figure 5.16. This oxidation–reduction capacity allows the molecule to perform its physiological function of electron transport.

BRIDGE

Coenzyme Q plays a role in Complexes I, II, and III of the electron transport chain. In Complex III, it is the main player in the Q cycle, which contributes to the formation of the proton-motive force across the inner mitochondrial membrane. The respiratory complexes are discussed in Chapter 10 of *MCAT Biochemistry Review.*

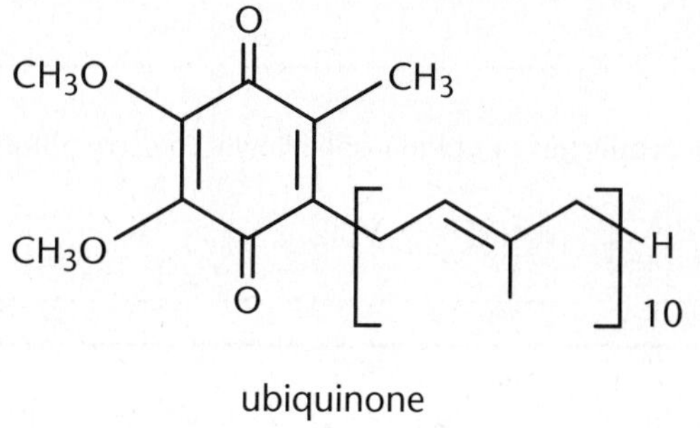

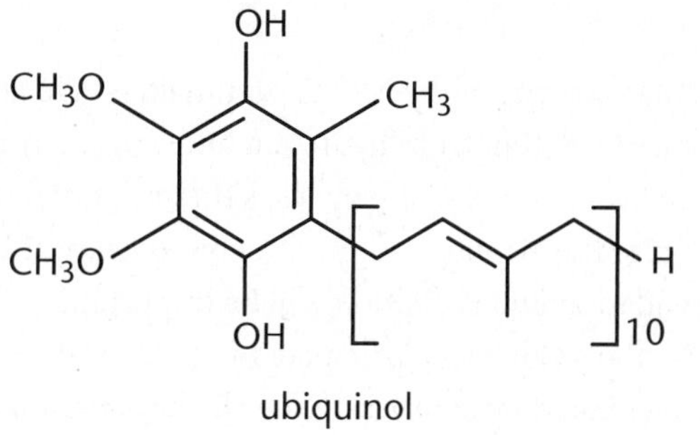

Figure 5.16 Ubiquinone (Coenzyme Q) and Ubiquinol
Ubiquinone is the oxidized form; when it picks up electrons, it is converted to its reduced form (ubiquinol).

The long alkyl chain of this molecule allows it to be lipid soluble, which allows it to act as an electron carrier within the phospholipid bilayer.

Other biological molecules that undergo oxidation–reduction reactions as part of their normal function include NADH, $FADH_2$, and NADPH. These molecules accept and donate electrons readily, similar to ubiquinone, and are discussed more thoroughly in Chapters 9 and 10 of *MCAT Biochemistry Review.*

MCAT CONCEPT CHECK 5.3

Before you move on, assess your understanding of the material with these questions.

1. How are quinones generally produced?

 ____

2. How are hydroxyquinones produced?

 ____

3. What chemical properties of ubiquinone allow it to carry out its biological functions?

 ____

Conclusion

Alcohols are a particular favorite of the MCAT test makers. We got our first look at the unique properties that stem from hydrogen bonding, an important ability of alcohols. Alcohols can be oxidized to aldehydes, ketones, or carboxylic acids depending on the substitution of the alcohol and the strength of the oxidizing agent. From this point forward, oxidation and reduction will be important reactions with all functional groups. Alcohols can also participate in nucleophilic substitution reactions, which may be facilitated by converting the alcohol into a mesylate or tosylate. Finally, phenols (and their oxidized counterparts, quinones and hydroxyquinones) are involved in a number of biochemical pathways. In particular, their utility is seen in processes that require rapid oxidation and reduction, such as photosynthesis and the electron transport chain.

Over the next four chapters, we'll explore other oxygen-containing compounds. Recognize that these chapters are put in a specific order: as you move further along in *MCAT Organic Chemistry Review*, the functional groups will become more oxidized and more reactive. First, we'll look at aldehydes and ketones (and their deprotonated forms, *enols* and *enolates*). Then, we'll explore carboxylic acids and their derivatives: amides, esters, and anhydrides.

You've reviewed the content, now test your knowledge and critical thinking skills by completing a test-like passage set in your online resources!

GO ONLINE

CONCEPT SUMMARY

Description and Properties

- **Alcohols** have the general form ROH and are named with the suffix *-ol*. If they are not the highest priority, they are given the prefix ***hydroxy-***.
- **Phenols** are benzene rings with hydroxyl groups. They are named for the relative positions of the hydroxyl groups: ***ortho-*** (adjacent carbons), ***meta-*** (separated by one carbon), or ***para-*** (on opposite sides of the ring).
- Alcohols can hydrogen bond, raising their boiling and melting points relative to corresponding alkanes. Hydrogen bonding also increases the solubility of alcohols.
- Phenols are more acidic than other alcohols because the aromatic ring can delocalize the charge of the conjugate base.
- Electron-donating groups like alkyl groups decrease acidity because they destabilize negative charges. Electron-withdrawing groups, such as electronegative atoms and aromatic rings, increase acidity because they stabilize negative charges.

Reactions of Alcohols

- Primary alcohols can be oxidized to aldehydes only by **pyridinium chlorochromate (PCC)**; they will be oxidized all the way to carboxylic acids by any stronger oxidizing agents.
- Secondary alcohols can be oxidized to ketones by any common oxidizing agent.
- Alcohols can be converted to mesylates or tosylates to make them better leaving groups for nucleophilic substitution reactions.
  - **Mesylates** contain the functional group $-SO_3CH_3$, which is derived from methanesulfonic acid.
  - **Tosylates** contain the functional group $-SO_3C_6H_4CH_3$, which is derived from toluenesulfonic acid.
- Aldehydes or ketones can be protected by converting them into acetals or ketals.
  - Two equivalents of alcohol or a dialcohol are reacted with the carbonyl to form an **acetal** (a primary carbon with two $-OR$ groups and a hydrogen atom) or **ketal** (a secondary carbon with two $-OR$ groups).
  - Other functional groups in the compound can be reacted (especially by reduction) without effects on the newly formed acetal or ketal.
  - The acetal or ketal can then be converted back to a carbonyl by catalytic acid, which is called **deprotection**.

Reactions of Phenols

- **Quinones** are synthesized through oxidation of phenols.
    - Quinones are resonance-stabilized electrophiles.
    - Vitamin K_1 (**phylloquinone**) and Vitamin K_2 (the **menaquinones**) are examples of biochemically relevant quinones.
- **Hydroxyquinones** are produced by oxidation of quinones, adding a variable number of hydroxyl groups.
- **Ubiquinone** (**coenzyme Q**) is another biologically active quinone that acts as an electron acceptor in Complexes I, II, and III of the electron transport chain. It is reduced to **ubiquinol**.

ANSWERS TO CONCEPT CHECKS

5.1

1. Phenols like *p*-ethylphenol have increased acidity due to resonance and the electron-withdrawing character of the phenol aromatic ring. Because *p*-ethylphenol is a stronger acid than ethanol, it will have a lower pK_a.
2. 1,6-Hexanediol will have the highest boiling point; a molecule with two hydroxyl moieties can have more hydrogen bonding. The 1-hexanol boiling point will be next, with 1-pentanol having the lowest boiling point. 1-Hexanol has a higher boiling point than 1-pentanol because the longer hydrocarbon chain has increased van der Waals forces.

5.2

1. In the presence of strong oxidizing agents, primary alcohols are completely oxidized to carboxylic acids. Secondary alcohols can only be oxidized to ketones.
2. Reacting 1-butanol with PCC results in the aldehyde, 1-butanal. Chromium trioxide is a stronger oxidizing agent that will produce the carboxylic acid, butanoic acid.
3. Mesylates and tosylates are used to convert an alcohol into a better leaving group. This is particularly useful for nucleophilic substitution reactions because it increases the stability of the product. They can also be used as protecting groups because many reagents (especially oxidizing agents) that would react with an alcohol cannot react with these compounds.
4. Aldehydes or ketones can be reacted with two equivalents of alcohol or a diol to form an acetal or ketal. Acetals and ketals are less reactive than aldehydes and ketones (especially to reducing agents), and can thus protect the functional group from reacting. The acetal or ketal can then be reverted back to the carbonyl by catalytic acid.

5.3

1. Quinones are produced by oxidation of phenols.
2. Hydroxyquinones are produced by the oxidation of quinones, adding a variable number of additional hydroxyl groups.
3. Ubiquinone has conjugated rings that stabilize the molecule when accepting electrons. Additionally, the long alkyl chain in the molecule allows for lipid solubility, which allows the molecule to function in the phospholipid bilayer.

SCIENCE MASTERY ASSESSMENT EXPLANATIONS

1. **B**

Alcohols have higher boiling points than their analogous hydrocarbons as a result of their polarized O—H bonds, in which oxygen is partially negative and hydrogen is partially positive. This enables the oxygen atoms of other alcohol molecules to be attracted to the hydrogen, forming a hydrogen bond. Heat is required to overcome these hydrogen bonds, thereby increasing the boiling point. The analogous hydrocarbons do not form hydrogen bonds and, therefore, vaporize at lower temperatures. **(A)** is irrelevant; oxygen's bond length is not a factor in determining a substance's boiling point. **(C)** and **(D)** are true statements, but are also irrelevant to boiling point determination.

2. **A**

Tertiary alcohols can be oxidized only under extreme conditions because their substrate carbons do not have spare hydrogens to give up. Alcohol oxidation involves the removal of such a hydrogen so that carbon can instead make another bond to oxygen. If no hydrogen is present, a carbon–carbon bond must be cleaved, which requires a great deal of energy and will, therefore, occur only under extreme conditions. **(B)** is incorrect because alcohols are not carbonyl-containing compounds and would more properly describe a carbonyl-containing compound that is unable to form an enolate. **(C)** is incorrect because the hydroxyl group of the tertiary carbon is still polarized. **(D)** is a false statement; tertiary alcohols are still involved in other reactions, such as S_N1 reactions.

3. **B**

Remember, diols are named after the parent alkane, with the position of the alcohols indicated, and ending in the suffix *-diol*. Here the carbon chain is three carbons, with a hydroxyl group on carbons 1 and 2. Thus, the name is propane-1,2-diol.

4. **B**

This molecule is a phenol, not a hexanol, because the cyclic group has aromatic double bonds rather than single bonds. The methyl group is separated from the hydroxyl carbon by one carbon in between, making this molecule *m*-methylphenol.

5. **C**

All else being equal, boiling points increase with increasing size of the alkyl chain because of increased van der Waals attractions. Isobutyl alcohol has the largest alkyl chain and will thus have the highest boiling point; methanol has the smallest chain and will thus have the lowest boiling point.

6. **B**

Phenols have significantly more acidic hydroxyl hydrogens than other alcohols because of resonance stabilization of the conjugate base, so this will be the most acidic hydroxyl hydrogen. The acidity of hexanol and cyclohexanol are close, but the hydroxyl hydrogen of hexanol is slightly more acidic because the ring structure of cyclohexanol is slightly electron-donating, which makes its hydroxyl hydrogen slightly less acidic.

7. **B**

$CH_3CH_2CH_2OH$ is 1-propanol, a primary alcohol. The desired end product, CH_3CH_2CHO, is propanal, an aldehyde. Of the available options, the only reactant capable of oxidizing primary alcohols to aldehydes is pyridinium chlorochromate (PCC). Chromic trioxide and dichromate salts will both oxidize primary alcohols to carboxylic acids.

8. **D**

Cyclohexanol is a secondary alcohol, so any of the oxidizing agents listed will convert it to a ketone.

9. **A**

Acidic conditions, provided by dilute sulfuric acid, are required to complete the Jones oxidation. This reaction is carried out in aqueous conditions, eliminating **(C)**. While heat may speed up the reaction, high temperatures are not required for this reaction, eliminating **(D)**.

10. **A**

Methylsulfonyl chloride serves as a protecting group for alcohols, which are converted into mesylates. Reacting with this reagent before continuing with what would normally be an oxidation reaction keeps the alcohol from reacting; when the protecting group is then removed using strong acid, the resultant product is the same as the initial reactant. Neither of the oxidation products in **(B)** or **(C)**, nor the reduction product in **(D)**, will be formed.

11. **A**

This reaction will create a ketal. This is the first step of the protection of aldehydes or ketones using dialcohols.

12. **D**

This is the Jones oxidation, which will convert a primary alcohol into a carboxylic acid. **(A)** is the original reacting molecule, and because the reaction will proceed, this is not correct. Because the reaction uses strong oxidizing agents, it won't stop at the aldehyde, **(B)**. This reaction also cannot make the ketone in **(C)** because it starts with a primary alcohol.

13. **B**

In order to convert phenols into hydroxyquinones, they must first be converted to quinones through an oxidation step; a second oxidation step is required to further oxidize quinones to hydroxyquinones.

14. **C**

The reaction that converts ubiquinone into ubiquinol is a reduction reaction in which two ketones are reduced to two hydroxyl groups.

15. **A**

An acetal can be converted to a carbonyl and a dialcohol by treatment with aqueous acid. This is the final step when using alcohols as protecting groups, called deprotection.

Consult your online resources for additional practice. GO ONLINE

SHARED CONCEPTS

Biochemistry Chapter 5
Lipid Structure and Function

General Chemistry Chapter 8
The Gas Phase

Organic Chemistry Chapter 1
Nomenclature

Organic Chemistry Chapter 4
Analyzing Organic Reactions

Organic Chemistry Chapter 6
Aldehydes and Ketones I

Organic Chemistry Chapter 8
Carboxylic Acids

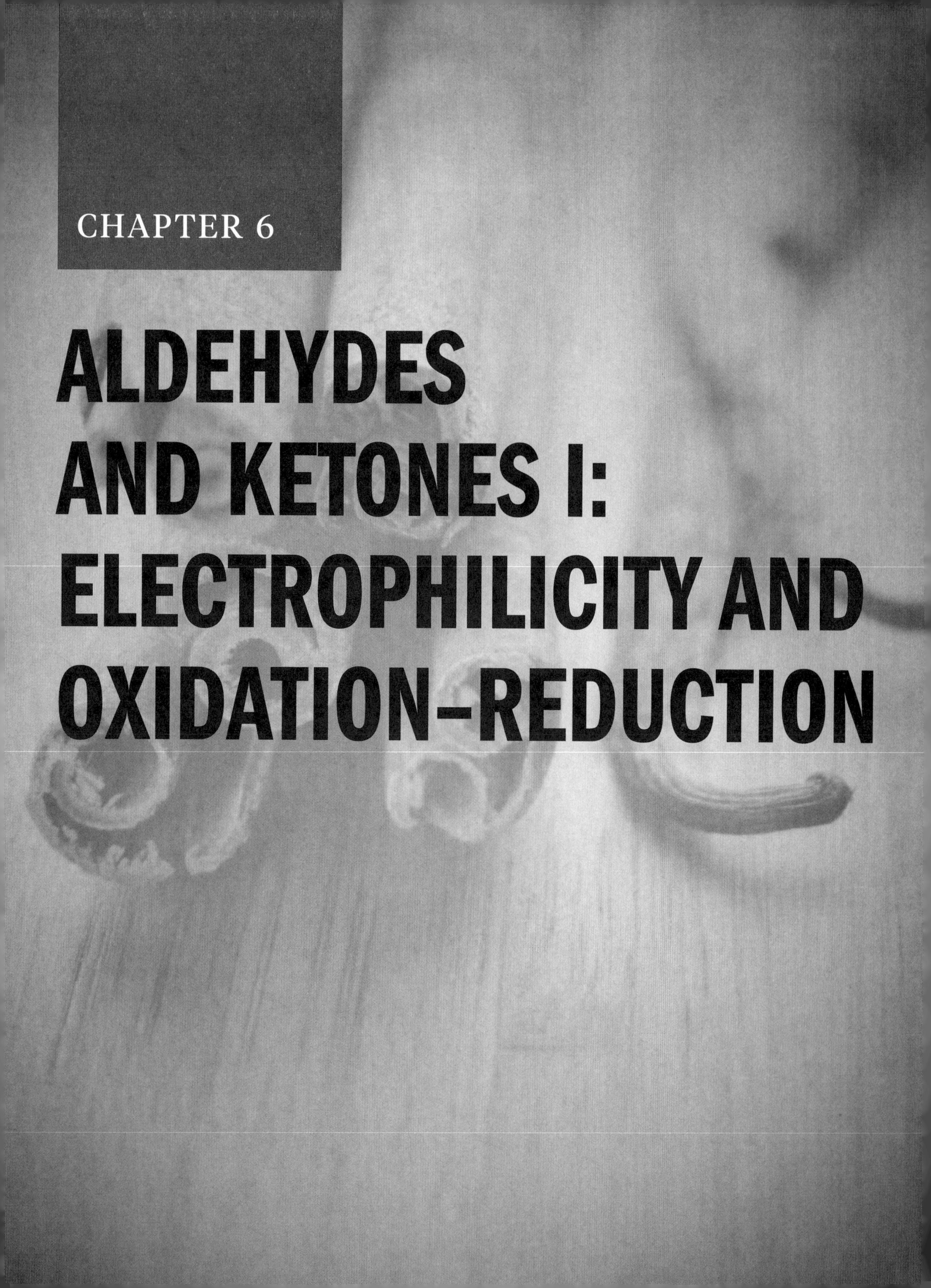

CHAPTER 6

ALDEHYDES AND KETONES I: ELECTROPHILICITY AND OXIDATION–REDUCTION

SCIENCE MASTERY ASSESSMENT

Every pre-med knows this feeling: there is so much content I have to know for the MCAT! How do I know what to do first or what's important?

While the high-yield badges throughout this book will help you identify the most important topics, this Science Mastery Assessment is another tool in your MCAT prep arsenal. This quiz (which can also be taken in your online resources) and the guidance below will help ensure that you are spending the appropriate amount of time on this chapter based on your personal strengths and weaknesses. Don't worry though—skipping something now does not mean you'll never study it. Later on in your prep, as you complete full-length tests, you'll uncover specific pieces of content that you need to review and can come back to these chapters as appropriate.

How to Use This Assessment

If you answer 0–7 questions correctly:

Spend about 1 hour to read this chapter in full and take limited notes throughout. Follow up by reviewing **all** quiz questions to ensure that you now understand how to solve each one.

If you answer 8–11 questions correctly:

Spend 20–40 minutes reviewing the quiz questions. Beginning with the questions you missed, read and take notes on the corresponding subchapters. For questions you answered correctly, ensure your thinking matches that of the explanation and you understand why each choice was correct or incorrect.

If you answer 12–15 questions correctly:

Spend less than 20 minutes reviewing all questions from the quiz. If you missed any, then include a quick read-through of the corresponding subchapters, or even just the relevant content within a subchapter, as part of your question review. For questions you got correct, ensure your thinking matches that of the explanation and review the Concept Summary at the end of the chapter.

1. All of the following are true with respect to carbonyls EXCEPT:
   A. the carbonyl carbon is electrophilic.
   B. the carbonyl oxygen is electron-withdrawing.
   C. a resonance structure of the functional group places a positive charge on the carbonyl carbon.
   D. the π electrons are mobile and are pulled toward the carbonyl carbon.

2. Order the following compounds by increasing boiling point: butane, butanol, butanone
   A. Butanol < butane < butanone
   B. Butane < butanone < butanol
   C. Butanone < butane < butanol
   D. Butane < butanol < butanone

3. What is the product of the reaction below?

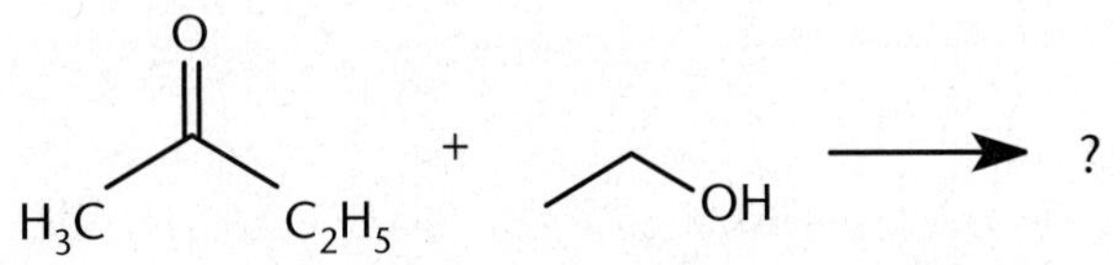

A. 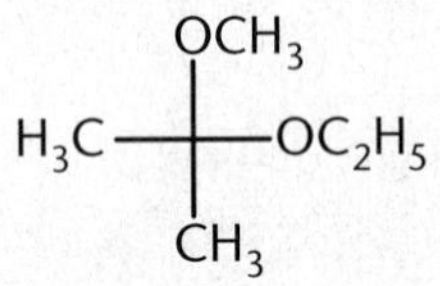

B. 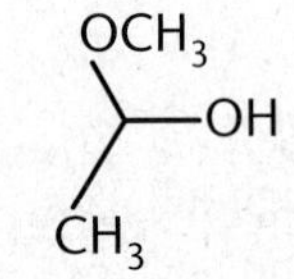

C. 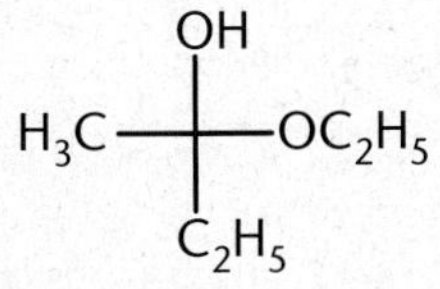

D. 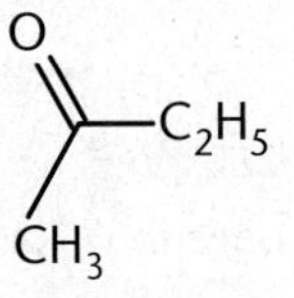

4. What is the product of the reaction below?

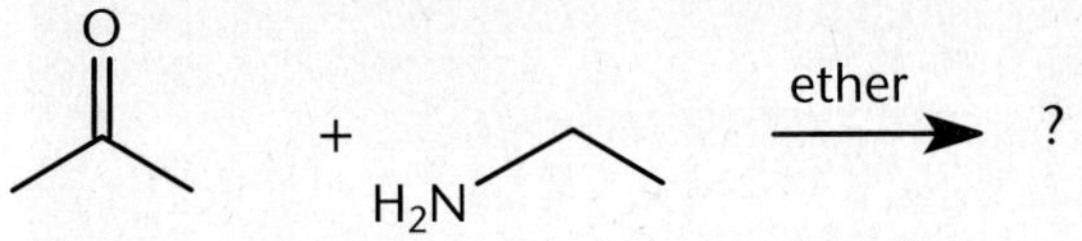

A. 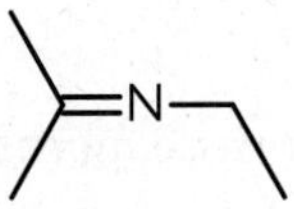

B. 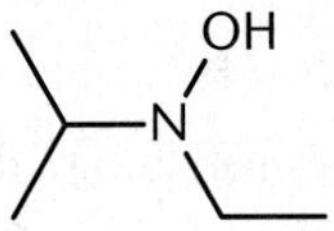

C. 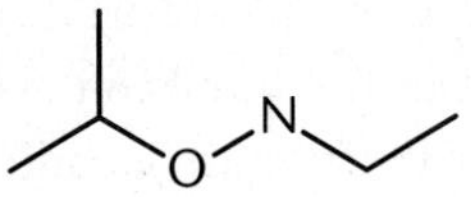

D. 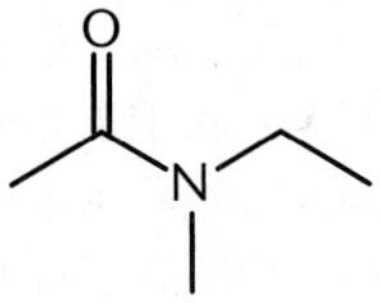

5. What is the product of the reaction below?

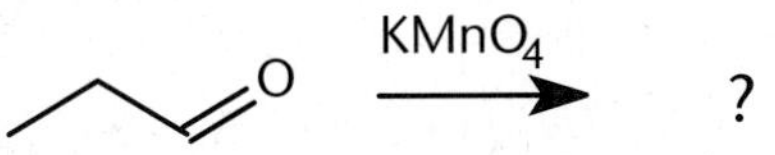

   A. C_3H_7OH
   B. C_2H_5COOH
   C. C_2H_5CHO
   D. CH_3COOH

6. What is the product of the reaction below?

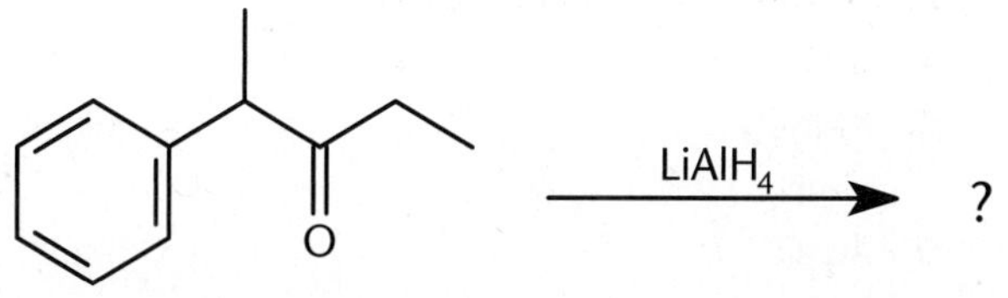

A. 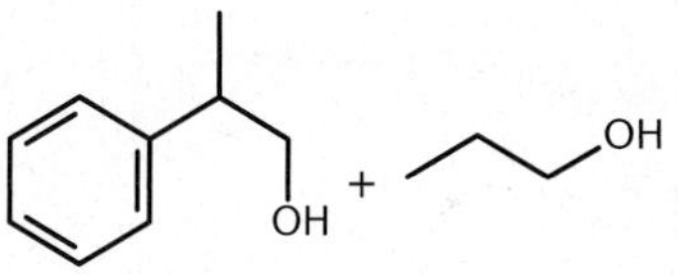

B. 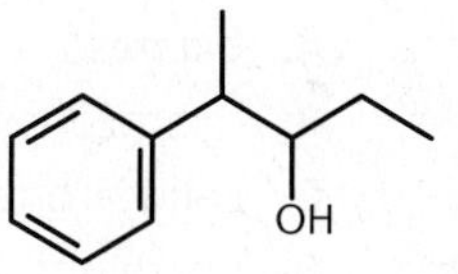

C. 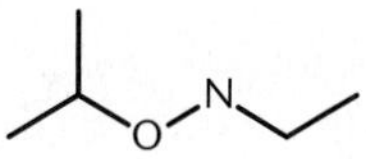

D. 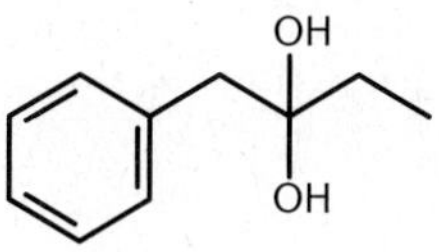

7. What is the product of the reaction between benzaldehyde and an excess of ethanol (CH_3CH_2OH) in the presence of anhydrous HCl?

A. 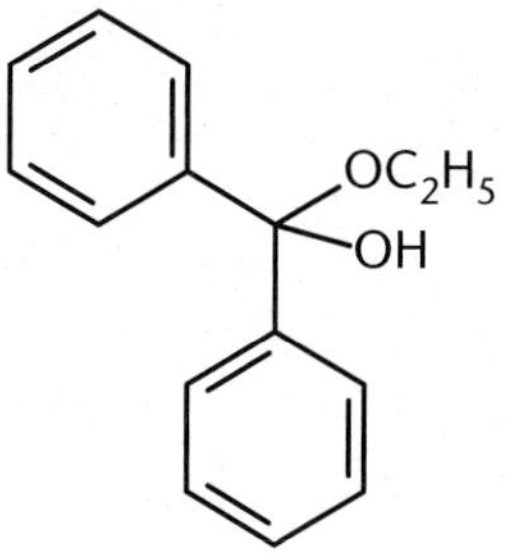

B. 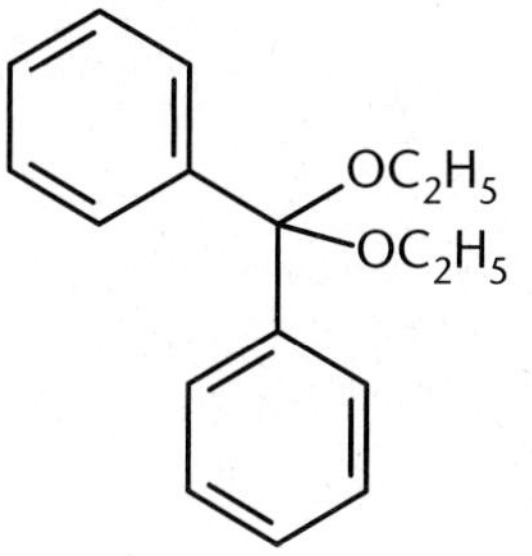

C. 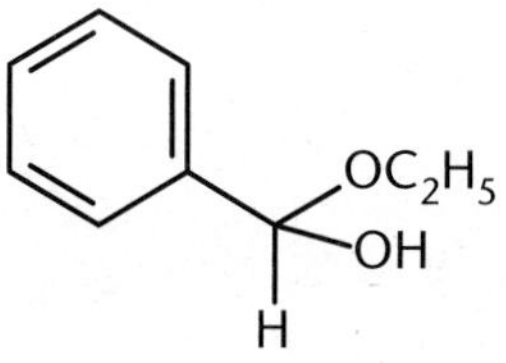

D. 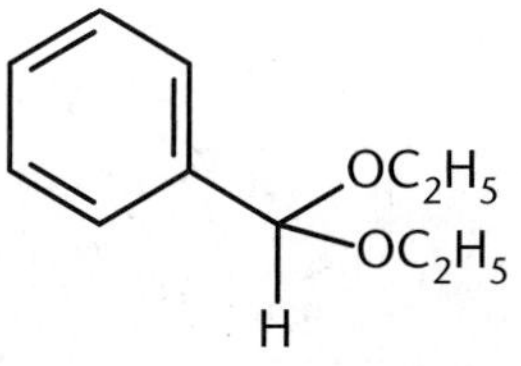

8. Hemiacetals and hemiketals usually keep reacting to form acetals and ketals. Why is it difficult to isolate hemiacetals and hemiketals?
   - **I.** These molecules are unstable.
   - **II.** The hydroxyl group is rapidly protonated and lost as water under acidic conditions, leaving behind a reactive carbocation.
   - **III.** The molecules are extremely basic and react rapidly with one another.

   A. I only
   B. I and II only
   C. II and III only
   D. I, II, and III

9. In a hemiacetal, the central carbon is bonded to:
   A. —OH, —OR, —H and —R.
   B. —H, —OR, —OR, and —R.
   C. —OH, —OR, —R, and —R.
   D. —OR, —OR, —R, and —R.

10. In a reaction between hydrogen cyanide, butyraldehyde, and ethylmethylketone, which compounds will come together to form the major product?
   A. Butyraldehyde and hydrogen cyanide
   B. Ethylmethylketone and butyraldehyde
   C. Hydrogen cyanide and ethylmethylketone
   D. No reaction will occur.

11. Which of the following describe(s) pyridinium chlorochromate (PCC)?
   - **I.** An oxidant that can form aldehydes from primary alcohols
   - **II.** An oxidant that can completely oxidize primary alcohols
   - **III.** An oxidant that can completely oxidize secondary alcohols

   A. I only
   B. I and II only
   C. I and III only
   D. I, II, and III

12. To form a geminal diol, which of the following could attack a carbonyl carbon?
   - **A.** Hydrogen peroxide
   - **B.** Water
   - **C.** Potassium dichromate
   - **D.** Ethanol

13. In a reaction between ammonia and glutaraldehyde, what is the major product?
   - **A.** An imine
   - **B.** A cyanohydrin
   - **C.** A semicarbazone
   - **D.** A hydrazone

14. Which of the following can be used to reduce a ketone to a secondary alcohol?
   - **A.** CrO_3
   - **B.** $KMnO_4$
   - **C.** $LiAlH_4$
   - **D.** Ag_2O

15. Imines naturally tautomerize to form:
   - **A.** oximes.
   - **B.** hydrazones.
   - **C.** semicarbazones.
   - **D.** enamines.

Answer Key follows on next page.

Answer Key

1. **D**
2. **B**
3. **C**
4. **A**
5. **B**
6. **B**
7. **D**
8. **B**
9. **A**
10. **A**
11. **C**
12. **B**
13. **A**
14. **C**
15. **D**

Detailed explanations can be found at the end of the chapter.

CHAPTER 6

ALDEHYDES AND KETONES I: ELECTROPHILICITY AND OXIDATION–REDUCTION

In This Chapter

CHAPTER PROFILE

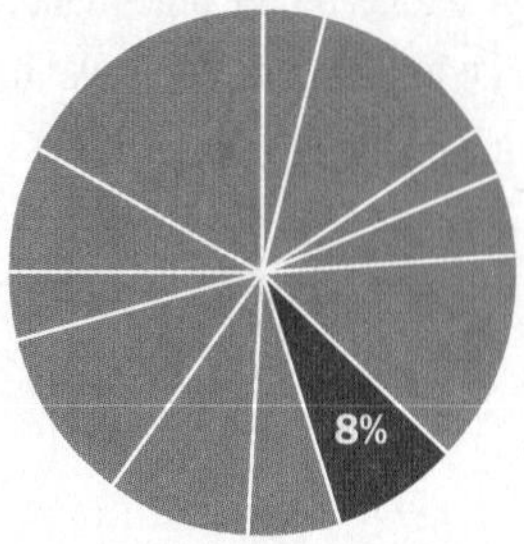

The content in this chapter should be relevant to about 8% of all questions about organic chemistry on the MCAT.

This chapter covers material from the following AAMC content category:

5D: Structure, function, and reactivity of biologically-relevant molecules

Introduction

This chapter focuses on an important functional group for the MCAT: the carbonyl. Aldehydes and ketones, the two functional groups highlighted here, have a lot in common because they both contain a **carbonyl**—a double bond between a carbon and an oxygen. The only difference between the two is what is attached to the carbonyl carbon.

The carbonyl group is one of the most common functional groups in organic chemistry for two reasons. First, the carbonyl is a component of many different functional groups. In addition to aldehydes and ketones, the carbonyl is found in carboxylic acids, esters, amides, anhydrides, and several other compounds. More importantly, the carbonyl has the unique ability to behave as either a nucleophile (as in condensation reactions) or an electrophile (as in nucleophilic addition reactions). In this chapter, we will investigate the overall properties of aldehydes and ketones, as well as their oxidation–reduction reactions and electrophilic properties. In the following chapter, we will investigate their nucleophilic properties through *enolate* chemistry.

6.1 Description and Properties

LEARNING OBJECTIVES

After Chapter 6.1, you will be able to:

- Name aldehydes and ketones using the proper suffixes
- Describe the reactivity of the carbonyl carbon
- Recognize common reactions used to form aldehydes and ketones
- Predict the boiling point of a compound based on its oxidation level

KEY CONCEPT

An aldehyde is a terminal functional group. A ketone, on the other hand, will always be internal and can never be a terminal functional group.

A **ketone** has two alkyl groups bonded to the carbonyl, whereas an **aldehyde** has one alkyl group and one hydrogen. This means that the carbonyl in a ketone is never a terminal group, whereas it always is in an aldehyde. Like many organic compounds, aldehydes and ketones are often strong-smelling compounds. Volatile carbonyls are found in many spices, including cinnamon (*cinnamaldehyde*), vanilla (*vanillin*), cumin (*cuminaldehyde*), dill (*carvenone*), and ginger (*zingerone*).

Nomenclature

Aldehydes are named by replacing the *–e* at the end of the alkane name with the suffix *–al*. Common names for the first five aldehydes, shown in Figure 6.1, are *formaldehyde, acetaldehyde, propionaldehyde, butyraldehyde,* and *valeraldehyde*. When aldehydes are named as substituents, use the prefix ***oxo–***.

MCAT EXPERTISE

Notice that these common names have a pattern that can help us: *form–* will also be seen in *formic acid* (a one-carbon carboxylic acid), and *acet–* is seen in many two-carbon compounds (*acetylene, acetic acid,* and *acetyl-CoA*).

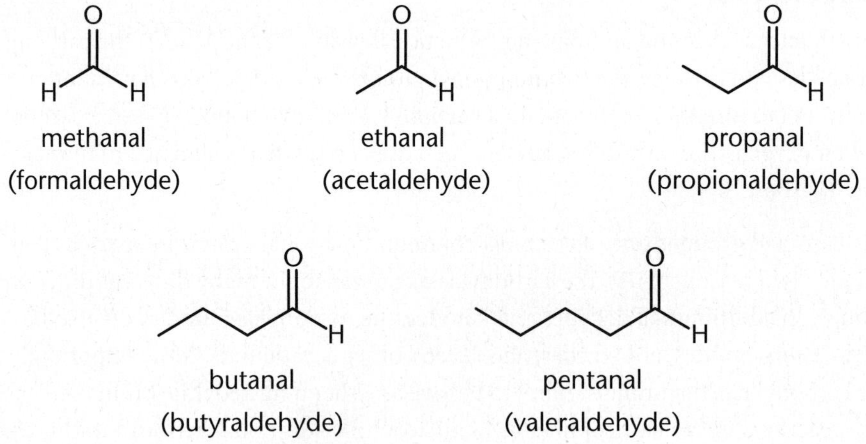

Figure 6.1 Naming Aldehydes

If the aldehyde is attached to a ring, the suffix *–**carbaldehyde*** is used instead. This is shown in Figure 6.2.

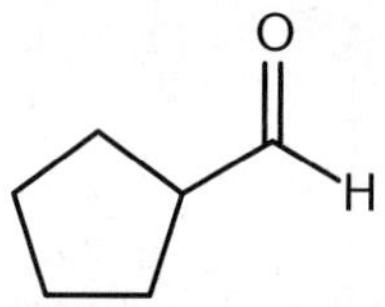

cyclopentanecarbaldehyde

Figure 6.2 Naming Cyclic Aldehydes

Ketones are named by replacing the –*e* with the suffix –***one***. When naming ketones by their common names, the two alkyl groups are named alphabetically, followed by –***ketone***. When ketones are named as substituents, use either the prefix ***oxo***– or ***keto***–. Figure 6.3 shows some examples of ketones.

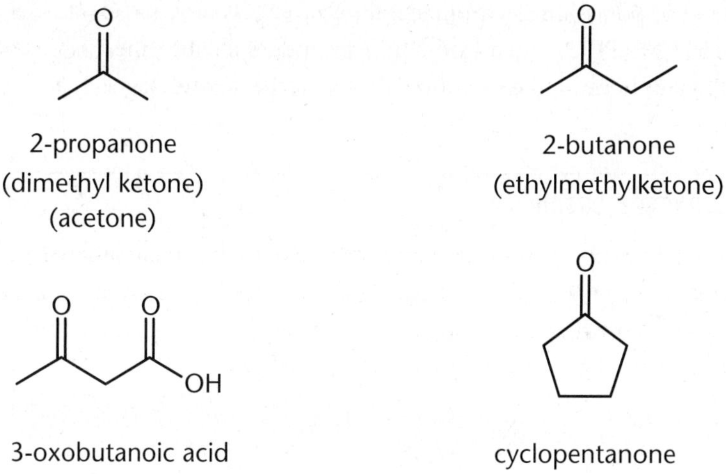

Figure 6.3 Naming Ketones

Physical Properties

The physical properties of aldehydes and ketones are governed by the presence of the carbonyl group. The dipole of the carbonyl is stronger than the dipole of an alcohol because the double-bonded oxygen is more electron-withdrawing than the single bond to oxygen in the hydroxyl group. In solution, the dipole moments associated with these polar carbonyl groups increase intermolecular attractions, causing an elevation in boiling point relative to their parent alkanes. However, even though aldehydes and ketones have dipoles more polar than those of alcohols, the elevation in boiling point is less than that in alcohols because no hydrogen bonding is present. In reactions, aldehydes and ketones both act as electrophiles, making good targets for nucleophiles. This is due to the electron-withdrawing properties of the carbonyl oxygen, which leaves a partial positive charge on the carbon, as shown in Figure 6.4. Generally, aldehydes are more reactive toward nucleophiles than ketones because they have less steric hindrance and fewer electron-donating alkyl groups.

KEY CONCEPT

While the dipole moment in the carbonyl group increases the intermolecular forces (and therefore boiling points) of aldehydes and ketones relative to alkanes, this is not as significant as the impact of hydrogen bonding seen in alcohols.

MCAT EXPERTISE

The carbonyl carbon is the most common electrophile you'll see on Test Day. Remember why this group has a dipole moment: oxygen is more electronegative and pulls electrons away from the carbon, making the carbon electrophilic and a good target for nucleophiles.

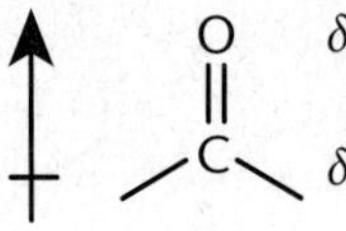

Figure 6.4 Polarity of the Carbonyl Group

Formation

Aldehydes and ketones can be produced by several mechanisms. An aldehyde can be obtained from the partial oxidation of a primary alcohol, although only by **pyridinium chlorochromate (PCC;** $C_5H_5NH[CrO_3Cl]$). With any stronger oxidants, aldehydes will continue to be oxidized to carboxylic acids. A ketone can be obtained from the oxidation of a secondary alcohol. This can be performed using reagents ranging from sodium or potassium dichromate salts ($Na_2Cr_2O_7$ or $K_2Cr_2O_7$) to chromium trioxide (CrO_3) to PCC. When oxidizing a secondary alcohol, there is no concern for oxidizing too far because the reaction will stop at the ketone stage.

MCAT CONCEPT CHECK 6.1

Before you move on, assess your understanding of the material with these questions.

1. Name the following two compounds:

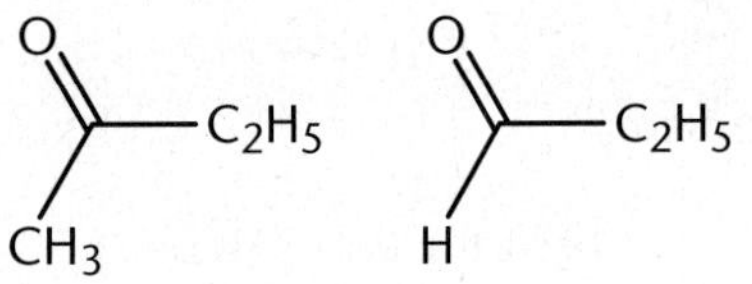

____

2. Given an alkane, an aldehyde, and an alcohol with equal-length carbon chains, which will have the highest boiling point? Why?

____

3. Is the carbon of a carbonyl electrophilic or nucleophilic? Why?

____

4. What is one method for forming an aldehyde? A ketone?

- Aldehyde:

____

- Ketone:

____

6.2 Nucleophilic Addition Reactions

LEARNING OBJECTIVES

After Chapter 6.2, you will be able to:

- Predict the products of reacting aldehydes or ketones with alcohols, in the presence or absence of acidic conditions
- Recall the functional group formed when nitrogen-containing derivatives react with aldehydes or ketones
- Predict the product of the reaction of HCN with aldehydes or ketones, including the reactivity of the product:

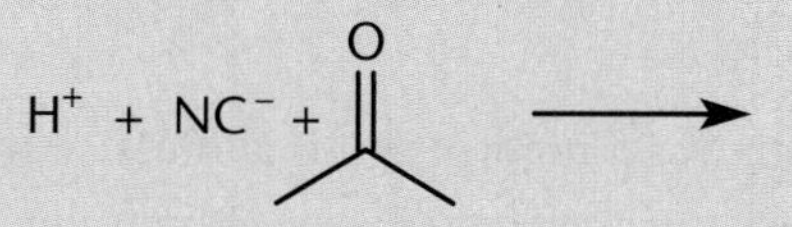

In each of the following reactions, the general reaction mechanism is the same: nucleophilic addition to a carbonyl. This is one of the most important reaction mechanisms on the MCAT, and many of the reactions of aldehydes, ketones, and more complex molecules share this general reaction mechanism. Rather than memorizing each reaction individually, focus on the overall pattern—then learn how a particular reaction exemplifies it.

As we have seen, the C=O bond is polarized, with a partial positive charge on the carbonyl carbon and a partial negative charge on the oxygen. This makes the carbonyl carbon an electrophile, ripe for nucleophilic attack.

When the nucleophile attacks, it forms a covalent bond to the carbon, breaking the π bond in the carbonyl. The electrons from the π bond are pushed onto the oxygen atom. Oxygen happily accepts extra electrons due to its electronegativity. Breaking the π bond forms a tetrahedral intermediate. Any time a carbonyl is opened, one should ask: *Can I reform the carbonyl?* If no good leaving group is present (as is the case with aldehydes and ketones), the carbonyl will not reform. Generally, O^- will accept a proton from the solvent to form a hydroxyl group, resulting in an alcohol. However, if a good leaving group is present (as is the case with carboxylic acids and their derivatives), the carbonyl double bond can reform, pushing off the leaving group. Figure 6.5 shows the reaction mechanism of nucleophilic addition for an aldehyde.

MCAT EXPERTISE

Memorizing one reaction may help you to get one question right on the MCAT, but understanding trends and overarching concepts will allow you to answer many more questions correctly. You will see that the carbonyl carbon is a great target for nucleophilic attack in many of the reactions in this chapter.

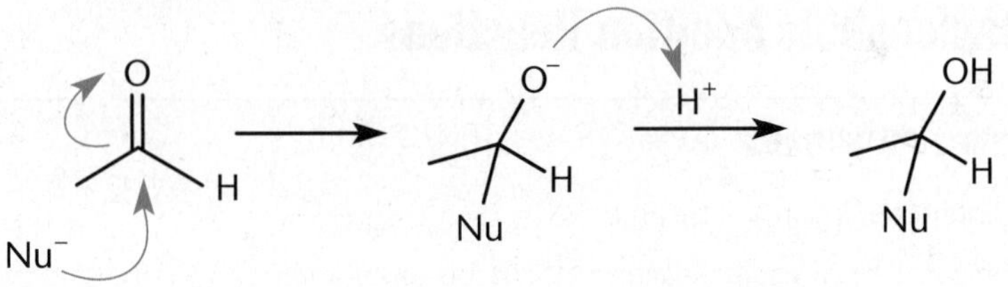

Figure 6.5 Nucleophilic Addition Reaction Mechanism
The nucleophile attacks the carbonyl carbon, opening the carbonyl. The carbonyl cannot reform because there is no good leaving group; thus, the O⁻ is protonated to generate an alcohol.

Hydration

In the presence of water, aldehydes and ketones react to form **geminal diols** (1,1-diols), as shown in Figure 6.6. In this case, the nucleophilic oxygen in water attacks the electrophilic carbonyl carbon. This hydration reaction normally proceeds slowly, but we can increase the rate by adding a small amount of catalytic acid or base.

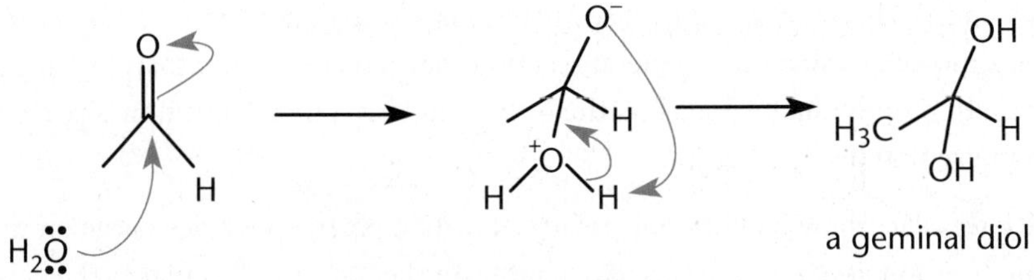

Figure 6.6 Hydration Reaction
The carbonyl is hydrated by water, then protonated, resulting in a geminal diol.

Acetals and Hemiacetals

A similar reaction occurs when aldehydes and ketones are treated with alcohols. When one equivalent of alcohol (the nucleophile in this reaction) is added to an aldehyde or ketone, the product is a **hemiacetal** or **hemiketal**, respectively, as shown in Figure 6.7. Hemiacetals and hemiketals can be recognized by the retention of the hydroxyl group. This "halfway" step (hence the *hemi–* prefix) is the endpoint in basic conditions.

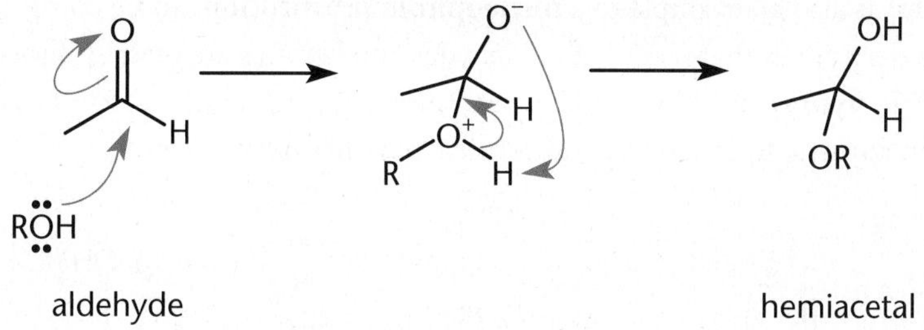

Figure 6.7 Hemiacetal Formation
The oxygen in the alcohol functions as the nucleophile, attacking the carbonyl carbon and generating a hemiacetal.

When two equivalents of alcohol are added, the reaction proceeds to completion, resulting in the formation of an **acetal** or **ketal**, as shown in Figure 6.8. This reaction proceeds by a nucleophilic substitution reaction (S_N1) and is catalyzed by anhydrous acid. The hydroxyl group of a hemiacetal or hemiketal is protonated under acidic conditions and lost as a molecule of water. A carbocation is thus formed, and another equivalent of alcohol attacks this carbocation, resulting in the formation of an acetal or ketal. Acetals and ketals, which are comparatively inert, are frequently used as protecting groups for carbonyl functionalities. Molecules with protecting groups can easily be converted back to carbonyls with aqueous acid and heat.

KEY CONCEPT

In the formation of hemiacetals and hemiketals, alcohol is the nucleophile and the carbonyl carbon is the electrophile. In the formation of acetals and ketals, alcohol is the nucleophile, and the carbocation carbon (formerly the carbonyl carbon) is the electrophile.

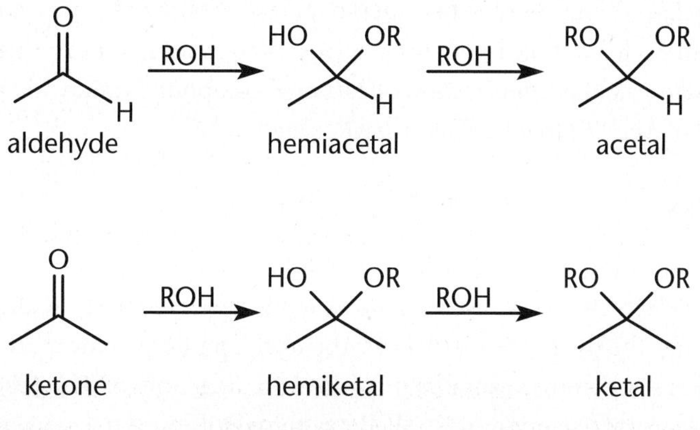

Figure 6.8 Acetal and Ketal Formation
Once a hemiacetal or hemiketal is formed, the hydroxyl group is protonated and released as a molecule of water; alcohol then attacks, forming an acetal or ketal.

Imines and Enamines

Nitrogen and nitrogen-based functional groups act as good nucleophiles due to the lone pair of electrons on nitrogen, and react readily with the electrophilic carbonyls of aldehydes and ketones. In the simplest case, ammonia adds to the carbon atom and water is lost, producing an **imine**, a compound with a nitrogen atom double-bonded to a carbon atom. This reaction is shown in Figure 6.9. Because a small molecule is lost during the formation of a bond between two molecules, this is an example of a **condensation reaction**. Because nitrogen replaces the carbonyl oxygen, this is also an example of a **nucleophilic substitution**. Some common ammonia derivatives that react with aldehydes and ketones are **hydroxylamine** ($H_2N{-}OH$), **hydrazine** ($H_2N{-}NH_2$), and **semicarbazide** ($H_2N{-}NH{-}C(O)NH_2$); these form **oximes**, **hydrazones**, and **semicarbazones**, respectively.

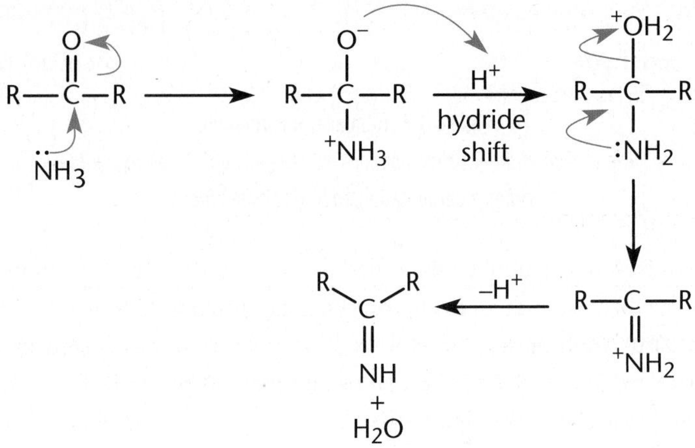

Figure 6.9 Imine Formation
Ammonia is added to the carbonyl, resulting in the elimination of water and generation of an imine.

Imines and related compounds can undergo tautomerization to form **enamines**, which contain both a double bond and a nitrogen-containing group. This is analogous to the *keto–enol* tautomerization of carbonyl compounds and will be explored in Chapter 7 of *MCAT Organic Chemistry Review*.

Cyanohydrins

Hydrogen cyanide (HCN) is a classic nucleophile on the MCAT. HCN has both triple bonds and an electronegative nitrogen atom, rendering it relatively acidic with a pK_a of 9.2. After the hydrogen dissociates, the nucleophilic cyanide anion can attack the carbonyl carbon atom, as shown in Figure 6.10. Reactions with aldehydes and ketones produce stable compounds called **cyanohydrins** once the oxygen has been reprotonated. The cyanohydrin gains its stability from the newly formed C–C bond.

KEY CONCEPT

In a reaction with HCN, $^{-}$CN is the nucleophile; the carbonyl carbon is the electrophile.

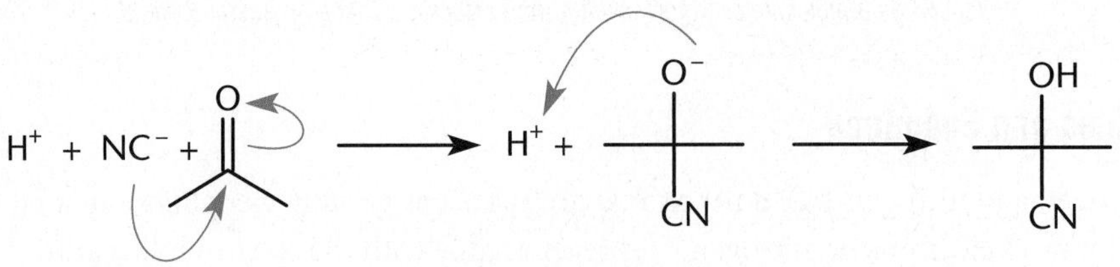

Figure 6.10 Cyanohydrin Formation
Cyanide functions as a nucleophile, attacking the carbonyl carbon and generating a cyanohydrin.

MCAT CONCEPT CHECK 6.2

Before you move on, assess your understanding of the material with these questions.

1. When an aldehyde or ketone is reacted with one equivalent of an alcohol, what occurs? What would be different if it were reacted with two equivalents in acidic conditions?

   - Aldehyde or ketone + 1 equivalent of alcohol:

   ____

   - Aldehyde or ketone + 2 equivalents of alcohol:

   ____

2. When nitrogen or nitrogen-containing derivatives react with aldehydes and ketones, what type of reaction happens, and what functional group is formed?

   ____

3. When HCN reacts with an aldehyde or ketone, what functional group is produced? Is the product stable?

   ____

6.3 Oxidation–Reduction Reactions

LEARNING OBJECTIVES

After Chapter 6.3, you will be able to:

- Recall common oxidizing and reducing agents used on aldehydes and ketones
- Predict the products of redox reactions involving aldehydes and ketones

Aldehydes occupy the middle of the oxidation–reduction spectrum; they are more oxidized than alcohols but less oxidized than carboxylic acids. Ketones, on the other hand, are as oxidized as secondary carbons can get.

Oxidation of Aldehydes

When aldehydes are further oxidized, they form carboxylic acids. Any oxidizing agent stronger than PCC can perform this reaction. Some examples include potassium permanganate ($KMnO_4$), chromium trioxide (CrO_3), silver(I) oxide (Ag_2O), and hydrogen peroxide (H_2O_2). This is shown in Figure 6.11.

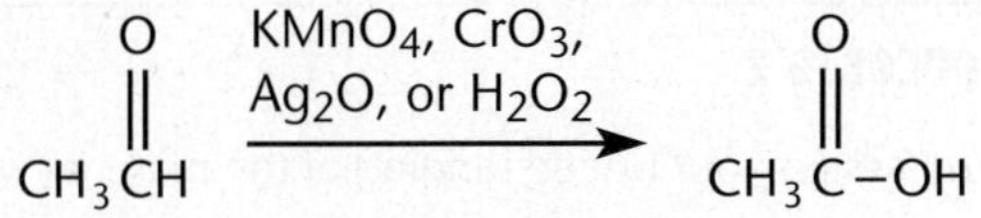

Figure 6.11 Aldehyde Oxidation
Most oxidizing agents will turn aldehydes into carboxylic acids; PCC, however, is anhydrous and is not strong enough to oxidize past the point of an aldehyde.

Reduction by Hydride Reagents

Aldehydes and ketones can also undergo reduction to form alcohols. This is often performed with **hydride reagents**. The most common of these seen on the MCAT are **lithium aluminum hydride** ($LiAlH_4$) and **sodium borohydride** ($NaBH_4$), which is often used when milder conditions are needed. This reaction is shown in Figure 6.12.

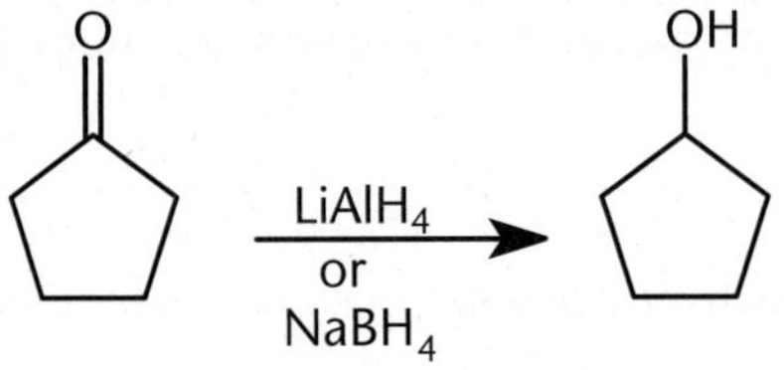

Figure 6.12 Ketone Reduction
Ketones are easily reduced to their respective alcohols using hydride reagents.

MCAT CONCEPT CHECK 6.3

Before you move on, assess your understanding of the material with these questions.

1. What functional group is formed when an aldehyde is oxidized? What are some common oxidizing agents that assist this reaction?
   - Functional group:
   - Oxidizing agents:
2. What functional group is formed when aldehydes and ketones are reduced? What are some common reducing agents that assist this reaction?
   - Functional group:
   - Reducing agents:
3. A chemistry student reacts butanone and butanal each with PCC and $KMnO_4$. What are the expected products of each reaction?
   - Butanone:
   - Butanal:

Conclusion

In this chapter, we have examined the properties of aldehydes and ketones. Specifically, we have taken a look at the reactivity of the carbonyl carbon in nucleophilic addition reactions and examined how aldehydes and ketones can be oxidized and reduced. Carbonyls are common reaction sites in many biosynthetic processes, which helps explain their importance on the MCAT.

In the following chapter, we will continue our exploration of aldehydes and ketones by looking at the chemistry of enolates, which are nucleophilic carbonyl-containing compounds.

GO ONLINE

You've reviewed the content, now test your knowledge and critical thinking skills by completing a test-like passage set in your online resources!

CONCEPT SUMMARY

Description and Properties

- **Aldehydes** are terminal functional groups containing a carbonyl bonded to at least one hydrogen. In nomenclature, they use the suffix *–**al*** and the prefix ***oxo***–. In rings, they are indicated by the suffix *–**carbaldehyde***.
- **Ketones** are internal functional groups containing a carbonyl bonded to two alkyl chains. In nomenclature, they use the suffix *–**one*** and the prefix ***oxo***– or ***keto***–.
- The reactivity of a **carbonyl** (C=O) is dictated by the polarity of the double bond. The carbon has a partial positive charge and is therefore electrophilic.
- Carbonyl-containing compounds have higher boiling points than equivalent alkanes because of dipole interactions. Alcohols have higher boiling points than carbonyls because of hydrogen bonding.
- Aldehydes and ketones are commonly produced by oxidation of primary and secondary alcohols, respectively.
  - Weaker, anhydrous oxidizing agents like **pyridinium chlorochromate** (**PCC**) must be used for synthesizing aldehydes, or the reaction will continue oxidizing to the level of the carboxylic acid.
  - Various oxidizing agents can be used for ketones, such as dichromate, chromium trioxide, or PCC because ketones are the most oxidized functional group for secondary carbons.

Nucleophilic Addition Reactions

- When a nucleophile attacks and forms a bond with a carbonyl carbon, electrons in the π bond are pushed to the oxygen atom.
  - If there is no good leaving group (aldehydes and ketones), the carbonyl will remain open and is protonated to form an alcohol.
  - If there is a good leaving group (carboxylic acids and derivatives), the carbonyl will reform and kick off the leaving group.
- In **hydration** reactions, water adds to a carbonyl, forming a **geminal diol**.
- When one equivalent of alcohol reacts with an aldehyde (via nucleophilic addition), a **hemiacetal** is formed. When the same reaction occurs with a ketone, a **hemiketal** is formed.
- When another equivalent of alcohol reacts with a hemiacetal (via nucleophilic substitution), an **acetal** is formed. When the same reaction occurs with a **hemiketal**, a ketal is formed.
- Nitrogen and nitrogen derivatives react with carbonyls to form **imines**, oximes, hydrazones, and semicarbazones. Imines can tautomerize to form **enamines**.
- Hydrogen cyanide reacts with carbonyls to form **cyanohydrins**.

Oxidation–Reduction Reactions

- Aldehydes can be oxidized to carboxylic acids using an oxidizing agent like $KMnO_4$, CrO_3, Ag_2O, or H_2O_2. They can be reduced to primary alcohols via **hydride reagents** ($LiAlH_4$, $NaBH_4$).
- Ketones cannot be further oxidized, but can be reduced to secondary alcohols using the same hydride reagents.

ANSWERS TO CONCEPT CHECKS

6.1

1. The molecule on the left is butanone. The molecule on the right is propanal.
2. The alkane will have the lowest boiling point, followed by the aldehyde, and then the alcohol. The boiling point of the aldehyde is elevated by its dipole, but the boiling point of an alcohol is further elevated by hydrogen bonding.
3. The carbon in a carbonyl is electrophilic; it is partially positively charged because oxygen is highly electron-withdrawing.
4. Aldehydes can be formed by the oxidation of primary alcohols, but can only be produced using weaker (and anhydrous) oxidizing agents like PCC—otherwise, they will oxidize fully to carboxylic acids. Ketones can be formed by the oxidation of secondary alcohols. Other methods can be used as well (ozonolysis, Friedel–Crafts acylation), but these are outside the scope of the MCAT.

6.2

1. With one equivalent of alcohol, aldehydes and ketones will form hemiacetals and hemiketals, respectively. With two equivalents of alcohol, the reaction will run to completion, forming acetals and ketals, respectively.
2. The reaction that occurs is a condensation reaction because a small molecule is lost, and also a nucleophilic substitution reaction. This reaction results in the formation of an imine (or, for nitrogen-containing derivatives: oximes, hydrazones, or semicarbazones).
3. When HCN reacts with an aldehyde or ketone, a cyanohydrin is produced, which is a stable product.

6.3

1. Oxidizing an aldehyde yields a carboxylic acid. Common oxidizing agents include $KMnO_4$, CrO_3, Ag_2O, and H_2O_2.
2. Reducing an aldehyde or ketone yields an alcohol. Under certain conditions not tested on the MCAT, aldehydes and ketones can be reduced all the way to alkanes. Common reducing agents include $LiAlH_4$ and $NaBH_4$.
3. Butanone reacts with neither PCC nor $KMnO_4$ because ketones cannot be oxidized with common oxidizing reagent that cannot break the carbon–carbon bond. Butanal is oxidized by $KMnO_4$ to form butanoic acid, but does not react with PCC, which is not a strong enough oxidant.

SCIENCE MASTERY ASSESSMENT EXPLANATIONS

1. **D**

The reactivity of the carbonyl can be attributed to the difference in electronegativity between the carbon and oxygen atoms. The more electronegative oxygen atom attracts the bonding electrons and is therefore electron-withdrawing. Thus, the carbonyl carbon is electrophilic. One resonance structure of the carbonyl pushes the π electrons onto the oxygen, resulting in a positively charged carbonyl carbon.

2. **B**

Assuming the length of the carbon chain remains the same, the alkane consistently has the lowest boiling point. The boiling point of the ketone is elevated by the dipole in the carbonyl. The boiling point of the alcohol is elevated further by hydrogen bonding.

3. **C**

The reaction between a ketone and one equivalent of alcohol produces a hemiketal. This has an –OR group, an –OH group, and two alkyl groups attached at the same carbon. **(A)** is a ketal, with two –OR groups and two –R groups. **(B)** is a hemiacetal, with an –OH group, an –OR group, one R group, and a hydrogen atom (not drawn). **(D)** is a ketone. Note that a hemiketal is a very unstable compound, and will react rapidly with a second equivalent of alcohol to form a ketal in acidic conditions.

4. **A**

Aldehydes and ketones react with ammonia and nitrogen-based derivatives to form imines—compounds with a double bond between carbon and nitrogen.

5. **B**

Aldehydes are easily oxidized to the corresponding carboxylic acids by $KMnO_4$. In **(A)**, the aldehyde has been reduced to an alcohol. In **(C)**, the molecule has not reacted. In **(D)**, the aldehyde has been oxidized, but a $-CH_2-$ group has been removed.

6. **B**

$LiAlH_4$ reduces aldehydes to primary alcohols and ketones to secondary alcohols. In this reaction, a ketone is converted to a secondary alcohol.

7. **D**

Because an excess of ethanol is present, the product of the reaction between this aldehyde and ethanol will be an acetal. The benzaldehyde will first be converted to a hemiacetal, shown in **(C)**, but will then proceed to completion as an acetal. **(A)** and **(B)** are incorrect because they show the presence of two benzene rings in the final product.

8. **B**

Hemiacetals and hemiketals are usually short-lived because the –OH group will rapidly become protonated in acidic conditions and is lost as water, leaving behind a carbocation that is very susceptible to attack by an alcohol. Once the alcohol has been added, the acetal or ketal becomes more stable because the newly added group is less likely to become protonated and leave as compared to –OH.

9. **A**

A hemiacetal is a molecule in which one equivalent of alcohol has been added to a carbonyl (–OR) and the carbonyl oxygen has been protonated (–OH). Otherwise, there is the same alkyl group (–R) and hydrogen atom (–H) as the parent aldehyde. **(B)** describes an acetal, **(C)** a hemiketal, and **(D)** a ketal.

10. **A**

Although both the aldehyde and ketone listed will be reactive with the strongly nucleophilic hydrogen cyanide, aldehydes are slightly more reactive toward nucleophiles than ketones for steric reasons, so the aldehyde and HCN will form the major product (which will be a cyanohydrin).

11. **C**

PCC is a mild anhydrous oxidant that can oxidize primary alcohols to aldehydes, and secondary alcohols to ketones. It is not strong enough to oxidize alcohols or aldehydes to carboxylic acids.

12. **B**

In a hydration reaction, water adds to a carbonyl, forming a geminal diol—a compound with two hydroxyl groups on the same carbon. Hydrogen peroxide and potassium dichromate are oxidizing agents that can convert an aldehyde to a carboxylic acid. Ethanol will react with a carbonyl compound to form an acetal or a ketal, if excess ethanol is available.

13. **A**

Ammonia, or NH_3, will react with an aldehyde like glutaraldehyde to form an imine. This is a condensation and a substitution reaction, as the C=O of the carbonyl will be replaced with a C=N bond.

14. **C**

Hydrides like $LiAlH_4$ and $NaBH_4$ are reducing agents; as such, they will reduce aldehydes and ketones to alcohols. The other reagents listed are oxidizing agents, which will not act on a ketone.

15. **D**

During tautomerization, the double bond between the carbon and nitrogen in an imine is moved to lie between two carbons. This results in an enamine—a compound with a double bond and an amine.

Consult your online resources for additional practice. GO ONLINE

SHARED CONCEPTS

Biochemistry Chapter 4
Carbohydrate Structure and Function

General Chemistry Chapter 11
Oxidation–Reduction Reactions

Organic Chemistry Chapter 1
Nomenclature

Organic Chemistry Chapter 4
Analyzing Organic Reactions

Organic Chemistry Chapter 7
Aldehydes and Ketones II

Organic Chemistry Chapter 8
Carboxylic Acids

CHAPTER 7

ALDEHYDES AND KETONES II: ENOLATES

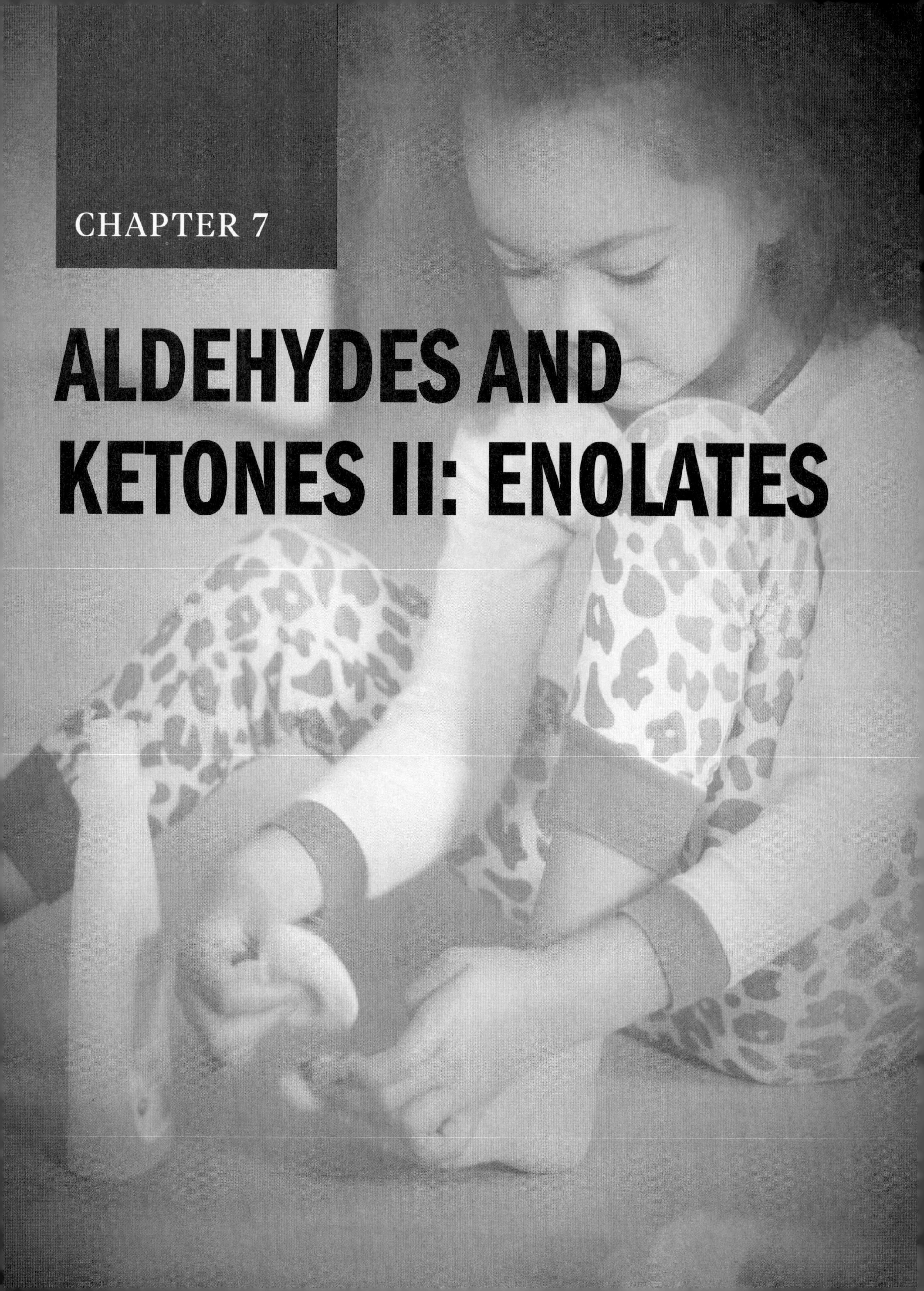

SCIENCE MASTERY ASSESSMENT

Every pre-med knows this feeling: there is so much content I have to know for the MCAT! How do I know what to do first or what's important?

While the high-yield badges throughout this book will help you identify the most important topics, this Science Mastery Assessment is another tool in your MCAT prep arsenal. This quiz (which can also be taken in your online resources) and the guidance below will help ensure that you are spending the appropriate amount of time on this chapter based on your personal strengths and weaknesses. Don't worry though—skipping something now does not mean you'll never study it. Later on in your prep, as you complete full-length tests, you'll uncover specific pieces of content that you need to review and can come back to these chapters as appropriate.

How to Use This Assessment

If you answer 0–7 questions correctly:

Spend about 1 hour to read this chapter in full and take limited notes throughout. Follow up by reviewing **all** quiz questions to ensure that you now understand how to solve each one.

If you answer 8–11 questions correctly:

Spend 20–40 minutes reviewing the quiz questions. Beginning with the questions you missed, read and take notes on the corresponding subchapters. For questions you answered correctly, ensure your thinking matches that of the explanation and you understand why each choice was correct or incorrect.

If you answer 12–15 questions correctly:

Spend less than 20 minutes reviewing all questions from the quiz. If you missed any, then include a quick read-through of the corresponding subchapters, or even just the relevant content within a subchapter, as part of your question review. For questions you got correct, ensure your thinking matches that of the explanation and review the Concept Summary at the end of the chapter.

1. What is the product of the reaction below?

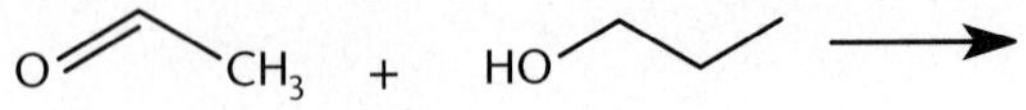

A. 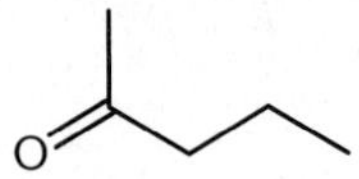

B. 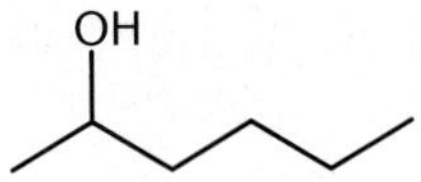

C. 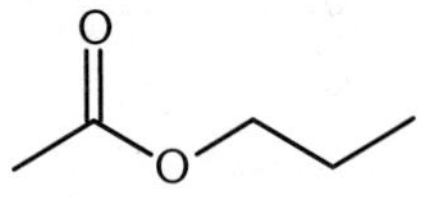

D. 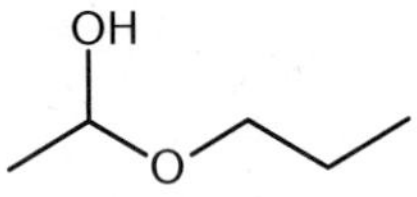

2. The reaction below is an example of:

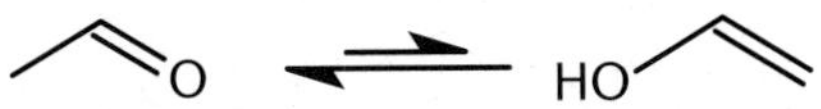

A. esterification.
B. tautomerization.
C. elimination.
D. dehydration.

3. Which of the following reactions would produce the compound below?

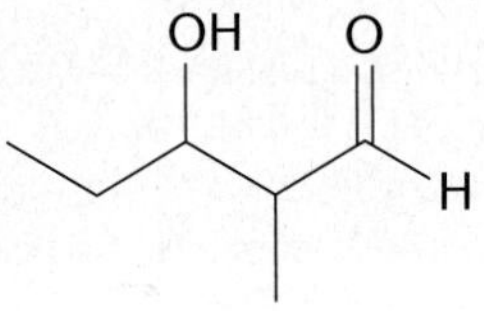

A. $CH_3CHO + CH_3CH_2CH_2CHO \rightarrow$
B. $CH_3COCH_3 + CH_3CH_2CH_2CHO \rightarrow$
C. $CH_3CH_2COCH_3 + CH_3CHO \rightarrow$
D. $CH_3CH_2CHO + CH_3CH_2CHO \rightarrow$

4. Why does the equilibrium between keto and enol tautomers lie far to the keto side?

I. The keto form is more thermodynamically stable.
II. The enol form is lower energy.
III. The enol form is more thermodynamically stable.

A. I only
B. III only
C. I and II only
D. II and III only

5. The aldol condensation is an example of which reaction type(s)?

I. Dehydration
II. Cleavage
III. Nucleophilic addition

A. I only
B. I and III only
C. II and III only
D. I, II, and III

6. Which of the hydrogens in the following molecule is the most acidic?

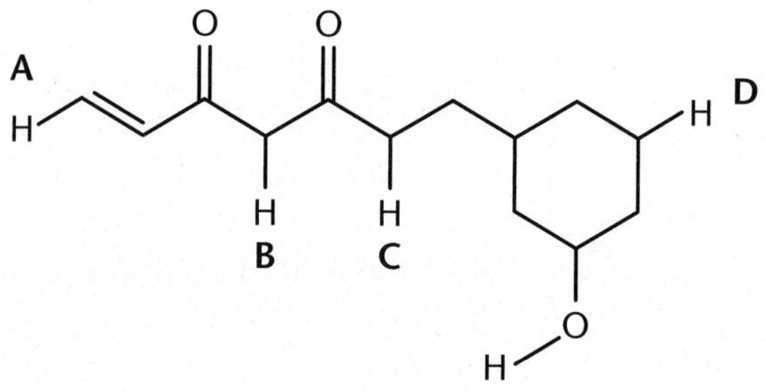

A. A
B. B
C. C
D. D

7. When reacted with ammonia (NH_3) at 200°C, which enolate of a carbonyl-containing compound would predominate?
A. Kinetic enolate
B. Thermodynamic enolate
C. Neither enolate; they would be present in roughly equal proportions.
D. Neither enolate; these reaction conditions would not form either enolate.

8. Which of the following compounds would be most reactive toward a nucleophile?
A. Pentanal
B. 3-Pentanone
C. Pentane
D. 2-Nonanone

9. α-hydrogens of a ketone are acidic due to:
I. resonance stabilization.
II. the electron-withdrawing properties of the alkyl groups.
III. the electronegative carbonyl oxygen.

A. I only
B. I and III only
C. II and III only
D. I, II, and III

10. Which of the following is considered a tautomer of the imine functional group?
A. Cyanohydrin
B. Hydrazone
C. Enamine
D. Semicarbazone

11. When succinaldehyde is treated with lithium diisopropylamide (LDA), it:
I. becomes more nucleophilic.
II. becomes less nucleophilic.
III. generates a carbanion.

A. I only
B. II only
C. I and III only
D. II and III only

12. Which of the following best describes the final product of an aldol condensation?
A. 1,3-dicarbonyl
B. 1,2-dicarbonyl
C. α,β-unsaturated carbonyl
D. β,γ-unsaturated carbonyl

13. When benzaldehyde is reacted with acetone, which will act as the nucleophile?
A. Benzaldehyde, after addition of strong acid
B. Benzaldehyde, after reaction with strong base
C. Acetone, after addition of strong acid
D. Acetone, after reaction with strong base

14. 3-Hydroxybutanal can be formed by the reaction of:
A. methanol in diethyl ether.
B. ethanal in base, then in acid.
C. butanal in strong acid.
D. methanal and ethanal in catalytic base.

15. The catalytic production of dihydroxyacetone and glyceraldehyde 3-phosphate (2-hydroxy-3-oxopropyl dihydrogen phosphate) from fructose-1,6-bisphosphate ([(2S,3S,4S,5R)-2,3,4-trihydroxy-5-(phosphonooxymethyl)oxolan-2-yl]methyl dihydrogen phosphate) is what type of reaction?
A. Aldol condensation
B. Retro-aldol reaction
C. Dehydration
D. Nucleophilic attack

Answer Key

1. **D**
2. **B**
3. **D**
4. **A**
5. **B**
6. **B**
7. **B**
8. **A**
9. **B**
10. **C**
11. **C**
12. **C**
13. **D**
14. **B**
15. **B**

Detailed explanations can be found at the end of the chapter.

CHAPTER 7

ALDEHYDES AND KETONES II: ENOLATES

In This Chapter

CHAPTER PROFILE

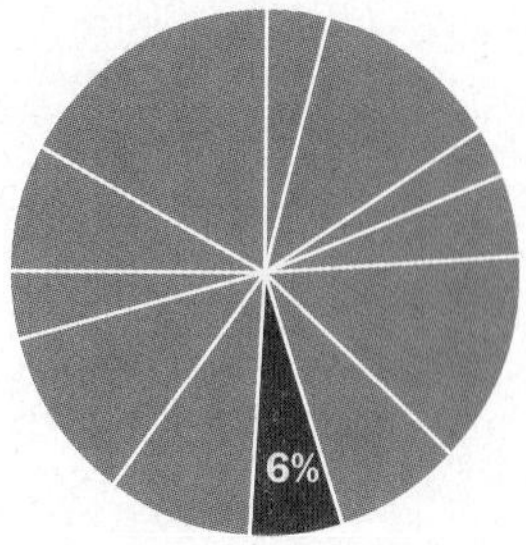

The content in this chapter should be relevant to about 6% of all questions about organic chemistry on the MCAT.

This chapter covers material from the following AAMC content category:

5D: Structure, function, and reactivity of biologically-relevant molecules

Introduction

In the previous chapter, we took a look at a few key properties and reactions of aldehydes and ketones. These molecules have highly predictable chemistry centered on their electrophilic, positively charged carbonyl carbon and will be sure to show up on Test Day. In this chapter, we take a look at several more properties of aldehydes and ketones, and focus on the reactivity of the α-hydrogen of carbonyl-containing compounds. The acidity of this α-hydrogen allows many aldehydes and ketones to act as both electrophiles and nucleophiles. Sometimes, they can even serve both functions in the same reaction. But don't worry—we'll also review some tips about how to understand when and how aldehydes and ketones will react.

7.1 General Principles

LEARNING OBJECTIVES

After Chapter 7.1, you will be able to:

- Explain the acidic nature of α-hydrogens on aldehydes and ketones
- Compare the acidity of the α-hydrogens of aldehydes to those of ketones
- Describe the relationship between steric hindrance and reactivity

In the previous chapter, we focused on how the electronegativity of the oxygen atom in a carbonyl pulls electrons away from the carbonyl carbon, making it partially positively charged. In this chapter, we take the electron-withdrawing characteristics of oxygen one bond further, focusing on the α-carbon in an aldehyde or ketone.

Acidity of α-Hydrogens

KEY CONCEPT

Electron-withdrawing groups like oxygen stabilize organic anions. Electron-donating groups like alkyl groups destabilize organic anions.

An **α-carbon** is adjacent to the carbonyl carbon, and the hydrogens connected to the α-carbon are termed **α-hydrogens**. Through induction, oxygen pulls some of the electron density out of these C—H bonds, weakening them. This makes it relatively easy to deprotonate the α-carbon of an aldehyde or ketone, as shown in Figure 7.1. The acidity of α-hydrogens is augmented by resonance stabilization of the conjugate base. Specifically, when the α-hydrogen is removed, the extra electrons that remain can resonate between the α-carbon, the carbonyl carbon, and the carbonyl oxygen. This increases the stability of this enolate intermediate, described in the next section. Through this resonance, the negative charge can be distributed to the more electronegative oxygen atom. The electron-withdrawing oxygen atom thereby helps stabilize the **carbanion** (a molecule with a negatively charged carbon atom). When in basic solutions, α-hydrogens will easily deprotonate.

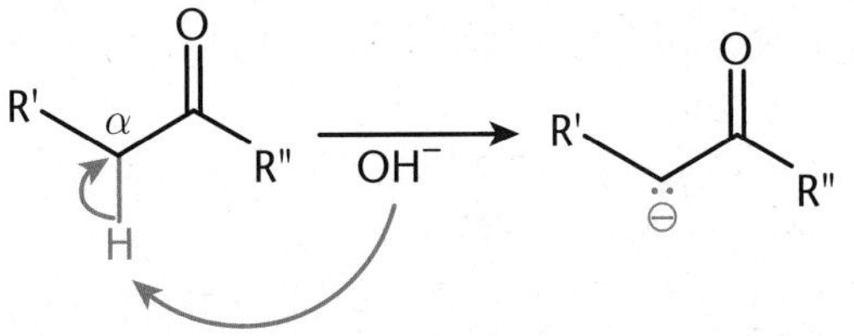

Figure 7.1 Deprotonation of an α-Carbon, Forming a Carbanion

The α-hydrogens of ketones tend to be slightly less acidic than those of aldehydes due to the electron-donating properties of the additional alkyl group in a ketone. This property is the same reason that alkyl groups help to stabilize carbocations—but in this case, they destabilize the carbanion.

Steric Hindrance

KEY CONCEPT

Ketones are slightly less likely to react with nucleophiles than aldehydes because the extra alkyl group destabilizes the carbanion and increases steric hindrance.

In reactions, aldehydes are slightly more reactive to nucleophiles than ketones. This is due in part to steric hindrance in the ketone, which arises from the additional alkyl group that ketones contain. When the nucleophile approaches the ketone or aldehyde in order to react, the additional alkyl groups on the ketone are in the way, more so than the single hydrogen of the aldehyde. This makes for a higher-energy, more crowded intermediate step. Remember, higher-energy intermediates mean that the reaction is less likely to proceed.

MCAT CONCEPT CHECK 7.1

Before you move on, assess your understanding of the material with these questions.

1. Why are the α-hydrogens of aldehydes and ketones acidic?

   ____

2. Which has a lower pK_a: 3-pentanone or pentanal? Why?

   ____

3. How does steric hindrance affect the relative reactivity of aldehydes and ketones?

   ____

7.2 Enolate Chemistry

LEARNING OBJECTIVES

After Chapter 7.2, you will be able to:

- Define tautomerization
- Predict the role of an enolate carbanion in a reaction
- Describe the conditions that favor keto and enol forms
- Identify the thermodynamically favored tautomer of an aldehyde or ketone:

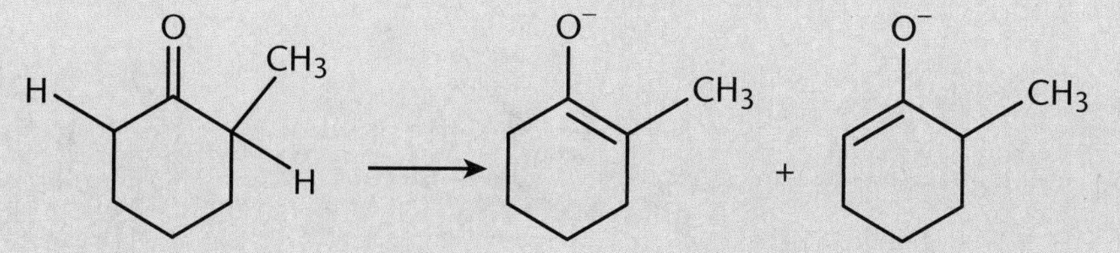

Due to the acidity of the α-hydrogen, aldehydes and ketones exist in solution as a mixture of two isomers: the familiar *keto* form, and the *enol* form.

Keto-Enol Tautomerization

The **enol** form gets its name from the presence of a carbon–carbon double bond (the *en–* component) and an alcohol (the *–ol* component). The two isomers, which differ in the placement of a proton and the double bond, are called **tautomers.** The equilibrium between the tautomers lies far to the keto side, so there will be many more keto isomers in solution. The process of interconverting from the keto to the enol tautomer, shown in Figure 7.2, is called **enolization**, or, more generally, **tautomerization**. By extension, any aldehyde or ketone with a chiral α-carbon will rapidly become a racemic mixture as the keto and enol forms interconvert, a phenomenon known as **α-racemization.**

KEY CONCEPT

Aldehydes and ketones exist in the traditional keto form (C=O) and as the less common enol tautomer (enol = *ene* + *ol*). The deprotonated enolate form can act as a nucleophile. Note that tautomers are *not* resonance structures because they differ in their connectivity of atoms.

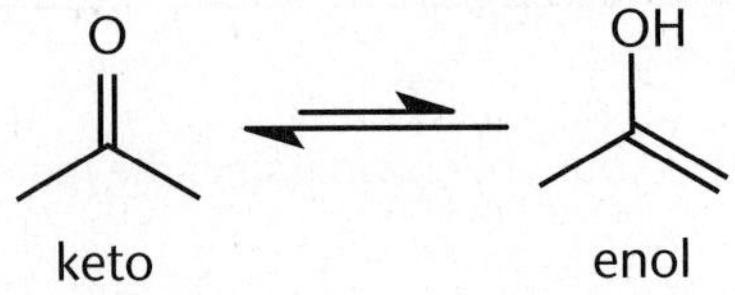

Figure 7.2 Enolization (Tautomerization)
On the left is the keto form, which is thermodynamically favored over the enol form on the right.

Enols are important intermediates in many reactions of aldehydes and ketones. The enolate carbanion results from the deprotonation of the α-carbon by a strong base, as described earlier. Common strong bases include the hydroxide ion, lithium diisopropyl amide (LDA), and potassium hydride (KH). A 1,3-dicarbonyl is particularly acidic because there are two carbonyls to delocalize negative charge and, as such, is often used to form enolate carbanions. Once formed, the nucleophilic carbanion reacts readily with electrophiles. We will see one example of this shortly in the aldol condensation. Another example of this type of reaction is a **Michael addition**, shown in Figure 7.3, in which the carbanion attacks an α,β-unsaturated carbonyl compound—a molecule with a multiple bond between the α- and β-carbons next to a carbonyl.

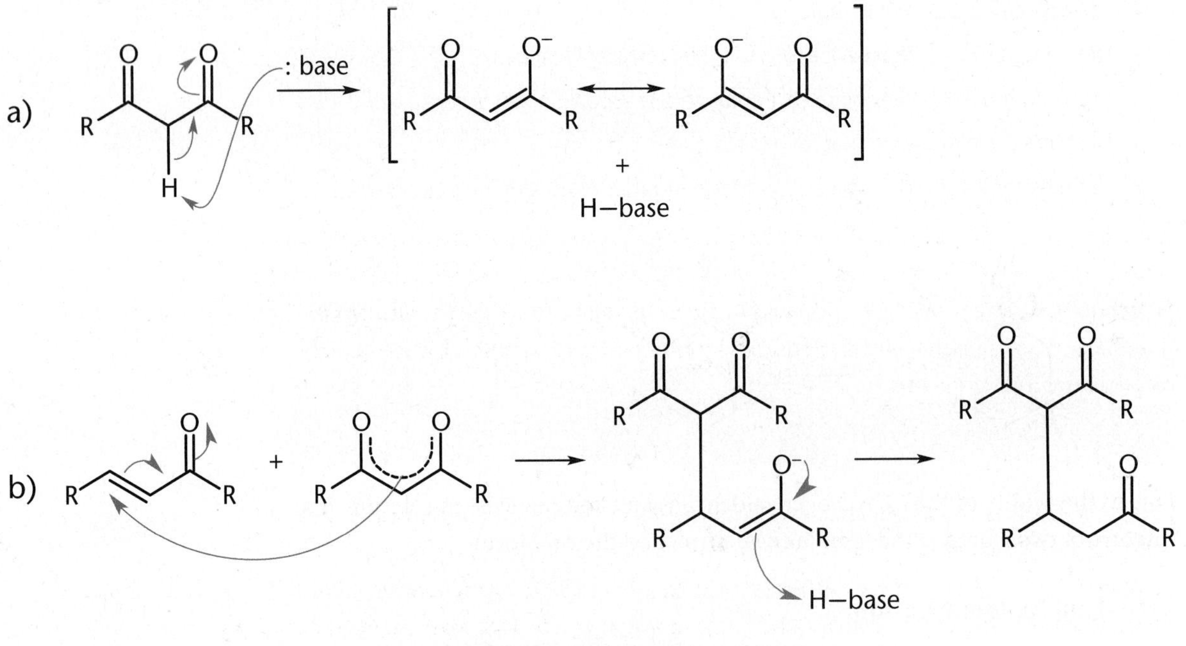

Figure 7.3 Michael Addition
(a) The base deprotonates the α-carbon, making it a good nucleophile;
(b) The carbanion attacks the double bond, resulting in a Michael addition.

This reaction proceeds as shown due to the resonance stabilization of the intermediates. The better you understand the resonance forms of molecules, the more you will be able to predict the specific location on a molecule where a reaction will occur.

Kinetic and Thermodynamic Enolates

Given a ketone that has two different alkyl groups, each of which may have α-hydrogens, two forms of the enolate can form, with the carbon–carbon double bond between the carbonyl carbon and either the more or less substituted carbon, as shown in Figure 7.4. The equilibrium between these forms is dictated by the kinetic and thermodynamic control of the reaction. The kinetically controlled product is formed more rapidly but is less stable. This form has the double bond to the less substituted α-carbon. As expected, this product is formed by the removal of the α-hydrogen from the less substituted α-carbon because it offers less steric hindrance. The thermodynamically controlled product is formed more slowly, but is more stable and features the double bond being formed with the more substituted α-carbon. Accordingly, this is formed by the removal of the α-hydrogen from the more substituted α-carbon.

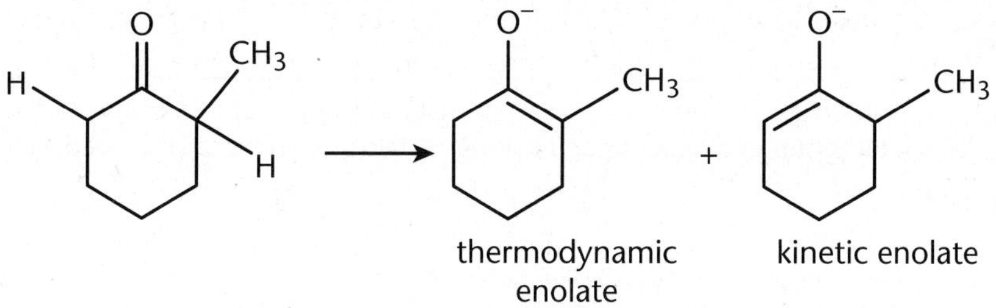

Figure 7.4 Kinetic and Thermodynamic Enolates
The kinetic enolate forms more quickly, but is less stable than the thermodynamic enolate.

Each of these two products is favored by different conditions. The kinetic product is favored in reactions that are rapid, irreversible, at lower temperatures, and with a strong, sterically hindered base. If the reaction is reversible, the kinetic product can revert to the original reactant and react again to form the thermodynamic product. The thermodynamic product is favored with higher temperatures; slow, reversible reactions; and weaker, smaller bases.

Enamines

Just as enols are tautomers of carbonyls, enamines are tautomers of imines. An imine is a compound that contains a C=N bond. The nitrogen in the imine may or may not be bonded to an alkyl group or other substituent. Through tautomerization (movement of a hydrogen and a double bond), imines can be converted into enamines, as shown in Figure 7.5.

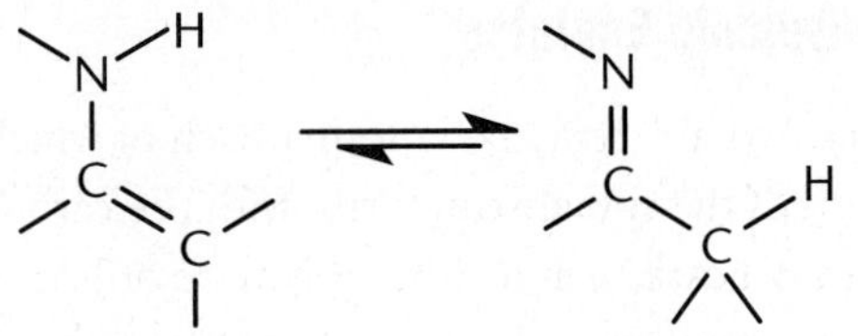

Figure 7.5 Enamination (Tautomerization)
On the right is the imine form, which is thermodynamically favored over the enamine form on the left.

MCAT CONCEPT CHECK 7.2

Before you move on, assess your understanding of the material with these questions.

1. What are tautomers?

____

2. Which tautomer of aldehydes and ketones is thermodynamically favored: keto or enol?

____

3. Which role does the enolate carbanion play in organic reactions: nucleophile, electrophile, oxidizing agent, or reducing agent?

____

4. In the following reaction, which product is the kinetic enolate? The thermodynamic? What conditions favor the formation of each?

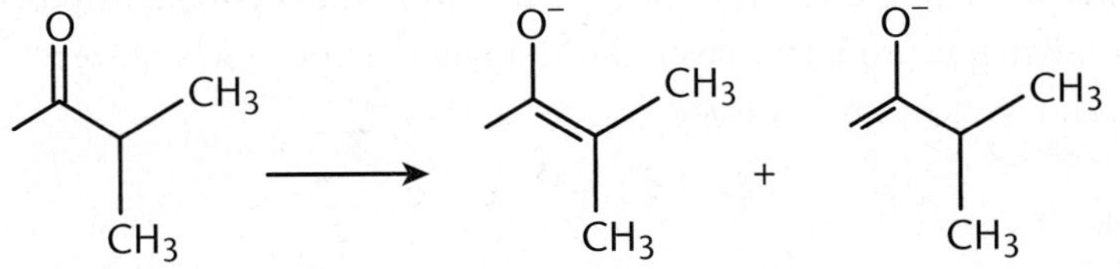

- Kinetic enolate:

____

- Thermodynamic enolate:

____

7.3 Aldol Condensation

LEARNING OBJECTIVES

After Chapter 7.3, you will be able to:

- Identify the species that act as nucleophiles and electrophiles in aldol condensations
- Describe the conditions, reactants, and products involved in a retro-aldol reaction
- List the reaction types associated with aldol condensation

The **aldol condensation** is another vital reaction for the MCAT. This reaction follows the same general mechanism of nucleophilic addition to a carbonyl as previously described. In this case, however, an aldehyde or ketone acts both as an electrophile (in its keto form) and a nucleophile (in its enolate form), and the end result is the formation of a carbon–carbon bond.

As shown in Figure 7.6, when acetaldehyde (ethanal) is treated with a catalytic amount of base, an enolate ion is produced. The enolate is more nucleophilic than the enol because it is negatively charged.

KEY CONCEPT

In aldol condensations, it's the same nucleophilic addition reaction that we have seen before with carbonyl compounds—just with the carbonyl-containing compound acting as both a nucleophile and an electrophile.

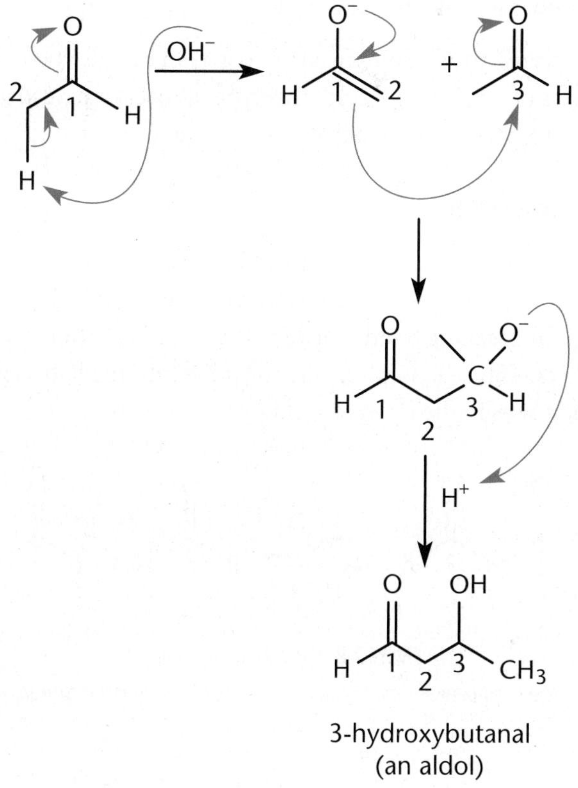

Figure 7.6 Aldol Condensation, Step 1: Forming the Aldol
An enolate ion is formed, which then attacks the carbonyl carbon, forming an aldol.

This nucleophilic enolate ion can react with the electrophilic carbonyl group of another acetaldehyde molecule. The key to this reaction is that both species are in the same flask. The product is 3-hydroxybutanal, which is an example of an **aldol** (a molecule that contains both **ald**ehyde and alcoh**ol** functional groups). Note that the mechanism is still called an aldol reaction even when the reactants are ketones.

With a strong base and high temperatures, dehydration occurs by an E1 or E2 mechanism: we kick off a water molecule and form a double bond, producing an α, β-unsaturated carbonyl, as shown in Figure 7.7.

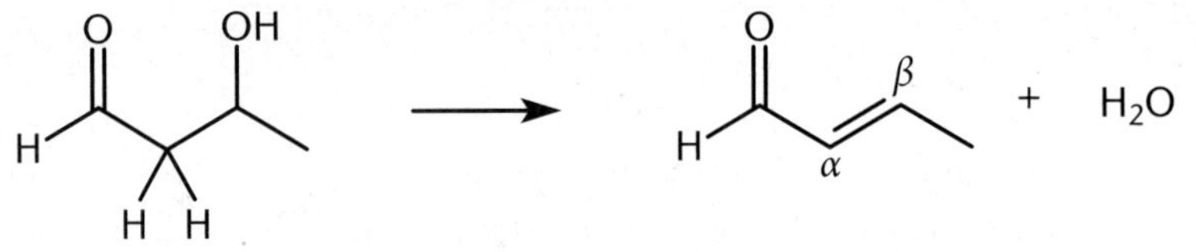

Figure 7.7 Aldol Condensation, Step 2: Dehydration of the Aldol
The —OH is removed as water (dehydration), forming a double bond.

Aldol condensations are most useful if we only use one type of aldehyde or ketone. If there are multiple aldehydes or ketones, we cannot easily control which will act as the nucleophile and which will act as the electrophile, and a mixture of products will result. This can be prevented if one of the molecules has no α-hydrogens because the α-carbons are quaternary (like benzaldehyde).

This reaction is referred to as a **condensation reaction** because two molecules are joined with the loss of a small molecule. This type of reaction is also a **dehydration reaction** because the small molecule that is lost is water.

The Retro-Aldol Reaction

KEY CONCEPT

In a retro-aldol reaction, a bond is broken between the α-and β-carbons of a carbonyl, forming two aldehydes, two ketones, or one aldehyde and one ketone.

The reverse of this reaction is called a **retro-aldol reaction**. To push the reaction in a retro-aldol direction, aqueous base is added and heat is applied. The retro-aldol reaction is useful for breaking bonds between the α-and β-carbons of a carbonyl, as shown in Figure 7.8. This reaction is facilitated if the intermediate can be stabilized in the enolate form, just as in the forward reaction.

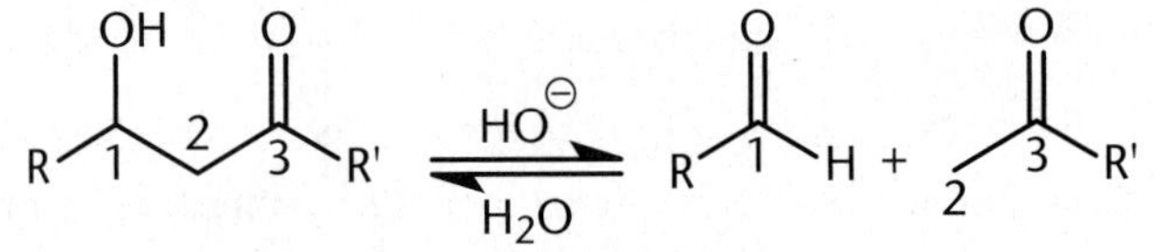

Figure 7.8 Retro-Aldol Reaction
The bond between the α- and β-carbons of a carbonyl is broken.

MCAT CONCEPT CHECK 7.3

Before you move on, assess your understanding of the material with these questions.

1. In the following reaction, an aldehyde is treated with a catalytic amount of base and an enolate ion is formed. The enolate then reacts with another aldehyde molecule leading to an aldol condensation. Identify the nucleophile and electrophile in the aldol condensation.

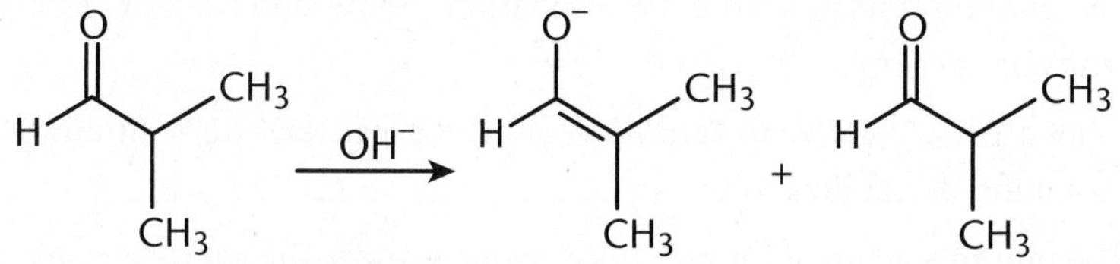

____

2. What is a retro-aldol reaction? What conditions favor retro-aldol reactions?

____

3. The aldol condensation can be classified under many categories of reactions. List some of these reaction types, and provide a short description of each.

____

Conclusion

In this second chapter on aldehydes and ketones, we've taken a look at the important resonance structures that the carbonyl of aldehydes and ketones allows. The high electronegativity of the oxygen atom in a carbonyl not only makes the carbonyl carbon electrophilic, but also weakens the C—H bonds on α-carbons. Deprotonation of this α-carbon results in an enolate, a nucleophilic version of carbonyl-containing compounds. Thus, while the carbonyl carbon dictates the electrophilic chemistry of carbonyls, it is the α-carbon, along with its acidic hydrogens, that dictates the nucleophilic chemistry of carbonyls.

Aldehydes and ketones are not the only carbonyl-containing compounds, of course. Carboxylic acids and their derivatives, including esters, anhydrides, and amides, also have chemistry controlled by a carbonyl. But there is one critical difference between aldehydes and ketones, and carboxylic acids and their derivatives: the absence or presence of a leaving group. While aldehydes and ketones lack leaving groups, carboxylic acids and carboxylic acid derivatives have leaving groups with varying degrees of stability. Over the next two chapters, we'll explore the chemistry of these interesting groups of compounds.

GO ONLINE

You've reviewed the content, now test your knowledge and critical thinking skills by completing a test-like passage set in your online resources!

CONCEPT SUMMARY

General Principles

- The carbon adjacent to the carbonyl carbon is termed an **α-carbon**; the hydrogens attached to the α-carbon are called **α-hydrogens**.
- α-hydrogens are relatively acidic and can be removed by a strong base.
  - The electron-withdrawing oxygen of the carbonyl weakens the C—H bonds on α-carbons.
  - The **enolate** resulting from deprotonation can be stabilized by resonance with the carbonyl.
- Ketones are less reactive toward nucleophiles because of steric hindrance and α-carbanion destabilization.
  - The presence of an additional alkyl group crowds the transition step and increases its energy.
  - The alkyl group also donates electron density to the carbanion, making it less stable.

Enolate Chemistry

- Aldehydes and ketones exist in the traditional **keto form** (C=O) and in the less common **enol form** (*ene* + *ol* = double bond + hydroxyl group).
  - **Tautomers** are isomers that can be interconverted by moving a hydrogen and a double bond. The keto and enol forms are tautomers of each other.
  - The enol form can be deprotonated to form an **enolate**. Enolates are good nucleophiles.
- In the **Michael addition**, an enolate attacks an α,β-unsaturated carbonyl, creating a bond.
- The **kinetic enolate** is favored by fast, irreversible reactions at lower temperatures with strong, sterically hindered bases. The **thermodynamic enolate** is favored by slower, reversible reactions at higher temperatures with weaker, smaller bases.
- **Enamines** are tautomers of imines. Like enols, enamines are the less common tautomer.

Aldol Condensation

- In the **aldol condensation**, the aldehyde or ketone acts as both nucleophile and electrophile, resulting in the formation of a carbon–carbon bond in a new molecule called an aldol.
  - An **aldol** contains both aldehyde and alcohol functional groups.
  - The nucleophile is the enolate formed from the deprotonation of the α-carbon.
  - The electrophile is the aldehyde or ketone in the form of the keto tautomer.
  - First, a **condensation reaction** occurs in which the two molecules come together.
  - After the aldol is formed, a **dehydration reaction** (loss of a water molecule) occurs. This results in an α, β-unsaturated carbonyl.
- **Retro-aldol reactions** are the reverse of aldol condensations.
  - Retro-aldol reactions are catalyzed by heat and base.
  - In these reactions, the bond between an α- and β-carbon is cleaved.

ANSWERS TO CONCEPT CHECKS

7.1

1. The α-hydrogens of aldehydes and ketones are acidic, or deprotonate easily, due to both inductive effects and resonance effects. The electronegative oxygen atom pulls electron density from the C—H bond, weakening it. Once deprotonated, the resonance stabilization of the negative charge between the α-carbon, carbonyl carbon, and electron-withdrawing carbonyl oxygen increases the stability of this form.
2. The α-hydrogens of aldehydes are slightly more acidic than those of ketones due to the electron-donating characteristics of the second alkyl group in ketones. This extra alkyl group destabilizes the carbanion, which slightly disfavors the loss of the α-hydrogens in ketones as compared to aldehydes. Therefore, pentanal is a stronger acid than 3-pentanone and will have a lower pK_a.
3. Steric hindrance is one of the two reasons that aldehydes are slightly more reactive than ketones. The additional alkyl group gets in the way and makes for a higher-energy, crowded intermediate.

7.2

1. Tautomers are isomers that can be interconverted by the movement of a hydrogen and a double bond.
2. The keto form is thermodynamically favored.
3. Enolate carbanions act as nucleophiles.
4. The product with the double bond to the less substituted α-carbon is the kinetically controlled product (the product shown on the right). The thermodynamically controlled product has the double bond formed with the more substituted α-carbon (the product on the left). Because the kinetic enolate forms rapidly and can interconvert with the thermodynamic form if given time, the kinetic form is favored by fast, irreversible reactions, such as with a strong, sterically hindered base, and lower temperatures. The thermodynamic form, on the other hand, is favored by slower, reversible reactions, with weaker or smaller bases, and higher temperatures.

7.3

1. In the aldol condensation reaction, the enolate carbanion (the deprotonated aldehyde or ketone) acts as the nucleophile and the keto form of the aldehyde or ketone acts as the electrophile.
2. A retro-aldol reaction is the reverse of an aldol reaction where instead a bond between the α-and β-carbons of a carbonyl is broken. This can be favored by the addition of base and heat. In this reaction, a bond between the α-and β-carbons of a carbonyl is broken.
3. An aldol condensation is a condensation reaction, in which two molecules are joined to form a single molecule with the loss of a small molecule; a dehydration reaction, in which a molecule of water is lost; and a nucleophile–electrophile reaction, in which a nucleophile pushes an electron pair to form a bond with an electrophile.

SCIENCE MASTERY ASSESSMENT EXPLANATIONS

1. **D**

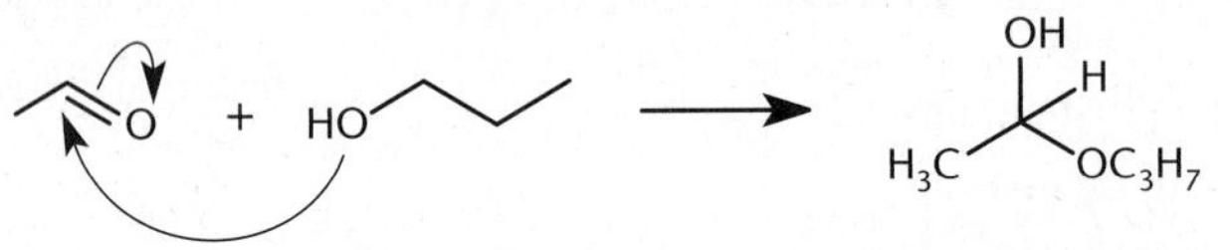

One mole of aldehyde reacts with one mole of alcohol via a nucleophilic addition reaction to form a product called a hemiacetal. In a hemiacetal, an –OH group, an –OR group, a hydrogen atom, and an –R group are attached to the same carbon atom.

2. **B**

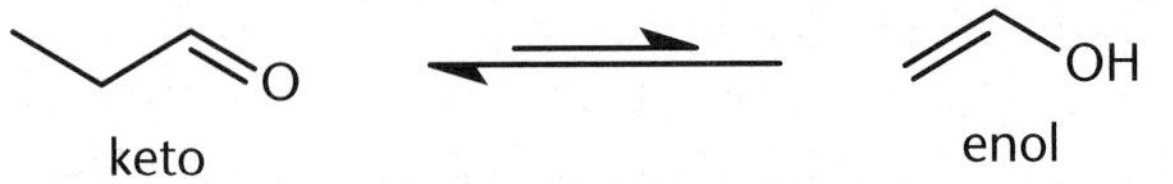

Tautomerization is the interconversion of two isomers in which a hydrogen and a double bond are moved. The keto and enol tautomers of aldehydes and ketones are common examples of tautomers seen on Test Day. Note that the equilibrium lies to the left because the keto form is more stable. Esterification, **(A)**, is the formation of esters from carboxylic acids and alcohols. Elimination, **(C)**, is a reaction in which a part of a reactant is removed and a new multiple bond is introduced. Dehydration, **(D)**, is a reaction in which a molecule of water is eliminated.

3. **D**

The reactions listed in the answer choices are examples of aldol condensations. In the presence of a base, the α-hydrogen is abstracted from an aldehyde, forming an enolate ion, $[CH_3CHCHO]^-$. This enolate ion then attacks the carbonyl group of the other aldehyde molecule, CH_3CH_2CHO, forming the pictured aldol.

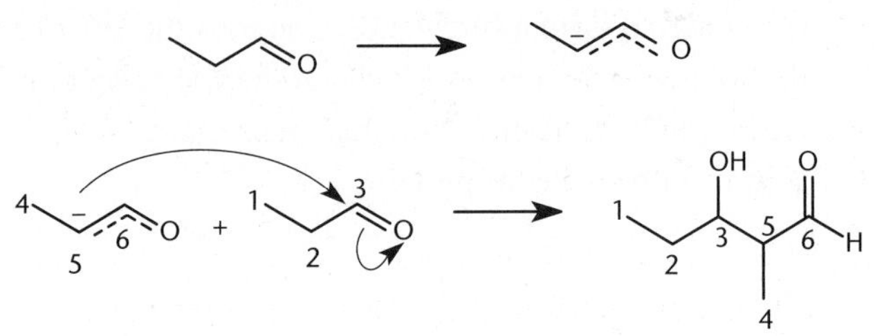

4. **A**

The keto–enol equilibrium lies far to the keto side because the keto form is significantly more thermodynamically stable than the enol form. This thermodynamic stability stems from the fact that the oxygen is more electronegative than the carbon, and the keto tautomer puts more electron density around the oxygen than the enol tautomer. If the enol tautomer is less thermodynamically stable, it is also higher energy than the keto tautomer.

5. **B**

The aldol condensation is both a dehydration reaction because a molecule of water is lost, and a nucleophilic addition reaction because the nucleophilic enolate attacks and bonds to the carbonyl carbon.

6. **B**

This hydrogen is on the carbon between two carbonyls, which means that it is particularly acidic. This is due to both the inductive effects of the two oxygen atoms in the carbonyls and the resonance stabilization of the anion between the carbonyl groups.

7. **B**

At high temperatures and with a weak base like NH_3, the thermodynamic enolate will be favored. The reaction proceeds slowly with the weak base, giving the kinetic enolate time to interconvert to the more stable thermodynamic enolate.

8. **A**

Aldehydes are generally more reactive than ketones because the additional alkyl group of a ketone is sterically hindering; this alkyl group is also electron-donating, destabilizing the carbanion intermediate. This eliminates **(B)** and **(D)**. The carbonyl carbon is highly electrophilic; alkanes lack any significant electrophilicity, eliminating **(C)**.

9. **B**

When α-carbons are deprotonated, the negative charge is resonance stabilized in part by the electronegative carbonyl oxygen, which is electron-withdrawing. Alkyl groups are actually electron-donating, which destabilizes carbanion intermediates; this invalidates statement II.

10. **C**

All of the answer choices are nitrogen-containing functional groups, but only enamines are tautomers of imines. Imines contain a double bond between a carbon and a nitrogen; enamines contain a double bond between two carbons as well as an amine.

11. **C**

When succinaldehyde (or any aldehyde or ketone with α-hydrogens) is treated with a strong base like lithium diisopropylamide (LDA), it forms the more nucleophilic enolate carbanion.

12. **C**

Aldol condensations contain two main steps. In the first step, the α-carbon of an aldehyde or ketone is deprotonated, generating the enolate carbanion. This carbanion can then attack another aldehyde or ketone, generating the aldol. In the second step, the aldol is dehydrated, forming a double bond. This double bond is between the α- and β-carbons, so the molecule is an α,β-unsaturated carbonyl.

13. **D**

Because benzaldehyde lacks an α-proton, it cannot be reacted with base to form the nucleophilic enolate carbanion. Therefore, acetone will act as our nucleophile, and both **(A)** and **(B)** can be eliminated. In order to perform this reaction, which is an aldol condensation, acetone will be reacted with a strong base—not a strong acid—in order to extract the α-hydrogen and form the enolate anion, which will act as a nucleophile.

14. **B**

This is an example of an aldol condensation, but stopped after aldol formation (before dehydration). After the aldol is formed using strong base, the reaction may be halted by the addition of acid. Butanal in strong acid, described in **(C)**, would be likely to deprotonate without gaining the hydroxyl group. Methanol in diethyl ether would not be reactive because diethyl ether is not a strong enough base to abstract the α-hydrogen, eliminating **(A)**. Reaction of the two aldehydes methanal and ethanal in catalytic base would form 3-hydroxypropanal (which would dehydrate to form propenal), not 3-hydroxybutanal.

15. **B**

The nomenclature in this question is well above what one needs to be able to draw on the MCAT; however, we can discern that we are forming a ketone and an aldehyde from a single molecule. The hallmark of a reverse aldol reaction is the breakage of a carbon–carbon bond, forming two aldehydes, two ketones, or one of each. In an aldol condensation, **(A)**, we would expect to form a single product by combining two aldehydes, two ketones, or one of each. A dehydration reaction, **(C)**, should release a water molecule, rather than breaking apart a large organic molecule into two smaller molecules. A nucleophilic attack, **(D)**, should feature the formation of a bond between a nucleophile and an electrophile; again, we would not expect to break apart a large organic molecule into two smaller molecules. Note that simply noting how many reactants and products are present in the reaction is sufficient to determine the answer.

Consult your online resources for additional practice. **GO ONLINE**

SHARED CONCEPTS

General Chemistry Chapter 5
Chemical Kinetics

Organic Chemistry Chapter 4
Analyzing Organic Reactions

Organic Chemistry Chapter 6
Aldehydes and Ketones I

Organic Chemistry Chapter 8
Carboxylic Acids

Organic Chemistry Chapter 9
Carboxylic Acid Derivatives

Organic Chemistry Chapter 10
Nitrogen- and Phosphorus-Containing Compounds

CHAPTER 8

CARBOXYLIC ACIDS

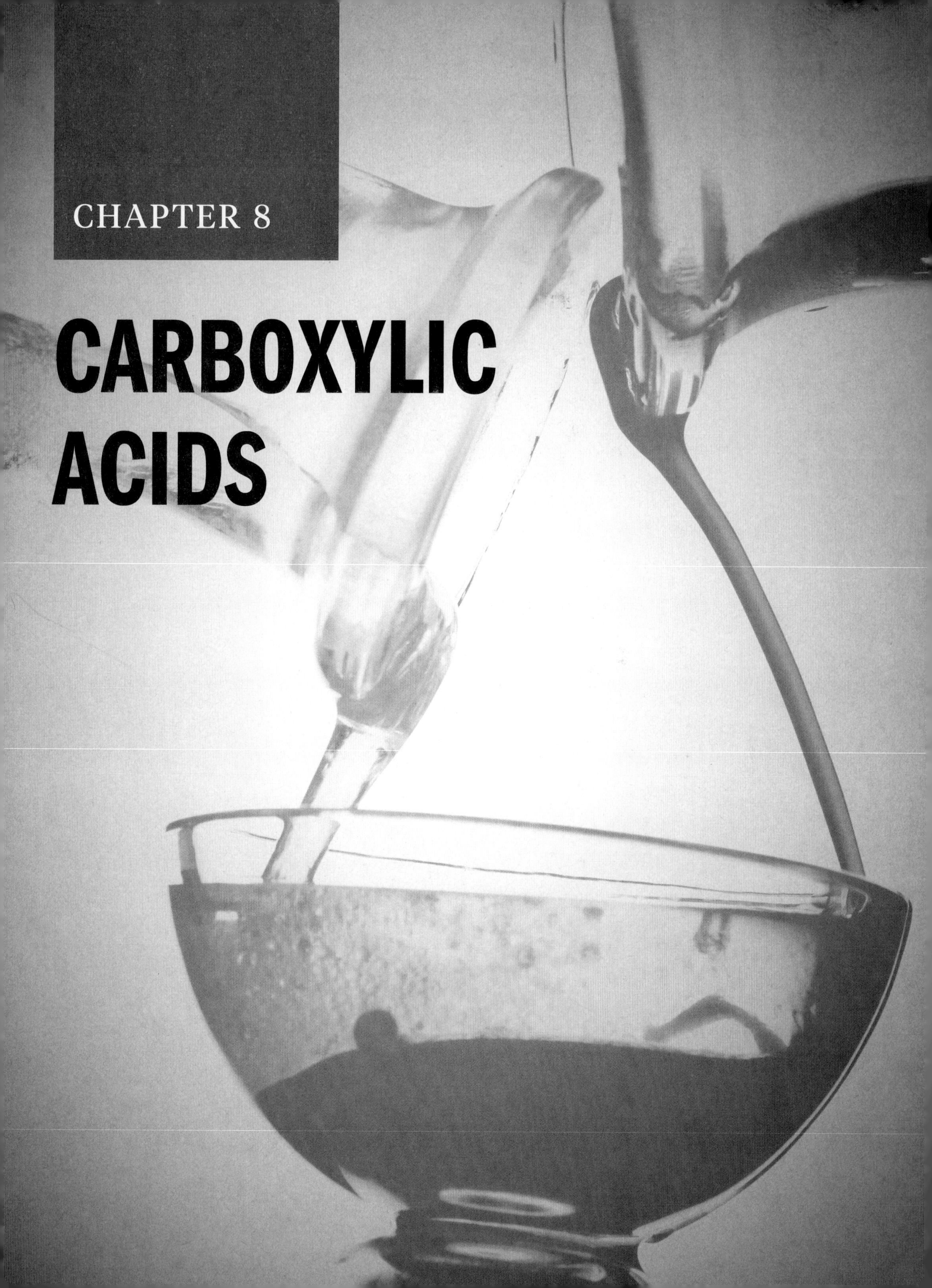

SCIENCE MASTERY ASSESSMENT

Every pre-med knows this feeling: there is so much content I have to know for the MCAT! How do I know what to do first or what's important?

While the high-yield badges throughout this book will help you identify the most important topics, this Science Mastery Assessment is another tool in your MCAT prep arsenal. This quiz (which can also be taken in your online resources) and the guidance below will help ensure that you are spending the appropriate amount of time on this chapter based on your personal strengths and weaknesses. Don't worry though—skipping something now does not mean you'll never study it. Later on in your prep, as you complete full-length tests, you'll uncover specific pieces of content that you need to review and can come back to these chapters as appropriate.

How to Use This Assessment

If you answer 0–7 questions correctly:

Spend about 1 hour to read this chapter in full and take limited notes throughout. Follow up by reviewing **all** quiz questions to ensure that you now understand how to solve each one.

If you answer 8–11 questions correctly:

Spend 20–40 minutes reviewing the quiz questions. Beginning with the questions you missed, read and take notes on the corresponding subchapters. For questions you answered correctly, ensure your thinking matches that of the explanation and you understand why each choice was correct or incorrect.

If you answer 12–15 questions correctly:

Spend less than 20 minutes reviewing all questions from the quiz. If you missed any, then include a quick read-through of the corresponding subchapters, or even just the relevant content within a subchapter, as part of your question review. For questions you got correct, ensure your thinking matches that of the explanation and review the Concept Summary at the end of the chapter.

1. Which of these compounds would be expected to decarboxylate when heated?

A. 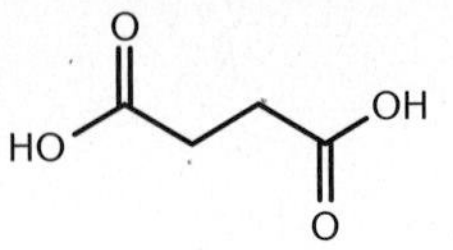

B. 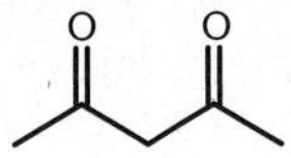

C. 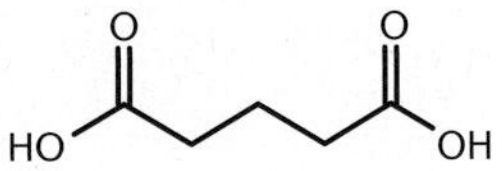

D. 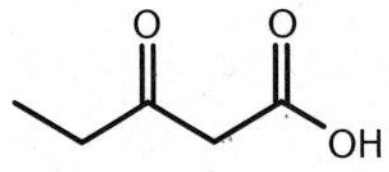

2. Carboxylic acids have higher boiling points than their corresponding alcohols primarily because:
   - **A.** molecular weight is increased by the additional carboxyl group.
   - **B.** the pH of the compound is lower.
   - **C.** acid salts are soluble in water.
   - **D.** hydrogen bonding is much stronger than in alcohols.

3. Which of the following carboxylic acids will be the most acidic?
   - **A.** $CH_3CHClCH_2COOH$
   - **B.** $CH_3CH_2CCl_2COOH$
   - **C.** $CH_3CH_2CHClCOOH$
   - **D.** $CH_3CH_2CH_2COOH$

4. Which of the following molecules could be classified as a soap?
   - **A.** $CH_3(CH_2)_{19}COOH$
   - **B.** CH_3COOH
   - **C.** $CH_3(CH_2)_{19}COO^-Na^+$
   - **D.** $CH_3COO^-Na^+$

5. What is the final product of the following reaction?

$$CH_3(CH_2)_4CH_2OH \xrightarrow[\text{acetone}]{CrO_3,\ H_2SO_4}$$

   - **A.** $CH_3(CH_2)_4CHO$
   - **B.** $CH_3(CH_2)_4COOH$
   - **C.** $CH_3(CH_2)_4CH_3$
   - **D.** $HOOC(CH_2)_4COOH$

6. Carboxylic acids can be reacted with one reagent (in addition to acid) to form all of the following compounds EXCEPT:
   - **A.** esters.
   - **B.** amides.
   - **C.** alkenes.
   - **D.** alcohols.

7. The reduction of a carboxylic acid using lithium aluminum hydride will yield what final product?
   - **A.** An aldehyde
   - **B.** An ester
   - **C.** A ketone
   - **D.** An alcohol

8. Which of the following is true with respect to a micelle in a hydrophilic environment?
   - **A.** The interior is hydrophilic.
   - **B.** The structure, as a whole, is hydrophobic.
   - **C.** It is composed of short-chain fatty acids with polar heads.
   - **D.** It can dissolve nonpolar molecules deep in its core.

9. In the presence of an acid catalyst, the major product of butanoic acid and 1-pentanol is:
   - **A.** 1-butoxy-1-pentanol.
   - **B.** butyl pentanoate.
   - **C.** 1-pentoxy-1-butanol.
   - **D.** pentyl butanoate.

10. The α-hydrogen of a carboxylic acid is:
   - **I.** more acidic than the hydroxyl hydrogen.
   - **II.** less acidic than the hydroxyl hydrogen.
   - **III.** relatively acidic, as organic compounds go.

   - **A.** I only
   - **B.** II only
   - **C.** I and III only
   - **D.** II and III only

11. The reaction of formic acid with sodium borohydride will yield what final product?
   - **A.** An aldehyde
   - **B.** A carboxylic acid
   - **C.** A ketone
   - **D.** An alcohol

12. The intramolecular reaction of 5-aminopentanoic acid through nucleophilic acyl substitution would result in a(n):
   - **A.** anhydride.
   - **B.** lactone.
   - **C.** lactam.
   - **D.** carboxylic acid.

13. Butanoic anhydride can be produced by the reaction of butanoic acid with which of the following compounds?
   - **A.** Butanoic acid
   - **B.** Ethanoic acid
   - **C.** Butanol
   - **D.** Methanal

14. Nucleophilic acyl substitution is favored by:
   - **I.** basic solution.
   - **II.** acidic solution.
   - **III.** leaving groups that are strong bases.

   - **A.** I only
   - **B.** II only
   - **C.** I and II only
   - **D.** I, II, and III

15. The reaction of ammonia with caprylic acid, found in coconuts, would produce a(n):
   - **A.** ester.
   - **B.** anhydride.
   - **C.** alcohol.
   - **D.** water molecule.

Answer Key

1. **D**
2. **D**
3. **B**
4. **C**
5. **B**
6. **C**
7. **D**
8. **D**
9. **D**
10. **D**
11. **B**
12. **C**
13. **A**
14. **C**
15. **D**

Detailed explanations can be found at the end of the chapter.

CHAPTER 8

CARBOXYLIC ACIDS

In This Chapter

CHAPTER PROFILE

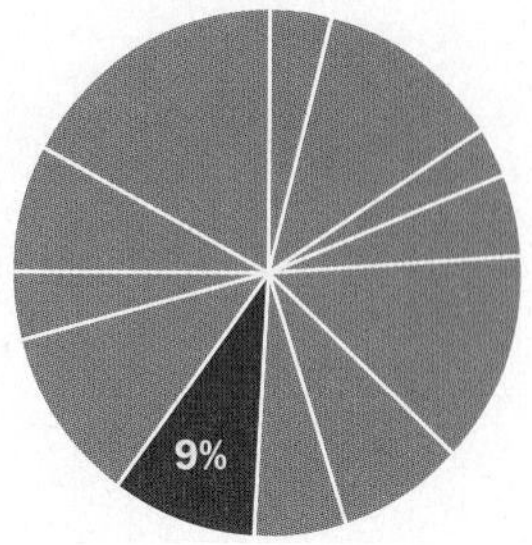

The content in this chapter should be relevant to about 9% of all questions about organic chemistry on the MCAT.

This chapter covers material from the following AAMC content category:

5D: Structure, function, and reactivity of biologically-relevant molecules

Introduction

Carboxylic acids, with both carbonyl and hydroxyl groups, are some of the most reactive organic molecules you'll encounter on Test Day. As we will see in this chapter, these molecules can react as acids (as their name suggests), nucleophiles, and electrophiles and are integral to many biological processes. Carboxylic acids are found in soaps, oils, preservatives, skin care products, clothing, and—most importantly for the MCAT—amino acids. Carboxylic acids often have strong, unpleasant odors. For example, acetic acid (ethanoic acid) is the main ingredient in vinegar; propionic acid (propanoic acid) gives Swiss cheese its smell; butyric acid (butanoic acid) is found in rancid butter and body odor.

So what makes carboxylic acids so interesting and versatile? First, they're acids, so they like to give away protons—particularly because when they do so, the remaining negative charge resonates between two oxygen atoms, making the anion very stable. This makes carboxylic acids some of the most acidic compounds encountered in organic chemistry, with pK_a values between 3 and 6. Compare this with alcohols, which have an average pK_a around 17. Carboxylic acids are also excellent at hydrogen bonding, which results in large intermolecular forces and high boiling points. Finally, carboxylic acids are ubiquitous in nature and are synthesized by all living organisms.

8.1 Description and Properties

LEARNING OBJECTIVES

After Chapter 8.1, you will be able to:

- Explain the underlying cause of the relatively high acidity of carboxylic acids
- Predict the effects of additional substituents on the acidity of a carboxylic acid
- Rank the acidity of comparable carboxylic acids based on their structure

A **carboxylic acid** contains both a carbonyl group and a hydroxyl group, bonded to the same carbon. With three bonds to oxygen atoms, this is one of the most oxidized functional groups encountered in organic chemistry. Carboxylic acids are always terminal groups.

Nomenclature

In the IUPAC system of nomenclature, carboxylic acids are named by adding the suffix ***–oic acid*** to the parent root when the carboxylic acid is the highest-priority functional group. When this is true, the carbonyl carbon becomes carbon number 1. Figure 8.1 shows two examples.

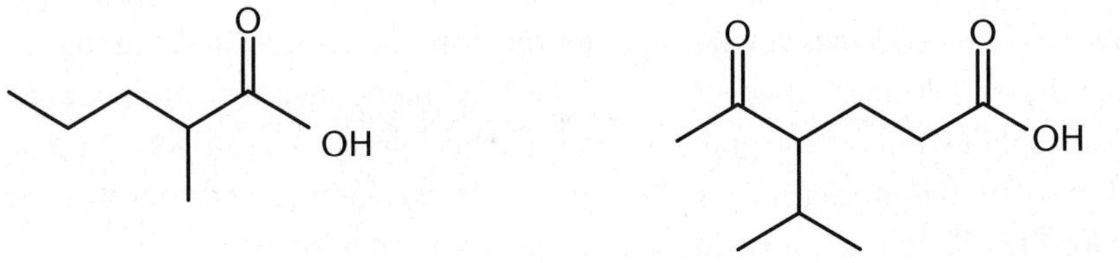

2-methylpentanoic acid — 4-isopropyl-5-oxohexanoic acid

Figure 8.1 IUPAC Names of Carboxylic Acids

Like the other functional groups, many carboxylic acids are also named by their common names. Make note of the common prefixes used in the examples in Figure 8.2.

MCAT EXPERTISE

The same common-name prefixes are used for both aldehydes and carboxylic acids: *form-* for one carbon, *acet-* for two, and *propion-* for three.

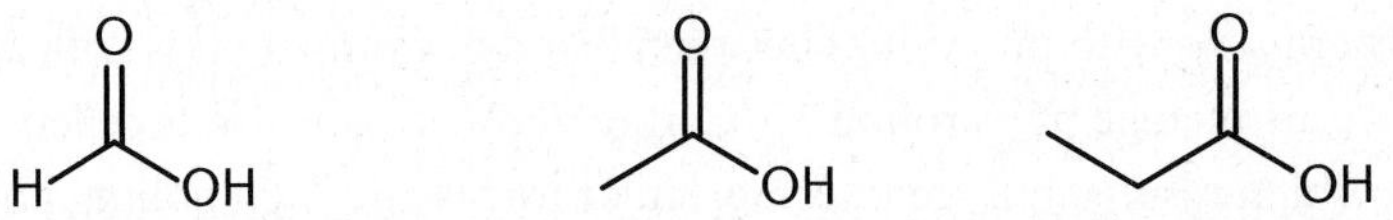

methanoic acid (formic acid) — ethanoic acid (acetic acid) — propanoic acid (propionic acid)

Figure 8.2 IUPAC and Common Names of Carboxylic Acids

Cyclic carboxylic acids are named by listing the cycloalkane with the suffix ***carboxylic acid***. Salts of carboxylic acids are named beginning with the cation, followed by the name of the acid with the ending ***–oate*** replacing ***–oic acid***. Typical examples are shown in Figure 8.3.

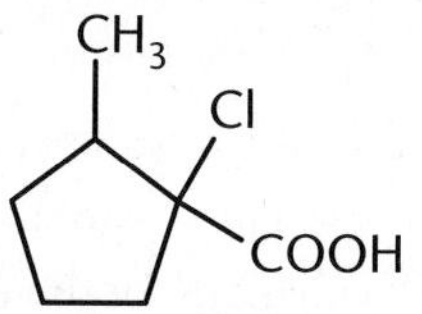

1-chloro-2-methylcyclo-
pentane carboxylic acid

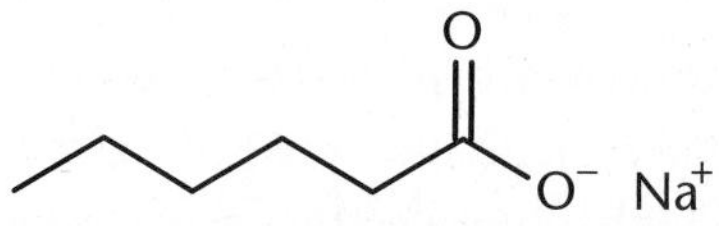

sodium hexanoate

Figure 8.3 Cyclic Carboxylic Acid and Carboxylic Acid Salt

Finally, **dicarboxylic acids**, which have a carboxylic acid group on each end of the molecule, are common in biological systems. The smallest dicarboxylic acid is *oxalic acid*, with two carbons. The next five straight-chain dicarboxylic acids are *malonic*, *succinic*, *glutaric*, *adipic*, and *pimelic* acids. Their IUPAC names have the suffix ***–dioic acid***: ethanedioic acid, propanedioic acid, butanedioic acid, pentanedioic acid, hexanedioic acid, and heptanedioic acid. Figure 8.4 shows several examples.

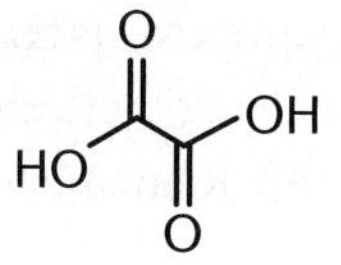

ethanedioic acid
(oxalic acid)

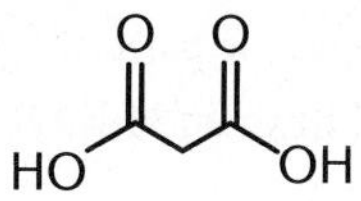

propanedioic acid
(malonic acid)

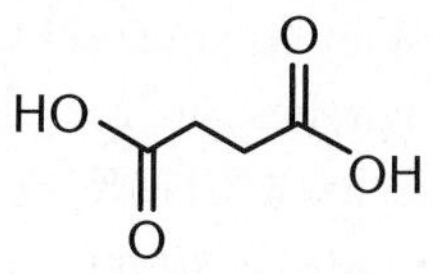

butanedioic acid
(succinic acid)

Figure 8.4 IUPAC and Common Names of Dicarboxylic Acids

Physical Properties

Many of the physical properties of carboxylic acids are similar to those of aldehydes and ketones because they both contain carbonyl groups. However, the additional hydroxyl group permits carboxylic acids to hydrogen bond and provides another acidic hydrogen that can participate in reactions.

Hydrogen Bonding

Carboxylic acids are polar because they contain a carbonyl group and can also form hydrogen bonds because they contain a hydrogen bonded to a very electronegative atom (in this case, the hydroxyl oxygen). Carboxylic acids display particularly strong intermolecular attractions because both the hydroxyl oxygen and carbonyl oxygen can participate in hydrogen bonding. As a result, carboxylic acids tend to form **dimers**: pairs of molecules connected by two hydrogen bonds. Multiple hydrogen bonds elevate the boiling and melting points of carboxylic acids past those of corresponding alcohols. Boiling points also increase with increasing molecular weight.

Acidity

KEY CONCEPT

Carboxylic acids are polar and can form hydrogen bonds. Their acidity is due to resonance stabilization and can be enhanced by the addition of electronegative groups or a greater ability to delocalize charge.

The hydroxyl hydrogen of a carboxylic acid is quite acidic. This results in a negative charge that remains after the hydrogen is removed and resonance stabilization occurs between both of the electronegative oxygen atoms. Delocalization of the negative charge results in a very stable carboxylate anion, which is demonstrated in Figure 8.5.

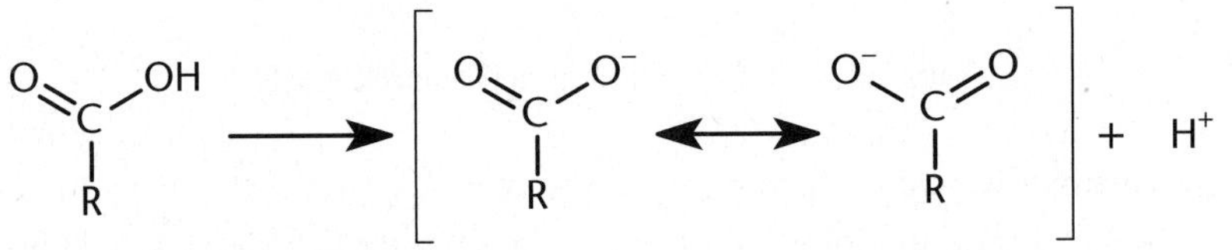

Figure 8.5 Carboxylate Anion Stability
The negative charge from deprotonation is stabilized through resonance.

The more stable the conjugate base is, the easier it is for the proton to leave, and thus, the stronger the acid. Carboxylic acids are relatively acidic, with pK_a values on the order of 4.8 for ethanoic acid and 4.9 for propanoic acid. However, keep in mind that although these are quite acidic for organic compounds, they do not compare to strong acids like HCl ($pK_a = -8.0$) or even HSO_4^- ($pK_a = 1.99$). Remember, lower pK_a values indicate stronger acids.

Substituents on carbon atoms near a carboxyl group influence anion stability and therefore affect acidity. Groups like $-NO_2$ or halides are electron-withdrawing and increase acidity. In contrast, $-NH_2$ or $-OCH_3$ are electron-donating groups that destabilize the negative charge, decreasing the acidity of the compound. The closer the substituent groups are to the carboxyl group, the greater the effect will be.

In dicarboxylic acids, each $-COOH$ group influences the other $-COOH$ group. Carboxylic acids are electron-withdrawing due to the electronegative oxygen atoms they contain. The net result is that dicarboxylic acids are more acidic than the analogous monocarboxylic acids. However, when one proton is removed from the molecule, the carboxylate anion is formed, resulting in an immediate decrease in the acidity of the remaining carboxylic acid. This makes sense because if the second group were deprotonated, it would create a doubly charged species with two negative charges repelling each other. Due to this instability, the second proton is actually *less* acidic (harder to remove) than the analogous proton of a monocarboxylic acid.

β-dicarboxylic acids are dicarboxylic acids in which each carboxylic acid is positioned on the β-carbon of the other; in other words, there are two carboxylic acids separated by a single carbon. These compounds are notable for the high acidity of the α-hydrogens located on the carbon between the two carboxyl groups ($pK_a \approx 9-14$). Loss of this acidic hydrogen atom produces a carbanion, which is stabilized by the electron-withdrawing effect of both carboxyl groups, as shown in Figure 8.6.

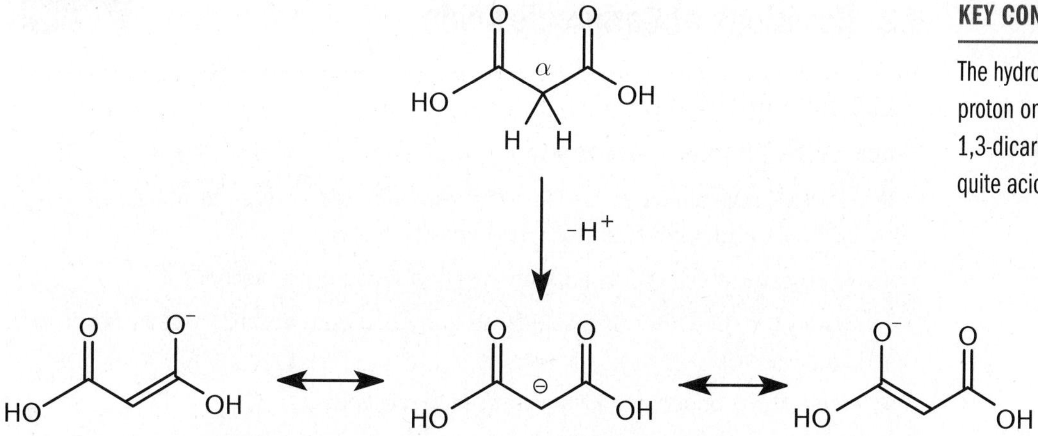

Figure 8.6 Acidity of the α-Hydrogen in β-Dicarboxylic Acids
Note that the α-hydrogen is less acidic than the hydroxyl hydrogens; the hydroxyl groups are left protonated in this example for demonstration purposes only.

KEY CONCEPT

The hydroxyl hydrogen is the most acidic proton on a carboxylic acid. However, in 1,3-dicarbonyls, the α-hydrogen is also quite acidic.

Note that this also applies to the α-hydrogens in a β-diketone, β-ketoacids, β-dialdehydes, and other molecules that share the 1,3-dicarbonyl structure shown in Figure 8.7.

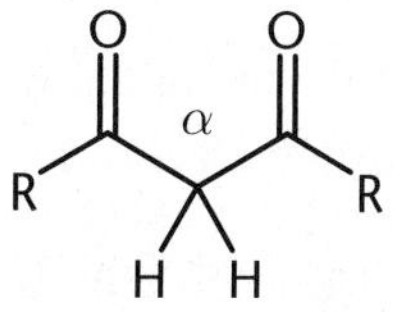

Figure 8.7 General Structure of 1,3-Dicarbonyl Compounds

MCAT CONCEPT CHECK 8.1

Before you move on, assess your understanding of the material with these questions.

1. What causes the relatively high acidity of carboxylic acids?

 ____

2. Among a monocarboxylic acid, a dicarboxylic acid, and a dicarboxylic acid that has been deprotonated once, which will be the most acidic? Why?

 ____

3. What effects do additional substituents have on the acidity of carboxylic acids?

 ____

8.2 Reactions of Carboxylic Acids

High-Yield

LEARNING OBJECTIVES

After Chapter 8.2, you will be able to:

- Recall the reactant types used in acyl substitution reactions to form the major carboxylic acid derivatives, such as amides and esters
- Describe the mechanism of nucleophilic acyl substitution reactions
- Identify the conditions that would lead to spontaneous decarboxylation of a carboxylic acid
- Predict the products of an acyl substitution reaction:

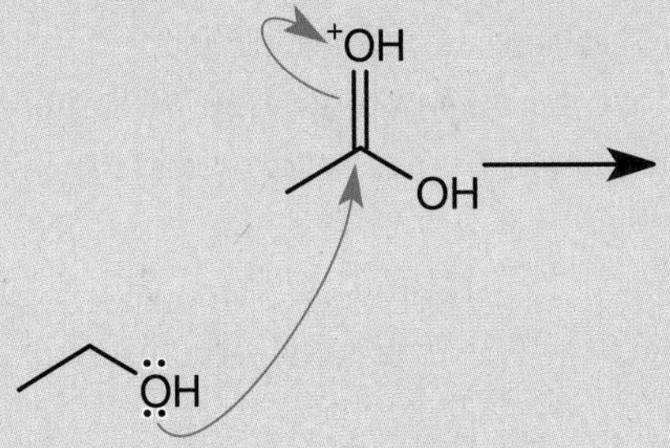

The properties of carboxylic acids make them highly reactive in a number of different categories. Several of the most important reactions are described here.

Synthesis of Carboxylic Acids

As described in earlier chapters, carboxylic acids can be prepared via oxidation of aldehydes and primary alcohols. The oxidant is often a dichromate salt ($Na_2Cr_2O_7$ or $K_2Cr_2O_7$), chromium trioxide (CrO_3), or potassium permanganate ($KMnO_4$), as shown in Figure 8.8, but several other oxidizing agents can also work. Remember that secondary and tertiary alcohols cannot be oxidized to carboxylic acids because they already have at least two bonds to other carbons.

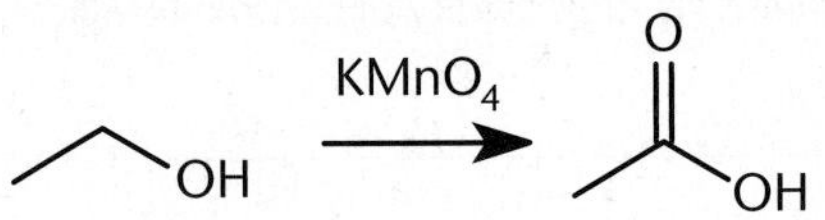

Figure 8.8 Synthesis of a Carboxylic Acid via Oxidation of a Primary Alcohol

There are many other methods of generating carboxylic acids, including organometallic reagents (Grignard reagents) and hydrolysis of nitriles (−C≡N), but these are outside the scope of the MCAT.

Nucleophilic Acyl Substitution

Many of the reactions in which carboxylic acids (and their derivatives) participate proceed via a single mechanism: nucleophilic acyl substitution. This mechanism is similar to nucleophilic addition to an aldehyde or ketone, which was discussed in

Chapters 6 and 7 of *MCAT Organic Chemistry Review*. The key difference, however, focuses on the existence of a leaving group in carboxylic acids and their derivatives. In this case, after opening the carbonyl via nucleophilic attack and forming a tetrahedral intermediate, the carbonyl can reform, thereby kicking off the leaving group. This reaction is shown in Figure 8.9.

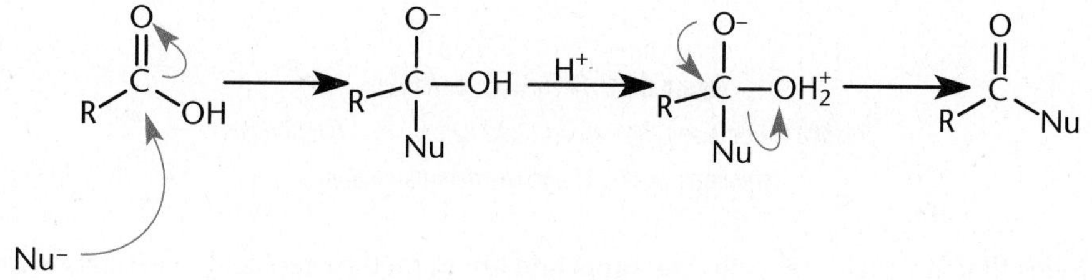

Figure 8.9 Nucleophilic Acyl Substitution
Step 1: Nucleophilic addition; Step 2: Elimination of the leaving group and reformation of the carbonyl.

In these reactions, the nucleophilic molecule replaces the leaving group of an acyl derivative. **Acyl derivatives** encompass all molecules with a carboxylic acid-derived carbonyl, including carboxylic acids, amides, esters, anhydrides, and others. These reactions are favored by a good leaving group. Remember, weak bases, which are often the conjugate bases of strong acids, make good leaving groups. These reactions are also favored in either acidic or basic conditions, which can alter the reactivity of the electrophile and nucleophile.

MCAT EXPERTISE

While you may have learned about other acyl derivatives in your organic chemistry classes, such as acyl halides and nitriles, the official content list for the MCAT restricts its focus to carboxylic acids, amides, esters, and anhydrides.

Amides

Carboxylic acids can be converted into amides if the incoming nucleophile is ammonia (NH_3) or an amine, as shown in Figure 8.10. This can be carried out in either an acidic or basic solution to drive the reaction forward.

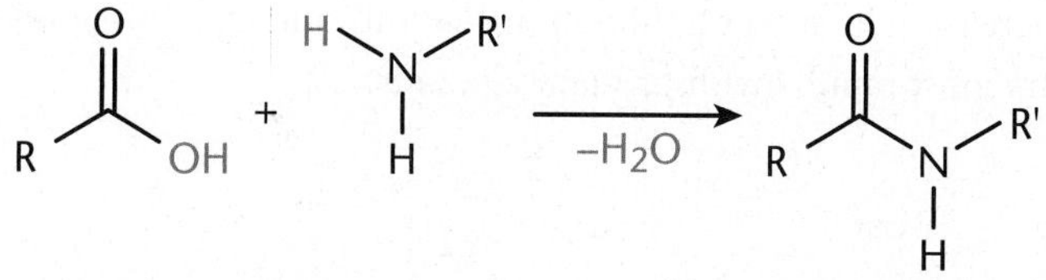

Figure 8.10 Formation of an Amide by Nucleophilic Acyl Substitution

Amides are named by replacing the *–oic acid* suffix with *–amide* in the name of the parent carboxylic acid. Any alkyl groups on the nitrogen are placed at the beginning of the name with the prefix *N*–. Amides exist in a resonance state where delocalization of electrons occurs between the oxygen and nitrogen atoms, as shown in Figure 8.11.

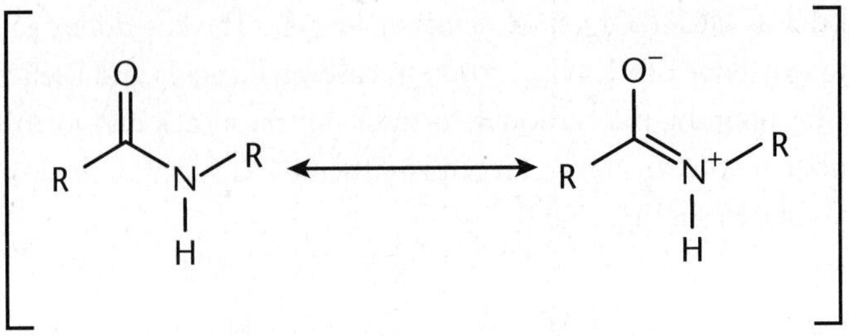

Figure 8.11 Resonance of Amides
Resonance between the carbonyl and lone pair on the nitrogen stabilizes this bond and restricts its motion.

Amides that are cyclic are called **lactams** and are named by replacing *–oic acid* with *–lactam*. They may also be named by indicating the specific carbon that is bonded during cyclization of the compound. Several examples are shown in Figure 8.12.

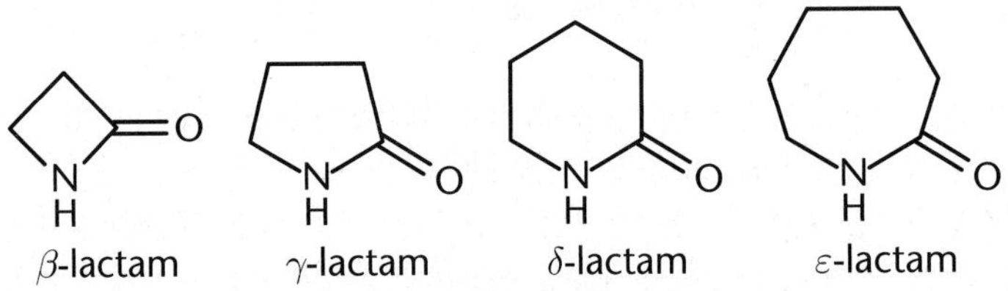

Figure 8.12 Examples of Lactams

Esters

Esters are a hybrid between a carboxylic acid and an ether (ROR′), which can be made by reacting carboxylic acids with alcohols under acidic conditions, as shown in Figure 8.13. **Esterification** is a **condensation** reaction with water as a side product. In acidic solutions, the carbonyl oxygen can be protonated, which enhances the polarity of the bond, thereby placing additional positive charge on the carbonyl carbon and increasing its susceptibility to nucleophilic attack. This condensation reaction occurs most rapidly with primary alcohols.

KEY CONCEPT

Protonating the C=O makes the electrophilic carbon even more ripe for nucleophilic attack.

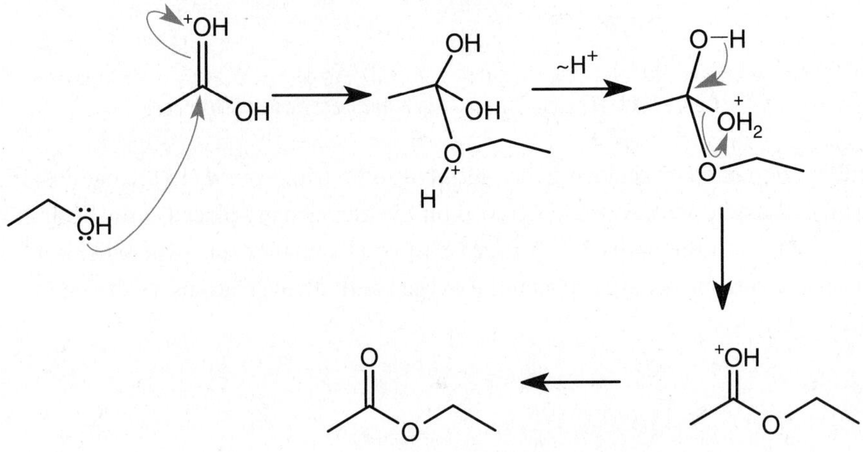

Figure 8.13 Esterification: Reaction of a Carboxylic Acid with an Alcohol

Esters are named in the same manner as salts of carboxylic acids. For example, the ester shown in the reaction in Figure 8.13 has the common name ethyl acetate, or the IUPAC name ethyl ethanoate.

Esters that are cyclic are called **lactones** and are named by replacing ***–oic acid*** with ***–lactone***. Several examples are shown in Figure 8.14.

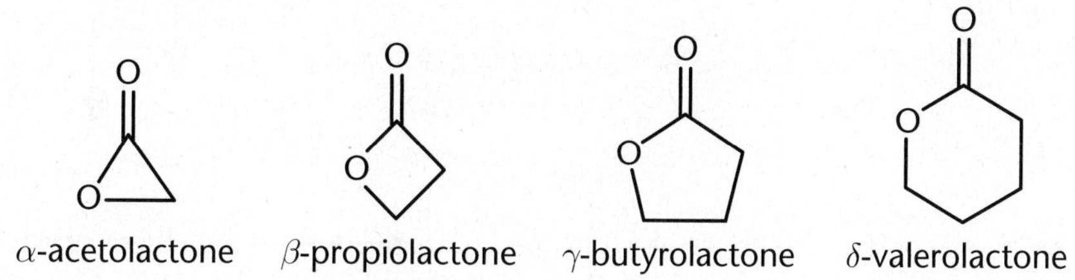

Figure 8.14 Examples of Lactones

Anhydrides

Anhydrides can be formed by the condensation of two carboxylic acids. They are named by replacing the ***acid*** at the end of the name of the parent carboxylic acid with ***anhydride***, whether cyclic or linear. One example is the condensation of two molecules of ethanoic acid to form ethanoic anhydride, as shown in Figure 8.15. Just like the above reactions, anhydride formation occurs via nucleophilic acyl substitution.

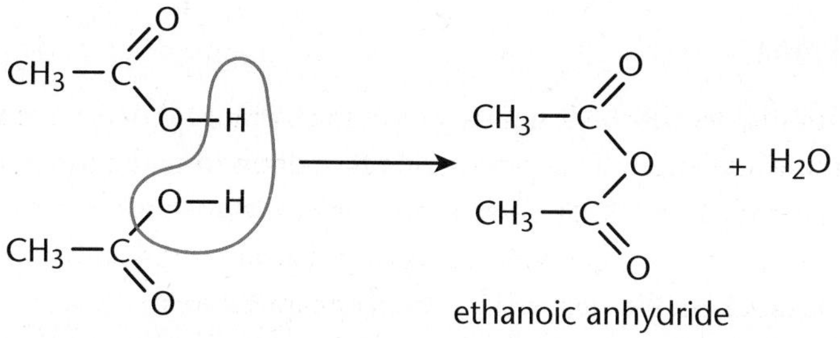

Figure 8.15 Synthesis of an Anhydride via Carboxylic Acid Condensation

Reduction

Carboxylic acids can be reduced to primary alcohols by the use of lithium aluminum hydride ($LiAlH_4$). Aldehyde intermediates may be formed in the course of this reaction, but they, too, will be reduced to the alcohol. The reaction occurs by nucleophilic addition of hydride to the carbonyl group. The reaction mechanism is shown in Figure 8.16.

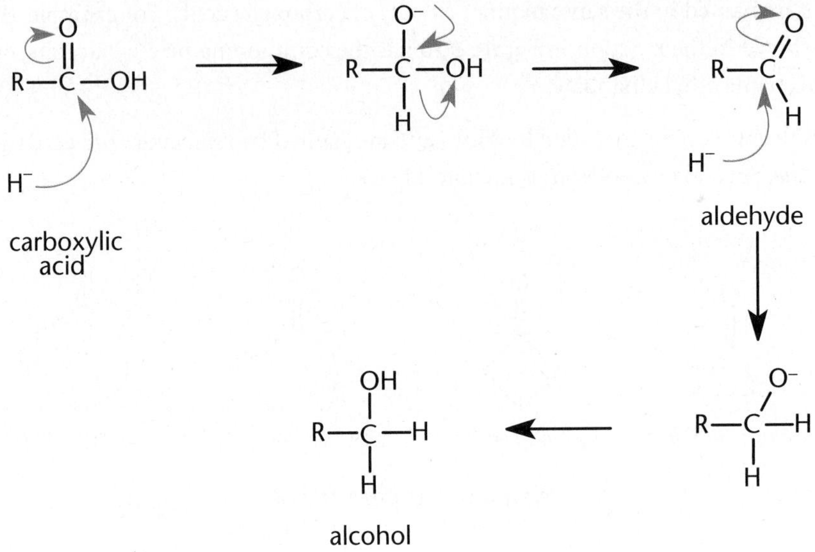

Figure 8.16 Reduction of a Carboxylic Acid to a Primary Alcohol
Reaction occurs by nucleophilic addition of hydride and proceeds through an aldehyde intermediate.

KEY CONCEPT

Carboxylic acids can be reduced by $LiAlH_4$, but not the less reactive $NaBH_4$.

Lithium aluminum hydride is a strong reducing agent that can successfully reduce a carboxylic acid; a gentler reducing agent like sodium borohydride ($NaBH_4$) is not strong enough to reduce carboxylic acids.

Decarboxylation

BRIDGE

Decarboxylation is common in biochemical pathways in the body. *Pyruvate dehydrogenase complex*, described in Chapter 10 of *MCAT Biochemistry Review*, carries out the decarboxylation of pyruvate to help form acetyl-CoA, which can feed into the citric acid cycle.

Decarboxylation describes the complete loss of the carboxyl group as carbon dioxide. This is a common way of getting rid of a carbon from the parent chain. 1,3-Dicarboxylic acids and other β-keto acids may spontaneously decarboxylate when heated. Under these conditions, the carboxyl group is lost and replaced with hydrogen. Because both the electrophile and nucleophile are in the same molecule, the reaction proceeds through a six-membered ring in its transition state, as shown in Figure 8.17. The enol that is initially formed from the destruction of the ring tautomerizes to the more stable keto form.

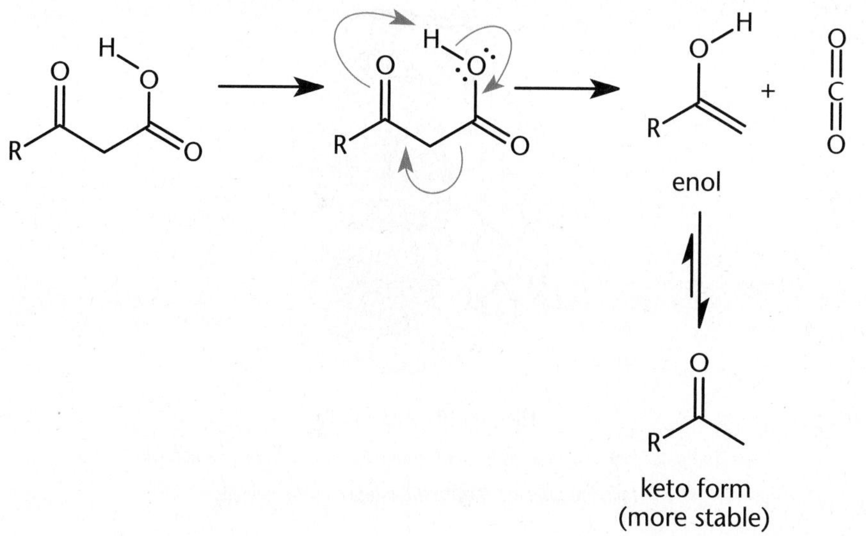

Figure 8.17 Decarboxylation of Carboxylic Acids: Loss of CO_2
The intramolecular reaction proceeds via a six-membered ring transition state, and the product tautomerizes from the enol to the more stable keto form.

Saponification

When long-chain carboxylic acids react with sodium or potassium hydroxide, a salt is formed. This process, called **saponification**, occurs by mixing fatty acids with lye (sodium or potassium hydroxide), resulting in the formation of a salt that we know as **soap**. Soaps can solvate nonpolar organic compounds in aqueous solutions because they contain both a nonpolar tail and a polar carboxylate head, as shown in Figure 8.18.

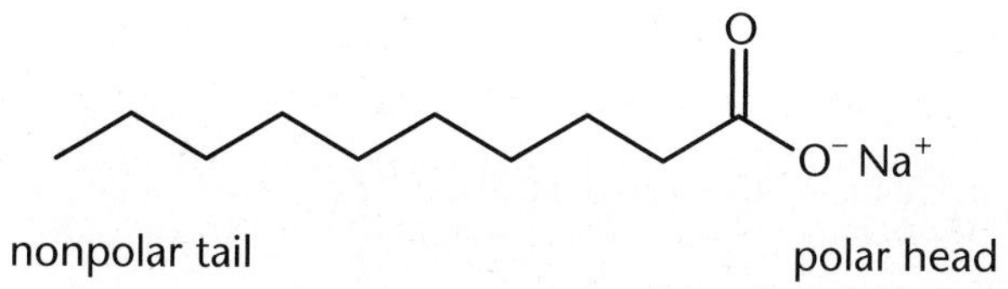

Figure 8.18 Carboxylic Acid Salt (Soap)

When placed in aqueous solution, soap molecules arrange themselves into spherical structures called **micelles**, as shown in Figure 8.19. The polar heads face outward, where they can be solvated by water, and the nonpolar hydrocarbon chains are oriented toward the inside of the sphere, protected from the solvent. Nonpolar molecules, such as grease, dissolve in the hydrocarbon interior of the spherical micelle; the micelle as a whole then dissolves in water due to the polarity of its exterior surface.

BRIDGE

The formation of the phospholipid bilayer, micelles, and liposomes are all contingent on the bipolar nature of carboxylic acids with long hydrocarbon chains. These structures are discussed in Chapter 5 of *MCAT Biochemistry Review*.

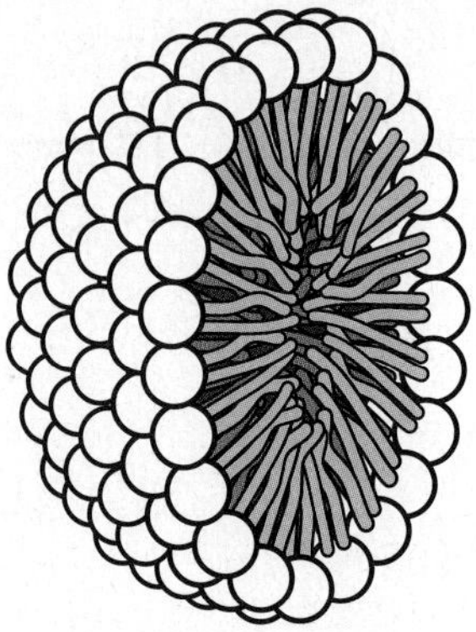

Figure 8.19 Soap Micelle
The polar heads interact with the hydrophilic environment; the nonpolar tails are oriented toward the interior of the micelle.

MCAT CONCEPT CHECK 8.2

Before you move on, assess your understanding of the material with these questions.

1. For each of the derivatives below, list the nucleophile used to form the derivative in an acyl substitution reaction and the name of the cyclic form of that functional group.

Carboxylic Acid Derivative	Formed by Reaction with:	Name of Cyclic Form:
Amide		
Ester		
Anhydride		

2. Briefly describe the mechanism of nucleophilic acyl substitution reactions.

___

3. What is the result when butanoic acid is reacted with sodium borohydride? With lithium aluminum hydride?
   - Sodium borohydride:

   ___

   - Lithium aluminum hydride:

   ___

4. Under what conditions will a carboxylic acid spontaneously decarboxylate?

___

Conclusion

Acids are an important concept on the MCAT: they can be tested in general chemistry, organic chemistry, and biochemistry. The underlying concept in all three subjects is the same: the more stable the conjugate base is, the more likely it is that the proton will leave. This stability is determined by three factors: periodic trends (electronegativity and, thus, induction), size of the anion, and resonance. Understanding these effects is a major key to success on Test Day. The reactions of carboxylic acids, in particular, are dictated by the polarity of the carbonyl group in conjunction with the ability of the hydroxyl group to act as a leaving group. This allows a diversity of reactions through nucleophilic acyl substitution, reduction by lithium aluminum hydride, decarboxylation, and saponification.

GO ONLINE

You've reviewed the content, now test your knowledge and critical thinking skills by completing a test-like passage set in your online resources!

CONCEPT SUMMARY

Description and Properties

- **Carboxylic acids** contain a carbonyl and a hydroxyl group connected to the same carbon. They are always terminal groups.
- Carboxylic acids are indicated with the suffix *–oic acid*. Salts are named with the suffix *–oate*, and **dicarboxylic acids** are ***–dioic acids***.
- Physical Properties
  - Carboxylic acids are polar and hydrogen bond very well, resulting in high boiling points. They often exist as **dimers** in solution.
  - The acidity of a carboxylic acid is enhanced by the resonance between its oxygen atoms.
  - Acidity can be further enhanced by substituents that are electron-withdrawing, and decreased by substituents that are electron-donating.
  - **β-dicarboxylic acids**, like other 1,3-dicarbonyl compounds, have an α-hydrogen that is also highly acidic.

Reactions of Carboxylic Acids

- Carboxylic acids can be made by the oxidation of primary alcohols or aldehydes using an oxidizing agent like potassium permanganate ($KMnO_4$), dichromate salts ($Na_2Cr_2O_7$ or $K_2Cr_2O_7$), or chromium trioxide (CrO_3).
- **Nucleophilic acyl substitution** is a common reaction in carboxylic acids.
  - A nucleophile attacks the electrophilic carbonyl carbon, opening the carbonyl and forming a tetrahedral intermediate.
  - The carbonyl reforms, kicking off the leaving group.
  - If the nucleophile is ammonia or an amine, an **amide** is formed. Amides are given the suffix ***–amide***. Cyclic amides are called **lactams**.
  - If the nucleophile is an alcohol, an **ester** is formed. Esters are given the suffix ***–oate***. Cyclic esters are called **lactones**.
  - If the nucleophile is another carboxylic acid, an **anhydride** is formed. Both linear and cyclic anhydrides are given the suffix ***anhydride***.
- Carboxylic acids can be reduced to a primary alcohol with a strong reducing agent like lithium aluminum hydride ($LiAlH_4$).
  - Aldehyde intermediates are formed, but are also reduced to primary alcohols.
  - Sodium borohydride ($NaBH_4$) is a common reducing agent for other organic reactions, but is not strong enough to reduce a carboxylic acid.
- β-dicarboxylic acids and other β-keto acids can undergo spontaneous **decarboxylation** when heated, losing a carbon as carbon dioxide. This reaction proceeds via a six-membered cyclic intermediate.

- Mixing long-chain carboxylic acids (fatty acids) with a strong base results in the formation of a salt we call **soap**. This process is called **saponification**.
  - Soaps contain hydrophilic carboxylate heads and hydrophobic alkyl chain tails.
  - Soaps organize in hydrophilic environments to form **micelles**. A micelle dissolves nonpolar organic molecules in its interior, and can be solvated with water due to its exterior shell of hydrophilic groups.

ANSWERS TO CONCEPT CHECKS

8.1

1. Carboxylic acids are particularly acidic due to the electron-withdrawing oxygen atoms in the functional group and the high stability of the carboxylate anion, which is resonance stabilized by delocalization with two electronegative oxygen atoms.
2. A dicarboxylic acid would be the most acidic, as the second carboxyl group is electron-withdrawing and therefore contributes to even higher stability of the anion after loss of the first hydrogen. However, a monocarboxylic acid is more acidic than a deprotonated dicarboxylic acid because the carboxylate anion is electron-donating and destabilizes the product of the second deprotonation step, resulting in decreased acidity.
3. Electron-withdrawing substituents make the anion more stable and therefore increase acidity. Electron-donating substituents, on the other hand, destabilize the anion, causing the carboxylic acid to be less acidic. The closer the substituent is to the carboxylic acid on the molecule, the stronger the effect will be.

8.2

1.

Carboxylic Acid Derivative	Formed by Reaction with:	Name of Cyclic Form:
Amide	Ammonia (NH_3) or an amine	Lactam
Ester	Alcohol	Lactone
Anhydride	Another carboxylic acid	Anhydride

2. Nucleophilic acyl substitution is the substitution of an attacking nucleophile for the leaving group of an acyl compound, which includes carboxylic acids, amides, esters, and anhydrides. The nucleophile attacks, opening the carbonyl and forming a tetrahedral intermediate. The carbonyl then reforms, kicking off the leaving group. This reaction is favored by acidic or basic conditions.
3. Sodium borohydride is not strong enough to reduce carboxylic acids so there will be no reaction. Lithium aluminum hydride, however, is strong enough to reduce carboxylic acids to primary alcohols—producing 1-butanol.
4. 1,3-Dicarboxylic acids will spontaneously decarboxylate when heated, due to the stable cyclic intermediate step.

SCIENCE MASTERY ASSESSMENT EXPLANATIONS

1. **D**

This compound is a β-keto acid: a carbonyl functional group at the β-position from a carboxyl group. Decarboxylation occurs with β-keto acids and β-dicarboxylic acids because they can form a cyclic transition state that permits simultaneous hydrogen transfer and loss of carbon dioxide. **(B)** is a diketone and does not have a single carboxyl group. **(A)** and **(C)** are γ- and δ-dicarboxylic acids, respectively, and can decarboxylate but with more difficulty.

2. **D**

The boiling points of compounds depend on the strength of the attractive forces between molecules. In both alcohols and carboxylic acids, the major form of intermolecular attraction is hydrogen bonding. However, hydrogen bonding is much stronger in carboxylic acids as compared to alcohols because carboxylic acids are more polar, and the carbonyl also contributes to hydrogen bonding in addition to the hydroxyl group. The stronger hydrogen bonds elevate the boiling points of carboxylic acids compared to alcohols. Boiling points also depend on molecular weight, **(A)**, but in this case, the difference in molecular weight is insignificant compared to the effect of hydrogen bonding. **(B)** and **(C)** are both true but do not explain the difference in boiling points.

3. **B**

The acidity of carboxylic acids is significantly increased by the presence of highly electronegative functional groups. Their electron-withdrawing effect increases the stability of the carboxylate anion, favoring proton dissociation. This effect increases as the number of electronegative groups on the chain increases, and it also increases as the distance between the acid functionality and electronegative group decreases. This answer has two halogens bonded to it at a smaller distance from the carboxyl group compared to the other answers.

4. **C**

Soap is a salt of a carboxylate anion with a long hydrocarbon tail. **(A)** and **(B)** are not salts of anionic compounds. **(D)** is sodium acetate, which is a salt but does not contain the long hydrocarbon tail needed to be considered a soap.

5. **B**

Jones reagent (chromium trioxide in aqueous sulfuric acid) is an oxidizing agent. As such, it oxidizes primary alcohols directly to carboxylic acids. This reagent is too strong an oxidant to give an aldehyde, so **(A)** is incorrect; remember that pyridinium chlorochromate (PCC) is a common oxidizing agent used to convert alcohols to aldehydes without progressing to a carboxylic acid. **(D)**, a dicarboxylic acid, cannot form because there is no functional group on the other end of the molecule for the reagent to attack, and it cannot attack an inert alkane. **(C)** represents reduction, not oxidation.

6. **C**

Carboxylic acids cannot be converted into alkenes with just one reagent. Esters, **(A)**, are formed in nucleophilic acyl substitution reactions with alcohols. Amides, **(B)**, are formed by nucleophilic acyl substitution reactions with ammonia. Alcohols, **(D)**, may be formed using a variety of reducing agents, most notably lithium aluminum hydride. To form alkenes, carboxylic acids may be reduced to alcohols, which can then be transformed into alkenes by elimination in a second step with addition of another reagent.

7. **D**

Lithium aluminum hydride ($LiAlH_4$ or LAH) is a strong reducing agent. LAH can completely reduce carboxylic acids to primary alcohols. Aldehydes are intermediate products of this reaction; therefore, **(A)** is incorrect. The other compounds are not created through the reduction of a carboxylic acid.

8. **D**

Micelles are self-assembled aggregates of soap in which the interior is composed of long hydrocarbon (fatty) tails, which can dissolve nonpolar molecules. The outer surface is covered with carboxylate groups, which makes the overall structure water-soluble. Soaps, in general, are salts of long-chain hydrocarbons with carboxylate head groups.

9. **D**

The reaction described is esterification, in which the nucleophilic oxygen atom of 1-pentanol attacks the electrophilic carbonyl carbon of butanoic acid, ultimately displacing water to form pentyl butanoate. The acid catalyst is regenerated from 1-pentanol's released proton. **(A)** reverses the carbon chains, considering the butyl tail to be the esterifying group. Ethers do not form under these conditions, so **(B)** and **(C)** are also incorrect.

10. **D**

The α-hydrogen of a carboxylic acid is relatively acidic as far as organic compounds go, due to resonance stabilization. However, the hydroxyl hydrogen is significantly more acidic because it is able to share the negative charge resulting from deprotonation between both electronegative oxygen atoms in the functional group.

11. **B**

The reaction of formic acid, which is a simple carboxylic acid, with sodium borohydride, which is a mild reducing agent, will result in no reaction, and therefore will result in maintenance of the carboxylic acid. Sodium borohydride is too mild to reduce carboxylic acids, and therefore cannot produce the primary alcohols that lithium aluminum hydride, a strong reducing agent, would.

12. **C**

5-aminopentanoic acid contains a carboxylic acid and an amine. If this molecule undergoes intramolecular nucleophilic acyl substitution, it will form a cyclic amide. These molecules are called lactams. Lactones, **(B)**, are cyclic esters, not amides.

13. **A**

Butanoic anhydride is an anhydride with two butane R groups. Anhydrides are produced by the reaction of two carboxylic acids with the loss of a water molecule. Therefore, butanoic anhydride would be produced by the reaction of two molecules of butanoic acid.

14. **C**

Nucleophilic acyl substitutions are favored in basic solution, which makes the nucleophile more nucleophilic; in acidic solution, which makes the electrophile more electrophilic; and by good leaving groups. However, strong bases do not make good leaving groups; weak bases do.

15. **D**

Based on its name, caprylic acid must be a carboxylic acid. The reaction between a carboxylic acid and ammonia (NH_3) would produce an amide—which is not one of the options listed. Instead, we should take a look at the type of reaction occurring. The production of an amide from a carboxylic acid and ammonia occurs through a condensation reaction in which a molecule of water is removed as a leaving group.

Consult your online resources for additional practice. GO ONLINE

SHARED CONCEPTS

Biochemistry Chapter 1
Amino Acids, Peptides, and Proteins

Biochemistry Chapter 5
Lipid Structure and Function

Organic Chemistry Chapter 1
Nomenclature

Organic Chemistry Chapter 4
Analyzing Organic Reactions

Organic Chemistry Chapter 6
Aldehydes and Ketones I

Organic Chemistry Chapter 9
Carboxylic Acid Derivatives

CHAPTER 9

CARBOXYLIC ACID DERIVATIVES

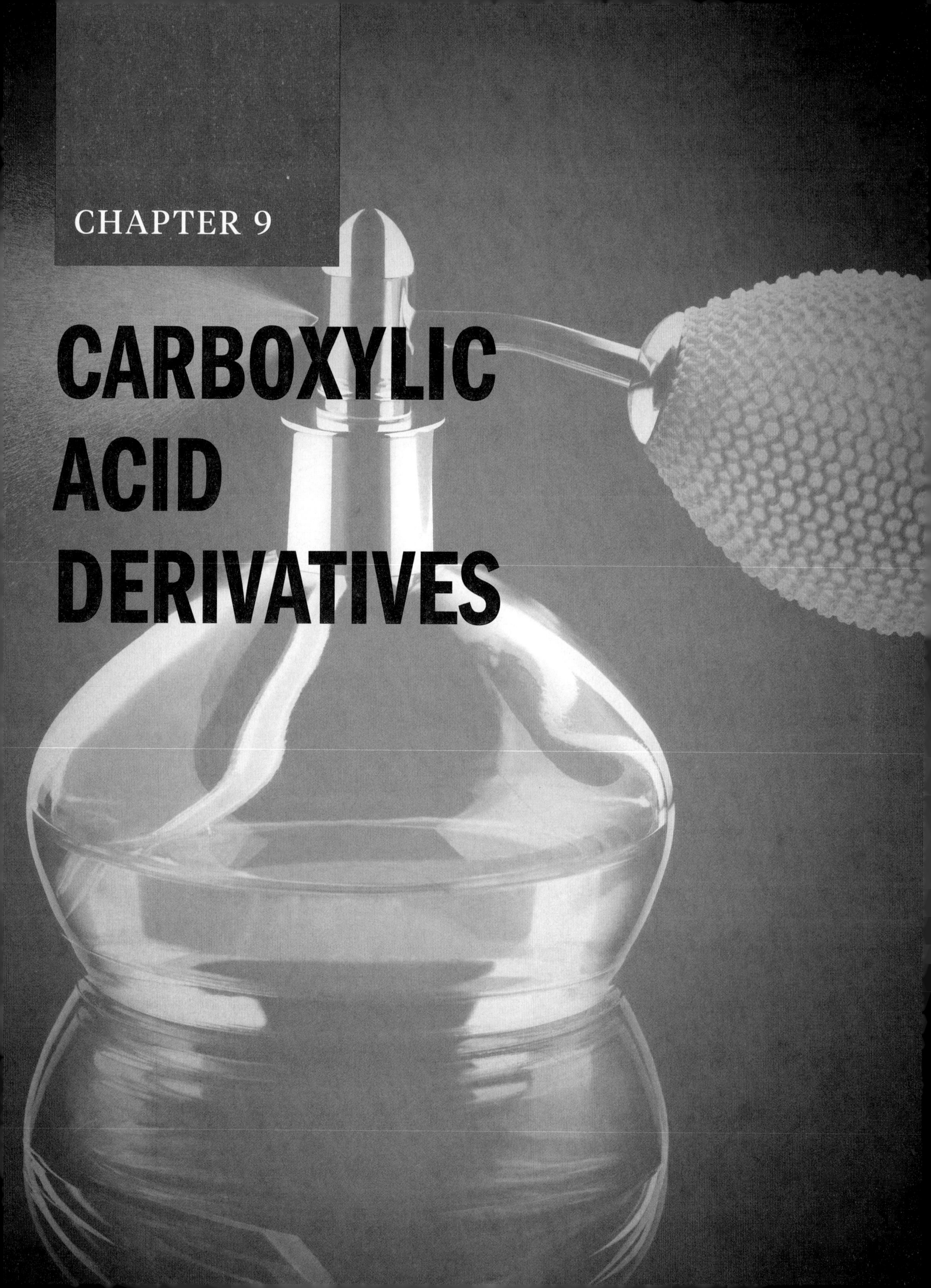

SCIENCE MASTERY ASSESSMENT

Every pre-med knows this feeling: there is so much content I have to know for the MCAT! How do I know what to do first or what's important?

While the high-yield badges throughout this book will help you identify the most important topics, this Science Mastery Assessment is another tool in your MCAT prep arsenal. This quiz (which can also be taken in your online resources) and the guidance below will help ensure that you are spending the appropriate amount of time on this chapter based on your personal strengths and weaknesses. Don't worry though—skipping something now does not mean you'll never study it. Later on in your prep, as you complete full-length tests, you'll uncover specific pieces of content that you need to review and can come back to these chapters as appropriate.

How to Use This Assessment

If you answer 0–7 questions correctly:

Spend about 1 hour to read this chapter in full and take limited notes throughout. Follow up by reviewing **all** quiz questions to ensure that you now understand how to solve each one.

If you answer 8–11 questions correctly:

Spend 20–40 minutes reviewing the quiz questions. Beginning with the questions you missed, read and take notes on the corresponding subchapters. For questions you answered correctly, ensure your thinking matches that of the explanation and you understand why each choice was correct or incorrect.

If you answer 12–15 questions correctly:

Spend less than 20 minutes reviewing all questions from the quiz. If you missed any, then include a quick read-through of the corresponding subchapters, or even just the relevant content within a subchapter, as part of your question review. For questions you got correct, ensure your thinking matches that of the explanation and review the Concept Summary at the end of the chapter.

1. Which of the following would be the best method of producing methyl propanoate?
   - **A.** Reacting propanoic acid and methanol in the presence of a mineral acid
   - **B.** Reacting methanoic acid and propanol in the presence of a mineral acid
   - **C.** Reacting propanoic anhydride with an aqueous base
   - **D.** Reacting propanoic acid with an aqueous base

2. What would be the product(s) of the reaction below?

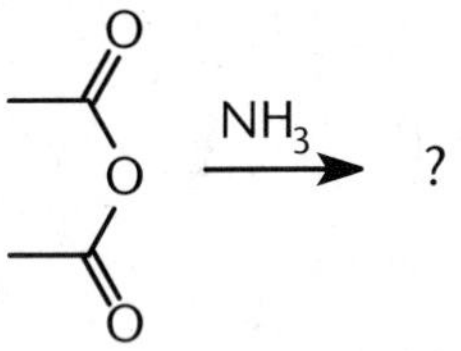

A. 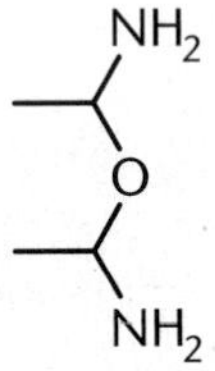

B. 2 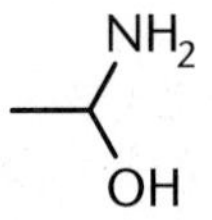

C. 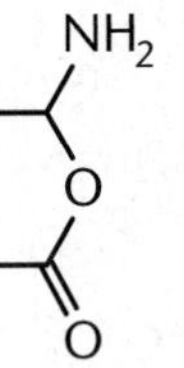

D. 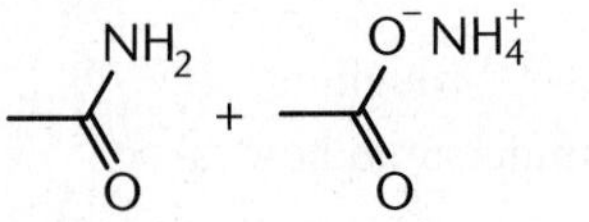

3. Which of the following undergoes a Fischer esterification most rapidly?

A. 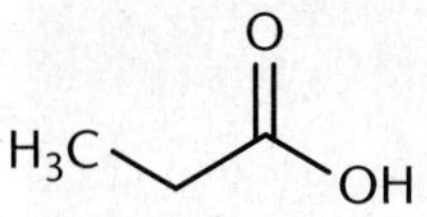

B. 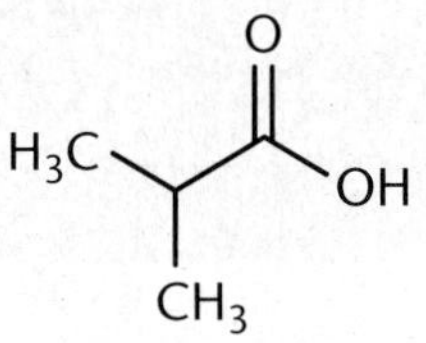

C. 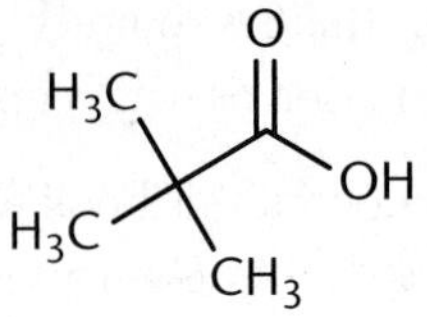

D. 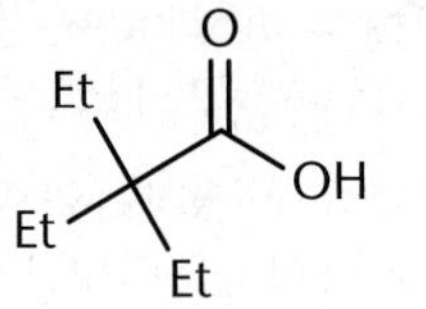

4. Each of the acyl compounds listed below contains a six-membered ring EXCEPT:
   - **A.** δ-lactam.
   - **B.** cyclohexane carboxylic acid.
   - **C.** γ-butyrolactone.
   - **D.** the anhydride formed from intramolecular ring closure of pentanedioic acid.

5. Which of the following would be most reactive toward nucleophiles?
   - **A.** Propyl ethanoate
   - **B.** Propanoic acid
   - **C.** Propanamide
   - **D.** Propanoic anhydride

6. How might succinic anhydride, shown below, be formed from succinic acid (butanedioic acid)?

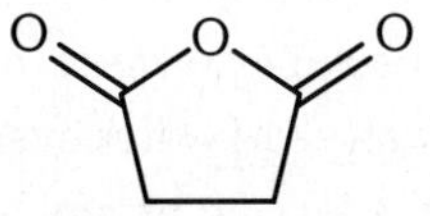

A. Catalytic acid
B. Catalytic base
C. Heat
D. Oxidation

7. Which of the following would react most readily with a carboxylic acid to form an amide?
A. Methylamine
B. Triethylamine
C. Diphenylamine
D. Ethylmethylamine

8. If propanamide were treated with water, what product(s) would be observed?
A. Propanamide
B. Propanoic acid
C. Equal concentrations of propanamide and propanoic acid
D. Propyl propanoate

9. β-lactams are:
I. cyclic forms of the least reactive type of carboxylic acid derivative.
II. more reactive than their straight-chain counterparts.
III. molecules with high levels of ring strain.

A. I only
B. II only
C. II and III only
D. I, II, and III

10. The acid-catalyzed conversion of propyl ethanoate to benzyl ethanoate is likely:
A. reduction.
B. hydrolysis.
C. transesterification.
D. oxidation.

11. The reaction shown, which is important for the breakdown of polypeptides, would be favored under what conditions?

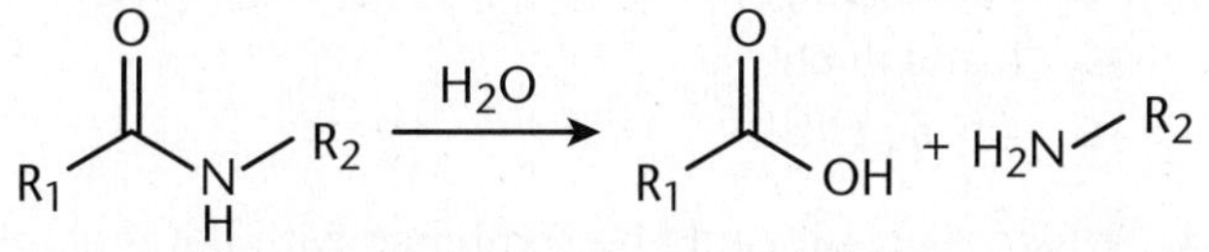

A. Mild heat
B. Acid environment
C. Anhydrous environment
D. Nonpolar solvent

12. A positive charge on the molecule shown would have greater stability than a positive charge on a straight-chain alkane version of the same molecule. What property most explains this effect?

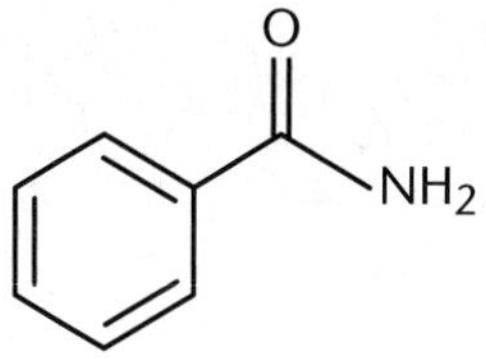

A. Steric hindrance
B. Nitrogen electronegativity
C. Induction
D. Conjugation

13. The molecule shown is:

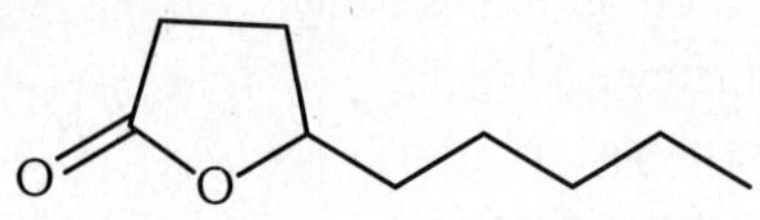

I. synthesizable from a γ-hydroxycarboxylic acid.
II. a lactone.
III. a form of an ester.

A. I only
B. I and II only
C. II and III only
D. I, II, and III

14. Which reactant could be combined with butanol to form butyl acetate?

A. $(CH_3CO)_2O$ and catalytic acid
B. $(CH_3CH_2CO)_2O$ and catalytic acid
C. $CH_3CH_2CONH_2$ and catalytic acid
D. CH_3CONH_2 and catalytic acid

15. Why should esterification reactions NOT be carried out in water?

A. Carboxylic acids, from which esters are made, are generally insoluble in water.
B. The polar nature of water overshadows the polar nature of the leaving group.
C. The extensive hydrogen bonding of water interferes with the nucleophilic addition mechanism.
D. Water molecules would hydrolyze the desired products back into the parent carboxylic acid.

Answer Key follows on next page.

Answer Key

1. **A**
2. **D**
3. **A**
4. **C**
5. **D**
6. **C**
7. **A**
8. **A**
9. **D**
10. **C**
11. **B**
12. **D**
13. **D**
14. **A**
15. **D**

Detailed explanations can be found at the end of the chapter.

CHAPTER 9

CARBOXYLIC ACID DERIVATIVES

In This Chapter

CHAPTER PROFILE

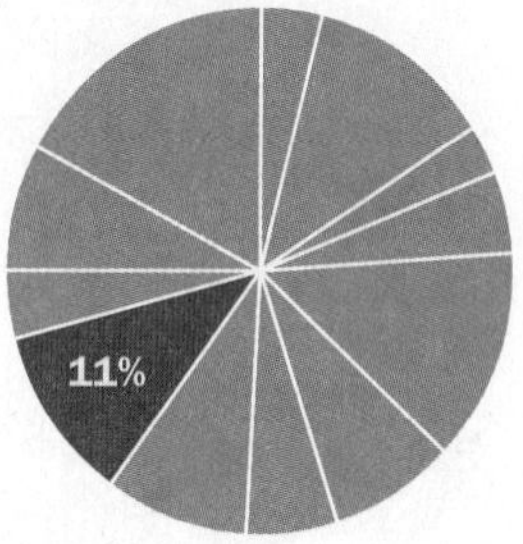

The content in this chapter should be relevant to about 11% of all questions about organic chemistry on the MCAT.

This chapter covers material from the following AAMC content categories:

1A: Structure and function of proteins and their constituent amino acids

5D: Structure, function, and reactivity of biologically-relevant molecules

Introduction

We saw in the previous three chapters that carbonyls are susceptible to attack by everything from water to amines to other carbonyl-containing compounds (in the enol or enolate form). These reactions often result in the formation of carboxylic acid derivatives. Our focus in this chapter will be on describing the carboxylic acid derivatives that appear on the MCAT: amides, esters, and anhydrides. Each of these molecules replaces the $-OH$ on the carboxyl group with another leaving group ($-NR_2$, $-OR$, and $-OCOR$, respectively). These each react in similar ways to carboxylic acids. Many of these functional groups are also critical for biochemical processes.

9.1 Amides, Esters, and Anhydrides

LEARNING OBJECTIVES

After Chapter 9.1, you will be able to:

- Apply the rules for naming carboxylic acid derivatives, including the nomenclature for the cyclic version of the molecule
- Describe a condensation reaction

Amides, esters, and anhydrides are all carboxylic acid derivatives. Each of these is formed by a **condensation** reaction with a carboxylic acid—a reaction that combines two molecules into one, while losing a small molecule. In this case, the small molecule is water, which is created from the hydroxyl group of the carboxylic acid and a hydrogen associated with the incoming nucleophile.

KEY CONCEPT

In a condensation reaction, two molecules are combined to form one, with the loss of a small molecule–water, in our case. Carboxylic acid derivatives are formed by this mechanism.

Descriptions

For each of the carboxylic acid derivatives described in this section, focus on the relevant nucleophile that forms the derivative and the nomenclature of the functional group. In the next section, we'll focus more directly on the relative reactivity of these compounds.

Amides

Amides are compounds with the general formula $RCONR_2$. They are named by replacing the *–oic acid* suffix with *–amide*. Alkyl substituents on the nitrogen atom are listed as prefixes, and their location is specified with the letter ***N*–**. Figure 9.1 shows a few examples.

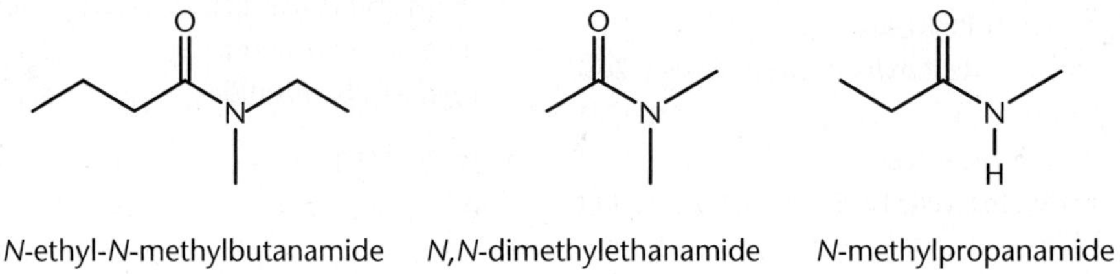

Figure 9.1 Naming Amides

KEY CONCEPT

Amides are formed by the condensation reaction of other carboxylic acid derivatives and ammonia or an amine.

Amides are generally synthesized by the reaction of other carboxylic acid derivatives with either ammonia or an amine. Note that loss of hydrogen from the nucleophile is required for this reaction to take place. Thus, only primary and secondary amines will undergo this reaction.

Cyclic amides are called **lactams**. These are named according to the carbon atom bonded to the nitrogen: β-lactams contain a bond between the β-carbon and the nitrogen, γ-lactams contain a bond between the γ-carbon and the nitrogen, and so forth. Structures of lactams are shown in Figure 9.2.

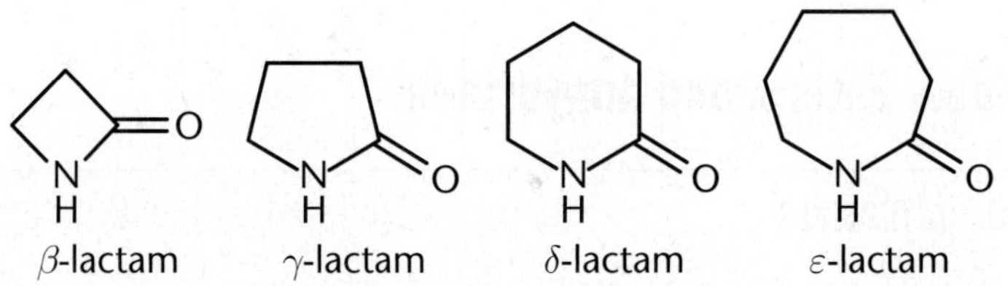

Figure 9.2 Examples of Lactams

Amides may or may not participate in hydrogen bonding depending on the number of alkyl groups they have bonded, and therefore their boiling points may be lower or on the same level as the boiling points of carboxylic acids.

Esters

Esters are the dehydration synthesis products of other carboxylic acid derivatives and alcohols. They are named by placing the **esterifying group** (the substituent bonded to the oxygen) as a prefix; the suffix *–oate* replaces *–oic acid*. Two examples are shown in Figure 9.3. As mentioned in the last chapter, ethyl acetate, derived from the condensation of acetic acid and ethanol, is called ethyl ethanoate according to IUPAC nomenclature.

KEY CONCEPT

Esters are formed by the condensation reaction of carboxylic acids or anhydrides with alcohols.

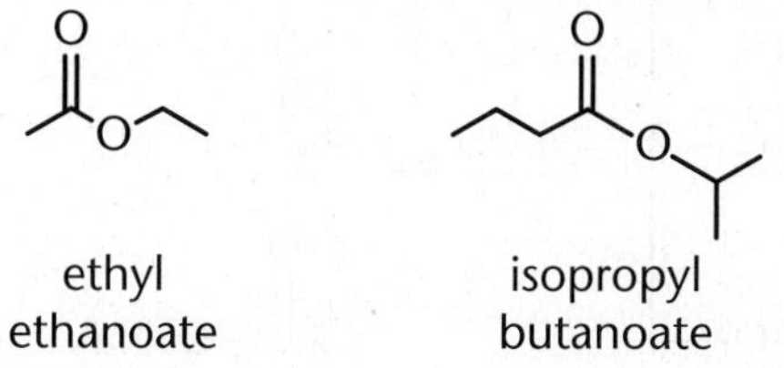

Figure 9.3 Naming Esters

Under acidic conditions, mixtures of carboxylic acids and alcohols will condense into esters. This reaction, called a **Fischer esterification**, is shown in Figure 9.4. Esters can also be obtained from the reaction of anhydrides with alcohols.

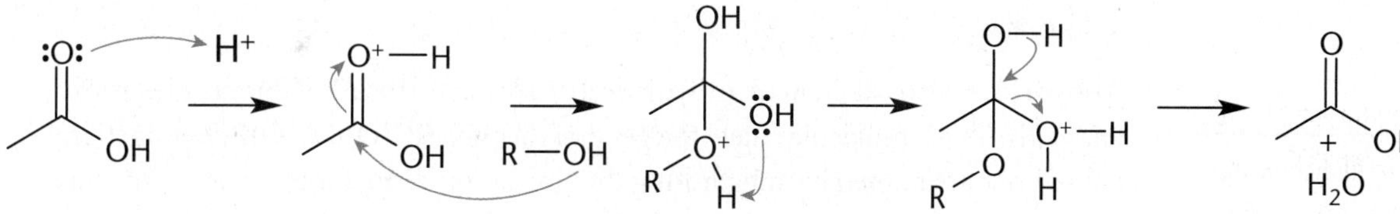

Figure 9.4 Fischer Esterification

Cyclic esters are called **lactones** and are named in the same manner as lactams, with the name of the precursor acid molecule also included. Examples are shown in Figure 9.5.

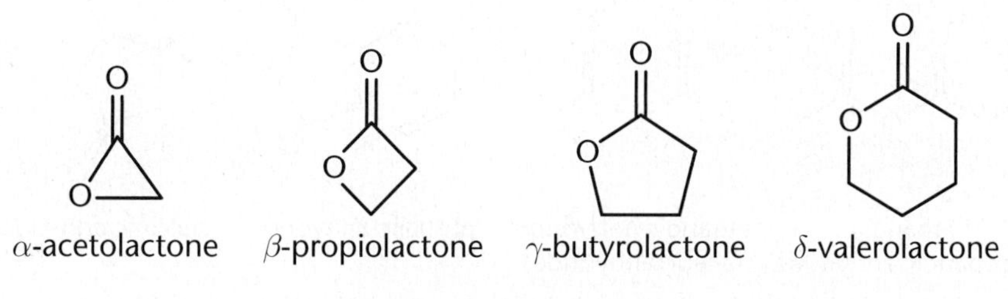

Figure 9.5 Examples of Lactones

Because they lack hydrogen bonding, esters usually have lower boiling points than their related carboxylic acids.

Triacylglycerols, the storage form of fats in the body, are esters of long-chain carboxylic acids (fatty acids) and *glycerol* (1,2,3-propanetriol). **Saponification** is the process by which fats are hydrolyzed under basic conditions to produce soap; saponification of a triacylglycerol is shown in Figure 9.6. Subsequent acidification of the soap regenerates the fatty acids.

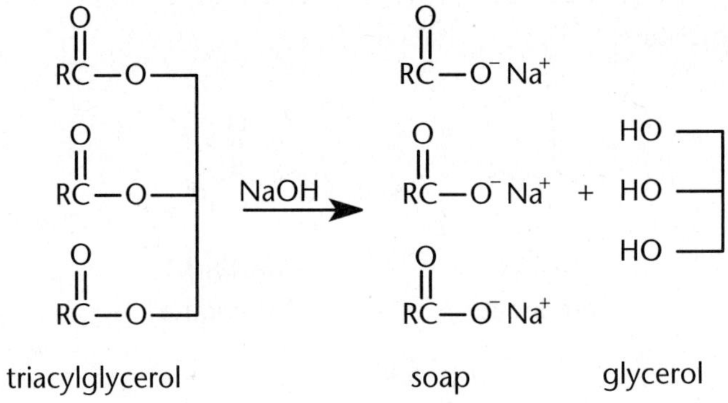

Figure 9.6 Saponification of a Triacylglycerol
Treating triacylglycerols with NaOH will produce fatty acid salts (soap) as well as glycerol.

Anhydrides

KEY CONCEPT

Anhydrides are usually formed by the condensation reaction of two carboxylic acids.

Anhydrides, also called **acid anhydrides**, are the condensation dimers of carboxylic acids. These molecules have the general formula RC(O)OC(O)R. Symmetrical anhydrides are named by substituting the word ***anhydride*** for the word ***acid*** in a carboxylic acid. When anhydrides are asymmetrical, simply name the two chains alphabetically, followed by ***anhydride***, as shown in Figure 9.7. Phthalic and succinic anhydrides are cyclic anhydrides arising from intramolecular condensation or dehydration of diacids; their structures need not be memorized, but recognize them as cyclic anhydrides.

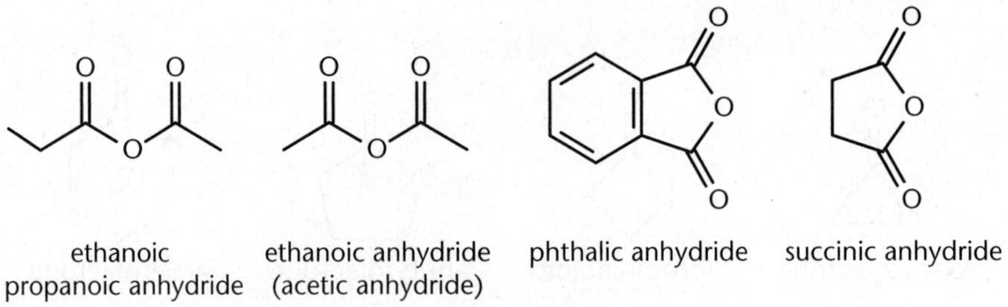

Figure 9.7 Naming Anhydrides

Acid anhydrides are synthesized, as mentioned previously, by a condensation reaction between two carboxylic acids, with one molecule of water lost in the condensation, as shown in Figure 9.8.

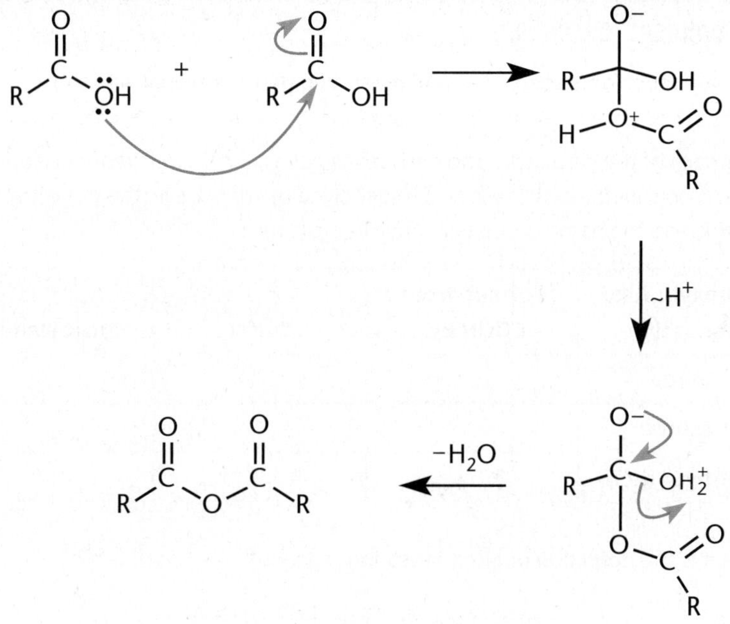

Figure 9.8 Synthesis of an Anhydride via Carboxylic Acid Condensation
Two molecules of carboxylic acid come together and lose a molecule of water in the formation of an anhydride.

Certain cyclic anhydrides can be formed simply by heating carboxylic acids, as shown in Figure 9.9. The reaction is driven forward by the increased stability of the newly formed ring; as such, only anhydrides with five- or six-membered rings are easily made. Just as with all anhydride formations, the hydroxyl group of one —COOH acts as the nucleophile, attacking the carbonyl on the other —COOH.

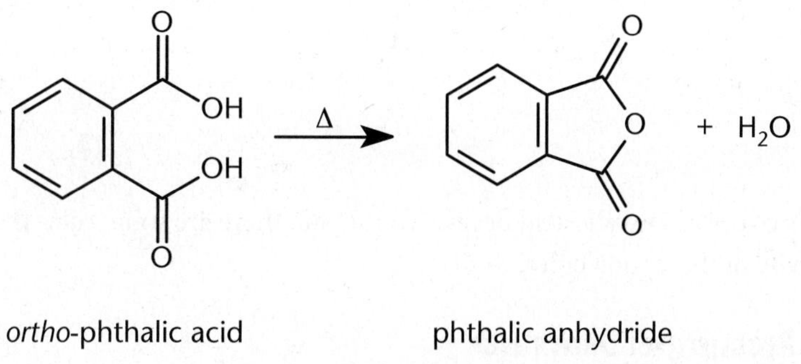

Figure 9.9 Intramolecular Anhydride Formation
Heat and the increased stability of the newly formed ring drive this intramolecular ring formation reaction forward.

Anhydrides often have higher boiling points than their related carboxylic acids, based solely on their much greater weight.

MCAT CONCEPT CHECK 9.1

Before you move on, assess your understanding of the material with these questions.

1. For each of the carboxylic acid derivatives below, list the relevant nucleophile that reacts with a carboxylic acid to generate the derivative, the derivative's suffix, and the name of the derivative in cyclic form.

Carboxylic Acid Derivative	Formed from –COOH by...	Suffix	Cyclic Naming
Amide			
Ester			
Anhydride			

2. What is the definition of a condensation reaction?

____

9.2 Reactivity Principles

LEARNING OBJECTIVES

After Chapter 9.2, you will be able to:

- Order carboxylic acid derivatives, including anhydrides, esters, and amides, based on their reactivity
- Explain the relatively high rate of hydrolysis in β-lactams
- Identify the properties of the carboxylic acid derivatives that cause their reactivities to differ

Regardless of the carboxylic acid derivative at hand, there are some rules that govern the reactivity of these molecules.

Relative Reactivity of Derivatives

KEY CONCEPT

When considering the reactivity of carboxylic acid derivatives toward nucleophilic attack, anhydrides are the most reactive, followed by esters and carboxylic acids, and then amides.

In a nucleophilic substitution reaction, the reactivity of the carbonyl is determined by its substituents. Anhydrides are most reactive, followed by esters (which are essentially tied with carboxylic acids), then finally amides. This can be explained by the structure of these molecules. Anhydrides, with their resonance stabilization and three electron-withdrawing oxygen atoms, are the most electrophilic. Esters, by comparison, lack one electron-withdrawing carbonyl oxygen and are slightly less reactive. Finally, amides, with an electron-donating amino group, are the least reactive toward nucleophiles.

Steric Effects

Steric hindrance is always worth keeping in mind when considering reactivity. **Steric hindrance** describes when a reaction does not proceed due to the size of the substituents. A good example of this is in S_N2 reactions, which will not occur at tertiary carbons. This effect, which might sound detrimental, can be used to our advantage—for example, if we want to push a reaction in an S_N1 direction, rather than S_N2, we can use a tertiary substrate. Another way that this is used synthetically is in the creation of protecting groups. As we saw in Chapter 6 of *MCAT Organic Chemistry Review*, aldehydes and ketones will readily react with strong reducing agents like $LiAlH_4$—but this can be prevented by first reacting the aldehyde or ketone with two equivalents of alcohol, producing a nonreactive acetal or ketal. After we complete the rest of the desired reactions, we can then regenerate the carbonyl with aqueous acid. In the context of carboxylic acid derivatives, the size and substitution of the leaving group can affect the ability of a nucleophile to access the carbonyl carbon, thus affecting the reactivity of the derivative to nucleophilic acyl substitution.

KEY CONCEPT

Steric hindrance can be used to control where a reaction occurs in a molecule. Protecting groups may make it too hard for a nucleophile, oxidizing agent, or reducing agent to access or react with a part of the molecule.

Electronic Effects

There are several electronic effects that must be considered in organic chemistry on the MCAT, and all of them come into play when considering carboxylic acid derivatives. **Induction** refers to the distribution of charge across σ bonds. Electrons are attracted to atoms that are more electronegative, generating a dipole across the σ bond. The less electronegative atom acquires a slightly positive charge, and the more electronegative atom acquires a slightly negative charge. This effect is relatively weak and gets increasingly weaker as one moves further away within the molecule from the more electronegative atom. This effect is responsible for the dipole character of the carbonyl group, as well as the increased dipole character (and, therefore, susceptibility to nucleophilic attack) of carboxylic acids—which contain an additional oxygen atom in their leaving group. This also explains the overall relative reactivity of anhydrides, esters, and amides toward nucleophilic attack. Anhydrides have two electron-withdrawing groups, which leave a significant partial positive charge on the electrophilic carbon. This effect is smaller in amides because nitrogen is less electronegative than oxygen, and the dipole is not as strong.

Resonance and conjugation also affect the reactivity of a molecule. **Conjugation** refers to the presence of alternating single and multiple bonds. This setup implies that all of the atoms involved in these bonds are either sp^2- or sp-hybridized—and therefore have unhybridized p-orbitals. When these p-orbitals align, they can delocalize π electrons through resonance, forming clouds of electron density above and below the plane of the molecule. This type of electron sharing is most commonly demonstrated using benzene, as shown in Figure 9.10.

KEY CONCEPT

Induction is the distribution of charge across σ bonds. Conjugation and resonance are much more powerful effects and occur in systems with alternating single and multiple bonds.

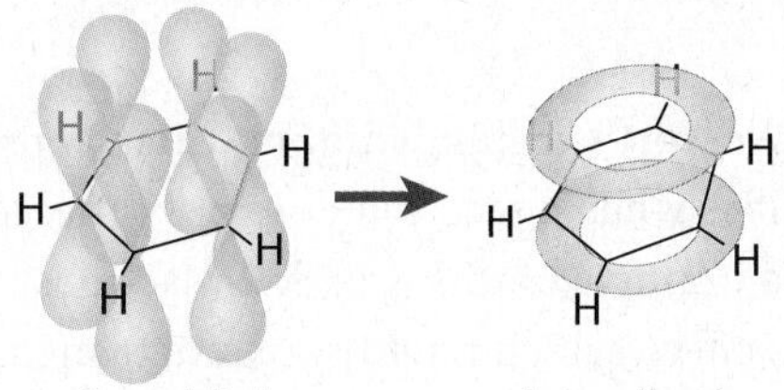

Figure 9.10 Conjugation in Benzene

Parallel unhybridized p-orbitals combine to form delocalized electron clouds above and below the plane of the molecule.

In carbonyl-containing compounds, conjugation can be established with the carbonyl group itself. α,β-unsaturated carbonyls or (**enones**) are common examples, as shown in Figure 9.11.

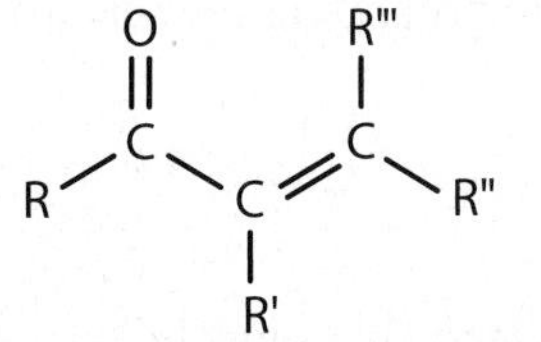

Figure 9.11 Conjugation in a Carbonyl-Containing Compound

This type of electron sharing makes for very stable compounds because these compounds have multiple resonance structures. This characteristic allows for the stabilization of a positive charge once the nucleophile has bonded, making these compounds more susceptible to nucleophilic attack.

Strain in Cyclic Derivatives

Lactams and lactones are cyclic amides and esters, respectively. Certain lactams and lactones are more reactive to hydrolysis because they contain more strain. β-lactams, for example, are four-membered cyclic amides and are highly reactive due to significant ring strain; four-membered rings have both torsional strain from eclipsing interactions and angle strain from compressing the normal sp^3 angle of 109.5°. These molecules are part of the core structure of several antibiotic families, as shown in Figure 9.12. The ring strain, and therefore the reactivity, is increased by fusion to a second ring. The four-membered structure of a β-lactam also forces a trigonal pyramidal bond geometry on the nitrogen atom in the ring, which reduces resonance, making hydrolysis more likely.

REAL WORLD

Many antibiotic families contain β-lactams, including the penicillin family, cephalosporins, carbapenems, and monobactams. Many bacteria have developed β-lactamases, which break β-lactam rings, as a resistance mechanism against these antibiotics. Therefore, β-lactams are sometimes given with β-lactamase inhibitors to increase their efficacy.

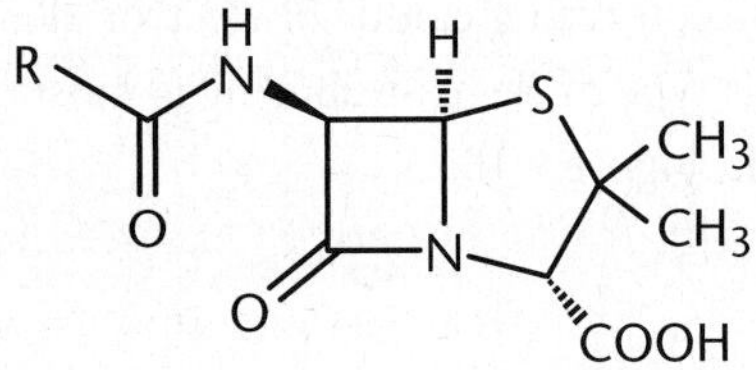

Figure 9.12 Penicillin, a β-Lactam-Containing Antibiotic

MCAT CONCEPT CHECK 9.2

Before you move on, assess your understanding of the material with these questions.

1. Rank the following molecules by decreasing reactivity to OR^-: acetamide, acetic anhydride, and ethyl acetate.

    1. ______________________________
    2. ______________________________
    3. ______________________________

2. What is responsible for the increased rate of hydrolysis in β-lactams?

    ____

3. What properties account for the differences in reactivity seen between anhydrides, esters, and amides with nucleophiles?

    ____

9.3 Nucleophilic Acyl Substitution Reactions

High-Yield

LEARNING OBJECTIVES

After Chapter 9.3, you will be able to:

- Describe the mechanism for transesterification reactions
- Explain how strong acid and strong base conditions would impact the mechanism of hydrolysis of an amide
- Identify the nucleophile and electrophile within nucleophilic acyl substitution reactions such as:

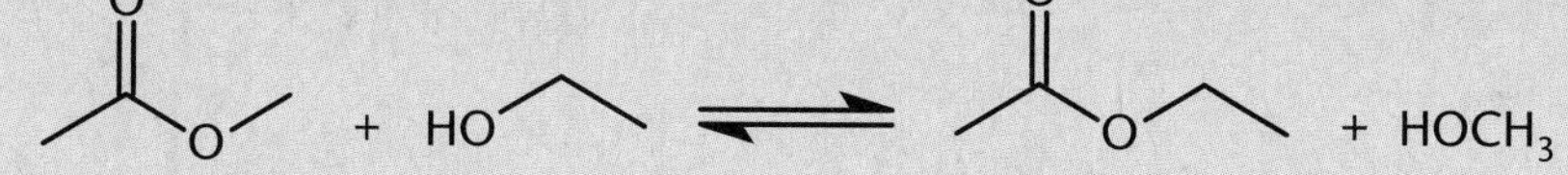

Although there are a seemingly infinite number of reactions in which carboxylic acid derivatives can participate, a much smaller group of reactions will appear on the MCAT. As we will observe, these reactions have much in common with those of carboxylic acids and other carbonyl-containing compounds. Many of the properties we have already discussed determine the ways in which these reactions proceed.

Anhydride Cleavage

As with carboxylic acids, nucleophilic acyl substitution involves nucleophilic attack of the carbonyl carbon with displacement of a leaving group. All carboxylic acid derivatives can participate in nucleophilic substitution reactions at different relative rates. Specifically, anhydrides are most reactive toward nucleophiles, followed by esters, and finally amides. One example of this is the formation of amides from the nucleophilic substitution reaction between ammonia and any carboxylic acid or derivative. The example shown in Figure 9.13 is not only a nucleophilic substitution reaction, but also a **cleavage reaction** because it splits an anhydride in two. In this reaction, ammonia acts as the nucleophile, one of the carbonyl carbons acts as the electrophile, and a carboxylic acid is the leaving group.

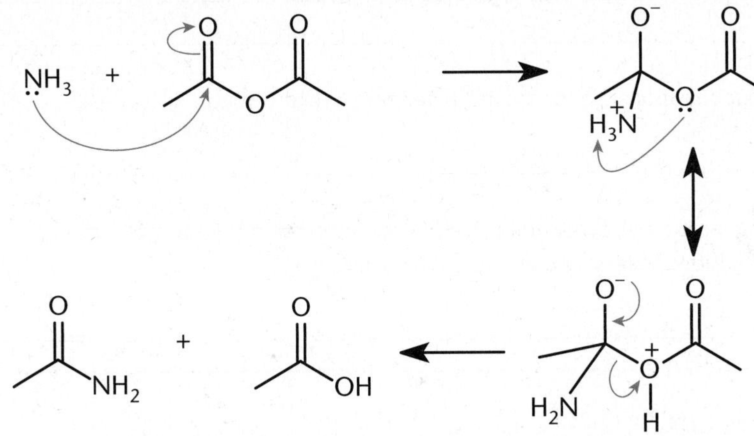

Figure 9.13 Nucleophilic Acyl Substitution: Anhydride to Amide and Carboxylic Acid

Alcohols can also act as nucleophiles toward anhydrides; this nucleophilic substitution reaction will result in the formation of esters and carboxylic acids, as shown in Figure 9.14.

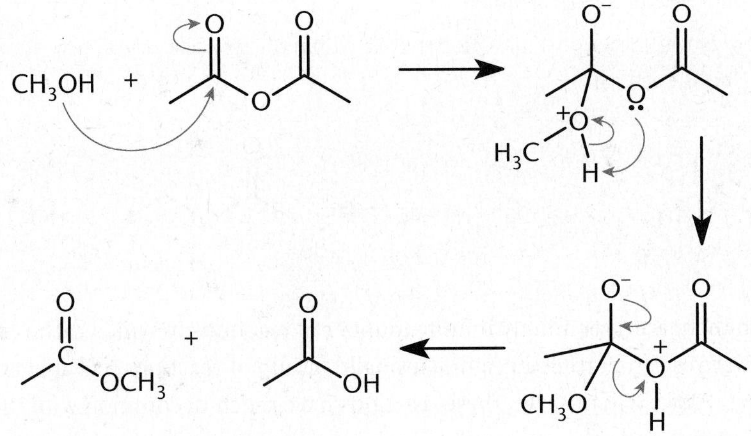

Figure 9.14 Nucleophilic Acyl Substitution: Anhydride to Ester and Carboxylic Acid

Anhydrides can also be reverted to carboxylic acids by exposing them to water, as shown in Figure 9.15. For these reactions to be useful, the anhydride should be symmetric; otherwise, one forms a mixture of products.

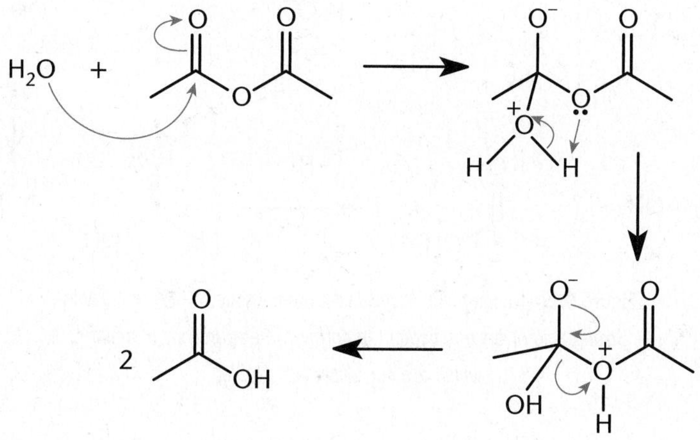

Figure 9.15 Nucleophilic Acyl Substitution: Anhydride to Carboxylic Acids

Transesterification

Alcohols can act as nucleophiles and displace the esterifying group on an ester. This process is called **transesterification**. In this reaction, one ester is simply transformed into another, as shown in Figure 9.16.

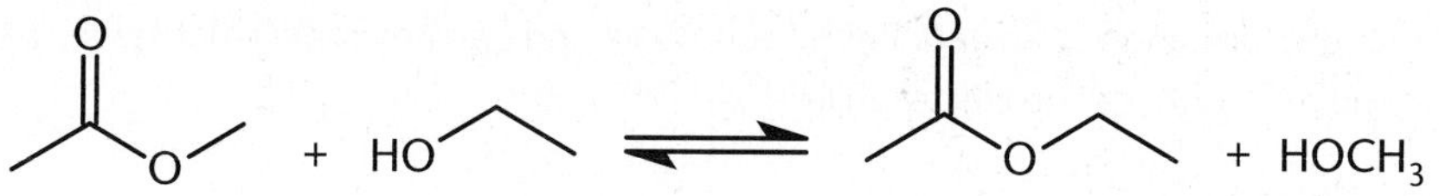

Figure 9.16 Nucleophilic Acyl Substitution: Transesterification
Different alcohol chains are swapped into and out of the esterifying group position.

Hydrolysis of Amides

Amides can be hydrolyzed under highly acidic conditions via nucleophilic substitution. The acidic conditions allow the carbonyl oxygen to become protonated, making the molecule more susceptible to nucleophilic attack by a water molecule. The product of this reaction is a carboxylic acid and ammonia. This should be no surprise because this is the reverse of the condensation reaction by which amides are formed. This reaction is shown in Figure 9.17.

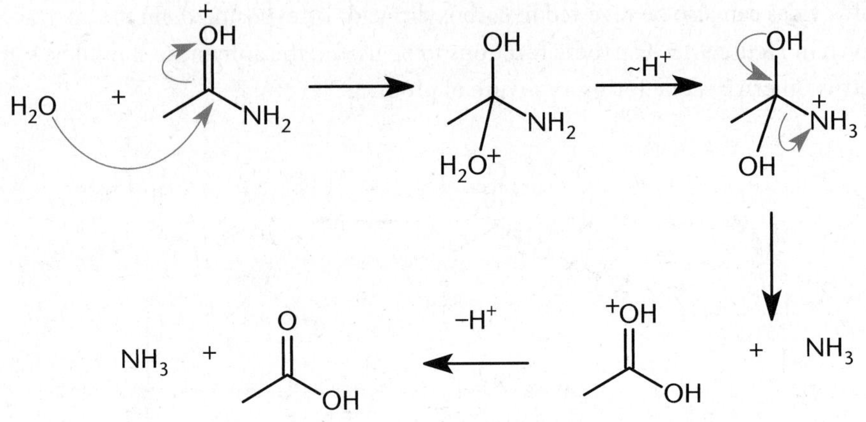

Figure 9.17 Nucleophilic Acyl Substitution: Amide to Carboxylic Acid
Strong acid or base is needed to catalyze the hydrolysis of amides, which are normally quite stable.

Hydrolysis can also occur if conditions are basic enough. The reaction is similar to an acid-catalyzed reaction, except that the carbonyl oxygen is not protonated and the nucleophile is a hydroxide ion. The product of this reaction would be the deprotonated carboxylate anion.

MCAT CONCEPT CHECK 9.3

Before you move on, assess your understanding of the material with these questions.

1. In the formation of an amide from ammonia and an anhydride, what serves as the nucleophile? The electrophile?
   - Nucleophile:
   - Electrophile:
2. What are the products of the transesterification reaction between isopropyl butanoate and ethanol?
3. How do strongly acidic and strongly basic conditions catalyze the hydrolysis of an amide?
   - Strongly acidic conditions:
   - Strongly basic conditions:

Conclusion

We're sure you've noticed that this chapter covers only a few reactions happening in a wide variety of contexts. The MCAT test makers don't want you to memorize all the possible reactions; they simply want you to truly understand the trends and the underlying reasons for these reactions. Make sure you know the order of reactivity of the derivatives (from anhydrides, the most, to amides, the least). Also, learn the special reactions of esters and amides. Your study of amides will pay off right away as we explore amino acids and other nitrogen- and phosphorus-containing compounds in the next chapter.

GO ONLINE

You've reviewed the content, now test your knowledge and critical thinking skills by completing a test-like passage set in your online resources!

CONCEPT SUMMARY

Amides, Esters, and Anhydrides

- **Amides** are the condensation products of carboxylic acids and ammonia or amines.
  - Amides are given the suffix *–amide*. The alkyl groups on a substituted amide are written at the beginning of the name with the prefix *N*–.
  - Cyclic amides are called **lactams**. Lactams are named by the Greek letter of the carbon forming the bond with the nitrogen (β-lactam, γ-lactam, and so on).
- **Esters** are the condensation products of carboxylic acids with alcohols (**Fischer esterification**).
  - Esters are given the suffix *–oate*. The **esterifying group** is written as a substituent, without a number.
  - Cyclic esters are called **lactones**. Lactones are named by the number of carbons in the ring and the Greek letter of the carbon forming the bond with the oxygen (α-acetolactone, β-propiolactone, and so on).
  - **Triacylglycerols**, which are a form of fat storage, include three ester bonds between glycerol and fatty acids. **Saponification** is the breakdown of fat using a strong base to form **soap** (salts of long-chain carboxylic acids).
- **Anhydrides** are the condensation dimers of carboxylic acids.
  - Symmetric anhydrides are named for the parent carboxylic acid, followed by ***anhydride***. Asymmetric anhydrides are named by listing the parent carboxylic acids alphabetically, followed by ***anhydride***.
  - Some cyclic anhydrides can be synthesized by heating dioic acids. Five- or six-membered rings are generally stable.

Reactivity Principles

- In nucleophilic substitution reactions, anhydrides are more reactive than esters, which are more reactive than amides.
- **Steric hindrance** describes when a reaction cannot proceed (or significantly slows) because of substituents crowding the reactive site. **Protecting groups**, such as acetals, can be used to increase steric hindrance or otherwise decrease the reactivity of a particular portion of a molecule.
- **Induction** refers to uneven distribution of charge across a σ bond because of differences in electronegativity. The more electronegative groups in a carbonyl-containing compound, the greater its reactivity.
- **Conjugation** refers to the presence of alternating single and multiple bonds, which creates delocalized π electron clouds above and below the plane of the molecule. Electrons experience **resonance** through the unhybridized *p*-orbitals, increasing stability. Conjugated carbonyl-containing compounds are more reactive because they can stabilize their transition states.

- Increased strain in a molecule can make it more reactive. **β-lactams** are prone to hydrolysis because they have significant ring strain. **Ring strain** is due to torsional strain from eclipsing interactions and angle strain from compressing bond angles below 109.5°.

Nucleophilic Acyl Substitution Reactions

- All carboxylic acid derivatives can undergo nucleophilic substitution reactions. The rates at which they do so are determined by their relative reactivities.
- Anhydrides can be **cleaved** by the addition of a nucleophile.
  - Addition of ammonia or an amine results in an amide and a carboxylic acid.
  - Addition of an alcohol results in an ester and a carboxylic acid.
  - Addition of water results in two carboxylic acids.
- **Transesterification** is the exchange of one esterifying group for another on an ester. The attacking nucleophile is an alcohol.
- **Amides** can be hydrolyzed to carboxylic acids under strongly acidic or basic conditions. The attacking nucleophile is water or the hydroxide anion.

ANSWERS TO CONCEPT CHECKS

9.1

1.

Carboxylic Acid Derivative	Formed from –COOH by...	Suffix	Cyclic Naming
Amide	Ammonia or an amine	*-amide*	Lactam
Ester	An alcohol	*-oate*	Lactone
Anhydride	Another carboxylic acid	*anhydride*	Anhydride

2. A condensation reaction is one in which two molecules are joined with the loss of a small molecule. In all of the examples in this section, the small molecule lost was water.

9.2

1. Anhydrides are the most reactive to nucleophiles, followed by esters, and then amides. Therefore, acetic anhydride will be the most reactive, followed by ethyl acetate, and finally acetamide.
2. β-lactams are susceptible to hydrolysis due to the high level of ring strain, which is due to both torsional strain (eclipsing interactions) and angle strain (deviation from 109.5°).
3. Electronic effects like induction have some effect on the reactivity of the carbonyl in these three functional groups. Differences in resonance also explain the increased reactivity of anhydrides, in particular. Steric effects could also be significant, depending on the specific leaving group present.

9.3

1. Ammonia acts as the nucleophile. One of the carbonyl carbons of the anhydride serves as the electrophile.
2. Transesterification is the exchange of one esterifying group for another in an ester. This reaction requires an alcohol as a nucleophile. In this case, the ethyl group of ethanol will replace the isopropyl group of isopropyl butanoate, resulting in ethyl butanoate and 2-propanol.
3. Strongly acidic conditions catalyze amide hydrolysis by protonating the oxygen in the carbonyl. This increases the electrophilicity of the carbon, making it more susceptible to nucleophilic attack. Strongly basic conditions greatly increase the concentration of OH^-, which can act as a nucleophile on amide carbonyls.

SCIENCE MASTERY ASSESSMENT EXPLANATIONS

1. **A**

Methyl propanoate is an ester; it can be synthesized by reacting a carboxylic acid with an alcohol in the presence of acid. Here, the parent chain is propanoate, and the esterifying group is a methyl group. **(B)** reverses the nomenclature and would form propyl methanoate. The other reactions listed would not form esters.

2. **D**

This question asks for the products when ammonia reacts with acetic anhydride. Recall from the chapter that an amide and a carboxylic acid will be formed. However, the carboxylic acid—an acid—is in the same environment as ammonia—a base. The two will react, forming the ammonium carboxylate shown.

3. **A**

A Fischer esterification involves reacting a carboxylic acid and an alcohol with an acid catalyst. Under these conditions, the carbonyl carbon is open to attack by the nucleophilic alcohol. The rate of this reaction depends on the amount of steric hindrance around the carbonyl carbon because there must be room for the alcohol to approach the carboxylic acid substrate. **(B)**, **(C)**, and **(D)** all have more crowding around the carbonyl carbon, which will decrease reactivity. The additional alkyl groups in these other choices also donate electron density to the carbonyl carbon, making it slightly less electrophilic.

4. **C**

This question requires knowledge of the nomenclature of cyclic molecules. A δ-lactam, **(A)**, has a bond between the nitrogen and the fourth carbon away from the carbonyl carbon. This ring will have six elements: the nitrogen, the carbonyl carbon, and the four carbons in between. Cyclohexane carboxylic acid, **(B)**, has cyclohexane, a six-membered cycloalkane. The anhydride formed from pentanedioic acid, **(D)**, will have the five carbons in the parent chain and one oxygen atom closing the ring, meaning there are still six elements. γ-butyrolactone will have five elements because it contains a bond between the ester oxygen and the third carbon away from the carbonyl carbon. The five elements will be the oxygen, the carbonyl carbon, and the three carbons in between.

5. **D**

With the same R groups, steric influence is the same in each case, so we can therefore rely solely on electronic effects. When this is all that is taken into account, reactivity toward nucleophiles is highest for anhydrides, followed by esters and carboxylic acids, then amides.

6. **C**

Anhydrides, particularly cyclic anhydrides, will form spontaneously from dicarboxylic acids when heated.

7. **A**

Methylamine would react readily to form an amide. The less substituted the nucleophile, the easier it will be for the nucleophile to attack the carbonyl carbon and form the amide. In fact, triethylamine, **(B)**, would not be able to form an amide at all because it does not have a hydrogen to lose while attaching to the carbonyl carbon.

8. **A**

Propanamide is an amide; as such, it is the least reactive of the carboxylic acid derivatives discussed in this chapter. Without a strong acid or base, propanamide will not be able to undergo nucleophilic acyl substitution and no reaction will occur.

9. **D**

β-lactams are amides in the form of four-membered rings; amides are generally the least reactive type of carboxylic acid derivative. β-lactams experience significant ring strain from both eclipsing interactions (torsional strain) and angle strain and are therefore more susceptible to hydrolysis than the linear form of the same molecule.

10. **C**

As far as we can tell, we are converting one ester to another in this reaction. The fact that this reaction is acid-catalyzed should confirm the suspicion that this is a transesterification reaction.

11. **B**

This reaction, which is the hydrolysis of an amide, is favored in strong acid. Acid protonates the carbonyl oxygen, which increases the electrophilicity of the carbonyl carbon. This allows water to serve as the nucleophile, attacking the bond and hydrolyzing the molecule.

12. **D**

This molecule is more stable with a positive charge than a straight-chain alkane due to the conjugation of the benzene ring. This permits delocalization of the charge through resonance. Although induction, **(C)**, does have an effect on the stabilization of the molecule, this effect is much less significant than the impact of having a conjugated system. The electronegativity of nitrogen, **(B)**, which primarily affects induction, is also not a vital component of the stabilization by this molecule of a positive charge because oxygen is more electronegative. Steric hindrance, **(A)**, would affect the reactivity of a molecule, but not its ability to stabilize charge.

13. **D**

The molecule shown, γ-nonalactone, is a cyclic ester, also called a lactone. This molecule could arise from intramolecular attack in a γ-hydroxycarboxylic acid.

14. **A**

In order to prepare butyl acetate from butanol, we need to perform a nucleophilic acyl substitution reaction. If the product is an ester, we need to start with a reactant that is more reactive than the ester itself, or the reaction will not proceed. Anhydrides are more reactive than esters, but amides are less reactive, eliminating **(C)** and **(D)**. Reaction with propanoic anhydride, as in **(B)**, would result in butyl propanoate.

15. **D**

The presence of water in an esterification reaction would likely revert some of the desired esters back into carboxylic acids. Small carboxylic acids, like formic or acetic acid, are easily dissolved in water, eliminating **(A)**. The polarity of water plays little role in affecting the leaving group; if anything, water can be used to increase the electrophilicity of the carbonyl carbon by protonating the carbonyl oxygen—eliminating **(B)**. Finally, this is a nucleophilic substitution mechanism, not a nucleophilic addition mechanism, as mentioned in **(C)**. Further, hydrogen bonding would likely augment the reaction.

Consult your online resources for additional practice. **GO ONLINE**

SHARED CONCEPTS

Biochemistry Chapter 11
Lipid and Amino Acid Metabolism

Organic Chemistry Chapter 1
Nomenclature

Organic Chemistry Chapter 3
Bonding

Organic Chemistry Chapter 4
Analyzing Organic Reactions

Organic Chemistry Chapter 6
Aldehydes and Ketones I

Organic Chemistry Chapter 8
Carboxylic Acids

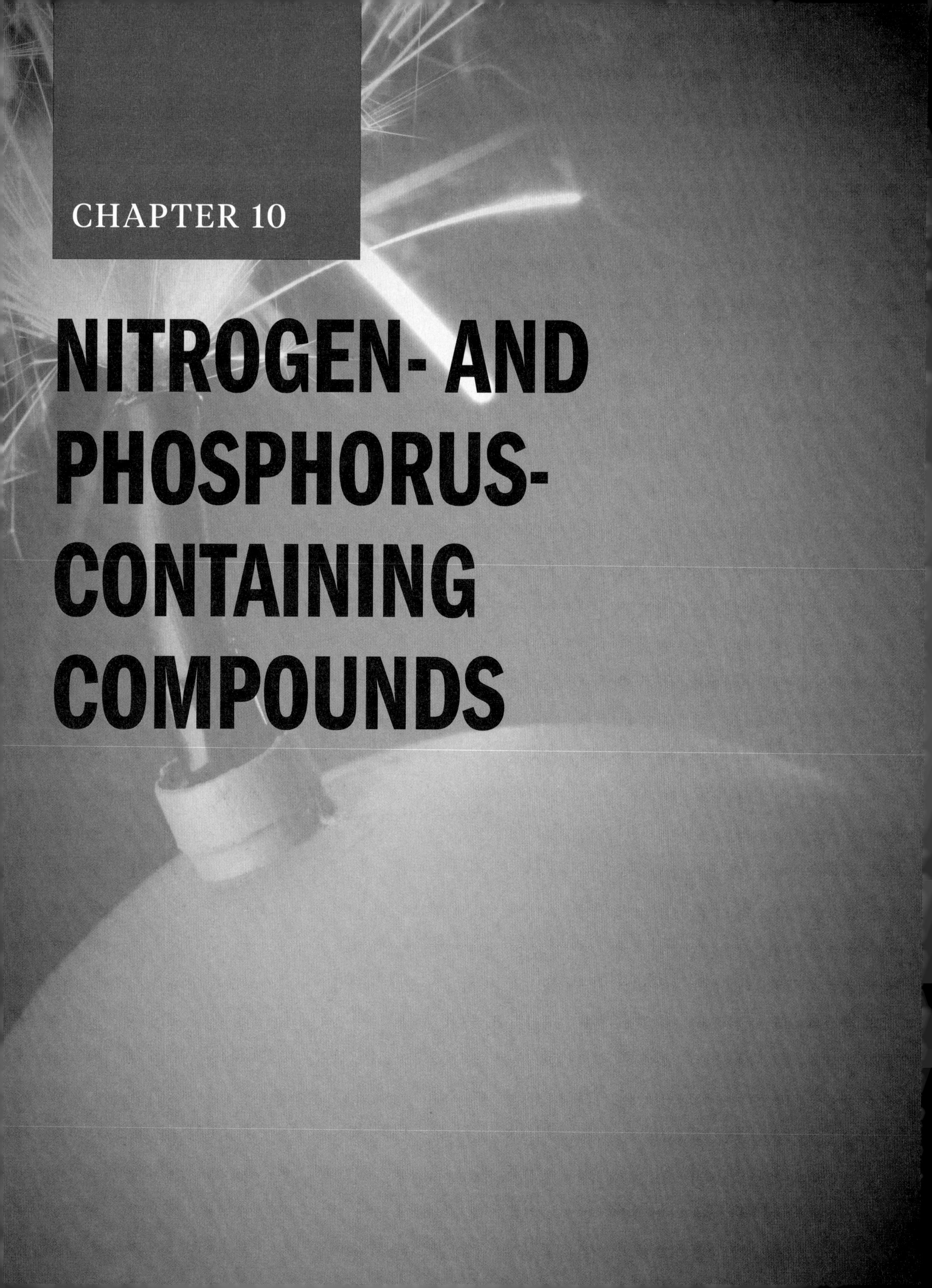

CHAPTER 10

NITROGEN- AND PHOSPHORUS-CONTAINING COMPOUNDS

SCIENCE MASTERY ASSESSMENT

Every pre-med knows this feeling: there is so much content I have to know for the MCAT! How do I know what to do first or what's important?

While the high-yield badges throughout this book will help you identify the most important topics, this Science Mastery Assessment is another tool in your MCAT prep arsenal. This quiz (which can also be taken in your online resources) and the guidance below will help ensure that you are spending the appropriate amount of time on this chapter based on your personal strengths and weaknesses. Don't worry though—skipping something now does not mean you'll never study it. Later on in your prep, as you complete full-length tests, you'll uncover specific pieces of content that you need to review and can come back to these chapters as appropriate.

How to Use This Assessment

If you answer 0–7 questions correctly:

Spend about 1 hour to read this chapter in full and take limited notes throughout. Follow up by reviewing **all** quiz questions to ensure that you now understand how to solve each one.

If you answer 8–11 questions correctly:

Spend 20–40 minutes reviewing the quiz questions. Beginning with the questions you missed, read and take notes on the corresponding subchapters. For questions you answered correctly, ensure your thinking matches that of the explanation and you understand why each choice was correct or incorrect.

If you answer 12–15 questions correctly:

Spend less than 20 minutes reviewing all questions from the quiz. If you missed any, then include a quick read-through of the corresponding subchapters, or even just the relevant content within a subchapter, as part of your question review. For questions you got correct, ensure your thinking matches that of the explanation and review the Concept Summary at the end of the chapter.

1. Which of the following amino acids does not have an L-enantiomer?
   - **A.** Cysteine
   - **B.** Threonine
   - **C.** Glutamic acid
   - **D.** Glycine

2. Which of the following would be formed if methyl bromide were reacted with phthalimide and followed by hydrolysis with an aqueous base?
   - **A.** $C_2H_5NH_2$
   - **B.** CH_3NH_2
   - **C.** $(C_2H_5)_3N$
   - **D.** $(CH_3)_4N^+Br^-$

3. Which of the following amino acids contain(s) sulfur?
   - **I.** Cysteine
   - **II.** Serine
   - **III.** Methionine

   - **A.** I only
   - **B.** I and III only
   - **C.** II and III only
   - **D.** I, II, and III

4. Nylon, a polyamide, is produced from hexanediamine and a substance, *X*. This substance, *X*, is most probably a(n):
   - **A.** amine.
   - **B.** carboxylic acid.
   - **C.** ketone.
   - **D.** alcohol.

5. Intermediates in the Strecker synthesis include all of the following nitrogen-containing functional groups EXCEPT a(n):
   - **A.** nitrile.
   - **B.** imine.
   - **C.** amide.
   - **D.** amine.

6. A biochemist is synthesizing valine, shown below, using the Strecker synthesis. Which of the following carbonyl-containing compounds would be an appropriate starting reactant in this synthesis?

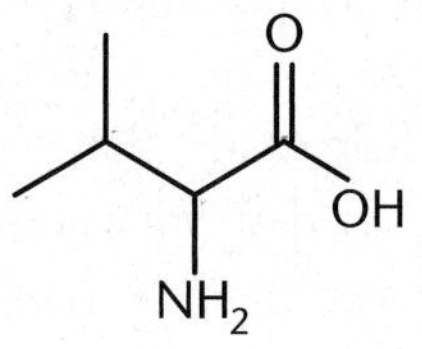

   - **A.** 2-Propanone
   - **B.** Propanal
   - **C.** 2-Methylpropanal
   - **D.** Butanal

7. Why is the C–N bond of an amide planar?
   - **I.** It has partial double-bond character.
   - **II.** It is sp^3-hybridized.
   - **III.** It has some sp^2 character.

   - **A.** I only
   - **B.** II only
   - **C.** I and II only
   - **D.** I and III only

8. Which of the primary methods of amino acid synthesis results in an optically active solution?

A. The Strecker synthesis only
B. The Gabriel synthesis only
C. Both the Strecker and Gabriel syntheses
D. Neither the Strecker nor the Gabriel syntheses

9. During the Gabriel synthesis, phthalimide serves as the:

A. nucleophile.
B. base.
C. leaving group.
D. electrophile.

10. Each of the following reaction types occurs during the Gabriel synthesis EXCEPT:

A. decarboxylation.
B. nucleophilic substitution.
C. dehydration.
D. hydrolysis.

11. At physiological pH, which two forms of phosphoric acid have the highest concentrations?

A. H_3PO_4 and $H_2PO_4^-$
B. $H_2PO_4^-$ and HPO_4^{2-}
C. HPO_4^{2-} and PO_4^{3-}
D. PO_4^{3-} and H_3PO_4

12. In aqueous solution, pyrophosphate will likely:

A. form insoluble complexes.
B. be stable and inert.
C. degrade into inorganic phosphate.
D. decrease the polarity of the solvent.

13. What would be the charge of aspartic acid at pH 7?

A. Neutral
B. Negative
C. Positive
D. There is not enough information to answer the question.

14. When a bond is created between two nucleotide triphosphates in DNA synthesis, the small molecule released from this reaction is:

A. pyrophosphate.
B. inorganic phosphate.
C. ATP.
D. organic phosphate.

15. The hydrogens of phosphoric acid have pK_a values that:

A. allow high buffering capacity over a small pH range.
B. allow moderate buffering capacity over a large pH range.
C. allow low buffering capacity over a small pH range.
D. do not allow buffering.

Answer Key

1. **D**
2. **B**
3. **B**
4. **B**
5. **C**
6. **C**
7. **D**
8. **D**
9. **A**
10. **C**
11. **B**
12. **C**
13. **B**
14. **A**
15. **B**

Detailed explanations can be found at the end of the chapter.

CHAPTER 10

NITROGEN- AND PHOSPHORUS-CONTAINING COMPOUNDS

In This Chapter

CHAPTER PROFILE

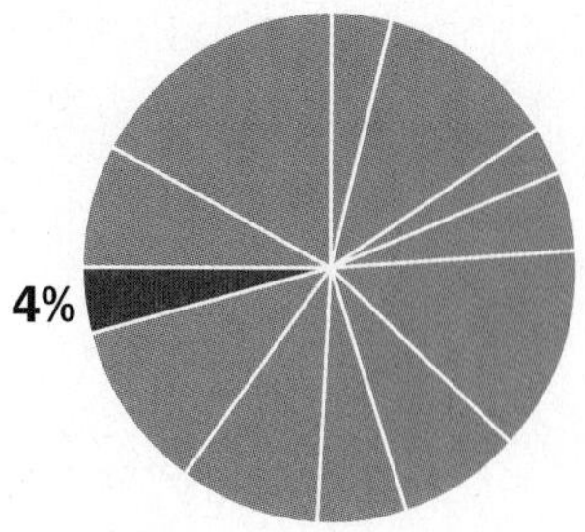

The content in this chapter should be relevant to about 4% of all questions about organic chemistry on the MCAT.

This chapter covers material from the following AAMC content categories:

1A: Structure and function of proteins and their constituent amino acids

5D: Structure, function, and reactivity of biologically-relevant molecules

Introduction

Organic chemistry is the study of carbon-containing molecules. But as you've seen, carbon is not the only element that plays a role in organic molecules; many of the functional groups we've explored up until this point also include hydrogen and oxygen. Together, these three elements make up 93% of the composition of the human body by weight. But other atoms also contribute to biomolecules: nitrogen comprises 3.2% of body weight and phosphorus 1.0%.

In this chapter, we'll take a look at some biologically important molecules that contain nitrogen and phosphorus. In addition to the amides explored in the previous chapter, amino acids also contain nitrogen. These building blocks of proteins are discussed in depth in Chapter 1 of *MCAT Biochemistry Review*; in this chapter, we review their structure and focus on laboratory methods for synthesizing amino acids. Finally, we turn our attention to phosphorus-containing molecules, which often are used to transfer energy—or store genetic information.

MCAT EXPERTISE

Note that, even though biological molecules–amino acids, proteins, and DNA–are called out in this chapter, the low percentage rating for this chapter only applies to non-biochemical reactions of these molecules. Mastery of these molecules in biological settings is still very important for Test Day success; that content is found in Chapters 1, 2, 3, 6, and 7 of *MCAT Biochemistry Review*.

10.1 Amino Acids, Peptides, and Proteins

LEARNING OBJECTIVES

After Chapter 10.1, you will be able to:

- Identify the functional groups that make amino acids amphoteric
- Recall the mechanisms for forming and cleaving peptide bonds
- Explain why the C–N bond of an amide is planar
- Recall the unique properties of glycine:

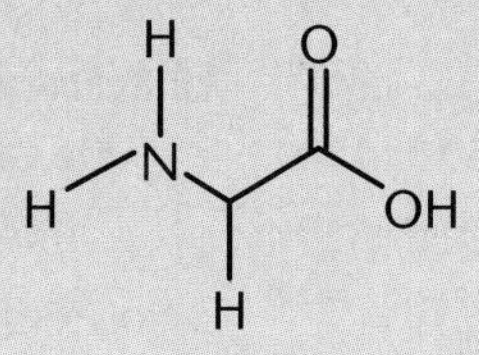

Amino acids are dipolar molecules that come together through a condensation reaction, forming peptides. Larger, folded peptide chains are considered proteins.

Description

Amino acids contain an amino group and a carboxyl group attached to a single carbon atom (the α-carbon). The other two substituents of the α-carbon are a hydrogen atom and a side chain referred to as the **R group**. This structure is shown in Figure 10.1.

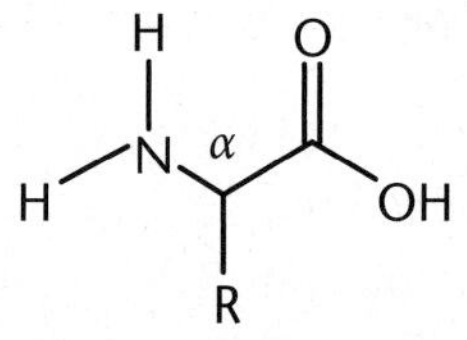

Figure 10.1 Amino Acid Structure

The α-carbon, with its four different groups, is a chiral (stereogenic) center. **Glycine**, the simplest amino acid, is an exception to this rule because its R group is a hydrogen atom. All naturally occurring amino acids in eukaryotes—except for glycine—are optically active, and all are L-isomers. Therefore, by convention, the Fischer projection for an amino acid is drawn with the amino group on the left, as shown in Figure 10.2. L-amino acids have (*S*) configurations, except for **cysteine**, which is (*R*) because of the change in priority caused by the sulfur in its R group.

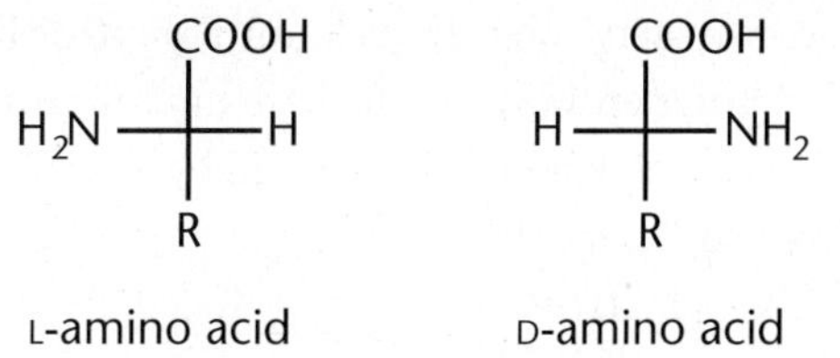

Figure 10.2 L- and D-Amino Acids

Properties

Amino acids, with their acidic carboxyl group and basic amino group, are **amphoteric** molecules. That is, they can act as both acids and bases. Amino groups can take on a positive charge by being protonated, and carboxyl groups can take on negative charges by being deprotonated. When an amino acid is put into solution, it will take on both of these charges, forming a dipolar ion or **zwitterion,** as shown in Figure 10.3. How an amino acid acts depends on the pH of the environment. In basic solutions, the amino acid can become fully deprotonated; in acidic solutions, it can become fully protonated.

BRIDGE

Amino acids are amphoteric molecules, just like water—they can act as both acids and bases. These acid-base characteristics (and titrations of amino acids) are discussed thoroughly in Chapter 1 of *MCAT Biochemistry Review*.

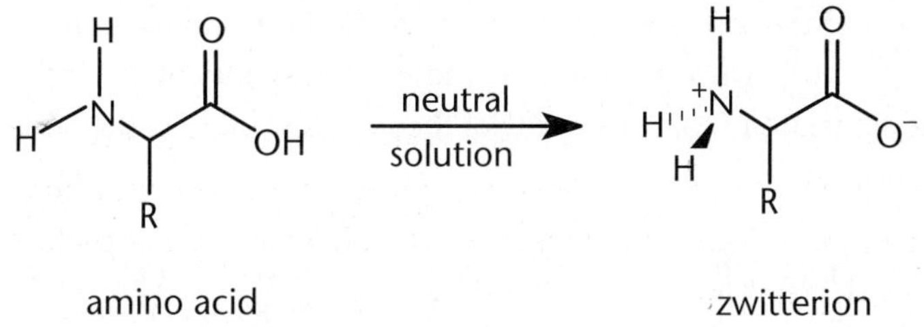

Figure 10.3 Amino Acids Exist as Zwitterions (Dipolar Ions) at Neutral pH

Aside from the zwitterionic properties common to every amino acid, each one has properties defined by its R group, or side chain. The 20 eukaryotic proteogenic amino acids are grouped into five categories: **nonpolar nonaromatic**, **aromatic**, **polar**, **negatively charged** (**acidic**), and **positively charged** (**basic**). Nonpolar nonaromatic amino acids tend to have side chains that are saturated hydrocarbons, like alanine, valine, leucine, and isoleucine; they also include glycine, proline (which is cyclic, with a secondary amine), and methionine (which contains sulfur). Aromatic amino acids include tryptophan, phenylalanine, and tyrosine. Nonpolar amino acids—both nonaromatic and aromatic—are also hydrophobic and tend to be sequestered in the interior of proteins. Polar amino acids tend to have terminal groups containing oxygen, nitrogen, or sulfur. These include serine, threonine, asparagine, glutamine, and cysteine. Negatively charged (acidic) amino acids include aspartic acid and glutamic acid. These amino acids have terminal carboxylate anions in their R groups. Finally, positively charged (basic) amino acids, including arginine, lysine, and histidine, have a protonated amino group in their R groups. Polar, acidic, and basic amino acids are all hydrophilic and tend to form hydrogen bonds with water in aqueous solution.

Amino acids undergo condensation reactions to form **peptide bonds**. The molecules these bonds form, called **polypeptides**, are the base unit of **proteins**. The reverse reaction, hydrolysis of the peptide bond, is catalyzed by a strong acid or base. Both of these reactions are shown in Figure 10.4.

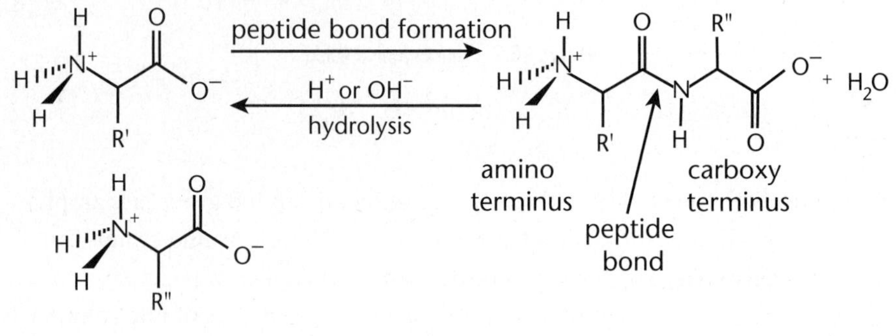

Figure 10.4 Peptide Bond Formation and Cleavage

KEY CONCEPT

Rotation is limited around the peptide bond because resonance gives the C—N bond partial double-bond character.

Like other carbonyl-containing functional groups, amides have two resonance structures, as shown in Figure 10.5. The true structure of the amide bond is therefore a hybrid of these two structures, with partial double-bond character between the nitrogen atom and the carbonyl carbon. This double-bond character limits rotation about the C—N bond, which adds to the rigidity and stability of the backbone of proteins. The single bonds on either side of the peptide bond, on the other hand, permit free rotation.

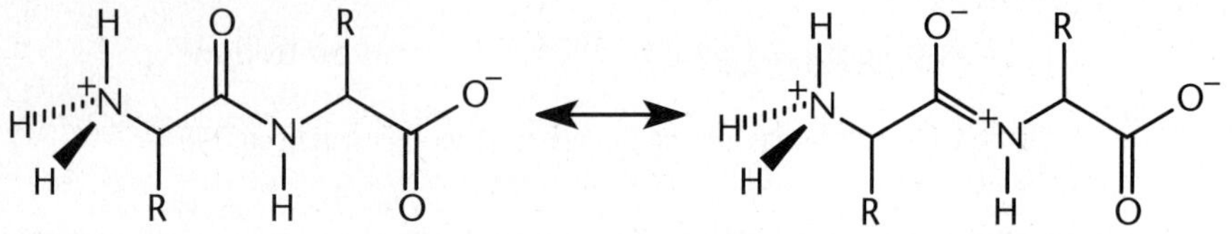

Figure 10.5 Resonance in the Peptide Bond

MCAT CONCEPT CHECK 10.1

Before you move on, assess your understanding of the material with these questions.

1. What makes glycine unique among the amino acids?

____

2. Amino acids are amphoteric. What does this mean? What functional groups give amino acids this characteristic?

____

3. How are peptide bonds formed and cleaved?

____

4. Why is the C–N bond of an amide planar?

____

10.2 Synthesis of α-Amino Acids

LEARNING OBJECTIVES

After Chapter 10.2, you will be able to:

- Recall the required reactants and product types for the Strecker and Gabriel synthesis reactions
- Identify the reaction types found in the Strecker and Gabriel synthesis reactions

Synthesis of amino acids occurs by an astonishing variety of mechanisms *in vivo*. In the lab, several simple reaction mechanisms are exploited to make amino acids neatly and efficiently.

Strecker Synthesis

In the **Strecker synthesis**, one starts with an aldehyde, ammonium chloride (NH_4Cl), and potassium cyanide (KCN), as shown in Figure 10.6. The carbonyl oxygen is protonated, increasing the electrophilicity of the carbonyl carbon. Then, as seen in Chapter 6 of *MCAT Organic Chemistry Review*, ammonia can attack the carbonyl carbon, forming an **imine**. The imine carbon is also susceptible to nucleophilic addition reactions; thus, the CN^- anion from KCN attacks, forming a **nitrile** group ($-C{\equiv}N$). The final molecule at the end of Step 1 is an ***aminonitrile***—a compound containing an amino group ($-NH_2$) and a nitrile group.

MNEMONIC

Ni**tri**les have a **tri**ple bond between nitrogen and carbon.

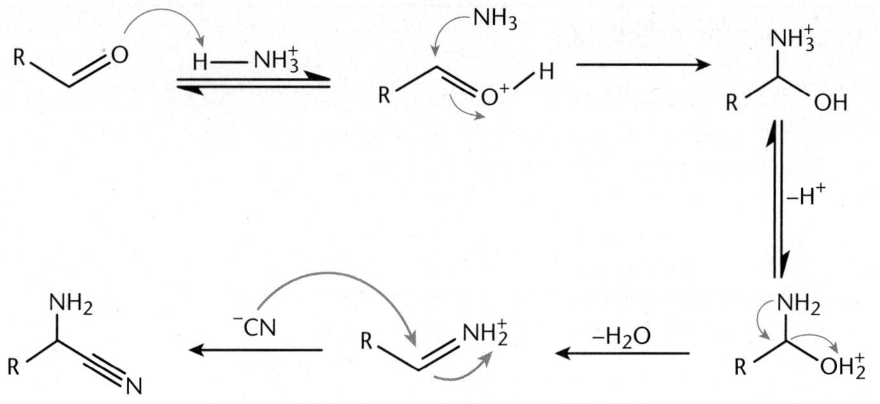

Figure 10.6 Strecker Synthesis: Step 1
An aminonitrile is generated from an aldehyde or ketone.

In Step 2, the nitrile nitrogen is protonated, increasing the electrophilicity of the nitrile carbon. This is similar to protonating the oxygen of a carbonyl. A water molecule attacks, leading to the creation of a molecule with both imine and hydroxyl moieties on the same carbon. This imine is attacked by another equivalent of water. A carbonyl is formed, kicking off ammonia and creating the carboxylic acid functionality. This step, shown in Figure 10.7, is performed in aqueous acid and can be accelerated by the use of heat.

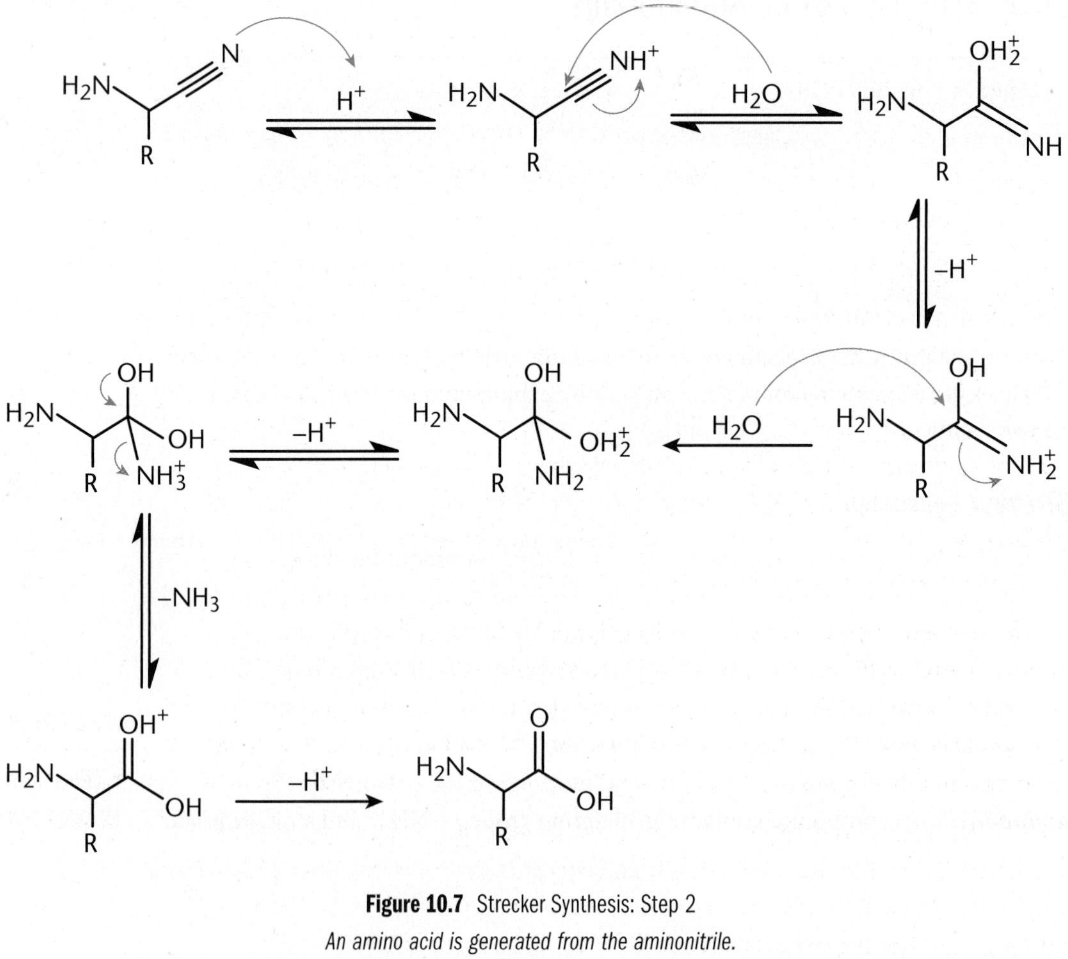

Figure 10.7 Strecker Synthesis: Step 2
An amino acid is generated from the aminonitrile.

The starting material for the Strecker synthesis is a planar carbonyl-containing compound; therefore, the product of this pathway is a racemic mixture. The incoming nucleophiles are equally able to attack from either side of the carbonyl; thus, both L- and D-amino acids can be generated through this process.

Gabriel Synthesis

Another way of synthesizing amino acids is the **Gabriel (malonic-ester) synthesis**, shown in Figure 10.8.

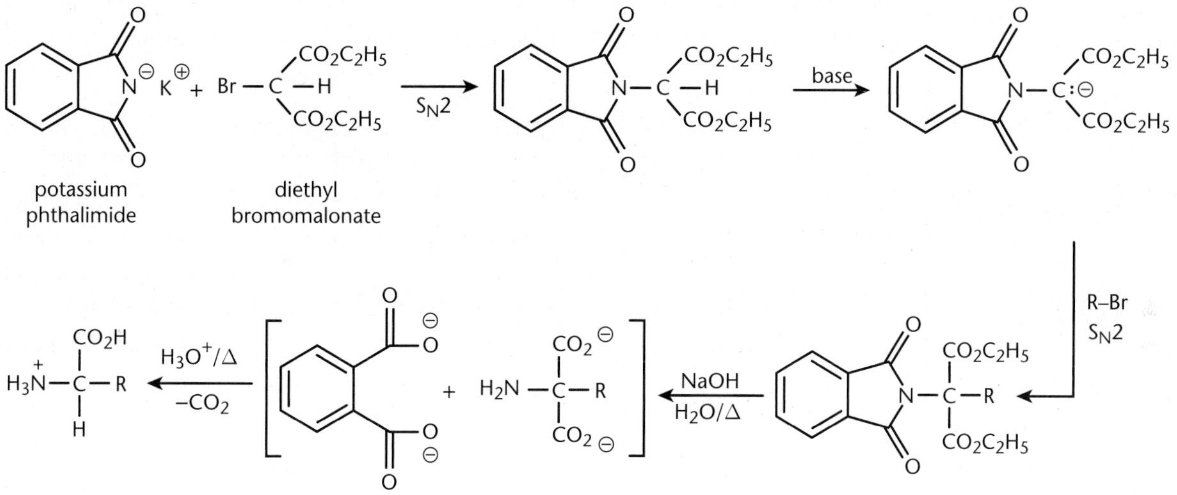

Figure 10.8 Gabriel Synthesis

An amino acid is generated from phthalimide and diethyl bromomalonate, using two S_N2 reactions, hydrolysis, and decarboxylation.

In this method, potassium phthalimide is reacted with diethyl bromomalonate. Phthalimide is acidic and exists in solution as a nucleophilic anion. Diethyl bromomalonate contains a secondary carbon bonded to bromine, a good leaving group. This setup should sound much like the S_N2 reactions discussed in Chapter 4 of *MCAT Organic Chemistry Review*. With phthalimide as the nucleophile, the (secondary) substrate carbon as the electrophile, and bromine as the leaving group, this reaction generates a phthalimidomalonic ester. Consider the benefits of using such a large nucleophile. The bulkiness of this group creates steric hindrance, which prevents the substrate carbon from undergoing multiple substitutions.

Instead, in the presence of base, this carbon (which is the α-carbon between two carbonyls) can easily be deprotonated. The molecule as a whole can then act as a nucleophile, attacking the substrate carbon of a bromoalkane. This is another example of an S_N2 reaction. The nucleophile is the large, deprotonated phthalimidomalonic ester, the electrophile is the substrate carbon, and the leaving group is the bromide anion.

Next, this molecule is hydrolyzed with strong base and heat. Much like converting a cyclic anhydride into a dioic acid, the phthalimide moiety is removed as phthalic acid (with two carboxylic acids). The malonic ester is hydrolyzed to a dicarboxylic acid with an amine on the α-carbon.

KEY CONCEPT

Both the Strecker and Gabriel synthesis methods result in a racemic mixture of amino acids.

Finally, this dicarboxylic acid, which is a 1,3-dicarbonyl, can be decarboxylated through the addition of acid and heat. The loss of a molecule of carbon dioxide results in the formation of the complete amino acid.

Like the Strecker synthesis, the Gabriel synthesis starts with a planar molecule; thus, the product is a racemic mixture of L- and D-amino acids.

MCAT CONCEPT CHECK 10.2

Before you move on, assess your understanding of the material with these questions.

1. What are the four reactants in the Strecker synthesis of an amino acid?
   - ____________________
   - ____________________
   - ____________________
   - ____________________
2. What are the reaction types used in the Strecker synthesis?

   ____
3. What are the four main reactants in the Gabriel synthesis of an amino acid?
   - ____________________
   - ____________________
   - ____________________
   - ____________________
4. What are the reactions types used in the Gabriel synthesis?

   ____

10.3 Phosphorus-Containing Compounds

LEARNING OBJECTIVES

After Chapter 10.3, you will be able to:

- Recognize the traits that make inorganic phosphate a useful molecule for energy transfer
- Explain why phosphoric acids are good buffers
- Recall what makes a molecule an organic phosphate

Phosphoric acid is an extremely important molecule biochemically. This molecule forms the high-energy bonds that carry energy in adenosine triphosphate (ATP).

Description

In a biochemical context, phosphoric acid is sometimes referred to as a **phosphate group** or **inorganic phosphate**, denoted $\mathbf{P_i}$. At physiological pH, inorganic phosphate includes molecules of both hydrogen phosphate (HPO_4^{2-}) and dihydrogen phosphate ($H_2PO_4^-$).

In addition to the energy-carrying nucleotide phosphates, phosphorus is also found in the backbone of DNA in **phosphodiester** bonds linking the sugar moieties of the nucleotides, as shown in Figure 10.9.

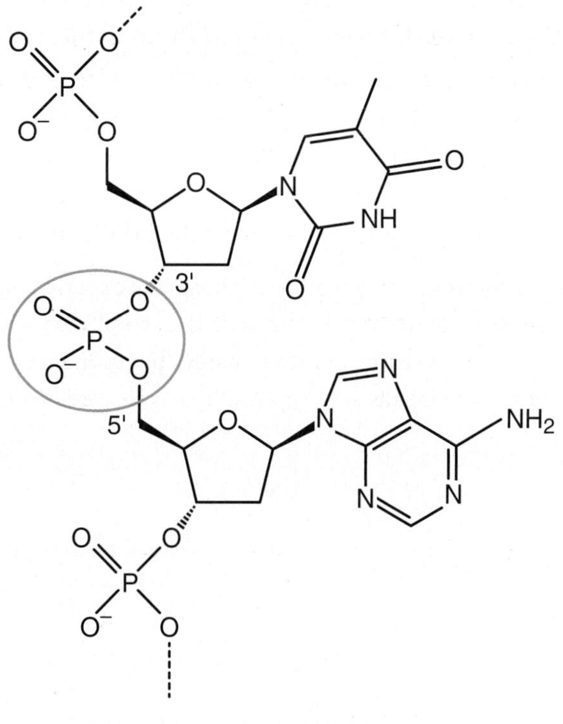

Figure 10.9 Phosphodiester Bond in DNA

BRIDGE

DNA replication is an important process for the MCAT. Nucleotide triphosphates are added to the growing daughter strand with the release of pyrophosphate, PP_i. The process of DNA synthesis is described in Chapter 6 of *MCAT Biochemistry Review*.

When a new nucleotide is joined to a growing strand of DNA by a *DNA polymerase*, it releases an ester dimer of phosphate, referred to as **pyrophosphate** ($P_2O_7^{4-}$), denoted $\mathbf{PP_i}$, and shown in Figure 10.10. The hydrolytic release of this molecule provides the energy for the formation of the new phosphodiester bond. Pyrophosphate is unstable in aqueous solution and is hydrolyzed to form two molecules of inorganic phosphate, which can then be recycled to form high-energy bonds in ATP or for other purposes.

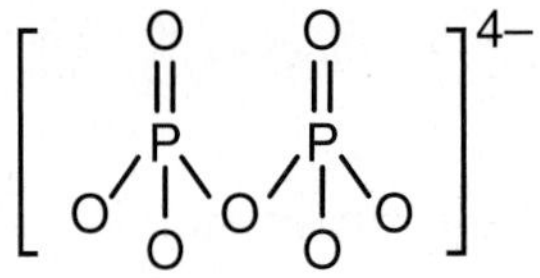

Figure 10.10 Pyrophosphate Anion

Nucleotides, such ATP, GTP, and those in DNA, are referred to as **organic phosphates** due to the presence of the phosphate group bonded to a carbon-containing molecule.

Properties

KEY CONCEPT

Phosphoric acid is an excellent buffer because it has three hydrogens with pK_a values that span nearly the entire pH scale.

Phosphoric acid is unique in that it has three acidic hydrogens, each with its own pK_a. Phosphoric acid most properly refers to the form that predominates in strongly acidic conditions, H_3PO_4. In mildly acidic conditions, it loses a proton to become dihydrogen phosphate, $H_2PO_4^-$; it will readily lose a second proton to become hydrogen phosphate, HPO_4^{2-} in weakly basic solutions. The form that exists in strongly basic solutions is phosphate, PO_4^{3-}. The pK_a for the loss of the first hydrogen is 2.15; for the second, 7.20; and for the third, 12.32. At a physiological pH of 7.4, this means that dihydrogen phosphate and hydrogen phosphate predominate in nearly equal proportions. This variety of pK_a values also makes phosphates good buffers because they can pick up or give off protons depending on the pH of the solution.

Adjacent phosphate groups on a nucleotide triphosphate experience a large amount of repulsion because they are negatively charged. This, combined with the ability of phosphate to stabilize up to three negative charges by resonance, means that the energy released when a phosphate or pyrophosphate is cleaved is quite high.

MCAT CONCEPT CHECK 10.3

Before you move on, assess your understanding of the material with these questions.

1. What characteristics make inorganic phosphate so useful for energy transfer biologically?

____

2. What is an organic phosphate?

____

3. What characteristics of phosphoric acids make them good buffers?

____

Conclusion

In this chapter, we spent a lot of time looking at biologically active molecules—but did you notice that these molecules are simply applications of the general principles that we have been learning throughout the chapters of this book? By applying your knowledge of the reactions and properties of different types of molecules, you can understand how biological processes work and how complex organic chemistry mechanisms work, like those of the Strecker and Gabriel syntheses. Many of these processes will fall into categories of reactions that we've seen before over and over—nucleophilic substitution, nucleophilic addition, and condensation reactions are just a few examples. The MCAT doesn't require you to memorize tables of reactants or regurgitate hundreds of named reactions from scratch. Instead, the MCAT asks you to look at the bigger picture and understand the trends—which you've now learned!

GO ONLINE

You've reviewed the content, now test your knowledge and critical thinking skills by completing a test-like passage set in your online resources!

CONCEPT SUMMARY

Amino Acids, Peptides, and Proteins

- The α-carbon of an amino acid is attached to four groups: an amino group, a carboxyl group, a hydrogen atom, and an **R group**. It is a chiral stereocenter in all amino acids except **glycine**.
- All amino acids in eukaryotes are L-amino acids. They all have (*S*) stereochemistry except **cysteine**, which is (*R*).
- Amino acids are **amphoteric**, meaning they can act as acids or bases.
  - Amino acids get their acidic characteristics from carboxylic acids and their basic characteristics from amino groups.
  - In a neutral solution, amino acids tend to exist as **zwitterions** (dipolar ions).
- Amino acids can be classified by their R groups.
  - **Nonpolar nonaromatic amino acids** include alanine, valine, leucine, isoleucine, glycine, proline, and methionine.
  - **Aromatic amino acids** include tryptophan, phenylalanine, and tyrosine. Both nonpolar nonaromatic and aromatic amino acids tend to be hydrophobic and reside in the interior of proteins.
  - **Polar amino acids** include serine, threonine, asparagine, glutamine, and cysteine.
  - **Negatively charged amino acids** contain carboxylic acids in their R groups and include aspartic acid and glutamic acid.
  - **Positively charged amino acids** contain amines in their R groups and include arginine, lysine, and histidine.
  - Nonpolar nonaromatic and aromatic amino acids tend to be hydrophobic and reside in the interior of proteins.
  - Polar, negatively charged (acidic), and positively charged (basic) amino acids tend to be hydrophilic and reside on the surface of proteins, making hydrogen bonds with the aqueous environment.
- **Peptide bonds** form by condensation reactions and can be cleaved hydrolytically.
  - Resonance of the peptide bond restricts motion about the C—N bond, which takes on partial double-bond character.
  - Strong acid or base is needed to cleave a peptide bond.
- **Polypeptides** are made up of multiple amino acids linked by peptide bonds. **Proteins** are large, folded, functional polypeptides.

Synthesis of α-Amino Acids

- Biologically, amino acids are synthesized in many ways. In the lab, certain standardized mechanisms are used.
- The **Strecker synthesis** generates an amino acid from an aldehyde.
  - An aldehyde is mixed with ammonium chloride (NH_4Cl) and potassium cyanide. The ammonia attacks the carbonyl carbon, generating an imine. The imine is then attacked by the cyanide, generating an aminonitrile.
  - The aminonitrile is hydrolyzed by two equivalents of water, generating an amino acid.
- The **Gabriel synthesis** generates an amino acid from potassium phthalimide, diethyl bromomalonate, and an alkyl halide.
  - Phthalimide attacks the diethyl bromomalonate, generating a phthalimidomalonic ester.
  - The phthalimidomalonic ester attacks an alkyl halide, adding an alkyl group to the ester.
  - The product is hydrolyzed, creating phthalic acid (with two carboxyl groups) and converting the esters into carboxylic acids.
  - One carboxylic acid of the resulting 1,3-dicarbonyl is removed by decarboxylation.

Phosphorus-Containing Compounds

- Phosphorus is found in **inorganic phosphate (P_i)**, a buffered mixture of hydrogen phosphate (HPO_4^{2-}) and dihydrogen phosphate ($H_2PO_4^-$).
- Phosphorus is found in the backbone of DNA, which uses **phosphodiester bonds**. In forming these bonds, a **pyrophosphate (PP_i**, $P_2O_7^{4-}$) is released. Pyrophosphate can then be hydrolyzed to two inorganic phosphates.
- Phosphate bonds are high energy because of large negative charges in adjacent phosphate groups and resonance stabilization of phosphates.
- **Organic phosphates** are carbon-containing compounds that also have phosphate groups. The most notable examples are nucleotide triphosphates (such as ATP or GTP) and DNA.
- Phosphoric acid has three hydrogens, each with a unique pK_a. This wide variety in pK_a values allows phosphoric acid to act as a buffer over a large range of pH values.

ANSWERS TO CONCEPT CHECKS

10.1

1. All amino acids, except glycine, have chiral α-carbons. Because the R group of glycine is a hydrogen atom, it is not chiral and therefore is not optically active.
2. Amphoteric molecules can act as acids or bases. Carboxylic acids give amino acids their acidic properties because they can be deprotonated. Amino groups give amino acids their basic properties because they can be protonated.
3. Peptide bonds are formed by a condensation reaction, in which water is lost, and cleaved hydrolytically by strong acid or base.
4. The C–N bond of an amide is planar because it has partial double-bond character due to resonance. Double bonds exist in a planar conformation and restrict movement.

10.2

1. An aldehyde, ammonium chloride (NH_4Cl), and potassium cyanide (KCN) are used to make the aminonitrile; water is used to hydrolyze the aminonitrile to form the amino acid.
2. Strecker synthesis is a condensation reaction (formation of an imine from a carbonyl-containing compound and ammonia, with loss of water), followed by nucleophilic addition (addition of the nitrile group), followed by hydrolysis.
3. Gabriel synthesis begins with potassium phthalimide and diethyl bromomalonate, followed by an alkyl halide. Water is then used to hydrolyze the resulting compound to form the amino acid. While acids and bases are used at various times as catalysts, they are not main reactants.
4. Gabriel synthesis proceeds through two S_N2 reactions, hydrolysis, and decarboxylation.

10.3

1. Inorganic phosphate contains a very negative charge. When bonded to other phosphate groups in a nucleotide triphosphate, this creates repulsion with adjacent phosphate groups, increasing the energy of the bond. Further, inorganic phosphate can be resonance-stabilized.
2. Organic phosphates are carbon-containing molecules with phosphate groups; the most common examples are nucleotides, like those in DNA, ATP, or GTP.
3. The three hydrogens in phosphoric acid have very different pK_a values. This allows phosphoric acid to pick up or give off protons in a wide pH range, making it a good buffer over most of the pH scale.

SCIENCE MASTERY ASSESSMENT EXPLANATIONS

1. **D**

Glycine's R group is a hydrogen atom; this amino acid is therefore achiral because the central carbon is not bonded to four different substituents. The other amino acids are all chiral and therefore have both L- and D-enantiomers.

2. **B**

This reaction is similar to the Gabriel synthesis. Phthalimide acts as a nucleophile, the methyl carbon acts as an electrophile, and bromide acts as the leaving group. Therefore, the reaction between methyl bromide and phthalimide results in the formation of methyl phthalimide. Subsequent hydrolysis then yields methylamine.

3. **B**

Cysteine is well known for containing a sulfur atom because it is able to form disulfide bridges; however, methionine also contains a sulfur atom in its R group.

4. **B**

An amide is formed from an amine and a carboxyl group or its acyl derivatives. In this question, an amine is already given; the compound to be identified must be an acyl compound. The only acyl compound among the choices given is a carboxylic acid.

5. **C**

During the Strecker synthesis, ammonia attacks a carbonyl, forming an imine, **(B)**. This imine is attacked by cyanide, forming an amine, **(D)**, and a nitrile, **(A)**. Amide bonds are formed between amino acids but do not appear during the Strecker synthesis.

6. **C**

The Strecker synthesis creates an amino acid from an aldehyde. The carbonyl carbon ultimately becomes the α-carbon of the amino acid. Any remaining alkyl chain becomes the R group, as shown below. The starting compound is therefore 2-methylpropanal (isobutyraldehyde).

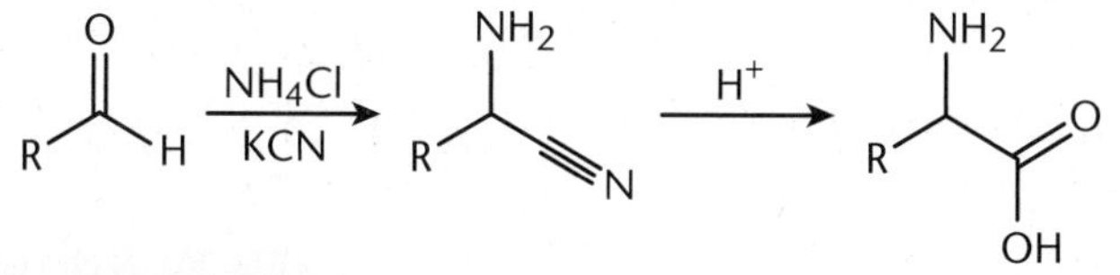

7. **D**

One resonance structure of a C—N bond in an amide has the double bond between the C and N, not between the C and O. Thus, the C—N bond of an amide has some sp^2 character, and sp^2-hybridized atoms exhibit planar geometry.

8. **D**

Both the Strecker and Gabriel syntheses contain planar intermediates, which can be attacked from either side by a nucleophile. This results in a racemic mixture of enantiomers, and the solution will therefore be optically inactive.

9. **A**

During the Gabriel synthesis, phthalimide attacks a secondary carbon in diethyl bromomalonate. The secondary carbon is the electrophile, **(D)**, and bromide is the leaving group, **(C)**.

10. **C**

The Gabriel synthesis includes two nucleophilic substitution steps, followed by hydrolysis and decarboxylation. Dehydration—the loss of a water molecule—is not a part of this reaction.

11. **B**

The pK_{a2} of phosphoric acid is close to physiological pH; therefore, $[H_2PO_4^-] \approx [HPO_4^{2-}]$ at this pH.

12. **C**

Pyrophosphate is unstable in aqueous solution and will degrade to form two equivalents of inorganic phosphate. The solvent is water, which should retain its polarity regardless of the presence of solutes, eliminating **(D)**. Pyrophosphate and inorganic phosphate are small, charged molecules which are relatively soluble, eliminating **(A)**.

13. **B**

The amino acid in question is aspartic acid, which is an acidic amino acid because it contains an extra carboxyl group. At neutral pH, both of the carboxyl groups are ionized, so there are two negative charges on the molecule. Only one of the charges is neutralized by the positive charge on the amino group, so the molecule has an overall negative charge.

14. **A**

As DNA is synthesized, it forms phosphodiester bonds, releasing pyrophosphate, PP_i. Pyrophosphate is an inorganic phosphate-containing molecule, but it is not the single phosphate group commonly referred to as inorganic phosphate, **(B)**. The DNA molecule itself is referred to as an organic phosphate, **(D)**.

15. **B**

Phosphoric acid has three hydrogens with pK_a values spread across the pH range. This allows some degree of buffering over almost the entire standard pH range from 0 to 14.

Consult your online resources for additional practice. GO ONLINE

SHARED CONCEPTS

Biochemistry Chapter 1
Amino Acids, Peptides, and Proteins

Biochemistry Chapter 6
DNA and Biotechnology

Biochemistry Chapter 9
Carbohydrate Metabolism I

General Chemistry Chapter 10
Acids and Bases

Organic Chemistry Chapter 4
Analyzing Organic Reactions

Organic Chemistry Chapter 8
Carboxylic Acids

CHAPTER 11

SPECTROSCOPY

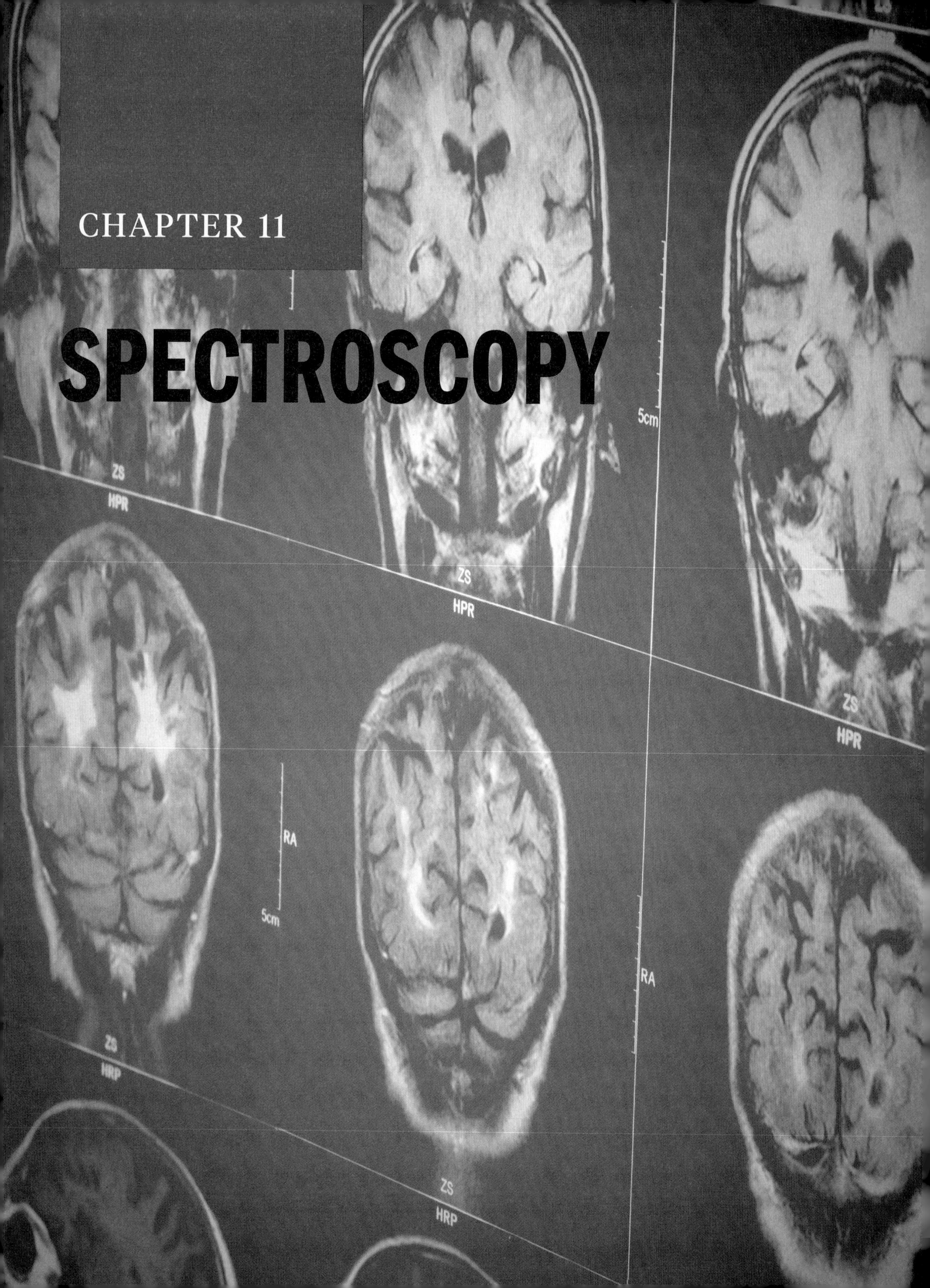

SCIENCE MASTERY ASSESSMENT

Every pre-med knows this feeling: there is so much content I have to know for the MCAT! How do I know what to do first or what's important?

While the high-yield badges throughout this book will help you identify the most important topics, this Science Mastery Assessment is another tool in your MCAT prep arsenal. This quiz (which can also be taken in your online resources) and the guidance below will help ensure that you are spending the appropriate amount of time on this chapter based on your personal strengths and weaknesses. Don't worry though—skipping something now does not mean you'll never study it. Later on in your prep, as you complete full-length tests, you'll uncover specific pieces of content that you need to review and can come back to these chapters as appropriate.

How to Use This Assessment

If you answer 0–7 questions correctly:

Spend about 1 hour to read this chapter in full and take limited notes throughout. Follow up by reviewing **all** quiz questions to ensure that you now understand how to solve each one.

If you answer 8–11 questions correctly:

Spend 20–40 minutes reviewing the quiz questions. Beginning with the questions you missed, read and take notes on the corresponding subchapters. For questions you answered correctly, ensure your thinking matches that of the explanation and you understand why each choice was correct or incorrect.

If you answer 12–15 questions correctly:

Spend less than 20 minutes reviewing all questions from the quiz. If you missed any, then include a quick read-through of the corresponding subchapters, or even just the relevant content within a subchapter, as part of your question review. For questions you got correct, ensure your thinking matches that of the explanation and review the Concept Summary at the end of the chapter.

1. IR spectroscopy is most useful for distinguishing:
   - **A.** double and triple bonds.
   - **B.** C–H bonds.
   - **C.** chirality of molecules.
   - **D.** relative percentage of enantiomers in mixtures.

2. Oxygen (O_2) does not exhibit an IR spectrum because:
   - **A.** it has no molecular motions.
   - **B.** it is not possible to record IR spectra of a gaseous molecule.
   - **C.** molecular vibrations do not result in a change in the dipole moment.
   - **D.** molecular oxygen contains four lone pairs overall.

3. If IR spectroscopy were employed to monitor the oxidation of benzyl alcohol to benzaldehyde, which of the following would provide the best evidence that the reaction was proceeding as planned?
   - **A.** Comparing the fingerprint region of the spectra of starting material and product
   - **B.** Noting the change in intensity of the peaks corresponding to the benzene ring
   - **C.** Noting the appearance of a broad absorption peak in the region of 3100–3500 cm^{-1}
   - **D.** Noting the appearance of a strong absorption in the region of 1750 cm^{-1}

4. Which of the following chemical shifts could correspond to an aldehydic proton signal in a ^1H–NMR spectrum?
   - **A.** 9.5 ppm
   - **B.** 7.0 ppm
   - **C.** 11.0 ppm
   - **D.** 1.0 ppm

5. The isotope ^{12}C is not useful for NMR because:
   - **A.** it is not abundant in nature.
   - **B.** its resonances are not sensitive to the presence of neighboring atoms.
   - **C.** it has no magnetic moment.
   - **D.** the signal-to-noise ratio in the spectrum is too low.

6. In ^1H–NMR, splitting of spectral lines is due to:
   - **A.** coupling between a carbon atom and protons attached to that carbon atom.
   - **B.** coupling between a carbon atom and protons attached to adjacent carbon atoms.
   - **C.** coupling between adjacent carbon atoms.
   - **D.** coupling between protons on adjacent carbon atoms.

7. Compared to IR and NMR spectroscopy, UV spectroscopy is preferred for detecting:
   - **A.** aldehydes and ketones.
   - **B.** unconjugated alkenes.
   - **C.** conjugated alkenes.
   - **D.** aliphatic acids and amines.

8. Considering only the 0 to 4.5 ppm region of a ^{1}H–NMR spectrum, how could ethanol and isopropanol be distinguished?

- **A.** They cannot be distinguished from ^{1}H–NMR alone.
- **B.** A triplet and quartet are observed for ethanol, whereas a doublet and septet are observed for isopropanol.
- **C.** A triplet and quartet are observed for isopropanol, whereas a doublet and septet are observed for ethanol.
- **D.** The alcohol hydrogen in ethanol will appear within that region, whereas the alcohol hydrogen in isopropanol will appear downfield of that region.

9. Before absorbing an ultraviolet photon, electrons can be found in:

- **A.** the HOMO only.
- **B.** the LUMO only.
- **C.** both the HOMO and the LUMO.
- **D.** neither the HOMO nor the LUMO.

10. In an IR spectrum, how does extended conjugation of double bonds affect the absorbance band of carbonyl (C=O) stretches compared with normal absorption?

- **A.** The absorbance band will occur at a lower wavenumber.
- **B.** The absorbance band will occur at a higher wavenumber.
- **C.** The absorbance band will occur at the same wavenumber.
- **D.** The absorbance band will disappear.

11. Wavenumber is directly proportional to:

- **A.** wavelength.
- **B.** frequency.
- **C.** percent transmittance.
- **D.** absorbance.

12. Two enantiomers will:

- **A.** have identical IR spectra because they have the same functional groups.
- **B.** have identical IR spectra because they have the same specific rotation.
- **C.** have different IR spectra because they are structurally different.
- **D.** have different IR spectra because they have different specific rotations.

13. In a molecule containing a carboxylic acid group, what would be expected in a ^{1}H–NMR spectrum?

- **A.** A deshielded hydrogen peak for the hydroxyl hydrogen, shifted left
- **B.** A deshielded hydrogen peak for the hydroxyl hydrogen, shifted right
- **C.** A shielded hydrogen peak for the hydroxyl hydrogen, shifted left
- **D.** A shielded hydrogen peak for the hydroxyl hydrogen, shifted right

14. The coupling constant, J, is:

- **A.** the value of $n + 1$ when determining splitting in NMR spectra.
- **B.** measured in parts per million (ppm).
- **C.** corrected for by calibration with tetramethylsilane.
- **D.** a measure of the degree of splitting caused by other atoms in the molecule.

15. The IR spectrum of a fully protonated amino acid would likely contain which of the following peaks?

- **I.** A sharp peak at 1750 cm^{-1}
- **II.** A sharp peak at 3300 cm^{-1}
- **III.** A broad peak at 3300 cm^{-1}

- **A.** I only
- **B.** I and II only
- **C.** II and III only
- **D.** I, II, and III

Answer Key

1. **A**
2. **C**
3. **D**
4. **A**
5. **C**
6. **D**
7. **C**
8. **B**
9. **A**
10. **A**
11. **B**
12. **A**
13. **A**
14. **D**
15. **B**

Detailed explanations can be found at the end of the chapter.

CHAPTER 11

SPECTROSCOPY

In This Chapter

CHAPTER PROFILE

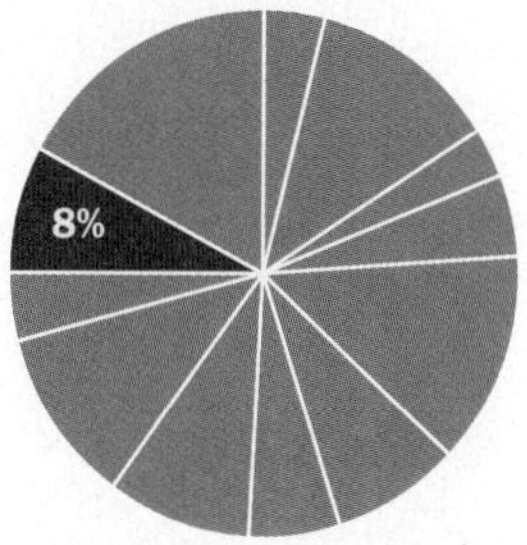

The content in this chapter should be relevant to about 8% of all questions about organic chemistry on the MCAT.

This chapter covers material from the following AAMC content category:

4D: How light and sound interact with matter

Introduction

If we are given an unknown compound, one of the most efficient ways to identify it and determine its properties is by using spectroscopy. **Spectroscopy** measures the energy differences between the possible states of a molecular system by determining the frequencies of electromagnetic radiation absorbed by the molecules. These possible states are quantized energy levels associated with different types of molecular motion, such as molecular rotation, vibration of bonds, electron absorption, and nuclear spin transitions. Different types of spectroscopy measure different types of molecular properties, allowing us to identify the presence of specific functional groups and to detect the connectivity (backbone) of a molecule.

In a medical context, spectroscopy is important in magnetic resonance imaging (MRI). MRI scanners actually measure ^{1}H–NMR spectra of water molecules in different environments in the body. They then convert these signals into greyscale, allowing excellent visualization of the body, especially soft tissue.

One of the big advantages of laboratory spectroscopy is that only a small quantity of a sample is needed. Also, the sample may be reused after a test is performed. The downside of spectroscopy is that it's difficult to do without special equipment—but as long as you have a chemistry lab available, these are some of the best techniques to identify compounds.

11.1 Infrared Spectroscopy

LEARNING OBJECTIVES

After Chapter 11.1, you will be able to:

- Predict the IR peaks for common organic functional groups, including ketones, carboxylic acids, and alcohols
- Recall the conditions in which IR spectroscopy is generally used, and what it is used to measure

Infrared (IR) spectroscopy measures molecular vibrations, which can be seen as bond stretching, bending, or combinations of different vibrational modes. To record an IR spectrum, infrared light is passed through a sample, and the absorbance is measured. By determining what bonds exist within a molecule, we hope to infer the functional groups in the molecule.

Intramolecular Vibrations and Rotations

KEY CONCEPT

Wavenumbers (cm^{-1}) are an analog of frequency. $f = \frac{c}{\lambda}$, whereas wavenumber $= \frac{1}{\lambda}$.

The infrared light range runs from $\lambda = 700$ nm to 1 mm, but the useful absorptions for spectroscopy occur at wavelengths of 2500 to 25,000 nm. On an IR spectrum, we use an analog of frequency called **wavenumber**. The standard range corresponding to 2500 to 25,000 nm is 4000 to 400 cm^{-1}. When light of these wavenumbers is absorbed, the molecules enter excited vibrational states. Four types of vibration that can occur are shown in Figure 11.1. Others include twisting and folding.

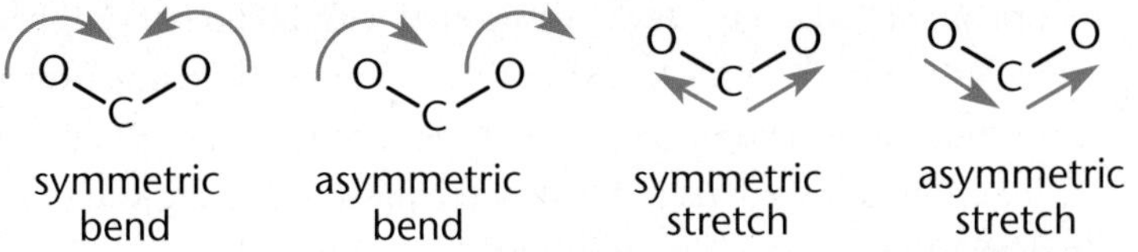

Figure 11.1 Molecular Vibrations Measured by Infrared (IR) Spectroscopy
Bond bending and stretching; twisting and folding can also occur.

More complex vibration patterns, caused by the motion of the molecule as a whole, can be seen in the 1500 to 400 cm^{-1} range. This is called the **fingerprint region** because the specific absorbance pattern is characteristic of each individual molecule. Spectroscopy experts can use this region to identify a substance, but you won't ever need to use it on the MCAT.

KEY CONCEPT

Symmetric stretches do not show up in IR spectra because they involve no net change in dipole movement.

For an absorption to be recorded, the vibration must result in a change in the bond dipole moment. This means that molecules that do not experience a change in dipole moment, such as those composed of atoms with the same electronegativity or molecules that are symmetrical, do not exhibit absorption. For example, we cannot get an absorption from O_2 or Br_2, but we can from HCl or CO. Symmetric bonds, such as the triple bond in acetylene (C_2H_2), will also be silent.

Characteristic Absorptions

For the MCAT, you only need to memorize a few absorptions. The first is the hydroxyl group, O—H, which absorbs with a broad (wide) peak at around one of two frequencies: 3300 cm^{-1} for alcohols, and 3000 cm^{-1} for carboxylic acids. The carbonyl of a carboxylic acid pulls some of the electron density out of the O—H bond, shifting the absorption to a lower wavenumber. The second is the carbonyl, which absorbs around 1700 cm^{-1} with a sharp (deep) peak. In Table 11.1, notice how the bond between any atom and hydrogen always has a relatively high absorption frequency and how, as we add more bonds between carbon atoms, the absorption frequency increases. N—H bonds are in the same region as O—H bonds (around 3300 cm^{-1}), but have a sharp peak instead of a broad one. You should be able to identify these three peaks in an IR spectrum. If you need to identify other peaks on Test Day, a list or table of peak wavenumbers will be provided.

FUNCTIONAL GROUP	WAVENUMBER (cm^{-1})	VIBRATION
Alkanes	2800-3000 1200	C—H C—C
Alkenes	3080-3140 1645	=C—H C=C
Alkynes	3300 2200	≡C—H C≡C
Aromatic	2900-3100 1475-1625	C—H C—C
Alcohols	3100-3500	O—H (broad)
Ethers	1050-1150	C—O
Aldehydes	2700-2900 1700-1750	(O)C—H C=O
Ketones	1700-1750	C=O
Carboxylic Acids	1700-1750 2800-3200	C=O O—H (broad)
Amines	3100-3500	N—H (sharp)

Table 11.1 Absorption Frequencies

MCAT EXPERTISE

Infrared spectroscopy is best used for identification of functional groups. The most important peaks to know are:

- O—H (broad around 3300 cm^{-1})
- N—H (sharp around 3300 cm^{-1})
- C=O (sharp around 1750 cm^{-1})

We can learn a great deal of information from an IR spectrum; for the MCAT, all of the information comes from the frequencies between 1400 and 4000 cm^{-1}. Everything lower (in the fingerprint region) is out of scope. IR spectra are plotted as percent **transmittance**, the amount of light that passes through the sample and reaches the detector, *vs.* wavenumber.

KEY CONCEPT

In an IR spectrum, percent transmittance is plotted *vs.* frequency. The equation relating absorbance, A, and percent transmittance, $\% T$, is $A = 2 - \log \%T$; this means that maximum absorptions appear as the bottoms of valleys on the spectrum.

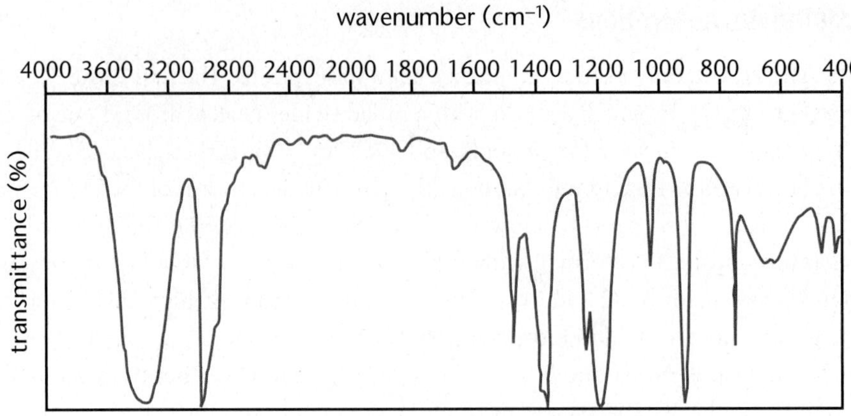

Figure 11.2 IR Spectrum of an Aliphatic Alcohol
Broad peak at 3300 cm^{-1}: —OH

Figure 11.2 shows the IR spectrum for an aliphatic alcohol: the large broad peak at 3300 cm^{-1} is due to the presence of a hydroxyl group, whereas the sharper peak at 3000 cm^{-1} is due to the carbon–hydrogen bonds in the alkane portion of the molecule, as listed in Table 11.1.

MCAT CONCEPT CHECK 11.1

Before you move on, assess your understanding of the material with these questions.

1. What does infrared (IR) spectroscopy measure? What is IR spectroscopy generally used for?

 ____

2. What two peaks would you expect to see in the IR spectrum of a carboxylic acid?

 - ______________________________
 - ______________________________

11.2 Ultraviolet Spectroscopy

LEARNING OBJECTIVES

After Chapter 11.2, you will be able to:

- Predict whether a given molecule can be detected via UV spectroscopy
- Describe the relationship between HOMO, LUMO, and absorption wavelength

Although you will never have to interpret **ultraviolet (UV) spectroscopy** data on the MCAT, it is fair game for discussion. A basic understanding of how it works and when it is used will suffice. UV spectra are obtained by passing ultraviolet light through a sample that is usually dissolved in an inert, nonabsorbing solvent, and recording the absorbance. The absorbance is then plotted against wavelength. The absorbance is caused by electronic transitions between orbitals. The biggest piece of information we get from this technique is the wavelength of maximum absorbance, which tells us the extent of conjugation within conjugated systems: the more conjugated the compound, the lower the energy of the transition and the greater the wavelength of maximum absorbance.

Electron Transitions

UV spectroscopy works because molecules with π-electrons or nonbonding electrons can be excited by ultraviolet light to higher-energy antibonding orbitals. Molecules with a lower energy gap between **highest occupied molecular orbital** (**HOMO**) and **lowest unoccupied molecular orbital** (**LUMO**) are more easily excited and can absorb longer wavelengths (lower frequencies) with lower energy.

MCAT EXPERTISE

UV spectroscopy is most useful for studying compounds containing double bonds or heteroatoms with lone pairs that create conjugated systems. For the MCAT, that is all you need to know.

Conjugated Systems

Conjugated molecules, or molecules with unhybridized *p*-orbitals, can also be excited by ultraviolet light. Conjugation shifts the absorption spectrum, resulting in higher maximum wavelengths (lower frequencies). For example, benzene has three broad absorbances, which mark the energy level transitions; these are found at 180, 200, and 255 nm wavelengths. Larger conjugated molecules may even absorb light in the visible range, leading to color. Because the technique for UV spectroscopy can also be used at visible wavelengths, it is sometimes called *UV–Vis spectroscopy*.

MCAT CONCEPT CHECK 11.2

Before you move on, assess your understanding of the material with these questions.

1. Which of the following molecules are detectable by UV spectroscopy: propane, propene, propanone?

   ____

2. In UV spectroscopy, what is the HOMO? What is the LUMO? How are they related to absorption wavelength?

   • HOMO:

   ____

   • LUMO:

   ____

   • Relation to absorption wavelength:

   ____

11.3 Nuclear Magnetic Resonance Spectroscopy

LEARNING OBJECTIVES

After Chapter 11.3, you will be able to:

- Describe what NMR spectroscopy measures and what it is generally used for
- Recall the units for chemical shift on standardized NMR
- Identify what deshielding and spin-spin coupling are, and how they impact NMR spectra
- Recognize key regions and peaks within an NMR spectrum
- Match a compound to a given NMR spectrum analysis:

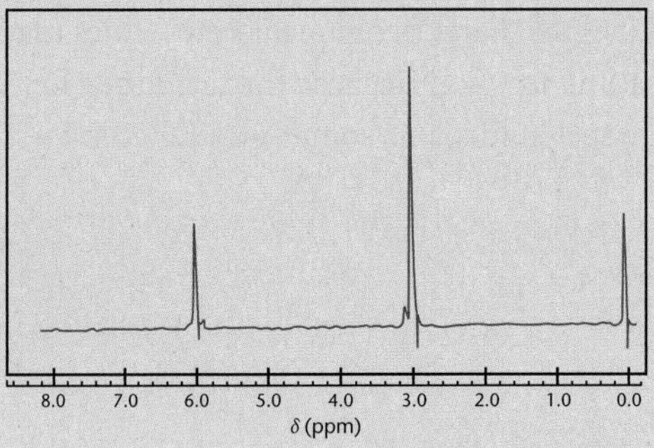

Nuclear magnetic resonance (NMR) spectroscopy is the most important spectroscopic technique to understand for the MCAT. NMR spectroscopy is based on the fact that certain atomic nuclei have magnetic moments that are oriented at random.

When such nuclei are placed in a magnetic field, their magnetic moments tend to align either with or against the direction of this applied field. Nuclei with magnetic moments that are aligned with the field are said to be in the **α-state** (lower energy). The nuclei can then be irradiated with radiofrequency pulses that match the energy gap between the two states, which will excite some lower-energy nuclei into the **β-state** (higher energy). The absorption of this radiation leads to excitation at different frequencies, depending on an atom's magnetic environment. In addition, the nuclear magnetic moments of atoms are affected by nearby atoms that also possess magnetic moments.

Magnetic resonance imaging (**MRI**) is a noninvasive diagnostic tool that uses proton NMR, as shown in Figure 11.3. Multiple cross-sectional scans of the patient's body are taken, and the various chemical shifts of absorbing protons are translated into specific shades of grey. This produces a picture that shows the relative density of specific types of protons; for instance, a dark area on a T1-weighted MRI tends to correspond to water, whereas a light area indicates fattier tissue. Comparison with a normal MRI then allows the diagnostician to detect abnormalities in the scanned region. We mention this to explain the relevance of NMR spectroscopy to medicine; the MCAT will not test you on the details of how MRI works.

An MRI machine combines a variety of NMR data to produce views of internal body tissues such as the brain.

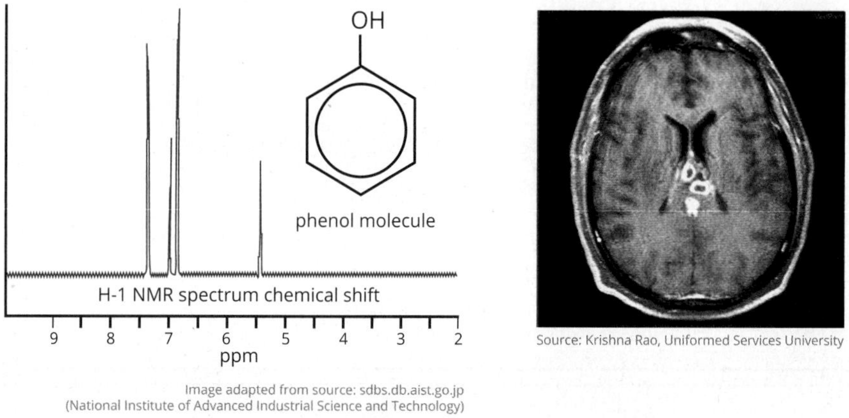

Figure 11.3 Magnetic Resonance Imaging (MRI)

A typical NMR spectrum is a plot of frequency *vs.* absorption of energy. Because different NMR spectrometers operate at different magnetic field strengths, a standardized method of plotting the NMR spectrum has been adopted. This standardized method, which is the only one seen on the MCAT, uses an arbitrary variable called **chemical shift** (**δ**), with units of **parts per million** (**ppm**) of spectrometer frequency. The chemical shift is plotted on the x-axis, and it increases toward the left (referred to as **downfield**). To make sure that we know just how far downfield compounds are, we use **tetramethylsilane** (**TMS**) as the calibration standard to mark 0 ppm; when counting peaks, make sure to skip the TMS peak.

KEY CONCEPT

TMS provides a reference peak. The signal for its ^1H atoms is assigned $\delta = 0$.

Nuclear magnetic resonance is most commonly used to study ^{1}H nuclei (protons), although any atom possessing a nuclear spin (with an odd atomic number, odd mass number, or both) can be studied, such as ^{13}C, ^{19}F, ^{17}O, ^{31}P, and ^{59}Co. The MCAT, however, only tests knowledge of ^{1}H–NMR.

BRIDGE

Nuclei with odd mass numbers, odd atomic numbers, or both, will have a magnetic moment when placed in a magnetic field. Not all nuclei have magnetic moments (^{12}C, for example). Atomic numbers and mass numbers are discussed in more detail in Chapter 1 of *MCAT General Chemistry Review*.

Proton NMR (^{1}H—NMR)

Most hydrogen (^{1}H) nuclei come into resonance 0 to 10 ppm downfield from TMS. Each distinct set of nuclei gives rise to a separate peak. This means that if multiple protons are **chemically equivalent**, having the same magnetic environment, they will lead to the same peak. For example, Figure 11.4 depicts the ^{1}H–NMR of dichloromethyl methyl ether, which has two distinct sets of ^{1}H nuclei. The single proton attached to the dichloromethyl group (H_a) is in a different magnetic environment from the three protons on the methyl group (H_b), so the two classes will resonate at different frequencies. The three protons on the methyl group are chemically equivalent and resonate at the same frequency because this group rotates freely, and, on average, each proton sees an identical magnetic environment.

MCAT EXPERTISE

To determine how many peaks will be in the spectrum, see if you can describe protons differently using words. In the dichloromethyl methyl ether shown in Figure 11.4, one could call H_a the *hydrogen on the carbon with two chlorides* and all three H_b hydrogens the *ones in the methyl group*. It would not be possible to describe each of these three hydrogens as distinct from each other because they rotate freely in space.

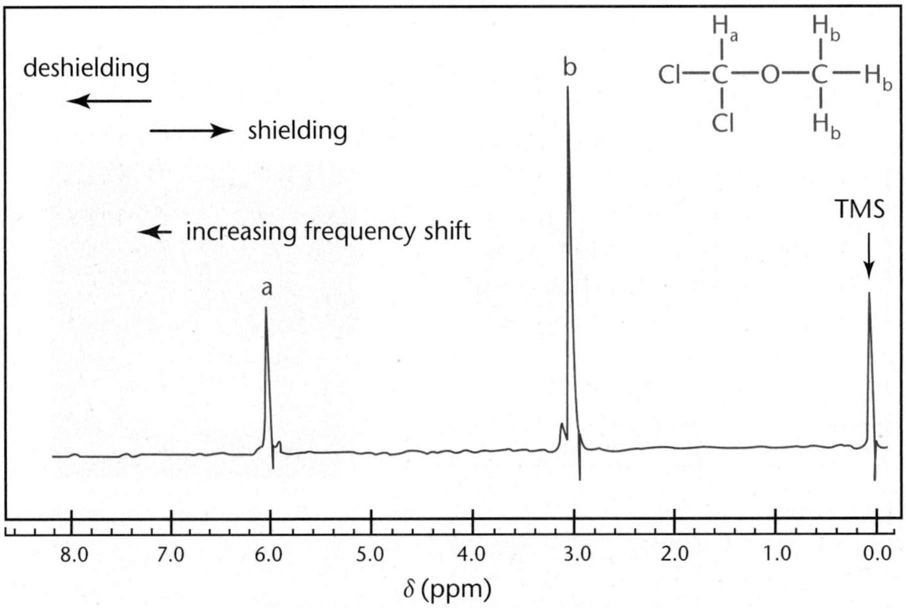

Figure 11.4 ^{1}H—NMR Spectrum of Dichloromethyl Methyl Ether
Peak a: Dichloromethyl proton; Peak b: Methyl protons.

The peak on the left (a) is from the single dichloromethyl proton, and the taller middle peak is from the three methyl protons (b). The height of each peak is proportional to the number of protons it contains. Specifically, if we were to analyze the area under the peaks, called the **integration**, we would find that the ratio of (a) to (b) is 1:3, corresponding exactly to the ratio of protons that produced each peak.

Now that we know which peak is which, let's talk about their respective positions on the spectrum. We can see that the peak for the single proton (a) is fairly far downfield compared with the other protons. This is because it is attached to a carbon with two electronegative chlorine atoms and an oxygen atom. These atoms pull electron density away from the surrounding atoms, thus **deshielding** the proton from the magnetic field. The more the proton's electron density is pulled away, the less it can shield itself from the applied magnetic field, resulting in a reading further downfield. With this same reasoning, we know that if we had an electron-donating group, such as the silicon atom in TMS, it would help shield the ^{1}H nuclei and give it a position further upfield. This is why tetramethylsilane is used as the reference or calibration peak; everything else in proton NMR will be more deshielded than it.

Now, let's make it a little more interesting. Consider a compound containing protons that are within three bonds of each other: in other words, a compound in which there are hydrogens on two adjacent atoms. When we have two protons in such close proximity to each other that are not magnetically identical, **spin–spin coupling (splitting)** occurs. Let's use the molecule in Figure 11.5 to demonstrate this concept.

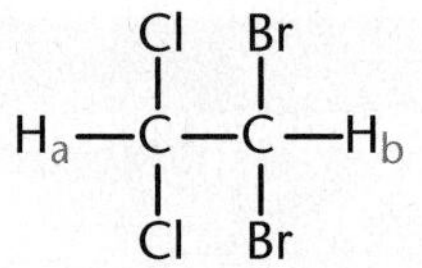

Figure 11.5 1,1-Dibromo-2,2-dichloroethane

Notice the two protons, H_a and H_b, on 1,1-dibromo-2,2-dichloroethane. Because of their proximity, the magnetic environment of H_a can be affected by H_b, and vice-versa. Thus, at any given time, H_a can experience two different magnetic environments because H_b can be in either the α- or the β-state. The different states of H_b influence the nucleus of H_a, causing slight upfield and downfield shifts. There is approximately a 50% chance that H_b will be in either of the two states, so the resulting absorption is a **doublet**: two peaks of identical intensity, equally spaced around the true chemical shift of H_a. H_a and H_b will both appear as doublets because each one is coupled with one other hydrogen. To determine the number of peaks present (as doublets, triplets, and so on), we use the ***n* + 1 rule**: if a proton has n protons that are three bonds away, it will be split into $n + 1$ peaks. (One caveat: do *not* include protons attached to oxygen or nitrogen.) The magnitude of this splitting, measured in hertz, is called the **coupling constant, *J***.

Let's try a molecule that has even more coupled protons. In 1,1-dibromo-2-chloroethane, shown in Figure 11.6, the H_a nucleus is affected by two nearby H_b nuclei, which together can be in one of four different states: $\alpha\alpha$, $\alpha\beta$, $\beta\alpha$, or $\beta\beta$.

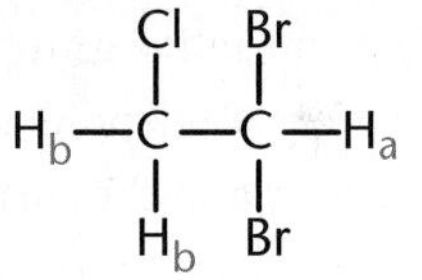

Figure 11.6 1,1-Dibromo-2-chloroethane

KEY CONCEPT

- Each peak or group of peaks that are part of a multiplet represents a single group of equivalent protons
- The relative area of each peak reflects the ratio of the protons producing each peak
- The position of the peak (upfield or downfield) is due to shielding or deshielding effects and reflects the chemical environment of the protons

MNEMONIC

When dealing with ^{1}H-NMR on the MCAT, think of a proton as being surrounded by a shield of electrons. As we add electronegative atoms or have resonance structures that pull electrons away from the proton, we **D**eshield and move **D**ownfield.

KEY CONCEPT

The splitting of the peak represents the number of adjacent hydrogens. A peak will be split into $n + 1$ subpeaks, where n is the number of adjacent hydrogens.

KEY CONCEPT

Proton NMR is good for:

- Determining the relative number of protons and their relative chemical environments
- Showing how many adjacent protons there are by splitting patterns
- Inferring certain functional groups

Although there are technically four different states, $\alpha\beta$ has the same effect as $\beta\alpha$, so both of these resonances occur at the same frequency. This means we will have three unique frequencies, $\alpha\alpha$, $\alpha\beta$ or $\beta\alpha$, and $\beta\beta$. H_a will thus appear as three peaks (a **triplet**) centered on the true chemical shift, with an area ratio of 1:2:1.

Now let's move on to H_b. Because both hydrogens are attached to the same carbon, which can freely rotate, they will be magnetically identical. These hydrogens are three bonds away from one other hydrogen, H_a. This means that they will appear as a doublet. Because there are two of them, the integration for the doublet representing H_b will be larger than the triplet for H_a.

Table 11.2 shows the ratios for up to seven adjacent hydrogens, but it isn't necessary to memorize this table for the MCAT. Just remember to follow the $n + 1$ rule for the proton of interest to determine the number of peaks. In addition, peaks that have more than four shifts will generally be referred to generically as a **multiplet**.

NUMBER OF ADJACENT HYDROGENS	TOTAL NUMBER OF PEAKS	AREA RATIOS
0	1	1
1	2	1:1
2	3	1:2:1
3	4	1:3:3:1
4	5	1:4:6:4:1
5	6	1:5:10:10:5:1
6	7	1:6:15:20:15:6:1
7	8	1:7:21:35:35:21:7:1

Table 11.2 Area Ratios for Peaks Split by Adjacent Hydrogens

Table 11.3 indicates the chemical shift ranges of several different types of protons. It is unnecessary to memorize this table, as it is fairly low-yield information. The values that are useful to memorize are the outliers like the deshielded aldehyde at 9 to 10 ppm, and the even more deshielded carboxylic acid between 10.5 and 12 ppm. Another popular peak on the MCAT is the hydrogen of an aromatic ring, which lies between 6.0 and 8.5 ppm. It is also worthwhile to know the general ranges for hydrogens on sp^3-hybridized carbons (0.0 to 3.0 ppm; higher if electron-withdrawing groups are present), sp^2-hybridized carbons (4.6 to 6.0 ppm), and sp-hybridized carbons (2.0 to 3.0 ppm). When electronegative groups are present, they pull electron density away from the protons. The more electron density that is pulled away from the proton, the more deshielded it will be and the further downfield the proton will appear.

TYPE OF PROTON	APPROXIMATE CHEMICAL SHIFT δ (ppm) DOWNFIELD FROM TMS
RCH_3	0.9
R_2CH_2	1.25
R_3CH	1.5
RC=CH	4.6-6.0
RC≡CH	2.0-3.0
Ar—H	6.0-8.5
RCHX	2.0-4.5
RCHOH/RCHOR	3.4-4.0
RCHO	9.0-10.0
$RCOCH_3$	2.0-2.5
RCHCOOH/RCHCOOR	2.0-2.6
ROH	1.0-5.5
ArOH	4.0-12.0
RCOOH	10.5-12.0
RNH_2	1.0-5.0

Table 11.3 Proton Chemical Shift Ranges

MCAT EXPERTISE

On Test Day, just counting the number of peaks and unique hydrogens may be enough to get you the correct answer. (Remember *not* to count the peak for TMS, though!) If you need to consider shifts, the main ones for Test Day are:

- Alkyl groups: 0 to 3 ppm
- Alkynes: 2 to 3 ppm
- Alkenes: 4.6 to 6 ppm
- Aromatics: 6 to 8.5 ppm
- Aldehydes: 9 to 10 ppm
- Carboxylic acids: 10.5 to 12 ppm

MCAT CONCEPT CHECK 11.3

Before you move on, assess your understanding of the material with these questions.

1. What does nuclear magnetic resonance (NMR) spectroscopy measure? What is NMR spectroscopy generally used for?

____

2. What are the units for chemical shift on a standardized NMR spectrum?

____

3. What does it mean for a proton to be deshielded? How does this affect its peak in NMR spectroscopy?

____

4. What is spin–spin coupling?

____

Conclusion

This chapter was full of numbers and values, but the most important thing to know about spectroscopy on the MCAT is that you don't need to know a lot of numbers. The numbers that you *do* need to know have already been stressed heavily in this chapter. Know that infrared (IR) spectroscopy is best for identifying the presence (or, more importantly, the absence) of functional groups. A cursory understanding of ultraviolet (UV) spectroscopy and its association with conjugation will suffice. Nuclear magnetic resonance (NMR) spectroscopy—specifically, proton (^1H) NMR—also helps us figure out the arrangement of functional groups. Know how to interpret IR and NMR spectra: IR spectra have three important peaks (O–H, C=O, and N–H), but NMR spectra can be far more complex. The MCAT can test the chemical shift of deshielded protons, which will be downfield, or toward the left of the spectrum. Make sure that you can interpret peak splitting, which is due to interference from neighboring hydrogens, and peak integration, which is proportional to the number of magnetically identical hydrogens.

Spectroscopy is often tested on the MCAT in the context of experiment-based passages. As you continue studying the reaction chemistry discussed in Chapters 4 through 10 of *MCAT Organic Chemistry Review*, consider what these products would yield in different spectroscopic modalities.

This chapter focused on one method of identifying compounds based on structural characteristics and interactions with electromagnetic energy, but spectroscopy is not the only method for characterizing organic molecules. In the next chapter, we explore another side of laboratory techniques: separation and purification schemes. These utilize physical differences between molecules to allow us to isolate and describe them.

You've reviewed the content, now test your knowledge and critical thinking skills by completing a test-like passage set in your online resources!

GO ONLINE

CONCEPT SUMMARY

Infrared Spectroscopy

- **Infrared (IR) spectroscopy** measures **absorption** of infrared light, which causes molecular vibration (stretching, bending, twisting, and folding).
- IR spectra are generally plotted as **percent transmittance** *vs.* **wavenumber** $\left(\frac{1}{\lambda}\right)$.
  - The normal range of a spectrum is 4000 to 400 cm^{-1}.
  - The **fingerprint region** is between 1500 and 400 cm^{-1}. It contains a number of peaks that can be used by experts to identify a compound.
- To appear on an IR spectrum, vibration of a bond must change the bond dipole moment. Certain bonds have characteristic absorption frequencies, which allow us to infer the presence (or absence) of particular functional groups.
  - The O–H peak is a broad peak around 3300 cm^{-1}. Molecules with O–H include alcohols, water, and carboxylic acids; the carboxylic acid O–H peak will be shifted around 3000 cm^{-1}.
  - The N–H peak is a sharp peak around 3300 cm^{-1}. Molecules with N–H include some amines, imines, and amides.
  - The C=O peak is a sharp peak around 1750 cm^{-1}. Molecules with C=O include aldehydes, ketones, carboxylic acids, amides, esters, and anhydrides.

Ultraviolet Spectroscopy

- Ultraviolet (UV) spectroscopy measures absorption of ultraviolet light, which causes movement of electrons between molecular orbitals.
- UV spectra are generally plotted as percent transmittance or absorbance *vs.* wavelength.
- To appear on a UV spectrum, a molecule must have a small enough energy difference between its **highest occupied molecular orbital (HOMO)** and its **lowest unoccupied molecular orbital (LUMO)** to permit an electron to move from one orbital to the other.
  - The smaller the difference between HOMO and LUMO, the longer the wavelengths a molecule can absorb.
  - **Conjugation** occurs in molecules with unhybridized *p*-orbitals. Conjugation shifts the absorption spectrum to higher maximum wavelengths (lower frequencies).

Nuclear Magnetic Resonance Spectroscopy

- **Nuclear magnetic resonance (NMR) spectroscopy** measures alignment of nuclear spin with an applied magnetic field, which depends on the magnetic environment of the nucleus itself. It is useful for determining the structure (connectivity) of a compound, including functional groups.
  - Nuclei may be in the lower-energy **α-state** or higher-energy **β-state**; radiofrequency pulses push the nucleus from the α-state to the β-state, and these frequencies can be measured.
- Magnetic resonance imaging (MRI) is a medical application of NMR spectroscopy.
- NMR spectra are generally plotted as frequency *vs.* absorption of energy. They are standardized by using **chemical shift** (δ), measured in parts per million (ppm) of spectrophotometer frequency.
  - NMR spectra are calibrated using **tetramethylsilane (TMS)**, which has a chemical shift of 0 ppm.
  - Higher chemical shifts are located to the left (**downfield**); lower chemical shifts are located to the right (**upfield**).
- Proton (^1H) NMR is the most common.
  - Each unique group of protons has its own peak.
  - The **integration** (area under the curve) of this peak is proportional to the number of protons contained under the peak.
  - **Deshielding** of protons occurs when electron-withdrawing groups pull electron density away from the nucleus, allowing it to be more easily affected by the magnetic field. Deshielding moves a peak further downfield.
  - When hydrogens are on adjacent atoms, they interfere with each other's magnetic environment, causing **spin–spin coupling (splitting)**. A proton's (or group of protons') peak is split into $n + 1$ subpeaks, where n is the number of protons that are three bonds away from the proton of interest.
  - Splitting patterns include **doublets**, **triplets**, and **multiplets**.
  - Protons on sp^3-hybridized carbons are usually in the 0 to 3 ppm range (but higher if electron-withdrawing groups are present). Protons on sp^2-hybridized carbons are usually in the 4.6 to 6.0 ppm range. Protons on sp-hybridized carbons are usually in the 2.0 to 3.0 ppm range.
  - Aldehydic hydrogens tend to appear between 9 and 10 ppm.
  - Carboxylic acid hydrogens tend to appear between 10.5 and 12 ppm.
  - Aromatic hydrogens tend to appear between 6.0 and 8.5 ppm.

ANSWERS TO CONCEPT CHECKS

11.1

1. IR spectroscopy measures absorption of infrared light by specific bonds that vibrate. These vibrations cause changes in the dipole moment of the molecule that can be measured. Once the bonds in a molecule are determined, one can infer the presence of a number of functional groups to determine the identity of the molecule.
2. A carboxylic acid would have a broad O–H peak around 2800–3200 cm^{-1} and a sharp carbonyl peak at 1700–1750 cm^{-1}.

11.2

1. Conjugated systems and other molecules with π or nonbonding electrons can give absorbances on a UV spectroscopy plot. Therefore, propane would not be detectable, but propene and propanone would.
2. HOMO is the highest occupied molecular orbital; LUMO is the lowest unoccupied molecular orbital. The smaller the difference in energy between the two, the longer the wavelengths that can be absorbed by the molecule.

11.3

1. NMR measures alignment of the spin of a nucleus with an applied magnetic field. It is most often used for identifying the different types and magnetic environments of protons in a molecule, which allows us to infer the connectivity (backbone) of a molecule.
2. The units for chemical shift on a standardized NMR spectrum are parts per million (ppm).
3. Deshielding occurs in molecules that have electronegative atoms that pull electron density away from the hydrogens being measured. This results in a downfield (leftward) shift of the proton peak.
4. Spin–spin coupling occurs when two protons close to one another have an effect on the other's magnetic environment. This results in the splitting of peaks into doublets, triplets, or multiplets, depending on the environment.

SCIENCE MASTERY ASSESSMENT EXPLANATIONS

1. **A**

Infrared spectroscopy is most useful for distinguishing between different functional groups. Almost all organic compounds have C—H bonds, **(B)**, so except for fingerprinting a compound, these absorptions are not useful. Little information about the optical properties of a compound, such as **(C)** and **(D)**, can be obtained by IR spectroscopy.

2. **C**

Because molecular oxygen is homonuclear (composed of only one element) and diatomic, there is no net change in its dipole moment during vibration or rotation; in other words, the compound does not absorb in a measurable way in the infrared region. IR spectroscopy is based on the principle that, when the molecule vibrates or rotates, there is a change in dipole moment. **(A)** is incorrect because oxygen does have molecular motions; they are just not detectable in IR spectroscopy. **(B)** is incorrect because it is possible to record the IR of a gaseous molecule as long as it shows a change in its dipole moment when it vibrates. **(D)** is incorrect because lone pairs do not have an effect on the ability to generate an IR spectrum of a compound.

3. **D**

In this reaction, the functional group is changing from a hydroxyl to an aldehyde. This means that a sharp peak will appear around 1750 cm^{-1}, which corresponds to the carbonyl functionality. **(C)** is the opposite of what occurs; the reaction will be characterized by the disappearance of the O—H peak at 3100 to 3500 cm^{-1}, not its appearance. Comparing the fingerprint regions, as in **(A)**, will provide evidence that a reaction is occurring, but it is not as useful for knowing that the reaction that occurred was indeed the one that was desired.

4. **A**

The peak at 9.5 ppm corresponds to an aldehydic proton. This signal lies downfield because the carbonyl oxygen is electron-withdrawing and deshields the proton. **(C)** corresponds to a carboxyl proton and is even further downfield because the acidic proton is deshielded to a greater degree than the aldehydic proton. **(B)** corresponds to aromatic protons. **(D)** is characteristic of an alkyl proton on an sp^3-hybridized carbon.

5. **C**

This isotope has no magnetic moment and will therefore not exhibit resonance with an applied magnetic field. Nuclei with odd mass numbers (^{1}H, ^{11}B, ^{13}C, ^{15}N, ^{19}F, and so on) or those with an even mass number but an odd atomic number (^{2}H, ^{10}B) will have a nonzero magnetic moment.

6. **D**

Spin–spin coupling (splitting) is due to influence on the magnetic environment of one proton by protons on the adjacent atom. These protons are three bonds away from each other. Splitting in other NMR spectra can include coupling with carbon atoms, but not in ^{1}H—NMR.

7. **C**

Most conjugated alkenes have an intense ultraviolet absorption. Aldehydes, ketones, acids, and amines, mentioned in **(A)** and **(D)**, all absorb in the ultraviolet range. However, other forms of spectroscopy (mainly IR and NMR) are more useful for precise identification. Isolated alkenes, **(B)**, can rarely be identified by UV spectroscopy.

8. **B**

The region in question often gives information about the types of alkyl groups present. Specifically, ethanol will give a characteristic triplet for the methyl group (which is coupled to $-CH_2-$) and a quartet for $-CH_2-$ (which is coupled to the methyl group). Isopropanol will have a septet for the $-CH-$ group (which is coupled to both methyl groups combined) and a doublet for the two methyl groups (which are coupled to $-CH-$). In both cases, the proton in the alcohol does not participate in coupling. The alcohol hydrogen likely lies downfield for both compounds because it is bonded to such an electronegative element.

9. **A**

The HOMO is the highest occupied molecular orbital. Only after absorbing ultraviolet light is an electron is excited from the HOMO to the LUMO, the lowest unoccupied molecular orbital.

10. **A**

Carbonyl groups (C=O) in conjugation with double bonds tend to absorb at lower wavenumbers because the delocalization of π electrons causes the C=O bond to lose double-bond character, shifting the stretching frequency closer to C–O stretches. Remember that higher-order bonds tend to have higher absorption frequencies, so loss of double-bond character should decrease the absorption frequency of the group.

11. **B**

Wavenumber $\left(\frac{1}{\lambda}\right)$ is directly proportional to frequency $\left(\frac{c}{\lambda}\right)$. It is inversely proportional to wavelength, **(A)**, and has no proportionality to percent transmittance or absorbance, **(C)** and **(D)**.

12. **A**

Enantiomers will have identical IR spectra because they have the same functional groups and will therefore have the exact same absorption frequencies. Enantiomers have opposite specific rotations, but specific rotation actually has no effect on the IR spectrum.

13. **A**

The oxygen of the hydroxyl group will deshield the hydroxyl hydrogen, shifting it downfield, or leftward. Hydrogens in carboxylic acids can have some of the most downfield absorbances, around 10.5 to 12 ppm.

14. **D**

The coupling constant is a measure of the degree of splitting introduced by other atoms in a molecule, and is the frequency of the distance between subpeaks. It is measured in hertz, eliminating **(B)**. The coupling constant is independent of the value of $n + 1$ and is not changed by calibration with tetramethylsilane, eliminating **(A)** and **(B)**.

15. **B**

Amino acids in their fully protonated form contain all three of the peaks that should be memorized for Test Day: C–O, N–H, and O–H. While statements I and II correctly give the peaks for the C=O bond (sharp peak at 1750 cm^{-1}) and the N–H bond (sharp peak at 3300 cm^{-1}), the peak for the O–H bond is in the wrong place. In a carboxylic acid, the C=O bond withdraws electron density from the O–H bond, shifting the absorption frequency down to about 3000 cm^{-1}. Statement III is therefore incorrect.

Consult your online resources for additional practice. GO ONLINE

SHARED CONCEPTS

General Chemistry Chapter 1
Atomic Structure

General Chemistry Chapter 3
Bonding and Chemical Interactions

Organic Chemistry Chapter 3
Bonding

Organic Chemistry Chapter 12
Separations and Purifications

Physics and Math Chapter 8
Light and Optics

Physics and Math Chapter 9
Atomic and Nuclear Phenomena

CHAPTER 12

SEPARATIONS AND PURIFICATIONS

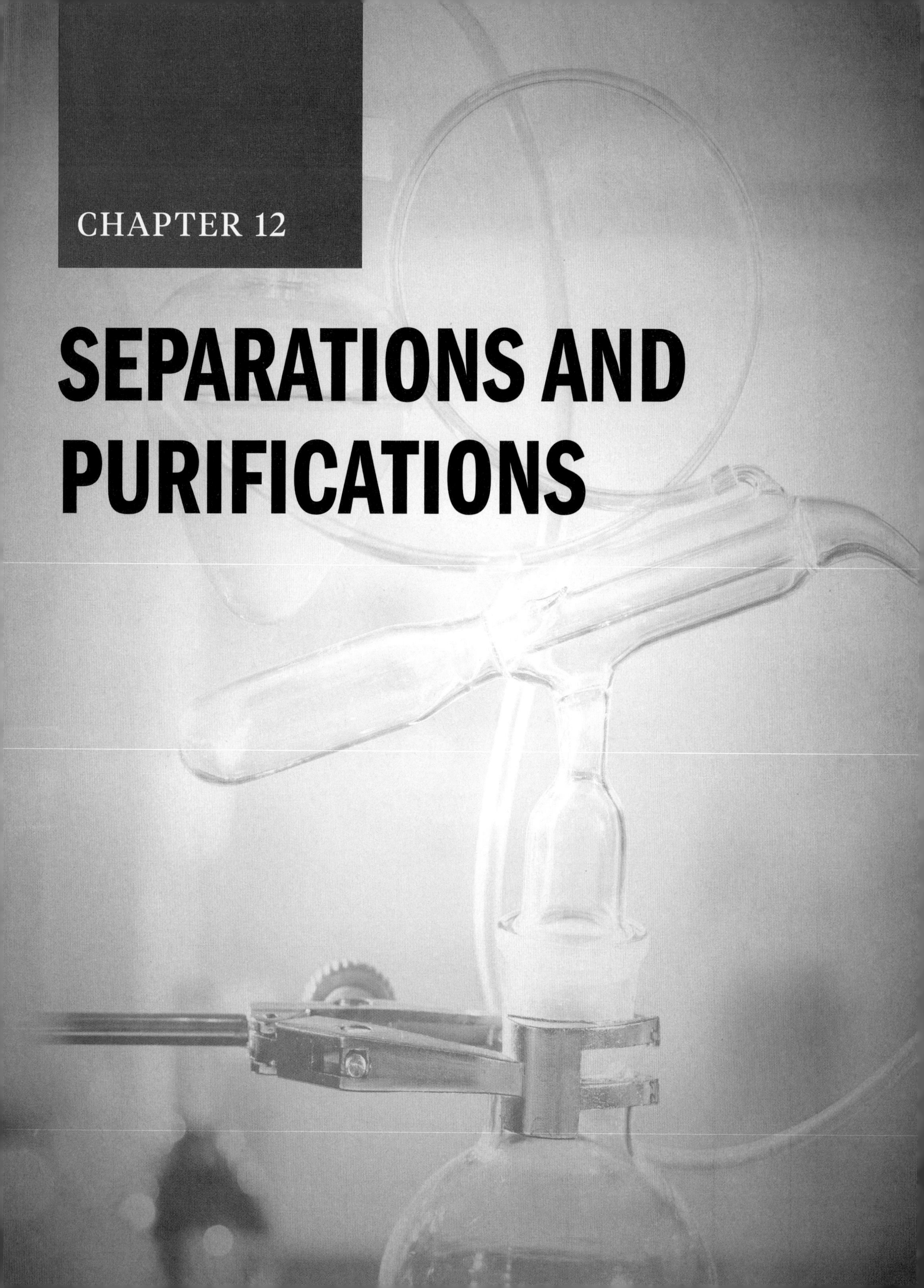

SCIENCE MASTERY ASSESSMENT

Every pre-med knows this feeling: there is so much content I have to know for the MCAT! How do I know what to do first or what's important?

While the high-yield badges throughout this book will help you identify the most important topics, this Science Mastery Assessment is another tool in your MCAT prep arsenal. This quiz (which can also be taken in your online resources) and the guidance below will help ensure that you are spending the appropriate amount of time on this chapter based on your personal strengths and weaknesses. Don't worry though—skipping something now does not mean you'll never study it. Later on in your prep, as you complete full-length tests, you'll uncover specific pieces of content that you need to review and can come back to these chapters as appropriate.

How to Use This Assessment

If you answer 0–7 questions correctly:

Spend about 1 hour to read this chapter in full and take limited notes throughout. Follow up by reviewing **all** quiz questions to ensure that you now understand how to solve each one.

If you answer 8–11 questions correctly:

Spend 20–40 minutes reviewing the quiz questions. Beginning with the questions you missed, read and take notes on the corresponding subchapters. For questions you answered correctly, ensure your thinking matches that of the explanation and you understand why each choice was correct or incorrect.

If you answer 12–15 questions correctly:

Spend less than 20 minutes reviewing all questions from the quiz. If you missed any, then include a quick read-through of the corresponding subchapters, or even just the relevant content within a subchapter, as part of your question review. For questions you got correct, ensure your thinking matches that of the explanation and review the Concept Summary at the end of the chapter.

1. Fractional distillation under atmospheric pressure would most likely be used to separate which of the following compounds?
   - **A.** Methylene chloride (boiling point of 40°C) and water (boiling point of 10°C)
   - **B.** Ethyl acetate (boiling point of 77°C) and ethanol (boiling point of 80°C)
   - **C.** Aniline (boiling point of 184°C) and benzyl alcohol (boiling point of 205°C)
   - **D.** Aniline (boiling point of 184°C) and water (boiling point of 100°C)

2. Which of the following compounds would be most effective in extracting benzoic acid from a diethyl ether solution?
   - **A.** Tetrahydrofuran
   - **B.** Aqueous hydrochloric acid
   - **C.** Aqueous sodium hydroxide
   - **D.** Water

3. Which of the following would be the best procedure for extracting acetaldehyde from an aqueous solution?
   - **A.** A single extraction with 100 mL of ether
   - **B.** Two successive extractions with 50 mL portions of ether
   - **C.** Three successive extractions with 33.3 mL portions of ether
   - **D.** Four successive extractions with 25 mL portions of ether

Questions 4 and 5 refer to the following table:

Compound	Retardation Factor in Ether
Benzyl alcohol	0.10
Benzyl acetate	0.26
p-Nitrophenol	0.23
1-Naphthalen-emethanol	0.40

4. What would be the effect on the R_f values if thin-layer chromatography (TLC) were run with hexane rather than ether as the eluent?
   - **A.** No effect
   - **B.** Increase tenfold
   - **C.** Double
   - **D.** Decrease

5. If these compounds were separated by column chromatography with ether on silica gel, which would elute first?
   - **A.** Benzyl alcohol
   - **B.** Benzyl acetate
   - **C.** *p*-Nitrophenol
   - **D.** 1-Naphthalenemethanol

6. Four compounds, I, II, III, and IV, are separated by chromatographic techniques. Compound III is the most polar, II the least polar, and I and IV have intermediate polarity. The solvent system is 85:15 ethanol:methylene chloride. Which spot on the card below likely belongs to compound III?

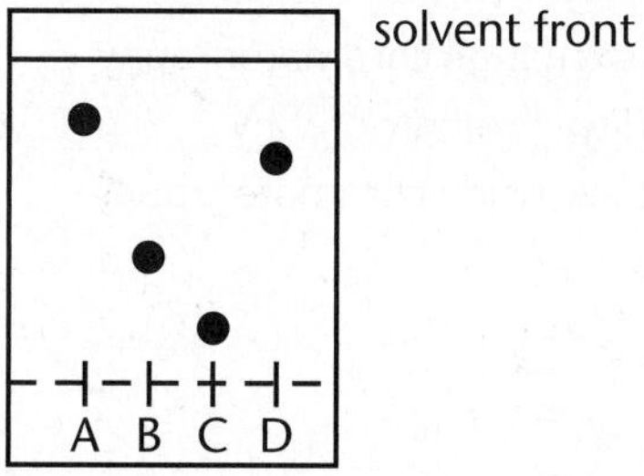

A. A
B. B
C. C
D. D

7. Suppose an extraction with methylene chloride $\left(\rho = 1.33\ \frac{g}{mL}\right)$ is performed, with the desired compound initially in brine $\left(\rho = 1.04\ \frac{g}{mL}\right)$. In a separatory funnel, which layer will be the organic layer?

A. The top layer
B. The bottom layer
C. No layers are observed; methylene chloride and brine are miscible.
D. More information is needed to answer the question.

8. Silica gel is often used in thin-layer chromatography. What property does silica gel probably possess that makes it useful for this purpose?

A. Acidity
B. Polarity
C. Specifically sized pores
D. Aqueous solubility

9. A mixture of sand, benzoic acid, and naphthalene in ether is best separated by:

A. filtration, followed by acidic extraction, followed by recrystallization.
B. filtration, followed by basic extraction, followed by evaporation.
C. extraction, followed by distillation, followed by gas chromatography.
D. filtration, followed by size-exclusion column chromatography, followed by extraction.

10. Simple distillation could be used to separate which of the following compounds?

A. Toluene (boiling point of 111°C) and water (boiling point of 100°C)
B. Naphthalene (boiling point of 218°C) and butyric acid (boiling point of 163°C)
C. Propionaldehyde (boiling point of 50°C) and acetic acid (boiling point of 119°C)
D. Benzene (boiling point of 80°C) and isopropyl alcohol (boiling point of 83°C)

11. In order to separate a biological effector from solution, which chromatographic technique would be the most effective?

A. Thin-layer chromatography
B. Ion-exchange chromatography
C. Affinity chromatography
D. Size-exclusion chromatography

12. Given a solution of insulin (molecular weight = 5.8 kD) and titin (molecular weight = 3816 kD), which chromatographic technique would be the most effective for separating out usable molecules of titin?

A. Thin-layer chromatography
B. Ion-exchange chromatography
C. Affinity chromatography
D. Size-exclusion chromatography

13. The gas eluent in gas chromatography and the liquid eluent in paper chromatography are examples of which component of these systems?
   - **A.** Stationary phase
   - **B.** Mobile phase
   - **C.** Column
   - **D.** Fraction

14. During gravity filtration, a student forgets to heat the solution before running it through the filter. After capturing the filtrate, the student analyzes the sample via infrared (IR) spectroscopy and finds none of the desired product in the filtrate. What likely occurred to the student's product?
   - **A.** The product degraded because of a prolonged filtration time.
   - **B.** The product evaporated with collection of the filtrate.
   - **C.** The product precipitated and is present in the residue.
   - **D.** The product was dissolved in the solvent.

15. Lactoferrin, a milk protein, is a valuable antimicrobial agent that is extracted from pasteurized, defatted milk utilizing a column containing a charged resin. This is an example of which of the following chromatographic techniques?
   - **A.** Thin-layer chromatography
   - **B.** Ion-exchange chromatography
   - **C.** Affinity chromatography
   - **D.** Size-exclusion chromatography

Answer Key follows on next page.

Answer Key

1. **B**
2. **C**
3. **D**
4. **D**
5. **D**
6. **A**
7. **B**
8. **B**
9. **B**
10. **C**
11. **C**
12. **D**
13. **B**
14. **C**
15. **B**

Detailed explanations can be found at the end of the chapter.

CHAPTER 12

SEPARATIONS AND PURIFICATIONS

In This Chapter

CHAPTER PROFILE

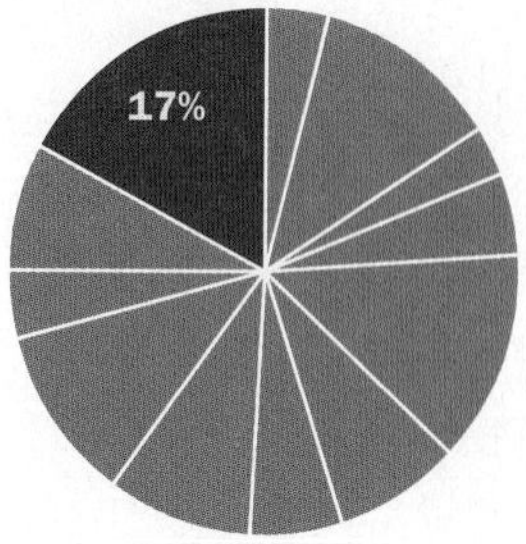

The content in this chapter should be relevant to about 17% of all questions about organic chemistry on the MCAT.

This chapter covers material from the following AAMC content category:

5C: Separation and purification methods

Introduction

We've spent a lot of time discussing how to theoretically get various products from a range of reagents. However, as we're sure you've learned in your organic chemistry labs, chemistry isn't as straightforward in the real world as it is on paper. Much of the time spent in the lab is dedicated to the isolation and purification of the desired product after the reaction has occurred. Throughout this chapter, we will discuss several techniques for this. Good news, though—there isn't a lab practical on the MCAT, of course! All you need to understand is when these techniques are used and how they work.

MCAT EXPERTISE

Purification and separation techniques are procedures that exploit different physical properties. These show up on the MCAT to test your knowledge of the basic principles of each of these techniques.

12.1 Solubility-Based Methods

LEARNING OBJECTIVES

After Chapter 12.1, you will be able to:

- Recall the conditions required for two solvents to be used together in an extraction
- Explain why repetition is important in extraction procedures
- Predict whether a given solute is more likely to dissolve in the aqueous or organic layer within a separatory funnel

One of the simplest ways to separate out a desired product is through **extraction**, the transfer of a dissolved compound (the desired product) from a starting solvent into a solvent in which the product is more soluble. Extraction is based on the fundamental concept that *like dissolves like*. This principle tells us that a polar substance will

KEY CONCEPT

Like dissolves like is a fundamental concept on the MCAT. Remember that polar substances will associate with other polar substances, and nonpolar with nonpolar.

dissolve best in polar solvents, and a nonpolar substance will dissolve best in nonpolar solvents. These characteristics can be taken advantage of in order to extract only the desired product, leaving most of the impurities behind in the first solvent.

Extraction

When we perform **extractions**, it is important to make sure that the two solvents are **immiscible**, meaning that they form two layers that do not mix, like water and oil. The two layers are temporarily mixed by shaking so that solute can pass from one solvent to the other. For example, in a solution of isobutyric acid and diethyl ether, shown in Figure 12.1, we can extract the isobutyric acid with water. Isobutyric acid, with its polar carboxyl group, is more soluble in a polar solvent like water than in a nonpolar solvent like ether. When the two solvents are mixed together, isobutyric acid will transfer to the water layer, which is called the **aqueous phase (layer)**. The nonpolar ether layer is called the **organic phase (layer)**.

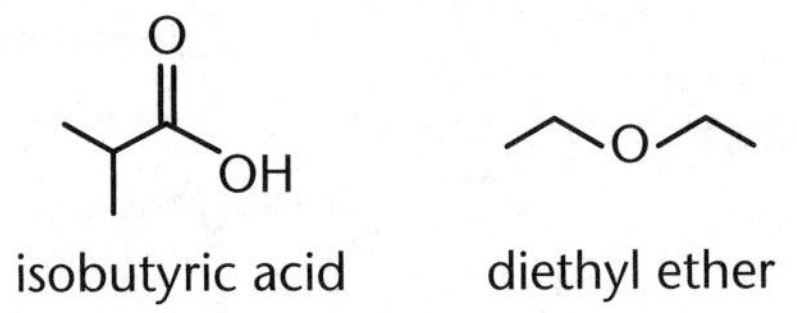

Figure 12.1 Isobutyric Acid and Diethyl Ether

Isobutyric acid is more polar than diethyl ether and can exhibit hydrogen bonding, so it will congregate in the aqueous layer; diethyl ether will remain in the organic layer.

MCAT EXPERTISE

Think of the organic and aqueous layers as being like the oil and water in salad dressings: you can shake the mixture to increase their interaction, but ultimately they will separate again.

After the two layers are mixed together, how do we then get the desired product out? The water (aqueous) and ether (organic) phases will separate on their own, given time to do so. In order to isolate these two phases, we use a piece of equipment called a **separatory funnel**, as shown in Figure 12.2. Gravitational forces cause the denser layer to sink to the bottom of the funnel, where it can then be removed by turning the stopcock at the bottom. It is more common for the organic layer to be on top, although the opposite can also occur. Remember that the position of the layers is determined by their relative densities.

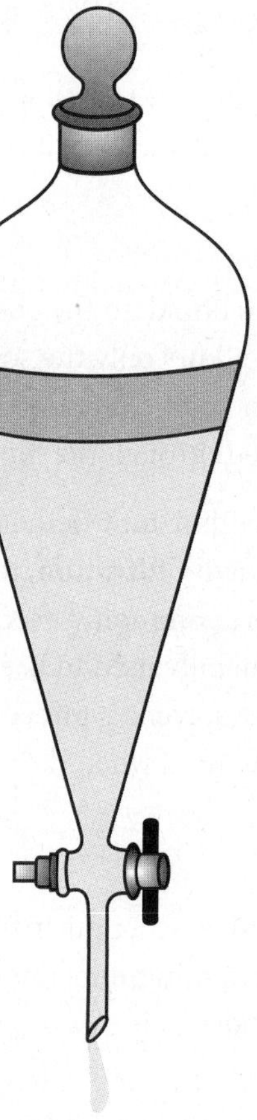

Figure 12.2 Separatory Funnel
Used to separate solvents based on their relative densities; the denser solvent is always drained first.

In this example, we'll assume that the aqueous layer is more dense and settles to the bottom of the separatory funnel. Once we drain the aqueous layer from the separatory funnel, we repeat the extraction several times. Additional water is added to the separatory funnel, it is shaken and allowed to settle, and the aqueous layer is once again drained off. This is done in order to extract as much of the isobutyric acid from the ether layer as possible because it does not completely transfer with the first extraction. Multiple extractions with fresh water are more effective for obtaining the most product, rather than a single extraction with a larger volume of water. You can imagine this as analogous to laundering dirty clothes several times, rather than laundering them with more water—the cleaner each volume of water is, the less dirt is likely to be left on the clothes afterward.

Once the desired product has been isolated in the solvent, we can obtain the product alone by evaporating the solvent, usually by using a **rotary evaporator** (**rotovap**).

Another way to take advantage of solubility properties is to perform the reverse of the extraction we just described in order to remove unwanted impurities. In this case, a small amount of solvent is used to extract and remove impurities, rather than the compound of interest. This process is called a **wash**.

KEY CONCEPT

Extraction depends on the rules of solubility and *like dissolves like.* Remember the three intermolecular forces that affect solubility:

1. Hydrogen bonding: Compounds that can do this, such as alcohols or acids, will move most easily into the aqueous layer
2. Dipole-dipole interactions: These compounds are less likely to move into the aqueous layer
3. Van der Waals (London) forces: With only these interactions, compounds are least likely to move into the aqueous layer

BRIDGE

You can use the properties of acids and bases to your advantage in extraction:

$$HA + \text{base} \longrightarrow A^- + H\text{—base}^+$$

When the acid dissociates, the anion formed will be more soluble in the aqueous layer than the original protonated acid because it is charged. Thus, adding a base will help to extract an acid into the aqueous phase.

Other Methods

In addition to extraction, filtration and recrystallization make use of solubility characteristics to separate compounds from a mixture.

Filtration

Filtration isolates a solid from a liquid. In the chemistry lab, one pours a liquid–solid mixture onto a paper filter that allows only the solvent to pass through, much like a coffee filter. At the end of filtration, one is left with the solid, called the **residue**, and the flask full of liquid that passed through the filter, known as the **filtrate**.

Filtration can be modified depending on whether the substance of interest is the solid or is dissolved in the filtrate. **Gravity filtration**, in which the solvent's own weight pulls it through the filter, is more commonly used when the product of interest is in the filtrate. Hot solvent is generally used to keep the product dissolved in liquid. **Vacuum filtration**, in which the solvent is forced through the filter by a vacuum connected to the flask, is more often used when the solid is the desired product.

Recrystallization

Recrystallization is a method for further purifying crystals in solution. In this process, we dissolve our product in a minimum amount of hot solvent and let it recrystallize as it cools. The solvent chosen for this process should be one in which the product is soluble only at high temperatures. Thus, when the solution cools, only the desired product will recrystallize out of solution, excluding the impurities.

MCAT CONCEPT CHECK 12.1

Before you move on, assess your understanding of the material with these questions.

1. What must be true about the two solvents used for an extraction to work?

____

2. When doing an extraction, would it be better to do three extractions with 10 mL of solvent, or one extraction with 30 mL?

____

3. Would acid dissolve better in an aqueous acid or aqueous base? Why?

____

12.2 Distillation

LEARNING OBJECTIVES

After Chapter 12.2, you will be able to:

- Differentiate between the separatory capabilities of simple, vacuum, and fractional distillation
- Recall the conditions in which distillation is a helpful separatory technique
- Select the best distillation technique for a given solute mixture

Extraction requires two solvents that are immiscible in order to separate the product. But what happens when the product itself is a liquid that is soluble in the solvent? This is where distillation comes in handy. **Distillation** takes advantage of differences in the boiling point to separate two liquids by evaporation and condensation. The liquid with the lower boiling point will vaporize first, and the vapors will rise up the distillation column to condense in a water-cooled condenser. This **condensate** then drips down into a vessel. The end product is called the **distillate**. The heating temperature is kept low so that the liquid with the higher boiling point will not be able to boil and therefore will remain liquid in the initial container. This is the process that is used to make liquor at a distillery. Because ethanol boils at a lower temperature than water, we can use distillation to make beverages with high ethanol contents.

Simple Distillation

Simple distillation, as the name indicates, is the least complex version of distillation. It proceeds precisely as described above. This technique should only be used to separate liquids that boil below 150°C and have at least a 25°C difference in boiling points. These restrictions prevent the temperature from becoming so high that the compounds degrade and provide a large enough difference in boiling points that the second compound won't accidentally boil off into the distillate. The apparatus for this technique consists of a **distilling flask** containing the combined liquid solution, a **distillation column** consisting of a thermometer and a **condenser**, and a **receiving flask** to collect the distillate. The setup is the same as that shown in Figure 12.3, sans the vacuum adapter. Sometimes an additional piece of equipment, such as a boiling chip, ebulliator, or magnetic stirrer, will be introduced to break surface tension and prevent superheating. **Superheating** occurs when a liquid is heated to a temperature above its boiling point without vaporization. Superheating situations occur when gas bubbles within a liquid are unable to overcome the combination of atmospheric pressure and surface tension.

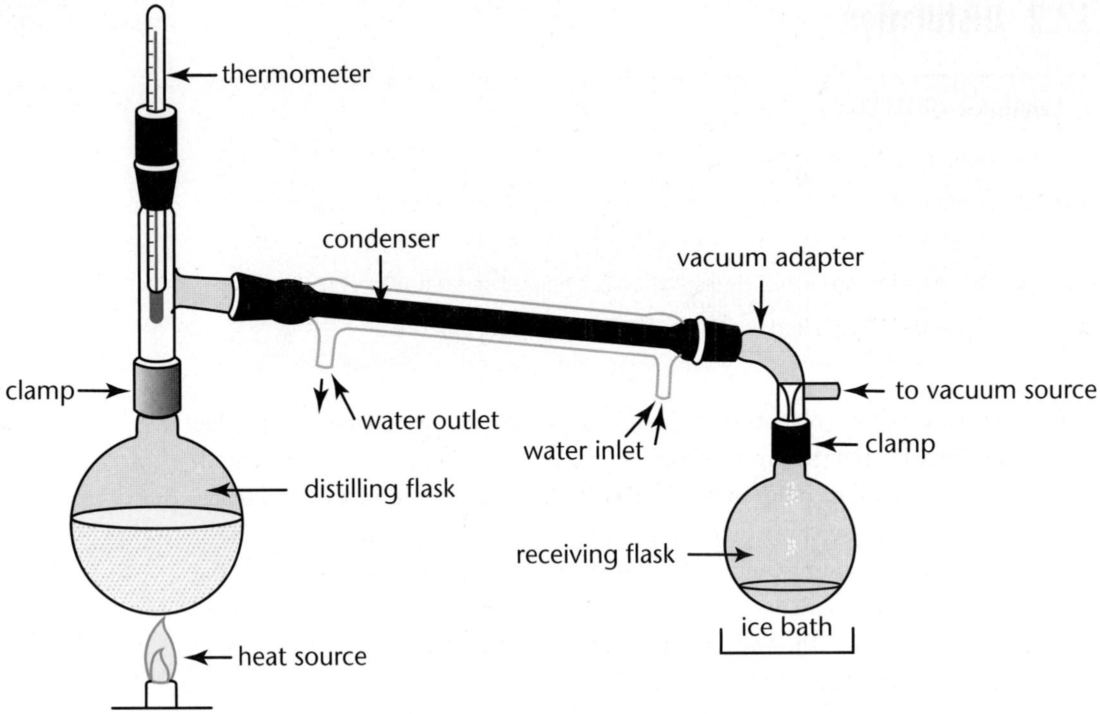

Figure 12.3 Vacuum Distillation

The initial solution is placed in the heated distilling flask, where the components of the solution with the lowest boiling points will vaporize first. The vapor then condenses in the water-cooled condenser, and this distillate drips into the receiving flask.

Vacuum Distillation

We use **vacuum distillation** whenever we want to distill a liquid with a boiling point over 150°C. By using a vacuum, we lower the ambient pressure, thereby decreasing the temperature that the liquid must reach in order to have sufficient vapor pressure to boil. This allows us to distill compounds with higher boiling points at lower temperatures so that we do not have to worry about degrading the product. The apparatus for vacuum distillation is shown above in Figure 12.3.

BRIDGE

Remember from Chapter 7 of *MCAT General Chemistry Review* that liquids boil when their vapor pressure equals ambient pressure. In vacuum distillation, we lower the ambient pressure so that the liquid can boil at lower temperatures.

Fractional Distillation

To separate two liquids with similar boiling points (less than 25°C apart), we use **fractional distillation**. In this technique, a fractionation column connects the distillation flask to the condenser, as shown in Figure 12.4. A fractionation column is a column in which the surface area is increased by the inclusion of inert objects like glass beads or steel wool. As the vapor rises up the column, it condenses on these surfaces and refluxes back down until rising heat causes it to evaporate again, only to condense again higher in the column. Each time the condensate evaporates, the vapor consists of a higher proportion of the compound with the lower boiling point. By the time the top of the column is reached, only the desired product drips down to the receiving flask.

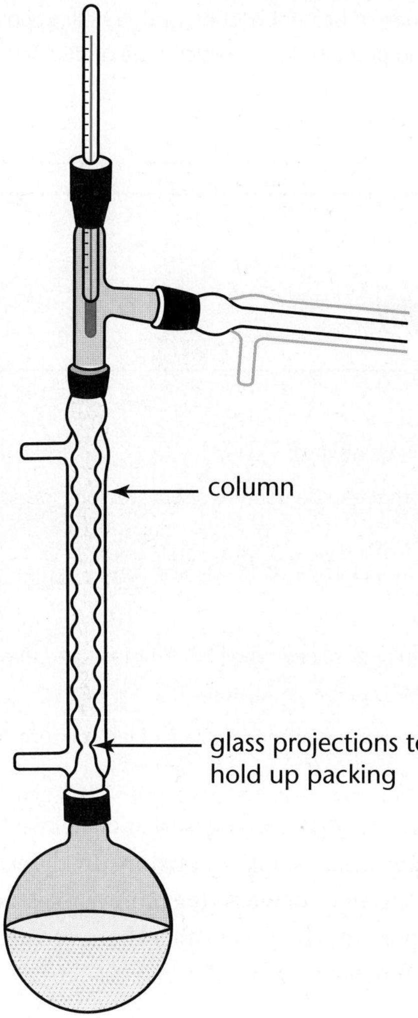

Figure 12.4 Fractional Distillation
With increased surface area in the distillation column, the distillate has more places to condense on its way up the column. This allows for more refined separation of liquids with fairly close boiling points.

MCAT CONCEPT CHECK 12.2

Before you move on, assess your understanding of the material with these questions.

1. Distillation separates compounds based on what property?

    ____

2. If we are given a solution of ether, with a boiling point of 308 K, and methylene chloride, with a boiling point of 313 K, which type of distillation should be used to separate them?

    ____

3. If we are given a solution of bromobenzene, with a boiling point of 156°C, and camphor, with a boiling point of 204°C, which type of distillation should be used to separate them?

____

12.3 Chromatography

High-Yield

LEARNING OBJECTIVES

After Chapter 12.3, you will be able to:

- Identify the properties that can be used to separate compounds through chromatography
- Differentiate between thin-layer, paper, column, gas, and high-performance liquid chromatography
- Describe the three main specialized types of columns used in column chromatography, and their methods for separation
- Predict the best chromatography method for a given mixture

Chromatography is another tool that uses physical and chemical properties to separate and identify compounds from a complex mixture. In all forms of chromatography discussed here, the concept is identical: the more similar a compound is to its surroundings (whether by polarity, charge, or other characteristics), the more it will stick to and move slowly through its surroundings.

KEY CONCEPT

Chromatography separates compounds based on how strongly they adhere to the solid, or stationary, phase (or in other words, how easily they come off into the mobile phase).

The process begins by placing the sample onto a solid medium called the **stationary phase**, or **adsorbent**. We then run the **mobile phase**, usually a liquid (or a gas in gas chromatography) through the stationary phase. This will displace (**elute**) the sample and carry it through the stationary phase. Depending on the characteristics of the substances in the sample and the polarity of the mobile phase, it will adhere to the stationary phase with differing strengths, causing the different substances to migrate at different speeds. This is called **partitioning**, and it represents an equilibrium between the two phases. Different compounds will have different **partitioning coefficients** and will elute at different rates. This results in separation within the stationary phase, allowing us to isolate each substance individually.

There are many different media that can be used as the stationary phase, each one exploiting different properties that allow us to separate out the desired compound. On the MCAT, the property most commonly used is polarity. For instance, thin-layer chromatography (TLC), which we will shortly discuss, uses silica gel, a highly polar substance, as its stationary phase. Cellulose, another polar substance, may also be used. This means that any polar compound will adhere well to the gel and thus move through (elute) slowly. When using column chromatography, size and charge both have a role in how quickly a compound moves through the stationary phase. Chromatography can use even strong interactions, such as antibody–ligand binding.

As mentioned earlier, chromatography is based on the speed at which compounds move through media. In practice, however, we will measure either how far each substance travels in a given amount of time (such as in TLC) or how long it takes to elute (as in column or gas chromatography).

The types of chromatography that we will discuss include thin-layer and paper chromatography, column chromatography, gas chromatography (also called gas–liquid chromatography), and high-performance liquid chromatography, or HPLC.

Thin-Layer and Paper Chromatography

Thin-layer chromatography and **paper chromatography** are extremely similar techniques, varying only in the medium used for the stationary phase. For thin-layer chromatography, a thin layer of silica gel or alumina adherent to an inert carrier sheet is used. For paper chromatography, as the name suggests, the medium used is paper, which is composed of cellulose.

For these techniques, the sample that we want to separate is placed directly onto the adsorbent itself; this is called **spotting** because we apply a small, well-defined spot of the sample directly onto the silica or paper plate. The plate is then **developed**, which involves placing the adsorbent upright in a developing chamber, usually a beaker with a lid or a wide-mouthed jar. At the bottom of this jar is a shallow pool of solvent, called the **eluent**. The spots of the sample must be above the level of the solvent, or else they will dissolve into the pool of solvent rather than running up the plate. When set up correctly, the solvent will creep up the plate by capillary action, carrying the various compounds in the sample with it at varying rates. When the solvent front nears the top of the plate, the plate is removed from the chamber and allowed to dry.

As mentioned before, TLC is often done with silica gel, which is polar and hydrophilic. The mobile phase, on the other hand, is usually an organic solvent of weak to moderate polarity, so it doesn't bind well to the gel. Because of this, nonpolar compounds dissolve in the organic solvent and move quickly as the solvent moves up the plate, whereas the more polar molecules stick to the gel. Thus, the more nonpolar the sample is, the further up the plate it will move, as shown in Figure 12.5.

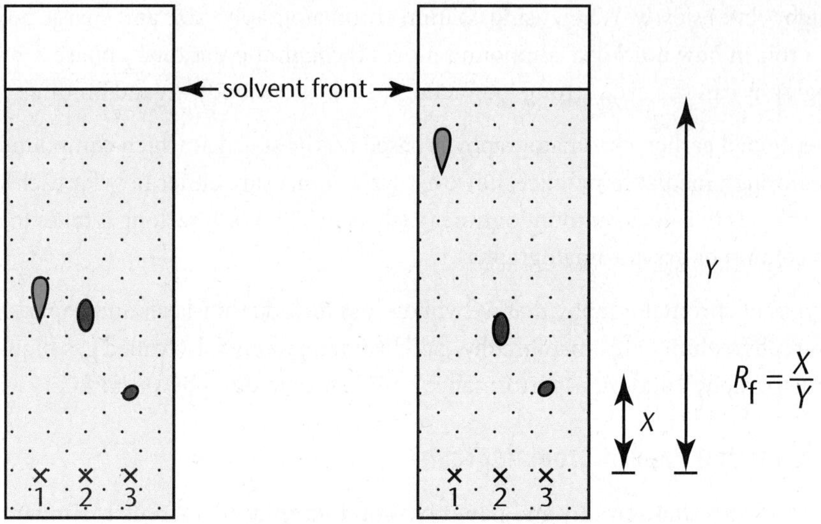

Figure 12.5 Thin-Layer Chromatography

Samples are placed at the "x" marks. As the nonpolar solvent moves up the plate via capillary action, the samples that are nonpolar move further up the plate along with the solvent, while the samples that are polar do not move as far.

Reverse-phase chromatography is the exact opposite. In this technique, the stationary phase used is nonpolar, so polar molecules move up the plate quickly, while nonpolar molecules stick more tightly to the stationary phase.

The spots of individual compounds are usually white, which makes them difficult or impossible to see on the white paper or TLC plate. To get around this problem, the developed plate can be placed under ultraviolet light, which will show any compounds that are ultraviolet-sensitive. Alternatively, iodine, phosphomolybdic acid, or vanillin can be used to stain the spots, although this will destroy the compounds such that they cannot be recovered.

When TLC is performed, compounds are generally identified using the **retardation factor (R_f)**, which is relatively constant for a particular compound in a given solvent. The R_f is calculated using the equation:

$$R_f = \frac{\text{distance spot moved}}{\text{distance solvent front moved}}$$

Equation 12.1

Because its value is relatively constant, the R_f value can be used to identify unknown compounds.

This technique is most frequently performed on a small scale to identify unknown compounds. It can also be used on a larger scale as a means of purification, a technique called **preparative TLC**. As the large plate develops, the larger spot of sample splits into bands of individual compounds, which can then be scraped off and washed to yield pure compounds.

Column Chromatography

The principles behind column chromatography are the same as for thin-layer chromatography, although there are some differences. First, **column chromatography** uses an entire column filled with silica or aluminum beads as an adsorbent, allowing for much greater separation. The setup for this is shown in Figure 12.6. In addition, thin-layer chromatography uses capillary action to move the solvent up the plate, whereas column chromatography uses gravity to move the solvent and compounds down the column. To speed up the process, one can force the solvent through the column using gas pressure, a technique called flash column chromatography. In column chromatography, the solvent polarity can also be changed to help elute the desired compound.

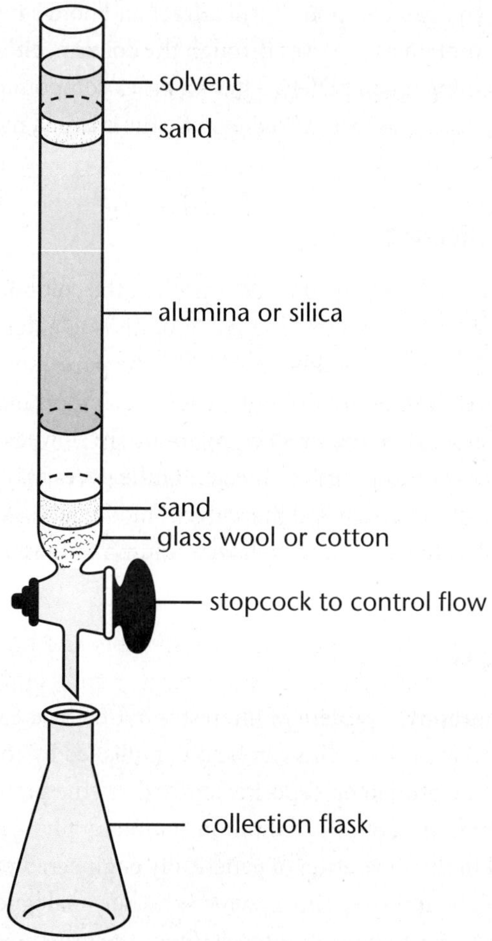

Figure 12.6 Column Chromatography

The sample is added to the top of the column, and a solvent is poured over it. The more similar the sample is to the mobile phase, the faster it elutes; the more similar it is to the stationary phase, the more slowly it will elute (if at all).

Eventually, the solvent drips out of the end of the column, and the different fractions that leave the column can be collected over time. Each fraction will contain different compounds. After collection, the solvent can be evaporated, leaving behind the compounds of interest. Column chromatography is particularly useful in biochemistry because it can be used to separate and collect macromolecules such as proteins or nucleic acids. There are several techniques that can be used to isolate specific materials, which are described in the following paragraphs, as well as in Chapter 3 of *MCAT Biochemistry Review*.

Ion-Exchange Chromatography

In **ion-exchange chromatography**, the beads in the column are coated with charged substances so that they attract or bind compounds that have an opposite charge. For instance, a positively charged compound will attract and hold a negatively charged backbone of DNA or protein as it passes through the column, either increasing its retention time or retaining it completely. After all other compounds have moved through the column, a salt gradient is used to elute the charged molecules that have stuck to the column.

Size-Exclusion Chromatography

In **size-exclusion chromatography**, the beads used in the column contain tiny pores of varying sizes. These tiny pores allow small compounds to enter the beads, thus slowing them down. Large compounds can't fit into the pores, so they will move around them and travel through the column faster. It is important to remember that in this type of chromatography, the small compounds are slowed down and retained longer—which may be counterintuitive. The size of the pores may be varied so that molecules with different molecular weights can be fractionated. A common approach in protein purification is to use an ion-exchange column followed by a size-exclusion column.

Affinity Chromatography

In **affinity chromatography**, a protein of interest is bound by creating a column with high affinity for that protein. This can be accomplished by coating beads with a receptor that binds the protein or a specific antibody to the protein; in either case, the protein is retained in the column. Common stationary phase molecules include nickel, which is used in the separation of genetically engineered proteins with histidine tags, antibodies or antigens, and enzyme substrate analogues, which mimic the natural substrate for an enzyme of interest. Once the protein is retained in the column, it can be eluted by washing the column with a free receptor (or target or antibody), which will compete with the bead-bound receptor and ultimately free the protein from the column. Eluents can also be created with a varying pH or salinity level that disrupts the bonds between the ligand and the protein of interest. The only drawback of the elution step is that the recovered substance can be bound to the eluent. If, for example, the eluent was an inhibitor of an enzyme, it could be difficult to remove.

Gas Chromatography

Gas chromatography (**GC**) is another method that can be used for qualitative separation. GC, also known as **vapor-phase chromatography** (**VPC**), is similar to the other types of chromatography and is shown in Figure 12.7. The main conceptual difference is that the eluent is a gas (usually helium or nitrogen) instead of a liquid. The adsorbent is a crushed metal or polymer inside a 30-foot column. This column is coiled and kept inside an oven to control its temperature. The mixture is then injected into the column and vaporized. The gaseous compounds travel through the column at different rates because they adhere to the adsorbent in the column to different degrees and will separate in space by the time they reach the end of the column. The injected compounds must be **volatile**: low melting-point, sublimable solids or vaporizable liquids. The compounds are registered by a detector, which records them as a peak on a chart.

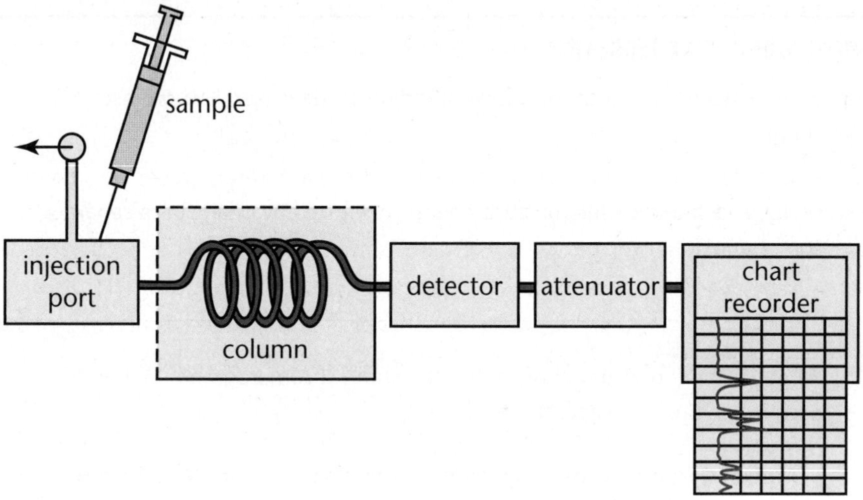

Figure 12.7 Gas Chromatography
The sample is injected into the column and moves with the gaseous mobile phase through a stationary liquid or solid phase; a computer identifies the sample components.

It is common to separate molecules using GC and then to inject the pure molecules into a **mass spectrometer** for molecular weight determination. **Mass spectrometry** involves the ionization and fragmentation of compounds; these fragments are then run through a magnetic field, which separates them by mass-to-charge ratio. The total molecular weight can thus be determined, or the relative concentrations of the different fragments can be calculated and compared against reference values to identify the compound.

High-Performance Liquid Chromatography

High-performance liquid chromatography (**HPLC**) was previously called high-pressure liquid chromatography. As the name suggests, the eluent is a liquid, and it travels through a column of a defined composition. There is a variety of stationary phases that can be chosen depending on the target molecule and the quantity of material that needs to be purified. This is fairly similar to column chromatography because the various compounds in solution will react differently with the adsorbent material. In the past, very high pressures were used, but recent advances allow for much lower pressures—hence the change in name. In HPLC, a small sample is injected into the column, and separation occurs as it flows through. The compounds pass through a detector and are collected as the solvent flows out of the end of the apparatus. The interface is similar to that used for GC because the entire process is computerized, but it uses liquid under pressure instead of gas. Because the whole process is under computer control, sophisticated solvent gradients as well as temperature can be applied to the column to help resolve the various compounds in the sample—hence the higher performance of HPLC over regular column chromatography.

MCAT CONCEPT CHECK 12.3

Before you move on, assess your understanding of the material with these questions.

1. What properties of molecules do thin-layer chromatography, paper chromatography, and standard column chromatography take advantage of to separate compounds?

   ____

2. What are the three specialized types of column chromatography? What does each use in order to separate the sample?

Type of Column Chromatography	Method for Separating Sample

3. In what way is gas chromatography distinct from all of the other techniques we have discussed?

   ____

4. What is the major historical distinction between HPLC and column chromatography? What is the major distinction now?
   - Historical distinction:

   ____

   - Current distinction:

   ____

Conclusion

Don't forget, the MCAT won't ask you to get into your lab coat and extract the product of a reaction! As long as you understand the principles governing these techniques and when you should apply them, you'll be in great shape. Remember that separation and purification techniques exploit physical properties of compounds, such as polarity, solubility, size and shape, and charge, to obtain a purified product. These properties can be traced back to intermolecular forces or properties of the molecules themselves. Having a variety of tools and methods to separate and collect a purified product is essential in practical organic chemistry, and choosing the proper techniques often requires knowledge and consideration of the desired product. When you look at the bigger picture, these methods may be easier to conceptualize than to actually apply in the lab!

Despite the subject's compelling relevance to everyday life, college organic chemistry often terrifies and alienates its students. The MCAT, on the other hand, doesn't ask you to memorize tables of reactants or regurgitate hundreds of named reactions from scratch. Instead, the MCAT asks you to look at the bigger picture, to know trends, and to participate in the logic of chemistry. We hope that studying for the MCAT has given you a chance to rediscover organic chemistry—to focus on the *how* and the *why*, instead of the *what*. Organic chemistry, like the MCAT as a whole, should be seen not as an obstacle but as an opportunity. So, work hard, have some fun along the way, and keep thinking about where you're heading—you can almost feel that white coat.

GO ONLINE

You've reviewed the content, now test your knowledge and critical thinking skills by completing a test-like passage set in your online resources!

CONCEPT SUMMARY

Solubility-Based Methods

- **Extraction** combines two immiscible liquids, one of which easily dissolves the compound of interest.
  - The polar (water) layer is called the **aqueous phase** and dissolves compounds with hydrogen bonding or polarity.
  - The nonpolar layer is called the **organic phase** and dissolves nonpolar compounds.
  - Extraction is carried out in a separatory funnel. One phase is collected, and the solvent is then evaporated.
  - Acid–base properties can be used to increase solubility.
- A **wash** is the reverse of extraction, in which a small amount of solvent that dissolves impurities is run over the compound of interest.
- **Filtration** isolates a solid (**residue**) from a liquid (**filtrate**).
  - **Gravity filtration** is used when the product of interest is in the filtrate. Hot solvent is used to maintain solubility.
  - **Vacuum filtration** is used when the product of interest is the solid. A vacuum is connected to the flask to pull the solvent through more quickly.
- In **recrystallization**, the product is dissolved in a minimum amount of hot solvent. If the impurities are more soluble, the crystals will reform while the flask cools, excluding the impurities.

Distillation

- **Distillation** separates liquids according to differences in their boiling points; the liquid with the lowest boiling point vaporizes first and is collected as the **distillate**.
- **Simple distillation** can be used if the boiling points are under 150°C and are at least 25°C apart.
- **Vacuum distillation** should be used if the boiling points are over 150°C to prevent degradation of the product.
- **Fractional distillation** should be used if the boiling points are less than 25°C apart because it allows more refined separation of liquids by boiling point.

Chromatography

- All forms of **chromatography** use two phases to separate compounds based on physical or chemical properties.
  - The **stationary phase** or **adsorbent** is usually a polar solid.
  - The **mobile phase** runs through the stationary phase and is usually a liquid or gas. This **elutes** the sample through the stationary phase.
  - Compounds with higher affinity for the stationary phase have smaller **retardation factors** and take longer to pass through, if at all; compounds with higher affinity for the mobile phase elute through more quickly. Compounds, therefore, get separated from each other, which is called **partitioning**.
- **Thin-layer** and **paper chromatography** are used to identify a sample.
  - The stationary phase is a polar material, such as silica, alumina, or paper.
  - The mobile phase is a nonpolar solvent, which climbs the card through capillary action.
  - The card is **spotted** and **developed**; R_f values can be calculated and compared to reference values.
  - **Reverse-phase chromatography** uses a nonpolar card with a polar solvent.
- **Column chromatography** utilizes polarity, size, or affinity to separate compounds based on their physical or chemical properties.
  - The stationary phase is a column containing silica or alumina beads.
  - The mobile phase is a nonpolar solvent, which travels through the column by gravity.
  - In **ion-exchange chromatography**, the beads are coated with charged substances to bind compounds with opposite charge.
  - In **size-exclusion chromatography**, the beads have small pores which trap smaller compounds and allow larger compounds to travel through faster.
  - In **affinity chromatography**, the column is made to have high affinity for a compound by coating the beads with a receptor or antibody to the compound.
- **Gas chromatography** separates vaporizable compounds according to how well they adhere to the adsorbent in the column.
  - The stationary phase is a coil of crushed metal or a polymer.
  - The mobile phase is a nonreactive gas.
  - Gas chromatography may be combined in sequence with **mass spectrometry**, which ionizes and fragments molecules and passes these fragments through a magnetic field to determine molecular weight or structure.
- **High-performance liquid chromatography** (HPLC) is similar to column chromatography but uses sophisticated computer-mediated solvent and temperature gradients. It is used if the sample size is small or if forces such as capillary action will affect results. It was formerly called high-pressure liquid chromatography.

ANSWERS TO CONCEPT CHECKS

12.1

1. The two solvents must be immiscible and must have different polarity or acid–base properties that allow a compound of interest to dissolve more easily in one than the other.
2. It is better to do three washes with 10 mL than to do one with 30 mL; more of the compound of interest would be extracted with multiple sequential extractions than one large one.
3. Acid dissolves better in an aqueous base because it will dissociate to form the conjugate base and, being more highly charged, will become more soluble. Note that *like dissolves like* applies to polarity; acids and bases dissolve more easily in solutions with the opposite acid–base characteristics.

12.2

1. Distillation takes advantage of differences in boiling points in order to separate solutions of miscible liquids.
2. A solution of ether and methylene chloride, which have very close boiling points, can be separated by using fractional distillation.
3. Vacuum distillation would be the best technique to separate two chemicals with such high boiling points because the decreased ambient pressure will allow them to boil at a lower temperature.

12.3

1. Each of these methods separates compounds using charge and polarity.
2.

Type of Column Chromatography	Method for Separating Sample
Ion-exchange	The column is given a charge, which attracts molecules with the opposite charge.
Size-exclusion	Small pores are used; smaller molecules are trapped, while larger molecules pass through the column.
Affinity	Specific receptors or antibodies can trap the target in the column; the target must then be washed out using other solutions.

3. As the name suggests, gas chromatography is simply the same technique of mobile and stationary phases performed with a gaseous eluent (instead of liquid). The stationary phase is usually a crushed metal or polymer.
4. Historically, HPLC was performed at high pressures, whereas column chromatography uses gravity to pull the solution through the column. Now, HPLC is performed with sophisticated and variable solvent and temperature gradients, allowing for much more specific separation of compounds than column chromatography; high pressures are no longer required.

SCIENCE MASTERY ASSESSMENT EXPLANATIONS

1. **B**

Fractional distillation is the most effective procedure for separating two liquids that boil within a few degrees of each other. Ethyl acetate and ethanol boil well within 25°C of each other and thus would be good candidates for fractional distillation. Fractional distillation could also be used for the liquids in **(C)**, but would require lower pressures because of their high boiling points.

2. **C**

By extracting with sodium hydroxide, benzoic acid will be converted to its sodium salt, sodium benzoate. Sodium benzoate, unlike its conjugate acid, will dissolve in an aqueous solution. The aqueous layer simply has to be acidified afterward to retrieve benzoic acid. **(A)** is incorrect because diethyl ether and tetrahydrofuran are both nonpolar and are miscible. Hydrochloric acid will not transform benzoic acid into a soluble salt, so **(B)** is incorrect. Finally, **(D)** is incorrect because protonated benzoic acid has limited solubility in water.

3. **D**

It is more effective to perform four successive extractions with small amounts of ether than to perform one extraction with a large amount of ether.

4. **D**

Hexane is less polar than ether and, therefore, is less likely to displace polar compounds adsorbed to the silica gel. This would decrease the distance these polar compounds would travel, decreasing R_f values.

5. **D**

In column chromatography, as in TLC, the less polar compound travels most rapidly. This means that 1-naphthalenemethanol, with the highest R_f value, would travel most rapidly and would be the first to elute from the column.

6. **A**

This is an example of reverse-phase chromatography. The solvent system is polar, which means that the most polar compound will travel the furthest up the card, resulting in the largest R_f. This gives compound III the largest R_f, which corresponds to spot A.

7. **B**

Because methylene chloride is denser than brine (salt water), the organic layer will settle at the bottom of the funnel. Methylene chloride is not soluble in water, eliminating **(C)**.

8. **B**

Silica gels are polar. Polarity is used to selectively attract specific solutes within a nonpolar solvent phase. Although silica gels have other properties, this is the most important to TLC.

9. **B**

In this question, three substances must be separated using a combination of techniques. The first step should be the most obvious: remove the sand by filtration. The remaining compounds—benzoic acid and naphthalene—are still dissolved in ether. If the solution is extracted with an aqueous base, the benzoate anion is formed and becomes dissolved in the aqueous layer, while naphthalene, a nonpolar compound, remains in the ether. Finally, evaporation of the ether will yield purified naphthalene.

10. **C**

This is the only option that would be effectively separated by a simple distillation. **(B)** would require vacuum distillation because the boiling points are over 150°C. In **(A)** and **(D)**, the boiling points are within 25°C of each other and would therefore require fractional distillation in order to be separated.

11. **C**

Affinity chromatography, using the target for the biological effector or a specific antibody, would work best in this case. It will specifically bind the protein of interest and keep it in the column.

12. **D**

Because this solution is composed of a much larger molecule and a much smaller molecule, size-exclusion chromatography would effectively remove the smaller insulin molecule into the fraction retained in the column and allow the titin to be eluted. Affinity chromatography, **(C)**, could also be used, but comes with a risk of rendering the titin unusable; the eluent run through an affinity chromatography column often binds to the target molecule.

13. **B**

Each of these is the mobile phase of the system, in which the solutes are dissolved and move. The stationary phase in gas chromatography is usually a crushed metal or polymer; the stationary phase in paper chromatography is paper.

14. **C**

Warm or hot solvent is generally used in gravity filtration to keep the desired product soluble. This allows the product to remain in the filtrate, which can then be collected. In this case, the student likely used solvent that was too cold, and the product crystallized out. The product should be present in the residue.

15. **B**

Because the lactoferrin proteins are likely to be charged, as is the resin described in the question, this is an example of ion-exchange chromatography. The charged protein molecules will stick to the column, while the remainder of the milk washes through and can later be washed off of the column and collected.

Consult your online resources for additional practice. GO ONLINE

EQUATIONS TO REMEMBER

(12.1) **Retardation factor:** $R_f = \frac{\text{distance spot moved}}{\text{distance solvent front moved}}$

SHARED CONCEPTS

Biochemistry Chapter 3
Nonenzymatic Protein Function and Protein Analysis

General Chemistry Chapter 7
Thermochemistry

General Chemistry Chapter 8
The Gas Phase

General Chemistry Chapter 9
Solutions

General Chemistry Chapter 10
Acids and Bases

Organic Chemistry Chapter 11
Spectroscopy

GLOSSARY

α-Carbon–The carbon adjacent to a carbonyl; in amino acids, the chiral stereocenter in all amino acids except glycine.

α-Hydrogen–Hydrogen atoms connected to α-carbons adjacent to carbonyls.

α-State–A magnetic state seen in NMR spectroscopy in which nuclei have magnetic moments that are aligned with an incident magnetic field, thus having lower energy.

Absolute conformation–The exact spatial arrangement of atoms or groups in a chiral molecule around a single chiral atom, designated by (*R*) or (*S*).

Acetal–A functional group that contains a carbon atom bonded to two —OR groups, an alkyl chain, and a hydrogen atom.

Achiral–A molecule that either does not contain a chiral center or contains chiral centers and a plane of symmetry; as such, it has a superimposable mirror image.

Acid dissociation constant (K_a)–A measurement of the strength of an acid in solution; the higher the K_a, the lower the pK_a and the stronger the acid.

Affinity chromatography–A special type of column chromatography in which a column is customized to bind a substance of interest.

Aldehyde–A functional group containing a carbonyl and a hydrogen (RCOH); always found at the end of a chain.

Aldol condensation–A reaction in which an aldehyde or ketone acts as both the electrophile and nucleophile, resulting in the formation of a carbon–carbon bond in a new molecule called an aldol.

Alkane–A simple hydrocarbon molecule with the formula C_nH_{2n+2}.

Amide–A functional group containing a carbonyl and an amino group ($RCONR_2$).

Amino acids–Dipolar compounds that contain an amine and a carboxylic acid attached to a single carbon (the α-carbon); the building blocks of peptides.

Amphoteric–Describes molecules that can act as both acids and bases.

Angle strain–Increased energy that results when bond angles deviate from their ideal values.

Anhydride–A functional group containing two carbonyls separated by an oxygen atom (RCOOCOR); often the condensation dimer of a carboxylic acid.

***Anti* conformation**–A type of staggered conformation in which the two largest groups are antiperiplanar to each other; the most energetically favorable conformation.

Antibonding orbital–A higher-energy, less stable orbital that results from the overlap of wave functions with opposite signs.

Antiperiplanar–A conformation in which substituents are in the same plane, but on opposite sides of a bond.

Axial–Describes groups on a cyclic molecule that are perpendicular to the plane of the molecule, pointing straight up or down.

Azimuthal quantum number (l)–Describes the subshell in which an electron is found; possible values range from 0 to $n - 1$, with $l = 0$ representing the *s* subshell, $l = 1$ representing *p*, $l = 2$ representing *d*, and $l = 3$ representing *f*.

β-lactam–Four-membered cyclic amides that are more reactive to hydrolysis than linear amides or larger cyclic amides; often used as the backbone for antibiotics.

β-state–A magnetic state seen in NMR spectroscopy in which nuclei have been irradiated with radiofrequency pulses to bring them to a higher-energy state.

Bonding orbital–A lower-energy, more stable orbital that results from the overlap of wave functions with the same sign.

Carbonyl–A double bond between a carbon and an oxygen.

Carboxylic acid–A functional group that contains a carbonyl and a hydroxyl group on the same carbon (RCOOH).

Carboxylic acid derivative–A compound that can be created from a carboxylic acid by nucleophilic acyl substitution; includes anhydrides, esters, amides, and others.

Chemical properties–Characteristics of compounds that change chemical composition during a reaction; determine how a molecule will react with other molecules.

Chemical shift (δ)–An arbitrary variable used to plot NMR spectra; measured in parts per million (ppm).

Chemoselectivity–A reaction's preference for one location over another within a molecule.

Chiral–A molecule or carbon atom bonded to four different groups and without a plane of symmetry; thus, it is not superimposable on its mirror image and has an enantiomer.

Chiral center–Atoms that are chiral within a molecule.

Chromatography–A tool used to separate compounds based on how strongly they adhere to a stationary phase or travel with a mobile phase.

Cis–A molecule in which the two substituents are on the same side of an immovable bond.

***Cis–trans* isomers**–Diastereomers with different arrangements of substituents around an immovable bond.

Column chromatography–A type of chromatography that uses a column filled with silica or alumina beads as an adsorbent, allowing for separation; uses gravity to move the solvent and compounds down the column.

Condensation reaction–A reaction that combines two molecules into one, with the loss of a small molecule.

Configuration–The spatial arrangement of the atoms or groups in a molecule.

Configurational isomers–Isomers that can only interconvert by breaking bonds; include enantiomers, diastereomers, and *cis–trans* isomers.

Conformational isomers–Isomers that are the same molecule, just at different points in their natural rotation about a σ bond.

Conjugation–Alternating single and multiple bonds that create a system of parallel unhybridized *p*-orbitals; thus, electrons can be shared between these orbitals, forming electron clouds above and below the plane of the molecule and stabilizing the molecule.

Constitutional isomers–Molecules that have the same molecular formulas but different connectivity; also called structural isomers.

Coordinate covalent bond–A covalent bond in which both electrons in the bond come from the same starting atom.

Coupling–In NMR spectroscopy, a phenomenon that occurs when there are protons in such close proximity to each other that their magnetic moments affect each other's appearance in the NMR spectrum by subdividing the peak into subpeaks; also called splitting.

Coupling constant (*J*)–The magnitude of splitting in NMR spectroscopy, measured in hertz.

Covalent–One of two types of chemical bonds in which electrons are shared between atoms.

Cyanohydrin–A functional group containing a nitrile ($-C{\equiv}N$) and a hydroxyl group.

***d*-orbital**–An atomic orbital that is composed of four symmetrical lobes and contains two nodes.

Decarboxylation–The complete loss of a carboxyl group as carbon dioxide.

Deprotection–Reversion of a protecting group to its original functional group.

Deprotonation–The removal of a hydrogen cation (H^+) from a molecule.

Deshielding–The phenomenon of atoms pulling electron density away from surrounding atoms; in NMR spectroscopy, pulls a group further downfield on the spectrum.

Developing chamber–A beaker with a lid or wide-mouthed jar used in thin-layer chromatography.

Dialcohols–Alcohols with two hydroxyl groups that are commonly used as protecting groups for aldehyde or ketone carbonyls; also called diols.

Diastereomers–Non-mirror-image configurational isomers that differ at at least one–but not all–chiral carbons; have different chemical and physical properties.

Distillate–The liquid evaporated, condensed, and collected during distillation.

Distillation–A separation and purification technique that takes advantage of differences in boiling point to separate two liquids by vaporization and condensation.

Doublet–Two peaks of identical intensity in an NMR spectrum that are equally spaced around the true chemical shift of a group of protons; it results from splitting by another hydrogen.

Downfield–Movement toward the left in an NMR spectrum.

Electron-donating–Describes groups that push additional electron density toward another atom; stabilizes positive charges and destabilizes negative charges while decreasing acidity.

Electron-withdrawing–Describes groups that pull electron density away from another atom; stabilizes negative charges and destabilizes positive charges while increasing acidity.

Electrophile–"Electron-loving" atoms with a positive charge or positive polarization that can accept an electron pair when forming new bonds with a nucleophile.

Eluent–The solvent used in chromatography, after it has passed through the stationary phase.

Elute–To displace with solvent, as in thin-layer chromatography.

Enantiomers–Nonsuperimposable mirror images of a chiral molecule; have all the same physical and chemical properties except for rotation of plane-polarized light and reactions in a chiral environment.

Enol–The resonance form of a carbonyl that has a carbon–carbon double bond (*ene*) and an alcohol (*–ol*).

Equatorial–Describes groups on a cyclic molecule that are in the plane of the molecule.

Ester–A functional group containing a carbonyl and an alkoxy group (RCOOR).

Extraction–The transfer of a dissolved compound from a starting solvent into a solvent in which the product is more soluble.

Fingerprint region–In an IR spectrum, the region of 1500 to 400 cm^{-1} where more complex vibration patterns, caused by the motion of the molecule as a whole, can be seen; it is characteristic of each individual molecule.

Fischer esterification–The formation of an ester from a carboxylic acid and an alcohol in acidic conditions.

Fischer projection–A system to represent three-dimensional molecules in which horizontal lines indicate bonds that project out from the plane of the page (wedges) and vertical lines indicate bonds going into the plane of the page (dashes); points of intersection represent carbon atoms.

Flash column chromatography–A technique that speeds up column chromatography by forcing the solvent through the column by increasing pressure with a nonreactive gas.

Fractional distillation–A modified form of distillation used to separate two liquids with similar boiling points (less than 25°C apart); uses a fractionation column, which contains inert materials onto which the liquids can condense and reflux back into the reaction vial, allowing more refined separation.

Fraction–A volume of eluted fluid from column chromatography; each fraction contains different compounds that are collected as they leave the column.

Gabriel (malonic-ester) synthesis–A method of synthesizing amino acids that uses potassium phthalimide and diethyl bromomalonate followed by an alkyl halide; two substitution reactions are followed by hydrolysis and decarboxylation.

Gas chromatography (GC)–A type of chromatography used to separate vaporizable compounds; the stationary phase is a crushed metal or polymer, and the mobile phase is a nonreactive gas.

***Gauche* conformation**–A type of staggered conformation in which the two largest groups are 60° apart.

Geminal diol–A functional group with two hydroxyl groups on the same carbon; also called a hydrate.

Hemiacetal–A functional group that contains a carbon atom bonded to one –OR group, one –OH group, an alkyl chain, and a hydrogen atom.

Hemiketal–A functional group that contains a carbon atom bonded to one –OR group, one –OH group, and two alkyl chains.

Heterolysis–Cleavage of a bond in which both electrons are given to the same atom.

High-performance liquid chromatography (HPLC)–A form of chromatography in which a small sample is put into a column that can be manipulated with sophisticated solvent gradients to allow very refined separation and characterization; formerly called high-pressure liquid chromatography.

Highest occupied molecular orbital (HOMO)–The highest-energy molecular orbital containing electrons; in UV spectroscopy, electrons are excited from the HOMO to the LUMO.

Hydride reagent–Reducing reagents containing hydride anions (H^-).

Hydrogen bonding–An intermolecular force that results from the extreme polarity of the bonds when hydrogen atoms are attached to highly electronegative atoms (N, O, or F).

Hydrolysis–The breaking of a molecule using water.

Hydroxyl group–An -OH group; seen in alcohols, hemiacetals and hemiketals, carboxylic acids, water, and other compounds.

Hydroxyquinone–A compound containing a quinone (conjugated ring with carbonyls) and a hydroxyl group.

Imine–A double bond between a carbon and a nitrogen.

Immiscible–Describes two solvents that will not mix with or dissolve each other.

Induction–The pull of electron density across sigma bonds.

Infrared (IR) spectroscopy–A technique that measures molecular vibrations at different frequencies, from which specific bonds can be determined; functional groups can be inferred based on this information.

Inorganic phosphate (P_i)–Derived from phosphoric acid, the molecule that forms high-energy bonds for energy transfer in nucleotide triphosphates like ATP; also used for enzyme regulation.

Ion-exchange chromatography–A special type of column chromatography in which the beads in the column are coated with charged substances so that they attract or bind compounds with an opposite charge.

Ionic–One of two types of chemical bonds in which electrons are transferred from one atom to another.

Isomers–Molecules with the same molecular formula but different chemical structures.

Jones oxidation–An oxidation reaction in which primary alcohols are oxidized to carboxylic acids and secondary alcohols are oxidized to ketones; requires CrO_3 dissolved with dilute sulfuric acid in acetone.

Ketal–A functional group that contains a carbon atom bonded to two –OR groups and two alkyl chains.

Ketone–A functional group containing a carbonyl with two alkyl groups (RCOR); always found within a chain.

Lactam–A cyclic amide; named according to the Greek letter of the carbon closing the ring.

Lactone–A cyclic ester; named according to the Greek letter of the carbon closing the ring and for the straight-chain form of the compound.

Leaving group–The molecular fragment that retains electrons after heterolysis; must be stable in solution.

Lewis acid–An electron acceptor in the formation of a covalent bond.

Lewis base–An electron donor in the formation of a covalent bond.

Lowest unoccupied molecular orbital (LUMO)–The lowest-energy molecular orbital that does not contain electrons; in UV spectroscopy, electrons are excited from the HOMO to the LUMO.

Magnetic quantum number (m_l)–Describes the orbital in which an electron is found; possible values range from $-l$ to $+l$.

***Meso* compound**–A molecule that has chiral centers but is not optically active because it has an internal plane of symmetry.

Mesylate–A compound containing the functional group $-SO_3CH_3$, derived from methanesulfonic acid.

Michael addition–A reaction in which a carbanion attacks an α,β-unsaturated carbonyl.

Mobile phase–A liquid (or a gas in gas chromatography) that is run through the stationary phase in chromatography.

Molecular orbital–The resulting electron structure when two atomic orbitals combine.

Multiplet–Peaks that have more than four shifts in NMR spectroscopy.

Newman projection–A method of visualizing a compound in which the line of sight is down a carbon–carbon bond axis.

Node–In orbital structure, an area where the probability of finding an electron is zero.

Nonbonded strain–Increased energy that results when nonadjacent atoms or groups compete for the same space; also called steric strain.

Nuclear magnetic resonance (NMR) spectroscopy–A technique that measures the alignment of magnetic moments from certain molecular nuclei with an external magnetic field; can be used to determine the connectivity and functional groups in a molecule.

Nucleophiles–"Nucleus-loving" atoms with either lone pairs or π bonds that can be used to form new bonds with electrophiles.

Nucleophilic acyl substitution–The substitution of a nucleophile for the leaving group of a carboxylic acid or carboxylic acid derivative.

Optical isomers–A type of configurational isomers that have different spatial arrangements of substituents, which affect the rotation of plane-polarized light.

Organic phosphates–Organic molecules–usually nucleotides–that have a variable number of phosphate groups attached.

Oxidation–Loss of electrons causing an increase in oxidation state; increasing bonds to oxygen or other heteroatoms in a molecule.

Oxidation state–An indication of the hypothetical charge that an atom would have if all of its bonds were completely ionic.

Oxidizing agent–An element or compound that accepts an electron from another species, thereby being reduced in the process.

***p*-orbital**–An atomic orbital that is composed of two lobes located symmetrically about the nucleus and contains a node.

Paper chromatography–A type of chromatography that uses paper as the stationary phase.

Partitioning–When components in a sample adhere differentially to the mobile and stationary phases of a chromatographic setup; this causes the different substances to migrate at different speeds through the stationary phase.

Peptide bond–An amide bond formed between two amino acids through a condensation (nucleophilic acyl substitution) reaction.

Phenol–An alcohol with an aromatic ring, which has slightly more acidic hydroxyl hydrogens than other alcohols.

Phosphodiester bond–The type of bond linking the sugar moieties of adjacent nucleotides in DNA.

Physical properties–Characteristics of compounds that do not change chemical composition, such as melting point, boiling point, solubility, odor, color, and density.

Pi (π) bond–The bonding molecular orbital formed when two parallel *p*-orbitals share electrons; exists as electrons clouds above and below the sigma (σ) bond between the two nuclei.

Polarity–An uneven distribution of charge caused by atoms in the same molecule having different electronegativities.

Polypeptide–A molecule formed from multiple amino acids connected by peptide bonds.

Preparative thin-layer chromatography–Large-scale use of thin-layer chromatography (TLC) as a means of purification; as the large plate develops, the larger spot of sample splits into bands of individual compounds, which can then be scraped off and washed to yield pure compounds.

Principal quantum number (*n*)–Describes the shell in which an electron is found; values range from 1 to ∞.

Protonation–The addition of a hydrogen cation (H^+) to a molecule.

Pyrophosphate (PP_i)–The ester dimer of phosphate $\left(P_2O_7^{4-}\right)$; released when a new nucleotide is joined to a growing strand of DNA by DNA polymerase.

Quinone–A compound produced by the oxidation of a phenol containing a conjugated ring with ketones.

R group–In general, an alkyl chain; in amino acid chemistry, the variable side chain on the α-carbon.

Racemic mixture–A mixture where both (+) and (−) enantiomers are present in equal concentrations.

Reduction–Gain of electrons causing a decrease in oxidation state; decreasing bonds to oxygen or other heteroatoms in a molecule.

Relative configuration–The spatial arrangement of groups in a chiral molecule compared to another chiral molecule.

Resonance–Delocalization of π electrons, which increases stability of a molecule.

Resonance structure–A possible arrangement of π electrons in a molecule; the actual electronic structure of a molecule is the weighted average of resonance structures, based on their stability.

Retardation factor (R_f)–A ratio used in thin-layer chromatography to identify a compound; calculated as how far the compound traveled relative to how far the solvent front traveled.

Retro-aldol reaction–The reverse of an aldol condensation reaction, in which a carbon–carbon bond is cleaved with heat and base, yielding two aldehydes, two ketones, or one of each.

Reverse-phase chromatography–The opposite of traditional thin-layer chromatography, in which the stationary phase is nonpolar and the mobile phase is polar.

Ring strain–Energy created in a cyclic molecule by angle strain, torsional strain, and nonbonded strain; determines if a ring is stable enough to stay intact.

***s*-orbital**–An atomic orbital that is spherical and symmetrical, centered on the nucleus.

Saponification–The process by which fats are hydrolyzed under basic conditions to produce soap.

Separatory funnel–A piece of laboratory equipment used in extraction; immiscible solvents are separated by gravity, causing the denser layer to sink to the bottom, where it can be removed by turning the stopcock at the bottom.

Shielding–The phenomenon of atoms pushing electron density toward surrounding atoms; in NMR spectroscopy, pulls a group further upfield on the spectrum.

Sigma (σ) bond–The bonding molecular orbital formed by head-to-head or tail-to-tail overlap of atomic orbitals; all single bonds are sigma bonds.

Simple distillation–Distillation without any special features; can be used to separate liquids that boil below 150°C and that have at least a 25°C difference in boiling points.

Size-exclusion chromatography–A special type of column chromatography in which the beads in the column contain tiny pores of varying sizes, slowing down small compounds that enter the beads.

sp–A hybrid orbital with 50% *s*-character and 50% *p*-character.

***sp*²**–A hybrid orbital with 33% *s*-character and 67% *p*-character.

***sp*³**–A hybrid orbital with 25% *s*-character and 75% *p*-character.

Specific rotation ($[\alpha]$)–A standardized measure of a compound's ability to rotate plane-polarized light.

Spectroscopy–Laboratory technique that relies on measurement of the energy differences between the possible states of a molecular system by determining the frequencies of electromagnetic radiation (light) absorbed by the molecules or response to a magnetic field.

Spin quantum number (m_s)–Describes the intrinsic spin of the two electrons in an orbital by arbitrarily assigning one of the electrons a spin of $+\frac{1}{2}$ and the other a spin of $-\frac{1}{2}$.

Spotting–In thin-layer chromatography, placing the sample directly onto the adsorbent as a small, well-defined spot.

Staggered conformation–When a molecule has no overlapping substituents along the line of sight between two carbons, as in a Newman projection.

Stationary phase–A solid medium onto which a sample is placed for chromatography; also called the adsorbent.

Stereogenic–Describes a chiral center in a molecule.

Stereoisomers–Isomers that have the same chemical formula and the same atomic connectivity, but differ in how atoms are arranged in space; any isomer that is not a structural isomer is a stereoisomer.

Stereoselective–A reaction that forms an unequal distribution of isomer products that is determined by stability of those products.

Stereospecific–A reaction that preferentially yields a specific conformation of product, such as S_N2 reactions.

Steric hindrance–The prevention of a reaction at a particular location in a molecule by substituent groups around the reactive site.

Steric protection–The prevention of the formation of alternative products using a protecting group.

Strecker synthesis–A method of synthesizing amino acids that uses condensation between an aldehyde and hydrogen cyanide, followed by hydrolysis.

Structural isomers–Molecules that have the same molecular formulas but different connectivity; also called constitutional isomers.

Substituent–Any functional group that is not part of the parent chain.

Tautomer–An isomer that differs from another by the placement of a proton and a double bond.

Tetramethylsilane (TMS)–The calibration standard that marks 0 ppm when plotting an NMR spectrum.

Thin-layer chromatography (TLC)–A type of chromatography that uses silica gel or alumina on a card as the medium for the stationary phase.

Torsional strain–Increased energy that results when molecules assume eclipsed or *gauche* staggered conformations.

Tosylate–A compound containing the functional group $-SO_3C_6H_4CH_3$, derived from toluenesulfonic acid.

Totally eclipsed conformation–A type of conformation in which the two largest groups are 0° apart; the most energetically unfavorable conformation.

Trans–A molecule in which the two substituents are on opposite sides of an immovable bond.

Transesterification–The process that transforms one ester to another when an alcohol acts as a nucleophile and displaces the alkoxy group on an ester.

Triacylglycerols–Esters of long-chain carboxylic acids (fatty acids) and glycerol (1,2,3-propanetriol); used as a storage form of energy.

Triplet–Three peaks with an area ratio of 1:2:1 in an NMR spectrum that are centered around the true chemical shift of a group of protons; results from splitting by two equivalent hydrogens.

Ubiquinone–A biologically active quinone that is a vital electron carrier in the electron transport chain; also called coenzyme Q.

Ultraviolet (UV) spectroscopy–A technique that measures absorbance of ultraviolet light of various wavelengths passing through a sample.

Upfield–Movement to the right in an NMR spectrum.

Vacuum distillation–A modified form of distillation used to separate two liquids with boiling points over 150°C; lowers the pressure to decrease the temperature at which a liquid will boil.

Vicinal diol–A dialcohol with hydroxyl groups on adjacent carbons.

Wash–The reverse of extraction, in which a small amount of solvent is poured over the compound of interest to dissolve and remove impurities.

Wavenumber–An analog of frequency used for infrared spectra instead of wavelength.

Zwitterion–A compound that contains charges but is overall neutral.

INDEX

G

H

I

J

K

L

M

N

O

P

ART CREDITS

Chapter 2 Cover—Image credited to Vladyslav Starozhylov. From Shutterstock.

Chapter 3 Cover—Image credited to FikMik. From Shutterstock.

Chapter 4 Cover—Image credited to Andrea Danti. From Shutterstock.

Chapter 5 Cover—Image credited to Wollertz. From Shutterstock.

Chapter 7 Cover—Image credited to Science Photo Library – Inti St Clair. From Getty Images.

Chapter 8 Cover—Image credited to Quayside. From Shutterstock.

Chapter 9 Cover—Image credited to Mike Laptev. From Shutterstock.

Chapter 11 Cover—Image credited to Oliver Sved. From Shutterstock.

Figure 11.3 (MRI) Source: Krishna Rao, Uniformed Services University (Illustration) Image adapted from source: sdbs.db.aist.go.jp (National Institute of Advanced Industrial Science and Technology)

Chapter 12 Cover—Image credited to luchschen. From Shutterstock.

Notes

Notes

Notes

Notes

Notes

Notes

Notes

KAPLAN

MCAT® BIOLOGY REVIEW 2024–2025

ONLINE + BOOK

Edited by Alexander Stone Macnow, MD

MCAT®
BIOLOGY REVIEW
2024–2025

ONLINE + BOOK

ACKNOWLEDGMENTS

Editor-in-Chief, 2024–2025 Edition
M. Dominic Eggert

Contributing Editors, 2024–2025 Edition
Christopher Durland; Charles Pierce, MD; Jason Selzer

Prior Edition Editorial Staff: Brandon Deason, MD; Christopher Durland; M. Dominic Eggert; Tyler Fara; Elizabeth Flagge; Adam Grey; Jason Selzer; Lauren K. White

Published by Kaplan North America, LLC dba Kaplan Publishing
1515 West Cypress Creek Road
Fort Lauderdale, Florida 33309

ISBN: 978-1-5062-8685-3

10 9 8 7 6 5 4 3

TABLE OF CONTENTS

GO ONLINE

kaptest.com/booksonline

THE *KAPLAN MCAT REVIEW* TEAM

Alexander Stone Macnow, MD
Editor-in-Chief

Áine Lorié, PhD
Editor

Pamela Willingham, MSW
Editor

Derek Rusnak, MA
Editor

Melinda Contreras, MS
Kaplan MCAT Faculty

Mikhail Alexeeff
Kaplan MCAT Faculty

Samantha Fallon
Kaplan MCAT Faculty

Laura L. Ambler
Kaplan MCAT Faculty

Jason R. Selzer
Kaplan MCAT Faculty

Krista L. Buckley, MD
Kaplan MCAT Faculty

M. Dominic Eggert
Editor

Kristen L. Russell, ME
Editor

MCAT faculty reviewers: Elmar R. Aliyev; James Burns; Jonathan Cornfield; Alisha Maureen Crowley; Brandon Deason, MD; Nikolai Dorofeev, MD; Benjamin Downer, MS; Colin Doyle; Christopher Durland; Marilyn Engle; Eleni M. Eren; Raef Ali Fadel; Elizabeth Flagge; Adam Grey; Tyra Hall-Pogar, PhD; Justine Harkness, PhD; Scott Huff; Samer T. Ismail; Aeri Kim, PhD; Elizabeth A. Kudlaty; Kelly Kyker-Snowman, MS; Ningfei Li; John P. Mahon; Brandon McKenzie; Matthew A. Meier; Nainika Nanda; Caroline Nkemdilim Opene; Kaitlyn E. Prenger; Uneeb Qureshi; Bela G. Starkman, PhD; Michael Paul Tomani, MS; Nicholas M. White; Allison Ann Wilkes, MS; Kerranna Williamson, MBA; MJ Wu; and Tony Yu.

Thanks to Rebecca Anderson; Jeff Batzli; Eric Chiu; Tim Eich; Tyler Fara; Owen Farcy; Dan Frey; Robin Garmise; Rita Garthaffner; Joanna Graham; Allison Gudenau; Allison Harm; Beth Hoffberg; Aaron Lemon-Strauss; Keith Lubeley; Diane McGarvey; Petros Minasi; Beena P V; John Polstein; Deeangelee Pooran-Kublall, MD, MPH; Rochelle Rothstein, MD; Larry Rudman; Srividhya Sankar; Sylvia Tidwell Scheuring; Carly Schnur; Aiswarya Sivanand; Todd Tedesco; Karin Tucker; Lee Weiss; Christina Wheeler; Kristen Workman; Amy Zarkos; and the countless others who made this project possible.

GETTING STARTED CHECKLIST

Getting Started Checklist

- [ ] Register for your free online assets—including full-length tests, Science Review Videos, and additional practice materials—at **www.kaptest.com/moreonline**.
- [ ] Create a study calendar that ensures you complete content review and sufficient practice by Test Day!
- [ ] As you finish a chapter and the online practice for that chapter, check it off on the table of contents.
- [ ] Register to take the MCAT at **www.aamc.org/mcat**.
- [ ] Set aside time during your prep to make sure the rest of your application—personal statement, recommendations, and other materials—is ready to go!
- [ ] Take a moment to admire your completed checklist, then get back to the business of prepping for this exam!

PREFACE

And now it starts: your long, yet fruitful journey toward wearing a white coat. Proudly wearing that white coat, though, is hopefully only part of your motivation. You are reading this book because you want to be a healer.

If you're serious about going to medical school, then you are likely already familiar with the importance of the MCAT in medical school admissions. While the holistic review process puts additional weight on your experiences, extracurricular activities, and personal attributes, the fact remains: along with your GPA, your MCAT score remains one of the two most important components of your application portfolio—at least early in the admissions process. Each additional point you score on the MCAT pushes you in front of thousands of other students and makes you an even more attractive applicant. But the MCAT is not simply an obstacle to overcome; it is an opportunity to show schools that you will be a strong student and a future leader in medicine.

We at Kaplan take our jobs very seriously and aim to help students see success not only on the MCAT, but as future physicians. We work with our learning science experts to ensure that we're using the most up-to-date teaching techniques in our resources. Multiple members of our team hold advanced degrees in medicine or associated biomedical sciences, and are committed to the highest level of medical education. Kaplan has been working with the MCAT for over 50 years and our commitment to premed students is unflagging; in fact, Stanley Kaplan created this company when he had difficulty being accepted to medical school due to unfair quota systems that existed at the time.

We stand now at the beginning of a new era in medical education. As citizens of this 21st-century world of healthcare, we are charged with creating a patient-oriented, culturally competent, cost-conscious, universally available, technically advanced, and research-focused healthcare system, run by compassionate providers. Suffice it to say, this is no easy task. Problem-based learning, integrated curricula, and classes in interpersonal skills are some of the responses to this demand for an excellent workforce—a workforce of which you'll soon be a part.

We're thrilled that you've chosen us to help you on this journey. Please reach out to us to share your challenges, concerns, and successes. Together, we will shape the future of medicine in the United States and abroad; we look forward to helping you become the doctor you deserve to be.

Good luck!

Alexander Stone Macnow, MD
Editor-in-Chief
Department of Pathology and Laboratory Medicine
Hospital of the University of Pennsylvania

BA, Musicology—Boston University, 2008
MD—Perelman School of Medicine at the University of Pennsylvania, 2013

ABOUT THE MCAT

Anatomy of the MCAT

Here is a general overview of the structure of Test Day:

Section	Number of Questions	Time Allotted
Test-Day Certification		4 minutes
Tutorial (optional)		10 minutes
Chemical and Physical Foundations of Biological Systems	59	95 minutes
Break (optional)		10 minutes
Critical Analysis and Reasoning Skills (CARS)	53	90 minutes
Lunch Break (optional)		30 minutes
Biological and Biochemical Foundations of Living Systems	59	95 minutes
Break (optional)		10 minutes
Psychological, Social, and Biological Foundations of Behavior	59	95 minutes
Void Question		3 minutes
Satisfaction Survey (optional)		5 minutes

The structure of the four sections of the MCAT is shown below.

Chemical and Physical Foundations of Biological Systems	
Time	95 minutes
Format	• 59 questions • 10 passages • 44 questions are passage-based, and 15 are discrete (stand-alone) questions. • Score between 118 and 132
What It Tests	• Biochemistry: 25% • Biology: 5% • General Chemistry: 30% • Organic Chemistry: 15% • Physics: 25%

Critical Analysis and Reasoning Skills (CARS)	
Time	90 minutes
Format	• 53 questions • 9 passages • All questions are passage-based. There are no discrete (stand-alone) questions. • Score between 118 and 132
What It Tests	Disciplines: • Humanities: 50% • Social Sciences: 50% Skills: • *Foundations of Comprehension*: 30% • *Reasoning Within the Text*: 30% • *Reasoning Beyond the Text*: 40%
Biological and Biochemical Foundations of Living Systems	
Time	95 minutes
Format	• 59 questions • 10 passages • 44 questions are passage-based, and 15 are discrete (stand-alone) questions. • Score between 118 and 132
What It Tests	• Biochemistry: 25% • Biology: 65% • General Chemistry: 5% • Organic Chemistry: 5%
Psychological, Social, and Biological Foundations of Behavior	
Time	95 minutes
Format	• 59 questions • 10 passages • 44 questions are passage-based, and 15 are discrete (stand-alone) questions. • Score between 118 and 132
What It Tests	• Biology: 5% • Psychology: 65% • Sociology: 30%
Total	
Testing Time	375 minutes (6 hours, 15 minutes)
Total Seat Time	447 minutes (7 hours, 27 minutes)
Questions	230
Score	472 to 528

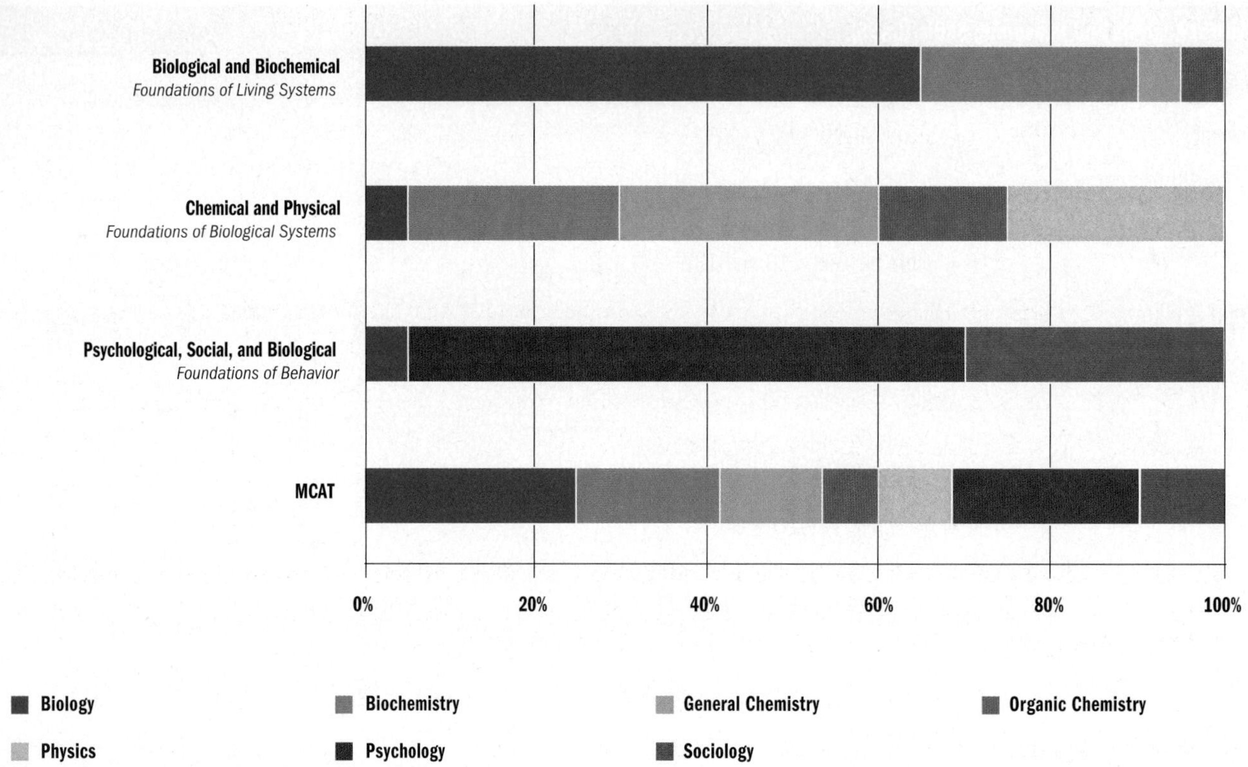

Scientific Inquiry and Reasoning Skills (SIRS)

The AAMC has defined four *Scientific Inquiry and Reasoning Skills* (SIRS) that will be tested in the three science sections of the MCAT:

1. *Knowledge of Scientific Concepts and Principles* (35% of questions)
2. *Scientific Reasoning and Problem-Solving* (45% of questions)
3. *Reasoning About the Design and Execution of Research* (10% of questions)
4. *Data-Based and Statistical Reasoning* (10% of questions)

Let's see how each one breaks down into more specific Test Day behaviors. Note that the bullet points of specific objectives for each of the SIRS are taken directly from the *Official Guide to the MCAT Exam*; the descriptions of what these behaviors mean and sample question stems, however, are written by Kaplan.

Skill 1: *Knowledge of Scientific Concepts and Principles*

This is probably the least surprising of the four SIRS; the testing of science knowledge is, after all, one of the signature qualities of the MCAT. Skill 1 questions will require you to do the following:

- Recognize correct scientific principles
- Identify the relationships among closely related concepts
- Identify the relationships between different representations of concepts (verbal, symbolic, graphic)
- Identify examples of observations that illustrate scientific principles
- Use mathematical equations to solve problems

At Kaplan, we simply call these Science Knowledge or Skill 1 questions. Another way to think of Skill 1 questions is as "one-step" problems. The single step is either to realize which scientific concept the question stem is suggesting or to take the concept stated in the question stem and identify which answer choice is an accurate application of it. Skill 1 questions are particularly prominent among discrete questions (those not associated with a passage). These questions are an opportunity to gain quick points on Test Day—if you know the science concept attached to the question, then that's it! On Test Day, 35% of the questions in each science section will be Skill 1 questions.

Here are some sample Skill 1 question stems:

- How would a proponent of the James–Lange theory of emotion interpret the findings of the study cited in the passage?
- Which of the following most accurately describes the function of FSH in the human menstrual cycle?
- If the products of Reaction 1 and Reaction 2 were combined in solution, the resulting reaction would form:
- Ionic bonds are maintained by which of the following forces?

Skill 2: *Scientific Reasoning and Problem-Solving*

The MCAT science sections do, of course, move beyond testing straightforward science knowledge; Skill 2 questions are the most common way in which it does so. At Kaplan, we also call these Critical Thinking questions. Skill 2 questions will require you to do the following:

- Reason about scientific principles, theories, and models
- Analyze and evaluate scientific explanations and predictions
- Evaluate arguments about causes and consequences
- Bring together theory, observations, and evidence to draw conclusions
- Recognize scientific findings that challenge or invalidate a scientific theory or model
- Determine and use scientific formulas to solve problems

Just as Skill 1 questions can be thought of as "one-step" problems, many Skill 2 questions are "two-step" problems, and more difficult Skill 2 questions may require three or more steps. These questions can require a wide spectrum of reasoning skills, including integration of multiple facts from a passage, combination of multiple science content areas, and prediction of an experiment's results. Skill 2 questions also tend to ask about science content without actually mentioning it by name. For example, a question might describe the results of one experiment and ask you to predict the results of a second experiment without actually telling you what underlying scientific principles are at work—part of the question's difficulty will be figuring out which principles to apply in order to get the correct answer. On Test Day, 45% of the questions in each science section will be Skill 2 questions.

Here are some sample Skill 2 question stems:

- Which of the following experimental conditions would most likely yield results similar to those in Figure 2?
- All of the following conclusions are supported by the information in the passage EXCEPT:
- The most likely cause of the anomalous results found by the experimenter is:
- An impact to a person's chest quickly reduces the volume of one of the lungs to 70% of its initial value while not allowing any air to escape from the mouth. By what percentage is the force of outward air pressure increased on a 2 cm^2 portion of the inner surface of the compressed lung?

Skill 3: *Reasoning About the Design and Execution of Research*

The MCAT is interested in your ability to critically appraise and analyze research, as this is an important day-to-day task of a physician. We call these questions Skill 3 or Experimental and Research Design questions for short. Skill 3 questions will require you to do the following:

- Identify the role of theory, past findings, and observations in scientific questioning
- Identify testable research questions and hypotheses
- Distinguish between samples and populations and distinguish results that support generalizations about populations
- Identify independent and dependent variables
- Reason about the features of research studies that suggest associations between variables or causal relationships between them (such as temporality and random assignment)
- Identify conclusions that are supported by research results
- Determine the implications of results for real-world situations
- Reason about ethical issues in scientific research

Over the years, the AAMC has received input from medical schools to require more practical research skills of MCAT test takers, and Skill 3 questions are the response to these demands. This skill is unique in that the outside knowledge you need to answer Skill 3 questions is not taught in any one undergraduate course; instead, the research design principles needed to answer these questions are learned gradually throughout your science classes and especially through any laboratory work you have completed. It should be noted that Skill 3 comprises 10% of the questions in each science section on Test Day.

Here are some sample Skill 3 question stems:

- What is the dependent variable in the study described in the passage?
- The major flaw in the method used to measure disease susceptibility in Experiment 1 is:
- Which of the following procedures is most important for the experimenters to follow in order for their study to maintain a proper, randomized sample of research subjects?
- A researcher would like to test the hypothesis that individuals who move to an urban area during adulthood are more likely to own a car than are those who have lived in an urban area since birth. Which of the following studies would best test this hypothesis?

Skill 4: *Data-Based and Statistical Reasoning*

Lastly, the science sections of the MCAT test your ability to analyze the visual and numerical results of experiments and studies. We call these Data and Statistical Analysis questions. Skill 4 questions will require you to do the following:

- Use, analyze, and interpret data in figures, graphs, and tables
- Evaluate whether representations make sense for particular scientific observations and data
- Use measures of central tendency (mean, median, and mode) and measures of dispersion (range, interquartile range, and standard deviation) to describe data
- Reason about random and systematic error

- Reason about statistical significance and uncertainty (interpreting statistical significance levels and interpreting a confidence interval)
- Use data to explain relationships between variables or make predictions
- Use data to answer research questions and draw conclusions

Skill 4 is included in the MCAT because physicians and researchers spend much of their time examining the results of their own studies and the studies of others, and it's very important for them to make legitimate conclusions and sound judgments based on that data. The MCAT tests Skill 4 on all three science sections with graphical representations of data (charts and bar graphs), as well as numerical ones (tables, lists, and results summarized in sentence or paragraph form). On Test Day, 10% of the questions in each science section will be Skill 4 questions.

Here are some sample Skill 4 question stems:

- According to the information in the passage, there is an inverse correlation between:
- What conclusion is best supported by the findings displayed in Figure 2?
- A medical test for a rare type of heavy metal poisoning returns a positive result for 98% of affected individuals and 13% of unaffected individuals. Which of the following types of errors is most prevalent in this test?
- If a fourth trial of Experiment 1 was run and yielded a result of 54% compliance, which of the following would be true?

SIRS Summary

Discussing the SIRS tested on the MCAT is a daunting prospect given that the very nature of the skills tends to make the conversation rather abstract. Nevertheless, with enough practice, you'll be able to identify each of the four skills quickly, and you'll also be able to apply the proper strategies to solve those problems on Test Day. If you need a quick reference to remind you of the four SIRS, these guidelines may help:

Skill 1 (**Science Knowledge**) questions ask:

- Do you remember this science content?

Skill 2 (**Critical Thinking**) questions ask:

- Do you remember this science content? And if you do, could you please apply it to this novel situation?
- Could you answer this question that cleverly combines multiple content areas at the same time?

Skill 3 (**Experimental and Research Design**) questions ask:

- Let's forget about the science content for a while. Could you give some insight into the experimental or research methods involved in this situation?

Skill 4 (**Data and Statistical Analysis**) questions ask:

- Let's forget about the science content for a while. Could you accurately read some graphs and tables for a moment? Could you make some conclusions or extrapolations based on the information presented?

Critical Analysis and Reasoning Skills (CARS)

The *Critical Analysis and Reasoning Skills* (CARS) section of the MCAT tests three discrete families of textual reasoning skills; each of these families requires a higher level of reasoning than the last. Those three skills are as follows:

1. *Foundations of Comprehension* (30% of questions)
2. *Reasoning Within the Text* (30% of questions)
3. *Reasoning Beyond the Text* (40% of questions)

These three skills are tested through nine humanities- and social sciences-themed passages, with approximately 5 to 7 questions per passage. Let's take a more in-depth look into these three skills. Again, the bullet points of specific objectives for each of the CARS are taken directly from the *Official Guide to the MCAT Exam*; the descriptions of what these behaviors mean and sample question stems, however, are written by Kaplan.

Foundations of Comprehension

Questions in this skill will ask for basic facts and simple inferences about the passage; the questions themselves will be similar to those seen on reading comprehension sections of other standardized exams like the SAT® and ACT®. *Foundations of Comprehension* questions will require you to do the following:

- Understand the basic components of the text
- Infer meaning from rhetorical devices, word choice, and text structure

This admittedly covers a wide range of potential question types including Main Idea, Detail, Inference, and Definition-in-Context questions, but finding the correct answer to all *Foundations of Comprehension* questions will follow from a basic understanding of the passage and the point of view of its author (and occasionally that of other voices in the passage).

Here are some sample *Foundations of Comprehension* question stems:

- **Main Idea**—The author's primary purpose in this passage is:
- **Detail**—Based on the information in the second paragraph, which of the following is the most accurate summary of the opinion held by Schubert's critics?
- **(Scattered) Detail**—According to the passage, which of the following is FALSE about literary reviews in the 1920s?
- **Inference (Implication)**—Which of the following phrases, as used in the passage, is most suggestive that the author has a personal bias toward narrative records of history?
- **Inference (Assumption)**—In putting together the argument in the passage, the author most likely assumes:
- **Definition-in-Context**—The word "obscure" (paragraph 3), when used in reference to the historian's actions, most nearly means:

Reasoning Within the Text

While *Foundations of Comprehension* questions will usually depend on interpreting a single piece of information in the passage or understanding the passage as a whole, *Reasoning Within the Text* questions require more thought because they will ask you to identify the purpose of a particular piece of information in the context of the passage, or ask how one piece of information relates to another. *Reasoning Within the Text* questions will require you to:

- Integrate different components of the text to draw relevant conclusions

The CARS section will also ask you to judge certain parts of the passage or even judge the author. These questions, which fall under the *Reasoning Within the Text* skill, can ask you to identify authorial bias, evaluate the credibility of cited sources, determine the logical soundness of an argument, identify the importance of a particular fact or statement in the context of the passage, or search for relevant evidence in the passage to support a given conclusion. In all, this category includes Function and Strengthen–Weaken (Within the Passage) questions, as well as a smattering of related—but rare—question types.

Here are some sample *Reasoning Within the Text* question stems:

- **Function**—The author's discussion of the effect of socioeconomic status on social mobility primarily serves which of the following functions?
- **Strengthen–Weaken (Within the Passage)**—Which of the following facts is used in the passage as the most prominent piece of evidence in favor of the author's conclusions?
- **Strengthen–Weaken (Within the Passage)**—Based on the role it plays in the author's argument, *The Possessed* can be considered:

Reasoning Beyond the Text

The distinguishing factor of *Reasoning Beyond the Text* questions is in the title of the skill: the word *Beyond*. Questions that test this skill, which make up a larger share of the CARS section than questions from either of the other two skills, will always introduce a completely new situation that was not present in the passage itself; these questions will ask you to determine how one influences the other. *Reasoning Beyond the Text* questions will require you to:

- Apply or extrapolate ideas from the passage to new contexts
- Assess the impact of introducing new factors, information, or conditions to ideas from the passage

The *Reasoning Beyond the Text* skill is further divided into Apply and Strengthen–Weaken (Beyond the Passage) questions, and a few other rarely appearing question types.

Here are some sample *Reasoning Beyond the Text* question stems:

- **Apply**—If a document were located that demonstrated Berlioz intended to include a chorus of at least 700 in his *Grande Messe des Morts*, how would the author likely respond?
- **Apply**—Which of the following is the best example of a "virtuous rebellion," as it is defined in the passage?
- **Strengthen–Weaken (Beyond the Passage)**—Suppose Jane Austen had written in a letter to her sister, "My strongest characters were those forced by circumstance to confront basic questions about the society in which they lived." What relevance would this have to the passage?
- **Strengthen–Weaken (Beyond the Passage)**—Which of the following sentences, if added to the end of the passage, would most WEAKEN the author's conclusions in the last paragraph?

CARS Summary

Through the *Foundations of Comprehension* skill, the CARS section tests many of the reading skills you have been building on since grade school, albeit in the context of very challenging doctorate-level passages. But through the two other skills (*Reasoning Within the Text* and *Reasoning Beyond the Text*), the MCAT demands that you understand the deep structure of passages and the arguments within them at a very advanced level. And, of course, all of this is tested under very tight timing restrictions: only 102 seconds per question—and that doesn't even include the time spent reading the passages.

Here's a quick reference guide to the three CARS skills:

Foundations of Comprehension questions ask:

- Did you understand the passage and its main ideas?
- What does the passage have to say about this particular detail?
- What must be true that the author did not say?

Reasoning Within the Text questions ask:

- What's the logical relationship between these two ideas from the passage?
- How well argued is the author's thesis?

Reasoning Beyond the Text questions ask:

- How does this principle from the passage apply to this new situation?
- How does this new piece of information influence the arguments in the passage?

Scoring

Each of the four sections of the MCAT is scored between 118 and 132, with the median at approximately 125. This means the total score ranges from 472 to 528, with the median at about 500. Why such peculiar numbers? The AAMC stresses that this scale emphasizes the importance of the central portion of the score distribution, where most students score (around 125 per section, or 500 total), rather than putting undue focus on the high end of the scale.

Note that there is no wrong answer penalty on the MCAT, so you should select an answer for every question—even if it is only a guess.

The AAMC has released the 2019–2021 correlation between scaled score and percentile, as shown on the following page. It should be noted that the percentile scale is adjusted and renormalized over time and thus can shift slightly from year to year. Percentile rank updates are released by the AAMC around May 1 of each year.

Total Score	Percentile	Total Score	Percentile
528	100	499	41
527	100	498	38
526	100	497	35
525	100	496	32
524	100	495	29
523	99	494	26
522	99	493	24
521	98	492	21
520	97	491	19
519	96	490	17
518	95	489	15
517	94	488	13
516	92	487	11
515	90	486	10
514	88	485	8
513	86	484	7
512	83	483	6
511	80	482	5
510	77	481	4
509	74	480	3
508	71	479	2
507	68	478	2
506	65	477	1
505	61	476	1
504	58	475	<1
503	55	474	<1
502	51	473	<1
501	48	472	<1
500	45		

Source: AAMC. 2022. *Summary of MCAT Total and Section Scores.* Accessed October 2022.
https://students-residents.aamc.org/mcat-research-and-data/percentile-ranks-mcat-exam

Further information on score reporting is included at the end of the next section (see *After Your Test*).

MCAT Policies and Procedures

We strongly encourage you to download the latest copy of *MCAT® Essentials*, available on the AAMC's website, to ensure that you have the latest information about registration and Test Day policies and procedures; this document is updated annually. A brief summary of some of the most important rules is provided here.

MCAT Registration

The only way to register for the MCAT is online. You can access AAMC's registration system at **www.aamc.org/mcat**.

The AAMC posts the schedule of testing, registration, and score release dates in the fall before the MCAT testing year, which runs from January into September. Registration for January through June is available earlier than registration for later dates, but see the AAMC's website for the exact dates each year. There is one standard registration fee, but the fee for changing your test date or test center increases the closer you get to your MCAT.

Fees and the Fee Assistance Program (FAP)

Payment for test registration must be made by MasterCard or VISA. As described earlier, the fee for rescheduling your exam or changing your testing center increases as one approaches Test Day. In addition, it is not uncommon for test centers to fill up well in advance of the registration deadline. For these reasons, we recommend identifying your preferred Test Day as soon as possible and registering. There are ancillary benefits to having a set Test Day, as well: when you know the date you're working toward, you'll study harder and are less likely to keep pushing back the exam. The AAMC offers a Fee Assistance Program (FAP) for students with financial hardship to help reduce the cost of taking the MCAT, as well as for the American Medical College Application Service (AMCAS®) application. Further information on the FAP can be found at **www.aamc.org/students/applying/fap**.

Testing Security

On Test Day, you will be required to present a qualifying form of ID. Generally, a current driver's license or United States passport will be sufficient (consult the AAMC website for the full list of qualifying criteria). When registering, take care to spell your first and last names (middle names, suffixes, and prefixes are not required and will not be verified on Test Day) precisely the same as they appear on this ID; failure to provide this ID at the test center or differences in spelling between your registration and ID will be considered a "no-show," and you will not receive a refund for the exam.

During Test Day registration, other identity data collected may include: a digital palm vein scan, a Test Day photo, a digitization of your valid ID, and signatures. Some testing centers may use a metal detection wand to ensure that no prohibited items are brought into the testing room. Prohibited items include all electronic devices, including watches and timers, calculators, cell phones, and any and all forms of recording equipment; food, drinks (including water), and cigarettes or other smoking paraphernalia; hats and scarves (except for religious purposes); and books, notes, or other study materials. If you require a medical device, such as an insulin pump or pacemaker, you must apply for accommodated testing. During breaks, you are allowed access to food and drink, but not to electronic devices, including cell phones.

Testing centers are under video surveillance and the AAMC does not take potential violations of testing security lightly. The bottom line: *know the rules and don't break them.*

Accommodations

Students with disabilities or medical conditions can apply for accommodated testing. Documentation of the disability or condition is required, and requests may take two months—or more—to be approved. For this reason, it is recommended that you begin the process of applying for accommodated testing as early as possible. More information on applying for accommodated testing can be found at **www.aamc.org/students/applying/mcat/accommodations.**

After Your Test

When your MCAT is all over, no matter how you feel you did, be good to yourself when you leave the test center. Celebrate! Take a nap. Watch a movie. Get some exercise. Plan a trip or outing. Call up all of your neglected friends or message them on social media. Go out for snacks or drinks with people you like. Whatever you do, make sure that it has absolutely nothing to do with thinking too hard—you deserve some rest and relaxation.

Perhaps most importantly, do not discuss specific details about the test with anyone. For one, it is important to let go of the stress of Test Day, and reliving your exam only inhibits you from being able to do so. But more significantly, the Examinee Agreement you sign at the beginning of your exam specifically prohibits you from discussing or disclosing exam content. The AAMC is known to seek out individuals who violate this agreement and retains the right to prosecute these individuals at their discretion. This means that you should not, under any circumstances, discuss the exam in person or over the phone with other individuals—including us at Kaplan—or post information or questions about exam content to Facebook, Student Doctor Network, or other online social media. You are permitted to comment on your "general exam experience," including how you felt about the exam overall or an individual section, but this is a fine line. In summary: *if you're not certain whether you can discuss an aspect of the test or not, just don't do it!* Do not let a silly Facebook post stop you from becoming the doctor you deserve to be.

Scores are typically released approximately one month after Test Day. The release is staggered during the afternoon and evening, ending at 5 p.m. Eastern Standard Time. This means that not all examinees receive their scores at exactly the same time. Your score report will include a scaled score for each section between 118 and 132, as well as your total combined score between 472 and 528. These scores are given as confidence intervals. For each section, the confidence interval is approximately the given score ± 1; for the total score, it is approximately the given score ± 2. You will also be given the corresponding percentile rank for each of these section scores and the total score.

AAMC Contact Information

For further questions, contact the MCAT team at the Association of American Medical Colleges:

MCAT Resource Center
Association of American Medical Colleges
www.aamc.org/mcat
(202) 828-0600
www.aamc.org/contactmcat

HOW THIS BOOK WAS CREATED

The *Kaplan MCAT Review* project began shortly after the release of the *Preview Guide for the MCAT 2015 Exam*, 2nd edition. Through thorough analysis by our staff psychometricians, we were able to analyze the relative yield of the different topics on the MCAT, and we began constructing tables of contents for the books of the *Kaplan MCAT Review* series. A dedicated staff of 30 writers, 7 editors, and 32 proofreaders worked over 5,000 combined hours to produce these books. The format of the books was heavily influenced by weekly meetings with Kaplan's learning science team.

In the years since this book was created, a number of opportunities for expansion and improvement have occurred. The current edition represents the culmination of the wisdom accumulated during that time frame, and it also includes several new features designed to improve the reading and learning experience in these texts.

These books were submitted for publication in April 2023. For any updates after this date, please visit www.kaptest.com/retail-book-corrections-and-updates.

If you have any questions about the content presented here, email KaplanMCATfeedback@kaplan.com. For other questions not related to content, email booksupport@kaplan.com.

Each book has been vetted through at least ten rounds of review. To that end, the information presented in these books is true and accurate to the best of our knowledge. Still, your feedback helps us improve our prep materials. Please notify us of any inaccuracies or errors in the books by sending an email to KaplanMCATfeedback@kaplan.com.

USING THIS BOOK

Kaplan MCAT Biology Review, and the other six books in the *Kaplan MCAT Review* series, bring the Kaplan classroom experience to you—right in your home, at your convenience. This book offers the same Kaplan content review, strategies, and practice that make Kaplan the #1 choice for MCAT prep.

This book is designed to help you review the biology topics covered on the MCAT. Please understand that content review—no matter how thorough—is not sufficient preparation for the MCAT! The MCAT tests not only your science knowledge but also your critical reading, reasoning, and problem-solving skills. Do not assume that simply memorizing the contents of this book will earn you high scores on Test Day; to maximize your scores, you must also improve your reading and test-taking skills through MCAT-style questions and practice tests.

Learning Objectives

At the beginning of each section, you'll find a short list of objectives describing the skills covered within that section. Learning objectives for these texts were developed in conjunction with Kaplan's learning science team, and have been designed specifically to focus your attention on tasks and concepts that are likely to show up on your MCAT. These learning objectives will function as a means to guide your study, and indicate what information and relationships you should be focused on within each section. Before starting each section, read these learning objectives carefully. They will not only allow you to assess your existing familiarity with the content, but also provide a goal-oriented focus for your studying experience of the section.

MCAT Concept Checks

At the end of each section, you'll find a few open-ended questions that you can use to assess your mastery of the material. These MCAT Concept Checks were introduced after numerous conversations with Kaplan's learning science team. Research has demonstrated repeatedly that introspection and self-analysis improve mastery, retention, and recall of material. Complete these MCAT Concept Checks to ensure that you've got the key points from each section before moving on!

Science Mastery Assessments

At the beginning of each chapter, you'll find 15 MCAT-style practice questions. These are designed to help you assess your understanding of the chapter before you begin reading the chapter. Using the guidance provided with the assessment, you can determine the best way to review each chapter based on your personal strengths and weaknesses. Most of the questions in the Science Mastery Assessments focus on the first of the *Scientific Inquiry and Reasoning Skills* (*Knowledge of Scientific Concepts and Principles*), although there are occasional questions that fall into the second or fourth SIRS (*Scientific Reasoning and Problem-Solving* and *Data-Based and Statistical Reasoning*, respectively). You can complete each chapter's assessment in a testing interface in your online resources, where you'll also find a test-like passage set covering the same content you just studied to ensure you can also apply your knowledge the way the MCAT will expect you to!

Guided Examples with Expert Thinking

Embedded in each chapter of this book is a Guided Example with Expert Thinking. These examples will be located adjacent to the content that they are related to, and contain an MCAT-like scientific article as a passage. Read through the passage as you would on the real MCAT, referring to the Expert Thinking material on the right to clarify the key information you should be gathering from each passage. Read and attempt to answer the associated question once you have worked through the passage. There is a full explanation, including the correct answer, following the question given. These passages and questions are designed to help build your critical thinking, experimental reasoning, and data interpretation skills as preparation for the challenges you will face on the MCAT.

Sidebars

The following is a guide to the five types of sidebars you'll find in *Kaplan MCAT Biology Review:*

- **Bridge:** These sidebars create connections between science topics that appear in multiple chapters throughout the *Kaplan MCAT Review* series.
- **Key Concept:** These sidebars draw attention to the most important takeaways in a given topic, and they sometimes offer synopses or overviews of complex information. If you understand nothing else, make sure you grasp the Key Concepts for any given subject.
- **MCAT Expertise:** These sidebars point out how information may be tested on the MCAT or offer key strategy points and test-taking tips that you should apply on Test Day.
- **Mnemonic:** These sidebars present memory devices to help recall certain facts.
- **Real World:** These sidebars illustrate how a concept in the text relates to the practice of medicine or the world at large. While this is not information you need to know for Test Day, many of the topics in Real World sidebars are excellent examples of how a concept may appear in a passage or discrete (stand-alone) question on the MCAT.

What This Book Covers

The information presented in the *Kaplan MCAT Review* series covers everything listed on the official MCAT content lists. Every topic in these lists is covered in the same level of detail as is common to the undergraduate and postbaccalaureate classes that are considered prerequisites for the MCAT. Note that your premedical classes may include topics not discussed in these books, or they may go into more depth than these books do. Additional exposure to science content is never a bad thing, but all of the content knowledge you are expected to have walking in on Test Day is covered in these books.

Chapter Profiles, on the first page of each chapter, represent a holistic look at the content within the chapter, and will include a pie chart as well as text information. The pie chart analysis is based directly on data released by the AAMC, and will give a rough estimate of the importance of the chapter in relation to the book as a whole. Further, the text portion of the Chapter Profiles includes which AAMC content categories are covered within the chapter. These are referenced directly from the AAMC MCAT exam content listing, available on the testmaker's website.

You'll also see new High-Yield badges scattered throughout the sections of this book:

In This Chapter

1.1 Amino Acids Found in Proteins

High-Yield

LEARNING OBJECTIVES

After Chapter 1.1, you will be able to:

These badges represent the top 100 topics most tested by the AAMC. In other words, according to the testmaker and all our experience with their resources, a High-Yield badge means more questions on Test Day.

This book also contains a thorough glossary and index for easy navigation of the text.

In the end, this is your book, so write in the margins, draw diagrams, highlight the key points—do whatever is necessary to help you get that higher score. We look forward to working with you as you achieve your dreams and become the doctor you deserve to be!

Studying with This Book

In addition to providing you with the best practice questions and test strategies, Kaplan's team of learning scientists are dedicated to researching and testing the best methods for getting the most out of your study time. Here are their top four tips for improving retention:

Review multiple topics in one study session. This may seem counterintuitive—we're used to practicing one skill at a time in order to improve each skill. But research shows that weaving topics together leads to increased learning. Beyond that consideration, the MCAT often includes more than one topic in a single question. Studying in an integrated manner is the most effective way to prepare for this test.

Customize the content. Drawing attention to difficult or critical content can ensure you don't overlook it as you read and re-read sections. The best way to do this is to make it more visual—highlight, make tabs, use stickies, whatever works. We recommend highlighting only the most important or difficult sections of text. Selective highlighting of up to about 10% of text in a given chapter is great for emphasizing parts of the text, but over-highlighting can have the opposite effect.

Repeat topics over time. Many people try to memorize concepts by repeating them over and over again in succession. Our research shows that retention is improved by spacing out the repeats over time and mixing up the order in which you study content. For example, try reading chapters in a different order the second (or third!) time around. Revisit practice questions that you answered incorrectly in a new sequence. Perhaps information you reviewed more recently will help you better understand those questions and solutions you struggled with in the past.

Take a moment to reflect. When you finish reading a section for the first time, stop and think about what you just read. Jot down a few thoughts in the margins or in your notes about why the content is important or what topics came to mind when you read it. Associating learning with a memory is a fantastic way to retain information! This also works when answering questions. After answering a question, take a moment to think through each step you took to arrive at a solution. What led you to the answer you chose? Understanding the steps you took will help you make good decisions when answering future questions.

Online Resources

In addition to the resources located within this text, you also have additional online resources awaiting you at **www.kaptest.com/booksonline**. Make sure to log on and take advantage of free practice and access to other resources!

Please note that access to the online resources is limited to the original owner of this book.

STUDYING FOR THE MCAT

The first year of medical school is a frenzied experience for most students. To meet the requirements of a rigorous work schedule, students either learn to prioritize their time or else fall hopelessly behind. It's no surprise, then, that the MCAT, the test specifically designed to predict success in medical school, is a high-speed, time-intensive test. The MCAT demands excellent time-management skills, endurance, and grace under pressure both during the test as well as while preparing for it. Having a solid plan of attack and sticking with it are key to giving you the confidence and structure you need to succeed.

Creating a Study Plan

The best time to create a study plan is at the beginning of your MCAT preparation. If you don't already use a calendar, you will want to start. You can purchase a planner, print out a free calendar from the Internet, use a built-in calendar or app on one of your smart devices, or keep track using an interactive online calendar. Pick the option that is most practical for you and that you are most likely to use consistently.

Once you have a calendar, you'll be able to start planning your study schedule with the following steps:

1. **Fill in your obligations and choose a day off.**

   Write in all your school, extracurricular, and work obligations first: class sessions, work shifts, and meetings that you must attend. Then add in your personal obligations: appointments, lunch dates, family and social time, etc. Making an appointment in your calendar for hanging out with friends or going to the movies may seem strange at first, but planning social activities in advance will help you achieve a balance between personal and professional obligations even as life gets busy. Having a happy balance allows you to be more focused and productive when it comes time to study, so stay well-rounded and don't neglect anything that is important to you.

   In addition to scheduling your personal and professional obligations, you should also plan your time off. Taking some time off is just as important as studying. Kaplan recommends taking at least one full day off per week, ideally from all your study obligations but at minimum from studying for the MCAT.

2. **Add in study blocks around your obligations.**

   Once you have established your calendar's framework, add in study blocks around your obligations, keeping your study schedule as consistent as possible across days and across weeks. Studying at the same time of day as your official test is ideal for promoting recall, but if that's not possible, then fit in study blocks wherever you can.

   To make your studying as efficient as possible, block out short, frequent periods of study time throughout the week. From a learning perspective, studying one hour per day for six days per week is much more valuable than studying for six hours all at once one day per week. Specifically, Kaplan recommends studying for no longer than three hours in one sitting. Within those three-hour blocks, also plan to take ten-minute breaks every hour. Use these breaks to get up from your seat, do some quick stretches, get a snack and drink, and clear your mind. Although ten minutes of break for every 50 minutes of studying may sound like a lot, these breaks will allow you to deal with distractions and rest your brain so that, during the 50-minute study blocks, you can remain fully engaged and completely focused.

3. **Add in your full-length practice tests.**

   Next, you'll want to add in full-length practice tests. You'll want to take one test very early in your prep and then spread your remaining full-length practice tests evenly between now and your test date. Staggering tests in this way allows you to form a baseline for comparison and to determine which areas to focus on right away, while also providing realistic feedback throughout your prep as to how you will perform on Test Day.

When planning your calendar, aim to finish your full-length practice tests and the majority of your studying by one week before Test Day, which will allow you to spend that final week completing a final, brief review of what you already know. In your online resources, you'll find sample study calendars for several different Test Day timelines to use as a starting point. The sample calendars may include more focus than you need in some areas, and less in others, and it may not fit your timeline to Test Day. You will need to customize your study calendar to your needs using the steps above.

The total amount of time you spend studying each week will depend on your schedule, your personal prep needs, and your time to Test Day, but it is recommended that you spend somewhere in the range of 300–350 hours preparing before taking the official MCAT. One way you could break this down is to study for three hours per day, six days per week, for four months, but this is just one approach. You might study six days per week for more than three hours per day. You might study over a longer period of time if you don't have much time to study each week. No matter what your plan is, ensure you complete enough practice to feel completely comfortable with the MCAT and its content. A good sign you're ready for Test Day is when you begin to earn your goal score consistently in practice.

How to Study

The MCAT covers a large amount of material, so studying for Test Day can initially seem daunting. To combat this, we have some tips on how to take control of your studying and make the most of your time.

Goal Setting

To take control of the amount of content and practice required to do well on the MCAT, break the content down into specific goals for each week instead of attempting to approach the test as a whole. A goal of "I want to increase my overall score by 5 points" is too big, abstract, and difficult to measure on the small scale. More reasonable goals are "I will read two chapters each day this week." Goals like this are much less overwhelming and help break studying into manageable pieces.

Active Reading

As you go through this book, much of the information will be familiar to you. After all, you have probably seen most of the content before. However, be very careful: Familiarity with a subject does not necessarily translate to knowledge or mastery of that subject. Do not assume that if you recognize a concept you actually know it and can apply it quickly at an appropriate level. Don't just passively read this book. Instead, read actively: Use the free margin space to jot down important ideas, draw diagrams, and make charts as you read. Highlighting can be an excellent tool, but use it sparingly: highlighting every sentence isn't active reading, it's coloring. Frequently stop and ask yourself questions while you read (e.g., *What is the main point? How does this fit into the overall scheme of things? Could I thoroughly explain this to someone else?*). By making connections and focusing on the grander scheme, not only will you ensure you know the essential content, but you also prepare yourself for the level of critical thinking required by the MCAT.

Focus on Areas of Greatest Opportunity

If you are limited by only having a minimal amount of time to prepare before Test Day, focus on your biggest areas of opportunity first. Areas of opportunity are topic areas that are highly tested and that you have not yet mastered. You likely won't have time to take detailed notes for every page of these books; instead, use your results from practice materials to determine which areas are your biggest opportunities and seek those out. After you've taken a full-length test, make sure you are using your performance report to best identify areas of opportunity. Skim over content matter for which you are already demonstrating proficiency, pausing to read more thoroughly when something looks unfamiliar or particularly difficult. Begin with the Science Mastery Assessment at the beginning of each chapter. If you can get all of those questions correct within a reasonable amount of time, you may be able to quickly skim through that chapter, but if the questions prove to be more difficult, then you may need to spend time reading the chapter or certain subsections of the chapter more thoroughly.

Practice, Review, and Tracking

Leave time to review your practice questions and full-length tests. You may be tempted, after practicing, to push ahead and cover new material as quickly as possible, but failing to schedule ample time for review will actually throw away your greatest opportunity to improve your performance. The brain rarely remembers anything it sees or does only once. When you carefully review the questions you've solved (and the explanations for them), the process of retrieving that information reopens and reinforces the connections you've built in your brain. This builds long-term retention and repeatable skill sets—exactly what you need to beat the MCAT!

One useful tool for making the most of your review is the How I'll Fix It (HIFI) sheet. You can create a HIFI sheet, such as the sample below, to track questions throughout your prep that you miss or have to guess on. For each such question, figure out why you missed it and supply at least one action step for how you can avoid similar mistakes in the future. As you move through your MCAT prep, adjust your study plan based on your available study time and the results of your review. Your strengths and weaknesses are likely to change over the course of your prep. Keep addressing the areas that are most important to your score, shifting your focus as those areas change. For more help with making the most of your full-length tests, including a How I'll Fix It sheet template, make sure to check out the videos and resources in your online syllabus.

Section	Q #	Type or Topic	Why I missed it	How I'll fix it
Chem/Phys	*42*	*Nuclear chem.*	*Confused electron absorption and emission*	*Reread Physics Chapter 9.2*
Chem/Phys	*47*	K_{eq}	*Didn't know right equation*	*Memorize equation for* K_{eq}
CARS	*2*	*Detail*	*Didn't read "not" in answer choice*	*Slow down when finding match*
CARS	*4*	*Inference*	*Forgot to research answer*	*Reread passage and predict first*

Where to Study

One often-overlooked aspect of studying is the environment where the learning actually occurs. Although studying at home is many students' first choice, several problems can arise in this environment, chief of which are distractions. Studying can be a mentally draining process, so as time passes, these distractions become ever more tempting as escape routes. Although you may have considerable willpower, there's no reason to make staying focused harder than it needs to be. Instead of studying at home, head to a library, quiet coffee shop, or another new location whenever possible. This will eliminate many of the usual distractions and also promote efficient studying; instead of studying off and on at home over the course of an entire day, you can stay at the library for three hours of effective studying and enjoy the rest of the day off from the MCAT.

No matter where you study, make your practice as much like Test Day as possible. Just as is required during the official test, don't have snacks or chew gum during your study blocks. Turn off your music, television, and phone. Practice on the computer with your online resources to simulate the computer-based test environment. When completing practice questions, do your work on scratch paper or noteboard sheets rather than writing directly on any printed materials since you won't have that option on Test Day. Because memory is tied to all of your senses, the more test-like you can make your studying environment, the easier it will be on Test Day to recall the information you're putting in so much work to learn.

CHAPTER 1

THE CELL

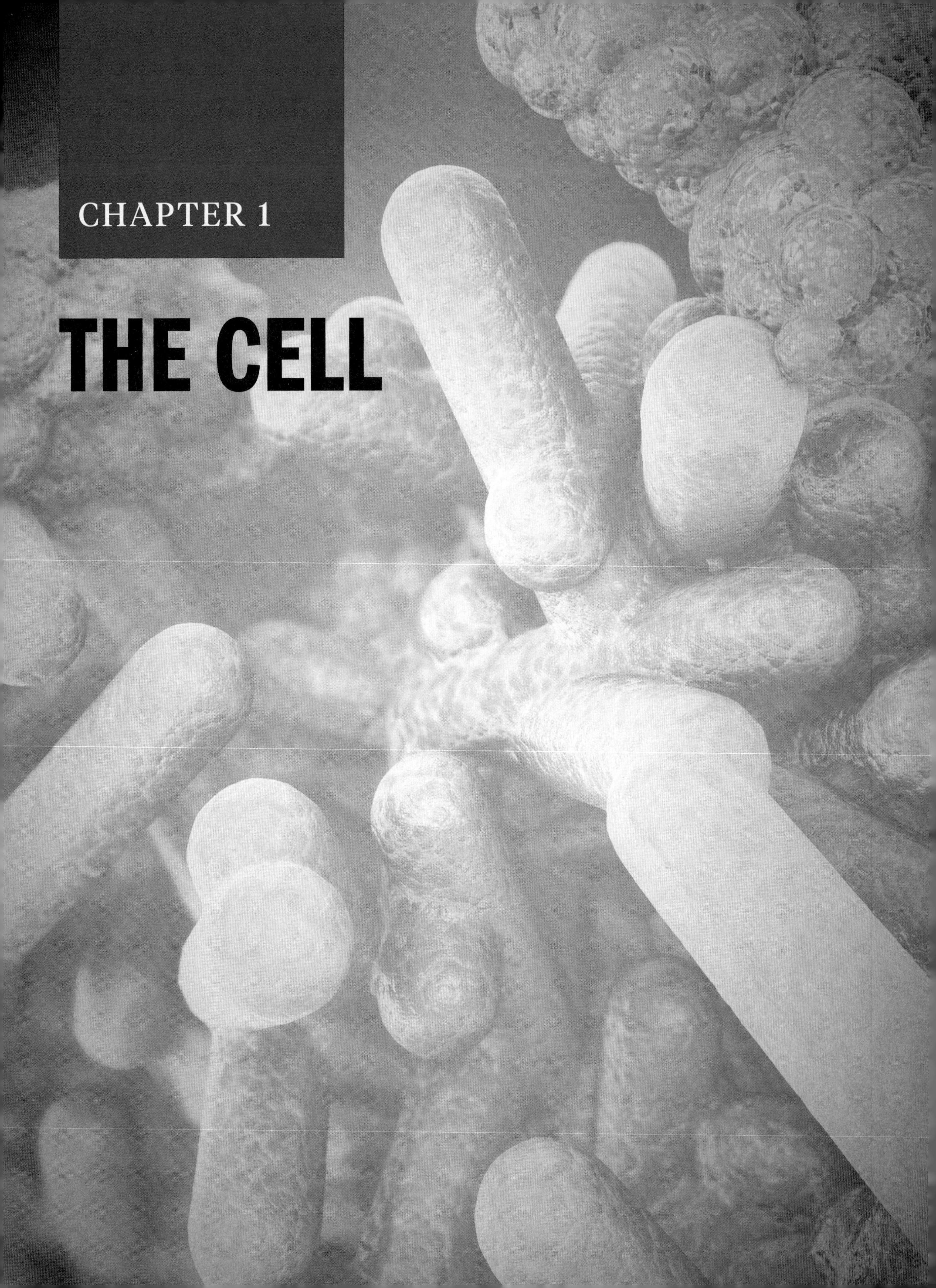

SCIENCE MASTERY ASSESSMENT

Every pre-med knows this feeling: there is so much content I have to know for the MCAT! How do I know what to do first or what's important?

While the high-yield badges throughout this book will help you identify the most important topics, this Science Mastery Assessment is another tool in your MCAT prep arsenal. This quiz (which can also be taken in your online resources) and the guidance below will help ensure that you are spending the appropriate amount of time on this chapter based on your personal strengths and weaknesses. Don't worry though—skipping something now does not mean you'll never study it. Later on in your prep, as you complete full-length tests, you'll uncover specific pieces of content that you need to review and can come back to these chapters as appropriate.

How to Use This Assessment

If you answer 0–7 questions correctly:

Spend about 1 hour to read this chapter in full and take limited notes throughout. Follow up by reviewing **all** quiz questions to ensure that you now understand how to solve each one.

If you answer 8–11 questions correctly:

Spend 20–40 minutes reviewing the quiz questions. Beginning with the questions you missed, read and take notes on the corresponding subchapters. For questions you answered correctly, ensure your thinking matches that of the explanation and you understand why each choice was correct or incorrect.

If you answer 12–15 questions correctly:

Spend less than 20 minutes reviewing all questions from the quiz. If you missed any, then include a quick read-through of the corresponding subchapters, or even just the relevant content within a subchapter, as part of your question review. For questions you answered correctly, ensure your thinking matches that of the explanation and review the Concept Summary at the end of the chapter.

1. Hyperbaric oxygen may be used as a treatment for certain types of bacterial infections. In this therapy, the patient is placed in a chamber in which the partial pressure of oxygen is significantly increased, increasing the partial pressure of oxygen in the patient's tissues. This treatment is most likely used for infections with:
   A. obligate aerobic bacteria.
   B. facultative anaerobic bacteria.
   C. aerotolerant anaerobic bacteria.
   D. obligate anaerobic bacteria.

2. Which of the following does NOT describe connective tissue cells?
   A. They account for most cells in muscles, bones, and tendons.
   B. They secrete substances to form the extracellular matrix.
   C. In organs, they tend to form the stroma.
   D. In organs, they provide support for epithelial cells.

3. Which of the following types of nucleic acid could form the genome of a virus?
   I. Single-stranded RNA
   II. Double-stranded DNA
   III. Single-stranded DNA

   A. I only
   B. II only
   C. I and II only
   D. I, II, and III

4. The theory of spontaneous generation states that living organisms can arise from nonliving material. In 1859, Pasteur demonstrated that no organisms emerged from sterilized growth media, weakening the theory of spontaneous generation and supporting which tenet of cell theory?
   A. All living things are composed of cells.
   B. The cell is the basic functional unit of life.
   C. Cells arise only from preexisting cells.
   D. Cells carry genetic information in the form of DNA.

5. Mitochondrial DNA is:
   I. circular.
   II. self-replicating.
   III. single-stranded.

   A. I only
   B. II only
   C. I and II only
   D. I, II, and III

6. Which of the following is NOT a function of the smooth endoplasmic reticulum?
   A. Lipid synthesis
   B. Poison detoxification
   C. Protein synthesis
   D. Transport of proteins

7. What is the main function of the nucleolus?
   A. Ribosomal RNA synthesis
   B. DNA replication
   C. Cell division
   D. Chromosome assembly

8. Which of the following organelles is surrounded by a single membrane?
   A. Lysosomes
   B. Mitochondria
   C. Nuclei
   D. Ribosomes

9. Which of the following is NOT a difference that would allow one to distinguish a prokaryotic and a eukaryotic cell?
A. Ribosomal subunit weight
B. Presence of a nucleus
C. Presence of a membrane on the outside surface of the cell
D. Presence of membrane-bound organelles

10. Which of the following does NOT contain tubulin?
A. Cilia
B. Flagella
C. Microfilaments
D. Centrioles

11. Herpes simplex virus (HSV) enters the human body and remains dormant in the nervous system until it produces an outbreak after exposure to heat, radiation, or other stimuli. Which of the following statements correctly describes HSV?
A. While it remains dormant in the nervous system, the virus is in its lytic cycle.
B. During an outbreak, the virus is in the lysogenic cycle.
C. Herpes simplex virus adds its genetic information to the genetic information of the cell.
D. The herpes simplex virus contains a tail sheath and tail fibers.

12. Resistance to antibiotics is a well-recognized medical problem. Which mechanisms can account for a bacterium's ability to increase its genetic variability and thus adapt itself to resist different antibiotics?
I. Binary fission
II. Conjugation
III. Transduction

A. I and II only
B. I and III only
C. II and III only
D. I, II, and III

13. A bacterial cell is noted to be resistant to penicillin. The bacterium is transferred to a colony that lacks the fertility factor, and the rest of the colony does not become resistant to penicillin. However, the penicillin-resistant cell has also started to exhibit other phenotypic characteristics, including secretion of a novel protein. Which of the following methods of bacterial recombination is NOT likely to account for this change?
A. Conjugation
B. Transformation
C. Transduction
D. Infection with a bacteriophage

14. In Alzheimer's disease, a protein called the amyloid precursor protein (APP) is cleaved to form a protein called β-amyloid. This protein has a β-pleated sheet structure and precipitates to form plaques in the brain. This mechanism of disease is most similar to which of the following pathogens?
A. Bacteria
B. Viruses
C. Prions
D. Viroids

15. After infection of a cell, a viral particle must transport itself to the nucleus in order to produce viral proteins. What is the likely genomic content of the virus?
A. Double-stranded DNA
B. Double-stranded RNA
C. Positive-sense RNA
D. Negative-sense RNA

Answer Key

1. **D**
2. **A**
3. **D**
4. **C**
5. **C**
6. **C**
7. **A**
8. **A**
9. **C**
10. **C**
11. **C**
12. **C**
13. **A**
14. **C**
15. **A**

Detailed explanations can be found at the end of the chapter.

CHAPTER 1

THE CELL

In This Chapter

Introduction

The human body contains approximately 37 trillion cells, with bacterial cells outnumbering the eukaryotic cells by about 10 to 1. Our cells create tissues that form organs, and each cell serves a purpose, communicating and carrying out the reactions that make life possible.

The sheer number of cells that make up the human body is not nearly as impressive as the numerous functions these cells can perform—from the conduction of impulses through the nervous system that allows for memory and learning, to the simultaneous contraction of cardiac myocytes that pump blood through the entire human body. In order to understand the human organism as a whole and how the human body reacts to various pathogens, a thorough understanding of cell biology is required. It is not enough to simply memorize each part of the cell; the MCAT requires an understanding of how each cell structure carries out its functions and affects the entire organism.

CHAPTER PROFILE

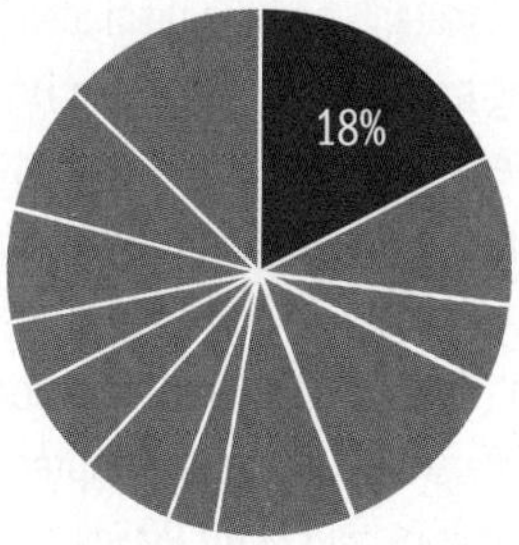

The content in this chapter should be relevant to about 18% of all questions about biology on the MCAT.

This chapter covers material from the following AAMC content categories:

1D: Principles of bioenergetics and fuel molecule metabolism

2A: Assemblies of molecules, cells, and groups of cells within single cellular and multicellular organisms

2B: The structure, growth, physiology, and genetics of prokaryotes and viruses

MCAT EXPERTISE

This chapter represents 18% of all biology questions you would see on Test Day. That makes the cell, specifically eukaryotic cell structure and function, one of the single highest-yield subjects within any of the review books. Make sure to work sufficient study of these materials into your study plan.

1.1 Cell Theory

LEARNING OBJECTIVE

After Chapter 1.1, you will be able to:

- Recall the four fundamental tenets of cell theory

BRIDGE

Robert Hooke, who invented the first crude microscopes to look at cork, is also known for his characterization of springs. Hooke's law, $F = -kx$, describes the relationship between elastic force, the spring constant, and the displacement of a spring from equilibrium. While Hooke's law does not appear on the official MCAT content lists, the related topic of elastic potential energy, $U = \frac{1}{2}kx^2$, is testable content. This equation and other forms of energy are discussed in Chapter 2 of *MCAT Physics and Math Review.*

Prior to the 1600s, organisms were perceived as being complete and inseparable into smaller parts. This was due in part to the inability to see smaller structures through simple optical instruments like magnifying glasses. In 1665, Robert Hooke assembled a crude compound microscope and tested its properties on a piece of cork. He noticed a honeycomb-like structure and compared the spaces within the cork to the small rooms of a monastery, known as cells. Because cork consists of desiccated non-living cells, Hooke was not able to see nuclei, organelles, or cell membranes. In 1674, Anton van Leeuwenhoek was the first to view a living cell under a microscope. Later researchers noted that cells could be separated, and that each cell was a distinct structure. Further research indicated that tissues were made of cells, and the function of a tissue was dependent upon the function of the cells that make up the tissue. Two centuries later, in 1850, Rudolph Virchow demonstrated that diseased cells could arise from normal cells in normal tissues.

The original form of the **cell theory** consisted of three basic tenets:

- All living things are composed of cells.
- The cell is the basic functional unit of life.
- Cells arise only from preexisting cells.

Through advances in molecular biology, a fourth tenet has been added to the theory:

- Cells carry genetic information in the form of deoxyribonucleic acid (DNA). This genetic material is passed on from parent to daughter cell.

Cell theory has created an interesting dilemma with respect to viruses. Viruses are small structures that contain genetic material, but are unable to reproduce on their own. This violates the third and fourth tenets of the cell theory because virions can only replicate by invading other organisms and because they may use ribonucleic acid (RNA) as their genetic information. Therefore, viruses, discussed later in this chapter, are not considered living organisms.

MCAT CONCEPT CHECK 1.1

Before you move on, assess your understanding of the material with this question.

1. What are the four fundamental tenets of the cell theory?
   -
   -
   -
   -

BRIDGE

Solutions to concept checks for a given chapter in *MCAT Biology Review* can be found near the end of the chapter in which the concept check is located, following the Concept Summary for that chapter.

1.2 Eukaryotic Cells

High-Yield

MCAT EXPERTISE

The "High-Yield" badge on this section indicates that the content is frequently tested on the MCAT.

LEARNING OBJECTIVES

After Chapter 1.2, you will be able to:

- Explain the importance of hydrogen peroxide to cellular function
- Identify the predominant proteins found in microfilaments, microtubules, and intermediate filaments
- Distinguish between the properties of different cytoskeletal structures
- Classify cell types as epithelial or connective tissue
- Recall the names and functions of cellular organelles:

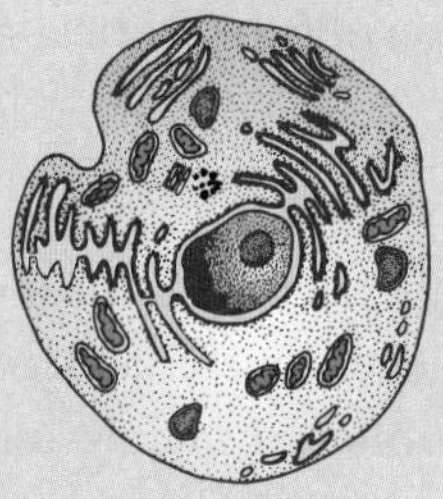

The first major distinction we can make between living organisms is whether they are composed of prokaryotic or eukaryotic cells. Prokaryotic organisms are always single celled, while eukaryotic organisms can be unicellular or multicellular. Whereas **eukaryotic cells** contain a true nucleus enclosed in a membrane, **prokaryotic cells** do not contain a nucleus. The major organelles are identified in the eukaryotic cell in Figure 1.1.

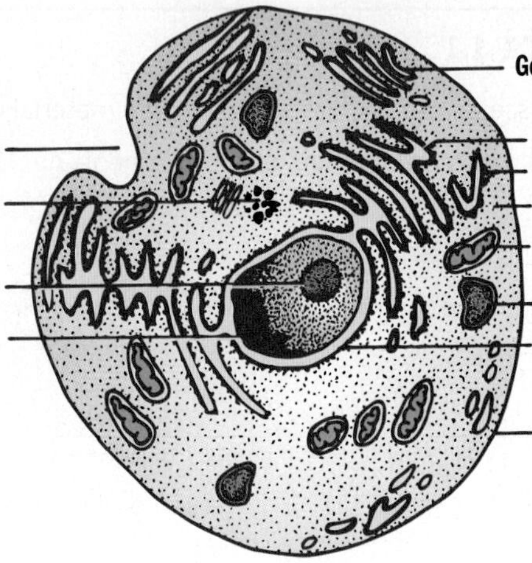

Figure 1.1 Eukaryotic Cell
Numerous membrane-bound organelles are found in the cytoplasm of a eukaryotic cell.

Membrane-Bound Organelles

Each cell has a membrane enclosing a semifluid cytosol in which the **organelles** are suspended. In eukaryotic cells, most organelles are membrane bound, allowing for compartmentalization of functions. Membranes of eukaryotic cells consist of a phospholipid bilayer. This membrane is unique in that its surfaces are hydrophilic, electrostatically interacting with the aqueous environments inside and outside of the cell, while its inner portion is hydrophobic, which helps to provide a highly selective barrier between the interior of the cell and the external environment. The cell membrane is such an important topic on the MCAT that an entire chapter—Chapter 8 of *MCAT Biochemistry Review*—is devoted solely to discussing the structure and physiology of biological membranes. The **cytosol** allows for the diffusion of molecules throughout the cell. Within the **nucleus**, genetic material is encoded in **deoxyribonucleic acid** (**DNA**), which is organized into **chromosomes**. Eukaryotic cells reproduce by **mitosis**, allowing for the formation of two identical daughter cells.

BRIDGE

The nuclear envelope creates two distinct environments within the cell because it separates the nucleus from the cytoplasm. This permits compartmentalization of transcription (the formation of hnRNA from DNA, which is subsequently processed to form mRNA) and translation (the formation of a peptide from mRNA). These processes are discussed in Chapter 7 of *MCAT Biochemistry Review*.

The Nucleus

As the control center of the cell, the **nucleus** is the most heavily tested organelle on the MCAT. It contains all of the genetic material necessary for replication of the cell. The nucleus is surrounded by the **nuclear membrane** or **envelope**, a double membrane that maintains a nuclear environment separate and distinct from the cytoplasm. **Nuclear pores** in the nuclear membrane allow selective two-way exchange of material between the cytoplasm and the nucleus.

The genetic material (DNA) contains coding regions called **genes**. Linear DNA is wound around organizing proteins known as **histones**, and is then further wound into linear strands called **chromosomes**. The location of DNA in the nucleus permits the compartmentalization of DNA transcription separate from RNA translation. Finally, there is a subsection of the nucleus known as the **nucleolus**, where the

ribosomal RNA (**rRNA**) is synthesized. The nucleolus actually takes up approximately 25 percent of the volume of the entire nucleus and can often be identified as a darker spot in the nucleus.

Mitochondria

Mitochondria, shown in Figure 1.2, are often called *the power plants of the cell*, in reference to their important metabolic functions. The mitochondrion contains two layers: the outer and inner membranes. The **outer membrane** serves as a barrier between the cytosol and the inner environment of the mitochondrion. The **inner membrane**, which is arranged into numerous infoldings called **cristae**, contains the molecules and enzymes of the electron transport chain. The cristae are highly convoluted structures that increase the surface area available for electron transport chain enzymes. The space between the inner and outer membranes is called the **intermembrane space**; the space inside the inner membrane is called the mitochondrial **matrix**. As described in Chapter 10 of *MCAT Biochemistry Review*, the pumping of protons from the mitochondrial matrix to the intermembrane space establishes the proton-motive force; ultimately, these protons flow through *ATP synthase* to generate ATP during oxidative phosphorylation.

REAL WORLD

The *serial endosymbiosis theory* attempts to explain the formation of some of the membrane-bound organelles; it posits that these organelles formed by the engulfing of one prokaryote by another and the establishment of a symbiotic relationship. In addition to mitochondria, chloroplasts in plant cells and organelles of motility (such as flagella) are believed to have originated from this process.

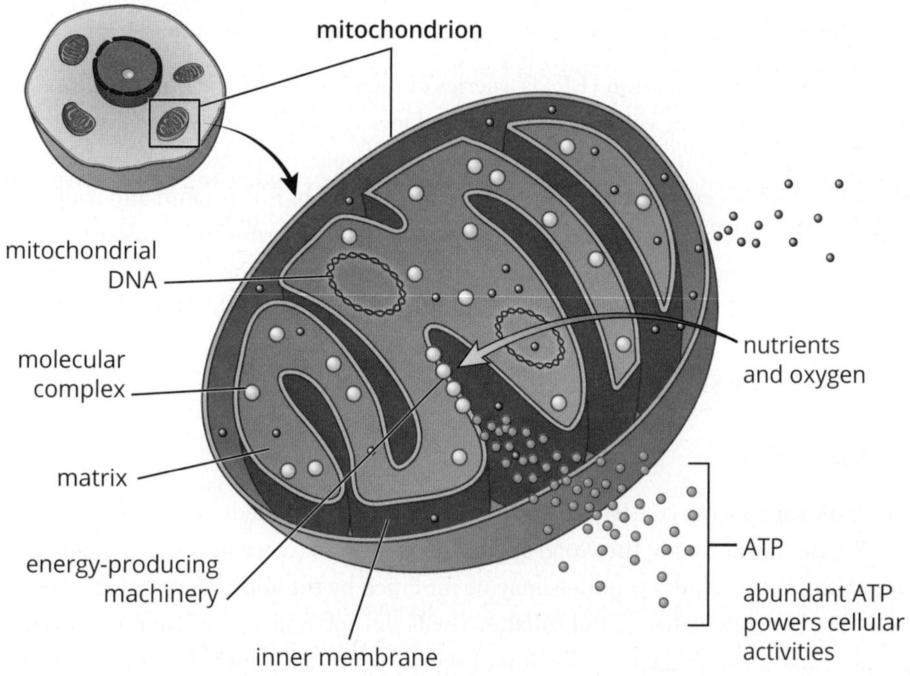

Figure 1.2 Mitochondrial Structure

Mitochondria are different from other parts of the cell in that they are semi-autonomous. They contain some of their own genes and replicate independently of the nucleus via binary fission. As such, they are paradigmatic examples of **cytoplasmic** or **extranuclear inheritance**—the transmission of genetic material independent of the nucleus. Mitochondria are thought to have originated when the engulfing of an aerobic prokaryote by an anaerobic prokaryote resulted in a symbiotic relationship.

In addition to keeping the cell alive by providing energy, the mitochondria are also capable of killing the cell by release of enzymes from the electron transport chain. This release kick-starts a process known as **apoptosis**, or programmed cell death.

Lysosomes

Lysosomes are membrane-bound structures containing hydrolytic enzymes that are capable of breaking down many different substrates, including substances ingested by endocytosis and cellular waste products. Lysosomes often function in conjunction with **endosomes**, which transport, package and sort cell material traveling to and from the membrane. Endosomes are capable of transporting materials to the *trans*-golgi, to the cell membrane, or to the lysosomal pathway for degradation. The lysosomal membrane sequesters these enzymes to prevent damage to the cell. However, release of these enzymes can occur in a process known as **autolysis**. Like mitochondria, when lysosomes release their hydrolytic enzymes, it results in apoptosis. In this case, the released enzymes directly lead to the degradation of cellular components.

KEY CONCEPT

Not all cells have the same relative distribution of organelles. Form will follow function. Cells that require a lot of energy for locomotion (such as sperm cells) have high concentrations of mitochondria. Cells involved in secretion (such as pancreatic islet cells and other endocrine tissues) have high concentrations of RER and Golgi apparatuses. Other cells, such as red blood cells, which primarily serve a transport function, have no organelles at all.

Endoplasmic Reticulum

The **endoplasmic reticulum** (**ER**) is a series of interconnected membranes that are actually contiguous with the nuclear envelope. The double membrane of the endoplasmic reticulum is folded into numerous invaginations, creating complex structures with a central lumen. There are two varieties of ER: smooth and rough. The **rough ER** (**RER**) is studded with **ribosomes**, which permit the translation of proteins destined for secretion directly into its lumen. On the other hand, the **smooth ER** (**SER**) lacks ribosomes and is utilized primarily for lipid synthesis (such as the phospholipids in the cell membrane) and the detoxification of certain drugs and poisons. The SER also transports proteins from the RER to the Golgi apparatus.

Golgi Apparatus

The **Golgi apparatus** consists of stacked membrane-bound sacs. Materials from the ER are transferred to the Golgi apparatus in vesicles. Once inside the Golgi apparatus, these cellular products may be modified by the addition of groups like carbohydrates, phosphates, and sulfates. The Golgi apparatus may also modify cellular products through the introduction of signal sequences, which direct the delivery of the product to a specific cellular location. After modification and sorting in the Golgi apparatus, cellular products are repackaged in vesicles, which are then directed to the correct cellular location. If the product is destined for secretion, the secretory vesicle merges with the cell membrane and its contents are released via **exocytosis**. The relationships between lysosomes, the ER, and the Golgi apparatus are shown in Figure 1.3.

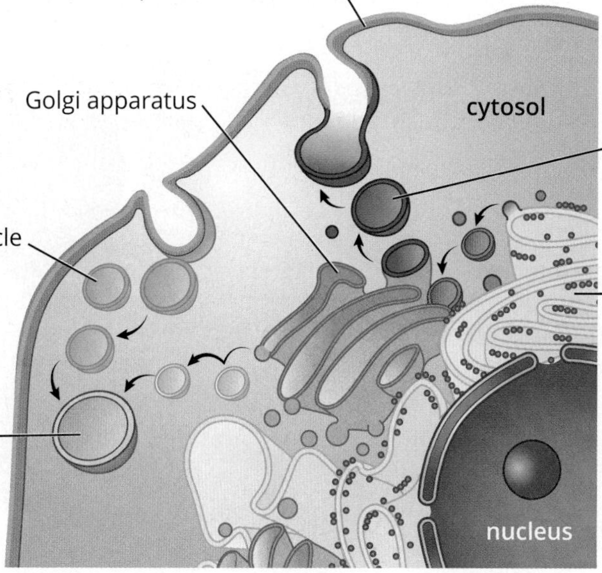

Figure 1.3 Lysosomes, the Endoplasmic Reticulum, and the Golgi Apparatus

Peroxisomes

Peroxisomes contain hydrogen peroxide. One of the primary functions of peroxisomes is the breakdown of very long chain fatty acids via β-oxidation. Peroxisomes participate in the synthesis of phospholipids and contain some of the enzymes involved in the pentose phosphate pathway, discussed in Chapter 9 of *MCAT Biochemistry Review.*

The Cytoskeleton

The **cytoskeleton**, shown in Figure 1.4, provides structure to the cell and helps it to maintain its shape. In addition, the cytoskeleton provides a conduit for the transport of materials around the cell. There are three components of the cytoskeleton: microfilaments, microtubules, and intermediate filaments.

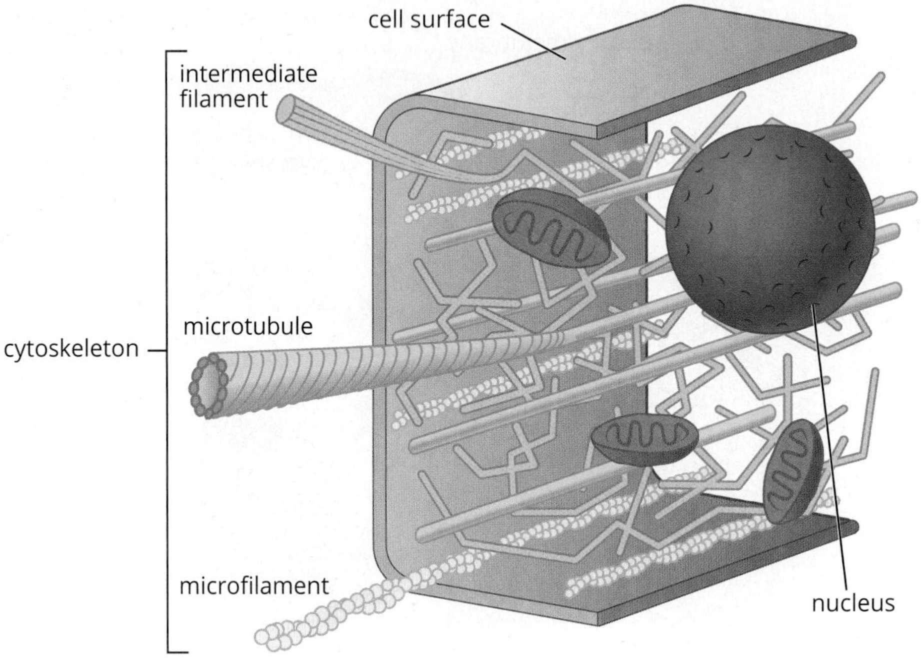

Figure 1.4 Cytoskeletal Elements

Microfilaments

Microfilaments are made up of solid polymerized rods of **actin**. The actin filaments are organized into bundles and networks and are resistant to both compression and fracture, providing protection for the cell. Actin filaments can also use ATP to generate force for movement by interacting with **myosin**, such as in muscle contraction.

Microfilaments also play a role in **cytokinesis**, or the division of materials between daughter cells. During mitosis, the **cleavage furrow** is formed from microfilaments, which organize as a ring at the site of division between the two new daughter cells. As the actin filaments within this ring contract, the ring becomes smaller, eventually pinching off the connection between the two daughter cells.

BRIDGE

Motor proteins like kinesin and dynein are classic examples of nonenzymatic protein function, along with binding proteins, cell adhesion molecules, immunoglobulins, and ion channels. Motor proteins often travel along cytoskeletal structures to accomplish their functions. Nonenzymatic protein functions are discussed in Chapter 3 of *MCAT Biochemistry Review.*

Microtubules

Unlike microfilaments, **microtubules** are hollow polymers of **tubulin** proteins. Microtubules radiate throughout the cell, providing the primary pathways along which motor proteins like ***kinesin*** and ***dynein*** carry vesicles.

Cilia and flagella are motile structures composed of microtubules. **Cilia** are projections from a cell that are primarily involved in the movement of materials along the surface of the cell; for example, cilia line the respiratory tract and are involved in the movement of mucus. **Flagella** are structures involved in the movement of the cell itself, such as the movement of sperm cells through the reproductive tract. Cilia and flagella share the same structure, composed of nine pairs of microtubules forming an outer ring, with two microtubules in the center, as shown in Figure 1.5. This is known as a **9 + 2 structure** and is seen only in eukaryotic organelles of motility. Bacterial flagella have a different structure with a different chemical composition, as discussed later in this chapter.

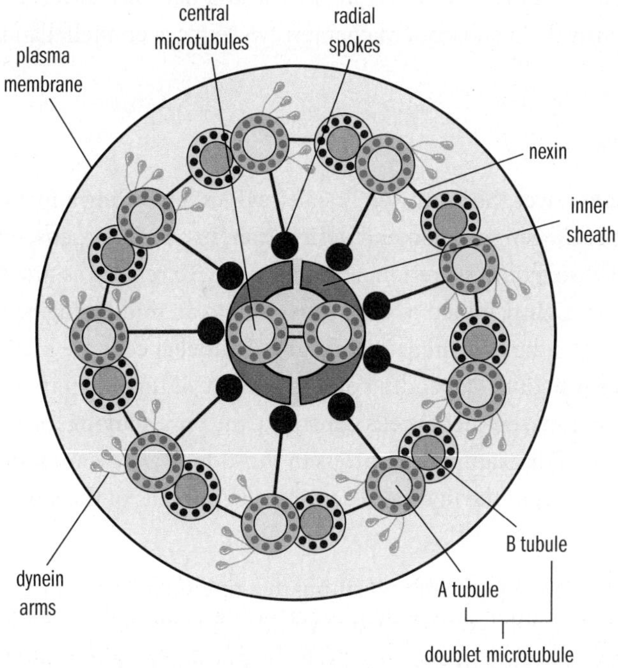

Figure 1.5 Cilium and Flagellum Structure
Microtubules are organized into a ring of 9 doublets with 2 central microtubules.

Centrioles are found in a region of the cell called the **centrosome**. They are the organizing centers for microtubules and are structured as nine triplets of microtubules with a hollow center. During mitosis, the centrioles migrate to opposite poles of the dividing cell and organize the mitotic spindle. The microtubules emanating from the centrioles attach to the chromosomes via complexes called **kinetochores** and exert force on the sister chromatids, pulling them apart.

Intermediate Filaments

Intermediate filaments are a diverse group of filamentous proteins, which includes keratin, desmin, vimentin, and lamins. Many intermediate filaments are involved in cell–cell adhesion or maintenance of the overall integrity of the cytoskeleton. Intermediate filaments are able to withstand a tremendous amount of tension, increasing the structural rigidity of the cell. In addition, intermediate filaments help anchor other organelles, including the nucleus. The identity of the intermediate filament proteins within a cell is specific to the cell and tissue type.

Tissue Formation

One of the unique characteristics of eukaryotic cells is the formation of tissues with division of labor, as different cells in a tissue may carry out different functions. For example, in the heart, some cells participate in the conduction pathways while others cause contraction; still others serve a supportive role like maintaining structural integrity of the organ. There are four tissue types: epithelial tissue, connective tissue, muscle tissue, and nervous tissue. While muscle and nervous tissue are considered more extensively in subsequent chapters, we explore epithelial and connective tissues below.

Epithelial Tissue

Epithelial tissues cover the body and line its cavities, providing a means for protection against pathogen invasion and desiccation. In certain organs, epithelial cells are involved in absorption, secretion, and sensation. To remain as one cohesive unit, epithelial cells are tightly joined to each other and to an underlying layer of connective tissue known as the **basement membrane**. Epithelial cells are highly diverse and serve numerous functions depending on the identity of the organ in which they are found; in most organs, epithelial cells constitute the **parenchyma**, or the functional parts of the organ. For example, nephrons in the kidney are composed of epithelial cells, and hepatocytes in the liver, and acid-producing cells of the stomach are epithelial cells.

Epithelial cells are often polarized, meaning that one side faces a lumen (the hollow inside of an organ or tube) or the outside world, while the other side interacts with underlying blood vessels and structural cells. For example, in the small intestine, one side of the cell will be involved in absorption of nutrients from the lumen, while the other side will be involved in releasing those nutrients into circulation for use in the rest of the body.

We can classify different epithelia according to the number of layers they have and the shape of their cells. **Simple epithelia** have one layer of cells; **stratified epithelia** have multiple layers; and **pseudostratified epithelia** appear to have multiple layers due to differences in cell height but are, in reality, only one layer. Turning to shape, cells may be classified as cuboidal, columnar, or squamous. As their names imply, **cuboidal** cells are cube-shaped and **columnar** cells are long and thin. **Squamous** cells are flat and scale-like.

Connective Tissue

Connective tissue supports the body and provides a framework for the epithelial cells to carry out their functions. Whereas epithelial cells contribute to the parenchyma of an organ, connective tissues are the main contributors to the **stroma** or support structure. Bone, cartilage, tendons, ligaments, adipose tissue, and blood are all examples of connective tissues. Most cells in connective tissues produce and secrete materials such as collagen and elastin to form the **extracellular matrix**.

MCAT CONCEPT CHECK 1.2

Before you move on, assess your understanding of the material with these questions.

1. Briefly describe the functions of each of the organelles listed below:
   - Nucleus:
   - Mitochondrion:
   - Lysosome:
   - Rough endoplasmic reticulum:
   - Smooth endoplasmic reticulum:
   - Golgi apparatus:
   - Peroxisome:
2. A child is diagnosed with an enzyme deficiency that prevents the production of hydrogen peroxide. What would the likely outcome be of such a deficiency?
3. What are the predominant proteins in each cytoskeletal element?
   - Microfilaments:
   - Microtubules:
   - Intermediate filaments:
4. How do the cytoskeletal structures of centrioles and flagella differ?

5. Classify each of the following cells as epithelial cells or connective tissue:
   - Fibroblasts, which produce collagen in a number of organs:

   - Endothelial cells, which line blood vessels:

   - α-cells, which produce glucagon in the pancreas:

   - Osteoblasts, which produce osteoid, the material that hardens into bone:

   - Chondroblasts, which produce cartilage:

1.3 Classification and Structure of Prokaryotic Cells

LEARNING OBJECTIVES

After Chapter 1.3, you will be able to:

- Compare and contrast archaea, bacteria, and eukaryotes
- Identify the three common bacterial shapes
- Explain the differences between gram-positive and gram-negative bacteria
- Detail the structural differences between eukaryotic and prokaryotic flagella
- Differentiate between the metabolic processes of aerobic and anaerobic bacteria

Prokaryotes are the simplest of all organisms and include all bacteria. Prokaryotes do not contain any membrane-bound organelles, and their genetic material is organized into a single circular molecule of DNA concentrated in an area of the cell called the **nucleoid region**. Despite the simplicity of prokaryotes, they are incredibly diverse, and knowledge of this diversity is essential for the study of medicine because many prokaryotes can cause infection. In fact, choosing the appropriate antibiotic to fight an infection requires knowledge about the basic structure of the bacteria causing the infection.

Prokaryotic Domains

There are three overarching domains into which all life is classified: Archaea, Bacteria, and Eukarya. Two of these—Archaea and Bacteria—contain prokaryotes. Initially, Archaea and Bacteria were classified together into the kingdom of Monera. However, modern genetics and biochemical techniques have indicated that the differences in the evolutionary pathways between Archaea and Bacteria are at least as significant as between either of these domains and Eukarya.

Archaea

Archaea are single-celled organisms that are visually similar to bacteria, but contain genes and several metabolic pathways that are more similar to eukaryotes than to bacteria. Historically, Archaea were considered **extremophiles**, in that they were most commonly isolated from harsh environments with extremely high temperatures, high salinity, or no light. More recent research has demonstrated a greater variety of habitats for these organisms, including the human body. Archaea are notable for their ability to use alternative sources of energy. While some are photosynthetic, many are chemosynthetic and can generate energy from inorganic compounds, including sulfur- and nitrogen-based compounds such as ammonia.

Due to the similarities of this domain to eukaryotes, it is hypothesized that eukaryotes and the Archaea share a common origin. Both eukaryotes and Archaea start translation with methionine, contain similar *RNA polymerases*, and associate their DNA with histones. However, Archaea contain a single circular chromosome, divide by binary fission or budding, and share a similar overall structure to bacteria. Interestingly, Archaea are resistant to many antibiotics.

Bacteria

All bacteria contain a **cell membrane** and **cytoplasm**, and some have **flagella** or **fimbriae** (similar to cilia), as shown in Figure 1.6. Because bacteria and eukaryotes often share analogous structures, it can be difficult to develop medicines that target only bacteria. However, in some cases, even seemingly similar structures have enough biochemical differences to allow the exclusive targeting of one kind of organism. For example, bacterial flagella and eukaryotic flagella are different enough that scientists are able to develop antibacterial vaccines that specifically target the bacterial flagellum. Also, many antibiotics target the bacterial ribosome, which is significantly smaller than the eukaryotic ribosome.

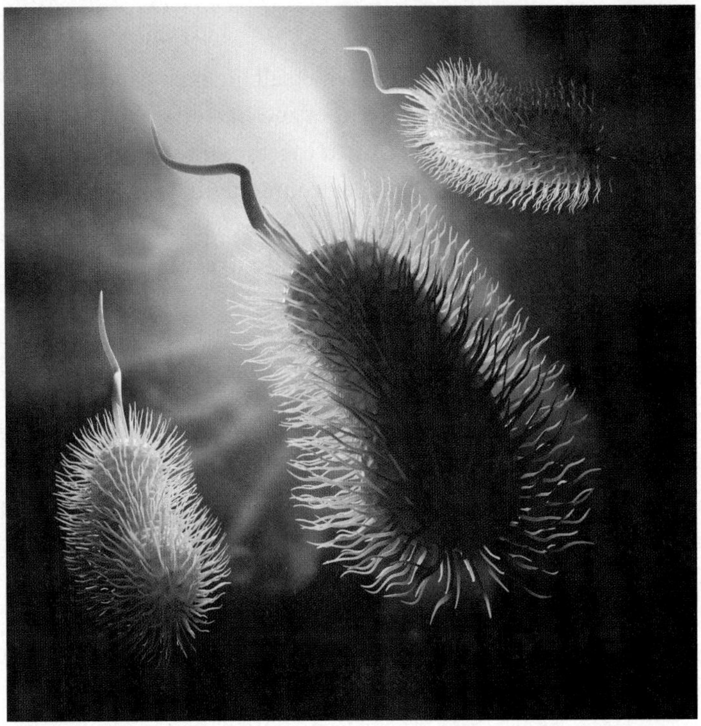

Figure 1.6 Prokaryotic Cell Specializations: Flagella and Fimbriae

REAL WORLD

Bacteria perform essential functions for human beings, including the production of vitamin K in the intestine. Vitamin K is required for production of the plasma proteins necessary for blood clotting. Newborn infants are not yet colonized by bacteria and cannot produce clotting factors, putting them at risk for hemorrhage. When babies are born, they are given an injection of vitamin K to aid in the production of clotting factors until they have been colonized with bacteria.

There are approximately 5×10^{30} bacteria on Earth, outnumbering all of the plants and animals combined. As mentioned in the introduction to this chapter, bacteria outnumber human cells in the body by 10:1. The relationship between the human body and bacteria is complex. Some bacteria are **mutualistic symbiotes**, meaning that both humans and the bacteria benefit from the relationship. Examples include the bacteria in the human gut that produce vitamin K and biotin (vitamin B_7), and which also prevent the overgrowth of harmful bacteria. Other bacteria are **pathogens** or **parasites**, meaning that they provide no advantage or benefit to the host, but rather cause disease. Pathogenic bacteria may live intracellularly or extracellularly. For example, *Chlamydia trachomatis*, a common sexually transmitted infection, lives inside cells of the reproductive tract; *Clostridium tetani*, the cause of tetanus, lives outside of cells and produces toxins that enter the bloodstream.

Classification of Bacteria by Shape

Classification of bacteria by shape provides scientists and pathologists (physicians who specialize in the identification and characterization of disease) a common language to talk about bacteria, as well as a way to identify different species of bacteria.

Most bacteria exist in one of three shapes, as shown in Figure 1.7. Spherical bacteria, known as **cocci**, include common pathogens such as *Streptococcus pyogenes*.

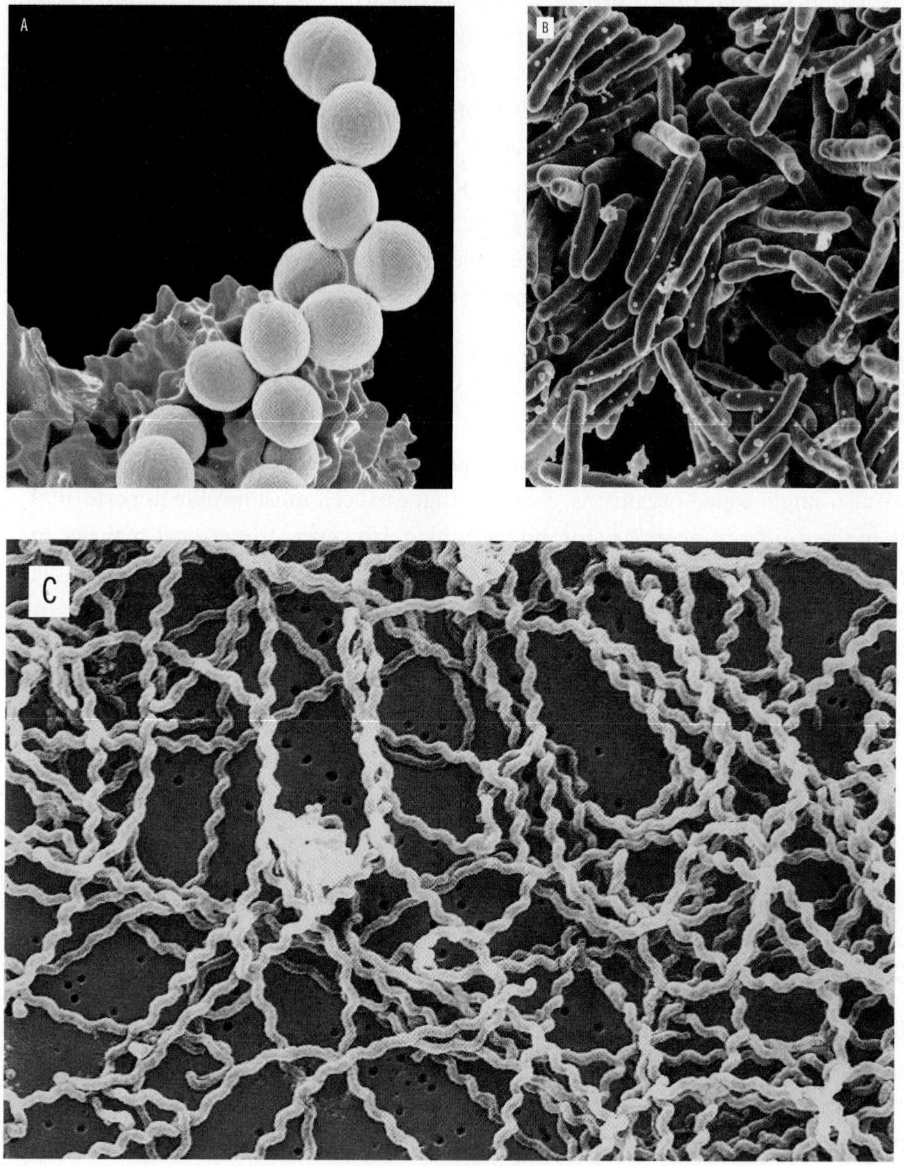

Figure 1.7 Prokaryotic Cell Shapes
(a) Cocci (Staphylococcus aureus), (b) Bacilli (Mycobacterium tuberculosis), (c) Spirilli (Leptospira interrogans)

REAL WORLD

Very few pathogenic bacteria are spiral shaped. The three most common are:

- *Treponema pallidum*, the cause of syphilis
- *Borrelia burgdorferi*, the cause of Lyme disease
- *Leptospira interrogans*, the cause of Weil's disease

Rod-shaped bacteria, like *Escherichia coli*, are known as **bacilli**. Finally, spiral-shaped bacteria, known as **spirilli**, include such species as *Treponema pallidum*, which causes syphilis.

Aerobes and Anaerobes

Some bacteria require oxygen for survival, while others do not. Bacteria that require oxygen for metabolism are termed **obligate aerobes**. Other bacteria that use fermentation, or some other form of cellular metabolism that does not require oxygen, are called **anaerobes**. There are different types of anaerobes. Anaerobes that cannot survive in an oxygen-containing environment are called **obligate anaerobes**; the presence of oxygen leads to the production of reactive oxygen-containing radicals in these species, which leads to cell death. Other bacteria can toggle between metabolic processes, using oxygen for aerobic metabolism if it is present, and switching to anaerobic metabolism if it is not. These bacteria are called **facultative anaerobes**. Finally, **aerotolerant anaerobes** are unable to use oxygen for metabolism, but are not harmed by its presence in the environment.

Prokaryotic Cell Structure

One of the main differences between prokaryotes and eukaryotes is that prokaryotes lack a nucleus and membrane-bound organelles, as shown in Figure 1.8. Prokaryotes are also single-celled organisms, meaning that each cell must be able to perform all of the functions necessary for life on its own. However, prokaryotes may live in colonies with other cells and may signal these cells to share information about the environment.

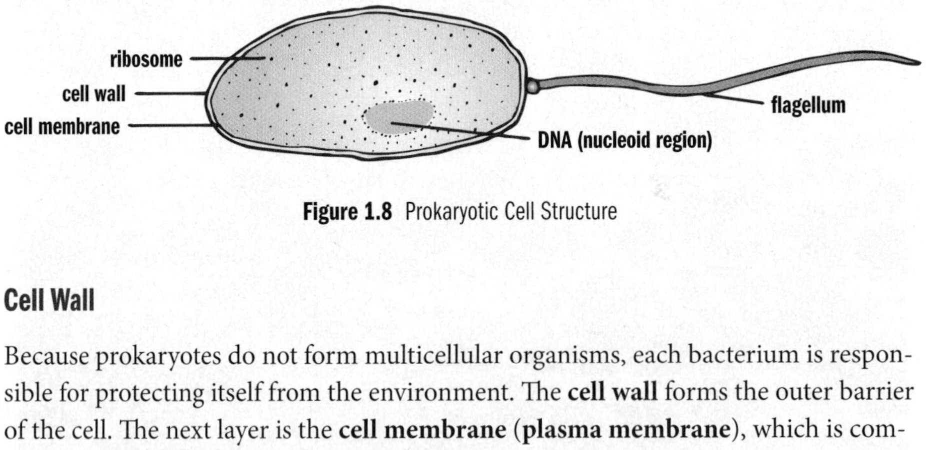

Figure 1.8 Prokaryotic Cell Structure

Cell Wall

Because prokaryotes do not form multicellular organisms, each bacterium is responsible for protecting itself from the environment. The **cell wall** forms the outer barrier of the cell. The next layer is the **cell membrane (plasma membrane)**, which is composed of phospholipids, similar to that of a eukaryote. Together, the cell wall and the cell membrane are known as the **envelope**.

The cell wall both provides structure and controls the movement of solutes into and out of the bacterium. This allows the cell to maintain a concentration gradient relative to the environment. In bacteria, there are two main types of cell wall: gram positive and gram negative. The type of cell wall is determined by the Gram staining process: a crystal violet stain, followed by a counterstain with a substance called *safranin.* If the envelope absorbs the crystal violet stain, it will appear deep purple, and the cell is said to be gram positive. If the envelope does not absorb the crystal violet stain, but absorbs the safranin counterstain, then the cell will appear pink-red, and it is said to be gram negative.

Gram-positive cell walls consist of a thick layer of **peptidoglycan**, a polymeric substance made from amino acids and sugars. In addition to its structural and barrier functions, the cell wall may also aid a bacterial pathogen by providing protection from a host organism's immune system. In addition to peptidoglycan, the gram-positive cell wall also contains **lipoteichoic acid**. It is not clear what role this acid serves for the bacterium, but the human immune system may be activated by exposure to these chemicals.

Gram-negative cell walls are very thin and also contain peptidoglycan, but in much smaller amounts. The peptidoglycan cell walls of these bacteria are adjacent to the cell membrane, and are separated from the membrane by the **periplasmic space**. In addition to the cell wall and cell membrane, gram-negative bacteria also have **outer membranes** containing phospholipids and **lipopolysaccharides**. Interestingly, lipopolysaccharides are the part of gram-negative bacteria that triggers an immune response in human beings; the inflammatory response to lipopolysaccharides is much stronger than the response to lipoteichoic acid.

KEY CONCEPT

Bacteria contain a cell wall, the composition of which is different in gram-positive and gram-negative bacteria. Specific components of the cell wall can trigger an inflammatory response.

REAL WORLD

The antibiotic penicillin targets the enzyme that catalyzes the cross-linking of peptidoglycan. If a gram-positive cell cannot cross-link its cell wall, it no longer serves as an effective barrier. The bacterium then becomes susceptible to osmotic damage and lyses. Most bacteria have developed resistance mechanisms to penicillin, although a few bacteria—including *Streptococcus pyogenes*, which causes strep throat and some skin infections, and *Treponema pallidum*, which causes syphilis—are still very sensitive to this antibiotic.

Flagella

Flagella are long, whip-like structures that can be used for propulsion; bacteria may have one, two, or many flagella, depending on the species. Flagella can be used to move toward food or away from toxins or immune cells. This ability of a cell to detect chemical stimuli and move toward or away from them is called **chemotaxis**. The flagella are composed of a filament, a basal body, and a hook, as shown in Figure 1.9. The **filament** is a hollow, helical structure composed of **flagellin**. The **basal body** is a complex structure that anchors the flagellum to the cytoplasmic membrane and is also the motor of the flagellum, which rotates at rates up to 300 Hz. The **hook** connects the filament and the basal body so that, as the basal body rotates, it exerts torque on the filament, which thereby spins and propels the bacterium forward. The overall structure of flagella is similar in both gram-positive and gram-negative bacteria, but there are slight differences due to the different physical structure and chemical composition of the envelope in gram-positive and gram-negative bacteria. Archaea also contain flagella, but the structure of their flagella is quite different from that of bacteria and is unlikely to be asked about on Test Day.

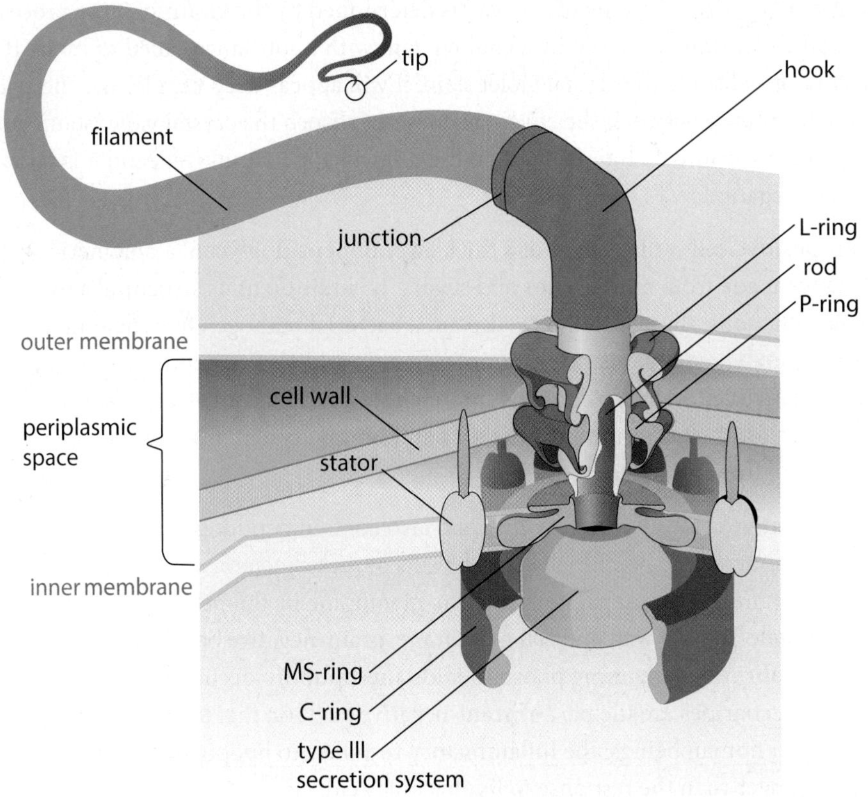

Figure 1.9 Prokaryotic Flagellum Structure
The hook connects the filament to the basal body (the complex structure of which is shown).

Other Organelles

As mentioned earlier, prokaryotes concentrate DNA in a region of the cell known as the nucleoid region, which does not contain a nuclear envelope. Prokaryotic DNA is carried on a single circular chromosome which can be found coiled around histone-like proteins in some bacteria. True histones are found in Archaea. In addition, DNA acquired from external sources may also be carried on smaller circular structures known as **plasmids**. Plasmids carry DNA that is not necessary for survival of the prokaryote—and therefore is not considered part of the genome of the bacterium—but may confer an advantage such as antibiotic resistance.

Prokaryotes lack several key organelles, such as mitochondria. Instead, the cell membrane is used for the electron transport chain and generation of ATP. Prokaryotes do contain a primitive cytoskeleton, but it is not nearly as complex as the one found in eukaryotes. Prokaryotes also contain ribosomes, but this ribosome is a different size from that found in eukaryotes: prokaryotic ribosomes contain 30S and 50S subunits, whereas eukaryotic ribosomes contain 40S and 60S subunits.

BRIDGE

The fact that prokaryotes and eukaryotes have different-sized ribosomes implies that they carry out protein synthesis in slightly different ways. These differences are highlighted in Chapter 7 of *MCAT Biochemistry Review*. This difference also allows us to target bacterial ribosomes with a number of antibiotics, including *tetracyclines*, *aminoglycosides*, and *macrolides*, while leaving the eukaryotic ribosome more or less unaffected.

MCAT CONCEPT CHECK 1.3

Before you move on, assess your understanding of the material with these questions.

1. In what ways are Archaea similar to bacteria? In what ways are Archaea similar to eukaryotes?
   - Similar to bacteria:

   - Similar to eukaryotes:

   ---

2. What are the three common shapes of bacteria?
   -

   -

   -

   ---

3. Compare and contrast the metabolisms of aerobic and anaerobic bacteria: (Note: Put "yes" or "no" in each box.)

	Oxygen Present		Oxygen Absent	
Type of Bacteria	**Can survive**	**Can carry out aerobic metabolism**	**Can survive**	**Can carry out anaerobic metabolism**
Obligate aerobe				
Facultative anaerobe				
Obligate anaerobe				
Aerotolerant anaerobe				

4. What difference between the envelopes of gram-positive and gram-negative bacteria make gram-positive bacteria more susceptible to antibiotics such as penicillin?

   ---

5. How do the structures of eukaryotic and prokaryotic flagella differ?
   - Eukaryotic:

   - Prokaryotic:

BIOLOGY GUIDED EXAMPLE WITH EXPERT THINKING

To investigate the collective resistance property of bacteria, co-colonization experiments were conducted. Eight-week-old female CD1 mice were infected intratracheally with chloramphenicol sensitive (Cm^S) pneumococci or an equivalent quantity of Cm^S:chloramphenicol resistant (Cm^R) pneumococci (1:1). One hour post-infection, mice were treated with one intraperitoneal injection of chloramphenicol (Cm) at a concentration of 75 mg kg^{-1}, followed by two additional doses spaced 5 hours apart. Control mice received vehicle injection only. Cm^R pneumococci are Cm resistant due to the expression of a resistance factor, chloramphenicol acetyltransferase (CAT).

Goal: investigate collective resistance of bacteria by comparing infection with one bacteria to a mixture of two bacteria

Experimental setup: Infect mice, then give intraperitoneal (IP) injections of chloramphenicol or vehicle only (vehicle is just the solvent without any antibiotic, probably saline)

Stable bacterial coexistence requires successful adjustment to several ecological constraints, such as limited resources and antibiotic concentration. To better quantify bacterial behavior under these conditions, in vitro population analysis was conducted.

Based on the experimental setup and this statement, collective resistance must be about the coexistence of bacterial types when only one is resistant to an antibiotic

Population analysis done to quantify collective resistance

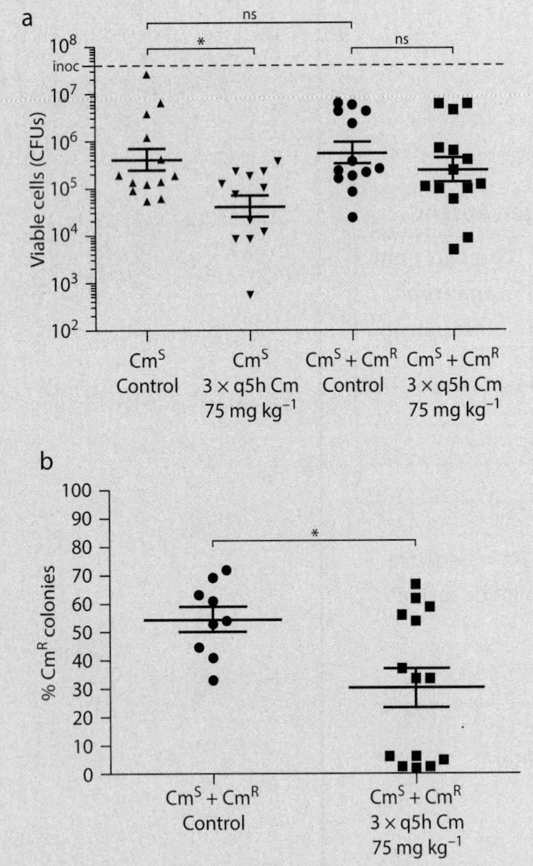

In figures always identify the variables and trends.

IVs: control or Cm administration, Cm^S or Cm^S/Cm^R bacteria

DVs: viable cells, percent Cm^R colonies

Trends: Cm^S bacteria have significantly fewer viable cells when treated with Cm. The percent of Cm^R colonies is significantly lower when Cm^S/Cm^R is treated with Cm.

Figure 1 Mixed Culture Experiment. (a) Antibiotic stress on Cm^S alone and $Cm^S + Cm^R$ co-colonization condition. (b) Co-colonization colonies analysis of Cm^S to Cm^R ratio.

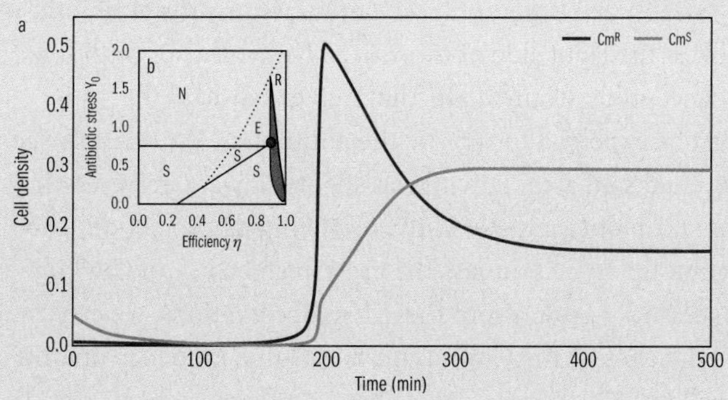

IVs: time, antibiotic stress

DVs: cell density, efficiency

Trends: highest cell density of Cm^R is at 200 min, Cm^S density levels off at 300 min. Based on the caption, the inner figure compares efficiency under several different conditions.

Figure 2 (a) Bacterial growth trajectories subject to antibiotic stress and resource competition. (b) Axes indicate co-colonization experiment parameters (efficiency refers to the growth rate efficiency of Cm^R cells). The dot indicates Figure 1 experiment antibiotic levels, with previous analysis establishing Cm^S only (area S), Cm^R only (area R), no bacterial growth (area N), and competition-induced extinction (area E, where Cm^S bacteria first outcompete Cm^R bacteria and are subsequently cleared by antibiotic).

Adapted from Sorg, R. A., Lin, L., Van Doorn, G. S., Sorg, M., Olson, J., Nizet, V., & Veening, J. W. (2016). Collective resistance in microbial communities by intracellular antibiotic deactivation. *PLoS Biology*, 14(12), e2000631.

Consider the following: For successful co-colonization with Cm^S, the growth efficiency of Cm^R must remain as a constant value in the presence or absence of antibiotic stress. Is this conclusion valid?

This question asks us to analyze a conclusion's validity. First, we must find where the key term is located in the passage. In this case, we are asked about growth efficiency, which can be found in the figure description of Figure 2b. According to the description, growth efficiency is a reference to the growth rate of Cm^R, and is depicted as the *x*-axis of the graph. The conclusion given in the question stem states that the growth efficiency is unchanged by the presence of antibiotics. To determine if this conclusion is valid, we first need to decipher what the graph represents.

The figure description can be a rich source of crucial information. According to that same Figure 2b description, each area on the graph depicts a different outcome of Cm^S and Cm^R co-colonization. To ensure we're drawing valid conclusions, we should examine the graph one axis at a time. To analyze a graph, hold one variable constant first. Assume no antibiotics are present, meaning that the antibiotic stress is zero, looking at the *x*-axis along the zero line, as the growth efficiency of Cm^R decreases, the Cm^S strain starts to outcompete it. In fact, unless the growth efficiency of Cm^R is at its highest, the susceptible strain (Cm^S) will always outcompete Cm^R.

Now let's hold the same variable at a different level. Let us assume the antibiotic stress is high, so we'll look to the right side of the *x*-axis. Under those conditions, there's no growth of the susceptible strain at all. That makes sense, as the susceptible strain wouldn't be expected to survive the antibiotics. We can also see that, for this *x*-axis value, there's an area, E, where at slightly lower Cm^R growth efficiency, the susceptible strain outcompetes Cm^R, removing all protection, and then succumbs to the antibiotic. In fact, unless the growth efficiency of Cm^R is high, no bacteria will successfully grow. From these two observations, we can observe that the growth efficiency of the Cm^R strain has a large influence on how the co-colonized strain will grow.

The shaded area of Figure 2b is not explained in the figure description, but we can deduce its meaning through context. All the other possibilities already have a designated area on the graph based on the figure label except for successful co-colonization. Also, the shaded area is between the area of Cm^S only and Cm^R only areas. From the figure description, we also learned that the large dot indicates the experiment conducted in Figure 1's conditions, and Figure 1's experiment demonstrates successful co-colonization. Thus, we can conclude that the shaded area is the region of successful co-colonization of the two strains.

The conclusion presented in the question stem claims that growth efficiency of Cm^R does not change with or without the antibiotic presence. To assess this, we simply need to compare those two conditions. With no antibiotics, we can see that successful co-colonization only occurs when the growth efficiency of the Cm^R is at 1. If the growth efficiency is not that high, then the Cm^S strain will outcompete it. When we raise the antibiotic level to that of the red dot, we can see that if the growth efficiency remains at 1, the Cm^R bacteria will outcompete the Cm^S bacteria. In order for the two strains to coexist under antibiotic stress, the resistance strain's growth efficiency has to be lower than 1. Thus, we can reasonably argue that the conclusion is not valid.

1.4 Genetics and Growth of Prokaryotic Cells

LEARNING OBJECTIVES

After Chapter 1.4, you will be able to:

- Describe bacterial genetic recombination via transformation, conjugation, or transduction
- Recall the four phases of a bacterial growth curve and the major features of each phase:

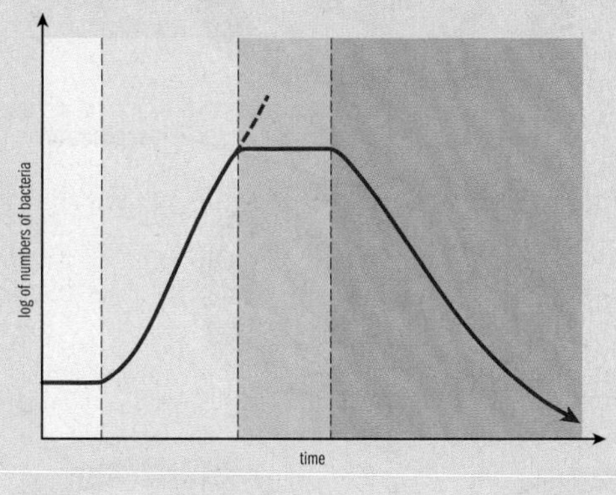

As we have seen, prokaryotic cells differ from eukaryotic cells both structurally and biochemically. Prokaryotes reproduce via asexual reproduction in the form of binary fission. In addition, prokaryotes are capable of acquiring and using genetic material from outside the cell.

Binary Fission

Binary fission, shown in Figure 1.10, is a simple form of asexual reproduction seen in prokaryotes. The circular chromosome attaches to the cell wall and replicates while the cell continues to grow in size. Eventually, the plasma membrane and cell wall begin to grow inward along the midline of the cell to produce two identical daughter cells. Because binary fission requires fewer events than mitosis, it can proceed more rapidly. In fact, some strains of *E. coli* can replicate every 20 minutes under ideal growth conditions.

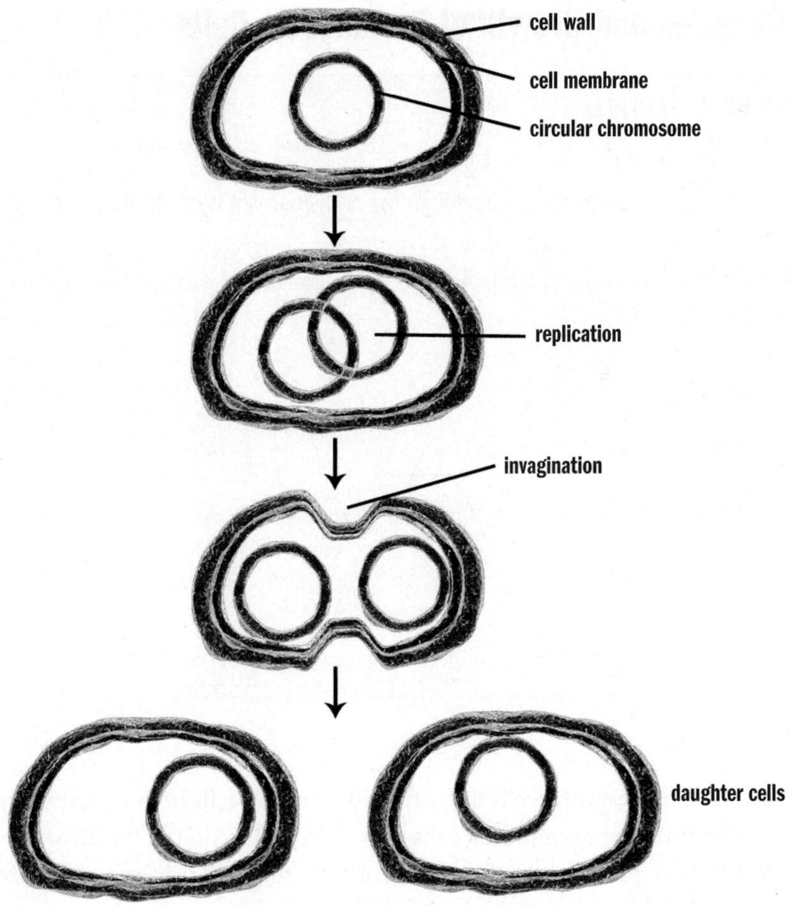

Figure 1.10 Stages of Binary Fission

Genetic Recombination

This single circular chromosome of a prokaryotic cell contains the information that is necessary for the cell to survive and reproduce. However, many bacteria also contain extrachromosomal (extragenomic) material known as **plasmids**. Plasmids often carry genes that impart some benefit to the bacterium, such as antibiotic resistance, some mechanisms of which are shown in Figure 1.11. Plasmids may also carry additional **virulence factors**, or traits that increase pathogenicity, such as toxin production, projections that allow attachment to certain kinds of cells, or features that allow evasion of the host's immune system. A subset of plasmids called **episomes** are capable of integrating into the genome of the bacterium.

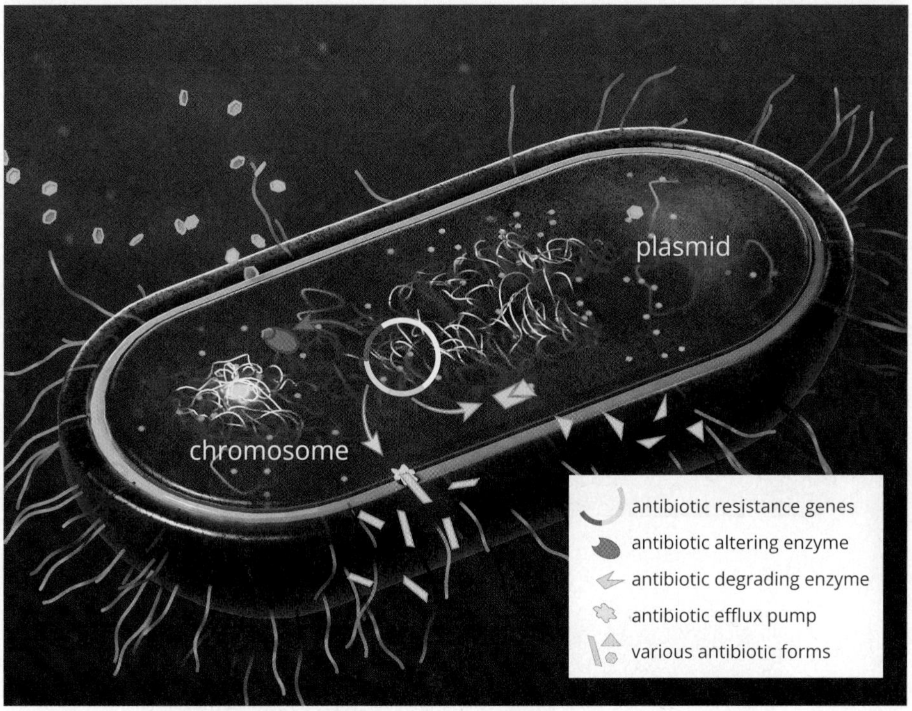

Figure 1.11 Mechanisms of Antibiotic Resistance

Bacterial genetic recombination helps increase bacterial diversity and thus permits evolution of a bacterial species over time. These recombination processes include transformation, conjugation, and transduction.

Transformation

Transformation results from the integration of foreign genetic material into the host genome. This foreign genetic material most frequently comes from other bacteria that, upon lysing, spill their contents into the vicinity of a bacterium capable of transformation. Many gram-negative rods are able to carry out this process.

Conjugation

Conjugation is the bacterial form of mating (sexual reproduction). It involves two cells forming a **conjugation bridge** between them that facilitates the transfer of genetic material. The transfer is unidirectional, from the **donor male** (+) to the **recipient female** (−). The bridge is made from appendages called **sex pili** that are found on the donor male. To form the pilus, bacteria must contain plasmids known as **sex factors** that contain the necessary genes. The best-studied sex factor is the **F (fertility) factor** in *E. coli*. Bacteria possessing this plasmid are termed F^+ cells; those without are called F^- cells. During conjugation the F^+ cell replicates its F factor and donates the copy to the F^- cell, converting it to an F^+ cell. This enables the cell obtaining the new plasmid to then transfer copies to other cells. This method of genetic recombination allows for rapid acquisition of antibiotic resistance or virulence factors throughout a colony because other plasmids can also be passed through the conjugation bridge. The process of conjugation is illustrated in Figure 1.12.

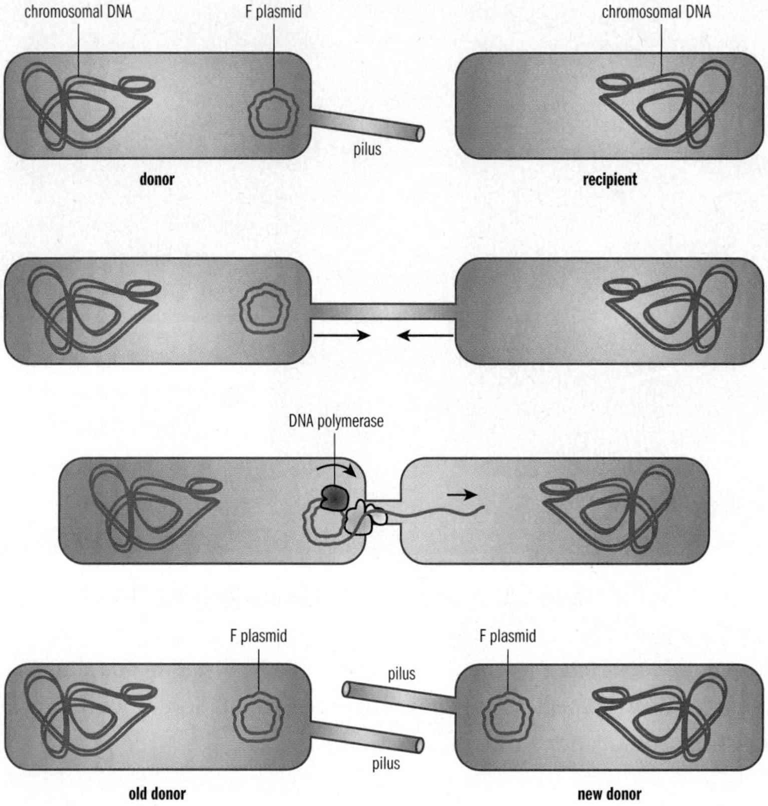

Figure 1.12 Bacterial Conjugation

The sex factor is a plasmid, but through processes such as transformation, it can become integrated into the host genome. In this case, when conjugation occurs, the entire genome replicates because it now contains the sex factor. The donor cell will then attempt to transfer an entire copy of its genome into the recipient; however, the bridge usually breaks before the full DNA sequence can be moved. Cells that have undergone this change are referred to by the abbreviation **Hfr** for **high frequency of recombination**.

Transduction

Transduction is the only genetic recombination process that requires a **vector**—a virus that carries genetic material from one bacterium to another. Viruses are obligate intracellular pathogens, which means that they cannot reproduce outside of a host cell. Because of this, **bacteriophages** (viruses that infect bacteria) can accidentally incorporate a segment of host DNA during assembly. When the bacteriophage infects another bacterium, it can release this trapped DNA into the new host cell. This transferred DNA can then integrate into the genome, giving the new host additional genes. The process of transduction is shown in Figure 1.13.

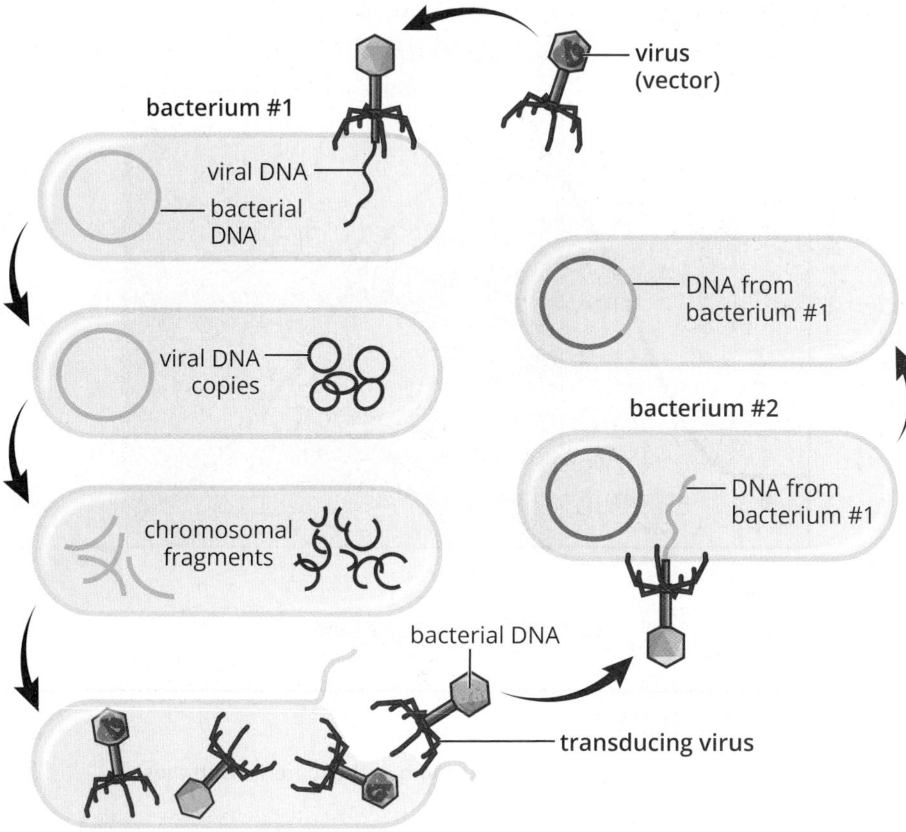

Figure 1.13 Bacterial Transduction

Transposons

Transposons are genetic elements capable of inserting and removing themselves from the genome. This phenomenon is not limited to prokaryotes; it has been seen in eukaryotes as well. If a transposon is inserted within a coding region of a gene, that gene may be disrupted.

Growth

As discussed previously, bacteria reproduce via binary fission. This implies that all of the bacteria are exactly the same in a local colony (assuming no mutations or genetic recombination), and that no bacteria are dividing faster than the others. Bacteria can be said to grow in a series of phases, as shown in Figure 1.14. In a new environment, bacteria first adapt to the new local conditions during the **lag phase**. As the bacteria adapt, the rate of division increases, causing an exponential increase in the number of bacteria in the colony during the **exponential phase**, also called the **log phase**. As the number of bacteria in the colony grows, resources are often reduced. The reduction of resources slows reproduction, and the **stationary phase** results. After the bacteria have exceeded the ability of the environment to support the number of bacteria, a **death phase** occurs, marking the depletion of resources.

REAL WORLD

One of the biggest challenges a doctor faces is patient compliance with treatment, especially antibiotics. Many patients fail to complete an entire course of antibiotics, often discontinuing the treatment because they feel better. Unfortunately, this breeds antibiotic resistance by killing off the bacteria that are nonresistant and leaving behind bacteria that are more resistant. These resistant bacteria then reproduce, resulting in recurrence of the infection. Over time, this practice has led to bacteria that are resistant to multiple antibiotics, making common infections more difficult to treat.

BRIDGE

The bacterial growth curve is an example of a semilog plot. The fact that the *y*-axis is logarithmic means that a straight line (as seen during the exponential phase) actually represents an exponential increase in the number of bacteria, not a linear increase. Semilog and log–log plots are discussed in Chapter 12 of *MCAT Physics and Math Review*.

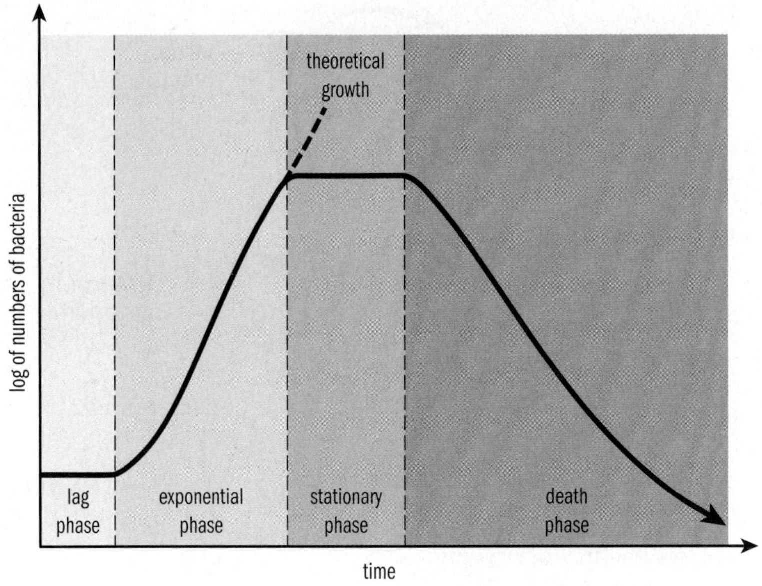

Figure 1.14 Bacterial Growth Curve

MCAT CONCEPT CHECK 1.4

Before you move on, assess your understanding of the material with these questions.

1. Briefly describe the three mechanisms of bacterial genetic recombination:
   - Transformation:

   ___

   - Conjugation:

   ___

   - Transduction:

   ___

2. What are the four phases of the bacterial growth curve? What are the features of each phase?

Phase	Features

1.5 Viruses and Subviral Particles

High-Yield

LEARNING OBJECTIVES

After Chapter 1.5, you will be able to:

- Explain why viruses are defined as "obligate intracellular parasites"
- Recall key virus terminology, including retrovirus and positive/negative sense
- Describe how viruses are able to produce progeny via infection of a host cell
- Compare and contrast the lytic and lysogenic cycles
- Describe how prions and viroids are able to cause disease

At the beginning of this chapter, we discussed the cell theory and noted that viruses do not fit the definition of living things because they are acellular. Viruses may be as small as 20 nm or as large as 300 nm. For reference, prokaryotes are 1–10 μm, and eukaryotes are about ten times larger. Unlike eukaryotic cells, viruses lack organelles and a nucleus.

Viral Structure

Viruses are composed of genetic material, a protein coat, and sometimes an envelope containing lipids. The genetic information may be circular or linear, single- or double-stranded, and composed of either DNA or RNA. The protein coat is known as a **capsid**, which may be surrounded by an envelope composed of phospholipids and virus-specific proteins. The envelope is very sensitive to heat, detergents, and desiccation; thus, enveloped viruses are easier to kill. On the other hand, viruses that do not have an envelope are more resistant to sterilization and are likely to persist on surfaces for an extended period of time.

Because viruses cannot reproduce independently, they are considered obligate intracellular parasites. Viruses must express and replicate genetic information within a **host cell** because they lack ribosomes to carry out protein synthesis. After hijacking a cell's machinery, a virus will replicate and produce viral progeny, called **virions**, which can be released to infect additional cells.

Bacteriophages are viruses that specifically target bacteria. They do not actually enter bacteria; rather, they simply inject their genetic material, leaving the remaining structures outside the infected cell. In addition to a capsid, bacteriophages contain a tail sheath and tail fibers, as shown in Figure 1.15. The **tail sheath** can act like a syringe, injecting genetic material into a bacterium. The **tail fibers** help the bacteriophage recognize and connect to the correct host cell.

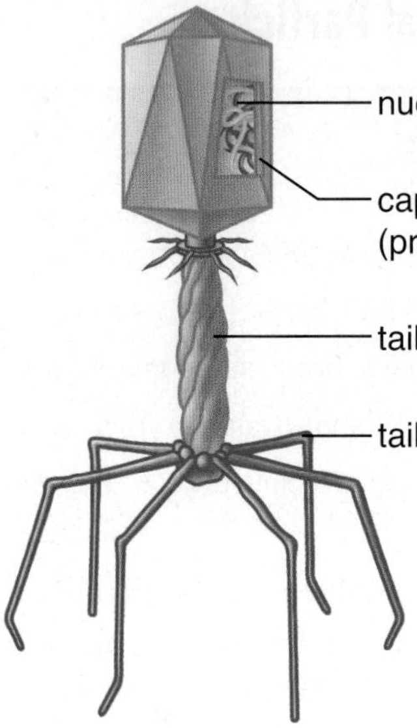

Figure 1.15 Structure of a Bacteriophage

Viral Genomes

Viral genomes come in a variety of shapes and sizes. Some are made of only a few genes, while others have several hundred. In addition, viral genomes may be made of either single- or double-stranded DNA or RNA.

Single-stranded RNA viruses may be positive sense or negative sense. **Positive sense** implies that the genome may be directly translated to functional proteins by the ribosomes of the host cell, just like mRNA. **Negative-sense** RNA viruses are a bit more complicated: the negative-sense RNA strand acts as a template for synthesis of a complementary strand, which can then be used as a template for protein synthesis. Negative-sense RNA viruses must carry an ***RNA replicase*** in the virion to ensure that the complementary strand is synthesized.

Retroviruses are enveloped, single-stranded RNA viruses in the family *Retroviridae*; usually, the virion contains two identical RNA molecules. These viruses carry an enzyme known as ***reverse transcriptase***, which synthesizes DNA from single-stranded RNA. The DNA then integrates into the host cell genome, where it is replicated and transcribed as if it were the host cell's own DNA. This is a clever mechanism because the integration of the genetic material into the host cell genome allows the cell to be infected indefinitely, so the only way to remove the infection is to kill the infected cell. The human immunodeficiency virus (HIV) is a retrovirus that utilizes this life cycle, which is one of the characteristics that make HIV so difficult to treat, as shown in Figure 1.16.

REAL WORLD

Both retroviruses and transduction are under investigation as methods of gene therapy. It is theorized that retroviral and transduction methods can deliver functional versions of missing or altered genes, so that the correct proteins can be synthesized and certain diseases can be treated. Gene therapy is discussed in Chapter 6 of *MCAT Biochemistry Review*.

1. The virus binds to CD4 and CCR5 proteins on the cell surface.
2. It then empties its contents into the cell as it fuses.
3. The reverse transcriptase enzyme makes a copy of the viral RNA and creates a double-stranded DNA.
4. This DNA is then inserted into the host cell's DNA by the viral enzyme, integrase.
5. When the infected cell divides it transcribes the viral DNA, making long chains of proteins.
6. Viral RNA and proteins move to the cell membrane to begin the process of the new virus creation.
7. The enzyme protease modifies protein chains aspart of the process in creating a mature virus.

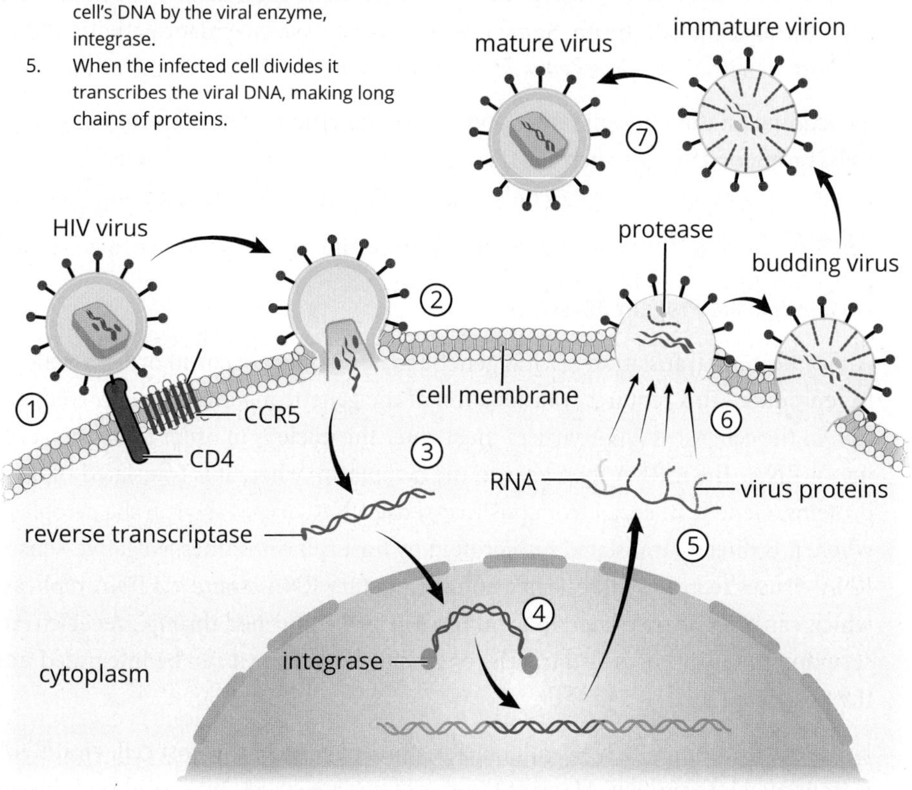

Figure 1.16 Life Cycle of the Human Immunodeficiency Virus (HIV)

Viral Life Cycle

As we have already discussed, viruses must infect a host cell and use the host cell's machinery in order to reproduce. Here, we will discuss the viral life cycle in detail.

Infection

REAL WORLD

HIV must bind to a receptor called CCR5 on white blood cells in order to infect them. Some people lack this receptor and are thus immune to HIV. There was recently a case in which an HIV-positive individual with leukemia received a bone marrow transplant from a donor that lacked CCR5. Not only was the leukemia cured, but the patient experienced remission of the HIV infection because the white blood cells from the newly acquired bone marrow were not susceptible to HIV infection.

Viruses can only infect a specific set of cells, because they must bind to specific receptors on the host cell. Without the proper receptors, a cell is essentially invisible to the virus. Once the virus binds the correct receptor, the virus and the cell are brought into close enough proximity to permit additional interactions. Enveloped viruses fuse with the plasma membrane of a cell, allowing entry of the virion into the host cell. Sometimes a host cell may mistake a virus bound to the membrane as nutrients or other useful molecules and will actually bring the virus into the cytoplasm via endocytosis. As mentioned earlier, bacteriophages use tail fibers to anchor themselves to the cell membrane and then inject their genome into the host bacterium through the tail sheath. Some tail fibers even have enzymatic activity, allowing for both penetration of the cell wall and the formation of pores in the cell membrane.

Depending on the virus, different portions of the virion will be inserted into host cells. Enveloped viruses such as HIV fuse with the membrane and enter the cell intact, whereas bacteriophages only insert their genetic material, leaving their capsids outside the host cell.

Translation and Progeny Assembly

After infection, translation of viral genetic material must occur in order for the virus to reproduce. This requires translocation of the genetic material to the correct location in the cell. Most DNA viruses must enter the nucleus in order to be transcribed into mRNA. The mRNA then goes to the cytoplasm, where it is translated into proteins. Genetic material from positive-sense RNA viruses stays in the cytoplasm, where it is directly translated into protein by host cell ribosomes. Negative-sense RNA viruses require synthesis of a complementary RNA strand via RNA replicase, which can then be translated to form proteins. DNA formed through reverse transcription in retroviruses also travels to the nucleus, where it can be integrated into the host genome.

Using the ribosomes, tRNA, amino acids, and enzymes of the host cell, viral RNA is translated into protein. Many of these proteins are structural capsid proteins and allow for the creation of new virions in the cytoplasm in the host cell. Once the viral genome has been replicated, it can be packaged within the capsid. Note that the viral genome must be returned to its original form before packaging; for example, retroviruses must transcribe new copies of their single-stranded RNA from the DNA that entered the host genome. A single virus may create anywhere from hundreds to many thousands of new virions within a single host cell.

Progeny Release

Viral progeny may be released in multiple ways. First, the viral invasion may initiate cell death, which results in spilling of the viral progeny. Second, the host cell may lyse as a result of being filled with extremely large numbers of virions. Lysis is actually a disadvantage for the virus because the virus can no longer use the cell to carry out its life cycle. Finally, a virus can leave the cell by fusing with its plasma membrane as shown in Figure 1.17, a process known as **extrusion**. This process keeps the host cell alive, and thus allows for the continued use of the host cell by the virus. A virus in this state is said to be in a **productive cycle**.

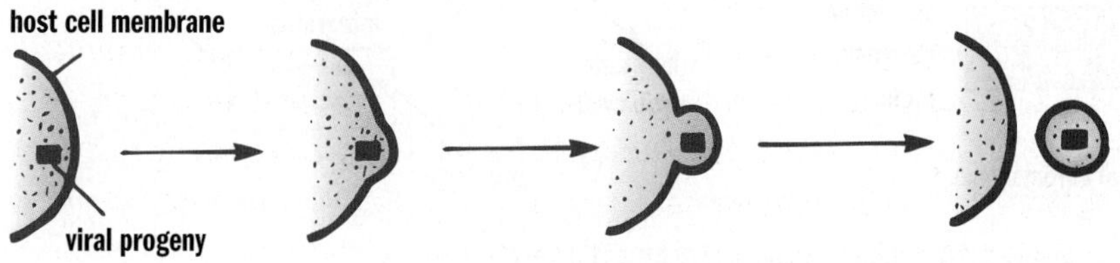

Figure 1.17 Viral Extrusion

Lytic and Lysogenic Cycles

Depending on growth conditions and the specific virus, bacteriophages may enter a lytic or lysogenic life cycle. These two phases are similar to the lysis and productive cycle methods of progeny release discussed above.

During a **lytic cycle**, the bacteriophage maximizes the use of the cell's machinery with little regard for the survival of the host cell. Once the host is swollen with new virions, the cell lyses, and other bacteria can be infected. Viruses in the lytic phase are termed **virulent**.

In the event that the virus does not lyse the bacterium, it may integrate into the host genome as a **provirus** or **prophage**, initiating the **lysogenic cycle**. In this case, the virus will be replicated as the bacterium reproduces because it is now a part of the host's genome. Although the virus may remain integrated into the host genome indefinitely, environmental factors (radiation, light, or chemicals) may cause the provirus to leave the genome and revert to a lytic cycle. As mentioned earlier, the provirus may extract bacterial genes as it leaves the genome, which allows transduction of genes from one bacterium to another. Although bacteriophages can kill their hosts, integration of the phage into the host genome may actually benefit the bacterium. Infection with one strain of phage generally makes the bacterium less susceptible to **superinfection** (simultaneous infection) with other phages. Because the provirus is relatively innocuous, this arrangement may confer an evolutionary advantage. The lytic and lysogenic cycles are contrasted in Figure 1.18.

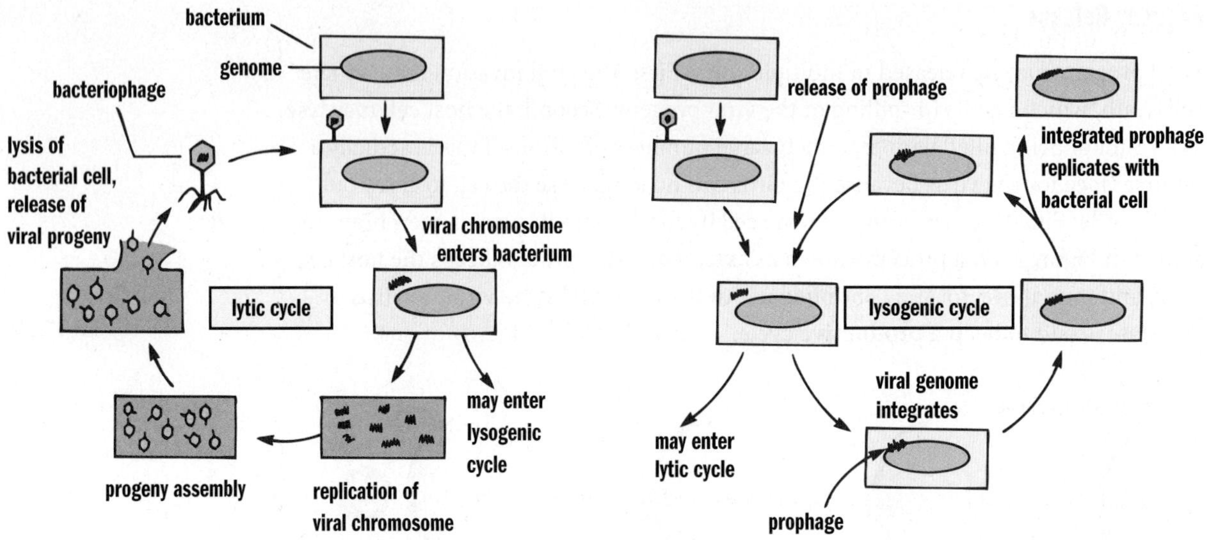

Figure 1.18 Lytic *vs.* Lysogenic Cycles of Bacteriophages

Prions and Viroids

Prions and viroids are very small (subviral) particles that can cause disease under certain circumstances.

Prions

Prions are infectious proteins and are, therefore, nonliving things. They cause disease by triggering misfolding of other proteins, usually through the conversion of a protein from an α-helical structure to a β-pleated sheet. This drastically reduces the solubility of the protein, as well as the ability of the cell to degrade the protein. Eventually, protein aggregates form, interfering with cell function. Prions are known to cause *bovine spongiform encephalopathy* (mad cow disease), *Creutzfeldt–Jakob disease*, and *familial fatal insomnia* in humans.

Viroids

Viroids are small pathogens consisting of a very short circular single-stranded RNA that infect plants. Viroids can bind to a large number of RNA sequences and can silence genes in the plant genome. This prevents synthesis of necessary proteins, resulting in metabolic disruption and structural damage to the cell. Viroids are classically thought of as plant pathogens, but a few examples of human viroids do exist, including the hepatitis D virus (HDV). Alone, HDV is innocuous; however, when coinfected with hepatitis B virus (HBV), HDV is able to exert its silencing effect on human hepatocytes.

MCAT CONCEPT CHECK 1.5

Before you move on, assess your understanding of the material with these questions.

1. Why are viruses considered obligate intracellular parasites?

____

2. A coronavirus, which causes the common cold, is described as an enveloped, single-stranded positive-sense RNA virus. What does this indicate about the virus?

____

3. Briefly describe the pathway of retroviral nucleic acids from infection of a host cell to release of viral progeny:

____

4. What are the differences between the lytic and lysogenic cycles?
   - Lytic cycle:

____

   - Lysogenic cycle:

____

5. How do prions cause disease?

____

Conclusion

Our first chapter introduced the basis of all biology: cell theory. All living things are made of prokaryotic or eukaryotic cells. Prokaryotes are simpler and do not contain membrane-bound organelles. Eukaryotes contain membrane-bound organelles with highly specialized functions. While eukaryotic organisms (especially humans!) will be the primary focus on Test Day, an understanding of prokaryotic structure and physiology is necessary to understand infectious disease. Viruses are nonliving infectious particles that must invade cells in order to reproduce. Finally, we discussed the smallest infectious particles, prions and viroids.

Our discussions from here on out will focus primarily on eukaryotes, but you will spend significant time in your clinical career battling the pathogens we've presented in this chapter. Vaccines are available for a number of bacteria (*Bacillus anthracis* [anthrax], *Corynebacterium diphtheriae* [diphtheria], *Haemophilus influenzae* type B [many upper respiratory and ear infections], *Neisseria meningitidis* [some cases of bacterial meningitis], *Streptoccocus pneumoniae* [many cases of bacterial pneumonia], *Clostridium tetani* [tetanus], *Salmonella typhi* [typhoid], and *Bordetella pertussis* [whooping cough]) and viruses (varicella-zoster virus [chickenpox and shingles], hepatitis A and B viruses, human papillomavirus [HPV], influenza, measles, mumps, polio, rabies, rotavirus, rubella, and yellow fever). Those for which we do not have vaccines may be targeted with antibiotic and antiviral therapies; the appropriate pharmacotherapy usually depends on an understanding of bacterial or viral physiology and the known resistance patterns in the local area. In other words, the principles presented in this chapter will show up in your everyday life as a physician!

We've discussed one method of cellular reproduction: the division of a bacterial cell into two cells by binary fission. Eukaryotic cells also must replicate, but use a different process: mitosis. In the next chapter, we will turn our attention to mitosis, as well as meiosis and human reproduction.

You've reviewed the content, now test your knowledge and critical thinking skills by completing a test-like passage set in your online resources!

GO ONLINE

CONCEPT SUMMARY

Cell Theory

- The **cell theory** has four basic tenets:
  - All living things are composed of cells.
  - The cell is the basic functional unit of life.
  - Cells arise only from preexisting cells.
  - Cells carry genetic information in the form of DNA. This genetic material is passed on from parent to daughter cell.
- Viruses are not considered living things because they are acellular, cannot reproduce without the assistance of a host cell, and may use RNA as their genetic material.

Eukaryotic Cells

- **Eukaryotes** have membrane-bound organelles, a nucleus, and may form multicellular organisms.
- The cell membrane and membranes of organelles contain phospholipids, which organize to form hydrophilic interior and exterior surfaces with a hydrophobic core.
- The **cytosol** suspends the organelles and allows diffusion of molecules throughout the cell.
- The eukaryotic organelles each serve specific functions:
  - The **nucleus** contains DNA organized into **chromosomes**. It is surrounded by the **nuclear membrane** or **envelope**, a double membrane that contains **nuclear pores** for two-way exchange of materials between the nucleus and cytosol. DNA is organized into coding regions called **genes**.
  - The **nucleolus** is a subsection of the nucleus in which ribosomal RNA (rRNA) is synthesized.
  - **Mitochondria** contain an outer and inner membrane. The **outer membrane** forms a barrier with the cytosol; the **inner membrane** is folded into **cristae** and contains enzymes for the electron transport chain. Between the membranes is the **intermembrane space**; inside the inner mitochondrial membrane is the mitochondrial **matrix**. Mitochondria can divide independently of the nucleus via binary fission and can trigger **apoptosis** by releasing mitochondrial enzymes into the cytoplasm.
  - **Lysosomes** contain hydrolytic enzymes that can break down substances ingested by endocytosis and cellular waste products. When these enzymes are released, **autolysis** of the cell can occur.
  - The **endoplasmic reticulum** (**ER**) is a series of interconnected membranes and is continuous with the nuclear envelope. The **rough ER** (**RER**) is studded with ribosomes, which permit translation of proteins destined for secretion. The **smooth ER** (**SER**) is used for lipid synthesis and detoxification.

- The **Golgi apparatus** consists of stacked membrane-bound sacs in which cellular products can be modified, packaged, and directed to specific cellular locations.
- **Peroxisomes** contain hydrogen peroxide and can break down very long chain fatty acids via β-oxidation. They also participate in phospholipid synthesis and the pentose phosphate pathway.

- The **cytoskeleton** provides stability and rigidity to the overall structure of the cell, while also providing transport pathways for molecules within the cell.
  - **Microfilaments** are composed of **actin**. They provide structural protection for the cell and can cause muscle contraction through interactions with **myosin**. They also help form the **cleavage furrow** during **cytokinesis** in mitosis.
  - **Microtubules** are composed of **tubulin**. They create pathways for motor proteins like **kinesin** and **dynein** to carry vesicles. They also contribute to the structure of **cilia** and **flagella**, where they are organized into nine pairs of microtubules in a ring with two microtubules at the center (**9 + 2 structure**). **Centrioles** are found in **centrosomes** and are involved in microtubule organization in the mitotic spindle.
  - **Intermediate filaments** are involved in cell–cell adhesion and maintenance of the integrity of the cytoskeleton; they help anchor organelles. Common examples include keratin and desmin.
- **Epithelial tissues** cover the body and line its cavities, protecting against pathogen invasion and desiccation. Some epithelial cells absorb or secrete substances, or participate in sensation.
  - In most organs, epithelial cells form the **parenchyma**, or the functional parts of the organ.
  - Epithelial cells may be polarized, with one side facing a lumen or the outside world, and the other side facing blood vessels and structural cells.
  - Epithelia can be classified by the number of layers: **simple epithelia** have one layer, **stratified epithelia** have many layers, and **pseudostratified epithelia** appear to have multiple layers due to differences in cell heights, but actually have only one layer.
  - Epithelia can be classified by the shapes of the cells: **cuboidal cells** are cube-shaped, **columnar cells** are long and narrow, and **squamous cells** are flat and scale-like.
- **Connective tissues** support the body and provide a framework for epithelial cells.
  - In most organs, connective tissues form the **stroma** or support structure by secreting materials to form an **extracellular matrix**.
  - Bone, cartilage, tendons, ligaments, adipose tissue, and blood are all connective tissues.

Classification and Structure of Prokaryotic Cells

- **Prokaryotes** do not contain membrane-bound organelles; they contain their genetic material in a single circular molecule of DNA located in the **nucleoid region**.
- There are three overarching domains of life; prokaryotes account for two of these:
  - **Archaea** are often extremophiles, living in harsh environments (high temperature, high salinity, no light) and often use chemical sources of energy (chemosynthesis) rather than light (photosynthesis). They have similarities to both eukaryotes (start translation with methionine, similar RNA polymerases, histones) and bacteria (single circular chromosome, divide by binary fission or budding).
  - **Bacteria** have many similar structures to eukaryotes, and have complex relationships with humans, including **mutualistic symbiosis** and **pathogenesis**.
  - **Eukarya** is the only non-prokaryotic domain.
- Bacteria can be classified by shape:
  - Spherical bacteria are called **cocci**.
  - Rod-shaped bacteria are called **bacilli**.
  - Spiral-shaped bacteria are called **spirilli**.
- Bacteria can be classified based on metabolic processes:
  - **Obligate aerobes** require oxygen for metabolism.
  - **Obligate anaerobes** cannot survive in oxygen-containing environments and can only carry out anaerobic metabolism.
  - **Facultative anaerobes** can survive in environments with or without oxygen and will toggle between metabolic processes based on the environment.
  - **Aerotolerant anaerobes** cannot use oxygen for metabolism, but can survive in an oxygen-containing environment.
- The cell wall and cell membrane of bacteria form the **envelope**. Together, they control the movement of solutes into and out of the cell.
  - Bacteria can be classified by the color their cell walls turn during Gram staining with a crystal violet stain, followed by a counterstain with safranin. Gram-positive bacteria turn purple, while gram-negative bacteria turn pink-red.
  - Gram-positive bacteria have a thick cell wall composed of **peptidoglycan** and **lipoteichoic acid**.
  - Gram-negative bacteria have a thin cell wall composed of peptidoglycan and an outer membrane containing phospholipids and **lipopolysaccharides**.

- Bacteria may have one, two, or many flagella that generate propulsion to move the bacterium toward food or away from immune cells. Moving in response to chemical stimuli is called **chemotaxis**. Bacterial flagella contain a filament composed of flagellin, a basal body that anchors and rotates the flagellum, and a hook that connects the two.
- Prokaryotes carry out the electron transport chain using the cell membrane.
- Prokaryotic ribosomes are smaller than eukaryotic ribosomes (30S and 50S, rather than 40S and 60S).

Genetics and Growth of Prokaryotic Cells

- Prokaryotes multiply through **binary fission**, in which the chromosome replicates while the cell grows in size, until the cell wall begins to grow inward along the midline of the cell and divides it into two identical daughter cells.
- In addition to the single circular chromosome in prokaryotes, extrachromosomal material can be carried in **plasmids**. Plasmids may contain antibiotic resistance genes or **virulence factors**. Plasmids that can integrate into the genome are called **episomes**.
- Bacterial genetic recombination increases bacterial diversity.
  - **Transformation** occurs when genetic material from the surroundings is taken up by a cell, which can incorporate this material into its genome.
  - **Conjugation** is the transfer of genetic material from one bacterium to another across a **conjugation bridge**; a plasmid can be transferred from **F^+ cells** to **F^- cells**, or a portion of the genome can be transferred from an **Hfr cell** to a recipient.
  - **Transduction** is the transfer of genetic material from one bacterium to another via a bacteriophage vector.
  - **Transposons** are genetic elements that can insert into or remove themselves from the genome.
- Bacterial growth follows a predictable pattern:
  - The bacteria adapt to new local conditions during the **lag phase**.
  - Growth then increases exponentially during the **exponential (log) phase**.
  - As resources are reduced, growth levels off during the **stationary phase**.
  - As resources are depleted, bacteria undergo a **death phase**.

Viruses and Subviral Particles

- Viruses contain genetic material, a protein coat (**capsid**), and sometimes a lipid-containing envelope.
- Viruses are obligate intracellular parasites, meaning that they cannot survive and replicate outside of a **host cell**. Individual virus particles are called **virions**.
- Bacteriophages are viruses that target bacteria. In addition to the other structures, they contain a **tail sheath**, which injects the genetic material into a bacterium, and **tail fibers**, which allow the bacteriophage to attach to the host cell.
- Viral genomes may be made of various nucleic acids:
  - They may be composed of DNA or RNA and may be single- or double-stranded.
  - Single-stranded RNA viruses may be **positive sense** (that can be translated by the host cell) or **negative sense** (which requires a complementary strand to be synthesized by **RNA replicase** before translation).
  - **Retroviruses** contain a single-stranded RNA genome, from which a complementary DNA strand is made using **reverse transcriptase**. The DNA strand can then be integrated into the genome.
- Viruses infect cells by attaching to specific receptors, and can then enter the cell by fusing with the plasma membrane, being brought in by endocytosis, or injecting their genome into the cell.
- The virus reproduces by replicating and translating genetic material using the host cell's ribosomes, tRNA, amino acids, and enzymes.
- Viral progeny are released through cell death, lysis, or **extrusion**.
- Bacteriophages have two specific life cycles:
  - In the **lytic cycle**, the bacteriophage produces massive numbers of new virions until the cell lyses. Bacteria in the lytic phase are termed **virulent**.
  - In the **lysogenic cycle**, the virus integrates into the host genome as a provirus or prophage, which can then reproduce along with the cell. The provirus can remain in the genome indefinitely, or may leave the genome in response to a stimulus and enter the lytic cycle.
- **Prions** are infectious proteins that trigger misfolding of other proteins, usually converting an α-helical structure to a β-pleated sheet. This decreases the solubility of the protein and increases its resistance to degradation.
- **Viroids** are plant pathogens that are small circles of complementary RNA that can turn off genes, resulting in metabolic and structural changes and, potentially, cell death.

ANSWERS TO CONCEPT CHECKS

1.1

1. All living things are made of cells. The cell is the basic functional unit of life. All cells arise from other cells. Genetic information is carried in the form of deoxyribonucleic acid (DNA) and is passed from parent to daughter cell.

1.2

1. The nucleus stores genetic information and is the site of transcription. The mitochondria are involved in ATP production and apoptosis. Lysosomes break down cellular waste products and molecules ingested through endocytosis, and can also be involved in apoptosis. The rough endoplasmic reticulum synthesizes proteins destined for secretion. The smooth endoplasmic reticulum is involved in lipid synthesis and detoxification. The Golgi apparatus packages, modifies, and distributes cellular products. Peroxisomes break down very long chain fatty acids, synthesize lipids, and contribute to the pentose phosphate pathway.
2. Peroxisomes are dependent on hydrogen peroxide for their functions, so an enzyme deficiency that results in an inability to form hydrogen peroxide would likely result in an inability to digest very long chain fatty acids. These fatty acids would build up in peroxisomes until they displaced cellular contents, ultimately resulting in cell death.
3. Microfilaments are composed of actin. Microtubules are composed of tubulin. Intermediate filaments differ by cell type, but may be composed of keratin, desmin, vimentin, and lamins.
4. Centrioles consist of nine triplets of microtubules around a hollow center, while flagella consist of nine doublets on the outside, with two microtubules on the inside.
5. Endothelial cells and α-cells are epithelial cells. Fibroblasts, osteoblasts, and chondroblasts are connective tissue cells.

1.3

1. Archaea are similar to bacteria in that both are single-celled organisms that lack a nucleus or membrane-bound organelles, contain a single circular chromosome, and divide by binary fission or budding. They are similar to eukaryotes in that they start translation with methionine, contain similar RNA polymerases, and contain DNA associated with histones.
2. The three common shapes of bacteria are spherical (cocci), rod-shaped (bacilli), and spiral-shaped (spirilli).

3.

Type of Bacteria	Oxygen Present		Oxygen Absent	
	Can survive	Can carry out aerobic metabolism	Can survive	Can carry out anaerobic metabolism
Obligate aerobe	Yes	Yes	No	No
Facultative anaerobe	Yes	Yes	Yes	Yes
Obligate anaerobe	No	No	Yes	Yes
Aerotolerant anaerobe	Yes	No	Yes	Yes

4. The antibiotic penicillin targets the enzyme that catalyzes the cross-linking of peptidoglycan. Gram-positive bacteria have a thick layer of peptidoglycan and lipoteichoic acid, and contain no outer membrane, whereas gram-negative bacteria have only a thin layer of peptidoglycan but also have an outer membrane containing lipopolysaccharides and phospholipids. Penicillin and antibiotics with similar function can more easily reach and weaken the peptidoglycan layer of gram-positive bacteria.
5. Eukaryotic flagella contain microtubules composed of tubulin, organized in a $9 + 2$ arrangement. Bacterial flagella are made of flagellin and consist of a filament, a basal body, and a hook.

1.4

1. Transformation is the acquisition of exogenous genetic material that can be integrated into the bacterial genome. Conjugation is the transfer of genetic material from one bacterium to another across a conjugation bridge; a plasmid can be transferred from F^+ cells to F^- cells, or a portion of the genome can be transferred from an Hfr cell to a recipient. Transduction is the transfer of genetic material from one bacterium to another by a bacteriophage.

2.

Phase	Features
Lag phase	Bacteria get used to environment; little growth
Exponential phase	Bacteria use available resources to multiply at an exponential rate
Stationary phase	Bacterial multiplication slows as resources are used up
Death phase	Bacteria die as resources become insufficient to support the colony

1.5

1. Viruses do not contain organelles such as ribosomes; therefore, in order to reproduce and synthesize proteins, viruses must infect cells and hijack their machinery.
2. This description indicates that the virus contains an outer layer of phospholipids with an inner capsid. Within the capsid, there is single-stranded RNA that can be immediately translated to protein by the ribosomes of the host cell.
3. The nucleic acid enters as single-stranded RNA, which undergoes reverse transcription (using reverse transcriptase) to form double-stranded DNA. This DNA enters the host genome and replicates with the host cell. The DNA is transcribed to mRNA, which can be used to make structural proteins. This mRNA doubles as the viral genome for new virions. Once new virions are assembled from the structural proteins and mRNA (single-stranded RNA) genome, the virions can be released to infect other cells.
4. In the lytic cycle, bacteriophages replicate in the host cell in extremely high numbers until the host cell lyses and releases the virions. In the lysogenic cycle, the bacteriophage genome enters the host genome and replicates with the host cell as a provirus. In response to an appropriate stimulus, the provirus may leave the host genome and can be used to synthesize new virions.
5. Prions cause disease by triggering a change in the conformation of a protein from an α-helix to a β-pleated sheet. This change reduces solubility of the protein and makes it highly resistant to degradation.

SCIENCE MASTERY ASSESSMENT EXPLANATIONS

1. **D**

Obligate anaerobes cannot survive in the presence of oxygen and would likely be killed by such a therapy, treating the infection. The other types of bacteria listed can all survive in the presence of oxygen, so infections involving these bacteria would likely not be treated using this therapy.

2. **A**

While bones and tendons are composed predominantly of connective tissue cells, muscle tissue is considered a different tissue type. Other examples of connective tissue include cartilage, ligaments, adipose tissue, and blood. Connective tissue often secretes substances to form the extracellular matrix, such as collagen and elastin, eliminating **(B)**. **(C)** and **(D)** are essentially identical and can both be eliminated: in organs, connective tissue often forms the support structure for epithelial cells, called the stroma.

3. **D**

In a virus, the nucleic acid can be either DNA or RNA and—in both cases—can be either single- or double-stranded. Therefore, all of the types of nucleic acids listed here could be used for a viral genome, making **(D)** the correct answer.

4. **C**

The process of sterilization kills all living cells. A lack of cellular growth in these conditions supports the idea that cells can only arise from preexisting cells, matching **(C)**. By contrast, since this experiment did not directly visualize the cells, nor did it analyze the genetic material, **(A)**, **(B)**, and **(D)** can be eliminated.

5. **C**

Mitochondria are thought to have evolved from an anaerobic prokaryote engulfing an aerobic prokaryote and establishing a symbiotic relationship; therefore, mitochondrial DNA, or mDNA, is likely to be similar to bacterial DNA. Both mDNA and bacterial DNA are organized into a single circular chromosome of double-stranded DNA that can replicate during binary fission. Therefore, Statements I and II are correct, while Statement III is incorrect.

6. **C**

The smooth endoplasmic reticulum is involved in the transport of materials throughout the cell, in lipid synthesis, and in the detoxification of drugs and poisons. Proteins from the rough ER can cross into the smooth ER, where they are secreted into cytoplasmic vesicles and transported to the Golgi apparatus. However, protein synthesis is not a function of the smooth ER, but rather of the free ribosomes or the ribosomes associated with the rough ER. **(C)** is therefore the correct answer.

7. **A**

The nucleolus (not to be confused with the nucleus) is a dense structure within the nucleus where ribosomal RNA (rRNA) is synthesized. **(A)** is therefore the correct answer.

8. **A**

Lysosomes are vesicular organelles that digest material using hydrolytic enzymes. They are surrounded by a single membrane. Both mitochondria and nuclei are surrounded by double membranes, eliminating **(B)** and **(C)**. Ribosomes must not be surrounded by membranes because they are found not only in eukaryotes but also in prokaryotes, which lack any membrane-bound organelles. This eliminates **(D)**.

9. **C**

Some of the main differences between prokaryotes and eukaryotes are that prokaryotes do not have a nucleus, while eukaryotes do, eliminating **(B)**; prokaryotes have ribosomal subunits of 30S and 50S, while eukaryotes have ribosomal subunits of 40S and 60S, eliminating **(A)**; and prokaryotes do not have membrane-bound organelles, whereas eukaryotes do, eliminating **(D)**. The presence of a membrane on the outer surface of the cell could not distinguish a prokaryotic cell from a eukaryotic one because both gram-negative bacteria and animal cells share this feature. Thus, **(C)** is the correct answer.

10. **C**

Tubulin is the primary protein in microtubules, which are responsible for the structure and movement of cilia and flagella, eliminating **(A)** and **(B)**. Centrioles organize microtubules into the mitotic spindle, eliminating **(D)**. Microfilaments are not composed of tubulin, but rather actin, making **(C)** the correct answer.

11. **C**

Viruses can exist in either the lytic or lysogenic cycle; they may even switch between them. During the lytic cycle, the virus's DNA takes control of the host cell's genetic machinery, manufacturing numerous progeny. In the end, the host cell bursts (lyses) and releases new virions, each capable of infecting other cells. In the lysogenic cycle, viral DNA is added to the host cell's genome, where it can remain dormant for days or years. Either spontaneously or as a result of environmental circumstances, the provirus can reactivate and enter a lytic cycle. Thus, **(A)** and **(B)** are incorrect because the terms are reversed. **(D)** describes features of bacteriophages, which are viruses that infect bacteria—not the human nervous system. **(C)** accurately describes how HSV operates during the lysogenic cycle, making it the correct answer.

12. **C**

Bacterial cells reproduce by binary fission, an asexual process in which the progeny is identical to the parent. Therefore, binary fission (Statement I) does not increase genetic variability. Conjugation can be described as sexual mating in bacteria; it is the transfer of genetic material between two bacteria that are temporarily joined. Transduction occurs when fragments of the bacterial chromosome accidentally become packaged into viral progeny produced during a viral infection and are introduced into another bacterium by the viral vector. Therefore, both conjugation and transduction (Statements II and III) increase bacterial genetic variability.

13. **A**

A bacterial cell that does not rapidly cause a phenotypic change in the rest of the colony is likely not F^+, meaning that this cell is not able to form a sex pilus for conjugation, making **(A)** correct. The expression of new phenotypic characteristics indicates that this bacterium may have acquired genetic material from the environment through transformation, **(B)**, or transduction (which occurs via bacteriophage infection), **(C)** and **(D)**.

14. **C**

Prions are infectious proteins that cause misfolding of other proteins. Prions generally cause a shift toward β-pleated sheet conformations, causing decreased solubility and increased resistance to degradation. This ultimately leads to disease. This mechanism is very similar to the one described here for Alzheimer's disease, making **(C)** the correct answer.

15. **A**

A virus that requires transport to the nucleus in order to produce viral proteins likely requires use of nuclear RNA polymerase in order to create mRNA that can be translated to protein. Therefore, only DNA viruses need to be transported to the nucleus to produce viral proteins, eliminating all answer choices but **(A)**.

Consult your online resources for additional practice. GO ONLINE

SHARED CONCEPTS

Biochemistry Chapter 3
Nonenzymatic Protein Function and Protein Analysis

Biochemistry Chapter 8
Biological Membranes

Biochemistry Chapter 10
Carbohydrate Metabolism II

Biology Chapter 2
Reproduction

Biology Chapter 8
The Immune System

Biology Chapter 12
Genetics and Evolution

CHAPTER 2

REPRODUCTION

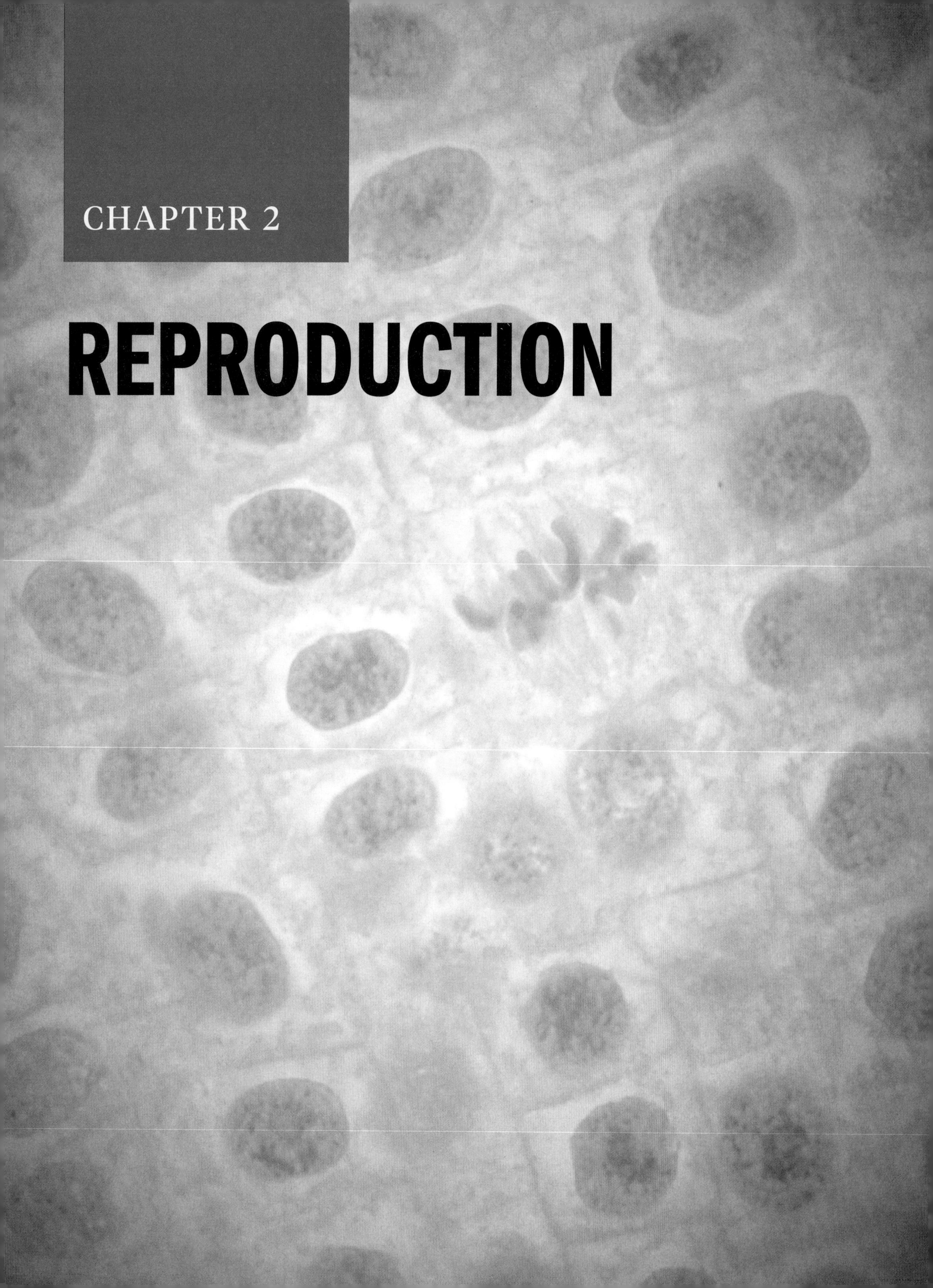

SCIENCE MASTERY ASSESSMENT

Every pre-med knows this feeling: there is so much content I have to know for the MCAT! How do I know what to do first or what's important?

While the high-yield badges throughout this book will help you identify the most important topics, this Science Mastery Assessment is another tool in your MCAT prep arsenal. This quiz (which can also be taken in your online resources) and the guidance below will help ensure that you are spending the appropriate amount of time on this chapter based on your personal strengths and weaknesses. Don't worry though—skipping something now does not mean you'll never study it. Later on in your prep, as you complete full-length tests, you'll uncover specific pieces of content that you need to review and can come back to these chapters as appropriate.

How to Use This Assessment

If you answer 0–7 questions correctly:

Spend about 1 hour to read this chapter in full and take limited notes throughout. Follow up by reviewing **all** quiz questions to ensure that you now understand how to solve each one.

If you answer 8–11 questions correctly:

Spend 20–40 minutes reviewing the quiz questions. Beginning with the questions you missed, read and take notes on the corresponding subchapters. For questions you answered correctly, ensure your thinking matches that of the explanation and you understand why each choice was correct or incorrect.

If you answer 12–15 questions correctly:

Spend less than 20 minutes reviewing all questions from the quiz. If you missed any, then include a quick read-through of the corresponding subchapters, or even just the relevant content within a subchapter, as part of your question review. For questions you answered correctly, ensure your thinking matches that of the explanation and review the Concept Summary at the end of the chapter.

1. Which of the following is the correct sequence of the development of a mature sperm cell?
   - **A.** Spermatid→1° spermatocyte→spermatogonium→2° spermatocyte→spermatozoan
   - **B.** Spermatogonium→1° spermatocyte→2° spermatocyte→spermatid→spermatozoan
   - **C.** Spermatozoan→1° spermatocyte→2° spermatocyte→spermatogonium→spermatid
   - **D.** Spermatogonium→1° spermatocyte→2° spermatocyte→spermatozoan→spermatid

2. Which of the following correctly pairs the stage of development of an egg cell with the relevant point in the life cycle?
   - **A.** From birth to menarche—prophase II
   - **B.** At ovulation—metaphase I
   - **C.** At ovulation—metaphase II
   - **D.** At fertilization—prophase II

3. Some studies suggest that, in patients who have Alzheimer's disease, there is a defect in the way the spindle apparatus attaches to the kinetochore fibers. At which stage of mitotic division would one first expect to be able to visualize this problem?
   - **A.** Prophase
   - **B.** Metaphase
   - **C.** Anaphase
   - **D.** Telophase

4. A researcher wishes to incorporate a radiolabeled deoxyadenine into the genome of one of the two daughter cells that would arise as a result of mitosis. What is the latest stage of cellular development during which the radiolabeled deoxyadenine could be added to achieve this result?
   - **A.** G_1
   - **B.** G_2
   - **C.** M
   - **D.** S

5. Certain ovarian tumors called granulosa cell tumors are known to produce excessive levels of estrogen. A physician who diagnoses a granulosa cell tumor should look for a secondary cancer in which of the following parts of the reproductive tract?
   - **A.** Fallopian tube
   - **B.** Cervix
   - **C.** Endometrium
   - **D.** Vagina

6. Upon ovulation, the oocyte is released into the:
   - **A.** fallopian tube.
   - **B.** follicle.
   - **C.** abdominal cavity.
   - **D.** uterus.

7. Cancer cells are cells in which mitosis occurs continuously, without regard to quality or quantity of the cells produced. For this reason, most chemotherapies attack rapidly dividing cells. At which point(s) in the cell cycle could chemotherapy effectively prevent cancer cell division?
   - **I.** S stage
   - **II.** Prophase
   - **III.** Metaphase

   - **A.** I only
   - **B.** I and II only
   - **C.** II and III only
   - **D.** I, II, and III

8. Which of the following INCORRECTLY pairs a structure of the male reproductive system with a feature of the structure?
   - **A.** Seminal vesicles—produce alkaline fructose-containing secretions
   - **B.** Prostate gland—surrounded by muscle to raise and lower the testes
   - **C.** Vas deferens—tube connecting the epididymis to the ejaculatory duct
   - **D.** Cowper's glands—produce a fluid to clear traces of urine in the urethra

9. What is the last point in the meiotic cycle in which the cell has a diploid number of chromosomes?
   - **A.** During interphase
   - **B.** During telophase I
   - **C.** During interkinesis
   - **D.** During telophase II

10. Which of the following does NOT likely contribute to genetic variability?
    - **A.** Random fertilization of an egg by a sperm
    - **B.** Random segregation of homologous chromosomes
    - **C.** Crossing over between homologous chromosomes during meiosis
    - **D.** Replication of the DNA during S stage

11. Which of the following statements correctly identifies a key difference between mitosis and meiosis?
    - **A.** In metaphase of mitosis, replicated chromosomes line up in single file; in metaphase II of meiosis, replicated chromosomes line up on opposite sides of the metaphase plate.
    - **B.** During anaphase of mitosis, homologous chromosomes separate; during anaphase of meiosis I, sister chromatids separate.
    - **C.** At the end of telophase of mitosis, the daughter cells are identical to each other; at the end of meiosis I, the daughter cells are identical to the parent cell.
    - **D.** During metaphase of mitosis, centromeres are present directly on the metaphase plate; during metaphase of meiosis I, there are no centromeres on the metaphase plate.

12. Which of the following is true regarding prophase?
    - **A.** The chromosomes separate and move to opposite poles of the cell.
    - **B.** The spindle apparatus disappears.
    - **C.** The chromosomes uncoil.
    - **D.** The nucleoli disappear.

13. An individual who is phenotypically female is found to have only one copy of a disease-carrying recessive allele on the X chromosome, yet demonstrates all of the classic symptoms of the disease. Geneticists determine that the individual has a genotype that likely arose from nondisjunction in one parent. What is the likely genotype of this individual?
    - **A.** 46,XX (46 chromosomes, with XX for sex chromosomes)
    - **B.** 46,XY
    - **C.** 45,X
    - **D.** 47,XXY

14. During which phase of the menstrual cycle does progesterone concentration peak?
    - **A.** Follicular phase
    - **B.** Ovulation
    - **C.** Luteal phase
    - **D.** Menses

15. Which of the following would NOT be seen during pregnancy?
    - **A.** High levels of hCG in the first trimester
    - **B.** High levels of progesterone throughout the pregnancy
    - **C.** Low levels of FSH in the first trimester
    - **D.** High levels of GnRH throughout the pregnancy

Answer Key

1. **B**
2. **C**
3. **A**
4. **D**
5. **C**
6. **C**
7. **D**
8. **B**
9. **B**
10. **D**
11. **D**
12. **D**
13. **C**
14. **C**
15. **D**

Detailed explanations can be found at the end of the chapter.

CHAPTER 2

REPRODUCTION

In This Chapter

CHAPTER PROFILE

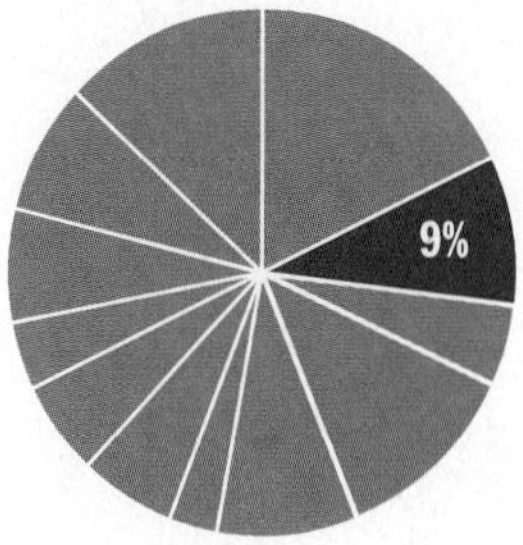

The content in this chapter should be relevant to about 9% of all questions about biology on the MCAT.

This chapter covers material from the following AAMC content categories:

1C: Transmission of heritable information from generation to generation and the processes that increase genetic diversity

2C: Processes of cell division, differentiation, and specialization

3B: Structure and integrative functions of the main organ systems

Introduction

All mammals share certain characteristics: milk-producing mammary glands, three bones in the middle ear and one in the lower jaw, fur or hair, heterodont dentition (different kinds of teeth), and both sebaceous (oil-producing) and sudoriferous (sweat) glands. What about placenta formation during embryonic development? This is a characteristic of humans, as we'll explore in Chapter 3 of *MCAT Biology Review*, but there are two groups of mammals that birth their young a bit differently: prototherians and metatherians.

Prototherians (monotremes), which include the duckbilled platypus and echidna (spiny anteater), encase their developing embryos within hard-shelled amniotic eggs and lay them to be hatched, like reptiles. This method of development is referred to as oviparity. Metatherians (marsupials) include koalas and kangaroos. A typical metatherian fetus (joey) undergoes some development in its mother's uterus and then climbs out of the birth canal and into her marsupium, or pouch. It might seem a bit strange that something as essential as reproduction can be so different between mammalian species, but there are, in fact, a wide variety of reproductive schemes in nature. Many organisms reproduce without a sexual partner. Others can reproduce sexually or asexually depending on environmental conditions. In Chapter 1 of *MCAT Biology Review*, we explored how bacteria and viruses reproduce. In this chapter, we'll explore eukaryotic reproductive systems.

2.1 The Cell Cycle and Mitosis

High-Yield

LEARNING OBJECTIVES

After Chapter 2.1, you will be able to:

- Describe the four phases of mitosis and the major events during each phase
- Identify the five stages of the cell cycle and the major events during each stage

In animals, autosomal cells are said to be **diploid** (**2*n***), which means that they contain two copies of each chromosome. Germ cells, on the other hand, are **haploid** (***n***), containing only one copy of each chromosome. In humans, these numbers are 46 and 23, respectively; we inherit 23 chromosomes from each parent. Eukaryotic cells replicate through the **cell cycle**, a specific series of phases during which a cell grows, synthesizes DNA, and divides. Derangements of the cell cycle can lead to unchecked cell division and may be responsible for the formation of cancer.

The Cell Cycle

The cell cycle, shown in Figure 2.1, is a perennial MCAT favorite. For actively dividing cells, the cell cycle consists of four stages: G_1, S, G_2, and M. The first three stages (G_1, S, and G_2) are known collectively as **interphase**. Interphase is the longest part of the cell cycle; even actively dividing cells spend about 90 percent of their time in interphase. Cells that do not divide spend all of their time in an offshoot of G_1 called G_0. During the **G_0 stage**, the cell is simply living and carrying out its functions, without any preparation for division.

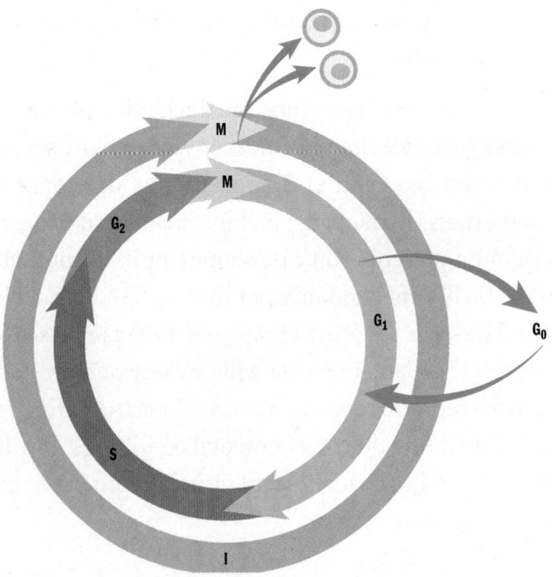

Figure 2.1 The Cell Cycle

During interphase, individual chromosomes are not visible with light microscopy because they are in a less condensed form known as **chromatin**. This is because the DNA must be available to *RNA polymerase* so that genes can be transcribed. During mitosis, however, it is preferable to condense the DNA into tightly coiled chromosomes to avoid losing any genetic material during cell division.

G_1 Stage: Presynthetic Gap

During the **G_1 stage**, cells create organelles for energy and protein production (mitochondria, ribosomes, and endoplasmic reticulum), while also increasing their size. In addition, passage into the S (synthesis) stage is governed by a **restriction point**. Certain criteria, such as containing the proper complement of DNA, must be met for the cell to pass the restriction point and enter the synthesis stage.

S Stage: Synthesis of DNA

During the **S stage**, the cell replicates its genetic material so that each daughter cell will have identical copies. After replication, each chromosome consists of two identical **chromatids** that are bound together at a specialized region known as the **centromere**, as shown in Figure 2.2. Note that the ploidy of the cell does not change even though the number of chromatids has doubled. In other words, humans in this stage still only have 46 chromosomes, even though 92 chromatids are present. Cells entering G_2 have twice as much DNA as cells in G_1.

KEY CONCEPT

Each chromatid is composed of a complete double-stranded molecule of DNA. Sister chromatids are identical copies of each other. The term *chromosome* may be used to refer to either a single chromatid before S phase or the pair of chromatids attached at the centromere after S phase.

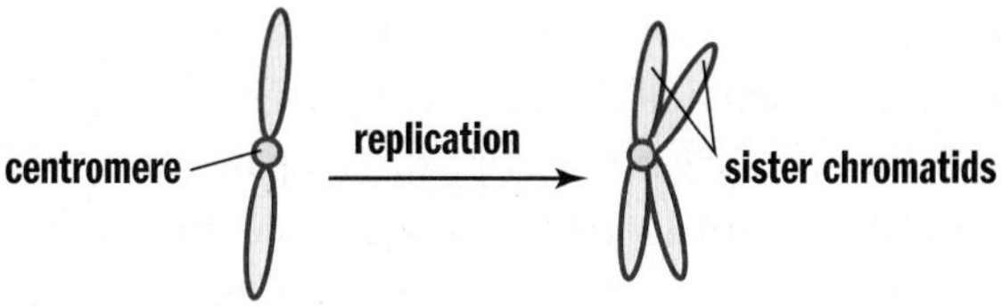

Figure 2.2 Chromosome Replication
A single chromatid replicates to form two sister chromatids.

G_2 Stage: Postsynthetic Gap

During the **G_2 stage**, the cell passes through another quality control checkpoint. DNA has already been duplicated, and the cell checks to ensure that there are enough organelles and cytoplasm for two daughter cells. Furthermore, the cell checks to make sure that DNA replication proceeded correctly to avoid passing on an error to daughter cells that may further pass on the error to their progeny.

M Stage: Mitosis

The **M stage** consists of mitosis itself along with cytokinesis. Mitosis is divided into four phases: prophase, metaphase, anaphase, and telophase. The features of each phase will be discussed in the next section. Cytokinesis is the splitting of the cytoplasm and organelles between the two daughter cells.

KEY CONCEPT

In autosomal cells, division results in two genetically identical daughter cells. In germ cells, the daughter cells are not equivalent.

Control of the Cell Cycle

The cell cycle is controlled by checkpoints, most notably between the G_1 and S phase and the G_2 and M phase. At the G_1/S checkpoint, the cell determines if the condition of the DNA is good enough for synthesis. As mentioned previously, this checkpoint is also known as the restriction point. If there has been damage to the DNA, the cell cycle goes into arrest until the DNA has been repaired. The main protein in control of this is **p53**.

At the G_2/M checkpoint, the cell is mainly concerned with ensuring that it has achieved adequate size and the organelles have been properly replicated to support two daughter cells. p53 also plays a role in the G_2/M checkpoint.

The molecules responsible for the cell cycle are known as **cyclins** and **cyclin-dependent kinases** (**CDK**). In order to be activated, CDKs require the presence of the right cyclins. During the cell cycle, concentrations of the various cyclins increase and decrease during specific stages. These cyclins bind to CDKs, creating an activated CDK–cyclin complex. This complex can then phosphorylate transcription factors. **Transcription factors** then promote transcription of genes required for the next stage of the cell cycle.

Cancer

Cell cycle control is essential to ensure that cells that are damaged or inadequately sized do not divide. When cell cycle control becomes deranged, and damaged cells are allowed to undergo mitosis, **cancer** may result. One of the most common mutations found in cancer is mutation of the gene that produces p53, called TP53. When this gene is mutated, the cell cycle is not stopped to repair damaged DNA. This allows mutations to accumulate, eventually resulting in a cancerous cell that divides continuously and without regard to the quality or quantity of the new cells produced. Often, cancer cells undergo rapid cell division, creating **tumors**. Eventually, if the cell begins to produce the right factors (such as proteases that can digest basement membranes or factors that encourage blood vessel formation), the damaged cells are then able to reach other tissues. This may include both local invasion as well as distant spread of cancerous cells through the bloodstream or lymphatic systems. The latter result is known as **metastasis**.

BRIDGE

Cancer-causing genes can often be classified into oncogenes (genes that, when mutated, actively promote cell division) and tumor suppressor genes (genes that, when mutated, lose their ability to regulate or arrest the cell cycle). Different cancer types are often associated with specific mutations in either oncogenes or tumor suppressor genes, or both. The biochemistry of these genes is discussed in Chapter 6 of *MCAT Biochemistry Review*.

Mitosis

Mitosis, shown in Figure 2.3, is the process by which two identical daughter cells are created from a single cell. Mitosis consists of four distinct phases—prophase, metaphase, anaphase, and telophase—and occurs in **somatic cells**, or cells that are not involved in sexual reproduction.

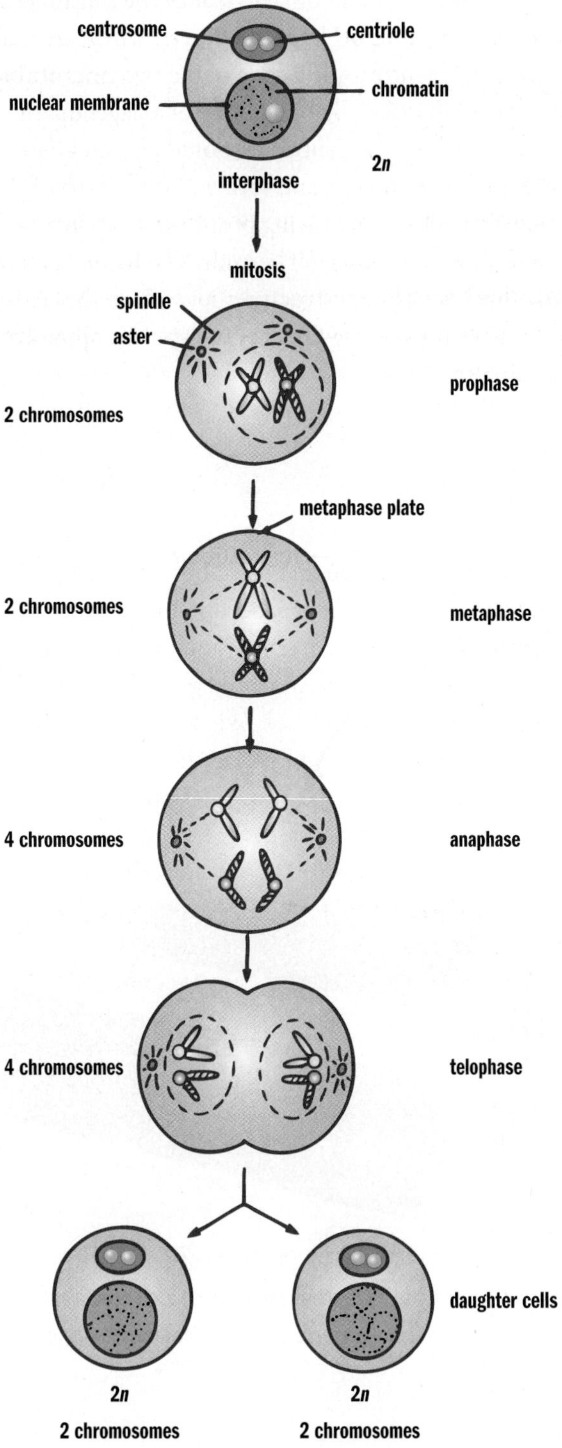

Figure 2.3 Mitosis

Mitosis results in two identical daughter cells.

Prophase

KEY CONCEPT

The phases of mitosis:

- Prophase—chromosomes condense, spindle forms
- Metaphase—chromosomes align
- Anaphase—sister chromatids separate
- Telophase—new nuclear membranes form

Prophase is the first phase in mitosis. The first step in prophase involves condensation of the chromatin into chromosomes. Also, the centriole pairs separate and move toward opposite poles of the cell. These paired cylindrical organelles, shown in Figure 2.4, are located outside the nucleus in a region known as the **centrosome** and are responsible for the correct division of DNA. Once the centrioles migrate to opposite poles of the cell, they begin to form **spindle fibers**, which are made of microtubules. This establishes the centrosome as one of the two **microtubule organizing centers** of the cell—the other being the basal body of a flagellum or cilium. Each of the fibers radiates outward from the centrioles. Some microtubules form **asters** that anchor the centrioles to the cell membrane. Others extend toward the middle of the cell. The nuclear membrane dissolves during prophase, allowing these spindle fibers to contact the chromosomes. The nucleoli become less distinct and may disappear completely. **Kinetochores** are protein structures located on the centromeres that serve as attachment points for specific fibers of the **spindle apparatus** (appropriately called **kinetochore fibers**).

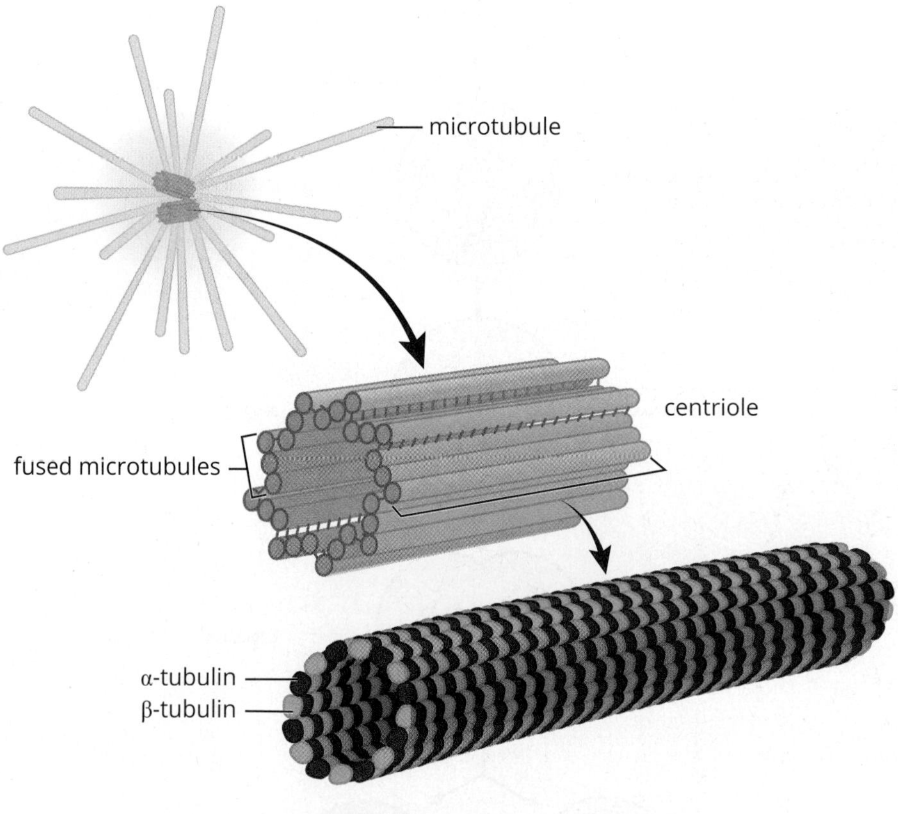

Figure 2.4 The Centrosome
Each centrosome contains two tubulin-based centrioles responsible for proper movement of the chromosomes during mitosis.

Metaphase

In **metaphase**, the centriole pairs are now at opposite ends of the cell. The kinetochore fibers interact with the fibers of the spindle apparatus to align the chromosomes at the **metaphase plate** (**equatorial plate**), which is equidistant from the two poles of the cell.

Anaphase

During **anaphase**, the centromeres split so that each chromatid has its own distinct centromere, thus allowing the sister chromatids to separate. The sister chromatids are pulled toward the opposite poles of the cell by the shortening of the kinetochore fibers.

Telophase and Cytokinesis

Telophase is essentially the reverse of prophase. The spindle apparatus disappears. A nuclear membrane reforms around each set of chromosomes, and the nucleoli reappear. The chromosomes uncoil, resuming their interphase form. Each of the two new nuclei receives a complete copy of the genome identical to the original genome and to each other.

Cytokinesis, which occurs at the end of telophase, is the separation of the cytoplasm and organelles, giving each daughter cell enough material to survive on its own. Each cell undergoes a finite number of divisions before programmed death; for human somatic cells, this is usually between 20 and 50. After that, the cell can no longer divide continuously.

BIOLOGY GUIDED EXAMPLE WITH EXPERT THINKING

The p53 tumor suppressor pathway has been heavily explored as a potential treatment for patients who have cancer. The p53 pathway induces growth arrest and apoptosis in response to cellular stress. Mutation of this pathway is thought to be nearly universal in human cancer.

Background on p53: mutation of pathway causes cancer

Researchers explored whether a retro-inverse p53C′ peptide (termed RI-TATp53C′) is a therapeutically effective means of activating the p53 tumor suppressor pathway in preclinical models of terminal metastatic cancer.

Hypothesis: Does RI-TATp53C′ activate the p53 pathway and thus treat cancer?

RI-TATp53C′ contains a protein transduction domain (PTD), which is capable of traversing the plasma membrane, and a functional sequence of the p53 C-terminus.

RI-TATp53C′ components: protein transduction domain (PTD) and functional C-terminus

A non-functional RI-TATp53C′ was developed by mutating the functional residues of the peptide.

They made a non-functional version of the treatment (RI-TATp53C′); this is going to be a negative control

Researchers exposed TA3/St mammary carcinoma cells to Wild-Type RI-TATp53C′ and the mutant peptide of RI-TATp53C′. The cells' DNA content was then analyzed to test if cell cycle arrest occurred (Figure 1).

Experiment IV: RI-TATp53C′ WT or mutant; DV: cell DNA content (determines cell cycle arrest)

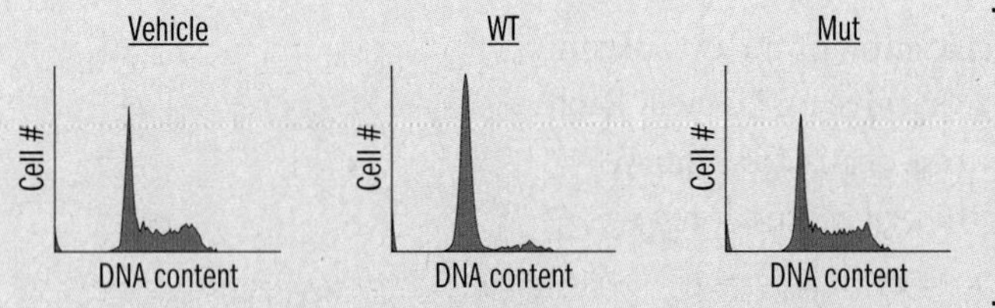

Figure 1

IV: Vehicle (no RI-TATp53C′), WT (RI-TATp53C′), or Mut (non-functional RI-TATp53C′)

DV: cell number and DNA content

Trend: Vehicle and Mut graphs have the same shape, while WT appears to make cells have less DNA

Researchers then explored the dependency of RI-TATp53C′ induction of growth arrest with endogenous p53 in cells (Figure 2). TA3/St and H1299 are both cancer cell lines.

Second experiment, asks: "Does RI-TATp53C′ depend on endogenous p53?" Probably going to manipulate endogenous p53 (IV) and measure RI-TATp53C′ effects (DV).

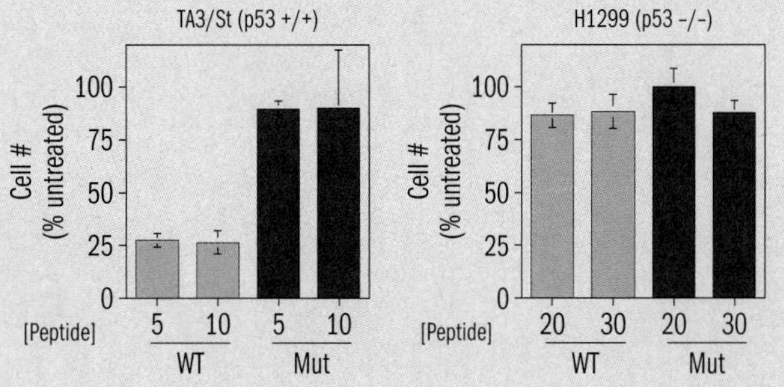

Figure 2

IV: cancer w/ endogenous p53 (TA3/St) or cancer w/ no p53 (H1299); WT or Mut; peptide concentration

DV: Cell # as % untreated

Trends: the WT peptide group produces a lower number of cells than Mut in TA3/St, but no difference in H1299; no effect with changes to peptide concentration

Adapted from: Snyder EL, Meade BR, Saenz CC, Dowdy SF (2004). Treatment of terminal peritoneal carcinomatosis by a transducible p53-activating peptide. *PLOS Biology* 2(2): e36. https://doi.org/10.1371/journal.pbio.0020036.

What stage of the cell cycle does RI-TATp53C′ arrest the cell in and does RI-TATp53C′-induced cell arrest require endogenous p53?

To answer this question we need to determine the relationship between RI-TATp53C′ and the cell cycle, as well as the relationship between RI-TATp53C′ and endogenous p53. With such an in-depth question it's worth considering the bigger picture to ensure that we understand the concepts and experiments in the passage. Start with the context: why are these experiments being done? As stated in paragraphs 1 and 2, p53 is a tumor-suppressing pathway that researchers are hoping to activate as a treatment to cancer. Both experiments, although distinct, will explore the activation of this pathway.

Keeping in mind the independent and dependent variables of the two experiments that we identified as we read, we can identify which experiment should be used to answer each question in the prompt. The first experiment has three conditions: Vehicle, WT, and Mut. The vehicle condition is something we should recognize as bio talk for "we did everything the same as the treatment condition, except the treatment," so this is a negative control. The WT condition, according to the second to last sentence in paragraph 2, is functional RI-TATp53C′. This is the treatment group! If the hypothesis at the start of the 2nd paragraph is correct we should see interesting data here. The Mut condition is described in the third to last and second to last sentences of paragraph 2 as a non-functional mutant RI-TATp53C′. In each of these conditions, the proportion of cells that have low/medium/high DNA content are measured, which, according to the last sentence of paragraph 2, determines if cell cycle arrest occurred. At this point, we know Exp 1 relates RI-TATp53C′ (IV) and the cell cycle (DV) and should, therefore, be used to answer the first question of the prompt.

Let's analyze the data from the first experiment. Looking at Figure 1, notice that the Vehicle and Mutant conditions are identical, while the WT (treatment) condition differs greatly. Specifically, the RI-TATp53C′ treatment (WT) results in a larger portion of cells having less DNA. Considering our background knowledge about the cell cycle and each phase's relative DNA content, we can deduce that G_1 has the lowest DNA content. This is because G_1 occurs after a division (decreases DNA) and before S phase (increases DNA). Thus, we can conclude RI-TATp53C′ must arrest the cell in G_1.

In order to answer the second question, the relationship between RI-TATp53C′ functionality and endogenous p53 must be determined. This aligns pretty well with paragraph 3's description of experiment 2, and is a solid indication that we need to analyze Figure 2. Looking at the titles of the graphs there are two different cancerous cell cultures, TA3/St (p53 +/+) and H1299 (p53 −/−), which differ in their expression of p53. This is the first independent variable. Analyzing the graphs further, there are two additional independent variables, WT (light blue) *vs.* Mut (dark blue) and peptide concentration, [Peptide]. The dependent variable in Figure 2 is the Cell # or % untreated. In other words, it's the number of cancerous cells that are unarrested and thus still cancerous after peptide exposure.

With an understanding of the variables, let's take a look at the data in Figure 2. Between the two graphs, the most striking difference is WT RI-TATp53C′ treatment in p53 +/+ cancerous cells results in a drastic drop in untreated (cancerous) cells (light blue, 1st graph), while in the p53 −/− condition WT RI-TATp53C′ cancerous cell levels remain constant (light blue, 2nd graph). This shows us that the ability of WT RI-TATp53C' to induce cell cycle arrest is dependent on endogenous p53. In addition, when both p53 +/+ and p53 −/− conditions are exposed to the mutant RI-TATp53C′ (non-functional), there is no drop in cancerous cells. This second point is to be expected, but is still worth noting, as it shows us that nothing unexpected occurred during the experiment. Thus, given the data in Figure 2, we can conclude that in order for RI-TATp53C′ to induce cell arrest, it requires endogenous p53 in the tumor.

Overall, Figure 1 shows that not only does WT RI-TATp53C′ induce cell arrest, but based on the increased proportion of cells with lower DNA content, it induces cell arrest in G_1. From Figure 2, we were able to determine that RI-TATp53C′ requires a functional p53 pathway in order to induce cell arrest due to the loss of RI-TATp53C′ functionality in the p53 −/− condition.

MCAT CONCEPT CHECK 2.1

Before you move on, assess your understanding of the material with these questions.

1. What are the five stages of the cell cycle? What happens in each stage?

Cell Cycle Stage	Features

2. What are the four phases of mitosis? What happens in each phase?

Mitotic Phase	Features

2.2 Meiosis

LEARNING OBJECTIVES

After Chapter 2.2, you will be able to:

- Predict the ploidy of daughter cells at the end of mitosis, meiosis I, and meiosis II
- Differentiate between homologous chromosomes and sister chromatids
- Compare and contrast mitosis and meiosis
- Explain the importance of crossing over events in relation to genetic diversity

Whereas mitosis occurs in somatic tissue and results in two identical daughter cells, meiosis occurs in **gametocytes** (**germ cells**) and results in up to four nonidentical sex cells (**gametes**). Meiosis shares some similarities with mitosis. In both processes, for instance, genetic material must be duplicated, chromatin is condensed to form chromosomes, and microtubules emanating from centrioles are involved in dividing genetic material. However, the MCAT tends to ask about the differences between these two processes.

In contrast to mitosis, which consists of one round each of replication and division, meiosis consists of one round of replication followed by two rounds of division, as shown in Figure 2.5. **Meiosis I** results in homologous chromosomes being separated, generating haploid daughter cells; this is known as **reductional division**. **Meiosis II** is similar to mitosis, in that it results in the separation of sister chromatids without a change in ploidy, and is therefore known as **equational division**.

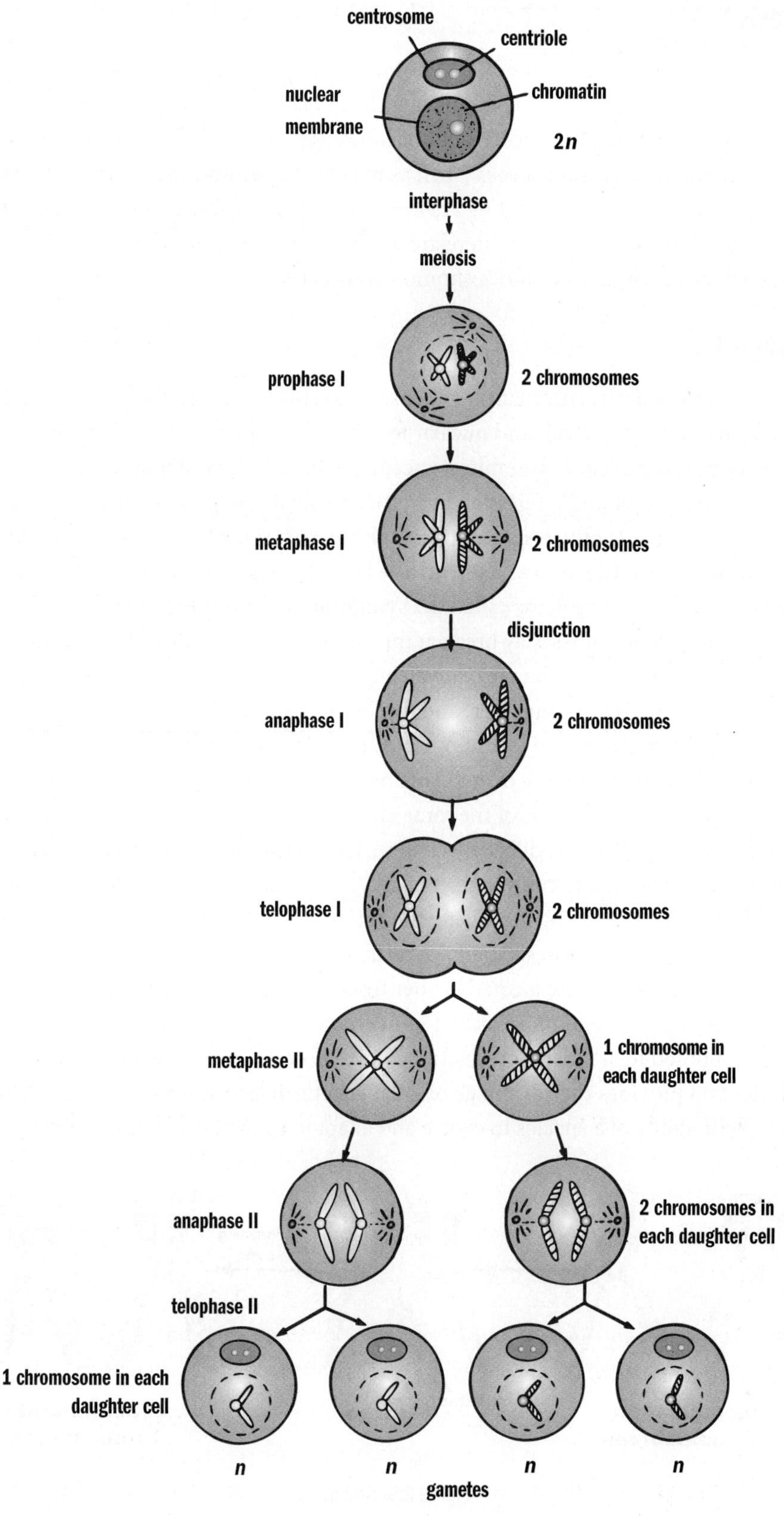

Figure 2.5 Meiosis

Meiosis results in up to four nonidentical daughter cells.

Meiosis I

The human genome is composed of 23 **homologous pairs** of chromosomes (**homologues**), each of which contains one chromosome inherited from each parent. This brings up an important note about terminology: whereas homologous pairs are considered separate chromosomes (such as maternal chromosome 15 and paternal chromosome 15), sister chromatids are identical strands of DNA connected at the centromere. Thus, after S phase, there are 92 chromatids organized into 46 chromosomes, which are organized into 23 homologous pairs.

Prophase I

During **prophase I**, the chromatin condenses into chromosomes, the spindle apparatus forms, and the nucleoli and nuclear membrane disappear. The first major difference between meiosis and mitosis occurs at this point: homologous chromosomes come together and intertwine in a process called **synapsis**. At this point, each chromosome consists of two sister chromatids, so each synaptic pair contains four chromatids and is referred to as a **tetrad**; the homologous chromosomes are held together by a group of proteins called the **synaptonemal complex**. Chromatids of homologous chromosomes may break at the point of contact, called the **chiasma** (plural: **chiasmata**) and exchange equivalent pieces of DNA, as shown in Figure 2.6. This process is called **crossing over**, and can be characterized by the number of crossover events that occur in one strand of DNA, including **single crossovers** and **double crossovers**. Note that crossing over occurs between homologous chromosomes and not between sister chromatids of the same chromosome—the latter are identical, so crossing over would not produce any change. Those chromatids involved are left with an altered but structurally complete set of genes. Such genetic **recombination** can unlink linked genes, thereby increasing the variety of genetic combinations that can be produced via gametogenesis. Linkage refers to the tendency for genes to be inherited together; genes that are located farther from each other physically are less likely to be inherited together, and more likely to undergo crossing over relative to each other. Thus, as opposed to asexual reproduction, which produces identical offspring, sexual reproduction provides the advantage of great genetic diversity, which is believed to increase the ability of a species to evolve and adapt to a changing environment.

REAL WORLD

The rate of gene unlinking is used to map differences between two genes on the same chromosome. The farther apart two genes are, the more likely they are to become unlinked during crossing over. These statistics can then be used to determine the distance between genes on the chromosome, measured in units called centimorgans.

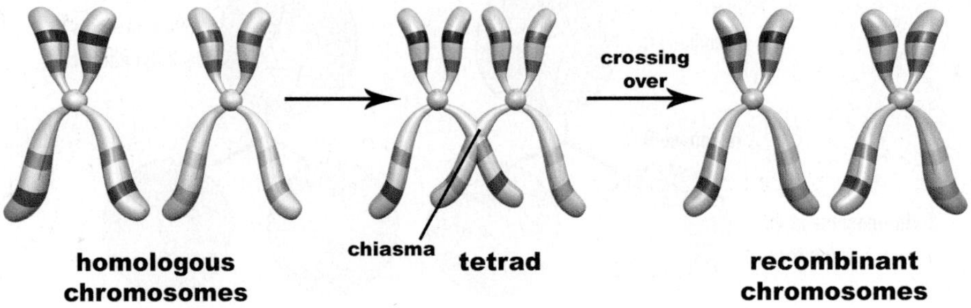

Figure 2.6 Synapsis
During prophase I, homologous chromosomes can exchange genetic material via crossing over.

Because of crossing over, each daughter cell will have a unique pool of alleles (genes coding for alternative forms of a given trait) from a random mixture of maternal and paternal origin. In classical genetics, crossing over explains **Mendel's second law (of independent assortment)**, which states that the inheritance of one allele has no effect on the likelihood of inheriting certain alleles for other genes.

Metaphase I

During **metaphase I**, homologous pairs (tetrads) align at the metaphase plate, and each pair attaches to a separate spindle fiber by its kinetochore. Note the difference from mitosis: in mitosis, each chromosome is lined up on the metaphase plate by two spindle fibers (one from each pole); in meiosis, homologous chromosomes are lined up across from each other at the metaphase plate and are held by one spindle fiber.

Anaphase I

During **anaphase I**, homologous pairs separate and are pulled to opposite poles of the cell. This process is called **disjunction**, and it accounts for **Mendel's first law (of segregation)**. During disjunction, each chromosome of paternal origin separates (or disjoins) from its homologue of maternal origin, and either chromosome can end up in either daughter cell. Thus, the distribution of homologous chromosomes to the two intermediate daughter cells is random with respect to parental origin. This separating of the two homologous chromosomes is referred to as **segregation**.

Telophase I

During **telophase I**, a nuclear membrane forms around each new nucleus. At this point, each chromosome still consists of two sister chromatids joined at the centromere. The cells are now haploid; once homologous chromosomes separate, only *n* chromosomes are found in each daughter cell (23 in humans). The cell divides into two daughter cells by cytokinesis. Between cell divisions, there may be a short rest period, or **interkinesis**, during which the chromosomes partially uncoil.

Meiosis II

Meiosis II is very similar to mitosis in that sister chromatids—rather than homologues—are separated from each other.

Prophase II

During **prophase II**, the nuclear envelope dissolves, nucleoli disappear, the centrioles migrate to opposite poles, and the spindle apparatus begins to form.

Metaphase II

During **metaphase II**, the chromosomes line up on the metaphase plate.

KEY CONCEPT

It is critical to understand how meiosis I is different from mitosis. The chromosome number is halved (reductional division) in meiosis I, and the daughter cells have the haploid number of chromosomes (23 in humans). Meiosis II is similar to mitosis in that sister chromatids are separated from one another; therefore, no change in ploidy is observed.

REAL WORLD

If, during anaphase I or II of meiosis, homologous chromosomes (anaphase I) or sister chromatids (anaphase II) fail to separate, one of the resulting gametes will have two copies of a particular chromosome and the other gamete will have none. Subsequently, during fertilization, the resulting zygote may have too many or too few copies of that chromosome. Nondisjunction can affect both autosomal chromosomes (such as trisomy 21, resulting in Down syndrome) and the sex chromosomes (such as Klinefelter and Turner syndromes).

Anaphase II

During **anaphase II**, the centromeres divide, separating the chromosomes into sister chromatids. These chromatids are pulled to opposite poles by spindle fibers.

Telophase II

During **telophase II**, a nuclear membrane forms around each new nucleus. Cytokinesis follows, and two daughter cells are formed. Thus, by completion of meiosis II, up to four haploid daughter cells are produced per gametocyte. We use the phrase *up to* because oogenesis, discussed later in this chapter, may result in fewer than four cells if an egg remains unfertilized after ovulation.

KEY CONCEPT

Mitosis	Meiosis
$2n \rightarrow 2n$	$2n \rightarrow n$
Occurs in all dividing cells	Occurs in sex cells only
Homologous chromosomes do not pair	Homologous chromosomes align on opposite sides of the metaphase plate
No crossing over	Crossing over can occur

MCAT CONCEPT CHECK 2.2

Before you move on, assess your understanding of the material with these questions.

1. What is the number and ploidy of the daughter cells produced from meiosis I? From meiosis II?
   - Meiosis I:

   ____
   - Meiosis II:

   ____
2. What is the difference between homologous chromosomes and sister chromatids?
   - Homologous chromosomes:

   ____
   - Sister chromatids:

   ____
3. For each phase of meiosis I listed below, what are the differences from the analogous phase of mitosis?

Meiotic Phase	Differences from Mitotic Phase
Prophase I	
Metaphase I	
Anaphase I	
Telophase I	

2.3 The Reproductive System

High-Yield

LEARNING OBJECTIVES

After Chapter 2.3, you will be able to:

- Recall the functions of the interstitial cells of Leydig and Sertoli cells
- Identify the phases of meiosis in which primary and secondary oocytes are arrested
- Describe the acrosome
- Differentiate between male and female sex organs and development
- Recall the phases of the menstrual cycle, including key features and relative hormone levels for each phase:

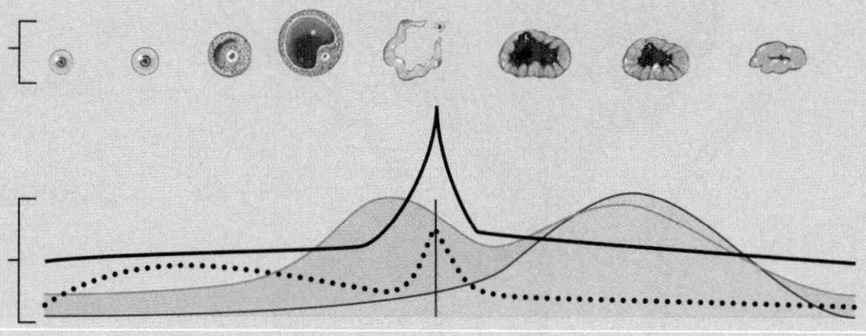

Chromosomal **sex** is determined by the 23rd pair of chromosomes, with XX being female and XY being male. Ova can only carry the X chromosome, while sperm can carry either the X or Y chromosome. The **X chromosome** carries a sizeable amount of genetic information; mutations in these genes can cause **sex-linked** (X-linked) disorders. Males are termed **hemizygous** with respect to many of the genes on the X chromosome because they only have one copy. Therefore, a male with a disease-causing allele on the unpaired part of X chromosome will necessarily express that allele. Females, on the other hand, may be homozygous or heterozygous with respect to genes on the X chromosome. Most X-linked disorders are recessively inherited; therefore, females express these disorders far less frequently than males. Females carrying a diseased allele on an X chromosome but not exhibiting the disease are said to be **carriers**.

Comparatively, the **Y chromosome** contains very little genetic information. One notable gene on the Y chromosome is ***SRY*** (**sex-determining region Y**), which codes for a transcription factor that initiates testis differentiation and, thus, the formation of male gonads. Therefore, in the absence of the Y chromosome, all zygotes will be female. In the presence of the Y chromosome a zygote will be male.

MNEMONIC

Se**x**-linked is **X**-linked.

REAL WORLD

There are actually a handful of Y-linked diseases, most of which result in reduced fertility. A father will pass a Y-linked disease to all of his sons, assuming fertility has not been lost. These diseases are extremely rare and are not included on the official MCAT content lists.

Male Reproductive Anatomy

The male reproductive system is shown in Figure 2.7.

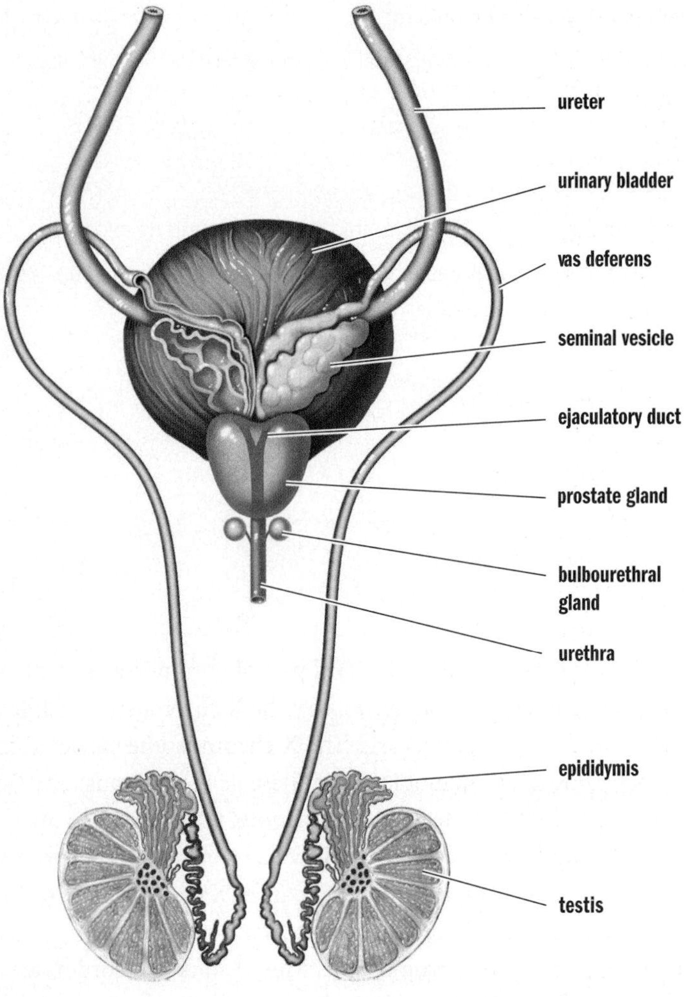

Figure 2.7 Male Reproductive System

In males, the primitive gonads develop into the **testes**. The testes have two functional components: the **seminiferous tubules** and the **interstitial cells of Leydig. Sperm** are produced in the highly coiled seminiferous tubules, where they are nourished by **Sertoli cells**. The cells of Leydig secrete **testosterone** and other male sex hormones (**androgens**). The testes are located in the **scrotum**, an external pouch that hangs below the **penis**, a position that allows it to maintain a temperature 2°C to 4°C lower than the body. In fact, there is a layer of muscle around the vas deferens (ductus deferens) that can raise and lower the testis to maintain the proper temperature for sperm development.

As sperm are formed they are passed to the **epididymis**, where their flagella gain motility, and they are then stored until **ejaculation**. During **ejaculation**, sperm travel through the **vas deferens** and enter the **ejaculatory duct** at the posterior edge of

MNEMONIC

Pathway of sperm through the male reproductive system: **SEVE(N) UP**

- **S**eminiferous tubules
- **E**pididymis
- **V**as deferens (also called the ductus deferens)
- **E**jaculatory duct
- (**N**othing)
- **U**rethra
- **P**enis

the prostate gland. The two ejaculatory ducts then fuse to form the **urethra**, which carries sperm through the penis as they exit the body. In males, the reproductive and urinary systems share a common pathway; this is not the case in females.

As sperm pass through the reproductive tract they are mixed with **seminal fluid**, which is produced through a combined effort by the seminal vesicles, prostate gland, and bulbourethral gland. The **seminal vesicles** contribute fructose to nourish sperm, and both the seminal vesicles and **prostate gland** give the fluid mildly alkaline properties so the sperm can survive in the relative acidity of the female reproductive tract. The **bulbourethral (Cowper's) glands** produce a clear viscous fluid that cleans out any remnants of urine and lubricates the urethra during sexual arousal. The combination of sperm and seminal fluid is known as **semen**.

REAL WORLD

The prostate often enlarges with age and frequently causes problems in older males, including a condition called *benign prostatic hyperplasia*. Because the prostate surrounds the urethra, classic symptoms of this condition include urinary frequency, urgency, and nighttime awakenings to use the bathroom.

Spermatogenesis

As mentioned above, **spermatogenesis**, the formation of haploid sperm through meiosis, occurs in the seminiferous tubules. In males, the diploid stem cells are known as **spermatogonia**. After replicating their genetic material (S stage), they develop into diploid **primary spermatocytes**. The first meiotic division will result in haploid **secondary spermatocytes**, which then undergo meiosis II to generate haploid **spermatids**. Finally, the spermatids undergo maturation to become mature **spermatozoa**. Spermatogenesis results in four functional sperm for each spermatogonium.

Mature sperm are very compact. They consist of a head (containing the genetic material), a midpiece (which generates ATP from fructose), and a flagellum (for motility), as shown in Figure 2.8. The **midpiece** is filled with mitochondria, which generate the energy for swimming through the female reproductive tract to reach the ovum in the fallopian tubes. Each sperm **head** is covered by a cap known as an **acrosome**. This structure is derived from the Golgi apparatus and is necessary to penetrate the **ovum**. Once a male reaches sexual maturity during puberty, approximately 3 million sperm are produced per day, which typically continues throughout the course of that individual's lifespan.

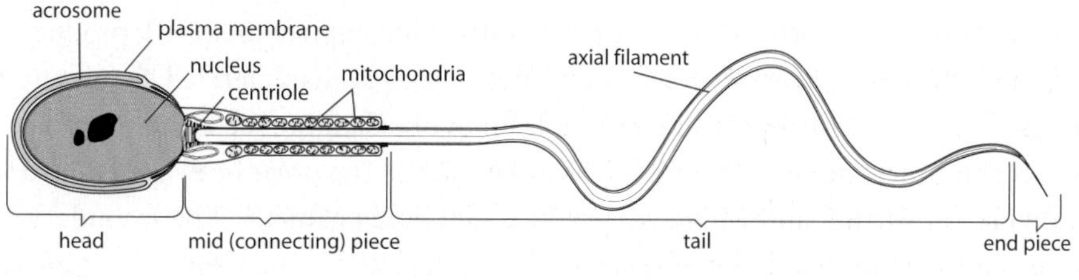

Figure 2.8 Structure of a Mature Sperm

Female Reproductive Anatomy

Female reproductive organs are primarily internal, as shown in Figure 2.9. The gonads, known as **ovaries**, produce estrogen and progesterone. The ovaries are located in the pelvic cavity; each consists of thousands of **follicles**, which are multilayered sacs that contain, nourish, and protect immature **ova** (eggs). Between puberty and menopause, one egg per month is **ovulated** into the **peritoneal sac**, which lines the abdominal cavity.

It is then drawn into the **fallopian tube** or **oviduct**, which is lined with cilia to propel the egg forward. The fallopian tubes are connected to the muscular **uterus**, which is the site of fetal development. The lower end of the uterus, known as the **cervix**, connects to the **vaginal canal**, where sperm are deposited during intercourse. The vagina is also the passageway through which childbirth can occur. The external parts of the female genital organs are known collectively as the **vulva**. As mentioned earlier, females have separate excretory and reproductive tracts.

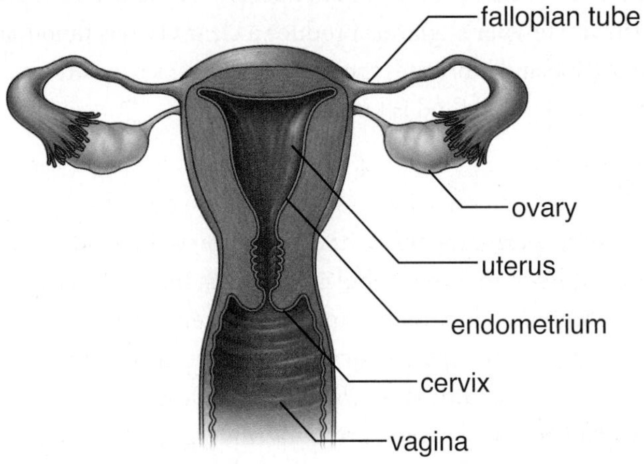

Figure 2.9 Female Reproductive System

Oogenesis

The production of female gametes is known as **oogenesis**. Although gametocytes undergo the same meiotic process in both females and males, there are some significant differences, too. First, there is no unending supply of stem cells analogous to spermatogonia in females; all of the oogonia a female will ever have are formed during fetal development. By birth, all of the oogonia have already undergone DNA replication and are considered **primary oocytes**. These cells are $2n$, like primary spermatocytes, and are actually arrested in prophase I. After **menarche** (the first menstrual cycle), one primary oocyte per month will complete meiosis I, producing a **secondary oocyte** and a polar body. The division is characterized by unequal cytokinesis, which distributes ample cytoplasm to one daughter cell (the secondary oocyte) and nearly none to the other (the polar body). The polar body generally does not divide any further and will never produce functional gametes. The secondary oocyte, on the other hand, remains arrested in metaphase II and does not complete the remainder of meiosis II unless fertilization occurs.

Oocytes are surrounded by two layers: the zona pellucida and the corona radiata. The **zona pellucida** surrounds the oocyte itself and is an acellular mixture of glycoproteins that protects the oocyte and contains compounds necessary for sperm cell binding. The **corona radiata** lies outside the zona pellucida and is a layer of cells that adheres to the oocyte during ovulation. Meiosis II is triggered when a sperm cell penetrates these layers with the help of acrosomal enzymes. The secondary oocyte undergoes the second meiotic division to split into a mature ovum and another polar body, which will eventually be broken down.

A mature ovum is a very large cell consisting of large quantities of cytoplasm and organelles. The ovum contributes nearly everything to the zygote (half of the DNA and all of the cytoplasm, organelles [including mitochondria], and RNA for early cellular processes), and sperm contribute half of the DNA. Upon completion of meiosis II, the haploid **pronuclei** of the sperm and the ovum join, creating a diploid **zygote**.

Sexual Development

The ability to reproduce is under hormonal control. Prior to puberty, the **hypothalamus** restricts production of **gonadotropin-releasing hormone** (**GnRH**). At the start of puberty, this restriction is lifted as the hypothalamus releases pulses of GnRH, which then triggers the **anterior pituitary gland** to synthesize and release **follicle-stimulating hormone** (**FSH**) and **luteinizing hormone** (**LH**). These hormones trigger the production of other sex hormones that develop and maintain the reproductive system.

Male Sexual Development

During the fetal period (from nine weeks after fertilization until birth), presence of the Y chromosome leads to production of androgens, resulting in male sexual differentiation. For the duration of infancy and childhood, androgen production is low. **Testosterone**, produced by the testes, increases dramatically during puberty, and sperm production begins. In order to achieve this, there is a delicate interplay of FSH and LH stimulation on two cell types in the testes. FSH stimulates the Sertoli cells and triggers sperm maturation, whereas LH causes the interstitial cells to produce testosterone. Testosterone not only develops and maintains the male reproductive system, but also results in the development of **secondary sexual characteristics** such as facial and axillary hair, deepening of the voice, and increased muscle and bone mass. Testosterone production remains high into adulthood and then declines with age. This hormone exerts negative feedback on the hypothalamus and anterior pituitary so that production is kept within an appropriate range.

REAL WORLD

If the receptors for testosterone are absent or defective, it cannot exert its effects. The result is a condition called *androgen insensitivity syndrome* (AIS), in which a chromosomal male (XY) has female secondary sexual characteristics. In complete androgen insensitivity, a chromosomal male will appear female at birth. Oftentimes the diagnosis of AIS is not made until puberty, when amenorrhea (failure to menstruate) manifests.

Female Sexual Development

The ovaries, which are derived from the same embryonic structures as the testes, are also under the control of FSH and LH secreted by the anterior pituitary. The ovaries produce estrogens and progesterone.

Estrogens are secreted in response to FSH and result in the development and maintenance of the female reproductive system and female secondary sexual characteristics (breast growth, widening of the hips, changes in fat distribution). In the embryo, estrogens stimulate development of the reproductive tract. In adults, estrogens lead to the thickening of the lining of the uterus (**endometrium**) each month in preparation for the implantation of a zygote.

MNEMONIC

Estrogen **est**ablishes and **pro**gesterone **pro**tects the endometrium.

Progesterone is secreted by the **corpus luteum**—the remains of the ovarian follicle following ovulation—in response to LH. Interestingly, progesterone is involved in the development and maintenance of the endometrium, but not in the initial thickening of the endometrium—this is the role of estrogen. This means that both estrogen and progesterone are required for the generation, development, and maintenance of an endometrium capable of supporting a zygote. By the end of the first trimester of a pregnancy, progesterone is supplied by the placenta, while the corpus luteum atrophies and ceases to function.

The Menstrual Cycle

During the reproductive years (from menarche to menopause), estrogen and progesterone levels rise and fall in a cyclic pattern. In response, the endometrial lining will grow and be shed. This is known as the **menstrual cycle** and can be divided into four events, as shown in Figure 2.10: the follicular phase, ovulation, the luteal phase, and menstruation.

MCAT EXPERTISE

The MCAT likes to test your ability to identify graphs of the blood concentrations of FSH, LH, estrogen, and progesterone throughout the menstrual cycle. Be sure to know when each peaks by studying Figure 2.10.

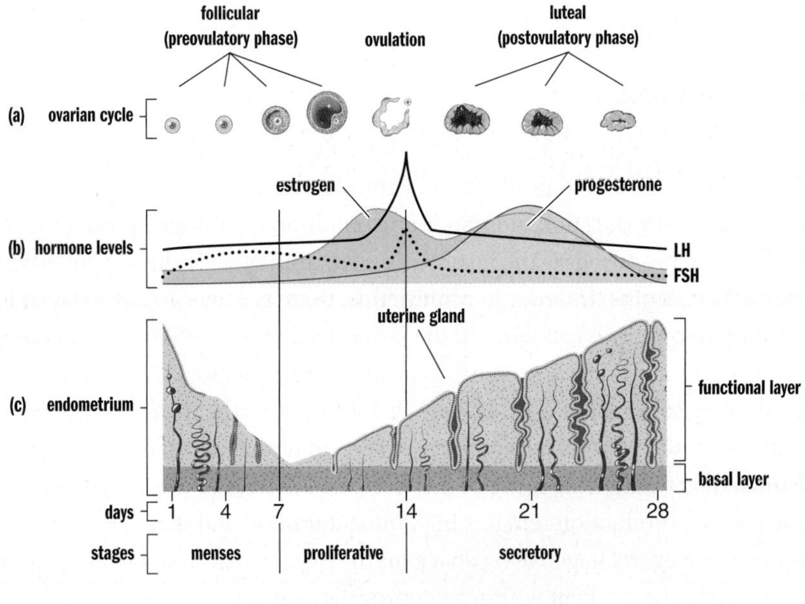

Figure 2.10 The Menstrual Cycle

(a) Follicle-stimulating hormone (FSH) facilitates the maturation of a single ovum; (b) The peak of luteinizing hormone (LH) around day 14 marks ovulation, the release of the oocyte from the follicle; (c) The endometrial lining of the uterus reaches its peak in the luteal phase and is shed at the beginning of the next cycle.

Follicular Phase

The **follicular phase** begins when the **menstrual flow**, which sheds the uterine lining of the previous cycle, begins. GnRH secretion from the hypothalamus increases in response to the decreased concentrations of estrogen and progesterone, which fall off toward the end of each cycle. The higher concentrations of GnRH cause increased secretions of both FSH and LH. These two hormones work in concert to develop several ovarian follicles. The follicles begin to produce estrogen, which has negative feedback effects and causes the GnRH, LH, and FSH concentrations to level off. Estrogen stimulates regrowth of the endometrial lining, stimulating vascularization and glandularization of the **decidua**.

Ovulation

Estrogen is interesting in that it can have both negative and positive feedback effects. Late in the follicular phase, the developing follicles secrete higher and higher concentrations of estrogen. Eventually, estrogen concentrations reach a threshold that paradoxically results in positive feedback, and GnRH, LH, and FSH levels spike. The surge in LH is important; it induces **ovulation**, the release of the ovum from the ovary into the abdominal (peritoneal) cavity.

Luteal Phase

After ovulation, LH causes the ruptured follicle to form the corpus luteum, which secretes progesterone. Remember that estrogen helps regenerate the uterine lining, but progesterone maintains it for implantation. Progesterone levels begin to rise, while estrogen levels remain high. The high levels of progesterone cause negative feedback on GnRH, FSH, and LH, preventing the ovulation of multiple eggs.

Menstruation

Assuming that implantation does not occur, the corpus luteum loses its stimulation from LH, progesterone levels decline, and the uterine lining is sloughed off. The loss of high levels of estrogen and progesterone removes the block on GnRH so that the next cycle can begin.

Pregnancy

On the other hand, if fertilization *has* occurred the resulting zygote will develop into a blastocyst that will implant in the uterine lining and secrete **human chorionic gonadotropin (hCG)**, an analog of LH—it looks very similar chemically and can stimulate LH receptors. This maintains the corpus luteum. hCG is critical during first trimester development because the estrogen and progesterone secreted by the corpus luteum keep the uterine lining in place. By the second trimester, hCG levels decline because the placenta has grown to a sufficient size to secrete enough progesterone and estrogen by itself. The high levels of estrogen and progesterone continue to serve as negative feedback on GnRH secretion.

Menopause

With aging, the ovaries become less sensitive to FSH and LH, resulting in ovarian atrophy. As estrogen and progesterone levels drop, the endometrium also atrophies, and menstruation stops. Also, because the negative feedback on FSH and LH is removed, the blood levels of these two hormones rise. This is called **menopause**.

REAL WORLD

Oral contraceptive pills (OCPs) are simply estrogen/progesterone (or progesterone-only) preparations. These block conception by inhibiting LH and FSH release through negative feedback, thereby inhibiting ovulation. When taking the placebo pills at the end of the month, withdrawal menstruation still occurs because estrogen and progesterone levels drop, but no egg passes with the menstrual flow.

KEY CONCEPT

Menstrual cycle:

- Follicles mature during the follicular phase (FSH, LH)
- LH surge at midcycle triggers ovulation
- Ruptured follicle becomes corpus luteum, which secretes estrogen and progesterone to build up uterine lining in preparation for implantation; LH and FSH are inhibited
- If fertilization does not occur, corpus luteum atrophies, progesterone and estrogen levels decrease, menses occurs, and LH and FSH levels begin to rise again

Profound physical and physiological changes usually accompany this process, including flushing, hot flashes, bloating, and headaches. Menopause usually occurs between the ages of 45 and 55.

MCAT CONCEPT CHECK 2.3

Before you move on, assess your understanding of the material with these questions.

1. What are the functions of interstitial cells of Leydig and Sertoli cells?
   - Interstitial cells of Leydig:

   ____

   - Sertoli cells:

   ____

2. During which phase of meiosis is a primary oocyte arrested? During which phase of meiosis is a secondary oocyte arrested?
   - Primary oocyte:

   ____

   - Secondary oocyte:

   ____

3. What is the acrosome? What organelle forms the acrosome?

   ____

4. Which hormones are key to sexual differentiation in a fetus with XY genotype? Describe the expected phenotype if receptors to these hormones are absent.

   ____

5. What are the four phases of the menstrual cycle? What are the features and relative hormone concentrations of each phase? (Note: Draw in symbols to signify the levels of each hormone, such as ↑, =, and ↓.)

Phase	Key Features	FSH	LH	Estrogen	Progesterone

Conclusion

In this chapter, we explored one of the key tenets of the cell theory—how cells produce more copies of themselves. We first examined mitosis, which results in genetically identical diploid daughter cells. We then moved on to meiosis, which results in genetically nonidentical haploid daughter cells, or gametes. We then looked at the male and female reproductive systems, which form these gametes, each of which contains half of the normal complement of genetic information. Finally, we explored basic reproductive endocrinology and saw how testosterone and estrogen are key in the development of the reproductive systems and the secondary sex characteristics that develop at puberty.

Formation of gametes is only half the story, of course. It serves us no good as a species to form sex cells if the cells cannot interact to form another human. Ultimately, gametes must accomplish their purpose: passing on the genes, the instructions for life, from one generation to another. Thus, we turn our attention in the next chapter to the next steps of fertilization, embryogenesis, and birth. Indeed, it is through the union of one egg and one sperm that every human being on the planet today—and since the beginning of the human race—came into existence.

GO ONLINE

You've reviewed the content, now test your knowledge and critical thinking skills by completing a test-like passage set in your online resources!

CONCEPT SUMMARY

The Cell Cycle and Mitosis

- **Diploid** ($2n$) cells have two copies of each chromosome; **haploid** (n) cells have one copy.
- The cell cycle contains five stages. The G_1, S, and G_2 stages are collectively called **interphase**, during which the DNA is uncoiled in the form of **chromatin**.
  - In the **G_1** stage (**presynthetic gap**), cells create organelles for energy and protein production, and increase their size. The **restriction point**, during which the DNA is checked for quality, must be passed for the cell to move into the S stage.
  - In the **S** stage (**synthesis**), DNA is replicated. The strands of DNA, called **chromatids**, are held together at the centromere.
  - In the **G_2** stage (**postsynthetic gap**), there is further cell growth and replication of organelles in preparation for mitosis. Another quality checkpoint must be passed for the cell to enter into mitosis.
  - In the **M** stage (**mitosis**), mitosis and cytokinesis occur.
  - In the **G_0** stage, the cell performs its functions without preparing for division.
- **p53** plays a role in the two major checkpoints of the cell cycle (G_1 to S, and G_2 to M).
- **Cyclins** and **cyclin-dependent kinases** (**CDK**) rise and fall during the cell cycle. Cyclins bind to CDKs, phosphorylating and activating **transcription factors** for the next stage of the cell cycle.
- **Cancer** occurs when cell cycle control becomes deranged, allowing damaged cells to undergo mitosis without regard to quality or quantity of the new cells produced. Cancerous cells may begin to produce factors that allow them to delocalize and invade adjacent tissues or **metastasize** elsewhere.
- Mitosis produces two genetically identical diploid daughter cells from a single cell and occurs in **somatic cells**.
- Mitosis has four phases:
  - In **prophase**, the chromosomes condense, the nuclear membrane dissolves, nucleoli disappear, centrioles migrate to opposite sides of the cell, and the **spindle apparatus** begins to form. The **kinetochore** of each chromosome is contacted by a spindle fiber.
  - In **metaphase**, chromosomes line up along the **metaphase plate** (**equatorial plate**).
  - In **anaphase**, sister chromatids are separated and pulled to opposite poles.
  - In **telophase**, the nuclear membrane reforms, spindle apparatus disappears, and cytosol and organelles are split between the two daughter cells through **cytokinesis**.

Meiosis

- **Meiosis** occurs in **gametocytes** (**germ cells**) and produces up to four nonidentical haploid sex cells (**gametes**).
- Meiosis has one round of replication and two rounds of division (the **reductional** and **equational** divisions).
- In **meiosis I**, homologous pairs of chromosomes (homologues) are separated from each other. **Homologues** are chromosomes that are given the same number, but are of opposite parental origin.
  - In **prophase I**, the same events occur as in prophase of mitosis, except that homologues come together and intertwine in a process called **synapsis**. The four chromatids are referred to as a **tetrad**, and **crossing over** exchanges genetic material between one chromatid and material from a chromatid in the homologous chromosome. This accounts for **Mendel's second law (of independent assortment)**.
  - In **metaphase I**, homologous chromosomes line up on opposite sides of the metaphase plate.
  - In **anaphase I**, homologous chromosomes are pulled to opposite poles of the cell. This accounts for **Mendel's first law (of segregation)**.
  - In **telophase I**, the chromosomes may or may not fully decondense, and the cell may enter **interkinesis** after cytokinesis.
- In **meiosis II**, sister chromatids are separated from each other in a process that is functionally identical to mitosis. **Sister chromatids** are copies of the same DNA held together at the centromere.

The Reproductive System

- Chromosomal sex is determined by the 23rd pair of chromosomes in humans, with XX being female and XY being male.
  - The **X chromosome** carries a sizeable amount of genetic information; mutations of X-linked genes can cause sex-linked disorders. Males are **hemizygous** with respect to the unpaired genes on the X chromosome, so they will express sex-linked disorders, even if they only have one recessive disease-carrying allele. Females with only one copy of the affected allele are called **carriers**.
  - The **Y chromosome** carries little genetic information, but does contain the ***SRY*** **(sex-determining region Y)** gene, which causes the gonads to differentiate into testes.
- The male reproductive system contains both internal and external structures.
  - **Sperm** develop in the **seminiferous tubules** in the **testes**. They are nourished by **Sertoli cells**.
  - **Interstitial cells of Leydig**, in the testes, secrete **testosterone** and other male sex hormones (**androgens**).

- The testes are located in the **scrotum**, which hangs outside of the abdominal cavity and has a temperature 2°C to 4°C lower than the rest of the body.
- Once formed, sperm gain motility in the **epididymis** and are stored there until ejaculation.
- During **ejaculation**, sperm travel through the **vas deferens** to the **ejaculatory duct**, and then to the **urethra** and out through the **penis**.
- The **seminal vesicles** contribute fructose to nourish sperm and produce alkaline fluid.
- The **prostate gland** also produces alkaline fluid.
- The **bulbourethral glands** produce a clear viscous fluid that cleans out any remnants of urine and lubricates the urethra during sexual arousal.
- **Semen** is composed of sperm and **seminal fluid** from the glands above.

- In **spermatogenesis**, four haploid sperm are produced from a **spermatogonium**.
  - After S stage, the germ cells are called **primary spermatocytes**.
  - After meiosis I, the germ cells are called **secondary spermatocytes**.
  - After meiosis II, the germ cells are called **spermatids**.
  - After maturation, the germ cells are called **spermatozoa**.
- Sperm contain a head, midpiece, and flagellum.
  - The **head** contains the genetic material and is covered with an **acrosome**—a modified Golgi apparatus that contains enzymes that help the sperm fuse with and penetrate the ovum.
  - The **midpiece** generates ATP from fructose and contains many mitochondria.
  - The **flagellum** promotes motility.
- The female reproductive system primarily contains internal structures.
  - **Ova** (eggs) are produced in **follicles** in the **ovaries**.
  - Once each month, an egg is **ovulated** into the **peritoneal sac** and is drawn into the **fallopian tube** or **oviduct**.
  - The fallopian tubes are connected to the **uterus**, the lower end of which is the **cervix**.
  - The **vaginal canal** lies below the cervix and is the site where sperm are deposited during intercourse.
  - The vaginal canal also can be the site of childbirth.
  - The external parts of the female genital organs are collectively known as the **vulva**.
- In **oogenesis**, one haploid ovum and a variable number of polar bodies are formed from an **oogonium**.
  - At birth, all oogonia have already undergone replication and are considered **primary oocytes**. They are arrested in prophase I.

- The ovulated egg each month is a **secondary oocyte**, which is arrested in metaphase II.
- If the oocyte is fertilized, it will complete meiosis II to become a true ovum.
- Cytokinesis is uneven in oogenesis. The cell receiving very little cytoplasm and organelles is called a **polar body**.
- Oocytes are surrounded by the **zona pellucida**, an acellular mixture of glycoproteins that protects the oocyte and contains the compounds necessary for sperm binding; and the **corona radiata**, which is a layer of cells that adheres to the oocyte during ovulation.

- **Gonadotropin-releasing hormone** (**GnRH**) from the **hypothalamus** causes the release of **follicle-stimulating hormone** (**FSH**) and **luteinizing hormone** (**LH**), the functions of which depend on the sex of the individual.
    - In males, FSH stimulates the Sertoli cells and triggers spermatogenesis, while LH causes the interstitial cells to produce testosterone. **Testosterone** is responsible for the maintenance and development of the male reproductive system and male secondary sex characteristics (facial and axillary hair, deepening of the voice, and increased bone and muscle mass).
    - In females, FSH stimulates development of the ovarian follicles, while LH causes ovulation. These hormones also stimulate production of estrogens and progesterone.
- The menstrual cycle is a periodic growth and shedding of the endometrial lining.
    - In the **follicular phase**, GnRH secretion stimulates FSH and LH secretion, which promotes follicle development. Estrogen is released, stimulating vascularization and glandularization of the **decidua**.
    - **Ovulation** is stimulated by a sudden surge in LH. This surge is triggered when estrogen levels reach a threshold and switch from negative to positive feedback effects.
    - In the **luteal phase**, LH causes the ruptured follicle to become the corpus luteum, which secretes progesterone that maintains the uterine lining. High estrogen and progesterone levels cause negative feedback on GnRH, LH, and FSH.
    - **Menstruation** occurs if there is no fertilization. As the estrogen and progesterone levels drop, the endometrial lining is sloughed off, and the block on GnRH production is removed.
    - If fertilization does occur, the blastula produces **human chorionic gonadotropin** (**hCG**) which, as an LH analog, can maintain the corpus luteum. Near the end of the first trimester, hCG levels drop as the placenta takes over progesterone production.
- **Menopause** occurs when the ovaries stop producing estrogen and progesterone, usually between ages 45 and 55. Menstruation stops and FSH and LH levels rise. Physical and physiological changes accompanying menopause include flushing, hot flashes, bloating, and headaches.

ANSWERS TO CONCEPT CHECKS

2.1

1.

Cell Cycle Stage	Features
G_1	Cell grows and performs its normal functions. DNA is examined and repaired.
S	DNA is replicated.
G_2	Cell continues to grow and replicates organelles in preparation for mitosis. Cell continues to perform its normal functions.
M	Mitosis (cell division) occurs.
G_0	The cell performs its normal functions and is not preparing to divide.

2.

Mitotic Phase	Features
Prophase	Chromosomes condense, nuclear membrane dissolves, nucleoli disappear, centrioles migrate to opposite poles and begin forming the spindle apparatus
Metaphase	Chromosomes gather along the metaphase plate in the center of the cell under the guidance of the spindle apparatus
Anaphase	Sister chromatids separate, and a copy of each chromosome migrates to opposite poles
Telophase and Cytokinesis	Chromosomes decondense, nuclear membrane reforms, nucleoli reappear, spindle apparatus breaks down, cell divides into two identical daughter cells

2.2

1. After meiosis I, there are two haploid daughter cells. After meiosis II, there are up to four haploid gametes.
2. Homologous chromosomes are related chromosomes of opposite parental origin (such as maternal chromosome 15 and paternal chromosome 15, or—in males—the X and Y chromosomes). Sister chromatids are identical copies of the same DNA that are held together at the centromere. After S phase, a cell contains 92 chromatids, 46 chromosomes, and 23 homologous pairs.

3.

Meiotic Phase	Differences from Mitotic Phase
Prophase I	Homologous chromosomes come together as tetrads during synapsis; crossing over
Metaphase I	Homologous chromosomes line up on opposite sides of the metaphase plate, rather than individual chromosomes lining up on the metaphase plate
Anaphase I	Homologous chromosomes separate from each other; centromeres do not break
Telophase I	Chromatin may or may not decondense; interkinesis occurs as the cell prepares for meiosis II

2.3

1. The interstitial cells of Leydig secrete testosterone and other male sex hormones (androgens). Sertoli cells nourish sperm during their development.
2. A primary oocyte is arrested in prophase I, while a secondary oocyte is arrested in metaphase II.
3. The acrosome contains enzymes that are capable of penetrating the corona radiata and zona pellucida of the ovum, permitting fertilization to occur. It is a modified Golgi apparatus.
4. Androgens, such as testosterone, lead to male sexual differentiation. Absence of androgen receptors, a condition known as androgen insensitivity syndrome, leads to an XY genotype with phenotypically female characteristics.

5.

Phase	Key Features	FSH	LH	Estrogen	Progesterone
Follicular	Egg develops, endometrial lining becomes vascularized and glandularized	↑	=	↓, then ↑	↓
Ovulation	Egg is released from follicle into peritoneal cavity	↑	↑↑	↑	↓
Luteal	Corpus luteum produces progesterone to maintain endometrium	↓	=	↑	↑
Menses	Shedding of endometrial lining	↓	↓	↓	↓

SCIENCE MASTERY ASSESSMENT EXPLANATIONS

1. **B**

Diploid cells called spermatogonia differentiate into primary spermatocytes, which undergo the first meiotic division to yield two haploid secondary spermatocytes. These undergo a second meiotic division to become immature spermatids. The spermatids then undergo a series of changes leading to the production of mature sperm, or spermatozoa.

2. **C**

From the time of birth until shortly before ovulation, all egg cells are arrested at the prophase stage of meiosis I. These cells are referred to as primary oocytes. At ovulation, the egg cell has completed meiosis I and is now arrested in metaphase II as a haploid cell called a secondary oocyte. When a sperm penetrates the outer layers of the secondary oocyte, it completes meiosis II to become a mature ovum.

3. **A**

The spindle apparatus first interacts with the kinetochore fibers near the end of prophase. While the spindle apparatus aligns the chromosomes at the equatorial plate during metaphase, **(B)**, the initial connection of the microtubule to the kinetochore occurs in prophase.

4. **D**

To ensure that the labeled deoxyadenine will be incorporated into the DNA of one of the daughter cells, we have to insert the nucleotide before DNA replication has been completed. Because replication occurs during S stage, we could introduce the deoxyadenine during G_1 or S stage. Because G_1 precedes S, the latest point at which the deoxyadenine could be added is the S stage.

5. **C**

Estrogen is known to cause growth of the endometrial lining during the follicular phase of the menstrual cycle, and its levels stay high during the luteal phase to promote vascularization and glandularization of this tissue. Excessive levels of estrogen may provide a strong enough signal for cell growth to promote tumor formation or even cancer. The other tissues listed in this question require estrogen for development, but are not strongly dependent on estrogen for growth.

6. **C**

This subtle point about ovulation is missed by most students and remains hard to believe until the organs are examined in anatomy class in medical school. The ruptured ovarian follicle releases an oocyte into the abdominal cavity, close to the entrance of the fallopian tube. With the aid of beating cilia, the oocyte is drawn into the fallopian tube, through which it travels until it reaches the uterus. If it is fertilized in the fallopian tube, it will implant in the uterine wall. If fertilization does not occur, it will be expelled along with the uterine lining during menstruation.

7. **D**

The question is asking us to determine at which points in the cell cycle we can prevent or at least lower the number of cells undergoing mitosis. One idea would be to prevent DNA synthesis during the S stage of the cell cycle. Without the DNA being replicated, two viable daughter cells could not be formed. Other ideas would be preventing the mitotic cycle from forming altogether in prophase by preventing spindle apparatus formation, preventing the nuclear membrane from dissolving, or interfering with other processes during this phase. Similarly, a treatment that would act on cells in the metaphase stage of the cell cycle would also interfere with the mitotic cycle. Therefore, any of the three solutions presented would be a viable option.

8. **B**

The prostate gland, along with the seminal vesicles and the bulbourethral gland, secretes seminal fluid that combines with sperm to produce semen. It is the cremaster muscle which surrounds the testes that raises and lowers the testes in response to changes in temperature.

9. **B**

The first meiotic division (reductional division) pulls homologous chromosomes to opposite poles of the cell during anaphase I. Near the end of telophase I, cytokinesis occurs, resulting in two haploid (n) daughter cells. Thus, during interkinesis and anaphase II, the daughter cells are already haploid, eliminating **(C)** and **(D)**. The cell is diploid during interphase, **(A)**, but remains diploid up until the end of telophase I.

10. **D**

The safest way to answer this question correctly is to go through each answer choice and eliminate the ones that contribute to genetic variability. The random fertilization of an egg by a sperm, the random segregation of homologous chromosomes during anaphase I, and crossing over between homologous chromosomes during prophase I all contribute to genetic variability during sexual reproduction because they result in novel combinations of genetic material, eliminating **(A)**, **(B)**, and **(C)**. S stage, **(D)**, should *not* cause increased genetic variability; the DNA should be copied precisely, without error, meaning that both strands of DNA should be identical.

11. **D**

The key differences between mitosis and meiosis primarily appear during meiosis I. Of note, synapsis and crossing over occur during prophase I, and homologous chromosomes are separated during meiosis I (rather than sister chromatids, as in mitosis). While the location of the centromeres relative to the metaphase plate may seem trivial, it is representative of the fact that homologous chromosomes line up on opposite sides of the equatorial plate in meiosis, in contrast to the positioning of each chromosome directly upon the metaphase plate in mitosis.

12. **D**

In prophase, the chromatin condenses into chromosomes, the spindle apparatus forms, and the nucleoli and nuclear membrane disappear. **(A)** describes anaphase, whereas **(B)** and **(C)** describe telophase.

13. **C**

Nondisjunction refers to the incorrect segregation of homologous chromosomes during anaphase I, or of sister chromatids during anaphase II. In either case, one daughter cell ends up with two copies of related genetic material, while the other receives zero. Immediately, this should eliminate **(A)** and **(B)**, which show a normal complement of chromosomes (46). An individual who has only one recessive disease-carrying allele, and yet still expresses the disease, likely does not have a dominant allele for the given trait. This is seen in males, who are hemizygous for many X-linked genes, and can also be seen in females who have Turner syndrome (45,X) and only one X chromosome. Thus, **(C)** is the answer.

14. **C**

Progesterone peaks during the luteal phase, as it supports the endometrium for potential implantation of a blastula. Progesterone levels are relatively low during the follicular phase and ovulation, eliminating **(A)** and **(B)**. Withdrawal of progesterone actually causes menses, eliminating **(D)**.

15. **D**

During the first trimester of pregnancy, the corpus luteum is preserved by human chorionic gonadotropin (hCG); hence, progesterone secretion by the corpus luteum is maintained during the first trimester. This eliminates **(A)**. During the second trimester, hCG levels decline, but progesterone levels rise because the hormone is now secreted by the placenta itself, eliminating **(B)**. High levels of progesterone and estrogen inhibit GnRH secretion, thus preventing FSH and LH secretion and the onset of a new menstrual cycle. This eliminates **(C)** and validates **(D)**.

GO ONLINE **Consult your online resources for additional practice.**

SHARED CONCEPTS

Behavioral Sciences Chapter 1
Biology and Behavior

Biochemistry Chapter 6
DNA and Biotechnology

Biology Chapter 1
The Cell

Biology Chapter 3
Embryogenesis and Development

Biology Chapter 5
The Endocrine System

Biology Chapter 12
Genetics and Evolution

CHAPTER 3

EMBRYOGENESIS AND DEVELOPMENT

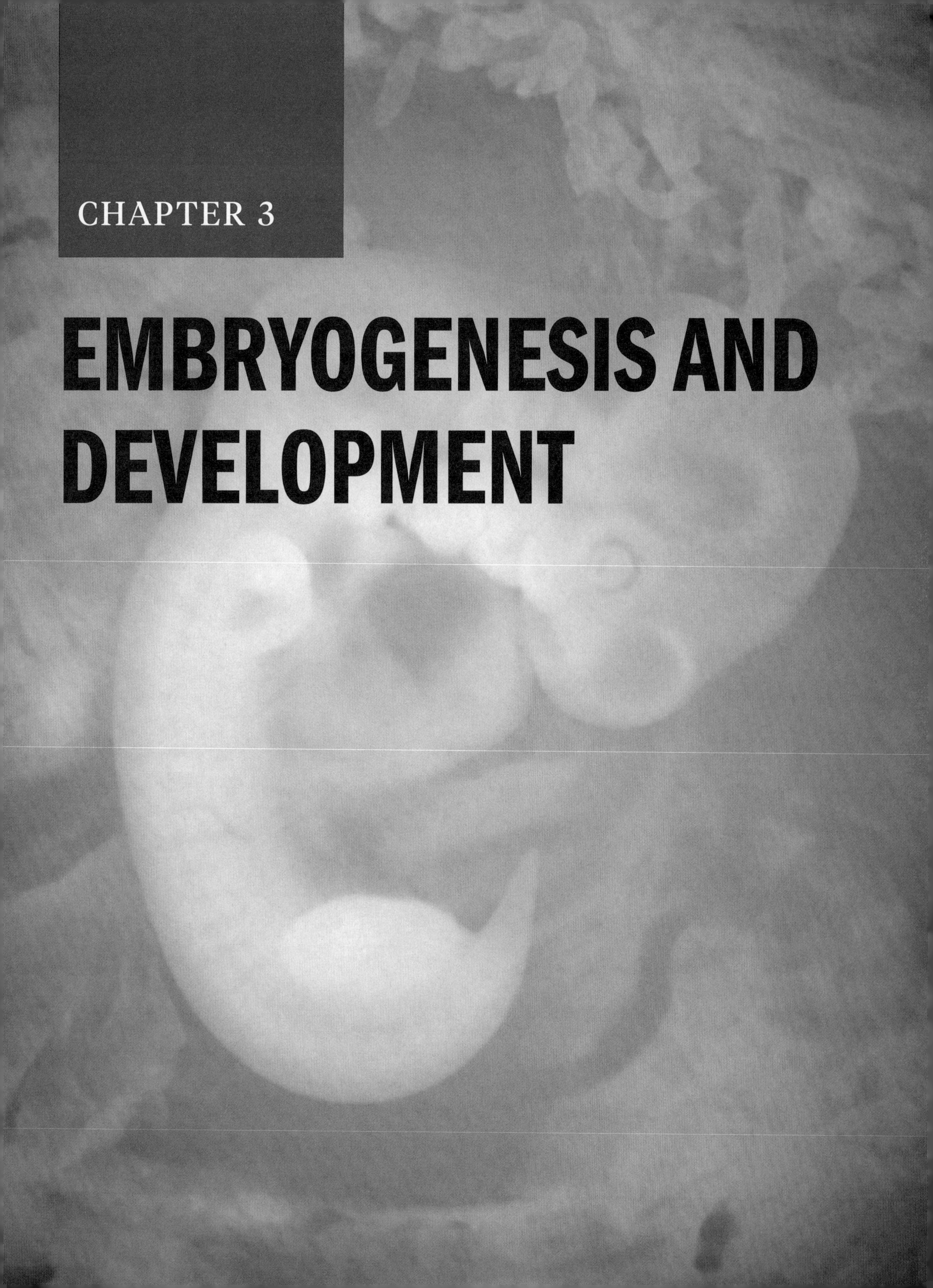

SCIENCE MASTERY ASSESSMENT

Every pre-med knows this feeling: there is so much content I have to know for the MCAT! How do I know what to do first or what's important?

While the high-yield badges throughout this book will help you identify the most important topics, this Science Mastery Assessment is another tool in your MCAT prep arsenal. This quiz (which can also be taken in your online resources) and the guidance below will help ensure that you are spending the appropriate amount of time on this chapter based on your personal strengths and weaknesses. Don't worry though—skipping something now does not mean you'll never study it. Later on in your prep, as you complete full-length tests, you'll uncover specific pieces of content that you need to review and can come back to these chapters as appropriate.

How to Use This Assessment

If you answer 0–7 questions correctly:

Spend about 1 hour to read this chapter in full and take limited notes throughout. Follow up by reviewing **all** quiz questions to ensure that you now understand how to solve each one.

If you answer 8–11 questions correctly:

Spend 20–40 minutes reviewing the quiz questions. Beginning with the questions you missed, read and take notes on the corresponding subchapters. For questions you answered correctly, ensure your thinking matches that of the explanation and you understand why each choice was correct or incorrect.

If you answer 12–15 questions correctly:

Spend less than 20 minutes reviewing all questions from the quiz. If you missed any, then include a quick read-through of the corresponding subchapters, or even just the relevant content within a subchapter, as part of your question review. For questions you answered correctly, ensure your thinking matches that of the explanation and review the Concept Summary at the end of the chapter.

1. Which of the following signaling molecules coordinate uterine contractions during childbirth?
   - **A.** Oxytocin and prolactin
   - **B.** Progesterone and prostaglandins
   - **C.** Oxytocin and progesterone
   - **D.** Oxytocin and prostaglandins

2. Which of the following associations of a primary germ layer and an adult organ is correct?
   - **A.** Endoderm—cardiac muscle
   - **B.** Endoderm—lens of the eye
   - **C.** Ectoderm—fingernails
   - **D.** Mesoderm—lining of digestive tract

3. From which of the following layers does the notochord form?
   - **A.** Ectoderm
   - **B.** Mesoderm
   - **C.** Endoderm
   - **D.** Archenteron

4. The influence of a specific group of cells on the differentiation of another group of cells is called:
   - **A.** competence.
   - **B.** senescence.
   - **C.** determination.
   - **D.** induction.

5. Which of the following is likely to be found in the blood of a person who is pregnant?
   - **A.** Immunoglobulins produced by the fetus
   - **B.** Fetal hemoglobin released from fetal red blood cells
   - **C.** Progesterone produced by placental cells
   - **D.** Carbon dioxide exhaled from fetal lungs

6. A cell releases a substance that diffuses through the environment, resulting in differentiation of a nearby cell. This is an example of what type of cell–cell communication?
   - **A.** Autocrine
   - **B.** Juxtacrine
   - **C.** Paracrine
   - **D.** Endocrine

7. A cancer cell is removed from a patient and cultured. The cells in this culture seem to be able to divide indefinitely with no cellular senescence. Which protein is likely activated in these cells that accounts for this characteristic?
   - **A.** Epidermal growth factor
   - **B.** Sonic hedgehog
   - **C.** Transforming growth factor beta
   - **D.** Telomerase

8. Anencephaly is a rare physiological abnormality in which the cerebrum fails to develop. During which trimester of pregnancy would this disorder manifest?
   - **A.** First trimester
   - **B.** Second trimester
   - **C.** Third trimester
   - **D.** Any trimester

9. Which of the following is FALSE with regard to adult stem cells?
   - **A.** They retain inherent pluripotency if harvested from selected organs.
   - **B.** They are less controversial than embryonic stem cells.
   - **C.** They require treatment with various transcription factors.
   - **D.** There is a reduced risk of rejection if the patient's own stem cells are used.

10. A child is born with an imperforate anus, in which the anal canal fails to form correctly and the rectum is not connected to the outside world. This pathology is most likely accounted for by a failure of:
    - **A.** cell differentiation.
    - **B.** cell determination.
    - **C.** apoptosis.
    - **D.** neurulation.

11. Following a myocardial infarction, the heart often heals by the creation of a scar by fibroblasts. This is an example of:

- **A.** complete regeneration.
- **B.** incomplete regeneration.
- **C.** competency.
- **D.** multipotency.

12. Neurofibromatosis type I, or von Recklinghausen's disease, is a disorder that causes formation of tumors in multiple nervous system structures as well as the skin. While all cells carry the same mutation on chromosome 17, selective transcription of the genome appears to cause the most significant tumorigenesis in which of the following primary germ tissue layers?

- **A.** Ectoderm
- **B.** Mesoderm
- **C.** Endoderm
- **D.** Notochord

13. Which of the following shows the correct order of early developmental milestones during embryogenesis?

- **A.** Blastula → gastrula → morula
- **B.** Morula → gastrula → blastula
- **C.** Morula → blastula → gastrula
- **D.** Gastrula → blastula → morula

14. A woman who is pregnant is accidentally given a single dose of a teratogenic drug late in the third trimester. The baby is born three days later. Which of the following is the most likely outcome?

- **A.** Complete failure of organ development and death of the fetus
- **B.** Partial failure of organ development with survival of the fetus
- **C.** Serious disfigurement of the fetus
- **D.** Respiratory distress at birth, but no long-term effects

15. Which of the following statements regarding fetal circulation is FALSE?

- **A.** In the umbilical cord, there are more arteries than veins.
- **B.** The foramen ovale is the only shunt that connects two chambers of the heart.
- **C.** Blood flow in the ductus arteriosus is from the aorta to the pulmonary artery.
- **D.** The ductus venosus is the only shunt that bypasses the liver.

Answer Key

1. **D**
2. **C**
3. **B**
4. **D**
5. **C**
6. **C**
7. **D**
8. **A**
9. **A**
10. **C**
11. **B**
12. **A**
13. **C**
14. **D**
15. **C**

Detailed explanations can be found at the end of the chapter.

CHAPTER 3

EMBRYOGENESIS AND DEVELOPMENT

In This Chapter

CHAPTER PROFILE

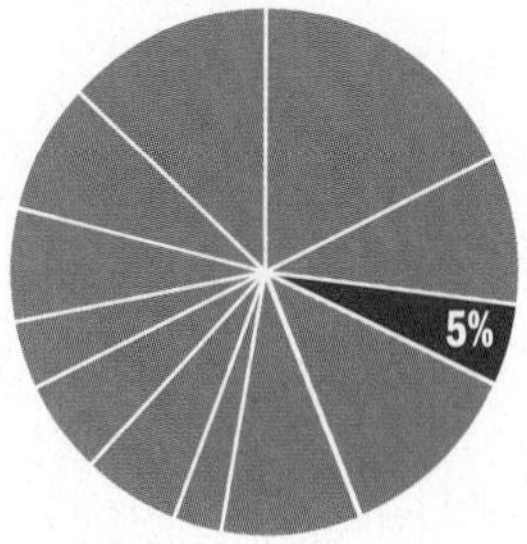

The content in this chapter should be relevant to about 5% of all questions about biology on the MCAT.

This chapter covers material from the following AAMC content categories:

1B: Transmission of genetic information from the gene to the protein

2C: Processes of cell division, differentiation, and specialization

3B: Structure and integrative functions of the main organ systems

7A: Individual influences on behavior

Introduction

Ultrasonography is a radiographic technique performed by placing a probe that emits high-frequency sound waves near the tissue to be examined. When used during pregnancy, the probe transduces an image onto a computer screen to determine gestational age, screen for multiple pregnancies or anomalies, and identify the baby's phenotypical sex. The latter typically cannot be determined before 16 to 17 weeks without a blood test, because ultrasonography equipment does not have high enough resolution.

In this chapter, we'll continue the discussion from Chapter 2 by beginning with fertilization, the formation of a diploid zygote from the union of a sperm and an ovum. We'll then follow development from this point until the birth of an autonomously breathing baby. We'll examine how the cells of a developing human divide and differentiate. We'll also explore some specific system differences that exist between developing fetuses and adults as we present an overview of the stages of pregnancy and childbirth.

3.1 Early Developmental Stages

LEARNING OBJECTIVES

After Chapter 3.1, you will be able to:

- Distinguish between determinate and indeterminate cleavage of a zygote
- Describe the process of implantation and the stage of development at which it occurs
- Connect the ectoderm, mesoderm, neural crest, and endoderm to the organs they will form
- Describe how induction influences development
- Recall the stages of embryonic development up to the gastrula:

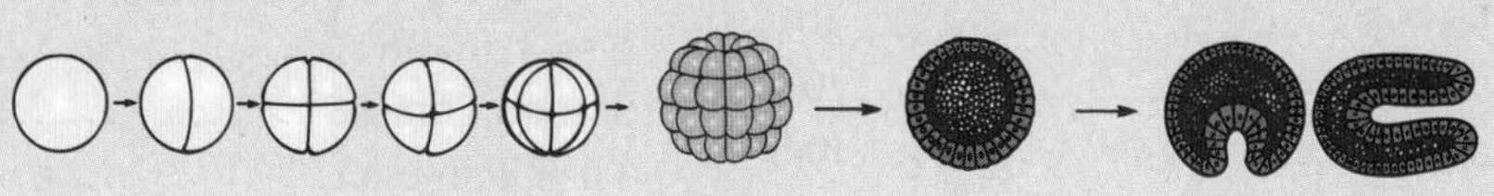

In this first section, we will explore development from the formation of a diploid zygote until neurulation, or the formation of the neural tube that will differentiate into the nervous system.

Fertilization

As discussed in Chapter 2 of *MCAT Biology Review*, a secondary oocyte is ovulated from the follicle on approximately day 14 of the menstrual cycle. The secondary oocyte travels into the fallopian tube, where it can be fertilized up to 24 hours after ovulation. Fertilization, shown in Figure 3.1, usually occurs in the widest part of the fallopian tube, called the **ampulla**. When the sperm meets the secondary oocyte in the fallopian tube, it binds to the oocyte and releases acrosomal enzymes that enable the head of the sperm to penetrate the corona radiata and zona pellucida. The first sperm to come into direct contact with the secondary oocyte's cell membrane forms a tube-like structure known as the **acrosomal apparatus**, which extends to and penetrates the cell membrane. Its pronucleus may then freely enter the oocyte once meiosis II has come to completion.

After penetration of the sperm through the cell membrane, the **cortical reaction**, a release of calcium ions, occurs. These calcium ions depolarize the membrane of the ovum, which serves two purposes: depolarization prevents fertilization of the ovum by multiple sperm cells, and the increased calcium concentration increases the metabolic rate of the newly formed diploid **zygote**. The now depolarized and impenetrable membrane is called the **fertilization membrane**.

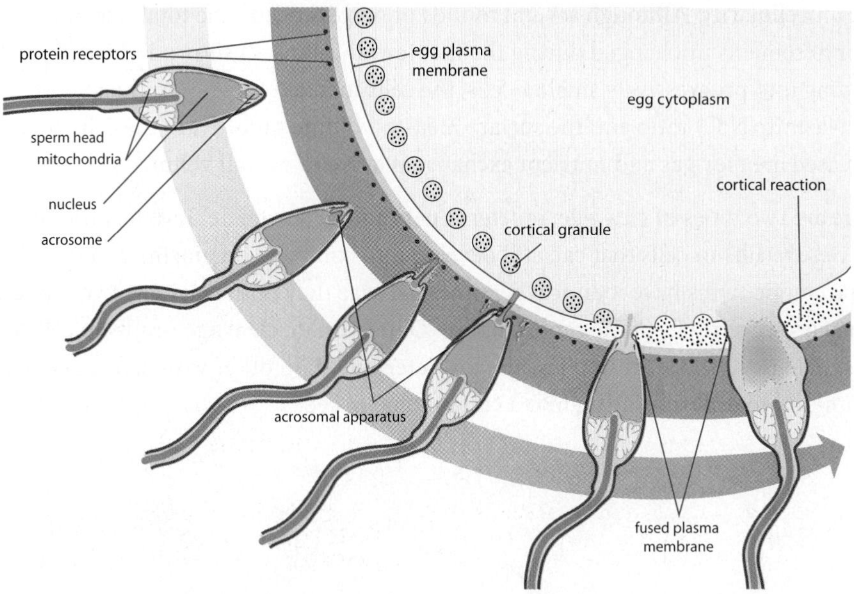

Figure 3.1 Fertilization

Twins

Twinning can occur by two different mechanisms. **Dizygotic (fraternal) twins** form from fertilization of two different eggs released during one ovulatory cycle by two different sperm. Each zygote will implant in the uterine wall, and each develops its own placenta, chorion, and amnion—these structures are discussed later in the chapter. If the zygotes implant close together, the placentas may grow onto each other. Fraternal twins are no more genetically similar than any other pair of siblings.

Monozygotic (identical) twins form when a single zygote splits into two. Because the genetic material is identical, the genomes of the offspring will be too. If division is incomplete, **conjoined twins** may result, where the two offspring are physically attached. Monozygotic twins can be classified by the number of structures they share. Monochorionic/monoamniotic twins share the same amnion and chorion. Monochorionic/diamniotic twins each have their own amnion, but share the same chorion. Dichorionic/diamniotic twins each have their own amnions and chorions. Which type of twinning occurs is a result of when the separation occurred. As more gestational structures are shared, there are more risks as the fetuses grow and develop.

Cleavage

After fertilization in the fallopian tubes, the zygote must travel to the uterus for implantation. If it arrives too late, there will no longer be an endometrium capable of supporting the embryo. As it moves to the uterus for implantation, the zygote undergoes rapid mitotic cell divisions in a process called **cleavage**. The first cleavage officially creates an embryo, as it nullifies one of the zygote's defining characteristics: unicellularity. Although several rounds of mitosis occur, the total size of the embryo remains unchanged during the first few divisions, as shown in Figure 3.2. By dividing into progressively smaller cells, the cells increase two ratios: the nuclear-to-cytoplasmic (N:C) ratio and the surface area-to-volume ratio. Thus, the cells achieve increased area for gas and nutrient exchange relative to overall volume.

There are two types of cleavage: indeterminate and determinate. **Indeterminate cleavage** results in cells that can still develop into complete organisms. In fact, monozygotic twins have identical genomes because they both originate from indeterminately cleaved cells of the same embryo. **Determinate cleavage** results in cells with fates that are, as the term implies, already determined. In other words, these cells are committed to **differentiating** into a certain type of cell.

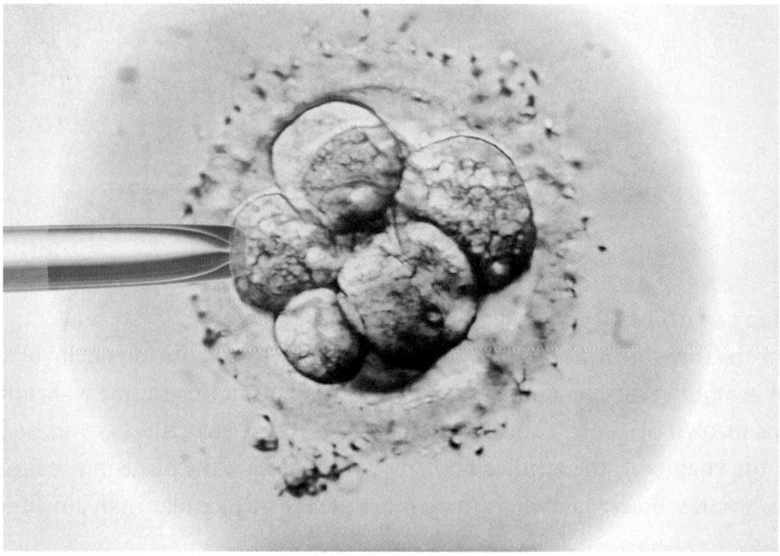

Figure 3.2 Embryo

Blastulation

Several divisions later, the embryo becomes a solid mass of cells known as a **morula**, as shown in Figure 3.3. This term comes from the Latin word for mulberry, which might help us grasp what an embryo at this stage looks like.

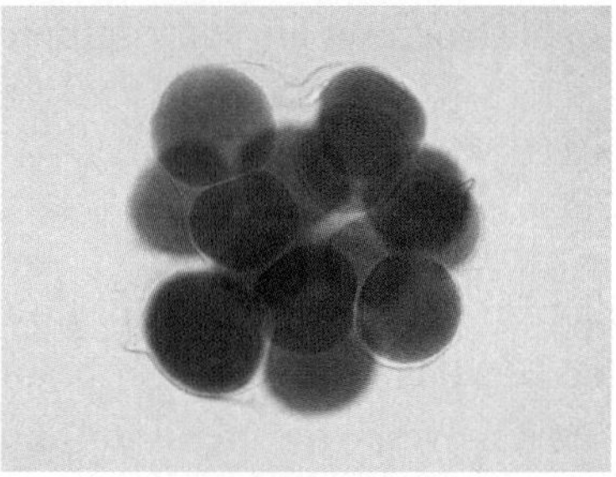

Figure 3.3 Morula
The morula is a solid ball of cells.

Once the morula is formed, it undergoes **blastulation**, which forms the **blastula**, a hollow ball of cells with a fluid-filled inner cavity known as a **blastocoel**. The mammalian blastula is known as a **blastocyst** and consists of two noteworthy cell groups, the trophoblast and inner cell mass (as shown in Figure 3.4). The **trophoblast cells** surround the blastocoel and give rise to the chorion and later the placenta, whereas the **inner cell mass** protrudes into the blastocoel and gives rise to the organism itself.

MNEMONIC

Remember that a **blast**ula is an embryo with a **blast**ed-out cavity.

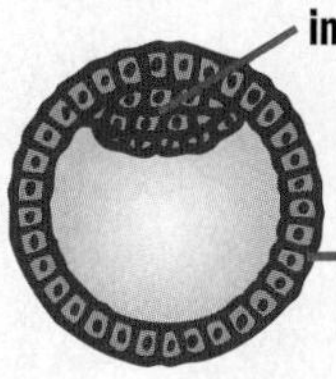

Figure 3.4 Blastula
The blastula contains a fluid-filled cavity called the blastocoel.

Implantation

The blastula moves through the fallopian tube to the uterus, where it burrows into the endometrium. The trophoblast cells are specialized to create an interface between the maternal blood supply and the developing embryo. These trophoblastic cells give rise to the **chorion**, an extraembryonic membrane that develops into the placenta. The trophoblasts form **chorionic villi**, which are microscopic finger-like projections that penetrate the endometrium. As these chorionic villi develop into the placenta they support maternal–fetal gas exchange. The embryo is connected to the placenta by the **umbilical cord**, which consists of two arteries and one vein encased in a gelatinous substance. The vein carries freshly oxygenated blood rich with nutrients from the placenta to the embryo. The umbilical arteries carry deoxygenated blood and waste to the placenta for exchange.

Until the placenta is functional, the embryo is supported by the **yolk sac**, which is also the site of early blood cell development. There are two other extraembryonic membranes that require discussion: the allantois and the amnion. The **allantois** is involved in early fluid exchange between the embryo and the yolk sac. Ultimately, the umbilical cord is formed from remnants of the yolk sac and the allantois. The allantois is surrounded by the **amnion**, a thin, tough membrane filled with amniotic fluid. This fluid serves as a shock absorber during pregnancy, lessening the impact of maternal motion on the developing embryo. In addition to forming the placenta, the chorion also forms an outer membrane around the amnion, adding an additional level of protection. The anatomy of these structures is shown in Figure 3.5.

REAL WORLD

Sometimes the blastula implants itself outside the uterus, a situation known as an ectopic pregnancy. Over 95% of ectopic pregnancies occur in the fallopian tube. Ectopic pregnancies are generally not viable because the narrow fallopian tube is not an environment in which an embryo can properly grow. If the embryo does not spontaneously abort, the tube may rupture and a considerable amount of hemorrhaging may result. In fact, a suspected ectopic pregnancy is often a surgical emergency.

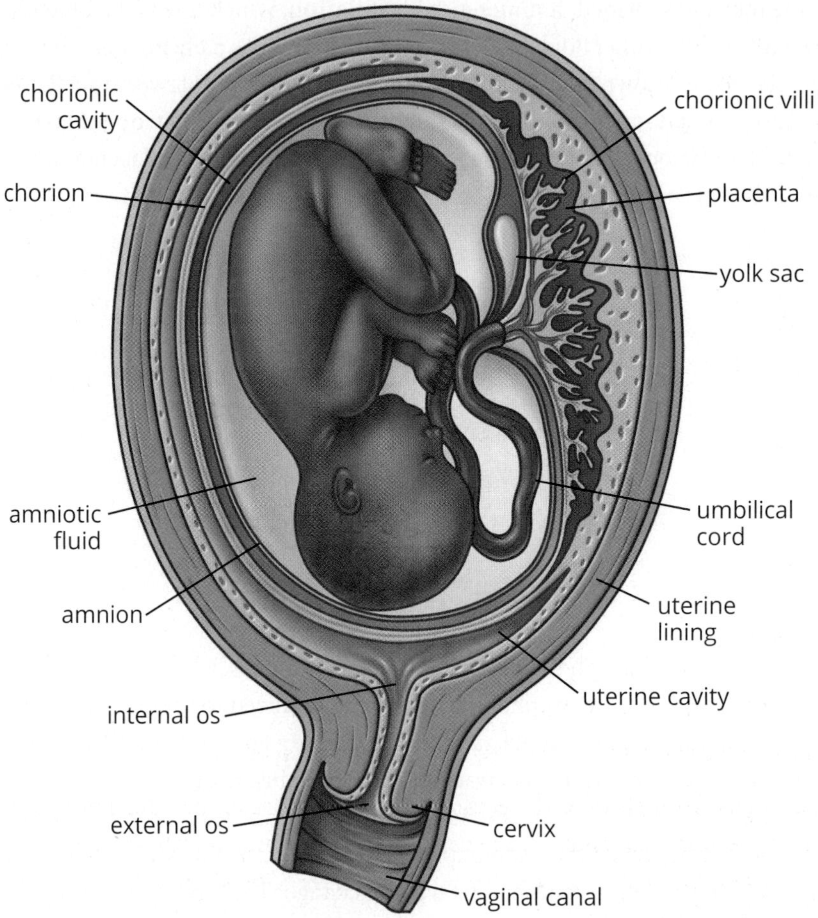

Figure 3.5 Anatomy of Pregnancy

REAL WORLD

Amniocentesis is the process of aspirating amniotic fluid by inserting a thin needle into the amniotic sac. The amniotic fluid contains fetal cells that can be examined for chromosomal abnormalities as well as sex determination. Amniocentesis is recommended for people who are over 35 and pregnant if earlier screening tests (blood tests and ultrasound) indicate a high chance of chromosomal abnormalities in the fetus. Individuals in this age group have a higher rate of meiotic nondisjunction, which can result in genetic deviations such as Down syndrome.

Gastrulation

Once the cell mass implants it can begin further developmental processes such as **gastrulation**, the generation of three distinct cell layers. The early developmental processes up to this point are shown in Figure 3.6. Much of today's understanding of development comes from the study of other organisms with varying degrees of similarity to human development. In sea urchins, gastrulation begins with a small invagination in the blastula. Cells continue moving toward the invagination, resulting in elimination of the blastocoel. To visualize this, imagine inflating a balloon and poking it with your finger. If you kept pushing, eventually the rubber from that side of the balloon would come into contact with the other side. If the two membranes could merge, as occurs in development, this would create a tube through the middle of the balloon. In living things, the result of this process is called a **gastrula**. The membrane invagination into the blastocoel is called the **archenteron**, which later develops into the gut. The opening of the archenteron is called the **blastopore**. In **deuterostomes**, such as humans, the blastopore develops into the anus. In **protostomes**, it develops into the mouth.

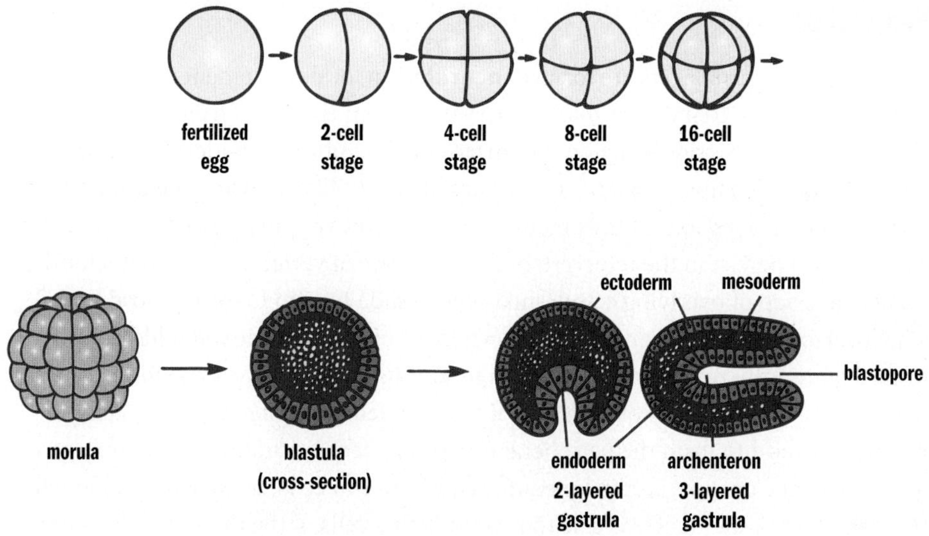

Figure 3.6 Early Stages of Embryonic Development

MNEMONIC

How can we remember the blastopore's fate in protostomes *vs.* deuterostomes? Think about how some adults talk to toddlers—*deuterostome* starts with *deu*, which looks like *duo*, meaning *two*. Thus, **deu**terostomes develop the anus—the orifice associated with "**number two**"—from the blastopore. Protostomes must start at the other end (the mouth).

Primary Germ Layers

Eventually, some cells will also migrate into what remains of the blastocoel. This establishes three layers of cells called **primary germ layers**.

The outermost layer is called the **ectoderm** and gives rise to the integument, including the epidermis, hair, nails, and the epithelia of the nose, mouth, and lower anal canal. The lens of the eye, nervous system (including adrenal medulla), and inner ear are also derived from ectoderm.

The middle layer is called the **mesoderm** and develops into several different systems including the musculoskeletal, circulatory, and most of the excretory systems. Mesoderm also gives rise to the gonads as well as the muscular and connective tissue layers of the digestive and respiratory systems and the adrenal cortex.

The innermost layer is called the **endoderm** and forms the epithelial linings of the digestive and respiratory tracts, including the lungs. The pancreas, thyroid, bladder, and distal urinary tracts, as well as parts of the liver, are derived from endoderm.

MNEMONIC

The primary germ layers:

- Ectoderm—"attracto"derm (things that attract us to others, such as cosmetic features and "smarts")
- Mesoderm—"means"oderm (the means of getting around as an organism, such as bones and muscle; the means of getting around in the body, such as the circulatory system; the means of *getting around*, such as the gonads)
- Endoderm—linings of "endernal" (internal) organs (the digestive and respiratory tract, and accessory organs attached to these systems)

Differentiation

So how is it that cells with the same genes are able to develop into such distinctly different cell types with highly specialized functions? Primarily, it is by **selective transcription** of the genome. In other words, only the genes needed for that particular cell type are transcribed. Thus, in pancreatic islet cells the genes to produce specific hormones (insulin, glucagon, or somatostatin) are turned on, while these same genes are turned off in other cell types. Selective transcription is often related to the concept of **induction**, which is the ability of one group of cells to influence the fate of nearby cells. This process is mediated by chemical substances called **inducers** which diffuse from the **organizing cells** to the **responsive cells**. These chemicals are responsible for processes such as the guidance of neuronal axons. Induction also ensures the proximity of different cell types that work together within an organ.

MCAT EXPERTISE

The MCAT likes to test on the dual embryonic origin of the adrenal glands. The adrenal cortex is derived from the mesoderm, but the adrenal medulla is derived from the ectoderm (because the adrenal medulla contains some nervous tissue).

Neurulation

Once the three germ layers are formed, **neurulation**, or development of the nervous system, can begin. Remember that the nervous system is derived from the ectoderm. How, then, do cells originating on the surface of the embryo (ectoderm) end up inside the final organism? First, a rod of mesodermal cells known as the **notochord** forms along the long axis of the organism like a primitive spine (in fact, remnants of notochord persist in the intervertebral discs between vertebrae). The notochord induces a group of overlying ectodermal cells to slide inward to form **neural folds**, which surround a **neural groove**, as shown in Figure 3.7. The neural folds grow toward one another until they fuse into a **neural tube**, which gives rise to the central nervous system. At the tip of each neural fold are **neural crest cells**. These cells migrate outward to form the peripheral nervous system (including the sensory ganglia, autonomic ganglia, adrenal medulla, and Schwann cells) as well as specific cell types in other tissues (such as calcitonin-producing cells of the thyroid, melanocytes in the skin, and others). Finally, ectodermal cells will migrate over the neural tube and crest to cover the rudimentary nervous system.

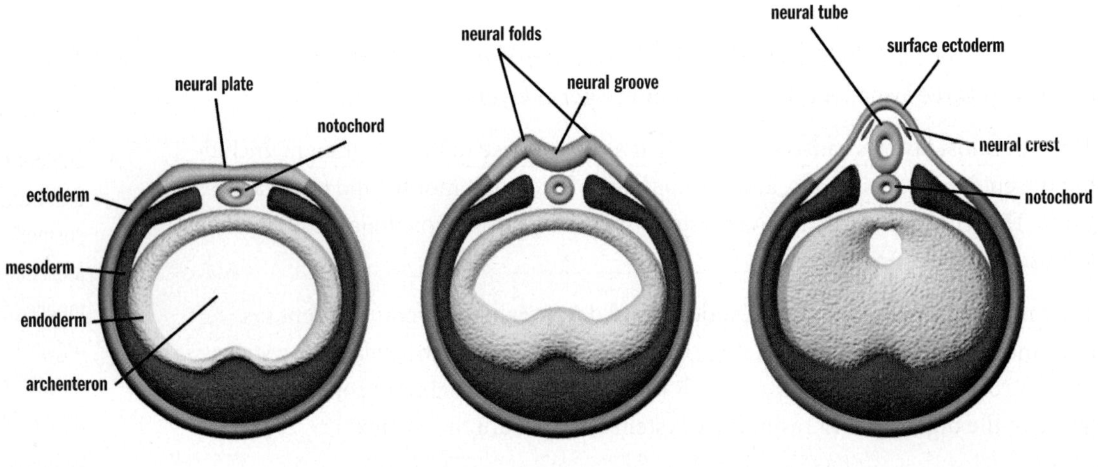

Figure 3.7 Formation of the Neural Tube

REAL WORLD

Failure of the neural tube to close results in either spina bifida (in which some or all of the spinal cord may be exposed to the outside world) or anencephaly (in which the brain fails to develop and the skull is left open). The severity of spina bifida's effects range from no significant distress to death, whereas anencephaly is universally fatal. Individuals who are likely to get pregnant are encouraged to take folate (folic acid) to prevent this complication; furthermore, it is recommended that all individuals who could become pregnant supplement their diets with folate because neurulation often occurs before pregnancy is detected.

Problems in Early Development

Early development is a highly sensitive time. During this stage, as the germ layers are forming and as organogenesis (the production of organs) begins, teratogens may have far-reaching and highly detrimental effects. **Teratogens** are substances that interfere with development, causing defects or even death of the developing embryo. However, each teratogen will not have the same effect on every embryo. It is believed that the unique genetics of the embryo influences the effects of the teratogen. In addition to genetics, the route of exposure, length of exposure, rate of placental transmission of the teratogen, and the exact identity of the teratogen will also affect the outcome. Some common teratogens include alcohol, prescription drugs, viruses, bacteria, and environmental chemicals including polycyclic aromatic hydrocarbons.

In addition to teratogens, maternal health can also influence development. Certain conditions may cause changes in the overall physiology of the person who is pregnant, resulting in overexposure or underexposure of the embryo or fetus to certain chemicals.

For example, pregnant individuals who have diabetes and hyperglycemia (high blood glucose) can have poor birth outcomes. Overexposure to sugar *in utero* can lead to a fetus that is too large to be delivered and that could become hypoglycemic soon after birth (due to synthesizing very high levels of insulin to compensate). Maternal folic acid deficiency may prevent complete closure of the neural tube, resulting in spina bifida, in which parts of the nervous system are exposed to the outside world or covered with a thin membrane, or anencephaly, in which the brain fails to develop. However, like teratogens, maternal health issues can have variable effects on the developing embryo or fetus. Spina bifida may be so severe as to result in profound disability, or may be completely asymptomatic and only detected by a tuft of hair overlying the area. Overall, trends and associations can certainly be found between various environmental conditions and genes during development; however, outcomes are somewhat unpredictable and highly variable.

MCAT CONCEPT CHECK 3.1

Before you move on, assess your understanding of the material with these questions.

1. What is the difference between determinate and indeterminate cleavage?
   - Determinate cleavage:

   ____

   - Indeterminate cleavage:

   ____

2. From zygote to gastrula, what are the various stages of development?

   ____

3. During which stage of development does implantation occur?

   ____

4. What are the primary germ layers, and what organs are formed from each?

Germ Layer	Organs

5. What is induction and how does it influence development?

   ____

6. What tissues do neural crest cells develop into?

   ____

3.2 Mechanisms of Development

High-Yield

LEARNING OBJECTIVES

After Chapter 3.2, you will be able to:

- Explain the difference between determination and differentiation
- Connect totipotency, pluripotency, and multipotency to their respective levels of differentiation
- Recall the four types of cell–cell communication
- Distinguish between apoptosis and necrosis

As described earlier, cells undergo determinate cleavage to commit to a particular cell line, and inducers can be used for communication between one group of differentiating cells and another. In this section, we take a more specific look at the biochemical properties of these developmental mechanisms, as well as a few others.

Cell Specialization

An adult human being is composed of approximately 37 trillion cells. These cells are organized into tissues that form organs within organ systems. In order to create an organism as complex as a human being, each cell must perform a specialized function. In addition, the cells in an organ must be organized such that the organ can function properly. For example, the pancreas must create both digestive enzymes (*trypsin*, *carboxypeptidases A* and *B*, *pancreatic lipase*, and others) and endocrine hormones (*insulin*, *glucagon*, and *somatostatin*). The cells that synthesize digestive enzymes must be located where cell products can enter ducts to ultimately empty into the duodenum. Likewise, the cells that synthesize endocrine hormones must be located near a blood vessel to put their products into systemic circulation. In order to accomplish this the cell must go through three stages: specification, determination, and differentiation.

Specification/Determination

The initial stage of cell specialization is **specification**, in which the cell is reversibly designated as a specific cell type. This is followed by **determination**, which was previously defined as the commitment of a cell to a particular function in the future. Prior to determination the cell can become any cell type, even if it has already gone through specification. After determination the cell is irreversibly committed to a specific lineage. There are multiple pathways by which determination may occur. During cleavage, where the existing mRNA and protein in the parent cell has been asymmetrically distributed between the daughter cells, the presence of specific mRNA and protein molecules may result in determination. Determination may also occur due to secretion of specific molecules from nearby cells. These molecules, also called **morphogens**, may cause neighboring cells to follow a particular developmental pathway. Determination is a commitment to a particular cell type, but note that the cell has not yet actually produced what it needs to carry out the functions of that cell type—that is the goal of differentiation.

Differentiation

After a cell's fate has been determined, the cell must begin to undertake changes that cause the cell to develop into the determined cell type. This includes changing the structure, function, and biochemistry of the cell to match the cell type, a process called **differentiation**.

Cells that have not yet differentiated or that give rise to *other* cells that will differentiate are known as **stem cells**. Stem cells exist in embryonic tissues as well as adult tissues. The tissues a particular stem cell can differentiate into are determined by its **potency**. Cells with the greatest potency are called **totipotent** and include embryonic stem cells; totipotent cells can differentiate into any cell type, either in the fetus or in placental structures. After the 16-cell stage, the cells of the morula begin to differentiate into two groups: the inner cell mass and the trophoblast. After a few more cycles of cell division these totipotent cells start to differentiate into the three germ cell layers. At this stage, the cells are said to be **pluripotent**; these cells can differentiate into any cell type except for those found in the placental structures. Finally, as the cells continue to become more specialized they are said to be **multipotent** stem cells, which can differentiate into multiple types of cells within a particular group. For example, hematopoietic stem cells are capable of differentiating into all of the cells found in blood, including the various types of white blood cells, red blood cells, and platelets—but not into skin cells, neurons, or muscle cells. While we use all of these different terms to describe potency, it is important to recognize that potency is a spectrum—not a series of strict definitions. Also, note that stem cells exist not only in embryos, but also in adults, who have stem cells that give rise to skin, blood, and the epithelial lining of the digestive tract, among others.

Over the last few decades, stem cell research has been a hotly contested issue. While harvesting of embryonic stem cells, as seen in Figure 3.8, ultimately results in termination of the embryo, it is thought that these cells could be used to regenerate human tissues, including the spinal cord (following injury) and the heart (following a heart attack). There are also immunologic concerns, as transplantation of stem cells of a different genetic makeup could evoke an immune response, resulting in rejection. In addition, once implanted, pluripotent cells may not necessarily differentiate into the desired tissue and may even become cancerous.

KEY CONCEPT

When a cell is determined, it is committed to a particular cell lineage. When the cell differentiates, it assumes the structure, function, and biochemistry of that cell type.

KEY CONCEPT

Stem cells are able to differentiate into different cell types. The potency of the stem cell determines how many different cell types a stem cell can become. As cells become more differentiated, the potency of the cell decreases (from totipotent to pluripotent to multipotent).

BRIDGE

Stem cells are a cornerstone of biotechnology. Gene studies can be performed by introducing altered embryonic stem cells that contain transgenes into mice. Stem cells lacking a particular gene can be used to create knockout mice. These processes are discussed in Chapter 6 of *MCAT Biochemistry Review*.

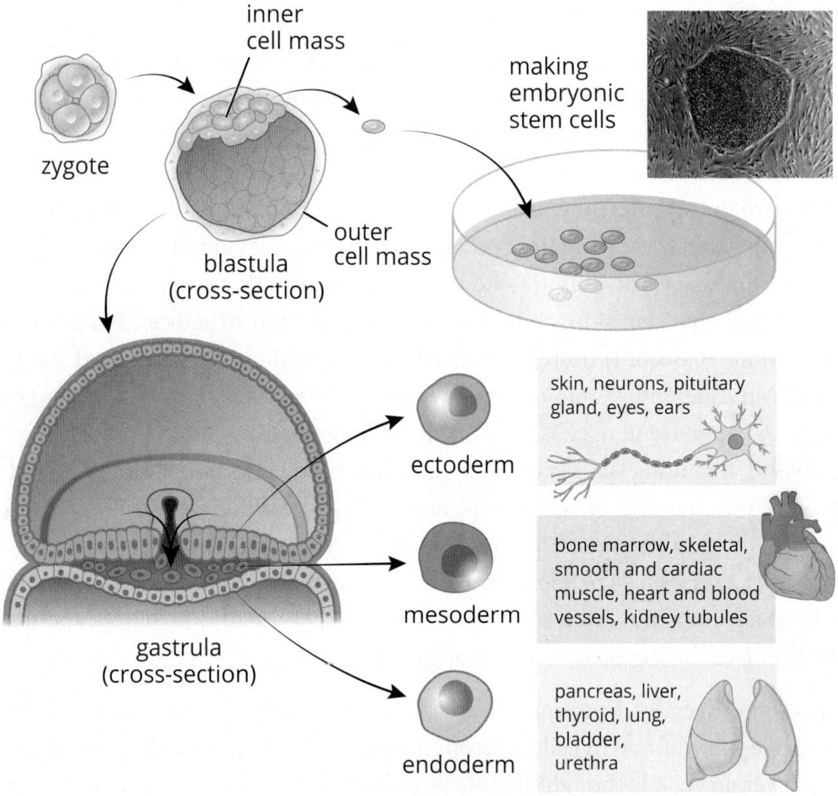

Figure 3.8 Embryonic Stem Cells

In order to address this controversy, many researchers have begun investigating adult stem cells. At best, these cells are multipotent, able to differentiate into only a few different cell types. Researchers may take adult stem cells and use various transcription factors to increase potency in these cells. One of the potential advantages of this approach is that a stem cell can be taken from a patient (usually from blood, bone marrow, or adipose tissue), induced to become a different tissue type, and then implanted into that same patient. This offers reduced risk of rejection of foreign tissue. However, it is challenging to induce differentiation into the correct cell type, and most organs have a complex structure that depends on a number of different cell types, each of which requires different signals. Research is ongoing and holds promise, despite limited success.

BIOLOGY GUIDED EXAMPLE WITH EXPERT THINKING

The role of microRNA-29b in controlling the differentiation of neuroectoderm cells into neural tube epithelial cells (NTE) and neural crest cells (NCC) remains unclear. To study the impact of microRNA-29b, researchers engineered microRNA sponges to contain multiple tandem binding sites for the target microRNA to competitively bind with microRNA-29b. In addition to the sponge, researchers also engineered microRNA-29b-overexpressed cells by inserting a microRNA-29b sequence into the embryonic stem cell genome. Both are driven by a CAG promoter and inserted into the ROSA26 site.

Study goal: clarify the role of microRNA-29b

It sounds like these sponges will "pick up" the microRNA-29b that is present

They made cells that overexpress microRNA-29b

The terms "CAG" and "ROSA26" are unfamiliar, but both have the same promoter and insertion site

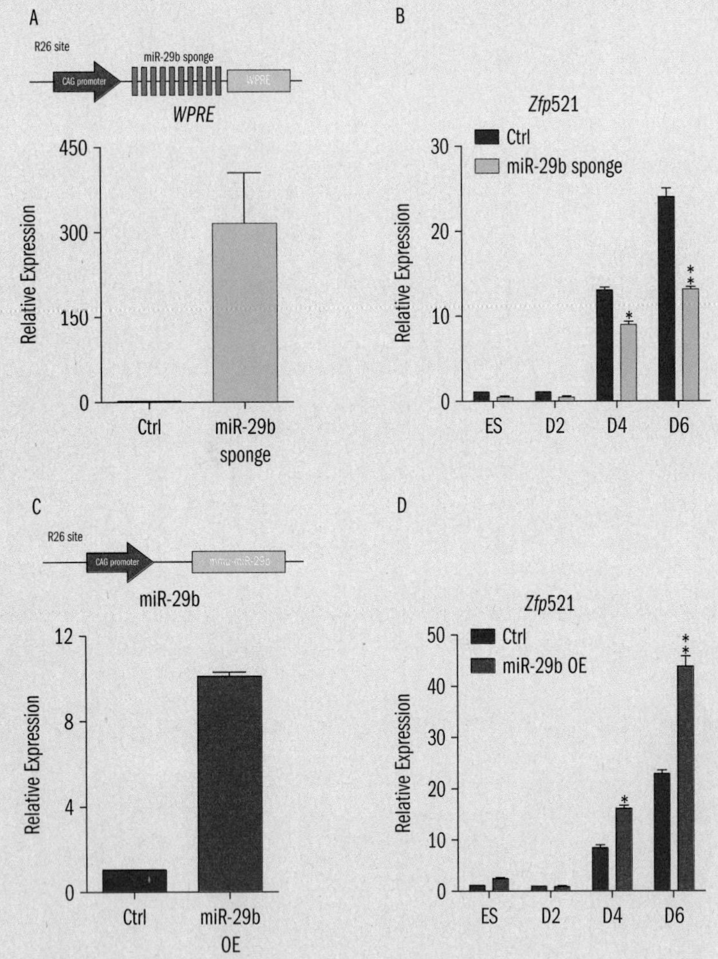

IVs: condition (control, sponge, overexpression)

DV: relative expression

Trends: (B) shows sponge is much lower than control, (D) shows OE is much higher than control

Figure 1 Neural tube epithelial cells differentiation experiment results. (A) The expression level of microRNA-29b sponge verified by qPCR. (B) qPCR results of NTE marker genes Zfp521 expression levels in microRNA-29b sponge condition. (C) The expression level of microRNA-29b verified by qPCR. (D) qPCR results of NTE marker genes Zfp521 in microRNA-29b overexpression condition.

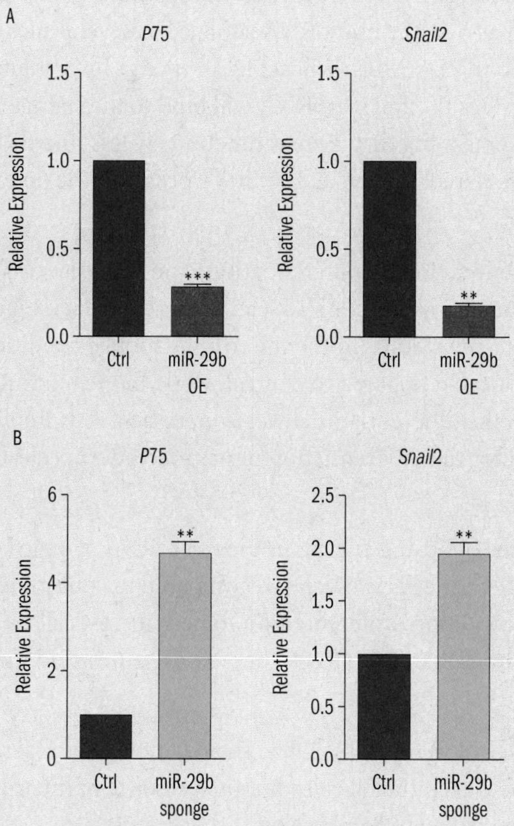

IVs: condition (control, sponge, OE)

DV: relative expression

Trends: (A) shows OE is much lower than control; (B) shows sponge is much higher than control

Figure 2 Neural crest cells differentiation experiment results. (A) qPCR results of NCC markers P75 and Snail2 expression in microRNA-29b overexpression condition. (B) qPCR results of NCC markers P75 and Snail3 expression in microRNA-29b sponge condition.

Adapted from Xi, J., Wu, Y., Li, G., Ma, L., Feng, K., Guo, X., ... Kang, J. (2017). Mir-29b mediates the neural tube versus neural crest fate decision during embryonic stem cell neural differentiation. *Stem Cell Reports*, 9(2), 571–586.

How does microRNA-29b influence the differentiation of neuroectoderm cells into neural epithelial cells and neural crest cells, respectively?

This question asks us to draw conclusions based on the data provided. To start, we'll want to define the terms in the question stem and make sure we're clear on exactly what we're being asked for. We are told in the first paragraph that the neuroectoderm cells will differentiate into two types of cells, the neural epithelial cells and the neural crest cells. We are also told that microRNA-29b influences this process, but we do not know how it impacts differentiation.

Now we must parse out how the target microRNA are being manipulated to see how those changes alter the neuroectoderm cells' differentiation. The researchers created two experimental conditions, the microRNA sponge and the microRNA overexpression. Recall that microRNA works by binding to complementary sites on mRNA, which blocks translation mechanisms and prevents the synthesis of the gene product. As stated in the passage, the microRNA sponge has several sites that are complementary to the microRNA, which will act like a sponge by grabbing all the microRNA in the cell. As a result, the microRNA will bind to the sponge instead of just binding to local RNA, meaning that there is functionally less microRNA-29b binding to the RNA as compared to normal. In other words, it is the opposite of the overexpressed condition.

Now that we know what our action is (differentiation) and what the two conditions are (overexpression and inhibition), we can analyze the data. Figure 1 shows the neural epithelial cell results. In the microRNA sponge condition, the differentiation level is reduced compared to control, while in the microRNA overexpression condition the differentiation level is increased. This implies that microRNA-29b is critical for the differentiation of neuroectoderm cells to neural epithelial cells.

Looking at Figure 2, we see opposing effects. In the microRNA sponge condition, differentiation into neural crest cells is increased compared to control. In the microRNA overexpression condition, differentiation to neural crest cells is reduced. From these data, we can infer that microRNA suppresses neuroectoderm cell differentiation to neural crest cells.

In conclusion, the presence of microRNA-29b is important for neuroectoderm cell differentiation into neural epithelial cells, but the presence of microRNA-29b suppresses differentiation into neural crest cells.

Cell–Cell Communication

The determination and differentiation of a cell depends on the location of the cell as well as the identity of the surrounding cells. The developing cell receives signals from organizing cells around it and may also secrete its own signaling molecules. As discussed previously, surrounding tissues induce a developing cell to become a particular cell type via inducers; the term *inducer* may also refer to the cell secreting the signal. The cell that is induced is called a **responder** (responsive cell); to be induced, a responder must be **competent**, or able to respond to the inducing signal.

Cell–cell communication can occur via autocrine, paracrine, juxtacrine, or endocrine signals. **Autocrine** signals act on the same cell that secreted the signal in the first place. **Paracrine** signals act on cells in the local area. **Juxtacrine** signals do not usually involve diffusion, but involve a cell directly stimulating receptors of an adjacent cell. Finally, **endocrine** signals involve secreted hormones that travel through the bloodstream to a distant target tissue.

Inducers

Inducers are often **growth factors**, which are peptides that promote differentiation and mitosis in certain tissues. Most growth factors only function on specific cell types or in certain areas, as determined by the competence of these cells. In this way, certain growth factors can code for particular tissues. For example, *PAX6* is expressed in the ectoderm of the head, but in no other location. Therefore, as the optic vesicle approaches the overlying ectoderm producing this factor, development of the lens of the eye is induced. Interestingly, induction is not always a one-way pathway. To that end, differentiation of the lens then triggers the optic vesicle to form the optic cup, which ultimately becomes the retina. This is known as **reciprocal development**. Most tissues will be exposed to multiple inducers during the course of development.

One of the main methods of signaling occurs via the use of gradients. Morphogens, or molecules that cause determination of cells, diffuse throughout the organism. Locations closer to the origin of the morphogen will be exposed to higher concentrations, while areas further away will have less exposure. Multiple morphogens are secreted simultaneously, resulting in unique combinations of morphogen exposure throughout the organism, which can thereby induce the differentiation of specific cell types. Some common morphogens include transforming growth factor beta (TGF-β), sonic hedgehog (Shh), and epidermal growth factor (EGF).

REAL WORLD

In development of the eyes, lateral outpocketings from the brain (optic vesicles) grow out and touch the overlying ectoderm. The optic vesicle induces the ectoderm to form the lens placode. The lens placode in turn induces the optic vesicle to create the optic cup. The optic cup then induces the lens placode to develop into the cornea and lens. Experiments with frog embryos show that if this ectoderm is subsequently transplanted to the trunk (after the optic vesicles have grown out), a lens will develop in the trunk. If, however, the ectoderm is transplanted before the outgrowth of the optic vesicles, it will not.

Cell Migration, Cell Death, and Regeneration

Induction and differentiation lead to the creation of different types of cells; however, these cells are not always in the right location to carry out their function. Further, the sculpting of various anatomic structures requires not only differentiation, but also the death of some cells. Certain organs also have the ability to recreate injured or surgically removed portions of tissue.

Cell Migration

Cells must be able to disconnect from adjacent structures and migrate to their correct location. For example, the anterior pituitary gland originates from a segment of oral ectoderm and must migrate from the top of the mouth to its final location just below the hypothalamus. Neural crest cells also undergo extensive migration. These cells form at the edge of the neural folds during neurulation and then migrate throughout the body to form many different structures including the sensory ganglia, autonomic ganglia, adrenal medulla, and Schwann cells, as well as specific cell types in other tissues such as calcitonin-producing cells of the thyroid, melanocytes in the skin, and others.

Cell Death

Apoptosis, or programmed cell death, occurs at various times in development. For example, the fingers are originally webbed during development of the hand. The cells of the webbing later undergo apoptosis, resulting in separation of each individual finger and toe. Apoptosis may occur via apoptotic signals or preprogramming.

During the process of apoptosis the cell undergoes changes in morphology and divides into many self-contained protrusions called **apoptotic blebs**, which can then be broken apart into **apoptotic bodies** and digested by other cells, as shown in Figure 3.9. This allows recycling of materials. Because the blebs are contained by a membrane, this also prevents the release of potentially harmful substances into the extracellular environment. This is different from **necrosis**, which is a process of cell death in which a cell dies as a result of injury. In necrosis, internal substances can be leaked, causing irritation of nearby tissues or even an immune response.

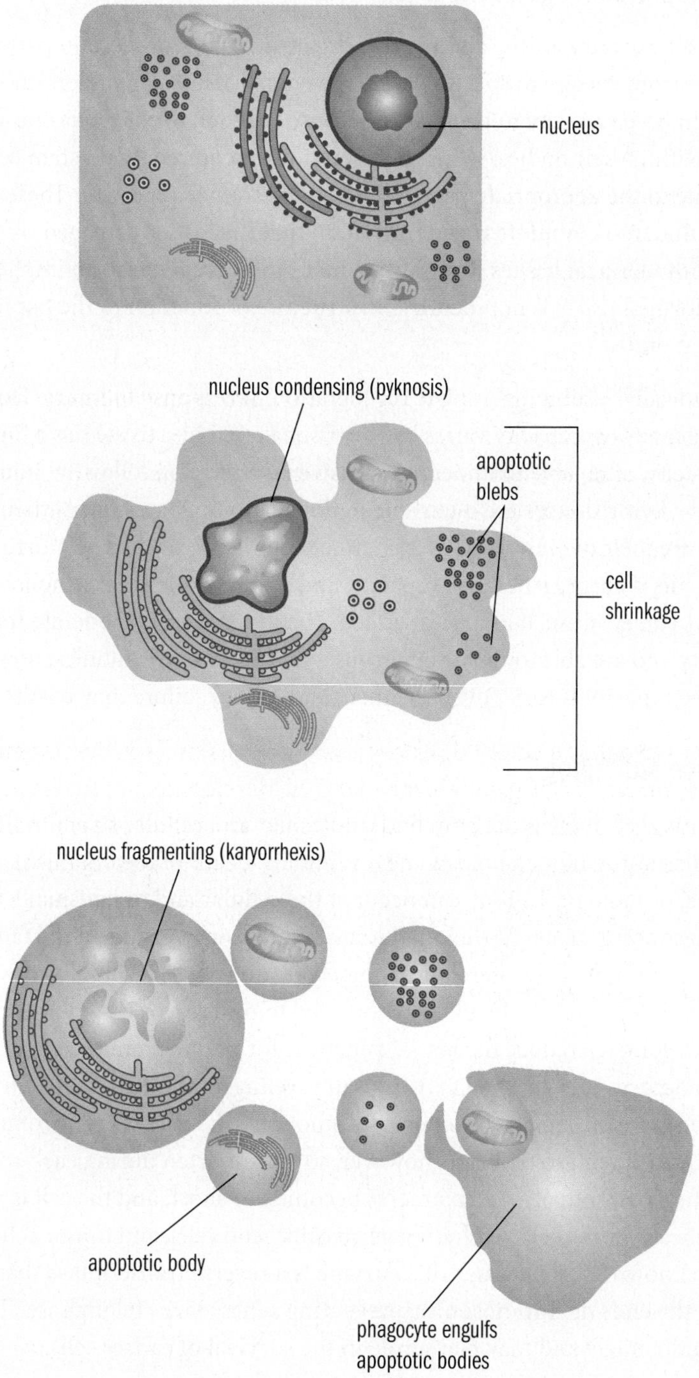

Figure 3.9 Apoptosis
An apoptotic cell disintegrates so that it can be absorbed and digested by other cells.

Regeneration

Regenerative capacity, or the ability of an organism to regrow certain parts of the body, varies from species to species. Some species, such as salamanders and newts, have an enhanced capacity to regenerate because they retain extensive clusters of stem cells within their bodies. When regeneration is required, these stem cells can then migrate to the appropriate part of the body to initiate regrowth. These species are said to undergo **complete regeneration**, in that the lost or damaged tissues are replaced with identical tissues. In contrast, **incomplete regeneration** implies that the newly formed tissue is not identical in structure or function to the tissue that has been injured or lost.

Humans typically exhibit incomplete regeneration in response to injury. However, in humans regenerative capacity varies by the tissue type. Liver tissue has a high regenerative capacity, often able to undergo extensive regeneration following injury or loss. For example, living donors are often able to donate up to 50 percent of their liver tissue because their own livers will regenerate the missing portion. Unfortunately, the heart has little, if any, regenerative capacity, and scarring often results following an injury due to an event such as a heart attack. The kidneys have moderate regenerative capacity and are able to repair nephrons after injury to the tubules; however this regenerative capacity is easily overwhelmed, and kidney failure may result.

Senescence and Aging

As organisms age, changes occur in both molecular and cellular structure. This results in disruption of metabolism and, eventually, death of the organism. **Senescence**, or biological aging, can occur at the cellular and organismal level as these changes accumulate. At the cellular level, senescence results in the failure of cells to divide, normally after approximately 50 divisions *in vitro*. Research has demonstrated that this may be due to shortened **telomeres**, or the ends of chromosomes. Telomeres reduce the loss of genetic information from the ends of chromosomes and help prevent the DNA from unraveling—their high concentration of guanine and cytosine enables telomeres to "knot off" the end of the chromosome. Telomeres are difficult to replicate, however, so they shorten during each round of DNA synthesis. Eventually, the telomeres become too short, and the cell is no longer able to replicate. Some cells, including germ cells, fetal cells, and tumor cells, express an enzyme known as *telomerase*. This enzyme is a reverse transcriptase that is able to synthesize the ends of chromosomes, preventing senescence. Telomerase allows cells to divide indefinitely and may play a role in the survival of cancer cells.

At the organismal level, senescence represents changes in the body's ability to respond to a changing environment. Aging is complex and often involves not only cellular senescence but also the accumulation of chemical and environmental damage over time.

MCAT CONCEPT CHECK 3.2

Before you move on, assess your understanding of the material with these questions.

1. What is the difference between determination and differentiation?
   - Determination:

   ____

   - Differentiation:

   ____

2. What are the three types of potency? What lineages can a cell of each type differentiate into?

Type of Potency	Cell Lineages

3. What are the four types of cell–cell communication?
   -
   ____
   -
   ____
   -
   ____
   -
   ____

4. What is the difference between apoptosis and necrosis?
   - Apoptosis:

   ____

   - Necrosis:

   ____

3.3 Fetal Circulation

LEARNING OBJECTIVES

After Chapter 3.3, you will be able to:

- Recall the oxygenation status of blood in umbilical arteries and umbilical veins
- Identify the three fetal shunts, their locations, and the organs they bypass

Recall that the placenta, shown in Figure 3.10, is the organ where nutrient, gas, and waste exchange occurs. It is crucial that maternal and fetal blood do not mix because they may be different blood types. The simplest method to move nutrients and waste products is by diffusion, the preferred method for water, glucose, amino acids, and inorganic salts. Diffusion requires a gradient, which implies there is a higher partial pressure of oxygen in maternal blood than in fetal blood. To further enhance the transfer of oxygen from maternal to fetal circulation, fetal blood cells contain **fetal hemoglobin** (**HbF**), which has a greater affinity for oxygen than adult hemoglobin (primarily HbA). This also assists with the transfer (and retention) of oxygen into the fetal circulatory system. Waste material and carbon dioxide move in the opposite direction.

KEY CONCEPT

Although the embryo obtains its nutrients and oxygen from the person who is pregnant, there is no actual mixing of the blood. Instead, the placenta depends on the close proximity of the embryonic and maternal bloodstreams, facilitating diffusion between them.

KEY CONCEPT

Remember, gas exchange in the fetus occurs across the placenta. Fetal lungs do not function until birth.

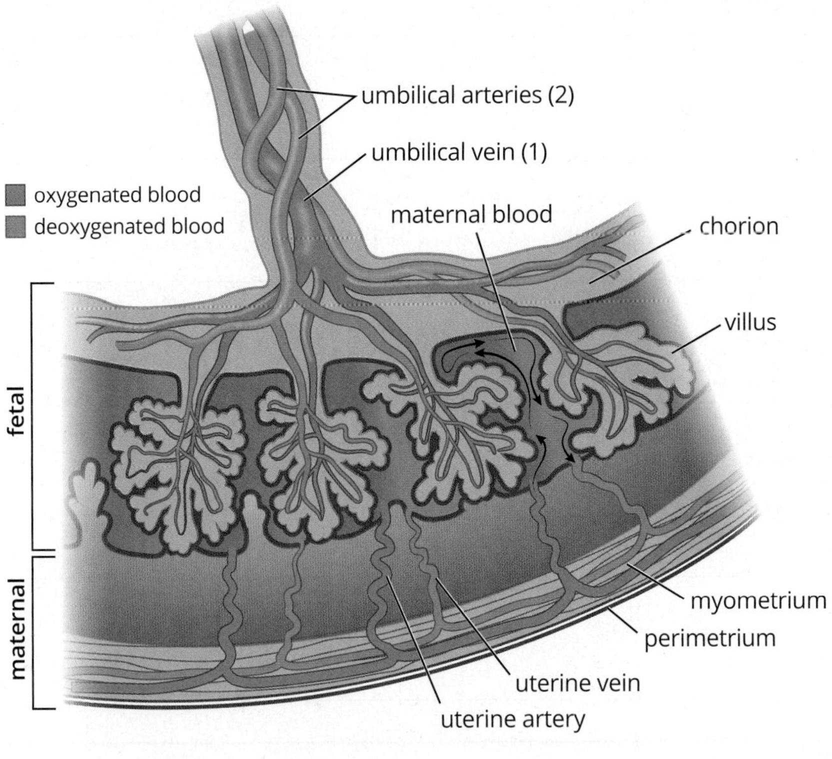

Figure 3.10 Placental Structure

The placental barrier also serves another function: immunity. The fetus is immunologically naïve because it has not yet been exposed to any pathogens; however, accidental exposure can happen *in utero*. Thus, the crossing of antibodies across the placental membrane serves a protective function. The placenta also qualifies as an endocrine organ because it produces progesterone, estrogen, and human chorionic gonadotropin (hCG), all which are essential for maintaining pregnancy.

The umbilical vessels are commonly tested on the MCAT because they demonstrate the need to understand the proper biological definitions of artery and vein. Like all other arteries that carry blood away from the heart, the **umbilical arteries** carry blood away from the fetus toward the placenta. And, like all of the other veins that carry blood toward the heart, the **umbilical vein** carries blood toward the fetus from the placenta. Remember that oxygenation occurs at the placenta, rather than in the fetal lungs. Therefore, the umbilical arteries carry deoxygenated blood and the umbilical vein carries oxygenated blood.

There are several key differences between fetal and adult circulation that demonstrate important characteristics of the developing organism. The lungs and liver both do not serve significant functions prior to birth. Gas exchange does not occur at the lungs, but rather at the placenta. Detoxification and metabolism are primarily controlled by the mother's liver, and nutrient and waste exchange occurs at the placenta as well. Thus, the fetus does not depend on its own lungs and liver. Notably, these two organs are both underdeveloped and sensitive to the high blood pressures they will receive in postnatal life; thus, the fetus constructs three **shunts** to actively direct blood away from these organs while they develop, as shown in Figure 3.11.

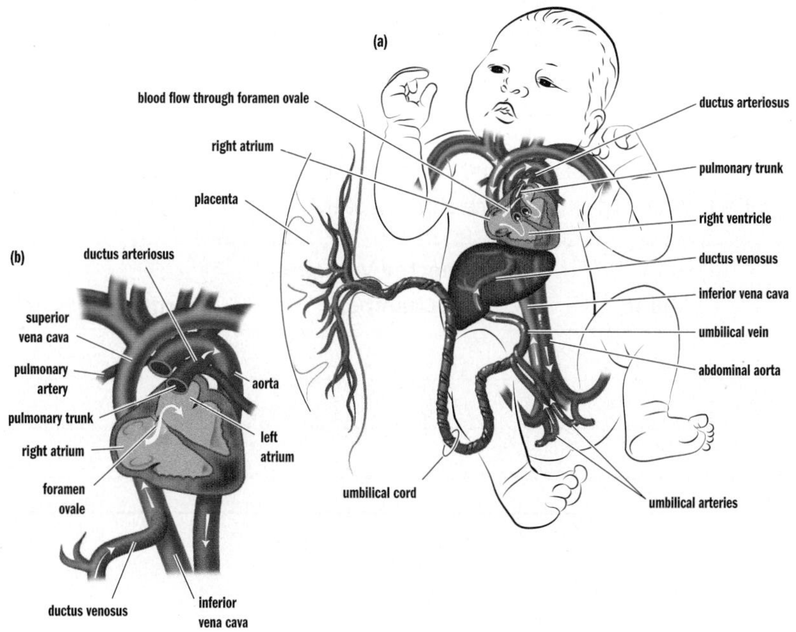

Figure 3.11 Fetal Circulation
(a) Systemic fetal circulation; (b) Enlarged view of fetal circulation highlighting the three fetal shunts

REAL WORLD

Many pathogens are too large to cross the placental barrier by diffusion, but a set of pathogens called TORCHES infections can cross this barrier and cause significant birth defects. Therefore, screening for (and sometimes immunization against) these infections is recommended in pregnancy. TORCHES stands for ***TO****xoplasma gondii*, **R**ubella, **C**ytomegalovirus, **HE**rpes or **H**IV, and **S**yphilis.

KEY CONCEPT

Unlike most other arteries, the umbilical arteries carry deoxygenated blood with waste products. Unlike most other veins, the umbilical vein carries oxygenated blood with nutrients.

Two different shunts are used to reroute blood from the lungs. The first, called the **foramen ovale**, is a one-way valve that connects the right atrium to the left atrium. This allows blood entering the right atrium from the inferior vena cava to flow into the left atrium instead of the right ventricle, and thereby be pumped through the aorta into systemic circulation directly. Unlike in adult circulation, the right side of the heart is at a higher pressure in the developing fetus than the left side, which pushes blood through the opening. After birth, this pressure differential reverses, shutting the foramen ovale. Second, the **ductus arteriosus** shunts leftover blood from the pulmonary artery to the aorta. Again, the pressure differential between the right and left sides of the heart pushes blood through this opening and into systemic circulation.

The liver is bypassed via the **ductus venosus**, which shunts blood returning from the placenta via the umbilical vein directly into the inferior vena cava. The liver still receives some blood supply from smaller hepatic arteries in the systemic circulation.

MCAT CONCEPT CHECK 3.3

Before you move on, assess your understanding of the material with these questions.

1. What is the oxygenation status of the blood in the umbilical arteries? In the umbilical vein?
   - Umbilical arteries:

   ____

   - Umbilical vein:

   ____

2. What are the three fetal shunts? What vessels or heart chambers do they connect? What organ does each shunt bypass?

Shunt	Connected Vessels or Chambers	Organ Bypassed

3.4 Gestation and Birth

LEARNING OBJECTIVES

After Chapter 3.4, you will be able to:

- Identify the major developmental features of each trimester
- Describe the three stages of birth
- Recall key concepts and terms used for the birth process, including parturition, prostaglandins, oxytocin, and afterbirth

Human gestation lasts an estimated 280 days, which are divided into three trimesters. As a general rule, the larger the animal, the longer the gestational period and the fewer the offspring per pregnancy. For example, elephants usually have one calf and gestate for 22 months. In contrast, mice have 10 to 12 offspring per litter and gestate for only 20 days. Although you don't need to know every detail of gestation for the MCAT, there are key developmental events in each trimester with which you should be familiar.

First Trimester

The major organs begin to develop during the first few weeks. The heart begins to beat at approximately 22 days, and soon afterward the eyes, gonads, limbs, and liver start to form. By five weeks the embryo is 10 mm in length, and by week six it has grown to 15 mm. The cartilaginous skeleton begins to harden into bone by the seventh week. By the end of eight weeks most of the organs have formed, the brain is fairly developed, and the embryo becomes known as a **fetus**. At the end of the third month the fetus is about 9 cm long.

Second Trimester

During the second trimester the fetus undergoes a tremendous amount of growth. It begins to move within the amniotic fluid, its face takes on a human appearance, and its toes and fingers elongate. By the end of the sixth month the fetus measures 30 to 36 cm long.

Third Trimester

The seventh and eighth months are characterized by continued rapid growth and further brain development. Antibodies are transported by highly selective active transport from the pregnant individual to the fetus for protection against foreign agents in preparation for life outside the womb; this transfer begins earlier in pregnancy, but is highest in the ninth month just before birth. The growth rate slows and the fetus becomes less active, as it has less room to move about.

REAL WORLD

Advances in medicine have allowed premature babies born as early as 24 weeks to survive—far short of the normal 40 weeks. While these neonates may survive, there are often severe complications because fetal development is not complete at 24 weeks. These problems are most apparent in the respiratory, gastrointestinal, and nervous systems.

Birth

Vaginal childbirth, or **parturition**, is accomplished by rhythmic contractions of uterine smooth muscle, coordinated by **prostaglandins** and the peptide hormone **oxytocin**. Birth consists of three basic phases. First, the cervix thins out and the amniotic sac ruptures, which is commonly called *water breaking*. Next, strong uterine contractions result in the birth of the fetus. Finally, the placenta and umbilical cord are expelled; these are often referred to as the **afterbirth**.

MCAT CONCEPT CHECK 3.4

Before you move on, assess your understanding of the material with these questions.

1. What are some of the key developmental features of each trimester?
    - First trimester:
    - Second trimester:
    - Third trimester:

2. What occurs in each of the three phases of birth?
    -
    -
    -

Conclusion

In this chapter, we have seen how a just-fertilized ovum (zygote) becomes an embryo. As organs develop and the body organizes into complex organ systems, that embryo will turn into a newborn baby. Development certainly does not stop there, however—humans nurture their young for years (sometimes decades!) as they undergo physical, cognitive, and sexual development. Embryonic development is extremely important because it lays the foundation for further development to proceed correctly. Most of the time, the process goes exactly as planned; however, this is not always the case. In medical school, you will study the wide spectrum of teratology—the study of birth defects.

Adult structures that arise from embryonic germ layers are of special importance to us because they are commonly tested on the MCAT. For the remainder of embryology—from the first cleavage event to the last uterine contraction—focus on the main terminology and highlights of each stage, in addition to the differences between fetal and adult physiology. Now that we have seen from where the organ systems derive, we will begin our survey of anatomy and physiology. For the next eight chapters (Chapters 4 to 11 of *MCAT Biology Review*), we will explore the cells, tissues, organs, and interactions of each of the major organ systems. Our discussion begins with the nervous system.

GO ONLINE

You've reviewed the content, now test your knowledge and critical thinking skills by completing a test-like passage set in your online resources!

CONCEPT SUMMARY

Early Developmental Stages

- **Fertilization** is the joining of a sperm and an ovum.
  - It usually occurs in the **ampulla** of the fallopian tube.
  - The sperm uses acrosomal enzymes to penetrate the corona radiata and zona pellucida.
  - Once it contacts the oocyte's plasma membrane, the sperm establishes the **acrosomal apparatus** and injects its pronucleus.
  - When the first sperm penetrates it causes a release of calcium ions, which prevents additional sperm from fertilizing the egg and increases the metabolic rate of the resulting diploid **zygote**. This is called the **cortical reaction**.
- **Fraternal** (**dizygotic**) **twins** result from the fertilization of two eggs by two different sperm. **Identical** (**monozygotic**) **twins** result from the splitting of a zygote in two. Monozygotic twins can be classified by the placental structures they share (mono- *vs.* diamniotic, mono- *vs.* dichorionic).
- **Cleavage** refers to the early divisions of cells in the embryo. These mitotic divisions result in a larger number of smaller cells, as the overall volume does not change.
  - The zygote becomes an embryo after the first cleavage because it is no longer unicellular.
  - **Indeterminate cleavage** results in cells that are capable of becoming any cell in the organism, while **determinate cleavage** results in cells that are committed to differentiating into a specific cell type.
- The **morula** is a solid mass of cells seen in early development.
- The **blastula** (**blastocyst**) has a fluid-filled center called a **blastocoel** and has two different structures: the **trophoblast** (which becomes placental structures) and the **inner cell mass** (which becomes the developing organism).
  - The blastula implants in the endometrial lining and forms the **placenta**.
  - The **chorion** contains **chorionic villi**, which penetrate the endometrium and create the interface between maternal and fetal blood.
  - Before the placenta is established, the embryo is supported by the **yolk sac**.
  - The **allantois** is involved in early fluid exchange between the embryo and the yolk sac.
  - The **amnion** lies just inside the chorion and produces amniotic fluid.
  - The developing organism is connected to the placenta via the **umbilical cord**.

- During **gastrulation**, the **archenteron** is formed with a **blastopore** at the end. As the archenteron grows through the blastocoel it contacts the opposite side, establishing three primary germ layers.
  - The **ectoderm** becomes epidermis, hair, nails, and the epithelia of the nose, mouth, and anal canal, as well as the nervous system (including adrenal medulla) and lens of the eye.
  - The **mesoderm** becomes much of the musculoskeletal, circulatory, and excretory systems. Mesoderm also gives rise to the gonads and the muscular and connective tissue layers of the digestive and respiratory systems, as well as the adrenal cortex.
  - The **endoderm** becomes much of the epithelial linings of the respiratory and digestive tracts and parts of the pancreas, thyroid, bladder, and distal urinary tracts.
- **Neurulation**, or development of the nervous system, begins after the formation of the three germ layers.
  - The **notochord** induces a group of overlying ectodermal cells to form **neural folds** surrounding a **neural groove**.
  - The neural folds fuse to form the **neural tube**, which becomes the central nervous system.
  - The tip of each neural fold contains **neural crest cells**, which become the peripheral nervous system (sensory ganglia, autonomic ganglia, adrenal medulla, and Schwann cells), as well as specific cell types in other tissues (calcitonin-producing cells of the thyroid, melanocytes in the skin, and others).
- Teratogens are substances that interfere with development, causing defects or even death of the developing embryo. Teratogens include alcohol, certain prescription drugs, viruses, bacteria, and environmental chemicals.
- Maternal conditions can affect development, including diabetes (increased fetal size and hypoglycemia after birth) and folic acid deficiency (neural tube defects).

Mechanisms of Development

- Cell specialization occurs as a result of determination and differentiation.
  - **Determination** is the commitment to a specific cell lineage, which may be accomplished by uneven segregation of cellular material during mitosis or with **morphogens**, which promote development down a specific cell line. To respond to a specific morphogen, a cell must have **competency**.
  - **Differentiation** refers to the changes a cell undergoes due to **selective transcription** to take on characteristics appropriate to its cell line.

- Stem cells are cells that are capable of developing into various cell types. They can be classified by potency.
  - **Totipotent cells** are able to differentiate into all cell types, including the three germ layers and placental structures.
  - **Pluripotent cells** are able to differentiate into all three of the germ layers and their derivatives.
  - **Multipotent cells** are able to differentiate only into a specific subset of cell types.
- Cells communicate through a number of different signaling methods. An **inducer** releases factors to promote the differentiation of a competent **responder**.
  - **Autocrine** signals act on the same cell that released the signal.
  - **Paracrine** signals act on local cells.
  - **Juxtacrine** signals act through direct stimulation of adjacent cells.
  - **Endocrine** signals act on distant tissues after traveling through the bloodstream.
  - These are often **growth factors**, which are peptides that promote differentiation and mitosis in certain tissues.
  - If two tissues both induce further differentiation in each other, this is **reciprocal induction**.
  - Signaling often occurs via gradients.
- Cells may need to migrate to arrive at their correct location.
- **Apoptosis** is programmed cell death via the formation of **apoptotic blebs** that can subsequently be absorbed and digested by other cells. Apoptosis can be used for sculpting certain anatomical structures, such as removing the webbing between digits.
- **Regenerative capacity** is the ability of an organism to regrow certain parts of the body. The liver has high regenerative capacity, while the heart has low regenerative capacity.
- **Senescence** is the result of multiple molecular and metabolic processes, most notably, the shortening of telomeres during cell division.

Fetal Circulation

- Nutrient, gas, and waste exchange occurs at the placenta.
- Oxygen and carbon dioxide are passively exchanged due to concentration gradients.
- **Fetal hemoglobin** (**HbF**) has a higher affinity for oxygen than adult hemoglobin (primarily HbA); this affinity assists in the transfer (and retention) of oxygen into the fetal circulatory system.

- The placental barrier also serves as immune protection against many pathogens, and antibodies are transferred from the pregnant individual to child.
- The placenta serves endocrine functions, secreting estrogen, progesterone, and human chorionic gonadotropin (hCG).
- The **umbilical arteries** carry deoxygenated blood from the fetus to the placenta; the **umbilical vein** carries oxygenated blood from the placenta back to the fetus.
- The fetal circulatory system differs from its adult version by having three shunts:
  - The **foramen ovale** connects the right atrium to the left atrium, bypassing the lungs.
  - The **ductus arteriosus** connects the pulmonary artery to the aorta, bypassing the lungs.
  - The **ductus venosus** connects the umbilical vein to the inferior vena cava, bypassing the liver.

Gestation and Birth

- In the first trimester, organogenesis occurs (development of heart, eyes, gonads, limbs, liver, brain).
- In the second trimester, tremendous growth occurs, movement begins, the face becomes distinctly human, and the digits elongate.
- In the third trimester, rapid growth and brain development continue, and there is transfer of antibodies to the fetus.
- During birth the cervix thins out and the amniotic sac ruptures. Then, uterine contractions, coordinated by prostaglandins and oxytocin, result in birth of the fetus. Finally, the placenta and umbilical cord are expelled.

ANSWERS TO CONCEPT CHECKS

3.1

1. Determinate cleavage refers to cell division that results in cells having definitive lineages; that is, at least one daughter cell is programmed to differentiate into a particular cell type. Indeterminate cleavage refers to cell division that results in cells that can differentiate into any cell type (or a whole organism).
2. Zygote → 2-, 4-, 8-, and 16-cell embryo → morula → blastula (blastocyst) → gastrula
3. Implantation occurs during the blastula (blastocyst) stage.
4.

Germ Layer	Organs
Ectoderm	Integument (including the epidermis, hair, nails, and epithelia of the nose, mouth, and anal canal), lens of the eye, nervous system (including adrenal medulla), inner ear
Mesoderm	Musculoskeletal system, circulatory system, excretory system, gonads, muscular and connective tissue layers of the digestive and respiratory systems, adrenal cortex
Endoderm	Epithelial linings of digestive and respiratory tracts, and parts of the liver, pancreas, thyroid, bladder, and distal urinary and reproductive tracts

5. Induction is the process by which nearby cells influence the differentiation of adjacent cells. This ensures proper spatial location and orientation of cells that share a function or have complementary functions.
6. Neural crest cells become the peripheral nervous system (including the sensory ganglia, autonomic ganglia, adrenal medulla, and Schwann cells) as well as specific cell types in other tissues (such as calcitonin-producing cells of the thyroid, melanocytes in the skin, and others).

3.2

1. Determination is the commitment of a cell to a particular lineage. Differentiation refers to the actual changes that occur in order for the cell to assume the structure and function of the determined cell type.
2.

Type of Potency	Cell Lineages
Totipotency	Any cell type in the developing embryo (primary germ layers) or in extraembryonic tissues (amnion, chorion, placenta)
Pluripotency	Any cell type in the developing embryo (primary germ layers)
Multipotency	Any cell type within a particular lineage (for example, hematopoietic stem cells)

3. Autocrine (the signal acts on the same cell that secreted it), paracrine (the signal acts on local cells), juxtacrine (a cell triggers adjacent cells through direct receptor stimulation), endocrine (the signal travels via the bloodstream to act on cells at distant sites)
4. Apoptosis is programmed cell death and results in contained blebs of the dead cell that can be picked up and digested by other cells. Necrosis is cell death due to injury and results in spilling of cytoplasmic contents.

3.3

1. The umbilical arteries carry deoxygenated blood. The umbilical vein carries oxygenated blood.
2.

Shunt	Connected Vessels or Chambers	Organ Bypassed
Foramen ovale	Right atrium to left atrium	Lungs
Ductus arteriosus	Pulmonary artery to aorta	Lungs
Ductus venosus	Umbilical vein to inferior vena cava	Liver

3.4

1. In the first trimester, organogenesis occurs (development of heart, eyes, gonads, limbs, liver, brain). In the second trimester, tremendous growth occurs, movement begins, the face becomes distinctly human, and the digits elongate. In the third trimester, rapid growth and brain development continue, and there is transfer of antibodies to the fetus.
2. In the first phase of birth, the cervix thins out and the amniotic sac ruptures. In the second phase, uterine contractions, coordinated by prostaglandins and oxytocin, result in birth of the fetus. In the third phase, the placenta and umbilical cord are expelled.

SCIENCE MASTERY ASSESSMENT EXPLANATIONS

1. **D**

Prostaglandins promote cervical dilation and the onset of contractions, and oxytocin promotes uterine contractions in a positive feedback loop. Oxytocin is also involved in milk letdown and helps the uterus to contract (shrink) following delivery. These factors together lead to **(D)** as the right answer. By contrast, prolactin, which promotes milk production, is produced following childbirth, which eliminates **(A)**, and progesterone maintains the pregnancy and actually inhibits uterine contractions, eliminating **(B)** and **(C)**.

2. **C**

To answer this question, it could be useful to review quickly the embryonic layers. The ectoderm gives rise to the integument (the epidermis, hair, nails, and the epithelia of the nose, mouth, and anal canal), the lens of the eye, and the nervous system (including the adrenal medulla). The endoderm gives rise to the epithelial linings of the digestive and respiratory tracts and parts of the liver, pancreas, thyroid, and bladder. Finally, the mesoderm gives rise to the musculoskeletal system, the circulatory system, the excretory system, the gonads, and the adrenal cortex. Therefore, the only correct association can be found in **(C)** because the fingernails are derived from ectoderm.

3. **B**

A rod of mesodermal cells called the notochord develops along the longitudinal axis just under the dorsal layer of ectoderm. Through inductive effects from the notochord, the overlying ectoderm starts bending inward and forms a groove on the dorsal surface of the embryo. The dorsal ectoderm will eventually pinch off and develop into the spinal cord and brain. While the neural tube forms from ectoderm, the notochord itself is mesodermal.

4. **D**

The influence of a specific group of cells on the differentiation of another group of cells is termed induction. For example, the eyes are formed through reciprocal induction between the brain and the ectoderm. Competence refers to the ability of a cell to respond to a given inducer, but not the influence of the group of organizing cells, eliminating **(A)**. Senescence is a term for biological aging, eliminating **(B)**. Determination may be the result of induction, but this term does not refer to the general concept of the effect of one group of cells on the differentiation of another group of cells, eliminating **(C)**.

5. **C**

During pregnancy, the placenta produces estrogen and progesterone to maintain the endometrium. These hormones are necessary for proper gestation of the fetus and should be measurable in maternal blood because they act on maternal organs. Prior to birth, the fetus is immunologically naïve and does not yet produce immunoglobulins, eliminating **(A)**. It is worth noting, though, that maternal immunoglobulins cross the placenta to enter fetal blood. Fetal hemoglobin is a large protein and, thus, cannot easily cross the placenta. Further, red blood cells are much too large to cross the barrier themselves, eliminating **(B)**. Carbon dioxide from fetal metabolism can be found in maternal blood, but the fetal lungs are nonfunctional prior to birth as the fetus is suspended in amniotic fluid. Carbon dioxide is transferred across the placenta directly from the fetal bloodstream, eliminating **(D)**.

6. **C**

The question stem states that a cell releases a substance that diffuses through the environment and causes differentiation of a nearby cell. Because the cell is acting on a nearby cell and the molecule spreads by diffusion, this is an example of paracrine signaling. Autocrine signaling, **(A)**, occurs when a molecule secreted by a cell acts on the same cell. Juxtacrine signaling, **(B)**, occurs between adjacent cells, but the signal does not spread by diffusion. In endocrine signaling, **(D)**, a molecule is secreted that travels via the bloodstream to a distant target.

7. **D**

Cells that are able to divide indefinitely with no senescence are not exhibiting normal cell behavior. Normally, somatic cells divide a limited number of times until the telomeres become too short to be effective protectors of genomic material. When this occurs, the cells stop dividing. However, in this case, the cells have continued to divide indefinitely. It is likely that the enzyme telomerase has been activated, which allows for synthesis of telomeres to counteract shortening during DNA replication.

8. **A**

Organogenesis primarily occurs during the first trimester of pregnancy; after 8 weeks of gestation, the brain is fairly developed and most of the organs have formed. The severity of anencephaly suggests a defect very early in fetal development, leading to **(A)** as the correct answer. The second and third trimesters are marked by significant growth and further development. Defects in these stages may cause structural abnormalities, but the absence of an organ is unlikely.

9. **A**

Embryonic stem cells are controversial because they require termination of an embryo to harvest, eliminating **(B)**. Adult stem cells are significantly less controversial, but require treatment with various transcription factors in order to increase the level of potency, eliminating **(C)**. Rejection is a concern when foreign cells are introduced into an individual; using one's own stem cells should remove this risk, eliminating **(D)**. Adult stem cells are not naturally pluripotent, unless pluripotency has been induced by strategic use of transcription factors. Therefore, **(A)** is the correct answer.

10. **C**

During development, programmed cell death occurs in multiple locations in order to ensure development of the correct adult structures. One of the places in which this occurs is between fingers and toes; another is the digestive tract, where a central lumen is formed. If apoptosis does not occur correctly in the digestive tract, an imperforate anus could result. Failure of determination or differentiation would likely result in the absence of anorectal structures altogether, eliminating **(A)** and **(B)**. Failure of neurulation would lead to the absence of a nervous system and would not be compatible with life, eliminating **(D)**.

11. **B**

After an injury, healing occurs by some sort of regenerative process. In humans, some tissues, such as the liver, are capable of regenerating tissue with much the same function and structure as the original tissue. However, the heart is not capable of this sort of regeneration, often forming a fibrous scar in an area of injury. This is an example of incomplete regeneration, in which newly formed tissues are not identical in structure or function to the tissues that have been injured or lost.

12. **A**

Here, the mutation affects the skin and the nervous system, both of which are derived from ectoderm. The other germ tissue layers do not lead to skin or nervous system formation, eliminating **(B)** and **(C)**. The notochord is not actually a primary germ tissue layer, and thus cannot be an answer to the question, eliminating **(D)**.

13. **C**

After the first cell divisions occur, the embryo consists of a solid ball of cells known as a morula. Then a hollow center forms, creating the blastula. Finally, as the cells begin to differentiate into the three germ layers, the embryo is considered a gastrula. **(C)** is therefore the correct answer.

14. **D**

The question stem states that the woman was given the drug three days before the baby was born. It is important to remember that organogenesis occurs during the first trimester. The last structure to become fully functional is the lungs. Because the organs were already largely formed prior to the administration of the teratogenic drug, it is likely that there was no major effect on the development of most organs as a result of exposure to the teratogen, eliminating **(A)**, **(B)**, and **(C)**. However, because lung tissues are so sensitive and because they mature so late, it is likely that the infant may have some respiratory distress at birth.

15. **C**

Blood flow in the ductus arteriosus is from the pulmonary artery to the aorta. The direction of flow is determined by the pressure differential between the right side of the heart (and pulmonary circulation) and the left side of the heart (and systemic circulation). Unlike in adults, the right side of the heart is at a higher pressure during prenatal life than the left side, so blood will shunt from the pulmonary circulation to the systemic circulation through both the foramen ovale and ductus arteriosus.

Consult your online resources for additional practice. **GO ONLINE**

SHARED CONCEPTS

Behavioral Sciences Chapter 1
Biology and Behavior

Biochemistry Chapter 3
Nonenzymatic Protein Function and Protein Analysis

Biochemistry Chapter 6
DNA and Biotechnology

Biology Chapter 1
The Cell

Biology Chapter 2
Reproduction

Biology Chapter 5
The Endocrine System

CHAPTER 4

THE NERVOUS SYSTEM

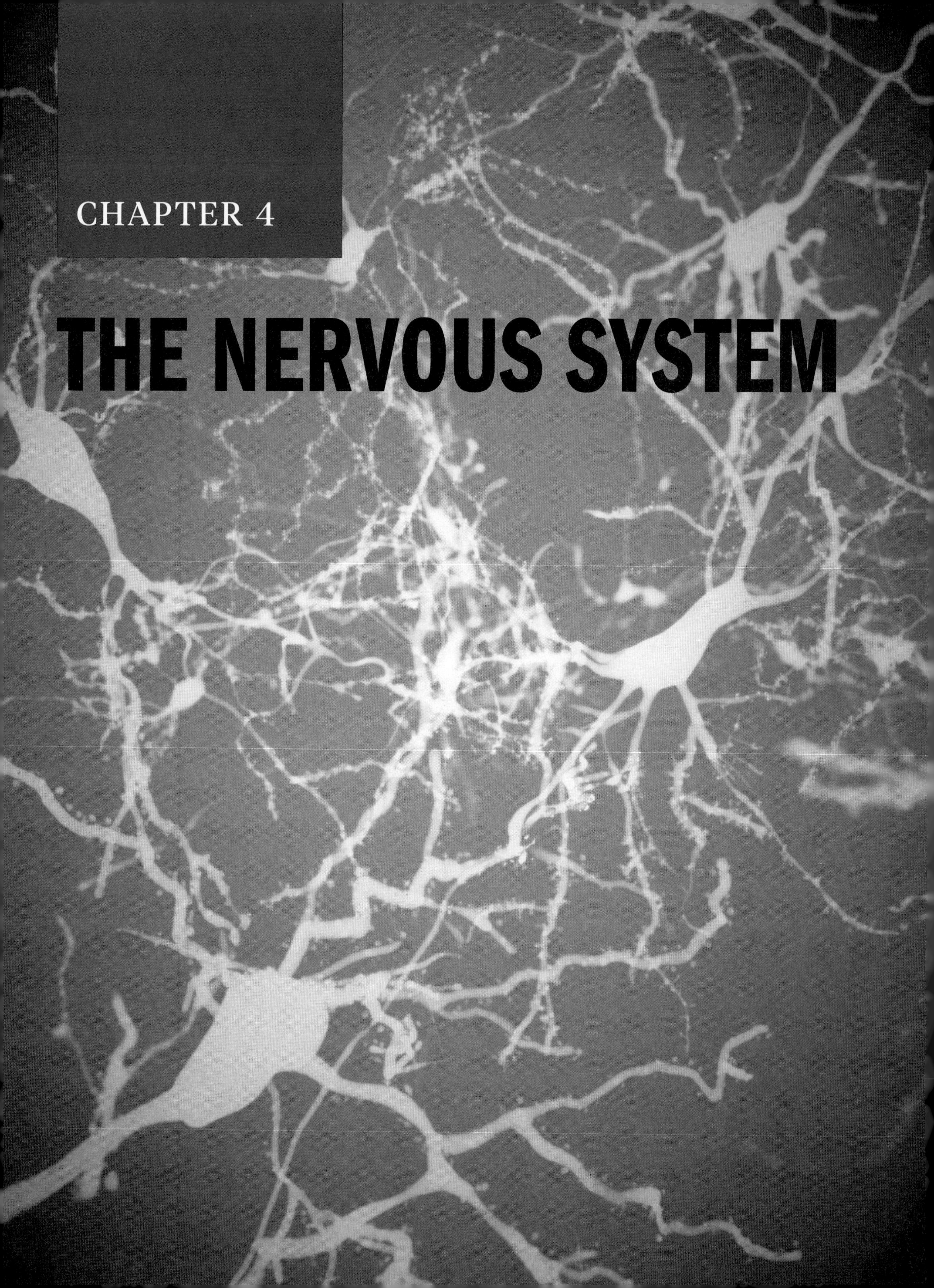

SCIENCE MASTERY ASSESSMENT

Every pre-med knows this feeling: there is so much content I have to know for the MCAT! How do I know what to do first or what's important?

While the high-yield badges throughout this book will help you identify the most important topics, this Science Mastery Assessment is another tool in your MCAT prep arsenal. This quiz (which can also be taken in your online resources) and the guidance below will help ensure that you are spending the appropriate amount of time on this chapter based on your personal strengths and weaknesses. Don't worry though—skipping something now does not mean you'll never study it. Later on in your prep, as you complete full-length tests, you'll uncover specific pieces of content that you need to review and can come back to these chapters as appropriate.

How to Use This Assessment

If you answer 0–7 questions correctly:

Spend about 1 hour to read this chapter in full and take limited notes throughout. Follow up by reviewing **all** quiz questions to ensure that you now understand how to solve each one.

If you answer 8–11 questions correctly:

Spend 20–40 minutes reviewing the quiz questions. Beginning with the questions you missed, read and take notes on the corresponding subchapters. For questions you answered correctly, ensure your thinking matches that of the explanation and you understand why each choice was correct or incorrect.

If you answer 12–15 questions correctly:

Spend less than 20 minutes reviewing all questions from the quiz. If you missed any, then include a quick read-through of the corresponding subchapters, or even just the relevant content within a subchapter, as part of your question review. For questions you answered correctly, ensure your thinking matches that of the explanation and review the Concept Summary at the end of the chapter.

1. Resting membrane potential depends on:
   I. differential distribution of ions across the axon membrane.
   II. the opening of voltage-gated calcium channels.
   III. active transport of ions across the membrane.
   A. I only
   B. I and II only
   C. I and III only
   D. II and III only

2. All of the following are associated with the myelin sheath EXCEPT:
   A. faster conduction of nerve impulses.
   B. nodes of Ranvier forming gaps along the axon.
   C. increased magnitude of the potential difference during an action potential.
   D. saltatory conduction of action potentials.

3. Which of the following is true with regard to the action potential?
   A. All hyperpolarized stimuli will be carried to the axon terminal without a decrease in size.
   B. The size of the action potential is proportional to the size of the stimulus that produced it.
   C. Increasing the intensity of the depolarization increases the size of the impulse.
   D. Once an action potential is triggered, an impulse of a given magnitude and speed is produced.

4. Which of the following correctly describes a difference between nerves and tracts?
   A. Nerves are seen in the central nervous system; tracts are seen in the peripheral nervous system.
   B. Nerves have cell bodies in nuclei; tracts have cell bodies in ganglia.
   C. Nerves may carry more than one type of information; tracts can only carry one type of information.
   D. Nerves contain only one neuron; tracts contain many neurons.

5. Which of the following accurately describes sensory neurons?
   A. Sensory neurons are afferent and enter the spinal cord on the dorsal side.
   B. Sensory neurons are efferent and enter the spinal cord on the dorsal side.
   C. Sensory neurons are afferent and enter the spinal cord on the ventral side.
   D. Sensory neurons are efferent and enter the spinal cord on the ventral side.

6. When a sensory neuron receives a stimulus that brings it to threshold, it will do all of the following EXCEPT:
   A. become depolarized.
   B. transduce the stimulus to an action potential.
   C. inhibit the spread of the action potential to other sensory neurons.
   D. cause the release of neurotransmitters onto cells in the central nervous system.

7. When the potential across the axon membrane is more negative than the normal resting potential, the neuron is said to be in a state of:
   A. depolarization.
   B. hyperpolarization.
   C. repolarization.
   D. polarization.

8. Which of the following statements concerning the somatic division of the peripheral nervous system is INCORRECT?
   A. Its pathways innervate skeletal muscle.
   B. Its pathways are usually voluntary.
   C. Some of its pathways are referred to as reflex arcs.
   D. Its pathways always involve more than two neurons.

9. Which of the following is a function of the parasympathetic nervous system?
   A. Increasing blood sugar during periods of stress
   B. Dilating the pupils to enhance vision
   C. Increasing oxygen delivery to muscles
   D. Decreasing heart rate and blood pressure

10. Which of the following neurotransmitters is used in the ganglia of both the sympathetic and parasympathetic nervous systems?
    - A. Acetylcholine
    - B. Dopamine
    - C. Norepinephrine
    - D. Serotonin

11. In which neural structure are ribosomes primarily located?
    - A. Dendrites
    - B. Soma
    - C. Axon hillock
    - D. Axon

12. An autoimmune disease attacks the voltage-gated calcium channels in the synaptic terminal of an excitatory neuron. What is a likely symptom of this condition?
    - A. Spastic paralysis (inability to relax the muscles)
    - B. Flaccid paralysis (inability to contract the muscles)
    - C. Inability to reuptake neurotransmitters once released
    - D. Retrograde flow of action potentials

13. A neuron only fires an action potential if multiple presynaptic cells release neurotransmitters onto the dendrites of the neuron. This is an example of:
    - A. saltatory conduction.
    - B. summation.
    - C. a feedback loop.
    - D. inhibitory transmission.

14. A disease results in the death of Schwann cells. Which portion of the nervous system is NOT likely to be affected?
    - A. Central nervous system
    - B. Somatic nervous system
    - C. Autonomic nervous system
    - D. Parasympathetic nervous system

15. A surgeon accidentally clips a dorsal root ganglion during a spinal surgery. What is a likely consequence of this error?
    - I. Loss of reflexes at that level
    - II. Loss of sensation at that level
    - III. Loss of cognitive function
    - A. I only
    - B. II only
    - C. I and II only
    - D. I, II, and III

Answer Key

1. **C**
2. **C**
3. **D**
4. **C**
5. **A**
6. **C**
7. **B**
8. **D**
9. **D**
10. **A**
11. **B**
12. **B**
13. **B**
14. **A**
15. **C**

Detailed explanations can be found at the end of the chapter.

CHAPTER 4

THE NERVOUS SYSTEM

In This Chapter

CHAPTER PROFILE

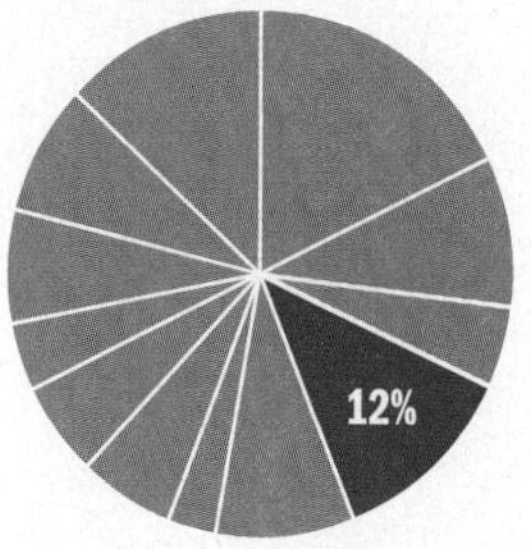

The content in this chapter should be relevant to about 12% of all questions about biology on the MCAT.

This chapter covers material from the following AAMC content categories:

2A: Assemblies of molecules, cells, and groups of cells within single cellular and multicellular organisms

3A: Structure and functions of the nervous and endocrine systems and ways in which these systems coordinate the organ systems

4C: Electrochemistry and electrical circuits and their elements

6A: Sensing the environment

Introduction

For generations, some indigenous peoples of South America used blow darts laced with a paralytic plant extract to hunt their prey. In the 1800s, English physicians who interacted with these indigenous South Americans recognized the possible uses of this paralytic agent, now known as *tubocurarine*, as an anesthetic agent for surgeries. Physicians noticed that animals under the influence of *tubocurarine* would become temporarily immobilized, but would recover after a period of paralysis. According to these physicians, this anesthetic agent would revolutionize surgery. To test the effectiveness of the new drug, one of the physicians volunteered to demonstrate its effectiveness by being tested for pain perception while under the influence of *tubocurarine*. While the drug was an effective paralyzing agent, it did not have any effect on the sensory receptors of the body—he felt every test without being able to move or express his discomfort.

Organisms sense pain, temperature, and all aspects of their environment through the nervous system, which also coordinates this sensory information and responds to stimuli. Specifically, the nervous system is responsible for the control of muscular movement, neuromuscular reflexes, and glandular secretions (such as salivation and lacrimation). In addition, the nervous system is responsible for higher-level thinking and mental function.

Despite all of its complex functions, the nervous system operates through basic electrical and chemical signals. Biomedical scientists have discovered much about the nervous system: its anatomical and functional divisions, the nature of the action potential, and its histological features under the microscope. However, there is so much more that we do not know. It is an inspirational challenge for future physicians to realize that the brain continues to be a vast frontier for human exploration and discovery.

4.1 Cells of the Nervous System

High-Yield

LEARNING OBJECTIVES

After Chapter 4.1, you will be able to:

- Recall the different terms used for myelin-producing cells in the peripheral and the central nervous systems
- Identify the functions of the five main categories of glial cells
- Describe the purpose of each major structure of the neuron

Neurons are specialized cells capable of transmitting electrical impulses and then translating those electrical impulses into chemical signals. In this section, we will consider the structure of the neuron as well as how neurons communicate with other parts of the nervous system.

Neurons

Each neuron has a shape that matches its function, as dictated by the other cells with which that neuron interacts. There are a variety of different types of neurons in the body, but they all share some specific features.

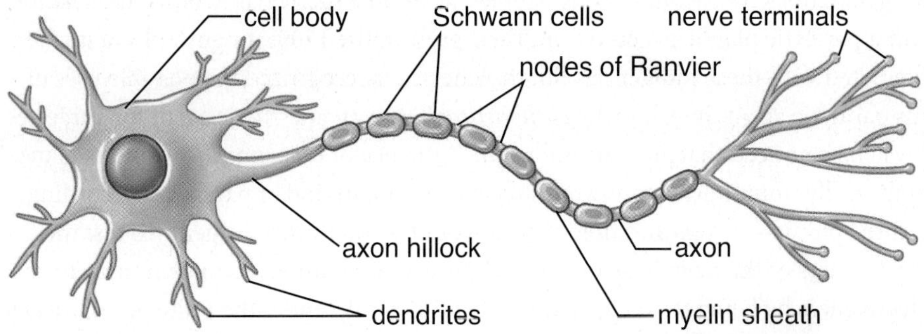

Figure 4.1 Structure of a Neuron

The anatomy of a neuron is shown in Figure 4.1. Like all other cells (besides mature red blood cells), neurons have nuclei. The nucleus is located in the **cell body**, also called the **soma**. The soma is also the location of the endoplasmic reticulum and ribosomes. The cell has many appendages emanating directly from the soma called **dendrites**, which receive incoming messages from other cells. The information received from the dendrites is transmitted through the cell body before it reaches the **axon hillock**, which integrates the incoming signals. The axon hillock plays an important role in **action potentials**, or the transmission of electrical impulses down the axon. Signals arriving from the dendrites can be either excitatory or inhibitory; the axon hillock sums up these signals, and if the result is excitatory enough (reaching threshold, as discussed later in this chapter), it will initiate an action potential. The **axon** is a long appendage that terminates in close proximity to a target structure (a muscle, a gland, or another neuron). Most mammalian nerve fibers are insulated

MNEMONIC

Axons carry neural signals away from the soma; dendrites carry signals toward the soma.

by **myelin**, a fatty membrane, to prevent signal loss or crossing of signals. Just like insulation prevents wires next to each other from accidentally discharging each other, the **myelin sheath** maintains the electrical signal within one neuron. In addition, myelin increases the speed of conduction in the axon. Myelin is produced by **oligodendrocytes** in the central nervous system and **Schwann cells** in the peripheral nervous system. At certain intervals along the axon, there are small breaks in the myelin sheath with exposed areas of axon membrane called **nodes of Ranvier**. As will be explored in the discussion of action potentials to follow, nodes of Ranvier are critical for rapid signal conduction. Finally, at the end of the axon is the **nerve terminal** or **synaptic bouton (knob)**. This structure is enlarged and flattened to maximize transmission of the signal to the next neuron and ensure proper release of **neurotransmitters**, the chemicals that transmit information between neurons.

Neurons are not physically connected to each other. Between the neurons, there is a small space into which the terminal portion of the axon releases neurotransmitters, which bind to the dendrites of the adjacent neuron (the postsynaptic neuron). This space is known as the **synaptic cleft**; together, the nerve terminal, synaptic cleft, and postsynaptic membrane are known as a **synapse**. Neurotransmitters released from the axon terminal traverse the synaptic cleft and bind to receptors on the postsynaptic neuron.

Multiple neurons may be bundled together to form a **nerve** in the peripheral nervous system. These nerves may be **sensory**, **motor**, or **mixed**, which refers to the type(s) of information they carry; mixed nerves carry both sensory and motor information. The cell bodies of neurons of the same type are clustered together into ganglia.

In the central nervous system, axons may be bundled together to form **tracts**. Unlike nerves, tracts only carry one type of information. The cell bodies of neurons in the same tract are grouped into **nuclei**.

REAL WORLD

Sometimes the body mounts an immune response against its own myelin, leading to the destruction of this insulating substance (demyelination). Because myelin speeds the conduction of impulses along a neuron, the absence of myelin slows down information transfer. A common demyelinating disorder is multiple sclerosis (MS). In MS, the myelin of the brain and spinal cord is selectively targeted. Because so many different kinds of neurons are demyelinated, patients who have MS experience a wide variety of symptoms including weakness, lack of balance, vision problems, and incontinence.

BIOLOGY GUIDED EXAMPLE WITH EXPERT THINKING

Huntington's disease (HD) is a devastating neurodegenerative condition caused by expansion of a CAG repeat in exon 1 of *IT15*, which encodes for the protein huntingtin. Although huntingtin is widely expressed, HD is associated with the neurodegeneration of the striatal medium spiny neurons. This particular vulnerability is hypothesized to result from transcriptional dysregulation within the cAMP and CREB signaling cascades in these neurons. Thus, a potential treatment would be to target phosphodiesterases (PDE) that inactivate cAMP and CREB cascades. To test this hypothesis, and the potential therapeutic approach, researchers investigated whether administration of TP-10, a highly specific phosphodiesterase inhibitor would alleviate neurological deficits in a highly utilized HD model system, the R6/2 mouse. Loss of reflexes, loss of body weight, and increased instances of clasping behavior in the mice were monitored in the TP-10 intervention group and the vehicle control group. Righting reflex is assessed by laying the mice on their side and monitoring their ability to get back to the upright position. Clasping is a behavior correlated to neurodegeneration.

Background: Huntington's disease

Hypothesis: dysregulation of transcription within cAMP and CREB leads to SMS neuron degeneration

Inactivate cAMP and CREB phosphodiesterase = they want to treat by increasing these cascades

IV: TP-10 (inhibitor), DV: neurological deficits reduced

Model system for HD = these mice have Huntington's-like symptoms

Behavior on these tests must correlate to symptom relief from HD

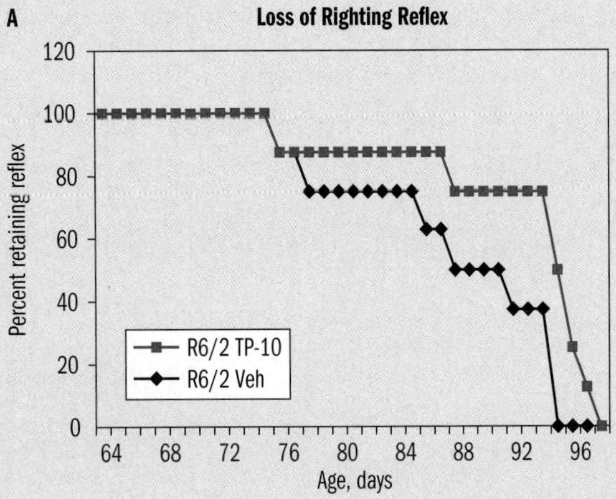

IV: age

DV: percent retaining reflex

Trend: treatment group (TP-10) loses reflex at a later age

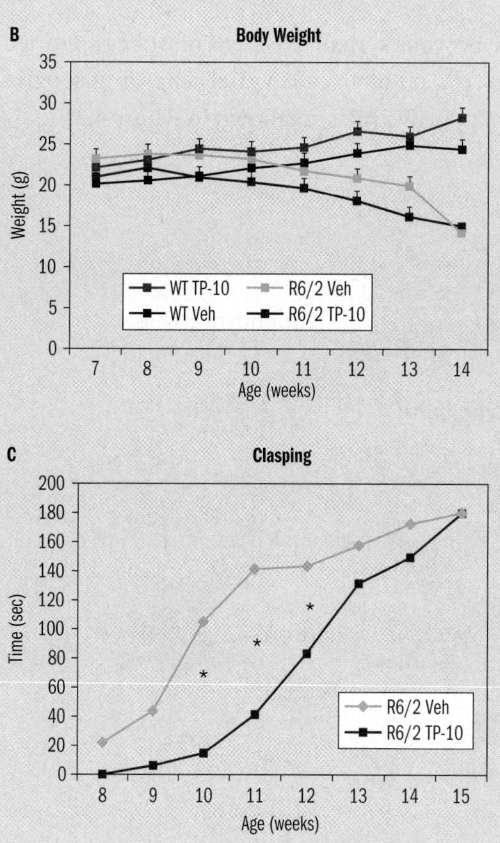

IV: age

DV: weight

Trend: wild-type (WT) gain weight toward the end of the experiment; R6/2 lose weight

IV: age

DV: time

Trend: vehicle group develops "clasping" before treatment (TP-10) group

Figure 1

Adapted from: Giampà, C., Laurenti, D., Anzilotti, S., Bernardi, G., Menniti, F. S., & Fusco, F. R. (2010). Inhibition of the striatal specific phosphodiesterase PDE10a ameliorates striatal and cortical pathology in R6/2 mouse model of Huntingtons disease. *PLoS One*, 5(10). doi:10.1371/journal.pone.0013417.

Does TP-10 treatment alleviate neurological deficits associated with Huntington's disease?

This question asks about the results of the associated study, so we are going to have to use the information in the article and the results in the figures in order to answer. The article says that TP-10 is a possible treatment for Huntington's disease (HD), and the second paragraph describes the dependent variables used to measure success in this experiment. There appears to be a figure associated with each dependent variable, so we will need to evaluate the results in each figure to reach a conclusion.

Based on the label and axes of the graph, Figure 1A shows the age at which mice lose their righting reflex. Specifically, we can see that that R6/2 TP-10 (red) retains their righting reflex longer than R6/2 Vehicle (black). According to the passage, the loss of the righting reflex indicates neurodegeneration; therefore, TP-10 appears to be alleviating this particular symptom. However, Figure 1B shows that mice who had the HD genetic condition lost weight in both treatment and vehicle conditions, meaning TP-10 doesn't appear to have helped with weight maintenance. Finally, Figure 1C shows that clasping occurs more readily in R6/2 Vehicle than R6/2 TP-10. The term clasping alone doesn't imply positive or negative effects on the brain, but the article tells us that clasping is a sign of neurodegeneration. Thus, the data showing that R6/2 TP-10-treated mice have later onset of clasping demonstrates that neurological deficits are being alleviated.

Overall, Figures 1A and 1C indicate that TP-10 may have potential to treat neurological deficits associated with Huntington's disease. Figure 1B, however, indicates that this treatment may not be addressing all aspects of the disease.

Other Cells in the Nervous System

Neurons are not the only cells in the nervous system. Neurons must be supported and myelinated by other cells. These cells are often called **glial cells**, or **neuroglia**. Glial cells play both structural and supportive roles, as shown in Figure 4.2.

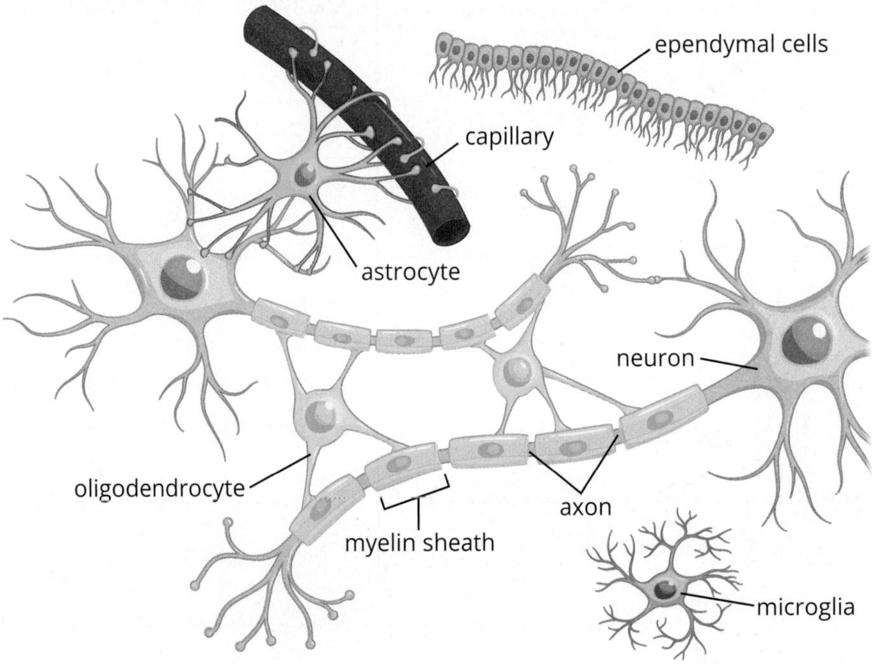

Figure 4.2 Glial Cells: Astrocytes and Oligodendrocytes

A detailed knowledge of these cell types is not necessary for the MCAT, so a familiarity with their basic functions will suffice:

- **Astrocytes** nourish neurons and form the blood–brain barrier, which controls the transmission of solutes from the bloodstream into nervous tissue.
- **Ependymal cells** line the ventricles of the brain and produce cerebrospinal fluid, which physically supports the brain and serves as a shock absorber.
- **Microglia** are phagocytic cells that ingest and break down waste products and pathogens in the central nervous system.
- **Oligodendrocytes** (CNS) and **Schwann cells** (PNS) produce myelin around axons.

MCAT CONCEPT CHECK 4.1

Before you move on, assess your understanding of the material with these questions.

1. For each of the following neuron structures, provide a brief description of its purpose:
   - Axon:

   ____

   - Axon hillock:

   ____

   - Dendrite:

   ____

   - Myelin sheath:

   ____

   - Soma:

   ____

   - Synaptic bouton:

   ____

2. What is a collection of cell bodies called in the CNS? In the PNS?
   - CNS:

   ____

   - PNS:

   ____

3. Which two types of glial cells, if not properly functioning, will make an individual most susceptible to a CNS infection?

   ____

4. Guillain-Barré syndrome (GBS) is an autoimmune disease that causes demyelination in the peripheral nervous system. What type of glial cell is being targeted in GBS?

   ____

4.2 Transmission of Neural Impulses

High-Yield

LEARNING OBJECTIVES

After Chapter 4.2, you will be able to:

- Explain the ion channels and regulatory steps involved in the process of initiating, propagating, and terminating an action potential
- Describe the resting membrane potential and how it is maintained
- Differentiate between temporal and spatial summation
- Identify the ion responsible for the fusion of neurotransmitter-containing vesicles at the nerve terminal membrane
- Recall the three main methods to block the action of a neurotransmitter
- Identify the ion channel changes that occur during the shifts in voltage associated with an action potential:

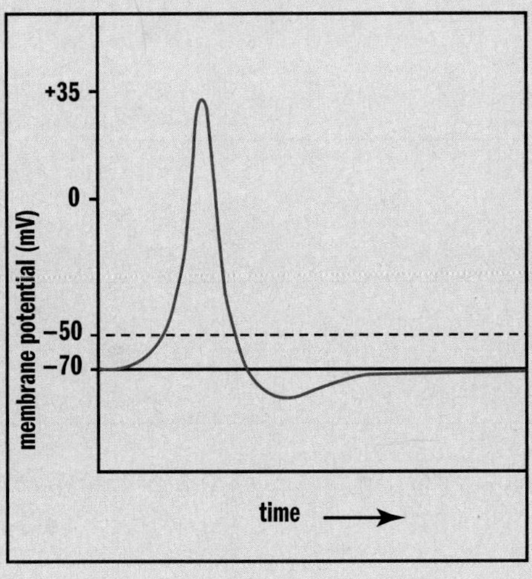

Now that we have discussed the basic anatomy of the neuron, we can turn to the physiology that underlies neuronal signaling.

The Action Potential

Neurons use all-or-nothing messages called **action potentials** to relay electrical impulses down the axon to the synaptic bouton. As we will explore in the following section, action potentials ultimately cause the release of neurotransmitters into the synaptic cleft.

Resting Potential

A cell's **resting membrane potential** is the net electric potential difference that exists across the cell membrane, created by movement of charged molecules across that membrane. For neurons, this potential is about −70 mV, with the inside of the neuron being negative relative to the outside. The two most important ions involved in generating and maintaining the resting potential are potassium (K^+) and sodium (Na^+).

The potassium concentration inside the cell averages about 140 mM, as compared to 4 mM outside of the cell. This concentration difference makes it favorable for potassium to move to the outside of the cell. To facilitate the outward movement of potassium, the cell membrane has transmembrane **potassium leak channels**, which allow the slow leak of potassium out of the cell. As potassium continually leaks out of the cell, the cell loses a small amount of positive charge, leaving behind a small amount of negative charge and making the outside of the cell slightly positively charged.

However, as negative charge builds up inside the cell, some potassium will be drawn back into the cell due to the attraction between the positive potassium ions and the negative potential building inside the cell. As the potential difference continues to grow, potassium will also be more strongly drawn back into the cell. And at a certain potential, each potassium cation that is pushed out due to the concentration gradient will be matched by another potassium cation pulled back in due to the electric potential. At this point, there is no more net movement of the ion, as the cell is in equilibrium with respect to potassium. The potential difference that represents this potassium equilibrium is called the **equilibrium potential of potassium**. Potassium's equilibrium potential is around −90 mV. The negative sign is assigned due to convention, and because a positive ion (potassium) is leaving the cell.

Next, let's consider in isolation the other important ion, sodium. Sodium's concentration gradient is the reverse of potassium's, with a concentration of about 12 mM inside and 145 mM outside of the cell, meaning there is a driving force pushing sodium into the cell. This movement is facilitated by **sodium leak channels**. The slow leak of sodium into the cell causes a buildup of electric potential. The **equilibrium potential of sodium** is around 60 mV, and is positive because sodium is moving into the cell.

In a living system, sodium and potassium are flowing across the cell's membrane at the same time. Potassium's concentration gradient causes potassium to leak out of the cell through potassium leak channels. At the same time, sodium is moving in the opposite direction, with the opposite effect. In a certain sense, sodium undoes the effect of potassium's movement. The resting potential is thus a tug-of-war: Potassium's movement pulls the cell potential toward −90 mV, while sodium's movement pulls the cell potential the opposite way, toward +60 mV. But neither ion ever "wins" the tug-of-war. Instead, a balance of these two effects is reached at around −70 mV for the average nerve cell, as can be seen in Figure 4.3. This balance, the net effect of sodium's and potassium's equilibrium potentials, is the **resting membrane potential**. The resting potential is significantly closer to potassium's equilibrium potential because the cell is much more permeable to potassium. Neither ion is ever able to establish its own equilibrium, so both ions continue leaking across the cell membrane.

REAL WORLD

Even though we may think of these influxes and effluxes as big events, only a very small amount of potassium needs to exit the cell before the resulting electrostatic force equals the force of the concentration gradient. In fact, during an action potential the change to potassium's intracellular concentration is so small that it cannot even be accurately measured using current devices! The action potential is reliant only on local voltage changes at the membrane itself, so this overall lack of change in intracellular ion concentration does not impact transmission. This is the reason why you see membrane potentials reported in units of voltage, which are easily measurable, instead of concentration change, which is almost negligible. Because so little potassium needs to exit, the equilibrium potential with respect to potassium is established almost instantly.

BRIDGE

The resting membrane potential is dependent on the intra- and extracellular ion concentrations, relative permeability of the membrane to these different ions, and charges of these ions. The Goldman-Hodgkin-Katz voltage equation brings together these different factors into one equation that predicts the resting membrane potential. This equation is discussed in Chapter 8 of *MCAT Biochemistry Review*.

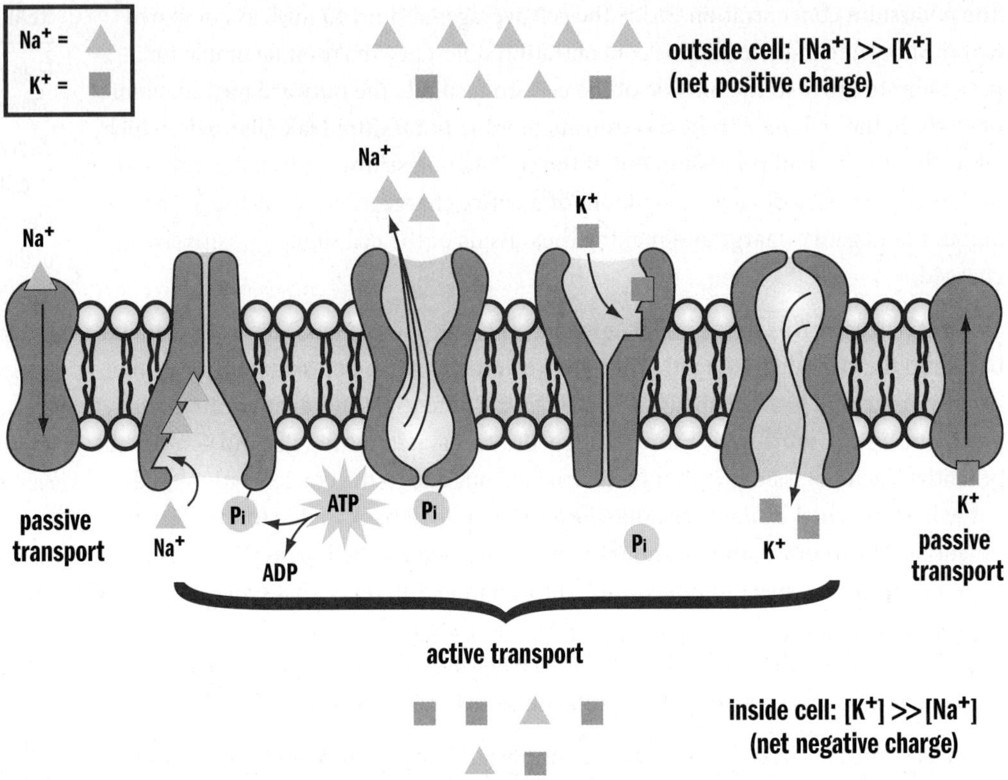

Figure 4.3 Maintenance of Resting Membrane Potential
The action of Na^+/K^+ ATPase, Na^+ leak channels, and K^+ leak channels creates and maintains a resting membrane potential of −70 mV.

MNEMONIC

To remember the direction of ion movement by Na^+/K^+ ATPase, think *pumpKin.*

Given the continual ion leaking at the membrane, there must be a means of moving both sodium and potassium ions back against their gradients if a resting potential is to be maintained. **Na^+/K^+ ATPase** continually pumps sodium and potassium back to where they started: potassium into the cell and sodium out of the cell, to maintain their respective gradients. In fact, in a person's body more ATP is spent by the Na^+/K^+ ATPase to maintain these gradients than for any other single purpose.

The Axon Hillock

Neurons can receive both excitatory and inhibitory input. Excitatory input causes **depolarization** (raising the membrane potential, V_m, from its resting potential) and thus makes the neuron more likely to fire an action potential. Inhibitory input causes **hyperpolarization** (lowering the membrane potential from its resting potential) and thus makes the neuron less likely to fire an action potential. If the axon hillock receives enough excitatory input to be depolarized to the **threshold** value (usually in the range of −55 mV to −40 mV), an action potential will be triggered.

This implies that not every stimulus necessarily generates a response. A small excitatory signal may not be sufficient to bring the axon hillock to threshold. Further, a postsynaptic neuron may receive information from several different presynaptic neurons, some of which are excitatory and some of which are inhibitory. The additive effect of multiple signals is known as **summation**.

There are two types of summation: temporal and spatial. In **temporal summation**, multiple signals are integrated during a relatively short period of time. A number of small excitatory signals firing at nearly the same moment could bring a postsynaptic cell to threshold, enabling an action potential. In **spatial summation**, the additive effects are based on the number and location of the incoming signals. A large number of inhibitory signals firing directly on the soma will cause more profound hyperpolarization of the axon hillock than the depolarization caused by a few excitatory signals firing on the dendrites of a neuron.

Ion Channels and Membrane Potential

A graph of membrane potential *vs.* time during an action potential is shown in Figure 4.4.

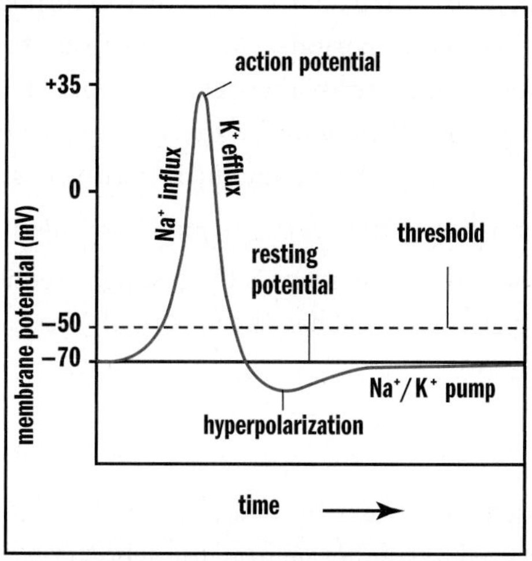

Figure 4.4 Action Potential Generation
Sufficient depolarization across the cell membrane to threshold leads to the generation of an action potential, followed by repolarization and hyperpolarization before returning to the resting membrane potential.

If the cell is brought to threshold, voltage-gated sodium channels open in the membrane. As the name implies, these ion channels open in response to the change in potential of the membrane (depolarization) and permit the passage of sodium ions. There is a strong **electrochemical gradient** that promotes the migration of sodium into the cell. From an electrical standpoint, the interior of the cell is more negative than the exterior of the cell, which favors the movement of positively charged sodium cations into the cell. From a chemical standpoint, there is a higher concentration of sodium outside the cell than inside, which also favors the movement of sodium into the cell. As sodium passes through these ion channels, the membrane potential becomes more positive; that is, the cell rapidly depolarizes. Sodium channels not only open in response to changes in membrane potential, but are also inactivated by them. When V_m approaches +35 mV, the sodium channels are **inactivated** and will have to be brought back near the resting potential to be **deinactivated**. Thus, these sodium channels can exist in three states: **closed** (before the cell reaches threshold, and after inactivation has been reversed), **open** (from threshold to approximately +35 mV), and **inactive** (from approximately +35 mV to the resting potential).

KEY CONCEPT

Na^+ wants to go into the cell because the cell is more negative inside (electrical gradient) and has a lower concentration of Na^+ inside (chemical gradient).

The positive potential inside the cell not only triggers the voltage-gated sodium channels to inactivate, but also triggers the voltage-gated potassium channels to open. Once sodium has depolarized the cell, there is an electrochemical gradient favoring the efflux of potassium from the neuron. As positively charged potassium cations are driven out of the cell, there will be a restoration of the negative membrane potential called **repolarization**. The efflux of K^+ causes an overshoot of the resting membrane potential, hyperpolarizing the neuron. This hyperpolarization serves an important function: it makes the neuron refractory to further action potentials. There are two types of **refractory periods**. During the **absolute refractory period**, no amount of stimulation can cause another action potential to occur. During the **relative refractory period**, there must be *greater than normal* stimulation to cause an action potential because the membrane is starting from a potential that is more negative than its resting value.

KEY CONCEPT

Action potentials rely on both electrical and chemical gradients. The neuron starts at the resting potential, around -70 mV. At the resting potential, potassium is high inside the cell and low outside the cell, while sodium is high outside the cell and low inside the cell. Once the cell reaches threshold, sodium channels open and sodium floods the cell, making it more positive inside (depolarization). Then, sodium channels are inactivated and the potassium channels open. This allows potassium to flow out of the cell, bringing the potential into the negative range (repolarization), and actually overshooting the resting potential (hyperpolarization). Na^+/K^+ ATPase then works to restore the resting potential.

The Na^+/K^+ ATPase acts to restore not only the resting potential, but also the sodium and potassium gradients that have been partially dissipated by the action potential.

Impulse Propagation

So far, we have discussed the movements of ions at one small segment of the axon. For a signal to be conveyed to another neuron, the action potential must travel down the axon and initiate neurotransmitter release. This movement is called **impulse propagation** and is shown in Figure 4.5. As sodium rushes into one segment of the axon, it will cause depolarization in the surrounding regions of the axon. This depolarization will bring subsequent segments of the axon to threshold, opening the sodium channels in those segments. Each of these segments then continues through the rest of the action potential in a wave-like fashion until the action potential reaches the nerve terminal. After the action potential has fired in one segment of the axon, that segment becomes momentarily refractory, as described previously. The functional consequence of this is that information can only flow in one direction.

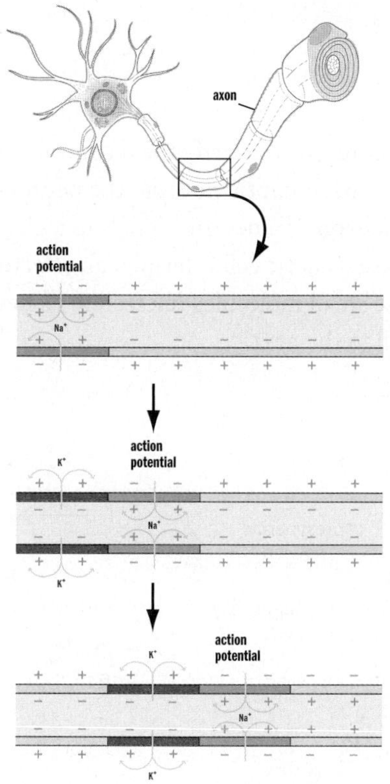

Figure 4.5 Action Potential Propagation

Action potentials are propagated down the axon when proximal sodium channels open and depolarize the membrane, inducing distal sodium channels to open as well; because of the refractory character of these channels, the action potential can move in only one direction.

The speed at which action potentials move depends on the length and cross-sectional area of the axon. Increased length of the axon results in higher resistance and slower conduction. Greater cross-sectional areas allow for faster propagation due to decreased resistance. The effect of cross-sectional area is more significant than the effect of length. In order to maximize the speed of transmission, mammals have myelin. Myelin is an extraordinarily good insulator, preventing the dissipation of the electric signal. The insulation is so effective that the membrane is only permeable to ion movement at the nodes of Ranvier. Thus, the signal "hops" from node to node—what is called **saltatory conduction.**

It is important to note that all action potentials within the same type of neuron have the same potential difference during depolarization. Increased intensity of a stimulus does not result in an increased potential difference of the action potential, but rather an increased frequency of firing.

REAL WORLD

A toxin called *tetrodotoxin* (TTX) is found in the pufferfish, a delicacy in some parts of the world. TTX blocks voltage-gated Na^+ channels, blocking neuronal transmission. This can rapidly cause death because the phrenic nerves innervating the diaphragm can no longer depolarize, leading to paralysis of the muscle and cessation of breathing. For this reason, chefs who prepare pufferfish must be specially trained and licensed.

REAL WORLD

Local anesthetics work by blocking voltage-gated Na^+ channels. These drugs work particularly well on sensory neurons and therefore block the transmission of pain. They favor pain neurons because these neurons have small axonal diameters and little or no myelin, allowing easy access to the sodium channels. Anesthetic concentrations are kept sufficiently low to block pain neurons without significant effects on other sensory modalities or motor function.

MNEMONIC

Saltatory conduction can be recalled by thinking of the Spanish verb *saltar*, to jump.

REAL WORLD

Insulation by myelin is extremely effective. A human spinal cord is about the thickness of a finger. Without this insulation, the cord would have to be almost as wide as a telephone pole to prevent signal loss.

The Synapse

As discussed previously, neurons are not actually in direct physical contact. There is a small space between neurons called the synaptic cleft into which neurotransmitters are secreted, as shown in Figure 4.6. To clarify the terminology, the neuron preceding the synaptic cleft is called the **presynaptic neuron**; the neuron after the synaptic cleft is called the **postsynaptic neuron**. If a neuron signals to a gland or muscle, rather than another neuron, the postsynaptic cell is termed an **effector**. Most synapses are **chemical** in nature; they use small molecules referred to as **neurotransmitters** to send messages from one cell to the next.

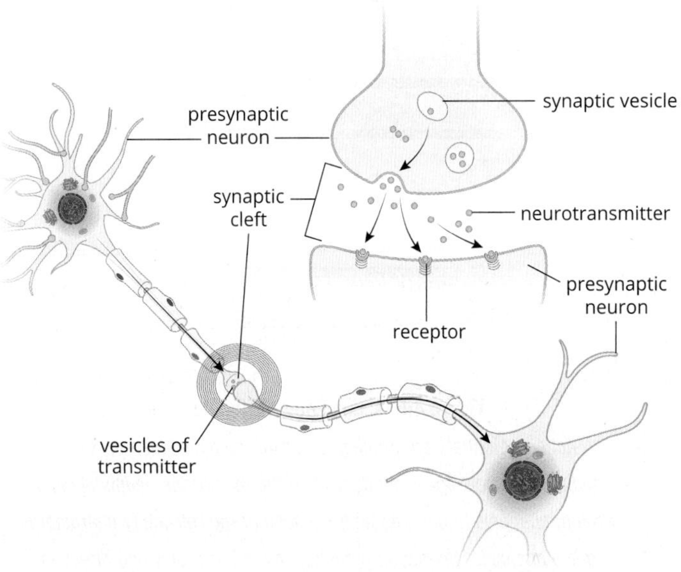

Figure 4.6 The Synapse
Synaptic vesicles are released from the presynaptic neuron and diffuse across the synaptic cleft to activate receptors on the postsynaptic neuron (or gland or muscle).

Neurotransmitters

Prior to release, neurotransmitter molecules are stored in membrane-bound vesicles in the nerve terminal. When the action potential reaches the nerve terminal, voltage-gated calcium channels open, allowing calcium to flow into the cell. This sudden increase in intracellular calcium triggers fusion of the membrane-bound vesicles with the cell membrane at the synapse, causing exocytosis of the neurotransmitter.

Once released into the synapse, the neurotransmitter molecules diffuse across the cleft and bind to receptors on the postsynaptic membrane. This allows the message to be passed from one neuron to the next. As stated earlier, neurons may be either excitatory or inhibitory; this distinction truly comes at the level of the neurotransmitter

KEY CONCEPT

It is critical to understand the difference between electrical and chemical transmission. Within a neuron, electricity is used to pass signals down the length of the axon. Between neurons, chemicals (neurotransmitters) are used to pass signals to the subsequent neuron (or gland or muscle).

receptors. If the receptor is a ligand-gated ion channel, the postsynaptic cell will either be depolarized or hyperpolarized. If it is a G protein–coupled receptor, it will cause either changes in the levels of cyclic AMP (cAMP) or an influx of calcium. Note that the physiology of receptors is further discussed in Chapter 3 of *MCAT Biochemistry Review*.

Neurotransmission must be regulated—there are almost no circumstances under which constant signaling to the postsynaptic cell would be desirable. Therefore, the neurotransmitter must be removed from the synaptic cleft. There are three main mechanisms to accomplish this goal. First, neurotransmitters can be broken down by enzymatic reactions. The breakdown of **acetylcholine** (**ACh**) by *acetylcholinesterase* (AChE), shown in Figure 4.7, is a classic example.

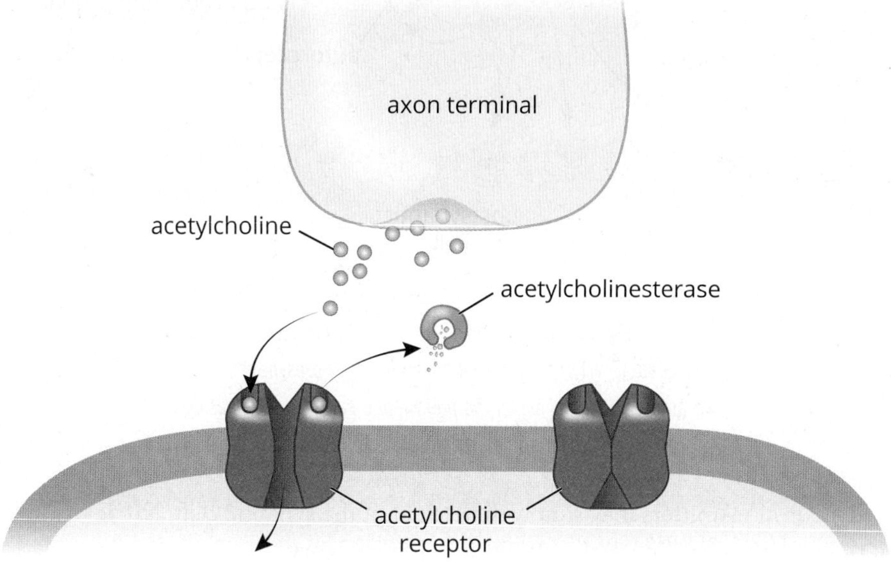

Figure 4.7 Breakdown of a Neurotransmitter by an Enzyme
Acetylcholine (ACh) can be broken down by acetylcholinesterase (AChE).

Second, neurotransmitters can be brought back into the presynaptic neuron using **reuptake carriers**. The reuptake of **serotonin** (**5-HT**), shown in Figure 4.8, is a classic example of this mechanism. **Dopamine** (**DA**) and **norepinephrine** (**NE**) also use reuptake carriers.

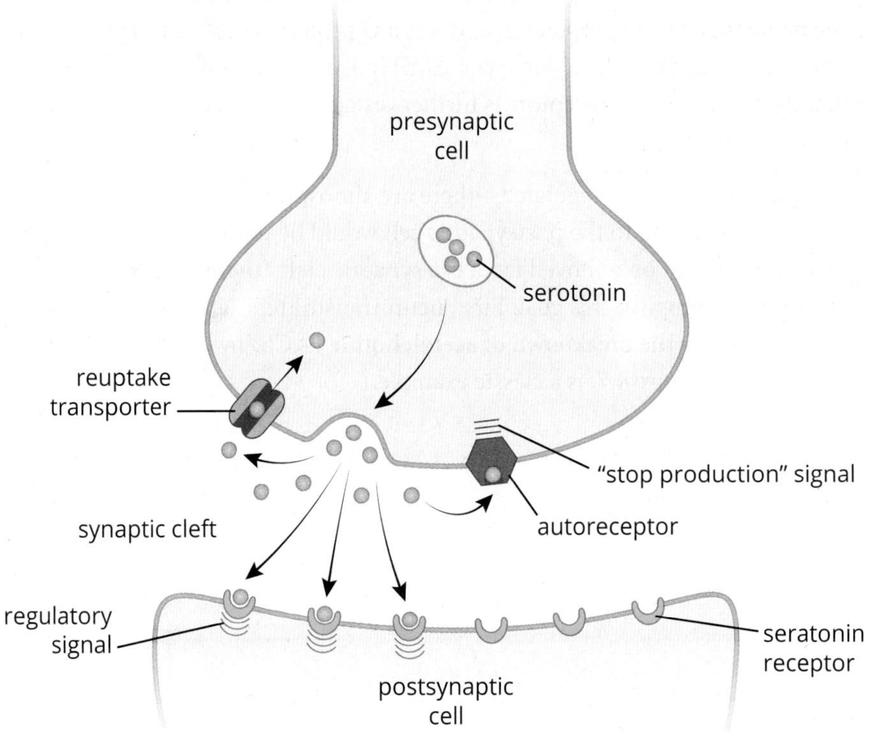

Figure 4.8 Reuptake of a Neurotransmitter
Serotonin (5-HT) can be taken back up by the presynaptic cell; an autoreceptor will signal the presynaptic cell to stop releasing serotonin and start the reuptake process.

REAL WORLD

Many common drugs modify processes that occur in the synapse. For instance, cocaine acts by blocking neuronal reuptake carriers, thus prolonging the action of neurotransmitters in the synapse. There are clinically useful drugs (some of which are used to treat Alzheimer's disease, glaucoma, and myasthenia gravis) that inhibit acetylcholinesterase, thereby elevating synaptic levels of acetylcholine. Nerve gases, which have been used in warfare and terrorism, are extremely potent acetylcholinesterase inhibitors. Nerve gas causes rapid death by preventing the relaxation of skeletal muscle (most importantly, the diaphragm), leading to respiratory arrest.

Third, neurotransmitters may simply diffuse out of the synaptic cleft. **Nitric oxide (NO)**, a gaseous signaling molecule, fits into this category.

MCAT CONCEPT CHECK 4.2

Before you move on, assess your understanding of the material with these questions.

1. What neural structure initiates the action potential?

___

2. What entity maintains the resting membrane potential? What is the approximate voltage of the resting membrane potential?

___

3. What is the difference between temporal and spatial summation?
   - Temporal summation:

   ___

   - Spatial summation:

   ___

4. During the action potential, which ion channel opens first? How is this ion channel regulated? What effect does the opening of this channel have on the polarization of the cell?
   - Ion channel:
   - Regulation:
   - Effect on polarization:

5. During the action potential, which ion channel opens second? How is this ion channel regulated? What effect does the opening of this channel have on the polarization of the cell?
   - Ion channel:
   - Regulation:
   - Effect on polarization:

6. What is the difference between the absolute and relative refractory period?
   - Absolute refractory period:
   - Relative refractory period:

7. What ion is primarily responsible for the fusion of neurotransmitter-containing vesicles with the nerve terminal membrane?

8. What are the three main methods by which a neurotransmitter's action can be stopped?
   -
   -
   -

4.3 Organization of the Human Nervous System

High-Yield

LEARNING OBJECTIVES

After Chapter 4.3, you will be able to:

- Classify elements of the nervous system as components of either the central nervous system or the peripheral nervous system
- Differentiate between afferent and efferent neurons
- Describe the functions of the somatic and autonomic nervous systems
- Recall the physiological effects of activating the sympathetic nervous system and the parasympathetic nervous system
- Distinguish between the neural pathways for a monosynaptic and a polysynaptic reflex

The nervous system is a remarkable collection of cells that governs both involuntary and voluntary behavior, while also maintaining **homeostasis**. Functions of the nervous system include:

- Sensation and perception
- Motor function
- Cognition (thinking) and problem solving
- Executive function and planning
- Language comprehension and creation
- Memory
- Emotion and emotional expression
- Balance and coordination
- Regulation of endocrine organs
- Regulation of heart rate, breathing rate, vascular resistance, temperature, and exocrine glands

The human nervous system is a complex web of over 100 billion cells that communicate, coordinate, and regulate signals for the rest of the body. Action occurs when the body can react to external stimuli using the nervous system. In this section, we will look at the nervous system and its basic organization.

Note: Much of the information contained in this section is also discussed in Chapter 1 of MCAT Behavioral Sciences Review.

MNEMONIC

Afferent neurons **a**scend in the spinal cord toward the brain; **e**fferent neurons **e**xit the spinal cord on their way to the rest of the body.

Central and Peripheral Nervous Systems

Generally speaking, there are three kinds of nerve cells in the nervous system: sensory neurons, motor neurons, and interneurons. **Sensory neurons** (also known as **afferent neurons**) transmit sensory information from sensory receptors to the spinal cord and brain. **Motor neurons** (also known as **efferent neurons**) transmit motor information from the brain and spinal cord to muscles and glands. **Interneurons** are found between other neurons and are the most numerous of the three types. Interneurons are located predominantly in the brain and spinal cord and are often linked to reflexive behavior.

Different types of information require different types of processing. Processing of stimuli and response generation may happen at the level of the spinal cord, or may require input from the brainstem or cerebral cortex. Reflexes, discussed later in this section, only require processing at the level of the spinal cord. For example, when a reflex hammer hits the patellar tendon, the sensory information goes to the spinal cord, where a motor signal is sent to the quadriceps muscles, causing the leg to jerk forward at the knee. No input from the brain is required. However, some scenarios require input from the brain or brainstem. When this happens, **supraspinal** circuits are used.

Let's turn to the overall structure of the human nervous system, which is diagrammed in Figure 4.9.

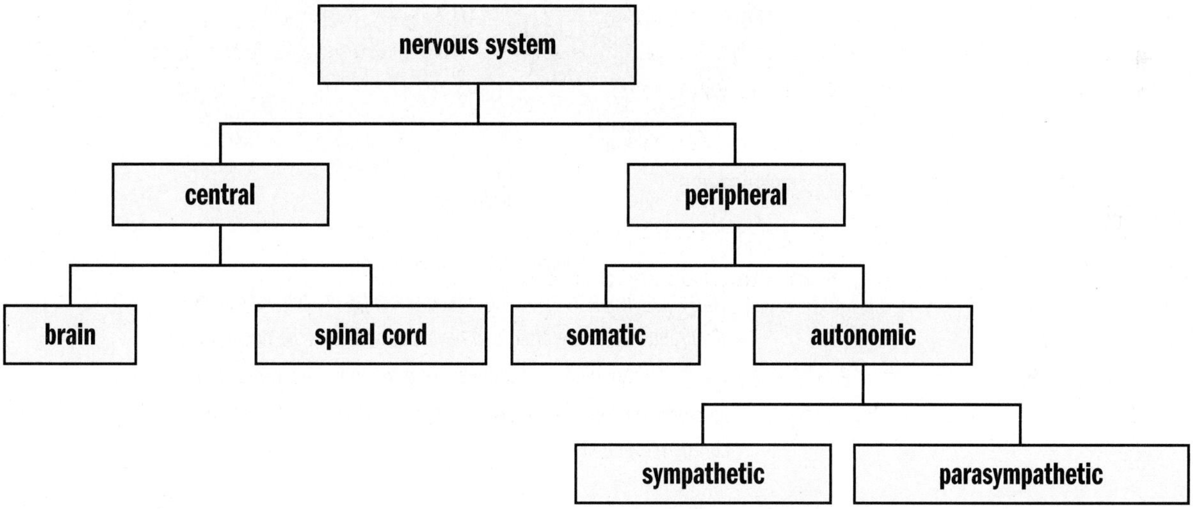

Figure 4.9 Major Divisions of the Nervous System

The nervous system can be broadly divided into two primary components: the central and peripheral nervous systems. The **central nervous system** (**CNS**) is composed of the brain and spinal cord. The brain consists of white matter and grey matter. The **white matter** consists of axons encased in myelin sheaths. The **grey matter** consists of unmyelinated cell bodies and dendrites. In the brain, the white matter lies deeper than the grey matter. At the base of the brain is the brainstem, which is largely responsible for basic life functions such as breathing. Note that the lobes of the brain and major brain structures are discussed in Chapter 1 of *MCAT Behavioral Sciences Review*.

The spinal cord extends downward from the brainstem and can be divided into four regions: **cervical**, **thoracic**, **lumbar**, and **sacral**. Almost all of the structures below the neck receive sensory and motor innervation from the spinal cord. The spinal cord is protected by the **vertebral column**, which transmits nerves at the space between adjacent vertebrae. Like the brain, the spinal cord also consists of white and grey matter. The white matter lies on the outside of the cord, and the grey matter is deep within it. The axons of motor and sensory neurons are in the spinal cord. The sensory neurons bring information in from the periphery and enter on the dorsal (back) side of the spinal cord. The cell bodies of these sensory neurons are found in the **dorsal root ganglia**. Motor neurons exit the spinal cord ventrally, or on the side closest to the front of the body. The structure of the spinal cord can be seen in Figure 4.10.

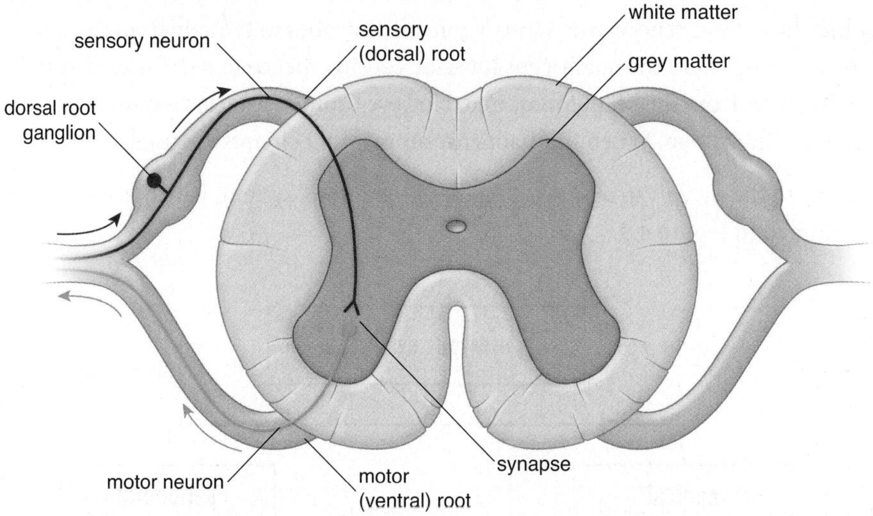

Figure 4.10 The Spinal Cord

Sensory neurons transmit information about pain, temperature, and vibration up to the brain and have cell bodies in the dorsal root ganglia toward the back of the spinal cord; the motor neurons run from the brain along the opposite side of the spinal cord and in the ventral root to control movements of skeletal muscle and glandular secretions.

The **peripheral nervous system (PNS)**, in contrast, is made up of nerve tissue and fibers outside the brain and spinal cord, including all 31 pairs of spinal nerves and 10 of the 12 pairs of cranial nerves (the olfactory and optic nerves are technically outgrowths of the central nervous system). The PNS thus connects the CNS to the rest of the body and can itself be subdivided into the somatic and autonomic nervous systems.

The **somatic nervous system** consists of sensory and motor neurons distributed throughout the skin, joints, and muscles. Sensory neurons transmit information through afferent fibers. Motor impulses, in contrast, travel along efferent fibers.

The **autonomic nervous system (ANS)** generally regulates heartbeat, respiration, digestion, and glandular secretions. In other words, the ANS manages the involuntary muscles associated with many internal organs and glands. The ANS also helps regulate body temperature by activating sweating or piloerection, depending on whether we are too hot or too cold, respectively. The main thing to understand about these functions is that they are automatic, or independent of conscious control. Note the similarity between the words autonomic and automatic. This association makes it easy to remember that the autonomic nervous system manages automatic functions such as heartbeat, respiration, digestion, and temperature control.

One primary difference between the somatic and autonomic nervous systems is that the peripheral component of the autonomic nervous system contains two neurons. By contrast, a motor neuron in the somatic nervous system goes directly from the spinal cord to the muscle without synapsing. In the autonomic nervous system, two neurons work in series to transmit messages from the spinal cord. The first neuron is known as the **preganglionic neuron**, whereas the second is the **postganglionic neuron**. The soma of the preganglionic neuron is in the CNS, and its axon travels to a ganglion in the PNS. Here it synapses on the cell body of the postganglionic neuron, which then stimulates the target tissue.

The Autonomic Nervous System

The ANS has two subdivisions: the sympathetic nervous system and the parasympathetic nervous system. These two branches often act in opposition to one another, meaning that they are antagonistic. For example, the sympathetic nervous system acts to accelerate heart rate and inhibit digestion, while the parasympathetic nervous system decelerates heart rate and promotes digestion.

The main role of the **parasympathetic nervous system** is to conserve energy. It is associated with resting and sleeping states and acts to reduce heart rate and constrict the bronchi. The parasympathetic nervous system is also responsible for managing digestion by increasing peristalsis and exocrine secretions. Acetylcholine is the neurotransmitter responsible for parasympathetic responses in the body and is released by both preganglionic and postganglionic neurons. The vagus nerve (cranial nerve X) is responsible for much of the parasympathetic innervation of the thoracic and abdominal cavity. The functions of the parasympathetic nervous system are summarized in Figure 4.11.

KEY CONCEPT

The first neuron in the autonomic nervous system is called the preganglionic neuron. The second neuron is the postganglionic neuron.

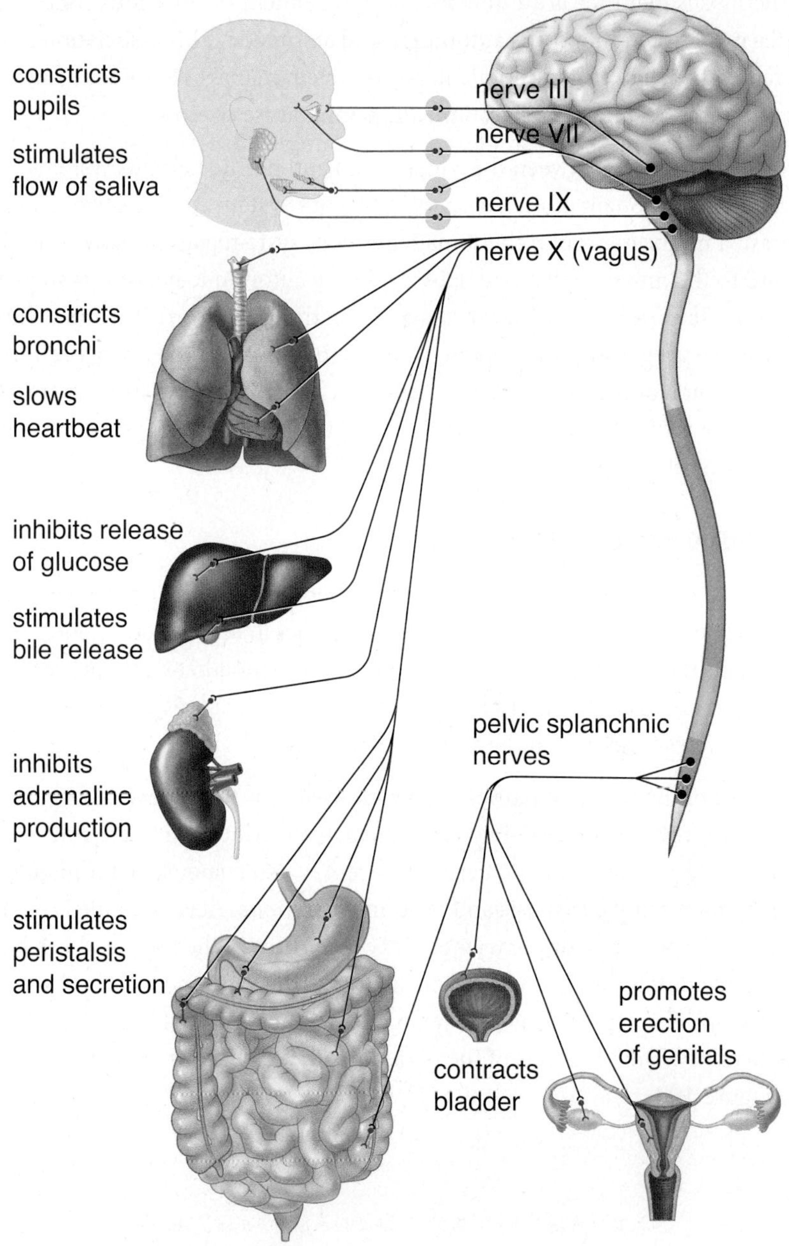

Figure 4.11 Functions of the Parasympathetic Nervous System

In contrast, the **sympathetic nervous system** is activated by stress. This can include everything from a mild stressor, such as keeping up with school or work deadlines, to emergencies that mean the difference between life and death. The sympathetic nervous system is closely associated with rage and fear reactions, also known as "fight-or-flight" reactions. When activated, the sympathetic nervous system:

- Increases heart rate
- Redistributes blood to muscles of locomotion
- Increases blood glucose concentration
- Relaxes the bronchi

MNEMONIC

Sympathetic and parasympathetic nervous systems:

- Sympathetic: "**fight**-or-**flight**"
- Parasympathetic: "**rest**-and-**digest**"

- Decreases digestion and peristalsis
- Dilates the eyes to maximize light intake
- Releases epinephrine into the bloodstream

The functions of the sympathetic nervous system are summarized in Figure 4.12. In the sympathetic nervous system, preganglionic neurons release acetylcholine, while most postganglionic neurons release norepinephrine.

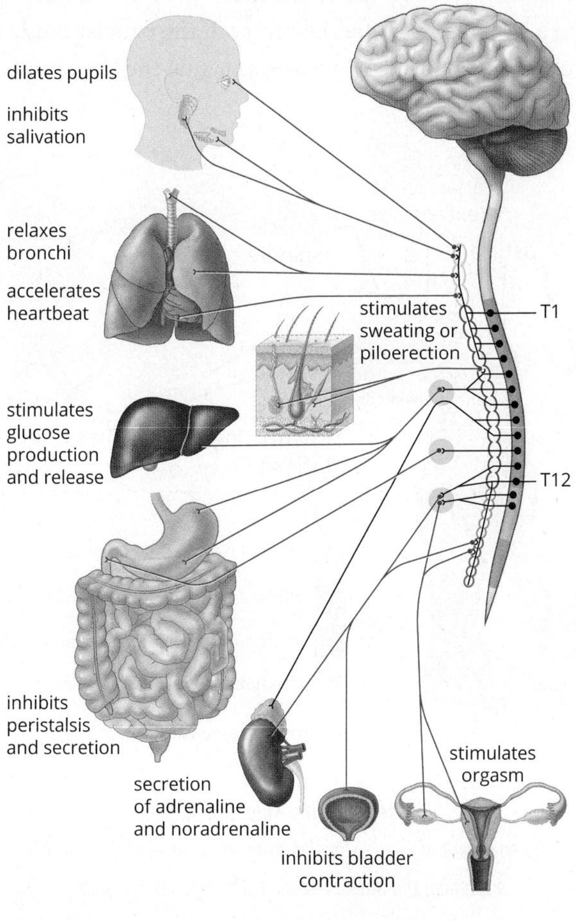

Figure 4.12 Functions of the Sympathetic Nervous System

Reflexes

Neural circuits called **reflex arcs** control reflexive behavior. For example, consider what occurs when someone steps on a nail. Receptors in the foot detect pain, and the pain signal is transmitted by sensory neurons up to the spinal cord. At that point, the sensory neurons connect with interneurons, which can then relay pain impulses up to the brain. Rather than wait for the brain to send out a signal, interneurons in the spinal cord can also send signals to the muscles of both legs directly, causing the individual to withdraw the foot with pain while supporting with the other foot. The original sensory information still makes its way up to the brain; however, by the time it arrives there, the muscles have already responded to the pain, thanks to the reflex arc. There are two types of reflex arcs: monosynaptic and polysynaptic.

KEY CONCEPT

Consider the purpose of reflexes. Although it may be amusing to watch your leg jump when a doctor tests your knee-jerk reflex, there is a more functional reason why this response occurs. The stretch on the patellar tendon makes the body think that the muscle may be getting overstretched. In response, the muscle contracts in order to prevent injury.

Monosynaptic

In a **monosynaptic reflex arc**, there is a single synapse between the sensory neuron that receives the stimulus and the motor neuron that responds to it. A classic example is the **knee-jerk reflex**, shown in Figure 4.13. When the patellar tendon is stretched, information travels up the sensory (afferent, presynaptic) neuron to the spinal cord, where it interfaces with the motor (efferent, postsynaptic) neuron that causes contraction of the quadriceps muscles. The net result is extension of the leg, which lessens the tension on the patellar tendon. Note that the reflex is simply a feedback loop and a response to potential injury. If the patellar tendon or quadriceps muscles are stretched too far, they may tear, damaging the knee joint. Thus, the reflex serves to protect the muscles.

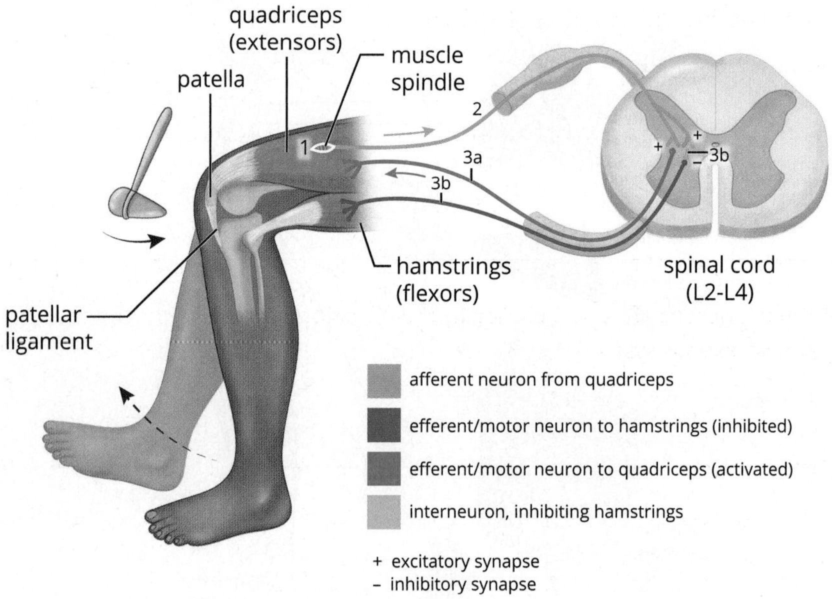

Figure 4.13 The Knee-Jerk Reflex
The knee-jerk or knee extension reflex may be elicited by swiftly stretching the patellar tendon with a reflex hammer.

Polysynaptic

In a **polysynaptic reflex arc**, there is at least one interneuron between the sensory and motor neurons. A real-life example is the reaction to stepping on a nail described earlier, which involves the **withdrawal reflex**. The extremity with which one steps on the nail will be stimulated to flex, using the hip muscles and hamstring muscles, pulling the foot away from the nail. This is a monosynaptic reflex, similar to the knee-jerk reflex described previously. However, if the person is to maintain balance, the other foot must be planted firmly on the ground. For this to occur, the motor neuron that controls the quadriceps muscles in the opposite limb must be stimulated, extending it. Interneurons in the spinal cord provide the connections from the incoming sensory information to the motor neurons in the supporting limb.

MCAT CONCEPT CHECK 4.3

Before you move on, assess your understanding of the material with these questions.

1. What parts of the nervous system are in the central nervous system (CNS)? Peripheral nervous system (PNS)?
   - CNS:
   - PNS:
2. What do afferent neurons do? Efferent neurons?
   - Afferent:
   - Efferent:
3. What functions are accomplished by the somatic nervous system? The autonomic nervous system?
   - Somatic:
   - Autonomic:
4. What are the effects of the sympathetic nervous system? The parasympathetic nervous system?
   - Sympathetic:
   - Parasympathetic:
5. What is the pathway of neural impulses in a monosynaptic reflex? In a polysynaptic reflex?
   - Monosynaptic reflex:
   - Polysynaptic reflex:

Conclusion

The nervous system is one of the most fascinating and complex systems of the human body; millions upon millions of cells allow for appropriate interactions in the everyday world. It is the seat of personality and, ultimately, the system that makes you *you*. In medical school, your courses on neuroscience will go into astounding detail about the nervous system, including the circuits that govern sensations such as pain and temperature, and circuits that allow your body to move and function.

In this chapter, we explored the nervous system at both the cellular and organizational level. Neurons are the primary cells of the nervous system, propagating impulses through both electrical and chemical means—action potentials and synaptic transmission, respectively. Neurons can be grouped together to form nerves, which are the primary organizational structures in one major branch of the nervous system, the peripheral nervous system. The central nervous system consists of the brain and spinal cord. The peripheral nervous system can be subdivided into the somatic and autonomic nervous systems, the latter of which can be further subdivided into the sympathetic and parasympathetic nervous systems.

The nervous system is heavily tested on the MCAT because it plays a role in the function of almost every other major organ system. Neurons cause muscles to move and digestive structures to carry food along through peristalsis, and they regulate breathing rate, heart rate, and glandular secretions. The nervous system is not the only system that has such a profound effect throughout the body, however. The endocrine system, which we will explore in the next chapter, serves a similar role—but through chemical messengers carried in the blood called hormones.

You've reviewed the content, now test your knowledge and critical thinking skills by completing a test-like passage set in your online resources!

GO ONLINE

CONCEPT SUMMARY

Cells of the Nervous System

- **Neurons** are highly specialized cells responsible for the conduction of impulses.
- Neurons communicate using both electrical and chemical forms of communication.
  - Electrical communication occurs via ion exchange and the generation of membrane potentials down the length of the axon.
  - Chemical communication occurs via neurotransmitter release from the presynaptic cell and the binding of these neurotransmitters to the postsynaptic cell.
- Neurons consist of many different parts.
  - **Dendrites** are appendages that receive signals from other cells.
  - The cell body or **soma** is the location of the nucleus as well as organelles such as the endoplasmic reticulum and ribosomes.
  - The **axon hillock** is where the cell body transitions to the axon, and where action potentials are initiated.
  - The **axon** is a long appendage down which an action potential travels.
  - The **nerve terminal** or **synaptic bouton** is the end of the axon from which neurotransmitters are released.
  - **Nodes of Ranvier** are exposed areas of myelinated axons that permit saltatory conduction.
  - The **synapse** consists of the nerve terminal of the presynaptic neuron, the membrane of the postsynaptic cell, and the space between the two, called the **synaptic cleft**.
- Many axons are coated in **myelin**, an insulating substance that prevents signal loss.
  - Myelin is created by **oligodendrocytes** in the central nervous system and **Schwann cells** in the peripheral nervous system.
  - Myelin prevents dissipation of the neural impulse and crossing of neural impulses from adjacent neurons.
- Individual axons are bundled into **nerves** or **tracts**.
  - A single nerve may carry multiple types of information, including sensory, motor, or both. Tracts contain only one type of information.
  - Cell bodies of neurons of the same type within a nerve cluster together in **ganglia** in the peripheral nervous system.
  - Cell bodies of the individual neurons within a tract cluster together in **nuclei** in the central nervous system.

- **Neuroglia** or **glial cells** are other cells within the nervous system in addition to neurons.
  - **Astrocytes** nourish neurons and form the blood–brain barrier, which controls the transmission of solutes from the bloodstream into nervous tissue.
  - **Ependymal cells** line the ventricles of the brain and produce cerebrospinal fluid, which physically supports the brain and serves as a shock absorber.
  - **Microglia** are phagocytic cells that ingest and break down waste products and pathogens in the central nervous system.
  - Oligodendrocytes (CNS) and Schwann cells (PNS) produce myelin around axons.

Transmission of Neural Impulses

- All neurons exhibit a **resting membrane potential** of approximately −70 mV.
  - Resting potential is maintained using selective permeability of ions as well as the Na^+/K^+ ATPase.
  - The **Na^+/K^+ ATPase** pumps three sodium ions out of the cell for every two potassium ions pumped in.
- Incoming signals can be either excitatory or inhibitory.
  - Excitatory signals cause depolarization of the neuron.
  - Inhibitory signals cause hyperpolarization of the neuron.
  - **Temporal summation** refers to the integration of multiple signals near each other in time.
  - **Spatial summation** refers to the addition of multiple signals near each other in space.
- An **action potential** is used to propagate signals down the axon.
  - When enough excitatory stimulation occurs, the cell is **depolarized** to the **threshold voltage** and voltage-gated sodium channels open.
  - Sodium flows into the neuron due to its strong **electrochemical gradient**. This continues depolarizing the neuron.
  - At the peak of the action potential (approximately +35 mV), sodium channels are inactivated and potassium channels open.
  - Potassium flows out of the neuron due to its strong electrochemical gradient, **repolarizing** the cell. Potassium channels stay open long enough to overshoot the resting potential, resulting in a **hyperpolarized** neuron; then, the potassium channels close.
  - The Na^+/K^+ ATPase brings the neuron back to the resting potential and restores the sodium and potassium gradients.
  - While the axon is hyperpolarized, it is in its **refractory period**. During the **absolute refractory period**, the cell is unable to fire another action potential. During the **relative refractory period**, the cell requires a larger than normal stimulus to fire an action potential.

- The impulse propagates down the length of the axon because the influx of sodium in one segment of the axon brings the subsequent segment of the axon to threshold. The fact that the preceding segment of the axon is in its refractory period means that the action potential can only travel in one direction.
- At the nerve terminal, neurotransmitters are released into the synapse.
  - When the action potential arrives at the nerve terminal, voltage-gated calcium channels open.
  - The influx of calcium causes fusion of vesicles filled with neurotransmitters with the presynaptic membrane, resulting in exocytosis of neurotransmitters into the synaptic cleft.
  - The neurotransmitters bind to receptors on the postsynaptic cell, which may be ligand-gated ion channels or G protein–coupled receptors.
- Neurotransmitters must be cleared from the postsynaptic receptors to stop the propagation of the signal. There are three ways this can happen:
  - The neurotransmitter can be enzymatically broken down.
  - The neurotransmitter can be absorbed back into the presynaptic cell by **reuptake channels**.
  - The neurotransmitter can diffuse out of the synaptic cleft.

Organization of the Human Nervous System

- There are three types of neurons in the nervous system: **motor** (**efferent**) neurons, **interneurons**, and **sensory** (**afferent**) neurons.
- The nervous system is made up of the **central nervous system** (**CNS**: brain and spinal cord) and **peripheral nervous system** (**PNS**: cranial and spinal nerves).
  - In the CNS, **white matter** consists of myelinated axons, and **grey matter** consists of unmyelinated cell bodies and dendrites. In the brain, white matter is deeper than grey matter. In the spinal cord, grey matter is deeper than white matter.
  - The PNS is divided into the **somatic** (voluntary) and **autonomic** (automatic) nervous systems.
  - The autonomic nervous system is further divided into the **parasympathetic** (rest-and-digest) and **sympathetic** (fight-or-flight) branches.
- **Reflex arcs** use the ability of interneurons in the spinal cord to relay information to the source of a stimulus while simultaneously routing it to the brain.
  - In a **monosynaptic reflex arc**, the sensory (afferent, presynaptic) neuron fires directly onto the motor (efferent, postsynaptic) neuron.
  - In a **polysynaptic reflex arc**, the sensory neuron may fire onto a motor neuron as well as interneurons that fire onto other motor neurons.

ANSWERS TO CONCEPT CHECKS

4.1

1. The axon transmits an electrical signal (the action potential) from the soma to the synaptic knob. The axon hillock integrates excitatory and inhibitory signals from the dendrites and fires an action potential if the excitatory signals are strong enough to reach threshold. Dendrites receive incoming signals and carry them to the soma. The myelin sheath acts as insulation around the axon and speeds conduction. The soma is the cell body and contains the nucleus, endoplasmic reticulum, and ribosomes. The synaptic bouton lies at the end of the axon and releases neurotransmitters.
2. A collection of cell bodies in the central nervous system is called a nucleus. In the peripheral nervous system, it is called a ganglion.
3. Astrocytes nourish neurons and form the blood–brain barrier, which helps protect the brain from foreign pathogens gaining entrance. Microglia ingest and break down waste products and pathogens. Disruption of either of these mechanisms would increase susceptibility to a CNS infection.
4. Oligodendrocytes produce myelin in the central nervous system while Schwann cells produce myelin in the peripheral nervous system. Since GBS causes demyelination in the PNS, it can be inferred that Schwann cells are targeted for immune destruction.

4.2

1. The action potential is initiated at the axon hillock.
2. The resting membrane potential is maintained by the Na^+/K^+ATPase at approximately −70 mV.
3. Temporal summation is the integration of multiple signals close to each other in time. Spatial summation is the integration of multiple signals close to each other in space.
4. The sodium channel opens first at threshold (around −50 mV). It is regulated by inactivation, which occurs around +35 mV. Inactivation can only be reversed by repolarizing the cell. The opening of the sodium channel causes depolarization.
5. The potassium channel opens second at approximately +35 mV. It is regulated by closing at low potentials (slightly below −70 mV). The opening of the potassium channel causes repolarization and, eventually, hyperpolarization.
6. During the absolute refractory period, the cell is unable to fire an action potential regardless of the intensity of a stimulus. During the relative refractory period, the cell can fire an action potential only with a stimulus that is stronger than normal.
7. Calcium is responsible for fusion of neurotransmitter vesicles with the nerve terminal membrane.
8. A neurotransmitter's action can be stopped by enzymatic degradation, reuptake, or diffusion.

4.3

1. The central nervous system includes the brain and spinal cord. The peripheral nervous system includes cranial and spinal nerves and sensory nerves.
2. Afferent (sensory) neurons bring signals from a sensor to the central nervous system. Efferent (motor) neurons bring signals from the central nervous system to an effector.
3. The somatic nervous system is responsible for voluntary actions—most notably, moving muscles. The autonomic nervous system is responsible for involuntary processes like heart rate, bronchial dilation, dilation of the pupils, exocrine gland function, and peristalsis.
4. The sympathetic nervous system promotes a "fight-or-flight" response, with increased heart rate and bronchial dilation, redistribution of blood to locomotor muscles, dilation of the pupils, and slowing of digestive and urinary function. The parasympathetic nervous system promotes "rest-and-digest" functions, slowing heart rate and constricting the bronchi, redistributing blood to the gut, promoting exocrine secretions, constricting the pupils, and promoting peristalsis and urinary function.
5. In a monosynaptic reflex, a sensory (afferent, presynaptic) neuron fires directly onto a motor (efferent, postsynaptic) neuron. In a polysynaptic reflex, a sensory neuron may fire directly onto a motor neuron, but interneurons are used as well. These interneurons fire onto other motor neurons.

SCIENCE MASTERY ASSESSMENT EXPLANATIONS

1. **C**

The polarization of the neuron at rest is the result of an uneven distribution of ions between the inside and outside of the cell. This difference is achieved through the active pumping of ions into and out of the neuron (using the Na^+/K^+ ATPase). Voltage-gated calcium channels are important in the nerve terminal, where the influx of calcium triggers the fusion of vesicles containing neurotransmitters with the membrane, but not in maintaining resting membrane potential.

2. **C**

Myelin is a white lipid-containing material surrounding the axons of many neurons in the central and peripheral nervous systems. It is arranged on the axon discontinuously; the gaps between the segments of myelin are called nodes of Ranvier, eliminating **(B)**. Myelin increases the conduction velocity by insulating segments of the axon so that the membrane is permeable to ions only at the nodes of Ranvier, eliminating **(A)**. The action potential jumps from node to node, a process known as saltatory conduction, eliminating **(D)**. Action potentials are often described as being "all-or-nothing"; the magnitude of the potential difference of an action potential is fixed, regardless of the intensity of the stimulus. Thus, myelin does not affect the magnitude of the potential difference in an action potential, making **(C)** the correct answer.

3. **D**

As in the previous question, the action potential is often described as an all-or-nothing response. This means that, whenever the threshold membrane potential is reached, an action potential with a consistent size and duration is produced. Neuronal information is coded by the frequency and number of action potentials, not the size of the action potential, eliminating **(B)** and **(C)** and making **(D)** the correct answer. Hyperpolarizing (inhibitory) signals are not transmitted to the nerve terminal, eliminating **(A)**.

4. **C**

Nerves are collections of neurons in the peripheral nervous system and may contain multiple types of information (sensory or motor); they contain cell bodies in ganglia. Tracts are collections of neurons in the central nervous system and contain only one type of information; they contain cell bodies in nuclei.

5. **A**

Sensory neurons are considered afferent (carrying signals from the periphery to the central nervous system) and enter the spinal cord on the dorsal side. Motor neurons are considered efferent (carrying signals from the central nervous system to the periphery) and exit the spinal cord on the ventral side.

6. **C**

When a sensory neuron receives a signal that is strong enough to bring it to threshold, one can assume that the receptor becomes depolarized, allowing it to transduce the stimulus to an action potential. The action potential will then be carried by sensory neurons to the central nervous system, where the cell will release neurotransmitters. Therefore, among the given choices, the only incorrect statement is found in **(C)**. If a receptor is stimulated, it will promote the spread of the action potential to postsynaptic sensory neurons in the spinal cord, which can send the signal toward the brain.

7. **B**

When the potential across the axon membrane is more negative than the normal resting potential, the neuron is referred to as hyperpolarized. Hyperpolarization occurs right after an action potential and is caused by excess potassium exiting the neuron.

8. **D**

The somatic division of the peripheral nervous system innervates skeletal muscles and is responsible for voluntary movement. Some of the pathways in this part of the nervous system are reflex arcs, which are reflexive responses to certain stimuli that involve only a sensory and a motor neuron. These neurons synapse in the spinal cord and do not require signaling from the brain. The pathways of the somatic division can involve two, three, or more neurons, depending on the type of signal. The correct answer therefore is **(D)**.

9. **D**

The parasympathetic nervous system governs the "rest-and-digest" response. The parasympathetic nervous system slows the heart rate, decreases blood pressure, promotes bloodflow to the GI tract, and constricts the pupils, among other functions. The sympathetic nervous system governs the fight-or-flight response, including increased heart rate and blood pressure, decreased bloodflow to the digestive tract, and increased bloodflow to the muscles. **(D)** is the only answer choice that represents a function of the parasympathetic nervous system.

10. **A**

Acetylcholine is the neurotransmitter released by the preganglionic neuron in both the sympathetic and parasympathetic nervous systems. The postganglionic neuron in the sympathetic nervous system usually releases norepinephrine, while the postganglionic neuron in the parasympathetic nervous system releases acetylcholine.

11. **B**

Neurons contain very specialized structures, including dendrites, axons, and the axon hillock. However, neurons are still cells and must carry out cellular functions including protein synthesis. The cell body or soma contains the nucleus, endoplasmic reticulum, and ribosomes.

12. **B**

First, consider the function of voltage-gated calcium channels. When the nerve terminal depolarizes, voltage-gated calcium channels open, allowing for influx of calcium. This influx of calcium triggers fusion of the synaptic vesicles containing neurotransmitters with the membrane of the neuron at the nerve terminal. This allows for exocytosis of the neurotransmitters into the synapse. If a disease blocked the influx of calcium, there would be no release of neurotransmitters. A lack of neurotransmitters means that the neuron cannot send excitatory signals. Thus, any symptoms resulting from this disease would be due to an inability of neurons to transmit excitatory signals to the muscle. If neurons cannot communicate, flaccid paralysis may be one of the results.

13. **B**

Some neurons require multiple instances of excitatory transmission to be brought to threshold. These excitatory signals may be close to each other in time (temporal) or in space (spatial); either way, this pattern of excitation is termed summation.

14. **A**

Schwann cells are responsible for myelination of cells in the peripheral nervous system. Thus, the central nervous system is unlikely to be affected. The peripheral nervous system includes the somatic nervous system and the autonomic nervous system. The autonomic nervous system is composed of both the parasympathetic and sympathetic nervous systems. Thus, **(A)** is the right answer.

15. **C**

The dorsal root ganglion contains cell bodies of sensory neurons only. If a dorsal root ganglion is disrupted at a certain level, there will be a loss of sensation at that level. Furthermore, reflexes rely on sensory afferents that are part of the dorsal root ganglion. As a result, reflex arcs will also be affected.

GO ONLINE **Consult your online resources for additional practice.**

SHARED CONCEPTS

Behavioral Sciences Chapter 1
Biology and Behavior

Behavioral Sciences Chapter 2
Sensation and Perception

Biochemistry Chapter 3
Nonenzymatic Protein Function and Protein Analysis

Biochemistry Chapter 8
Biological Membranes

Biology Chapter 11
The Musculoskeletal System

General Chemistry Chapter 12
Electrochemistry

CHAPTER 5

THE ENDOCRINE SYSTEM

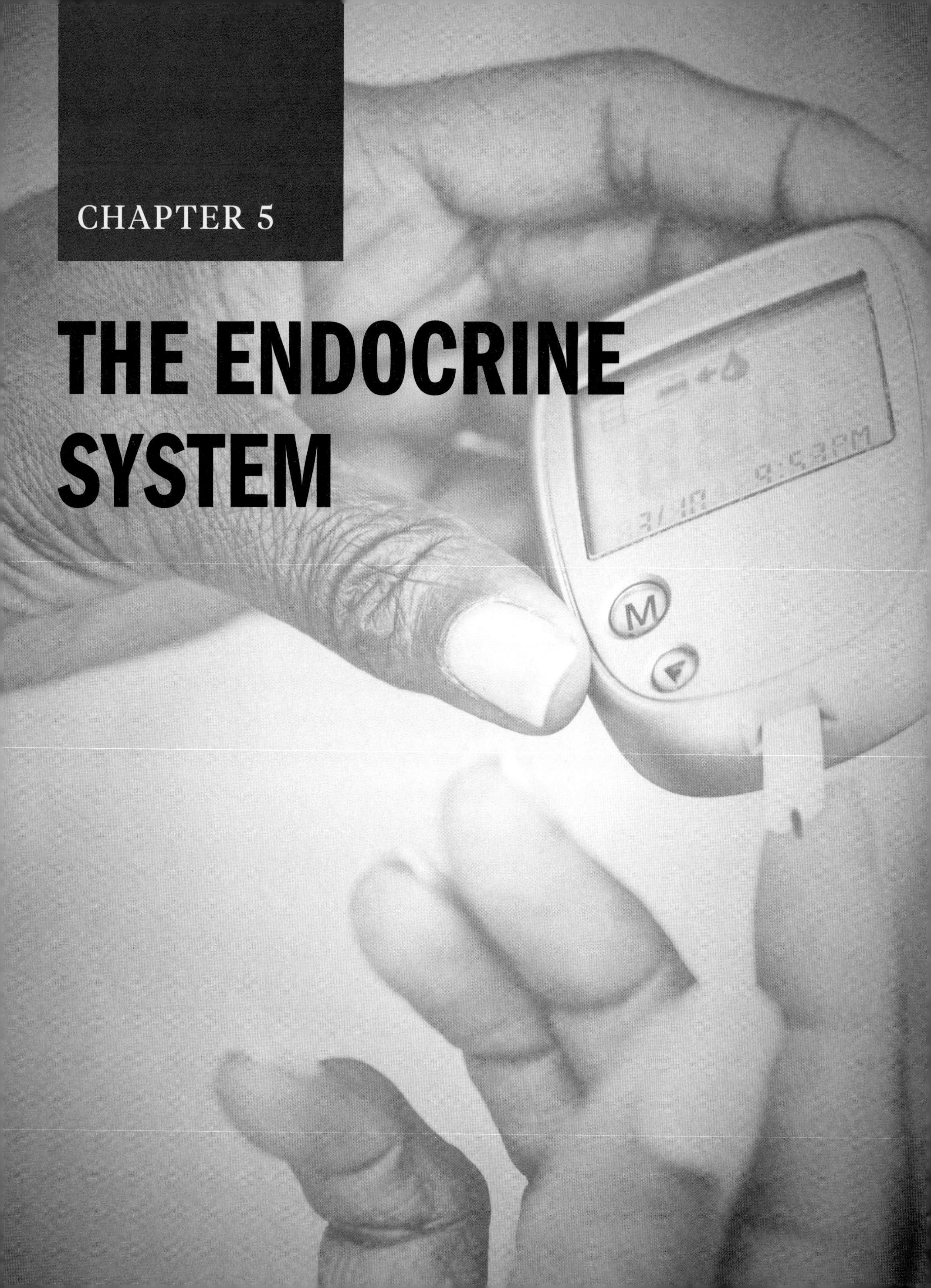

SCIENCE MASTERY ASSESSMENT

Every pre-med knows this feeling: there is so much content I have to know for the MCAT! How do I know what to do first or what's important?

While the high-yield badges throughout this book will help you identify the most important topics, this Science Mastery Assessment is another tool in your MCAT prep arsenal. This quiz (which can also be taken in your online resources) and the guidance below will help ensure that you are spending the appropriate amount of time on this chapter based on your personal strengths and weaknesses. Don't worry though—skipping something now does not mean you'll never study it. Later on in your prep, as you complete full-length tests, you'll uncover specific pieces of content that you need to review and can come back to these chapters as appropriate.

How to Use This Assessment

If you answer 0–7 questions correctly:

Spend about 1 hour to read this chapter in full and take limited notes throughout. Follow up by reviewing **all** quiz questions to ensure that you now understand how to solve each one.

If you answer 8–11 questions correctly:

Spend 20–40 minutes reviewing the quiz questions. Beginning with the questions you missed, read and take notes on the corresponding subchapters. For questions you answered correctly, ensure your thinking matches that of the explanation and you understand why each choice was correct or incorrect.

If you answer 12–15 questions correctly:

Spend less than 20 minutes reviewing all questions from the quiz. If you missed any, then include a quick read-through of the corresponding subchapters, or even just the relevant content within a subchapter, as part of your question review. For questions you answered correctly, ensure your thinking matches that of the explanation and review the Concept Summary at the end of the chapter.

1. Which of the following associations between a hormone and its category is INCORRECT?
   A. Aldosterone—mineralocorticoid
   B. Testosterone—cortical sex hormone
   C. ADH—mineralocorticoid
   D. Cortisone—glucocorticoid

2. Which of the following hormones directly stimulates a target tissue that is NOT an endocrine organ?
   A. ACTH
   B. TSH
   C. LH
   D. GH

3. Increased synthetic activity of the parathyroid glands would lead to:
   A. an increase in renal calcium reabsorption.
   B. a decrease in the rate of bone resorption.
   C. a decrease in basal metabolic rate.
   D. a decrease in blood glucose concentration.

4. Which of the following best describes the structure and mechanism of action of a peptide hormone?
   A. Cholesterol derivative that binds to a receptor on the cell surface
   B. Chain of amino acids that signals through a second messenger
   C. Chain of amino acids that directly binds to DNA to alter gene expression
   D. Cholesterol derivative that binds to an intracellular receptor and alters gene expression

5. Iodine deficiency may result in:
   A. galactorrhea.
   B. cretinism.
   C. gigantism.
   D. hyperthyroidism.

6. A patient has a very high TSH level. Which of the following would NOT cause a high TSH level?
   A. Autoimmune destruction of thyroid cells that produce T_3 and T_4
   B. A tumor in the hypothalamus that secretes high levels of TRH
   C. High levels of T_4 from thyroid replacement medications
   D. Cancerous growth of parafollicular cells in the thyroid, destroying other cell types in the organ

7. Testing of a novel hormone indicates nuclear localization and a composition of carbon, hydrogen, and oxygen. Based on these findings, how would this hormone most likely be classified?
   A. Peptide hormone
   B. Steroid hormone
   C. Amino acid derivative
   D. Direct hormone

8. Which of the following is true regarding pancreatic somatostatin?
   A. Its secretion is increased by low blood glucose.
   B. It is always inhibitory.
   C. It is regulated by cortisol levels.
   D. It stimulates insulin and glucagon secretion.

9. Destruction of all β-cells in the pancreas would cause:
   A. glucagon secretion to stop and an increase in blood glucose concentration.
   B. glucagon secretion to stop and a decrease in blood glucose concentration.
   C. insulin secretion to stop and an increase in blood glucose concentration.
   D. insulin secretion to stop and a decrease in blood glucose concentration.

10. Which of the following is FALSE regarding aldosterone regulation?

- **A.** Renin converts the plasma protein angiotensinogen to angiotensin I.
- **B.** Angiotensin II stimulates the adrenal cortex to secrete aldosterone.
- **C.** Angiotensin I is converted to angiotensin II by angiotensin-converting enzyme.
- **D.** A decrease in blood oxygen concentrations stimulates renin production.

11. A scientist discovers a new hormone that is relatively large in size and triggers the conversion of ATP to cAMP. Which of the following best describes the type of hormone that was discovered?

- **A.** Amino acid–derivative hormone
- **B.** Peptide hormone
- **C.** Steroid hormone
- **D.** Tropic hormone

12. A patient presents with muscle weakness, slow movement, and calcium deposits in some tissues. A blood test reveals very low calcium levels in the blood. Administration of which of the following would be an appropriate treatment for the blood test findings?

- **A.** Calcitonin
- **B.** Parathyroid hormone
- **C.** Aldosterone
- **D.** Thymosin

13. Oxytocin and antidiuretic hormone are:

- **A.** peptide hormones produced and released by the pituitary.
- **B.** steroid hormones produced and released by the pituitary.
- **C.** peptide hormones produced by the hypothalamus and released by the pituitary.
- **D.** steroid hormones produced by the hypothalamus and released by the pituitary.

14. Excessive levels of dopamine in the brain are associated with psychosis. Accordingly, many antipsychotic medications block dopamine receptors. Which of the following effects may be seen in an individual taking antipsychotics?

- **A.** Increased secretion of growth hormone
- **B.** Decreased secretion of growth hormone
- **C.** Increased secretion of prolactin
- **D.** Decreased secretion of prolactin

15. A genotypically female infant is born with ambiguous genitalia. Soon after birth, the infant suffers from hyponatremia, or low blood concentrations of sodium. Which endocrine organ is most likely to be affected?

- **A.** Hypothalamus
- **B.** Pituitary
- **C.** Kidneys
- **D.** Adrenal cortex

Answer Key

1. **C**
2. **D**
3. **A**
4. **B**
5. **B**
6. **C**
7. **B**
8. **B**
9. **C**
10. **D**
11. **B**
12. **B**
13. **C**
14. **C**
15. **D**

Detailed explanations can be found at the end of the chapter.

CHAPTER 5

THE ENDOCRINE SYSTEM

In This Chapter

CHAPTER PROFILE

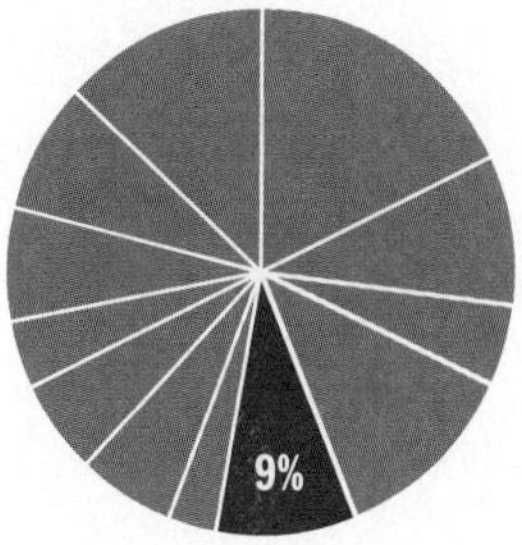

The content in this chapter should be relevant to about 9% of all questions about biology on the MCAT.

This chapter covers material from the following AAMC content categories:

3A: Structure and functions of the nervous and endocrine systems and ways in which these systems coordinate the organ systems

3B: Structure and integrative functions of the main organ systems

Introduction

The human body consists of many trillions of cells that must work together to sustain life. In order to work effectively, fuel resources must be conserved or used appropriately, such as when responding to stressful situations. In addition, organs must be able to communicate with the brain to cause changes in behavior and physiology to maintain homeostasis. As the messengers in the endocrine system, hormones play an essential role in this communication. For example, the pancreas produces insulin and glucagon. Insulin induces the transport of glucose into organs and the storage of excess glucose when blood glucose concentrations are high. Conversely, glucagon triggers the release of sugar stores which raises blood glucose concentration. Working together, these hormones ensure that there are adequate levels of glucose for organ function, but that glucose levels are not so high as to cause damage to organ systems.

Diabetes mellitus is one of the most common diseases in the United States and a major cause of morbidity and mortality. Type 1 diabetes mellitus is an autoimmune disease in which insulin-producing cells in the islets of Langerhans are destroyed. Type 2 diabetes mellitus is caused by end-organ insensitivity to insulin. In both cases, blood glucose concentrations rise to dangerous levels (sometimes up to ten times the normal concentration), which can cause significant damage to organs, including the retina of the eye, the glomeruli of the kidneys, the coronary vessels of the heart and cerebral vessels of the brain, and peripheral nerves. Left untreated (or, to be frank, even if treated in many cases), diabetes can lead to blindness, kidney failure, heart attacks, strokes, and limb amputations. Regardless of the field you enter, you will spend a significant amount of time working with diabetic patients and will have to think about the effects of this disease on other conditions and their treatment.

In this chapter, we will explore the different types of hormones and how they work. We'll survey the various endocrine organs and discuss the hormones each one produces. This is an extremely high-yield chapter: the MCAT frequently tests not only the makeup of the endocrine system (hormones and their functions), but also the processes of the endocrine system (feedback loops and their regulation). Return to this chapter frequently; a thorough knowledge of this system will definitely pay off on Test Day.

5.1 Mechanisms of Hormone Action

High-Yield

LEARNING OBJECTIVES

After Chapter 5.1, you will be able to:

- Compare and contrast the traits and actions of peptide *vs.* steroid hormones
- Recall the process for synthesizing amino acid–derivative hormones
- Distinguish between direct and tropic hormones

The endocrine system consists of organs, known as **glands**, that secrete hormones. **Hormones** are signaling molecules that are secreted directly into the bloodstream to distant target tissues At target tissues, hormones bind to receptors, inducing a change in gene expression or cellular functioning. Not all hormones share the same structure and function. In order to understand how each hormone functions, it is first important to understand basic hormone structure.

Classification of Hormones by Chemical Structure

Hormones can be subdivided into categories based on different criteria. First, hormones can be classified by their chemical identities. Hormones can be **peptides**, **steroids**, or **amino acid derivatives**.

Peptide Hormones

Peptide hormones are made up of amino acids, ranging in size from quite small (such as anti-diuretic hormone, ADH) to relatively large (such as insulin). Peptide hormones are all derived from larger precursor polypeptides that are cleaved during posttranslational modification. These smaller units are transported to the Golgi apparatus for further modifications that activate the hormones and direct them to the correct locations in the cell. Such hormones are released by exocytosis after being packaged into vesicles.

Because peptide hormones are charged and cannot pass through the plasma membrane, they must bind to an extracellular receptor. The peptide hormone is considered the **first messenger**; it binds to the receptor and triggers the transmission of a second signal, known as the **second messenger**. There are many different receptor subtypes, and the type of receptor determines what happens once the hormone has stimulated the receptor.

The connection between the hormone at the surface and the effect brought about by second messengers within the cell is known as a **signaling cascade**. At each step, there is the possibility of **amplification**. For example, one hormone molecule may bind to multiple receptors before it is degraded. Also, each receptor may activate multiple enzymes, each of which will trigger the production of large quantities of second messengers. Thus, each step can result in an increase in signal intensity. Some common second messengers are **cyclic adenosine monophosphate (cAMP)**, **inositol triphosphate (IP_3)**, and calcium. The activation of a G protein–coupled receptor is shown in Figure 5.1. In this system, the binding of a peptide hormone triggers the receptor to either activate or inhibit an enzyme called ***adenylate cyclase***, raising or lowering the levels of cAMP accordingly. cAMP can bind to intracellular targets, such as *protein kinase A*, which phosphorylates transcription factors like cAMP response element-binding protein (CREB) to exert the hormone's ultimate effect. Keep in mind that protein kinase A can modify other enzymes as well as transcription factors, and therefore it can have a rapid or slow effect on the cell.

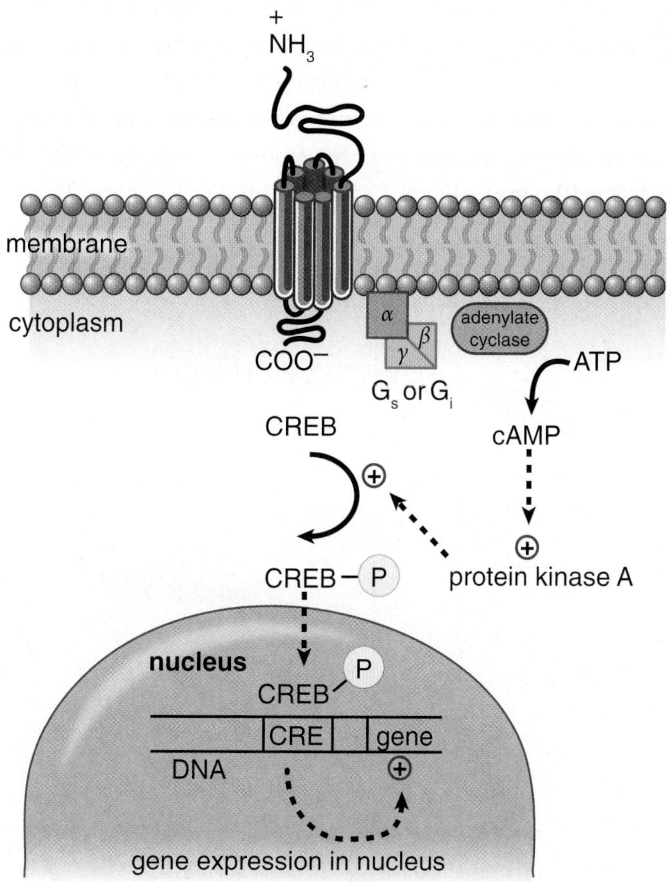

Figure 5.1 Mechanism of Action of a Peptide Hormone

Peptide hormones bind to membrane-bound receptors to intiate a signal cascade, using second messengers like cAMP.

The effects of peptide hormones are usually rapid but short lived because these hormones act through second messenger cascades, which are transient. It is quicker to turn them on and off, compared with steroid hormones, but their effects do not last without relatively constant stimulation.

Because peptides are generally water-soluble, peptide hormones can travel freely in the bloodstream and usually do not require carriers. This is in stark contrast to steroid hormones, which are lipid-soluble.

KEY CONCEPT

Peptide hormones have surface receptors and act via second messenger systems. Steroid hormones bind to intracellular receptors and function by binding to DNA to alter gene transcription.

Steroid Hormones

Steroid hormones are derived from cholesterol and are produced primarily by the gonads and adrenal cortex. Because steroid hormones are derived from nonpolar molecules, they can easily cross the cell membrane. Hence, their receptors are usually intracellular (in the cytosol) or intranuclear (in the nucleus). Upon binding to the receptor, steroid hormone–receptor complexes undergo conformational changes. The receptor can then bind directly to DNA, resulting in either increased or decreased transcription of particular genes, depending on the identity of the hormone, as shown in Figure 5.2. One common form of conformational change is **dimerization**, or pairing of two receptor–hormone complexes. The effects of steroid hormones are slower but longer lived than peptide hormones because steroid hormones participate in gene regulation, causing alterations in the amount of mRNA and protein present in a cell by direct action on DNA.

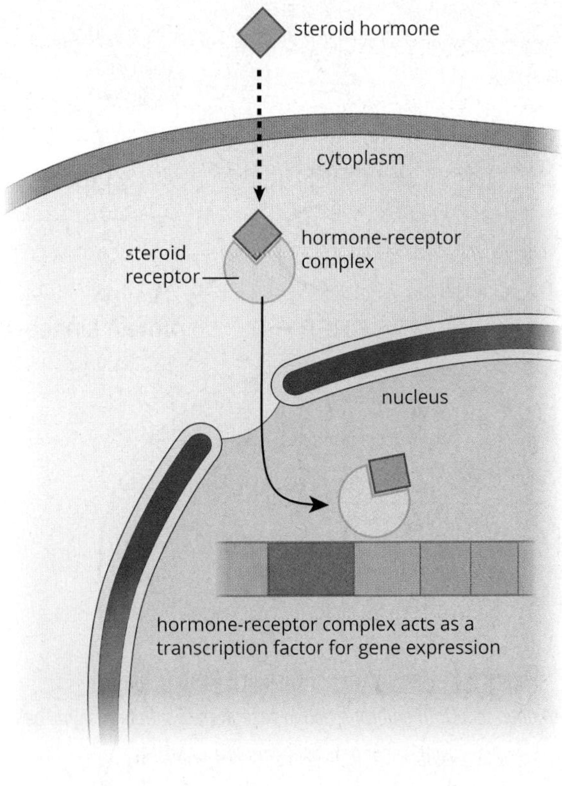

Figure 5.2 Mechanism of Action of a Steroid Hormone
Steroid hormones influence cell behavior by modifying transcription.

Steroid hormones are not water-soluble, so they must be carried by proteins in the bloodstream to travel around the body. Some of these proteins are very specific and carry only one hormone (such as *sex hormone-binding globulin*), while other proteins are nonspecific (such as ***albumin***). Note that hormones are generally inactive while attached to a carrier protein and must dissociate from the carrier to function. Therefore, levels of carrier proteins can change the levels of *active* hormone. For example, some conditions increase the quantity of a protein that carries thyroid hormones, *thyroxine-binding globulin* (TBG). This causes the body to perceive a lower level of thyroid hormone because the increased quantity of TBG binds a larger proportion of the hormone, meaning there is less free hormone available.

Amino Acid-Derivative Hormones

Finally, **amino acid–derivative hormones** are less common than peptide and steroid hormones, but include some of the most important hormones discussed in this chapter, including epinephrine, norepinephrine, triiodothyronine, and thyroxine. These hormones are derived from one or two amino acids, usually with a few additional modifications. For example, thyroid hormones are made from tyrosine modified by the addition of several iodine atoms.

The chemistry of this family of hormones is considerably less predictable and is one of the few instances where overt memorization may be the best strategy. For instance, the **catecholamines** (epinephrine and norepinephrine) bind to G protein–coupled receptors, while thyroid hormones bind intracellularly.

Classification of Hormones by Target Tissue

Some hormones, known as **direct hormones**, are secreted and then act directly on a target tissue. For example, insulin released by the pancreas causes increased uptake of glucose by muscles. Other hormones, known as **tropic hormones**, require an intermediary to act. For example, as discussed in Chapter 2 of *MCAT Biology Review*, gonadotropin-releasing hormone (GnRH) from the hypothalamus stimulates the release of luteinizing hormone (LH) and follicle-stimulating hormone (FSH). LH then acts on the gonads to stimulate testosterone production in males and estrogen production in females. GnRH and LH do not cause direct changes in the physiology of muscle, bone, and hair follicles; rather, they stimulate the production of another hormone by another endocrine gland that acts on these target tissues. Tropic hormones usually originate in the brain and anterior pituitary gland, allowing for the coordination of multiple processes within the body.

MNEMONIC

Insulin is a peptide hormone, and it has to be released at every meal in order to be active. Thus, it has fast onset but is short-acting (like most peptide hormones). Estrogen and testosterone are steroid hormones that promote sexual maturation. This is a slower, but longer-lasting change (as is true for most steroid hormones).

REAL WORLD

During pregnancy, high levels of estrogen and progesterone cause increased production of TBG, thyroxine-binding globulin. In order to compensate, people who are pregnant secrete much higher levels of the thyroid hormones. Thus, in order to diagnose thyroid disease during pregnancy, different reference values must be used.

MCAT EXPERTISE

The mechanism of action of the amino acid–derivative hormones should be memorized because it is so unpredictable. Epinephrine and norepinephrine have extremely fast onset but are short-lived, like peptide hormones—think of an *adrenaline rush*. Thyroxine and triiodothyronine, on the other hand, have slower onset but a longer duration, like steroid hormones—they regulate metabolic rate over a long period of time.

MNEMONIC

Most peptide and amino acid–derivative hormones have names that end in ***-in*** or ***-ine*** (insul***in***, vasopress***in***, thyrox***ine***, triiodothyron***ine***, and so on). Most steroid hormones have names that end in ***-one***, ***-ol***, or ***-oid*** (testoster***one***, aldoster***one*** and other mineralocortic***oid***s, cortis***ol*** and other glucocortic***oid***s, and so on). This is not exhaustive, but may help you identify the chemistry of a hormone on Test Day.

MCAT CONCEPT CHECK 5.1

Before you move on, assess your understanding of the material with these questions.

1. Compare and contrast peptide and steroid hormones based on the following criteria:

Criterion	Peptide Hormones	Steroid Hormones
Chemical precursor		
Location of receptor		
Mechanism of action		
Method of travel in the bloodstream		
Speed of onset		
Duration of action		

2. How are amino acid–derivative hormones synthesized?

____

3. What is the difference between a direct and a tropic hormone?

   - Direct hormone:

____

   - Tropic hormone:

____

5.2 Endocrine Organs and Hormones

High-Yield

LEARNING OBJECTIVES

After Chapter 5.2, you will be able to:

- Recall the hormones involved in calcium homeostasis and their impact on blood calcium
- Identify the tissue that synthesizes catecholamines and the major catecholamines it produces
- List the pancreatic hormones, their regulators, and their impact on blood glucose concentration
- Recall details about the hormones involved in water homeostasis, including their production, action, and ultimate impact on blood volume and osmolarity
- Recall the releasing hormones produced by the hypothalamus, their pituitary targets, and the end result of each signaling pathway on the final target organ:

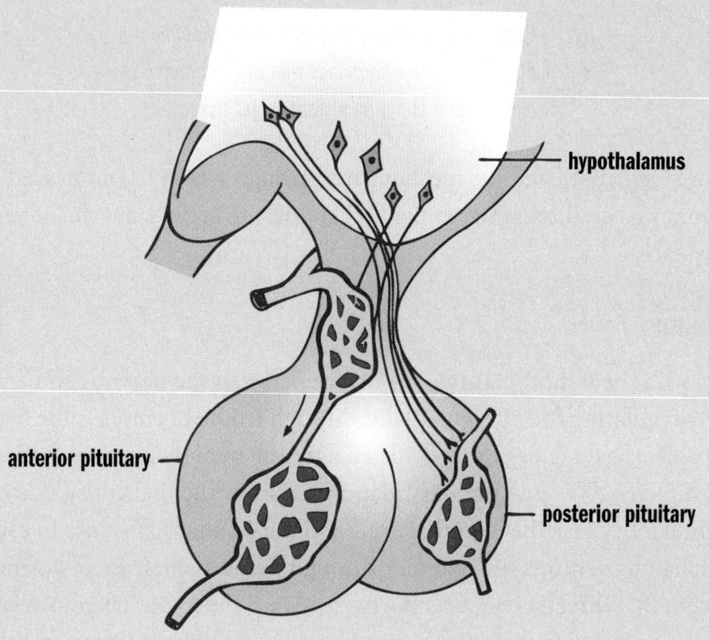

The hypothalamus, the pituitary, the thyroid, the parathyroid glands, the adrenal glands, the pancreas, the gonads (testes and ovaries), and the pineal gland are all endocrine glands, as shown in Figure 5.3. Each of these organs is capable of synthesizing and secreting one or more hormones. Furthermore, there are collections of cells within organs, such as the kidneys, gastrointestinal glands, heart, and thymus, that serve important endocrine roles. The organs in this second group are traditionally not called endocrine organs because hormone production is not their main function.

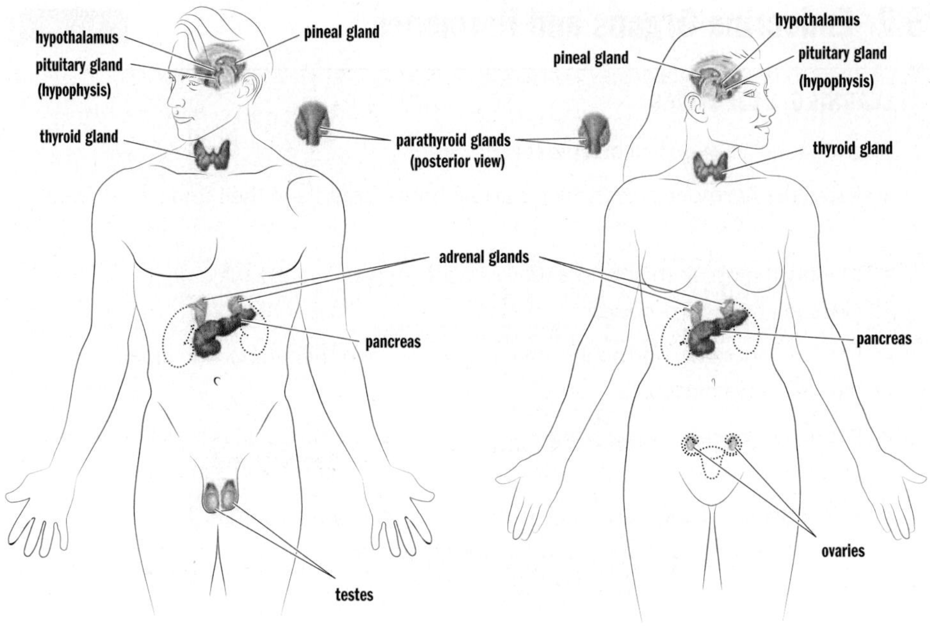

Figure 5.3 Organs of the Endocrine System
Endocrine organs produce hormones that are secreted into the bloodstream to act on distant target tissues.

Now that we have discussed the mechanisms through which hormones act and their classification, we can discuss the individual endocrine organs and the hormones secreted by each.

BRIDGE

The hypothalamus contains a number of nuclei in its three sections, called the lateral, ventromedial, and anterior hypothalamus. These nuclei play roles in emotional experience, aggressive behavior, sexual behavior, metabolism, temperature regulation, and water balance. The parts of the hypothalamus are discussed in Chapter 1 of *MCAT Behavioral Sciences Review*.

Hypothalamus

Let's begin with the **hypothalamus**, the bridge between the nervous and endocrine systems. By regulating the pituitary gland through tropic hormones, the hypothalamus is capable of having organism-wide effects. The hypothalamus is located in the forebrain, directly above the pituitary gland and below the thalamus (hence the name *hypo*thalamus). Because the hypothalamus and the pituitary are close to each other, the hypothalamus controls the pituitary through paracrine release of hormones into a portal system that directly connects the two organs. The hypothalamus receives input from a wide variety of sources. For example, a part of the hypothalamus called the *suprachiasmatic nucleus* receives some of the light input from the retinae and helps to control sleep–wake cycles. Other parts of the hypothalamus respond to increases in blood osmolarity. Still other parts of the hypothalamus regulate appetite and satiety.

The release of hormones by the hypothalamus is regulated by negative feedback. **Negative feedback** occurs when a hormone (or product) later in the pathway inhibits hormones (or enzymes) earlier in the pathway. This type of feedback maintains homeostasis and conserves energy by restricting production of substances that are already present in sufficient quantities. The hypothalamus and pituitary gland are inextricably linked. The pituitary gland has an anterior and posterior component, each with a unique interaction with the hypothalamus. We will discuss each in turn.

Interactions with the Anterior Pituitary

The hypothalamus secretes compounds into the **hypophyseal portal system**, which is a blood vessel system that directly connects the hypothalamus with the anterior pituitary, as shown in Figure 5.4. Thus, hormones released from the hypothalamus travel directly to the anterior pituitary and cannot be found in appreciable concentrations in the systemic circulation. Note that **hypophysis** is an alternative term for the pituitary. Once hormones have been released from the hypothalamus into this portal bloodstream, they travel down the pituitary stalk and bind to receptors in the anterior pituitary, stimulating the release of other hormones.

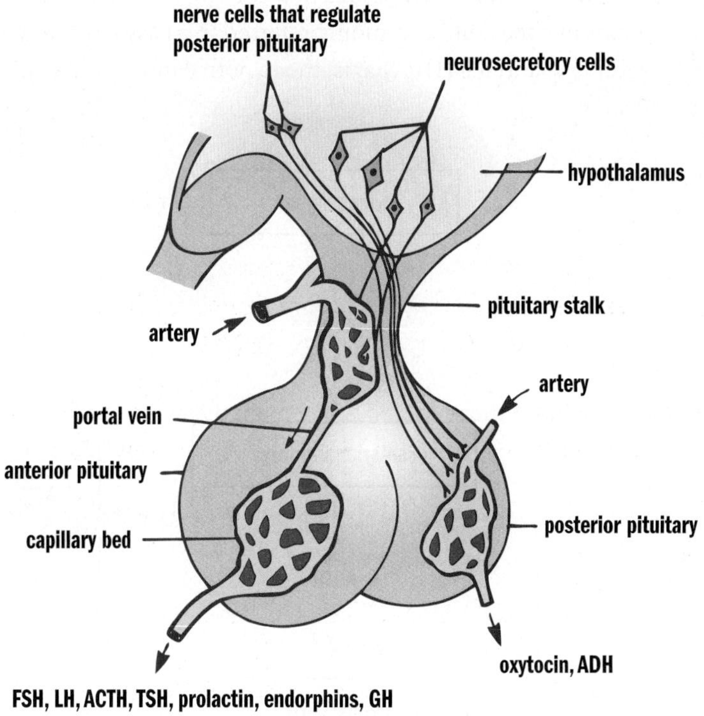

Figure 5.4 The Hypophyseal Portal System
A system of blood vessels connects the hypothalamus to the pituitary.

The hypothalamus secretes several different tropic hormones. The following indicates each hormone released by the hypothalamus and the hormone(s) released by the anterior pituitary in response:

- Gonadotropin-releasing hormone (GnRH) → follicle-stimulating hormone (FSH) and luteinizing hormone (LH)
- Growth hormone–releasing hormone (GHRH) → growth hormone (GH)
- Thyroid-releasing hormone (TRH) → thyroid-stimulating hormone (TSH)
- Corticotropin-releasing factor (CRF) → adrenocorticotropic hormone (ACTH)

There is one exception to this pattern—prolactin-inhibiting factor (PIF), which is actually dopamine, is released by the hypothalamus and causes a *decrease* in prolactin secretion.

KEY CONCEPT

Although it seems as if the anterior pituitary has all the power in the endocrine system, it is controlled by the hypothalamus, which is located directly above it.

KEY CONCEPT

Whereas most of the hormones in the anterior pituitary require a factor from the hypothalamus to be released, prolactin is the exception. As long as the hypothalamus releases PIF (which is actually dopamine), no prolactin will be released. It is the *absence* of PIF that allows prolactin to be released.

Each of the tropic hormones then causes the release of another hormone from an endocrine gland that has negative feedback effects. For example, release of CRF from the hypothalamus will stimulate the anterior pituitary to secrete ACTH. ACTH will then cause the adrenal cortex to increase the level of **cortisol** being secreted into the blood. However, cortisol is detrimental when levels become too high. To prevent excess cortisol secretion, cortisol inhibits the hypothalamus and anterior pituitary from releasing CRF and ACTH, respectively, as shown in Figure 5.5. This makes sense because CRF and ACTH have already accomplished their desired effect: getting more cortisol into the blood. What does this mean in terms of receptors in the hypothalamus and pituitary? Cortisol receptors must be present in these organs; otherwise, they wouldn't be able to recognize that cortisol levels had increased. Three-organ systems like these are commonly referred to as **axes**; for example, the hypothalamic–pituitary–adrenal (HPA) axis, the hypothalamic–pituitary–ovarian (HPO) axis, and so on.

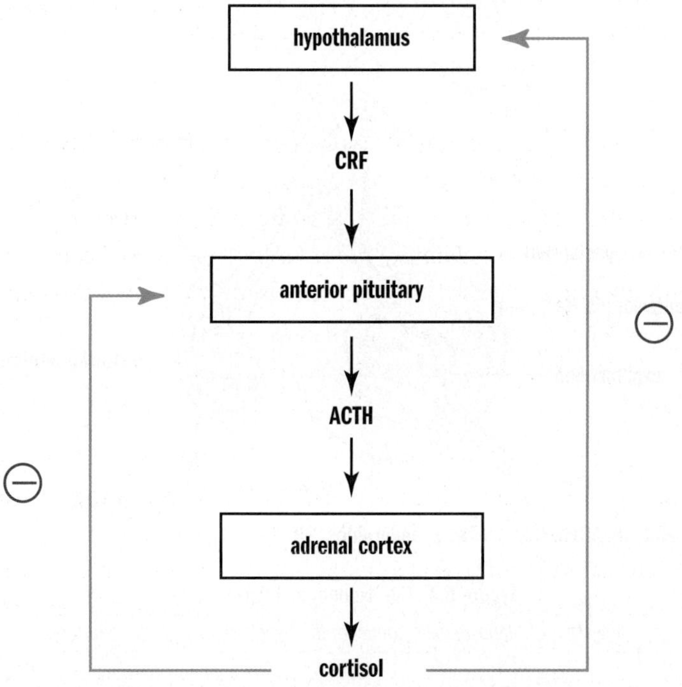

Figure 5.5 Hypothalamic Negative Feedback Mechanism

Interactions with the Posterior Pituitary

The posterior pituitary does not receive tropic hormones through the hypophyseal portal system. Rather, neurons in the hypothalamus send their axons down the pituitary stalk directly into the posterior pituitary, which can then release oxytocin and antidiuretic hormone. **Oxytocin** stimulates uterine contractions during labor, as well as milk letdown during lactation. There is evidence that oxytocin is also involved in bonding behavior. **Antidiuretic hormone** (**ADH**, also called **vasopressin**) increases reabsorption of water in the collecting ducts of the kidneys. ADH is secreted in response to increased plasma osmolarity, or increased concentration of solutes within the blood.

Anterior Pituitary

As described earlier, the pituitary gland is divided into anterior and posterior sections. Because this distinction has already been covered, our discussion of the pituitary gland here will focus on the hormones released by each section.

The **anterior pituitary** synthesizes and secretes seven different products. Four of these are tropic hormones, while the other three are direct hormones.

Tropic Hormones

We are going to mention the tropic hormones only briefly here. These hormones work by causing the release of another hormone at the organ level. Thus, we will discuss the tropic hormones in tandem with the endocrine organ on which they act. The release of both follicle-stimulating hormone (FSH) and luteinizing hormone (LH) is stimulated by gonadotropin-releasing hormone (GnRH) from the hypothalamus. These two hormones act on the gonads (testes and ovaries). The release of adrenocorticotropic hormone (ACTH) is stimulated by corticotropin-releasing factor (CRF) from the hypothalamus; ACTH acts on the adrenal cortex. The release of thyroid-stimulating hormone (TSH) is stimulated by thyroid-releasing hormone (TRH) from the hypothalamus; TSH acts on the thyroid.

Direct Hormones

Prolactin is more important in females than in males; it stimulates milk production in the **mammary glands**. Milk production in the male is always pathologic. During pregnancy, estrogen and progesterone levels are high. In addition, prolactin, a hormone that increases milk production, is also secreted by the anterior pituitary. Prolactin is an unusual hormone in that the release of dopamine from the hypothalamus *decreases* its secretion. The high levels of estrogen and progesterone allow for the development of milk ducts in preparation for lactation, but it is not until shortly after the expulsion of the placenta, when estrogen, progesterone, and dopamine levels drop, that the block on milk production is removed and lactation actually begins.

Milk ejection occurs when the newborn infant latches on to the breast. Nipple stimulation causes activation of the hypothalamus, resulting in two different reactions. First, oxytocin is released from the posterior pituitary, resulting in contraction of the smooth muscle of the breast and ejection of milk through the nipple. Second, the hypothalamus stops releasing dopamine onto the anterior pituitary, which allows prolactin release, causing production of milk and regulation of the milk supply.

REAL WORLD

A tumor of the pituitary gland may result in compression of the portal system that connects the pituitary to the hypothalamus. This will block the ability of PIF to reach the pituitary and exert its effect. Thus, more prolactin will be released. This may result in lactation (galactorrhea), even in males. Thus, milk production in a male or nonpregnant female should lead a physician to suspect the presence of a pituitary tumor.

MNEMONIC

Products of the anterior pituitary:

FLAT PEG

- **F**ollicle-stimulating hormone (FSH)
- **L**uteinizing hormone (LH)
- **A**drenocorticotropic hormone (ACTH)
- **T**hyroid-stimulating hormone (TSH)
- **P**rolactin
- **E**ndorphins
- **G**rowth hormone (GH)

Additionally, the four hormones in **FLAT** are all tropic hormones, while the three hormones in **PEG** are all direct hormones.

Endorphins decrease the perception of pain. For example, after completing a marathon, many people will say they are on an endorphin "high" or "rush." Endorphins mask the pain from having run 26.2 miles and can even induce a sense of euphoria. Many pharmaceutical agents, such as morphine, mimic the effect of these naturally occurring painkillers.

Growth hormone (**GH**) is named for exactly what it does: it promotes the growth of bone and muscle. This sort of growth is energetically expensive and requires large quantities of glucose. Growth hormone prevents glucose uptake in certain tissues (those that are not growing) and stimulates the breakdown of fatty acids. This increases the availability of glucose overall, allowing muscle and bone to use it. GH release is stimulated by growth hormone–releasing hormone (GHRH) from the hypothalamus.

Bone growth originates in special regions of the bone known as epiphyseal plates, which seal shut during puberty. An excess of GH released in childhood (before this closure) can cause **gigantism**, and a deficit results in **dwarfism**. In adults, the situation is slightly different. Because the long bones are sealed, GH still has an effect, but it is primarily in the smaller bones. The resulting medical condition is known as **acromegaly**. The bones most commonly affected are those in the hands, feet, and head. Patients with acromegaly tend to seek medical help because they have had to buy larger shoes, cannot wear their rings, and can no longer fit into their hats.

Posterior Pituitary

The **posterior pituitary** contains the nerve terminals of neurons with cell bodies in the hypothalamus. As mentioned earlier, the posterior pituitary receives and stores two hormones produced by the hypothalamus: ADH and oxytocin.

ADH is secreted in response to low blood volume (as sensed by baroreceptors) or increased blood osmolarity (as sensed by osmoreceptors), shown in Figure 5.6. Its action is at the level of the collecting duct, where it increases the permeability of the duct to water. This increases the reabsorption of water from the filtrate in the nephron. This results in greater retention of water, which results in increased blood volume and higher blood pressure.

Oxytocin is secreted during childbirth and allows for coordinated contraction of uterine smooth muscle. Its secretion may also be stimulated by suckling, as it promotes milk ejection through contraction of smooth muscle in the breast. Finally, oxytocin may be involved in bonding behavior. Oxytocin is unusual in that it has a **positive feedback** loop: the release of oxytocin promotes uterine contraction, which promotes more oxytocin release, which promotes stronger uterine contractions, and so on. Positive feedback loops can usually be identified by a "spiraling forward" scheme and usually have a definitive endpoint—in this case, delivery.

KEY CONCEPT

The two hormones released from the posterior pituitary are actually synthesized in the hypothalamus and simply released from the posterior pituitary gland. The posterior pituitary does not synthesize any hormones itself.

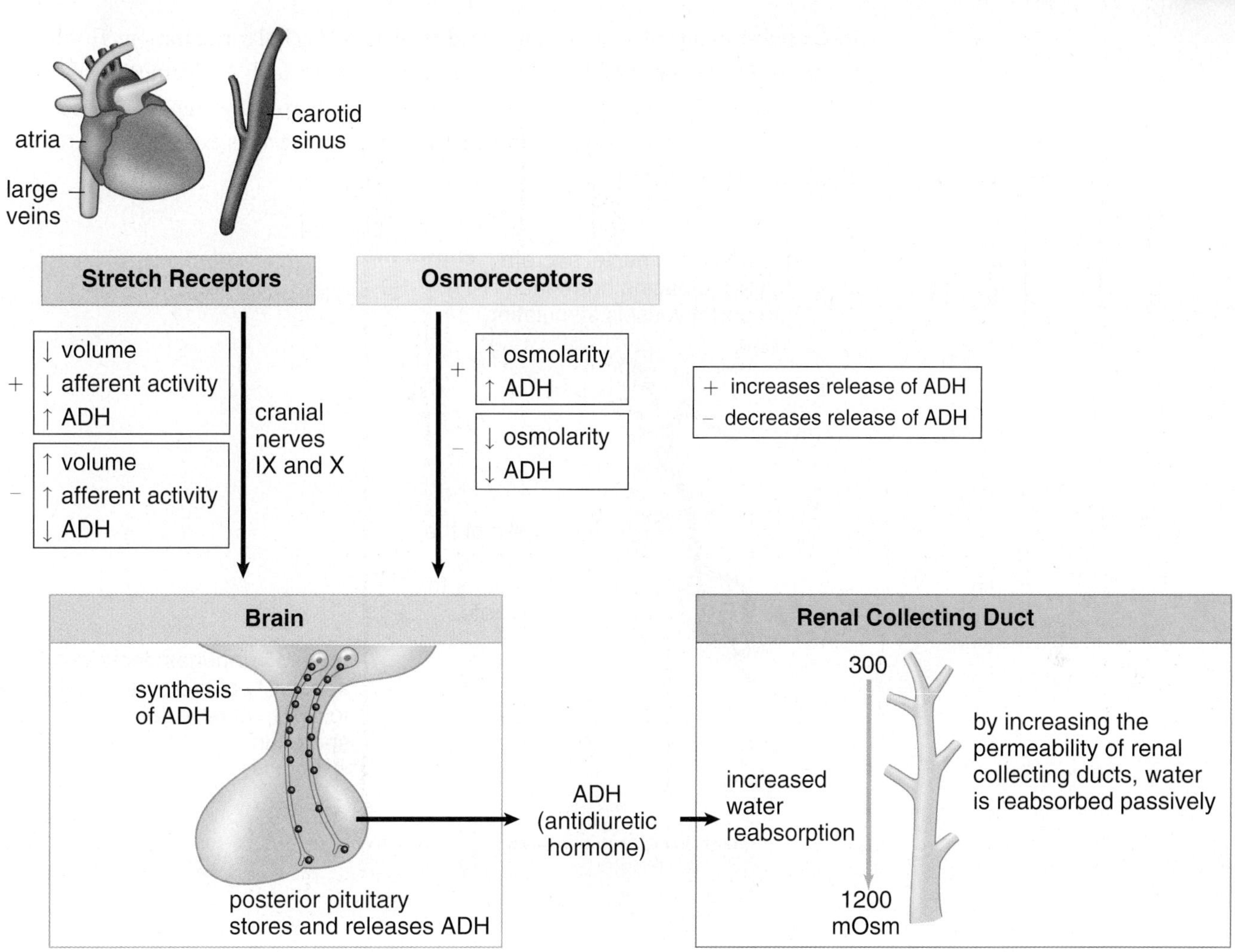

Figure 5.6 Antidiuretic Hormone (ADH)

Thyroid

The **thyroid** is controlled by **thyroid-stimulating hormone** from the anterior pituitary. The thyroid is on the front surface of the trachea; it can be palpated (felt) as an organ near the base of the neck that moves up and down with swallowing. The thyroid has two major functions: setting basal metabolic rate and promoting calcium homeostasis. It mediates the first effect by releasing triiodothyronine (T_3) and thyroxine (T_4), while it carries out the second effect through the release of calcitonin.

Triiodothyronine and Thyroxine

Triiodothyronine (T_3) and **thyroxine** (T_4) are both produced by the iodination of the amino acid tyrosine in the **follicular cells** of the thyroid. The numbers 3 and 4 refer to the number of iodine atoms attached to the tyrosine. Thyroid hormones are capable of resetting the basal metabolic rate of the body by making energy production more or less efficient, as well as altering the utilization of glucose and fatty acids.

Increased amounts of T_3 and T_4 will lead to increased cellular respiration. This leads to increased protein and fatty acid turnover by speeding up both synthesis and degradation of these compounds. High plasma levels of thyroid hormones will lead to decreased TSH and TRH synthesis; negative feedback prevents excessive secretion of T_3 and T_4, as shown in Figure 5.7.

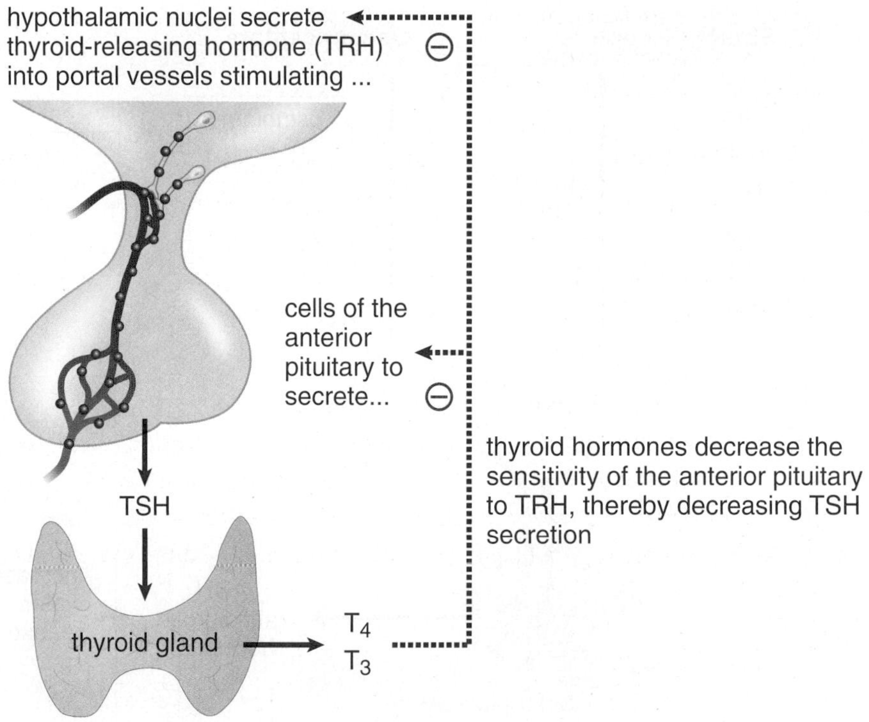

Figure 5.7 Thyroid Hormone Negative Feedback Mechanism

A deficiency of iodine or inflammation of the thyroid may result in **hypothyroidism**, in which thyroid hormones are secreted in insufficient amounts or not at all. The condition is characterized by lethargy, decreased body temperature, slowed respiratory and heart rate, cold intolerance, and weight gain. Thyroid hormones are required for appropriate neurological and physical development in children. Most children are tested at birth for appropriate levels because a deficiency will result in intellectual disability and developmental delay (**cretinism**).

An excess of thyroid hormone, which may result from a tumor or thyroid overstimulation, is called **hyperthyroidism**. We can predict the clinical course of this syndrome by considering the opposite of each of the effects seen in hypothyroidism: heightened activity level, increased body temperature, increased respiratory and heart rate, heat intolerance, and weight loss.

Calcitonin

If we were to examine thyroid tissue under a light microscope, we would see two distinct cell populations within the gland. Follicular cells produce thyroid hormones and **C-cells** (also called **parafollicular cells**) produce **calcitonin**.

MNEMONIC

Calci**ton**in **ton**es down calcium levels in the blood.

Calcitonin decreases plasma calcium levels in three ways: by increasing calcium excretion from the kidneys, by decreasing calcium absorption from the gut, and by increasing storage of calcium in the bone. High levels of calcium in the blood stimulate secretion of calcitonin from the C-cells.

Parathyroid Glands

The parathyroids are four small pea-sized structures that sit on the posterior surface of the thyroid. The hormone produced by the parathyroid glands is aptly named **parathyroid hormone** (**PTH**). PTH serves as an antagonistic hormone to calcitonin, raising blood calcium levels; specifically, it decreases excretion of calcium by the kidneys, increases absorption of calcium in the gut (via vitamin D), and increases bone resorption, thereby freeing up calcium, as shown in Figure 5.8. Like the hormones we have already seen, PTH is also subject to feedback inhibition. As levels of plasma calcium rise, PTH secretion is decreased. Parathyroid hormone also promotes phosphorus homeostasis by increasing the resorption of phosphate from bone and reducing reabsorption of phosphate in the kidney (thus promoting its excretion in the urine).

PTH also activates **vitamin D**, which is required for the absorption of calcium and phosphate in the gut. The overall effect of parathyroid hormone, therefore, is a significant increase in blood calcium levels with little effect on phosphate (the absorption of phosphate in the gut and its excretion in the kidney somewhat cancel each other).

KEY CONCEPT

Calcium is an exceptionally important ion. The critically important functions of calcium include:

- Bone structure and strength
- Release of neurotransmitters from neurons
- Regulation of muscle contraction
- Clotting of blood (calcium is a cofactor)

In addition, calcium also plays a role in cell movement and exocytosis of cellular materials.

KEY CONCEPT

Just like glucagon and insulin, PTH and calcitonin are antagonistic to each other. We should think of these hormones as a pair with the primary function of regulating calcium levels in the blood. PTH increases serum calcium levels, whereas calcitonin decreases calcium levels.

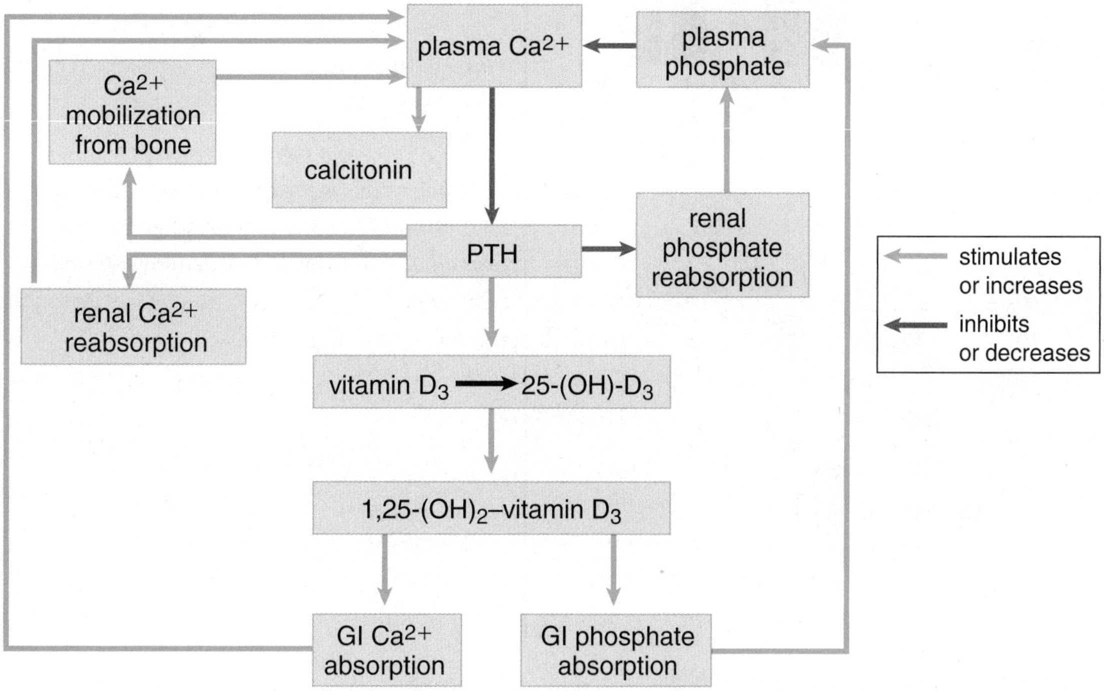

Figure 5.8 Calcium and Phosphorus Homeostasis

BIOLOGY GUIDED EXAMPLE WITH EXPERT THINKING

Patients with mutations of the THRA (thyroid hormone receptor alpha) gene exhibit classical features of hypothyroidism. Researchers created a mouse expressing a mutated TRα1 (denoted as PV; Thra1PV/+ mouse) that faithfully reproduces the classical hypothyroidism seen in patients. TRα1PV is a dominant negative mutant and cannot bind T3. Researchers then rendered Thra1PV/+ mice hypothyroidic by treating them with propylthiouracil (PTU). PTU is a medication used to treat hyperthyroidism by inhibiting the enzyme thyroperoxidase. PTU-treated mice were then treated with T3 to induce symptoms of hyperthyroidism. Results are summarized in Figure 1. These findings are consistent with earlier reports that the feedback loop in the pituitary-thyroid axis is not affected by expressing TRα1PV mutant in Thra1PV/+ mice.

Topic: hypothyroidism; some outside knowledge of the endocrine system might be necessary

Specific mutation of THRA cannot bind T3 and mice with mutation have hypothyroidism

PTU: medicine to treat hyperthryoidism, used to induce hypothyroidism in these mice

Findings are consistent with idea that the feedback loop is not affected

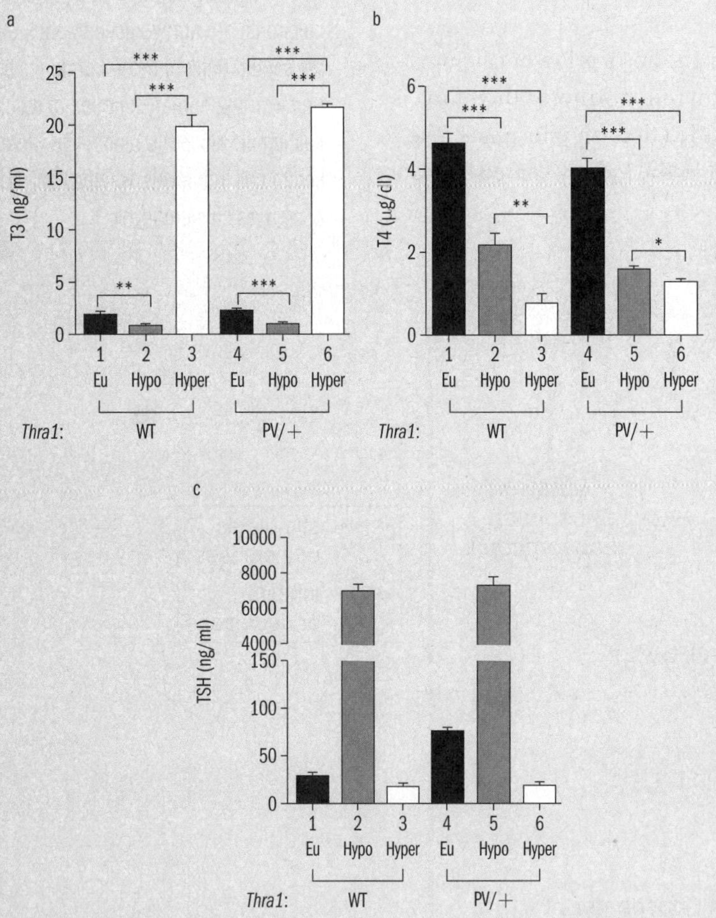

Figure 1 Thyroid experiment results. Eu = euthyroid condition.

IVs: Eu, Hypo, Hyper

DVs: T3, T4, TSH

Trends: Euthryoid means the thyroid is kept normal, so this is the control. The changes in T3, T4, and TSH are pretty consistent for each condition (Eu, Hypo, Hyper) between WT and PV/+ mice.

Adapted from Park, S., Han, C. R., Park, J. W., Zhao, L., Zhu, X., Willingham, M., ... Cheng, S. Y. (2017). Defective erythropoiesis caused by mutations of the thyroid hormone receptor α gene. *PLoS Genetics*, 13(9), e1006991. doi:10.1371/journal.pgen.1006991.

Why are TSH levels elevated in mice given propylthiouracil (PTU)?

A question like this is asking us to explain the underlying biological cause for an observed phenomenon. The MCAT often tests our ability to reason with a concept or mechanism that we are already familiar with. For this question, the stated change to the system is "propylthiouracil" and the effect observed is "elevated TSH levels". It is now our job to determine how the two are related.

First, we'll want to identify what information we'll need, both from the passage and from our science background. MCAT questions will often intentionally include terms that we aren't familiar with. The key to answering these questions, even if we're not familiar with the phenomenon described, is finding the relevant information from the passage and using that information in conjunction with our scientific understanding to solve the problem. We already identified the change to the system in this question as the application of PTU. According to the passage, PTU is a medication that inhibits thyroperoxidase and it is used to treat hyperthyroidism. In the experiment, they used PTU to "render[ed] Thra1PV/+ mice hypothyroidic". If we look to Figure 1A, we can see that in the T3 and T4 graphs, the hypothyroid (gray) bar is significantly smaller than the euthyroid (black) bar. If we weren't sure what euthyroid referred to, we could infer that, given that the other two categories in each graph are hypothyroid and hyperthyroid, this must be wild-type or normal function. Based on these data and the context from the passage, it is reasonable to infer that PTU is a drug that functions by lowering the production of thyroid hormone (T3 and T4).

Now we must consider how having low thyroid hormones would be related to elevated TSH levels. TSH is a tropic hormone released from the anterior pituitary, and it is regulated by a negative feedback mechanism involving thyroid hormone. Specifically, we should know that the hypothalamus releases thyroid-releasing hormone (TRH), which causes the anterior pituitary to release thyroid-stimulating hormone (TSH). TSH acts upon the thyroid to stimulate the release of thyroid hormone triiodothyronine (T3) and thyroxine (T4). T3 and T4 then act as negative feedback on the hypothalamus and the pituitary gland, lowering TRH and TSH levels. We can reason that, if T3 and T4 levels were low, TRH and TSH would be continuously produced, as they would not be inhibited by the presence of T3 and T4.

The mice in the experiment have normally functioning endocrine glands prior to treatment. We can always assume this to be the case unless the passage explicitly states otherwise: subjects should be assumed to be healthy individuals with normal hormone levels. When PTU is administered, the thyroid hormone levels in the mice decreased. As a result, there is now less thyroid hormone in circulation. As we predicted, there is now little to no negative feedback on the hypothalamus and the anterior pituitary gland. TRH and TSH levels in the mice would be elevated as a result of this lack of feedback. Normally, that would work to create more T3 and T4, but in this case, the mice are under the influence of PTU, and despite TSH stimulation, the thyroid will not be able to produce more T3 and T4. The cycle will continue, and more TRH and TSH will be secreted.

In short, the reason why TSH level is elevated in mice administered with PTU is that there is no T3 or T4 to activate the negative feedback mechanism on TSH and TRH, which "tricks" the brain into secreting more TSH (and TRH).

Adrenal Cortex

The **adrenal glands** are located on top of the kidneys. Adrenal actually translates to *near* or *next to the kidney*. Each adrenal gland consists of a cortex and a medulla. This distinction is more than anatomical. Each part of the gland is responsible for the secretion of different hormones. The **adrenal cortex** secretes **corticosteroids**. These are steroid hormones that can be divided into three functional classes: **glucocorticoids**, **mineralocorticoids**, and **cortical sex hormones**.

REAL WORLD

Many people who suffer from joint pain are treated with glucocorticoid injections into the joint space to decrease inflammation. In addition, glucocorticoids are used to treat systemic inflammation caused by allergic reactions or autoimmune disease.

Glucocorticoids

Glucocorticoids are steroid hormones that regulate glucose levels. In addition, these hormones also affect protein metabolism. The two glucocorticoids most likely to be tested on the MCAT are **cortisol** and **cortisone**. These hormones raise blood glucose by increasing gluconeogenesis and decreasing protein synthesis. Cortisol and cortisone can also decrease inflammation and immunologic responses. Cortisol is known as a stress hormone because it is released in times of physical or emotional stress. This increases blood sugar and provides a ready source of fuel in case the body must react quickly to a dangerous stimulus.

Glucocorticoid release is under the control of adrenocorticotropic hormone (ACTH) as described earlier. Corticotropin-releasing factor (CRF) from the hypothalamus promotes release of adrenocorticotropic hormone (ACTH) from the anterior pituitary, which promotes release of glucocorticoids from the adrenal cortex.

REAL WORLD

In addition to stimulating the secretion of aldosterone, which increases blood volume and hence blood pressure, angiotensin II also increases blood pressure directly through a powerful vasoconstrictive effect and increases heart rate. Angiotensin-converting enzyme (ACE) inhibitors block the conversion of angiotensin I to angiotensin II, inhibiting vasoconstriction. Therefore, ACE inhibitors are frequently prescribed for the treatment of high blood pressure and congestive heart failure. In the latter case, vasodilation helps reduce vascular resistance, decreasing the pressure against which the failing heart must pump. ACE inhibitors' generic names end with *-pril* (*lisinopril*, *enalapril*, *ramipril*).

Mineralocorticoids

Mineralocorticoids are used in salt and water homeostasis; their most profound effects are on the kidneys. The most noteworthy mineralocorticoid is **aldosterone**, which increases sodium reabsorption in the distal convoluted tubule and collecting duct of the nephron. Water follows the sodium cations into the bloodstream, increasing blood volume and pressure. Since water and sodium ions flow together, plasma osmolarity remains unchanged; this is in contrast to ADH, which only increases water reabsorption (decreasing plasma osmolarity). Aldosterone also decreases the reabsorption of potassium and hydrogen ions in these same segments of the nephron, promoting their excretion in the urine.

Unlike the glucocorticoids, aldosterone is primarily under the control of the **renin–angiotensin–aldosterone** system, as shown in Figure 5.9. Decreased blood pressure causes the **juxtaglomerular cells** of the kidney to secrete **renin**, which cleaves an inactive plasma protein, **angiotensinogen**, to its active form, **angiotensin I**. Angiotensin I is then converted to **angiotensin II** by **angiotensin-converting enzyme (ACE)** in the lungs. Angiotensin II stimulates the adrenal cortex to secrete aldosterone. Once blood pressure is restored, there is a decreased drive to stimulate renin release, thus serving as the negative feedback mechanism for this system.

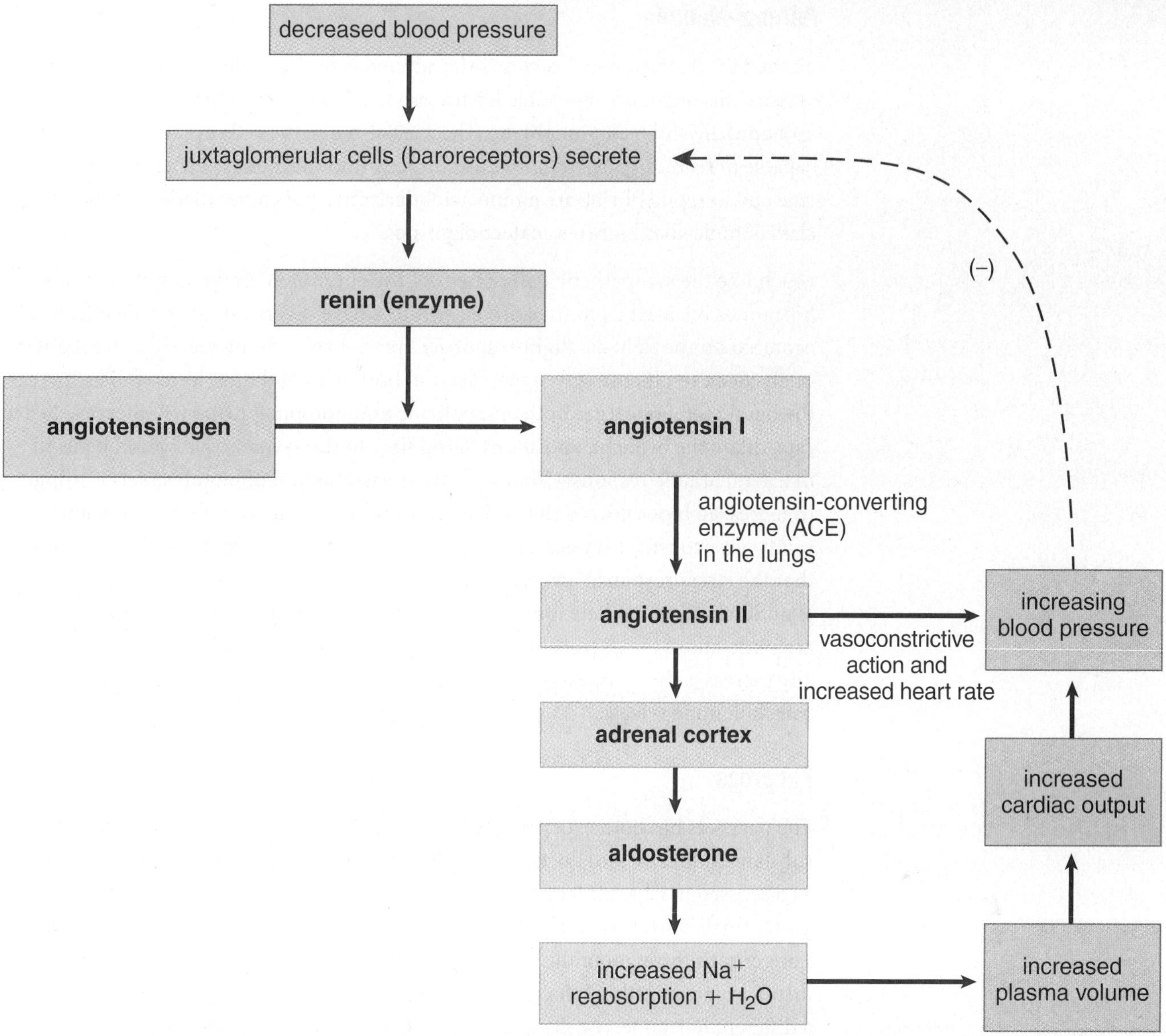

Figure 5.9 The Renin-Angiotensin-Aldosterone System

Cortical Sex Hormones

The adrenal glands also make **cortical sex hormones** (**androgens** and **estrogens**). Because the testes already secrete large quantities of androgens, adrenal testosterone plays a relatively small role in male physiology. But because the ovaries secrete far smaller amounts of androgens, females are much more sensitive to disorders of cortical sex hormone production. For example, certain enzyme deficiencies in the synthetic pathways of other adrenal cortex hormones result in excess androgen production in the adrenal cortex. Such a deficiency would result in no obvious phenotypic effects in a male fetus; however, a genotypic female may be born with ambiguous or masculinized genitalia due to the presence of excess cortical sex hormones. Males can be affected by similar disorders if they lead to excessive production of estrogens.

MNEMONIC

Functions of the corticosteroids:

The 3 **S**'s

- **S**alt (mineralocorticoids)
- **S**ugar (glucocorticoids)
- **S**ex (cortical sex hormones)

Adrenal Medulla

Nestled inside the adrenal cortex is the adrenal medulla. A derivative of the nervous system, this organ is responsible for the production of the sympathetic hormones **epinephrine** and **norepinephrine**. The specialized nerve cells in the medulla are capable of secreting these compounds directly into the bloodstream. Both epinephrine and norepinephrine are amino acid–derivative hormones that belong to a larger class of molecules known as **catecholamines**.

Much like the sympathetic component of the autonomic nervous system, the hormones released from the adrenal medulla have diverse system-wide effects, all centered on the fight-or-flight response. Epinephrine can increase the breakdown of glycogen to glucose (glycogenolysis) in both liver and muscle, as well as increase the basal metabolic rate. Both epinephrine and norepinephrine will increase heart rate, dilate the bronchi, and shunt blood flow to the systems that would be used in a sympathetic response. That is, there is vasodilation of blood vessels leading to increased bloodflow to the skeletal muscle, heart, lungs, and brain. Concurrently, vasoconstriction decreases bloodflow to the gut, kidneys, and skin. Note that the stress response involves both cortisol and epinephrine. Classically, cortisol is understood to mediate long-term (slow) stress responses, while catecholamines are understood to control short-term (fast) stress responses. In fact, cortisol actually increases the synthesis of catecholamines as well, resulting in an increase in catecholamine release.

Pancreas

The pancreas has both exocrine and endocrine functions. Exocrine tissues secrete substances directly into ducts; the pancreas produces a number of digestive enzymes, as discussed in Chapter 9 of *MCAT Biology Review*. From an endocrine standpoint, small clusters of hormone-producing cells are grouped together into **islets of Langerhans** throughout the pancreas, as shown in Figure 5.10. Islets contain three distinct types of cells: **alpha (α)**, **beta (β)**, and **delta (δ) cells**. Each cell type secretes a different hormone: α-cells secrete **glucagon**, β-cells secrete **insulin**, and δ-cells secrete **somatostatin**.

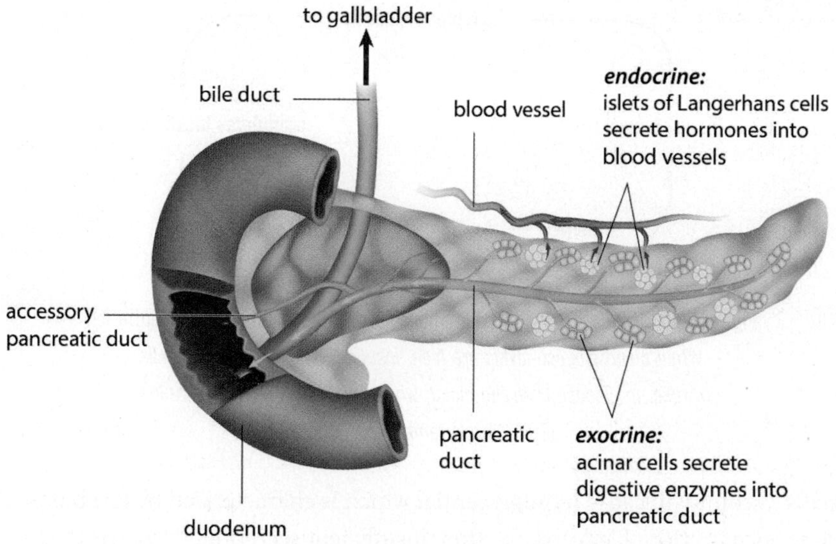

Figure 5.10 Anatomy of the Pancreas
Islets of Langerhans are scattered throughout the pancreas and carry out the endocrine function of the organ.

Glucagon

Glucagon is secreted during times of fasting. When glucose levels are low, glucagon increases glucose production by triggering glycogenolysis, gluconeogenesis, and the degradation of protein and fat. In addition to low blood glucose concentrations, certain gastrointestinal hormones (such as cholecystokinin and gastrin) increase glucagon release from α-cells. When blood glucose concentrations are high, glucagon release is inhibited.

MNEMONIC

Glucagon levels are high when **glucose** is **gone**.

Insulin

Insulin is antagonistic to glucagon and is therefore secreted when blood glucose levels are high, as shown in Figure 5.11. Insulin induces muscle and liver cells to take up glucose and store it as glycogen for later use. In addition, because it is active when glucose levels are high, insulin stimulates anabolic processes such as fat and protein synthesis.

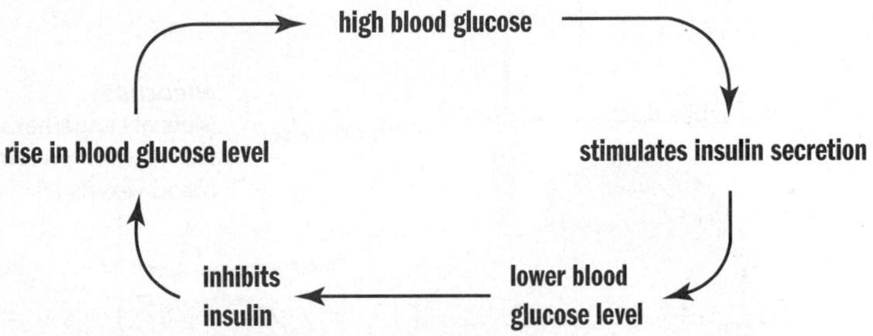

Figure 5.11 Insulin Has a Direct Relationship with Blood Glucose Concentration
When blood glucose levels are high, insulin levels rise, causing cells to take up glucose from the blood; when blood glucose levels are low, insulin levels remain low as well.

In excess, insulin will cause **hypoglycemia**, which is characterized by low blood glucose concentration. Underproduction, insufficient secretion, or insensitivity to insulin all can result in **diabetes mellitus**, which is clinically characterized by **hyperglycemia** (excess glucose in the blood). In the kidneys, excessive glucose in the filtrate will overwhelm the nephron's ability to reabsorb glucose, resulting in its presence in the urine. Because it is an osmotically active particle and does not readily cross the cell membrane, the presence of glucose in the filtrate leads to excess excretion of water and an increase—that is sometimes quite dramatic—in the urine volume. Therefore, patients who have diabetes often report **polyuria** (increased frequency of urination) and **polydipsia** (increased thirst). There are two types of diabetes mellitus. **Type I** (insulin-dependent) diabetes mellitus is caused by autoimmune destruction of the β-cells of the pancreas, resulting in low or absent insulin production. People who have type I diabetes require regular injections of insulin to prevent hyperglycemia and to permit uptake of glucose into cells. **Type II** (non-insulin-dependent) diabetes mellitus is the result of receptor-level resistance to the effects of insulin. Type II diabetes mellitus is partially inherited and partially due to environmental factors, such as high-carbohydrate diets and obesity. Certain pharmaceutical agents can be taken orally to help the body more effectively use the insulin it produces. These individuals require insulin only when their bodies can no longer control glucose levels, even when aided by these medications.

KEY CONCEPT

Insulin decreases plasma glucose. Glucagon increases plasma glucose. Growth hormone, glucocorticoids, and epinephrine are also capable of increasing plasma glucose. These hormones that raise blood glucose levels are commonly called counterregulatory hormones.

Somatostatin

Somatostatin is an inhibitor of both insulin and glucagon secretion. High blood glucose and amino acid concentrations stimulate its secretion. Somatostatin is also produced by the hypothalamus, where it decreases growth hormone secretion in addition to its effects on insulin and glucagon.

Gonads

Because reproductive endocrinology is discussed in detail in Chapter 2 of *MCAT Biology Review*, we offer only a brief overview in this chapter. The **testes** secrete testosterone in response to stimulation by gonadotropins (LH and FSH). Testosterone causes sexual differentiation of the male during gestation and also promotes the development and maintenance of secondary sex characteristics in males, such as axillary and pubic hair, deepening of the voice, and muscle growth.

The **ovaries** secrete estrogen and progesterone in response to gonadotropins. Estrogen is involved in development of the female reproductive system during gestation and also promotes the development and maintenance of secondary sex characteristics in females, such as axillary and pubic hair, breast growth, and body fat redistribution. These two steroid hormones also govern the menstrual cycle as well as pregnancy.

Pineal Gland

The **pineal gland** is located deep within the brain, where it secretes the hormone **melatonin**. The precise mechanism of this hormone is unclear, although it has been demonstrated to be involved in **circadian rhythms**. Blood levels of melatonin are at least partially responsible for the sensation of sleepiness. The pineal gland receives projections directly from the retina, but is not involved in vision; it is hypothesized that the pineal gland responds to decreases in light intensity by releasing melatonin.

REAL WORLD

Melatonin has enjoyed somewhat of a wonder drug status over the past decade as it is touted as a remedy for everything from jet lag to aging. Certainly, one effect of melatonin is to cause profound drowsiness, hence its use in "resetting" one's daily rhythm. Melatonin is available over the counter in health food stores, but the long-term effects of melatonin therapy are currently unknown.

Other Organs

In addition to the organs listed above, specific cells and tissues in other organs exhibit endocrine functions. In the gastrointestinal tract, endocrine tissue can be found in both the stomach and intestine. Many gastrointestinal peptides have been identified; important ones include secretin, gastrin, and cholecystokinin. The specific functions of these hormones are discussed in Chapter 9 of *MCAT Biology Review*, but as we might expect for the digestive system, the stimulus for release of most of these peptides is the presence of specific nutrients.

The kidneys play a role in water balance. As mentioned earlier, ADH increases water permeability in the collecting duct, and the renin–angiotensin–aldosterone system increases sodium and water reabsorption in the distal convoluted tubule and collecting duct. The kidneys also produce **erythropoietin**, which stimulates bone marrow to increase production of erythrocytes (red blood cells). It is secreted in response to low oxygen levels in the blood.

The heart releases **atrial natriuretic peptide** (**ANP**) to help regulate salt and water balance. When cells in the atria are stretched from excess blood volume, they release ANP. This hormone promotes excretion of sodium and therefore increases urine volume. This effect is functionally antagonistic to aldosterone because it lowers blood volume and pressure, and has no effect on blood osmolarity.

The thymus, located directly behind the sternum, releases **thymosin**, which is important for proper T-cell development and differentiation. The thymus atrophies by adulthood, and thymosin levels drop accordingly. The function of T-cells is discussed in Chapter 8 of *MCAT Biology Review*.

A full list of hormones and their actions can be found in Table 5.1 below.

SOURCE	HORMONE	TYPE	ACTION
Anterior pituitary	Follicle-stimulating hormone (FSH)	Peptide	Stimulates follicle maturation in females; spermatogenesis in males
	Luteinizing hormone (LH)	Peptide	Stimulates ovulation in females; testosterone synthesis in males
	Adrenocorticotropic hormone (ACTH)	Peptide	Stimulates the adrenal cortex to synthesize and secrete glucocorticoids
	Thyroid-stimulating hormone (TSH)	Peptide	Stimulates the thyroid to produce thyroid hormones
	Prolactin	Peptide	Stimulates milk production and secretion
	Endorphins	Peptide	Decrease sensation of pain; can promote euphoria
	Growth hormone (GH)	Peptide	Stimulates bone and muscle growth; raises blood glucose levels
Hypothalamus (released by posterior pituitary)	Antidiuretic hormone (ADH; vasopressin)	Peptide	Stimulates water reabsorption in kidneys by increasing permeability of collecting duct
	Oxytocin	Peptide	Stimulates uterine contractions during labor and milk secretion during lactation; may promote bonding behavior
Thyroid (follicular cells)	Triiodothyronine (T_3) and thyroxine (T_4)	Amino acid-derivative	Stimulate metabolic activity
Thyroid (parafollicular or C cells)	Calcitonin	Peptide	Decreases blood calcium concentrations
Parathyroids	Parathyroid hormone (PTH)	Peptide	Increases blood calcium concentrations
Adrenal cortex	Glucocorticoids (cortisol and cortisone)	Steroid	Increase blood glucose concentrations; decrease protein synthesis; anti-inflammatory
	Mineralocorticoids (aldosterone)	Steroid	Increase water reabsorption in the kidneys by increasing sodium reabsorption; promote potassium and hydrogen ion excretion

Table 5.1 Major Hormones in Humans

Adrenal medulla	Epinephrine and norepinephrine	Amino acid-derivative	Increase blood glucose concentrations and heart rate; dilate bronchi; alter blood flow patterns
Pancreas (α-cells)	Glucagon	Peptide	Stimulates glycogen breakdown (glycogenolysis); increases blood glucose concentrations
Pancreas (β-cells)	Insulin	Peptide	Lowers blood glucose concentrations and promotes anabolic processes
Pancreas (δ-cells)	Somatostatin	Peptide	Suppresses secretion of glucagon and insulin
Testis (and adrenal cortex)	Testosterone	Steroid	Induces the development and maintenance of male reproductive system and male secondary sex characteristics
Ovary (and placenta)	Estrogen	Steroid	Induces the development and maintenance of female reproductive system and female secondary sex characteristics
	Progesterone	Steroid	Promotes maintenance of the endometrium
Pineal gland	Melatonin	Peptide	Involved in circadian rhythms
Kidney	Erythropoietin	Peptide	Stimulates bone marrow to produce erythrocytes
Heart (atria)	Atrial natriuretic peptide (ANP)	Peptide	Promotes salt and water excretion
Thymus	Thymosin	Peptide	Stimulates T-cell development

Table 5.1 (Continued)

MCAT CONCEPT CHECK 5.2

Before you move on, assess your understanding of the material with these questions.

1. For each of the hypothalamic releasing hormones listed below, what hormone(s) does each affect in the anterior pituitary? On which organ does each pituitary hormone act? What hormone(s) are released by the target organs?

Hypothalamic Releasing Hormone	Hormone(s) from Anterior Pituitary	Target Organ	Hormone(s) Released by Target Organ
Gonadotropin-releasing hormone (GnRH)			
Corticotropin-releasing factor (CRF)			
Thyroid-releasing hormone (TRH)			
Dopamine			N/A
Growth hormone–releasing hormone (GHRH)			N/A

2. Which two hormones are primarily involved in calcium homeostasis? Where does each come from, and what effect does each have on blood calcium concentrations?

    •

    ____

    ____

    •

    ____

    ____

3. Which endocrine tissue synthesizes catecholamines? What are the two main catecholamines it produces?

    ____

4. Which two pancreatic hormones are the major drivers of glucose homeostasis? Where does each come from, and what effect does each have on blood glucose concentrations?

   •

   ____

   ____

   •

   ____

   ____

5. Which three hormones are primarily involved in water homeostasis? Where does each come from, and what effect does each have on blood volume and osmolarity?

   •

   ____

   ____

   •

   ____

   ____

   •

   ____

   ____

Conclusion

The endocrine system is unique because its organs are not anatomically related. Hormones are produced in a wide variety of locations and can have far-reaching effects throughout the entire organism. The endocrine system allows for integration and execution of the homeostatic parameters that are necessary to ensure proper functioning of the body. For example, we learned that calcium levels are maintained within a narrow concentration range in the plasma by the antagonistic actions of calcitonin and parathyroid hormone (and vitamin D). Each hormone manipulates the steady state of the organism. As you continue your study of the human body, you will find that the endocrine system has effects on every system of the body by regulating fuel metabolism, blood flow, growth, and development.

In the last section of this chapter, there was a small note on erythropoietin, the hormone that stimulates the production of red blood cells in the bone marrow. Don't interpret this brief mention as an indication that it is relatively unimportant. In fact, every cell of the body (except red blood cells themselves) needs a constant supply of oxygen to accomplish its function. Our bodies take in this oxygen through the respiratory system and then distribute the oxygen to tissues via the circulatory system. In the next two chapters, we will explore each of these systems separately. Recognize, however, that this division is artificial; indeed, like the body as a whole, the respiratory and circulatory systems are inseparable as they serve a common function: providing oxygen for every working cell in the body.

You've reviewed the content, now test your knowledge and critical thinking skills by completing a test-like passage set in your online resources!

GO ONLINE

CONCEPT SUMMARY

Mechanisms of Hormone Action

- Endocrine signaling involves the secretion of **hormones** directly into the bloodstream. The hormones travel to distant target tissues, where they bind to receptors and induce a change in gene expression or cell function.
- **Peptide hormones** are composed of amino acids and are derived from larger precursor proteins that are cleaved during posttranslational modification.
  - Peptide hormones are polar and cannot pass through the plasma membrane.
  - These hormones bind to extracellular receptors, where they trigger the transmission of a **second messenger**.
  - Each step of the **signaling cascade** can induce **amplification** of the signal.
  - Peptide hormones exert effects that usually have rapid onset but are short lived.
  - These hormones are water-soluble, so they travel freely in the bloodstream and do not require a special carrier.
- **Steroid hormones** are derived from cholesterol.
  - Steroid hormones are minimally polar and can pass through the plasma membrane.
  - These hormones bind to and promote a conformational change in cytosolic or intranuclear receptors; the hormone–receptor complex binds to DNA, altering the transcription of a particular gene.
  - Steroid hormones exert effects that usually have slow onset but are long-lived.
  - Because these hormones are lipid-soluble, they cannot dissolve in the bloodstream and must be carried by specific proteins.
- **Amino acid–derivative hormones** are modified amino acids.
  - Their chemistry shares some features with peptide hormones and some features with steroid hormones; different amino acid–derivative hormones share different features with these other hormone classes.
  - Common examples are epinephrine, norepinephrine, triiodothyronine, and thyroxine.
- Hormones can be classified by their target tissues.
  - **Direct hormones** have major effects on non-endocrine tissues.
  - **Tropic hormones** have major effects on other endocrine tissues.

Endocrine Organs and Hormones

- The hypothalamus is the bridge between the nervous and endocrine systems.
  - The release of hormones from the hypothalamus is mediated by a number of factors, including projections from other parts of the brain, chemo- and baroreceptors in the blood vessels, and negative feedback from other hormones.
  - In **negative feedback**, the final hormone (or product) of a pathway inhibits hormones (or enzymes) earlier in the pathway, maintaining **homeostasis**.
  - The hypothalamus stimulates the anterior pituitary gland through paracrine release of hormones into the hypophyseal portal system, which directly connects the two organs.
  - **Gonadotropin-releasing hormone** (**GnRH**) promotes the release of follicle-stimulating hormone (FSH) and luteinizing hormone (LH).
  - **Growth hormone–releasing hormone** (**GHRH**) promotes the release of growth hormone.
  - **Thyroid-releasing hormone** (**TRH**) promotes the release of thyroid-stimulating hormone (TSH).
  - **Corticotropin-releasing factor** (**CRF**) promotes the release of adrenocorticotropic hormone (ACTH).
  - **Prolactin-inhibiting factor** (**PIF** or **dopamine**) inhibits the release of prolactin.
  - Interactions with the posterior pituitary occur via the axons of nerves projected by the hypothalamus. Antidiuretic hormone (ADH or vasopressin) and oxytocin are synthesized in the hypothalamus and then travel down these axons to the posterior pituitary, where they are released into the bloodstream.
- The **anterior pituitary** releases hormones in response to stimulation from the hypothalamus. Four of these (FSH, LH, ACTH, and TSH) are tropic hormones, while three (prolactin, endorphins, and growth hormone) are direct hormones.
  - **Follicle-stimulating hormone** (**FSH**) promotes the development of ovarian follicles in females and spermatogenesis in males.
  - **Luteinizing hormone** (**LH**) promotes ovulation in females and testosterone production in males.
  - **Adrenocorticotropic hormone** (**ACTH**) promotes the synthesis and release of glucocorticoids from the adrenal cortex.
  - **Thyroid-stimulating hormone** (**TSH**) promotes the synthesis and release of triiodothyronine and thyroxine from the thyroid.
  - **Prolactin** promotes milk production.
  - **Endorphins** decrease perception of pain and can produce euphoria.
  - **Growth hormone** (**GH**) promotes growth of bone and muscle and shunts glucose to these tissues. It raises blood glucose concentrations.

- The **posterior pituitary** releases two hormones produced in the hypothalamus.
  - **Antidiuretic hormone** (**ADH** or **vasopressin**) is secreted in response to low blood volume or increased blood osmolarity and increases reabsorption of water in the collecting duct of the nephron, increasing blood volume and decreasing blood osmolarity.
  - **Oxytocin** is secreted during childbirth and promotes uterine contractions. It also promotes milk ejection and may be involved in bonding behavior. It is unusual in that it has a **positive feedback** loop, not negative.
- The **thyroid** is located at the base of the neck in front of the trachea; it produces three key hormones.
  - **Triiodothyronine** (**T_3**) and **thyroxine** (**T_4**) are produced by **follicular cells** and contain iodine. They increase basal metabolic rate and alter the utilization of glucose and fatty acids. Thyroid hormones are required for proper neurological and physical development in children.
  - **Calcitonin** is produced by **parafollicular (C) cells**. It decreases plasma calcium concentration by promoting calcium excretion in the kidneys, decreasing calcium absorption in the gut, and promoting calcium storage in bone.
- The **parathyroid glands** release **parathyroid hormone** (**PTH**), which increases blood calcium concentration.
  - PTH decreases excretion of calcium by the kidneys and increases bone resorption directly to increase blood calcium concentration.
  - PTH activates vitamin D, which is necessary for calcium and phosphate absorption from the gut.
  - PTH promotes resorption of phosphate from bone and reduces reabsorption of phosphate in the kidney, but vitamin D promotes absorption of phosphate from the gut; these two effects on phosphate concentration somewhat cancel each other out.
- The **adrenal cortex** produces three classes of steroid hormones.
  - **Glucocorticoids** such as **cortisol** and **cortisone** increase blood glucose concentration, reduce protein synthesis, inhibit the immune system, and participate in the stress response. Glucocorticoid release is stimulated by ACTH.
  - **Mineralocorticoids** such as **aldosterone** promote sodium reabsorption in the distal convoluted tubule and collecting duct, thus increasing water reabsorption. Aldosterone also increases potassium and hydrogen ion excretion. Aldosterone activity is regulated by the **renin–angiotensin–aldosterone system**, not ACTH.
  - **Cortical sex hormones** include **androgens** (like **testosterone**) and **estrogens** in both males and females.

- The **adrenal medulla** is derived from the nervous system and secretes catecholamines into the bloodstream.
    - **Catecholamines** include **epinephrine** and **norepinephrine**, which are involved in the fight-or-flight (sympathetic) response.
    - These hormones promote glycogenolysis, increase the basal metabolic rate, increase heart rate, dilate the bronchi, and alter blood flow.
- The endocrine **pancreas** produces hormones that regulate glucose homeostasis.
    - **Glucagon** is produced by **α-cells** and raises blood glucose levels by stimulating protein and fat degradation, glycogenolysis, and gluconeogenesis.
    - **Insulin** is produced by **β-cells** and lowers blood glucose levels by stimulating glucose uptake by cells and promoting anabolic processes, like glycogen, fat, and protein synthesis.
    - **Somatostatin** is produced by **δ-cells** and inhibits insulin and glucagon secretion.
- The gonads produce hormones that are involved in the development and maintenance of the reproductive systems and secondary sex characteristics.
    - The **testes** secrete **testosterone**.
    - The **ovaries** secrete **estrogen** and **progesterone**.
- The **pineal gland** releases **melatonin**, which helps to regulate **circadian rhythms**.
- Other organs may release hormones, even if they are not primarily considered part of the endocrine system.
    - Cells in the stomach and intestine produce hormones like **secretin**, **gastrin**, and **cholecystokinin**.
    - The kidneys secrete **erythropoietin**, which stimulates bone marrow to produce erythrocytes (red blood cells) in response to low oxygen levels in the blood.
    - The atria of the heart secrete **atrial natriuretic peptide** (**ANP**), which promotes excretion of salt and water in the kidneys in response to stretching of the atria (high blood volume).
    - The thymus secretes **thymosin**, which is important for proper T-cell development and differentiation.

ANSWERS TO CONCEPT CHECKS

5.1

1.

Criterion	Peptide Hormones	Steroid Hormones
Chemical precursor	Amino acids (polypeptides)	Cholesterol
Location of receptor	Extracellular (cell membrane)	Intracellular or intranuclear
Mechanism of action	Stimulates a receptor (usually a G protein–coupled receptor), affecting levels of second messengers (commonly cAMP). Initiates a signal cascade	Binds to a receptor, induces conformational change, and regulates transcription at the level of the DNA
Method of travel in the bloodstream	Dissolves and travels freely	Binds to a carrier protein
Speed of onset	Quick	Slow
Duration of action	Short lived	Long lived

2. Amino acid–derivative hormones are made by modifying amino acids, such as the addition of iodine to tyrosine (in thyroid hormone production).
3. Direct hormones are secreted into the bloodstream and travel to a target tissue, where they have direct effects. Tropic hormones cause secretion of another hormone that then travels to the target tissue to cause an effect.

5.2

1.

Hypothalamic Releasing Hormone	Hormone(s) from Anterior Pituitary	Target Organ	Hormone(s) Released by Target Organ
Gonadotropin-releasing hormone (GnRH)	Follicle-stimulating hormone (FSH) and luteinizing hormone (LH)	Gonads (testes or ovaries)	Testosterone (testes) or estrogen and progesterone (ovaries)
Corticotropin-releasing factor (CRF)	Adrenocortico-tropic hormone (ACTH)	Adrenal cortex	Glucocorticoids (cortisol and cortisone)
Thyroid-releasing hormone (TRH)	Thyroid-stimulating hormone (TSH)	Thyroid	Triiodothyronine (T_3), thyroxine (T_4)
Dopamine	Prolactin*	Breast tissue	N/A
Growth hormone–releasing hormone (GHRH)	Growth hormone	Bone, muscle	N/A

*Note that a *decrease* in dopamine from the hypothalamus promotes prolactin secretion.

2. Calcitonin from the parafollicular (C-) cells of the thyroid decreases blood calcium concentration. Parathyroid hormone from the parathyroid glands increases blood calcium concentration.
3. The adrenal medulla synthesizes catecholamines, including epinephrine and norepinephrine.
4. Glucagon from the α-cells of the pancreas increases blood glucose concentration. Insulin from the β-cells of the pancreas decreases blood glucose concentration.
5. Antidiuretic hormone (ADH or vasopressin) from the hypothalamus (released by the posterior pituitary) increases blood volume and decreases blood osmolarity. Aldosterone from the adrenal cortex increases blood volume with no effect on blood osmolarity. Atrial natriuretic peptide (ANP) from the heart decreases blood volume with no effect on blood osmolarity.

SCIENCE MASTERY ASSESSMENT EXPLANATIONS

1. **C**

Unlike the other hormones listed here, ADH is not secreted by the adrenal cortex and is therefore not a *–corticoid*. Rather, ADH is a peptide hormone produced by the hypothalamus and released by the posterior pituitary that promotes water reabsorption. The other associations are all correct.

2. **D**

A hormone that directly stimulates a non-endocrine target tissue is referred to as a direct hormone. Glancing at the answer choices, we notice that all of the hormones are secreted by the anterior pituitary gland. The direct hormones secreted by the anterior pituitary are prolactin, endorphins, and growth hormone (GH). All of the other answer choices are tropic hormones. The tropic hormones of the anterior pituitary include follicle-stimulating hormone (FSH), luteinizing hormone (LH), adrenocorticotropic hormone (ACTH), and thyroid-stimulating hormone (TSH).

3. **A**

The parathyroid glands secrete parathyroid hormone (PTH), a hormone that functions to increase blood calcium levels. An increase in synthetic activity of the parathyroid glands would lead to an increase in PTH and, therefore, an increase in blood calcium levels through three mechanisms: increased calcium reabsorption in the kidneys (decreased excretion), increased bone resorption, and increased absorption of calcium from the gut (via activation of vitamin D).

4. **B**

Peptide hormones are composed of chains of amino acids and, though they vary in size, are generally too large, charged, and polar to cross the cell membrane. Instead, these hormones bind to extracellular receptors and rely on second messengers to mediate their effects. All of these observations justify **(B)**.

5. **B**

Inflammation of the thyroid or iodine deficiency can cause hypothyroidism, in which the thyroid hormones are undersecreted or not secreted at all. Hypothyroidism in newborn infants causes cretinism, which is characterized by poor neurological and physical development (including intellectual disabilities, short stature, and coarse facial features). While iodine deficiency can result in a swelling of the thyroid gland (called a goiter), which can also be seen in causes of hyperthyroidism, iodine deficiency does not cause hyperthyroidism, eliminating **(D)**. Galactorrhea, **(A)**, is associated with prolactin; gigantism, **(C)**, is associated with growth hormone.

6. **C**

The hypothalamic–pituitary–thyroid axis includes the secretion of thyroid-releasing hormone (TRH) from the hypothalamus triggering the secretion of thyroid-stimulating hormone (TSH) from the anterior pituitary, which stimulates the secretion of triiodothyronine (T_3) and thyroxine (T_4) from the thyroid. Overproduction of TRH would promote overproduction of TSH, eliminating **(B)**. Destruction of the follicular cells that produce T_3 and T_4 would remove negative feedback, allowing TSH levels to rise, eliminating **(A)** and **(D)**. High levels of T_4 would cause too much negative feedback and lower TSH levels, making **(C)** the correct answer.

7. **B**

Steroid hormones are nonpolar cholesterol derivatives and bind to internal receptors. Importantly, as cholesterol derivatives, these hormones generally lack nitrogen and are composed primarily of carbon, hydrogen, and oxygen. All of these factors support **(B)** as the right answer. By contrast, **(A)** can be eliminated because peptide hormones would localize to the cell surface. And, while amino acid derivatives can signal like steroid hormones, **(C)** can be eliminated since the chemical composition given in the question stem indicates a lack of nitrogen. **(D)** can be eliminated since the term "direct" refers to the hormone target, and data about the target of the hormone are not given in this question stem.

8. **B**

Pancreatic somatostatin secretion is increased by high blood glucose or amino acid levels, leading to decreased insulin and glucagon secretion, eliminating **(A)** and **(D)**. Somatostatin is thus always an inhibitory hormone, confirming **(B)**. The stimuli for somatostatin release include high blood glucose or amino acids, as mentioned above, as well as high levels of certain gastrointestinal hormones, as discussed in Chapter 9 of *MCAT Biology Review*—but not cortisol, eliminating **(C)**.

9. **C**

β-cells are responsible for insulin production. The function of insulin is to lower blood glucose levels by promoting the influx of glucose into cells and by stimulating anabolic processes, such as glycogenesis or fat and protein synthesis. Thus, destruction of the β-cells would result in a cessation of insulin production, which would lead to hyperglycemia, or high blood glucose concentration.

10. **D**

The stimulus for renin production is low blood pressure, which causes the juxtaglomerular cells of the kidney to produce renin, an enzyme that converts the plasma protein angiotensinogen to angiotensin I. Angiotensin I is then converted to angiotensin II by an enzyme in the lungs; angiotensin II then stimulates the adrenal cortex to secrete aldosterone. Aldosterone helps to restore blood volume by increasing sodium reabsorption in the kidney, leading to an increase in water reabsorption. This removes the initial stimulus for renin production. Thus, **(A)**, **(B)**, and **(C)** correctly describe the renin–angiotensin–aldosterone system, while **(D)** describes the stimulus for erythropoietin secretion.

11. **B**

The question stem indicates that the newly discovered hormone functions as a first messenger, stimulating the conversion of ATP to cAMP; cAMP functions as a second messenger, triggering a signaling cascade in the cell. Hormones that act via second messengers and are relatively large in size (short peptides or complex polypeptides) are peptide hormones. This hormone could be a tropic hormone, but it is also entirely possible for it to be a direct hormone; thus, **(D)** can be eliminated.

12. **B**

Regardless of the cause, the low levels of calcium in the blood require treatment. While other therapies are more frequently used to treat hypocalcemia (low blood calcium levels), such as calcium gluconate or calcium chloride, administration of parathyroid hormone would also raise blood calcium concentration. Calcitonin would be a poor choice in this case, as this hormone lowers blood calcium concentrations, eliminating **(A)**. Aldosterone and thymosin play no role in calcium homeostasis, eliminating **(C)** and **(D)**.

13. **C**

Both oxytocin and vasopressin (another name for antidiuretic hormone) end with the suffix *–in*; this should hint that they are peptide or amino acid–derivative hormones. These two hormones are both synthesized by the hypothalamus, but released by the posterior pituitary. Remember that the posterior pituitary does not actually synthesize any hormones itself; rather, it contains the axons that originate in cells in the hypothalamus and is the site of release for these hormones.

14. **C**

Dopamine is used in a number of neurological systems; most relevant to the endocrine system is the fact that dopamine secretion prevents prolactin release. Thus, an individual taking medications that block dopamine receptors would lose this inhibition on prolactin release and have elevated prolactin levels.

15. **D**

The question stem states that an infant who is genotypically female is born with ambiguous genitalia, meaning that the genitalia do not appear to be specifically female or specifically male. In a genotypic female, this indicates that the infant was exposed to androgens during the fetal period. In addition, the infant is also losing sodium, causing hyponatremia. This indicates two issues: excess androgens and a lack of aldosterone, a hormone required for proper reuptake of sodium in the kidneys. Both of these hormones are synthesized in the adrenal cortex, making **(D)** the correct answer. Note that neither of these hormones is regulated by the hypothalamic–pituitary–adrenal axis, eliminating **(A)** and **(B)**.

Consult your online resources for additional practice. **GO ONLINE**

SHARED CONCEPTS

Behavioral Sciences Chapter 5
Motivation, Emotion, and Stress

Biochemistry Chapter 3
Nonenzymatic Protein Function and Protein Analysis

Biochemistry Chapter 8
Biological Membranes

Biochemistry Chapter 12
Bioenergetics and Regulation of Metabolism

Biology Chapter 4
The Nervous System

Biology Chapter 10
Homeostasis

CHAPTER 6

THE RESPIRATORY SYSTEM

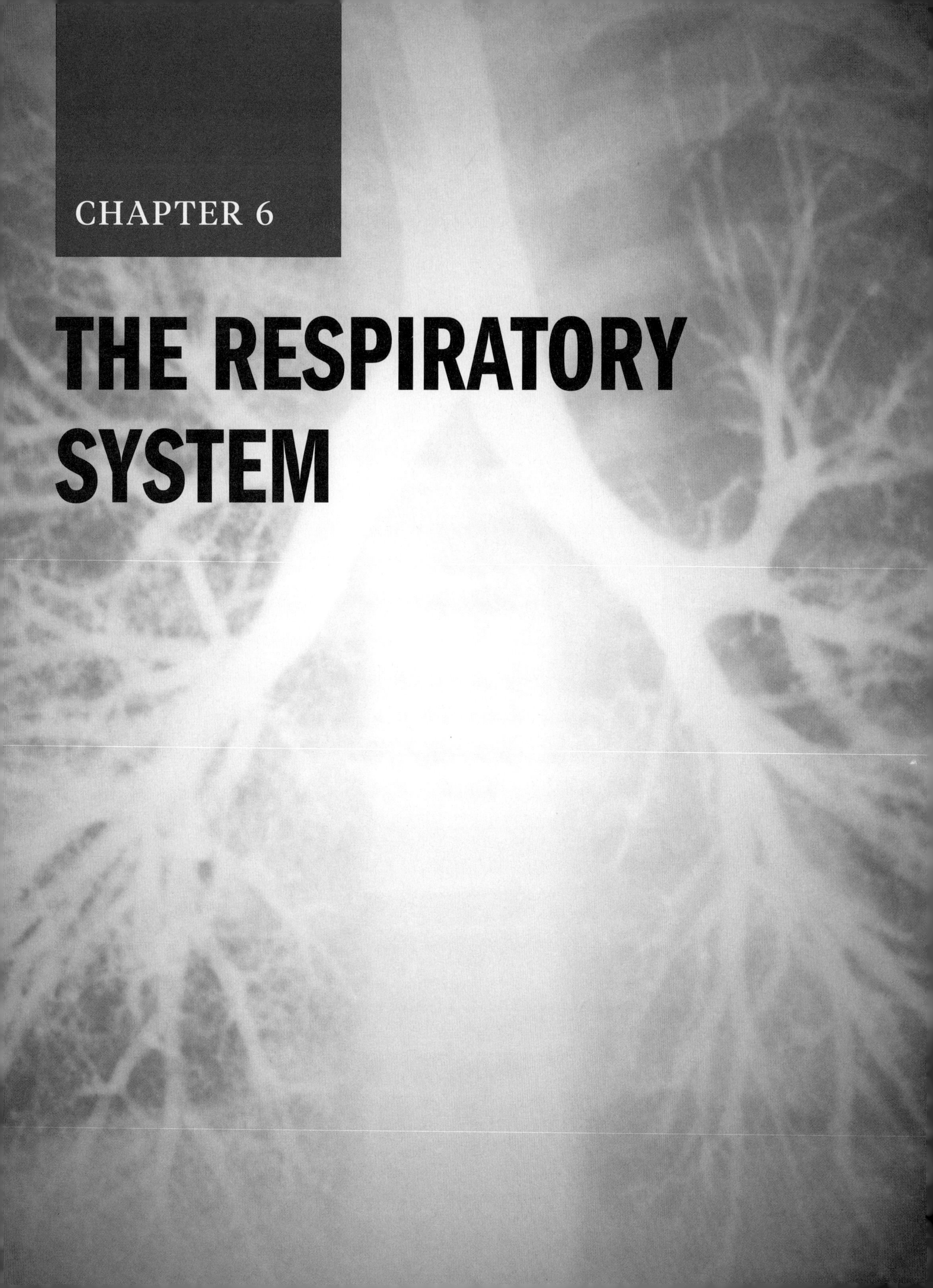

SCIENCE MASTERY ASSESSMENT

Every pre-med knows this feeling: there is so much content I have to know for the MCAT! How do I know what to do first or what's important?

While the high-yield badges throughout this book will help you identify the most important topics, this Science Mastery Assessment is another tool in your MCAT prep arsenal. This quiz (which can also be taken in your online resources) and the guidance below will help ensure that you are spending the appropriate amount of time on this chapter based on your personal strengths and weaknesses. Don't worry though—skipping something now does not mean you'll never study it. Later on in your prep, as you complete full-length tests, you'll uncover specific pieces of content that you need to review and can come back to these chapters as appropriate.

How to Use This Assessment

If you answer 0–7 questions correctly:

Spend about 1 hour to read this chapter in full and take limited notes throughout. Follow up by reviewing **all** quiz questions to ensure that you now understand how to solve each one.

If you answer 8–11 questions correctly:

Spend 20–40 minutes reviewing the quiz questions. Beginning with the questions you missed, read and take notes on the corresponding subchapters. For questions you answered correctly, ensure your thinking matches that of the explanation and you understand why each choice was correct or incorrect.

If you answer 12–15 questions correctly:

Spend less than 20 minutes reviewing all questions from the quiz. If you missed any, then include a quick read-through of the corresponding subchapters, or even just the relevant content within a subchapter, as part of your question review. For questions you answered correctly, ensure your thinking matches that of the explanation and review the Concept Summary at the end of the chapter.

1. All of the following facilitate gas exchange in the lungs EXCEPT:
   - **A.** thin alveolar walls.
   - **B.** multiple subdivisions of the respiratory tree.
   - **C.** differences in the partial pressures of O_2 and CO_2.
   - **D.** active transporters in alveolar cells.

2. Which of the following associations correctly pairs a stage of respiration with the muscle actions occurring during that stage?
   - **A.** Inhalation—diaphragm relaxes
   - **B.** Inhalation—internal intercostal muscles contract
   - **C.** Exhalation—diaphragm contracts
   - **D.** Exhalation—external intercostal muscles relax

3. Total lung capacity is equal to the vital capacity plus the:
   - **A.** tidal volume.
   - **B.** expiratory reserve volume.
   - **C.** residual volume.
   - **D.** inspiratory reserve volume.

4. The intrapleural pressure is necessarily lower than the atmospheric pressure during:
   - **A.** inhalation, because the expansion of the chest cavity causes compression of the intrapleural space, decreasing its pressure.
   - **B.** inhalation, because the expansion of the chest cavity causes expansion of the intrapleural space, decreasing its pressure.
   - **C.** exhalation, because the compression of the chest cavity causes compression of the intrapleural space, decreasing its pressure.
   - **D.** exhalation, because the compression of the chest cavity causes expansion of the intrapleural space, decreasing its pressure.

5. A patient presents to the emergency room with a stab wound to the left side of the chest. On a chest X-ray, blood is noted to be collecting in the chest cavity, causing collapse of both lobes of the left lung. The blood is most likely located between:
   - **A.** the parietal pleura and the chest wall.
   - **B.** the parietal pleura and the visceral pleura.
   - **C.** the visceral pleura and the lung.
   - **D.** the alveolar walls and the lung surface.

6. Each of the following statements regarding the anatomy of the respiratory system is true EXCEPT:
   - **A.** the epiglottis covers the glottis during swallowing to ensure that food does not enter the trachea.
   - **B.** the trachea and bronchi are lined by ciliated epithelial cells.
   - **C.** the pharynx contains two vocal cords, which are controlled by skeletal muscle and cartilage.
   - **D.** the nares are lined with vibrissae, which help filter out particulate matter from inhaled air.

7. Which of the following is a correct sequence of passageways through which air travels during inhalation?
   - **A.** Pharynx → trachea → bronchioles → bronchi → alveoli
   - **B.** Pharynx → trachea → larynx → bronchi → alveoli
   - **C.** Larynx → pharynx → trachea → bronchi → alveoli
   - **D.** Pharynx → larynx → trachea → bronchi → alveoli

8. Idiopathic pulmonary fibrosis (IPF) is a disease in which scar tissue forms in the alveolar walls, making the lung tissue significantly more stiff. Which of the following findings would likely be detected through spirometry in a patient with IPF?
   - **I.** Decreased total lung capacity
   - **II.** Decreased inspiratory reserve volume
   - **III.** Increased residual volume

   - **A.** I only
   - **B.** II only
   - **C.** I and II only
   - **D.** I, II, and III

9. Studies have indicated that premature babies are often deficient in lysozyme. What is a possible consequence of this deficiency?
   - **A.** Respiratory distress and alveolar collapse shortly after birth
   - **B.** Increased susceptibility to certain infections
   - **C.** Inability to humidify air as it passes through the nasal cavity
   - **D.** Slowing of the respiratory rate in response to acidemia

10. Some forms of pneumonia cause an excess of fluids such as mucus or pus to build up within an entire lobe of the lung. How will this affect the diffusion of gases within the affected area?

- **A.** Carbon dioxide can diffuse out, but oxygen will not be able to enter the blood.
- **B.** Oxygen can diffuse into the blood, but carbon dioxide cannot diffuse out.
- **C.** No change in diffusion will occur.
- **D.** No diffusion will occur in the affected area.

11. Some people with anxiety disorders respond to stress by hyperventilating. It is recommended that they breathe into a paper bag and then rebreathe this air. Why is this treatment appropriate?

- **A.** Hyperventilation causes an increase in blood carbon dioxide, and breathing the air in the bag helps to readjust blood levels of carbon dioxide.
- **B.** Hyperventilation causes a decrease in blood carbon dioxide, and breathing the air in the bag helps to readjust blood levels of carbon dioxide.
- **C.** Hyperventilation causes an increase in blood oxygen, and breathing the air in the bag helps to readjust blood levels of oxygen.
- **D.** Hyperventilation causes a decrease in blood oxygen, and breathing the air in the bag helps to readjust blood levels of oxygen.

12. A patient presents to the emergency room with an asthma attack. The patient has been hyperventilating for the past hour and has a blood pH of 7.52. The patient is given treatment and does not appear to respond, but a subsequent blood pH reading is 7.41. Why might this normal blood pH NOT be a reassuring sign?

- **A.** The patient's kidneys may have compensated for the alkalemia.
- **B.** The normal blood pH reading is likely inaccurate.
- **C.** The patient may be descending into respiratory failure.
- **D.** The patient's blood should ideally become acidemic for some time to compensate for the alkalemia.

13. Premature infants with respiratory distress are often placed on ventilators. Often, the ventilators are set to provide positive end-expiratory pressure. Why might this setting be useful for a premature infant?

- **A.** Premature infants lack surfactant.
- **B.** Premature infants lack lysozyme.
- **C.** Premature infants cannot thermoregulate.
- **D.** Premature infants are unable to control pH.

14. In emphysema, the alveolar walls are destroyed, decreasing the recoil of the lung tissue. Which of the following changes may be seen in a patient with emphysema?

- **A.** Increased residual volume
- **B.** Decreased total lung capacity
- **C.** Increased blood concentration of oxygen
- **D.** Decreased blood concentration of carbon dioxide

15. Allergic reactions occur due to an overactive immune response to a substance. Which cells within the respiratory tract play the largest role in the generation of allergic reactions?

- **A.** Alveolar epithelial cells
- **B.** Macrophages
- **C.** Mast cells
- **D.** Ciliated epithelial cells

Answer Key

1. **D**
2. **D**
3. **C**
4. **B**
5. **B**
6. **C**
7. **D**
8. **B**
9. **B**
10. **D**
11. **B**
12. **C**
13. **A**
14. **A**
15. **C**

Detailed explanations can be found at the end of the chapter.

CHAPTER 6

THE RESPIRATORY SYSTEM

In This Chapter

Introduction

Coughing. Fever. Shortness of breath. Hypoxia. All are symptoms of a number of pulmonary diseases, from a flareup of *chronic obstructive pulmonary disease* (COPD), to *Streptococcus pneumoniae* (pneumococcal) pneumonia, to a type of hypersensitivity pneumonitis known as *extrinsic allergic alveolitis* (EAA). This last example is a bit more esoteric and can be brought on by hypersensitivity to anything from dried grass, to rat urine, to mold that grows in hot tubs—what is sometimes called *hot tub lung*. Not all cases of hot tub lung are severe, but certainly none are enjoyable. They are often misdiagnosed as asthma or bronchitis and may be treated with steroids, which quell the immune system and reduce inflammation. Because hot tub lung can potentially go away by itself, antibiotic therapy is not always recommended. As a physician, you may end up simply having to tell your patients that the best way to avoid hot tub lung is to make sure that the tub is cleaned properly and routinely before use.

The lesson here isn't to avoid hot tubs. It's that the lungs are essential, sensitive organs with delicate membranes that must be protected. Many types of stressors (pathogens, particles, or chemicals) can irritate them and cause respiratory distress. In this chapter, we'll look at the structure of the lungs and the microanatomy of respiration. We'll also talk about the mechanics of breathing, as well as the overall function of the lungs.

CHAPTER PROFILE

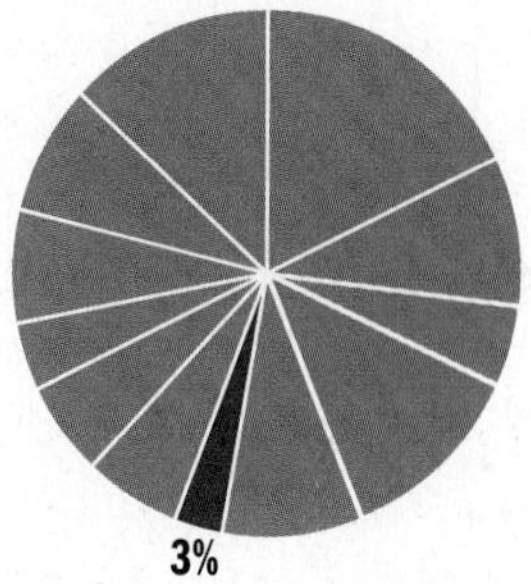

The content in this chapter should be relevant to about 3% of all questions about biology on the MCAT.

This chapter covers material from the following AAMC content category:

3B: Structure and integrative functions of the main organ systems

MCAT EXPERTISE

You may be surprised at the low percentage of questions associated with this chapter, given that this chapter touches on several classic MCAT topics including pressure, gases, and equilibrium. And you may see questions on your MCAT that relate to the work done on air in the lungs, for example. However, such a question would depend much more on your general knowledge of work, energy, and gases (regardless of context) than your knowledge of the respiratory system specifically.

6.1 Anatomy and Mechanism of Breathing

LEARNING OBJECTIVES

After Chapter 6.1, you will be able to:

- Identify the muscles involved in inhalation and exhalation
- Explain the purpose and function of surfactant
- Recall the mathematical relationships between vital capacity, inspiratory reserve volume, expiratory reserve volume, and tidal volume
- Predict how the brain will alter respiratory rate in response to changing blood levels of O_2 and CO_2
- Order the structures in the pathway that air uses to enter the body, from the nares to the alveoli

The lungs are located in the **thoracic cavity**, the structure of which is specially designed to perform breathing.

Anatomy

KEY CONCEPT

The nose and mouth serve several important roles in breathing by removing dirt and particulate matter from the air and warming and humidifying it before it reaches the lungs.

The anatomy of the respiratory system is summarized in Figure 6.1. Gas exchange occurs in the lungs. Air enters the respiratory tract through the external **nares** of the nose and then passes through the nasal cavity, where it is filtered by mucous membranes and nasal hairs (**vibrissae**).

Next, air passes into the pharynx and the larynx. The **pharynx** resides behind the nasal cavity and at the back of the mouth; it is a common pathway for both air destined for the lungs and food destined for the esophagus. In contrast, the **larynx** lies below the pharynx and is only a pathway for air. To keep food out of the respiratory tract, the opening of the larynx (**glottis**) is covered by the **epiglottis** during swallowing. The larynx contains two **vocal cords** that are maneuvered using skeletal muscle and cartilage. From the larynx, air passes into the cartilaginous **trachea** and then into one of the two mainstem **bronchi**. The bronchi and trachea contain ciliated epithelial cells to catch material that has made it past the mucous membranes in the nose and mouth.

In the **lungs**, the bronchi continue to divide into smaller structures known as **bronchioles**, which divide further until they end in the tiny balloon-like structures in which gas exchange occurs (**alveoli**). Each alveolus is coated with **surfactant**, a detergent that lowers surface tension and prevents the alveolus from collapsing on itself. A network of capillaries surrounds each alveolus to carry oxygen and carbon dioxide. The branching and minute size of the alveoli allow for an exceptionally large surface area for gas exchange—approximately 100 m^2 in total.

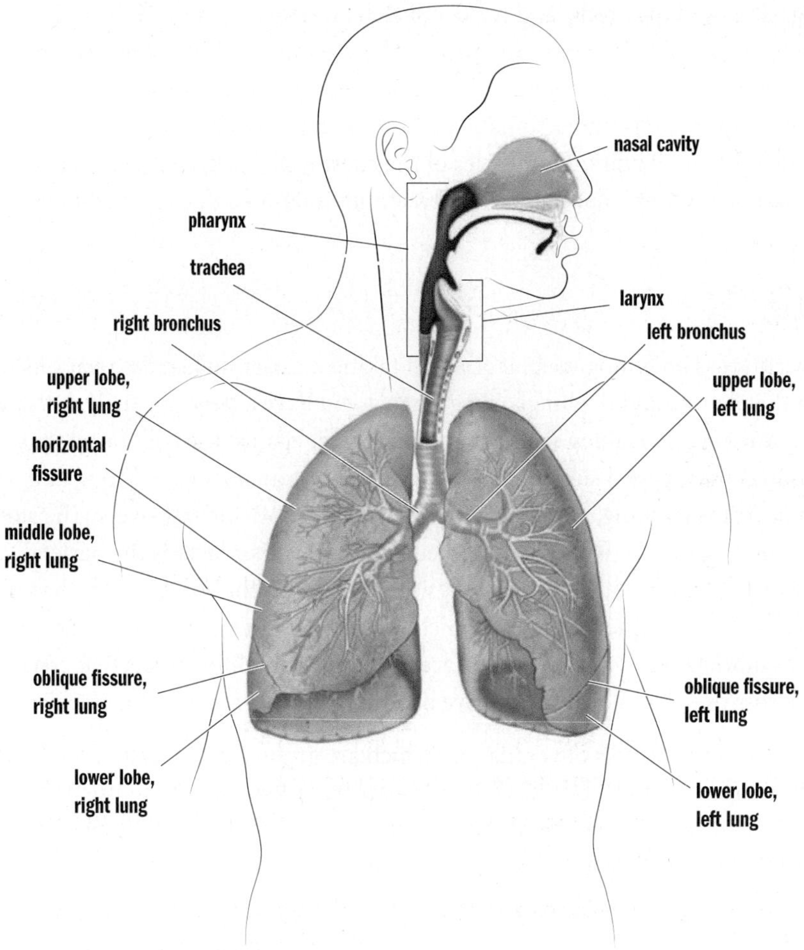

Figure 6.1 Anatomy of the Respiratory System

REAL WORLD

The left lung has a small indentation, making it slightly smaller than the right lung. It also contains only two lobes, while the right lung contains three. Why might this be? It is due to the position of the heart in the thoracic cavity.

The lungs themselves are contained in the thoracic cavity, which also contains the heart. The chest wall forms the outside of the thoracic cavity. Membranes known as **pleurae** surround each lung, as shown in Figure 6.2. The pleura forms a closed sac against which the lung expands. The surface adjacent to the lung is the **visceral pleura**, and the outer part is the **parietal pleura**.

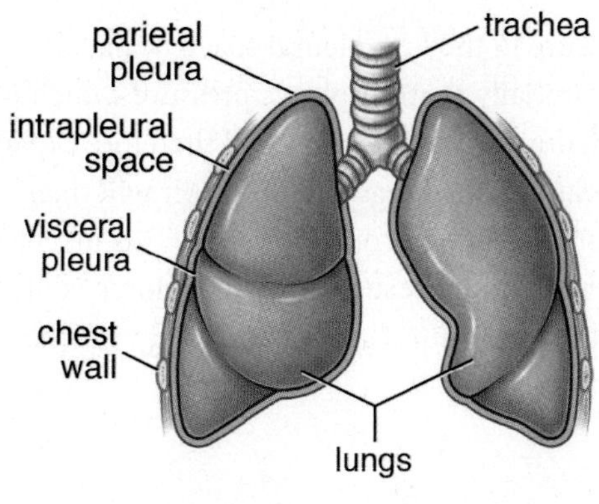

Figure 6.2 Lung Membranes

The lungs do not fill passively, and require skeletal muscle to generate the negative pressure for expansion. The most important of these muscles is the **diaphragm**, a thin, muscular structure that divides the thoracic (chest) cavity from the abdominal cavity. The diaphragm is under somatic control, even though breathing itself is under autonomic control. In addition, muscles of the chest wall, back, and neck may also participate in breathing, especially when breathing is labored due to a pathologic condition.

Breathing

REAL WORLD

The intrapleural space is an example of a potential space—a space that is normally empty or collapsed. In some pathologic states, that potential space can be expanded by fluid or air that accumulates between the two pleural layers. For example, in a pleural effusion, fluid accumulates in the intrapleural space. In a pneumothorax, air collects here. Each of these states disturbs the normal mechanics of the breathing apparatus and can cause atelectasis, or lung collapse.

Before we discuss breathing itself, it is worth taking a closer look at the relationship between the pleurae and the lungs. Imagine that you have a large, partially deflated balloon. Now, imagine taking your fist and pushing it against the balloon so that the balloon comes up and surrounds your hand. This is analogous to a lung and its pleura. Our fist is the lung, and the balloon represents both pleural layers. The side directly touching our fist is the visceral pleura, and the outer layer is the parietal pleura, which is associated with the chest wall in real life. The space within the sac is referred to as the **intrapleural space**, which contains a thin layer of fluid. This pleural fluid helps lubricate the two pleural surfaces. The pressure differentials that can be created across the pleura ultimately drive breathing, as we explore in the next section.

Let's turn to the mechanics of ventilation, which are grounded in physics. As discussed in Chapters 2 and 3 of *MCAT Physics and Math Review*, we can use pressure to do useful work in a system. Here, we use pressure differentials between the intrapleural space and the lungs to drive air into the lungs.

Inhalation

BRIDGE

Boyle's law states that, at a constant temperature, the pressure and volume of gases are inversely related. This is the principle underlying negative-pressure breathing: as the chest wall expands, the pressure in the lungs drops, and air is drawn into the lungs.

Inhalation is an active process. We use our diaphragm as well as the **external intercostal muscles** (one of the layers of muscles between the ribs) to expand the thoracic cavity, as shown in Figure 6.3. As the diaphragm flattens and the chest wall expands outward, the **intrathoracic volume** (the volumc of the chest cavity) increases. Specifically, because the intrapleural space most closely abuts the chest wall, its volume increases first. Can we predict what will happen to intrapleural pressure? From our understanding of Boyle's law, an increase in intrapleural volume leads to a *decrease* in intrapleural pressure.

Now we have low pressure in the intrapleural space. What about inside the lungs? The gas in the lungs is initially at atmospheric pressure, which is now higher than the pressure in the intrapleural space. The lungs will therefore expand into the intrapleural space, and the pressure in the lungs will drop. Air will then be sucked in from a higher-pressure environment—the outside world. This mechanism is referred to as **negative-pressure breathing** because the driving force is the lower (relatively negative) pressure in the intrapleural space compared with the lungs.

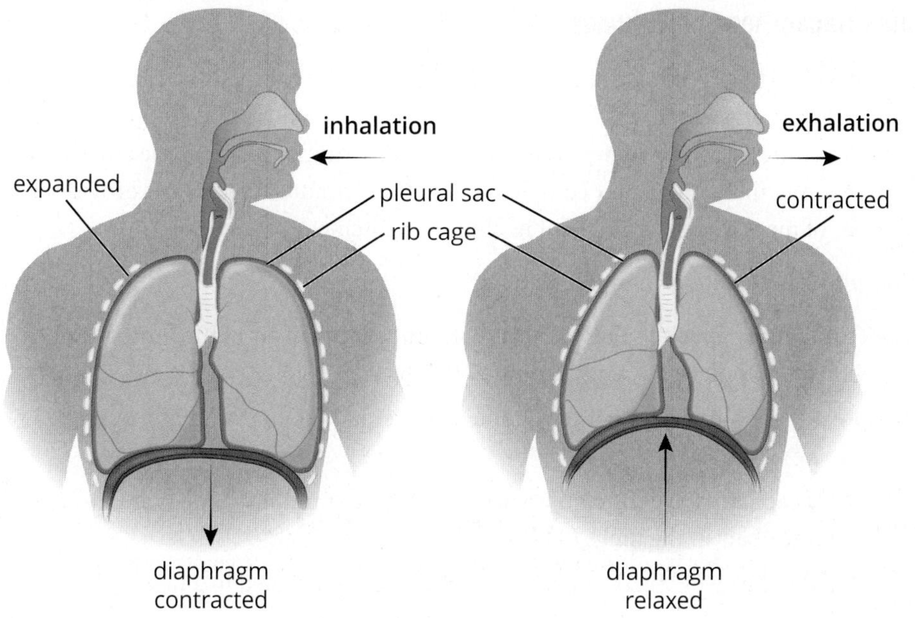

Figure 6.3 Stages of Ventilation
The diaphragm contracts during inhalation and relaxes during exhalation.

Exhalation

Unlike inhalation, exhalation does not have to be an active process. Simple relaxation of the external intercostal muscles will reverse the processes we discussed in the last paragraph. As the diaphragm and external intercostals relax, the chest cavity decreases in volume. What will happen to pressure in the intrapleural space? It will go up, again explained by Boyle's law. Now pressure in the intrapleural space is higher than in the lungs, which is still at atmospheric pressure. Thus, air will be pushed out, resulting in exhalation. During active tasks, we can speed this process up by using the **internal intercostal muscles** and abdominal muscles, which oppose the external intercostals and pull the rib cage down. This actively decreases the volume of the thoracic cavity. Finally, recall that surfactant prevents the complete collapse of the alveoli during exhalation by reducing surface tension at the alveolar surface.

Remember the balloon analogy from before. The lungs have a resilient, elastic quality and are attached via the pleurae to the chest wall. The chest wall expands on inhalation, pulling the lungs with it and creating the pressure differential required for inhalation. As the chest wall relaxes, the lungs recoil due to the intrinsic elastic quality of the lungs and surface tension in the alveoli, accentuating the relaxation process. When the lungs recoil, their volume becomes smaller, and the pressure increases. Now the pressure inside the lungs is higher than the outside pressure, and exhalation occurs. Note that the indirect connection of the lungs to the chest wall also prevents them from collapsing completely on recoil, like surfactant.

KEY CONCEPT

Inhalation and exhalation require different amounts of energy expenditure. Muscle contraction is required to create the negative pressure in the thoracic cavity that forces air into the lungs during inspiration. Expiration during calm states is entirely due to elastic recoil of the lungs and the musculature. During more active states, the muscles can be used to force air out and speed up the process of ventilation.

REAL WORLD

Emphysema is a disease characterized by the destruction of the alveolar walls. This results in reduced elastic recoil of the lungs, making the process of exhalation extremely difficult. Most cases of emphysema are caused by cigarette smoking.

Lung Capacities and Volumes

In pulmonology (the medical field associated with the lungs and breathing), we frequently must assess lung capacities and volumes. One instrument used to measure these quantities is a **spirometer**. While a spirometer cannot measure the amount of air remaining in the lung after complete exhalation (residual volume), it provides a number of measures that are useful in clinical medicine.

Commonly tested lung volumes include:

- **Total lung capacity** (**TLC**): The maximum volume of air in the lungs when one inhales completely; usually around 6 to 7 liters
- **Residual volume** (**RV**): The volume of air remaining in the lungs when one exhales completely
- **Vital capacity** (**VC**): The difference between the minimum and maximum volume of air in the lungs (TLC – RV)
- **Tidal volume** (**TV**): The volume of air inhaled or exhaled in a normal breath
- **Expiratory reserve volume** (**ERV**): The volume of additional air that can be forcibly exhaled after a normal exhalation
- **Inspiratory reserve volume** (**IRV**): The volume of additional air that can be forcibly inhaled after a normal inhalation

These different lung volumes and capacities can be seen in Figure 6.4.

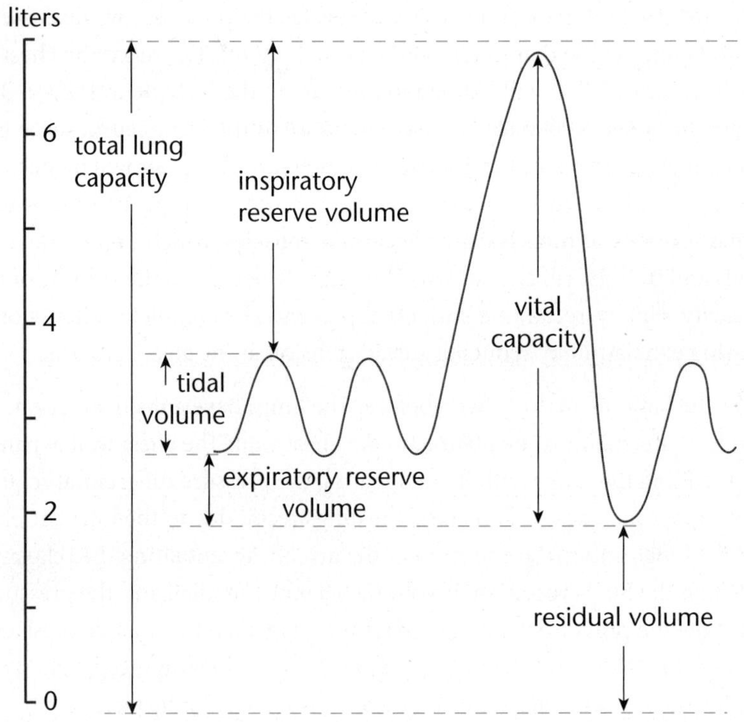

Figure 6.4 Lung Volumes

Regulation of Breathing

Breathing requires input from our nervous control center. Ventilation is primarily regulated by a collection of neurons in the medulla oblongata called the **ventilation center** that fire rhythmically to cause regular contraction of respiratory muscles. These neurons contain **chemoreceptors** that are primarily sensitive to carbon dioxide concentration. As the partial pressure of carbon dioxide in the blood rises (**hypercarbia** or **hypercapnia**), the **respiratory rate** will increase so that more carbon dioxide is exhaled, causing carbon dioxide levels in the blood to fall. These cells also respond to changes in oxygen concentration, although this tends to have significance only during periods of significant **hypoxemia** (low oxygen concentration in the blood).

We can, to a limited extent, control our breathing consciously. We can choose to breathe more rapidly or slowly; however, extended periods of hypoventilation would lead to increased carbon dioxide levels and an override by the medulla oblongata (which would jump-start breathing). The opposite process (hyperventilation) would blow off too much carbon dioxide and ultimately inhibit ventilation.

MCAT CONCEPT CHECK 6.1

Before you move on, assess your understanding of the material with these questions.

1. List the structures in the respiratory pathway, from where air enters the nares to the alveoli.

____

2. Which muscle(s) are involved in inhalation? Exhalation?
    - Inhalation:

____

    - Exhalation:

____

3. What is the purpose of surfactant?

____

4. What is the mathematical relationship between vital capacity (VC), inspiratory reserve volume (IRV), expiratory reserve volume (ERV), and tidal volume (TV)?

____

5. If blood levels of CO_2 become too low, how does the brain alter the respiratory rate to maintain homeostasis?

____

6.2 Functions of the Respiratory System

LEARNING OBJECTIVES

After Chapter 6.2, you will be able to:

- Describe the mechanisms used in the respiratory system to prevent infection
- Recall the chemical equation for the bicarbonate buffer system
- Predict how blood pH will change in response to changing concentrations of O_2 or CO_2

No organ system functions alone. The lungs function in gas exchange, but this is only part of the respiratory story. The lungs are lined with a tremendous number of capillaries that can also be used in thermoregulation. The lungs also represent a pathway into the body and serve an immune function to prevent invaders from gaining access to the bloodstream. Finally, the lungs also allow for control of blood pH by controlling carbon dioxide concentrations. Therefore, the lungs are integrated with many other body systems, including the cardiovascular, immune, renal, and nervous systems.

REAL WORLD

Diffusion of gases occurs across a very thin membrane between the alveolus and the capillary. However, certain diseases may cause fibrosis, or scarring, of this membrane, resulting in less effective diffusion. Other diseases may cause a limitation of ventilation (gas flow) or perfusion (blood flow) to the lung. All of these mechanisms can cause hypoxia—low blood oxygen levels—although they accomplish that same end result through different means.

Gas Exchange

Gas exchange is, of course, the primary function of the lungs. Each alveolus is surrounded by a network of capillaries. The capillaries bring deoxygenated blood from the **pulmonary arteries**, which originate from the right ventricle of the heart. The walls of the alveoli are only one cell thick, which facilitates the diffusion of carbon dioxide from the blood into the lungs, and oxygen into the blood. The oxygenated blood returns to the left atrium of the heart via the **pulmonary veins**.

The driving force for gas exchange is the pressure differential of the gases. When it initially arrives at the alveoli, blood has a relatively low partial pressure of oxygen and a relatively high partial pressure of carbon dioxide, facilitating transfer of each down its respective concentration gradient, as shown in Figure 6.5. Because the gradient between the blood and air in the lungs is already present as the blood enters the lungs, no energy is required for gas transfer.

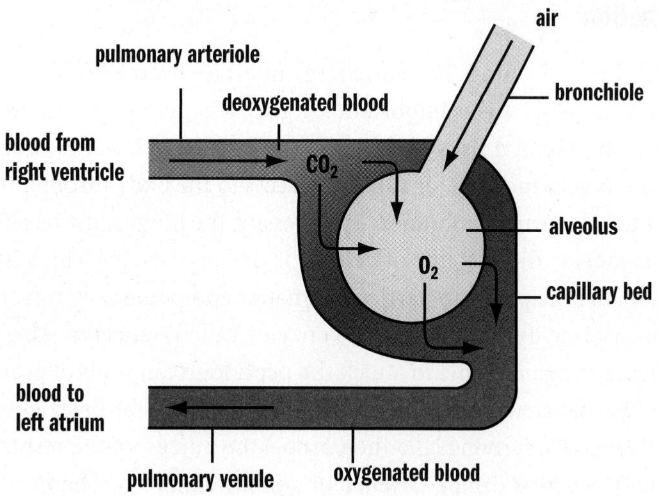

Figure 6.5 Gas Exchange in the Alveolus

KEY CONCEPT

O_2 in the alveoli flows down its partial pressure gradient from the alveoli into the pulmonary capillaries, where it can bind to hemoglobin for transport. Meanwhile, CO_2 flows down its partial pressure gradient from the capillaries into the alveoli for expiration.

How would our respiratory systems adjust if we moved to higher altitudes where less oxygen is available? First, we would breathe more rapidly to try to avoid hypoxia; second, the binding dynamics of hemoglobin to oxygen would be altered to facilitate the unloading of oxygen at the tissues. As we will discuss in Chapter 7 of *MCAT Biology Review*, the natural response of hemoglobin to the decreased carbon dioxide concentration in the environment would actually be to *decrease* the unloading of oxygen to tissues, so other mechanisms must counteract and override this phenomenon. In the short term, the body can make more red blood cells to ensure the adequate delivery of oxygen. In the long term, the body could develop more blood vessels (vascularization), which would facilitate the distribution of oxygen to tissues.

Thermoregulation

In order to maximize gas exchange, there is a tremendous surface area over which the alveoli and capillaries interact. Because the entire respiratory tract is highly vascular, it can also be used for **thermoregulation**, or the regulation of body temperature. Heat—the transfer of thermal energy—is regulated via the body surfaces by **vasodilation** and **vasoconstriction**. As capillaries expand, more blood can pass through these vessels, and a larger amount of thermal energy can be dissipated. As capillaries contract, less blood can pass through them, conserving thermal energy. Nasal and tracheal capillaries are most frequently used for these purposes within the respiratory system. While these capillary beds provide a mechanism for thermoregulation, humans predominantly regulate temperature using capillaries and sweat glands in the skin, or rapid muscle contraction (shivering). The respiratory system can also transfer heat to the environment through evaporation of water in mucous secretions. Other animals, such as dogs, take advantage of this cooling mechanism by **panting**.

Immune Function

As mentioned above, the lungs provide a large interface for the body to interact with the outside world. While this is important for gas exchange and thermoregulation, it also comes with potential risks—pathogens such as bacteria, viruses, and fungi can cause infections in the lung, or can gain access to the body through the rich vascularity of the alveolar membranes. By necessity, the lungs must be able to fight off potential invaders. The first line of defense is the nasal cavity, which has small hairs (vibrissae) that help to trap particulate matter and potentially infectious particles. The nasal cavity also contains an enzyme called ***lysozyme***. Also found in tears and saliva, lysozyme is able to attack the peptidoglycan walls of gram-positive bacteria. The internal airways are lined with mucus, which traps particulate matter and larger invaders. Underlying cilia then propel the mucus up the respiratory tract to the oral cavity, where it can be expelled or swallowed; this mechanism is called the **mucociliary escalator**.

The lungs, especially the alveoli, also contain numerous immune cells, including macrophages. **Macrophages** can engulf and digest pathogens and signal to the rest of the immune system that there is an invader. Mucosal surfaces also contain IgA antibodies that help to protect against pathogens that contact the mucous membranes. Finally, **mast cells** also populate the lungs. These cells have preformed antibodies on their surfaces. When the right substance attaches to the antibody, the mast cell releases inflammatory chemicals into the surrounding area to promote an immune response. Unfortunately, these antibodies are often reactive to substances such as pollen and molds, so mast cells also provide the inflammatory chemicals that mediate allergic reactions.

Control of pH

The respiratory system plays a role in pH balance through the **bicarbonate buffer system** in the blood:

$$CO_2\ (g) + H_2O\ (l) \rightleftharpoons H_2CO_3\ (aq) \rightleftharpoons H^+\ (aq) + HCO_3^-\ (aq)$$

Questions regarding the bicarbonate buffer system are MCAT favorites, and you are very likely to see it in some form on Test Day. This equation represents an opportunity for the MCAT to test understanding of basic chemistry concepts, such as Le Châtelier's principle, as well as how disturbances in pH may affect respiration.

The body attempts to maintain a pH between 7.35 and 7.45. When the pH is lower, and hydrogen ion concentration is higher (**acidemia**), acid-sensing chemoreceptors just outside the blood–brain barrier send signals to the brain to increase the respiratory rate. Further, an increasing hydrogen ion concentration will cause a shift in the bicarbonate buffer system, generating additional carbon dioxide. As described earlier, the respiratory centers in the brain are sensitive to this increasing partial pressure of carbon dioxide and will also promote an increase in respiratory rate.

MCAT EXPERTISE

The division within the sciences is largely artificial; the MCAT often contains questions that integrate multiple science disciplines. A question located in the *Biological and Biochemical Foundations of Living Systems* section may require knowledge of general chemistry. In fact, 10% of this section is chemistry: 5% general chemistry and 5% organic chemistry.

REAL WORLD

Pneumonia is an infection of the lung most often caused by bacteria or viruses. *Atypical pneumonia*, commonly called walking pneumonia (because the infection does not require hospitalization and does not leave the patient bedridden), is often caused by a very small bacterium called *Mycoplasma pneumoniae*. This bacterium causes a prolonged cough because it damages epithelial cells lining the lung and paralyzes the cilia lining the respiratory tract. The lack of cilia makes it much more difficult to clear mucus from the lungs. The cough lasts until the respiratory epithelial cells have recovered and the cilia are once again functional.

REAL WORLD

Metabolic acidosis–a condition of excess acid by any mechanism besides hypoventilation–is a common occurrence in medicine. Anaerobic respiration can generate lactic acid; individuals with type 1 diabetes mellitus can produce ketoacids when they are hypoinsulinemic; certain poisons, like methanol and formaldehyde, can produce organic acids. In each of these cases, one of the primary methods of compensation is increasing respiration rate.

As the respiratory rate increases, more carbon dioxide is blown off. This will also push the buffer equation to the left, but notice the difference: the shift to the left in the previous paragraph was caused by an increase in hydrogen ion concentration, which elevated the concentration of carbon dioxide. Here, the removal of carbon dioxide causes a shift to the left that allows the hydrogen ion concentration to drop back to normal.

If the blood is too basic (**alkalemia**), then the body will seek to increase acidity. How can the lungs contribute to this? If the respiratory rate is slowed, then more carbon dioxide will be retained, shifting the buffer equation to the right and producing more hydrogen ions and bicarbonate ions. This results in a lower pH.

Overall, the lungs play a role in the immediate adjustment of carbon dioxide levels and, by extension, hydrogen ion levels. However, the lungs do not work alone to maintain proper pH. The kidneys also play a role by modulating secretion and reabsorption of acid and base within the nephron. This is a much slower response, however, and represents long-term compensation. For more information on kidney function and homeostasis, see Chapter 10 of *MCAT Biology Review*.

BRIDGE

If H^+ is an acid and HCO_3^- is a base, then why doesn't increasing both of them yield a constant pH? The reason is that H^+ is a strong acid, while HCO_3^- is a weak base. Just like a titration, discussed in Chapter 10 of *MCAT General Chemistry Review*, this combination will shift the pH of the solution toward the acidic range.

KEY CONCEPT

This equation is essential to Test Day success:

$$CO_2\,(g) + H_2O\,(l) \rightleftharpoons H_2CO_3\,(aq) \rightleftharpoons H^+\,(aq) + HCO_3^-\,(aq)$$

It is likely to be tested in both the *Biological and Biochemical Foundations of Living Systems* and the *Chemical and Physical Foundations of Biological Systems* sections.

BIOLOGY GUIDED EXAMPLE WITH EXPERT THINKING

Chronic inhalation of crystalline silica has been shown to result in silicosis and pulmonary fibrosis and may also play a role in the development of pulmonary hypertension. The mechanism by which these pathologies develop is not clearly understood, but oxidant/antioxidant imbalances have been suggested. Extracellular superoxide dismutase (Sod3) is one of the most abundant antioxidant enzymes in the pulmonary vasculature. To study the role of Sod3 in the development of silica-mediated pathologies, scientists injected a crystalline silica suspension into the trachea of WT and Sod3–/– mice. 28 days later, a pressure catheter was inserted into the right ventricle through the jugular vein to measure the right ventricular systolic pressure (RVSP) (Figure 1). Elevated RVSP is associated with pulmonary hypertension. Following the RVSP measurement, mice were sacrificed. mRNA was extracted from lung tissue and assayed for Sod3 expression (Figure 2). Lung sections were stained with Mason's trichrome to visualize collagen, a marker of pulmonary fibrosis (Figure 3).

Background info: silica damages the lungs, maybe through oxidants

Researcher thought process: this enzyme is most prevalent in the blood vessels around the lungs, so let's test it first!

Experimental set up: compare silica-induced lung pathologies between WT and Sod3–/– (knockout) mice

Exp 1: measured RVSP; high RVSP = pulmonary hypertension

Exp 2: measuring Sod3 gene expression

Exp 3: quantifying collagen content in the lungs; increased collagen in lungs = fibrosis

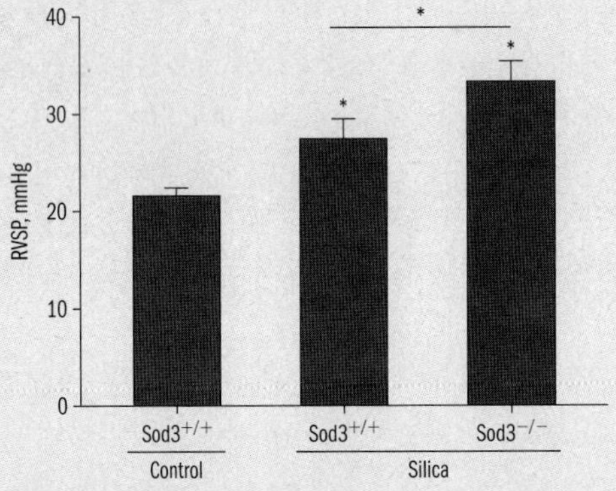

Figure 1

In all three figures, IV = silica treatment and presence or absence of Sod3

Figure 1 DV: RVSP

Trend: RVSP appears highest in Sod3 KO mice treated with silica

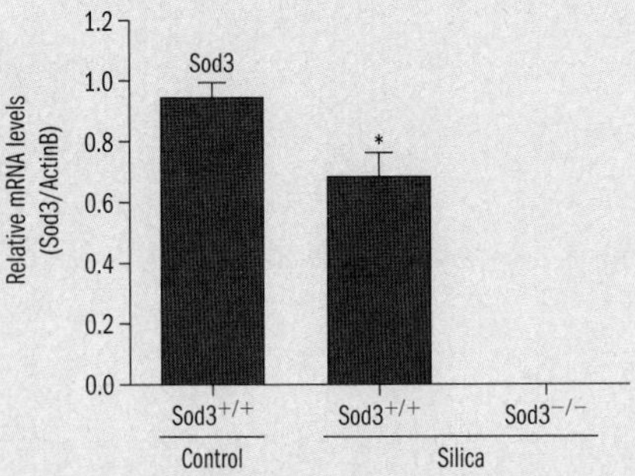

Figure 2

DV: Sod3 expression

Trend: silica treatment decreases Sod3 expression in normal mice

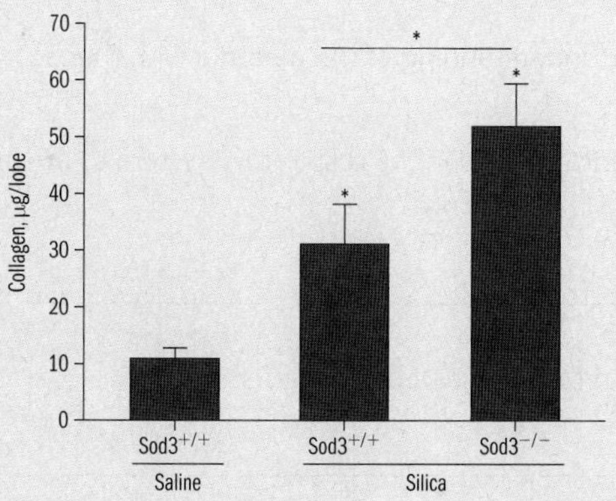

DV: collagen in lungs

Trend: highest in Sod3 KO mice treated with silica

Figure 3

Adapted from Zelko, I. N., Zhu, J., & Roman, J. (2018). Role of SOD3 in silica-related lung fibrosis and pulmonary vascular remodeling. *Respiratory Research, 19*(1), 221. doi:10.1186/s12931-018-0933-6.

Based on the findings of this study, does Sod3 protect against or exacerbate crystalline silica-induced pathologies?

This question is really testing our understanding of how the presence or absence of Sod3 affects the development of silica-induced lung pathologies. Finding an answer will require a strong understanding of the experimental design and careful analysis of the data. Let's start with the experimental design. Paragraph 2 tells us that we have three experimental groups: normal mice not treated with silica, normal mice treated with silica, and Sod3 knockout (KO) mice treated with silica. The normal mice lacking treatment serve as a negative control, whereas the normal mice treated with silica serve as the positive control. Paragraph 1 tells us that crystalline silica has already been shown to cause pulmonary fibrosis and silicosis, so we should expect to see indicators of these pathologies in normal mice treated with silica, but not in the untreated mice. If Sod3 has a protective role, deleting it should lead to an increase in lung damage. If Sod3 exacerbates silica-induced lung damage, deleting it should lead to a decrease in lung damage.

Time to analyze the data! Figure 1 shows that in normal mice, exposure to silica leads to an increase in RVSP, indicating a potential role for silica in the development of pulmonary hypertension. Furthermore, deletion of Sod3 leads to a greater elevation in RVSP, suggesting that Sod3 may have a protective role. Figure 2 shows the expression of the Sod3 transcript in lung tissue. The Sod3 KO mice show no expression, which is consistent with a gene knockout. We also note that the silica exposure leads to a decrease in Sod3 expression. Figure 3 shows an elevation in collagen content in the lungs of silica-treated mice compared to untreated mice. This elevation is significantly higher in Sod3 KO mice. Taken together, these results suggest that Sod3 protects against both silica-induced pulmonary fibrosis and pulmonary hypertension.

Because knockout of Sod3 lead to an increase in pulmonary fibrosis and pulmonary hypertension after exposure to crystalline silica, Sod3 most likely serves a protective role in the lungs against silica-mediated damage.

MCAT CONCEPT CHECK 6.2

Before you move on, assess your understanding of the material with these questions.

1. What are some of the mechanisms used in the respiratory system to prevent infection?

____

2. What is the chemical equation for the bicarbonate buffer system?

____

3. Respiratory failure refers to inadequate ventilation to provide oxygen to the tissues. How would the pH change in respiratory failure?

____

Conclusion

As we learn about the human body, it may be easy to reduce the complex and varied functions of the lungs to breathing and providing a supply of oxygen. The lungs do indeed perform gas exchange, which relies on differences in partial pressures of gases between the alveoli and the blood. Oxygen is taken up by the blood, while carbon dioxide is released for exhalation. Inhalation and exhalation also require pressure differentials created by anatomical structures such as the chest wall, diaphragm, pleurae, and lungs.

However, the lungs are so much more than just *bags of air*; gas exchange is not the only function of the respiratory system. The respiratory system also serves essential roles in thermoregulation, immunity, and pH regulation. As we go through the individual systems within the human body, take special note of how each system is integrated with the other systems. One of the more clear connections is the binding of oxygen to hemoglobin in the lungs and in the rest of the circulatory system—a concept we will expand upon in the next chapter, along with the effects of altitude, pH, and chemicals on this binding.

You've reviewed the content, now test your knowledge and critical thinking skills by completing a test-like passage set in your online resources!

GO ONLINE

CONCEPT SUMMARY

Anatomy and Mechanism of Breathing

- Air is drawn in through the **nares**, and through the nasal cavity and **pharynx**, where it is warmed and humidified. It is filtered by nasal hairs (**vibrissae**) and mucous membranes. It then enters the **larynx**, followed by the **trachea**. The trachea divides into two mainstem **bronchi**, which divide into **bronchioles**, which divide into continually smaller passages until they reach the alveoli.
- **Alveoli** are small sacs that interface with the pulmonary capillaries, allowing gases to diffuse across a one-cell-thick membrane.
- **Surfactant** in the alveoli reduces surface tension at the liquid–gas interface, preventing collapse.
- The pleurae cover the lungs and line the chest wall.
  - The **visceral pleura** lies adjacent to the lung itself.
  - The **parietal pleura** lines the chest wall.
  - The **intrapleural space** lies between these two layers and contains a thin layer of fluid that lubricates the two pleural surfaces.
- The **diaphragm** is a thin skeletal muscle that helps to create the pressure differential required for breathing.
- Inhalation is an active process.
  - The diaphragm and **external intercostal muscles** expand the thoracic cavity, increasing the volume of the intrapleural space. This decreases the intrapleural pressure.
  - This pressure differential ultimately expands the lungs, dropping the pressure within and drawing in air from the environment. This mechanism is termed **negative-pressure breathing**.
- Exhalation may be passive or active.
  - In passive exhalation, relaxation of the muscles of inspiration and elastic recoil of the lungs allow the chest cavity to decrease in volume, reversing the pressure differentials seen in inhalation.
  - In active exhalation, the internal intercostal muscles and abdominal muscles can be used to forcibly decrease the volume of the thoracic cavity, pushing out air.
- A **spirometer** can be used to measure lung capacities and volumes.
  - **Total lung capacity** (TLC) is the maximum volume of air in the lungs when one inhales completely.
  - **Residual volume** (RV) is the volume of air remaining in the lungs when one exhales completely.
  - **Vital capacity** (VC) is the difference between the minimum and maximum volume of air in the lungs.

    - **Tidal volume** (**TV**) is the volume of air inhaled or exhaled in a normal breath.
    - **Expiratory reserve volume** (**ERV**) is the volume of additional air that can be forcibly exhaled after a normal exhalation.
    - **Inspiratory reserve volume** (**IRV**) is the volume of additional air that can be forcibly inhaled after a normal inhalation.
- Ventilation is regulated by the **ventilation center**, a collection of neurons in the medulla oblongata.
    - **Chemoreceptors** respond to carbon dioxide concentrations, increasing the respiratory rate when there is a high concentration of carbon dioxide in the blood (**hypercarbia** or **hypercapnia**).
    - The ventilation center can also respond to low oxygen concentrations in the blood (**hypoxemia**) by increasing ventilation rate.
    - Ventilation can also be controlled consciously through the cerebrum, although the medulla oblongata will override the cerebrum during extended periods of hypo- or hyperventilation.

Functions of the Respiratory System

- The lungs perform gas exchange with the blood through simple diffusion across concentration gradients.
    - Deoxygenated blood with a high carbon dioxide concentration is brought to the lungs via the **pulmonary arteries**.
    - Oxygenated blood with a low carbon dioxide concentration leaves the lungs via the **pulmonary veins**.
- The large surface area of interaction between the alveoli and capillaries allows the respiratory system to assist in thermoregulation through **vasodilation** and **vasoconstriction** of capillary beds.
- The respiratory system must be protected from potential pathogens.
    - Multiple mechanisms, including vibrissae, mucous membranes, and the **mucociliary escalator**, help filter the incoming air and trap particulate matter.
    - **Lysozyme** in the nasal cavity and saliva attacks peptidoglycan cell walls of gram-positive bacteria.
    - **Macrophages** can engulf and digest pathogens and signal to the rest of the immune system that there is an invader.
    - Mucosal surfaces are covered with IgA antibodies.
    - **Mast cells** have antibodies on their surface that, when triggered, can promote the release of inflammatory chemicals. Mast cells are often involved in allergic reactions as well.

- The respiratory system is involved in pH control through the bicarbonate buffer system.
  - When blood pH decreases, respiration rate increases to compensate by blowing off carbon dioxide. This causes a left shift in the buffer equation, reducing hydrogen ion concentration.
  - When blood pH increases, respiration rate decreases to compensate by trapping carbon dioxide. This causes a right shift in the buffer equation, increasing hydrogen ion concentration.

ANSWERS TO CONCEPT CHECKS

6.1

1. Nares → nasal cavity → pharynx → larynx → trachea → bronchi → bronchioles → alveoli
2. Inhalation uses the diaphragm and external intercostal muscles; in labored breathing, muscles of the neck and back may also be involved. Passive exhalation uses the recoil of these same muscles; active exhalation also uses the internal intercostal muscles and abdominal muscles.
3. Surfactant reduces surface tension at the air–liquid interface in the alveoli. This prevents their collapse.
4. Vital capacity is the sum of the inspiratory reserve volume, expiratory reserve volume, and tidal volume: $VC = IRV + ERV + TV$
5. When CO_2 levels become too low, the brain can decrease the respiratory rate in order to raise CO_2 levels.

6.2

1. Immune mechanisms in the respiratory system include vibrissae in the nares, lysozyme in the mucous membranes, the mucociliary escalator, macrophages in the lungs, mucosal IgA antibodies, and mast cells.
2. $CO_2\ (g) + H_2O\ (l) \rightleftharpoons H_2CO_3\ (aq) \rightleftharpoons H^+\ (aq) + HCO_3^-\ (aq)$
3. In respiratory failure, ventilation slows, and less carbon dioxide is blown off. As this occurs, the buffer equation shifts to the right, and more hydrogen ions are generated. This results in a lower pH of the blood.

SCIENCE MASTERY ASSESSMENT EXPLANATIONS

1. **D**

Gas exchange in the lungs relies on passive diffusion of oxygen and carbon dioxide. This is accomplished easily because there is always a difference in the partial pressures of these two gases and because the subdivision of the respiratory tree creates a large surface area of interaction between the alveoli and the circulatory system. In addition, the thin alveolar walls allow for fast diffusion and gas exchange. Therefore, **(A)**, **(B)**, and **(C)** can be eliminated. **(D)** is the correct answer because active transport is not used in the gas exchange process in the lungs.

2. **D**

The muscles involved in ventilation are the diaphragm, which separates the thoracic cavity from the abdominal cavity, and the intercostal muscles. During inhalation, the diaphragm contracts and flattens, while the external intercostal muscles contract, pulling the rib cage up and out. These actions cause an overall increase in the volume of the thoracic cavity. During exhalation, both the diaphragm and the external intercostals relax, causing a decrease in the volume of the thoracic cavity because of the recoil of these tissues. In forced exhalation, the internal intercostals and abdominal muscles may contract to force out air. Thus, the only correct association from the given answers is **(D)**.

3. **C**

Total lung capacity is equal to the vital capacity (the maximum volume of air that can be forcibly inhaled and exhaled from the lungs) plus the residual volume (the air that always remains in the lungs, preventing the alveoli from collapsing).

4. **B**

During inhalation, the chest cavity expands, causing expansion of the intrapleural space. According to Boyle's law, an increase in volume at a constant temperature is accompanied by a decrease in pressure. When the intrapleural pressure (and, by extension, the alveolar pressure) is less than atmospheric pressure, air enters the lungs. During exhalation, these pressure gradients reverse; thus, during exhalation, intrapleural pressure is higher than atmospheric pressure, not lower.

5. **B**

The intrapleural space, bounded by the parietal and visceral pleurae, is a potential space. As such, it is normally collapsed and contains a small amount of fluid. However, introduction of fluid or air into the intrapleural space can fill the space, causing collapse of the lung. The other options listed are too firmly apposed to permit blood to collect in these spaces.

6. **C**

The pharynx, which lies behind the nasal cavity and oral cavity, is a common pathway for food entering the digestive system and air entering the respiratory system. It is the larynx that contains the vocal cords, not the pharynx.

7. **D**

Air enters the respiratory tract through the external nares (nostrils) and travels through the nasal cavities. It then passes through the pharynx and into the larynx. Ingested food also passes through the pharynx on its way to the esophagus; to ensure that food does not accidentally enter the larynx, the epiglottis covers the larynx during swallowing. After the larynx, air goes to the trachea, which eventually divides into two bronchi, one for each lung. The bronchi branch into smaller bronchioles, which terminate in clusters of alveoli. From the given sequences, only **(D)** correctly describes the sequence of the passages through which air travels.

8. **B**

In a patient with IPF, the increased stiffness of the lungs would likely decrease the volume of air the individual could inhale, which would decrease both the total lung capacity and inspiratory reserve volume. However, spirometry cannot measure the total lung capacity accurately because it cannot determine the residual volume—the volume of air left in the lungs when an individual has maximally exhaled. Because the residual volume makes up a portion of the total lung capacity (total lung capacity = vital capacity + residual volume), a spirometer cannot be used to determine the total lung capacity. Therefore, while Statement I is a true statement about individuals with IPF, it cannot appear in the answer choice. Finally, increased stiffness of the lungs would be expected to decrease the residual volume, not increase it; further, residual volume, as described above, cannot be measured with a spirometer.

9. **B**

Lysozyme is an enzyme present in the nasal cavity, saliva, and tears that degrades peptidoglycan, preventing infection by gram-positive bacteria. Thus, premature infants who lack lysozyme are more likely to suffer from infections with these organisms.

10. **D**

If an area of the lung becomes filled with mucus and inflammatory cells, the area will not be able to participate in gas exchange. Because no air will enter or leave the area, the concentration gradient will no longer exist, and neither oxygen nor carbon dioxide will be able to diffuse across the alveolar wall.

11. **B**

When people hyperventilate, their respiratory rate increases. When the respiratory rate increases, more carbon dioxide is blown off. This causes a shift to the left in the bicarbonate buffer equation, and the blood becomes more alkaline. Breathing into the bag allows some of this carbon dioxide to be returned to the bloodstream in order to maintain the proper pH.

12. **C**

When a patient who has an asthma attack does not respond to treatment and has been hyperventilating for over an hour, the patient may become fatigued and may not be able to maintain hyperventilation. In this case, the patient's breathing rate starts to decrease, and the patient fails to receive adequate oxygen. By extension, carbon dioxide is trapped in the blood, and the pH begins to drop. Despite the fact that this pH is normal at the moment, this patient is crashing and may start demonstrating acidemia in the near future. While the kidneys should compensate for alkalemia, this is a slow process and would not normalize the blood pH within an hour; further, adequate compensation by the kidneys would actually be a reassuring sign, eliminating **(A)**. There is no evidence to suggest that the measurement was inaccurate, eliminating **(B)**. Finally, after treatment, the patient should return to a normal blood pH with adequate ventilation and would not be expected to overcompensate by becoming acidemic, eliminating **(D)**.

13. **A**

This question requires a few different levels of thinking. The question stem states that premature infants often require ventilation using positive end-expiratory pressures. While you are not expected to know ventilator settings for the MCAT, you should be able to decode what this phrase means: at the end of expiration, the ventilator will provide a higher pressure than normal, which forces extra air into the alveoli. This pressure must be used to prevent alveolar collapse, which should remind you that surfactant serves the same purpose by reducing surface tension. Thus, it makes sense that if premature babies lack surfactant, providing extra air pressure at the end of expiration would be beneficial.

14. **A**

The intrinsic elastic properties of the lung are important during exhalation as the passive recoil of lung tissue helps decrease lung volume. With decreased recoil, the patient will have difficulty exhaling completely, increasing the residual volume. The total lung capacity would be expected to increase in this case because there would be less recoil opposing inhalation, eliminating **(B)**. With decreased alveolar surface area, one would expect decreased gas exchange, which would decrease blood concentrations of oxygen while increasing blood concentrations of carbon dioxide, eliminating **(C)** and **(D)**.

15. **C**

Allergic reactions occur when a substance binds to an antibody and promotes an overactive immune response with inflammatory chemicals. The antibody is already attached to a mast cell. Thus, when the substance binds to the antibody, the mast cell can release the inflammatory mediators that cause allergic reactions.

Consult your online resources for additional practice. GO ONLINE

SHARED CONCEPTS

Biology Chapter 7
The Cardiovascular System

Biology Chapter 10
Homeostasis

General Chemistry Chapter 6
Equilibrium

General Chemistry Chapter 8
The Gas Phase

General Chemistry Chapter 10
Acids and Bases

Physics and Math Chapter 3
Thermodynamics

CHAPTER 7

THE CARDIOVASCULAR SYSTEM

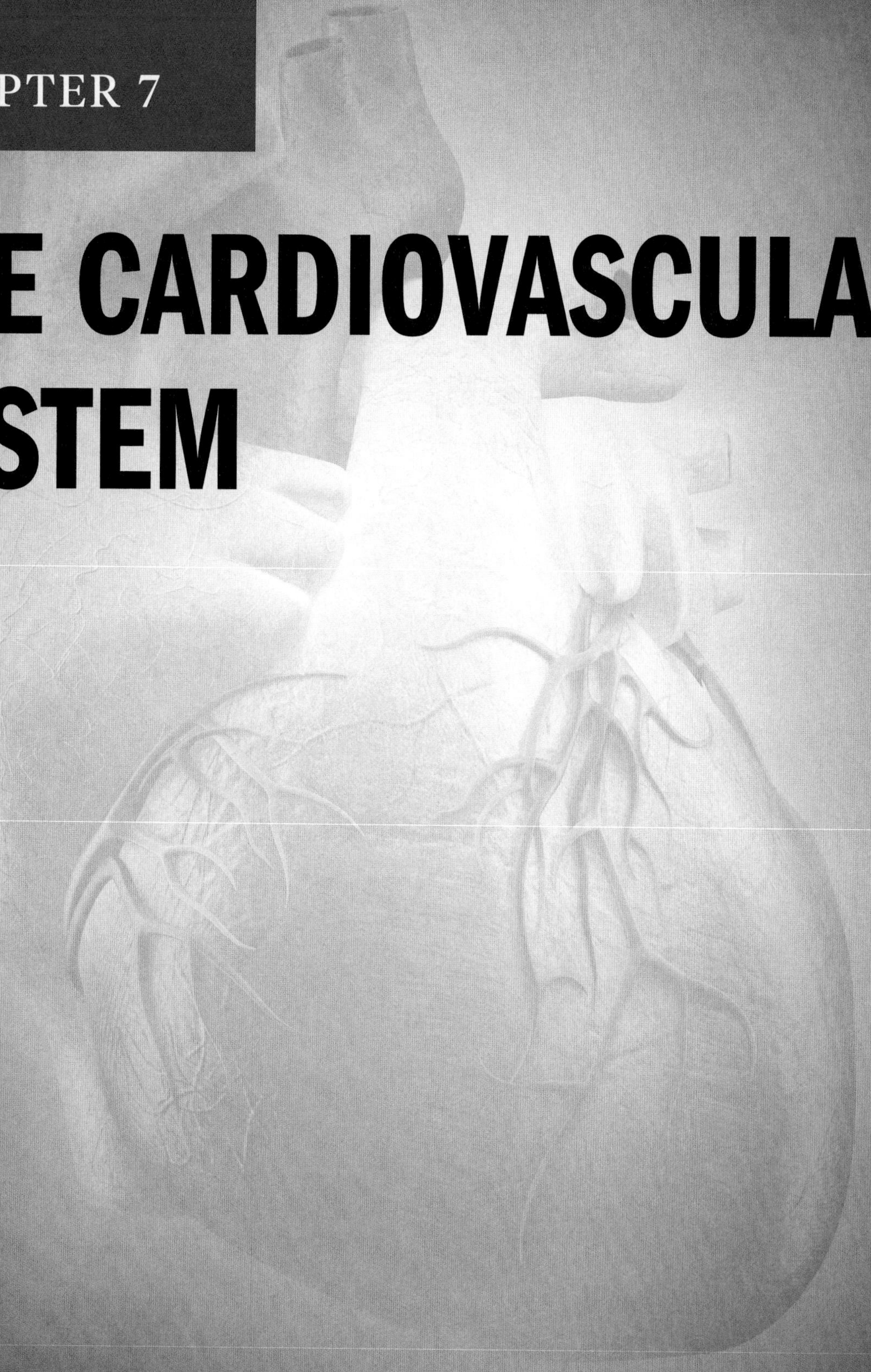

SCIENCE MASTERY ASSESSMENT

Every pre-med knows this feeling: there is so much content I have to know for the MCAT! How do I know what to do first or what's important?

While the high-yield badges throughout this book will help you identify the most important topics, this Science Mastery Assessment is another tool in your MCAT prep arsenal. This quiz (which can also be taken in your online resources) and the guidance below will help ensure that you are spending the appropriate amount of time on this chapter based on your personal strengths and weaknesses. Don't worry though—skipping something now does not mean you'll never study it. Later on in your prep, as you complete full-length tests, you'll uncover specific pieces of content that you need to review and can come back to these chapters as appropriate.

How to Use This Assessment

If you answer 0–7 questions correctly:

Spend about 1 hour to read this chapter in full and take limited notes throughout. Follow up by reviewing **all** quiz questions to ensure that you now understand how to solve each one.

If you answer 8–11 questions correctly:

Spend 20–40 minutes reviewing the quiz questions. Beginning with the questions you missed, read and take notes on the corresponding subchapters. For questions you answered correctly, ensure your thinking matches that of the explanation and you understand why each choice was correct or incorrect.

If you answer 12–15 questions correctly:

Spend less than 20 minutes reviewing all questions from the quiz. If you missed any, then include a quick read-through of the corresponding subchapters, or even just the relevant content within a subchapter, as part of your question review. For questions you answered correctly, ensure your thinking matches that of the explanation and review the Concept Summary at the end of the chapter.

1. Which of the following is a FALSE statement regarding erythrocytes?
   - **A.** Erythrocytes contain hemoglobin.
   - **B.** Erythrocytes are anaerobic.
   - **C.** The nuclei of erythrocytes are located in the middle of the biconcave disc.
   - **D.** Erythrocytes are phagocytized in the spleen and liver after a certain period of time.

2. Which of the following is the correct sequence of a cardiac impulse?
   - **A.** SA node → AV node → Purkinje fibers → bundle of His → ventricles
   - **B.** AV node → bundle of His → Purkinje fibers → ventricles → atria
   - **C.** SA node → atria → AV node → bundle of His → Purkinje fibers → ventricles
   - **D.** SA node → AV node → atria → bundle of His → Purkinje fibers → ventricles

3. Hemoglobin's affinity for O_2:
   - **A.** increases in exercising muscle tissue.
   - **B.** decreases as blood P_aCO_2 decreases.
   - **C.** decreases as blood pH decreases.
   - **D.** is higher in maternal blood than in fetal blood.

4. Which of the following correctly traces the circulatory pathway?
   - **A.** Superior vena cava → right atrium → right ventricle → pulmonary artery → lungs → pulmonary veins → left atrium → left ventricle → aorta
   - **B.** Superior vena cava → left atrium → left ventricle → pulmonary artery → lungs → pulmonary veins → right atrium → right ventricle → aorta
   - **C.** Aorta → right atrium → right ventricle → pulmonary artery → lungs → pulmonary veins → left atrium → left ventricle → superior vena cava
   - **D.** Superior vena cava → right atrium → right ventricle → pulmonary veins → lungs → pulmonary artery → left atrium → left ventricle → aorta

5. At the venous end of a capillary bed, the osmotic pressure:
   - **A.** is greater than the hydrostatic pressure.
   - **B.** results in a net outflow of fluid.
   - **C.** is significantly higher than the osmotic pressure at the arterial end.
   - **D.** causes proteins to enter the interstitium.

6. A patient's chart indicates a cardiac output of 7500 mL per minute and a stroke volume of 50 mL. What is the patient's pulse, in beats per minute?
   - **A.** 50
   - **B.** 100
   - **C.** 150
   - **D.** 400

7. An unconscious patient is rushed into the emergency room and needs an immediate blood transfusion. Because there is no time to check the patient's medical history or determine blood type, which type of blood should the patient receive?
   - **A.** AB^+
   - **B.** AB^-
   - **C.** O^+
   - **D.** O^-

8. Which of the following is true regarding arteries and veins?
   - **A.** Arteries are thin-walled, muscular, and elastic, whereas veins are thick-walled and inelastic.
   - **B.** Arteries always conduct oxygenated blood, whereas veins always carry deoxygenated blood.
   - **C.** The blood pressure in the aorta is always higher than the pressure in the superior vena cava.
   - **D.** Arteries facilitate blood transport by using skeletal muscle contractions, whereas veins make use of the pumping of the heart to push blood.

9. At any given time, there is more blood in the venous system than the arterial system. Which of the following features of veins allows for this?
   - **A.** Relative lack of smooth muscle in the wall
   - **B.** Presence of valves
   - **C.** Proximity of veins to lymphatic vessels
   - **D.** Thin endothelial lining

10. Which of the following is involved in the body's primary blood-buffering mechanism?
   A. Fluid intake
   B. Absorption of nutrients in the gastrointestinal system
   C. Carbon dioxide produced from metabolism
   D. Hormones released by the kidneys

11. Due to kidney disease, a person is losing albumin into the urine. What effect is this likely to have within the capillaries?
   A. Increased oncotic pressure
   B. Increased hydrostatic pressure
   C. Decreased oncotic pressure
   D. Decreased hydrostatic pressure

12. The tricuspid valve prevents backflow of blood from the:
   A. left ventricle into the left atrium.
   B. aorta into the left ventricle.
   C. pulmonary artery into the right ventricle.
   D. right ventricle into the right atrium.

13. The world record for the longest-held breath is 22 minutes and 0 seconds. If a sample were taken from this individual during the last minute of breath-holding, which of the following might be observed?
   A. Increased hemoglobin affinity for oxygen
   B. Decreased P_aCO_2
   C. Increased hematocrit
   D. Decreased pH

14. A person has a heart attack that primarily affects the wall between the two ventricles. Which portion of the electrical conduction system is most likely affected?
   A. AV node
   B. SA node
   C. Bundle of His
   D. Left ventricular muscle

15. Which vascular structure creates the most resistance to blood flow?
   A. Aorta
   B. Arterioles
   C. Capillaries
   D. Veins

Answer Key

1. **C**
2. **C**
3. **C**
4. **A**
5. **A**
6. **C**
7. **D**
8. **C**
9. **A**
10. **C**
11. **C**
12. **D**
13. **D**
14. **C**
15. **B**

Detailed explanations can be found at the end of the chapter.

CHAPTER 7

THE CARDIOVASCULAR SYSTEM

In This Chapter

CHAPTER PROFILE

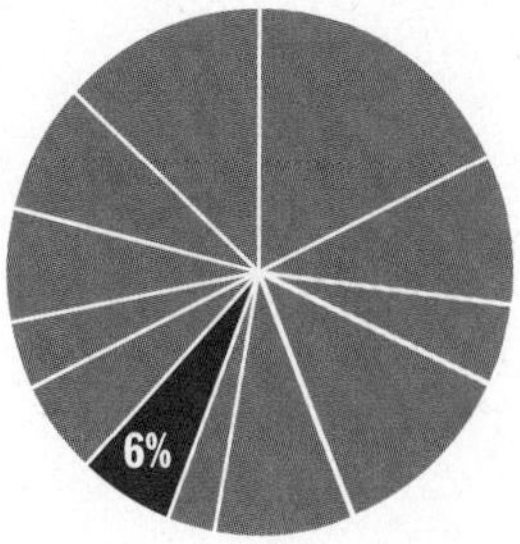

The content in this chapter should be relevant to about 6% of all questions about biology on the MCAT.

This chapter covers material from the following AAMC content category:

3B: Structure and integrative functions of the main organ systems

Introduction

As late as the 19th century, physicians adhered to a doctrine of health known as *humoralism.* This theory, developed by Greek and Roman physicians and philosophers and adopted by Islamic physicians, remained dominant in medical thought and practice until it was displaced by modern medical research in the 1800s. The theory of humoralism holds that the human body is composed of four fluids or substances called humors: black bile, yellow bile, phlegm, and blood. In the healthy state, these four humors are in balance, but excess or deficiency of any one of them would cause illness, disease, and even maladaptive personality characteristics. Over the course of a lifetime the levels of each of the four humors would rise and fall in accordance with diet and activity, resulting in maladies reflective of the imbalance. Treatments were intended to restore this balance.

Perhaps one of the most well-known treatments associated with humoralism is the practice of bloodletting. Because many diseases were associated with an excess of blood, physicians would withdraw significant amounts of blood from their patients to restore balance to the four humors. Methods for bloodletting were many, and some were dramatic—including drawing blood from major veins in the arm or neck and puncturing arteries. Devices known as scarificators were developed to cut into the superficial vessels. Most famously, leeches were used (especially in the early 19th century) to draw out excess blood. In fact, in the early decades of the 1800s, hundreds of millions of leeches were used by European physicians; in the 1830s, France alone imported about 40 million leeches per year for medical treatments.

While the humoral theory has been completely discredited by modern science, some practices associated with humoralism are still being used, albeit based on very different medical understanding and for different purposes. For example, new research has shown that medicinal leeches can be used effectively in microsurgery to help prevent blood coagulation, and in reconstructive surgery to stimulate circulation to the reattached tissue.

The cardiovascular system is one of the most commonly tested organ systems on the MCAT. It serves a variety of functions, including the movement of respiratory gases, nutrients, and wastes. We will review the structures and functional anatomy of the cardiovascular system and then discuss blood and its functional components. We'll also trace the pathways created by the electrically excitable cells that initiate and spread contractions through the heart. A quick recap of genetics and inheritance will help explain the consequences of ABO and Rh antigens. In addition, the binding of oxygen and carbon dioxide to hemoglobin will be discussed in detail.

7.1 Anatomy of the Cardiovascular System

High-Yield

LEARNING OBJECTIVES

After Chapter 7.1, you will be able to:

- Recall the names of the chambers and valves of the heart
- Describe the chain of events in the conduction system of the heart that leads to heartbeat generation
- Identify autonomic inputs into the heart and their effects
- Distinguish between arteries, capillaries, and veins
- Explain why the right side of the heart is less muscular than the left side
- Trace the flow of blood through the heart:

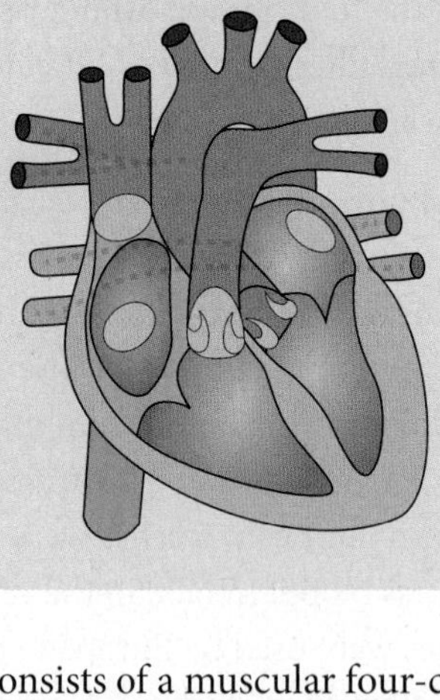

The **cardiovascular system** consists of a muscular four-chambered **heart**, **blood vessels**, and **blood**, as shown in Figure 7.1. The heart acts as a pump, distributing blood through the vasculature. The vasculature consists of arteries, capillaries, and veins.

After blood travels through veins, it is returned to the right side of the heart where it is pumped to the lungs to be reoxygenated. Then, the oxygenated blood returns to the left side of the heart where it is once again pumped to the rest of the body.

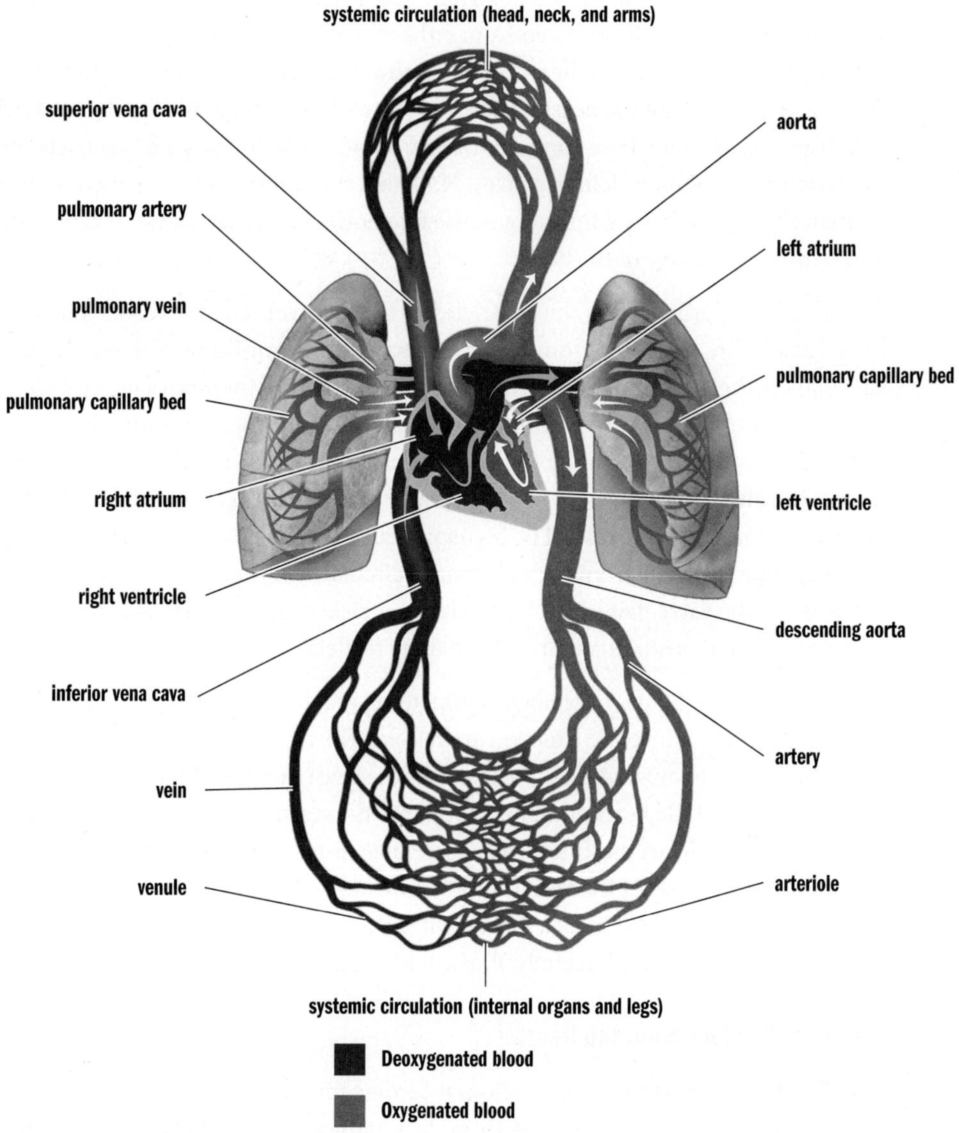

Figure 7.1 Anatomy of the Cardiovascular System

The Heart

The **heart** is a four-chambered structure composed predominantly of cardiac muscle. We often speak of the heart as a pump, supporting a single circulatory system. However, the heart is actually composed of two pumps supporting two different circulations in series. The right side of the heart accepts deoxygenated blood returning from the body and moves it to the lungs by way of the pulmonary arteries;

this constitutes the first pump (**pulmonary circulation**). The second pump is the left side of the heart, which receives oxygenated blood from the lungs by way of the pulmonary veins and forces it out to the body through the aorta (**systemic circulation**).

Each side of the heart consists of an atrium and a ventricle. The **atria** are thin-walled structures where blood is received from either the **venae cavae** (deoxygenated blood entering the right side of the heart) or the **pulmonary veins** (oxygenated blood entering the left side of the heart). The atria contract to push blood into the **ventricles**. After the ventricles fill, they contract to send blood to the lungs (right ventricle) and the systemic circulation (left ventricle). Note that the ventricles are far more muscular than the atria, allowing for more powerful contractions that are necessary to push blood through the rest of the body.

MNEMONIC

Atrioventricular valves: **LAB RAT**

Left **A**trium = **B**icuspid

Right **A**trium = **T**ricuspid

The atria are separated from the ventricles by the **atrioventricular valves**. Likewise, the ventricles are separated from the vasculature by the **semilunar valves**. These valves allow the heart muscle to create the pressure within the ventricles necessary to propel the blood forward within the circulation, while also preventing backflow of blood. The valve between the right atrium and the right ventricle is known as the **tricuspid valve** (three leaflets), while the valve between the left atrium and the left ventricle is known as the **mitral** or **bicuspid valve** (two leaflets). The valve that separates the right ventricle from the pulmonary circulation is known as the **pulmonary valve**, while the valve that separates the left ventricle from the aorta is known as the **aortic valve**. Both semilunar valves have three leaflets.

One of the central themes in biology is something that we've touched on already in previous chapters: structure and function are related. The right and left sides of the heart are two different pumps, with the right side of the heart pumping blood to the lungs, and the left side of the heart pumping blood into the systemic circulation. Blood leaving the left side of the heart must travel a considerable distance, so blood pressure must be maintained as far away as the feet. Thus, the left side of the heart is more muscular than the right side of the heart. In fact, if the right side of the heart were as muscular as the left and pumped blood as forcefully, this would damage the lungs.

Electrical Conduction in the Heart

The coordinated, rhythmic contraction of cardiac muscle originates in an electrical impulse generated by and traveling through a pathway formed by four electrically excitable structures, as shown in Figure 7.2. This commonly tested pathway consists of, in order of excitation: the sinoatrial (SA) node, the atrioventricular (AV) node, the bundle of His (AV bundle) and its branches, and the Purkinje fibers. Impulse initiation occurs at the **SA node**, which generates 60–100 signals per minute without requiring any neurological input. This small collection of cells is located in the wall of the right atrium. As the depolarization wave spreads from the SA node, it causes the two atria to contract simultaneously. While most ventricular filling is passive (that is, blood moves from the atria to the ventricles based solely on ventricular relaxation), atrial **systole** (contraction) results in an increase in atrial pressure that forces a little more blood into the ventricles. This additional volume of blood is called the **atrial kick** and accounts for about 5–30 percent of cardiac output. Next, the signal reaches the **AV node**, which sits at the junction of the atria and ventricles. The signal is delayed here to allow the ventricles to fill completely before they contract. The signal then travels down the **bundle of His** and its branches, embedded in the **interventricular septum** (wall), and to the **Purkinje fibers**, which distribute the electrical signal through the ventricular muscle. The muscle cells are connected by **intercalated discs**, which contain many gap junctions directly connecting the cytoplasm of adjacent cells. This allows for coordinated ventricular contraction.

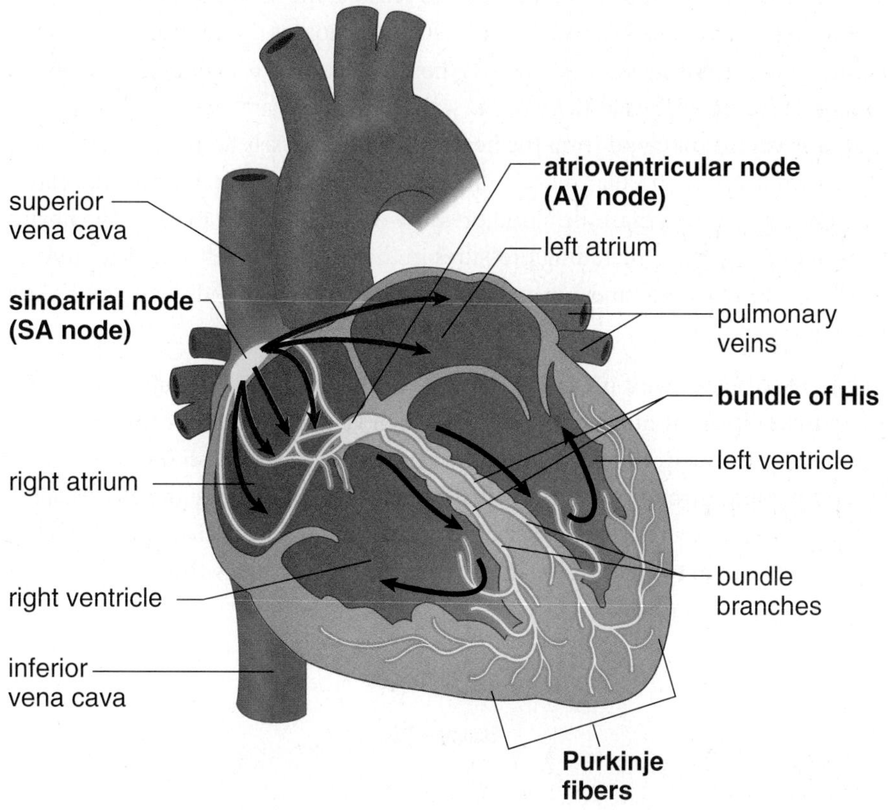

Figure 7.2 Electrical Conduction System of the Heart
Electrical impulses travel from the SA node to the AV node, through the bundle of His, and finally to the Purkinje fibers.

The SA node has an intrinsic rhythm of 60–100 signals per minute, so the normal human heart rate is 60–100 beats per minute. Highly conditioned athletes may have heart rates significantly lower than 60, in the range of 40–50 beats per minute. Stress, exercise, excitement, surprise, or danger can cause the heart rate to rise significantly above 100.

KEY CONCEPT

Cardiac muscle has myogenic activity, meaning that it can contract without any neurological input. The SA node generates about 60-100 beats per minute, even if all innervation to the heart is cut. The neurological input to the heart is important in speeding up and slowing the rate of contraction, but not generating it in the first place.

REAL WORLD

The heart's electrical impulses can be detected on the body's surface by placing electrodes on the skin on opposite sides of the heart. A recording of these currents is called an electrocardiogram (ECG or EKG; the *K*, by the way, reflects the German spelling). Electrocardiograms are incredibly powerful tools for assessing the status of a patient's heart. A normal EKG is shown below.

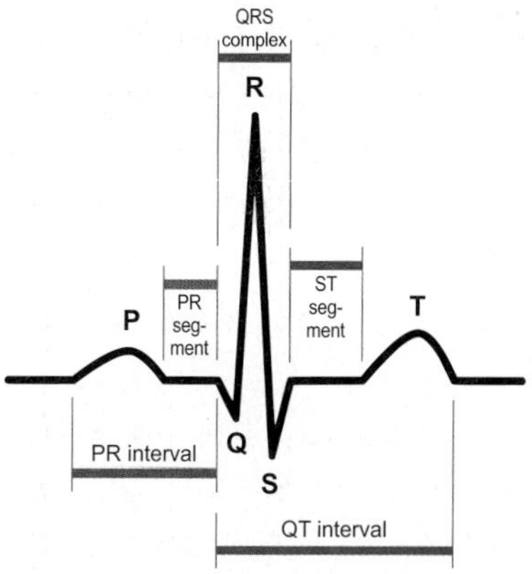

Depolarization precedes cardiac muscle contraction, so the electrical spikes of the EKG occur just before a cardiac contractile event. The P-wave occurs immediately before the atria contract, and the QRS complex occurs just before the ventricles contract. The T-wave represents ventricular repolarization.

The circulatory system is under autonomic control. The autonomic system consists of the sympathetic ("fight-or-flight") and parasympathetic ("rest-and-digest") branches, controls the heart and affects the vasculature. Sympathetic signals speed up the heart rate and increase the contractility of cardiac muscle, while parasympathetic signals, provided by the **vagus nerve**, slow down the heart rate.

Contraction

The heart is a muscle that must contract in order to move blood. Each heartbeat is composed of two phases, known as systole and diastole. During **systole**, ventricular contraction and closure of the AV valves occurs and blood is pumped out of the ventricles. During **diastole**, the ventricles are relaxed, the semilunar valves are closed, and blood from the atria fills the ventricles. Contraction of the ventricles generates a higher pressure during systole, whereas their relaxation during diastole causes the pressure to decrease. The elasticity of the walls of the large arteries, which stretch to receive the volume of blood from the heart, allows the vessels to maintain sufficient pressure while the ventricular muscles are relaxed. In fact, if it weren't for the elasticity of the large arteries, diastolic blood pressure would plummet to zero. The normal events of one heartbeat, including pressures in the left atrium, left ventricle, and aorta; left ventricular volume; normal and pathologic heart sounds; and an EKG are shown in Figure 7.3.

A measure to be aware of is **cardiac output**, or the total blood volume pumped by a ventricle in a minute. Does it matter which ventricle one chooses? As mentioned previously, the two pumps are connected in series, so the volumes of blood passing through each side must be the same, much like the electrical current between two resistors in series must be the same. Cardiac output (CO) is the product of **heart rate** (HR, beats per minute) and **stroke volume** (SV, volume of blood pumped per beat):

$$CO = HR \times SV$$

Equation 7.1

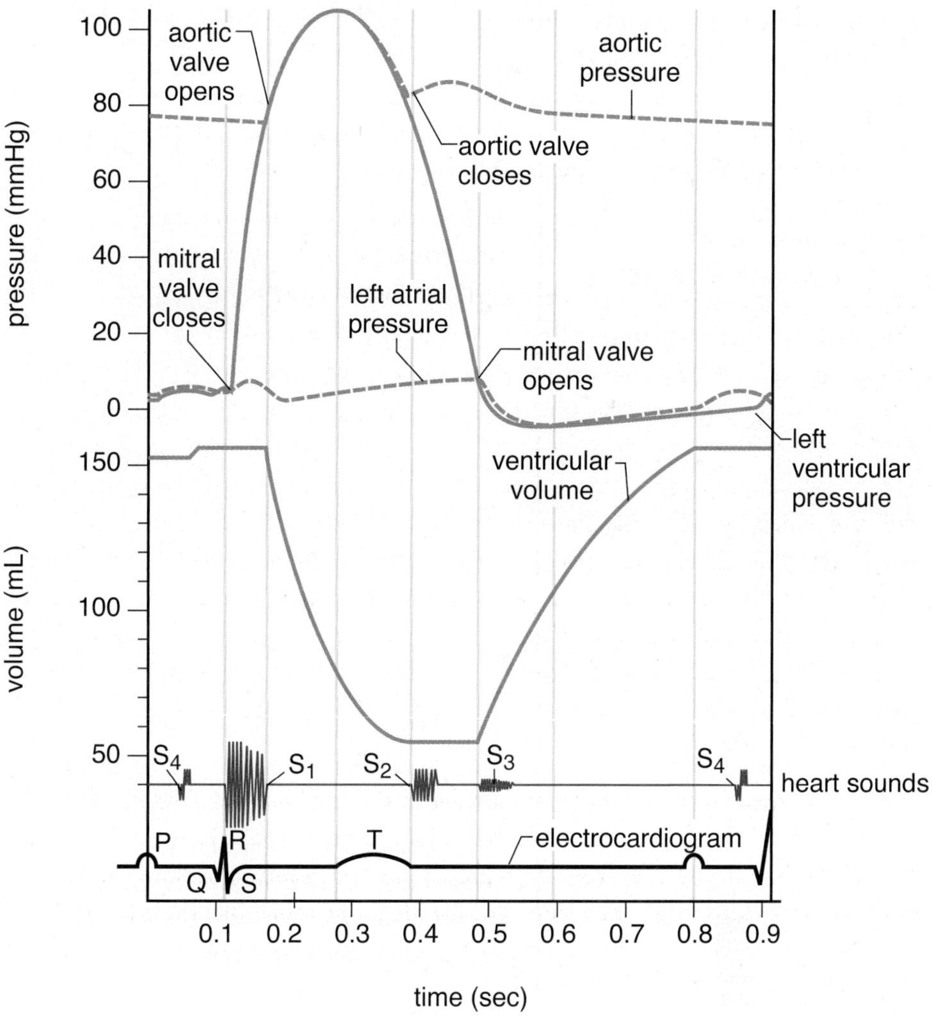

Figure 7.3 The Cardiac Cycle

The MCAT will not expect a thorough understanding of every detail of this diagram; it is more important to see how the changes in valves (open or closed), pressures, and volumes are related.

For humans, cardiac output is about 5 liters per minute. During periods of exercise or rest, the autonomic nervous system will increase (sympathetic) or decrease (parasympathetic) cardiac output, respectively.

REAL WORLD

The rhythmic impulses we hear when we listen to someone's heart with a stethoscope (*lub dub*) are referred to as the heart sounds. The first sound, S_1, is produced when the two AV valves close at the start of systole to prevent backflow into the atria. The second sound, S_2, is produced when the two semilunar valves close at the end of systole to prevent backflow into the ventricles. Extra heart sounds (S_3 and S_4) can result from stiffness of the heart muscle or high blood pressure. Heart murmurs, which may be so loud as to be audible without a stethoscope, may arise when the valves malfunction and become either narrow and stiff or wide and floppy, resulting in abnormal flow patterns across the valve.

REAL WORLD

There is a limit to how fast the heart can beat and still pump blood effectively. Because the heart fills with blood when it is relaxing (diastole), the faster it beats, the less time there is for blood to enter the heart during relaxation. Thus, a faster heartbeat means diminishing returns in terms of the amount of blood supplied to the body. A dangerous condition called ventricular tachycardia (often abbreviated *v-tach*) features a very rapid rate of ventricular contraction. The heart in v-tach cannot properly fill with blood and, paradoxically, stops pumping blood despite its fast rate. Systemic pressures drop precipitously. Death will result unless the heart is forced out of this abnormal rhythm.

BIOLOGY GUIDED EXAMPLE WITH EXPERT THINKING

To further investigate the effects of atorvastatin on post-myocardial infarction recovery, left ventricular myocardial infarction was artificially induced in rats. Rats were randomly assigned to atorvastatin or vehicle treatment. After four weeks, the left ventricles of all rats were examined. Results are summarized in Figures 1A–F below.

This isn't the full article, just the results! This is fairly common on the MCAT.

Vehicle means to give the base solution without the active ingredient itself. A lot of times it is just saline, and serves as a control.

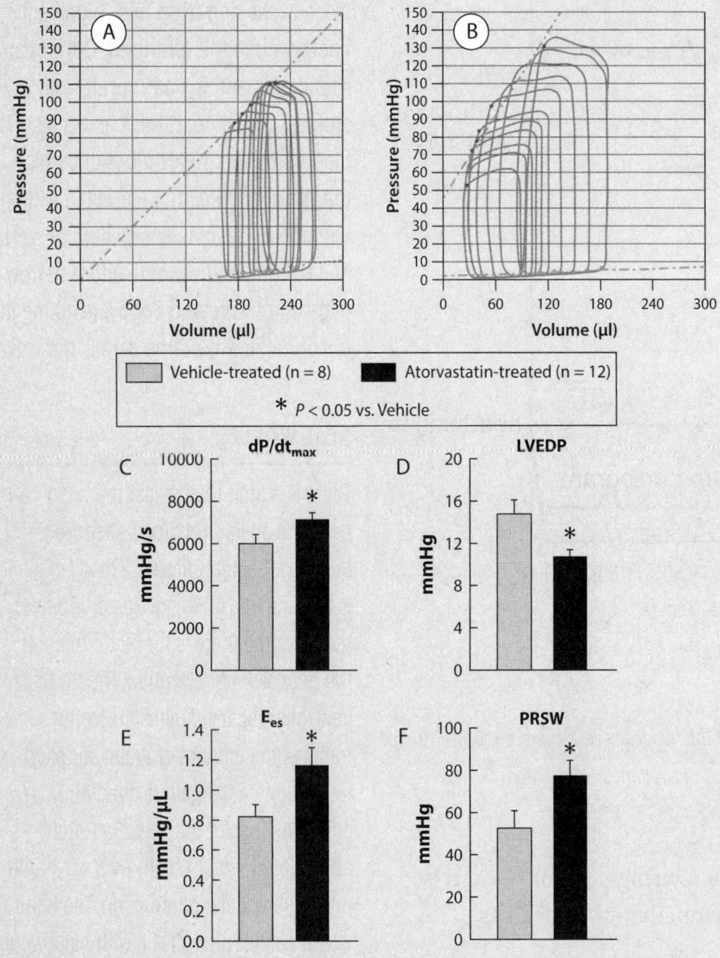

IVs: vehicle or atorvastatin treatment

DVs: pressure-volume cardiac cycle, hemodynamic variables (dP/dt, LVEDP, E_{es}, and PRSW)

Trend: Atorvastatin treatment widens the volume range in pressure-volume cardiac cycle loops. Atorvastating treatment increases dP/dt, E_{es}, and PRSW and decreases LVEDP.

Figure 1 Representative pressure-volume cardiac cycle loops from a vehicle-treated rat (A) and an atorvastatin-treated rat (B) recorded during preload manipulation by a brief period of inferior vena cava occlusion. Panels C–F illustrate the quantitative analysis of hemodynamic variables of the rats including dP/dt (C), LV end-diastolic pressure (D), end-systolic elastance (E), and preload recruitable stroke work (F).

Adapted from Tang X-L, Sanganalmath SK, Sato H, Bi Q, Hunt G, Vincent RJ, et al. (2011) Atorvastatin therapy during the peri-infarct period attenuates left ventricular dysfunction and remodeling after myocardial infarction. *PLoS One* 6(9): e25320. https://doi.org/10.1371/journal.pone.0025320.

Which treatment condition is correlated with a greater stroke volume in rats following myocardial infarction?

This question asks us to interpret the given figure in order to determine which condition is associated with a particular outcome. The MCAT will require us to bring in testable content knowledge, but it will also expect us to know how to use logical reasoning to analyze an experiment.

The first step is to think about what the question is asking for us to analyze from within the given passage and figure. We know from our outside content knowledge that stroke volume is defined as the volume of blood pumped per heartbeat. Simply speaking, all we need to do is to identify what information on the figure is related to the volume of blood pumped.

If we're not sure how to do this, a good place to start is to look at the units of each graph in the figure. In a novel figure, units can serve as a great clue as to what the figure is about. Since we're looking for stroke volume, we should be looking for units of volume like liters or cm^3. Parts C through F have units of pressure per seconds, pressure, or pressure per volume, which are not what we are looking for. We'll need to refer to images A and B, both of which have a unit of volume on their *x*-axes.

According to the figure label, graph A shows the vehicle-treated rat, and graph B shows the atorvastatin-treated rat. The label also tells us that these graphs show pressure-volume cardiac cycle loops of two rats, one in each condition. Now we must relate these graphs to stroke volume. Remember that stroke volume is the volume of blood pumped per heartbeat. In other words, it is the amount of blood pumped after one cardiac cycle. On a pressure-volume graph, a cardiac cycle is seen here as a rectangular loop, with the height and width of the loop representing the pressure change and volume change, respectively. Looking at the two graphs in the figure, we must compare the changes in the volume of the loops of the two conditions. Even without explicitly measuring the dimensions, we can see that the atorvastatin graph has much wider loops, and thus a greater stroke volume.

Based on parts A and B of Figure 1, we can reasonably conclude that treatment with atorvastatin is correlated with greater stroke volume in rats post-infarction as compared to the control (vehicle) treatment.

MNEMONIC

Arteries carry blood **away** from the heart.

REAL WORLD

A heart attack, or myocardial infarction, is caused by a lack of bloodflow through the coronary arteries, which results in decreased oxygen delivery to the cardiac muscle itself. Anaerobic respiration cannot produce enough ATP to keep up with demand, so the muscle tissue begins to die. A person suffering a heart attack is often given a β-blocker, which blocks the sympathetic stimulation of the heart, resulting in lower heart rate and lower contractility. With a β-blocker, the heart does not work as hard, so its oxygen demand is diminished, which helps to prevent further damage to cardiac tissue.

The Vasculature

In order to deliver blood to the entire body, the circulatory system utilizes vessels of different sizes. The three major types of vessels are arteries, veins, and capillaries. Blood travels away from the heart in **arteries**, the largest of which is the aorta (in the systemic circulation). Major arteries, such as the common carotids, subclavians, and renal arteries, branch off of the aorta to distribute the bloodflow toward different peripheral tissues. Arteries then undergo further divisions and name changes as they divert blood to specific tissues and organs until, upon reaching their target, they branch into **arterioles**, which ultimately lead to **capillaries** that perfuse the tissues. There is also a set of coronary arteries at the base of the aorta that sends blood to perfuse the heart musculature. On the venous side of a capillary network, the capillaries join together into **venules**, which join to form **veins**. Venous blood empties into the superior and inferior venae cavae for entry into the right side of the heart. All blood vessels are lined with **endothelial cells**. This special type of cell helps to maintain the vessel by releasing chemicals that aid in vasodilation and vasoconstriction. In addition, endothelial cells can allow white blood cells to pass through the vessel wall and into the tissues during an inflammatory response. Finally, endothelial cells release certain chemicals when damaged that are involved in the formation of blood clots to repair the vessel and stop bleeding.

Cross sections of the different blood vessels are shown in Figure 7.4. Don't worry about the names of the layers; simply be able to recognize that the same types of cells comprise the different vessels and that arteries have much more smooth muscle than veins.

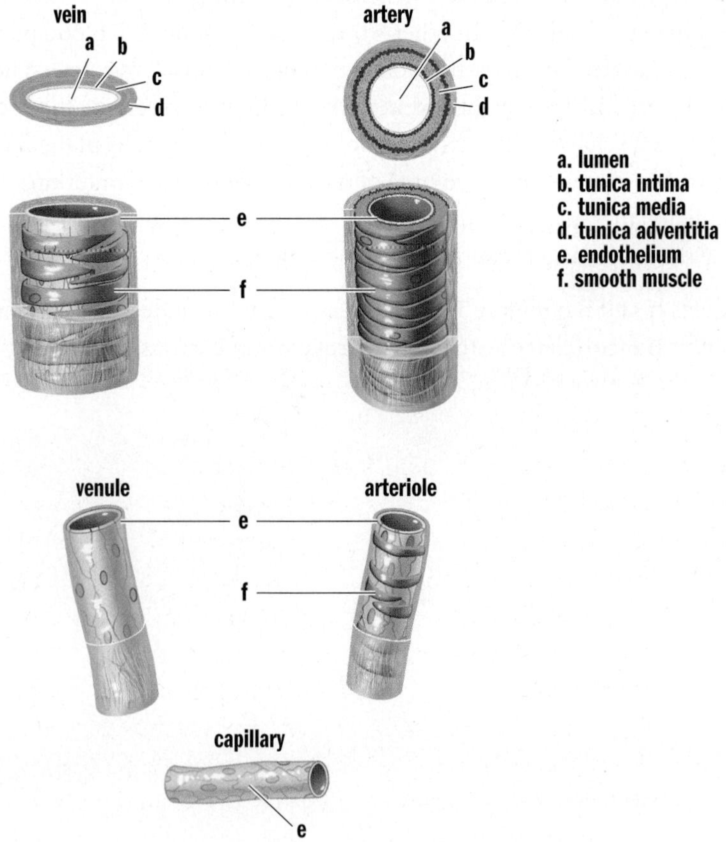

Figure 7.4 Structure of Blood Vessels

Arteries

Arteries move blood away from the heart to the lungs and other parts of the body. Most arteries contain oxygenated blood; in fact, only the pulmonary arteries and umbilical arteries contain deoxygenated blood. Smaller, muscular arteries are known as arterioles.

Arteries are highly muscular and elastic, creating tremendous resistance to the flow of blood. This is one of the reasons why the left side of the heart must generate much higher pressures: to overcome the resistance caused by systemic arteries. After arteries are filled with blood, the elastic recoil from their walls maintains a high pressure and forces blood forward.

Capillaries

Capillaries are vessels with a single endothelial cell layer and are so small that red blood cells must pass through the capillaries in a single-file line. The thin wall of the capillary allows easy diffusion of gases (O_2 and CO_2), nutrients (most notably, glucose), and wastes (ammonia and urea, among others). Capillaries are therefore the interface for communication of the circulatory system with the tissues. Remember, too, that blood also carries hormones, so capillaries allow endocrine signals to arrive at their target tissues.

Capillaries can be quite delicate. When capillaries are damaged, blood can leave the capillaries and enter the interstitial space. If this occurs in a closed space, it results in a bruise.

Veins

Veins are thin-walled, inelastic vessels that transport blood to the heart. Except for the pulmonary and umbilical veins, all veins carry deoxygenated blood. **Venules** are smaller venous structures that connect capillaries to the larger veins of the body.

The smaller amount of smooth muscle in the walls of veins gives them less recoil than arteries. Furthermore, veins are able to stretch to accommodate larger quantities of blood. Indeed, three-fourths of our total blood volume may be in venous circulation at any one time. Note that, even though the volume of arterial blood is normally much less than the volume of venous blood, the total volume passing through either side of the heart per unit time (cardiac output) is the same.

Given that the heart is located in the chest, bloodflow in most veins is upward from the lower body back to the heart, against gravity. In the inferior vena cava, this translates into a large amount of blood in a vertical column. The pressure at the bottom of this venous column in the large veins of the legs can be quite high. In fact, it can exceed systolic pressure (120 mmHg), going as high as 200 mmHg or more. Thus, veins must have structures to push the blood forward and prevent backflow. Larger veins contain valves; as blood flows forward in the veins, the valves open. When blood tries to move backward, the valves will slam shut. Failure of the venous valves can result in the formation of varicose veins, which are distended where blood has pooled. People who are pregnant are especially susceptible to the formation of varicose veins due to an increase in the total blood volume during pregnancy and compression of the inferior vena cava by the fetus.

REAL WORLD

Blood clots may form in the deep veins of the legs as a result of injury, inactivity (blood stasis), or a hypercoagulable state (a tendency for the blood to clot excessively). The clots may dislodge and travel through the right atrium and right ventricle, through the pulmonary artery, and into the lungs. Such clots, called pulmonary emboli (or, more specifically, thromboemboli), block segments of the pulmonary arteries and produce rapid, labored breathing and chest pain. Death may occur if the thromboemboli are large.

REAL WORLD

Many patients may be immobile following a surgical procedure or during a long hospital stay. This introduces the threat of DVT and pulmonary emboli, which are very undesirable complications in someone who is already sick. Thus, in hospitals, special wraps are placed on the legs that contract rhythmically in order to prevent pooling of blood and the formation of blood clots. In addition, many patients receive medications like *heparin* or *warfarin* to prevent the formation of clots.

In addition to high pressure in the lower extremities, the small amount of smooth muscle also creates a challenge for propelling blood forward. Thus, the veins must rely on an external force to generate the pressure to push blood toward the heart. Most veins are surrounded by skeletal muscles, which squeeze the veins as the muscles contract, forcing the blood up against gravity in much the same way that squeezing the bottom of a tube of toothpaste causes the contents to be expelled through the top of the tube. This is why sitting motionless for long periods of time, such as in the cramped middle seat on a long transoceanic flight or after surgery, can increase the risk of blood clot formation in the veins of the legs and pelvis. Blood pools in the lower extremities, and sluggish blood coagulates more easily. A clot in the deep veins of the leg is called a deep vein thrombosis (DVT). This clot may become dislodged and travel through the right side of the heart to the lungs, where it can cause a life-threatening condition called a pulmonary embolus.

Circulation

Circulation is, by definition, circular. Let's return to the anatomy of the heart and vasculature, shown in Figure 7.1, to trace the flow of blood through the body. A closeup of bloodflow through the heart is also shown in Figure 7.5. Here, we begin with the return of blood to the right atrium. Blood returns to the heart from the body via the venae cavae, which are divided into the **superior vena cava (SVC)** and the **inferior vena cava (IVC)**. The superior vena cava returns blood from the portions of the body above the heart, while the inferior vena cava returns blood from portions of the body below the heart. Deoxygenated blood enters the right atrium, travels through the tricuspid valve, and enters the right ventricle. On contraction, the blood from the right ventricle passes through the pulmonary valve and enters the pulmonary arteries, where it travels to the lungs and breaks up into continuously smaller vessels. Once the blood reaches the capillaries that line the alveoli, it participates in gas exchange, with carbon dioxide leaving the blood and oxygen entering the blood. The blood then travels into pulmonary venules and into the pulmonary veins, which carry the blood to the left side of the heart. Oxygenated blood enters the left atrium, travels through the mitral valve, and enters the left ventricle. On contraction, the blood from the left ventricle passes through the aortic valve and enters the aorta. From the aorta, blood enters arteries, then arterioles, and then capillaries. After gas and nutrient exchange occurs at the capillaries, the blood enters the venules, which lead to the larger veins. The veins then empty into either the SVC or IVC for return to the right side of the heart.

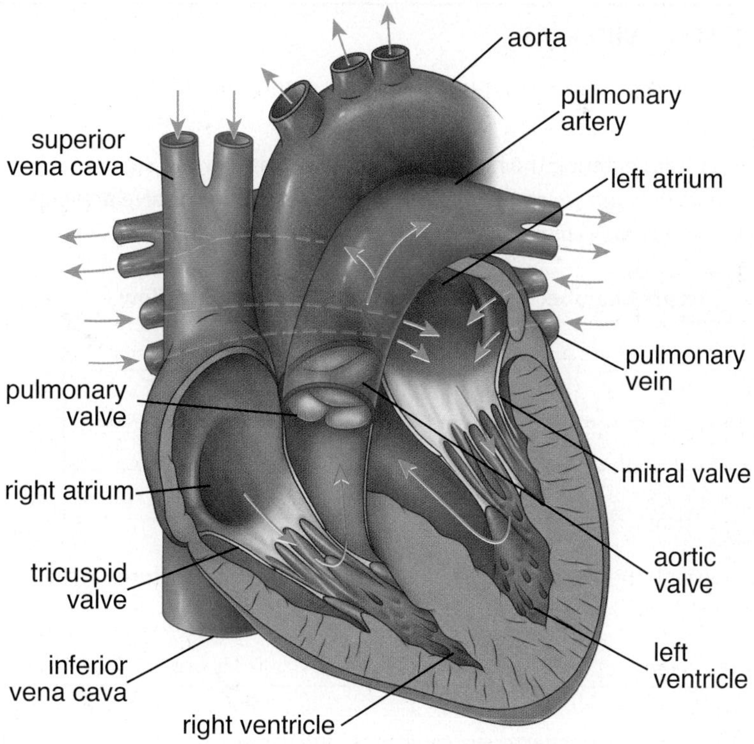

Figure 7.5 Bloodflow through the Heart

Written in shorthand, the pathway appears like this:

$$\text{right atrium} \xrightarrow[\text{valve}]{\text{tricuspid}} \text{right ventricle} \xrightarrow[\text{valve}]{\text{pulmonary}} \text{pulmonary artery} \rightarrow \text{lungs} \rightarrow$$

$$\text{pulmonary veins} \rightarrow \text{left atrium} \xrightarrow[\text{valve}]{\text{mitral}} \text{left ventricle} \xrightarrow[\text{valve}]{\text{aortic}} \text{aorta} \rightarrow \text{arteries}$$

$$\rightarrow \text{arterioles} \rightarrow \text{capillaries} \rightarrow \text{venules} \rightarrow \text{veins} \rightarrow \text{venae cavae} \rightarrow \text{right atrium}$$

In most cases, blood will pass through only one capillary bed before returning to the heart. However, there are three **portal systems** in the body, in which blood will pass through two capillary beds in series before returning to the heart. In the **hepatic portal system**, blood leaving capillary beds in the walls of the gut passes through the hepatic portal vein before reaching the capillary beds in the liver. In the **hypophyseal portal system**, blood leaving capillary beds in the hypothalamus travels to a capillary bed in the anterior pituitary to allow for paracrine secretion of releasing hormones. In the **renal portal system**, blood leaving the glomerulus travels through an efferent arteriole before surrounding the nephron in a capillary network called the vasa recta.

REAL WORLD

While *bicuspid valve* is an acceptable alternative name for *mitral valve*, it is rarely used in medicine. Most practitioners will refer to valves by one-letter abbreviations (*M* for mitral). The name *mitral* refers to a *miter*, which is the name for a ceremonial headdress worn by some religious leaders. The two large leaflets of the mitral valve somewhat resemble this headdress.

MCAT CONCEPT CHECK 7.1

Before you move on, assess your understanding of the material with these questions.

1. Starting from entering the heart from the venae cavae, what are the four chambers through which blood passes in the heart? Which valve prevents backflow into each chamber?

Heart Chamber	Valve That Prevents Backflow

2. Starting with the site of impulse initiation, what are the structures in the conduction system of the heart?

3. Compare and contrast arteries, capillaries, and veins:

Vessel	Carries Blood in Which Direction?	Relative Wall Thickness	Smooth Muscle Present?	Contains Valves?
Artery				
Capillary				
Vein				

4. Why does the right side of the heart contain less cardiac muscle than the left side?

5. If all autonomic input to the heart were cut, what would happen?

7.2 Blood

LEARNING OBJECTIVES

After Chapter 7.2, you will be able to:

- Recall the components of plasma
- Predict compatible blood types given a blood type
- Identify the purpose of hematocrit measurements, as well as the relevant unit of measurement
- Recognize the different types of leukocytes and their functions
- Describe how platelets are produced
- Distinguish between cell types within blood that contain or do not contain a nucleus

Now that we have examined the pump and the pipes through which blood travels, let's take a look at this fluid.

Composition

In the pathology lab, we frequently study the composition of the blood using a centrifuge. By spinning the blood at a rapid rate, we can separate this complex fluid into its components based on density. By volume, blood is about 55% liquid and 45% cells, as shown in Figure 7.6. **Plasma** is the liquid portion of blood, an aqueous mixture of nutrients, salts, respiratory gases, hormones, and blood proteins. Plasma can be further refined via the removal of clotting factors into serum. The cellular portion of blood consists of three major categories: **erythrocytes**, **leukocytes**, and **platelets**. All blood cells are formed from hematopoietic stem cells, which originate in the bone marrow.

REAL WORLD

Serum (plural sera) is used in a variety of medical testing procedures such as antibody testing and blood typing. Serum is considered preferable to plasma for many applications due to the lack of clotting factors and fibrinogens.

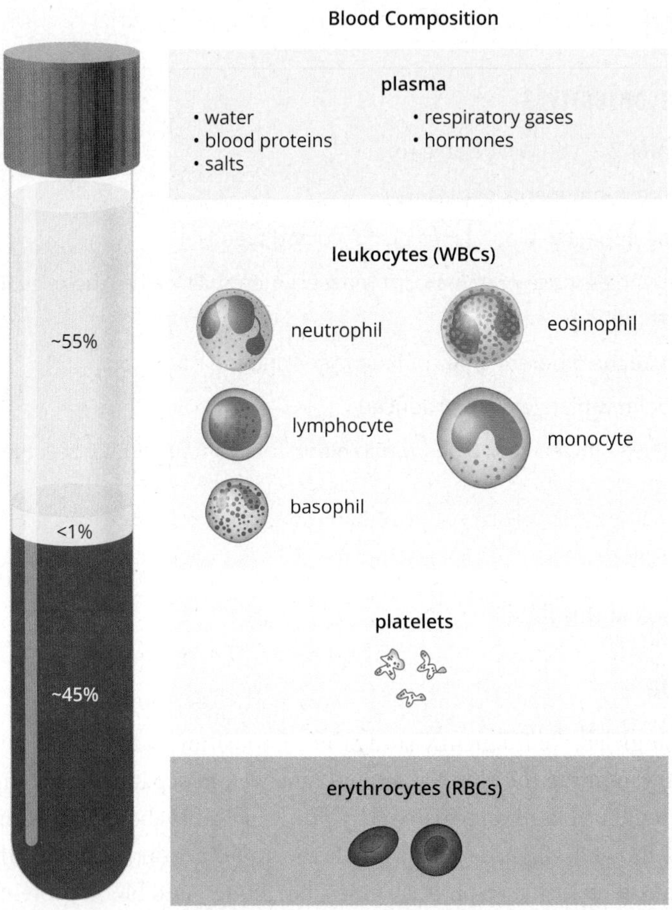

Figure 7.6 The Composition of Blood

Erythrocytes—Red Blood Cells

In the body, oxygen and nutrients are delivered to the peripheral tissues, and carbon dioxide and other wastes (such as hydrogen ions and ammonia) are picked up from the peripheral tissues and delivered to the organs that process this waste: the lungs, liver, and kidneys. The **erythrocyte** or **red blood cell** is a specialized cell designed for oxygen transport. Oxygen does not simply dissolve in the cytoplasm of the red blood cell—remember, molecular oxygen is nonpolar and therefore has low solubility in aqueous environments. Rather, each erythrocyte contains about 250 million molecules of **hemoglobin**, each of which can bind four molecules of oxygen. Therefore, each red blood cell can carry approximately 1 billion molecules of oxygen.

Red blood cells are unique in a number of ways, and their modifications reflect the special role they play in the human body. Red blood cells are biconcave, or indented on both sides, which serves a dual purpose. First, this shape assists them in traveling through tiny capillaries. Second, it increases the cell's surface area, which increases gas exchange. Red blood cells are also unique in that, when they mature, the nuclei, mitochondria, and other membrane-bound organelles are lost. The loss of organelles makes space for the molecules of hemoglobin. In addition, the loss of mitochondria in particular means that the red blood cell does not consume the oxygen it is carrying before it is delivered to peripheral tissues. In other words, red blood cells do not carry out oxidative phosphorylation to generate ATP; rather, they rely entirely on glycolysis for ATP, with lactic acid (arising from fermentation) as the main byproduct. Because red blood cells lack nuclei, they are unable to divide. Erythrocytes can live for 120 days in the bloodstream before cells in the liver and spleen phagocytize senescent (old) red blood cells to recycle them for their parts.

In medicine, a complete blood count measures the quantity of each cell type in the blood. For red blood cells, two commonly given measures are the hemoglobin and hematocrit. Hemoglobin, of course, measures the quantity of hemoglobin in the blood, giving a result in grams per deciliter. Hematocrit is a measure of how much of the blood sample consists of red blood cells, given as a percentage. A normal hemoglobin is considered to be between 13.5 and 17.5 $\frac{g}{dL}$ for phenotypical males and between 12.0 and 16.0 $\frac{g}{dL}$ for phenotypical females. A normal hematocrit is considered to be between 41 and 53% for males and between 36 and 46% for females. For example, a patient may have a hemoglobin of 13.8 $\frac{g}{dL}$ and a hematocrit of 41.2%.

Leukocytes—White Blood Cells

Leukocytes or **white blood cells** usually comprise less than 1 percent of total blood volume. This translates into about 4,500–11,000 leukocytes per microliter of blood, which is a small number relative to the erythrocyte concentration. This number can massively increase under certain conditions when we need more white blood cells, most notably during infection. White blood cells are a crucial part of the immune system, acting as our defenders against pathogens, foreign cells, cancer, and other materials not recognized as *self*. Let's briefly discuss five basic types of leukocytes, which are all categorized into two classes: granulocytes and agranulocytes.

The granular leukocytes or **granulocytes** (**neutrophils**, **eosinophils**, and **basophils**) are so named because they contain cytoplasmic granules that are visible by microscopy. These granules contain a variety of compounds that are toxic to invading microbes; these compounds can be released through exocytosis. Granular leukocytes are involved in inflammatory reactions, allergies, pus formation, and destruction of bacteria and parasites. The specific functions of the three granulocytes are discussed in Chapter 8 of *MCAT Biology Review*.

The agranulocytes, which do not contain granules that are released by exocytosis, consist of **lymphocytes** and **monocytes**. Lymphocytes are important in the **specific immune response**, the body's targeted fight against particular pathogens, such as viruses and bacteria. Some lymphocytes act as primary responders against an infection, while others function to maintain a long-term memory bank of pathogen recognition. These cells, in a very real sense, help our body learn from experience and are prepared to mount a fast response upon repeated exposure to familiar pathogens.

Many vaccines work by training these cells. Through exposure to a weakened pathogen, or an antigenic protein (a protein that can be recognized by the immune system) of the pathogen, memory cells can be created. For example, most children in the United States receive the varicella (chickenpox) vaccine, which includes a live but weakened strain of the varicella-zoster virus that causes chickenpox. When the vaccine is administered, the virus is recognized as foreign and an immune response is activated. During this process, certain immune cells form a memory of the virus; in other words, our body learns to remember the virus and prepares itself to ward off the virus if it appears again later in life.

Lymphocyte maturation takes place in one of three locations. Lymphocytes that mature in the bone marrow are referred to as B-cells, and those that mature in the thymus are called T-cells. B-cells are responsible for antibody generation, whereas T-cells kill virally infected cells and activate other immune cells. The details of these two components of the specific immune response are discussed in Chapter 8 of *MCAT Biology Review*.

The other agranulocytes are monocytes, which phagocytize foreign matter such as bacteria. Most organs of the body contain a collection of these phagocytic cells; once they leave the bloodstream and enter an organ, monocytes are renamed **macrophages**. Each organ's macrophage population may have a specific name, as well. In the central nervous system, for example, they are called **microglia**; in the skin, they are called **Langerhans cells**; in bone, they are called **osteoclasts**.

Thrombocytes—Platelets

Thrombocytes or **platelets** are cell fragments or shards released from cells in bone marrow known as **megakaryocytes**. Their function is to assist in blood clotting and they are present in high concentrations (150,000–400,000 per microliter of blood). The enzymatic reactions involved in the formation of a clot (the clotting cascade) will be discussed shortly.

As mentioned above, all of the cellular elements of blood originate in the bone marrow. The production of blood cells and platelets is called **hematopoiesis**, and is triggered by a number of hormones, growth factors, and cytokines. The most notable of these are **erythropoietin**, which is secreted by the kidney and stimulates mainly red blood cell development, and **thrombopoietin**, which is secreted by the liver and kidney and stimulates mainly platelet development. The hematopoietic pathways are shown in Figure 7.7.

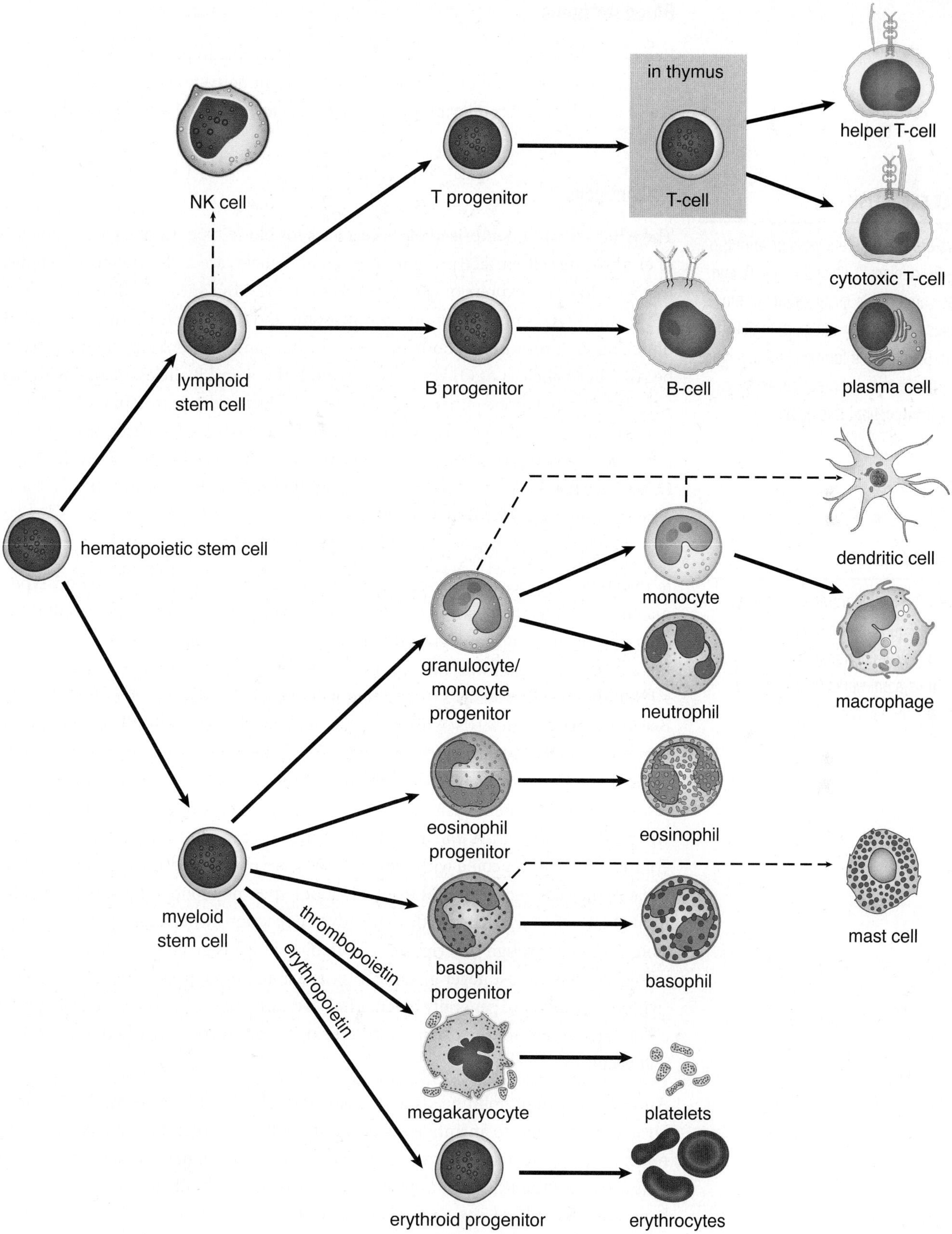

Figure 7.7 Hematopoiesis

Blood Antigens

Red blood cells express surface proteins called **antigens**. In general, an antigen is any specific target (usually a protein) to which the immune system can react. The two major antigen families relevant for blood groups are the **ABO antigens** and the **Rh factor**.

ABO Antigens

The ABO system is comprised of three alleles for blood type. In this particular class of erythrocyte cell-surface proteins, the A and B alleles are codominant, which means that a person may express one, both, or none of the ABO antigens. If the A allele (I^A or simply A) is present on one chromosome and the B allele (I^B or B) is present on the other chromosome, both will be expressed, and the person's blood type will be AB. The O allele (i or O) is recessive to both the A and B alleles. People with type O blood do not express either variant (A or B antigen) of this protein and have a homozygous recessive genotype. The naming system of blood types is based on the presence or absence of these protein variants. The four blood types are: A, B, AB, and O. Because the A and B alleles are dominant, the genotypes for A may be I^AI^A or I^Ai, while the genotypes for B may be I^BI^B or I^Bi.

MCAT EXPERTISE

There are two different ways of writing the ABO alleles: I^A, I^B, and i; or A, B, and O. Be comfortable using either system because the MCAT could show one or the other. Because the former system is more common in medical practice, we'll be using it throughout this book.

The ABO classification has important implications for medical practice; it is critical to match blood types for transfusions. It is no exaggeration to say that blood-type matching is a life and death matter, given the severe hemolysis that can result if the donor blood antigen is recognized as foreign by the recipient's immune system. For example, a person who has type A blood will recognize the type A protein as *self* but the type B protein as *foreign* and will make antibodies to types B and AB. Because type O blood cells express neither antigen variant, they will not initiate any immune response, regardless of the recipient's actual blood type; people with type O blood are therefore considered **universal donors** because their blood will not cause ABO-related hemolysis in any recipient. However, a recipient who is type O will produce both anti-A *and* anti-B antibodies and can only receive type O blood. On the other hand, people with type AB blood are considered **universal recipients** because they can receive blood from all blood types: no blood antigen is foreign to individuals who have AB blood, so no adverse reactions will occur upon transfusion. A more thorough description of each blood type is given in Table 7.1. Note that whole blood is almost never given in a transfusion; rather, packed red blood cells (with no plasma) are generally given. Thus, we care only about the donor's red blood cell antigens (and not the plasma antibodies) when determining whether hemolysis will occur.

MCAT EXPERTISE

You are almost guaranteed to see at least one question on blood groups on Test Day. It is critical that you learn how the system works (I^A and I^B are codominant, i is recessive).

Another important point needs to be made here about antibodies. Antibodies are created in response to an antigen, and they specifically target that antigen. You would not expect to have antibodies to the Ebola virus if you had never been exposed to it. This is true for the Rh factor as well—an individual who is Rh-negative would not have anti-Rh antibodies prior to exposure to Rh-positive blood. Why, then, does an individual lacking the A allele automatically have an anti-A antibody? The reason may lie in the gut: research has demonstrated that *E. coli* that inhabit the colon may have proteins that match the A and B alleles. This would serve as a source of exposure and would allow one to develop anti-A (or anti-B) antibodies prior to exposure to another person's blood. This is why ABO compatibility is so important during blood transfusions—giving the wrong ABO blood type would lead to rapid hemolysis.

BLOOD TYPE	GENOTYPE(S)	ANTIGENS PRODUCED	ANTIBODIES PRODUCED	CAN DONATE TO...	CAN RECEIVE FROM...
A	I^AI^A, I^Ai	A	anti-B	A, AB	A, O
B	I^BI^B, I^Bi	B	anti-A	B, AB	B, O
AB	I^AI^B	A and B	none	AB only	A, B, AB, O (universal recipient)
O	ii	none	anti-A and anti-B	A, B, AB, O (universal donor)	O only

Table 7.1 ABO Blood Types

Rh Factor

The **Rh factor** (so named because it was first described in rhesus monkeys) is also a surface protein expressed on red blood cells. Although at one time it was thought to be a single antigen, it has since been found to exist as several variants. When left unmodified, Rh-positive (Rh^+) or Rh-negative (Rh^-) refers to the presence or absence of a specific allele called D. The presence or absence of D can also be indicated with a plus or minus superscript on the ABO blood type (such as O^+ or AB^-). Rh-positivity follows autosomal dominant inheritance; one positive allele is enough for the protein to be expressed.

The Rh factor status is particularly important in obstetric medicine. Exposure to at least a small amount of fetal blood during childbirth is inevitable, no matter how good the obstetrician is. If a person who is pregnant is Rh^- and the fetus is Rh^+, the person will become sensitized to the Rh factor, and the person's immune system will begin making antibodies against it. This is not a problem for the first child; by the time the person starts producing antibodies, the child has already been born. However, any subsequent pregnancy in which the fetus is Rh^+ will present a problem because maternal anti-Rh antibodies can cross the placenta and attack the fetal blood cells, resulting in hemolysis of the fetal cells. This condition is known as **erythroblastosis fetalis** and can be fatal to the fetus. Today, we can use medicine to prevent this condition. There is less concern with maternal-fetal ABO mismatching because antibodies against AB antigens are of a class called IgM, which does not readily cross the placenta (unlike anti-Rh IgG antibodies, which can).

KEY CONCEPT

Antigens are the stimuli for B-cells to make antibodies. After exposure of a B-cell to its specific antigen, the cell becomes an antibody-producing factory.

REAL WORLD

The most common blood type in the United States is O^+. The least common is AB^-.

REAL WORLD

In blood bank pathology, the Rh factor is often referred to as D. Note that while the A, B, and D proteins are the most important for blood typing, dozens of other antigens can (and should) be matched as well, including C, E, Kell, Lewis, Duffy, and others. The more antigens that are correctly matched, the lower the probability of hemolysis.

REAL WORLD

When a person who is Rh^- is pregnant with a first Rh^+ fetus, the risk of erythroblastosis fetalis in subsequent Rh-mismatched pregnancies can usually be avoided by giving the Rh^- parent Rh-immunoglobulin (RhoGAM) during pregnancy and immediately after delivery. Administration of immunoglobulin (which is a type of passive immunization) will absorb the fetus's Rh^+ cells, preventing the production of anti-Rh antibodies by the parent.

MCAT CONCEPT CHECK 7.2

Before you move on, assess your understanding of the material with these questions.

1. What are the components of plasma?

____

2. An individual with B^+ blood is in an automobile accident and requires a blood transfusion. What blood types could this person receive? After recovery, the same individual, thankful for the transfusion, decides to donate blood. To which blood types could this person donate?
   - Could receive from:

____

   - Could donate to:

____

3. What does a hematocrit measure? What are the units for hematocrit?

____

4. Which types of leukocytes are involved in the specific immune response?

____

5. Where do platelets come from?

____

6. Which cell type(s) in blood contain nuclei? Which do not?
   - Contain nuclei:

____

   - Do not contain nuclei:

____

7.3 Physiology of the Cardiovascular System

LEARNING OBJECTIVES

After Chapter 7.3, you will be able to:

- Predict the impact of changing bloodflow through arteries, capillaries, and veins on blood pressure and heart function
- Recall the bicarbonate buffer chemical equation, including its catalyzing enzyme
- Explain how the oxyhemoglobin dissociation curve can be shifted to the left or right
- Recall the series of events and compounds in a coagulation cascade
- Identify the regions of the body associated with different parts of the oxyhemoglobin dissociation curve:

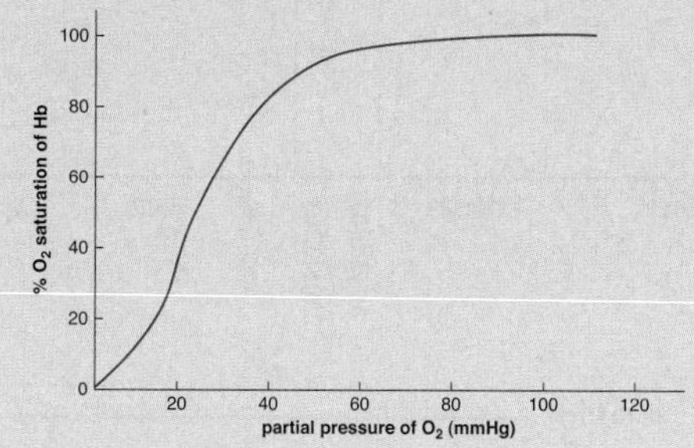

The cardiovascular system transports many compounds, including gases, nutrients, and waste products, to and from the body's tissues via red blood cells and plasma. Furthermore, it serves an important role in immunity through specialized cells, such as leukocytes, which help the body fight localized or systemic pathogens. Capillaries within the body can dilate and constrict to maintain proper body temperature. In addition, the circulatory system mediates the formation of blood clots to repair damaged vessels. These functions reflect the important jobs of the cardiovascular system, which include maintenance of blood pressure, gas and solute exchange, coagulation, and thermoregulation.

Blood Pressure

Before we can even discuss gas and solute exchange, it is important to recognize that, for the circulatory system to serve its predominant functions, blood pressure must be kept sufficiently high to propel blood forward. Blood pressure, therefore, provides healthcare professionals with information regarding the health of the circulatory system. In addition, high blood pressure, or *hypertension*, is a pathological state that may result in damage to the blood vessels and organs. Blood pressure is a measure of the force per unit area exerted on the wall of the blood vessels and is measured with a **sphygmomanometer**. Sphygmomanometers measure the gauge pressure in the systemic circulation, which is the pressure above and beyond atmospheric pressure (760 mmHg at sea level), as discussed in Chapter 4 of *MCAT Physics and Math Review*. Blood pressure is expressed as a ratio of the systolic (ventricular contraction) to diastolic (ventricular relaxation) pressures. Pressure gradually drops from the arterial to venous circulation, with the largest drop occurring across the arterioles, as shown in Figure 7.8. Normal blood pressure is considered to be between 90/60 and 120/80.

KEY CONCEPT

The largest drop in blood pressure occurs across the arterioles. This is critical because the capillaries are thin-walled and unable to withstand the pressure of the arterial side of the vasculature.

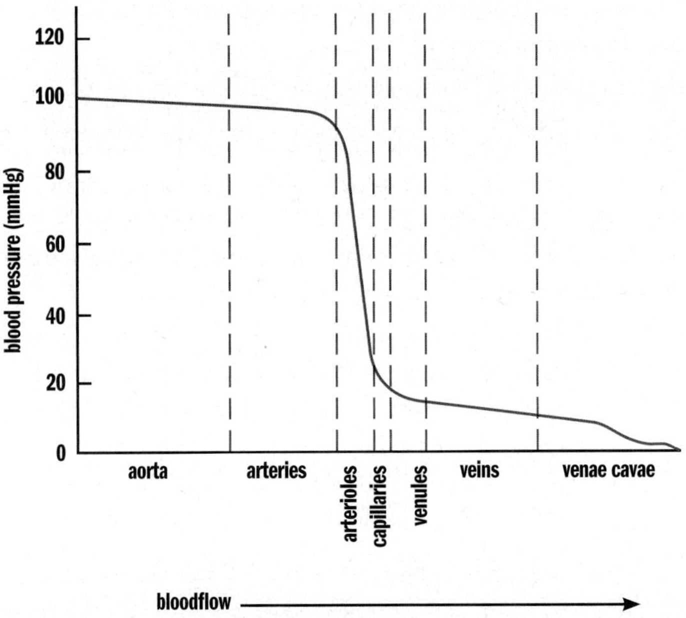

Figure 7.8 Mean Arterial Pressure at Different Locations in the Cardiovascular System

An analogy can be drawn between circulation and an electric circuit. Much like an electromotive force (voltage) drives a current through a given electrical resistance, the pressure gradient across the circulatory system drives cardiac output through a given vascular resistance. This analogy is an important one to remember because the equations of electric circuits can be applied to the cardiovascular system. For example, Ohm's law ($V = IR$) can be translated into the following equation for circulation:

$$\Delta P = \text{CO} \times \text{TPR}$$

Equation 7.2

where ΔP is the pressure differential across the circulation, CO is the cardiac output, and TPR is the total peripheral (vascular) resistance.

It is also important to note that arterioles and capillaries act much like resistors in a circuit. When electricity travels through a wire, the wire itself provides an intrinsic level of resistance that limits the flow of electricity through it. Resistance is based on three factors: resistivity, length, and cross-sectional area. Resistivity has no obvious correlate in physiology, but the other two factors certainly do. The longer a blood vessel is, the more resistance it offers. The larger the cross-sectional area of a blood vessel, the less resistance it offers. In addition, arteries are highly muscular and are able to expand and contract as needed to change vascular resistance and maintain blood pressure. Arterioles can also contract to limit the amount of blood entering a given capillary bed (much like increasing resistance will decrease current flow to a given branch in a circuit). Finally, with the exception of the three portal systems, all systemic capillary beds are in parallel with each other. Therefore, opening capillary beds will decrease vascular resistance (like adding another resistor in parallel) and, assuming the body can compensate, increase cardiac output.

Blood pressure is regulated using baroreceptors in the walls of the vasculature. Baroreceptors are specialized neurons that detect changes in the mechanical forces on the walls of the vessel. When the blood pressure is too low, they can stimulate the sympathetic nervous system, which causes vasoconstriction, thereby increasing the blood pressure. In addition, chemoreceptors can sense when the osmolarity of the blood is too high, which could indicate dehydration. This promotes the release of antidiuretic hormone (ADH or vasopressin), a peptide hormone made in the hypothalamus but stored in the posterior pituitary, which increases the reabsorption of water, thereby increasing blood volume and pressure (while also diluting the blood). Low perfusion to the juxtaglomerular cells of the kidney stimulates aldosterone release through the renin–angiotensin–aldosterone system; aldosterone increases the reabsorption of sodium and, by extension, water, thereby increasing the blood volume and pressure.

So, what if blood pressure is too high? Neurologically, sympathetic impulses could decrease, permitting relaxation of the vasculature with a concurrent drop in blood pressure. Within the heart, specialized atrial cells are able to secrete a hormone called **atrial natriuretic peptide** (**ANP**). This hormone aids in the loss of salt within the nephron, acting as a natural diuretic with loss of fluid. Interestingly, ANP is a fairly weak diuretic. Some fluid is lost, but it is often not enough to counter the effects of a high-salt diet on blood pressure. Indeed, the human body has many different ways to raise blood pressure, but very few ways to lower it.

REAL WORLD

Vital signs include temperature, heart rate, respiratory rate, and blood pressure. They provide a quick snapshot of a person's condition at a given moment. High blood pressure may indicate clinical hypertension, anxiety, catecholamine-producing tumors, or stimulant use, while low blood pressure may indicate hemorrhage, a heart attack, sepsis (severe bloodstream infection), or neurological damage. These are very broad differential diagnoses; however, vital signs combined with a quick clinical history provide a way for clinicians to identify the patients that require immediate intervention.

Gas and Solute Exchange

Blood pressure ensures sufficient forward flow of blood through the system. However, what happens when the blood reaches the capillaries? Here, oxygen and nutrients diffuse out of the blood into tissues, while waste products like carbon dioxide, hydrogen ions, urea, and ammonia diffuse into the blood. In addition, hormones are secreted into the capillaries, travel with the circulation, and diffuse into their target tissue. Ions and fluid must also be returned to the blood to ensure that no area becomes too swollen with fluid. Regardless of the substance being exchanged, there is one fundamental concept to be considered in this process: concentration gradients. In each case, one side of the capillary wall has a higher concentration of a given substance than the other. This allows for movement of gases and solutes by diffusion.

Oxygen

Oxygen is carried primarily by **hemoglobin** in the blood. Hemoglobin is a protein composed of four cooperative subunits, each of which has a prosthetic heme group that binds to an oxygen molecule. The binding of oxygen occurs at the heme group's central iron atom, which can undergo changes in its oxidation state. The binding or releasing of oxygen to or from the iron atom in the heme group is an oxidation–reduction reaction. It is also important to note that some oxygen does diffuse into the blood and dissolve into the plasma, but this amount is negligible compared to the quantity of oxygen bound to hemoglobin. The level of oxygen in the blood is often measured as the partial pressure of O_2 within the blood, or P_aO_2. A normal P_aO_2 is approximately 70–100 mmHg. However, taking this measurement is inconvenient because it involves taking a sample of blood from an artery. By contrast, **oxygen saturation**—that is, the percentage of hemoglobin molecules carrying oxygen—is easily measured using a finger probe. A healthy oxygen saturation level is above 97 percent.

In the lungs, oxygen diffuses into the alveolar capillaries. As the first oxygen binds to a heme group, it induces a conformational shift in the shape of hemoglobin from taut to relaxed. This shift increases hemoglobin's affinity for oxygen, making it easier for subsequent molecules of oxygen to bind to the remaining three unoccupied heme groups. As other heme groups acquire an oxygen molecule, the affinity continues to increase, thus creating a positive feedback-like (spiraling forward) mechanism. Once all of the hemoglobin subunits are bound to oxygen, the removal of one molecule of oxygen will induce a conformational shift, decreasing the overall affinity for oxygen, and making it easier for the other molecules of oxygen to leave the heme groups. This is again a positive feedback process; as oxygen molecules leave hemoglobin, it becomes progressively easier for more oxygen to be removed. This phenomenon is a form of allosteric regulation referred to as **cooperative binding** and results in the classic sigmoidal (S-shaped) oxyhemoglobin dissociation curve shown in Figure 7.9.

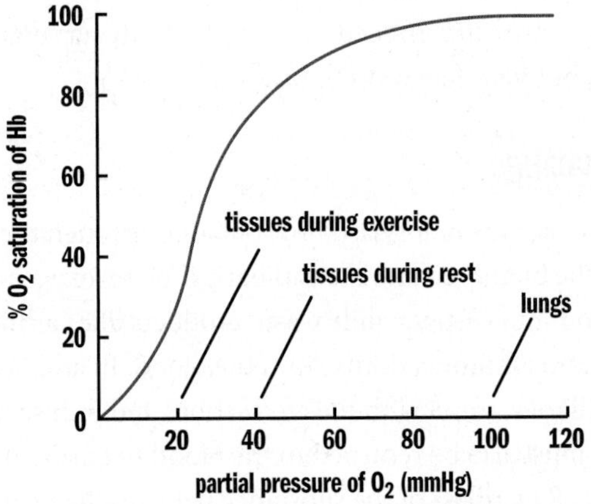

Figure 7.9 Oxyhemoglobin Dissociation Curve

Before looking at shifts in this curve, let's make sure we understand what everything means. According to the curve, the blood is 100 percent saturated in the lungs, at a partial pressure of 100 mmHg O_2. The tissues are at a lower partial pressure of oxygen, around 40 mmHg during rest; at this lower partial pressure, the hemoglobin is approximately 80 percent saturated. Therefore, about $100 - 80 = 20\%$ of the oxygen has been released from the hemoglobin. Where did this oxygen go? Into the tissues, of course.

During exercise, the partial pressure of oxygen in the tissues is even lower—around 20 mmHg. At this lower partial pressure, the hemoglobin is approximately 30 percent saturated. Therefore, about $100 - 30 = 70\%$ of the oxygen has been released to the tissues. In reality, unloading of oxygen is also facilitated by shifts in the hemoglobin curve that occur during exercise, as described later.

Carbon Dioxide

Delivering oxygen to tissues is only part of the job of transporting respiratory gases; removing carbon dioxide gas (CO_2), the primary waste product of cellular respiration, is also important. Carbon dioxide gas, like oxygen gas, is nonpolar and therefore has low solubility in the aqueous plasma; only a small percentage of the total CO_2 being transported in the blood to the lungs will be dissolved in the plasma. Carbon dioxide can be carried by hemoglobin, but hemoglobin has a much lower affinity for carbon dioxide than for oxygen. The vast majority of CO_2 exists in the blood as the bicarbonate ion (HCO_3^-). When CO_2 enters a red blood cell, it encounters the enzyme *carbonic anhydrase*, which catalyzes the combination reaction between carbon dioxide and water to form carbonic acid (H_2CO_3). Carbonic acid, a weak acid, will dissociate into a proton and the bicarbonate anion. The hydrogen ion (proton) and bicarbonate ion both have high solubilities in water, making them a more effective method of transporting metabolic waste products to the lungs for excretion. Upon reaching the alveolar capillaries in the lungs, the same reactions that led to the formation of the proton and bicarbonate anion can be reversed, allowing us to breathe out carbon dioxide:

$$CO_2(g) + H_2O(l) \underset{\text{carbonic anhydrase}}{\rightleftharpoons} H_2CO_3(aq) \rightleftharpoons H^+(aq) + HCO_3^-(aq)$$

This chemical reaction is important, not only because it provides an effective means of ridding the body's tissues of carbon dioxide gas, but also because the concentration of free protons in the blood affects pH; the pH, in turn, can have allosteric effects on the oxyhemoglobin dissociation curve. Increased carbon dioxide production will cause a right shift in the bicarbonate buffer equation, resulting in increased $[H^+]$ (decreased pH). These protons can bind to hemoglobin, reducing hemoglobin's affinity for oxygen. This decreased affinity can be seen in the oxyhemoglobin curve as a shift to the right; this is known as the **Bohr effect**. Note that the triggers for this right shift (increased P_aCO_2, increased $[H^+]$, decreased pH) are often associated with oxygen demand; higher rates of cellular metabolism result in increased carbon dioxide production and accumulation of lactic acid, both of which decrease pH. This decreased affinity allows more oxygen to be unloaded at the tissues, as shown in Figure 7.10. Looking at the red and green lines, we see that hemoglobin is nearly 100 percent saturated in the lungs (at a partial pressure of 100 mmHg O_2) for both lines. However, the green line is significantly lower than the red one when we reach a partial pressure of 20 mmHg O_2, around that of exercising muscle. Therefore, the right shift represents greater unloading of oxygen into the tissues.

MNEMONIC

Causes of a **right** shift of the oxyhemoglobin curve: **Exercise** is the **right** thing to do.

The following occur during **exercise**:

- Increased P_aCO_2
- Increased $[H^+]$ (decreased pH)
- Increased temperature

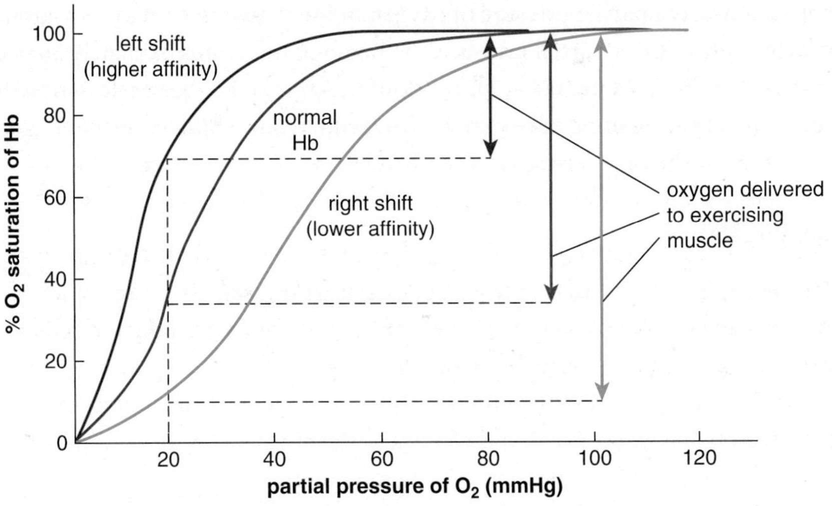

Figure 7.10 Shifts in the Oxyhemoglobin Dissociation Curve

Other causes of a right shift in the oxyhemoglobin curve include increased temperature and increased 2,3-bisphosphoglycerate (2,3-BPG), a side product of glycolysis in red blood cells.

KEY CONCEPT

Fetal hemoglobin has a higher affinity for oxygen than adult hemoglobin, and therefore has a left-shifted curve compared to adult hemoglobin.

A left shift, like the blue line in Figure 7.10, may occur due to decreased P_aCO_2, decreased $[H^+]$, increased pH, decreased temperature, and decreased 2,3-BPG. In addition, **fetal hemoglobin (HbF)** has a higher affinity for oxygen than **adult hemoglobin (HbA)**. This should make sense because fetal red blood cells must literally pull oxygen off of maternal hemoglobin and onto fetal hemoglobin.

The bicarbonate buffer system is also important because it links the respiratory and renal systems. Disturbances in either of these systems can lead to changes in the pH of the blood. For example, if an individual hyperventilates, excess CO_2 will be blown off, shifting the bicarbonate buffer system to the left and decreasing the concentration of protons. This leads to an increase in pH, or what is known as respiratory alkalosis. The kidney can compensate for this change by increasing excretion of bicarbonate, which brings the pH back to normal. In contrast, in *renal tubular acidosis type I*, the kidney is unable to excrete acid effectively. This leads to a buildup of protons in the blood (metabolic acidosis), which causes the buffer system to shift to the left. The excess CO_2 formed in the process can be exhaled, and the person may increase respiratory rate to compensate, bringing the pH back to normal.

Nutrients, Waste, and Hormones

In addition to respiratory gases, blood also carries nutrients, waste products, and hormones to the appropriate location for use or disposal. As discussed earlier, concentration gradients guide much of the movement of these substances to and from the tissues.

Carbohydrates and amino acids are absorbed into the capillaries of the small intestine and enter the systemic circulation via the hepatic portal system. Fats are absorbed into lacteals in the small intestine, bypassing the hepatic portal circulation to enter systemic circulation via the thoracic duct. When released from intestinal cells, fats are packaged into lipoproteins, which are water-soluble. The absorption of nutrients is covered more extensively in Chapter 9 of *MCAT Biology Review*.

Wastes, such as carbon dioxide, ammonia, and urea, enter the bloodstream by traveling down their respective concentration gradients from the tissues to the capillaries. The blood eventually travels to the kidneys, where these waste products are filtered or secreted for elimination from the body.

Hormones enter the circulation in or near the organ where the hormone is produced. This usually occurs by exocytosis, allowing for secretion of hormones into the bloodstream. Certain hormones are carried by proteins in the blood and are released under specific conditions. Once hormones reach their target tissues, they can activate cell-surface receptors (peptide hormones) or diffuse into the cell to activate intracellular or intranuclear receptors (steroid hormones).

Fluid Balance

In the bloodstream, two pressure gradients are essential for maintaining a proper balance of fluid volume and solute concentrations between the blood and the interstitium (the cells surrounding the blood vessels). These are the opposing but related hydrostatic and osmotic (oncotic) pressures.

Hydrostatic pressure is the force per unit area that the blood exerts against the vessel walls. This is generated by the contraction of the heart and the elasticity of the arteries, and can be measured upstream in the large arteries as blood pressure. Hydrostatic pressure pushes fluid out of the bloodstream and into the interstitium through the capillary walls, which are somewhat leaky by design. **Osmotic pressure**, on the other hand, is the "sucking" pressure generated by solutes as they attempt to draw water into the bloodstream. Because most of this osmotic pressure is attributable to plasma proteins, it is usually called **oncotic pressure**.

At the arteriole end of a capillary bed, hydrostatic pressure (pushing fluid out) is much larger than oncotic pressure (drawing fluid in), and there is a net efflux of water from the circulation, as shown in Figure 7.11. As fluid moves out of the vessels, the hydrostatic pressure drops significantly, but the osmotic pressure stays about the same. Therefore, at the venule end of the capillary bed, hydrostatic pressure (pushing fluid out) has dropped below oncotic pressure (drawing fluid in), and there is a net influx of water back into the circulation.

KEY CONCEPT

Hydrostatic pressure *pushes* fluid *out* of vessels and is dependent on blood pressure generated by the heart and the elastic arteries. Osmotic pressure *pulls* fluid back *into* the vessels and is dependent on the number of particles dissolved in the plasma; most are proteins, so we often refer to this as oncotic pressure.

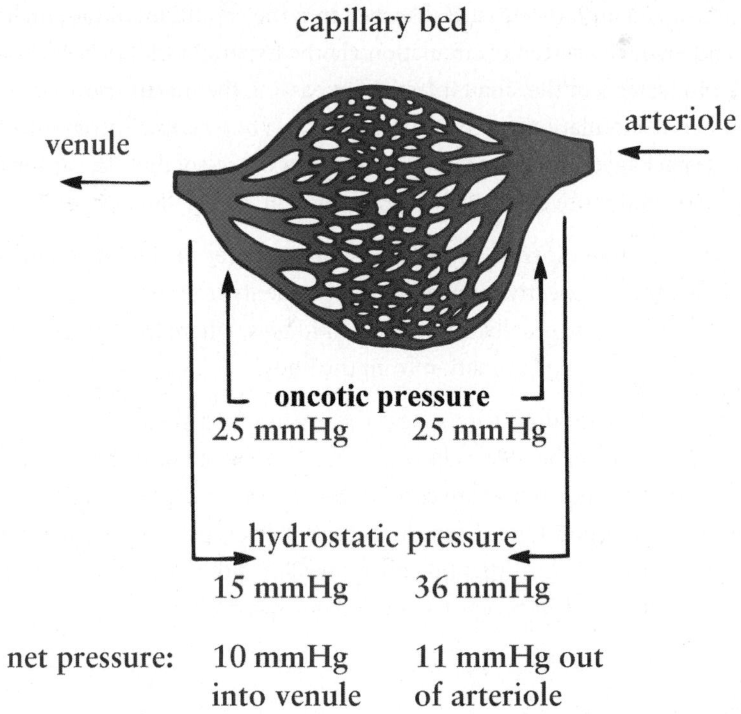

Figure 7.11 Starling Forces at a Capillary Bed

The balance of these opposing pressures, also called **Starling forces**, is essential for maintaining the proper fluid volumes and solute concentrations inside and outside the vasculature. Imbalance of these pressures can result in too much or too little fluid in the tissues. For example, accumulation of excess fluid in the interstitium results in a condition called **edema**. We should note that some interstitial fluid is also taken up by the lymphatic system. Most lymphatic fluid (**lymph**) is returned to the central circulatory system by way of a channel called the **thoracic duct**. Blockage of lymph nodes by infection or surgery can also result in edema. Although you do not need to learn or memorize the Starling equation, which quantifies the net filtration rate between two fluid compartments, you should understand that the movement of solutes and fluid at the capillary level is governed by pressure differentials, just like the movement of carbon dioxide and oxygen in the lungs.

Coagulation

We have now covered most of the functions of red blood cells and plasma. We've briefly touched on white blood cells, which we'll explore more extensively in Chapter 8 of *MCAT Biology Review*. This leaves us with platelets, which protect the vascular system in the event of damage by forming a clot. **Clots** are composed of both coagulation factors (proteins) and platelets, and they prevent (or at least minimize) blood loss. When the endothelium of a blood vessel is damaged, it exposes the underlying connective tissue, which contains collagen and a protein called **tissue factor**. When platelets come into contact with exposed collagen, they sense this as evidence of injury. In response, they release their contents and begin to aggregate, or clump together. Simultaneously, **coagulation factors**, most of which are secreted

REAL WORLD

Certain genetic diseases, such as hemophilia, cause malfunctions in the cascade of clotting reactions and increase the risk of life-threatening blood loss from even relatively minor injuries. Hemophilia A is the most common form and, as a sex-linked trait, is far more common in genotypical males than genotypical females.

by the liver, sense tissue factor and initiate a complex activation cascade. While the details of the coagulation cascade are beyond the scope of the MCAT, it is important to know that the endpoint of the cascade is the activation of **prothrombin** to form **thrombin** by ***thromboplastin***. Thrombin can then convert **fibrinogen** into **fibrin**. Fibrin ultimately forms small fibers that aggregate and cross-link into a woven structure, like a net, that captures red blood cells and other platelets, forming a stable clot over the area of damage, as shown in Figure 7.12. A clot that forms on a surface vessel that has been cut is called a scab.

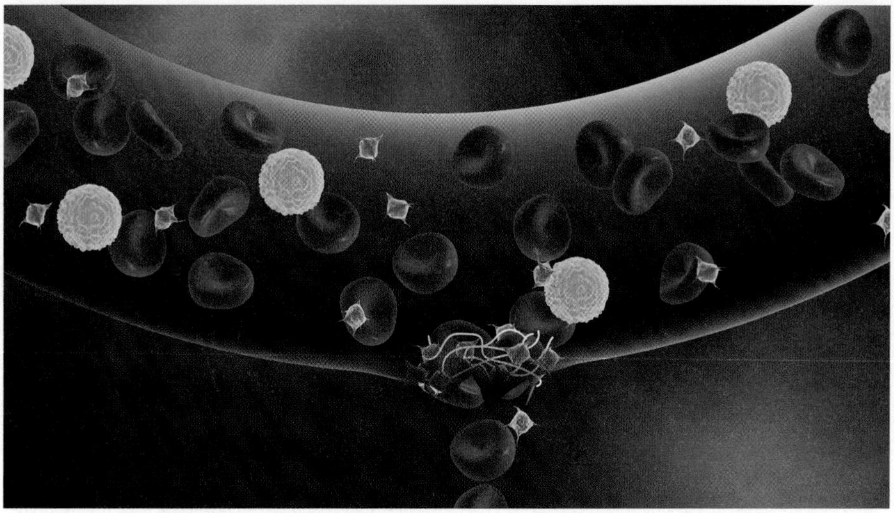

Figure 7.12 Thrombus (Clot) Formation

Thrombus formation, or blood clotting, occurs when blood vessels are injured. The process begins when platelets attach to the matrix that becomes exposed when the endothelial cells lining blood vessels are disrupted. This attachment then activates quiescent $\alpha_{IIb}\beta_3$ integrin molecules, causing them to adhere to circulating proteins—including fibrinogen, which forms bridges to additional platelets. Together the cells and proteins ultimately form a network of cells and fibers dense enough to plug the injury and prevent blood loss until the wound can be repaired.

Ultimately, the clot will have to be broken down. This task is accomplished predominantly by **plasmin**, which is generated from **plasminogen**.

MCAT CONCEPT CHECK 7.3

Before you move on, assess your understanding of the material with these questions.

1. In bacterial sepsis (overwhelming bloodstream infection), a number of capillary beds throughout the body open simultaneously. What effect would this have on the blood pressure? Besides the risk of infection, why might sepsis be dangerous for the heart?

    ____

2. What is the chemical equation for the bicarbonate buffer system? What enzyme catalyzes this reaction?

    ____

3. Where should you look on the oxyhemoglobin dissociation curve to determine the amount of oxygen that has been delivered to tissues?

    ____

4. What direction does the oxyhemoglobin dissociation curve shift as a result of exercise? What physiological changes cause this shift and why?

    ____

5. Exposure of which subendothelial compounds start the coagulation cascade? What protein helps stabilize the clot?

    - Starts the cascade:

      ____

    - Stabilizes the clot:

      ____

Conclusion

The cardiovascular system is one of the most commonly tested MCAT topics. You should be familiar with its basic structure: a system with two pumps in series. The right ventricle pumps blood into the pulmonary circulation, while the left ventricle pumps blood into the systemic circulation. We discussed the myogenic activity of cardiac muscle and the pathway that electricity follows in the heart through the SA node, AV node, bundle of His, and Purkinje fibers. The movement of blood through the vascular system is a result of the heart's pumping to generate pressure. Blood pressure is a measure of the blood's force per unit area on the vessel walls and is recorded as a gauge pressure (pressure above and beyond atmospheric pressure). We discussed the differences in structure between arteries, capillaries, and veins, and how these anatomical differences are reflective of their different functions. We then reviewed the composition of blood along with the three major blood cell types. We examined the ABO and Rh antigen systems, which frequently appear on the MCAT due to their widespread clinical relevance. The blood's ability to carry oxygen and carbon dioxide was also described; recall that carbon dioxide is primarily carried as bicarbonate ions in the blood. The conversion of carbon dioxide to and from this ion is accomplished by the enzyme carbonic anhydrase.

In this chapter, we focused on the functions of red blood cells, plasma, and platelets. We briefly examined the immune system, which is primarily driven by the actions of white blood cells and their products. Immunology is considered one of the most challenging courses in medical school, as you'll learn about dozens of cytokines, clusters of differentiation (CD), and specialized cell types. In the next chapter, we'll focus on the basics of immunology, discussing the major components of the innate (nonspecific) and adaptive (specific) immune responses.

GO ONLINE

You've reviewed the content, now test your knowledge and critical thinking skills by completing a test-like passage set in your online resources!

CONCEPT SUMMARY

Anatomy of the Cardiovascular System

- The **cardiovascular system** consists of a muscular four-chambered heart, blood vessels, and blood.
- The **heart** is composed of **cardiac muscle** and supports two different circulations: the **pulmonary circulation** and the **systemic circulation**.
    - Each side of the heart consists of an **atrium** and a **ventricle**.
    - The atria are separated from the ventricles by the **atrioventricular valves** (**tricuspid** on the right, bicuspid [mitral] on the left).
    - The ventricles are separated from the vasculature by the **semilunar valves** (**pulmonary** on the right, **aortic** on the left).
    - The pathway of blood is: right atrium $\xrightarrow[\text{valve}]{\text{tricuspid}}$ right ventricle $\xrightarrow[\text{valve}]{\text{pulmonary}}$ pulmonary artery → lungs → pulmonary veins → left atrium $\xrightarrow[\text{valve}]{\text{mitral}}$ left ventricle $\xrightarrow[\text{valve}]{\text{aortic}}$ aorta → arteries → arterioles → capillaries → venules → veins → venae cavae → right atrium
    - The left side of the heart contains more muscle than the right side because the systemic circulation has a much higher resistance and pressure.
    - Electrical conduction of the heart starts at the **sinoatrial (SA) node** and then goes to the **atrioventricular (AV) node**. From the AV node, electrical impulses travel to the **bundle of His** before traveling through the **Purkinje fibers**.
    - **Systole** refers to the period during ventricular contraction when the AV valves are closed. During **diastole**, the heart is relaxed and the semilunar valves are closed.
    - The **cardiac output** is the product of **heart rate** and **stroke volume**.
    - The sympathetic nervous system increases the heart rate and contractility. The parasympathetic nervous system decreases heart rate.
- The vasculature consists of arteries, veins, and capillaries.
    - **Arteries** are thick, highly muscular structures with an elastic quality. This allows for recoil and helps to propel blood forward within the system. Small muscular arteries are **arterioles**, which control flow into capillary beds.
    - **Capillaries** have walls that are one cell thick, making them so narrow that red blood cells must travel through them single file. Capillaries are the sites of gas and solute exchange.
    - **Veins** are inelastic, thin-walled structures that transport blood to the heart. They are able to stretch in order to accommodate large volumes of blood but do not have recoil capability. Veins are compressed by surrounding skeletal muscles and have **valves** to maintain one-way flow. Small veins are called **venules**.

- A portal system is one in which blood passes through two capillary beds in series.
  - In the **hepatic portal system**, blood travels from the gut capillary beds to the liver capillary bed via the hepatic portal vein.
  - In the **hypophyseal portal system**, blood travels from the capillary bed in the hypothalamus to the capillary bed in the anterior pituitary.
  - In the **renal portal system**, blood travels from the glomerulus to the vasa recta through an efferent arteriole.

Blood

- Blood is composed of cells and plasma, an aqueous mixture of nutrients, salts, respiratory gases, hormones, and blood proteins.
- **Erythrocytes** (**red blood cells**) lack mitochondria, a nucleus, and organelles in order to make room for **hemoglobin**, a protein that carries oxygen. Common measurements include hemoglobin concentration and **hematocrit**, the percentage of blood composed of erythrocytes.
- **Leukocytes** (**white blood cells**) are formed in the bone marrow. They are a crucial part of the immune system.
  - Granular leukocytes such as neutrophils, eosinophils, and basophils play a role in nonspecific immunity.
  - Agranulocytes, including lymphocytes and monocytes, also play a role in immunity, with lymphocytes playing a large role in specific immunity.
- **Thrombocytes** (**platelets**) are cell fragments from **megakaryocytes** that are required for coagulation.
- Blood antigens include the surface antigens A, B, and O, as well as Rh factor (D).
  - The I^A (A) and I^B (B) alleles are codominant, while the i (O) allele is recessive. People have antibodies for any AB alleles they do not have.
  - Positive Rh factor is dominant. An Rh-negative individual will only create anti-Rh antibodies after exposure to Rh-positive blood.

Physiology of the Cardiovascular System

- **Blood pressure** refers to the force per unit area that is exerted on the walls of blood vessels by blood. It is divided into systolic and diastolic components.
  - It must be high enough to overcome the resistance created by arterioles and capillaries, but low enough to avoid damaging the vasculature and surrounding structures.
  - It can be measured with a **sphygmomanometer**.
  - Blood pressure is maintained by baroreceptor and chemoreceptor reflexes. Low blood pressure promotes **aldosterone** and **antidiuretic hormone** (**ADH** or **vasopressin**) release. High blood osmolarity also promotes ADH release. High blood pressure promotes **atrial natriuretic peptide** (**ANP**) release.

- Gas and solute exchange occurs at the level of the capillaries and relies on the existence of concentration gradients to facilitate diffusion across the capillary walls. Capillaries are also leaky, which aids in the transport of gases and solutes.
  - **Starling forces** consist of **hydrostatic pressure** and **osmotic** (**oncotic**) **pressure**. Hydrostatic pressure is the pressure of the fluid within the blood vessel, while osmotic pressure is the "sucking" pressure drawing water toward solutes. Oncotic pressure is osmotic pressure due to proteins. Hydrostatic pressure forces fluid out at the arteriolar end of a capillary bed; oncotic pressure draws it back in at the venule end.
  - Oxygen is carried by hemoglobin, which exhibits **cooperative binding**. In the lungs, there is a high partial pressure of oxygen, resulting in loading of oxygen onto hemoglobin. In the tissues, there is a low partial pressure of oxygen, resulting in unloading. With cooperative binding, each successive oxygen bound to hemoglobin increases the affinity of the other subunits, while each successive oxygen released decreases the affinity of the other subunits.
  - Carbon dioxide is largely carried in the blood in the form of carbonic acid, or bicarbonate and hydrogen ions. Carbon dioxide is nonpolar and not particularly soluble, while bicarbonate, hydrogen ions, and carbonic acid are polar and highly soluble.
  - A high P_aCO_2, high $[H^+]$, low pH, high temperature, and high concentration of 2,3-BPG can cause a right shift in the **oxyhemoglobin dissociation curve**, reflecting a decreased affinity for oxygen.
  - In addition to the opposites of the causes of a right shift, a left shift can also be seen in the dissociation curve for fetal hemoglobin compared to adult hemoglobin.
  - Nutrients, wastes, and hormones are carried in the bloodstream to tissues for use or disposal.
- **Coagulation** results from an activation cascade.
  - When the endothelial lining of a blood vessel is damaged, the collagen and **tissue factor** underlying the endothelial cells are exposed. This results in a cascade of events known as the **coagulation cascade**, ultimately resulting in the formation of a clot over the damaged area.
  - Platelets bind to the collagen and are stabilized by **fibrin**, which is activated by **thrombin**.
  - Clots can be broken down by **plasmin**.

ANSWERS TO CONCEPT CHECKS

7.1

1.

Heart Chamber	Valve That Prevents Backflow
Right atrium	Tricuspid valve
Right ventricle	Pulmonary valve
Left atrium	Mitral (bicuspid) valve
Left ventricle	Aortic valve

2. Sinoatrial (SA) node → atrioventricular (AV) node → bundle of His (AV bundle) and its branches → Purkinje fibers

3.

Vessel	Carries Blood Which Direction?	Relative Wall Thickness	Smooth Muscle Present?	Contains Valves?
Artery	Away from heart	Thick	Yes, a lot	No
Capillary	From arterioles to venules	Very thin (one cell layer)	No	No
Vein	Toward heart	Thin	Yes, a little	Yes

4. The right side of the heart pumps blood into a lower-resistance circuit and must do so at lower pressures; therefore, it requires less muscle. The left side of the heart pumps blood into a higher-resistance circuit at higher pressures; therefore, it requires more muscle.
5. If all autonomic innervation to the heart were lost, the heart would continue beating at the intrinsic rate of the pacemaker (SA node). The individual would be unable to modify heart rate via the sympathetic or parasympathetic nervous system, but the heart would not stop beating.

7.2

1. Plasma is an aqueous mixture of nutrients, salts, respiratory gases, hormones, and blood proteins (clotting proteins, immunoglobulins, and so on).
2. A person with B^+ blood could receive B^+, B^-, O^+, or O^- blood. A person with B^+ blood could donate to people with B^+ or AB^+ blood.
3. Hematocrit measures the percentage of a blood sample occupied by red blood cells. It is measured in percentage points.
4. Lymphocytes are involved in specific immune defense.
5. Platelets are cellular fragments or shards that are given off by megakaryocytes in the bone marrow.
6. Only leukocytes (including neutrophils, eosinophils, basophils, monocytes/macrophages, and lymphocytes) contain nuclei. Erythrocytes and platelets do not.

7.3

1. Opening up more capillary beds (which are in parallel) will decrease the overall resistance of the circuit. The cardiac output will therefore increase in an attempt to maintain constant blood pressure. This is a risk to the heart because the increased demand on the heart can eventually tire it, leading to a heart attack or a precipitous drop in blood pressure.
2. The bicarbonate buffer system equation is

   $$CO_2\ (g) + H_2O\ (l) \rightleftharpoons H_2CO_3\ (aq) \rightleftharpoons H^+\ (aq) + HCO_3^-\ (aq).$$

   The combining of carbon dioxide and water is catalyzed by carbonic anhydrase.
3. The amount of oxygen delivery can be seen as a drop in the *y*-value (percent hemoglobin saturation) on an oxyhemoglobin dissociation curve. For example, if the blood is 100% saturated while in the lungs (at 100 mmHg O_2) and only 80% saturated while in tissues (at 40 mmHg O_2), then 20% of the oxygen has been released to tissues.
4. The oxyhemoglobin curve shifts to the right during exercise in response to increased arterial CO_2, increased $[H^+]$, decreased pH, and increased temperature. This right shift represents hemoglobin's decreased affinity for oxygen, which allows more oxygen to be unloaded at the tissues.
5. The coagulation cascade can be started by the exposure of collagen and tissue factor to platelets and coagulation factors. The clot is stabilized by fibrin.

SCIENCE MASTERY ASSESSMENT EXPLANATIONS

1. **C**

Erythrocytes, or red blood cells, are produced in the red bone marrow and circulate in the blood for about 120 days, after which they are phagocytized in the spleen and the liver, eliminating **(D)**. Red blood cells have a disc-like shape and lose their membranous organelles (like mitochondria and nuclei) during maturation. This makes **(C)** the correct answer. Erythrocytes are filled with hemoglobin; their lack of mitochondria makes their metabolism solely anaerobic, eliminating **(A)** and **(B)**.

2. **C**

An ordinary cardiac contraction originates in, and is regulated by, the sinoatrial (SA) node. The impulse travels through both atria, stimulating them to contract simultaneously. The impulse then arrives at the atrioventricular (AV) node, which momentarily slows conduction, allowing for completion of atrial contraction and ventricular filling. The impulse is then carried by the bundle of His and its branches through the Purkinje fibers in the walls of both ventricles, generating a strong contraction.

3. **C**

According to the Bohr effect, decreasing the pH in the blood decreases hemoglobin's affinity for O_2. This makes **(C)** the correct answer. The affinity is generally lowered in exercising muscle to facilitate unloading of oxygen to tissues, eliminating **(A)**. A decrease in the P_aCO_2 would cause a decrease in $[H^+]$ or increased pH—which increases hemoglobin's affinity for O_2, eliminating **(B)**. Finally, **(D)** is incorrect because hemoglobin's affinity for O_2 is higher in fetal blood than in adult blood.

4. **A**

Blood drains from the superior and inferior venae cavae into the right atrium. It passes through the tricuspid valve and into the right ventricle, and then through the pulmonary valve into the pulmonary artery, which leads to the lungs. Oxygenated blood returns to the left atrium via the pulmonary veins. It flows through the mitral valve into the left ventricle. From the left ventricle, it is pumped through the aortic valve into the aorta for distribution throughout the body.

5. **A**

The exchange of fluid is greatly influenced by the differences in the hydrostatic and osmotic pressures of blood and tissues. The osmotic (oncotic) pressure remains relatively constant; however, the hydrostatic pressure at the arterial end is greater than the hydrostatic pressure at the venous end. As a result, fluid moves out of the capillaries at the arterial end and back in at the venous end. Fluid is reabsorbed at the venous end because the osmotic pressure exceeds the hydrostatic pressure. Proteins should not cross the capillary wall under normal circumstances.

6. **C**

The first step in solving this problem is to define cardiac output: cardiac output = heart rate × stroke volume. We can therefore divide the cardiac output by the stroke volume to determine heart rate:

$$HR = \frac{CO}{SV} = \frac{7500\ \frac{\text{mL}}{\text{min}}}{50\ \frac{\text{mL}}{\text{beat}}} = 150\ \frac{\text{beats}}{\text{min}}$$

Note that this heart rate is actually pathologically fast; a normal heart rate is considered to be between 60 and 100 beats per minute.

7. **D**

Without knowing a patient's blood type, the only type of transfusion that we can safely give is O^-. People with O^- blood are considered universal donors because their blood cells contain no surface antigens. Therefore, O^- blood can be given to anyone without potentially life-threatening consequences from ABO or Rh incompatibility.

8. **C**

The only answer choice that correctly describes arteries and veins is **(C)**; the pressure in the aorta usually ranges between 120 and 80 mmHg, depending on whether the heart is in systole or diastole, whereas the pressure in the superior vena cava is near zero. **(A)** is incorrect because arteries are thick-walled and veins are thin-walled. **(B)** is also incorrect; this relationship is reversed in pulmonary and umbilical circulation. **(D)** is reversed as well; arteries make use of the pumping of the heart and the "snapping back" of their elastic walls to transport blood, whereas venous blood is propelled along by skeletal muscle contractions.

9. **A**

The relative lack of smooth muscle in venous walls allows stretching to store most of the blood in the body. Valves in the veins allow for one-way flow of blood toward the heart, not stretching. Both arteries and veins are close to lymphatic vessels, which has no bearing on their relative difference in volume. Both arteries and veins have a single-cell endothelial lining.

10. **C**

Carbon dioxide is a byproduct of metabolism in cells that later combines with water to form bicarbonate in a reaction catalyzed by carbonic anhydrase. This system is blood plasma's most important buffer system. Food and fluid absorption are not significant sources of buffering, eliminating **(A)** and **(B)**. While the kidneys can be involved in acid–base balance, they carry out this function through their filtration, secretion, and reabsorption mechanisms, not through hormone release, eliminating **(D)**.

11. **C**

In circulation, plasma proteins play an important role in generating osmotic (oncotic) pressure. This allows water that is displaced at the arterial end of a capillary bed by hydrostatic pressure to be reabsorbed at the venule end. Loss of these plasma proteins would cause a decrease in the plasma osmotic (oncotic) pressure.

12. **D**

The atrioventricular valves are located between the atria and the ventricles on both sides of the heart. Their role is to prevent backflow of blood into the atria. The valve on the right side of the heart has three cusps and is called the tricuspid valve. It prevents backflow of blood from the right ventricle into the right atrium.

13. **D**

Holding one's breath for a prolonged period would result in a drop in oxygenation and an increase in P_aCO_2. The increased carbon dioxide would associate with water to form carbonic acid, which would dissociate into a proton and a bicarbonate anion. Further, the low oxygen saturation would eventually lead to anaerobic metabolism in some tissues, causing an increase in lactic acid. These would all lead to a decreased pH.

14. **C**

The cardiac conduction system starts at the SA node, which is located near the top of the right atrium, and continues down to the AV node, which is located between the two AV valves. The bundle of His is located within the wall between the ventricles, and is likely to be affected if the wall between the ventricles has been damaged by a heart attack. This may affect the left ventricle, but the left ventricular muscle itself is not part of the cardiac conduction system.

15. **B**

The greatest amount of resistance is provided by the arterioles. Arterioles are highly muscular and have the ability to contract and dilate in order to regulate blood pressure.

Consult your online resources for additional practice. **GO ONLINE**

EQUATIONS TO REMEMBER

(7.1) **Cardiac output:** $CO = HR \times SV$

(7.2) **Ohm's law applied to circulation:** $\Delta P = CO \times TPR$

SHARED CONCEPTS

Biochemistry Chapter 9
Carbohydrate Metabolism I

Biology Chapter 6
The Respiratory System

Biology Chapter 8
The Immune System

General Chemistry Chapter 12
Electrochemistry

Physics and Math Chapter 4
Fluids

Physics and Math Chapter 6
Circuits

CHAPTER 8

THE IMMUNE SYSTEM

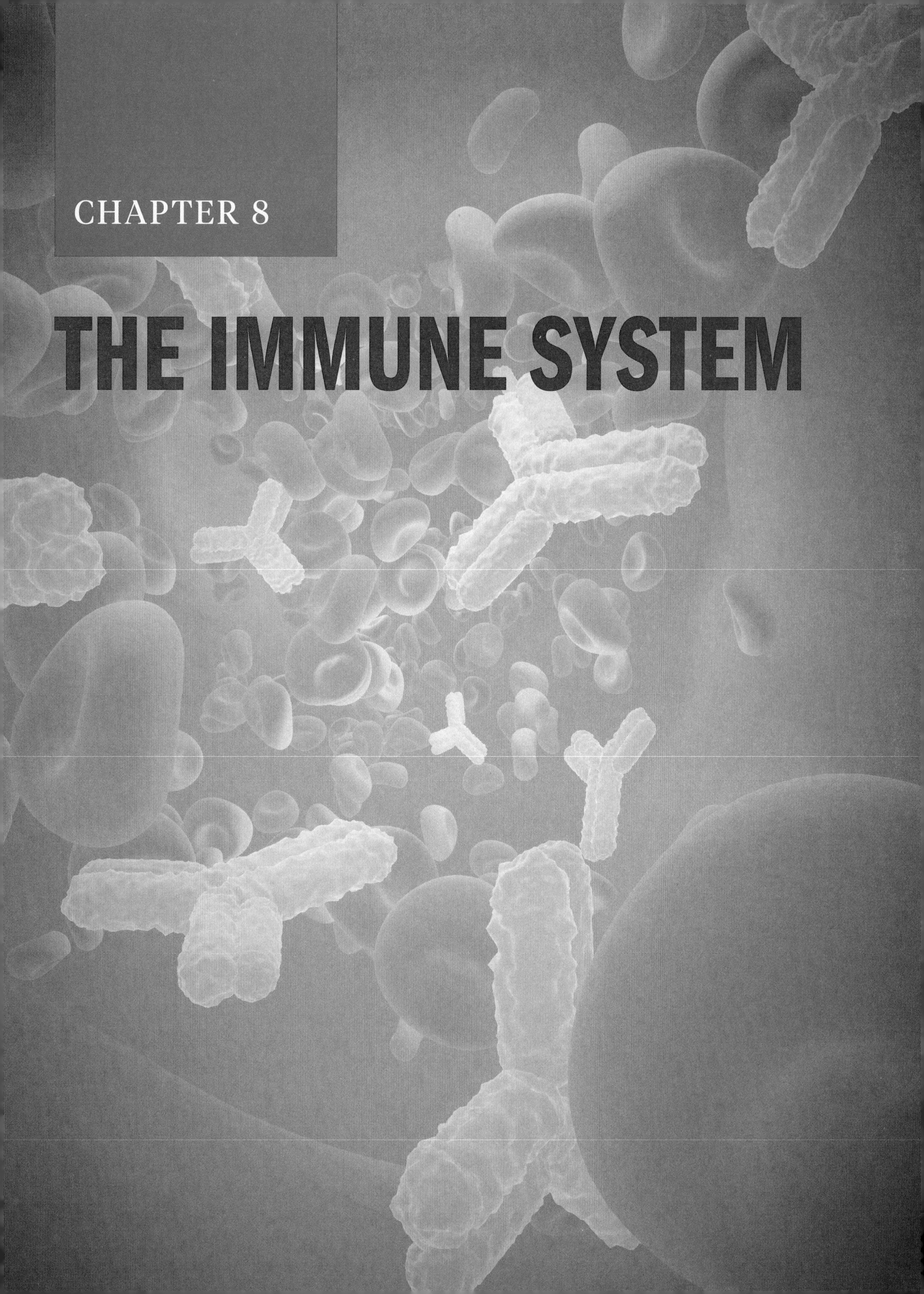

SCIENCE MASTERY ASSESSMENT

Every pre-med knows this feeling: there is so much content I have to know for the MCAT! How do I know what to do first or what's important?

While the high-yield badges throughout this book will help you identify the most important topics, this Science Mastery Assessment is another tool in your MCAT prep arsenal. This quiz (which can also be taken in your online resources) and the guidance below will help ensure that you are spending the appropriate amount of time on this chapter based on your personal strengths and weaknesses. Don't worry though—skipping something now does not mean you'll never study it. Later on in your prep, as you complete full-length tests, you'll uncover specific pieces of content that you need to review and can come back to these chapters as appropriate.

How to Use This Assessment

If you answer 0–7 questions correctly:

Spend about 1 hour to read this chapter in full and take limited notes throughout. Follow up by reviewing **all** quiz questions to ensure that you now understand how to solve each one.

If you answer 8–11 questions correctly:

Spend 20–40 minutes reviewing the quiz questions. Beginning with the questions you missed, read and take notes on the corresponding subchapters. For questions you answered correctly, ensure your thinking matches that of the explanation and you understand why each choice was correct or incorrect.

If you answer 12–15 questions correctly:

Spend less than 20 minutes reviewing all questions from the quiz. If you missed any, then include a quick read-through of the corresponding subchapters, or even just the relevant content within a subchapter, as part of your question review. For questions you answered correctly, ensure your thinking matches that of the explanation and review the Concept Summary at the end of the chapter.

1. In DiGeorge syndrome, the thymus can be completely absent. The absence of the thymus would leave an individual unable to mount specific defenses against which of the following types of pathogens?
   - **A.** Viruses
   - **B.** Bacteria
   - **C.** Parasites
   - **D.** Fungi

2. Which of the following are NOT involved in cell-mediated immunity?
   - **A.** Memory cells
   - **B.** Plasma cells
   - **C.** Cytotoxic cells
   - **D.** Suppressor cells

3. The lymphatic system:
   - **A.** transports hormones throughout the body.
   - **B.** transports chylomicrons to the circulatory system.
   - **C.** causes extravasation of fluid into tissues.
   - **D.** is the site of mast cell activation.

4. Which of the following are involved in antibody production?
   - **A.** Plasma cells
   - **B.** Memory cells
   - **C.** Helper T-cells
   - **D.** Cytotoxic cells

5. Which of the following is NOT true of the innate immune system?
   - **A.** Includes macrophages to mediate inflammation
   - **B.** Is always active against infection
   - **C.** Recognizes unique features of a pathogen
   - **D.** Contains cells derived from a hematopoietic stem cell

6. Which of the following is an example of adaptive immunity?
   - **A.** PRRs recognize that a pathogen is an invasive parasite and eosinophils are recruited to the area.
   - **B.** Complement is activated, causing osmotic instability in a bacterium.
   - **C.** Memory B-cells generated through vaccination are activated when their antigen is encountered.
   - **D.** Dendritic cells sample bacteria within a laceration and travel to the lymph nodes to present the antigen.

7. Which of the following is true regarding passive and active immunity?
   - **A.** Active immunity requires weeks to build, whereas passive immunity is acquired immediately.
   - **B.** Active immunity is short lived, whereas passive immunity is long lived.
   - **C.** Active immunity may be acquired during pregnancy through the placenta.
   - **D.** Passive immunity may be acquired through vaccination.

8. Where are most self-reactive T-cells eliminated?
   - **A.** Spleen
   - **B.** Lymph nodes
   - **C.** Bone marrow
   - **D.** Thymus

9. What is the response of the immune system to downregulation of MHC molecules on somatic cells?
   - **A.** B-cells are activated and antibodies are released.
   - **B.** T-cells are activated, resulting in a cytotoxic response.
   - **C.** Natural killer cells induce apoptosis of affected cells.
   - **D.** Macrophages engulf the pathogen and display its antigens.

10. Which of the following correctly indicates the response of $CD8^+$ T-cells when activated?
    A. Secretion of cytotoxic chemicals
    B. Causing isotype switching
    C. Presentation of antigens
    D. Activation of B-cells

11. Lymphoma is cancer of the cells of lymphoid lineage. These cells often reside within lymph nodes. What type of cell is NOT likely to cause a lymphoma?
    A. $CD8^+$ T-cells
    B. B-cells
    C. Macrophages
    D. T_h1 cells

12. Upon encountering an antigen, only T-cells with a specific T-cell receptor are activated. This is an example of:
    A. innate immunity.
    B. a cytotoxic T-cell response.
    C. humoral immunity.
    D. clonal selection.

13. Which cell type is a phagocyte that attacks bacterial pathogens in the bloodstream?
    A. Neutrophils
    B. Eosinophils
    C. Basophils
    D. Dendritic cells

14. What type of immunity is likely to be affected by removal of the spleen?
    A. Cytotoxic immunity
    B. Humoral immunity
    C. Innate immunity
    D. Passive immunity

15. Which of the following is NOT an example of a nonspecific defense mechanism?
    A. Skin provides a physical barrier against invasion.
    B. Macrophages engulf and destroy foreign particles.
    C. An inflammatory response is initiated in response to physical damage.
    D. Cytotoxic T-cells destroy cells displaying foreign antigens.

Answer Key

1. **A**
2. **B**
3. **B**
4. **A**
5. **C**
6. **C**
7. **A**
8. **D**
9. **C**
10. **A**
11. **C**
12. **D**
13. **A**
14. **B**
15. **D**

Detailed explanations can be found at the end of the chapter.

CHAPTER 8

THE IMMUNE SYSTEM

In This Chapter

CHAPTER PROFILE

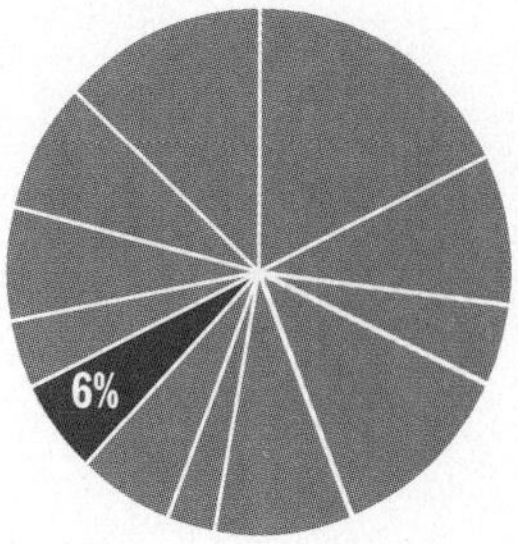

The content in this chapter should be relevant to about 6% of all questions about biology on the MCAT.

This chapter covers material from the following AAMC content category:

3B: Structure and integrative functions of the main organ systems

Introduction

Over the past few decades, the public's imagination has been captured by alarming reports of "flesh-eating" bacteria and diseases. While these bacteria do not actually eat flesh, that doesn't make them any less dangerous. "Flesh-eating" bacteria cause a condition called *necrotizing fasciitis*, a serious disease that requires aggressive medical and surgical treatment including intravenous antibiotics, surgical debridement (removal) of the necrotic tissue, and sometimes even amputation. Many different types of bacteria, including group A *Streptococcus*, *Clostridium perfringens*, and methicillin-resistant *Staphylococcus aureus* (MRSA), can cause necrotizing fasciitis. The massive destruction of skin, muscle, and connective tissue by the release of bacterial toxins called superantigens is life-threatening. These superantigens cause the immune system to become nonspecifically overactivated. Necrotizing fasciitis is dangerous not only because of the bacteria and subsequent inflammatory response, but also because the destruction of skin—a nonspecific immune defense—leaves the body susceptible to superinfection (infection with another pathogen).

In this chapter, we will consider this type of nonspecific defense, as well as specific immune defenses. The human body relies on the interaction between the innate (nonspecific) and adaptive (specific) immune systems in order to protect itself from disease. However, the immune system is not always perfect in its responses. Sometimes the immune system may become nonspecifically overactivated, as is the case with necrotizing fasciitis, or it may become activated against the same human it is supposed to protect. We will discuss the individual parts of the immune system and how these parts work together to protect from disease. In addition, we will discuss the concept of autoimmunity, or disease that results from immune attack against oneself. We'll briefly touch on vaccines, which take advantage of our understanding of the immune system to protect us from life-threatening infections. The immune system is largely integrated with the lymphatic system, which will be discussed in this chapter as well.

8.1 Structure of the Immune System

LEARNING OBJECTIVES

After Chapter 8.1, you will be able to:

- Distinguish between innate and adaptive immunity
- Draw comparisons between B- and T-cells, including their development, maturation, functions, specificity, and control mechanisms
- Identify immune cells as granulocytes or agranulocytes

MCAT EXPERTISE

The immune system is a topic where cell biology, biochemistry, anatomy, and biology interact. Thus, it is a topic that allows the MCAT to ask questions that integrate these four topics. As we discuss these complex ideas, focus on the big picture first, creating a mental image to help you put these concepts together. Then go back and plug in the details. This approach will foster your ability to associate structure with function and to think critically about the topic on Test Day.

Each day, the human body is exposed to numerous bacteria, viruses, fungi, and even parasites. Yet our bodies are able to protect us from infection most of the time. Even when we do get sick, the immune system is usually able to contain and eliminate the infection.

Innate and Adaptive Immunity

In order to fight infection, the human body has two different divisions of the immune system: innate and adaptive immunity, compared in Figure 8.1. **Innate immunity** is composed of defenses that are always active against infection, but lack the ability to target specific invaders; for this reason, it is also called **nonspecific immunity**. **Adaptive** or **specific immunity** refers to the defenses that target a specific pathogen. This system is slower to act, but can maintain immunological memory of an infection to mount a faster attack in subsequent infections.

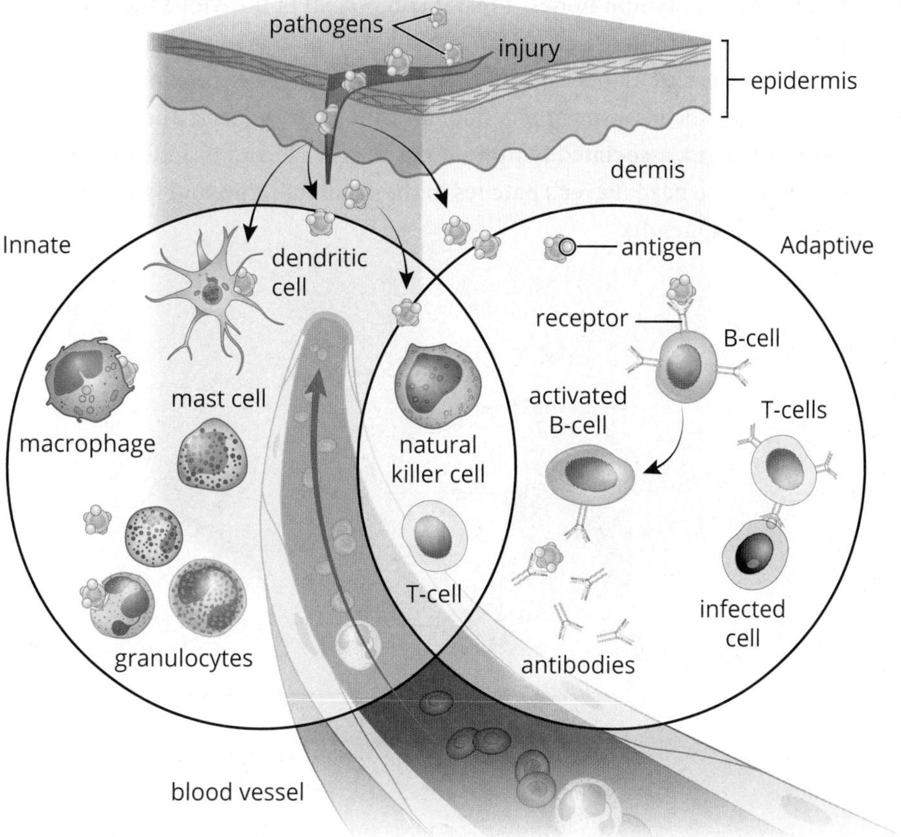

Figure 8.1 Divisions of the Immune System

Anatomy

The immune system is not housed in a single organ, as shown in Figure 8.2. The structure and components that serve as nonspecific defenses often serve functions in other organ systems. The **bone marrow** produces all of the **leukocytes** (**white blood cells**) that participate in the immune system through the process of hematopoiesis, discussed in Chapter 7 of *MCAT Biology Review*. The **spleen** is a location of blood storage and activation of **B-cells**, which turn into **plasma cells** to produce antibodies as part of adaptive immunity. Note that when B-cells leave the bone marrow, they are considered mature but naïve (because they have not yet been exposed to an antigen). Because these antibodies dissolve and act in the blood (rather than within cells), this division of adaptive immunity is called **humoral immunity**. **T-cells**, another class of adaptive immune cells, mature in the **thymus**, a small gland just in front of the pericardium, the sac that protects the heart. T-cells are the agents of **cell-mediated immunity** because they coordinate the immune system and directly kill virally

REAL WORLD

Lay people not involved in medicine often say that their "glands" are swollen when they feel a sensation of fullness around the throat. From a biological standpoint, lymph nodes are not glands—they do not secrete products into the bloodstream (endocrine) or ducts (exocrine). What they are actually experiencing is known medically as *lymphadenopathy*, or the swelling of the lymph nodes that occurs with activation of the immune system.

infected cells. Finally, **lymph nodes**, a major component of the lymphatic system, provide a place for immune cells to communicate and mount an attack; B-cells can be activated here as well. Other immune tissue is found in close proximity to the digestive system, which is a site of potential invasion by pathogens. These tissues are commonly called **gut-associated lymphoid tissue** (**GALT**) and include the **tonsils** and **adenoids** in the head, **Peyer's patches** in the small intestine, and lymphoid aggregates in the **appendix**.

KEY CONCEPT

Organs of the immune system:

- Lymph nodes filter lymph and are a site where immune responses can be mounted.
- Bone marrow is the site of immune cell production.
- The thymus is the site of T-cell maturation.
- The spleen acts as a storage area for white blood cells and platelets, a recycling center for red blood cells, and a filter of blood and lymph for the immune system.

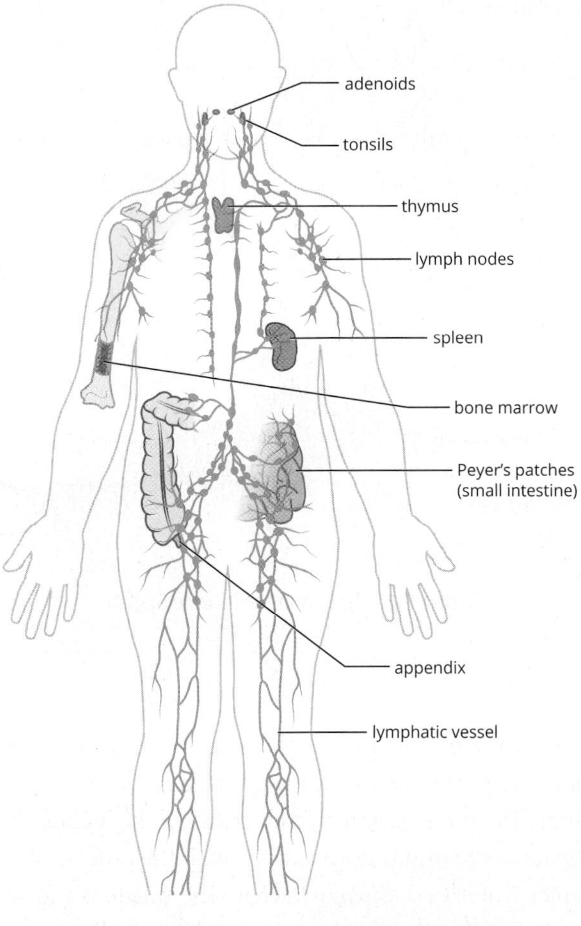

Figure 8.2 Anatomy of the Immune and Lymphatic Systems

Leukocytes are produced in the bone marrow through hematopoiesis, shown in Figure 8.3. (Note: This is the same image shown in Figure 7.7, but is copied here for convenience.) Leukocytes are divided into two groups of cells: **granulocytes** and **agranulocytes**. These names refer to the presence or absence of **granules** in the cytoplasm. These granules contain toxic enzymes and chemicals, which can be released by exocytosis, and are particularly effective against bacterial, fungal, and parasitic pathogens. Both granulocytes and agranulocytes come from a common precursor: **hematopoietic stem cells**. Remember from Chapter 7 of *MCAT Biology Review* that hematopoietic stem cells are also the cell type that gives rise to red blood cells and platelets. Granulocytes include cells such as **neutrophils**, **eosinophils**, and **basophils**. The names of these cells actually refer to the way that the cells appear after

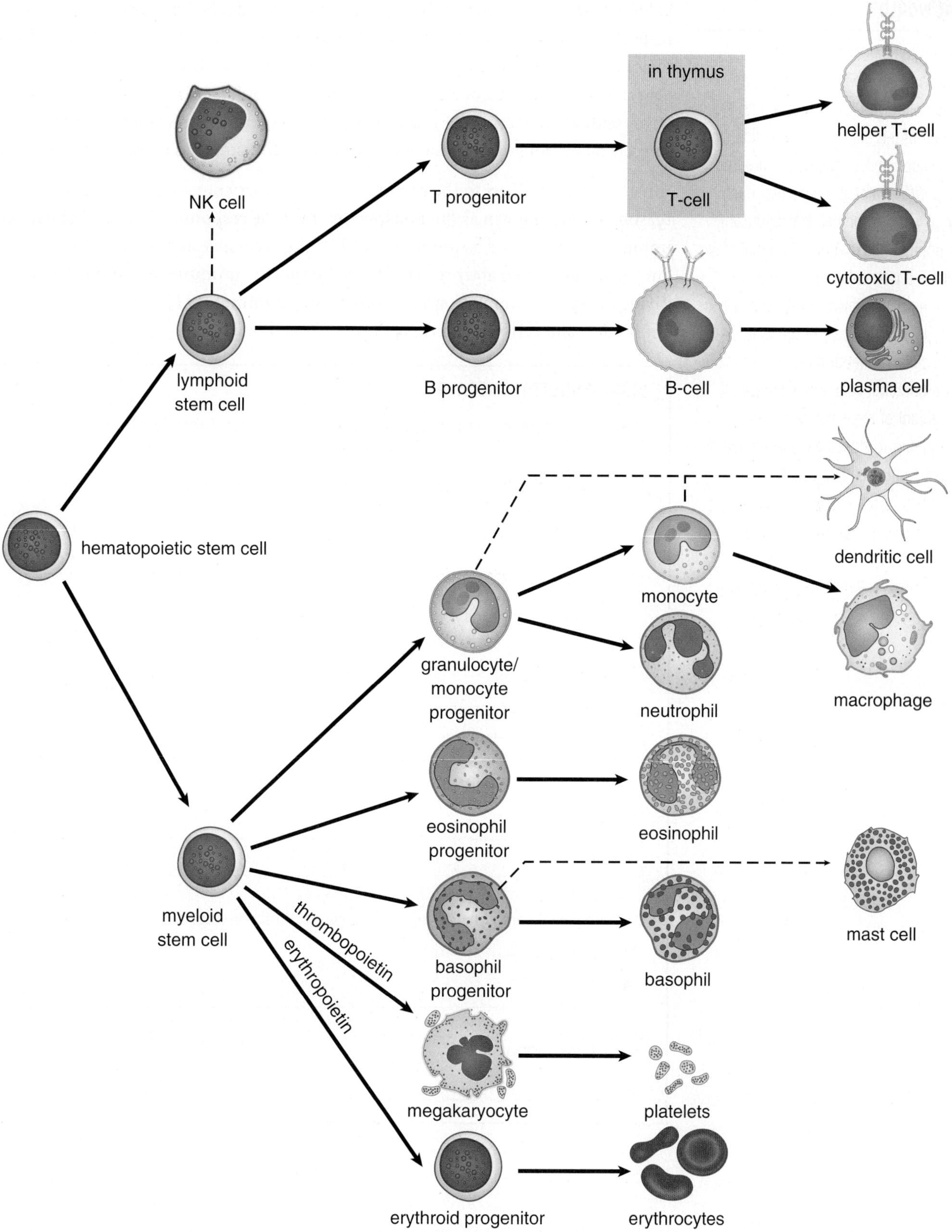

Figure 8.3 Hematopoiesis

staining with certain chemicals. Agranulocytes include the **lymphocytes**, which are responsible for antibody production, immune system modulation, and targeted killing of infected cells. **Monocytes**, which are phagocytic cells in the bloodstream, are also considered agranulocytes. They become **macrophages** in tissues; many tissues have resident populations of macrophages with specific names (such as **microglia** in the central nervous system, **Langerhans cells** in the skin, and **osteoclasts** in bone).

Innate immunity refers to the responses cells can carry out without learning; for this reason, it is also known as the **nonspecific immune response**. Conversely, adaptive immunity is developed as immune cells learn to recognize and respond to particular antigens, and is often aptly referred to as the **specific immune response**. We can also divide the specific immune system into **humoral immunity** (driven by B-cells and antibodies) and **cell-mediated immunity** (driven by T-cells).

REAL WORLD

One of the tests often ordered by physicians is known as a complete blood count (CBC). This test counts the number of red blood cells, platelets, and white blood cells. If the CBC is ordered with a *differential*, it means that each type of white blood cell is counted. Any cell populations that are abnormal may indicate a particular type of infection given the right clinical conditions. For example, if 90 percent of the white blood cells are neutrophils, it is possible that a bacterial infection is present. If 20 percent of the white blood cells are eosinophils, it is possible that an invasive parasitic infection is present.

MCAT CONCEPT CHECK 8.1

Before you move on, assess your understanding of the material with these questions.

1. What are the differences between innate and adaptive immunity?
   - Innate immunity:

   ____

   - Adaptive immunity:

   ____

2. Compare and contrast B- and T-cells:

Cell Type	Site of Development	Site of Maturation	Major Functions	Specific or Nonspecific?	Humoral or Cell-Mediated?
B-cell					
T-cell					

3. Which cells are considered granulocytes? Which are considered agranulocytes?
   - Granulocytes:

   ____

   - Agranulocytes:

   ____

8.2 The Innate Immune System

LEARNING OBJECTIVES

After Chapter 8.2, you will be able to:

- Describe the immunologic functions of each of the noncellular nonspecific immune defenses, including defensins and mucus
- Identify the immune cell type used for antigen presentation
- Differentiate between MHC-I and MHC-II
- Recall the stimuli required for activating natural killer cells, neutrophils, eosinophils, basophils, and mast cells

The innate immune system consists of cells and structures that offer nonspecific protection.

Noncellular Nonspecific Defenses

Our first line of defense is the **skin (integument)**. In Chapter 10 of *MCAT Biology Review*, we will discuss the specific homeostatic functions of the skin; for now, we'll focus on how skin protects the body. The skin provides a physical barrier between the outside world and our internal organs, preventing most bacteria, viruses, fungi, and parasites from entering the body. Additionally, antibacterial enzymes called **defensins** can be found on the skin. Sweat also has antimicrobial properties. The skin is an important first line of defense: a cut or abrasion on the skin provides an entry point for pathogens into the body. Deeper wounds allow pathogens to penetrate deeper into the body.

As discussed in Chapter 6 of *MCAT Biology Review*, the respiratory system also has mechanisms to prevent pathogens from entering the body. The respiratory passages are mucous membranes, lined with cilia to trap particulate matter and push it up toward the oropharynx, where it can be swallowed or expelled. While mucus helps to trap particulates like smoke and dirt, it also helps to prevent bacteria and viruses from gaining access to the lung tissue below. Several other mucous membranes, including those around the eye and in the oral cavity, produce a nonspecific bacterial enzyme called **lysozyme**, which is secreted in tears and saliva, respectively.

The Gastrointestinal Tract

The gastrointestinal tract also plays a role in nonspecific immunity. First, the stomach secretes acid, resulting in the elimination of most pathogens. In addition, the gut is colonized by bacteria. Most of these bacteria lack the necessary characteristics to cause infection. Because there is already such a large bacterial population in the gut, many potential invaders are not able to compete and are thus kept at bay. Many antibiotics reduce the population of gut flora, providing an opportunity for the growth of pathogens resistant to that antibiotic.

REAL WORLD

The GI tract of a newborn baby is particularly susceptible to infection because the newborn's immune system is underdeveloped and the GI tract is not yet colonized. Breast milk contains a family of antibodies that are particularly effective on mucosal surfaces and help to defend newborn babies against gastrointestinal infections.

Complement

The **complement** system consists of a number of proteins in the blood that act as a nonspecific defense against bacteria. Complement can be activated through a **classical pathway** (which requires the binding of an antibody to a pathogen) or an **alternative pathway** (which does not require antibodies). The complement proteins punch holes in the cell walls of bacteria, making them osmotically unstable. Despite the association with antibodies, complement is considered a nonspecific defense because it cannot be modified to target a specific organism over others.

Interferons

To protect against viruses, cells that have been infected with viruses produce **interferons**, proteins that prevent viral replication and dispersion. Interferons cause nearby cells to decrease production of both viral and cellular proteins. They also decrease the permeability of these cells, making it harder for a virus to infect them. In addition, interferons upregulate MHC class I and class II molecules, resulting in increased antigen presentation and better detection of the infected cells by the immune system, as described in the next section. Interferons are responsible for many "flu-like" symptoms that occur during viral infection, including malaise, tiredness, muscle soreness, and fever.

Cells of the Innate Immune System

So, what happens when bacteria, viruses, fungi, or parasites breach noncellular defenses? The cells of the innate immune system are always poised and ready to attack.

Macrophages

Macrophages, a type of agranulocyte, reside within the tissues. These cells derive from blood-borne **monocytes** and can become a **resident population** within a tissue (becoming a permanent, rather than transient, cell group in the tissue). Many of these resident macrophages are highlighted throughout *MCAT Biology Review*, including microglia in the central nervous system, Langerhans cells in the skin, and osteoclasts in bone. When a bacterial invader enters a tissue, the macrophages become activated. The activated macrophage does three things. First, it phagocytizes the invader through endocytosis. Then, it digests the invader using enzymes. Finally, it presents little pieces of the invader (mostly peptides) to other cells using a protein called **major histocompatibility complex** (**MHC**). MHC binds to a pathogenic peptide (also called an **antigen**) and carries it to the cell surface, where it can be recognized by cells of the adaptive immune system. In addition, macrophages release **cytokines**, chemical substances that stimulate inflammation and recruit additional immune cells to the area.

MHC molecules come in two main classes: class I and class II. All nucleated cells in the body display **MHC class I** molecules. Any protein produced within a cell can be loaded onto MHC-I and presented on the surface of the cell, as shown in Figure 8.4.

This allows the immune system to monitor the health of these cells and to detect if the cells have been infected with a virus or another intracellular pathogen; only those cells that are infected would be expected to present an unfamiliar (nonself) protein on their surfaces. Therefore, the MHC-I pathway is often called the **endogenous pathway** because it binds antigens that come from inside the cell. Cells that have been invaded by intracellular pathogens can then be killed by a certain group of T-cells (cytotoxic T-lymphocytes) to prevent infection of other cells.

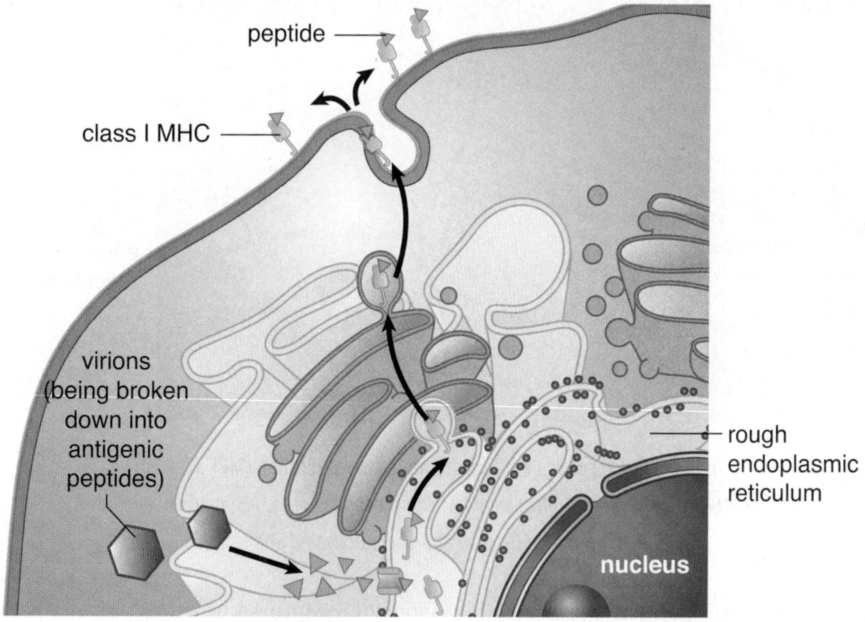

Figure 8.4 Endogenous Pathway for Antigen Presentation (MHC Class I)
MHC-I exists in all nucleated cells.

MHC class II molecules are mainly displayed by professional **antigen-presenting cells** like macrophages, as shown in Figure 8.5. Remember that these phagocytic cells pick up pathogens from the environment, process them, and then present them on MHC-II. An **antigen** is a substance (usually a pathogenic protein) that can be targeted by an antibody. While antibody production is the domain of the adaptive immune system, it is important to understand that cells of the innate immune system also present antigens. Because these antigens originated outside the cell, the MHC-II pathway is often called the **exogenous pathway**. The presentation of an antigen by an immune cell may result in the activation of both the innate and adaptive immune systems. Professional antigen-presenting cells include macrophages, **dendritic cells** in the skin, some B-cells, and certain activated epithelial cells.

REAL WORLD

MHC molecules are highly variable among humans, but can usually be divided into particular subtypes. People with certain MHC subtypes have different susceptibility to disease, and individuals with certain subtypes are considerably more susceptible to autoimmune diseases. It is also important to match the MHC types of the donor and recipient as closely as possible during transplants to avoid rejection.

KEY CONCEPT

Major histocompatibility complex molecules are joined with antigens. The MHC–antigen complex then goes to the cell surface to display the antigen. This allows the immune system to monitor the health of cells. MHC-I is in all nucleated cells and presents endogenous antigens. MHC-II is in antigen-presenting cells and presents exogenous antigens.

KEY CONCEPT

The innate immune cells are nonspecific and form the first line of defense against pathogens.

Innate Immunity

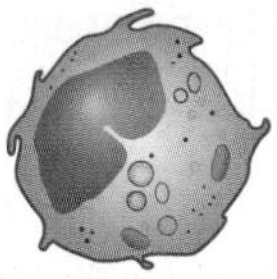

Macrophages envelop pathogens and break them down.

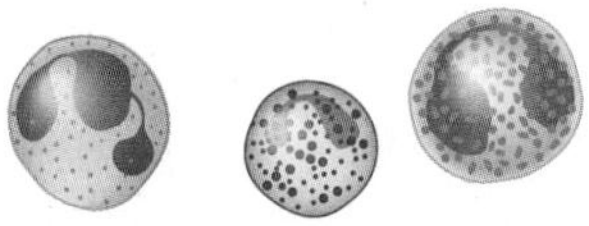

Granulocytes contain granules and also contribute to inflammation. The three types of granulocytes are neutrophils, eosinophils, and basophils.

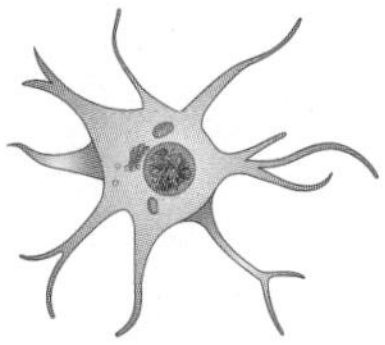

Dendritic cells induce adaptive immune cells to attack pathogens by presenting them with antigens from those pathogens.

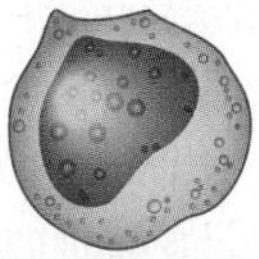

Natural killer cells destroy cancer cells and body cells infected with pathogens.

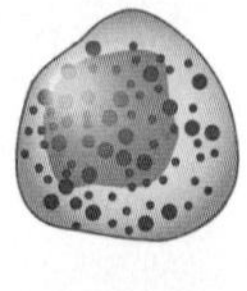

Mast cells release histamine and other inflammatory agents.

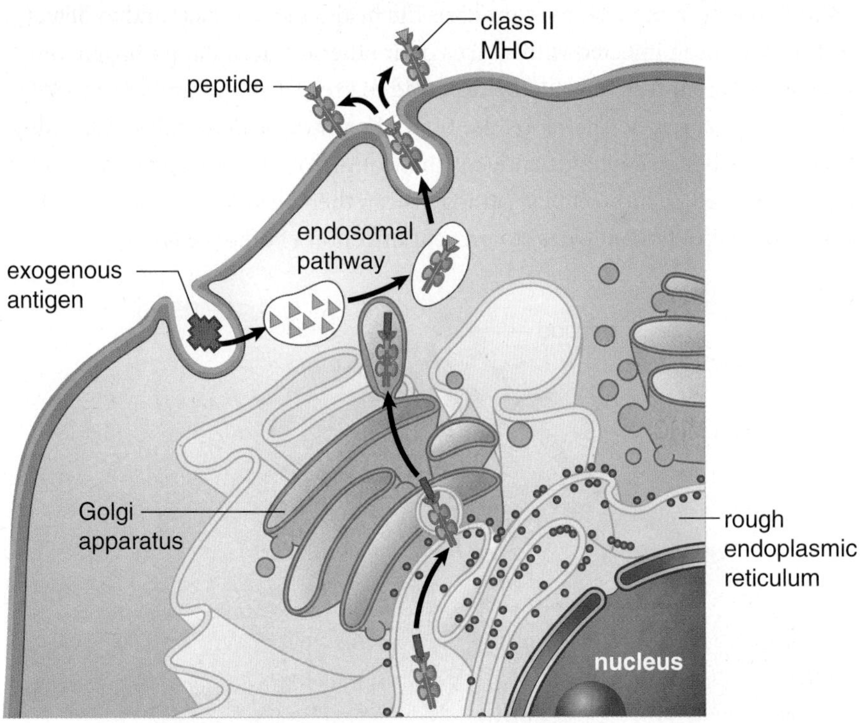

Figure 8.5 Exogenous Pathway for Antigen Presentation (MHC Class II)
MHC-II exists only in professional antigen-presenting cells, like macrophages, dendritic cells, some B-cells, and some activated epithelial cells.

Macrophages and dendritic cells also have special receptors known as **pattern recognition receptors** (**PRR**), the best-described of which are **toll-like receptors** (**TLR**). PRRs are able to recognize the category of the invader (bacterium, virus, fungus, or parasite). This allows for the production of appropriate cytokines to recruit the right type of immune cells; each immune cell has different weapons that can target particular groups of pathogens.

Natural Killer Cells

In the arms race between the human immune system and pathogens, some pathogens have found ways to avoid certain defenses. For example, some viruses cause downregulation of MHC molecules, making it harder for T-cells to recognize the presence of an infection. **Natural killer** (**NK**) **cells**, a type of nonspecific lymphocyte, are able to detect the downregulation of MHC and induce apoptosis in these virally infected cells. Cancer cells may also downregulate MHC production, so NK cells also offer protection from the growth of cancer as well.

Granulocytes

In addition to macrophages, the granulocytes, which include neutrophils, eosinophils, and basophils (and closely related mast cells), are also involved in nonspecific defense. **Neutrophils** are the most populous leukocyte in blood and are very short lived (a bit more than five days). These cells are phagocytic, like macrophages, and target bacteria. Neutrophils can follow bacteria using chemotaxis—the movement of an organism according to chemical stimuli; in this case, the neutrophil senses products given off by bacteria, moving up the concentration gradient to the source. Neutrophils can also detect bacteria once they have been **opsonized** (marked with an antibody from a B-cell). Other cells, like natural killer cells, macrophages, monocytes, and eosinophils, also contain receptors for antibodies and can attack opsonized bacteria. Dead neutrophil collections are responsible for the formation of **pus** during an infection.

Eosinophils contain bright red-orange granules and are primarily involved in allergic reactions and invasive parasitic infections. Upon activation, eosinophils release large amounts of **histamine**, an inflammatory mediator. This results in vasodilation and increased leakiness of the blood vessels, allowing additional immune cells (especially macrophages and neutrophils) to move out of the bloodstream and into the tissue. **Inflammation** is particularly useful against extracellular pathogens, including bacteria, fungi, and parasites.

KEY CONCEPT

Histamine causes inflammation by inducing vasodilation and the movement of fluid and cells from the bloodstream into tissues.

Finally, **basophils** contain large purple granules and are involved in allergic responses. They are the least populous leukocyte in the bloodstream under normal conditions. **Mast cells** are closely related to basophils, but have smaller granules and exist in the tissues, mucosa, and epithelium. Both basophils and mast cells release large amounts of histamine in response to allergens, leading to inflammatory responses.

MCAT CONCEPT CHECK 8.2

Before you move on, assess your understanding of the material with these questions.

1. For each of the noncellular nonspecific immune defenses listed below, provide a brief description of its immunologic function:
   - Skin:
   - Defensins:
   - Lysozyme:
   - Mucus:
   - Stomach acid:
   - Normal gastrointestinal flora:
   - Complement:
2. Which cells are professional antigen-presenting cells?
3. What are the differences between MHC-I and MHC-II?
   - MHC-I:
   - MHC-II:

4. What stimulus activates each of the following types of cells?
   - Natural killer cells:
   ____
   - Neutrophils:
   ____
   - Eosinophils:
   ____
   - Basophils and mast cells:
   ____

8.3 The Adaptive Immune System

High-Yield

LEARNING OBJECTIVES

After Chapter 8.3, you will be able to:

- Recall the major classes of lymphocytes and their functions
- Describe the three main effects that circulating antibodies can have on a pathogen
- Describe the effects of positive and negative selection on T-cell maturation
- Explain why the secondary response to a pathogen is more efficient than the primary response
- Differentiate between passive and active immunity
- Explain how antibodies become specific for a given antigen

The adaptive immune system can identify specific invaders and mount an attack against that pathogen. The response is variable and depends on the identity of the pathogen. The adaptive immune system can be divided into two divisions: humoral immunity and cell-mediated (cytotoxic) immunity. Each involves the identification of the specific pathogen and organization of an appropriate immune response.

Cells of the Adaptive Immune System

The adaptive immune system consists mainly of two types of lymphocytes, B-cells and T-cells. B-cells govern the humoral response, while T-cells mount the cell-mediated response. All cells of the immune system are created in the bone marrow, but B- and T-cells mature in different locations. B-cells mature in the bone marrow and spleen (although the B in their name originally stood for the bursa of Fabricius, an organ found in birds), and T-cells mature in the thymus. When we are exposed to a pathogen, it may take a few days for the physical symptoms to be relieved. This occurs because the adaptive immune response takes time to form specific defenses against the pathogen.

KEY CONCEPT

B-cells mature in the **b**one marrow.
T-cells mature in the **t**hymus.

Humoral Immunity

Humoral immunity, which involves the production of **antibodies**, may take as long as a week to become fully effective after initial infection. These antibodies are specific to the antigens of the invading microbe. Antibodies are produced by B-cells, which are lymphocytes that originate and mature in the bone marrow and are activated in the spleen and lymph nodes.

Antibodies (also called **immunoglobulins** [**Ig**]) can carry out many different jobs in the body. Just as antigens can be displayed on the surface of cells or can float freely in blood, chyle (lymphatic fluid), or air, so too can antibodies be present on the surface of a cell or secreted into body fluids. When an antibody binds to an antigen, the response will depend on the location. For antibodies secreted into body fluids, there are three main possibilities: first, once bound to a specific antigen, antibodies may attract other leukocytes to phagocytize those antigens immediately. This is called opsonization, as described earlier. Second, antibodies may cause pathogens to clump together or **agglutinate**, forming large insoluble complexes that can be phagocytized. Third, antibodies can block the ability of a pathogen to invade tissues, essentially neutralizing it. For cell-surface antibodies, the binding of antigen to a B-cell causes activation of that cell, resulting in its proliferation and formation of plasma and memory cells, as described later in this chapter. In contrast, when antigen binds to antibodies on the surface of a mast cell, it causes **degranulation** (exocytosis of granule contents), releasing histamine and causing an inflammatory allergic reaction.

Antibodies are Y-shaped molecules that are made up of two identical **heavy chains** and two identical **light chains**, as shown in Figure 8.6. Disulfide linkages and noncovalent interactions hold the heavy and light chains together. Each antibody has an **antigen-binding region** at the end of which is called the **variable region** (**domain**), at the tips of the Y. Within this region, there are specific polypeptide sequences that will bind one, and only one, specific antigenic sequence. Part of the reason it takes so long to initiate the antibody response is that each B-cell undergoes **hypermutation** of its antigen-binding region, trying to find the best match for the antigen. Only those B-cells that can bind the antigen with high affinity survive, providing a mechanism for generating specificity called **clonal selection**. The remaining part of the antibody molecule is known as the **constant region** (**domain**). It is this region that cells such as natural killer cells, macrophages, monocytes, and eosinophils have receptors for, and that can initiate the complement cascade. Each B-cell makes only one type of antibody, but we have many B-cells, so our immune system can recognize many antigens. Further, antibodies come in five different isotypes (IgM, IgD, IgG, IgE, and IgA). While the specific purposes of each antibody isotype is outside the scope of the MCAT, you should know that the different types can be used at different times during the adaptive immune response, for different types of pathogens, or in different locations in the body. Cells can change which isotype of antibody they produce when stimulated by specific cytokines in a process called **isotype switching**.

KEY CONCEPT

The adaptive immune cells target invaders with greater specificity, but respond slower since they are replicated in response to an antigen.

Adaptive Immunity

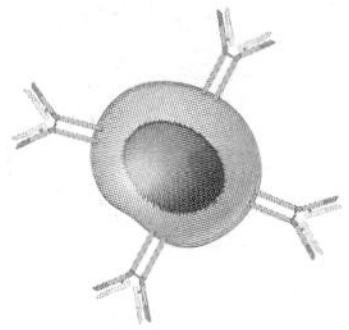

B-cells respond to antigens by dividing and making antibodies that can neutralize pathogens directly or indirectly with the help of other leukocytes.

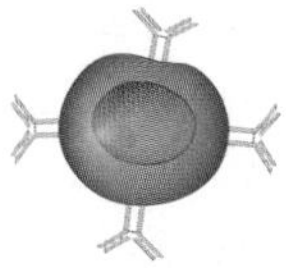

T-cells have a variety of functions in adaptive immune response. Cytotoxic T-cells detect specific antigens and destroy the infected cells that present them. Suppressor and helper T-cells play coordinating roles in immune response. Memory T-cells prepare for potential reinfections.

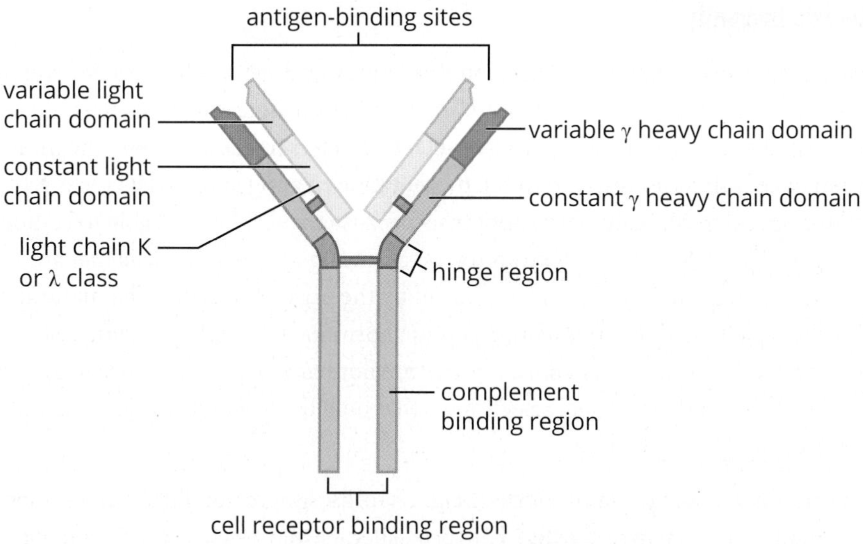

Figure 8.6 Structure of an Antibody Molecule

Not all B-cells that are generated actively or constantly produce antibodies. Antibody production is an energetically expensive process, and there is no reason to expend energy to produce antibodies that are not needed. Instead, **naïve** B-cells (those that have not yet been exposed to an antigen) wait in the lymph nodes for their particular antigen to come along. Upon exposure to the correct antigen, a B-cell will proliferate and produce two types of daughter cells. **Plasma cells** produce large amounts of antibodies, whereas **memory B-cells** stay in the lymph node, awaiting reexposure to the same antigen. This initial activation takes approximately seven to ten days and is known as the **primary response**. The plasma cells will eventually die, but the memory cells may last the lifetime of the organism. If the same microbe is ever encountered again, the memory cells rapidly proliferate and differentiate into plasma cells to produce antibodies specific to that pathogen. This immune response, called the **secondary response**, will be more rapid and robust. The development of these lasting memory cells is the basis of the efficacy of **vaccination**.

Cytotoxic Immunity

Whereas humoral immunity is based on the activity of B-cells, cell-mediated immunity involves the T-cells. T-cells mature in the thymus, where they undergo both positive and negative selection. **Positive selection** refers to allowing only the maturation of cells that can respond to the presentation of antigen on MHC (cells that cannot respond to MHC undergo apoptosis because they will not be able to respond in the periphery). **Negative selection** refers to causing apoptosis in cells that are self-reactive (activated by proteins produced by the organism itself). The maturation of T-cells is facilitated by **thymosin**, a peptide hormone secreted by thymic cells. Once the T-cell has left the thymus, it is mature but naïve. Upon exposure to antigen, T-cells will also undergo clonal selection so that only those with the highest affinity for a given antigen proliferate.

There are three major types of T-cells: helper T-cells, suppressor T-cells, and killer (cytotoxic) T-cells. **Helper T-cells (T_h)**, also called **$CD4^+$ T-cells**, coordinate the immune response by secreting chemicals known as **lymphokines**. These molecules are capable of recruiting other immune cells (such as plasma cells, cytotoxic T-cells, and macrophages) and increasing their activity. The loss of these cells, as occurs in **human immunodeficiency virus** (**HIV**) infection, prevents the immune system from mounting an adequate response to infection; in advanced HIV infection, also called **acquired immunodeficiency syndrome** (**AIDS**), even weak pathogens can cause devastating consequences as opportunistic infections. $CD4^+$ T-cells respond to antigens presented on MHC-II molecules. Because MHC-II presents exogenous antigens, $CD4^+$ T-cells are most effective against bacterial, fungal, and parasitic infections.

Cytotoxic T-cells (T_c or **CTL**, for cytotoxic T-lymphocytes), also called **$CD8^+$ T-cells**, are capable of directly killing virally infected cells by injecting toxic chemicals that promote apoptosis into the infected cell. $CD8^+$ T-cells respond to antigens presented on MHC-I molecules. Because MHC-I presents endogenous antigens, $CD8^+$ T-cells are most effective against viral (and intracellular bacterial or fungal) infections.

Suppressor or **regulatory T-cells** (T_{reg}) also express CD4, but can be differentiated from helper T-cells because they also express a protein called *Foxp3*. These cells help to tone down the immune response once infection has been adequately contained. These cells also turn off self-reactive lymphocytes to prevent autoimmune diseases: this is termed **self-tolerance**.

Finally, **memory T-cells** can be generated. Similar to memory B-cells, these cells lie in wait until the next exposure to the same antigen. When activated, they carry out a more robust and rapid response.

REAL WORLD

"CD" in immunology stands for *cluster of differentiation* and includes cell-surface markers that can be detected by the lab technique called flow cytometry; these markers give an indication of the types of leukocytes under investigation, how many are present, and their state of maturity.

KEY CONCEPT

$CD4^+$ T-cells are better at fighting extracellular infections, while $CD8^+$ T-cells are better at targeting intracellular infections.

MNEMONIC

CD $\times$ MHC = 8

$CD4^+$ cells respond to MHC-**II**
($4 \times 2 = 8$)

$CD8^+$ cells respond to MHC-**I**
($8 \times 1 = 8$)

REAL WORLD

Many suppressor T-cells were formerly self-reactive T-cells that have been turned off. When a suppressor T-cell inactivates another lymphocyte, it can either target it for destruction or promote its conversion into another suppressor T-cell.

A summary of the different types of lymphocytes in adaptive (specific) immunity is shown in Figure 8.7.

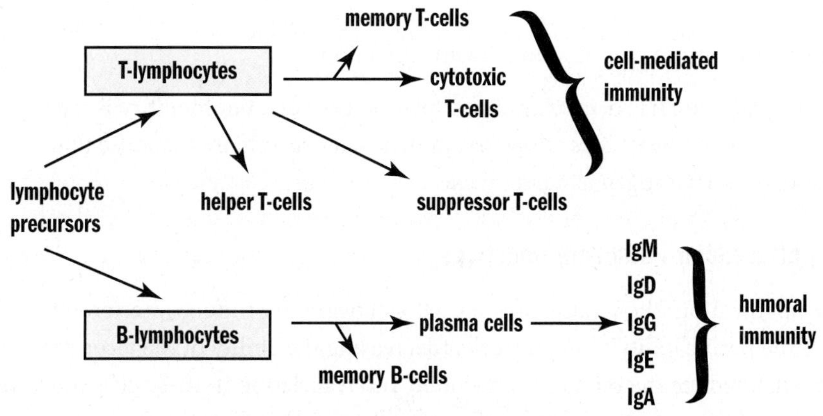

Figure 8.7 Lymphocytes of Specific Immunity
This diagram shows the differentiation of lymphocyte precursors and the cell types involved in specific immunity.

Activation of the Adaptive Immune System

It is important to note that the innate and adaptive immune systems are not really disparate entities that function separately. The proper functioning of the entire immune system depends on the interactions between these two systems. There are five types of infectious pathogens: bacteria, viruses, fungi, parasites (including protozoa, worms, and insects), and prions (for which there are no immune defenses). While the immune system's response depends on the specific identity of the pathogen, we present two classic examples: a bacterial (extracellular pathogen) infection and a viral (intracellular pathogen) infection. Keep in mind that this categorization is imperfect; for example, some bacteria, like *Mycobacterium tuberculosis* and *Listeria monocytogenes*, are actually intracellular pathogens.

Bacterial (Extracellular Pathogen) Infections

Macrophages are like the sentinels of the human body, always on the lookout for potential invaders. Let's say a person suffers a laceration and bacteria are introduced into the body via this laceration. First, macrophages (and other antigen-presenting cells) engulf the bacteria and subsequently release inflammatory mediators. These cells also digest the bacteria and present antigens from the pathogen on their surfaces in conjunction with MHC-II. The cytokines attract inflammatory cells, including neutrophils and additional macrophages. Mast cells are activated by the inflammation and degranulate, resulting in histamine release and increased leakiness of the capillaries. This augments the ability of the immune cells to leave the bloodstream to travel to the affected tissue. The dendritic cell then leaves the affected tissue and travels to the nearest lymph node, where it presents the antigen to B-cells. B-cells that produce the correct antibody proliferate through clonal selection to create plasma cells and memory cells. Antibodies then travel through the bloodstream to the affected tissue, where they tag the bacteria for destruction.

At the same time, dendritic cells are also presenting the antigen to T-cells, activating a T-cell response. In particular, $CD4^+$ T-cells are activated. These cells come in two types, called T_h1 and T_h2. T_h1 cells release interferon gamma (IFN-γ), which activates macrophages and increases their ability to kill bacteria. T_h2 cells help activate B-cells and are more common in parasitic infections.

After the pathogen has been eliminated, plasma cells die, but memory B- and T-cells remain. These memory cells allow for a much faster secondary response upon exposure to the pathogen at a later time.

Viral (Intracellular Pathogen) Infections

In a viral infection, the virally infected cell will begin to produce interferons, which reduce the permeability of nearby cells (decreasing the ability of the virus to infect these cells), reduce the rate of transcription and translation in these cells (decreasing the ability of the virus to multiply), and cause systemic symptoms (malaise, muscle aching, fever, and so on). These infected cells also present intracellular proteins on their surface in conjunction with MHC-I; in a virally infected cell, at least some of these intracellular proteins will be viral proteins.

$CD8^+$ T-cells will recognize the MHC-I and antigen complex as foreign and will inject toxins into the cell to promote apoptosis. In this way, the infection can be shut down before it is able to spread to nearby cells. In the event that the virus downregulates the production and presentation of MHC-I molecules, natural killer cells will recognize the absence of MHC-I and will accordingly cause apoptosis of these cells.

Again, once the pathogen has been cleared, memory T-cells will be generated that can allow a much faster response to be mounted upon a second exposure.

REAL WORLD

Autoimmune diseases can result in destruction of tissues, which may cause various deficiencies. Type I diabetes mellitus results from autoimmune destruction of the β-cells of the pancreas. This results in an inability to produce insulin, characterized by high blood sugars and excessive utilization of fats and proteins for energy. Other examples of autoimmune diseases include multiple sclerosis, myasthenia gravis, psoriasis, systemic lupus erythematosus, rheumatoid arthritis, Graves' disease, and Guillain-Barré syndrome.

Recognition of Self and Nonself

Self-antigens are the proteins and carbohydrates present on the surface of every cell of the body. Under normal circumstances, these self-antigens signal to immune cells that the cell is not foreign and should not be attacked. However, when the immune system fails to make the distinction between *self* and *foreign*, it may attack cells expressing particular self-antigens, a condition known as **autoimmunity**. Note that autoimmunity is only one potential problem with immune functioning: another problem arises when the immune system misidentifies a foreign antigen as dangerous when, in fact, it is not. Pet dander, pollen, and peanuts are not inherently threatening to human life, yet some people's immune systems are hypersensitive to these antigens and become overactivated when these antigens are encountered. This is called an allergic reaction. Allergies and autoimmunity are part of a family of immune reactions classified as **hypersensitivity reactions**.

The human body strives to prevent autoimmune reactions very early in T-cell and B-cell maturation processes. T-cells are educated in the thymus. Part of this education involves the elimination of T-cells that respond to self-antigens, called negative selection. Immature B-cells that respond to self-antigens are eliminated before they leave the bone marrow. However, this process is not perfect, and occasionally a cell that responds to self-antigens is allowed to survive. Most autoimmune diseases can be treated with a number of therapies; one common example is administration of **glucocorticoids** (modified versions of cortisol), which have potent immunosuppressive qualities.

Immunization

Often, diseases can have significant, long-term consequences. Infection with the poliovirus, for example, can cause permanent paralysis. Polio used to be a widespread illness; however, today we hardly hear about outbreaks of polio because of a highly effective vaccination program that led to the elimination of polio from many parts of the world.

Immunization can be achieved in an active or passive fashion. In **active immunity**, the immune system is stimulated to produce antibodies against a specific pathogen. The means by which we are exposed to this pathogen may either be natural or artificial. Through natural exposure, antibodies are generated by B-cells once an individual becomes infected. Artificial exposure (through vaccines) also results in the production of antibodies; however, the individual never experiences true infection. Instead, the individual receives an injection or intranasal spray containing an antigen that will activate B-cells to produce antibodies to fight the specific infection. The antigen may be a weakened or killed form of the microbe, or it may be a part of the microbe's protein structure.

Immunization may also be achieved passively. **Passive immunity** results from the transfer of antibodies to an individual. The immunity is transient because only the antibodies, and not the plasma cells that produce them, are given to the individual. Natural examples are the transfer of antibodies across the placenta during pregnancy to protect the fetus and the transfer of antibodies from a mother to her nursing infant through breast milk. In some cases of exposure, such as to the rabies virus or tetanus, intravenous immunoglobulin may be given to prevent the pathogen from spreading.

REAL WORLD

In 1998, a paper published in *The Lancet* claimed to have found a link between vaccines and autism. This paper was withdrawn from *The Lancet* after it was demonstrated that the primary author had an undisclosed conflict of interest and that the results were scientifically inaccurate. In fact, no well-designed scientific study has yet shown this link to exist. Nevertheless, reporting of this unsubstantiated connection in the lay media has influenced some parents and guardians to avoid immunizing their children. Since 1998, outbreaks of measles and mumps in the United States and other industrialized nations have raised concerns about the resurgence of illnesses that were previously thought to have been eliminated from these countries. Vaccines do carry risks, including rare cases of encephalitis (brain inflammation) and Guillain-Barré syndrome (an autoimmune disease in which the myelin of peripheral nerves is attacked), but so too do the pathogens these vaccines protect against.

BIOLOGY GUIDED EXAMPLE WITH EXPERT THINKING

The development of immune-mediated liver failure during viral hepatitis has recently been linked to the action of $CD8^+$ T-cells. Several effector mechanisms have been identified in preclinical models, including the cytokines interferon (IFN) and tumor necrosis factor (TNF), as well as apoptosis-inducing molecules such as Fas Ligand (FasL) and perforin-1 (Prf1). To better study these factors, a mouse model of acute hepatitis was developed by immunizing mice with OVA epitope (a short peptide sequence derived from the protein ovalbumin) and then infected with recombinant adenovirus expressing OVA peptide 30 days later. Acute liver damage was observed, marked by an increase in serum alanine aminotransferase (sALT), a marker of liver damage, and a decrease in body weight.

Topic: $CD8^+$ T-cells and hepatitis

These are all components of the immune system that may lead to immune-mediated liver failure

New model to study immune-mediated liver damage during acute hepatitis

Damage to liver = elevated sALT, decrease in body weight

To study the contribution of FasL and TNF to liver pathology, mice were injected with Anti-FasL, anti-TNF, or IgG control antibodies before adenovirus challenge. Researchers measured sALT levels and body weight in the days post challenge (Figure 1). To better elucidate the role of perforin-1, OVA-specific T-cells (OT-1 cells) with either WT perforin or perforin-1 KO (OT-1 x Prf1-/- cells), were injected into naive mice prior to adenovirus challenge. Serum ALT and weight measurements were taken following infection (Figure 2).

Exp 1: test FasL and TNF contribution, antibodies added that will prevent factors from exerting their normal biological function

Exp 2: test role of perforin-1, add T-cells with and without perforin-1, measure sALT and body mass

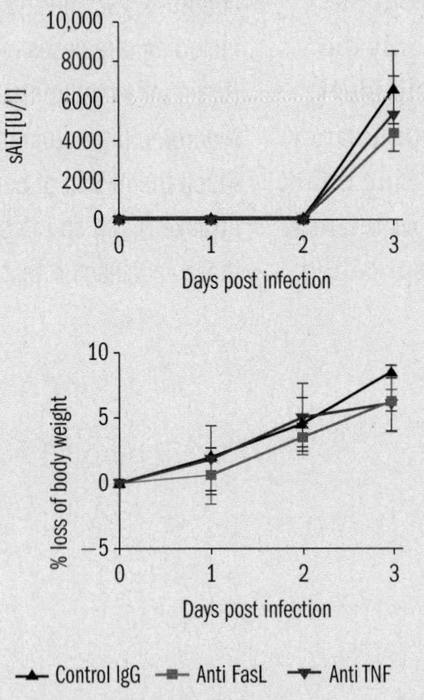

Figure 1

Figure 1 = antibody study

IV: antibody treatment

DVs: sALT levels and % loss of body weight

Trend: in both graphs, the three groups have overlapping error bars

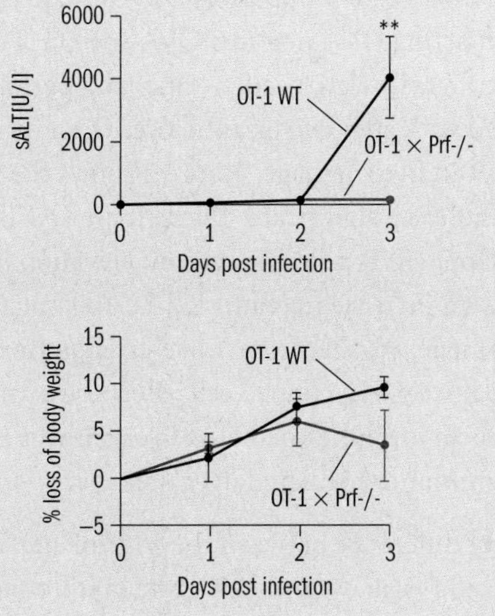

Figure 2

Figure 2 = cell transfer study

IV: presence or absence of perforin-1

DVs: same as previous

Trends: mice given perforin-1 knockout cells have no increase in sALT and lose less weight compared to controls

Adapted from Welz, M., Eickhoff, S., Abdullah, Z., Trebicka, J., Gartlan, K. H., Spicer, J. A., & Kastenmüller, W. (2018). Perforin inhibition protects from lethal endothelial damage during fulminant viral hepatitis. *Nature Communications*, *9*(1), 4805. doi:10.1038/s41467-018-07213-x.

Based on the results, which of the three parameters tested, FAS Ligand, Tumor Necrosis Factor, or Perforin, is most likely involved in the destruction of liver tissue during acute infection?

This question is really testing our understanding of the experimental design and comprehension of the results. Let's start with the experimental design. Paragraph 1 tells us that there are four main factors that are believed to be involved in immune-mediated liver damage: FasL, TNF, perforin-1, and INF. To test the involvement of these factors, the researchers designed a new experimental model. They first injected mice with OVA peptide to induce a primary immune response and the development of memory cells. Thirty days later, the researchers infected the mice with adenovirus expressing OVA. This will result in activation of memory cells and a secondary immune response, which the researchers showed was able to induce immune-controlled liver damage.

In the first experiment, the mice were injected with antibodies against FasL and TNF prior to adenovirus infection. These antibodies will bind to FasL and TNF, rendering them unable to function, similar to knocking out the gene (but significantly cheaper than developing transgenic mice!). Figure 1 shows the results. We notice that there is no significant difference in sALT levels nor body weight loss between mice treated with the control antibody and mice treated with either FasL or TNF antibody. We see the same increase in sALT and the same decrease in weight loss, indicating that removing TNF and FasL function did not prevent liver damage. This suggests that these two factors are not required for the immune-mediated liver damage.

In the second experiment, we test the involvement of perforin-1. The experimental setup is slightly different. Instead of injecting OVA peptide, OVA specific T-cells were injected into mice. Two different types of cells were used, normal and perforin-1 knockout. The mice were then infected with adenovirus as before. This enables us to examine the contribution of perforin-1 in liver damage. Figure 2 shows the results of the experiment. We can note that there is a significant difference in sALT levels between control and perforin-1 knockout (KO) cells. There is no elevation in sALT in the knockout cells, whereas there is an increase in control cells. This suggests that perforin-1 contributes to liver damage. Furthermore, mice given perforin-1 KO cells lose less weight compared to mice given control cells. Because a knockout of the perforin-1 gene led to a decrease in immune-mediated liver damage in mice, perforin-1 plays an important role in immune-mediated liver damage.

Because the results show no significant difference between the control and TNF and FasL antibody treated mice, TNF and FasL do not play a role in immune-mediated liver damage. However, a statistically significant difference between control and perforin-1 knockout cells was observed, indicating a role for perforin-1 in immune-mediated liver damage.

MCAT CONCEPT CHECK 8.3

Before you move on, assess your understanding of the material with these questions.

1. For each of the lymphocytes listed below, what are its main functions?
   - Plasma cell:
   - Memory B-cell:
   - Helper T-cell:
   - Cytotoxic T-cell:
   - Suppressor (regulatory) T-cell:
   - Memory T-cell:

2. What are the three main effects circulating antibodies can have on a pathogen?
   -
   -
   -

3. How do antibodies become specific for a given antigen?

4. A T-cell appropriately passes through positive selection, but then inappropriately passes through negative selection. What will this T-cell be reactive toward?

5. Which cells account for the fact that the secondary response to a pathogen is much more rapid and robust than the primary response?

____

6. What is the difference between active and passive immunity?
   - Active immunity:

____

   - Passive immunity:

____

8.4 The Lymphatic System

LEARNING OBJECTIVES

After Chapter 8.4, you will be able to:

- Predict how a blockage of flow from a lymph node would impact the lymphatic system and the body as a whole
- Describe the factors and structures linking lymphatic and cardiovascular circulation

The immune system and the lymphatic system are intimately related. B-cells proliferate and develop within the lymphatic system, especially the lymph nodes. This system also serves other functions for the body.

Structure

The lymphatic system, along with the cardiovascular system, is a type of circulatory system. It is made up of one-way vessels that become larger as they move toward the center of the body. These vessels carry lymphatic fluid (**lymph**) and most join to form a large **thoracic duct** in the posterior chest, which then delivers the fluid into the left subclavian vein (near the heart).

Lymph nodes are small, bean-shaped structures along the lymphatic vessels. Lymph nodes contain a lymphatic channel, as well as an artery and a vein. The lymph nodes provide a space for the cells of the immune system to be exposed to possible pathogens.

REAL WORLD

Certain cancers, especially breast cancer, are prone to spread via lymphatic channels. Mastectomy, a surgery that removes the breast, is one of the treatments for breast cancer. In order to ensure that all of the cancer has been removed, local lymph nodes are often removed at the same time.

Function

The lymphatic system serves many different purposes for the body by providing a secondary system for circulation.

Equalization of Fluid Distribution

At the capillaries, fluid leaves the bloodstream and goes into the tissues. The quantity of fluid that leaves the tissues at the arterial end of the capillary bed depends on both hydrostatic and oncotic pressures (Starling forces). Remember that the oncotic pressure of the blood draws water back into the vessel at the venule end, once hydrostatic pressure has decreased. Because the net pressure drawing fluid in at the venule end is slightly less than the net pressure pushing fluid out at the arterial end, a small amount of fluid remains in the tissues. Lymphatic vessels drain these tissues and subsequently return the fluid to the bloodstream.

The lymphatics offer some protection against pathology. For example, if the blood has a low concentration of albumin (a key plasma protein), the oncotic pressure of the blood is decreased, and less water is driven back into the bloodstream at the venule end. Thus, this fluid will collect in the tissues. Provided that the lymphatic channels are not blocked, much of this fluid may eventually return to the bloodstream via the lymphatics. Only when the lymphatics are overwhelmed does **edema** occur—swelling due to fluid collecting in tissue.

Transportation of Biomolecules

The lymphatic system also transports fats from the digestive system into the bloodstream. **Lacteals,** small lymphatic vessels, are located at the center of each villus in the small intestine. Fats, packaged into chylomicrons by intestinal mucosal cells, enter the lacteal for transport. Lymphatic fluid carrying many chylomicrons takes on a milky white appearance and is called **chyle**.

Immunity

As stated previously in this chapter, lymph nodes are a place for antigen-presenting cells and lymphocytes to interact. B-cells proliferate and mature in the lymph nodes in collections called **germinal centers**.

MCAT CONCEPT CHECK 8.4

Before you move on, assess your understanding of the material with these questions.

1. *Filariasis* is the name for an infection with a member of a certain group of parasites, most notably *Wuchereria bancrofti*. This parasite resides in lymph nodes and causes blockage of flow. If an individual had a *W. bancrofti* infection in the lymph nodes of the thigh, what would likely happen?

   ____

   ____

2. What structure is primarily responsible for returning materials from lymphatic circulation to the cardiovascular system?

   ____

Conclusion

The ability to fend off microbial invasion is critical to our survival. The immune system is throughout the body and involves multiple different organs and cell types. Nonspecific mechanisms, such as intact skin, mucous membranes, defensins, lysozyme, complement, interferons, natural killer cells, neutrophils, eosinophils, basophils, and monocytes/macrophages, constitute a complex first line of defense; these mechanisms comprise the innate immune system, which is capable of an immediate response but cannot target a specific pathogen or maintain immunologic memory. The adaptive immune system, comprised of B- and T-cells (lymphocytes), allows our immune system to target specific pathogens and learn from past exposure. Thus, once we are infected with a certain strain of virus, activation of specific immunity confers long-term protection against that particular virus. We take advantage of this secondary response through immunization, and we can see the problems specificity can have when a self-antigen is labeled as foreign, leading to autoimmune disease.

If the immune system is focused on destroying pathogens, including bacteria, then it's an interesting transition we make in the next chapter. We're going from a "sterilization" system to one in which bacterial colonization is the norm. From oral flora to the normal gut bacteria, our ability to digest and absorb nutrients is intimately linked to symbiotic bacteria throughout the digestive tract. In the next chapter, we will explore the anatomy and physiology of the digestive system, which provides us with the raw materials to generate energy, build proteins, and carry out activities of daily living.

You've reviewed the content, now test your knowledge and critical thinking skills by completing a test-like passage set in your online resources!

GO ONLINE

CONCEPT SUMMARY

Structure of the Immune System

- The immune system can be divided into innate and adaptive immunity.
  - **Innate immunity** is composed of defenses that are always active, but that cannot target a specific invader and cannot maintain immunologic memory; also called **nonspecific immunity**.
  - **Adaptive immunity** is composed of defenses that take time to activate, but that target a specific invader and can maintain immunologic memory; also called **specific immunity**.
- The immune system is dispersed in the body.
  - Immune cells come from the **bone marrow**.
  - The **spleen** and **lymph nodes** are sites where immune responses can be mounted, and in which B-cells are activated.
  - The **thymus** is the site of T-cell maturation.
  - **Gut-associated lymphoid tissue (GALT)** includes the **tonsils** and **adenoids**.
- **Leukocytes**, or white blood cells, are involved in immune defenses.

The Innate Immune System

- Many of the nonspecific defenses are noncellular.
  - The **skin** acts as a physical barrier and secretes antimicrobial compounds, like **defensins**.
  - **Mucus** on mucous membranes traps pathogens; in the respiratory system, the mucus is propelled upward by cilia and can be swallowed or expelled.
  - Tears and saliva contain **lysozyme**, an antibacterial compound.
  - The stomach produces acid, killing most pathogens. Colonization of the gut helps prevent overgrowth by pathogenic bacteria through competition.
  - The **complement** system can punch holes in the cell walls of bacteria, making them osmotically unstable.
  - **Interferons** are given off by virally infected cells and help prevent viral replication and dispersion to nearby cells.
- Many of the nonspecific defenses are also cellular.
  - **Macrophages** ingest pathogens and present them on **major histocompatibility complex** (MHC) molecules. They also secrete **cytokines**.
  - **MHC class I** (**MHC-I**) is present in all nucleated cells and displays **endogenous antigen** (proteins from within the cell) to cytotoxic T-cells ($CD8^+$ cells).
  - **MHC class II** (**MHC-II**) is present in professional antigen-presenting cells (macrophages, dendritic cells, some B-cells, and certain activated epithelial cells) and displays **exogenous antigen** (proteins from outside the cell) to helper T-cells ($CD4^+$ cells).

- **Dendritic cells** are antigen-presenting cells in the skin.
- **Natural killer cells** attack cells not presenting MHC molecules, including virally infected cells and cancer cells.
- **Granulocytes** include neutrophils, eosinophils, and basophils.
- **Neutrophils** ingest bacteria, particularly opsonized bacteria (those marked with antibodies). They can follow bacteria using **chemotaxis**.
- **Eosinophils** are used in allergic reactions and invasive parasitic infections. They release **histamine**, causing an inflammatory response.
- **Basophils** are used in allergic reactions. **Mast cells** are related cells found in the skin.

The Adaptive Immune System

- **Humoral immunity** is centered on antibody production by plasma cells, which are activated **B-cells**.
  - **Antibodies** target a particular **antigen**. They contain two heavy chains and two light chains. They have a **constant region** and a **variable region**; the tip of the variable region is the **antigen-binding region**.
  - When activated, the antigen-binding region undergoes **hypermutation** to improve the specificity of the antibody produced. Cells may be given signals to switch **isotypes** of antibody (IgM, IgD, IgG, IgE, IgA).
  - Circulating antibodies can **opsonize** pathogens (mark them for destruction), cause **agglutination** (clumping) into insoluble complexes that are ingested by phagocytes, or neutralize pathogens.
  - Cell-surface antibodies can activate immune cells or mediate allergic reactions.
  - **Memory B-cells** lie in wait for a second exposure to a pathogen and can then mount a more rapid and vigorous immune response (**secondary response**).
- **Cell-mediated (cytotoxic) immunity** is centered on the functions of **T-cells**.
  - T-cells undergo maturation in the thymus through **positive selection** (only selecting for T-cells that can react to antigen presented on MHC) and **negative selection** (causing apoptosis in self-reactive T-cells). The peptide hormone **thymosin** promotes T-cell development.
  - **Helper T-cells (T_h or $CD4^+$)** respond to antigen on MHC-II and coordinate the rest of the immune system, secreting **lymphokines** to activate various arms of immune defense. **T_h1 cells** secrete **interferon gamma**, which activates macrophages. **T_h2 cells** activate B-cells, primarily in parasitic infections.
  - **Cytotoxic T-cells (T_c, CTL, or $CD8^+$)** respond to antigen on MHC-I and kill virally infected cells.
  - **Suppressor (regulatory) T-cells (T_{reg})** tone down the immune response after an infection and promote self-tolerance.
  - **Memory T-cells** serve a similar function to memory B-cells.

- In **autoimmune** conditions, a self-antigen is identified as foreign, and the immune system attacks the body's own cells.
- In **allergic** reactions, nonthreatening exposures incite an inflammatory response.
- Immunization is a method of inducing **active immunity** (activation of B-cells that produce antibodies to an antigen) prior to exposure to a particular pathogen.
- **Passive immunity** is the transfer of antibodies to an individual.

The Lymphatic System

- The **lymphatic system** is a circulatory system that consists of one-way vessels with intermittent lymph nodes.
- The lymphatic system connects to the cardiovascular system via the **thoracic duct** in the posterior chest.
- The lymphatic system equalizes fluid distribution, transports fats and fat-soluble compounds in **chylomicrons**, and provides sites for mounting immune responses.

ANSWERS TO CONCEPT CHECKS

8.1

1. Innate immunity consists of defenses that are always active against pathogens, but that are not capable of targeting specific invaders. It takes longer to mount a response with adaptive immunity, but the response targets a specific pathogen and maintains immunologic memory of the infection to mount a faster response during subsequent infections.

2.

Cell Type	Site of Development	Site of Maturation	Major Functions	Specific or Nonspecific?	Humoral or Cell-Mediated?
B-cell	Bone marrow	Bone marrow (but are activated in spleen or lymph nodes)	Produce antibodies	Specific	Humoral
T-cell	Bone marrow	Thymus	Coordinate immune system and directly kill infected cells	Specific	Cell-mediated

3. Granulocytes include neutrophils, eosinophils, and basophils. Agranulocytes include B- and T-cells (lymphocytes) and monocytes (macrophages).

8.2

1. Skin provides a physical barrier and secretes antimicrobial enzymes. Defensins are examples of antibacterial enzymes on the skin. Lysozyme is antimicrobial and is present in tears and saliva. Mucus is present on mucous membranes and traps incoming pathogens; in the respiratory system, cilia propel the mucus upward so it can be swallowed or expelled. Stomach acid is an antimicrobial substance in the digestive system. The normal gastrointestinal flora provides competition, making it hard for pathogenic bacteria to grow in the gut. Complement is a set of proteins in the blood that can create holes in bacteria.
2. Professional antigen-presenting cells include macrophages, dendritic cells in the skin, some B-cells, and certain activated epithelial cells.
3. MHC-I is found in all nucleated cells and presents pieces of proteins (peptides) created within the cell (endogenous antigens); this can allow for detection of cells infected with intracellular pathogens (especially viruses). MHC-II is only found in antigen-presenting cells and presents proteins that result from the digestion of extracellular pathogens that have been brought in by endocytosis (exogenous antigens).

4. Natural killer cells are activated by cells that do not present MHC (such as virally infected cells and cancer cells). Neutrophils are activated by bacteria, especially those that have been opsonized (tagged with an antibody on their surface). Eosinophils are activated by invasive parasites and allergens. Basophils and mast cells are activated by allergens.

8.3

1. Plasma cells form from B-cells exposed to antigen and produce antibodies. Memory B-cells also form from B-cells exposed to antigen and lie in wait for a second exposure to a given antigen to mount a rapid, robust response. Helper T-cells coordinate the immune system through lymphokines and respond to antigen bound to MHC-II. Cytotoxic T-cells directly kill virally infected cells and respond to antigen bound to MHC-I. Suppressor (regulatory) T-cells quell the immune response after a pathogen has been cleared and promote self-tolerance. Memory T-cells, like memory B-cells, lie in wait until a second exposure to a pathogen to mount a rapid, robust response.
2. Circulating antibodies can mark a pathogen for destruction by phagocytic cells (opsonization), cause agglutination of the pathogen into insoluble complexes that can be taken up by phagocytic cells, or neutralize the pathogen by preventing it from invading tissues.
3. B-cells originally mature in the bone marrow and have some specificity at that point; however, antibodies that can respond to a given antigen undergo hypermutation, or rapid mutation of their antigen-binding sites. Only those B-cells that have the highest affinity for the antigen survive and proliferate, increasing the specificity for the antigen over time.
4. Positive selection occurs when T-cells in the thymus that are able to respond to antigen presented on MHC are allowed to survive (those that do not respond undergo apoptosis). Negative selection occurs when T-cells that respond to self-antigens undergo apoptosis before leaving the thymus. A T-cell that appropriately passes through positive selection, but then inappropriately passes through negative selection will be reactive to self-antigens.
5. Memory cells allow the immune system to carry out a much more rapid and robust secondary response.
6. Active immunity refers to the stimulation of the immune system to produce antibodies against a pathogen. Passive immunity refers to the transfer of antibodies to prevent infection, without stimulation of the plasma cells that produce these antibodies.

8.4

1. Fluid would be unable to return from the lower leg, and edema would result. This infection leads to *elephantiasis*, severe swelling of the limb with thickening of the skin.
2. The thoracic duct carries lymphatic fluid into the left subclavian vein.

SCIENCE MASTERY ASSESSMENT EXPLANATIONS

1. **A**

T-lymphocytes, which mature in the thymus, are the only specific defense against intracellular pathogens. While some bacteria, fungi, and parasites can live intracellularly, viruses—by definition—must replicate within cells. The absence of T-cells would leave an individual unable to fight viral infections with specific defenses.

2. **B**

The lymphocytes involved in cell-mediated immunity are the T-lymphocytes, or T-cells. There are four types of T-cells, each playing a different role in cell-mediated immunity: cytotoxic T-cells, helper T-cells, memory T-cells, and suppressor T-cells. Thus, from the answer choices, the only cells not involved in cell-mediated immunity are the plasma cells, which are differentiated immunoglobulin-secreting B-lymphocytes involved in humoral immunity. **(B)** is therefore the correct answer.

3. **B**

The main function of the lymphatic system is to collect excess interstitial fluid and return it to the circulatory system, maintaining the balance of body fluids. However, this is not one of the answer choices. In addition, the lymphatic system accepts chylomicrons from the small intestine and delivers them to the cardiovascular circulation. Transport of hormones is a function of the cardiovascular system, eliminating **(A)**. The lymphatic system absorbs fluid that has been pushed into tissues, but does not cause the extravasation of the fluid, eliminating **(C)**. Mast cells reside in (and are activated in) the skin and mucous membranes, eliminating **(D)**.

4. **A**

Antibodies are produced by plasma cells derived from B-lymphocytes. The other cells are all types of T-lymphocytes, although memory B-cells can also exist. Upon secondary antigen exposure, memory B-cells rapidly proliferate and differentiate into plasma cells to produce antibodies. Memory B-cells do not directly produce antibodies.

5. **C**

In this question, true statements should be eliminated. The innate immune system does include phagocytes like macrophages, which can activate an inflammatory response to recruit additional immune cells, eliminating **(A)**. The innate immune system acts near entry points into the body and is always active, eliminating **(B)**. Furthermore, all blood cells, including all cells of the immune system, are derived from hematopoietic stem cells in the bone marrow, eliminating **(D)**. By contrast, the innate immune system does not recognize specific antigens on a pathogen, making **(C)** correct.

6. **C**

Adaptive immunity involves the activation of B-cells and T-cells specific to the encountered antigen. Any choice that conforms to this paradigm will be correct. **(C)** indicates that B-cells are activated. Pattern recognition receptors, or PRRs, in **(A)** recognize patterns common to certain pathogens, but do not identify the specific pathogen. Complement is an example of a blood-borne nonspecific defense against bacteria, eliminating **(B)**. Dendritic cells traveling to the lymph nodes **(D)** are a part of the interaction between the innate and adaptive immune systems, but the dendritic cells themselves are nonspecific.

7. **A**

Active immunity refers to the production of antibodies during an immune response. Active immunity may be conferred on an individual by vaccination, such as when an individual is injected with a weakened, inactive, or modified form of a particular antigen that stimulates the immune system to produce antibodies. Active immunity may require weeks to build. Passive immunity, on the other hand, involves the transfer of antibodies through, for example, breast milk. Another example of passive immunity would be during pregnancy, when some maternal antibodies cross the placenta and enter fetal circulation, conferring passive immunity to the fetus. Although passive immunity is acquired immediately, it is very short lived, lasting only as long as the antibodies circulate in blood.

8. **D**

T-cells mature in the thymus, where they are "educated." This education involves the elimination of T-cells with improper binding to MHC–antigen complexes (positive selection) and self-reactive T-cells (negative selection). Thus, self-reactive T-cells are eliminated in the thymus.

9. **C**

Healthy cells exhibit MHC class I molecules. Natural killer cells monitor the expression of MHC molecules on the surface of cells. Viral infection and cancer often cause a reduction in the expression of MHC class I molecules on the cell surface. Natural killer cells detect this lack of MHC and induce apoptosis in the affected cells.

10. **A**

$CD8^+$ T-cells are largely responsible for the cytotoxic immune response. By releasing toxic chemicals into virally infected cells, $CD8^+$ T-cells are able to kill these cells in an effort to contain viral infections. Isotype switching refers to changes in the isotype of antibody produced, which is not caused by $CD8^+$ cells, eliminating **(B)**. Antigens are presented by macrophages, dendritic cells, certain epithelial cells, and some B-cells, eliminating **(C)**. B-cells are not activated by cytotoxic T-lymphocytes, eliminating **(D)**.

11. **C**

Lymphocytes arise from the lymphoid lineage, which includes B-cells and T-cells. Thus, all types of B- and T-cells are capable of causing lymphoma. Macrophages, however, are not lymphocytes and are not likely to cause lymphoma.

12. **D**

When the adaptive immune system encounters an antigen, only the cells with antibodies or T-cell receptors specific to that antigen are activated. This is known as clonal selection. While a T-cell response may be a cytotoxic response, it could also be the activation of helper T-cells; plus, this does not explain the specificity of the response, eliminating **(B)**.

13. **A**

The only phagocytes that attack bacteria on this list are neutrophils and dendritic cells. Dendritic cells are able to sample and present any type of material, and reside in the skin. Neutrophils, on the other hand, are present in the bloodstream and can attack bacteria present there or in tissues. Eosinophils and basophils are involved in the development of allergies; eosinophils also defend against parasites.

14. **B**

The spleen is a location where B-cells mature and proliferate. Therefore, removal of the spleen is likely to result in a reduction of humoral immunity. In fact, many people receive vaccinations prior to removal of the spleen in order to bolster their immunity.

15. **D**

The body employs a number of nonspecific defense mechanisms against foreign invasion. The skin and mucous membranes provide a physical barrier against bacterial invasion. In addition, sweat contains enzymes that attack bacterial cell walls. Certain passages, such as the respiratory tract, are lined with ciliate mucus-coated epithelia, which filter and trap foreign particles. Macrophages engulf and destroy foreign particles. The inflammatory response is initiated in response to physical damage. The only choice that is not a nonspecific defense mechanism is **(D)**, the correct answer. Cytotoxic T-cells are involved in (specific) cell-mediated immunity.

GO ONLINE **Consult your online resources for additional practice.**

SHARED CONCEPTS

Biochemistry Chapter 3
Nonenzymatic Protein Function and Protein Analysis

Biology Chapter 1
The Cell

Biology Chapter 6
The Respiratory System

Biology Chapter 7
The Cardiovascular System

Biology Chapter 9
The Digestive System

Biology Chapter 10
Homeostasis

CHAPTER 9

THE DIGESTIVE SYSTEM

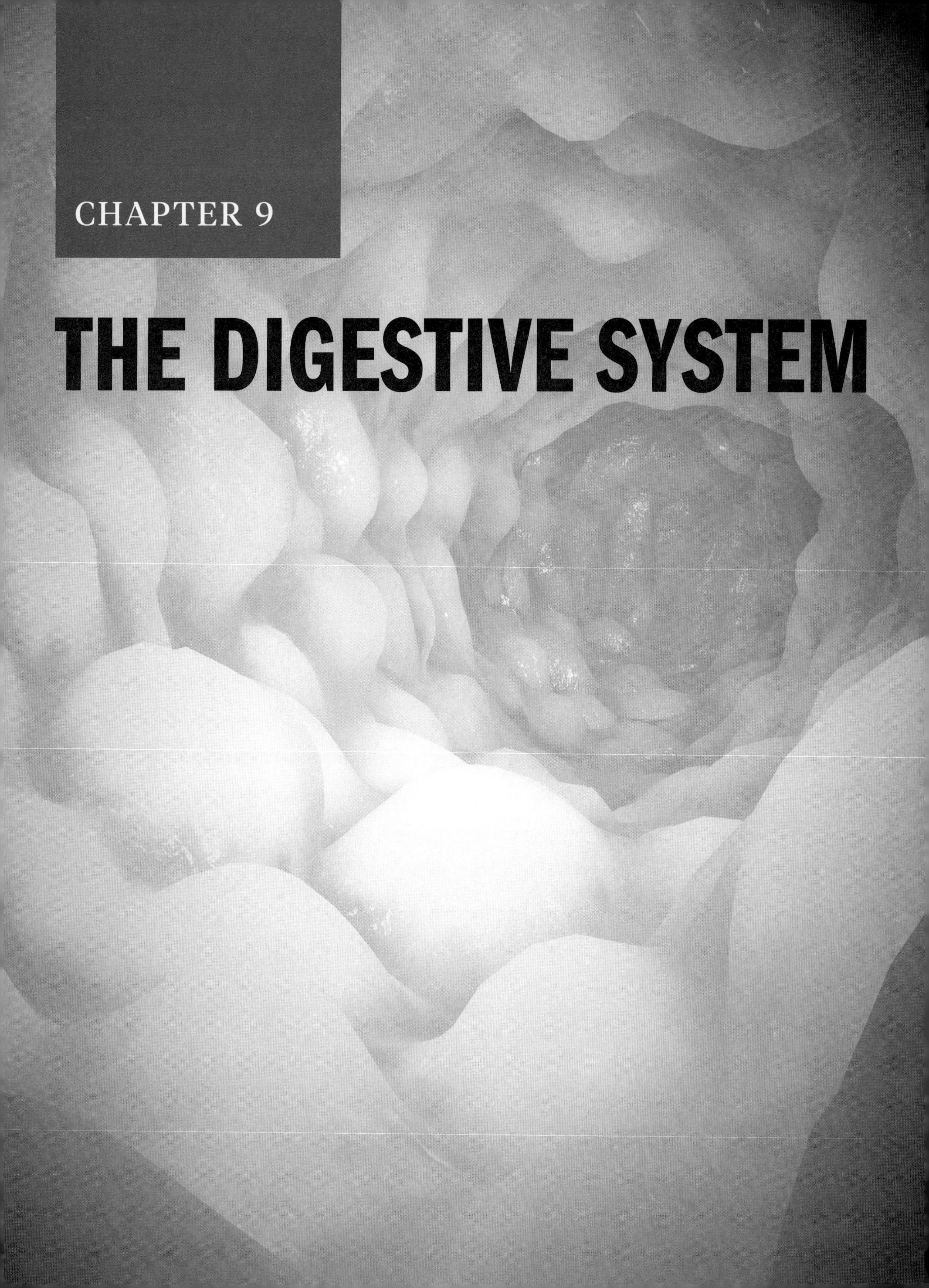

SCIENCE MASTERY ASSESSMENT

Every pre-med knows this feeling: there is so much content I have to know for the MCAT! How do I know what to do first or what's important?

While the high-yield badges throughout this book will help you identify the most important topics, this Science Mastery Assessment is another tool in your MCAT prep arsenal. This quiz (which can also be taken in your online resources) and the guidance below will help ensure that you are spending the appropriate amount of time on this chapter based on your personal strengths and weaknesses. Don't worry though—skipping something now does not mean you'll never study it. Later on in your prep, as you complete full-length tests, you'll uncover specific pieces of content that you need to review and can come back to these chapters as appropriate.

How to Use This Assessment

If you answer 0–7 questions correctly:

Spend about 1 hour to read this chapter in full and take limited notes throughout. Follow up by reviewing **all** quiz questions to ensure that you now understand how to solve each one.

If you answer 8–11 questions correctly:

Spend 20–40 minutes reviewing the quiz questions. Beginning with the questions you missed, read and take notes on the corresponding subchapters. For questions you answered correctly, ensure your thinking matches that of the explanation and you understand why each choice was correct or incorrect.

If you answer 12–15 questions correctly:

Spend less than 20 minutes reviewing all questions from the quiz. If you missed any, then include a quick read-through of the corresponding subchapters, or even just the relevant content within a subchapter, as part of your question review. For questions you answered correctly, ensure your thinking matches that of the explanation and review the Concept Summary at the end of the chapter.

1. Which of the following associations correctly matches a gastric cell with a compound it secretes?
   A. G-cells—HCl
   B. Chief cells—pepsinogen
   C. Parietal cells—alkaline mucus
   D. Mucous cells—intrinsic factor

2. Which of the following is NOT part of the small intestine?
   A. Ileum
   B. Cecum
   C. Jejunum
   D. Duodenum

3. In an experiment, enteropeptidase secretion was blocked. As a direct result, levels of all of the following active enzymes would likely be affected EXCEPT:
   A. trypsin.
   B. aminopeptidase.
   C. chymotrypsin.
   D. carboxypeptidase A.

4. Which of the following INCORRECTLY pairs a digestive enzyme with its function?
   A. Trypsin—hydrolyzes specific peptide bonds
   B. Lactase—hydrolyzes lactose to glucose and galactose
   C. Pancreatic amylase—hydrolyzes starch to maltose
   D. Lipase—emulsifies fats

5. Which of the following correctly lists two organs in which proteins are digested?
   A. Mouth and stomach
   B. Stomach and large intestine
   C. Stomach and small intestine
   D. Small intestine and large intestine

6. Which of the following choices INCORRECTLY pairs a digestive enzyme with its site of secretion?
   A. Sucrase—salivary glands
   B. Carboxypeptidase—pancreas
   C. Trypsin—pancreas
   D. Lactase—duodenum

7. A two-week-old infant is brought to the emergency room. The infant's caregiver reports that the infant has been unable to keep any milk down; shortly after nursing, the infant has sudden projectile vomiting. During exam, an olive-shaped mass can be felt in the infant's upper abdomen. It is determined that there is a constriction in the digestive system that prevents food from reaching the small intestine from the stomach. Which structure is most likely the site of the problem?
   A. Cardiac sphincter
   B. Pyloric sphincter
   C. Ileocecal valve
   D. Internal anal sphincter

8. Many medications have anticholinergic side effects, which block the activity of parasympathetic neurons throughout the body. Individuals who are older may be on many such medications simultaneously, exacerbating the side effects. Which of the following would NOT be expected in an individual taking medications with anticholinergic activity?
   A. Dry mouth
   B. Diarrhea
   C. Slow gastric emptying
   D. Decreased gastric acid production

9. The two graphs below show the relative activities of two enzymes in solutions of varying pH. Which of the following choices correctly identifies the two enzymes?

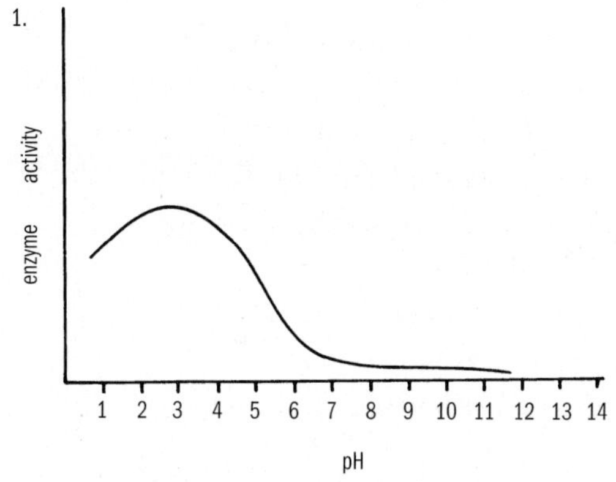

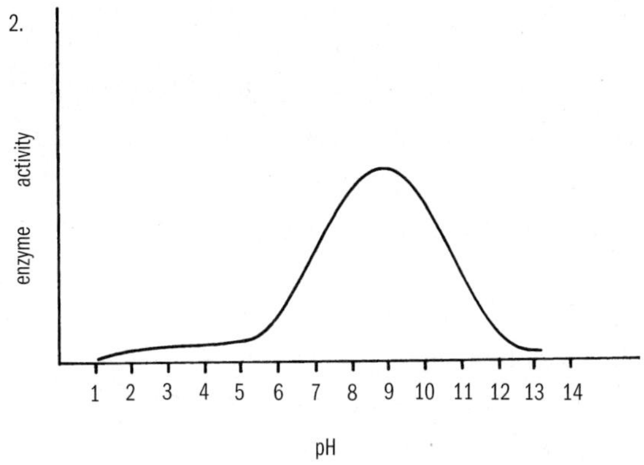

A. 1—chymotrypsin; 2—pepsin
B. 1—pepsin; 2—carboxypeptidase B
C. 1—lactase; 2—aminopeptidase
D. 1—enteropeptidase; 2—amylase

10. Which of the following would NOT likely lead to elevated levels of bilirubin in the blood?
A. Cholangiocarcinoma, a cancer of the bile ducts that can ultimately lead to full occlusion of the duct lumen
B. Autoimmune hemolytic anemia, a disease in which the red blood cells are attacked by antibodies and are lysed
C. Ménétrier's disease, in which rugae thicken and overlying glands lose secretory ability
D. Acetaminophen (Tylenol) overdose, in which the accumulation of toxic metabolites can cause rapid liver failure

11. Which of the following correctly pairs the molecule with its primary site of absorption?
A. Chylomicrons—lacteals
B. Amino acids—large intestine
C. Vitamins A and E—stomach
D. Cholesterol—ascending colon

12. The cleavage of fats into glycerol and fatty acids catalyzed by lipases in the lumen of the duodenum is best described as:
A. mechanical digestion.
B. chemical digestion.
C. intracellular digestion.
D. absorption.

13. Which of the following biomolecules does NOT drain into the liver before arriving at the right side of the heart?
A. Cholecalciferol (vitamin D)
B. Threonine (an amino acid)
C. Fructose (a monosaccharide)
D. Pantothenic acid (vitamin B_5)

14. Which of the following hormones increases feeding behavior?
A. Leptin
B. Cholecystokinin
C. Ghrelin
D. Gastrin

15. Which of the following is likely to be seen in a patient with liver failure?
A. High concentrations of urea in the blood
B. High concentrations of albumin in the blood
C. Low concentrations of ammonia in the blood
D. Low concentrations of clotting factors in the blood

Answer Key

1. **B**
2. **B**
3. **B**
4. **D**
5. **C**
6. **A**
7. **B**
8. **B**
9. **B**
10. **C**
11. **A**
12. **B**
13. **A**
14. **C**
15. **D**

Detailed explanations can be found at the end of the chapter.

CHAPTER 9

THE DIGESTIVE SYSTEM

In This Chapter

CHAPTER PROFILE

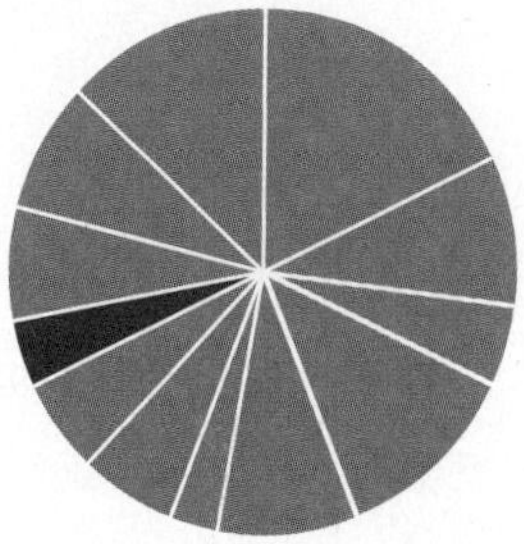

The content in this chapter should be relevant to about 4% of all questions about biology on the MCAT.

This chapter covers material from the following AAMC content category:

3B: Structure and integrative functions of the main organ systems

Introduction

As we continue our survey of organ systems, we now come to the digestive system. As with our previous reviews of other organ systems, we will start with a basic anatomical overview of the organs of digestion (including the accessory organs) and then move on to discuss how these organs function to provide nutrition to the individual. The food we eat is complex, incorporating meats, grains, vegetables and fruits, dairy products, and nuts. The job of the digestive system is to take these complex foods—composed of polysaccharides, fats, and proteins—and turn large macromolecules into smaller, simpler monosaccharides, fatty acids, and amino acids. In order to cleave all of these bonds, the body requires a complex system of mechanical and chemical agents. These compounds can then be absorbed from the gut, transported to the tissues by the circulatory system, and used by cells. In this chapter, we will consider the organs that make up the digestive system as well as the processes by which the foods we eat become the fuel we need for energy, growth, development, and maintenance of other essential activities.

9.1 Anatomy of the Digestive System

LEARNING OBJECTIVES

After Chapter 9.1, you will be able to:

- Describe mechanical and chemical digestion and differentiate between them
- Identify the interactions between the sympathetic and parasympathetic nervous systems and the digestive system
- Trace the path of food through the body, naming major organs and valves in the digestive tract

There are two types of digestion that occur. First, **intracellular digestion**, as a part of **metabolism**, involves the oxidation of glucose and fatty acids for energy. However, our diets do not consist of pure glucose and fatty acids; rather, these substances must be extracted from our food. The process by which these nutrients are obtained from food occurs within the lumen of the **alimentary canal** and is known as **extracellular digestion**. This is technically "outside" the body, because the lumen of the gastrointestinal tract communicates directly with the outside world. The alimentary canal runs from the **mouth** to the **anus** and is sectioned off by **sphincters**, or circular smooth muscles around the canal that can contract to allow compartmentalization of function.

The human digestive tract has specialized sections with different functional roles. The most basic functional distinction is between digestion and absorption. **Digestion** involves the breakdown of food into its constituent organic molecules: starches and other carbohydrates into monosaccharides, lipids (fats) into free fatty acids and glycerol, and proteins into amino acids. Digestion can be subdivided into mechanical and chemical processes. **Mechanical digestion** is the physical breakdown of large food particles into smaller food particles, but does not involve breaking chemical bonds. **Chemical digestion** is the enzymatic cleavage of chemical bonds, such as the peptide bonds of proteins or the glycosidic bonds of starches. **Absorption** involves the transport of products of digestion from the digestive tract into the circulatory system for distribution to the body's tissues and cells.

The digestive tract, shown in Figure 9.1, begins with the **oral cavity** (mouth) followed by the **pharynx**, a shared pathway for both food entering the digestive system and air entering the respiratory system. From the pharynx, food enters the **esophagus**, which transports it to the **stomach**. From the stomach, food travels to the **small intestine**, and then to the **large intestine**. Finally, waste products of digestion enter the **rectum**, where feces are stored until an appropriate time of release. In addition to the digestive tract itself, the **salivary glands**, **pancreas**, **liver**, and **gallbladder** help to provide the enzymes and lubrication necessary to aid in the digestion of food.

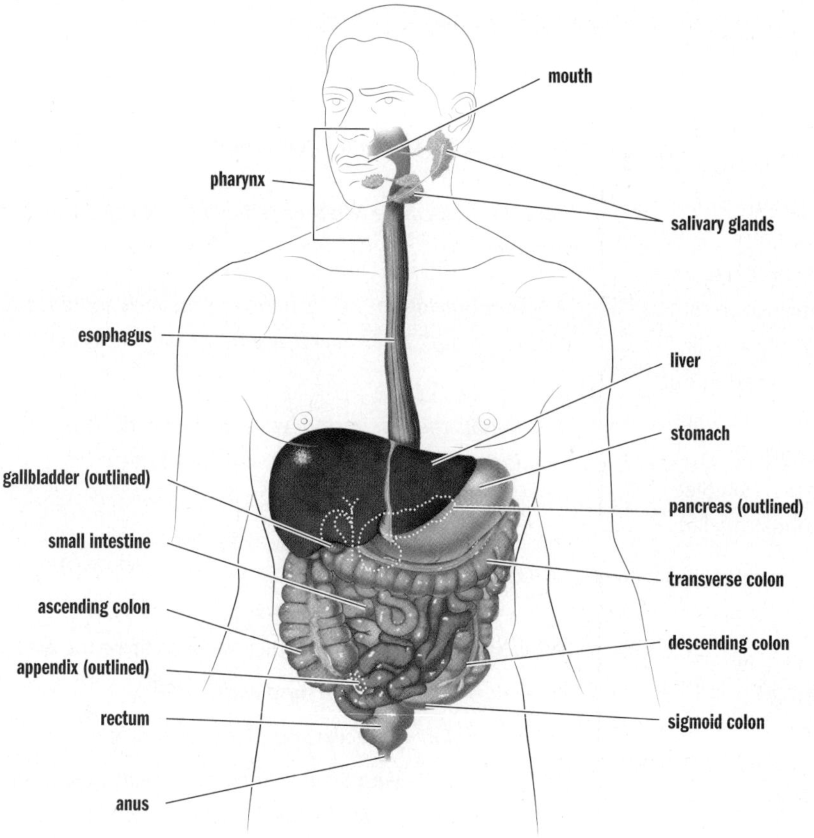

Figure 9.1 Anatomy of the Digestive System

The **enteric nervous system** is a collection of one hundred million neurons that govern the function of the gastrointestinal system. These neurons are present in the walls of the digestive tract and trigger **peristalsis**, or rhythmic contractions of the gut tube, in order to move materials through the system. This system can function independently of the brain and spinal cord, although it is heavily regulated by the autonomic nervous system. The parasympathetic division is involved in stimulation of digestive activities, increasing secretions from exocrine glands and promoting peristalsis. The sympathetic division is involved in the inhibition of these activities. The fact that so often we feel sleepy and lethargic after eating a big meal (often called a *food coma* colloquially) is due, in part, to parasympathetic activity. On the other hand, during periods of high sympathetic activity, bloodflow is decreased to the digestive tract, and gut motility slows significantly.

KEY CONCEPT

All of the glands of the body (except sweat glands) are innervated by the parasympathetic nervous system.

BIOLOGY GUIDED EXAMPLE WITH EXPERT THINKING

Bile acids are crucial for the intestinal absorption of dietary fatty acids, of cholesterol, and of fat-soluble vitamins. To determine whether the interruption of the enterohepatic circulation of bile acids alters triglyceride and glucose metabolism, researchers tested ileal sodium-dependent bile acid transporter (Slc10a2) KO mice. Over 95% of intestinal bile acid is absorbed and returned to the liver; thus, knocking out Slc10a2 should dramatically reduce the total pool of bile acid in the body (approx. 80% reduction). In addition, some mice were fed a sucrose-rich (SR) diet to simulate the metabolic stress of an unhealthy diet.

This is just background information

Purpose: determine whether removing bile acids changes metabolism

A new abbreviation "KO" is here, but the next sentence says "knocking out", so I know this must stand for "Knock Out"

This details the IVs: normal vs reduced bile acids and regular vs sugary diet

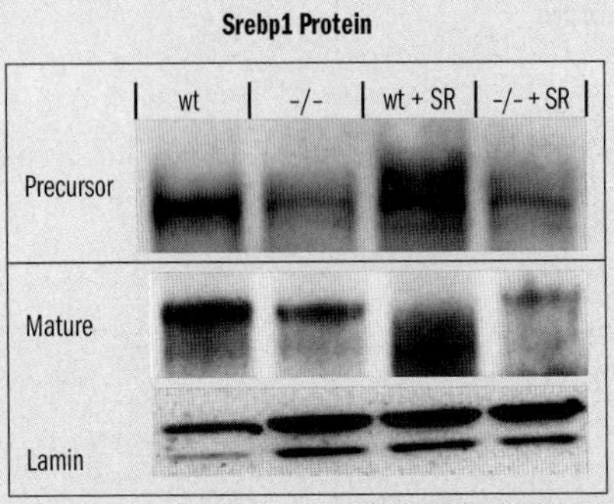

WT is wild-type and -/- is the KO, so SR must be the diet

IV: Srebp1 in WT, KO, with and without SR

DV: expression of precursor and mature protein

Trends: WT mice with SR have increased levels of protein; there is no noticeable change for KO mice with or without SR

Figure 1 Expression of sterol regulatory element-binding protein 1 (Srebp1) Protein Immunoblot. The transcription factor Srebp1c is crucial for optimal activation of most genes in fatty acid synthesis and gluconeogenesis.

This is testing for a new protein involved in fatty acid synthesis and gluconeogenesis (metabolic protein)

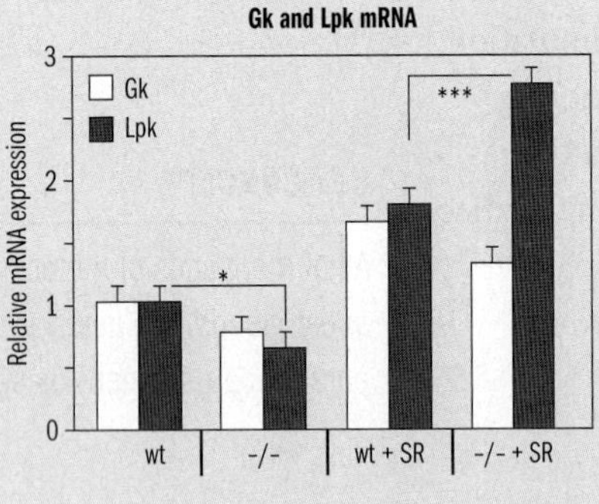

IVs: Gk and Lpk in WT and KO with and without diet (SR)

DV: relative mRNA expression

Trend: Lpk is signficantly lower in KO mice without the diet and significantly higher in KO mice with the diet

Figure 2 Hepatic mRNA expression of Glucokinase (Gk) and Liver Pyruvate Kinase (Lpk)

Adapted from Lundåsen T, Andersson E-M, Snaith M, Lindmark H, Lundberg J, Östlund-Lindqvist A-M, et al. (2012) Inhibition of intestinal bile acid transporter Slc10a2 improves triglyceride metabolism and normalizes elevated plasma glucose levels in mice. *PLoS One* 7(5): e37787. https://doi.org/10.1371/journal.pone.0037787.

Would reducing the total pool of bile acid be a good strategy to combat the hypertriglyceridemia and diabetes induced by an unhealthy diet?

This question asks whether an action, reducing the total pool of bile acid, would have a specified impact on two conditions, hypertriglyceridemia and diabetes. To answer this question, we must assess the data we are given in the article regarding how changing bile acid quantity affects traits and outcomes associated with those conditions.

We should start by making sure we're comfortable with the terms used in the question, relying on either the article or our critical thinking skills to fill our knowledge gaps. Hypertriglyceridemia is a condition when blood triglyceride levels are too high, and diabetes is a condition when blood glucose levels are too high. However, that information wasn't given to us in the passage, and it's not entirely in scope for Test Day—so how could we figure out what we need to know to answer this question? Even if we didn't know this, though, we know the mice were fed food to simulate an unhealthy diet that would supply them with too much sugar, and we should recognize at least diabetes as a metabolic disorder linked with sugar metabolism. We should also recognize that triglycerides are fats, so this is probably a condition involving fat metabolism. Thus, we can assume that any action that lowers blood triglycerides (relating to hypertriglyceridemia) and blood glucose (relating to diabetes) could constitute a potentially beneficial therapy for these two conditions. So, when we look at the data for the experimental mice as compared to controls, we should be looking for changes related to these two metabolic pathways to determine if there are possible treatment implications for reducing bile salt concentrations in order to treat these conditions.

According to the passage, the knockout mice do not have the bile acid transporter, meaning that the pool of available bile acid in their system should be significantly lower. There's also a second variable, diet, which should be simulating mice that are experiencing metabolic stressors in the sucrose-rich condition as compared to normal metabolic function. Figure 1 shows the concentration of a protein involved in fatty acid synthesis in the KO mice versus wild-type mice, with both normal and sucrose-rich diets. In the wild-type mice, we can see that the addition of a metabolically stressful, high-sugar diet (lane 3) leads to a big increase in production of that protein as compared to regular diet (lane 1). However, in the knockout mice, there's no perceivable change from the regular diet (lane 2) to the sucrose-rich diet (lane 4). This is true both for the actual protein and the precursor, which means that the KO mouse is just not transcribing as much of that metabolic protein. The lamin lane down at the bottom seems like it's just a control for protein expression, and it looks pretty much the same across the board, so we can ignore it in our data analysis. Based on this figure, which is all about a metabolic protein in the fatty acid synthesis chain, it looks like the knockout mice just aren't experiencing the same amount of metabolic stress; they're not trying to turn that extra sucrose into fatty acids. Based on this piece of data, it looks like reducing bile acid might be one way to relieve the metabolic stress associated with hypertriglyceridemia, or at least, it's worth more investigation!

Moving on, Figure 2 shows the same conditions, but is measuring mRNA production of two different proteins: glucokinase and pyruvate kinase. Even if we aren't exactly sure of what those enzymes do, they have glucose and pyruvate in their names, so it sounds like they are probably involved in the sugar metabolism pathway. Looking at the figure, we can see in the first two pairs of columns that wild-type mice are expressing more mRNA for both of these proteins than KO mice. After metabolic stress is added, it looks like pyruvate kinase production specifically spikes within the KO mice. That seems to indicate that these mice are responding to the metabolic stress to an even greater extent (in terms of Lpk) than the wild-type mice. Without directly measuring the level of blood glucose, we cannot determine whether that increased metabolic response represents a positive or negative trend. So, unlike the data in Figure 1, it looks like bile salt reduction may not be a good treatment option for diabetic individuals, and we may even need to reevaluate whether it would be truly helpful for those with triglyceridemia, as the energetic processing of fats can't be considered as fully separate from the processing of sugars.

Overall, our takeaway is that we have mixed results. Figure 1 made the reduction of bile salts look like a promising treatment for triglyceridemia, but Figure 2 indicates that reducing bile salts may not be effective in treating diabetes. We can conclude that more data is needed to assess this therapy's effect on sugar and lipid metabolism.

MCAT CONCEPT CHECK 9.1

Before you move on, assess your understanding of the material with these questions.

1. What is the difference between mechanical and chemical digestion?
   - Mechanical digestion:
   ____
   - Chemical digestion:
   ____
2. Trace the path of food through the body, starting with ingestion and ending with excretion of feces:
   ____
3. What effect does the parasympathetic nervous system have on the digestive system? What effect does the sympathetic nervous system have?
   - Parasympathetic nervous system:
   ____
   - Sympathetic nervous system:
   ____

9.2 Ingestion and Digestion

LEARNING OBJECTIVES

After Chapter 9.2, you will be able to:

- Identify the secretory cells of the digestive tract, their secretions, and the function of their secretions
- Explain how bile and pancreatic lipase work together to digest fats
- Recall the key digestive enzymes and hormones produced in saliva, the stomach, and the intestines, and summarize the function of each

To supply the body with nutrients, we must **ingest** (eat) food. Several hormones are involved with feeding behavior, including antidiuretic hormone (ADH or vasopressin), aldosterone, glucagon, ghrelin, leptin, and cholecystokinin. ADH and aldosterone trigger the sensation of thirst, encouraging the behavior of fluid consumption. Glucagon, secreted by the pancreas, and ghrelin, secreted by the stomach and pancreas, stimulate feelings of hunger. Leptin and cholecystokinin do the opposite, stimulating feelings of satiety. Digestion begins in the oral cavity and continues in the stomach and the first part of the small intestine, known as the duodenum.

Oral Cavity

The **oral cavity** plays a role in both mechanical and chemical digestion of food. Mechanical digestion in the mouth involves the breaking up of large food particles into smaller particles using the teeth, tongue, and lips. This process is called **mastication** (chewing). Chewing helps to increase the surface area-to-volume ratio of the food, creating more surface area for enzymatic digestion as it passes through the gut tube. It also moderates the size of food particles entering the lumen of the alimentary canal; food particles that are too large create an obstruction risk in the tract.

Chemical digestion is the breakdown of chemical bonds in the macromolecules that make up food. This relies on enzymes from **saliva** produced by the three pairs of **salivary glands**. Saliva also aids mechanical digestion by moistening and lubricating food. The salivary glands, like all glands of the digestive tract, are innervated by the parasympathetic nervous system. The presence of food in the oral cavity triggers a neural circuit that ultimately leads to increased parasympathetic stimulation of these glands. Salivation can also be triggered by signals that food is near, such as smell or sight. Saliva contains *salivary amylase*, also known as *ptyalin*, and *lipase*. **Salivary amylase** is capable of hydrolyzing starch into smaller sugars (maltose and dextrins), while **lipase** catalyzes the hydrolysis of lipids. The amount of chemical digestion that occurs in the mouth is minimal, though, because the food does not stay in the mouth for long. Our muscular tongue forms the food into a **bolus**, which is forced back to the pharynx and swallowed.

KEY CONCEPT

The chemical digestion of carbohydrates occurs in both the mouth and small intestine, with the two amylases targeting complementary starches. Salivary amylase (active in the mouth) has a higher specificity for rapidly soluble starches, while pancreatic amylase (active in the small intestine) has a higher specificity for less soluble, more nonpolar starches.

REAL WORLD

There are three pairs of major salivary glands: the parotid, submandibular, and sublingual glands. Other microscopic salivary glands are scattered throughout the upper digestive system. While the parasympathetic nervous system is responsible for promoting salivation, the sympathetic nervous system has some input into the glands as well. The sympathetic nervous system increases the viscosity of saliva, which is why dry mouth and even a tacky sensation in the mouth occurs during a fight-or-flight response.

Pharynx

The **pharynx** is the cavity that leads from the mouth and posterior nasal cavity to the esophagus. The pharynx connects not only to the esophagus, but also to the larynx, which is a part of the respiratory tract. The pharynx can be divided into three parts: the **nasopharynx** (behind the nasal cavity), the **oropharynx** (at the back of the mouth), and the **laryngopharynx** (above the vocal cords). Food is prevented from entering the larynx during swallowing by the **epiglottis**, a cartilaginous structure that folds down to cover the laryngeal inlet. Failure of this mechanism can lead to aspiration of food and choking.

Esophagus

The **esophagus** is a muscular tube that connects the pharynx to the stomach. The top third of the esophagus is composed of skeletal muscle, the bottom third is composed of smooth muscle, and the middle third is a mix of both. What does this mean in terms of nervous control? While the top of the esophagus is under somatic (voluntary) motor control, the bottom—and most of the rest of the gastrointestinal tract, for that matter—is under autonomic (involuntary) nervous control. The rhythmic contraction of smooth muscle that propels food toward the stomach is called **peristalsis**. Under normal circumstances, peristalsis proceeds down the digestive tract. However, certain factors such as exposure to chemicals, infectious agents, physical stimulation in the posterior pharynx, and even cognitive stimulation, can lead to reversal of peristalsis in the process of **emesis** (**vomiting**).

Swallowing is initiated in the muscles of the oropharynx, which constitute the **upper esophageal sphincter**. Peristalsis squeezes, pushes, and propels the bolus toward the stomach. As the bolus approaches the stomach, a muscular ring known as the **lower esophageal sphincter** (**cardiac sphincter**) relaxes and opens to allow the passage of food.

Stomach

There are three main energy sources: carbohydrates, fats, and proteins. As mentioned earlier, the chemical digestion of carbohydrates and fats is initiated in the mouth. No mechanical or chemical digestion takes place in the esophagus, except for the continued enzymatic activity initiated in the mouth by salivary enzymes. Thus, digestion that occurs prior to the entrance of the bolus into the stomach is minimal compared to the digestion that occurs in the stomach and small intestine.

The **stomach** is a highly muscular organ with a capacity of approximately two liters. In humans, the stomach is located in the upper left quadrant of the abdominal cavity, underneath the diaphragm. This organ uses hydrochloric acid and enzymes to digest food, creating a fairly harsh environment. Therefore, its mucosa is quite thick to prevent autodigestion. The stomach can be divided into four main anatomical divisions, as shown in Figure 9.2: the **fundus** and **body**, which contain mostly gastric glands, and the **antrum** and **pylorus,** which contain mostly pyloric glands. The internal curvature of the stomach is called the **lesser curvature**; the external curvature is called the **greater curvature**. The lining of the stomach is thrown into folds called **rugae**.

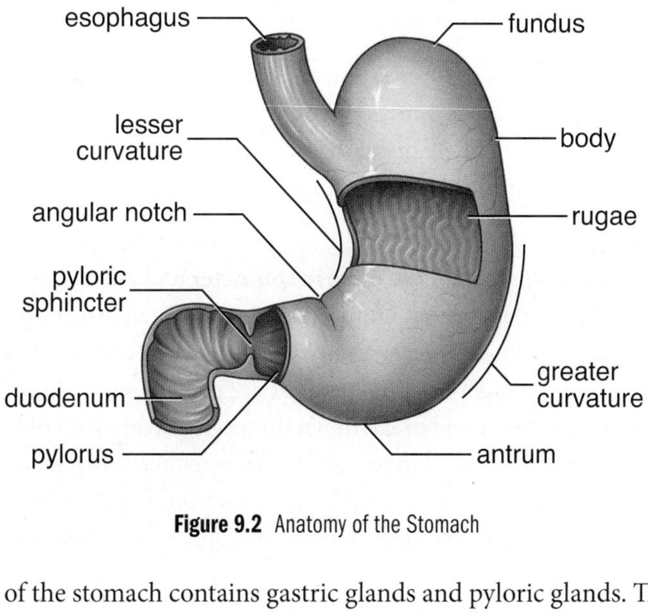

Figure 9.2 Anatomy of the Stomach

The mucosa of the stomach contains gastric glands and pyloric glands. The **gastric glands** respond to signals from the **vagus nerve** of the parasympathetic nervous system, which is activated by the brain in response to the sight, taste, and smell of food. Gastric glands have three different cell types: mucous cells, chief cells, and parietal cells. **Mucous cells** produce the bicarbonate-rich mucus that protects the muscular wall from the harshly acidic (pH = 2) and proteolytic environment of the stomach.

REAL WORLD

Weakness in the lower esophageal sphincter is a key feature of gastroesophageal reflux disease (GERD), which causes classic heartburn symptoms after eating. As food and acid reflux into the lower esophagus, they irritate the less-protected mucosa, stimulating pain receptors. These receptors localize pain poorly, so a general burning sensation is felt in the lower chest—leading to the common term *heartburn*.

REAL WORLD

Nonsteroidal anti-inflammatory drugs (NSAIDs), such as ibuprofen, naproxen, and aspirin, are very common drugs. However, these drugs are not without side effects. One such side effect is the disruption of mucus production within the stomach. This leaves the mucosa of the stomach unprotected, and irritation results. This irritation can be in the form of *gastritis*, inflammation of the mucosa of the stomach, or *gastric ulcers*, deep wounds in the lining of the stomach.

KEY CONCEPT

The stomach secretes six products:

1. HCl (kills microbes, denatures proteins, and converts pepsinogen into pepsin)
2. Pepsinogen (cleaved in the stomach to pepsin; an enzyme that partially digests proteins)
3. Mucus (protects mucosa)
4. Bicarbonate (protects mucosa)
5. Water (dissolves and dilutes ingested material)
6. Intrinsic factor (required for normal absorption of vitamin B_{12})

REAL WORLD

Zollinger-Ellison syndrome is a rare disease resulting from a gastrin-secreting tumor (gastrinoma). Typically, this tumor is found in the pancreas. The excess gastrin leads to excessive HCl production by parietal cells. Not surprisingly, one of the most common signs of Zollinger-Ellison syndrome is the presence of intractable ulcer disease.

Gastric juice is a combination of secretions from the other two cell types in the gastric glands: chief cells and parietal cells. The **chief cells** secrete ***pepsinogen***. This is the inactive, **zymogen** form of *pepsin*, a proteolytic enzyme. Hydrogen ions in the stomach, secreted by **parietal cells** as hydrochloric acid, cleave pepsinogen to pepsin. **Pepsin** digests proteins by cleaving peptide bonds near aromatic amino acids, resulting in short peptide fragments. Because pepsin is activated by the acidic environment, it follows that pepsin is most active at a low pH. This is a unique characteristic among human enzymes, as most human enzymes are most active at physiological pH. Stomach acid also kills most harmful bacteria (with the exception of *Helicobacter pylori*, infection with which is usually asymptomatic but can cause inflammation, ulcers, and even certain gastric cancers). The acidic environment also helps to denature proteins and can break down some intramolecular bonds that hold food together. In addition to HCl, parietal cells secrete **intrinsic factor**, a glycoprotein involved in the proper absorption of vitamin B_{12}.

The **pyloric glands** contain **G-cells** that secrete gastrin, a peptide hormone. **Gastrin** induces the parietal cells in the stomach to secrete more HCl and signals the stomach to contract, mixing its contents. The digestion of solid food in the stomach results in an acidic, semifluid mixture known as **chyme**. The combined mechanical and chemical digestive activities of the stomach result in a significant increase in the surface area of the now unrecognizable food particles, so when the chyme reaches the small intestine, the absorption of nutrients from it can be maximized. There are a few substances that are absorbed directly from the stomach (such as alcohol and aspirin), but the stomach is mainly an organ of digestion.

Duodenum

The **small intestine** consists of three segments: the duodenum, the jejunum, and the ileum. The small intestine is quite long, up to seven meters. The duodenum is responsible for the majority of chemical digestion and has some minor involvement in absorption. However, most of the absorption in the small intestine takes place in the jejunum and ileum.

Food leaves the stomach through the **pyloric sphincter** and enters the duodenum. The presence of chyme in the duodenum causes the release of brush-border enzymes like *disaccharidases* (*maltase*, *isomaltase*, *lactase*, and *sucrase*) and *peptidases* (including *dipeptidase*). **Brush-border enzymes** are present on the luminal surface of cells lining the duodenum and break down dimers and trimers of biomolecules into absorbable monomers. The duodenum also secretes *enteropeptidase*, which is involved in the activation of other digestive enzymes from the accessory organs of digestion. Finally, it secretes hormones like secretin and cholecystokinin (CCK) into the bloodstream.

The **disaccharidases** digest disaccharides. **Maltase** digests maltose, **isomaltase** digests isomaltose, **lactase** digests lactose, and **sucrase** digests sucrose. Lack of a particular disaccharidase causes an inability to break down the corresponding disaccharide. Then bacteria in the intestines are able to hydrolyze that disaccharide, producing methane gas as a byproduct. In addition, undigested disaccharides can have an osmotic effect, pulling water into the stool and causing diarrhea. This is why people who are lactose intolerant have symptoms of bloating, flatulence, and possibly diarrhea after ingesting dairy products.

Peptidases break down proteins (or peptides, as the name implies). **Aminopeptidase** is a peptidase secreted by glands in the duodenum that removes the N-terminal amino acid from a peptide. **Dipeptidases** cleave the peptide bonds of dipeptides to release free amino acids. Unlike carbohydrates, which must be broken down into monosaccharides for absorption, proteins can be broken down into di- and even tripeptides and can be absorbed across the small intestine wall.

Enteropeptidase (formerly called ***enterokinase***) is an enzyme critical for the activation of ***trypsinogen***, a pancreatic protease, to ***trypsin***. Trypsin then initiates an activation cascade, as described later in this chapter. Enteropeptidase can also activate ***procarboxypeptidases A*** and ***B*** to their active forms.

Secretin is a peptide hormone that causes pancreatic enzymes to be released into the duodenum. It also regulates the pH of the digestive tract by reducing HCl secretion from parietal cells and increasing bicarbonate secretion from the pancreas. Secretin is also an **enterogastrone**, a hormone that slows motility through the digestive tract. Slowing of motility allows increased time for digestive enzymes to act on chyme—especially fats.

Finally, **cholecystokinin (CCK)** is secreted in response to the entry of chyme (specifically, amino acids and fat in the chyme) into the duodenum. This peptide hormone stimulates the release of both bile and pancreatic juices and also acts in the brain, where it promotes satiety. **Bile** is a complex fluid composed of bile salts, pigments, and cholesterol. **Bile salts** are derived from cholesterol. They are not enzymes and therefore do not directly perform chemical digestion (the enzymatic cleavage of chemical bonds). However, bile salts serve an important role in the mechanical digestion of fats and ultimately facilitate the chemical digestion of lipids. Bile salts have hydrophobic and hydrophilic regions, allowing them to serve as a bridge between aqueous and lipid environments. In fact, bile salts are much like the common soaps and detergents we use to wash our hands, clothes, and dishes. In the small intestine, bile salts **emulsify** fats and cholesterol into **micelles**. Without bile, fats would spontaneously separate out of the aqueous mixture in the duodenum and would not be accessible to *pancreatic lipase*, which is water-soluble. In addition, these micelles increase the surface area of the fats, increasing the rate at which lipase can act. Ultimately, proper fat digestion depends on both bile and lipase. Bile gets the fats into the solution and increases their surface area by placing them in micelles (mechanical digestion). Then, lipase can come in to hydrolyze the ester bonds holding the lipids together (chemical digestion).

CCK also promotes the secretion of pancreatic juices into the duodenum, as shown in Figure 9.3. **Pancreatic juices** are a complex mixture of several enzymes in a bicarbonate-rich alkaline solution. This bicarbonate helps to neutralize acidic chyme, as well as provide an ideal working environment for the digestive enzymes, which

REAL WORLD

Celiac disease results from an immune reaction against gluten, a protein found in grains, especially wheat. In this condition, the immune system develops antibodies against certain components of gluten. These antibodies then cross-react with elements of the small intestine, causing damage to the mucosa. This results in diarrhea and discomfort. Sometimes, this condition also results in malabsorptive syndromes, including the inability to absorb fat and fat-soluble vitamins. Contrary to popular belief, celiac disease and gluten sensitivity are immune conditions, but not true allergies.

are most active around pH 8.5. Pancreatic juices contain enzymes that can digest all three types of nutrients: carbohydrates, fats, and proteins. The identities and functions of these enzymes will be discussed in the next section of this chapter.

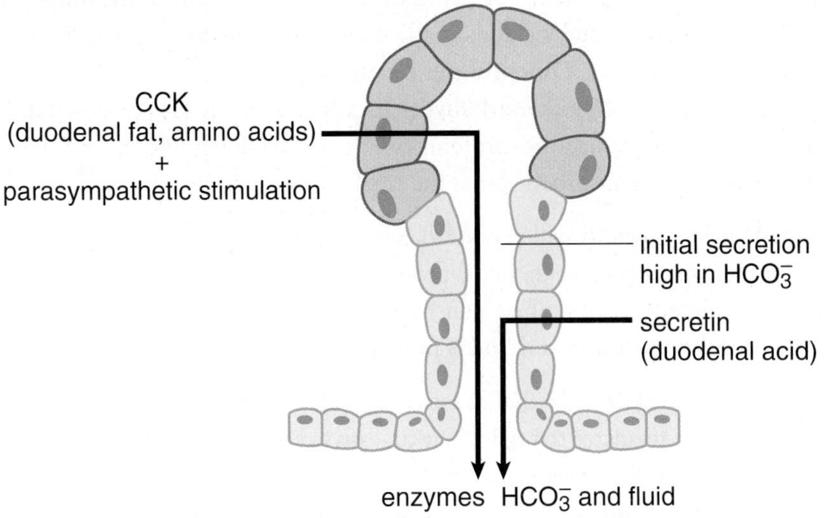

Figure 9.3 Hormonal Control of the Exocrine Pancreas

BRIDGE

The acidic environment of the stomach and basic environment of the duodenum point out the important correlation between pH and enzyme activity. Pepsin is active in the stomach and works best at pH 2. Pancreatic enzymes are active in the duodenum and work best at pH 8.5. pH, temperature, and salinity can all affect enzyme function, as highlighted in Chapter 2 of *MCAT Biochemistry Review*.

MCAT CONCEPT CHECK 9.2

Before you move on, assess your understanding of the material with these questions.

1. What two main enzymes are found in saliva? What do these enzymes do?

   •

   •

   ---

2. For each of the cell types below, list the major secretions of the cell and the functions of these secretions.

Cell	Secretions	Functions
Mucous cell		
Chief cell		
Parietal cell		
G-cell		

3. For each of the following substances, determine whether it is a digestive enzyme or a hormone and briefly summarize its functions.

Substance	Enzyme or Hormone?	Functions
Sucrase		
Secretin		
Dipeptidase		
Cholecystokinin		
Enteropeptidase		

4. How do bile and pancreatic lipase work together to digest fats?

____

9.3 Accessory Organs of Digestion

LEARNING OBJECTIVES

After Chapter 9.3, you will be able to:

- Recall the pancreatic enzymes and the molecules they help to digest
- Describe the significance and the function of bile, including its production, components, and release
- List the major functions of the liver
- Associate the accessory organs of digestion with their germ layer of origin

Digestion is a complex process that requires the release of enzymes not only from the cells directly lining the alimentary canal, but also from the pancreas, liver, and gallbladder. Collectively, these organs—which all originate as outgrowths of endoderm from the gut tube during development—are called **accessory organs of digestion**.

Pancreas

The pancreas serves two quite different roles in the body, reflecting its exocrine and endocrine functions. As discussed in Chapter 5 of *MCAT Biology Review*, the endocrine functions of the pancreas include the release of insulin, glucagon, and somatostatin—peptide hormones necessary for the maintenance of proper blood sugar levels. The hormonal function of the pancreas is limited to cells residing in islets of Langerhans scattered throughout the organ. The bulk of the pancreas, however, is made of exocrine cells called **acinar cells** that produce pancreatic juices. As mentioned earlier, pancreatic juices are bicarbonate-rich alkaline secretions containing many digestive enzymes that work on all three classes of biomolecules. ***Pancreatic amylase*** breaks down large polysaccharides into small disaccharides and is therefore responsible for carbohydrate digestion. The pancreatic peptidases

REAL WORLD

Pancreatitis, or inflammation of the pancreas, is usually caused by gallstones or excessive consumption of alcohol. Regardless of the cause, pancreatitis results from premature activation of pancreatic enzymes and autodigestion of the pancreatic tissue. This is a very painful condition that may result in a long hospital stay and long-term consequences such as diabetes and the reduced digestion of proteins and fats.

(***trypsinogen***, ***chymotrypsinogen***, and ***carboxypeptidases A*** and ***B***) are released in their zymogen form, but once activated are responsible for protein digestion. Enteropeptidase, produced by the duodenum, is the master switch. It converts trypsinogen to trypsin, which can then activate the other zymogens, and also activates procarboxypeptidases A and B. Finally, the pancreas secretes ***pancreatic lipase***, which is capable of breaking down fats into free fatty acids and glycerol.

Pancreatic juices are transferred to the duodenum via a duct system that runs along the middle of the pancreas, as shown in Figure 9.4. Like all exocrine cells, acinar cells secrete their products into ducts. These ducts then empty into the duodenum through the **major** and **minor duodenal papillae**.

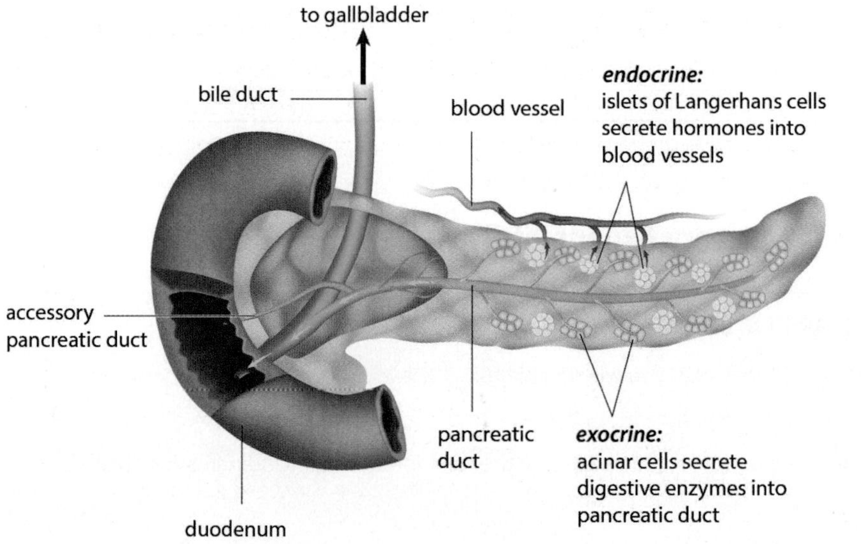

Figure 9.4 Anatomy of the Pancreas

KEY CONCEPT

The functions of the liver include processing and synthesis of nutrients (glycogenesis and glycogenolysis, storage and mobilization of fats, gluconeogenesis), production of urea, detoxification of chemicals, production of bile, and synthesis of albumin and clotting factors.

Liver

The **liver** is located in the upper right quadrant of the abdomen and contains two unique structures for communicating with the digestive system. First, **bile ducts** connect the liver with both the gallbladder and small intestine. Bile is produced in the liver and travels down these bile ducts where it may be stored in the gallbladder or secreted into the duodenum. The liver also receives all blood draining from the abdominal portion of the digestive tract through the **hepatic portal vein**. This nutrient-rich blood can be processed by the liver before draining into the inferior vena cava on its way to the right side of the heart. For example, the liver takes up excess sugar to create **glycogen**, the storage form of glucose, and stores fats as **triacylglycerols**. The liver can also reverse these processes, producing glucose for the rest of the body through **glycogenolysis** and **gluconeogenesis** and mobilizing fats in **lipoproteins**. The liver detoxifies both endogenous compounds (those made in the body) and exogenous compounds (those brought in from the environment). For example, the liver converts ammonia, a toxic waste product of amino acid metabolism, into urea, which can be excreted by the kidneys. The liver also detoxifies and metabolizes alcohol and medications. Some drugs actually require activation by the enzymes of the liver. In addition, some drugs cannot be taken orally because modification of these drugs by the liver renders them inactive.

Bile production is one of the most significant jobs of the liver *vis-à-vis* the digestive system. As mentioned earlier, bile is composed of bile salts, pigments, and cholesterol. Bile salts are amphipathic molecules that can emulsify fat in the digestive system. The major pigment in bile is **bilirubin**, which is a byproduct of the breakdown of hemoglobin. Bilirubin travels to the liver, where it is **conjugated** (attached to a protein) and secreted into the bile for excretion. If the liver is unable to process or excrete bilirubin (due to liver damage, excessive red blood cell destruction, or blockage of the bile ducts), **jaundice** or yellowing of the skin may occur.

In addition to bile production, processing of nutrients, and detoxification and drug metabolism, the liver also synthesizes certain proteins necessary for proper body function. These proteins include **albumin**, a protein that maintains plasma oncotic pressure and also serves as a carrier for many drugs and hormones, and **clotting factors** used during blood coagulation.

KEY CONCEPT

The major components of bile are bile salts, which emulsify fats; pigments (especially bilirubin, from the breakdown of hemoglobin); and cholesterol.

REAL WORLD

Cirrhosis of the liver can result from many different processes, including chronic alcohol consumption, hepatitis C infection, autoimmune hepatitis, and fatty liver disease. However, the outcome is the same. Cirrhosis is scarring of the liver, and this scar tissue builds up, creating increased resistance within the portal vein, resulting in portal hypertension. This causes a backup of fluid within the portal system, resulting in swollen veins in the digestive system, especially the esophagus, which may rupture and cause life-threatening bleeding. This often manifests as *hematemesis*, or vomiting of blood. Cirrhosis also causes bleeding disorders because production of clotting factors is disrupted. The inability to properly dispose of ammonia results in increased ammonia in the blood, which affects mentation. Finally, cirrhosis may also cause hepatocellular carcinoma, or cancer of the hepatocytes.

BRIDGE

Stone formation is nothing more than precipitation of a solid once its concentration has reached the K_{sp} of the compound. This is particularly common in the gallbladder because bile is concentrated there. Solubility and K_{sp} are discussed in Chapter 9 of *MCAT General Chemistry Review*.

Gallbladder

The **gallbladder** is located just beneath the liver and both stores and concentrates bile. Upon release of CCK, the gallbladder contracts and pushes bile out into the **biliary tree**. The bile duct system merges with the pancreatic duct, as shown in Figure 9.4 earlier, before emptying into the duodenum.

The gallbladder is a common site of cholesterol or bilirubin stone formation. This painful condition causes inflammation of the gallbladder. The stones may also travel into the bile ducts and get stuck in the biliary tree. In some cases, stones can get caught just before entering the duodenum, resulting in blockage of not only the biliary tree, but the pancreatic duct as well, causing pancreatitis.

The functions of the various digestive enzymes (and bile) are summarized in Table 9.1.

NUTRIENT	ENZYME	SITE OF PRODUCTION	SITE OF FUNCTION	FUNCTION
Carbohydrates	Salivary amylase (ptyalin)	Salivary glands	Mouth	Hydrolyzes starch to maltose and dextrins
	Pancreatic amylase	Pancreas (acinar cells)	Duodenum	Hydrolyzes starch to maltose and dextrins
	Maltase	Intestinal glands	Duodenum	Hydrolyzes maltose to two glucose molecules
	Isomaltase	Intestinal glands	Duodenum	Hydrolyzes isomaltose to two glucose molecules
	Sucrase	Intestinal glands	Duodenum	Hydrolyzes sucrose to glucose and fructose
	Lactase	Intestinal glands	Duodenum	Hydrolyzes lactose to glucose and galactose
Proteins	Pepsin(ogen)	Gastric glands (chief cells)	Stomach	Hydrolyzes specific peptide bonds; activated by HCl
	Trypsin(ogen)	Pancreas (acinar cells)	Duodenum	Hydrolyzes specific peptide bonds; converts chymotrypsinogen to chymotrypsin; activated by enteropeptidase
	Chymotrypsin (ogen)	Pancreas (acinar cells)	Duodenum	Hydrolyzes specific peptide bonds; activated by trypsin
	(Pro)carboxy peptidases A and B	Pancreas (acinar cells)	Duodenum	Hydrolyzes terminal peptide bond at carboxy end; activated by enteropeptidase
	Aminopeptidase	Intestinal glands	Duodenum	Hydrolyzes terminal peptide bond at amino end
	Dipeptidases	Intestinal glands	Duodenum	Hydrolyzes pairs of amino acids
	Enteropeptidase	Intestinal glands	Duodenum	Converts trypsinogen to trypsin and procarboxypeptidases A and B to carboxypeptidases A and B
Lipids	Bile*	Liver (stored in gallbladder)	Duodenum	Emulsifies fat
	Lipase	Pancreas (acinar cells)	Duodenum	Hydrolyzes lipids

*Note: Bile is not an enzyme, but is involved in mechanical digestion of fats.

Table 9.1 Digestive Enzymes

A summary of the digestion of each major class of biomolecules is provided in Figure 9.5.

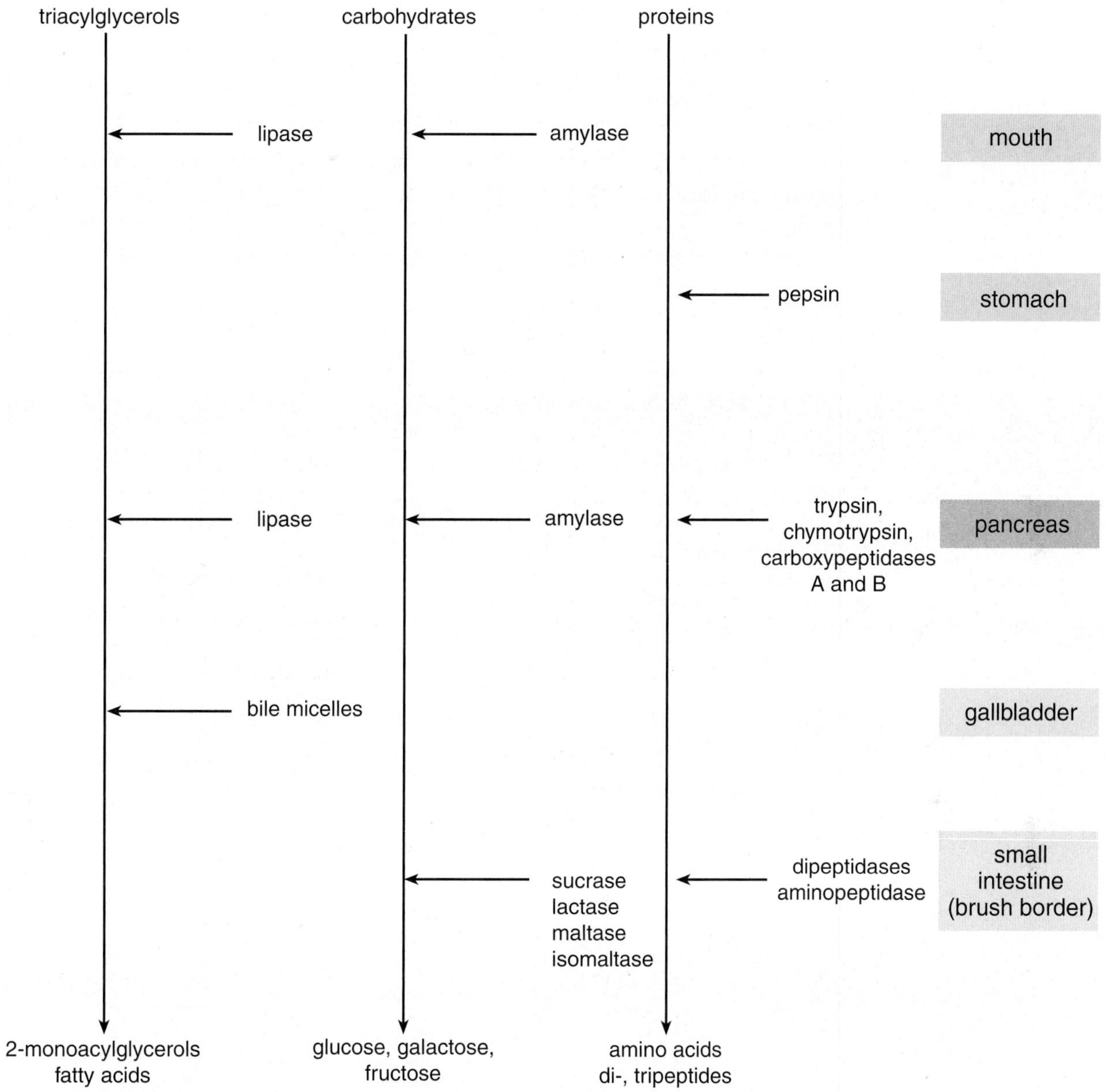

Figure 9.5 Summary of Digestive Processes

MCAT CONCEPT CHECK 9.3

Before you move on, assess your understanding of the material with these questions.

1. List at least one pancreatic enzyme that digests each of the three major classes of biomolecules:
   - Carbohydrates: __________
   - Proteins: __________
   - Fats: __________

2. What are the main components of bile?

____

3. Where is bile synthesized? Where is bile stored? Where does bile carry out its digestive function?
   - Synthesized: __________
   - Stored: __________
   - Carries out function: __________

4. List at least four functions of the liver:
   - __________
   - __________
   - __________
   - __________

5. The accessory organs of digestion originate from which primary germ layer?

____

9.4 Absorption and Defecation

LEARNING OBJECTIVES

After Chapter 9.4, you will be able to:

- Recall the four fat-soluble vitamins
- Order the three sections of the small intestine and the three sections of the large intestine
- Predict the portions of the gut impacted by a disease when given a digestive symptom, such as watery stool
- Identify the biomolecules typically absorbed into each vessel of the villus:

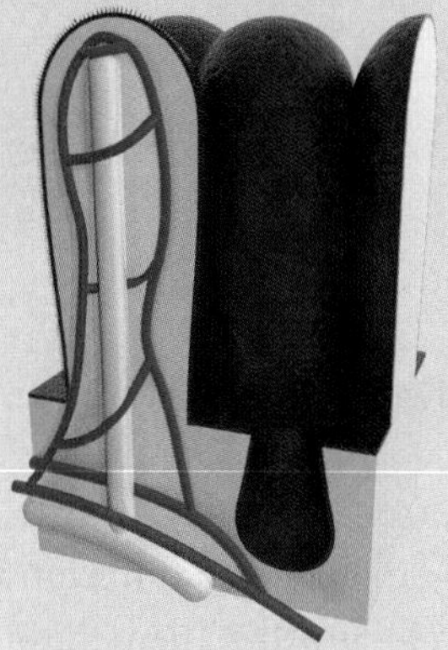

Absorption of nutrients primarily occurs in the small intestine, especially in the jejunum and ileum. The large intestine largely absorbs water.

Jejunum and Ileum

The small intestine consists of three segments: the duodenum, the jejunum, and the ileum. As discussed previously, the **duodenum** is primarily involved in digestion. The **jejunum** and **ileum** are involved in the absorption of nutrients. The small intestine is lined with **villi**, which are small, finger-like projections from the epithelial lining, as shown in Figure 9.6. Each villus has many **microvilli**, drastically increasing the surface area available for absorption. In addition, at the middle of each villus there is a capillary bed for the absorption of water-soluble nutrients and a **lacteal**, a lymphatic channel that takes up fats for transport into the lymphatic system.

MNEMONIC

Segments of the small intestine: **D**ow **J**ones **I**ndustrial

- **D**uodenum
- **J**ejunum
- **I**leum

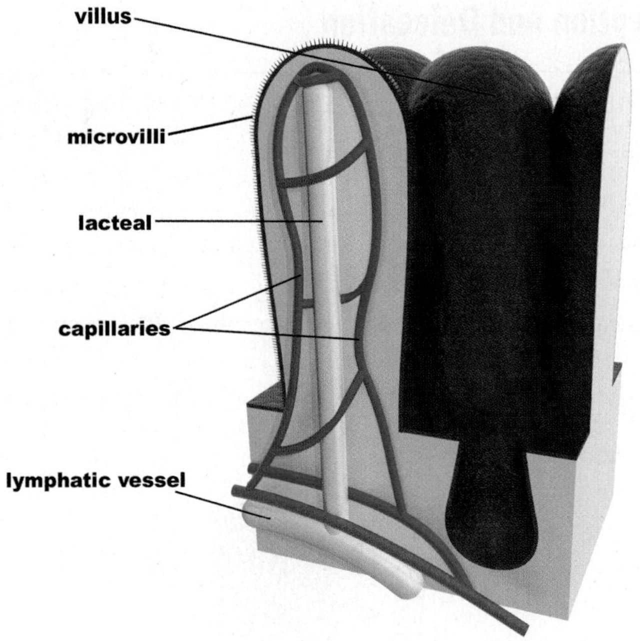

Figure 9.6 Structure of a Villus

Simple sugars, such as glucose, fructose, and galactose, and amino acids are absorbed by secondary active transport and facilitated diffusion into the epithelial cells lining the small intestine, as shown in Figure 9.7. Then, these substances move across the epithelial cell membrane into the intestinal capillaries. Blood is constantly passing by the epithelial cells, carrying the carbohydrate and amino acid molecules away. This creates a concentration gradient such that the blood always has a lower concentration of monosaccharides and amino acids than inside the epithelial cells. Thus, simple carbohydrates and amino acids diffuse from the epithelial cells into the capillaries. The absorbed molecules then go to the liver via the hepatic portal circulation.

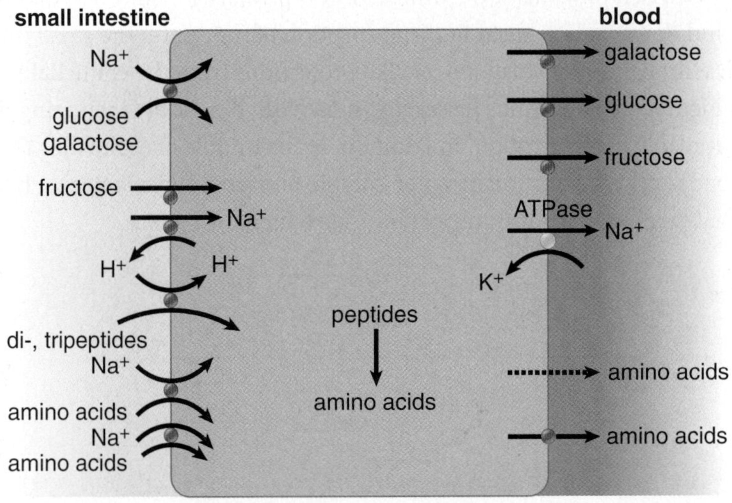

Figure 9.7 Absorption of Carbohydrates and Amino Acids in the Small Intestine

What about fats? Short-chain fatty acids will follow the same process as carbohydrates and amino acids by diffusing directly into the intestinal capillaries. These fatty acids do not require transporters because they are nonpolar, so they can easily traverse the cellular membrane. Larger fats, glycerol, and cholesterol move separately into the intestinal cells but then reform into triglycerides, as shown in Figure 9.8. The triglycerides and esterified cholesterol molecules are packaged into **chylomicrons**. Rather than entering the bloodstream, chylomicrons enter the lymphatic circulation through **lacteals**, small vessels that form the beginning of the lymphatic system. These lacteals converge and enter the venous circulation at the **thoracic duct** in the base of the neck, which empties into the left subclavian vein.

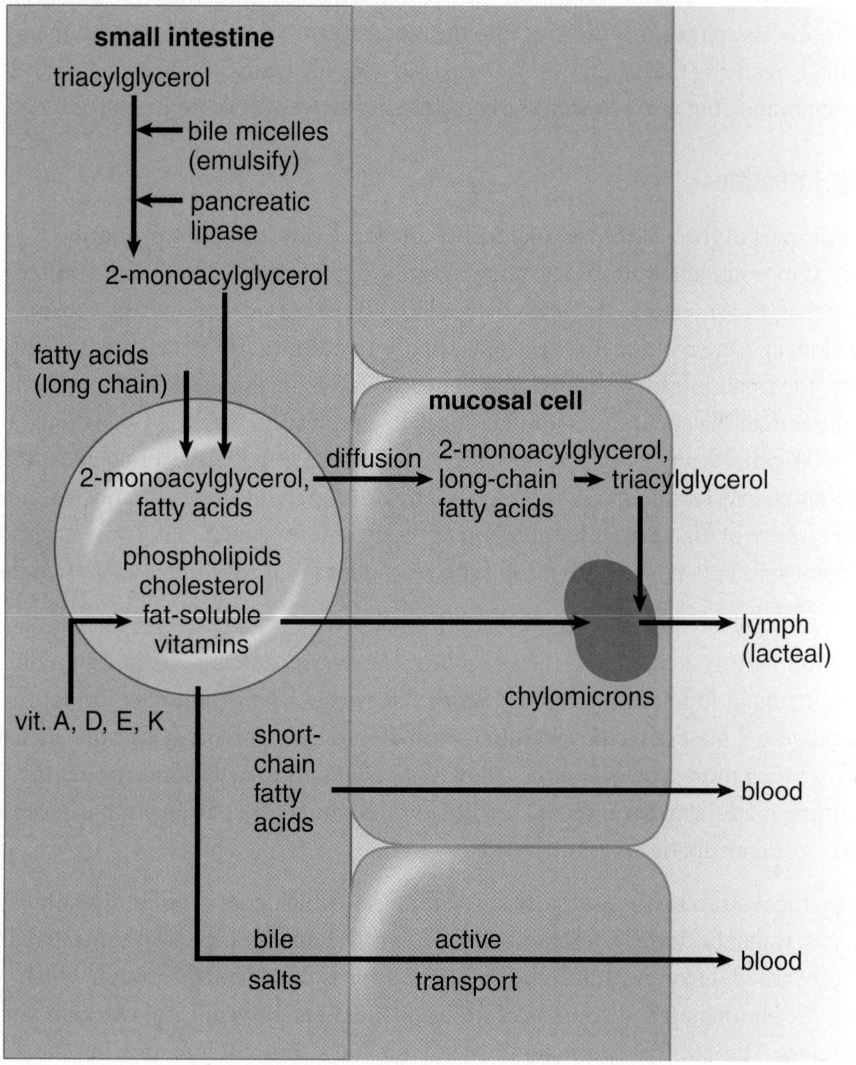

Figure 9.8 Absorption of Lipids

Vitamins are also absorbed in the small intestine. Vitamins can be categorized as either fat-soluble or water-soluble. Because there are only four **fat-soluble vitamins** (A, D, E, and K), these can be easily memorized. All other vitamins (B complex and C) are water-soluble. Fat-soluble vitamins dissolve directly into chylomicrons to enter the lymphatic circulation. Failure to digest and absorb fat properly, which can be due to pathologies in the liver, gallbladder, pancreas, or small intestine, may lead to deficiencies of fat-soluble vitamins. The **water-soluble vitamins** are taken up, along with water, amino acids, and carbohydrates, across the endothelial cells of the small intestine, passing directly into the plasma.

In addition to fats, carbohydrates, amino acids, and vitamins, the small intestine also absorbs water. Much of the water in chyme is actually the result of secretions. On average, a person may consume up to two liters of fluid per day, but secretions into the upper gastrointestinal tract may total up to seven liters of fluid per day. In order to maintain proper fluid levels within the body, much of this fluid must be reabsorbed by osmosis. As solutes are absorbed into the bloodstream, water is drawn with them, eventually reaching the capillaries. Water passes not only **transcellularly** (across the cell membrane), but also **paracellularly** (squeezing between cells) to reach the blood.

Large Intestine

The final part of the gastrointestinal tract is the **large intestine**. It is primarily involved in water absorption. The large intestine has a larger diameter but shorter length than the small intestine. It is divided into three major sections: the cecum, the colon, and the rectum. The **cecum** is simply an outpocketing that accepts fluid exiting the small intestine through the **ileocecal valve** and is the site of attachment of the **appendix**. The appendix is a small finger-like projection that was once thought to be **vestigial**. Recent evidence, however, suggests that it may have a role in warding off certain bacterial infections and repopulating the large intestine with normal flora after episodes of diarrhea. Inflammation of the appendix (appendicitis) is a surgical emergency; in fact, it is the most common reason for an unscheduled surgery in the United States.

The **colon** itself is divided into the ascending, transverse, descending, and sigmoid colons. Its main function is to absorb water and salts (such as sodium chloride) from the undigested material left over from the small intestine. The small intestine actually absorbs much more water than the colon, so the colon primarily concentrates the remaining material to form **feces**. Too little or too much water absorption can cause diarrhea or constipation, respectively.

BRIDGE

Note the similarity between the muscles that control voiding of urine and feces. In both cases, there is an internal sphincter under autonomic control (internal urethral sphincter and internal anal sphincter) and an external sphincter under somatic control (external urethral sphincter and external anal sphincter). Urination is discussed in Chapter 10 of *MCAT Biology Review*.

Finally, the rectum serves as a storage site for feces, which consists of indigestible material, water, bacteria (*E. coli* and others), and certain digestive secretions that are not reabsorbed (enzymes and some bile). The **anus** is the opening through which wastes are eliminated and consists of two sphincters: the **internal** and **external anal sphincters**. The external sphincter is under voluntary control (somatic), but the internal sphincter is under involuntary control (autonomic).

The large intestine—and even the small intestine—is home to many different species of bacteria. In fact, 30 percent of the dry matter in stool consists of bacteria. Most of these bacteria are anaerobes, but the cecum is also home to many aerobic bacteria. The presence of bacteria in the colon represents a symbiotic relationship:

the bacteria are provided with a steady source of food, and the byproducts produced by the bacteria are beneficial to humans. For example, bacteria in the gut produce vitamin K, which is essential for the production of clotting factors, and biotin (vitamin B_7), which is a coenzyme for many metabolic enzymes.

MCAT CONCEPT CHECK 9.4

Before you move on, assess your understanding of the material with these questions.

1. What are the two circulatory vessels in a villus? What biomolecules are absorbed into each?

   •
   ____

   •
   ____

2. What are the four fat-soluble vitamins?

   ____

3. What are the three sections of the small intestine, in order? What are the three sections of the large intestine, in order?

   • Small intestine: __________, __________, __________
   • Large intestine: __________, __________, __________

4. *Vibrio cholera* causes a severe infection in the intestines, leading to massive volumes of watery diarrhea—up to 20 liters per day. Given these symptoms, does cholera likely impact the small intestine or the large intestine?

   ____

Conclusion

In this chapter, we have reviewed a lot of information about the digestive system that we can use to our advantage on Test Day. We began with an overview of the anatomy, keeping in mind that the system is designed to carry out extracellular digestion. Considering that all our foodstuffs are made up of fats, proteins, and carbohydrates, these compounds have to be broken down to their simplest molecular forms before they can be absorbed and distributed to the tissues and cells of the body. As we moved through the gastrointestinal tract, we discussed whether each organ was a site of absorption, digestion, or both. We spent a good bit of time discussing each of the enzymes involved in digestion and their specific purposes. While digestion occurs primarily in the oral cavity, stomach, and duodenum, absorption occurs primarily in the jejunum and ileum, where the method of transport into the circulatory system is slightly different depending on the compound. Finally, we discussed the three segments of the large intestine and their roles in water and salt absorption, as well as the temporary storage of waste products. Although the amount of information about the digestive system may seem overwhelming, the underlying concepts are relatively straightforward, and a systematic approach (such as charts, tables, or flashcards) will help you manage this content.

In the end, the digestive system's main purpose is to break down energy-containing compounds and get them into the circulation so they can be used by the rest of the body. Equally important are the systems the body has for getting rid of compounds from the blood. Buildup of waste products like ammonia, urea, potassium, and hydrogen ions can lead to serious pathology. For instance, hyperammonemia (buildup of ammonia in the blood) can lead to severe, permanent neurological damage. Hyperkalemia (buildup of potassium in the blood) can quickly cause a fatal heart attack. Temperature regulation is similarly important; both hyperthermia and hypothermia can lead to organ dysfunction and, ultimately, death. In the next chapter, we turn our attention to these regulatory systems: the renal system and the skin.

You've reviewed the content, now test your knowledge and critical thinking skills by completing a test-like passage set in your online resources!

GO ONLINE

CONCEPT SUMMARY

Anatomy of the Digestive System

- **Intracellular digestion** involves the oxidation of glucose and fatty acids to make energy. **Extracellular digestion** occurs in the lumen of the **alimentary canal.**
  - **Mechanical digestion** is the physical breakdown of large food particles into smaller food particles.
  - **Chemical digestion** is the enzymatic cleavage of chemical bonds, such as the peptide bonds of proteins or the glycosidic bonds of starches.
- The pathway of the digestive tract is: oral cavity → pharynx → esophagus → stomach → small intestine → large intestine → rectum
- The **accessory organs of digestion** are the salivary glands, pancreas, liver, and gallbladder.
- The **enteric nervous system** is in the wall of the alimentary canal and controls peristalsis. Its activity is upregulated by the parasympathetic nervous system and downregulated by the sympathetic nervous system.

Ingestion and Digestion

- Multiple hormones regulate feeding behavior, including antidiuretic hormone (ADH or vasopressin) and aldosterone, which promote thirst; glucagon and ghrelin, which promote hunger; and leptin and cholecystokinin, which promote satiety.
- In the **oral cavity, mastication** starts the mechanical digestion of food, while **salivary amylase** and **lipase** start the chemical digestion of food. Food is formed into a **bolus** and swallowed.
- The **pharynx** connects the mouth and posterior nasal cavity to the esophagus.
- The **esophagus** propels food to the stomach using peristalsis. Food enters the stomach through the **lower esophageal (cardiac) sphincter**.
- The stomach has four parts: **fundus**, **body**, **antrum**, and **pylorus**. The stomach has a **lesser** and **greater curvature** and is thrown into folds called **rugae**. Numerous secretory cells line the stomach.
  - **Mucous cells** produce bicarbonate-rich mucus to protect the stomach.
  - **Chief cells** secrete **pepsinogen**, a protease activated by the acidic environment of the stomach.
  - **Parietal cells** secrete hydrochloric acid and **intrinsic factor**, which is needed for vitamin B_{12} absorption.
  - **G-cells** secrete **gastrin**, a peptide hormone that increases HCl secretion and gastric motility.

- After mechanical and chemical digestion in the stomach, the food particles are now called **chyme**. Food passes into the duodenum through the **pyloric sphincter**.
- The **duodenum** is the first part of the small intestine and is primarily involved in chemical digestion.
    - **Disaccharidases** are brush-border enzymes that break down maltose, isomaltose, lactose, and sucrose into monosaccharides.
    - Brush-border **peptidases** include **aminopeptidase** and **dipeptidases**.
    - **Enteropeptidase** activates trypsinogen and procarboxypeptidases, initiating an activation cascade.
    - **Secretin** stimulates the release of pancreatic juices into the digestive tract and slows motility.
    - **Cholecystokinin** stimulates bile release from the gallbladder, release of pancreatic juices, and satiety.

Accessory Organs of Digestion

- **Acinar cells** in the pancreas produce pancreatic juices that contain bicarbonate, **pancreatic amylase**, pancreatic peptidases (**trypsinogen**, **chymotrypsinogen**, **carboxypeptidases A** and **B**), and **pancreatic lipase**.
- The **liver** synthesizes **bile**, which can be stored in the gallbladder or secreted into the duodenum directly.
    - Bile emulsifies fats, making them soluble and increasing their surface area.
    - The main components of bile are **bile salts**, pigments (especially **bilirubin** from the breakdown of hemoglobin), and cholesterol.
- The liver also processes nutrients (through glycogenesis and glycogenolysis, storage and mobilization of fats, and gluconeogenesis), produces urea, detoxifies chemicals, activates or inactivates medications, produces bile, and synthesizes albumin and clotting factors.
- The **gallbladder** stores and concentrates bile.

Absorption and Defecation

- The **jejunum** and **ileum** of the small intestine are primarily involved in absorption.
    - The small intestine is lined with **villi**, which are covered with **microvilli**, increasing the surface area available for absorption.
    - Villi contain a capillary bed and a **lacteal**, a vessel of the lymphatic system.
    - Water-soluble compounds, such as monosaccharides, amino acids, water-soluble vitamins, small fatty acids, and water, enter the capillary bed.
    - Fat-soluble compounds, such as fats, cholesterol, and fat-soluble vitamins, enter the lacteal.

- The **large intestine** absorbs water and salts, forming semisolid feces.
  - The **cecum** is an outpocketing that accepts fluid from the small intestine through the **ileocecal valve** and is the site of attachment of the **appendix**.
  - The **colon** is divided into ascending, transverse, descending, and sigmoid portions.
  - The **rectum** stores feces, which are then excreted through the **anus**.
  - Gut bacteria produce vitamin K and biotin (vitamin B_7).

ANSWERS TO CONCEPT CHECKS

9.1

1. Mechanical digestion, such as chewing, physically breaks down food into smaller pieces. Chemical digestion involves hydrolysis of bonds and breakdown of food into smaller biomolecules.
2. Oral cavity (mouth) → pharynx → esophagus → stomach → small intestine → large intestine → rectum → anus
3. The parasympathetic nervous system increases secretions from all of the glands of the digestive system and promotes peristalsis. The sympathetic nervous system slows peristalsis.

9.2

1. Saliva contains salivary amylase (ptyalin), which digests starch into smaller sugars (maltose and dextrin); and lipase, which digests fats.
2.

Cell	Secretions	Functions
Mucous cell	Mucus	Protects lining of stomach, increases pH (bicarbonate)
Chief cell	Pepsinogen	Digests proteins, activated by H^+
Parietal cell	HCl, intrinsic factor	HCl: decreases pH, kills microbes, denatures proteins, carries out some chemical digestion; intrinsic factor: absorption of vitamin B_{12}
G-cell	Gastrin	Increases HCl production, increases gastric motility

3.

Substance	Enzyme or Hormone?	Functions
Sucrase	Enzyme	Brush-border enzyme; breaks down sucrose into monosaccharides
Secretin	Hormone	Increases pancreatic secretions, especially bicarbonate; reduces HCl secretion; decreases motility
Dipeptidase	Enzyme	Brush-border enzyme; breaks down dipeptides into free amino acids
Cholecystokinin	Hormone	Recruits secretions from gallbladder and pancreas; promotes satiety
Enteropeptidase	Enzyme	Activates trypsinogen, which initiates an activation cascade

4. Bile accomplishes mechanical digestion of fats, emulsifying them and increasing their surface area. Pancreatic lipase accomplishes chemical digestion of fats, breaking their ester bonds.

9.3

1. Carbohydrates: pancreatic amylase; proteins: trypsin, chymotrypsin, carboxypeptidases A and B; fats: pancreatic lipase
2. Bile is composed of bile salts (amphipathic molecules derived from cholesterol that emulsify fats), pigments (especially bilirubin from the breakdown of hemoglobin), and cholesterol.
3. Bile is synthesized in the liver, stored in the gallbladder, and serves its function in the duodenum.
4. The liver processes nutrients (through glycogenesis and glycogenolysis, storage and mobilization of fats, and gluconeogenesis), produces urea, detoxifies chemicals, activates or inactivates medications, produces bile, and synthesizes albumin and clotting factors.
5. As outgrowths of the gut tube, the accessory organs of digestion arise from embryonic endoderm.

9.4

1. The two circulatory vessels are capillaries and lacteals. The capillary absorbs water-soluble nutrients like monosaccharides, amino acids, short-chain fatty acids, water-soluble vitamins, and water itself. The lacteal absorbs fat-soluble nutrients, like fats, cholesterol, and fat-soluble vitamins.
2. The fat-soluble vitamins are A, D, E, and K.
3. The small intestine consists of the duodenum, jejunum, and ileum. The large intestine consists of the cecum, colon, and rectum.
4. While the large intestine's main function is to absorb water, the small intestine actually absorbs a much larger volume of water. Thus, massive volumes of watery diarrhea are more likely to arise from infections in the small intestine than in the large intestine.

SCIENCE MASTERY ASSESSMENT EXPLANATIONS

1. **B**

Chief cells secrete pepsinogen, a protease secreted as a zymogen that is activated by the acidic environment of the stomach. G-cells secrete gastrin, parietal cells secrete hydrochloric acid and intrinsic factor, and mucous cells secrete alkaline mucus, eliminating the other answer choices.

2. **B**

The small intestine is divided into three sections: the duodenum, the jejunum, and the ileum. The cecum is part of the large intestine, making **(B)** the correct answer.

3. **B**

Aminopeptidase is a brush-border peptidase secreted by the cells lining the duodenum; it does not require enteropeptidase for activation. Both trypsinogen and procarboxypeptidases A and B are activated by enteropeptidase, eliminating **(A)** and **(D)**. Once activated, trypsin can activate chymotrypsinogen; if trypsinogen cannot be activated, then chymotrypsinogen will not be activated either, eliminating **(C)**.

4. **D**

Lipase is involved in the digestion of fats, but its function is not to emulsify fats—this is the job of bile. Rather, lipase chemically digests fats in the duodenum, allowing them to be brought into duodenal cells and packaged into chylomicrons. The other associations given here are all correct.

5. **C**

Protein digestion begins in the stomach, where pepsin (secreted as pepsinogen) hydrolyzes specific peptide bonds. Protein digestion continues in the small intestine as trypsin (secreted as trypsinogen), chymotrypsin (secreted as chymotrypsinogen), carboxypeptidases A and B (secreted as procarboxypeptidases A and B), aminopeptidase, and dipeptidases hydrolyze specific parts of the peptide. No protein digestion occurs in the mouth or large intestine.

6. **A**

Sucrase is a brush-border enzyme found on duodenal cells and is not secreted by the salivary glands. This enzyme hydrolyzes sucrose (a disaccharide) to form glucose and fructose (monosaccharides). The other associations are all correct.

7. **B**

The question is basically asking us to identify the structure that lies between the stomach and the small intestine. This is the pyloric sphincter; the presentation given in the question is a classic example of what is called pyloric stenosis, in which the pyloric sphincter is thickened and cannot relax to permit chyme through. The cardiac sphincter, **(A)**, lies between the esophagus and the stomach. The ileocecal valve, **(C)**, lies between the ileum of the small intestine and the cecum of the large intestine. The internal anal sphincter, **(D)**, lies at the end of the rectum.

8. **B**

The parasympathetic nervous system has many roles in the digestive system. It promotes motility of the gut tube and secretion from glands. Therefore, blocking the parasympathetic nervous system would likely result in dry mouth (from reduced secretion of saliva), slow gastric emptying (from decreased peristalsis), and decreased gastric acid production (from reduced HCl secretion from the parietal cells in the gastric glands), eliminating **(A)**, **(C)**, and **(D)**. **(B)** is the correct answer because we would expect constipation in such an individual, not diarrhea: slowed motility through the colon would lead to increased water reabsorption, making the feces too firm and causing constipation.

9. **B**

The first graph shows maximal activity at a very acidic pH, implying that this is an enzyme acting in the stomach. The second graph shows maximal activity around pH 8.5, implying that this is an enzyme acting in the duodenum. The only choice that matches the first graph with a stomach enzyme (pepsin) and the second with a duodenal enzyme (carboxypeptidase B) is **(B)**.

10. **C**

Elevated bilirubin implies a blockage to bile flow, increased production of bilirubin (from massive hemoglobin release), or an inability of the liver to produce bile. If the bile duct were occluded, as in **(A)**, then bile would not be able to flow into the digestive tract and would build up, increasing bilirubin levels in the blood. If many red blood cells were lysed, as in **(B)**, then bilirubin levels would rise in accordance with the increased hemoglobin release. If liver failure occurred, as in **(D)**, then the liver would be unable to produce bile, and bilirubin would again build up. **(C)** refers to a pathology in the stomach—the key word given here is rugae, which are the folds in the stomach wall. Lack of gastric function would have no effect on bilirubin levels, making this the correct choice.

11. **A**

Chylomicrons contain triacylglycerols, cholesteryl esters, and fat-soluble vitamins and are secreted by intestinal cells into lacteals. Amino acids, fat-soluble vitamins (like vitamins A and E), and cholesterol are all absorbed in the small intestine.

12. **B**

The cleavage of a fat described in this question stem refers to the breakdown of triacylglycerides, which is a hydrolysis reaction in which water is added across the ester linkage of the fatty acids to the glycerol backbone, breaking these bonds. For this reason, chemical digestion, **(B)**, is correct. Note that, the location of this reaction occurs in the lumen of a digestive organ, so this reaction could also be classified as an extracellular reaction. This observation is important because it eliminates **(C)**.

13. **A**

While the capillaries from the intestine come together to form the portal vein, which drains to the liver, the lacteals come together to form the thoracic duct, which drains directly into the left subclavian vein. Therefore, fat-soluble compounds do not pass through the liver before reaching the right side of the heart. Only **(A)**, vitamin D, is fat-soluble.

14. **C**

Ghrelin promotes a sensation of hunger, increasing feeding behavior. Both leptin and cholecystokinin promote satiety, decreasing feeding behavior—eliminating **(A)** and **(B)**. Gastrin increases acid production and gastric motility, but does not have any significant relationship with feeding behavior, eliminating **(D)**.

15. **D**

The liver serves many functions, including carrying out metabolic processes (glycogenesis and glycogenolysis, fat storage, and gluconeogenesis), detoxification or activation of medications, and synthesis of bile. Germane to this question are the roles of converting ammonia into urea through the urea cycle and synthesis of proteins, including albumin and clotting factors. A patient with liver failure would thus not be able to convert ammonia into urea and would have high concentrations of ammonia and low concentrations of urea in the blood, eliminating **(A)** and **(C)**. With decreased synthetic activity, both albumin and clotting factor concentrations would be low, eliminating **(B)** and making **(D)** the correct answer.

Consult your online resources for additional practice. **GO ONLINE**

SHARED CONCEPTS

Biochemistry Chapter 2
Enzymes

Biochemistry Chapter 9
Carbohydrate Metabolism I

Biochemistry Chapter 11
Lipid and Amino Acid Metabolism

Biology Chapter 5
The Endocrine System

Biology Chapter 7
The Cardiovascular System

Biology Chapter 8
The Immune System

CHAPTER 10

HOMEOSTASIS

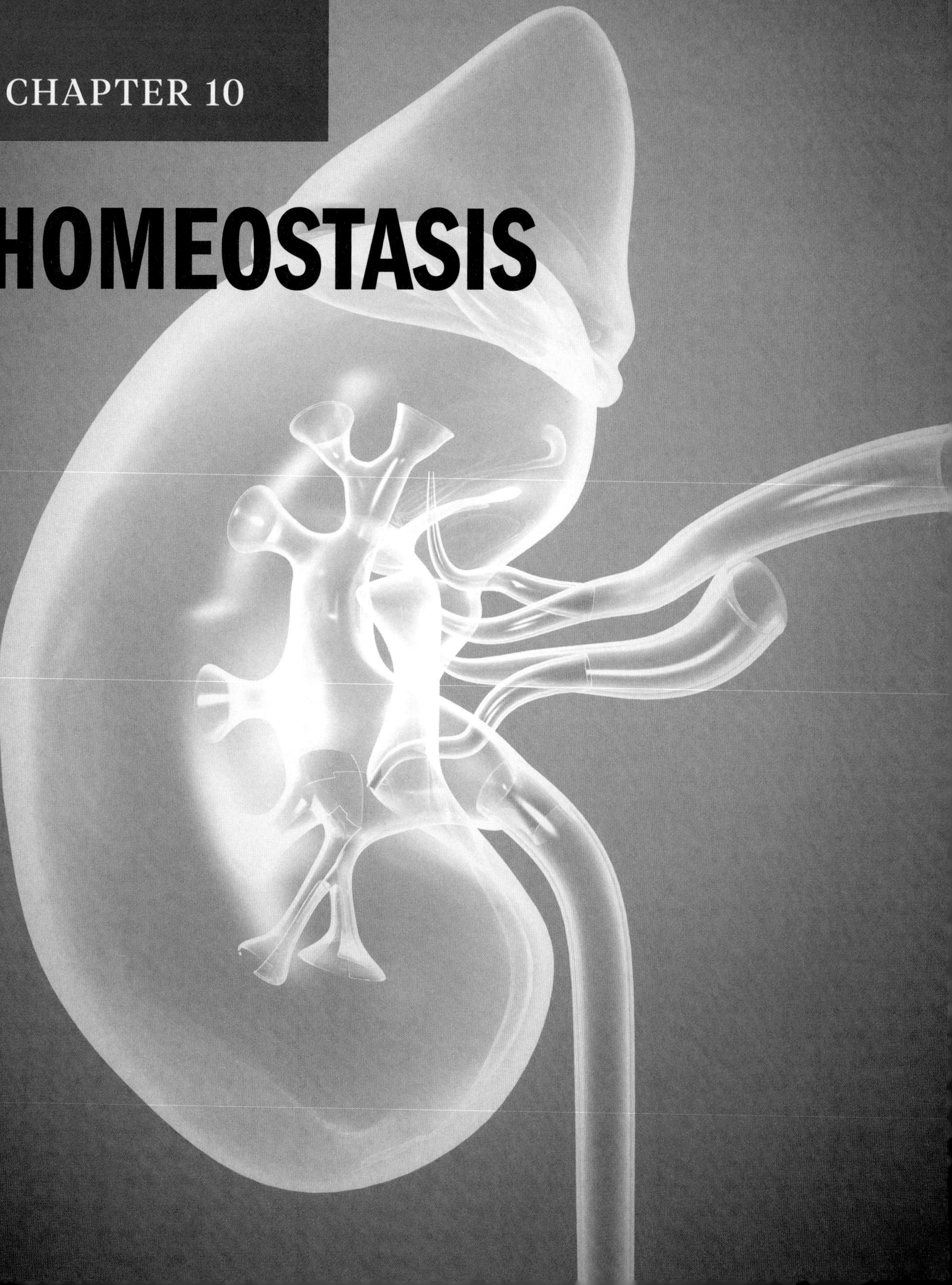

SCIENCE MASTERY ASSESSMENT

Every pre-med knows this feeling: there is so much content I have to know for the MCAT! How do I know what to do first or what's important?

While the high-yield badges throughout this book will help you identify the most important topics, this Science Mastery Assessment is another tool in your MCAT prep arsenal. This quiz (which can also be taken in your online resources) and the guidance below will help ensure that you are spending the appropriate amount of time on this chapter based on your personal strengths and weaknesses. Don't worry though—skipping something now does not mean you'll never study it. Later on in your prep, as you complete full-length tests, you'll uncover specific pieces of content that you need to review and can come back to these chapters as appropriate.

How to Use This Assessment

If you answer 0–7 questions correctly:

Spend about 1 hour to read this chapter in full and take limited notes throughout. Follow up by reviewing **all** quiz questions to ensure that you now understand how to solve each one.

If you answer 8–11 questions correctly:

Spend 20–40 minutes reviewing the quiz questions. Beginning with the questions you missed, read and take notes on the corresponding subchapters. For questions you answered correctly, ensure your thinking matches that of the explanation and you understand why each choice was correct or incorrect.

If you answer 12–15 questions correctly:

Spend less than 20 minutes reviewing all questions from the quiz. If you missed any, then include a quick read-through of the corresponding subchapters, or even just the relevant content within a subchapter, as part of your question review. For questions you answered correctly, ensure your thinking matches that of the explanation and review the Concept Summary at the end of the chapter.

1. Which of the following would most likely be filtered through the glomerulus into Bowman's space?
   - **A.** Erythrocytes
   - **B.** Monosaccharides
   - **C.** Platelets
   - **D.** Proteins

2. In which of the following segments of the nephron is sodium NOT actively transported out of the nephron?
   - **A.** Proximal convoluted tubule
   - **B.** Thin portion of the ascending limb of the loop of Henle
   - **C.** Distal convoluted tubule
   - **D.** Thick portion of the ascending limb of the loop of Henle

3. Which region of the kidney has the lowest solute concentration under normal physiological circumstances?
   - **A.** Cortex
   - **B.** Outer medulla
   - **C.** Inner medulla
   - **D.** Renal pelvis

4. Which of the following sequences correctly shows the passage of blood through the vessels of the kidney?
   - **A.** Renal artery → afferent arterioles → glomerulus → efferent arterioles → vasa recta → renal vein
   - **B.** Afferent arterioles → renal artery → glomerulus → vasa recta → renal vein → efferent arterioles
   - **C.** Glomerulus → renal artery → afferent arterioles → efferent arterioles → renal vein → vasa recta
   - **D.** Renal vein → efferent arterioles → glomerulus → afferent arterioles → vasa recta → renal artery

5. Which of the following statements is FALSE?
   - **A.** ADH increases water reabsorption in the kidney.
   - **B.** Aldosterone indirectly increases water reabsorption in the kidney.
   - **C.** ADH acts directly on the proximal convoluted tubule.
   - **D.** Aldosterone stimulates reabsorption of sodium from the collecting duct.

6. In the nephron, amino acids enter the vasa recta via the process of:
   - **A.** filtration.
   - **B.** secretion.
   - **C.** excretion.
   - **D.** reabsorption.

7. On a very cold day, a person waits for over an hour at the bus stop. Which of the following structures helps the person's body set and maintain a normal temperature?
   - **A.** Hypothalamus
   - **B.** Kidneys
   - **C.** Posterior pituitary
   - **D.** Brainstem

8. Glucose reabsorption in the nephron occurs in the:
   - **A.** loop of Henle.
   - **B.** distal convoluted tubule.
   - **C.** proximal convoluted tubule.
   - **D.** collecting duct.

9. Under normal physiological circumstances, the primary function of the nephron is to create urine that is:
   - **A.** hypertonic to the blood.
   - **B.** hypotonic to the blood.
   - **C.** isotonic to the filtrate.
   - **D.** hypotonic to the vasa recta.

10. Diabetic nephropathy is commonly detected by finding protein in the urine of a patient. In such a disease, where is the likely defect in the nephron?
    - **A.** Glomerulus
    - **B.** Proximal convoluted tubule
    - **C.** Loop of Henle
    - **D.** Collecting duct

11. A laceration cuts down into a layer of loose connective tissue in the skin. Which layer of the skin is this?
    - **A.** Stratum corneum
    - **B.** Stratum lucidum
    - **C.** Papillary layer
    - **D.** Reticular layer

12. When the pH of the blood is high, which substance is likely to be excreted in larger quantities in the urine?
    - **A.** Urea
    - **B.** Ammonia
    - **C.** Hydrogen ions
    - **D.** Bicarbonate ions

13. In which layer of the skin can the stem cells of keratinocytes be found?
    - **A.** Stratum lucidum
    - **B.** Stratum granulosum
    - **C.** Stratum basale
    - **D.** Stratum corneum

14. A drug is used that prevents the conversion of angiotensin I to angiotensin II. What is a likely effect of this drug?
    - **A.** Increased sodium reabsorption
    - **B.** Increased potassium reabsorption
    - **C.** Increased blood pressure
    - **D.** Increased blood pH

15. Sarin is a potent organophosphate that can be used in chemical warfare. As an inhibitor of acetylcholinesterase, sarin causes excessive buildup of acetylcholine in all synapses where it is the neurotransmitter. Which of the following symptoms would most likely be seen in an individual with sarin poisoning?
    - **A.** Increased urination and increased sweating
    - **B.** Increased urination and decreased sweating
    - **C.** Decreased urination and increased sweating
    - **D.** Decreased urination and decreased sweating

Answer Key

1. **B**
2. **B**
3. **A**
4. **A**
5. **C**
6. **D**
7. **A**
8. **C**
9. **A**
10. **A**
11. **C**
12. **D**
13. **C**
14. **B**
15. **A**

Detailed explanations can be found at the end of the chapter.

CHAPTER 10

HOMEOSTASIS

In This Chapter

CHAPTER PROFILE

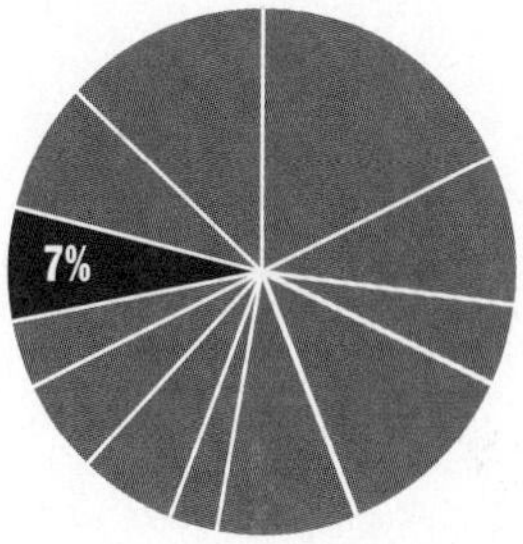

The content in this chapter should be relevant to about 7% of all questions about biology on the MCAT.

This chapter covers material from the following AAMC content category:

3B: Structure and integrative functions of the main organ systems

Introduction

Have a headache? Take an ibuprofen. Backache? Works for that, too. Ibuprofen, which has been around for over 50 years, is a relatively inexpensive, over-the-counter, nonsteroidal anti-inflammatory drug (NSAID). Ibuprofen is known as an analgesic, or pain reliever. When used in moderation, ibuprofen carries relatively little risk. However, taking multiple doses for many years can profoundly affect the kidneys. Years of analgesic use (usually as self-therapy) can lead to kidney failure, known as analgesic nephropathy. If untreated, kidney failure is universally fatal.

If kidney failure is detected, however, dialysis (or a kidney transplant) could save an individual's life. How does dialysis save a patient with kidney failure? Dialyzing fluid has many of the same solutes as blood, in strategic concentrations, and it is kept separate from blood by a semipermeable membrane. As blood is filtered through the dialysis machine, fluid and solutes diffuse down their concentration gradients, limited only by size (as determined by the membrane). The dialysis machine therefore performs filtration to purify the blood and excrete wastes, a crucial function that the kidneys would normally perform.

In this chapter, we'll learn more about filtration, as well as reabsorption and secretion. These processes are collectively responsible for osmoregulation. Osmoregulation is just one mechanism the body uses to maintain homeostasis in its fluids and tissues. We'll also discuss the skin, which plays a significant role in temperature homeostasis (thermoregulation).

10.1 The Excretory System

High-Yield

LEARNING OBJECTIVES

After Chapter 10.1, you will be able to:

- List the structures of the secretory pathway
- Order the vessels in the renal vascular pathway
- Identify the nervous system components used to control the detrusor muscle
- Describe the processes by which components of the kidney are able to exchange solutes between the filtrate and the blood
- Identify the function(s) of each segment of the nephron:

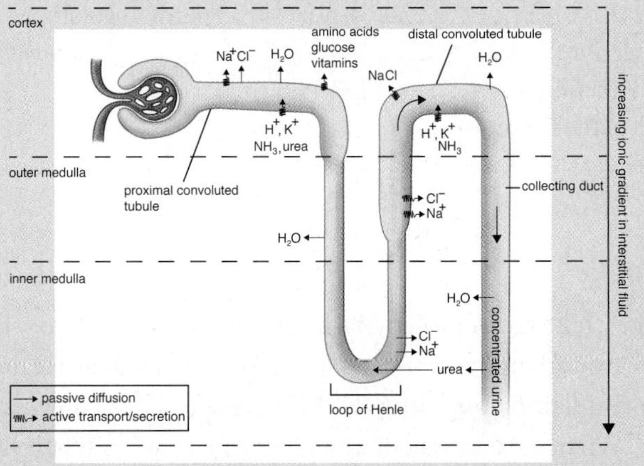

The **excretory system** serves many functions, including the regulation of blood pressure, blood osmolarity, acid–base balance, and removal of nitrogenous wastes. The kidneys play an essential role in these functions.

Anatomy of the Excretory System

The excretory system consists of the kidneys, ureters, bladder, and urethra, as shown in Figure 10.1. The kidneys are two bean-shaped structures located behind the digestive organs at the level of the bottom rib. The functional unit of the kidney is the nephron; each kidney has approximately 1 million nephrons. All of the nephrons eventually empty into the renal pelvis, which narrows to form the the ureter. Urine travels through the ureter to the bladder. From the bladder, urine is transported through the urethra to exit the body.

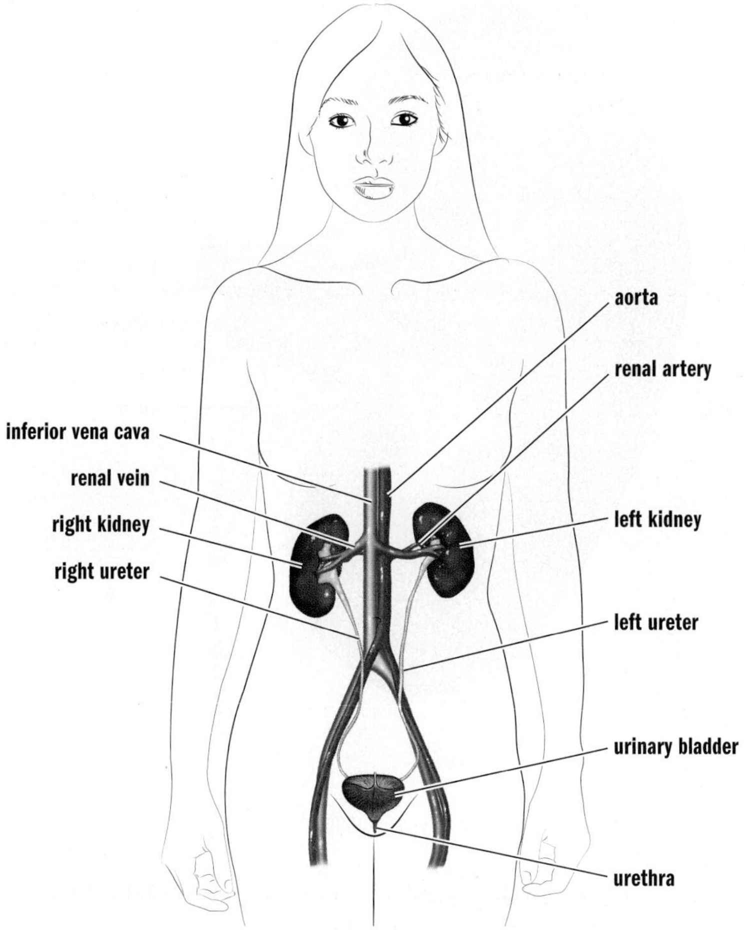

Figure 10.1 The Excretory System
Once it leaves the kidneys, urine moves through the ureters to be stored in the urinary bladder until it is excreted through the urethra.

Kidney Structure

Each kidney is subdivided into a cortex and a medulla, as shown in Figure 10.2. The **cortex** is the kidney's outermost layer, while the **medulla** of the kidney sits within the cortex. Each kidney also has a renal **hilum**, which is a deep slit in the center of its medial surface. The widest part of the ureter, the **renal pelvis**, spans almost the entire width of the renal hilum. The **renal artery**, **renal vein**, and **ureter** enter and exit through the renal hilum.

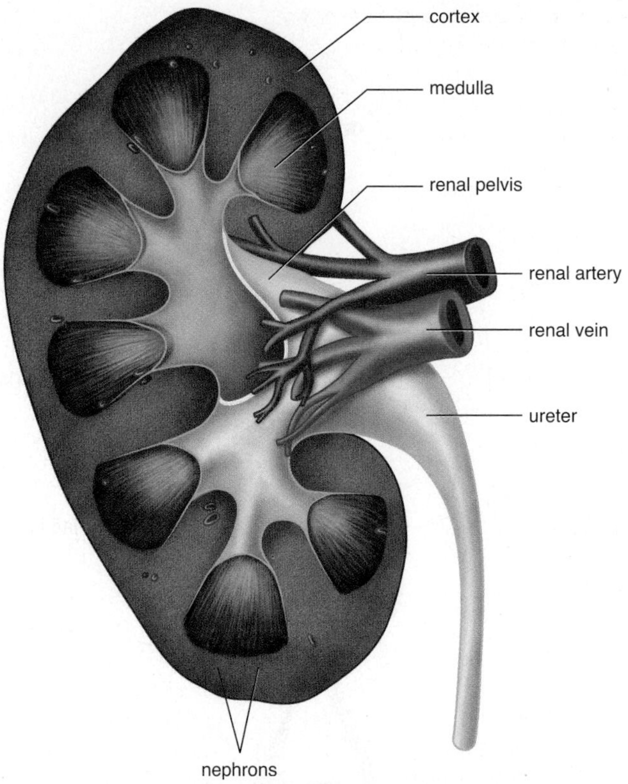

Figure 10.2 Gross Anatomy of the Kidney

BRIDGE

The portal system in the kidney is one of three major portal systems in the body. The other two are the hypophyseal portal system, which connects the hypothalamus and the anterior pituitary (discussed in Chapter 5 of *MCAT Biology Review*), and the hepatic portal system, which connects the gut tube and the liver (discussed in Chapter 9 of *MCAT Biology Review*). In each case, blood passes through two capillary beds before returning to the heart.

The kidney has one of the few portal systems in the body. A **portal system** consists of two capillary beds in series through which blood must travel before returning to the heart. The renal artery branches out, passes through the medulla, and enters the cortex as **afferent arterioles**. The highly convoluted capillary tufts derived from these afferent arterioles are known as **glomeruli**. After blood passes through a glomerulus, the **efferent arterioles** then form a second capillary bed. These capillaries surround the loop of Henle and are known as **vasa recta**. The renal vascular system is shown in Figure 10.3.

Also visible in Figure 10.3 is the structure of the nephron. Around the glomerulus is a cup-like structure known as **Bowman's capsule**. Bowman's capsule leads to a long tubule with many distinct areas; in order, these are the proximal convoluted tubule, descending and ascending limbs of the Loop of Henle, distal convoluted tubule, and collecting duct. The kidney's ability to excrete waste is intricately tied to the specific placement of these structures and their physiology.

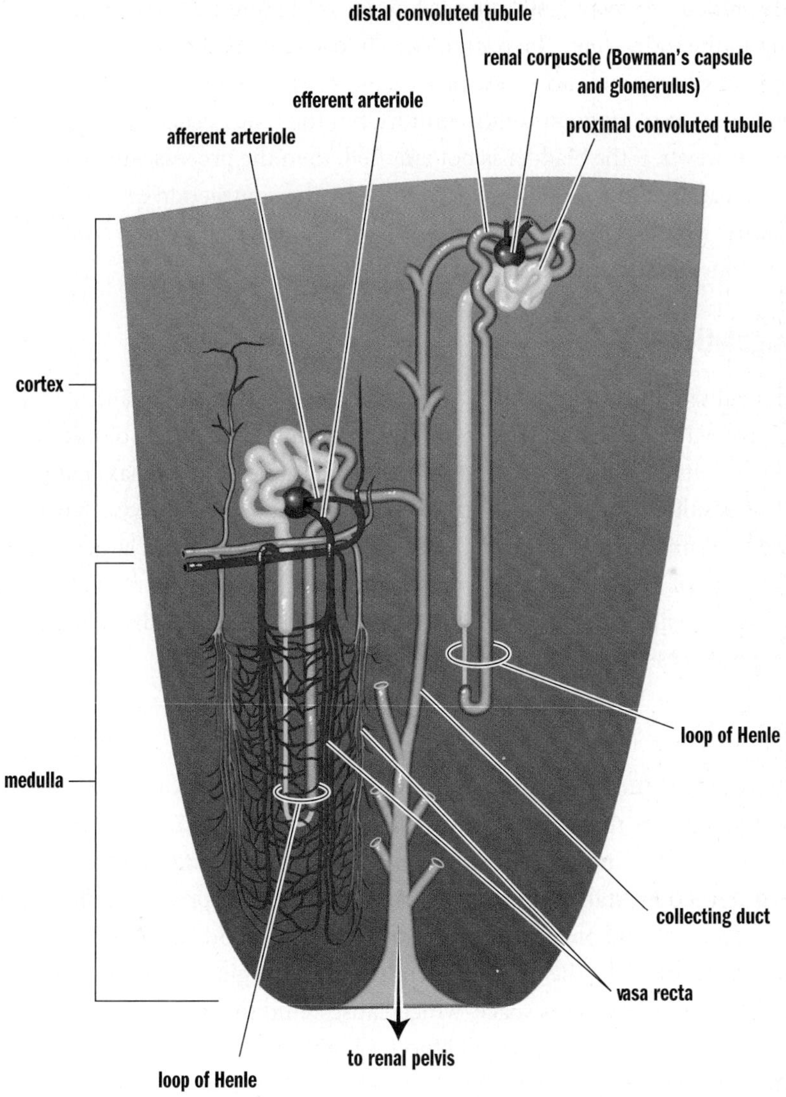

Figure 10.3 Microanatomy of the Renal Vascular System and the Nephron

BRIDGE

Our discussion of neurons in Chapter 4 of *MCAT Biology Review* used some of the same terms as those that describe the organization of blood vessels in the kidney. Afferent neurons carry sensory information toward the central nervous system much as afferent arterioles carry blood toward the glomeruli. Efferent neurons relay signals away from the central nervous system just as efferent arterioles carry blood away from the glomerulus.

Bladder Structure

The bladder has a muscular lining known as the **detrusor muscle**. Parasympathetic activity causes the detrusor muscle to contract. However, in order to leave the body, urine must pass through two sphincters—the internal and external urethral sphincters. The **internal urethral sphincter**, consisting of smooth muscle, is contracted in its normal state. Because the internal sphincter is made of smooth muscle, it is under involuntary control. The **external urethral sphincter** consists of skeletal muscle and is under voluntary control. When the bladder is full, stretch receptors convey to the nervous system that the bladder requires emptying. This causes parasympathetic neurons to fire, and the detrusor muscle contracts. This contraction also causes the internal sphincter to relax. This reflex is known as the **micturition reflex**. The next step is up to the individual. The person can choose to relax the external sphincter to urinate, or can maintain the tone of the external sphincter to prevent urination. This can cause a few moments of discomfort, but the reflex usually dissipates in a few minutes. However, if the bladder is not emptied, then the process will begin anew shortly thereafter. Urination itself is facilitated by the contraction of the abdominal musculature, which increases pressure within the abdominal cavity, resulting in compression of the bladder and increased urine flow rate.

Osmoregulation

The kidney filters the blood to form urine. The composition and quantity of urine is determined by the present state of the body. For example, if blood volume is low and blood osmolarity is high, then it is most beneficial to the body to maximally retain water. This results in low-volume, highly concentrated urine. Likewise, a patient receiving large amounts of intravenous fluids is likely to produce a larger volume of less concentrated urine. Thus, the primary job of the kidneys is to regulate blood volume and osmolarity. In order to do this, kidney function may be divided into three different processes: filtration, secretion, and reabsorption.

Filtration

The nephron's first function is **filtration**. In the kidneys, approximately 20 percent of the blood that passes through the glomerulus is filtered as fluid into Bowman's space. The collected fluid is known as the **filtrate**. The movement of fluid into Bowman's space is governed by **Starling forces**, which account for the pressure differentials in both hydrostatic and oncotic pressures between the blood and Bowman's space, as shown in Figure 10.4. The hydrostatic pressure in the glomerulus is significantly higher than that in Bowman's space, which causes fluid to move into the nephron. On the other hand, the osmolarity of blood is higher than that of Bowman's space, resulting in pressure opposing the movement of fluid into the nephron. However, the hydrostatic pressure is much larger than the oncotic pressure, so the net flow is still from blood into the nephron.

BRIDGE

Like the electromotive force discussed in Chapter 6 of *MCAT Physics and Math Review*, Starling *forces* are really a misnomer. Rather than forces, it is a pressure differential that causes the net movement of fluid from the glomerulus to Bowman's space. Pressure is discussed in Chapter 4 of *MCAT Physics and Math Review*.

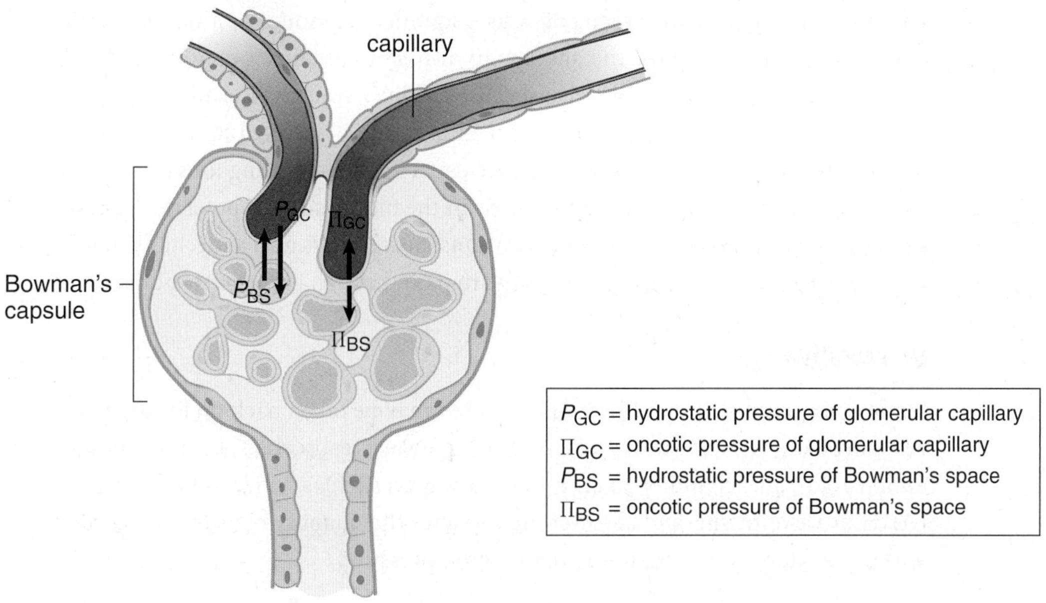

Figure 10.4 Starling Forces
The relative hydrostatic and oncotic pressure gradients determine the direction and rate of filtration.

Under most circumstances, fluid will flow from the glomerulus into Bowman's space. However, various pathologies can cause derangements of this flow. Consider what might happen if the ureter was obstructed by a kidney stone. An obstruction would result in a buildup of urine behind the stone. Eventually, enough fluid will build up and cause distention of the renal pelvis and the nephrons. What will happen to filtration in this case? The hydrostatic pressure in Bowman's space would increase to the point that filtration could no longer occur because there would be excessive pressure opposing movement of fluid into the nephron.

The filtrate is similar in composition to blood but does not contain cells or proteins due to the filter's ability to select based on size. In other words, molecules or cells that are larger than glomerular pores will remain in the blood. As described earlier, the blood remaining in the glomerulus then travels into the efferent arterioles, which empty into the vasa recta. The filtrate is isotonic to blood so that neither the capsule nor the capillaries swell. Our kidneys filter about 180 liters per day, which is approximately 36 times our blood volume. This means that the entire volume of a person's blood is filtered about every 40 minutes.

Secretion

In addition to filtering blood, the nephrons are able to **secrete** salts, acids, bases, and urea directly into the tubule by either active or passive transport. The quantity and identity of the substances secreted into the nephron are directly related to the needs of the body at that time. For example, a diet heavy in meat results in the intake of

KEY CONCEPT

Imagine that the glomerulus is like a sieve or colander. Small molecules dissolved in the blood will pass through the tiny pores (such as glucose, which is later reabsorbed), whereas large molecules such as proteins and blood cells will not. If blood cells or proteins are found in the urine, this indicates a health problem at the level of the glomerulus.

KEY CONCEPT

- Filtration: movement of solutes from blood to filtrate at Bowman's capsule
- Secretion: movement of solutes from blood to filtrate anywhere besides Bowman's capsule
- Reabsorption: movement of solutes from filtrate to blood

large amounts of protein, which contains a significant amount of nitrogen. Ammonia (NH_3) is a byproduct of the metabolism of nitrogen-containing compounds and, as a base, can disturb the pH of blood and cells. The liver converts the ammonia to **urea**, a neutral compound, which travels to the kidney and is secreted into the nephron for excretion in the urine. The kidneys are capable of eliminating ions or other substances when present in relative excess in the blood, such as potassium cations, hydrogen ions, or metabolites of medications. Secretion is also a mechanism for excreting wastes that are simply too large to pass through glomerular pores.

Reabsorption

Some compounds that are filtered or secreted may be taken back up for use via **reabsorption**. Certain substances are almost always reabsorbed, such as glucose, amino acids, and vitamins. In addition, hormones such as antidiuretic hormone (ADH or vasopressin) and aldosterone can alter the quantity of water reabsorbed within the kidney in order to maintain blood pressure.

Nephron Function

The kidney uses mechanisms such as filtration, secretion, and reabsorption to produce urine and to regulate the blood volume and osmolarity. However, the function of the nephron isn't quite that simple. In fact, renal physiology is often considered one of the most difficult topics covered in medical school.

In order to simplify this topic, it is important to understand that the kidney has two main goals: keep what the body needs and lose what it doesn't, and concentrate the urine to conserve water. The kidney allows the human body to reabsorb certain materials for reuse, while also selectively eliminating waste. For example, glucose and amino acids are not usually present in the urine because the kidney is able to reabsorb these substances for later use. On the contrary, waste products like hydrogen and potassium ions, ammonia, and urea remain in the filtrate and are excreted. Finally, water is reabsorbed in large quantities in order to maintain blood pressure and adequate hydration.

KEY CONCEPT

Anything that makes it into the filtrate and that is not reabsorbed will be lost from the body in the urine.

In order to understand this complex organ, we will study the nephron piece-by-piece, discussing exactly what is occurring in each segment. Follow along with the nephron diagram shown in Figure 10.5. As a theme, note that segments that are horizontal in the diagram (Bowman's capsule, the proximal convoluted tubule, and the distal convoluted tubule) are primarily focused on the *identity* of the particles in the urine (*keep what the body needs and lose what it doesn't*). In contrast, the segments that are vertical in the diagram (the loop of Henle and collecting duct) are primarily focused on the volume and concentration of the urine (*concentrate the urine to conserve water*).

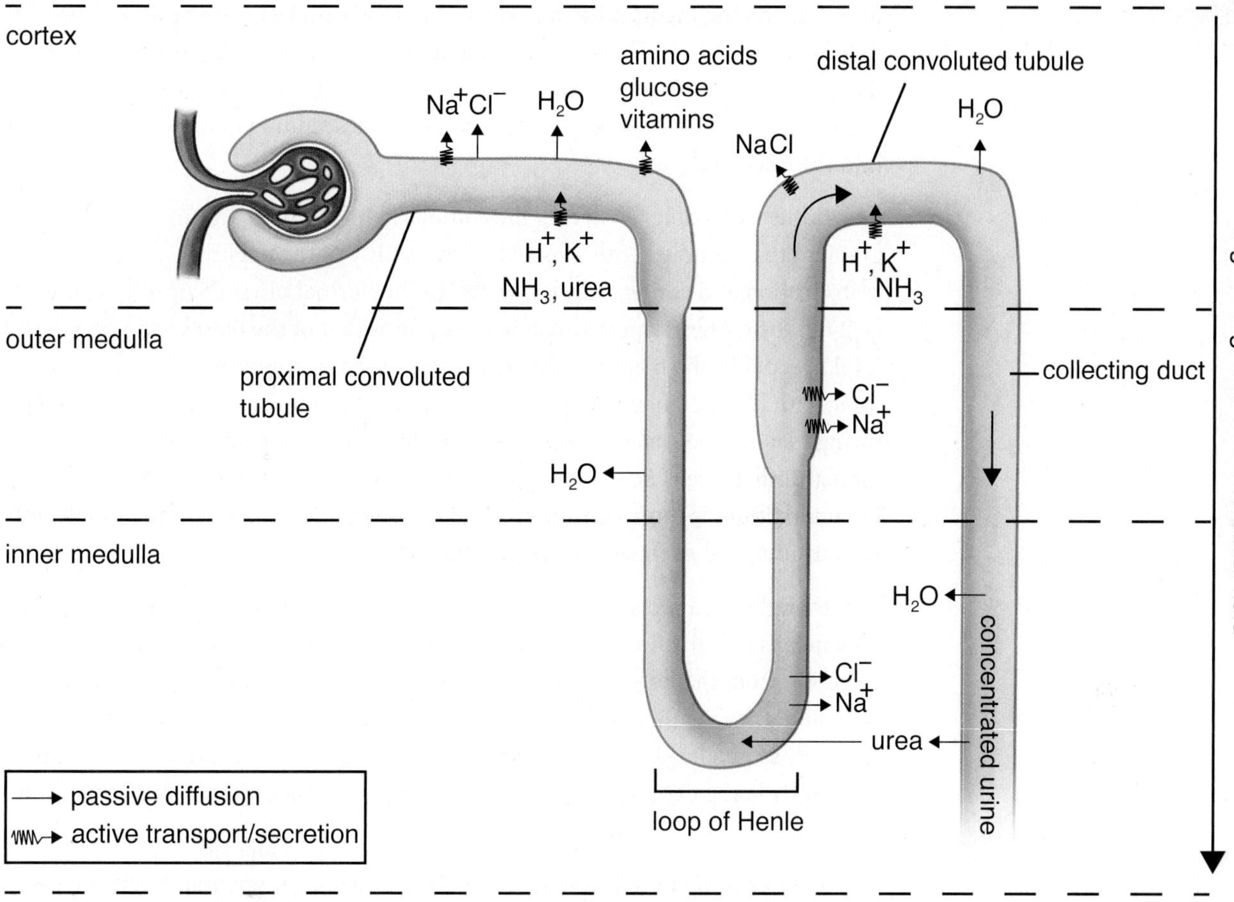

Figure 10.5 Reabsorption and Secretion in the Nephron

Proximal Convoluted Tubule

The filtrate first enters the **proximal convoluted tubule** (**PCT**). In this region, amino acids, glucose, water-soluble vitamins, and the majority of salts are reabsorbed along with water. Almost 70 percent of filtered sodium will be reabsorbed here, but the filtrate remains isotonic to the interstitium, as other solutes and a large volume of water are also reabsorbed. Solutes that enter the **interstitium**—the connective tissue surrounding the nephron—are picked up by the vasa recta to be returned to the bloodstream for reuse within the body. The PCT is also the site of secretion for a number of waste products, including hydrogen ions, potassium ions, ammonia, and urea.

MNEMONIC

Major waste products excreted in the urine: **Dump** the **HUNK**

- **H**$^+$
- **U**rea
- **N**H_3
- **K**$^+$

Loop of Henle

Filtrate from the proximal convoluted tubule then enters the **descending limb of the loop of Henle**, which dives deep into the medulla before turning around to become the **ascending limb of the loop of Henle**. The descending limb is permeable only to water, and the medulla has an ever-increasing osmolarity as the descending limb travels deeper into it. Think for a moment how this would affect the flow of water. As the descending limb traverses deeper into the medulla, the increasing interstitial concentration favors the outflow of water from the descending limb, which is reabsorbed into the vasa recta.

The kidney is capable of altering the osmolarity of the interstitium. This creates a gradient that, coupled with selective permeability of the nephron, allows maximal reabsorption and conservation of water. In the normal physiological state, the osmolarity in the cortex is approximately the same as that of the blood and remains at that level. Deeper in the medulla, the osmolarity in the interstitium can range from isotonic with blood (when trying to excrete water) to four times as concentrated (when trying to conserve water). If the concentration is the same in the tubule and in the interstitium, there is no driving force (gradient), and the water will be lost in urine. If the interstitium is more concentrated, then water will move out of the tubule, into the interstitium, and eventually back into the blood.

Together, the vasa recta and nephron create a **countercurrent multiplier system**. This means that the flow of filtrate through the loop of Henle is in the opposite direction from the flow of blood through the vasa recta. If the two flowed in the same direction, they would quickly reach equilibrium and the kidney would be unable to reabsorb as much water. By making the two flow in opposite directions, the filtrate is constantly being exposed to hypertonic blood, which allows maximal reabsorption of water.

As the descending limb transitions to become the ascending limb of the loop of Henle, a change in permeability occurs. The ascending limb is only permeable to salts and is impermeable to water. So while the descending limb maximizes water reabsorption by taking advantage of increasing medullary osmolarity, the ascending limb maximizes salt reabsorption by taking advantage of *decreasing* medullary osmolarity.

At the transition from the inner to outer medulla, the loop of Henle becomes thicker in what is termed the **diluting segment**. This is not because the lumen within the tube has enlarged, but because the cells lining the tube are larger. These cells contain large amounts of mitochondria, which allow the reabsorption of sodium and chloride by active transport. Indeed, because so much salt is reabsorbed while water is stuck in the nephron, the filtrate actually becomes hypotonic compared to the interstitium. While we tend to focus on the concentrating abilities of the nephron, this segment is noteworthy because it is the only portion of the nephron that can produce urine that is more dilute than the blood. This is important during periods of *overhydration* and provides a mechanism for eliminating excess water.

At the beginning of the loop of Henle, the filtrate is isotonic to the interstitium. Thus, from the beginning of the loop of Henle to the end, there is a slight degree of dilution. Far more important, however, is the fact that the volume of the filtrate has been significantly reduced, demonstrating a net reabsorption of a large volume of water.

Distal Convoluted Tubule

Next, the filtrate enters the **distal convoluted tubule (DCT)**. The DCT responds to aldosterone, which promotes sodium reabsorption. Because sodium ions are osmotically active particles, water will follow the sodium, concentrating the urine and decreasing its volume. The DCT is also a site of waste product secretion, like the PCT.

REAL WORLD

In certain conditions, such as congestive heart failure, the body accumulates excess fluid in the lungs or peripheral tissues (edema). The judicious use of a diuretic drug can help the body get rid of excess fluid. Diuretics typically inhibit the reabsorption of sodium in one or more regions of the nephron, thereby increasing sodium excretion. As an osmotically active particle, sodium will pull water with it, thereby relieving the body of some of its excess fluid.

Collecting Duct

The final concentration of the urine will depend largely on the permeability of the collecting duct, which is responsive to both aldosterone and antidiuretic hormone (ADH or vasopressin). As permeability of the collecting duct increases, so too does water reabsorption, resulting in further concentration of the urine. The reabsorbed water enters the interstitium and makes its way to the vasa recta, where it reenters the bloodstream to once again become part of the plasma. The collecting duct almost always reabsorbs water, but the amount is variable. When the body is very well hydrated, the collecting duct will be fairly impermeable to salt and water. When in conservation mode, ADH and aldosterone will each act to increase reabsorption of water in the collecting duct, allowing for greater water retention and more concentrated urine output.

Ultimately, anything that is not reabsorbed from the tubule by the end of the collecting duct will be excreted; the collecting duct is the point of no return. After that, there are no further opportunities for reabsorption. As the filtrate leaves the tubule, it collects in the renal pelvis. The fluid, which carries mostly urea, uric acid, and excess ions (sodium, potassium, magnesium, and calcium), flows through the ureter to the bladder where it is stored until voiding.

Functions of the Excretory System

The kidneys use osmolarity gradients and selective permeability to filter, secrete, and reabsorb materials in the process of making urine. However, these processes have larger implications for the human body as a whole. The selective elimination of water and solutes allows the kidneys, in conjunction with the endocrine, cardiovascular, and respiratory systems, to control blood pressure, blood osmolarity, and acid–base balance.

Blood Pressure

In Chapter 5 of *MCAT Biology Review*, we discussed two hormones that are very important for the maintenance of proper blood pressure: aldosterone and antidiuretic hormone (ADH or vasopressin).

Aldosterone is a steroid hormone that is secreted by the adrenal cortex in response to decreased blood pressure. Decreased blood pressure stimulates the release of **renin** from **juxtaglomerular cells** in the kidney. Renin then cleaves **angiotensinogen**, a liver protein, to form **angiotensin I**. This peptide is then metabolized by **angiotensin-converting enzyme** in the lungs to form **angiotensin II**, which promotes the release of aldosterone from the adrenal cortex.

REAL WORLD

Aldosterone increases blood pressure by increasing the reabsorption of sodium. In medicine, we exploit this characteristic by using drugs that actually block angiotensin-converting enzyme or the angiotensin II receptor. In Chapter 5 of *MCAT Biology Review*, we mentioned the ACE inhibitors, which mostly end with *-pril*. The angiotensin II receptor blockers mostly end with *-sartan* (*losartan*, *valsartan*, *irbesartan*). Blocking this receptor limits aldosterone release, which limits salt and water reabsorption, and therefore results in lowered blood pressure.

KEY CONCEPT

ADH only governs water reabsorption and thus results in a lower blood osmolarity. Aldosterone causes both salt and water reabsorption and does not change blood osmolarity.

Aldosterone works by altering the ability of the distal convoluted tubule and collecting duct to reabsorb sodium. Remember that water does not move on its own, but rather travels down its osmolarity gradient. Thus, if we reabsorb more sodium, water will flow with it. This reabsorption of isotonic fluid has the net effect of increasing blood volume and therefore blood pressure. Aldosterone will also increase potassium and hydrogen ion excretion.

Antidiuretic hormone (**ADH**, also known as **vasopressin**) is a peptide hormone synthesized by the hypothalamus and released by the posterior pituitary in response to high blood osmolarity. It directly alters the permeability of the collecting duct, allowing more water to be reabsorbed by making the cell junctions of the duct leaky. Increased concentration in the interstitium (hypertonic to the filtrate) will then cause the reabsorption of water from the tubule. Alcohol and caffeine both inhibit ADH release and lead to the frequent excretion of dilute urine.

In addition to the kidneys, the cardiovascular system also regulates blood pressure, specifically by vasoconstricting or vasodilating in order to maintain blood pressure. Constriction of the afferent arteriole will lead to a lower pressure of blood reaching the glomeruli, which are adjacent to the juxtaglomerular cells. Therefore, this vasoconstriction will secondarily lead to renin release, which will also help raise blood pressure.

Osmoregulation

The osmolarity of the blood must be tightly controlled to ensure correct oncotic pressures within the vasculature. A note on terminology: **osmotic pressure** is the "sucking" pressure that draws water into the vasculature caused by all dissolved particles. **Oncotic pressure**, on the other hand, is the osmotic pressure that is attributable to dissolved proteins specifically. Blood osmolarity is usually maintained at approximately 290 milliosmoles (mOsm) per liter. As described earlier, the kidneys control osmolarity by modulating the reabsorption of water and by filtering and secreting dissolved particles. When blood osmolarity is low, excess water will be excreted, while solutes will be reabsorbed in higher concentrations. In contrast, when blood osmolarity is high, water reabsorption increases and solute excretion increases.

Acid-Base Balance

The **bicarbonate buffer system** is the major regulator of blood pH. Remind yourself of the buffer equation:

$$CO_2\ (g) + H_2O\ (l) \rightleftharpoons H_2CO_3\ (aq) \rightleftharpoons H^+\ (aq) + HCO_3^-\ (aq)$$

In Chapter 6 of *MCAT Biology Review*, we talked about how the respiratory system can contribute to acid–base balance by increasing or decreasing the respiratory rate. If the blood pH is too low, then increasing the respiratory rate blows off more CO_2 and favors the conversion of H^+ and HCO_3^- to water and carbon dioxide, increasing the pH. If the blood pH is too high, then decreasing the respiratory rate causes the opposite effects. The respiratory system can react to derangements of pH quickly. What can the excretory system do to contribute? The kidneys are able to selectively increase or decrease the secretion of hydrogen ions and bicarbonate. When blood pH is too low, the kidneys excrete more hydrogen ions and increase reabsorption of bicarbonate, resulting in a higher pH. Likewise, when blood pH is too high, the kidneys can excrete more bicarbonate and increase the reabsorption of hydrogen ions. This is slower than the respiratory response, but it is a highly effective way for the body to maintain acid–base balance.

BIOLOGY GUIDED EXAMPLE WITH EXPERT THINKING

Carbonic anhydrases are a group of zinc metalloenzymes that catalyze the reversible hydration of carbon dioxide into carbonic acid, which in solution rapidly dissociates into bicarbonate and a proton. The second isoform, carbonic anhydrase II (CAII) is soluble and is expressed in most tissues including red blood cells, osteoclasts, and the kidney. CAII physically and functionally interacts with aquaporin-1 (AQP1) to increase permeability of AQP1 to water. AQP1 is expressed in the lumen facing and the interstitium facing membranes of the proximal tubule, as well as the thin descending limb (TDL) of the loop of Henle. Our observation that CAII augments water flux through AQP1 led us to posit that CAII may contribute to water reabsorption and consequently to urinary concentrating ability. To test this hypothesis, we examined water homeostasis in CAII-deficient (CAII def) mice. These mice were found to be polydipsic (high water intake) and polyuric (high urine volume). Analysis of the osmolarity of the urine is seen in Figure 1. We also measured the following properties in the interstitium of the renal cortex, inner strip of the outer medulla (ISOM), which lies between the cortex and the medulla, and the inner medulla (IM): osmolarity (Figure 2) and sodium ion concentration (Figure 3). *Represents $p < 0.05$

CA = enzyme that catalyzes CO_2 into bicarbonate ion

CAII isoform is expressed in most tissues

CAII interacts with AQP1 → more water reabsorption

APQ1 is found in the proximal convoluted tubule and descending limb of loop of Henle

Hypothesis: CAII helps with water resorption and concentrating urine

Knocked out CAII in mice, looked at water homeostasis

CAII-def mice drank lots of water, had high volume of urine

Fig 1: urine osmolarity

Looked at three different kidney areas: cortex, between cortex and medulla, and medulla

Fig 2: osmolarity in three kidney regions

Fig 3: sodium ion concentration in three kidney regions

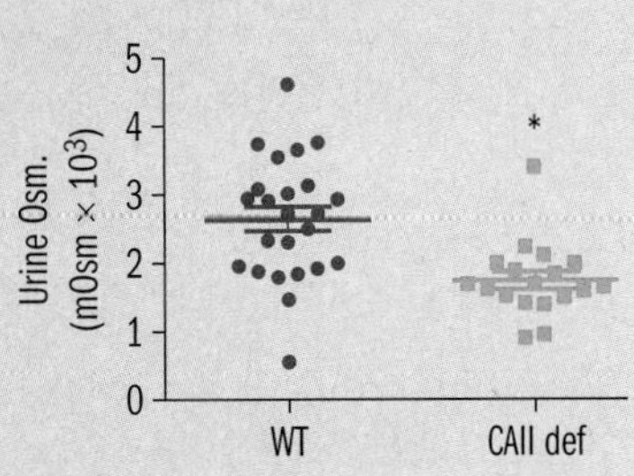

Figure 1

IV: wild-type or CAII-def mice

DV: urine osmolarity

Trend: CAII-def mice have significantly lower urine osmolarity

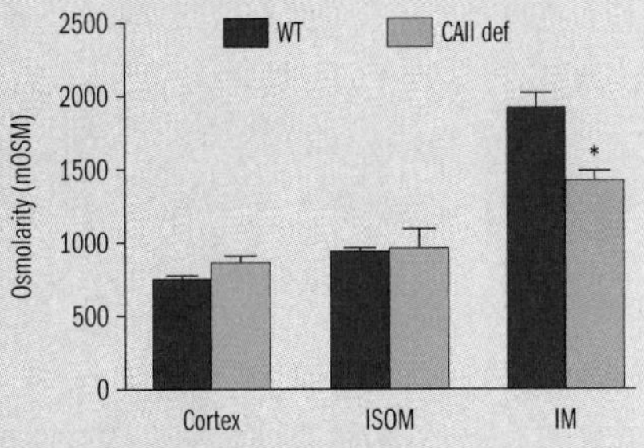

Figure 2

IV: region of kidney, type of mice (WT or CAII-def)

DV: interstitium osmolarity

Trend: inner medulla of kidney interstitium has significantly lower osmolarity in CAII-def mice compared to WT

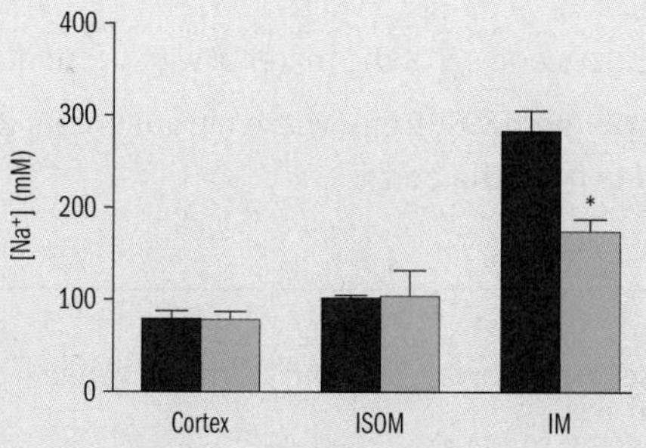

Figure 3

IV: region of kidney, type of mice (WT or CAII-def)

DV: interstitium sodium concentration

Trend: inner medulla of kidney interstitium has significantly lower sodium concentration in CAII-def mice compared to WT

Adapted from Krishnan, D., Pan, W., Beggs, M. R., Trepiccione, F., Chambrey, R., Eladari, D., Cordat, E., Dimke, H., ... Alexander, R. T. (2018). Deficiency of carbonic anhydrase II results in a urinary concentrating defect. *Frontiers in Physiology* 8, 1108. doi:10.3389/fphys.2017.01108.

According to the data, lack of CAII has the greatest impact on which portion of the nephron?

Since the question is asking us to use the data to pinpoint a specific area of the nephron being affected, it's important to understand the experimental setup and the results, and to be prepared to use our outside content knowledge. The researcher's goal is to better understand the role CAII plays in water resorption through its interaction with AQP1. We should know from our content background that aquaporin (AQP) is a water-specific membrane channel found in many parts of the nephron, and AQP availability on the membrane allows for movement of water from the filtrate back into the body. We're also given some information about CAII—it's the enzyme responsible for creating bicarbonate ions, and we're told it interacts with AQP1 to increase water permeability.

In creating mice with deficient CAII, the researchers are looking for a change in the osmolarity of the urine and the kidney. We're told in paragraph 2 that the CAII-deficient mice have a high urine volume and high water intake, supporting the hypothesis that the mice are not reabsorbing enough water, but instead are excreting it as urine. Figure 1 also supports this conclusion by showing that urine is more dilute in CAII-deficient mice than in wild-type (controls). However, this data doesn't answer the question of where specifically in the nephron lack of CAII is having the greatest impact. Figures 2 and 3 both have information about specific parts of the kidney, which is where our answer is going to come from. Recall that cortex refers to the outer region of the organ, while medulla refers to the inner part. We're given an additional area called the ISOM, which is the boundary between the cortex and medulla. We can see from those two figures that the osmolarity of the interstitium in the inner medulla (IM) is significantly lower than in normal mice, indicating that the part of the nephron existing in the inner medulla is the problem area. Paragraph 1 states that AQP1 is found in the proximal tubule and the thin descending limb of the loop of Henle. The proximal tubule would be in the outer part of the kidney in the cortex, and the thin descending limb would go deep into the kidney, moving into the inner medulla, making the descending limb the part of the nephron that is being most affected. While this satisfies the requirements of the question, this brings up another issue: why does less water being reabsorbed into the interstitium result in less osmolarity? Shouldn't the expected result be a higher osmolarity? This ultimately comes down to how the nephron works as a whole to concentrate your urine. Lack of water being reabsorbed by the thin descending limb will result in a decrease of ions being passively reabsorbed in the ascending limb, giving us that drop in osmolarity.

Using the results of the data, we can conclude that the CAII-deficient mice are being most impacted by the reduced efficacy of AQP1 in the thin descending limb of the loop of Henle.

MCAT CONCEPT CHECK 10.1

Before you move on, assess your understanding of the material with these questions.

1. List the structures in the excretory pathway, from where filtrate enters the nephron to the excretion of urine from the body.

____

2. List the vessels in the renal vascular pathway, starting from the renal artery and ending at the renal vein.

____

3. What arm of the nervous system is responsible for contraction of the detrusor muscle?

____

4. What are the three processes by which solutes are exchanged between the filtrate and the blood? What happens in each process?

    -
    ____
    -
    ____
    -
    ____

5. For each segment of the nephron listed below, what are its major functions?

    - Bowman's capsule:
    ____
    - Proximal convoluted tubule:
    ____
    - Descending limb of the loop of Henle:
    ____
    - Ascending limb of the loop of Henle:
    ____
    - Distal convoluted tubule:
    ____
    - Collecting duct:
    ____

10.2 Skin

LEARNING OBJECTIVES

After Chapter 10.2, you will be able to:

- Recall the predominant cell type in the epidermis
- Order the layers of the epidermis and dermis
- Describe the mechanisms the body uses to regulate temperature using the integument

By both weight and size, the **skin** (**integument**) is the largest organ in our bodies. It makes up about 16 percent of total body weight, on average. Skin is one of the major components of nonspecific immune defense, protecting us from exposure to the elements and invasion by pathogens.

Structure

The skin has several layers. Starting from the deepest layer and working outward, these layers are the **hypodermis** (**subcutaneous** layer), **dermis**, and **epidermis**, as shown in Figure 10.6. Skin is derived from the ectoderm.

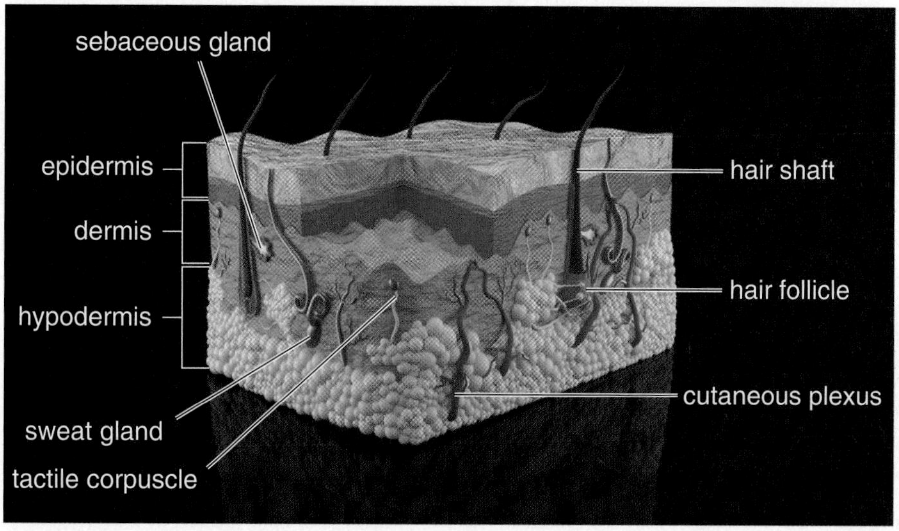

Figure 10.6 Anatomy of the Skin and Subcutaneous Tissue

The Epidermis

The **epidermis** is also subdivided into layers called **strata**. From the deepest layer outward, these are the stratum basale, stratum spinosum, stratum granulosum, stratum lucidum, and stratum corneum, as shown in Figure 10.7. The **stratum basale** contains stem cells and is responsible for proliferation of **keratinocytes**, the predominant cells of the skin, that produce **keratin**. In the **stratum spinosum**, these cells become connected to each other; this layer is also the site of Langerhans cells, described below. In the **stratum granulosum**, the keratinocytes die and lose their nuclei. The **stratum lucidum** is only present in thick, hairless skin, such as the skin on the sole of the foot or the palms, and is nearly transparent. Finally, the **stratum corneum** contains up to several dozen layers of flattened keratinocytes, forming a barrier that prevents invasion by pathogens and that helps to prevent loss of fluids and salt. Hair projects above the skin, and there are openings for sweat and sebaceous glands.

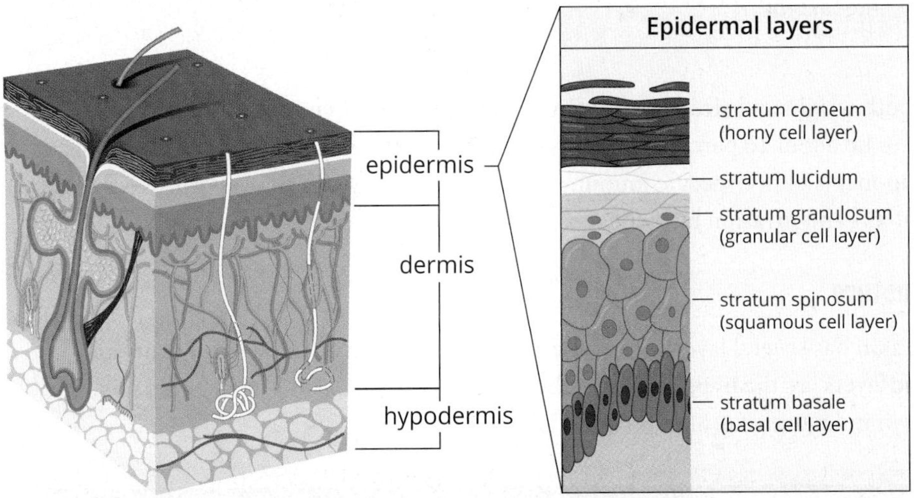

Figure 10.7 Layers of the Epidermis

Other Cells of the Epidermis

In the epidermis, the main cells are keratinocytes. Keratin, mentioned above, is resistant to damage and provides protection against injury, water, and pathogens. **Calluses** form from excessive keratin deposition in areas of repeated strain due to friction; they provide protection to avoid damage in the future. **Fingernails** and **hair** are also formed from keratin and are produced by specialized cells in the skin.

Melanocytes are a cell type derived from neural crest cells and found in the stratum basale. These cells produce **melanin**, a pigment that serves to protect the skin from DNA damage caused by ultraviolet radiation. Once produced, the pigment is transferred to the keratinocytes. All humans have comparable numbers of melanocytes; skin color is caused by varying levels of activity of the melanocytes. More active melanocytes result in darker skin tones. Upon exposure to ultraviolet radiation, melanocytes increase activity, resulting in a darker skin color.

Langerhans cells are actually special macrophages that reside within the stratum spinosum. These cells are capable of presenting antigens to T-cells in order to activate the immune system.

MNEMONIC

Layers of the skin (superficial to deep): **C**ome, **L**et's **G**et **S**un **B**urned

- Stratum **c**orneum
- Stratum **l**ucidum
- Stratum **g**ranulosum
- Stratum **s**pinosum
- Stratum **b**asale

REAL WORLD

People who have albinism suffer from a genetic metabolic disorder characterized by the inability to synthesize melanin. Typically, albinism is inherited in an autosomal recessive fashion. As would be expected, patients with albinism are extremely sensitive to the harmful effects of the sun. Depigmentation can also occur in vitiligo, an autoimmune disorder in which melanocytes are killed by the individual's immune system.

The Dermis

The dermis also consists of multiple layers. The upper layer (right below the epidermis) is the **papillary layer**, which consists of loose connective tissue. Below the papillary layer is the denser **reticular layer**. Sweat glands, blood vessels, and hair follicles originate in the dermis.

Most sensory receptors are also located in the dermis. **Merkel cells (discs)**, for example, are sensory receptors present at the epidermal–dermal junction. These cells are connected to sensory neurons and are responsible for deep pressure and texture sensation within the skin. Other sensory organs in the skin include free nerve endings, which respond to pain; **Meissner's corpuscles**, which respond to light touch; **Ruffini endings**, which respond to stretch; and **Pacinian corpuscles**, which respond to deep pressure and vibration.

BRIDGE

Evaporation is an endothermic process and, thus, substances absorb energy from the surroundings to undergo this phase change. Further, the presence of dissolved solutes in sweat increases the boiling point of sweat slightly in comparison to pure water; this allows the absorption of even more heat energy. Boiling point elevation is a colligative property that is discussed in Chapter 9 of *MCAT General Chemistry Review.*

The Hypodermis

Finally, the **hypodermis** is a layer of connective tissue that connects the skin to the rest of the body. This layer contains fat and fibrous tissue.

Thermoregulation

We have already mentioned that the skin protects us from the elements and microbes. It also has other functions, including ultraviolet protection (via melanin) and transduction of sensory information from the outside world. In this section, we look at another function of the skin: thermoregulation.

Thermoregulation is achieved by sweating, piloerection, vasodilation, and vasoconstriction. **Sweating** is an excellent cooling mechanism that is controlled by the autonomic nervous system. When body temperature rises above the set point determined by the hypothalamus, thermoregulation processes must occur in order to rid the body of heat. Postganglionic sympathetic neurons that utilize acetylcholine innervate sweat glands and promote the secretion of water with certain ions onto the skin. Heat is then absorbed from the body as the water molecules undergo a phase change to evaporate. The production of sweat itself is not the main mechanism of cooling; it is the evaporation of water from the skin which absorbs body heat. At the same time, arteriolar vasodilation occurs to maximize heat loss. This brings a large quantity of blood to the skin, which accelerates the evaporation of sweat by maximizing the heat energy available for the liquid–gas phase change.

BRIDGE

The neurons that innervate sweat glands are actually very unusual. Unlike all other postganglionic sympathetic neurons, these neurons are cholinergic—not noradrenergic (that is, they release acetylcholine, not norepinephrine). All preganglionic neurons in the autonomic nervous system and postganglionic neurons in the parasympathetic nervous system are cholinergic as well. These neurons are discussed in Chapter 4 of *MCAT Biology Review.*

In cold conditions, **arrector pili** muscles contract, causing the hairs of the skin to stand up on end (**piloerection**). This helps to trap a layer of heated air near the skin. The arterioles that feed the capillaries of the skin constrict, limiting the quantity of blood reaching the skin. Skeletal muscle may also begin to contract rapidly, causing shivering. **Shivering** requires a sizeable amount of ATP; however, a significant portion of the energy from ATP is converted into thermal energy. In addition to these mechanisms, humans possess a layer of fat just below the skin. This fat helps to insulate the body. In addition to this fat, which is called **white fat**, **brown fat** may also be present, especially in infants. Brown fat has a much less efficient electron transport chain, which means that more heat energy is released as fuel is burned.

The skin also helps to maintain the osmolarity of the body. This is because the skin is relatively impermeable to water. This prevents not only the entrance of water through the skin, but also the loss of water from the tissues. This becomes very important in cases such as burns or large losses of skin as dehydration of the tissues becomes a real threat to survival.

MCAT CONCEPT CHECK 10.2

Before you move on, assess your understanding of the material with these questions.

1. What is the predominant cell type in the epidermis?

____

2. What are the layers of the epidermis, from superficial to deep?
   - ______________________________
   - ______________________________
   - ______________________________
   - ______________________________
   - ______________________________

3. What are the layers of the dermis, from superficial to deep?
   - ______________________________
   - ______________________________

4. What are some mechanisms the body uses to cool itself? What are some mechanisms the body uses to retain heat?
   - Cooling:
   ____
   - Retaining heat:
   ____

Conclusion

Two main organ systems were discussed in this chapter: the excretory system and the skin. Both of these systems play an essential role in homeostasis. However, this chapter also demonstrated a very MCAT-worthy concept: no system works alone. Multiple systems participate in homeostasis. While the kidneys are the major players in salt, water, and acid–base balance, their function depends on the endocrine system, circulatory system, and respiratory system. While the skin is an important immune organ in and of itself, its function as a thermoregulatory organ is dependent on the nervous system—and it also sends sensory signals *to* the nervous system. As you move on to the last organ system in the next chapter—the musculoskeletal system—notice how each system interacts with other systems in order to produce a fully functioning organism. The MCAT is far more focused on how you conceptualize the big picture, and not on how many details you memorize. As you study, focus on understanding these systems and how each system influences the rest of the body.

GO ONLINE

You've reviewed the content, now test your knowledge and critical thinking skills by completing a test-like passage set in your online resources!

CONCEPT SUMMARY

The Excretory System

- The **excretory system** serves many functions, including the regulation of blood pressure, blood osmolarity, acid–base balance, and removal of nitrogenous wastes.
- The **kidney** produces urine, which flows into the **ureter** at the **renal pelvis.** Urine is then collected in the **bladder** until it is excreted through the **urethra**.
- The kidney contains a cortex and a medulla. Each kidney has a **hilum**, which contains a renal artery, renal vein, and ureter.
- The kidney contains a **portal system** with two capillary beds in series.
  - Blood from the renal artery flows into **afferent arterioles**, which form **glomeruli** in Bowman's capsule (the first capillary bed).
  - Blood then flows through the **efferent arteriole** to the **vasa recta** (the second capillary bed), which surround the nephron, before leaving the kidney through the renal vein.
- The bladder has a muscular lining known as the **detrusor muscle**, which is under parasympathetic control. It also has two muscular sphincters.
  - The **internal urethral sphincter** consists of smooth muscle and is under involuntary (parasympathetic) control.
  - The **external urethral sphincter** consists of skeletal muscle and is under voluntary control.
- The kidney participates in solute movement through three processes:
  - **Filtration** is the movement of solutes from blood to filtrate at Bowman's capsule. The direction and rate of filtration is determined by **Starling forces**, which account for the hydrostatic and oncotic pressure differentials between the glomerulus and Bowman's space.
  - **Secretion** is the movement of solutes from blood to filtrate anywhere other than Bowman's capsule.
  - **Reabsorption** is the movement of solutes from filtrate to blood.
- Each segment of the nephron has a specific function.
  - The **proximal convoluted tubule** (**PCT**) is the site of bulk reabsorption of glucose, amino acids, soluble vitamins, salt, and water. It is also the site of secretion for hydrogen ions, potassium ions, ammonia, and urea.
  - The **descending limb of the loop of Henle** is permeable to water but not salt; therefore, as the filtrate moves into the more osmotically concentrated renal medulla, water is reabsorbed from the filtrate. The vasa recta and nephron flow in opposite directions, creating a **countercurrent multiplier system** that allows maximal reabsorption of water.

  - The **ascending limb of the loop of Henle** is permeable to salt but not water; therefore, salt is reabsorbed both passively and actively. The **diluting segment** is in the outer medulla; because salt is actively reabsorbed in this site, the filtrate actually becomes hypotonic compared to the blood.
  - The **distal convoluted tubule** (**DCT**) is responsive to aldosterone and is a site of salt reabsorption and waste product excretion, like the PCT.
  - The **collecting duct** is responsive to both aldosterone and antidiuretic hormone and has variable permeability, which allows reabsorption of the right amount of water depending on the body's needs.
- The kidney is under hormonal control. When blood pressure (and volume) are low, two different hormonal systems are activated.
  - **Aldosterone** is a steroid hormone regulated by the renin–angiotensin–aldosterone system that increases sodium reabsorption in the distal convoluted tubule and collecting duct, thereby increasing water reabsorption. This results in an increased blood volume (and pressure), but no change in blood osmolarity.
  - **Antidiuretic hormone** (**ADH** or **vasopressin**) is a peptide hormone synthesized by the hypothalamus and released by the posterior pituitary. Its release is stimulated not only by low blood volume but also by high blood osmolarity. It increases the permeability of the collecting duct to water, increasing water reabsorption. This results in an increased blood volume (and pressure) and a decreased blood osmolarity.
- The kidney can regulate pH by selective reabsorption or secretion of bicarbonate or hydrogen ions.

Skin

- The skin acts as a barrier, protecting us from the elements and invasion by pathogens.
- The skin is composed of three major layers: the **hypodermis** (**subcutaneous** layer), **dermis**, and **epidermis**.
  - The epidermis is composed of five layers: the **stratum basale**, **stratum spinosum**, **stratum granulosum**, **stratum lucidum**, and **stratum corneum**. The stratum basale contains stem cells that proliferate to form keratinocytes. Keratinocyte nuclei are lost in the stratum granulosum, and many thin layers form in the stratum corneum.
  - **Melanocytes** produce **melanin**, which protects the skin from DNA damage caused by ultraviolet radiation; melanin is passed to keratinocytes.
  - **Langerhans cells** are special macrophages that serve as antigen-presenting cells in the skin.

- The dermis is composed of two layers: the **papillary layer** and the **reticular layer**.
- Many sensory cells are located in the dermis, including **Merkel cells** (deep pressure and texture), free nerve endings (pain), **Meissner's corpuscles** (light touch), **Ruffini endings** (stretch), and **Pacinian corpuscles** (deep pressure and vibration).
- The hypodermis contains fat and connective tissue and connects the skin to the rest of the body.

- The skin is important for thermoregulation, or the maintenance of a constant internal temperature.
  - Cooling mechanisms include **sweating**, which draws heat from the body through evaporation of water from sweat, and vasodilation. Sweat glands are innervated by postganglionic cholinergic sympathetic neurons.
  - Warming mechanisms include: piloerection, in which arrector pili muscles contract, causing hairs to stand on end (trapping a layer of warmed air around the skin); vasoconstriction; shivering; and insulation provided by fat.
- The skin also prevents dehydration and salt loss from the body.

ANSWERS TO CONCEPT CHECKS

10.1

1. Bowman's space → proximal convoluted tubule → descending limb of the loop of Henle → ascending limb of the loop of Henle → distal convoluted tubule → collecting duct → renal pelvis → ureter → bladder → urethra
2. Renal artery → afferent arteriole → glomerulus → efferent arteriole → vasa recta → renal vein
3. The parasympathetic nervous system causes contraction of the detrusor muscle.
4. Filtration is the movement of solutes from blood into filtrate at Bowman's capsule. Secretion is the movement of solutes from blood into filtrate anywhere besides Bowman's capsule. Reabsorption is the movement of solutes from filtrate into blood.
5. Bowman's capsule is the site of filtration, through which water, ions, amino acids, vitamins, and glucose pass (essentially everything besides cells and proteins). The proximal convoluted tubule controls solute identity, reabsorbing vitamins, amino acids, and glucose, while secreting potassium and hydrogen ions, ammonia, and urea. The descending limb of the loop of Henle is important for water reabsorption, and uses the medullary concentration gradient. The ascending limb of the loop of Henle is important for salt reabsorption and dilution of the urine in the diluting segment. The distal convoluted tubule, like the PCT, is important for solute identity by reabsorbing salts while secreting potassium and hydrogen ions, ammonia, and urea. The collecting duct is important for urine concentration; its variable permeability allows water to be reabsorbed based on the needs of the body.

10.2

1. Keratinocytes are the primary cells of the epidermis.
2. Stratum corneum, stratum lucidum, stratum granulosum, stratum spinosum, stratum basale
3. The papillary layer and the reticular layer
4. The body can cool itself through sweating and vasodilation. The body can warm itself through vasoconstriction, piloerection, and shivering.

SCIENCE MASTERY ASSESSMENT EXPLANATIONS

1. **B**

The glomerulus functions like a sieve; small molecules dissolved in the fluid will pass through the glomerulus, including glucose, which is later reabsorbed. Large molecules, such as proteins, and cells, such as erythrocytes and platelets, will not be able to pass through the glomerular filter.

2. **B**

Sodium is actively transported out of the nephron in the proximal and distal convoluted tubules, where the concentration of sodium outside of the nephron is higher than inside; thus, energy is required to transport the sodium molecules against their concentration gradient, eliminating **(A)** and **(C)**. In the inner medulla, however, sodium and other ions (such as chloride) diffuse passively down their concentration gradients at the thin ascending limb of the loop of Henle, making **(B)** the correct answer. The thick ascending limb of the loop of Henle is thick because its cells contain many mitochondria—which produce the ATP needed for active transport of sodium and chloride out of the filtrate, eliminating **(D)**.

3. **A**

The region of the kidney that has the lowest solute concentration is the cortex, where the proximal convoluted tubule and a part of the distal convoluted tubule are found. The solute concentration increases as one descends into the medulla, and concentrated urine can be found in the renal pelvis.

4. **A**

Blood enters the kidney through the renal artery, which divides into many afferent arterioles that run through the medulla and into the cortex. Each afferent arteriole branches into a convoluted network of capillaries called a glomerulus. Rather than converging directly into a vein, the capillaries converge into an efferent arteriole, which divides into a fine capillary network known as the vasa recta. The vasa recta capillaries envelop the nephron tubule, where they reabsorb various ions, and then converge into the renal vein. The arrangement of tandem capillary beds is known as a portal system.

5. **C**

All of the answer choices describe ADH or aldosterone. These two hormones ultimately act to increase water reabsorption in the kidney; their respective mechanisms of action, however, are different. ADH increases water reabsorption by increasing the permeability of the collecting duct to water, whereas aldosterone stimulates reabsorption of sodium from the distal convoluted tubule and collecting duct. Using this knowledge, we can now evaluate the answer choices. **(C)** is the correct answer because ADH does not act on the proximal convoluted tubule, but rather on the collecting duct.

6. **D**

Essential substances, such as glucose, salts, amino acids, and water, are reabsorbed from the filtrate and returned to the blood in the vasa recta. In general, reabsorption refers to the movement of solutes from the filtrate back into the blood.

7. **A**

The hypothalamus functions as a thermostat that regulates body temperature. When it's cold outside, nervous stimulation to the blood vessels in the skin is increased, causing the vessels to constrict. This constriction diminishes blood flow to the skin surface and prevents heat loss. Sweat glands are turned off to prevent heat loss through evaporation. Skeletal muscles are stimulated to shiver (rapidly contract), which increases the metabolic rate and produces heat. The hypothalamus is also involved in other processes, including the release of endocrine hormones, regulation of appetite, and circadian rhythms.

8. **C**

The filtrate enters Bowman's capsule and then flows into the proximal convoluted tubule, where virtually all glucose, amino acids, and other important organic molecules are reabsorbed via active transport.

9. **A**

The kidneys function to eliminate wastes such as urea, while reabsorbing various important substances such as glucose and amino acids for reuse by the body. Generation of a solute concentration gradient from the cortex to the medulla allows a considerable amount of water to be reabsorbed. Excretion of concentrated urine serves to limit water losses from the body and helps to preserve blood volume. Thus, the primary function of the nephron is to create urine that is hypertonic to the blood, making **(A)** the correct answer and eliminating **(B)** and **(D)**. Water should be reabsorbed from the filtrate, so urine should be hypertonic to the filtrate, eliminating **(C)**.

10. **A**

The glomerulus is the most likely location of pathology if large proteins are detected in the urine. This is because large proteins should not be able to pass through the filter of the glomerulus in the first place. Once large proteins are in the filtrate, no other nephron structure can reabsorb them. Thus, the only likely source of protein in the urine is glomerular pathology.

11. **C**

The layer of the skin that is predominantly loose connective tissue is the papillary layer of the dermis. The stratum corneum and stratum lucidum, **(A)** and **(B)**, contain dead keratinocytes, while the reticular layer, **(D)**, consists of dense connective tissue.

12. **D**

When the pH of the blood is high, this indicates that the blood is alkalemic. In order to correct the pH of the blood, the kidney will increase the excretion of a base, namely bicarbonate. Excretion of urea would have little effect on the pH, eliminating **(A)**. While ammonia is a base, it is quite toxic and is generally converted into urea before excretion, eliminating **(B)**. Excretion of hydrogen ions would exacerbate the alkalemia, eliminating **(C)**.

13. **C**

The stratum basale contains the stem cells that proliferate to form keratinocytes, which then ascend through the other layers of skin until they are shed from the stratum corneum.

14. **B**

Normally, angiotensin II causes secretion of aldosterone from the adrenal cortex. Aldosterone serves to increase reabsorption of sodium, while promoting excretion of potassium and hydrogen ions. Thus, blocking the release of aldosterone should result in decreased reabsorption of sodium, while decreasing excretion of potassium and hydrogen ions. This eliminates **(A)** and **(D)** and makes **(B)** the correct answer. In the absence of aldosterone, less sodium reabsorption will occur, leading to less water reabsorption, eliminating **(C)**.

15. **A**

An excess of acetylcholine will lead to activation of all parasympathetic neurons, preganglionic sympathetic neurons, and the postganglionic sympathetic neurons that innervate sweat glands. Because the parasympathetic nervous system causes contraction of the bladder, one would expect increased urination. The increased activation of sweat glands would lead to increased sweating as well.

GO ONLINE **Consult your online resources for additional practice.**

SHARED CONCEPTS

Behavioral Sciences Chapter 2
Sensation and Perception

Biochemistry Chapter 8
Biological Membranes

Biology Chapter 6
The Respiratory System

Biology Chapter 7
The Cardiovascular System

Biology Chapter 8
The Immune System

General Chemistry Chapter 9
Solutions

CHAPTER 11

THE MUSCULOSKELETAL SYSTEM

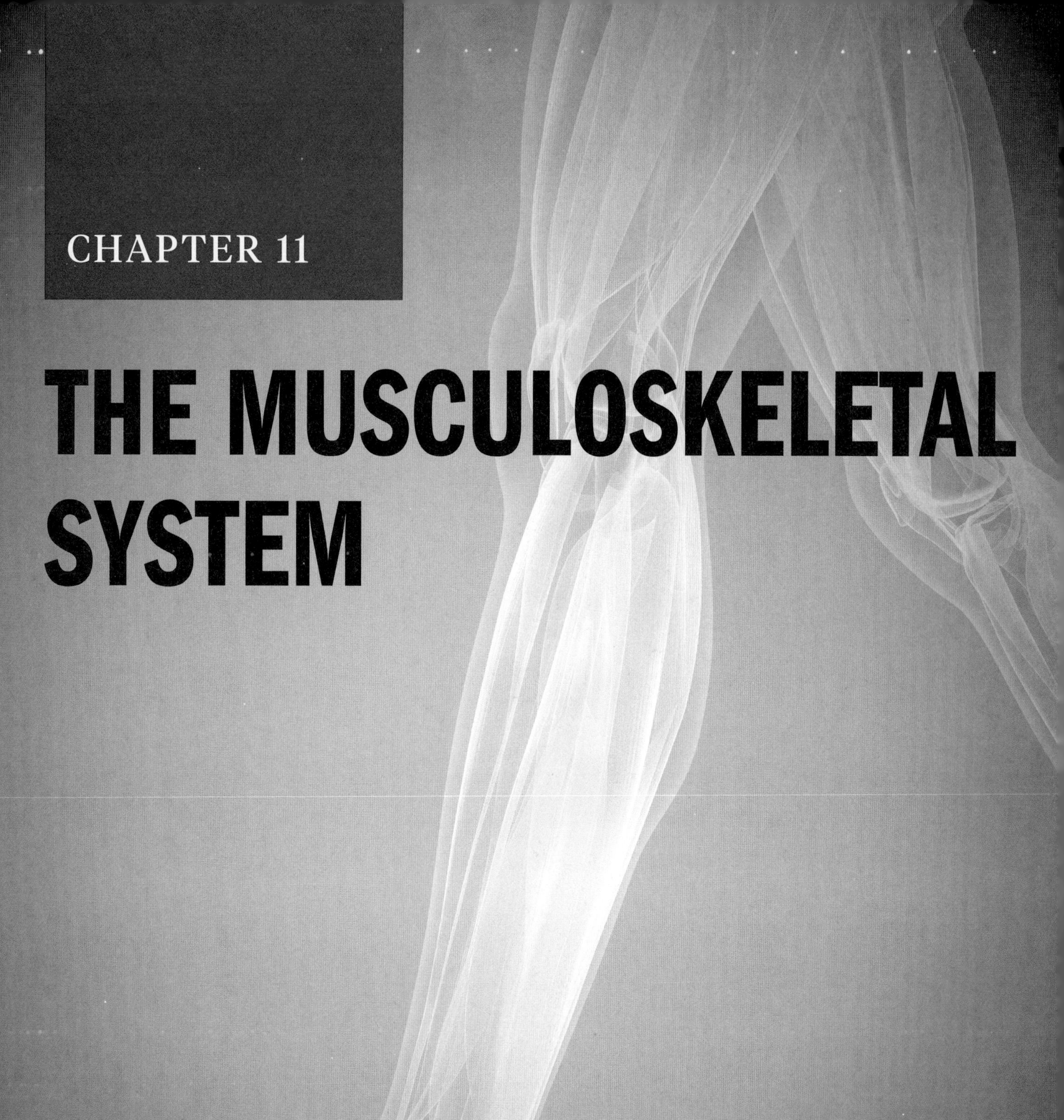

SCIENCE MASTERY ASSESSMENT

Every pre-med knows this feeling: there is so much content I have to know for the MCAT! How do I know what to do first or what's important?

While the high-yield badges throughout this book will help you identify the most important topics, this Science Mastery Assessment is another tool in your MCAT prep arsenal. This quiz (which can also be taken in your online resources) and the guidance below will help ensure that you are spending the appropriate amount of time on this chapter based on your personal strengths and weaknesses. Don't worry though—skipping something now does not mean you'll never study it. Later on in your prep, as you complete full-length tests, you'll uncover specific pieces of content that you need to review and can come back to these chapters as appropriate.

How to Use This Assessment

If you answer 0–7 questions correctly:

Spend about 1 hour to read this chapter in full and take limited notes throughout. Follow up by reviewing **all** quiz questions to ensure that you now understand how to solve each one.

If you answer 8–11 questions correctly:

Spend 20–40 minutes reviewing the quiz questions. Beginning with the questions you missed, read and take notes on the corresponding subchapters. For questions you answered correctly, ensure your thinking matches that of the explanation and you understand why each choice was correct or incorrect.

If you answer 12–15 questions correctly:

Spend less than 20 minutes reviewing all questions from the quiz. If you missed any, then include a quick read-through of the corresponding subchapters, or even just the relevant content within a subchapter, as part of your question review. For questions you answered correctly, ensure your thinking matches that of the explanation and review the Concept Summary at the end of the chapter.

Questions 1, 2, and 3 are based on the following diagram:

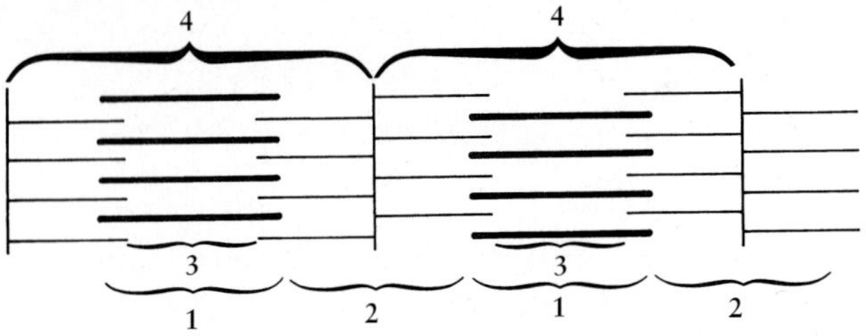

1. During muscle contraction, which of the following regions decrease(s) in length?
   - **A.** 1 only
   - **B.** 1 and 2 only
   - **C.** 3 and 4 only
   - **D.** 2, 3, and 4 only

2. Region 1 refers to:
   - **A.** the thick filaments only.
   - **B.** the thin filaments only.
   - **C.** the A-band.
   - **D.** the I-band.

3. Which region represents one sarcomere?
   - **A.** 1
   - **B.** 2
   - **C.** 3
   - **D.** 4

4. With which of the following molecules does Ca^{2+} bind after its release from the sarcoplasmic reticulum to regulate muscle contraction?
   - **A.** Myosin
   - **B.** Actin
   - **C.** Troponin
   - **D.** Tropomyosin

5. Which of the following cells is correctly coupled with its definition?
   - **A.** Osteoblasts—bone cells involved in the secretion of bone matrix
   - **B.** Osteoclasts—immature bone cells
   - **C.** Osteocytes—polynucleated cells actively involved in bone resorption
   - **D.** Chondrocytes—undifferentiated bone marrow cells

6. An X-ray of the right femur in a child shows that it is shorter than the opposite femur, and below the average length for a child of this age. Which region of the bone is most likely to have caused this abnormality?
   - **A.** Diaphysis
   - **B.** Metaphysis
   - **C.** Epiphysis
   - **D.** Periosteum

7. Which of the following INCORRECTLY pairs a type of muscle fiber with a characteristic of that fiber?
   - **A.** Red fibers—rich in mitochondria
   - **B.** Red fibers—high levels of myoglobin
   - **C.** White fibers—fast-twitching
   - **D.** White fibers—predominantly use aerobic respiration

8. When the knee moves back and forth during walking, what prevents the surfaces of the leg bones from rubbing against each other?
   - **A.** Articular cartilage
   - **B.** Epiphyses
   - **C.** Synovial fluid
   - **D.** Smooth muscle

9. Which type(s) of muscle is/are always multinucleated?
   - **I.** Cardiac muscle
   - **II.** Skeletal muscle
   - **III.** Smooth muscle

   - **A.** I only
   - **B.** II only
   - **C.** III only
   - **D.** I and II only

10. Which type(s) of muscle has/have myogenic activity?

- **I.** Cardiac muscle
- **II.** Skeletal muscle
- **III.** Smooth muscle

- **A.** I only
- **B.** II only
- **C.** III only
- **D.** I and III only

11. Red bone marrow is involved in erythrocyte formation. In contrast, yellow bone marrow:

- **A.** is involved in leukocyte formation.
- **B.** is responsible for drainage of lymph.
- **C.** causes the formation of spicules.
- **D.** contains predominantly adipose tissue.

12. Which of the following statements regarding the periosteum is INCORRECT?

- **A.** The periosteum serves as a site of attachment of bone to muscle.
- **B.** Cells of the periosteum may differentiate into osteoblasts.
- **C.** The periosteum is a fibrous sheath that surrounds long bones.
- **D.** The periosteum secretes fluid into the joint cavity.

13. Which of the following bones is NOT a part of the appendicular skeleton?

- **A.** The triquetrum, one of the carpal bones
- **B.** The calcaneus, which forms the heel
- **C.** The ischium, one of the fused pelvic bones
- **D.** The sternum, or breastbone

14. To facilitate the process of birth, an infant's head is somewhat flexible. This flexibility is due in part to the two fontanelles, which are soft spots of connective tissue in the infant's skull. With time, the fontanelles will close through a process known as:

- **A.** endochondral ossification.
- **B.** intramembranous ossification.
- **C.** bone resorption.
- **D.** longitudinal growth.

15. A young patient presents to the emergency room with a broken hip. The patient denies any recent history of trauma to the joint. Blood tests reveal a calcium concentration of 11.5 $\frac{\text{mg}}{\text{dL}}$ (normal: 8.4–10.2). Which tissue is likely responsible for these findings?

- **A.** Thyroid
- **B.** Cartilage
- **C.** Parathyroid
- **D.** Smooth muscle

Answer Key

1. **D**
2. **C**
3. **D**
4. **C**
5. **A**
6. **C**
7. **D**
8. **A**
9. **B**
10. **D**
11. **D**
12. **D**
13. **D**
14. **B**
15. **C**

Detailed explanations can be found at the end of the chapter.

CHAPTER 11

THE MUSCULOSKELETAL SYSTEM

In This Chapter

CHAPTER PROFILE

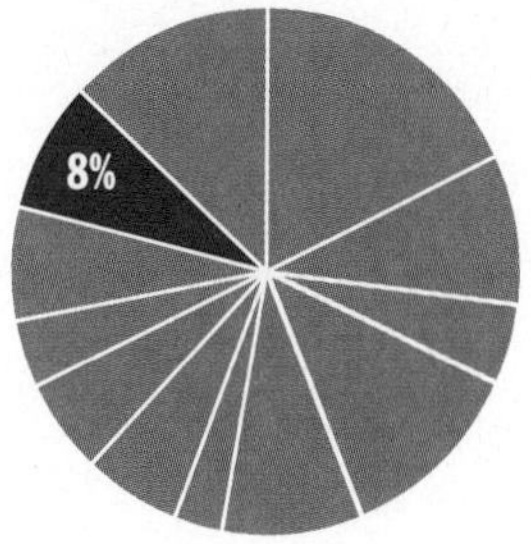

The content in this chapter should be relevant to about 8% of all questions about biology on the MCAT.

This chapter covers material from the following AAMC content category:

3B: Structure and integrative functions of the main organ systems

Introduction

Large disasters or traumatic events like wars or earthquakes can deeply affect the health of populations, which also has an impact on the practice of medicine, sometimes leading to the discovery of new medical conditions. During World War II, Nazi Germany bombed London for 57 consecutive days during the beginning of what came to be known as the *Blitzkrieg*, or an eight-month "lightning war." Victims of the Blitz, as it is known in London, included those afflicted with a specific set of symptoms: pain and swelling with accompanying effects of depleted blood volume (shock, weakness, low blood pressure, and decreased urine output). Less obvious was acute kidney failure, which could lead quickly to death if left untreated.

What caused the Blitz victims to suffer from these symptoms? Extreme physical trauma to muscles—namely, compression—destroys skeletal muscle tissue. This condition is called *rhabdomyolysis* (*rhabdo–* refers to striation, *myo–* to muscle, and *–lysis* to breakdown). The products of skeletal muscle destruction, some of which are toxic, circulate in the blood until they are filtered out. *Creatine kinase* is one of these products; in fact, rhabdomyolysis is diagnosed with a creatine kinase level five times the normal upper limit. Myoglobin is another. Much like hemoglobin, myoglobin uses heme to carry oxygen; it is not, however, housed within a red blood cell. Thus, an erythrocyte-free urine sample that tests positive for heme points compellingly toward rhabdomyolysis. Myoglobin oxygen reserves are just one of the specialized features of muscles, as we will see in this chapter.

Skeletal muscles are only able to exert an effect on the body by moving bony structures around joints. Further, skeletal muscle isn't the only form of muscle in the body; smooth muscle plays roles in the cardiovascular, respiratory, reproductive, and digestive systems, and cardiac muscle comprises the contractile tissue of the heart.

Bones are more than simply a support structure, however; they also provide protection to internal organs, serve as a storage reserve of calcium and other minerals, and are the site of hematopoiesis. In this chapter, we'll explore the biology of all of these tissues, completing our tour of systems anatomy and physiology.

11.1 The Muscular System

High-Yield

LEARNING OBJECTIVES

After Chapter 11.1, you will be able to:

- Categorize muscles as skeletal, smooth, or cardiac based on their innervation and structure
- Order the series of events in muscular contraction
- Explain the relationship between ATP binding and muscular contraction
- Recall the meaning of the terms summation, simple twitch, and tetanus
- Identify the zones and bands within a sarcomere and predict their length changes during contraction:

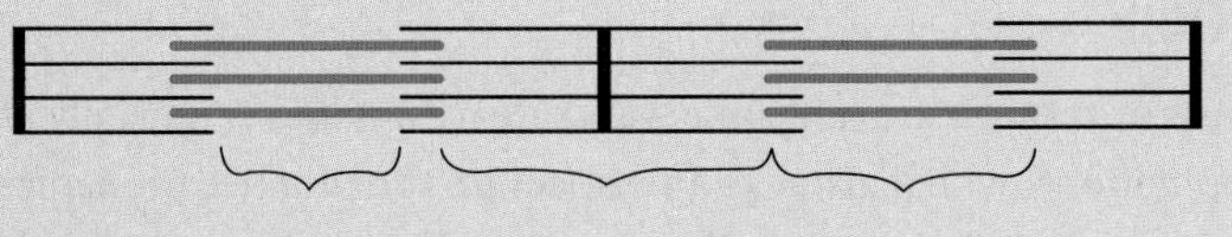

The muscular system is composed of not only skeletal muscle, but also smooth muscle and cardiac muscle. Skeletal muscle is essential for supporting the body and facilitating movement. The contraction of skeletal muscle also compresses venous structures and helps propel blood through the low-pressure venous system toward the heart, as well as lymph through the lymphatic system. Rapid muscle contraction also leads to shivering, which is important in thermoregulation. Smooth muscle is responsible for involuntary movement, such as the rhythmic contractions of smooth muscle in the digestive system called peristalsis. Smooth muscle also aids in the regulation of blood pressure by constricting and relaxing the vasculature. Cardiac muscle is a special type of muscle that is able to maintain rhythmic contraction of the heart without nervous system input. In this section, we will discuss each type of muscle as well as the physiology of muscles.

Types of Muscle

Muscle can be divided into the three different subtypes: skeletal muscle, smooth muscle, and cardiac muscle. Each muscle type performs specific functions, although they share some similarities. All muscle is capable of contraction, which relies on calcium ions. All muscle is innervated, although—as we will see—the part of the nervous system that innervates the muscle and the ability of the muscle to contract without nervous input varies from type to type.

Skeletal Muscle

Skeletal muscle is responsible for voluntary movement and is therefore innervated by the somatic nervous system. Due to the arrangement of actin and myosin into repeating units called **sarcomeres**, it appears striped or **striated** when viewed microscopically. Skeletal muscle is multinucleated because it is formed as individual muscle cells fuse into long rods during development.

There are multiple different types of fibers within skeletal muscle. **Red fibers**, also known as **slow-twitch fibers**, have high myoglobin content and primarily derive their energy aerobically. **Myoglobin** is an oxygen carrier that uses iron in a heme group to bind oxygen, imparting a red color. Red fibers also contain many mitochondria to carry out oxidative phosphorylation. **White fibers**, also known as **fast-twitch fibers**, contain much less myoglobin. Because there is less myoglobin, and therefore less iron, the color is lighter. These two types of fibers can be mixed in muscles. Muscles that contract slowly, but that can sustain activity (such as the muscles that support posture), contain a predominance of red fibers. Muscles that contract rapidly, but fatigue quickly, contain mostly white fibers.

REAL WORLD

Poultry provides a great example of the difference between red and white fibers. Most muscles of support, such as the thigh, are considered dark meat and contain a high concentration of red fibers. The pectoral muscles (breast meat), used by some poultry for only short bursts of flight, are considered white meat and have a high concentration of white fibers.

Smooth Muscle

Smooth muscle is responsible for involuntary action. Thus, smooth muscle is controlled by the autonomic nervous system. It is found in the respiratory tree, digestive tract, bladder, uterus, blood vessel walls, and many other locations. Smooth muscle cells have a single nucleus located in the center of the cell. Just like skeletal muscle, smooth muscle cells contain actin and myosin, but the fibers are not as well organized, so striations cannot be seen. Compared to skeletal muscle, smooth muscle is capable of more sustained contractions; a constant state of low-level contraction, as may be seen in the blood vessels, is called **tonus**. Smooth muscle can actually contract without nervous system input in what is known as **myogenic activity**. In this case, the muscle cells contract directly in response to stretch or other stimuli.

MCAT EXPERTISE

The MCAT loves to test the fact that both smooth and cardiac muscle exhibit myogenic activity. These muscle cells will respond to nervous input, but do not require external signals to undergo contraction.

Cardiac Muscle

Cardiac muscle has characteristics of both smooth and skeletal muscle types. Cardiac muscle is primarily uninucleated, but cells may contain two nuclei. Like smooth muscle, cardiac muscle contraction is involuntary and innervated by the autonomic nervous system. Unlike smooth muscle, cardiac muscle appears striated like skeletal.

One of the unique characteristics of cardiac muscle is how each cardiac myocyte communicates. Cardiac muscle cells are connected by **intercalated discs**, which contain many **gap junctions**. These gap junctions are connections between the cytoplasm of adjacent cells, allowing for the flow of ions directly between cells. This allows for rapid and coordinated depolarization of muscle cells and efficient contraction of cardiac muscle.

Cardiac muscle cells are able to define and maintain their own rhythm, termed myogenic activity. Starting at the **sinoatrial (SA) node**, depolarization spreads using conduction pathways to the **atrioventricular (AV) node**. From there, the depolarization spreads to the **bundle of His** and its branches, and then to the **Purkinje fibers**. The gap junctions allow for progressive depolarizations to spread via ion flow across the gap junctions between cells. The nervous and endocrine systems also play a role in the regulation of cardiac muscle contraction. The vagus nerve provides parasympathetic outflow to the heart and slows the heart rate. Norepinephrine from sympathetic neurons or epinephrine from the adrenal medulla binds to adrenergic receptors in the heart, causing an increased heart rate and greater contractility. One of the ways epinephrine does this is by increasing intracellular calcium levels within cardiac myocytes. Ultimately, cardiac contraction—like that of all types of muscle—relies on calcium.

The main characteristics of each muscle type are summarized in Table 11.1.

SKELETAL MUSCLE	CARDIAC MUSCLE	SMOOTH MUSCLE
Striated	Striated	Nonstriated
Voluntary	Involuntary	Involuntary
Somatic innervation	Autonomic innervation	Autonomic innervation
Many nuclei per cell	1-2 nuclei per cell	1 nucleus per cell
Ca^{2+} required for contraction	Ca^{2+} required for contraction	Ca^{2+} required for contraction

Table 11.1 Types of Muscle

Microscopic Structure of Skeletal Muscle

Each type of muscle has a specific microscopic structure. However, the MCAT tends to focus on the contractile elements and microscopic structure of skeletal muscle. In order to accurately answer those questions on Test Day, let's take a moment to discuss skeletal muscle in detail.

The Sarcomere

The **sarcomere** is the basic contractile unit of skeletal muscle. Sarcomeres are made of **thick** and **thin filaments**. The thick filaments are organized bundles of **myosin**, whereas the thin filaments are made of **actin** along with two other proteins: **troponin** and **tropomyosin**. These proteins help to regulate the interaction between the actin and myosin filaments. Another protein, **titin**, acts as a spring and anchors the actin and myosin filaments together, preventing excessive stretching of the muscle.

Each sarcomere is divided into different lines, zones, and bands, as shown in Figure 11.1. **Z-lines** define the boundaries of each sarcomere. The **M-line** runs down the center of the sarcomere, through the middle of the myosin filaments. The **I-band** is the region containing exclusively thin filaments, whereas the **H-zone** contains only thick filaments. The **A-band** contains the thick filaments in their entirety, including any overlap with thin filaments. During contraction, the H-zone, I-band, the distance between Z-lines, and the distance between M-lines all become smaller, whereas the A-band's size remains constant.

MNEMONIC

To remember which filament is associated with **t**roponin and **t**ropomyosin, remember that ac**t**in has a **T** in it.

MNEMONIC

To remember which is the thin and thick filament, remember **acthin**: **actin** filaments are **thin** (while myosin filaments are thick).

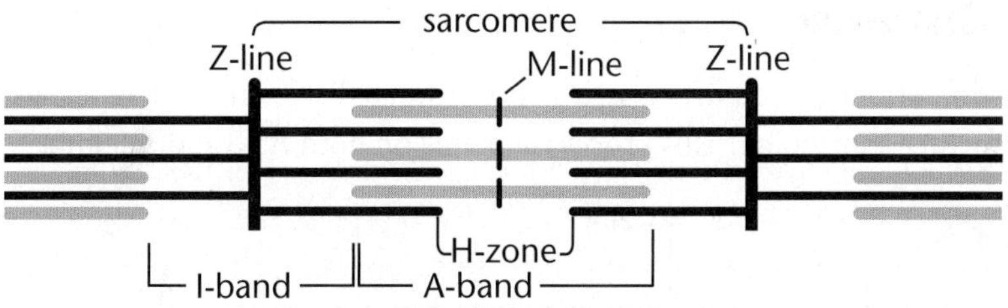

Figure 11.1 The Sarcomere
Sarcomeres are the functional units of striated muscle.

Gross Structure of Myocytes

Sarcomeres are attached end-to-end to form **myofibrils**. Myofibrils are surrounded by a covering known as the **sarcoplasmic reticulum (SR)**, a modified endoplasmic reticulum that contains a high concentration of Ca^{2+} ions. The **sarcoplasm** is a modified cytoplasm located just outside the sarcoplasmic reticulum. The cell membrane of a myocyte is known as the **sarcolemma**. The sarcolemma is capable of propagating an action potential and can distribute the action potential to all sarcomeres in a muscle using a system of **transverse tubules (T-tubules)** that are oriented perpendicularly to the myofibrils, as shown in Figure 11.2. Each **myocyte**, or muscle cell, contains many myofibrils arranged in parallel and can also be called a **muscle fiber**. The nuclei, of which there are many, are usually found at the periphery of the cell. Finally, many myocytes in parallel form a muscle.

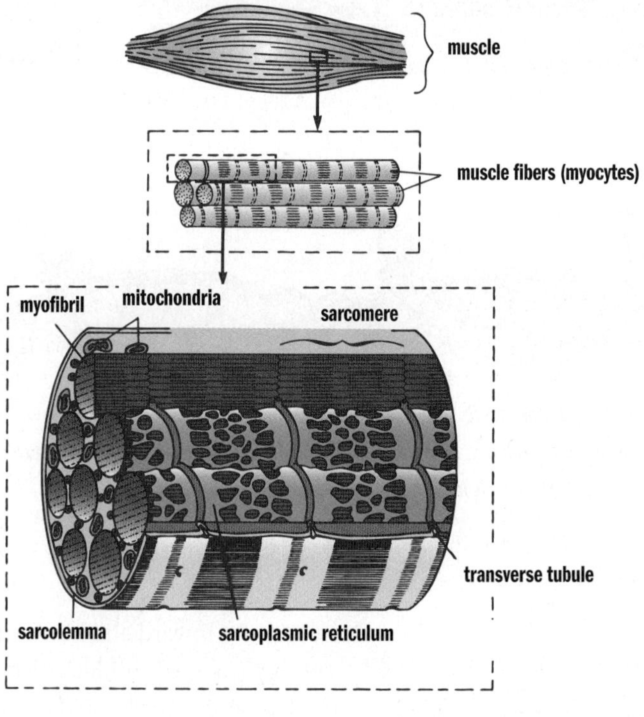

Figure 11.2 Architecture of Skeletal Muscle
A muscle is composed of parallel myocytes (muscle fibers), which are composed of parallel myofibrils.

MNEMONIC

Parts of the sarcomere:

- **Z–Z** is the end of the alphabet, and the end of the sarcomere
- **M–M**iddle of the **m**yosin filaments
- **I–I** is a **thin** letter (**thin** filaments only)
- **H–H** is a **thick** letter (**thick** filaments only)
- **A–A**ll of the thick filament, whether or not it is overlapping

KEY CONCEPT

The sarcoplasmic reticulum is just a fancy name for the specialized endoplasmic reticulum in muscle cells.

KEY CONCEPT

A myofibril is an arrangement of many sarcomeres in series. A muscle fiber (or myocyte, or muscle cell) contains many myofibrils within it, arranged in parallel. A muscle is made up of parallel muscle fibers. These names are very similar; pay careful attention to terminology when reading about muscle structure!

Muscle Contraction

Contraction of muscle requires a series of coordinated steps that are repeated to induce further shortening. This process depends on both ATP and calcium.

Initiation

Contraction starts at the **neuromuscular junction**, where the nervous system communicates with muscles via **motor (efferent) neurons**. This signal travels down the neuron until it reaches the **nerve terminal (synaptic bouton)**, where acetylcholine is released into the synapse. In the case of the neuromuscular junction, the nerve terminal can also be called the **motor end plate**. Acetylcholine binds to receptors on the sarcolemma, causing depolarization. Each nerve terminal controls a group of myocytes; together, the nerve terminal and its myocytes constitute a **motor unit**.

Depolarization triggers an action potential, which spreads down the sarcolemma to the T-tubules. The action potential travels down the T-tubules into the muscle tissues to the sarcoplasmic reticulum. When the action potential reaches the sarcoplasmic reticulum, Ca^{2+} is ultimately released. The calcium ions bind to a regulatory subunit in troponin, triggering a change in the confirmation of tropomyosin, to which troponin is bound. This change exposes the **myosin-binding sites** on the actin thin filament, as shown in Figure 11.3.

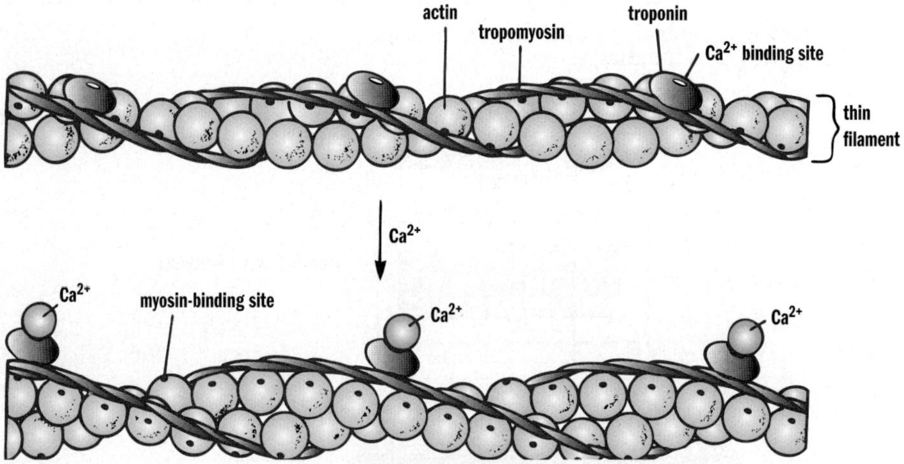

Figure 11.3 Regulation of Contraction with Calcium
Calcium binds to troponin, leading to a conformational change in tropomyosin, which exposes the myosin-binding sites of actin.

Shortening of the Sarcomere

The free globular heads of the myosin molecules move toward and bind with the exposed sites on actin. The newly formed actin–myosin cross bridges then allow myosin to pull on actin, which draws the thin filaments toward the M-line, resulting in shortening of the sarcomere. The actin–myosin cross-bridge cycle is illustrated in Figure 11.4.

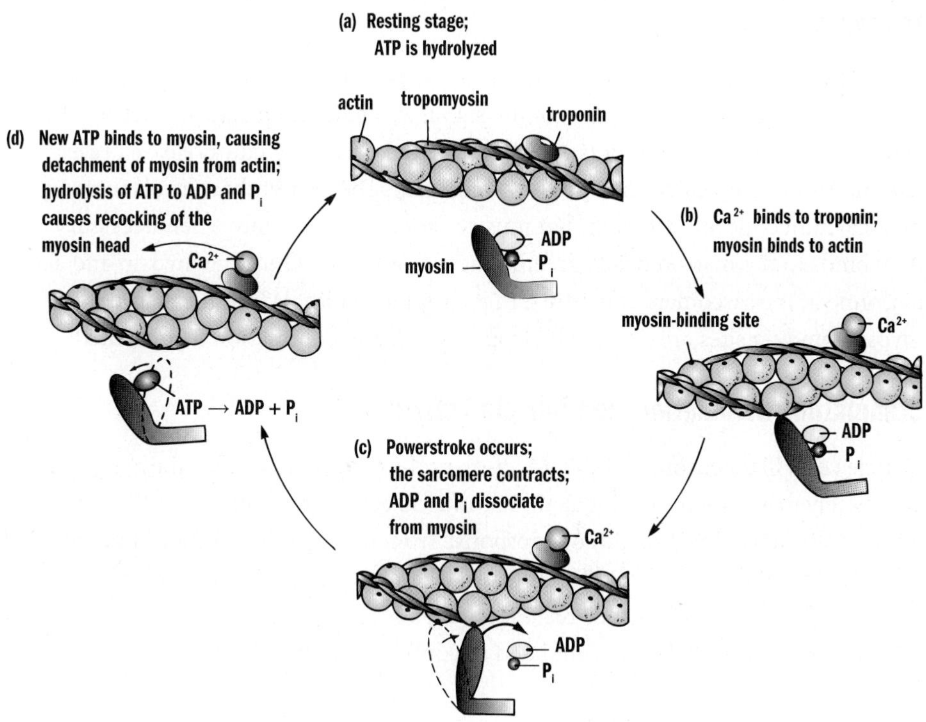

Figure 11.4 The Actin-Myosin Cross-Bridge Cycle
Calcium and ATP are essential for muscle contraction and relaxation.

Starting at the top of the diagram, myosin carrying hydrolyzed ATP (ADP and an inorganic phosphate, P_i) is able to bind with the myosin-binding site. The release of the inorganic phosphate and ADP in rapid succession provides the energy for the powerstroke and results in sliding of the actin filament over the myosin filament. Then, ATP binds to the myosin head, releasing it from actin. This ATP is hydrolyzed to ADP and P_i, which **recocks** the myosin head so that it is in position to initiate another cross-bridge cycle. The repetitive binding and releasing of myosin heads on actin filaments allows the thin filament to slide along the thick filament, causing sequential shortening of the sarcomere. This is known as the **sliding filament model**, as shown in Figure 11.5.

KEY CONCEPT

It is the dissociation of ADP and P_i from myosin that is responsible for the powerstroke, not the hydrolysis of ATP. The binding of ATP is required for releasing the myosin head from the actin filament.

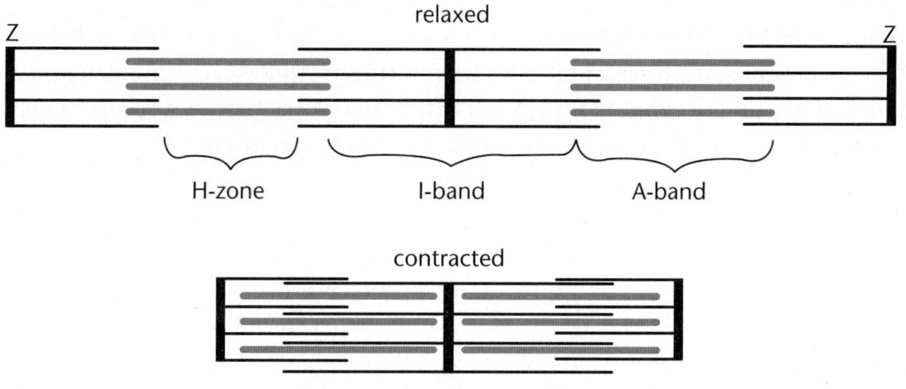

Figure 11.5 Sarcomere Contraction
When a sarcomere contracts, both the H-zone and I-band shorten, while the A-band is unchanged.

Relaxation

Acetylcholine is degraded in the synapse by the enzyme known as ***acetylcholinesterase***. This results in termination of the signal at the neuromuscular junction and allows the sarcolemma to repolarize. As the signal decays, calcium release ceases, and the SR takes up calcium from the sarcoplasm. The SR tightly controls intracellular calcium concentrations so that muscles are contracted only when necessary. ATP binds to the myosin heads, freeing them from actin. Once the myosin and actin disconnect, the sarcomere can return to its original width. Without calcium, the myosin-binding sites are covered by tropomyosin and contraction is prevented.

REAL WORLD

After death, ATP production ceases. Myosin heads cannot detach from actin, making it impossible for muscles to relax and lengthen. This condition is known as rigor mortis.

Stimulation, Summation, and Muscle Fatigue

Muscle cells, like neurons, exhibit an all-or-nothing response; either they respond completely to a stimulus or not at all. For muscle cells to respond, stimuli must reach a threshold value. The strength of a response from one muscle cell cannot be changed because the only options are all or nothing. Therefore, nerves control overall force by the number of motor units they recruit to respond. Maximal response occurs when all fibers within a muscle are stimulated to contract simultaneously.

BRIDGE

Why do muscle fibers contract in an all-or-nothing fashion? Because they are innervated by neurons that deliver signals using action potentials, which are all-or-nothing phenomena as well. Action potentials are discussed in Chapter 4 of *MCAT Biology Review*.

Simple Twitch

A simple twitch is the response of a single muscle fiber to a brief stimulus at or above threshold, as shown in Figure 11.6a. It consists of a latent period, contraction period, and relaxation period. The **latent period** is the time between reaching threshold and the onset of contraction. It is during this time that the action potential spreads along the muscle and allows for calcium to be released from the sarcoplasmic reticulum. The muscle then contracts, and, assuming calcium is cleared from the sarcoplasm, it then relaxes.

Summation and Tetanus

If a muscle fiber is exposed to frequent and prolonged stimulation, it will have insufficient time to relax. The contractions will combine, become stronger and more prolonged. This is known as **frequency summation**, as shown in Figure 11.6b. If the contractions become so frequent that the muscle is unable to relax at all, this is known as **tetanus**. Prolonged tetanus will result in muscle fatigue, explained below. Note that tetanus (the disease) includes tetanus (the physiological phenomenon) as one of its primary clinical features, but that tetanic physiology also occurs under normal circumstances with multiple simple twitches in succession.

REAL WORLD

The disease *tetanus* is caused by a bacterium called *Clostridium tetani* that releases the toxin *tetanospasmin*. Tetanospasmin blocks the release of GABA from the neurons that *inhibit* motor neurons, making the motor neurons overexcitable. This leads to constant contraction of muscles, which can be so strong as to fracture bones. Tetanus can usually be prevented after exposure by administration of a tetanus immunoglobulin.

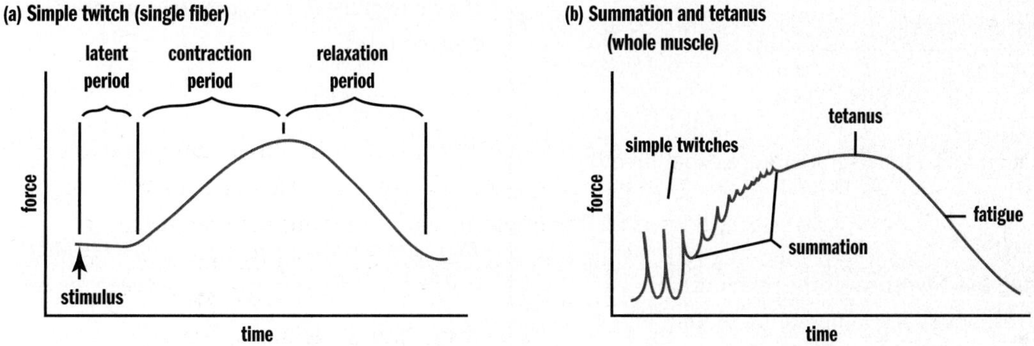

Figure 11.6 Force of Muscle Contraction Due to a Simple Twitch and Tetanus
(a) A simple twitch contraction; (b) Summation of frequent simple twitches can lead to tetanus.

BIOLOGY GUIDED EXAMPLE WITH EXPERT THINKING

Study 1

Previous research has shown muscle tension generation is influenced by temperature of the muscle fibers. To further establish the connection between how temperature interacts with muscle tension generation, researchers measured the rate of tension rise at various temperatures. More specifically, researchers established change in the rate of tension rise is different at high temperatures (25°C to 35°C) and low temperatures (20°C to 10°C).

IV: temperature

DV: muscle tension generation

Experiment is trying to test the connection between temperature and tension

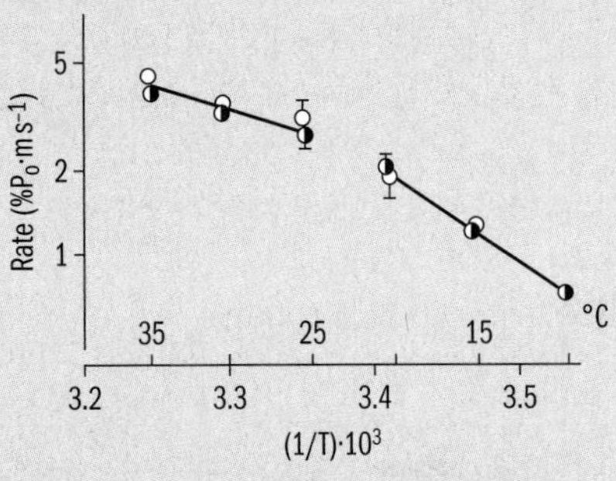

Figure 1 Tension generation rate versus temperature experiment results.

Trend: Tension generation rate is lower and the slope of the line is more steep at lower temperatures

Study 2

Another study is conducted that investigates the relationship between tetanic tension responses and temperature of the same type of muscle fibers. In this experiment, researchers directly observe the tension generation of the muscle plotted over time with electromyography sensor.

There are two studies in the passage, the MCAT will likely ask for comparisons between the two

IV: temperature again

DV: tetanic tension responses (tetanic must be another type of tension)

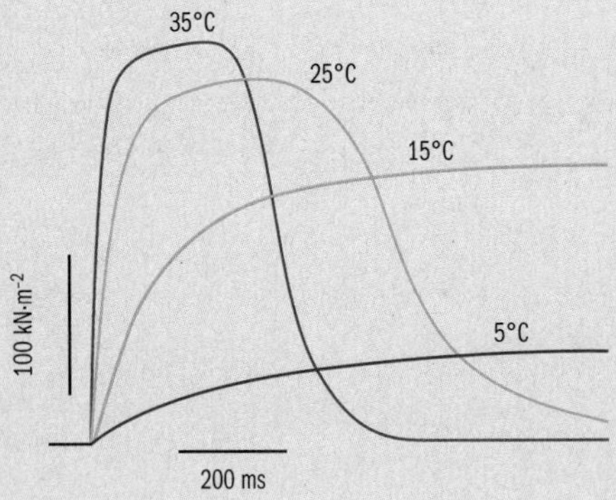

Figure 2 Tetanic tension responses obtained from one intact fiber bundle at four different temperatures, using suitable stimulation frequencies and duration.

Trend: as temperature decreases, the curve flattens out (i.e., change in tension remains low)

Adapted from Ranatunga K. W. (2018). Temperature effects on force and actin–myosin interaction in muscle: a look back on some experimental findings. *International Journal of Molecular Sciences*, 19(5), 1538. doi:10.3390/ijms19051538.

Does Study 2's data conflict with Study 1's data?

This question asks us whether two sets of data conflict with one another. To analyze this relationship, we need to draw the proper conclusions from each data set, and see how these two data sets are related. Conflict is when one data set reveals a relationship that is either not validated by similar data sets, or directly contradicted by similar data sets.

To start, we'll want to make sure we can understand each data set separately. The first study seeks to investigate how temperature affects the rate of tension generation by the muscle tissues. The results of this experiment are displayed as a line graph. One of the first things to look at when analyzing any figure are axes labels and their corresponding units. On the *y*-axis, we see the rate of tension rise. So, a higher value on that axis means the muscle can generate tension faster, or in other words, have a higher rate. For the *x*-axis, things are a bit more confusing. The axis displays temperature, but in two ways. Technically, it is the reciprocal of temperature, but fortunately for us the graph is also labeled with the corresponding real temperature location. Because of the reciprocal, higher temperatures are found closer to the left, and temperature decreases going toward the right. Besides this complication, the graph shows a pretty straightforward relationship. At higher temperatures (close to physiological temperature), the rate of tension rise is high, with the drop in rate from 35°C to 25°C being relatively minor. At lower temperatures, the rate of tension rise is much lower, and the change in rate as temperature decreases is more dramatic.

Study 2 examined a similar relationship between temperature and muscle tension. Here the graph shows a more visual representation of how the tension is generated in those muscles. From the shape of the curve, it appears that the measurement is for one stimulation, as the tension rises once and quickly tapers off. From the graph, we can make some quick observations. At higher temperatures, the max tension generated is higher, as well as the time required to reach peak tension. When temperature is lowered, muscle tension generation drops significantly.

To evaluate whether Study 2's data conflicts with Study 1's data, we need to compare and assess how the two data sets are related. Both of these graphs have temperature as the independent variable, so we must look at what each data set demonstrates with that change in temperature. Study 1 shows a rise in rate of tension. While Study 2 does not report rate of tension rise explicitly, it does show tension over time, which is essentially rate! At 35°C and 25°C, the slope of tension increase is sharp, meaning that the rate of tension increase is high. At lower temperature, the slope is more gentle, and tension generation takes significantly longer. This means that Study 2 corroborates Study 1's data in that higher temperature is correlated with a higher rate, while lower temperature is correlated with lower rate.

What about the *change* in rate? How is that visualized? Study 1 shows that change in the rate of tension rise at high temperature is more mild than the change in rate at lower temperatures. From Study 2's graph, we can see that from 35°C to 25°C, the change in the slope (and therefore rate) of the tension is rather small. However, the change in slope between 15°C and 5°C is much more dramatic. Since we know that the slope represents the rate of tension rise, the change in slope must represent the change in rate.

Thus, Study 2 does not conflict with Study 1. In fact, the two studies corroborate each other!

Oxygen Debt and Muscle Fatigue

Muscles require ATP to function. Slow-twitch (red) muscle fibers have high levels of mitochondria and thus use oxidative phosphorylation to make ATP. However, this means that high concentrations of oxygen are required to generate the large amounts of ATP muscle cells need. There are two supplemental energy reserves in muscle. **Creatine phosphate** is created by transferring a phosphate group from ATP to creatine during times of rest. This reaction can then be reversed during muscle use to quickly generate ATP from ADP:

$$\text{creatine} + \text{ATP} \rightleftharpoons \text{creatine phosphate} + \text{ADP}$$

Muscle also contains myoglobin, which binds oxygen with high affinity. As exercising muscles run out of oxygen, they use myoglobin reserves to keep aerobic metabolism going. Fast-twitch (white) muscle fibers have fewer mitochondria and must rely on glycolysis and fermentation to make ATP under most circumstances. When a person exercises, heart rate and respiratory rate increase in order to move more oxygen to actively respiring muscles. The oxyhemoglobin dissociation curve undergoes a right shift in the presence of increased carbon dioxide concentration, increased hydrogen ion concentration (decreased pH), and increased temperature. However, even with these adaptations, muscle use can quickly overwhelm the ability of the body to deliver oxygen. Then, even red muscle fibers must switch to anaerobic metabolism and produce lactic acid, at which point the muscle begins to fatigue. The difference between the amount of oxygen needed by the muscles and the actual amount present is called the **oxygen debt**. After the cessation of strenuous exercise, the body must metabolize all of the lactic acid it has produced. Most lactic acid is converted back into pyruvate, which can enter the citric acid cycle. This process requires oxygen, and the amount of oxygen required to recover from strenuous exercise is equal to the oxygen debt.

MCAT CONCEPT CHECK 11.1

Before you move on, assess your understanding of the material with these questions.

1. What type(s) of muscle (skeletal, smooth, or cardiac) does each of the following describe? (Note: Circle the correct response(s) next to each item.)

• Striated:	Skeletal	Smooth	Cardiac
• Always uninucleated:	Skeletal	Smooth	Cardiac
• Always polynucleated:	Skeletal	Smooth	Cardiac
• Voluntary:	Skeletal	Smooth	Cardiac
• Innervated by the autonomic nervous system:	Skeletal	Smooth	Cardiac
• Exhibits myogenic activity:	Skeletal	Smooth	Cardiac

2. Which zone or band in the sarcomere does NOT change its length during muscle contraction? Why?

3. What are the events that initiate muscle contraction, in order? Start with neurotransmitter release and trace the pathway to the point where myosin binds with actin.

4. What role does the binding of ATP to the myosin head play in the cross-bridge cycle? What about the dissociation of ADP and inorganic phosphate from the myosin head?
   - Binding of ATP:
   - Dissociation of ADP and inorganic phosphate:

5. What is tetanus (the physiological phenomenon, not the disease)?

11.2 The Skeletal System

LEARNING OBJECTIVES

After Chapter 11.2, you will be able to:

- Distinguish between compact and spongy bone
- Identify the three structural parts of a bone and their relative contributions to growth
- Recall the major chemical component of bone
- Describe the function(s) of osteoblasts, osteoclasts, and chondrocytes
- Name the substance that lubricates movable joints and where it is produced

There are two types of skeletons: exoskeletons and endoskeletons. **Exoskeletons** encase whole organisms and are usually found in arthropods, such as crustaceans and insects. Vertebrates, including humans, have **endoskeletons**. Endoskeletons are internal, but are not able to protect the soft tissue structures as well as exoskeletons. However, exoskeletons must be shed and regrown to accommodate growth. Endoskeletons are much better able to accommodate the growth of a larger organism.

Skeletal Structure

The components of our skeletal system are divided into axial and appendicular skeletons. The **axial skeleton** consists of the skull, vertebral column, rib cage, and hyoid bone (a small bone in the anterior neck used for swallowing); it provides the basic central framework for the body. The **appendicular skeleton** consists of the bones of the limbs (humerus, radius and ulna, carpals, metacarpals, and phalanges in the upper limb; and femur, tibia and fibula, tarsals, metatarsals, and phalanges in the lower limb); the pectoral girdle (scapula and clavicle); and pelvis. Both skeleton types are covered by other structures (muscle, connective tissue, and vasculature). The structure of the skeleton is shown in Figure 11.7, with many of the bones labeled (individual bones are labeled in red).

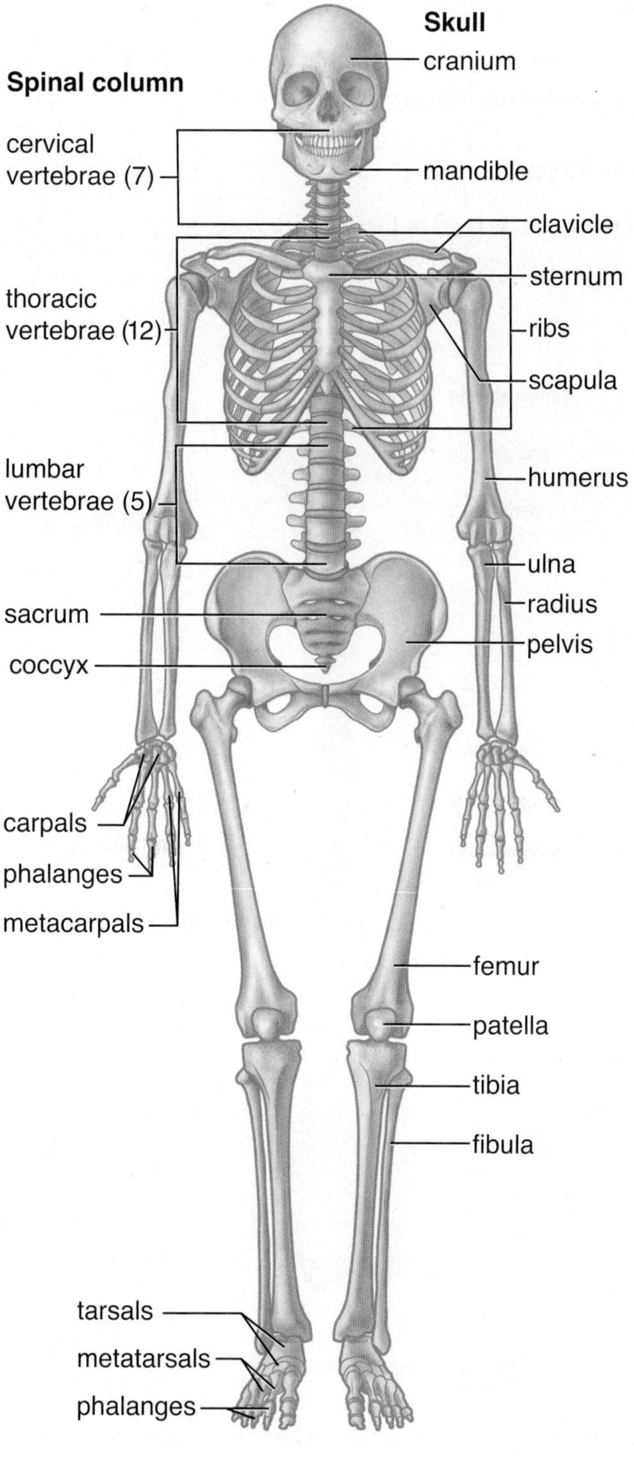

Figure 11.7 Anatomy of the Human Skeleton

The skeleton is created from two major components: bone and cartilage.

REAL WORLD

An adult human has 206 bones. Over 100 of these are in the hands and feet.

Bone Composition

Bone is a connective tissue derived from embryonic mesoderm. Bone is much harder than cartilage, but is relatively lightweight.

Macroscopic Bone Structure

The structure of bone can be seen in Figure 11.8.

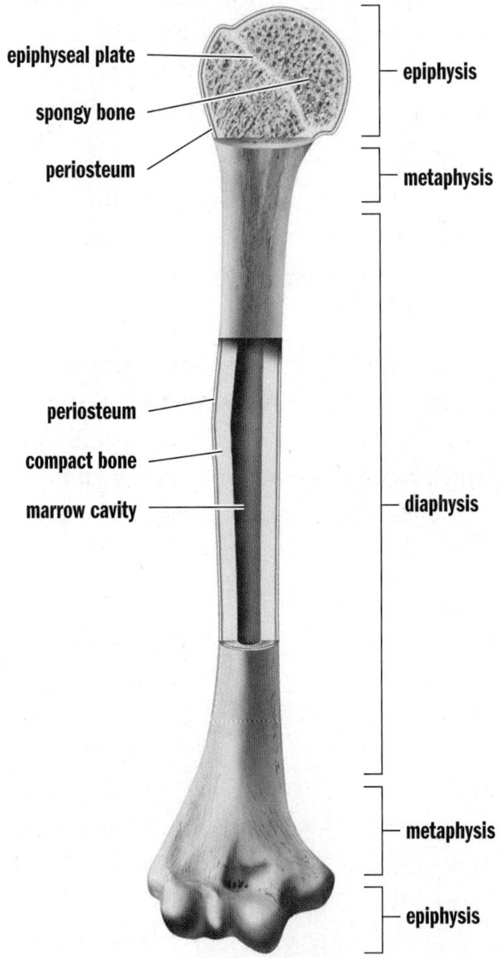

Figure 11.8 Anatomy of a Long Bone (Humerus)

Bone's characteristic strength comes specifically from **compact bone**. It lives up to its name, as it is both dense and strong. The other type of bone structure is **spongy** or **cancellous** bone. The lattice structure of spongy bone is visible under microscopy and consists of bony spicules (points) known as **trabeculae**. The cavities between trabeculae are filled with **bone marrow**, which may be either red or yellow. **Red marrow** is filled with hematopoietic stem cells, which are responsible for the generation of all the cells in our blood; **yellow marrow** is composed primarily of fat and is relatively inactive.

Bones in the appendicular skeleton are typically **long bones**, which are characterized by cylindrical shafts called **diaphyses** that swell at each end to form **metaphyses**, and that terminate in **epiphyses**. The outermost portions of bone are composed of compact bone, whereas the internal core is made of spongy bone. Long bone diaphyses and metaphyses are full of bone marrow. The epiphyses, on the other hand, use their spongy cores for more effective dispersion of force and pressure at the joints. At the internal edge of the epiphysis is an **epiphyseal (growth) plate**, which is a cartilaginous structure and the site of longitudinal growth. Prior to adulthood, the epiphyseal plate is filled with mitotic cells that contribute to growth; during puberty, these epiphyseal plates close and vertical growth is halted. Finally, a fibrous sheath called the **periosteum** surrounds the long bone to protect it as well as serve as a site for muscle attachment. Some periosteal cells are capable of differentiating into bone-forming cells; a healthy periosteum is necessary for bone growth and repair.

BRIDGE

The root *lig-* comes from Latin, where it means to "to tie; bind." Think of *DNA ligase*, discussed in Chapter 6 of *MCAT Biochemistry Review*. Think of ligands in complex ions, discussed in Chapter 9 of *MCAT General Chemistry Review*. In this case, ligaments tie bones to each other to stabilize joints.

Structures in the musculoskeletal system are held together with dense connective tissue. **Tendons** attach muscle to bone and **ligaments** hold bones together at joints.

Microscopic Bone Structure

The strength of compact bone comes from the **bone matrix**, which has both organic and inorganic components. The organic components include collagen, glycoproteins, and other peptides. The inorganic components include calcium, phosphate, and hydroxide ions, which harden together to form **hydroxyapatite** crystals ($Ca_{10}(PO_4)_6(OH)_2$). Minerals such as sodium, magnesium, and potassium are also stored in bone.

Strong bones require uniform distribution of organic and inorganic materials. The bony matrix is ordered into structural units known as **osteons** or **Haversian systems**, as shown in Figure 11.9. Each of these osteons contains concentric circles of bony matrix called **lamellae** surrounding a central microscopic channel. Longitudinal channels (those with an axis parallel to the bone) are known as **Haversian canals**, while transverse channels (those with an axis perpendicular to the bone) are known as **Volkmann's canals**. These canals contain the blood vessels, nerve fibers, and lymph vessels that maintain the health of the bone. Between the lamellar rings are small spaces called **lacunae**, which house mature bone cells known as **osteocytes**. The lacunae are interconnected by tiny channels called **canaliculi** that allow for the exchange of nutrients and wastes between osteocytes and the Haversian and Volkmann's canals.

KEY CONCEPT

Bone appears to be rigid and static, but it is actually quite dynamic. It is both vascular and innervated, which is why it hurts so much to break a bone. In addition, bone remains in a vigorous equilibrium between construction and destruction, known as bone remodeling.

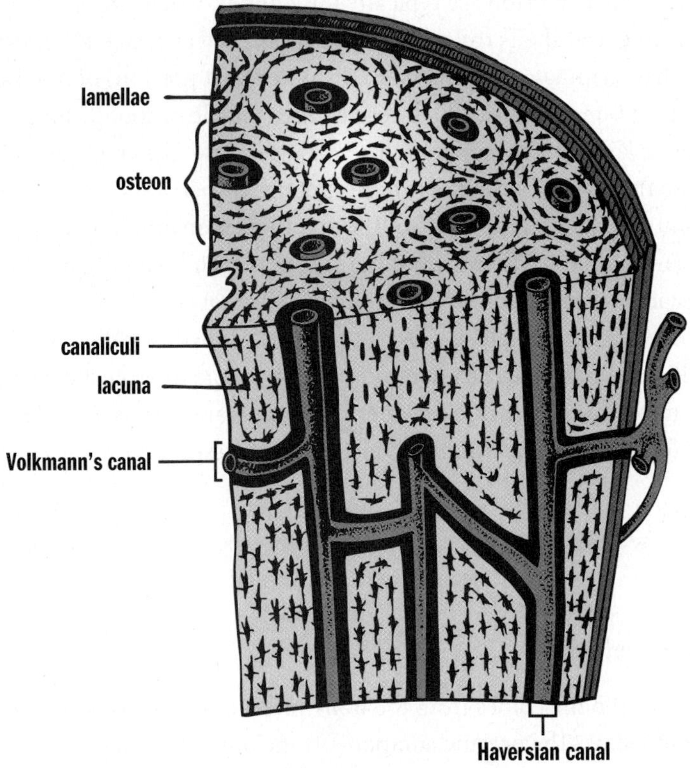

Figure 11.9 Bone Matrix
Cross-sectional and longitudinal views highlighting Haversian systems

REAL WORLD

Osteoporosis is the most common bone disease in the United States. It is thought to be the result of increased osteoclast resorption and some concomitant slowing of bone formation, both of which lead to loss of bone mass. Estrogen is believed to help prevent osteoporosis by stimulating osteoblast activity.

Bone Remodeling

Two cell types are largely responsible for building and maintaining strong bones: osteoblasts and osteoclasts. **Osteoblasts** build bone, whereas **osteoclasts**, polynucleated resident macrophages of bone, resorb it. These processes together contribute to the constant turnover of bone, as shown in Figure 11.10. During bone formation, essential ingredients such as calcium and phosphate are obtained from the blood. During bone resorption, these ions are released back into the bloodstream. Bone remodeling occurs in response to stress, and bone actually remodels in such a way as to accommodate the repetitive stresses faced by the body. Endocrine hormones may also affect bone metabolism. **Parathyroid hormone**, a peptide hormone released by the parathyroid glands in response to low blood calcium, promotes resorption of bone, increasing the concentration of calcium and phosphate in the blood. **Vitamin D**, which is activated by parathyroid hormone, also promotes the resorption of bone. This may seem counterintuitive at first—isn't vitamin D used to promote bone growth? Indeed, the resorption of bone in response to vitamin D actually encourages the growth of new, stronger bone, thus overcompensating for the effect of resorbing bone in the first place. Finally, **calcitonin**, a peptide hormone released by the parafollicular cells of the thyroid in response to high blood calcium, promotes bone formation, lowering blood calcium levels.

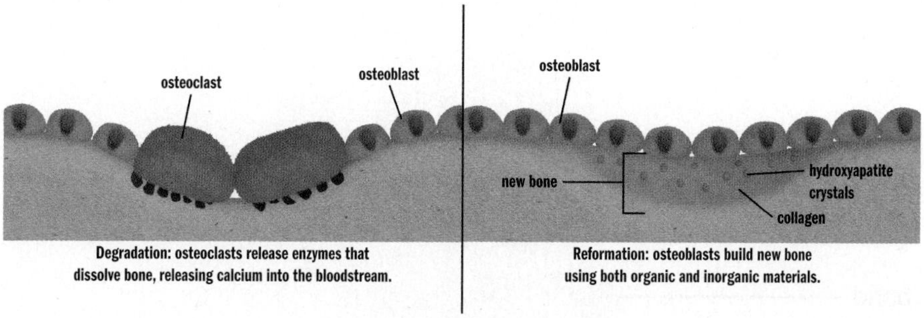

Figure 11.10 Bone Remodeling

MNEMONIC

Osteo**b**lasts **b**uild bone. Osteo**c**lasts **c**hew bone.

Cartilage

Cartilage is softer and more flexible than bone. Cartilage consists of a firm but elastic matrix called **chondrin** that is secreted by cells called **chondrocytes**. Fetal skeletons are mostly made up of cartilage. This is advantageous because fetuses must grow and develop in a confined environment and then must traverse the birth canal. Adults have cartilage only in body parts that need a little extra flexibility or cushioning (external ear, nose, walls of the larynx and trachea, intervertebral discs, and joints). Cartilage also differs from bone in that it is avascular (without blood and lymphatic vessels) and is not innervated.

Most of the bones of the body are created by the hardening of cartilage into bone. This process is known as **endochondral ossification** and is responsible for the formation of most of the long bones of the body. Bones may also be formed through **intramembranous ossification**, in which undifferentiated embryonic connective tissue (**mesenchymal tissue**) is transformed into, and replaced by, bone. This occurs in bones of the skull.

Joints and Movement

Like bone and cartilage, joints are also made of connective tissue and come in two major varieties: immovable and movable. **Immovable joints** consist of bones that are fused together to form **sutures** or similar fibrous joints. These joints are found primarily in the head, where they anchor bones of the skull together.

Movable joints, structures of which are shown in Figure 11.11, include hinge joints (like the elbow or knee), ball-and-socket joints (like the shoulder or hip), and others. They permit bones to shift relative to one another. Movable joints are strengthened by **ligaments**, which are pieces of fibrous tissue that connect bones to one another, and consist of a **synovial capsule**, which encloses the actual **joint cavity** (**articular cavity**). A layer of soft tissue called the **synovium** secretes **synovial fluid**, which lubricates the movement of structures in the joint space. The **articular cartilage** contributes to the joint by coating the articular surfaces of the bones so that impact is restricted to the lubricated joint cartilage, rather than to the bones.

REAL WORLD

Degradation of articular cartilage (cartilage in joints) can lead to medical issues like osteoarthritis. Osteoarthritis (or "arthritis" in the lay population) is painful because a lack of cartilage in joints leads to bones rubbing directly on one another.

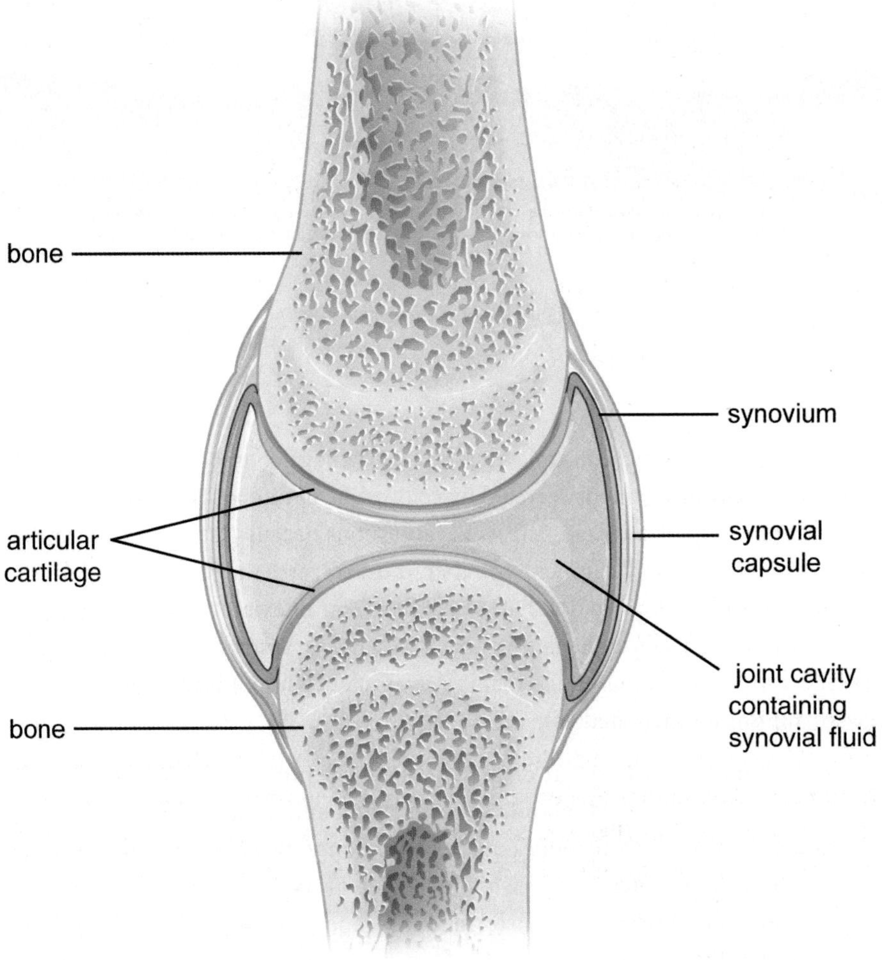

Figure 11.11 Structures in a Movable Joint

When a muscle is attached to two bones, its contraction will cause one of the bones to move. The end of the muscle with a larger attachment to bone (usually the proximal connection) is called the **origin**. The end with the smaller attachment to bone (usually the distal connection) is called the **insertion**. Often, our muscles work in **antagonistic pairs**; one relaxes while the other contracts. Such is the case in the arm, where the biceps brachii and triceps brachii work antagonistically, as shown in Figure 11.12. When the biceps contracts and the triceps relaxes, the elbow is flexed; when the triceps contracts and the biceps relaxes, the elbow is extended. Muscles can also be **synergistic**—working together to accomplish the same function.

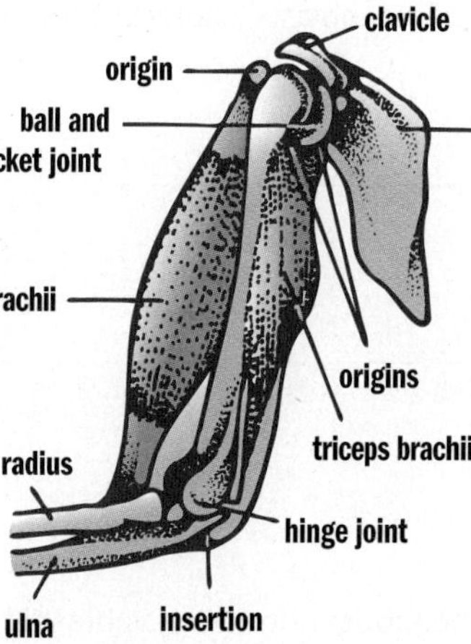

Figure 11.12 Antagonistic Muscle Pairs
The biceps brachii and triceps brachii are an example of a muscle pair that works antagonistically; the contraction of one causes the other to elongate.

Muscles may also be classified by the types of movements they coordinate. A **flexor** muscle decreases the angle across a joint (like the biceps brachii); an **extensor** increases or straightens this angle (like the triceps brachii). An **abductor** moves a part of the body away from the midline (like the deltoid); an **adductor** moves a part of the body toward the midline (like the pectoralis major). **Medial** and **lateral rotation** describe motions that occur in limbs; a medial rotator rotates the axis of the limb toward the midline (like the subscapularis), whereas a lateral rotator rotates the axis of the limb away from the midline (like the infraspinatus).

MCAT CONCEPT CHECK 11.2

Before you move on, assess your understanding of the material with these questions.

1. What is the difference between compact and spongy bone?
    - Compact bone:

    ____

    - Spongy bone:

    ____

2. What are the three structural parts of a bone? Which part contributes most to linear growth?

    ____

3. What chemical forms most of the inorganic component of bone?

    ____

4. What are the functions of osteoblasts, osteoclasts, and chondrocytes?
    - Osteoblast:

    ____

    - Osteoclast:

    ____

    - Chondrocyte:

    ____

5. What liquid provides the lubrication for movable joints? What tissue produces it?

    ____

Conclusion

One concept that has been emphasized throughout the past eight chapters on anatomy and physiology is the notion that organ systems work together in order to achieve a desired effect. The musculoskeletal system is no different. Usually, we think of the musculoskeletal system as being responsible for movement, but to limit the musculoskeletal system to that function would be shortsighted. The bones are reservoirs of calcium and other minerals that can be released through hormonal signaling. They protect the internal organs and provide support for the body. Muscle tissue not only moves these bones, but pumps blood through the body and is key to the function of a number of other systems, including respiration, digestion, blood pressure and vascular tone, and reproduction and childbirth. As you review anatomy and physiology and master the fundamentals of each organ system, be sure to pay special attention to how each organ system interacts with the others. While the MCAT expects you to understand each individual organ system, it will also challenge you by asking you to think critically about how one system impacts another. By spending some time in your studies looking at these interactions, you will be one step ahead on Test Day.

In our final chapter of *MCAT Biology Review*, we will switch gears and look at the transfer of information from generation to generation. This picks up on a discussion from the first three chapters of the book in which we explored the organization of cells and their genetic material, reproduction, and embryogenesis and development. In the next chapter, we'll describe classical (Mendelian) inheritance and conclude with a note on how the gene pool can change over time with the topic of evolution.

You've reviewed the content, now test your knowledge and critical thinking skills by completing a test-like passage set in your online resources!

GO ONLINE

CONCEPT SUMMARY

The Muscular System

- There are three main types of muscle: skeletal muscle, smooth muscle, and cardiac muscle.
  - **Skeletal muscle** is involved in support and movement, propulsion of blood in the venous system, and thermoregulation. It appears **striated**, is under voluntary (somatic) control, is polynucleated, and can be divided into **red (slow-twitch) fibers** that carry out oxidative phosphorylation and **white (fast-twitch) fibers** that rely on anaerobic metabolism.
  - **Smooth muscle** is in the respiratory, reproductive, cardiovascular, and digestive systems. It appears nonstriated, is under involuntary (autonomic) control, and is uninucleated. It can display **myogenic activity**, or contraction without neural input.
  - **Cardiac muscle** comprises the contractile tissue of the heart. It appears striated, is under involuntary (autonomic) control, and is uninucleated (sometimes binucleated). It can also display myogenic activity. Cells are connected with **intercalated discs** that contain **gap junctions**.
- The **sarcomere** is the basic contractile unit of striated muscle.
  - Sarcomeres are made of thick (**myosin**) and thin (**actin**) filaments.
  - **Troponin** and **tropomyosin** are found on the thin filament and regulate actin–myosin interactions.
- The sarcomere can be divided into different lines, zones, and bands.
  - The boundaries of each sarcomere are defined by **Z-lines.**
  - The **M-line** is located in the middle of the sarcomere.
  - The **I-band** contains only thin filaments.
  - The **H-zone** consists of only thick filaments.
  - The **A-band** contains the thick filaments in their entirety. It is the only part of the sarcomere that maintains a constant size during contraction.
- Sarcomeres attach end-to-end to become **myofibrils**, and each **myocyte** (muscle cell or **muscle fiber**) contains many myofibrils.
  - Myofibrils are surrounded by the **sarcoplasmic reticulum**, a calcium-containing modified endoplasmic reticulum, and the cell membrane of a myocyte is known as the **sarcolemma**.
  - A system of **T-tubules** is connected to the sarcolemma and oriented perpendicularly to the myofibrils, allowing the action potential to reach all parts of the muscle.
- Muscle contraction begins at the **neuromuscular junction**, where the motor neuron releases acetylcholine that binds to receptors on the sarcolemma, causing depolarization.
  - This depolarization spreads down the sarcolemma to the T-tubules, triggering the release of calcium ions.

  - Calcium binds to troponin, causing a shift in tropomyosin and exposure of the myosin-binding sites on the actin thin filament.
  - Shortening of the sarcomere occurs as myosin heads bind to the exposed sites on actin, forming cross bridges and pulling the actin filament along the thick filament, which results in contraction. This is known as the **sliding filament model**.
  - The muscle relaxes when acetylcholine is degraded by acetylcholinesterase, terminating the signal and allowing calcium to be brought back into the SR. ATP binds to the myosin head, allowing it to release from actin.
- Muscle cells exhibit an all-or-nothing response called a **simple twitch**.
  - Addition of multiple simple twitches before the muscle has an opportunity to fully relax is called **frequency summation**.
  - Simple twitches that occur so frequently as to not let the muscle relax at all can lead to **tetanus**, a more prolonged and stronger contraction.
- Muscle cells have additional energy reserves to reduce **oxygen debt** (the difference between the amount of oxygen needed and the amount present) and forestall fatigue.
  - **Creatine phosphate** can transfer a phosphate group to ADP, forming ATP.
  - **Myoglobin** is a heme-containing protein that is a muscular oxygen reserve.

The Skeletal System

- Internal skeletons (like those in humans) are called **endoskeletons**; external skeletons (like those in arthropods) are called **exoskeletons**.
- The human skeletal system can be divided into axial and appendicular skeletons.
  - The **axial skeleton** consists of structures in the midline such as thc skull, vertebral column, rib cage, and hyoid bone.
  - The **appendicular skeleton** consists of the bones of the limbs, the pectoral girdle, and the pelvis.
- Bone is derived from embryonic mesoderm and includes both compact and spongy (cancellous) types.
  - **Compact bone** provides strength and is dense.
  - **Spongy** or **cancellous bone** has a lattice-like structure consisting of bony spicules known as **trabeculae**. The cavities are filled with bone marrow.
  - Long bones contain shafts called **diaphyses** that flare to form **metaphyses** and terminate in **epiphyses**. The epiphysis contains an **epiphyseal (growth) plate** that causes linear growth of the bone.
  - Bone is surrounded by a layer of connective tissue called **periosteum**.
  - Bones are attached to **muscles** by tendons and to each other by **ligaments**.

- **Bone matrix** has both organic components, like collagen, glycoproteins, and other peptides; and inorganic components, like **hydroxyapatite**.
  - Bone is organized into concentric rings called **lamellae** around a central **Haversian** or **Volkmann's canal**. This structural unit is called an **osteon** or **Haversian system**.
  - Between lamellar rings are **lacunae**, where osteocytes reside, which are connected with **canaliculi** to allow for nutrient and waste transfer.
- Bone remodeling is carried out by osteoblasts and osteoclasts. **Osteoblasts** build bone, while **osteoclasts** resorb bone.
  - **Parathyroid hormone** increases resorption of bone, increasing calcium and phosphate concentrations in the blood.
  - **Vitamin D** also increases resorption of bone, leading to increased turnover and, subsequently, the production of stronger bone.
  - **Calcitonin** increases bone formation, decreasing calcium concentrations in the blood.
- Cartilage is a firm, elastic material secreted by **chondrocytes**. Its matrix is called **chondrin**.
  - Cartilage is usually found in areas that require more flexibility or cushioning.
  - Cartilage is avascular and is not innervated.
- In fetal life, bone forms from cartilage through **endochondral ossification**. Some bones, especially those of the skull, form directly from undifferentiated tissue (**mesenchyme**) in **intramembranous ossification**.
- Joints may be classified as immovable or movable.
  - **Immovable joints** are fused together to form sutures or similar fibrous joints.
  - **Movable joints** are usually strengthened by ligaments and contain a **synovial capsule**.
  - **Synovial fluid**, secreted by the **synovium**, aids in motion by lubricating the joint.
  - Each bone in the joint is coated with **articular cartilage** to aid in movement and provide cushioning.
- Muscles that serve opposite functions come in **antagonistic pairs**; when one muscle contracts, the other lengthens.

ANSWERS TO CONCEPT CHECKS

11.1

1. Skeletal and cardiac muscle are striated. Smooth muscle is always uninucleated. Skeletal muscle is always polynucleated. Skeletal muscle is voluntary. Smooth and cardiac muscle are innervated by the autonomic nervous system. Smooth and cardiac muscle exhibit myogenic activity.
2. The A-band does not change length during muscle contraction because it is the entire length of the myosin filament. The filaments do not change length, but rather slide over each other; thus, the A-band should remain a constant length during contraction.
3. Release of acetylcholine from motor neuron → activation of acetylcholine receptors in sarcolemma → depolarization of sarcolemma → spreading of signal using T-tubules → release of calcium from sarcoplasmic reticulum (SR) → binding of calcium to troponin → conformational shift in tropomyosin → exposure of myosin-binding sites → myosin binds to actin
4. ATP binding allows the myosin filament to disconnect from actin. Dissociation of ADP and inorganic phosphate from myosin causes the powerstroke.
5. Tetanus is the summation of multiple simple twitches that occur too quickly for the muscle to relax. This leads to a stronger and more prolonged contraction of the muscle.

11.2

1. Compact bone is dense and is used for its strength; it forms most of the outer layers of a bone. Spongy (cancellous) bone has many spaces between bony spicules called trabeculae and is the site of marrow production. It is found in the interior core of the bone and also helps distribute forces or pressures on the bone.
2. The three parts of a bone are the diaphysis, metaphysis, and epiphysis. Growth plates are found in epiphyses and contribute to linear growth.
3. Most inorganic bone is composed of hydroxyapatite crystals.
4. Osteoblasts build bone. Osteoclasts "chew" bone (break it down). Chondrocytes form cartilage.
5. Synovial fluid, produced by the synovium, lubricates movable joints.

SCIENCE MASTERY ASSESSMENT EXPLANATIONS

1. **D**

We are given a diagram of a sarcomere and asked to determine which regions shorten during muscle contraction. All bands and zones of the sarcomere shorten during contraction except the A-band, which is the full length of the thick filaments. In this diagram, that is region 1. Thus, the remaining regions all shorten, making **(D)** the correct answer. Region 2 represents the I-band, region 3 represents the H-zone, and region 4 is the length of the sarcomere between Z-lines.

2. **C**

Region 1 contains both thick and thin filaments overlapping each other. This region refers to the A-band and is measured from one end of the thick filaments to the other. This is also the only portion of the sarcomere that does not change length during muscle contraction.

3. **D**

The sarcomere is the contractile unit in striated muscle cells. One sarcomere is represented by the area between the two vertical lines, referred to as the Z-lines. In addition, the Z-lines anchor the thin filaments. In the diagram, a sarcomere is therefore defined by region 4.

4. **C**

Calcium is released from the sarcoplasmic reticulum into the sarcoplasm. It binds the troponin molecules on the thin filaments, causing the strands of tropomyosin to shift, thereby exposing the myosin-binding sites on the thin filaments.

5. **A**

Let's quickly define each one of the four cells discussed in the answer choices. Osteoblasts are bone cells involved in the secretion of bone matrix, as **(A)** states. Osteoclasts are large, polynucleated cells involved in bone resorption. Osteocytes are mature bone cells that eventually become surrounded by their matrix; their primary role is bone maintenance. Finally, chondrocytes are cells that secrete chondrin, an elastic matrix that makes up cartilage.

6. **C**

This question is essentially asking where longitudinal growth occurs in bones. The most likely site of abnormalities in this child's femur is the epiphyseal plate, a disc of cartilaginous cells at the internal border of the epiphysis, because the epiphyseal plate is the site of longitudinal growth. Damage to the epiphysis (with or without metaphysis involvement) can imply damage to the epiphyseal plate.

7. **D**

Red fibers are slow-twitching fibers that have high levels of myoglobin and many mitochondria. They derive their energy from aerobic respiration and are capable of sustained vigorous activity. This eliminates **(A)** and **(B)**. White fibers, on the other hand, are fast-twitching fibers and contain lower levels of myoglobin and fewer mitochondria. Because of their composition, they derive more of their energy anaerobically and fatigue more easily. This eliminates **(C)** and makes **(D)** the correct answer.

8. **A**

The articular surfaces of the bones are covered with a layer of smooth articular cartilage. The epiphysis is a portion of the bone itself, eliminating **(B)**. Synovial fluid lubricates the movement in the joint space, but does not stop the bones from contacting one another; this is the job of articular cartilage, eliminating **(C)**. There is no appreciable function for smooth muscle in the joint space, eliminating **(D)**.

9. **B**

The only type of muscle that is always multinucleated is skeletal muscle, making **(B)** the correct answer. Cardiac muscle may contain one or two centrally located nuclei, so Statement I is incorrect. Smooth muscle, on the other hand, always has only one centrally located nucleus.

10. **D**

Myogenic activity refers to the ability of a muscle to contract without nervous stimulation, such as in response to other stimuli like stretching. Smooth and cardiac muscle both possess myogenic activity.

11. **D**

Yellow marrow is largely inactive and is infiltrated by adipose tissue, making **(D)** the correct answer.

12. **D**

The periosteum, a fibrous sheath that surrounds long bones, is the site of attachment to muscle tissue. Some periosteum cells are capable of differentiating into bone-forming cells called osteoblasts. This eliminates **(A)**, **(B)**, and **(C)**. It is the synovium that secretes fluid into the joint cavity (joint space), not the periosteum, making **(D)** the correct answer.

13. **D**

The axial skeleton includes the skull, vertebral column, rib cage, and hyoid bone. The sternum is a point of attachment of the rib cage and is thus a part of the axial, not appendicular, skeleton. The limb bones, pectoral girdle, and pelvis are all part of the appendicular skeleton.

14. **B**

Bones form in one of two ways: endochondral ossification and intramembranous ossification. Endochondral ossification is the replacement of cartilage with bone and occurs mostly in long bones, eliminating **(A)**. Intramembranous ossification is the formation of bone from undifferentiated connective tissue cells (mesenchyme) and occurs mostly in the skull, making **(B)** the correct answer. Bone resorption is the breakdown of bone, not its formation, eliminating **(C)**. Longitudinal growth occurs in long bones and is responsible for increasing height over time, but does not play a role in fontanelle ossification, eliminating **(D)**.

15. **C**

An unprovoked fracture of the hip is not a normal finding in a person who is younger. Given that the patient has a high calcium level, it is likely that the patient has an increased level of bone resorption that is causing the bones to be more fragile. Parathyroid hormone causes calcium release from bones. If this patient had an overactive parathyroid gland—or even cancer in this gland—then it is likely that calcium could still be resorbed from the bones even though blood calcium levels are already high.

Consult your online resources for additional practice. **GO ONLINE**

SHARED CONCEPTS

Biology Chapter 4
The Nervous System

Biology Chapter 5
The Endocrine System

Biology Chapter 6
The Respiratory System

Biology Chapter 7
The Cardiovascular System

General Chemistry Chapter 9
Solutions

Physics and Math Chapter 1
Kinematics and Dynamics

CHAPTER 12

GENETICS AND EVOLUTION

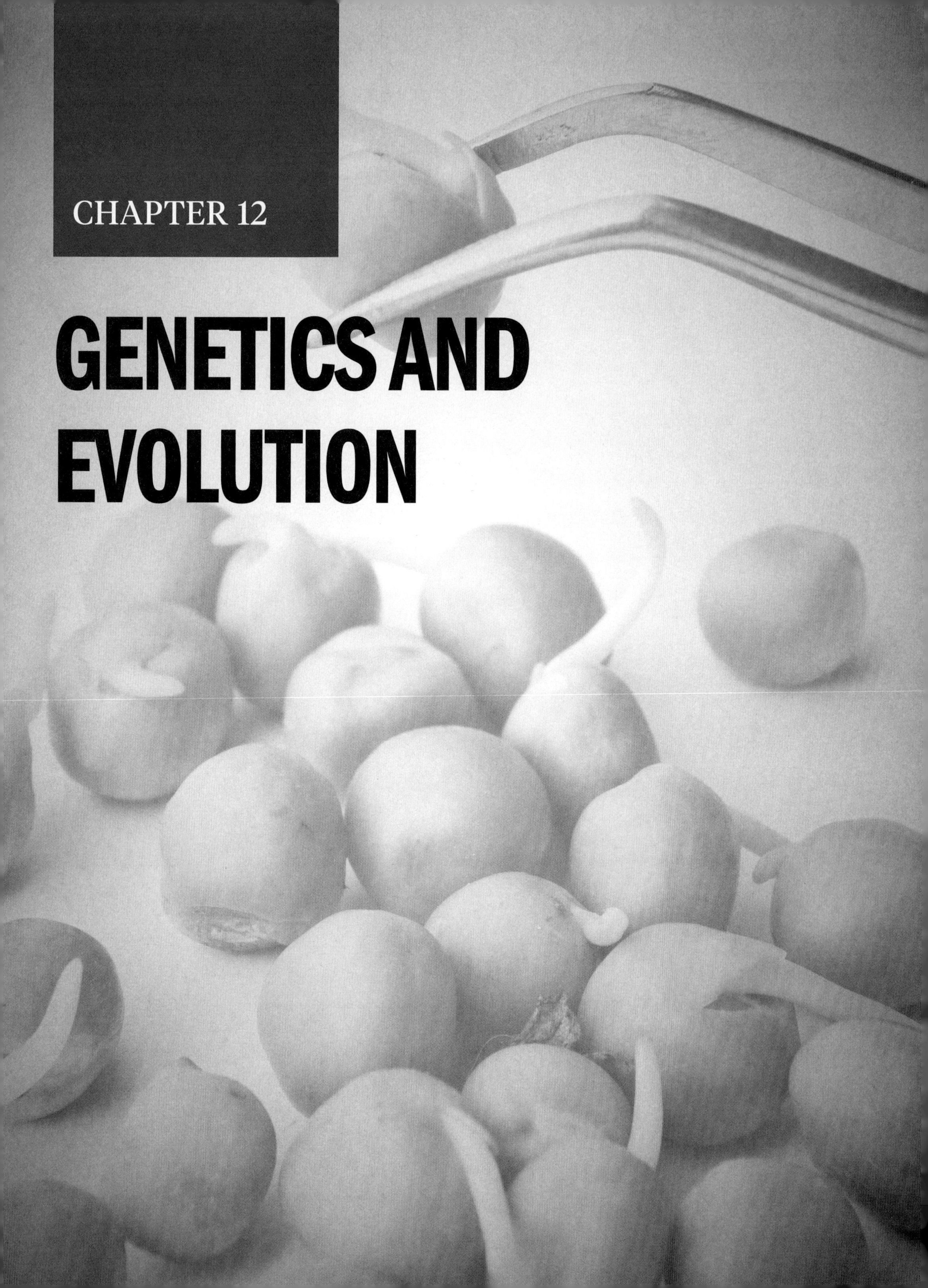

SCIENCE MASTERY ASSESSMENT

Every pre-med knows this feeling: there is so much content I have to know for the MCAT! How do I know what to do first or what's important?

While the high-yield badges throughout this book will help you identify the most important topics, this Science Mastery Assessment is another tool in your MCAT prep arsenal. This quiz (which can also be taken in your online resources) and the guidance below will help ensure that you are spending the appropriate amount of time on this chapter based on your personal strengths and weaknesses. Don't worry though—skipping something now does not mean you'll never study it. Later on in your prep, as you complete full-length tests, you'll uncover specific pieces of content that you need to review and can come back to these chapters as appropriate.

How to Use This Assessment

If you answer 0–7 questions correctly:

Spend about 1 hour to read this chapter in full and take limited notes throughout. Follow up by reviewing **all** quiz questions to ensure that you now understand how to solve each one.

If you answer 8–11 questions correctly:

Spend 20–40 minutes reviewing the quiz questions. Beginning with the questions you missed, read and take notes on the corresponding subchapters. For questions you answered correctly, ensure your thinking matches that of the explanation and you understand why each choice was correct or incorrect.

If you answer 12–15 questions correctly:

Spend less than 20 minutes reviewing all questions from the quiz. If you missed any, then include a quick read-through of the corresponding subchapters, or even just the relevant content within a subchapter, as part of your question review. For questions you answered correctly, ensure your thinking matches that of the explanation and review the Concept Summary at the end of the chapter.

1. What is the gene order of linked genes M, N, O, and P, given the following recombination frequencies?

MN: 6%	NO: 18%
MO: 12%	NP: 1%
MP: 5%	OP: 17%

A. MOPN
B. NPMO
C. ONPM
D. PNMO

2. Suppose that in a mammalian species, the allele for black hair (B) is dominant to the allele for brown hair (b), and the allele for curly hair (C) is dominant to the allele for straight hair (c). When an organism of unknown genotype is crossed against one with straight, brown hair, the phenotypic ratio is as follows:
I. 25% curly black hair
II. 25% straight black hair
III. 25% curly brown hair
IV. 25% straight brown hair

What is the genotype of the unknown parent?
A. BbCC
B. bbCc
C. Bbcc
D. BbCc

3. If a genotypical male who has hemophilia (X_hY) is crossed with a genotypical female carrier of both color blindness and hemophilia (X_cX_h), what is the probability that a genotypically female child would be born without either condition?
A. 0%
B. 25%
C. 50%
D. 100%

4. If a test cross on a species of plant reveals the appearance of a recessive phenotype in the offspring, what must be true of the phenotypically dominant parent?
A. It must be genotypically heterozygous.
B. It must be genotypically homozygous.
C. It could be either genotypically heterozygous or homozygous.
D. It must have the same genotype as the test cross control parent.

5. Which of the following definitions is FALSE?
A. Penetrance—the percentage of individuals in the population carrying the allele who actually express the phenotype associated with it
B. Expressivity—the percentage of individuals in the population carrying the allele who do not express the phenotype associated with it
C. Incomplete dominance—occurs when the phenotype of the heterozygote is an intermediate of the phenotypes of the homozygotes
D. Codominance—occurs when multiple alleles exist for a given gene and more than one of them is dominant

6. In a species of plant, a homozygous red flower (RR) is crossed with a homozygous yellow flower (rr). If the F_1 generation is self-crossed and the F_2 generation has a phenotypic ratio of red:orange:yellow of 1:2:1, which characteristic accounts for these results?
A. Codominance
B. Incomplete dominance
C. Penetrance
D. Expressivity

7. Which of the following statements is INCORRECT regarding inheritance of traits according to the modern synthesis model?
A. A mutation due to excessive amounts of ultraviolet light occurs in an unfertilized egg; this will affect the child who is born from that egg.
B. The muscular strength gained by a weight lifter over a lifetime is inherited by the weight lifter's children.
C. A green-feathered bird that survived all of the predators in the forest will pass on the green feather genes to its offspring.
D. A flower with a tasty nectar eaten by a butterfly is more likely to pass on its genes through the pollen spread by the butterfly than a flower with less desirable nectar.

8. Which of the following statements is FALSE based on Darwin's theory of natural selection?
   A. Natural selection is the driving force for evolution.
   B. Favorable genetic variations become more and more common in individuals throughout their lives.
   C. Natural selection can drive organisms living in groups to ultimately become distinct species.
   D. Fitness is measured by reproductive success.

9. Which of the following is NOT a necessary condition for Hardy–Weinberg equilibrium?
   A. Large population size
   B. No mutations
   C. Monogamous mating partners
   D. No migration into or out of the population

10. As the climate became colder during the Ice Age, a particular species of mammal evolved a thicker layer of fur. What kind of selection occurred in this population?
    A. Stabilizing selection
    B. Directional selection
    C. Disruptive selection
    D. Speciation selection

11. At what point are two populations descended from the same ancestral stock considered to be separate species?
    A. When they can no longer produce viable, fertile offspring
    B. When they look significantly different from each other
    C. When they can interbreed successfully and produce offspring
    D. When their habitats are separated by a significantly large distance so that they cannot meet

12. In a nonevolving population, there are two alleles, R and r, which code for the same trait. The frequency of R is 30 percent. What are the frequencies of all the possible genotypes?
    A. 49% RR, 42% Rr, 9% rr
    B. 30% RR, 21% Rr, 49% rr
    C. 0.09% RR, 0.42% Rr, 0.49% rr
    D. 9% RR, 42% Rr, 49% rr

13. In a particular Hardy–Weinberg population, there are only two eye colors: brown and blue. Of the population, 36% have blue eyes, the recessive trait. What percentage of the population is heterozygous?
    A. 24%
    B. 48%
    C. 60%
    D. 64%

14. Tay-Sachs disease is an autosomal recessive disorder characterized by defective hexosaminidase A. Proteomic analysis of a cell affected by this condition revealed a shortened protein with an abnormal amino acid sequence at the C-terminus. Based on this information, which mutation is mostly likely?
    A. Silent mutation
    B. Missense mutation
    C. Nonsense mutation
    D. Frameshift mutation

15. A child is born with a number of rare phenotypic features and genetic testing is performed. The child is determined to have partial trisomy 21, with three copies of some segments of DNA from chromosome 21, and partial monosomy 4, with only one copy of some segments of DNA from chromosome 4. Which of the following mutations could have occurred in one of the parental gametes during development to explain both findings?
    A. Deletion
    B. Insertion
    C. Translocation
    D. Inversion

Answer Key

1. **B**
2. **D**
3. **C**
4. **A**
5. **B**
6. **B**
7. **B**
8. **B**
9. **C**
10. **B**
11. **A**
12. **D**
13. **B**
14. **D**
15. **C**

Detailed explanations can be found at the end of the chapter.

CHAPTER 12

GENETICS AND EVOLUTION

In This Chapter

CHAPTER PROFILE

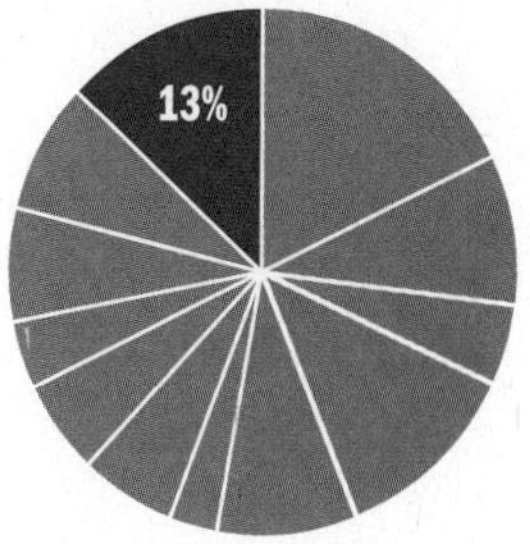

The content in this chapter should be relevant to about 13% of all questions about biology on the MCAT.

This chapter covers material from the following AAMC content category:

1C: Transmission of heritable information from generation to generation and the processes that increase genetic diversity

Introduction

For generations, European royal families practiced what is known as royal intermarriage. For purposes of establishing or continuing political alliances, maintaining bloodline purity, or smoothing out diplomatic relations, marriages between royal families were arranged, resulting in such an interweaving of bloodlines that eventually much of European royalty was—and still is—genetically related.

Such marriage unions led to rather severe restrictions on the gene pool, or all the alleles represented in the royal family lines. Offspring of parents who were also related to each other through blood lineage (consanguinity) came to have greater similarities in their genotypes, and certain alleles became so frequent that their phenotypic expression became almost a hallmark of royal descent. The House of Habsburg, which ruled a number of European kingdoms from the 11th century until the late 18th century, was perhaps the most infamous for its inbreeding practices. Members of this royal family bore the unmistakable mark of their restricted genes through a jaw malformation that even came to be known as the *Habsburg lip*. Medically termed *prognathism* (Greek: "forward jaw"), the condition is a misalignment of the mandible and maxilla. The Habsburg family portraits present individuals with prominent, forward-thrusting lower jaws and chins characteristic of mandibular prognathism. The genetic condition has more than just aesthetic implications; it can lead to serious disfigurement and disability. Charles II of Spain suffered from the worst case of the Habsburg lip on record—his lower teeth protruded so much farther than his upper teeth that he was not able to chew his food.

In this chapter, we will explore the concepts of classical genetics, which were originally described in the mid-1800s. Consider this chapter in tandem with the discussions of molecular genetics in Chapters 6 and 7 of *MCAT Biochemistry Review*. Then, we will explore the changes in the gene pool that occur over time with a discussion of evolution. We'll also quantify the genetics of populations that are *not* undergoing evolution with the Hardy–Weinberg principle.

12.1 Fundamental Concepts of Genetics

High-Yield

LEARNING OBJECTIVES

After Chapter 12.1, you will be able to:

- Recall what traits make alleles dominant or recessive
- Differentiate between homozygous, heterozygous, and hemizygous genotypes
- Compare and contrast complete dominance, codominance, and incomplete dominance
- Explain the difference between penetrance and expressivity
- Connect Mendel's laws with the phase of meiosis to which they are most closely correlated

BRIDGE

Blood type A individuals carry the A antigen on their erythrocytes and have circulating anti-B antibodies. Blood type B individuals carry the B antigen on their erythrocytes and have circulating anti-A antibodies. Those with type AB have both antigens and neither antibody; those with type O have neither antigen and both antibodies. That makes type O individuals universal donors and type AB individuals universal recipients. Blood typing is discussed in Chapter 7 of *MCAT Biology Review*.

The physical and biochemical characteristics of every living organism are determined by **genes**, which are DNA sequences that code for heritable traits that can be passed from one generation to the next. Taken together, all genes (as well as a large supply of noncoding DNA) are organized into **chromosomes** to ensure that genetic material is passed easily to daughter cells during mitosis and meiosis. Each gene may have alternative forms called **alleles**. We've already explored the ABO blood antigens as an example of three alleles for the same gene (I^A, I^B, and i). The genetic combination possessed by an individual is known as a **genotype**, and the manifestation of a given genotype as an observable trait is known as a **phenotype**.

Human beings typically possess two copies of each chromosome, called **homologues**, with the exception of the sex chromosomes of genotypical males, who have one X chromosome and one Y chromosome. Each gene has a particular **locus**, or location on a specific chromosome. The normal locus of a particular gene is consistent among human beings—a gene can be described by its location. Because each chromosome is part of a homologous pair, a person will inherit two alleles for all genes (again, except for male sex chromosomes). Alleles can be categorized based on their expression. If only one copy of an allele is needed to express a given phenotype, the allele is said to be **dominant** and is usually represented with a capital letter. If two copies are needed, the allele is said to be **recessive** and is usually represented with a lowercase letter. If both alleles are the same for a given gene, the individual is said to have a **homozygous** genotype. If the alleles are different, the individual has a **heterozygous** genotype. A **hemizygous** genotype describes a situation in which only one allele is present for a given gene, as is the case for parts of the X chromosome in genotypical males.

Patterns of Dominance

When only one dominant and one recessive allele exist for a given gene, there is said to be **complete dominance**. In this case, the presence of one dominant allele will mask the recessive allele, if present. When more than one dominant allele exists for a given gene, there is **codominance**. For example, a person with one allele for the A blood antigen and one allele for the B blood antigen will express both antigens simultaneously. Finally, **incomplete dominance** occurs when a heterozygote expresses a phenotype that is intermediate between the two homozygous genotypes. A classic example of incomplete dominance is the mating of certain flowers, in which a red flower crossed with a white flower results in pink flowers, as shown in Figure 12.1.

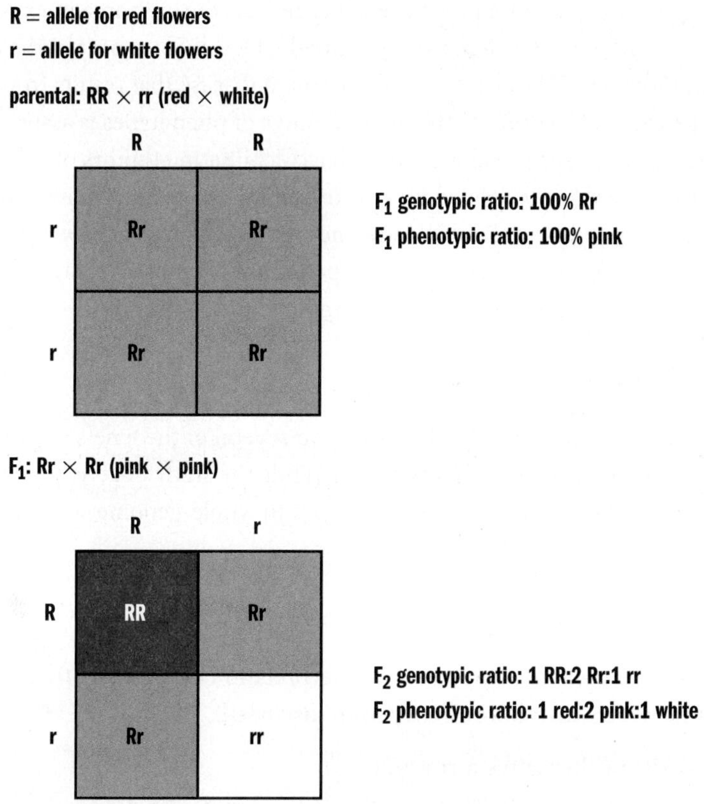

Figure 12.1 Incomplete Dominance
Snapdragons display incomplete dominance, in which neither allele is dominant and the heterozygous phenotype is a mixture of the two homozygous phenotypes.

Penetrance and Expressivity

Penetrance and expressivity both reveal the complex interplay between genes and the environment. **Penetrance** is a population measure defined as the proportion of individuals in the population carrying the allele who actually express the phenotype. In other words, it is the probability that, given a particular genotype, a person will express the phenotype. Alleles can be classified by their degree of penetrance; Huntington's disease, caused by an expansion of a repetitive sequence in the *huntingtin* gene, is a classic example. Individuals with more than 40 sequence repeats have **full penetrance**—100 percent of individuals with this allele show symptoms of Huntington's disease. Individuals with fewer sequence repeats show **high penetrance**, wherein most (but not all) of those with the allele show symptoms of the disease. With fewer sequence repeats, the gene comes to have **reduced penetrance**, **low penetrance**, or even **nonpenetrance**.

KEY CONCEPT

- **Penetrance**–the proportion of the population with a given genotype who actually express the phenotype
- **Expressivity**–the different manifestations of the same genotype across the population

A related but distinct concept is **expressivity**, which is defined as varying phenotypes despite identical genotypes. If expressivity is **constant**, then all individuals with a given genotype express the same phenotype. However, if expressivity is **variable**, then individuals with the same genotype may have different phenotypes. Whereas penetrance is a population parameter (what percentage of individuals with a given genotype express the phenotype?), expressivity reflects the gray area in expression and is more commonly considered at the individual level. For example, the disease *neurofibromatosis type II* is an autosomal dominant disease that results from a mutation of the gene *NF2* (*merlin*). Interestingly, a range of phenotypes is associated with carrying the defective allele. Many patients have debilitating tumors of the vestibulocochlear nerve, which is needed for hearing and balance. Some have cataracts, while others have tumors in the skin called neuromas; still others have spinal lesions. A small proportion of the population is nonpenetrant. The disease shows variable expressivity because presentations range from no clinical effect to severe disability.

Mendelian Concepts

Gregor Mendel, an Augustinian friar, developed several of the tenets of genetics in the 1860s based on his work with pea plants. While the study of genetics has come a long way, from pedigree analysis to DNA probes to whole-genome sequencing, many of Mendel's original ideas still hold.

Mendel's First Law: Law of Segregation

There are four basic tenets of the modern interpretation of **Mendel's first law (of segregation)**, some which have already been discussed:

- Genes exist in alternative forms (alleles).
- An organism has two alleles for each gene—one inherited from each parent.
- The two alleles segregate during meiosis, resulting in gametes that carry only one allele for any inherited trait.
- If two alleles of an organism are different, only one will be fully expressed and the other will be silent. The expressed allele is said to be dominant, while the silent allele is recessive. (Keep in mind that codominance and incomplete dominance are exceptions to this rule.)

The key cellular correlate to draw here is the separation of homologous chromosomes during anaphase I of meiosis. By separating—segregating—these chromosomes into different cells, each gamete carries only one allele for any given trait.

Mendel's Second Law: Law of Independent Assortment

Mendel's second law (**of independent assortment**) states that the inheritance of one gene does not affect the inheritance of another gene. Remember from Chapter 2 of *MCAT Biology Review* that spermatogonia and oogonia undergo genome replication before meiosis I. The daughter DNA strand is held to the parent strand at the **centromere**. Together, these DNA strands are known as **sister chromatids**. During prophase I of meiosis, homologous chromosomes pair up to form **tetrads**, which derive their name from the four chromatids involved (two chromatids in each of two homologous chromosomes). Small segments of genetic material are swapped between chromatids in homologous chromosomes, resulting in novel combinations of alleles that were not present in the original chromosomes (**recombination**). This allows the inheritance of one gene to be independent of the inheritance of all others.

Mendel's second law has been complicated by the discovery of linked genes. We will discuss nonindependent assortment and linkage later in this chapter in the section on analytical approaches in genetics.

Both segregation of homologous chromosomes and independent assortment of alleles increase the genetic diversity of gametes and, subsequently, the genetic diversity of offspring. This has been demonstrated to improve the ability of a species to evolve and adapt to environmental stresses.

KEY CONCEPT

Segregation of chromosomes and independent assortment of alleles allow for greater genetic diversity in the offspring.

DNA as Genetic Material

While Mendel noticed there were certain patterns of inheritance, what he did not know was that DNA was the genetic material transferred to offspring and that genes were made of DNA. In fact, the scientific community rejected Mendel's initial papers on inheritance. It wasn't until the early 1900s that his work was rediscovered. In the early to mid-1900s, it was largely believed that protein was the heritable material. In the mid-1900s, there were three experiments conducted that largely pointed to DNA's role in genetic inheritance.

BRIDGE

The transforming principle described in Griffith's experiment is the same as bacterial transformation discussed in Chapter 1 of *MCAT Biology Review*. Remember that transformation is one of three main ways bacteria increase genetic variability; the other two are conjugation and transduction.

In the 1920s, Frederick Griffith was a scientist working for the British government, studying *Streptococcus pneumoniae,* a bacteria that causes pneumonia. Two strains of *S. pneumoniae* were identified: a virulent (disease-causing) strain and a nonvirulent strain. In successive trials, Griffith exposed mice to these strains of bacteria under different conditions and observed whether the mice lived or died, as shown in Figure 12.2. The virulent *S. pneumonia* has a smooth capsule that helps the bacterium evade the immune system and cause disease. He injected this strain into mice, which resulted in death of the mice. Naturally, if the virulent bacteria were killed prior to injection, no disease resulted. Likewise, exposure of the mice to the nonvirulent strain, which has a rough capsule, did not cause disease. However, when both dead virulent bacteria and live nonvirulent bacteria were injected into the mouse, the mouse died and live bacteria with smooth capsules could be found in the mice. He theorized that the live, nonvirulent bacteria must have acquired the ability to form smooth capsules from the dead virulent bacteria. This was known as the *transforming principle.*

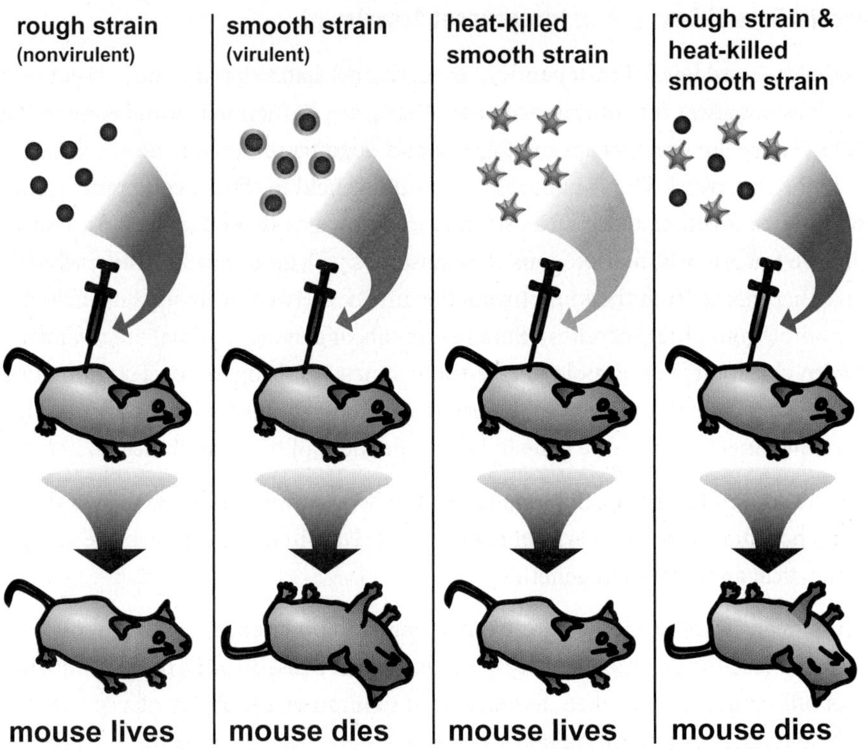

Figure 12.2 The Griffith Experiment

Researchers at the Rockefeller Institute confirmed the transformation principle. Three American scientists—Oswald Avery, Colin MacLeod, and Maclyn McCarty—were attempting to identify the exact material underlying the transformation principle. These scientists purified a very large quantity of heat-killed virulent *S. pneumoniae* bacteria and separated the subcellular components of the bacteria into different extracts. It was noted that the addition of one particular extract to nonvirulent *S. pneumoniae* transformed the bacteria and enabled them to kill the mouse when injected. When this substance was treated with enzymes known to degrade DNA, the bacteria were not transformed and the mice lived. However, when the substance was treated with enzymes known to degrade proteins, the bacteria were still transformed and the mice died. Thus, the group concluded that the transforming substance must be DNA.

BRIDGE

Radiolabeling sulfur was an appropriate choice to tag proteins in the Hershey-Chase experiment. Recall from Chapter 1 of *MCAT Biochemistry Review* that two amino acids—cysteine and methionine—contain sulfur in their R group, while no nucleotides contain any sulfur.

In 1952 (one year before the description of the Watson–Crick model), Alfred Hershey and Martha Chase worked to confirm the idea that DNA could independently carry genetic information. These scientists created bacteriophages with radiolabeled DNA and protein. One group of bacteriophages contained radiolabeled sulfur, which is found in protein but not in DNA. Another group contained radiolabeled phosphorus, which is found in DNA but not in protein. Each of these bacteriophages was permitted to infect a group of nonlabeled bacteria. Recall from Chapter 1 of *MCAT Biology Review* that when bacteriophages infect a bacterium, they inject their genetic material into the cell and leave their capsid outside. After the phages and bacteria were incubated, the sample was centrifuged to separate the material that remained outside the cell from the bacterial cells themselves. It was determined that while no radiolabeled protein entered the cells, radiolabeled DNA had. It was known that viruses must enter a cell to cause disease and replicate, so this experiment once again helped confirm that DNA was the heritable genetic material.

Epigenetics

Epigenetics is a general term for changes in DNA that do not involve an alteration to the nucleotide sequence. The prefix *epi–* is Greek for "over" or "above," so the name suggests regulatory mechanisms that are in addition to the traditional features of inheritance. Epigenetic modifications can include the covalent attachment of different chemical groups to nucleotides and histone proteins, including but not limited to methylation or acetylation. These modifications can be temporary and function to increase or decrease the expression of specific genes. In general, modifications like methylation of DNA promoter regions tends to decrease the expression of specific genes, whereas modifications of lysines and/or arginines on histones have variable effects on the expression of genes.

BRIDGE

Methylation of DNA is commonly used for transcriptional regulation. Recall from Chapter 7 of the *MCAT Biochemistry Review* that the addition of methyl groups to adenine and cytosine is linked to gene silencing.

Because almost all cells in the body contain the same genetic code, epigenetics allows cells to undergo differentiation, where different cells are able to express certain genes while silencing others. One prominent example of this is X-inactivation in cells that have two X chromosomes, in which one of the two X chromosomes is transcriptionally silenced via methylation; the inactive X chromosome is called a **Barr body**.

Epigenetic changes can have significant clinical impact. Hypermethylation of tumor suppressor genes and hypomethylation of oncogenes have been implicated in some forms of cancer. Furthermore, studies have shown that epigenetic changes can be a mechanism by which organisms' responses to their changing environment can be passed down to their progeny. Indeed, the Överkalix study found that the grandchildren of those who had experienced food scarcity had different health outcomes compared to the grandchildren of those who had not experienced famine.

Another important concept is **imprinting**, an epigenetic process in which gene expression is determined by the contributing parent. There are certain genes that are differentially methylated when inherited from one parent; one of the most well known examples of imprinting comes from a region on the long arm of chromosome 15. If the deletion of this region of the chromosome occurs on the paternal chromosome and the maternal copy is heavily methylated, it leads to a developmental disorder called *Prader-Willi syndrome*. Deletion of the same genomic region on the maternal chromosome and paternal methylation leads to a different outcome, *Angelman syndrome*.

MCAT CONCEPT CHECK 12.1

Before you move on, assess your understanding of the material with these questions.

1. What does it mean for an allele to be dominant? Recessive?
   - Dominant:

   ____

   - Recessive:

   ____

2. What does it mean for a genotype to be homozygous? Heterozygous? Hemizygous?
    - Homozygous:
    - Heterozygous:
    - Hemizygous:

3. What is the difference between complete dominance, codominance, and incomplete dominance?
    - Complete dominance:
    - Codominance:
    - Incomplete dominance:

4. What is the difference between penetrance and expressivity?
    - Penetrance:
    - Expressivity:

5. With which phase of meiosis does each of Mendel's laws most closely correlate?
    - Mendel's first law:
    - Mendel's second law:

12.2 Changes in the Gene Pool

LEARNING OBJECTIVES

After Chapter 12.2, you will be able to:

- Identify the three main types of point mutations and the genetic changes they are associated with
- Recall the two main types of frameshift mutation
- Explain why genetic leakage would increase within the last century
- Describe the relationship between genetic drift, small population, and the founder effect
- Identify the main types of chromosomal mutation and the impact they have at the chromosomal level:

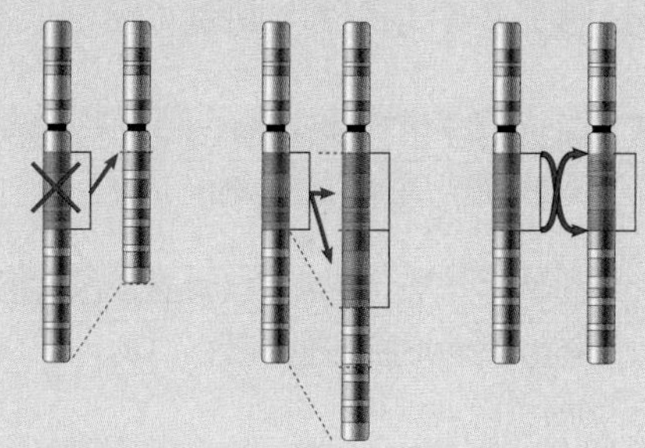

All of the alleles that exist within a species are known as the **gene pool**. When mutations or genetic leakage occur, new genes are introduced into the gene pool. Genetic variability is essential for the survival of a species because it allows it to evolve to adapt to changing environmental stresses. Certain traits may be more desirable than others and confer a selective advantage that allows for an individual to produce more viable, fertile offspring. In this section, we will consider genetic diversity and mutations, leakage, and genetic drift, which cause changes to the alleles or their frequency in the gene pool.

Mutations

A **mutation** is a change in DNA sequence, and it results in a mutant allele. Mutant alleles can be contrasted with their **wild-type** counterparts, which are alleles that are considered "normal" or "natural" and are ubiquitous in the study population. New mutations may be introduced in a variety of ways. Ionizing radiation, such as ultraviolet rays from the sun, and chemical exposures can damage DNA; substances that can cause mutations are called **mutagens**. *DNA polymerase* is subject to making mistakes during DNA replication, albeit at a very low rate; proofreading mechanisms help prevent mutations from occurring through this mechanism. Elements known as **transposons** can insert and remove themselves from the genome. If a transposon inserts in the middle of a coding sequence, the mutation will disrupt the gene.

Flawed proteins can arise in other ways without an underlying change in DNA sequence. Incorrect pairing of nucleotides during transcription or translation, or a tRNA molecule charged with the incorrect amino acid for its anticodon, can result in derangements of the normal amino acid sequence.

The major types of nucleotide-level mutations are discussed in great detail in Chapter 7 of *MCAT Biochemistry Review*, so we offer just a brief overview here of each type.

Nucleotide-Level Mutations

Many mutations occur at the level of a single nucleotide (or a very small number of nucleotides). These mutations are shown in Figure 12.3 and are summarized below.

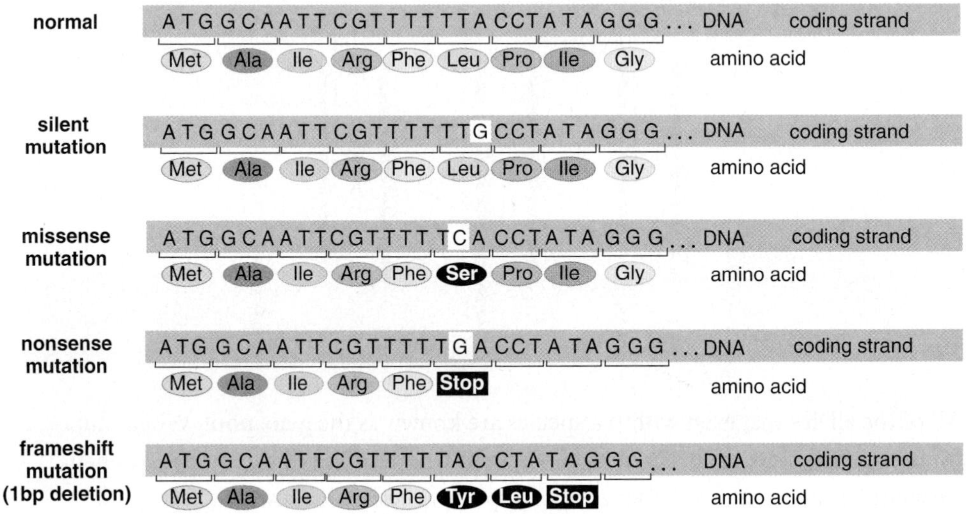

Figure 12.3 Common Nucleotide-Level Mutations

Point mutations occur when one nucleotide in DNA (A, C, T, or G) is swapped for another. These can be subcategorized as silent, missense, or nonsense mutations:

- **Silent mutations** occur when the change in nucleotide has no effect on the final protein synthesized from the gene. This most commonly occurs when the changed nucleotide is transcribed to be the third nucleotide in a codon because there is **degeneracy** (**wobble**) in the genetic code.
- **Missense mutations** occur when the change in nucleotide results in substituting one amino acid for another in the final protein.
- **Nonsense mutations** occur when the change in nucleotide results in substituting a **stop codon** for an amino acid in the final protein.

Frameshift mutations occur when nucleotides are inserted into or deleted from the genome. Because mRNA transcribed from DNA is always read in three-letter sequences called **codons**, insertion or deletion of nucleotides can shift the **reading frame**, usually resulting in either changes in the amino acid sequence or premature truncation of the protein (due to the generation of a nonsense mutation). These can be subcategorized as **insertion** or **deletion mutations**.

Chromosomal Mutations

Chromosomal mutations are larger-scale mutations in which large segments of DNA are affected, as demonstrated in Figure 12.4 and summarized below.

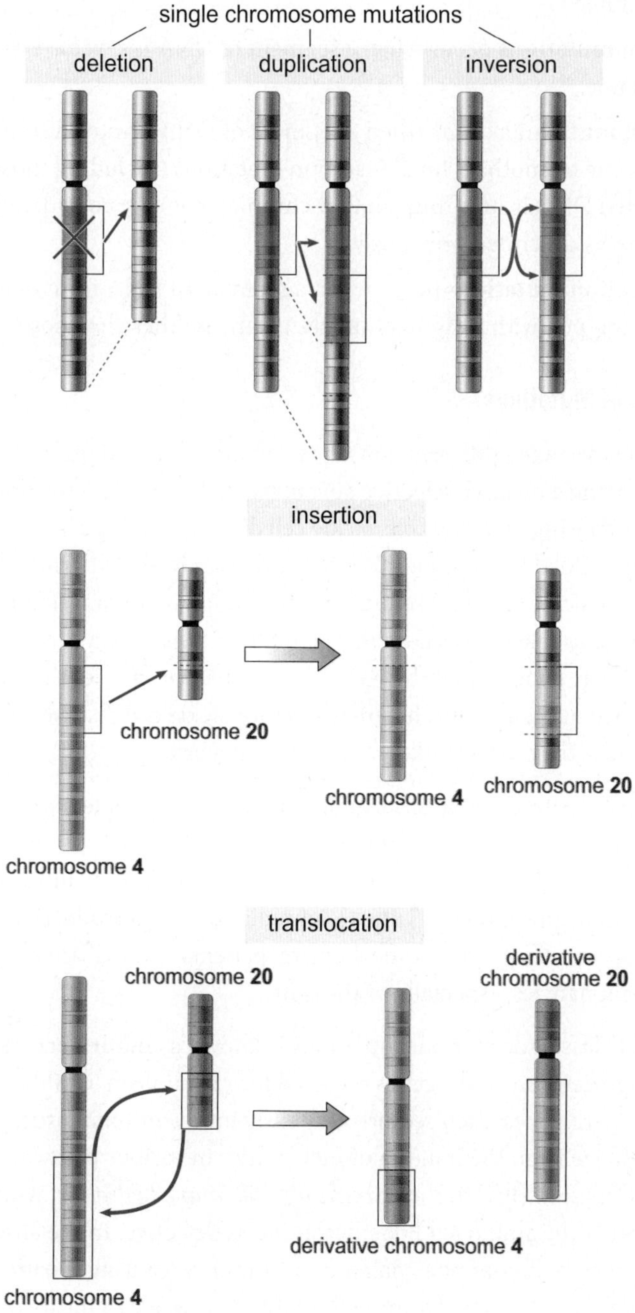

Figure 12.4 Common Chromosomal Mutations

- **Deletion mutations** occur when a large segment of DNA is lost from a chromosome. Small deletion mutations are considered frameshift mutations, as described previously.
- **Duplication mutations** occur when a segment of DNA is copied multiple times in the genome.
- **Inversion mutations** occur when a segment of DNA is reversed within the chromosome.
- **Insertion mutations** occur when a segment of DNA is moved from one chromosome to another. Small insertion mutations (including those where the inserted DNA is not from another chromosome) are considered frameshift mutations, as described previously.
- **Translocation mutations** occur when a segment of DNA from one chromosome is swapped with a segment of DNA from another chromosome.

Consequences of Mutations

Mutations can have many different consequences. Some mutations can be **advantageous**, conferring a positive selective advantage that may allow the organism to produce fitter offspring. For example, sickle cell disease is a single nucleotide mutation that causes sickled hemoglobin. While the disease itself is detrimental to life, heterozygotes for sickle cell disease usually have minor symptoms, if any, and have natural resistance to malaria because their red blood cells have a slightly shorter lifespan—just short enough that the parasitic *Plasmodium* species that causes malaria cannot reproduce in them. Thus, heterozygotes for sickle cell disease have a selective advantage because they are less likely to die from malaria.

On the other hand, some mutations can be detrimental or **deleterious**. For example, *xeroderma pigmentosum* (XP) is an inherited defect in the nucleotide excision repair mechanism. In patients with XP, DNA that has been damaged by ultraviolet radiation cannot be repaired appropriately. Ultraviolet radiation can introduce cancer-causing mutations; since they lack a repair mechanism, patients with XP are frequently diagnosed with malignancies, especially of the skin.

One important class of deleterious mutations is known as **inborn errors of metabolism**. These are deficiencies in genes required for metabolism. Children born with these deficient genes often require very early intervention in order to prevent permanent damage from the buildup of metabolites in various pathways. For example, in *phenylketonuria* (PKU), the enzyme *phenylalanine hydrolase*, which completes the metabolism of the amino acid phenylalanine, is defective. In the absence of this enzyme, toxic metabolites of phenylalanine accumulate, causing seizures, impairment of cerebral function, and learning disabilities, as well as a musty odor to bodily secretions. However, if the disease is discovered shortly after birth, then dietary phenylalanine can be eliminated and treatments can be administered to aid in metabolizing any remaining phenylalanine.

Leakage

Genetic **leakage** is a flow of genes between species. In some cases, individuals from different (but closely related) species can mate to produce **hybrid** offspring. Many hybrid offspring, such as the mule (hybrid of a male horse and a female donkey), are not able to reproduce because they have odd numbers of chromosomes—horses have 64 chromosomes and donkeys have 62, so mules, with 63 chromosomes, cannot undergo normal homologous pairing in meiosis and cannot form gametes. In some cases, however, a hybrid can reproduce with members of one species or the other, such as the *beefalo* (a cross between cattle and American bison). The hybrid carries genes from both parent species, so this can result in a net flow of genes from one species to the other.

Genetic Drift

Genetic drift refers to changes in the composition of the gene pool due to chance. Genetic drift tends to be more pronounced in small populations. The **founder effect** is a more extreme case of genetic drift in which a small population of a species finds itself in reproductive isolation from other populations as a result of natural barriers, catastrophic events, or other **bottlenecks** that drastically and suddenly reduce the size of the population available for breeding. Because the breeding group is small, **inbreeding**, or mating between two genetically related individuals, may occur in later generations. Inbreeding encourages homozygosity, which increases the prevalence of both homozygous dominant and recessive genotypes. Ultimately, genetic drift, the founder effect, and inbreeding cause a reduction in genetic diversity, which is often the reason why a small population may have increased prevalence of certain traits and diseases. For example, *branched-chain ketoacid dehydrogenase deficiency* (also called *maple syrup urine disease*) is especially common in Mennonite communities; this implies a common origin of the mutation, which may have been in a very small original population.

This loss of genetic variation may cause reduced fitness of the population, a condition known as **inbreeding depression**. On the opposite end of the spectrum, **outbreeding** or **outcrossing** is the introduction of unrelated individuals into a breeding group. Theoretically, this could result in increased variation within a gene pool and increased fitness of the population.

MCAT CONCEPT CHECK 12.2

Before you move on, assess your understanding of the material with these questions.

1. What are the three main types of point mutations? What change occurs in each?
   -
   -
   -
2. What are the two main types of frameshift mutations?
   -
   -
3. What are the three main types of chromosomal mutations that do NOT share their name with a type of frameshift mutation? What change occurs in each?
   -
   -
   -
4. Why would genetic leakage in animals be rare prior to the last century?
5. Why is genetic drift more common in small populations? What relationship does this have to the founder effect?

12.3 Analytical Approaches in Genetics

LEARNING OBJECTIVES

After Chapter 12.3, you will be able to:

- Predict the phenotype ratio in the offspring of a cross, such as AaBB × AAbb
- Order genes on a chromosome given their recombination frequencies
- Recall the five criteria of the Hardy–Weinberg principle and the underlying population characteristic each one implies
- Solve calculation problems requiring use of the Hardy–Weinberg equations: $p + q = 1$, and $p^2 + 2pq + q^2 = 1$

Genetics is a field in which a number of **biometric techniques**, or quantitative approaches to biological data, have been developed. These range from the Punnett square to mapping of chromosomes with recombinant frequencies to Hardy–Weinberg equilibrium.

Punnett Squares

Punnett squares are diagrams that predict the relative genotypic and phenotypic frequencies that will result from the crossing of two individuals. The alleles of the two parents are arranged on the top and side of the square, with the genotypes of the progeny represented at the intersections of these alleles. The genotypes of the progeny will be the product of the two parental alleles.

MCAT EXPERTISE

Pedigree (or family tree) analysis was once a mainstay of MCAT passages and questions. While this topic no longer appears on the exam, it will appear in your medical school genetics studies. The symbology of pedigree analysis is complex and intricate, but a great deal of information can be gleaned from a well-drawn pedigree.

Monohybrid Cross

In genetics problems, including those on the MCAT, dominant alleles are assigned capital letters and recessive alleles are assigned lowercase letters. If both copies of the allele are the same, that individual is said to be homozygous; if they are different, the individual is heterozygous.

A cross in which only one trait is being studied is said to be **monohybrid**. The **parent** or **P generation** refers to the individuals being crossed; the offspring are the **filial** or **F generation**. Multiple generations can be denoted F generations by using numeric subscripts. If you think of your grandparents as the P generation, then your parents are in the F_1 generation, and you are in the F_2 generation.

Mendel worked with pea plants that had either purple or white flowers. Before crossing the different plants, each group contained homozygotes; subsequent experimentation revealed that the allele for purple color was dominant (P) and the allele for white color was recessive (p). Thus, crossing a homozygous purple flower with a white flower would be crossing PP with pp, resulting in an F_1 generation that contained 100 percent Pp or heterozygotes, as shown in Figure 12.5. All of the flowers in this generation would be purple because P is a dominant allele.

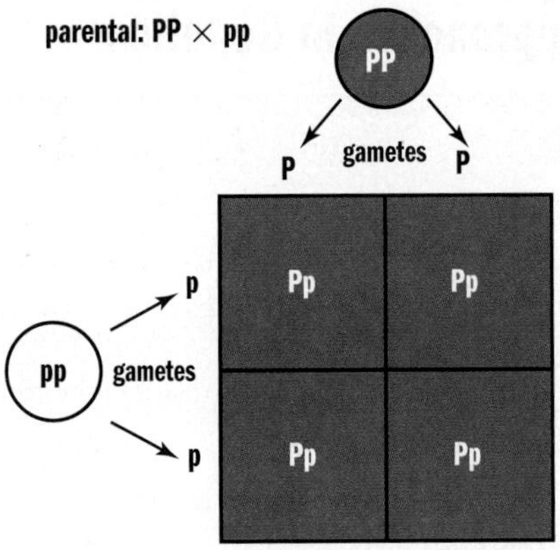

F_1 genotypic ratio: 100% Pp (heterozygous)

F_1 phenotypic ratio: 100% purple

Figure 12.5 Punnett Square of Homozygous Parents

KEY CONCEPT

Crossing two heterozygotes for a trait with complete dominance results in a 1:2:1 ratio of genotypes and a 3:1 ratio of phenotypes. Know these ratios cold for Test Day!

MCAT EXPERTISE

The ability to create and read a Punnett square quickly on Test Day is one of the most useful skills for questions involving Mendelian inheritance. Often, an entire passage in the *Biological and Biochemical Foundations of Living Systems* section will be devoted to classical and molecular genetics and will require the use of at least one Punnett square.

If two members of the F_1 generation were crossed, the resulting offspring in the F_2 generation would be more genotypically and phenotypically diverse than their parents. Crossing two plants with the genotype Pp would result in 25 percent PP, 50 percent Pp, and 25 percent pp offspring, as shown in Figure 12.6. Phenotypically, this would be a 3:1 distribution because both the homozygous dominant and heterozygous dominant offspring would be purple-flowering plants. Thus, crossing two heterozygotes in a case of complete dominance will result in a 1:2:1 distribution of genotypes (homozygous dominant:heterozygous dominant:homozygous recessive) and a 3:1 distribution of phenotypes (dominant:recessive). These ratios are, of course, theoretical probabilities and will not always hold true—especially in a small population of offspring. Usually, the more offspring parents have, the closer their phenotypic ratios will be to the expected ratios.

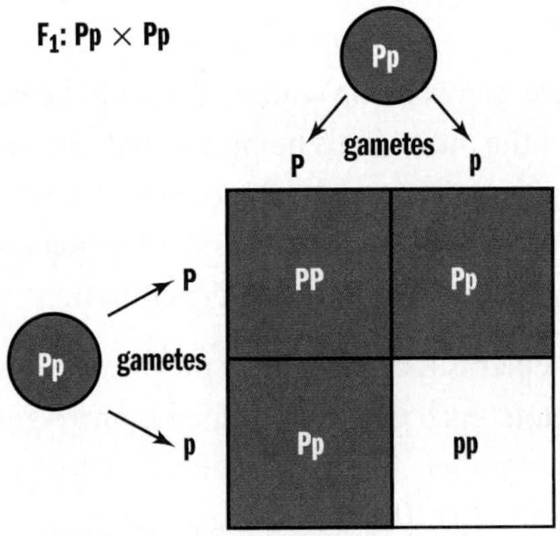

F_2 genotypic ratio: 1:2:1; 1 PP: 2 Pp:1 pp

F_2 phenotypic ratio: 3:1; 3 purple:1 white

Figure 12.6 Punnett Square of Heterozygous Parents

Test Cross

A **test cross** is used to determine an unknown genotype, as shown in Figure 12.7. In a test cross, the organism with an unknown genotype is crossed with an organism known to be homozygous recessive. If all of the offspring (100 percent) are of the dominant phenotype, then the unknown genotype is likely to be homozygous dominant. If there is a 1:1 distribution of dominant to recessive phenotypes, then the unknown genotype is likely to be heterozygous. Because a test cross is used to determine the genotype of the parent based on the phenotypes of its offspring, test crosses are sometimes called **back crosses**.

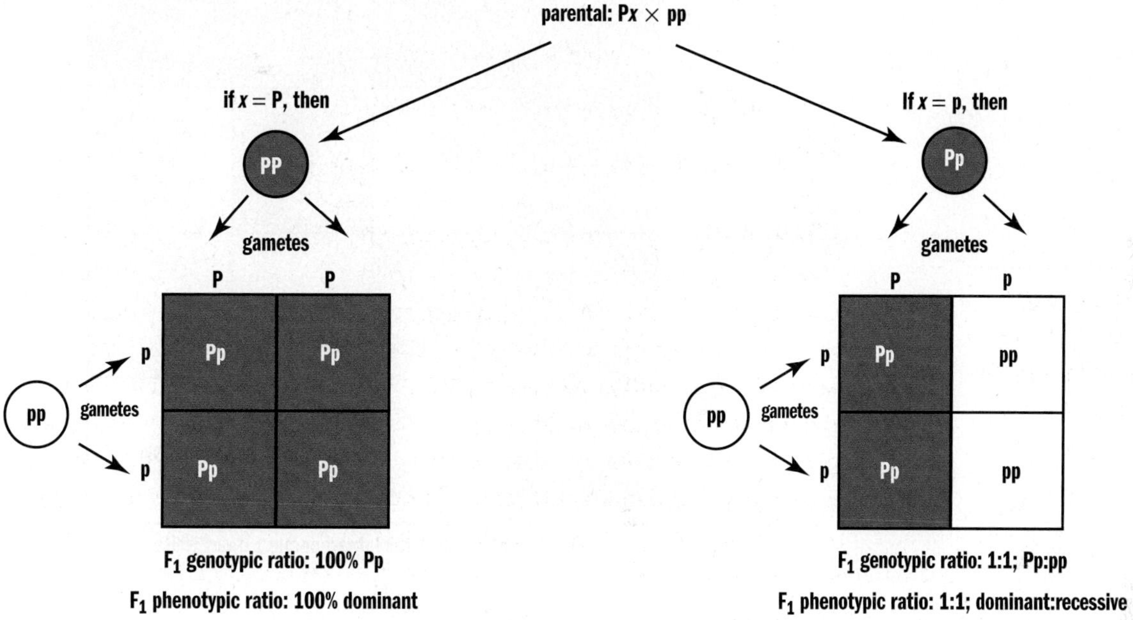

Figure 12.7 Test Cross

An organism with an unknown genotype is crossed with a homozygous recessive organism to identify the unknown genotype using the phenotypes of the resulting offspring.

Dihybrid Cross

We can extend a Punnett square to account for the inheritance of two different genes using a **dihybrid cross**. Remember, according to Mendel's second law (of independent assortment) the inheritance of one gene is independent of the inheritance of the other. This will hold true for **unlinked genes**, although it will be more complicated for linked genes, as described later in this chapter.

If we expand the previous crosses to consider not only flower color, but also plant height, then we can create a 4 × 4 Punnett square as shown in Figure 12.8. Remember that purple is dominant (P) and white is recessive (p); similarly, tall is dominant (T) and short or dwarf is recessive (t). If we cross two plants that are heterozygous for both traits, then the offspring have a phenotypic ratio of 9:3:3:1 (9 tall and purple:3 tall

MCAT EXPERTISE

Just as with the 3:1 phenotypic ratio of a monohybrid cross, it is worth memorizing the 9:3:3:1 distribution for dihybrid crosses between two heterozygotes with complete dominance.

and white:3 dwarf and purple:1 dwarf and white). Note that the 3:1 phenotypic ratio still holds for each trait (12 tall:4 dwarf and 12 purple:4 white), reflecting Mendel's second law.

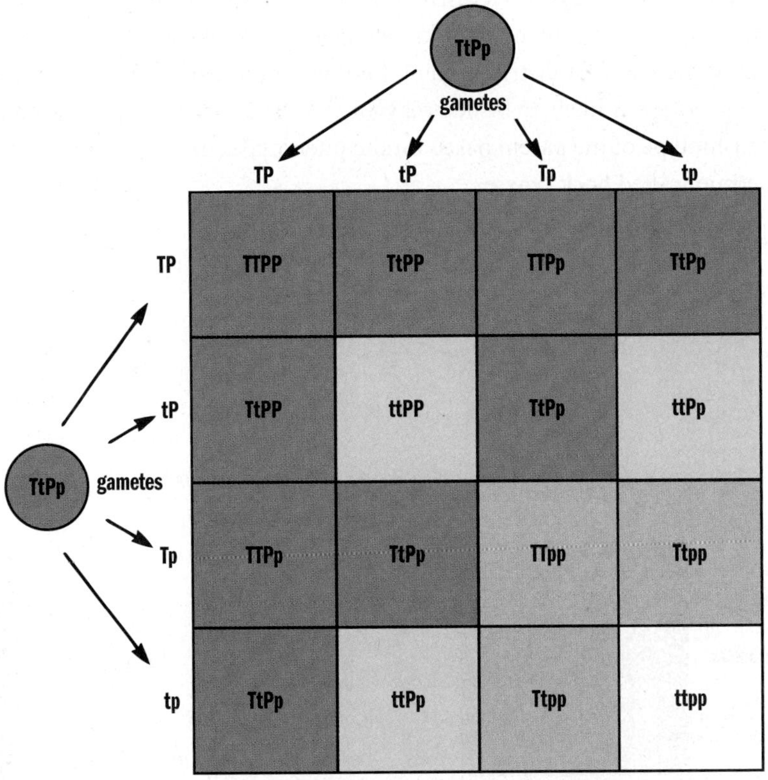

Figure 12.8 Dihybrid Cross

MNEMONIC

On the MCAT, se**x**-linked is **X**-linked. Y-linked diseases exist, but are exceedingly rare. Further, unless told otherwise, assume that sex-linked traits are recessive.

Sex-Linked Crosses

When considering **sex-linked (X-linked) traits**, a slightly different system is used to symbolize the various alleles because genotypical females have two X chromosomes and thus may be homozygous or heterozygous for a condition carried on the X chromosome. Genotypical males have only one X chromosome (and one Y chromosome) and are hemizygous for many genes carried on the X chromosome. This is why sex-linked traits are much more common in genotypical males; having only one recessive allele is sufficient for expression of the recessive phenotype.

When writing genotypes for sex-linked traits, we use X and Y to symbolize normal X and Y chromosomes. An X chromosome carrying a defective allele is commonly given a subscript, such as X_h, to indicate the presence of the disease-carrying allele. Hemophilia is a particularly common example of a sex-linked trait; Punnett squares for a heterozygous (**carrier**) female and both an unaffected (normal) male and affected (hemophiliac) male are shown in Figure 12.9.

KEY CONCEPT

Because an egg necessarily carries an X chromosome, the sperm determines the chromosomal or genotypical sex of a child. It follows that, for genotypical males with a sex-linked trait, genotypically female offspring will either carry the trait or express it, but genotypically male offspring will do neither (unless the X chromosome in the egg contains the affected allele, in which case they will express it).

cross between a carrier female (X_hX) and a normal male (XY)

	X_h	X
X	X_hX	XX
Y	X_hY	XY

offspring

25% X_hX = 25% carrier female
25% XX = 25% normal female
25% X_hY = 25% hemophiliac male
25% XY = 25% normal male

cross between a carrier female (X_hX) and a hemophiliac male (X_hY)

	X_h	X
X_h	X_hX_h	X_hX
Y	X_hY	XY

offspring

25% X_hX_h = 25% hemophiliac female
25% X_hX = 25% carrier female
25% X_hY = 25% hemophiliac male
25% XY = 25% normal male

Figure 12.9 Sex-Linked Cross
Unless stated otherwise, assume that all sex-linked traits on the MCAT are X-linked recessive.

Gene Mapping

Genes are organized in a linear fashion on chromosomes. As discussed earlier, crossing over during prophase I of meiosis causes alleles to be swapped between homologous chromosomes, supporting Mendel's second law (of independent assortment). However, genes that are located very close together on a chromosome are less likely to be separated from each other during crossing over. In other words, the further apart two genes are, the more likely it is that there will be a point of crossing over, called a **chiasma**, between them. The likelihood that two alleles are separated from each other during crossing over, called the **recombination frequency** (θ), is roughly proportional to the distance between the genes on the chromosome. We can also describe the strength of linkage between genes based on the recombination frequency: tightly linked genes have recombination frequencies close to 0 percent; weakly linked genes have recombination frequencies approaching 50 percent, as expected from independent assortment.

By analyzing recombination frequencies, a **genetic map** representing the relative distance between genes on a chromosome can be constructed. By convention, one **map unit** or **centimorgan** corresponds to a 1 percent chance of recombination occurring between two genes. Thus, if two genes were 25 map units apart, we would expect 25 percent of the total gametes examined to show recombination somewhere between these two genes. Recombination frequencies can be added in a crude approximation to determine the order of genes in the chromosome, as shown in Figure 12.10.

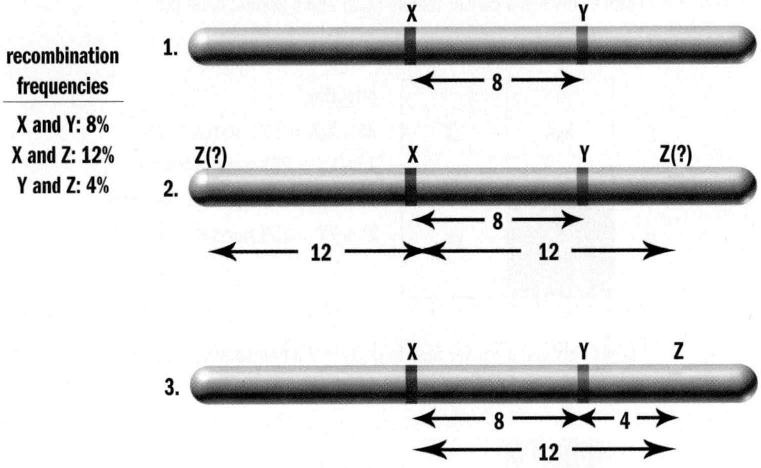

Figure 12.10 Genetic Maps from Recombination Frequencies

If the recombination frequencies are known, one can deduce the order of genes on the chromosome because map units are roughly additive.

Hardy-Weinberg Principle

How often an allele appears in a population is known as its **allele frequency**. For example, if we took a one-cell sample from 50 of Mendel's plants, we could collect 100 copies of alleles for flower color (two from each cell). If 75 of these alleles were the dominant allele, we could say that the allele frequency of P is $75 \div 100 = 0.75$. Note that this does not indicate which flowers contain the allele or if those flowers are homozygous or heterozygous; it only tells us the representation of the allele across all chromosomes in the population. Evolution results from changes in these gene frequencies in reproducing populations over time. However, when the gene frequencies of a population are not changing, the gene pool is stable and evolution is ostensibly *not* occurring. The following five criteria are mandatory for this to be possible:

- The population is very large (no genetic drift).
- There are no mutations that affect the gene pool.
- Mating between individuals in the population is random (no sexual selection).
- There is no migration of individuals into or out of the population.
- The genes in the population are all equally successful at being reproduced.

Provided that all of these conditions are met, the population is said to be in **Hardy–Weinberg equilibrium**, and a pair of equations can be used to predict the allelic and phenotypic frequencies.

Let us define a particular gene as having only two possible alleles, T and t. We will define p to be the frequency of the dominant allele T and q to be the frequency of the recessive allele t. Because there are only these two choices at the same gene locus, $p + q = 1$. That is, the combined allele frequencies of T and t must equal 100 percent. If we square both sides of the equation, we get:

$$(p + q)^2 = 1^2$$
$$p^2 + 2pq + q^2 = 1$$

where p^2 is the frequency of the TT (homozygous dominant) genotype, $2pq$ is the frequency of the Tt (heterozygous dominant) genotype, and q^2 is the frequency of the tt (homozygous recessive) genotype. Note that the sum $p^2 + 2pq$ would represent the frequency of the dominant *phenotype* (both homozygous and heterozygous dominant genotypes).

For Test Day, you should know the two key Hardy–Weinberg equations demonstrated above:

$$p + q = 1$$
$$p^2 + 2pq + q^2 = 1$$

Equation 12.1

KEY CONCEPT

All you need to know to solve any MCAT Hardy–Weinberg problem is the value of p (or p^2) or q (or q^2). From there, you can calculate everything else using $p + q = 1$ and $p^2 + 2pq + q^2 = 1$.

Each equation provides us with different information. The first tells us about the frequency of *alleles* in the population, whereas the second provides information about the frequency of *genotypes* and *phenotypes* in the population.

These equations can also be used to demonstrate that evolution is *not* occurring in a population. Assuming that the conditions listed earlier are met, the allele frequencies will remain constant from generation to generation. For example, imagine that we have a population of Mendel's pea plants in which the frequency of the tall allele, T, is 0.80. This value is represented by p. This means that q (the short allele, t) is 0.20 by subtraction. Setting up our F_1 cross for two heterozygotes, we can see the results of such a mating:

KEY CONCEPT

The Hardy–Weinberg equations allow you to find two pieces of information: first, the relative frequency of alleles in a population, and second, the frequency of a given genotype or phenotype in the population. Remember that there will be twice as many alleles as individuals in a population because each individual has two autosomal copies of each gene.

	$p = 0.80$ (T = 80%)	$q = 0.20$ (t = 20%)
$p = 0.80$ (T = 80%)	$p^2 = 0.64$ (TT = 64%)	$pq = 0.16$ (Tt = 16%)
$q = 0.20$ (t = 20%)	$pq = 0.16$ (Tt = 16%)	$q^2 = 0.04$ (tt = 4%)

We see that the filial generation contains 64 percent homozygous tall, 32 percent heterozygous tall, and 4 percent homozygous short plants. These are the genotypic frequencies. We can determine the allele frequencies in this generation as follows:

$$\begin{array}{rcl} 64\%\ TT = 64\%\ T & \text{and} & 0\%\ t \\ 32\%\ Tt = 16\%\ T & \text{and} & 16\%\ t \\ 4\%\ tt = 0\%\ T & \text{and} & 4\%\ t \\ \hline \text{allele frequencies} = 80\%\ T & \text{and} & 20\%\ t \end{array}$$

Notice that the allele frequencies are unchanged compared to the parent generation. T is still 0.80 and t is still 0.20. Populations in Hardy–Weinberg equilibrium will exhibit this property.

MCAT CONCEPT CHECK 12.3

Before you move on, assess your understanding of the material with these questions.

1. For each of the crosses below, what is the phenotypic ratio seen in the offspring?

Cross	Phenotypic Ratio
Bb × Bb	
Aa × aa	
DdEe × ddEE	
$X_qX \times XY$	
$X_rX \times X_rY$	

2. If genes Q and R have a recombination frequency of 2%, genes R and S have a recombination frequency of 6%, genes S and T have a recombination frequency of 23%, and genes Q and T have a recombination frequency of 19%, then what is the order of these four genes in the chromosome?

___

3. All five criteria of the Hardy–Weinberg principle are required to imply what characteristic of the study population?

___

4. Assume that a population is in Hardy–Weinberg equilibrium. If 9% of the population is homozygous dominant, then solve for the following:

   - The frequency of the dominant allele:

   ____

   - The frequency of the recessive allele:

   ____

   - The portion of the population that is heterozygous:

   ____

   - The portion of the population with a homozygous recessive genotype:

   ____

   - The portion of the population with a dominant phenotype:

   ____

12.4 Evolution

LEARNING OBJECTIVES

After Chapter 12.4, you will be able to:

- Describe the key tenets of the major theories of evolution, including punctuated equilibrium, natural selection, inclusive fitness, and the modern synthesis model
- Identify the three patterns of selection and the changes they create in the population phenotype
- Recall the three patterns of evolution between species and the outcome of each
- Recall the biological definition of a species

Evolutionary thought has a relatively short history; the first theories suggesting that new species may arise from older ones were proposed in the 19th century. Significant alterations to these initial theories have been made since then.

Natural Selection

Natural selection, sometimes called *survival of the fittest*, is the theory that certain characteristics or traits possessed by individuals within a species may help those individuals have greater reproductive success, thus passing on those traits to offspring. This theory was originally proposed by Charles Darwin in his 1859 publication *On the Origin of Species*. His theory was built on several basic tenets:

- Organisms produce offspring, few of which survive to reproductive maturity.
- Chance variations within individuals in a population may be heritable. If these variations give an organism even a slight survival advantage, the variation is termed **favorable**.
- Individuals with a greater preponderance of these favorable variations are more likely to survive to reproductive age and produce offspring; the overall result will be an increase in these traits in future generations. This level of reproductive success is termed **fitness**, and an organism's fitness is directly related to the relative genetic contribution of this individual to the next generation.

Darwin's theory was ultimately proven to be correct in many ways—although not completely. In the 20th century, modern genetics led to the development of the currently accepted theory.

Modern Theories

The **modern synthesis model**, sometimes called **neo-Darwinism**, adds knowledge of genetic inheritance and changes in the gene pool to Darwin's original theory. Once scientists showed that inheritance occurs through the passing of genes from parent to child and that genes ultimately change due to mutation or recombination, Darwin's theory was updated to its current form: when mutation or recombination results in a change that is favorable to the organism's reproductive success, that change is more likely to pass on to the next generation. The opposite is also true. This process is termed **differential reproduction**. Over time, those traits passed on by the more successful organisms will become ubiquitous in the gene pool. Because the gene pool changes over time, it is important to note that populations evolve, not individuals.

KEY CONCEPT

Evolution is not equivalent to natural selection. The MCAT likes to test your ability to understand that natural selection is simply a mechanism for evolution. Natural selection is, however, equivalent to *survival of the fittest*.

Also germane to the modernization of Darwin's theory is a shift in scope to focus on inclusive fitness over the fitness of an individual organism. **Inclusive fitness** is a measure of an organism's success in the population, based on the number of offspring, success in supporting offspring, and the ability of the offspring to then support others. Early descriptions of evolutionary success, like those of Darwin, were based solely on the number of viable offspring of an organism. However, contemporary theories take into account the benefits of certain behaviors on the population at large. For example, the existence of altruism could be supported by the observation that close relatives of an individual will share many of the same genes; thus, promoting the reproduction and survival of related or similar individuals can also lead to genetic success. Other species show examples of inclusive fitness by protecting the offspring of the group at large. By endangering themselves to protect the young, these organisms ensure the passing of genes to future generations. Inclusive fitness therefore promotes the idea that altruistic behavior can improve the fitness and success of a species as a whole.

One final theory to consider was proposed as a result of research into the fossil record. Upon examination, it was discovered that little evolution would occur within a lineage of related lifeforms for long periods of time, followed by an explosion in evolutionary change. Niles Eldredge and Stephen Jay Gould proposed the theory of **punctuated equilibrium** to explain this in 1972. In contrast to Darwin's theory, punctuated equilibrium suggests that changes in some species occur in rapid bursts rather than evenly over time.

Modes of Natural Selection

Natural selection may occur as stabilizing selection, directional selection, or disruptive selection, as shown in Figure 12.11.

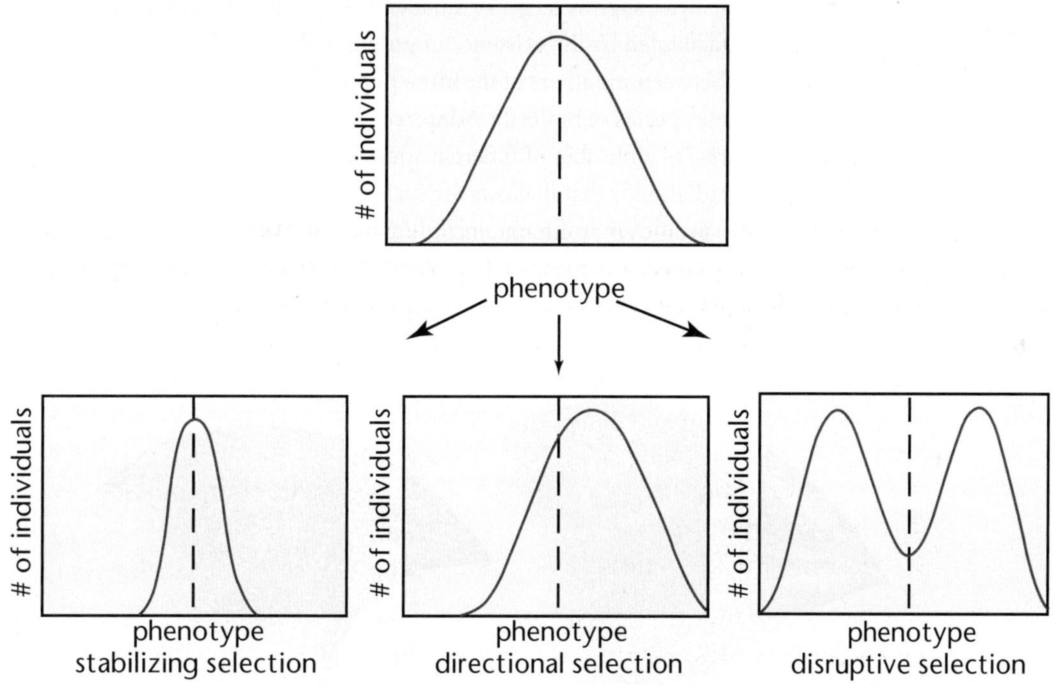

Figure 12.11 Modes of Natural Selection

Stabilizing selection keeps phenotypes within a specific range by selecting against extremes. For instance, human birth weight is maintained within a narrow band by stabilizing selection. Fetuses that weigh too little may not be healthy enough to survive, and fetuses that weigh too much can experience trauma during delivery through the relatively narrow birth canal. In addition, the larger the fetus, the more maternal resources it requires. For all of these reasons, there is a fitness advantage to keeping birth weights within a narrow range.

Adaptive pressure can lead to the emergence and dominance of an initially extreme phenotype through **directional selection**. For example, if we have a heterogeneous plate of bacteria, very few may have resistance to antibiotics. If the plate is then treated with *ampicillin* (an antibiotic), only those colonies that exhibit resistance to this antibiotic will survive. A new standard phenotype emerges as a result of differential survivorship. Natural selection is the history of differential survivorship over time. The emergence of mosquitoes resistant to *dichlorodiphenyltrichloroethane* (DDT), a type of pesticide, is attributed to directional selection.

In **disruptive selection**, two extreme phenotypes are selected over the norm. When Darwin studied finches on the Galapagos Islands, he noted that although there were many species, all the species arguably had a common ancestor, given their similar appearances. However, when he compared beak sizes they were all either large or small, as shown in Figure 12.12. No animals exhibited the intermediate phenotype of medium-size beaks. Darwin hypothesized that the sizes of seeds on the island (the finches' food) led to this effect. Seeds were either quite large or fairly small, requiring a large or small beak, respectively. Thus, if the original ancestor had a medium-size beak, over time the animals with slightly larger or smaller beaks would be selected for. Disruptive selection is facilitated by the existence of **polymorphisms**—naturally occurring differences in form between members of the same population, such as light and dark coloration in the same species of butterfly. **Adaptive radiation** is a related concept that describes the rapid rise of a number of different species from a common ancestor. The benefit of adaptive radiation is that it allows for various species to occupy different niches. A **niche** is a specific environment, including habitat, available resources, and predators, for which a species is specifically adapted. Adaptive radiation is favored by environmental changes or isolation of small groups of the ancestral species.

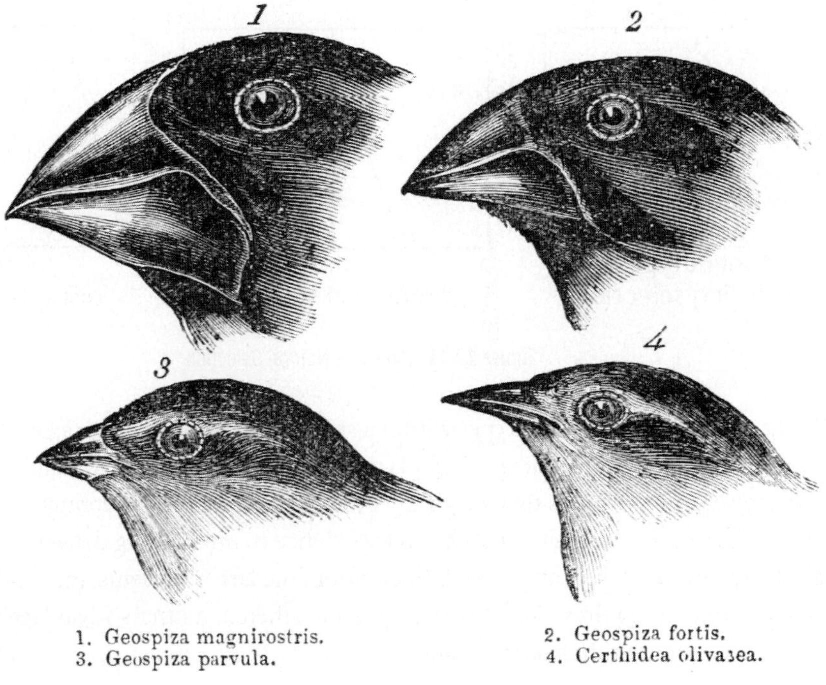

Figure 12.12 Darwin's Finches
Image of Darwin's finches as drawn by John Gould

Speciation

A **species** is defined as the largest group of organisms capable of breeding to form fertile offspring; the formation of a new species through evolution is called **speciation**. If we took two populations from the same species and separated them geographically for a long period of time, different evolutionary pressures would lead to different adaptive changes. If enough time passed, the changes would be sufficient to lead to **isolation**, which means the progeny of these populations could no longer freely interbreed. We would now consider the two groups separate species.

Reproductive isolation may occur either prezygotically or postzygotically. **Prezygotic mechanisms** prevent formation of the zygote completely; **postzygotic mechanisms** allow for gamete fusion but yield either nonviable or sterile offspring. Examples of prezygotic mechanisms include temporal isolation (breeding at different times), ecological isolation (living in different niches within the same territory), behavioral isolation (a lack of attraction between members of the two species due to differences in pheromones, courtship displays, and so on), reproductive isolation (incompatibility of reproductive anatomy), or gametic isolation (intercourse can occur, but fertilization cannot). Postzygotic mechanisms include hybrid inviability (formation of a zygote that cannot develop to term), hybrid sterility (forming hybrid offspring that cannot reproduce), and hybrid breakdown (forming first-generation hybrid offspring that are viable and fertile, but second-generation hybrid offspring that are inviable or infertile). As described earlier in this chapter, mules are an example of postzygotic hybrid sterility. Although a horse and donkey can produce a viable mule, the mule will be sterile and thus unable to establish a self-perpetuating mule lineage.

Patterns of Evolution

When we look at similarities between two species, we must be careful to determine whether those similarities are due to sharing a common ancestor or sharing a common environment with the same evolutionary pressures. When analyzing species this way, three patterns of evolution emerge: divergent evolution, parallel evolution, and convergent evolution, as shown in Figure 12.13.

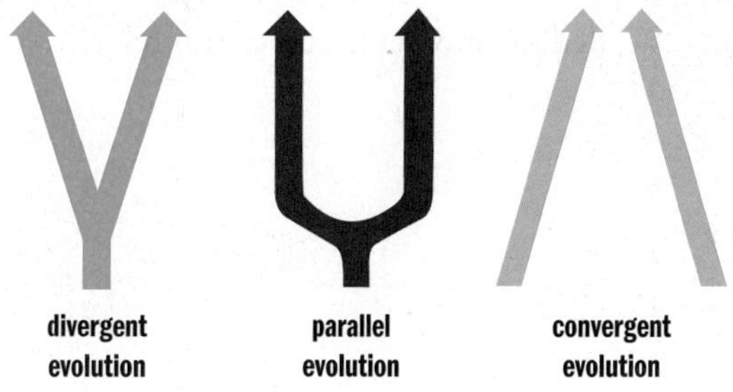

Figure 12.13 Patterns of Evolution

Divergent evolution refers to the independent development of dissimilar characteristics in two or more lineages sharing a common ancestor. For example, seals and cats are both mammals in the order Carnivora, yet they differ markedly in general appearance. These two species live in very different environments and adapted to different selection pressures while evolving.

Parallel evolution refers to the process whereby related species evolve in similar ways for a long period of time in response to analogous environmental selection pressures.

Convergent evolution refers to the independent development of similar characteristics in two or more lineages not sharing a recent common ancestor. For example, fish and dolphins have come to resemble one another physically, though they belong to different classes of vertebrates. They evolved certain similar features in adapting to the conditions of aquatic life.

Measuring Evolutionary Time

Evolution is a slow process, featuring changes in the environment and subsequent changes in genotypes and phenotypes of a population over time. The rate of evolution is measured by the rate of change of a genotype over a period of time and is related to the severity of the evolutionary pressures on the species. In other words, if a species is already perfectly suited to its habitat and there are no changes to the conditions in which it lives, the rate of evolution will be exceedingly slow—although there will still be some small base rate of genetic mutation. On the other hand, if an organism lives in a rapidly changing environment, the rate of evolution will be greater, as selection for and against certain traits will be actively occurring within that population.

By comparing DNA sequences between different species, scientists can quantify the degree of similarity between two organisms. For example, chimpanzees share over 95 percent of their genome with humans, whereas mice share only about 70 percent. As species become more taxonomically distant, the proportion of the shared genome will decrease. Molecular evolutionists correlate the degree of genomic similarity with the amount of time since two species split off from the same common ancestor; the more similar the genomes, the more recently the two species separated from each other. This is sometimes called the **molecular clock model**.

MCAT CONCEPT CHECK 12.4

Before you move on, assess your understanding of the material with these questions.

1. What are the key tenets of each of the following theories of evolution?
   - Natural selection:
   - Modern synthesis model:
   - Inclusive fitness:
   - Punctuated equilibrium:

2. What are the three patterns of selection? What changes would each create to the population phenotype?

Pattern of Selection	Change to Population Phenotype

3. What are the three patterns of evolution between species? What is the outcome of each one?

Pattern of Evolution	Outcome

4. What is the biological definition of a species?

BIOLOGY GUIDED EXAMPLE WITH EXPERT THINKING

While the genus *Saccharomyces* is best known for the model and industrial yeast *S. cerevisiae*, it also includes eight closely related additional species.

Saccharomyces has 9 related species

The repeated isolation of *S. cerevisiae* from wine, beer, and other fermented beverages, and the difficulty in finding its truly natural habitats, has led to the common view that this species was a product of domestication. However, the unusual degree of shared physiological characteristics among *Saccharomyces* species along with the recent isolation of *S. cerevisiae* from a natural environment suggests *S. cerevisiae* may be a result of natural evolution.

Issue: Is the formation of S. cervevisiae due to domestication or natural evolution?

In the present work we used a comparative genomics approach and publicly available complete genome sequences of five *Saccharomyces* species to search for proteins exhibiting molecular patterns of evolution. We used the dN/dS ratio [rate of nonsynonymous substitutions per nonsynonymous site (dN)/rate of synonymous substitutions per synonymous site (dS)] of the complete *Saccharomyces* ORFeomes to measure protein divergence and corrected for phylogenetic distance. From this data, we created the phylogenetic tree shown in Figure 1 and searched for genes associated with

There's a lot of technical jargon here, so to rephrase, the key takeaway is that the researchers used comparative genomics to create the phylogenic tree in Figure 1

divergence. Some of the identified genes had been previously associated with adaptation to growth at suboptimal temperatures. This prompted us to examine catabolic fluxes at different temperatures in *Saccharomyces* species with different growth temperature preferences. Figure 1 depicts schematically the phylogenetic relationships of the species in the genus *Saccharomyces* and assigns them to the thermotolerant or cryotolerant groups.

After creating the tree, the researchers saw that optimal growth temperature was a pattern that corresponded to the phylogeny

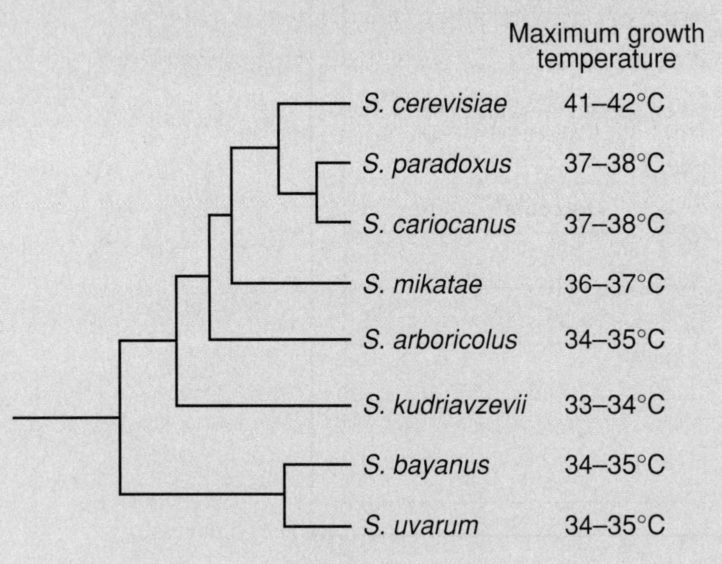

Trend: maximum growth temperature is highest at the top of the tree, and generally descends in order

Figure 1

Adapted from Gonçalves, P., Valério, E., Correia, C., de Almeida, J. M., & Sampaio, J. P. (2011). Evidence for divergent evolution of growth temperature preference in sympatric Saccharomyces species. *PloS One*, 6(6), e20739.

Based on the information provided, could temperature have provided the selective pressure for the divergent evolution of *Saccharomyces* species?

The question is asking us if there is support in the passage and figure for the hypothesis that temperature can explain the divergence of the various *Saccharomyces* species in the phylogenetic tree. Notice the phrasing of the question—it's not asking if we have proof that the evolution was due to temperature selection. This analysis is retrospective, so we would have no way to verify whether or not the relationship between growth and temperature leading up to speciation was causal.

In paragraph 2, the researchers used fairly complex techniques to analyze the genomes of *Saccharomyces* species and arranged them in the phylogenetic tree. We don't need to understand all of the details behind this method. The takeaway is that the phylogeny was generated prior to the analysis of optimal growth temperatures. The researchers then searched for genes associated with divergence and noticed that some of those genes corresponded to adaptations for growth at nonideal temperatures. Finally, an analysis of the optimal growth temperature for the listed *Saccharomyces* species gave us a workable pattern—species that are close together on the tree also have very similar optimal growth temperatures. We know from content background that changes in environment can definitely apply selection pressures strong enough to lead to speciation, or the formation of new species. Recall also that divergent evolution is the development of species with different characteristics despite a shared common ancestor.

Since temperature is an environmental factor, we can say that based on the given information, there is plausible evidence to support that temperature could have provided the selection pressure for divergent evolution of *Saccharomyces* species.

Conclusion

Genetics and the mechanisms of evolution are becoming increasingly important in medicine, as we unintentionally breed strains of highly resistant bacteria. Antibiotic stewardship, or the use of the appropriate antibiotics only as necessary, is very important as the medical community seeks to preserve the effectiveness of antibiotics. In order to understand and apply the concepts of antibiotic stewardship, one must understand that creating environmental pressures leads to directional selection in microorganisms which can increase the frequency of the resistant phenotype. In this chapter, we covered genetics and mutations, as well as evolution. We also gave you some tools to analyze the biometric (statistical) side of genetics through the use of Punnett squares, recombinant frequencies, and the Hardy–Weinberg equations.

It seems fitting to complete this book with a discussion of evolution. You've spent hundreds of pages (and hours!) preparing for the MCAT, learning the basics of cell biology, embryogenesis and development, anatomy and physiology, genetics, and evolution. Our understanding of these topics relies on generations and generations of scientists who came before us, who passed down their knowledge through books, letters, articles, lectures, and—more recently—television, film, and popular media. But science is a field that is constantly evolving itself. At the beginning of medical school, students are often told that no more than 25 percent of what they learn during the first year will remain true by the time they enter practice. We're not sure if this statistic actually holds, but it does speak to the importance of staying on top of the latest research—not only as a medical student, but also as a practitioner. Every day, new discoveries about the human body and the practice of medicine are being made—soon, you'll be one of those making these very discoveries and bringing them to your practice, improving your patients' lives. And at the end of it all, as a provider, an attending physician, or a researcher, you too will pass on your knowledge to future generations of physicians who will also help medical science to evolve and improve. The human body is astoundingly complex. Take a moment to genuinely think about that—*the human body is astoundingly complex*. There's so much more to learn. Medical school and your future awaits!

You've reviewed the content, now test your knowledge and critical thinking skills by completing a test-like passage set in your online resources!

GO ONLINE

CONCEPT SUMMARY

Fundamental Concepts of Genetics

- **Chromosomes** contain **genes** in a linear sequence.
- **Alleles** are alternative forms of a gene.
  - A **dominant** allele requires only one copy to be expressed.
  - A **recessive** allele requires two copies to be expressed.
- A **genotype** is the combination of alleles one has at a given genetic **locus**.
  - Having two of the same allele is termed **homozygous**.
  - Having two different alleles is termed **heterozygous**.
  - Having only one allele is termed **hemizygous** (such as in male sex chromosomes).
  - A **phenotype** is the observable manifestation of a genotype.
- There are different patterns of dominance.
  - **Complete dominance** occurs when the effect of one allele completely masks the effect of another.
  - **Codominance** has more than one dominant allele.
  - **Incomplete dominance** has no dominant alleles; heterozygotes have intermediate phenotypes.
- **Penetrance** is the proportion of a population with a given genotype who express the phenotype.
- **Expressivity** refers to the varying phenotypic manifestations of a given genotype.
- The modern interpretations of Mendel's laws help explain the inheritance of genes from parent to offspring.
  - **Mendel's first law (of segregation)** states that an organism has two alleles for each gene, which segregate during meiosis, resulting in gametes carrying only one allele for a trait.
  - **Mendel's second law (of independent assortment)** states that the inheritance of one allele does not influence the probability of inheriting an allele for a different trait.
- Support for DNA as genetic material came through a number of experiments.
  - The Griffith experiment demonstrated the transforming principle, converting nonvirulent live bacteria into virulent bacteria by exposure to heat-killed virulent bacteria.
  - The Avery–MacLeod–McCarty experiment demonstrated that DNA is the genetic material because degradation of DNA led to a cessation of bacterial transformation.
  - The Hershey–Chase experiment confirmed that DNA is the genetic material because only radiolabeled DNA could be found in bacteriophage-infected bacteria.

Changes in the Gene Pool

- All of the alleles in a given population constitute the **gene pool**.
- **Mutations** are changes in DNA sequence.
- Nucleotide mutations include **point mutations** (the substituting of one nucleotide for another) and **frameshift mutations** (moving the three-letter transcriptional reading frame).
  - A **silent mutation** has no effect on the protein.
  - A **missense mutation** results in the substitution of one amino acid for another.
  - A **nonsense mutation** results in the substitution of a stop codon for an amino acid.
  - **Insertions** and **deletions** result in a shift in the **reading frame**, leading to changes for all downstream amino acids.
- Chromosomal mutations include larger-scale mutations affecting whole segments of DNA.
  - **Deletion mutations** occur when a large segment of DNA is lost.
  - **Duplication mutations** occur when a segment of DNA is copied multiple times.
  - **Inversion mutations** occur when a segment of DNA is reversed.
  - **Insertion mutations** occur when a segment of DNA is moved from one chromosome to another.
  - **Translocation mutations** occur when a segment of DNA is swapped with a segment of DNA from another chromosome.
- Genetic **leakage** is a flow of genes between species through hybrid offspring.
- **Genetic drift** occurs when the composition of the gene pool changes as a result of chance.
- The **founder effect** results from **bottlenecks** that suddenly isolate a small population, leading to **inbreeding** and increased prevalence of certain homozygous genotypes.

Analytical Approaches in Genetics

- **Punnett squares** visually represent the crossing of gametes from parents to show relative genotypic and phenotypic frequencies.
  - The **parent generation** is represented by P; **filial** (offspring) **generations** are represented by F_1, F_2, and so on in sequence.
  - A **monohybrid cross** accounts for one gene; a **dihybrid cross** accounts for two genes.
  - In **sex-linked crosses**, sex chromosomes are usually used to indicate sex as well as genotype.

- The **recombination frequency** (θ) is the likelihood of two alleles being separated during crossing over in meiosis. **Genetic maps** can be made using recombination frequency as the scale in **centimorgans**.
- The **Hardy–Weinberg principle** states that if a population meets certain criteria (aimed at a lack of evolution), then the **allele frequencies** will remain constant (**Hardy–Weinberg equilibrium**).

Evolution

- **Natural selection** states that chance variations exist between individuals and that advantageous variations—those that increase an individual's **fitness** for survival or adaptation to the environment—afford the most opportunities for reproductive success.
- The **modern synthesis model** (**neo-Darwinism**) accounts for mutation and recombination as mechanisms of variation and considers **differential reproduction** to be the mechanism for reproductive success.
- **Inclusive fitness** considers an organism's success to be based on the number of offspring, success in supporting offspring, and the ability of the offspring to then support others; survival of offspring or relatives ensures appearance of genes in subsequent generations.
- **Punctuated equilibrium** considers evolution to be a very slow process with intermittent rapid bursts of evolutionary activity.
- Different types of selection lead to changes in phenotypes.
  - **Stabilizing selection** keeps phenotypes in a narrow range, excluding extremes.
  - **Directional selection** moves the average phenotype toward one extreme.
  - **Disruptive selection** moves the population toward two different phenotypes at the extremes and can lead to **speciation**.
  - **Adaptive radiation** is the rapid emergence of multiple species from a common ancestor, each of which occupies its own ecological **niche**.
- A **species** is the largest group of organisms capable of breeding to form fertile offspring. Species are **reproductively isolated** from each other by **pre**- or **postzygotic mechanisms**.
- Two species can evolve with different relationship patterns.
  - **Divergent evolution** occurs when two species sharing a common ancestor become more different.
  - **Parallel evolution** occurs when two species sharing a common ancestor evolve in similar ways due to analogous selection pressures.
  - **Convergent evolution** occurs when two species not sharing a recent ancestor evolve to become more similar due to analogous selection pressures.
- According to the **molecular clock model**, the degree of difference in the genome between two species is related to the amount of time since the two species broke off from a common ancestor.

ANSWERS TO CONCEPT CHECKS

12.1

1. A dominant allele is one that requires only one copy for expression. A recessive allele requires two copies for expression.
2. A homozygous genotype is one in which the two alleles are the same. A heterozygous genotype is one in which the two alleles are different. A hemizygous genotype is one in which only one allele is present for a given gene (such as parts of the X chromosome in males).
3. Complete dominance occurs when one allele (the dominant one) completely masks the expression of the other (the recessive one). Codominance occurs when a gene has more than one dominant allele, and two different dominant alleles can be expressed simultaneously. Incomplete dominance occurs when a gene has no dominant alleles, and heterozygotes have phenotypes that are intermediate between homozygotes.
4. Penetrance describes the proportion of the population that expresses a phenotype, given a particular genotype. Expressivity describes the differences in expression (severity, location, and so on) of a phenotype in individuals.
5. Mendel's first law (of segregation) most aligns with anaphase I of meiosis. Mendel's second law (of independent assortment) most aligns with prophase I of meiosis.

12.2

1. Silent point mutations occur when one nucleotide is changed for another, but there is no change in the protein coded for by this DNA sequence (due to redundancy in the genetic code). Missense mutations occur when one nucleotide is changed for another, and one amino acid is substituted for another in the final protein. Nonsense mutations occur when one nucleotide is changed for another, and a stop codon substitutes for an amino acid in the final protein.
2. The two types of frameshift mutations are insertion and deletion mutations.
3. Duplication mutations occur when a segment of DNA is copied multiple times in the genome. Inversion mutations occur when a segment of DNA is reversed in the genome. Translocation mutations occur when a segment of DNA from one chromosome is swapped with a segment of DNA from another chromosome.
4. Genetic leakage requires the formation of a hybrid organism that can then mate with members of one or the other parent species. While hybrids existed historically (especially mules), fertile hybrids were certainly rare before a more modern understanding of genetics (and before a commercial, financial, or academic impetus existed to create these organisms).
5. Genetic drift occurs due to chance, so its effects will be more pronounced with a smaller sample size (in smaller populations). The founder effect occurs when a small group is reproductively isolated from the larger population, allowing certain alleles to take on a higher prevalence in the group than in the rest of the population.

12.3

1.

Cross	Phenotypic Ratio
Bb × Bb	3 dominant:1 recessive
Aa × aa	1 dominant:1 recessive
DdEe × ddEE	1 dominant (for D)/dominant (for E): 1 recessive (for D)/dominant (for E)
$X_qX \times XY$	Female: all unaffected; male: 1 unaffected:1 affected
$X_rX \times X_rY$	Both male and female: 1 unaffected:1 affected

2. The genes must be in the order SQRT:

$$S \xleftrightarrow{4\%} Q \xleftrightarrow{2\%} R \xleftrightarrow{17\%} T$$

3. The criteria for the Hardy–Weinberg principle all imply that the study population is *not* undergoing evolution; thus, the allele frequencies will remain stable over time.
4. The frequency of the dominant allele (p) is 0.3. The frequency of the recessive allele (q) is 0.7. The fraction of the population with a heterozygous genotype ($2pq$) is $2 \times 0.3 \times 0.7 = 0.42$ (42%). The fraction of the population with a homozygous recessive genotype (q^2) is $(0.7)^2 = 0.49$ (49%). The fraction of the population with a dominant phenotype ($p^2 + 2pq$) is $0.09 + 0.42 = 0.51 = 51\%$.

12.4

1. Natural selection states that certain traits that arise from chance are more favorable for reproductive success in a given environment, and that those traits will be passed on to future generations. The modern synthesis model takes natural selection and explains that selection is for specific alleles, which are passed on to future generations through formation of gametes; the alleles for these favorable traits arise from mutations. Inclusive fitness explains that the reproductive success of an organism is not only due to the number of offspring it creates, but also the ability to care for young (that can then care for others); it explains changes not only at the individual level, but changes based on the survival of the species (and that individual's alleles within the species, including in other related individuals). Punctuated equilibrium states that for some species, little evolution occurs for a long period, which is interrupted by rapid bursts of evolutionary change.

2.

Pattern of Selection	Change to Population Phenotype
Stabilizing	Loss of extremes, maintenance of phenotype in a small window
Directional	Movement toward one extreme or the other
Disruptive	Movement toward both extremes with loss of the norm; speciation may occur

3.

Pattern of Evolution	Outcome
Divergent	Two species with a common ancestor become less similar because of different evolutionary pressures
Parallel	Two species with a common ancestor remain similar because of similar evolutionary pressures
Convergent	Two species with no recent common ancestor become more similar because of similar evolutionary pressures

4. A species is defined as the largest group of organisms capable of breeding to form fertile offspring.

SCIENCE MASTERY ASSESSMENT EXPLANATIONS

1. **B**

This is a gene-mapping problem. Because there is a correlation between the frequency of recombination and the distance between genes on a chromosome, if we are given the frequencies, we can determine gene order. Remember that one map unit equals 1 percent recombination frequency. The easiest way to begin is to determine the two genes that are farthest apart; in this case, N and O recombine with a frequency of 18%, so they are 18 map units apart on the chromosome:

$$N \xleftrightarrow{18\%} O$$

N and P recombine with 1% frequency, and P and O recombine with 17% frequency, so P must be between N and O:

$$N \xleftrightarrow{1\%} P \xleftrightarrow{17\%} O$$

Finally, M and P recombine with 5% frequency, and M and O recombine with 12% frequency, so M must be between P and O:

$$N \xleftrightarrow{1\%} P \xleftrightarrow{5\%} M \xleftrightarrow{12\%} O$$

2. **D**

In this dihybrid problem, a doubly recessive individual is crossed with an individual of unknown genotype; this is known as a test cross. The straight- and brown-haired organism has the genotype bbcc and can thus only produce gametes carrying bc. Looking at the F_1 offspring, there is a 1:1:1:1 phenotypic ratio. The fact that both the dominant and recessive traits are present in the offspring means that the unknown parental genotype must contain both dominant and recessive alleles for each trait. The unknown parental genotype must therefore be BbCc. If you want to double-check the answer, you can work out the Punnett square for the cross BbCc × bbcc:

	BC	Bc	bC	bc
bc	BbCc	Bbcc	bbCc	bbcc
bc	BbCc	Bbcc	bbCc	bbcc
bc	BbCc	Bbcc	bbCc	bbcc
bc	BbCc	Bbcc	bbCc	bbcc
	25% black curly	25% black straight	25% brown curly	25% brown straight

3. **C**

The female in this example is a carrier of two sex-linked traits; based on the genotype, the affected alleles are found on different X chromosomes. Drawing out a Punnett square, we see that 25% of the offspring will be female hemophiliacs (X_hX_h) and 25% will be female carriers of both alleles (X_cX_h). This question is asking what percentage of females will have a phenotype with no hemophilia or color blindness, which would be half of the females (those who are carriers for both traits).

	X_c	X_h
X_h	X_cX_h	X_hX_h
Y	X_cY	X_hY

offspring
25% female hemophiliac
25% female carrier of both traits (phenotypically normal)
25% male hemophiliac
25% male colorblind

4. **A**

The control parent in a test cross is always recessive. Therefore, if the test parent is phenotypically dominant, yet can provide a recessive allele (as evidenced by the presence of recessive children), then the parent must have both a dominant and recessive allele. Therefore, this test parent must be heterozygous.

5. **B**

The definition given here for expressivity is a much better match for defining penetrance (or, really, one minus the penetrance). Expressivity refers to the variable manifestations of a given genotype as different phenotypes; the degree to which various phenotypes are expressed. All of the other definitions given are accurate.

6. **B**

Some progeny in the second generation are apparently blends of the parental phenotypes. The orange color is the result of the combined effects of the red and yellow alleles. An allele is incompletely dominant if the phenotype of the heterozygotes is an intermediate of the phenotypes of the homozygotes.

7. **B**

To find the correct answer, we have to read each choice and eliminate the ones that fit with the modern-day theories of inheritance, which state that the genes that make an organism most fit for its environment will be passed to offspring. This can be seen in **(C)** and **(D)**, both of which demonstrate that an organism with improved fitness will pass those genes to offspring. **(A)** mentions a gamete being exposed to mutagens; a zygote created from this gamete would contain any mutations that were present in the egg and would be affected by them. Thus, **(B)** must be the correct answer: indeed, acquired characteristics not encoded in the genome should not be passed to offspring according to the modern synthesis model.

8. **B**

Darwin's theory of natural selection argues that chance variations between organisms can help certain organisms survive to reproductive age and produce many offspring, transmitting their variations to the next generation. Thus, natural selection would drive the process of evolution forward, enabling the persistence of characteristics that impart an advantage in the environment, eliminating **(A)**. In Darwin's theory, fitness is measured in terms of reproductive success, as **(D)** states. Through natural selection, organisms may be separated into groups depending on environmental pressures, and these groups can eventually separate to the point of becoming distinct species, eliminating **(C)**. **(B)** is the correct answer because the theory of natural selection applies to a population of organisms, not to a particular individual. As such, favorable genetic variations become more and more common from generation to generation, not during the lifetime of an individual.

9. **C**

Hardy–Weinberg equilibrium exists under certain ideal conditions that, when satisfied, allow one to calculate the gene frequencies within a population. The Hardy–Weinberg equation can be applied only under these five conditions: (1) the population is very large; (2) there are no mutations that affect the gene pool; (3) mating between individuals in the population is random; (4) there is no migration of individuals into or out of the population; (5) the genes in the population are all equally successful at being reproduced. Thus, from the given choices, only **(C)** is false: monogamy is not a necessary condition for Hardy–Weinberg equilibrium.

10. **B**

The situation described in the question stem is an example of directional selection. In directional selection, the phenotypic norm of a particular species shifts toward an extreme to adapt to a selective pressure, such as an increasingly colder environment. Only those individuals with a thicker layer of fur were able to survive during the Ice Age, thus shifting the phenotypic norm.

11. **A**

A species is defined as the largest group of organisms that can interbreed to produce viable, fertile offspring. Therefore, two populations are considered separate species when they can no longer do so.

12. **D**

Let's use the information provided by the question stem to set up our equations. We are told that the frequency of R equals 30%, and as such, $p = 0.30$. The frequency of the recessive gene is $r = 100\% - 30\% = 70\%$; thus, $q = 0.70$. The frequency of the genotypes, according to the Hardy–Weinberg equilibrium, are given by $p^2 = RR$, $2pq = Rr$, and $q^2 = rr$. Therefore, the frequency of the genotypes are $(0.3)^2 = 0.09 = 9\%$ RR, $2 \times 0.3 \times 0.7 = 0.42 = 42\%$ Rr, and $(0.7)^2 = 0.49 = 49\%$ rr.

13. **B**

Using the information given in the question stem, we can determine that the percentage of the population with blue eyes (genotype bb) $= 36\% = 0.36 = q^2$; therefore, $q = 0.6$. Because this is a Hardy–Weinberg population, we can assume that $p + q = 1$, so $p = 1 - 0.6 = 0.4$. The frequency of heterozygous brown eyes is therefore $2pq = 2 \times 0.4 \times 0.6 = 0.48 = 48\%$.

14. **D**

Frameshift mutations include insertions and deletions of nucleotides that change the triplet reading frame. In such a mutation, the amino acid sequence preceding the mutation is normal, yielding a normal N terminal end. However, the triplet reading frame after the mutation is changed, yielding a drastically different C terminal sequence that often includes a premature stop codon. These factors together support **(D)** as the correct answer. Note that nonsense mutations also introduce premature stop codons. However, **(C)** can be eliminated since a nonsense mutation will create a stop codon directly and will not change the identity of the amino acids before the stop codon.

15. **C**

This scenario—a deletion of some DNA and a duplication of other DNA—would be consistent with a translocation between chromosomes 4 and 21 during development of an egg or sperm. If part of chromosome 21 was swapped with part of chromosome 4, then a gamete resulting from meiosis in this cell would result in a daughter cell with two copies of some of the DNA from 21 and no copies of some of the DNA from 4. Therefore, after fertilization, there would be partial trisomy 21 and partial monosomy 4. While a deletion or insertion could explain one of the findings, it cannot explain both, eliminating **(A)** and **(B)**. An inversion should not lead to partial trisomy or partial monosomy because the DNA is simply reversed, eliminating **(D)**.

GO ONLINE **Consult your online resources for additional practice.**

EQUATIONS TO REMEMBER

(12.1) **Hardy–Weinberg equations:** $p + q = 1$

$$p^2 + 2pq + q^2 = 1$$

SHARED CONCEPTS

Behavioral Sciences Chapter 10
Social Thinking

Biochemistry Chapter 6
DNA and Biotechnology

Biochemistry Chapter 7
RNA and the Genetic Code

Biology Chapter 1
The Cell

Physics and Math Chapter 11
Reasoning About the Design and Execution of Research

Physics and Math Chapter 12
Data-Based and Statistical Reasoning

GLOSSARY

Abductor–A muscle that moves a limb away from the center of the body.

Absorption–The process by which substances are taken up into or across tissues.

Acetylcholine–A neurotransmitter found throughout the nervous system (somatic motor neurons, preganglionic parasympathetic and sympathetic nerves, and postganglionic parasympathetic neurons); metabolized by acetylcholinesterase.

Acrosome–The large vesicle at the head of a sperm cell containing enzymes that degrade the ovum cell membrane to allow fertilization.

Actin–A protein found in the cytoskeleton and muscle cells; it is the principal constituent of the thin filaments and microfilaments.

Action potential–An abrupt change in the membrane potential of a nerve or muscle caused by changes in membrane ionic permeability; results in conduction of an impulse in nerves or contraction in muscles.

Active immunity–An immune response (antibody production or cellular immunity) acquired in response to exposure to an antigen.

Active site–Substrate-binding region of an enzyme.

Adaptation–The development of characteristics that enable an organism to survive and reproduce in its habitat.

Adaptive immunity–Highly specific form of immunity that retains chemical memory of each invader encountered and is able to tailor the immune response to the specific pathogen.

Adaptive radiation–The evolutionary process by which one species gives rise to several species, each specialized for different niches.

Adductor–A muscle that moves a limb toward the center of the body.

Adenine–A purine base present in DNA and RNA; it forms hydrogen bonds with thymine and uracil.

Adenosine triphosphate (ATP)–A nucleotide molecule consisting of adenine, ribose, and three phosphate moieties; the outer two phosphates are bound by high-energy bonds.

Adipose–Refers to fatty tissue, fat-storing tissue, or fat within cells.

Aerobic–Refers to a biological process that occurs in the presence of molecular oxygen (O_2) or to organisms that cannot live without molecular oxygen.

Afferent (sensory) neuron–A neuron that picks up impulses from sensory receptors and transmits them toward the central nervous system.

Agranulocyte–Type of leukocyte that does not contain cytoplasmic granules, including lymphocytes and monocytes.

Albumin–Protein synthesized in the liver that maintains the oncotic pressure of the blood and serves as a carrier for many drugs and hormones.

Allantois–One of four embryonic membranes; it contains the growing embryo's waste products.

Allele–Alternative forms of the same gene coding for a particular trait; alleles segregate during meiosis.

Allergy–A type of autoimmunity in which a person's immune system becomes overactivated by common substances in the environment.

Alveolus–Basic functional unit of the lung; a tiny sac specialized for passive gas exchange between the lungs and the blood.

Amino acids–The building blocks of proteins, each containing an amino group, a carboxylic acid group, and a side chain (or R group) attached to the α-carbon.

Amnion–The innermost fluid-filled embryonic membrane; it forms a protective sac surrounding the embryos of birds, reptiles, and mammals.

Amplification–Characteristic of a signaling cascade, in which the binding of a single peptide hormone to a membrane-bound receptor results in a signal that increases in strength through the signaling cascade.

Anaerobic–Refers to a biological process that can occur without oxygen or to organisms that can live without molecular oxygen.

Anaphase–The stage of mitosis or meiosis characterized by the migration of chromatids or homologous chromosomes to opposite poles of the dividing cell.

Androgen–Any male sex hormone, such as testosterone.

Antibiotic–Substance that kills or inhibits the growth of bacteria or fungi (usually by disrupting cell wall assembly or by binding to ribosomes, thus inhibiting protein synthesis).

Antibody–Immune or protective protein whose synthesis is induced by the presence of foreign substances (antigens) in the body; each antibody binds to a specific antigen in an immune response; also called immunoglobulin.

Antigen–A substance that binds to an antibody; may be foreign or a self-antigen.

Antigen-binding region–Portion of an antibody that is specific for a particular antigen; the area of the antibody to which the antigen binds.

Aortic valve–One of the semilunar valves, separating the left ventricle from the aorta.

Apoptosis–Process by which a cell undergoes programmed cell death in a highly organized manner in response to either external or internal signals.

Appendicular skeleton–Peripheral portion of the skeleton consisting of arms, legs, and pelvic and pectoral girdles.

Archenteron–The central cavity in the gastrula stage of embryological development; it is lined by endoderm and ultimately gives rise to the adult digestive tract.

Arterioles–Small arterial structures that link the arteries to the capillaries.

Artery–Thick-walled, muscular blood vessel that generally carries blood away from the heart.

Articular cartilage–Cartilaginous coating at the ends of bones that provides a smooth surface for articulation of bones within a joint.

Asexual reproduction–Any reproductive process that does not involve the fusion of gametes (such as budding).

Asters–Star-shaped structures that form around the centrosome during mitosis.

Atrium–One of two paired structures on either side of the heart, into which blood returning from either the body (right atrium) or the lungs (left atrium) flows.

Autocrine–Form of cell–cell communication in which a cell releases a substance that then binds to the membrane of the releasing cell to either inhibit or activate a cellular activity.

Autoimmunity–Inappropriate immune response that targets self-antigens.

Autonomic nervous system–Subdivision of the peripheral nervous system responsible for involuntary activities, which is further subdivided into the parasympathetic and sympathetic nervous systems.

Autosome–Any chromosome other than a sex chromosome.

Axial skeleton–Midline structures of the skeleton including the skull, vertebral column, and rib cage; provides the central framework of the body.

Axon–The long fiber of a neuron; it conducts impulses away from the cell body toward the synapse.

Axon hillock–Transition point between the cell body (soma) and the axon of a neuron; the site of action potential initiation.

Bacillus–Rod-shaped bacterium.

Bacteriophage–A virus that invades bacteria and sometimes uses bacterial RNA and ribosomes to self-replicate.

Barr body–In cells that contain 2 X chromosomes and undergo X-inactivation, the X chromosome that is transcriptionally silenced by methylation.

Basophil–Type of granulocytic leukocyte that largely participates in allergic reactions and local inflammation.

Bile–A solution of salts, pigments, and cholesterol produced by the liver and stored in the gallbladder; it emulsifies large fat droplets when secreted into the small intestine via the bile duct.

Bilirubin–Product of the breakdown of hemoglobin that is modified to a more soluble form in the liver.

Binary fission–A type of asexual reproduction characteristic of prokaryotes in which there is equal nuclear and cytoplasmic division.

Blastocoel–The fluid-filled central cavity of the blastula.

Blastocyst–A mammalian blastula, consisting of the trophoblastic cells and an inner cell mass.

Blastopore–Opening of the archenteron to the external environment in the gastrula stage of embryonic development.

Blastula–The early embryonic stage during which the embryo is a hollow, fluid-filled sphere of undifferentiated cells.

Blastulation–Process by which a solid mass of early embryonic cells, known as the morula, becomes the blastula, a hollow fluid-filled sphere of undifferentiated cells.

Bohr effect–Changes in the affinity of hemoglobin for oxygen caused by changes in the environment; when pH is low (increased concentration of hydrogen ions), the oxyhemoglobin dissociation curve shifts right, indicating a decreased affinity of hemoglobin for oxygen and more efficient off-loading of oxygen from hemoglobin.

Bolus–An initial dose of medication; in the digestive system, chewed food leaving the mouth, traveling through the esophagus, and entering the stomach.

Bone marrow–Central portion of bones, especially long bones, that contains fat and developing blood cells, including erythrocytes, leukocytes, and megakaryocytes.

Bone matrix–Organic and inorganic minerals that provide strength to compact bone; organic components include collagen, glycoproteins, and other peptides; inorganic components include calcium, phosphate, and hydroxide ions (in hydroxyapatite).

Bowman's capsule–The cup-like structure of the nephron; it collects the glomerular filtrate and channels it into the proximal convoluted tubule.

Bronchi–Tube-like passages for air that connect the trachea to the bronchioles.

Bronchioles–Passageways for air that start at the bronchi, dividing into continuously smaller passageways that eventually lead to the alveoli, where gas exchange occurs.

Brush-border enzymes–Group of enzymes present on the luminal surface of cells lining the duodenum that break down larger biomolecules into monomers that are able to be absorbed.

Bundle of His–Part of the conduction system of the heart; it carries impulses from the AV node to the ventricles.

Callus–Area of excessive deposition of keratin in response to repeated strain due to friction.

Canaliculi–Small canals connecting lacunae within the bone matrix with Haversian canals, allowing for the flow of nutrients and wastes.

Capillary–Small, thin-walled blood vessel where gas, nutrient, and waste exchange occurs between blood and tissues.

Capsid–Protein coat surrounding a virus.

Cardiac output–Total blood volume pumped by the left ventricle in one minute, found by multiplying the heart rate by the stroke volume.

Cartilage–A firm, elastic, translucent connective tissue produced by cells called chondrocytes.

Catabolism–The chemical breakdown of complex substances (macromolecules) to yield simpler substances and energy.

Cecum–The first part of the large intestine; accepts material flowing through the ileocecal valve and is the point of attachment of the appendix.

Cell body–Portion of a neuron where the nucleus, endoplasmic reticulum, and ribosomes are located; also known as the soma.

Cell theory–A foundational belief in modern biology that all living things are composed of cells, that the cell is the basic functional unit of life, that all cells arise from preexisting cells, and that DNA is the genetic material.

Cell-mediated immunity–Type of immunity that uses cytotoxic chemicals released from cells to cause death of cells that have been infected by viruses.

Central nervous system (CNS)–The brain and spinal cord.

Centriole–A small organelle in the cytoplasm of animal cells; it organizes the spindle apparatus during mitosis or meiosis.

Centromere–The area of a chromosome where sister chromatids are joined; it is also the point of attachment to the spindle fiber during mitosis and meiosis.

Centrosomes–Paired cylindrical organelles, located in the cytoplasm, that contain the centrioles.

Cerebellum–The section of the mammalian hindbrain that controls muscle coordination and equilibrium.

Cerebral cortex–The outer layer of the forebrain, consisting of grey matter; it is the site of higher cognitive functions in humans.

Cervix–Lower end of the uterus that marks the transition between the vagina and the uterus.

Chemical digestion–Enzymatic cleavage of chemical bonds within foodstuffs, resulting in smaller molecules.

Chemotaxis–Movement of cells toward or away from a chemical within the environment.

Chiasmata–Sites where crossing over occurs between homologous chromosomes during meiosis.

Chief cells–Cells within the stomach that secrete pepsinogen, a zymogen that is converted to its active form, pepsin, by the acidic environment of the stomach.

Chondrin–Elastic cartilage matrix substance secreted by chondrocytes.

Chondrocyte–A differentiated cartilage cell that synthesizes the cartilaginous matrix.

Chromatid–Each of the two chromosomal strands formed by DNA replication in the S phase of the cell cycle; held together by the centromere.

Chromosome–A filamentous body found within the nucleus of a eukaryotic cell or nucleoid region of a prokaryotic cell, composed of DNA.

Chylomicron–Soluble lipid molecule that consists of triglycerides and esterified cholesterol molecules; absorbed into lacteals from the digestive tract.

Chyme–Aqueous mixture of food and secretions that leaves the stomach to enter the duodenum.

Cilia–Projection from a cell involved in movement of materials on the outside of the cell.

Circadian rhythm–A behavioral pattern based on a 24-hour cycle, related to cycling of hormones such as cortisol and melatonin.

Cleavage–A series of mitotic divisions of the zygote immediately following fertilization, resulting in progressively smaller cells with increased nucleus-to-cytoplasm ratios.

Clonal selection–Phenomenon in which only B- or T-cells specific to a particular pathogen are activated.

Coccus–Spherically shaped bacterium.

Codominance–A genetic effect in which the phenotype of a heterozygote is a distinct reflection of both alleles at a particular locus.

Competent–Describes a cell capable of responding to induction signals.

Conjugation–The temporary joining of two organisms via a tube called a pilus, through which genetic material is exchanged; a form of sexual reproduction used by bacteria.

Connective tissue–Animal tissue composed of cells lying in an extracellular proteinaceous network that supports, connects, and surrounds the organs and structures of the body.

Constant region–Portion of an antibody molecule that is not variable and participates in the binding of other immune modulators.

Convergent evolution–The process by which unrelated organisms living in a similar environment develop analogous structures.

Corona radiata–Layer of cells surrounding an oocyte that aids in the development of the ovum.

Corpus luteum–The remnant of the ovarian follicle, which after ovulation continues to secrete progesterone. Its degeneration leads to menstruation; it also maintains the uterine lining during pregnancy.

Cortex–The external layer found in many organs of the body, including the brain, adrenal glands, and kidney.

Cortical reaction–Release of calcium ions by an ovum after fertilization, resulting in the creation of a fertilization membrane, a structure that prevents fertilization of an ovum by multiple sperm cells.

Corticosteroids–Steroid hormones produced in the adrenal cortex, including glucocorticoids (cortisol), mineralocorticoids (aldosterone), and cortical sex hormones.

Crossing over–The exchange of genetic material between homologous chromosomes during meiosis.

Cyclic adenosine monophosphate (cAMP)–An intracellular second messenger in the signaling cascade initiated by a peptide hormone; synthesized from ATP by adenylate cyclase.

Cytokine–Chemical substance that stimulates inflammation and recruits additional immune cells to a specific area.

Cytokinesis–The division and distribution of parent cell cytoplasm to the two daughter cells during mitotic and meiotic cell division.

Cytoplasm–The fluid and solutes within a cell membrane, external to the nucleus and cellular organelles.

Cytotoxic T-cell–T-cell that seeks out infected cells and induces apoptosis in these cells to prevent spread of the pathogen.

Deletion–A type of genetic mutation in which some variable amount of DNA is removed.

Dendrite–The portion of a neuron that receives stimuli and conveys them toward the cell body.

Dermis–The layer of skin cells under the epidermis. Contains sweat glands, hair follicles, fat, and blood vessels.

Determinate cleavage–Rapid mitotic divisions occurring in an embryo that result in cells with predetermined fates; these cells are only capable of differentiating into certain kinds of tissues within an organism.

Determination–Designation of a cell within an embryo as having a particular future function.

Diaphragm–Thin, muscular structure that divides the thorax from the abdomen and provides the driving force for inhalation.

Diaphysis–Cylindrical shaft of a long bone.

Diastole–The period of relaxation of cardiac muscle during which the atrioventricular valves open and the ventricles fill with blood.

Differentiation–The process by which unspecialized cells become specialized. Involves selective transcription of the genome.

Digestion–The breakdown of macromolecular nutrient material via mechanical and chemical means to simple molecular building blocks; this facilitates absorption.

Diploid–Having two chromosomes of each type per cell; symbolized by $2n$.

Direct hormone–Substance secreted into the bloodstream that causes a change in the physiological activity of cells without requiring an intermediary.

Directional selection–Selective pressures favor the development of an extreme phenotype that provides a selective advantage; this phenotype emerges as the primary phenotype over time.

Disruptive selection–Type of selection in which selective pressures favor extreme phenotypes over the norm.

Divergent evolution–A process of change whereby organisms with a common ancestor evolve dissimilar structures (such as dolphin flippers and human arms).

Dominant–Refers to an allele that requires only one copy for expression.

Ductus arteriosus–Fetal structure that shunts blood from the pulmonary artery to the aorta to bypass the developing lungs.

Ductus venosus–Shunt from the umbilical vein to the inferior vena cava, allowing oxygenated blood returning from the placenta to bypass the liver and enter the systemic circulation.

Duodenum–First segment of the small intestine; the contents of the stomach and the pancreatic and bile ducts empty into it; site of digestion and some absorption.

Ectoderm–Outermost embryonic germ layer; it gives rise to the skin, nervous system, inner ear, lens of the eye, and other structures.

Effector–An organ, muscle, or gland used by an organism to respond to a stimulus.

Efferent (motor) neuron–A neuron that transmits nervous impulses from the central nervous system to an effector.

Embryo–An organism at the early developmental stage; in humans, the term refers to the first eight weeks after fertilization.

Endocrine–A form of cell–cell communication that involves the secretion of hormones into the bloodstream by ductless glands; these hormones then travel to distant locations within the organism to cause a change in cellular activity.

Endoderm–Innermost embryonic germ layer; it later gives rise to the linings of the alimentary canal and of the digestive and respiratory organs.

Endometrium–Uterine lining that is regenerated each month in preparation for implantation of an embryo; absence of an embryo results in sloughing off of the endometrium in a process known as menstruation.

Endoplasmic reticulum–Membrane-bound channels in the cytoplasm that transport proteins and lipids to various parts of the cell.

Endothelium–Lining of blood vessels consisting of endothelial cells.

Enteric nervous system–Collection of neurons within the gastrointestinal tract that governs peristalsis.

Eosinophil–Type of granulocytic leukocyte that largely participates in the immune response against parasites; also involved in the pathogenesis of allergies.

Epidermis–The outermost layer of the skin.

Epididymis–The coiled tube in which sperm gain motility and are stored after production in the testes.

Epigenetics–The study of changes to genes other than alterations to nucleotide sequences.

Epiglottis–The small flap of cartilage that covers the glottis during swallowing, preventing food from entering the larynx.

Epinephrine–A hormone synthesized by the adrenal medulla; it stimulates the fight-or-flight response; also a neurotransmitter in the sympathetic nervous system.

Epiphyseal plate–Cartilaginous structure in the epiphysis where growth occurs.

Epiphysis–Dilated end of a long bone.

Episomes–A specialized subset of plasmids capable of integrating into the genome of bacteria under specific circumstances.

Epithelium–The cellular layer that covers internal and external surfaces of body structures and cavities.

Erythrocyte–Red blood cell; a biconcave, disc-shaped cell that contains hemoglobin and has no nucleus.

Esophagus–Portion of the alimentary canal connecting the pharynx and the stomach.

Eukaryote–A unicellular or multicellular organism composed of cells that contain a membrane-bound nucleus and other membrane-bound organelles.

Evolution–The changes in the gene pool from one generation to the next caused by mutation, nonrandom mating, natural selection, and genetic drift.

Exocrine glands–Glands that release their secretions into ducts (such as the parts of the liver and sweat glands).

Expressivity–Varying expression of disease symptoms despite identical genotypes.

Extensor–A muscle used in the straightening of a limb.

Facultative anaerobes–Prokaryotes that can exist with or without oxygen.

Fertilization–Fusion of two gametes.

Fertilization membrane–Structure created by the cortical reaction after fertilization of an ovum by a sperm cell; prevents fertilization of an ovum by multiple sperm cells.

Fetus–A developing organism that has passed the early developmental stages. In humans, the term refers to an embryo from the ninth week after fertilization until birth.

Fibrin–The insoluble protein that forms the bulk of a blood clot.

Filial generation–Offspring in a genetic cross; may be supplemented with a subscript to show how many generations out from the parents.

Filtration–In the nephron, the process by which blood plasma is forced (under high pressure) out of the glomerulus into Bowman's capsule.

Fitness–Reproductive success of an individual, measured in increased number and survival of offspring.

Flagellum–A microscopic, whip-like filament that functions in the locomotion of sperm cells and some unicellular organisms; composed of microtubules.

Flexor–A muscle used in the bending of a limb.

Follicle–The set of cells surrounding a developing or mature ovum. Secretes nutrients and estrogen and atrophies into the corpus luteum after ovulation.

Foramen ovale–Shunt within the fetal heart between the right and left atria that allows the circulation to largely bypass the developing lungs.

Gallbladder–Organ below the liver that stores bile; contracts in response to stimulation by cholecystokinin, resulting in release of bile into the biliary system and eventually into the duodenum.

Gamete–Sperm or ovum; a cell that has half the number of chromosomes of a somatic cell (haploid) and can fuse with another gamete to form a zygote.

Ganglion–A mass of neuron cell bodies outside the central nervous system.

Gastrula–The embryonic stage characterized by the presence of ectoderm, mesoderm, and endoderm.

Gene–The basic unit of heredity; a region on a chromosome that codes for a specific product.

Gene pool–All of the alleles for every gene in every individual in a given population.

Genetic drift–Variations in the gene pool caused by chance.

Genetic map–A diagrammatic representation of a chromosome indicating distance between two genes on a chromosome as determined by recombination frequencies.

Genome–An organism's complete set of chromosomes.

Genotype–The genetic composition of an entire organism or in reference to a particular trait.

Glomerulus–The network of capillaries encapsulated by Bowman's capsule. Acts as a filter for blood entering the nephron.

Glottis–The opening to the trachea.

Golgi apparatus–Organelle that plays a role in the packaging and secretion of proteins and other molecules produced intracellularly.

Gonad–Ovary or testis; the reproductive organ in which gametes are produced.

Gram staining–A process of staining bacterial cells such that cells containing large amounts of peptidoglycan within the cell wall are stained purple, while cells with less peptidoglycan within their cell walls appear pink-red after counterstaining.

Granulocyte–Type of leukocyte with cytoplasmic granules that are visible under a microscope, such as neutrophils, basophils, or eosinophils.

Grey matter–Any region in the central nervous system that consists largely of neuron cell bodies, dendrites, and synapses.

Growth factors–Substances that cause induction during embryonic development and ensure the development of the correct structure in the right location.

Haploid–Having only one of each type of chromosome per cell; symbolized by *n*.

Hardy–Weinberg principle–States that gene ratios and allelic frequencies remain constant through the generations in a non-evolving population.

Haversian canal–Central channel within the osteon (Haversian system) containing blood vessels, nerve fibers, and lymph vessels.

Heavy chain–One of two types of chains, made of peptides, that create an antibody; each antibody consists of two heavy chains and two light chains.

Helper T-cells–Type of T-cell that secretes lymphokines; the specific combination of lymphokines secreted will determine the nature of the immune response; activation of T_h1 cells will result in a cytotoxic response, while a T_h2 response will rely on B-cells.

Hematocrit–Measurement of how much of a blood sample consists of red blood cells, expressed as a percentage.

Hemoglobin–Iron-containing protein found in red blood cells that binds O_2 and transports it throughout the body.

Heterozygous–Having two different alleles for a particular trait.

Hilum–Area of an organ where large vessels or other structures enter or exit; the renal hilum is where the renal artery enters the kidney, the renal vein leaves the kidney, and the ureter exits the kidney to transport urine to the bladder.

Histamine–An inflammatory mediator that causes vasodilation and results in increased movement of fluid and cells out of the blood vessels and into the tissues.

Homeostasis–Maintenance of a stable internal physiological environment in an organism.

Homologous chromosomes–Chromosomes in a diploid cell that carry corresponding genes for the same traits at corresponding loci.

Homozygous–Having two identical alleles for a given trait.

Hormones–Chemical messengers secreted by cells of one part of the body and carried by the bloodstream to cells elsewhere in the body, where they regulate biochemical activity.

Humoral immunity–Form of adaptive immunity that takes place within body fluids, driven by B-cells and antibodies.

Hybrid–The resultant offspring of a cross (mating) either between two different gene types or between two different species.

Hypodermis–Subcutaneous layer beneath the dermis in the skin.

Hypothalamus–The region of the vertebrate forebrain that controls the autonomic nervous system and is the control center for hunger, thirst, body temperature, and other visceral functions; also secretes factors that stimulate or inhibit pituitary secretions.

Ileum–The terminal portion of the small intestine.

Imprinting–An epigenetic process in which gene expression is determined by only one parent.

Impulse propagation–Movement of an action potential down an axon, resulting in neurotransmitter release at the synaptic bouton and transmission of the impulse to the target neuron or organ.

Inborn error of metabolism–Genetic mutation that causes a change in an enzyme required for metabolism; early intervention is necessary to prevent the development of life-threatening conditions; some inborn errors of metabolism are ultimately incompatible with life.

Incomplete dominance–A genetic effect in which the phenotype of a heterozygote is a mixture of the two parental phenotypes.

Independent assortment–Unlinked genes within a primary germ cell separate randomly during gametogenesis.

Indeterminate cleavage–Rapid mitotic divisions resulting in cells that are individually capable of becoming complete organisms.

Inducer–A chemical substance passed from an organizing cell to a responsive cell, resulting in differentiation of the responsive cell.

Induction–The initiation of cell differentiation in a developing embryo due to the influence of other cells.

Innate immunity–Form of immunity that is nonspecific and does not require learning.

Integument–The outer layer of the body (skin); provides function for thermoregulation and innate immunity.

Intermediate filament–Collection of fibers that help to maintain the overall integrity of the cytoskeleton.

Interneuron–A neuron that has its cell body and nerve terminals confined to one specific area; often involved in spinal reflexes.

Interphase–The stage between successive nuclear divisions; it is divided into the G_1, S, and G_2 stages; cell growth and DNA replication occur during interphase.

Intracellular digestion–Oxidation of fatty acids and glucose for energy within cells.

Intrapleural space–Fluid-filled potential space between the parietal and visceral pleura that lubricates the two pleural surfaces and allows for a pressure differential between the intrapleural space and the lungs.

Inversion–A chromosomal mutation in which a section of a chromosome breaks off, flips over, and then reattaches in its original spot.

Isolation–Mechanism that prevents genetic exchange between individuals of different species or populations.

Jejunum–The middle portion of the small intestine.

Joint cavity–Space between two bones in a joint; enclosed and maintained by fibrous tissues.

Juxtacrine–A form of cell–cell communication in which a cell releases a substance that binds to receptors on cells directly adjacent to the releasing cell.

Keratin–Protein present in the outermost layer of the skin that is largely responsible for preventing the loss of fluids and salts as well as the entry of foreign substances into the body; also present as an intermediate filament within cells.

Keratinocytes–Cells within the epidermis that produce keratin.

Kidney–Vertebrate organ that regulates water and salt concentration in the blood and is responsible for urine formation.

Kinetochore–A protein structure, located at the centromere, that provides a place for spindle fibers to attach to the chromosome.

Lacteal–Small lymphatic vessel that runs in the center of the villi in the small intestine; site of lipid absorption into the lymphatic system.

Lacunae–Small spaces within the bone matrix where osteocytes reside.

Lamellae–Concentric circles of bony matrix within the Haversian systems of bone.

Langerhans cells–Specialized macrophages that reside within the skin.

Large intestine–Tube-like structure, shorter but wider than the small intestine, largely responsible for resorption of water and the formation of semisolid feces; consists of the cecum, ascending colon, transverse colon, descending colon, sigmoid colon, and rectum.

Larynx–Pathway for air between the pharynx and the trachea. The epiglottis closes to prevent food from entering the larynx.

Latent period–The short interval between the application of a stimulus to a muscle and the contraction of the muscle.

Leakage–Flow of genes between closely related species.

Leukocytes–White blood cells; can be subdivided into granulocytes and agranulocytes.

Ligament–Connective tissue that joins two bones.

Light chain–One of two types of chains, made of peptides, that create antibodies; each antibody consists of two heavy chains and two light chains.

Linkage–Tendency for certain alleles to be inherited together due to proximity on the same chromosome.

Lipase–Enzyme that specifically cleaves the bonds in lipids.

Locus–In genetics, an area or region of a chromosome.

Loop of Henle–The U-shaped section of a mammalian nephron.

Lower esophageal sphincter–Ring-shaped muscular structure that separates the esophagus from the stomach; also known as the cardiac sphincter.

Lumen–The space within a tube or a sac.

Lymph–Clear fluid derived from blood plasma and transported through lymph vessels to the lymphatic ducts, which empty into the circulatory system.

Lymph node–Small, bean-shaped structure that provides a location for antigen presentation and mounting of an attack by the adaptive immune system.

Lymphocyte–A type of white blood cell involved in an organism's specific immune response.

Lysogenic cycle–Bacteriophage infection involving the integration of viral DNA into the bacterial genome without disrupting or destroying the host. The virus may subsequently reemerge and enter a lytic cycle.

Lysosome–A membrane-bound organelle that stores hydrolytic enzymes.

Lytic cycle–Bacteriophage infection involving the destruction (lysis) of the host bacterium.

Macrophage–A phagocytic white blood cell.

Map unit–A unit used to denote a 1 percent recombination frequency between two genes when creating a genetic map; corresponds to one centimorgan.

Mast cell–A granulocyte that releases histamine and causes inflammation.

Mastication–Breaking up of large food particles using the teeth, tongue, and lips; chewing.

Maternal–Of or relating to an individual who is pregnant. (As used in this text, it implies nothing about the gender identity of pregnant individuals.)

Mechanical digestion–Physical breakdown of large food particles into smaller food particles.

Medulla–The internal section of an organ (such as the adrenal glands and the kidney); may generally refer to the medulla oblongata of the mammalian hindbrain.

Medulla oblongata–The part of the brainstem closest to the spinal cord. It controls vital functions, such as breathing and heartbeat.

Megakaryocyte–Precursor cell that gives off platelets.

Meiosis–A process of cell division in which two successive nuclear divisions produce up to four haploid gametes from one diploid germ cell.

Melanin–Skin pigment produced by melanocytes that protects the skin from UV radiation and provides color to skin.

Melanocytes–Melanin-producing cells of the skin.

Memory cell–Lymphocyte of B- or T-cell lineage that remains after an infection is gone in order to recognize the previous invader and rapidly induce a humoral immune response.

Menstruation–The shedding of the uterine lining that occurs every four weeks in phenotypically female individuals who are not presently pregnant but are capable of becoming pregnant.

Mesoderm–The middle embryonic germ layer; it gives rise to the muscular, skeletal, urogenital, and circulatory systems.

Metabolism–The sum of all biochemical reactions that occur in an organism.

Metaphase–The stage of mitosis or meiosis during which single chromosomes or tetrads line up on the central axis of the dividing cell and become attached to spindle fibers.

Microfilaments–Small polymerized rods of actin that participate in muscle contraction, movement of material within the cellular membrane, and amoeboid movement.

Microglia–Phagocytic white blood cells that reside in the central nervous system.

Microtubule–A small, hollow tube composed of two types of protein subunits; serves numerous functions in the cell, such as comprising the internal structures of cilia and flagella and allowing vesicle movement in the cell.

Missense mutation–Type of mutation that results in the substitution of one amino acid for another.

Mitochondria–Membrane-bound cellular organelles in which the reactions of aerobic respiration and ATP synthesis occur.

Mitosis–Cellular division that results in the formation of two daughter cells that are genetically identical to each other and to the parent cell.

Mitral valve–The atrioventricular valve separating the left atrium from the left ventricle.

Mixed nerve–Nerve carrying both afferent (sensory) and efferent (motor) fibers.

Monocyte–A white blood cell that transforms into a macrophage or dendritic cell once it enters tissues.

Monohybrid cross–A cross between two members of a species that seeks to study only one trait.

Monosaccharide–A sugar consisting of one monomer (glucose, fructose, or galactose).

Morphogen–Molecule that causes nearby cells to proceed in a specific developmental pathway during embryonic development.

Morula–The solid ball of cells that results from the early stages of cleavage in an embryo.

Mucosa–The type of epithelial tissue that lines moist body cavities; a mucous membrane.

Mucous cells–Type of epithelial cell that secretes mucus.

Multipotent–Stem cell that is able to differentiate into various cells within a particular lineage.

Mutagen–An agent, either chemical or physical, that can cause mutations.

Mutation–A change in DNA sequence.

Myelin–The white, lipid-containing material surrounding the axons of many neurons in the central and peripheral nervous systems.

Myogenic activity–Ability of a muscle cell to contract without input from the nervous system; found in smooth and cardiac muscle types.

Myoglobin–Heme-containing protein that binds molecular oxygen in muscle cells.

Myosin–A protein found in muscle cells that functions in muscle contraction; myosin fibers are also called thick filaments.

Natural selection–An ongoing evolutionary process resulting in changes in gene frequencies, leading to the differential development of phenotypes in a population.

Negative sense–Describes the genome of an RNA virus that contains an RNA sequence that is complementary to the actual transcript for viral protein synthesis.

Nephron–The functional unit of the vertebrate kidney.

Nerve–A bundle of neurons.

Nerve impulse–The self-propagating change in electrical potential across the axon membrane.

Nerve terminal–End of the axon from which neurotransmitter molecules are released; also called a synaptic bouton.

Neural crest cells–Cells that originate at the tip of the neural fold and then migrate outward to form the peripheral nervous system, melanocytes, C-cells of the thyroid, and others.

Neural fold–Group of ectodermal cells that slide together to create a fold, which later becomes the neural tube.

Neural tube–Embryonic hollow tube that subsequently gives rise to the central nervous system.

Neuroglia–Support cells for neurons; responsible for functions such as holding neurons in place, supplying neurons with oxygen and nutrients, insulating neurons from other neurons, destroying pathogens, and removing dead neurons.

Neuron–A cell that conducts electrical impulses; the functional unit of the nervous system.

Neurotransmitter–A chemical agent released into the synaptic cleft by the synaptic bouton of a neuron; binds to receptor sites on postsynaptic neurons or effector membranes to alter activity.

Neutrophil–Type of granulocytic leukocyte that largely participates in the nonspecific immune response against bacteria.

Niche–The specific way of life occupied by a given organism within the environment, including its interactions with other organisms and with the physical environment.

Nodes of Ranvier–Points on a myelinated axon that are not covered by myelin.

Nondisjunction–Failure of homologous chromosomes to separate during meiosis.

Nonsense mutation–A change in nucleotide sequence of DNA that results in a premature stop codon in the mRNA sequence.

Norepinephrine–A hormone synthesized by the adrenal medulla; it stimulates the fight-or-flight response; also, a neurotransmitter in the sympathetic nervous system.

Notochord–A supportive rod running just ventral to the neural tube in vertebrate embryos that induces neurulation.

Nuclear membrane–Double membrane enveloping the nucleus, interrupted periodically by pores; found in eukaryotic cells only; also known as the nuclear envelope.

Nuclear pore–Small hole in the nuclear membrane that allows for two-way exchange of material between the cytoplasm and nucleus.

Nucleoid region–Location in prokaryotic cells where the chromosome is found.

Nucleolus–Dense body visible in a nondividing nucleus; site of ribosomal RNA synthesis.

Nucleus–The eukaryotic membrane-bound organelle that contains the cell's chromosomes; in neuroscience, a collection of cell bodies in the central nervous system.

Oligodendrocyte–Myelin-producing cells in the central nervous system.

Oocyte–An undifferentiated cell that undergoes meiosis to produce an egg cell (ovum).

Oogenesis–Gametogenesis in the ovary leading to the formation of mature ova.

Osmotic pressure–A "sucking" pressure generated by the presence of solutes drawing in water.

Osteoblast–Bone cell responsible for the generation of new bone due to bone remodeling or storage of minerals within the bone matrix.

Osteoclast–Bone cell responsible for the resorption of bone due to bone remodeling or mobilization of minerals from the bone matrix.

Osteocytes–Mature bone cells housed within the bone matrix.

Ovary–The female egg-producing gonad.

Oviduct–The tube leading from the ovary to the uterus; generally, the site of fertilization; also called the fallopian tube.

Ovulation–The release of the mature ovum from the ovarian follicle.

Ovum–The female gamete; egg cell.

Oxygen debt–The amount of oxygen needed to reconvert lactic acid to pyruvate following strenuous exercise; the difference between the amount of oxygen needed by the tissue and the amount of oxygen available.

Pancreas–A gland that secretes digestive enzymes into the duodenum via a duct and synthesizes and secretes the hormones insulin, glucagon, and somatostatin; located between the stomach and the duodenum.

Papillary layer–Upper layer of the dermis, right below the epidermis, that consists of loose connective tissue.

Paracrine–A form of cell–cell communication in which a cell releases a substance into the extracellular fluid and the substance binds to receptors on nearby cells to cause a change in cellular activities.

Parasympathetic nervous system–The subdivision of the autonomic nervous system involved in rest and homeostasis; it is generally antagonistic to the sympathetic nervous system.

Parathyroid glands–Two pairs of glands located on the thyroid that secrete hormones that regulate calcium and phosphorous metabolism.

Parietal cells–Cells within the stomach that are responsible for the secretion of acid into the lumen of the stomach.

Passive immunity–Immunity conferred by the transfer or injection of previously formed antibodies.

Pathogen–An infectious disease-causing agent; includes bacteria, viruses, fungi, parasites, and prions.

Pattern recognition receptor–Type of receptor on macrophages and dendritic cells that is able to recognize the nature of the invader (bacteria, virus, or fungi) and release the appropriate cytokines to attract the right immune cells to the area.

Penetrance–Percent of individuals with a particular genotype that actually express the associated phenotype.

Peptidase–Enzyme that cleaves peptide bonds.

Periosteum–Fibrous sheath surrounding long bones.

Peripheral nervous system–Includes all neurons outside the central nervous system, including sensory and motor neurons; it is subdivided into the somatic and autonomic nervous systems.

Peristalsis–Rhythmic waves of muscular contraction that move a substance through a tube (most commonly, food through the digestive tract).

Peroxisome–Organelle that contains hydrogen peroxide and participates in the breakdown of very long chain fatty acids.

Pharynx–Pathway for food from the mouth to the esophagus, and for air from the nose and mouth to the larynx.

Phenotype–The physical manifestation of an organism's genotype.

Pineal gland–Structure within the brain that secretes melatonin, a hormone that aids in the regulation of sleep–wake cycles.

Pituitary–The bilobed endocrine gland that lies just below the hypothalamus; because many of its hormones regulate other endocrine glands, it is known as the "master gland."

Placenta–The structure formed by the wall of the uterus and the chorion of the embryo; contains a network of capillaries through which exchange between maternal and fetal circulation occurs.

Plasma–The fluid component of blood containing dissolved solutes, minus the cells.

Plasma cells–Derived from B-lymphocytes; have the ability to produce and secrete antibodies.

Plasmid–Small circular ring of extrachromosomal DNA found in bacteria.

Platelets–Small, enucleated, disc-shaped shards of blood cells that play an important role in clotting.

Pleura–Connective tissue that surrounds each lung and aids in providing attachment of the lungs to the chest wall; the parietal pleura lies along the chest wall, while the visceral pleura is adherent to the lungs.

Pluripotent–Stem cell that has undergone gastrulation and is able to differentiate into any cell type within the same primary germ layer.

Polar body–A small, nonfunctional haploid cell created during oogenesis.

Population–A group of organisms of the same species living together in a given location.

Portal system–A circuit of blood in which there are two capillary beds in tandem connected by an artery or vein; examples include the hypophyseal, hepatic, and renal portal systems.

Positive sense–Describes the genome of an RNA virus containing RNA that serves directly as the transcript for viral protein production.

Potency–Term used to describe the ability or inability of a stem cell to differentiate into different cell types.

Primary response–Humoral immune response against an invader during the first encounter; takes seven to ten days to become effective.

Prion–Infectious protein that causes disease by causing changes in the three-dimensional structure of other proteins from α-helices to β-pleated sheets.

Prokaryote–Cell lacking a nuclear membrane and membrane-bound organelles, such as a bacterium.

Prophase–The stage of mitosis or meiosis during which the DNA strands condense to form visible chromosomes; during prophase I of meiosis, homologous chromosomes align.

Prostate–A gland in phenotypically male mammals that secretes alkaline seminal fluid.

Pulmonary valve–One of the semilunar valves, separating the right ventricle from the pulmonary arteries.

Purkinje fibers–The terminal fibers of the heart's conduction system; located in the walls of ventricles.

Pyloric sphincter–The valve that regulates the flow of chyme from the stomach into the small intestine.

Recessive–An allele that requires two copies to be expressed.

Recombination–New gene combinations achieved by sexual reproduction or crossing over in eukaryotes and by transformation, transduction, or conjugation in prokaryotes.

Recombination frequency–Measurement of how often genes recombine in different combinations; genes that are closer together have lower recombination frequencies.

Rectum–Terminal portion of the large intestine, where feces is stored until defecation.

Reflex–An involuntary nervous pathway consisting of sensory neurons, interneurons, motor neurons, and effectors; it occurs in response to a specific stimulus.

Refractory period–The period of time following an action potential during which the neuron is incapable of depolarization.

Releasing hormones–Proteins synthesized and secreted by the hypothalamus that stimulate the pituitary to synthesize and release its hormones. Also known as tropic hormones.

Renal pelvis–The widest part of the ureter, located within the kidney; location into which all collecting ducts eventually empty.

Renin–angiotensin–aldosterone system–Hormonal pathway that, among other functions, raises blood pressure.

Repolarization–Restoration of the resting membrane potential in neurons from being depolarized by both active and passive processes.

Respiration–In biochemistry, the series of oxygen-requiring biochemical reactions that lead to ATP synthesis; in physiology, the inhalation and exhalation of gases and their exchange in the lungs.

Responder–Embryonic cell that is undergoing induction.

Resting potential–The electrical potential of a cell at rest, approximately −70 mV in most excitable cells.

Restriction point–A point in the cell cycle that prevents the cell from entering the next portion of the cell cycle unless certain criteria are met.

Reticular layer–Lower layer of the dermis, consisting of dense connective tissue.

Retrovirus–An RNA virus that contains the enzyme reverse transcriptase, which transcribes RNA into DNA.

Rh factor–An antigen on a red blood cell, the presence or absence of which is indicated by + or −, respectively, in blood type notation; may also be called the D allele.

Ribosome–Organelle composed of RNA and protein; it translates mRNA during protein synthesis.

Rough endoplasmic reticulum–Portion of the endoplasmic reticulum that appears rough microscopically due to the presence of ribosomes attached to the outer surface; site of protein synthesis for proteins destined to be membrane-bound or secreted.

Saltatory conduction–Process by which an electrical signal jumps across the nodes of Ranvier to travel down the axon.

Sarcolemma–Muscle cell membrane capable of propagating action potentials.

Sarcomere–The functional contractile unit of striated muscle.

Sarcoplasmic reticulum–The endoplasmic reticulum of a muscle cell; it envelops myofibrils.

Schwann cell–Myelin-producing cell in the peripheral nervous system.

Second messenger–Substance that is mobilized within a cell after the binding of a hormone to its receptor.

Secondary response–Humoral immune response against a previously encountered invader; results in activation of memory cells and an immediate response.

Semen–Fluid released during ejaculation consisting of sperm cells suspended in seminal fluid.

Seminal vesicle–A gland found in phenotypically male mammals that produces seminal fluid.

Sex factor–Plasmid containing genetic material for the formation of a sex pili, required for conjugation.

Sex pilus–Appendage extending from the donor male (+) bacterial cell to the recipient female (−), allowing for the formation of the cytoplasmic bridge and transfer of genetic material.

Sex-linked gene–A gene located only on a sex chromosome (almost always the X chromosome); such genes exhibit different inheritance patterns in genotypical males and genotypical females.

Sexual reproduction–Any reproductive process that involves the fusion of gametes, resulting in the passage of combined genetic information to offspring.

Silent mutation–Change of one nucleotide for another that does not result in a change in the protein due to the degenerative nature of the genetic code (multiple codons code for the same amino acid).

Small intestine–Long tube-like structure; longer, but narrower than the large intestine, largely responsible for chemical digestion of foodstuffs and absorption of nutrients; consists of the duodenum, jejunum, and ileum.

Smooth endoplasmic reticulum–Portion of the endoplasmic reticulum that lacks ribosomes on its surface; location of lipid synthesis and detoxification of drugs and poisons.

Somatic cells–All cells in the body except germ cells and gametes.

Somatic nervous system–Subdivision of the peripheral nervous system that governs all voluntary actions.

Species–The largest group of organisms capable of mating to produce viable, fertile offspring.

Specific immune response–An organism's targeted fight against a specific pathogen using both antibodies and cytotoxic immunity.

Sperm–The mature male gamete or sex cell.

Spermatids–Immature haploid sperm cells.

Spermatogenesis–Gametogenesis in the testes leading to sperm formation.

Spermatogonia–Diploid stem cells in males that eventually give rise to sperm cells.

Spermatozoa–Mature haploid sperm cells.

Sphincter–A ring-shaped muscle that closes and opens a tube (such as the pyloric sphincter).

Sphygmomanometer–Device used to measure blood pressure, consisting of an inflatable cuff and a gauge that measures pressure.

Spindle–A structure within dividing cells composed of microtubules; it is involved in the separation of chromosomes during mitosis and meiosis.

Spirilli–Spiral-shaped bacteria.

Spleen–Highly vascular organ in the left upper quadrant of the abdomen; serves as a location for disposal of aged red blood cells and the presentation of antigens to B-cells.

Stabilizing selection–Selective pressure resulting in the elimination of extremes.

Starling forces–A sum of the forces generated by hydrostatic and osmotic pressures; results in a greater attraction of fluid to one side of a membrane.

Stroke volume–Amount of blood ejected from a ventricle with each heartbeat.

Summation–Process that occurs when the postsynaptic neuron or target organ requires stimulation from multiple presynaptic neurons in order to respond to the stimulus; may be spatial or temporal.

Suppressor T-cells–Also known as regulatory T-cells (T_{reg}), these T-cells limit the immune response to prevent detrimental immune reactions, such as autoimmunity.

Surfactant–A detergent that lowers surface tension and prevents collapse of the alveoli.

Symbiote–Organism living closely with a host and engaging in a mutually beneficial relationship.

Sympathetic nervous system–The subdivision of the autonomic nervous system that produces the "fight-or-flight" response.

Synapse–The junction between two neurons into which neurotransmitters are released.

Synapsis–The pairing of homologous chromosomes during prophase I of meiosis.

Synovial capsule–Fluid-filled space between bones in a joint; enclosed by fibrous tissue; synovial fluid lubricates the joint.

Systole–The period of the cardiac cycle during which the ventricles contract and pump blood into the aorta and pulmonary arteries.

T-cells–Type of leukocyte that matures in the thymus and participates in adaptive immunity.

Telophase–The final stage of mitosis or meiosis during which the chromosomes uncoil, nuclear membranes reform, and cytokinesis occurs.

Tendon–A fibrous connective tissue that connects a bone to a muscle.

Test cross–A cross between an organism showing a dominant trait and an organism showing a recessive trait to determine whether the former organism is homozygous or heterozygous for that trait.

Testis–The sperm-producing organ; also secretes testosterone.

Tetanus–Sustained muscle contraction that results from continuous stimulation.

Tetrad–A pair of homologous chromosomes synapsing during prophase I of meiosis. Each chromosome consists of two sister chromatids; thus, each tetrad consists of four chromatids.

Thermoregulation–Process by which an organism regulates its internal temperature by using the respiratory, integumentary, and circulatory systems.

Thoracic duct–The main lymphatic vessel that empties lymph into the bloodstream.

Threshold–The lowest magnitude of stimulus strength that will induce a response.

Thrombin–An enzyme that participates in blood clotting; it converts fibrinogen into fibrin.

Thymus–A ductless gland in the upper chest region of vertebrates; it functions in the development of the immune system.

Thyroid–A vertebrate endocrine gland located in the neck that synthesizes triiodothyronine, thyroxine, and calcitonin.

Tissue–A mass of similar cells and support structures organized into a functional unit.

Tonus–A continuous state of low-level muscle contraction.

Totipotent–Type of stem-cell potency describing cells that are able to differentiate into all cell types within an organism.

Trachea–The tube that connects the pharynx to the bronchi.

Transduction–The transposition of genetic material from one organism to another by a virus.

Transformation–Uptake and incorporation of DNA from the environment by a recipient bacterial cell.

Transposon–Genetic element capable of inserting and removing itself from the genome.

Tricuspid valve–One of the atrioventricular valves, separating the right atrium from the right ventricle.

Trophoblast–Embryonic cells that line the blastocoel and give rise to the chorion and the placenta.

Tropic hormone–Hormone that is secreted and travels to a target cell or organ, where it triggers release of another hormone, which causes changes in the physiological activity of target cells.

Tubulin–Protein constituent of microtubules.

Universal donor–A person (O^- blood) whose blood is able to be given to all types without inducing an immune response.

Universal recipient–A person (AB^+ blood) who is able to receive all blood types without undergoing an immune response.

Urea–A nitrogenous waste product produced in the liver from ammonia.

Ureter–The tube that carries urine from the kidneys to the bladder.

Urethra–The tube that carries urine from the bladder to the exterior.

Urine–Liquid waste resulting from the filtration, reabsorption, and secretion of filtrate in the nephron.

Uterus–Organ in the mammalian female reproductive system that is the site of embryonic development.

Vaccine–A solution of fractionated, dead, or attenuated live pathogenic material that is introduced into an individual for the purpose of stimulating a primary immune response or "boosting" a previously produced anamnestic state.

Vagina–Passageway through which childbirth occurs; location into which sperm is deposited during sexual intercourse.

Vagus nerve–The tenth cranial nerve; it innervates the palate, pharynx, larynx, heart, lungs, and abdominal viscera; responsible for maintaining homeostatic activity through the parasympathetic response.

Vas deferens–The tube carrying sperm from the testis to the urethra in phenotypically male mammals.

Vasa recta–Second capillary bed within the kidney that removes substances from the interstitium of the kidney to be returned to the systemic circulation.

Vein–Thin-walled blood vessel that carries blood toward the heart.

Venae cavae–Two large veins (superior and inferior) that return deoxygenated blood from the periphery to the right atrium of the heart.

Ventilation center–Groups of neurons in the medulla oblongata that regulate respiration.

Ventricles–The chambers of the heart that pump blood into pulmonary and systemic circulation.

Venule–Small venous structure that links the capillaries to the veins.

Vestigial–Referring to an organ or limb that has no apparent function now, but was functional at some time in the organism's evolutionary past.

Villus–A small projection from the wall of the small intestine that increases the surface area for digestion and absorption.

Viroid–A small plant pathogen consisting of a very short, circular, single strand of RNA.

Virus–A tiny, organism-like particle composed of protein-encased nucleic acid; viruses are obligate parasites.

Vitamin–An organic nutrient that an organism cannot produce itself and that is required by the organism in small amounts to aid in proper metabolic functioning; vitamins often function as cofactors for enzymes.

White matter–The portion of the central nervous system consisting primarily of myelinated axons.

Zona pellucida–One of two layers of cells surrounding an oocyte.

Zygote–The diploid ($2n$) cell that results from the fusion of two haploid (n) gametes.

Zymogen–An inactive enzyme precursor that is converted into an active enzyme.

INDEX

Note: Material in figures or tables is indicated by italic *f* or *t* after the page number.

A

C

F

G

H

K

L

M

N

O

P

R

S

T

U

V

W

X

Y

Z

ART CREDITS

Chapter 1 Cover—Image credited to MichaelTaylor3d. From Shutterstock.

Figure 1.6—Image credited to Mopic. From Shutterstock.

Figure 1.11—Image credited to NANOCLUSTERING/SCIENCE PHOTO LIBRARY. From Getty Images. Modified from source.

Chapter 2 Cover—Image credited to Jose Luis Calvo. From Shutterstock.

Figure 3.2—Image credited to Science Photo Library - ZEPHYR. From Getty Images.

Figure 3.3—Image credited to Ed Reschke. From Getty Images.

Figure 3.8—Image credited to Callista Images. From Getty Images.

Chapter 4 Cover—Image credited to Juane Gaertner. From Shutterstock.

Figure 4.2—Image credited to Vitalii Dumma. From Getty Images. Modified from source.

Figure 4.11—Image credited to Alila Medical Media. From Shutterstock.

Figure 4.12—Image credited to Alila Medical Media. From Shutterstock.

Chapter 5 Cover—Image credited to Vitapix. From Getty Images.

Figure 5.10—Image credited to Alila Medical Media. From Shutterstock.

Chapter 6 Cover—Image credited to Guzel Studio. From Shutterstock.

Chapter 7 Cover—Image credited to decade3d. From Shutterstock.

Figure 7.12—Image credited to Stocktrek Images. From Getty Images.

Chapter 9 Cover—Image credited to Juan Gaertner. From Shutterstock.

Figure 9.4—Image credited to User: BruceBlaus. From Wikimedia Commons. Copyright © 2013. Used under license: CC-BY-3.0.

Figure 10.6—Image credited to Anton Nalivayko. From Shutterstock.

Figure 10.7—Image credited to User: Blamb. From Shutterstock. Modified from source.

Chapter 11 Cover—Image credited to SEBASTIAN KAULITZKI. From Getty Images.

Figure 11.11—Image credited to OpenStax College. In: Anatomy & Physiology, Connexions website. Copyright © 2013. Used under license: CC-BY-3.0.

Notes

Notes

Notes

Notes

Notes

Notes

Notes

Notes

Notes

Notes

Notes

Notes

Notes

Notes

Notes

KAPLAN

MCAT® BEHAVIORAL SCIENCES REVIEW 2024–2025

ONLINE + BOOK

Edited by Alexander Stone Macnow, MD

ACKNOWLEDGMENTS

Editor-in-Chief, 2024–2025 Edition
M. Dominic Eggert

Contributing Editors, 2024–2025 Edition
Christopher Durland; Charles Pierce, MD; Jason Selzer

Prior Edition Editorial Staff: Brandon Deason, MD; Christopher Durland; M. Dominic Eggert; Tyler Fara; Elizabeth Flagge; Adam Grey; Lauren K. White

Published by Kaplan North America, LLC dba Kaplan Publishing
1515 West Cypress Creek Road
Fort Lauderdale, Florida 33309

ISBN: 978-1-5062-8656-3

10 9 8 7 6 5 4 3

Kaplan Publishing print books are available at special quantity discounts to use for sales promotions, employee premiums, or educational purposes. For more information or to purchase books, please call the Simon & Schuster special sales department at 866-506-1949.

TABLE OF CONTENTS

GO ONLINE
kaptest.com/booksonline

THE *KAPLAN MCAT REVIEW* TEAM

Alexander Stone Macnow, MD
Editor-in-Chief

Áine Lorié, PhD
Editor

Derek Rusnak, MA
Editor

Mikhail Alexeeff
Kaplan MCAT Faculty

Laura L. Ambler
Kaplan MCAT Faculty

Krista L. Buckley, MD
Kaplan MCAT Faculty

Kristen L. Russell, ME
Editor

Pamela Willingham, MSW
Editor

Melinda Contreras, MS
Kaplan MCAT Faculty

Samantha Fallon
Kaplan MCAT Faculty

Jason R. Selzer
Kaplan MCAT Faculty

M. Dominic Eggert
Editor

Faculty Reviewers and Editors: Elmar R. Aliyev; James Burns; Jonathan Cornfield; Alisha Maureen Crowley; Nikolai Dorofeev, MD; Benjamin Downer, MS; Colin Doyle; Christopher Durland; Marilyn Engle; Eleni M. Eren; Raef Ali Fadel; Elizabeth Flagge; Adam Grey; Rohit Gupta, Jonathan Habermacher; Tyra Hall-Pogar, PhD; Justine Harkness, PhD; Scott Huff; Samer T. Ismail; Ae-Ri Kim, PhD; Elizabeth A. Kudlaty; Kelly Kyker-Snowman, MS; Ningfei Li; John P. Mahon; Brandon McKenzie; Matthew A. Meier; Nainika Nanda; Caroline Nkemdilim Opene; Kaitlyn E. Prenger; Uneeb Qureshi; Jason Selzer; Allison St. Clair; Bela G. Starkman, PhD; Chris Sun; Michael Paul Tomani, MS; Bonnie Wang; Ethan Weber; Lauren K. White; Nicholas M. White; Allison Ann Wilkes, MS; Kerranna Williamson, MBA; and Tony Yu

Thanks to Rebecca Anderson; Jeff Batzli; Eric Chiu; Tim Eich; Tyler Fara; Owen Farcy; Dan Frey; Robin Garmise; Rita Garthaffner; Joanna Graham; Allison Gudenau; Allison Harm; Beth Hoffberg; Aaron Lemon-Strauss; Keith Lubeley; Diane McGarvey; Petros Minasi; Beena P V; John Polstein; Deeangelee Pooran-Kublall, MD, MPH; Rochelle Rothstein, MD; Larry Rudman; Srividhya Sankar; Sylvia Tidwell Scheuring; Carly Schnur; Aiswarya Sivanand; Todd Tedesco; Karin Tucker; Lee Weiss; Christina Wheeler; Kristen Workman; Amy Zarkos; and the countless others who made this project possible.

GETTING STARTED CHECKLIST

Getting Started Checklist

- [ ] Register for your free online assets—including full-length tests, Science Review Videos, and additional practice materials—at **www.kaptest.com/moreonline**.
- [ ] Create a study calendar that ensures you complete content review and sufficient practice by Test Day!
- [ ] As you finish a chapter and the online practice for that chapter, check it off on the table of contents.
- [ ] Register to take the MCAT at **www.aamc.org/mcat**.
- [ ] Set aside time during your prep to make sure the rest of your application—personal statement, recommendations, and other materials—is ready to go!
- [ ] Take a moment to admire your completed checklist, then get back to the business of prepping for this exam!

PREFACE

And now it starts: your long, yet fruitful journey toward wearing a white coat. Proudly wearing that white coat, though, is hopefully only part of your motivation. You are reading this book because you want to be a healer.

If you're serious about going to medical school, then you are likely already familiar with the importance of the MCAT in medical school admissions. While the holistic review process puts additional weight on your experiences, extracurricular activities, and personal attributes, the fact remains: along with your GPA, your MCAT score remains one of the two most important components of your application portfolio—at least early in the admissions process. Each additional point you score on the MCAT pushes you in front of thousands of other students and makes you an even more attractive applicant. But the MCAT is not simply an obstacle to overcome; it is an opportunity to show schools that you will be a strong student and a future leader in medicine.

We at Kaplan take our jobs very seriously and aim to help students see success not only on the MCAT, but as future physicians. We work with our learning science experts to ensure that we're using the most up-to-date teaching techniques in our resources. Multiple members of our team hold advanced degrees in medicine or associated biomedical sciences, and are committed to the highest level of medical education. Kaplan has been working with the MCAT for over 50 years and our commitment to premed students is unflagging; in fact, Stanley Kaplan created this company when he had difficulty being accepted to medical school due to unfair quota systems that existed at the time.

We stand now at the beginning of a new era in medical education. As citizens of this 21st-century world of healthcare, we are charged with creating a patient-oriented, culturally competent, cost-conscious, universally available, technically advanced, and research-focused healthcare system, run by compassionate providers. Suffice it to say, this is no easy task. Problem-based learning, integrated curricula, and classes in interpersonal skills are some of the responses to this demand for an excellent workforce—a workforce of which you'll soon be a part.

We're thrilled that you've chosen us to help you on this journey. Please reach out to us to share your challenges, concerns, and successes. Together, we will shape the future of medicine in the United States and abroad; we look forward to helping you become the doctor you deserve to be.

Good luck!

Alexander Stone Macnow, MD
Editor-in-Chief
Department of Pathology and Laboratory Medicine
Hospital of the University of Pennsylvania

BA, Musicology—Boston University, 2008
MD—Perelman School of Medicine at the University of Pennsylvania, 2013

ABOUT THE MCAT

Anatomy of the MCAT

Here is a general overview of the structure of Test Day:

Section	Number of Questions	Time Allotted
Test-Day Certification		4 minutes
Tutorial (optional)		10 minutes
Chemical and Physical Foundations of Biological Systems	59	95 minutes
Break (optional)		10 minutes
Critical Analysis and Reasoning Skills (CARS)	53	90 minutes
Lunch Break (optional)		30 minutes
Biological and Biochemical Foundations of Living Systems	59	95 minutes
Break (optional)		10 minutes
Psychological, Social, and Biological Foundations of Behavior	59	95 minutes
Void Question		3 minutes
Satisfaction Survey (optional)		5 minutes

The structure of the four sections of the MCAT is shown below.

Chemical and Physical Foundations of Biological Systems	
Time	95 minutes
Format	• 59 questions • 10 passages • 44 questions are passage-based, and 15 are discrete (stand-alone) questions. • Score between 118 and 132
What It Tests	• Biochemistry: 25% • Biology: 5% • General Chemistry: 30% • Organic Chemistry: 15% • Physics: 25%

Critical Analysis and Reasoning Skills (CARS)	
Time	90 minutes
Format	• 53 questions • 9 passages • All questions are passage-based. There are no discrete (stand-alone) questions. • Score between 118 and 132
What It Tests	Disciplines: • Humanities: 50% • Social Sciences: 50% Skills: • *Foundations of Comprehension*: 30% • *Reasoning Within the Text*: 30% • *Reasoning Beyond the Text*: 40%
Biological and Biochemical Foundations of Living Systems	
Time	95 minutes
Format	• 59 questions • 10 passages • 44 questions are passage-based, and 15 are discrete (stand-alone) questions. • Score between 118 and 132
What It Tests	• Biochemistry: 25% • Biology: 65% • General Chemistry: 5% • Organic Chemistry: 5%
Psychological, Social, and Biological Foundations of Behavior	
Time	95 minutes
Format	• 59 questions • 10 passages • 44 questions are passage-based, and 15 are discrete (stand-alone) questions. • Score between 118 and 132
What It Tests	• Biology: 5% • Psychology: 65% • Sociology: 30%
Total	
Testing Time	375 minutes (6 hours, 15 minutes)
Total Seat Time	447 minutes (7 hours, 27 minutes)
Questions	230
Score	472 to 528

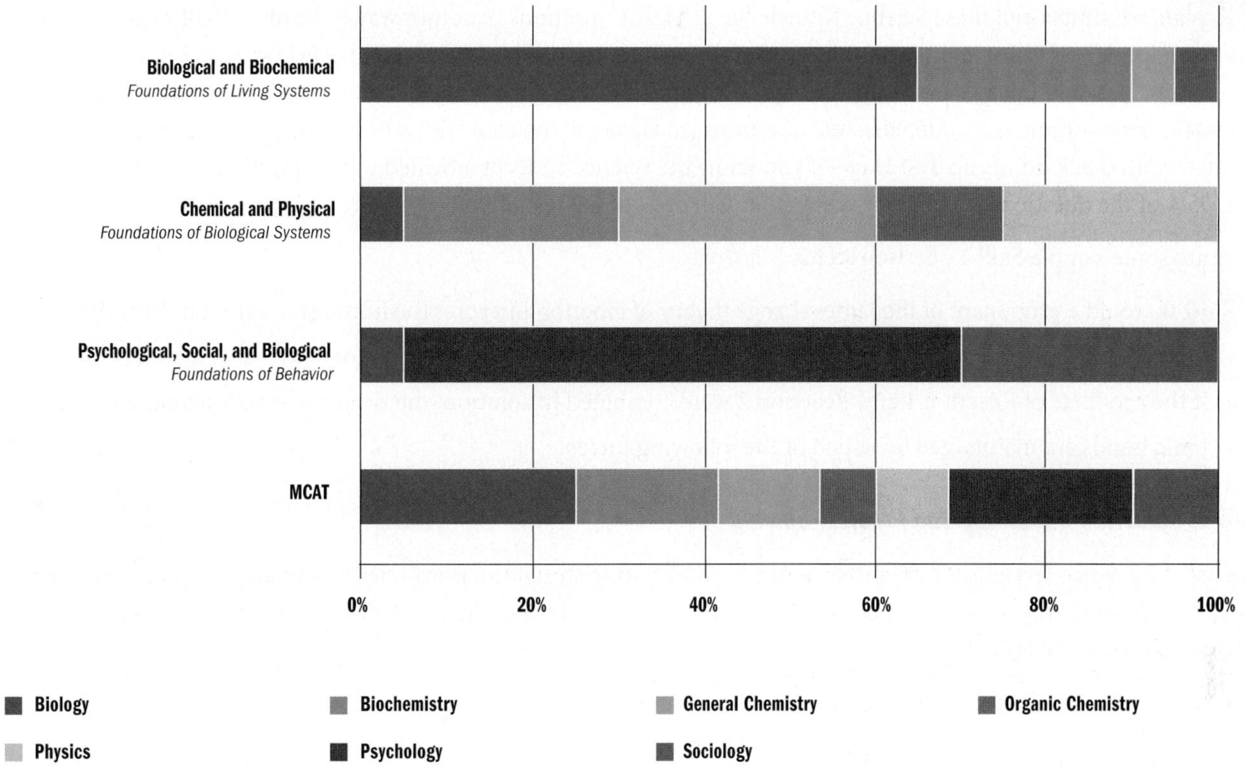

Scientific Inquiry and Reasoning Skills (SIRS)

The AAMC has defined four *Scientific Inquiry and Reasoning Skills* (SIRS) that will be tested in the three science sections of the MCAT:

1. *Knowledge of Scientific Concepts and Principles* (35% of questions)
2. *Scientific Reasoning and Problem-Solving* (45% of questions)
3. *Reasoning About the Design and Execution of Research* (10% of questions)
4. *Data-Based and Statistical Reasoning* (10% of questions)

Let's see how each one breaks down into more specific Test Day behaviors. Note that the bullet points of specific objectives for each of the SIRS are taken directly from the *Official Guide to the MCAT Exam*; the descriptions of what these behaviors mean and sample question stems, however, are written by Kaplan.

Skill 1: *Knowledge of Scientific Concepts and Principles*

This is probably the least surprising of the four SIRS; the testing of science knowledge is, after all, one of the signature qualities of the MCAT. Skill 1 questions will require you to do the following:

- Recognize correct scientific principles
- Identify the relationships among closely related concepts
- Identify the relationships between different representations of concepts (verbal, symbolic, graphic)
- Identify examples of observations that illustrate scientific principles
- Use mathematical equations to solve problems

At Kaplan, we simply call these Science Knowledge or Skill 1 questions. Another way to think of Skill 1 questions is as "one-step" problems. The single step is either to realize which scientific concept the question stem is suggesting or to take the concept stated in the question stem and identify which answer choice is an accurate application of it. Skill 1 questions are particularly prominent among discrete questions (those not associated with a passage). These questions are an opportunity to gain quick points on Test Day—if you know the science concept attached to the question, then that's it! On Test Day, 35% of the questions in each science section will be Skill 1 questions.

Here are some sample Skill 1 question stems:

- How would a proponent of the James–Lange theory of emotion interpret the findings of the study cited in the passage?
- Which of the following most accurately describes the function of FSH in the human menstrual cycle?
- If the products of Reaction 1 and Reaction 2 were combined in solution, the resulting reaction would form:
- Ionic bonds are maintained by which of the following forces?

Skill 2: *Scientific Reasoning and Problem-Solving*

The MCAT science sections do, of course, move beyond testing straightforward science knowledge; Skill 2 questions are the most common way in which it does so. At Kaplan, we also call these Critical Thinking questions. Skill 2 questions will require you to do the following:

- Reason about scientific principles, theories, and models
- Analyze and evaluate scientific explanations and predictions
- Evaluate arguments about causes and consequences
- Bring together theory, observations, and evidence to draw conclusions
- Recognize scientific findings that challenge or invalidate a scientific theory or model
- Determine and use scientific formulas to solve problems

Just as Skill 1 questions can be thought of as "one-step" problems, many Skill 2 questions are "two-step" problems, and more difficult Skill 2 questions may require three or more steps. These questions can require a wide spectrum of reasoning skills, including integration of multiple facts from a passage, combination of multiple science content areas, and prediction of an experiment's results. Skill 2 questions also tend to ask about science content without actually mentioning it by name. For example, a question might describe the results of one experiment and ask you to predict the results of a second experiment without actually telling you what underlying scientific principles are at work—part of the question's difficulty will be figuring out which principles to apply in order to get the correct answer. On Test Day, 45% of the questions in each science section will be Skill 2 questions.

Here are some sample Skill 2 question stems:

- Which of the following experimental conditions would most likely yield results similar to those in Figure 2?
- All of the following conclusions are supported by the information in the passage EXCEPT:
- The most likely cause of the anomalous results found by the experimenter is:
- An impact to a person's chest quickly reduces the volume of one of the lungs to 70% of its initial value while not allowing any air to escape from the mouth. By what percentage is the force of outward air pressure increased on a 2 cm^2 portion of the inner surface of the compressed lung?

Skill 3: *Reasoning About the Design and Execution of Research*

The MCAT is interested in your ability to critically appraise and analyze research, as this is an important day-to-day task of a physician. We call these questions Skill 3 or Experimental and Research Design questions for short. Skill 3 questions will require you to do the following:

- Identify the role of theory, past findings, and observations in scientific questioning
- Identify testable research questions and hypotheses
- Distinguish between samples and populations and distinguish results that support generalizations about populations
- Identify independent and dependent variables
- Reason about the features of research studies that suggest associations between variables or causal relationships between them (such as temporality and random assignment)
- Identify conclusions that are supported by research results
- Determine the implications of results for real-world situations
- Reason about ethical issues in scientific research

Over the years, the AAMC has received input from medical schools to require more practical research skills of MCAT test takers, and Skill 3 questions are the response to these demands. This skill is unique in that the outside knowledge you need to answer Skill 3 questions is not taught in any one undergraduate course; instead, the research design principles needed to answer these questions are learned gradually throughout your science classes and especially through any laboratory work you have completed. It should be noted that Skill 3 comprises 10% of the questions in each science section on Test Day.

Here are some sample Skill 3 question stems:

- What is the dependent variable in the study described in the passage?
- The major flaw in the method used to measure disease susceptibility in Experiment 1 is:
- Which of the following procedures is most important for the experimenters to follow in order for their study to maintain a proper, randomized sample of research subjects?
- A researcher would like to test the hypothesis that individuals who move to an urban area during adulthood are more likely to own a car than are those who have lived in an urban area since birth. Which of the following studies would best test this hypothesis?

Skill 4: *Data-Based and Statistical Reasoning*

Lastly, the science sections of the MCAT test your ability to analyze the visual and numerical results of experiments and studies. We call these Data and Statistical Analysis questions. Skill 4 questions will require you to do the following:

- Use, analyze, and interpret data in figures, graphs, and tables
- Evaluate whether representations make sense for particular scientific observations and data
- Use measures of central tendency (mean, median, and mode) and measures of dispersion (range, interquartile range, and standard deviation) to describe data
- Reason about random and systematic error

- Reason about statistical significance and uncertainty (interpreting statistical significance levels and interpreting a confidence interval)
- Use data to explain relationships between variables or make predictions
- Use data to answer research questions and draw conclusions

Skill 4 is included in the MCAT because physicians and researchers spend much of their time examining the results of their own studies and the studies of others, and it's very important for them to make legitimate conclusions and sound judgments based on that data. The MCAT tests Skill 4 on all three science sections with graphical representations of data (charts and bar graphs), as well as numerical ones (tables, lists, and results summarized in sentence or paragraph form). On Test Day, 10% of the questions in each science section will be Skill 4 questions.

Here are some sample Skill 4 question stems:

- According to the information in the passage, there is an inverse correlation between:
- What conclusion is best supported by the findings displayed in Figure 2?
- A medical test for a rare type of heavy metal poisoning returns a positive result for 98% of affected individuals and 13% of unaffected individuals. Which of the following types of error is most prevalent in this test?
- If a fourth trial of Experiment 1 was run and yielded a result of 54% compliance, which of the following would be true?

SIRS Summary

Discussing the SIRS tested on the MCAT is a daunting prospect given that the very nature of the skills tends to make the conversation rather abstract. Nevertheless, with enough practice, you'll be able to identify each of the four skills quickly, and you'll also be able to apply the proper strategies to solve those problems on Test Day. If you need a quick reference to remind you of the four SIRS, these guidelines may help:

Skill 1 (**Science Knowledge**) questions ask:

- Do you remember this science content?

Skill 2 (**Critical Thinking**) questions ask:

- Do you remember this science content? And if you do, could you please apply it to this novel situation?
- Could you answer this question that cleverly combines multiple content areas at the same time?

Skill 3 (**Experimental and Research Design**) questions ask:

- Let's forget about the science content for a while. Could you give some insight into the experimental or research methods involved in this situation?

Skill 4 (**Data and Statistical Analysis**) questions ask:

- Let's forget about the science content for a while. Could you accurately read some graphs and tables for a moment? Could you make some conclusions or extrapolations based on the information presented?

Critical Analysis and Reasoning Skills (CARS)

The *Critical Analysis and Reasoning Skills* (CARS) section of the MCAT tests three discrete families of textual reasoning skills; each of these families requires a higher level of reasoning than the last. Those three skills are as follows:

1. *Foundations of Comprehension* (30% of questions)
2. *Reasoning Within the Text* (30% of questions)
3. *Reasoning Beyond the Text* (40% of questions)

These three skills are tested through nine humanities- and social sciences-themed passages, with approximately 5 to 7 questions per passage. Let's take a more in-depth look into these three skills. Again, the bullet points of specific objectives for each of the CARS are taken directly from the *Official Guide to the MCAT Exam*; the descriptions of what these behaviors mean and sample question stems, however, are written by Kaplan.

Foundations of Comprehension

Questions in this skill will ask for basic facts and simple inferences about the passage; the questions themselves will be similar to those seen on reading comprehension sections of other standardized exams like the SAT® and ACT®. *Foundations of Comprehension* questions will require you to do the following:

- Understand the basic components of the text
- Infer meaning from rhetorical devices, word choice, and text structure

This admittedly covers a wide range of potential question types including Main Idea, Detail, Inference, and Definition-in-Context questions, but finding the correct answer to all *Foundations of Comprehension* questions will follow from a basic understanding of the passage and the point of view of its author (and occasionally that of other voices in the passage).

Here are some sample *Foundations of Comprehension* question stems:

- **Main Idea**—The author's primary purpose in this passage is:
- **Detail**—Based on the information in the second paragraph, which of the following is the most accurate summary of the opinion held by Schubert's critics?
- **(Scattered) Detail**—According to the passage, which of the following is FALSE about literary reviews in the 1920s?
- **Inference (Implication)**—Which of the following phrases, as used in the passage, is most suggestive that the author has a personal bias toward narrative records of history?
- **Inference (Assumption)**—In putting together the argument in the passage, the author most likely assumes:
- **Definition-in-Context**—The word "obscure" (paragraph 3), when used in reference to the historian's actions, most nearly means:

Reasoning Within the Text

While *Foundations of Comprehension* questions will usually depend on interpreting a single piece of information in the passage or understanding the passage as a whole, *Reasoning Within the Text* questions require more thought because they will ask you to identify the purpose of a particular piece of information in the context of the passage, or ask how one piece of information relates to another. *Reasoning Within the Text* questions will require you to:

- Integrate different components of the text to draw relevant conclusions

In other words, questions in this skill often ask either *How do these two details relate to one another?* or *What else must be true that the author didn't say?* The CARS section will also ask you to judge certain parts of the passage or even judge the author. These questions, which fall under the *Reasoning Within the Text* skill, can ask you to identify authorial bias, evaluate the credibility of cited sources, determine the logical soundness of an argument, identify the importance of a particular fact or statement in the context of the passage, or search for relevant evidence in the passage to support a given conclusion. In all, this category includes Function and Strengthen–Weaken (Within the Passage) questions, as well as a smattering of related—but rare—question types.

Here are some sample *Reasoning Within the Text* question stems:

- **Function**—The author's discussion of the effect of socioeconomic status on social mobility primarily serves which of the following functions?
- **Strengthen–Weaken (Within the Passage)**—Which of the following facts is used in the passage as the most prominent piece of evidence in favor of the author's conclusions?
- **Strengthen–Weaken (Within the Passage)**—Based on the role it plays in the author's argument, *The Possessed* can be considered:

Reasoning Beyond the Text

The distinguishing factor of *Reasoning Beyond the Text* questions is in the title of the skill: the word *Beyond*. Questions that test this skill, which make up a larger share of the CARS section than questions from either of the other two skills, will always introduce a completely new situation that was not present in the passage itself; these questions will ask you to determine how one influences the other. *Reasoning Beyond the Text* questions will require you to:

- Apply or extrapolate ideas from the passage to new contexts
- Assess the impact of introducing new factors, information, or conditions to ideas from the passage

The *Reasoning Beyond the Text* skill is further divided into Apply and Strengthen–Weaken (Beyond the Passage) questions, and a few other rarely appearing question types.

Here are some sample *Reasoning Beyond the Text* question stems:

- **Apply**—If a document were located that demonstrated Berlioz intended to include a chorus of at least 700 in his *Grande Messe des Morts*, how would the author likely respond?
- **Apply**—Which of the following is the best example of a "virtuous rebellion," as it is defined in the passage?
- **Strengthen–Weaken (Beyond the Passage)**—Suppose Jane Austen had written in a letter to her sister, "My strongest characters were those forced by circumstance to confront basic questions about the society in which they lived." What relevance would this have to the passage?
- **Strengthen–Weaken (Beyond the Passage)**—Which of the following sentences, if added to the end of the passage, would most WEAKEN the author's conclusions in the last paragraph?

CARS Summary

Through the *Foundations of Comprehension* skill, the CARS section tests many of the reading skills you have been building on since grade school, albeit in the context of very challenging doctorate-level passages. But through the two other skills (*Reasoning Within the Text* and *Reasoning Beyond the Text*), the MCAT demands that you understand the deep structure of passages and the arguments within them at a very advanced level. And, of course, all of this is tested under very tight timing restrictions: only 102 seconds per question—and that doesn't even include the time spent reading the passages.

Here's a quick reference guide to the three CARS skills:

Foundations of Comprehension questions ask:

- Did you understand the passage and its main ideas?
- What does the passage have to say about this particular detail?
- What must be true that the author did not say?

Reasoning Within the Text questions ask:

- What's the logical relationship between these two ideas from the passage?
- How well argued is the author's thesis?

Reasoning Beyond the Text questions ask:

- How does this principle from the passage apply to this new situation?
- How does this new piece of information influence the arguments in the passage?

Scoring

Each of the four sections of the MCAT is scored between 118 and 132, with the median at approximately 125. This means the total score ranges from 472 to 528, with the median at about 500. Why such peculiar numbers? The AAMC stresses that this scale emphasizes the importance of the central portion of the score distribution, where most students score (around 125 per section, or 500 total), rather than putting undue focus on the high end of the scale.

Note that there is no wrong answer penalty on the MCAT, so you should select an answer for every question—even if it is only a guess.

The AAMC has released the 2019–2021 correlation between scaled score and percentile, as shown on the following page. It should be noted that the percentile scale is adjusted and renormalized over time and thus can shift slightly from year to year. Percentile rank updates are released by the AAMC around May 1 of each year.

Total Score	Percentile	Total Score	Percentile
528	100	499	41
527	100	498	38
526	100	497	35
525	100	496	32
524	100	495	29
523	99	494	26
522	99	493	24
521	98	492	21
520	97	491	19
519	96	490	17
518	95	489	15
517	94	488	13
516	92	487	11
515	90	486	10
514	88	485	8
513	86	484	7
512	83	483	6
511	80	482	5
510	77	481	4
509	74	480	3
508	71	479	2
507	68	478	2
506	65	477	1
505	61	476	1
504	58	475	<1
503	55	474	<1
502	51	473	<1
501	48	472	<1
500	45		

Source: AAMC. 2022. Summary of MCAT Total and Section Scores. Accessed October 2022.
https://students-residents.aamc.org/mcat-research-and-data/percentile-ranks-mcat-exam

Further information on score reporting is included at the end of the next section (see *After Your Test*).

MCAT Policies and Procedures

We strongly encourage you to download the latest copy of *MCAT® Essentials*, available on the AAMC's website, to ensure that you have the latest information about registration and Test Day policies and procedures; this document is updated annually. A brief summary of some of the most important rules is provided here.

MCAT Registration

The only way to register for the MCAT is online. You can access AAMC's registration system at **www.aamc.org/mcat**.

The AAMC posts the schedule of testing, registration, and score release dates in the fall before the MCAT testing year, which runs from January into September. Registration for January through June is available earlier than registration for later dates, but see the AAMC's website for the exact dates each year. There is one standard registration fee, but the fee for changing your test date or test center increases the closer you get to your MCAT.

Fees and the Fee Assistance Program (FAP)

Payment for test registration must be made by MasterCard or VISA. As described earlier, the fee for rescheduling your exam or changing your testing center increases as one approaches Test Day. In addition, it is not uncommon for test centers to fill up well in advance of the registration deadline. For these reasons, we recommend identifying your preferred Test Day as soon as possible and registering. There are ancillary benefits to having a set Test Day, as well: when you know the date you're working toward, you'll study harder and are less likely to keep pushing back the exam. The AAMC offers a Fee Assistance Program (FAP) for students with financial hardship to help reduce the cost of taking the MCAT, as well as for the American Medical College Application Service (AMCAS®) application. Further information on the FAP can be found at **www.aamc.org/students/applying/fap**.

Testing Security

On Test Day, you will be required to present a qualifying form of ID. Generally, a current driver's license or United States passport will be sufficient (consult the AAMC website for the full list of qualifying criteria). When registering, take care to spell your first and last names (middle names, suffixes, and prefixes are not required and will not be verified on Test Day) precisely the same as they appear on this ID; failure to provide this ID at the test center or differences in spelling between your registration and ID will be considered a "no-show," and you will not receive a refund for the exam.

During Test Day registration, other identity data collected may include: a digital palm vein scan, a Test Day photo, a digitization of your valid ID, and signatures. Some testing centers may use a metal detection wand to ensure that no prohibited items are brought into the testing room. Prohibited items include all electronic devices, including watches and timers, calculators, cell phones, and any and all forms of recording equipment; food, drinks (including water), and cigarettes or other smoking paraphernalia; hats and scarves (except for religious purposes); and books, notes, or other study materials. If you require a medical device, such as an insulin pump or pacemaker, you must apply for accommodated testing. During breaks, you are allowed access to food and drink, but not to electronic devices, including cell phones.

Testing centers are under video surveillance and the AAMC does not take potential violations of testing security lightly. The bottom line: *know the rules and don't break them.*

Accommodations

Students with disabilities or medical conditions can apply for accommodated testing. Documentation of the disability or condition is required, and requests may take two months—or more—to be approved. For this reason, it is recommended that you begin the process of applying for accommodated testing as early as possible. More information on applying for accommodated testing can be found at **www.aamc.org/students/applying/mcat/accommodations**.

After Your Test

When your MCAT is all over, no matter how you feel you did, be good to yourself when you leave the test center. Celebrate! Take a nap. Watch a movie. Get some exercise. Plan a trip or outing. Call up all of your neglected friends or message them on social media. Go out for snacks or drinks with people you like. Whatever you do, make sure that it has absolutely nothing to do with thinking too hard—you deserve some rest and relaxation.

Perhaps most importantly, do not discuss specific details about the test with anyone. For one, it is important to let go of the stress of Test Day, and reliving your exam only inhibits you from being able to do so. But more significantly, the Examinee Agreement you sign at the beginning of your exam specifically prohibits you from discussing or disclosing exam content. The AAMC is known to seek out individuals who violate this agreement and retains the right to prosecute these individuals at their discretion. This means that you should not, under any circumstances, discuss the exam in person or over the phone with other individuals—including us at Kaplan—or post information or questions about exam content to Facebook, Student Doctor Network, or other online social media. You are permitted to comment on your "general exam experience," including how you felt about the exam overall or an individual section, but this is a fine line. In summary: *if you're not certain whether you can discuss an aspect of the test or not, just don't do it!* Do not let a silly Facebook post stop you from becoming the doctor you deserve to be.

Scores are typically released approximately one month after Test Day. The release is staggered during the afternoon and evening, ending at 5 p.m. Eastern Standard Time. This means that not all examinees receive their scores at exactly the same time. Your score report will include a scaled score for each section between 118 and 132, as well as your total combined score between 472 and 528. These scores are given as confidence intervals. For each section, the confidence interval is approximately the given score ± 1; for the total score, it is approximately the given score ± 2. You will also be given the corresponding percentile rank for each of these section scores and the total score.

AAMC Contact Information

For further questions, contact the MCAT team at the Association of American Medical Colleges:

MCAT Resource Center
Association of American Medical Colleges
www.aamc.org/mcat
(202) 828-0600
www.aamc.org/contactmcat

HOW THIS BOOK WAS CREATED

The *Kaplan MCAT Review* project began shortly after the release of the *Preview Guide for the MCAT 2015 Exam*, 2nd edition. Through thorough analysis by our staff psychometricians, we were able to analyze the relative yield of the different topics on the MCAT, and we began constructing tables of contents for the books of the *Kaplan MCAT Review* series. A dedicated staff of 30 writers, 7 editors, and 32 proofreaders worked over 5,000 combined hours to produce these books. The format of the books was heavily influenced by weekly meetings with Kaplan's learning science team.

In the years since this book was created, a number of opportunities for expansion and improvement have occurred. The current edition represents the culmination of the wisdom accumulated during that time frame, and it also includes several new features designed to improve the reading and learning experience in these texts.

These books were submitted for publication in April 2023. For any updates after this date, please visit www.kaptest.com/retail-book-corrections-and-updates.

If you have any questions about the content presented here, email KaplanMCATfeedback@kaplan.com. For other questions not related to content, email booksupport@kaplan.com.

Each book has been vetted through at least ten rounds of review. To that end, the information presented in these books is true and accurate to the best of our knowledge. Still, your feedback helps us improve our prep materials. Please notify us of any inaccuracies or errors in the books by sending an email to KaplanMCATfeedback@kaplan.com.

USING THIS BOOK

Kaplan MCAT Behavioral Sciences Review, and the other six books in the *Kaplan MCAT Review* series, bring the Kaplan classroom experience to you—right in your home, at your convenience. This book offers the same Kaplan content review, strategies, and practice that make Kaplan the #1 choice for MCAT prep.

This book is designed to help you review the behavioral sciences topics covered on the MCAT. Please understand that content review—no matter how thorough—is not sufficient preparation for the MCAT! The MCAT tests not only your science knowledge but also your critical reading, reasoning, and problem-solving skills. Do not assume that simply memorizing the contents of this book will earn you high scores on Test Day; to maximize your scores, you must also improve your reading and test-taking skills through MCAT-style questions and practice tests.

Learning Objectives

At the beginning of each section, you'll find a short list of objectives describing the skills covered within that section. Learning objectives for these texts were developed in conjunction with Kaplan's learning science team, and have been designed specifically to focus your attention on tasks and concepts that are likely to show up on your MCAT. These learning objectives will function as a means to guide your study, and indicate what information and relationships you should be focused on within each section. Before starting each section, read these learning objectives carefully. They will not only allow you to assess your existing familiarity with the content, but also provide a goal-oriented focus for your studying experience of the section.

MCAT Concept Checks

At the end of each section, you'll find a few open-ended questions that you can use to assess your mastery of the material. These MCAT Concept Checks were introduced after numerous conversations with Kaplan's learning science team. Research has demonstrated repeatedly that introspection and self-analysis improve mastery, retention, and recall of material. Complete these MCAT Concept Checks to ensure that you've got the key points from each section before moving on!

Science Mastery Assessments

At the beginning of each chapter, you'll find 15 MCAT-style practice questions. These are designed to help you assess your understanding of the chapter before you begin reading the chapter. Using the guidance provided with the assessment, you can determine the best way to review each chapter based on your personal strengths and weaknesses. Most of the questions in the Science Mastery Assessments focus on the first of the *Scientific Inquiry and Reasoning Skills* (*Knowledge of Scientific Concepts and Principles*), although there are occasional questions that fall into the second or fourth SIRS (*Scientific Reasoning and Problem-Solving* and *Data-Based and Statistical Reasoning*, respectively). You can complete each chapter's assessment in a testing interface in your online resources, where you'll also find a test-like passage set covering the same content you just studied to ensure you can also apply your knowledge the way the MCAT will expect you to!

Guided Examples with Expert Thinking

Embedded in each chapter of this book is a Guided Example with Expert Thinking. Each of these guided examples will be located in the same section as the content used in that example. Each example will feature an MCAT-level scientific article, that simulates an MCAT experiment passage. Read through the passage as you would on the real MCAT, referring to the Expert Thinking material to the right of the passage to clarify the key information you should be gathering from each paragraph. Read and attempt to answer the associated question once you have worked through the passage. There is a full explanation, including the correct answer, following the given question. These passages and questions are designed to help build your critical thinking, experimental reasoning, and data interpretation skills as preparation for the challenges you will face on the MCAT.

Sidebars

The following is a guide to the five types of sidebars you'll find in *Kaplan MCAT Behavioral Sciences Review:*

- **Bridge:** These sidebars create connections between science topics that appear in multiple chapters throughout the *Kaplan MCAT Review* series.
- **Key Concept:** These sidebars draw attention to the most important takeaways in a given topic, and they sometimes offer synopses or overviews of complex information. If you understand nothing else, make sure you grasp the Key Concepts for any given subject.
- **MCAT Expertise:** These sidebars point out how information may be tested on the MCAT or offer key strategy points and test-taking tips that you should apply on Test Day.
- **Mnemonic:** These sidebars present memory devices to help recall certain facts.
- **Real World:** These sidebars illustrate how a concept in the text relates to the practice of medicine or the world at large. While this is not information you need to know for Test Day, many of the topics in Real World sidebars are excellent examples of how a concept may appear in a passage or discrete (stand-alone) question on the MCAT.

What This Book Covers

The information presented in the *Kaplan MCAT Review* series covers everything listed on the official MCAT content lists. Every topic in these lists is covered in the same level of detail as is common to the undergraduate and postbaccalaureate classes that are considered prerequisites for the MCAT. Note that your premedical classes may include topics not discussed in these books, or they may go into more depth than these books do. Additional exposure to science content is never a bad thing, but all of the content knowledge you are expected to have walking in on Test Day is covered in these books.

Chapter profiles, on the first page of each chapter, represent a holistic look at the content within the chapter, and will include a pie chart as well as text information. The pie chart analysis is based directly on data released by the AAMC, and will give a rough estimate of the importance of the chapter in relation to the book as a whole. Further, the text portion of the Chapter Profiles includes which AAMC content categories are covered within the chapter. These are referenced directly from the AAMC MCAT exam content listing, available on the testmaker's website.

You'll also see new High-Yield badges scattered throughout the sections of this book:

In This Chapter

1.1 Amino Acids Found in Proteins

High-Yield

LEARNING OBJECTIVES

After Chapter 1.1, you will be able to:

These badges represent the top 100 topics most tested by the AAMC. In other words, according to the testmaker and all our experience with their resources, a High-Yield badge means more questions on Test Day.

This book also contains a thorough glossary and index for easy navigation of the text.

In the end, this is your book, so write in the margins, draw diagrams, highlight the key points—do whatever is necessary to help you get that higher score. We look forward to working with you as you achieve your dreams and become the doctor you deserve to be!

Studying with This Book

In addition to providing you with the best practice questions and test strategies, Kaplan's team of learning scientists are dedicated to researching and testing the best methods for getting the most out of your study time. Here are their top four tips for improving retention:

Review multiple topics in one study session. This may seem counterintuitive—we're used to practicing one skill at a time in order to improve each skill. But research shows that weaving topics together leads to increased learning. Beyond that consideration, the MCAT often includes more than one topic in a single question. Studying in an integrated manner is the most effective way to prepare for this test.

Customize the content. Drawing attention to difficult or critical content can ensure you don't overlook it as you read and re-read sections. The best way to do this is to make it more visual—highlight, make tabs, use stickies, whatever works. We recommend highlighting only the most important or difficult sections of text. Selective highlighting of up to about 10 percent of text in a given chapter is great for emphasizing parts of the text, but over-highlighting can have the opposite effect.

Repeat topics over time. Many people try to memorize concepts by repeating them over and over again in succession. Our research shows that retention is improved by spacing out the repeats over time and mixing up the order in which you study content. For example, try reading chapters in a different order the second (or third!) time around. Revisit practice questions that you answered incorrectly in a new sequence. Perhaps information you reviewed more recently will help you better understand those questions and solutions you struggled with in the past.

Take a moment to reflect. When you finish reading a section for the first time, stop and think about what you just read. Jot down a few thoughts in the margins or in your notes about why the content is important or what topics came to mind when you read it. Associating learning with a memory is a fantastic way to retain information! This also works when answering questions. After answering a question, take a moment to think through each step you took to arrive at a solution. What led you to the answer you chose? Understanding the steps you took will help you make good decisions when answering future questions.

Online Resources

In addition to the resources located within this text, you also have additional online resources awaiting you at **www.kaptest.com/booksonline**. Make sure to log on and take advantage of free practice and other resources!

Please note that access to the online resources is limited to the original owner of this book.

STUDYING FOR THE MCAT

The first year of medical school is a frenzied experience for most students. To meet the requirements of a rigorous work schedule, students either learn to prioritize their time or else fall hopelessly behind. It's no surprise, then, that the MCAT, the test specifically designed to predict success in medical school, is a high-speed, time-intensive test. The MCAT demands excellent time-management skills, endurance, and grace under pressure both during the test as well as while preparing for it. Having a solid plan of attack and sticking with it are key to giving you the confidence and structure you need to succeed.

Creating a Study Plan

The best time to create a study plan is at the beginning of your MCAT preparation. If you don't already use a calendar, you will want to start. You can purchase a planner, print out a free calendar from the Internet, use a built-in calendar or app on one of your smart devices, or keep track using an interactive online calendar. Pick the option that is most practical for you and that you are most likely to use consistently.

Once you have a calendar, you'll be able to start planning your study schedule with the following steps:

1. **Fill in your obligations and choose a day off.**

   Write in all your school, extracurricular, and work obligations first: class sessions, work shifts, and meetings that you must attend. Then add in your personal obligations: appointments, lunch dates, family and social time, etc. Making an appointment in your calendar for hanging out with friends or going to the movies may seem strange at first, but planning social activities in advance will help you achieve a balance between personal and professional obligations even as life gets busy. Having a happy balance allows you to be more focused and productive when it comes time to study, so stay well-rounded and don't neglect anything that is important to you.

   In addition to scheduling your personal and professional obligations, you should also plan your time off. Taking some time off is just as important as studying. Kaplan recommends taking at least one full day off per week, ideally from all your study obligations but at minimum from studying for the MCAT.

2. **Add in study blocks around your obligations.**

   Once you have established your calendar's framework, add in study blocks around your obligations, keeping your study schedule as consistent as possible across days and across weeks. Studying at the same time of day as your official test is ideal for promoting recall, but if that's not possible, then fit in study blocks wherever you can.

   To make your studying as efficient as possible, block out short, frequent periods of study time throughout the week. From a learning perspective, studying one hour per day for six days per week is much more valuable than studying for six hours all at once one day per week. Specifically, Kaplan recommends studying for no longer than three hours in one sitting. Within those three-hour blocks, also plan to take ten-minute breaks every hour. Use these breaks to get up from your seat, do some quick stretches, get a snack and drink, and clear your mind. Although ten minutes of break for every 50 minutes of studying may sound like a lot, these breaks will allow you to deal with distractions and rest your brain so that, during the 50-minute study blocks, you can remain fully engaged and completely focused.

3. **Add in your full-length practice tests.**

   Next, you'll want to add in full-length practice tests. You'll want to take one test very early in your prep and then spread your remaining full-length practice tests evenly between now and your test date. Staggering tests in this way allows you to form a baseline for comparison and to determine which areas to focus on right away, while also providing realistic feedback throughout your prep as to how you will perform on Test Day.

When planning your calendar, aim to finish your full-length practice tests and the majority of your studying by one week before Test Day, which will allow you to spend that final week completing a final review of what you already know. In your online resources, you'll find sample study calendars for several different Test Day timelines to use as a starting point. The sample calendars may include more focus than you need in some areas, and less in others, and it may not fit your timeline to Test Day. You will need to customize your study calendar to your needs using the steps above.

The total amount of time you spend studying each week will depend on your schedule, your personal prep needs, and your time to Test Day, but it is recommended that you spend somewhere in the range of 300–350 hours preparing before taking the official MCAT. One way you could break this down is to study for three hours per day, six days per week, for four months, but this is just one approach. You might study six days per week for more than three hours per day. You might study over a longer period of time if you don't have much time to study each week. No matter what your plan is, ensure you complete enough practice to feel completely comfortable with the MCAT and its content. A good sign you're ready for Test Day is when you begin to earn your goal score consistently in practice.

How to Study

The MCAT covers a large amount of material, so studying for Test Day can initially seem daunting. To combat this, we have some tips for how to take control of your studying and make the most of your time.

Goal Setting

To take control of the amount of content and practice required to do well on the MCAT, break the content down into specific goals for each week instead of attempting to approach the test as a whole. A goal of "I want to increase my overall score by 5 points" is too big, abstract, and difficult to measure on the small scale. More reasonable goals are "I will read two chapters each day this week." Goals like this are much less overwhelming and help break studying into manageable pieces.

Active Reading

As you go through this book, much of the information will be familiar to you. After all, you have probably seen most of the content before. However, be very careful: Familiarity with a subject does not necessarily translate to knowledge or mastery of that subject. Do not assume that if you recognize a concept you actually know it and can apply it quickly at an appropriate level. Don't just passively read this book. Instead, read actively: Use the free margin space to jot down important ideas, draw diagrams, and make charts as you read. Highlighting can be an excellent tool, but use it sparingly: highlighting every sentence isn't active reading, it's coloring. Frequently stop and ask yourself questions while you read (e.g., *What is the main point? How does this fit into the overall scheme of things? Could I thoroughly explain this to someone else?*). By making connections and focusing on the grander scheme, not only will you ensure you know the essential content, but you also prepare yourself for the level of critical thinking required by the MCAT.

Focus on Areas of Greatest Opportunity

If you are limited by only having a minimal amount of time to prepare before Test Day, focus on your biggest areas of opportunity first. Areas of opportunity are topic areas that are highly tested and that you have not yet mastered. You likely won't have time to take detailed notes for every page of these books; instead, use your results from practice materials to determine

which areas are your biggest opportunities and seek those out. After you've taken a full-length test, make sure you are using your performance report to best identify areas of opportunity. Skim over content matter for which you are already demonstrating proficiency, pausing to read more thoroughly when something looks unfamiliar or particularly difficult. Begin with the Science Mastery Assessment at the beginning of each chapter. If you can get all of those questions correct within a reasonable amount of time, you may be able to quickly skim through that chapter, but if the questions prove to be more difficult, then you may need to spend time reading the chapter or certain subsections of the chapter more thoroughly.

Practice, Review, and Tracking

Leave time to review your practice questions and full-length tests. You may be tempted, after practicing, to push ahead and cover new material as quickly as possible, but failing to schedule ample time for review will actually throw away your greatest opportunity to improve your performance. The brain rarely remembers anything it sees or does only once. When you carefully review the questions you've solved (and the explanations for them), the process of retrieving that information reopens and reinforces the connections you've built in your brain. This builds long-term retention and repeatable skill sets—exactly what you need to beat the MCAT!

One useful tool for making the most of your review is the How I'll Fix It (HIFI) sheet. You can create a HIFI sheet, such as the sample below, to track questions throughout your prep that you miss or have to guess on. For each such question, figure out why you missed it and supply at least one action step for how you can avoid similar mistakes in the future. As you move through your MCAT prep, adjust your study plan based on your available study time and the results of your review. Your strengths and weaknesses are likely to change over the course of your prep. Keep addressing the areas that are most important to your score, shifting your focus as those areas change. For more help with making the most of your full-length tests, including a How I'll Fix It sheet template, make sure to check out the videos and resources in your online syllabus.

Section	Q #	Type/Topic	Why I missed it	How I'll fix it
Chem/Phys	*42*	*Nuclear chem.*	*Confused electron absorption and emission*	*Reread Physics Chapter 9.2*
Chem/Phys	*47*	K_{eq}	*Didn't know right equation*	*Memorize equation for* K_{eq}
CARS	*2*	*Detail*	*Didn't read "not" in answer choice*	*Slow down when finding match*
CARS	*4*	*Inference*	*Forgot to research answer*	*Reread passage and predict first*

Where to Study

One often-overlooked aspect of studying is the environment where the learning actually occurs. Although studying at home is many students' first choice, several problems can arise in this environment, chief of which are distractions. Studying can be a mentally draining process, so as time passes, these distractions become ever more tempting as escape routes. Although you may have considerable willpower, there's no reason to make staying focused harder than it needs to be. Instead of studying at home, head to a library, quiet coffee shop, or another new location whenever possible. This will eliminate many of the usual distractions and also promote efficient studying; instead of studying off and on at home over the course of an entire day, you can stay at the library for three hours of effective studying and enjoy the rest of the day off from the MCAT.

No matter where you study, make your practice as much like Test Day as possible. Just as is required during the official test, don't have snacks or chew gum during your study blocks. Turn off your music, television, and phone. Practice on the computer with your online resources to simulate the computer-based test environment. When completing practice questions, do your work on scratch paper or noteboard sheets rather than writing directly on any printed materials since you won't have that option on Test Day. Because memory is tied to all of your senses, the more test-like you can make your studying environment, the easier it will be on Test Day to recall the information you're putting in so much work to learn.

CHAPTER 1

BIOLOGY AND BEHAVIOR

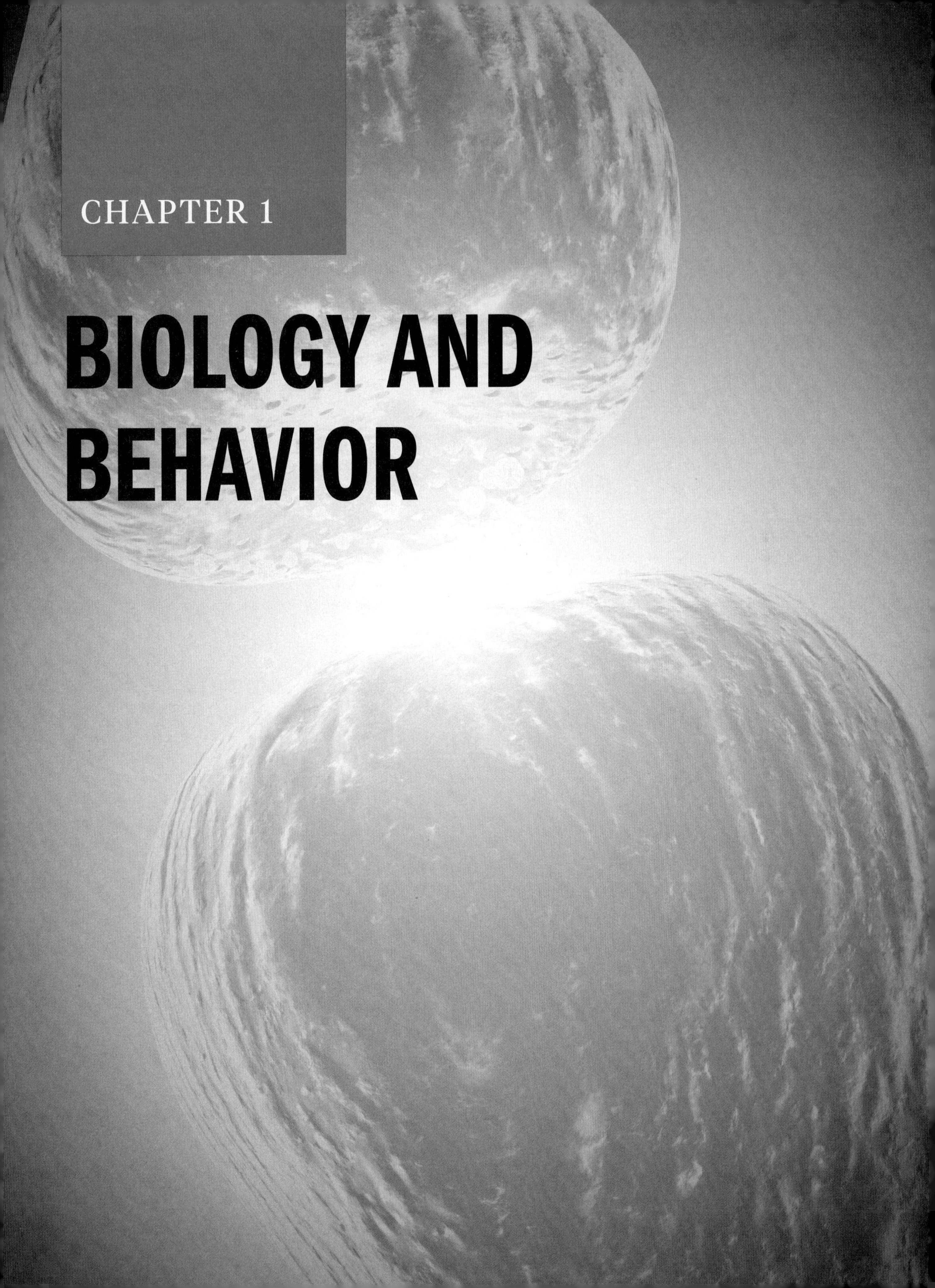

SCIENCE MASTERY ASSESSMENT

Every pre-med knows this feeling: there is so much content I have to know for the MCAT! How do I know what to do first or what's important?

While the high-yield badges throughout this book will help you identify the most important topics, this Science Mastery Assessment is another tool in your MCAT prep arsenal. This quiz (which can also be taken in your online resources) and the guidance below will help ensure that you are spending the appropriate amount of time on this chapter based on your personal strengths and weaknesses. Don't worry though—skipping something now does not mean you'll never study it. Later on in your prep, as you complete full-length tests, you'll uncover specific pieces of content that you need to review and can come back to these chapters as appropriate.

How to Use This Assessment

If you answer 0–7 questions correctly:

Spend about 1 hour to read this chapter in full and take limited notes throughout. Follow up by reviewing **all** quiz questions to ensure that you now understand how to solve each one.

If you answer 8–11 questions correctly:

Spend 20–40 minutes reviewing the quiz questions. Beginning with the questions you missed, read and take notes on the corresponding subchapters. For questions you answered correctly, ensure your thinking matches that of the explanation and you understand why each choice was correct or incorrect.

If you answer 12–15 questions correctly:

Spend less than 20 minutes reviewing all questions from the quiz. If you missed any, then include a quick read-through of the corresponding subchapters, or even just the relevant content within a subchapter, as part of your question review. For questions you answered correctly, ensure your thinking matches that of the explanation and review the Concept Summary at the end of the chapter.

1. A researcher deletes a gene from an organism to determine the gene's function. This approach is most analogous to the work of which of the following scientists?
   - **A.** Paul Broca
   - **B.** Pierre Flourens
   - **C.** Franz Gall
   - **D.** Sir Charles Sherrington

2. Which component of the nervous system is NOT involved in the initial reflexive response to pain?
   - **A.** Spinal cord
   - **B.** Cerebral cortex
   - **C.** Interneuron
   - **D.** Motor neuron

3. A child has experienced nervous system damage and can no longer coordinate the movements to dribble a basketball, although the child can still walk in an uncoordinated fashion. Which region of the central nervous system was most likely affected?
   - **A.** Forebrain
   - **B.** Midbrain
   - **C.** Hindbrain
   - **D.** Spinal cord

4. The temporal lobe deals with all of the following EXCEPT:
   - **A.** language comprehension.
   - **B.** memory.
   - **C.** emotion.
   - **D.** motor skills.

5. Which part of the brain deals with both homeostasis and emotions?
   - **A.** Cerebellum
   - **B.** Pons
   - **C.** Hypothalamus
   - **D.** Thalamus

6. Which of the following activities would most likely be completed by the right hemisphere of a left-handed person?
   - **A.** Finding a car in a parking lot
   - **B.** Learning a new language
   - **C.** Reading a book for pleasure
   - **D.** Jumping rope with friends

7. Which of the following is/are true with regard to neurulation?
   - **I.** The neural tube differentiates from endoderm.
   - **II.** The neural tube becomes the peripheral nervous system.
   - **III.** Neural crest cells migrate from their original site.

   - **A.** I only
   - **B.** III only
   - **C.** II and III only
   - **D.** I, II, and III

8. Which of the following neurotransmitters is NOT classified as a catecholamine?
   - **A.** Epinephrine
   - **B.** Norepinephrine
   - **C.** Dopamine
   - **D.** Acetylcholine

9. If the amount of acetylcholinesterase, an enzyme that breaks down acetylcholine, is increased, which of the following would likely be the result?
   - **A.** Weakness of muscle movements
   - **B.** Excessive pain or discomfort
   - **C.** Mood swings and mood instability
   - **D.** Auditory and visual hallucinations

10. The adrenal glands do all of the following EXCEPT:
    - **A.** promote the fight-or-flight response via estrogen.
    - **B.** produce stress responses via cortisol.
    - **C.** produce both hormones and neurotransmitters.
    - **D.** release estrogen in males and testosterone in females.

11. A disorder of the pineal gland would most likely result in which of the following disorders?
    - **A.** High blood pressure
    - **B.** Diabetes
    - **C.** Insomnia
    - **D.** Hyperthyroidism

12. Which of the following conclusions would William James most likely support?
    - **A.** Mental processes help individuals adapt to their environments.
    - **B.** Psychological attributes could be measured by feeling the skull.
    - **C.** Specific functional impairments can be linked to specific lesions in the brain.
    - **D.** Synaptic transmission is an electrical process.

13. A scientist designs a study to determine if different regions of the brain are activated when a person speaks their native language vs. a second language. Which of the following methods would the scientist most likely choose?
    - **A.** MRI
    - **B.** CT scan
    - **C.** fMRI
    - **D.** EEG

14. During a physical examination, a physician brushes the bottom of the foot of a patient who is fifty years old with multiple sclerosis. The patient's toes are observed to curl toward the bottom of the foot, with no fanning of the toes. This response is:
    - **A.** abnormal, and evidence that the patient is exhibiting a primitive reflex.
    - **B.** normal, and evidence that the patient is exhibiting a primitive reflex.
    - **C.** abnormal, and evidence that the patient is not exhibiting a primitive reflex.
    - **D.** normal, and evidence that the patient is not exhibiting a primitive reflex.

15. Which of the following fine motor tasks would one expect to see first in an infant?
    - **A.** Grasping for objects with two fingers
    - **B.** Following objects with the eyes
    - **C.** Scribbling with a crayon
    - **D.** Moving a toy from one hand to the other

Answer Key

1. **B**
2. **B**
3. **C**
4. **D**
5. **C**
6. **A**
7. **B**
8. **D**
9. **A**
10. **A**
11. **C**
12. **A**
13. **C**
14. **D**
15. **B**

Detailed explanations can be found at the end of the chapter.

CHAPTER 1

BIOLOGY AND BEHAVIOR

In This Chapter

CHAPTER PROFILE

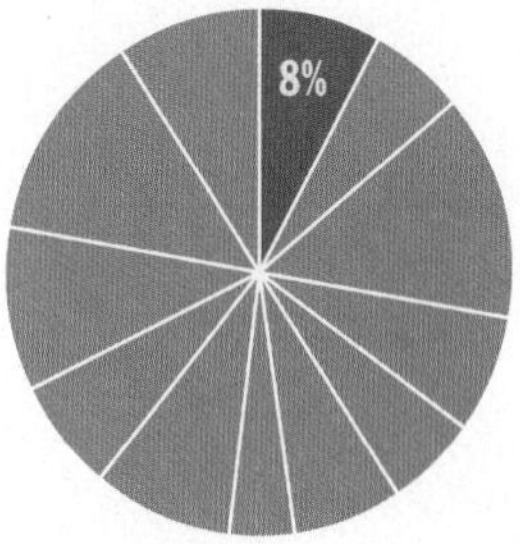

The content in this chapter should be relevant to about 8% of all questions about the behavioral sciences on the MCAT.

This chapter covers material from the following AAMC content categories:

3A: Structure and functions of the nervous and endocrine systems and ways in which these systems coordinate the organ systems

7A: Individual influences on behavior

Introduction

When you woke up this morning and got ready to start reading *MCAT Behavioral Sciences Review*, you almost certainly had specific feelings about it—perhaps you were excited to crack open the book and start learning some of the material that will get you that top score on the MCAT; perhaps you dreaded the size and rich detail of the information in the book. Either way, your body began to respond to these impulses from your mind: increasing heart rate, increasing breathing rate, dilating the eyes, and slowing down digestion. This link between the mind and the body is still a hot topic in medicine, although we've been exploring the effects of psychology on well-being for almost two centuries now.

In this chapter, we'll begin our exploration of psychology and sociology by looking at the biological side of psychology. After a quick survey of the history of neuropsychology, we'll look at the structure and organization of the human nervous system, communication between the nervous and endocrine systems, the effects of genes and environment on behavior, and some aspects of psychological development.

1.1 A Brief History of Neuropsychology

LEARNING OBJECTIVES

After Chapter 1.1, you will be able to:

- Recall the major contributions to early neuropsychology
- Connect the major contributors of early neuropsychology to their contributions

Researchers in the 19th century began to think about behavior from a physiological perspective. Many of these early thinkers formed the foundation of current knowledge about neuroanatomy, linking the functions of specific areas of the brain with thought and behavior.

Franz Gall (1758–1828) had one of the earliest theories that behavior, intellect, and even personality might be linked to brain anatomy. He developed the doctrine of phrenology. The basic idea was that if a particular trait was well-developed, then the part of the brain responsible for that trait would expand. This expansion, according to Gall, would push the area of the skull that covered that part of the brain outward and therefore cause a bulge on the head. Gall believed that one could thus measure psychological attributes by feeling or measuring the skull. Although phrenology was shown to be false, it did generate serious research on brain functions and was the impetus for the work of other psychologists through the remainder of the 19th century.

Pierre Flourens (1794–1867) was the first person to study the functions of the major sections of the brain. He did this by **extirpation**, also known as **ablation**, on rabbits and pigeons. In extirpation, various parts of the brain are surgically removed and the behavioral consequences are observed. Flourens's work led to his assertion that specific parts of the brain had specific functions, and that the removal of one part weakens the whole brain.

William James (1842–1910), known as the founder of American psychology, studied how the mind adapts to the environment. His views formed the foundation for the system of thought in psychology known as **functionalism**, which studies how mental processes help individuals adapt to their environments.

John Dewey (1859–1952) is another important name in functionalism because his 1896 article is seen as its inception. This article criticized the concept of the reflex arc, which breaks the process of reacting to a stimulus into discrete parts. Dewey believed that psychology should focus on the study of the organism as a whole as it functioned to adapt to the environment.

Around 1860, **Paul Broca** (1824–1880) added to the knowledge of physiology by examining the behavioral deficits of people with brain damage. He was the first person to demonstrate that specific functional impairments could be linked with specific brain lesions. Broca studied a person who was unable to speak and discovered that the person's disability was due to a lesion in a specific area on the left side of the person's brain. This area of the brain is now referred to as Broca's area.

Hermann von Helmholtz (1821–1894) was the first to measure the speed of a nerve impulse. He also related the measured speed of such impulses to reaction time, providing an important early link between behavior and underlying nervous system activity. Because Helmholtz provided one of the earliest measurable links between psychology and physiology, he is often credited with the transition of psychology out of the realm of philosophy and into the realm of quantifiable natural science.

Around the turn of the century, **Sir Charles Sherrington** (1857–1952) first inferred the existence of synapses. Many of his conclusions have held over time—except for one. He thought that synaptic transmission was an electrical process, but we now know that it is primarily a chemical process.

MCAT CONCEPT CHECK 1.1

Before you move on, assess your understanding of the material with this question.

1. Briefly list the main contributions of each of the following scientists to neuropsychology.
   - Franz Gall:

   - Pierre Flourens:

   - William James:

   - John Dewey:

   - Paul Broca:

   - Hermann von Helmholtz:

   - Sir Charles Sherrington:

BRIDGE

Solutions to concept checks for a given chapter in *MCAT Behavioral Sciences Review* can be found near the end of the chapter in which the concept check is located, following the Concept Summary for that chapter.

1.2 Organization of the Human Nervous System

High-Yield

MCAT EXPERTISE

The "High-Yield" badge on this section indicates that the content is frequently tested on the MCAT.

LEARNING OBJECTIVES

After Chapter 1.2, you will be able to:

- Correctly associate regions of the nervous system with the CNS or PNS
- Distinguish between afferent and efferent neurons
- Describe the functions of the somatic and autonomic nervous systems, as well as the sympathetic and parasympathetic nervous systems:

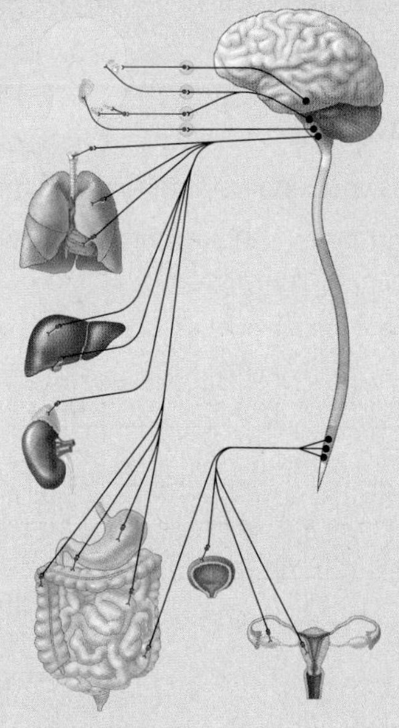

The human nervous system is a complex web of over 100 billion cells that communicate, coordinate, and regulate signals for the rest of the body. Mental and physical action occurs when the body can react to external stimuli using the nervous system. In this section, we will look at the nervous system and its basic organization.

Note: Much of the information contained in this section is also discussed in Chapter 4 of MCAT Biology Review.

Central and Peripheral Nervous Systems

MNEMONIC

Afferent neurons **a**scend in the cord toward the brain; **e**fferent neurons **e**xit the cord on their way to the rest of the body.

There are three kinds of nerve cells in the nervous system: sensory neurons, motor neurons, and interneurons. **Sensory neurons** (also known as **afferent neurons**) transmit sensory information from receptors to the spinal cord and brain. **Motor neurons** (also known as **efferent neurons**) transmit motor information from the brain and spinal cord to muscles and glands. **Interneurons** are found between other neurons and are the most numerous of the three types of neurons. Interneurons are located predominantly in the brain and spinal cord and are often linked to reflexive behavior. Neural circuits called **reflex arcs** control this type of reflexive behavior. For example, consider what occurs when someone steps on a nail. Receptors in the foot detect pain and the pain signal is transmitted by sensory neurons up to the spinal cord. At that point, the sensory neurons connect with interneurons, which then relay pain impulses up to the brain. However, rather than waiting for the brain to send out a signal, interneurons in the spinal cord send signals to the muscles of both legs directly, causing the individual to reflexively withdraw the foot in pain while simultaneously reflexively transferring weight to the other foot. The original sensory information still makes its way up to the brain; however, by that time, the muscles have already responded to the pain, thanks to the cooperation of these several reflex arcs.

Let's turn to the overall structure of the human nervous system, which is diagrammed in Figure 1.1. The nervous system can be broadly divided into two primary components: the central and peripheral nervous systems. The **central nervous system** (**CNS**) is composed of the brain and spinal cord. The **peripheral nervous system** (**PNS**), in contrast, is made up of nerve tissue and fibers outside the brain and spinal cord. Note that the peripheral nervous system includes all 31 pairs of nerves emanating from the spinal cord, which are called **spinal nerves**, and 12 pairs of nerves emanating directly from the brain, called **cranial nerves**. The olfactory and optic nerves (cranial nerves I and II) are structurally outgrowths of the central nervous system, but are still considered components of the peripheral nervous system. The PNS thus connects the CNS to the rest of the body.

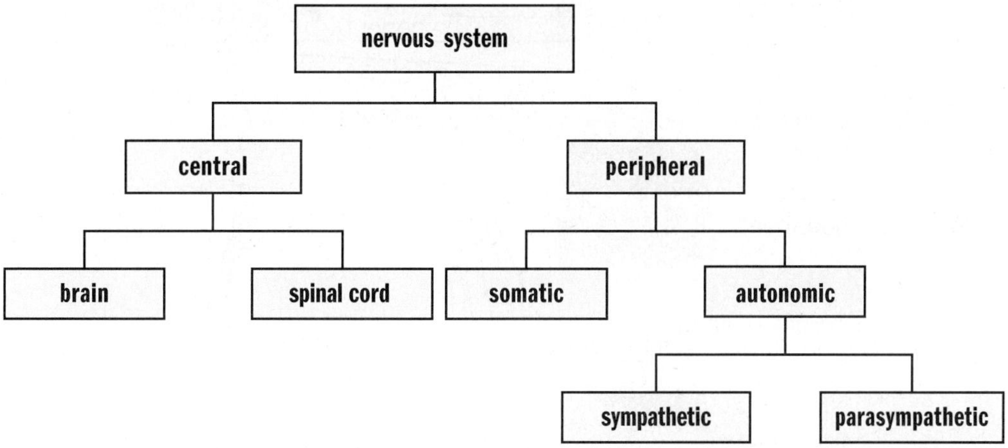

Figure 1.1 Major Divisions of the Nervous System

The peripheral nervous system is further subdivided into the somatic and autonomic nervous systems. The **somatic nervous system** consists of sensory and motor neurons distributed throughout the skin, joints, and muscles. Sensory neurons transmit information toward the CNS through afferent fibers. Motor impulses, in contrast, travel from the CNS back to the body along efferent fibers.

The **autonomic nervous system** (**ANS**) generally regulates heartbeat, respiration, digestion, and glandular secretions. In other words, the ANS manages the involuntary muscles associated with many internal organs and glands. The ANS also helps regulate body temperature by activating sweating or piloerection, depending on whether the body is too hot or too cold. The main thing to understand about all of these functions is that they are automatic, or independent of conscious control. Note the similarity between the words autonomic and automatic. This association makes it easy to remember that the autonomic nervous system manages automatic functions such as heartbeat, respiration, digestion, and temperature control.

The Autonomic Nervous System

The ANS has two subdivisions: the sympathetic nervous system and the parasympathetic nervous system. These two branches often act in opposition to one another, meaning they are antagonistic. For example, the sympathetic nervous system acts to accelerate heart rate and inhibit digestion, while the parasympathetic nervous system decelerates heart rate and increases digestion.

The main role of the **parasympathetic nervous system** is to conserve energy. It is associated with resting and sleeping states, and acts to reduce heart rate and constrict the bronchi. The parasympathetic nervous system is also responsible for managing digestion by increasing peristalsis and exocrine secretions. Acetylcholine is the neurotransmitter responsible for parasympathetic responses in the body. The functions of the parasympathetic nervous system are summarized in Figure 1.2.

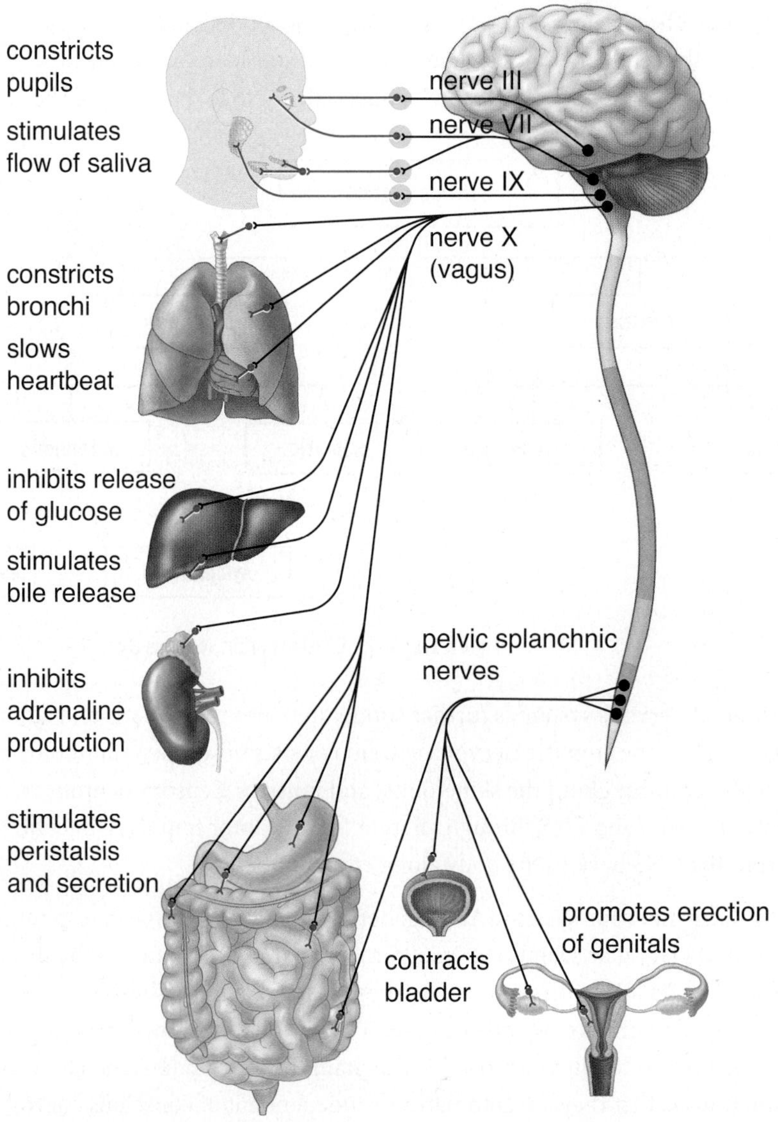

Figure 1.2 Functions of the Parasympathetic Nervous System

In contrast, the **sympathetic nervous system** is activated by stress. This can include everything from a mild stressor, such as keeping up with schoolwork, to emergencies that mean the difference between life and death. The sympathetic nervous system is closely associated with rage and fear reactions, also known as "fight-or-flight" reactions.

When activated, the sympathetic nervous system:

- Increases heart rate
- Redistributes blood to muscles of locomotion
- Increases blood glucose concentration
- Relaxes the bronchi
- Decreases digestion and peristalsis
- Dilates the eyes to maximize light intake
- Releases epinephrine into the bloodstream

The functions of the sympathetic nervous system are summarized in Figure 1.3.

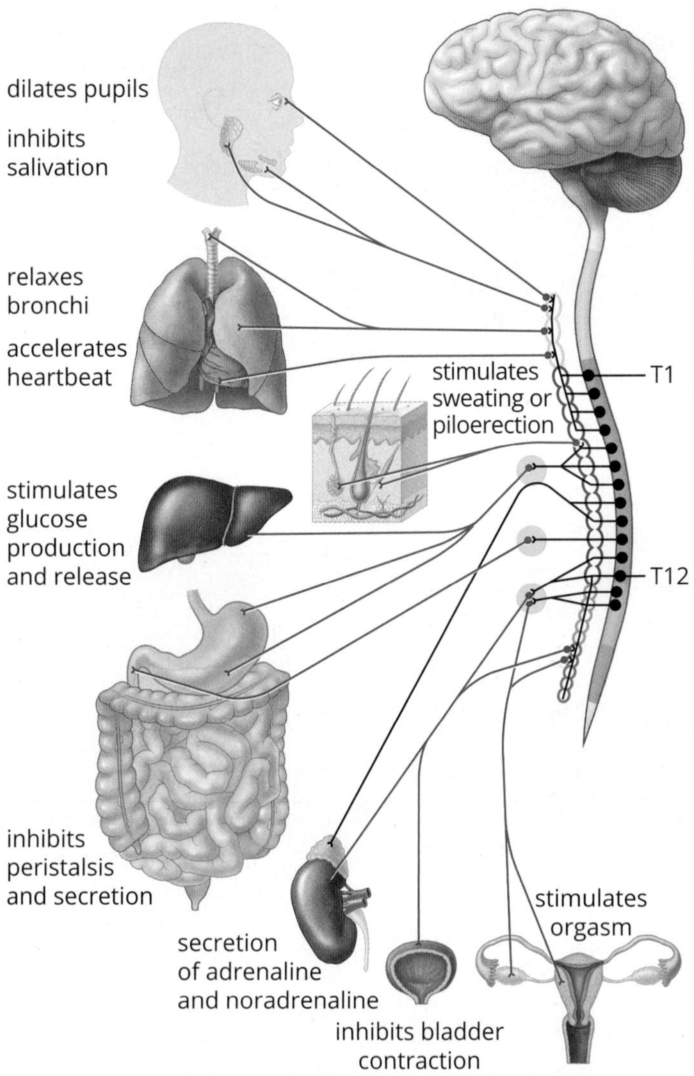

Figure 1.3 Functions of the Sympathetic Nervous System

MNEMONIC

Sympathetic and parasympathetic nervous systems:

- Sympathetic: "**fight**-or-**flight**"
- Parasympathetic: "**rest**-and-**digest**"

MCAT CONCEPT CHECK 1.2

Before you move on, assess your understanding of the material with these questions.

1. What parts of the nervous system are in the central nervous system (CNS)? Peripheral nervous system (PNS)?
   - CNS:

   - PNS:

   ---

2. What do afferent neurons do? Efferent neurons?
   - Afferent:

   - Efferent:

   ---

3. What functions are accomplished by the somatic nervous system? The autonomic nervous system?
   - Somatic:

   - Autonomic:

   ---

4. What are the effects of the sympathetic nervous system? The parasympathetic nervous system?
   - Sympathetic:

   - Parasympathetic:

1.3 Organization of the Brain

High-Yield

LEARNING OBJECTIVES

After Chapter 1.3, you will be able to:

- Describe the major functions of the hindbrain, midbrain, and forebrain
- Recognize the most commonly used methods for mapping the brain
- Identify the structures protecting and surrounding the brain

Throughout this section, refer to Figure 1.4, which identifies various anatomical structures inside the human brain. As we discuss different parts of the brain, it's important to remember the functions of these brain structures. Different parts of the brain perform remarkably different functions. For instance, one part of the brain processes sensory information while an entirely different part of the brain maintains activities of the internal organs. For complex functions such as playing a musical instrument, several brain regions work together. For the MCAT, you will need to know some of the basics about how the brain integrates input from different regions.

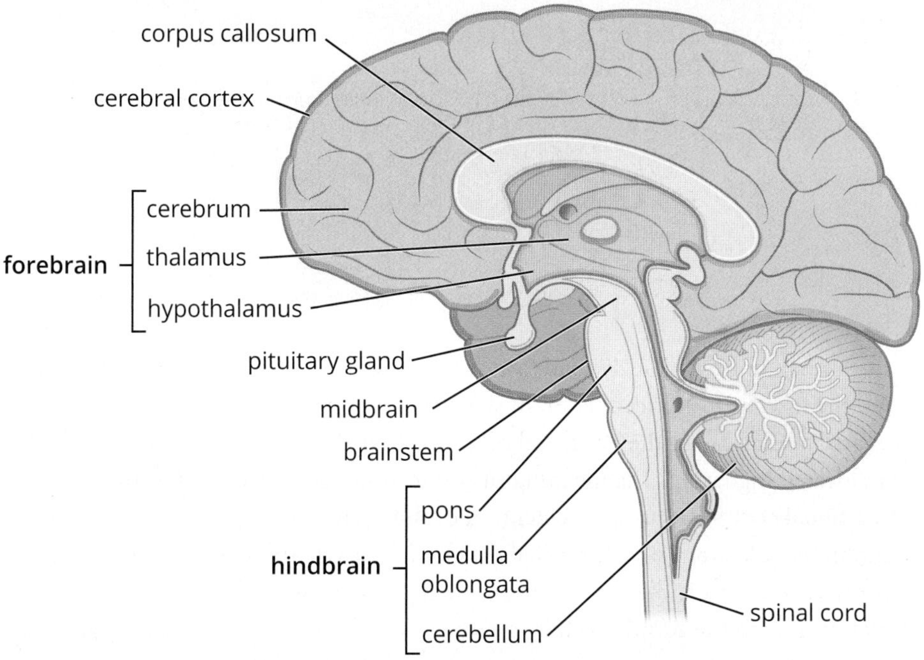

Figure 1.4 Anatomical Structures Inside the Human Brain

The brain is covered with a thick, three-layered sheath of connective tissue collectively called the **meninges**. The outer layer of connective tissue is the **dura mater**, and is connected directly to the skull. The middle layer is a fibrous, weblike structure called **arachnoid mater**. And the inner layer, connected directly to the brain, is known as the **pia mater**. These three layers of connective tissue are shown in Figure 1.5. The meninges help protect the brain by keeping it anchored within the skull, and the meninges also resorb **cerebrospinal fluid**, which is the aqueous solution that nourishes the brain and spinal cord and provides a protective cushion. Cerebrospinal fluid is produced by specialized cells that line the **ventricles** (internal cavities) of the brain.

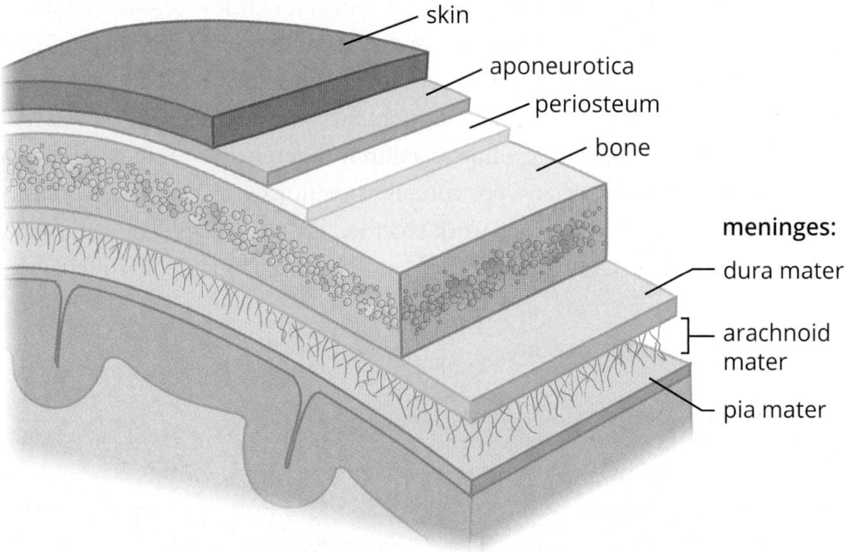

Figure 1.5 Layers of the Meninges

The human brain can be divided into three basic parts: the hindbrain, the midbrain, and the forebrain. Notice that brain structures associated with basic survival are located at the base of the brain and brain structures with more complex functions are located higher up. The meaningful connection between brain location and functional complexity is no accident. In evolutionary terms, the hindbrain and midbrain were brain structures that developed earlier. Together they form the **brainstem**, which is the most primitive region of the brain. The forebrain developed later, including the **limbic system**, a group of neural structures primarily associated with emotion and memory. Aggression, fear, pleasure, and pain are all related to the limbic system. The most recent evolutionary development of the human brain is the **cerebral cortex**, which is the outer covering of the cerebral hemispheres. In humans, the cerebral cortex is associated with everything from language processing to problem solving, and from impulse control to long-term planning. Most of the key brain regions described in the following sections are summarized in Table 1.1.

MAJOR DIVISIONS AND PRINCIPAL STRUCTURES	FUNCTIONS
Forebrain	
Cerebral cortex	Complex perceptual, cognitive, and behavioral processes
Basal ganglia	Movement
Limbic system	Emotion and memory
Thalamus	Sensory relay station
Hypothalamus	Hunger and thirst; emotion
Midbrain	Sensorimotor reflexes
Inferior and superior colliculi	
Hindbrain	
Cerebellum	Refined motor movements
Medulla oblongata	Heart, vital reflexes (vomiting, coughing)
Reticular formation	Arousal and alertness
Pons	Communication within the brain, breathing

Table 1.1 Anatomical Subdivisions of the Brain

In prenatal life, the brain develops from the neural tube. At first, the tube is composed of three swellings, which correspond to the hindbrain, midbrain, and forebrain. Both the hindbrain and forebrain later divide into two swellings, creating five total swellings in the mature neural tube. The embryonic brain is diagrammed in Figure 1.6, and its subdivisions are described further in the following sections. Understanding the relationship between the structures of the developing brain and the fully developed brain is important. So the following sections describe both the structures of the developing brain and what those structures develop into.

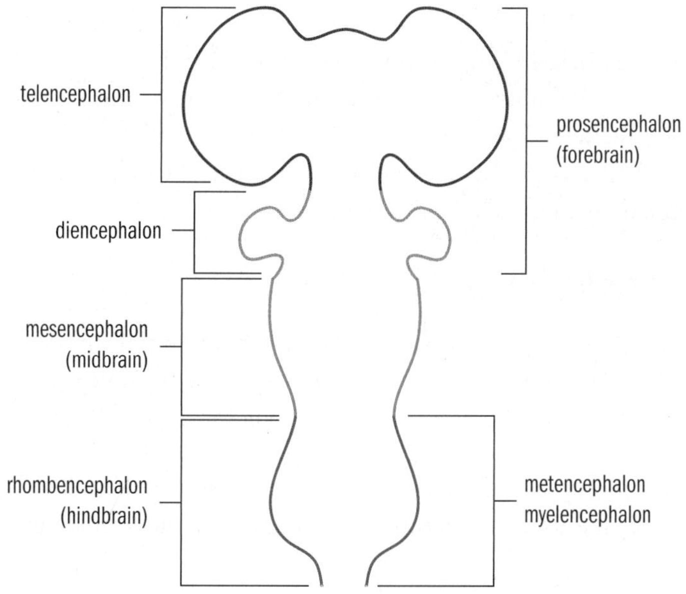

Figure 1.6 Subdivisions of the Embryonic Brain

Hindbrain

Located where the brain meets the spinal cord, the **hindbrain** (**rhombencephalon**) controls balance, motor coordination, breathing, digestion, and general arousal processes such as sleeping and waking. In short, the hindbrain manages vital functioning necessary for survival. During embryonic development, the rhombencephalon divides to form the **myelencephalon** (which becomes the medulla oblongata) and the **metencephalon** (which becomes the pons and cerebellum). In the developed brain, the **medulla oblongata** is a lower brain structure that is responsible for regulating vital functions such as breathing, heart rate, and digestion. The **pons** lies above the medulla and contains sensory and motor pathways between the cortex and the medulla. At the top of the hindbrain, mushrooming out of the back of the pons, is the **cerebellum**, a structure that helps maintain posture and balance and coordinates body movements. Damage to the cerebellum causes clumsiness, slurred speech, and loss of balance. Notably, alcohol impairs the functioning of the cerebellum, and consequently affects speech and balance.

Midbrain

Just above the hindbrain is the **midbrain** (**mesencephalon**), which receives sensory and motor information from the rest of the body. The midbrain is associated with involuntary reflex responses triggered by visual or auditory stimuli. There are several prominent nuclei in the midbrain, two of which are collectively called **colliculi**. The **superior colliculus** receives visual sensory input, and the **inferior colliculus** receives sensory information from the auditory system. The inferior colliculus has a role in reflexive reactions to sudden loud noises.

Forebrain

Above the midbrain is the **forebrain** (**prosencephalon**), which is associated with complex perceptual, cognitive, and behavioral processes. Among its other functions, the forebrain is associated with emotion and memory; it is the forebrain that has the greatest influence on human behavior. Its functions are not absolutely necessary for survival, but are associated instead with the intellectual and emotional capacities most characteristic of humans. During prenatal development, the prosencephalon divides to form the **telencephalon** (which forms the cerebral cortex, basal ganglia, and limbic system) and the **diencephalon** (which forms the thalamus, hypothalamus, posterior pituitary gland, and pineal gland).

Methods of Mapping the Brain

Neuropsychology refers to the study of functions and behaviors associated with specific regions of the brain. It is most often applied in research settings, where researchers attempt to associate very specific areas in the brain to behavior. Neuropsychology is also applied in clinical settings with evaluations of patient cognitive and behavioral functioning, as well as the diagnosis and treatment of brain disorders. Neuropsychology has its own experimental methodology and technology.

Studying human patients with brain lesions is one way that researchers have determined the functions of the brain. In order to conclude that a specific structure of the brain is responsible for a specific function, researchers look for patients that exhibit damage to that structure coupled with a loss of the function. One problem in studying human brain lesions, however, is that such lesions are rarely isolated to specific brain structures. When several brain structures are damaged, the impairment could be attributed to any of the damaged structures, and pinpointing a specific link between brain structure and function becomes difficult.

One method for studying the relationship of brain regions and behaviors is to study brain lesions in lab animals. The advantage of this approach is that precisely defined brain lesions can be created in animals by extirpation. Researchers can also produce lesions by inserting tiny electrodes inside the brain and then selectively applying intense heat, cold, or electricity to specific brain regions. Such electrodes can be placed with great precision by using stereotactic instruments, which provide high-resolution, three-coordinate images of the brain. Ethical or cruelty concerns notwithstanding, such studies have greatly increased our understanding of comparable neural structures in humans.

Another neuropsychology method involves electrically stimulating the brain and recording consequent brain activity. While operating on the brain, a surgeon can stimulate a patient's cortex with a small electrode. This stimulation causes groups of neurons to fire, thereby activating the behavioral or perceptual processes associated with those neurons. For instance, if the electrode stimulates neurons in the motor cortex, the stimulation can lead to specific muscle movements. If the electrode stimulates the visual cortex, the patient may "see" flashes of light that are not really there. By using electrical stimulation, neurosurgeons can thus create **cortical maps**. This method relies on the assistance of the patient, who is awake and alert. Because there are no pain receptors in the brain, only local anesthesia is required. Electrodes have also been used in lab animals to study deeper regions of the brain. Depending on where these electrodes are implanted, they can elicit sleep, sexual arousal, rage, or terror. Once the electrode is turned off, these behaviors cease.

Electrodes can also be used to record electrical activity produced by the brain itself. In some studies, individual neurons are recorded by inserting ultrasensitive microelectrodes into individual brain cells and recording their electrical activity. Electrical activity generated by larger groups of neurons can be studied using an **electroencephalogram (EEG)**, which involves placing several electrodes on the scalp. Broad patterns of electrical activity can thus be detected and recorded. Because this procedure is noninvasive (it does not cause any damage), electroencephalograms are commonly used with human subjects. In fact, research on sleep, seizures, and brain lesions relies heavily on EEGs, like the one shown in Figure 1.7.

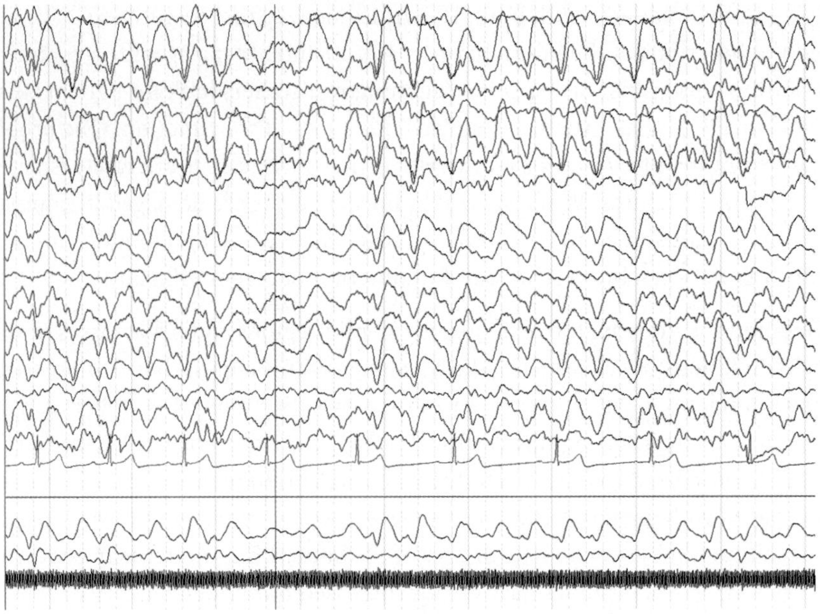

Figure 1.7 Electroencephalogram (EEG) during REM Sleep

Another noninvasive mapping procedure is **regional cerebral blood flow (rCBF)**, which detects broad patterns of neural activity based on increased blood flow to different parts of the brain. rCBF relies on the assumption that blood flow increases to regions of the brain that are engaged in cognitive function. For example, listening to music may increase blood flow to the right auditory cortex because music is processed in that region in most individuals' brains. To measure blood flow, the patient inhales a harmless radioactive gas; a special device that can detect radioactivity in the bloodstream can then correlate radioactivity levels with regional cerebral blood flow. This research method uses noninvasive computerized scanning devices.

Some of the other common scanning devices and methods of visualization used for brain imaging include:

- **CT (computed tomography)**, also known as **CAT (computed axial tomography) scan**, in which multiple X-rays are taken at different angles and processed by a computer to produce cross-sectional images of the tissue.
- **PET (positron emission tomography) scan**, in which a radioactive sugar is injected and absorbed into the body, and its dispersion and uptake throughout the target tissue is imaged.
- **MRI (magnetic resonance imaging)**, in which a magnetic field that interacts with hydrogen atoms is used to map out hydrogen dense regions of the body.
- **fMRI (functional magnetic resonance imaging)**, which uses the same base technique as MRI, but specifically measures changes associated with blood flow. fMRI is especially useful for monitoring neural activity, since increased blood flow to a region of the brain is typically coupled with its neuronal activation.

BRIDGE

MRI techniques are dependent on the reaction of hydrogen to a magnetic field, and the scientific principles behind MRI scans are also applied in NMR techniques, which can be found in Chapter 11 of *MCAT Organic Chemistry Review.*

MCAT CONCEPT CHECK 1.3

Before you move on, assess your understanding of the material with these questions.

1. What are the main functions of the hindbrain? Midbrain? Forebrain?

Subdivision	Functions
Hindbrain	
Midbrain	
Forebrain	

2. What are some of the methods used for mapping the brain?

____

3. What structures surround and protect the brain?

____

BEHAVIORAL SCIENCES GUIDED EXAMPLE WITH EXPERT THINKING

Multiple sclerosis is a demyelinating disease that results in a host of neurological and physiological symptoms including muscle weakness, numbness, spasms, visual problems, pain, unstable mood, and fatigue. This last symptom is interesting because it is effort-independent; patients express a subjective feeling of fatigue as a result of performing physical tasks that are not typically physically or mentally taxing. To investigate a mechanism for this phenomenon, researchers used the following fMRI mask to highlight regions of interest in measuring neural resource use with respect to subjective fatigue in patients who have MS:

MS symptoms. The author finds fatigue interesting because it is subjective. Used fMRI to investigate.

Independent Variable (IV): MS (probably versus control)

Dependent Variable (DV): fMRI activity detection differences

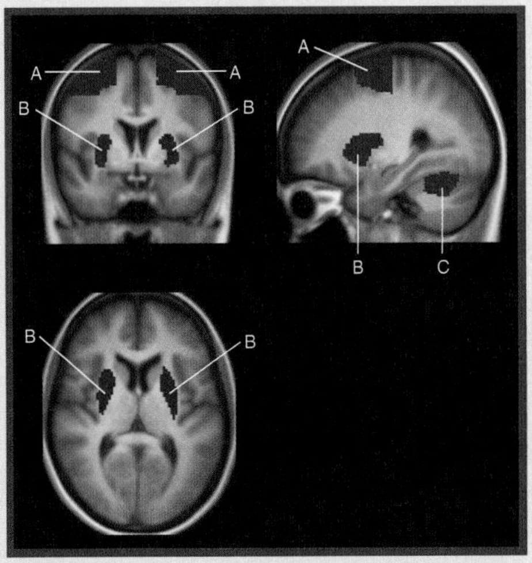

Figure 1 fMRI mask

Mask shows regions of interest for the study

Region B is a structure called the putamen, a part of the basal ganglia. It is connected to and provides pathways of communication for many structures in the brain, and generally influences and regulates motor behaviors such as planning, learning, preparation, and execution of motor sequences.

Region B = putamen: communication and motor behaviors

Researchers found no difference in activity in region B between patients with relapsing-remitting MS and controls. However, it was found that region C showed increased activation over the course of a non-fatiguing tonic grip task in patients who have MS. This increased activation correlated positively with subjective fatigue, and was not present in healthy control subjects. Furthermore, control subjects showed increased activation in region A over the course of the task, and no such activation occurred in patients who have MS.

Results: region B not implicated in MS-related fatigue, but C shows more activity and A shows less.

Adapted from: Svolgaard O, Andersen KW, Bauer C, Madsen KH, Blinkenberg M, Selleberg F, et al. (2018) Cerebellar and premotor activity during a non-fatiguing grip task reflects motor fatigue in relapsing-remitting multiple sclerosis. *PLoS ONE* 13(10): e0201162. https://doi.org/10.1371/journal.pone.0201162

Based on the functions of the regions studied, what do these results suggest about the nature of subjective fatigue in patients who have MS compared to healthy participants?

Our first step in answering this question is to identify the regions presented in the study that are referenced in the question stem. For this particular question, we don't have to worry too much about the structure of the experiment, as most of the information we need is in the results and the description of the regions. The authors give us the name and function of region B: the putamen, described in paragraph 2. This information is helpful because the actual brain isn't color coded and labeled, and due to the low structural resolution of the image, it's tough to tell exactly what region B is from the shape of the mask. On Test Day, using the image alone, we might be able to infer that region B is part of the midbrain and therefore, like other structures of the midbrain, it is probably involved in some kind of relay system. But the additional information in the passage text gives us insight that the picture alone just cannot provide. The passage also says that activity in region B is the same in patients who have MS and controls, allowing us to infer that difficulties in relaying motor signals are probably not the cause of subjective fatigue.

Based on our outside content knowledge, region C is the cerebellum, which we know is responsible for coordinating movement and for maintaining posture and balance. A differential increase in activity here implies that patients with MS may need more resources to perform motor tasks the longer these tasks are maintained.

Region A is in the forebrain. If we've studied the regions of the cerebrum, we might recognize this region as the premotor cortex, which is responsible for higher-level motor control and motivation. However, even without the specifics, we can guess that this region of the forebrain has something to do with executive motor control because of its general location. From the noted activity pattern in the final paragraph, we can guess that increased activity in region A helps to prevent subjective fatigue; thus, for patients who have MS, a lack of activation in this region may contribute to their experience of increased subjective fatigue.

We now have enough information to form a general picture of events here. In patients who have MS, the cerebellum is more active, presumably consuming more resources during maintained motor movements than the cerebellum of their healthy counterparts. This increase in resource consumption could be the patient's brain attempting to accommodate for functions from other regions that have been lost as a result of disease, or could indicate a greater overall demand on cognitive processes involving movement. This overtaxing of cerebellar resources is most likely related to the increase in subjective fatigue experienced by patients who have MS.

1.4 Parts of the Forebrain

LEARNING OBJECTIVES

After Chapter 1.4, you will be able to:

- Link the regions of the forebrain to their functions
- Describe the laterality of brain–body communication and the role of hemispheric dominance
- Describe the functions of the four lobes of the cerebral cortex:

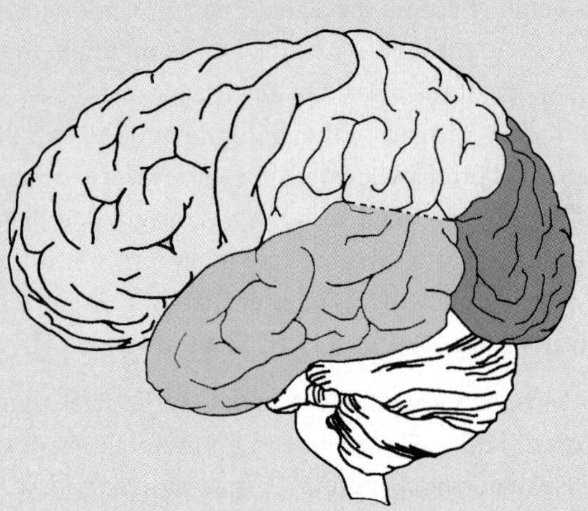

The forebrain is the most "modern" portion of the brain, and—in humans—forms the largest portion of the brain by weight and volume. The forebrain contains regions derived from the diencephalon, such as the thalamus, hypothalamus, posterior pituitary, and pineal gland; it also includes derivatives of the telencephalon, such as the cerebral cortex, basal ganglia, and limbic system.

Thalamus

The **thalamus** is a structure within the forebrain that serves as an important relay station for incoming sensory information, including all senses except for smell. After receiving incoming sensory impulses, the thalamus sorts and transmits them to the appropriate areas of the cerebral cortex. The thalamus is therefore a sensory "way station."

Hypothalamus

The **hypothalamus**, subdivided into the lateral hypothalamus, ventromedial hypothalamus, and anterior hypothalamus, serves homeostatic functions, and is a key player in emotional experiences during high arousal states, aggressive behavior, and sexual behavior. The hypothalamus also helps control some endocrine functions, as well as the autonomic nervous system. The hypothalamus serves many homeostatic functions, which are self-regulatory processes that maintain a stable balance within the body. Receptors in the hypothalamus regulate metabolism, temperature, and water balance. When any of these functions are out of balance, the hypothalamus

MNEMONIC

Functions of the Hypothalamus—The Four **F**s:

- **F**eeding
- **F**ighting
- **F**lighting
- (Sexual) **F**unctioning

detects the problem and signals the body to correct the imbalance; for example, osmoreceptors in the hypothalamus may trigger the release of antidiuretic hormone to increase water reabsorption as part of fluid balance. The hypothalamus is also the primary regulator of the autonomic nervous system and is important in drive behaviors: hunger, thirst, and sexual behavior.

The **lateral hypothalamus** (LH) is referred to as the hunger center because it has special receptors thought to detect when the body needs more food or fluids. In other words, the LH triggers eating and drinking. When this part of the hypothalamus is removed in lab rats, they refuse to eat and drink and must be force-fed with tubes to survive.

The **ventromedial hypothalamus** (VMH) is identified as the "satiety center," and provides signals to stop eating. Brain lesions to this area usually lead to obesity.

The **anterior hypothalamus** controls sexual behavior. When the anterior hypothalamus is stimulated, lab animals will mount just about anything (including inanimate objects). In many species, damage to the anterior hypothalamus leads to permanent inhibition of sexual activity. The anterior hypothalamus also regulates sleep and body temperature.

MNEMONIC

When the **L**ateral **H**ypothalamus (**LH**) is removed, one **L**acks **H**unger.

MNEMONIC

When the **V**entro**M**edial **H**ypothalamus (**VMH**) is destroyed, one is **V**ery **M**uch **H**ungry.

Other Parts of the Diencephalon

The diencephalon also differentiates to form the posterior pituitary gland, pineal gland, and connecting pathways to other brain regions. The **posterior pituitary** is comprised of axonal projections from the hypothalamus and is the site of release for the hypothalamic hormones **antidiuretic hormone** (**ADH**, also called **vasopressin**) and **oxytocin**. The functions of these hormones are described in Chapter 5 of *MCAT Biology Review*. The **pineal gland** is the key player in several biological rhythms. Most notably, the pineal gland secretes a hormone called **melatonin**, which regulates circadian rhythms. The pineal gland receives direct signals from the retina for coordination with sunlight.

Basal Ganglia

In the middle of the brain are a group of structures known as the basal ganglia. The **basal ganglia** coordinate muscle movement as they receive information from the cortex and relay this information (via the extrapyramidal motor system) to the brain and the spinal cord. The **extrapyramidal system** gathers information about body position and carries this information to the central nervous system, but does not function directly through motor neurons. Essentially, the basal ganglia help make our movements smooth and our posture steady. **Parkinson's disease** is one chronic illness associated with destruction of portions of the basal ganglia. This disease is characterized by jerky movements and uncontrolled resting tremors. The basal ganglia may also play a role in schizophrenia and obsessive–compulsive disorder.

REAL WORLD

In the early 1920s, researchers first discovered the hypothalamus's role in rage and fighting through classic experiments conducted with cats. When researchers removed the cat's cerebral cortex but left the hypothalamus in place, the cat displayed a pattern of pseudoaggressive behavior that was called "sham rage"—lashing of the tail, arching of the back, clawing, and biting—except that rage was spontaneous or triggered by the mildest touch. The researchers concluded that the cortex typically inhibits this type of response. When the researchers removed the cat's cortex and hypothalamus together, the outcome was very different. The cat no longer showed any signs of sham rage, and much rougher stimulation was required before the cats showed any defensive behavior at all.

Limbic System

The **limbic system**, diagrammed in Figure 1.8, comprises a group of interconnected structures looping around the central portion of the brain and is primarily associated with emotion and memory. Its primary components include the septal nuclei, amygdala, hippocampus, and anterior cingulate cortex. In Chapter 5 of *MCAT Behavioral Sciences Review*, we will also explore the roles of the thalamus, hypothalamus, and cortex in the limbic system.

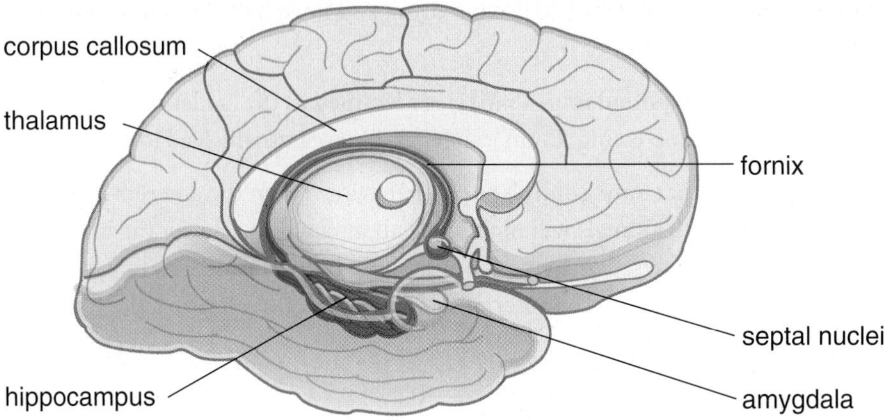

Figure 1.8 The Limbic System

Septal Nuclei

The **septal nuclei** contain one of the primary pleasure centers in the brain. Mild stimulation of the septal nuclei is reported to be intensely pleasurable; there is an association between these nuclei and addictive behavior.

REAL WORLD

James Olds and Peter Milner discovered the association between the septal nuclei and addictive behavior in the 1950s. They demonstrated that when rats could stimulate their septal regions at will by pushing a lever, they found it so pleasurable that they preferred it to eating or any other activities, even after going 24 hours without food or sleep.

Amygdala

The **amygdala** is a structure that plays an important role in defensive and aggressive behaviors, including fear and rage. Researchers base this observation on studies of animals and humans with brain lesions. When the amygdala is damaged, aggression and fear reactions are markedly reduced. Lesions to the amygdala result in docility and hypersexual states.

REAL WORLD

Heinrich Klüver and Paul Bucy performed studies that linked the amygdala with defensive and aggressive behavior in monkeys. When the amygdala of the Rhesus monkey was removed, they noted increased sexual behavior, decreased fear responses, and hyperorality, or the examination of inanimate or animate objects by mouth. These symptoms are now referred to as Klüver–Bucy syndrome.

Hippocampus

The **hippocampus** plays a vital role in learning and memory processes; specifically, the hippocampus helps consolidate information to form long-term memories, and can redistribute remote memories to the cerebral cortex. The hippocampus communicates with other portions of the limbic system through a long projection called the **fornix**. Researchers originally discovered the connection between memory and the hippocampus through a famous patient named Henry Molaison (known as H.M. in the scientific literature until his death in 2008). Parts of H.M.'s temporal lobes—including the amygdala and hippocampus—were removed in an effort to control epileptic seizures. After surgery, H.M.'s intelligence was largely intact but he suffered a drastic and irreversible loss of memory for any new information. This kind of memory loss is called **anterograde amnesia** and is characterized by not being able to establish new long-term memories, whereas memory for events that occurred before brain injury is usually intact. The opposite kind of memory loss, **retrograde amnesia**, refers to memory loss of events that transpired before brain injury.

BRIDGE

Learning and memory are discussed thoroughly in Chapter 3 of *MCAT Behavioral Sciences Review.*

Anterior Cingulate Cortex

Due to the connection with the frontal and parietal lobes, the **anterior cingulate cortex** functions in higher order cognitive processes, including regulation of impulse control and decision-making. It also maintains connections to other parts of the limbic system, and thus plays a role in emotion and motivation.

Cerebral Cortex

The outer surface of the brain is called the **cerebral cortex**. The cortex is sometimes called the **neocortex**, a reminder that the cortex is the most recent brain region to evolve. Rather than having a smooth surface, the cortex has numerous bumps and folds called **gyri** and **sulci**, respectively. The convoluted structure of the brain provides increased surface area. The cerebrum is divided into two halves, called **cerebral hemispheres**. The surface of the cortex is divided into four lobes—the frontal lobe, parietal lobe, occipital lobe, and temporal lobe. These lobes are identified in Figure 1.9, which shows a side view of the left cerebral hemisphere.

MNEMONIC

Lobes of the brain: **F-POT**

- **F**rontal
- **P**arietal
- **O**ccipital
- **T**emporal

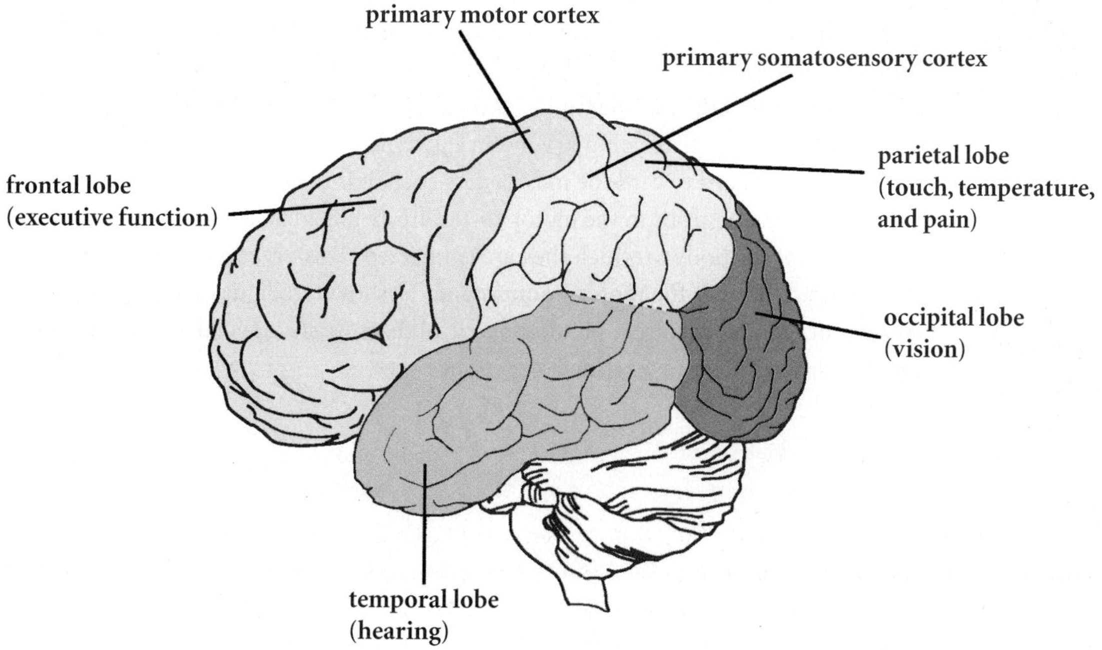

Figure 1.9 Lobes of the Brain

Frontal Lobe

The **frontal lobe** is comprised of two basic regions: the prefrontal cortex and the motor cortex. The **prefrontal cortex** manages executive function by supervising and directing the operations of other brain regions. To regulate attention and alertness, the prefrontal cortext communicates with the reticular formation in the brainstem, telling an individual either to wake up or to relax, depending on the situation. This region also supervises processes associated with perception, memory, emotion, impulse control, and long-term planning. In memory, for instance, the role of the prefrontal cortex is not to store any memory traces, but rather to remind individuals that they have something to remember at all.

Damage to the prefrontal cortex impairs its overall supervisory functions. People with prefrontal lesions may be more impulsive and generally less in control of their behavior. As a result, these individuals can have an increased tendency towards angry outbursts, as well as a higher predisposition to crying. Additionally, it is not unusual for someone with a prefrontal lesion to make vulgar and inappropriate sexual remarks, or to be apathetic to the emotional responses of others.

Because the prefrontal cortex integrates information from different cortical regions, the prefrontal cortex is a good example of an **association area**, which is an area that integrates input from diverse regions of the brain. For example, multiple inputs may be necessary to solve a complex puzzle, to plan ahead for the future, or to reach a difficult decision.

Association areas are generally contrasted with **projection areas**, which perform more rudimentary perceptual and motor tasks. An example of a projection area is the **primary motor cortex**, which is located on the **precentral gyrus**, just in front of the **central sulcus** that divides the frontal and parietal lobes. The function of the primary motor cortex is to initiate voluntary motor movements by sending neural impulses down the spinal cord toward the muscles. As such, it is considered a projection area in the brain. The neurons in the motor cortex are arranged systematically according to the parts of the body to which they are connected. This organizational pattern can be visualized through the **motor homunculus**, as shown in Figure 1.10. Because certain sets of muscles require finer motor control than others, they take up additional space in the cortex relative to their size in the body.

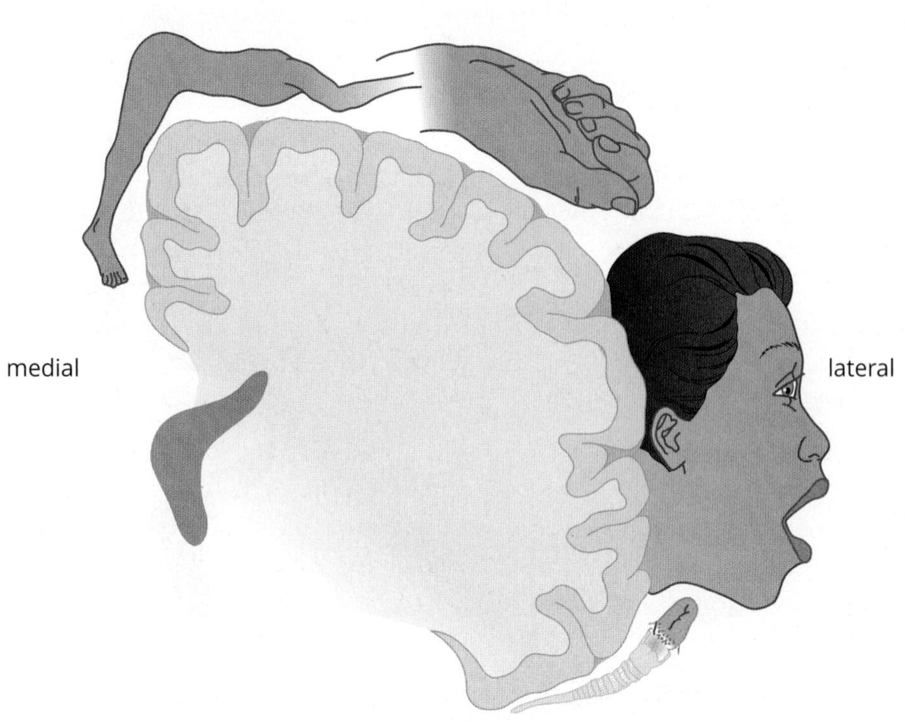

Figure 1.10 Motor Homunculus on the Precentral Gyrus of the Frontal Lobe

A third important part of the frontal lobe is **Broca's area**, which is vitally important for speech production. Broca's area is usually found in only one hemisphere, the so-called "dominant" hemisphere; for most people—both right- and left-handed—this is the left hemisphere.

Parietal Lobe

The **parietal lobe** is located to the rear of the frontal lobe. The **somatosensory cortex** is located on the **postcentral gyrus** (just behind the central sulcus) and is involved in somatosensory information processing. This projection area is the destination for all incoming sensory signals for touch, pressure, temperature, and pain. Despite certain differences, the somatosensory cortex and motor cortex are very closely related. In fact, they are so interrelated they sometimes are described as a single unit: the sensorimotor cortex. The somatosensory homunculus is shown in Figure 1.11. The central region of the parietal lobe is associated with spatial processing and manipulation. This region makes it possible to orient oneself and other objects in three-dimensional space, to do spatial manipulation of objects, and to apply spatial orientation skills such as those required for map reading.

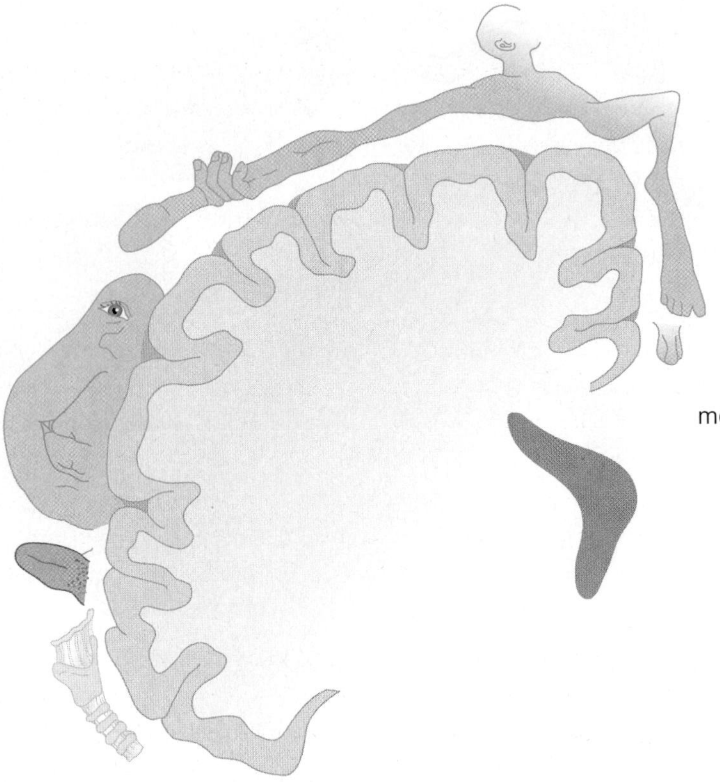

Figure 1.11 Somatosensory Homunculus on the Postcentral Gyrus of the Parietal Lobe

Occipital Lobe

The **occipital lobes**, at the very rear of the brain, contain the **visual cortex**, which is sometimes called the **striate cortex**. *Striate* means furrowed or striped, which is how the visual cortex appears when examined under a microscope. The visual cortex is one of the best-understood brain regions, owing to the large amount of research that has been done on visual processing. Sensation and perception of visual information are discussed thoroughly in Chapter 2 of *MCAT Behavioral Sciences Review*. Areas in the occipital lobe have also been implicated in learning and motor control.

Temporal Lobe

The **temporal lobes** are associated with a number of functions. The auditory cortex and Wernicke's area are located in the temporal lobe. The **auditory cortex** is the primary site of most sound processing, including speech, music, and other sound information. **Wernicke's area** is associated with language reception and comprehension. The temporal lobe also functions in memory processing, emotion, and language. Studies have shown that electrical stimulation of the temporal lobe can evoke memories for past events. This makes sense because the hippocampus is located deep inside the temporal lobe. It is important to note that the lobes, although having seemingly independent functions, are not truly independent of one another. Often, a sensory modality may be represented in more than one area.

REAL WORLD

Several techniques have been developed to assess the function of brain regions, especially those associated with language and auditory processing. One such technique is called **speech shadowing**, which is a technique used to research both stuttering and speech perception. Speech shadowing involves participants reciting along with auditory inputs, which can be presented to one or both ears. If different messages are presented to each ear, as in a dichotic listening test, speech shadowing can ensure that the participant is paying attention to the auditory input to the correct ear. This seemingly simple experimental task requires successful functioning of the temporal lobe, parietal lobe, and frontal cortex!

Cerebral Hemispheres and Laterality

In most cases, one side of the brain communicates with the opposite side of the body. In such cases, we say a cerebral hemisphere communicates **contralaterally**. For example, the motor neurons on the left side of the brain activate movements on the right side of the body. In other cases (for instance, hearing), cerebral hemispheres communicate with the same side of the body. In such cases, the hemispheres communicate **ipsilaterally**.

We distinguish between dominant and nondominant hemispheres. The dominant hemisphere is typically defined as the one that is more heavily stimulated during language reception and production. In the past, hand dominance was used as a proxy for hemispheric dominance; that is, right-handed individuals were assumed to have left-dominant brains and left-handed individuals were assumed to have right-dominant brains (because the brain communicates contralaterally with the hand). However, this correlation has not held up under scrutiny; 95 percent of right-handed individuals are indeed left brain dominant, but only 18 percent of left-handed individuals are right brain dominant.

The **dominant hemisphere** (usually the left) is primarily analytic in function, making it well-suited for managing details. For instance, language, logic, and math skills are all located in the dominant hemisphere. Again, language production (Broca's area) and language comprehension (Wernicke's area) are primarily driven by the dominant hemisphere.

The **nondominant hemisphere** (usually the right) is associated with intuition, creativity, music cognition, and spatial processing. The nondominant hemisphere simultaneously processes the pieces of a stimulus and assembles them into a holistic image. The nondominant hemisphere serves a less prominent role in language. It is more sensitive to the emotional tone of spoken language, and permits us to recognize others' moods based on visual and auditory cues, which adds to communication. The dominant hemisphere thus screens incoming language to analyze its content, and the nondominant hemisphere interprets it according to its emotional tone. The roles of the dominant and nondominant hemispheres are summarized in Table 1.2; remember that the left hemisphere is the dominant hemisphere in most individuals, regardless of handedness.

REAL WORLD

The **corpus callosum** connects and shares information between the two cerebral hemispheres; its function was discovered in patients who have epilepsy whose corpora callosa were severed in a last-ditch effort to limit their convulsive seizures. In these "split-brain" patients, in whom the corpus callosum has been severed, each hemisphere has its own function and specialization that is no longer accessible by the other. As an example of the result: an object felt only by the left hand (which projects to the right hemisphere) could not be named (because language function is usually in the left hemisphere).

FUNCTION	DOMINANT HEMISPHERE	NONDOMINANT HEMISPHERE
Visual system	Letters, words	Faces
Auditory system	Language-related sounds	Music
Language	Speech, reading, writing, arithmetic	Emotions
Movement	Complex voluntary movement	-
Spatial processes	-	Geometry, sense of direction

Table 1.2 Comparison of Dominant and Nondominant Hemispheres' Functions

MCAT CONCEPT CHECK 1.4

Before you move on, assess your understanding of the material with these questions.

1. Match the parts of the brain below to their functions:

1. Basal ganglia	A. Smooth movement
2. Cerebellum	B. Sensory relay station
3. Cerebral cortex	C. Sensorimotor reflexes
4. Hypothalamus	D. Arousal and alertness
5. Inferior and superior colliculi	E. Hunger and thirst; emotion
6. Limbic system	F. Complex perceptual, cognitive, and behavioral processes
7. Medulla oblongata	G. Vital function (breathing, digestion)
8. Reticular formation	H. Coordinated movement
9. Thalamus	I. Emotion and memory

2. What are the four lobes of the cerebral cortex, and what is the function of each?

Lobe	Function

3. What is the difference between ipsilateral and contralateral communication between the brain and the body?

____

4. How is the dominant hemisphere typically defined?

____

1.5 Influences on Behavior

High-Yield

LEARNING OBJECTIVES

After Chapter 1.5, you will be able to:

- Associate major neurotransmitters with their common functions
- Detail the links between the endocrine system and the brain
- Explain the nature *vs.* nurture debate and the different study types used to explore this question

Merely describing the functions of brain regions does not fully explain the wide variety of human behaviors that are possible. Other influences on behavior include chemical controls (neurotransmitters, hormones in the endocrine system), heredity, and the environment.

Neurotransmitters

A **neurotransmitter** is a chemical used by neurons to send signals to other neurons; more than 100 neurotransmitters have been identified. Several of the most important are described in this section and are summarized in Table 1.3. Some drugs mimic the action of neurotransmitters by binding to the same receptor to produce the same biological response. A drug that mimics the action of some neurotransmitter is called an **agonist**. Drugs can also act by blocking the action of neurotransmitters, and such drugs are called **antagonists**.

Acetylcholine

Acetylcholine is a neurotransmitter found in both the central and peripheral nervous systems. In the peripheral nervous system, acetylcholine is used to transmit nerve impulses to the muscles. It is the neurotransmitter used by the parasympathetic nervous system and a small portion of the sympathetic nervous system (in ganglia and for innervating sweat glands). In the central nervous system, acetylcholine has been linked to attention and arousal. In fact, loss of cholinergic neurons connecting with the hippocampus is associated with Alzheimer's disease, an illness resulting in progressive and incurable memory loss.

KEY CONCEPT

Acetylcholine is the neurotransmitter used by the efferent limb of the somatic nervous system and the parasympathetic nervous system. Acetylcholine can act as an excitatory or inhibitory neurotransmitter in muscle cells, dependent on the type of receptor found on the cell. For example, acetylcholine will transmit an inhibitory response in cardiac muscle cells, but it can also transmit an excitatory response if acting on skeletal muscle cells. Acetylcholine within the central nervous system largely functions as an excitatory neurotransmitter.

Epinephrine and Norepinephrine

Epinephrine, norepinephrine, and dopamine are three closely related neurotransmitters known as **catecholamines**. Due to similarities in their molecular composition, these three transmitters are also classified as **monoamines** or **biogenic amines**. The most important thing to know about the catecholamines is that they all play important roles in the experience of emotions.

Epinephrine (**adrenaline**) and **norepinephrine** (**noradrenaline**) are involved in controlling alertness and wakefulness. As the primary neurotransmitter of the sympathetic nervous system, they promote the fight-or-flight response. Whereas norepinephrine more commonly acts at a local level as a neurotransmitter, epinephrine is more often secreted from the adrenal medulla to act systemically as a hormone. Low levels of norepinephrine are associated with depression; high levels are associated with anxiety and mania.

Dopamine

Dopamine is another catecholamine that plays an important role in movement and posture. High concentrations of dopamine are normally found in the basal ganglia, which help smooth movements and maintain postural stability.

Imbalances in dopamine transmission have been found to play a role in **schizophrenia**. An important theory about the origin of this mental illness is called the **dopamine hypothesis of schizophrenia**. The dopamine hypothesis argues that delusions, hallucinations, and agitation associated with schizophrenia arise from either too much dopamine or from an oversensitivity to dopamine in the brain. Although the dopamine hypothesis of schizophrenia is an important theory, it does not account for all of the findings of the disease.

Parkinson's disease is associated with a loss of dopaminergic neurons in the basal ganglia. These disruptions of dopamine transmission lead to resting tremors and jerky movements, as well as to postural instability.

REAL WORLD

The role of dopamine in both schizophrenia and Parkinson's disease can be seen in their treatment. Antipsychotic medications used in schizophrenia are dopamine blockers, and can cause motor disturbances ("extrapyramidal symptoms") as a side effect. Parkinson's disease can be treated with L-DOPA, which increases dopamine levels in the brain; an overdose of L-DOPA can lead to psychotic symptoms similar to schizophrenia.

Serotonin

Along with the catecholamines, serotonin is classified as a monoamine or biogenic amine neurotransmitter. **Serotonin** is generally thought to play roles in regulating mood, eating, sleeping, and dreaming. Like norepinephrine, serotonin is thought to play a role in depression and mania. An oversupply of serotonin is thought to produce manic states; an undersupply is thought to produce depression.

GABA, Glycine, and Glutamate

The neurotransmitter **γ-aminobutyric acid (GABA)** produces inhibitory postsynaptic potentials and is thought to play an important role in stabilizing neural activity in the brain. GABA exerts its effects by causing hyperpolarization of the postsynaptic membrane.

Glycine may be better known as one of the twenty proteinogenic amino acids, but it also serves as an inhibitory neurotransmitter in the central nervous system by increasing chloride influx into the neuron. This hyperpolarizes the postsynaptic membrane, similar to the function of GABA.

Finally, **glutamate**, another of the twenty proteinogenic amino acids, also acts as a neurotransmitter in the central nervous system. In contrast to glycine, however, it is an excitatory neurotransmitter.

Peptide Neurotransmitters

Studies suggest that peptides are also involved in neurotransmission. The synaptic action of these **neuromodulators** (also called **neuropeptides**) involves a more complicated chain of events in the postsynaptic cell than that of regular neurotransmitters. Neuromodulators are therefore relatively slow and have longer effects on the postsynaptic cell than neurotransmitters. The **endorphins**, which are natural painkillers produced in the brain, are the most important peptides to know. Endorphins (and their relatives, **enkephalins**) have actions similar to morphine or other opioids in the body.

NEUROTRANSMITTER	BEHAVIOR
Acetylcholine	Voluntary muscle control, parasympathetic nervous system, attention, alertness
Epinephrine and Norepinephrine	Fight-or-flight responses, wakefulness, alertness
Dopamine	Smooth movements, postural stability
Serotonin	Mood, sleep, eating, dreaming
GABA and Glycine	Brain "stabilization"
Glutamate	Brain excitation
Endorphins	Natural painkillers

Table 1.3 Neurotransmitters and Their Functions

The Endocrine System

We've already discussed the relatively fast communication network—the nervous system—that uses chemical messages called neurotransmitters. The **endocrine system** is the other internal communication network in the body, and it uses chemical messengers called **hormones**. The endocrine system is somewhat slower than the nervous system because hormones travel to their target destinations through the bloodstream. The endocrine system is covered extensively in Chapter 5 of *MCAT Biology Review*, so our focus here will be on the role of certain endocrine organs on behavior.

The hypothalamus links the endocrine and nervous systems and, in addition to the roles described earlier, regulates the hormonal function of the pituitary gland. The hypothalamus and pituitary gland are spatially close to each other, and control is maintained through endocrine release of hormones into the **hypophyseal portal system** that directly connects the two organs, as shown in Figure 1.12.

BRIDGE

The entire endocrine system is covered in Chapter 5 of *MCAT Biology Review.*

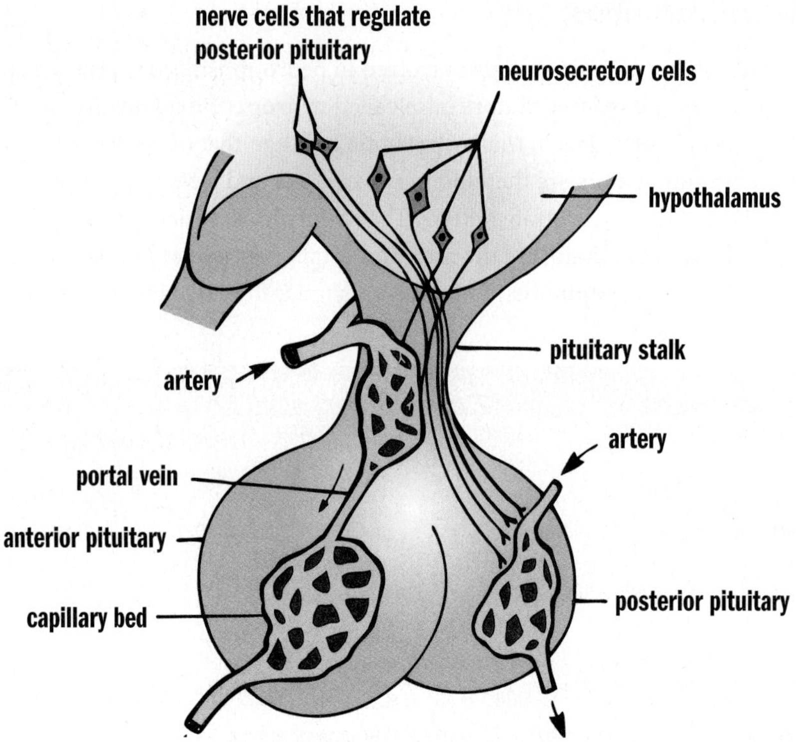

Figure 1.12 The Hypophyseal Portal System

The **pituitary gland**, sometimes referred to as the "master" gland, is located at the base of the brain and is divided into two parts: anterior and posterior. It is the **anterior pituitary** that is the "master" because it releases hormones that regulate activities of endocrine glands elsewhere in the body. However, the anterior pituitary itself is controlled by the hypothalamus. The pituitary secretes various hormones into the bloodstream that travel to other endocrine glands located elsewhere in the body to activate them. Once activated by the pituitary, a given endocrine gland manufactures and secretes its own characteristic hormone into the bloodstream.

The **adrenal glands** are located on top of the kidneys and are divided into two parts: the adrenal medulla and adrenal cortex. The **adrenal medulla** releases epinephrine and norepinephrine as part of the sympathetic nervous system. The **adrenal cortex** produces many hormones called **corticosteroids**, including the stress hormone **cortisol**. The adrenal cortex also contributes to sexual functioning by producing sex hormones, such as **testosterone** and **estrogen**.

The **gonads** are the sex glands of the body—ovaries in females and testes in males. These glands produce sex hormones in higher concentrations, leading to increased levels of testosterone in males and increased levels of estrogen in females. These sex hormones increase **libido** and contribute to mating behavior and sexual function. Higher levels of testosterone also increase aggressive behavior.

Genetics and Behavior

Just as physical traits are inherited from parents, behavioral traits can be inherited as well. Evidence for the inherited nature of behavior comes from the fact that many behaviors are species specific. For example, many animals exhibit mating behaviors only seen within their species. Behaviors can also be bred into a species; many breeds of dog have been bred for certain traits and behaviors. Behaviors are also seen to run in families. Often times, violence and aggression are observed passing along a family line, as are mental illnesses.

Innate behavior is genetically programmed as a result of evolution and is seen in all individuals regardless of environment or experience. In contrast, other behaviors are considered learned. **Learned behaviors** are not based on heredity but instead are based on experience and environment. **Adaptive value** is the extent to which a trait or behavior positively benefits a species by influencing the evolutionary fitness of the species, thus leading to **adaptation** through **natural selection**.

How much of an individual's behavior is based on genetic makeup and how much is based on environment and experiences? This controversial question is often referred to as the **nature *vs.* nurture** question. Here, **nature** is the influence of inherited characteristics on behavior. **Nurture** refers to the influence of environment and physical surroundings on behavior. There is no easy answer to this long-debated question. An individual's behavior is not only influenced by both genetics and environment, but also by how these two factors may influence each other. For example, hereditary traits may make a certain person more likely to have an addictive personality. But, the individual would still have to be exposed to drugs, alcohol, or gambling to develop an addiction.

To determine the degree of genetic influence on behavior, researchers often use one of three methods: family studies, twin studies, and adoption studies. **Family studies** rely on the fact that genetically related individuals are more similar genotypically than unrelated individuals. Researchers may compare rates of a given trait among family members to rates of that trait among unrelated individuals. For example, family studies have determined that the risk of developing schizophrenia for children of a patient who has schizophrenia is 13 times higher than in the general population. For siblings of a patient who has schizophrenia, the rate is 9 times higher. Observations such as these have led psychologists to conclude that schizophrenia has a hereditary component. Family studies are limited, however, because families share both genetics and environment. Family studies cannot distinguish shared environmental factors from shared genetic factors. For example, what if the increased rates of schizophrenia in families are a result of experiencing the same emotional climate in the home rather than genetically shared characteristics?

Twin studies, comparing concordance rates for a trait between **monozygotic** (**MZ**; identical) and **dizygotic** (**DZ**; fraternal) twins, are better able to distinguish the relative effects of shared environment and genetics. **Concordance rates** refer to the likelihood that both twins exhibit the same trait. MZ twins are genetically identical, sharing 100 percent of their genes, whereas DZ twins share approximately 50 percent of their genes. The assumption made by twin studies is that the two individuals in each MZ or DZ twin pair share the same environment; thus, differences between MZ

REAL WORLD

Bipolar disorder is considered one of the most heritable disorders, including medical illnesses. In one study, having a monozygotic (identical) twin with bipolar disorder was associated with a 43% risk of being diagnosed with the same disorder.

BRIDGE

Natural selection is discussed in greater detail in Chapter 12 of *MCAT Biology Review*.

and DZ twins are thought to reflect hereditary factors. Twin studies can also be used to measure genetic effects relative to environmental effects. In this version of the twin study, researchers compare traits in twins raised together versus twins raised apart. For example, one study of personality characteristics showed that MZ (identical) twins raised in separate families were still more similar than DZ (fraternal) twins raised together. Such a result offers convincing evidence for a strong genetic component to personality.

Finally, **adoption studies** also help us understand environmental and genetic influences on behavior. These studies compare the similarities between biological relatives and the child who was adopted to similarities between adoptive relatives and the child. For example, researchers have found that the IQ of children who were adopted is more similar to their biological parents' IQ than to their adoptive parents' IQ. This research suggests that IQ is heritable. Criminal behavior among teenagers shows a similar pattern of heritability.

MCAT CONCEPT CHECK 1.5

Before you move on, assess your understanding of the material with these questions.

1. Match the neurotransmitters below to their functions:

1. Acetylcholine	A. Wakefulness and alertness, fight-or-flight responses
2. Dopamine	B. Brain "stabilizer"
3. Endorphins	C. Mood, sleep, eating, dreaming
4. Epinephrine/norepinephrine	D. Natural painkiller
5. GABA/glycine	E. Smooth movements and steady posture
6. Glutamate	F. Voluntary muscle control
7. Serotonin	G. Brain excitation

2. Which endocrine organs influence behavior? What hormones do they use, and what do they accomplish?

____

3. Briefly discuss the influence of nature *vs.* nurture on behavior.

____

4. In each of the study types below, what is the sample group? The control group?

Study	Sample Group	Control Group
Family study		
Twin study		
Adoption study		

1.6 Development

LEARNING OBJECTIVES

After Chapter 1.6, you will be able to:

- Describe the process of neurulation
- Link the primitive reflexes with the behaviors to which they correspond
- Identify the main themes that dictate stages of motor development in children

The developmental process begins at the moment of conception. Physiological changes are rapid from embryonic to fetal stages, and well into infancy. Children exhibit surprisingly consistent patterns of motor abilities, as well as physiological changes based on age. Understanding these changes and when they occur is important in the discussion of developmental psychology. There are specific periods in development where children are particularly susceptible to environmental factors, called **critical periods**. Absence of the appropriate environmental factors may result in failure to learn a given skill or trait during the critical period, which may also mean learning that skill later on is difficult or even impossible.

Prenatal

The development of the nervous system starts with neurulation, at three to four weeks' gestational age. **Neurulation** occurs when the ectoderm overlying the notochord begins to furrow, forming a **neural groove** surrounded by two **neural folds**, as shown in Figure 1.13. Cells at the leading edge of the neural fold are called the **neural crest**, and will migrate throughout the body to form disparate tissues, including dorsal root ganglia, melanocytes (pigment-producing cells), and calcitonin-producing cells of the thyroid. The remainder of the furrow closes to form the **neural tube**, which will ultimately form the central nervous system (CNS). The neural tube has an **alar plate**, which differentiates into sensory neurons, and a **basal plate**, which differentiates into motor neurons. Over time, the neural tube invaginates and folds on itself many times; the embryonic brain begins as three swellings (prosencephalon, mesencephalon, rhombencephalon) that become five swellings (telencephalon, diencephalon, mesencephalon, metencephalon, myelencephalon) as it becomes the mature brain, as demonstrated in Figure 1.6 earlier in this chapter.

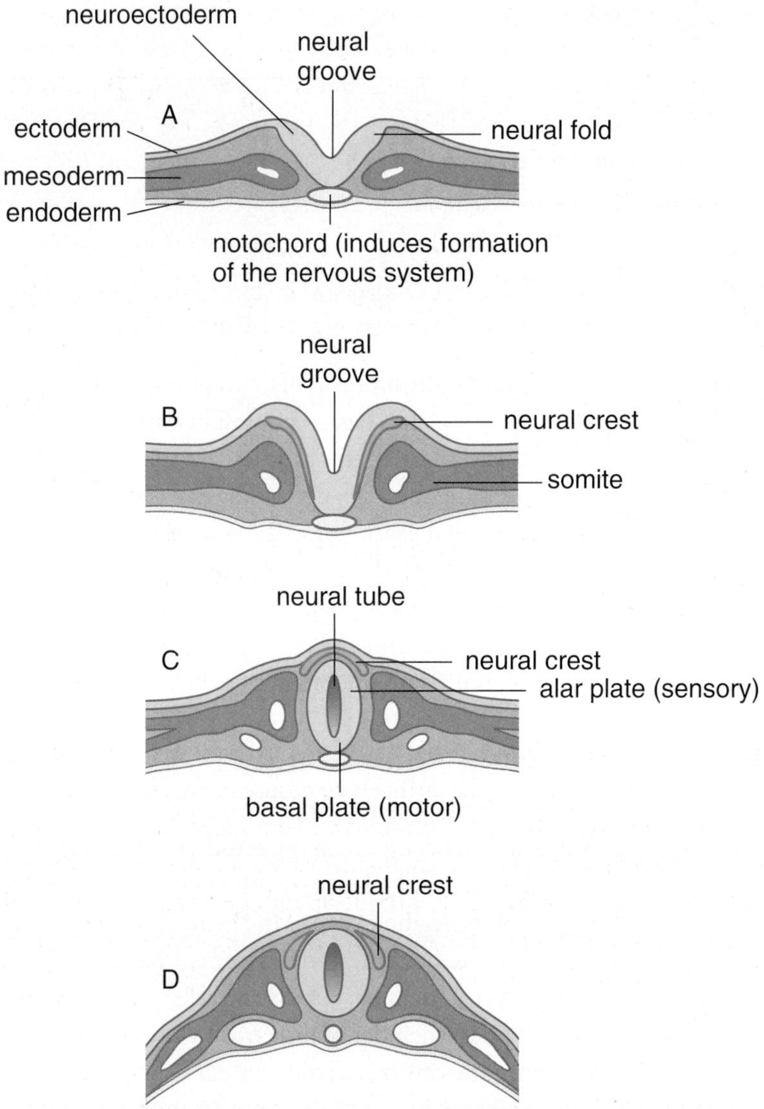

Figure 1.13 Development of the Nervous System

Prenatal development does not occur in a vacuum, of course, but in the mother's uterus. Within this environment, temperature, chemical balance, orientation of the fetus with respect to gravity, and atmospheric pressure are all carefully controlled and remain relatively constant. The fetus is attached to the uterine wall and placenta by the **umbilical cord**. The **placenta** transmits food, oxygen, and water to the fetus while returning water and waste to the mother. Maternal blood supplies many of the proteins and amino acids needed for growth, although the embryo begins to produce its own proteins and amino acids as well.

A variety of external influences can have deleterious effects on the development of the fetus. A number of viruses or bacteria can cross the placenta and cause damage to the developing fetus, including rubella (German measles), which may cause cataracts, deafness, heart defects, and intellectual disability. Other viral infections—such as measles, mumps, hepatitis, influenza, varicella (chickenpox), and herpes—have been linked to various birth defects.

An unfortunate side effect of the revolution in pharmaceutical development is that many drugs that help the mother can have damaging effects on the fetus she carries. The most notorious of these drugs is *thalidomide*, which was prescribed in the late 1950s and early 1960s to reduce morning sickness. Mothers who took this drug while pregnant often gave birth to babies with missing and malformed limbs and defects of the heart, eyes, ears, digestive tract, and kidneys. Antiepileptic medications are associated with neural tube defects, in which the neural tube fails to close completely, leading to malformations such as *spina bifida* or *anencephaly*.

A host of environmental factors and exposures may also affect maturation. Maternal malnutrition is considered to be a leading cause of abnormal development. Protein deficiency can slow growth, lead to intellectual disability, and reduce immunity to disease. Maternal narcotic addiction produces chemically dependent infants who must undergo severe withdrawal after birth. Regular cigarette smoking can lead to slowed growth, increased fetal heart rate, and a greater chance of premature birth. Daily use of alcohol also leads to slowed growth, both physically and psychologically. Finally, prenatal exposure to X-rays has been strongly linked to intellectual disabilities; defects of the skull, spinal cord, and eyes; cleft palate; and limb deformities.

Motor

Although they may seem helpless, infants are equipped with well-developed somatic structures and a broad array of reflexes that help ensure survival. A **reflex** is a behavior that occurs in response to a given stimulus without higher cognitive input. While motor and startle reflexes exist in adults, infants have a number of **primitive reflexes** that disappear with age. For example, the **rooting reflex** is the automatic turning of the head in the direction of a stimulus that touches the cheek—such as a nipple during feeding. Sucking and swallowing when an object is placed in the mouth are also examples of reflexes related to feeding.

Other primitive reflexes may have served an adaptive purpose in earlier stages of human evolution, but are currently used mainly in assessing infant neurological development. By comparing the point in time at which each of these reflexes disappears relative to the established norms, it is possible to tell whether neurological development is taking place in a normal fashion. One such reflex is the **Moro reflex**, illustrated in Figure 1.14. Infants react to abrupt movements of their heads by flinging out their arms, then slowly retracting their arms and crying. It has been speculated that this reflex may have developed during a time when our prehuman ancestors lived in trees and falling could have been prevented by instinctive clutching. The Moro reflex usually disappears after four months and its continuation at one year is a strong suggestion of developmental difficulties. Asymmetry of the Moro reflex may hint at underlying neuromuscular problems.

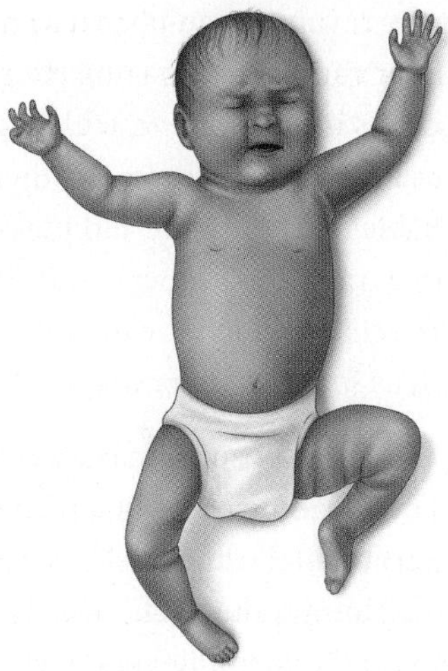

Figure 1.14 The Moro Reflex
The infant extends the arms, then slowly withdraws them and cries.

The **Babinski reflex** causes the toes to spread apart automatically when the sole of the foot is stimulated, as seen in Figure 1.15. The **grasping reflex** occurs when infants close their fingers around an object placed in the hand. Adults with neurological diseases may exhibit these primitive reflexes, especially in illnesses that cause demyelination (loss of the myelin sheath).

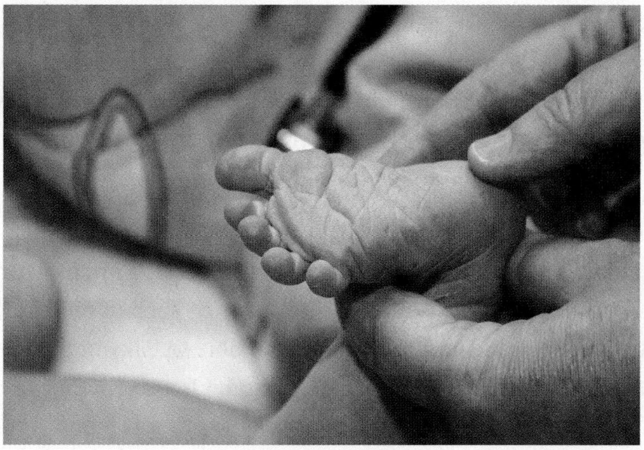

Figure 1.15 The Babinski Reflex
The big toe extends while the other toes fan outward.

Although reflexive behavior dominates the repertoire of the neonate, other behaviors occur as well. Newborn infants also kick, turn, and wave their arms. These uncoordinated, unconnected behaviors form the basis for later, more coordinated movements.

Infants typically develop motor skills at about the same age, in the same order. Due to this pattern, most psychologists and doctors agree that these are innately programmed abilities for human infants. However, the educational richness of the environment has been observed to affect the rate of learning, with more enriched environments promoting quicker development.

Motor skills are broken down into two classes: gross and fine motor skills. **Gross motor skills** incorporate movement from large muscle groups and whole body motion, such as sitting, crawling, and walking. **Fine motor skills** involve the smaller muscles of the fingers, toes, and eyes, providing more specific and delicate movement. Fine motor abilities include tracking motion, drawing, catching, and waving.

Social

In addition to motor skills, social development occurs in infancy and through adolescence. At birth, the parental figure becomes the center of the infant's world, and as the infant ages, **stranger anxiety** (a fear and apprehension of unfamiliar individuals) and **separation anxiety** (a fear of being separated from the parental figure) develop at approximately seven months and one year, respectively. During this time, play style progresses from solitary to onlooker, and at two years develops into **parallel play**, in which children will play alongside each other without influencing each other's behavior. At age three, children have an awareness of their assigned gender at birth, engage in gender-stereotyped play, and know their full name.

By age five, conformity to peers and romantic feelings for others begin to develop. From ages six through twelve, friend circles tend to be of the same gender without expression of romantic feelings. In the teenage years, children become more self-sufficient, and often express their desire for independence by rebelling against their parents. Inter-gender friendships become more common. Individuals also become more aware of their gender identity and sexual orientation and may begin sexual relationships.

In this chapter we have described several abilities and behaviors that are expected to emerge at particular times in a person's development. These skills are known as **developmental milestones**. The developmental milestones of the first three years of life are listed in Table 1.4. While this is a general timetable based on averages, most children fall within plus or minus two months of the chart. The goal is not to memorize this chart, but to recognize some themes. For example, gross motor skills progress in a head-to-toe order: children first develop the ability to lift the head, then to stabilize the trunk, and finally to walk. There is also a correlation between the development of motor skills and proximity to the center of the body, with skills being developed at the core prior to extremities. Social skills move from being parent-oriented to self-oriented to other-oriented. Language skills, discussed in Chapter 4 of *MCAT Behavioral Sciences Review*, become more complex and structured.

AGE	PHYSICAL AND MOTOR DEVELOPMENTS	SOCIAL DEVELOPMENTS	LANGUAGE DEVELOPMENTS
1st year of life	• Puts everything in mouth • Sits with support (4 mo) • Stands with help (8 mo) • Crawls, fear of falling (9 mo) • Pincer grasp (10 mo) • Follows objects to midline (4 wk) • One-handed approach/grasp of toy • Feet in mouth (5 mo) • Bang and rattle stage • Changes hands with toy (6 mo)	• Parental figure central • Issues of trust are key • Stranger anxiety (7 mo) • Play is solitary and exploratory • Pat-a-cake, peek-a-boo (10 mo)	• Laughs aloud (4 mo) • Repetitive responding (8 mo) • "mama, dada" (10 mo)
Age 1	• Walks alone (13 mo) • Climbs stairs alone (18 mo) • Emergence of hand preference (18 mo) • Kicks ball, throws ball • Pats pictures in book • Stacks three cubes (18 mo)	• Separation anxiety (12 mo) • Dependency on parental figure • Onlooker play	• Great variation in timing of language development • Uses 10 words
Age 2	• High activity level • Walks backward • Can turn doorknob, unscrew jar lid • Scribbles with crayon • Stacks six cubes (24 mo) • Stands on tiptoes (30 mo) • Able to aim thrown ball	• Selfish and self-centered • Imitates mannerisms and activities • May be aggressive • Recognizes self in mirror • "No" is favorite word • Parallel play	• Use of pronouns • Parents understand most • Two-word sentences • Uses 250 words • Identifies body parts by pointing
Age 3	• Rides tricycle • Stacks nine cubes (36 mo) • Alternates feet going up stairs • Bowel and bladder control (toilet training) • Draws recognizable figures • Catches ball with arms • Cuts paper with scissors • Unbuttons buttons	• Awareness of assigned gender • Gender-stereotyped play • Understands "taking turns" • Knows full name	• Complete sentences • Uses 900 words • Understands 3600 words • Strangers can understand • Recognizes common objects in pictures • Can answer, "Tell me what we wear on our feet?" "Which block is bigger?"

Table 1.4 Child Development Milestones

MCAT CONCEPT CHECK 1.6

Before you move on, assess your understanding of the material with these questions.

1. Describe the process of neurulation.

____

2. For each of the primitive reflexes below, briefly describe the observed behavior.

Primitive Reflex	Behavior
Rooting	
Moro	
Babinski	
Grasping	

3. What are the two main themes that dictate the stages of motor development in early childhood?

    1. ____
    2. ____

Conclusion

Behavioral psychology is the study of all physical and mental actions based on the response of the body to external stimuli, specifically the activity of the nervous and endocrine systems. The nervous system is a complex organization of structures and neurons that communicate and coordinate information. The endocrine system, in conjunction with the nervous system, controls human behavior. Aside from neurotransmitter and hormonal control of behavior, certain behaviors are genetically passed from generation to generation, as are many other physical traits. The genetic aspects of behavior are thought to interact with the learned components of behavior. Human behavior is also studied as it correlates to the development from embryo to fetus to infant and well into adolescence and adulthood. The development of motor skills and social behavior is seen to progress at a consistent rate across the species.

In the next chapter, our focus will be on the neurological systems used to interact with the world—most notably, those systems that exist for sensation and perception of the environment. These include vision, hearing, smell and taste, somatosensation, and others.

GO ONLINE

You've reviewed the content, now test your knowledge and critical thinking skills by completing a test-like passage set in your online resources!

CONCEPT SUMMARY

A Brief History of Neuropsychology

- **Neuropsychology** is the study of the connection between the nervous system and behavior. It most often focuses on the functions of various brain regions.

Organization of the Human Nervous System

- There are three types of neurons in the nervous system: **sensory** (**afferent**) neurons, **motor** (**efferent**) neurons, and **interneurons**.
- **Reflex arcs** use the ability of interneurons in the spinal cord to relay information to the source of stimuli while simultaneously routing it to the brain.
- The nervous system is made up of the **central nervous system** (**CNS**; brain and spinal cord) and **peripheral nervous system** (**PNS**; most cranial and spinal nerves).
  - The PNS is divided into the **somatic** (voluntary) and **autonomic** (automatic) divisions.
  - The autonomic system is further divided into the **parasympathetic** (rest-and-digest) and **sympathetic** (fight-or-flight) branches.

Organization of the Brain

- The brain has three subdivisions: hindbrain, midbrain, and forebrain.
  - The **hindbrain** contains the cerebellum, medulla oblongata, and reticular formation.
  - The **midbrain** contains the inferior and superior colliculi.
  - The **forebrain** contains the thalamus, hypothalamus, basal ganglia, limbic system, and cerebral cortex.
- Methods of studying the brain include studying humans and animals with lesions, electrical stimulation and activity recording (including **electroencephalography** [EEG]), and **regional cerebral blood flow**.

Parts of the Forebrain

- The **thalamus** is a relay station for sensory information.
- The **hypothalamus** maintains homeostasis and integrates with the endocrine system through the **hypophyseal portal system** that connects it to the **anterior pituitary**.
- The **basal ganglia** smoothen movements and help maintain postural stability.
- The **limbic system**, which contains the septal nuclei, amygdala, and hippocampus, controls emotion and memory.
  - The **septal nuclei** are involved with feelings of pleasure, pleasure-seeking behavior, and addiction.

  - The **amygdala** controls fear and aggression.
  - The **hippocampus** consolidates memories and communicates with other parts of the limbic system through an extension called the **fornix**.
- The **cerebral cortex** is divided into four lobes: frontal, parietal, occipital, and temporal.
  - The **frontal lobe** controls executive function, impulse control, long-term planning, motor function, and speech production.
  - The **parietal lobe** controls sensations of touch, pressure, temperature, and pain; spatial processing; orientation; and manipulation.
  - The **occipital lobe** controls visual processing.
  - The **temporal lobe** controls sound processing, speech perception, memory, and emotion.
- The brain is divided into two **cerebral hemispheres**, left and right. In most individuals, the left hemisphere is the dominant hemisphere for language.

Influences on Behavior

- **Neurotransmitters** are released by neurons and carry a signal to another neuron or effector (a muscle fiber or a gland).
  - **Acetylcholine** is used by the somatic nervous system (to move muscles), the parasympathetic nervous system, and the central nervous system (for alertness).
  - **Dopamine** maintains smooth movements and steady posture.
  - **Endorphins** and **enkephalins** act as natural painkillers.
  - **Epinephrine** and **norepinephrine** maintain wakefulness and alertness and mediate fight-or-flight responses. Epinephrine tends to act as a hormone, and norepinephrine tends to act more classically as a neurotransmitter.
  - **γ-Aminobutyric acid** (**GABA**) and **glycine** act as brain "stabilizers."
  - **Glutamate** acts as an excitatory neurotransmitter in the brain.
  - **Serotonin** modulates mood, sleep patterns, eating patterns, and dreaming.
- The endocrine system is tied to the nervous system through the hypothalamus and the anterior pituitary, as well as a few other hormones.
  - **Cortisol** is a stress hormone released by the adrenal cortex.
  - **Testosterone** and **estrogen** mediate libido; testosterone also increases aggressive behavior. Both are released by the adrenal cortex. In males, the testes also produce testosterone. In females, the ovaries also produce estrogen.
  - **Epinephrine** and **norepinephrine** are released by the adrenal medulla and cause physiological changes associated with the sympathetic nervous system.

- **Nature *vs.* nurture** is a classic debate regarding the relative contributions of genetics (nature) and environment (nurture) to an individual's traits. For most traits, both nature and nurture play a role. The relative effects of each can be studied.
  - **Family studies** look at the relative frequency of a trait within a family compared to the general population.
  - **Twin studies** compare concordance rates between monozygotic (identical) and dizygotic (fraternal) twins.
  - **Adoption studies** compare similarities between children who were adopted and their adoptive parents, relative to similarities with their biological parents.

Development

- The nervous system develops through neurulation, in which the notochord stimulates overlying ectoderm to fold over, creating a **neural tube** topped with **neural crest** cells.
  - The **neural tube** becomes the central nervous system (CNS).
  - The **neural crest** cells spread out throughout the body, differentiating into many different tissues.
- **Primitive reflexes** exist in infants and should disappear with age. Most primitive reflexes serve (or served, in earlier times) a protective role. They can reappear in certain nervous system disorders.
  - In the **rooting reflex**, infants turn their heads toward anything that brushes the cheek.
  - In the **Moro reflex**, the infant extends the arms, then slowly retracts them and cries in response to a sensation of falling.
  - In the **Babinski reflex**, the big toe is extended and the other toes fan in response to the brushing of the sole of the foot.
  - In the **grasping reflex**, infants grab anything put into their hands.
- Developmental milestones give an indication of what skills and abilities a child should have at a given age. Most children adhere closely to these milestones, deviating by only one or two months.
  - Gross and fine motor abilities progress head to toe and core to periphery.
  - Social skills shift from parent-oriented to self-oriented to other-oriented.
  - Language skills become increasingly complex.

ANSWERS TO CONCEPT CHECKS

1.1

1. - Franz Gall: phrenology; associated development of a trait with growth of its relevant part of the brain.
   - Pierre Flourens: extirpation/ablation; concluded that different brain regions have specific functions.
   - William James: "founder of American psychology"; pushed for importance of studying adaptations of the individual to the environment.
   - John Dewey: credited with the landmark article on functionalism; argued for studying the entire organism as a whole.
   - Paul Broca: correlated pathology with specific brain regions, such as speech production from Broca's area.
   - Hermann von Helmholtz: measured speed of a nerve impulse.
   - Sir Charles Sherrington: inferred the existence of synapses.

1.2

1. The central nervous system includes the brain and spinal cord. The peripheral nervous system includes most of the cranial and spinal nerves and sensors.
2. Afferent (sensory) neurons bring signals from a sensor to the central nervous system. Efferent (motor) neurons bring signals from the central nervous system to an effector.
3. The somatic nervous system is responsible for voluntary actions; most notably, moving muscles. The autonomic nervous system is responsible for involuntary actions, like heart rate, bronchial dilation, dilation of the eyes, exocrine gland function, and peristalsis.
4. The sympathetic nervous system promotes a fight-or-flight response, with increased heart rate and bronchial dilation, redistribution of blood to locomotor muscles, dilation of the eyes, and slowing of digestive and urinary functions. The parasympathetic nervous system promotes rest-and-digest functions, slowing heart rate and constricting the bronchi, redistributing blood to the gut, promoting exocrine secretions, constricting the pupils, and promoting peristalsis and urinary function.

1.3

1.

Subdivision	Functions
Hindbrain	Balance, motor coordination, breathing, digestion, general arousal processes (sleeping and waking); "vital functioning"
Midbrain	Receives sensory and motor information from the rest of the body; reflexes to auditory and visual stimuli
Forebrain	Complex perceptual, cognitive, and behavioral processes; emotion and memory

2. Methods used for mapping the brain include studying humans with brain lesions, extirpation, stimulation or recording with electrodes (cortical mapping, single-cell electrode recordings, electroencephalogram [EEG]), and regional cerebral blood flow (rCBF).
3. From most deep to most superficial, the structures surrounding the brain are the meninges, bone, periosteum, and skin.

1.4

1. 1–A, 2–H, 3–F, 4–E, 5–C, 6–I, 7–G, 8–D, 9–B
2.

Lobe	Function
Frontal	Executive function, impulse control, long-term planning (prefrontal cortex), motor function (primary motor cortex), speech production (Broca's area)
Parietal	Sensation of touch, pressure, temperature, and pain (somatosensory cortex); spatial processing, orientation, and manipulation
Occipital	Visual processing
Temporal	Sound processing (auditory cortex), speech perception (Wernicke's area), memory, and emotion (limbic system)

3. Ipsilateral communication occurs when cerebral hemispheres communicate with the same side of the body. Contralateral communication occurs when cerebral hemispheres communicate with the opposite side of the body.
4. The dominant hemisphere is typically defined as the one that is more heavily stimulated during language reception and production.

1.5

1. 1–F, 2–E, 3–D, 4–A, 5–B, 6–G, 7–C
2. The hypothalamus controls release of pituitary hormones; the pituitary is the "master gland" that triggers hormone secretion in many other endocrine glands. The adrenal medulla produces adrenaline (epinephrine), which causes sympathetic nervous system effects throughout the body. The adrenal cortex produces cortisol, a stress hormone. The adrenal cortex and testes produce testosterone, which is associated with libido.
3. Nature is defined as heredity, or the influence of inherited characteristics on behavior. Nurture refers to the influence of environment and physical surroundings on behavior. It has long been debated whether nature or nurture has the larger influence; it is a complicated situation, but for most traits, both exert some influence.
4.

Study	Sample Group	Control Group
Family study	Family of genetically related individuals	Unrelated individuals (general population)
Twin study	Monozygotic (MZ, identical) twins	Dizygotic (DZ, fraternal) twins
Adoption study	Adoptive family (relative to child who was adopted)	Biological family (relative to child who was adopted)

1.6

1. Neurulation occurs when a furrow is produced from ectoderm overlying the notochord and consists of the neural groove and two neural folds. As the neural folds grow, the cells at their leading edge are called neural crest cells. When the neural folds fuse, this creates the neural tube, which will form the CNS.
2.

Primitive Reflex	Behavior
Rooting	Turns head toward direction of any object touching the cheek
Moro	In response to sudden head movement, arms extend and slowly retract; baby usually cries
Babinski	Extension of big toe and fanning of other toes in response to brushing the sole of the foot
Grasping	Holding onto any object placed in the hand

3. Gross motor development proceeds from head to toe, and from the core to the periphery.

SCIENCE MASTERY ASSESSMENT EXPLANATIONS

1. **B**

Creating knockouts to study gene function is similar to ablation, or extirpation, in which specific parts of an organism's anatomy are removed. This approach was used by Pierre Flourens to show that specific parts of the brain served particular functions, supporting **(B)** as the correct answer. Unlike Pierre, Paul Broca, choice **(A)**, did not ablate regions of the brain; rather he studied the functional impairments in individuals with different brain lesions.

2. **B**

The cerebral cortex is not involved in the initial reflexive response to pain. Instead, the sensory receptors send information to the interneurons in the spinal cord, which stimulate a motor neuron to allow quick withdrawal. While the brain does ultimately get the signal, the reflexive withdrawal has already occurred by that time.

3. **C**

The hindbrain is responsible for balance and motor coordination, which would be necessary for dribbling a basketball. The midbrain, **(B)**, manages sensorimotor reflexes that also promote survival. The forebrain, **(A)**, is associated with emotion, memory, and higher-order cognition. The spinal cord, **(D)**, is likely not damaged as the child can still walk.

4. **D**

The temporal lobes have many functions, but motor skills are not associated with this area. The temporal lobes contain Wernicke's area, which is responsible for language comprehension, **(A)**. The temporal lobes also function in memory and emotion, **(B)** and **(C)**, because they contain the hippocampus and amygdala. Motor skills are associated with the frontal lobe (primary motor cortex), basal ganglia (smooth movements), and cerebellum (coordination).

5. **C**

The hypothalamus is responsible for homeostatic and emotional functions. The cerebellum, **(A)**, is responsible for maintaining posture and balance while the pons, **(B)**, is above the medulla and contains sensory and motor tracts between the cortex and the medulla. The thalamus, **(D)**, acts as a relay station for sensory information.

6. **A**

The right hemisphere is usually the nondominant hemisphere, even in left-handed individuals. Sense of direction is an ability of the nondominant hemisphere. The other answer choices are all abilities attributed to the dominant hemisphere.

7. **B**

Neurulation occurs when the notochord causes differentiation of overlying ectoderm into the neural tube and neural crest cells. The neural tube ultimately becomes the central nervous system (brain and spinal cord), and neural crest cells migrate to other sites in the body to differentiate into a number of different tissues. Thus, only statement III is true.

8. **D**

Catecholamines are the hormones produced by the adrenal glands during the fight-or-flight response, and include epinephrine, norepinephrine, and dopamine. Acetylcholine is produced by cholinergic neurons and is, thus, not a catecholamine.

9. **A**

If there were increased amounts of acetylcholinesterase, more acetylcholine would be degraded, lowering acetylcholine levels in the body. Low levels of acetylcholine would result in weakness or paralysis of muscles. Pain, **(B)**, could result if one were injured and endorphins were found in low levels. Mood swings, **(C)**, could be a result of varying levels of serotonin. Hallucinations, **(D)**, have been seen to result from high levels of dopamine.

10. **A**

The adrenal glands do promote the fight-or-flight response, but through epinephrine and norepinephrine, not estrogen. The adrenal cortex produces both estrogen and testosterone in both sexes, as mentioned in **(D)**, thus serving as a source of estrogen in males and testosterone in females.

11. **C**

The pineal gland is responsible for producing melatonin, which controls the body's circadian rhythm. Insomnia would be a disturbance of this circadian rhythm, and may be attributable to a pineal gland disorder in some cases. Hypertension, diabetes, and hyperthyroidism would be unrelated to issues with the pineal gland.

12. **A**

William James studied how the mind adapts to the environment and formed the foundation of functionalism. Thus, **(A)** is correct. The remaining wrong answer choices can be ascribed to other scientists. Answer **(B)** describes phrenology, the theory of Franz Gall. Answer **(C)** describes the conclusions of Paul Broca. Answer **(D)** describes one of the conclusions of Sir Charles Sherrington (although we now know that his conclusion was false).

13. **C**

Activity in different regions of the brain is assumed to positively correlate with blood flow. Thus, regions that are more active should have increased blood flow. Changes in blood flow can be measured via fMRI, supporting **(C)** as the preferred methodology. On the other hand, MRI and CT scans are used to image tissues, ruling out **(A)** and **(B)**, and EEGs are useful in measuring broad brain activity and not specific brain regions, eliminating **(D)**.

14. **D**

The Babinski reflex is a primitive reflex that refers to an extension of the big toe accompanied by fanning of the other toes. It is normal in infants, but should disappear with time—certainly by the time a child begins to walk. In a person who is fifty years old, the Babinski reflex would be abnormal. However, despite having a neurological illness, this patient is exhibiting a normal response to the brushing of the foot; that is, the patient is not showing the Babinski reflex.

15. **B**

Motor skills tend to develop from the core toward the periphery. Following objects with the eyes occurs around four weeks of age. The other actions all require movements of the hand, which do not occur in an organized fashion until later.

Consult your online resources for additional practice. **GO ONLINE**

SHARED CONCEPTS

Behavioral Sciences Chapter 2
Sensation and Perception

Behavioral Sciences Chapter 3
Learning and Memory

Behavioral Sciences Chapter 4
Cognition, Consciousness, and Language

Biology Review Chapter 3
Embryogenesis and Development

Biology Review Chapter 4
The Nervous System

Biology Review Chapter 5
The Endocrine System

CHAPTER 2

SENSATION AND PERCEPTION

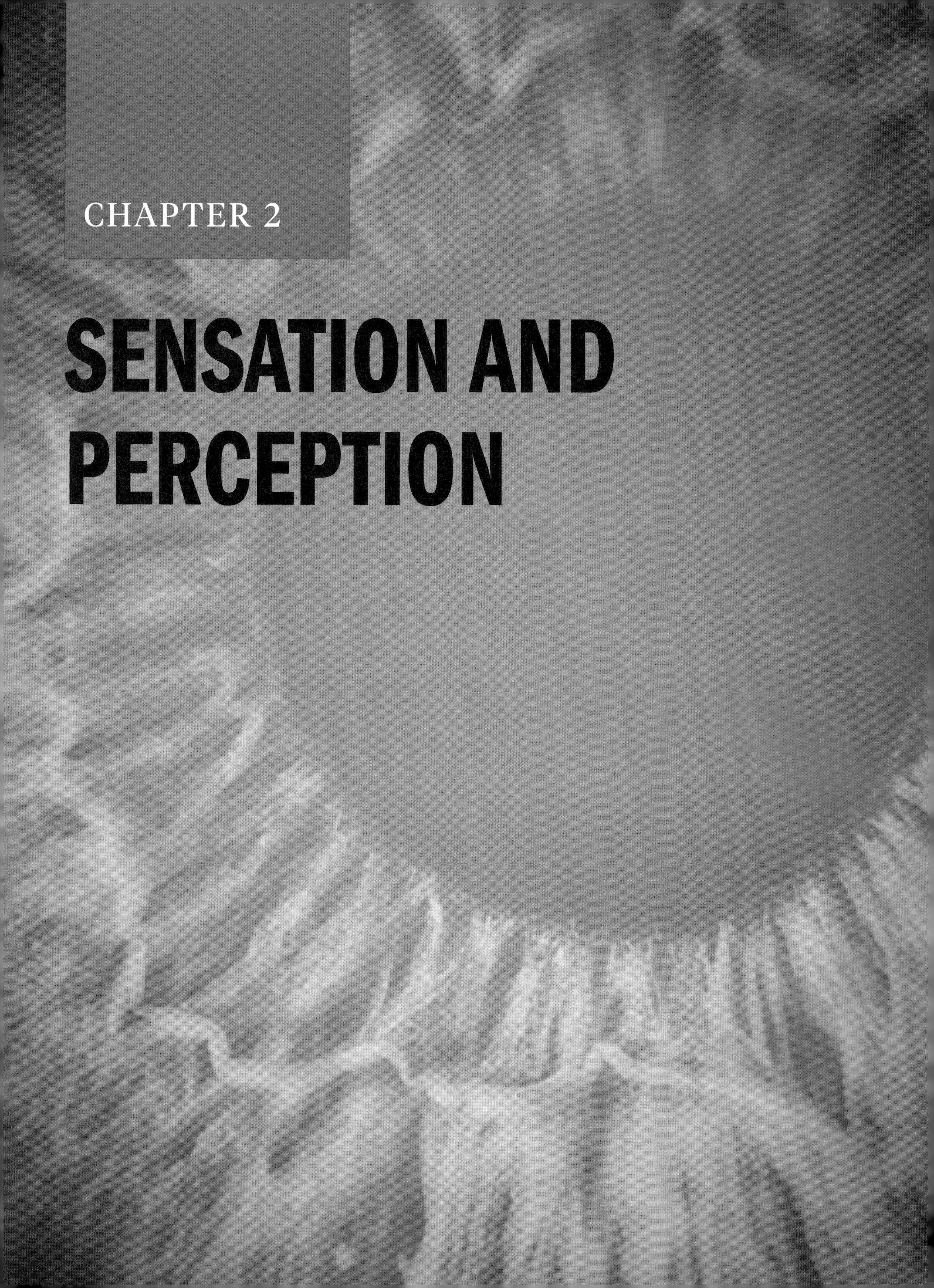

SCIENCE MASTERY ASSESSMENT

Every pre-med knows this feeling: there is so much content I have to know for the MCAT! How do I know what to do first or what's important?

While the high-yield badges throughout this book will help you identify the most important topics, this Science Mastery Assessment is another tool in your MCAT prep arsenal. This quiz (which can also be taken in your online resources) and the guidance below will help ensure that you are spending the appropriate amount of time on this chapter based on your personal strengths and weaknesses. Don't worry though—skipping something now does not mean you'll never study it. Later on in your prep, as you complete full-length tests, you'll uncover specific pieces of content that you need to review and can come back to these chapters as appropriate.

How to Use This Assessment

If you answer 0–7 questions correctly:

Spend about 1 hour to read this chapter in full and take limited notes throughout. Follow up by reviewing **all** quiz questions to ensure that you now understand how to solve each one.

If you answer 8–11 questions correctly:

Spend 20–40 minutes reviewing the quiz questions. Beginning with the questions you missed, read and take notes on the corresponding subchapters. For questions you answered correctly, ensure your thinking matches that of the explanation and you understand why each choice was correct or incorrect.

If you answer 12–15 questions correctly:

Spend less than 20 minutes reviewing all questions from the quiz. If you missed any, then include a quick read-through of the corresponding subchapters, or even just the relevant content within a subchapter, as part of your question review. For questions you answered correctly, ensure your thinking matches that of the explanation and review the Concept Summary at the end of the chapter.

1. A weight lifter is just able to tell the difference between 100 and 125 pounds. According to Weber's law, the lifter would notice a difference between:
   A. 125 and 150 pounds.
   B. 5 and 6 pounds.
   C. 25 and 35 pounds.
   D. 225 and 275 pounds.

2. A person is at a party with a friend. There is loud music in the background and the location is crowded. While listening to the music, the person hears what seems like the friend's laughter and turns around to investigate. The person is exhibiting:
   A. feature detection.
   B. bottom-up processing.
   C. vestibular sense.
   D. signal detection.

3. A person is at a restaurant and orders a spicy entrée. After the first bite, the person experiences burning in the mouth and becomes concerned that the food is too hot. The next few bites are similarly uncomfortable, but after a while the spiciness seems to subside somewhat, and by the end of the meal, the person doesn't notice the spice level. The end of the meal experience is best described as:
   A. adaptation.
   B. signal detection.
   C. a difference threshold.
   D. pain perception.

4. Which sensory receptors send signals in response to tissue damage?
   A. Chemoreceptors
   B. Nociceptors
   C. Osmoreceptors
   D. Photoreceptors

5. Which part of the eye is responsible for gathering and focusing light?
   A. Cornea
   B. Pupil
   C. Iris
   D. Retina

6. A person is looking for change to do laundry and decides to look under the seats of the household car. Even using a flashlight allows no more than an obscured look at the space below. There are various items such as wrappers and papers, but the person sees the glint of silver from an object laying flat and determines it to be a coin. To make this determination, this person used:
   A. signal detection.
   B. sensory adaptation.
   C. feature detection.
   D. kinesthetic sense.

7. Upon which part of the eye are images projected and transduced into electrical signals?
   A. Cornea
   B. Pupil
   C. Retina
   D. Lens

8. The ability to sense stimuli against one's own skin is known as:
   A. somatosensation.
   B. kinesthetic sense.
   C. vestibular sense.
   D. chemoreception.

9. Which of the following is NOT a taste modality?

- **A.** Sweet
- **B.** Floral
- **C.** Savory
- **D.** Bitter

10. Which of the following best describes the difference between endolymph and perilymph?

- **A.** Endolymph is found in the vestibule, while perilymph is found in the cochlea.
- **B.** Endolymph is found in the cochlea, while perilymph is found in the vestibule.
- **C.** Endolymph is found in the membranous labyrinth, while perilymph is found in the bony labyrinth.
- **D.** Endolymph is found in the bony labyrinth, while perilymph is found in the membranous labyrinth.

11. Chemicals that compel behavior after binding with chemoreceptors are known as:

- **A.** pheromones.
- **B.** olfactory receptors.
- **C.** somatostimuli.
- **D.** papillae.

12. Prolonged vitamin B_{12} deficiency can be associated with subacute combined degeneration of the spinal cord. Patients with this disease have difficulty walking because they lose the ability to feel where their feet are in space. This represents a loss of:

- **A.** vestibular sense.
- **B.** kinesthetic sense.
- **C.** parallel processing.
- **D.** feature detection.

13. A person proofreading a paper reads over a long, misspelled word in which an "e" is replaced with an "o." The person does not recognize the error and reads the word as correct. Which of the following could explain why the proofreader read the word as correct?

- **A.** Parallel processing
- **B.** Feature detection
- **C.** Top-down processing
- **D.** Bottom-up processing

14. A corporate logo uses five unconnected angles equally spaced in a circular fashion. When viewed, it appears to be a star. Which of the following is the logo artist using to create a complete pattern to viewers?

- **A.** Bottom-up processing
- **B.** Top-down processing
- **C.** Gate theory
- **D.** Gestalt principles

15. A patient comes in with a tumor of the pituitary gland which has grown upward into the optic chiasm and caused a visual field defect. The most likely defect from compression of the optic chiasm is:

- **A.** complete blindness in one eye.
- **B.** loss of the upper visual fields in both eyes.
- **C.** loss of the nasal visual fields in both eyes.
- **D.** loss of the temporal visual fields in both eyes.

Answer Key

1. **C**
2. **D**
3. **A**
4. **B**
5. **A**
6. **C**
7. **C**
8. **A**
9. **B**
10. **C**
11. **A**
12. **B**
13. **C**
14. **D**
15. **D**

Detailed explanations can be found at the end of the chapter.

CHAPTER 2

SENSATION AND PERCEPTION

In This Chapter

CHAPTER PROFILE

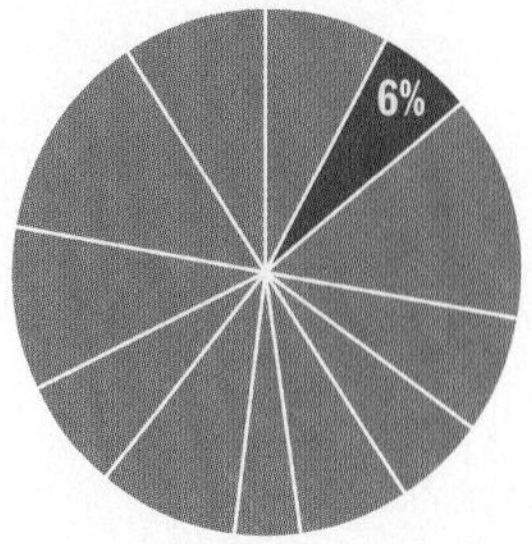

The content in this chapter should be relevant to about 6% of all questions about the behavioral sciences on the MCAT.

This chapter covers material from the following AAMC content category:

6A: Sensing the environment

Introduction

It's your first time visiting a new city. You can't wait to explore the area, try out a new café or restaurant, and see famous landmarks there. You want to take in the sights and sounds of this new place—you want to have a sensory experience. To truly experience any location, your sensory receptors—for vision, hearing, taste, smell, and somatosensation—gather all of the information from the world around you, and your brain filters and processes that information to focus on the most salient details. This activity involves a complex interplay between sensory processes, neural tracts, and the brain itself.

You finally arrive in the new city and begin to explore. You turn the corner on one street and are suddenly overwhelmed with an odd feeling of familiarity. *But . . . I've never been here before!* you think as the strange sensation of *déjà vu* sets in. Everything just seems "right": the signs are in the proper place, the cars look familiar, and everything is bizarrely where you expect it to be. *Déjà vu* (French for "already seen") comes from many sources, including processing information faster than expected. When you process an image (or other sensory input) for the first time, it actually takes longer than the next time you are exposed to that same stimulus. Thus, an exposure to the same scenery at an earlier time through a movie or television show may have primed you for *déjà vu*.

But we don't feel *déjà vu* every time we see an image again; that's where memory comes in—a topic we'll discuss in Chapter 3 of *MCAT Behavioral Sciences Review*. Indeed, this phenomenon of *déjà vu* comes from the brain's sensory receptors saying, *Yes, you have seen this before!* in tandem with the memory system saying, *But I don't know when or where!*

In this chapter, we will focus on the concept of sensation and its associated receptors, including the eyes and hair cells in the ear, as well as perception and the complex brain functions associated with processing sensory information. We'll briefly touch on the other sensory modalities, including vestibular sense, taste, smell, somatosensation, and kinesthetic sense, and consider the roles these senses play in helping us interact with the world.

2.1 Sensation *vs.* Perception

LEARNING OBJECTIVES

After Chapter 2.1, you will be able to:

- Explain the pathway for a stimulus to reach conscious perception
- Connect the common sensory receptors to their functions
- Describe absolute threshold, threshold of conscious perception, and difference threshold
- Explain Weber's law and signal detection theory
- Describe how sensory adaptation affects a difference threshold

In common parlance, we often use the terms "sensation" and "perception" interchangeably, as synonyms. However, in the field of psychology, these two terms have very specific definitions and are commonly contrasted. **Sensation** more appropriately aligns with **transduction**, which means taking the physical, electromagnetic, auditory, and other information from our internal and external environment and converting this information into electrical signals in the nervous system. Sensation is performed by receptors in the peripheral nervous system, which forward the stimuli to the central nervous system in the form of action potentials and neurotransmitters. Sensation can therefore be thought of as a raw signal, which is unfiltered and unprocessed until it enters the central nervous system.

Perception, on the other hand, refers to processing this information within the central nervous system in order to make sense of the information's significance. The complex manipulations involved in perception include both the external sensory experience and the internal activities of the brain and spinal cord. Perception thus helps us make sense of the world. The difference between sensation and perception is key to the challenge of creating artificial intelligence: we can easily create sensors for robots to pick up information from their environment, but teaching them how to comprehend and respond to that information is far more challenging.

Sensory processing is a common topic on the MCAT; you should not only understand the definitions of these terms, but also be able to apply the concepts herein to your own day-to-day sensory experiences.

Sensory Receptors

Sensory receptors are neurons that respond to stimuli by triggering electrical signals that carry information to the central nervous system. Physical objects outside of the body are referred to as **distal stimuli**. These objects often produce photons, sound waves, heat, pressure, or other stimuli that directly interact with sensory receptors; these sensory-stimulating byproducts are called **proximal stimuli**. For example, a campfire is a distal stimulus. The photons that are emitted by the fire, the sounds of crackling and popping, and the energetic gas particles that transfer heat energy are all proximal stimuli. So, proximal stimuli directly interact with and affect the sensory receptors, and thereby inform the observer about the presence of distal stimuli. Sensory receptors may encode multiple aspects of a stimulus. For example, photoreceptors respond to light and can encode not only the brightness of the light, but also its color and shape. The relationship between the physical nature of stimuli and the sensations and perceptions these stimuli evoke is studied in the field of **psychophysics**.

MNEMONIC

Distal = in the **dista**nce

Proximal = in close **proxim**ity

In order to inform the central nervous system, the signals from these stimuli must pass through specific sensory pathways. In each case, different types of receptors—generally nerve endings or specific sensory cells—receive the stimulus, transduce the stimulus into electrical signals, and transmit the data to the central nervous system through sensory ganglia. **Ganglia** are collections of neuron cell bodies found outside the central nervous system. Once transduction from these sensory ganglia occurs, the electrochemical energy is sent along neural pathways to various **projection areas** in the brain, which further analyze the sensory input.

Sensory receptors differ from one sense to another. There are over a dozen recognized sensory receptors, but the MCAT is unlikely to test even half of those. The most heavily tested receptors include:

- Photoreceptors: respond to electromagnetic waves in the visible spectrum (sight)
- Mechanoreceptors: respond to pressure or movement. Hair cells, for example, respond to movement of fluid in the inner ear structures (movement, vibration, hearing, rotational and linear acceleration)
- Nociceptors: respond to painful or noxious stimuli (somatosensation)
- Thermoreceptors: respond to changes in temperature (thermosensation)
- Osmoreceptors: respond to the osmolarity of the blood (water homeostasis)
- Olfactory receptors: respond to volatile compounds (smell)
- Taste receptors: respond to dissolved compounds (taste)

Thresholds

Perception, like sensation, is closely tied to the biology and physiology of interpreting the world around us. However, unlike sensation, perception is inextricably linked to experience as well as to internal and external biases. Sensations are relayed to the brain, which perceives the significance of the stimulus. To illustrate the significance of perception, keep in mind that all sensory information is sent to the central nervous system in the form of action potentials, which the central nervous system must then interpret and act upon. For example, the central nervous system must determine whether incoming action potentials from thermoreceptors are indicating whether an object is hot or is cold, and whether that temperature difference is enough to cause us harm. Moreover, the same sensation can produce radically different perceptions in different people, and because these variations must be explained by central nervous system activity, perception is considered a part of psychology.

MCAT EXPERTISE

On the MCAT, thresholds will frequently be used in conjunction with subjects in studies. Be on the lookout for experimental design questions when thresholds appear in a passage.

A good example of the psychological element of perception is a **threshold**—the minimum amount of a stimulus that renders a difference in perception. For example, the temperature may noticeably change from warm to cool when the sun sets, but subtle fluctuations in temperature throughout the day are generally unnoticeable because they are below the difference threshold. If sound volume increases 10 dB (ten times the sound intensity), the change is usually very obvious; but, if volume increases only 0.1 dB, the change might be too small to detect. There are three main types of thresholds: the absolute threshold, the threshold of conscious perception, and the difference threshold.

KEY CONCEPT

The absolute threshold is the minimum intensity at which a stimulus will be transduced (converted into action potentials).

Absolute Threshold

The **absolute threshold** is the minimum of stimulus energy that is needed to activate a sensory system. This threshold is therefore a threshold in sensation, not in perception. While most human sensory systems are extremely sensitive, all systems also have an absolute threshold below which the stimulus will not be transduced into action potentials, and the information will therefore never be sent to the central nervous system. For example, sounds of extremely low intensity may still cause slight vibrations in the sensory receptors of the inner ear, but these vibrations might not be significant enough to open ion channels linked to these sensory receptors. The absolute threshold for sweet taste is a teaspoon of sucrose dissolved in two gallons of water. On a clear, dark night with no other lights shining, the eye can just detect the light of one candle burning thirty miles away. When we are talking about an absolute threshold, we're talking about how bright, loud, or intense a stimulus must be before it is sensed.

BRIDGE

You may already know one of the absolute thresholds from the discussion of sound in Chapter 7 of *MCAT Physics and Math Review*. Remember that $I_0\ (10^{-12}\frac{\text{W}}{\text{m}^2})$ in the equation for sound level is the absolute threshold of normal human hearing.

Threshold of Conscious Perception

It is possible for sensory systems to send signals to the central nervous system without a person perceiving these signals. This lack of conscious perception may be because the stimulus is too subtle to demand our attention, or may last for too brief a duration for the brain to fully process the information. The level of intensity that a stimulus must pass in order to be consciously perceived by the brain is the **threshold of conscious perception**. By way of contrast, information that is received by the central nervous system but that does not cross this threshold is called **subliminal perception**. Note the difference between the absolute threshold and the threshold for conscious perception: a stimulus below the absolute threshold will not be transduced, and thus never reaches the central nervous system. A stimulus below the threshold of conscious perception arrives at the central nervous system, but does not reach the higher-order

REAL WORLD

The Latin word for "thresholds" is *limina*. Hence, something that is "subliminal" is literally "below threshold." The threshold referred to in the term "subliminal perception" is the threshold of conscious perception. So, signals that are "subliminal" are strong enough to pass the absolute threshold, but not strong enough to pass the threshold of conscious perception.

brain regions that control attention and consciousness. Contrary to common thinking, there is actually little practical value to using subliminal perception to sell products.

Difference Threshold

A third commonly studied threshold is the **difference threshold**, sometimes called the **just-noticeable difference (jnd)** between two stimuli. The difference threshold refers to the minimum change in magnitude required for an observer to perceive that two different stimuli are, in fact, different. If the difference between stimuli is below the difference threshold, the two stimuli will seem to the observer to be the same. For example, imagine two sound waves are played one after the other, the first having frequency 440 Hz and then the second having frequency 441 Hz. These sounds are different. But without formal ear training, most individuals cannot hear the difference. In this range of sound frequencies, the just-noticeable difference for most listeners is about 3 Hz. So, for the average person to hear a difference in pitch, the sound waves need to be 440 Hz and 443 Hz. Below this difference threshold, the two pitches will sound the same.

The previous example illustrates one common experimental technique researchers use to explore the difference threshold. The technique is called psychophysical discrimination testing, or sometimes just **discrimination testing**. In a common discrimination testing experiment, a participant is presented with a stimulus. The stimulus is then varied slightly and researchers ask the participant to report whether they perceive a change. Often, the difference continues to be increased until the participant reports they notice the change, and this interval is recorded as the just noticeable difference.

Returning to the example of two sounds: The difference between a 440 Hz sound and a 443 Hz sound is just noticeable for most people. But, by using discrimination testing, researchers have discovered that the absolute difference (3 Hz, in this case) is far less important than the percent difference. For this reason, the just noticeable difference is usually reported as a fraction or a percent. To compute this percent, divide the change in stimulus by the magnitude of the original stimulus. In our example, we would compute 3 Hz / 440 Hz = 0.0068 = 0.68%. To illustrate why percentages are used, consider a 1000 Hz sound. An increase of 0.68% results in a sound of frequency 1007 Hz. So, to the average person, the difference in pitch from 1000 Hz to 1007 Hz would be just noticeable. By contrast, the difference from 1000 Hz to 1003 Hz would not be noticeable. While a 3 Hz difference was noticeable in the lower frequency range, that same 3 Hz difference is not noticeable in the higher frequency range.

Ernst Heinrich Weber (1795–1878) is often credited with the observation that difference thresholds are proportional and must be computed as percentages. This idea is therefore often called **Weber's law**. Weber's law applies to the perception of a number of senses, including the perception of loudness and pitch of sounds, the perception of brightness of light, and the perception of weight of objects.

MCAT EXPERTISE

When the MCAT brings up Weber's law, questions will usually give a numerical relationship and then ask for it to be applied; typically, the solution simply amounts to applying a ratio.

Signal Detection Theory

Perception of stimuli can also be affected by nonsensory factors, such as experiences (memory), motives, and expectations. **Signal detection theory** studies how internal (psychological) and external (environmental) factors influence thresholds of sensation and perception. For example, how loud would someone need to yell your name in a crowd to get your attention? The answer depends on environmental factors, like the size of the crowd; social factors, like the makeup of the crowd and your comfort with the individuals around you; psychological factors, like whether or not you are expecting to have your name called; and personality factors, like your level of introversion or extroversion. In signal detection theory, these factors are treated like independent variables. For example, researchers can measure how likely a person is to hear their name called when the person is informed that at some point their name will be called, versus when the person is left uninformed.

A basic signal detection experiment consists of many trials; during each trial, a stimulus (signal) may or may not be presented. Trials in which the signal is presented are called **noise trials**, whereas those in which the signal is not presented are called **catch trials**. After each trial, the subject is asked to indicate whether or not a signal was presented. There are therefore four possible outcomes for each trial, as illustrated in Figure 2.1. A **hit** is a trial in which the signal is presented and the subject correctly perceives the signal; a **miss** is a trial in which the subject fails to perceive the presented signal. A **false alarm** is a trial in which the subject indicates perceiving the signal, even though the signal was not presented; a **correct negative** is a trial in which the subject correctly identifies that no signal was presented. By tracking the rates of these various outcomes, researchers are able to identify factors that influence perception.

Subject's Response

	"Yes"	"No"
Signal Present	Hit	Miss
Signal Absent	False alarm	Correct negative

Figure 2.1 Possible Outcomes from a Signal Detection Experiment Trial

REAL WORLD

On the surface, signal detection experiments would appear to be easy tasks—shouldn't individuals easily be able to tell if they perceived something or not? However, consider the thought processes that occur when you're quietly studying in the library with your phone on silent and you suddenly think you may have heard a buzz. *Is my phone ringing?* you wonder. You freeze in place and wait for another buzz; even if it doesn't come, you may still be so convinced you heard a signal that you still check your phone. Perception is not a passive matter!

Adaptation

Our ability to detect a stimulus can change over time through **adaptation**. Adaptation can have both a physiological (sensory) component and a psychological (perceptual) component. For example, the pupils of the eyes will dilate in the dark and constrict in the light, which illustrates physiological adaptation. Similarly, in loud environments, small muscles in the middle ear will reflexively contract in order to dampen the vibration of the ossicles, reducing sound intensity. We also adapt to somatosensory stimuli; cold water no longer seems so cold once our bodies "get used to it." Once we're dressed, we stop feeling the clothes on our bodies until we have a reason to think about them. Adaptation is one way the mind and body try to focus attention on only the most relevant stimuli, which are usually changes in the environment around us.

MCAT CONCEPT CHECK 2.1

Before you move on, assess your understanding of the material with these questions.

1. What is the pathway for a stimulus to reach conscious perception?

____

2. Match each sensory receptor to its function:

1. Hair cell	A. Sense painful or bothersome physical stimuli
2. Nociceptor	B. Sense changes in temperature
3. Olfactory receptor	C. Sense electromagnetic radiation in the visible range
4. Osmoreceptor	D. Sense changes in blood concentration
5. Photoreceptor	E. Sense volatile chemicals
6. Taste receptor	F. Sense motion of fluid in the inner ear
7. Thermoreceptor	G. Sense dissolved chemicals

3. For each of the thresholds below, provide a brief description:
   - Absolute threshold:

   ____

   - Threshold of conscious perception:

   ____

   - Difference threshold:

   ____

4. What aspect of thresholds do Weber's law and signal detection theory focus on?
   - Weber's law:

   ____

   - Signal detection theory:

   ____

5. How does sensory adaptation affect a difference threshold?

____

2.2 Vision

High-Yield

LEARNING OBJECTIVES

After Chapter 2.2, you will be able to:

- List the functions of the parts of the eye, including the cornea, pupil, iris, ciliary body, canal of Schlemm, lens, retina, and sclera
- Describe parallel processing
- Identify the cell types responsible for color, shape, and motion detection
- Recall the structures in the visual pathway:

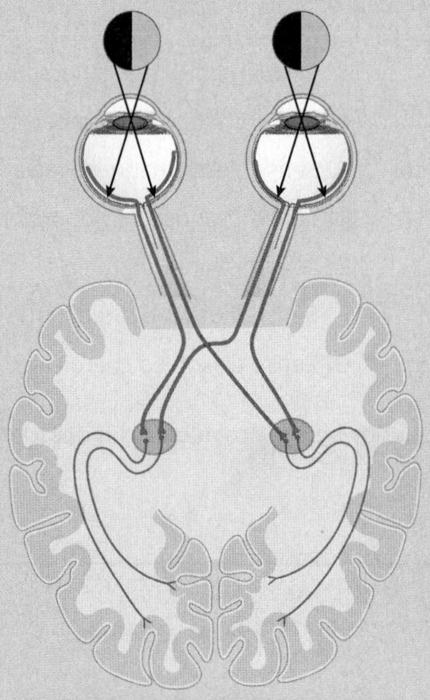

Vision is a highly adapted sense in human beings. With the ability to sense brightness, color, shape, and movement, and then to integrate this information to create a cohesive three-dimensional model of the world, the visual pathways are extremely important to everyday life. In fact, vision is the only sense to which an entire lobe of the brain is devoted: the occipital lobe. While some individuals experience vision differently, such as those who are color deficient or partially sighted, the MCAT focuses primarily on the details of unimpaired vision.

Structure and Function of the Eye

The anatomy of the eye is shown in Figure 2.2.

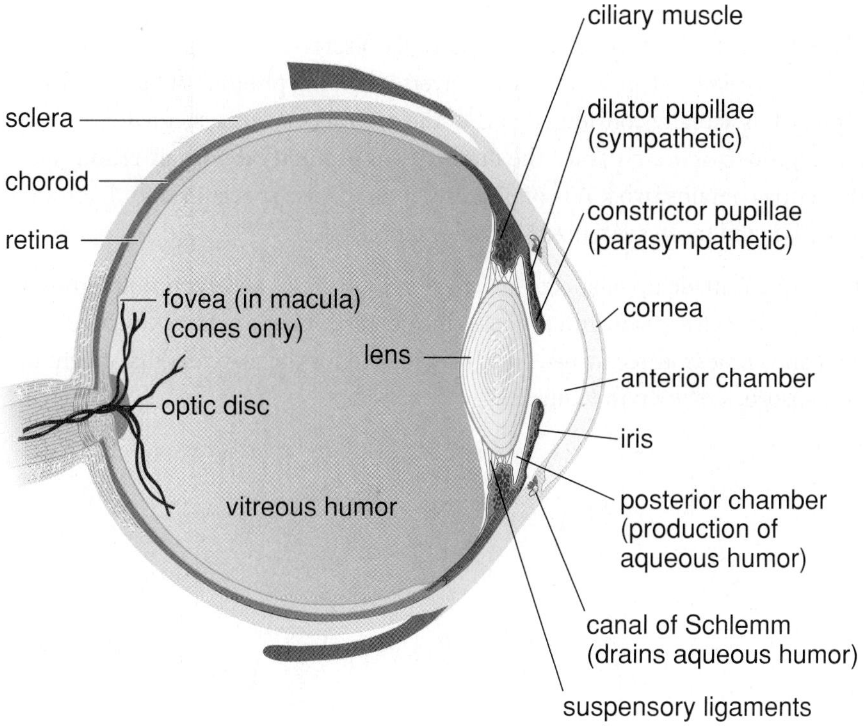

Figure 2.2 Anatomy of the Eye

The eye is a specialized organ used to detect light in the form of photons. Most of the exposed portion of the eye is covered by a thick structural layer known as the **sclera**, or the white of the eye. The sclera does not cover the frontmost portion of the eye, the cornea. The eye is supplied with nutrients by two sets of blood vessels: the **choroidal vessels**, a complex intermingling of blood vessels between the sclera and the retina, and the **retinal vessels**. The innermost layer of the eye is the **retina**, which contains the actual photoreceptors that transduce light into electrical information the brain can process.

When entering the eye, light passes first through the **cornea**, a clear, domelike window in the front of the eye, which gathers and focuses the incoming light. The front of the eye is divided into the **anterior chamber**, which lies in front of the iris, and the **posterior chamber** between the iris and the lens. The **iris**, which is the colored part of the eye, is composed of two muscles: the **dilator pupillae**, which opens the pupil under sympathetic stimulation; and the **constrictor pupillae**, which constricts the pupil under parasympathetic stimulation. The iris is continuous with the **choroid**, which is a vascular layer of connective tissue that surrounds and provides nourishment to the retina. The iris is also continuous with the the **ciliary body**, which produces the **aqueous humor** that bathes the front part of the eye before draining into the **canal of Schlemm**. The **lens** lies right behind the iris and helps control the refraction of the incoming light. Contraction of the **ciliary muscle**, a component of the ciliary body, is under parasympathetic control. As the muscle contracts, it pulls on the **suspensory ligaments** and changes the shape of the lens to focus on an image as the distance varies, a phenomenon known as **accommodation**. Behind the lens lies the **vitreous humor**, a transparent gel that supports the retina.

The **retina** is in the back of the eye and is like a screen consisting of neural elements and blood vessels. Its function is to convert incoming photons of light to electrical signals. It is actually considered part of the central nervous system and develops as an outgrowth of brain tissue. The **duplexity** or **duplicity theory of vision** states that the retina contains two kinds of photoreceptors: those specialized for light-and-dark detection and those specialized for color detection.

The retina is made up of approximately 6 million cones and 120 million rods. **Cones** are used for color vision and to sense fine details. Cones are most effective in bright light and come in three forms, which are named for the wavelengths of light they best absorb, as shown in Figure 2.3.

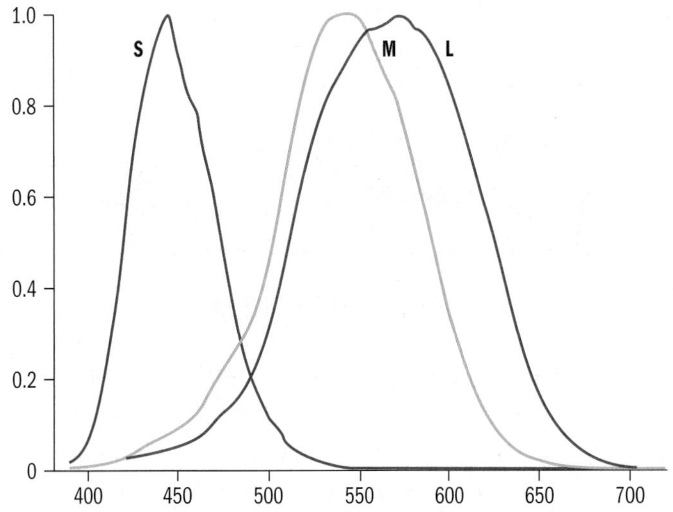

Figure 2.3 Relative Absorption of the Three Types of Cones at Different Wavelengths
The cones are named for the wavelengths at which they have highest light absorption: short (S, also called blue), medium (M, green), and long (L, red).

MNEMONIC

Cones are for **c**olor vision. **Rods** function best in "**rod**uced" light.

In reduced illumination, **rods** are more functional than cones because each rod cell is highly sensitive to photons and is somewhat easier to stimulate than a cone cell. In part, the sensitivity of rods has to do with the fact that all rods contain only a single pigment type called **rhodopsin**. In general, color vision requires far more light because each cone responds only to certain wavelengths of light. By contrast, a rod can be stimulated by light of any color. However, while rods permit vision in reduced light, the tradeoff is that rods only allow sensation of light and dark. Also, even though individual rods are highly sensitive to light, as a whole they are less useful for detecting fine details because rods are spread over a much larger area of the retina.

While there are many more rods than cones in the human eye, the central section of the retina, called the **macula**, has a high concentration of cones; in fact, the center-most region of the macula, called the **fovea**, contains only cones. As one moves further away from the fovea, the concentration of rods increases while the concentration of cones decreases. Therefore, visual acuity is best at the fovea, and the fovea is most sensitive in normal daylight vision. Some distance away from the center of the retina, the optic nerve leaves the eye. This region of the retina, which is devoid of photoreceptors, is called the optic disk, and gives rise to a **blind spot**, as shown in Figure 2.4.

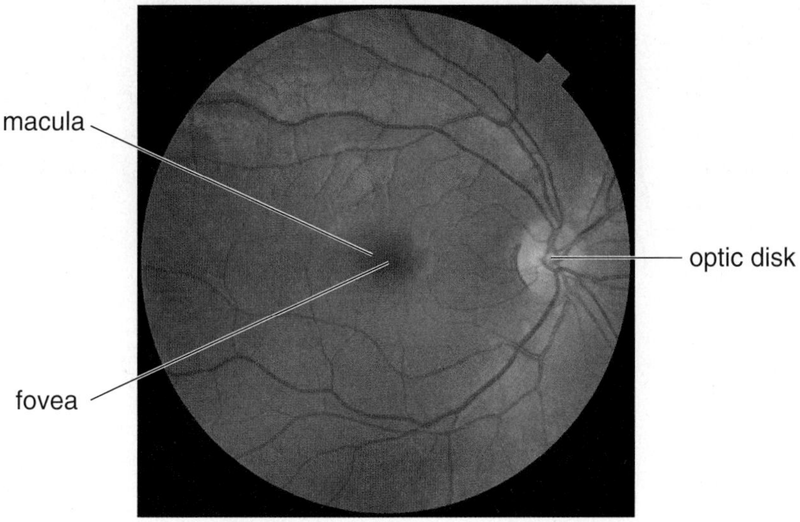

Figure 2.4 Specialized Regions of the Retina

Rods and cones are specialized neurons and, like most neurons, connect with other neurons through synapses. However, rods and cones do not connect directly to the optic nerve. Rather, there are several layers of neurons in between, as shown in Figure 2.5. Rods and cones synapse directly with **bipolar cells**, which highlight gradients between adjacent rods or cones. Bipolar cells then synapse with **ganglion cells**, the axons of which group together to form the **optic nerve**. These bipolar and ganglion cells not only fall "in between" the rods and cones and the optic nerve, but also the bipolar and ganglion cells are actually located in front of the rods and cones, closer to the front of the eye. This arrangement means that a photon must actually navigate past several layers of cells to reach the rods and cones at the "back" of the retina; the information is then transmitted "forward" (in the form of action potentials) from the rod and cone cells until the signal reaches the ganglion cells. Observe in Figure 2.5 that there are significantly more photoreceptor cells than ganglion cells, so the output from each ganglion cell represents the combined activity of many rods and cones. The result is a pruning of details as information from the photoreceptors is combined. As the number of receptors that converge through the bipolar neurons onto one ganglion cell increases, the resolution decreases. On average, the number of cones converging onto an individual ganglion cell is smaller than for rods. This arrangement helps explain why color vision has a greater sensitivity to fine detail than black-and-white vision does.

Also shown in Figure 2.5 are **amacrine** and **horizontal cells**, which receive input from multiple retinal cells in the same area before the information is passed on to ganglion cells. Amacrine and horizontal cells can thereby accentuate slight differences between the visual information in each bipolar cell. For example, these cells are important for edge detection, as they increase our perception of contrasts.

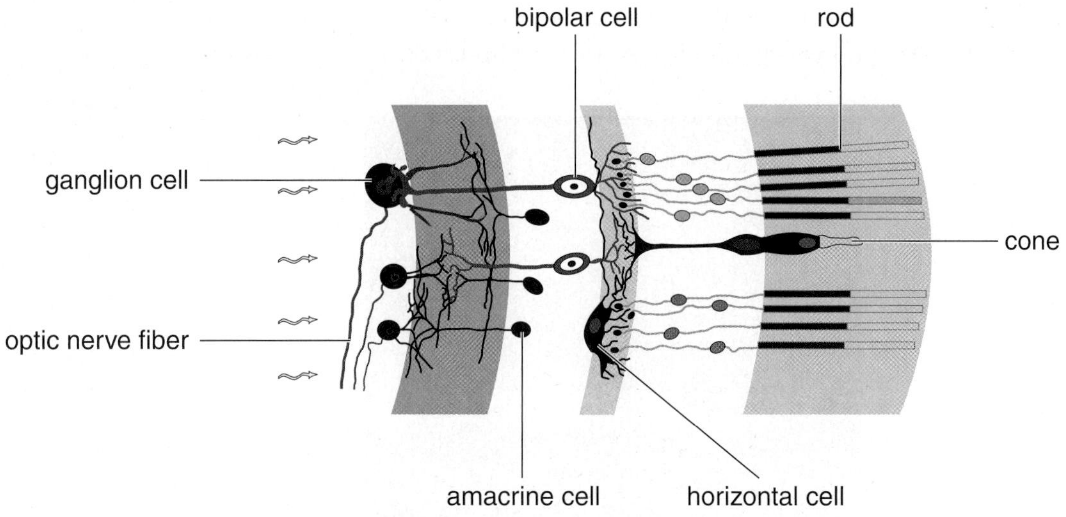

Figure 2.5 Cells of the Retina

Visual Pathways

Visual pathways refer to both the anatomical connections between the eyes and brain and to the flow of visual information along these connections. These pathways are illustrated in Figure 2.6. The terminology for these pathways can seem confusing. So here is a simple rule of thumb to start: If an object is to your left, then photons from that object stimulate the right side of the retina in each eye. To help visualize this result, look at Figure 2.6. In this figure, an object to your left is represented by the black patches. Photons from that object enter each eye and stimulate the retinal fibers that are illustrated using the color orange. This result is due to simple geometry! If an object is to your left, then photons from that object must travel to the right to reach your eyes, and in so doing, these photons enter your eyes and continue travelling to the right, thereby stimulating the right side of each of your eyes' retinas. From there, retinal fibers from each eye project to the right side of your brain. All of this leads to a famous result: Visual information from objects to your left is processed by the right side of your brain. Similarly, if an object is to your right (the blue patches in the figure), then photons from this object stimulate the left side of each retina (the green nerves), and this visual data is sent to the left side of your brain.

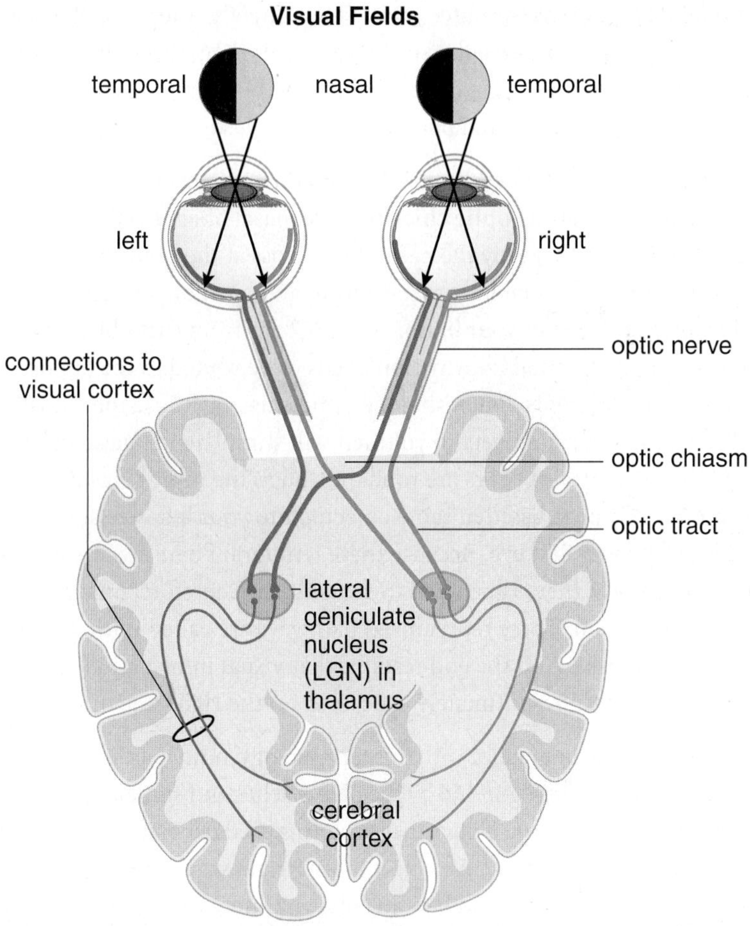

Figure 2.6 Visual Pathways

To help describe these phenomena with more specificity, scientists use the terms **temporal** and **nasal retinal fibers**. Here's an example. Consider an object to your left, which, again, is represented in Figure 2.6 by the black patches. In each eye, photons from this object strike the retinal fibers that are illustrated in Figure 2.6 using the color orange. But notice: In the right eye, those orange fibers are on the lateral side of the retina, closer to your temple, and so these fibers are called the temporal fibers of the right eye. In the left eye, the orange fibers are medial, closer to your nose, and so are called the nasal fibers of the left eye.

Scientists also describe the placement of the object in space, relative to your eyes, using the terms "temporal" and "nasal," but now referring to the **temporal** and **nasal visual fields**. Again, this terminology is best explained by example. Imagine an object is a little to your left. Then photons from that object must cross in front of your nose in order to reach your right eye. So, this object is described as being in the nasal field of your right eye. Think carefully about what happens to these photons next. They enter your right eye, continue heading to the right, and ultimately strike the temporal fibers on the right side of your right eye. Pay close attention to the terminology: We're saying that an object in the *nasal field* of the right eye stimulates the *temporal fibers* of that eye! This mixing of terminology—nasal field stimulates temporal fibers—illustrates the crossing over of visual information. By contrast, for that same object, which, remember, is

MNEMONIC

If photons from an object would need to cross your nose to reach your eye (or if the object is right in front of your nose) then the object is said to be in the nasal visual field for that eye.

spatially to your left, photons can enter your left eye directly. Therefore, this object is described as being in the temporal field of your left eye. Then, these photons strike the nasal fibers of the left eye. So again, there is mixing of the terminology—the object is in the *temporal field* of the left eye, and photons strike the *nasal fibers* of the left eye.

As the retinal fibers from each eye travel through the optic nerves toward the brain, a significant event occurs at the **optic chiasm**. Here, nasal fibers from the left and right eyes cross paths. Notice that only the nasal fibers cross at the optic chiasm. Again, an example helps illustrate: Visual information from an object to your left is ultimately processed by the right side of your brain. So if photons from that object are captured by the left eye, then this visual information needs to be routed to the opposite side of your brain. That routing is done using the optic chiasm. To use the "nasal" and "temporal" terminology: An object to your left will stimulate the nasal fibers of your left eye, and then these nasal fibers are routed through the optic chiasm to the right side of your brain. By contrast, that same object, off to your left, will stimulate the temporal fibers of your right eye. Because these temporal fibers are already on the right side of your body, there is no need to cross them. Therefore, only nasal fibers cross at the optic chiasm. These reorganized pathways are called **optic tracts** after leaving the optic chiasm. And the end result is that visual information emanating from an object to your left is ultimately processed on the right side of your brain.

MNEMONIC

For each eye, the temporal visual field stimulates the nasal retinal fibers. The nasal visual field stimulates the temporal retinal fibers.

To summarize, and to gain practice with this terminology, now consider an object off to your right, represented in Figure 2.6 by the blue patches and stimulating the fibers illustrated using the color green. Notice that the terms used depend on which eye is considered. Let's start with the left eye. An object to your right would be in the nasal field of your left eye, because photons would have to cross your nose to reach your left eye. These photons would stimulate the temporal fibers of the left eye—nasal field stimulates temporal fibers. Then, because these temporal fibers are already on the left side of your body, they would be routed directly back to the left side of your brain. Now consider the right eye. An object spatially to your right is in the temporal field of your right eye, and stimulates the nasal fibers of that eye. Then, in order to bring this visual information to the left side of your brain, these nasal fibers are routed through the optic chiasm. Through all of this, keep these two trends in mind: First, the temporal field of each eye stimulates the nasal fibers of each eye, and vice versa. Second, the nasal fibers cross at the optic chiasm.

REAL WORLD

When there is a sudden, bright flash of light, the superior colliculus aligns the eyes with the likely stimulus. In other words, it's the superior colliculus (as well as the sympathetic nervous system) that gives us the "deer in the headlights" appearance during the startle response.

From the optic chiasm, the information goes to several different places in the brain: some nerve fibers pass to the **lateral geniculate nucleus (LGN)** of the **thalamus** where they synapse with nerves that then pass through radiations in the temporal and parietal lobes to the **visual cortex** in the **occipital lobe**. This connectivity makes sense because the thalamus is a well-known connecting and routing center of the forebrain. Other nerve fibers branch off from the optic tracts, skip the thalamus, and head directly to the **superior colliculi** in the midbrain, which control some reflexive responses to visual stimuli and reflexive eye movements.

Processing

The ability to sense light information in the environment around us is useful in its own right. But, to effectively interact with the environment, we must also be able to make sense of visual stimuli. The connections between optic tract, LGN, and visual cortex help create a cohesive image of the world through a phenomenon known as parallel processing. Visual **parallel processing** is the brain's ability to analyze information regarding color, form, motion, and depth simultaneously, i.e. "in parallel," using independent pathways in the brain. For example, most people can quickly and easily recognize a moving car from a distance. The speed of recognition is facilitated, in part, by the fact that the form of the car (i.e. its shape) and the motion of the car are processed simultaneously in separate, parallel pathways in the brain.

Now let's explore where each of these four aspects of vision is processed and the specialized cells that contribute to their detection. As described previously, cones are responsible for our perception of color. **Form** refers not only to the shape of an object, but also our ability to discriminate an object of interest from the background by detecting its boundaries. Neurons carrying information from the fovea and surrounding central portion of the retina synapse with **parvocellular cells** in the lateral geniculate nucleus. These cells have very high color **spatial resolution**; that is, these cells permit us to detect very fine detail when thoroughly examining an object. However, parvocellular cells can only work with stationary or slow-moving objects because these cells have very low **temporal resolution**.

Conversely, **magnocellular cells** are well-suited for detecting motion because these cells have very high temporal resolution. Reflecting the fact that form and motion are processed in parallel, magnocellular cells and parvocellular cells are located in distinct layers of the lateral geniculate nucleus. Also, magnocellular cells predominantly receive inputs from the periphery of our vision, allowing more rapid detection of objects approaching us from the sides. However, magnocellular cells have low spatial resolution, so much of the rich detail of an object can no longer be seen once the object is motion. Magnocellular cells therefore provide a blurry but moving image of an object.

MNEMONIC

Magnocellular cells specialize in **m**otion detection.

Depth perception, our ability to discriminate the three-dimensional shape of our environment and judge the distance of objects within it, is largely based on discrepancies between the inputs the brain receives from our two eyes (more on this to follow in *MCAT Behavioral Sciences Review*, Section 2.5, Object Recognition). Specialized cells in the visual cortex known as **binocular neurons** are responsible for comparing the inputs to each hemisphere and detecting these differences.

Finally, our brains wouldn't be very good at processing visual information if they didn't learn to associate certain patterns of stimuli with expected behaviors or outcomes. To assist in this, a whole slew of even more specialized cells called **feature detectors** exist in the visual cortex. Each feature detector cell type detects a very particular, individual feature of an object in the visual field. For example, if we were to look at a stop sign we would activate: a feature detector for the color red, while another feature detector would respond to the white border and letters. Yet another type of feature detector would recognize the horizontal lines, while still others would be activated by the angled lines of the octagon. Rather than needing to individually process each of these features every time, the overall combination of feature detectors become activated in parallel. Finally, our response to the stop sign, i.e. to STOP, also is stored for future retrieval.

MCAT CONCEPT CHECK 2.2

Before you move on, assess your understanding of the material with these questions.

1. List the functions of the various parts of the eye:
   - Cornea:
   - Pupil:
   - Iris:
   - Ciliary body:
   - Canal of Schlemm:
   - Lens:
   - Retina:
   - Sclera:
2. List the structures in the visual pathway, from where light enters the cornea to the visual projection areas in the brain.
3. What is parallel processing?

4. In feature detection, what type of cells are responsible for color? Form? Motion? Depth?
   - Color:
   - Form:
   - Motion:
   - Depth:

2.3 Hearing and Vestibular Sense

LEARNING OBJECTIVES

After Chapter 2.3, you will be able to:

- Identify the structures used to detect linear acceleration and rotational acceleration
- Explain how the structural features of the cochlea and the hair cells are able to transmit information about pitch of an incoming sound to the brain
- List the structures in the auditory pathway

The ear is a complex organ responsible not only for our sense of hearing, but also for our **vestibular sense**, which is our ability to both detect rotational and linear acceleration and to use this information to inform our sense of balance and spatial orientation. These senses are critically important to our ability to get around in the world, and their associated structures are encased in some of the densest bone of the body to protect these structures from damage. While recognizing that individuals can differ in their hearing and vestibular senses, as with vision, the MCAT primarily focuses on the standard healthy operations of these senses.

Structure and Function of the Ear

The ear is divided into three parts, as shown in Figure 2.7: the outer, middle, and inner ear. A sound wave first reaches the cartilaginous outside part of the ear, called the **pinna** or **auricle**. The main function of the pinna is to channel sound waves into the **external auditory canal**, which directs the sound waves to the **tympanic membrane (eardrum)**. The membrane vibrates in phase with the incoming sound waves. The frequency of the sound wave determines the rate at which the tympanic membrane vibrates: it moves back and forth at a high rate for high-frequency sounds and more slowly for low-frequency sounds. Louder sounds have greater **intensity**, which corresponds to an increased amplitude of vibration.

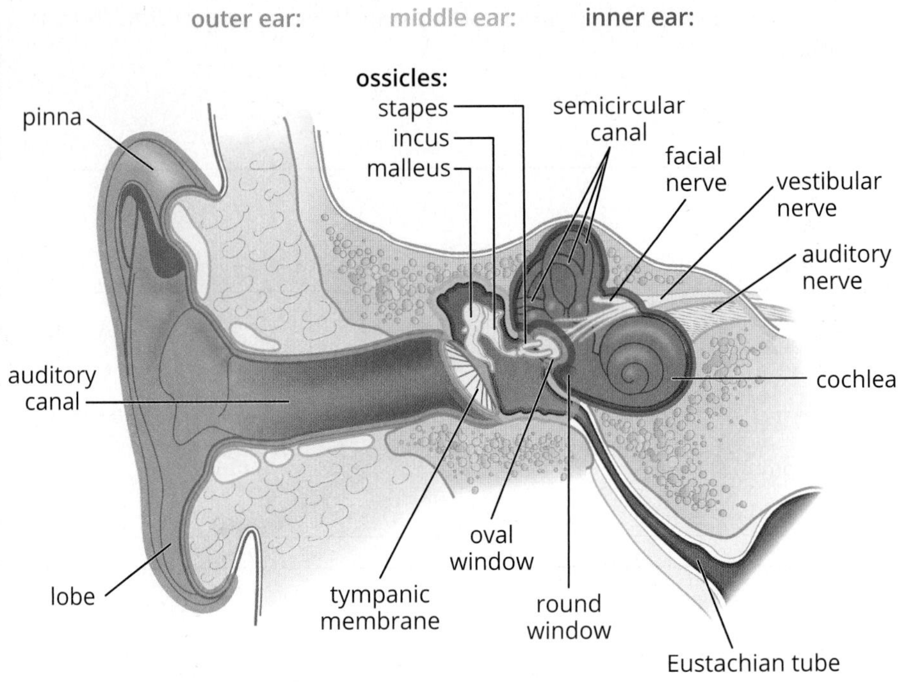

Figure 2.7 Anatomy of the Ear

BRIDGE

Remember that sound is a longitudinal wave carried through air (or another medium), which causes displacement of particles parallel to the axis of sound propagation. In other words, when a sound wave hits your eardrum, it literally causes it to oscillate back and forth because of moving air particles. Sound is discussed in Chapter 7 of *MCAT Physics and Math Review*.

The tympanic membrane divides the outer ear from the middle ear. The middle ear houses the three smallest bones in the body, called **ossicles**. The ossicles help transmit and amplify the vibrations from the tympanic membrane to the inner ear. The **malleus** (**hammer**) is affixed to the tympanic membrane; it acts on the **incus** (**anvil**), which acts on the **stapes** (**stirrup**). The baseplate of the stapes rests on the oval window of the cochlea, which is the entrance to the inner ear. The middle ear is connected to the nasal cavity via the **Eustachian tube**, which helps equalize pressure between the middle ear and the environment.

The inner ear sits within a **bony labyrinth**, which is a hollow region of the temporal bone containing the cochlea, vestibule, and semicircular canals, as shown in Figure 2.8. Inside the bony labyrinth rests a continuous collection of tubes and chambers called the **membranous labyrinth**. This collection of structures contains receptors for the sense of equilibrium and hearing. The membranous labyrinth is filled by a potassium-rich fluid called **endolymph**, and is suspended within the bony labyrinth by a thin layer of another fluid called perilymph. **Perilymph** simultaneously transmits vibrations from the outside world and cushions the inner ear structures.

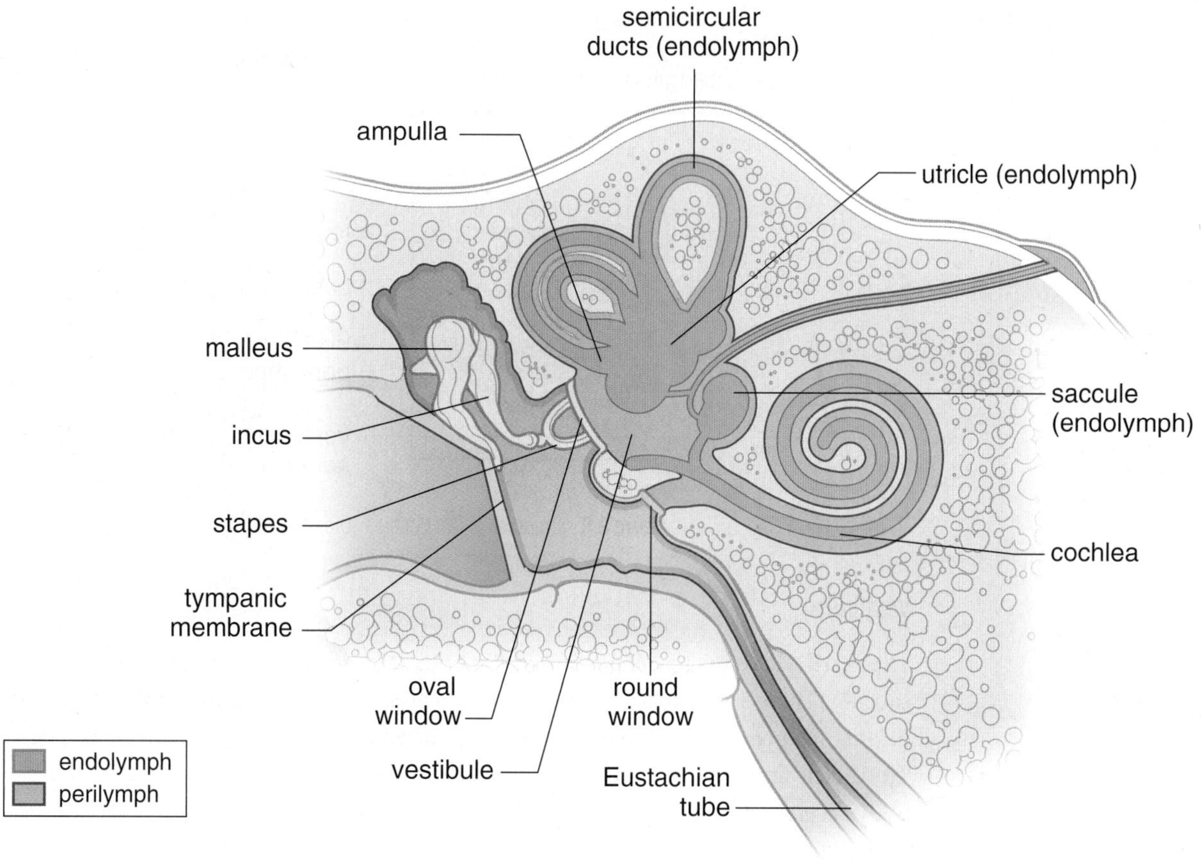

Figure 2.8 The Membranous and Bony Labyrinth
The membranous labyrinth is filled with endolymph (blue); it is suspended within the bony labyrinth, which is filled with perilymph (purple).

Cochlea

The **cochlea** is a spiral-shaped organ that contains the receptors for hearing; it is divided into three parts called **scalae**, as shown in Figure 2.9. All three scalae run the entire length of the cochlea. The middle scala houses the actual hearing apparatus, called the **organ of Corti**, which rests on a thin, flexible membrane called the **basilar membrane**. The organ of Corti is composed of thousands of hair cells, which are bathed in endolymph. On top of the organ of Corti is a relatively immobile membrane called the **tectorial membrane**. The other two scalae, filled with perilymph, surround the hearing apparatus and are continuous with the oval and round windows of the cochlea. Thus, sound entering the cochlea through the oval window causes vibrations in perilymph, which are transmitted to the basilar membrane. Because fluids are essentially incompressible, the **round window**, a membrane-covered hole in the cochlea, permits the perilymph to actually move within the cochlea. Like the rods and cones of the eye, the hair cells in the organ of Corti transduce the physical stimulus into an electrical signal, which is carried to the central nervous system by the **auditory** (**vestibulocochlear**) **nerve**.

BRIDGE

The junction between the stapes and the oval window is extremely similar to a thermodynamic gas-piston system, as described in Chapter 3 of *MCAT Physics and Math Review*. However, fluids are not as compressible as gases; therefore, the round window must be present to allow the perilymph in the cochlea to actually move back and forth with the stapedial footplate.

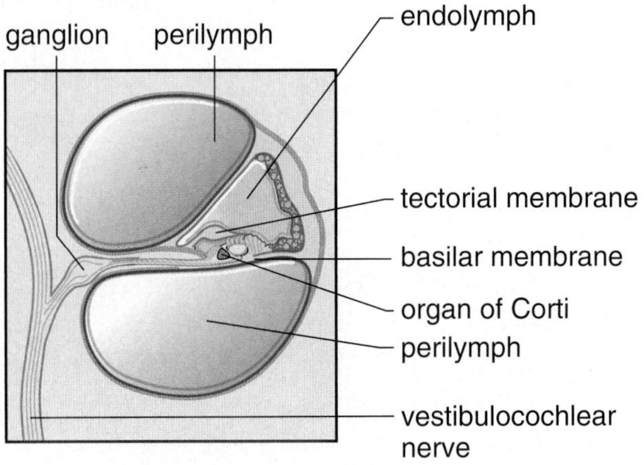

Figure 2.9 Structure of the Cochlea (Cross-Section)

Vestibule

The **vestibule** refers to the portion of the bony labyrinth that contains the **utricle** and **saccule**. These structures are sensitive to linear acceleration, so are used as part of the balancing apparatus and to determine one's orientation in three-dimensional space. The utricle and saccule contain modified hair cells covered with **otoliths**. As the body accelerates, these otoliths will resist that motion. This bends and stimulates the underlying hair cells, which send a signal to the brain.

Semicircular Canals

While the utricle and saccule are sensitive to linear acceleration, the three **semicircular canals** are sensitive to rotational acceleration. The semicircular canals are arranged perpendicularly to each other, and each ends in a swelling called an **ampulla**, where hair cells are located. When the head rotates, endolymph in the semicircular canal resists this motion, bending the underlying hair cells, which send a signal to the brain.

MNEMONIC

The **l**ateral geniculate nucleus (**L**GN) is for **l**ight; the **m**edial geniculate nucleus (**M**GN) is for **m**usic.

Auditory Pathways

The **auditory pathways** in the brain are a bit more complex than the visual pathways. Most sound information passes through the vestibulocochlear nerve to the brainstem, where it ascends to the **medial geniculate nucleus** (**MGN**) of the thalamus. From there, nerve fibers project to the **auditory cortex** in the temporal lobe for sound processing. Some information is also sent to the **superior olive**, which localizes the sound, and the **inferior colliculus**, which is involved in the startle reflex and helps keep the eyes fixed on a point while the head is turned (vestibulo–ocular reflex).

Hair Cells

Hair cells are named for the long tufts of **stereocilia** on their top surface, shown in Figure 2.10. As vibrations reach the basilar membrane underlying the organ of Corti, the stereocilia adorning the hair cells begin to sway back and forth within the endolymph. The swaying causes the opening of ion channels, which cause a receptor potential. Certain hair cells are also directly connected to the immobile tectorial membrane; these hair cells are involved in amplifying the incoming sound.

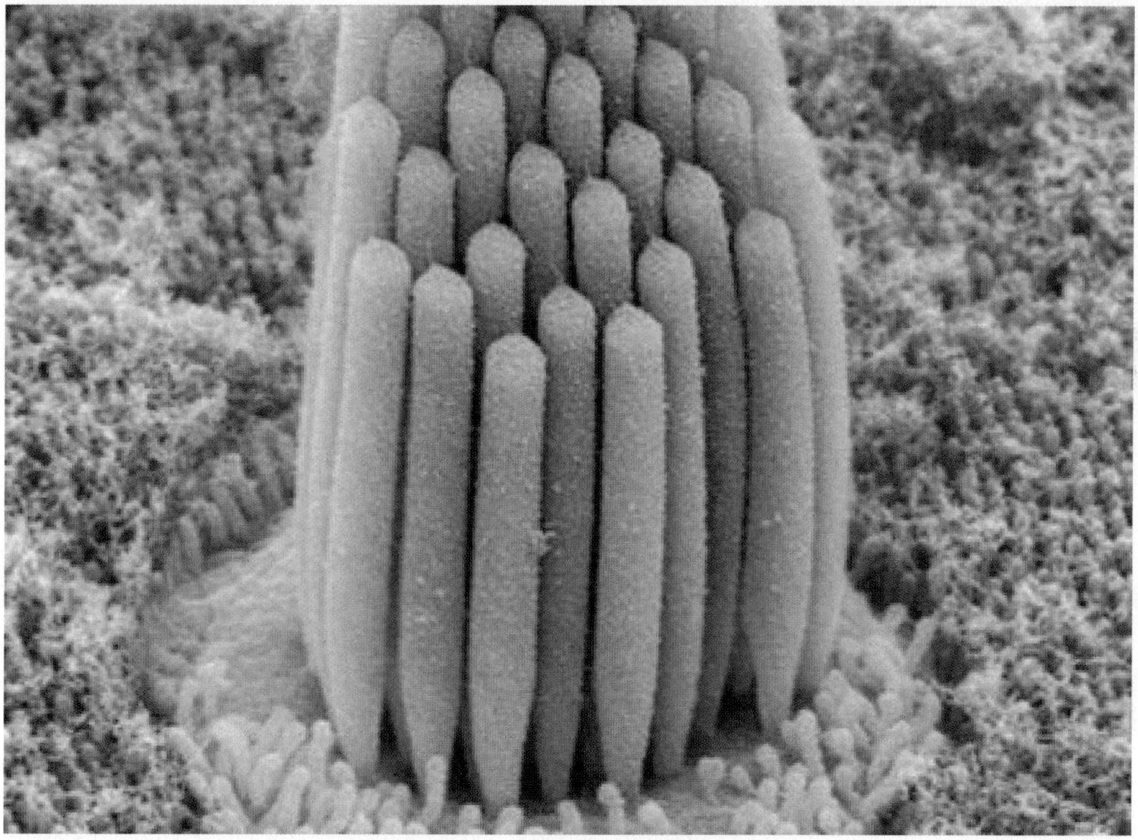

Figure 2.10 Stereocilia of a Hair Cell
Movement of fluid inside the cochlea leads to depolarization of the neuron associated with the hair cell.

The basilar membrane changes thickness depending on its location in the cochlea. The accepted theory on sound perception is **place theory**, which states that the location of a hair cell on the basilar membrane determines the perception of pitch when that hair cell is vibrated. The highest-frequency pitches cause vibrations of the basilar membrane very close to the oval window, whereas low-frequency pitches cause vibrations at the apex, away from the oval window. Thus, the cochlea is **tonotopically** organized: which hair cells are vibrating gives the brain an indication of the pitch of the sound.

BEHAVIORAL SCIENCES GUIDED EXAMPLE WITH EXPERT THINKING

Researchers sought to explain a puzzling phenomenon: that differences in frequency of auditory stimuli sometimes correspond with greater than proportional increases in perceived pitch, even when taking Weber's law into account.

Translated: even if a noise "should" sound high (high frequency), it isn't necessarily perceived as high (high pitch). This is a reference to my outside knowledge: I'll need to recall what Weber's law is!

The researchers hypothesized that differences in pitch specifically for sounds that are familiar, such as human speech, would be amplified perceptually when compared to those of unfamiliar sounds. Participants listened to recordings of both human vocalizations and synthesized tones at 165 Hz and 175 Hz.

There are a couple of independent variables here: type of sound and frequency. The dependent variable must be what the participants report hearing.

Adapted from: Monson BB, Han S, Purves D (2013) Are Auditory Percepts Determined by Experience? *PLoS ONE* 8(5): e63728. https://doi.org/10.1371/journal.pone.0063728

What results would help to support the researchers' hypothesis? What effect would these results have on the place theory of sound perception?

When we encounter experimental passages on the MCAT, there are a few things we should always be on the lookout for: what is the hypothesis, and what are the independent and dependent variables? What results are presented, and what effect do they have on the hypothesis? What conclusion did the researchers come to, and is this conclusion reasonable given the results? If any of these pieces are missing, we should anticipate questions asking us to identify possibilities that would fit with the passage and our outside content knowledge. Here, we are given a hypothesis without results, and the question asks us for results that would support the hypothesis. We'll need to dive into the scenario to identify what is being tested and why, and then use that information in conjunction with our content knowledge to answer this question.

The researchers hypothesized that differences in perceived pitch are amplified for more commonly encountered sounds. Take a moment to consider what the researchers should expect if this hypothesis is correct. It would stand to reason that the difference between perceived pitch for the 165 Hz and 175 Hz samples would be larger for voices (which we hear all the time) than for synthesized tones (which we don't hear too often). In other words, a result that would help support the researchers' hypothesis would be experimental evidence that human vocalizations sounded more different in pitch than the synthesized tones, despite the absolute difference in frequency remaining the same.

For the second part of the question, we need to recall that place theory predicts that perceived pitch results directly from the location of the hair cells that are vibrated when exposed to that frequency; higher frequencies vibrate hair cells closer to the oval window, and lower frequencies vibrate hair cells that are farther away. What is important here is that, according to place theory, the type of sound is irrelevant; sounds of the same frequency should be perceived in the same way. However, the hypothesis of this study (and the hypothetical results we've just imagined in support of that hypothesis), call place theory into question as, according to the passage, similar changes in vibrations are not perceived as the same change in pitch. According to this study, the perceived pitch instead depends at least in part on the nature of the sound perceived by the listener. Note that this new finding wouldn't affect a place theory of sound sensation/detection, which could still be accurate: this experiment is specifically about how sounds are *perceived*, not about how they are *sensed*.

In sum, to support the researchers, the results must find a greater perceived difference in pitch between the vocal samples as compared to the synthesized audio samples. This finding would contradict the place theory of sound perception.

MCAT CONCEPT CHECK 2.3

Before you move on, assess your understanding of the material with these questions.

1. What structures are used to detect linear acceleration? Rotational acceleration?
   - Linear acceleration:

   ____

   - Rotational acceleration:

   ____

2. List the structures in the auditory pathway, from where sound enters the pinna to the auditory projection areas in the brain.

   ____

3. How does the organization of the cochlea indicate the pitch of an incoming sound?

   ____

2.4 Other Senses

High-Yield

LEARNING OBJECTIVES

After Chapter 2.4, you will be able to:

- List the structures in the olfactory pathway
- Distinguish between the chemicals detected by the nose and mouth
- Recall the four main modalities of somatosensation

While vision and hearing are, by far, the most heavily tested senses on the MCAT, the other senses are still considered fair game on Test Day. These include the chemical senses of smell and taste; somatosensation, which includes all of the modalities of "touch"; and kinesthetic sense.

REAL WORLD

Smell is an impressive motivator for behavior. Food aromas may make a person hungry, a familiar fragrance may remind a person of a significant other from years ago, and an unpleasant smell may signify that an unknown bottle contains a dangerous chemical rather than water. Smell is the only sense that does not pass through the thalamus, but rather travels—unfiltered—into higher-order brain centers.

Smell

Smell is considered one of the chemical senses, which means that it responds to incoming chemicals from the outside world. Specifically, smell responds to volatile or aerosolized compounds. **Olfactory chemoreceptors** (**olfactory nerves**) are located in olfactory epithelium in the upper part of the nasal cavity. Chemical stimuli must bind to their respective chemoreceptors to cause a signal. There are a tremendous number of specific chemoreceptors, which allows us to recognize subtle differences in similar scents, such as lavender and jasmine.

Smell can also carry interpersonal information through the medium of **pheromones**, which are chemicals secreted by one animal, and which, once bonded with chemoreceptors, compel or urge another animal to behave in a specific way. Pheromones have debatable effects on humans, but play an enormous role in many animals' social, foraging, and sexual behaviors.

As is true with all senses, there is a defined **olfactory pathway** to the brain. Odor molecules are inhaled into the nasal passages and then contact the olfactory nerves in the olfactory epithelium. These receptor cells are activated, sending signals to the **olfactory bulb**. These signals are then relayed via the **olfactory tract** to higher regions of the brain, including the limbic system.

Taste

As a sense, taste is often simpler than we imagine. There are five basic tastes: sweet, sour, salty, bitter, and umami (savory). Flavor is not synonymous with taste, but rather refers to the complex interplay between smell and taste, which can be affected by nonchemical stimuli like texture and the individual's mood.

Tastes are detected by **chemoreceptors**, which are sensitive to dissolved compounds. Saltiness, for example, is a reaction to alkali metals, and is generally triggered by the sodium found in table salt. Sourness, on the other hand, is a reaction to acid, such as lemon juice or vinegar. Sweet, bitter, and savory flavors are also triggered by specific molecules binding to receptors. The receptors for taste are groups of cells called **taste buds**, which are found in little bumps on the tongue called **papillae**. Taste information travels from taste buds to the brainstem, and then ascends to the **taste center** in the thalamus before traveling to higher-order brain regions.

Somatosensation

Somatosensation is often reduced to "touch" when listed as a sense, but is actually quite complex. Somatosensation is usually described as having four modalities: pressure, vibration, pain, and temperature. At least five different types of receptor receive tactile information, including:

- **Pacinian corpuscles:** respond to deep pressure and vibration
- **Meissner corpuscles:** respond to light touch
- **Merkel cells** (**discs**)**:** respond to deep pressure and texture
- **Ruffini endings:** respond to stretch
- **Free nerve endings:** respond to pain and temperature

Transduction occurs in the receptors, which send the signal to the central nervous system where it eventually travels to the **somatosensory cortex** in the parietal lobe.

There are three additional concepts related to touch perception that are important to know: two-point thresholds, physiological zero, and gate theory of pain. A **two-point threshold** refers to the minimum distance necessary between two points of stimulation on the skin such that the points will be felt as two distinct stimuli. Below the two-point threshold, the two stimuli will be felt as one. The size of the two-point threshold depends on the density of nerves in the particular area of skin being tested.

REAL WORLD

Pain and temperature actually use a different pathway than pressure and vibration through the spinal cord. This can be seen in Brown-Séquard syndrome, in which half of the spinal cord is severed. Patients lose pressure and vibration sense on the same side as the lesion, but lose pain and temperature sensation on the opposite side.

Temperature is judged relative to **physiological zero**, or the normal temperature of the skin (between 86° and 97°F). Thus, an object feels "cold" because it is under physiological zero; an object feels "warm" because it is above physiological zero.

REAL WORLD

The gate theory of pain explains why rubbing an injury (like bumping your knee on a table) seems to reduce the pain of the injury.

Pain perception is part of the somatosensory system and can result from signals sent from a variety of sensory receptors, most commonly **nociceptors**. Pain also relies on thresholds, which may vary greatly from person to person. For example, the temperature of water that is perceived to be "so hot it hurts" may vary by several degrees between individuals. The **gate theory of pain** proposes that a special "gating" mechanism can turn pain signals on or off, affecting whether or not we perceive pain. In this theory, the spinal cord is able to preferentially forward the signals from other touch modalities (pressure, temperature) to the brain, thus reducing the sensation of pain. Gate theory has been superseded by other theories, but is still a useful model for understanding how touch is processed at the spinal cord.

Kinesthetic Sense

Kinesthetic sense is also called **proprioception** and refers to the ability to tell where one's body is in space. For example, even with your eyes closed, you could still describe the location and position of your hand. The receptors for proprioception, called **proprioceptors**, are found mostly in muscle and joints, and play critical roles in hand–eye coordination, balance, and mobility.

MCAT CONCEPT CHECK 2.4

Before you move on, assess your understanding of the material with these questions.

1. List the structures in the olfactory pathway, from where odor molecules enter the nose to where olfactory signals project in the brain.

___

___

2. Both smell and taste are sensitive to chemicals. What is different about the types of chemicals each one can sense?

___

___

3. What are the four main modalities of somatosensation?

   1. ___
   2. ___
   3. ___
   4. ___

2.5 Object Recognition

High-Yield

LEARNING OBJECTIVES

After Chapter 2.5, you will be able to:

- Compare and contrast bottom-up processing and top-down processing
- Describe each of the Gestalt principles: proximity, similarity, good continuation, subjective contours, closure, and prägnanz

Modern theories of object recognition assume at least two major types of psychological processing: bottom-up processing and top-down processing. **Bottom-up (data-driven) processing** refers to object recognition by parallel processing and feature detection, as described earlier. Essentially, the brain takes the individual sensory stimuli and combines them together to create a cohesive image before determining what the object is. **Top-down (conceptually driven) processing** is driven by memories and expectations that allow the brain to recognize the whole object and then recognize the components based on these expectations. In other words, top-down processing allows us to quickly recognize objects without needing to analyze their specific parts. Neither system is sufficient by itself: if we only performed bottom-up processing, we would be extremely inefficient at recognizing objects; every time we looked at an object, it would be like looking at the object for the first time. On the other hand, if we only performed top-down processing, we would have difficulty discriminating slight differences between similar objects. This distinction is also partially responsible for the feeling of *déjà vu* described in the introduction to this chapter: when we believe we are experiencing something for the first time, we expect to rely on bottom-up processing; however, when the mind is able to recognize an experience more quickly than expected (through top-down processing), the mind searches for a reason for this recognition. In other words, *déjà vu* is often evoked when we have recognition without an obvious reason: *I know that person from somewhere . . . but where?* The distinction between top-down and bottom-up processing is relevant for all senses, but is most commonly applied in the context of vision.

Perceptual organization refers to the ability to create a complete picture or idea by combining top-down and bottom-up processing with all of the other sensory clues gathered from an object. Most of the images we see in everyday life are incomplete; often, we may only be able to see a part of an object and we must infer what the rest of the object looks like. By using what information is available in terms of depth, form, motion, constancy, and other clues, we can often "fill in the gaps" using Gestalt principles (described below).

Depth perception relies on a number of visual cues that are interpreted by the brain to deduce an object's distance. These visual cues are separated into monocular and binocular cues. **Monocular cues** only require one eye and include relative size, interposition, linear perspective, motion parallax, and other minor cues. **Relative size** refers to the idea that objects appear larger the closer they are. **Interposition** means that when two objects overlap, the one in front is closer. **Linear perspective** refers to the convergence of parallel lines at a distance: the greater the convergence, the further the distance. **Motion parallax** is the perception that objects closer to us seem to move faster when we change our field of vision (look at something else).

REAL WORLD

If you've ever looked out the side window of a car, bus, or train on a clear night, you've experienced motion parallax. Parallax is the reason why the objects on the side of the road are a blur as you go past, why objects further away move more slowly as you pass them, and why the moon seems to follow you as you ride along.

Binocular cues primarily involve **retinal disparity** which refers to the slight difference in images projected on the two retinas. This feature of depth perception is exploited in virtual reality (VR) devices: the images supplied to each eye are slightly different, giving the perception of depth even though the VR device displays 2D images. A secondary binocular cue is **convergence**, in which the brain detects the angle between the two eyes required to bring an object into focus. If a person was looking at a distant object, both of their eyes would stare straight ahead. However if they were looking at something nearby (perhaps their own nose!) the left and right eyes would be held at an extreme angle. This difference in the degree of convergence is used to perceive distance.

The form of an object is usually determined through parvocellular cells and feature detection, and the motion of an object is perceived through magnocellular cells, as described earlier. **Constancy** refers to our ability to perceive that certain characteristics of objects remain the same, despite changes in the environment. For example, we perceive a white piece of paper as essentially the same color whether the paper is illuminated by fluorescent lights, incandescent bulbs, or sunlight—this type of constancy is called color constancy. We also have constancy for brightness, size, and shape, depending on context.

Gestalt Principles

The brain constantly uses incomplete information to try to create a complete picture of the environment. **Gestalt principles** are a set of general rules that account for the fact that the brain tends to view incomplete stimuli in organized, patterned ways. There are dozens of Gestalt principles, but the highest-yield are summarized below and can be visualized in Figure 2.11.

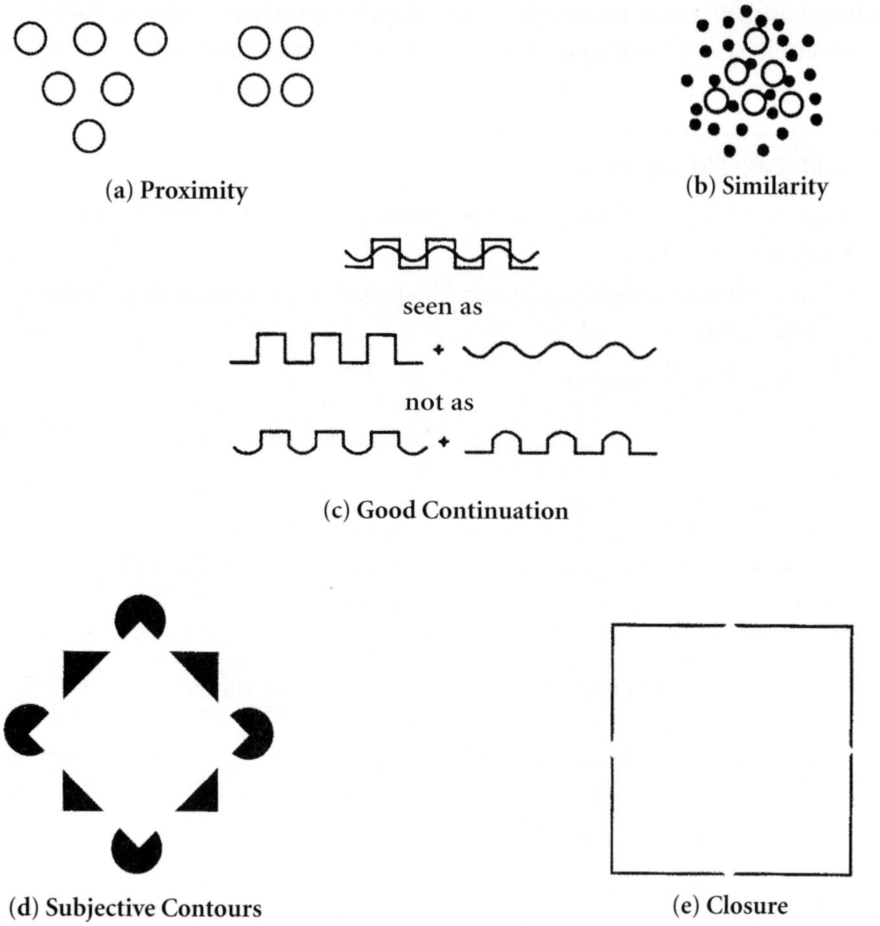

Figure 2.11 Gestalt Principles

The **law of proximity** says that elements close to one another tend to be perceived as a unit. In Figure 2.11a, we do not see ten unrelated dots; rather, we see a triangle and a square, each composed of a certain number of dots. The **law of similarity** says that objects that are similar tend to be grouped together. In Figure 2.11b, we see the big hollow dots as being distinct from the others, forming a triangle against a background of small filled-in dots. The **law of good continuation** says that elements that appear to follow in the same pathway tend to be grouped together. That is, there is a tendency to perceive continuous patterns in stimuli rather than abrupt changes. As seen in Figure 2.11c, our mind tends to break down this complex figure into a sawtooth line and a wavy line, rather than two lines that contain both sawtooth and wavy elements. Some researchers have argued that the phenomena of subjective contours may arise from this law. **Subjective contours** have to do with perceiving contours and, therefore, shapes that are not actually present in the stimulus. In Figure 2.11d, subjective contours lead to the perception of a white diamond on a black square with its corners lying on the four circles. Finally, the **law of closure** says that when a space is enclosed by a contour, the space tends to be perceived as a complete figure. Closure also refers to the fact that certain figures tend to be perceived as more complete (or closed) than they really are. In Figure 2.11e, we don't see four right angles; instead, we see a square, even though the four sides aren't complete. All these laws operate to create the most stable, consistent, and simplest figures possible within a given visual field. Taken altogether, the Gestalt principles are governed by the **law of prägnanz**, which says that perceptual organization will always be as regular, simple, and symmetric as possible.

MCAT CONCEPT CHECK 2.5

Before you move on, assess your understanding of the material with these questions.

1. How is sensory information integrated in bottom-up processing? Top-down processing?

    - Bottom-up processing:

    ____

    - Top-down processing:

    ____

2. Briefly describe each of the Gestalt principles below:

Gestalt Principle	Description
Proximity	
Similarity	
Good continuation	
Subjective contours	
Closure	
Prägnanz	

Conclusion

The sensory systems described in this chapter are key to your success on Test Day. Not only are the eye, ear, and other senses high-yield in their own right, but connections to topics in physics, biology, research design, and other concepts in the behavioral sciences make these key topics for passages. But sensation is only one part of the system; we must then take this raw information and process it in the brain to truly perceive the world around us. We use complex neurological pathways to integrate and sort sensory information. We then process sensory information through multiple systems, analyzing individual features and components of the environment while building expectations based on our memories and past experiences. We fill in gaps in our sensorium using Gestalt principles. And what reaches our conscious awareness is the final product: a cohesive concept of the world around us.

You've completed your visit to the new city. You used your rods and cones to see the sites, your chemoreceptors to taste and smell the local food, your hair cells to listen to the local sounds, and your kinesthetic and vestibular senses to help navigate through physical space. As you get ready to head home, all you're left with are your memories—a topic we'll turn to in the next chapter.

GO ONLINE

You've reviewed the content, now test your knowledge and critical thinking skills by completing a test-like passage set in your online resources!

CONCEPT SUMMARY

Sensation *vs.* Perception

- **Sensation** is the conversion, or transduction, of physical, electromagnetic, auditory, and other information from the internal and external environment into electrical signals in the nervous system.
- **Perception** is the processing of sensory information to make sense of its significance.
- **Sensory receptors** are nerves that respond to stimuli and trigger electrical signals.
  - Sensory neurons are associated with **sensory ganglia**: collections of cell bodies outside the central nervous system.
  - Sensory stimuli are transmitted to **projection areas** in the brain, which further analyze the sensory input.
  - Common sensory receptors include photoreceptors, hair cells, nociceptors, thermoreceptors, osmoreceptors, olfactory receptors, and taste receptors.
- A **threshold** is the minimum stimulus that causes a change in signal transduction.
  - The **absolute threshold** is the minimum of stimulus energy that is needed to activate a sensory system.
  - The **threshold of conscious perception** is the minimum of stimulus energy that will create a signal large enough in size and long enough in duration to be brought into awareness.
  - The **difference threshold** or **just-noticeable difference** (**jnd**) is the minimum difference in magnitude between two stimuli before one can perceive this difference.
  - **Weber's law** states that the jnd for a stimulus is proportional to the magnitude of the stimulus, and that this proportion is constant over most of the range of possible stimuli.
  - **Signal detection theory** refers to the effects of nonsensory factors, such as experiences, motives, and expectations, on perception of stimuli.
  - Signal detection experiments allow us to look at **response bias**. In a signal detection experiment, a stimulus may or may not be given, and the subject is asked to state whether or not the stimulus was given. There are four possible outcomes: hits, misses, false alarms, or correct negatives.
- **Adaptation** refers to a decrease in response to a stimulus over time.

Vision

- The eye is an organ specialized to detect light in the form of photons.
  - The **cornea** gathers and filters incoming light.
  - The **iris** divides the front of the eye into the **anterior** and **posterior chambers**. It contains two muscles, the **dilator** and **constrictor pupillae**, which open and close the **pupil**.
  - The **lens** refracts incoming light to focus it on the retina and is held in place by **suspensory ligaments** connected to the **ciliary muscle**.
  - The ciliary body produces **aqueous humor**, which drains through the **canal of Schlemm**.
  - The retina contains rods and cones. **Rods** detect light and dark; **cones** come in three forms (short-, medium-, and long-wavelength) to detect colors.
  - The retina contains mostly cones in the **macula**, which corresponds to the central visual field. The center of the macula is the **fovea**, which contains only cones.
  - Rods and cones synapse on **bipolar cells**, which synapse on **ganglion cells**. Integration of the signals from ganglion cells and edge-sharpening is performed by **horizontal** and **amacrine cells**.
  - The bulk of the eye is supported by the **vitreous** on the inside and the **sclera** and **choroid** on the outside.
- The visual pathway starts from the eye, and travels through the **optic nerves**, **optic chiasm**, **optic tracts**, **lateral geniculate nucleus** (**LGN**) of the thalamus, and **visual radiations** to get to the **visual cortex**.
  - The optic chiasm contains fibers crossing from the nasal side of the retina (temporal visual fields) of both eyes.
  - The visual radiations run through the temporal and parietal lobes.
  - The visual cortex is in the occipital lobe.
- Vision, like all senses, is processed through **parallel processing**: the ability to simultaneously analyze and combine information regarding color, form, motion, and depth.
  - Color is detected by **cones**.
  - Form is detected by **parvocellular cells**, with high spatial resolution and low temporal resolution.
  - Motion is detected by **magnocellular cells**, with low spatial resolution and high temporal resolution.
  - Depth is detected by **binocular neurons**.

Hearing and Vestibular Sense

- The ear is divided into the outer, middle, and inner ear.
  - The **outer ear** consists of the **pinna** (**auricle**), **external auditory canal**, and **tympanic membrane**.
  - The **middle ear** consists of the **ossicles**: **malleus** (hammer), **incus** (anvil), and **stapes** (stirrup). The footplate of the stapes rests on the **oval window** of the cochlea. The middle ear is connected to the nasal cavity by the **Eustachian tube**.
  - The **inner ear** contains the **bony labyrinth**, within which is the **membranous labyrinth**. The bony labyrinth is filled with **perilymph**; the membranous labyrinth is filled with **endolymph**. The membranous labyrinth consists of the **cochlea**, which detects sound; **utricle** and **saccule**, which detect linear acceleration; and **semicircular canals**, which detect rotational acceleration.
- The auditory pathway starts from the cochlea and travels through the **vestibulocochlear nerve** and **medial geniculate nucleus** (**MGN**) of the thalamus to get to the **auditory cortex** in the temporal lobe.
- Sound information also projects to the **superior olive**, which localizes the sound, and the **inferior colliculus**, which is involved in the startle reflex.

Other Senses

- Smell is the detection of volatile or aerosolized chemicals by the **olfactory chemoreceptors** (**olfactory nerves**) in the olfactory epithelium.
  - The olfactory pathway starts from the olfactory nerves and travels through the **olfactory bulb** and **olfactory tract** to get to higher-order brain areas, such as the limbic system.
  - Pheromones are chemicals given off by animals that have an effect on social, foraging, and sexual behavior in other members of that species.
- Taste is the detection of dissolved compounds by **taste buds** in **papillae**. It comes in five modalities: sweet, sour, salty, bitter, and umami (savory).
- **Somatosensation** refers to the four touch modalities: pressure, vibration, pain, and temperature.
  - A **two-point threshold** is the minimum distance necessary between two points of stimulation on the skin such that the points will be felt as two distinct stimuli.
  - **Physiological zero** is the normal temperature of the skin to which objects are compared to determine if they feel "warm" or "cold."
  - **Nociceptors** are responsible for pain perception. The **gate theory of pain** states that pain sensation is reduced when other somatosensory signals are present.
- **Kinesthetic sense** (**proprioception**) refers to the ability to tell where one's body is in three-dimensional space.

Object Recognition

- **Bottom-up (data-driven) processing** refers to recognition of objects by parallel processing and feature detection. It is slower, but less prone to mistakes.
- **Top-down (conceptually driven) processing** refers to recognition of an object by memories and expectations, with little attention to detail. It is faster, but more prone to mistakes.
- Perceptual organization refers to our synthesis of stimuli to make sense of the world, including integration of depth, form, motion, and constancy.
- **Gestalt principles** are ways that the brain can infer missing parts of a picture when a picture is incomplete.
  - The **law of proximity** says that elements close to one another tend to be perceived as a unit.
  - The **law of similarity** says that objects that are similar appear to be grouped together.
  - The **law of good continuation** says that elements that appear to follow the same pathway tend to be grouped together.
  - **Subjective contours** refer to the perception of nonexistent edges in figures, based on surrounding visual cues.
  - The **law of closure** says that when a space is enclosed by a group of lines, it is perceived as a complete or closed line.
  - The **law of prägnanz** says that **perceptual organization** will always be as regular, simple, and symmetric as possible.

ANSWERS TO CONCEPT CHECKS

2.1

1. Sensory receptor → afferent neuron → sensory ganglion → spinal cord → brain (projection areas)
2. 1–F, 2–A, 3–E, 4–D, 5–C, 6–G, 7–B
3. Absolute threshold is the minimum stimulus that can evoke an action potential in a sensory receptor. Threshold of conscious perception is the minimum stimulus that can evoke enough action potentials for a long enough time that the brain perceives the stimulus. The difference threshold (just-noticeable difference) is the minimum difference between two stimuli that can be detected by the brain.
4. Weber's law explains that just-noticeable differences are best expressed as a ratio, which is constant over most of the range of sensory stimuli. Signal detection theory concerns the threshold to sense a stimulus, given obscuring internal and external stimuli.
5. Adaptation generally raises the difference threshold for a sensory response; as one becomes used to small fluctuations in the stimulus, the difference in stimulus required to evoke a response must be larger.

2.2

1. Cornea: gathers and focuses the incoming light
   Pupil: allows passage of light from the anterior to posterior chamber
   Iris: controls the size of the pupil
   Ciliary body: produces aqueous humor; accommodation of the lens
   Canal of Schlemm: drains aqueous humor
   Lens: refracts the incoming light to focus it on the retina
   Retina: detects images
   Sclera: provides structural support
2. Cornea → pupil → lens → vitreous → retina (rods and cones → bipolar cells → ganglion cells) → optic nerve → optic chiasm → optic tract → lateral geniculate nucleus (LGN) of thalamus → radiations through parietal and temporal lobes → visual cortex (occipital lobe)
3. Parallel processing is the ability to simultaneously analyze color, shape, and motion of an object and to integrate this information to create a cohesive image of the world. Parallel processing also calls on memory systems to compare a visual stimulus to past experiences to help determine the object's identity.
4. Cones are responsible for color. Parvocellular cells are responsible for form. Magnocellular cells are responsible for motion. Binocular neurons are responsible for depth.

2.3

1. Linear acceleration is detected by the utricle and saccule. Rotational acceleration is detected by the semicircular canals.
2. Pinna → external auditory canal → tympanic membrane → malleus → incus → stapes → oval window → perilymph in cochlea → basilar membrane → hair cells → vestibulocochlear nerve → brainstem → medial geniculate nucleus (MGN) of thalamus → auditory cortex (temporal lobe)
3. The basilar membrane is tonotopically organized: high-pitched sounds cause vibrations at the base of the cochlea, whereas low-pitched sounds cause vibrations at the apex of the cochlea.

2.4

1. Nostril → nasal cavity → olfactory chemoreceptors (olfactory nerves) on olfactory epithelium → olfactory bulb → olfactory tract → higher-order brain regions, including limbic system
2. Smell is sensitive to volatile or aerosolized compounds; taste is sensitive to dissolved compounds.
3. The four main modalities of somatosensation are pressure, vibration, pain, and temperature.

2.5

1. Bottom-up processing requires each component of an object to be interpreted through parallel processing and then integrated into one cohesive whole. Top-down processing starts with the whole object and, through memory, creates expectations for the components of the object.
2.

Gestalt Principle	Description
Proximity	Components close to one another tend to be perceived as a unit.
Similarity	Components that are similar (in color, shape, size) tend to be grouped together.
Good continuation	Components that appear to follow in the same pathway tend to be grouped together; abrupt changes in form are less likely than continuation of the same pattern.
Subjective contours	Edges or shapes that are not actually present can be implied by the surrounding objects (especially if good continuation is present).
Closure	A space enclosed by a contour tends to be perceived as a complete figure; such figures tend to be perceived as more complete (or closed) than they really are.
Prägnanz	Perceptual organization will always be as regular, simple, and symmetric as possible.

SCIENCE MASTERY ASSESSMENT EXPLANATIONS

1. **C**

Weber's law posits that thresholds are proportional. Going from 100 to 125 pounds is a 25 percent increase. **(C)** is a 40 percent increase while all the rest are all under 25 percent.

2. **D**

The person is discerning a specific noise within a field of many noises. This is the definition of signal detection. In an experimental setup, the person's response would be considered a hit if the friend was indeed laughing; it would be considered a false alarm if the friend was not laughing.

3. **A**

The spicy food can be considered an extreme stimulus because it eclipses what the person believes can be handled in terms of heat. However, after experiencing the stimulus over and over, the experience of spice drops to barely perceptible. This is sensory adaptation: a reduction in response to a stimulus over time.

4. **B**

Nociceptors are important for pain sensation, which would be expected during tissue damage. Chemoreceptors, **(A)**, respond to chemicals, whether volatile or aerosolized (olfaction) or dissolved (taste). Osmoreceptors, **(C)**, respond to changes in blood osmolarity, and photoreceptors, **(D)**, respond to light.

5. **A**

The cornea is responsible for gathering and focusing light. The pupil and iris, **(B)** and **(C)**, are both involved in regulating the amount of light coming into the eye but not in focusing it. The retina, **(D)**, transduces the light into electrical signals that are sent to the brain. The lens serves a similar function to the cornea and would also be a valid answer to this question.

6. **C**

This person was able to distinguish the coin from other items by recognizing specific features of the coin; in this case, it was the glint of the metal surface and its position in the car. This phenomenon is called feature detection.

7. **C**

The retina is the part of the eye upon which images are projected. Rods and cones in the retina then convert the electromagnetic radiation into electrical signals.

8. **A**

Somatosensation refers to the various modalities of touch: pressure, vibration, temperature, and pain. Kinesthetic sense, **(B)**, refers to the ability to tell where one's body is in space. Vestibular sense, **(C)**, refers to the detection of linear and rotational acceleration in the middle ear. Finally, chemoreception, **(D)**, refers to sensing chemicals in the environment.

9. **B**

The five tastes are sweet, sour, salty, bitter, and umami. Floral would be related to smell rather than taste.

10. **C**

Endolymph is the potassium-rich fluid that bathes the hair cells of the inner ear, all of which are found within the membranous labyrinth. Perilymph is found in the space between the membranous labyrinth and the bony labyrinth. Both the membranous labyrinth and bony labyrinth contribute to the cochlea and the vestibule, eliminating **(A)** and **(B)**.

11. **A**

Pheromones are the volatile chemicals given off by organisms that bind with olfactory chemoreceptors and influence behavior. It is debatable if pheromones serve a role in humans, but they are known to affect foraging and sexual behavior in some animals.

12. **B**

Kinesthetic sense, or proprioception, refers to the ability to tell where body parts are in three-dimensional space. The sensors for proprioception are found predominantly in the muscles and joints. Loss of vestibular sense, **(A)**, would also cause difficulty walking, but this would be due to a sense of dizziness or vertigo, not an inability to feel one's feet.

13. **C**

The proofreader used a larger pattern to identify the word and expected to see an "e," thus missing the error. This is related to top-down processing; the proofreader used recognition and expectations, which led to missing a detail. Bottom-up processing, **(D)**, would be the analysis of each detail individually before creating a cohesive image.

14. **D**

Gestalt principles are the basis for many optical illusions and include the tendency of people to see continuity even when lines are unconnected. Specifically, this logo appears to rely on the law of closure to create one complete star from five nontouching angles.

15. **D**

The optic chiasm houses the crossing fibers from each optic nerve. Specifically, the fibers coming from the nasal half of the retina in each eye cross in the chiasm to join the optic tract on the opposite side. Remember that the lens of the eye causes inversion, so images on the nasal half of the retina actually originate in the temporal visual field. This condition is called bitemporal hemianopsia.

Consult your online resources for additional practice. GO ONLINE

SHARED CONCEPTS

Behavioral Sciences Chapter 1
Biology and Behavior

Biology Chapter 4
The Nervous System

Biology Chapter 10
Homeostasis

Physics and Math Chapter 3
Thermodynamics

Physics and Math Chapter 7
Waves and Sound

Physics and Math Chapter 8
Light and Optics

CHAPTER 3

LEARNING AND MEMORY

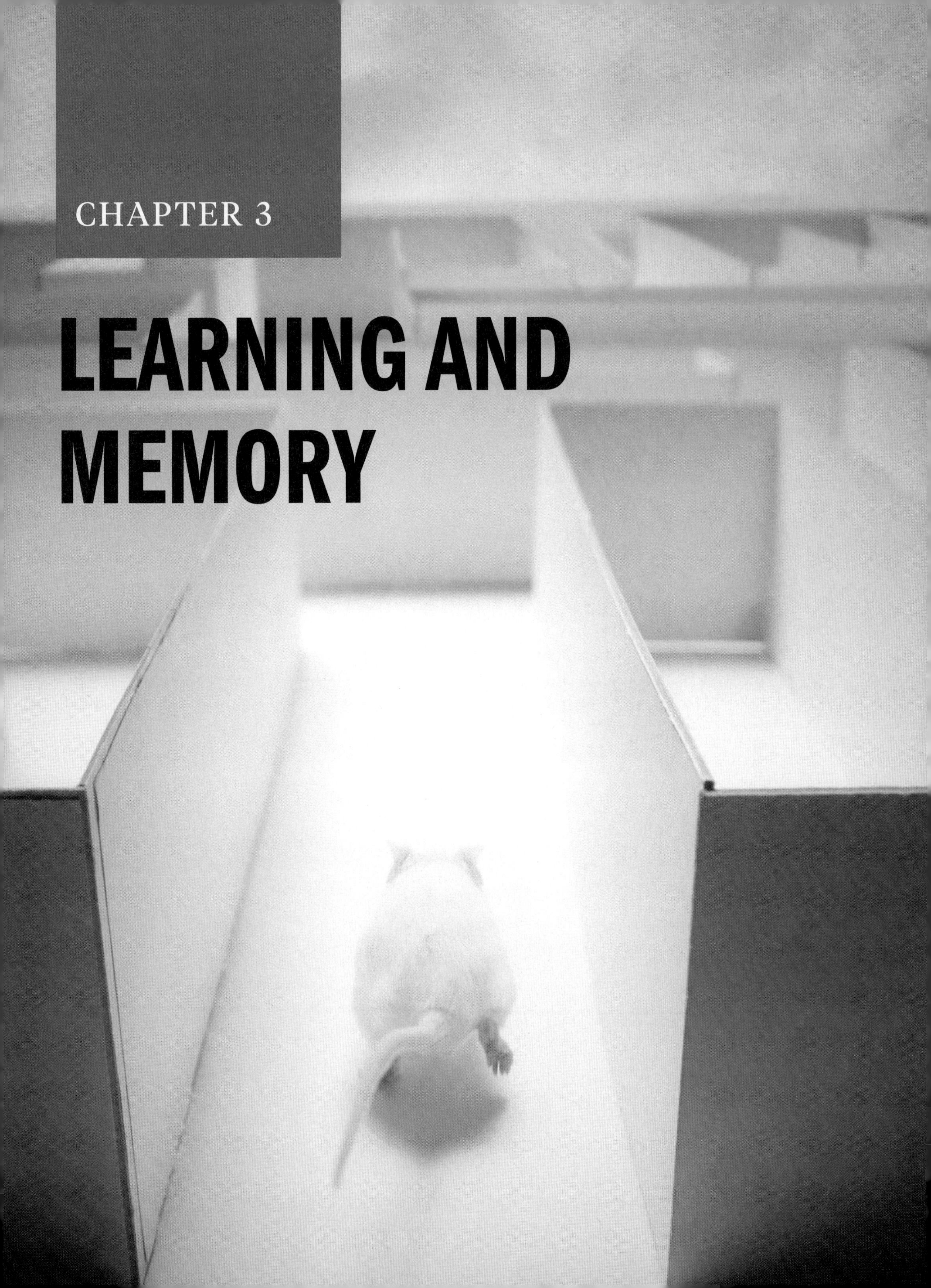

SCIENCE MASTERY ASSESSMENT

Every pre-med knows this feeling: there is so much content I have to know for the MCAT! How do I know what to do first or what's important?

While the high-yield badges throughout this book will help you identify the most important topics, this Science Mastery Assessment is another tool in your MCAT prep arsenal. This quiz (which can also be taken in your online resources) and the guidance below will help ensure that you are spending the appropriate amount of time on this chapter based on your personal strengths and weaknesses. Don't worry though—skipping something now does not mean you'll never study it. Later on in your prep, as you complete full-length tests, you'll uncover specific pieces of content that you need to review and can come back to these chapters as appropriate.

How to Use This Assessment

If you answer 0–7 questions correctly:

Spend about 1 hour to read this chapter in full and take limited notes throughout. Follow up by reviewing **all** quiz questions to ensure that you now understand how to solve each one.

If you answer 8–11 questions correctly:

Spend 20–40 minutes reviewing the quiz questions. Beginning with the questions you missed, read and take notes on the corresponding subchapters. For questions you answered correctly, ensure your thinking matches that of the explanation and you understand why each choice was correct or incorrect.

If you answer 12–15 questions correctly:

Spend less than 20 minutes reviewing all questions from the quiz. If you missed any, then include a quick read-through of the corresponding subchapters, or even just the relevant content within a subchapter, as part of your question review. For questions you answered correctly, ensure your thinking matches that of the explanation and review the Concept Summary at the end of the chapter.

1. Researchers repeatedly startle a participant with a loud buzzer. After some time, the participant stops being startled by the buzzer. If the researchers interrupt the study with the sound of pans banging together, which of the following would likely be observed?
   - **A.** Increased startle response to the buzzer
   - **B.** Decreased startle response to the buzzer
   - **C.** No change in the response to the buzzer
   - **D.** Generalization to previously nonaversive stimuli

2. Many pets will run toward the kitchen when they hear the sound of a can opener opening a can of pet food. The sound of the can opener is a(n):
   - **A.** conditioned response.
   - **B.** unconditioned response.
   - **C.** conditioned stimulus.
   - **D.** unconditioned stimulus.

3. A person suffers from food poisoning after eating a spoiled orange and later finds that the smell of lemon and other citrus fruits causes a feeling of nausea. This is an example of:
   - **A.** acquisition.
   - **B.** generalization.
   - **C.** discrimination.
   - **D.** negative reinforcement.

4. Which of the following processes would increase the likelihood of a behavior?
   - **A.** Extinction
   - **B.** Negative punishment
   - **C.** Positive punishment
   - **D.** Avoidance learning

5. The presynaptic neuron becomes more efficient at releasing neurotransmitters while receptor density increases on the postsynaptic neuron. These changes are consistent with:
   - **A.** long term potentiation.
   - **B.** synaptic pruning.
   - **C.** an increase in neuroplasticity.
   - **D.** amnesia.

6. A rat is trained to press a lever to obtain food under a fixed-interval schedule. Which of the following behaviors would the rat most likely exhibit?
   - **A.** Pressing the lever continuously whenever it is hungry.
   - **B.** Pressing the lever exactly once and waiting for the food pellet before pressing it again.
   - **C.** Pressing the lever slowly at first, but with increasing frequency as the end of the interval approaches.
   - **D.** None of the above; the association formed by fixed-interval schedules is too weak to increase behavior.

7. Which of the following is true of teaching an animal a complicated, multistage behavior?
   - **I.** The individual parts of the behavior should not run counter to the animal's natural instincts.
   - **II.** The behaviors must be tied to a food reward of some kind.
   - **III.** Rewarding individual parts of the behavior on their own interferes with reinforcement of the entire behavior.

   - **A.** I only
   - **B.** I and III only
   - **C.** II and III only
   - **D.** I, II, and III

8. Which of the following is true of controlled processing?
   - **A.** It is the means through which information enters short-term memory.
   - **B.** Information that requires controlled processing cannot become automatic.
   - **C.** It always requires active attention to the information being encoded.
   - **D.** Most information we can later recall is encoded using controlled processing.

9. Which of the following methods of encoding is most conducive to later recall?

A. Semantic
B. Visual
C. Iconic
D. Acoustic

10. A hemisphere of the brain can be removed to prevent the recurrence of severe seizures. How would the ability of the other hemisphere to adopt functionalities of the removed section differ between a two year old and a twenty year old?

A. The brain of the twenty year old would be more adaptable due to higher neuroplasticity.
B. The brain of the twenty year old would be more adaptable due to lower neuroplasticity.
C. The brain of the two year old would be more adaptable due to higher neuroplasticity.
D. The brain of the two year old would be more adaptable due to lower neuroplasticity.

11. An individual memorizes a shopping list by associating each item with an image that corresponds with a number. This individual is using which of the following mnemonics?

A. Clustering
B. Method of loci
C. Elaborative rehearsal
D. Peg-words

12. A researcher uses a partial-report procedure after presenting participants with an array of nine numbers for a fraction of a second. Which of the following is the most likely result of this procedure?

A. The participants will be able to recall any of the rows or columns in great detail but only immediately after presentation.
B. The participants will only be able to recall the first few numbers in the array due to the serial position effect.
C. The participants will be able to recall approximately seven of the numbers for a few seconds following presentation of the stimulus.
D. The participants will not be able to recall any of the numbers verbally, but will be able to draw the full array under hypnosis.

13. Which of the following is an example of a semantic memory?

A. Having the ability to drive a car
B. Knowing the parts of a car engine
C. Remembering the experience of learning to drive
D. Associating a car with other vehicles in a semantic network

14. Which of the following is an example of a circumstance that could cause a state-dependent recall effect?

I. The individual is outside on a rainy day.
II. The individual is intoxicated on cannabis.
III. The individual is experiencing a manic episode.

A. I only
B. III only
C. II and III only
D. I, II, and III

15. Which of the following would an older adult be most likely to have trouble recalling?

A. The circumstances of meeting a significant other in college
B. A doctor's appointment scheduled for 1:00 p.m.
C. The names of the characters in a favorite television show
D. That a library book needs to be returned when passing by the library on a morning walk

Answer Key

1. **A**
2. **C**
3. **B**
4. **D**
5. **A**
6. **C**
7. **A**
8. **C**
9. **A**
10. **C**
11. **D**
12. **A**
13. **B**
14. **C**
15. **B**

Detailed explanations can be found at the end of the chapter.

CHAPTER 3

LEARNING AND MEMORY

In This Chapter

Introduction

A college student sits hunched over a desk in a quiet library, poring over a small stack of textbooks. It's 11 p.m. the night before the organic chemistry midterm, and there seems to be a near endless list of reactions to commit to memory before tomorrow. The situation seems bleak, but the student has been here before and has taken every precaution to make sure that this study session will be successful: drinking coffee will increase alertness, while the quiet of the library will reduce distractions to aid concentration. It's stressful, to be sure, but the student has been able to study this way before and do quite well, reinforcing this current set of behaviors. The student works through a set of flashcards—reactants on one side, products on the other—and is able to identify most of them but misses a few. Those cards are placed in a separate pile to be reviewed later. Sure, this rehearsal will most likely help for the exam tomorrow, but will the student be able to recall this information again for the final in two months? The student takes another sip of coffee and tries to put everything else out of mind, focusing intently on the book sitting open on the desk.

Sound familiar? If you're like most students, you've found yourself in a similar scenario at least once. This chapter will discuss the ways in which you both memorize new information and learn new behaviors. This will not only help you to directly prepare to answer MCAT questions about this content, but also to learn a few new tricks about how to effectively commit all of the MCAT content to memory. This is a skill that will be helpful both now and later in your career as a doctor.

CHAPTER PROFILE

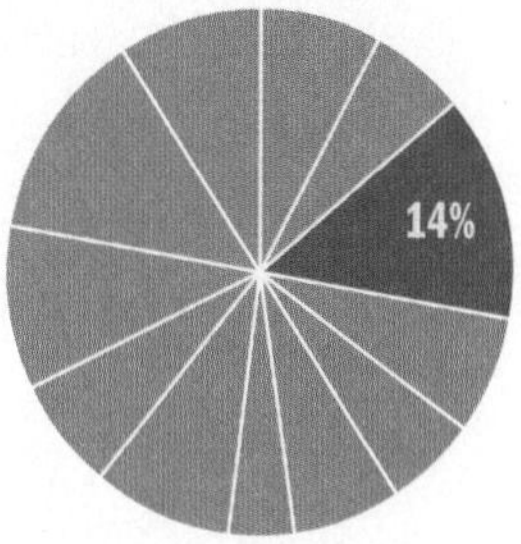

The content in this chapter should be relevant to about 14% of all questions about the behavioral sciences on the MCAT.

This chapter covers material from the following AAMC content categories:

6B: Making sense of the environment

7C: Attitude and behavior change

3.1 Learning

High-Yield

LEARNING OBJECTIVES

After Chapter 3.1, you will be able to:

- Apply principles of habituation, dishabituation, and sensitization to real-life scenarios
- Identify the conditioned stimulus, unconditioned stimulus, conditioned response, and unconditioned response in a Pavlovian learning paradigm
- Distinguish between negative reinforcement, positive reinforcement, negative punishment, and positive punishment
- Predict how reinforcement schedule will affect relative frequency of behavioral response in an operant conditioning scenario:

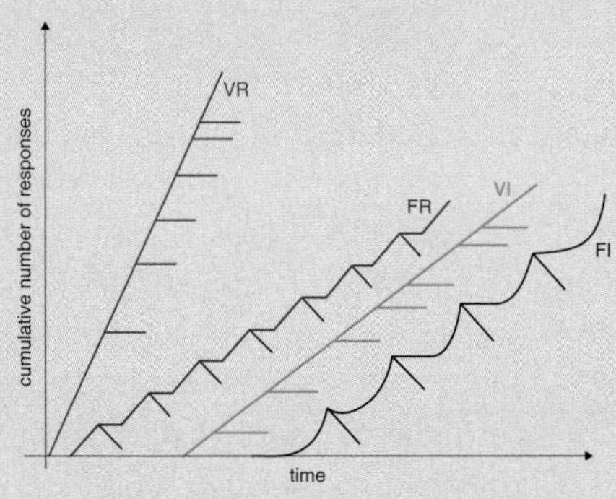

To a psychologist, **learning** refers specifically to the way in which we acquire new behaviors. To understand learning, we must start with the concept of a stimulus. A **stimulus** can be defined as anything to which an organism can respond, including all of the sensory inputs we discussed in Chapter 2 of *MCAT Behavioral Sciences Review*. The combination of stimuli and responses serves as the basis for all behavioral learning.

Responses to stimuli can change over time depending on the frequency and intensity of the stimulus. For instance, repeated exposure to the same stimulus can cause a decrease in response called **habituation**. This is seen in many first-year medical students: students often have an intense physical reaction the first time they see a cadaver or treat a severe laceration, but as they get used to these stimuli, the reaction lessens until they are unbothered by these sights. Note that a stimulus too weak to elicit a response is called **subthreshold** stimulus.

KEY CONCEPT

Dishabituation is the recovery of a response to a stimulus, usually after a different stimulus has been presented. Note that the term refers to changes in response to the original stimulus, not the new one.

The opposite process can also occur. **Dishabituation** is defined as the recovery of a response to a stimulus after habituation has occurred. Dishabituation is often noted when, late in the habituation of a stimulus, a second stimulus is presented. The second stimulus interrupts the habituation process and thereby causes an increase in response to the original stimulus. Imagine, for example, that you're taking a long car trip and driving for many miles on a highway. After a while, your brain will get used to the sights, sounds, and sensations of highway driving: the dashed lines dividing the lanes, the sound of the engine and the tires on the road, and so on. Habituation has occurred. At some point you use an exit ramp, and these sensations change. As you merge onto the new highway, you pay more attention to the sensory stimuli coming in. Even if the stimuli are more or less the same as on the previous highway, the presentation of a different stimulus (using the exit ramp) causes dishabituation and a new awareness of—and response to—these stimuli. Dishabituation is temporary and always refers to changes in response to the original stimulus, not the new one.

Learning, then, is a change in behavior that occurs in response to a stimulus. While there are many types of learning, the MCAT focuses on two types: associative learning and observational learning.

Associative Learning

Associative learning is the creation of a pairing, or association, either between two stimuli or between a behavior and a response. On the MCAT, you'll be tested on two kinds of associative learning: classical and operant conditioning.

Classical Conditioning

Classical conditioning is a type of associative learning that takes advantage of biological, instinctual responses to create associations between two unrelated stimuli. For many people, the first name that comes to mind for research in classical conditioning is Ivan Pavlov. His experiments on dogs were not only revolutionary, but also provide a template for the way the MCAT will test classical conditioning.

Classical conditioning works, first and foremost, because some stimuli cause an innate or reflexive physiological response. For example, we reflexively salivate when we smell bread baking in an oven, or we may jump or recoil when we hear a loud noise. Any stimulus that brings about such a reflexive response is called an **unconditioned stimulus**, and the innate or reflexive response is called an **unconditioned response**. Many stimuli do not produce a reflexive response and are known as **neutral stimuli**.

In Pavlov's experiment, the unconditioned stimulus was meat, which would cause the dogs to salivate reflexively, and the neutral stimulus was a ringing bell. Through the course of the experiment, Pavlov repeatedly rang the bell before placing meat in the dogs' mouths. Initially, the dogs did not react much when they only heard the bell ring without receiving meat. However, after this procedure was repeated several times, the dogs began to salivate when they heard the bell ring. In fact, the dogs would salivate even if Pavlov only rang the bell and did not deliver any meat. Pavlov thereby turned a neutral stimulus into a **conditioned stimulus**: a normally neutral stimulus that, through association, now causes a reflexive response called a **conditioned response**. The process of using a reflexive, unconditioned stimulus to turn a neutral stimulus into a conditioned stimulus is termed **acquisition**, as shown in Figure 3.1.

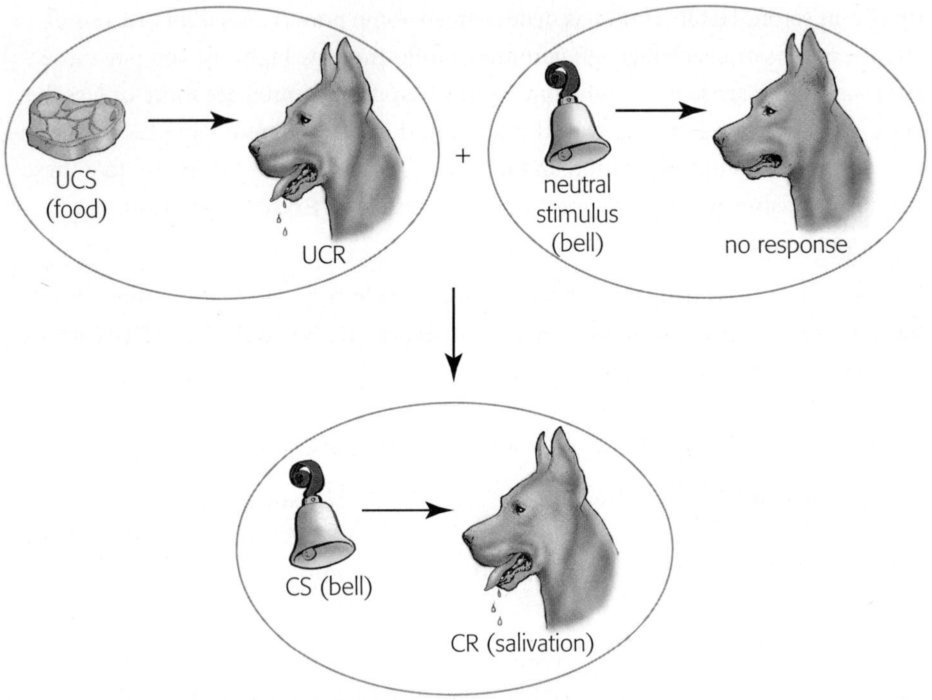

Figure 3.1 Acquisition in Classical Conditioning
UCS = unconditioned stimulus, UCR = unconditioned response, CS = conditioned stimulus, CR = conditioned response

MCAT EXPERTISE

On the MCAT, the key to telling conditioned and unconditioned responses apart will be to look at which stimulus is causing them: unconditioned stimuli cause an unconditioned response, while conditioned stimuli cause a conditioned response.

Notice that the stimuli change in this experiment, but the response is the same throughout. Because salivation in response to food is natural and requires no conditioning, it is an unconditioned response in this context. On the other hand, when paired with the conditioned stimulus of the bell, salivation is considered a conditioned response.

However, it is important to recognize that just because a conditioned response has been acquired, that does not mean that the conditioned response is permanent. **Extinction** refers to the loss of a conditioned response, and can occur if the conditioned stimulus is repeatedly presented without the unconditioned stimulus. Applying this concept to the Pavlov example, if the bell rings often enough without the dog getting meat, the dog may stop salivating when the bell sounds. Interestingly, this extinction of a response is not always permanent; after some time, presenting subjects again with an extinct conditioned stimulus will sometimes produce a weak conditioned response, a phenomenon called **spontaneous recovery**.

There are a few processes that can modify the response to a conditioned stimulus after acquisition has occurred. **Generalization** is a broadening effect by which a stimulus similar enough to the conditioned stimulus can also produce the conditioned response. In one famous experiment, researchers conditioned a child called Little Albert to be afraid of a white rat by pairing the presentation of the rat with a loud noise. Subsequent tests showed that Little Albert's conditioning had generalized such that he also exhibited a fear response to a white stuffed rabbit, a white sealskin coat, and even a man with a white beard.

Finally, in **stimuli discrimination** (sometimes referred to as just **discrimination**), an organism learns to distinguish between similar stimuli. Discrimination is the opposite of generalization. Pavlov's dogs could have been conditioned to discriminate between bells of different tones by having one tone paired with meat, and another tone presented without meat. In this case, association could have occurred with one tone but not the other.

MCAT EXPERTISE

Classical conditioning is a favorite topic on the MCAT. Expect at least one question to describe a Pavlovian experiment and ask you to identify the role of one of the stimuli or responses described.

Operant Conditioning

Whereas classical conditioning is concerned with instincts and biological responses, the study of **operant conditioning** examines the ways in which consequences of voluntary behaviors change the frequency of those behaviors. Just as the MCAT will test you on the difference between conditioned and unconditioned responses and stimuli, it will ask you to distinguish between reinforcement and punishment too. Operant conditioning is associated with B. F. Skinner, who is considered one of the founders of **behaviorism**, the theory that all behaviors are conditioned. The four possible relationships between stimulus and behavior are summarized in Figure 3.2.

Behavior	Stimulus: Added	Stimulus: Removed
Continues	Positive reinforcement	Negative reinforcement
Stops	Positive punishment	Negative punishment

Figure 3.2 Terminology of Operant Conditioning

Reinforcement

Almost all animals will innately search for resources in their environment. These **reward-seeking behaviors**, such as foraging and approach behaviors, are modified over time as the animal interacts with various stimuli and adjusts its behaviors accordingly. **Reinforcement** is the process of increasing the likelihood that an animal will perform a behavior. Reinforcers are divided into two categories. **Positive reinforcers** increase the frequency of a behavior by adding a positive consequence or incentive following the desired behavior. Money is an example of a common and

REAL WORLD

This concept of learning by consequence forms the foundation for behavioral therapies for many disorders including phobias, anxiety disorders, and obsessive-compulsive disorder.

strong positive reinforcer: employees will continue to work if they are paid. **Negative reinforcers** act similarly in that they increase the frequency of a behavior, but they do so by removing something unpleasant. For example, taking an aspirin reduces a headache, so the next time you have a headache, you are more likely to take one. Negative reinforcement is often confused with punishment, which will be discussed in the next section, but remember that the frequency of the behavior is the distinguishing factor: any reinforcement—positive or negative—increases the likelihood that a behavior will be performed.

Negative reinforcement can be subdivided into escape learning and avoidance learning, which differ in whether the unpleasant stimulus occurs or not. **Escape learning** describes a situation where the animal experiences the unpleasant stimulus and, in response, displays the desired behavior in order to trigger the removal of the stimulus. So, in this type of learning, the desired behavior is used to escape the stimulus. In contrast, **avoidance learning** occurs when the animal displays the desired behavior in anticipation of the unpleasant stimulus, thereby avoiding the unpleasant stimulus.

Avoidance learning often develops from multiple experiences of escape learning. An example of this progression from escape learning to avoidance learning is the seat belt warning in a car. If a driver begins driving without buckling the seat belt, then the car will produce an annoying beeping noise, which only ends when the seat belt is buckled. In this example, the desired behavior is to buckle the seat belt. This behavior is reinforced by the removal of an unpleasant stimulus (the audible beeping), so this type of learning is negative reinforcement. More specifically, this example illustrates escape learning, since the driver first experiences the unpleasant stimulus, then exhibits the desired behavior in order to escape the unpleasant stimulus. However, after forgetting to buckle the seat belt several times, the driver will eventually learn to preemptively buckle up before driving the car in order to avoid the beeping sound. At that point, the escape learning has progressed to avoidance learning. Finally, this example illustrates an important misconception about the term *negative reinforcement:* Buckling one's seat belt is generally considered a "positive" behavior, in that it protects one's health. Nevertheless, the terms "positive" and "negative" in operant conditioning only refer to the addition or removal of a stimulus. So even though buckling up is a "good" thing, this example illustrates several types of negative reinforcement!

Classical and operant conditioning can be used hand-in-hand. For example, some dog trainers take advantage of reinforcers when training dogs to perform tricks. Sometimes, the trainers will feed the dog a bit of meat after it performs a trick. The meat can be said to be a **primary reinforcer** because the meat is a treat that the dog responds to naturally. Dog trainers also use tiny handheld devices that emit a clicking sound. This clicker would not normally be a reinforcer on its own, but the trainers use classical conditioning to pair the clicker with meat to elicit the same response. The clicker is thus a **conditioned reinforcer**, which is sometimes called a **secondary reinforcer**. Eventually, the dog may even associate the presence of the trainer with the possibility of reward, making the presence of the trainer a **discriminative stimulus**. A discriminative stimulus indicates that reward is potentially available in an operant conditioning paradigm.

Punishment

In contrast to reinforcement, **punishment** uses conditioning to reduce the occurrence of a behavior. **Positive punishment** adds an unpleasant consequence in response to a behavior to reduce that behavior; for example, receiving a ticket and having to pay a fine for parking illegally. Because positive punishment involves using something unpleasant to discourage a behavior, it is sometimes referred to as **aversive conditioning**. By contrast, **negative punishment** is removing a stimulus in order to cause reduction of a behavior. For example, a parent or guardian may forbid a child from watching television as a consequence for bad behavior, with the goal of preventing the behavior from happening again.

Reinforcement Schedules

The presence or absence of reinforcing or punishing stimuli is just a part of the story. The rate at which desired behaviors are acquired is also affected by the **reinforcement schedule** being used to deliver the stimuli. There are two key factors to reinforcement schedules: whether the schedule is fixed or variable, and whether the schedule is based on a ratio or an interval.

- **Fixed-ratio (FR) schedules** reinforce a behavior after a specific number of performances of that behavior. For example, in a typical operant conditioning experiment, researchers might reward a rat with a food pellet every third time it presses a bar in its cage. **Continuous reinforcement** is a fixed-ratio schedule in which the behavior is rewarded every time it is performed.
- **Variable-ratio (VR) schedules** reinforce a behavior after a varying number of performances of the behavior, but such that the average number of performances to receive a reward is relatively constant. With this type of reinforcement schedule, researchers might reward a rat first after two button presses, then eight, then four, then finally six.
- **Fixed-interval (FI) schedules** reinforce the first instance of a behavior after a specified time period has elapsed. For example, once our rat gets a pellet, it has to wait 60 seconds before it can get another pellet. The first lever press after 60 seconds gets a pellet, but subsequent presses during those 60 seconds accomplish nothing.
- **Variable-interval (VI) schedules** reinforce a behavior the first time that behavior is performed after a varying interval of time. Instead of waiting exactly 60 seconds, for example, our rat might have to wait 90 seconds, then 30 seconds, then three minutes. In each case, once the interval elapses, the next press gets the rat a pellet.

Of these schedules, variable-ratio works the fastest for learning a new behavior, and is also the most resistant to extinction. The effectiveness of the various reinforcement schedules is demonstrated in Figure 3.3.

KEY CONCEPT

Negative reinforcement is often confused with positive punishment. Negative reinforcement is the *removal* of a bothersome stimulus to *encourage* a behavior; positive punishment is the *addition* of a bothersome stimulus to *reduce* a behavior.

BRIDGE

Sociological institutions often rely on punishments and rewards to adjust behavior. Within a society, **formal sanctions**, or rules and laws, can be used to reinforce or punish behavior. Likewise, **informal sanctions**, such as ostracization, praise, and shunning, can be used to reinforce or punish social behavior without depending on rules established by social institutions. Socialization and social institutions are discussed in Chapters 8 and 11 of *MCAT Behavioral Sciences Review*, respectively.

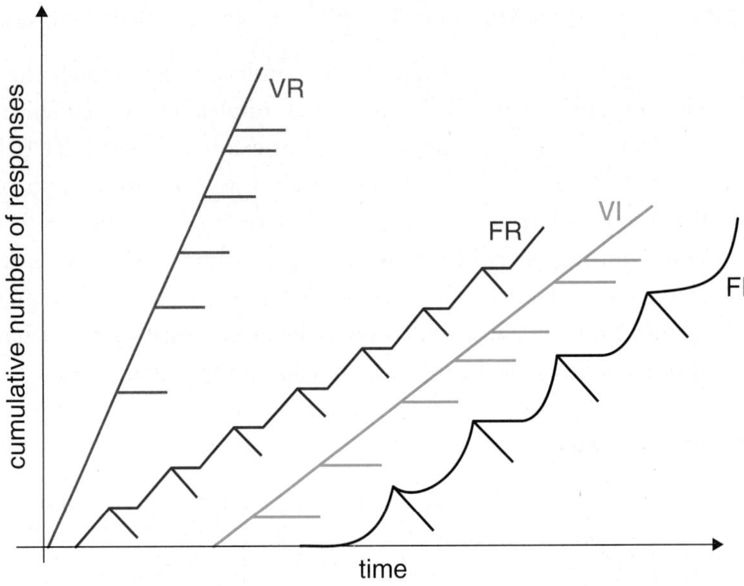

Figure 3.3 Reinforcement Schedules
Hatches correspond to instances of reinforcement. The start of each line corresponds to time zero for that schedule.

MNEMONIC

VR stands for **V**ariable-**R**atio, but it can also stand for **V**ery **R**apid and **V**ery **R**esistant to extinction.

REAL WORLD

Gambling (and gambling addiction) is so difficult to extinguish because most gambling games are based on variable-ratio schedules. While the probability of winning the jackpot on any individual pull of a slot machine is the same, we get caught in the idea that the next pull will be the "right one."

There are a few things to note in this graph. First, variable-ratio schedules have the fastest response rate: the rat will continue pressing the bar quickly with the hope that the next press will be the "right one." Also note that fixed schedules (fixed-ratio and fixed-interval) often have a brief moment of no responses after the behavior is reinforced: the rat will stop hitting the lever until it wants another pellet, once it has figured out what behavior is necessary to receive the pellet.

One final idea associated with operant conditioning is the concept of **shaping**, which is the process of rewarding increasingly specific behaviors that become closer to a desired response. For example, if you wanted to train a bird to spin around in place and then peck a key on a keyboard, you might first give the bird a treat for turning slightly to the left, then only for turning a full 90 degrees, then 180, and so on, until the bird has learned to spin around completely. Then you might only reward this behavior if done near the keyboard until eventually the bird is only rewarded once the full set of behaviors is performed. While it may take some time, the use of shaping in operant conditioning can allow for the training of extremely complicated behaviors.

Cognitive and Biological Factors in Associative Learning

It would be incorrect to say that classical and operant conditioning are the only factors that affect behavior, nor would it be correct to say that we are all mindless and robotic, unable to resist the rewards and punishments that occur in our lives. Since Skinner's initial perspectives, it has been found that many cognitive and biological factors are at work that can change the effects of associative learning or allow us to resist them altogether.

Many organisms undergo **latent learning**, which is learning that occurs without a reward but that is spontaneously demonstrated once a reward is introduced. The classic experiment associated with latent learning involves rats running a maze. Rats that were simply carried through the maze and then incentivized with a food reward for completing the maze on their own performed just as well—and in some cases better—than those rats that had been trained to run the maze using more standard operant conditioning techniques by which they were rewarded along the way.

Problem solving is another method of learning that steps outside the standard behaviorist approach. Think of the way young children put together a jigsaw puzzle: often, they will take pieces one-by-one and try to make them fit together until they find the correct match. Many animals will also use this kind of trial-and-error approach, testing behaviors until they yield a reward. As we get older, we gain the ability to analyze the situation and respond correctly the first time, as when we seek out the correct puzzle piece and orientation based on the picture we are forming. Humans and chimpanzees alike will often avoid trial-and-error learning and instead take a step back, observe the situation, and take decisive action to solve the challenges they face.

Not all behaviors can be taught using operant conditioning techniques. Many animals are predisposed to learn (or not learn) behaviors based on their own natural abilities and instincts. Animals are most able to learn behaviors that coincide with their natural behaviors: birds naturally peck when searching for food, so rewarding them with food in response to a pecking-based behavior works well. This predisposition is known as **preparedness**. Similarly, it can be very difficult to teach animals behaviors that work against their natural instincts. When animals revert to an instinctive behavior after learning a new behavior that is similar, the animal has undergone **instinctive** (or **instinctual**) **drift**. For example, researchers used behavioral techniques to train raccoons to place coins in a piggy bank. Their efforts were ultimately unsuccessful as the learned behaviors were only temporary. Eventually, rather than placing the coins in the bank, the raccoons would pick up the coins, rub them together, and dip them into the bank before pulling them back out. The researchers concluded that the task they were trying to train the raccoons to perform was conflicting with their natural food-gathering instinct, which was to rub seeds together and wash them in a stream to clean them before eating. The researchers had far better luck training the raccoons to place a ball in a basketball net, as the ball was too large to trigger the food-washing instinct.

Observational Learning

Observational learning is the process of learning a new behavior or gaining information by watching others. The most famous and perhaps most controversial study into observational learning is Albert Bandura's Bobo doll experiment, in which children watched an adult in a room full of toys punching and kicking an inflatable clown toy. When the children were later allowed to play in the room, many of them ignored the other toys in the room and inflicted similar violence on the Bobo doll

REAL WORLD

The connection between violent video games and aggressive behavior is still under active debate. While there are many interest groups on both sides of the controversy, the American Academy of Pediatrics (a major medical society) published one report in which they attributed a 13 to 22% increase in aggressive behavior to observational learning from video games.

just as they had seen the adult do. It's important to note that observational learning is not simply imitation because observational learning can be used to teach individuals to avoid behavior as well. In later iterations of the Bobo doll experiment, children who watched the adult get scolded after attacking the Bobo doll were less likely to be aggressive toward the Bobo doll themselves.

Like associative learning, there are a few neurological factors that affect observational learning. The most important of these are **mirror neurons**. These neurons are located in the frontal and parietal lobes of the cerebral cortex and fire both when an individual performs an action and when that individual observes someone else performing that action. Mirror neurons are largely involved in motor processes, but additionally are thought to be related to empathy and vicarious emotions; some mirror neurons fire both when we experience an emotion and also when we observe another experiencing the same emotion. Mirror neurons also play a role in imitative learning by a number of primates, as shown in Figure 3.4.

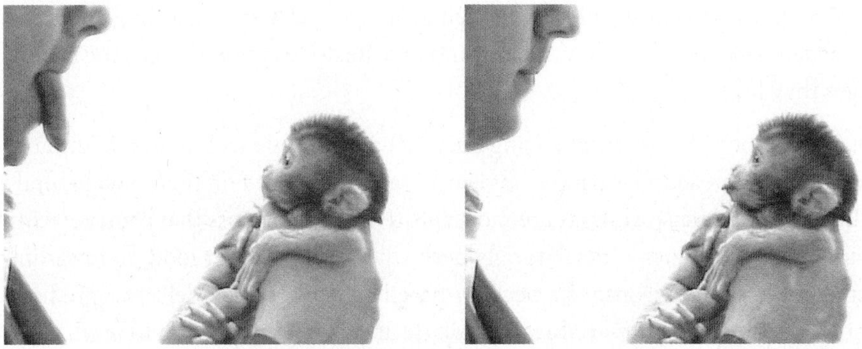

Figure 3.4 Use of Mirror Neurons in a Macaque
Many neonatal primates imitate facial expressions using mirror neurons.

Research suggests that observational learning through **modeling** is an important factor in determining people's behavior throughout their lifetime. People learn what behaviors are acceptable by watching others perform them. Much attention is focused on violent media as a model for antisocial behavior, but prosocial modeling can be just as powerful. Of course, observational learning is strongest when a model's words are consistent with actions. Many parents and guardians adopt a *Do as I say, not as I do* approach when teaching their children, but research suggests that children will disproportionately imitate what the model *did*, rather than what the model *said*.

MCAT CONCEPT CHECK 3.1

Before you move on, assess your understanding of the material with these questions.

1. Which of the following might cause a person to eat more food during a meal: eating each course separately and moving to the next only when finished with the current course, or interrupting the main course several times by eating side dishes?

___

2. A college student plays a prank on a roommate by popping a balloon behind the roommate's head after every time making popcorn. Before long, the smell of popcorn makes the roommate nervous. Which part of the story corresponds to each of the classical conditioning concepts below?
   - Conditioned stimulus:

   ___

   - Unconditioned stimulus:

   ___

   - Conditioned response:

   ___

   - Unconditioned response:

   ___

3. What is the difference between negative reinforcement and positive punishment? Provide an example of each.
   - Negative reinforcement:

   ___

   ___

   - Positive punishment:

   ___

   ___

3.2 Memory

High-Yield

LEARNING OBJECTIVES

After Chapter 3.2, you will be able to:

- Order the three modes of encoding from strongest to weakest
- Distinguish between maintenance rehearsal and elaborative rehearsal
- Predict how learning environments may impact recall
- Describe factors and phenomena that can lead to flaws in memory
- Define each type of human memory:

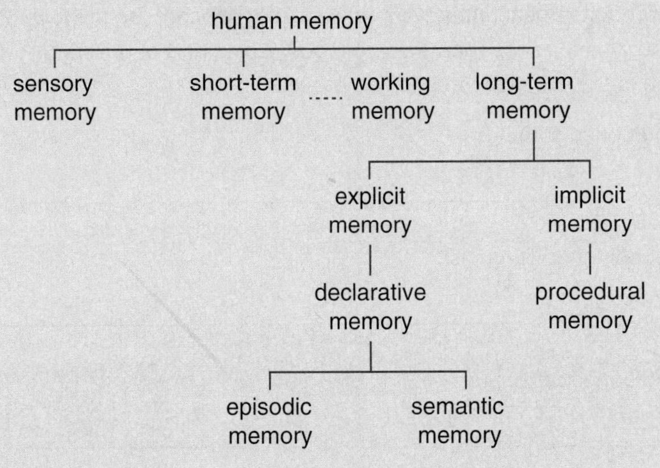

While learning is mostly concerned with behavior, the study of memory focuses on how we gain the knowledge that we accumulate over our lifetimes. The formation of memories can be divided into three major processes: encoding, storage, and retrieval.

Encoding

Encoding refers to the process of putting new information into memory. Information gained without any effort is the result of **automatic processing**. This type of cognitive processing is unintentional, and information is passively absorbed from the environment. As you walk down the street, you are constantly bombarded with information that seeps into your brain: you notice the temperature; you keep track of the route that you're taking; you might stop for coffee and realize that the same cashier has been working each day this week.

There are, however, times when we must actively work to gain information. In studying for the MCAT, for example, you may create flashcards to memorize the enzymes of digestion or the functions of endocrine hormones. This active memorization is known as **controlled (effortful) processing**.

MCAT EXPERTISE

Do not allow yourself to study for the MCAT using automatic processing! Just reading the text "to get through it" won't cut it for the MCAT. Engage with the text: fill out the MCAT Concept Checks, write notes in the margins, ask yourself questions. Scientific studies of learning have demonstrated, time and time again, that controlled processing improves comprehension, retention, and speed and accuracy on Test Day.

With practice, controlled processing can become automatic. Think back to a time when you were learning a foreign language. At first, each word required a great deal of processing to decipher: you had to hear the word and consciously translate it into your native language in order to understand what was being said. This process took an amount of time and effort that was probably difficult to maintain for prolonged periods. However, as you gained more experience with the language, this process became easier until you may have been able to understand those same words intuitively, without having to think very hard about them at all. At that point, this skill that once required controlled processing became automatic.

There are a few different ways that we encode the meaning of information when controlled processing is required. We can visualize information (**visual encoding**), store the way it sounds (**acoustic encoding**), link it to knowledge that is already in memory (**elaborative encoding**), or put it into a meaningful context (**semantic encoding**). Of these, semantic encoding is the strongest and visual encoding is the weakest. When using semantic encoding, the more vivid the context, the better. In fact, we tend to recall information best when we can put it into the context of our own lives, a phenomenon called the **self-reference effect**.

REAL WORLD

The purpose of the Real World sidebars in your *MCAT Review* books is semantic encoding: by putting content into a meaningful context, retention of the information is improved. Most of our Real World sidebars are related to medicine because of the self-reference effect.

Of course, grouping information into a meaningful context is only one trick that we can use to aid in encoding. Another such aid is **maintenance rehearsal**, which is the repetition of a piece of information to either keep it within working memory (to prevent forgetting) or to store it in short-term and eventually long-term memory—topics discussed in the next section.

Mnemonics are another common way to memorize information, particularly lists. As you've seen in your Kaplan study materials, mnemonics are often acronyms or rhyming phrases that provide a vivid organization of the information we are trying to remember. Two other mnemonic techniques are commonly employed by memory experts. The **method of loci** involves associating each item in a list with a location along a route through a building that has already been memorized. For example, in memorizing a grocery list, someone might picture a carton of eggs sitting on their doorstep, a person spilling milk in the front hallway, a giant stick of butter in the living room, and so on. Later, when the person wishes to recall the list, they simply take a mental walk through the locations and recall the images they formed earlier. Similarly, the **peg-word system** associates numbers with items that rhyme with or resemble the numbers. For example, one might be associated with the sun, two with a shoe, three with a tree, and so on. As groundwork, the individual memorizes their personal peg-list. When another list needs to be memorized, the individual can simply pair each item in the list with their peg-list. In this example, the individual may visualize eggs being fried by the sun (1), a pair of shoes (2) filled with milk, and a tree (3) with leaves made of butter. Because of the serial nature of both the method-of-loci and peg-word systems, they are very useful for memorizing large lists of objects in order.

REAL WORLD

Many feats of memory are accomplished via mnemonic techniques. In fact, the method of loci is a favorite among participants in the World Memory Championships.

Finally, **chunking** (sometimes referred to as **clustering**) is a memory trick that involves taking individual elements of a large list and grouping them together into groups of elements with related meaning. For example, consider the following list of 16 letters: E-N-A-L-P-K-C-U-R-T-R-A-C-S-U-B. Memorizing the list in order by rote might prove difficult until we realize that we can reverse the items and group them into meaningful chunks: BUS, CAR, TRUCK, PLANE.

Storage

Following encoding, information must be stored if it is to be remembered. There are several types of memory storage.

Sensory Memory

MCAT EXPERTISE

Sensory memory theoretically encompasses all five major senses, but studies have been mostly limited to sight, hearing, and touch (haptic memory).

The first and most fleeting kind of memory storage is **sensory memory**, which preserves information in its original sensory form (auditory, visual, etc.) with high accuracy and lasts only a very short time, generally less than one second. Sensory memory consists of both **iconic memory** (fast-decaying memory of visual stimuli) and **echoic memory** (fast-decaying memory of auditory stimuli). Sensory memories are maintained by the major projection areas of each sensory system, such as the occipital lobe for vision and the temporal lobe for hearing. Of course, sensory memory fades very quickly, so unless the information is attended to, it will be lost.

MCAT EXPERTISE

Eidetic memory refers to the ability to recall, with high precision, an image after only a brief exposure. It is hypothesized that eidetic memory represents an extreme example of iconic memory that endures for a few minutes. Although generally not observed in adults, it is reported to occur in a small percentage of children.

The nature of sensory memory can be demonstrated experimentally. Consider the following procedure: a research participant is presented with a three-by-three array of letters, such as that presented in Figure 3.5, that is flashed onto a screen for a mere fraction of a second. When asked to list all of the letters in the array, the participant is able to correctly identify three or four (a procedure known as **whole-report**). However, when asked to list the letters of a particular row immediately after the presentation of the stimulus (known as **partial-report**), the participant can do so with 100 percent accuracy, no matter which row is chosen. This is iconic memory in action: in the time it takes to list out a few of the items, the entire list fades; yet it is clear that all of the letters do make their way into iconic memory because any small subset can be recalled at will.

B	X	O
R	T	P
W	Q	L

Figure 3.5 A Sample 3-by-3 Array for Studying Sensory Memory

Short-Term Memory

Of course, we do pay attention to some of the information that we are exposed to, and that information enters our **short-term memory**. Similar to sensory memory, short-term memory fades quickly, over the course of approximately 30 seconds without rehearsal. In addition to having a limited duration, the number of items we can hold in our short-term memory at any given time, our **memory capacity**, is limited to approximately seven items, usually stated as the 7 ± 2 rule. As discussed in the previous section, the capacity of short-term memory can be increased by clustering information, and the duration can be extended using maintenance rehearsal. Short-term memory is housed primarily in the **hippocampus**, which is also responsible for the consolidation of short-term memory into long-term memory.

Working Memory

Working memory is closely related to short-term memory and is similarly supported by the hippocampus. It enables us to keep a few pieces of information in our con sciousness simultaneously and to manipulate that information. To do this, one must integrate short-term memory, attention, and executive function; accordingly, the frontal and parietal lobes are also involved. This is the form of memory that allows us to do simple math in our heads.

REAL WORLD

Have you ever looked at a picture of a simple unfinished puzzle, and been able to fit the pieces together mentally? This skill is explained by one of the major theories that underlies working memory, which includes the concept of a visuospatial sketchpad. The visuospatial sketchpad was proposed by Baddeley and Hitch as part of their three-part working memory model along with the other two components they proposed: the central executive and the phonological loop. The visuospatial sketchpad explains our ability to not only store visual and spatial information, but to manipulate it as well.

Long-Term Memory

With enough rehearsal, information moves from short-term to **long-term memory**, an essentially limitless warehouse for knowledge that we are then able to recall on demand, sometimes for the rest of our lives. One of the ways that information is consolidated into long-term memory is **elaborative rehearsal**. Unlike maintenance rehearsal, which is simply a way of keeping the information at the forefront of consciousness, elaborative rehearsal is the association of the information to knowledge already stored in long-term memory. Elaborative rehearsal is closely tied to the self-reference effect noted earlier; those ideas that we are able to relate to our own lives are more likely to find their way into our long-term memory. While long-term memory is primarily controlled by the hippocampus, it should be noted that memories are moved, over time, back to the cerebral cortex. Thus, very long-term memories—our names and birthdates, the faces of our parents—are generally not affected by damage to the hippocampus.

BEHAVIORAL SCIENCES GUIDED EXAMPLE WITH EXPERT THINKING

A musical melody is a series of tones played in succession that form a coherent musical idea. Melodies can be played in many different keys: absolute pitch of each of the notes changes as one changes keys, but as long as the relative pitches remain the same, the melody should still be recognizable. For example, the familiar melody of the song "Happy Birthday" should sound the same regardless of whether the first note is a C, an F, or a B-flat. While most people cannot name the key of a piece of music just by listening to it, they might still implicitly remember the way it "is supposed to sound" such that they could distinguish between the same melody played in different keys.

The passage provides the definition of melody, and the difference between absolute and relative pitch. Helpful if I'm not a musician, but really just setting the stage for the experiment.

Researchers interested in musical memory conducted an experiment with three groups of participants: 7- to 8-year-olds, 9- to 11-year-olds, and adults. Twenty-four British and Irish folk melodies were selected to be used as stimuli. The researchers expected that because these melodies share the sorts of patterns that are common in much North American and European music, they should thereby be recognizable as melodies rather than simply a series of tones. It was also expected that these melodies were uncommon enough to be unfamiliar to the participants prior to the beginning of the study.

Setup: Three groups, two children, one adult, presented with melodies. The melodies were intended to be unfamiliar.

IV: age

In the exposure phase, participants were presented with twelve of the twenty-four melodies to listen to. In the recognition phase, all twenty-four melodies were presented. Of the melodies that were presented in the exposure phase, six were then presented in the recognition phase transposed to a higher or lower key. Participants were asked to rate whether each melody they heard in the recognition phase had been presented in the exposure phase, and rated this recognition on a scale from 1 ("definitely new") to 6 ("definitely heard before").

Finally, the description of the procedure. I'll want to parse this carefully. In the second phase, some melodies were heard earlier and some weren't. Some of those that have been heard before were presented in a different key.

Second IV: transposition

DV: recognition

To eliminate bias, researchers used an Area Under the Curve (AUC) score, which measures the relative difference in recognition rather than the absolute difference. If all of the recognition scores for old melodies are higher than the recognition scores for new melodies for a given participant, the AUC score is 1.0, which represents perfect discrimination. A score of 0.5 represents chance performance, such that the old and new melodies are indistinguishable.

I've never heard of an AUC score before, but the passage explains it. I'll probably need this to interpret the results.

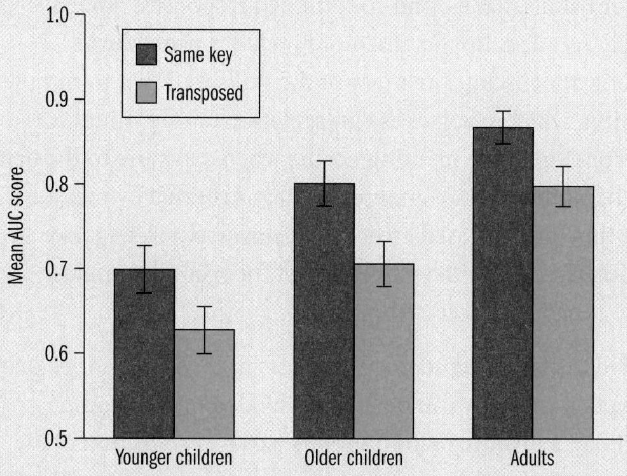

Figure 1 Mean AUC score for each group

IV: age and transposition

DV: recognition (AUC)

Higher AUC means better recognition, so it looks like people get better as they get older. It also seems people were slightly worse at recognizing the transposed melodies.

Adapted from: Schellenberg EG, Poon J, Weiss MW (2017) Memory for melody and key in childhood. *PLoS ONE* 12(10): e0187115. https://doi.org/10.1371/journal.pone.0187115

What do these results suggest about between-group and within-group trends with respect to explicit and implicit memory for music?

To answer this question, we're going to have to make use of the results of this study, but we'll also have to recall and apply content knowledge from outside this passage. The prompt asks about differences in explicit and implicit memory, so we'll want to start by figuring out how these terms apply in this general context, then apply these ideas specifically to the experiment. For the MCAT, we should know that explicit and implicit memory are both subdivisions of long-term memory. Explicit memory is the encoding of facts, and particularly relevant to the present study is episodic memory, the kind of explicit memory that involves experiences. The question "have I heard this melody before?" is answered by accessing an explicit memory. The relevance of implicit memory is more difficult here, since we typically think of implicit memories as procedural, involving skills and conditioned responses. Whenever we're not sure of how a concept in a question is related to the passage, we should go back to the passage and search for clues. The passage does provide a clue: in the first paragraph, the author describes the memory of the key of a melody as implicit rather than explicit. Now that we know what we're looking for, we can examine the results of the study with these concepts, and the way in which they relate to the passage, already in mind.

The AUC score system used by the researchers might be unfamiliar, but the concept isn't that much different from what we might normally see in a study like this one. A score of 0.5 represents random chance, and a score higher than that means that the participants were able to distinguish the melodies they'd heard from the ones they hadn't. The higher the score, the better the recognition. From the figure, we can see two trends: as participants get older, recognition gets better, but when the melody is transposed, recognition gets worse for all participants by approximately the same amount.

We must apply the memory vocabulary words to these trends. We can conclude from these results that explicit memory for music improved by age across groups. Further, within each group, implicit memory did play a significant role in recognition, because melodies that matched those heard earlier explicitly but not implicitly (i.e., they were the same melody but transposed to a different key) were less readily recognized. The role of implicit memory on recognition seems to be consistent between groups.

There are two types of long-term memory. **Implicit memory** (also called **nondeclarative memory**) consists of our skills, habits, and conditioned responses, none of which need to be consciously recalled. Implicit memory includes **procedural memory**, which relates to our unconscious memory of the skills required to complete procedural tasks, and **priming**, which involves the presentation of one stimulus affecting perception of a second. **Positive priming** occurs when exposure to the first stimulus improves processing of the second stimulus, as demonstrated by measures such as decreased response time or decreased error rate. Conversely, in **negative priming** the first stimulus interferes with the processing of the second stimulus, resulting in slower response times and more errors.

MCAT EXPERTISE

Although semantic and episodic memory are differentiated and can be separate, they can also co-occur. One type of explicit memory with components of both episodic and semantic memory is **flashbulb memory**, which is the detailed recollection of stimuli immediately surrounding an important (or emotionally arousing) event. Flashbulb memory helps you answer the question "Do you remember where you were when...?"

Explicit memory (also called **declarative memory**) consists of those memories that require conscious recall. Explicit memory can be further divided into episodic memory and semantic memory. **Episodic memory** refers to our recollection of life experiences. By contrast, **semantic memory** refers to ideas, concepts, or facts that we know, but are not tied to specific life experiences. **Autobiographical memory** is the name given to our explicit memories about our lives and ourselves, and includes all of our episodic memories of our own life experiences, but also includes semantic memories that relate to our personal traits and characteristics. Interestingly, memory disorders can affect one type of memory but leave others alone. For example, a patient who has amnesia might not remember learning to ride a bicycle (episodic memory) or the names of the parts of a bicycle (semantic memory), but may, surprisingly, retain the skill of riding a bicycle when given one (procedural memory). The various major categories of memory are summarized in Figure 3.6.

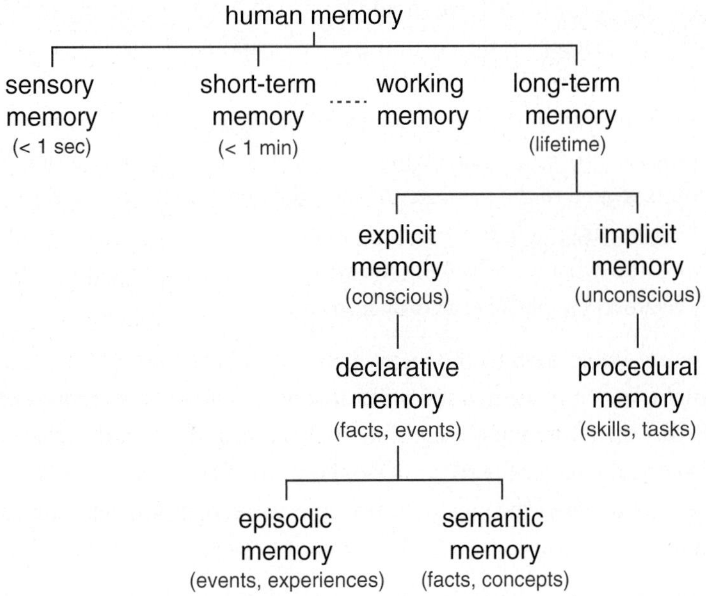

Figure 3.6 Types of Memory

Retrieval

Of course, memories that are stored are of no use unless we can pull them back out to use them. **Retrieval** is the name given to the process of demonstrating that something that has been learned has been retained. Most people think about retrieval in terms of **recall**, or the retrieval and statement of previously learned information, but learning can be additionally demonstrated by recognizing or quickly relearning information.

Recognition, the process of merely identifying a piece of information that was previously learned, is far easier than recall. This difference is something you can take advantage of because the MCAT, as a multiple-choice test, is largely based on recognizing information. If the MCAT were a fill-in-the-blank style exam, your approach to studying would have to be vastly different and far more in-depth.

REAL WORLD

Think back to elementary school. How many of your classmates do you think you could list? Chances are, not many. On the other hand, glancing through your class photo, you would probably recognize the vast majority of your former classmates. This gap is the difference between recall and recognition.

Relearning is another way of demonstrating that information has been stored in long-term memory. In studying the memorization of lists, Hermann Ebbinghaus found that his recall of a list of short words he had learned the previous day was often quite poor. However, he was able to rememorize the list much more quickly the second time through. Ebbinghaus interpreted this to mean that the information had been stored, even though it wasn't readily available for recall. Through additional research, he discovered that the longer the amount of time between sessions of relearning, the greater the retention of the information later on. Ebbinghaus dubbed this phenomenon the **spacing effect**, and it helps to explain why cramming is not nearly as effective as spacing out studying over an extended period of time.

Recalling a fact at a moment's notice can be difficult. Fortunately, the brain has ways of organizing information so that it can take advantage of environmental cues to tell it where to find a given memory. Psychologists think of memory not as simply a stockpile of unrelated facts, but rather as a network of interconnected ideas. The brain organizes ideas into a **semantic network**, as shown in Figure 3.7, in which concepts are linked together based on similar meaning, not unlike an Internet encyclopedia wherein each page includes links for similar topics. For example, the concept of *red* might be closely linked to other colors, like *orange* and *green*, as well as objects, like *fire engine* and *roses*. When one node of our semantic network is activated, such as seeing the word *red* on a sign, the other linked concepts around it are also unconsciously activated, a process known as **spreading activation**. Spreading activation is at the heart of the previously mentioned positive priming, as recall is aided by first being presented with a word or phrase, a **recall cue**, that is close to the desired semantic memory.

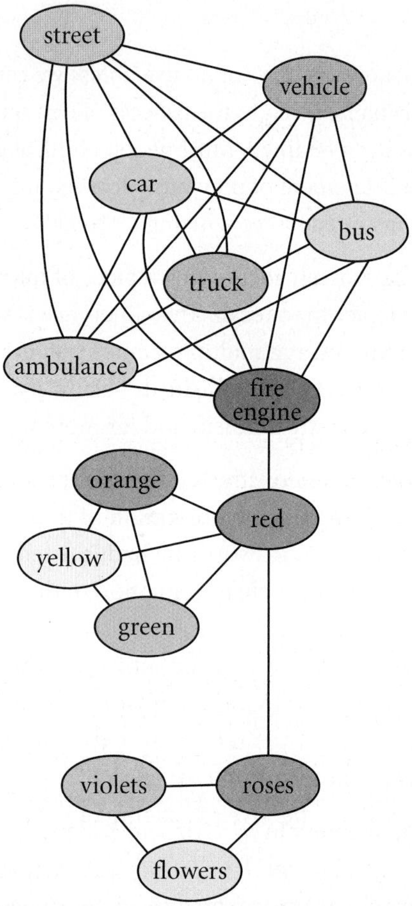

Figure 3.7 An Example Semantic Network

In spreading activation, the concept of red will also unconsciously activate other linked concepts.

Another common retrieval cue is **context effect**, where memory is aided by being in the physical location where encoding took place. Psychologists have shown a person will score better when they take an exam in the same room in which they learned the information. Context effects can go even further than this; facts learned underwater are better recalled when underwater than when on land. Similarly, **source monitoring** is a part of the retrieval process that involves determining the origin of memories, and whether they are factual (real and accurate) or fictional (from a dream, novel, or movie).

A person's mental state can also affect their ability to recall. **State-dependent memory,** alternately referred to as a **state-dependent effect**, is a retrieval cue based on performing better when in the same mental state as when the information was learned. People who learn facts or skills while intoxicated, for example, will show better recall or proficiency when performing those same tasks while intoxicated as compared to performing them while sober. Emotions work in a similar way: being in a foul mood primes negative memories, which in turn work to sustain the foul mood. So not only will memory be better for information learned when in a similar mood, but recall of negative or positive memories will lead to the persistence of the mood.

Finally, studies on list memorization have indicated that an item's position in the list affects participants' ability to recall, which Ebbinghaus termed the **serial-position effect**. When researchers give participants a list of items to memorize, the participants have much higher recall for both the first few and last few items on the list. The tendency to remember early and late items in the list is known as the **primacy** and **recency effect**, respectively. However, when asked to remember the list later, people show strong recall for the first few items while recall of the last few items fades. Psychologists interpret this to mean that the recency effect is a result of the last items still being in short-term memory on initial recall.

Forgetting

Unfortunately, even long-term memory is not always permanent. Several phenomena can result in **amnesia**, a significant loss of memorized information. The inability to remember where, when, or how one has obtained knowledge is called **source amnesia**.

Brain Disorders

There are several disorders that can lead to decline in memory. The most common is **Alzheimer's disease**, which is a degenerative brain disorder thought to be linked to a loss of acetylcholine in neurons that link to the hippocampus, although its exact causes are not well understood. Alzheimer's is marked by progressive **dementia** (a loss of cognitive function) and memory loss, with atrophy of the brain, as shown in Figure 3.8. While not perfectly linear, memory loss in Alzheimer's disease tends to proceed in a retrograde fashion, with loss of recent memories before distant memories. Microscopic findings of Alzheimer's include **neurofibrillary tangles** and **β-amyloid plaques**. One common phenomenon that occurs in individuals with middle- to late-stage Alzheimer's is **sundowning**, an increase in dysfunction in the late afternoon and evening.

BRIDGE

The β-amyloid plaques of Alzheimer's disease are incorrectly folded copies of the amyloid precursor protein, in which insoluble β-pleated sheets form and then deposit in the brain. Protein folding is discussed in detail in Chapter 1 of *MCAT Biochemistry Review*.

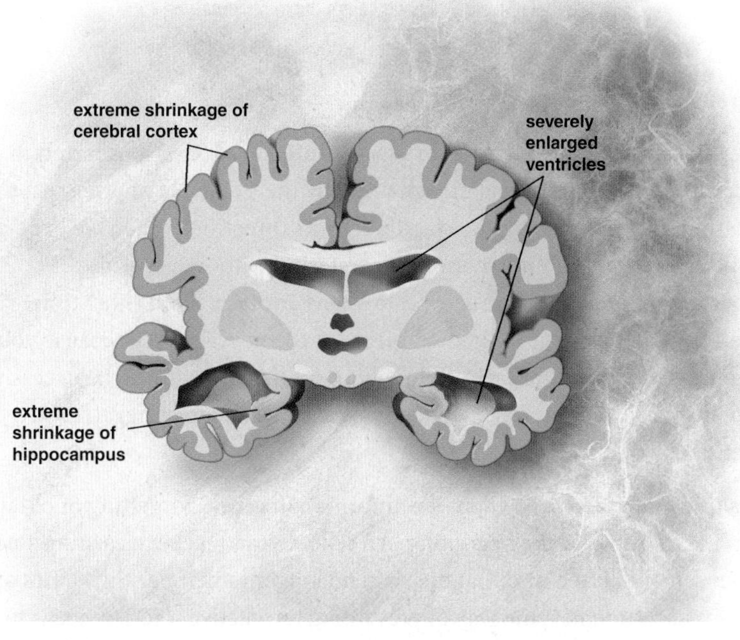

Figure 3.8 Findings of Alzheimer's Disease

Korsakoff's syndrome is another form of memory loss caused by thiamine deficiency in the brain. The disorder is marked by both **retrograde amnesia** (the loss of previously formed memories) and **anterograde amnesia** (the inability to form new memories). Another common symptom is **confabulation**, or the process of creating vivid but fabricated memories, typically thought to be an attempt made by the brain to fill in the gaps of missing memories.

Agnosia is the loss of the ability to recognize objects, people, or sounds, though usually only one of the three. Agnosia is usually caused by physical damage to the brain, such as that caused by a stroke or a neurological disorder such as multiple sclerosis.

Decay

Of course, not all memory loss is due to a disorder. Through a process known as **decay**, memories are simply lost naturally over time as the neurochemical trace of a short-term memory fades. In his word memorization experiment, Ebbinghaus noted what he called a "curve of forgetting," formally called the **retention function**, as shown in Figure 3.9. For a day or two after learning the list, recall fell sharply but then leveled off.

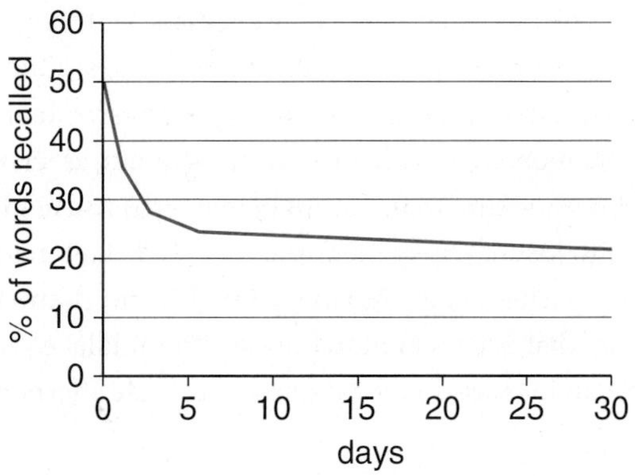

Figure 3.9 Ebbinghaus's Curve of Forgetting

Interference

Another common reason for memory loss is **interference** (also referred to as an **interference effect**), a retrieval error caused by the existence of other, usually similar, information. Interference can be classified by its direction. When we experience **proactive interference**, old information is interfering with new learning. For example, think back to a time when you moved to a new address. For a short time, you may have had trouble recalling individual pieces of the new address because you were so used to the old one. Similarly, Ebbinghaus found that with each successive list he learned, his recall for new lists decreased over time, an effect he attributed to interference caused by older lists.

Retroactive interference is when new information causes forgetting of old information. For example, at the beginning of a school year, teachers learning a new set of students' names often find that they can no longer remember the names of the previous year's students. One way of preventing retroactive interference is to reduce the number of interfering events, which is why it is often best to study in the evening about an hour before falling asleep (although this also depends on your personal style!).

Aging and Memory

Contrary to popular belief, aging does not necessarily lead to significant memory loss; while there are many individuals whose memory fades in old age, this is not always the case. In fact, studies show that there is a larger range of memory ability for 70-year-olds than there is for 20-year-olds. There are, however, some trends that can be demonstrated when evaluating the memories of older individuals. When asked about the most pivotal events in their lives, people in their 70s and 80s tend to say that their most vivid memories are of events that occurred in their teens and 20s, a fact that psychologists interpret to mean that this time is a peak period for encoding in a person's life.

Even for older adults, certain types of memory remain quite strong. People tend not to demonstrate much degeneration in recognition or skill-based memory as they age. Even certain types of recall will remain strong for most people; semantically meaningful material can be easily learned and recalled, most likely due to older individuals having a larger semantic network than their younger counterparts. **Prospective memory** (remembering to perform a task at some point in the future) remains mostly intact when it is event-based—that is, primed by a trigger event, such as remembering to buy milk when walking past the grocery store. On the other hand, time-based prospective memory, such as remembering to take a medication every day at 7:00 a.m., does tend to decline with age.

Memory Reconstruction

We often think of memory as a record of our experiences or a kind of video recording that is stored to be accessed later; this accurate recall of past events is defined as **reproductive memory**. Nothing could be further from the truth. **Reconstructive memory** is a theory of memory recall in which cognitive processes such as imagination, semantic memory, and perception affect the act of remembering. This theory explains how two people can recall the same event as occurring in completely different ways. A memory that incorrectly recalls actual events or recalls events that never occurred is known as a **false memory**. Despite their unsettling nature, false memories are common and are to be expected when we consider the many factors that can affect memory. Most memories are encoded with little detail, only focusing on the details deemed important in the moment. Also, as previously discussed, if a person repeatedly rehearses the memory in their mind, then that person may fill in missing details with unreliable information. Repressed memories, memories stored in the unconscious mind and blocked from recall, have also been a topic of controversy. Some psychologists believe repressed memories can be brought back into our conscious mind either spontaneously or through psychotherapy. Such memories are called **recovered memories**. However, it is not possible to distinguish between false memories and recovered memories without evidence and some research psychologists believe psychotherapy is more likely to lead to the creation of false memories. So, the act of recalling a memory can result in the production of a false memory.

False memory production is not only limited to internal factors. Memories can also be affected by outside sources as well. In a famous experiment, participants were shown several pictures including one picture of a car stopped at a yield sign. Later, these participants were presented with written descriptions of the pictures, and some of these descriptions contained misinformation, such as a description of a car stopped at a stop sign. When asked to recall the details of the pictures, many participants insisted they had seen a stop sign in the picture. This example illustrates the **misinformation effect**, where a person's recall of an event becomes less accurate due to the injection of outside information into the memory.

The misinformation effect can also be seen at the point of recall. In another experiment, participants were shown a video of an automobile accident. Some participants were then asked, *How fast were the cars moving when they collided?*, while others were asked about the accident using more descriptive language such as *How fast were the cars moving when they crashed?* Those participants who were asked the question with leading language were much more likely to overstate the severity of the accident than those who had been asked the question with less descriptive language.

Intrusion errors refers to false memories that have included a false detail into a particular memory. This is similar to the misinformation effect but distinct in that the intrusion error is not from an outside source. Instead, the intruding memory is injected into original memory due to both memories being related or sharing a theme. Upon memory recall, the brain incorrectly associates the intruding memory with the source memory, leading to a false memory. For example, if over the years you've attended multiple New Year's Eve celebrations in two different cities, then your memories of the two cities are linked. A possible intrusion error could be recalling that a particular restaurant is located in Vancouver, because you recall eating at the restaurant on New Year's Eve and celebrating New Year's Eve in Vancouver. However, the restaurant is really in Toronto, where you have also celebrated on New Year's.

Source-monitoring error involves confusion between semantic and episodic memory: a person remembers the details of an event, but confuses the context under which those details were gained. Source-monitoring error often manifests when a person hears a story of something that happened to someone else, and later recalls the story as a personal memory.

REAL WORLD

During a Congressional Medal of Honor ceremony in 1983, Ronald Reagan relayed a vivid story about a heroic World War II pilot who received a posthumous medal. Skeptical reporters, unaware of any incident matching the details of Reagan's story, checked into the story and found that the pilot had existed—in the 1944 movie *A Wing and a Prayer*. Reagan had remembered the details of the pilot's heroic actions but had forgotten their source.

MCAT CONCEPT CHECK 3.2

Before you move on, assess your understanding of the material with these questions.

1. List the three modes in which information can be encoded, from strongest to weakest.

   1. ____________________
   2. ____________________
   3. ____________________

2. In what ways is maintenance rehearsal different from elaborative rehearsal?

   ____

3. In terms of recall, why might it be a bad idea to study for the MCAT while listening to music?

   ____

4. What are some factors that might cause eyewitness courtroom testimony to be unreliable?

   ____

3.3 Neurobiology of Learning and Memory

LEARNING OBJECTIVES

After Chapter 3.3, you will be able to:

- Describe neuroplasticity and changes that occur throughout the human life span
- Recall the terms involved with removing and strengthening memory connections

Even as you read this text, your brain is changing. Memory, and therefore learning, involves changes in brain physiology, such that with each new concept you learn your brain is altering its synaptic connections in response. You may have heard that it is far easier for children to learn a new language than it is for adults. Indeed, the saying *you can't teach an old dog new tricks*, while not strictly true, does have its roots in neurobiology.

As infants, we are born with many more neurons than we actually need. As our brains develop, neural connections form rapidly in response to stimuli via a phenomenon called **neuroplasticity** (also known as **neural plasticity**). In fact, the brains of young children are so plastic that they can reorganize drastically in response to injury, as evidenced by studies of children who have had entire hemispheres of their brains removed to prevent severe seizures. The remaining hemisphere will change to take over functions of the missing parts of the brain, allowing these children to grow up to lead unimpaired lives. While our brains do maintain a degree of plasticity throughout our lives, adult brains display nowhere near the degree of plasticity as those of a child. Another way our brains change is through a process called **synaptic pruning**. As we grow older, weak neural connections are broken while strong ones are bolstered, increasing the efficiency of our brains' ability to process information.

MCAT EXPERTISE

Recent research has begun to elucidate the mechanism of long-term potentiation. It has been observed that a specific type of glutamate receptor, the **NMDA receptor**, is required for the strengthening of synaptic connections.

MNEMONIC

The word *potentiate* means to increase the potency or strength of something. Long-term potentiation can be thought of as the strengthening of a "long-term" synaptic connection.

This concept of plasticity is important because it is closely linked to learning and memory. As you learned in Chapter 4 of *MCAT Biology Review*, stimuli cause activation of neurons, which release their neurotransmitters into the **synaptic cleft**, the gap between a neuron and a target cell. These neurotransmitters continue to stimulate activity until degradation, reuptake, or diffusion out of the synaptic cleft. In the interim, this neural activity forms a memory trace that is thought to be the cause of short-term memory. As discussed earlier, if the stimulus isn't repeated or rehearsed, the memory trace disappears, and the consequence is the loss of the short-term memory. However, as the stimulus is repeated, the stimulated neurons become more efficient at releasing their neurotransmitters and at the same time receptor sites on the other side of the synapse increase, increasing receptor density. The strengthening of neural connections through repeated use is known as **long-term potentiation**, and is believed to be the neurophysiological basis of long-term memory.

As described in the previous section, a memory begins its life as a sensory memory in the projection area of a given sensory modality. This sensory memory is brief, unless maintained in consciousness and moved, as a short-term memory, into the hippocampus in the temporal lobe. The memory can then be manipulated through working memory while in the hippocampus (in tandem with the frontal and parietal lobes), and even stored for later recall. Over very long periods of time, memories are gradually moved from the hippocampus back to the cerebral cortex. Note that this general pathway is a drastic oversimplification of the complex interplay of brain regions involved in memory, but is a useful paradigm for Test Day.

MCAT CONCEPT CHECK 3.3

Before you move on, assess your understanding of the material with these questions.

1. What is neuroplasticity? How does neuroplasticity change during life?

____

____

2. What is the term for removing weak neural connections? What is the term for strengthening memory connections through increased neurotransmitter release and receptor density?
   - Removing weak connections:

   ____

   - Strengthening connections:

   ____

Conclusion

In this chapter, we discussed two very important ways that we react to our environments. We are constantly receiving input from the world around us, and the way we memorize that information depends greatly on both the nature of the information and its importance to us individually. That information can also have a profound effect on us, causing us to increase or decrease the frequency of certain behaviors, sometimes without our conscious knowledge. Because the concepts of learning and memory are both used heavily in research, we can expect the MCAT to place many of its passages testing these topics within an experimental context.

GO ONLINE

You've reviewed the content, now test your knowledge and critical thinking skills by completing a test-like passage set in your online resources!

CONCEPT SUMMARY

Learning

- **Habituation** is the process of becoming used to a stimulus. **Dishabituation** can occur when a second stimulus intervenes, causing a resensitization to the original stimulus.
- **Associative learning** is a way of pairing together stimuli and responses, or behaviors and consequences.
- In **classical conditioning**, an unconditioned stimulus that produces an instinctive, unconditioned response is paired with a neutral stimulus. With repetition, the neutral stimulus becomes a conditioned stimulus that produces a conditioned response.
- In **operant conditioning**, behavior is changed through the use of consequences.
  - **Reinforcement** increases the likelihood of a behavior.
  - **Punishment** decreases the likelihood of a behavior.
  - The schedule of reinforcement affects the rate at which the behavior is performed. Schedules can be based either on a ratio of behavior to reward or on an amount of time, and can be either fixed or variable. Behaviors learned through variable-ratio schedules are the hardest to extinguish.
- **Observational learning**, or **modeling**, is the acquisition of behavior by watching others.

Memory

- **Encoding** is the process of putting new information into memory. It can be **automatic** or **effortful**. Semantic encoding is stronger than both acoustic and visual encoding.
- **Sensory** and **short-term memory** are transient and are based on neurotransmitter activity. **Working memory** requires short-term memory, attention, and executive function to manipulate information.
- **Long-term memory** requires elaborative rehearsal and is the result of increased neuronal connectivity.
  - **Explicit** (**declarative**) **memory** stores facts and stories.
  - **Implicit** (**nondeclarative**) **memory** stores skills and conditioning effects.
- Facts are stored via **semantic networks**.
- **Recognition** of information is stronger than **recall**.
- **Retrieval** of information is often based on **priming** interconnected nodes of the semantic network.

- Memories can be lost through disorders such as Alzheimer's disease, Korsakoff's syndrome, or agnosia; decay; or interference.
- Memories are highly subject to influence by outside information and mood both at the time of encoding and at recall.

Neurobiology of Learning and Memory

- Both learning and memory rely on changes in brain chemistry and physiology, the extent of which depends on **neuroplasticity**, which decreases as we age.
- **Long-term potentiation**, responsible for the conversion of short-term to long-term memory, is the strengthening of neuronal connections resulting from increased neurotransmitter release and adding of receptor sites.

ANSWERS TO CONCEPT CHECKS

3.1

1. Eating each course of a meal before moving on to the next causes habituation; each bite causes less pleasurable stimulation, so people feel less desire to keep eating. On the other hand, mixing up the courses of a meal causes dishabituation for taste, which would cause people to eat more overall.
2. The conditioned stimulus is the smell of popcorn. The unconditioned stimulus is the popping of the balloon. The conditioned response is nervousness (fear) in response to the presence of popcorn. The unconditioned response is fear in response to the popping of the balloon.
3. Negative reinforcement causes an increase of a given behavior by removing something unpleasant, while positive punishment reduces behavior by adding something unpleasant. Examples will vary, but common negative reinforcers include medicines that reduce pain or avoiding uncomfortable situations to reduce anxiety. Common examples of positive punishments include having to pay a fine for speeding while driving or getting detention in school for bad behavior.

3.2

1. Of the three modes in which information can be encoded, semantic is the strongest, followed by acoustic. Visual is the weakest.
2. Maintenance rehearsal is the repetition of information to keep it within short-term memory for near-immediate use. Elaborative rehearsal is the association of information to other stored knowledge and is a more effective way to move information from short-term to long-term memory.
3. Because you will be taking the MCAT in a quiet room, studying under similar circumstances will aid recall due to context effects. Music may also compete for attention, reducing your ability to focus on the relevant study material.
4. Several factors can affect the accuracy of eyewitness testimony, including the manner in which questions are asked; the nature of information shared with the witness by police, lawyers, and other witnesses following the event; the misinformation effect; source-monitoring error; and the amount of time elapsed between the event and the trial. Even watching crime dramas, watching the news, or witnessing similar events can cause source-monitoring error.

3.3

1. Neuroplasticity is the ability of the brain to form new connections rapidly. The brain is most plastic in young children, and plasticity quickly drops off after childhood.
2. Pruning is the term for removing weak neural connections. Long-term potentiation is the strengthening of memory connections through increased neurotransmitter release and receptor density.

SCIENCE MASTERY ASSESSMENT EXPLANATIONS

1. **A**

After a while, the participant became habituated to the sound of the buzzer. Introducing a new stimulus, such as the banging pans, should dishabituate (resensitize) the original stimulus, causing a temporary increase in response to the sound of the buzzer.

2. **C**

The sound of a can opener would not normally produce a response on its own, making it a stimulus that must have been conditioned by association with food.

3. **B**

Generalization is the process by which similar stimuli can produce the same conditioned response. Here, the response to the taste and smell of oranges has generalized to that of all citrus.

4. **D**

Avoidance learning is a type of negative reinforcement in which a behavior is increased to prevent an unpleasant future consequence. Extinction, **(A)**, is a decreased response to a conditioned stimulus when it is no longer paired with an unconditioned stimulus. Punishment, **(B)** and **(C)**, leads to decreased behaviors in operant conditioning.

5. **A**

Long term potentiation is believed to be the neurophysiological basis of long-term memory, making **(A)** the correct answer. As synapses are reinforced, the neuroplasticity of the brain decreases, eliminating **(C)**. Also, synaptic pruning, **(B)**, refers to the removal of infrequently used synapses, which is not consistent with the description in the question stem.

6. **C**

In a fixed-interval schedule, the desired behavior is rewarded the first time it is exhibited after the fixed interval has elapsed. Both fixed-interval and fixed-ratio schedules tend to show this phenomenon: almost no response immediately after the reward is given, but the behavior increases as the rat gets close to receiving the reward.

7. **A**

Complicated, multistage behaviors are typically taught through shaping, so statement III must not be part of the correct answer. Reinforcers do not necessarily need to be food-based, and instinctive drift can interfere with learning of complicated behaviors; therefore, only statement I is accurate.

8. **C**

This is the definition of controlled processing and is the only answer choice that is necessarily true of controlled processing. Effortful processing is used to create long-term memories, and—with practice—can become automatic, invalidating **(A)** and **(B)**. Most of our day-to-day activities are processed automatically, making **(D)** incorrect.

9. **A**

Semantic encoding, or encoding based on the meaning of the information, is the strongest of the methods of encoding. Visual encoding, **(B)**, is the weakest, and acoustic encoding, **(D)**, is intermediate between the two. Iconic memory, **(C)**, is a type of sensory memory.

10. **C**

We are born with an overabundance of neurons and quickly form many new synapses in the first few years of life. As we age, the plasticity of our brains decreases, although we do retain some plasticity throughout adulthood. Thus, the brain of a two year old, due to its higher neuroplasticity, would better adapt, supporting **(C)** as the correct answer.

11. **D**

The association of words on a list to a preconstructed set of ideas is common to both the method-of-loci and peg-word mnemonics. Method-of-loci systems, **(B)**, associate items with locations, while peg-word systems use images associated with numbers.

12. **A**

Partial-report procedures, in which the individual is asked to recall a specific portion of the stimulus, are incredibly accurate, but only for a very brief time. This is a method of studying sensory (specifically, iconic) memory. Both the serial position effect, **(B)**, and the 7 ± 2 rule, **(C)**, are characteristics of short-term memory.

13. **B**

Semantic memory is the category of long-term memory that refers to recall of facts, rather than experiences or skills. Be careful not to confuse semantic memory with semantic networks, **(D)**, which are the associations of similar concepts in the mind to aid in their retrieval.

14. **C**

State-dependent recall is concerned with the internal rather than external states of the individual. As such, both statements II and III are examples of state-dependent circumstances, while statement I might cause a context effect instead.

15. **B**

Older adults may have trouble with time-based prospective memory, which is remembering to do an activity at a particular time. Other forms of memory are generally preserved, or may decline slightly but less significantly than time-based prospective memory.

Consult your online resources for additional practice. **GO ONLINE**

SHARED CONCEPTS

Behavioral Sciences Chapter 1
Biology and Behavior

Behavioral Sciences Chapter 2
Sensation and Perception

Behavioral Sciences Chapter 4
Cognition, Consciousness, and Language

Behavioral Sciences Chapter 5
Motivation, Emotion, and Stress

Behavioral Sciences Chapter 7
Psychological Disorders

Biology Chapter 4
The Nervous System

CHAPTER 4

COGNITION, CONSCIOUSNESS, AND LANGUAGE

SCIENCE MASTERY ASSESSMENT

Every pre-med knows this feeling: there is so much content I have to know for the MCAT! How do I know what to do first or what's important?

While the high-yield badges throughout this book will help you identify the most important topics, this Science Mastery Assessment is another tool in your MCAT prep arsenal. This quiz (which can also be taken in your online resources) and the guidance below will help ensure that you are spending the appropriate amount of time on this chapter based on your personal strengths and weaknesses. Don't worry though—skipping something now does not mean you'll never study it. Later on in your prep, as you complete full-length tests, you'll uncover specific pieces of content that you need to review and can come back to these chapters as appropriate.

How to Use This Assessment

If you answer 0–7 questions correctly:

Spend about 1 hour to read this chapter in full and take limited notes throughout. Follow up by reviewing **all** quiz questions to ensure that you now understand how to solve each one.

If you answer 8–11 questions correctly:

Spend 20–40 minutes reviewing the quiz questions. Beginning with the questions you missed, read and take notes on the corresponding subchapters. For questions you answered correctly, ensure your thinking matches that of the explanation and you understand why each choice was correct or incorrect.

If you answer 12–15 questions correctly:

Spend less than 20 minutes reviewing all questions from the quiz. If you missed any, then include a quick read-through of the corresponding subchapters, or even just the relevant content within a subchapter, as part of your question review. For questions you answered correctly, ensure your thinking matches that of the explanation and review the Concept Summary at the end of the chapter.

1. Which of the following terms describes how existing schemata are modified to incorporate new information?
   - **A.** Assimilation
   - **B.** Adaptation
   - **C.** Affirmation
   - **D.** Accommodation

2. After completing final exams, a student reports to student health complaining of paranoia, lack of appetite, and elevated heart rate. After some questioning, the student admits to having been awake for over 48 hours after having bought pills from another student in the library. Which of the following drugs has this student likely taken?
   - **A.** Phenobarbitol
   - **B.** Dextroamphetamine
   - **C.** Oxycodone
   - **D.** Lysergic acid diethylamide

3. A student is volunteering in a hospital with a stroke center. When asked what the prevalence of stroke is among those greater than 65 years old, the student states that it is probably about 40% even though data analysis indicates that it is significantly lower. What accounts for this error?
   - **A.** Deductive reasoning
   - **B.** Representativeness heuristic
   - **C.** Base rate fallacy
   - **D.** Confirmation bias

4. Which of the following types of intelligence is NOT described by Gardner's theory of multiple intelligences?
   - **A.** Fluid intelligence
   - **B.** Bodily-kinesthetic intelligence
   - **C.** Visual–spatial intelligence
   - **D.** Linguistic intelligence

5. EEG waveforms during REM sleep most resemble which of the following states of consciousness?
   - **A.** Alertness
   - **B.** Slow-wave sleep
   - **C.** Stage 1 sleep
   - **D.** Meditation

6. Which of the following indicates the pattern of sleep stages during a complete sleep cycle early in the night?
   - **A.** 1–2–3–4–1–2–REM
   - **B.** 1–2–3–4–3–2–REM
   - **C.** 4–3–2–1–2–3–REM
   - **D.** 4–3–2–4–3–1–REM

7. Which of the following best explains a student's ability to sit on the couch and watch reruns of a favorite TV show while studying for a chemistry exam?
   - **A.** Selective attention
   - **B.** Divided attention
   - **C.** Shadowing
   - **D.** Parallel processing

8. Which theory of dreaming states that dreams and thoughts during wakeful periods use the same stream-of-consciousness system?
   - **A.** Activation–synthesis theory
   - **B.** Problem solving theory
   - **C.** Cognitive process theory
   - **D.** Neurocognitive theory

9. A 19-year-old college student with bloodshot eyes is picked up by campus police after shoplifting a large bag of corn chips and a dozen ice cream sandwiches. During questioning, the student cannot stop giggling and repeatedly asks for water, complaining of dryness in the mouth. What is the psychoactive substance in the drug this student has most likely recently taken?
   - **A.** Alprazolam
   - **B.** 3,4-Methylenedioxy-*N*-methylamphetamine
   - **C.** Diacetylmorphine
   - **D.** Tetrahydrocannabinol

10. Language consists of multiple components. Which of the following involves the order in which words are put together?
    - **A.** Phonology
    - **B.** Semantics
    - **C.** Syntax
    - **D.** Pragmatics

11. A child speaks in sentences of at least 3 words, but makes grammatical errors including misuse of the past tense. How old is this child likely to be?
    - **A.** 14 months
    - **B.** 22 months
    - **C.** 30 months
    - **D.** 5 years

12. Which language theory states that language development occurs due to preferential reinforcement of certain phonemes by parents and caregivers?
    - **A.** Nativist theory
    - **B.** Learning theory
    - **C.** Social interactionist theory
    - **D.** Neurocognitive theory

13. A stroke patient comprehends speech but cannot properly move the mouth to form words. Which of the following brain areas is likely affected?
    - **A.** Broca's area
    - **B.** Wernicke's area
    - **C.** Arcuate fasciculus
    - **D.** Superior temporal gyrus

14. A person sits at a terminal of the airport and works on a challenging sudoku puzzle. The individual ignores most of the intercom announcements but, after an announcement indicates that boarding for the flight has begun, quickly gets in line. Which of the following best explains the person's rapid response for boarding?
    - **A.** Cocktail party phenomenon
    - **B.** Divided attention
    - **C.** Automatic processing
    - **D.** Effortful processing

15. During which of the following stages does dreaming occur?
    - **I.** Stage 3
    - **II.** Stage 4
    - **III.** REM

    - **A.** I only
    - **B.** II only
    - **C.** III only
    - **D.** I, II, and III

Answer Key

1. **D**
2. **B**
3. **C**
4. **A**
5. **A**
6. **B**
7. **B**
8. **C**
9. **D**
10. **C**
11. **C**
12. **B**
13. **A**
14. **A**
15. **D**

Detailed explanations can be found at the end of the chapter.

CHAPTER 4

COGNITION, CONSCIOUSNESS, AND LANGUAGE

In This Chapter

CHAPTER PROFILE

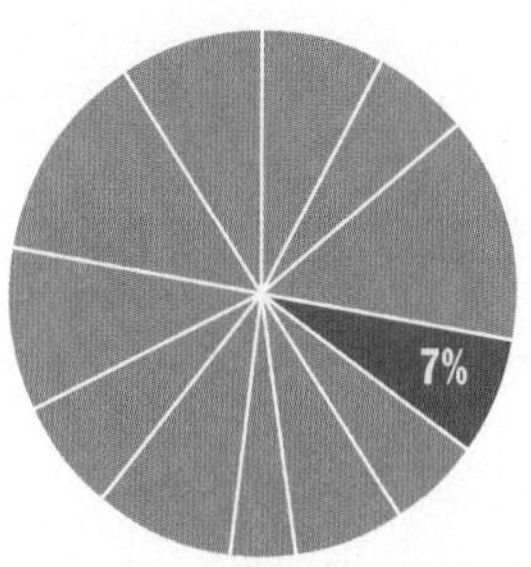

The content in this chapter should be relevant to about 7% of all questions about the behavioral sciences on the MCAT.

This chapter covers material from the following AAMC content category:

6B: Making sense of the environment

Introduction

As you think and move through the world, you often take your brain for granted. As you read, speak, ponder, make decisions, and perform complex motor functions, your brain is rapidly using electrical and chemical impulses to encode, store, and retrieve information. Most of these processes occur without your awareness or conscious thought. Imagine going to the grocery store. You fill your cart while comparing prices, assessing the produce, and planning what meals to make in the near future. After the cashier totals your purchases, you pull out a debit card, punch in a PIN, and leave with your groceries. While you were shopping in that grocery store, your brain was busy taking in all of the information around it and deciding which stimuli required attention. At the same time, you were making conscious decisions about your purchases, likely daydreaming, and maybe even singing along to music playing in the background. But, to your awareness, this was still just a simple trip to the store because most of the time, you don't even notice the tremendous processing power of your brain as you navigate the world.

But in some ways, this capacity for simultaneous conscious thinking, daydreaming, and decision making is what makes us human. Many of these functions are under the province of the frontal lobe, which—in comparison to other species on this planet—is disproportionately large in *H. sapiens sapiens*. Your frontal lobe enables you to eschew instantaneous reward and to seek out delayed gratification, like studying for the MCAT to get that high score you deserve. The frontal lobe also controls your production of language, which permits you to transmit ideas between individuals, cultures, and time. Finally, the frontal lobe helps you coordinate your thinking by deciding which stimuli deserve your attention. These are functions that are indispensable to your daily functioning and will be the focus of this chapter.

4.1 Cognition

High-Yield

LEARNING OBJECTIVES

After Chapter 4.1, you will be able to:

- List the steps in the information processing model of cognition
- Describe the effects of aging, heredity, and environment on cognitive function
- Recall Piaget's four stages of cognitive development and their key features

The study of **cognition** looks at how our brains process and react to the incredible information overload presented to us by the world. Cognition, overall, is not a uniquely human trait, but we are certainly the most advanced species on the planet in terms of complex thought. As described in the introduction, the frontal lobe is disproportionately large in our subspecies; a comparison to our recent anthropological ancestors demonstrates that our skull is shaped to accommodate this enlarged lobe, as shown in Figure 4.1.

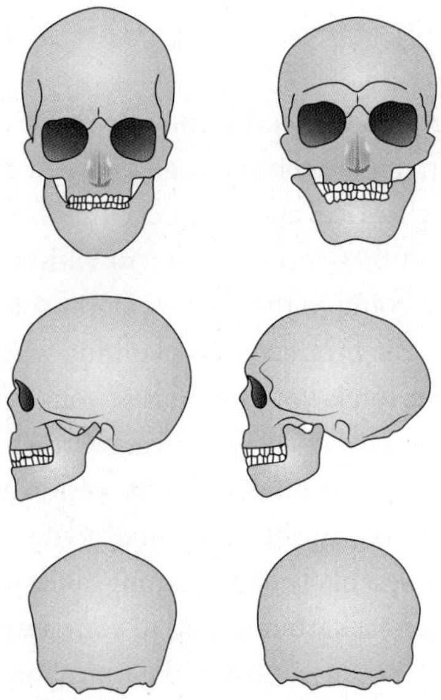

Figure 4.1 Skulls of *H. sapiens* (left) and *H. neanderthalensis* (right)

Information Processing Model

In the 1950s, much of science and engineering turned toward the production of computers and artificial intelligence. It was noted that certain steps were required in order to use a computer to store and process information. First, the information must be encoded in a language that the computer understands. Then, the information must be stored in such a way that it can be found later. Finally, the computer must be able to retrieve that information when required.

Psychologists took this model of information processing and applied it to the human brain. They theorized that the brain is somewhat like a computer. It must encode information into a series of chemical and electrical signals. Then, the brain must be able to store this information such that it can be retrieved when needed. Then, there must be a process by which the brain is able to retrieve information.

The manner in which information is encoded, stored, and retrieved has been a consistent source of debate. One prominent theory, Paivio's **dual-coding theory**, states that both verbal association and visual images are used to process and store information. For example, the word "tree" can recall some information, and a picture of a tree can recall that same information. The fact that we can code this information in two different ways builds redundancy and increases the chance that the information can be retrieved and used effectively when cued, much like search engine optimization within a computer program.

However, the human brain is not a computer. While the computer analogy creates a simple paradigm by which information is processed by the brain, it does not tell the whole story. The human brain doesn't just handle information in the form of facts: it also handles emotions, sensations such as smell and taste, as well as memories. As discussed in Chapter 3 of *MCAT Behavioral Sciences Review*, encoding, storage, and retrieval are often flavored by context and emotion.

BRIDGE

The key memory processes of encoding, storage, and retrieval are covered in Chapter 3 of *MCAT Behavioral Sciences Review.*

The **information processing model** has four key components, or pillars:

- Thinking requires sensation, encoding, and storage of stimuli.
- Stimuli must be analyzed by the brain (rather than responded to automatically) to be useful in decision making.
- Decisions made in one situation can be extrapolated and adjusted to help solve new problems (also called situational modification).
- Problem solving is dependent not only on the person's cognitive level, but also on the context and complexity of the problem.

Cognitive Development

Cognitive development is the development of one's ability to think and solve problems across the life span. Interestingly, during childhood, cognitive development is limited by the pace of brain maturation. Early cognitive development includes learning control of one's own body as well as learning how to interact with and manipulate the environment. Early cognitive development is characterized by mastering the

REAL WORLD

Abstract thought, the ability to think about things that are not physically present, can be lost in some mental disorders. For example, a common cognitive test with patients who have schizophrenia is to ask them to interpret a cliché, such as *Don't count your chickens before they hatch*. These patients have concrete thinking and will give an answer focused on the chickens themselves—not the underlying concept.

KEY CONCEPT

Piaget's stages of cognitive development:

- Sensorimotor
- Preoperational
- Concrete operational
- Formal operational

physical environment. As physical tasks are mastered, a new challenge looms for a developing child: abstract thinking. As discussed in Chapter 1 of *MCAT Behavioral Sciences Review*, social skills also develop during the lifetime.

As you will see during our review of Piaget's stages of cognitive development, the development of the ability to think abstractly is developed throughout childhood. The development of abstract thinking is also dependent upon increases in working memory and mental capacities. As the brain develops, the ability to process information in an abstract manner also develops.

Piaget's Stages of Cognitive Development

Jean Piaget was one of the most influential figures in developmental psychology. Piaget's model of cognitive development proposes that there are qualitative differences between the way that children and adults think, and that these differences can be explained by dividing the life span into four stages of cognitive development: sensorimotor, preoperational, concrete operational, and formal operational. Piaget believed that passage through each of these stages was a continuous and sequential process in which completion of each stage prepares the individual for the stage that follows.

Before delving into the actual stages, we have to look at how Piaget explained learning. According to Piaget, infants learn mainly through instinctual interaction with the environment. For example, infants possess a grasping reflex. Through experience with this reflex, the infant learns that it is possible to grasp objects. Piaget referred to these organized patterns of behavior and thought as schemata. A **schema** can include a concept (What is a *dog*?), a behavior (What do you do when someone asks you your name?), or a sequence of events (What do you normally do in a sit-down restaurant?). As a child proceeds through the stages, new information has to be placed into the different schemata. Piaget theorized that new information is processed via **adaptation**. According to Piaget, adaptation to information comes about by two complementary processes: assimilation and accommodation. **Assimilation** is the process of classifying new information into existing schemata. If the new information does not fit neatly into existing schemata, then accommodation occurs. **Accommodation** is the process by which existing schemata are modified to encompass this new information.

The first stage in Piaget's model is the **sensorimotor stage**, starting at birth and lasting until about two years of age. In this stage, a child learns to manipulate the environment in order to meet physical needs and learns to coordinate sensory input with motor actions (hence the name *sensorimotor*). To explore their surroundings, infants in the sensorimotor stage begin to exhibit two types of behavior patterns called **circular reactions**, named for their repetitive natures. **Primary circular reactions** are repetitions of body movements that originally occurred by chance, such as sucking the thumb. Usually such behaviors are repeated because the child finds these behaviors soothing. **Secondary circular reactions** occur when manipulation is focused on something outside the body, such as repeatedly throwing toys from a high chair. These behaviors are often repeated because the child gets a response from the environment, such as a parent picking up the dropped toy. The key milestone that ends the sensorimotor stage is the development of **object permanence**, which is the understanding that objects continue to exist even when out of view. Object permanence is the idea behind "peek-a-boo," shown in Figure 4.2. This game is so entertaining to young infants because they lack object permanence. Each time an adult reveals the face from behind hands, the child interprets it as though the adult has just come into existence. Object permanence marks the beginning of **representational thought**, in which the child has begun to create mental representations of external objects and events.

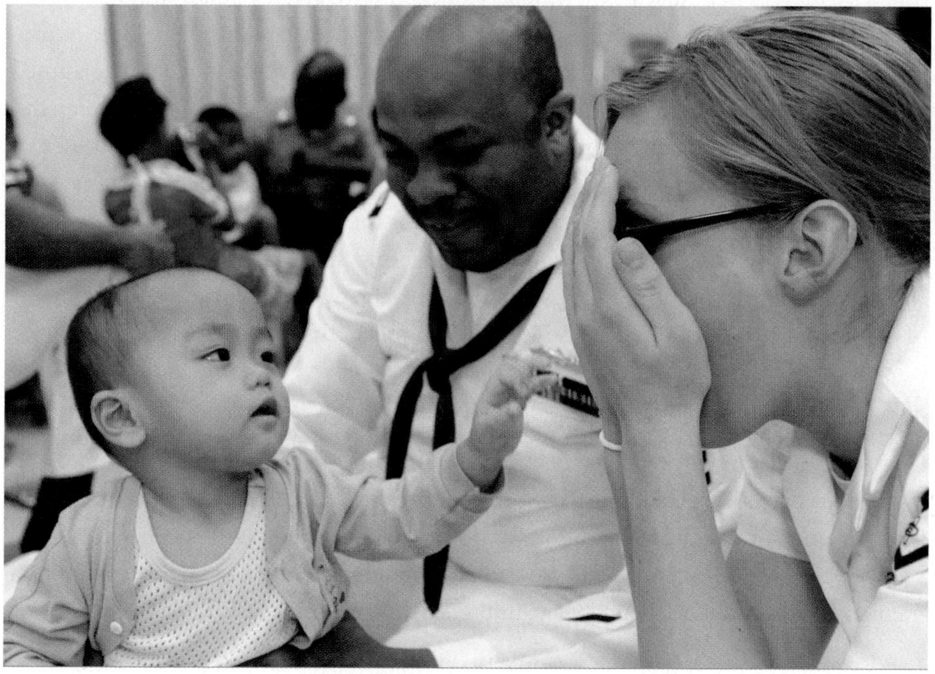

Figure 4.2 Peek-a-Boo
This game depends on the child being in the sensorimotor stage, prior to the development of object permanence.

The **preoperational stage** lasts from about two to seven years of age and is characterized by symbolic thinking and egocentrism. **Symbolic thinking** refers to the ability to pretend, play make-believe, and have an imagination. **Egocentrism** refers to the inability to imagine what another person may think or feel. The preoperational stage also includes the inability to grasp the concept of **conservation**, which is the understanding that a physical amount remains the same, even if there is a change in shape or appearance. For example, imagine a child presented with two equal quantities of pizza. On one plate is a single large slice, while the other plate has the exact same quantity in two slices. A child in the preoperational stage will be unable to tell that the quantities are equal and will focus mainly on the number of slices on the plate rather than the actual quantity. Piaget believed that this flaw in cognition was due to **centration**, which is the tendency to focus on only one aspect of a phenomenon, for example the number of slices, while ignoring other important elements.

The **concrete operational stage** lasts from about 7 to 11 years of age. In this stage, children can understand conservation and consider the perspectives of others. This consideration results in the loss of egocentrism. Additionally, they are able to engage in logical thought as long as they are working with concrete objects or information that is directly available. These children have not yet developed the ability to think abstractly.

The **formal operational stage** starts around 11 years of age, and is marked by the ability to think logically about abstract ideas. Generally coinciding with adolescence, this stage is marked by the ability to reason about abstract concepts and problem solve. The difference between this type of thought and concrete operations is illustrated by Piaget's pendulum experiment. Children were given a pendulum in which they could vary the length of the string, the weight of the pendulum, the force of the push, and the initial angle of the swing. They were asked to find out what determined the frequency of the swing. Children in the concrete operational stage manipulated the variables at random and even distorted the data to fit preconceived hypotheses. Adolescents, on the other hand, were able to hold all variables but one constant at a given time, proceeding methodically to discover that only the length of the string affects the frequency. The ability to mentally manipulate variables in a number of ways, generally within the scope of scientific experiments, is an important component of the formal operational stage, and is termed **hypothetical reasoning**.

BRIDGE

Culture has profound effects on cognitive development, as well as social structure, rules, and mores. Culture is discussed in detail in Chapter 11 of *MCAT Behavioral Sciences Review.*

BRIDGE

Lev Vygotsky is also a key figure in the psychology of identity. Along with Kohlberg, Freud, and Erikson, he proposed a staged system of identity formation. These theorists are discussed in Chapter 6 of *MCAT Behavioral Sciences Review.*

Role of Culture in Cognitive Development

Cognitive development is very much related to culture, as one's culture will determine what one is expected to learn. Some cultures will place a higher value on social learning, including cultural traditions and roles, while other cultures will value knowledge. In addition, one's culture will also influence the rate of cognitive development as children can be treated very differently from culture to culture.

Lev Vygotsky, a prominent educational psychologist, proposed that the engine driving cognitive development is children's internalization of their culture, including interpersonal and societal rules, symbols, and language. As children develop, their skills and abilities are still in formative stages. With help from adults or other children, those skills can develop further. That help may come in the form of instruction from a teacher or even watching another child perform the skill.

Cognitive Changes in Late Adulthood

Aging brings about many changes in cognition. Reaction time increases steadily in early adulthood, while time-based prospective memory—the ability to remember to perform a task at a specific time in the future—declines with age. Intellectual changes also occur; however, IQ changes have been found to be misleading. Early research into the field of intelligence and aging indicated that a substantial decline in IQ occurs between the ages of 30 and 40. In order to further elucidate what specific changes were occurring, intelligence itself was separated into two subtypes: fluid intelligence and crystallized intelligence. **Fluid intelligence** consists of solving new or novel problems, possibly using creative methods. Figuring out how to navigate through a new video game world involves the usage of fluid intelligence. **Crystallized intelligence** is more related to solving problems using acquired knowledge, and often can be procedural. For instance, working through a General Chemistry stoichiometry problem requires crystallized intelligence since it involves recall of the proper equations and the steps taken to work through the calculations. Fluid intelligence was shown to peak in early adulthood but decline with age, while crystallized intelligence peaked in middle adulthood and remains stable with age.

Decline in intellectual abilities in adulthood has been linked with how long an older adult retains the ability to function in what are known as **activities of daily living** (eating, bathing, toileting, dressing, and ambulation). It appears, however, that this decline is not uniform. Certain characteristics, such as higher level of education, more frequent performance of intellectual activities, socializing, and a stimulating environment have been found to be protective against intellectual decline.

Intellectual decline is not always benign. Some types of intellectual decline are very common and indicate a progressive loss of function beyond that of old age. Disorders and conditions that are characterized by a general loss of cognitive function are collectively known as **dementia**. Dementia often begins with impaired memory, but later progresses to impaired judgment and confusion. Personality changes are also very common as dementia progresses. The most common cause of dementia is Alzheimer's disease. Vascular (multi-infarct) dementia, caused by high blood pressure and repeated microscopic clots in the brain, is also a very common cause. It is also important to note that people with dementia often require full-time supportive care in order to carry out activities of daily living. This causes tremendous stress on families, including children and spouses of those with dementia, as the care for the person with dementia often falls on family members.

REAL WORLD

Alzheimer's disease accounts for approximately 60 to 80% of all dementia cases.

Heredity, Environment, and Biologic Factors

Cognition can be affected by a wide variety of conditions. These may include actual problems with the brain itself (organic brain disorders), genetic and chromosomal conditions, metabolic derangements, and long-term drug use. The environment can also affect both cognitive development and day-to-day cognition.

Parenting styles may influence cognitive development by reward, punishment, or indifference for an emerging skill. In addition, genetics can predispose to a state that may make cognitive development difficult. For example, many genetic and chromosomal diseases such as Down syndrome and Fragile X syndrome are associated with delayed cognitive development. Antisocial personality disorder has also been shown to have a strong genetic component. The presence of genes for this disorder may make it difficult for a child to appreciate the rights of others.

Intellectual disabilities in children can also be caused by chemical exposures, illness, injury, or trauma during birth. Alcohol use during pregnancy can cause fetal alcohol syndrome, which results in slowed cognitive development and distinct craniofacial features, shown in Figure 4.3. Infections in the brain may result in electrical abnormalities and slowed development. Complications during birth—especially those causing reduced oxygen delivery to the brain—may also affect cognition. Finally, reduced cognition can also occur following trauma to the brain, as occurs with shaken baby syndrome.

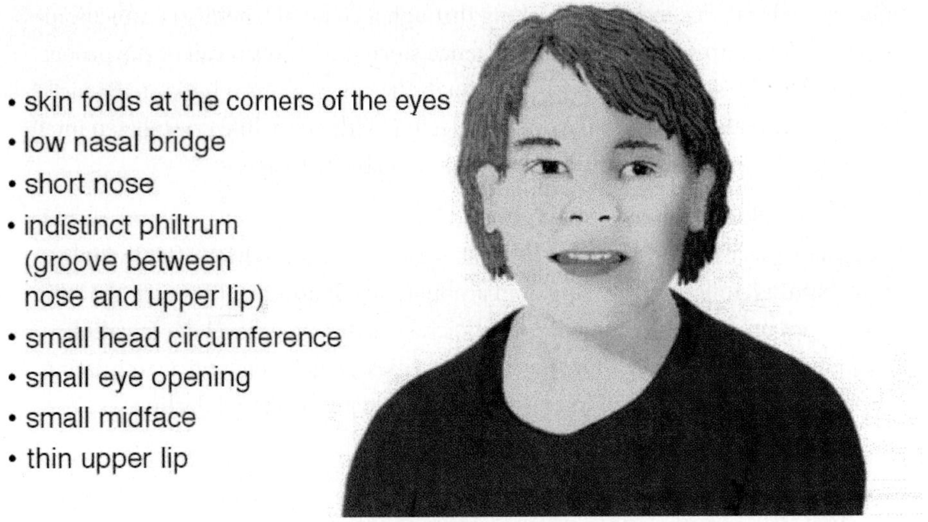

Figure 4.3 Craniofacial Features of Fetal Alcohol Syndrome

However, not all cognitive decline in adulthood is slow. If there has been a rapid decline in cognition, this may be the result of delirium. **Delirium** is rapid fluctuation in cognitive function that is reversible and caused by medical (nonpsychological) causes. It can be caused by a variety of issues, including electrolyte and pH disturbances, malnutrition, low blood sugar, infection, a drug reaction, alcohol withdrawal, and pain.

REAL WORLD

The delirium associated with alcohol withdrawal, called *delirium tremens*, can be life threatening. As a depressant, alcohol is the only major drug of abuse in which both overdose and withdrawal can be lethal.

MCAT CONCEPT CHECK 4.1

Before you move on, assess your understanding of the material with these questions.

1. The three steps in the information processing model are:

    1. ______________________________
    2. ______________________________
    3. ______________________________

2. A person brings a parent, who is an older adult, to the doctor. During the past two days, the parent has been overheard speaking to a spouse who has been deceased for four years. Prior to that, the parent was completely normal. The parent most likely has:

____

3. List Piaget's four stages of cognitive development and the key features of each.

Stage	Key Features

4.2 Problem Solving and Decision Making

High-Yield

LEARNING OBJECTIVES

After Chapter 4.2, you will be able to:

- Identify examples of functional fixedness, mental sets, trial-and-error problem solving, algorithms, and deductive reasoning
- Recall key fallacies and biases, including base rate fallacy, disconfirmation principle, confirmation bias, overconfidence, and belief perseverance
- Describe models of intellectual functioning and tests of intellectual ability
- Explain the availability and representativeness heuristics

Every day you are faced with problems. Many of these problems you solve without any real conscious thought about what is happening. However, much like the scientific method, problem solving itself has a process. First, we must frame the problem; that is, we create a mental image or schematic of the issue. Then, we generate potential solutions and begin to test them. These potential solutions may be derived from a **mental set**, which is the tendency to approach similar problems in the same way. Once solutions have been tested, we evaluate the results, considering other potential solutions that may have been easier or more effective in some way.

KEY CONCEPT

The first step in problem solving (framing the problem) may seem obvious; however, when we get "stuck" on a problem, it is most often because the manner in which we have framed the problem is inefficient or not useful.

Problem solving can be impeded by an inappropriate mental set, as well as by functional fixedness, which is demonstrated by Duncker's candle problem. Consider the following scenario: You walk into a room and see a box of matches, some tacks, and a candle. Your task is to mount the candle on the wall so that it can be used without the wax dropping on the floor. Before reading on, try to solve the problem.

Most people find the task challenging. You might have thought of tacking the candle to the wall, but that solution doesn't work because the wax would still drop to the floor. The key is to realize that the matchbox can serve not just as a container for the matches, but as a holder for the candle. The solution, therefore, is to tack the box to the wall and put the candle in the box. **Functional fixedness** can thus be defined as the inability to consider how to use an object in a nontraditional manner.

Types of Problem Solving

In psychology, different approaches to problem solving include trial-and-error, algorithms, deductive reasoning, and inductive reasoning.

Trial-and-Error

Trial-and-error is a less sophisticated type of problem solving in which various solutions are tried until one is found that seems to work. While an educated approach may be used, this type of problem solving is usually only effective when there are relatively few possible solutions.

Algorithms

An **algorithm** is a formula or procedure for solving a certain type of problem. Algorithms can be mathematical or a set of instructions, designed to automatically produce the desired solution.

Deductive Reasoning

Deductive (top-down) reasoning starts from a set of general rules and draws conclusions from the information given. An example of deductive reasoning is a logic puzzle, as shown in Figure 4.4. In these puzzles, one has to synthesize a list of logical rules to come up with the single possible solution to the problem.

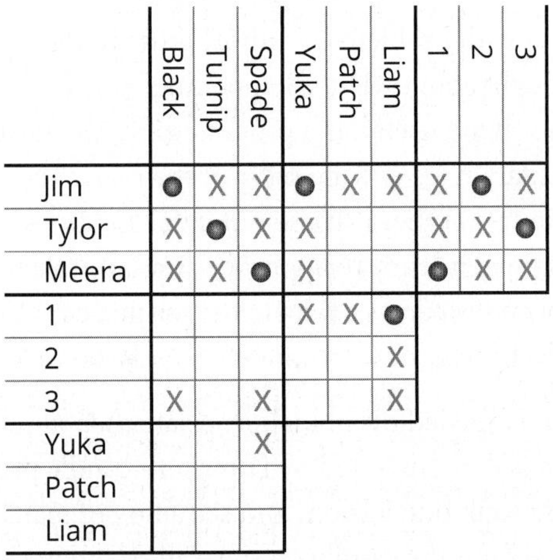

Figure 4.4 A Logic Puzzle Grid
Logic puzzles are applications of deductive reasoning in which only one possible solution can be deduced based on the information given.

MCAT EXPERTISE

Remember that a deduction is a solution that *must* be true based on the information given. This is why answers on the MCAT that merely *might* be true (but don't *have* to be) are never the correct answer.

Inductive Reasoning

Inductive (bottom-up) reasoning seeks to create a theory via generalizations. This type of reasoning starts with specific instances, and then draws a conclusion from them.

Heuristics, Biases, Intuition, and Emotion

We make decisions every day. Some are related to our daily routines: *What should I wear today?* Others concern our broader life goals: *Where am I going to apply to medical school?* Decision making is a complicated process, but we use a number of tools, such as heuristics, biases, intuition, and emotions, to speed up or simplify the process. While useful from a time and complexity standpoint, these tools can also lead us to short-sighted or problematic solutions.

Heuristics

Heuristics are simplified principles used to make decisions; they are colloquially called "rules of thumb." The **availability heuristic** is a heuristic used when we base the likelihood of an event on how easily examples of that event come to mind. Often, the use of this heuristic leads us to a correct decision, but not always. As an example, answer the following question: *Are there more words in the English language that start with the letter "K" or that have "K" as their third letter?*

Most people respond that there are more words that begin with the letter "K" than have "K" as their third letter. In fact, there are actually at least twice as many words in English that have "K" as the third letter than begin with "K." Most people approach this question by trying to think of words that fit into each category. Because we so often classify words by their first letter, most people can easily think of words beginning with "K." However, most people have a harder time thinking of words with "K" as their third letter. Thus, in this case, the availability heuristic tends to lead to an incorrect answer.

The **representativeness heuristic** involves categorizing items on the basis of whether they fit the prototypical, stereotypical, or representative image of the category. For example, consider a standard coin that is flipped ten times in a row and lands on heads every time. What is the probability of the coin landing on heads the next time? Mathematically, the probability must still be 50 percent, but most individuals will either overestimate the probability based on the pattern that has been established, or underestimate the probability with the logic that the number of heads and tails must "even out." Hence, like the availability heuristic, the use of the representativeness heuristic can sometimes lead us astray. Using prototypical or stereotypical factors while ignoring actual numerical information is called the **base rate fallacy**.

While heuristics can lead us astray, they are essential to speedy and effective decision making. Heuristics are often used by experts in a given field. For instance, to win at chess, one must be able to think several moves ahead. On any particular turn, there may be 15 or 20 possible moves, each one of which may have multiple consequences; analyzing every possibility would take far too long. There are heuristics, however, that can quickly rule out some of the possible moves: the king must be protected, it is generally good to control the center squares, and pieces should not be put in danger when possible. In this way, heuristics provide a more efficient—although sometimes inaccurate—method for problem solving.

MCAT EXPERTISE

Detail questions on the MCAT often have wrong answer choices that are stated in the passage, but that fail to answer the question posed. According to the availability heuristic, students who do not truly problem solve on MCAT questions will be tempted by these familiar-sounding answers merely because they can recall that statement being mentioned in the passage. Don't forget to use your Distillation effectively, as described in Chapter 6 of *MCAT Critical Analysis and Reasoning Skills Review*!

Bias and Overconfidence

When a potential solution to a problem fails during testing, this solution should be discarded. This is known as the **disconfirmation principle**: the evidence obtained from testing demonstrated that the solution does not work. However, the presence of a confirmation bias may prevent an individual from eliminating this solution. **Confirmation bias** is the tendency to focus on information that fits an individual's beliefs, while rejecting information that goes against them. Confirmation bias also contributes to **overconfidence**, or a tendency to erroneously interpret one's decisions, knowledge, and beliefs as infallible. An additional type of bias is **hindsight bias**, which is the tendency for people to overestimate their ability to predict the outcome of events that already happened. The similar phenomenon of **belief perseverance** refers to the inability to reject a particular belief despite clear evidence to the contrary. Together, confirmation bias, overconfidence, hindsight bias, and belief perseverance can seriously impede a person's analysis of available evidence.

Intuition

Intuition can be defined as the ability to act on perceptions that may not be supported by available evidence. Often, people may have beliefs that are not necessarily supported by evidence, but that a person "feels" to be correct. Intuition is often developed by experience. For example, an emergency room physician, over the course of seeing thousands of patients with chest pain, may develop a keen sense of which patients are actually having a heart attack without even looking at an electrocardiogram (EKG) or a patient's vital signs. This intuition can be more accurately described by the **recognition-primed decision model**: the doctor's brain is actually sorting through a wide variety of information to match a pattern. Over time, the doctor has gained an extensive level of experience that can be accessed without awareness.

Emotion

Emotion is the subjective experience of a person in a certain situation. How a person feels often influences how a person thinks and makes decisions. For example, a person who is angry is often more likely to engage in more risky decision making. In addition, emotions in decision making are not limited to the emotion experienced while the decision is being made; emotions that a person *expects* to feel from a particular decision are also involved. For example, if people believe a car will make them feel more powerful, they may be more likely to purchase that car.

Intellectual Functioning

Intellectual functioning is a highly studied area of psychology. How is intelligence defined? What makes someone more intelligent than someone else? These are multifaceted questions that are difficult to answer; however, theorists have proposed models for some aspects of intelligence.

Theories of Intelligence

There has been much debate concerning the definition of intelligence. Howard Gardner's theory of **multiple intelligences** is one of the most all-encompassing definitions, with at least eight defined types of intelligence: linguistic, logical–mathematical, musical, visual–spatial, bodily–kinesthetic, interpersonal, intrapersonal, and naturalist. Gardner argues that some cultures value the first two abilities over the others. After all, linguistic ability and logical–mathematical ability are the two abilities tested on traditional intelligence quotient (IQ) tests. Despite not being the central focus of the cultures Gardner discusses, people's interpersonal and intrapersonal intelligence can heavily impact their quality of life. **Interpersonal intelligence** is the ability to detect and navigate the moods and motivations of others. Gardner believed that people with high interpersonal intelligence would make great sales representatives and therapists. While intrapersonal intelligence centers around being mindful of one's own emotions, strengths, and weaknesses, which can provide clear guidance what role one should take in a group or society.

KEY CONCEPT

Gardner's multiple intelligences include linguistic, logical-mathematical, musical, visual-spatial, bodily-kinesthetic, interpersonal, intrapersonal, and naturalist.

Robert Sternberg pioneered a cognitive perspective that focused on how people use their intelligence, rather than taking the traditional approach of trying to measure an individual's level of intelligence. More specifically, Sternberg's triarchic theory of human intelligence defines three subtypes: **analytical intelligence**, which involves the ability to evaluate and reason; **creative intelligence**, which is the ability to solve problems using novel methods; and **practical intelligence**, which involves dealing with everyday problems at home or at work.

Successful navigation of our social world also requires us to have a good understanding of both our own emotions and the emotions of those around us. The theory of **emotional intelligence** addresses our emotional awareness in four components: the ability to express and perceive emotions in ourself and others, the ability to comprehend and analyze our emotions, the ability to regulate our emotions, and awareness of how emotions shape our thoughts and decisions. Empathy is often given as an example of emotional intelligence because empathy requires individuals to understand their own emotions well enough to recognize those emotions in other people.

Variations in Intellectual Ability

There are a number of tests and studies that have historically attempted to quantify intelligence. A founding concept behind these tests is Charles Spearman's "g factor," or general intelligence factor. The theory behind the existence of a g factor is based on the observation that performance on different cognitive tasks is in many cases positively correlated, indicating an underlying factor or variable is playing a role. This underlying variable of intelligence is often measured with standardized tests that generate an **intelligence quotient** (**IQ**) for the test taker. IQ tests were largely pioneered by Alfred Binet in the early twentieth century. A professor at Stanford University took Binet's work and created what is known as the **Stanford–Binet IQ test**.

BEHAVIORAL SCIENCES GUIDED EXAMPLE WITH EXPERT THINKING

Many decisions we make use the affect heuristic; that is, we make quick judgments that depend on our emotional state as well as the emotional content of the decision. Specifically, options that provoke positive emotions are more likely to be chosen than those that evoke negative emotions when the choices are quantitatively identical, and even in cases in which the choice associated with negative feelings is quantitatively better. The following three studies were conducted:

Definition of new term: affect heuristic

Study 1: Researchers provided participants with quantitative information about one of two issues: violent crime (steadily declining) and deer overpopulation (steadily increasing). The participants were asked to rate the severity of each problem on a scale from "very bad" to "very good."

Two problems which differ in severity and emotional content.

IV: issue

DV: rating

Study 2: Participants were asked to set a price for a listing of retail electronics. One listing included ten unused items and another included 18 items, 14 of which were unused and 4 of which were described as being used and in "poor working order."

Comparison between two sets of items, varying in content.

IV: list contents (broken items)

DV: price

Study 3: Participants were asked to determine punishments for a number of hypothetical college students who had committed some form of academic dishonesty. The participants were provided a photograph and description for each student. The same student was used, but one group of participants was provided a picture of the student smiling, and the other group was provided a picture of the student with a neutral expression.

Meting out punishment for people, some of whom are smiling in pictures.

IV: photograph

DV: punishment

Adapted from: Wilson, Robyn S.; Arvai, Joseph L. (March 2006). "When Less Is More: How Affect Influences Preferences When Comparing Low and High-risk Options". *Journal of Risk Research.* **9** (2): 165–178.

LaFrance, M.; Hecht, M.A. (March 1995). "Why Smiles Generate Leniency". *Personality and Social Psychology Bulletin.* **21** (3): 207–214.

If the affect heuristic is shown to be a factor in each of the studies described, what can be predicted about the results of each?

When the MCAT asks us to predict the outcome of an experiment, we want to first consider any content, either from the passage or from our outside knowledge, that might be relevant. Fortunately, this passage provides us with what we need: a definition of the affect heuristic in paragraph one. For each study, then, you'll want to select the result that prioritizes emotional content. For Study 1, the notion of "violent crime" likely provokes a strong negative feeling, while for most people, the idea of "deer overpopulation" would not be expected to be associated with the same emotional response. It is likely, then, that participants would rate violent crime as a worse problem than deer overpopulation regardless of the actual outcome of analyzing the quantitative impact of each issue. The same heuristic explains why people are more afraid of being attacked by a shark at the beach than of other, more likely causes of death, even though statistically injury or death by shark attack is extremely unlikely.

In Study 2, we would predict that the broken items would cause the second listing to be valued the same as or lower than the first listing, even though the second listing actually contains more items that are unused. This is because the additional broken items would be expected to provoke a negative feeling about the second listing. In fact, further research supports the idea that participants do not add up the value of each item separately, but rather evaluate heuristically what they perceive as an average value of the set of items as a whole.

Finally, in Study 3, we should expect that the smiling students were judged less harshly than those presented with a neutral expression. This is based on the same decision-making heuristic we've been using all along: the smiling student is more likely to be associated with positive emotions, and the decision is likely to be altered based on this emotional input.

To summarize: we should predict based on the affect heuristic that in Study 1 the violent crime will be rated as the more problematic of the two issues, that in Study 2 the batch of items containing broken goods will be rated as less valuable, and that in Study 3 the smiling student will be judged less harshly than the neutral student.

While later iterations of the test use different methodologies to arrive at a score, it is useful to know the original formula for calculating IQ:

$$IQ = \frac{\text{mental age}}{\text{chronological age}} \times 100$$

Equation 4.1

Using this equation, a four-year-old with intelligence abilities at the level of the average six-year-old would have an IQ of 150. The distribution of IQ scores from the original study of the Stanford–Binet IQ test is shown in Figure 4.5.

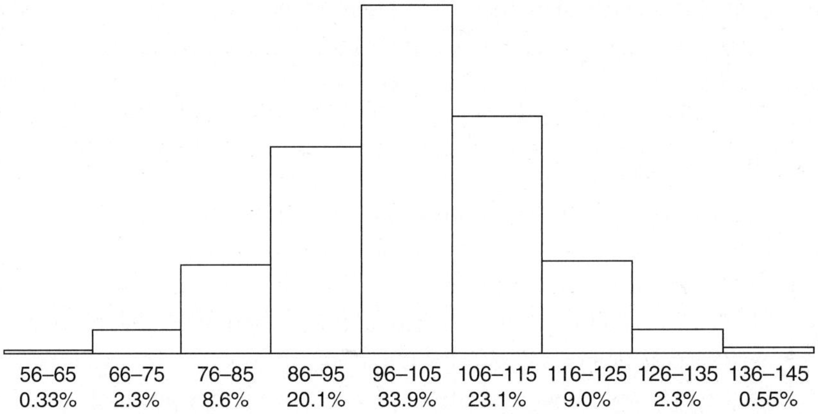

Figure 4.5 Distribution of IQ Scores for Children 5 to 14 Years of Age
Mean = 100; SD = 15

Some theorists have argued heavily for intelligence as a hereditary trait, most notably Galton in his novel *Hereditary Genius.* In reality, variations in intellectual ability can be attributed to many determinants, including genes, environment, and educational experiences. Intellectual ability does appear to run in families, which may be due to both genetics and the environment; some environments are simply more enriching than others. Parental expectations, socioeconomic status, and nutrition have all been shown to correlate with intelligence.

The educational system plays a significant role in the development of intelligence. Children who attend school tend to have greater increases in IQ, and IQ actually decreases slightly during summer vacations. Early intervention in childhood also improves IQ, especially for children in low-enrichment environments. Finally, both children with high IQs and those with cognitive disabilities benefit from specialized educational environments. For students with cognitive disabilities, this is often defined as the least restrictive environment, in which they are encouraged to participate as much as possible in the regular mainstream classroom, with individualized help as needed.

REAL WORLD

The Stanford-Binet IQ test, while still popular, has been found to have variable levels of success in assessing intelligence with different ages and cultural groups. In practice, a variety of intelligence assessments can be found in use around the world. Some of these tests still use measures similar to IQ but are specialized for a subpopulation, such as the Wechsler Intelligence Scale for Children (WISC) exam. Other assessments eschew the concept of IQ entirely and instead follow alternative theories, including Gardner's theory of multiple intelligences.

MCAT CONCEPT CHECK 4.2

Before you move on, assess your understanding of the material with these questions.

1. A child plays with a tool set, noting that a nail can only be hit with a hammer. When a friend suggests that the handle of a screwdriver can be used to hit a nail, the child passionately objects. This is an example of:

 ____

2. A doctor uses a flowchart to treat a patient with sepsis. Given its use in problem solving, a flowchart is an example of a(n):

 ____

3. A patient in a mental health facility believes that the sky is pink. Despite several trips outside, the patient still declares the sky is pink. Which psychological principle does this represent?

 ____

4. Provide a brief definition of the availability and representativeness heuristics.
   - Availability heuristic:

 ____

   - Representativeness heuristic:

 ____

4.3 Consciousness

High-Yield

LEARNING OBJECTIVES

After Chapter 4.3, you will be able to:

- Identify the two hormones most associated with circadian rhythms
- Distinguish between dyssomnia and parasomnia
- Associate the stages of sleep with their EEG waveforms and other main features:

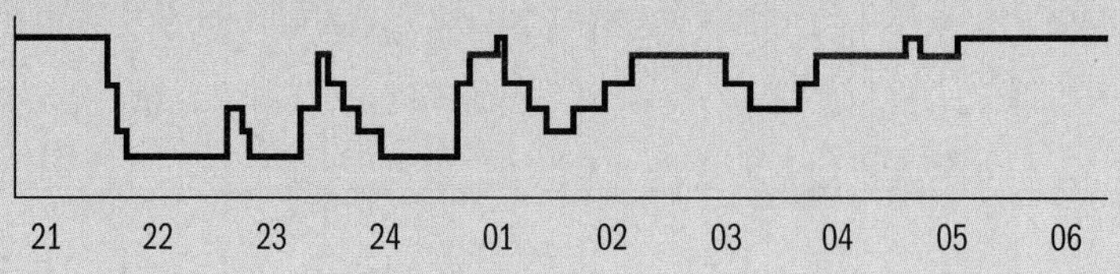

Consciousness is one's level of awareness of both the world and one's own existence within that world.

States of Consciousness

The accepted states of consciousness are alertness, sleep, dreaming, and altered states of consciousness. Technically, sleep and dreaming are also considered altered states, but we will consider these states separately from hypnosis, meditation, and drug-induced altered states of consciousness. Altered states of consciousness may also result from sickness, dementia, delirium, and coma.

Alertness

Alertness is a state of consciousness in which we are awake and able to think. In this state, we are able to perceive, process, access, and verbalize information. In the alert state, we also experience a certain level of **physiological arousal**, which is characterized by physiological reactions such as increased heart rate, breathing rate, blood pressure, and so on. Cortisol levels tend to be higher, and electroencephalogram (EEG) waves indicate a brain in the waking state.

Alertness is maintained by neurological circuits in the prefrontal cortex at the very front of the brain. Fibers from the prefrontal cortex communicate with the **reticular formation** (reticular activation system), a neural structure located in the brainstem, to keep the cortex awake and alert. A brain injury that results in disruption of these connections results in coma.

MCAT EXPERTISE

One of the best ways to enhance your recall and test performance is to maintain a regular schedule of sleep. Regular sleep, exercise, and a healthy diet help to make Test Day successful.

Sleep

Sleep is important to consider while studying for the MCAT or any other major exam. While it may be tempting to pull all-nighters in an attempt to maximize your test score, this may not be the best strategy for success. In fact, long-term sleep deprivation has been linked with diminished cognitive performance as well as the development of chronic diseases such as diabetes and obesity.

Stages of Sleep

Sleep is studied by recording brain wave activity occurring during the course of a night's sleep. This is done with **electroencephalography**, or **EEG**, which records an average of the electrical patterns within different portions of the brain. There are four characteristic EEG patterns correlated with different stages of waking and sleeping: beta, alpha, theta, and delta waves. There is a fifth wave that corresponds to REM sleep, which is the time during the night when we have most of our dreams. These sleep stages form a complete cycle lasting about 90 minutes.

Beta and alpha waves characterize brain wave activity when we are awake and are shown in Figure 4.6. **Beta waves** have a high frequency and occur when the person is alert or attending to a mental task that requires concentration. Beta waves occur when neurons are randomly firing. **Alpha waves** occur when we are awake but relaxing with our eyes closed, and are somewhat slower than beta waves. Alpha waves are also more synchronized than beta waves.

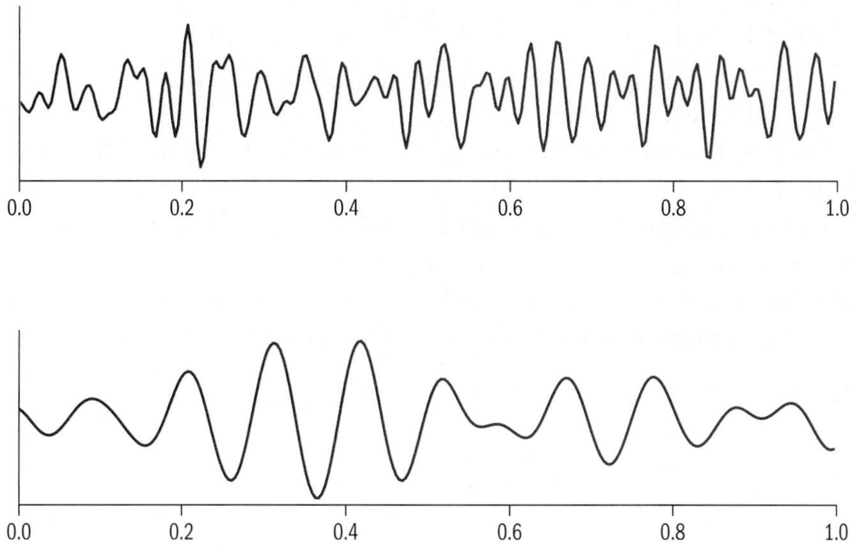

Figure 4.6 Beta (top) and Alpha (bottom) Waves on EEG
Beta and alpha waves are seen during alertness.

As soon as you doze off, you enter **Stage 1** (also known as NREM1), which is detected on the EEG by the appearance of **theta waves**, shown in Figure 4.7. At this point, EEG activity is characterized by irregular waveforms with slower frequencies and higher voltages.

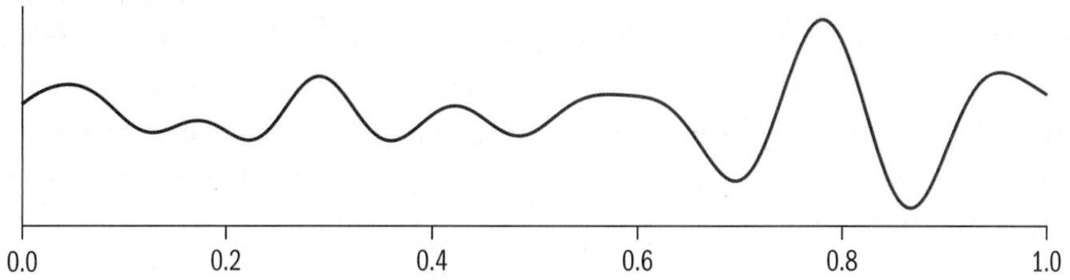

Figure 4.7 Theta Waves
Theta waves are seen during Stage 1 and 2 sleep.

REAL WORLD

An electroencephalogram (EEG) is a test used to monitor electrical activity in the brain. It consists of 19 recording electrodes placed on the scalp for 20 to 40 minutes, or continuously in the inpatient setting. This technique is used to study sleep and to identify areas of unusual brain activity, as seen during seizures.

As you fall more deeply asleep, you enter **Stage 2** (NREM2). The EEG shows theta waves along with **sleep spindles**, which are bursts of high-frequency waves, and **K complexes**, which are singular high-amplitude waves, shown in Figure 4.8.

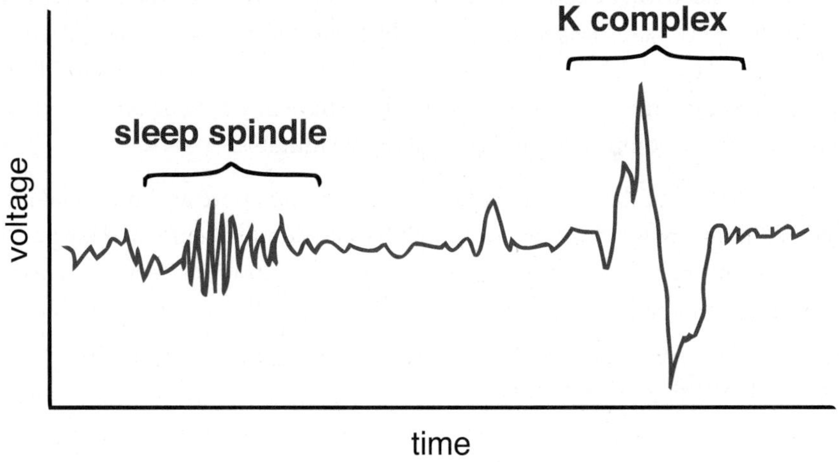

Figure 4.8 Sleep Spindle and K Complex in Stage 2 Sleep

As you fall even more deeply asleep, you enter **Stage 3** (NREM3), also known as **slow-wave sleep (SWS)**. EEG activity grows progressively slower until only a few sleep waves per second are seen. These low-frequency, high-voltage sleep waves are called **delta waves**, shown in Figure 4.9. During this stage, rousing someone from sleep becomes exceptionally difficult. SWS has been associated with cognitive recovery and memory consolidation, as well as increased growth hormone release.

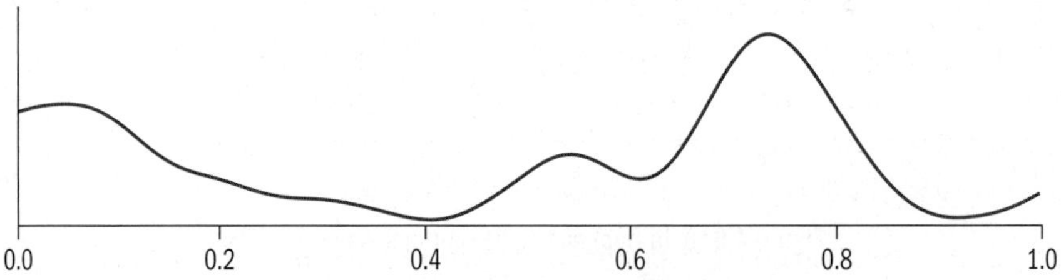

Figure 4.9 Delta Waves of Slow-Wave Sleep

MNEMONIC

Remember the sequential order of these brain waves—**b**eta, **a**lpha, **t**heta, **d**elta—by combining their first letters to form **BAT-D** and remember that a **bat** sleeps during the **d**ay.

The stages above are collectively called **non-rapid eye movement sleep**, which is where the acronym *NREM* comes from. Interspersed between cycles of the NREM stages is **rapid eye movement** (**REM**) **sleep**. In REM sleep, arousal levels reach that of wakefulness, but the muscles are paralyzed. REM sleep is also called **paradoxical sleep** because one's heart rate, breathing patterns, and EEG mimic wakefulness, but the individual is still asleep. This is the stage in which dreaming is most likely to occur and is also associated with memory consolidation. Recent studies have associated REM more with procedural memory consolidation and SWS with declarative memory consolidation.

Sleep Cycles and Changes to Sleep Cycles

A **sleep cycle** refers to a single complete progression through the sleep stages. The makeup of a sleep cycle changes during the course of the night, as shown in Figure 4.10. Early in the night, SWS predominates as the brain falls into deep sleep and then into more wakeful states. Later in the night, REM sleep predominates.

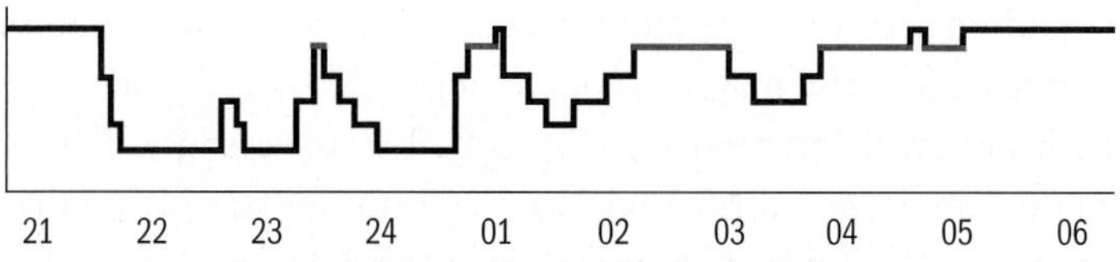

Figure 4.10 Hypnogram of Sleep Cycles

Over the life span, the length of the sleep cycle increases from approximately 50 minutes in children to 90 minutes in adults. Children also spend more time in SWS than adults. Changes to sleep cycles from disrupted sleep or disordered work schedules can cause many health problems. Disruption of SWS and REM can result in diminished memory. Sleep deprivation also causes diminished cognitive performance, although the person who is sleep-deprived is unlikely to recognize that performance has been subpar. Sleep deprivation also negatively affects mood, problem solving, and motor skills.

Sleep and Circadian Rhythms

Our daily cycle of waking and sleeping is regulated by internally generated rhythms or **circadian rhythms**. In humans and other animals, the circadian rhythm approximates a 24-hour cycle that is somewhat affected by external cues such as light. Biochemical signals underlie circadian rhythms. Sleepiness can partially be attributed to blood levels of **melatonin**, a serotonin-derived hormone from the **pineal gland**. The retina has direct connections to the hypothalamus, which controls the pineal gland; thus, decreasing light can cause the release of melatonin.

Cortisol, a steroid hormone produced in the **adrenal cortex**, is also related to the sleep–wake cycle. Its levels slowly increase during early morning because increasing light causes the release of **corticotropin-releasing factor** (**CRF**) from the hypothalamus. CRF causes release of **adrenocorticotropic hormone** (**ACTH**) from the anterior pituitary, which stimulates cortisol release. Cortisol contributes to wakefulness.

MNEMONIC

Melatonin **mell**ows you out. Corti**sol** helps you get up with the sun (*sol* is Latin for sun).

Dreaming

Philosophers and those interested in the human experience have hypothesized about the purpose, meaning, and function of dreaming since antiquity. The ancient Egyptians believed that dreams were messages sent from the supernatural world to tell of future events. In ancient Greece, people believed dreams to carry messages from the gods, but the dream required the help of a priest to interpret. Dreams have long been a subject of wonder.

BRIDGE

The hypothalamic-pituitary-adrenal axis is an example of how the endocrine system can regulate behavior. The endocrine system is discussed in Chapter 5 of *MCAT Biology Review.*

Most dreaming occurs during REM; however, soon after we enter Stage 2 sleep, our mental experience starts to shift to a dreamlike state. Throughout the night, approximately 75% of dreaming occurs during REM. REM dreams tend to be longer and more vivid than those experienced during NREM sleep.

BRIDGE

Other psychologists have proposed explanations for dreams. One of the most notable is Freud, who separated dreams into their *manifest content* (what one actually sees and hears) and their *latent content* (the underlying significance of these dream elements). Freud's model of personality is discussed in Chapter 6 of *MCAT Behavioral Sciences Review.*

While the purpose and meaning of dreams is not fully understood, a few theories have been proposed. In the **activation–synthesis theory**, dreams are caused by widespread, random activation of neural circuitry. This activation can mimic incoming sensory information, and may also consist of pieces of stored memories, current and previous desires, met and unmet needs, and other experiences. The cortex then tries to stitch this unrelated information together, resulting in a dream that is both bizarre and somewhat familiar. In the **problem solving dream theory**, dreams are a way to solve problems while you are sleeping. Dreams are untethered by the rules of the real world, and thus allow interpretation of obstacles differently than during waking hours. Finally, in the **cognitive process dream theory**, dreams are merely the sleeping counterpart of stream-of-consciousness. Just as you may be thinking about an upcoming weekend trip when your consciousness quickly shifts to your upcoming MCAT Test Day, so too does the content of a dream rapidly shift and change. Ultimately, the question is less *Which group is right?* and more *How can we unify these theories?* The study of dreaming is limited by the difference between the brain and the mind: dreaming must have a neurological component, but is still highly subjective. **Neurocognitive models of dreaming** seek to unify biological and psychological perspectives on dreaming by correlating the subjective, cognitive experience of dreaming with measurable physiological changes.

Sleep-Wake Disorders

Sleep-wake disorders are divided into two categories: dyssomnias and parasomnias. **Dyssomnias** refer to disorders that make it difficult to fall asleep, stay asleep, or avoid sleep, and include insomnia, narcolepsy, and sleep apnea. **Parasomnias** are abnormal movements or behaviors during sleep, and include night terrors and sleepwalking. Most sleep-wake disorders occur during NREM sleep.

MNEMONIC

Hypna**go**gic hallucinations occur when one is **go**ing to bed. Hypno**pom**pic hallucinations occur when one is **pop**ping up out of bed.

Insomnia is difficulty falling asleep or staying asleep. It is the most common sleep-wake disorder and may be related to anxiety, depression, medications, or disruption of sleep cycles and circadian rhythms. **Narcolepsy**, in contrast, is a condition characterized by lack of voluntary control over the onset of sleep. The symptoms of narcolepsy are unique and include **cataplexy**, a loss of muscle control and sudden intrusion of REM sleep during waking hours, usually caused by an emotional trigger; **sleep paralysis**, a sensation of being unable to move despite being awake; and **hypnagogic** and **hypnopompic hallucinations**, which are hallucinations when going to sleep or awakening. Another dyssomnia is **sleep apnea**, which is an inability to breathe during sleep. People with this disorder awaken often during the night in order to breathe. Sleep apnea can be either obstructive or central. Obstructive sleep apnea occurs when a physical blockage in the pharynx or trachea prevents airflow; central sleep apnea occurs when the brain fails to send signals to the diaphragm to breathe.

Night terrors, which are most common in children, are periods of intense anxiety that occur during slow-wave sleep. Children will often thrash and scream during these terrors, and will show signs of sympathetic overdrive, with a high heart rate and rapid breathing. Because these usually occur during SWS, the child experiencing the episode is very difficult to wake, and usually does not remember the dream the next morning. **Sleepwalking**, or **somnambulism**, also usually occurs during SWS. Some people who sleepwalk may eat, talk, have sexual intercourse, or even drive great distances while sleeping with absolutely no recollection of the event. Most return to their beds and awake in the morning, with no knowledge of their nighttime activities. Contrary to popular belief, awakening a person who is sleepwalking will not harm the person; however, it is generally suggested to quietly guide the individual back to bed to avoid disturbing SWS.

Sleep deprivation can result from as little as one night without sleep, or from multiple nights with poor-quality, short-duration sleep. Sleep deprivation results in irritability, mood disturbances, decreased performance, and slowed reaction time. Extreme deprivation can cause psychosis. While one cannot make up for lost sleep, people who are permitted to sleep normally after sleep deprivation often exhibit **REM rebound**, an earlier onset and greater duration of REM sleep compared to normal.

Hypnosis

Hypnosis, named after the ancient Greek god of sleep, *Hypnos*, was first documented in the eighteenth century. **Hypnosis** can be defined as a state in which a person appears to be in control of normal functions, but is in a highly suggestible state. In other words, a hypnotized person easily succumbs to the suggestions of others. Hypnosis starts with **hypnotic induction**, in which the hypnotist seeks to relax the subject and increase the subject's level of concentration. Then, the hypnotist can suggest perceptions or actions to the hypnotized person. In practice, hypnosis is not the same as its sensationalized version in the media, in which a hypnotist will snap his fingers and cause an individual to exhibit bizarre behavior. Rather, hypnosis has been used successfully for pain control, psychological therapy, memory enhancement, weight loss, and smoking cessation. Brain imaging has indicated that hypnotic states are indeed real; however, effective hypnosis requires a willing personality and lack of skepticism on the part of the patient.

BRIDGE

Hypnosis has been used to recover repressed memories of trauma; however, these memories are not admissible in a court of law. This is because the suggestible state of hypnotism makes an individual vulnerable to creating false memories, which can be perceived as completely real. False memories are discussed in Chapter 3 of *MCAT Behavioral Sciences Review*.

Meditation

Defining **meditation** can be tricky and is highly dependent on the practitioners of meditation and their beliefs. Meditation has been a central practice in many religions. Meditation usually involves quieting of the mind for some purpose, whether spiritual, religious, or related to stress reduction. In the secular Western tradition, meditation is often used for counseling and psychotherapy because it produces a sense of relaxation and relief from anxiety and worrying. To that end, meditation causes physiological changes such as decreased heart rate and blood pressure. On EEG, meditation resembles Stage 1 sleep with theta and slow alpha waves.

MCAT EXPERTISE

Recent studies have demonstrated that mindful meditation not only improves psychological well-being, but may even help improve test scores and student performance. Take time for yourself while studying for the MCAT; keep your mind calm to keep it sharp.

MCAT CONCEPT CHECK 4.3

Before you move on, assess your understanding of the material with these questions.

1. For each of the sleep stages below, list its EEG waveforms and main features.

Stage	EEG Waves	Features
Awake		
Stage 1		
Stage 2		
Stage 3		
Stage 4		
REM		

2. Which two hormones are most associated with maintaining circadian rhythms?

   -

   -

3. What is the difference between a dyssomnia and a parasomnia? Provide an example of each.

   - Dyssomnia:

   - Parasomnia:

4.4 Consciousness-Altering Drugs

LEARNING OBJECTIVES

After Chapter 4.4, you will be able to:

- List the drugs (or drug classes) known to increase GABA activity in the brain
- Recall the drugs (or drug classes) known to upregulate dopamine, norepinephrine, or serotonin activity
- Identify the three main structures in the mesolimbic reward pathway and the primary neurotransmitter of the pathway:

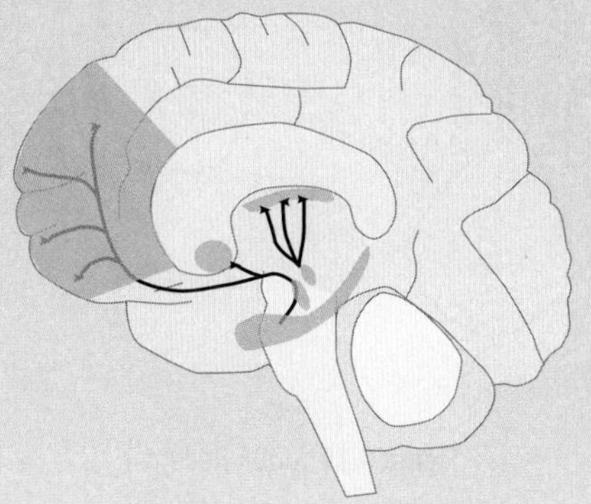

Consciousness-altering drugs, also known as psychoactive drugs, are generally described in four different groups: depressants, stimulants, opiates, and hallucinogens. Biologically speaking, marijuana has depressant, stimulant, and hallucinogenic effects, and will be considered separately.

Depressants

Depressants reduce nervous system activity, resulting in a sense of relaxation and reduced anxiety. Of the depressants, alcohol is certainly the most common. Another is sedatives, or "downers," which calm and induce sleep.

Alcohol

Alcohol has several different effects on the brain. It increases activity of the GABA receptor, a chloride channel that causes hyperpolarization of the membrane, as shown in Figure 4.11. This hyperpolarization causes generalized brain inhibition at the physiological level, resulting in diminished arousal at moderate doses. The changes in brain activity also cause changes in outward behavior. For example, excessive consumption of alcohol may be associated with a notable a lack of self-control known as **disinhibition**, which occurs because the centers of the brain that prevent inappropriate behavior are also depressed. Alcohol also increases dopamine levels, causing a sense of mild euphoria. At higher doses, brain activity becomes more disrupted. Logical reasoning and motor skills are affected, and fatigue may result. One of the main effects on logical reasoning is the inability to recognize consequences of actions, creating a short-sighted view of the world called **alcohol myopia**.

Alcohol use is implicated in many automobile accidents, homicides (for both perpetrator and victim), and hospital admissions. Intoxication with alcohol is often measured using blood alcohol level.

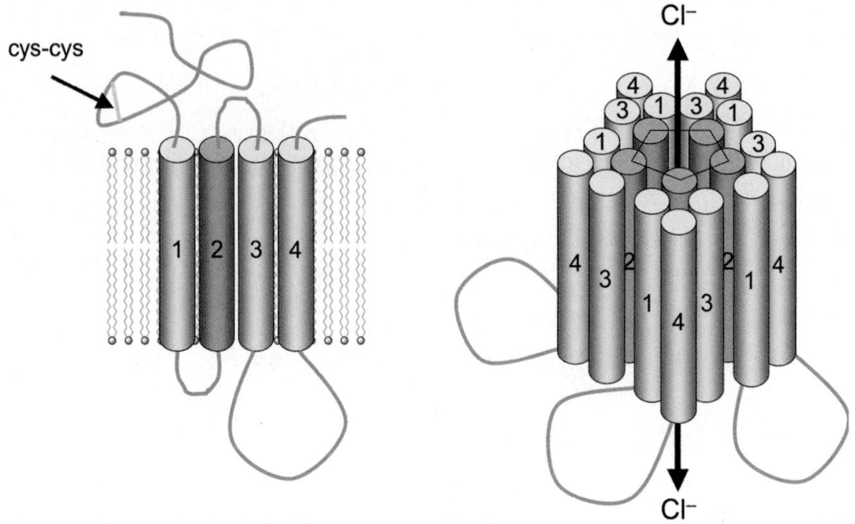

Figure 4.11 GABA Receptor

GABA is the primary inhibitory neurotransmitter in the brain; its receptor is a chloride channel that causes hyperpolarization of the membrane.

Alcohol is one of the most widely abused drugs. Alcoholism rates tend to be higher for those of lower socioeconomic status (SES), but people with a lower SES who have alcoholism tend to enter recovery sooner and at higher rates. Alcoholism tends to run in families, and children of people with alcoholism are also likely to suffer from major depressive disorder. Long-term consequences of alcoholism include cirrhosis and liver failure, pancreatic damage, gastric or duodenal ulcers, gastrointestinal cancer, and brain disorders including **Wernicke–Korsakoff syndrome**, caused by a deficiency of thiamine (vitamin B_1) and characterized by severe memory impairment with changes in mental status and loss of motor skills.

Sedatives

Sedatives tend to depress central nervous system activity, resulting in feelings of calm, relaxation, and drowsiness. Two types of sedatives are barbiturates and benzodiazepines. **Barbiturates** were historically used as anxiety-reducing (anxiolytic) and sleep medications, but have mostly been replaced by **benzodiazepines**, which are less prone to overdose. Barbiturates include *amobarbital* and *phenobarbital*; benzodiazepines include *alprazolam*, *lorazepam*, *diazepam*, and *clonazepam*. These drugs also increase GABA activity, causing a sense of relaxation. However, both of these drug types can be highly addictive. If taken with alcohol, overdoses of barbiturates or benzodiazepines may result in coma or death.

Stimulants

Stimulants cause an increase in arousal in the nervous system. Each drug increases the frequency of action potentials, but does so by different mechanisms.

Amphetamines

Amphetamines cause increased arousal by increasing release of dopamine, norepinephrine, and serotonin at the synapse and decreasing their reuptake. This increases arousal and causes a reduction in appetite and decreased need for sleep. Physiological effects include an increase in heart rate and blood pressure. Psychological effects include euphoria, hypervigilance (being "on edge"), anxiety, delusions of grandeur, and paranoia. Prolonged use of high doses of amphetamines can result in stroke or brain damage. People who take amphetamines often suffer from withdrawal after discontinuation, leading to depression, fatigue, and irritability.

Cocaine

Cocaine originates from the coca plant, grown in the high-altitude regions of South America. Cocaine can be purified from these leaves or created synthetically. Similar to amphetamines, cocaine also acts on dopamine, norepinephrine, and serotonin synapses, but cocaine decreases reuptake of the neurotransmitters instead. Hence, the effects of cocaine intoxication and withdrawal are therefore similar to amphetamines, as listed above. Cocaine also has anesthetic and vasoconstrictive properties, and is therefore sometimes used in surgeries in highly vascularized areas, such as the nose and throat. These vasoconstrictive properties can also lead to heart attacks and strokes when used recreationally. **Crack** is a form of cocaine that can be smoked. With quick and potent effects, this drug is highly addictive.

Ecstasy (3,4-methylenedioxy-*N*-methylamphetamine, MDMA)

Ecstasy, commonly called "E," acts as a hallucinogen combined with an amphetamine. As a designer amphetamine, its mechanism and effects are similar to other amphetamines. Physiologically, ecstasy causes increased heart rate, increased blood pressure, blurry vision, sweating, nausea, and hyperthermia. Psychologically, ecstasy causes feelings of euphoria, increased alertness, and an overwhelming sense of well-being and connectedness. Ecstasy is an example of a club or rave drug, and is often packaged in colorful pills, as shown in Figure 4.12.

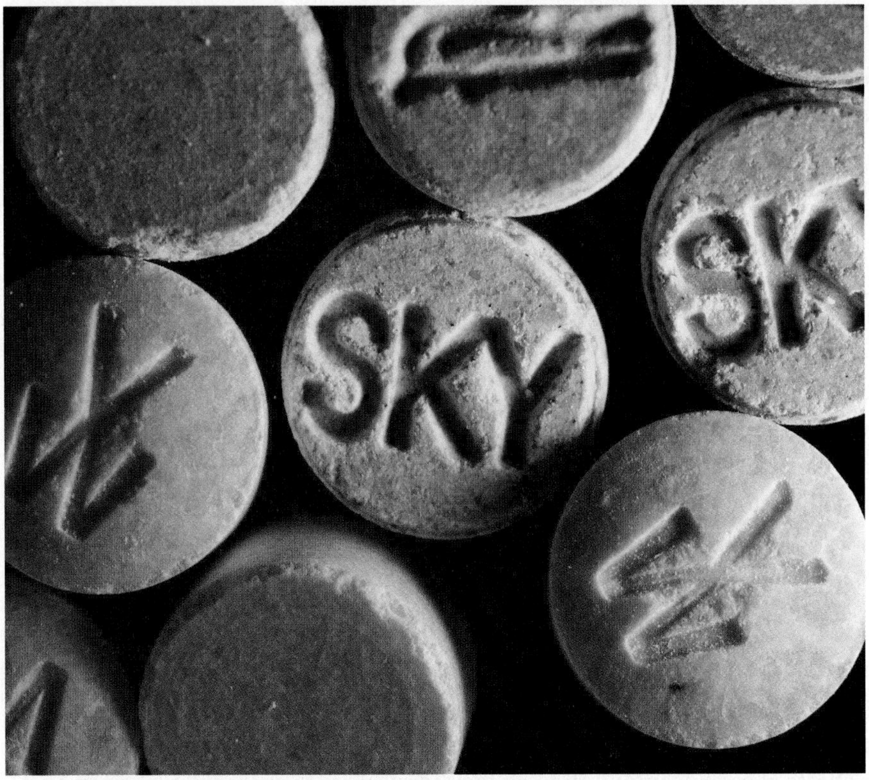

Figure 4.12 Pills of Ecstasy (MDMA)

Opiates and Opioids

Opiates and opioids are types of narcotics, also known as painkillers. Derived from the poppy plant, **opium** has been used and abused for centuries. Today, we have numerous drugs, used both recreationally and therapeutically, derived from opium. Naturally occurring forms, called **opiates**, include *morphine* and *codeine*. Semisynthetic derivatives, called **opioids**, include *oxycodone, hydrocodone*, and *heroin*. These compounds bind to opioid receptors in the peripheral and central nervous system. They act as endorphin agonists and cause a decreased reaction to pain and a sense of euphoria. Overdose, however, can cause death by respiratory suppression, in which the brain stops sending signals to breathe.

Heroin, or *diacetylmorphine*, was originally created as a substitute for morphine. Once injected, the body rapidly metabolizes heroin to morphine. Usually smoked or injected, heroin was once the most widely abused opioid; however, this designation has shifted to prescription opioids like oxycodone and hydrocodone. Treatment for opioid addiction may include use of *methadone*, a long-acting opioid with lower risk of overdose.

Hallucinogens

Hallucinogens are drugs which typically cause introspection, distortions of reality and fantasy, and enhancement of sensory experiences. Physiologic effects include increased heart rate and blood pressure, dilation of pupils, sweating, and increased body temperature. Examples of hallucinogens include **lysergic acid diethylamide (LSD)**, shown in Figure 4.13, *peyote, mescaline, ketamine*, and *psilocybin*-containing mushrooms. The exact mechanism of most hallucinogens is unknown, but is thought to be a complex interaction between various neurotransmitters, especially serotonin.

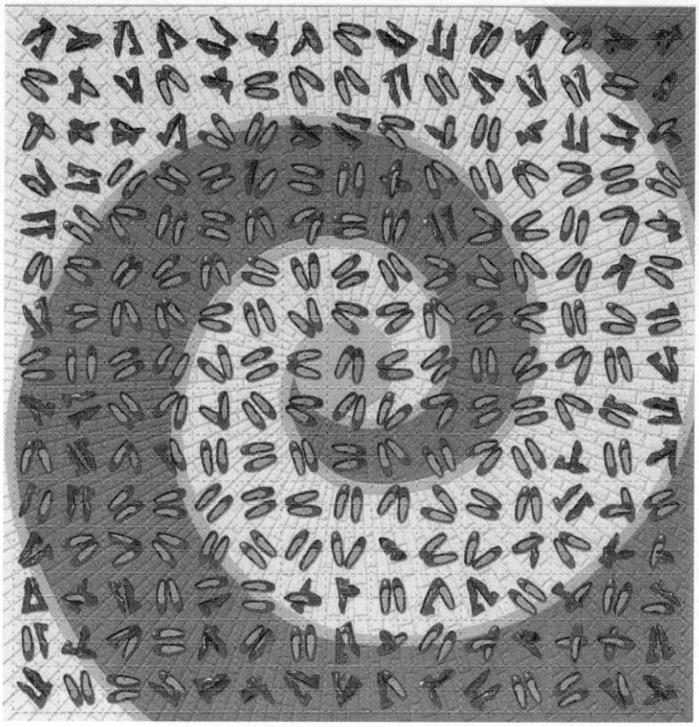

Figure 4.13 Sheet of LSD Blotter Paper
LSD is often sold on colorful paper, reflecting the fact that, like ecstasy, LSD is considered a club drug.

Marijuana

Marijuana, shown in Figure 4.14, primarily refers to the leaves and flowers of two plant species: *Cannabis sativa* and *Cannabis indica*. It has been the subject of many news reports in the last few years as many states move toward the legalization of marijuana for medical or recreational use. While talks about the legal status of marijuana in the United States are fairly recent, marijuana has been used for centuries, with the earliest known accounts originating from approximately 3 B.C.E.

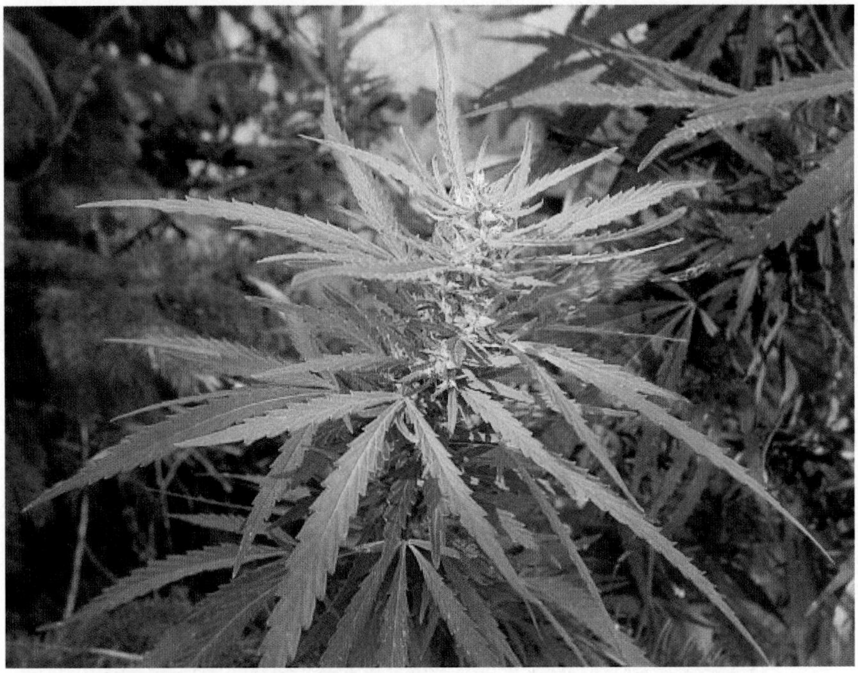

Figure 4.14 Cannabis

The active chemical in marijuana is known as **tetrahydrocannabinol** (**THC**). THC exerts its effects by acting at cannabinoid receptors, glycine receptors, and opioid receptors. How these receptors interact to create the "high" achieved from marijuana use is unknown. It is known, however, that THC inhibits GABA activity and indirectly increases dopamine activity (causing pleasure). Physiological effects are mixed, including eye redness, dry mouth, fatigue, impairment of short-term memory, increased heart rate, increased appetite, and lowered blood pressure. Psychologically, effects seem to fall into the categories of stimulant, depressant, and hallucinogen.

Drug Addiction

Drug addiction is highly related to the **mesolimbic reward pathway**, one of four dopaminergic pathways in the brain, as shown in Figure 4.15. This pathway includes the **nucleus accumbens** (**NAc**), the **ventral tegmental area** (**VTA**), and the connection between them called the **medial forebrain bundle** (**MFB**). This pathway is normally involved in motivation and emotional response, and its activation accounts for the positive reinforcement of substance use. This addiction pathway is activated by all substances that produce psychological dependence. Gambling and falling in love also activate this pathway.

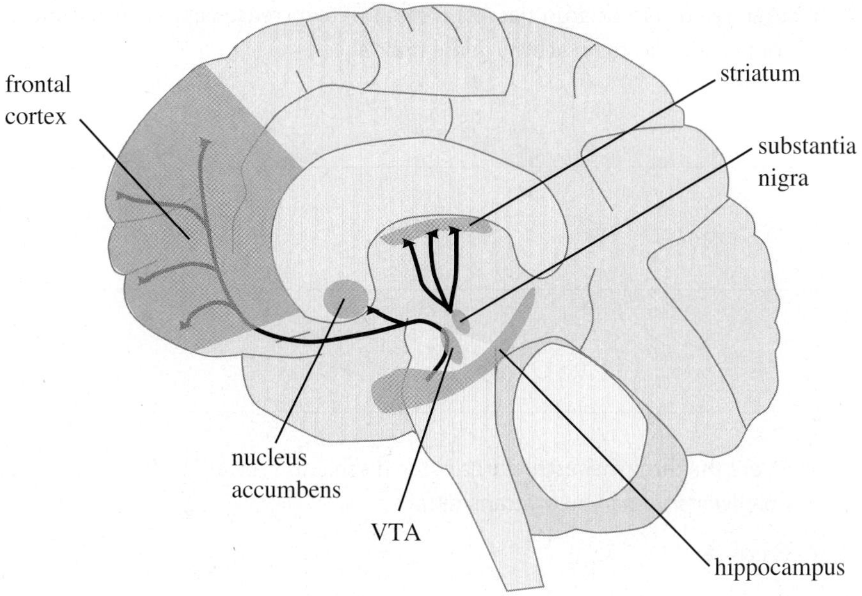

Figure 4.15 Dopaminergic Pathways in the Brain
The reward pathway is composed of the nucleus accumbens, ventral tegmental area (VTA), and the medial forebrain bundle between them (not labeled).

MCAT CONCEPT CHECK 4.4

Before you move on, assess your understanding of the material with these questions.

1. Which three drugs (or drug classes) are known to increase GABA activity in the brain?

 - ______________________________

 - ______________________________

 - ______________________________

2. Which three drugs (or drug classes) are known to increase dopamine, norepinephrine, and serotonin activity in the brain?
   -
   -
   -

3. What are the three main structures in the mesolimbic reward pathway? What is this pathway's primary neurotransmitter?
   - Structure:
   - Structure:
   - Structure:
   - Neurotransmitter:

4.5 Attention

LEARNING OBJECTIVES

After Chapter 4.5, you will be able to:

- Compare and contrast controlled processing and automatic processing
- Describe the role of the "filter" used in selective attention

Attention refers to concentrating on one aspect of the sensory environment, or **sensorium**. While this definition is straightforward, an understanding of how attention works and the mechanism by which we can shift our attention from one set of stimuli to another is still somewhat unclear.

Selective Attention

Selective attention is focusing on one part of the sensorium while ignoring other stimuli. It therefore acts as a filter between sensory stimuli and our processing systems. If a stimulus is attended to, it is passed through a filter and analyzed further. If the stimulus is not attended to, it is lost. In its original conceptualization, selective attention was viewed as an all-or-nothing process: if we choose a particular stimulus to give our attention to, the other stimuli are lost. However, recent evidence indicates that this is not the case.

Imagine this: You are at a party, talking with a friend. However, your ears perk up when you hear your name spoken halfway across the room. Even though you were engaged in conversation and presumably paying attention, you were able to perceive your name being mentioned. This is sometimes called the **cocktail party phenomenon** and is evidence of a different interpretation of selective attention. Selective attention is probably more of a filter that allows us to focus on one thing while allowing other stimuli to be processed in the background. Only if the other stimuli are particularly important—one's name being mentioned, a sudden flash of light, pain—do we shift our attention to them.

Dichotic listening tests are designed to test selective attention. Participants are given headphones that have distinct auditory stimuli going to each ear. Participants are then asked to pay attention to either or both stimuli, then asked to repeat out loud what they heard in the attended ear, which is termed **shadowing**. This task tests selective attention because participants are asked to filter out information from the unattended ear. Alternatively, the task can test whether participants can subconsciously gain information from the unattended ear.

Divided Attention

Divided attention is the ability to perform multiple tasks at the same time. Most new or complex tasks require undivided attention and utilize **controlled (effortful) processing**, discussed in Chapter 3 of *MCAT Behavioral Sciences Review*. In contrast, familiar or routine actions can be performed with **automatic processing**, which permits the brain to focus on other tasks with divided attention. Consider learning to drive: at first, drivers intensely grip the steering wheel and pay undivided attention to the road ahead. But as you become more accustomed to driving, you can relegate some aspects of driving—like knowing how hard to push on the pedal—to automatic processing. This lets a driver perform secondary tasks such as changing the radio station. That being said, automatic processing is far from perfect. It does not allow for innovation or rapid response to change, which may contribute to the high incidence of car accidents that result from distracted driving.

MCAT CONCEPT CHECK 4.5

Before you move on, assess your understanding of the material with these questions.

1. Compare and contrast controlled (effortful) processing and automatic processing:
   - Controlled (effortful) processing:

   ____

   - Automatic processing:

   ____

2. Briefly describe the function of the "filter" used in selective attention:

   ____

   ____

4.6 Language

High-Yield

LEARNING OBJECTIVES

After Chapter 4.6, you will be able to:

- Recall the expected milestones of language development and the ages at which they should occur
- Identify the primary characteristics of the nativist, behaviorist, and social interactionist theories of language development
- Describe the symptoms and brain regions associated with Broca's, Wernicke's, and conduction aphasia:

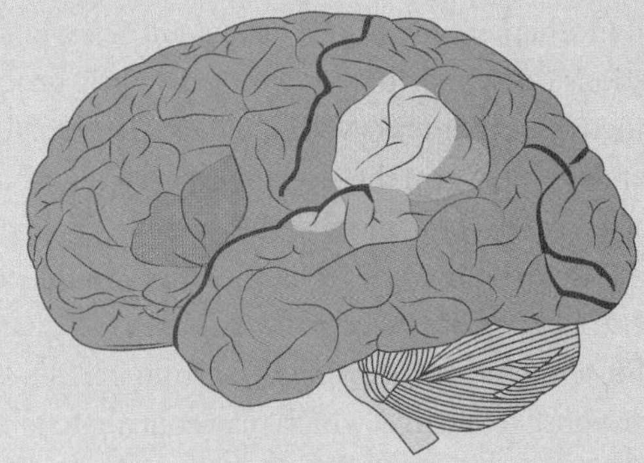

Whether it is written, spoken, or signed, **language** is fundamental to the creation of communities. As humans began to live in groups, the ability to communicate became essential. Division of labor and a sense of shared history require that the meaning of the language be the same for all speakers of the language.

Components of Language

There are five basic components of language: phonology, morphology, semantics, syntax, and pragmatics.

Phonology

Phonology refers to the actual sound of language. There are about 40 speech sounds or **phonemes** in English, although many more exist in other languages, as shown in Figure 4.16. Children must learn to produce and recognize the sounds of language, separating them from environmental noises and other human-created sounds, like coughing. Additionally, when a language has subtle differences in speech sounds that represent a change in meaning, children learn to distinguish those phonemes; this ability is called **categorical perception**. The ability to recognize a word as being the same, even if the pronunciation of the word varies between people is an auditory example of **constancy**, which is described in Chapter 2 of *MCAT Behavioral Sciences Review*.

International Phonetic Alphabet

Plosive

Name	Text
Voiceless bilabial	p
Voiced bilabial	b
Voiceless alveolar	t
Voiced alveolar	d
Voiceless retroflex	ʈ
Voiced retroflex	ɖ
Voiceless palatal	c
Voiced palatal	ɟ
Voiceless velar	k
Voiced velar	ɡ
Voiceless uvular	q
Voiced uvular	ɢ
Voiceless glottal	ʔ

Nasal

Name	Text
Voiced bilabial	m
Voiced labiodental	ɱ
Voiced alveolar	n
Voiced retroflex	ɳ
Voiced palatal	ɲ
Voiced velar	ŋ
Voiced uvular	ɴ

Trill

Name	Text
Voiced bilabial	ʙ
Voiced alveolar	r
Voiced uvular	ʀ

Tap or Flap

Name	Text
Voiced alveolar	ɾ
Voiced retroflex	ɽ

Fricative

Name	Text
Voiceless bilabial	ɸ
Voiced bilabial	β
Voiceless labiodental	f
Voiced labiodental	v
Voiceless dental	θ
Voiced dental	ð
Voiceless alveolar	s
Voiced alveolar	z
Voiceless postalveolar	ʃ
Voiced postalveolar	ʒ
Voiceless retroflex	ʂ
Voiced retroflex	ʐ
Voiceless palatal	ç
Voiced palatal	ʝ
Voiceless velar	x
Voiced velar	ɣ
Voiceless uvular	χ
Voiced uvular	ʁ
Voiceless pharyngeal	ħ
Voiced pharyngeal	ʕ
Voiceless glottal	h
Voiced glottal	ɦ
Voiceless dorso-palatal	ɧ

Lateral Fricative

Name	Text
Voiceless alveolar	ɬ
Voiced alveolar	ɮ

Approximant

Name	Text
Voiced labiodental	ʋ
Voiced alveolar	ɹ
Voiced retroflex	ɻ
Voiced palatal	j
Voiced velar	ɰ

Lateral Approximant

Name	Text
Voiced alveolar	l
Voiced retroflex	ɭ
Voiced palatal	ʎ
Voiced velar	ʟ

Clicks

Name	Text
Bilabial	ʘ
Dental	ǀ
(Post)alveolar	ǃ
Palatoalveolar	ǂ
Alveolar lateral	ǁ

Figure 4.16 A Section of the International Phonetic Alphabet
The IPA is an unambiguous system of writing all of the known phonemes of all human languages.

Morphology

Morphology refers to the structure of words. Many words are composed of multiple building blocks called **morphemes**, each of which connotes a particular meaning. Consider the word *redesigned*, which can be broken into three morphemes: *re–*, indicating *to do again*; *–design–*, the verb root; and *–ed*, indicating an action in the past.

Semantics

Semantics refers to the association of meaning with a word. A child must learn that certain combinations of phonemes represent certain physical objects or events, and that words may refer to entire categories, such as *animal*, while others refer to specific members of categories, such as *doggy*. One can see this skill developing in young children as they may refer to all animals as *doggy*.

Syntax

Syntax refers to how words are put together to form sentences. A child must notice the effects of word order on meaning: *Nathan has only three pieces of candy* has a very different meaning than *Only Nathan has three pieces of candy*.

Pragmatics

Finally, **pragmatics** refers to the dependence of language on context and preexisting knowledge. In other words, the manner in which we speak may differ depending on the audience and our relationship to that audience. Imagine asking to share a seat on a bus. Depending on whom we ask, we may word this request in wildly different ways. To a stranger, we may be more formal: *Pardon me, do you mind if I share this seat?* To a close friend, we may be less so: *Hey, move over!* Pragmatics are also affected by **prosody**—the rhythm, cadence, and inflection of our voices.

Language Development

To effectively interact with society, a child must learn to communicate through language, whether oral or signed. An important precursor to language is **babbling**. Almost without exception, children—including children who are hearing impaired—spontaneously begin to babble during their first year. For children who can hear, babbling reaches its highest frequency between nine and twelve months. For children who are hearing impaired or deaf, verbal babbling often ceases soon after it begins.

KEY CONCEPT

Timeline of language acquisition:

- 9 to 12 months: babbling
- 12 to 18 months: about one word per month
- 18 to 20 months: "explosion of language" and combining words
- 2 to 3 years: longer sentences (3 words or more)
- 5 years: language rules largely mastered

The timeline of language acquisition is fairly consistent among children. From 12 to 18 months, children add about one word per month. Starting around 18 months, an explosion of language begins. During this **naming explosion**, the child quickly learns dozens of words, and uses each word with varying inflection and gestures to convey a desired meaning. For example, a child may ask, *Apple?* while pointing at an apple in a bowl of fruit, in an effort to request the apple. During this naming explosion, children may also frequently fall into **overextension**, in which they inappropriately apply a term to an object that bears cursory similarities to the term. For example, in an attempt to request a kiwi from a fruit bowl, a child might point at the kiwi and ask, *Apple?* For children at this age, gestures, inflection, and context are essential for the parent or caregiver to identify the meaning.

Between 18 and 20 months of age, children begin to combine words. For example, children may say, *Eat apple* to indicate that they would like to eat an apple. In the grocery store, the same children may ask, *That apple?* to distinguish between fruit. In this way, context and gesture becomes less important as the ability to assemble sentences develops.

By the age of two or three years, children can speak in longer sentences. Vocabulary grows exponentially. As a child creates longer sentences, grammatical errors increase as the child internalizes the complex rules of grammar. These include **errors of growth** in which a child applies a grammatical rule (often a morpheme) in a situation where it does not apply: *runned* instead of *ran*, or *funner* instead of *more fun*. Interestingly, caregivers are less likely to correct errors of grammar than errors of word choice.

For the most part, language is substantially mastered by the age of five. The acquisition of language appears easy for most children, which has led to significant speculation on exactly how this occurs.

REAL WORLD

Pediatricians often monitor language development to determine if there is a developmental delay. For example, a two-year-old child who uses fewer than 10 words has a significant developmental delay and should be referred for speech therapy. This would also prompt a search for other developmental issues.

Nativist (Biological) Theory

The **nativist (biological) theory**, largely credited to linguist Noam Chomsky, advocates for the existence of some innate capacity for language. Chomsky is known for his study of **transformational grammar**. He focused on syntactic transformations, or changes in word order that retain the same meaning; for example, *I took the MCAT* vs. *The MCAT was taken by me*. Chomsky noted that children learn to make such transformations effortlessly at an early age. He therefore concluded that this ability must be innate. In this theory, this innate ability is called the **language acquisition device (LAD)**, a theoretical pathway in the brain that allows infants to process and absorb language rules.

Nativists believe in a **critical period** for language acquisition between two years and puberty. If no language exposure occurs during this time, later training is largely ineffective. This idea came to light through an unfortunate test case: a victim of child abuse. This child had been isolated from all human contact from age two to thirteen, when she was discovered by authorities. Even with later language exposure, she was unable to master many rules of language, although she was able to learn some aspects of syntax. The fact that this child was able to learn some rules may indicate that there is a sensitive period for language development, rather than a critical period. A **sensitive period** is a time when environmental input has maximal effect on the development of an ability. Most psychologists consider the sensitive period for language development to be before the onset of puberty.

Learning (Behaviorist) Theory

The **learning (behaviorist) theory**, proposed by B. F. Skinner, explained language acquisition by operant conditioning. Very young babies are capable of distinguishing between phonemes of all human languages, but by six months of age show a strong preference for phonemes in the language spoken by their parents. Skinner explained language acquisition by **reinforcement**. That is, caregivers repeat and reinforce sounds that sound most like the language they speak. Thus, over time, the infant perceives that certain sounds have little value and are not reinforced, while other sounds have value and are reliably reinforced by caregivers. While this may account for the development of words and speech, many psycholinguists point out that this theory cannot fully explain the explosion in vocabulary that occurs during early childhood.

Social Interactionist Theory

The **social interactionist theory** of language development focuses on the interplay between biological and social processes. That is, language acquisition is driven by the child's desire to communicate and behave in a social manner, such as interacting with caretakers and other children. Interactionist theory allows for the role of brain development in the acquisition of language. As the biological foundation for language develops and children are exposed to language, the brain groups sounds and meanings together. Then, as the child interacts with others, certain brain circuits are reinforced, while others are de-emphasized, resulting in atrophy of those circuits.

Influence of Language on Cognition

Psycholinguistics has long focused on the relationship between language and thinking. Linguist Benjamin Whorf proposed the **Whorfian hypothesis**, also called the **linguistic relativity hypothesis**, which suggests that our perception of reality—the way we think about the world—is determined by the content of language. In essence, language affects the way we think rather than the other way around. For instance, some Inuit dialects have a wide variety of names for different types of snow, whereas the English language has very few. Therefore, according to the Whorfian hypothesis, people who speak one of those Inuit dialects are better at discriminating subtleties between different types of snow than English speakers are. This is a somewhat controversial notion that depends on the definition of "a word" but most linguists agree that language can influence how we think to some degree. Word choice, inflection, context, and speaker all play a role in our perception of a message. In addition, language often provides an original framework for understanding information. A more expansive framework with more specific vocabulary allows for more sophisticated processing of that information and enhanced communication of that information to others.

Brain Areas and Language

Two different areas of the brain are responsible for speech production and language comprehension, as shown in Figure 4.17. Both, however, are located in the dominant hemisphere, which is usually the left hemisphere. **Broca's area**, located in the inferior frontal gyrus of the frontal lobe, controls the motor function of speech via connections with the motor cortex. **Wernicke's area**, located in the superior temporal gyrus of the temporal lobe, is responsible for language comprehension. Broca's area and Wernicke's area are connected by the **arcuate fasciculus**, a bundle of axons that allows appropriate association between language comprehension and speech production.

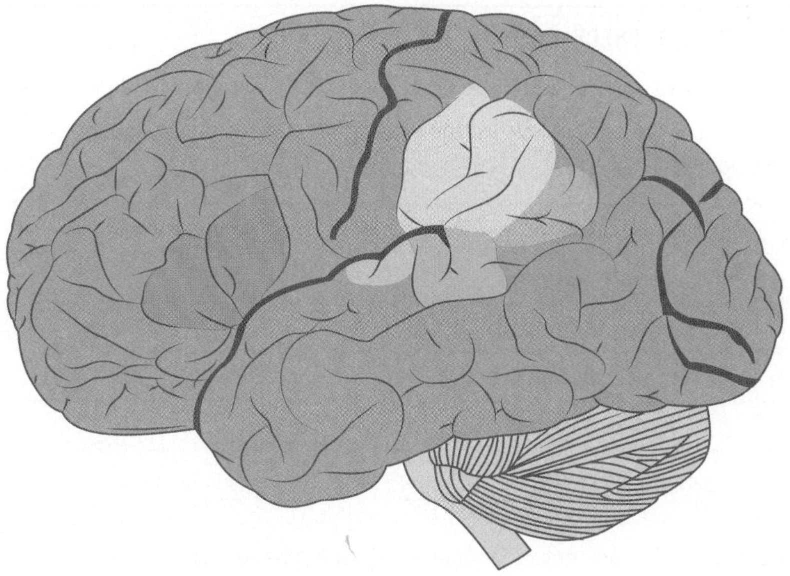

Figure 4.17 Brain Areas Associated with Language
Blue = Broca's area; Green = Wernicke's area. Other colored regions are associated with other aspects of language beyond the scope of the MCAT (yellow = supramarginal gyrus; orange = angular gyrus; light pink = primary auditory cortex).

Aphasia is a deficit of language production or comprehension. Much of what we know regarding language and aphasia is through observations of people with damage to speech-related areas. When damage occurs to Broca's area, speech comprehension is intact but the patient will have a reduced or absent ability to produce spoken language. This is known as **Broca's (expressive) aphasia**. These patients are often very frustrated because they are stuck with the sensation of having every word on the tip of their tongue.

On the other hand, when Wernicke's area is damaged, motor production and fluency of speech is retained but comprehension of speech is lost. This is known as **Wernicke's (receptive) aphasia**. Because speech comprehension is lost, these patients speak nonsensical sounds and inappropriate word combinations devoid of meaning. Patients with Wernicke's aphasia often believe that they are speaking and understanding perfectly well, even though the people around them have no comprehension of what is being said. This can also be very frustrating to patients.

Finally, if the arcuate fasciculus is affected, the resulting aphasia is known as **conduction aphasia**. Because Broca's and Wernicke's areas are unaffected, speech production and comprehension are intact. However, the patient is unable to repeat something that has been said because the connection between these two regions has been lost. This is a very rare form of aphasia.

MCAT CONCEPT CHECK 4.6

Before you move on, assess your understanding of the material with these questions.

1. For each of the ages below, list the expected milestone(s) of language development:

Age	Milestone(s)
9 to 12 months	
12 to 18 months	
18 to 20 months	
2 to 3 years	
5 years	

2. For each of the theories of language acquisition below, what is the primary motivation or trigger for language development?
   - Nativist (Biological):
   - Learning (Behaviorist):
   - Social interactionist:

3. Briefly describe the clinical features of each type of aphasia listed below:
   - Broca's aphasia:
   - Wernicke's aphasia
   - Conduction aphasia:

Conclusion

One of the biggest questions that psychology and biology seek to answer is how the brain, an organ consisting of lipids, water, and neurotransmitters, becomes the mind. Cognition and consciousness allow us to think about who we are, where we are, and what we are doing at a given moment, and this all occurs due to a complex interaction between individual neurons within the brain. Not only do we experience consciousness, but our behaviors are also intricately intertwined with physiological brain function. Language is one of the most complex cognitive processes, requiring intact comprehension and production mechanisms and an understanding of the rules of our native language.

As much as we research what the mind is and how it works, there is as much interest in *why* we do what we do and how we *feel* about it. This is the function of motivation (both internal and external) and emotion, which we will explore in detail in the next chapter.

GO ONLINE

You've reviewed the content, now test your knowledge and critical thinking skills by completing a test-like passage set in your online resources!

CONCEPT SUMMARY

Cognition

- Thought is more than just that of which we are conscious. The brain processes and makes decisions about the importance of various stimuli below the level of conscious awareness.
- The **information processing model** states that the brain encodes, stores, and retrieves information much like a computer.
- The ability to think abstractly develops over the life span. Early cognitive development is limited by brain maturation. Culture, genes, and environment also influence cognitive development.
- **Piaget's stages of cognitive development** are sensorimotor, preoperational, concrete operational, and formal operational.
  - The **sensorimotor stage** focuses on manipulating the environment to meet physical needs through **circular reactions**. **Object permanence** ends this stage.
  - The **preoperational stage** focuses on **symbolic thinking**, **egocentrism**, and **centration**.
  - The **concrete operational stage** focuses on understanding the feelings of others and manipulating physical (concrete) objects.
  - The **formal operational stage** focuses on abstract thought and problem solving.
- A mild level of cognitive decline while aging is normal; significant changes in cognition may signify an underlying disorder.
- Biological factors that affect cognition include organic brain disorders, genetic and chromosomal conditions, metabolic derangements, and drug use.

Problem Solving and Decision Making

- **Problem solving** requires identification and understanding of the problem, generation of potential solutions, testing of potential solutions, and evaluation of results.
  - A **mental set** is a pattern of approach for a given problem. An inappropriate mental set may negatively impact problem solving.
  - **Functional fixedness** is the tendency to use objects only in the way they are normally utilized, which may create barriers to problem solving.
- Types of problem solving include **trial-and-error**, **algorithms**, **deductive reasoning** (deriving conclusions from general rules), and **inductive reasoning** (deriving generalizations from evidence).
- Heuristics, biases, intuition, and emotions may assist decision making but may also lead to erroneous or problematic decisions.

- **Heuristics** are shortcuts or rules of thumb used to make decisions.
- **Biases** exist when an experimenter or decision maker is unable to objectively evaluate information.
- **Intuition** is a "gut feeling" regarding a particular decision. However, intuition can often be attributed to experience with similar situations.
- Emotional state often plays a role in decision making.

- Gardner's theory of **multiple intelligences** proposes at least eight areas of intelligence including: linguistic, logical–mathematical, musical, visual–spatial, bodily–kinesthetic, interpersonal, intrapersonal, and naturalist.
- Variations in intellectual ability can be attributed to combinations of environment, education, and genetics.

Consciousness

- States of consciousness include alertness, sleep, dreaming, and altered states of consciousness.
- **Alertness** is the state of being awake and able to think, perceive, process, and express information. **Beta** and **alpha waves** predominate on **electroencephalography** (**EEG**).
- **Sleep** is important for health of the brain and body.
    - **Stage 1** is light sleep and is dominated by **theta waves** on EEG. **Stage 2** is slightly deeper and includes theta waves, **sleep spindles**, and **K complexes**.
    - **Stages 3** and **4** are deep (**slow-wave**) sleep (**SWS**). **Delta waves** predominate on EEG. Most sleep-wake disorders occur during Stage 3 and 4 **non-rapid eye movement** (**NREM**) **sleep**. Dreaming in SWS focuses on consolidating declarative memories.
    - **Rapid eye movement** (**REM**) **sleep** is sometimes called **paradoxical sleep**: the mind appears close to awake on EEG, but the person is asleep. Eye movements and body paralysis occur in this stage. Dreaming in REM focuses on consolidating procedural memories.
    - The **sleep cycle** is approximately 90 minutes for adults; the normal cycle is Stage 1–2–3–4–3–2–REM or just 1–2–3–4–REM, although REM becomes more frequent toward the morning.
    - Changes in light in the evening trigger release of **melatonin** by the **pineal gland**, resulting in sleepiness. **Cortisol** levels increase in the early morning and help promote wakefulness. **Circadian rhythms** normally trend around a 24-hour day.
    - Most **dreaming** occurs during REM, but some dreaming occurs during other sleep stages. There are many different models that attempt to account for the content and purpose of dreaming.
    - Sleep-wake disorders include **dyssomnias**, such as insomnia, narcolepsy, sleep apnea, and sleep deprivation; and **parasomnias**, such as night terrors and sleepwalking (somnambulism).

- **Hypnosis** is a state of consciousness in which individuals appear to be in control of their normal faculties but are in a highly suggestible state. Hypnosis is often used for pain control, psychological therapy, memory enhancement, weight loss, and smoking cessation.
- **Meditation** involves a quieting of the mind and is often used for relief of anxiety. It has also played a role in many of the world's religions.

Consciousness-Altering Drugs

- Consciousness-altering drugs are grouped by effect into depressants, stimulants, opiates, and hallucinogens.
    - **Depressants** include alcohol, barbiturates, and benzodiazepines. They promote or mimic GABA activity in the brain.
    - **Stimulants** include amphetamines, cocaine, and ecstasy. They increase dopamine, norepinephrine, and serotonin concentration at the synaptic cleft.
    - **Opiates** and **opioids** include heroin, morphine, opium, and prescription pain medications such as oxycodone and hydrocodone. They can cause death by respiratory depression.
    - **Hallucinogens** include lysergic acid diethylamide (LSD), peyote, mescaline, ketamine, and psilocybin-containing mushrooms.
    - **Marijuana** has depressant, stimulant, and hallucinogenic effects. Its active ingredient is **tetrahydrocannabinol**.
- Drug addiction is mediated by the **mesolimbic pathway**, which includes the **nucleus accumbens**, **medial forebrain bundle**, and **ventral tegmental area**. Dopamine is the main neurotransmitter in this pathway.

Attention

- **Selective attention** allows one to pay attention to a particular stimulus while determining if additional stimuli in the background require attention.
- **Divided attention** uses **automatic processing** to pay attention to multiple activities at one time.

Language

- Language consists of phonology, morphology, semantics, syntax, and pragmatics.
    - **Phonology** refers to the actual sound of speech.
    - **Morphology** refers to the building blocks of words, such as rules for pluralization (–*s* in English), past tense (–*ed*), and so forth.
    - **Semantics** refers to the meaning of words.
    - **Syntax** refers to the rules dictating word order.
    - **Pragmatics** refers to the changes in language delivery depending on context.

- Theories of language development focus on different reasons or motivations for language acquisition.
  - The **nativist (biological) theory** explains language acquisition as being innate and controlled by the **language acquisition device (LAD)**.
  - The **learning (behaviorist) theory** explains language acquisition as being controlled by operant conditioning and reinforcement by caregivers.
  - The **social interactionist theory** explains language acquisition as being caused by a motivation to communicate and interact with others.
- The **Whorfian (linguistic relativity) hypothesis** states that the lens through which we view and interpret the world is created by language.
- Speech areas in the brain are found in the dominant hemisphere, which is usually the left.
  - The motor function of speech is controlled by **Broca's area**. Damage results in **Broca's aphasia**, a nonfluent aphasia in which generating each word requires great effort.
  - Language comprehension is controlled by **Wernicke's area**. Damage results in **Wernicke's aphasia**, a fluent, nonsensical aphasia with lack of comprehension.
  - The **arcuate fasciculus** connects Wernicke's area and Broca's area. Damage results in **conduction aphasia**, marked by the inability to repeat words heard despite intact speech generation and comprehension.

ANSWERS TO CONCEPT CHECKS

4.1

1. The three steps in the information processing model are encoding, storage, and retrieval.
2. The older adult most likely has delirium. The time course is incompatible with the slow decline of dementia.
3.

Stage	Key Features
Sensorimotor	Focuses on manipulating environment for physical needs; circular reactions; ends with object permanence
Preoperational	Symbolic thinking, egocentrism, and centration
Concrete operational	Understands conservation and the feelings of others; can manipulate concrete objects logically
Formal operational	Can think abstractly and problem solve

4.2

1. Functional fixedness
2. Algorithm
3. Belief perseverance
4. The availability heuristic is used for making decisions based on how easily similar instances can be imagined. The representativeness heuristic is used for making decisions based on how much a particular item or situation fits a given prototype or stereotype.

4.3

1.

Stage	EEG Waves	Features
Awake	Beta and alpha	Able to perceive, process, access information, and express that information verbally
Stage 1	Theta	Light sleep and dozing
Stage 2	Theta	Sleep spindles and K complexes
Stage 3	Delta	Slow-wave sleep; dreams; declarative memory consolidation; sleep-wake disorders occur in this stage
Stage 4	Delta	Slow-wave sleep; dreams; declarative memory consolidation; sleep-wake disorders occur in this stage
REM	Mostly beta	Appears awake physiologically; dreams; procedural memory consolidation; body is paralyzed

2. The two hormones most associated with maintaining circadian rhythms are melatonin and cortisol.
3. Dyssomnias are disorders in which the duration or timing of sleep is disturbed. Examples include insomnia, narcolepsy, and sleep apnea. Parasomnias are disorders in which abnormal behaviors occur during sleep. Examples include night terrors and sleepwalking (somnambulism).

4.4

1. Drugs known to increase GABA activity in the brain include alcohol, barbiturates, and benzodiazepines. Note that marijuana inhibits GABA activity.
2. Drugs known to increase dopamine, norepinephrine, and serotonin activity in the brain include amphetamines, cocaine, and ecstasy (MDMA). Ecstasy is a designer amphetamine; it is mentioned separately here because of its hallucinogenic properties.
3. The three main structures in the mesolimbic reward pathway are the nucleus accumbens, medial forebrain bundle, and ventral tegmental area. The neurotransmitter of this pathway is dopamine.

4.5

1. Controlled (effortful) processing is used when maintaining undivided attention on a task, and is usually used for new or complex actions. Automatic processing is used for less critical stimuli in divided attention, and is usually used for familiar or repetitive actions.
2. The filter in selective attention permits us to focus on one set of stimuli while scanning other stimuli in the background for important information (such as our name or a significant change in the environment).

4.6

1.

Age	Milestone(s)
9 to 12 months	Babbling
12 to 18 months	Increase of about one word per month
18 to 20 months	"Explosion of language" and combining words (two-word sentences)
2 to 3 years	Longer sentences of three or more words
5 years	Language rules largely mastered

2. The primary trigger in the nativist theory is an innate ability to pick up language via the language acquisition device. In the learning theory, it is operant conditioning with reinforcement by caregivers. In the social interactionist theory, it is a desire to communicate and act socially.
3. Broca's aphasia is marked by difficulty producing language, with hesitancy and great difficulty coming up with words. Wernicke's aphasia is fluent, but includes nonsensical sounds and words devoid of meaning; language comprehension is lost. Conduction aphasia is marked by difficulty repeating speech, with intact speech production and comprehension.

SCIENCE MASTERY ASSESSMENT EXPLANATIONS

1. **D**

Jean Piaget hypothesized that new information is processed by adaptation, **(B)**. Adaptation is too broad of an answer because it includes both assimilation, **(A)**, and accommodation, **(D)**. Assimilation is incorporation of new information into existing schemata. If the new information doesn't fit, then accommodation occurs. Accommodation is the modification of existing schemata to account for new information and is thus the correct answer.

2. **B**

While many drugs can cause paranoia, the elevation in heart rate combined with prolonged alertness and a decrease in appetite suggests amphetamines, matching choice **(B)**.

3. **C**

The base rate fallacy occurs when prototypical or stereotypical factors are used for analysis rather than actual data. Because the student is volunteering in a hospital with a stroke center, the student sees more patients who have experienced a stroke than would be expected in a hospital without a stroke center. Thus, this experience changes the student's perception and results in base rate fallacy. Deductive reasoning, **(A)**, refers to drawing conclusions by integrating different pieces of evidence. The representativeness heuristic, **(B)**, involves categorization and classification based on how well an individual example fits its category. Confirmation bias, **(D)**, occurs when people only seek information that reinforces their opinions.

4. **A**

Fluid intelligence consists of problem-solving skills and is not one of Gardner's eight multiple intelligences. Gardner's theory lists linguistic, logical–mathematical, musical, visual–spatial, bodily–kinesthetic, interpersonal, intrapersonal, and naturalist intelligences.

5. **A**

EEG during REM is composed mainly of beta waves, which are present during alertness. SWS, **(B)**, consists mainly of delta waves, which are not typically present during REM sleep. Stage 1 sleep, **(C)**, consists mainly of theta waves. Meditation, **(D)**, is quieting of the mind, and consists mainly of slow alpha and theta waves.

6. **B**

Early in the evening, sleep cycles include deepening of sleep (Stages 1–2–3–4), followed either by lightening of sleep (Stages 4–3–2) and then REM, or just directly moving from Stage 4 into REM. Later in the evening, the cycle may be shortened as slow-wave sleep becomes less common.

7. **B**

Divided attention is the ability to perform several tasks simultaneously. Routine actions, such as rewatching familiar episodes of a favorite TV show, are completed via automatic processing which allows the brain to focus on other tasks. Working on two tasks simultaneously means the student is using divided attention, supporting **(B)** as the correct answer. By contrast, parallel processing, **(D)**, refers to the brain's ability to analyze imagery by processing several aspects of the image (shape, color, motion, etc.) independently and simultaneously.

8. **C**

Cognitive theorists proposed in the cognitive process dream theory that wakeful and dreaming states use the same mental systems within the brain, particularly stream-of-consciousness. The activation–synthesis theory, **(A)**, states that dreams are caused by widespread, random activation of neural circuitry. The problem solving dream model, **(B)**, indicates that dreams are used to solve problems while sleeping due to untethering of dreams from obstacles perceived while awake. The neurocognitive theorists, **(D)**, seek to unify cognitive and biological perspectives by correlating the subjective dream experience with the physiological experience of dreaming.

9. **D**

The description of the student matches the clinical features of marijuana (cannabis) use: hunger (presumably, based on what was shoplifted), redness of the eyes, dry mouth, and euphoria. Marijuana may also cause an increased heart rate, short-term memory loss, paranoia, and—in high doses—hallucinations. Tetrahydrocannabinol is the primary active substance in marijuana.

10. **C**

Syntax refers to how words are put together to form sentences and create meaning. Phonology, **(A)**, refers to the actual sounds of a language. Semantics, **(B)**, refers to the association of meaning with a word. Pragmatics, **(D)**, refers to changes in usage, wording, and inflection based on context.

11. **C**

A child who speaks in three-word sentences but has not yet mastered most of the fundamental rules of language, including past tense, is likely to be between two and three years old.

12. **B**

Learning theory, largely based on the work of B. F. Skinner, states that parents reinforce phonemes that sound most like their language, resulting in preferential preservation of these phonemes. Nativist theory, **(A)**, posits a critical period during which language acquisition occurs. Social interactionist theory, **(C)**, indicates that language develops via interaction with parents and caregivers as well as a desire of the child to communicate. Neurocognitive theory, **(D)**, is concerned with the subjective experience of dreaming and the physiology of dreaming.

13. **A**

Broca's area governs the motor function of language. A stroke that affects Broca's area will leave receptive language intact, but word formation will be affected. A stroke affecting Wernicke's area, **(B)**, will make it so the individual is unable to comprehend speech. A stroke affecting the arcuate fasciculus, **(C)**, will result in an inability to repeat words heard but spontaneous language production is intact. The superior temporal gyrus, **(D)**, is where Wernicke's area is located.

14. **A**

With selective attention, a person focuses on a specific task while filtering out background stimuli. In this way, the individual in the airport ignored most of the background noise while working on a puzzle. However, the brain can shift attention quickly when a stimulus is particularly important, such as the specific call for boarding the flight. This shift is known as the cocktail party phenomenon, named for a person's ability to quickly reorient their focus when they hear their name at a party. Thus, **(A)** is the correct answer. By contrast, while effortful processing, **(D)**, describes this person's intense focus on the puzzle, it does not explain the ability to respond quickly to the boarding announcement. Similarly, divided attention, **(B)**, works best on simple tasks and the question stem uses the word "challenging" to describe the puzzle.

15. **D**

About 75% of dreaming occurs during REM, but dreams occur in all other stages of sleep as well. More bizarre dreams are likely to occur during REM.

Consult your online resources for additional practice. **GO ONLINE**

EQUATION TO REMEMBER

(4.1) **Stanford–Binet intelligence quotient:** $IQ = \frac{\text{mental age}}{\text{chronological age}} \times 100$

SHARED CONCEPTS

Behavioral Sciences Chapter 1
Biology and Behavior

Behavioral Sciences Chapter 3
Learning and Memory

Behavioral Sciences Chapter 6
Identity and Personality

Behavioral Sciences Chapter 11
Social Structure and Demographics

Biology Chapter 4
The Nervous System

Critical Analysis and Reasoning Skills Chapter 6
Formal Logic

CHAPTER 5

MOTIVATION, EMOTION, AND STRESS

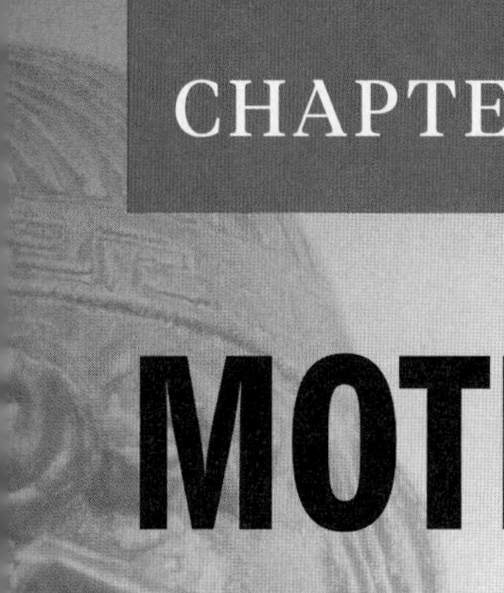
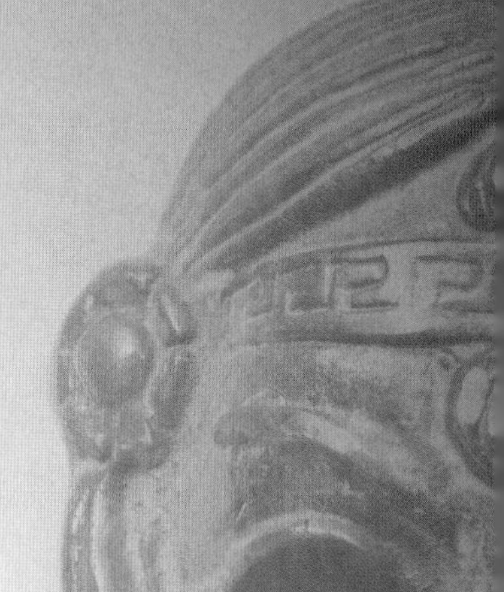

SCIENCE MASTERY ASSESSMENT

Every pre-med knows this feeling: there is so much content I have to know for the MCAT! How do I know what to do first or what's important?

While the high-yield badges throughout this book will help you identify the most important topics, this Science Mastery Assessment is another tool in your MCAT prep arsenal. This quiz (which can also be taken in your online resources) and the guidance below will help ensure that you are spending the appropriate amount of time on this chapter based on your personal strengths and weaknesses. Don't worry though—skipping something now does not mean you'll never study it. Later on in your prep, as you complete full-length tests, you'll uncover specific pieces of content that you need to review and can come back to these chapters as appropriate.

How to Use This Assessment

If you answer 0–7 questions correctly:

Spend about 1 hour to read this chapter in full and take limited notes throughout. Follow up by reviewing **all** quiz questions to ensure that you now understand how to solve each one.

If you answer 8–11 questions correctly:

Spend 20–40 minutes reviewing the quiz questions. Beginning with the questions you missed, read and take notes on the corresponding subchapters. For questions you answered correctly, ensure your thinking matches that of the explanation and you understand why each choice was correct or incorrect.

If you answer 12–15 questions correctly:

Spend less than 20 minutes reviewing all questions from the quiz. If you missed any, then include a quick read-through of the corresponding subchapters, or even just the relevant content within a subchapter, as part of your question review. For questions you answered correctly, ensure your thinking matches that of the explanation and review the Concept Summary at the end of the chapter.

1. A college student strives for excellent grades and hopes to graduate with a better GPA than an older sibling. This type of motivation is considered:
   - **A.** extrinsic motivation.
   - **B.** intrinsic motivation.
   - **C.** a primary drive.
   - **D.** a secondary drive.

2. When practicing a recital song at home, a student sounds perfectly in pitch to family and friends. However, when performing at the recital in front of a large audience of peers, strangers, and coaches, the student's pitch and tone are off, resulting in a poor performance. This second performance is best explained by:
   - **A.** drive reduction theory.
   - **B.** instinct approach theory.
   - **C.** Maslow's hierarchy of needs.
   - **D.** the Yerkes–Dodson law.

3. Seeking homeostasis to reduce an uncomfortable internal state is associated with which motivational theory?
   - **A.** Drive reduction theory
   - **B.** Instinct theory
   - **C.** Arousal theory
   - **D.** Incentive theory

4. People from cultures around the world can identify which of the following emotions?
   - **A.** Happiness, sadness, and surprise
   - **B.** Happiness, anger, and apathy
   - **C.** Sadness, anticipation, and happiness
   - **D.** Excitement, anger, and disgust

5. Experiencing emotion involves three components, which are:
   - **A.** behavioral, reactionary, and cognitive.
   - **B.** emotional, physical, and mental.
   - **C.** physiological, cognitive, and behavioral.
   - **D.** emotional, cognitive, and behavioral.

6. The statement "I noticed my heart racing and breathing rate increasing when I saw a bear, so I am afraid" corresponds most closely with which theory of emotion?
   - **A.** Schachter–Singer theory
   - **B.** Yerkes–Dodson theory
   - **C.** Cannon–Bard theory
   - **D.** James–Lange theory

7. Which theory of motivation is most significantly informed by Darwin's theory of evolution?
   - **A.** Arousal theory
   - **B.** Drive reduction theory
   - **C.** Instinct theory
   - **D.** Incentive theory

8. Simultaneous processing of conscious emotions and physiological activation is the defining feature of which theory of emotion?
   - **A.** Schachter–Singer theory
   - **B.** James–Lange theory
   - **C.** Incentive theory
   - **D.** Cannon–Bard theory

9. All of the following brain regions are primarily responsible for the experience of emotions EXCEPT the:

- **A.** amygdala.
- **B.** prefrontal cortex.
- **C.** basal ganglia.
- **D.** thalamus.

10. A person with high left frontal lobe activity is most likely experiencing which emotion?

- **A.** Happiness
- **B.** Sadness
- **C.** Surprise
- **D.** Disgust

11. Determination of the intensity and risk of a stressor occurs during which stage(s) of stress appraisal?

- **A.** Primary appraisal only
- **B.** Secondary appraisal only
- **C.** Both primary and secondary appraisal
- **D.** Neither primary nor secondary appraisal

12. A medical student is feeling a high level of stress due to upcoming exams and pressure from family to engage in activities at home. The student chooses to go to the gym for a workout to help relax. This workout is which type of stress?

- **A.** Hassle
- **B.** Frustration
- **C.** Distress
- **D.** Eustress

13. Which type of conflict is associated with the LEAST amount of stress?

- **A.** Approach–approach conflict
- **B.** Avoidance–avoidance conflict
- **C.** Approach–avoidance conflict
- **D.** Avoidance–escape conflict

14. While cleaning your house, you notice a large spider on the wall by your head and feel your heart rate jump up and your skin temperature grow warm. Which stage of stress response are you experiencing?

- **A.** Alarm
- **B.** Resistance
- **C.** Exhaustion
- **D.** Homeostasis

15. Each of the following responses to stress is considered maladaptive EXCEPT:

- **A.** drug use.
- **B.** social withdrawal.
- **C.** progressive muscle relaxation.
- **D.** avoiding the stressor.

Answer Key

1. **A**
2. **D**
3. **A**
4. **A**
5. **C**
6. **D**
7. **C**
8. **D**
9. **C**
10. **A**
11. **B**
12. **D**
13. **A**
14. **A**
15. **C**

Detailed explanations can be found at the end of the chapter.

CHAPTER 5

MOTIVATION, EMOTION, AND STRESS

In This Chapter

CHAPTER PROFILE

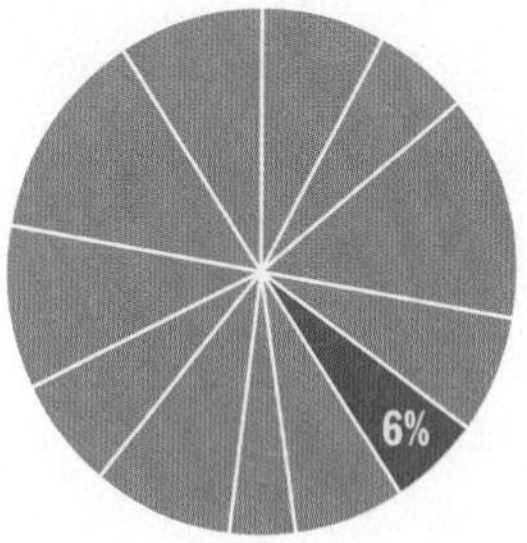

The content in this chapter should be relevant to about 6% of all questions about the behavioral sciences on the MCAT.

This chapter covers material from the following AAMC content categories:

6C: Responding to the world

7A: Individual influences on behavior

Introduction

A heart condition, substantial bone density decreases, esophageal and stomach ulcers, a loss of 25 percent of body mass—these are some of the possible consequences of anorexia nervosa. Sometimes those who develop this condition have been put under extreme pressure in their work or personal lives to look a certain way. Over time, this pressure can motivate weight loss in an unhealthy manner. Patients are sometimes motivated by feelings of disgust and guilt that go directly against the body's basic needs. A combination of stress from job and peers, intrinsic and extrinsic motivation, and negative emotions can result in what could be a life-threatening condition.

In this chapter, we'll discuss motivation, emotion, and stress. We will look at factors that influence motivation, the components of emotion, and the stressors that lead to the stress response. We will also look at theories used to explain these processes and associated behaviors. The physiological, cognitive, and behavioral elements will be examined in order to understand the role that these topics play in everyday life. Exploring these ideas will enable us to tackle any question related to these concepts on Test Day.

5.1 Motivation

High-Yield

LEARNING OBJECTIVES

After Chapter 5.1, you will be able to:

- Describe the sources of motivation posited by instinct theory, arousal theory, drive reduction theory, and the need-based theories
- Order Maslow's proposed hierarchy of needs from most to least essential
- Apply opponent-process theory to drug use and withdrawal

Motivation is the purpose, or driving force, behind our actions. The word derives from the Latin *movere*, meaning "to move." There are many examples of motivation in our everyday lives. As you sit, studying for the MCAT, you realize you are thirsty, so you reach for your water bottle. When you realize it is empty, the need to quench your thirst drives you to get up, walk to the kitchen, and fill the bottle with water. Thus, the physical state of thirst motivated an action. The desire to go to medical school and become a physician has motivated you to complete required undergraduate coursework, strive for a competitive GPA, participate in extracurricular activities, and dedicate your time to study for a standardized test. The goal of staying fit and healthy motivates many to spend hours in the gym, while the initial discomfort of physical activity might motivate others to stay sedentary. Motivation can be directed toward minimizing pain, maximizing pleasure, or it can be rooted in the desire, or **appetite**, to fullfil a physical need. Though the term appetite is commonly used to refer to a need for food, this term can more generally be applied to any need such as eating, drinking, sleeping, or social acceptance.

REAL WORLD

Intrinsic motivation can be reduced by introducing external reward into a scenario. In one study, children were given art supplies and told to draw. Some children were told they would receive a gold ribbon for their drawing, while others were not. Those who knew of the potential reward were driven by extrinsic motivation and spent less time drawing, acting only to receive the reward. Children who did not know about the reward drew for the sake of drawing—by intrinsic motivation—and spent more time drawing.

Motivation can manifest from external forces, such as rewards and punishments, or internal forces, where the behavior is personally gratifying. External forces, coming from outside oneself, create extrinsic motivation. **Extrinsic motivation** can include rewards for showing a desired behavior or avoiding punishment if the desired behavior is not achieved. Examples of such motivation include working hard at your job for praise from your boss, practicing regularly for a sport so that you will perform strongly in an upcoming game, or studying for months on end to achieve a high score on the MCAT. Each of these acts results in external, tangible rewards. Extrinsic motivation can also include doing chores to avoid punishment and working to avoid being fired. Competition is a strong form of external motivation because people are is incentivized to beat others and not only to win, perform, or achieve for themselves. Motivation that comes from within oneself is referred to as **intrinsic motivation**. This can be driven by interest in a task or pure enjoyment. A student who takes interest in the subject matter at hand and has the goal of mastering the content is driven by intrinsic motivation, while the goal of achieving high grades is considered extrinsic.

The primary views of motivation focus on instincts that elicit natural behavior, the desire to maintain optimal levels of arousal, the drive to reduce uncomfortable states, and the goal of satisfying physiological and psychological needs.

Instinct Theory

Early attempts to understand the basis of motivation focused on **instincts**, which are innate, fixed patterns of behavior. For example, wolves are instinctively pack creatures that naturally follow the alpha male of their group. Additionally, they are highly territorial creatures, protecting areas that are much larger than needed to hunt and dwell. This protection includes scent-marking, howling, and direct aggressive attacks on intruders. Humans also have instinctive behavior; for example, thumb sucking is an instinctual response to stress in babies that is aimed at self-soothing. As discussed in Chapter 1 of *MCAT Behavioral Sciences Review*, primitive reflexes like the grasp reflex, shown in Figure 5.1, are also instinctual. Note that some instincts last for the entire lifetime, while others may appear or disappear with age.

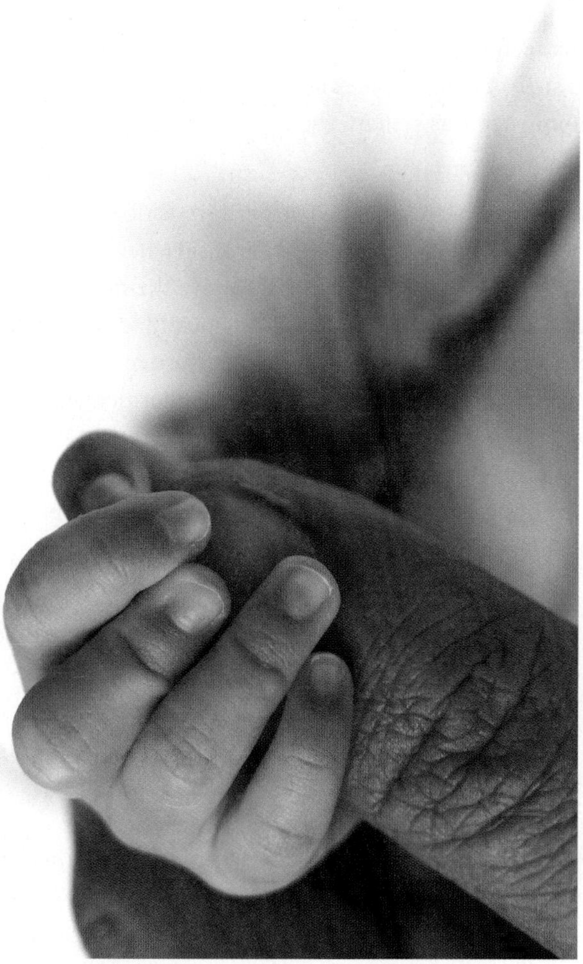

Figure 5.1 The Grasp Reflex
Primitive reflexes are examples of instincts seen in infants that extinguish with age.

According to the **instinct theory** of motivation, certain behaviors are based on evolutionarily programmed instincts. This theory was one of the first to describe motivation and was derived from Darwin's theory of evolution. William James, the father of modern psychology, was one of the first to write about human instincts in his 1890 publication of *Principles of Psychology*. He stated that humans were motivated by many instincts, possibly more than any other animal studied. James suggested that human actions are derived from 20 physical instincts, including suckling and locomotion, and 17 mental instincts, including curiosity and fearfulness. However, he said that many of these instincts were in direct conflict with each other and could be overridden by experience. Arguably the greatest proponent of instinct theory was William McDougall, who proposed that humans were led to all thoughts and behaviors by 18 distinctive instincts, including flight and acquisition. James and McDougall postulated that the instincts of suckling and carrying food to the mouth result in naturally motivating one to eat.

KEY CONCEPT

An instinct is an innate, fixed pattern of behavior. It may be consistent throughout life, or it may appear or disappear with time.

Arousal Theory

Another factor that influences motivation is **arousal**, the psychological and physiological state of being awake and reactive to stimuli. Arousal involves the brainstem, autonomic nervous system, and endocrine system and plays a vital role in behavior and cognition.

Arousal theory states that people perform actions in order to maintain an optimal level of arousal: seeking to increase arousal when it falls below their optimal level, and to decrease arousal when it rises above their optimum level. Additionally, the **Yerkes–Dodson law** postulates a U-shaped function between the level of arousal and performance. This law states that performance is worst at extremely high and low levels of arousal and optimal at some intermediate level, as depicted in Figure 5.2. The optimal level of arousal varies between different types of tasks: lower levels are optimal for highly cognitive tasks, while higher levels are optimal for activities that require physical endurance and stamina. Further, simple tasks generally require slightly higher arousal than complex tasks.

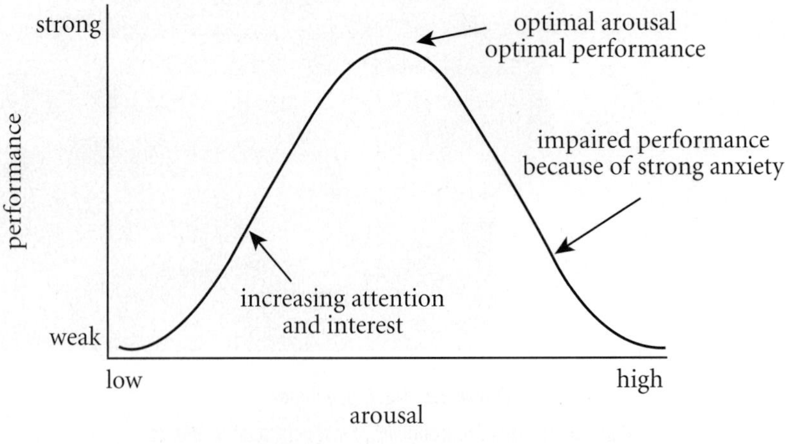

Figure 5.2 Yerkes–Dodson Law

REAL WORLD

While a moderate level of arousal is optimal for performance, certain individuals seek out higher levels of arousal. Such people may seek out dangerous activities, such as skydiving or bungee jumping. These individuals are sometimes found to have lower levels of monoamine oxidase (MAO), which breaks down catecholamines. Low levels of MAO result in higher neurotransmitter levels, which may lead to motivation to experience high levels of arousal.

Drive Reduction Theory

Drives are defined as internal states of tension that activate particular behaviors focused on goals. Drives are thought to originate within an individual without requiring any external factors to motivate behavior. In other words, drives help humans survive by creating an uncomfortable state, ensuring motivation to eliminate this state or to relieve the internal tension created by unmet needs. **Primary drives**, including the need for food, water, and warmth, motivate us to sustain bodily processes in homeostasis. **Homeostasis** is the regulation of the internal environment to maintain an optimal, stable set of conditions. In homeostatic regulation, external factors are encountered, and the system will react to push the system back to its optimal state.

Homeostasis is usually controlled by **negative feedback** loops. A common real-life example of a negative feedback loop is a thermostat. A thermostat is set to a desired temperature, and then sensors monitor the air temperature in relation to this desired temperature. If the air temperature gets too cold, the heater will turn on; if the temperature gets too warm, the heater will turn off. Negative feedback loops in the body operate the same way. Likewise when our bodies are lacking nutrients and energy, feedback systems release hormones like ghrelin that create hunger and motivate eating. After we consume food, feedback is sent to the brain to turn off the hunger drive through hormones like leptin. Hunger is a complex feedback system involving these hormones, receptors in the walls of the stomach, levels of glucose (maintained by the liver), and insulin and glucagon levels (released by the pancreas). The concentrations of many hormones of the endocrine system are regulated by three-organ "axes," such as the hypothalamic–pituitary–adrenal axis shown in Figure 5.3.

REAL WORLD

One well-characterized drive is the hunger (food) drive, which has been studied for more than 60 years. The hunger drive is a primary drive, in that food is necessary for life. Given the necessity of food to life, many species possess multiple processes that drive the individual to consume food. These biological processes include tie-ins to the sense of smell and taste, which were demonstrated by many studies, notably those of Janowitz and Grossman.

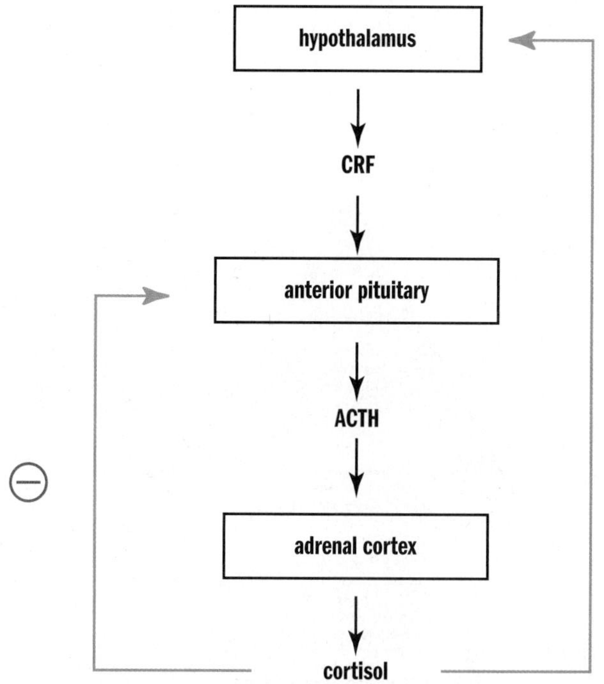

Figure 5.3 Negative Feedback in the Endocrine System

Additional drives that are not directly related to biological processes are called **secondary drives**. These drives are thought to stem from learning. The drive to matriculate into medical school and become a physician is an example of a secondary drive. Secondary drives also include certain emotions, such as the desire for nurturing, love, achievement, and aggression.

Drive reduction theory explains that motivation is based on the goal of eliminating uncomfortable states. Theorists hypothesize that certain physiological conditions result in a negative internal environment. This internal environment then drives motivation and seeks homeostasis in order to reduce the uncomfortable internal state.

KEY CONCEPT

Primary drives are those that motivate us to sustain necessary biological processes. Secondary drives are those that motivate us to fulfill nonbiological, emotional, or "learned" desires.

BRIDGE

Drive reduction theory can be applied to motivation in terms of learning, and is commonly used to define motivational states within behavioral conditioning. Conditioning and learning are discussed in Chapter 3 of *MCAT Behavioral Sciences Review*.

Need-Based Theories

In need-based theories of motivation, energy and resources are allocated to best satisfy human needs. These needs may be **primary needs**, which are generally physiological needs such as the need for food, water, sleep, and shelter. Or these needs might be **secondary needs**, which are generally mental states, like a desire for power, achievement, or social belonging.

MCAT EXPERTISE

Knowing the four primary factors that influence motivation is key for Test Day: instincts, arousal, drives, and needs. The MCAT will expect you to know the common theories for explaining motivation.

Abraham Maslow defined **needs** as relatively long-lasting feelings that require relief or satisfaction and tend to influence action. He observed that certain needs will yield a greater influence on our motivation and he established what is referred to as **Maslow's hierarchy of needs**. Maslow classified needs into five groups, and assigned different levels of priority to each group. The hierarchy is typically displayed as a pyramid, as shown in Figure 5.4, where the most primitive, essential, and important needs are at the base. The first four levels of the pyramid correspond to physiological needs, safety and security, love and belonging, and self-esteem. The highest level of the pyramid corresponds to **self-actualization**, or the need to realize one's fullest potential. Maslow theorized that if the lowest level of need is not met, motivation to meet that need will be the highest priority. Once the lowest level of needs is met, if additional needs exist, they will be satisfied based on priority. For example, a person's most basic motivation will be to satisfy physiological needs, followed by the need to establish a safe and secure environment.

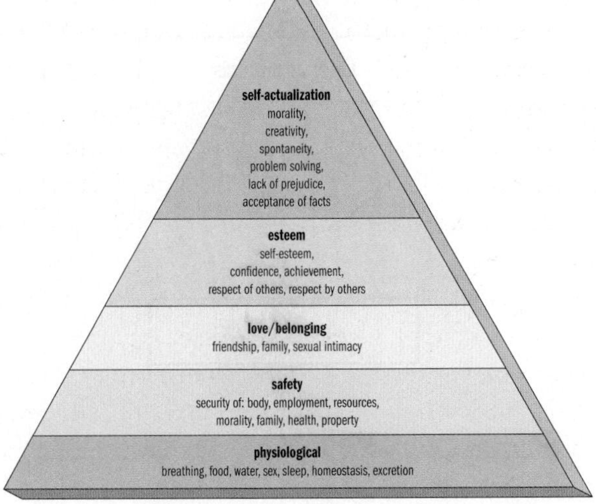

Figure 5.4 Maslow's Hierarchy of Needs

Another need-based motivational theory is the **self-determination theory** (**SDT**), which emphasizes the role of three universal needs: autonomy, the need to be in control of one's actions and ideas; competence, the need to complete and excel at difficult tasks; and relatedness, the need to feel accepted and wanted in relationships. Theorists explain that these three needs must be met in order to develop healthy relationships with oneself and others.

Additional Theories and Applications

There are a few other theories of motivation that you should know for the MCAT: opponent-process theory, sexual motivation, incentive theory, and expectancy-value theory. Opponent-process theory and sexual motivation will be discussed in more detail below. **Incentive theory** explains that behavior is motivated not by need or arousal, but by the desire to pursue rewards and to avoid punishments. **Expectancy–value theory** states that the amount of motivation needed to reach a goal is the result of both the individual's expectation of success in reaching the goal and the degree to which the individual values succeeding at the goal.

There are many motivations that stem from biology but that are impacted by additional psychological and sociocultural factors. One of the strongest natural motivations is hunger. However, people often eat for the sheer pleasure of the act, a motivation that may contribute to obesity occurring at alarming rates in the United States. Societal and cultural norms can determine what types of foods one eats and when. For example, some cultures have a traditional diet that is very high in fat and participate in many social activities involving food. At the other extreme, anorexia nervosa is also correlated to biological and cultural factors. It has been observed that those suffering from the disease are more likely to suffer from personality disorders as well. The prevalence of anorexia in the United States has increased significantly in the last several decades as the societal concept of beauty has changed from more full-bodied idols to extremely thin cultural icons.

Opponent-Process Theory

Motivations are considered destructive if they result in harm to oneself. For example, drug abusers can be motivated to take drugs by the pleasure experienced when taking the drug or by the removal of withdrawal symptoms. Most recreational drugs in the United States are psychoactive substances such as narcotics, sedatives, stimulants (e.g. caffeine and nicotine), hallucinogens, cannabis, and alcohol. A theory of motivation that explains continuous drug use is the **opponent-process theory**. This theory explains that when a drug is taken repeatedly, the body will attempt to counteract the effects of the drug by changing its physiology. For example, the body will counteract repeated use of alcohol, a depressant, by increasing arousal. The problem with this reaction is that it will last longer than the drug, resulting in withdrawal symptoms that are exactly opposite the effects of alcohol: sensations of anxiety, jitteriness, and irritability. The withdrawal created by this mechanism can create a physical dependence on the drug. Opponent-process theory can also explain **tolerance**, a decrease in perceived drug effect over time. Cultural and demographic factors also affect drug use. Young adults are the most likely age group to smoke, with a decline in smoking rates seen as the group ages. Smoking is also seen more commonly in disadvantaged socioeconomic groups. Across the globe, smoking rates are highest in Eastern Europe; this creates visibility, leading to additional pressure or desire to smoke in these communities.

BEHAVIORAL SCIENCES GUIDED EXAMPLE WITH EXPERT THINKING

Researchers conducting a meta-analysis of the literature on intrinsic and extrinsic motivation examined the following two studies:

Intrinsic vs. extrinsic motivation

Study 1:
Undergraduate university students ($n = 27$) were recruited to perform a weekly filing task over four weeks at the university library. Participants were randomly divided into three groups: one group received $20 per week, one group received a general education credit for finishing all four weeks, and one group received no compensation. Participants completed a survey designed to measure their baseline engagement and enjoyment of the tasks they were asked to perform. At the end of the four weeks, the survey was administered again, and each participant was invited to continue the weekly tasks on a volunteer basis. No further compensation was offered. Results are shown in Figure 1.

This article has multiple studies that appear complex. I'll need to make sure to keep track of all variables.

IV: compensation ($)

DV: engagement in/enjoyment of task

2nd DV: 2nd survey + willingness to volunteer

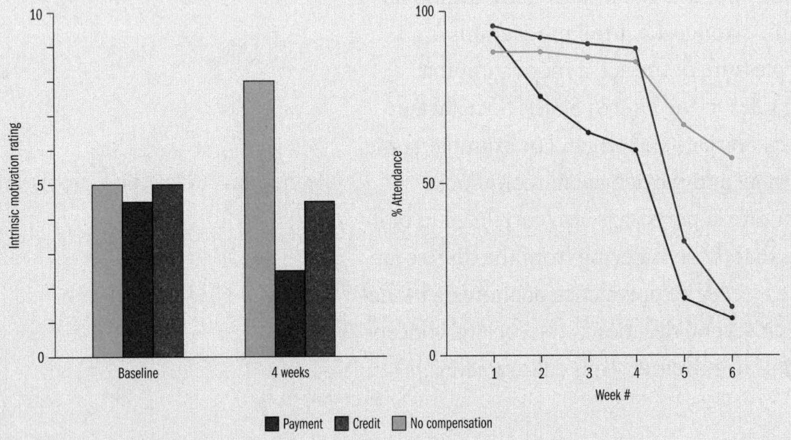

Figure 1 Enjoyment survey results and participation

The no-compensation group seemed to enjoy the task much more than the other two groups compared to baseline, and more of them continued to volunteer after the study was over.

Study 2:
A sample of men identified as being at high risk of heart disease ($n = 128$) were recruited for a multifaceted intervention program which required attending a clinic once per week for medication, physical exercise, and counseling. Participants came from both medium and low socioeconomic status (SES) households. All individuals in the low SES group experienced food insecurity. Participants in each SES group were divided into three conditions: monetary compensation for attendance, grocery credit for attendance, and no compensation for attendance. Compensation was offered for a six-month period. Participants completed an inventory designed to measure baseline intrinsic motivation to improve their health, with items such as "The reason I am participating in this course of treatment as prescribed is because participation in this treatment is consistent with my life goals." The inventory was administered again at six months and at twelve months. Results are shown in Figure 2.

IVs: SES and compensation for attendance

DV: intrinsic motivation, measured by survey

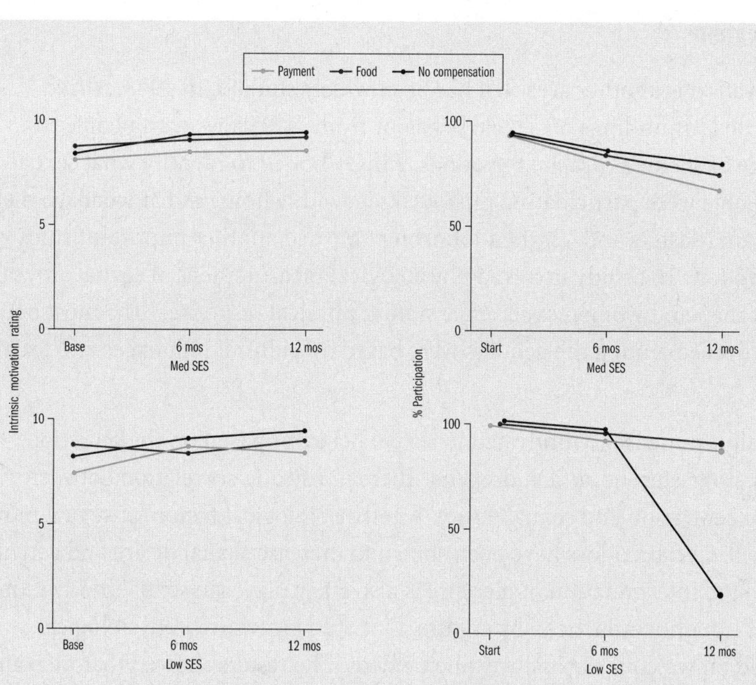

Motivation is high for all groups, as is participation, with the exception of the no-compensation low SES group once compensation ends.

Figure 2 Motivation and participation over 12 months

Adapted from: Czaicki NL, Dow WH, Njau PF, McCoy SI (2018) Do incentives undermine intrinsic motivation? Increases in intrinsic motivation within an incentive-based intervention for people living with HIV in Tanzania. *PLoS ONE* 13(6): e0196616. https://doi.org/10.1371/journal.pone.0196616

What do the results of these two studies suggest about the role of intrinsic and extrinsic factors in motivation?

This question is asking for a fairly high-level analysis of the three different conditions across the two studies. To answer, first we will need to consider what was being tested and the results from each study. Identifying the variables as we read the studies will make this task much more manageable and, as we have seen in guided examples from other chapters, is a generally good approach to reading any study. In Study 1, the only difference between groups is the offer of compensation, which is an extrinsic motivator. The results are consistent with conventional wisdom (and our outside content knowledge) that when an extrinsic motivator is introduced, intrinsic motivation decreases. Therefore, when the compensation is removed, participation declines. We can specifically see this within the data: groups receiving compensation see a substantial decline in intrinsic motivation and attendance as compared to the no-compensation group. Additionally, the lack of an extrinsic motivator increases intrinsic motivation, as demonstrated by the volunteerism rate in the no-compensation group.

Given the results of Study 1, Study 2 may seem surprising. Based on the results in the figure for Study 2, for the medium SES and low SES groups receiving compensation, intrinsic motivation remained consistent throughout the study. For the low SES group, however, participation declined sharply for the non-compensated group.

Fortunately, on Test Day we will never be asked to write an essay explaining these results, so we are not responsible for coming up with an explanation on our own. Among the answer choices will be an explanation that is consistent with both the scientific content we studied and the analysis of the results we conducted.

If a question like this shows up on the real MCAT, take a moment to consider what we know and what we've learned from the passage, and make a general prediction that targets the *kind* of information a correct answer could provide. In this case we are looking for a difference between the low and medium SES groups that might explain the observed difference in the no-compensation group. We might consider the implications of SES generally, but the passage provided a potential clue when it mentioned that the low SES group had food insecurity. Given what we know about Maslow's hierarchy of needs we might anticipate an answer that implies motivation to obtain food is more important than reducing the risk of heart disease.

Sexual Motivation

Sexual motivation is another area that has been widely studied. In 1948, Alfred Kinsey reported his findings on sexual behavior from interviews with people from a broad range of sociocultural backgrounds. Kinsey hoped to identify what sexual behaviors people were participating in, how often, with whom, and at what age they began. William Masters and Virginia Johnson published another important study of sexual motivation. The study involved physiological measurement of sexual arousal, proving that men and women experience similar physical responses. The most notable differences seen among the genders were based on cultural influences and learned behavior.

Physiologically, humans are motivated to sexual behavior based on the secretion of estrogens, progesterone, and androgens. There is a strong correlation between hormone concentration and sexual desire. Another biological factor for sexual motivation is smell. Certain odors have been shown to increase sexual desire and activity. Pleasure and the interpretation of pleasure is also a key player in sexual motivation and one that is highly influenced by culture. One study measured physiological arousal based on watching sexually explicit videos. The results showed that men and women experienced the same levels of arousal, but women more often reported being unaroused or having feelings of disgust based on subjective interviews. This study demonstrated that cognition plays a role in sexual motivation. Additionally, culture and society influence what is deemed appropriate sexual behavior, the age at which it is deemed appropriate, and with whom. Cultural norms and conditioning influence the desire for sexual interaction, or lack thereof.

MCAT CONCEPT CHECK 5.1

Before you move on, assess your understanding of the material with these questions.

1. For each of the theories listed below, what creates motivation?

Theory	Factor for Motivation
Instinct theory	
Arousal theory	
Drive reduction theory	
Need-based theories	

2. List Maslow's hierarchy of needs in decreasing priority:

-

-

-

-

-

3. Based on opponent-process theory, what clinical features would be expected with withdrawal from cocaine use?

5.2 Emotion

High-Yield

LEARNING OBJECTIVES

After Chapter 5.2, you will be able to:

- Describe the three elements of emotion: psychological response, behavioral response, and cognitive response
- Recall the seven universal facially expressed emotions
- Compare and contrast the James–Lange, Cannon–Bard, and Schachter–Singer theories of emotion
- Identify the names and functions of the parts of the limbic system

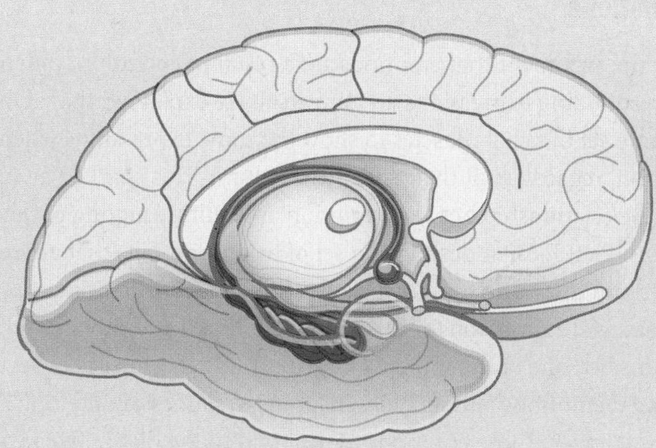

Emotion is a natural instinctive state of mind derived from one's circumstances, mood, or relationships with others. The word emotion is derived from the same Latin word as motivation.

Three Elements of Emotion

There are three elements of an emotion: the physiological response, the behavioral response, and the cognitive response.

Physiological Response

When a feeling is first experienced, arousal is stimulated by the autonomic nervous system. The physiological component includes changes in heart rate, breathing rate, skin temperature, and blood pressure. While it may be hard to recognize these changes and associate them with an emotion in everyday life, these changes have been detected in laboratory settings. Some emotions, such as fear, aggression, and embarrassment, are associated with more pronounced physiological changes than others.

Behavioral Response

The behavioral component of an emotion includes facial expressions and body language. For example, a smile, a friendly hand gesture, or even a subtle head tilt toward someone are commonly recognized as warm and happy signals. On the other hand, a frown, slumping of the shoulders, and looking downward are recognized as sad or downtrodden signals.

Cognitive Response

Finally, the cognitive component of emotion is the subjective interpretation of the feeling being experienced. Determination of one's emotion is an evaluative process largely based on memories of past experiences and perception of the cause of the emotion.

MCAT EXPERTISE

The AAMC lists fear, anger, happiness, surprise, joy, disgust, and sadness as universal emotions. Given the lack of consensus in the scientific community, the MCAT is more likely to test the topic conceptually than specifically.

Universal Emotions

Darwin made the argument that emotions are a result of evolution; thus, emotions and their corresponding expressions are universal. He explained that all humans evolved the same set of facial muscles to show the same expressions when communicating emotion, regardless of their society or culture. This sparked an ongoing discussion of the relationship between emotion and culture among psychologists and sociologists. Paul Ekman described a set of basic emotions that are recognized by societies around the world and further identified that six emotions are associated with consistent facial expressions across cultures. Ekman and other psychologists have revised this list; one of the more well-recognized sets consists of seven universal facially expressed emotions and includes: happiness, sadness, contempt, surprise, fear, disgust, and anger. These emotions correspond to the distinctive facial expressions explained in Table 5.1 and depicted in Figure 5.5.

EMOTION	FACIAL EXPRESSION CUES
Happiness	Smile, wrinkling around eyes, raised cheeks
Sadness	Frown, inner eyebrows pulled up and together
Contempt	One corner of the mouth pulled upwards
Surprise	Eyes widen, eyebrows pulled up and curved, jaw opens
Fear	Eyes widen, eyebrows pulled up and together, lips pulled toward ears
Disgust	Nose wrinkling and/or raising of upper lip
Anger	Glaring, eyebrows pulled down and together, lips pressed together

Table 5.1 Seven Universal Emotions

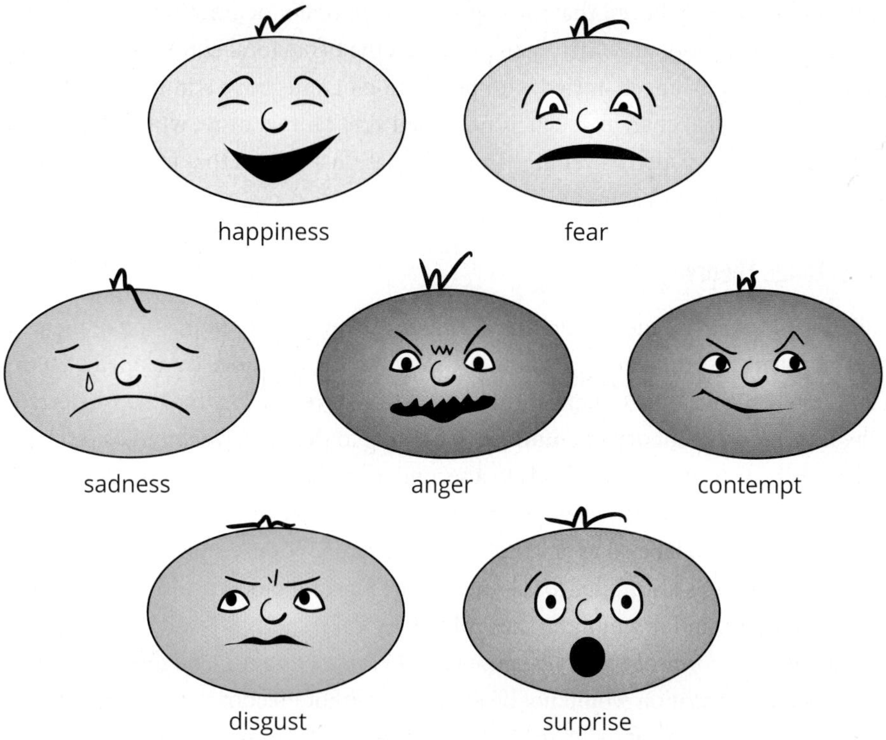

Figure 5.5 Seven Universal Emotions

While emotions are experienced universally, it is argued that they can be affected greatly by culture. Cultural dissimilarities in emotion include varying reactions to similar events, differences in the emotional experience itself, the behavior exhibited in response to an emotion, and the perception of that emotion by others within the society.

Adaptive Role of Emotion

In accordance with Darwin's thoughts on universal emotion, the **evolutionary perspective** states that everything we do, think, and feel is based on specialized functional programs designed for any problem we encounter. These programs are functionally coordinated in order to produce a cohesive response. Emotions are thought to be evolutionary adaptations due to situations encountered over the evolutionary history of the human species that guide sensory processing, physiological response, and behavior. Further, different emotions are thought to have evolved during different periods in history. Among the earliest to develop were primal emotions, such as fear; other, more evolutionarily progressive emotions include social emotions, such as guilt and pride.

Theories of Emotion

Early psychologists believed that the cognitive component of emotion led to the physiological component, which then produced the behavioral component. In other words, the feeling of anger started with perception of a negative stimulus, which caused physiological changes, such as increased skin temperature, which then resulted in behavior, such as yelling. This explanation assumes that feeling precedes arousal, which precedes action.

James–Lange Theory

William James, the founder of functionalist theory, viewed the progression of these emotional elements differently. Around the same time, Carl Lange developed a theory of emotion similar to that of James. The explanation developed by the two is referred to as the **James–Lange theory of emotion**. According to the theory, a stimulus results first in physiological arousal, which leads to a secondary response in which the emotion is labeled. James believed that when peripheral organs receive information and respond, that response is then labeled as an emotion by the brain. For example, a car cutting you off on the highway is a stimulus for elevated heart rate and blood pressure, increased skin temperature, and dry mouth. These physiological responses result in the cognitive labeling of anger: *I must be angry because my skin is hot and my blood pressure is high.* By extension, an emotion would not be processed without feedback from the peripheral organs; this theory predicts that individuals who cannot mount a sympathetic response, like patients with spinal cord injuries, should show decreased levels of emotion. Subsequent studies have proven this claim to be false; spinal cord injury subjects continue to show the same level of emotion after their injuries as before.

Cannon–Bard Theory

Walter Cannon and Philip Bard developed another scheme for explaining emotional components, referred to as the Cannon–Bard theory of emotion. In an attempt to test the James–Lange theory, Cannon studied the expression of emotion and its relationship to feedback from the sympathetic nervous system using cats whose afferent nerves had been severed. He hypothesized that physiological arousal and feeling an emotion occur at the same time, not in sequence. Thus, severing the feedback should not alter the emotion experienced. In this theory, a person will respond with action after experiencing the emotion both mentally and physically. Bard, a student of Cannon's, further explained that when exposed to a stimulus, sensory information is received and sent to both the cortex and the sympathetic nervous system simultaneously by the thalamus. Thus, the **Cannon–Bard theory of emotion**, depicted in Figure 5.6, states that the conscious experience of emotion and physiological arousal occur simultaneously, and then the behavioral component of emotion (i.e., action) follows: *I see a snake, so I feel afraid and my heart is racing . . . Let me out of here!*

While critics of the James–Lange theory cite the severed afferent nerve study as support for the Cannon–Bard theory, there are also weaknesses in this theory. The Cannon–Bard theory fails to explain the vagus nerve, a cranial nerve that functions as a feedback system, conveying information from the peripheral organs back to the central nervous system.

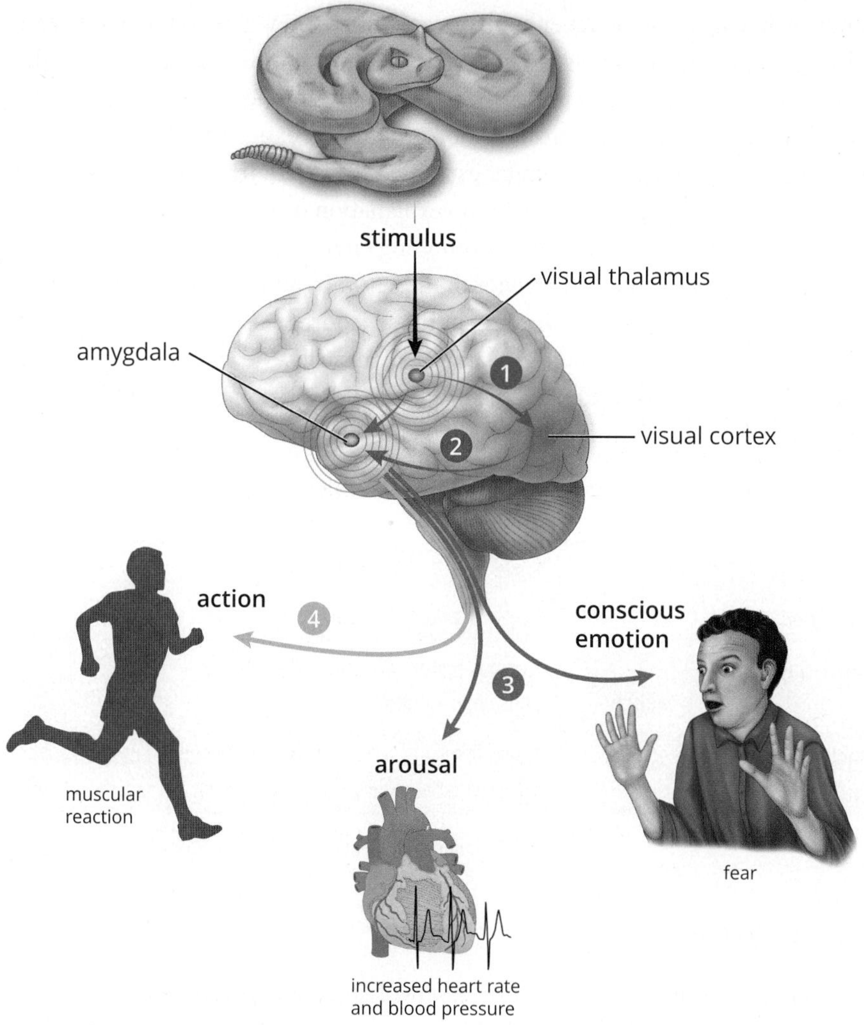

Figure 5.6 Cannon-Bard Theory of Emotion

Visual stimuli pass through the thalamus, and rough information is sent to the amygdala (fear) and the sympathetic nervous system (arousal). Action (muscle contraction) quickly follows. The visual cortex can either strengthen or quell this fear response once it has identified the stimulus.

MCAT EXPERTISE

The MCAT will expect that you have a solid understanding of the differences in emotional processing described by each of the three theories of emotion. It is best to mentally sort these theories by "first response" and "second response" to the stimulus.

Schachter-Singer Theory

A third theory is the **Schachter–Singer theory of emotion**, also termed the **cognitive arousal theory** or the **two-factor theory**, which states that two factors (physiological arousal and a cognitive label) are needed to experience emotion. According to this theory, physiological arousal alone is insufficient to elicit an emotional response. To feel an emotion, the mind must also identify the environmental stimulus causing that physiological arousal: *I am excited because my heart is racing and everyone else is happy.*

What is unique to the Schachter–Singer theory is this aspect of cognitive appraisal: to feel an emotion, one must consciously analyze the environment in relation to nervous system arousal. To study this phenomenon, Stanley Schachter and Jerome Singer gave injections of epinephrine or placebo to groups of subjects that were either informed, ignorant, or misinformed. They also manipulated external cues in the study by having an actor act either happy or angry. They observed that epinephrine did result in increased physiological arousal; however, they also discovered that the environment and cognitive processing affected the emotion experienced by the subjects. The groups who were misinformed or ignorant experienced the highest levels of emotion. Schachter and Singer explained this result by stating that subjects experiencing physiological arousal with no explanation or with a misleading explanation will attribute that arousal to the surrounding environment, and label themselves as happy or angry based on the behavior of the actor. In other words, the presence of unexpected arousal plus an environment that encourages a particular emotion is sufficient to create that emotion in the subject. Contrarily, the informed group knew to expect physiological arousal from the drug, and thus attributed their feelings to side effects of the epinephrine, rather than to emotions.

The three theories of emotion discussed in this section are summarized in Table 5.2.

THEORY		FIRST RESPONSE	SECOND RESPONSE
James-Lange	**Stimulus**	Nervous system arousal	Conscious emotion
Cannon-Bard	**Stimulus**	Nervous system arousal and conscious emotion	Action
Schachter-Singer	**Stimulus**	Nervous system arousal and cognitive appraisal	Conscious emotion

Table 5.2 Theories of Emotion

The Limbic System

Experiencing emotion is a complex process involving many parts of the brain. The most notable of these circuits is the **limbic system**, a complex set of structures that reside below the cerebrum on either side of the thalamus, as shown in Figure 5.7. The system is made up of the amygdala, thalamus, hypothalamus, hippocampus and fornix, septal nuclei, and parts of the cerebral cortex; it plays a large role in both motivation and emotion.

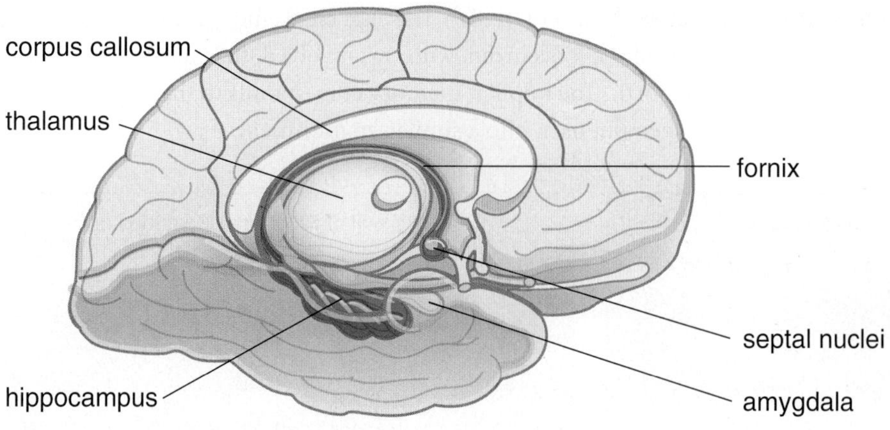

Figure 5.7 The Limbic System

REAL WORLD

When specific areas of the limbic system are stimulated during brain surgery, patients have described sensations such as happiness, contentment, and pleasure; in other areas, they report fear and anxiety.

The **amygdala** is a small round structure that signals the cortex about stimuli related to attention and emotions. The amygdala processes the environment, detects external cues, and learns from the person's surroundings in order to produce emotion. This region is associated with fear and also plays a role in human emotion through interpretation of facial expressions.

REAL WORLD

Research on rats has shown that when the amygdalae are damaged, the rats can no longer be classically conditioned to establish new fears. Similar effects have also been seen in humans wherein damage to this region prevents fear conditioning. This has been measured by autonomic nervous system responses as well as functional imaging.

The **thalamus** functions as a preliminary sensory processing station and routes information to the cortex and other appropriate areas of the brain. The **hypothalamus**, located below the thalamus, synthesizes and releases a variety of neurotransmitters. It serves many homeostatic functions, and is involved in modulating emotion. Indeed, by controlling the neurotransmitters that affect mood and arousal, the hypothalamus largely dictates emotional states.

The **hippocampus**, within the temporal lobe, is primarily involved in creating long-term memories. Along with the functions of the amygdala and hypothalamus, the storage and retrieval of emotional memories is key in producing an emotional response. The hippocampus also aids in creating context for stimuli to lead to an emotional experience. As described in Chapter 3 of *MCAT Behavioral Sciences Review*, memory systems can be divided into two categories: explicit and implicit. When an emotion is experienced, sensory systems transmit this information into both the explicit memory system, primarily controlled by the hippocampus in the medial temporal lobe, and the implicit memory system, controlled by the amygdala. Both memory systems are used for both the formation and retrieval of emotional memories, as shown in Figure 5.8. The conscious (explicit) memory is the memory of experiencing the actual emotion: remembering that you were happy at your high school graduation or that you were sad when you lost a loved one is explicit memory. Note that these are episodic memories: they are more properly considered memories *about* emotions than stored emotions. The unconscious (implicit) memory is referred to as **emotional memory**; this is the storage of the actual feelings of emotion associated with an event. When experiencing a similar event later on, these emotions may be retrieved. Thus, explicit memory of the emotion produces a conscious memory of the experience, and implicit memory determines the expression of past emotions. This distinction can be further identified when looking at individuals with posttraumatic stress disorder (PTSD). The explicit memory is the "story" of the event: what happened, where it occurred, who was involved, the fact that the scenario was traumatic, and so forth. The implicit memory corresponds to the sensations of unease and anxiety when put back into a similar environment.

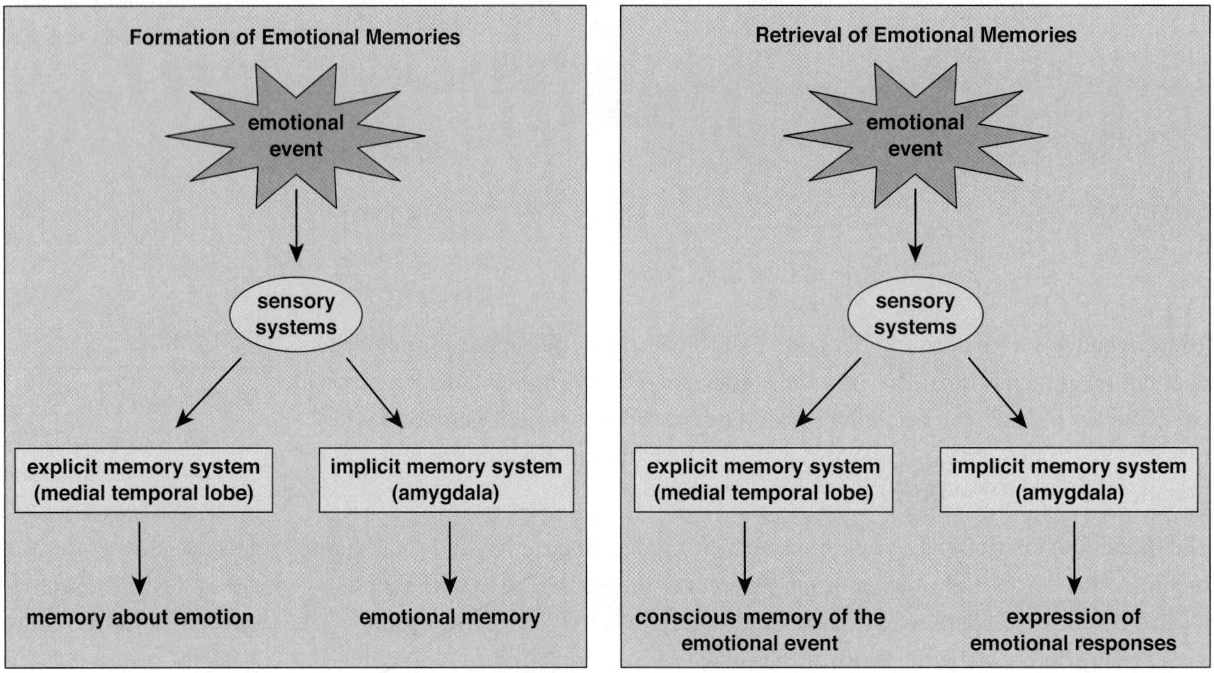

Figure 5.8 Formation and Retrieval of Emotional Memories

The ability to distinguish and interpret others' facial expressions is primarily controlled by the temporal lobe, with some input from the occipital lobe. This function is lateralized: the right hemisphere is more active when discerning facial expressions than the left. There are also gender differences: women demonstrate more activation of these brain areas than men. This ability is present but weak in children and develops into adulthood; adults are much more effective at identifying both positive and negative emotions.

REAL WORLD

One of the most notable studies on prefrontal cortex function is that of Phineas Gage. Gage was involved in an accident in which a metal rod pierced his brain, destroying the left frontal lobe. Gage's memory, speech, and motor skills were unaffected, but his personality was dramatically altered. Post-accident, Gage displayed irritable and impatient behavior, which inhibited his ability to complete simple tasks.

The **prefrontal cortex** is the anterior portion of the frontal lobes and is associated with planning intricate cognitive functions, expressing personality, and making decisions. The prefrontal cortex also receives arousal input from the brainstem, coordinating arousal and cognitive states. It has been demonstrated that the left prefrontal cortex is associated with positive emotions and the right prefrontal cortex with negative emotions. The **dorsal prefrontal cortex** is associated with attention and cognition, while the **ventral prefrontal cortex** connects with regions of the brain responsible for experiencing emotion. Specifically, the **ventromedial prefrontal cortex**, shown in Figure 5.9, is thought to play a substantial role in decision making and controlling emotional responses from the amygdala.

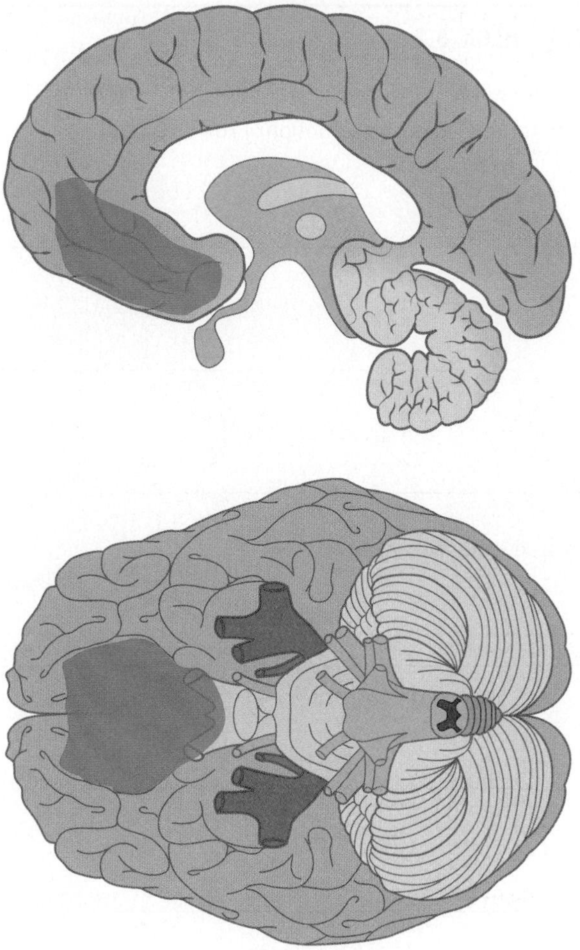

Figure 5.9 Ventromedial Prefrontal Cortex
The ventromedial prefrontal cortex is highlighted in blue.

As described earlier, the **autonomic nervous system** is also related to emotion; specific physiological reactions are associated with specific emotions. Skin temperature, heart rate, breathing rate, and blood pressure are all affected when experiencing emotion. Decreased skin temperature is detected in subjects experiencing fear, while increased skin temperature is associated with anger. Increased heart rate is observed in subjects experiencing both anger and fear, while decreased heart rate is observed in subjects who are feeling happiness. Heart rate variability is another factor used to determine emotion. Decreased heart rate variability is associated with stress, frustration, and anger. Blood pulse volume increases with anger or stress and decreases with sadness or relaxation. Skin conductivity is directly correlated with sympathetic arousal; however, a specific emotion cannot be identified by skin response. Diastolic blood pressure is increased to the greatest degree by anger, followed by fear, sadness, and happiness.

MCAT CONCEPT CHECK 5.2

Before you move on, assess your understanding of the material with these questions.

1. What are the three elements of emotion? Provide a brief description of each.
   -
   -
   -

2. What are the seven universal emotions?
   -
   -
   -
   -
   -
   -
   -

3. Compare and contrast the James–Lange, Cannon–Bard, and Schachter–Singer theories of emotion:

James–Lange Theory	Cannon–Bard Theory	Schachter–Singer Theory

4. What is the function of each part of the limbic system listed below?
   - Amygdala:

   ____

   - Thalamus:

   ____

   - Hypothalamus:

   ____

   - Hippocampus:

   ____

   - Ventromedial prefrontal cortex:

   ____

5.3 Stress

High-Yield

LEARNING OBJECTIVES

After Chapter 5.3, you will be able to:

- Distinguish between primary and secondary appraisals of stress
- Recall the three stages of general adaptation syndrome and the physiological changes associated with each stage
- Recognize common stressors and effective techniques for management of stress

In all aspects of life, at all times of day, we must make decisions, overcome challenges, and continue forward. While some of these decisions are small, others require planning and adaptation to new circumstances. Behavior of others and the perception of our surroundings affect our behavior and mental state, at times in a negative manner. It is our response to challenging events, be they physical, emotional, cognitive, or behavioral, that defines **stress**.

Cognitive Appraisal of Stress

Cognitive appraisal is the subjective evaluation of a situation that induces stress. This process consists of two stages. Stage 1, or **primary appraisal**, is the initial evaluation of the environment and the associated threat. This appraisal can be identified as irrelevant, benign–positive, or stressful. If primary appraisal reveals a threat, stage 2 appraisal begins. **Secondary appraisal** is directed at evaluating whether the organism can cope with the stress. This appraisal involves the evaluation of three things: harm,

MCAT EXPERTISE

The MCAT will expect you to know the two stages of stress appraisal: primary and secondary. Primary appraisal is the initial examination, which results in the identification of the stress as irrelevant, benign-positive, or stressful. If identified as a threat, secondary appraisal is an evaluation of one's ability to cope with the stress.

or damage caused by the event; threat, or the potential for future damage caused by the event; and challenge, or the potential to overcome and possibly benefit from the event. Individuals who perceive themselves as having the ability to cope with the event experience less stress than those who don't. In general, appraisal and stress level are personal, as individuals have different skills, abilities, and coping mechanisms. For example, while a spider might incite fear and stress in some, it would result in irrelevant appraisal in others. Some situations require ongoing monitoring through constant **reappraisal**, such as the perception of being followed.

Types of Stressors

A **stressor** is a biological element, external condition, or event that leads to a stress response. The severity of stressors can range from minimal or irritating hassles, like temporarily lost keys, to catastrophic scenarios, such as an impending natural disaster. Common stressors include:

- Environmental factors: uncomfortable temperature, loud sounds, inclement weather
- Daily events: running late, losing items, unexpected occurrences
- Workplace or academic setting: assignments, hierarchical interactions, time management
- Social expectations: demands placed on oneself by society, family, and friends
- Chemical and biological stressors: diet, alcohol, drugs, viruses, allergies, medications, medical conditions

Stressors are classified as either causing distress or causing eustress. **Distress** occurs when a stressor is perceived as unpleasant (e.g., a threat), whereas **eustress** is the result of a positively-perceived stressor (e.g., a challenge). Eustress can include life events such as graduating from college, studying to achieve a high score on the MCAT, getting married, or buying a house. While these events are largely positive, any event requiring individuals to change or adapt their lifestyle leads to stress. Stress level can be measured in "life change units" in a system called the **social readjustment rating scale**.

Stressors can also be psychological. Pressure, control, predictability, frustration, and conflict are all forms of psychological stress. Pressure is experienced when expectations or demands are put in place from external sources; this produces a feeling of urgency to complete tasks, perform actions, or display particular behaviors. The ability to control one's surroundings typically reduces stress levels; the inability to control a situation or event increases stress. In a study of nursing home patients, it was observed that those who had the most control of their daily environment displayed more active, positive, and social behavior. Predictability also plays a role in stress levels. For example, firefighters and police officers who cannot predict their daily scenarios experience higher levels of stress on the job. Frustration, which occurs when attaining a goal or need is prevented, increases stress. These frustration stresses can be external, such as not getting a raise, or internal, such as a disability interfering with everyday life. Finally, conflict stresses arise from the need to make a choice.

Approach–approach conflict refers to the need to choose between two desirable options. Avoidance–avoidance conflicts are choices between two negative options. Approach–avoidance conflicts deal with only one choice, goal, or event, but the outcome could have both positive and negative elements. For instance, while a job promotion might mean more money or status, it also comes with increased responsibility, potential for longer working hours, and increased pressure.

Physiological Response to Stressors

When subjected to stress, the body initially responds via the sympathetic nervous system. The "fight-or-flight" response initiates an increase in heart rate and decrease in digestion, with all available energy being reserved for reacting to the stressful event. The sequence of physiological responses developed by Hans Selye is called the **general adaptation syndrome** and consists of three distinct stages, as shown in Figure 5.10.

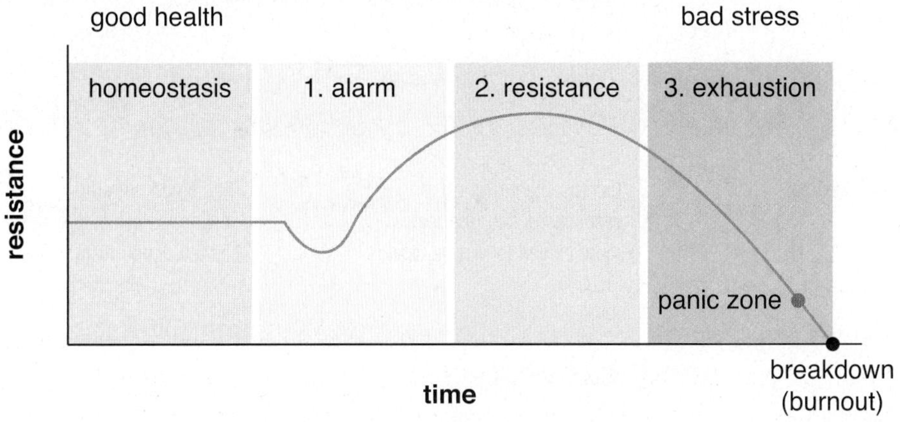

Figure 5.10 Three Stages of Stress Response

First is **alarm**, or the initial reaction to a stressor and the activation of the sympathetic nervous system. Shortly thereafter, the hypothalamus stimulates the pituitary to secrete adrenocorticotropic hormone (ACTH). This hormone stimulates the adrenal glands to produce cortisol, which maintains the steady supply of blood sugar needed to respond to stressful events. The hypothalamus also activates the adrenal medulla, which secretes epinephrine and norepinephrine to activate the sympathetic nervous system. The next stage is **resistance**, in which the continuous release of hormones allows the sympathetic nervous system to remain engaged to fight the stressor. Last, a person will experience **exhaustion** when the body can no longer maintain an elevated response with sympathetic nervous system activity. At this point, individuals become more susceptible to illnesses and medical conditions (such as ulcers and high blood pressure), organ systems can begin to deteriorate (with effects including heart disease), and in extreme cases, death can result. Some of the positive and negative effects of stress are shown in Figure 5.11.

Organ System	Acute Stress	Chronic Stress
Nervous system	Increased alertness, decreased pain perception	Memory problems, heightened risk of depressive disorders
Endocrine system	Adrenals secrete cortisol and other hormones to increase available energy	Slowed recovery from stress response due to high levels of cortisol and other hormones
Immune system	Thymus and other glands and tissues primed for immune response	Diminished immune response
Circulatory system	Increased heart rate, vasoconstriction to direct more oxygen to muscle tissue	High blood pressure, heightened risk of cardiovascular disorders
Reproductive system	Temporary suppression of functions	Heightened risk of infertility or miscarriage

Figure 5.11 Positive and Negative Effects of Stress

Emotional and Behavioral Responses to Stress

Beyond the effects on the human body, stress also takes a psychological toll on people who are unable to reduce their stress levels. On the emotional level, elevated stress can result in individuals feeling irritable, moody, tense, fearful, and helpless. They may also have difficulties with concentration and memory. Negative behavior responses to stress include withdrawing from others, difficulties at work or at school, substance use, aggression, and suicide. Additionally, chronic stress can lead to mental health disorders, such as anxiety and depression.

Coping and Stress Management

Strategies for coping with stress fall into two groups. Problem-focused strategies involve working to overcome a stressor, such as reaching out to family and friends for social support, confronting the issue head-on, and creating and following a plan of problem-solving actions. Emotionally focused strategies center on changing one's feelings about a stressor. They include taking responsibility for the issue, engaging in self-control, distancing oneself from the issue, engaging in wishful thinking, and using positive reappraisal to focus on positive outcomes instead of the stressor. Some coping strategies are adaptive, and reduce stress in a healthy way. A person who is feeling stressed could, for example, reach out to a loved one for help as a support-seeking coping strategy. However, coping strategies may also be maladaptive and include detrimental tactics, such as turning to drugs or alcohol.

Individuals can also engage in stress management to reduce their stress levels. Exercise is a powerful stress management tool that not only improves health and well-being, but also enhances mood. Exercise releases endorphins, opioid neuropeptides that act as "feel-good" neurotransmitters. Relaxation techniques, including meditation, diaphragmatic breathing, and progressive muscle relaxation have also been found to reduce stress. Additionally, studies have shown that engaging in a spiritual practice helps to manage stress.

BRIDGE

Maladaptiveness is a key factor in determining whether a behavior should be considered a disorder. Maladaptive behaviors are discussed in more detail in Chapter 7 of *MCAT Behavioral Sciences Review*.

MCAT EXPERTISE

Use these coping and stress management techniques to boost your performance (and mood) on Test Day!

MCAT CONCEPT CHECK 5.3

Before you move on, assess your understanding of the material with these questions.

1. What are the key features of primary and secondary cognitive appraisal of stress?
   - Primary appraisal:

   - Secondary appraisal:

   ---

2. What are the three stages of the general adaptation syndrome? What physiological changes are evident in each stage?

Stage	Physiological Changes

3. What are some common stressors? What are some effective techniques for managing stress?
    - Common stressors:

    ____

    - Stress management techniques:

    ____

    ____

    ____

Conclusion

The ability to strive for our goals and desires, be it for internal or external reasons, is an important aspect of psychology and behavior. Motivation is the mechanism used to meet our needs, act toward an end goal, and ultimately survive. While there are many factors that influence motivation, including instincts, arousal, drives, and needs, they all result in action to obtain perceived rewards, fulfill needs, or avoid perceived punishments. Emotion is a complex process resulting in physiological, cognitive, and behavioral elements, described in different fashions by the James–Lange, Cannon–Bard, and Schachter–Singer theories of emotion. Many components of the nervous system play a role in experiencing emotions, including the seven universal emotions. The response of the body and mind to challenges defines stress. Stress appraisal has phases that identify and allow the body to respond to the stressor encountered. The physical and mental response to stress can be severe, but there are many management and coping mechanisms commonly used to reduce the level of stress experienced.

Hopefully this chapter has left you motivated to keep working toward that goal of an excellent MCAT score and becoming the doctor you deserve to be. Studying for the MCAT certainly introduces a significant stress, but effective stress management techniques and a solid foundation in MCAT content and strategy will turn Test Day into eustress. Just keep your eyes on that white coat, an important garment that will someday be part of your identity—a topic we'll explore in the next chapter.

You've reviewed the content, now test your knowledge and critical thinking skills by completing a test-like passage set in your online resources!

GO ONLINE

CONCEPT SUMMARY

Motivation

- **Motivation** is the purpose, or driving force, behind our actions.
- Motivation can be **extrinsic**, based on external circumstances; or **intrinsic**, based on internal drive or perception.
- The primary factors that influence motivation are instincts, arousal, drives, and needs.
    - **Instincts** are innate, fixed patterns of behavior. In the **instinct theory** of motivation, people perform certain behaviors because of these evolutionarily programmed instincts.
    - In the **arousal theory**, people perform actions to maintain **arousal**, the state of being awake and reactive to stimuli, at an optimal level. The **Yerkes–Dodson law** shows that performance is optimal at a medium level of arousal.
    - **Drives** are internal states of tension that beget particular behaviors focused on goals. Primary drives are related to bodily processes; secondary drives stem from learning and include accomplishments and emotions. **Drive reduction theory** states that motivation arises from the desire to eliminate drives, which create uncomfortable internal states.
    - Satisfying **needs** may also motivate. **Maslow's hierarchy of needs** prioritizes needs into five categories: physiological needs (highest priority), safety and security, love and belonging, self-esteem, and self-actualization (lowest priority).
    - **Self-determination theory** emphasizes the role of three universal needs: autonomy, competence, and relatedness.
- **Incentive theory** explains motivation as the desire to pursue rewards and avoid punishments.
- **Expectancy–value theory** states that the amount of motivation for a task is based on the individual's expectation of success and the amount that success is valued.
- **Opponent-process theory** explains motivation for drug use: as drug use increases, the body counteracts its effects, leading to tolerance and uncomfortable withdrawal symptoms.
- Sexual motivation is related to hormones as well as cultural and social factors.

Emotion

- **Emotion** is a state of mind, or feeling, that is subjectively experienced based on circumstances, mood, and relationships.
- The three components of emotion are **cognitive** (subjective), **behavioral** (facial expressions and body language), and **physiological** (changes in the autonomic nervous system).

- The **seven universal emotions** are happiness, sadness, contempt, surprise, fear, disgust, and anger.
- There are multiple theories of emotion, based on the interactions of the three components of emotion.
  - In the **James–Lange theory**, nervous system arousal leads to an emotional experience.
  - In the **Cannon–Bard theory**, arousal of the nervous system and the experience of emotion occur simultaneously.
  - In the **Schachter–Singer theory**, nervous system arousal is combined with cognition to create the experience of emotion.
- The **limbic system** is the primary nervous system component involved in experiencing emotion.
  - The **amygdala** is involved with attention and fear, helps interpret facial expressions, and is part of the intrinsic memory system for emotional memory.
  - The **thalamus** is a sensory processing station.
  - The **hypothalamus** releases neurotransmitters that affect mood and arousal.
  - The **hippocampus** creates long-term explicit (episodic) memories.
  - The **prefrontal cortex** is involved with planning, expressing personality, and making decisions. The **ventral prefrontal cortex** is critical for experiencing emotion; the **ventromedial prefrontal cortex**, specifically, is involved in controlling emotional responses from the amygdala and decision making.

Stress

- The physiological and cognitive response to challenges or life changes is defined as **stress**.
- Stress appraisal has two stages:
  - **Primary appraisal** is classifying a potential stressor as irrelevant, benign–positive, or stressful.
  - **Secondary appraisal** is directed at evaluating if the organism can cope with the stress, based on harm, threat, and challenge.
- A **stressor** is anything that leads to a stress response and can include environment, daily events, workplace or academic settings, social expectations, chemicals, and biological stressors. Psychological stressors include pressure, control, predictability, frustration, and conflict.
- Stressors can lead to **distress** or **eustress**.
- The three stages of the **general adaptation syndrome** are alarm, resistance, and exhaustion.
- Stress management can include psychological, behavioral, and spiritual aspects.

ANSWERS TO CONCEPT CHECKS

5.1

1.

Theory	Factor for Motivation
Instinct theory	Instincts: innate, fixed patterns of behavior in response to stimuli
Arousal theory	Maintaining a constant level of arousal, the psychological and physiological state of being awake and reactive to stimuli
Drive reduction theory	Drives: internal states of tension or discomfort that can be relieved with a particular action
Need-based theories	Needs: factors necessary for physiological function or emotional fulfillment

2. Physiological needs, safety and security, love and belonging, self-esteem, self-actualization
3. Cocaine is a stimulant, causing euphoria, restlessness, increased heart rate, increased temperature, and anxiety. According to opponent-process theory, cocaine withdrawal should be the opposite: depressed mood, fatigue, decreased heart rate, decreased temperature, and apathy.

5.2

1. The three elements of emotion are as follows:
    - Physiological response (autonomic nervous system): heart rate, breathing rate, skin temperature, blood pressure
    - Behavioral response: facial expressions, body language
    - Cognitive response: subjective interpretation, memories of past experiences, perception of cause of emotion
2. The seven universal emotions are happiness, sadness, contempt, surprise, fear, disgust, and anger.

3.

James–Lange Theory	Cannon–Bard Theory	Schachter–Singer Theory
• Stimulus leads to physiological arousal • Arousal leads to the conscious experience of emotion • *My skin is hot and my blood pressure is high so I must be angry* • Requires connection between sympathetic nervous system and brain	• Stimulus leads to physiological arousal and feeling of emotion • Thalamus processes sensory information, sends it to cortex and sympathetic nervous system • Action is secondary response to stimulus • *I see a snake, so I am afraid and my heart is racing…Let me out of here!* • Does not explain vagus nerve	• Both arousal and labeling based on environment are required to experience an emotion • *I am excited because my heart is racing and everyone else is happy*

4. The amygdala is involved with attention and emotions (specifically fear), helps interpret facial expressions, and is part of the intrinsic memory system for emotional memory. The thalamus is a sensory processing station. The hypothalamus releases neurotransmitters that affect mood and arousal. The hippocampus creates long-term explicit memories (episodic memories). The ventromedial prefrontal cortex is involved in decision making and controlling emotional responses from the amygdala.

5.3

1. Primary appraisal is categorizing the stressor as irrelevant, benign–positive, or stressful. Secondary appraisal is the evaluation of the ability of the organism to cope with that stress.

2.

Stage	Physiological Changes
Alarm	Activation of sympathetic nervous system, release of ACTH and cortisol, stimulation of adrenal medulla to secrete epinephrine and norepinephrine
Resistance	Continuous release of hormones activates sympathetic nervous system
Exhaustion	Can no longer maintain elevated sympathetic nervous system activity, more susceptible to illness and medical conditions, organ systems deteriorate, death

3. Common stressors include environmental or physical discomfort, daily events, workplace or academic setting, social expectations, and chemical and biological stressors. Effective stress management techniques include exercise, relaxation techniques (meditation, diaphragmatic breathing, progressive muscle relaxation), spiritual practice, and many more.

SCIENCE MASTERY ASSESSMENT EXPLANATIONS

1. **A**

Due to the competitive nature of the motivation, this is considered extrinsic motivation. Extrinsic motivation is based on external conditions, including perceived reward or fear of punishment. In this case, the reward is beating the sibling. There is no suggestion of an uncomfortable internal state or tension, which is an aspect of drives, eliminating **(C)** and **(D)**.

2. **D**

The Yerkes–Dodson law states that there is an optimal level of arousal necessary to perform. If levels of arousal are too high, poor performance can result. In the case of this student performing at a recital, arousal level is very high as a result of nervousness and anxiety, resulting in a poor performance.

3. **A**

Drive reduction theory is the theory that one will act to eliminate uncomfortable internal states known as drives. The body will push toward equilibrium, or homeostasis.

4. **A**

The seven universal emotions are happiness, sadness, contempt, surprise, fear, disgust, and anger.

5. **C**

The three components of emotion are the physiological (changes in the autonomic nervous system), cognitive (subjective interpretation of an emotion), and behavioral (facial expressions and body language) responses.

6. **D**

Experiencing a physiological reaction to a stimulus and then labeling that response as emotion is in line with the James–Lange theory of emotion. In the statement, seeing the bear is the stimulus, an increase in heart rate and breathing rate is the physiological reaction, and identifying this as fear is the emotion experienced.

7. **C**

According to Darwin's theory of evolution, all species have instincts that help them survive. The instinct theory of motivation states that people are motivated to act based on instincts that they are programmed to exhibit.

8. **D**

The Cannon–Bard theory of emotion is based on the premise that conscious feelings and physiological components of emotion are experienced at exactly the same time. In this theory, this combination then leads to action. This is commonly confused with the Schachter–Singer theory, **(A)**, in which nervous system arousal occurs and then is labeled based on the context provided by the environment.

9. **C**

The amygdala, prefrontal cortex, and thalamus all play a role in the experience of emotions. The basal ganglia are involved in smooth movement and are not primarily responsible for the experience of emotions.

10. **A**

The left frontal lobe is associated with positive feelings, corresponding with joy and happiness. The right frontal lobe is associated with negative feelings, such as sadness and disgust, **(B)** and **(D)**.

11. **B**

Secondary appraisal of stress is the stage at which the ability of the organism to cope with the stressor is evaluated. This is based on the harm, threat, and challenge of the stressor, which are all correlated with its intensity. Primary appraisal is simply the initial determination of whether there is a negative association at all, not its intensity.

12. **D**

A positive stressor creates eustress. Because working out is used to relax, it is considered a eustress. Hassle, **(A)**, and frustration, **(B)**, are both types of distress, **(C)**, or negative stressors.

13. **A**

Approach–approach conflict is one in which both results are good outcomes. While one must be chosen, neither choice results in a negative outcome: for example, choosing between two desserts. Avoidance–escape conflict, **(D)**, is not a recognized form of conflict; these two terms are related to types of negative reinforcers.

14. **A**

The initial reaction to stress, which is activation of the sympathetic nervous system, is the alarm stage of stress response.

15. **C**

Progressive muscle relaxation is a relaxation technique demonstrated to help reduce stress in a manner that is beneficial to the body and psyche. The other methods described here, including avoidance of the stressor, **(D)**, serve to increase stress or merely change the source of the stress.

Consult your online resources for additional practice. GO ONLINE

SHARED CONCEPTS

Behavioral Sciences Chapter 1
Biology and Behavior

Behavioral Sciences Chapter 3
Learning and Memory

Behavioral Sciences Chapter 7
Psychological Disorders

Biology Chapter 4
The Nervous System

Biology Chapter 5
The Endocrine System

Biology Chapter 10
Homeostasis

CHAPTER 6

IDENTITY AND PERSONALITY

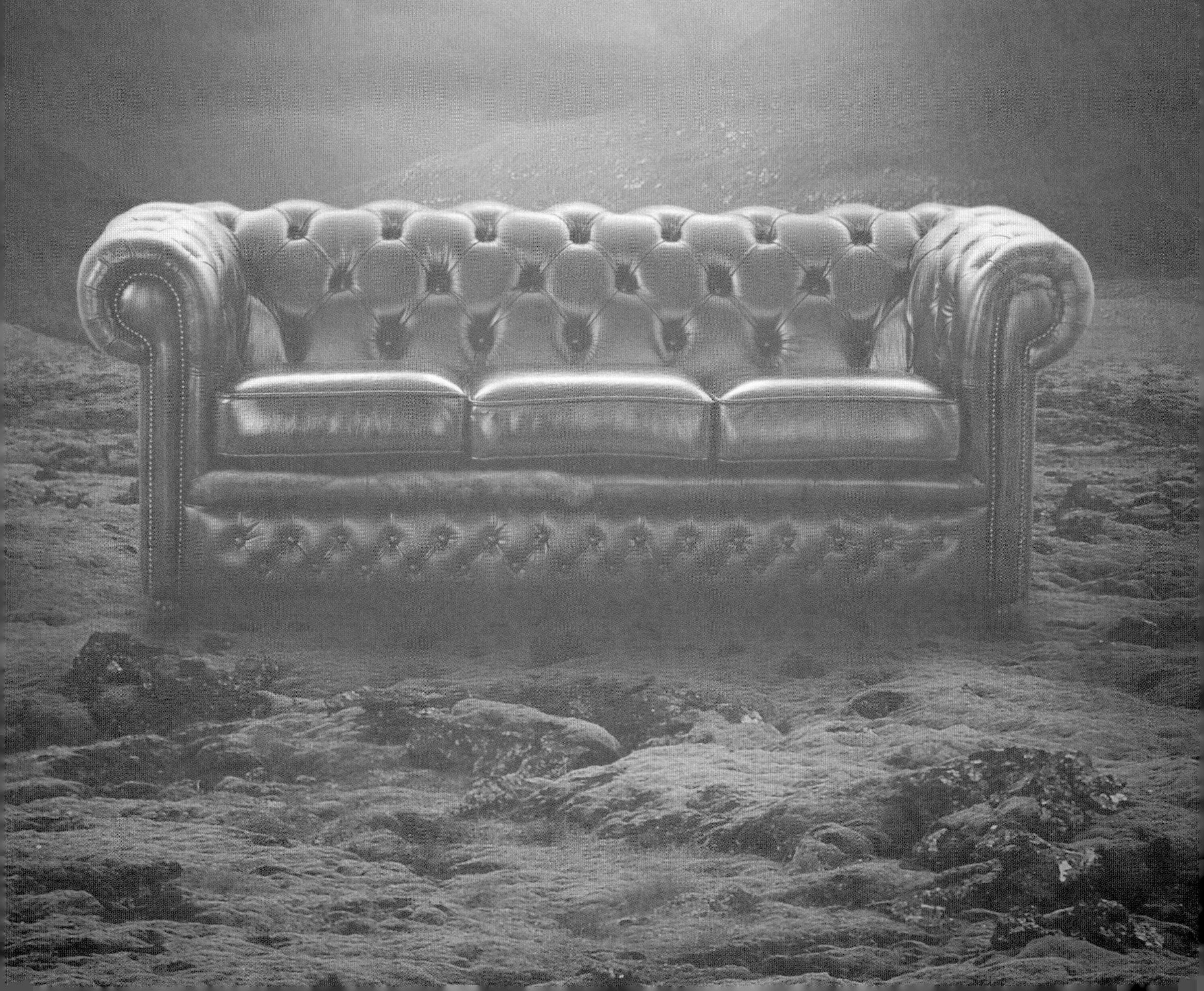

SCIENCE MASTERY ASSESSMENT

Every pre-med knows this feeling: there is so much content I have to know for the MCAT! How do I know what to do first or what's important?

While the high-yield badges throughout this book will help you identify the most important topics, this Science Mastery Assessment is another tool in your MCAT prep arsenal. This quiz (which can also be taken in your online resources) and the guidance below will help ensure that you are spending the appropriate amount of time on this chapter based on your personal strengths and weaknesses. Don't worry though—skipping something now does not mean you'll never study it. Later on in your prep, as you complete full-length tests, you'll uncover specific pieces of content that you need to review and can come back to these chapters as appropriate.

How to Use This Assessment

If you answer 0–7 questions correctly:

Spend about 1 hour to read this chapter in full and take limited notes throughout. Follow up by reviewing **all** quiz questions to ensure that you now understand how to solve each one.

If you answer 8–11 questions correctly:

Spend 20–40 minutes reviewing the quiz questions. Beginning with the questions you missed, read and take notes on the corresponding subchapters. For questions you answered correctly, ensure your thinking matches that of the explanation and you understand why each choice was correct or incorrect.

If you answer 12–15 questions correctly:

Spend less than 20 minutes reviewing all questions from the quiz. If you missed any, then include a quick read-through of the corresponding subchapters, or even just the relevant content within a subchapter, as part of your question review. For questions you answered correctly, ensure your thinking matches that of the explanation and review the Concept Summary at the end of the chapter.

1. Each of the following is considered a part of a person's self-concept EXCEPT:
   - **A.** the past self.
   - **B.** the ought self.
   - **C.** the future self.
   - **D.** self-schemata.

2. As a gender identity, androgyny is defined as:
   - **A.** low femininity, low masculinity.
   - **B.** high femininity, low masculinity.
   - **C.** low femininity, high masculinity.
   - **D.** high femininity, high masculinity.

3. A high school student struggles consistently with math and feels that no amount of studying will help because "I just don't get it." Which of the following is the most likely short-term result with respect to the student's ability to do math?
   - **A.** Low self-esteem
   - **B.** Low self-efficacy
   - **C.** Learned helplessness
   - **D.** An external locus of control

4. A district attorney with an internal locus of control wins an important court trial. Which of the following best represents the lawyer's attribution of the events?
   - **A.** "I won because I made great arguments and had more experience than the defense."
   - **B.** "I won because the jury was on my side from the beginning and believed my arguments."
   - **C.** "I won because the defense did not adequately present their side of the case."
   - **D.** "I shouldn't have won because I don't deserve to be successful."

5. A person keeps an extremely tidy desk and becomes very nervous whenever things are disorganized or out of place. In which of the following stages would a psychodynamic therapist say this person had become fixated?
   - **A.** The oral stage
   - **B.** The anal stage
   - **C.** The phallic stage
   - **D.** The genital stage

6. According to Erikson's stages of psychosocial development, which of the following would be the most important for a recent college graduate to accomplish?
   - **A.** Figuring out what identities are most important personally
   - **B.** Feeling like a contributing member of society
   - **C.** Forming an intimate relationship with a significant other
   - **D.** Finding a feeling of accomplishment in life

7. Matt and Cati discuss the reasons why they avoid driving above the speed limit. Matt cites wanting to avoid a traffic fine, while Cati says that speeding is dangerous and, if everyone did it, there would be more accidents and people would get hurt. According to Kohlberg, which of the following describes the phases of moral reasoning demonstrated by Matt and Cati, respectively?
   - **A.** Preconventional; conventional
   - **B.** Preconventional; postconventional
   - **C.** Conventional; preconventional
   - **D.** Postconventional; conventional

8. A child cannot make an origami swan alone, but is able to do so when observing and being assisted by an adult. This scenario is described in the ideas of which of the following theorists?

- **A.** Albert Bandura
- **B.** Alfred Adler
- **C.** B. F. Skinner
- **D.** Lev Vygotsky

9. Which of the following is a conclusion that can be made from research in role-taking and observational learning?

- **A.** Young children will only model actions performed by their parents.
- **B.** Celebrities and athletes are an adolescent's most important role models.
- **C.** Children who role-take identities that are not gender typical are more likely to take on those roles later in life.
- **D.** A female child is more likely to model the behavior of another female than a male.

10. A person feels extremely guilty after having an extramarital affair. According to the psychodynamic perspective, which of the following is responsible for this anxiety?

- **A.** The id
- **B.** The ego
- **C.** The superego
- **D.** The libido

11. A woman advances through the ranks of a company, eventually becoming the CEO. Which of the following Jungian archetypes reflects this woman's drive to be successful within the company?

- **A.** The persona
- **B.** The anima
- **C.** The animus
- **D.** The shadow

12. Researchers discover that polymorphisms in the *DRD2* gene can be associated with thrill-seeking behavior, and that individuals with certain forms of the gene are more likely to become extreme athletes and have more dangerous hobbies. Which of the following theories is supported by this discovery?

- **I.** The social cognitive perspective
- **II.** The behavioral perspective
- **III.** The biological perspective

- **A.** I only
- **B.** III only
- **C.** I and III only
- **D.** II and III only

13. A person who works as an EMT identifies as a bit of a rebel, but is highly sociable and is able to keep calm in an emergency. This person would likely score in the lower range of which of the following traits?

- **A.** Psychoticism
- **B.** Neuroticism
- **C.** Extraversion
- **D.** Conscientiousness

14. Stockholm syndrome is a phenomenon in which people who are kidnapped or held hostage may begin to identify with or even feel affection for their captors. A psychoanalyst might explain Stockholm syndrome by citing which of the following defense mechanisms?

- **A.** Reaction formation
- **B.** Regression
- **C.** Projection
- **D.** Displacement

15. Having struggled for years through an economic recession, a young professional begins to buy lottery tickets every Friday. "If I won the lottery," the individual reasons, "I'd finally have the life I've always wanted. All my stress would go away and I could live comfortably." These thoughts regarding winning the lottery are most representative of:

- **A.** a cardinal trait.
- **B.** fictional finalism.
- **C.** functional autonomy.
- **D.** unconditional positive regard.

Answer Key

1. **B**
2. **D**
3. **B**
4. **A**
5. **B**
6. **C**
7. **A**
8. **D**
9. **D**
10. **C**
11. **C**
12. **C**
13. **B**
14. **A**
15. **B**

Detailed explanations can be found at the end of the chapter.

CHAPTER 6

IDENTITY AND PERSONALITY

In This Chapter

CHAPTER PROFILE

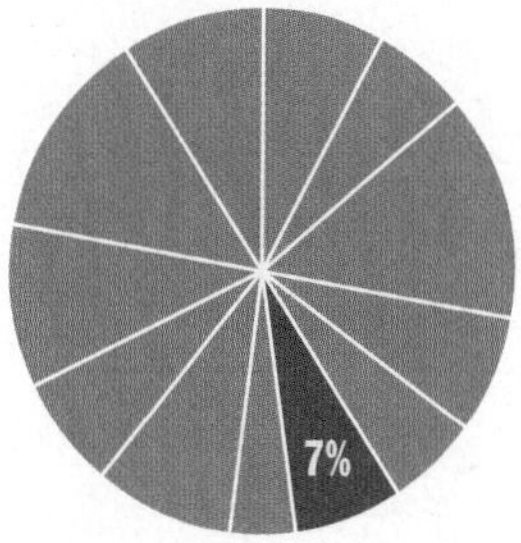

The content in this chapter should be relevant to about 7% of all questions about the behavioral sciences on the MCAT.

This chapter covers material from the following AAMC content categories:

7A: Individual influences on behavior

8A: Self-identity

Introduction

Social psychologists are concerned with how our social lives influence the ways in which we perceive ourselves. Specifically, researchers have focused on the influence that other people's views, our social roles, and our group memberships have on our perceptions of who we are.

Who are you? If you're like most people, you could probably answer that question in many different ways. You might list your physical characteristics, your family relationships, your emotional tendencies, or your skills and talents. In fact, many introductory psychology courses include an exercise in which students are asked to make a list of answers to the question *Who am I?* Completing this list gives each student a glimpse into their identity and personality. These ideas form the core of the study of psychology, in which the central goal is explaining our thoughts and behaviors. In this chapter, we'll discuss this and review the key theorists and their approaches to answering the question of who we are.

6.1 Self-Concept and Identity

High-Yield

LEARNING OBJECTIVES

After Chapter 6.1, you will be able to:

- Distinguish between self-concept and identity
- Recall the factors that contribute to different types of identity, such as gender and ethnicity
- Predict how a person would explain an event to themselves based on their locus of control

When you look in the mirror, whom do you see? If you're studying to take the MCAT, chances are some descriptors that come to mind include *student, intelligent, future doctor*, and so on. Our awareness of ourselves as distinct from others and our own internal list of answers to the question *Who am I?* form our **self-concept**. Many of the ways in which we define ourselves fall under the classification of a **self-schema**; that is, a self-given label that carries with it a set of qualities. For example, the *athlete* self-schema usually carries the qualities of youth, physical fitness, and dressing and acting in certain ways, although these qualities may change depending on culture, socioeconomic status, and personal beliefs. The idea of self-concept goes beyond these self-schemata; it also includes our appraisal of who we used to be and who we will become.

Sometimes the terms *self-concept* and *identity* are used interchangeably, but psychologists generally use them to refer to two different but closely related ideas. Social scientists define **identity** as the individual components of our self-concept related to the groups to which we belong. Whereas we have one self-concept, we have multiple identities that define who we are and how we should behave within any given context. Religious affiliation, sexual orientation, personal relationships, and membership in social groups are just a few of the identities that sum to create our self-concept. In fact, our individual identities do not always need to be compatible. Are you the same person when interacting with your friends as you are when you interact with coworkers or family? For most people the answer is *no*; they take on particular identities in different social situations.

Types of Identity

While there are many different types of identity, the MCAT—for historical or social reasons—tends to focus on some forms of identity more than others.

Gender Identity

Gender identity describes people's appraisals of themselves on scales of masculinity and femininity. While these concepts were long thought to be two extremes on a single continuum, theorists have reasoned that they must be two separate dimensions because an individual can achieve high scores on scales of both masculinity and femininity. **Androgyny** is defined as the state of being simultaneously very masculine and very feminine, while those who achieve low scores on both scales are referred to as **undifferentiated**. An initial sense of gender identity is usually established by age three, although it may morph and change over time. Some theories, such as the theory of **gender schema**, hold that key components of gender identity are transmitted through cultural and societal means.

Keep in mind that gender identity is not necessarily tied to biological sex or sexual orientation, although in many cultures these concepts are seen as closely related. While it is typical of many cultures to view gender as a strictly binary concept, some cultures recognize three or more genders. For example, some peoples of Samoa refer to androgynous but phenotypically male individuals as *fa'afafine*. To these Samoans, the *fa'afafine* are seen as an important social caste and are accepted as equals, although this is not always the case for all genders across all cultures.

REAL WORLD

Individuals who are transgender are those for whom gender identity does not match sex assigned at birth. They have been a heavily stigmatized group in American culture. In fact, it was not until the publication of the DSM-5 in 2013 that gender identity disorder was formally removed as a diagnosis. The DSM-5 includes the diagnosis gender dysphoria, which is given only to individuals for whom gender identity causes significant psychological stress.

Ethnic and National Identity

Ethnic identity refers to the part of one's identity associated with membership in a particular racial/ethnic group. Members in a given ethnic group often share a common ancestry, cultural heritage, and language. Many social psychologists study the ways in which our ethnic identity influences our perspectives of ourselves. In a 1947 study, Kenneth and Mamie Clark explored ethnic self-concepts among children who were ethnically White and Black using a doll preference task: the experimenter showed each child a Black doll and a White doll and asked the child a series of questions about how the child felt about the dolls. The majority of children, both White and Black, preferred the White doll. This study was important because it highlighted the negative effects of racism and underrepresented group status on the self-concept of Black children at the time. However, subsequent research using improved methodology (for example, randomizing the ethnicity of the experimenter), has shown that children who are Black hold more positive views of their own ethnicity; this may also represent societal changes at large.

While ethnicity is largely an identity into which we are born, **nationality** is based on political borders. National identity is the result of shared history, media, cuisine, and national symbols such as a country's flag. Nationality need not be tied to one's ethnicity or even to legal citizenship. Symbols play an important role in both ethnic and national identity. Some examples of symbols, representing American nationality, are shown in Figure 6.1.

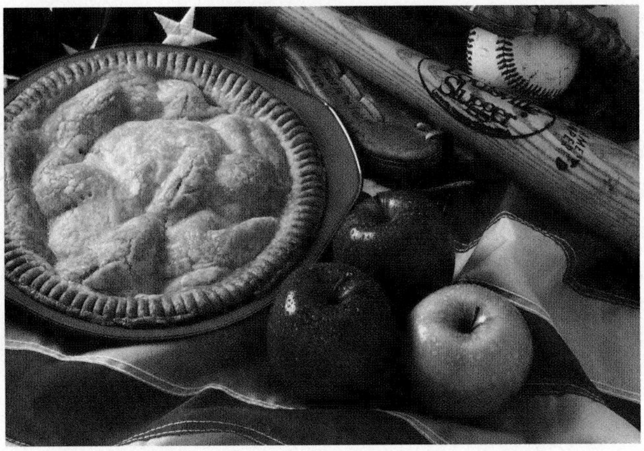

Figure 6.1 Examples of National Symbols
Symbols commonly associated with residents of the United States of America

Other Types of Identity

Of course, there are many more categories through which we evaluate our identity. We compare ourselves to others in terms of age, class, religious affiliation, sexual orientation, and so on. Aspects of these other identities are explored in other parts of *MCAT Behavioral Sciences Review.*

It is important to know that there are several factors that determine which identity will be enacted in particular situations. It is believed that our identities are organized according to a **hierarchy of salience**, such that we let the situation dictate which identity holds the most importance for us at any given moment. For instance, male and female college students in same-gender groups are less likely to list gender in their self-descriptions than students in mixed-gender groups. Furthermore, researchers have found that the more salient the identity, the more we conform to the role expectations of the identities. Salience is determined by a number of factors, including the amount of work we have invested into the identity, the rewards and gratification associated with the identity, and the amount of self-esteem we have associated with the identity.

Self-Evaluation

BRIDGE

Remember that *esteem* is one of Maslow's hierarchy of needs (#4 in priority). This model is discussed in Chapter 5 of *MCAT Behavioral Sciences Review.*

Our individual self-concept plays a very important role in the way we evaluate and feel about ourselves. **Self-discrepancy theory** maintains that each of us has three selves and that perceived differences between these selves lead to negative feelings. Our self-concept makes up our **actual self**, the way we see ourselves as we currently are. Our **ideal self** is the person we would like to be, and our **ought self** is our representation of the way others think we should be. Generally, the closer these three selves are to one another, the higher our **self-esteem** or self-worth will be.

Those with low self-esteem don't necessarily view themselves as worthless, but they will be far more critical of themselves. As a result, they take criticism from others poorly and typically believe that people will only accept them if they are successful. Research also shows that they are more likely to use drugs, to be pessimistic, and to give up when facing frustration than their counterparts with high self-esteem.

While self-esteem is the measure of how we feel about ourselves, **self-efficacy** is our belief in our ability to succeed. Self-efficacy can vary by activity for individuals; we all can think of situations in which we hold the belief that we are able to be effective and, conversely, those in which we feel powerless. Of course, we are more motivated to pursue those tasks for which our self-efficacy is high, but we can get into trouble when it is too high. **Overconfidence** can lead us to take on tasks for which we are not ready, leading to frustration, humiliation, or sometimes even personal injury. On the other hand, self-efficacy can also be depressed; an individual can develop a perceived lack of control over the outcome of a situation, a phenomenon called **learned helplessness**. Learned helplessness has been found to be strongly related to clinical depression.

Locus of control is another core self-evaluation that is closely related to self-concept. **Locus of control** refers to the way we characterize the influences in our lives. People with an internal locus of control view themselves as controlling their own fate, whereas those with an external locus of control feel that the events in their lives are caused by luck or outside influences. For example, a runner who loses a race may attribute the cause of the loss internally (*I didn't train hard enough*) or externally (*My shoes didn't fit and the track was wet*).

All of these ideas work hand-in-hand to influence the way we feel about ourselves. The happiest among us are those who have high self-esteem, view themselves as effective people, feel that they are in control of their destinies, and see themselves as living up to their own expectations of who they would like to be.

BRIDGE

Locus of control and cognitive dissonance are integral to attribution theory. In order to preserve self-esteem, we often see our successes as a direct result of our efforts and our failures as the result of uncontrollable outside influences. Attribution theory is discussed in Chapter 10 of *MCAT Behavioral Sciences Review.*

MCAT EXPERTISE

Effective MCAT students review full-length exams with an internal locus of control: *What can I do to prepare myself better for the next practice test?* An external locus of control prevents students from actually gaining anything from their practice: *Oh, that was just a stupid question.*

MCAT CONCEPT CHECK 6.1

Before you move on, assess your understanding of the material with these questions.

1. What is the difference between self-concept and identity?

____

2. List three factors that contribute to a person's ethnic identity. How are these factors different from those that determine national identity?

   1. _______________
   2. _______________
   3. _______________

   - National identity:

____

3. A high school student fails a history test. How might a student with an internal locus of control interpret this event? What about a student with an external locus of control?

   - Internal:

____

   - External:

____

6.2 Formation of Identity

High-Yield

LEARNING OBJECTIVES

After Chapter 6.2, you will be able to:

- Identify the three major phases of Kohlberg's theory of moral development and their central tenets
- Explain, and distinguish between, the theories of identity of Erikson, Freud, Vygotsky, and Kohlberg

Psychologists generally agree that we are not born with our self-concept and identity in place and fully developed. As young children, our identities are largely defined by our relationship to our caregivers. As we move into adolescence, we begin to develop into unique individuals, deciding who we want to be when on our own. Several theorists have proposed stages through which we develop. They vary in scope with respect to both the aspects of our identity they describe and their time span, but they all have one thing in common: the MCAT loves to test your mastery of these theories!

Freud: Psychosexual Development

Sigmund Freud was a pioneer in charting personality and emotional growth. For Freud, human psychology and human sexuality were inextricably linked. In fact, Freud made the assertion that far from lying dormant until puberty, the **libido** (sex drive) is present at birth. Freud believed that libidinal energy and the drive to reduce libidinal tension were the underlying dynamic forces that accounted for human psychological processes.

Freud hypothesized five distinct stages of psychosexual development, summarized in Table 6.1 at the end of this section. In each stage, children are faced with a conflict between societal demands and the desire to reduce the libidinal tension associated with different erogenous zones of the body. Each stage differs in the manner in which libidinal energy is manifested and the way in which the libidinal drive is met. **Fixation** occurs when a child is overindulged or overly frustrated during a stage of development. In response to the anxiety caused by fixation, the child forms a personality pattern based on that particular stage, which persists into adulthood as a functional mental disorder known as a **neurosis**.

The first stage is the **oral stage**, spanning from 0 to 1 year of age. During this stage, gratification is obtained primarily through putting objects into the mouth, biting, and sucking. Libidinal energy is centered on the mouth. An adult who is orally fixated would be expected to exhibit excessive dependency.

Next is the **anal stage**, from 1 to 3 years, during which the libido is centered on the anus and gratification is gained through the elimination and retention of waste materials. Toilet training occurs during this stage. Fixation during this stage would lead to either excessive orderliness (*anal-retentiveness*) or sloppiness in the adult.

The **phallic stage**, sometimes known as the **Oedipal stage**, is the third of Freud's stages of psychosexual development. Generally, children aged 3 to 5 years are in this developmental stage. This stage centers on resolution of the **Oedipal conflict** for male children or the analogous **Electra conflict** for female children. In Freud's view, the male child envies his father's intimate relationship with his mother and fears castration

MCAT EXPERTISE

Though revolutionary at the time, Freud's theories have largely been discredited. They do, however, provide an interesting window into the history of personality theory. Expect the MCAT to test these ideas from a historical context, usually prefaced by *According to Freud's theory of psychosexual development . . .*

BRIDGE

Freud's stages of psychosexual development are based on the same principles as drive reduction theory, as discussed in Chapter 5 of *MCAT Behavioral Sciences Review:* libidinal energy creates internal tension, which we aim to reduce through certain behaviors.

at his father's hands. He wishes to eliminate his father and possess his mother, but the child feels guilty about these wishes. To successfully resolve the conflict, he deals with his guilty feelings by identifying with his father, establishing his sexual identity, and internalizing moral values. Also, the child to a large extent de-eroticizes, or **sublimates** his libidinal energy. This may be expressed through collecting objects or focusing on schoolwork. Freud did not elaborate much on the Electra conflict, although he theorized a similar desire. Because females cannot have castration fear (instead, they are theorized to have **penis envy**), female children are expected to exhibit less stereotypically female behavior and to be less morally developed in this theory.

Once the libido is sublimated, the child has entered the **latency stage**, which lasts until puberty is reached.

For Freud, the final stage is the **genital stage**, beginning in puberty and lasting through adulthood. According to Freud, if prior development has proceeded correctly, the person should enter into healthy heterosexual relationships at this point. Freud claimed, however, that if sexual traumas of childhood have not been resolved, such behaviors as homosexuality, asexuality, or fetishism may result.

STAGE	DESCRIPTION
Oral	Libidinal energy centered on the mouth; fixation can lead to excessive dependency
Anal	Toilet training occurs during this time; fixation can lead to excessive orderliness or messiness
Phallic	Oedipal or Electra conflict is resolved during this stage
Latency	Libido is largely sublimated during this stage
Genital	Begins at puberty; in theory, if previous stages have been successfully resolved, the person will enter into heterosexual relationships

Table 6.1 Freud's Stages of Psychosexual Development

Erikson: Psychosocial Development

Erik **Erikson's theory of psychosocial development** theorizes that personality development is driven by the successful resolution of a series of social and emotional conflicts. For example, the first such conflict is that of **trust** *vs.* **mistrust**, which occurs during the first year of life. Newborn humans are quite helpless and unsure of their environment. A newborn depends on their caregivers for support. So, the psychosocial conflict that a newborn faces is whether or not to trust caregivers to reliably provide that support. If caregivers do reliably care for the newborn, then the newborn will learn trust, which is a social skill. In different circumstances, the newborn could fail to learn to trust. However, according to Erikson's theory, such an individual may nevertheless move on to the next stage of psychosocial development, and may even learn trust later in life.

This example illustrates three key features of Erikson's theory. First, the conflicts that Erikson describes arise because an individual lacks some critical social or emotional skill. Each conflict therefore represents an opportunity to learn a new social or emotional skill, which, according to Erikson, is the mechanism for psychosocial development. Second, each conflict has either a positive or negative resolution. For example, a newborn can learn to be mistrustful. This outcome does represent a resolution of the trust *vs.* mistrust conflict. However, this outcome would be a negative outcome and, in Erikson's view, would represent a failure to develop. Psychosocial development means not only resolving each conflict, but obtaining a positive resolution. However, the third key idea is that, in Erikson's theory, an individual who fails to obtain a positive resolution at one stage can still advance to later stages and, later in life, may even learn the skill that they failed to learn during the developmental conflict.

The second conflict is **autonomy** *vs.* **shame and doubt** (1 to 3 years), where children begin to explore their surroundings and develop their interests. The favorable outcome here is feeling able to exert control over the world and to exercise choice as well as self-restraint. However, if children are overly controlled and criticized, the unfavorable outcome is a sense of doubt and a persistent external locus of control.

The next conflict confronted is **initiative** *vs.* **guilt** (3 to 6 years), in which children learn basic cause and effect principles in physics, and starting and finishing out tasks for a purpose. Favorable outcomes include a sense of purpose, the ability to initiate activities, and the ability to enjoy accomplishment. If guilt wins out, children will be so overcome by the fear of punishment that they may either unduly restrict themselves or may overcompensate by showing off.

Next is the conflict of **industry** *vs.* **inferiority** (6 to 12 years), where pre-adolescents are becoming aware of themselves as individuals. If resolved favorably, children will feel competent, be able to exercise their abilities and intelligence in the world, and be able to affect the world in the way that they desire. Unfavorable resolution results in a sense of inadequacy, a sense of inability to act in a competent manner, and low self-esteem.

During adolescence (12 to 20 years), individuals experience **identity** *vs.* **role confusion**. During this conflict, adolescents explore their independence to determine who they are and what their purpose is in society. At this stage, individuals either form a single identity or become unsure about their place in society. The favorable outcome is fidelity, the ability to see oneself as a unique and integrated person with sustained loyalties. Unfavorable outcomes are confusion about one's identity and an amorphous personality that shifts from day to day.

The main crisis of young adulthood (20 to 40 years) is **intimacy** *vs.* **isolation**, where people focus on creating long-lasting bonds with others. Favorable outcomes are love, the ability to have intimate relationships with others, and the ability to commit oneself to another person and to one's own goals. If this crisis is not favorably resolved, there will be an avoidance of commitment, alienation, and distancing of oneself from others and one's ideals. Isolated individuals are either withdrawn or capable of only superficial relationships with others.

The conflict of middle age (40 to 65 years) is **generativity** *vs.* **stagnation**, where the focus is on advancing present and future society. The successful resolution of this conflict results in an individual capable of being a productive, caring, and contributing member of society. If this crisis is not overcome, one acquires a sense of stagnation and may become self-indulgent, bored, and self-centered with little care for others.

REAL WORLD

The conflict of identity *vs.* role confusion has some positive effects: teenagers identifying their interests, gravitating toward friends who share these interests, and creating a sense of who they want to be. On the other hand, this conflict can lead to the formation of cliques, bullying, and significant peer pressure. The increase of online and in-person bullying among adolescents has led to a number of programs to ease this crisis, such as *StopBullying.gov* and the *It Gets Better* campaign.

Finally, old age (above 65 years) brings about the crisis of **integrity** *vs.* **despair**, where the focus tends to be reflective and contemplative. If favorably resolved, we will see wisdom, which Erikson defined as detached concern with life itself, with assurance in the meaning of life, dignity, and an acceptance of the fact that one's life has been worthwhile, along with a readiness to face death. If not resolved favorably, there will be feelings of bitterness about one's life, a feeling that life has been worthless, and at the same time, fear over one's own impending death.

ERIKSON'S STAGE (CRISIS)	AGE	EXISTENTIAL QUESTION
Trust *vs.* mistrust	0 to 1 year	Can I trust the world?
Autonomy *vs.* shame and doubt	1 to 3 years	Is it okay to be me?
Initiative *vs.* guilt	3 to 6 years	Is it okay for me to do, move, and act?
Industry *vs.* inferiority	6 to 12 years	Can I make it in the world of people and things?
Identity *vs.* role confusion	12 to 20 years	Who am I? What can I be?
Intimacy *vs.* isolation	20 to 40 years	Can I love?
Generativity *vs.* stagnation	40 to 65 years	Can I make my life count?
Integrity *vs.* despair	65 years to death	Is it okay to have been me?

Table 6.2 Erikson's Stages of Psychosocial Development

Kohlberg: Moral Reasoning

Lawrence Kohlberg's theory of personality development focuses not on urges or on resolving conflicts, but rather on the development of moral thinking. For this reason, this theory is often called **Kohlberg's theory of moral reasoning**. Kohlberg reasoned that, as our cognitive abilities grow, we are able to think about the world in more complex and nuanced ways, and this directly affects the ways in which we resolve moral dilemmas and perceive the notion of right and wrong.

Kohlberg's observations about moral reasoning were based on responses of subjects to hypothetical moral dilemmas. One often-cited example is the *Heinz dilemma*. In this scenario, a man named Heinz has a wife who is dying of a rare disease. There is a druggist in the town who invented a drug that could cure the disease. It costs him $200 to produce, yet he sells it for $2000. Heinz cannot afford this price, so he goes to the druggist and asks him if he would lower the price, a request that the druggist refuses. Desperate to save his wife, Heinz breaks into the druggist's office one night and steals the medication. Kohlberg presented dilemmas such as this one to volunteers and asked them to explain whether the characters in the story acted morally and why or why not. Kohlberg wasn't interested in the participants' appraisal of the actions as right or wrong, as he believed either answer could be justified. Instead, he was far more interested in the reasoning behind the appraisal. Based on the participants' responses, Kohlberg organized moral reasoning into six distinct stages ranging from the concrete to the abstract. He then organized these stages into three phases consisting of two stages each. Kohlberg's stages are summarized in Table 6.3.

Preconventional morality, the first of these phases, is typical of preadolescent thinking and places an emphasis on the consequences of the moral choice. Stage one (**obedience**) is concerned with avoiding punishment (*If I steal the drug, I'll go to jail*), while stage two (**self-interest**) is about gaining rewards (*I need to save my wife because I want to spend more of my life with her*). Stage two is often called the **instrumental relativist stage** because it is based on the concepts of reciprocity and sharing: *I'll scratch your back, you scratch mine.*

The second phase is **conventional morality**, which begins to develop in early adolescence when individuals begin to see themselves in terms of their relationships to others. This phase is based on understanding and accepting social rules. Stage three (**conformity**) places emphasis on the "nice person" orientation in which an individual seeks the approval of others (*I should not steal the drug because stealing is wrong*). Stage four (**law and order**) maintains the social order in the highest regard (*If everyone stole things they couldn't afford, people who produce those items would not be able to continue their business*).

KEY CONCEPT

Conventional morality corresponds to average adult moral reasoning. Preconventional is therefore expected in children, and postconventional is expected in a smaller subset of adults with more advanced moral reasoning skills than the average population.

The third phase is **postconventional morality**, which describes a level of reasoning that Kohlberg claimed not everyone was capable of and is based on social mores, which may conflict with laws. Stage five (**social contract**) views moral rules as conventions that are designed to ensure the greater good, with reasoning focused on individual rights (*Everyone has a right to live; businesses have a right to profit from their products*). Finally, stage six (**universal human ethics**) reasons that decisions should be made in consideration of abstract principles (*It is wrong for one person to hold another's life for ransom*).

Kohlberg viewed these stages as a progression in which each stage is adopted and then abandoned for the next as the individual progresses. In other words, we all begin in stage one and progress to varying degrees as our thinking matures.

Kohlberg is not without his critics. Some argue that postconventional morality describes views that are more prevalent in individualistic societies and is therefore biased against collectivist cultures. Similarly, Kohlberg's research was only performed using male subjects, which may cloud differences in reasoning patterns that may exist between genders.

PHASE	AGE	STAGES
Preconventional morality	Preadolescence	1: Obedience 2: Self-interest
Conventional morality	Adolescence to adulthood	3: Conformity 4: Law and order
Postconventional morality	Adulthood (if at all)	5: Social contract 6: Universal human ethics

Table 6.3 Kohlberg's Stages of Moral Development

Vygotsky: Cultural and Biosocial Development

BRIDGE

Kohlberg and Vygotsky's theories of cognitive development were both heavily influenced by Piaget's work in this area, discussed in Chapter 4 of *MCAT Behavioral Sciences Review.*

Like Kohlberg, Lev Vygotsky's work was focused on understanding cognitive development. For Vygotsky, the engine driving cognitive development was the child's internalization of various aspects of culture: rules, symbols, language, and so on. As the child internalized these various interpersonal and cultural rules, cognitive activity developed accordingly.

Vygotsky is known for his concept of the **zone of proximal development**, referring to those skills and abilities that have not yet fully developed but are in the process of development. Gaining these skills successfully requires the help of a "more knowledgeable other," typically an adult. For example, children may struggle to ride a bicycle on their own, but with the help and guidance of an adult may be successful. Vygotsky would say that this skill is currently within the children's zone of proximal development.

The Influence of Others on Identity

Our personalities do not form in a vacuum; we are as much a product of those around us as a product of our own internal growth and development. Albert Bandura, who was also the psychologist behind the Bobo doll experiment described in Chapter 3 of *MCAT Behavioral Sciences Review*, claimed that observational learning contributes greatly to our future behaviors.

Young children observe and encode the behaviors they see in others, and may later imitate these behaviors. Children are more likely to imitate behaviors performed by someone who is like them: for example, young children will reliably mimic behaviors performed by their same-gender siblings. Children's first models are their caregivers, but as children grow and form more relationships, other role models emerge. Siblings, teachers, and the media all play an important role in modeling behavior for a developing child, but by adolescence, peers become the most important role models in a person's life.

As children grow, they become more able to see the identities of others as different from their own. They might experiment with other identities by taking on the roles of others, such as when children play *house* or *school*. Such **role-taking** is good practice for later in life, when a child begins to understand the perspectives and roles of others. Eventually, children become able to see how others perceive them and to imagine themselves from the outside. The ability to sense how another's mind works—for example, understanding how a friend is interpreting a story while you tell it—is referred to as **theory of mind**. Once we develop a theory of mind, we begin to recognize and react to how others think about us. We become aware of judgments from the outside world and react to these judgments. Our reactions to how others perceive us can be varied—maintaining, modifying, downplaying, or accentuating different aspects of our personality. Our understanding of how others see us, which relies on perceiving a reflection of ourselves based on the words and actions of others, is appropriately called the **looking-glass self**.

A related concept is a **reference group**, the group that we use as a standard to evaluate ourselves. Our self-concept often depends on whom we are comparing ourselves to. For example, in 2012, the average annual salary for a physician in the United States was about $200,000. Compared to the national median household salary (approximately $50,000), these individuals were quite well off. However, only 11 percent considered themselves "rich." Why? Many physicians live in higher socioeconomic areas and regularly interact with other physicians, and their responses may thus be biased by comparison to those around them.

MCAT CONCEPT CHECK 6.2

Before you move on, assess your understanding of the material with these questions.

1. Each of the following theorists evaluates an individual and determines that the person has failed in completing one of the theorist's developmental stages. What would each say is the most likely outcome for this person?
   - Freud:

   ____

   - Erikson:

   ____

   - Kohlberg:

   ____

2. Name and briefly describe the three major phases of Kohlberg's theory of moral development.

Phase	Description

3. How could Vygotsky's concept of zone of proximal development be applied to standardized test preparation?

   ____

6.3 Personality

High-Yield

LEARNING OBJECTIVES

After Chapter 6.3, you will be able to:

- Describe how personality is defined by the psychoanalytic, humanistic, type, behaviorist, social cognitive, biological, and trait perspectives
- List the traits described by Eysenck's PEN theory
- List the Big Five personality traits
- Recall the roles of the id, ego, and superego in the psychoanalytic perspective of personality

We've seen that identity is the way we define ourselves. **Personality**, while similar, describes the set of thoughts, feelings, traits, and behaviors that are characteristic of an individual across time and location. In a way, identity describes who we are, while personality describes how we act and react to the world around us. There are many different theories of personality, and different theorists within each category espouse sometimes conflicting views in an attempt to describe behavior. Like the various theories of development discussed earlier in this chapter, some of these ideas have been discredited, and so will only be tested on the MCAT from a historical perspective.

We can categorize theories of personality into four areas: psychoanalytic (psychodynamic), humanistic (phenomenological), type and trait, and behaviorist. There are great differences between and within these divisions in how personality is defined and how abnormal personalities are explained.

MCAT EXPERTISE

The psychoanalytic perspective, much like other Freudian and Jungian theories within psychology, is not backed by more modern understandings of personality and has fallen from use in professional circles, though it remains prevalent in popular culture. However, the psychoanalytic perspective is useful as a contrast to other theories of personality, and is included within testable materials as laid out by the AAMC.

The Psychoanalytic Perspective

The **psychoanalytic** or **psychodynamic theories of personality** contain some of the most widely varying perspectives on behavior, but they all have in common the assumption of unconscious internal states that motivate the overt actions of individuals and determine personality. The most noteworthy supporter of the psychoanalytic theory is Freud.

Sigmund Freud

Freud's contribution to the study of personality was his structural model, which involved three major entities: the id, ego, and superego, illustrated in Figure 6.2.

REAL WORLD

If a person is hungry and food is unavailable, wish fulfillment—fantasizing or daydreaming about food—helps relieve some of the tension created by the pleasure principle.

The **id** consists of all the basic, primal, inborn urges to survive and reproduce. It functions according to the **pleasure principle**, in which the aim is to achieve immediate gratification to relieve any pent-up tension. The **primary process** is the id's response to frustration based on the pleasure principle: *obtain satisfaction now, not later*. Mental imagery, such as daydreaming or fantasy, that fulfills this need for satisfaction is termed **wish fulfillment**.

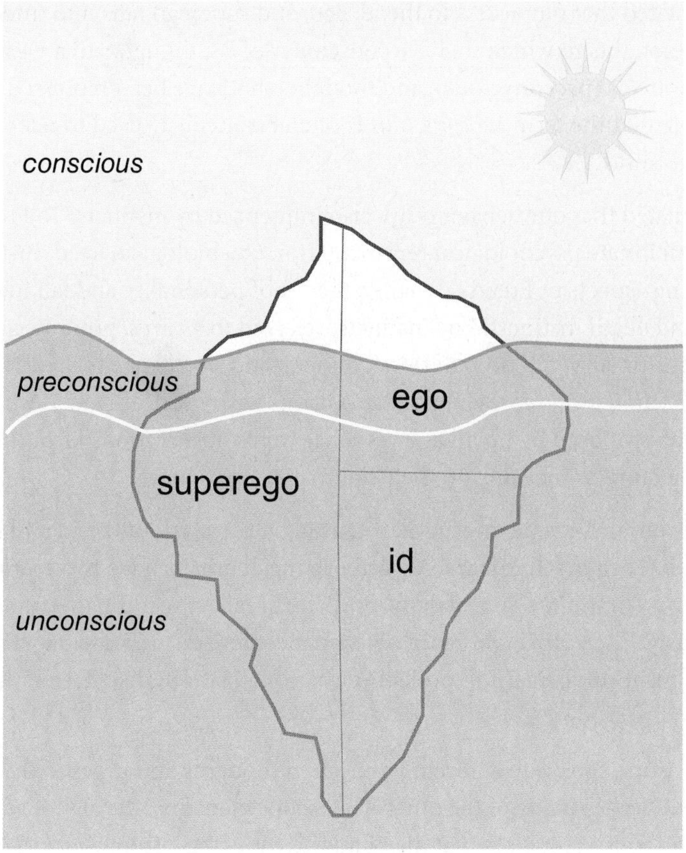

Figure 6.2 Freud's Topographic Model of the Mind

Because this mental image cannot effectively reduce tension on a permanent basis, the **ego** comes into play. The ego operates according to the **reality principle**, taking into account objective reality as it guides or inhibits the activity of the id and the id's pleasure principle. This guidance is referred to as the **secondary process**. The aim of the reality principle is to postpone the pleasure principle until satisfaction can actually be obtained. It must be emphasized that while the ego suspends the workings of the primary process, it does so only to meet the demands of objective reality. The mutual give and take of the ego and reality promotes the growth of perception, memory, problem solving, thinking, and reality testing. The ego can be understood to be the organizer of the mind: it receives its power from—and can never be fully independent of—the id.

The ego is also responsible for moderating the desires of the superego. Whereas the id's desires are basic needs, those of the superego are refined and focused on the ideal self. The **superego** is the personality's perfectionist, judging our actions and responding with pride at our accomplishments and guilt at our failures. The superego can be divided into two subsystems, both of which are a reflection of the morals taught to children by their caregivers. The **conscience** is a collection of the improper actions for which a child is punished, and the **ego-ideal** consists of those proper actions for which a child is rewarded. Ultimately, a system of right and wrong substitutes for caregivers' rewards and punishments.

REAL WORLD

When stuck in traffic, our id may desire to honk loudly at the cars in front of us, or to even pull over to the shoulder of the highway and drive recklessly past the congestion. Our ego knows that this would be unwise, and may advise us to breathe deeply and change the radio station to something calming instead.

Freud also stated that our access to the id, ego, and superego falls into three main categories: thoughts to which we have conscious access, thoughts that we aren't currently aware of (**preconscious**), and thoughts that have been repressed (**unconscious**). Note that the term *subconscious* is often erroneously used to refer to Freud's unconscious mind.

Freud postulated that our behaviors are also influenced by instincts. To Freud, an **instinct** is an innate psychological representation of a biological need. Instincts are the propelling aspects of Freud's dynamic theory of personality and fall into two types: life and death instincts. Life instincts, referred to as *Eros*, promote an individual's quest for survival through thirst, hunger, and sexual needs. Death instincts, referred to as *Thanatos*, represent an unconscious wish for death and destruction. *Thanatos* was proposed by Freud as a response to his observations of victims of trauma reenacting or focusing on their traumatic experiences.

The ego's recourse for relieving anxiety caused by the clash of the id and superego is through **defense mechanisms**. All defense mechanisms have two common characteristics: first, they deny, falsify, or distort reality; second, they operate unconsciously. There are eight main defense mechanisms: repression, suppression, regression, reaction formation, projection, rationalization, displacement, and sublimation.

KEY CONCEPT

While repression is unconscious forgetting (such as that which may occur after traumatic events), suppression is a conscious form of forgetting: *I'm not going to think about that right now.*

Repression is the ego's way of forcing undesired thoughts and urges to the unconscious and underlies many of the other defense mechanisms, the aim of which is to disguise threatening impulses that may find their way back from the unconscious. While repression is mostly an unconscious forgetting, **suppression** is a more deliberate, conscious form of forgetting.

Regression is reversion to an earlier developmental state. Faced with stress, older children may return to earlier behaviors such as thumb sucking, throwing temper tantrums, or clinging to their caregivers.

Reaction formation occurs when an individual suppresses urges by unconsciously converting these urges into their exact opposites. For example, a person pining after an inaccessible celebrity may outwardly express hatred for the celebrity as a way of reducing the stress caused by these unrequited feelings.

Projection is the defense mechanism by which individuals attribute their undesired feelings to others. *I hate my parents* might, for example, turn into *My parents hate me.* Projection is an important part of personality analysis. Tests that make use of projection to gain insight into a client's mind are common in psychoanalytic therapy. For example, the **Rorschach inkblot test**, shown in Figure 6.3, relies on the assumption that clients project their unconscious feelings onto the shape.

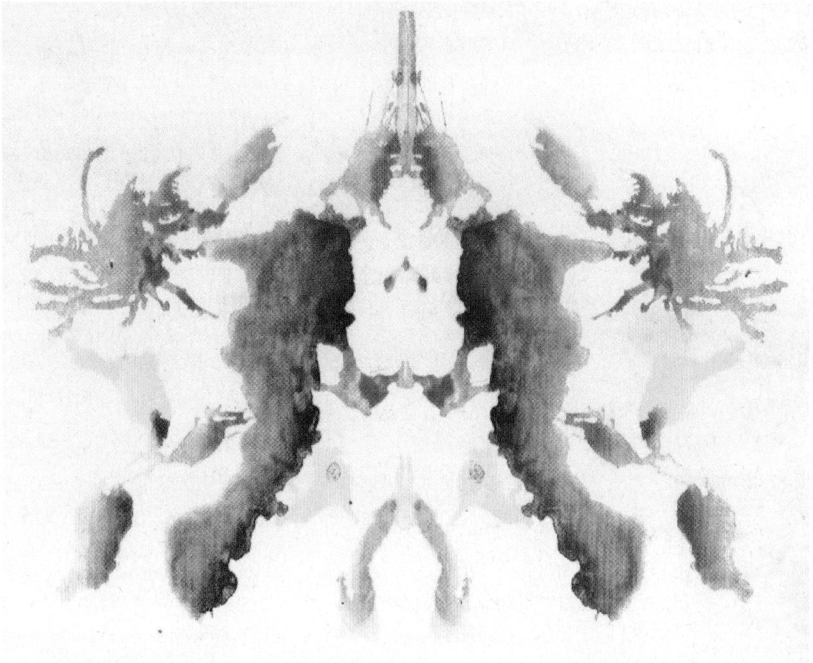

Figure 6.3 Card #10 from the Rorschach Inkblot Test

Similarly, the **thematic apperception test** consists of a series of pictures that are presented to the client, who is asked to make up a story about each one. The story, presumably, will elucidate the client's own unconscious thoughts and feelings.

Rationalization is the justification of behaviors in a manner that is acceptable to the self and society. Drivers who engage in reckless feats such as the Cannonball Run (a cross-country race from Los Angeles to New York) might justify their dangerous pursuits by saying, both to themselves and others: *I'm in complete control, and besides, there are plenty of dangerous drivers on the road. What difference will one more make?*

Displacement describes the transference of an undesired urge from one person or object to another. Someone angry at a supervisor at work may remain quiet there but snap at a family member at home.

Finally, **sublimation** is the transformation of unacceptable urges into socially acceptable behaviors. Freud might say that pent-up sexual urges may be sublimated into a drive for business success or artistic creativity.

The descriptions of the most commonly tested defense mechanisms, as well as examples, are provided in Table 6.4.

DEFENSE MECHANISM	DESCRIPTION	EXAMPLE
Repression	Unconsciously removing an idea or feeling from consciousness	A person who survived six months in a concentration camp cannot recall anything about life during that time period
Suppression	Consciously removing an idea or feeling from consciousness	A terminally ill cancer patient puts aside feelings of anxiety to enjoy a family gathering
Regression	Returning to an earlier stage of development	A person speaks to a significant other in "baby talk" when relaying bad news
Reaction formation	An unacceptable impulse is transformed into its opposite	Two coworkers fight all the time because they are actually very attracted to each other
Projection	Attribution of wishes, desires, thoughts, or emotions to someone else	A person who has committed adultery is convinced the spouse is cheating, despite a lack of evidence
Rationalization	Justification of attitudes, beliefs, or behaviors	A murderer who claims that, while killing is wrong, this particular victim "deserved it"
Displacement	Changing the target of an emotion, while the feelings remain the same	When sent to their room as punishment, children begin to punch and kick their pillows
Sublimation	Channeling of an unacceptable impulse in a socially acceptable direction	A boss who is attracted to an employee becomes that employee's mentor and advisor

Table 6.4 Commonly Tested Defense Mechanisms

Carl Jung

Later psychoanalytic theories have given more emphasis to interpersonal, sociological, and cultural influences, while maintaining their link with the psychoanalytic tradition. Carl Jung preferred to think of libido as psychic energy in general, not just psychic energy rooted in sexuality. Jung identified the ego as the conscious mind, and he divided the unconscious into two parts: the **personal unconscious**, similar to Freud's notion of the unconscious, and the collective unconscious. The **collective unconscious** is a powerful system that is shared among all humans and considered to be a residue of the experiences of our early ancestors. Its building blocks are images of common experiences, such as having caregivers as children. These images invariably have an emotional element, and are referred to as **archetypes** in Jung's theory. You can see an example of two archetypal images in Figure 6.4: God and the Devil.

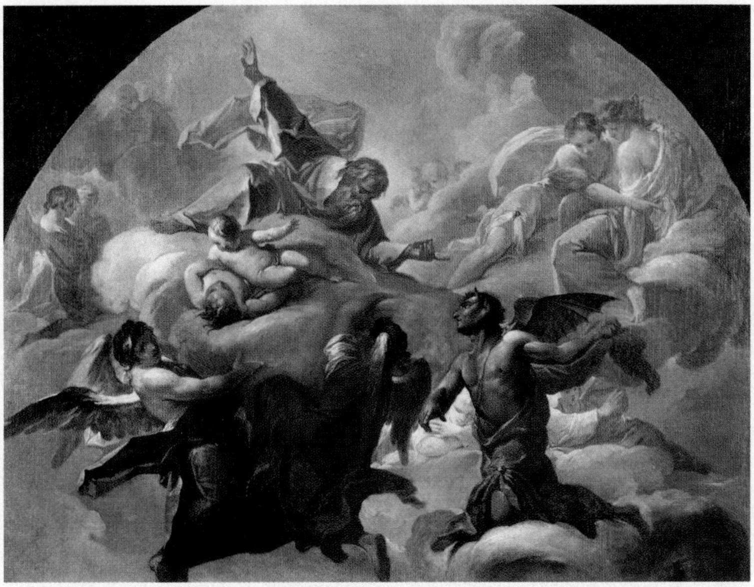

Figure 6.4 Jungian Archetypes: God and the Devil
Archetypes are underlying forms or concepts that give rise to archetypal images, which may differ somewhat between cultures.

There are several important Jungian archetypes. The **persona** is likened to a mask that we wear in public, and is the part of our personality that we present to the world. Like our identity, Jung described the persona as adaptive to our social interactions, emphasizing those qualities that improve our social standing and suppressing our other, less desirable qualities. The **anima** (feminine) and the **animus** (masculine) describe gender-inappropriate qualities—in other words, feminine behaviors in males and masculine behaviors in females. For example, in Jung's theory, the anima is the suppressed female quality in males that explains emotional behavior (described by Jung as a *man's inner woman*), while the animus is the analogous male quality of females that explains power-seeking behavior (*a woman's inner man*). The **shadow** archetype is responsible for the appearance of unpleasant and socially reprehensible thoughts, feelings, and actions experienced in the unconscious mind.

The **self**, to Jung, was the point of intersection between the collective unconscious, the personal unconscious, and the conscious mind. The self strives for unity. Jung symbolized the self as a *mandala* (Sanskrit: "circle"), shown in Figure 6.5. Jung saw the mandala, a symbol of the universe in Buddhism and Hinduism, as the mythic expression of the self: the reconciler of opposites and the promoter of harmony. Jung also developed **word association testing** to assess how unconscious elements may be influencing the conscious mind and thus the self. In word association testing, patients respond to a single word with the first word that comes to mind. Jung believed that patient responses, in combination with evaluating mood and speed of response, would reveal elements of the unconscious.

KEY CONCEPT

Important Jungian archetypes:

- Persona—the aspect of our personality we present to the world
- Anima—a "man's inner woman"
- Animus—a "woman's inner man"
- Shadow—unpleasant and socially reprehensible thoughts, feelings, and actions experienced in the unconscious mind

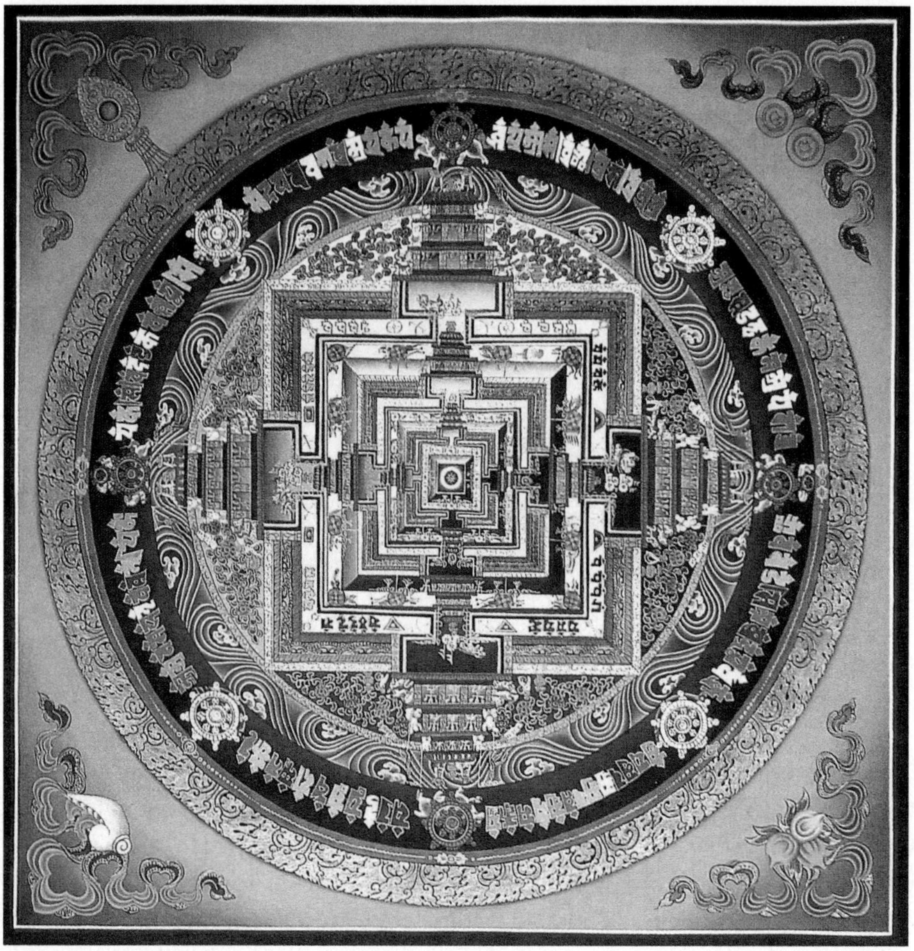

Figure 6.5 Tibetan Mandala

Jung saw the self as a mandala: the promoter of unity, balance, and harmony between the conscious mind, personal unconscious, and collective unconscious.

Jung described three dichotomies of personality:

- Extraversion (E, orientation toward the external world) *vs.* introversion (I, orientation toward the inner, personal world)
- Sensing (S, obtaining objective information about the world) *vs.* intuiting (N, working with information abstractly)
- Thinking (T, using logic and reason) *vs.* feeling (F, using a value system or personal beliefs)

In most individuals, both sides of each dichotomy are present to some degree, but one tends to dominate. Jung's work laid the groundwork for creation of the **Myers–Briggs Type Inventory** (**MBTI**), a classic personality test. Each of Jung's three dichotomies, and a fourth—judging (J, preferring orderliness) *vs.* perceiving (P, preferring spontaneity)—is labeled as a specific personality type, as shown in Figure 6.6.

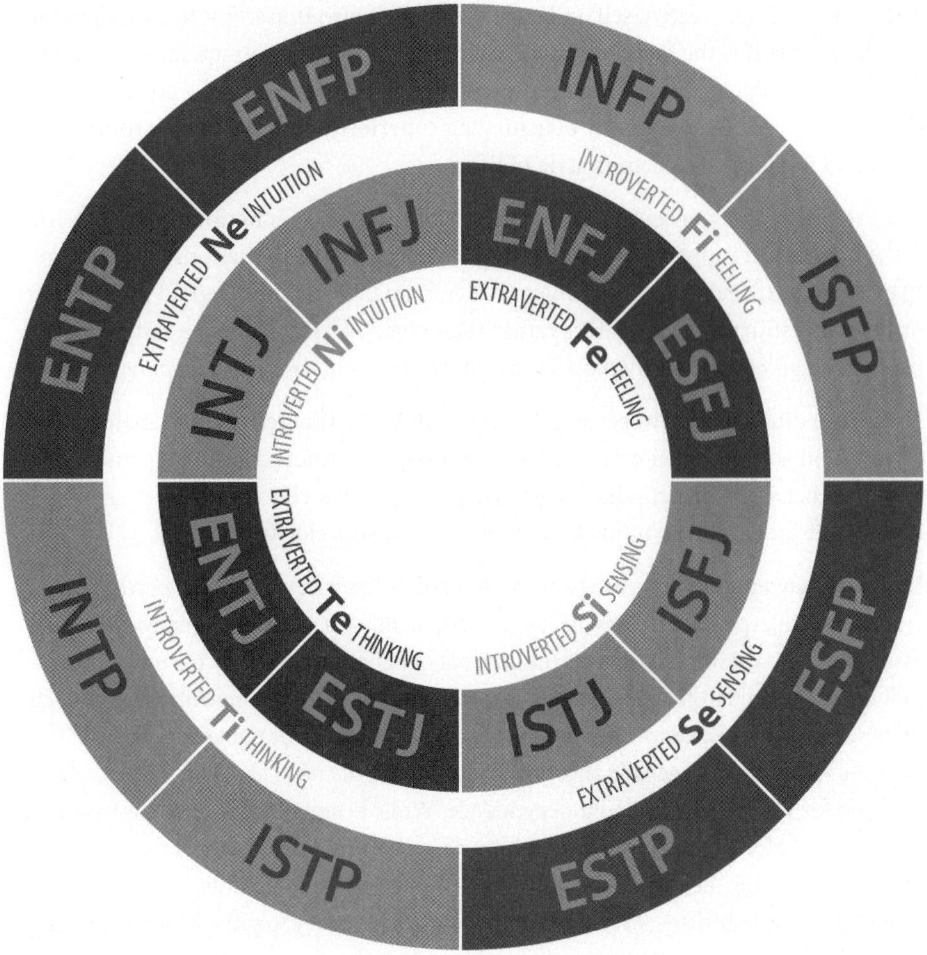

Figure 6.6 Myers-Briggs Type Inventory Personality Types

Other Psychoanalysts

As with most psychological movements, psychoanalysis gained a following of theorists who learned from and often disagreed with its original tenets. In opposition to many of Freud's key ideas, later psychoanalysts often emphasized social rather than sexual motivations for behavior. Jung can be counted among these, as can Alfred Adler, whose theory focused on the immediate social imperatives of family and society and their effects on unconscious factors.

Adler was the originator of the concept of the **inferiority complex**: an individual's sense of incompleteness, imperfection, and inferiority both physically and socially. According to Adler, striving for superiority drives the personality. This striving enhances the personality when it is oriented toward benefiting society, but yields disorder when it is selfish.

The notions of the creative self and style of life were also important to Adler's theory. The **creative self** is the force by which individuals shape their uniqueness and establish their personality. **Style of life** represents the manifestation of the creative self and describes a person's unique way of achieving superiority. The family environment is crucial in molding the person's style of life.

Another important concept in Adler's theory of personality is **fictional finalism**. This is the notion that individuals are motivated more by their expectations of the future than by past experiences. According to Adler, human goals are based on the subjective or fictional estimate of life's values rather than objective data from the past. Fictional finalism can often be summed up by the phrase *Life would be perfect if only...*

Notice the difference between Freud, Jung, and Adler. Whereas Freud's major assumption is that behavior is motivated by inborn instincts and Jung's principal axiom is that a person's conduct is governed by inborn archetypes, Adler assumes that people are primarily motivated by striving for superiority.

Karen Horney, another dissenting student of Freud's, likewise argued that personality is a result of interpersonal relationships, and adamantly disagreed with many of Freud's assumptions about women, such as the concept of penis envy. Horney postulated that individuals with neurotic personalities are governed by one of ten **neurotic needs**. Each of these needs is directed toward making life and interactions bearable. Examples of these neurotic needs are the need for affection and approval, the need to exploit others, and the need for self-sufficiency and independence. While healthy people have these needs to some degree, Horney emphasized that these needs become problematic if they fit at least one of four criteria: they are disproportionate in intensity, they are indiscriminate in application, they partially disregard reality, or they have a tendency to provoke intense anxiety. For instance, someone with a neurotic need for self-sufficiency and independence would go to great extremes to avoid being obligated to someone else in any way. As the central focus of the person's life, it would be a neurotic need and not a healthy one.

Horney's primary concept is that of basic anxiety. This is based on the premise that children's early perception of self is important and stems from their relationship with their caregivers. Inadequate caregiving can cause vulnerability and helplessness, which Horney termed **basic anxiety**, while neglect and rejection cause anger known as **basic hostility**. To overcome basic anxiety or basic hostility and attain a degree of security, children use three strategies in their relationships with others: moving toward people to obtain the goodwill of people who provide security; moving against people, or fighting them to obtain the upper hand; and moving away, or withdrawing, from people. These three strategies are the general headings under which the ten neurotic needs fall. Healthy people use all three strategies, depending on the situation. However, the highly threatened child will use one of these strategies rigidly and exclusively, and carries this strategy into adulthood.

Object relations theory also falls under the realm of psychodynamic theories of personality. In this context, *object* refers to the representation of caregivers based on subjective experiences during early infancy. These objects then persist into adulthood and impact our interactions with others, including the social bonds we create and our predictions of others' behavior.

The Humanistic Perspective

In direct contrast to the psychoanalysts, who focus on "sick" individuals and their troubling urges, **humanistic** or **phenomenological theorists** focus on the value of individuals and take a more person-centered approach, describing those ways in which healthy people strive toward self-realization. Humanism is often associated with **Gestalt therapy**, in which practitioners tend to take a holistic view of the self, seeing each individual as a complete person rather than reducing the person to individual behaviors or drives. For the humanists, our personality is the result of the conscious feelings we have for ourselves as we attempt to attain our needs and goals.

Kurt Lewin's **force field theory** puts very little stock in constraints on personalities such as fixed traits, habits, or structures such as the id, ego, and superego. Further, Lewin focused little on an individual's past or future, focusing instead on situations in the present. Lewin defined the field as one's current state of mind, which was simply the sum of the forces (influences) on the individual at that time. If the focus of humanistic psychology is exploring how an individual reaches self-realization, then these forces could be divided into two large groups: those assisting in our attainment of goals and those blocking the path to them.

Abraham Maslow, whose hierarchy of needs is discussed in Chapter 5 of *MCAT Behavioral Sciences Review*, was a humanist who studied the lives of individuals such as Ludwig van Beethoven, Albert Einstein, and Eleanor Roosevelt, who he felt were self-actualizers and had lived rich and productive lives. He identified several characteristics that these people had in common, including a nonhostile sense of humor, originality, creativity, spontaneity, and a need for some privacy. According to Maslow, self-actualized people are more likely than people who are not self-actualized to have what he called **peak experiences**: profound and deeply moving experiences in a person's life that have important and lasting effects on the individual.

George Kelly used himself as a model to theorize about human nature, and set aside the traditional concepts of motivation, unconscious emotion, and reinforcement in his descriptions of **personal construct psychology**. Kelly thought of the individual as a scientist, a person who devises and tests predictions about the behavior of significant people in the individual's life. The individual constructs a scheme of anticipation of what others will do, based on knowledge, perception, and relationships with these other people. Thus, the anxious person, rather than being the victim of inner conflicts and pent-up energy (as in psychodynamic theory), is one who is having difficulty constructing and understanding the variables in the environment. According to Kelly, psychotherapy is a process of insight whereby people acquire new constructs that will allow them to successfully predict troublesome events. Then, the individual will be able to integrate these new constructs into already existing ones.

Carl Rogers is most known for his psychotherapy technique known as **client-centered**, **person-centered**, or **nondirective** therapy. Rogers believed that people have the freedom to control their own behavior, and are neither slaves to the unconscious (as the psychoanalysts would suggest), nor subjects of faulty learning (as the behaviorists would say). Rather than providing solutions or diagnoses, the person-centered therapist helps clients reflect on problems, make choices, generate solutions, take positive action, and determine their own destiny. Rogers was the originator of the concepts of the real and ideal self discussed earlier in the chapter, and his therapeutic techniques aimed to help clients reconcile the differences between the various selves and reduce stress-inducing incongruence. Rogers also pioneered the concept of **unconditional positive regard**, a therapeutic technique by which the therapist accepts the client completely and expresses empathy in order to promote a positive therapeutic environment.

The Type and Trait Perspectives

The type and trait theorists were also borne out of dissatisfaction with psychoanalysis. **Type theorists** attempt to create a taxonomy of personality types, while **trait theorists** prefer to describe individual personality as the sum of a person's characteristic behaviors. For our purposes, we will consider them together.

Early attempts at personality types are generally discredited today. The ancient Greeks, for example, devised **personality types** based on **humors** or body fluids, an imbalance of which could lead to various personality disorders, as shown in Figure 6.7.

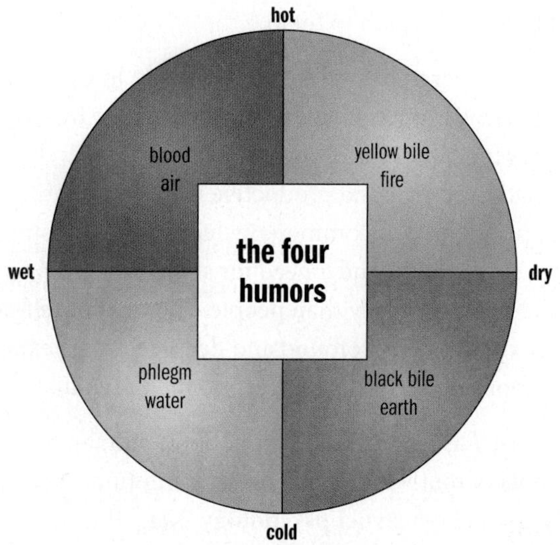

Figure 6.7 The Four Humors
Each humor was correlated with an element, an imbalance of which could lead to different personalities: blood (sanguine; impulsive and charismatic), bile (choleric; aggressive and dominant), black bile (melancholic; depressive and cautious), and phlegm (phlegmatic; relaxed and affectionate).

In the early 20th century, William Sheldon proposed personality types based on body type called **somatotypes**. Sheldon presumed that all short, stocky people were jolly, all tall people were high-strung and aloof, and people in between were strong and well-adjusted. One well-known type theory divides personalities into Types A and B. Individuals with **Type A** personalities are characterized by behavior that tends to be competitive and compulsive, while someone described as **Type B** is generally laid-back and relaxed. Not surprisingly, people with Type A personalities are more prone to heart disease than those with Type B personalities, although there is not much evidence to suggest that people with Type A personalities have a higher mortality rate.

The Myers–Briggs Type Inventory, described earlier in this chapter, also stands as a well-known example of a type theory.

Trait theorists instead use clusters of behaviors to describe individuals. Hans and Sybil Eysenck used factor analysis to group behaviors that typically occur together and assigned labels to those groups. These groups of behaviors are often also called **traits**. For example, people who are more reserved and less outspoken in groups also tend to enjoy solitary activities and avoid overstimulation. These behaviors fall under the label of introversion. The Eysencks described three traits in the **PEN model**: **Psychoticism** is a measure of nonconformity or social deviance. **Extraversion** is a measure of tolerance for social interaction and stimulation. **Neuroticism** is a measure of emotional arousal in stressful situations.

Negative affect, though not directly included in the PEN model, is related to neuroticism and describes how a person thinks of themselves and experiences negative emotions. High negative affect corresponds with neuroticism and anxiety, and is associated with several mood disorders. The Eysencks reasoned that people could be distinguished from one another based on where they fell in each of these three dimensions. More recently, the PEN theory has been expanded to what is known as the Five Factor Model, the **Big Five**, which as the name would suggest, uses dimensions of five traits: openness, conscientiousness, extraversion, agreeableness, and neuroticism. In this theory, **openness** describes openness to experience, or willingness to engage with the world and desire to try new things. Low openness is associated with persevering in tasks and difficulty with abstraction. **Conscientiousness** is in some ways analogous to self control, with high conscientiousness associated with high impulse control and low conscientiousness associated with spontaneity. **Agreeableness** refers to the degree to which a person is concerned about maintaining peace and harmony in their interactions with others.

MNEMONIC

The Big Five Traits of Personality: **OCEAN**

- **O**penness
- **C**onscientiousness
- **E**xtraversion
- **A**greeableness
- **N**euroticism

Gordon Allport, primarily a trait theorist, listed three basic types of traits or dispositions: cardinal, central, and secondary. **Cardinal traits** are traits around which people organize their lives. For instance, Mother Teresa's cardinal trait may have been self-sacrifice. While not everyone develops a cardinal trait, everyone does have central and secondary traits. **Central traits** represent major characteristics of the personality that are easy to infer, such as honesty or charisma. **Secondary traits** are other personal characteristics that are more limited in occurrence: aspects of one's personality that only appear in close groups or specific social situations. A major part of Allport's theory is the concept of **functional autonomy**, in which a behavior continues despite satisfaction of the drive that originally created the behavior. A hunter, for example, may have originally hunted to obtain food to eat. However, the hunter may continue even after there is enough food simply for the enjoyment of the hunt: that which began as a means to obtain a goal became the goal itself.

David McClelland identified a personality trait that is referred to as the need for achievement (N-Ach). People who are rated high in N-Ach tend to be concerned with achievement and have pride in their accomplishments. These individuals avoid high risks (to avoid failing) and low risks (because easy tasks will not generate a sense of achievement). Additionally, they set realistic goals, and stop striving toward a goal if success is unlikely.

BEHAVIORAL SCIENCES GUIDED EXAMPLE WITH EXPERT THINKING

Flow is a psychological state marked by high but subjectively effortless attention to a task that usually is accompanied by feelings of complete immersion, enjoyment, and loss of a sense of time. Feelings of flow are maximal in cases in which the task provides a significant challenge, but the individual's skill allows them to meet that challenge.

New term: flow. Challenge and task tell me this may be related to Yerkes–Dodson. I'll be on the lookout for more relationships between these concepts.

Flow proneness, the likelihood that an individual will enter a flow state given an appropriate compatibility between skill and demand, correlates positively with psychological well-being, self-esteem, life satisfaction, coping strategies, and conscientiousness. It has also been shown that flow proneness correlates negatively with traits related to neuroticism, such as trait anxiety.

New term: flow proneness. Self-esteem stands out here as a component of identity. I also see conscientiousness and neuroticism, which opens the door for the MCAT to ask about the Big Five.

Behavioral inhibition is a temperamental trait associated with fear and avoidance of novel experience. Because behavioral inhibition is also associated with anxiety and neurotic introversion, it would be reasonable to expect that low behavioral inhibition correlates with flow proneness.

Yet another new term: behavioral inhibition (BI). I want to keep these relationships straight. BI is related to the same OCEAN traits that correspond with low flow proneness (FP), so FP should relate to low BI.

Since the feelings of happiness and enjoyment related to flow derive from intrinsic motivation and rewards, it has also been shown that flow proneness is also correlated with an internal locus of control. Indeed, those with an internal locus of control are more sensitive to differences between individual skill and task challenge but are more likely to experience flow when performing tasks in which skill and challenge are compatible. Locus of control has also been shown to relate to high conscientiousness and low neuroticism.

More relationships: locus of control (LoC) is related in several ways to FP, and one of those ways involves the OCEAN traits again. High FP = Internal LoC = Low BI

Researchers analyzed data from a web-based survey of approximately 11,000 twins registered with the Swedish Twin Registry. This survey included a flow proneness questionnaire, a locus of control scale, and a measure of behavioral inhibition.

Twin study = genetics.
IV: genetic relationship
DV: survey results

These results confirmed a low but statistically significant correlation between flow proneness, low behavioral inhibition, and internal locus of control.

Analyzing relationship between dependent variables (survey results). Confirms relationship that correlation is low but significant.

Analysis also showed a strong relationship between specific genetic markers and all three measures, indicating that a specific set of genes account for a significant amount of the variance in these traits between individuals, possibly through dopaminergic pathways. The data support a dominant inheritance pattern.

Genetics confirmed. Summary: a few genes related to dopamine might be behind incidence of all of these traits.

Adapted from: Mosing MA, Pedersen NL, Cesarini D, Johannesson M, Magnusson PKE, Nakamura J, et al. (2012) Genetic and Environmental Influences on the Relationship between Flow Proneness, Locus of Control and Behavioral Inhibition. *PLoS ONE* 7(11): e47958. https://doi.org/10.1371/journal.pone.0047958

Which theory of personality is most supported by this experiment, and in what way do concepts from the study of both identity and personality contribute to this support?

The question demands that we integrate the data from the study with our outside knowledge of theories of personality. This passage blends quite a few topics together, so we'll want to read strategically and identify where and when new topics are introduced and explained; any time the passage alludes to content that we've studied we want to be ready to answer at least one question about that topic, so it's worth taking a few seconds to remind ourselves of what we know. Trait theory is definitely included, since the passage makes explicit reference to two of the Big Five: conscientiousness, which is the tendency to be organized, self-disciplined, and achievement focused; and neuroticism, the tendency to be prone to psychological stress and quickness to experience unpleasant emotions such as anger and anxiety. Two more Big Five traits are hinted at in the discussion of behavioral inhibition, which mentions avoidance of novel experience (low openness to experience) and introversion (the opposite of extraversion). If we're careful to look for these types of links as we read the first time, it will save us quite a lot of time on Test Day.

The passage also mentions self-esteem and locus of control, two ideas related to self-concept, and states that they are related to the traits discussed. With all this talk of traits, it would be reasonable to think that the passage is supporting trait theory, but the phrasing of the question stem is key here. We are asked about the experiment specifically, which is only located in the last paragraph of the study. In fact, while we've included a lot of analysis for the sake of completeness, a particularly astute test taker might even avoid some of this analysis and focus solely on analyzing the experiment to answer this question. By tying genetics to personality traits, the experiment in the passage most strongly supports the biological perspective. Overall, the results demonstrate a correlation between the genes regulating dopamine and reward pathways and the traits relating to rewards such as discipline, motivation, and locus of control. Then those traits are linked to the tendency in question in the study, flow proneness.

In summary, while the passage discusses other theories of personality and does provide some support for trait theory, the experiment and data provided most directly support the biological perspective of personality theory.

Other Theories of Personality

Of course, entire textbooks can be (and in fact are) devoted to personality theorists and their ideas. The MCAT tests only the key ideas of each theory, or the concepts that overlap heavily with other topics in this text.

The **behaviorist** perspective, championed by B. F. Skinner, is based heavily on the concepts of operant conditioning, discussed in Chapter 3 of *MCAT Behavioral Sciences Review*. Skinner reasoned that personality is simply a reflection of behaviors that have been reinforced over time. Therapy, then, should focus on learning skills and changing behaviors through operant conditioning techniques. **Token economies**, for example, are often used in inpatient therapeutic settings: positive behavior is rewarded with tokens that can be exchanged for privileges, treats, or other reinforcers.

The **social cognitive** perspective takes behaviorism one step further, focusing not just on how our environment influences our behavior, but also on how we interact with that environment. Albert Bandura's concept of reciprocal determinism is a central idea to this perspective. **Reciprocal determinism** refers to the idea that our thoughts, feelings, behaviors, and environment all interact with each other to determine our actions in a given situation. People choose environments that suit their personalities, and their personalities determine how they will feel about and react to events in those environments. Locus of control is another important concept in the social cognitive perspective: some people feel more in control of their environment while others feel that their environment controls them. For a social cognitive theorist, the best predictor of future behavior is past behavior in similar situations.

On the other end of the spectrum lies the **biological** perspective, which holds that personality can be explained as a result of genetic expression in the brain. The biological and trait perspectives are closely linked, as biological theorists maintain that many traits can be shown to result from genes or differences in brain anatomy.

The dichotomy presented by the social cognitive and biological perspectives of personality is similar to another debate in psychology: whether behavior is primarily determined by an individual's personality (the **dispositional approach**) or by the environment and context (the **situational approach**). This division is investigated in depth in the section on attribution theory in Chapter 10 of *MCAT Behavioral Sciences Review.*

MCAT CONCEPT CHECK 6.3

Before you move on, assess your understanding of the material with these questions.

1. For each of the following perspectives, briefly describe how each would define personality.
    - Psychoanalytic:
    - Humanistic:
    - Type:
    - Trait:
    - Behaviorist:
    - Social cognitive:
    - Biological:
2. What are the roles of the id, ego, and superego, according to the psychoanalytic perspective?
    - Id:
    - Ego:
    - Superego:

3. What are the traits described by the Eysencks' PEN theory, and what does each describe?
   - P:
   - E:
   - N:

4. What are the Big Five personality traits?
   1. ______
   2. ______
   3. ______
   4. ______
   5. ______

Conclusion

In this chapter, we discussed two concepts that are central to the study of psychology: identity, which describes who we are, and personality, which describes the set of thoughts, feelings, traits, and behaviors that are characteristic of each of us across time and different locations. We discussed a variety of approaches to both, each with their own theorists and critics. The ideas presented in this chapter are ripe for the MCAT to test; expect questions on Test Day to ask you to identify the various perspectives and the differences between them as they apply to behavior and research.

Many of the theories of personality focus on problems in everyday life: how we cope with stresses, anxiety, and depression. In medical school, your focus will be primarily on these pathologic states of mind, or psychological disorders. It is to this extremely important topic—abnormal psychology—that we turn our attention in the next chapter.

You've reviewed the content, now test your knowledge and critical thinking skills by completing a test-like passage set in your online resources!

GO ONLINE

CONCEPT SUMMARY

Self-Concept and Identity

- **Self-concept** is the sum of the ways in which we describe ourselves: in the present, who we used to be, and who we might be in the future.
- Our **identities** are individual components of our self-concept related to the groups to which we belong. Religious affiliation, sexual orientation, and ethnic and national affiliations are examples of identities.
- **Self-esteem** describes our evaluation of ourselves. Generally, the closer our **actual self** is to our **ideal self** (who we want to be) and our **ought self** (who others want us to be), the higher our self-esteem will be.
- **Self-efficacy** is the degree to which we see ourselves as being capable at a given skill or in a given situation. When placed in a consistently hopeless scenario, self-efficacy can be diminished to the point where **learned helplessness** results.
- **Locus of control** is a self-evaluation that refers to the way we characterize the influences in our lives. People with an internal locus of control see their successes and failures as a result of their own characteristics and actions, while those with an external locus of control perceive outside factors as having more of an influence in their lives.

Formation of Identity

- Freud's psychosexual stages of personality development are based on the tensions caused by the **libido**. Failure at any given stage leads to **fixation** that causes personality disorders. Freud's phases (oral, anal, phallic [Oedipal], latent, and genital) are based on the erogenous zones that are the focus of each phase of development.
- Erikson's stages of psychosocial development stem from conflicts that occur throughout life (trust *vs.* mistrust, autonomy *vs.* shame and doubt, initiative *vs.* guilt, industry *vs.* inferiority, identity *vs.* role confusion, intimacy *vs.* isolation, generativity *vs.* stagnation, integrity *vs.* despair). These conflicts are the result of decisions we are forced to make about ourselves and the environment around us at each phase of our lives.
- Kohlberg's stages of moral development describe the approaches of individuals to resolving moral dilemmas. Kohlberg believed that we progress through six stages divided into three main phases: **preconventional**, **conventional**, and **postconventional**.
- Vygotsky described development of language, culture, and skills. He proposed the idea of the **zone of proximal development**, which describes those skills that a child has not yet mastered and require a **more knowledgeable other** to accomplish.

- **Imitation** and **role-taking** are common ways children learn from others. Children first reproduce the behaviors of role models, and later learn to see the perspectives of others and practice taking on new roles.
- Our self-concept depends in part on our **reference group**, or the group to which we compare ourselves. Two individuals with the same qualities might see themselves differently depending on how those qualities compare to their reference groups.

Personality

- The **psychoanalytic** perspective views personality as resulting from unconscious urges and desires.
  - Freud's theories are based on the **id** (base urges of survival and reproduction), the **superego** (the idealist and perfectionist), and the **ego** (the mediator between the two and the conscious mind). The ego makes use of **defense mechanisms** to reduce stress caused by the urges of the id and the superego.
  - Jung assumed a **collective unconscious** that links all humans together. He viewed the personality as being influenced by **archetypes**.
  - Other psychoanalysts such as Adler and Horney have distanced themselves from Freud's theories, claiming that the unconscious is motivated by social rather than sexual urges.
- The **humanistic** perspective emphasizes the internal feelings of healthy individuals as they strive toward happiness and self-realization. Maslow's **hierarchy of needs** and Rogers's therapeutic approach of **unconditional positive regard** flow from the humanistic view of personality.
- **Type** and **trait** theorists believe that personality can be described as a number of identifiable traits that carry characteristic behaviors.
  - Type theories of personality include the ancient Greek notion of humors, Sheldon's **somatotypes**, division into **Types A** and **B**, and the **Myers–Briggs Type Inventory**.
  - The Eysencks identified three major traits which could be used to describe all individuals. The acronym for these traits is PEN: **psychoticism** (nonconformity), **extraversion** (tolerance for social interaction and stimulation), and **neuroticism** (arousal in stressful situations). Later trait theorists expanded these traits to the **Big Five**: openness, conscientiousness, extraversion, agreeableness, and neuroticism.
  - Allport identified three basic types of traits: cardinal, central, and secondary. **Cardinal traits** are the traits around which people organize their lives; not everyone develops a cardinal trait. **Central traits** represent major characteristics of the personality and **secondary traits** are more personal characteristics and are limited in occurrence.
  - McClelland identified the personality trait of the need for achievement (N-Ach).

- The **social cognitive** perspective holds that individuals interact with their environment in a cycle called **reciprocal determinism**. People mold their environments according to their personalities, and those environments in turn shape our thoughts, feelings, and behaviors.
- The **behaviorist** perspective, based on the concept of operant conditioning, holds that personality can be described as the behaviors one has learned from prior rewards and punishments.
- **Biological** theorists claim that behavior can be explained as a result of genetic expression.

ANSWERS TO CONCEPT CHECKS

6.1

1. Self-concept describes the sum of all of the phrases that come to mind when we think of who we are, who we used to be, and who we may become in the future. Identity, on the other hand, describes a set of behaviors and labels we take on when in a specific group.
2. Ethnic identity is determined by common ancestry, cultural heritage, and language, among other similarities. Rather than being determined by birth, national identity is determined by the political borders of where one lives and the cultural identity of that nation.
3. A student with an internal locus of control will look for internal factors, such as not having studied hard enough. A student with an external locus of control will blame external factors such as bad luck or the test being too difficult.

6.2

1. Freud would say that the individual has become fixated in that stage and will display the personality traits of that fixation for life. Erikson would say that the individual will still move through subsequent phases, but will be lacking the skills and virtues granted by successful resolution of that stage. Kohlberg would say that the individual was incapable of reasoning at the level of failure, and that the individual would use the reasoning described in previous stages to resolve moral dilemmas.
2.

Phase	Description
Preconventional	Reasoning is based on individual rewards and punishments
Conventional	Reasoning is based on the relationship of the individual to society
Postconventional	Reasoning is based on abstract principles

3. Zone of proximal development does not just apply to children, but rather the acquisition of new skills and abilities at any age. Standardized tests require students to utilize many skills that they may not yet have fully developed, but are in the process of development. This is why results can be improved by getting the help of those with more knowledge about the exam, such as expert instructors and authors.

6.3

1. Psychoanalytic: Personality is the result of unconscious urges and desires.

   Humanistic: Personality comes from conscious feelings about oneself resulting from healthy striving for self-realization.

   Type: Personalities are sets of distinct qualities and dispositions into which people can be grouped.

   Trait: Personalities are assembled from having different degrees of certain qualities and dispositions.

   Behaviorist: Personality is the result of behavioral responses to stimuli based on prior rewards and punishments.

   Social cognitive: Personality comes from the interactions between individuals and their environment.

   Biological: Personality is based on genetic influences and brain anatomy.
2. The id is the sum of our basic urges to reproduce and survive, while the superego is our sense of perfectionism and idealism. The ego mediates the anxieties caused by the actions of the id and superego by using defense mechanisms.
3. Psychoticism: nonconformity or social deviance

   Extraversion: tolerance for social interaction and stimulation

   Neuroticism: emotional arousal in stressful situations
4. The Big Five personality traits are openness, conscientiousness, extraversion, agreeableness, and neuroticism.

SCIENCE MASTERY ASSESSMENT EXPLANATIONS

1. **B**

Self-concept is defined as the sum of all of the ways in which we see ourselves, including who we are, as in **(D)**, who we were in the past, **(A)**, and who we may become in the future, **(C)**. The ought self, while closely related to self-esteem, is our appraisal of how others see us and is not a part of our self-concept.

2. **D**

Androgyny is defined as scoring highly on scales of both femininity and masculinity. Achieving a low score on both scales, **(A)**, would be considered undifferentiated, while **(B)** and **(C)** would be described as feminine and masculine, respectively.

3. **B**

Because there is nothing in the question stem to suggest that this situation will fundamentally change this student's attitudes in the short term, **(A)** and **(D)** can be eliminated. **(C)** is unlikely in the short term, as learned helplessness requires a repeated inability to have any effect on a situation over a long period of time and is much more severe, usually manifesting as depression. It is far more likely that the student will simply feel ineffective when it comes to math, which is low self-efficacy.

4. **A**

Because we know the lawyer has an internal locus of control, we expect belief in being in control of the events happening in life. Both **(B)** and **(C)** attribute success to outside factors, representing an external locus of control. While **(D)** perhaps represents an attribution that could correlate to low self-esteem, it is not indicative of locus of control.

5. **B**

Both excessive organization and excessive sloppiness are indicative of fixation in the anal stage of psychosexual development—what is commonly referred to as anal-retentiveness.

6. **C**

As a postadolescent young adult, this person would be described by Erikson as experiencing the conflict of intimacy *vs.* isolation, and so forming significant relationships with others would be a primary goal. **(B)** and **(D)** represent the next two stages in life (generativity *vs.* stagnation and integrity *vs.* despair, respectively), while **(A)** is the conflict that Erikson would say should have been resolved in adolescence (identity *vs.* role confusion).

7. **A**

Matt's reasoning reflects a desire to avoid punishment, which reflects stage one in Kohlberg's preconventional phase (obedience). Cati's reasoning takes into account social order, reflecting stage four in the conventional phase (law and order).

8. **D**

This situation is best described by Lev Vygotsky's zone of proximal development theory, which holds that children are often unable to perform tasks by themselves, but can complete the task with the help of a more knowledgeable other.

9. **D**

(C) has no support from role-taking research and can be eliminated. **(A)** and **(B)** are both inaccurate; the Bobo doll experiment shows young children modeling behavior not performed by their parents, and teens are most influenced by their peers, not celebrities and athletes. The research does suggest, however, that children are more likely to engage in behavior modeled by individuals who are like themselves; thus, a female child is more likely to imitate behavior by another female.

10. **C**

The superego is responsible for moral guilt when we do not live up to our ideals. While the id and the libido, **(A)** and **(D)**, may be responsible for the urge to have an affair, the superego is responsible for the anxiety one feels afterward.

11. **C**

Jung saw the drive for power and success as typically male traits, so Jung would say this woman is exercising her "inner man." The animus is the archetype that most closely reflects this quality.

12. **C**

This research supports a link between genetic expression and behavior, which is a central tenet of the biological perspective. The social cognitive perspective also holds that people's behaviors and traits shape their environments, which in turn have an effect on their identity, so the discovery also supports this perspective. Behaviorism is not supported, as the discovery is not related to rewards and punishments.

13. **B**

As a rebel and a sociable person, this individual would score highly on both psychoticism and extraversion, respectively. Neuroticism is associated with high emotional arousal in stressful situations, so being able to keep calm in an emergency is a sign of low neuroticism. Conscientiousness, a trait associated with being hardworking and organized instead of impulsive, is not described by the question stem.

14. **A**

Reaction formation is a defense mechanism that converts unwanted feelings into their exact opposite. A psychodynamic theorist would say that the terror and hatred victims feel toward their captors might be unconsciously turned into affection in an effort to reduce the stress of the situation.

15. **B**

Fictional finalism is comprised of internal, idealistic beliefs about the future. The assumption that winning the lottery will solve all of life's problems is representative of this form of thinking. Cardinal traits, **(A)**, are the traits around which individuals organize their entire life. Functional autonomy, **(C)**, is when a behavior continues after the drive behind the behavior has ceased; for example, if this young professional continued purchasing lottery tickets after winning simply for enjoyment, then this behavior would have gained functional autonomy. Unconditional positive regard, **(D)**, is used in some forms of humanistic therapy in which the therapist believes in the internal good of the client and does not judge the client negatively for any words or actions.

Consult your online resources for additional practice. GO ONLINE

SHARED CONCEPTS

Behavioral Sciences Chapter 3
Learning and Memory

Behavioral Sciences Chapter 4
Cognition, Consciousness, and Language

Behavioral Sciences Chapter 5
Motivation, Emotion, and Stress

Behavioral Sciences Chapter 7
Psychological Disorders

Behavioral Sciences Chapter 9
Social Interaction

Behavioral Sciences Chapter 10
Social Thinking

CHAPTER 7

PSYCHOLOGICAL DISORDERS

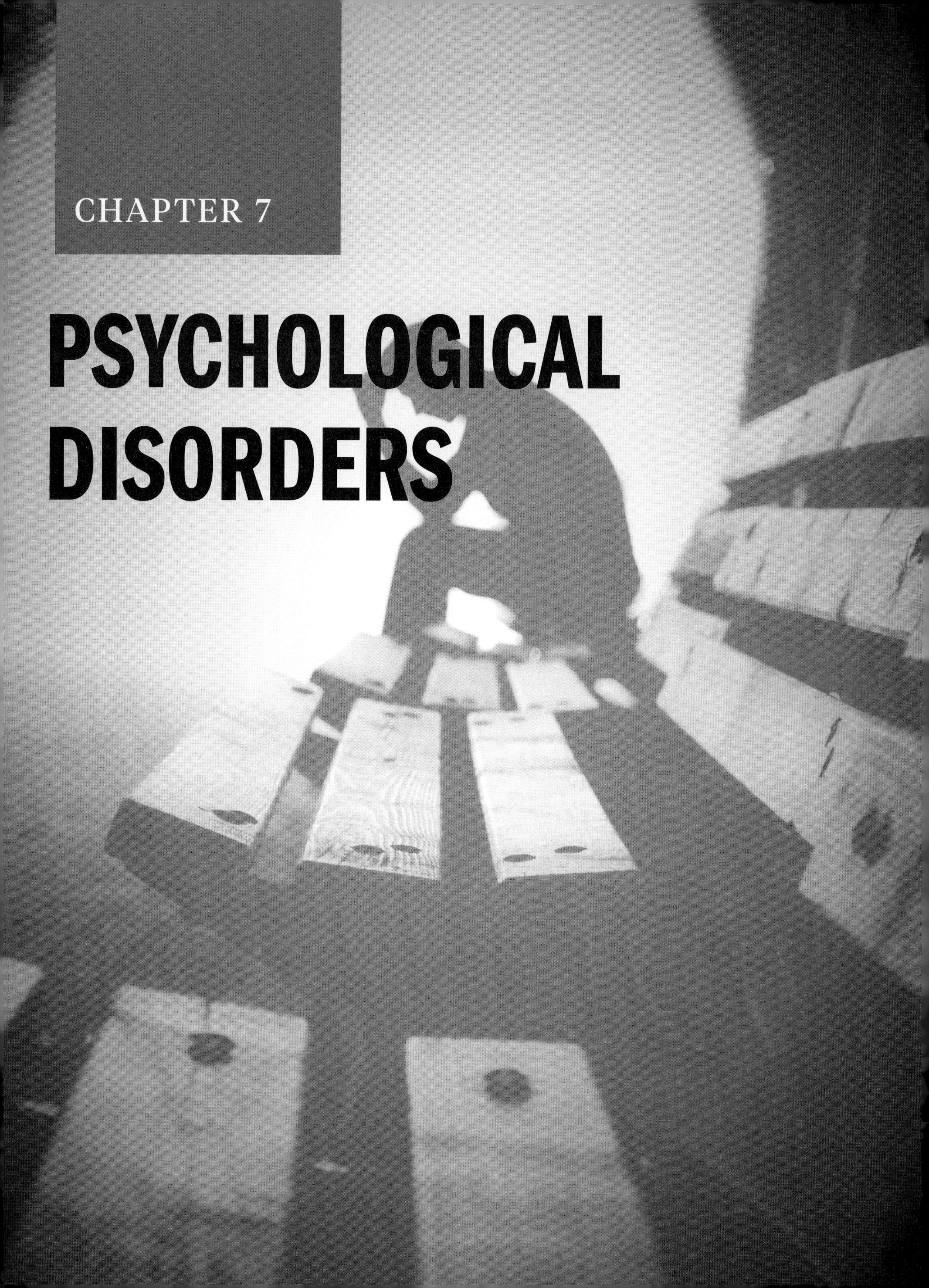

SCIENCE MASTERY ASSESSMENT

Every pre-med knows this feeling: there is so much content I have to know for the MCAT! How do I know what to do first or what's important?

While the high-yield badges throughout this book will help you identify the most important topics, this Science Mastery Assessment is another tool in your MCAT prep arsenal. This quiz (which can also be taken in your online resources) and the guidance below will help ensure that you are spending the appropriate amount of time on this chapter based on your personal strengths and weaknesses. Don't worry though—skipping something now does not mean you'll never study it. Later on in your prep, as you complete full-length tests, you'll uncover specific pieces of content that you need to review and can come back to these chapters as appropriate.

How to Use This Assessment

If you answer 0–7 questions correctly:

Spend about 1 hour to read this chapter in full and take limited notes throughout. Follow up by reviewing **all** quiz questions to ensure that you now understand how to solve each one.

If you answer 8–11 questions correctly:

Spend 20–40 minutes reviewing the quiz questions. Beginning with the questions you missed, read and take notes on the corresponding subchapters. For questions you answered correctly, ensure your thinking matches that of the explanation and you understand why each choice was correct or incorrect.

If you answer 12–15 questions correctly:

Spend less than 20 minutes reviewing all questions from the quiz. If you missed any, then include a quick read-through of the corresponding subchapters, or even just the relevant content within a subchapter, as part of your question review. For questions you answered correctly, ensure your thinking matches that of the explanation and review the Concept Summary at the end of the chapter.

1. Which of the following is an example of a negative symptom seen in schizophrenia?
   - **A.** Auditory hallucinations
   - **B.** Disorganized behavior
   - **C.** Disturbance of affect
   - **D.** Delusions

2. During an interview with a schizophrenic patient, a psychiatrist notices that the patient keeps repeating what the psychiatrist says. This phenomenon is known as:
   - **A.** echolalia.
   - **B.** echopraxia.
   - **C.** loosening of associations.
   - **D.** neologisms.

3. A 42-year-old patient has always been extremely neat and tidy. This person works as a secretary and stays long after normal working hours to check the punctuation and spelling of letters prepared during the day. The patient was referred for counseling by a supervisor after repeatedly getting into fights with coworkers. "They don't take the job to heart," the patient says. "They just joke around all day." The most likely preliminary diagnosis for this patient is:
   - **A.** obsessive–compulsive personality disorder.
   - **B.** antisocial personality disorder.
   - **C.** narcissistic personality disorder.
   - **D.** borderline personality disorder.

4. Which of the following is true with regard to a major depressive episode?
   - **A.** It may last less than two weeks.
   - **B.** It must involve thoughts of suicide or a suicide attempt.
   - **C.** It may involve a decrease in sleep.
   - **D.** It must involve feelings of sadness.

5. A young person moves to a new city to start work on an accelerated degree program. After a few months this individual visits the doctor complaining of stress and isolation and is diagnosed with depression. The doctor ascribes the cause to low levels of serotonin and prescribes an SSRI for treatment. Which of the following best describes the physician's approach to diagnosis and treatment?
   - **A.** Biomedical approach with indirect therapy
   - **B.** Biomedical approach with direct therapy
   - **C.** Biopsychosocial approach with indirect therapy
   - **D.** Biopsychosocial approach with direct therapy

6. A young person of unknown age is brought by the Philadelphia police to the local emergency department for evaluation after being found wandering in a park. The patient carries no identification and is unable to provide a first or last name or any life details, except that the name Phoenix seems familiar. The police in Arizona are contacted and find a missing persons report matching the patient's description. Based on this information, the most likely diagnosis for this patient is:
   - **A.** depersonalization/derealization disorder.
   - **B.** dissociative identity disorder.
   - **C.** somatic symptom disorder.
   - **D.** dissociative amnesia with dissociative fugue.

7. In addition to being a freestanding diagnosis, agoraphobia is most often seen in association with which other psychiatric diagnosis?
   - **A.** Obsessive–compulsive disorder
   - **B.** Avoidant personality disorder
   - **C.** Generalized anxiety disorder
   - **D.** Panic disorder

8. A researcher is interested in studying fear responses to a variety of different stimuli. To rule out potential confounding variables, the research excludes individuals with phobias from the study. In a sample of 50 participants, how many will likely be excluded from the study, assuming that the sample is representative of the overall population?
   - **A.** 45
   - **B.** 15
   - **C.** 10
   - **D.** 5

Questions 9–10 refer to the scenario described below.

A physician is attempting to diagnose a patient's mental disorder based on a set of symptoms. The confirmed symptoms currently include appetite disturbance, substantial weight change, decreased energy, a feeling of worthlessness, and excessive guilt.

9. What two disorders could these symptoms indicate?
   - **A.** Major depressive and bipolar disorders
   - **B.** Dissociative amnesia and depersonalization/derealization disorder
   - **C.** Alzheimer's disease and Parkinson's disease
   - **D.** Specific phobia and panic disorder

10. What should the physician ask about to distinguish between the two possible disorders affecting that patient?
   - **A.** Whether the patient has amnesia
   - **B.** Whether the patient has also had manic episodes
   - **C.** Whether the patient is irrationally afraid of anything
   - **D.** Whether the patient has experienced difficulty performing familiar tasks

11. All of the following are risk factors or diagnostic criteria for Alzheimer's disease EXCEPT:
   - **A.** Extra copies of the β-amyloid precursor protein gene.
   - **B.** Decreased abundance of serotonin and norepinephrine.
   - **C.** Neurofibrillary tangles of hyperphosphorylated tau protein.
   - **D.** Deficient blood flow to the parietal lobes.

12. Splitting is a defense mechanism commonly seen with which personality disorder?
   - **A.** Antisocial personality disorder
   - **B.** Borderline personality disorder
   - **C.** Histrionic personality disorder
   - **D.** Narcissistic personality disorder

13. A patient comes to the doctor with a two-week history of complete paralysis of the left arm. The patient has had no injury to the extremity, and full neurological workup fails to demonstrate any underlying cause. The patient seems surprisingly unconcerned about the paralysis, and seems more worried about an argument that happened one month ago in which the patient hit a family member. Based on this information, the patient's most likely diagnosis is:
   - **A.** conversion disorder.
   - **B.** generalized anxiety disorder.
   - **C.** illness anxiety disorder.
   - **D.** histrionic personality disorder.

14. A patient is taken to the doctor after starting to move the fingers in such a way that it looks like rolling something, despite nothing actually being there. The patient also exhibits slowed movement and a shuffling gait. Which neurotransmitter is likely to be present in decreased levels in the patient's brain?
   - **A.** Epinephrine
   - **B.** Histamine
   - **C.** Dopamine
   - **D.** Serotonin

15. Which of the following is/are true regarding bipolar disorders?
   - **I.** They have little, if any, genetic heritability.
   - **II.** They are associated with increased levels of serotonin in the brain.
   - **III.** They all require at least one depressive episode for diagnosis.

   - **A.** I only
   - **B.** II only
   - **C.** I and III only
   - **D.** II and III only

Answer Key

1. **C**
2. **A**
3. **A**
4. **C**
5. **B**
6. **D**
7. **D**
8. **D**
9. **A**
10. **B**
11. **B**
12. **B**
13. **A**
14. **C**
15. **B**

Detailed explanations can be found at the end of the chapter.

CHAPTER 7

PSYCHOLOGICAL DISORDERS

In This Chapter

CHAPTER PROFILE

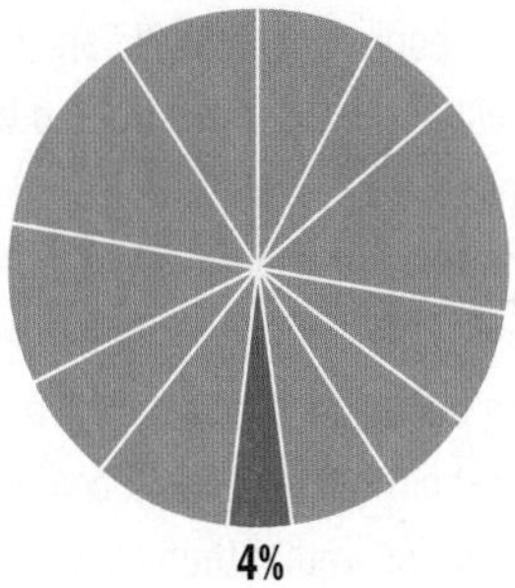

The content in this chapter should be relevant to about 4% of all questions about the behavioral sciences on the MCAT.

This chapter covers material from the following AAMC content category:

7A: Individual influences on behavior

Introduction

The progress in our understanding of hysteria has come largely through the elaboration of the so-called mechanisms by which the symptoms arise. These mechanisms have been declared to reside or to have their origin in the subconsciousness or coconsciousness. The mechanisms range all the way from the conception of Janet that the personality is disintegrated owing to lowering of the psychical tension to that of Freud, who conceives all hysterical symptoms as a result of dissociation arising through conflicts between repressed sexual desires and experiences and the various censors organized by the social life.

The above is an excerpt from the *Journal of Abnormal Psychology* in 1915. Merely a century ago, our understanding of psychological disorders was in its infancy. Hysteria—the antiquated name for conversion disorder—was thought to result from marital discord and repressed sexual desires. We are now beginning to understand the underlying psychological and biological factors at play in a number of mental illnesses. In this chapter, we will focus on several different types of psychological disorders, their classification, causes, and frequencies.

MCAT EXPERTISE

If you've taken a glance at the rest of this book, you might have noticed that this chapter has a low percentage of relevant content as compared to the rest of the chapters within *MCAT Behavioral Sciences Review*. While Chapter 7 materials will be tested less often than the other materials in this book, there are so many psychology questions on the MCAT that even lower-yield topics within the behavioral sciences will get you points!

7.1 Understanding Psychological Disorders

LEARNING OBJECTIVES

After Chapter 7.1, you will be able to:

- Compare and contrast the biomedical and the biopsychosocial models of psychological disorders
- Recall the most common psychological disorders in the United States

REAL WORLD

Thomas Szasz, an outspoken critic of labeling people "mentally ill," argues that most of the disorders treated by clinicians are not really illnesses. Rather, they are traits or behaviors that differ from the cultural norm. Szasz argues that labeling people as mentally ill is a way to force them to change and conform to societal norms rather than allowing them to attack the societal causes of their problems.

MCAT EXPERTISE

The biopsychosocial model was originally theorized in a 1977 *Science* article and has grown in breadth, depth, and applicability since it was first described. In fact, the increased recognition of psychological and social factors on patient care was one of the primary drivers for the creation of the *Psychological, Social, and Biological Foundations of Behavior* section of the MCAT!

Psychological disorders are characteristic sets of thoughts, feelings, or actions that cause noticeable distress to the sufferer, are considered deviant by the individual's culture, or cause **maladaptive** functioning in society, meaning that some aspect of the individual's behavior negatively impacts others or leads to self-defeating outcomes. Many disorders can be treated once diagnosed. The process of defining these disorders varies, and there are two main classification systems you'll need to know for the MCAT.

Biomedical *vs.* Biopsychosocial Approaches

The first classification system to know for the MCAT is the **biomedical approach** to psychological disorders. Biomedical therapy emphasizes interventions that rally around symptom reduction of psychological disorders. In other words, this approach assumes that any disorder has roots in biomedical disturbances, and thus the solution should also be of a biomedical nature. This view is thought of as narrower than other approaches because it fails to take into account many of the other sources of disorders, such as lifestyle and socioeconomic status. For example, heart disease clearly has roots within the mechanisms of the cardiac muscle, but the causes of these malfunctions have as much to do with biomedical causes (such as genetics) as they do with lifestyle causes (such as a diet rich in salty, fatty foods; smoking; and alcohol use). Similarly, this biomedical approach can miss some underlying sources of psychological disorders and is often more effective when supplemented with a broader approach to diagnosis and treatment.

A broader classification system commonly used for these psychological disorders is the **biopsychosocial approach**. This method assumes that there are biological, psychological, and social components to an individual's disorder. The biological component of a disorder is something in the body, like having a particular genetic syndrome. The psychological component of a disorder stems from the individual's thoughts, emotions, or behaviors. Finally, the disorder's social component results from the individual's surroundings and can include issues of perceived class in society and even discrimination or stigmatization. All three of these aspects of a disorder are considered in the biopsychosocial approach for both diagnosis and treatment.

To better understand the biopsychosocial approach, consider depression. Certain genetic factors can make an individual more or less susceptible to depressive tendencies, showing a purely biological influence on the disorder. However, from a psychological perspective, the levels of stress that the individual experiences can also contribute to the severity of the depression experienced. Finally, the social environment may provide additional stressors or support from one's career, family, and friends. Accordingly, in the biopsychosocial model, the goal is often to provide not only **direct therapy**—treatment that acts directly on the individual, such as medication or periodic meetings with a psychologist—but also **indirect therapy**, which aims to increase social support by educating and empowering family and friends of the affected individual.

Classifying Psychological Disorders

To aid clinicians in considering these factors, the ***Diagnostic and Statistical Manual of Mental Disorders*** (**DSM**) was created. Originally, the manual was written to collect statistical data in the United States. It is now used as a diagnostic tool in the United States and various other countries. The manual is currently in its fifth edition, which was published in May 2013, so the common abbreviation seen is DSM-5. This manual is a compilation of many known psychological disorders. The DSM-5's classification scheme is not based on theories of etiology (cause) or treatments of different disorders. Rather, it is based on descriptions of symptoms. It is used by clinicians to fit lists of compiled symptoms from a patient into a category and thus to diagnose that patient. The DSM-5 has 20 diagnostic classes of mental disorders; those that will be tested on the MCAT are discussed in this chapter.

REAL WORLD

David Rosenhan studied whether it was possible to be judged sane if you are in an "insane place" (a psychiatric hospital). Rosenhan and seven other "sane" people were admitted into psychiatric hospitals by reporting auditory hallucinations. Each of these pseudopatients was diagnosed to have either schizophrenia or bipolar disorder, and each was admitted. Once admitted, they acted completely normal—but it still took an average of three weeks to be discharged, and each was still given the diagnosis of schizophrenia in remission. Once labeled, it is very hard to distance oneself from the diagnosis of mental illness.

Rates of Psychological Disorders

Suffering from a mental disorder can be a lonely experience because the disorder usually occurs only in the mind of the patient. However, the rates of these psychological disorders are higher than this experience would otherwise suggest. Table 7.1 covers these rates in detail.

MCAT EXPERTISE

The MCAT tests many, but not all, categories of mental disorder described within the DSM-5. Neurodevelopmental disorders, eating disorders, impulse control disorders, sleeping disorders, and others are not listed within the AAMC's guide to MCAT content, and as such are not included within this text.

DISORDER	PERCENTAGE AFFECTED	NUMBER AFFECTED (IN MILLIONS)
Any mental disorder	18.3	44.7
Specific phobia	9.1	22.2
Social anxiety disorder	7.1	17.3
Major depressive disorder	6.7	16.4
Posttraumatic stress disorder	3.6	8.8
Bipolar disorder	2.8	6.8
Generalized anxiety disorder	2.7	6.6
Panic disorder	2.7	6.6
Borderline personality disorder	1.4	3.4
Obsessive-compulsive disorder	1.2	2.9
Agoraphobia	0.9	2.2
Anorexia nervosa	0.6	1.5
Schizophrenia	0.6	1.5
All cancers*	6.1	15.1
Diabetes*	9.4	23.0

*Note: These nonpsychological conditions are included for comparison.

All data from this website: https://www.nimh.nih.gov/health/statistics/index.shtml

Table 7.1 One-Year Prevalence Rates for Psychological Disorders in the United States

MCAT CONCEPT CHECK 7.1

Before you move on, assess your understanding of the material with these questions.

1. What is the difference between the biomedical and biopsychosocial models of psychological disorders?

2. Name three psychological disorders with greater than 2% one-year prevalence in the United States (affecting more than 1 in 50 people per year). Refer to Table 7.1 if you get stuck.

•

•

•

7.2 Types of Psychological Disorders

High-Yield

LEARNING OBJECTIVES

After Chapter 7.2, you will be able to:

- List the major positive symptoms and major negative symptoms of schizophrenia and psychotic disorders
- Recall the features of major depressive episodes, manic and hypomanic episodes
- Distinguish between the testable mood disorders
- Relate obsessions and compulsions to the symptoms of obsessive–compulsive disorder
- Describe and explain the symptoms of posttraumatic stress disorder (PTSD)
- Describe and distinguish dissociative and somatic symptom disorders
- Describe the features and individual disorders that fall under cluster A, B, and C personality disorders

As mentioned earlier, the DSM-5 categorizes common symptoms into 20 diagnostic classes. Many of these classes represent significant revisions from the DSM-5's immediate predecessor, the DSM-IV-TR. The most heavily tested diagnostic classes on the MCAT are schizophrenia spectrum and other psychotic disorders, bipolar and related disorders, depressive disorders, anxiety disorders, obsessive–compulsive and related disorders, trauma- and stressor-related disorders, dissociative disorders, somatic symptom and related disorders, and personality disorders.

Schizophrenia and Other Psychotic Disorders

According to the DSM-5, individuals with a **psychotic disorder** present with one or more of the following symptoms: delusions, hallucinations, disorganized thought, disorganized behavior, catatonia, and negative symptoms. Like most psychological categories, psychotic disorders are on a spectrum. To delineate the psychotic disorders as described in the DSM-5, psychotic symptoms must be understood.

REAL WORLD

The term schizophrenia is a relatively recent term, coined in 1911 by Eugen Bleuler. Before Bleuler, schizophrenia was called *dementia praecox*. Schizophrenia literally means "split mind" because the disorder is characterized by distortions of reality and disturbances in the content and form of thought, perception, and affect. Unfortunately, this has led to confusion with dissociative identity disorder (formerly multiple personality disorder). By *split mind*, Bleuler did not mean that the mind is split into different personalities, but that the mind is split from reality.

Psychotic symptoms are divided into positive and negative types. **Positive symptoms** are behaviors, thoughts, or feelings added to normal behavior. In other words, positive symptoms are features that are experienced in individuals with psychotic disorders that are not present in the general population. Examples include delusions and hallucinations, disorganized thought, and disorganized or catatonic behavior. Positive symptoms are considered by some to be two distinct dimensions—the psychotic dimension (delusions and hallucinations) and the disorganized dimension (disorganized thought and behavior)—perhaps with different underlying causes. **Negative symptoms** are those that involve the absence of normal or desired behavior, such as disturbance of affect and avolition.

Positive Symptoms

MCAT EXPERTISE

The fact that delusions must be considered deviant from the society in which an individual lives provides an excellent opportunity for the MCAT to integrate mental illness and sociology. For example, a belief in shamanism—which is common in the Caribbean, Central and South America, Africa, and in some American Indian tribes—would not be considered a delusion within societies that endorse shamanic medicine.

Delusions are false beliefs discordant with reality and not shared by others in the individual's culture. These delusions are maintained often in spite of strong evidence to the contrary. Common delusions include delusions of reference, persecution, and grandeur. **Delusions of reference** involve the belief that common elements in the environment are directed toward the individual. For example, people with delusions of reference may believe that characters in a TV show are talking to them directly. **Delusions of persecution** involve the belief that the person is being deliberately interfered with, discriminated against, plotted against, or threatened. **Delusions of grandeur**, also common in bipolar I disorder, involve the belief that the person is remarkable in some significant way, such as being an inventor, historical figure, or religious icon. Other common delusions involve the concept of **thought broadcasting**, which is the belief that one's thoughts are broadcast directly from one's head to the external world, **thought withdrawal**, the belief that thoughts are being removed from one's head, and **thought insertion**, the belief that thoughts are being placed in one's head.

Hallucinations are perceptions that are not due to external stimuli but which nevertheless seem real to the person perceiving them. The most common form of hallucination is auditory, involving voices that are perceived as coming from inside or outside the patient's head. Visual and tactile hallucinations are less common, but may be seen in drug use or withdrawal.

BRIDGE

Word salad can be seen in severe schizophrenia as well as Wernicke's (receptive) aphasia. Patients will string together unrelated words, although the prosody of the speech (its rhythm, stress, and intonation) remains intact. Aphasias are discussed in Chapter 3 of *MCAT Behavioral Sciences Review*.

Disorganized thought is characterized by loosening of associations. This may be exhibited as speech in which ideas shift from one subject to another in such a way that a listener would be unable to follow the train of thought. A patient's speech may be so disorganized that it seems to have no structure—as though it were just words thrown together incomprehensibly. This is sometimes called **word salad**. In fact, a person with schizophrenia may even invent new words, called **neologisms**.

Disorganized behavior refers to an inability to carry out activities of daily living, such as paying bills, maintaining hygiene, and keeping appointments. **Catatonia** refers to certain motor behaviors characteristic of some people with schizophrenia. The patient's spontaneous movement and activity may be greatly reduced or the patient may maintain a rigid posture, refusing to be moved. At the other extreme, catatonic behavior may include useless and bizarre movements not caused by any external stimuli, **echolalia** (repeating another's words), or **echopraxia** (imitating another's actions).

Negative Symptoms

The classic negative symptoms of schizophrenia and related psychotic disorders are disturbance of affect and avolition. **Affect** refers to the experience and display of emotion, so disturbance of affect is any disruption to these abilities. Affective symptoms may include **blunting**, in which there is a severe reduction in the intensity of affect expression; **emotional flattening** (**flat affect**), in which there are virtually no signs of emotional expression; or **inappropriate affect**, in which the affect is clearly discordant with the content of the individual's speech. For example, a patient with inappropriate affect may begin to laugh hysterically while describing a parent's death. Interestingly, it has become more difficult to assess the affective aspects of schizophrenia because the antipsychotic medications used in treatment frequently blunt and flatten affect as well. Finally, **avolition** is marked by decreased engagement in purposeful, goal-directed actions.

Schizophrenia

Schizophrenia is the prototypical psychotic disorder in this category of disorders. **Schizophrenia** is characterized by a break between an individual and reality. In fact, the term *schizophrenia* literally means "split mind." Eugen Bleuler coined the term in reference to the splitting of one's mind from reality. To be given the diagnosis of schizophrenia, an individual must show continuous signs of the disturbance for at least six months, and this six-month period must include at least one month of positive symptoms (delusions, hallucinations, or disorganized speech).

MCAT EXPERTISE

When the MCAT tests schizophrenia, it is likely to include a connection to sociology through the *downward drift hypothesis*, which states that schizophrenia causes a decline in socioeconomic status, leading to worsening symptoms, which sets up a negative spiral for the patient toward poverty and psychosis. This is why rates of schizophrenia are much, much higher among homeless and indigent people.

Phases of Schizophrenia

The diagnosis and course of schizophrenia typically follows a specific path, termed the phases of schizophrenia. Before schizophrenia is diagnosed, a patient often goes through a phase characterized by poor adjustment. This phase is called the **prodromal phase**. The prodromal phase is exemplified by clear evidence of deterioration, social withdrawal, role functioning impairment, peculiar behavior, inappropriate affect, and unusual experiences. This is followed by the **active phase** in which pronounced psychotic symptoms are displayed. If schizophrenia development is slow, correct diagnosis is difficult and the prognosis is especially poor. If the onset of symptoms is intense and sudden, the diagnosis is readily made and the prognosis is better. Diagnosis usually occurs during the active phase. The **residual phase,** also called the **recovery phase,** occurs after an active episode and is characterized by mental clarity often resulting in concern or depression as the individual becomes aware of previous behavior.

Other Psychotic Disorders

Other psychotic disorders differ from schizophrenia by the presence, severity, and duration of psychotic symptoms. As a general trend, the *other psychotic disorders* present symptoms to a lesser degree in comparison to schizophrenia.

- **Schizotypal Personality Disorder**: Include both personality disorder and psychotic symptoms, with the personality symptoms having been already established before psychotic symptoms present. This condition is covered in greater detail in *Personality Disorders.*

- **Delusion Disorder**: Psychotic symptoms are limited to delusions and are present for at least a month.
- **Brief Psychotic Disorder**: Positive psychotic symptoms are present for at least a day, but less than a month.
- **Schizophreniform Disorder**: Same diagnostic criteria as schizophrenia except in duration; the required duration for this diagnosis is only 1 month.
- **Schizoaffective Disorder**: Major mood episodes (major depressive episodes and manic episodes) while also presenting psychotic symptoms.

Depressive Disorders

Sadness is a natural part of life, especially in response to stressful life events like the death of a loved one. During periods of sadness, people might call themselves depressed. However, periodic sadness in response to life events is not a mental disorder. **Depressive disorders**, in contrast, are conditions characterized by feelings of sadness that are severe enough, in both magnitude and duration, to meet specific diagnostic criteria.

To understand the DSM-5's categorization of the spectrum of depressive disorders, we must first discuss the 9 **depressive symptoms** defined in the DSM-5. These symptoms can be recalled with the mnemonic **sadness + SIG E. CAPS**:

- **Sadness**: Depressed mood, feelings of sadness and emptiness
- Sleep: Insomnia or hypersomnia
- Interest: Loss of interest and pleasure in activities that previously sparked joy, termed **anhedonia**
- Guilt: A feeling of inappropriate guilt or worthlessness
- Energy: Lower levels of energy throughout the day
- Concentration: Decrease in ability to concentrate (self described, or observed by others)
- Appetite: Pronounced change in appetite (increase or decrease) resulting in a significant change (5%+) in weight.
- Psychomotor symptoms: Psychomotor retardation (slowed thoughts and physical movements) and psychomotor agitation (restlessness resulting in undesired movement)
- Suicidal thoughts: Recurrent suicidal thoughts

In addition to depressive symptoms, the DSM-5 also categorizes depressive disorders based on duration, timing, and cause of depressive symptoms.

Major Depressive Disorder

The key diagnostic feature of **major depressive disorder (MDD)** is the presence of major depressive episodes. A **major depressive episode** is defined as a 2-week (or longer) period in which 5 of the 9 defined depressive symptoms are encountered, which must include either depressed mood or **anhedonia** (inability to feel and anticipate pleasure). In addition, the symptoms must be severe enough to impair one's daily social- or work-related activities.

MNEMONIC

Symptoms of a major depressive episode: **SIG E. CAPS**

Sadness +

- **S**leep
- **I**nterest
- **G**uilt
- **E**nergy
- **C**oncentration
- **A**ppetite
- **P**sychomotor symptoms
- **S**uicidal thoughts

Persistent Depressive Disorder

Considering the difference in naming between major depressive disorder and persistent depressive disorder, it may seem reasonable to assume that persistent depressive disorder is a lesser form of major depressive disorder. However, this is not the case. In fact, major depressive episodes can coincide with persistent depressive disorder. A diagnosis of **persistent depressive disorder (PDD)**, also known as **dysthymia**, is given when an individual experiences a period, lasting at least 2 years, in which they experience a depressed mood on the majority of days. With the primary diagnostic feature of PDD being time, a patient can receive both the PDD and MDD diagnosis if they meet both the duration and severity requirements of both disorders.

BRIDGE

The most common first-line treatment for depression is the class of medications called selective serotonin reuptake inhibitors (SSRIs). These block the reuptake of serotonin by the presynaptic neuron, resulting in higher levels of serotonin in the synapse and relief of symptoms. The nervous system is outlined in Chapter 1 of *MCAT Behavioral Sciences Review* and Chapter 4 of *MCAT Biology Review*.

Other Depressive Disorders

Whereas major depressive disorder and persistent depressive disorder are characterized by severity and duration of depressive symptoms, other depressive disorders can be characterized by their age of incidence and apparent cause.

Children often exhibit more dramatic emotional responses than adults and, in previous editions of the DSM, this led to the potential overdiagnosis of bipolar disorders in children. To address this concern the DSM-5 includes **disruptive mood dysregulation disorder**, which is typically diagnosed between the ages of 6 and 10, and has the key diagnostic feature of persistent and recurrent emotional irritability in multiple environments (school, home, etc.).

Depressive symptoms can also arise in response to specific times and situations; if these symptoms meet certain diagnostic criteria then they are considered disorders. **Premenstrual dysphoric disorder** is characterized by mood changes, often depressed mood, occurring a few days before menses and resolving after menses onset.

Although not freestanding diagnoses in the DSM-5, both seasonal affective disorder and postpartum depression are conditions that have an apparent cause. In **seasonal affective disorder (SAD)**, the dark winter months are believed to be the source of depressive symptoms and thus the disorder is best categorized as major depressive disorder with seasonal onset, while in **postpartum depression** the rapid change in hormone levels just after giving birth is the cause of the depressive symptoms. In the case of seasonal affective disorder, depressive symptoms are present only in the winter months. This disorder may be related to abnormal melatonin metabolism; it is often treated with **bright light therapy**, where the patient is exposed to a bright light for a specified amount of time each day, as demonstrated with a plant in Figure 7.1.

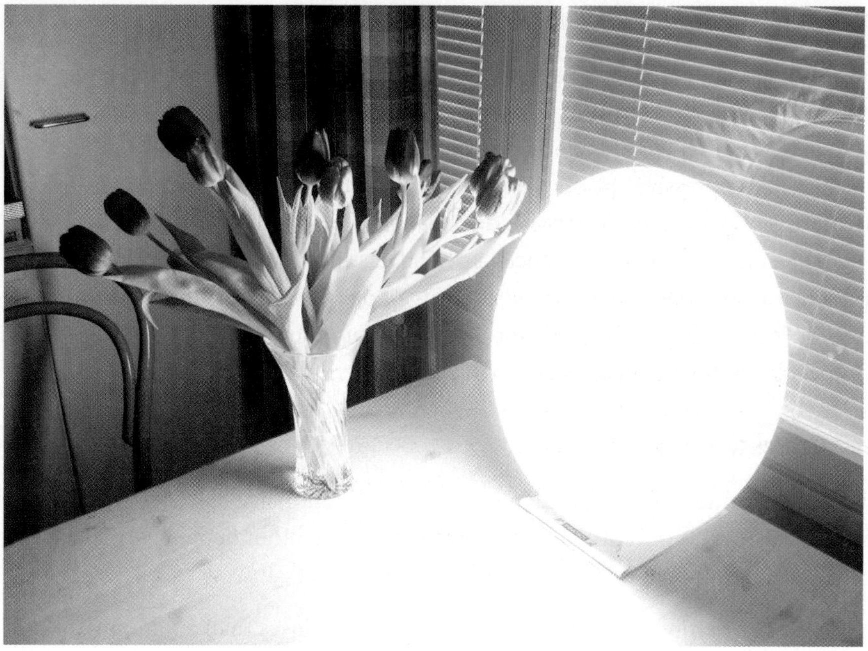

Figure 7.1 Bright Light Therapy for Seasonal Affective Disorder

Bipolar and Related Disorders

This category of disorders is characterized by the presence of manic and depressive symptoms, which if severe and persistent enough can be labelled as episodes. **Manic symptoms** are associated with an exaggerated elevation in mood, accompanied by an increase in goal-directed activity and energy. Put simply, manic symptoms can be thought of as the prolonged and exaggerated emotion of happiness or joy. According to the DSM-5, there are 7 manic symptoms. These symptoms can be recalled with the mnemonic **DIG FAST**:

- **D**istractibility: Inability to remain focused on an activity
- **I**rresponsibility: Engaging in risky activities without considering future consequences
- **G**randiosity: Exaggerated and unrealistic increase in self-esteem
- **F**light of thoughts: Racing thoughts, self-reported or revealed through rapid speech
- **A**ctivity or agitation: Increase in goal-oriented work or social activities
- **S**leep: Decreased need for sleep, e.g. sleeping for only a couple hours but feeling rested
- **T**alkative: Exaggerated desire to speak

The presence of manic symptoms are considered a **hypomanic episode** if the symptoms are present for at least 4 days and include at least 3 or more of the 7 defined manic symptoms, yet the symptoms are not severe enough to impair the person's social or work activities. However, the diagnosis progresses to a **manic episode** if the manic symptoms (3 or more of the defined 7) are severe enough to impair a person's social or work activities and persist for at least 7 days.

In addition to manic symptoms and their associated episodes, the presence or absence of depressive symptoms and their associated episodes are also used to differentiate bipolar and related disorders. Specifically, these disorders are classified by the presence or absence of manic, hypomanic, and major depressive episodes. Depressive symptoms were covered in *Depressive Disorders.*

Bipolar I Disorder

When manic episodes are present, a diagnosis of **bipolar I disorder** is likely to be made, as the key diagnostic feature of this disorder is the presence of manic episodes. While most diagnoses of bipolar I disorder also include depressive symptoms, often major depressive episodes, they are not a requirement. To illustrate this point consider two hypothetical patients: Patient A only experiences manic episodes, while Patient B regularly experiences both manic and major depressive episodes, cycling between the two regularly. Despite both patients presenting very differently, both fit the categorization of bipolar I disorder.

Bipolar II Disorder

The key feature of a **bipolar II disorder** diagnosis is the presence of both a major depressive episode and an accompanying hypomanic episode, but not a manic episode. To avoid confusion, it is worth noting that if a patient has experienced both major depressive episodes and manic episodes, a diagnosis of bipolar I disorder will likely be made. In addition, if a person experiences only major depressive symptoms (absence of hypomanic and manic episodes), then a diagnosis of major depressive disorder is likely to be made. Thus, the diagnosis of bipolar II only captures individuals who experience major depressive episodes and the lesser, hypomanic episodes.

Cyclothymic Disorder

The diagnostic features of cyclothymic disorder are the presence of both manic and depressive symptoms that are not severe enough to be considered episodes. In other words, the patient has not experienced major depressive, manic, or hypomanic episodes. Or, more specifically, the patient has never experienced *3 or more of the 7 manic symptoms in a 4 day period* (diagnostic criteria for hypomanic episode) and has never experienced *5 or more of the 9 depressive symptoms in a 2-week period* (diagnostic criteria for a major depressive episode). Considering the relatively low threshold of symptom requirements, it may seem that everyone would be diagnosed with cyclothymic disorder. However despite the relatively low symptom requirements, the duration requirements for this disorder are high. For a diagnosis of **cyclothymic disorder** to be made, a person must have experienced numerous periods of manic and depressive symptoms for the majority of time over a 2-year (or longer) period.

Before moving on to anxiety disorders, a brief discussion of proposed neurological etiologies of mood disorders is warranted. The most common explanation revolves around the neurotransmitters norepinephrine and serotonin. These two are often linked together into what is called the **monoamine** or **catecholamine theory of depression**. This theory holds that too much norepinephrine and serotonin in the

REAL WORLD

Depressive and manic episodes are essentially two sides of the same coin: Depression is associated with low norepinephrine and serotonin levels, and manic episodes are associated with high levels of these neurotransmitters. When patients are put on treatment for depression, they must be watched for signs of mania because antidepressant medications may trigger manic symptoms or episodes.

synapse leads to mania, while too little leads to depression. Although more recent research has shown that it is not that simple, you should be aware of this theory for the MCAT.

Anxiety Disorders

BRIDGE

For all anxiety disorders, clinicians must rule out hyperthyroidism—excessive levels of the thyroid hormones triiodothyronine (T_3) and thyroxine (T_4)—because increasing the whole body's metabolic rate will create anxiety-like symptoms. Thyroid function is discussed in Chapter 5 of *MCAT Biology Review*.

From an evolutionary perspective, emotions served to direct and modulate behavior based on environmental stimuli. As seen in bipolar and depressive disorders, when the regulation of emotions, such as happiness or sadness, are insufficient, then symptoms arise. In the case of anxiety, fear is the associated emotion. Fear is often defined as an emotional response to an immediate threat, while **anxiety** can be viewed as fear of an upcoming or future event. Like fear, anxiety is healthy and important in one's life. It is only considered an **anxiety disorder** when irrational and excessive fear or anxiety affects an individual's daily functioning.

There are more than 10 disorders listed in the anxiety disorders portion of the DSM-5. These disorders are categorized by the situation or stimulus that induces anxiety.

Specific Phobias

The most common type of anxiety disorder is a phobia. A **phobia** is an irrational fear of something that results in a compelling desire to avoid it. Most of the phobias that you are likely familiar with are what the DSM-5 calls specific phobias. A **specific phobia** is one in which fear and anxiety are produced by a specific object or situation. Unlike other sources of anxiety, specific phobias lack a specific ideation or thought pattern and instead present as an immediate and irrational fear response to the specific object or situation. For example, *claustrophobia* is an irrational fear of closed places, *acrophobia* is an irrational fear of heights, and *arachnophobia* is an irrational fear of spiders.

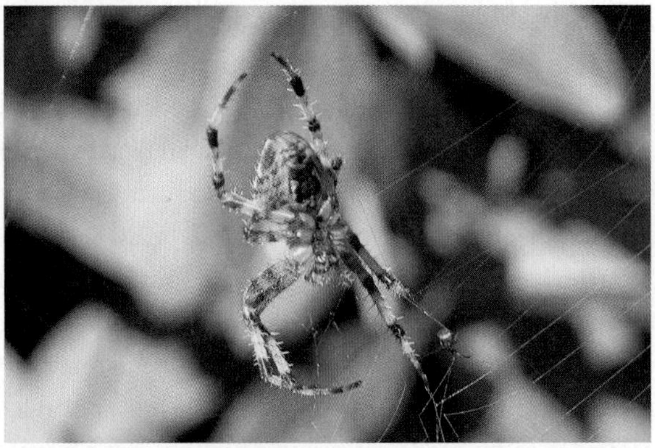

Figure 7.2 Specific Phobia
Arachnophobia, the fear of spiders, is a common example of a specific phobia.

Separation Anxiety Disorder

Separation anxiety is the excessive fear of being separated from one's caregivers or home environment. Although some separation anxiety is common and to be expected in young children, when this anxiety is excessive and persists beyond the age where it is deemed developmentally appropriate, the person may be diagnosed with **separation anxiety disorder**. This diagnosis is accompanied by the ideation that when separated, the caregiver or the individual themselves will be harmed (e.g. kidnapping, getting sick). These persistent beliefs may result in avoidant behaviors such as refusal to leave the home, shadowing the caregiver, etc.

Social Anxiety Disorder

On the surface, social anxiety disorder can be viewed as a social phobia, that is, fear and anxiety towards social situations and encounters. However, unlike previously discussed specified phobias, social anxiety disorder has an accompanying ideation in which individuals think that they will be perceived negatively by others. Thus, the key diagnostic feature of **social anxiety disorder** is fear or anxiety towards social situations with the belief that the individual will be exposed, embarrassed, or simply negatively perceived by others.

Like other anxiety disorders, avoidant behaviors are often conditioned as a means to reduce the associated anxiety. In the case of social anxiety, this can be as broad as avoiding social situations entirely or as narrow as avoiding handshakes out of fear of sweaty palms. Avoidant behavior to the point of social or occupational impairment is necessary for a social anxiety disorder diagnosis.

Selective Mutism

Although categorized as a separate anxiety disorder, **selective mutism** is heavily associated with social anxiety disorder and characterized by the consistent inability to speak in situations where speaking is expected. However, in situations that are more relaxed or when communication is not expected, speaking is unaffected. From this perspective, selective mutism may be conceptualized as a patient's fear of being negatively evaluated for what the patient might say.

Panic Disorder

The key diagnostic feature of **panic disorder** is the recurrence of unexpected panic attacks. To understand panic disorder, we must first cover panic attacks. From a physiological perspective, a panic attack is the misfiring of the sympathetic nervous system resulting in an unwanted *fight or flight* response. From a psychological perspective, a panic attack includes the associated emotions that accompany the sympathetic response, such as intense fear and *a sense of impending doom/danger*. Combining these two perspectives, a **panic attack** is the sudden surge of fear in which individuals feel that they are losing control of their body and/or that they are dying. The occurrence of an individual's attacks may be associated with specific triggers, in which case the attacks are termed **expected panic attacks**. If there is no clear trigger and the panic attacks are seemingly random, they are termed **unexpected panic attacks**.

BRIDGE

Notice that a large number of the symptoms of panic disorder are caused by excess activation of the sympathetic nervous system (autonomic overdrive). These include trembling, sweating, hyperventilation, shortness of breath, a racing heart rate, and palpitations. The autonomic nervous system is discussed in Chapter 1 of *MCAT Behavioral Sciences Review* and Chapter 4 of *MCAT Biology Review*.

The diagnosis of panic disorder requires the recurrence of *unexpected* panic attacks. The unexpected panic attacks themselves can produce an associated anxiety. In other words, an individual may become anxious at the thought of having an unexpected panic attack. If this anxiety impairs one's daily functions and persists for at least a month, then the diagnosis of panic disorder is made.

It is worth noting that panic attacks themselves are not considered a psychological disorder. They may occur in the absence of physiological disorders or may be associated with anxiety disorders in which there is a clear trigger. For instance, an individual with arachnophobia may experience expected panic attacks when encountering a spider.

Agoraphobia

Agoraphobia is an anxiety disorder characterized by a fear of being in places or situations where it might be difficult for an individual to escape. This fear may stem from the thought that the individual may experience a panic attack or similar event in which they would need to escape to avoid embarrassment. People who have agoraphobia tend to be uncomfortable leaving their homes, using public transport, being in open spaces, waiting in lines, or simply being in crowds. Due to agoraphobia's association with panic attacks and fear of being negatively evaluated by others, it is often comorbid with panic disorder, social anxiety disorder, and specific phobias.

Generalized Anxiety Disorder

As previously mentioned, the DSM-5 categorizes anxiety disorders based on the stimulus that induces fear or anxiety. For instance, anxiety towards social interactions is termed social anxiety; anxiety at the thought of separation from one's caregivers is termed separation anxiety. On the other hand, some individuals have more anxious temperaments, making them susceptible to anxiety triggered by a multitude of stimuli. It is for this reason that specific anxiety disorders are often comorbid with one another, resulting in patients having multiple diagnoses. However, a better diagnosis for some patients with many triggers for anxiety might be generalized anxiety disorder.

Generalized anxiety disorder (GAD) is defined as a disproportionate and persistent worry about many different things—making mortgage payments, doing a good job at work, returning emails, political issues, and so on—for at least six months. In addition, the worrying is difficult to control, even in cases where the individual knows that their worrying and fear is irrational. These individuals often have physical symptoms like fatigue, muscle tension, and sleep problems that accompany the worry. General anxiety disorder is relatively common in the US population, with approximately 3% of the population experiencing GAD in a 12-month period. Furthermore, over the course of a lifetime, individuals have a 1 in 10 chance of meeting the diagnostic criteria for general anxiety disorder.

Obsessive–Compulsive and Related Disorders

Formerly classified under anxiety and somatic symptom disorders, the disorders in this group were relabeled as obsessive–compulsive and related disorders in the DSM-5.

The reason for this organizational change reveals the common feature among these conditions. Across all of the following disorders, individuals perceive a particular need and respond to the need by completing a particular action. Disorders in this category are differentiated by the compulsiveness of the need to be met as well as the nature of the action.

Obsessive–Compulsive Disorder

Obsessive–compulsive disorder (**OCD**) is characterized by obsessions (persistent, intrusive thoughts and impulses), which produce tension, and compulsions (repetitive tasks) that relieve tension but cause significant impairment in a person's life. The relationship between the two is key: obsessions raise the individual's stress level, and the compulsions relieve this stress. Obsessions and their compulsions are ego-dystonic, meaning that the individual knows that their behavior is irrational, but the anxiety that arises when compulsions are not performed cannot be ignored.

Obsessions are perceived needs with the accompanying ideation that if a particular need is not met, then disastrous events will follow. Actions paired with obsessions are termed **compulsions**. As individuals with OCD attempt to satisfy their obsessions, rituals or sets of rules are developed for how their compulsions must be performed. For example, individuals may need to wash their hands for a specific length of time or else the intrusive thought of getting sick occurs. Alternatively, individuals may need to check if their door is locked a specific number of times or else worry obsessively about getting robbed. To be diagnosed with OCD, the compulsions must impair one's daily activities, for instance by taking up a lot of time during the day.

Body Dysmorphic Disorder

In **body dysmorphic disorder**, a person has an unrealistic negative evaluation of personal appearance and attractiveness, usually directed toward a certain body part. This is known as a **preoccupation**, a type of worry which lacks the disastrous ideation that accompanies obsessions. Patients with this disorder see their nose, skin, or stomach as ugly or even horrific when actually ordinary in appearance. This body–focused preoccupation also disrupts day-to-day life, and the sufferer may seek multiple plastic surgeries or other extreme interventions. A common association with this disorder is **muscle dysmorphia**, in which individuals believe that their body is too small or unmuscular (a preoccupation) and respond through working out. Like body dysmorphic disorder in general, this belief persists even with clear evidence to the contrary.

Hoarding Disorder

Hoarding disorder presents as a need to save or keep items and is often paired with excessive acquisition of objects. This behavior stems from several possible sources, ranging from the belief that kept items will eventually be useful to the feeling that the patient has a responsibility to care for the items. As a result, individuals with hoarding disorder often fill their homes with seemingly useless items even past the point where the accumulation of belongings impairs daily life.

Obsessive–Compulsive and Related Disorders with Body-Focused Repetitive Behaviors

Trichotillomania and excoriation are two obsessive–compulsive and related disorders that both present with body-focused compulsions. In the case of **trichotillomania**, individuals are compelled to pull out their hair, while with **excoriation disorder,** individuals are compelled to pick at their skin. A required diagnostic feature in both of these disorders is that patients have previously attempted to stop their body-focused compulsions but have so far failed.

Trauma- and Stressor-Related Disorders

This category captures disorders where a traumatic event is the source of the symptoms and thus is a diagnostic requirement in these disorders. The typical response to traumatic events includes fear, helplessness, and perhaps anxiety. In trauma and stressor related disorders, however, individuals also present with maladaptive symptoms like anhedonia, dysphoria (generalized dissatisfaction with life), aggression, or dissociation.

By far, the most notable disorder in this category is **posttraumatic stress disorder** (**PTSD**). PTSD occurs after experiencing or witnessing a traumatic event, such as war, a home invasion, rape, or a natural disaster, and consists of intrusion symptoms, arousal symptoms, avoidance symptoms, and negative cognitive symptoms.

- **Intrusion symptoms** include recurrent reliving of the event, flashbacks, nightmares, and prolonged distress.
- **Arousal symptoms** include an increased startle response, irritability, anxiety, self-destructive or reckless behavior, and sleep disturbances.
- **Avoidance symptoms** include deliberate attempts to avoid the memories, people, places, activities, and objects associated with the trauma.
- **Negative cognitive symptoms** include an inability to recall key features of the event, negative mood or emotions, feeling distanced from others, and a persistent negative view of the world.

To meet the criteria of PTSD, a particular number of these symptoms must be present for at least one month. If the same symptoms last for less than one month (but more than three days), it may be called **acute stress disorder**.

From a behaviorist perspective, symptoms of PTSD can be explained by the traumatic event and one's reaction to it. *Intrusion* and *arousal symptoms* can be explained by associative learning, specifically classical conditioning, in which the event has become associated with traumatic triggers and has generalized to include everyday stimuli. *Avoidance symptoms* can be explained through operant conditioning, specifically avoidance learning, in which an individual learns behavior to avoid unpleasant stimuli, or involuntary responses in the case of PTSD. Finally, negative cognitive symptoms can be viewed as a form of dissociation, which is a defense mechanism to avoid unpleasant stimuli. Dissociation will be covered in greater detail in *Dissociative Disorders.*

Dissociative Disorders

Patients with **dissociative disorders** avoid stress by escaping from parts of their identity. Such patients otherwise still have an intact sense of reality. Examples of dissociative disorders include dissociative amnesia, dissociative identity disorder (formerly multiple personality disorder), and depersonalization/derealization disorder.

Dissociative Amnesia

Dissociative amnesia is characterized by an inability to recall past experiences. The qualifier *dissociative* simply means that the amnesia is not due to a neurological disorder. This disorder is often linked to trauma. Some individuals with this disorder may also experience **dissociative fugue**: a sudden, unexpected move or purposeless wandering away from one's home or location of usual daily activities. Individuals in a fugue state are confused about their identity and can even assume a new identity. Significantly, they may actually believe that they are someone else, with a complete backstory.

Dissociative Identity Disorder

In **dissociative identity disorder** (**DID**, formerly multiple personality disorder), there are two or more personalities that recurrently take control of the patient's behavior, as represented in Figure 7.3. This disorder results when the components of identity fail to integrate. In most cases, patients have suffered severe physical or sexual abuse as young children. After much therapy, the personalities can sometimes be integrated into one. The existence of dissociative identity disorder is justifiably debated within the medical community, but its characteristics are still important to recognize on Test Day.

REAL WORLD

One of the first and most famous cases of dissociative identity disorder in the media is Shirley Ardell Mason, also known as "Sybil," who claimed to have at least 13 separate personalities. Mason underwent years of therapy in an attempt to combine her personalities into a single one. Two separate TV movies, both called *Sybil,* have been produced to tell the story of Sybil's struggle with this disorder.

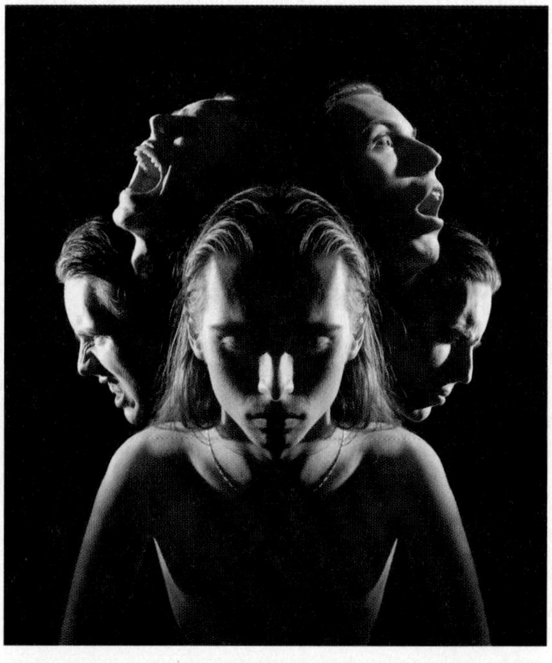

Figure 7.3 Dissociative Identity Disorder (DID)
One artist's interpretation of many personalities seen in DID.

Depersonalization/Derealization Disorder

In **depersonalization/derealization disorder**, individuals feel detached from their own minds and bodies (**depersonalization**) or from their surroundings (**derealization**). This often presents as a feeling of automation, and can include symptoms like a failure to recognize one's reflection. An out-of-body experience is an example of depersonalization. Derealization is often described as giving the world a dreamlike or insubstantial quality. Such patients may also experience depersonalization and derealization simultaneously. These feelings cause significant impairment of regular activities. However, even during these times, such patients do not display psychotic symptoms like delusions or hallucinations.

Somatic Symptom and Related Disorders

Diagnoses in this category are marked by somatic (bodily) symptoms that cause significant stress or impairment.

Somatic Symptom Disorder

Individuals with **somatic symptom disorder** have at least one somatic symptom, which may or may not be linked to an underlying medical condition, and that is accompanied by disproportionate concerns about its seriousness, devotion of an excessive amount of time and energy to it, or elevated levels of anxiety.

Illness Anxiety Disorder

Illness anxiety disorder is characterized by being consumed with thoughts about having or developing a serious medical condition. Individuals with this disorder are quick to become alarmed about their health, and either excessively check themselves for signs of illness or avoid medical appointments altogether. Most patients classified under hypochondriasis in the DSM-IV-TR now fit into either somatic symptom disorder if somatic symptoms are present, or illness anxiety disorder if they are not.

Conversion Disorder

Conversion disorder, also known as **functional neurological symptom disorder**, is characterized by symptoms affecting voluntary motor or sensory functions that are incompatible with the patient's neurophysiological condition. The symptoms generally begin soon after the individual experiences high levels of stress or a traumatic event, but may not develop until some time has passed after the initiating experience. Examples include paralysis or blindness without evidence of neurological damage. The patient may be surprisingly unconcerned by the symptom—what is called ***la belle indifférence***. Conversion disorder was historically called *hysteria*. The symptoms seen in conversion disorder may sometimes be connected with the inciting event in a literal or poetic way; for example, a parent going blind shortly after watching a child die tragically.

Personality Disorders

A **personality disorder** is a pattern of behavior that is inflexible and maladaptive, causing distress or impaired functioning in at least two of the following: cognition, emotions, interpersonal functioning, or impulse control. Personality disorders are considered **ego-syntonic**, meaning that individuals perceive their behavior as correct, normal, or in harmony with their goals. This is in contrast to the other disorders covered in this chapter that are **ego-dystonic**, meaning that individuals see the illness as something thrust upon them that is intrusive and bothersome. In addition to **general personality disorder** (which fits the diagnostic criteria described above), there are ten personality disorders grouped into three clusters: cluster A (paranoid, schizotypal, and schizoid), cluster B (antisocial, borderline, histrionic, and narcissistic), and cluster C (avoidant, dependent, and obsessive–compulsive). Personality disorder criteria will continue changing over time; the DSM-5 includes a section specifically devoted to research models for redefining personality disorders.

REAL WORLD

The distinction between **ego-syntonic** and **ego-dystonic** symptoms is a key feature in differential diagnosis of disorders in the DSM-5. For instance, social anxiety disorder shares many of the same symptoms as avoidant personality disorder, such as anxiety directed towards social interactions and maladaptive avoidance behavior. The distinction between these disorders is that individuals with social anxiety disorder often know that their fear of being ridiculed is irrational (ego-dystonic), while individuals with avoidant personality disorder actually believe they are inferior and that their fear of ridicule is valid (ego-syntonic).

Cluster A (Paranoid, Schizotypal, and Schizoid Personality Disorders)

The **cluster A personality disorders** are all marked by behavior that is labeled as odd or eccentric by others. Its three examples include paranoid, schizotypal, and schizoid personality disorders.

Paranoid personality disorder is marked by a pervasive distrust of others and suspicion regarding their motives. In some cases, these patients may actually be in the prodromal phase of schizophrenia and are termed premorbid.

Schizotypal personality disorder refers to a pattern of odd or eccentric thinking. These individuals may have ideas of reference (similar to delusions of reference, but not as extreme in intensity) as well as magical thinking, such as superstitiousness or a belief in clairvoyance.

Finally, **schizoid personality disorder** is a pervasive pattern of detachment from social relationships and a restricted range of emotional expression. People with this disorder show little desire for social interactions, have few or no close friends, and have poor social skills. It should be noted that neither schizotypal nor schizoid personality disorder are the same as schizophrenia.

Cluster B (Antisocial, Borderline, Histrionic, and Narcissistic Personality Disorders)

The **cluster B personality disorders** are all marked by behavior that is labeled as dramatic, emotional, or erratic by others. Its four examples include antisocial, borderline, histrionic, and narcissistic personality disorders.

Antisocial personality disorder is three times more common in males than in females. The essential feature of the disorder is a pattern of disregard for and violations of the rights of others. This is evidenced by repeated illegal acts, deceitfulness, aggressiveness, or a lack of remorse for said actions. Many serial killers and career criminals who show no guilt for their actions have this disorder. Additionally, people with this disorder comprise about 20 to 40 percent of prison populations.

Borderline personality disorder is two times more common in females than in males. In this disorder, there is pervasive instability in interpersonal behavior, mood, and self-image. Interpersonal relationships are often intense and unstable. There may be profound identity disturbance with uncertainty about self-image, sexual identity, long-term goals, or values. There is often intense fear of abandonment. Individuals with borderline personality disorder may use **splitting** as a defense mechanism, in which they view others as either all good or all bad (an *angel* vs. *devil* mentality). Suicide attempts and self-mutilation (cutting or burning) are common.

Histrionic personality disorder is characterized by constant attention-seeking behavior. These individuals often wear colorful clothing, are dramatic, and are exceptionally extroverted. They may also use seductive behavior to gain attention.

In **narcissistic personality disorder**, the patient has a grandiose sense of self-importance or uniqueness, preoccupation with fantasies of success, a need for constant admiration and attention, and characteristic disturbances in interpersonal relationships such as feelings of entitlement. As used in everyday language, narcissism refers to those who like themselves too much. However, people with narcissistic personality disorder have very fragile self-esteem and are constantly concerned with how others view them. There may be marked feelings of rage, inferiority, shame, humiliation, or emptiness when these individuals are not viewed favorably by others.

Cluster C (Avoidant, Dependent, and Obsessive–Compulsive Personality Disorders)

The **cluster C personality disorders** are all marked by behavior that is labeled as anxious or fearful by others. Its three examples include avoidant, dependent, and obsessive–compulsive personality disorders.

In **avoidant personality disorder**, the affected individual has extreme shyness and fear of rejection. Individuals who have this disorder will see themselves as socially inept and are often socially isolated, despite an intense desire for social affection and acceptance. These individuals tend to stay in the same jobs, life situations, and relationships despite wanting to change.

Dependent personality disorder is characterized by a continuous need for reassurance. Individuals with dependent personality disorder tend to remain dependent on one specific person, such as a caregiver or significant other, to take actions and make decisions.

In **obsessive–compulsive personality disorder** (**OCPD**), the individual is perfectionistic and inflexible, tending to like rules and order. Other characteristics may include an inability to discard worn-out objects, lack of desire to change, excessive stubbornness, lack of a sense of humor, and maintenance of careful routines. Note that obsessive–compulsive personality disorder is not the same as obsessive–compulsive disorder. Whereas OCD has obsessions and compulsions that are focal and acquired, OCPD is lifelong. OCD is also ego-dystonic (*I can't stop washing my hands because of the germs!*), whereas OCPD is ego-syntonic (*I just like rules and order!*).

KEY CONCEPT

Obsessive-compulsive disorder (OCD) and obsessive-compulsive personality disorder (OCPD) are not synonymous. OCD is marked by obsessions (intrusive thoughts causing tension) and compulsions (repetitive tasks that relieve this tension but cause significant impairment). OCPD is a personality disorder in which individuals are perfectionistic and inflexible.

BEHAVIORAL SCIENCES GUIDED EXAMPLE WITH EXPERT THINKING

The following individuals are patients at an inpatient mental health facility.

Patient A's hospitalization is the result of an intense argument with a family member that involved threats of violence, which prompted the police to be called. For the first two weeks of her stay, Patient A spoke often about plans to start several online business ventures, saying that she felt she was a "business genius" and that she would be a billionaire by the end of the year. She slept very little and was irritable, often becoming angry with clinic staff when they tried to reason with her about the soundness of her plans. In the following weeks of Patient A's stay, her mood leveled and she expressed regret over her treatment of her family.

A: Elevated mood, irritable, rapid speech. Lasts 2 weeks.

Patient B arrived at the clinic as a result of complaints from his neighbors. When police entered his apartment, they found it in complete disrepair, and it was clear that he had stopped attending to his personal hygiene long ago. During the first few weeks of his stay, Patient B made no effort to speak to staff or other patients. When he did respond to questions, his answers were short phrases, sometimes unrelated to the question, and sometimes simply a repetition of a few words from the question. He spent his days isolated, often sitting, immobile and unresponsive to occurrences around him.

B: Not taking care of himself, not talking or reacting to others.

Based only on the information provided, what diagnosis from the DSM-5 is most likely for each of these patients?

If you're asked to make a diagnosis for a hypothetical patient, make a checklist of the symptoms described in the passage or question, and then match them to what you know about the disorders that are within the scope of the MCAT. It is worth taking a moment to consider the severity of the symptoms as well, since it can help to differentiate between similar disorders (depression and dysthymic disorder, for example).

Patient A exhibits grandiose self-esteem, rapid speech, a lack of need for sleep, and irritability, which are all symptoms of mania and together are sufficient to apply the label of manic episode. The described transition out of mania into a different mood state suggests bipolar disorder. Specifically, the presence of a full manic episode rules out bipolar II and would lead to a diagnosis of bipolar I, which does not require a depressive episode to follow.

Patient B is trickier, but consider that the writers of the MCAT know that you are not a trained psychiatrist and so will not require a nuanced diagnosis from you. The symptoms that they present will be straightforward and should add up to a description of a disorder that you are familiar with. For patient B, those symptoms are avolition (an inability to perform basic goal-directed activities), flat or blunted affect (lack of emotional expression), and alogia (reduction in speaking). These are all negative symptoms of schizophrenia. The description of patient B also includes echolalia (repetition of words or short phrases), which is a positive symptom and is a signal to you as a test taker that this is indeed schizophrenia, rather than a case of severe depression. While there is still the possibility that Patient B has another, related disorder, the MCAT would not present you with a choice that would require you to distinguish between, say, schizophrenia and schizoid personality disorder without substantial additional information allowing that decision to be made.

In summary, patient A is most likely experiencing bipolar I disorder, and patient B is most likely experiencing schizophrenia or a related disorder.

MCAT CONCEPT CHECK 7.2

Before you move on, assess your understanding of the material with these questions.

1. A schizophrenic patient is started on the atypical antipsychotic *risperidone*, which is effective for treatment of the positive symptoms of schizophrenia, but not the negative symptoms. Which of the patient's symptoms are likely to improve, and which are not?

____

____

____

2. What are the features of a major depressive episode? Of a manic episode?
   - Major depressive episode:

____

   - Manic episode:

____

3. For each of the following disorders, briefly describe their makeup with respect to depressive episodes, manic episodes, and other mood disturbances:
   - Major depressive disorder:

____

   - Bipolar I disorder:

____

   - Bipolar II disorder:

____

   - Cyclothymic disorder:

____

4. A patient with obsessive–compulsive disorder believes that the latch on the apartment door must be checked five times before it is okay to go to bed. Without checking the latch five times, the patient cannot sleep for fear that someone will break into the apartment. Identify the patient's obsession, the patient's compulsion, and how they are related in obsessive–compulsive disorder.
   - Obsession:

   ____

   - Compulsion:

   ____

   - Relationship:

   ____

5. What features describe each cluster of personality disorders? Which personality disorders fall into each cluster?

Cluster	Features	Personality Disorders
A		
B		
C		

7.3 Biological Basis of Nervous System Disorders

High-Yield

LEARNING OBJECTIVES

After Chapter 7.3, you will be able to:

- Describe the impact of depression on hormone and neurotransmitter levels
- Recall the general features and risk factors for Alzheimer's disease
- Explain the role of dopamine in schizophrenia and Parkinson's disease

In addition to knowing the psychological and sociological components of these diagnoses, the MCAT also expects you to know the biological basis of a few mental disorders. These disorders include schizophrenia, depression, Alzheimer's disease, and Parkinson's disease. Research into how to stop the progression of the biological component of these diseases is widespread and will also be something to stay apprised of as a medical student and a physician.

Schizophrenia

Schizophrenia is an area of active research, though some biological factors have been isolated. Most potential causes are genetic, but trauma at birth, especially hypoxemia (low oxygen concentrations in the blood), is also considered to be a risk factor. Other exposures may also play a role; excessive marijuana use in adolescence is associated with increased risk. There is significant data to indicate that schizophrenia is partially inherited. If a person has this disorder, the risk that first-degree relatives will also have the disorder is ten times that of an unrelated person in the general population; this measurement controls for environmental effects.

Schizophrenia may be associated with structural changes in the brain, but more research is needed to determine their significance and prevalence within the affected population. Schizophrenia is highly associated with an excess of dopamine in the brain; many medications used to treat schizophrenia, such as neuroleptics, block dopamine receptors. The term **neuroleptic** means that these medications depress nerve function. Neuroleptics are also known as **antipsychotics**.

Depressive and Bipolar Disorders

There are a host of markers associated with depression:

- Abnormally high glucose metabolism in the amygdala
- Hippocampal atrophy after a long duration of illness
- Abnormally high levels of glucocorticoids (cortisol)
- Decreased norepinephrine, serotonin, and dopamine (monoamine theory of depression)

It has been found that both these neurotransmitters and their metabolites are decreased in depressed patients, meaning that their actual production is decreased (rather than production staying the same and their degradation increasing).

For bipolar disorders, there exists a different set of biological factors and genetic corollaries that contribute to the disease:

- Increased norepinephrine and serotonin (monoamine theory)
- Higher risk if parent has bipolar disorder
- Higher risk for persons with multiple sclerosis

Alzheimer's Disease

Alzheimer's disease is a type of dementia characterized by gradual memory loss, disorientation to time and place, problems with abstract thought, and a tendency to misplace things. Later stages of the disease are associated with changes in mood or behavior, changes in personality, difficulty with procedural memory, poor judgment, and loss of initiative. Now, each of these symptoms alone doesn't necessarily point to Alzheimer's; however, when all or almost all of these symptoms are seen in one person, and especially when the symptoms end up inhibiting normal daily function, this points to Alzheimer's disease. This disease is most common in patients older than 65, and women are at greater risk than men. Family history is a significant risk factor and, interestingly, there is a lower risk of developing the disease with higher levels of education.

There is a genetic component to Alzheimer's disease. Research shows that mutations in the *presenilin* genes on chromosomes 1 and 14 contribute to having the disease, and mutations in the *apolipoprotein E* gene on chromosome 19 can also alter the likelihood of acquiring the disease. Finally, the *β-amyloid precursor protein* gene on chromosome 21 is known to contribute to Alzheimer's disease, explaining the much higher risk of Alzheimer's in individuals with Down syndrome.

While the precise biological cause of Alzheimer's disease is unknown, there are many biological markers that are found in patients with the disease. Don't worry about understanding each of these markers in depth, but rather be able to recognize these factors if you see them on the MCAT:

- Diffuse atrophy of the brain on CT or MRI
- Flattened sulci in the cerebral cortex
- Enlarged cerebral ventricles, shown in Figure 7.4(a)
- Deficient blood flow in parietal lobes, which is correlated with cognitive decline
- Reduction in levels of acetylcholine
- Reduction in *choline acetyltransferase* (ChAT), the enzyme that produces acetylcholine
- Reduced metabolism in temporal and parietal lobes
- Senile plaques of ***β*-amyloid** (a misfolded protein in β-pleated sheet form), shown in Figure 7.4(b)
- Neurofibrillary tangles of hyperphosphorylated tau protein, shown in Figure 7.4(c)

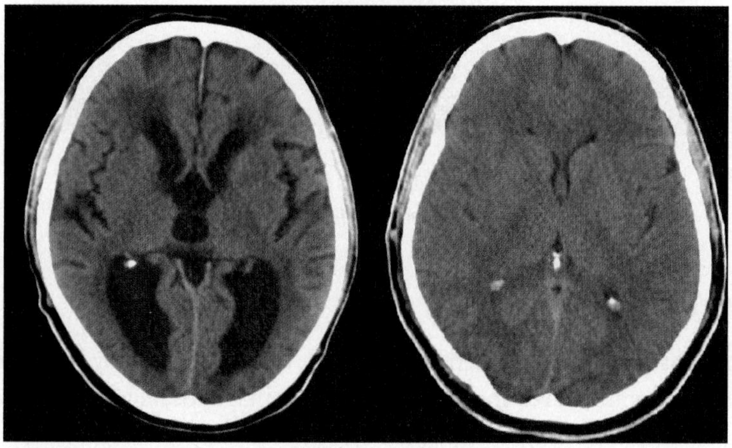

Figure 7.4(a) Symptoms of Alzheimer's Disease
Enlarged cerebral ventricles (left) vs. normal cerebral ventricles (right)

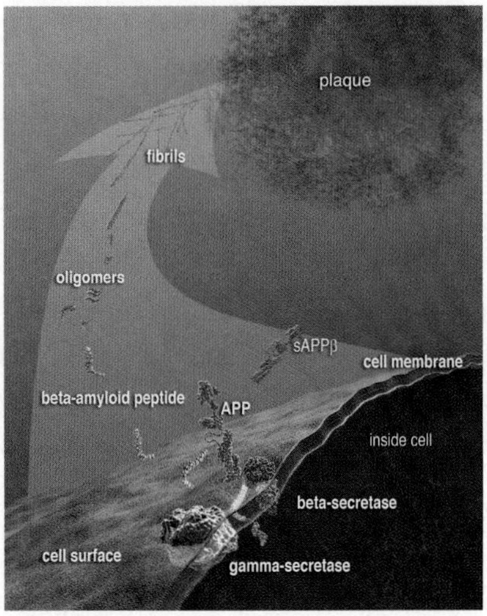

Figure 7.4(b) Symptoms of Alzheimer's Disease
Formation of senile plaques of β-amyloid

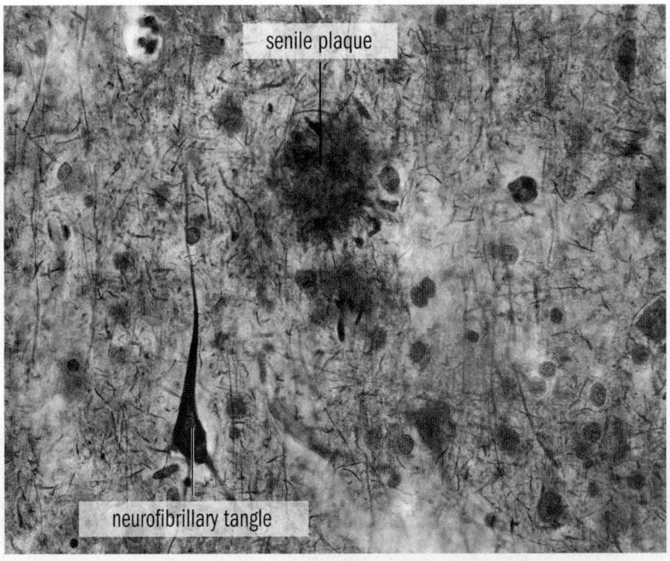

Figure 7.4(c) Symptoms of Alzheimer's Disease
Neurofibrillary tangles of hyperphosphorylated tau protein (magenta)

Parkinson's Disease

Parkinson's disease, demonstrated in Figure 7.5, is characterized by **bradykinesia** (slowness in movement), **resting tremor** (a tremor that appears when muscles are not being used), **pill-rolling tremor** (flexing and extending the fingers while moving the thumb back and forth, as if rolling something in the fingers), **masklike facies** (static and expressionless facial features, staring eyes, and a partially open mouth), **cogwheel rigidity** (muscle tension that intermittently halts movement as an examiner attempts to manipulate a limb), and a **shuffling gait** with stooped posture. A common but not characteristic symptom is depression. Dementia is also common in Parkinson's disease.

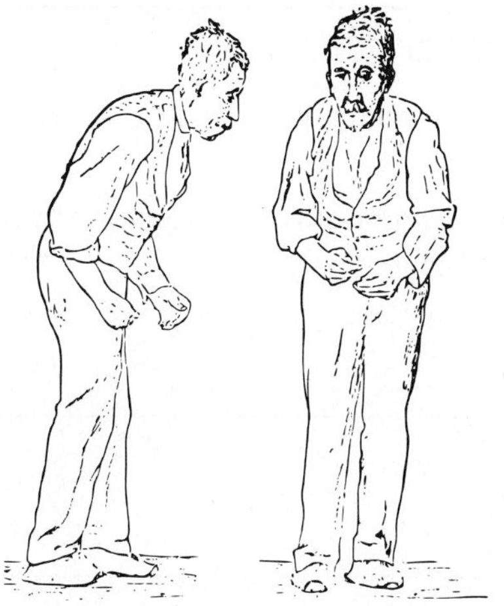

Figure 7.5 Findings of Parkinson's Disease
Note the masklike facies, shuffling gait, and stooped posture.

The biological basis of this disease is decreased dopamine production in the **substantia nigra**, a layer of cells in the brain that functions to produce dopamine to permit proper functioning of the **basal ganglia**, as shown in Figure 7.6. The basal ganglia are critical for initiating and terminating movements, as well as sustaining repetitive motor tasks and smoothening motions; thus, the symptoms of Parkinson's disease flow logically from its underlying cause. This condition can be partially managed, therefore, with **L-DOPA**, a precursor that is converted to dopamine once in the brain, replacing that which is lost due to Parkinson's disease. There have also been attempts to regenerate dopaminergic neurons in the substantia nigra using stem cells placed into the central nervous system. Similar stem cell-based therapies have been used in other contexts, such as after a spinal cord injury or stroke to attempt to regenerate function in the central nervous system, with limited results.

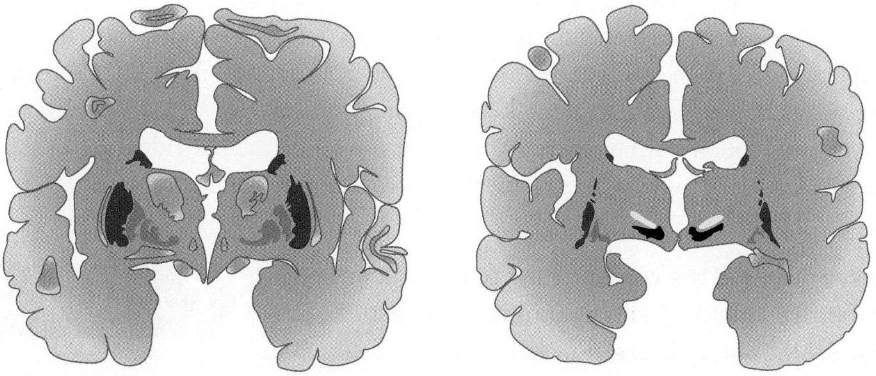

Figure 7.6 The Basal Ganglia
The substantia nigra in the midbrain (black) releases dopamine to activate the other regions of the basal ganglia (blue, red, and yellow).

REAL WORLD

Note the connection between schizophrenia and psychosis (caused by an excess of dopamine) and Parkinson's disease (caused by a deficit of dopamine). Antipsychotic medications often lead to "parkinsonian" side effects, like muscle rigidity and flattened affect. Medications used in Parkinson's disease often lead to psychotic side effects, such as hallucinations and delusions.

MCAT CONCEPT CHECK 7.3

Before you move on, assess your understanding of the material with these questions.

1. Which hormone and neurotransmitter concentrations are elevated in depression? Which ones are reduced?
   - Elevated:

   ____

   - Reduced:

   ____

2. Provide an example of a genetic factor that appears to increase risk of Alzheimer's disease.

   ____

3. How are dopamine levels related in schizophrenia and Parkinson's disease?

   ____

Conclusion

The content covered in this chapter will allow you to score more points on the MCAT—and to prepare for your clinical clerkships in psychiatry. This chapter is unique in that it covers not how the mind normally works, as we see in the other chapters in this book, but rather how the mind works when it is functioning abnormally. The MCAT tests critical thinking; one common way to do this is to ask what happens when a system—like the mind—is not functioning normally. Thus, this chapter covered high-yield information that is likely to appear on the MCAT because it connects all three subjects of the *Psychological, Social, and Biological Foundations of Behavior* section. In the next chapter, we move away from the individual as we begin to explore social psychology; from there, we'll continue expanding outward as we move into sociology.

You've reviewed the content, now test your knowledge and critical thinking skills by completing a test-like passage set in your online resources!

GO ONLINE

CONCEPT SUMMARY

Understanding Psychological Disorders

- The **biomedical approach** to psychological disorders takes into account only the physical and medical causes of a psychological disorder. Thus, treatments in this approach are of a biomedical nature.
- The **biopsychosocial approach** considers the relative contributions of biological, psychological, and social components to an individual's disorder. Treatments also fall into these three areas.
- The ***Diagnostic and Statistical Manual of Mental Disorders*** is used to diagnose psychological disorders. Its current version is DSM-5 (published May 2013). It categorizes mental disorders based on symptom patterns.
- Psychological disorders, especially anxiety, depressive, and substance use disorders, are very common in the population.

Types of Psychological Disorders

- **Schizophrenia** is the prototypical disorder with psychosis as a feature. It contains positive and negative symptoms.
  - **Positive symptoms** add something to behavior, cognition, or affect and include delusions, hallucinations, disorganized speech, and disorganized behavior.
  - **Negative symptoms** are the loss of something from behavior, cognition, or affect and include disturbance of affect and avolition.
- **Depressive disorders** include major depressive disorder, dysthymia, and seasonal affective disorder.
  - **Major depressive disorder** contains at least one major depressive episode.
  - **Persistent depressive disorder (dysthymia)** is the presence of depressive symptoms for at least two years that do not meet criteria for major depressive disorder.
- **Bipolar and related disorders** have manic or hypomanic episodes.
  - **Bipolar I disorder** contains at least one manic episode.
  - **Bipolar II disorder** contains at least one major depressive episode and least one hypomanic episode.
  - **Cyclothymic disorder** describes periods of manic and depressive symptoms that are not severe enough to be labeled an episode. These symptoms must persist for at least 2 years and be present the majority of that time.
- **Anxiety disorders** capture conditions in which excessive fear or anxiety impairs one's daily functions. Anxiety disorders are differentiated by the stimuli that induces anxiety.
  - **Specific phobias** are irrational fears of specific objects or situations.

- **Separation anxiety disorder** is anxiety due to separation from one's caregivers, often with the ideation that if separated, either the caregiver or the patient will be harmed.
- **Social anxiety disorder** is anxiety due to social or performance situations with the ideation that the patient will be negatively evaluated.
- **Selective mutism** disorder is the impairment of speech in situations where speaking is expected.
- **Panic disorder** is marked by recurrent panic attacks: intense, overwhelming fear and sympathetic nervous system activity with no clear stimulus. It may lead to agoraphobia.
- **Agoraphobia** is a fear of places or situations where it is hard for an individual to escape.
- **Generalized anxiety disorder** is a disproportionate and persistent worry about many different things for at least six months.

- **Obsessive–compulsive disorder and related disorders** are characterized by perceived needs (obsessions or preoccupations) and paired actions to meet those needs (compulsions).
  - **Obsessive–compulsive disorder** is characterized by **obsessions** (persistent, intrusive thoughts and impulses) and **compulsions** (repetitive tasks that relieve tension but cause significant impairment in a person's life).
  - **Body dysmorphic disorder** is characterized by an unrealistic negative evaluation of one's appearance or a specific body part. The individual often takes extreme measures to correct the perceived imperfection.
  - **Hoarding disorder** is characterized by the reluctance of giving up one's physical possessions. Often this behavior is associated with excessive acquisition of physical items.
- **Posttraumatic stress disorder** (**PTSD**) is characterized by intrusion symptoms (reliving the event, flashbacks, nightmares), avoidance symptoms (avoidance of people, places, objects associated with trauma), negative cognitive symptoms (amnesia, negative mood and emotions), and arousal symptoms (increased startle response, irritability, anxiety). These symptoms can be explained from the behaviorist perspective.
- **Dissociative disorders** include dissociative amnesia, dissociative identity disorder, and depersonalization/derealization disorder.
  - **Dissociative amnesia** is an inability to recall past experience without an underlying neurological disorder. In severe forms, it may involve **dissociative fugue**, a sudden change in location that may involve the assumption of a new identity.
  - **Dissociative identity disorder** is the occurrence of two or more personalities that take control of a person's behavior.
  - **Depersonalization/derealization disorder** involves feelings of detachment from the mind and body or from the environment.

- **Somatic symptom and related disorders** involve significant bodily symptoms.
  - **Somatic symptom disorder** involves at least one somatic symptom, which may or may not be linked to an underlying medical condition, that causes disproportionate concern.
  - **Illness anxiety disorder** is a preoccupation with thoughts about having, or coming down with, a serious medical condition.
  - **Conversion disorder** involves unexplained symptoms affecting motor or sensory function and is associated with prior trauma.
- **Personality disorders (PD)** are patterns of inflexible, maladaptive behavior that cause distress or impaired functioning in at least two of the following: cognition, emotions, interpersonal functioning, or impulse control. They occur in three **clusters**: **A** (odd, eccentric), **B** (dramatic, emotional, erratic), and **C** (anxious, fearful).
  - Cluster A includes paranoid, schizotypal, and schizoid PDs. Cluster B includes antisocial, borderline, histrionic, and narcissistic PDs. Cluster C includes avoidant, dependent, and obsessive–compulsive PDs.
  - **Paranoid PD** involves a pervasive distrust and suspicion of others.
  - **Schizotypal PD** involves ideas of reference, magical thinking, and eccentricity.
  - **Schizoid PD** involves detachment from social relationships and limited emotion.
  - **Antisocial PD** involves a disregard for the rights of others.
  - **Borderline PD** involves instability in relationships, mood, and self-image. **Splitting** is characteristic, as are recurrent suicide attempts.
  - **Histrionic PD** involves constant attention-seeking behavior.
  - **Narcissistic PD** involves a grandiose sense of self-importance and need for admiration.
  - **Avoidant PD** involves extreme shyness and fear of rejection.
  - **Dependent PD** involves a continuous need for reassurance.
  - **Obsessive–compulsive PD** involves perfectionism, inflexibility, and preoccupation with rules.

Biological Basis of Nervous System Disorders

- Schizophrenia may be associated with genetic factors, birth trauma, adolescent marijuana use, and family history. There are high levels of dopaminergic transmission.
- Depression is accompanied by high levels of glucocorticoids and low levels of norepinephrine, serotonin, and dopamine.

- Bipolar disorders are accompanied by high levels of norepinephrine and serotonin. They are also highly heritable.
- Alzheimer's disease is associated with genetic factors, brain atrophy, decreases in acetylcholine, senile plaques of **β-amyloid**, and **neurofibrillary tangles** of hyperphosphorylated tau protein.
- **Parkinson's disease** is associated with **bradykinesia**, **resting tremor**, **pill-rolling tremor**, **masklike facies**, **cogwheel rigidity**, and a **shuffling gait**. There is decreased production of dopamine by cells in the **substantia nigra**.

ANSWERS TO CONCEPT CHECKS

7.1

1. Whereas the biomedical model considers only the physical, pathological mechanisms that underlie mental illness, the biopsychosocial model considers the contributions of these biological factors along with psychology (thoughts, emotions, or behaviors) and social situation (environment, social class, discrimination, or stigmatization).
2. The following disorders occur in greater than 2 percent of the United States population per year: specific phobia, social anxiety disorder, major depressive disorder, posttraumatic stress disorder, bipolar disorder, generalized anxiety disorder, and panic disorder.

7.2

1. Positive symptoms of schizophrenia, including delusions, hallucinations (usually auditory), disorganized thought, and disorganized behavior, are likely to improve from treatment with an antipsychotic medication. Negative symptoms, including disturbance of affect and avolition, are largely unaffected by antipsychotic medications.
2. Major depressive episodes include a two-week duration of at least five of the following symptoms: depressed mood, loss of interest (anhedonia), sleep disturbance, feelings of guilt, lack of energy, difficulty concentrating, changes in appetite, psychomotor symptoms, and suicidal thoughts. At least one of the symptoms must be depressed mood or anhedonia. Manic episodes include a one-week duration of at least three of the following symptoms: elevated or expansive mood, distractibility, decreased need for sleep, grandiosity, flight of ideas or racing thoughts, agitation, pressured speech, and engagement in risky behavior.
3. Major depressive disorder contains at least one major depressive episode with no manic episodes. Bipolar I disorder has at least one manic episode with or without depressive episodes. Bipolar II disorder has at least one hypomanic episode with at least one major depressive episode. Cyclothymic disorder has hypomanic episodes and dysthymia that is not severe enough to be a major depressive episode.
4. Obsessions are persistent, intrusive thoughts and impulses that produce tension. In this case, the obsession is the patient's thought that someone will break into the apartment. Compulsions are repetitive tasks that relieve tension but cause significant impairment in a person's life. This patient's compulsion is having to check the latch on the apartment door five times before going to bed. Their relationship is that obsessions raise tension while compulsions relieve that tension.

5.

Cluster	Features	Personality Disorders
A	Odd or eccentric	Paranoid, schizotypal, schizoid
B	Dramatic, emotional, or erratic	Antisocial, borderline, histrionic, narcissistic
C	Anxious or fearful	Avoidant, dependent, obsessive–compulsive

7.3

1. In depression, levels of cortisol are increased. Many neurotransmitter levels are reduced, including norepinephrine, serotonin, and dopamine.
2. Mutations in the *presenilin* genes (chromosomes 1 and 14) and β-amyloid precursor protein gene (chromosome 21) are associated with increased risk for Alzheimer's disease.
3. Dopamine levels are elevated in schizophrenia and reduced in Parkinson's disease. Thus, treatments for one disorder may cause symptoms similar to those of the other.

SCIENCE MASTERY ASSESSMENT EXPLANATIONS

1. **C**

Negative symptoms are the absence of normal or desired behavior, which include disturbance of affect and avolition. Positive symptoms are the addition of abnormal behavior, including hallucinations, **(A)**, disorganized behavior, **(B)**, and delusions, **(D)**.

2. **A**

Echolalia is an involuntary repetition of others' words and utterances and may be seen in schizophrenia. Echopraxia, **(B)**, is imitation of others' actions. Loosening of associations, **(C)**, is a type of disordered thought in which the patient moves between remotely related ideas. Neologisms, **(D)**, are newly invented words.

3. **A**

Focusing on details, loving routine, having a sense that there is only one right way to do things, and lack of humor suggests an obsessive–compulsive personality disorder.

4. **C**

Depression is marked by a period of at least two weeks in which the patient has five of nine cardinal symptoms, one of which must be depressed mood or lack of interest (anhedonia). While decreased need for sleep is commonly seen in manic episodes, it may also appear in depression, as sleep disturbance is one of the nine cardinal symptoms. Not all depressed individuals are suicidal, as in **(B)**. In older individuals, depression may often manifest as anhedonia without feelings of sadness, invalidating **(D)**.

5. **B**

The doctor is using the biomedical approach since the focus is on only the biological cause of the patient's symptoms. Furthermore, since the treatment centers only on the patient, the doctor is using direct therapy. This combination of approach and therapy matches **(B)** as the correct answer. By contrast, a doctor using the biopsychosocial approach would likely consider the patient's recent move, stresses associated with the accelerated program, and lack of support structure as potential causes of depression. Additionally, treatment using the biopsychosocial approach includes indirect therapy which focuses on increasing social support.

6. **D**

Dissociative fugue is characterized by sudden travel or change in normal day-to-day activities and occurs in some cases of dissociative amnesia. Symptoms include an inability to recall one's past or confusion about one's identity. Thus, the described patient is most likely to be suffering dissociative amnesia accompanied by dissociative fugue.

7. **D**

Agoraphobia, or a fear of places or situations in which it would be difficult to escape, is commonly seen in panic disorder. Concern about having a panic attack in public may make these individuals fearful of leaving their home.

8. **D**

Phobias affect approximately 9% of the population, meaning that on average 9 in 100 individuals will have some sort of phobia. In a sample of 50 people, 4 or 5 people will need to be excluded, assuming that the sample is representative of the larger population. Thus, **(D)** is correct.

9. **A**

The symptoms listed indicate a major depressive episode. However, depressive episodes can be a part of bipolar disorders, which also contain manic episodes. Thus, if manic episodes have not yet been asked about, one cannot distinguish between depression or bipolar disorder as the correct diagnosis yet.

10. **B**

To determine if this patient has major depressive disorder or a bipolar disorder, the presence of manic (or hypomanic) episodes should be confirmed. Bipolar disorders contain manic (or hypomanic) episodes, while major depressive disorder does not.

11. **B**

The correct answer should be a statement that is not relevant to Alzheimer's disease. Choice **(B)**, a decreased abundance of serotonin and norepinephrine, describes the monoamine theory of depression. These neurochemical changes are not known risk factors or diagnostic criteria for Alzheimer's disease, making **(B)** the correct answer. The remaining choices are either risk factors or diagnostic criteria for Alzheimer's disease. Choice **(A)** describes the increased risk of Alzheimer's disease in individuals with Down syndrome, as the gene for β-amyloid precursor is on chromosome 21. Choices **(C)** and **(D)** both describe biological markers of Alzheimer's disease.

12. **B**

Splitting, the consideration of others as either "all good" or "all bad," is characteristic of borderline personality disorder.

13. **A**

Conversion disorder is marked by a motor or sensory symptom in the absence of an underlying physical or neurological cause. It is associated with an inciting event that, in this case, may have been the argument with the family member. The patient's lack of concern over the deficit is referred to as *la belle indifférence*.

14. **C**

The symptoms indicate that the patient likely has Parkinson's disease. This disease is caused by decreased dopamine production in the substantia nigra.

15. **B**

Bipolar disorders have been shown to be highly heritable and are associated with increased levels of norepinephrine and serotonin in the brain. Bipolar I disorder can be diagnosed with a single manic episode and does not require a major depressive episode. Bipolar II disorder requires at least one hypomanic episode and one major depressive episode. Cyclothymic disorder contains at least one hypomanic episode and dysthymia.

Consult your online resources for additional practice. **GO ONLINE**

SHARED CONCEPTS

Behavioral Sciences Chapter 1
Biology and Behavior

Behavioral Sciences Chapter 3
Learning and Memory

Behavioral Sciences Chapter 12
Social Stratification

Biology Chapter 4
The Nervous System

Biology Chapter 5
The Endocrine System

Biology Chapter 12
Genetics and Evolution

CHAPTER 8

SOCIAL PROCESSES, ATTITUDES, AND BEHAVIOR

SCIENCE MASTERY ASSESSMENT

Every pre-med knows this feeling: there is so much content I have to know for the MCAT! How do I know what to do first or what's important?

While the high-yield badges throughout this book will help you identify the most important topics, this Science Mastery Assessment is another tool in your MCAT prep arsenal. This quiz (which can also be taken in your online resources) and the guidance below will help ensure that you are spending the appropriate amount of time on this chapter based on your personal strengths and weaknesses. Don't worry though—skipping something now does not mean you'll never study it. Later on in your prep, as you complete full-length tests, you'll uncover specific pieces of content that you need to review and can come back to these chapters as appropriate.

How to Use This Assessment

If you answer 0–7 questions correctly:

Spend about 1 hour to read this chapter in full and take limited notes throughout. Follow up by reviewing **all** quiz questions to ensure that you now understand how to solve each one.

If you answer 8–11 questions correctly:

Spend 20–40 minutes reviewing the quiz questions. Beginning with the questions you missed, read and take notes on the corresponding subchapters. For questions you answered correctly, ensure your thinking matches that of the explanation and you understand why each choice was correct or incorrect.

If you answer 12–15 questions correctly:

Spend less than 20 minutes reviewing all questions from the quiz. If you missed any, then include a quick read-through of the corresponding subchapters, or even just the relevant content within a subchapter, as part of your question review. For questions you answered correctly, ensure your thinking matches that of the explanation and review the Concept Summary at the end of the chapter.

1. The behavior of the individuals in the Stanford prison experiment is best explained by which of the following terms?
   I. Bystander effect
   II. Deindividuation
   III. Internalization
   IV. Social loafing

   A. I only
   B. III only
   C. II and III only
   D. II and IV only

2. A jury member who initially feels that a strict penalty should be placed on the defendant votes for an even stricter penalty after deliberation with the other jury members. This behavior is best described by which social phenomenon?
   A. Social facilitation
   B. Group polarization
   C. Assimilation
   D. Socialization

3. Which of the following would decrease the likelihood of a bystander lending aid to a victim?
   A. Increasing the number of people in the room
   B. Increasing the degree of danger experienced by the victim
   C. Making the victim an acquaintance instead of a stranger
   D. Being alone in the room with the victim

4. During groupthink, members of the group do all of the following EXCEPT:
   A. stereotype members outside of the group.
   B. withhold opposing views.
   C. ignore warnings against the ideas of the group.
   D. create a sense of negativity against risk taking.

5. Adult prison systems may attempt to change the behavior of inmates through all of the following mechanisms of socialization EXCEPT:
   A. primary socialization.
   B. secondary socialization.
   C. anticipatory socialization.
   D. resocialization.

6. Your neighbors ask you to collect their mail while they are out of town and you agree. Later that day, they ask you to water their plants as well. What technique for compliance are they using in this scenario?
   A. Lowball technique
   B. That's-not-all technique
   C. Foot-in-the-door technique
   D. Door-in-the-face technique

7. Which of the following statements represents the affective component of an attitude?
   A. "I love action movies."
   B. "I'm going to see a new action movie at the theater."
   C. "Action movies are much better than comedies."
   D. "Tomorrow, I'm going to rent an action movie."

8. After sitting in a lecture, determining that a professor is a bad teacher based on the professor's unprofessional attire and monotone speech is an example of which type of processing?
   A. Knowledge route processing
   B. Adaptive route processing
   C. Central route processing
   D. Peripheral route processing

9. In the Milgram shock experiment, many subjects were willing to give the maximal voltage shock because they were influenced by which psychological principle?
   A. Deviance
   B. Obedience
   C. Conformity
   D. Compliance

10. Each individual in a group of teenagers is asked to estimate the height of a tree. One individual estimates the height to be 25 feet, but after discussing with the group is convinced that the height is likely closer to 40 feet. Which type of conformity is seen here?
    A. Normative
    B. Identification
    C. Internalization
    D. Compliance

11. Which of the following is NOT a component of the functional attitudes theory?
    A. Knowledge
    B. Acceptance
    C. Ego defense
    D. Ego expression

12. The swimming times for all members of a swim team are tracked over a six-month period in team-only practices and at public meets. For 14 of the 16 members, top times were clocked at the meets. What social phenomenon does this evidence support?
    A. Social facilitation
    B. Peer pressure
    C. Identification
    D. Group polarization

13. An 18-year-old is completing the final months of high school and begins to wake up early each day to run five miles in preparation for joining the Army. What type of socialization is this young person experiencing?
    A. Normative socialization
    B. Informative socialization
    C. Resocialization
    D. Anticipatory socialization

14. Which of the following best reflects the difference between social action and social interaction?
    A. Social action refers to positive changes one makes in their society; social interaction refers to the route by which these changes occur.
    B. Social action refers to the effects of a group on an individual's behavior; social interaction refers to the effects that multiple individuals all have on each other.
    C. Social action refers to changes in behavior caused by internal factors; social interaction refers to changes in behavior caused by external factors.
    D. Social action refers to changes in behaviors that benefit only the individual; social interaction refers to changes in behavior that benefit others.

15. In the group setting, the mentality of "If you aren't with us, you're against us" is most representative of which factor of groupthink?
    A. Illusion of invulnerability
    B. Illusion of morality
    C. Pressure for conformity
    D. Self-censorship

Answer Key

1. **C**
2. **B**
3. **A**
4. **D**
5. **A**
6. **C**
7. **A**
8. **D**
9. **B**
10. **C**
11. **B**
12. **A**
13. **D**
14. **B**
15. **C**

Detailed explanations can be found at the end of the chapter.

CHAPTER 8

SOCIAL PROCESSES, ATTITUDES, AND BEHAVIOR

In This Chapter

CHAPTER PROFILE

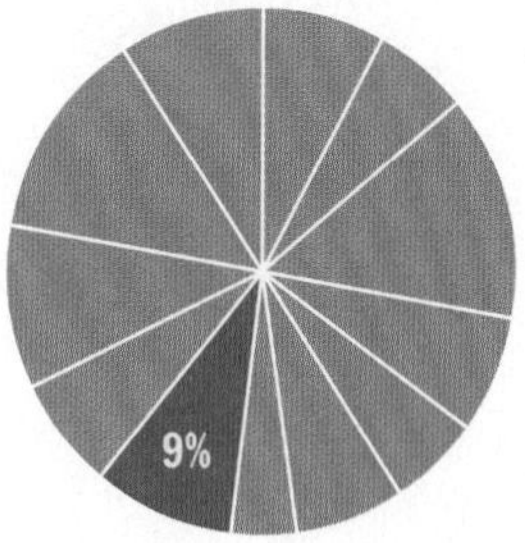

The content in this chapter should be relevant to about 9% of all questions about the behavioral sciences on the MCAT.

This chapter covers material from the following AAMC content categories:

7A: Individual influences on behavior

7B: Social processes that influence human behavior

7C: Attitude and behavior change

Introduction

The renowned Italian painter and sculptor Michelangelo Buonarroti stated that a sculptor simply releases and uncovers the ideal figures that are hidden within stone. This idea has led psychologists and sociologists to describe what is known as the **Michelangelo phenomenon**. The concept of self is made up of both the intrapersonal self, the ideas that individuals have regarding their own abilities, traits, and beliefs, and the interpersonal self, the manner in which others influence creation of the ideal self. In the Michaelangelo phenomenon, a close relationship between two individuals 'sculpts' both individuals' skills and traits. This development occurs because of each individual's perceptions of the other, and their behaviors in response to one another.

In this chapter, you will learn about the social processes and interactions that develop this self. The behavior and attitudes of individuals are highly influenced by the people with whom they interact, the society in which they live, and the culture in which they are immersed. Humans, being naturally social creatures, learn how to behave and react based on their relationships and experiences. The following pages will give us an in-depth look at the ways behavior is affected by the presence of others, group processes, culture, and socialization, as well as how attitudes are formed and how they impact behavior.

8.1 Group Psychology

High-Yield

LEARNING OBJECTIVES

After Chapter 8.1, you will be able to:

- Describe social facilitation, deindividuation, the bystander effect, social loafing, and peer pressure
- Compare and contrast group polarization and groupthink
- Distinguish between assimilation and multiculturalism

Understanding social processes and interaction has long been a goal of sociologists, notably Max Weber, who was one of the first sociologists to study this interaction. Weber attempted to understand and describe **social action**, which he defined as actions and behaviors that individuals are performing or modulating because others are around. The idea is that humans will behave in different ways based on their social environment and how their behavior will affect those around them. If individuals predict a negative reaction from those around them, they will often modify their behavior.

Social Action

Social action should be contrasted with social interaction. Social action considers just the individual that is surrounded by others. When examining social interaction, we will look at the behavior and actions of two or more individuals who take one another into account.

Social Facilitation

It has been observed that people tend to perform better on simple tasks when in the presence of others. This tendency is known as **social facilitation**, and it supports the idea that people naturally exhibit a performance response when they know they are being watched. Although being in the presence of others does not necessarily constitute an evaluation, the theory suggests that performance sparks a perceived evaluation in the individual performing. According to the **Yerkes–Dodson law of social facilitation**, being in the presence of others will significantly raise arousal, which enhances the ability to perform tasks one is already good at (or **simple tasks**), and hinders the performance of less familiar tasks (or **complex tasks**). For example, an expert pianist may perform better in concert than when alone in practice sessions. However, someone with very limited knowledge of music would perform worse in a social setting than when alone. This is demonstrated in Figure 8.1.

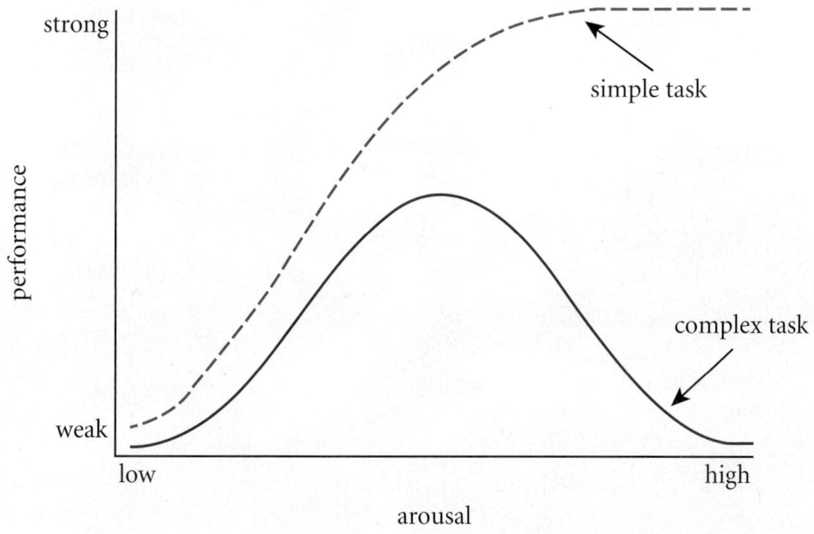

Figure 8.1 Yerkes-Dodson Law

Note the difference between Figure 5.2 (in Chapter 5 of *MCAT Behavioral Sciences Review*) and Figure 8.1. Whereas Figure 5.2 focuses solely on new or less-familiar tasks, Figure 8.1 also includes simple tasks, which are not adversely affected by heightened arousal. Social facilitation reflects the idea that performance is not solely influenced by individual ability, but also by social environment and awareness of that environment.

BRIDGE

The Yerkes-Dodson law is also used to describe the relationship between stress or sympathetic arousal and performance. Just as social facilitation can enhance the ability to perform tasks, so can moderate levels of arousal. Arousal can also be an effect of being surrounded by others and feeling pressure to perform: if there's too much pressure, performance drops. Motivation and stress are discussed in Chapter 5 of *MCAT Behavioral Sciences Review.*

Deindividuation

Deindividuation describes the loss of one's self-awareness in a group setting and the associated adoption of a more group oriented identity. This phenomenon is sometimes called mob mentality, as the individuals of the group lose their own sense of morals and judgment and follow along with the actions of the group. To explain this phenomenon social psychologists have cited group cohesion and individual anonymity as factors impacting deindividuation. If an individual can relate to the group, perhaps through a sports team or political affiliation, then the likelihood of that person adopting the group identity increases. In addition, group settings increase anonymity and thus diffuse the sense of individual responsibility for the actions of the group. Thus, as group anonymity increases, so does the strength of deindividuation. Applied to the real world, deindividuation often leads to **antinormative behavior**, that is, behavior not socially acceptable in most social circumstances; behavior "against the norm." A commonly cited example of antinormative behavior in the context of deindividuation is the violence seen in crowds and riots. Large, homogenous groups are postulated to increase deindividuation effects, particularly when relative anonymity is a factor due to the group's size. These factors can be further enhanced when a group is in uniform or masked, as shown in Figure 8.2.

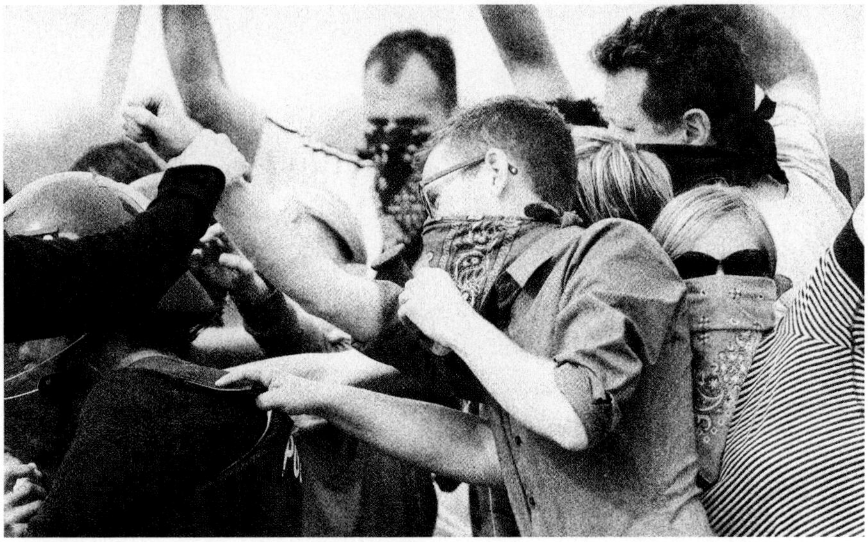

Figure 8.2 Deindividuation
Being masked or in uniform facilitates anonymity in a crowd.

Bystander Effect

The **bystander effect** is another observed phenomenon that occurs in social groups wherein individuals do not intervene to assist those who are in perceived need when other people are present. The likelihood and timeliness of response is inversely related to the number of bystanders. In other words, the more people standing by, the less likely any one of those people is to help. There are several factors at play in the bystander effect. First, when in groups, people are less likely to notice danger or anything out of the ordinary. Additionally, when in groups, humans take cues from others. If other people are not responding to a situation, an individual is less likely to perceive the situation as a threat or emergency. The degree of emergency or the perceived danger plays a role in response. In low-danger scenarios, bystanders are less likely to provide aid; in high-danger scenarios, bystanders are more likely to intervene. Another factor is the degree of responsibility felt by the bystanders. This is determined by the competency of the bystanders, their relationship to the at risk individual(s), and whether they consider considers the person(s) at risk to be deserving of aid. Finally, cohesiveness of the group has been shown to influence responsiveness. In groups made up of strangers, the likelihood of a response, and the speed of that response, is much slower than in a group of well-acquainted individuals.

REAL WORLD

The violent 1964 murder of Kitty Genovese outside her home in Queens created interest in the bystander effect after her murder and a lack of response by neighbors were reported in the newspaper. Kitty reportedly cried out while being attacked in her apartment parking lot. One neighbor called out the window for the attacker to leave her alone. The attacker left, but returned ten minutes later and found Kitty barely conscious just outside the back door. Genovese was attacked again for over half an hour and ultimately died en route to the hospital. Of the 38 witnesses (bystanders), it was reported that no one had called the police. Later investigation determined this not to be true, but the misreported incident was nevertheless influential for promoting the idea of the bystander effect.

Social Loafing

Social loafing refers to the tendency of individuals to reduce effort when in a group setting. This phenomenon may apply in many contexts: physical effort, such as carrying a heavy object; mental effort, such as working on a group project; or initiative, such as coming up with the solution to a problem.

Peer Pressure

From a sociology perspective, **peers** are individuals who are regarded as equals within a social group. **Peer pressure** refers to the social influence placed on an individual by one's peers. Peer pressure exists at all ages. This pressure can come in many forms, including religious ideals, appearance, values, and sexual behavior. It can be positive or negative; certain types of peer pressure can benefit the individual experiencing the influence. In children, social acceptance is associated with being most like the social norm of the group, regardless of positive or negative connotations.

In adolescence, peers play an extremely important role in determining lifestyle, appearance, and social activities. While caregivers and other adults provide the foundation for development of beliefs and values, peers become very important as teenagers become independent from their parental figures. The pressure exerted by peers can cause changes in behavior, attitudes, or beliefs to conform to the norms of the group. Stress and the presence of peers can lead to poor choices and potentially facilitate **risky behaviors** such as binge eating, reckless driving, and violent activities.

Changes in beliefs or behavior due to peer pressure can be explained by the **identity shift effect**. When an individual's state of harmony is disrupted by a threat of social rejection, the individual will often conform to the norms of the group. Upon doing so, however, the individual will begin to experience internal conflict because the behavior is outside the normal character of the individual. To eliminate the sense of internal conflict, individuals experience an identify shift wherein they adopt the standards of the group as their own. The identity shift effect also highlights a larger theme in psychology: **cognitive dissonance**, the simultaneous presence of two opposing thoughts or opinions. This generally leads to an internal state of discomfort, which may manifest as anxiety, fear, anger, or confusion. Individuals will try to reduce this discomfort by changing, adding to, or minimizing one of these dissonant thoughts.

Solomon Asch's conformity experiment showed that individuals will often conform to an opinion held by the group. In this experiment, male college students participated in simple tasks of perception. The study was set up to have one individual who made observations in the presence of confederates, or actors who were pretending to be a part of the experiment. The point of the study was to examine if the behavior of the individual was influenced by the confederates. The participants were shown two cards like those in Figure 8.3. They were then asked to say aloud which line on the second card, labeled A, B, or C, matched the length of the line on the first card. Prior to the experiment, the confederates were secretly told to unanimously respond correctly or incorrectly to the question. When the confederates answered correctly, the error rate for the real participants was less than 1 percent. However, when the confederates answered incorrectly, it was seen that the real participants answered incorrectly up to one-third of the time. Thus, Asch concluded, individuals will sometimes provide answers they know to be untrue if it avoids going against the group: the urge toward conformity could outweigh the desire to provide the correct answer.

MCAT EXPERTISE

The MCAT can ask about psychological experiments by name, so you should be familiar with some of the landmark experiments in social psychology. For example, a question may refer to the Asch conformity experiment by name, or it may include a similar experiment without a direct reference and ask you to draw conclusions using your content knowledge.

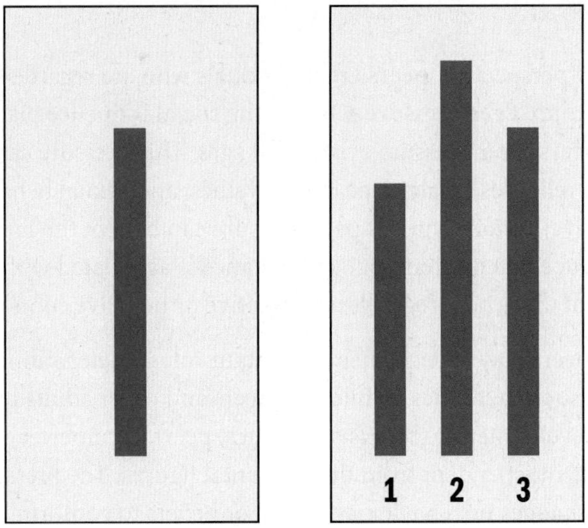

Figure 8.3 Example of Cards Used in the Asch Conformity Experiment

Group Processes

In contrast to social action, **social interaction** explores the ways in which two or more individuals can both shape each other's behavior. These include group processes and establishment of culture.

Group Polarization

Group polarization describes the tendency for groups to collaboratively make decisions that are more extreme than the individual ideas and inclinations of the members within the group. Thus, polarization can lead to riskier or more cautious decisions based on the initial tendencies of the group members toward risk or caution. This phenomenon has shown that individuals in groups will form opinions that are more extreme than the opinions they would reach in isolation. The hypothesis underlying polarization is that initial ideas tend not to be extreme, but that through discussion within the group, these ideas tend to become more and more extreme. This concept was originally termed **risky shift** because it was noted that groups tended to make riskier decisions than individuals. However, when psychologists began to realize that groups could also shift toward caution, the term became **choice shift**. Choice shift and group polarization refer to very similar concepts. However, choice shift refers specifically to measured changes in decisions before and after group interaction, whereas group polarization refers more generally to the tendency of a group to move to more extreme conclusions and decisions as a result of interaction.

Group polarization explains many real-life scenarios, including policy making, violence, and terrorism. For example, members of the same political party may espouse the same ideals and opinions in the group setting, but may waver slightly on issues when alone. This kind of polarization is also seen in jury deliberation. In the case of punitive damages (monetary penalties for a certain behavior), jurors who initially favor a high punishment may deliberate and decide upon an even higher punishment after discussion. As social media has exploded in recent decades, research has shown that the group does not necessarily need to be together physically in order for polarization to occur. Simply reading others' ideas on social media sites can result in more extreme ideas from individuals.

Groupthink

Groupthink refers to a social phenomenon in which desire for harmony or conformity results in a group of people coming to an incorrect or poor decision. In an attempt to eliminate or minimize conflict among the group members, consensus decisions are reached without alternative ideas being assessed. In these cases, the desire to agree with the group causes a loss of independent critical thinking. The group also begins to isolate and ignore external viewpoints, seeing its own ideas as correct without question.

Groupthink can have a large impact on group decision making and is influenced by a variety of factors, including group cohesiveness, group structure, leadership, and situational context. Irving Janis conducted the first research on the theory in the 1970s. Janis studied the effect of extreme stress on group cohesiveness and its resulting effect on groupthink. Janis further investigated the decision making of groups that had led to disastrous American foreign policy decisions, including the Bay of Pigs invasion. Janis specifically examined eight factors that are indicative of groupthink:

- **Illusion of invulnerability:** Members encourage risks, ignore possible pitfalls and are too optimistic.
- **Collective rationalization:** Members ignore expressed concerns about group approved ideas.
- **Illusion of morality:** Members believe ideas produced by the group are morally correct, disregarding evidence to the contrary.
- **Excessive stereotyping:** Members construct stereotypes of those expressing outside opinions.
- **Pressure for conformity:** Members feel pressured not to express opinions that disagree with the group, and view opposition as disloyal.
- **Self-censorship:** Members withhold ideas and opinions that disagree with the group.
- **Illusion of unanimity:** Members believe the decisions and judgments of the group to be without disagreement, even if it does exist.
- **Mindguards:** Some members may decide to take on a role protecting the group against opposing views.

Many of these factors, including illusion of morality, excessive stereotyping, pressure for conformity, and mindguards can be seen in Figure 8.4, a propaganda poster from the United States during the McCarthy era. The poster draws on antisemitic stereotypes and fear of Communist influence to argue against public health measures like water fluoridation, polio vaccines, and mental healthcare.

REAL WORLD

The Bay of Pigs Invasion and Cuban Missile Crisis were used by Janis as case studies. When JFK took over the White House, the administration inherited a CIA Cuban invasion plan, and it was accepted without critique. When Senator Fulbright and Secretary Schlesinger expressed objections, they were ignored by the Kennedy team. Over time, Fulbright and Schlesinger started to perform self-censorship. After the invasion, it was revealed that there were many inaccuracies in the CIA plan, including underestimation of the Cuban air force and the assumption that Castro would not have the ability to quell uprisings.

At the Sign of THE UNHOLY THREE

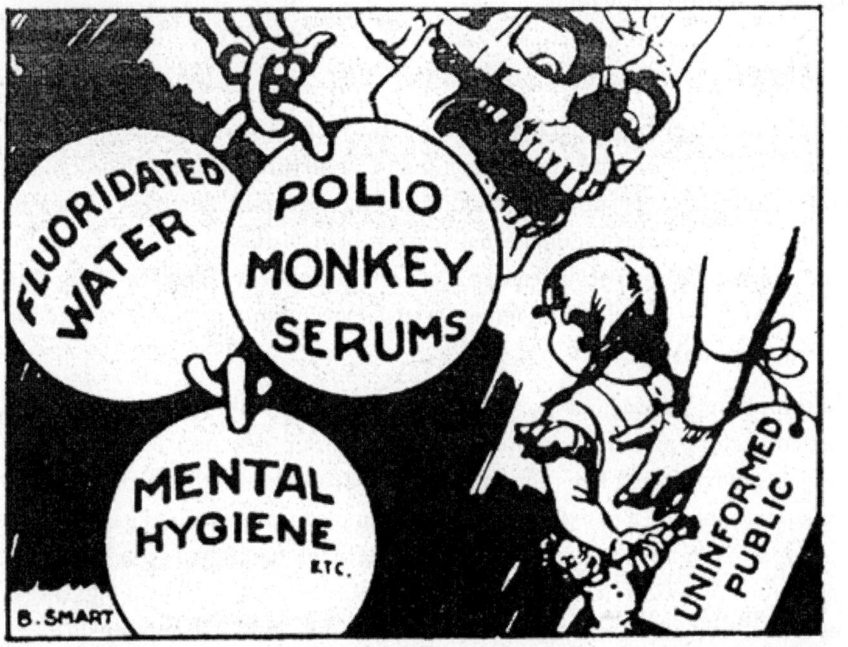

Are you willing to PUT IN PAWN to the UNHOLY THREE all of the material, mental and spiritual resources of this GREAT REPUBLIC?

FLUORIDATED WATER

1—Water containing Fluorine (rat poison—no antidote) is already the only water in many of our army camps, making it very easy for saboteurs to wipe out an entire camp personel. If this happens, every citizen will be at the mercy of the enemy—already within our gates.

POLIO SERUM

2—Polio Serum, it is reported, has already killed and maimed children; its future effect on minds and bodies cannot be guaged. This vacciné drive is the entering wedge for nation-wide socialized medicine, by the U. S. Public Health Service, (heavily infiltrated by Russian-born doctors, according to Congressman Clare Hoffman.) In enemy hands it can destroy a whole generation.

MENTAL HYGIENE

3—Mental Hygiene is a subtle and diabolical plan of the enemy to transform a free and intelligent people into a cringing horde of zombies.

Rabbi Spitz in the American Hebrew, March 1, 1946: "American Jews must come to grips with our contemporary anti-Semites; we must fill our insane asylums with anti-Semitic lunatics."

FIGHT COMMUNISTIC WORLD GOVERNMENT by destroying THE UNHOLY THREE ! ! ! It is later than you think!

KEEP AMERICA COMMITTEE
Box 3094, Los Angeles 54, Calif. H. W. Courtois, Secy. May 16, 1955

Figure 8.4 Groupthink as Seen in McCarthy-Era Propaganda

Similar patterns of thinking, in which a group arrives at a common (but often extreme) consensus also underlie many cultural phenomena, including riots, fads, and mass hysteria. Antinormative behavior in riots was described previously in the section on deindividuation. Still, like groupthink, a shared political or social motivation may urge groups to engage in potentially violent and destructive behavior. A **fad** is a behavior that is transiently viewed as popular and desirable by a large community. Fads can include owning certain objects (such as pet rocks in the 1970s, Rubik's cubes in the 1980s, and pogs in the 1990s) or engaging in certain behaviors (using catchphrases, altering clothing in some way, or engaging in particular types of media such as viral videos). Finally, **mass hysteria** refers to a shared, intense concern about the threats to society. In mass hysteria, many features of groupthink—collective rationalization, illusion of morality, excessive stereotyping, and pressure for conformity, in particular—lead to a shared delusion that is augmented by distrust, rumors, propaganda, and fear mongering. Perhaps the most notable historical case of mass hysteria was the Salem witch trials in colonial Massachusetts, which led to the execution of twenty individuals for fears of witchcraft.

Culture

Culture can be defined as the beliefs, behaviors, actions, and characteristics of a group or society of people. Culture is learned by living within a society, observing behaviors and traits, and adopting them. Culture is also passed down from generation to generation. While a "cultured" individual is often thought of as someone who has knowledge of the arts and expensive taste, sociology considers all people to be cultured by living within a society and participating in its culture. Culture is universal throughout humanity; while many animals exhibit purely instinctual behavior, humans show variable behaviors based on the cultures in which they reside. For example, while all wolf parents care for their pups in the same manner, human parents show vast differences in their caregiving. In some cultures, children are breastfed for years, while in others, infants are breastfed for mere months or not at all. Some groups have multiple caregivers who are not a parent, while others allow only a parent to care for the child. Even within a given culture, beliefs about the correct way to respond to infants crying can vary dramatically: some groups instantly comfort crying children and others let them "cry it out." The beliefs held by an individual are typically based on learned behavior, expectations, and pressure from the group one is in. Cultural differences include everything from typical jobs, common dwellings, and diet to what time of day one eats and where one travels on vacation, if at all. When traveling outside of one's own society, these cultural differences can seem quite dramatic and are often referred to as **culture shock**.

BRIDGE

A discussion of culture in the context of social structure is described in Chapter 11 of *MCAT Behavioral Sciences Review.*

Assimilation and Multiculturalism

Cultural **assimilation** is the process by which an individual's or group's behavior and culture begin to resemble that of another group. This can also mean that groups with different cultures begin to merge. Assimilation integrates new aspects of a society and culture with old ones, transforming the culture itself. While one society melds into another, it is typically not an even blend. One group will generally have more power and influence than the other, resulting in more traits of that culture being displayed after transformation. Four primary factors are sometimes used to assess the degree of assimilation in immigrant communities: socioeconomic status, geographic distribution, language attainment, and intermarriage.

One alternative to assimilation is the creation of **ethnic enclaves**, which are locations (usually neighborhoods) with a high concentration of one specific ethnicity, as shown in Figure 8.5. These are most common in urban areas and often have names like Chinatown or Little Italy.

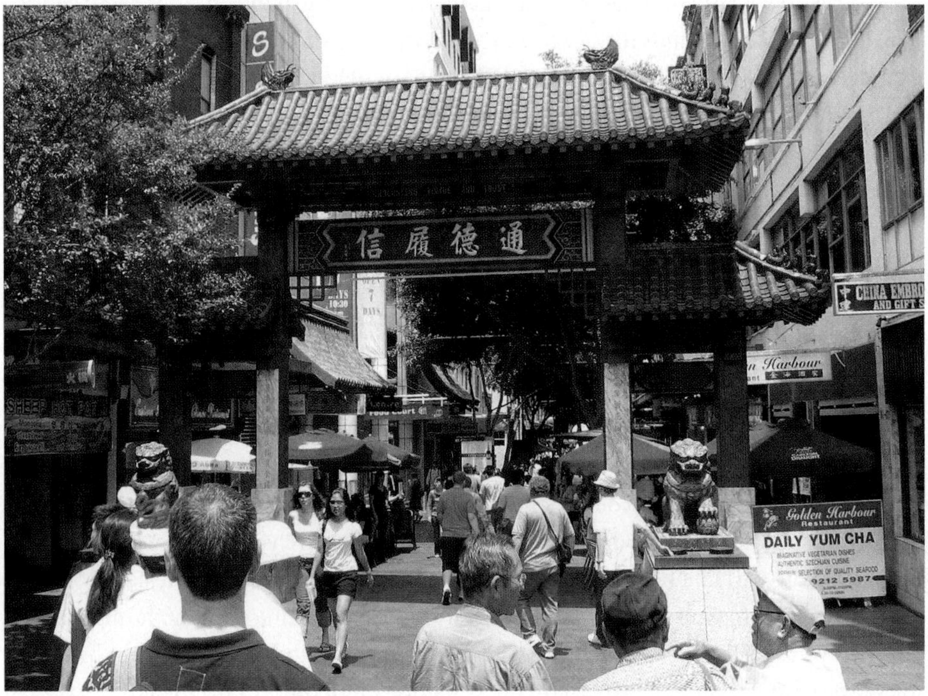

Figure 8.5 An Ethnic Enclave
Entrance to Chinatown, Sydney, Australia

KEY CONCEPT

- Assimilation—(usually uneven) merging of cultures; a melting pot
- Multiculturalism—celebration of coexisting cultures; a cultural mosaic

Multiculturalism, also known as **cultural diversity**, refers to communities or societies containing multiple cultures or ethnic groups. From a sociology perspective, multiculturalism encourages, respects, and celebrates cultural differences, as shown in Figure 8.6. This view can enhance acceptance of cultures within society, which contrasts with the concept of assimilation. While multiculturalism is often described as a creating a *cultural mosaic*, or mixture of cultures and ethnic groups that coexist in society, assimilationism is described as creating a *melting pot*, or melting together of different elements of culture into one homogeneous culture.

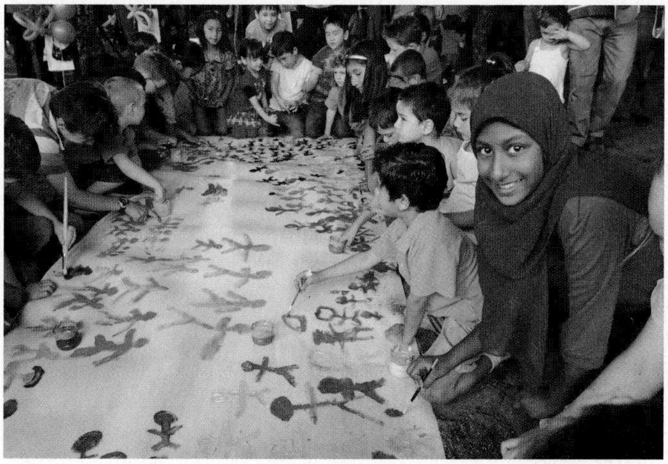

Figure 8.6 Multiculturalism
Multiculturalism may be celebrated through holidays and festivals, such as Harmony Day in Australia, shown here.

Subcultures

Subcultures refer to groups of people within a culture that distinguish themselves from the primary culture to which they belong. When studying subcultures, symbolic attachment to things such as clothing or music can differentiate the group from the majority. Subcultures can be formed based on race, gender, ethnicity, sexuality, and other differentiating factors from the whole of society.

Subcultures can be perceived as negative when they subvert the majority culture's definitions of normalcy. In the case of **counterculture**, the subculture group gravitates toward an identity that is at odds with the majority culture and deliberately opposes the prevailing social mores.

MCAT CONCEPT CHECK 8.1

Before you move on, assess your understanding of the material with these questions.

1. Provide a brief definition for the following social phenomena:
   - Social facilitation:
   - Deindividuation:
   - Bystander effect:
   - Social loafing:
   - Peer pressure:
2. What are the similarities and differences between group polarization and groupthink?
3. What are the differences between assimilation and multiculturalism?

8.2 Socialization

High-Yield

LEARNING OBJECTIVES

After Chapter 8.2, you will be able to:

- Distinguish between conformity, compliance, and obedience
- Compare and contrast primary and secondary socialization
- Describe compliance techniques, such as foot-in-the-door, door-in-the-face, lowball, and that's-not-all

More than any other animal, humans use social experiences to learn acceptable behavior in the culture in which they live. Sociologists and psychologists use the term **socialization** when discussing the process of developing, inheriting, and spreading norms, customs, and beliefs. Individuals gain the knowledge, skills, habits, and behaviors that are necessary for inclusion in society. Widely held views in a society become the accepted viewpoints and are generally adopted by the majority of individuals within that society. Beliefs, customs, and cultural norms are often passed down from one generation to another within a society in a process called **cultural transmission** or **cultural learning**. Spread of norms, customs, and beliefs from one culture to another can also occur, and is called **cultural diffusion**.

Socialization can be further categorized. **Primary socialization** occurs during childhood when we initially learn acceptable actions and attitudes in our society, primarily through observation of our caregivers and other adults in close proximity. In children, this sets the stage for future socialization and provides the foundation for creating personal opinions. **Secondary socialization** is the process of learning appropriate behavior within smaller sections of the larger society. This type of socialization occurs outside of the home and is based on learning the rules of specific social environments. For example, the behavior necessary to thrive in school is different from that in the home setting, and also from that which is acceptable on a sports field or in a church. Secondary socialization is typically associated with adolescents and adults and includes smaller changes and refinements to behavior that were established in primary socialization. Secondary socialization can also occur when moving to a new region or changing schools or professions. **Anticipatory socialization** is the process by which a person prepares for future changes in occupations, living situations, or relationships. A premedical student shadowing physicians to assimilate and practice appropriate behaviors in expectation of one day becoming a doctor is an example of anticipatory socialization. **Resocialization** is another process by which one discards old behaviors in favor of new ones, typically through intensive retraining, and can have positive or negative connotations. The method by which members of the armed forces are trained to obey orders and commands without hesitation is a prime example of resocialization, but so is attracting and indoctrinating members into a cult.

REAL WORLD

Cults that have become a mainstay in media today are often "Doomsday cults." This term refers both to groups that prophesy catastrophe and apocalypse and to those who attempt to bring it about. In December of 2012, nearly 1000 members of the Chinese cult Church of Almighty God were arrested for broadcasting fears of apocalypse and encouraging the overthrow of the Communist Party.

Norms

Sociologists define **norms** as societal rules that define the boundaries of acceptable behavior. **Mores** are widely observed social norms. While norms are not laws, they do provide a mechanism for regulating the behavior of individuals and groups and thereby serve as a means of **social control**. Penalties for misconduct or rewards for appropriate behavior, called **sanctions**, can also be used to maintain social control. Negative sanctions punish behaviors that deviate from norms, while positive sanctions reward behaviors that comply with norms. Sanctions can also be categorized as formal or informal. **Formal sanctions** are enforced by formal social institutions like governments or employers and can include receiving a promotion (positive) or a jail sentence (negative). By contrast, **informal sanctions** are enforced by social groups. Informal sanctions might include being allowed to sit at a particular table in the school cafeteria (positive) or exclusion from a social group (negative).

Norms provide us with a sense of what is appropriate, what we should do, and what is considered **taboo**—socially unacceptable, disgusting, or reprehensible. Norms exist for behavior, speech, dress, home life, and more and can differ between groups within a society, and also between different cultures. For example, many Americans tend to be extraverted and talkative, even among strangers, while Japanese culture sometimes teaches that showing too much of oneself in a public setting is a sign of weakness. Thus, a very quiet person who does not make eye contact could seem odd in America but may fit in perfectly in Japan. **Folkways** are norms that refer to behavior that is considered polite in particular social interactions, such as shaking hands after a sports match, as seen in Figure 8.7.

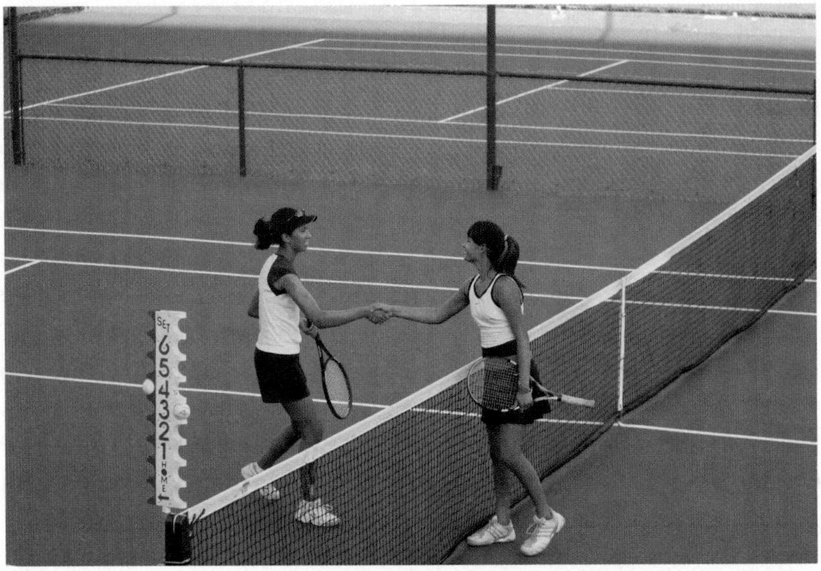

Figure 8.7 Folkways
An act as simple as shaking hands after a sporting match is an example of a folkway.

Agents of Socialization

Any part of society that is important when learning social norms and values is called an **agent of socialization**. For children, the primary agents of socialization are caregivers, often parents or other family members. Direct family remains an important agent of socialization for adolescents, but social circles—including friends, peers, and teachers—become important agents as well. For adults, colleagues and bosses can also act as agents of socialization. Aside from personal relationships, the environment is another agent of socialization. For example, when entering college, some teenagers may experience a complete lifestyle change and are in nearly constant interaction with people of their own age. This new environment creates a shift in acceptable behavior that can include late nights out with friends or all-night study sessions. When entering the workforce, another change in environment leads to socialization within the organization. Ethnic background, religion, and government also play a role in learned behavior, and are therefore also important agents of socialization. And geography at the national, regional, and neighborhood levels also dictates norms of behavior: acceptable behavior in downtown Manhattan is not identical to acceptable behavior in rural Montana.

Furthermore, the media are an important agent of socialization through their influence on what is accepted within a particular society. **Popular culture**, i.e. common

REAL WORLD

A study published in 2002 examined the link between television and violence. In the study, the researchers followed 707 subjects for 17 years. Study subjects who watched more than one hour of TV per day were approximately four times more likely to act aggressively toward others later in life than those who watched less than one hour of TV. Of those who watched more than three hours of TV per day, nearly 30% were involved in assaults, robberies, or other aggressive behaviors. While this is an interesting link, remember that it shows correlation—not causation!

trends and beliefs prevalent at a given point in time, is heavily influenced by the media. The media can determine what is considered important in a particular society. Mass media is most commonly accessed through television, radio, newspapers, and the Internet. It delivers impersonalized communication to a vast audience, and can thereby establish trends in American or international popular culture. Many of the agents of socialization are summarized in Figure 8.8.

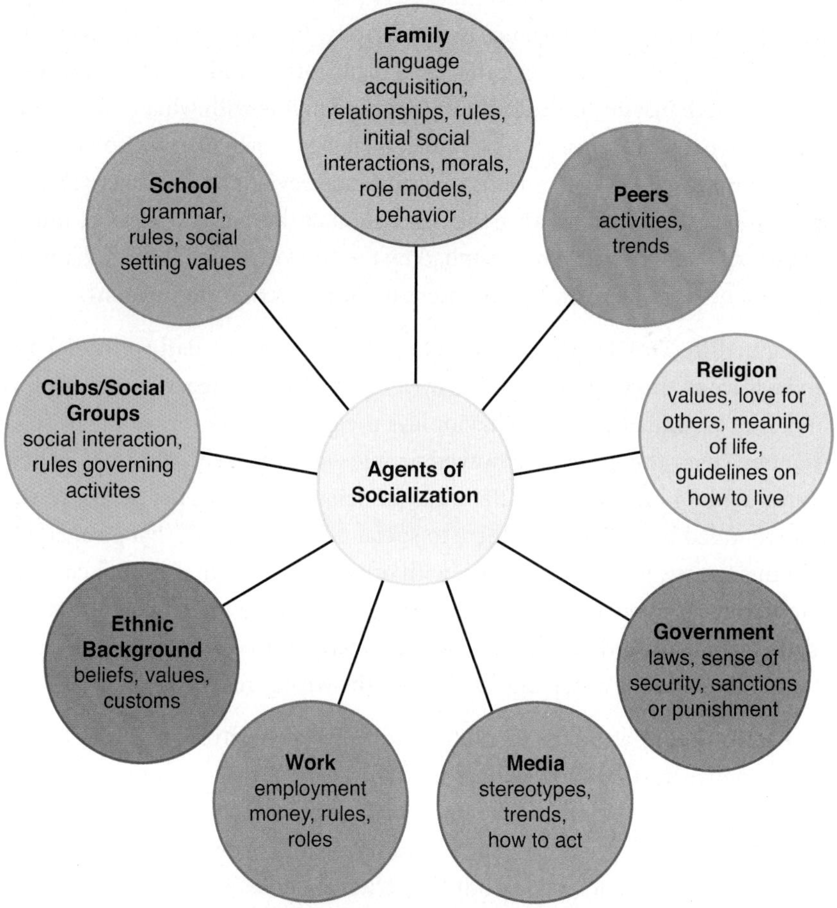

Figure 8.8 Agents of Socialization

Deviance and Stigma

Deviance refers to any violation of norms, rules, or expectations within a society. It is important to note that using the term *deviant* is often associated with strongly negative connotations; however, in the sociological context, it simply refers to any act that goes against societal norms. Deviance can vary in severity, from something as simple as jaywalking to something as serious as committing murder. Deviance also includes any act that meets with disapproval from the larger society.

Social stigma is the extreme disapproval or dislike of a person or group based on perceived differences from the rest of society. These deviations from the norm can include differences in beliefs, abilities, behaviors, and appearance. Certain medical conditions such as HIV, achondroplasia (dwarfism), and obesity can also be stigmatized. Stigma can

BRIDGE

Mental illness has long been stigmatized in American society. While this is slowly changing, the potential stigma associated with a mental health diagnosis continues to be a hurdle to many patients seeking out or receiving care. Many common psychological disorders are discussed in Chapter 7 of *MCAT Behavioral Sciences Review*.

also spread to affect others who are associated with a particular individual. For example, family members of an alleged or convicted murderer or rapist can be stigmatized. Stigma also evolves over time: whereas divorce was stigmatized in the early twentieth century, it no longer has such strong negative connotations.

Deviance, stigmatization, and reputation are strongly linked with the **labeling theory**. This theory posits that the labels given to a person affect not only how others respond to that person, but also affect that person's self-image. Labels can lead to channeling of behavior into deviance or conformity. For example, if members of society label a person as a criminal, this label could either lead to further criminality or to a change in behavior toward something more in line with what is accepted in that society. In many instances, we resist being labeled, particularly with labels we perceive as negative. However, groups may embrace deviant labels. Biker gangs, for example, utilize labeling to enhance the perception of their own subgroup. Internalizing a label and assuming the role implied by the label may lead to the assumed role taking over a person's identity, a phenomenon known as **role engulfment**.

According to **differential association theory**, deviance, particularly criminal behavior, can be learned through interactions with others. In this theory, intimate exposure to others who engage in deviant behavior lays the groundwork for people to engage in deviant behavior themselves. However, people will also likely come into contact with norm-abiding individuals. Differential association, then, is the degree to which one is surrounded by ideals that adhere to social norms *vs.* ideals that go against them. In this theory, when associations with others engaging in deviant behavior are more numerous or intense than those engaging in normative behavior, individuals begins to gravitate toward deviant behavior themselves. In common language, we might describe someone as having "fallen into the wrong group."

Finally, **strain theory** attempts to explain deviance as a natural reaction to the disconnect between social goals and social structure. One common example in strain theory is the American dream, which refers to acquiring wealth and personal stability through achievement and hard work. The American dream is considered a desirable social goal, but the structure of society is unable to guarantee the education and opportunity needed to achieve this goal to all citizens. Therefore, deviant behavior such as theft may arise as an attempt to achieve the social goal *outside* of the limiting social structure.

While deviance is often associated with negative behavior such as crime, functional theorists argue that it is necessary for social order. These theorists argue that deviance provides a clear perception of social norms and acceptable boundaries, encourages unity within society, and can even promote social change.

Conformity, Compliance, and Obedience

While deviance is defined as going against societal norms, conformity, compliance, and obedience are manners of adhering to social expectations or others' requests.

Conformity

Conformity is matching one's attitudes, beliefs, and behaviors to group or societal norms. The pressure to conform can be real or imagined: an actual pressure from others, or a perceived pressure or expectation. Conformity is also known as **majority influence**. The Asch experiments, described earlier, showed the strength of social influence on **normative conformity**, the desire to fit into a group because of fear of rejection.

There are distinct types of conformity, including internalization and identification. **Internalization** involves changing one's behavior to fit with a group while also privately agreeing with the ideas of the group. **Identification** refers to the outward acceptance of others' ideas without personally taking on these ideas.

A classic experiment looking at internalization was Philip Zimbardo's Stanford Prison Experiment. Zimbardo advertised for a role-playing experiment in which he recruited 21 male college students. The study participants were randomly assigned the role of prisoner or guard. The prisoners were arrested in their homes and taken to a "prison" created in the Stanford University psychology building. Guards were issued uniforms, including whistles, handcuffs, and dark glasses to prevent eye contact. The prisoners and guards quickly fell into their roles and displayed related behaviors almost immediately. Guards began to taunt and harass prisoners, appearing to enjoy their role. Prisoners also adopted their new role, taking the prison rules very seriously, and becoming more and more dependent on the guards. As the guards became more aggressive, the prisoners became more submissive, although they also attempted to mount a revolt. The study had to be ended after six days because the guards had begun to physically abuse the prisoners so severely that ethical concerns were raised. After the study ended, Zimbardo interviewed each participant. The guards and prisoners, who had internalized their roles, were both shocked by their behavior during the experiment.

The likelihood of conformity differs among cultures. For instance, individualist cultures tend to value independent thought and unique ideas and are thus less likely to conform; in collectivist cultures, group mentality often supersedes the individual. The latter type of society tends toward conformity.

Compliance

Compliance is a change in behavior based on a direct request. The person or group that asks the individual to make the change typically has no actual power or authority to command the individual, yet will ask the individual to change behavior. There are several notable techniques used to gain compliance of others, particularly within the marketing arena. The **foot-in-the-door** technique begins with a small request, and after gaining compliance, a larger request is made. An example of this scenario could be a fellow classmate asking to borrow your notes after missing class. You agree and offer to share the notes at the next class session. Later in the day, when you see the student again, you're asked if you would be willing to make copies of your notes too. Many people will still agree at this point, as the first request opened the door to continued compliance.

KEY CONCEPT

Internalization and identification both deal with accepting others' ideas, but whereas internalization also reflects a change in internal thoughts to agree with the idea, identification is acceptance of the idea on the surface level without internalizing it.

REAL WORLD

In recent years, design flaws in the Stanford Prison Experiment have come to light. These include sampling biases, ethical concerns, lack of controls, and active participation in the experiment by Zimbardo himself.

The next technique is called the **door-in-the-face technique**. This is the opposite of the foot-in-the-door technique, wherein a large request is made at first and, if refused, a second, smaller request is made. Often, this smaller request is the actual goal of the requester. Using this technique, a fellow student might ask you to make a copy of your notes from class and bring them to the next class. If you deny the request, the student might follow up with a smaller request, asking to borrow your notes to make personal copies. The second, more reasonable request may be granted.

Another common method of achieving compliance is the **lowball technique**. In this technique, the requestor will get an initial commitment from an individual, and then raise the cost of the commitment. It is important to note that cost need not only include money, but can also include effort and time. An example of this technique is a scenario in which you are asked by your boss to head a committee with a time commitment of five hours per month of meetings. You agree to head the committee, but later discover that the commitment also includes written reports from each meeting and a quarterly presentation.

Yet another technique used to gain compliance is the **that's-not-all technique**. In this method, an individual is made an offer, but before making a decision, is told the deal is even better than expected. This method is frequently seen in infomercials: *We can offer you these earrings for the stunningly low price of $19.99. But wait! If you buy them, you'll also receive our matching necklace, normal retail value $49.99, absolutely free.*

Obedience

While compliance deals with requests made by people without actual authority over an individual, **obedience** is changing one's behavior in response to a direct order or expectation expressed by an authority figure. While a classmate has no authority to demand notes from you, an authority figure has social power over other individuals. For instance, if a teacher demands that you hand over your notes from class, you would be obeying rather than complying. People are far more likely to obey than comply due to the real or perceived social power of the individual.

One of the most notable obedience experiment series was conducted by Stanley Milgram. In this classic set of studies, Milgram claimed to be recruiting participants for a study to test the effects of punishment on learning behavior. Participants were told they would be randomly assigned to be the "teacher" or "learner"; however, the "learner" was actually a paid actor (confederate). The teachers were told that they would be controlling an electrical panel that would administer shocks to the learners if they made mistakes. Prior to giving the first shock, the teachers were given a sample 45 V shock to make them aware of what they would be doing to the learners. The teachers were then told that they would need to increase the voltage by 15 V each time an incorrect response was given. The learners, who received no actual shock, were provided with scripts telling them to show pain, ask to stop the experiment, scream, and even feign passing out. As the learners acted more and more uncomfortable, the teachers became less willing to increase the shock voltage. However, by using increasingly demanding language (from *Please continue* to *You have no other choice, you must go on*), the researchers were able to get 65 percent of the participants to administer shocks to the maximum of 450 V, even if they showed discomfort in doing so. Milgram and other researchers were surprised at the level of obedience the participants showed during the experiment. This type of experiment has been repeated many times and has consistently shown that more than 60 percent of people will obey even if they do not wish to continue.

MCAT CONCEPT CHECK 8.2

Before you move on, assess your understanding of the material with these questions.

1. What is the difference between primary and secondary socialization?

___

2. What are conformity, compliance, and obedience?
   - Conformity:

   ___

   - Compliance:

   ___

   - Obedience:

   ___

3. For each of the compliance techniques listed below, provide a brief description:
   - Foot-in-the-door:

   ___

   - Door-in-the-face:

   ___

   - Lowball:

   ___

   - That's-not-all:

   ___

8.3 Attitudes and Behavior

High-Yield

LEARNING OBJECTIVES

After Chapter 8.3, you will be able to:

- Recall the three components of attitude
- Describe the four functional areas of the functional attitude theory
- Identify the roles of central route and peripheral route processing in the elaboration likelihood model
- Recall the three interactive factors of Bandura's triadic reciprocal causation

Social cognition focuses on the ways in which people think about others and how these ideas impact behavior. Our attitudes—the ways in which we perceive others—impact the ways we behave toward them.

Components of Attitudes

An **attitude** is the expression of positive or negative feeling toward a person, place, thing, or scenario. Attitudes develop from experiences with others who affect our opinions and behaviors. Even prior to meeting someone, past experiences and information from others can influence your attitude toward a person.

MNEMONIC

Components of Attitude: **ABC**

- **A**ffective
- **B**ehavioral
- **C**ognitive

There are three primary components of attitude: affective, behavioral, and cognitive. The **affective** component of attitude refers to the way a person feels toward something, and is the emotional component of attitude. *Snakes scare me* and *I love my family* are both affective expressions of attitude. The **behavioral** component of attitude is the way a person acts with respect to something. For example, avoiding snakes and spending time with one's family would reflect the behavioral component of the attitudes described earlier. Finally, the **cognitive** component of attitude is the way an individual thinks about something, which is usually the justification for the other two components. In the snake example above, knowing that snakes can be dangerous (and sometimes venomous) provides a reason to be afraid of snakes and to avoid them.

Theories of Attitudes

The **functional attitudes theory** states that attitudes serve four functions: knowledge, ego expression, adaptation, and ego defense. The **knowledge function** can be summarized as follows: attitudes help provide organization to thoughts and experiences, and knowing the attitudes of others helps to predict their behavior. For example, one would predict that an individual who cares about political action would vote in an upcoming election. Attitudes facilitate being **ego-expressive**, allowing us to communicate and solidify our self-identity. For instance, if a person strongly identifies with a sports team, that person might wear a team hat to identify as having a positive attitude towards that team. **Adaptive** attitude is the idea that expressed socially acceptable attitudes will lead to acceptance. For example, a person declaring to a social group that they enjoyed a popular movie can help to build social bonds.

Lastly, attitudes are **ego-defensive** if they protect our self-esteem or justify actions that we know are wrong. For example, a child who has difficulty doing math may develop a negative attitude toward the subject.

Learning theory posits that attitudes are developed through different forms of learning. Direct contact with the object of an attitude can influence attitude towards that object. For example, children form a positive attitude toward sweets almost immediately after tasting them. Direct instruction from others can also influence attitudes. For instance, a child who is taught by caregivers not to use curse words can form a negative attitude toward curse words and, indirectly, a negative attitude toward those who use curse words. Our attitudes can also be influenced by others' attitudes. For example, teenagers may begin to have a positive attitude toward smoking if they notice that all of their friends smoke. Finally, attitudes may be formed through classical conditioning, operant conditioning, or observational learning, all of which are discussed in Chapter 3 of *MCAT Behavioral Sciences Review*.

The **elaboration likelihood model** is a theory of attitude formation and attitude change that separates individuals on a continuum based on how they process persuasive information. At one extreme are those who elaborate extensively, that is, those who think deeply about information, scrutinize its meaning and purpose, and draw conclusions or make decisions based on this analysis. Deep thinking in this manner is referred to as **central route processing**. When an attempt to influence attitudes uses information that appeals to central route processing, this attempt is said to be using the **central route to persuasion**. A scientific paper would be one example of an attempt to influence attitudes that uses the central route to processing. At the other extreme are those who do not elaborate and focus instead on superficial details such as the appearance of the person delivering the argument, catchphrases and slogans, and credibility. This type of processing is known as **peripheral route processing**. When attempts to influence attitudes appeal to peripheral route processing, these attempts are said to be using the **peripheral route to persuasion**. An advertisement with just a logo that contains a visually appealing image is one example of an attempt to influence attitudes that uses the peripheral route to persuasion. To contrast these two types of processing, consider two voters watching a well-informed and charismatic politician speak: One voter might be swayed by the cogent arguments made by the politician, and this illustrates high elaboration, central route processing. The other voter might be swayed by the perception that the speaker is likable and a good person, illustrating low elaboration, peripheral route processing. Most individuals fall in the middle of this continuum, and the degree to which we elaborate on information can vary depending on the specific situation.

KEY CONCEPT

- Central route processing (high elaboration)—scrutinizing and analyzing the content of persuasive information
- Peripheral route processing (low elaboration)—focusing on superficial details of persuasive information, such as appearances, catchphrases and slogans, and credibility

Social cognitive theory postulates that people learn how to behave and shape attitudes by observing the behaviors of others. According to this theory, behavior is not learned by trial-and-error, but develops through direct observation and replication of the actions of others. This learning is influenced by personal factors (such as thoughts about the behavior) and the environment in which the behavior is observed. These three factors—behavior, personal factors, and environment—are not independent concepts, but influence each other, as shown in Bandura's triadic

BEHAVIORAL SCIENCES GUIDED EXAMPLE WITH EXPERT THINKING

Corporate researchers conducted a longitudinal study of gym members at ten locations in the second week of January for five consecutive years. Participants engaged in a short series of physical activities and measurements assessing physical fitness, then responded to questions about attitudes and fitness. Participants who were present for at least three of the five years and received consistent, low scores in physical fitness measures were associated with the following: lower self-reported gym attendance, lower perceived value of exercise, and low expressed regard for those who attended the gym with a frequency greater than five visits/week. These participants also reported high levels of seasonal motivation (New Year's resolutions).

This is giving me context on a specific set of beliefs involving consistent behavior over time. With a consistent social behavior (high motivation and low adherence) I'm expecting questions about social psychology.

In response to these data, gym owners established a social media group devoted to creating small local workout groups meeting 3–4 days per week with regular check-ins for their members and invited gym attendees within this demographic set to join.

Social psychology: it sounds like the gym owner is trying for positive peer pressure.

How might the group who received consistent low scores in physical fitness measures respond to the new initiative if they choose to participate? How do the results of the five year study inform predictions of their adherence to the 3–4 day per week workout plan?

The writers of the MCAT will hint at a concept in the passage or question stem and then ask us a question about recognizing or applying that concept to the situation described. We'll want to be familiar enough with the content that when the question tells a story or mentions some specific example, we can say to ourselves "Oh, that's ________!"

In order to answer this question, we're going to have to dive into the scenario and identify factors that will influence behavioral outcomes. In the first paragraph, these gym members have maintained the same low level of fitness and low gym attendance for five years, which should remind us of attribution theory: consistent behaviors tend to have dispositional rather than situational explanations. Despite the finding of high seasonal motivation to engage with exercise, it's likely that this group of individuals aren't already in shape because of their attitudes towards themselves or working out ("I'm nervous people will judge me at the gym" or "I just don't enjoy lifting weights"), rather than situational barriers ("My preferred gym is being renovated" or "I'm just super busy this year"). In other words, such attributions are about "who they are" instead of "what has happened to them." We also get a hint in this direction with the finding about low regard for people who attend the gym very regularly. The cause/effect relationship for this set of findings and past behaviors is difficult to assess with the information provided, and may differ between participants. It could be that for some, the thoughts on gym enthusiasts influence their avoidance of the gym in an effort not to adopt similar behaviors. But for others, it could also be that their inability to get to the gym regularly might be influencing their attitudes about those who do in order to protect their egos.

Things are different this year, thanks to the creation of the new fitness group by the gym owners. Some subset of this group of participants have now joined a group of people who will be going to the gym together and will hold each other accountable. We should identify a specific social phenomenon as soon as we read that sentence: peer pressure!

Now that we've identified the important information in the scenario, we should return to the question itself. The question asks how the information we already have about this group of participants might predict their behaviors, which are the three factors of social-cognitive theory. Social-cognitive theory says that all of these things influence one another. If we put together everything we've learned, we see that the attitudes expressed in this group make it less likely that they'll stick to working out, but they've also taken steps to change their environment by opting to join a new peer group for themselves, which makes it more likely that their behaviors may change. While it's impossible to tell which of these influences will win out over the other, it is possible that putting themselves into this new environment and changing their behaviors will in fact change their attitudes over time to be more accepting of those people (now including themselves!) who go to the gym often.

In short, our answer is: the data on this group indicates a possible disposition that makes it less likely they will consistently go and work out at the gym. However, there is now a competing influence to go to the gym that applies to them based on peer pressure from their new group.

reciprocal causation in Figure 8.9. For example, the work ethic of employees in a company (behavior) is affected by how hard their colleagues work, their previous attitudes toward hard work (personal), and the systems and infrastructure of the company (environment). Reciprocally, this behavior may create a change in the employees' attitude toward work (personal) and the systems within the company (environment).

MCAT EXPERTISE

MCAT passages tend to describe an experiment or a scenario and drop in sentences or even short phrases that hint at related scientific content that is then used in questions. The better you are at recognizing this content, the more ready you will be to answer these questions quickly and correctly. But don't feel like you need to scour each passage for every single concept that could appear in the question set.

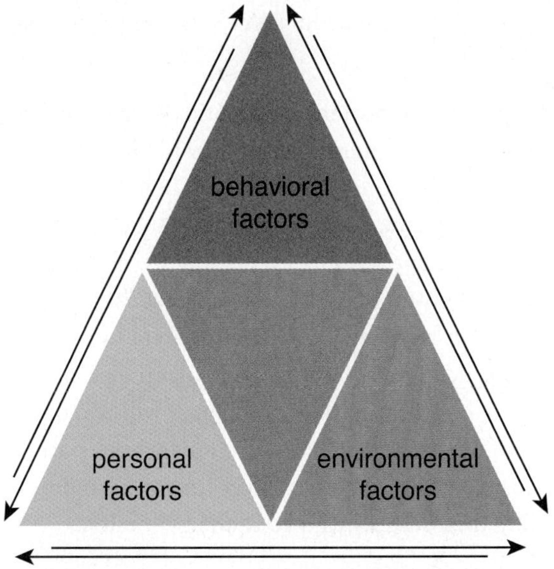

Figure 8.9 Bandura's Triadic Reciprocal Causation

MCAT CONCEPT CHECK 8.3

Before you move on, assess your understanding of the material with these questions.

1. What are the three components of attitude?

    •
    •
    •

2. What are the four functional areas of the functional attitudes theory?

    •
    •
    •
    •

3. What are the routes of processing used to explain the elaboration likelihood model? Which is associated with high elaboration?

    •
    •

4. What are the three interactive factors of Bandura's triadic reciprocal causation?
   -
   -
   -

Conclusion

Human behavior is learned and influenced by those around us. Simply being around others can lead to changes in behavior from how we act when alone. Pressure from others can also lead to changes in behavior when people crave acceptance: inclusion in a group can lead to changes in thought processes and decision making. Social norms, which are learned through experience and observation, can be rejected by individuals, leading to deviance and stigmatization. However, the need to fit in can lead to conformity, compliance, and obedience. Attitudes are also developed through observations, experiences, and interactions with others, and there are multiple theories explaining their specific methods of formation.

This chapter focused primarily on how groups influence an individual's behavior. In the next chapter, we'll look at the structure of these groups and how we present ourselves to the larger society. We'll explore methods of communication between individuals—both verbal and nonverbal—and consider how we encourage others to gain certain impressions about us.

You've reviewed the content, now test your knowledge and critical thinking skills by completing a test-like passage set in your online resources!

GO ONLINE

CONCEPT SUMMARY

Group Psychology

- **Social facilitation** describes the tendency of people to perform at a different level based on the fact that others are around.
- **Deindividuation** is a loss of self-awareness in large groups, which can lead to drastic changes in behavior.
- The **bystander effect** describes the observation that when in a group, individuals are less likely to respond to a person in need.
- **Peer pressure** refers to the social influence placed on individuals by others they consider equals.
- Group decision making may differ from individual decision making.
  - Group **polarization** is the tendency toward making decisions in a group that are more extreme than the thoughts of the individual group members.
  - **Groupthink** is the tendency for groups to make decisions based on ideas and solutions that arise within the group without considering outside ideas. Ethics may be disturbed as pressure is created to conform and remain loyal to the group.
- **Culture** describes the beliefs, ideas, behaviors, actions, and characteristics of a group or society of people.
  - **Assimilation** is the process by which a group or individual's culture begins to melt into another culture.
  - **Multiculturalism** refers to the encouragement of multiple cultures within a community to enhance diversity.
  - **Subcultures** refer to a group of people within a culture that distinguish themselves from the primary culture to which they belong.

Socialization

- **Socialization** is the process of developing and spreading norms, customs, and beliefs.
- **Norms** are what determine the boundaries of acceptable behavior within society.
- Agents of socialization include family, peers, school, religious affiliation, and other groups that promote socialization.
- **Stigma** is the extreme disapproval or dislike of a person or group based on perceived differences from the rest of society.
- **Deviance** refers to any violation of norms, rules, or expectations within a society.
- **Conformity** is changing beliefs or behaviors in order to fit into a group or society.

- **Compliance** occurs when individuals change their behavior based on the requests of others. Methods of gaining compliance include the foot-in-the-door technique, door-in-the-face technique, lowball technique, and that's-not-all technique, among others.
- **Obedience** is a change in behavior based on a command from someone seen as an authority figure.

Attitudes and Behavior

- **Attitudes** are tendencies toward expression of positive or negative feelings or evaluations of something.
- There are affective, behavioral, and cognitive components to attitudes.
- The **functional attitudes theory** states that there are four functional areas of attitudes that serve individuals in life: knowledge, ego expression, adaptability, and ego defense.
- The **learning theory** states that attitudes are developed through forms of learning: direct contact, direct interaction, direct instruction, and conditioning.
- The **elaboration likelihood model** states that attitudes are formed and changed through different routes of information processing based on the degree of elaboration (**central route processing**, **peripheral route processing**).
- The **social cognitive theory** states that attitudes are formed through observation of behavior, personal factors, and environment.

ANSWERS TO CONCEPT CHECKS

8.1

1. Social facilitation describes the tendency of people to perform at a different level based on the fact that others are around. Deindividuation is the idea that people will lose a sense of self-awareness and can act dramatically different because of the influence of a group. The bystander effect describes the observation that individuals are less likely to respond to a person in need when in a group. Social loafing refers to a decrease in effort seen when individuals are in a group. Peer pressure refers to the social influence placed on individuals by others they consider their equals.
2. Group polarization and groupthink are both social processes that occur when groups make decisions. Group polarization is the tendency toward extreme decisions in a group. Groupthink is the tendency for groups to make decisions based on ideas and solutions that arise within the group without considering outside ideas, given the pressure to conform and remain loyal to the group.
3. Societies that contain multiple cultures can exhibit multiculturalism or assimilation. Assimilation is the process by which multiple cultures begin to merge into one, typically with an unequal blending of ideas and beliefs. Multiculturalism refers to the idea that multiple cultures should be encouraged and respected without one culture becoming dominant overall.

8.2

1. Primary socialization refers to the initial learning of acceptable behaviors and societal norms during childhood, which is facilitated mostly by caregivers and other adults. Secondary socialization refers to learning the norms of specific subgroups or situations during adolescence and adulthood.
2. Conformity is changing beliefs or behaviors in order to fit into a group or society. Compliance occurs when individuals change their behavior based on the request of others who do not wield authority over the individual. Obedience is a change in behavior because of a request from an authority figure.
3. The foot-in-the-door technique refers to asking for favors that increase in size with each subsequent request. The door-in-the-face technique refers to making a large request and then, if refused, making a smaller request. The lowball technique refers to gaining compliance without revealing the full cost (money, effort, or time) of the favor. The that's-not-all technique refers to increasing the reward for a request before an individual has the chance to make a decision.

8.3

1. The three components of attitude are affective, behavioral, and cognitive.
2. The four functional areas of the functional attitudes theory are knowledge, ego expression, adaptation, and ego defense.
3. The routes of processing used to explain the elaboration likelihood model are central route processing and peripheral route processing. Central route processing is associated with high elaboration.
4. The three interactive factors of Bandura's triadic reciprocal causation are behavior, personal factors, and environment.

SCIENCE MASTERY ASSESSMENT EXPLANATIONS

1. **C**

When fulfilling particular roles, an individual's behavior can be very out of character. The changing of one's behavior (and internal ideas) to match a group is called internalization conformity. This was a key part of the experiment. The experiment also involved deindividuation, the loss of self-identity in the group setting that can lead to antinormative or violent behavior.

2. **B**

The fact that individual opinions became more extreme during group discussion is explained by group polarization. The jury member initially felt that a strict penalty should be given, but this opinion became more extreme after conversation with the rest of the group.

3. **A**

It has been observed that increasing the number of bystanders decreases the likelihood that any of them will aid a victim. Increasing the degree of danger experienced by the victim, **(B)**, making the victim an acquaintance instead of a stranger, **(C)**, and being alone in the room with the victim, **(D)**, would increase the likelihood that the bystander would help the victim.

4. **D**

With groupthink, a member would perform all of the actions described by the answer choices except create a sense of negativity against risk taking; in fact, there is optimism and encouragement toward risk taking in groupthink.

5. **A**

Primary socialization is the teaching of acceptable actions and attitudes during childhood, which would occur too early to be part of the adult prison system. Resocialization, **(D)**, is the process by which one changes behaviors by discarding old routines and patterns and transitions to new behaviors necessary for a life change. The prison environment is designed to change unlawful behavior into desired behavior, making this an incorrect choice. When entering prison, an inmate must also undergo secondary socialization, **(B)**, learning the rules of the specific social environment of the prison. Finally, if the inmate is not incarcerated for life, attempts at anticipatory socialization, **(C)**, must be made before releasing the inmate in preparation for life outside of the prison.

6. **C**

This is a prime example of the foot-in-the-door technique. The neighbors first ask for a small favor and, after receiving commitment, ask for a larger favor.

7. **A**

The affective component of attitude consists of feelings and emotions toward something.

8. **D**

Peripheral route processing deals with processing information that is not based on content, but instead on superficial parameters such as boring speech patterns or appearance of the speaker. Central route processing, **(C)**, is the processing of information through analysis of its content.

9. **B**

The Milgram shock experiment showed that individuals would obey orders from authority figures even if they were not comfortable with the task at hand. Conformity and compliance, **(C)** and **(D)**, also deal with changes in individual behavior, but are not based on the requests of an authority figure.

10. **C**

Internalization refers to the type of conformity in which individuals change their outward opinion to match the group and also personally agree with those ideas.

11. **B**

The four functional areas of the functional attitudes theory are knowledge, adaptability, ego expression, and ego defense. Acceptance into a group may influence attitudes or opinions; however, this is not a part of the functional attitudes theory.

12. **A**

For 14 out of the 16 members, the record times were obtained during public meets. The fact that the team members performed better when in front of a crowd supports the notion of social facilitation.

13. **D**

This young person is preparing to spend time in a new social setting. The process of preparing for future changes in environment is considered anticipatory socialization.

14. **B**

Social action is best described as the effects that a group has on individual behavior, including social facilitation, deindividuation, the bystander effect, social loafing, and peer pressure. Social interaction describes how two or more individuals influence each other's behavior, including group polarization and groupthink.

15. **C**

Placing spoken or unspoken expectations on individuals to agree with the ideas of the group is best described as pressure for conformity.

Consult your online resources for additional practice. GO ONLINE

SHARED CONCEPTS

Behavioral Sciences Chapter 5
Motivation, Emotion, and Stress

Behavioral Sciences Chapter 6
Identity and Personality

Behavioral Sciences Chapter 9
Social Interaction

Behavioral Sciences Chapter 10
Social Thinking

Behavioral Sciences Chapter 11
Social Structure and Demographics

Physics and Math Chapter 11
Reasoning About the Design and Execution of Research

CHAPTER 9

SOCIAL INTERACTION

SCIENCE MASTERY ASSESSMENT

Every pre-med knows this feeling: there is so much content I have to know for the MCAT! How do I know what to do first or what's important?

While the high-yield badges throughout this book will help you identify the most important topics, this Science Mastery Assessment is another tool in your MCAT prep arsenal. This quiz (which can also be taken in your online resources) and the guidance below will help ensure that you are spending the appropriate amount of time on this chapter based on your personal strengths and weaknesses. Don't worry though—skipping something now does not mean you'll never study it. Later on in your prep, as you complete full-length tests, you'll uncover specific pieces of content that you need to review and can come back to these chapters as appropriate.

How to Use This Assessment

If you answer 0–7 questions correctly:

Spend about 1 hour to read this chapter in full and take limited notes throughout. Follow up by reviewing **all** quiz questions to ensure that you now understand how to solve each one.

If you answer 8–11 questions correctly:

Spend 20–40 minutes reviewing the quiz questions. Beginning with the questions you missed, read and take notes on the corresponding subchapters. For questions you answered correctly, ensure your thinking matches that of the explanation and you understand why each choice was correct or incorrect.

If you answer 12–15 questions correctly:

Spend less than 20 minutes reviewing all questions from the quiz. If you missed any, then include a quick read-through of the corresponding subchapters, or even just the relevant content within a subchapter, as part of your question review. For questions you answered correctly, ensure your thinking matches that of the explanation and review the Concept Summary at the end of the chapter.

1. Which of the following best describes the sociological definition of a status?
   - **A.** The emotional state of a social interaction
   - **B.** Expectations that are associated with a specific title in society
   - **C.** A position in society used to classify an individual
   - **D.** A means to describe one's peers

2. Becoming a college graduate requires hard work and diligence in academics. As such, being a college graduate could be considered a(n):
   - **A.** ascribed status.
   - **B.** achieved status.
   - **C.** master status.
   - **D.** cardinal status.

3. A bureaucracy is a specific example of a(n):
   - **A.** immediate network.
   - **B.** primary group.
   - **C.** organization.
   - **D.** reference group.

4. Which of the following is NOT characteristic of a bureaucracy?
   - **A.** Rigidly defined work procedures
   - **B.** Requirement for officials to hold an advanced degree
   - **C.** Regular salary increases
   - **D.** Election by constituents

5. Which of the following is a form of verbal communication?
   - **A.** Facial expressions
   - **B.** Eye contact
   - **C.** Written text
   - **D.** Body language

6. Which of the following best describes the impression management strategy of aligning actions?
   - **A.** Adhering to the behaviors that are expected for a given role in society
   - **B.** Relieving tension brought about by holding conflicting views in one's head
   - **C.** Providing socially acceptable reasons to explain unexpected behavior
   - **D.** Dictating that members of a group should follow similar practices to one another

7. While on the phone, a friend says: "A good friend would let me borrow the bike." This friend is using which impression management strategy?
   - **A.** Managing appearances
   - **B.** Alter-casting
   - **C.** Ingratiation
   - **D.** Self-disclosure

8. Which of the following is an example of a *Gesellschaft*?
   - **A.** A large corporation
   - **B.** A small rural neighborhood
   - **C.** Members of the same family
   - **D.** An ethnic enclave in a large city

9. In some cultures, it is considered taboo for one to show too much sadness at a funeral. In other cultures, wailing and crying loudly is expected. These cultures differ in their:
   - **A.** characteristic institutions.
   - **B.** display rules.
   - **C.** authentic selves.
   - **D.** peer groups.

10. Which of the following is NOT a dimension of the system for multiple level observation of groups (SYMLOG)?

A. Friendliness *vs.* unfriendliness
B. Dominance *vs.* submission
C. Conformity *vs.* contrast
D. Instrumentally controlled *vs.* emotionally expressive

11. Political campaign ads often focus on "exposing" an opposing candidate's negative characteristics. In the dramaturgical approach, one would describe this as:

A. bringing the front stage self to the back stage.
B. bringing the back stage self to the front stage.
C. removing the front stage self.
D. removing the back stage self.

12. In the context of impression management, which of the following selves is most similar to the ought self?

A. The ideal self
B. The tactical self
C. The authentic self
D. The presented self

13. The evolutionary role of emotions has been used as support for which model(s) of emotional expression?

A. The basic model only
B. The social construction model only
C. Both the basic model and social construction model
D. Neither the basic model nor the social construction model

14. Which of the following is an example of intraspecific animal communication?

A. A dog who barks when a stranger enters the house
B. An anglerfish that uses a bioluminescent appendage to attract prey
C. Bats using echolocation to detect the surrounding environment
D. A cat who uses scent glands to mark his territory for other cats

15. Primary groups differ from secondary groups in that:

A. primary groups are shorter-lived than secondary groups.
B. primary groups are larger than secondary groups.
C. primary groups are formed of stronger bonds than secondary groups.
D. primary groups are assigned while secondary groups are chosen.

Answer Key

1. **C**
2. **B**
3. **C**
4. **D**
5. **C**
6. **C**
7. **B**
8. **A**
9. **B**
10. **C**
11. **B**
12. **B**
13. **A**
14. **D**
15. **C**

Detailed explanations can be found at the end of the chapter.

CHAPTER 9

SOCIAL INTERACTION

In This Chapter

CHAPTER PROFILE

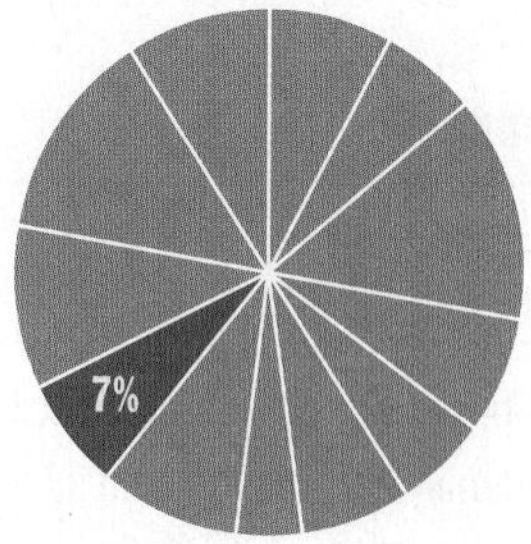

The content in this chapter should be relevant to about 7% of all questions about the behavioral sciences on the MCAT.

This chapter covers material from the following AAMC content categories:

7B: Social processes that influence human behavior

8C: Social interactions

Introduction

Every day, you present yourself to others and interact with society. You interact with others in a number of ways, using emotional expression, verbal communication, and cultural norms. You may also interact with nonhuman animals on a day-to-day basis. This interaction can be just as complex and meaningful to your emotional state and life experience. What shapes and molds your interactions? How do you know the appropriate way to connect with other members of society?

9.1 Elements of Social Interaction

High-Yield

LEARNING OBJECTIVES

After Chapter 9.1, you will be able to:

- Identify the meaning of social interaction terms such as status, role, group, network, and organization
- List the three types of status and provide an example of each

Society has developed out of necessity for human beings to survive and develop. Social interaction is the basis of social life and helps humans reach their full potential. Social interaction is facilitated by preexisting commonalities between individuals and shared understanding or experiences, such as a shared language. Through our social interactions, we develop culture.

Statuses

In most human societies, people do not view every individual as an equal. Instead, we create a hierarchical structure with inequalities of material goods, social opportunities, social acceptance, and skills. Some are wealthy, and some are impoverished; some are talented in sports, while others are not. Some are admired by others, most are liked, and some are disliked or even stigmatized. **Social statuses** are perceived positions in society that are used to classify individuals. Being a premed student, for example, is considered a status. Most statuses exist in relation to other statuses: being a premed student does not have meaning unless there are other statuses with which to compare it, such as *medical student* or *resident*. It is important to note that not all personal characteristics are considered to be social statuses. For example, being left-handed is not considered a status.

KEY CONCEPT

Types of statuses:

- Ascribed—given involuntarily, based on race, ethnicity, sex, family background, and so on
- Achieved—gained as a result of one's efforts or choices
- Master—status by which one is most identified; is pervasive in that person's life

There are three key types of statuses: ascribed, achieved, and master statuses. An **ascribed status** is one that is given involuntarily (usually at birth), due to such factors as race, ethnicity, sex, and family background. An **achieved status** is a status that is gained as a result of one's efforts or choices, such as being a doctor. A person can hold multiple statuses at the same time (collectively known as one's status set), but one's **master status** is the status by which a person is most identified. This status is typically the most important status the individual holds and affects all aspects of that person's life. It is also generally how people view themselves and often holds a symbolic value. Master statuses can also cause pigeonholing: we may view individuals only through the lens of their master status, without regard to any other personal characteristics (such as with a president or other major political figure).

Roles

Each status is associated with **roles**, or sets of beliefs, values, attitudes, and norms that define expectations for those who hold the status. **Role performance** is the carrying out of behaviors associated with a given role. Individuals can vary in how successful they are at performing a role. For example, part of a doctor's role is to translate medical information into language their patients can understand; however, some doctors are far better at this skill than others. Role performance can also change depending on the social situation and context of the interaction. When doctors interact with each other, the pertinent parts of their roles are quite different than when interacting with patients. Behaviors and expectations thus change as a result of the **role partner**—the person with whom one is interacting. Doctors have many role partners: patients, nurses, patients' relatives, other doctors, residents, and hospital administration. The various roles associated with a status are referred to as a **role set**.

REAL WORLD

A great example of role conflict is a single parent who also works a full-time job. Both of these roles carry a very large set of expectations, which are often at odds with each other.

Through our lives, we each take on numerous statuses, each of which may contain a variety of roles. Additionally, we are often playing several roles at one time. Due to the complex nature of statuses and role sets, it is not surprising that conflict, challenges, uncertainty, and ambivalence arise as we try to navigate the many expectations of day-to-day life. **Role conflict** is the difficulty in satisfying the requirements or expectations of multiple roles, whereas **role strain** is the difficulty in satisfying multiple requirements of the same role. **Role exit** is the dropping of one identity for another.

Groups

Another major component of social interaction involves groups. In sociological terms, a **group** (also known as a **social group**) consists of two or more people who share any number of similar characteristics as well as a sense of unity. The simplest of social groups is called a **dyad** (two people), followed by a **triad** (three people). As group size increases, the group trades intimacy for stability. Social groups are more complex than a group of individuals who happen to be in the same physical space. For example, people waiting to cross the street at a crosswalk do not constitute a social group. Common characteristics shared by social groups include values, interests, ethnicity, social background, family ties, and political representation. Many sociologists see social interaction as the most important characteristic that strengthens a social group.

We center most of our lives around social groups, from the camaraderie of teammates to the complexity of governments. Social groups also meet many of the needs we have; these groups provide an opportunity to belong and be accepted and they offer protection, safety, and support. Many people also learn, earn a living, and practice religion in groups. Groups can also be a source of conflict, including discrimination, persecution, oppression, and war. These conflicts sprout from the relationships within and between groups.

An **in-group** is a social group with which a person experiences a sense of belonging or identifies as a member. An **out-group**, on the other hand, refers to a social group with which an individual does not identify. An in-group can form based on a variety of identifying characteristics, including but not limited to race, culture, gender, religion, profession, or education. Out-groups can sometimes compete with or oppose in-groups, creating **group conflict**. Notably, negative feelings toward an out-group are not necessarily based on a sense of dislike toward the characteristics of the out-group; rather, they can be based on favoritism for the in-group and the absence of favoritism for the out-group.

A **peer group** is a group that consists of self-selected equals associated by similar interests, ages, or statuses. Peer groups provide an opportunity for friendship and feelings of belonging. A **family group**, by contrast, is not self-selected but determined by birth, adoption, and marriage. It joins members of various ages, genders, and generations through emotional ties. The family group can be filled with conflict at times; this is often true in adolescence when peer groups begin to compete with family groups for time and loyalty. Family groups may also struggle with cultural gaps and social differences between generations, such as speaking in different languages.

Another important type of group is a **reference group**. These are groups that individuals use as a standard for evaluating themselves. For example, to determine how strong a medical school applicant you are, you might compare yourself to the reference group of all medical school applicants.

Primary and Secondary Groups

Groups can also be categorized into primary and secondary groups. In a **primary group**, interactions between members of the group are direct, with close bonds providing warm, personal, and intimate relationships to members. These groups often last a long period of time and may include a core circle of friends, a tightly knit family, or members of a team. In a **secondary group**, the interactions are impersonal and businesslike, with few emotional bonds and with the goal of accomplishing a specific purpose. Secondary groups typically last for a short period of time, and they form and dissolve without any special significance to those involved, an example being students working together on a group project.

Community and Society

The German sociologist Ferdinand Tönnies distinguished two major types of groups. His theory is known as ***Gemeinschaft und Gesellschaft***, which translates to *community and society*. *Gemeinschaft* (community) refers to groups unified by feelings of togetherness due to shared beliefs, ancestry, or geography. Families and neighborhoods are examples of *Gemeinschaften*. *Gesellschaft* (society) refers to less personal groups that are formed out of mutual self-interests working together toward the same goal. Companies and countries are examples of *Gesellschaften*.

Observing and Analyzing Groups

Group size may vary; the smallest size a group can be is two people. Smaller group sizes, like dyads or triads, allow individuals to present more of themselves to the group. **Interaction process analysis** is a technique for observing, classifying, and measuring the interactions within small groups. In the 1970s, it was revised to the **system for multiple level observation of groups** (**SYMLOG**), which is based on the belief that there are three fundamental dimensions of interaction: dominance *vs.* submission, friendliness *vs.* unfriendliness, and instrumentally controlled *vs.* emotionally expressive.

Extensive research on groups has revealed that a group holds power over its members, creating group pressure that can ultimately shape members' behaviors. This is called **group conformity**; individuals are compliant with the group's goals, even when the group's goals may be in direct contrast to the individual's goal. Individuals conform in an attempt to fit in and be accepted by the group. Individuals will often participate in behaviors they normally would not.

Groupthink is related to group conformity and occurs when members focus on reaching a consensus at the cost of critical evaluation of relevant information. This can lead to groups not exploring all sides of an issue and may limit the group's options or views; further, group members may self-censor by not expressing their beliefs. A more extensive discussion of the effects of groups on individual behavior (social action) and group dynamics is explored in Chapter 8 of *MCAT Behavioral Sciences Review*.

Networks

The term **network** is used to describe the observable pattern of social relationships among individuals or groups. Patterns of relationship can be determined by mapping the interactions between individual units, the nature of which can be highly variable. For example, a sociologist may look at the patterns in the interactions between friends, family members, or societal institutions. Researchers often display networks with maps containing a series of points, with each point representing a unit in the network. They connect the points with lines to display the interactions between units, as shown in Figure 9.1. Not all contact points within a network are necessarily unique.

If there are overlapping connections with the same individual, it is referred to as **network redundancy**. Network analysis can be used to gain understanding of the actions of individuals and groups and to study the broader social structure.

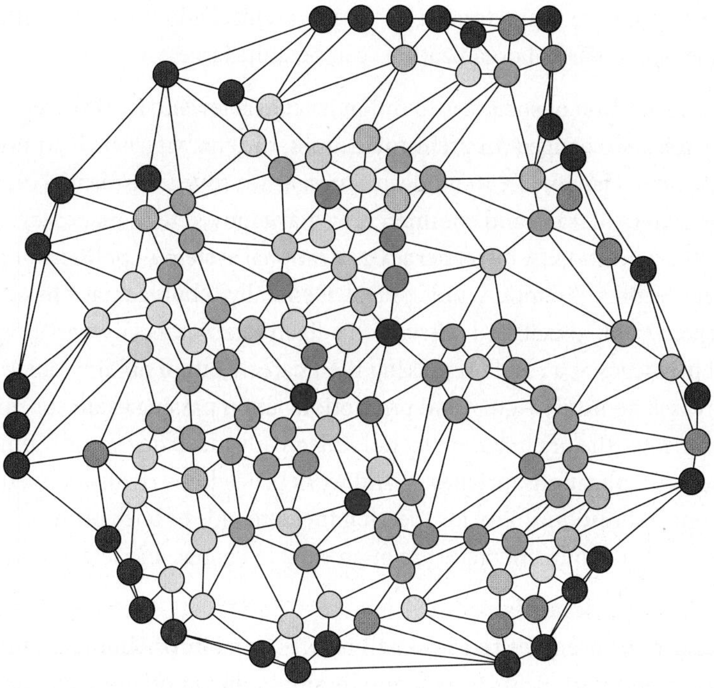

Figure 9.1 Example of a Social Network Diagram

Individuals in networks face the demands and expectations of other members, constraining what they are able to do. They also may have access to resources through the network. An example of a network is a university's alumni association: the members are held to certain standards and commitments, but also may reap the benefits of the network when searching for a job. **Immediate networks** are dense with strong ties, whereas **distant networks** are looser and contain weaker ties; immediate networks may be composed of friends, whereas distant networks may include acquaintances. The combination of immediate and distant networks provide the most benefit to individuals, which is augmented if the networks work complementarily to provide different resources.

BRIDGE

A genetic pedigree can be thought of as a specific type of network map, in which geneticists can track genetic patterns. The lines in genetic pedigrees represent mating patterns, parent-child relationships, and other familial structures. While pedigree analysis does not appear on the MCAT, the related topic of genetics is discussed in Chapter 12 of *MCAT Biology Review*.

Organizations

In sociology, **organizations** are complex secondary groups that are set up to achieve specific goals and are characterized by having a structure and a culture. We have all been members of multiple organizations, such as schools, companies, music groups, sports teams, fraternities and sororities, political organizations, community action committees, and so on. The study of organizations is at the heart of sociology because of the importance that organizations have throughout a person's life.

The modern **formal organization** developed during the Industrial Revolution as a way to maximize efficiency. The formal aspect derives from the explicit goals that guide the members and their activities. Furthermore, formal organizations have enforcement procedures that seek to control the activities of their members. Lastly, these organizations are characterized by the hierarchical allotment of formal roles or duties to members. Formal organizations can be quite large.

The basic organization of society is found in its **characteristic institution**. Throughout history this has changed. In prehistoric times, the characteristic institution was primarily the kin, clan, or sib. In modern times, as we have transformed our cities into urban centers of trade and commerce, we have moved to bureaucracy as the characteristic institution. A **bureaucracy** is a rational system of political organization, administration, discipline, and control. Generally, a bureaucracy has these six characteristics: paid, nonelected officials on a fixed salary; officials who are provided rights and privileges as a result of making their careers out of holding office; regular salary increases, seniority rights, and promotions upon passing exams or milestones; officials who enter the organization by holding an advanced degree or training; responsibilities, obligations, privileges, and work procedures rigidly defined by the organization; and responsibility for meeting the demands of one's position. Due to these characteristics, bureaucracies are often slow to change and less efficient than other organizations.

Bureaucracies have been criticized over time. The **iron law of oligarchy** states that democratic or bureaucratic systems naturally shift to being ruled by an elite group. This shift is due to a number of factors, including the necessity of a core body of individuals to carry out the day-to-day activities of the organization, increased need for specialization, and leadership characteristics of certain members of the group. Thus, even a group established with democratic principles and complete egalitarianism will ultimately centralize, placing power in the hands of a few key leaders.

McDonaldization is commonly used to refer to a shift in focus toward efficiency, predictability, calculability, and control in societal practices. While the original model for McDonaldization was, of course, the fast-food restaurant and its push towards efficiency, examples of these same characteristics can be seen in many other institutions. For example, 24-hour news channels, which feature running footers of the latest news stories as "bite-size" headlines, demonstrate efficient and predictable sources of information. Corporations may mine "big data" to make business decisions using controlled, standardized methods, allowing the business to focus on the calculable outcomes of a choice such as profit and loss analysis and market share.

MCAT CONCEPT CHECK 9.1

Before you move on, assess your understanding of the material with these questions.

1. List the three types of statuses and provide an example of each:

Status	Example

2. For each of the sociological terms below, provide a brief definition:
   - Status:

   ____

   - Role:

   ____

   - Group:

   ____

   - Network:

   ____

   - Organization:

   ____

9.2 Self-Presentation and Interacting with Others

High-Yield

LEARNING OBJECTIVES

After Chapter 9.2, you will be able to:

- Classify forms of communication as verbal or nonverbal
- Distinguish between front-stage self and back-stage self
- Identify examples of body language, facial expression, visual display, scent, and vocalization in communication

To Erving Goffman, the sociologist who developed the dramaturgical perspective, every interaction we have with other people is a theatrical performance in which we consciously or unconsciously use the "scene," our "costume," and the role that we "perform" to influence the way others think or feel. Whenever we try to influence others' perception with respect to a person, object, or event, we are engaging in impression management. One form of impression management is **self-presentation**, the process of displaying ourselves to society both visually (through clothing, grooming, etc.) and through our actions, often to make sure others see us in the best possible light.

Expressing and Detecting Emotions

Expressed emotions include both verbal and nonverbal behaviors that communicate internal states. We can express emotions with or without conscious awareness.

The **basic model of emotional expression** was first established by Charles Darwin. Darwin stated that emotional expression involves a number of components: facial expressions, behaviors, postures, vocal changes, and physiological changes. Darwin claimed that expression is consistent with his theories on evolution and should be similar across cultures. Darwin also stated that primates and animals exhibit rudimentary muscle actions that are similar to those used by humans for facial expressions. Since Darwin, many researchers have found that a number of basic human emotions are universally experienced and that their corresponding facial expressions are universally recognized. The **appraisal model** is closely related, and accepts that there are biologically predetermined expressions once an emotion is experienced, but that there is a cognitive antecedent to emotional expression.

BRIDGE

Paul Ekman's work with universal emotions, as detailed in Chapter 5 of *MCAT Behavioral Sciences Review*, was a key development in the basic model of emotional expression. Individuals knowledgeable about Ekman's work are capable of detecting very subtle and transient facial expressions that may indicate that an individual is trying to be deceptive about the emotions being conveyed.

Three of the primary models that describe individual emotion (James–Lange, Cannon–Bard, and Schachter–Singer) were discussed in Chapter 5 of *MCAT Behavioral Sciences Review*. In this chapter, we will look at how emotions are shaped by social context and culture.

The **social construction model** assumes that there is no biological basis for emotions. Instead, emotions are based on experiences and the situational context alone. It also suggests that certain emotions can only exist within social encounters and that emotions are expressed differently—and thus play different roles—across cultures. In this model, one must be familiar with social norms for a certain emotion to perform the corresponding emotional behaviors in a given social situation.

Culture provides the foundation to understand and interpret behaviors. Studies have suggested that cultural differences can lead to very different social consequences when emotions are expressed. Cultural expectations of emotions are often referred to as **display rules**. For example, in Utkuhikhalik Inuit society, anger is rarely expressed; individuals who demonstrate anger are considered social pariahs. Display rules govern which emotions can be expressed and to what degree. They may differ as a function of the culture, gender, or family background of an individual. Emotional expressions can be managed in several different ways: by simulating feelings one does not actually feel; by qualifying, amplifying, or deamplifying feelings; by masking an emotion with another emotion; or by neutralizing any emotional expression whatsoever.

A **cultural syndrome** is a shared set of beliefs, attitudes, norms, values, and behaviors among members of the same culture that are organized around a central theme. Cultural syndromes influence the rules for expressing or suppressing emotions and can even influence the ways emotions are experienced. For example, happiness is generally considered a positive emotion across cultures. However, in countries with more individualistic cultural syndromes, like the United States, happiness is viewed as infinite, attainable, and internally experienced. In contrast, in countries with a more collectivist cultural syndrome, such as Japan, happiness is a very rational emotion and generally applied to collective experiences more than to individual successes or experiences. This difference is illustrated in the contrast between the phrases *I am happy* and *I am sharing happiness with others*.

Gender can also play an important role in emotional expression. Research on the expression of emotion in the United States has shown that women are expected to express anger in public less often than men, while men are expected to repress the expression of sadness. Research also supports the conclusion that women are better at detecting subtle differences in emotional expression than men.

Impression Management

Impression management refers to our attempts to influence how others perceive us. This is done by regulating or controlling information we present about ourselves in social interactions. Impression management is often used synonymously with self-presentation. When describing impression management, theorists describe three "selves": the authentic self, the ideal self, and the tactical self. The **authentic self** describes who the person actually is, including both positive and negative attributes. The **ideal self**, as described in Chapter 6 of *MCAT Behavioral Sciences Review*, refers to who we would like to be under optimal circumstances. The **tactical self** refers to who we market ourselves to be when we adhere to others' expectations of us. This is similar to the ought self described in Chapter 6 of *MCAT Behavioral Sciences Review.*

People use a number of impression management strategies when in the presence of others. Some common strategies are summarized in Table 9.1, with examples of each.

STRATEGY	DEFINITION	EXAMPLE(S)
Self-disclosure	Giving information about oneself to establish an identity	Disclosing that you are a premedical student
Managing appearances	Using props, appearance, emotional expression, or associations with others to create a positive image	Wearing a white coat, keeping calm while dealing with a difficult patient, mentioning associations with important researchers during an interview
Ingratiation	Using flattery or conforming to expectations to win someone over	Blindly agreeing to someone else's opinion, complimenting a friend before asking for a favor
Aligning actions	Making questionable behavior acceptable through excuses	Justifications for missing deadlines, blaming a bad grade on too little sleep
Alter-casting	Imposing an identity onto another person	Any example in this course that says *As a good MCAT student, you should*...in which Kaplan is assigning *you* the role of *good MCAT student*

Table 9.1 Impression Management Strategies

Erving Goffman described impression management through the **dramaturgical approach**, using the metaphor of a theatrical performance to describe how individuals create images of themselves in various situations. In this analogy, Goffman relates a person's attempts to manage the impressions of others to an actor's performance in a play. A person's **front stage self** is the persona they present to an audience. A person will adapt their front stage self depending on the social situation, similar to an actor on stage in front of an audience performing according to the setting, role, and script of the play. In contrast, when an actor is back stage, the actor is hidden from the audience and is free to act in ways that may not be congruent with the actor's character in the play. According to Goffman, the **back stage self** is the persona adopted when not in a social situation and there is no concern about upholding the performance of a desired public image.

Another theory comes from George Herbert Mead, who described the self in two parts called the *Me* and the *I*. The part of self that is developed through interaction with society is the ***Me***. The development of the *Me* comes from considering the **generalized other**, which is based on a person's established perceptions of the expectations of society. Any time that a person tries to imagine what is expected of them in a social situation, they are taking on the perspective of the generalized other. And by considering the perspective of the generalized other and adapting one's behavior appropriately, the *Me* develops. By contrast, the ***I*** is the individual's own impulses. However, the *I* is not totally independent of the *Me*. Rather, a person's impulses are shaped by their interpretation of society's expectations. In short, the *Me* shapes the *I*.

MCAT EXPERTISE

Many of the sociological theories tested on the MCAT are far more extensive than the knowledge base the AAMC expects of test takers. The dramaturgical approach, for example, describes over twenty sociological concepts in theatrical terms; however, the MCAT only expects you to know front stage *vs.* back stage self.

BRIDGE

Mead's description of *Me* and *I* formed the foundation for the sociological theory of symbolic interactionism, which is described in Chapter 11 of *MCAT Behavioral Science Review.*

BEHAVIORAL SCIENCES GUIDED EXAMPLE WITH EXPERT THINKING

Researchers conducted two experiments in an effort to investigate social behavior.

Experiment 1:
Five-year-old children participated in one of four conditions. In all four conditions, the children played a game in which they received a sheet of paper with five symbols drawn on it. The children were also given a sheet of stickers, some of which matched the symbols, and were given 90 seconds to find the appropriate stickers and affix them to the sheet of paper over their matching symbols. Also on the table was a second set of materials, which the children were told was for another child who would be playing the game later.

Exp. 1: Sticker matching game

In the stealing condition, the participant's sticker sheet was missing one of the five symbols necessary to complete the game, while the sticker could be found on the second sheet. In the helping condition, the second sheet was conspicuously missing one of the stickers needed to complete the game, and the participant's sheet included an extra of those stickers, which participants were told they could keep or give to the next child. In some trials, the experimenter left the child alone while the child completed the task (the unobserved case), and in others, another child who was participating in the study but not part of the same experimental group was seated near the child during the task (the observed case).

Two conditions: children need to steal to complete their task; children can give to another child who is missing stickers.

IVs: steal or help condition; observation

DV: behavior

In the stealing condition, 4% of subjects stole in the observed case and 24% stole in the unobserved case ($p = .02$). In the helping condition, 28% of subjects helped in the observed case and 11% helped in the unobserved case ($p = .07$). Results are summarized in Figure 1.

The percentages are stated here, but are summarized in the figure. Missing from the figure are the p-values. Looks like the stealing condition was significant and the helping condition wasn't, but we could call it a trend.

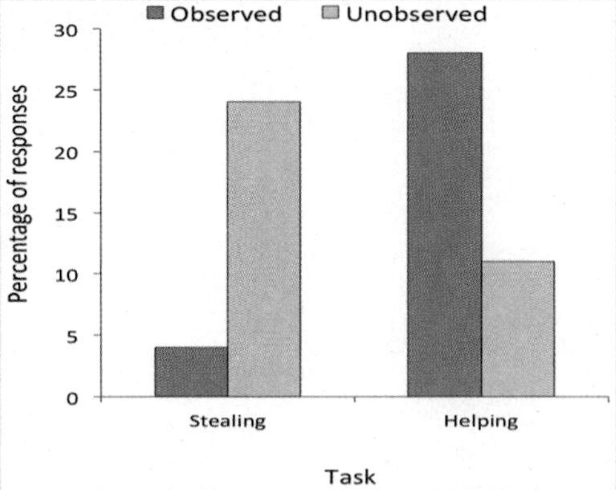

Figure 1 Stealing and helping behavior for children in their respective conditions.

Children helped when people were watching and stole when no one was.

Experiment 2:
Two chimpanzees were placed in separate cages. One of the chimps had access to a rope attached to a tray that contained food. In the stealing condition, the food was placed such that the other chimp could reach it, but pulling the rope moved the tray out of reach of both chimps. In the helping condition, the food was placed out of reach of both chimps, but pulling the rope moved the tray within reach of the second chimp. The subject chimps were not able to see the recipient chimps during the experiment, but were taught what the rope mechanism did prior to testing. Just as in Experiment 1, each of these conditions was carried out in one of two cases: either the chimps were alone in the experimental room, or a third dominant male chimp was present, observing the interaction. It is known that in chimpanzees, fitness improves with relationships to dominant group members. Results are summarized in Figure 2.

Similar conditions here. IVs: help or hurt, observation; DV: behavior.

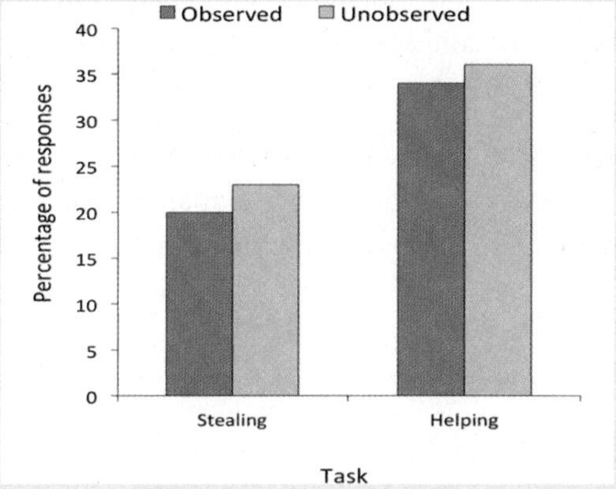

This is different from the children. Observation didn't seem to matter.

Figure 2 Stealing and helping behavior for chimps in their respective conditions.

Adapted from: Engelmann JM, Herrmann E, Tomasello M (2012) Five-Year Olds, but Not Chimpanzees, Attempt to Manage Their Reputations. *PLoS ONE* 7(10): e48433. https://doi.org/10.1371/journal.pone.0048433

What conclusion can be drawn based on these studies about the differences between human children and chimpanzees in social settings?

The question asks for a conclusion, so our plan should be to summarize the results of the studies and relate them to outside knowledge. Fortunately, once we understand the design of the two studies, the results aren't difficult to interpret. In Experiment 1, it looks like the children were more likely to steal when they were alone and more likely to help when they were being observed. From the *p*-values, it looks like that first result is statistically significant and the second result would count as merely a trend. Chimpanzees, on the other hand, showed no such concern for the presence of others. If this were a multiple-choice question, we would look for an answer that explained both results.

Knowing exactly what bit of content to tie these results to might be tricky without answer choices, but the passage does provide a clue. In Experiment 2, we're told that it is adaptive for chimpanzees to gain the favor of dominant group members, so these researchers are likely interested in the way individuals may change their behavior in order to gain the favor of others. This could be called self-presentation, reputation management, or impression management.

Applying this concept to the results of the study, we can conclude that children have at least some capacity for acting in a prosocial manner to manage impressions, but chimpanzees in the given situation are incapable of or unconcerned with doing the same.

Verbal and Nonverbal Communication

Communication is the ability to convey information by speech, writing, signals, or behavior. It is the foundation of social interaction and is often used to elicit changes, generate action, create understanding, share a point of view, or inform. Effective communication occurs when the desired message is received by the recipient.

Verbal communication is the transmission of information via the use of words, whether spoken, written, or signed. It is tied to nonverbal communication and is often dependent on nonverbal cues for the receiver to understand the sender's full meaning. While face-to-face conversations are rich with nonverbal communication, even phone conversations include nonverbal means of communication, such as pauses and changes in tone.

Nonverbal communication refers to how people communicate, intentionally or unintentionally, without words. Some examples of nonverbal communication are facial expressions, tone of voice, body position and movement, touches, and eye positioning. Gestures involving the hands and other parts of the body are often nonverbal, but the formal signs of a sign language count as verbal communication. Nonverbal cues serve a number of functions in communication, including expression of emotions, as shown in Figure 9.2, conveyance of attitudes and personality traits, and facilitation of verbal communication. Nonverbal communication is often dictated by culture. For example, in US culture, people can be suspicious of someone who does not make eye contact, as this is sometimes considered to be a sign of lying. However, in many other cultures, direct eye contact is used far less often than in the United States. For example, many children in Thailand are taught not to make eye contact with teachers and adults in order to show respect. Some types of verbal and nonverbal communication are listed in Table 9.2.

BRIDGE

Strong communication skills are tested everywhere on the MCAT, but are particularly important in the *Critical Analysis and Reasoning Skills* section. See Chapter 2 of *MCAT Critical Analysis and Reasoning Skills Review* for a discussion of analyzing rhetoric.

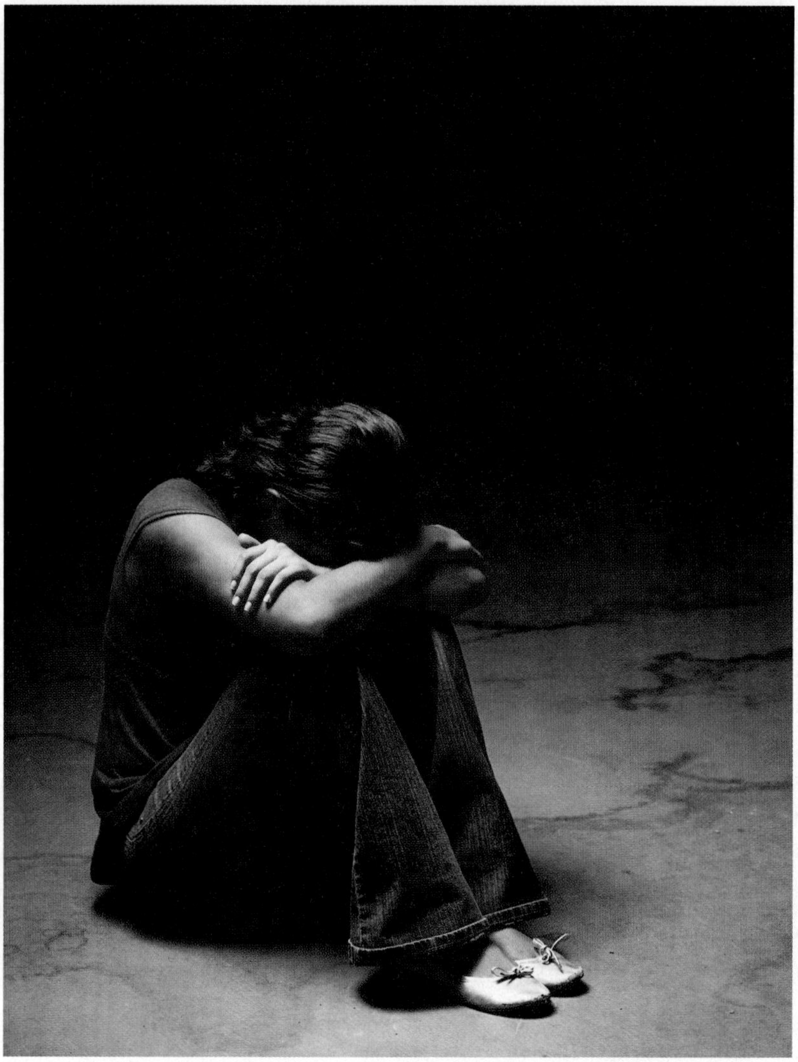

Figure 9.2 Human Body Language
Sadness is associated with drooping upper eyelids, staring into the distance, frowning, and slumping of shoulders, the last of which is seen here.

VERBAL	NONVERBAL
Spoken language	Facial expressions
Written language (print and electronic)	Body language (posture)
Sign languages (American Sign Language)	Gestures
Tactile languages (Braille alphabet)	Tone of voice (prosody)
	Eye contact
	Amount of personal space

Table 9.2 Verbal and Nonverbal Communication

Animal Signals and Communication

We not only communicate with other people, but also with other living creatures. **Animal communication** is defined as any behavior of one animal that affects the behavior of another.

Nonhuman animals communicate with one another in order to convey information such as emotions, intent, status, health, and the location of resources. They communicate with one another through a variety of nonverbal means, including body language, rudimentary facial expressions, visual displays, scents, and vocalizations.

The use of body language is common across a number of species. Body language can indicate that an animal is frightened, as shown in Figure 9.3, aggressive, relaxed, or even embarrassed; dogs often tuck their tails between their legs when scolded or fearful. Body language can also have significance for reproduction, as many animals will get into certain positions to signify readiness to mate.

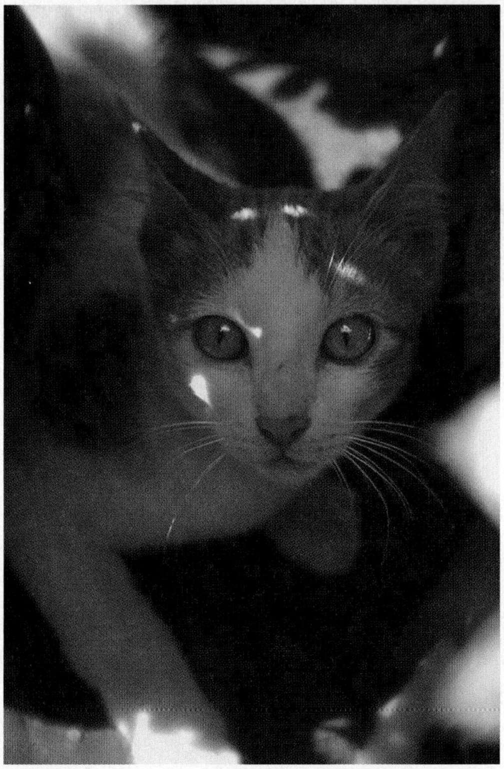

Figure 9.3 Animal Body Language
When surprised or scared, cats will recoil, crouch, and remain relatively motionless.

While humans possess far finer motor control of the muscles of facial expression, many animals (especially mammals) use facial expressions to indicate similar emotions to body language. It is noteworthy, however, that facial expressions appear to be more highly conserved between species than body language. For example, baring teeth and lunging forward, as shown in Figure 9.4, are perceived almost universally as signs of aggression or readiness to attack.

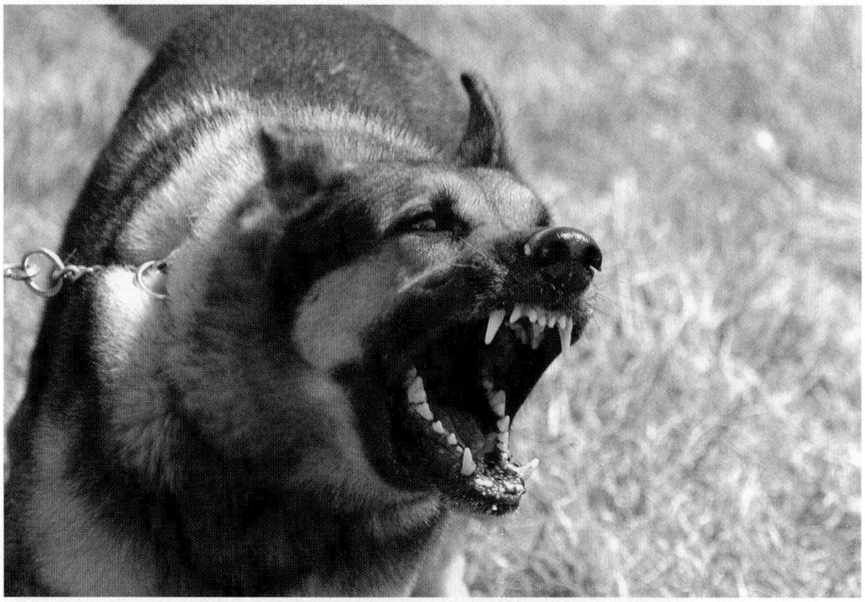

Figure 9.4 Animal Facial Expressions
Baring teeth and lunging forward are recognized by many animals as signs that an attack is imminent.

Animals may also use visual displays for communication. This is common for sex discrimination in birds; females are often less colorful than males because it permits them a greater degree of camouflage and protection when caring for their young. However, this also serves as communication between birds, as sex is readily apparent from the bird's appearance. Other visual displays include bioluminescence (the production of light), colorful plumage (as in peacocks), and dancing. Bees are well-known for communicating through dancing, as shown in Figure 9.5.

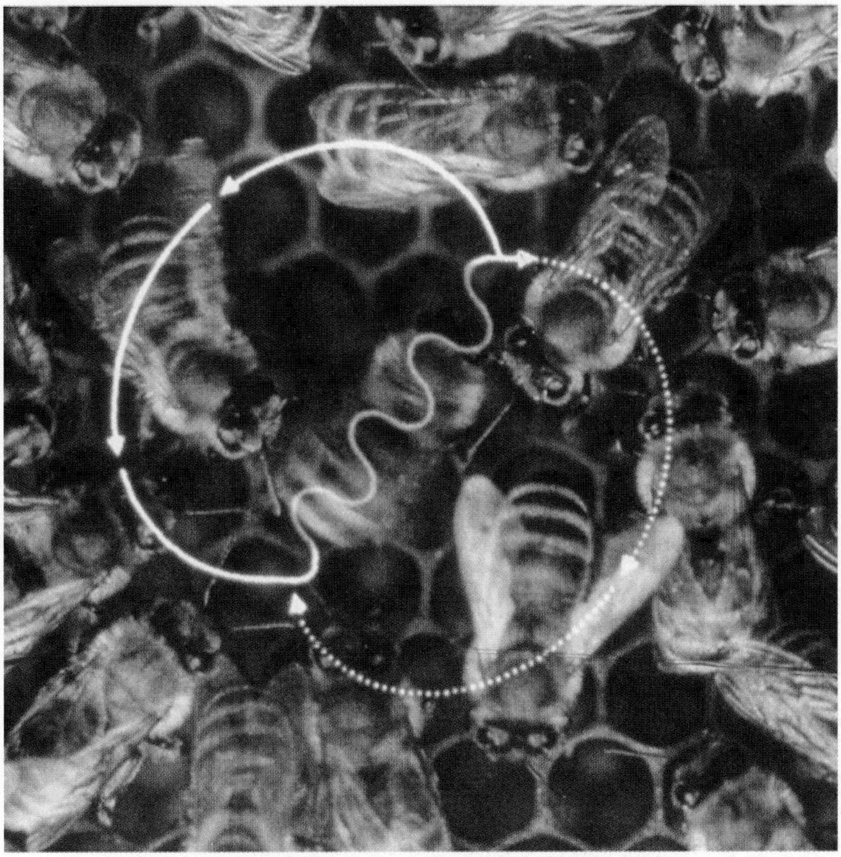

Figure 9.5 Bee Communication through Movement
The "waggle dance," illustrated here, indicates the location of food relative to the hive.

Many animals use scents to communicate both intraspecifically (between members of the same species) and interspecifically (between members of different species). Pheromones are a common example and are given off by members of a species to attract a mate. Scents can be used to mark an animal's territory or as a method of defense, such as in skunks.

Finally, animals also communicate through vocalizations with various levels of sophistication. For example, research has shown that prairie dogs have different "words" for specific predators, and can even create new words for novel objects. Bird calls are species specific and are used to attract a mate or warn of a threat.

In addition to interacting in the wild, humans use both verbal and nonverbal communication when interacting with domesticated animals, as is often seen between owners and their pets. Dog owners may use vocal commands to tell their pets to come, stay, or sit. Additionally, just as tone of voice can express joy or anger to a person, it can communicate the same information to a pet. Pets can be scolded with a look or a gesture. Communication works in the opposite direction as well, as a pet's body language and expressions convey information to its owner.

BRIDGE

It is debatable if pheromones actually have an effect on humans because we lack many of the genes necessary for function of the vomeronasal organ, an accessory olfactory organ seen in other animals. Olfaction and scent detection is discussed in Chapter 2 of *MCAT Behavioral Sciences Review*.

Communication between humans and animals is not confined strictly to pets. One of the most famous examples of animal communication is Koko, a gorilla who was able to communicate with humans through the use of American Sign Language. Koko's vocabulary included more than one thousand words.

MCAT CONCEPT CHECK 9.2

Before you move on, assess your understanding of the material with these questions.

1. Classify the following forms of communication as verbal or nonverbal:

• American Sign Language	Verbal	Nonverbal
• Turning your body away from another person	Verbal	Nonverbal
• Text messages	Verbal	Nonverbal
• Giving a "high five"	Verbal	Nonverbal
• Frowning	Verbal	Nonverbal

2. What is the front stage self? The back stage self?

   • Front stage self:

   ____

   ____

   • Back stage self:

   ____

   ____

3. For each of the methods of animal communication below, provide one example:

Method of Communication	Example
Body language	
Facial expressions	
Visual displays	
Scents	
Vocalizations	

Conclusion

Skunks are unique in how they communicate with other animals they perceive as threats. Their anal glands are capable of producing high concentrations of thiol-containing compounds, which create a distinctive malodorous scent. But it is noteworthy that skunks only carry five or six sprays' worth of material at a time—thus, they tend to use other forms of animal communication, such as body language, hissing, and foot stamping before resorting to spraying. The spray, however, is an ultimate defense: intense, caustic, and very sticky. Animals who are sprayed quickly learn that the skunk is not an animal to mess with.

Humans also use many methods of communication. While they may certainly not follow the same patterns as skunks, humans use combinations of vocalization, body language, facial expressions, and gestures to interact with each other socially. The field of sociology flows from these interactions as we create groups, networks, and organizations; organize our society into hierarchies with statuses; and fulfill the roles dictated by our statuses. We put much of our energy into controlling how we communicate with others, trying to create the optimal image of ourselves through impression management.

The content of this chapter plays a large role in your day-to-day life. Every day you interact with other people, and how you interact is largely determined by the culture and society in which you live. In the next chapter, we begin to analyze specific types of interactions, like attraction and altruism, and then examine the dark side of human society: bias, prejudice, discrimination, and stereotypes.

GO ONLINE

You've reviewed the content, now test your knowledge and critical thinking skills by completing a test-like passage set in your online resources!

CONCEPT SUMMARY

Elements of Social Interaction

- A **status** is a perceived position in society used to classify individuals.
    - An **ascribed status** is involuntarily assigned to an individual based on race, ethnicity, gender, family background, and so on.
    - An **achieved status** is voluntarily earned by an individual.
    - A **master status** is the status by which an individual is primarily identified.
- A **role** is a set of beliefs, values, and norms that define the expectations of a certain status in a social situation.
    - **Role performance** refers to carrying out the behaviors of a given role.
    - A **role partner** is a person with whom one is interacting who helps define the roles within the relationship.
    - A **role set** contains all of the different roles associated with a status.
    - **Role conflict** occurs when one has difficulty in satisfying the requirements of multiple roles simultaneously; **role strain** occurs when one has difficulty satisfying multiple requirements of the same role simultaneously.
- **Groups** are made up of two or more individuals with similar characteristics that share a sense of unity.
    - A **peer group** is a self-selected group formed around similar interests, ages, or statuses.
    - A **family group** is the group into which an individual is born, adopted, or married.
    - An **in-group** is a social group with which a person experiences a sense of belonging or identifies as a member.
    - An **out-group** is a social group with which an individual does not identify.
    - **Group conflict** occurs when an out-group competes with or opposes an in-group.
    - A **reference group** is a group to which individuals compare themselves.
    - **Primary groups** are those that contain strong, emotional bonds.
    - **Secondary groups** are often temporary and contain fewer emotional bonds and weaker bonds overall.
    - ***Gemeinschaft*** **(community)** is a group unified by feelings of togetherness due to shared beliefs, ancestry, or geography.
    - ***Gesellschaft*** **(society)** is a group unified by mutual self-interests in achieving a goal.
    - **Groupthink** occurs when members begin to conform to one another's views without critical evaluation.
- A **network** is an observable pattern of social relationships between individuals or groups.
- **Organizations** are bodies of people with a structure and culture designed to achieve specific goals.

Self-Presentation and Interacting with Others

- Various models have been proposed for how we express emotion in social situations.
    - The **basic model** states that there are universal emotions, along with corresponding expressions that can be understood across cultures.
    - The **social construction model** states that emotions are solely based on the situational context of social interactions.
- **Display rules** are unspoken rules that govern the expression of emotion.
- A **cultural syndrome** is a shared set of beliefs, norms, values, and behaviors organized around a central theme, as is found among people sharing the same language and geography.
- **Impression management** refers to the maintenance of a public image, which is accomplished through various strategies.
    - **Self-disclosure** is sharing factual information.
    - **Managing appearances** refers to using props, appearance, emotional expression, or associations to create a positive image.
    - **Ingratiation** is using flattery or conformity to win over someone else.
    - **Aligning actions** is the use of excuses to account for questionable behavior.
    - **Alter-casting** is imposing an identity onto another person.
- The **dramaturgical approach** says that individuals create images of themselves in the same way that actors perform a role in front of an audience.
    - The **front stage** is where individuals are seen by the audience and where they strive to preserve their desired image.
    - The **back stage** is where individuals are not in front of an audience and where they are free to act outside of their desired image.
- Communication includes both verbal and nonverbal elements.
    - **Verbal communication** is the conveyance of information through spoken, written, or signed words.
    - **Nonverbal communication** is the conveyance of information by means other than the use of words, such as body language, prosody, facial expressions, and gestures.
    - **Animal communication** takes place not only between nonhuman animals, but between humans and other animals as well. Animals use body language, rudimentary facial expressions, visual displays, scents, and vocalizations to communicate.

ANSWERS TO CONCEPT CHECKS

9.1

1.

Status	Example
Ascribed	Any status given involuntarily, due to factors such as race, ethnicity, gender, and family background
Achieved	Any status that is gained as a result of one's efforts or choices
Master	Any status by which a person would be most readily identified and that pervades all aspects of an individual's life

2. Statuses are perceived positions in society used to classify individuals. Roles are the behaviors and expectations associated with a status in a particular context. A group is a collection of at least two individuals. A network is a more formal illustration of the relationships between individuals, usually through graphic representation. An organization is a body with a specific set of goals, a structure, and a culture; organizations are complex secondary groups that are set up to achieve specific goals.

9.2

1. Verbal: American Sign Language, text messages

   Nonverbal: turning your body away (body language), giving a "high five" (gesture), frowning (facial expression)
2. The front stage self refers to when we are on stage and performing. This requires us to live up to the roles and expectations assumed by our status. The back stage self is when we are away from others and may include behaviors that would not be appropriate or consistent with the front stage self.
3. Examples may vary.

Method of Communication	Example
Body language	Dogs: tail between the legs
Facial expressions	Various animals: baring teeth
Visual displays	Peacocks: colorful plumage
Scents	Insects (and others): pheromones
Vocalizations	Birds: birdcalls

SCIENCE MASTERY ASSESSMENT EXPLANATIONS

1. **C**

A status is a position in society used to classify a person and exists in relation to other statuses. The specific behaviors associated with this status, **(B)**, best describe a role.

2. **B**

An achieved status is one that is acquired through personal efforts. This is in contrast to an ascribed status, **(A)**, in which the status is involuntarily given based on race, ethnicity, gender, family background, and so on. A master status, **(C)**, is one that influences all aspects of an individual's life. While being a college graduate is an important aspect of day-to-day life, it does not usually pervade every part of one's life.

3. **C**

A bureaucracy is an example of an organization, specifically one with the goal of performing complex tasks as efficiently as possible. Immediate networks and primary groups, **(A)** and **(B)**, are characterized by strong, intimate bonds, which are not commonly seen in bureaucracies. Reference groups, **(D)**, are those groups to which we compare ourselves for various characteristics.

4. **D**

Generally, bureaucracies are marked by six characteristics: paid officials on a fixed salary; nonelected officials who are provided rights and privileges as a result of making their career out of holding office; regular salary increases, seniority rights, and promotions upon passing exams or milestones, **(C)**; officials who enter the organization by holding an advanced degree or training, **(B)**; responsibilities, obligations, privileges, and work procedures rigidly defined by the organization, **(A)**; and responsibility for meeting the obligations of the office one holds.

5. **C**

Verbal communication uses words (whether spoken, written, or signed). Nonverbal communication uses other means of signaling emotions or ideas, such as body language, **(D)**, facial expressions, **(A)**, eye contact, **(B)**, prosody, and personal space. Hand gestures and other bodily movements are also often nonverbal communication, but can be verbal when used as part of a sign language.

6. **C**

Aligning actions is an impression management technique in which one provides socially acceptable reasons for unexpected behavior. This may manifest as providing an excuse for poor performance or laughing off an inappropriate comment as a joke. Tension created from having conflicting thoughts or opinions, as mentioned in **(B)**, refers to cognitive dissonance.

7. **B**

Imposing a role on another person (in this case, "good friend") is the hallmark of alter-casting. This example is also the opposite of ingratiation, **(C)**, because the implication behind the statement is that not lending the bike makes one a "bad friend"; ingratiation is the use of flattery or conformity to win over someone else.

8. **A**

A *Gesellschaft* (society) is one in which individuals are working toward the same goal, such as a company or country. *Gemeinschaften* (communities), on the other hand, are those that are bonded together by beliefs, ancestry, or geography.

9. **B**

Display rules are those that dictate cultural expectations of emotion. In some cultures, sadness is considered personal and internal; in others, sadness is shared externally with the community.

10. **C**

SYMLOG is a method for analyzing group dynamics and considers groups along three dimensions: dominant *vs.* submissive, friendliness *vs.* unfriendliness, and instrumentally controlled *vs.* emotionally expressive.

11. **B**

If a candidate is "exposed," then personal characteristics that are usually shielded from public view have been brought in front of the public. This would be pulling aspects of the back stage self to the front stage. It would not be considered removing the front stage self, **(C)**, because the candidate still has a public image, even if it has been tarnished.

12. **B**

The ought self is who others think we should be: the expectations imposed by others on us. This is most similar to the tactical self, which is the self we present to others when we adhere to their expectations. The presented self, **(D)**, is a combination of the authentic, ideal, and tactical selves.

13. **A**

The basic model of emotion, as proposed by Charles Darwin, states that emotions serve an evolutionary purpose and thus are similar across cultures. The seven universal emotions have also been used as support for this theory. The social construction model states that emotions are always a product of the current social situation and does not posit any biological basis for emotions, implying a lack of a role for emotions in evolution.

14. **D**

Intraspecific communication refers to communication between members of the same species. Interspecific communication, on the other hand, refers to communication between members of different species. Echolocation, **(C),** is not an example of intraspecific communication because the sender of the signal and the recipient are the same organism; this would be considered autocommunication.

15. **C**

Primary groups have direct and close bonds between members, providing warm, personal, and intimate relationships to its members. Secondary groups, in contrast, form superficial bonds and tend to last for a shorter period of time.

Consult your online resources for additional practice. GO ONLINE

SHARED CONCEPTS

Behavioral Sciences Chapter 3
Learning and Memory

Behavioral Sciences Chapter 5
Motivation, Emotion, and Stress

Behavioral Sciences Chapter 6
Identity and Personality

Behavioral Sciences Chapter 8
Social Processes, Attitudes, and Behavior

Behavioral Sciences Chapter 10
Social Thinking

Behavioral Sciences Chapter 11
Social Structure and Demographics

CHAPTER 10

SOCIAL THINKING

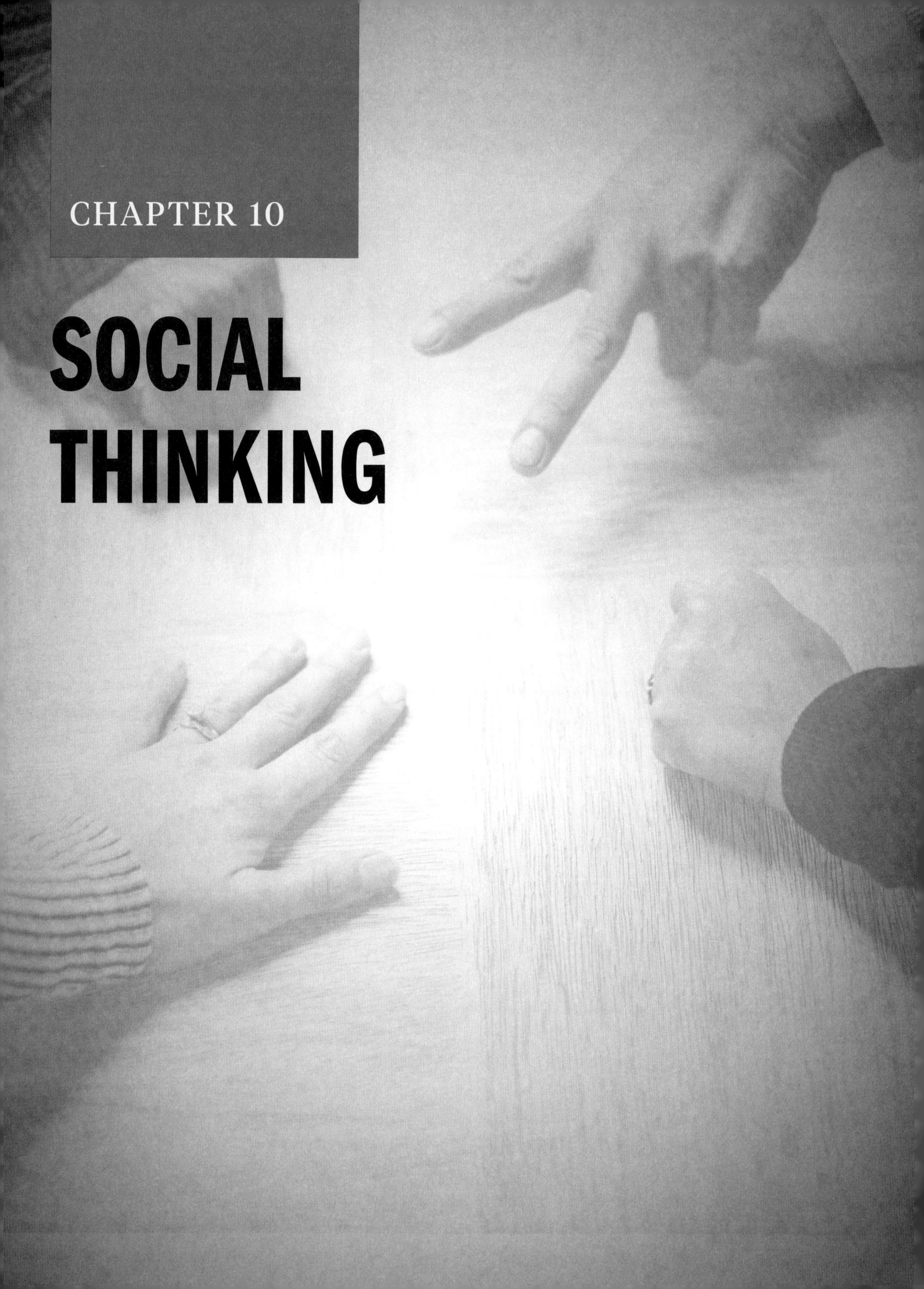

SCIENCE MASTERY ASSESSMENT

Every pre-med knows this feeling: there is so much content I have to know for the MCAT! How do I know what to do first or what's important?

While the high-yield badges throughout this book will help you identify the most important topics, this Science Mastery Assessment is another tool in your MCAT prep arsenal. This quiz (which can also be taken in your online resources) and the guidance below will help ensure that you are spending the appropriate amount of time on this chapter based on your personal strengths and weaknesses. Don't worry though—skipping something now does not mean you'll never study it. Later on in your prep, as you complete full-length tests, you'll uncover specific pieces of content that you need to review and can come back to these chapters as appropriate.

How to Use This Assessment

If you answer 0–7 questions correctly:

Spend about 1 hour to read this chapter in full and take limited notes throughout. Follow up by reviewing **all** quiz questions to ensure that you now understand how to solve each one.

If you answer 8–11 questions correctly:

Spend 20–40 minutes reviewing the quiz questions. Beginning with the questions you missed, read and take notes on the corresponding subchapters. For questions you answered correctly, ensure your thinking matches that of the explanation and you understand why each choice was correct or incorrect.

If you answer 12–15 questions correctly:

Spend less than 20 minutes reviewing all questions from the quiz. If you missed any, then include a quick read-through of the corresponding subchapters, or even just the relevant content within a subchapter, as part of your question review. For questions you answered correctly, ensure your thinking matches that of the explanation and review the Concept Summary at the end of the chapter.

1. The tendency to become close friends with neighbors rather than people in other neighborhoods is most strongly related to which of the following factors?
   - **A.** Proximity
   - **B.** Reciprocity
   - **C.** Self-disclosure
   - **D.** Similarity

2. Which of the following would be associated with high levels of aggression?
   - **I.** Increased amygdala activity
   - **II.** Decreased amygdala activity
   - **III.** Increased prefrontal cortex activity
   - **IV.** Decreased prefrontal cortex activity

   - **A.** I and III only
   - **B.** I and IV only
   - **C.** II and III only
   - **D.** II and IV only

3. A child who cries when a caregiver departs and smiles and runs to the caregiver upon return is displaying which type of attachment pattern?
   - **A.** Avoidant attachment
   - **B.** Ambivalent attachment
   - **C.** Disorganized attachment
   - **D.** Secure attachment

4. Elephant seal males mate with multiple females each mating season, while females only have one mate each. What type of mating system is this?
   - **A.** Polyandry
   - **B.** Polygyny
   - **C.** Monogamy
   - **D.** Promiscuity

5. A person with a ventromedial hypothalamus injury will likely show which behavior?
   - **A.** Increased empathy
   - **B.** Decreased empathy
   - **C.** Increased food intake
   - **D.** Decreased food intake

6. Female great reed warblers are attracted to males with larger song repertoires because they tend to produce offspring with higher viability. This is an example of which of the following?
   - **A.** Runaway selection
   - **B.** Sensory bias
   - **C.** Direct phenotypic benefits
   - **D.** Indirect phenotypic benefits

7. In several species of shrimp, the larger adults will sacrifice themselves to protect the younger, smaller shrimp. How is this behavior best explained?
   - **A.** Inclusive fitness
   - **B.** Direct benefit
   - **C.** Sensory bias
   - **D.** Foraging

8. Which of the following is NOT a component of social perception?
   - **A.** The target
   - **B.** The situation
   - **C.** The perceiver
   - **D.** The process

9. When you first meet Dustin, he is very rude to you. You run into him twice more and he is very friendly, but you still dislike him because of your first meeting. What impression bias does this describe?

- **A.** Primacy effect
- **B.** Recency effect
- **C.** Reliance on central traits
- **D.** Proximity

10. Mei brings cookies to work. Although you have not yet tasted them, you say to another coworker, "Mei is such a great person; I'm sure these cookies are fantastic!" What type of bias is this?

- **A.** Reliance on central traits
- **B.** Direct benefits
- **C.** Halo effect
- **D.** Similarity

11. A friend wins a tennis game and says, "I trained so hard—that was a great win!" After losing a subsequent match, the friend says, "My baby brother kept me up all night crying; I was tired for the match." These statements reflect which of the following principles?

- **A.** Just-world hypothesis
- **B.** Fundamental attribution error
- **C.** Self-serving bias
- **D.** Esteem bias

12. Carlos is always happy and smiling. Today, you notice he seems down and think something must have happened to upset him. What types of attribution are you making?

- **I.** Internal
- **II.** External
- **III.** Situational
- **IV.** Dispositional

- **A.** I and III only
- **B.** I and IV only
- **C.** II and III only
- **D.** II and IV only

13. A group of men and women are going to be rated on their driving abilities. The role of gender is emphasized in the experiment and the women perform worse than the men. In another experiment, the role of gender is not mentioned and the ratings are comparable between the two groups. Which principle do these results support?

- **A.** Institutional discrimination
- **B.** Stereotype threat
- **C.** Prejudice
- **D.** The just-world hypothesis

14. The behavior that accompanies the negative attitudes a person has toward a group or individual is referred to as:

- **A.** stereotyping.
- **B.** cultural relativism.
- **C.** prejudice.
- **D.** discrimination.

15. Game theory is designed to study:

- **A.** reliance on central traits.
- **B.** behavior attribution.
- **C.** decision-making behavior.
- **D.** self-enhancement.

Answer Key

1. **A**
2. **B**
3. **D**
4. **B**
5. **C**
6. **D**
7. **A**
8. **D**
9. **A**
10. **C**
11. **C**
12. **C**
13. **B**
14. **D**
15. **C**

Detailed explanations can be found at the end of the chapter.

CHAPTER 10

SOCIAL THINKING

In This Chapter

Introduction

Social psychology is concerned with social behavior, including the ways people influence each other's attitudes and behavior. It looks at the impact that individuals have on one another, that social groups have on individual group members, that individual group members have upon the social group, and that social groups have on other social groups. In this chapter, we will continue our discussion of social psychology, highlighting its close relationship to sociology and the other fields within psychology, theoretical perspectives on human behavior within the social environment, and key concepts and classical studies in the field of social psychology. But whereas the last two chapters focused on how individuals are affected by groups and how individuals interact within groups, we will turn our attention in this chapter to specific behaviors seen across human beings, including attraction, aggression, attachment, and the need for social support. We'll also take a look at the dark side of social psychology as we look at patterns of blame in attribution theory and the misappropriation of social structure for prejudice and discrimination. This will be highly relevant for you as a physician, as many patients face prejudice based on their diagnoses or are discriminated against because of personal characteristics, including age, sex, race, ethnicity, socioeconomic status, sexual orientation, gender identity, and more.

CHAPTER PROFILE

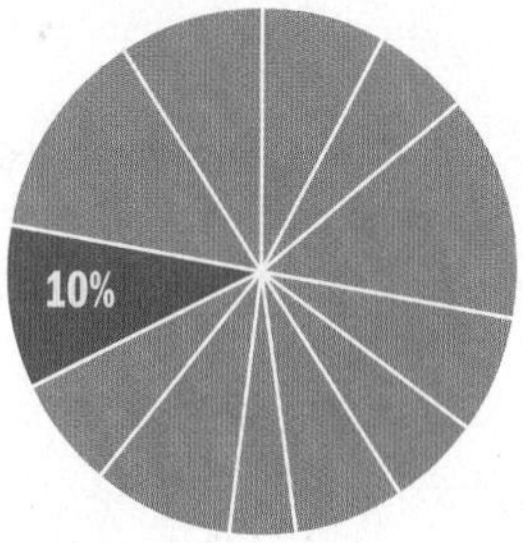

The content in this chapter should be relevant to about 10% of all questions about the behavioral sciences on the MCAT.

This chapter covers material from the following AAMC content categories:

8B: Social thinking

8C: Social interactions

10.1 Social Behavior

High-Yield

LEARNING OBJECTIVES

After Chapter 10.1, you will be able to:

- Describe interpersonal attraction, including the factors that influence interpersonal attraction
- Recall the meaning of the term *aggression*, including examples of aggressive behaviors
- List the four types of attachment and how they affect childhood behavior
- Identify the common types of social support
- Explain the relationship between altruism and inclusive fitness

Social behaviors involve interactions with others. These may flow from positive feelings, such as attraction or attachment, or they may flow from negative feelings, such as aggression.

Attraction

KEY CONCEPT

Interpersonal attraction is influenced by many factors, including physical characteristics, similarity, self-disclosure, reciprocity, and proximity.

Have you ever wondered what makes some people friends and others enemies? How second graders choose their best friends? Why you keep eyeing that attractive person in your physics class? Social psychologists call this phenomenon of individuals liking each other **interpersonal attraction**. Researchers have found several factors that affect attraction, including similarity, self-disclosure, reciprocity, and proximity. Outward appearance also plays a role; the more symmetric someone's face is, the more physically attractive people tend to perceive that person to be. Humans are also attracted to individuals with certain body proportions approximating the **golden ratio** (1.618:1).

We tend to be attracted to people who are similar to us in attitudes, intelligence, education, height, age, religion, appearance, and socioeconomic status. One reason for this may be convenience: it's easier to spend time together if you both want to go on a bike ride or if you both enjoy Thai food. Also, people are drawn to having their values and choices validated by another person. So why is there a cliché about opposites attracting? Social psychologists find that attraction also occurs if opposing qualities match up with each other; for example, a nurturer is attracted to someone who craves being nurtured. Notably, successful complementary relationships still have fundamental similarities in some attitudes that make the complementary aspects of the relationship work.

Another component of attraction lies in the opportunity for **self-disclosure**, or sharing one's fears, thoughts, and goals with another person and being met with nonjudgmental empathy. Engaging in this behavior deepens attraction and friendship. This must be a reciprocal behavior, however. Revealing one's innermost secrets creates a sense of vulnerability that, if not met by the other person, can be interpreted as being taken advantage of. Reciprocity is important in other aspects of interpersonal attraction as well. **Reciprocal liking** is the phenomenon whereby people like others better when they believe the other person likes them. Researchers have shown that even if we disagree with others on important issues, we will have increased interest in them if we have indications that they like us.

Finally, **proximity**, or just being physically close to someone, plays a factor in attraction to a person. Studies have shown that we are more likely to form friendships with people in the same dorm as us or with the people who sit closest to us in class. Part of this is convenience; it's easier to have conversations and make plans with people in the same area. Another explanation is the **mere exposure effect** or **familiarity effect**, the tendency for people to prefer stimuli that they have been exposed to more frequently. You may have observed this in your everyday life: Have you disliked a song the first time you heard it, only to find yourself singing along and saying, *I like this song!* after hearing it many more times? This principle is also used in marketing: the more people hear the name of a product, the more likely they are to be attracted to and purchase that product.

Aggression

Aggression is defined as a behavior that intends to cause harm or increase social dominance. Aggression can take the form of physical actions as well as verbal or nonverbal communication. Ethologists study aggression in terms of the interactions between animals in natural settings. Aggression in these settings can include bodily contact, as seen in Figure 10.1, but most displays of aggression are settled by threat and withdrawal without actual bodily harm. Threat displays are common in both animals and humans. Before a fight, someone might puff up the chest or pull back a fist to threaten another person. This display may or may not result in physical harm or violence. Other examples of aggression include a bully hurling insults at another child or a gang member making threatening gestures to a member of another gang.

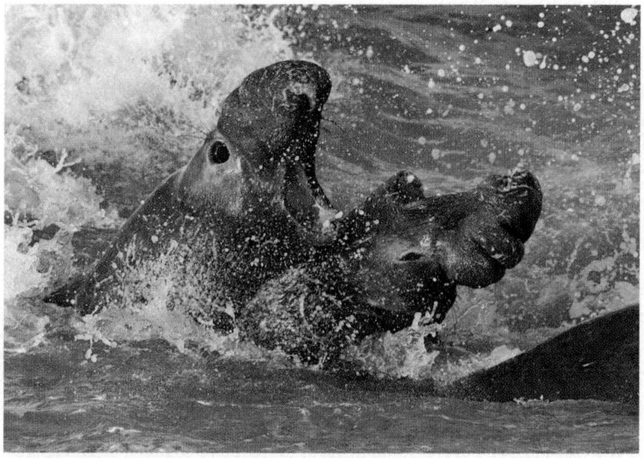

Figure 10.1 Aggression Following Threat Displays of Elephant Seals
While threat displays may lead to violence, as seen here, threat displays commonly lead to withdrawal to prevent fights.

What is the purpose of aggressive behavior if it causes so much destruction? Evolutionarily, aggression offers protection against perceived and real threats. Aggression helped our ancestors fight off predators. It also helps organisms gain access to resources such as food, additional territory, or mates. In cases of limited resources, aggression could be the deciding factor that allows one to pass on genes.

BRIDGE

The prefrontal cortex is critically important to managing the limbic system, which is important in managing emotion and stress. These roles of the prefrontal cortex are discussed in Chapter 5 of *MCAT Behavioral Sciences Review.*

From a biological perspective, multiple parts of the brain contribute to violent behavior. The **amygdala** is the part of the brain responsible for associating stimuli and their corresponding rewards or punishments. In short, it is responsible for telling us whether or not something is a threat. If the amygdala is activated, this increases aggression. However, higher-order brain structures, such as the prefrontal cortex, can hit the brakes on a revved-up amygdala, reducing emotional reactivity and impulsiveness. Reduced activity in the prefrontal cortex has been linked to increased aggressive behavior.

REAL WORLD

Alcohol has been shown to increase aggressive behavior. Alcohol impairs judgment and limits one's ability to control aggressive reactions. It also makes one feel less inhibited by social mores that would normally restrict aggressive behavior.

Aggression is also under hormonal control. Higher levels of testosterone have been linked to more aggressive behavior in humans irrespective of sex or gender. Some speculate that the higher levels of testosterone in phenotypical males compared to phenotypical females may explain the trend that males are generally more aggressive than females across cultures and that males commit a disproportionate majority of violent crimes.

Beyond the biological contributions to aggressive behavior, studies have found many psychological and situational predictors of aggression. Do you find yourself snapping at people more when you're in pain? Have you ever gotten annoyed with a waiter when you were extremely hungry? Such responses are accounted for by the **cognitive neoassociation model**, which states that we are more likely to respond to others aggressively whenever we are feeling negative emotions, such as being tired, sick, frustrated, or in pain. This can also be seen on a large scale: riots are more likely to happen on hot days than cool ones; drivers without air conditioning are more likely to honk at other drivers than those with air conditioning.

Another factor that contributes to aggressive behavior is exposure to violent behavior. The effects on children of media portrayals of violence continue to be a hot topic. Research findings are mixed but tend to show that viewing violent behavior indeed correlates to an increase in aggressive behavior. The contribution of modeling to violence in children was also explored in Albert Bandura's Bobo doll experiment, described in Chapter 3 of *MCAT Behavioral Sciences Review.*

Attachment

KEY CONCEPT

In attachment, a secure base is a caregiver who is consistent, available, comforting, and responsive.

Attachment is an emotional bond between a caregiver and a child that begins to develop during infancy. While parental figures are most common, emotional bonds can occur with any caregiver who is sensitive and responsive during social interaction. After World War II, psychiatrist John Bowlby noticed the negative effects of isolation on social and emotional development in orphaned children and started the study of attachment. In the 1970s, psychologist Mary Ainsworth expounded on this theory, saying that infants need a secure base, in the form of a consistent caregiver during the first six months to two years of life, from which to explore the world and develop appropriately. Four main types of attachment styles have been described: secure, avoidant, ambivalent, and disorganized.

Secure Attachment

Secure attachment is seen when a child has a consistent caregiver and is able to go out and explore, knowing that there is a secure base to return to. The child will be upset at the departure of the caregiver and will be comforted by the return of the caregiver. The child trusts that the caregiver will be there for comfort, and while the child can be comforted by a stranger, the child will clearly prefer the caregiver. Having a secure attachment pattern is thought to be a vital aspect of a child's social development. Children with avoidant, ambivalent, or disorganized attachment can have deficits in social skills. Collectively, these attachment types are known as **insecure attachment**.

Avoidant Attachment

Avoidant attachment results when the caregiver has little or no response to a distressed child. Given the choice, these children will show no preference between a stranger and the caregiver. They show little or no distress when the caregiver leaves and little or no relief when the caregiver returns.

Ambivalent Attachment

Ambivalent attachment occurs when a caregiver has an inconsistent response to a child's distress, sometimes responding appropriately, sometimes neglectfully. As such, the child is unable to form a secure base because the child cannot consistently rely on the caregiver's response. The child will be very distressed on separation from the caregiver but has a mixed response when the caregiver returns, often displaying ambivalence. This is sometimes referred to as **anxious–ambivalent attachment** because the child is always anxious about the reliability of the caregiver.

Disorganized Attachment

Children with **disorganized attachment** show no clear pattern of behavior in response to the caregiver's absence or presence, but instead can show a mix of different behaviors. These can include avoidance or resistance; seeming dazed, frozen, or confused; or repetitive behaviors like rocking. Disorganized attachment is often associated with erratic behavior and social withdrawal by the caregiver. It may also be a red flag for abuse.

REAL WORLD

As a physician, you will be a mandated reporter. This means that you are required by law to report suspected cases of child abuse. Remember: It is better to report and be incorrect than to miss a potentially fatal scenario.

BEHAVIORAL SCIENCES GUIDED EXAMPLE WITH EXPERT THINKING

The Strange Situation is an experimental procedure used to assess attachment in infants who are between 9 and 18 months old. The procedure occurs over the course of twenty-one minutes and progresses as follows:

1. The parent and child are introduced to the experimental room.
2. The parent and child are left alone in the room. The infant is allowed to explore the room. The parent does not participate.
3. A stranger enters the room, converses with the parent, and attempts to engage with the child.
4. The parent conspicuously leaves the room, and the child is left with the stranger.
5. The parent returns and comforts the child.
6. Both the parent and the stranger leave, and the child is left alone.
7. The stranger returns and attempts to engage with the child.
8. The parent returns and comforts the child, and the stranger conspicuously leaves.

Researchers observe the amount of exploration the child engages in, reactions to the stranger, reactions to the absence of the parent, and the child's behavior upon reunion with the parent.

Experimental procedure. I'll take a brief moment to picture each step, but I'll have to return to this list if a question asks for details.

Not a traditional experiment so no real IV, the differing input is the child and the relationship to the parent, and the output is the child's behavior/attachment style.

This procedure has been replicated with nonhuman animals. In particular, it has been shown that dogs tend to form secure attachments with their owners. This procedure has been attempted with cats, but it appears that cats' behaviors may not serve the same function as behaviors of humans, and as such it is difficult to use procedures developed for humans to assess cat attachment. Furthermore, individual cats' behaviors are inconsistent throughout the procedure, possibly because the experimental procedure is a scenario that cats do not frequently encounter outside the laboratory.

Attachment in nonhuman animals.

Dogs are secure and cats are complicated.

Adapted from: Potter A, Mills DS (2015) Domestic Cats (*Felis silvestris catus*) Do Not Show Signs of Secure Attachment to Their Owners. *PLoS ONE* 10(9): e0135109. https://doi.org/10.1371/journal.pone.0135109

A child exposed to the Strange Situation was uninterested in exploring the room in the presence of either parent or stranger, and did not emotionally engage with either individual. In what ways do dogs' attachment behaviors and style differ from those of the child? What experimental limitations do the researchers point out regarding assessing attachment in cats?

The beginning of the question stem presents a scenario in which a child was reluctant to explore the surroundings, regardless of who was present. This description will have to be matched to our outside content knowledge regarding attachment. The different attachment styles are content we should know for the MCAT, and avoidant attachment is characterized by children who show no substantial behavioral change based on the presence or absence of a parent. Behaviorally, we can conclude the child described is displaying an avoidant attachment style. Dogs were described in the article as demonstrating secure attachment, so we'll want to recall the characteristics of a secure attachment and apply them to this situation. In secure attachment, the subject may or may not show distress when left with a stranger, but will definitely prefer the caregiver. The dogs must have displayed distress when left alone but were easily comforted when the caregiver returned. Specifically, then, the difference between the child and a typical dog should be twofold: the dogs should show greater engagement and positive response with their caregiver as compared to this child, and the dogs should show more distress when left alone without the caregiver as compared to the child.

The answer to the second question requires that we approach the problem in a similar way, this time applied to experimental design. We'll need to consider the description we were given and attempt to match the description to a vocabulary word or concept we've studied. Here, the researchers noted two issues. The first was that the behaviors measured in cats did not serve a function with respect to attachment. Since cats aren't social animals, trying to evaluate their behavior in a social context might be inappropriate. The experiment might not actually be measuring what it seeks to measure, which is a problem with internal validity. The author also mentions that the scenario presented in the experiment might not have a real-world analogue. When an experimental procedure might not actually apply to situations outside the lab, the experiment can be said to lack external validity.

In sum, the dog displayed secure attachment, while the infant displayed avoidant attachment. The application of this methodology to cats potentially lacks both internal (not measuring the targeted variable) and external (not bearing relevance to real-world analogues) validity.

Social Support

In psychology, **social support** is the perception or reality that one is cared for by a social network. Social support can be divided into many different categories: emotional, esteem, material, informational, and network support. While social support is present at all times, it is often most pronounced—and necessary—when someone suffers a personal or family tragedy.

Emotional support is listening, affirming, and empathizing with someone's feelings. It's the *I'm sorry for your loss* condolence card or a trip to the hospital to visit a sick relative. Many people equate social support with emotional support, but other forms of support exist as well.

Esteem support is similar, but touches more directly on affirming the qualities and skills of a person. Reminding others of the skills they possess to tackle a problem can bolster their confidence. For example, consider a friend who has missed a significant amount of school due to illness. Calling that friend a smart and efficient worker who should have no problem making up the work would be providing esteem support.

Material support, also called **tangible support**, is any type of financial or material contribution to another person. It can come in the form of making a meal for friends after they have lost a loved one or donating money to a person in need.

Informational support refers to providing information that will help someone. You will spend much of your career providing informational support to patients as you explain their diagnoses, potential treatment options, and risks and benefits of those treatment options.

Network support is the type of social support that gives a person a sense of belonging. This can be shown physically, as demonstrated in Figure 10.2, or can be accomplished through gestures, group activities, and shared experiences.

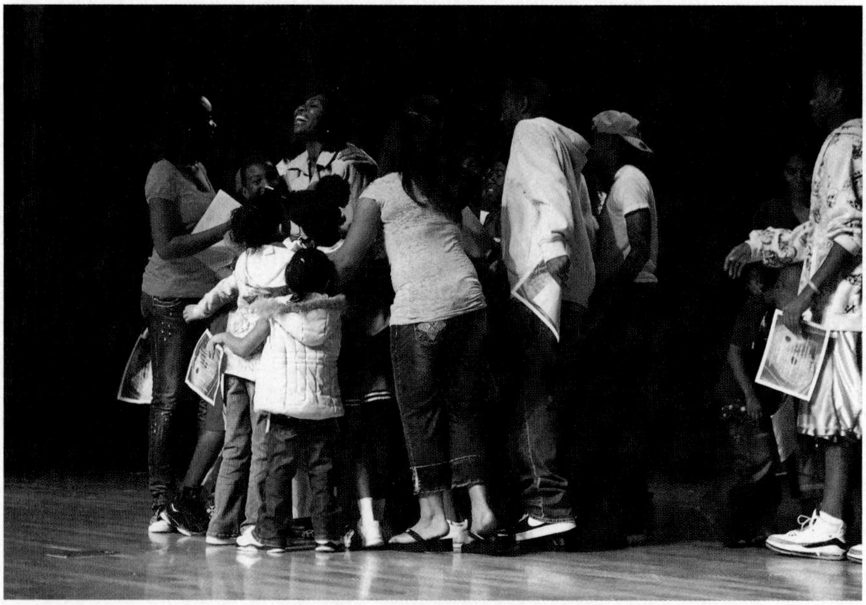

Figure 10.2 Network Support
A group hug creates a sense of belonging.

No matter the form, all of these social supports offer many different types of health benefits. Social support helps reduce psychological distress such as anxiety and depression. People with low social support show higher levels of major mental disorders, alcohol and drug use, and suicidal ideation. Beyond these intuitive improvements in mental health, there are also improvements to our physical health. Studies have found that people with low social support have a higher mortality risk from many different diseases, including diabetes, cardiovascular disease, and cancer. Strong social support appears to correlate with immunological health, too: those with higher social support are less likely to get colds and recover faster when they do.

Social Behaviors and Evolutionary Fitness

Many behaviors have neurological corollaries. Here, we will look at some specific behaviors and the brain regions that are implicated in causing them.

Foraging

The behavior of **foraging**, or seeking out and eating food, is driven by biological, psychological, and social influences. Biologically, hunger is driven by a complex pathway involving both neurotransmitters and hormones. The sensation of hunger is controlled by the **hypothalamus**. Specifically, the lateral hypothalamus promotes hunger, while the ventromedial hypothalamus responds to cues that we are full and promotes satiety. Thus, damage to the lateral hypothalamus will cause a person to lose all interest in eating; meanwhile, damage to the ventromedial hypothalamus will result in obesity because the individual never feels satiated. Foraging is also impacted by genetics. Certain genes play a role in the onset of foraging behavior and the division of tasks between members of the same group. Some species forage together while others engage in solitary foraging.

Cognitive skills play a role in the success of both solitary and group foraging. These skills include spatial awareness, memory, and decision making. In species that forage as a group, foraging is primarily a learned behavior. Young individuals learn through observing how to find and consume food and how to determine what is safe to eat, as shown in Figure 10.3. Animals also learn how to hunt by watching others. Some animals, such as wolves, hunt in packs that have strict rules regarding the order in which individuals are allowed to eat after a successful hunt.

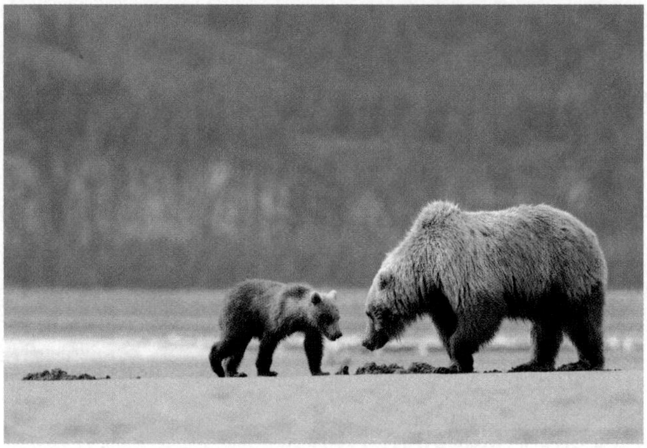

Figure 10.3 Foraging Is Learned through Observational Learning

Mating and Mate Choice

A **mating system** describes the organization of a group's sexual behavior. Mating systems seen among animals include monogamy, polygamy, and promiscuity. **Monogamy** refers to an exclusive mating relationship. **Polygamy** means having exclusive relationships with multiple partners. Having exclusive relationships with multiple females is called **polygyny** and with multiple males is called **polyandry**. **Promiscuity** refers to a member of one sex mating with others without exclusivity. In most animal species, there is one dominant mating system; however, humans exhibit more flexibility. In humans, mating behavior is highly influenced by both biological and social factors. Humans also differ from animals by having formal relationships to correspond with mate choice. Mating may or may not be associated with these social relationships, such as marriage or dating.

Mate choice, or **intersexual selection**, is the selection of a mate based on attraction. **Mate bias** refers to how choosy members of the species are while choosing a mate. This bias is an evolutionary mechanism aimed at increasing the fitness of the species. It may carry **direct benefits** by providing material advantages, protection, or emotional support, or **indirect benefits** by promoting better survival in offspring.

KEY CONCEPT

Direct benefits provide advantages to the mate. Indirect benefits provide advantages to offspring.

There are five recognized mechanisms of mate choice:

- **Phenotypic benefits:** observable traits that make a potential mate more attractive to the opposite sex. Usually, these traits indicate increased production and survival of offspring. For example, males that appear more nurturing are more likely to care for, and promote the survival of, their offspring.
- **Sensory bias:** development of a trait to match a preexisting preference that exists in the population. For example, fiddler crabs are naturally attracted to structures that break up the level horizon because they may indicate a food source; male crabs take advantage of this fact by building pillars around their territory to attract mates.

- **Fisherian** or **runaway selection:** a positive feedback mechanism in which a particular trait that has no effect or a negative effect on survival becomes more and more exaggerated over time. In this model, a trait is deemed sexually desirable and thus is more likely to be passed on. This increases the attractiveness of the trait, which in turn increases the likelihood that it continues to be passed on. The bright plumage of the peacock, shown in Figure 10.4, is the prototypical example of Fisherian selection.

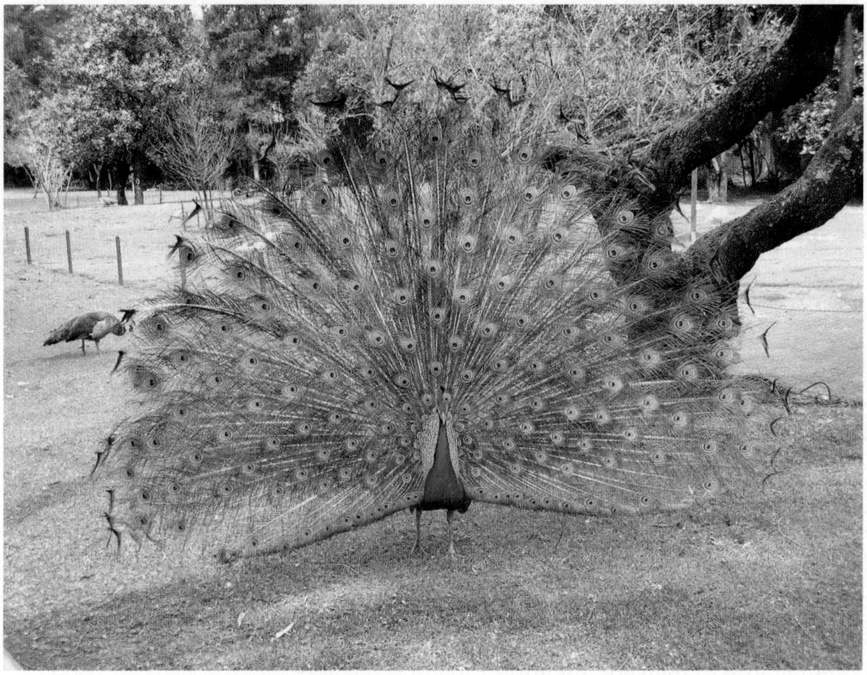

Figure 10.4 Fisherian Selection

The exaggerated plumage of the peacock is the prototypical example of Fisherian selection, in which the attractiveness of a trait that imparts a survival disadvantage leads to its continuation and exaggeration within the species.

- **Indicator traits:** traits that signify overall good health and well-being of an organism, increasing its attractiveness to mates. Notably, these traits may or may not be genetic in origin. For example, female cats are more attracted to male cats with clean and shiny coats; a dirty and dull coat may be related to an underlying genetic problem, or to malnutrition or infection.
- **Genetic compatibility:** the creation of mate pairs that, when combined, have complementary genetics. This theory provides a mechanism for the reduced frequency of recessive genetic disorders in the population: attraction to others who have starkly different genetic makeups reduces the probability of offspring being homozygotic for a disease-carrying allele.

REAL WORLD

Altruism creates a bit of a problem for the traditional Darwinist model of evolution. Why would an organism sacrifice its own fitness for the fitness of another? Evolutionary biologists still wrestle with this question, but inclusive fitness offers at least one potential solution.

Altruism

Altruism is a form of helping behavior in which the individual's intent is to benefit another at some cost to the self. Helping behavior can be motivated by selflessness, but can also be motivated by egoism or ulterior motives, such as public recognition. **Empathy** is the ability to vicariously experience the emotions of another, and it is thought by some social psychologists to be a strong influence on helping behavior. The **empathy–altruism hypothesis** is one explanation for the relationship between empathy and helping behavior. According to this theory, one individual helps another person when feeling empathy for the other person, regardless of the cost. This theory has been heavily debated, and more recent conceptions of altruism posit that an individual will help another person only when the benefits outweigh the costs for the individual.

Game Theory

Game theory attempts to explain decision-making behavior. The theory was originally used in economics and mathematics to predict interaction based on game characteristics, including strategy, winning and losing, rewards and punishments, and profits and cost. A game is defined by its players, the information and actions available to each player at decision points, and the payoffs associated with each outcome.

In the context of biology, game payoffs refer to fitness. Game theorists studying sex ratios in various species developed the concept of the **evolutionary stable strategy (ESS)**. When an ESS is adopted by a given population in a specific environment, natural selection will prevent alternative strategies from arising. The strategies are thus inherited traits passed along with the population, with the object of the game being becoming more fit than competitors.

One of the classic evolutionary games is the Hawk–Dove game. The game focuses on access to shared food resources. In each round, a player chooses one of two strategies: hawk or dove. The hawk exhibits a fighter strategy, displaying aggression and fighting until he wins or is injured. The dove exhibits a fight avoidance strategy, displaying aggression at first but retreating if the fight escalates. If not faced with a fight, the dove will attempt to share the food resources. There are three potential outcomes. If two hawks compete, one will win and one will lose. If a hawk and a dove compete, the hawk will invariably win. If two doves compete, they will share the food resources. The payoff in this case is based on both the value of the reward and the cost of fighting: If the reward is significantly larger than the cost of fighting, then hawks have an advantage. If the cost of fighting is significantly larger, doves have an advantage. There thus exists an equilibrium point where, based on the magnitude of the reward and the cost of fighting, the hawk and dove strategies can coexist as evolutionary stable strategies.

The Hawk–Dove game represents pure competition between individuals. However, social influences apply in nature and can result in four possible alternatives for competitors when dealing with strategic interactions. The four alternatives are shown in Figure 10.5 and are:

- **Altruism:** the donor provides a benefit to the recipient at a cost to the donor
- **Cooperation:** both the donor and recipient benefit by cooperating
- **Spite:** both the donor and recipient are negatively impacted
- **Selfishness:** the donor benefits while the recipient is negatively impacted

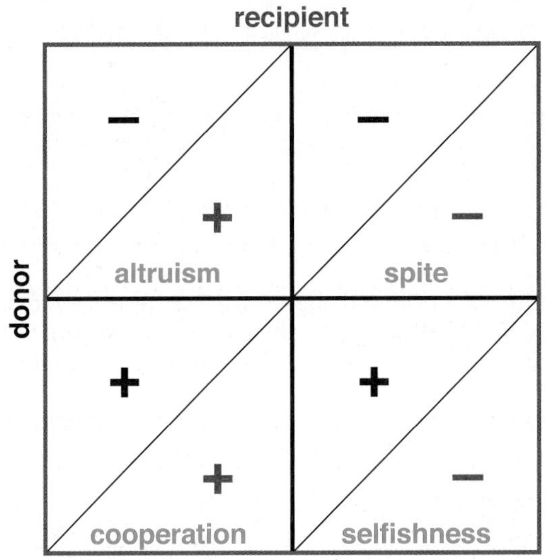

Figure 10.5 Strategic Alternatives for Socially Influenced Competitors

Other common strategy games, like rock–paper–scissors and chicken, can also be explained by game theory.

Inclusive Fitness

In evolutionary psychology, **inclusive fitness** is a measure of an organism's success in the population. This is based on the number of offspring, success in supporting offspring, and the ability of the offspring to then support others. Early descriptions of evolutionary success were based solely on the number of viable offspring of an organism. However, contemporary theories take into account the benefits of certain behaviors on the population at large. For example, the existence of altruism could be supported by the observation that close relatives of an individual will share many of the same genes; thus, promoting the reproduction and survival of related or similar individuals can also lead to genetic success. Other species show examples of inclusive fitness by protecting the offspring of the group at large. By sacrificing themselves to protect the young, these organisms ensure the passing of genes to future generations. Inclusive fitness therefore promotes the idea that altruistic behavior can improve the fitness and success of a species as a whole.

MCAT CONCEPT CHECK 10.1

Before you move on, assess your understanding of the material with these questions.

1. What is interpersonal attraction, and what are three factors that influence this attraction?

   •

   •

   •

2. For a behavior to be considered aggressive, is it necessary to have the intent to do harm? Does the behavior have to be physical in nature?

3. What are the four types of attachment? How does a child with each form of attachment act with regard to the caregiver?

Type of Attachment	Response to Caregiver

4. What is social support? List three of the common types of social support.

   •

   •

   •

5. What is altruism?

____

____

10.2 Social Perception and Behavior

High-Yield

LEARNING OBJECTIVES

After Chapter 10.2, you will be able to:

- Describe the primacy effect, recency effect, halo effect, fundamental attribution error, attribute substitution, just-world hypothesis, and self-serving bias
- Contrast dispositional and situational attributions, and what factors can make each one more likely
- Identify examples of attribution and attribution biases in real-world examples

Social perception is the name social psychologists give to how we form impressions about the characteristics of individuals and groups of people. We form impressions of others through observation of their behavior, past experiences, and personal beliefs and attitudes. We also feel the need to be able to explain and understand the behavior of others, a process we perform through attribution.

BRIDGE

Social perception is highly linked to attitudes; social perception focuses on how we form attitudes about specific characteristics of individuals and groups. Attitudes are discussed in detail in Chapter 8 of *MCAT Behavioral Sciences Review.*

Social Perception

Social perception is also referred to as **social cognition**, and provides the tools to make judgments and impressions regarding other people. These judgments and impressions include assessments of social roles, relationships, characteristics such as trustworthiness or friendliness, and **attributions**, which are explanations for the causes of a person's actions.

Components of Social Perception

There are three primary components of social perception: the perceiver, the target, and the situation. The **perceiver** is influenced by experience, motives, and emotional state. Past experiences affect our attitudes toward current and future experiences and can lead to particular expectations of events. Our motives influence what information we deem important and what we choose to ignore. Finally, emotional state can flavor our interpretation of an event. The **target** refers to the person about which the perception is made. Knowledge of the target can include past experiences or specific information that affect perception. When little information is available, there is a need for greater observation and interpretation by the perceiver. Finally, the **situation** is also important in developing perception. A given social context can determine what information is available to the perceiver.

Impression Bias

One model of social perception focuses on our selection of cues to form interpretations of others that are consistent over time. When coming into contact with an unfamiliar target, a perceiver takes in all cues from the target and environment, unfiltered. After becoming more familiar with a given target, the perceiver uses these cues to categorize the target: friend *vs.* enemy, caring *vs.* standoffish, open-minded *vs.* bigoted, and so on. Additional time spent with the target in the situational context will lead the perceiver to confirm the categorization. After this point, the perception of additional cues becomes selective in order to paint a picture of the target that is consistent with the perceptions the perceiver has already made. This theory is consistent with the **primacy effect**, which is the idea that first impressions are often more important than subsequent impressions. Sometimes, however, it is actually the most recent information we have about an individual that is the most important in forming our impressions; this is called the **recency effect**.

Individuals tend to organize the perception of others based on traits and personal characteristics of the target that are most relevant to the perceiver. This idea is referred to as the **reliance on central traits**. People may also project their own beliefs, opinions, ideas, and actions onto others. The categories we place others in during impression formation is based on **implicit personality theory**. This theory states that there are sets of assumptions people make about how different types of people, their traits, and their behavior are related. Making assumptions about people based on the category in which they are placed is known as **stereotyping**, and will be discussed in detail in the next section.

Halo Effect

The **halo effect** is a cognitive bias in which judgments about a specific aspect of an individual can be affected by one's overall impression of the individual. It is the tendency to allow a general impression about a person (*I like Jin*) to influence other, more specific evaluations about a person (*Jin is a good person, Jin is trustworthy, Jin can do no wrong*). The halo effect explains why people are often inaccurate when evaluating people that they either believe to be generally good or those that they believe to be generally bad. An individual's attractiveness has also been seen to produce the halo effect. As described earlier, attractiveness can be determined by a variety of traits, and the perception of these traits can impact the view of an individual's personality. It has been shown that people who are perceived as attractive are also more likely to be perceived as trustworthy and friendly.

Just-World Hypothesis

Another cognitive bias during impression formation is the **just-world hypothesis**. In a so-called just world, good things happen to good people and bad things happen to bad people; noble actions are rewarded and evil actions are punished. Consequences may be attributed to a universal restoring force; in some religions and cultures, this force is referred to as *karma*. A strong belief in a just world increases the likelihood of "blaming the victim" or stating that victims *get what they deserve* because such a worldview denies the possibility of innocent victims.

Self-Serving Bias

Self-identity and perception can be skewed through **self-serving bias**, also known as **self-serving attributional bias**, which refers to the fact that individuals credit their own successes to internal factors and blame their failures on external factors. The tendency to attribute good outcomes to our good traits or behaviors and to attribute bad outcomes to situational factors is used to protect our self-esteem. For example, students who earn a good grade on a test may attribute their success to their intelligence or to how intensely they studied. However, if they received a bad grade, they might attribute this outcome to poor teaching by the professor, unfair questions, or too long a test for the allotted time. These types of attributions have been found to occur in many settings including the workplace, school, interpersonal relationships, and athletics. Self-serving bias is influenced by motivational processes, like self-enhancement and self-verification. **Self-enhancement** focuses on the need to maintain self-worth, which can be accomplished in part by the self-serving bias. **Self-verification** suggests people will seek the companionship of others who see them as they see themselves, thereby validating a person's self-serving bias. Self-serving bias is also influenced by cognitive processes. For example, emotion is a factor in self-serving bias because emotion can impact self-esteem, which influences the need to protect one's self-identity. Individuals with higher self-esteem are more likely to protect this image and thus more likely to exhibit self-serving bias. Relationships to others also determine the likelihood of the bias: Individuals who have close relationships are less likely to attribute failures to one another, and instead will make joint attributions. On the other hand, strangers are much more likely to self-serve by placing blame for a failure on each other.

REAL WORLD

People with depression often have a reversed attributional bias, viewing their successes as caused by external factors (*I got lucky this time*) and failures as caused by internal factors (*It was all my fault*).

In-group *vs.* Out-group Bias

As suggested in Chapter 9 of *MCAT Behavioral Sciences Review* on social interaction, humans naturally come together to form groups, which results in the subjective categorization of in-group and out-group. In-group refers to other members of one's social group, while out-group refers to those who are not in the group. Given the propensity for humans to form groups, it's understandable that how an individual perceives members within their group (in-group) versus people outside their group (out-group) is heavily biased. Specifically, **in-group bias** refers to the inclination to view members in one's group more favorably, while **out-group bias** refers to the inclination to view individuals outside one's group harshly.

Attribution Theory

Another aspect of social cognition is explaining the behavior of others. It is human nature to observe and try to understand why others act the way they do. **Attribution theory** describes how individuals infer the causes of other people's behavior.

Dispositional and Situational Causes

Fritz Heider, one of the founders of attribution theory, divided the causes for attribution into two main categories: dispositional (internal) and situational (external). **Dispositional** (**internal**) attributions are those that relate to the person whose behavior is being considered, including beliefs, attitudes, and personality characteristics. **Situational** (**external**) attributions are those that relate to features of the surroundings, such as threats, money, social norms, and peer pressure. For instance, suppose you hear that a friend has been nominated for an academic award. Believing that the friend has been nominated because of hard work and personal effort would be a dispositional attribution. Contrarily, chalking up the nomination to luck would be a situational attribution. Situational attributions, therefore, consider the characteristics of the social context rather than the characteristics of the individual as the primary cause.

Cues

KEY CONCEPT

- Consistency cues—has consistent behavior over time
- Consensus cues—matches others' behavior
- Distinctiveness cues—uses similar behavior in similar situations

In order to understand the behavior of others, a variety of cues are used. These include consistency cues, consensus cues, and distinctiveness cues. **Consistency cues** refer to the behavior of a person over time. The more regular the behavior, the more we associate that behavior with the motives of the person. **Consensus cues** relate to the extent to which a person's behavior differs from others. If a person deviates from socially expected behavior, we are likely to form a dispositional attribution about the person's behavior. **Distinctiveness cues** refer to the extent to which a person engages in similar behavior across a series of scenarios. If a person's behavior varies in different scenarios, we are more likely to form a situational attribution to explain it.

MCAT EXPERTISE

Actor-observer asymmetry (or **bias**) results from the self-serving bias (by the actor) and the fundamental attribution error (by the observer). Actor-observer bias holds that, due to our unique knowledge about our own actions, we are more likely to make situational attributions for the self as compared to others. If you, rather than another person, failed to complete an assignment, for example, you would be far more likely to consider the situational factors involved in your behavior because you are intimately aware of them. This effect is most commonly seen with negative behaviors.

The **correspondent inference theory** takes this concept one step further by focusing on the intentionality of others' behavior. When an individual unexpectedly performs a behavior that helps or hurts us, we tend to explain the behavior by dispositional attribution. Thus, we may correlate these unexpected actions with the person's personality.

Fundamental Attribution Error

The **fundamental attribution error** posits that we are generally biased toward making dispositional attributions rather than situational attributions when judging the actions of others. For example, suppose that on a team project, other team members were unable to complete their assignments. According to the fundamental attribution error, our immediate response might be to assume that these team members are lazy or unreliable—both of which are dispositional attributions. We may ignore the possibility that the team members got ill, had too many concurrent assignments, or suffered a personal tragedy—all of which are situational attributions. The fundamental attribution error can present itself in positive contexts as well. Imagine if you observed someone getting out of their car to help an older adult across the road. According to the fundamental attribution error, you would likely make a dispositional attribution like, "What a kind stranger!" rather than a situational attribution like, "Oh, maybe that's their grandparent." Notice that in these examples, the dispositional attributions often provide simpler explanations than the situational attributions. This difference in complexity is actually the source of the fundamental attribution error: Assuming that a person's behaviors accurately portray who they are as a person is easier than speculating about what circumstances might have caused the observed behavior.

Attribute Substitution

Attribute substitution occurs when individuals must make judgments that are complex, but instead they substitute a simpler solution or apply a heuristic. When making automatic or intuitive judgments on difficult questions or scenarios, an individual may address a different question or scenario without even realizing a substitution has been made. In one study, individuals were asked to envision a sphere that could just fit inside a cube. They were then asked what percentage of the volume of the cube would be taken up by the sphere. This is challenging to envision, so most individuals likely simplified the problem in their minds to imagine a circle inside a square. The answers given in this study averaged around 74 percent, which is approximately the area of a square taken up by a circumscribed circle (79%), but significantly higher than the volume of a cube taken up by a circumscribed sphere (52%).

Attribute substitution can take place in far simpler setups as well. A classic example used in many psychology classes is the following question: *A pencil and an eraser cost $1.10 together. If the pencil costs one dollar more than the eraser, how much does the eraser cost?* Most individuals respond instinctively with the answer *ten cents*. It is easy to recognize that the pencil costs more, and to integrate the information given in the question stem (*$1.10* and *one dollar*) incorrectly.

This process is also common when dealing with size and color in optical illusions. For instance, when judging the size of figures in an image with perspective, the apparent sizes shown in the image can be distorted by three-dimensional context, as shown in Figure 10.6. The expected three-dimensional size of the figure, based on perspective cues, substitutes for the actual two-dimensional size of the birds within the image. It is interesting to note that painters and photographers with experience in two-dimensional images are less likely to substitute due to the fact that two-dimensional size is more understandable to their perception.

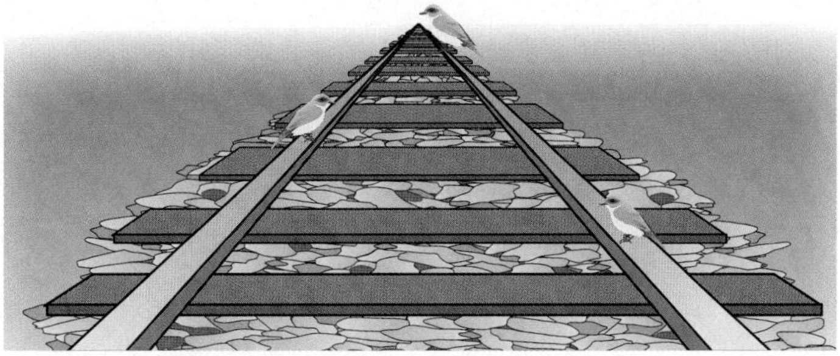

Figure 10.6 Attribute Substitution for Size in Optical Illusions
The birds are of identical size, but three-dimensional cues affect our interpretation of the image.

Shadows, patterns, the position of the sun, and other visual cues can also cause attribute substitution for color, as shown in Figure 10.7.

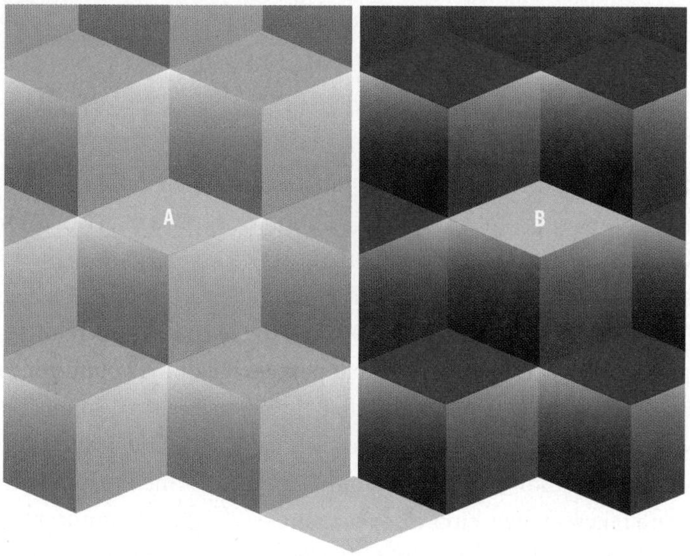

Figure 10.7 Attribute Substitution for Color in Optical Illusions
The central boxes labeled A and B are of identical color, but shadow cues affect our interpretation of the image.

Cultural Attribution

Another important factor in attribution is culture. The type of culture an individual belongs to plays a major role in the types of attributions the individual makes. Individualist cultures put high value on the individual, personal goals, and independence. Collectivist cultures view individuals as members of a group and place high value on conformity and interdependence. Individualists tend to make more fundamental attribution errors than those in collectivist cultures. Individualists are also more likely to attribute behavior to dispositional factors, whereas collectivists are more likely to attribute behavior to situational factors.

MCAT CONCEPT CHECK 10.2

Before you move on, assess your understanding of the material with these questions.

1. For each of the social cognitive biases below, provide a brief description:
   - Primacy effect:
   - Recency effect:
   - Halo effect:
   - Just-world hypothesis:
   - Self-serving bias:
2. What is attribution theory? What are the two types of attribution?
   -
   -
3. What is the fundamental attribution error?
4. What is attribute substitution?

10.3 Stereotypes, Prejudice, and Discrimination

High-Yield

LEARNING OBJECTIVES

After Chapter 10.3, you will be able to:

- Distinguish between stereotypes, prejudice, and discrimination
- List the types of social inequality that can influence prejudice
- Compare and contrast ethnocentrism and cultural relativism

KEY CONCEPT

- Stereotypes are cognitive
- Prejudices are affective
- Discrimination is behavioral

While stereotypes, prejudice, and discrimination are terms that are related and often used together, they are very different concepts. Stereotypes are viewed as cognitive, prejudice as affective, and discrimination as behavioral. **Stereotypes** refer to the expectations, impressions, and opinions about the characteristics of members of a group. Prejudice reflects the overall attitude and emotional response to a group. Discrimination refers to differences in actions toward different groups.

Note: Kaplan Test Prep does not endorse or encourage any of the stereotypes mentioned in this chapter; they are included only as examples.

Stereotypes

Despite their negative connotations, stereotypes often appear in everyday life, and can be beneficial when not directed toward other human beings. In a psychological sense, the purpose of a stereotype is to make sense of a complex world by categorizing and systematizing information in order to better identify items, predict their behavior, and react. In the context of stereotyping what different items of furniture look like, how different types of stores operate, or how different cuisines taste, stereotypes are extremely useful in defining categories and determining what does or does not fit into that category. However, when stereotypes are used to develop prejudices toward others and to discriminate, they are being appropriated for negative uses.

In the context of sociology, **stereotypes** occur when attitudes and impressions are based on limited and superficial information about a person or a group of individuals. The content of stereotypes are the attributes that people believe define and characterize a group. The **stereotype content model** attempts to classify stereotypes with respect to a hypothetical in-group using two dimensions: warmth and competence. Warm groups are those that are not in direct competition with the in-group for resources; competent groups are those that have high status within society. The four possible combinations of warmth and competence are shown in Figure 10.8 and are associated with distinct emotions.

Warmth		Competence: low	Competence: high
	high	**paternalistic stereotype** low status, not competitive	**admiration stereotype** high status, not competitive
	low	**contemptuous stereotype** low status, competitive	**envious stereotype** high status, competitive

Figure 10.8 Classifications of Stereotypes in the Stereotype Content Model
Adapted from Fiske et al. (2002)

Paternalistic stereotypes are those in which the group is looked down upon as inferior, dismissed, or ignored. **Contemptuous** stereotypes are those in which the group is viewed with resentment, annoyance, or anger. **Envious** stereotypes are those in which the group is viewed with jealousy, bitterness, or distrust. **Admiration** stereotypes are those in which the group is viewed with pride and other positive feelings.

Self-Fulfilling Prophecy

Stereotypes can lead to expectations of certain groups of individuals. These expectations can create conditions that then cause the expectations to become reality, a process referred to as **self-fulfilling prophecy**. For example, some medical students experience a self-fulfilling prophecy during their first days of surgery clerkship in medical school: During their first year in the wards, new students are stereotyped as being unable to quickly and efficiently throw knots during a surgery. With this knowledge in mind, these students are nervous to suture for the first time and may struggle with every step of the knot-tying process. This struggle validates the stereotype and thus completes the self-fulfilling prophecy.

Stereotype Threat

In some social situations, a person might be concerned or anxious about inadvertently confirming a negative stereotype about their social group. This concern is known as **stereotype threat**. Unfortunately, the feeling of stereotype threat often results in a self-fulfilling prophesy: People experiencing stereotype threat often exhibit stress arousal and are preoccupied by monitoring their own performance on a task, and these distractions can then lead to reduced performance on the task. An example of a well-studied group that often experiences stereotype threat is women

KEY CONCEPT

Stereotype threat is concern or anxiety about confirming a negative stereotype about one's group. This may hinder performance, which may actually create a self-fulfilling prophecy.

in mathematics. A study showed that women taking a math exam scored lower when the only other test takers in the room were men. The researchers concluded that when taking an exam with only men present, women test subjects were more concerned about stereotype threat, and performed more poorly as a result of their concerns. Researchers theorize that stereotype threat may be a contributing factor to long-standing racial and gender gaps in certain careers and in academic performance.

Prejudice

From a social psychology approach, **prejudice** is defined as an irrational positive or negative attitude toward a person, group, or thing, prior to an actual experience with that entity. The process of socialization results in the formation of attitudes regarding our own groups and a sense of identity as an individual and a group member. Prejudice can form in response to dissimilarities among groups, races, ethnicities, or even environments. While racial and ethnic prejudices against individuals are at the forefront of most people's minds, prejudices exist against objects and places as well. For instance, people have attitudes toward different regions of the country based on culture, weather, and history; which car manufacturers are the most reliable; what types of food are considered unhealthy; and even what types of animals make good pets. Prejudicial attitudes can run the gamut from hate to love, contempt to admiration, and indifference to loyalty.

Prejudices may be kept internally or shared with the larger community. **Propaganda** is a common way by which large organizations and political groups attempt to create prejudices in others. Propaganda posters often invoke messages of fear, and depictions of the target group are often exaggerated to an absurd degree.

Power, Prestige, and Class

There are a variety of social factors that influence prejudice. Three of the most important are power, prestige, and class. **Power** refers to the ability of people or groups to achieve their goals despite any obstacles, and their ability to control resources. **Prestige** is the level of respect shown to a person by others. **Class** refers to socioeconomic status. Social inequality, or the unequal distribution of power, resources, money, or prestige, can result in the grouping of *haves* and *have-nots*. *Have-nots* may develop a negative attitude toward *haves* based on envy. *Haves* may develop a negative attitude toward *have-nots* as a defense mechanism to justify the fact that they have more.

Ethnocentrism

Ethnocentrism refers to the practice of making judgments about other cultures based on the values and beliefs of one's own culture, especially when it comes to language, customs, and religion. Ethnocentrism can manifest in many ways, from innocent displays of ethnic pride to violent supremacy groups. Because of this, ethnocentrism is closely tied to the previously discussed concepts of in-group *vs.* out-group biases and group conflict.

Cultural Relativism

In order to avoid ethnocentrism, the concept of cultural relativism has been employed by sociologists to compare and understand other cultures. **Cultural relativism** is the recognition that social groups and cultures should be studied on their own terms. When studying a culture, social relativism acknowledges that the values, mores, and rules make sense in the context of that culture, and should not be judged against the norms of another culture. In other words, while one group may follow a given set of rules (say, the dietary rules of *kashrut* or *halal*), cultural relativism holds that those rules should not be perceived as superior or inferior to those of other cultures—just different.

Discrimination

Discrimination occurs when prejudicial attitudes cause individuals of a particular group to be treated differently from others. While prejudice is an attitude, discrimination is a behavior. As prejudice typically refers to a negative attitude, discrimination typically refers to a negative behavior. It is also important to note that prejudice does not always result in discrimination. For instance, a person might have strong feelings against a particular race (prejudice), but may not express those feelings or act on them. As social inequality influences prejudice, the same idea applies to discrimination. The unequal distribution of power, prestige, and class influence discrimination.

Individual *vs.* Institutional Discrimination

Discrimination can be either individual or institutional. **Individual discrimination** refers to one person discriminating against a particular person or group, whereas **institutional discrimination** refers to the discrimination against a particular person or group by an entire institution. Individual discrimination is considered to be conscious and obvious, and can be eliminated by removing the person who is displaying the behavior. Sociologists have begun to stress the need to focus on institutional discrimination, as it is discrimination built into the structure of society, so it is far more covert and harder to extricate. Because it is part of society, it is perpetuated by simply maintaining the status quo.

The United States has a long history of institutional discrimination against myriad groups. Perhaps the most overt example was that of racial segregation that existed in the early to mid-twentieth century. Even today, there are still concerns of institutional discrimination against individuals based on their race, ethnicity, gender identity, sexual orientation, religion, and other characteristics.

MCAT CONCEPT CHECK 10.3

Before you move on, assess your understanding of the material with these questions.

1. What are the distinctions between stereotypes, prejudice, and discrimination?
   - Stereotypes:
   - Prejudice:
   - Discrimination:
2. List three types of social inequality that can influence prejudice:
   -
   -
   -
3. What is the difference between ethnocentrism and cultural relativism?

Conclusion

Social psychology focuses on social behavior and the attitudes, perceptions, and influences of others that impact behavior. In this chapter, we first looked at social behaviors, including attraction, aggression, attachment, and social support. We also looked at the biological explanations of specific social behaviors, including foraging, mate choice, altruism, game theory, and inclusive fitness. We further defined the components of social perception and impression biases. The way we view ourselves also influences the way we view others and how we attribute behavior to others. Finally, we took a look at stereotypes, prejudice, and discrimination.

These last few topics demonstrate a negative side of classifying individuals. We can use classification to create hierarchies, inequities in opportunity and finances, as well as to silence or suppress communities. But classification can also serve a positive purpose. In social science, we often classify populations to study interactions between groups, changes in population makeup over time, and to track migration patterns. These classifications are considered in the field of demographics, which we will explore in the next chapter.

GO ONLINE

You've reviewed the content, now test your knowledge and critical thinking skills by completing a test-like passage set in your online resources!

CONCEPT SUMMARY

Social Behavior

- **Interpersonal attraction** is what makes people like each other and is influenced by multiple factors:
  - Physical attractiveness, which is increased with symmetry and proportions close to the **golden ratio**
  - Similarity of attitudes, intelligence, education, height, age, religion, appearance, and socioeconomic status
  - **Self-disclosure**, which includes sharing fears, thoughts, and goals with another person and being met with empathy and nonjudgment
  - **Reciprocity**, in which we like people who we think like us
  - **Proximity**, or being physically close to someone
- **Aggression** is a physical, verbal, or nonverbal behavior with the intention to cause harm or increase social dominance.
- **Attachment** is an emotional bond to another person, and usually refers to the bond between a child and a caregiver. There are four types of attachment:
  - **Secure attachment** requires a consistent caregiver so the child is able to go out and explore, knowing there is a secure base to return to; the child will show strong preference for the caregiver.
  - **Avoidant attachment** occurs when a caregiver has little or no response to a distressed, crying child; the child shows no preference for the caregiver compared to strangers.
  - **Ambivalent attachment** occurs when a caregiver has an inconsistent response to a child's distress, sometimes responding appropriately, sometimes neglectfully; the child will become distressed when the caregiver leaves and is ambivalent when the caregiver returns.
  - **Disorganized attachment** occurs when a caregiver is erratic or abusive; the child shows no clear pattern of behavior in response to the caregiver's absence or presence and may show repetitive behaviors.
- **Social support** is the perception or reality that one is cared for by a social network.
  - **Emotional support** includes listening to, affirming, and empathizing with someone's feelings.
  - **Esteem support** affirms the qualities and skills of the person.
  - **Material support** is providing physical or monetary resources to aid a person.
  - **Informational support** is providing useful information to a person.
  - **Network support** is providing a sense of belonging to a person.

- **Foraging** is searching for and exploiting food resources.
- A **mating system** describes the way in which a group is organized in terms of sexual behavior.
  - **Monogamy** consists of exclusive mating relationships.
  - **Polygamy** consists of multiple exclusive relationships, including **polygyny** (with multiple females) and **polyandry** (with multiple males).
  - **Promiscuity** means mating without exclusivity.
- **Mate choice**, or **intersexual selection**, is the selection of a mate based on attraction and traits.
- **Altruism** is a form of helping behavior in which people's intent is to benefit someone else at some cost to themselves.
- **Game theory** attempts to explain decision making between individuals as if they are participating in a game.
- **Inclusive fitness** is a measure of an organism's success in the population. This is based on the number of offspring, success in supporting offspring, and the ability of the offspring to then support others.

Social Perception and Behavior

- **Social perception** or **social cognition** is the way by which we generate impressions about people in our social environment. It contains a **perceiver**, a **target**, and the **situation** or social context of the scenario.
- **Implicit personality theory** states that people make assumptions about how different types of people, their traits, and their behavior are related.
- Certain cognitive biases impact our perceptions of others.
  - The **primacy effect** refers to when first impressions are more important than subsequent impressions.
  - The **recency effect** is when the most recent information we have about an individual is most important in forming our impressions.
  - A **reliance on central traits** is the tendency to organize the perception of others based on traits and personal characteristics that matter to the perceiver.
  - The **halo effect** is when judgments of an individual's character can be affected by the overall impression of the individual.
  - The **just-world hypothesis** is the tendency of individuals to believe that good things happen to good people and bad things happen to bad people.
  - **Self-serving bias** refers to the fact that individuals will view their own successes as being based on internal factors, while viewing failures as being based on external factors.

- **Attribution theory** focuses on the tendency for individuals to infer the causes of other people's behavior.
  - **Dispositional** (**internal**) causes are those that relate to the features of the person whose behavior is being considered.
  - **Situational** (**external**) causes are related to features of the surroundings or social context.
- **Correspondent inference theory** is used to describe attributions made by observing the intentional (especially unexpected) behaviors performed by another person.
- **Fundamental attribution error** is the bias toward making dispositional attributions rather than situational attributions in regard to the actions of others.
- **Attribute substitution** occurs when individuals must make judgments that are complex but instead substitute a simpler solution or heuristic.
- Attributions are highly influenced by the culture in which one resides.

Stereotypes, Prejudice, and Discrimination

- **Stereotypes** occur when attitudes and impressions are made based on limited and superficial information about a person or a group of individuals.
- Stereotypes can lead to expectations of certain groups, which can create conditions that lead to confirmation of the stereotype, a process referred to as **self-fulfilling prophecy**.
- **Stereotype threat** is concern or anxiety about confirming a negative stereotype about one's social group.
- **Prejudice** is defined as an irrational positive or negative attitude toward a person, group, or thing prior to an actual experience.
- **Ethnocentrism** refers to the practice of making judgments about other cultures based on the values and beliefs of one's own culture.
- **Cultural relativism** refers to the recognition that social groups and cultures should be studied on their own terms.
- **Discrimination** is when prejudicial attitudes cause individuals of a particular group to be treated differently from others.
  - **Individual discrimination** refers to one person discriminating against a particular person or group.
  - **Institutional discrimination** refers to the discrimination against a particular person or group by an entire institution.

ANSWERS TO CONCEPT CHECKS

10.1

1. Interpersonal attraction is what makes people like each other and is influenced by at least five factors discussed in the chapter: physical attractiveness, similarity, self-disclosure, reciprocity, and proximity.
2. No, in addition to behavior with the intent to cause harm, aggression can also be a behavior that increases relative social dominance. Aggression can be physical, verbal, or nonverbal.
3.

Type of Attachment	Response to Caregiver
Secure	Upset at departure of caregiver, comforted by return; trusts caregiver, who is viewed as a secure base
Avoidant	Shows no preference for a stranger or caregiver; shows little distress at departure and little relief by return of caregiver
Ambivalent	Distressed by departure of caregiver with mixed reactions at return
Disorganized	No clear pattern of behavior; sometimes exhibits repetitive behaviors or seems dazed, frozen, or confused

4. Social support is the perception or reality that one is cared for by a social network. There are five types discussed in this chapter: emotional support, esteem support, material support, informational support, and network support.
5. Altruism is a form of helping behavior in which people's intent is to benefit someone else at some cost to themselves.

10.2

1. The primacy effect is the power of first impressions over later impressions of an individual. The recency effect is weighing the most recent information of a person as the most important. The halo effect occurs when one applies general feelings about a person (usually, "good" or "bad") to specific characteristics of that person. The just-world hypothesis is the belief that good things happen to good people and bad things happen to bad people. Self-serving bias is the tendency to attribute our successes to internal factors and our failures to external factors.
2. Attribution theory focuses on the tendency of individuals to infer the causes of other people's behavior. Attributions are divided into two types: dispositional (internal) causes, which relate to the features of the target, and situational (external) causes, which relate to features of the surroundings or context.
3. Fundamental attribution error is the general bias toward making dispositional attributions rather than situational attributions about the behavior of others, especially in negative contexts.
4. Attribute substitution occurs when individuals must make judgments that are complex but instead substitute a simpler solution or heuristic.

10.3

1. Stereotypes occur when attitudes and impressions are made based on limited and superficial information about a person or a group of individuals and are cognitive. Prejudice is defined as an irrational negative, or occasionally positive, attitude toward a person, group, or thing, which is formed prior to an actual experience and is affective. Discrimination is when prejudicial attitudes cause individuals of a particular group to be treated differently than others and is behavioral.
2. Power, prestige, and class all influence prejudice through unequal distribution of wealth, influence, and resources.
3. Ethnocentrism refers to the practice of making judgments about other cultures based on the values and beliefs of one's own culture. Cultural relativism refers to the recognition that social groups and cultures must be studied on their own terms. In both cases, an individual perceives another group to which that individual does not belong; however, it is the reaction to that other group that determines which paradigm is being used.

SCIENCE MASTERY ASSESSMENT EXPLANATIONS

1. **A**

Each of the answer choices influences social attraction; however, proximity deals with the tendency to be attracted to those who are physically close by.

2. **B**

Aggression is influenced both by the amygdala and prefrontal cortex activity. Activity of the amygdala increases aggression. The prefrontal cortex should control aggression; decreased activity in the prefrontal cortex, therefore, is associated with increased aggression.

3. **D**

This attachment pattern is representative of secure attachment. Secure attachment is seen when a child has a consistent caregiver and is able to go out and explore, knowing there is a secure base to return to. The child will be upset at the departure of the caregiver and will be comforted and resume exploring upon the return of the caregiver.

4. **B**

Polygamy involves having exclusive relationships with several partners, several females (polygyny), or several males (polyandry), **(A)**. Monogamy, **(C)**, consists of exclusive mating relationships. Promiscuity, **(D)**, refers to mating with others without exclusivity.

5. **C**

A person with a ventromedial hypothalamus injury will never feel satiated when eating and will therefore never feel the sensation to stop eating. A person with a lateral hypothalamus injury will never feel hunger and will have decreased food intake, **(D)**.

6. **D**

Phenotypic benefits refer to observed traits in an individual that make them more attractive to other members of their species. Benefits associated with increased fitness through direct material advantages are direct benefits, **(C)**, while indirect benefits involve increased genetic fitness for offspring.

7. **A**

In evolutionary psychology, inclusive fitness is a measure of the number of offspring an individual has, how they support their offspring, and how their offspring can support others. Inclusive fitness promotes the idea that altruistic behavior can improve the fitness and success of a species; the behavior in this scenario can be described as altruism: benefiting another at one's own expense.

8. **D**

There are three primary components of perception: the perceiver, the target, and the situation.

9. **A**

The impressions we form when meeting others are influenced by a number of perceptual biases. The primacy effect refers to those occasions when first impressions are more important than subsequent impressions.

10. **C**

The halo effect is a cognitive bias in which judgments of an individual's character can be affected by the overall impression of the individual.

11. **C**

Self-serving bias refers to the fact that individuals will view their own successes as being based on internal factors, while viewing their failures as being based on external factors.

12. **C**

Types of attribution fall into two main categories: dispositional (internal) and situational (external). Dispositional (internal) causes are related to the features of the person whose behavior is being considered. Situational (external) causes are related to features of the surroundings.

13. **B**

Stereotype threat refers to the phenomenon of people being concerned or anxious about confirming a negative stereotype of their social group. Stereotype threat can hinder performance, creating a self-fulfilling prophecy.

14. **D**

Discrimination is when prejudicial attitudes cause individuals of a particular group to be treated differently than others. While prejudice is an attitude, discrimination is a behavior.

15. **C**

Game theory was originally designed to study decision-making behavior in economics and mathematics; it has since been used to describe decision making in politics, biology, philosophy, and other fields.

Consult your online resources for additional practice. GO ONLINE

SHARED CONCEPTS

Behavioral Sciences Chapter 5
Motivation, Emotion, and Stress

Behavioral Sciences Chapter 6
Identity and Personality

Behavioral Sciences Chapter 8
Social Processes, Attitudes, and Behavior

Behavioral Sciences Chapter 9
Social Interaction

Behavioral Sciences Chapter 11
Social Structure and Demographics

Behavioral Sciences Chapter 12
Social Stratification

CHAPTER 11

SOCIAL STRUCTURE AND DEMOGRAPHICS

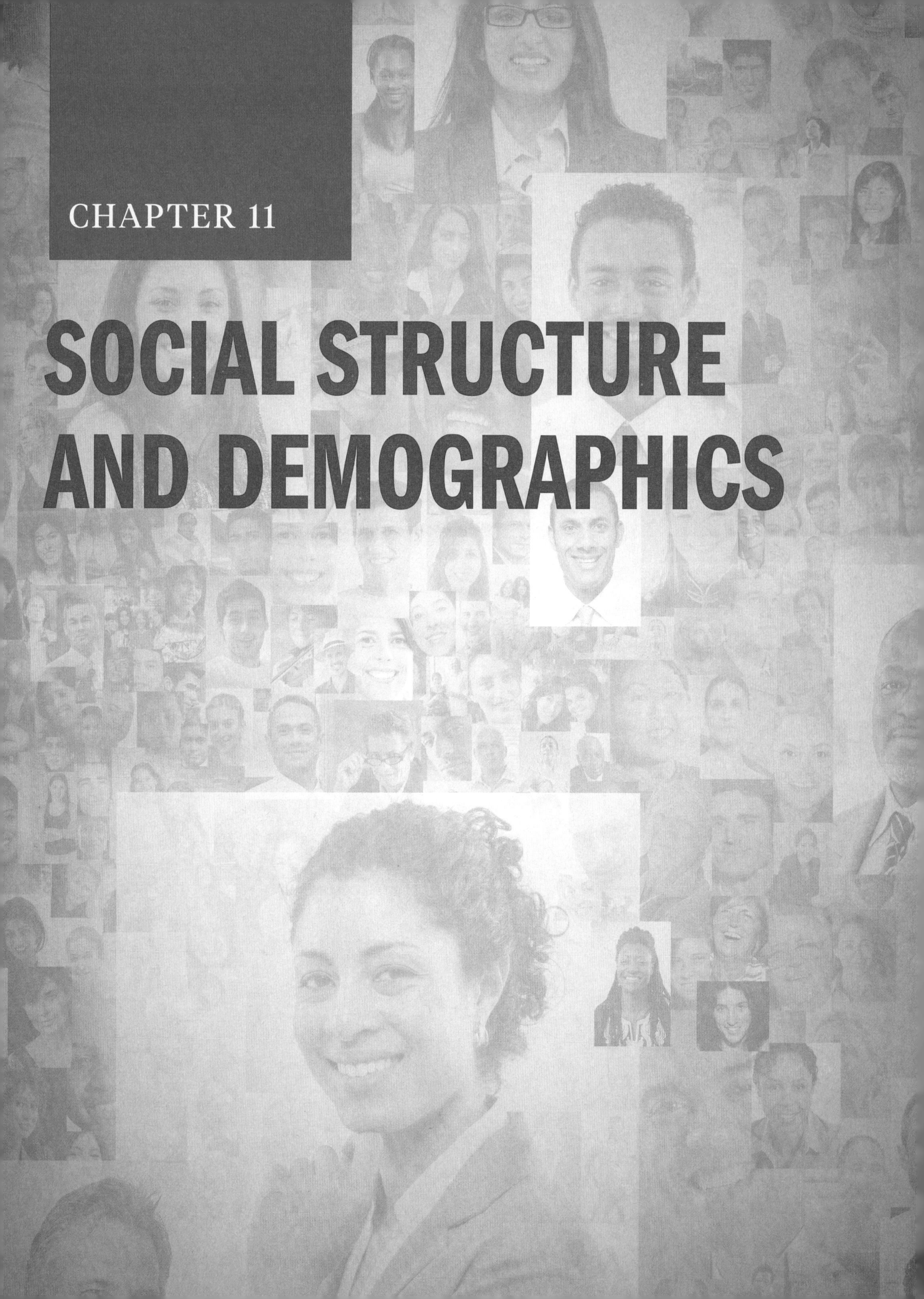

SCIENCE MASTERY ASSESSMENT

Every pre-med knows this feeling: there is so much content I have to know for the MCAT! How do I know what to do first or what's important?

While the high-yield badges throughout this book will help you identify the most important topics, this Science Mastery Assessment is another tool in your MCAT prep arsenal. This quiz (which can also be taken in your online resources) and the guidance below will help ensure that you are spending the appropriate amount of time on this chapter based on your personal strengths and weaknesses. Don't worry though—skipping something now does not mean you'll never study it. Later on in your prep, as you complete full-length tests, you'll uncover specific pieces of content that you need to review and can come back to these chapters as appropriate.

How to Use This Assessment

If you answer 0–7 questions correctly:

Spend about 1 hour to read this chapter in full and take limited notes throughout. Follow up by reviewing **all** quiz questions to ensure that you now understand how to solve each one.

If you answer 8–11 questions correctly:

Spend 20–40 minutes reviewing the quiz questions. Beginning with the questions you missed, read and take notes on the corresponding subchapters. For questions you answered correctly, ensure your thinking matches that of the explanation and you understand why each choice was correct or incorrect.

If you answer 12–15 questions correctly:

Spend less than 20 minutes reviewing all questions from the quiz. If you missed any, then include a quick read-through of the corresponding subchapters, or even just the relevant content within a subchapter, as part of your question review. For questions you answered correctly, ensure your thinking matches that of the explanation and review the Concept Summary at the end of the chapter.

1. Which of the following best describes a manifest function?
   - **A.** An intended positive effect on a system
   - **B.** An intended negative effect on a system
   - **C.** An unintended positive effect on a system
   - **D.** An unintended negative effect on a system

2. Studying why a nod means "yes" in many cultures is most representative of which of the following sociological concepts?
   - **A.** Demographic transition
   - **B.** Expectancy theory
   - **C.** Symbolic interactionism
   - **D.** Demographic shift

3. Which of the following ethical principles states that physicians should avoid using treatments with greater potential for harm than benefit?
   - **A.** Autonomy
   - **B.** Beneficence
   - **C.** Justice
   - **D.** Nonmaleficence

4. A Cuban-American man living in the United States has the dominant physical features of a Black man. He speaks Spanish, prefers Latin foods, and listens to Latin music. His preferences are best defined through which of the following attributes?
   - **I.** Race
   - **II.** Ethnicity
   - **III.** Culture

   - **A.** I only
   - **B.** II only
   - **C.** II and III only
   - **D.** I, II, and III

5. A patient who resides in the United States says, "I love you," and hugs the doctor after every routine visit. This behavior violates:
   - **A.** personal beliefs.
   - **B.** patient autonomy.
   - **C.** social values.
   - **D.** social norms.

6. Which of the following demographics can be measured in events per 1000 people per year?
   - **I.** Birth rate
   - **II.** Fertility rate
   - **III.** Mortality rate

   - **A.** I only
   - **B.** I and III only
   - **C.** II and III only
   - **D.** I, II, and III

7. Because there are more than 500 American Indian tribes, there are several different healing practices among them. Some tribes may have ceremonies that include chanting, singing, body painting, dancing, and even use of mind-altering substances to persuade the spirits to heal the sick person. These ceremonies are examples of:
   - **A.** latent functions.
   - **B.** rituals.
   - **C.** cultural barriers.
   - **D.** social movements.

8. Over the last few decades, the United States population has become:
   - **A.** bigger, older, and more diverse.
   - **B.** bigger, younger, and more diverse.
   - **C.** smaller, older, and less diverse.
   - **D.** smaller, older, and more diverse.

9. Which of the following is NOT an example of material culture?
- **A.** Traditional Kenyan clothing
- **B.** Japanese cuisine
- **C.** American values
- **D.** American Indian sand paintings

10. During which stage of demographic transition are both birth rates and mortality rates low?
- **A.** Stage 1
- **B.** Stage 2
- **C.** Stage 3
- **D.** Stage 4

11. Shortly after a state legalizes gambling in casinos, a formal coalition forms to oppose the building of any casinos in the major cities of the state. This scenario includes:
- **I.** conflict theory.
- **II.** social institutions.
- **III.** a social movement.

- **A.** I only
- **B.** I and III only
- **C.** II and III only
- **D.** I, II, and III

12. A young adult male claims to have had sexual relationships mostly with other men, although he has been attracted to women at times. What would be his most likely score on the Kinsey scale?
- **A.** 0
- **B.** 1
- **C.** 5
- **D.** 6

13. Which of the following demographic variables is known to be biologically determined?
- **A.** Gender
- **B.** Sex
- **C.** Ethnicity
- **D.** Sexual orientation

14. Which of the following would contribute to increasing population growth over time?
- **A.** A fertility rate less than 2
- **B.** An immigration rate larger than emigration rate
- **C.** An increase in mortality rate
- **D.** A decrease in birth rate

15. Urbanization can cause all of the following negative effects EXCEPT:
- **A.** decreased opportunity for social interaction.
- **B.** increased transmission of infectious disease.
- **C.** decreased air quality and sanitation.
- **D.** increased rates of violent crime.

Answer Key

1. **A**
2. **C**
3. **D**
4. **C**
5. **D**
6. **B**
7. **B**
8. **A**
9. **C**
10. **D**
11. **D**
12. **C**
13. **B**
14. **B**
15. **A**

Detailed explanations can be found at the end of the chapter.

CHAPTER 11

SOCIAL STRUCTURE AND DEMOGRAPHICS

In This Chapter

CHAPTER PROFILE

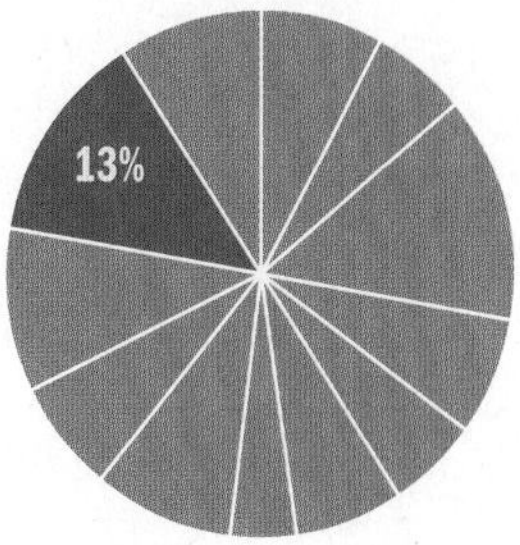

The content in this chapter should be relevant to about 13% of all questions about the behavioral sciences on the MCAT.

This chapter covers material from the following AAMC content categories:

7B: Social processes that influence human behavior

9A: Understanding social structure

9B: Demographic characteristics and processes

Introduction

A frail, older man is admitted to the Intensive Care Unit at a local hospital. He is gaunt, weighing just over 100 pounds, in severe respiratory distress, and nearing circulatory collapse. The intensive care team works to stabilize the patient by starting intravenous lines and pumping fluids. The patient screams statements in a language the team doesn't speak and is eventually sedated so they can intubate and ventilate him. They begin to run tests and discover that the man has widespread metastatic lung cancer that is unlikely to be cured or even controlled through chemotherapy or radiation. The patient's wife and children visit the next morning and are told of the bad news. After crying for some time, they turn to the intensive care team and ask them not to inform the patient of this grave diagnosis. They explain that in their culture family members are expected to make healthcare decisions for the ill to avoid burdening them with such matters. The members of the medical team, however, feel that they must adhere to the tenets of local medical ethics—and their country's laws—and allow the patient to make his own healthcare decisions. As the head of the hospital ethics committee, you get a call from the team to help them make this decision. What would you do?

Ethicists and sociologists alike wrestle with medical dilemmas like these. As a clinician in an ever-diversifying society, you will certainly run into challenging situations like these, where you must try to balance a patient's cultural beliefs with the processes and protocols of the healthcare system in which you work. In this chapter, we'll explore some of the sociological topics on the MCAT, focusing on theoretical models and the key institutions on which you are likely to be tested. We'll then explore culture itself. Finally, we'll describe demographics, the mathematical and statistical modeling of sociological concepts.

11.1 Sociology: Theories and Institutions

High-Yield

LEARNING OBJECTIVES

After Chapter 11.1, you will be able to:

- Recall the primary theses of major sociological theories, including functionalism, conflict theory, symbolic interactionism, social constructionism, rational choice theory, and feminist theory
- Contrast manifest and latent functions of given elements of a sociological system
- List the four key tenets of American medical ethics

Sociology is the study of society: how we create society, how we interact within and change society, and how we define what is normal and abnormal in society. Whereas psychologists focus on the behaviors of individuals, sociologists focus on the way groups organize and interact. Of course, it would be difficult to describe society as a whole since human society is not completely uniform and is instead made up of distinct cultures, subcultures, groups, and institutions, each with its own structure, patterns, and interests. As a result, sociologists study the subject at different levels: The **micro** level consists of family groups and local communities. The **meso** level consists of organizations, institutions, and ethnic subcultures. And the **macro** level consists of national and international systems.

Theoretical Approaches

Because human interaction is so complex, sociologists have proposed many models, called **theoretical approaches to sociology**, to help analyze and explain aspects of human social behavior. Sociologists don't necessarily disagree about which model is "best." Rather, each model was created to explain certain aspects of sociology, and is inadequate for explaining other aspects. For example, one theoretical approach we will examine is symbolic interactionism, which studies how humans interact and communicate using language, writing, and other symbols. By contrast, another approach, called conflict theory, examines how groups with little power in society can rise up and create more equality. These two models are not necessarily competing explanations. Rather, they examine such vastly different aspects of human interaction that both models are necessary!

As you read this section, keep track of which aspects of human behavior each model explains, and what the weaknesses of each model are. For example, approaches such as symbolic interactionism, social constructionism, and rational choice (exchange) theory tend to focus on society at the micro- and meso-levels. On the other hand, conflict theory, structural-functionalism, and feminist theory are more applicable at the macro-level.

Symbolic Interactionism

Communication among humans stretches far beyond just language, spoken, signed, or written. Our bodies are tools of communication through our posture, facial expressions, and informal hand gestures. We recognize and put meaning into images like the smiley face, traffic signs, or corporate logos. Sacred emblems like the cross, the Star of David, or the star and crescent communicate deep religious significance. Even our clothing can communicate meaning. Any object, image, sound, or action that carries meaning to humans is a **symbol**. Importantly, according to this definition, while many physical objects are symbols, a symbol need not be a physical object. For example, spoken words are symbols, and so are meaningful grunts. Body language and hand gestures are symbols. Anything that carries meaning beyond its own existence is a symbol.

Symbolic interactionism is an approach to sociology pioneered by influential sociologist George Herbert Mead that attempts to understand human action and interaction by studying the symbols we use to communicate. This theoretical approach makes three main assumptions about human behavior:

- Humans act toward symbols based on the meanings that these symbols carry.
- The meanings symbols carry come from social interaction.
- Humans interpret the meaning of symbols, and this interpretation influences action.

Therefore, according to symbolic interactionism, humans are different from lower animals in that lower animals simply respond to stimuli, while humans have the capability to interpret the stimulus first, then react. For example, a dog might bare its teeth, which is a gesture that other dogs always interpret as a symbol of aggression. Lower animals are not able to conceive of alternative meanings to gestures. By contrast, the thumbs up gesture in American culture generally signifies approval. In a different context, however, it could be used sarcastically to communicate disapproval. And in some Middle Eastern countries, it is an offensive gesture. The meaning of the thumbs up symbol therefore depends not only on social and cultural understanding, but also on a person's interpretation.

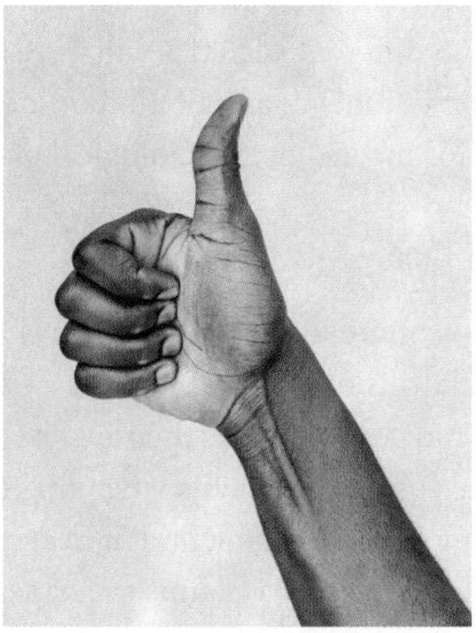

Figure 11.1 Symbolic Interactionism
Hand gestures do not always carry the same meaning across cultures. The thumbs-up is a sign of approval in American culture; in some Middle Eastern countries, it is an offensive gesture.

Not only do hand gestures carry different meanings in different cultures, but different cultures have unique languages and slang, alphabets and number systems, traffic signs, and so on. In fact, the meaning of a symbol might differ even from group to group within a culture. The shared understanding of symbols is therefore a micro- or meso-level phenomenon. One major limitation to the symbolic interactionist approach is that it overlooks macro-level structures, like cultural norms or class interactions.

Social Constructionism

KEY CONCEPT

Symbolic interactionism reflects on how we use symbols to interact with each other. Social constructionism reflects on how we, as a society, construct concepts and principles.

The agreed-upon meaning of symbols can change. For example, the peace sign, which today is a symbol signifying peace and freedom in general, originally was used to indicate support for nuclear disarmament specifically. Society's interpretation of the peace sign has therefore broadened over time. This example shows that the meaning of a symbol does not come from the symbol itself, but from implicit social agreement. Symbols are therefore examples of social constructs. A **social construct** is any idea that has been created and accepted by the people in a society. **Social constructionism** is the attempt to understand a society through the study of the society's social constructs.

Symbols are not the only type of social construct. Abstract ideas might also be social constructs. For example, the definitions of concepts like honor and justice rely on group agreement among individuals within a given society, and these concepts are therefore social constructs. Sociologists also apply social constructionism to physical objects, such as money. Paper money and coinage do not inherently have significant value; it is only because we, as a society, imbue these objects with value that they can be used to trade for goods and services. Other examples of social constructs include work ethic, acceptable dress, and gender roles.

As with symbolic interactionism, social constructionism is useful for explaining micro- and meso-level sociological phenomena. Any social construct depends on the society being studied, and different societies will have different social constructs. Therefore, like symbolic interactionism, a limitation of social constructionism is that this theory cannot account for macro-level sociological phenomena.

Rational Choice (Exchange) Theory

Rational choice theory is one more micro- to meso-level approach to sociology. This theory focuses on individual decision making. According to rational choice theorists, humans will make rational choices to further their own self-interests. This theory claims that people weigh the costs and benefits when making choices, ranking their options based on maximizing perceived benefit. For example, when deciding to purchase a new laptop, rational choice theory claims that a person will gather information about characteristics such as cost, performance, brand recognition, and so on, and then will rank their options and choose the best one.

This laptop example illustrates that rational choice theory is influenced by the study of economics. Rational choice theory becomes a model of sociology when this idea of rational transactions is applied to the social interaction. The rational choice perspective views all social interactions as transactions that take into consideration the benefits and harms to the individual. Every outcome in a given social interaction can be associated with particular social rewards (such as accolades, honor, prestige, or social approval) and with particular punishments (such as embarrassment, humiliation, sanctions, or stigmatization). From the rational choice perspective, an individual carefully considers all of the possible rewards and punishments of each social action and chooses the option that results in the greatest social benefit.

Moreover, according to rational choice theorists, people evaluate whether there is reciprocity and balance in social relationships: People stay in relationships because they get something from the exchange, and they leave relationships when there are more social costs than benefits. Due to this view of relationships as exchanges of social value, rational choice theory is sometimes called **social exchange theory**, or just **exchange theory** for short.

Rational choice (exchange) theory is acceptable for explaining some micro- and meso-level sociological phenomena. However, rational choice (exchange) theory does not easily explain charitable, illogical, unselfish, or altruistic behavior.

Conflict Theory

Conflict theory is a macro theory that attempts to understand society by examining the inevitable conflicts between groups in society. Conflict theory has its origins in the writings of Karl Marx, a 19th century social philosopher who examined the influence of capitalism on 19th century society. **Capitalism** is an economic system in which individuals and corporations, rather than governments, own and control what Marx called the means of production, meaning property, machinery, factories, or any other means of creating a saleable good or service. According to Marx, such private ownership naturally leads to a small, wealthy **capitalist (bourgeoisie) class**, who control the means of production. In Marx's model, the rest of society is relegated to a lower **worker (proletariat) class** that performs manual labor. Because the capitalist class owns the means of production, this class has power over the worker class, and the disparity in power and resources between these two groups leads to conflict. According to Marx, the conflict in such a society would be a physical one: Eventually, the worker class would rise up and overthrow the capitalist class and form a new, classless society.

Where Marx focused specifically on conflict between capitalists and workers, modern conflict theory expands this idea to examine any conflict between groups with more power and those with less. For example, conflict might exist between people of different generations, different religions, or different regions of a country. According to conflict theory, in any such conflict, individuals in the group with more power attempt to preserve their power by shaping the structure of society itself. The group

REAL WORLD

Conflict theory can be applied to healthcare and medicine. Conflict theorists would not deny that modern healthcare can help people maintain or restore their health; however, they may ask who holds the power in the healthcare system. Is it the patient? The doctor? Hospitals? Pharmaceutical companies? Insurance companies? The government? This is an issue the United States continues to grapple with.

with more power uses their influence to dictate the laws, customs, and cultural norms of the society. However, according to conflict theorists, if people in lower-status positions recognize this power differential and see that others share a common dissatisfaction, then these individuals can organize to form **interest groups**, through which they can use tools such as protesting or voting to enact change and equalize power. In short, according to conflict theory, for the more powerful in society, maintenance of the status quo is usually desirable, and for the less powerful, change comes through disruption and revolution.

While conflict theory is a useful model for describing many large-scale changes and other macro-level societal phenomena, it is not very effective for explaining the choices of individuals in society. Also, conflict theorists tend to focus on social stress and disharmony, so conflict theory is less effective than some other models at explaining social cohesion, cooperation, and altruism.

Structural-Functionalism

In some ways, **structural-functionalism** is the inverse of conflict theory. The founder of structural-functionalism, Émile Durkheim, was interested in how large societies survive over long time periods, and was therefore concerned with social cohesion and stability. Durkheim compared society to an organism and proposed that each group in society has a role to play in the overall health and operation of society. These roles might be very different, in the same way that different organs or even different cells have very different functions within an organism, but each is important. Durkheim called each social group's role its **function**: the contribution made by that group to the system. According to structural-functionalist theory, the different groups of society work together in an unconscious, almost automatic way toward maintenance of equilibrium.

In structural-functionalism, functions can either be manifest or latent. A **manifest function** is an intended consequence of the actions of a group within a society. When an organization or institution has unintended but beneficial consequences, these are called **latent functions**. For example, annual meetings of medical societies have the manifest function of educating a group of physicians, sharing research findings, and setting goals for the next year. Such meetings also create stronger interpersonal bonds between physicians and provide a sense of identity for the group, both of which are latent functions. On the other hand, while both manifest and latent functions provide a benefit to society, **dysfunctions** are negative consequences of the existence of an institution, organization, or interaction.

Because structural-functionalism focuses on social cohesion and equilibrium, this approach is not well suited for explaining social change. Additionally, while structural-functionalism attempts to explain how groups interact with other groups, it does not explain how individuals interact *within* a group. To understand those kinds of micro-level interactions, other models are better suited.

Feminist Theory

Feminist theory critiques the institutional power structures that disadvantage women in society. Feminist theory was originally an offshoot of conflict theory. From a conflict theory perspective, feminist theory describes society as inherently **patriarchal**, with men seeking to preserve their position of power over women through societal privilege and institutional discrimination. For example, some feminist theorists argue that the study of sociology itself has been historically dominated by a male perspective.

In developed countries, gender stratification and inequality typically lessens, often as a result of the activism of feminist interest groups. However, imbalances of power still exist. In the workplace, for example, the term **glass ceiling** refers to processes that limit the progress of women to the highest job positions because of invisible social barriers to promotion. In contrast, even in cases where men do not seek to climb the job ladder, invisible social forces sometimes push men up to higher positions, a phenomenon called the **glass escalator**. The glass escalator is especially prevalent for men working in traditionally female occupations.

BEHAVIORAL SCIENCES GUIDED EXAMPLE WITH EXPERT THINKING

In societies facing increasing amounts of migration and ethnic integration, concerns about intergroup conflicts have prompted research into the effects of diversity on a society as a whole. Previous studies suggest that ethnic diversity negatively impacts social cohesion, but critics have pointed out that historic measures of social cohesion have focused on single indicators such as trust or volunteering.

Older studies demonstrated a negative relationship between diversity and social cohesion, but those are in doubt.

The current study sought to operationalize social cohesion across a more comprehensive set of indicators. Ethnic diversity was found to be associated with lower social cohesion with respect to some indicators, particularly volunteering and feelings of safety, but this trend could not be generalized when including a larger scope of indicators of social cohesion, such as neighborhood social capital or belonging. When heterogeneous groups showed increased contact with one another, subject assessment via survey showed a significant increase in feelings of trust, safety, and social capital.

Several results here. Not only were previous studies possibly wrong, but new results show that integration increases *cohesion. Not an experiment so no experimenter-controlled IV, looking at association only.*

Adapted from: McKenna S, Lee E, Klik KA, Markus A, Hewstone M, Reynolds KJ (2018) Are diverse societies less cohesive? Testing contact and mediated contact theories. *PLoS ONE* 13(3): e0193337. https://doi.org/10.1371/journal.pone.0193337

How does conflict theory relate to the results of this study?

This question at first might seem tough, as the results of the study seem to suggest that there is less conflict than one would expect in more diverse societies. When faced with a question that asks us to apply a concept to a new situation, it's useful to think critically about the definition of that concept. According to conflict theory, institutions arise as a result of power differentials between individuals, and those institutions seek to maintain that power differential.

So where is the conflict in this situation? According to the study, there can be a great deal of diversity in an area that has low interaction between different groups. In those situations, some measures of social cohesion decrease, including feelings of safety. So when people are in close quarters with diverse others, particularly when not interacting with those others regularly, perceived threat to the establishment and maintenance of the power differential will increase, which increases the conflict between groups.

However, the study also found that when people in close quarters with a diverse population interact more with diverse others, they report increased feelings of trust, safety, and social capital, indicating a reduction in perceived threat from other groups. We could infer that this increased interaction may counter the conflict theory effects noted earlier: increased trust and safety reduces fear of others, generally, and fear of loss of power, specifically. With a reduction in perceived threat and increased social cohesion, motivation for conflict should decrease, as power differentials are less threatened or groups are actively integrated into the existing power structure.

So, in summary, conflict theory provides some explanation as to why those who are not interacting with their diverse society may experience more perceived threat and conflict motivation. The study further indicates the perceived threat effect, and possibly societal conflict overall, can be countered by increased social interaction.

Social Institutions

Social institutions are well-established social structures that dictate certain patterns of behavior or relationships and are accepted as a fundamental part of culture. Social institutions regulate the behavior of individuals in core areas of society. For example, family is a social institution that encourages learning of acceptable behavior, socialization, and bonding.

Institutions exist at the meso-level of sociological analysis because they are a part of society, but are not dependent upon the individuals involved—in the United States, the idea of "government" stays basically the same even as the president, senators, representatives, and other officials change. The exact nature of each institution differs from culture to culture, although each institution performs a similar role regardless of culture. Often, institutions are dependent upon and support one another, though competition over resources can bring institutions into conflict. A summary of six of the major social institutions is provided in Table 11.1 at the end of this section.

Family

The definition of **family** differs greatly from culture to culture. For some, the term means "those people to whom I maintain close ties and who are related to me by blood." For others, family is simply "the people who live in my house." In fact, even terms for different family members (such as *sister*, *father*, *cousin*, and so on) are not conserved across time and culture; different **patterns of kinship** may be reflected by these terms. For example, it is common in Hawaiian culture to refer to all family members as *cousins*, while this term would not be used by many other Americans to describe one's mother's brother (the term *uncle* being preferred by many continental Americans). Different patterns of kinship between societies have bearing on responsibility for child rearing, familial loyalty, and even the boundaries of what is considered incest.

Regardless of the definition, family is the most basic of institutions. It is the institution most closely tied to the individual and helps to meet many of our most basic needs, especially when we are young, providing food, shelter, emotional and physical security, and intimacy. Additionally, many life rituals and rites of passage, such as marriage, funerals, and graduations occur in the context of family.

BRIDGE

Families help to meet many of the basic needs at the base of Maslow's hierarchy pyramid. Maslow's hierarchy of needs is discussed in chapter 5 of *MCAT Behavioral Science Review*.

Sociologists studying family relationships may examine the stages of coupling (courtship, cohabitation, engagement, and marriage), changes in relationships between spouses through time, or parenting. Parenting is a complex topic that involves socialization of children; varied definitions of the role of father, mother, and child; and single parenting, same-sex parenting, adoption, and foster parenting. Not all families are composed of a mother, a father, and children. Alternative forms exist, including single-parent families; families that cohabitate with other family members beyond the nuclear family, such as grandparents, aunts, uncles, cousins, godparents, and surrogate kin; and families with marital disunions (divorce). A number of different family structures are illustrated in Figure 11.2.

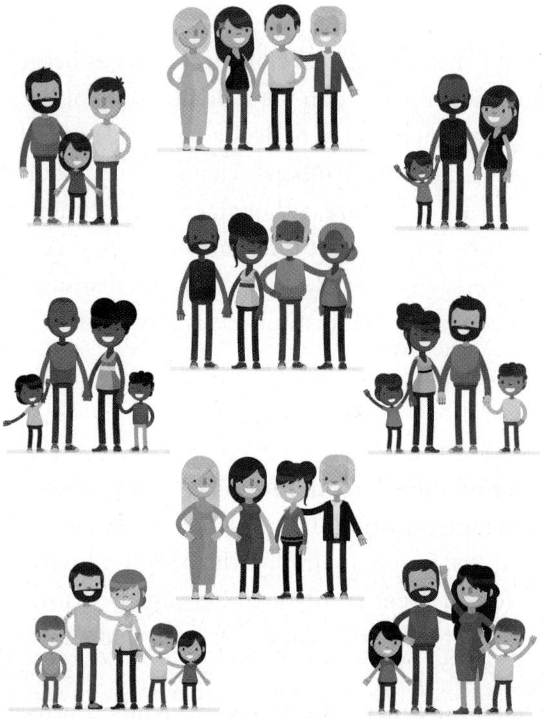

Figure 11.2 Various Family Structures

MCAT EXPERTISE

The MCAT will not expect you to know any specific demographic numbers for the exam, but you should be familiar with some of the recent trends seen in the United States population.

Divorce rates in the United States rose significantly in the second half of the twentieth century but have started to drop over the last two decades.

While the family can be a source of joy and support, it can also be a source of violence. Spousal abuse (**domestic violence**) is seen across all social classes and genders and can include not only physical violence, but sexual abuse, emotional abuse, and financial abuse. Domestic violence is the #1 cause of injury to American women, and is most common in families with drug abuse, especially alcoholism. Victims of domestic violence may find it challenging to leave the abusive relationship for a variety of reasons, including lack of a safe haven to escape to, financial restrictions, and psychological disorders (consider the connection to learned helplessness, described in Chapter 6 of *MCAT Behavioral Sciences Review*). **Elder abuse** is also seen across all socioeconomic classes, and most commonly manifests as neglect of an older relative—although physical, psychological, and financial abuse may occur as well. The caretaker of the individual is most commonly the source of abuse. Finally, **child abuse** also most commonly manifests as neglect, although physical, sexual, and psychological abuse are also common. During medical school, you will be trained to recognize certain signs suggestive of nonaccidental trauma, such as a broken femur in a child who is too young to have begun walking or burn marks on the buttocks from placing a child in scalding water. As a physician, you will be considered a **mandated reporter**, which means that you are legally required to report suspected cases of elder or child abuse. Domestic abuse does not fall under mandated reporting laws, but counseling and information about shelters for victims of intimate partner violence should be provided.

Education

Education, as an institution, aims to provide a population with a set of skills that will be useful to them or to society. In many societies, education is formal—in other words, it takes place in a setting designated for educational purposes using a prescribed curriculum. The function of formal education is to teach skills, facts, and mental processes, but the system also has a social latent function, providing opportunities for peer socialization and reinforcing social stratification, both within individual schools and through comparisons between schools. Education, therefore, includes not only the information and cognitive skills students learn but also the **hidden curriculum** of transmitting social norms, attitudes, and beliefs to students. Sociological investigations into education may focus on the ethics, morals, practices, political influence, finances, and values of an education system. Sociologists also explore educational trends, including grade inflation and deflation, adult education, online education, and accessibility of education.

Performance in the education system depends not only on a student's intrinsic abilities, but also on the education system itself. **Teacher expectancy** refers to the idea that teachers tend to get what they expect from students. Thus, a teacher who places high demands on students—but who also believes that students can rise to the challenge—will more often see students succeed than a teacher who places the same demands but doubts that the students can achieve them. This is an example of a self-fulfilling prophecy, discussed in Chapter 10 of *MCAT Behavioral Sciences Review*, and may be due to differences in how teachers motivate, interact, and offer feedback to their students.

Education is susceptible to inequalities across socioeconomic class. Lower socioeconomic status is associated with decreased accessibility to and quality of education. This is not an easy trend to reverse. Low funding, deprioritization of education, and poor historical performance can make it challenging for a failing school district to acquire resources and improve education to its students.

As mentioned earlier, institutions are intentionally or unintentionally connected, and there is a well-known, persistent association between education and medicine. Health disparities between more educated and less educated individuals are significant, and lack of education may be a hurdle to accessing or trusting healthcare providers.

Religion

As an institution, **religion** is a pattern of social activities organized around a set of beliefs and practices that seek to address the meaning of existence. **Religiosity** refers to how religious one considers oneself to be, and includes strength of religious beliefs, engagement in religious practices, and attitudes about religion itself.

More than 80% of the global population identifies with a religion. Most follow either Christianity or Islam; other world religions include Hinduism, Buddhism, Sikhism, and Judaism. These religions are generally divided into multiple **denominations** or **sects** that may share certain beliefs and practices but not others. A denomination is simply a part of a **church**, a term which can refer both to a large, universal religious group and to the building in which the congregation of such a group meets. Orthodox and Reform are examples of Jewish denominations, and the Sunni and Shia are examples of Islamic denominations. Denominations often coexist, but can come into conflict when their religious beliefs promote opposing values. Whereas the word *sect* was historically a pejorative term, it now refers more properly to a religious group that has chosen to break off from the parent religion. The Amish would be considered a sect of Christianity. In rare cases, a religious sect may take on extreme or deviant philosophies and transform into a **cult**.

As the twenty-first century continues, religious groups—many of which have existed in more or less the same form for thousands of years—grapple with finding a place in contemporary society. For many religious groups, this is reflected by a shift toward modernization within the religion and relaxing historical practices. For others, there is a shift away from religion as society **secularizes**, or moves from a world dominated by religion toward rationality and scientific thinking. For other groups, maintenance of strict adherence to religious code, or **fundamentalism**, predominates.

While spirituality and religion are not equivalent terms, they are often linked to each other because they both seek to understand the meaning of existence and to identify what is sacred. Spirituality and religion may play a role in a patient's understanding of disease, may impact healthcare decisions, and can be an essential component of the patient's coping mechanisms.

Government and Economy

Government and **economy** can be defined as systematic arrangements of political and capital relationships, activities, and social structures that affect rule making, representation of the individual in society, rights and privileges, division of labor, and production of goods and services. Notably, political and economic institutions impact all other institutions to some extent. That is, the government may sanction or define specific family structures, may finance and regulate education, may recognize some religions but not others, and may play a key role in funding and certifying healthcare and medicine. The effects of the economy on institutions can also be viewed from the individual level. For example, when the economy takes a downturn, large swaths of the population may have trouble supporting their families and paying for health insurance. Note that this institutional influence is bidirectional: because of the economic downturn and changes in family, education, or health, an individual may choose to vote a new political candidate into office, or to support or oppose a particular piece of legislation.

While an in-depth exploration of the American (or any other) government is outside the scope of the MCAT, you could be asked to distinguish between different types of government. A **democracy** allows every citizen a political voice, usually through electing representatives to office (i.e., a representative democracy). **Monarchies** include a royal ruler (a king or queen), although the ruler's powers may be significantly limited by the presence of a constitution, a parliamentary system, or some other legislative body. A **dictatorship** is a system where a single person holds power, and usually includes mechanisms to quell threats to this power. A **theocracy** is a system where power is held by religious leaders. Many of these systems of leadership are based around a **charismatic authority** (a leader with a compelling personality).

In comparative economics, the largest division is between capitalist and socialist economies. **Capitalist** economies focus on free market trade and laissez-faire policies, where success or failure in business is primarily driven by consumerism with as little intervention from central governing bodies as possible. In capitalism, a private owner or corporation maintains and profits from the success of the business. Capitalist societies encourage **division of labor**, where specific components of a larger task (say, developing, manufacturing, quality testing, and marketing goods) are separated and assigned to skilled and trained individuals. This promotes specialization and efficiency. **Socialist** economies, on the other hand, treats large industries as collective, shared businesses, and compensation is provided based on the work contribution of each individual into the system. Profit, then, is distributed equally to the workforce. There are many other forms of government and economy, but these would be defined and explained if necessary on Test Day.

Healthcare and Medicine

The institutions of **healthcare** and **medicine** are aimed at maintaining or improving the health status of the individual, family, community, and society as a whole. Healthcare is an ever-changing field, but some of the key goals in American healthcare over the past few decades include:

- Increased access to care
- Decreased costs of healthcare
- Prevention of disease before it occurs
- Association of patients with a primary care physician or a patient-centered medical home
- Increased education for the public with public health outreach
- Decreased paternalism (*doctor knows best* mentality)
- Reduced economic conflicts of interest for physicians
- **Life course approach to health** (maintaining and considering a comprehensive view of the patient's history beyond the immediate presenting symptoms)

There has also been a shift in the role of the patient in the medical system. In the mid-twentieth century, sociologists believed that a patient who is ill takes on what was called the **sick role**. These sociologists believed that such patients are not responsible for their illness and are exempt from normal social roles. But on the other hand, these sociologists also believed that a patient had the obligation to want to become well and to seek out competent help. While this paradigm still exists, patients are now expected to take more ownership of their health through diet, exercise, seeking help before it is needed (through annual primary care visits and screenings), and so on. Modern sociologists also recognize that the notion that patients should feel an obligation to want to become better does not fit patients with chronic, long-term, or permanent conditions.

Even our understanding of disease has shifted over time. On the one hand, many ordinary parts of the human condition, including the full range of sexual orientations and gender identities, are no longer defined as medical conditions, as they misguidedly were in earlier editions of the DSM. On the other hand, other types of behaviors have become **medicalized**, meaning that they are now defined and treated as medical conditions.This latter shift can be seen in the addition of a number of diagnostic entities to the DSM-5, such as hoarding disorder and binge eating disorder.

The medical community also now recognizes that health is not only characterized by physiological wellness or disease, but also by a person's subjective experience of their health. The phrase **illness experience** refers to the ways in which people, rather than doctors, define and adjust to changes in their health. For example, people can experience disease without illness, as is the case for someone living a full and productive life with a manageable condition such as HIV. People can also experience illness without disease, such as when a person experiences somatic symptoms as a result of psychological stress.

Sociologists studying healthcare are often interested in **social epidemiology**. Epidemiology is the study of health and its determinants within a society (discussed in detail in Chapter 12 of *MCAT Behavioral Sciences Review*); social epidemiology is specifically the study of the effects of institutions, social structures, and relationships on health. Social epidemiologists study the effects of racial and economic inequality or government safety net legislation on health and access to healthcare. They might also be interested in how social conditions early in life affect healthcare outcomes later.

In addition, many sociologists investigate medical ethics. In the United States, physicians are expected to adhere to four key tenets of medical ethics:

- **Beneficence:** the physician has a responsibility to act in the patient's best interest.
- **Nonmaleficence:** *do no harm*; the physician has a responsibility to avoid treatments or interventions in which the potential for harm outweighs the potential for benefit.
- **Respect for patient autonomy:** the physician has a responsibility to respect patients' decisions and choices about their own healthcare. While there are exceptions to this rule (significant psychiatric illness interfering with decision-making capacity, children, public health threats), patients do have the right to refuse life-saving therapies.
- **Justice:** the physician has a responsibility to treat similar patients with similar care, and to distribute healthcare resources fairly.

SOCIAL INSTITUTION	NEEDS MET BY INSTITUTION	STATUSES	VALUES	NORMS
Education	Transmit knowledge and skills across generations	Teacher, student, dean, principal	Academic honesty, good grades	Doing homework, preparing for lectures, being kind to other students
Family	Regulate reproduction, socialize and protect children	Father, mother, son, daughter, brother, sister, uncle, aunt, grandparent	Sexual fidelity, providing for children, keeping a clean home, respect for caregivers	Having as many children as one desires, being faithful to one's spouse
Religion	Concerns about life and death, the meaning of suffering and loss, desire to connect with a creator	Clergy, worshipper, teacher, disciple, missionary, prophet, convert	God and holy texts should be honored	Going to services, following teachings of the religion, applying beliefs outside of worship
Government	Maintain social order, enforce laws	President, senator, lobbyist, voter, candidate	Transparency, accountability, professionalism	Acting in the best interest of constituents, debating political issues
Economy	Organize money, goods, and services	Worker, boss, buyer, seller, creditor, debtor, advertiser	Making money, paying bills on time, producing efficiently	Maximizing profits, *the customer is always right*, working hard
Medicine	Heal the sick and injured, care for the dying	Doctor, nurse, pharmacist, insurer, patient	Hippocratic oath, staying in good health, following care providers' recommendations	Beneficence, nonmaleficence, respect for autonomy, justice

Table 11.1 Social Institutions

MCAT CONCEPT CHECK 11.1

Before you move on, assess your understanding of the material with these questions.

1. What are manifest and latent functions?
   - Manifest functions:

   - Latent functions:

   ---

2. For each of the theoretical approaches listed below, what is the primary thesis or idea of the theory?

Theoretical Approach	Primary Thesis or Idea
Functionalism	
Conflict theory	
Symbolic interactionism	
Social constructionism	
Rational choice-exchange theory	
Feminist theory	

3. What are the four key tenets of American medical ethics? Provide a short description of each.

Ethical Principle	Description

11.2 Culture

LEARNING OBJECTIVES

After Chapter 11.2, you will be able to:

- Distinguish between material and symbolic culture
- Recall the definitions of, and the differences between, the values, beliefs, norms, and rituals of a culture

The study of culture is likely the most diverse and complex dimension within sociology. **Culture** can be defined as encompassing the entire lifestyle for a given group. It binds our nation-states, political institutions, marketplaces, religions, and ideologies. Culture flavors our interpretations of the world, and is generally passed through familial lines. In short, culture is what makes human societies unique from one another.

Material and Symbolic Culture

Sociologists view culture according to two different categories: material culture and symbolic culture.

Material Culture

One can discern a lot about people by looking at their **artifacts**: material items that they make, possess, and value. This examination surrounds **material culture**, which includes the physical items one associates with a given group, such as artwork, emblems, clothing, jewelry, foods, buildings, and tools. Sociologists explore the meaning of these objects to a given society.

An example of material culture in the United States is the American flag. This item is used to reinforce a sense of belonging via shared American citizenship. Other symbols that are considered traditionally American include barbecue, baseball, apple pie, and rock and roll.

Material culture is often most visible during ceremonies, such as birthdays, weddings, and funerals. Some artifacts of traditional Indian material culture are shown in Figure 11.3.

BRIDGE

A description of culture in the context of group processes is described in Chapter 8 of *MCAT Behavioral Sciences Review*

MCAT EXPERTISE

Ethnography is the study of cultures and customs, and **ethnographic methods** are experimental methods used to study the ethnicity or culture of a group.

BRIDGE

Symbols are also discussed in Chapter 6 of *MCAT Behavioral Sciences Review*

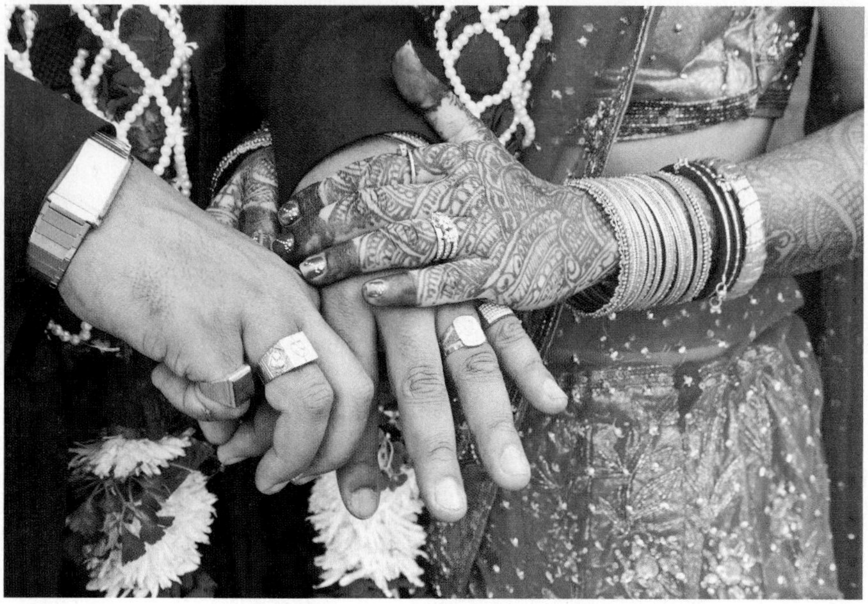

Figure 11.3 Material Culture

Material culture includes objects important to a group, including clothing, jewelry, cuisine, ceremonial objects, and so on.

Symbolic Culture

KEY CONCEPT

Material culture is associated with artifacts (objects). Symbolic culture is associated with ideas.

Symbolic culture, also called **nonmaterial culture**, focuses on the ideas that represent a group of people. These may be encoded in mottos, songs, or catchphrases, or may simply be themes that are pervasive in the culture. Phrases like *free enterprise* and *life, liberty, and the pursuit of happiness* are examples of American symbolic culture. Material culture is often the tangible embodiment of the underlying ideas of symbolic culture.

For any social group to remain connected over time, there must be a culture that binds its members together. In times of war and crisis, governments often draw upon symbolic culture to rally people to action, using songs, parades, discussion of heroes past, and so on, as shown in Figure 11.4. It is not a coincidence that most high schools have a school mascot, school colors, and a school song. Such cultural artifacts are in place to help create a shared sense of identity, loyalty, and belonging. Symbolic culture includes both cognitive and behavioral components; that is, it informs cultural values and beliefs, as well as cultural norms and communication styles.

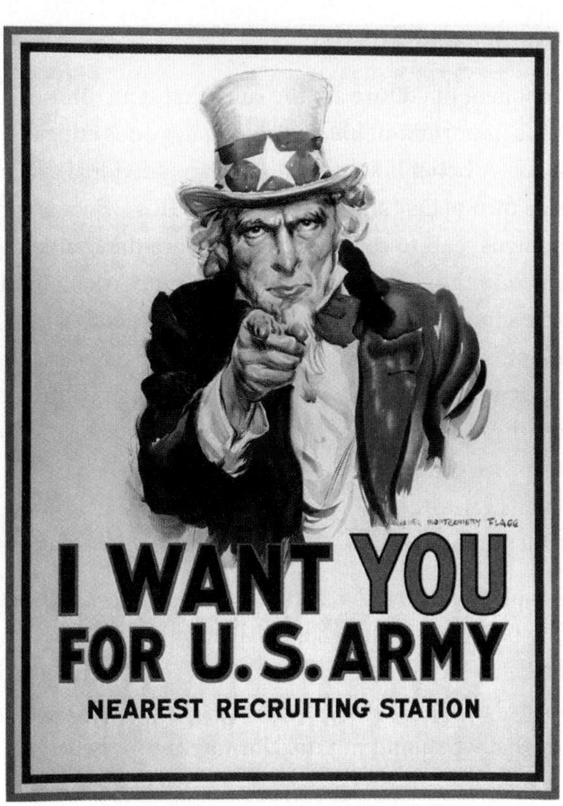

Figure 11.4 Symbolic Culture
Symbolic culture includes ideas that identify a culture; it may be drawn upon to encourage loyalty or patriotism, as shown here.

Symbolic culture is usually slower to change than material culture, which can lead to the phenomenon of **culture lag**. The expansion of devices and technology in contemporary times are prototypical examples of culture lag: whereas American culture still prizes individuality and privacy, the development of smartphones and social media push toward a more community-oriented and less private world. Still, there is evidence that symbolic culture is beginning to change in response to these technological (material) innovations: younger generations appear to be less concerned about what personal information is publicly accessible than older generations.

Language

Language is the most highly developed and complex symbol system used by most cultures. Language consists of spoken, written, or signed symbols, which are regulated according to certain rules of grammar and syntax. Language enables us to share our ideas, thoughts, experiences, discoveries, fears, plans, and desires with others. Written language extends our capacity to communicate across both spatial and temporal boundaries. Without language, it would be difficult to transmit culture. Understanding a group's language is critical to understanding its culture.

BRIDGE

Language is critically important in the transmission of culture. It requires a complex interplay of multiple brain circuits, which are discussed in Chapter 4 of *MCAT Behavioral Sciences Review*.

Values, Beliefs, Norms, and Rituals

An important component of culture are the rules that structure society. **Values** are what a person deems important in life, which dictates one's ethical principles and standards of behavior. A **belief** is something that an individual accepts to be truth. Every culture has its own beliefs and value systems. This will be important in your future career, as patients tend to carry their beliefs into the healthcare system. For example, as described in the chapter introduction, some Asian cultures believe that healthcare decisions should be the responsibility of a patient's family, which avoids burdening the patient (who is already ill) with having to make such a decision. This belief is in direct contrast to the American belief that patient autonomy should be prized and that healthcare decisions should be made by a patient whenever possible. These conflicts can prove challenging to healthcare professionals, and there is not always one correct answer to such dilemmas. Such situations—when a cultural difference impedes interaction with others—are called **cultural barriers**.

REAL WORLD

Many health systems have an ethics board to deal with conflicts that may arise from differences in belief systems between patient and practitioner, among other ethical issues. These committees tend to facilitate discussion, rather than simply issuing a decision.

As described in Chapter 8 of *MCAT Behavioral Sciences Review*, **norms** are societal rules that define the boundaries of acceptable behavior. While norms are not laws, they do govern the behavior of many individuals in society and provide a sense of social control. Norms are what provide us with a sense of what is appropriate, what we should do, and what we should not do. Norms exist for behavior, speech, dress, home life, and more.

A **ritual** is a formalized ceremony that usually involves specific material objects, symbolism, and additional mandates on acceptable behavior. Rituals tend to have a prescribed order of events or routine. These rituals can be associated with specific milestones, such as a baby-naming, graduation ceremony, wedding, or funeral; with holidays, such as a Thanksgiving dinner, trick-or-treating on Halloween, or a Passover seder, shown in Figure 11.5; or with regular activities, such as a Catholic mass, a pregame pep rally, or even just getting ready in the morning (showering, brushing teeth, eating breakfast, and so on).

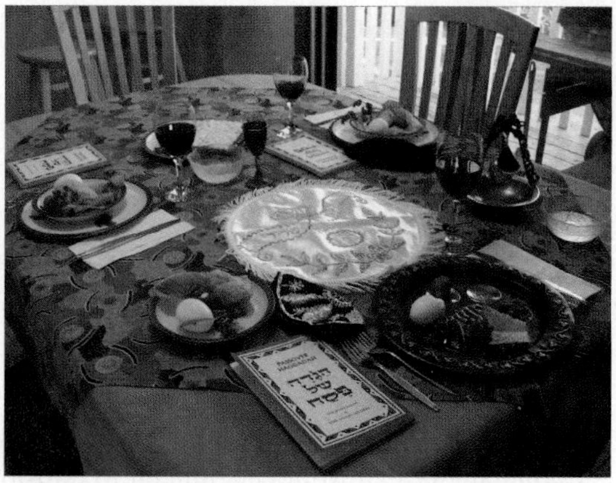

Figure 11.5 A Passover Seder Is an Example of a Ritual
Seder means "order" in Hebrew; most rituals have a specific order of events.

Evolution and Human Culture

Evolution may have selected for the development of culture. Culture serves as a method of passing down information from generation to generation; in prehistoric times, the transmission of information through culture served to teach future generations how to create tools, hunt, domesticate animals, and grow crops. Culture also creates a sense of loyalty and allegiance, which, as described in Chapter 10 of *MCAT Behavioral Sciences Review*, may help explain altruistic behavior. Finally, culture creates a sense of *us* vs. *them*, which presumably served a role in the dispersion of populations across the globe in different environmental niches.

Culture, in turn, may also influence evolution. There is evidence that some genetic traits may have been favored because of cultural values and beliefs. For example, human beings—at least those who are not lactose intolerant—are the only animals that are able to digest milk after adolescence; they are also the only animals that ingest another animal's milk. These evolutionary adaptations may have arisen out of Northern European cultures, which relied heavily on cattle farming for sustenance. A mutation permitting digestion of milk into adulthood presumably imparted a nutritional and survival advantage to certain individuals, and would thus be retained within the population.

MCAT CONCEPT CHECK 11.2:

Before you move on, assess your understanding of the material with these questions.

1. What are material and symbolic culture?
   - Material culture:

   ____

   - Symbolic culture:

   ____

2. What is the difference between a value and a belief?

   ____

11.3 Demographics

High-Yield

LEARNING OBJECTIVES

After Chapter 11.3, you will be able to:

- Distinguish between race and ethnicity
- Describe symbolic ethnicity
- Describe fertility rate, birth rate, and mortality rate and how they shift during a demographic transition
- Recall examples of proactive and reactive social movements and how the two types of movements differ

Demographics refer to the statistics of populations and are the mathematical applications of sociology. Demographics can be gathered informally, such as a professor asking how many freshmen, sophomores, juniors, and seniors are in a given course, or may be gathered formally. For example, the United States Census Bureau gathers demographic data about every individual in the country every ten years.

Common Demographic Categories

Demographers can classify individuals based on hundreds of different criteria. The MCAT will not expect you to know advanced topics within demographics, but familiarity with some of the common demographic categories as well as their implications on society and healthcare are important. In this section, we'll explore age, gender, race and ethnicity, sexual orientation, and immigration status.

Age

Aging is a inevitable process experienced by all people around the world. In this section we will explore the implications of an individual's age on healthcare, then dive deeper into its implications on society.

Considering an individual's age and cumulative life experiences when analyzing their personality, social status, health, and other social metrics is known as the **life course perspective** (sometimes referred to as the **life course approach**). For example, in healthcare, a psychiatrist may consider a patient's early life events and how those events continue to impact a patient's condition. Or perhaps a general practitioner chooses to conduct additional lung screenings on a patient who previously worked in a coal mine. In both these examples, the physician is incorporating the life course perspective into the treatment of the patient.

With the potentially large difference in the experiences between age cohorts, prejudice or discrimination based on a person's age can arise. This is known as **ageism** and can be seen at all ages. For example, young professionals entering the workplace are often viewed as being inexperienced, and their opinions and ideas may therefore be ignored or downplayed. Older individuals may be perceived as frail, vulnerable, or less intelligent, and may thus be treated with less respect.

In order to understand and analyze age-related differences, researchers can group individuals based on their age or birth year; these groupings are known as **age cohorts** (sometimes called generational cohorts). The utility of age cohorts goes beyond understanding the differences of an individual's life course, as they allow researchers to look at a population at a macroscopic level. An analysis of a population's distribution among its age cohorts can predict demographic shifts, such as an aging population, the shift from a developing to developed economy, or a stable population. We'll explore examples of each below.

In the United States, many sociologists document a "graying of America" as the Baby Boomer generation ages. The term Baby Boomer stems from the large spike in fertility rates (birth rates) after World War II, or in other words, a "boom of babies." Due to the baby boom spanning from the 1940s to 1960s, over 70 million Americans will be 65 or older by 2030, representing nearly 20 percent of the population. Thus, the fastest-growing age cohort in the United States is the 85-or-older group. This has profound effects on healthcare: more than 40 percent of adult patients in acute care hospital beds are 65 or older. Considering this shift in demographics, government programs such as Medicare and Social Security will experience increased demand, which may pose challenges for these programs.

This situation is an application of the **dependency ratio**, which is the ratio of the number of members of a population that are not in the workforce to the number of members that are in the workforce. This ratio depends on two components, the youth ratio and age dependency ratio. The **youth ratio** is defined by the number of people under the age of 15 divided by the number of people aged 15–65. The **age dependency ratio** is defined by the number of people over 65 divided by the number of people aged 15–65. Applied to societies, the dependency ratio quantifies the economic burden felt by the working age population (15–65) in order to support the portion of the population outside of the workforce (under 15 and over 65).

In contrast to the United States, developing countries, such as Uganda, see the reverse trend with 48% of the population being under the age of 15 years old, resulting in a dependency ratio of about 1 (2% of the population is 65 years and over, which means the dependent population roughly equals the working age population). This can be explained by the country's steadily dropping infant mortality rate over the last several decades. Forecasting the next 10 to 20 years for Uganda would predict a large proportion of the population entering the working-age age cohort. Although this may lead to an increase in the country's economic productivity, this demographic shift must be matched with job growth. If that does not occur, unemployment rates will increase, which could lead to civil unrest or other negative outcomes. This shift from developing to developed country is explained by demographic transition theory, covered later in this chapter.

Finally, when a population's fertility rate and mortality rate remain relatively consistent over a long period of time, the distribution of the population among the age cohorts remains fairly constant. This is known as a **stable population**.

REAL WORLD

The demographic tool of age cohorts has woven its way into our everyday language. If you've heard terms like the Silent Generation, Baby Boomers, Generation X, Millennial (Generation Y), and Generation Z, then you've encountered age cohorts. These generational terms group individuals by their birth year. However, age cohorts can be used to group individuals based on their current age, such as 0-14, 15-30, etc.

Gender

Sex and gender are not synonymous terms. **Sex** is a biological category. In many species, including humans, a phenotypical female is an individual that produces the larger gamete (the ovum) and carries offspring. **Gender** refers to a society's notions of femininity, masculinity, and other sexual identities. Gender is therefore a socially constructed set of ideas about what it means to be male, female, or otherwise in a given culture. A culture's ideas about gender usually include expected behavioral traits associated with a particular sex. These expected behavioral traits are known as **gender roles**. As such, gender roles are also social constructs. Once an individual understands these socially constructed behavioral expectations, an individual can adopt behaviors that project the gender that individual wishes to portray, which is known as the individual's **gender identity**.

Gender segregation is the separation of individuals based on perceived gender. Such segregation includes divisions of male, female, and gender-neutral bathrooms, or separating male and female sports teams. Differences between genders and the phenomenon of gender segregation do not necessarily imply inequality, although inequality can occur. **Gender inequality** is the intentional or unintentional empowerment of one gender to the detriment of others. In the presence of gender inequality, gender stratification may occur. **Gender stratification** is defined as any inequality in access to social resources that is based on gender, and is an example of social stratification in general, which will be studied in Chapter 12 of *MCAT Behavioral Sciences Review*. To illustrate the difference between gender segregation and gender stratification: Single-gender schools are an example of gender segregation. Children enrolled in such schools do not necessarily receive unequal qualities of education. However, if there is a systemic difference in resource allocation between single-gender schools, the result is uneven access to resources, leading to gender stratification.

Race and Ethnicity

REAL WORLD

Certain racial and ethnic groups have a higher incidence of specific health problems. For example, the Chinese population accounts for a disproportionate number of chronic hepatitis B infections and liver cancer. Mediterranean and African populations have a significantly higher rate of hemoglobinopathies (diseases related to hemoglobin). The Ashkenazi Jewish population has a higher rate of autoimmune diseases. Some American Indian populations are associated with gallbladder and biliary tree diseases. Being of a particular race or ethnicity is not necessary for the development of any disease, but may certainly be associated with increased risk.

The definition of race has changed through recent history, and continues to change. The term originally referred to speakers of a common language, and later indicated national origin. However, the term has also historically been used to denote certain shared phenotypic similarities between people. The five racial categories currently recognized by the U.S. Census exemplify these shifting definitions of race. These categories are: White, Black, Asian, American Indian or Alaskan native, and Native Hawaiian/Pacific Islander. Observe that some of these racial categories, like White and Black, describe phenotypic similarities, while other categories, like American Indian and Pacific Islander, are based on national origin. Furthermore, no other country uses these same five racial labels, and in fact the officially recognized races differ in each country. So, there is no uniform agreement about racial categories; rather each society generates its own racial labels, making race a social construct.

If race is not consistently defined, then why do sociologists concern themselves with this concept? The answer is that racial labels, though socially constructed, do materially affect the lives of people through institutionalized practices of preference and discrimination. In order to define race more scientifically, sociologists specify that the term **race** refers to socially constructed groupings of people based specifically on inherited phenotypic characteristics. Note that the human history of migration and mixing of populations means that there are few if any genetically isolated people left on earth. So sociologists recognize that scientifically categorizing people by genetic differences is not possible. Nevertheless, societies continue to generate racial labels based on perceived phenotypic differences, and so sociologists study how each society treats its socially defined racial groups.

An important takeaway from the above discussion is that sociologists narrow the definition of the term race to refer specifically to attempts to group people by phenotypic difference. However, sociologists recognize that societies also group people by shared language, cultural heritage, religion, and/or national origin. The term sociologists use for these types of groupings is **ethnicity**. While certain ethnicities are often associated with certain racial labels, race and ethnicity are distinct. Here is an illustration of the difference: African American individuals, African immigrants, and West Indian immigrants speak different languages and express different cultural norms. These three groups represent three different ethnicities. However, due to some phenotypic similarities shared by some members of these groups, individuals in these groups would generally be given the same racial label. Like race, ethnicity is also a social construct, in that ethnic labels and the criteria for inclusion in a certain ethnic group change from society to society and change over time.

Symbolic ethnicity describes a specific connection to one's ethnicity in which ethnic symbols and identity remain important, even when ethnic identity does not play a significant role in everyday life. For example, many Irish Americans in the United States celebrate their heritage only one day per year: St. Patrick's Day. In all other facets of life, these individuals' Irish-American ethnicity does not play a significant role. Other examples include attending folk festivals, visiting specific cultural locales for holidays, or participating in an ethnic celebration.

It is important to consider how race and ethnicity may affect one's ability to receive proper healthcare. The Agency for Healthcare Research and Quality (AHRQ), a government agency, reports that race and ethnicity influence a patient's chance of receiving many specific procedures and treatments. Whether due to conscious or unconscious bias, there is evidence that different races are not always offered the same level of care escalation in a medical emergency.

BRIDGE

Many public health outreach efforts are aimed at closing the gap in health disparities between populations. Health and healthcare disparities are discussed in Chapter 12 of *MCAT Behavioral Sciences Review*.

On the other hand, there are a number of public health outreach projects that target at-risk racial or ethnic populations through education, screening, and treatment. These specific strategies are geared to close gaps in health disparities. Many large university health systems run free clinics in local neighborhoods and may target specific populations; for example, some of these clinics will staff Spanish-speaking doctors and medical students to cater to the Hispanic immigrant population.

Sexual Orientation

Sexual orientation can be defined as the direction of one's sexual interest. In scientific and healthcare communities, sexual orientation has historically been divided into three categories:

- **Heterosexual**: attraction to individuals of a different sex
- **Bisexual** (or pansexual): attraction to members of multiple sexes
- **Homosexual**: attraction to individuals of the same sex

Sexual orientation involves a person's sexual feelings and may or may not be a significant contributor to that person's sense of identity. It may or may not be evident in the person's appearance or behavior. Disclosure of minority sexual orientations, sometimes called *coming out of the closet*, can be a major milestone in the absorption of sexuality into one's identity. This disclosure has also been shown sometimes to have therapeutic effects: coming out is associated with decreases in depressive and anxious symptoms linked to cortisol levels and stress.

Human sexuality continues to be an important area of research for psychologists, sociologists, and biologists alike, but evidence shows that sexuality is likely more fluid than previously believed. Alfred Kinsey was a pioneer in this area, and—in addition to a number of other models and publications—described sexuality on a zero to six scale, with zero representing exclusive heterosexuality and six representing exclusive homosexuality. When ranked on this **Kinsey scale**, few people actually fell into the categories of zero and six, with a significant proportion of the population falling somewhere between the two.

Sexual and gender identity minorities are often grouped together under the umbrella term **LGBTQ** (lesbian, gay, bisexual, transgender, and queer or questioning). In some cases, this acronym has been expanded to include other self-definitions of sexuality and sexual identity, including I (intersex) or A (asexual).

Several health disparities have been recognized within the LGBTQ community. The most significant historical disparity is HIV, which disproportionately affected individuals who are gay in urban environments during the early 1980s. While the prevalence of HIV is still slightly higher in men who have sex with men (MSM), it exists in all populations. Efforts to encourage safe sex and increase screening have helped to slow the epidemic of HIV, as has increased awareness of those with HIV/AIDS with projects like the AIDS Memorial Quilt, shown in Figure 11.6. Within the healthcare system, individuals who are lesbian receive less screening for cervical cancer and may not be screened for other sexually transmitted infections. Individuals who are transgender have multiple areas of increased risk, including off-label or unsupervised use of "street hormones" without proper counseling on their side effects.

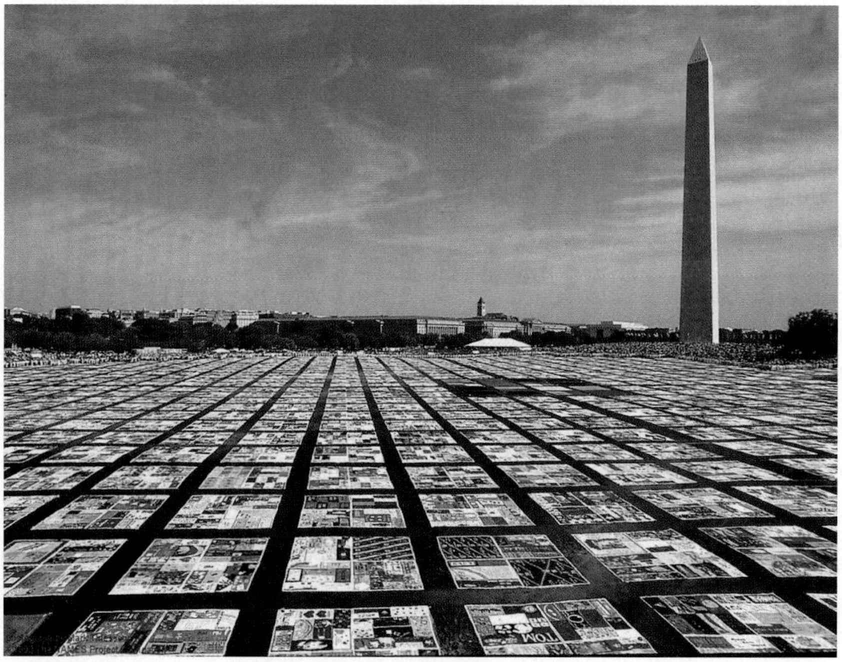

Figure 11.6 The AIDS Memorial Quilt

Mental health disparities are also common in the LGBTQ community. LGBTQ youth are at significantly higher risk for bullying, victimization, and violence, and have higher rates of suicide. In adults, the LGBTQ population has a higher prevalence of depression and anxiety than their heterosexual and cisgender counterparts. In addition, men who are gay have an increased rate of eating disorders as compared to men who are heterosexual. A host of campaigns and outreach efforts have begun to target these disparities.

Immigration Status

According to the US Census Bureau, the nation's total recent immigrant population is growing rapidly; it was quantified at 40.4 million in 2011 and is expected to increase by roughly 20 million in the next two decades. This tells us that immigrants, whether documented or undocumented, are interwoven into every social structure and institution in the United States. The nativity of immigrant populations changes over time; in the most recent census, the largest proportions of immigrants had emigrated from Mexico, the Caribbean, and India. **Generational status** refers to the place of birth of a specific person or that person's parents. For instance, first generation refers to someone who is born outside of their place of residence. Second generation refers to a person that has at least one parent that is foreign-born.

Considering the number of immigrant communities, there are often barriers that affect interactions with social structures and institutions. The complex organization of the United States healthcare system is starkly different from those of most other nations, and this may present a barrier to use for immigrants. Language barriers may also make it difficult for immigrants to access healthcare or to take control of their healthcare decisions; telephone translation services have been created to help facilitate the conversation between clinician and patient. Racial and ethnic identity may be more apparent in first-generation immigrants, and the biases and prejudices against certain racial and ethnic groups might be compounded by the individual's immigrant status; this interplay between multiple demographic factors—especially when it leads to discrimination or oppression—is termed **intersectionality**. Finally, undocumented status presents a major barrier for many immigrants to access healthcare for fear of reporting and deportation.

Demographic Shifts and Social Change

Since 1950, the United States population has roughly doubled. In addition to increasing in size, the makeup of the American population has changed significantly. The average age in the United States has increased, and the population is continuing to become more racially and ethnically diverse. These are examples of **demographic shifts**: changes in the makeup of a population over time. These shifts can be measured by considering the **population density**, which counts the number of people per square kilometer of land area.

Population projections attempt to predict changes in population size over time, and can be assisted by historical measures of growth, understanding of changes in social structure, and analysis of other demographic information. To aid in the construction of population projections, **population pyramids** provide a histogram of the population size of various age cohorts, as shown in Figure 11.7.

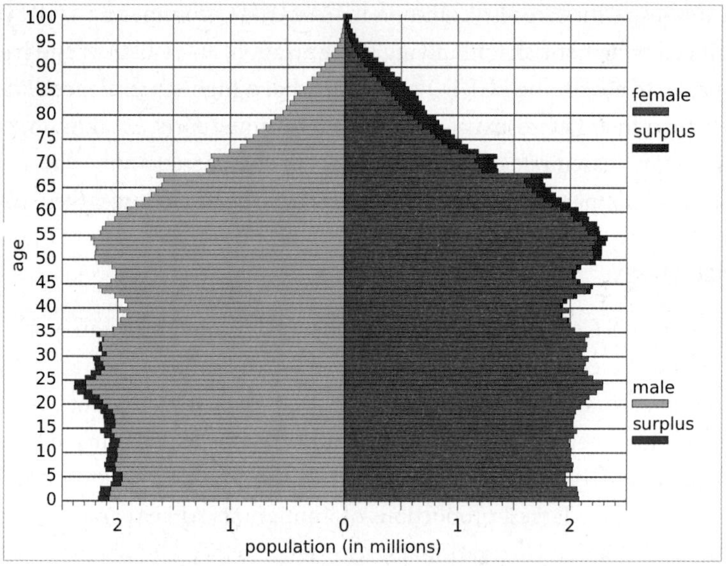

Figure 11.7 U.S. Population Pyramid, 2014

Surplus occurs when one gender has a larger population than another.

Fertility, Mortality, and Migration

KEY CONCEPT

Demographic statistics:

- Fertility rate = children per woman per lifetime
- Birth rate = children per 1000 people per year
- Mortality rate = deaths per 1000 people per year
- Migration rate = immigration rate minus emigration rate

The increased population of the United States is due to a number of factors that center around fertility, mortality, and migration. **Fertility rate** refers to the average number of children born to a woman over a lifetime in a population. In many parts of the world, fertility rate is the primary driver of population expansion; for example, in some parts of Africa, the average fertility rate is between four and eight children per woman, as seen in Figure 11.8. In the United States, fertility rates have trended downward over time; in 2013, the rate was still above two, indicating that fertility rates were still contributing to population growth.

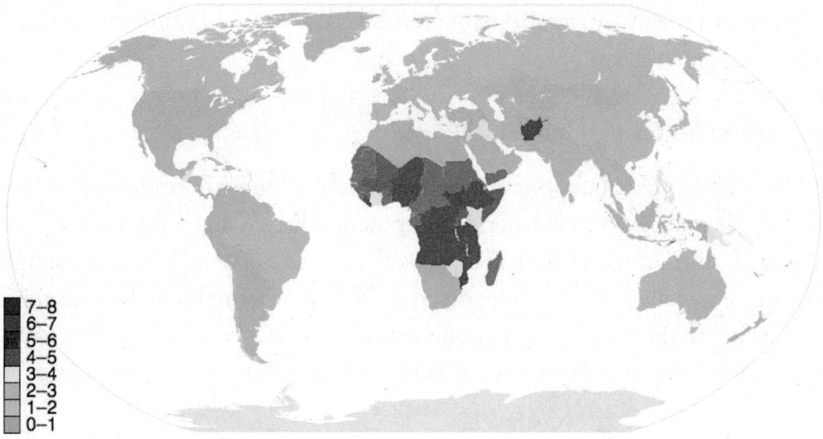

Figure 11.8 Fertility Rates around the World, 2013

Based on data from the CIA World Factbook; measured in children born per woman in the population

Mortality rates refer to the number of deaths in a population per unit time. Usually, this rate is measured in deaths per 1000 people per year. With advancements in healthcare and access, the mortality rate in the United States has dropped significantly over the past century. However, mortality rates are a significant brake on population growth in many parts of the world, as demonstrated in Figure 11.9. The decreased mortality rate in the United States is one contributor to the increase in average age of the population, as is a decreased fertility rate. In addition, the aging of the Baby Boomer generation, one of the largest generations in United States history, increases this average age. Both birth and mortality rates can be reported in multiple forms: the total rate for a population, the **crude rate** (adjusted to a certain population size over a specific period of time and multiplied by a constant to give a whole number), or age-specific rates.

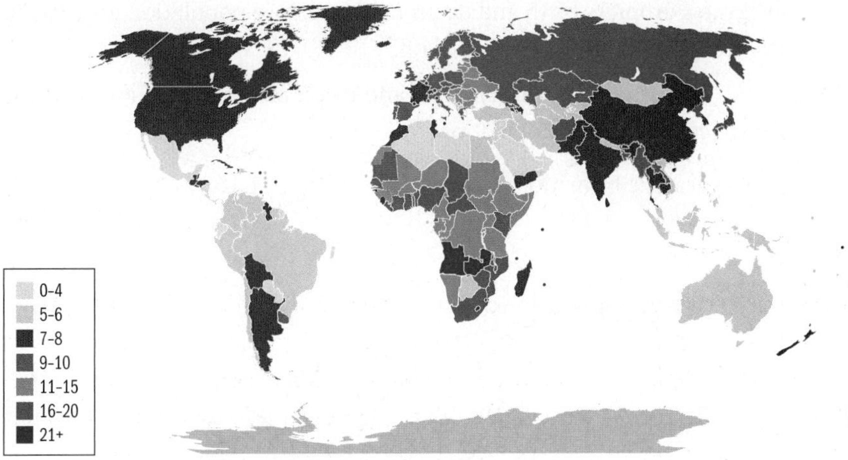

Figure 11.9 Mortality Rates around the World, 2009
Based on data from the CIA World Factbook; measured in deaths per 1000 individuals per year

Finally, **migration** is a contributor to population growth. **Immigration** is defined as movement into a new geographic space, whereas **emigration** is movement away from a geographic space. As described earlier, the United States continues to have larger net immigration than emigration, driving an increase in the population size. Immigration also increases the racial and ethnic diversity of the United States, as do increased mobility within the country and increases in intermarriage between different races and ethnicities. Migration can be motivated by both **pull factors**, which are positive attributes of the new location that attract new residents, and **push factors**, which are negative attributes of the old location that encourage existing residents to leave.

KEY CONCEPT

The United States population is getting bigger, older (average age has increased), and more diverse (through immigration, mobility, and intermarriage).

Demographic Transition Theory

While demographic shift refers to general changes in population makeup over time, **demographic transition** is a specific example of a demographic shift that occurs as a country develops from a preindustrial to an industrial economic system. Demographic transition has been seen in the United States since the Industrial Revolution and is currently occurring in many developing countries.

Demographic transition theory explains this link between economic development and demographic shift in four stages:

- **Stage 1**: Preindustrial society; birth and death rates are both high, resulting in a stable population.
- **Stage 2**: Economic progress leads to improvements to healthcare, nutrition, sanitation, and wages, causing a decrease in death rates. Thus, total population increases.
- **Stage 3**: Improvements in contraception, women's rights, and a shift from an agricultural to an industrial economy cause birth rates to drop. For example, with an industrializing society, children must go to school for many years to be productive in society and may need to be supported by parents for a longer period of time than was formerly the case. Thus families have fewer children, and birth rates drop. As birth and death rates equalize, population growth hits an inflection point and begins to level off.
- **Stage 4**: An industrialized society; birth and death rates are both low, resulting in a relative constant total population.

KEY CONCEPT

During demographic transition, mortality rate drops before birth rate. Therefore, the population grows at first while mortality rate is dropping, and then plateaus as the birth rate decreases as well.

A model of demographic transition can be seen in Figure 11.10.

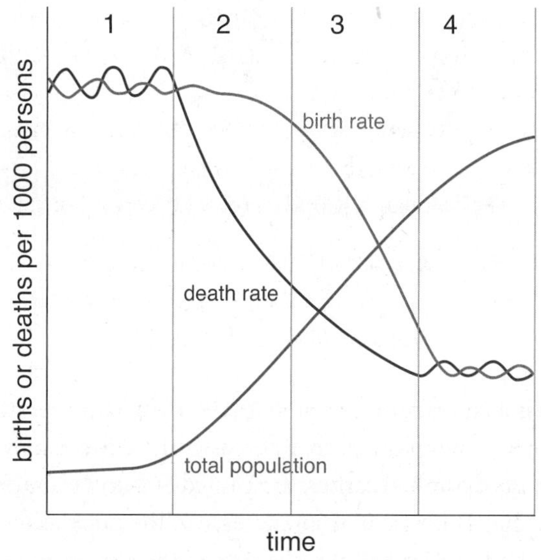

Figure 11.10 Demographic Transition

Recently, sociologists have described a fifth stage of demographic transition theory in which birth rates continue to drop and fall below the death rate, resulting in a decline of total population. Japan and Germany are currently experiencing demographic shifts expected in this theorized fifth stage.

Malthusian theory focuses on how the exponential growth of a population can outpace growth of the food supply and lead to social degradation and disorder. For example, some theorists predict that demographic transition among developing nations might cause growth in the world's population to outpace the world's ability to generate food. The resulting hypothetical mass starvation is called the Malthusian catastrophe. This result is similar to the death phase of bacterial growth, when resources in the environment have been depleted, as described in Chapter 1 of *MCAT Biology Review*.

Social Movements

Social movements are organized either to promote or to resist social change. These movements are often motivated by a group's perceived **relative deprivation**, which is a decrease in resources, representation, or agency relative to the whole of society, or relative to what the group is accustomed to from the past. Social movements that promote social change are termed **proactive**; those that resist social change are **reactive**. Members of social movements work to correct what they perceive as social injustices. Some examples of proactive movements include the civil rights movement, women's rights movement, gay rights movement, animal rights movement, and environmentalism movement. Some examples of reactive movements include the White supremacist movement, counterculture movement, antiglobalization movement, and anti-immigration movement. To further their goals, social movements may establish coordinated organizations. For example, some organizations associated with the proactive movements above include the National Association for the Advancement of Colored People (NAACP), American Civil Liberties Union (ACLU), Human Rights Campaign (HRC), Humane Society, and Greenpeace. Social movements may also seek to share their message through the media and demonstrations. Political involvement is also common through lobbying and donations.

Globalization

Globalization is the process of merging of the separate nations of the world into a single sociocultural entity, and is a relatively recent phenomenon spurred on by improvements in global communication technology and economic interdependence. Globalization leads to a decrease in the geographical constraints on social and cultural exchanges and can lead to both positive and negative effects. For example, the availability of foods (especially produce) from around the world during the entire calendar year can only be accomplished through trade with an extremely large number of world markets. However, significant worldwide unemployment, rising prices, increased pollution, civil unrest (particularly in unindustrialized or undemocratic nations), and global terrorism are negative effects of globalization.

Traditionally, the health sector has been organized at the national, state, or local level, but this is beginning to change. Groups such as the World Health Organization (WHO), the American Red Cross, and Doctors Without Borders supply aid to populations in need around the globe. Many medical schools are also increasing opportunities for medical students to complete rotations in other countries.

Urbanization

Urbanization refers to dense areas of population creating a pull for migration. In other words, cities are formed as individuals move into and establish residency in these new urban centers. Urbanization is not a new phenomenon; ancient populations established cities in Jerusalem, Athens, Timbuktu, and other locations. The economic opportunities offered in cities and creation of a large number of "world cities" has fueled an increase in urbanization during the last few decades. Currently, more than half of the world's populations live in what are considered urban areas. Sociologists and other professionals have found links between urban societies and health challenges related to water sanitation, air quality, environmental hazards, violence and injuries, infectious diseases, unhealthy diets, and physical inactivity.

Cities are rarely homogenous with respect to their population makeup. Most cities have areas that are more socioeconomically well-off and others that are more impoverished. Sometimes, members of specific racial, ethnic, or religious groups are concentrated in particular areas, usually due to social or economic inequities. In the most extreme cases, as shown in Figure 11.11, there arises an extremely densely populated area of a city with low-quality, often informal housing and poor sanitation.

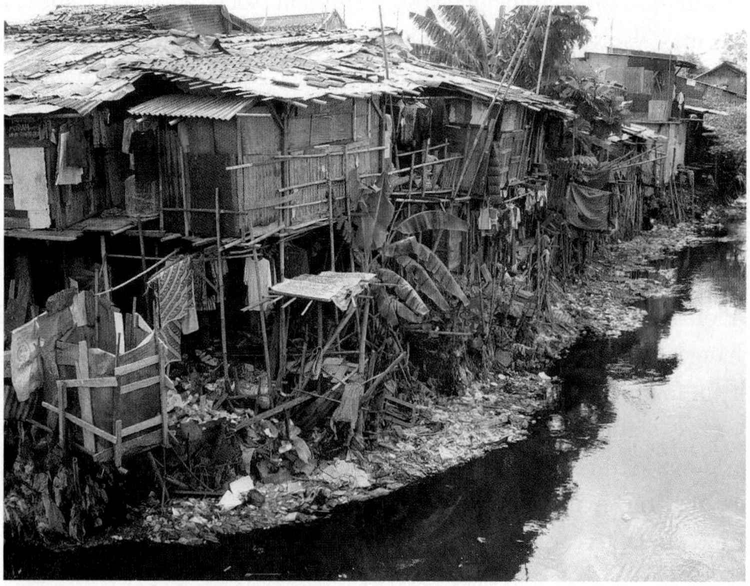

Figure 11.11 A Disadvantaged Area in Jakarta, Indonesia

MCAT CONCEPT CHECK 11.3

Before you move on, assess your understanding of the material with these questions.

1. What is the difference between race and ethnicity?

____

2. What is symbolic ethnicity?

____

3. Define the following demographic statistics:

    - Fertility rate:

    ____

    - Birth rate:

    ____

    - Mortality rate:

    ____

4. During demographic transition, what happens to the mortality rate? To the birth rate?

    - Mortality rate:

    ____

    - Birth rate:

    ____

5. What are the two types of social movements? How do they differ?

    - ____
    - ____

Conclusion

There are three major trends that are changing our nation's healthcare needs and our patient population. First, the increased diversity in the American population as a whole (from immigration, increased social and academic mobility, and interconnectedness through technology) puts us in front of patients whose thoughts and beliefs about health and well-being may be starkly different from our own. Second, increased access to healthcare through reform legislation has allowed millions of Americans to reach providers for the first time. Finally, our successes in medicine and public health have increased survival rates of many formerly fatal conditions and have enabled us to live longer. This leaves us with an aging population, in which individuals may be coping with multiple illnesses simultaneously.

To arm physicians of the future with the skills needed to take care of this population, many medical schools are increasing their coursework in interpersonal skills (*Doctor–Patient Relationship*; *Doctoring*; or *Physician, Patient, and Society* are such courses at various schools), as well as **cultural sensitivity**, the recognition and respect of differences between cultures, and research ethics. This is part of the biopsychosocial model of medicine described in Chapter 7 of *MCAT Behavioral Sciences Review*. Knowledge of the structure of society and how it shifts over time, as explained in this chapter, will enhance your ability to communicate with patients. Unlike the old model of *doctor knows best* (often referred to as the paternalistic approach to medicine), today's doctors must work together with patients to find solutions to their health problems. By working with patients on their own terms, you will be able to help maintain and improve their health status and begin to correct the health inequities that exist in today's population. In the next chapter—the last of *MCAT Behavioral Sciences Review*—we will explore these inequities in resources, health status, and healthcare.

You've reviewed the content, now test your knowledge and critical thinking skills by completing a test-like passage set in your online resources!

GO ONLINE

CONCEPT SUMMARY

Sociology: Theories and Institutions

- Theoretical approaches provide frameworks for the interactions we observe within society.
  - **Functionalism** focuses on the function of each component of society and how those components fit together. **Manifest functions** are deliberate actions that serve to help a given system; **latent functions** are unexpected, unintended, or unrecognized positive consequences of manifest functions.
  - **Conflict theory** focuses on how power differentials are created and how these differentials contribute to the maintenance of social order.
  - **Symbolic interactionism** is the study of the ways individuals interact through a shared understanding of words, gestures, and other symbols.
  - **Social constructionism** explores the ways in which individuals and groups make decisions to agree upon a given social reality.
  - **Rational choice theory** states that individuals will make decisions that maximize potential benefit and minimize potential harm; **exchange theory** applies rational choice theory within social groups.
  - **Feminist theory** critiques the institutional power structures that disadvantage women in society.
- **Social institutions** are well-established social structures that dictate certain patterns of behavior or relationships and are accepted as a fundamental part of culture. Common social institutions include the family, education, religion, government and the economy, and health and medicine.
- There are four key ethical tenets of American medicine.
  - **Beneficence** refers to acting in the patient's best interest.
  - **Nonmaleficence** refers to avoiding treatments for which risk is larger than benefit.
  - **Respect for autonomy** refers to respecting patients' rights to make decisions about their own healthcare.
  - **Justice** refers to treating similar patients similarly and distributing healthcare resources fairly.

Culture

- **Culture** encompasses the lifestyle of a group of people and includes both material and symbolic elements.
  - **Material culture** includes the physical items one associates with a given group, such as artwork, emblems, clothing, jewelry, foods, buildings, and tools.
  - **Symbolic culture** includes the ideas associated with a cultural group.
- **Cultural lag** refers to the idea that material culture changes more quickly than symbolic culture.
- A **cultural barrier** is a social difference that impedes interaction.
- **Language** consists of spoken, signed, or written symbols combined into a system and governed by rules.
- A **value** is what a person deems important in life.
- A **belief** is something a person considers to be true.
- A **ritual** is a formalized ceremonial behavior in which members of a group or community regularly engage. It is governed by specific rules, including appropriate behavior and a predetermined order of events.
- **Norms** are societal rules that define the boundaries of acceptable behavior.
- There is evidence that culture flows from evolutionary principles, and that culture can also influence evolution.

Demographics

- **Demographics** refer to the statistics of populations and are the mathematical applications of sociology. One can analyze hundreds of demographic variables; some of the most common are age, gender, race and ethnicity, sexual orientation, and immigration status.
  - **Ageism** is prejudice or discrimination on the basis of a person's age.
  - **Gender** is the set of behavioral, cultural, or psychological traits typically associated with a biological sex. **Gender inequality** is the intentional or unintentional empowerment of one gender to the detriment of the other.
  - **Race** is a social construct based on phenotypic differences between groups of people; these may be either real or perceived differences.
  - **Ethnicity** is also a social construct that sorts people by cultural factors, including language, nationality, religion, and other factors. **Symbolic ethnicity** is recognition of an ethnic identity that is only relevant on special occasions or in specific circumstances and does not specifically impact everyday life.
  - **Sexual orientation** can be defined by one's sexual interest toward members of same or different genders.
  - **Immigration** is the movement into a new geographic area. **Emigration** is the movement away from a geographic area.

- A **fertility rate** is the average number of children born to a woman over a lifetime in a population. A **birth rate** is relative to a population size over time, usually measured as the number of births per 1000 people per year.
- A **mortality rate** is the average number of deaths per population size over time, usually measured as the number of deaths per 1000 people per year.
- **Migration** refers to the movement of people from one geographic location to another.
- **Demographic transition** is a model used to represent drops in birth and death rates as a result of industrialization.
- **Social movements** are organized to either promote (**proactive**) or resist (**reactive**) social change.
- **Globalization** is the process of integrating a global economy with free trade and tapping of foreign labor markets.
- **Urbanization** refers to the process of dense areas of population creating a pull for migration or, in other words, creating cities.

ANSWERS TO CONCEPT CHECKS

11.1

1. Manifest functions are actions that are intended to help some part of a system. Latent functions are unintended, unstated, or unrecognized positive consequences of these actions on society.

2.

Theoretical Approach	Primary Thesis or Idea
Functionalism	Each part of society serves a function; when these functions work together correctly, society overall can function normally
Conflict theory	Power differentials are created when groups compete for economic, social, and political resources; these differentials contribute to the maintenance of social order
Symbolic interactionism	Humans communicate through words, gestures, and other symbols to which we attach meaning
Social constructionism	Individuals and groups make decisions to agree upon a given social reality
Rational choice theory	Individuals will make decisions that maximize potential benefit and minimize potential harm
Feminist theory	Critiques the institutional power structures that disadvantage women in society

3.

Ethical Principle	Description
Beneficence	Act in the patient's best interest
Nonmaleficence	*Do no harm*; avoid interventions where the potential for harm outweighs the potential for benefit
Respect for autonomy	Respect patients' decisions and choices about their own healthcare
Justice	Treat similar patients with similar care; distribute healthcare resources fairly

11.2

1. Material culture focuses on the artifacts associated with a group: the physical objects, such as artwork, emblems, clothing, jewelry, foods, buildings, and tools. Symbolic culture focuses on the ideas and principles that belong to a particular group.
2. A value is what a person deems to be important; a belief is what a person deems to be true. While these terms are often used interchangeably in everyday life, they have specific definitions in the social sciences.

11.3

1. Race is based on phenotypic differences between groups of people. Ethnicity is based on common language, religion, nationality, or other cultural factors.
2. Symbolic ethnicity is recognition of an ethnic identity on special occasions or in specific circumstances, but not during everyday life.
3. Fertility rate is the average number of children a woman has over a lifetime in a population. Birth rate is the number of births in a population per unit time, usually measured as births per 1000 people per year. Mortality rate is the number of deaths in a population per unit time, usually measured as deaths per 1000 people per year.
4. During demographic transition, both the mortality and birth rates decrease.
5. Proactive social movements are in favor of a specific social change. Reactive social movements run against a specific social change.

SCIENCE MASTERY ASSESSMENT EXPLANATIONS

1. **A**

A manifest function is an intended positive effect on a system. A latent function is an unintended positive effect on a system, **(C)**. A negative effect on a system, **(B)** and **(D)**, is termed a dysfunction.

2. **C**

Symbolic interactionism studies how individuals interact through a shared understanding of words, gestures, and other symbols. A nod is thus a symbol in many cultures that signifies "yes."

3. **D**

The principle of nonmaleficence states that physicians must not only act in their patient's best interest (beneficence, **(B)**), but must also avoid treatments where the potential for harm outweighs the potential for benefit.

4. **C**

Although one's dominant physical features are associated with race, this man's preferences are those of Latino ethnicity and culture. Ethnicity is a social construct that considers language, religion, nationality, and cultural factors. Culture relates to a group's way of life; the preferences listed in the question are examples of material and symbolic culture.

5. **D**

In the United States, it is not a common practice to say, "I love you," and hug one's physician after each routine checkup; therefore, this behavior could be considered deviant, going against the social norm. Values, **(C)**, are what an individual deems to be important.

6. **B**

Both birth rate and mortality rate can be measured per 1000 people per year. Fertility rate is measured in number of children per woman over a lifetime.

7. **B**

Rituals are formalized ceremonial behaviors in which members of a group or community regularly engage. Therefore, these activities are examples of rituals performed for healing.

8. **A**

With a decrease in mortality rate and a higher immigration rate than emigration rate, the United States population continues to grow, with an increasing average age and increasing racial and ethnic diversity.

9. **C**

Material culture includes any cultural artifact—an object to which meaning is assigned. Values are ideas, which are associated with symbolic culture.

10. **D**

During demographic transition, both birth rates and mortality rates are high in stage 1, **(A)**. Mortality rates drop during stage 2, **(B)**, and then birth rates drop during stage 3, **(C)**. In stage 4, both birth rates and mortality rates are low.

11. **D**

In this scenario, a group is fighting for social power, which is an aspect of conflict theory. Further, this group is an example of a reactive social movement because it is running counter to social change. The fact that gambling had been legalized implies the involvement of the government, a social institution.

12. **C**

This man is describing his sexuality as mostly homosexual, although he has also had some heterosexual attractions. The Kinsey scale scores a 6, **(D)**, as exclusively homosexual. A score of 3 would equate to bisexuality. Thus, this man would likely score a 4 or 5.

13. **B**

Sex is determined by one's genotype, and therefore is biologically determined. Gender, **(A)**, may or may not match biological sex and therefore is not biologically determined. Ethnicity, **(C)**, is a social construct that sorts people by cultural factors, and therefore is not biologically determined. Sexual orientation, **(D)**, may have some biological component, but the relative role of biology and environment is not yet known.

14. **B**

If the immigration rate in a geographic area is larger than the emigration rate, then there is a larger influx than efflux of people. This will increase the population of that area.

15. **A**

Urbanization is the migration of people into urban centers to create cities. The increased population density should provide additional opportunities for social interaction, not decreased opportunities.

Consult your online resources for additional practice. GO ONLINE

SHARED CONCEPTS

Behavioral Sciences Chapter 6
Identity and Personality

Behavioral Sciences Chapter 8
Social Processes, Attitudes, and Behavior

Behavioral Sciences Chapter 9
Social Interaction

Behavioral Sciences Chapter 10
Social Thinking

Behavioral Sciences Chapter 12
Social Stratification

Biology Chapter 12
Genetics and Evolution

CHAPTER 12

SOCIAL STRATIFICATION

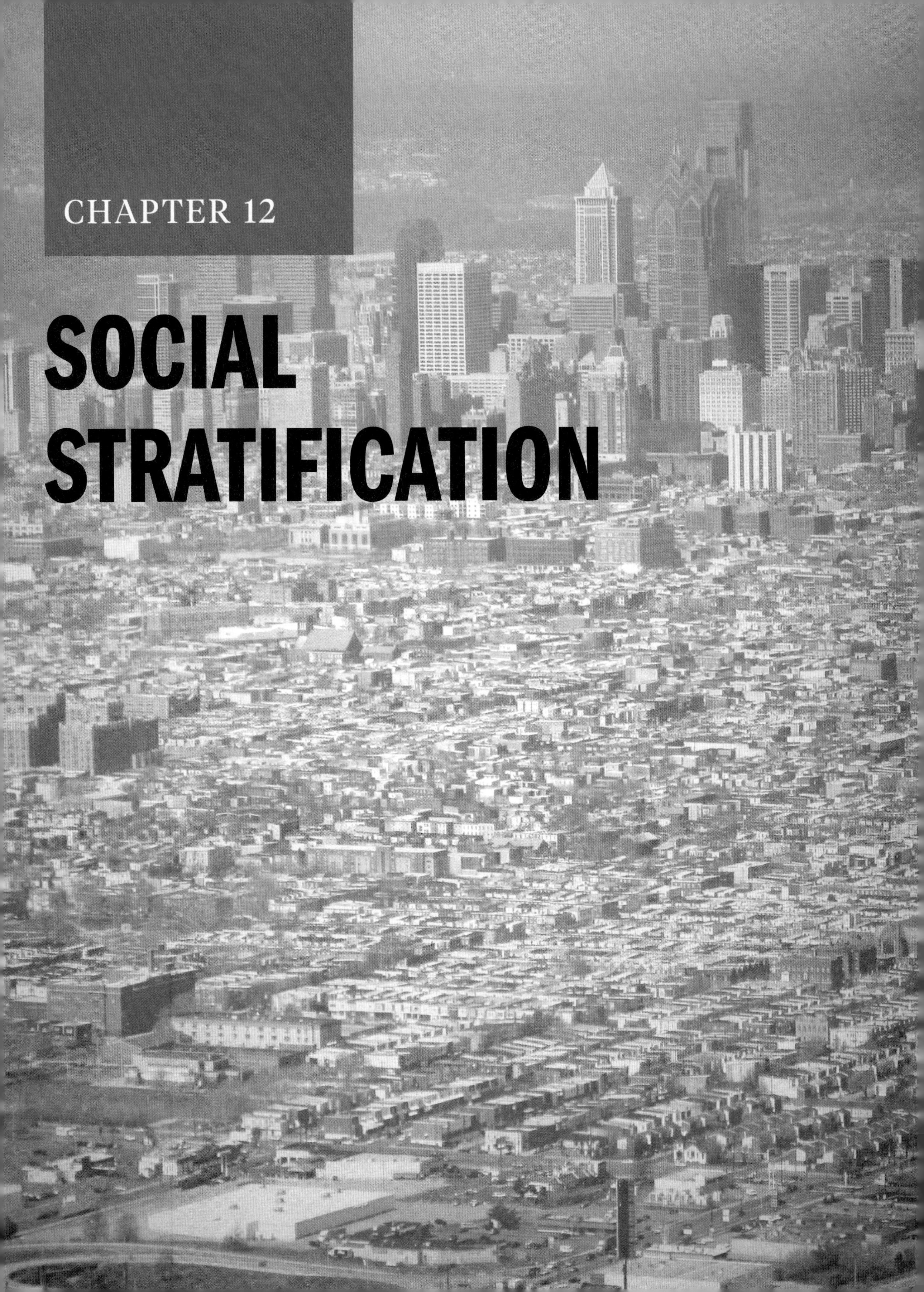

SCIENCE MASTERY ASSESSMENT

Every pre-med knows this feeling: there is so much content I have to know for the MCAT! How do I know what to do first or what's important?

While the high-yield badges throughout this book will help you identify the most important topics, this Science Mastery Assessment is another tool in your MCAT prep arsenal. This quiz (which can also be taken in your online resources) and the guidance below will help ensure that you are spending the appropriate amount of time on this chapter based on your personal strengths and weaknesses. Don't worry though—skipping something now does not mean you'll never study it. Later on in your prep, as you complete full-length tests, you'll uncover specific pieces of content that you need to review and can come back to these chapters as appropriate.

How to Use This Assessment

If you answer 0–7 questions correctly:

Spend about 1 hour to read this chapter in full and take limited notes throughout. Follow up by reviewing **all** quiz questions to ensure that you now understand how to solve each one.

If you answer 8–11 questions correctly:

Spend 20–40 minutes reviewing the quiz questions. Beginning with the questions you missed, read and take notes on the corresponding subchapters. For questions you answered correctly, ensure your thinking matches that of the explanation and you understand why each choice was correct or incorrect.

If you answer 12–15 questions correctly:

Spend less than 20 minutes reviewing all questions from the quiz. If you missed any, then include a quick read-through of the corresponding subchapters, or even just the relevant content within a subchapter, as part of your question review. For questions you answered correctly, ensure your thinking matches that of the explanation and review the Concept Summary at the end of the chapter.

1. Which of the following best describes the component of socioeconomic status attributable to direct individual efforts?
   - **A.** Ascribed status
   - **B.** Meritocratic competition
   - **C.** Anomic condition
   - **D.** Achieved status

2. Which of the following displays a correct association?
   - **A.** High social networking and low social capital
   - **B.** High social mobility and low social capital
   - **C.** Low social class and low social capital
   - **D.** Low social networking and high social capital

3. Which of the following phenomena are LEAST likely to coincide?
   - **A.** Hazardous waste facilities and low-income neighborhoods
   - **B.** Tuberculosis and poor living conditions
   - **C.** Environmental pollution and populations of underrepresented groups
   - **D.** Globalization and global equality

4. Which of the following trends is most likely FALSE?
   - **A.** Mortality rates are increased in groups with low income.
   - **B.** Life expectancy is decreased in groups with high income.
   - **C.** Birth weights are decreased in children of low-income women.
   - **D.** Rates of lung cancer are increased in low-income groups.

Questions 5–6 refer to the scenario described below.

A small town has 1000 residents, including 500 males and 500 females. In this town, 20 of the males have prostate cancer. During a calendar year, 10 more males are diagnosed with prostate cancer. Assume none of the males are cured or die during the year.

5. What is the prevalence of prostate cancer in the population that can develop the condition at the end of the year?
   - **A.** $10 \div 480$
   - **B.** $10 \div 1000$
   - **C.** $20 \div 500$
   - **D.** $30 \div 500$

6. What is the incidence of prostate cancer in this population during the year?
   - **A.** $10 \div 480$
   - **B.** $10 \div 1000$
   - **C.** $20 \div 500$
   - **D.** $30 \div 1000$

7. A low-income single parent works a part-time job and lives in a small apartment in the city. When the single parent's children grow up, they take similar jobs and live in similar housing. This is an example of:
   - **A.** upward social mobility.
   - **B.** downward social mobility.
   - **C.** social exclusion.
   - **D.** social reproduction.

8. Which of the following is true with regard to relative poverty?
   - **A.** Individuals in relative poverty have incomes below the poverty line.
   - **B.** Individuals in relative poverty exhibit downward social mobility.
   - **C.** Individuals in relative poverty may be in the upper class.
   - **D.** Individuals in relative poverty exhibit upward social mobility.

9. In comparison to urban centers, suburbs tend to have:
   - **A.** larger racially and ethnically underrepresented populations.
   - **B.** higher rates of poverty.
   - **C.** larger upper- and middle-class populations.
   - **D.** higher rates of crime and homicide.

10. Which of the following terms refers to the burden or degree of disease associated with a given illness?
    - **A.** Morbidity
    - **B.** Mortality
    - **C.** Second sickness
    - **D.** Chronicity

11. Compared to White Americans, which of the following racial or ethnic groups tends to have a better overall health profile?
    - **A.** African Americans
    - **B.** Asian Americans
    - **C.** Hispanic Americans
    - **D.** American Indians

12. Which of the following best describes the populations targeted by Medicare and Medicaid, respectively?
    - **A.** Medicare: mostly patients without employer-guaranteed healthcare; Medicaid: mostly patients who have recently immigrated
    - **B.** Medicare: mostly patients who have recently immigrated; Medicaid: mostly patients without employer-guaranteed healthcare
    - **C.** Medicare: mostly patients in older age groups; Medicaid: mostly patients with low socioeconomic status
    - **D.** Medicare: mostly patients with low socioeconomic status; Medicaid: mostly patients in older age groups

13. Morbidity is increased in low-income groups because of all of the following EXCEPT:
    - **A.** higher rates of obesity.
    - **B.** less access to healthcare.
    - **C.** higher rates of homicide.
    - **D.** lower rates of physical activity.

14. Hypertension (high blood pressure) can be diagnosed by having two or more blood pressure readings higher than 140/90 on two different occasions, separated by a week. Suppose that the criteria were changed to include anyone with a reading higher than 130/80 on at least one occasion. How would this change the prevalence of diagnosed hypertension in the population?
    - **A.** The prevalence would increase.
    - **B.** The prevalence would decrease.
    - **C.** The prevalence would remain the same.
    - **D.** There is not enough information to determine the change in prevalence.

15. Which of the following trends regarding healthcare disparities has NOT been documented?
    - **A.** Females are more likely to be insured than males.
    - **B.** Primary care use is more likely among males than females.
    - **C.** Low-income individuals have more difficulty accessing care than high-income individuals.
    - **D.** LGBTQ individuals have more barriers to healthcare than other individuals.

Answer Key

1. **D**
2. **C**
3. **D**
4. **B**
5. **D**
6. **A**
7. **D**
8. **C**
9. **C**
10. **A**
11. **B**
12. **C**
13. **C**
14. **A**
15. **B**

Detailed explanations can be found at the end of the chapter.

CHAPTER 12

SOCIAL STRATIFICATION

In This Chapter

CHAPTER PROFILE

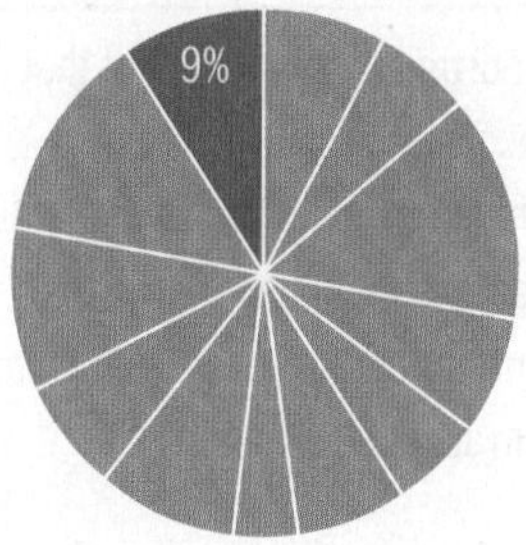

The content in this chapter should be relevant to about 9% of all questions about the behavioral sciences on the MCAT.

This chapter covers material from the following AAMC content categories:

8B: Social thinking

8C: Social interactions

10A: Social inequality

Introduction

The wonderfully witty Oscar Wilde once said, "Work is the curse of the drinking classes." While this quote is intended to be humorous, it does speak to the stereotypical characteristics associated with socioeconomic class. Some Americans think that class and social stratification are nonissues in our society. Unlike earlier feudal societies, most Americans are not royals or gentry, possessing inherited titles, land, or palaces; we're often considered to be a much more equality-oriented society, in keeping with our constitutional ideals. Yet how do we explain such differences in wealth, power, and privilege as a Manhattan lawyer driving a shiny Porsche past a homeless person rooting through a trash can? Such scenes make it hard to ignore the uneven distributions of material wealth and the overall social inequality in the United States.

To understand social inequalities in America and how such disparities impact health and healthcare services, we will examine several aspects of social stratification in terms of class, status, and social capital and how these intersect with race, gender, and age. We will also focus on patterns of social mobility and how poverty and location play major roles in health and illness. Later, we will connect how race, gender, and socioeconomic inequalities impact health profiles and access to quality healthcare.

12.1 Social Class

High-Yield

LEARNING OBJECTIVES

After Chapter 12.1, you will be able to:

- Explain how socioeconomic status of an individual or a community is determined
- Define social capital and social cohesion
- Identify groups that suffer disproportionate social inequality
- Describe the relationship between social mobility and merit

KEY CONCEPT

It's important to keep in mind that socioeconomic status is not only determined by merit (achieved status), but also external characteristics or outward appearances like skin color and gender (ascribed status).

BRIDGE

There are three major types of status: ascribed, achieved, and master status. While ascribed and achieved statuses are described here, remember that a master status is one that pervades all aspects of an individual's life. The role of statuses in social interaction is discussed in Chapter 9 of *MCAT Behavioral Sciences Review*.

A **social class** is defined as a category of people who share a similar socioeconomic position in society, and can be identified by looking at the economic opportunities, job positions, lifestyles, attitudes, and behaviors of a given slice of society. **Social cohesion**, or social integration, refers to the solidarity and sense of connectedness among different social groups and social classes in society.

Aspects of Social Stratification

Social stratification focuses on social inequalities and studies the basic question of who gets what and why. Social stratification is thus related to one's **socioeconomic status (SES)**, which may depend on ascribed or achieved status, and causes the emergence of status hierarchies. **Ascribed status** derives from clearly identifiable characteristics, such as age, gender, and skin color; **achieved status** is acquired via direct, individual efforts. In other words, ascribed status is involuntary, while achieved status is obtained through hard work or merit. An important factor in achieved status is **educational attainment**, which is the highest degree obtained, or number of years of education completed. Caste and estate systems stratify by ascribed SES, while class systems stratify by achieved SES. After breaking free from British colonial rule, the United States moved toward a class-based system of social stratification.

Class, Status, and Power

There are three major classes—upper, middle, and lower—although these vary to different degrees in different locations. The upper class consists of those who have great wealth, along with recognized reputations and lifestyles, and have a larger influence on society's political and economic systems. In other words, the upper class has a high concentration of prestige and power. The middle class can be further divided into three levels: upper-middle, middle-middle, and lower-middle class. The middle class includes successful business and professional people (upper-middle), those who have been unable to achieve the upper-middle lifestyle because of educational and economic shortcomings (middle-middle), and those who are skilled and semiskilled workers with fewer luxuries (lower-middle). The lower class includes people who have lower incomes, and has a greatly reduced amount of sociopolitical power. The proportional improvement in healthcare as one moves up in socioeconomic status is called the **socioeconomic gradient** in health and development.

Prestige refers to the amount of positive regard society has for a given person or idea. Certain occupations, such as physicians, are broadly viewed with high levels of status, respect, and importance. Particular educational institutions, organizations, awards, and accolades may also be considered prestigious.

Power can be described as the ability to affect others' behavior through real or perceived rewards and punishments, and is based on the unequal distribution of valued resources. At its core, power defines the relationship between individuals, groups, and social institutions. Power relationships function to maintain order, organize economic systems, conduct warfare, and rule over and exploit people. As a result, power creates worldwide social inequalities as people tend to fall somewhere within the *haves* and the *have-nots*.

You may recall from Chapter 11 of *MCAT Behavioral Sciences Review* that Marxist theory, also called conflict theory, proposes that the *have-nots*, called the proletariat, could overthrow the *haves*, called the bourgeoisie, as well as the entire capitalist economy by developing class consciousness. **Class consciousness** refers to the organization of the working class around shared goals and recognition of a need for collective political action. By working together as one unit, the proletariat could revolt and take control of the political and economic system, laying the groundwork for a socialist state. The one major barrier to class consciousness, however, is **false consciousness**, a misperception of one's actual position within society. Members of the proletariat either do not see just how bad conditions are, do not recognize the commonalities between their own experiences and others, or otherwise are too clouded to assemble into the revolutionaries Marx envisioned.

Even in developed countries of the modern, globalized world, social inequality persists. Early sociologists explained that social inequality is further accelerated by what is called **anomie**, which refers to a lack of widely accepted social norms and the breakdown of social bonds between an individual and society. **Strain theory** focuses on how anomic conditions can lead to deviance. Anomic conditions include excessive individualism, social inequality, and isolation; these all erode **social solidarity**, which is the sense of community and social cohesion. Other sociologists have focused on the importance of social trust in the proper functioning of civil society. Social trust comes from two primary sources: social norms of reciprocity (*I'll scratch your back if you scratch mine*) and social networks. In the past several decades, as some societies have become more urbanized, self-oriented, and materialistic, associational ties have diminished and consequently have led to a decline in social capital. But what is the relationship between social stratification, social capital, and power?

KEY CONCEPT

Anomic conditions in postindustrial modern life have accelerated the decline of social inclusion and, as a result, have further obstructed opportunities to acquire social capital.

Social Capital

Essentially, **social capital** is the investment people make in their society in return for economic or collective rewards; the greater the investment, the higher the level of **social integration**, which is the movement of new or underrepresented populations into a larger culture while maintaining their ethnic identities. One of the main forms of social capital is the social network. Social networks can create two types of social inequality: situational (socioeconomic advantage) and positional (based on how connected one is within a network and one's centrality within that network). Inequality in networks creates and reinforces **privilege**, which is inequality in opportunity. Moreover, low social capital leads to greater social inequality. As social capital refers to the benefits one receives from group association, **cultural capital** refers to the benefits one receives from knowledge, abilities, and skills.

REAL WORLD

People who experience poor mental health are one of the largest disadvantaged groups to lack both strong and weak ties. Due to repercussions of social exclusion, these individuals may find that social capital is out of their reach. Consequently, this group is personally and socially disempowered, further propelling a cycle of exclusion. Social exclusion has huge financial repercussions on healthcare, with greater morbidity rates.

Communities are joined together through what are called strong and weak ties. **Strong ties** refer to peer group and kinship contacts, which are quantitatively small but qualitatively powerful. **Weak ties** refer to social connections that are personally superficial, such as associates, but that are large in number and provide connections to a wide range of other individuals. Social networking websites—especially those focusing on professional relationships—are examples of groups of weak ties. People without multiple weak ties, such as disadvantaged groups, may find accessing and contributing to social capital extremely difficult.

Intersections with Race, Gender, and Age

Social stratification, or, more properly, social inequality, remains higher among certain disadvantaged groups than others, including groups who are racially and ethnically underrepresented (especially Hispanic and African American people), households headed by women, and older adults. Think about who you know that may fall into these underprivileged or underserved groups. Your friends? Your relatives? Yourself? Socioeconomic inequalities remain in the United States. As described in Chapter 11 of *MCAT Behavioral Sciences Review*, this continued socioeconomic inequality is partially due to **intersectionality**—the compounding of disadvantage seen in individuals who belong to more than one underserved group.

Patterns of Social Mobility

Unlike a caste-based or estate-based system of social stratification, people in North America generally have the ability to move up or down from one class to another. In a class system, **social mobility**, also known as **structural mobility**, is typically the result of an economic and occupational structure that allows one to acquire higher-level employment opportunities given proper credentials and experience requirements. In the United States, the class system encourages this type of ambition through dedication and hard work, an ethos embodied in the phrase *The American Dream*.

Intergenerational and Intragenerational Mobility

Social mobility can either occur within a generation or across generations. **Intragenerational mobility** refers to changes in social status that happen within a person's lifetime, while **intergenerational mobility** refers to changes in social status from parents to children. Many people consider the United States to be *the land of opportunity*, where intragenerational and intergenerational mobility can easily occur. However, others argue that opportunities for social mobility are diminishing because the gap between the upper class and the middle and lower classes continues to widen.

MCAT EXPERTISE

For the guided example that follows, we were able to answer part of the question very quickly. On Test Day, all questions are multiple choice, so as soon as you have even part of the answer to a question, you can look at the answers and eliminate any that aren't a match.

BEHAVIORAL SCIENCES GUIDED EXAMPLE WITH EXPERT THINKING

Social class differences are related to health and mortality outcomes as a result of differences in stress, financial strain, and working conditions, among others. The present study focused on incidence of psychiatric disorder and its relation to social class, and social mobility as compared to parental social status in predicting mental health outcomes.

Purpose: evaluate relationship between psych disorders and socioeconomic status/social mobility

Researchers conducted a longitudinal study to target this relationship. Participants were adults born between 1949 and 1959. Participants' adult social class between 1980 and 1990 was coded by occupation type and compared to parental social class at participants' birth. Researchers then noted participants' psychiatric admissions between 1990 and 2005. Results are summarized in Figures 1 and 2.

Standard longitudinal study: collected outcome data over 15 years.

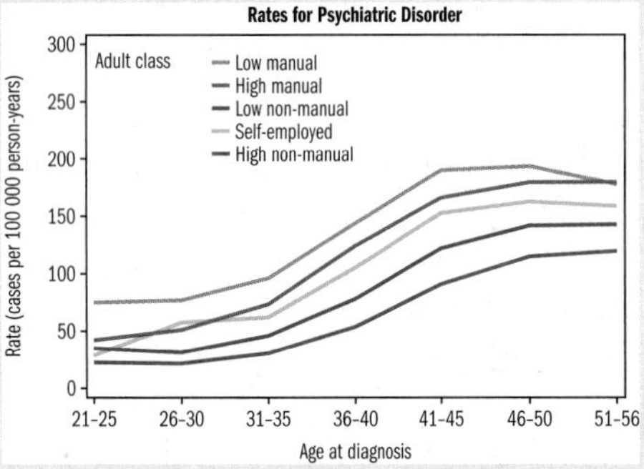

Figure 1 Incidence of psychiatric disorder by social class

IV: age, class

DV: rate of psychiatric cases

Results agree with the trend from the introduction, though not sure how self-employed fits.

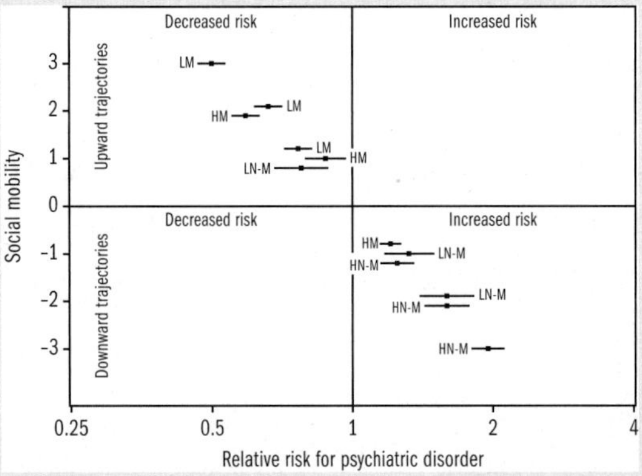

This figure is challenging, I will have to make sure to use the variable descriptions from the figure label to interpret. It looks like the LM (low manual) line in the top right corner means that this person's parents were LM and their own mobility is +3, which would put them at HN-M (high non-manual). These individuals have a 0.5 relative risk compared to LM individuals whose parents were LM, meaning that they're half as likely to develop mental health issues. The overall trend is linear and seems strong: higher upward mobility means lower risk.

Figure 2 Risk for psychiatric disorder resulting from social mobility compared to that of subjects who were socially stable. Social mobility scale and labels for confidence intervals are based on parental status, in order from high to low: high non-manual, low non-manual, high manual, low manual.

Figure label defines the variables, but I'll have to identify the relationship between them. The first letter of each word is the label in the graph.

Adapted from: Tiikkaja S, Sandin S, Malki N, Modin B, Sparén P, Hultman CM (2013) Social Class, Social Mobility and Risk of Psychiatric Disorder—A Population-Based Longitudinal Study. *PLoS ONE* 8(11): e77975. https://doi.org/10.1371/journal.pone.0077975

Researchers examined the records of three individuals: Person A (HM, parental class HN-M), Person B (LM, parental class LN-M), and Person C (HM, parental class HM). What can be predicted about the comparative risk of psychiatric disorder for A, B, and C?

This question is asking for a direct application of the results of the study, so the first thing to do to answer the question is to take a deeper look at the figures and determine what can be learned about these three individuals. Figure 1 gives overall incidence of mental health diagnoses for each class, and it looks like risk is inversely proportional to social class: people in lower social classes have a higher risk for psychiatric disorder. We can use this information alone to answer part of the question: Because the social class of person A is HM, i.e. "high manual," and the social class of person B is LM, i.e. "low manual," person B is in a lower social class and is therefore overall more likely to develop a psychiatric disorder.

Figure 2 is a little tougher to interpret, but we can start by finding the region of the graph where persons A and B would be located. Person A has parents in the HN-M class, but is in the HM class, for a mobility of −2. Person B has the same mobility, −2, from LN-M to LM. Looking at the data for individuals at −2 mobility, both persons A and B are about 1.75 times more likely to develop a psychiatric disorder than members of their respective social class with stable mobility. So, although person A will have a lower overall risk compared to person B due to social class, both persons A and B will have an elevated risk compared to socially stable members of their respective social class.

By contrast, person C shares a social class with their parents, meaning no additional risk is conferred to person C by downward social mobility. Given that persons A and C are in the same social class, but person C did not experience intergenerational downward mobility, person C would be expected to have a lower risk of disorder than person A.

Therefore, in order of risk, person C is at the lowest risk for psychiatric disorder based on the results of this study, followed by person A, with person B at the highest risk for psychiatric disorder based on both social status and downward social mobility.

Meritocracy

One of the largest factors driving American social mobility has been meritocratic competition or a merit-based system of social mobility. **Meritocracy** is a social structure in which intellectual talent and achievement are means for a person to advance up the social ladder. Given the rising levels of social inequality and concentration of wealth in the United States, some argue that motivation, a strong work ethic, a conscientious drive, and mastery of skills no longer offer the same opportunities for advancement. Some fear that the US meritocratic system is quickly becoming a **plutocracy**, or a rule by the upper classes. Nonetheless, merit still plays a key role in many segments of society, but merit does not always guarantee positive social mobility.

Upward and Downward Mobility

Social mobility usually occurs in one of two directions: up or down. Upward and downward mobility both refer to patterns of **vertical mobility**, or movement from one social class to another. **Upward mobility** is a positive change in a person's social status, resulting in a higher position. **Downward mobility** is the opposite: a negative change in a person's social status, wherein they fall to a lower position. Social mobility is often directly correlated with education, although other factors can contribute to upward mobility as well. Some of the best examples of upward mobility are seen with professional athletes, professional musicians, and entrepreneurs. So, in addition to education, athletics, music, and greater opportunities for small businesses may offer disadvantaged individuals more potential ladders to a higher social status.

Horizontal Mobility

Horizontal mobility is a change in occupation or lifestyle by an individual that keeps that individual within the same social class. For example, a construction worker who switches jobs to work in custodial services or mechanical maintenance has made a shift in occupation but typically remains in the lower-middle class.

Poverty

Poverty is defined by low socioeconomic status and a lack of possessions or financial resources. Poverty can be handed down from generation to generation, and can be defined on its own terms or in comparison to the rest of the population.

Social Reproduction

Social inequality, especially poverty (but also inherited wealth), can be reproduced or passed on from one generation to the next. This idea is referred to as **social reproduction**. Some consider social reproduction to be a cycle-of-poverty explanation for social inequality. In other words, the lifestyle of poverty, powerlessness, isolation, and even apathy is handed down from one generation to another as a feature of the society. However, there are many other factors that contribute to poverty, including where one lives and an emphasis on present orientation, in which people do not plan for the future. One theory, that of **structural poverty**, is based on the concept of "holes" in the structure of society being more responsible for poverty than the actions of any individual. Proponents of structural poverty argue that the same individuals do not by necessity occupy these "holes" from year to year, but the percentage of a society that falls under the poverty line stays relatively constant due to their existence. To understand how poverty is reproduced, it may be helpful to examine what types of poverty exist.

Absolute and Relative

On an **absolute** level, poverty is a socioeconomic condition in which people do not have enough money or resources to maintain a quality of living that includes basic life necessities such as shelter, food, clothing, and water. This absolute poverty view applies across locations, countries, and cultures. Poverty can also be defined as **relative**, in which people have less income and wealth in comparison to the larger population in which they live. For example, surviving on a low teaching salary while living in the Upper East Side of Manhattan may very well be considered poor relative to the other, far wealthier residents of that neighborhood.

In the United States, the official definition of the **poverty line** is derived from the government's calculation of the minimum income requirements for families to acquire the minimum necessities of life. Poverty is highly related to geography, as can be seen in Figure 12.1. One of the main problems with the official poverty line is that it is not contextualized according to geographic location and, as a result, does not take into account the cost of living in different communities. For example, the price of renting an apartment in a major urban center is much higher than the cost of rent in a rural small town. Some conceive of poverty as a form of powerlessness or a sociological and psychological condition of hopelessness, indifference, and distrust. In other words, poverty can be the result of the inability to control events that shape a person's life, often leading to a large degree of dependency on others.

KEY CONCEPT

In the United States, poverty is determined by the government's estimation of the minimum income requirements for families to acquire their minimum needs, such as shelter, food, water, and clothing. The problem with this official definition is that it fails to take into account geographical variables that impact the value of money in different locations. Certain areas are more costly to live in than others.

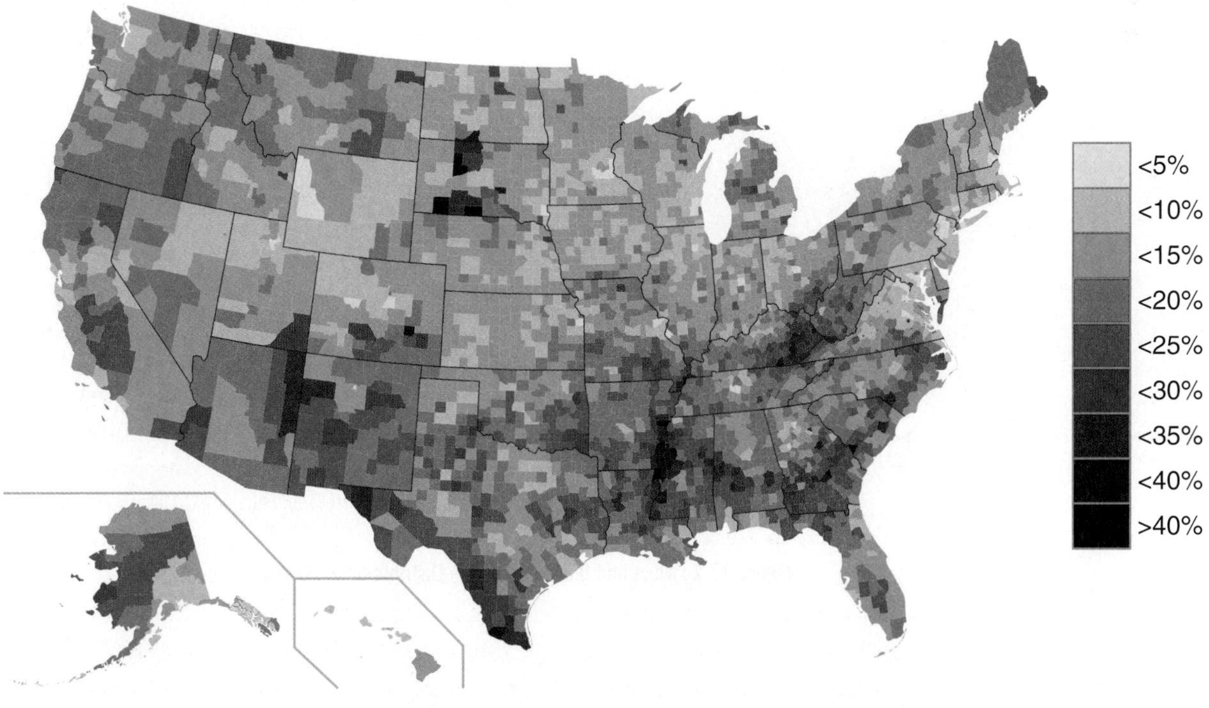

Figure 12.1 Percentage of Population Living below the Poverty Line by County, 2009

Social Exclusion

Social exclusion can arise from a sense of powerlessness when individuals who are poor or otherwise disadvantaged feel segregated and isolated from society. This feeling can create further obstacles to achieving self-help, independence, and self-respect. Disadvantaged groups, such as the racially and ethnically underrepresented, can experience magnified feelings of alienation and powerlessness when living in an affluent community. These feelings are similar to anomic conditions, which tend to further accelerate social inequality.

Spatial Inequality

Another important factor influencing poverty is the spatial setting of one's social life. In other words, where one lives plays a major role in the distribution of valuable resources. Does a person living in a low-income neighborhood in Mumbai have the same access to clean water and electricity as someone living in the posh neighborhood of London's West End? **Spatial inequality** focuses on social stratification across territories and their populations. Examining space helps to illuminate social inequalities because it attends to how geography influences social processes. Social categories such as gender, ethnicity and race, and class are distributed across spaces differently, as shown in Figure 12.2. In turn, these groups use spaces differently. For example, some cultures consider the home the center of family life, culture, and entertainment, while other cultures may view the home as merely a stop-off point for eating and sleeping while spending most of their time outside of the home.

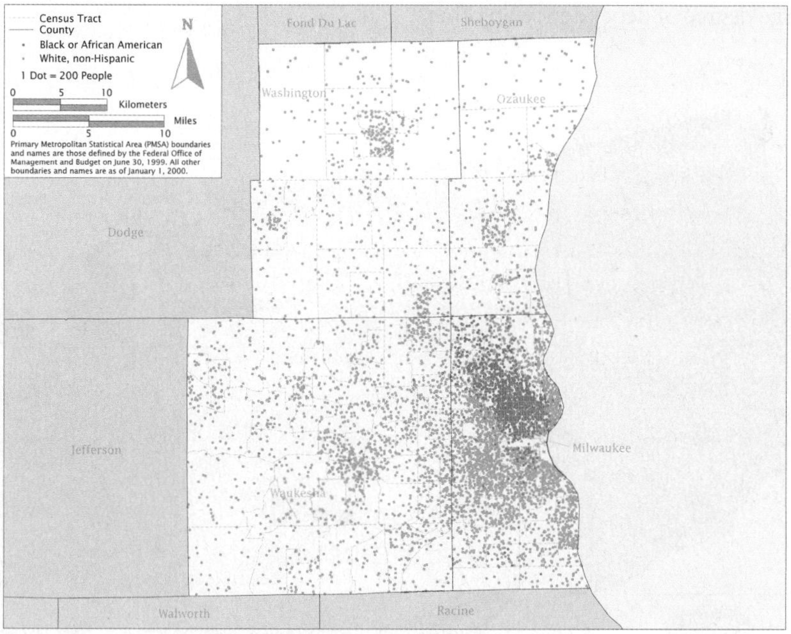

Figure 12.2 White and Black Population Distribution in Milwaukee County, WI

Space can be used to reinforce existing inequalities and can even amplify their effects, particularly poverty, leading to population segregation and the formation or expansion of destitute neighborhoods. Space can also be used to create social inequalities. In other words, social relationships between different agents, such as capitalists, laborers, the government, and citizens, result in spatially-varied social structures, built environments, and unequal regional development. For example, poorer neighborhoods tend to have less political and social influence than more affluent neighborhoods; as a result, "undesirable" buildings, like water refineries, trash-smoldering plants, and chemical manufacturers, tend to be placed in low-income areas, as shown in Figure 12.3. Citizens of these areas may lack the social resources to fight government and industry. To further understand spatial inequality, we must explore this idea on three levels: residential, environmental, and global.

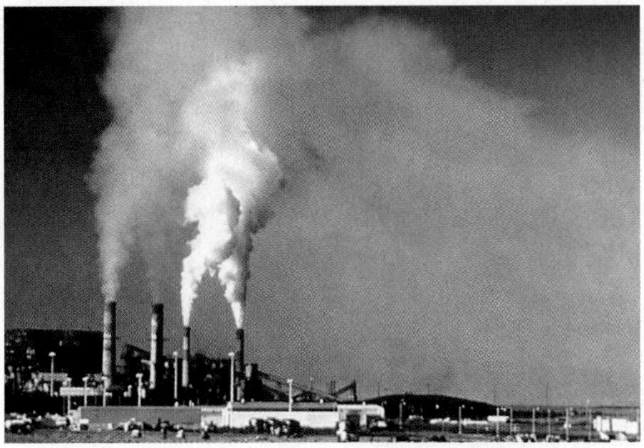

Figure 12.3 Industrial Park in a Low Socioeconomic Area

Residential Segregation

Where one resides—an urban, suburban, or rural environment, and which neighborhood in that environment—has a substantial effect on how people interact, cooperate, and advance. The cultural diversity and anonymity of urban neighborhoods offer a person a greater range of opportunities than normally found in rural areas. For example, in urban environments, people are less likely to fall into their occupations and social positions because of familial ties. In rural environments, this is more likely to occur: *My parents were farmers, my grandparents were farmers, my great-grandparents were farmers; therefore, I will take up the family business when it's handed down to me.* People in urban areas tend to have more career options to choose from and can more easily improve their SES through such avenues as education, career choice, and marriage. In rural environments, these choices exist, but are less universally available. Such opportunities also do not always extend across urban environments. The neighborhood in which one lives plays a major role: affluent neighborhoods tend to have more homeowners, professionals and managers, college graduates, and higher-quality schools. Low-income neighborhoods tend to have greater poverty, unemployment rates, lower-quality schools, and higher rates of homelessness. Low-income neighborhoods are also less safe, with higher rates of violent crime, organized crime, and gang activity. These key attributes stratify neighborhoods and create unequal chances for people who live in these communities. The overall greater concentration of individuals who are poor in urban centers helps to explain **suburbanization**, or the migration pattern of the middle classes to suburban communities, as shown in Figure 12.4. The suburbs have become more attractive as they are generally cleaner and less crowded, have lower crime rates, and often have better school systems. Unlike the middle or upper classes, members of the lower class are often less able to relocate to areas that might offer them better opportunities. Many disadvantaged groups therefore remain in urban centers under poor living conditions. To make matters worse, this type of environment can easily expose low-income groups to illness and disease. Suburbanization can also lead to **urban decay**, in which a previously functional portion of a city deteriorates and becomes decrepit over time. Interestingly, this process can spontaneously reverse in the process of **urban renewal**, in which city land is reclaimed and renovated for public or private use. Urban renewal is often fueled by **gentrification**, when upper- and middle-class populations begin to purchase and renovate neighborhoods in deteriorated areas, displacing the low-SES population.

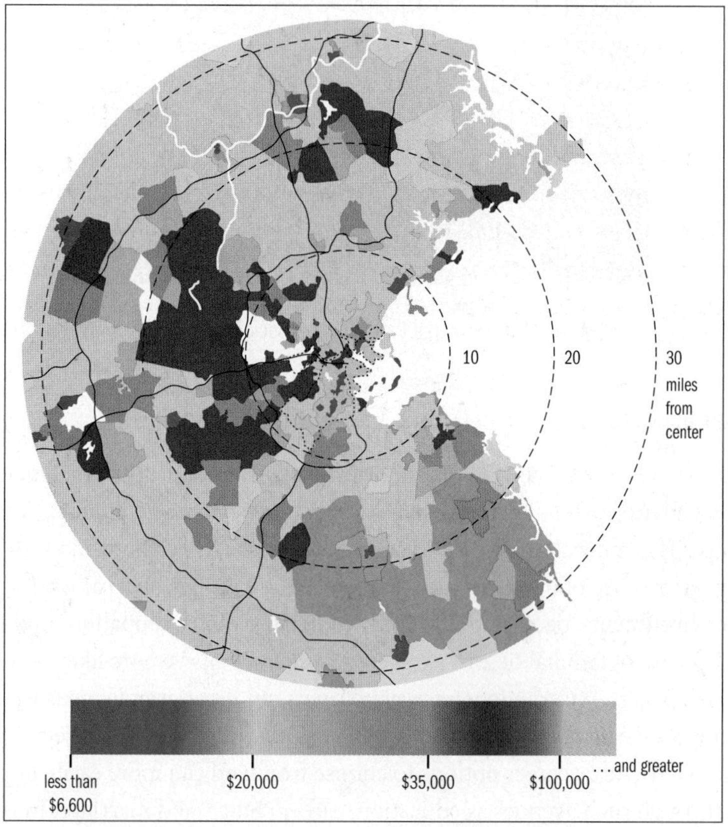

Figure 12.4 The Boston "Doughnut" of Income and Socioeconomic Status
Urban centers tend to contain lower-SES communities, surrounded by a ring of middle- to upper-SES suburbs. Further out are lower-SES exurbs and rural areas.

Environmental Justice

Poor living conditions and dangerous environmental conditions can result in an increase in illness and disease. Many low-income and underrepresented groups tend to reside closer to sites of environmental pollution because these areas are usually cheaper housing markets. Environmental risks, such as hazardous waste-producing plants and toxic waste dumps, tend to be located in low-income areas with a high concentration of groups who are racially and ethnically underrepresented. It is no surprise that inadequate housing, heating, and sanitation, in concert with toxin exposure, can contribute to acute medical problems. Illnesses such as influenza, pneumonia, substance use disorders, tuberculosis, and whooping cough are much more common among people living in poor-quality conditions. As mentioned earlier, these low-income areas also may lack the social and political power to prevent environmental risks from encroaching on their communities.

Global Inequalities

Poverty and social inequalities are not limited to hierarchies within a country. The **world system theory** categorizes countries and emphasizes the inequalities of the division of labor at the global level. **Core nations** focus on higher skills and higher paying productions while exploiting **peripheral nations** for their lower-skilled productions. **Semi-peripheral nations** are midway between the two—these nations work toward becoming core nations, while having many characteristics of peripheral nations. Much of the world, especially within semi-peripheral and peripheral nations, lives on less than the equivalent of $1.25 per day. Such rates of poverty are especially prevalent in parts of India, sub-Saharan Africa, and South Central Asia, as shown in Figure 12.5.

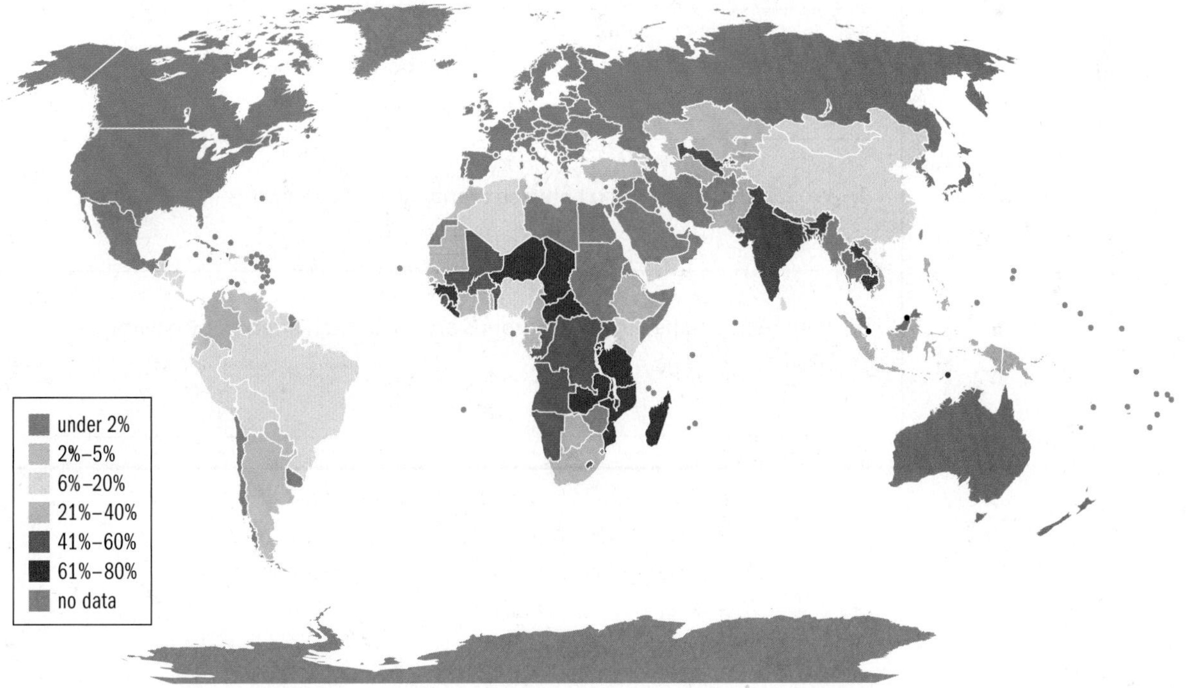

Figure 12.5 Percentage of Population Living on Less than $1.25 per Day, 2008

Largely due to the effects of globalization, massive restructuring of industry and trade patterns have had a major impact on local communities, specifically because of the production of cheap goods at suppressed rates for the global market. This reconfiguration obstructs or limits access to power and resources as the production of goods constantly shifts from location to location. Social inequalities have increased on a worldwide level as local communities become more and more subject to the ebb and flow of the global market. Since the advent of globalization, with the development of world cities, international communication chains, and global immigration, interaction between industrialized and developing nations has had more of an impact on peoples and regions within the state, and has thereby led to further inequalities in space, food and water, energy, housing, and education. Global inequality has been further exacerbated by an unprecedented large population spike, placing strain on the world's resources. The majority of the world also has limited access to healthcare. Consequently, many people around the globe suffer from malnutrition and parasitic and infectious diseases, and have higher rates of morbidity and mortality.

MCAT CONCEPT CHECK 12.1

Before you move on, assess your understanding of the material with these questions.

1. How is socioeconomic status (SES) determined?

   ____

2. How does social capital affect social cohesion?

   ____

3. What are some groups that suffer disproportionate social inequality?

   ____

4. What is the relationship between merit and social mobility?

   ____

5. With regard to health, which groups are most often affected by environmental hazards?

   ____

12.2 Epidemiology and Disparities

LEARNING OBJECTIVES

After Chapter 12.2, you will be able to:

- Identify the causes of Waitzkin's "second sickness"
- Explain why women are more likely to have better health profiles than men
- Describe the links between class, ethnicity, and healthcare disparities

An old saying intones that *Your health is your wealth*. This same correlation certainly holds true in reverse: the wealthier tend to have better health and better access to healthcare. Wherever there is low social capital, high urban degradation, interpersonal violence, and low social trust, the social environment is poor, and there is less protection against disease. As a result, class gradients often increase. Poor health conditions and lower life expectancy, as shown in Figure 12.6, are some of the many consequences of social stratification. Low-income groups are significantly worse off than the middle or upper classes when it comes to health disparities, meaning they tend to be sicker than others. **Social epidemiology** is a branch of epidemiology that studies the ways in which health and disease correlate to social advantages and disadvantages.

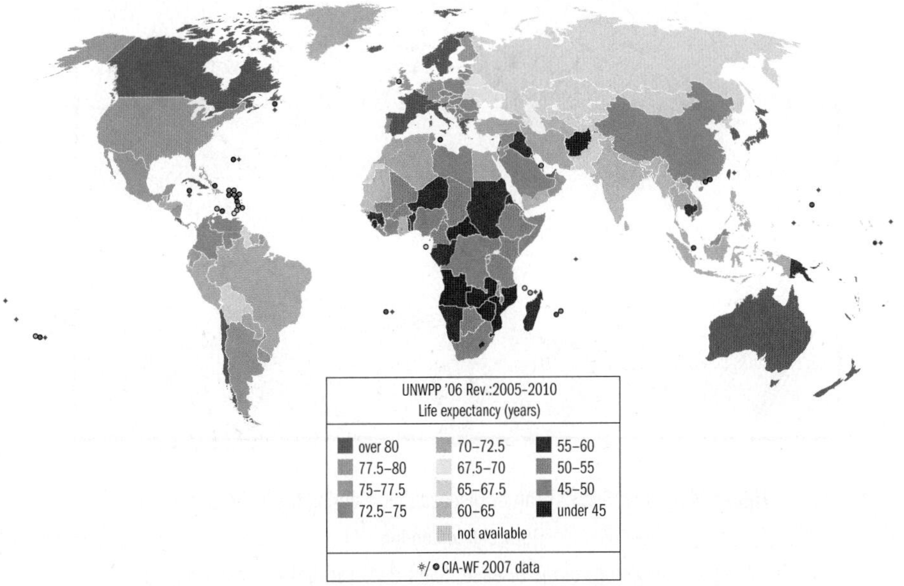

Figure 12.6 Life Expectancy at Birth, 2005-2010

To understand health statistics, it is important to define a few epidemiological terms. **Incidence** is defined as the number of new cases of an illness per population at risk in a given amount of time; for example, the number of new cases of lung cancer per 1000 at-risk people per year. **Prevalence** is a measure of the number of cases of an illness overall—whether new or chronic—per population in a given amount of time; for example, the number of people with new or chronic

KEY CONCEPT

Epidemiology statistics:

- Incidence = new cases/population at risk/time
- Prevalence = total cases/total population/time

Note that incidence is relative to the population at risk, not the total population; if you already have the illness, you are no longer at risk!

lung cancer per 1000 people per year. Health statistics are also given in terms of morbidity and mortality. **Morbidity** is the burden or degree of illness associated with a given disease, while **mortality** refers to deaths caused by a given disease.

Inequities in Health

Science has clearly demonstrated that poor environmental and social factors negatively impact health. This correlation was first demonstrated in the nineteenth century through public health efforts. One landmark example linking geography with disease was John Snow's investigation of a cholera outbreak in London in 1854. Snow tracked cases of cholera on a map, as shown in Figure 12.7, and was able to deduce that a water pump in the neighborhood was causing the spread of the infectious agent (a bacterium called *Vibrio cholerae*).

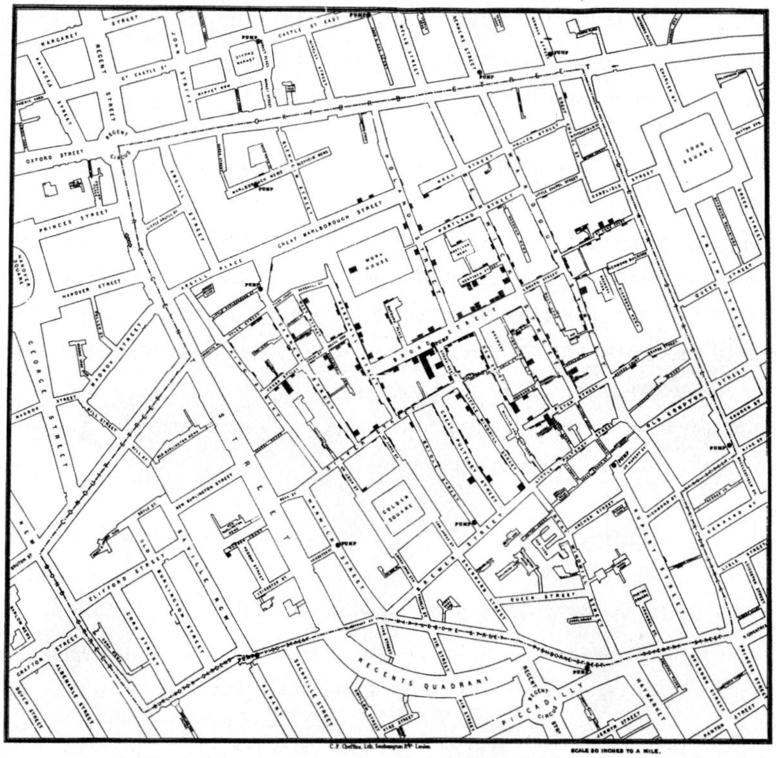

Figure 12.7 John Snow's Map of Disease Cases during the 1854 Cholera Outbreak in London

By tracing the geography of the disease, Snow deduced that a water pump was responsible for cholera transmission.

Health is dependent not only on geography, but also on social and economic factors. Over time, socioeconomic improvements lead to greater general health in the population, and the best health outcomes are generally seen in egalitarian societies. However, despite the ambitions of the modern **welfare state** (the system of government that protects the health and well-being of its citizens), the Black Report of 1980 showed that class differences in health still exist, with professional groups having longer life expectancies than working-class people. Howard Waitzkin described this outcome as the **second sickness**, which is an exacerbation of health outcomes caused by social injustice. As the Centers for Disease Control and Prevention (CDC) have shown, low-income groups are more likely to have poorer health, be uninsured, and die younger than middle- or upper-class adults. Poverty, in combination with a culture of inequality, leads to worse health outcomes, and this effect runs across gender, age, and racial and ethnic boundaries. For example, low-income women are more likely to deliver babies with low birth weights, thereby placing these babies at risk for numerous physical and cognitive problems in life. Similarly, impoverished members of racially and ethnically underrepresented groups have lower life expectancies. Members of the lower class, overall, are four times more likely to view themselves in worse health compared with affluent groups. Low-income groups are much more likely to develop life-shortening diseases such as lung cancer, diabetes, heart disease, and other degenerative illnesses. These groups are also more likely to commit suicide and die from homicide in comparison to wealthier adults. The infant mortality rate among the poor is also much higher; in some populations of the United States, the infant mortality rate can approximate that of developing countries. However, because of the correlation between poverty and racially and ethnically underrepresented groups, many of these characteristics apply to particular ethnic groups more than others.

When it comes to health and illness among racially and ethnically underrepresented groups, Asian Americans and Pacific Islanders have some of the best health profiles. Reports illustrate that, in comparison to White Americans, these groups have a lower rate of death associated with cancer, heart disease, diabetes, and infant mortality. African Americans appear to have a worse health profile in comparison to White Americans, showing higher rates of death linked to cancer, heart disease, diabetes, drug and alcohol use, infant mortality, and HIV/AIDS. African American infants have twice the infant mortality rate of White infants. Specifically, African American males have the lowest life expectancy of any racial or gender category. Hispanic Americans have a mixed profile in comparison to White Americans, in that they have lower mortality rates attributable to cancer, heart disease, and infant mortality, but higher mortality rates attributable to diabetes, alcohol and drug use, and HIV/AIDS. Hispanic Americans also have a high mortality rate from influenza, pneumonia, and accidents. American Indians also have a mixed profile in this regard, showing higher rates of death from diabetes, alcohol and drug use, and infant mortality, but lower mortality rates compared to White Americans from cancer, heart disease, and HIV/AIDS. American Indians also show some of the highest rates of death by suicide in comparison to the general population. This group also has some of the highest mortality rates linked to diabetes compared to any racial category.

MCAT EXPERTISE

The MCAT will not expect you to be able to rattle off the relative rates of these illnesses across racial groups, but a sensitivity to these differences between groups may be important in passages related to sociology and public health.

KEY CONCEPT

Low-income groups, especially those who are racially and ethnically underrepresented, have an overall worse health profile in terms of morbidity and mortality rates.

When it comes to gender-related health disparities, most statistical information shows that women have better health profiles than men. This trend is true throughout the world. Female life expectancy has been consistently higher than male life expectancy since records began. While the gap in life expectancy is beginning to narrow in the United States, most countries still have higher life expectancies for female citizens than male citizens, as shown in Figure 12.8.

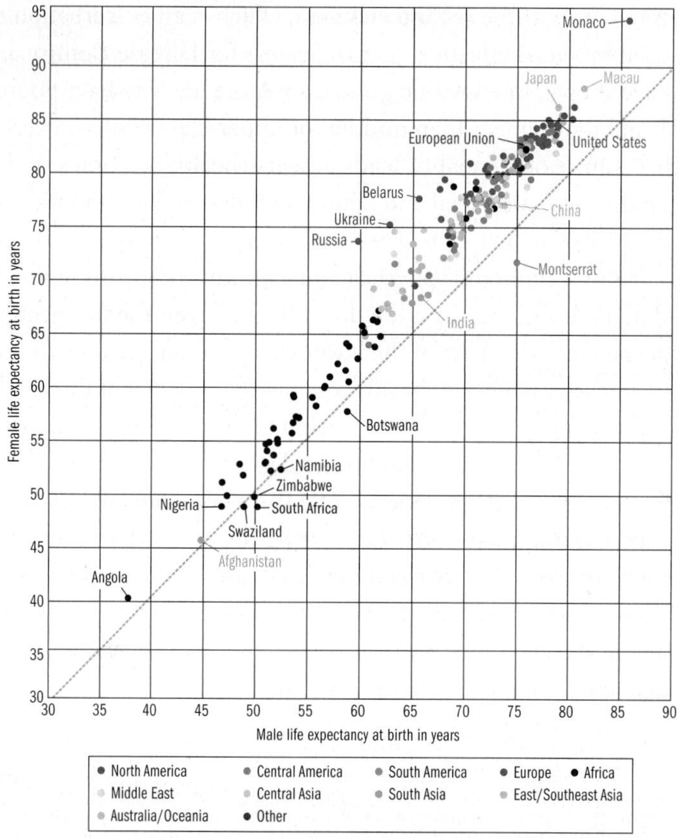

Figure 12.8 Male and Female Life Expectancies by Region and Country *Note that female life expectancies are almost universally higher than male life expectancies. Based on data from the CIA World Factbook.*

Mortality rates from heart disease, cancer, chronic lower respiratory diseases, and diabetes are higher for men than women. Men are also three times more likely than women to die from accidents, suicide, and homicide. Men are far less likely to seek medical attention than women. Men, especially those raised to have hypermasculine behaviors, may try to "tough it out" rather than go to a doctor. When men do seek healthcare, they are less likely to comply with medical instructions or adhere to medical advice.

KEY CONCEPT

In comparison to women, men tend to have worse mortality rates. However, women have higher morbidity rates. Differences in male and female health profiles are both biologically and sociologically determined, the latter being the result of factors like risk-taking behavior, hypermasculinity, and dangerous employment.

While women show better mortality rates, this is not the case when it comes to morbidity rates for certain acute and chronic diseases. More women than men suffer from infectious and parasitic diseases, digestive problems, respiratory conditions, high blood pressure (hypertension), arthritis, diabetes, and inflammatory bowel diseases (colitis). Women tend to suffer more from illnesses and disabilities than men, but their conditions are less often life threatening.

The reasons that men tend to have lower life expectancy rates are both sociological and biological. Sociologically, men are considered to be bigger risk takers, and therefore more likely to expose themselves to accidents and unintentional injuries. This is especially true of young men. Men are also more likely to be employed in dangerous jobs, such as the police force, steel industry, and coal mining. Men also have higher rates of alcohol use, speeding, and participation in potentially violent sports. Biologically speaking, men are at a disadvantage from infancy onward. Throughout life, men are more likely to come down with diseases that are life threatening.

Inequities in Healthcare

While the United States has one of the most advanced healthcare systems in the world, quality healthcare and services are not always extended to all. Like many institutions, quality healthcare favors those in higher social classes. Many people are frustrated by the way healthcare is delivered in the United States, especially with regard to health insurance. Further, the healthcare system of the United States is one of the few among industrialized nations that is not organized and planned by a central (governmental) system.

Passage of the Affordable Care Act (ACA) in 2010 was an attempt in the United States to increase coverage and affordability of insurance for all Americans, and also to reduce the overall costs of healthcare. Medicare and Medicaid are also programs that attempt to increase access to healthcare in the United States. **Medicare** covers patients over the age of 65, those with end-stage renal disease, and those with amyotrophic lateral sclerosis (ALS). **Medicaid** covers patients who are in significant financial need. However, disadvantaged groups, especially those who are poor, are still affected by disparities in healthcare both in terms of access and quality. Even those individuals who have Medicare or Medicaid may lack access, as many physicians will not accept such public insurance programs. Additionally, some doctors will not open practices in low-income neighborhoods, making access even harder for populations with low socioeconomic status. Consequently, individuals in the lower class are less likely to seek medical assistance until they are seriously ill; by then, intervention may be too late.

KEY CONCEPT

Medicare covers patients over 65, those with end-stage renal disease, and those with amyotrophic lateral sclerosis (ALS). Medicaid covers patients in significant financial need.

Some of the primary reasons low-income groups have higher mortality rates include poor access to quality medical care, poor nutrition, and feeling less in control of life circumstances. Those who are poor are more likely to smoke and be overweight or obese; they are less likely to engage in physical activity. In addition to socioeconomic status, race and ethnicity can create barriers to care. In race-concordant patient-physician relationships, the patient and physician are of the same race, whereas they are of different races in race-discordant relationships. Sometimes, culture and non-native language are viewed as contributors to pathology because they can act as obstacles to diagnosis and treatment. Also, despite efforts to systemically address unequal treatment of underrepresented populations by physicians, there are still inequalities and disparities in treatment relative to race and ethnicity over a wide range of medical specialties. In other words, underrepresented and low-income groups tend to face greater barriers to care, and poorer quality of care when they receive it. To be specific, it has been demonstrated that African Americans, Asian Americans, American Indians, and Hispanic Americans receive worse care than White Americans.

Quality of preventative care, acute treatment, and chronic disease management also differ regionally. States in New England and the Mid-Atlantic are shown to be in the top quartile of healthcare quality while states in the South are in the bottom quartile.

Outside of race and ethnicity, other identifiable characteristics may have a large impact on how patients are treated by their providers. One of the most common biases is discrimination against overweight and obese patients. This bias can apply to any individual who is overweight, regardless of socioeconomic status, gender, age, and racial and ethnic background, although there is a higher prevalence of obesity in low-income groups. Doctors may assume that being overweight or obese is the only cause of a patient's health problems, which can sometimes lead to misdiagnoses and ineffective treatments. This, in turn, damages the trust necessary to form a strong doctor–patient relationship. As a result, patients who are overweight or obese are more likely than other patients to switch doctors repeatedly. When one does not have a consistent primary care doctor, continuity of care is nearly nonexistent. Additionally, patients who are overweight or obese are less likely to have quality preventative care and screenings, including screenings for breast and colon cancer.

In terms of gender, women tend to be favored by the healthcare system. As a whole, women tend to fare better when it comes to accessing healthcare, largely because women are more likely to be insured. Women tend to utilize healthcare services more than men, with more examinations, blood pressure checks, lab tests, drug prescriptions, and physician visits per year. Women also receive more services per visit than men do. Healthcare use is likely more common among women due to higher morbidity rates among women for many illnesses, thereby facilitating the need to seek medical attention. On the other hand, women are more likely to be delayed or unable to obtain necessary medical care, dental care, and prescription medicines. Also, for LGBTQ individuals, discrimination and decreased access to healthcare are quite common, often due to homophobia and other prejudices.

MCAT CONCEPT CHECK 12.2

Before you move on, assess your understanding of the material with these questions.

1. What is Waitzkin's second sickness?

2. What is the relationship between class, ethnicity, and health?

3. Why are women more likely to have better health profiles than men?

4. What are some of the factors that contribute to healthcare disparities between classes?

Conclusion

So what have we learned? We do not live in a perfect world where valuable materials and resources are unlimited and evenly distributed. In the United States and on a worldwide level, social stratification is an unfortunate reality. In a class-based economic system such as ours, status and power are inextricably linked, which can either facilitate or hinder access to social capital and its associated rewards. This is especially the case for certain disadvantaged groups based on categories of class, race, gender, and age. While not perfect, our class system does tend to allow for upward social mobility either in one's lifetime or across generations. At the heart of America's socioeconomic values is the principle of meritocracy, which means that through hard work, credentials, and dedication, one can move up in society. However, many people in the United States remain impoverished. Social inequality and social exclusion make it increasingly difficult for low-income groups to improve their socioeconomic condition. Some hold that social inequalities such as poverty remain because these inequalities are passed down from one generation to another. While there is some truth to the social reproduction of poverty, one's situational context also plays a role through spatial inequality. Where one lives in this world has an impact on one's position in life, especially in terms of accessing key resources and prosperous opportunities. Spatial inequality remains at the residential, environmental, and global level.

But how do such social inequalities influence health and healthcare disparities? Well, as is the case with many facets of life, wealth matters. Those with greater income typically have access to better quality healthcare. This is especially the case in the U.S. healthcare system because of uneven levels of coverage and high healthcare costs. Socioeconomic status or class greatly impacts one's ability to navigate the system and procure healthcare in the United States. Low-income racially and ethnically underrepresented groups tend to be worse off, having both poorer health and poorer access to healthcare. Women, despite being more prone to chronic and degenerative diseases, tend to fare better than men when it comes to overall health and accessing and utilizing healthcare resources.

While the U.S. healthcare system is undergoing a significant reorientation and taking on a more preventative approach, it is more important now than ever to place a greater emphasis on sociological issues to understand the relationship between social stratification and health and healthcare disparities. Illness and disease are a product of social as well as psychological and physiological issues. This chapter is the last chapter in *MCAT Behavioral Sciences Review*; you have therefore covered all of the psychology and sociology content required for the MCAT. This is a fitting chapter to finish this discussion, and we leave you with a charge: as you prepare for the MCAT, medical school, and life as the physician you deserve to be, think about the changes that are needed in the U.S. healthcare system. Serve your local, national, and international community and improve the health status of those around you, while contributing to a future where everyone can access quality healthcare.

GO ONLINE

You've reviewed the content, now test your knowledge and critical thinking skills by completing a test-like passage set in your online resources!

CONCEPT SUMMARY

Social Class

- Social stratification is based on **socioeconomic status (SES)**. Socioeconomic status depends on ascribed status and achieved status.
  - **Ascribed status** is involuntary and derives from clearly identifiable characteristics, such as age, gender, and skin color.
  - **Achieved status** is acquired through direct, individual efforts.
- A **social class** is a category of people with shared socioeconomic characteristics. The three main social classes are upper, middle, and lower class. These groups also have similar lifestyles, job opportunities, attitudes, and behaviors.
- **Prestige** is the respect and importance tied to specific occupations or associations.
- **Power** is the capacity to influence people through real or perceived rewards and punishments. It often depends on the unequal distribution of valued resources. Power differentials create social inequality.
- **Anomie** is a state of normlessness. Anomic conditions erode social solidarity by means of excessive individualism, social inequality, and isolation.
- **Social capital** is the investment people make in their society in return for economic or collective rewards. Social networks, either situational or positional, are one of the most powerful forms of social capital and can be achieved through establishing strong and weak social ties.
- **Meritocracy** refers to a society in which advancement up the social ladder is based on intellectual talent and achievement.
- **Social mobility** allows one to acquire higher-level employment opportunities by achieving required credentials and experience. Social mobility can either occur in a positive upward direction or a negative downward direction depending on whether one is promoted or demoted in status.
- **Poverty** is a socioeconomic condition. In the United States, the poverty line is determined by the government's calculation of the minimum income requirements for families to acquire the minimum necessities of life.
- **Social reproduction** refers to the passing on of social inequality, especially poverty, from one generation to the next.
- Poverty can either be absolute or relative.
  - **Absolute poverty** is when people do not have enough resources to acquire basic life necessities, such as shelter, food, clothing, and water.
  - **Relative poverty** is when one is poor in comparison to a larger population.
- **Social exclusion** is a sense of powerlessness when individuals feel alienated from society.

- **Spatial inequality** is a form of social stratification across territories and their populations, and can occur along residential, environmental, and global lines.
  - Urban areas tend to have more diverse economic opportunities and more ability for social mobility than rural areas. Urban areas also tend to have more neighborhoods that are low-income and racially and ethnically underrepresented than do rural areas.
  - Formation of higher-income suburbs is a common occurrence, and is due in part to the limited mobility of lower-income groups in urban centers.
  - **Environmental injustice** refers to an uneven distribution of environmental hazards in communities. Lower-income neighborhoods may lack the social and political power to prevent the placement of environmental hazards in their neighborhoods.
- **Globalization** has led to further inequalities in space, food and water, energy, housing, and education as the production of goods shifts to cheaper and cheaper labor markets. This has led to significant economic hardship in industrializing nations.

Epidemiology and Disparities

- **Incidence** is calculated as the number of new cases of a disease per population at risk in a given period of time: for example, new cases per 1000 at-risk people per year.
- **Prevalence** is calculated as the number of cases of a disease per population in a given period of time: for example, cases per 1000 people per year.
- **Morbidity** is the burden or degree of illness associated with a given disease.
- **Mortality** refers to deaths caused by a given disease.
- Health is dependent on geographic, social, and economic factors.
  - The **second sickness** refers to an exacerbation of health outcomes caused by social injustice.
  - Poverty is associated with worse health outcomes, including decreased life expectancy, higher rates of life-shortening diseases, higher rates of suicide and homicide, and higher infant mortality rates.
  - Certain racially and ethnically underrepresented groups have worse health profiles than others. African Americans have the worst health profiles; White Americans, American Indians, and Hispanic Americans have health profiles in the middle; and Asian Americans and Pacific Islanders have the best health profiles.
  - Females have better health profiles than males, including higher life expectancy, lower rates of life-threatening illnesses, and higher rates of accessing and utilizing health resources. However, females have higher rates of chronic diseases and higher morbidity rates.
- Efforts to improve healthcare for underserved populations include the **Affordable Care Act** (ACA) and the **Medicare** and **Medicaid** programs.

- Healthcare access and quality differ across the population.
    - Low-income groups and racially and ethnically underrepresented groups (specifically, African Americans, Asian Americans, American Indians, and Hispanic Americans) receive worse care than high-income groups and White Americans, respectively.
    - Biases against overweight or obese patients are associated with lower-quality treatment, including less preventative care and fewer screenings.
    - Women tend to have better access to healthcare and utilize more healthcare resources than men.
    - LGBTQ individuals may have barriers to care due to prejudices, discrimination, homophobia, and transphobia.

ANSWERS TO CONCEPT CHECKS

12.1

1. SES is determined by two factors: it can be ascribed according to physical or external characteristics such as age, gender, or skin color, or acquired through direct efforts such as hard work or merit.
2. The less social capital a person has (reduced network equality and equality of opportunity), the more social inequality. This, in turn, decreases social cohesion.
3. Social inequality is highest among racially and ethnically underrepresented groups (especially African Americans and Hispanic Americans), households headed by women, and older adults. It is also most prevalent among those living in poverty.
4. Social mobility can be dependent on intellectual talent and achievement (meritocratic competition) but can also be obstructed by concentrated power as well as discrimination based on ethnicity, gender, age, or other identifiable characteristics.
5. Environmental hazards tend to be located in low-income areas with a higher population of racially and ethnically underrepresented groups. Poor living conditions can result in increased illness and disease among these groups of people.

12.2

1. The second sickness refers to the fact that health outcomes are exacerbated by social inequalities and social injustice. As a result, higher-income groups have longer life expectancies than lower-income groups.
2. Low-income racially and ethnically underrepresented groups have higher morbidity rates and overall worse health compared to the middle and upper classes. The lower class also has higher infant mortality rates, homicide rates, and suicide rates in comparison to wealthier classes.
3. Women typically have longer life expectancies and an overall better health profile in comparison to men. This can be attributed to both biological and sociological causes: women are less likely to have life-threatening conditions, although they do have higher morbidity rates. Women are also more likely to seek care and to utilize healthcare services than men.
4. Low-income groups have less access to healthcare services and often experience lower quality healthcare. Poor Americans are less likely to be insured and consequently are less likely to seek medical attention until conditions have become extremely serious, thereby limiting available interventions. As a result, morbidity and mortality rates are highest among low-income groups.

SCIENCE MASTERY ASSESSMENT EXPLANATIONS

1. **D**

Social stratification based on direct efforts, such as merit, is a form of achieved socioeconomic status. Ascribed socioeconomic status, **(A)**, is based on identifiable external characteristics. Achieved status may be due to meritocratic competition, **(B)**, but other individual efforts can also be associated with achieved status. Anomic conditions, **(C)**, are those that cause a breakdown between the individual and society and erode social solidarity.

2. **C**

Low social class may lead to low social capital. Members of the lower class often have smaller numbers of weak ties in social networks, and therefore have less opportunity to invest in society and reap its benefits.

3. **D**

Globalization does not typically lead to global equality; rather, globalization tends to create further global inequalities. In regard to environmental justice, higher numbers of hazardous waste facilities tend to be found in low-income neighborhoods, **(A)**. Poor living conditions tend to be associated with greater health problems, including tuberculosis, **(B)**. Finally, environmental pollution is more prevalent in areas with larger populations of underrepresented groups, especially when low-income, **(C)**.

4. **B**

Groups with high income tend to have increased life expectancy rates, not decreased. People with low income have higher mortality rates than those with high income, **(A)**. Low-income women tend to have children with lower birth weights, **(C)**. Finally, rates of various diseases, including lung cancer, are increased among low-income groups, **(D)**.

5. **D**

Prevalence is defined as the total number of cases divided by the possibly affected population during a period of time. Here, the period of time is defined as one point: the end of the year. At the end of the year, there are 30 total cases in a population of 1000 individuals, but only 500 of those individuals can develop prostate cancer, meaning the prevalence is $30 \div 500$.

6. **A**

Incidence is defined as the total number of new cases divided by the at-risk population during a period of time. Here, the period of time is one year. There were 10 new cases in this year, and the at-risk population will be only the males who do not already have prostate cancer; the 20 males already diagnosed and the 500 females should not be included in the at-risk population. Therefore, the incidence in this population is $10 \div 480$.

7. **D**

In this scenario, the children remain in the same socioeconomic class as their parent, indicating a lack of social mobility, **(A)** and **(B)**. Rather, this is an example of social reproduction, in which social inequality, especially poverty, is passed from one generation to the next.

8. **C**

Relative poverty is a comparative term: it describes being poorer than those in the surrounding population. Members of the upper class can live in relative poverty compared to others in their neighborhood if they are not as well-off as their neighbors. Relative poverty is not directly associated with upward or downward social mobility, eliminating **(B)** and **(D)**; individuals living in relative poverty could exhibit mobility in either direction or no social mobility at all.

9. **C**

Suburbs tend to have larger upper- and middle-class populations than urban centers; urban centers tend to have larger low-socioeconomic status populations than suburbs. This is due, in part, to the increased mobility seen in upper- and middle-class populations, which permits their migration into the suburbs.

10. **A**

Morbidity refers to the burden of illness, or the severity or degree of illness. Mortality, **(B)**, refers to deaths caused by a given illness. Second sickness, **(C)**, is a term used to describe the exacerbation of health outcomes due to social injustice. Chronicity, **(D)**, refers to the duration of a disease, not its severity or significance for the patient.

11. **B**

In comparison to White Americans, Asian Americans tend to have better overall health profiles. African Americans, **(A)**, tend to have worse overall health profiles. Hispanic Americans and American Indians, **(C)** and **(D)**, both have mixed health profiles in comparison to White Americans: they are better off in some categories and worse off in others. However, Hispanic Americans and American Indians do not have better overall health profiles than White Americans.

12. **C**

Medicare covers patients over the age of 65 (older age groups), those with end-stage renal disease, and those with amyotrophic lateral sclerosis (ALS). Medicaid covers patients below a certain socioeconomic level.

13. **C**

Morbidity refers to the burden or severity of disease. All of the factors listed are true with regard to low-socioeconomic status populations; however, high homicide rates cause increases in mortality, not morbidity.

14. **A**

If the threshold for hypertension (high blood pressure) were lowered, more individuals would be fit the criteria for the disease. If the number of individuals with the disease increases and the population stays the same overall, there will be an increased prevalence of the disease.

15. **B**

In comparison to females, males visit primary care doctors less frequently. All of the other trends listed here have been documented.

Consult your online resources for additional practice. **GO ONLINE**

SHARED CONCEPTS

Behavioral Sciences Chapter 5
Motivation, Emotion, and Stress

Behavioral Sciences Chapter 6
Identity and Personality

Behavioral Sciences Chapter 7
Psychological Disorders

Behavioral Sciences Chapter 8
Social Processes, Attitudes, and Behavior

Behavioral Sciences Chapter 10
Social Thinking

Behavioral Sciences Chapter 11
Social Structure and Demographics

GLOSSARY

Absolute poverty–Poverty wherein people do not have enough resources to acquire basic life necessities such as shelter, food, clothing, and water.

Absolute threshold–The minimum stimulus energy needed to activate a sensory system.

Accommodation–Process by which existing schemata are modified to encompass new information.

Acetylcholine–A neurotransmitter associated with voluntary muscle control.

Achieved status–A status gained as a result of direct, individual action.

Acquisition–In classical conditioning, the process of taking advantage of reflexive responses to turn a neutral stimulus into a conditioned stimulus.

Actor-observer bias–The tendency to make situational attributions about the self, but dispositional attributions about others, regarding similar behaviors.

Adaptation–In perception, a decrease in stimulus perception after a long duration of exposure; in learning, the process by which new information is processed; consists of assimilation and accommodation.

Adaptive value–The extent to which a trait benefits a species by influencing the evolutionary fitness of the species.

Affect–The experience and display of emotion. Can be described as a scale, with both positive and negative affect having separate scales.

Afferent neuron–Sensory neurons which transmit information to the brain from the body in response to sensory input.

Ageism–Prejudice or discrimination on the basis of a person's age.

Agent of socialization–Any part of society that is important when learning social norms and values.

Aggression–A behavior with the intention to cause harm or increase relative social dominance; can be physical or verbal.

Agnosia–The loss of the ability to recognize objects, people, or sounds, though typically just one of the three.

Alcohol myopia–The inability to think about consequences and possible outcomes of one's actions due to alcohol intoxication.

Alertness–State of consciousness in which one is aware, able to think, and able to respond to the environment; nearly synonymous with arousal.

Algorithm–A formula or procedure for solving a certain type of problem.

Aligning actions–An impression management strategy in which one makes questionable behavior acceptable through excuses.

Alter-casting–An impression management strategy in which one imposes an identity onto another person.

Altruism–A form of helping behavior in which people's intent is to benefit someone else at a cost to themselves.

Alzheimer's disease–Degenerative brain disorder that is characterized by dementia and memory loss. Neurofibrillary tangles and β-amyloid plaques are phenomena found in the brains of Alzheimer's patients.

Amphetamine–A central nervous system stimulant that increases activity of both dopamine and norepinephrine in the brain.

Amygdala–A portion of the limbic system that is important for memory and emotion, especially fear.

Anomie–A state of normlessness; anomic conditions erode social solidarity by means of excessive individualism, social inequality, and isolation.

Anterograde amnesia–Form of memory loss in which new long-term memories cannot be established.

Anxiety disorders–Disorders that involve worry, unease, fear, and apprehension about future uncertainties based on real or imagined events that can impair physical and psychological health.

Aphasia–Deficit of language production or comprehension.

Appraisal model–A similar theory to the basic model, accepting that there are biologically predetermined expressions once an emotion is experienced; accepts that there is a cognitive antecedent to emotional expression.

Archetype–In Jungian psychoanalysis, a thought or image that has an emotional element and is a part of the collective unconsciousness.

Arcuate fasciculus–A bundle of axons that connects Wernicke's area (language comprehension) with Broca's area (motor function of speech).

Arousal–A psychological and physiological state of being awake or reactive to stimuli; nearly synonymous with alertness.

Arousal theory–A theory of motivation that states there is a particular level of arousal required in order to perform actions optimally; summarized by the Yerkes–Dodson law.

Ascribed status–A status that one is given at birth, such as race, ethnicity, or sex.

Assimilation–In psychology, the process by which new information is interpreted in terms of existing schemata; in sociology, the process by which the behavior and culture of a group or an individual begins to merge with that of another group.

Associative learning–The process by which a connection is made between two stimuli or a stimulus and a response; examples include classical conditioning and operant conditioning.

Attachment–An emotional bond to another person, particularly a parent or caregiver. The four main attachment styles are: secure, avoidant, ambivalent, and disorganized.

Attitude–A tendency toward expression of positive or negative feelings or evaluations of a person, place, thing, or situation.

Attribute substitution–A phenomenon observed when individuals must make judgments that are complex but instead substitute a simpler solution or perception.

Attribution theory–A theory that focuses on the tendency for individuals to infer the causes of other people's behavior.

Auditory cortex–Region of the temporal lobe devoted to sound processing.

Auditory pathway–After entering the brain, sound is processed by several regions, including the MGN, auditory cortex, superior olive, and inferior colliculus.

Authentic self–Who someone actually is, including both positive and negative attributes.

Automatic processing–The brain process most closely resembling autopilot, enabling performance of multiple activities at the same time.

Autonomic nervous system–The involuntary branch of the peripheral nervous system that controls involuntary functions such as heart rate, bronchial dilation, temperature, and digestion.

Autonomy–The ethical tenet that the physician has the responsibility to respect patients' choices about their own healthcare.

Availability heuristic–A shortcut in decision making that relies on the information that is most readily available, rather than the total body of information on a subject.

Avoidance learning–A form of negative reinforcement in which one avoids the unpleasantness of something that has yet to happen.

Babbling–Precursor to language known to spontaneously occur in children.

Back stage–In the dramaturgical approach, the setting where players are free from their role requirements and not in front of the audience; back stage behaviors may not be deemed appropriate or acceptable and are thus kept invisible from the audience.

Barbiturate–A drug that acts as a central nervous system depressant; often used for anxiety, for insomnia, and as an antiseizure medication.

Basal ganglia–A portion of the forebrain that coordinates muscle movement and routes information from the cortex to the brain and spinal cord.

Base-rate fallacy–Using prototypical or stereotypical factors while ignoring actual numerical information when making a decision.

Basic model–First established by Charles Darwin, a theory that states that emotional expression involves a number of systems: facial expression as well as behavioral and physical responses; claims that emotions are universal and should be similar across cultures.

Behaviorism–B. F. Skinner's theory that all behaviors are conditioned. Behaviorism can be applied across many bodies of psychological thought, including theories of development, of identity, and of personality.

Belief–An acceptance that a statement is true or that something exists.

Belief perseverance–The inability to reject a particular belief despite clear evidence to the contrary.

Beneficence–The ethical tenet that the physician has a responsibility to act in the patient's best interest.

Benzodiazepine–A central nervous system depressant that is often used to reduce anxiety or promote sleep.

Biomedical approach–An approach to psychological disorders that considers only pathophysiological causes and offers pharmaceutical and medical solutions for symptom alleviation.

Biopsychosocial approach–An approach to psychological disorders that considers conditions and treatments to be dependent on biological, psychological, and social causes. Treatment under this approach includes both direct and indirect therapy.

Bipolar disorders–Class of mood disorders characterized by both depression and mania.

Birth rate–The number of births per population in a period of time; usually the number of births per 1000 people per year.

Bisexual–A sexual orientation wherein individuals are attracted to members of multiple sexes.

Bottom-up processing–Object recognition by parallel processing and feature detection in response to sensory stimuli.

Brainstem–The most primitive portion of the brain, which includes the midbrain and hindbrain; controls the autonomic nervous system and communication between the spinal cord, cranial nerves, and brain.

Broca's aphasia–Loss of the motor function of speech, resulting in intact understanding with an inability to correctly produce spoken language.

Broca's area–A brain region located in the inferior frontal gyrus of the frontal lobe (usually in the left hemisphere); largely responsible for the motor function of speech.

Bureaucracy–A formal organization with the goal of performing complex tasks as efficiently as possible by dividing work among a number of bureaus.

Bystander effect–The observation that, when in a group, individuals are less likely to respond to a person in need.

Cannon–Bard theory–A theory of emotion that states that a stimulus is first received and is then simultaneously processed physiologically and cognitively, allowing for the conscious emotion to be experienced.

Cataplexy–Loss of muscle control with intrusion of REM sleep during waking hours, usually caused by an emotional trigger.

Catatonia–Disorganized motor behavior characterized by various unusual physical movements or stillness.

Central nervous system (CNS)–The portion of the nervous system composed of the brain and spinal cord.

Cerebellum–A portion of the hindbrain that maintains posture and balance and coordinates body movements.

Cerebral cortex–The outermost layer of the cerebrum, responsible for complex perceptual, behavioral, and cognitive processes.

Cerebrospinal fluid (CSF)–An aqueous solution in which the brain and spinal cord rest; produced by cells lining the ventricles of the brain.

Cerebrum–A portion of the brain that contains the cerebral cortex, limbic system, and basal ganglia.

Characteristic institution–The social structure or institution about which societies are organized.

Chemoreceptors–Sensory neurons that respond to chemical stimuli.

Choice shift–This term is analogous to group polarization, but describes the behavior change of the group as a whole rather than the individual.

Circadian rhythm–The alignment of physiological processes with the 24-hour day, including sleep–wake cycles and some elements of the endocrine system.

Circular reaction–A repetitive action that achieves a desired response; seen during Piaget's sensorimotor stage.

Class consciousness–In Marxist theory, the organization of the working class around shared goals and recognition of a need for collective political action.

Classical conditioning–A form of associative learning in which a neutral stimulus becomes associated with an unconditioned stimulus such that the neutral stimulus alone produces the same response as the unconditioned stimulus; the neutral stimulus thus becomes a conditioned stimulus.

Cocaine–Drug that decreases reuptake of dopamine, norepinephrine, and serotonin, with effects similar to amphetamines.

Cognition–The process of acquiring knowledge and understanding through thought, experiences, and the senses; how we think and respond to the world.

Cognitive appraisal–The subjective evaluation of a situation that induces stress, consisting of both an initial primary appraisal and a potential secondary appraisal if a threat is revealed during primary appraisal.

Cognitive development–The development of one's ability to think and solve problems across the life span.

Cognitive dissonance–The simultaneous presence of two opposing thoughts or opinions.

Cognitive reassociation model–A model of aggression which states that we are more likely to respond aggressively when experiencing negative emotions.

Collective unconscious–In Jungian psychoanalysis, the part of the unconscious mind that is shared among all humans and is a result of our common ancestry.

Colliculi–Two structures in the midbrain involved in sensorimotor reflexes; the superior colliculus receives visual sensory input, and the inferior colliculus receives auditory sensory input.

Compliance–A change of behavior of an individual at the request of another.

Concordance rates–In twin studies, the presence of a trait in both twins.

Conditioned response–In classical conditioning paradigms, the reflexive response caused by a conditioned stimulus.

Conditioned stimulus–In classical conditioning paradigms, this is an initially neutral stimulus that is paired with an unconditioned stimulus to train a behavioral response, rendering the previously neutral stimulus a conditioned stimulus.

Conduction aphasia–A speech disorder characterized by the inability to repeat words with intact spontaneous speech production and comprehension; usually due to injury to the arcuate fasciculus.

Confirmation bias–A cognitive bias in which one focuses on information that supports a given solution, belief, or hypothesis and ignores evidence against it.

Conflict theory–A theoretical framework that emphasizes the role of power differentials in producing social order.

Conformity–The changing of beliefs or behaviors in order to fit into a group or society.

Consciousness–Awareness of oneself; can be used to describe varying levels of awareness that occur with wakefulness, sleep, dreaming, and drug-induced states.

Conservation–Concept seen in quantitative analysis performed by a child; develops when a child is able to identify the difference between quantity by number and actual amount, especially when faced with identical quantities separated into varying pieces.

Constancy–In sensory perception, perceiving certain characteristics of object to remain the same despite differences in the environment.

Context effect–A retrieval cue by which memory is aided when a person is in the location where encoding took place.

Contralateral–On the opposite side of the body, relative to something else (usually a side of the brain).

Controlled (conscious) processing–Processing method used when a task requires complete attention.

Correspondent inference theory–A theory that states that people pay closer attention to intentional behavior than accidental behavior when making attributions, especially if the behavior is unexpected.

Cortical homunculus–A "map" that relates regions of the brain to the anatomical regions of the body.

Critical period–A time during development during which exposure to language is essential for eventual development of the effective use of language; occurs between two years of age and puberty.

Crystallized intelligence–Cognitive capacity to understand relationships or solve problems using information acquired during schooling and other experiences.

Cues–In understanding the behavior of others, indicators of the underlying cause of a behavior. This includes consistency cues, consensus cues, and difference cues.

Cultural capital–The benefits one receives from knowledge, abilities, and skills.

Cultural diffusion–The spread of norms, cultures, and beliefs throughout a culture.

Cultural relativism–The theory that social groups and cultures must be studied on their own terms to be understood.

Cultural sensitivity–Recognizing and respecting the differences between cultures.

Cultural syndrome–A shared set of beliefs, attitudes, norms, values, and behaviors organized around a central theme and found among people who speak the same language and share a geographic region.

Cultural transmission–The means by which a society socializes its members.

Culture–The beliefs, behaviors, actions, and characteristics of a group or society of people.

Culture shock–Cultural differences that are seen as quite dramatic when travelling outside of one's own society.

Deductive reasoning–A form of cognition that starts with general information and narrows down that information to create a conclusion.

Defense mechanism–In Freudian psychoanalysis, a technique used by the ego that denies, falsifies, or distorts reality in order to resolve anxiety caused by undesirable urges of the id and superego.

Deindividuation–The idea that people will lose a sense of self-awareness and can act dramatically differently based on the influence of a group.

Delirium–Rapid fluctuation in cognitive function that is reversible and has a nonpsychological cause.

Delusions–Fixed, false beliefs that are discordant with reality and not shared by one's culture, and are maintained in spite of strong evidence to the contrary.

Dementia–Intellectual decline starting with impaired memory and progressing to impaired judgment and confusion.

Demographic shift–A change in the makeup of a population over time.

Demographic transition–The transition from high birth and mortality rates to lower birth and mortality rates, seen as a country develops from a preindustrial to an industrialized economic system.

Demographics–The statistical arm of sociology, which attempts to characterize and explain populations by quantitative analysis.

Depressant–Any substance that reduces nervous system function.

Depressive disorder–Sadness meeting certain conditions of severity and duration such that a diagnosis of a mental health issue is warranted. Depressive disorders include, among others: major depression, dysthymic disorder, and seasonal affective disorder.

Depressive episode–A period of at least two weeks in which there is a prominent and persistent depressed mood or lack of interest and at least four other depressive symptoms.

Deviance–The violation of norms, rules, or expectations within a society.

***Diagnostic and Statistical Manual of Mental Disorders* (DSM)**–The guide by which most psychological disorders are characterized, described, and diagnosed; currently in its fifth edition (DSM-5, published May 2013).

Diencephalon–A portion of the prosencephalon that becomes the thalamus, hypothalamus, posterior pituitary gland, and pineal gland.

Differential association theory–Theory that deviance can be learned through interactions with others who engage in deviant behavior, provided those interactions outnumber interactions with those who conform to social norms in number and/or importance.

Disconfirmation principle–The idea that states that if evidence obtained during testing does not confirm a hypothesis, then the hypothesis is discarded or revised.

Discrimination–In classical conditioning, the process by which two similar but distinct conditioned stimuli produce different responses; in sociology, when individuals of a particular group are treated differently than others based on their group.

Discriminative stimulus–In behavioral conditioning, a stimulus whose presence indicates the opportunity for reward.

Dishabituation–A sudden increase in response to a stimulus, usually due to a change in the stimulus or addition of another stimulus; sometimes called resensitization.

Displacement–A defense mechanism by which undesired urges are transferred from one target to another, more acceptable one.

Display rules–Cultural expectations of how emotions can be expressed.

Dispositional (internal) attributions–Attributions that relate to the decisions or personality of the person whose behavior is being considered.

Dissociative disorders–Disorders that involve a perceived separation from identity or the environment.

Distal stimulus–Part of the outside world that serves as a source for stimuli that reach the sensory neurons.

Distant networks–Networks that are looser and composed of weaker ties.

Distress–The stress response to unpleasant stressors.

Divided attention–The ability to attend to multiple stimuli simultaneously and to perform multiple tasks at the same time.

Dizygotic twins–Fraternal twins who share approximately 50% of their genes, as with most siblings.

Dominant hemisphere–The side of the brain that provides analytic, language, logic, and math skills; in most individuals, the left hemisphere.

Dopamine–A neurotransmitter associated with smooth movements, steady posture, the reward pathway, and psychosis.

Dramaturgical approach–An impression management theory that represents the world as a stage and individuals as actors performing to an audience.

Dreaming–Phenomenon which mostly occurs during REM sleep. Theories proposed to explain this phenomenon include activation-synthesis theory, problem-solving dream theory, and cognitive process dream theory.

Drive reduction theory–A theory that explains motivation as being based on the goal of eliminating uncomfortable internal states.

Drives–Deficiencies that activate particular behaviors focused on a goal, which can be further subdivided into either primary (body-sustaining) or secondary (not biologically necessary) drives.

Dual-coding theory–A cognitive theory that states that both visual and verbal associations are used to encode and retrieve information.

Duplicity theory of vision–A theory which holds that the retina contains two types of specialized photoreceptors: rods specialized for light and dark perception and cones specialized for color perception.

Dyssomnia–A sleep disorder in which one has difficulty falling asleep, staying asleep, or avoiding sleep.

Ecstasy–Common name for MDMA (3,4-methylenedioxy-*N*-methylamphetamine); a central nervous system stimulant with effects similar to both amphetamines and hallucinogens.

Efferent neurons–Motor neurons that transmit information from the central nervous system to the periphery.

Ego–In Freudian psychoanalysis, the part of the unconscious mind that mediates the urges of the id and superego; operates under the reality principle.

Egocentrism–Self-centered view of the world in which one is not necessarily able to understand the experience of another person; seen in Piaget's preoperational stage.

Elaboration likelihood model–A theory in which attitudes are formed and changed through different routes of information processing based on the degree of deep thought given to persuasive information. There are two possible processing routes within this model: central route processing (deep thinking or elaborative) and peripheral route processing (non-elaborative).

Elaborative rehearsal–The association of information in short-term memory to information already stored in long-term memory; aids in long-term storage.

Electroencephalography (EEG)–A test used to study the electrical patterns of the brain under varying conditions; consists of multiple electrodes placed on the scalp. Characteristic EEG patterns include beta, alpha, theta, and delta waves, as well as patterns associated with REM sleep.

Emotion–A feeling and state of mind derived from circumstances, mood, or relationships.

Emotional support–Listening to, affirming, and empathizing with someone's feelings as part of social support.

Empathy–The ability to vicariously experience the emotions of another.

Empathy-altruism hypothesis–Theory that one individual helps another when they feel empathy for the other person.

Encoding–The process of receiving information and preparing it for storage; can be automatic or effortful.

Endorphins–Natural painkillers produced by the brain.

Epinephrine–A neurotransmitter associated with the fight-or-flight response.

Errors of growth–Misuse of grammar characterized by universal application of a rule, regardless of exceptions; seen in children during language development.

Escape learning–A form of negative reinforcement in which one reduces the unpleasantness of something that already exists.

Esteem support–Affirming qualities and skills of the person as part of social support.

Ethnic enclave–Locations with a high concentration of one specific ethnicity that can often slow assimilation.

Ethnicity–A social construct that sorts people by cultural factors, including language, nationality, religion, and other factors.

Ethnocentrism–The practice of making judgments about other cultures based on the values and beliefs of one's own culture.

Eustress–The stress response to positive conditions.

Evolutionary stable strategy–A strategy that, once adopted, will use natural selective pressure to prevent alternate strategies from arising.

Exchange theory–In social structure, an extension of rational choice theory that focuses on interactions in groups. Exchange theory holds that behavior is engaged in based on expectancy of future rewards and/or punishments.

Expectancy-value theory–The amount of motivation needed to reach a goal is the result of both expectation of success in reaching the goal and degree to which reaching the goal is valued.

Explicit memory–Memory that requires conscious recall, divided into facts (semantic memory) and experiences (episodic memory); also known as declarative memory.

Extinction–In classical conditioning, the decrease in response resulting from repeated presentation of the conditioned stimulus without the presence of the unconditioned stimulus.

Extrapyramidal system–Part of the basal ganglia that modulates motor activity.

Extraversion–In trait theory, the degree to which an individual is able to tolerate social interaction and stimulation.

Extrinsic motivation–Motivation that is external, or outside the self, including rewards and punishments.

False consciousness–In Marxist theory, a misperception of one's actual position within society.

Family group–A group determined by birth, adoption, and marriage rather than self-selection (as in a peer group).

Fertility rate–The average number of children born to a woman during her lifetime in a population.

Fisherian selection–Also called runaway selection, this is a positive feedback mechanism in which a trait with no impact (or a negative impact) on survival becomes more and more exaggerated over time, especially if the trait is deemed sexually desirable.

Fixation–In Freudian psychoanalysis, the result of overindulgence or frustration during a psychosexual stage causing a neurotic pattern of personality based on that stage.

Flat affect–Behavior characterized by showing virtually no signs of emotion or affective expression.

Fluid intelligence–Ability to quickly identify relationships and connections, and then use those relationships and connections to make correct deductions.

Foraging–The act of searching for and exploiting food resources.

Forebrain–A portion of the brain that is associated with complex perceptual, cognitive, and behavioral processes such as emotion and memory.

Fornix–A long projection from the hippocampus that connects to other nuclei in the limbic system.

Front stage–In the dramaturgical approach, the setting where players are in front of an audience and perform roles that are in keeping with the image they hope to project about themselves.

Frontal lobe–A portion of the cerebral cortex that includes the prefrontal cortex and the motor cortex; it controls motor processing, executive function, and the integration of cognitive and behavioral processes.

Functional attitudes theory–Theory that attitudes serve four functions: knowledge, ego expression, adaptation, and ego defense.

Functional fixedness–The inability to identify uses for an object beyond its usual purpose.

Functionalism–A theoretical framework that explains how parts of society fit together to create a cohesive whole, via both manifest (intended to help some part of the system) and latent (unintended positive) functions.

Fundamental attribution error–The general bias toward making dispositional attributions rather than situational attributions when analyzing another person's behavior.

Game theory–A model that explains social interaction and decision making as a game, including strategies, incentives, and punishments.

γ-aminobutyric acid (GABA)–A neurotransmitter associated with stabilizing and quelling brain activity.

Ganglia–Collections of neuron cell bodies found outside the central nervous system.

Gemeinschaft und Gesellschaft–Theory that distinguishes between two major types of groups: communities (*Gemeinschaften*), which share beliefs, ancestry, or geography; and societies (*Gesellschaften*), which work together toward a common goal.

Gender–The set of behavioral, cultural, or psychological traits typically associated with a biological sex.

Gender inequality–The intentional or unintentional empowerment of one gender to the detriment of others.

Gender segregation–The separation of individuals based on perceived gender.

General adaptation syndrome–Sequence of physiological responses developed by Selye in response to stress, initiating with alarm, followed by resistance, and finally exhaustion.

Generalization–In classical conditioning, the process by which two distinct but similar stimuli come to produce the same response.

Genotype–The genetic makeup of an individual.

Gentrification–The process of renewal of low income areas by upper-class populations, ultimately displacing the lower income residents.

Gestalt principles–Governed by the law of prägnanz, ways for the brain to infer missing parts of a picture when a picture is incomplete.

Globalization–The process of integrating the global economy with free trade and tapping of foreign labor markets.

Glutamate–An excitatory neurotransmitter in the central nervous system.

Glycine–An inhibitory neurotransmitter in the central nervous system.

Group–A social entity that involves at least two people, usually those sharing common characteristics.

Group conformity–Compliance with a group's goals, even when the group's goals may be in direct contrast to an individual's goals.

Group polarization–The tendency toward decisions that are more extreme than the individual inclinations of the group members.

Groupthink–The tendency for groups to make decisions based on ideas and solutions that arise within the group without considering outside ideas and ethics; based on pressure to conform and remain loyal to the group.

Gyrus–A ridge of the cerebral cortex.

Habituation–A decrease in response caused by repeated exposure to a stimulus.

Hallucinations–Perceptions that are not due to external stimuli but have a compelling sense of reality.

Hallucinogens–A group of drugs that cause distortions of reality in users, including lysergic acid diethylamide (LSD) and psilocybin-containing mushrooms.

Halo effect–A cognitive bias in which judgments of an individual's character can be affected by the overall impression of the individual.

Heterosexual–A sexual orientation wherein individuals are attracted to members of a different sex.

Heuristic–A rule of thumb or shortcut that is used to make decisions.

Hidden curriculum–In education, the transmission to students of social norms, attitudes, and beliefs.

Hierarchy of salience–Theory of identity organization that posits that we let situations dictate which identity holds the most importance at any given moment.

Hindbrain–A portion of the brain that controls balance, motor coordination, breathing, digestion, and general arousal processes.

Hippocampus–A portion of the limbic system that is important for memory and learning.

Homosexual–A sexual orientation wherein individuals are attracted to members of the same sex.

Humanistic theory–The set of theories that hold that personality is the result of the conscious feelings we have for ourselves as we attempt to attain our needs and goals. The theories of Kelly, Maslow, Lewin, and others fall into this category.

Hypnagogic hallucinations–Hallucinations that occur when going to sleep; seen in narcolepsy.

Hypnopompic hallucinations–Hallucinations that occur when awakening from sleep; seen in narcolepsy.

Hypnosis–An altered state of consciousness in which a person appears to be awake but is, in fact, in a highly suggestible state in which another person or event may trigger action by the person.

Hypothalamus–A portion of the forebrain that controls homeostatic and endocrine functions by controlling the release of pituitary hormones.

Id–In Freudian psychoanalysis, the part of the unconscious resulting from basic, instinctual urges for sexuality and survival; operates under the pleasure principle and seeks instant gratification.

Ideal self–The person one would optimally like to be.

Identity–A piece of an individual's self-concept based on the groups to which that person belongs and relationships to others.

Identity shift effect–When an individual's state of harmony is disrupted by a threat of social rejection, the individual will often conform to the norms of the group, followed by a corresponding identity shift to reduce cognitive dissonance.

Immediate networks–Networks that are dense with strong ties; generally overlap with distant networks.

Implicit memory–Memory that does not require conscious recall; consists of skills and conditioned behaviors.

Implicit personality theory–A theory that states that people tend to associate traits and behavior in others, and that people have the tendency to attribute their own beliefs, opinions, and ideas onto others.

Impression management–Behaviors that are intended to influence the perceptions of other people about a person, object, or event.

Incentive–A reward intended to motivate particular behaviors.

Incentive theory–Theory that behavior is motivated by the desire to pursue rewards and avoid punishments.

Incidence–The number of new cases of a disease per population at risk in a given period of time; usually, new cases per 1000 at-risk people per year.

Inclusive fitness–A measure of reproductive success; depends on the number of offspring an individual has, how well they support their offspring, and how well their offspring can support others.

Individual discrimination–One person discriminating against a particular person or group.

Inductive reasoning–A form of cognition that utilizes generalizations to develop a theory.

Inferior colliculus–Region of the midbrain that receives and integrates sensory input from the auditory system, and is involved in reflexive reactions to auditory input.

Information processing model–Model of human cognition containing four key components: information intake, information analysis, situational modification, and content/complexity of problem.

Informational support–Support given by providing information to help another person.

Ingratiation–An impression management strategy that uses flattery to increase social acceptance.

In-group–A social group to which people experience a sense of belonging or one in which they identify as a member.

Innate behavior–A behavior that is genetically programmed or instinctive.

Insomnia–Sleep disorder characterized by either an inability to fall asleep or difficulty staying asleep.

Instinct–An innate behavioral response to stimuli.

Instinct theory–In motivation, the theory that people are driven to engage in behaviors based on evolutionarily preprogrammed instincts.

Instinctive drift–The tendency of animals to resist learning when a conditioned behavior conflicts with the animal's instinctive behaviors.

Institutional discrimination–Discrimination against a particular person or group by an entire institution.

Intelligence quotient–Numerical measurement of intelligence, usually accomplished by some form of standardized testing.

Interaction process analysis–A technique of observing and immediately classifying the activities of small groups.

Interference–A retrieval error caused by the learning of information; can be proactive (old information causes difficulty learning new information) or retroactive (new information interferes with older learning).

Internalization–Changing one's behavior to fit with a group while also privately agreeing with the ideas of the group.

Interneuron–A neuron found between sensory and motor neurons; involved in the reflex arc.

Interpersonal attraction–The force that makes people like each other.

Intersectionality–The interconnected nature of social categorizations as they apply to a given individual/group, especially when they lead to discrimination or oppression.

Intrinsic motivation–Motivation that is internal or that comes from within.

Intuition–Perceptions about a situation that may or may not be supported by available evidence, but are nonetheless perceived as information that may be used to make a decision.

Ipsilateral–On the same side of the body, relative to something else (usually a side of the brain).

Iron law of oligarchy–Democratic or bureaucratic systems naturally shift to being ruled by an elite group.

James–Lange theory–A theory of emotion that states that a stimulus results in physiological arousal, which then leads to a secondary response in which emotion is consciously experienced.

Justice–In medical ethics, the tenet that the physician has a responsibility to treat similar patients with similar care and to distribute healthcare resources fairly.

Just-noticeable difference (jnd)–The minimum difference in magnitude between two stimuli before one can perceive this difference; also called a difference threshold.

Just-world hypothesis–The cognitive bias that good things happen to good people, and bad things happen to bad people.

Labeling theory–Theory that labels given to people affect not only how others respond to that person, but also the person's self-image.

Language–Spoken or written symbols (verbal and nonverbal symbols), which are regulated according to certain rules of conduct or social norms and used for communication.

Language acquisition device (LAD)–An innate capacity for language acquisition that is triggered by exposure to language; part of the nativist (biological) perspective of language acquisition.

Latent learning–Learning that occurs without a reward but that is spontaneously demonstrated once a reward is introduced.

Learned helplessness–A state of hopelessness and resignation resulting from being unable to avoid repeated negative stimuli; often used as a model of depression.

Learning–In psychology, the way in which new behaviors are acquired.

Learning (behaviorist) theory–A theory that attitudes are developed through forms of learning (direct contact, direct interaction, direct instruction, and conditioning).

Libido–In Freudian psychoanalysis, the sex or life drive.

Life course approach to health–An analysis of health and probable outcomes that includes consideration of the patient's entire history.

Limbic system–A portion of the cerebrum that is associated with emotion and memory and includes the amygdala and hippocampus.

Linguistic relativity hypothesis–A hypothesis suggesting that one's perception of reality is largely determined by the content, form, and structure of language; also known as the Whorfian hypothesis.

Locus of control–The characterization of the source of influences on the events in one's life; can be internal or external.

Long-term memory–The relatively limitless form of memory reserved for information that is sufficiently rehearsed or of sufficient impact. There are both implicit and explicit forms of long-term memory.

Long-term potentiation–The strengthening of neural connections due to rehearsal or relearning; thought to be the neurophysiological basis of long-term memory.

Looking-glass self–Social psychological construct stating that the self is developed through interpersonal reactions, specifically through a person's understanding of the perception others have of them.

Magnocellular cells–In vision processing, cells that have high temporal resolution and detect motion.

Maintenance rehearsal–Repetition of a piece of information either to keep it within working memory or to store it.

Malthusian theory–Theory of demographic transition that focuses on how population growth can outpace food supply growth and lead to social degradation and disorder.

Managing appearances–An impression management strategy in which one uses props, appearance, emotional expression, or associations with others to create a positive image.

Manic episode–A period of at least one week with prominent and persistent elevated or expansive mood and at least two other manic symptoms.

Maslow's hierarchy of needs–Abraham Maslow's theory that certain needs will yield a greater influence on motivation. Maslow's hierarchy consists of five "levels" of need.

Mass hysteria–A shared, intense concern about the threats to society.

Master status–A status with which a person is most identified.

Mate bias–A measure of how choosy members of a species are in choosing a mate, based upon both direct and indirect benefits of mate selection.

Mate choice–The selection of a mate based on attraction and traits.

Material culture–The physical items one associates with a given cultural group.

Material support–Providing economic or other physical resources to aid a person as part of social support.

Mating system–The way in which a group organizes its sexual behavior and sexual relationships.

McDonaldization–A shift in focus toward efficiency, predictability, calculability, and control in societies.

Meditation–A state of consciousness entered voluntarily, characterized by a decreased level of physiological arousal and a quieting of the mind.

Medulla oblongata–A portion of the brainstem that regulates vital functions, including breathing, heart rate, and blood pressure.

Melatonin–A serotonin derivative secreted by the pineal gland that is associated with sleepiness.

Meninges–A thick layer of connective tissue that covers and protects the brain; composed of the dura mater, arachnoid mater, and pia mater.

Mental set–A tendency to repeat solutions that have yielded positive results at some time in the past.

Mere exposure effect–An explanation of attraction, also called the familiarity effect, which holds that people prefer stimuli that they have been exposed to more frequently.

Meritocracy–A society in which advancement up the social ladder is based on intellectual talent and achievement.

Mesencephalon–The embryonic portion of the brain that becomes the midbrain.

Mesolimbic reward pathway–Dopaminergic pathway in the brain including the nucleus accumbens, ventral tegmental area, and the medial forebrain bundle. This pathway is normally involved in motivation and emotional response, and is involved in drug addiction.

Metencephalon–The embryonic portion of the brain that becomes the pons and cerebellum.

Midbrain–A portion of the brainstem that manages sensorimotor reflexes to visual and auditory stimuli and gives rise to some cranial nerves.

Migration–The movement of people from one population to another, including immigration and emigration.

Mirror neurons–Neurons located in the frontal and parietal lobes and which fire both when an individual performs an action and when an individual sees that action performed.

Misinformation effect–A phenomenon in which memories are altered by misleading information provided at the point of encoding or recall.

Mnemonic–A technique that aids in memory recall.

Monogamy–An exclusive mating relationship.

Monozygotic twins–Identical twins, sharing the same genetic material.

Mood disorder–A mental health diagnosis category containing disorders primarily characterized by disturbance in mood. This includes depressive disorders, substance-induced, and bipolar disorders.

Moral reasoning–Kohlberg's theory of personality evelopment, which is focused on the development of moral thinking through preconventional, conventional, and postconventional stages.

Morbidity–The burden or degree of illness associated with a given disease.

Morphology–The structure of words, including their building blocks (prefixes, suffixes, and so on).

Mortality rate–The number of deaths in a population per unit time.

Motivation–The process of psychological and physical requirements, goals, or desires causing behavior.

Motor neuron–A neuron that transmits motor information from the spinal cord and brain to the periphery.

Multiculturalism–The encouragement of multiple cultures in a society to enhance diversity. Also referred to as cultural diversity.

Multiple intelligences–The idea that intelligence may exist in multiple areas, not just in the areas typically assessed by traditional intelligence quotient tests.

Myelencephalon–The embryonic portion of the brain that becomes the medulla oblongata.

Narcolepsy–A sleep disorder characterized by a lack of voluntary control over the onset of sleep; also involves cataplexy and hypnagogic and hypnopompic hallucinations.

Nativist theory (of language)–Theory credited to Noam Chomsky that posits the existence of an innate capacity for language, referred to as the language acquisition device.

Needs–Physiological and psychological requirements that motivate and influence behavior.

Negative symptoms–In mental illness, symptoms characterized by the absence of normal or desired behaviors.

Neologism–Coining a new word; seen in schizophrenia.

Network–A term used to describe the observable pattern of social relationships among individual units of analysis.

Network redundancy–Overlapping contact points within a social network.

Network support–Providing a sense of belonging as part of social support.

Neurocognitive models of dreaming–Models of dreaming that correlate subjective, cognitive experiences of dreaming with measurable physiological changes.

Neuroleptics (antipsychotics)–A class of drugs used to treat schizophrenia by blocking dopamine receptors.

Neuromodulator–Peptides that act as signaling molecules in the central nervous system; they are slower to act and longer lasting than neurotransmitters.

Neuroplasticity–Change in neural connections caused by learning or a response to injury.

Neuropsychology–The study of functions and behaviors associated with specific regions of the brain.

Neurosis–In Freudian theory, a disorder that occurs in response to the anxiety of a fixation during childhood that impacts personality development.

Neuroticism–In trait theory, the degree to which an individual is prone to emotional arousal in stressful situations.

Neurotransmitter–A chemical that transmits signals from a neuron to a target cell across a synapse.

Neurulation–Stage in development in which the ectoderm furrows over the notochord, forming the neural crest and neural tube.

Night terror–An experience of intense anxiety during sleep, causing the sleeper to scream in terror with no recall of the event in the morning; occurs during slow-wave sleep.

Nondominant hemisphere–The side of the brain associated with sensitivity to the emotional tone of language, intuition, creativity, music, and spatial processing; in most individuals, the right hemisphere.

Nonmaleficence–The ethical tenet that the physician has a responsibility to avoid interventions in which the potential for harm outweighs the potential for benefit.

Non-rapid eye movement (NREM) sleep–Stages 1 through 4 of sleep; contains ever-slowing brain waves as one gets deeper into sleep.

Nonverbal communication–How people communicate, intentionally or unintentionally, without using words; examples include body language, gestures, and facial expressions.

Norepinephrine–A neurotransmitter associated with wakefulness and alertness.

Norms–Societal rules that define the boundaries of acceptable behavior.

Obedience–The changing of behavior of an individual based on a command from someone seen as an authority figure.

Object permanence–Knowledge that an object does not cease to exist even when the object cannot be seen; a milestone in cognitive development.

Observational learning–A form of learning in which behavior is modified as a result of watching others.

Obsessive-compulsive disorders–This category, which also includes related disorders, describes the set of disorders where people feel the need to check things repeatedly or have certain thoughts repeatedly, without the ability to control these thoughts or activities.

Occipital lobe–A portion of the cerebral cortex that controls visual processing.

Operant conditioning–A form of associative learning in which the frequency of a behavior is modified using reinforcement or punishment.

Opiates–A drug family consisting of naturally occurring, highly addictive, pain-reducing drugs used in both medical and recreational settings; opioids are synthetic versions of these drugs.

Opponent-process theory–A theory that states that the body will adapt to counteract repeated exposure to stimuli, such as seeing afterimages or ramping up the sympathetic nervous system in response to a depressant.

Organization–A specific type of group characterized by five traits: formality, hierarchy of ranked positions, large size, complex division of labor, and continuity beyond its members.

Ought self–The representation of the way others think one should be.

Out-group–A social group with which an individual does not identify.

Overconfidence–A tendency to interpret one's decisions, knowledge, or beliefs as infallible.

Parallel play–Play style in which children can play alongside each other without interfering in each other's behavior.

Parallel processing–The ability to simultaneously analyze and combine information regarding multiple aspects of a stimulus, such as color, shape, and motion.

Parasomnia–A sleep disorder characterized by abnormal movements or behaviors during sleep.

Parasympathetic nervous system–A branch of the autonomic nervous system that promotes resting and digesting; associated with relaxed states, reductions in heart and respiration rates, and promotion of digestion.

Parietal lobe–A portion of the cerebral cortex that controls somatosensory and spatial processing.

Parkinson's disease–A disease characterized by slowness in movement, resting tremor, pill-rolling tremor, masklike facies, cogwheel rigidity, and a shuffling gait; caused by destruction of dopaminergic neurons in the substantia nigra.

Parvocellular cells–In visual processing, cells which have very high spatial resolution and detect shape.

Peer group–A group of self-selected equals that forms around common interests, ideas, preferences, and beliefs.

Peer pressure–The social influence placed on an individual by other individuals who are perceived as equals.

Perception–Processing of incoming information to comprehend and respond to the current incoming stimuli.

Peripheral nervous system (PNS)–The portion of the nervous system composed of nerve tissue and fibers outside the central nervous system.

Personality–The set of thoughts, feelings, traits, and behaviors that are characteristic of an individual across time and different locations.

Personality disorders–Disorders that involve patterns of behavior that are inflexible and maladaptive, causing distress or impaired function in at least two of the following: cognition, emotion, interpersonal functioning, or impulse control.

Phenotype–The expressed traits of an individual based on their genotype.

Phoneme–Individual speech sound associated with a language.

Phonology–The set of sounds that compose a language.

Piaget's theory–Piaget's theory of cognitive development divided the life span into sensorimotor, preoperational, concrete operational, and formal operational stages.

Pineal gland–A brain structure located near the thalamus that secretes melatonin.

Pituitary gland–The "master gland" of the endocrine system that triggers hormone release in other endocrine glands.

Place theory–Theory of sound conduction in the ear that holds that vibration on particular areas of the basilar membrane determines perception of pitch, also referred to as tonotopical organization.

Polyandry–A mating system in which an individual has exclusive relationships with several males.

Polygamy–A mating system in which an individual has multiple exclusive relationships.

Polygyny–A mating system in which an individual has exclusive relationships with several females.

Pons–A portion of the brainstem that relays information between the cortex and medulla, regulates sleep, and carries some motor and sensory information from the face and neck.

Positive symptoms–Behaviors, thoughts, or feelings added to normal behavior.

Poverty–A socioeconomic condition of low resource availability; in the United States, the poverty line is determined by the government's calculation of the minimum income requirements for families to acquire the minimum necessities of life.

Power–The capacity to influence people through the real or threatened use of rewards and punishments; often based on unequal distribution of valued resources.

Pragmatics–The ways in which use of language can be altered, depending on social context.

Prejudice–An irrational positive or negative attitude toward a person, group, or thing, formed prior to actual experience.

Prestige–In sociology, the amount of positive regard society has for a given person or idea.

Prevalence–The number of cases of a disease per population in a given period of time; usually, cases per 1000 people per year.

Primacy effect–The phenomenon of first impressions of a person being more important than subsequent impressions.

Primary group–A group wherein the interactions are direct, with close bonds, providing relationships to members that are very warm, personal, and intimate.

Primary stress appraisal–An initial evaluation of the environment to determine if there is an associated threat.

Priming–A retrieval cue by which recall is aided by a word or phrase that is semantically related to the desired memory.

Primitive reflexes–Reflexes present in infants that disappear with age.

Prodromal phase–A phase of poor adjustment that precedes the full onset of schizophrenia.

Projection–A defense mechanism by which individuals attribute their undesired feelings to others.

Projection area–A portion of the cerebral cortex that analyzes sensory input.

Promiscuity–A mating system in which an individual mates with others without exclusivity.

Proprioception–The ability to tell where one's body is in space.

Prosencephalon–The embryonic portion of the brain that becomes the forebrain.

Prosody–The rhythm, cadence, and inflection of speech.

Prospective memory–Remembering to perform a task at some point in a future.

Proximal stimulus–A stimulus that directly interacts with and affects sensory receptors.

Proximity–An aspect of interpersonal attraction based on being physically close to someone.

Psychoanalytic theory–In personality theory, the set of theories based on the assumption that unconscious internal states motivate overt actions and determine personality. The theories of several psychologists, including both Freud and Jung, fall into this category.

Psychological disorder–A set of thoughts, feelings, or actions that are considered deviant by the culture at hand and that cause noticeable distress to the sufferer.

Psychophysics–The study of the relationship between the physical nature of stimuli and the sensations/perceptions they evoke.

Psychosocial development–Erikson's theory of personality development, which is based in the concept that personality is developed based on a series of crises deriving from conflicts between needs and social demands.

Psychoticism–In trait theory, the measure of nonconformity or social deviance of an individual.

Punishment–In operant conditioning, the use of an aversive stimulus designed to decrease the frequency of an undesired behavior.

Race–A social construct based on phenotypic differences between groups of people; these may be either real or perceived differences.

Racial formation theory–Theory that racial identity is fluid and dependent on political, economic, and social factors.

Racialization–The definition or establishment of a group as a particular race.

Rapid eye movement (REM) sleep–Sleep stage in which the eyes move rapidly back and forth and physiological arousal levels are more similar to wakefulness than sleep; dreaming occurs during this stage.

Rational choice theory–In social structure, the theory that individuals consider benefits and harms to themselves in any given social interaction and choose the best possible action.

Rationalization–A defense mechanism by which individuals explain undesirable behaviors in a way that is self-justifying and socially acceptable.

Reaction formation–A defense mechanism by which individuals suppress urges by unconsciously converting them into their exact opposites.

Reappraisal–Process for ongoing monitoring of a continuing source of stress that cannot be dealt with via the normal 2-step appraisal method.

Recency effect–The phenomenon in which the most recent information we have about an individual is most important in forming our impressions.

Reciprocal determinism–In the social cognitive perspective, the notion that thoughts, feelings, behaviors, and environment interact to determine behavior in a given situation.

Reciprocal liking–The phenomenon whereby people like others better when they believe the other person likes them.

Reciprocity–An aspect of interpersonal attraction based on the idea that we like people who we think like us.

Recognition-primed decision model–A decision-making model in which experience and recognition of similar situations one has already experienced play a large role in decision making and actions; also one of the explanations for the experience of intuition.

Reference group–The group to which individuals compare themselves for a given identity.

Reflex–A behavior that occurs in response to a given stimulus without higher cognitive input.

Reflex arc–A neural pathway that controls reflex actions.

Regional cerebral blood flow (rCBF)–A technique used to record patterns of neural activity based on blood flow to different areas of the brain measured using detection of inhaled radioactive markers.

Regression–A defense mechanism by which an individual deals with stress by reverting to an earlier developmental state.

Reinforcement–In operant conditioning, the use of a stimulus designed to increase the frequency of a desired behavior.

Reinforcement schedule–The schedule by which reinforcement is administered for behavior in operant conditioning; reinforcement schedules can be fixed or variable, and can be based on a ratio or an interval between rewards.

Relative poverty–Poverty in comparison to the larger surrounding population.

Reliance on central traits–The tendency to organize the perception of others based on traits and personal characteristics of the target that matter to the perceiver.

REM rebound–Phenomenon in which one spends an increased time in REM sleep following a period of sleep deprivation.

Representativeness heuristic–A shortcut in decision making that relies on categorizing items on the basis of whether they fit the prototypical, stereotypical, or representative image of the category.

Repression–A defense mechanism by which the ego forces undesired thoughts and urges to the unconscious mind.

Response bias–The tendency of subjects to respond systematically to a stimulus in a particular way due to nonsensory factors.

Reticular formation–A structure in the brainstem that is responsible for alertness.

Retrieval–The process of demonstrating that information has been retained in memory; includes recall, recognition, and relearning.

Retrograde amnesia–A form of memory loss that impacts long-term memories of events prior to the time of injury.

Rhombencephalon–The embryonic portion of the brain that becomes the hindbrain.

Ritual–A formalized ceremony that usually involves specific material objects, symbolism, and additional mandates on acceptable behavior.

Role–A set of beliefs, values, attitudes, and norms that define expectations for behavior associated with a particular status.

Role conflict–A difficulty in satisfying role requirements or expectations among various roles.

Role engulfment–Internalizing a label and assuming the role implied by the label leads to the assumed role taking over a person's identity.

Role partner–The person with whom one interacts while playing a particular role; each role partner provides a different set of behavioral expectations.

Role performance–Carrying out the behaviors associated with a given role.

Role set–A group of role partners relative to a given status.

Role strain–Difficulty in satisfying multiple requirements of the same role.

Role-taking–Roleplaying, by which children come to understand the perspectives of others and the ways in which these perspectives may differ from their own.

Sanction–A societally enforced punishment or reward for behavior. Formal sanctions are those enforced by social institutions (laws), and informal sanctions are enforced by social behaviors (ostracization, etc.).

Schachter–Singer theory–A theory of emotion that states that both physiological arousal and cognitive appraisal must occur before an emotion is consciously experienced.

Schema–An organized pattern of thought and behavior; one of the central concepts of Piaget's stages of cognitive development.

Schizophrenia–A psychotic disorder characterized by gross distortions of reality and disturbances in the content and form of thought, perception, and behavior.

Second sickness–The concept proposed by Howard Waitzkin that poor health outcomes are exacerbated by social injustice.

Secondary group–Groups wherein interactions are based on weaker, impersonal bonds.

Secondary stress appraisal–The interpretation of primary stress appraisal to determine emotional response to a given threat.

Selective attention–The ability to focus on a single stimulus even while other stimuli are occurring simultaneously.

Self-concept–The sum of the thoughts and feelings about oneself; includes self-schemata and appraisal of one's past and future self.

Self-determination theory–Need-based motivational theory that emphasizes the importance of autonomy, competence, and relatedness.

Self-disclosure–An aspect of interpersonal attraction or impression management in which one shares fears, thoughts, and goals with another person in the hopes of being met with empathy and nonjudgment.

Self-discrepancy theory–Theory that each of us has three selves: the actual self, the ideal self, and the ought self.

Self-efficacy–The degree to which individuals see themselves as being capable at a given skill or in a particular situation.

Self-enhancement–In self-serving bias, the need to maintain self worth through internal attribution of success and external attribution of failure.

Self-esteem–An individual's feelings of self-worth.

Self-fulfilling prophecy–The phenomenon of a stereotype creating an expectation of a particular group, which creates conditions that lead to confirmation of this stereotype.

Self-handicapping–An impression management strategy wherein people create obstacles to avoid self-blame when they do not meet expectations.

Self-presentation–The process of displaying oneself to society through culturally accepted actions and behaviors.

Self-reference effect–The tendency for individuals to best recall information that they can relate to their own experiences.

Self-schema–A self-given label that carries with it a set of qualities.

Self-serving bias–The idea that individuals will view their own success as being based on internal factors, while viewing failures as being based on external factors.

Semantic network–Organization of information in the brain by linking concepts with similar characteristics and meaning.

Semantics–The association of meaning with a word.

Sensation–Transduction of physical stimuli into neurologic signals.

Sensitive period–A time during which environmental input has a maximal impact on the development of a particular ability.

Sensory memory–Visual (iconic) and auditory (echoic) stimuli briefly stored in memory; fades very quickly unless attention is paid to the information.

Sensory neuron–A neuron that transmits information from sensory receptors to the central nervous system.

Septal nuclei–Part of the limbic system and one of the pleasure centers of the brain.

Serial position effect–The tendency to better remember items presented at the beginning or end of a list; related to the primacy and recency effects.

Serotonin–A neurotransmitter associated with mood, sleep, eating, and dreaming.

Sexual orientation–The direction of one's sexual interest.

Shadowing–An experimental technique in which participants recite speech immediately after hearing it.

Shaping–In operant conditioning, the process of conditioning a complicated behavior by rewarding successive approximations of the behavior.

Short-term memory–Memory which fades quickly, over about 30 seconds without rehearsal, and which is limited in capacity by the 7 ± 2 rule.

Sick role–Theory that a person who is ill enters a role of "sanctioned deviance," in which they are not responsible for the illness and are exempt from social norms.

Signal detection theory–A theory of perception in which internal (psychological) and external (environmental) context both play a role in the perception of stimuli.

Similarity–An aspect of interpersonal attraction based on being alike in attitudes, intelligence, education, height, age, religion, appearance, or socioeconomic status.

Situational (external) attributions–Attributions that relate to features of the surroundings, such as threats, money, social norms, and peer pressure, rather than to features of the individual.

Sleep apnea–Sleep disorder in which a person may cease to breathe while sleeping; may be due to obstruction or a central (neurological) cause.

Sleep cycle–A single complete progression through each stage of sleep.

Slow-wave sleep–Consists of NREM sleep stages 3 and 4; also called delta-wave sleep.

Social action–Actions and behaviors that individuals are conscious of and performing because others are around.

Social capital–The investment people make in their society in return for economic or collective rewards.

Social class–A category of people with a shared socioeconomic background that exhibit similar lifestyles, job opportunities, attitudes, and behaviors.

Social cognitive theory–A theory that attitudes are formed through observation of behavior, cognition, and the environment.

Social construction model–A theory of emotional expression that assumes there are no biologically wired emotions; rather, they are based on experiences and situational context alone.

Social constructionism–A theoretical approach that uncovers the ways in which individuals and groups participate in the formation of their perceived social reality.

Social control–Regulating the behavior of individuals and groups within a society.

Social exclusion–The sense of being separated from and powerless in society when impoverished.

Social facilitation–The tendency of people to perform at a different level based on the fact that others are around.

Social institutions–Well-established, structured patterns of behavior or relationships that are accepted as a fundamental part of a culture.

Social interaction–The ways in which two or more individuals can shape each other's behavior.

Social interactionist theory–In language development, the theory that language acquisition is driven by the desire to communicate. This theory includes both biological and social processes.

Social loafing–The tendency of individuals to put in less effort in group settings as compared to an individual setting.

Social mobility–The movement of individuals in the social hierarchy through changes in income, education, or occupation.

Social movements–Philosophies that drive large numbers of people to organize to promote or resist social change.

Social perception–Understanding the thoughts and motives of other people present in the social world; also referred to as social cognition.

Social reproduction–The concept that social inequality, especially poverty, can be reproduced and passed on from one generation to the next.

Social stratification–Organization of societies into a hierarchical system, usually based on socioeconomic status and social class.

Social structure–A system of people within a society organized by a characteristic pattern of relationships.

Social support–The perception or reality that one is cared for by a social network.

Socialization–The process of developing and spreading norms, customs, and beliefs.

Socioeconomic status–Social standing or class of an individual or group, determined as a combination of education, income, and occupation.

Sociology–The study of society, including how it is created, interacted with, defined, and institutionalized.

Somatic nervous system–The voluntary branch of the peripheral nervous system, which consists of sensory and motor neurons used to control bodily movements.

Somatic symptom disorders–Mental health disorders marked by bodily symptoms that cause significant stress or impairment. This category of disorder also includes related disorders, such as illness anxiety and conversion disorders.

Somatosensation–The sense of touch, which contains multiple modalities: pressure, vibration, pain, and temperature.

Somatosensory cortex–Region of the parietal lobe located on the postcentral gyrus and involved in somatosensory information processing.

Somnambulism–Sleep disorder in which one carries out actions while asleep; also called sleepwalking.

Source-monitoring error–A memory error by which a person remembers the details of an event but confuses the context by which the details were gained; often causes people to remember events that happened to someone else as having happened to themselves.

Spacing effect–The phenomenon of retaining larger amounts of information when the amount of time between sessions of relearning is increased.

Spatial inequality–A form of social stratification across territories and their populations that can involve residential, environmental, or global components.

Spontaneous recovery–The reappearance of a conditioned response previously determined to be extinct.

Spreading activation–The unconscious activation of closely linked nodes of a semantic network.

State-dependent memory–A retrieval cue by which memory is aided when a person is in the same state of emotion or intoxication as when encoding took place.

Status–A position in society used to classify individuals.

Stereocilia–Structures on hair cells in the ear that sway with the movement of endolymph, causing receptor potential in the hair cells and ultimately leading to detection of incoming sound.

Stereotype content model–A model that classifies stereotypes using two dimensions: warmth and competence.

Stereotype threat–A feeling of anxiety about confirming a negative stereotype about one's social group.

Stereotypes–Attitudes and impressions that are made based on limited and superficial information about a person or a group of individuals.

Stigma–The extreme disapproval or dislike of a person or group based on perceived differences in social characteristics from the rest of society.

Stimulant–A drug that causes an increase in central nervous system arousal.

Stimulus–Any energy pattern that is sensed in some way by the body; includes visual, auditory, and physical sensations, among others.

Storage–The retention of encoded information; divided into sensory, short-term, and long-term memory.

Strain theory–Theory that explains deviance as a natural reaction to the disconnect between social goals and social structure.

Stress–The response to significant events, challenges, and decisions.

Stressors–Biological elements, external conditions, or events that lead to a stress response.

Structural poverty–Theory that poverty is due to inadequacies in societal and economic structure.

Subcultures–Groups of people within a culture that distinguish themselves from the primary culture to which they belong.

Sublimation–A defense mechanism by which unacceptable urges are transformed into socially acceptable behaviors.

Subliminal perception–Perception of a stimulus below a threshold (usually the threshold of conscious perception).

Substantia nigra–Part of the basal ganglia responsible for dopamine release that permits proper functioning of the rest of the basal ganglia.

Sulcus–A fold in the cerebral cortex.

Superego–In Freudian psychoanalysis, the part of the unconscious mind focused on idealism, perfectionism, and societal norms.

Superior colliculus–Structure in the midbrain that receives visual input and impacts eye movements and object oriented behaviors.

Symbolic culture–The nonmaterial culture that represents a group of people; expressed through ideas and concepts.

Symbolic ethnicity–An ethnic identity that is only relevant on special occasions or in specific circumstances and that does not impact everyday life.

Symbolic interactionism–A theoretical framework that studies the way individuals interact through a shared understanding of words, gestures, and other symbols.

Sympathetic nervous system–The branch of the autonomic nervous system that controls the fight-or-flight response; associated with stressful situations that increase heart and respiration rates and decrease digestion.

Synaptic pruning–Adjustment of neural connections throughout life, involving breaking of weak neural connections and bolstering of strong neural connections.

Syntax–The way in which words are organized to create meaning.

System for multiple level observation of groups (SYMLOG)–A method of studying group dynamics; focuses on three fundamental dimensions of interaction: dominance *vs.* submission, friendliness *vs.* unfriendliness, and instrumentally controlled *vs.* emotionally expressive.

Tactical self–In impression management, the person one markets oneself to be when adhering to others' expectations.

Telencephalon–A portion of the prosencephalon that becomes the cerebrum.

Temporal lobe–A portion of the cerebral cortex that controls auditory processing, memory processing, emotional control, and language.

Tetrahydrocannabinol (THC)–The main active ingredient in marijuana.

Thalamus–A portion of the forebrain that serves as a relay and sorting station for sensory information, and then transmits the information to the cerebral cortex.

Theory of mind–The ability to sense how another's mind works.

Threshold–Also called limina; the minimum amount of a stimulus that renders a difference in perception.

Tolerance–Decreased response to a drug after physiological adaptation.

Top-down processing–Object recognition driven by memories and expectations that allow the brain to first recognize the whole object, and then recognize components based on existing expectations.

Trait theory–Personality theory that is focused on describing individual personalities as the sum of characteristic behaviors.

Transduction–Conversion of physical, electromagnetic, auditory, and other stimuli to electrical signals in the nervous system.

Transformational grammar–A linguistic theory that focuses on how changes in word order affect meaning.

Two-point threshold–The minimum distance necessary between two points of stimulation on the skin such that the points will be felt as two distinct stimuli.

Type theory–Theorifes of personality that are focused on creating taxonomies, or finite lists, of personality types.

Unconditioned response–In classical conditioning paradigms, the innate response brought about by an unconditioned stimulus prior to any conditioning.

Unconditioned stimulus–In classical conditioning paradigms, a stimulus that brings about an innate response.

Universal emotions–Emotions that are recognized by all cultures; include happiness, sadness, contempt, surprise, fear, disgust, and anger.

Urbanization–The process whereby large numbers of people migrate to and establish residence in relatively dense areas of population.

Value–What one deems important in life.

Ventricle–An internal cavity within the brain; cells lining the ventricles produce cerebrospinal fluid.

Verbal communication–The use of spoken or signed language.

Vestibular sense–One of the functions of the ear, the detection of rotational and linear acceleration to maintain awareness of body rotation and movement.

Visual cortex–Region of the occipital lobe devoted to processing visual information.

Visual pathways–Term which refers to both anatomical connections between eyes and brain and the flow of information from eyes to brain. The visual pathway contains several brain regions including the LGN, the visual cortex, and the superior colliculus.

Vygotsky theory–In cognitive development, the theory that the engine driving cognitive development is childhood internalization of culture.

Weber's law–A theory of perception that states that there is a constant ratio between the change in stimulus magnitude needed to produce a just noticeable difference and the magnitude of the original stimulus.

Wernicke-Korsakoff Syndrome–A condition resulting from chronic thiamine (vitamin B_1) deficiency, which is common in individuals who have alcoholism; characterized by severe memory impairment with changes in mental status and loss of coordination.

Wernicke's aphasia–Loss of language comprehension, resulting in fluid production of language without meaning.

Wernicke's area–A brain region located in the superior temporal gyrus of the temporal lobe (usually in the left hemisphere); largely responsible for language comprehension.

Working memory–Form of memory that allows limited amounts of information in short-term memory to be manipulated.

World system theory–World system theory argues there are global level inequalities in the division of labor between core, semi-peripheral, and peripheral nations.

Yerkes-Dodson law–A theory that there is a U shaped function relating arousal level and performance, dictating that performance is worst at the extreme high and low ends of arousal and optimal at intermediate arousal levels. This law is the basis of the Yerkes-Dodson law of social facilitation, a specific application of the Yerkes-Dodson law.

Zone of proximal development–Those skills that a child has not yet mastered but can accomplish with the help of a more knowledgeable other.

INDEX

Note: Material in figures or tables is indicated by italic *f* or *t* after the page number.

B

C

D

R

T

ART CREDITS

Chapter 1 Cover—Image credited to nobeastsofierce. From Shutterstock.

Figure 1.2—Image credited to Alila Medical Media. From Shutterstock.

Figure 1.3—Image credited to Alila Medical Media. From Shutterstock.

Figure 1.7—Image credited to User: _moep_. From Wikimedia Commons.

Figure 1.15—From Shutterstock.

Chapter 2 Cover—Image credited to Phatic Photography. From Shutterstock.

Chapter 3 Cover—Image credited to Fer Gregory. From Shutterstock.

Figure 3.4—Image credited to Public Library of Science. From Wikimedia Commons. Copyright © 2006. Used under license: CC-BY-2.5.

Chapter 4 Cover—Image credited to Igor Zh. From Shutterstock.

Figure 4.10—Image credited to User: Nitramas. From Wikimedia Commons.

Figure 4.13—Image credited to William Rafti. From Wikimedia Commons. Copyright © 2006. Used under license: CC-BY-2.5.

Figure 4.14—Image credited to User: Saxo. From Wikimedia Commons.

Chapter 5 Cover—Image credited to A.B.G. From Shutterstock.

Figure 5.1—Image credited to Mohd Fuad Salleh/EyeEm. From Getty Images.

Chapter 6 Cover—Image credited to Kanea. From Shutterstock.

Chapter 7 Cover—Image credited to hikrcn. From Shutterstock.

Figure 7.3—Image credited to User: Stepan Kapl. From Shutterstock.

Figure 7.4c—Image credited to Jose Luis Calvo. From Shutterstock.

Chapter 8 Cover—Image credited to file404. From Shutterstock.

Figure 8.2—Image credited to RonTech2000. From Getty Images.

Figure 8.5—Image credited to Newhoggy-commonswiki. From Wikimedia Commons.

Figure 8.6—Image credited to User: russavia. From Wikimedia Commons. Copyright © 2013. Used under license: CC-BY-2.0.

Figure 8.7—Image credited to User: kance. From Wikimedia Commons. Copyright © 2006. Used under license: CC-BY-2.0.

Chapter 9 Cover—Image credited to 10'000 Hours. From Getty Images.

Figure 9.2—Image credited to aldomurillo. From Getty Images.

Figure 9.3—Image credited to Tobertz Chavez. From Wikimedia Commons. Copyright © 2006.
Used under license: CC-BY-2.0.

Figure 9.4—Image credited to Josh Plueger. From Wikimedia Commons.

Figure 9.5—Image credited to J. Tautz and M. Kleinheinz. From the Public Library of Science. Copyright © 2004.
Used under license: CC-BY-2.5.

Chapter 10 Cover—Image credited to eyecrave productions. From Getty Images.

Figure 10.1—Image credited to Michael L. Baird. From Wikimedia Commons. Copyright © 2008.
Used under license: CC-BY-2.0.

Figure 10.3—Image credited to AndreAnita. From Shutterstock.

Figure 10.4—Image credited to Alex Pronove. From Wikimedia Commons. Copyright © 2011.
Used under license: CC-BY-2.5.

Chapter 11 Cover—Image credited to John M Lund Photography Inc. From Getty Images.

Figure 11.1—Image credited to Yana Iskayeva. From Getty Images.

Figure 11.2—Image credited to Baluchis. From Getty Images.

Figure 11.3—Image credited to arfabita. From Shutterstock.

Figure 11.10—Image credited to User: NikNaks93. From Wikimedia Commons.

Figure 11.11—Image credited to User: Jonathan McIntosh. From Wikimedia Commons.

Chapter 12 Cover—Image credited to Olivier Le Queinec. From Shutterstock.

Figure 12.1—Image credited to User: TastyCakes. From Wikimedia Commons. Copyright © 2009.
Used under license: CC-BY-3.0.

Figure 12.3—Image credited to the National Park Service. From Wikimedia Commons.

Notes

Notes

Notes

Notes

Notes

Notes

Notes

Notes

Notes

Notes

Notes

Notes

MCAT® PHYSICS AND MATH REVIEW 2024–2025

ONLINE + BOOK

Edited by Alexander Stone Macnow, MD

ACKNOWLEDGMENTS

Editor-in-Chief, 2024–2025 Edition
M. Dominic Eggert

Contributing Editors, 2024–2025 Edition
Christopher Durland; Charles Pierce, MD; Jason Selzer

Prior Edition Editorial Staff: Brandon Deason, MD; Christopher Durland; M. Dominic Eggert; Tyler Fara; Elizabeth Flagge; Adam Grey; Jason Selzer; Lauren White

Published by Kaplan North America, LLC dba Kaplan Publishing
1515 West Cypress Creek Road
Fort Lauderdale, Florida 33309

ISBN: 978-1-5062-8701-0

10 9 8 7 6 5 4 3

Kaplan Publishing print books are available at special quantity discounts to use for sales promotions, employee premiums, or educational purposes. For more information or to purchase books, please call the Simon & Schuster special sales department at 866-506-1949.

TABLE OF CONTENTS

GO ONLINE

kaptest.com/booksonline

THE *KAPLAN MCAT REVIEW* TEAM

Alexander Stone Macnow, MD
Editor-in-Chief

Áine Lorié, PhD
Editor

Derek Rusnak, MA
Editor

Mikhail Alexeeff
Kaplan MCAT Faculty

Laura L. Ambler
Kaplan MCAT Faculty

Krista L. Buckley, MD
Kaplan MCAT Faculty

Kristen L. Russell, ME
Editor

Pamela Willingham, MSW
Editor

Melinda Contreras, MS
Kaplan MCAT Faculty

Samantha Fallon
Kaplan MCAT Faculty

Jason R. Selzer
Kaplan MCAT Faculty

M. Dominic Eggert
Editor

Faculty Reviewers and Editors: Elmar R. Aliyev; James Burns; Jonathan Cornfield; Alisha Maureen Crowley; Brandon Deason, MD; Nikolai Dorofeev, MD; Benjamin Downer, MS; Colin Doyle; Christopher Durland; Marilyn Engle; Eleni M. Eren; Raef Ali Fadel; Elizabeth Flagge; Adam Grey; Tyra Hall-Pogar, PhD; Scott Huff; Samer T. Ismail; Ae-Ri Kim, PhD; Elizabeth A. Kudlaty; Kelly Kyker-Snowman, MS; Ningfei Li; John P. Mahon; Matthew A. Meier; Nainika Nanda; Caroline Nkemdilim Opene; Kaitlyn E. Prenger; Uneeb Qureshi; Sadije Redzovic, PhD; Bela G. Starkman, PhD; Rebecca Stover, MS; Kyle Swerdlow; Michael Paul Tomani, MS; Lauren K. White; Nicholas M. White; Allison Ann Wilkes, MS; Kerranna Williamson, MBA; and Tony Yu

Thanks to Rebecca Anderson; Jeff Batzli; Eric Chiu; Tim Eich; Tyler Fara; Owen Farcy; Dan Frey; Robin Garmise; Rita Garthaffner; Joanna Graham; Allison Gudenau; Allison Harm; Beth Hoffberg; Aaron Lemon-Strauss; Keith Lubeley; Diane McGarvey; Petros Minasi; Beena P V; John Polstein; Deeangelee Pooran-Kublall, MD, MPH; Rochelle Rothstein, MD; Larry Rudman; Srividhya Sankar; Sylvia Tidwell Scheuring; Carly Schnur; Aiswarya Sivanand; Todd Tedesco; Karin Tucker; Lee Weiss; Christina Wheeler; Kristen Workman; Amy Zarkos; and the countless others who made this project possible.

GETTING STARTED CHECKLIST

Getting Started Checklist

- [ ] Register for your free online assets—including full-length tests, Science Review Videos, and additional practice materials—at **www.kaptest.com/moreonline**.
- [ ] Create a study calendar that ensures you complete content review and sufficient practice by Test Day!
- [ ] As you finish a chapter and the online practice for that chapter, check it off on the table of contents.
- [ ] Register to take the MCAT at **www.aamc.org/mcat**.
- [ ] Set aside time during your prep to make sure the rest of your application—personal statement, recommendations, and other materials—is ready to go!
- [ ] Take a moment to admire your completed checklist, then get back to the business of prepping for this exam!

PREFACE

And now it starts: your long, yet fruitful journey toward wearing a white coat. Proudly wearing that white coat, though, is hopefully only part of your motivation. You are reading this book because you want to be a healer.

If you're serious about going to medical school, then you are likely already familiar with the importance of the MCAT in medical school admissions. While the holistic review process puts additional weight on your experiences, extracurricular activities, and personal attributes, the fact remains: along with your GPA, your MCAT score remains one of the two most important components of your application portfolio—at least early in the admissions process. Each additional point you score on the MCAT pushes you in front of thousands of other students and makes you an even more attractive applicant. But the MCAT is not simply an obstacle to overcome; it is an opportunity to show schools that you will be a strong student and a future leader in medicine.

We at Kaplan take our jobs very seriously and aim to help students see success not only on the MCAT, but as future physicians. We work with our learning science experts to ensure that we're using the most up-to-date teaching techniques in our resources. Multiple members of our team hold advanced degrees in medicine or associated biomedical sciences, and are committed to the highest level of medical education. Kaplan has been working with the MCAT for over 50 years and our commitment to premed students is unflagging; in fact, Stanley Kaplan created this company when he had difficulty being accepted to medical school due to unfair quota systems that existed at the time.

We stand now at the beginning of a new era in medical education. As citizens of this 21st-century world of healthcare, we are charged with creating a patient-oriented, culturally competent, cost-conscious, universally available, technically advanced, and research-focused healthcare system, run by compassionate providers. Suffice it to say, this is no easy task. Problem-based learning, integrated curricula, and classes in interpersonal skills are some of the responses to this demand for an excellent workforce—a workforce of which you'll soon be a part.

We're thrilled that you've chosen us to help you on this journey. Please reach out to us to share your challenges, concerns, and successes. Together, we will shape the future of medicine in the United States and abroad; we look forward to helping you become the doctor you deserve to be.

Good luck!

Alexander Stone Macnow, MD
Editor-in-Chief
Department of Pathology and Laboratory Medicine
Hospital of the University of Pennsylvania

BA, Musicology—Boston University, 2008
MD—Perelman School of Medicine at the University of Pennsylvania, 2013

ABOUT THE MCAT

Anatomy of the MCAT

Here is a general overview of the structure of Test Day:

Section	Number of Questions	Time Allotted
Test-Day Certification		4 minutes
Tutorial (optional)		10 minutes
Chemical and Physical Foundations of Biological Systems	59	95 minutes
Break (optional)		10 minutes
Critical Analysis and Reasoning Skills (CARS)	53	90 minutes
Lunch Break (optional)		30 minutes
Biological and Biochemical Foundations of Living Systems	59	95 minutes
Break (optional)		10 minutes
Psychological, Social, and Biological Foundations of Behavior	59	95 minutes
Void Question		3 minutes
Satisfaction Survey (optional)		5 minutes

The structure of the four sections of the MCAT is shown below.

Chemical and Physical Foundations of Biological Systems	
Time	95 minutes
Format	• 59 questions • 10 passages • 44 questions are passage-based, and 15 are discrete (stand-alone) questions. • Score between 118 and 132
What It Tests	• Biochemistry: 25% • Biology: 5% • General Chemistry: 30% • Organic Chemistry: 15% • Physics: 25%

Critical Analysis and Reasoning Skills (CARS)	
Time	90 minutes
Format	• 53 questions • 9 passages • All questions are passage-based. There are no discrete (stand-alone) questions. • Score between 118 and 132
What It Tests	Disciplines: • Humanities: 50% • Social Sciences: 50% Skills: • *Foundations of Comprehension:* 30% • *Reasoning Within the Text:* 30% • *Reasoning Beyond the Text:* 40%
Biological and Biochemical Foundations of Living Systems	
Time	95 minutes
Format	• 59 questions • 10 passages • 44 questions are passage-based, and 15 are discrete (stand-alone) questions. • Score between 118 and 132
What It Tests	• Biochemistry: 25% • Biology: 65% • General Chemistry: 5% • Organic Chemistry: 5%
Psychological, Social, and Biological Foundations of Behavior	
Time	95 minutes
Format	• 59 questions • 10 passages • 44 questions are passage-based, and 15 are discrete (stand-alone) questions. • Score between 118 and 132
What It Tests	• Biology: 5% • Psychology: 65% • Sociology: 30%
Total	
Testing Time	375 minutes (6 hours, 15 minutes)
Total Seat Time	447 minutes (7 hours, 27 minutes)
Questions	230
Score	472 to 528

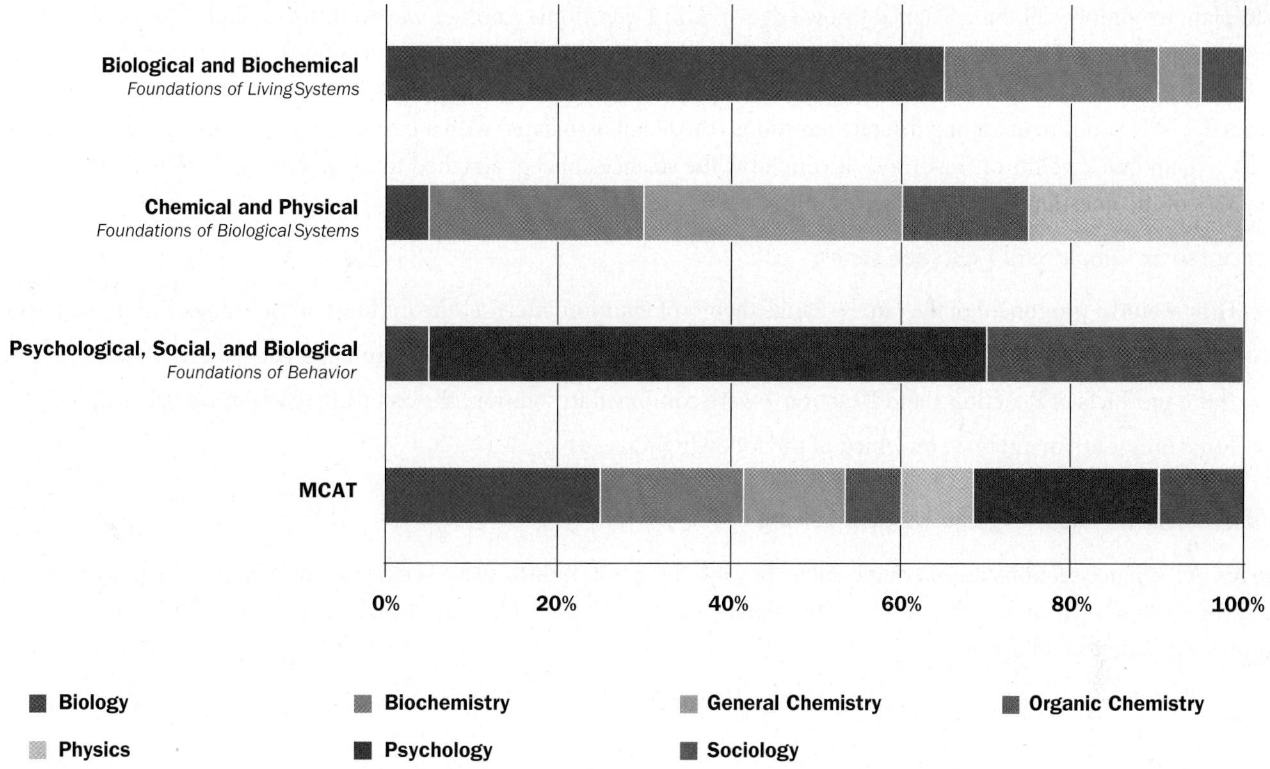

Scientific Inquiry and Reasoning Skills (SIRS)

The AAMC has defined four *Scientific Inquiry and Reasoning Skills* (SIRS) that will be tested in the three science sections of the MCAT:

1. *Knowledge of Scientific Concepts and Principles* (35% of questions)
2. *Scientific Reasoning and Problem-Solving* (45% of questions)
3. *Reasoning About the Design and Execution of Research* (10% of questions)
4. *Data-Based and Statistical Reasoning* (10% of questions)

Let's see how each one breaks down into more specific Test Day behaviors. Note that the bullet points of specific objectives for each of the SIRS are taken directly from the *Official Guide to the MCAT Exam*; the descriptions of what these behaviors mean and sample question stems, however, are written by Kaplan.

Skill 1: *Knowledge of Scientific Concepts and Principles*

This is probably the least surprising of the four SIRS; the testing of science knowledge is, after all, one of the signature qualities of the MCAT. Skill 1 questions will require you to do the following:

- Recognize correct scientific principles
- Identify the relationships among closely related concepts
- Identify the relationships between different representations of concepts (verbal, symbolic, graphic)
- Identify examples of observations that illustrate scientific principles
- Use mathematical equations to solve problems

At Kaplan, we simply call these Science Knowledge or Skill 1 questions. Another way to think of Skill 1 questions is as "one-step" problems. The single step is either to realize which scientific concept the question stem is suggesting or to take the concept stated in the question stem and identify which answer choice is an accurate application of it. Skill 1 questions are particularly prominent among discrete questions (those not associated with a passage). These questions are an opportunity to gain quick points on Test Day—if you know the science concept attached to the question, then that's it! On Test Day, 35% of the questions in each science section will be Skill 1 questions.

Here are some sample Skill 1 question stems:

- How would a proponent of the James–Lange theory of emotion interpret the findings of the study cited in the passage?
- Which of the following most accurately describes the function of FSH in the human menstrual cycle?
- If the products of Reaction 1 and Reaction 2 were combined in solution, the resulting reaction would form:
- Ionic bonds are maintained by which of the following forces?

Skill 2: *Scientific Reasoning and Problem-Solving*

The MCAT science sections do, of course, move beyond testing straightforward science knowledge; Skill 2 questions are the most common way in which it does so. At Kaplan, we also call these Critical Thinking questions. Skill 2 questions will require you to do the following:

- Reason about scientific principles, theories, and models
- Analyze and evaluate scientific explanations and predictions
- Evaluate arguments about causes and consequences
- Bring together theory, observations, and evidence to draw conclusions
- Recognize scientific findings that challenge or invalidate a scientific theory or model
- Determine and use scientific formulas to solve problems

Just as Skill 1 questions can be thought of as "one-step" problems, many Skill 2 questions are "two-step" problems, and more difficult Skill 2 questions may require three or more steps. These questions can require a wide spectrum of reasoning skills, including integration of multiple facts from a passage, combination of multiple science content areas, and prediction of an experiment's results. Skill 2 questions also tend to ask about science content without actually mentioning it by name. For example, a question might describe the results of one experiment and ask you to predict the results of a second experiment without actually telling you what underlying scientific principles are at work—part of the question's difficulty will be figuring out which principles to apply in order to get the correct answer. On Test Day, 45% of the questions in each science section will be Skill 2 questions.

Here are some sample Skill 2 question stems:

- Which of the following experimental conditions would most likely yield results similar to those in Figure 2?
- All of the following conclusions are supported by the information in the passage EXCEPT:
- The most likely cause of the anomalous results found by the experimenter is:
- An impact to a person's chest quickly reduces the volume of one of the lungs to 70% of its initial value while not allowing any air to escape from the mouth. By what percentage is the force of outward air pressure increased on a 2 cm^2 portion of the inner surface of the compressed lung?

Skill 3: *Reasoning About the Design and Execution of Research*

The MCAT is interested in your ability to critically appraise and analyze research, as this is an important day-to-day task of a physician. We call these questions Skill 3 or Experimental and Research Design questions for short. Skill 3 questions will require you to do the following:

- Identify the role of theory, past findings, and observations in scientific questioning
- Identify testable research questions and hypotheses
- Distinguish between samples and populations and distinguish results that support generalizations about populations
- Identify independent and dependent variables
- Reason about the features of research studies that suggest associations between variables or causal relationships between them (such as temporality and random assignment)
- Identify conclusions that are supported by research results
- Determine the implications of results for real-world situations
- Reason about ethical issues in scientific research

Over the years, the AAMC has received input from medical schools to require more practical research skills of MCAT test takers, and Skill 3 questions are the response to these demands. This skill is unique in that the outside knowledge you need to answer Skill 3 questions is not taught in any one undergraduate course; instead, the research design principles needed to answer these questions are learned gradually throughout your science classes and especially through any laboratory work you have completed. It should be noted that Skill 3 comprises 10% of the questions in each science section on Test Day.

Here are some sample Skill 3 question stems:

- What is the dependent variable in the study described in the passage?
- The major flaw in the method used to measure disease susceptibility in Experiment 1 is:
- Which of the following procedures is most important for the experimenters to follow in order for their study to maintain a proper, randomized sample of research subjects?
- A researcher would like to test the hypothesis that individuals who move to an urban area during adulthood are more likely to own a car than are those who have lived in an urban area since birth. Which of the following studies would best test this hypothesis?

Skill 4: *Data-Based and Statistical Reasoning*

Lastly, the science sections of the MCAT test your ability to analyze the visual and numerical results of experiments and studies. We call these Data and Statistical Analysis questions. Skill 4 questions will require you to do the following:

- Use, analyze, and interpret data in figures, graphs, and tables
- Evaluate whether representations make sense for particular scientific observations and data
- Use measures of central tendency (mean, median, and mode) and measures of dispersion (range, interquartile range, and standard deviation) to describe data
- Reason about random and systematic error

- Reason about statistical significance and uncertainty (interpreting statistical significance levels and interpreting a confidence interval)
- Use data to explain relationships between variables or make predictions
- Use data to answer research questions and draw conclusions

Skill 4 is included in the MCAT because physicians and researchers spend much of their time examining the results of their own studies and the studies of others, and it's very important for them to make legitimate conclusions and sound judgments based on that data. The MCAT tests Skill 4 on all three science sections with graphical representations of data (charts and bar graphs), as well as numerical ones (tables, lists, and results summarized in sentence or paragraph form). On Test Day, 10% of the questions in each science section will be Skill 4 questions.

Here are some sample Skill 4 question stems:

- According to the information in the passage, there is an inverse correlation between:
- What conclusion is best supported by the findings displayed in Figure 2?
- A medical test for a rare type of heavy metal poisoning returns a positive result for 98% of affected individuals and 13% of unaffected individuals. Which of the following types of error is most prevalent in this test?
- If a fourth trial of Experiment 1 was run and yielded a result of 54% compliance, which of the following would be true?

SIRS Summary

Discussing the SIRS tested on the MCAT is a daunting prospect given that the very nature of the skills tends to make the conversation rather abstract. Nevertheless, with enough practice, you'll be able to identify each of the four skills quickly, and you'll also be able to apply the proper strategies to solve those problems on Test Day. If you need a quick reference to remind you of the four SIRS, these guidelines may help:

Skill 1 (Science Knowledge) questions ask:

- Do you remember this science content?

Skill 2 (Critical Thinking) questions ask:

- Do you remember this science content? And if you do, could you please apply it to this novel situation?
- Could you answer this question that cleverly combines multiple content areas at the same time?

Skill 3 (Experimental and Research Design) questions ask:

- Let's forget about the science content for a while. Could you give some insight into the experimental or research methods involved in this situation?

Skill 4 (Data and Statistical Analysis) questions ask:

- Let's forget about the science content for a while. Could you accurately read some graphs and tables for a moment? Could you make some conclusions or extrapolations based on the information presented?

Critical Analysis and Reasoning Skills (CARS)

The *Critical Analysis and Reasoning Skills* (CARS) section of the MCAT tests three discrete families of textual reasoning skills; each of these families requires a higher level of reasoning than the last. Those three skills are as follows:

1. *Foundations of Comprehension* (30% of questions)
2. *Reasoning Within the Text* (30% of questions)
3. *Reasoning Beyond the Text* (40% of questions)

These three skills are tested through nine humanities- and social sciences–themed passages, with approximately 5 to 7 questions per passage. Let's take a more in-depth look into these three skills. Again, the bullet points of specific objectives for each of the CARS are taken directly from the *Official Guide to the MCAT Exam*; the descriptions of what these behaviors mean and sample question stems, however, are written by Kaplan.

Foundations of Comprehension

Questions in this skill will ask for basic facts and simple inferences about the passage; the questions themselves will be similar to those seen on reading comprehension sections of other standardized exams like the SAT® and ACT®. *Foundations of Comprehension* questions will require you to do the following:

- Understand the basic components of the text
- Infer meaning from rhetorical devices, word choice, and text structure

This admittedly covers a wide range of potential question types including Main Idea, Detail, Inference, and Definition-in-Context questions, but finding the correct answer to all *Foundations of Comprehension* questions will follow from a basic understanding of the passage and the point of view of its author (and occasionally that of other voices in the passage).

Here are some sample *Foundations of Comprehension* question stems:

- **Main Idea**—The author's primary purpose in this passage is:
- **Detail**—Based on the information in the second paragraph, which of the following is the most accurate summary of the opinion held by Schubert's critics?
- **(Scattered) Detail**—According to the passage, which of the following is FALSE about literary reviews in the 1920s?
- **Inference (Implication)**—Which of the following phrases, as used in the passage, is most suggestive that the author has a personal bias toward narrative records of history?
- **Inference (Assumption)**—In putting together the argument in the passage, the author most likely assumes:
- **Definition-in-Context**—The word "obscure" (paragraph 3), when used in reference to the historian's actions, most nearly means:

Reasoning Within the Text

While *Foundations of Comprehension* questions will usually depend on interpreting a single piece of information in the passage or understanding the passage as a whole, *Reasoning Within the Text* questions require more thought because they will ask you to identify the purpose of a particular piece of information in the context of the passage, or ask how one piece of information relates to another. *Reasoning Within the Text* questions will require you to:

- Integrate different components of the text to draw relevant conclusions

In other words, questions in this skill often ask either *How do these two details relate to one another?* or *What else must be true that the author didn't say?* The CARS section will also ask you to judge certain parts of the passage or even judge the author. These questions, which fall under the *Reasoning Within the Text* skill, can ask you to identify authorial bias, evaluate the credibility of cited sources, determine the logical soundness of an argument, identify the importance of a particular fact or statement in the context of the passage, or search for relevant evidence in the passage to support a given conclusion. In all, this category includes Function and Strengthen–Weaken (Within the Passage) questions, as well as a smattering of related—but rare—question types.

Here are some sample *Reasoning Within the Text* question stems:

- **Function**—The author's discussion of the effect of socioeconomic status on social mobility primarily serves which of the following functions?
- **Strengthen–Weaken (Within the Passage)**—Which of the following facts is used in the passage as the most prominent piece of evidence in favor of the author's conclusions?
- **Strengthen–Weaken (Within the Passage)**—Based on the role it plays in the author's argument, *The Possessed* can be considered:

Reasoning Beyond the Text

The distinguishing factor of *Reasoning Beyond the Text* questions is in the title of the skill: the word *Beyond.* Questions that test this skill, which make up a larger share of the CARS section than questions from either of the other two skills, will always introduce a completely new situation that was not present in the passage itself; these questions will ask you to determine how one influences the other. *Reasoning Beyond the Text* questions will require you to:

- Apply or extrapolate ideas from the passage to new contexts
- Assess the impact of introducing new factors, information, or conditions to ideas from the passage

The *Reasoning Beyond the Text* skill is further divided into Apply and Strengthen–Weaken (Beyond the Passage) questions, and a few other rarely appearing question types.

Here are some sample *Reasoning Beyond the Text* question stems:

- **Apply**—If a document were located that demonstrated Berlioz intended to include a chorus of at least 700 in his *Grande Messe des Morts*, how would the author likely respond?
- **Apply**—Which of the following is the best example of a "virtuous rebellion," as it is defined in the passage?
- **Strengthen–Weaken (Beyond the Passage)**—Suppose Jane Austen had written in a letter to her sister, "My strongest characters were those forced by circumstance to confront basic questions about the society in which they lived." What relevance would this have to the passage?
- **Strengthen–Weaken (Beyond the Passage)**—Which of the following sentences, if added to the end of the passage, would most WEAKEN the author's conclusions in the last paragraph?

CARS Summary

Through the *Foundations of Comprehension* skill, the CARS section tests many of the reading skills you have been building on since grade school, albeit in the context of very challenging doctorate-level passages. But through the two other skills (*Reasoning Within the Text* and *Reasoning Beyond the Text*), the MCAT demands that you understand the deep structure of passages and the arguments within them at a very advanced level. And, of course, all of this is tested under very tight timing restrictions: only 102 seconds per question—and that doesn't even include the time spent reading the passages.

Here's a quick reference guide to the three CARS skills:

Foundations of Comprehension questions ask:

- Did you understand the passage and its main ideas?
- What does the passage have to say about this particular detail?
- What must be true that the author did not say?

Reasoning Within the Text questions ask:

- What's the logical relationship between these two ideas from the passage?
- How well argued is the author's thesis?

Reasoning Beyond the Text questions ask:

- How does this principle from the passage apply to this new situation?
- How does this new piece of information influence the arguments in the passage?

Scoring

Each of the four sections of the MCAT is scored between 118 and 132, with the median at approximately 125. This means the total score ranges from 472 to 528, with the median at about 500. Why such peculiar numbers? The AAMC stresses that this scale emphasizes the importance of the central portion of the score distribution, where most students score (around 125 per section, or 500 total), rather than putting undue focus on the high end of the scale.

Note that there is no wrong answer penalty on the MCAT, so you should select an answer for every question—even if it is only a guess.

The AAMC has released the 2019–2021 correlation between scaled score and percentile, as shown on the following page. It should be noted that the percentile scale is adjusted and renormalized over time and thus can shift slightly from year to year. Percentile rank updates are released by the AAMC around May 1 of each year.

Total Score	Percentile	Total Score	Percentile
528	100	499	41
527	100	498	38
526	100	497	35
525	100	496	32
524	100	495	29
523	99	494	26
522	99	493	24
521	98	492	21
520	97	491	19
519	96	490	17
518	95	489	15
517	94	488	13
516	92	487	11
515	90	486	10
514	88	485	8
513	86	484	7
512	83	483	6
511	80	482	5
510	77	481	4
509	74	480	3
508	71	479	2
507	68	478	2
506	65	477	1
505	61	476	1
504	58	475	<1
503	55	474	<1
502	51	473	<1
501	48	472	<1
500	45		

Source: AAMC. 2022. *Summary of MCAT Total and Section Scores*. Accessed October 2022.
https://students-residents.aamc.org/mcat-research-and-data/percentile-ranks-mcat-exam

Further information on score reporting is included at the end of the next section (see *After Your Test*).

MCAT Policies and Procedures

We strongly encourage you to download the latest copy of *MCAT® Essentials*, available on the AAMC's website, to ensure that you have the latest information about registration and Test Day policies and procedures; this document is updated annually. A brief summary of some of the most important rules is provided here.

MCAT Registration

The only way to register for the MCAT is online. You can access AAMC's registration system at **www.aamc.org/mcat**.

The AAMC posts the schedule of testing, registration, and score release dates in the fall before the MCAT testing year, which runs from January into September. Registration for January through June is available earlier than registration for later dates, but see the AAMC's website for the exact dates each year. There is one standard registration fee, but the fee for changing your test date or test center increases the closer you get to your MCAT.

Fees and the Fee Assistance Program (FAP)

Payment for test registration must be made by MasterCard or VISA. As described earlier, the fee for rescheduling your exam or changing your testing center increases as one approaches Test Day. In addition, it is not uncommon for test centers to fill up well in advance of the registration deadline. For these reasons, we recommend identifying your preferred Test Day as soon as possible and registering. There are ancillary benefits to having a set Test Day, as well: when you know the date you're working toward, you'll study harder and are less likely to keep pushing back the exam. The AAMC offers a Fee Assistance Program (FAP) for students with financial hardship to help reduce the cost of taking the MCAT, as well as for the American Medical College Application Service (AMCAS®) application. Further information on the FAP can be found at **www.aamc.org/students/applying/fap**.

Testing Security

On Test Day, you will be required to present a qualifying form of ID. Generally, a current driver's license or United States passport will be sufficient (consult the AAMC website for the full list of qualifying criteria). When registering, take care to spell your first and last names (middle names, suffixes, and prefixes are not required and will not be verified on Test Day) precisely the same as they appear on this ID; failure to provide this ID at the test center or differences in spelling between your registration and ID will be considered a "no-show," and you will not receive a refund for the exam.

During Test Day registration, other identity data collected may include: a digital palm vein scan, a Test Day photo, a digitization of your valid ID, and signatures. Some testing centers may use a metal detection wand to ensure that no prohibited items are brought into the testing room. Prohibited items include all electronic devices, including watches and timers, calculators, cell phones, and any and all forms of recording equipment; food, drinks (including water), and cigarettes or other smoking paraphernalia; hats and scarves (except for religious purposes); and books, notes, or other study materials. If you require a medical device, such as an insulin pump or pacemaker, you must apply for accommodated testing. During breaks, you are allowed access to food and drink, but not to electronic devices, including cell phones.

Testing centers are under video surveillance and the AAMC does not take potential violations of testing security lightly. The bottom line: *know the rules and don't break them.*

Accommodations

Students with disabilities or medical conditions can apply for accommodated testing. Documentation of the disability or condition is required, and requests may take two months—or more—to be approved. For this reason, it is recommended that you begin the process of applying for accommodated testing as early as possible. More information on applying for accommodated testing can be found at **www.aamc.org/students/applying/mcat/accommodations**.

After Your Test

When your MCAT is all over, no matter how you feel you did, be good to yourself when you leave the test center. Celebrate! Take a nap. Watch a movie. Get some exercise. Plan a trip or outing. Call up all of your neglected friends or message them on social media. Go out for snacks or drinks with people you like. Whatever you do, make sure that it has absolutely nothing to do with thinking too hard—you deserve some rest and relaxation.

Perhaps most importantly, do not discuss specific details about the test with anyone. For one, it is important to let go of the stress of Test Day, and reliving your exam only inhibits you from being able to do so. But more significantly, the Examinee Agreement you sign at the beginning of your exam specifically prohibits you from discussing or disclosing exam content. The AAMC is known to seek out individuals who violate this agreement and retains the right to prosecute these individuals at their discretion. This means that you should not, under any circumstances, discuss the exam in person or over the phone with other individuals—including us at Kaplan—or post information or questions about exam content to Facebook, Student Doctor Network, or other online social media. You are permitted to comment on your "general exam experience," including how you felt about the exam overall or an individual section, but this is a fine line. In summary: *if you're not certain whether you can discuss an aspect of the test or not, just don't do it!* Do not let a silly Facebook post stop you from becoming the doctor you deserve to be.

Scores are typically released approximately one month after Test Day. The release is staggered during the afternoon and evening, ending at 5 p.m. Eastern Standard Time. This means that not all examinees receive their scores at exactly the same time. Your score report will include a scaled score for each section between 118 and 132, as well as your total combined score between 472 and 528. These scores are given as confidence intervals. For each section, the confidence interval is approximately the given score ± 1; for the total score, it is approximately the given score ± 2. You will also be given the corresponding percentile rank for each of these section scores and the total score.

AAMC Contact Information

For further questions, contact the MCAT team at the Association of American Medical Colleges:

MCAT Resource Center
Association of American Medical Colleges
www.aamc.org/mcat
(202) 828-0600
www.aamc.org/contactmcat

HOW THIS BOOK WAS CREATED

The *Kaplan MCAT Review* project began shortly after the release of the *Preview Guide for the MCAT 2015 Exam*, 2nd edition. Through thorough analysis by our staff psychometricians, we were able to analyze the relative yield of the different topics on the MCAT, and we began constructing tables of contents for the books of the *Kaplan MCAT Review* series. A dedicated staff of 30 writers, 7 editors, and 32 proofreaders worked over 5,000 combined hours to produce these books. The format of the books was heavily influenced by weekly meetings with Kaplan's learning science team.

In the years since this book was created, a number of opportunities for expansion and improvement have occurred. The current edition represents the culmination of the wisdom accumulated during that time frame, and it also includes several new features designed to improve the reading and learning experience in these texts.

These books were submitted for publication in April 2023. For any updates after this date, please visit www.kaptest.com/retail-book-corrections-and-updates.

If you have any questions about the content presented here, email KaplanMCATfeedback@kaplan.com. For other questions not related to content, email booksupport@kaplan.com.

Each book has been vetted through at least ten rounds of review. To that end, the information presented in these books is true and accurate to the best of our knowledge. Still, your feedback helps us improve our prep materials. Please notify us of any inaccuracies or errors in the books by sending an email to KaplanMCATfeedback@kaplan.com.

USING THIS BOOK

Kaplan MCAT Physics and Math Review, and the other six books in the *Kaplan MCAT Review* series, bring the Kaplan classroom experience to you—right in your home, at your convenience. This book offers the same Kaplan content review, strategies, and practice that make Kaplan the #1 choice for MCAT prep.

This book is designed to help you review the physics and math topics covered on the MCAT. Please understand that content review—no matter how thorough—is not sufficient preparation for the MCAT! The MCAT tests not only your science knowledge but also your critical reading, reasoning, and problem-solving skills. Do not assume that simply memorizing the contents of this book will earn you high scores on Test Day; to maximize your scores, you must also improve your reading and test-taking skills through MCAT-style questions and practice tests.

Learning Objectives

At the beginning of each section, you'll find a short list of objectives describing the skills covered within that section. Learning objectives for these texts were developed in conjunction with Kaplan's learning science team, and have been designed specifically to focus your attention on tasks and concepts that are likely to show up on your MCAT. These learning objectives will function as a means to guide your study, and indicate what information and relationships you should be focused on within each section. Before starting each section, read these learning objectives carefully. They will not only allow you to assess your existing familiarity with the content, but also provide a goal-oriented focus for your studying experience of the section.

MCAT Concept Checks

At the end of each section, you'll find a few open-ended questions that you can use to assess your mastery of the material. These MCAT Concept Checks were introduced after numerous conversations with Kaplan's learning science team. Research has demonstrated repeatedly that introspection and self-analysis improve mastery, retention, and recall of material. Complete these MCAT Concept Checks to ensure that you've got the key points from each section before moving on!

Science Mastery Assessments

At the beginning of each chapter, you'll find 15 MCAT-style practice questions. These are designed to help you assess your understanding of the chapter before you begin reading the chapter. Using the guidance provided with the assessment, you can determine the best way to review each chapter based on your personal strengths and weaknesses. Most of the questions in the Science Mastery Assessments focus on the first of the *Scientific Inquiry and Reasoning Skills* (*Knowledge of Scientific Concepts and Principles*), although there are occasional questions that fall into the second or fourth SIRS (*Scientific Reasoning and Problem-Solving* and *Data-Based and Statistical Reasoning*, respectively). You can complete each chapter's assessment in a testing interface in your online resources, where you'll also find a test-like passage set covering the same content you just studied to ensure you can also apply your knowledge the way the MCAT will expect you to!

Sidebars

The following is a guide to the five types of sidebars you'll find in *Kaplan MCAT Physics and Math Review:*

- **Bridge:** These sidebars create connections between science topics that appear in multiple chapters throughout the *Kaplan MCAT Review* series.
- **Key Concept:** These sidebars draw attention to the most important takeaways in a given topic, and they sometimes offer synopses or overviews of complex information. If you understand nothing else, make sure you grasp the Key Concepts for any given subject.
- **MCAT Expertise:** These sidebars point out how information may be tested on the MCAT or offer key strategy points and test-taking tips that you should apply on Test Day.
- **Mnemonic:** These sidebars present memory devices to help recall certain facts.
- **Real World:** These sidebars illustrate how a concept in the text relates to the practice of medicine or the world at large. While this is not information you need to know for Test Day, many of the topics in Real World sidebars are excellent examples of how a concept may appear in a passage or discrete (stand-alone) question on the MCAT.

What This Book Covers

The information presented in the *Kaplan MCAT Review* series covers everything listed on the official MCAT content lists. Every topic in these lists is covered in the same level of detail as is common to the undergraduate and postbaccalaureate classes that are considered prerequisites for the MCAT. Note that your premedical classes may include topics not discussed in these books, or they may go into more depth than these books do. Additional exposure to science content is never a bad thing, but all of the content knowledge you are expected to have walking in on Test Day is covered in these books.

Chapter profiles, on the first page of each chapter, represent a holistic look at the content within the chapter, and will include a pie chart as well as text information. The pie chart analysis is based directly on data released by the AAMC, and will give a rough estimate of the importance of the chapter in relation to the book as a whole. Further, the text portion of the Chapter Profiles includes which AAMC content categories are covered within the chapter. These are referenced directly from the AAMC MCAT exam content listing, available on the testmaker's website.

You'll also see new High-Yield badges scattered throughout the sections of this book:

In This Chapter

1.1 Amino Acids Found in Proteins

High-Yield

LEARNING OBJECTIVES

After Chapter 1.1, you will be able to:

- Recognize common abbreviations for amino acids, such as Glu and Y

These badges represent the top 100 topics most tested by the AAMC. In other words, according to the testmaker and all our experience with their resources, a High-Yield badge means more questions on Test Day.

This book also contains a thorough glossary and index for easy navigation of the text.

In the end, this is your book, so write in the margins, draw diagrams, highlight the key points—do whatever is necessary to help you get that higher score. We look forward to working with you as you achieve your dreams and become the doctor you deserve to be!

Studying with This Book

In addition to providing you with the best practice questions and test strategies, Kaplan's team of learning scientists are dedicated to researching and testing the best methods for getting the most out of your study time. Here are their top four tips for improving retention:

Review multiple topics in one study session. This may seem counterintuitive—we're used to practicing one skill at a time in order to improve each skill. But research shows that weaving topics together leads to increased learning. Beyond that consideration, the MCAT often includes more than one topic in a single question. Studying in an integrated manner is the most effective way to prepare for this test.

Customize the content. Drawing attention to difficult or critical content can ensure you don't overlook it as you read and re-read sections. The best way to do this is to make it more visual—highlight, make tabs, use stickies, whatever works. We recommend highlighting only the most important or difficult sections of text. Selective highlighting of up to about 10 percent of text in a given chapter is great for emphasizing parts of the text, but over-highlighting can have the opposite effect.

Repeat topics over time. Many people try to memorize concepts by repeating them over and over again in succession. Our research shows that retention is improved by spacing out the repeats over time and mixing up the order in which you study content. For example, try reading chapters in a different order the second (or third!) time around. Revisit practice questions that you answered incorrectly in a new sequence. Perhaps information you reviewed more recently will help you better understand those questions and solutions you struggled with in the past.

Take a moment to reflect. When you finish reading a section for the first time, stop and think about what you just read. Jot down a few thoughts in the margins or in your notes about why the content is important or what topics came to mind when you read it. Associating learning with a memory is a fantastic way to retain information! This also works when answering questions. After answering a question, take a moment to think through each step you took to arrive at a solution. What led you to the answer you chose? Understanding the steps you took will help you make good decisions when answering future questions.

Online Resources

In addition to the resources located within this text, you also have additional online resources awaiting you at **www.kaptest.com/booksonline**. Make sure to log on and take advantage of free practice and other resources!

Please note that access to the online resources is limited to the original owner of this book.

STUDYING FOR THE MCAT

The first year of medical school is a frenzied experience for most students. To meet the requirements of a rigorous work schedule, students either learn to prioritize their time or else fall hopelessly behind. It's no surprise, then, that the MCAT, the test specifically designed to predict success in medical school, is a high-speed, time-intensive test. The MCAT demands excellent time-management skills, endurance, and grace under pressure both during the test as well as while preparing for it. Having a solid plan of attack and sticking with it are key to giving you the confidence and structure you need to succeed.

Creating a Study Plan

The best time to create a study plan is at the beginning of your MCAT preparation. If you don't already use a calendar, you will want to start. You can purchase a planner, print out a free calendar from the Internet, use a built-in calendar or app on one of your smart devices, or keep track using an interactive online calendar. Pick the option that is most practical for you and that you are most likely to use consistently.

Once you have a calendar, you'll be able to start planning your study schedule with the following steps:

1. **Fill in your obligations and choose a day off.**

   Write in all your school, extracurricular, and work obligations first: class sessions, work shifts, and meetings that you must attend. Then add in your personal obligations: appointments, lunch dates, family and social time, etc. Making an appointment in your calendar for hanging out with friends or going to the movies may seem strange at first, but planning social activities in advance will help you achieve a balance between personal and professional obligations even as life gets busy. Having a happy balance allows you to be more focused and productive when it comes time to study, so stay well-rounded and don't neglect anything that is important to you.

   In addition to scheduling your personal and professional obligations, you should also plan your time off. Taking some time off is just as important as studying. Kaplan recommends taking at least one full day off per week, ideally from all your study obligations but at minimum from studying for the MCAT.

2. **Add in study blocks around your obligations.**

   Once you have established your calendar's framework, add in study blocks around your obligations, keeping your study schedule as consistent as possible across days and across weeks. Studying at the same time of day as your official test is ideal for promoting recall, but if that's not possible, then fit in study blocks wherever you can.

   To make your studying as efficient as possible, block out short, frequent periods of study time throughout the week. From a learning perspective, studying one hour per day for six days per week is much more valuable than studying for six hours all at once one day per week. Specifically, Kaplan recommends studying for no longer than three hours in one sitting. Within those three-hour blocks, also plan to take ten-minute breaks every hour. Use these breaks to get up from your seat, do some quick stretches, get a snack and drink, and clear your mind. Although ten minutes of break for every 50 minutes of studying may sound like a lot, these breaks will allow you to deal with distractions and rest your brain so that, during the 50-minute study blocks, you can remain fully engaged and completely focused.

3. **Add in your full-length practice tests.**

   Next, you'll want to add in full-length practice tests. You'll want to take one test very early in your prep and then spread your remaining full-length practice tests evenly between now and your test date. Staggering tests in this way allows you to form a baseline for comparison and to determine which areas to focus on right away, while also providing realistic feedback throughout your prep as to how you will perform on Test Day.

When planning your calendar, aim to finish your full-length practice tests and the majority of your studying by one week before Test Day, which will allow you to spend that final week completing a final review of what you already know. In your online resources, you'll find sample study calendars for several different Test Day timelines to use as a starting point. The sample calendars may include more focus than you need in some areas, and less in others, and it may not fit your timeline to Test Day. You will need to customize your study calendar to your needs using the steps above.

The total amount of time you spend studying each week will depend on your schedule, your personal prep needs, and your time to Test Day, but it is recommended that you spend somewhere in the range of 300–350 hours preparing before taking the official MCAT. One way you could break this down is to study for three hours per day, six days per week, for four months, but this is just one approach. You might study six days per week for more than three hours per day. You might study over a longer period of time if you don't have much time to study each week. No matter what your plan is, ensure you complete enough practice to feel completely comfortable with the MCAT and its content. A good sign you're ready for Test Day is when you begin to earn your goal score consistently in practice.

How to Study

The MCAT covers a large amount of material, so studying for Test Day can initially seem daunting. To combat this, we have some tips for how to take control of your studying and make the most of your time.

Goal Setting

To take control of the amount of content and practice required to do well on the MCAT, break the content down into specific goals for each week instead of attempting to approach the test as a whole. A goal of "I want to increase my overall score by 5 points" is too big, abstract, and difficult to measure on the small scale. More reasonable goals are "I will read two chapters each day this week." Goals like this are much less overwhelming and help break studying into manageable pieces.

Active Reading

As you go through this book, much of the information will be familiar to you. After all, you have probably seen most of the content before. However, be very careful: Familiarity with a subject does not necessarily translate to knowledge or mastery of that subject. Do not assume that if you recognize a concept you actually know it and can apply it quickly at an appropriate level. Don't just passively read this book. Instead, read actively: Use the free margin space to jot down important ideas, draw diagrams, and make charts as you read. Highlighting can be an excellent tool, but use it sparingly: highlighting every sentence isn't active reading, it's coloring. Frequently stop and ask yourself questions while you read (e.g., *What is the main point? How does this fit into the overall scheme of things? Could I thoroughly explain this to someone else?*). By making connections and focusing on the grander scheme, not only will you ensure you know the essential content, but you also prepare yourself for the level of critical thinking required by the MCAT.

Focus on Areas of Greatest Opportunity

If you are limited by only having a minimal amount of time to prepare before Test Day, focus on your biggest areas of opportunity first. Areas of opportunity are topic areas that are highly tested and that you have not yet mastered. You likely won't have time to take detailed notes for every page of these books; instead, use your results from practice materials to determine

which areas are your biggest opportunities and seek those out. After you've taken a full-length test, make sure you are using your performance report to best identify areas of opportunity. Skim over content matter for which you are already demonstrating proficiency, pausing to read more thoroughly when something looks unfamiliar or particularly difficult. Begin with the Science Mastery Assessment at the beginning of each chapter. If you can get all of those questions correct within a reasonable amount of time, you may be able to quickly skim through that chapter, but if the questions prove to be more difficult, then you may need to spend time reading the chapter or certain subsections of the chapter more thoroughly.

Practice, Review, and Tracking

Leave time to review your practice questions and full-length tests. You may be tempted, after practicing, to push ahead and cover new material as quickly as possible, but failing to schedule ample time for review will actually throw away your greatest opportunity to improve your performance. The brain rarely remembers anything it sees or does only once. When you carefully review the questions you've solved (and the explanations for them), the process of retrieving that information reopens and reinforces the connections you've built in your brain. This builds long-term retention and repeatable skill sets—exactly what you need to beat the MCAT!

One useful tool for making the most of your review is the How I'll Fix It (HIFI) sheet. You can create a HIFI sheet, such as the sample below, to track questions throughout your prep that you miss or have to guess on. For each such question, figure out why you missed it and supply at least one action step for how you can avoid similar mistakes in the future. As you move through your MCAT prep, adjust your study plan based on your available study time and the results of your review. Your strengths and weaknesses are likely to change over the course of your prep. Keep addressing the areas that are most important to your score, shifting your focus as those areas change. For more help with making the most of your full-length tests, including a How I'll Fix It sheet template, make sure to check out the videos and resources in your online syllabus.

Section	Q #	Topic or Type	Why I missed it	How I'll fix it
Chem/Phys	*42*	*Nuclear chem.*	*Confused electron absorption and emission*	*Reread Physics Chapter 9.2*
Chem/Phys	*47*	K_{eq}	*Didn't know right equation*	*Memorize equation for* K_{eq}
CARS	*2*	*Detail*	*Didn't read "not" in answer choice*	*Slow down when finding match*
CARS	*4*	*Inference*	*Forgot to research answer*	*Reread passage and predict first*

Where to Study

One often-overlooked aspect of studying is the environment where the learning actually occurs. Although studying at home is many students' first choice, several problems can arise in this environment, chief of which are distractions. Studying can be a mentally draining process, so as time passes, these distractions become ever more tempting as escape routes. Although you may have considerable willpower, there's no reason to make staying focused harder than it needs to be. Instead of studying at home, head to a library, quiet coffee shop, or another new location whenever possible. This will eliminate many of the usual distractions and also promote efficient studying; instead of studying off and on at home over the course of an entire day, you can stay at the library for three hours of effective studying and enjoy the rest of the day off from the MCAT.

No matter where you study, make your practice as much like Test Day as possible. Just as is required during the official test, don't have snacks or chew gum during your study blocks. Turn off your music, television, and phone. Practice on the computer with your online resources to simulate the computer-based test environment. When completing practice questions, do your work on scratch paper or noteboard sheets rather than writing directly on any printed materials since you won't have that option on Test Day. Because memory is tied to all of your senses, the more test-like you can make your studying environment, the easier it will be on Test Day to recall the information you're putting in so much work to learn.

CHAPTER 1

KINEMATICS AND DYNAMICS

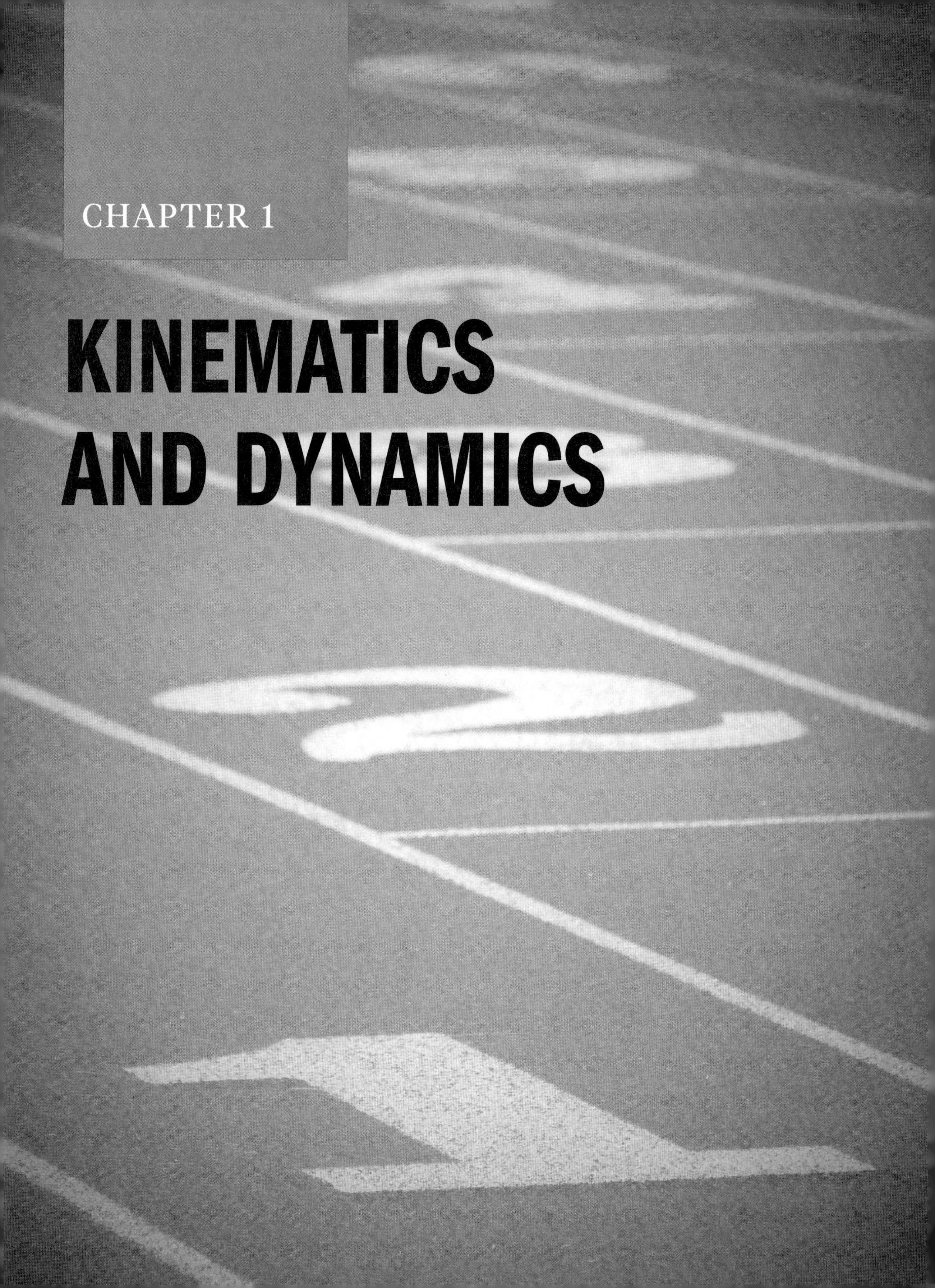

SCIENCE MASTERY ASSESSMENT

Every pre-med knows this feeling: there is so much content I have to know for the MCAT! How do I know what to do first or what's important?

While the high-yield badges throughout this book will help you identify the most important topics, this Science Mastery Assessment is another tool in your MCAT prep arsenal. This quiz (which can also be taken in your online resources) and the guidance below will help ensure that you are spending the appropriate amount of time on this chapter based on your personal strengths and weaknesses. Don't worry though—skipping something now does not mean you'll never study it. Later on in your prep, as you complete full-length tests, you'll uncover specific pieces of content that you need to review and can come back to these chapters as appropriate.

How to Use This Assessment

If you answer 0–7 questions correctly:

Spend about 1 hour to read this chapter in full and take limited notes throughout. Follow up by reviewing **all** quiz questions to ensure that you now understand how to solve each one.

If you answer 8–11 questions correctly:

Spend 20–40 minutes reviewing the quiz questions. Beginning with the questions you missed, read and take notes on the corresponding subchapters. For questions you answered correctly, ensure your thinking matches that of the explanation and you understand why each choice was correct or incorrect.

If you answer 12–15 questions correctly:

Spend less than 20 minutes reviewing all questions from the quiz. If you missed any, then include a quick read-through of the corresponding subchapters, or even just the relevant content within a subchapter, as part of your question review. For questions you got correct, ensure your thinking matches that of the explanation and review the Concept Summary at the end of the chapter.

1. A person walks 30 m east and then 40 m north. What is the difference between the traveled distance and the displacement?
   - **A.** 0 m
   - **B.** 20 m
   - **C.** 50 m
   - **D.** 70 m

2. A 1000 kg rocket ship, travelling at 100 $\frac{\text{m}}{\text{s}}$, is acted upon by an average force of 20 kN applied in the direction of its motion for 8 s. What is the change in velocity of the rocket?
   - **A.** 160 $\frac{\text{m}}{\text{s}}$
   - **B.** 260 $\frac{\text{m}}{\text{s}}$
   - **C.** 160,000 $\frac{\text{m}}{\text{s}}$
   - **D.** 260,000 $\frac{\text{m}}{\text{s}}$

3. A car is traveling at 40 $\frac{\text{km}}{\text{hr}}$ and the driver puts on the brakes, bringing the car to rest in a time of 6 s. What is the magnitude of the average acceleration of the car?
   - **A.** 240 $\frac{\text{km}}{\text{hr}^2}$
   - **B.** 12,000 $\frac{\text{km}}{\text{hr}^2}$
   - **C.** 24,000 $\frac{\text{km}}{\text{hr}^2}$
   - **D.** 30,000 $\frac{\text{km}}{\text{hr}^2}$

4. An elevator is designed to carry a maximum weight of 9800 N (including its own weight), and to move upward at a speed of 5 $\frac{\text{m}}{\text{s}}$ after an initial period of acceleration. What is the relationship between the maximum tension in the elevator cable and the maximum weight of the elevator while the elevator is accelerating upward?
   - **A.** The tension is greater than 9800 N.
   - **B.** The tension is less than 9800 N.
   - **C.** The tension equals 9800 N.
   - **D.** It cannot be determined from the information given.

5. A student must lift a mass of 4 kg a distance of 0.5 m. The ambient temperature is 298 K and the student must lift the mass in 30 seconds. Which of the following values is NOT necessary to calculate power?
   - **A.** Mass
   - **B.** Distance
   - **C.** Temperature
   - **D.** Time

6. A firefighter jumps horizontally from a burning building with an initial speed of 1.5 $\frac{\text{m}}{\text{s}}$. At what time is the angle between the firefighter's velocity and acceleration vectors the greatest?
   - **A.** The instant the firefighter jumps
   - **B.** When the firefighter reaches terminal velocity
   - **C.** Halfway through the firefighter's fall
   - **D.** Right before the firefighter lands on the ground

7. A 10 kg wagon rests on an inclined plane. The plane makes an angle of 30° with the horizontal. Approximately how large is the force required to keep the wagon from sliding down the plane (Note: $\sin 30° = 0.5$, $\cos 30° = 0.866$)?
   - **A.** 10 N
   - **B.** 49 N
   - **C.** 85 N
   - **D.** 98 N

8. Which of the following expressions correctly illustrates the SI base units for each of the variables in the formula below?

$$m\Delta\mathbf{v} = \mathbf{F}\Delta t$$

   - **A.** $\text{lb} \times \text{mph} = \text{ft} \times \text{lb} \times \text{s}$
   - **B.** $\text{kg} \times \frac{\text{m}}{\text{s}} = \text{N} \times \text{s}$
   - **C.** $\text{kg} \times \frac{\text{m}}{\text{s}} = \frac{\text{kg}\cdot\text{m}}{\text{s}^2} \times \text{s}$
   - **D.** $\text{g} \times \frac{\text{m}}{\text{s}} = \frac{\text{g}\cdot\text{m}}{\text{s}^2} \times \text{s}$

9. The diagram below shows two vectors.

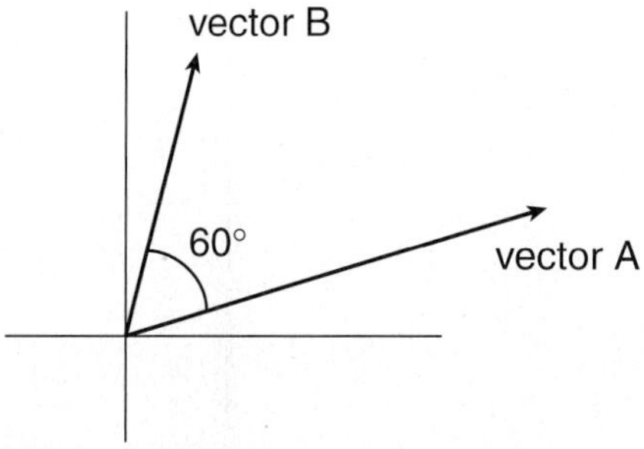

If a student uses the formula $ab \cdot sin\,(60°)$, where a and b are the magnitudes of the respective vectors A and B, then which of the following best describes the computed value?

A. Positive scalar
B. Negative scalar
C. Vector into the page
D. Vector out of the page

10. Which of the following quantities is NOT a vector?
A. Velocity
B. Force
C. Displacement
D. Distance

11. A 30 kg child sits on a seesaw at a distance of 2 m from the fulcrum. Where must the child's parent sit to balance the seesaw if the parent has a mass of 90 kg?
A. 67 cm from the child
B. 67 cm from the fulcrum
C. 133 cm from the child
D. 267 cm from the fulcrum

12. A physics major builds a potato launcher and tests it in an open field. The student launches a potato with a velocity of 12 m/s at an angle of 30°. The potato is found 60 meters from the launch site. Which of the following represents the maximum height achieved by the potato? (Note: $\cos(60°) = 0.5$)
A. 0.3 m
B. 1.8 m
C. 5 m
D. 18 m

13. A rock ($m = 2$ kg) is shot up vertically at the same time that a ball ($m = 0.5$ kg) is projected horizontally. If both start from the same height:
A. the rock and ball will reach the ground at the same time.
B. the rock will reach the ground first.
C. the ball will reach the ground first.
D. the rock and ball will collide in the air before reaching the ground.

14. Centrifugal force is an apparent outward force during circular motion. It has been described as a reaction force according to Newton's third law. Which of the following statements is most likely to be correct regarding centrifugal force?
A. Centrifugal force exists only for uniform circular motion, not nonuniform circular motion.
B. Centrifugal force exists only when tension or a normal force provides centripetal acceleration.
C. Centrifugal force always acts antiparallel to the centripetal force vector.
D. Centrifugal force is result of repulsive electrostatic interactions.

15. Which of the following statements is true of movement on a plane with friction?
I. Acceleration is a function of applied force only.
II. More force is needed to accelerate a stationary object than an identical moving object.
III. The force of friction is independent of the mass of objects.

A. I only
B. II only
C. I and II only
D. I and III only

Answer Key

1. **B**
2. **A**
3. **C**
4. **A**
5. **C**
6. **A**
7. **B**
8. **C**
9. **D**
10. **D**
11. **B**
12. **B**
13. **C**
14. **C**
15. **B**

Detailed explanations can be found at the end of the chapter.

CHAPTER 1

KINEMATICS AND DYNAMICS

In This Chapter

CHAPTER PROFILE

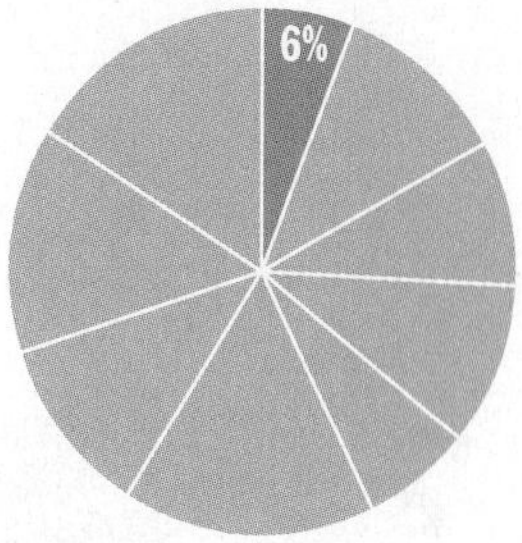

The content in this chapter should be relevant to about 6% of all questions about physics on the MCAT.

This chapter covers material from the following AAMC content category:

4A: Translational motion, forces, work, energy, and equilibrium in living systems

Introduction

A professor once said: *Biology is chemistry. Chemistry is physics. Physics is life.* Not surprisingly, this was the claim of a physics professor.

Walking into MCAT preparation, many students think of physics as the least applicable science to medicine, reflecting on calculus-heavy premedical classes. But even in the medical field, physics is all around us. When we treat patients at a rehab hospital, we often talk about motion, forces, and bone strength. An ophthalmologist may draw diagrams to help students better understand myopia and hyperopia. When we talk about mitochondria functioning as the batteries of the cell, we mean that fairly literally.

This first chapter reviews the three systems of units encountered on the MCAT: MKS (meter–kilogram–second), CGS (centimeter–gram–second), and SI (International System of Units). We'll take a few moments to review the geometry of physics questions, especially vector mathematics. Next, we'll move into true physics content as we consider kinematics—the equations that deal with the motion of objects—and Newtonian mechanics and dynamics—the study of forces and their effects.

REAL WORLD

Natural phenomena occur on many scales, as shown in Figure 1.1. We often assume that the fine details have little bearing on the larger scale of the universe, but the rapid inflation of the universe allows the infinitesimally small to affect the astronomically big.

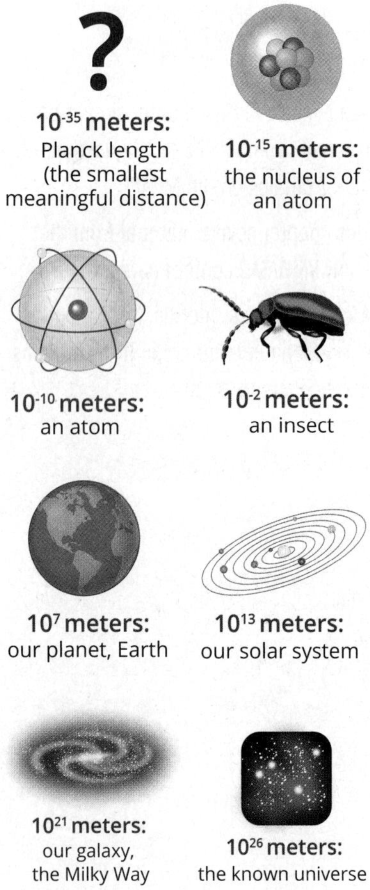

Figure 1.1 Size of Natural Phenomena

1.1 Units

LEARNING OBJECTIVES

After Chapter 1.1, you will be able to:

- Recall the fundamental measurements and their units
- Order a given set of units that measure the same type of quantity from smallest to largest

Before we begin our discussion of motion, we must define a consistent vocabulary for our discussion of physics throughout this book. Physics relies on the language of mathematics to convey important descriptions and explanations of the world around us. Yet those numbers would themselves be meaningless—or vague at best—without the labels of units.

Fundamental Measurements

Over the years, various systems of units have been developed for specific purposes. Some of these systems are commonly used in everyday life but rarely in science. The **British** or **Imperial system** (foot–pound–second or **FPS**) is used commonly in the United States but virtually nowhere else—not even in Britain. Basic units for length, weight, and time are the **foot** (**ft**), the **pound** (**lb**), and the **second** (**s**), respectively. Because weight, and not mass, is used, the British system later derived the **slug** as a unit of mass. The MCAT rarely—if ever—utilizes FPS in passages or questions.

The most common system of units is the metric system, which is the basis for the SI units used on the MCAT. Depending on the context of a passage or question, the **metric system** may be given in meters, kilograms, and seconds (**MKS**) or centimeters, grams, and seconds (**CGS**). **SI units** include the MKS system as well as four other base units, as shown in Table 1.1.

QUANTITY	UNIT	SYMBOL
Length	meter	m
Mass (*not* weight)	kilogram	kg
Time	second	s
Current	ampère (coulomb/second)	A
Amount of Substance	mole	mol
Temperature	kelvin	K
Luminous Intensity	candela	cd

Table 1.1 SI Units

In each measurement system, there are base units and derived units. **Base units** are the standard units around which the system itself is designed. **Derived units**, as the name implies, are created by associating base units with each other. For example, the newton—a unit of force—is derived from kilograms, meters, and seconds: $1\text{ N} = 1\ \frac{\text{kg}\cdot\text{m}}{\text{s}^2}$. Table 1.2 contains examples of important derived units from each of the systems described above. Prefixes for metric units and conversions between metric and Imperial units are discussed in Chapter 10 of *MCAT Physics and Math Review.*

QUANTITY	FPS	CGS	MKS (SI)
Mass	slug $\left(\frac{\text{lb}\cdot\text{s}^2}{\text{ft}}\right)$ or blob $\left(\frac{\text{lb}\cdot\text{s}^2}{\text{in}}\right)$		
Force		dyne $\left(\frac{\text{g}\cdot\text{cm}}{\text{s}^2}\right)$	newton $\left(\frac{\text{kg}\cdot\text{m}}{\text{s}^2}\right)$
Work and Energy	foot-pound (ft · lb)	erg $\left(\frac{\text{g}\cdot\text{cm}^2}{\text{s}^2}\right)$	joule $\left(\frac{\text{kg}\cdot\text{m}^2}{\text{s}^2}\right)$
Power	foot-pound per second	erg per second	watt $\left(\frac{\text{kg}\cdot\text{m}^2}{\text{s}^3}\right)$

Table 1.2 Derived Units in Various Systems of Measurement

At the molecular, atomic, or subatomic level, different units may be given that are easier to work with at such a small scale. For example, length may be given in **ångströms** ($1\text{ Å} = 10^{-10}\text{ m}$) or nanometers ($1\text{ nm} = 10^{-9}\text{ m}$). Energy on the atomic scale can be expressed in **electron–volts** ($1\text{ eV} = 1.6 \times 10^{-19}\text{ J}$), which represent the amount of energy gained by an electron accelerating through a potential difference of one volt.

MCAT EXPERTISE

While it is good to be aware of the various systems of measurement, the only system that you are required to memorize for the MCAT is the SI system.

BRIDGE

Solutions to concept checks for a given chapter in *MCAT Physics and Math Review* can be found near the end of the chapter in which the concept check is located, following the Concept Summary for that chapter.

MCAT CONCEPT CHECK 1.1

Before you move on, assess your understanding of the material with these questions.

1. If the newton is the product of kilograms and meters/second^2, what units comprise the pound?

____

2. Order the following units from smallest to largest: centimeter, angstrom, inch, mile, foot.

__________ < __________ < __________ < __________ < __________

1.2 Vectors and Scalars

LEARNING OBJECTIVES

After Chapter 1.2, you will be able to:

- Explain the importance of order when performing vector calculations
- Calculate a scalar or a vector as a product of two vectors, using the right-hand rule when applicable:

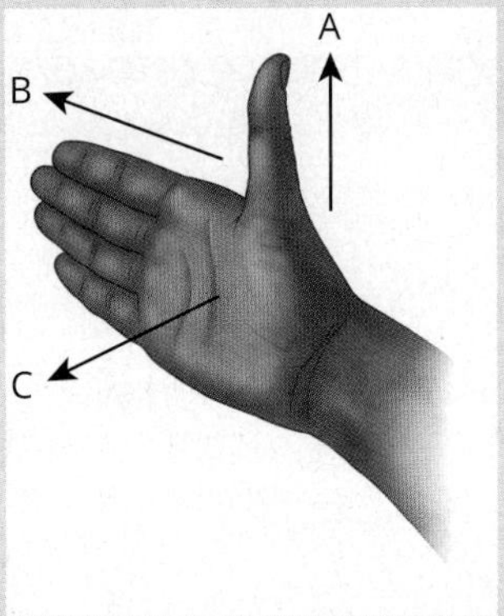

Vectors are numbers that have magnitude and direction. Vector quantities include displacement, velocity, acceleration, and force. **Scalars** are numbers that have magnitude only and no direction. Scalar quantities include distance, speed, energy, pressure, and mass. The difference between a vector and scalar quantity can be quite pronounced when there is a nonlinear path involved. For example, in the course of a year, the Earth travels a distance of roughly 940 million kilometers. However, because this is a circular path, the displacement of the Earth in one year is zero kilometers. This difference between distance and displacement can be further illustrated with vector representations.

Vectors may be represented by arrows; the direction of the arrow indicates the direction of the vector. The length of the arrow is usually proportional to the magnitude of the vector quantity. Common notations for a vector quantity are either an arrow or boldface. For example, the straight-line path from *here* to *there* might be represented by a vector identified as $\vec{\mathbf{A}}$ or **A**. The magnitude of the displacement between the two positions can be represented as $|\vec{\mathbf{A}}|$, $|\mathbf{A}|$, or A. Scalar quantities are generally represented with italic type: the distance between two points could be represented by d.

In this book (and all books of the *Kaplan MCAT Review* series), we will consistently use **boldface** to represent a vector quantity and *italic* to represent the magnitude of a vector or a scalar quantity.

Vector Addition

KEY CONCEPT

When adding vectors, always add tip-to-tail!

The sum or difference of two or more vectors is called the **resultant** of the vectors. One way to find the sum or resultant of two vectors **A** and **B** is to place the tail of **B** at the tip of **A** without changing either the length or the direction of either arrow. In this **tip-to-tail method**, the lengths of the arrows must be proportional to the magnitudes of the vectors. The vector sum **A** + **B** is the vector joining the tail of **A** to the tip of **B** and pointing toward the tip of **B**. Vector addition is demonstrated in Figure 1.2 below.

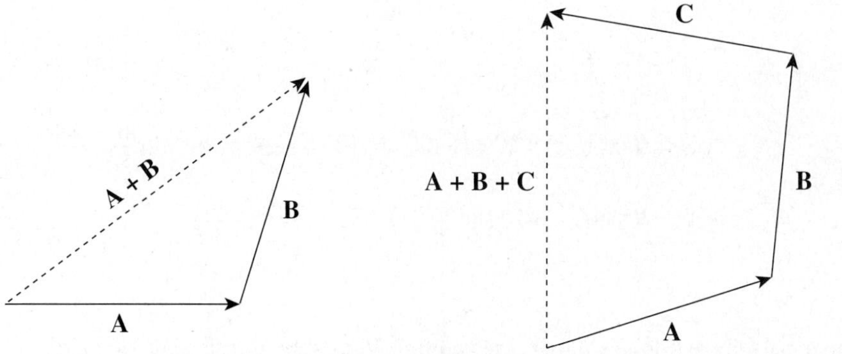

Figure 1.2 The Tip-to-Tail Method of Vector Addition
*(left) Vectors **A** and **B** with resultant **A** + **B**; (right) Vectors **A, B,** and **C** with resultant **A** + **B** + **C***

Another method for finding the resultant of several vectors involves breaking each vector into perpendicular **components**. In most cases, these components are horizontal and vertical (***x***- and ***y***-components, respectively); however, in some instances—such as inclined planes—it may make more sense to define the components as parallel and perpendicular ($\|$ and $\perp$, respectively) to some other surface.

Given any vector **V**, we can find the *x*- and *y*-components (**X** and **Y**) by drawing a right triangle with **V** as the hypotenuse, as shown in Figure 1.3.

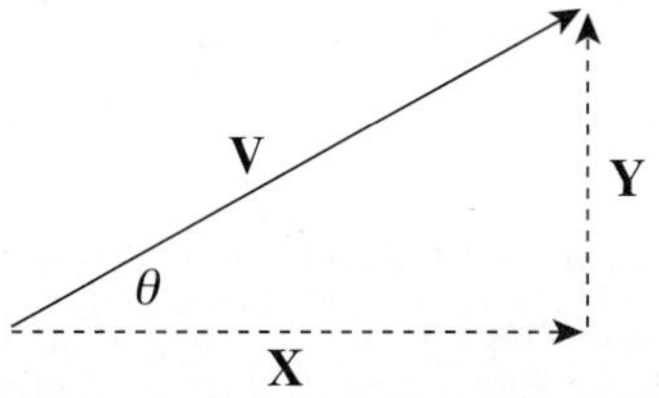

Figure 1.3 Splitting a Vector into Components

If θ is the angle between **V** and the *x*-component, then $\cos\theta = \frac{\mathbf{X}}{\mathbf{V}}$ and $\sin\theta = \frac{\mathbf{Y}}{\mathbf{V}}$. In other words:

$$\mathbf{X} = \mathbf{V}\cos\theta$$

$$\mathbf{Y} = \mathbf{V}\sin\theta$$

Equation 1.1

Example: Find the *x*- and *y*-components of the following vector

$$\mathbf{V} = 10\ \frac{\text{m}}{\text{s}}$$

$$\theta = 30^\circ$$

Solution:

$$\mathbf{X} = \mathbf{V}\cos(\theta) = 10\cos(30^\circ) = 10 \times \frac{\sqrt{3}}{2} = 5\sqrt{3}\ \frac{\text{m}}{\text{s}}$$

$$\mathbf{Y} = \mathbf{V}\sin(\theta) = 10\sin(30^\circ) = 10 \times \frac{1}{2} = 5\ \frac{\text{m}}{\text{s}}$$

Conversely, if we know **X** and **Y**, we can find **V**, as shown in Figure 1.4 below.

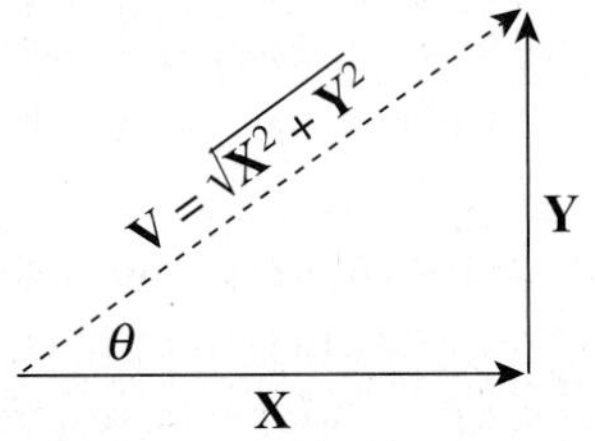

Figure 1.4 Using the Pythagorean Theorem to Determine the Magnitude of the Resultant Vector

Calculating the magnitude of **V** requires use of the **Pythagorean theorem**:

$$\mathbf{X}^2 + \mathbf{Y}^2 = \mathbf{V}^2 \quad \text{or} \quad \mathbf{V} = \sqrt{\mathbf{X}^2 + \mathbf{Y}^2}$$

Equation 1.2

The angle of the resultant vector can also be calculated by knowing inverse trigonometric functions, discussed in Chapter 10 of *MCAT Physics and Math Review* (Note: This inverse tangent calculation is beyond the scope of the MCAT):

$$\theta = \tan^{-1}\frac{\mathbf{Y}}{\mathbf{X}}$$

Equation 1.3

Example: What is the magnitude of the vector with the following components?

$$\mathbf{X} = 3\ \frac{\text{m}}{\text{s}}$$

$$\mathbf{Y} = 4\ \frac{\text{m}}{\text{s}}$$

Solution:

$$\mathbf{V} = \sqrt{3^2 + 4^2} = \sqrt{25} = 5\ \frac{\text{m}}{\text{s}}$$

The x-component of a resultant vector is simply the sum of the x-components of the vectors being added. Similarly, the y-component of a resultant vector is simply the sum of the y-components of the vectors being added. This is illustrated in Figure 1.5.

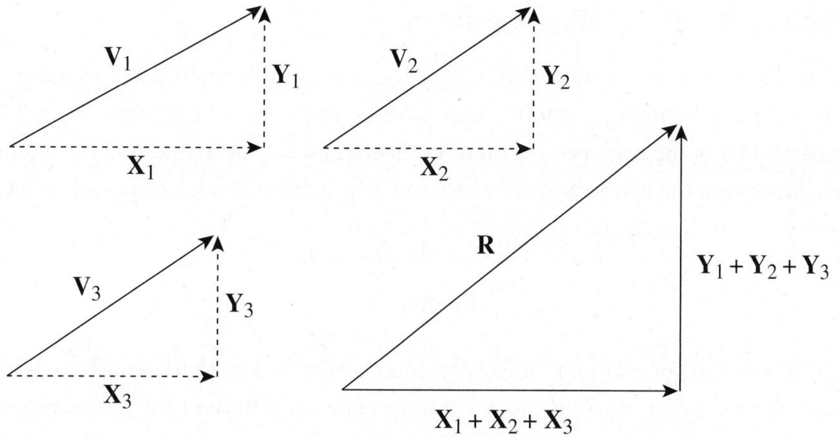

Figure 1.5 Finding the Resultant (R) of $V_1 + V_2 + V_3$

To find the resultant (**R**) using the components method, follow these steps:

1. Resolve the vectors to be added into their x- and y-components.
2. Add the x-components to get the x-component of the resultant ($\mathbf{R}_x$). Add the y-components to get the y-component of the resultant ($\mathbf{R}_y$).
3. Find the magnitude of the resultant by using the Pythagorean theorem. If $\mathbf{R}_x$ and $\mathbf{R}_y$ are the components of the resultant, then $R = \sqrt{R_x^2 + R_y^2}$.
4. Find the direction (θ) of the resultant by using the relationship $\theta = \tan^{-1} \frac{R_y}{R_x}$.

Vector Subtraction

Subtracting one vector from another can be accomplished by adding a vector with equal magnitude—but opposite direction—to the first vector. This can be expressed mathematically as $\mathbf{A} - \mathbf{B} = \mathbf{A} + (-\mathbf{B})$, where $-\mathbf{B}$ represents a vector with the same magnitude as **B**, but pointing in the opposite direction. Vector subtraction may also be performed on the component vectors first and then combined to create a final vector. As with vector addition, the x-component of the resultant vector is the difference of the x-components of the vectors being subtracted. Similarly, the y-component of the resultant vector is the difference of the y-components of the vectors being subtracted.

KEY CONCEPT

Notice that when you subtract vectors, you are simply flipping the direction of the vector being subtracted and then following the same rules as normal: adding tip-to-tail.

Multiplying Vectors by Scalars

When a vector is multiplied by a scalar, its magnitude will change. Its direction will be either parallel or antiparallel to its original direction. If a vector **A** is multiplied by the scalar value n, a new vector, **B**, is created such that $\mathbf{B} = n\mathbf{A}$. To find the magnitude of the new vector, **B**, simply multiply the magnitude of **A** by $|n|$, the absolute value of n. To determine the direction of the vector **B**, we must look at the sign on n. If n is a positive number, then **B** and **A** are in the same direction. However, if n is a negative number, then **B** and **A** point in opposite directions. For example, if vector **A** is multiplied by the scalar +3, then the new vector **B** is three times as long as **A**, and points in the same direction. If vector **A** is multiplied by the scalar −3, then **B** would still be three times as long as **A** but would now point in the opposite direction.

Multiplying Vectors by Other Vectors

In some circumstances, we want to be able to use two vector quantities to generate a third vector or a scalar by multiplication. To generate a scalar quantity like work, we multiply the magnitudes of the two vectors of interest (force and displacement) and the cosine of the angle between the two vectors. In vector calculus, this is called the **dot product** ($\mathbf{A} \cdot \mathbf{B}$):

$$\mathbf{A} \cdot \mathbf{B} = |\mathbf{A}|\ |\mathbf{B}| \cos \theta$$

Equation 1.4

In contrast, when generating a third vector like torque, we need to determine both its magnitude and direction. To do so, we multiply the magnitudes of the two vectors of interest (force and lever arm) and the sine of the angle between the two vectors. Once we have the magnitude, we use the **right-hand rule** to determine its direction. In vector calculus, this is called the **cross product** ($\mathbf{A} \times \mathbf{B}$):

$$\mathbf{A} \times \mathbf{B} = |\mathbf{A}|\ |\mathbf{B}| \sin \theta$$

Equation 1.5

The resultant of a cross product will always be perpendicular to the plane created by the two vectors. Because the MCAT is a two-dimensional test, this usually means that the vector of interest will be going into or out of the page (or screen).

There are multiple versions of the right-hand rule that can be used to determine the direction of a cross product resultant vector. Figure 1.6 shows one method considering a resultant **C** where $\mathbf{C} = \mathbf{A} \times \mathbf{B}$:

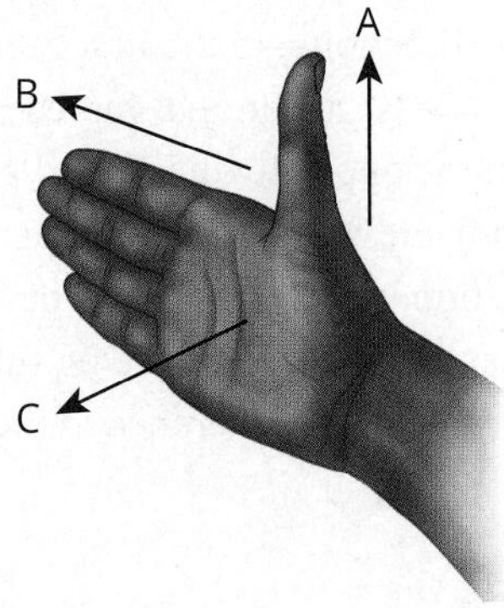

Figure 1.6 Applying the Right-Hand Rule

1. Start by pointing your thumb in the direction of vector **A**.
2. Extend your fingers in the direction of vector **B**. You may need to rotate your wrist to get the correct configuration of thumb and fingers.
3. Your palm establishes the plane between the two vectors. The direction your palm points is the direction of the resultant **C**.

Note that you may have learned a version of the right-hand rule that is different from what is described here. For example, some students learn to point the right index finger in the direction of **A** and the right middle finger in the direction of **B**; when one holds the thumb perpendicular to these two fingers, it points in the direction of **C**. It makes no difference which version of the right-hand rule you use, as long as you are comfortable with it and are skilled in its proper use.

Example: What are the magnitudes and directions of the resultant vectors from the following cross products: **C** = **A** × **B** and **D** = **B** × **A**?

$$\mathbf{A}: \mathbf{X} = -3\text{ N}, \mathbf{Y} = 0$$

$$\mathbf{B}: \mathbf{X} = 0, \mathbf{Y} = +4\text{ m}$$

Solution: The magnitude of the resultant vector is simply the product of the magnitudes of the factor vectors and the sine of the angle between them. In this case, because one is oriented in the *x*-direction and the other is in the *y*-direction, the angle between them is 90°.

$$|\mathbf{A}| \times |\mathbf{B}| \times \sin 90^\circ = 3\text{ N} \times 4\text{ m} \times 1 = 12\text{ N·m}$$

The magnitude is therefore 12 N·m.

Now, to determine the direction of **C**, start by pointing your right thumb toward the left (negative *x*-direction). Your fingers will point toward the top of the page (positive *y*-direction). Your palm is therefore pointing into the page.

Now, to determine the direction of **D**, start by pointing your right thumb toward the top of the page (positive *y*-direction). Your fingers will point toward the left (negative *x*-direction). Your palm is therefore pointing out of the page.

Therefore, **C** is 12 N·m [⊗ (into the page)] and **D** is 12 N·m [⊙ (out of the page)].

MCAT EXPERTISE

There are several different methods for determining the direction of a cross product resultant vector. Choose whichever method you prefer and stick with it—it's more important to be skilled in using one method than to be only somewhat familiar with multiple methods.

KEY CONCEPT

For cross products and the right-hand rule, order matters! Unlike scalar multiplication, which is commutative ($3 \times 4 = 4 \times 3$), vector multiplication is not commutative ($\mathbf{A} \times \mathbf{B} \neq \mathbf{B} \times \mathbf{A}$)!

MCAT CONCEPT CHECK 1.2

Before you move on, assess your understanding of the material with these questions.

1. When calculating the sum of vectors **A** and **B** (**A** + **B**), we put the tail of **B** at the tip of **A**. What would be the effect of reversing this order (**B** + **A**)?

---

2. When calculating the difference of vectors **A** and **B** (**A** – **B**), we invert **B** and put the tail of this new vector at the tip of **A**. What would be the effect of reversing this order (**B** – **A**)?

---

3. How is a scalar calculated from the product of two vectors? How is a vector calculated?
   - Scalar:

   - Vector:

---

4. True or False: If **C** = **A** × **B**, where **A** is directed toward the right side of the page and **B** is directed to the top of the page, then **C** is directed midway between **A** and **B** at a 45° angle.

1.3 Displacement and Velocity

LEARNING OBJECTIVES

After Chapter 1.3, you will be able to:

- Describe the relationship between the average and instantaneous versions of velocity and speed
- Distinguish between total distance and total displacement
- Connect displacement and velocity with an equation

Now that we've covered the basic geometry that serves as the foundation of physics, we can examine the related physical quantities. The basic quantities that relate to kinematics are displacement, velocity, and acceleration.

Displacement

An object in motion may experience a change in its position in space, known as **displacement** (**x** or **d**). This is a vector quantity and, as such, has both magnitude and direction. The displacement vector connects (in a straight line) the object's initial position and its final position. Understand that displacement does not account for the actual pathway taken between the initial and the final positions—only the net change in position from initial to final. **Distance** (d) traveled, on the other hand, considers the pathway taken and is a scalar quantity.

Example: What is the displacement of a person who walks 2 km east, then 2 km north, then 2 km west, and then 2 km south?

Solution: While the total distance traveled is 8 km, the displacement is a vector quantity that represents the change in position. In this case, the displacement is zero because the person ends up back at the start, as shown below.

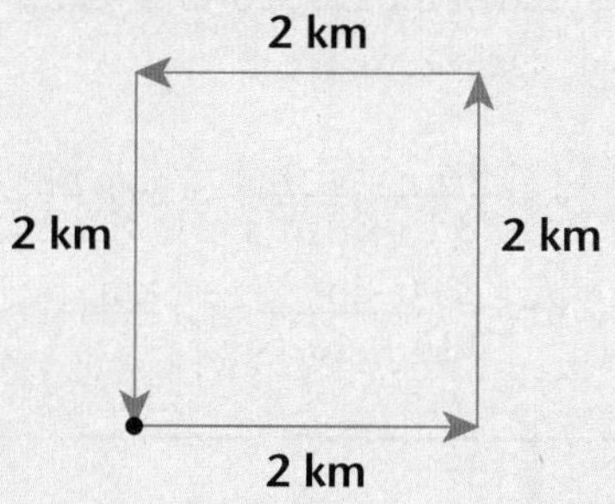

Velocity

As was mentioned earlier, **velocity** (**v**) is a vector. Its magnitude is measured as the rate of change of displacement in a given unit of time, and its SI units are meters per second. The direction of the velocity vector is necessarily the same as the direction of the displacement vector. **Speed** (v) is the rate of actual distance traveled in a given unit of time.

The distinction is subtle, so let's examine this a little more carefully. The **instantaneous speed** of an object will always be equal to the magnitude of the object's **instantaneous velocity**, which is a measure of the average velocity as the change in time (Δt) approaches zero:

$$\mathbf{v} = \lim_{\Delta t \to 0} \frac{\Delta \mathbf{x}}{\Delta t}$$

Equation 1.6

where **v** is the instantaneous velocity, $\Delta\mathbf{x}$ is the change in position, and Δt is the change in time. As a measure of speed, instantaneous speed is a scalar number. Average speed will not necessarily always be equal to the magnitude of the average velocity. This is because average velocity is the ratio of the displacement vector over the change in time (and is a vector), whereas average speed (which is scalar) is the ratio of the total distance traveled over the change in time. Average speed accounts for actual distance traveled, whereas average velocity does not:

$$\bar{\mathbf{v}} = \frac{\Delta \mathbf{x}}{\Delta t}$$

Equation 1.7

where $\bar{\mathbf{v}}$ is the average velocity, $\Delta \mathbf{x}$ is the change in position, and Δt is the change in time.

Consider the example given earlier regarding the Earth's orbit. In one year, the Earth travels roughly 940 million kilometers, but its displacement is zero:

$$d = 9.4 \times 10^8 \text{ km}$$
$$\mathbf{x} = 0 \text{ km}$$

The average speed is a measure of distance traveled in a given period of time; the average velocity is a measure of the displacement of an object over a given period of time. While the average speed of the Earth over a year is about 30 kilometers per second, its average velocity is again zero:

$$v = \frac{9.4 \times 10^8 \text{ km}}{3.16 \times 10^7 \text{ s}} = 29.8 \frac{\text{km}}{\text{s}}$$
$$\bar{\mathbf{v}} = \frac{0 \text{ km}}{3.16 \times 10^7 \text{ s}} = 0 \frac{\text{km}}{\text{s}}$$

MCAT CONCEPT CHECK 1.3

Before you move on, assess your understanding of the material with these questions.

1. What is the relationship between instantaneous velocity and instantaneous speed? Between average velocity and average speed?

2. True or False: Total distance traveled can never be less than the total displacement.

3. Provide a definition for displacement or velocity in terms of the other variable.

1.4 Forces and Acceleration

LEARNING OBJECTIVES

After Chapter 1.4, you will be able to:

- Calculate a frictional force and predict its direction
- Describe the relationship between force, velocity, and acceleration
- Identify common forces, including frictional and gravitational forces
- Explain the concept of normal forces and how they impact a system

Every change in velocity is motivated by a push or a pull—a **force**. In this section, we'll examine how forces interact with one another, as well as how acceleration results from those forces.

Forces

Force (F) is a vector quantity that is experienced as pushing or pulling on objects. Forces can exist between objects that are not even touching. While it is common for forces to be exerted by one object pushing on another, there are even more instances in which forces exist between objects nowhere near each other, such as gravity or electrostatic forces between point charges. The SI unit for force is the **newton (N)**, which is equivalent to one $\frac{\text{kg}\cdot\text{m}}{\text{s}^2}$.

Gravity

When Newton observed apples falling out of trees, he was struck by the fact that they always fell perpendicularly to the ground, rather than sideways or even away from the ground. Furthermore, Newton began to wonder about the farthest reaches of gravity. If the apple feels this attractive pull toward the Earth, then what about the Moon? This force is what Newton would later term "universal gravitation."

Gravity is an attractive force that is felt by all forms of matter. We usually think of gravity as acting on us to keep us from floating off of the Earth's surface, or for holding the planets of our solar system in orbit. However, all objects exert gravitational forces on each other; there is a small (but measurable) force of gravity between you and this *MCAT Physics and Math Review* book, the chair you're sitting on, and all the objects around you. Gravitational forces usually do not have much significance on a small scale because other forces tend to be much larger in magnitude. Only on the planetary level do gravitational forces really take on a significant value.

The magnitude of the **gravitational force** between two objects is

$$F_g = \frac{Gm_1m_2}{r^2}$$

Equation 1.8

MCAT EXPERTISE

Acceleration due to gravity, g, decreases with height above the Earth and increases the closer one gets to the Earth's center of mass. Near the Earth's surface, use $g = 10\ \frac{\text{m}}{\text{s}^2}$.

REAL WORLD

Newton's third law states that the force of gravity on m_1 from m_2 is equal and opposite to the force of gravity on m_2 from m_1. This means that the force of gravity on you from the Earth is equal and opposite to the force of gravity from you on the Earth. Because the forces are equal but the masses are very different, the accelerations must also be very different, from $\mathbf{F} = m\mathbf{a}$ (discussed later in this chapter). Because your mass is very small compared to the Earth, you experience a large acceleration from it. In contrast, because the Earth is massive, it experiences a tiny acceleration from the same magnitude of force.

where G is the universal gravitational constant $\left(6.67 \times 10^{-11} \frac{\text{N}\cdot\text{m}^2}{\text{kg}^2}\right)$, m_1 and m_2 are the masses of the two objects, and r is the distance between their centers of mass. This equation is commonly tested in the context of proportionalities. For instance, the magnitude of the gravitational force is inversely related to the square of the distance (that is, if r is halved, then F_g will quadruple). The magnitude of the gravitational force is also directly related to the masses of the objects (that is, if m_1 is tripled, then F_g will triple).

Example: Find the gravitational force between an electron and a proton that are 10^{-11} m apart. (Note: Mass of a proton $= 1.67 \times 10^{-27}$ kg; mass of an electron $= 9.11 \times 10^{-31}$ kg)

Solution: Use Newton's law of gravitation:

$$F_g = \frac{Gm_1m_2}{r^2}$$

$$= \frac{\left(6.67 \times 10^{-11} \frac{\text{N}\cdot\text{m}^2}{\text{kg}^2}\right)(1.67 \times 10^{-27}\ \text{kg})(9.11 \times 10^{-31}\ \text{kg})}{(10^{-11}\ \text{m})^2}$$

$$F_g \approx \frac{\left(\frac{20}{3} \times 10^{-11}\right)\left(\frac{5}{3} \times 10^{-27}\right)(9 \times 10^{-31})}{10^{-22}} = \frac{\frac{100 \times 9}{9} \times 10^{-69}}{10^{-22}}$$

$$= \frac{10^{-67}}{10^{-22}} = 10^{-45}\ \text{N}\ (\text{actual} = 1.02 \times 10^{-45}\ \text{N})$$

Friction

Friction is a type of force that opposes the movement of objects. Unlike other kinds of forces, such as gravity or electromagnetic force, which can cause objects either to speed up or slow down, friction forces always oppose an object's motion and cause it to slow down or become stationary. There are two types of friction: static and kinetic.

Static friction (f_s) exists between a stationary object and the surface upon which it rests. The inequality that describes the magnitude of static friction is

$$0 \leq f_s \leq \mu_s N$$

Equation 1.9

where μ_s is the coefficient of static friction and N is the magnitude of the normal force. The **coefficient of static friction** is a unitless quantity that is dependent on the two materials in contact. The **normal force** is the component of the force between two objects in contact that is perpendicular to the plane of contact between the object and the surface upon which it rests.

Note the less-than-or-equal-to signs in the equation. These signify that there is a range of possible values for static friction. The minimum, of course, is zero. This would be the case if an object were resting on a surface with no applied forces. The maximum value of static friction can be calculated from the right side of the previous equation. One should not assume that objects that are stationary are experiencing a maximal static force of friction.

Consider trying to push a heavy piece of luggage. When a 25 N force is applied, the bag does not move. When a 50 N force is applied, the bag still does not move. When a 100 N force is applied, the bag slides a meter or so and slows to a rest. This setup implies that the maximal value of static friction is somewhere between 50 and 100 N; any applied force less than this threshold will not be sufficient to move the bag as there will be an equal but opposite force of static friction opposing the bag's motion.

Kinetic friction (f_k) exists between a sliding object and the surface over which the object slides. Sometimes, students misidentify the presence of kinetic friction. A wheel, for example, that is rolling along a road does not experience kinetic friction because the tire is not actually sliding against the pavement. The tire maintains an instantaneous point of static contact with the road and, therefore, experiences static friction. Only when the tire begins to slide on, say, an icy patch will kinetic friction come into play. Any time two surfaces slide against each other, kinetic friction will be present and its magnitude can be measured according to this equation:

$$f_k = \mu_k N$$

Equation 1.10

where μ_k is the coefficient of kinetic friction and N is the normal force. There are two important distinctions between this equation for kinetic friction and the previous equation for static friction. First, the kinetic friction equation has an equals sign. This means that kinetic friction will have a constant value for any given combination of a coefficient of kinetic friction and normal force. It does not matter how much surface area is in contact or even the velocity of the sliding object. Second, the two equations have a different coefficient of friction. The value of μ_s is always larger than the value of μ_k. Therefore, the maximum value for static friction will always be greater than the constant value for kinetic friction: objects will "stick" until they start moving, and then will slide more easily over one another.

As previously mentioned in the discussion of static friction, pay close attention to the conditions set in an MCAT passage or question. Does it say that friction can be assumed to be negligible, or does it provide the coefficient of friction values, which will most likely need to be used in a calculation of friction? Friction will be incorporated into our examination of translational equilibrium later in this chapter.

Mass and Weight

Mass and weight are not the same. **Mass** (m) is a measure of a body's inertia—the amount of matter in the object. Mass is a scalar quantity, and, as such, has magnitude only. The SI unit for mass is the kilogram, which is independent of gravity. One kilogram of material on Earth will have the same mass as one kilogram of material on the Moon. **Weight** ($\mathbf{F}_g$), on the other hand, is a measure of gravitational force (usually that of the Earth) on an object's mass. Because weight is a force, it is a vector quantity with units in newtons (N).

KEY CONCEPT

Contact points are the places where friction occurs between two rough surfaces sliding past each other. If the normal load—the force that squeezes the two together—rises, the total area of contact increases. That increase, more than the surface's roughness, governs the degree of friction. This is illustrated in Figure 1.7 below.

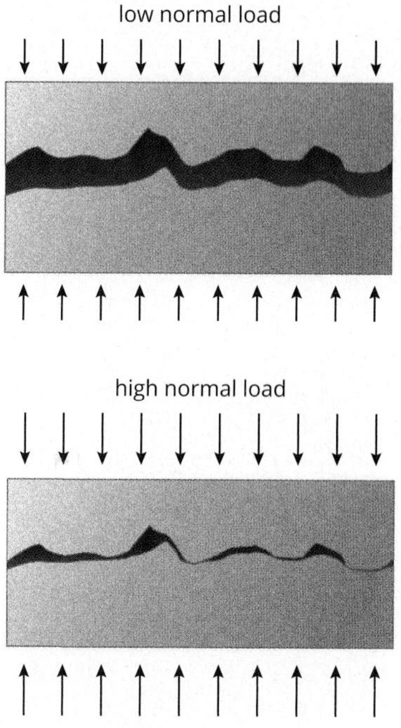

Figure 1.7 Increases in Contact Area Increase Frictional Forces

KEY CONCEPT

The coefficient of static friction will always be larger than the coefficient of kinetic friction. It always requires more force to get an object to start sliding than it takes to keep an object sliding.

While mass and weight are not synonymous, they are related by the equation:

$$\mathbf{F}_g = m\mathbf{g}$$

Equation 1.11

where $\mathbf{F}_g$ is the weight of the object, m is its mass, and $\mathbf{g}$ is acceleration due to gravity, $9.8\ \frac{\text{m}}{\text{s}^2}$ (usually rounded to $10\ \frac{\text{m}}{\text{s}^2}$).

The weight of an object can be thought of as being applied at a single point in that object called the **center of mass** or **gravity**. The MCAT will not directly test your ability to determine center of mass; however, such a calculation may be an important step in a problem with the larger focus of Newtonian mechanics.

To illustrate this concept and calculation, consider a tennis racket that has been thrown into the air. Each part of the racket moves in its own pathway, so it's not possible to represent the motion of the whole racket as a single particle. However, one point within the racket moves in a simple parabolic path, very similar to the flight of a ball. It is this point within the racket that is known as the center of mass. This is clearly shown in Figure 1.8.

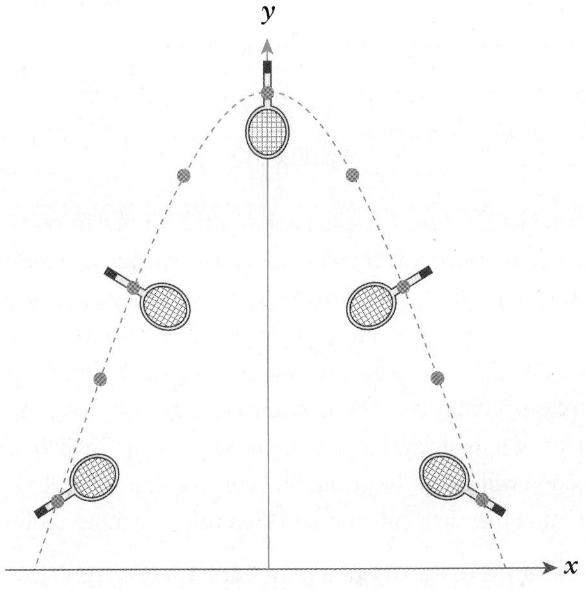

Figure 1.8 Center of Mass of a Tennis Racket
The center of mass of a racket thrown into the air travels along a parabolic pathway.

For a system in which particles are distributed in all three dimensions, the center of mass is defined by the three coordinates:

$$x = \frac{m_1 x_1 + m_2 x_2 + m_3 x_3 + \cdots}{m_1 + m_2 + m_3 + \cdots}$$

$$y = \frac{m_1 y_1 + m_2 y_2 + m_3 y_3 + \cdots}{m_1 + m_2 + m_3 + \cdots}$$

$$z = \frac{m_1 z_1 + m_2 z_2 + m_3 z_3 + \cdots}{m_1 + m_2 + m_3 + \cdots}$$

Equation 1.12

where m_1, m_2, and m_3 are the three sample masses, and the x-, y-, and z-values are coordinates. The center of gravity is related and corresponds to the single point at which one can conceptualize gravity acting on an object. Only for a homogeneous body (with symmetrical shape and uniform density) should one expect the center of gravity to be located at its geometric center. For example, we can approximate the center of gravity for a metal ball as the geometric center of the sphere. The same cannot be said, however, for a human body, television, or any asymmetrical, non-uniform object.

KEY CONCEPT

The center of mass of a uniform object is at the geometric center of the object.

Acceleration

Acceleration (a) is the rate of change of velocity that an object experiences as a result of some applied force. Acceleration, like velocity, is a vector quantity and is measured in SI units of meters per second squared. Acceleration in the direction opposite the initial velocity may be called **deceleration. Average acceleration** is defined as

$$\bar{\mathbf{a}} = \frac{\Delta \mathbf{v}}{\Delta t}$$

Equation 1.13

where $\bar{\mathbf{a}}$ is the average acceleration, $\Delta \mathbf{v}$ is the change in velocity, and Δt is the change in time.

Instantaneous acceleration is defined as the average acceleration as Δt approaches zero.

$$\mathbf{a} = \lim_{\Delta t \to 0} \frac{\Delta \mathbf{v}}{\Delta t}$$

Equation 1.14

On a graph of velocity *vs.* time, the tangent to the graph at any time t, which corresponds to the slope of the graph at that time, indicates the instantaneous acceleration. If the slope is positive, then the acceleration is positive and in the same direction as the velocity. If the slope is negative, then the acceleration is negative and in the opposite direction of the velocity (this is a deceleration).

MCAT CONCEPT CHECK 1.4

Before you move on, assess your understanding of the material with these questions.

1. When calculating frictional forces, how is directionality assigned?

____

2. When no force is being applied, the velocity must be:

____

3. True or False: The Earth creates a larger force on you than you create on the Earth.

4. Name two forces in addition to mechanical manipulation (pushing or pulling forces created by contact with an object):

- ______________________________
- ______________________________

1.5 Newton's Laws

LEARNING OBJECTIVES

After Chapter 1.5, you will be able to:

- Describe Newton's three laws of motion

Now that we have a clear understanding of force, mass, and acceleration, let's examine how they relate to each other. While it is unlikely that Newton "discovered" gravity by having an apple fall on his head, he did record that he was indeed inspired by watching apples fall from trees. His observations about objects in motion and at rest are the basis for the branch of physics that we now know as mechanics. Newton's laws, which are expressed as equations, concisely describe the effects forces have on objects that have mass.

First Law

$$\mathbf{F}_{\text{net}} = m\mathbf{a} = 0$$

Equation 1.15

where $\mathbf{F}_{\text{net}}$ is the net force, m is the mass, and $\mathbf{a}$ is the acceleration.

A body either at rest or in motion with constant velocity will remain that way unless a net force acts upon it. This is also known as the law of **inertia**. Newton's first law ought to be thought of as a special case of his second law, which is described next.

Second Law

$$\mathbf{F}_{\text{net}} = m\mathbf{a}$$

Equation 1.16

where $\mathbf{F}_{\text{net}}$ is the net force, m is the mass, and $\mathbf{a}$ is the acceleration.

What Newton's second law states is actually a corollary of the first: *An object of mass m will accelerate when the vector sum of the forces results in some nonzero resultant force vector.* No acceleration will occur when the vector sum of the forces results in a cancellation of those forces. Note that the net force and acceleration vectors necessarily point in the same direction.

Third Law

$$\mathbf{F}_{\text{AB}} = -\mathbf{F}_{\text{BA}}$$

Equation 1.17

This law is also known as the law of action and reaction: *To every action, there is always an opposed but equal reaction.* More formally, the law states that for every force exerted by object A on object B, there is an equal but opposite force exerted by object B on object A. For example, when you hit your hand against your desk, your hand exerts a force on the desk. Simultaneously, the desk exerts a force of equal magnitude in the opposite direction on your hand. Physical contact is not necessary for Newton's third law; the mutual gravitational pull between the Earth and the Moon traverses hundreds of thousands of kilometers of space.

MCAT CONCEPT CHECK 1.5

Before you move on, assess your understanding of the material with this question.

1. In your own words, provide a description of Newton's laws of motion:
   1. ______________________________
      ____
   2. ______________________________
      ____
   3. ______________________________
      ____

2. During a test crash, a 500 kg car is driven at a constant velocity of 50 mph until it hits a wall without braking. Apply all three of Newton's laws to this situation.
   1. ______________________________
   2. ______________________________
   3. ______________________________

1.6 Motion with Constant Acceleration

LEARNING OBJECTIVES

After Chapter 1.6, you will be able to:

- Identify which forces are active during different types of motion, including free fall and projectile motion
- Predict the angle of launch necessary to maximize horizontal or vertical displacement
- Recall the equation used to calculate centripetal acceleration

Objects can undergo only two types of motion—that which is constant (with no acceleration) or that which is changing (with acceleration). If an object's motion is changing, as indicated by a change in velocity, then the object is experiencing acceleration, and that acceleration may be constant or itself changing. A moving object that experiences constant acceleration presents a relatively simple case for analysis. The MCAT tends to restrict kinematics problems to those that involve motion with constant acceleration.

Linear Motion

In **linear motion**, the object's velocity and acceleration are along the line of motion, so the pathway of the moving object continues along a straight line. Linear motion does not need to be limited to vertical or horizontal paths; the inclined surface of a ramp will provide a path for linear motion at some angle. On the MCAT, the most common presentations of linear motion problems involve objects, such as balls, being dropped to the ground from some starting height.

Falling objects exhibit linear motion with constant acceleration. This one-dimensional motion can be fully described by the following equations:

$$\mathbf{v} = \mathbf{v}_0 + \mathbf{a}t$$

$$\mathbf{x} = \mathbf{v}_0 t + \frac{\mathbf{a}t^2}{2}$$

$$\mathbf{v}^2 = \mathbf{v}_0^2 + 2\mathbf{a}\mathbf{x}$$

$$\mathbf{x} = \overline{\mathbf{v}}t$$

Equations 1.18 to 1.21

where **x**, **v**, and **a** are the displacement, velocity, and acceleration vectors, respectively; $\mathbf{v}_0$ is the initial velocity; $\overline{\mathbf{v}}$ is the average velocity; and *t* is time. When the motion is vertical, we often use **y** instead of **x** for displacement.

MCAT EXPERTISE

When dealing with free fall problems, you can choose to make *down* either positive or negative. However, for the sake of simplicity, get in the habit of always making *up* positive and *down* negative.

To demonstrate the typical setup of a kinematics problem on the MCAT, we will consider an object falling through the air. For now, we will assume air resistance to be negligible, meaning that the only force acting on the object would be the gravitational force causing it to fall. Consequently, the object would fall with constant acceleration—the **acceleration due to gravity** $\left(\mathbf{g} = 9.8\ \frac{\text{m}}{\text{s}^2}\right)$—and would not reach **terminal velocity**. This is called **free fall**. Under these conditions of a free-falling object that has not reached terminal velocity, which are typical for Test Day, we could analyze the fall, using the relevant kinematics equations.

Example: A ball is thrown vertically up into the air from a window ledge 30 meters above the ground with an initial velocity of 10 $\frac{m}{s}$.

A. Find the velocity and position of the ball after two seconds.
B. Find the distance and time at which the ball reaches its maximum height above the window ledge.

Solution:

A. Remember that velocity and acceleration are vector quantities. For this question, let's call the ball's initial position, $\mathbf{y}_0$, zero. If we consider *up* to be positive, then the initial velocity, $\mathbf{v}_0$, is $+10\ \frac{m}{s}$, and the acceleration, g, is $-9.8\ \frac{m}{s^2}$. Note that g is negative because it's oriented downward. Velocity after two seconds can be found using Equation 1.18:

$$\mathbf{v} = \mathbf{v}_0 + \mathbf{a}t$$
$$= \left(+10\ \frac{m}{s}\right) + \left(-9.8\ \frac{m}{s^2}\right)(2\ s)$$
$$= 10\ \frac{m}{s} - 19.6\ \frac{m}{s} = -9.6\ \frac{m}{s}$$

After two seconds, the position of the ball is found using Equation 1.19:

$$\mathbf{y} = \mathbf{v}_0 t + \frac{\mathbf{a}t^2}{2}$$
$$= \left(10\ \frac{m}{s}\right)(2\ s) + \frac{\left(-9.8\ \frac{m}{s^2}\right)(2\ s)^2}{2}$$
$$= 20 - 19.6 = 0.4\ \text{m (above the ledge)}$$

B. When the ball is at its maximum height, the velocity, which has been decreasing on the way up, is now zero. We can find the maximum height the ball reaches using Equation 1.20:

$$\mathbf{v}^2 = \mathbf{v}_0^2 + 2\ \mathbf{ay}$$
$$0^2 = \left(10\ \frac{m}{s}\right)^2 + 2\left(-9.8\ \frac{m}{s^2}\right)(\mathbf{y})$$
$$19.6\mathbf{y} = 100$$
$$\mathbf{y} \approx 5\ \text{m (actual} = 5.1\ \text{m)}$$

The time at which the ball reaches its maximum height can be found from Equation 1.18:

$$\mathbf{v} = \mathbf{v}_0 + \mathbf{a}t$$
$$0 = \left(+10\ \frac{m}{s}\right) + \left(-9.8\ \frac{m}{s^2}\right)(t)$$
$$t \approx 1\ \text{s (actual} = 1.02\ \text{s)}$$

Let's now consider what happens when air resistance is *not* negligible. **Air resistance**, like friction, opposes the motion of an object. Its value increases as the speed of the object increases. Therefore, an object in free fall will experience a growing **drag force** as the magnitude of its velocity increases. Eventually, this drag force will be equal in magnitude to the weight of the object, and the object will fall with constant velocity according to Newton's first law. This velocity is called the **terminal velocity**.

Projectile Motion

Projectile motion is motion that follows a path along two dimensions. The velocities and accelerations in the two directions (usually horizontal and vertical) are independent of each other and must, accordingly, be analyzed separately. Objects in projectile motion on Earth, such as cannonballs, baseballs, or footballs, experience the force and acceleration of gravity only in the vertical direction (along the *y*-axis). This means that $\mathbf{v}_y$ will change at the rate of **g** but $\mathbf{v}_x$ will remain constant. In fact, on the MCAT, you will generally be able to assume that the horizontal velocity, $\mathbf{v}_x$, will be constant because we usually assume that air resistance is negligible and, therefore, no measurable force is acting along the *x*-axis.

Example: A projectile is fired from ground level with an initial velocity of 50 $\frac{\text{m}}{\text{s}}$ and an initial angle of elevation of 37°, as shown below. Assuming $\mathbf{g} = -10\ \frac{\text{m}}{\text{s}^2}$, find the following: (Note: sin 37° = 0.6; cos 37° = 0.8)

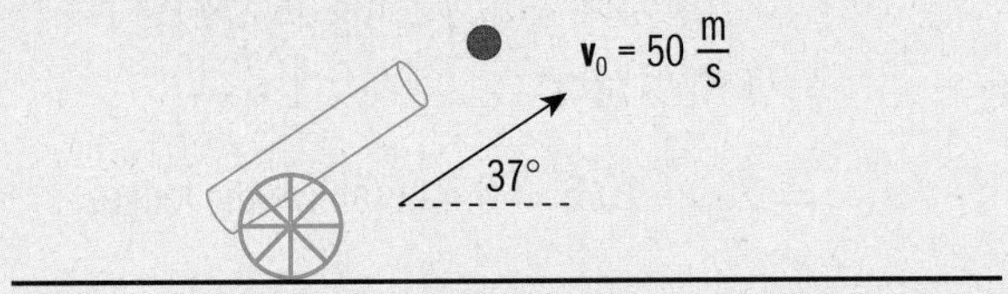

A. The projectile's total time in flight
B. The total horizontal distance traveled

Solution:

A. Let **y** equal the vertical displacement, and *up* be the positive direction. If we are going to use the vertical displacement and acceleration due to gravity (which is also in the *y*-direction), we must use the *y*-component of velocity in this part of the problem:

$$v_{0_y} = v_0 \sin 37° = \left(50\ \frac{\text{m}}{\text{s}}\right)(0.6) = 30\ \frac{\text{m}}{\text{s}}$$

MCAT EXPERTISE

The amount of time that an object takes to get to its maximum height is the same time it takes for the object to fall back down to the starting height (assuming air resistance is negligible); this fact makes solving these problems much easier. Because you can solve for the time to reach maximum height by setting your final velocity to zero, you can then multiply your answer by two, getting the total time in flight—as long as the object ends at the same height at which it started. Because the only force acting on the object after it is launched is gravity, the velocity it has in the *x*-direction will remain constant throughout its time in flight. By multiplying the time by the velocity in the *x*-direction, one can find the horizontal distance traveled.

KEY CONCEPT

Note that gravity is set in bold, indicating it has a vector value. Gravity is unique in that it is used as both a constant and as a vector in calculations. Though gravity is not always bolded, you should recall for Test Day that gravity has a direction.

Now we can plug in:

$$\mathbf{y} = v_{0_y} t + \frac{\mathbf{a}_y t^2}{2}$$

$$0 = \left(30 \frac{\text{m}}{\text{s}}\right)(t) + \frac{\left(-10 \frac{\text{m}}{\text{s}^2}\right)(t)^2}{2}$$

$$0 = (30)(t) - 5(t)^2$$

$$5(t)^2 = 30\,t$$

$$t^2 = 6\,t$$

$$t = 0 \text{ s or } 6 \text{ s}$$

The height of the ball is zero at 0 seconds (its initial position) and 6 seconds (when it hits the ground again).

B. Now that we know the time, we can find the horizontal distance traveled. Here, we will need to consider only the *x*-component of the velocity:

$$v_{0_x} = v_0 \cos 37° = \left(50 \frac{\text{m}}{\text{s}}\right)(0.8) = 40 \frac{\text{m}}{\text{s}}$$

Now we can plug in:

$$\mathbf{x} = \mathbf{v}_x t + \frac{\mathbf{a}_x t^2}{2} = \left(40 \frac{\text{m}}{\text{s}}\right)(6 \text{ s}) + 0 = 240 \text{ m}$$

Note: There is only acceleration in the vertical direction due to gravity, $a_x = 0$.

Inclined Planes

Inclined planes are another example of motion in two dimensions. When working with an inclined plane question, it is often best to divide force vectors into components that are parallel and perpendicular to the plane. Most often, gravity must be split into components for these calculations. These components can be defined as:

$$\mathbf{F}_{g,||} = mg \sin \theta$$

$$\mathbf{F}_{g,\perp} = mg \cos \theta$$

Equation 1.22

where $\mathbf{F}_{g,||}$ is the component of gravity parallel to the plane (oriented down the plane), $\mathbf{F}_{g,\perp}$ is the component of gravity perpendicular to the plane (oriented into the plane), m is the mass, g is acceleration due to gravity, and θ is the angle of the incline. Otherwise, the same kinematics equations can be used in these problems.

Example: A 5 kg block slides down a frictionless incline at 30°. Find the normal force and acceleration of the block. (Note: sin 30° = 0.5, sin 60° = 0.866, cos 30° = 0.866, cos 60° = 0.5)

Solution: The block in this example has two forces acting on it: the normal force, which is perpendicular to the surface, and gravity, which points straight down:

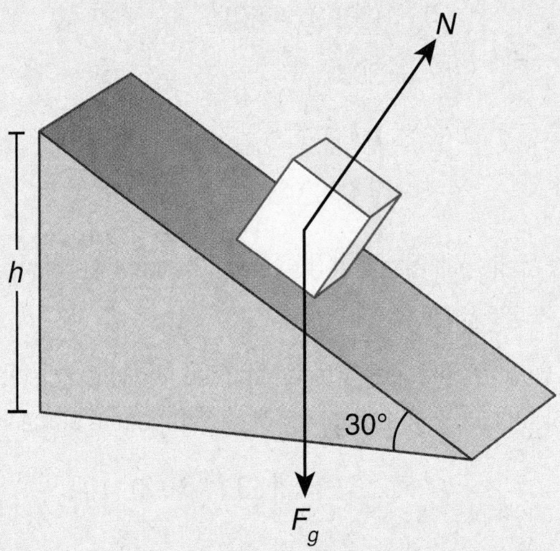

Because gravity is not in the same coordinate system as the normal force, one of the two forces must be split into components. In this case, because we are concerned with magnitude of the normal force (which is perpendicular to the plane) and the acceleration (which is parallel to the plane), we should split the force of gravity into parallel and perpendicular components:

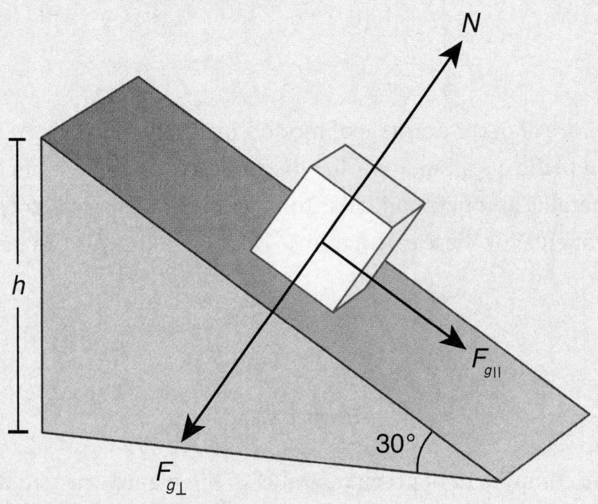

Because there is no acceleration in the perpendicular dimension, the magnitude of the normal force must be equal to that of the perpendicular component of gravity:

$$|\mathbf{N}| = |\mathbf{F}_{g,\perp}| = mg\cos\theta = (5\text{ kg})\left(9.8\,\frac{\text{m}}{\text{s}^2}\right)\cos 30° \approx 50(0.866)$$
$$= 43.3\text{ N (actual} = 42.4\text{ N)}$$

The acceleration can then be determined in the parallel direction. Because the only force in this dimension is the parallel component of the force of gravity, it is the net force:

$$\mathbf{F}_{\mathbf{net},\parallel} = \mathbf{F}_{g,\parallel} = ma_{\parallel}$$
$$mg\sin(\theta) = ma_{\parallel}$$
$$g\sin(\theta) = a_{\parallel} = \left(9.8\,\frac{m}{s^2}\right)\sin(30) = \left(9.8\,\frac{m}{s^2}\right)(0.5) = 4.9\,\frac{m}{s^2}$$

Circular Motion

Circular motion occurs when forces cause an object to move in a circular pathway. Upon completion of one cycle, the displacement of the object is zero. Although the MCAT focuses on uniform circular motion, in which case the speed of the object is constant, recognize that there is also nonuniform circular motion.

In **uniform circular motion**, the instantaneous velocity vector is always tangent to the circular path, as shown in Figure 1.9. What this means is that the object moving in the circular path has a tendency (inertia) to break out of its circular pathway and move in a linear direction along the tangent. It is kept from doing so by a **centripetal force**, which always points radially inward. In all circular motion, we can resolve the forces into radial and tangential components. In uniform circular motion, the tangential force is zero because there is no change in the speed of the object.

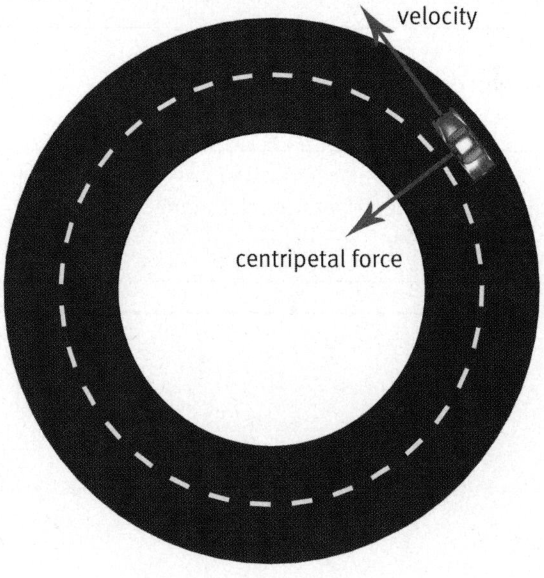

Figure 1.9 Uniform Circular Motion

As a force, the centripetal force generates **centripetal acceleration**. Remember from the discussion of Newton's laws that both force and acceleration are vectors and the acceleration is always in the same direction as the net force. Thus, it is this acceleration generated by the centripetal force that keeps an object in its circular pathway. When the centripetal force is no longer acting on the object, it will simply exit the circular pathway and assume a path tangential to the circle at that point. The equation that describes circular motion is

$$F_c = \frac{mv^2}{r}$$

Equation 1.23

where F_c is the magnitude of the centripetal force, m is the mass, v is the speed, and r is the radius of the circular path. Note that the centripetal force can be caused by tension, gravity, electrostatic forces, or other forces.

MCAT CONCEPT CHECK 1.6

Before you move on, assess your understanding of the material with these questions.

1. How do the forces acting in free fall and projectile motion differ?

____

2. At what angle of launch is a projectile going to have the greatest horizontal displacement? What angle will result in the greatest vertical displacement, assuming a level surface?
   - Greatest horizontal displacement:

____

   - Greatest vertical displacement:

____

3. What is the equation for centripetal acceleration?

____

1.7 Mechanical Equilibrium

LEARNING OBJECTIVES

After Chapter 1.7, you will be able to:

- Identify whether an object is in equilibrium
- Calculate torque within a system:

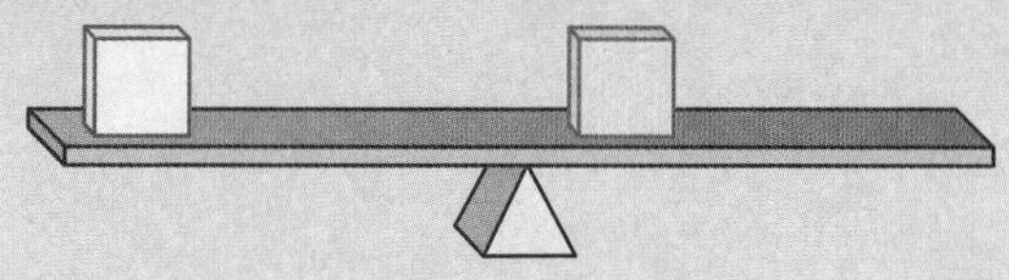

So far we've been paying attention to kinematics and the special cases of linear and projectile motion. However, many times the MCAT will require you to eliminate acceleration, or otherwise maintain a system in equilibrium. To accomplish this, you must be familiar with analyzing forces, especially with free body diagrams, as well as with the special conditions for translational and rotational equilibrium. The study of forces and torques is called **dynamics**.

Free Body Diagrams

While we all have an intuitive sense of forces (and their effects) in everyday life, students often struggle to represent them diagrammatically. Drawing **free body diagrams** takes some practice but will be a valuable tool on the MCAT. On Test Day, make sure to draw a free body diagram for any problem in which you must perform calculations on forces.

MCAT EXPERTISE

When dealing with dynamics questions, always draw a quick picture of what is happening in the problem; this will keep everything in its proper relative position and help prevent you from making simple mistakes.

Example: Three people are pulling on ropes tied to a tire with forces of 100 N, 125 N, and 125 N as shown below. Find the magnitude and direction of the resultant force. (Note: sin 30° = 0.5, cos 30° = 0.866, sin 37° = 0.6, cos 37° = 0.8)

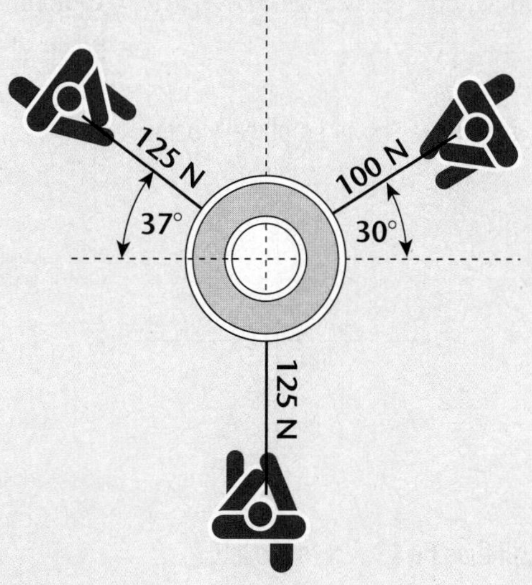

Solution: First, draw a free body diagram that shows the forces acting on the tire. Its purpose is to identify and visualize the acting forces.

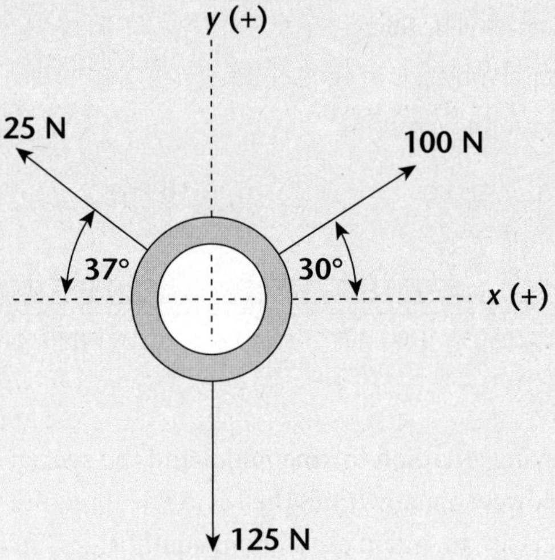

The resultant force is simply the sum of the forces. To find the resultant force vector, we need the sum of the force components, shown below.

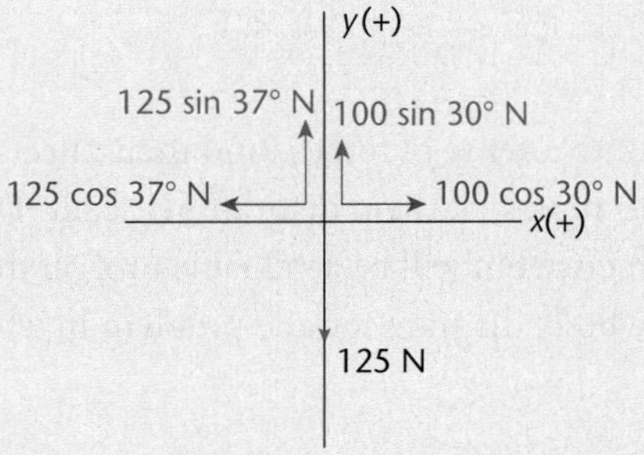

$$\mathbf{F}_{\text{net},x} = \sum F_x = 100\cos(30°) - 125\cos(37) = 100(0.866) - 125(0.8)$$
$$= 86.6 - 100 = -13.4 \text{ N}$$

$$\mathbf{F}_{\text{net},y} = \sum F_y = 100\sin(30°) + 125\sin(37) - 125 = 100(0.5) + 125(0.6) - 125$$
$$= 50 + 75 - 125 = 0 \text{ N}$$

The net component vectors are shown graphically below.

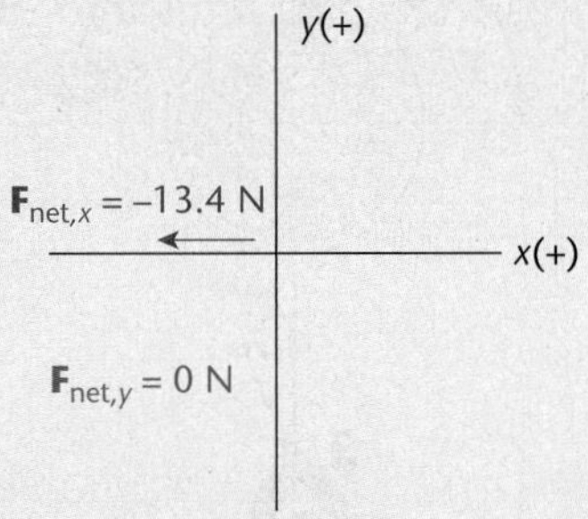

The resultant force will thus be 13.4 N to the left.

Translational Equilibrium

Translational motion occurs when forces cause an object to move without any rotation. The simplest pathways may be linear, such as when a child slides down a snowy hill on a sled, or parabolic, as in the case of a cannonball shot out of a cannon. Any problem regarding translational motion in the *Chemical and Physical Foundations of Biological Systems* section can be solved using free body diagrams and Newton's three laws.

Equilibrium Conditions

Translational equilibrium exists only when the vector sum of all of the forces acting on an object is zero. This is called the **first condition of equilibrium**, and it is merely a reiteration of Newton's first law. Remember that when the resultant force upon an object is zero, the object will not accelerate; that may mean that the object is stationary, but it could just as well mean that the object is moving with a constant nonzero velocity. Thus, an object experiencing translational equilibrium will have a constant velocity: both a constant speed (which could be zero or a nonzero value) and a constant direction.

KEY CONCEPT

If there is no acceleration, then there is no net force on the object. This means that any object with a constant velocity has no net force acting on it. However, just because the net force equals zero does not mean the velocity equals zero.

Example: Two blocks are in static equilibrium, as shown below:

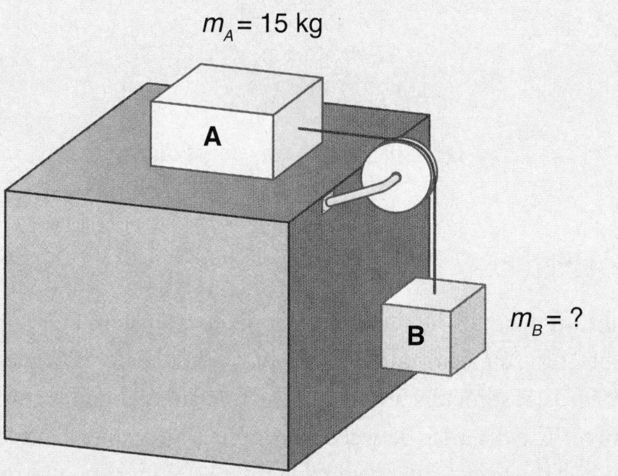

If block A has a mass of 15 kg and the coefficient of static friction between block A and the surface is 0.2, what is the maximum mass of block B?

Solution: Start by making a free body diagram of each block:

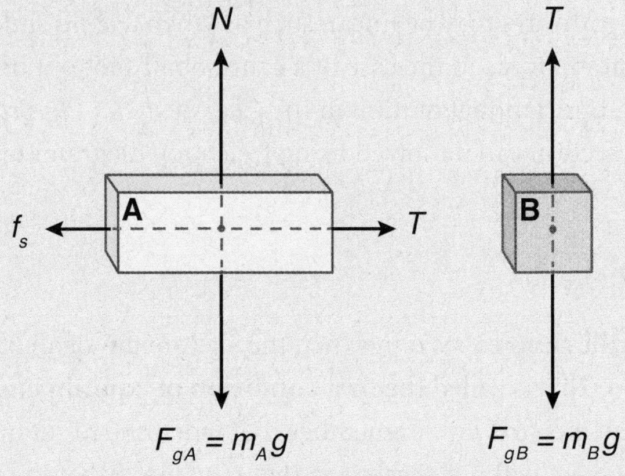

Both blocks have a net force of zero because they are in equilibrium. Therefore, the magnitude of **T** is equal to that of $\mathbf{F}_{g,B}$. Asking for the maximum mass of block B means that the force of static friction is maximized ($f_s = \mu_s N$); further, because block A is in equilibrium, $\mathbf{f}_s$ is equal in magnitude to **T** and $\mathbf{F}_{g,A}$ is equal in magnitude to **N**. Therefore:

$$f_s = T \text{ and } T = F_{g,B}$$
$$f_s = F_{g,B}$$
$$\mu_s N = m_B g$$
$$\mu_s m_A g = m_B g$$
$$\mu_s m_A = m_B$$
$$(0.2)(15 \text{ kg}) = m_B = 3.0 \text{ kg}$$

Rotational Equilibrium

Rotational motion occurs when forces are applied against an object in such a way as to cause the object to rotate around a fixed pivot point, also known as the **fulcrum**. Application of force at some distance from the fulcrum generates **torque** ($\boldsymbol{\tau}$) or the **moment of force**. The distance between the applied force and the fulcrum is termed the **lever arm**. It is the torque that generates rotational motion, not the mere application of the force itself. This is because torque depends not only on the magnitude of the force but also on the length of the lever arm and the angle at which the force is applied. The equation for torque is a cross product:

$$\boldsymbol{\tau} = \mathbf{r} \times \mathbf{F} = rF \sin \theta$$

Equation 1.24

where r is the length of the lever arm, F is the magnitude of the force, and θ is the angle between the lever arm and force vectors.

KEY CONCEPT

Remember that $\sin 90° = 1$. This means that torque is greatest when the force applied is 90 degrees (perpendicular) to the lever arm. Knowing that $\sin 0° = 0$ tells us that there is no torque when the force applied is parallel to the lever arm.

Equilibrium Conditions

Rotational equilibrium exists only when the vector sum of all the torques acting on an object is zero. This is called the **second condition of equilibrium**. Torques that generate clockwise rotation are considered negative, while torques that generate counterclockwise rotation are positive. Thus, in rotational equilibrium, it must be that all of the positive torques exactly cancel out all of the negative torques. Similar to the behavior defined by translational equilibrium, there are two possibilities of motion in the case of rotational equilibrium.

Either the object is not rotating at all (that is, it is stationary), or it is rotating with a constant angular velocity. The MCAT almost always takes rotational equilibrium to mean that the object is not rotating at all.

Example: A seesaw with a mass of 5 kg has one block of mass 10 kg two meters to the left of the fulcrum and another block 0.5 m to the right of the fulcrum, as shown below.

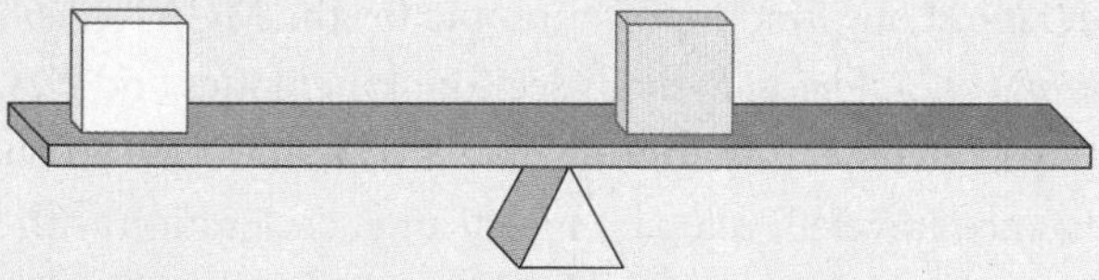

If the seesaw is in equilibrium, find the mass of block 2 and the force exerted by the fulcrum.

Solution: If the seesaw is balanced, this implies rotational equilibrium. Therefore, the positive (counterclockwise) torque exerted by block 1 is equal in magnitude to the negative (clockwise) torque exerted by block 2. Use the fulcrum as the pivot point; because the fulcrum is centered under the seesaw, both the normal force and the weight of the seesaw will be eliminated from the equation because their lever arms are 0.

$$\tau_1 = \tau_2$$
$$r_1 F_{g_1} \sin\theta_1 = r_2 F_{g_2} \sin\theta_2$$
$$r_1(m_1 g)\sin 90^\circ = r_2(m_2 g)\sin 90^\circ$$
$$r_1 m_1 = r_2 m_2 \rightarrow m_2 = \frac{r_1 m_1}{r_2} = \frac{(2\text{ m})(10\text{ kg})}{0.5\text{ m}} = 40\text{ kg}$$

To find the normal force exerted by the fulcrum, consider that the seesaw is not only in rotational equilibrium but also in translational equilibrium. Therefore, the combined weight of the seesaw and blocks (pointing down) is equal in magnitude to the normal force (pointing up):

$$N = F_{g,\text{ seesaw + blocks}}$$
$$= (m_{\text{seesaw}} + m_1 + m_2)\,g$$
$$\approx (5\text{ kg} + 10\text{ kg} + 40\text{ kg})\left(10\,\frac{\text{m}}{\text{s}^2}\right) = 550\text{ N (actual} = 539\text{ N)}$$

MCAT CONCEPT CHECK 1.7

Before you move on, assess your understanding of the material with these questions.

1. Can a moving object be in equilibrium? Why or why not?

____

2. If you have an object three times as heavy as you can lift, how could a lever be used to lift the object? Where would the fulcrum need to be placed?

____

Conclusion

In this chapter, we've equipped you with the math—the language of physics—necessary to understand our first important topic for the MCAT *Chemical and Physical Foundations of Biological Systems* section: kinematics and Newtonian mechanics. This study of objects in motion allows us to describe an object's position, displacement, distance traveled, velocity, speed, and acceleration with respect to time. We now understand how to use the four key kinematics equations when objects experience constant acceleration, a relatively simple scenario presented on Test Day.

We also learned that different kinds of forces act on objects to cause them to move in certain ways. Application of forces may cause objects to accelerate or decelerate according to Newton's second law. If the vector sum of all the forces acting on an object is equal to zero, the forces cancel out, and the object experiences no acceleration, a condition known as translational equilibrium. This is expressed in Newton's first law. Even when objects aren't touching, they can still exert forces between them, as described by Newton's third law. We considered linear motion, projectile motion, inclined planes, and circular motion. We also considered the special conditions of translational and rotational equilibrium.

We hope that you will come to appreciate the relevance that these concepts and principles have for your performance not only on the MCAT but also in medical school, residency training, and your career as a physician. Your careful consideration of the discussion topics in this chapter and your practice with the kinds of problems demonstrated here will earn you many points on Test Day.

You've reviewed the content, now test your knowledge and critical thinking skills by completing a test-like passage set in your online resources!

GO ONLINE

CONCEPT SUMMARY

Units

- The MCAT will test the **SI units** that are related to the metric system. The SI units include meter, kilogram, second, ampère, mole, kelvin, and candela.

Vectors and Scalars

- **Vectors** are physical quantities that have both magnitude and direction. Vector quantities include displacement, velocity, acceleration, and force, among others.
- **Scalars** are quantities without direction. Scalar quantities may be the magnitude of vectors, like speed, or may be dimensionless, like coefficients of friction.
- Vector addition may be accomplished using the tip-to-tail method or by breaking a vector into its components and using the Pythagorean theorem.
- Vector subtraction is accomplished by changing the direction of the subtracted vector and then following the procedures for vector addition.
- Multiplying a vector by a scalar changes the magnitude and may reverse the direction.
- Multiplying two vectors using the **dot product** results in a scalar quantity. The dot product is the product of the vectors' magnitudes and the cosine of the angle between them.
- Multiplying two vectors using the **cross product** results in a vector quantity. The cross product is the product of the vectors' magnitudes and the sine of the angle between them. The right-hand rule is used to determine the resultant vector's direction.

Displacement and Velocity

- **Displacement** is the vector representation of a change in position. It is path independent and is equivalent to the straight-line distance between the start and end locations.
- **Distance** is a scalar quantity that reflects the path traveled.
- **Velocity** is the vector representation of the change in displacement with respect to time.
  - **Average velocity** is the total displacement divided by the total time.
  - **Average speed** is the total distance traveled divided by the total time.
  - **Instantaneous velocity** is the limit of the change in displacement over time as the change in time approaches zero.
  - **Instantaneous speed** is the magnitude of the instantaneous velocity vector.

Forces and Acceleration

- A **force** is any push or pull that has the potential to result in an acceleration.
- **Gravity** is the attractive force between two objects as a result of their masses.
- **Friction** is a force that opposes motion as a function of electrostatic interactions at the surfaces of two objects.
  - **Static friction** exists between two objects that are not in motion relative to each other.
  - **Kinetic friction** exists between two objects that are in motion relative to each other.
  - Whereas static friction can take on many values depending on the magnitude of an applied force, kinetic friction is a constant value.
  - The **coefficient of friction** depends on the two materials in contact. The coefficient of static friction is always higher than the coefficient of kinetic friction.
- Mass and weight are not synonymous.
  - **Mass** is a measure of the inertia of an object—its amount of material.
  - **Weight** is the force experienced by a given mass due to its gravitational attraction to the Earth.
- **Acceleration** is the vector representation of the change in velocity over time. Average or instantaneous acceleration may both be considered, similar to velocity.

Newton's Laws

- **Newton's first law**, or the **law of inertia**, states that an object will remain at rest or move with a constant velocity if there is no net force on the object.
- **Newton's second law** states that any acceleration is the result of the sum of the forces acting on the object and its mass.
- **Newton's third law** states that any two objects interacting with one another experience equal and opposite forces as a result of their interaction.

Motion with Constant Acceleration

- **Linear motion** includes **free fall** and motion in which the velocity and acceleration vectors are parallel or antiparallel.
- **Projectile motion** contains both an *x*- and *y*-component. Assuming negligible air resistance, the only force acting on the object is gravity.
- **Inclined planes** are another example of two-dimensional movement. It is often easiest to consider the dimensions as being parallel and perpendicular to the surface of the plane.
- **Circular motion** is best thought of as having radial and tangential dimensions. In **uniform circular motion**, the only force is the **centripetal force**, pointing radially inward. The instantaneous velocity vector always points tangentially.

Mechanical Equilibrium

- **Free body diagrams** are representations of the forces acting on an object. They are useful for equilibrium and dynamics problems.
- **Translational equilibrium** occurs in the absence of any net forces acting on an object. An object in translational equilibrium has a constant velocity, and may or may not also be in rotational equilibrium.
- **Rotational equilibrium** occurs in the absence of any net **torques** acting on an object. Rotational motion may consider any pivot point, but the center of mass is most common. An object in rotational equilibrium has a constant angular velocity; on the MCAT, the angular velocity is usually zero.

ANSWERS TO CONCEPT CHECKS

1.1

1. Force will obey the same relationship with mass and acceleration, regardless of the unit system. Force is always the product of mass and acceleration, so one pound (lb) must be equal to one $\frac{\text{slug}\cdot\text{ft}}{\text{s}^2}$.
2. ångström < centimeter < inch < foot < mile

1.2

1. Vector addition, unlike vector multiplication, is a commutative function. The resultant of $\mathbf{A} + \mathbf{B}$ is the same as $\mathbf{B} + \mathbf{A}$, so there would be no difference between the two resultants.
2. Vector subtraction, like vector multiplication, is not a commutative function. The resultant of $\mathbf{A} - \mathbf{B}$ has the same magnitude as $\mathbf{B} - \mathbf{A}$, but is oriented in the opposite direction.
3. A scalar is calculated from two vectors by using the dot product: $\mathbf{A} \cdot \mathbf{B} = |\mathbf{A}|\ |\mathbf{B}| \cos\theta$. A vector is calculated by using the cross product: $\mathbf{A} \times \mathbf{B} = |\mathbf{A}|\ |\mathbf{B}| \sin\theta$.
4. False. This would be true of an addition problem in which both vectors have equal magnitude, but it is never true for vector multiplication. To find the direction of **C**, we must use the right-hand rule. If the thumb points in the direction of **A**, and the fingers point in the direction of **B**, then our palm, **C**, points out of the page.

1.3

1. Instantaneous speed is the magnitude of the instantaneous velocity vector. Average speed and average velocity may be unrelated because speed does not depend on displacement, but is rather the total distance traveled divided by time.
2. True. Displacement considers the most direct route between two points. Distance will always be equal to or larger in magnitude than displacement.
3. Velocity is the rate of change of the displacement of an object. Displacement is a function of velocity acting over a period of time.

1.4

1. The direction of the frictional force always opposes movement. Once the instantaneous velocity vector is known (or net force, in the case of static friction), the frictional force must be in the opposite direction.
2. If there is no net force acting on an object, then that object is not experiencing an acceleration and it has a constant velocity.
3. False. Forces are always reciprocal in nature. When the Earth exerts a force on a person, the person also exerts a force of the same magnitude on the Earth (in the opposite direction). The difference in masses gives the Earth an apparent acceleration of zero.
4. Gravity and frictional forces were discussed in this chapter. Electrostatic, magnetic, elastic, weak nuclear, and strong nuclear forces are other examples of forces.

1.5

1. Any answer which is similar to the following is acceptable:
    1. In the absence of any forces—or when the net force is zero—there will be no change in velocity.
    2. Acceleration results from the sum of the force vectors.
    3. For any two interacting objects, all forces acting on one object have an equal and opposing force acting on the other object.
2. Any answer which is similar to the following is acceptable:
    1. Prior to the collision, the vehicle is travelling at constant velocity, which (according to Newton's first law) indicates that there is no acceleration and no net force.
    2. The collision with the wall creates a sudden deceleration. Because there is acceleration, there must be a net force. The value of the net force can be calculated by multiplying the mass of the car times the acceleration.
    3. When the car collides with the wall, the car exerts a force on the wall. Simultaneously, the wall exerts a force of equal magnitude in the opposite direction on the car.

1.6

1. The only force acting in both free fall and projectile motion is gravity.
2. The product of sine and cosine is maximized when the angle is 45°. Because horizontal displacement relies on both measurements, the maximum horizontal displacement will also be achieved at this angle. Vertical displacement will always be zero as the object returns to the starting point. Objects launched vertically will experience the greatest vertical *distance*.
3. If the equation for centripetal force is $F_c = \frac{mv^2}{r}$ and force is simply mass times acceleration (from Newton's second law), then $a_c = \frac{v^2}{r}$.

1.7

1. A moving object can be in either translational or rotational equilibrium (or both). Translational equilibrium only requires the net force on an object be zero—its velocity is constant. The corresponding condition in rotational equilibrium is that net torque equals zero—its angular velocity is constant.
2. One could place the fulcrum one quarter of the way across the lever, closer to the object. The ratio of the lever arms would then be 3:1, which means that only one-third of the original force is necessary. (Alternatively, the fulcrum could be placed at the end with the object one-third of the way across the lever. This would again result in a 3:1 ratio of lever arms, meaning that only one-third of the original force is necessary.)

SCIENCE MASTERY ASSESSMENT EXPLANATIONS

1. **B**

Using the Pythagorean theorem, calculate the magnitude of the person's displacement:

$$x = \sqrt{30^2 + 40^2} = 50 \text{ m}$$

The total distance traveled is equal to $30 + 40 = 70$ m. Therefore, the difference between these two is 20 m.

2. **A**

The average force on the rocket equals its mass times the average acceleration; the average acceleration equals the change in velocity divided by the time over which the change occurs. So, the change in velocity equals the average force times the time divided by the mass:

$$\mathbf{F} = m\mathbf{a} \rightarrow \mathbf{a} = \frac{\mathbf{F}}{m}$$

$$\mathbf{a} = \frac{\Delta \mathbf{v}}{\Delta t} \rightarrow \Delta \mathbf{v} = \mathbf{a}\Delta t = \frac{\mathbf{F}\Delta t}{m} = \frac{(20 \times 10^3 \text{ N})(8 \text{ s})}{1000 \text{ kg}}$$

$$= 160 \ \frac{\text{m}}{\text{s}}$$

(B) represents the new velocity of the rocket, not its change in velocity. **(C)** and **(D)** neglect dividing by the mass of the rocket.

3. **C**

The magnitude of the average acceleration is the change in velocity divided by the time. The velocity changes by $-40 \ \frac{\text{km}}{\text{hr}}$ because the car comes to rest. The time, in hours, is $6 \text{ s} \times \left[\frac{1 \text{ hr}}{3600 \text{ s}}\right] = \frac{1}{600}$ hr. The average acceleration is then

$$\bar{\mathbf{a}} = \frac{\Delta \mathbf{v}}{\Delta t} = \frac{-40 \ \frac{\text{km}}{\text{hr}}}{\frac{1}{600} \text{ hr}} = -24{,}000 \ \frac{\text{km}}{\text{hr}^2}$$

This question asked for the magnitude of this acceleration, which is $24{,}000 \ \frac{\text{km}}{\text{hr}^2}$.

4. **A**

The forces on the elevator are the tension upward and the weight downward, so the net force on the elevator is the difference between the two. For the elevator to accelerate upwards, the tension in the cable will have to be greater than the maximum weight so that there is a net force directed upwards.

5. **C**

The unit of power is the Watt, which breaks down to $\text{kg} \cdot \text{m}^2/\text{s}^2$. Because there is no unit of temperature in this formulation, the ambient temperature is extra information, supporting **(C)** as the correct answer. Note that mass, distance, and time are all used to compute power, eliminating **(A)**, **(B)**, and **(D)**.

6. **A**

The firefighter's acceleration is always directed downward, whereas the firefighter's velocity starts out horizontal and gradually rotates downwards as the downward velocity increases. Therefore, as time progresses, the angle between the velocity and acceleration decreases, which means that the maximum angle occurs at the instant the firefighter jumps.

7. **B**

The static force of friction acts parallel to the plane and is in the opposite direction from the parallel component of gravity in this setup. Because the wagon is in equilibrium, these two forces are equal in magnitude. Remember that gravity is often split into components in inclined plane problems. Rather than splitting into x- and y-components, however, it is more convenient to split the gravity vector into parallel and perpendicular components. The parallel component of gravity is given by the expression $mg \sin \theta$. Plugging in the values from the question, both the parallel component of gravity and static force of friction must be equal to $(10 \text{ kg})\left(9.8 \ \frac{\text{m}}{\text{s}^2}\right)(\sin 30°) = 49$ N.

8. **C**

In SI units, mass is measured in kilograms (kg), velocity in meters per second $\left(\frac{\text{m}}{\text{s}}\right)$, and time in seconds (s). The newton is a derived unit, and is not considered to be a base unit of the SI system. A newton is equal to a $\frac{\text{kg} \cdot \text{m}}{\text{s}^2}$.

9. **D**

Since the equation uses the sine of the angle, this equation computes a cross product. The output of the cross product is another vector quantity. To find the direction of the resultant vector, use the right hand rule. The thumb of the right hand points in the direction of vector A, the fingers point in the direction of vector B, and the palm reveals the direction of the vector product. In this problem, the right hand rule indicates that the direction of the resulting vector is out of the page, consistent with **(D)**. Note that since the cross product always produces another vector, choices **(A)** and **(B)** can be immediately eliminated.

10. **D**

A vector is characterized by both magnitude and direction. From the given answer choices, all are vectors except for distance. Distance is a scalar because it has only a numerical value and lacks direction.

11. **B**

In order for the seesaw to be balanced, the torque due to the child (τ_c) must be exactly counteracted by the torque due to the parent (τ_p). In other words, the magnitudes of these torques must be equal ($\tau_c = \tau_p$):

$$r_c F_c \sin\theta_c = r_p F_p \sin\theta_p$$

$$r_c m_c g \sin 90° = r_p m_p g \sin 90°$$

$$(2\text{m})(30\text{ kg}) = r_p(90\text{ kg})$$

$$0.67\text{ m} = r_p$$

Because r represents the distance of each person from the fulcrum, the parent must sit 67 cm from the fulcrum.

12. **B**

The maximum height depends only on the y-component of the velocity, so the horizontal distance can be ignored. The initial y-velocity can be calculated by: $v_f = 12 \cdot \sin(30°) = 6\text{ m/s}$. To solve for max height, use the equation: $v_f^2 = v_i^2 + 2ax$, where, at the maximum height, the vertical velocity is equal to 0 m/s. Plugging in values yields the equation $0 = 36 - 20x$. Solving for x gives $x = 1.8$ m, matching **(B)**.

13. **C**

We only need to analyze the motion in the vertical dimension to answer this question. If both the rock and ball began with no vertical velocity, they would reach the ground at the same time. However, because the rock begins with an upward component of velocity, it will take time to reach a maximum height before falling back toward the ground. Functionally, the rock's free fall thus starts higher and later than the ball's. The rock will necessarily hit the ground after the ball.

14. **C**

Because the question stem indicates that centrifugal force is reactionary and acts outwardly away from the center of rotation, we can draw the conclusion that it is a reaction to the centripetal force. According to Newton's third law, these forces must have equal magnitude and opposite directions (antiparallel).

15. **B**

The presence of friction does not change the impact of Newton's laws. A net force must still be applied to cause motion. This net force is not necessarily equal to an applied force, as friction and gravity also act on the object; thus, statement I is eliminated. Static friction opposes the movement of stationary objects, and is necessarily greater than the force of kinetic friction; thus, statement II is correct. Statement III is false because the normal force is related to mass, and friction is related to the normal force.

Consult your online resources for additional practice. **GO ONLINE**

EQUATIONS TO REMEMBER

(1.1) **Component vectors:** $\mathbf{X} = \mathbf{V}\cos\theta$

$$\mathbf{Y} = \mathbf{V}\sin\theta$$

(1.2) **Pythagorean theorem:** $\mathbf{X}^2 + \mathbf{Y}^2 = \mathbf{V}^2$ or $\mathbf{V} = \sqrt{\mathbf{X}^2 + \mathbf{Y}^2}$

(1.3) **Determination of direction from component vectors:** $\theta = \tan^{-1}\frac{\mathbf{Y}}{\mathbf{X}}$

(1.4) **Dot product:** $\mathbf{A}\cdot\mathbf{B} = |\mathbf{A}|\,|\mathbf{B}|\cos\theta$

(1.5) **Cross product:** $\mathbf{A}\times\mathbf{B} = |\mathbf{A}|\,|\mathbf{B}|\sin\theta$

(1.6) **Instantaneous velocity:** $\mathbf{v} = \lim_{\Delta t\to 0}\frac{\Delta \mathrm{x}}{\Delta t}$

(1.7) **Average velocity:** $\bar{\mathbf{v}} = \frac{\Delta \mathrm{x}}{\Delta t}$

(1.8) **Universal gravitation equation:** $F_{\mathrm{g}} = \frac{Gm_1m_2}{r^2}$

(1.9) **Static friction:** $0 \leq f_{\mathrm{s}} \leq \mu_{\mathrm{s}}N$

(1.10) **Kinetic friction:** $f_{\mathrm{k}} = \mu_{\mathrm{k}}N$

(1.11) **Force of gravity (weight on Earth):** $\mathbf{F}_{\mathrm{g}} = m\mathbf{g}$

(1.12) **Center of mass:**

$$x = \frac{m_1x_1 + m_2x_2 + m_3x_3 + \cdots}{m_1 + m_2 + m_3 + \cdots}$$

$$y = \frac{m_1y_1 + m_2y_2 + m_3y_3 + \cdots}{m_1 + m_2 + m_3 + \cdots}$$

$$z = \frac{m_1z_1 + m_2z_2 + m_3z_3 + \cdots}{m_1 + m_2 + m_3 + \cdots}$$

(1.13) **Average acceleration:** $\bar{\mathbf{a}} = \frac{\Delta \mathbf{v}}{\Delta t}$

(1.14) **Instantaneous acceleration:** $\mathbf{a} = \lim_{\Delta t\to 0}\frac{\Delta \mathbf{v}}{\Delta t}$

(1.15) **Newton's first law:** $\mathbf{F}_{\mathrm{net}} = m\mathbf{a} = 0$

(1.16) **Newton's second law:** $\mathbf{F}_{\mathrm{net}} = m\mathbf{a}$

(1.17) **Newton's third law:** $\mathbf{F}_{\mathrm{AB}} = -\mathbf{F}_{\mathrm{BA}}$

(1.18) **Kinematics (no displacement):** $\mathbf{v} = \mathbf{v}_0 + \mathbf{a}t$

(1.19) **Kinematics (no final velocity):** $\mathbf{x} = \mathbf{v}_0t + \frac{\mathbf{a}t^2}{2}$

(1.20) **Kinematics (no time):** $\mathbf{v}^2 = \mathbf{v}_0^2 + 2\mathbf{ax}$

(1.21) **Kinematics (no acceleration):** $\mathbf{x} = \bar{\mathbf{v}}t$

(1.22) **Components of gravity on an inclined plane:** $\mathbf{F}_{g,||} = mg \sin \theta$

$\mathbf{F}_{g,\perp} = mg \cos \theta$

(1.23) **Centripetal force:** $F_c = \frac{mv^2}{r}$

(1.24) **Torque:** $\boldsymbol{\tau} = \mathbf{r} \times \mathbf{F} = rF \sin \theta$

SHARED CONCEPTS

General Chemistry Chapter 1
Atomic Structure

General Chemistry Chapter 3
Bonding and Chemical Interactions

Physics and Math Chapter 2
Work and Energy

Physics and Math Chapter 4
Fluids

Physics and Math Chapter 5
Electrostatics and Magnetism

Physics and Math Chapter 10
Mathematics

CHAPTER 2

WORK AND ENERGY

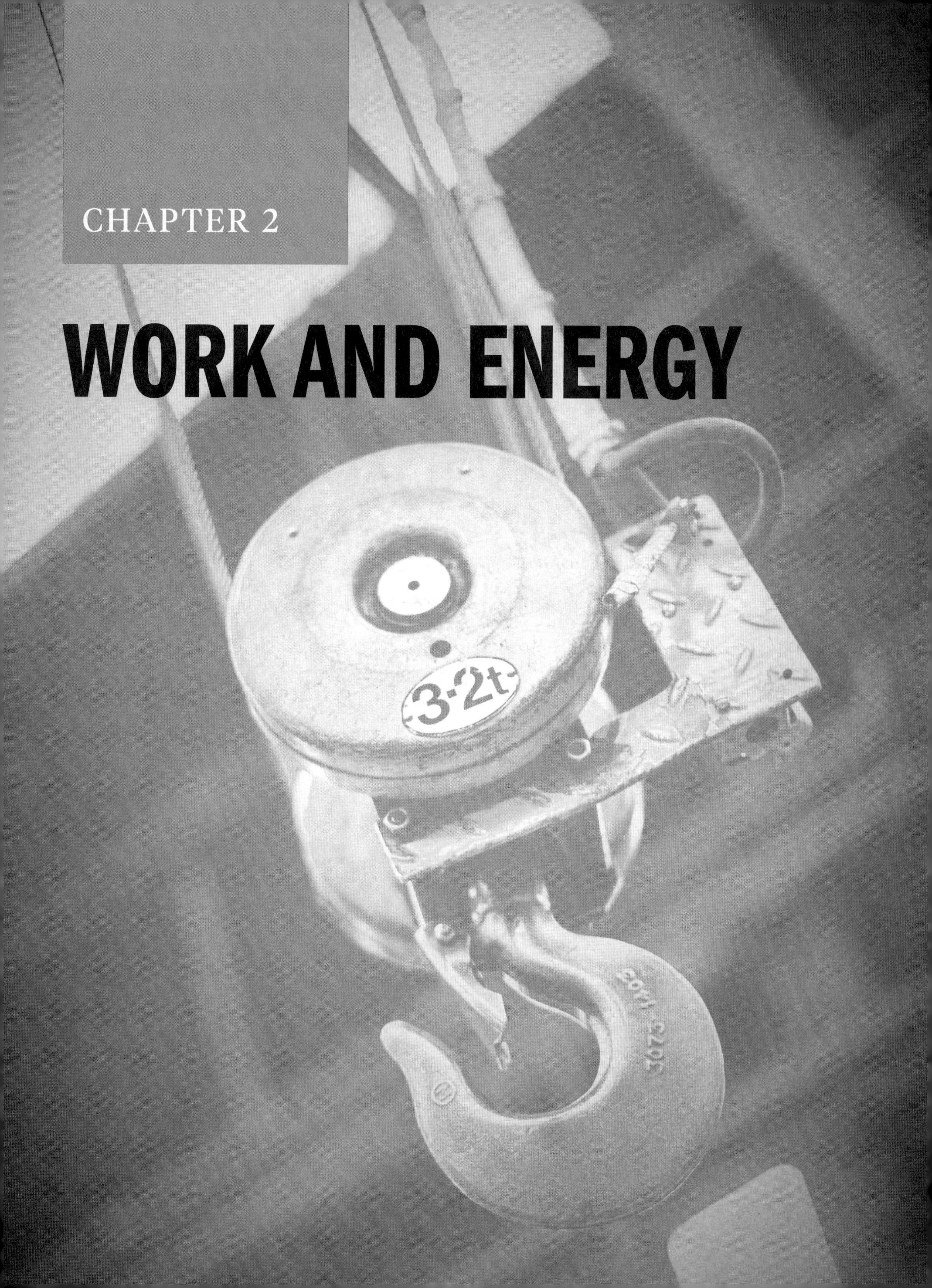

SCIENCE MASTERY ASSESSMENT

Every pre-med knows this feeling: there is so much content I have to know for the MCAT! How do I know what to do first or what's important?

While the high-yield badges throughout this book will help you identify the most important topics, this Science Mastery Assessment is another tool in your MCAT prep arsenal. This quiz (which can also be taken in your online resources) and the guidance below will help ensure that you are spending the appropriate amount of time on this chapter based on your personal strengths and weaknesses. Don't worry though—skipping something now does not mean you'll never study it. Later on in your prep, as you complete full-length tests, you'll uncover specific pieces of content that you need to review and can come back to these chapters as appropriate.

How to Use This Assessment

If you answer 0–7 questions correctly:

Spend about 1 hour to read this chapter in full and take limited notes throughout. Follow up by reviewing **all** quiz questions to ensure that you now understand how to solve each one.

If you answer 8–11 questions correctly:

Spend 20–40 minutes reviewing the quiz questions. Beginning with the questions you missed, read and take notes on the corresponding subchapters. For questions you answered correctly, ensure your thinking matches that of the explanation and you understand why each choice was correct or incorrect.

If you answer 12–15 questions correctly:

Spend less than 20 minutes reviewing all questions from the quiz. If you missed any, then include a quick read-through of the corresponding subchapters, or even just the relevant content within a subchapter, as part of your question review. For questions you got correct, ensure your thinking matches that of the explanation and review the Concept Summary at the end of the chapter.

1. A weightlifter lifts a 275 kg barbell from the ground to a height of 2.4 m. How much work has the weightlifter done in lifting the barbell, and how much work is required to hold the weight at that height?
   - **A.** 3234 J and 0 J, respectively
   - **B.** 3234 J and 3234 J, respectively
   - **C.** 6468 J and 0 J, respectively
   - **D.** 6468 J and 6468 J, respectively

2. A tractor pulls a log with a mass of 500 kg along the ground for 100 m. The rope (between the tractor and the log) makes an angle of 30° with the ground and is acted on by a tensile force of 5000 N. How much work does the tractor perform in this scenario? (Note: $\sin 30° = 0.5$, $\cos 30° = 0.866$, $\tan 30° = 0.577$)
   - **A.** 250 kJ
   - **B.** 289 kJ
   - **C.** 433 kJ
   - **D.** 500 kJ

3. A 2000 kg experimental car can accelerate from 0 to 30 $\frac{\text{m}}{\text{s}}$ in 6 s. What is the average power of the engine needed to achieve this acceleration?
   - **A.** 150 W
   - **B.** 150 kW
   - **C.** 900 W
   - **D.** 900 kW

4. A 40 kg block is resting at a height of 5 m off the ground. If the block is released and falls to the ground, which of the following is closest to its total mechanical energy at a height of 2 m, assuming negligible air resistance?
   - **A.** 0 J
   - **B.** 400 J
   - **C.** 800 J
   - **D.** 2000 J

5. 5 m^3 of a gas are brought from an initial pressure of 1 kPa to a pressure of 3 kPa through an isochoric process. During this process, the work performed by the gas is:
   - **A.** −10 kJ
   - **B.** −10 J
   - **C.** 0 J
   - **D.** +10 kJ

6. In the pulley system shown below, which of the following is closest to the tension force in each rope if the mass of the object is 10 kg and the object is accelerating upwards at 2 $\frac{\text{m}}{\text{s}^2}$?

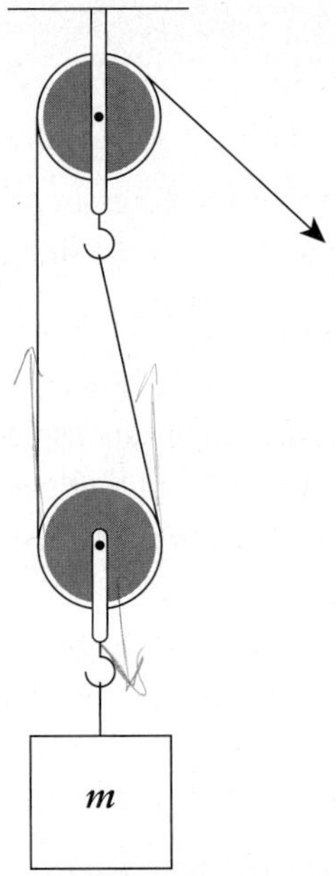

   - **A.** 50 N
   - **B.** 60 N
   - **C.** 100 N
   - **D.** 120 N

7. Which of the following is a conservative force?
   - **A.** Air resistance
   - **B.** Friction
   - **C.** Gravity
   - **D.** Convection

8. During uniform circular motion, which of the following relationships is necessarily true?
   - **A.** No work is done.
   - **B.** The centripetal force does work.
   - **C.** The velocity does work.
   - **D.** Potential energy depends on position of the object around the circle.

9. Which of the following best characterizes the work–energy theorem?
   - **A.** The work done by any force is proportional only to the magnitude of that force.
   - **B.** The total work done on any object is equal to the change in kinetic energy for that object.
   - **C.** The work done on an object by any force is proportional to the change in kinetic energy for that object.
   - **D.** The work done by an applied force on an object is equal to the change in kinetic energy of that object.

10. A massless spring initially compressed by a displacement of two centimeters is now compressed by four centimeters. How has the potential energy of this system changed?
   - **A.** The potential energy has not changed.
   - **B.** The potential energy has doubled.
   - **C.** The potential energy has increased by two joules.
   - **D.** The potential energy has quadrupled.

11. Josh, who has a mass of 80 kg, and Sarah, who has a mass of 50 kg, jump off a 20 m tall building and land on a fire net. The net compresses, and they bounce back up at the same time. Which of the following statements is NOT true?
   - **A.** Sarah will bounce higher than Josh.
   - **B.** For Josh, the change in speed from the start of the jump to contacting the net is 20 $\frac{m}{s}$.
   - **C.** Josh will experience a greater force upon impact than Sarah.
   - **D.** The energy in this event is converted from potential to kinetic to elastic to kinetic.

12. A parachutist jumps from a plane. Beginning at the point when the jumper reaches terminal velocity (constant velocity during freefall), which of the following is/are true?
   - **I.** The jumper is in translational equilibrium.
   - **II.** The jumper is not being acted upon by any forces.
   - **III.** There is an equal amount of work being done by gravity and air resistance.
   - **A.** I only
   - **B.** I and III only
   - **C.** II and III only
   - **D.** I, II, and III

13. Mechanical advantage and efficiency are both ratios. Which of the following is true regarding the quantities used in these ratios?
   - **A.** Mechanical advantage compares values of work; efficiency compares values of power.
   - **B.** Mechanical advantage compares values of forces; efficiency compares values of work.
   - **C.** Mechanical advantage compares values of power; efficiency compares values of energy.
   - **D.** Mechanical advantage compares values of work; efficiency compares values of forces.

14. If the gravitational potential energy of an object has doubled in the absence of nonconservative forces, which of the following must be true, assuming the total mechanical energy of the object is constant?
   - **A.** The object has been lifted to twice its initial height.
   - **B.** The kinetic energy of the object has been halved.
   - **C.** The kinetic energy has decreased by the same quantity as the potential energy has increased.
   - **D.** The mass of the object has doubled.

15. A consumer is comparing two new cars. Car A exerts 250 horsepower, while Car B exerts 300 horsepower. The consumer is most concerned about the peak velocity that the car can reach. If nonconservative forces can be ignored, which of the following statements is true? (Note: 1 horsepower = 745.7 W)
   - **A.** Car A and Car B both have unlimited velocities.
   - **B.** Car A will reach its peak velocity more quickly than Car B.
   - **C.** Car A will dissipate less energy to the surroundings than Car B.
   - **D.** Car A will have a lower peak velocity than Car B.

Answer Key

1. **C**
2. **C**
3. **B**
4. **D**
5. **C**
6. **B**
7. **C**
8. **A**
9. **B**
10. **D**
11. **A**
12. **B**
13. **B**
14. **C**
15. **A**

Detailed explanations can be found at the end of the chapter.

CHAPTER 2

WORK AND ENERGY

In This Chapter

CHAPTER PROFILE

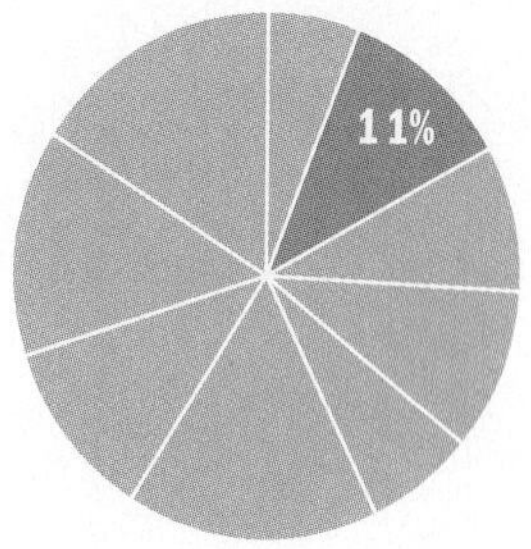

The content in this chapter should be relevant to about 11% of all questions about physics on the MCAT.

This chapter covers material from the following AAMC content category:

4A: Translational motion, forces, work, energy, and equilibrium in living systems

Introduction

The Greek myth of Sisyphus is a tale of unending, pointless work. For eternity, Sisyphus was sentenced to roll a large, heavy rock up a steep hill as penance for his crimes. Just as Sisyphus would nearly reach the top of the hill, the rock would roll back again to the bottom. The cycle continued for eternity: Sisyphus would near the top of the hill, and the boulder—enchanted by Zeus—would roll back down, forcing Sisyphus to restart his task.

This is a story of work and mechanical energy transfer. Pushing that boulder up the hill, Sisyphus exerted forces that performed work on the rock, resulting in an increase in the rock's gravitational potential energy. When the rock escaped from his grasp and rolled backwards, its energy changed from gravitational potential energy into kinetic energy. While Sisyphus's punishment was futile work, it serves as a strong model of the exchange of mechanical energy between its two forms: potential and kinetic. Although a number of other forms of energy exist (thermal energy, sound, light, chemical potential energy, and electrical potential energy, to name a few), mechanical energy specifically focuses on objects in motion.

This chapter reviews the fundamental concepts of energy and work. The work–energy theorem is a powerful expression of the relationship between energy and work that is often a simpler approach to kinematics questions on Test Day. Finally, we'll discuss the topic of mechanical advantage, and we'll examine how a pulley or ramp might be helpful in raising heavy objects. We hope to convince you throughout the Kaplan MCAT program that your preparation for Test Day is in no way a Sisyphean task.

2.1 Energy

LEARNING OBJECTIVES

After Chapter 2.1, you will be able to:

- Describe kinetic energy and potential energy
- Compare and contrast conservative and nonconservative forces

Energy refers to a system's ability to do work or—more broadly—to make something happen. This broad definition helps us understand that different forms of energy have the capacity to perform different actions. For example, mechanical energy can cause objects to move or accelerate. An ice cube sitting on the kitchen counter at room temperature will absorb thermal energy through heat transfer and eventually melt into water, undergoing a phase transformation from solid to liquid. Nuclear binding energy can be released during fission reactions to run power plants. Let's turn our attention to the different forms that energy can take. After that, we will discuss the two ways in which energy can be transferred from one system to another.

Kinetic Energy

KEY CONCEPT

Kinetic energy is incredibly important on the MCAT; any time an object has a speed, think about kinetic energy and link its kinetic energy to the related concepts of work and conservation of mechanical energy.

Kinetic energy is the energy of motion. Objects that have mass and that are moving with some speed will have an associated amount of kinetic energy, calculated as follows:

$$K = \frac{1}{2} mv^2$$

Equation 2.1

where K is kinetic energy, m is the mass in kilograms, and v is speed in meters per second. The SI unit for kinetic energy, as with all forms of energy, is the **joule (J)**, which is equal to $\frac{\text{kg}\cdot\text{m}^2}{\text{s}^2}$.

KEY CONCEPT

Kinetic energy is related to speed, not velocity. An object has the same kinetic energy regardless of the direction of its velocity vector.

Recall the falling objects in Chapter 1. Such objects have kinetic energy while they fall. The faster they fall, the more kinetic energy they have. Be mindful of the fact that the MCAT is interested in testing students' comprehension of the relationship between kinetic energy and speed. From the equation, we can see that the kinetic energy is a function of the square of the speed. If the speed doubles, the kinetic energy will quadruple, assuming the mass is constant. Also note that kinetic energy is related to speed—not velocity. An object has the same kinetic energy regardless of the direction of its velocity vector.

Falling objects have kinetic energy, but so do objects that are moving in other ways. For example, the kinetic energy of a fluid flowing at some speed can be measured indirectly as the dynamic pressure, which is one of the terms in Bernoulli's equation—discussed in Chapter 4 of *MCAT Physics and Math Review*. Objects that slide down inclined planes gain kinetic energy as their speeds increase down the ramp.

Example: A 15 kg block, initially at rest, slides down a frictionless incline and comes to the bottom with a speed of 7 $\frac{m}{s}$, as shown below. What is the kinetic energy of the object at the top and bottom of the ramp?

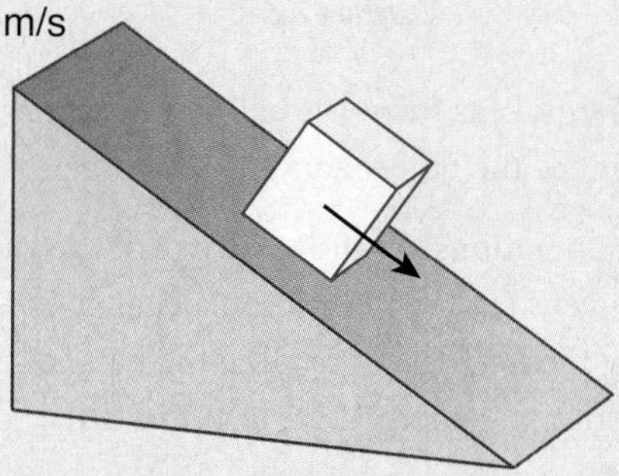

Solution: At the top, $v = 0$, so the kinetic energy is

$$K = \frac{1}{2}mv^2 = \frac{1}{2}(15\text{ kg})\left(0\,\frac{\text{m}}{\text{s}}\right)^2 = 0\text{ J}$$

At the bottom, the kinetic energy is

$$K = \frac{1}{2}mv^2 = \frac{1}{2}(15\text{ kg})\left(7\,\frac{\text{m}}{\text{s}}\right)^2 \approx 15 \times 25 = 375\text{ J (actual} = 367.5\text{ J)}$$

Potential Energy

Potential energy refers to energy that is associated with a given object's position in space or other intrinsic qualities of the system. Potential energy is often said to have the *potential* to do work, and can take named forms. Energy can be stored as chemical potential energy—this is the energy we absorb from the food we eat when we digest and metabolize it. Electrical potential energy, which is discussed in Chapter 5 of *MCAT Physics and Math Review*, is based on the electrostatic attractions between charged particles. In this chapter, we'll examine the types of potential energy that are dissipated as movement: gravitational potential energy and elastic potential energy.

Gravitational Potential Energy

Gravitational potential energy depends on an object's position with respect to some level identified as the **datum** ("ground" or the zero potential energy position). This zero potential energy position is usually chosen for convenience. For example, you may find it convenient to consider the potential energy of the pencil in your hand with respect to the floor if you are holding the pencil above the floor, or with respect to a desktop if you are holding the pencil over a desk. The equation that we use to calculate gravitational potential energy is

$$U = mgh$$

Equation 2.2

where U is the potential energy, m is the mass in kilograms, g is the acceleration due to gravity, and h is the height of the object above the datum.

Potential energy has a direct relationship with all three of the variables, so changing any one of them by some given factor will result in a change in the potential energy by the same factor. Tripling the height—or tripling the mass of the object—will increase the gravitational potential energy by a factor of three.

MCAT EXPERTISE

The height used in the potential energy equation is relative to whatever the problem states is the ground level. It will often be simply the distance to the ground, but it doesn't need to be. The zero potential energy position may be a ledge, a desktop, or a platform. Just pay attention to the question stem and use the height that is discussed.

Example: An 80 kg diver leaps from a 10 m cliff into the sea, as shown below. Find the diver's potential energy at the top of the cliff and when the diver is two meters underwater, using sea level as the datum.

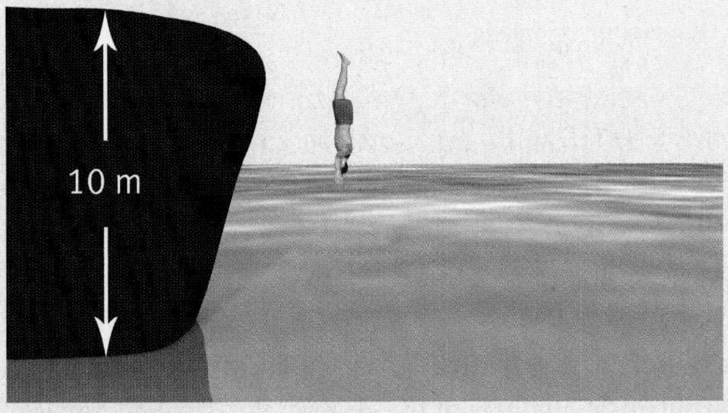

Solution: At the top of the cliff:

$$U = mgh = (80\text{ kg})\left(9.8\,\frac{\text{m}}{\text{s}^2}\right)(10\text{ m}) \approx 8000\text{ J (actual} = 7840\text{ J)}$$

When the diver is two meters underwater:

$$U = mgh = (80\text{ kg})\left(9.8\,\frac{\text{m}}{\text{s}^2}\right)(-2\text{ m}) \approx -1600\text{ J (actual} = -1568\text{ J)}$$

Elastic Potential Energy

Springs and other elastic systems act to store energy. Every spring has a characteristic length at which it is considered relaxed, or in equilibrium. When a spring is stretched or compressed from its **equilibrium length**, the spring has **elastic potential energy**, which can be determined by

$$U = \frac{1}{2}kx^2$$

Equation 2.3

where U is the potential energy, k is the **spring constant** (a measure of the stiffness of the spring), and x is the magnitude of displacement from equilibrium. Note the similarities between this equation and the formula for kinetic energy.

Total Mechanical Energy

The sum of an object's potential and kinetic energies is its **total mechanical energy**. The equation is

$$E = U + K$$

Equation 2.4

where E is total mechanical energy, U is potential energy, and K is kinetic energy. The **first law of thermodynamics** accounts for the **conservation of mechanical energy**, which posits that energy is never created nor destroyed—it is merely transferred from one form to another. This does not mean that the total mechanical energy will necessarily remain constant, though. You'll notice that the total mechanical energy equation accounts for potential and kinetic energies but not for other forms of energy, such as thermal energy that is transferred as a result of friction (heat). If frictional forces are present, some of the mechanical energy will be transformed into thermal energy and will be "lost"—or, more accurately, dissipated from the system and not accounted for by the equation. Note that there is no violation of the first law of thermodynamics, as a full accounting of all the forms of energy (kinetic, potential, thermal, sound, light, and so on) would reveal no net gain or loss of total energy, but merely the transformation of some energy from one form to another.

Conservation of Mechanical Energy

In the absence of nonconservative forces, such as frictional forces, the sum of the kinetic and potential energies will be constant. **Conservative forces** are those that are path independent and that do not dissipate energy. Conservative forces also have potential energies associated with them. On the MCAT, the two most commonly encountered conservative forces are gravitational and electrostatic. Elastic forces can also be approximated to be conservative in many cases, although the MCAT may include spring problems in which frictional forces are *not* ignored (in actuality, springs heat up as they move back and forth due to the friction between the particles of the spring material). There are two equivalent ways to determine whether a force is conservative, as demonstrated in Figure 2.1.

BRIDGE

The transfer of energy from one form to another is a key feature of bioenergetics and metabolism, discussed in Chapters 9 through 12 of *MCAT Biochemistry Review*. When looking at carbohydrate metabolism, one can see the chemical potential energy in the bonds in glucose being converted into electrical potential energy in the high-energy electrons of NADH and $FADH_2$, which is dissipated along the electron transport chain to generate the proton-motive force (another example of electrical potential energy). This force fuels ATP synthase, trapping the energy in high-energy phosphate bonds in ATP.

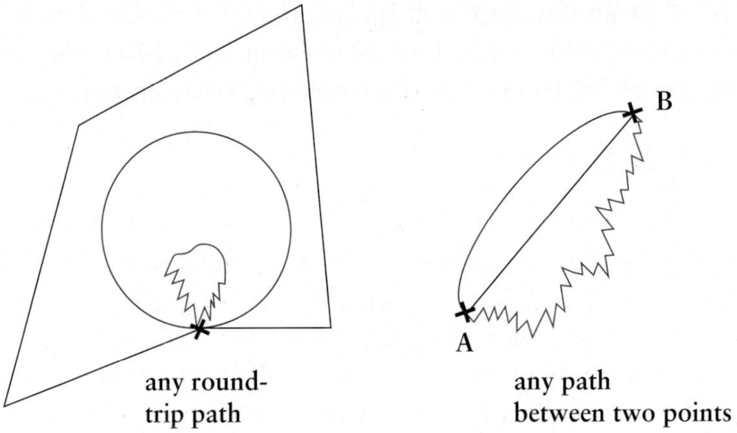

Figure 2.1 Determining if a Force Is Conservative
If the change in energy around any round-trip path is zero—or if the change in energy is equal despite taking any path between two points—then the force is conservative.

One method is to consider the change in energy of a system in which the system is brought back to its original setup. In mechanical terms, this means that an object comes back to its starting position. If the net change in energy is zero regardless of the path taken to get back to the initial position, then the forces acting on the object are conservative. Basically, this means that a system that is experiencing only conservative forces will be "given back" an amount of usable energy equal to the amount that had been "taken away" from it in the course of a closed path. For example, an object that falls through a certain displacement in a vacuum will lose some measurable amount of potential energy but will gain exactly that same amount of potential energy when it is lifted back to its original height, regardless of whether the return pathway is the same as that of the initial descent. Furthermore, at all points during the fall through the vacuum, there will be a perfect conversion of potential energy into kinetic energy, with no energy lost to nonconservative forces such as air resistance. Of course, in real life, nonconservative forces are impossible to avoid.

The other method is to consider the change in energy of a system moving from one setup to another. In mechanical terms, this means an object undergoes a particular displacement. If the energy change is equal regardless of the path taken, then the forces acting on the object are again all conservative.

KEY CONCEPT

Conservative forces (such as gravity and electrostatic forces) conserve mechanical energy. Nonconservative forces (such as friction and air resistance) dissipate mechanical energy as thermal or chemical energy.

When the work done by nonconservative forces is zero, or when there are no nonconservative forces acting on the system, the total mechanical energy of the system $(U + K)$ remains constant. The conservation of mechanical energy can be expressed as

$$\Delta E = \Delta U + \Delta K = 0$$

Equation 2.5

where ΔE, ΔU, and ΔK are the changes in total mechanical energy, potential energy, and kinetic energy, respectively.

When **nonconservative forces**, such as friction, air resistance, or viscous drag (a resistance force created by fluid viscosity) are present, total mechanical energy is not conserved. The equation is

$$W_{\text{nonconservative}} = \Delta E = \Delta U + \Delta K$$

Equation 2.6

where $W_{\text{nonconservative}}$ is the work done by the nonconservative forces only. The work done by the nonconservative forces will be exactly equal to the amount of energy "lost" from the system. In reality, this energy is simply transformed into another form of energy, such as thermal energy, that is not accounted for in the mechanical energy equation. Nonconservative forces, unlike conservative forces, are path dependent. The longer the distance traveled, the larger the amount of energy dissipated.

Example: A baseball of mass 0.25 kg is thrown in the air with an initial speed of 30 $\frac{\text{m}}{\text{s}}$, but because of air resistance, the ball returns to the ground with a speed of 27 $\frac{\text{m}}{\text{s}}$. Find the work done by air resistance.

Solution: Air resistance is a nonconservative force. To solve this problem, the energy equation for a nonconservative system is needed. The work done by air resistance is:

$$W_{\text{nonconservative}} = \Delta E = \Delta U + \Delta K$$

In this case, $\Delta U = 0$ because the initial and final heights are the same. Therefore,

$$\begin{aligned} W_{\text{nonconservative}} &= 0 + \Delta K \\ &= \frac{1}{2}mv_f^2 - \frac{1}{2}mv_i^2 \\ &= \frac{1}{2}(0.25\text{ kg})\left[\left(27\,\frac{\text{m}}{\text{s}}\right)^2 - \left(30\,\frac{\text{m}}{\text{s}}\right)^2\right] \\ &= \frac{1}{8}(729 - 900) \approx \frac{-160}{8} \\ &= -20\text{ J (actual} = -21.4\text{ J)} \end{aligned}$$

The negative sign in the answer indicates that energy is being dissipated from the system.

MCAT CONCEPT CHECK 2.1

Before you move on, assess your understanding of the material with these questions.

1. Define kinetic energy and potential energy.
    - Kinetic energy:

    ____

    - Potential energy:

    ____

2. Compare and contrast conservative and nonconservative forces:

	Conservative Forces	Nonconservative Forces
What happens to total mechanical energy of the system?		
Does the path taken matter?		
What are some examples?		

2.2 Work

High-Yield

MCAT EXPERTISE

The "High-Yield" badge on this section indicates that the content is frequently tested on the MCAT.

LEARNING OBJECTIVES

After Chapter 2.2, you will be able to:

- Recall the units used for work
- Distinguish between work and energy
- Calculate the work done on or by a system

KEY CONCEPT

Work is not energy but a measure of energy transfer. The other form of energy transfer is heat.

Often, the term work is used erroneously to mean another form of energy. After all, the SI unit for work is the joule (J), which is the same SI unit for all forms of energy. Nevertheless, to say that work is just another form of energy is to miss something important: **work** is not actually a form of energy itself, but a process by which energy is transferred from one system to another. In fact, it is one of only two ways in which energy can be transferred. The other transfer of energy is called heat, which we will focus on quite a bit in Chapter 3 of *MCAT Physics and Math Review*.

The transfer of energy by work or heat is the only way by which anything occurs. We are familiar with both processes from everyday life. For example, as discussed in the introduction to this chapter, every time King Sisyphus pushed the rock up the hill, the rock gained kinetic and potential energy. That energy came from Sisyphus's muscles, in which the potential energy contained in the high-energy phosphate bonds of ATP molecules was converted to the mechanical energy of the contracting muscles, which exerted forces against the rock, causing it to accelerate and move up the hill.

On a chemical level, the potential energy in the ATP was harnessed by heat transfer. In fact, at the molecular level, this is no different from work because it involves the movement of molecules, atoms, and electrons, each of which exert forces that do work on other molecules and atoms. Like any transfer of energy, it's not a perfectly efficient process, and some of the energy is lost as thermal energy. Our muscles quite literally warm up when we contract them repeatedly.

Force and Displacement

Energy is transferred through the process of work when something exerts forces on or against something else. This is expressed mathematically by the equation

$$W = \mathbf{F} \cdot \mathbf{d} = Fd \cos \theta$$

Equation 2.7

where W is work, F is the magnitude of the applied force, d is the magnitude of the displacement through which the force is applied, and θ is the angle between the applied force vector and the displacement vector. You'll notice that work is a dot product; as such, it is a function of the cosine of the angle between the vectors. This also means that only forces (or components of forces) parallel or antiparallel to the displacement vector will do work (that is, transfer energy). We've already said that the SI unit for work is the joule. While this suggests that work and energy are the same thing, remember they are not: work is the process by which a quantity of energy is moved from one system to another.

Pressure and Volume

As described above, work is a process of energy transfer. In mechanics, we think of work as application of force through some distance. We will learn in our discussion of fluids in Chapter 4 of *MCAT Physics and Math Review* that pressure can be thought of as an "energy density." In systems of gases, we therefore approach work as a combination of pressure and volume changes. In Chapter 3 of *MCAT Physics and Math Review*, we'll examine how these changes also relate to heat.

For a gas system contained in a cylinder with a movable **piston**, we can analyze the relationship between pressure, volume, and work. When the gas expands, it pushes up against the piston, exerting a force that causes the piston to move up and the volume of the system to increase. When the gas is compressed, the piston pushes down on the gas, exerting a force that decreases the volume of the system. We say that work has been done when the volume of the system has changed due to an applied pressure. Gas expansion and compression processes can be represented in graphical form with volume on the x-axis and pressure on the y-axis. Such graphs, as shown in Figure 2.2, are termed **P–V graphs**.

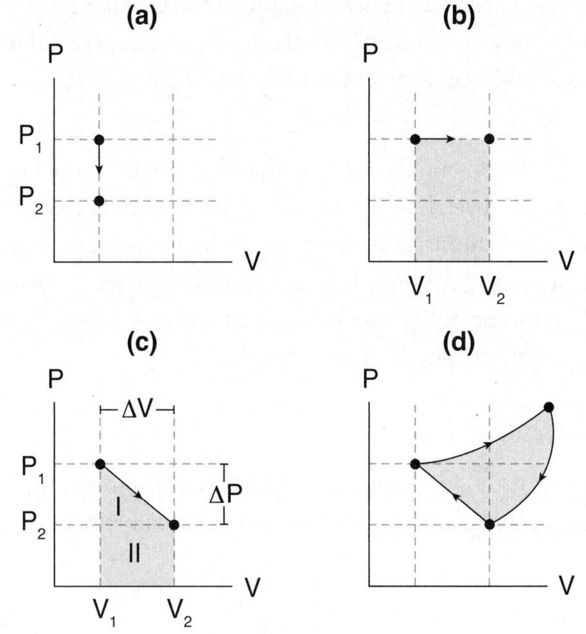

Figure 2.2 Pressure-Volume (P-V) Curves
The work done on or by a system undergoing a thermodynamic process can be determined by finding the area enclosed by the corresponding pressure-volume curve.

KEY CONCEPT

When work is done *by* a system (the gas expands), the work is said to be positive. When work is done *on* a system (the gas compresses), the work is said to be negative. The MCAT will not expect you to calculate the integral of a P-V graph using calculus, but you are expected to be able to calculate the area under a straight-line graph if necessary.

When a gas expands, we say that work was done by the gas and the work is positive; when a gas is compressed, we say that work was done on the gas and the work is negative. There are an infinite number of paths between an initial and final state. Different paths require different amounts of work. You can calculate the work done on or by a system by finding the area under the pressure–volume curve. Note that if volume stays constant as pressure changes (that is, $\Delta V = 0$), then no work is done because there is no area to calculate. This is the case in Figure 2.2a above, and is called an **isovolumetric** or **isochoric process**. On the other hand, if pressure remains constant as volume changes (that is, $\Delta P = 0$), then the area under the curve is a rectangle of length P and width ΔV as shown in Figure 2.2b. For processes in which pressure remains constant (**isobaric processes**), the work can be calculated as

$$W = P\Delta V$$

Equation 2.8

Figure 2.2c shows a process in which neither pressure nor volume is held constant. The total area under the graph (Regions I and II) gives the work done.

Region I is a triangle with base ΔV and height ΔP, so the area is

$$A_{\text{I}} = \frac{1}{2}\,\Delta V \Delta P$$

Region II is a rectangle with base ΔV and height P_2, so its area is

$$A_{II} = P_2 \Delta V$$

The work done is the sum of the areas of regions I and II:

$$W = A_I + A_{II}$$

Figure 2.2d shows a closed cycle in which, after certain interchanges of work and heat, the system returns to its initial state. Because work is positive when the gas expands and negative when the gas is compressed, the work done is the area enclosed by the curve. Calculating the work done in this situation would require calculus, but the MCAT does not test calculus-based physics.

Power

Power refers to the rate at which energy is transferred from one system to another. It is calculated with the equation

$$P = \frac{W}{t} = \frac{\Delta E}{t}$$

Equation 2.9

where P is power, W is work (which is equal to ΔE, the change in energy), and t is the time over which the work is done. The SI unit for power is the **watt (W)**, which is equal to $\frac{\text{J}}{\text{s}}$. In Chapter 6 of *MCAT Physics and Math Review*, we will identify additional ways to calculate power in electric circuits. For now, note that many of the devices we use every day—toaster ovens, light bulbs, phones, cars, and so on—are quantified by the rate at which these appliances transform electrical potential energy into other forms, such as thermal, light, sound, and kinetic energy.

BRIDGE

Power is calculated in many different situations, especially those involving circuits, resistors, and capacitors. The equation for electric power is $P = IV$, where P is power, I is current, and V is electrical potential difference (voltage). This equation is discussed in Chapter 6 of *MCAT Physics and Math Review*. Power is always a measure of the rate of energy consumption, transfer, or transformation per unit time.

Work–Energy Theorem

The **work–energy theorem** is a powerful expression of the relationship between work and energy. In its mechanical applications, it offers a direct relationship between the work done by all the forces acting on an object and the change in kinetic energy of that object. The net work done by forces acting on an object will result in an equal change in the object's kinetic energy. In other words:

$$W_{\text{net}} = \Delta K = K_{\text{f}} - K_{\text{i}}$$

Equation 2.10

This relationship is important to understand, as it allows one to calculate work without knowing the magnitude of the forces acting on an object or the displacement through which the forces act. If one calculates the change in kinetic energy experienced by an object, then—by definition—the net work done on or by an object is the same. Pressing the brake pedal in your car puts the work–energy theorem into practice. The brake pads exert frictional forces against the rotors, which are attached to the wheels. These frictional forces do work against the wheels, causing them to decelerate and bringing the car to a halt. The net work done by all these forces is equal to the change in kinetic energy of the car.

In more general iterations, the work–energy theorem can be applied to changes in other forms of energy. In fact, the first law of thermodynamics is essentially a reiteration of the work–energy theorem, in which the change in internal energy (ΔU) is equal to the heat transferred into the system (Q) minus the mechanical work done by the system (W).

Example: A lead ball of mass 0.125 kg is thrown straight up in the air with an initial velocity of 30 $\frac{m}{s}$. Assuming no air resistance, find the work done by the force of gravity by the time the ball is at its maximum height.

Solution: The answer could be calculated using kinematics and determining the maximum height of the ball ($W = Fd \cos \theta$), but it is simpler to use the work-energy theorem:

$$\begin{aligned} W_{net} &= K_f - K_i \\ &= 0 - \frac{1}{2} m v_i^2 \\ &= -\left(\frac{1}{2}\right)\left(\frac{1}{8}\text{ kg}\right)\left(30 \frac{m}{s}\right)^2 = -\frac{900}{16} \approx -\frac{900}{15} \\ &= -60 \text{ J (actual} = -56.25 \text{ J)} \end{aligned}$$

MCAT CONCEPT CHECK 2.2

Before you move on, assess your understanding of the material with these questions.

1. What are the units for work? How are work and energy different?

    ___

2. Provide three methods for calculating the work done on or by a system.
    - ___
    - ___
    - ___

3. While driving a vehicle at constant velocity on a flat surface, the accelerator must be slightly depressed to overcome resistive forces. How does the amount of work done by the engine (via the accelerator) compare to the amount of work done by resistance?

    ___

2.3 Mechanical Advantage

LEARNING OBJECTIVES

After Chapter 2.3, you will be able to:

- Explain how work can be lost in a system that is not 100% efficient
- Recall the meaning of mechanical advantage
- Recognize the six simple machines
- Predict the impact of changing effort values on effort distance in a pulley system, assuming work output remains the same:

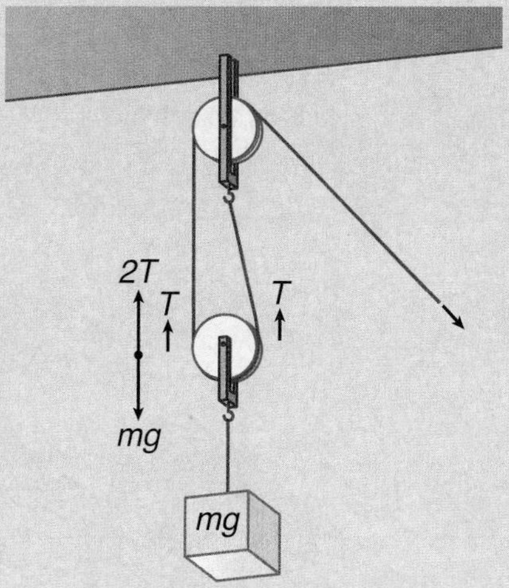

Would it make a difference whether Sisyphus lifted the rock vertically to its final position or rolled it there along an incline? The difference between these two scenarios is mechanical advantage, a measure of the increase in force accomplished by using a tool. Sloping inclines, such as hillsides and ramps, make it easier to lift objects because they distribute the required work over a larger distance, decreasing the required force. For a given quantity of work, any device that allows for work to be accomplished through a smaller applied force is thus said to provide mechanical advantage. In addition to the inclined plane, five other devices are considered the classic **simple machines** which are designed to provide mechanical advantage: wedge (two merged inclined planes), wheel and axle, lever, pulley, and screw (rotating inclined plane). Of these, the inclined plane, lever, and pulley are most frequently tested on the MCAT.

Mechanical advantage is the ratio of magnitudes of the force exerted on an object by a simple machine (F_{out}) to the force actually applied on the simple machine (F_{in}):

$$\text{Mechanical advantage} = \frac{F_{out}}{F_{in}}$$

Equation 2.11

The mechanical advantage, because it is a ratio, is dimensionless.

Reducing the force needed to accomplish a given amount of work does have a cost associated with it; however, the distance through which the smaller force must be applied in order to do the work must be increased. Inclined planes, levers, and pulleys do not magically change the amount of work necessary to move an object from one place to another. Because displacement is pathway independent, the actual distance traveled from the initial to final position does not matter, assuming all forces are conservative. Therefore, applying a lesser force over a greater distance to achieve the same change in position (displacement) accomplishes the same amount of work. We've already considered the dynamics of inclined planes and levers in Chapter 1 of *MCAT Physics and Math Review*. Here, we look at the work associated with inclined planes.

Example: A block weighing 100 N is pushed up a frictionless incline over a distance of 20 m to a height of 10 m as shown below.

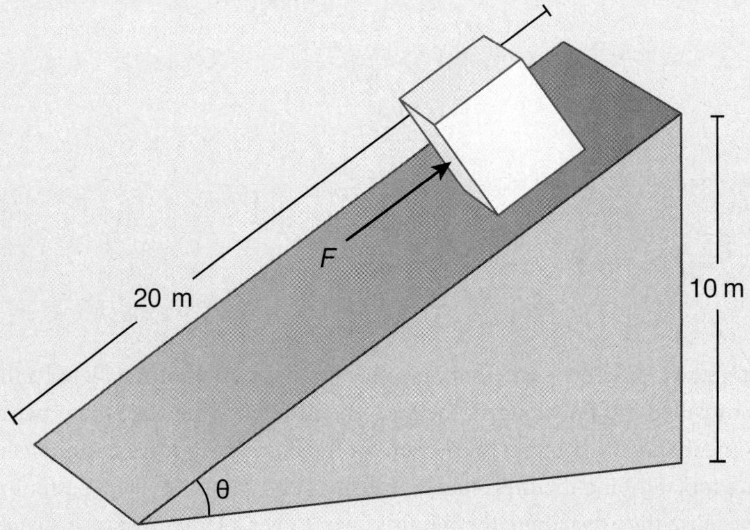

Find:

A. The minimum force required to push the block

B. The work done by the force

C. The force required and the work done by the force if the block were simply lifted vertically 10 m

Solution:

A. To find the minimum force required to push the block, we must draw a free body diagram of the situation:

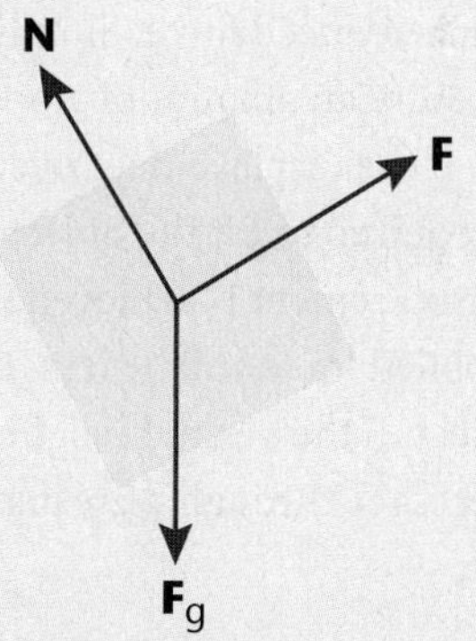

The minimum force needed is a force that will push the block with no acceleration parallel to the surface of the incline. This means the magnitude of the applied force is equal to that of the parallel component of gravity:

$$F = mg \sin \theta$$

mg represents the weight of the object, which is 100 N. Using trigonometry, $\sin \theta$ is ratio of the length of the opposite side to the hypotenuse, which is $\frac{10}{20}$. Therefore,

$$F = (100 \text{ N})\left(\frac{10}{20}\right) = 50 \text{ N}$$

B. The work done by **F** is

$$W = Fd \cos \theta$$

In this case, θ represents the angle between the force and displacement vectors, *not* the angle of the inclined plane. Because the force and displacement vectors are parallel, $\theta = 0$ and $\cos \theta = 1$. Therefore,

$$W = (50 \text{ N})(20 \text{ m})(1) = 1000 \text{ J}$$

C. To raise the block vertically, an upward force equal to the object's weight (100 N) would have to be generated. The work done by the lifting force is

$$W = Fd \cos \theta = (100 \text{ N})(10 \text{ m})(1) = 1000 \text{ J}$$

The same amount of work is required in both cases, but twice the force is needed to raise the block vertically compared with pushing it up the incline.

Pulleys

Pulleys utilize the same paradigm to provide mechanical advantage as the inclined plane: a reduction of necessary force at the cost of increased distance to achieve a given value of work or energy transference. In practical terms, pulleys allow heavy objects to be lifted using a much-reduced force. Simply lifting a heavy object of mass m to a height of h will require an amount of work equal to mgh—its change in gravitational potential energy. If the displacement occurs over a distance equal to the displacement, then the force required to lift the object will equal mg. If, however, the distance through which the displacement is achieved is greater than the displacement (an indirect path), then the applied force will be less than mg. In other words, we've been able to lift this heavy object to the desired height by using a smaller force, but we've had to apply that smaller force through a greater distance in order to lift this heavy object to its final height.

Before examining how pulleys create this mechanical advantage, let's consider first the heavy block in Figure 2.3, suspended from two ropes. Because the block is not accelerating, it is in translational equilibrium, and the force that the block exerts downward (its weight) is cancelled by the sum of the tensions in the two ropes. For a symmetrical system, the tensions in the two ropes are the same and are each equal to half the weight of the block.

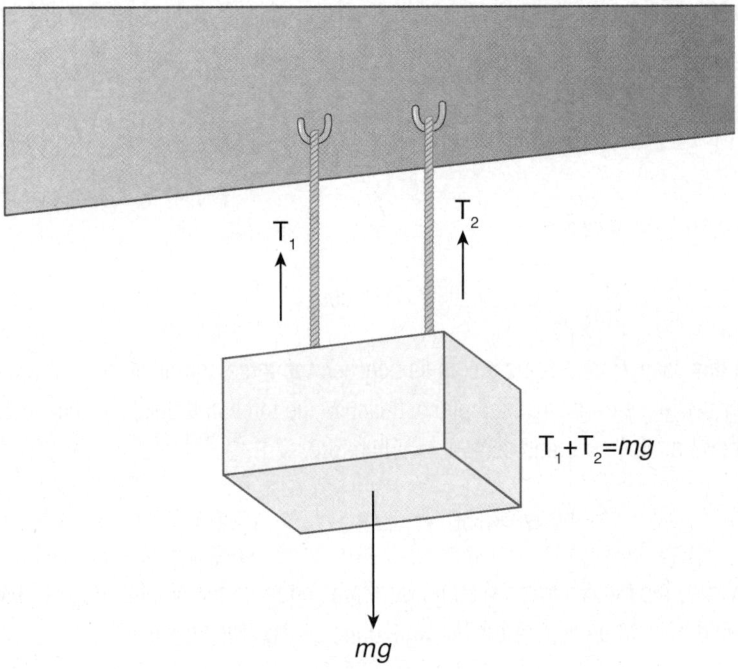

Figure 2.3 Block Suspended by Two Ropes
If the block is in translational equilibrium, the tension in each rope is equal to half the weight of the block.

Now let's imagine the heavy block in Figure 2.4 represents a heavy crate that must be lifted. Assuming that the crate is momentarily being held stationary in midair, we again have a system in translational equilibrium: the weight (the **load**) is balanced by the total tension in the ropes. The tensions in the two vertical ropes are equal to each other; if they were unequal, the pulleys would turn until the tensions were equal on both sides. Therefore, each rope supports one-half of the crate's total weight. By extension, only half the force (**effort**) is required to lift the crate. This decrease in effort is the mechanical advantage provided by the pulley, but as we've already discussed, mechanical advantage comes at the expense of distance. To lift an object to a certain height in the air (the **load distance**), one must pull through a length of rope (the **effort distance**) equal to twice that displacement. If, for example, the crate must be lifted to a shelf 3 meters above the ground, then both sides of the supporting rope must shorten by 3 meters, and the only way to accomplish this is by pulling through 6 meters of rope.

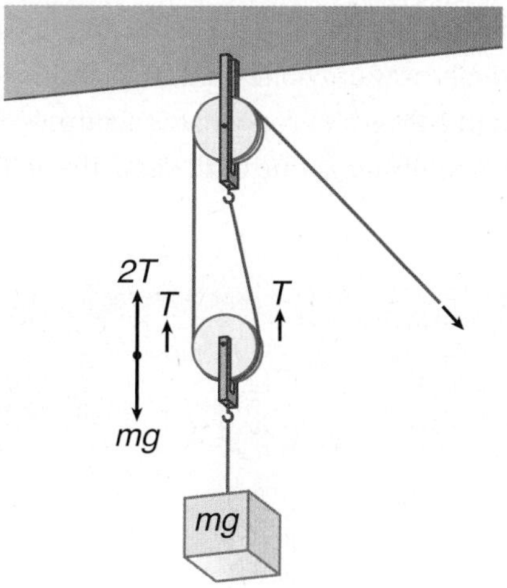

Figure 2.4 Two-Pulley System
The block is suspended from two ropes, each of which bears half of the block's weight.

All simple machines can be approximated as conservative systems if we ignore the (usually) small amount of energy that is lost due to external forces, such as friction. The idealized pulley is massless and frictionless, and under these theoretical conditions, the work put into the system (the exertion of force through a distance of rope) will exactly equal the work that comes out of the system (the displacement of the mass to some height). Real pulleys—and all real machines, for that matter—fail to conform to these idealized conditions and, therefore, do not achieve 100 percent **efficiency** in conserving energy output to input. We can define work input as the

KEY CONCEPT

When considering simple machines, load and effort are both forces. The load determines the necessary output force. From the output force and mechanical advantage, we can determine the necessary input force.

product of effort and effort distance; likewise, we can define work output as the product of load and load distance. Comparing the two as a ratio defines the efficiency of the simple machine:

$$\text{Efficiency} = \frac{W_{\text{out}}}{W_{\text{in}}} = \frac{(\text{load})(\text{load distance})}{(\text{effort})(\text{effort distance})}$$

Equation 2.12

Efficiency is often expressed as a percentage by multiplying the efficiency ratio by 100 percent. The efficiency of a machine gives a measure of the amount of useful work generated by the machine for a given amount of work put into the system. A corollary of this definition is that the percentage of the work put into the system that becomes unusable is due to nonconservative or external forces.

The pulley system in Figure 2.5 illustrates the fact that adding more pulleys further increases mechanical advantage: for each additional pair of pulleys, we can reduce the effort further still. In this case, the load has been divided among six lengths of rope, so the effort required is now only one-sixth the total load. Remember that we would need to pull through a length of rope that is six times the desired displacement, and that efficiency will decrease due to the added weight of each pulley and the additional friction forces.

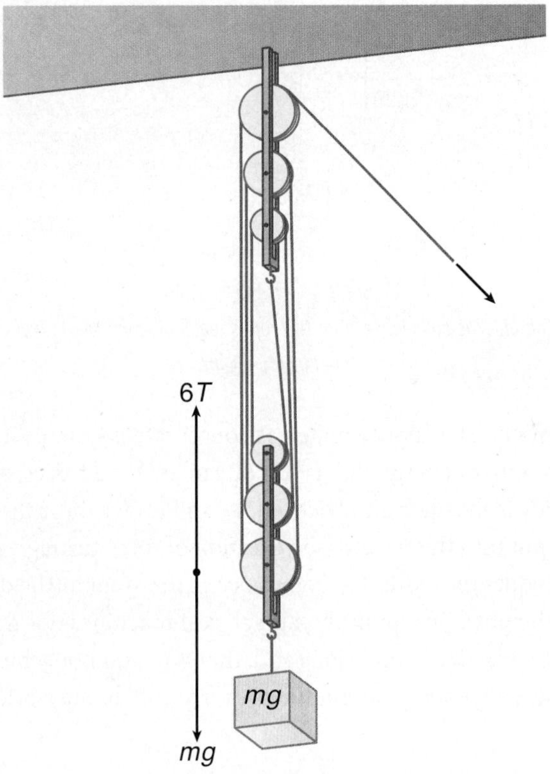

Figure 2.5 System of Six Pulleys
Increasing the number of pulleys decreases the tension in each segment of rope; this leads to an increase in the mechanical advantage of the setup.

Example: The pulley system in Figure 2.5 has an efficiency of 80 percent. A person is lifting a mass of 200 kg with the pulley.

Find:

A. The distance through which the effort must move to raise the load a distance of 4 m
B. The effort required to lift the load
C. The work done by the person lifting the load through a height of 4 m

Solution:

A. For the load to move through a vertical distance of 4 m, all six of the supporting ropes must also shorten 4 m. This may only be accomplished by pulling $6 \times 4 =$ 24 m of rope through the setup. Therefore, the effort must move through a distance of 24 m.
B. To calculate the effort required, the equation for efficiency should be used. The load is the weight of the object being lifted and is equal to the mass of the object times the acceleration due to gravity g. The effort distance, calculated in part A, is 24 m.

$$\text{Efficiency} = \frac{(\text{load})(\text{load distance})}{(\text{effort})(\text{effort distance})}$$

$$0.8 = \frac{\left(200 \text{ kg} \times 9.8 \frac{\text{m}}{\text{s}^2}\right)(4 \text{ m})}{(\text{effort})(24 \text{ m})}$$

$$\text{effort} \approx \frac{2000 \times 4}{0.8 \times 24} \approx \frac{8000}{20} = 400 \text{ N (actual} = 408 \text{ N)}$$

C. The work done by the person is

$$W_{\text{in}} = (\text{effort})(\text{effort distance}) = 408 \text{ N} \times 24$$

$$\approx 9600 \text{ J (actual} = 9800 \text{ J)}$$

MCAT CONCEPT CHECK 2.3

Before you move on, assess your understanding of the material with these questions.

1. As the length of an inclined plane increases, what happens to the force required to move an object the same displacement?

___

2. As the effort decreases in a pulley system, what happens to the effort distance to maintain the same work output?

___

3. What accounts for the difference between work input and work output in a system that operates at less than 100% efficiency?

___

4. What does it mean for a device to provide mechanical advantage?

___

5. Name the six simple machines:

    - ___
    - ___
    - ___
    - ___
    - ___
    - ___

Conclusion

The conceptualization of energy as the capacity to do something or make something happen is a very broad definition. However, such an all-encompassing definition allows us to understand everything from pushing a rock up a hill to melting an ice cube, from stopping a car at an intersection to harnessing the energy of biomolecules in metabolism, to all the forms of energy transfer. Indeed, energy on its own has little significance without considering the *transfer* of energy, either through work or heat. The work–energy theorem is a powerful expression that will guide our approach to many problems in the *Chemical and Physical Foundations of Biological Systems* section. We also covered the application of energy and work with simple machines, such as levers, inclined planes, and pulleys. These devices assist us in accomplishing work by reducing the forces necessary for displacing objects.

Preparing for the MCAT is hard (mental) work, but you are well on your way to achieving success on Test Day. This *MCAT Physics and Math Review* book (and all the materials provided in your Kaplan program) is part of a set of tools—your simple machines, if you will—that will provide you with the mechanical advantage to ease your efforts toward a higher score.

GO ONLINE

You've reviewed the content, now test your knowledge and critical thinking skills by completing a test-like passage set in your online resources!

CONCEPT SUMMARY

Energy

- **Energy** is the property of a system that enables it to do something or make something happen, including the capacity to do work. The SI units for all forms of energy are joules (J).
- **Kinetic energy** is energy associated with the movement of objects. It depends on mass and speed squared (not velocity).
- **Potential energy** is energy stored within a system. It exists in gravitational, elastic, electrical, and chemical forms.
  - **Gravitational potential energy** is related to the mass of an object and its height above a zero-point, called a **datum**.
  - **Elastic potential energy** is related to the **spring constant** (a measure of the stiffness of a spring) and the degree of stretch or compression of a spring squared.
  - **Electrical potential energy** exists between charged particles.
  - **Chemical potential energy** is the energy stored in the bonds of compounds.
- The total **mechanical energy** of a system is the sum of its kinetic and potential energies.
- **Conservative forces** are path independent and do not dissipate the mechanical energy of a system.
  - If only conservative forces are acting on an object, the total mechanical energy is conserved.
  - Examples of conservative forces include gravity and electrostatic forces. Elastic forces, such as those created by springs, are nearly conservative.
- **Nonconservative forces** are path dependent and cause dissipation of mechanical energy from a system.
  - While total energy is conserved, some mechanical energy is lost as thermal or chemical energy.
  - Examples of nonconservative forces include friction, air resistance, and viscous drag.

Work

- **Work** is a process by which energy is transferred from one system to another.
  - Work may be expressed as the dot product of force and displacement, or the product of force and distance traveled with the cosine of the angle between the two.
  - Work may also be expressed as the area under a **pressure–volume (P–V) curve**.
- **Power** is the rate at which work is done or energy is transferred. The SI unit for power is the watt (W).
- The **work–energy theorem** states that when net work is done on or by a system, the system's kinetic energy will change by the same amount. In more general applications, the work done on or by a system can be transferred to other forms of energy as well.

Mechanical Advantage

- **Mechanical advantage** is the factor by which a simple machine multiplies the input force to accomplish work.
- The six **simple machines** are the inclined plane, wedge, wheel and axle, lever, pulley, and screw. Simple machines provide the benefit of mechanical advantage.
- Mechanical advantage makes it easier to accomplish a given amount of work because the input force necessary to accomplish the work is reduced; the distance through which the reduced input force must be applied, however, is increased by the same factor (assuming 100% efficiency).
- The **load** is the output force of a simple machine, which acts over a given **load distance** to determine the work output of the simple machine. The **effort** is the input force of a simple machine, which acts over a given **effort distance** to determine the work input of the simple machine.
- **Efficiency** is the ratio of the machine's work output to work input when nonconservative forces are taken into account.

ANSWERS TO CONCEPT CHECKS

2.1

1. Kinetic energy is the energy of motion. It is related to the mass of an object, as well as its speed squared. Potential energy is energy associated with a given position or intrinsic property of a system; it is stored in gravitational, electrical, elastic, or chemical forms. Gravitational potential energy is directly related to the mass of the object and its height above a reference point.

2.

	Conservative Forces	Nonconservative Forces
What happens to total mechanical energy of the system?	Remains constant	Decreases (energy is dissipated)
Does the path taken matter?	No	Yes; more energy is dissipated with a longer path
What are some examples?	Gravity Electrostatic forces Elastic forces (approximately conservative)	Friction Air resistance Viscous drag

2.2

1. The unit of work is the joule, which is also the unit for energy. Work and energy are related concepts. By performing work, the energy of a system is changed. Work, along with heat, is a form of energy transfer.
2. Three methods for calculating work discussed in this chapter are:
    1. $W = Fd \cos \theta$ (the dot product of the force and displacement vectors)
    2. $W = P\Delta V$ (the area under a pressure–volume curve)
    3. $W_{net} = \Delta K$ (the work–energy theorem)
3. Begin by thinking about how each form of work is affecting the vehicle. While we could try to work through what may be happening in terms of forces and displacements, this gets very tricky when considering moving engine parts. In this case, it is simpler to think about each work in terms of kinetic energy. The work done by the engine increases the kinetic energy of the car, so it's positive. Conversely, the work done by resistance decreases the kinetic energy of the car, meaning the work done on the car is negative. If the engine does more work than friction, then there is a positive change in kinetic energy. If resistance does more work, then the change is negative. If they do equal amounts of work, then there is no change in kinetic energy. We are given that the vehicle maintains a constant velocity; thus, there is no change in kinetic energy. Therefore, according to the work–energy theorem, the net work must also be zero, and we can infer that the amount of positive work done by the engine must be equal to the amount of negative work done by resistance.

2.3

1. As the length of an inclined plane increases, the amount of force necessary to perform the same amount of work (moving the object the same displacement) decreases.
2. As the effort (required force) decreases in a pulley system, the effort distance increases to generate the same amount of work.
3. The decrease in work output is due to nonconservative or external forces that generate or dissipate energy.
4. When a device provides mechanical advantage, it decreases the input force required to generate a particular output force. Generally, this is accomplished at the expense of increased distance over which the force must act.
5. The six simple machines are: inclined plane, wedge, wheel and axle, lever, pulley, and screw.

SCIENCE MASTERY ASSESSMENT EXPLANATIONS

1. **C**

Because the weight of the barbell (force acting downward) is $mg = 275 \text{ kg} \times 10 \frac{\text{m}}{\text{s}^2}$, or about 2750 N, it follows that the weightlifter must exert an equal and opposite force of 2750 N on the barbell. The work done in lifting the barbell is therefore $W = Fd \cos \theta = (2750 \text{ N})(2.4 \text{ m})(\cos 0) \approx 7000 \text{ J}$. Using the same equation, it follows that the work done to hold the barbell in place is $W = Fd \cos \theta = (2750 \text{ N})(0 \text{ m})(\cos \theta) = 0 \text{ J}$. Because the barbell is held in place and there is no displacement, the work done is zero. This is closest to **(C)**.

2. **C**

The work done by the tractor can be calculated from the equation $W = Fd \cos \theta = (5000 \text{ N})(100 \text{ m})(\cos 30°) = (5000)(100)(0.866) \approx 5000 \times 90 = 450{,}000 \text{ J} = 450 \text{ kJ}$. This is closest to **(C)**. Since we estimated by rounding 0.866 up to 0.9, we can expect the actual answer to be less than the calculated answer.

3. **B**

The work done by the engine is equal to the change in kinetic energy of the car: $W = \Delta K = \frac{1}{2} m\left(v_f^2 - v_i^2\right) = \frac{1}{2}(2000 \text{ kg})\left(900 \frac{\text{m}^2}{\text{s}^2} - 0\right) = 900{,}000 \text{ J}$. The average power therefore is

$$P = \frac{W}{t} = \frac{900{,}000 \text{ J}}{6 \text{ s}} = 150{,}000 \text{ W} = 150 \text{ kW}.$$

4. **D**

Assuming negligible air resistance, conservation of energy states that the total mechanical energy of the block is constant as it falls. At the starting height of 5 m, the block only has potential energy equal to $U = mgh \approx 40 \text{ kg} \times 10 \frac{\text{m}}{\text{s}^2} \times 5 \text{ m} = 2000 \text{ J}$. Because the kinetic energy at this point is 0 J, the total mechanical energy is 2000 J at any point during the block's descent.

5. **C**

An isochoric process, by definition, is one in which the gas system undergoes no change in volume. If the gas neither expands nor is compressed, then no work is performed. Remember that work in a thermodynamic system is the area under a P–V curve; if the change in volume is 0, then the area under the curve is also 0.

6. **B**

To calculate the tension force in each rope, first draw a free body diagram:

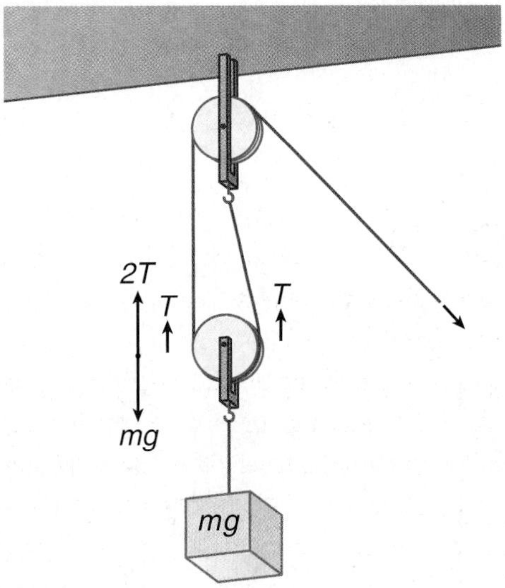

From the force diagram, notice that there are two tension forces pulling the mass up. The net force for this system ($\mathbf{F}_{net}$) is equal to $2\mathbf{T} - m\mathbf{g}$. Now we can use Newton's second law:

$$\mathbf{F}_{net} = m\mathbf{a}$$
$$2\mathbf{T} - m\mathbf{g} = m\mathbf{a}$$
$$\mathbf{T} = \frac{m(\mathbf{a} + \mathbf{g})}{2} \approx \frac{(10 \text{ kg})\left(2 \frac{\text{m}}{\text{s}^2} + 10 \frac{\text{m}}{\text{s}^2}\right)}{2}$$
$$= 5 \times 12 = 60 \text{ N}$$

7. **C**

Gravity is a conservative force because it is pathway independent and it does not dissipate mechanical energy. Air resistance and friction—**(A)** and **(B)**—are nonconservative forces that dissipate energy thermally. Convection is not a force, but a method of heat transfer, eliminating **(D)**.

8. **A**

In uniform circular motion, the displacement vector and force vector are always perpendicular; therefore, no work is done. Potential energy is constant for an object in uniform circular motion, whether it is the gravitational potential energy of a satellite orbiting the Earth or the electrical potential energy of an electron orbiting the nucleus of an idealized atom. In both cases, potential energy does not change and does not depend on the position of the object around the circle, eliminating **(D)**.

9. **B**

The work–energy theorem relates the total work done on an object by all forces to the change in kinetic energy experienced by the same object. While the work done by a force is indeed proportional to the magnitude of the force, it is also proportional to the displacement of the object, eliminating **(A)**. The change in kinetic energy is equal—not proportional—to the total work done on the object; further, it is the net force, not *any* force, that relates to the work done on an object, eliminating **(C)**. Finally, the change in kinetic energy of the object is equal to the work done by all of the forces acting on the object combined, not just the applied force, which eliminates **(D)**.

10. **D**

Elastic potential energy, like kinetic energy, is related to the square of another variable, as shown by the equation $U = \frac{1}{2}kx^2$. Increasing the displacement by a factor of 2 increases the potential energy by a factor of $2^2 = 4$.

11. **A**

Sarah will not bounce higher than Josh. Assuming that mechanical energy is conserved, Sarah and Josh will start with a given amount of potential energy, which is converted into kinetic energy, then elastic potential energy, then kinetic energy again with no loss of energy from the system, eliminating **(D)**. By this logic, both individuals should return to the same starting height. Josh starts with $U = mgh \approx 80 \text{ kg} \times 10 \frac{\text{m}}{\text{s}^2} \times 20 \text{ m} = 16{,}000 \text{ J}$ of potential energy. At the moment Josh hits the net, all of this potential energy has been converted into kinetic energy. Therefore:

$$K = \frac{1}{2}mv^2 \rightarrow v = \sqrt{\frac{2K}{m}}$$

$$= \sqrt{\frac{2 \times 16{,}000}{80}} = \sqrt{400} = 20 \frac{\text{m}}{\text{s}}$$

eliminating **(B)**. Josh will experience a greater force upon impact because the net exerts a force proportional to weight; the higher the weight, the larger the force exerted by the net, eliminating **(C)**.

12. **B**

At terminal velocity, the force of gravity and force of air resistance are equal in magnitude, leading to translational equilibrium. Thus, statement I is true. If these forces have the same magnitude and act over the same displacement, then the work performed is the same as well, making statement III true. Even though the net force is equal to zero, there are still forces acting on the parachutist, making statement II false.

13. **B**

Mechanical advantage is a ratio of the output force generated given a particular input force. Efficiency is a ratio of the useful work performed by a system compared to the work performed on the system.

14. **C**

In the absence of nonconservative forces, all changes in potential energy must be met by an equal change in kinetic energy. Note that it is the difference in potential energy that is the same as the difference in kinetic energy, not the proportionality, eliminating **(B)**. Both **(A)** and **(D)** could be true statements but do not necessarily have to be—the object's mass could have been quadrupled while its height was halved.

15. **A**

Horsepower is a unit of power, as evidenced by the name and the conversion factor given in the question stem. Power is a rate of energy expenditure over time. Given unlimited time, both cars are capable of unlimited increases in (kinetic) energy, meaning that they have unlimited maximum velocities. The fact that Car B has a higher power rating means that it will reach any given velocity faster than Car A, eliminating **(B)**. There is not enough information to make any judgments on the efficiency of the cars, eliminating **(C)**. While it may take longer for Car A to reach a given velocity, both cars have unlimited maximum velocities, eliminating **(D)**.

Consult your online resources for additional practice. GO ONLINE

EQUATIONS TO REMEMBER

(2.1) **Kinetic energy:** $K = \frac{1}{2}mv^2$

(2.2) **Gravitational potential energy:** $U = mgh$

(2.3) **Elastic potential energy:** $U = \frac{1}{2}kx^2$

(2.4) **Total mechanical energy:** $E = U + K$

(2.5) **Conservation of mechanical energy:** $\Delta E = \Delta U + \Delta K = 0$

(2.6) **Work done by nonconservative forces:** $W_{\text{nonconservative}} = \Delta E = \Delta U + \Delta K$

(2.7) **Definition of work (mechanical):** $W = \mathbf{F} \cdot \mathbf{d} = Fd\cos\theta$

(2.8) **Definition of work (isobaric gas–piston system):** $W = P\Delta V$

(2.9) **Definition of power:** $P = \frac{W}{t} = \frac{\Delta E}{t}$

(2.10) **Work–Energy theorem:** $W_{\text{net}} = \Delta K = K_{\text{f}} - K_{\text{i}}$

(2.11) **Mechanical advantage:** Mechanical advantage $= \frac{F_{\text{out}}}{F_{\text{in}}}$

(2.12) **Efficiency:** Efficiency $= \frac{W_{\text{out}}}{W_{\text{in}}} = \frac{(\text{load})(\text{load distance})}{(\text{effort})(\text{effort distance})}$

SHARED CONCEPTS

Biochemistry Chapter 6
DNA and Biotechnology

Biochemistry Chapter 9
Carbohydrate Metabolism I

Biochemistry Chapter 12
Bioenergetics and Regulation of Metabolism

General Chemistry Chapter 7
Thermochemistry

Physics and Math Chapter 1
Kinematics and Dynamics

Physics and Math Chapter 3
Thermodynamics

CHAPTER 3

THERMODYNAMICS

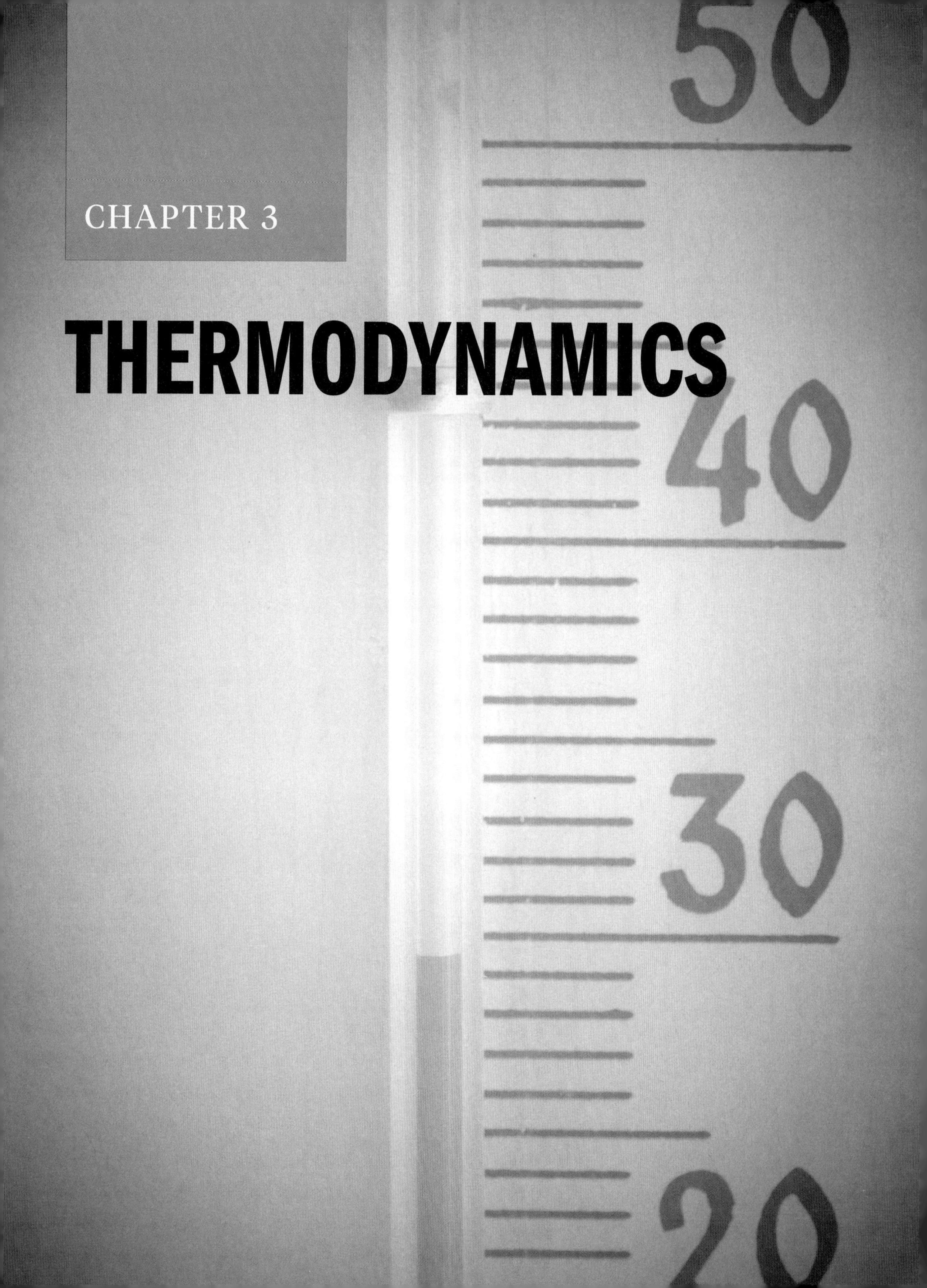

SCIENCE MASTERY ASSESSMENT

Every pre-med knows this feeling: there is so much content I have to know for the MCAT! How do I know what to do first or what's important?

While the high-yield badges throughout this book will help you identify the most important topics, this Science Mastery Assessment is another tool in your MCAT prep arsenal. This quiz (which can also be taken in your online resources) and the guidance below will help ensure that you are spending the appropriate amount of time on this chapter based on your personal strengths and weaknesses. Don't worry though—skipping something now does not mean you'll never study it. Later on in your prep, as you complete full-length tests, you'll uncover specific pieces of content that you need to review and can come back to these chapters as appropriate.

How to Use This Assessment

If you answer 0–7 questions correctly:

Spend about 1 hour to read this chapter in full and take limited notes throughout. Follow up by reviewing **all** quiz questions to ensure that you now understand how to solve each one.

If you answer 8–11 questions correctly:

Spend 20–40 minutes reviewing the quiz questions. Beginning with the questions you missed, read and take notes on the corresponding subchapters. For questions you answered correctly, ensure your thinking matches that of the explanation and you understand why each choice was correct or incorrect.

If you answer 12–15 questions correctly:

Spend less than 20 minutes reviewing all questions from the quiz. If you missed any, then include a quick read-through of the corresponding subchapters, or even just the relevant content within a subchapter, as part of your question review. For questions you got correct, ensure your thinking matches that of the explanation and review the Concept Summary at the end of the chapter.

1. If an object with an initial temperature of 300 K increases its temperature by 1°C every minute, by how many degrees Fahrenheit will its temperature have increased in 10 minutes?
   - **A.** 6°F
   - **B.** 10°F
   - **C.** 18°F
   - **D.** 30°C

2. Which of the following choices correctly identifies the following three heat transfer processes?
   - **I.** Heat transferred from the Sun to the Earth
   - **II.** A metal spoon heating up when placed in a pot of hot soup
   - **III.** A rising plume of smoke from a fire

   - **A.** I. Radiation; II. Conduction; III. Convection
   - **B.** I. Conduction; II. Radiation; III. Convection
   - **C.** I. Radiation; II. Convection; III. Conduction
   - **D.** I. Convection; II. Conduction; III. Radiation

3. A 20 m steel rod at 10°C is dangling from the edge of a building and is 2.5 cm from the ground. If the rod is heated to 110°C, will the rod touch the ground? (Note: $\alpha = 1.1 \times 10^{-5}\ \text{K}^{-1}$)
   - **A.** Yes, because it expands by 3.2 cm.
   - **B.** Yes, because it expands by 2.6 cm.
   - **C.** No, because it expands by 2.2 cm.
   - **D.** No, because it expands by 1.8 cm.

4. What is the final temperature of a 3 kg wrought iron fireplace tool that is left in front of an electric heater, absorbing heat energy at a rate of 100 W for 10 minutes? Assume the tool is initially at 20°C and that the specific heat of wrought iron is $500\ \frac{\text{J}}{\text{kg}\cdot\text{K}}$.
   - **A.** 40°C
   - **B.** 50°C
   - **C.** 60°C
   - **D.** 70°C

5. How much heat is required to completely melt a pair of gold earrings weighing 500 g, given that their initial temperature is 25°C? (The melting point of gold is 1064°C, its heat of fusion is $6.37 \times 10^4\ \frac{\text{J}}{\text{kg}}$, and its specific heat is $126\ \frac{\text{J}}{\text{kg}\cdot\text{K}}$.)
   - **A.** 15 kJ
   - **B.** 32 kJ
   - **C.** 66 kJ
   - **D.** 97 kJ

6. Given the cycle shown, what is the total work done by the gas during the cycle?

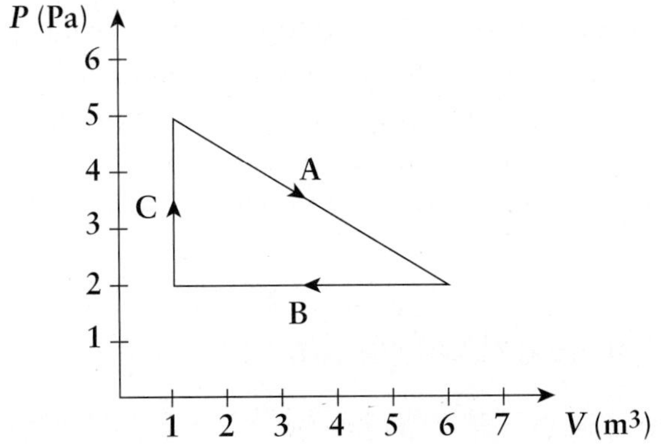

   - **A.** −10 J
   - **B.** 0 J
   - **C.** 7.5 J
   - **D.** 17.5 J

7. In an adiabatic compression process, the internal energy of the gas:
   - **A.** increases because the work done on the gas is negative.
   - **B.** increases because the work done on the gas is positive.
   - **C.** decreases because the work done on the gas is negative.
   - **D.** decreases because the work done on the gas is positive.

8. The entropy of a system can:
   - **A.** never decrease.
   - **B.** decrease when the entropy of the surroundings increases by at least as much.
   - **C.** decrease when the system is isolated and the process is irreversible.
   - **D.** decrease during an adiabatic reversible process.

9. A student making a coffee cup calorimeter fails to use a second coffee cup and inadequately seals the lid. What was the student's initial goal, and what was the result of this mistake?
   - **A.** The student was trying to create an isolated system but created an open system instead.
   - **B.** The student was trying to create an isolated system but created a closed system instead.
   - **C.** The student was trying to create a closed system but created an open system instead.
   - **D.** The student was trying to create a closed system but created an isolated system instead.

10. A certain substance has a specific heat of $1 \frac{\text{J}}{\text{mol} \cdot \text{K}}$ and a melting point of 350 K. If one mole of the substance is currently at a temperature of 349 K, how much energy must be added in order to melt it?
    - **A.** More than 1 J
    - **B.** Exactly 1 J
    - **C.** Less than 1 J but more than 0 J
    - **D.** Less than 0 J

11. Which of the following is NOT a state function?
    - **A.** Internal energy
    - **B.** Heat
    - **C.** Temperature
    - **D.** Entropy

12. The figure shown depicts a thick metal container with two compartments. Compartment A is full of a hot gas, while compartment B is full of a cold gas. What is the primary mode of heat transfer in this system?

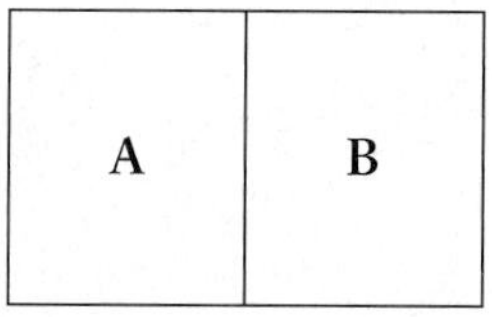

    - **A.** Radiation
    - **B.** Convection
    - **C.** Conduction
    - **D.** Enthalpy

13. Substances A and B have the same freezing and boiling points. If solid samples of both substances are heated in the exact same way, substance A boils before substance B. Which of the following would NOT explain this phenomenon?
    - **A.** Substance B has a higher specific heat.
    - **B.** Substance B has a higher heat of vaporization.
    - **C.** Substance B has a higher heat of fusion.
    - **D.** Substance B has a higher internal energy.

14. In experiment A, a student mixes ink with water and notices that the two liquids mix evenly. In experiment B, the student mixes oil with water; in this case, the liquids separate into two different layers. The entropy change is:
    - **A.** positive in experiment A and negative in experiment B.
    - **B.** positive in experiment A and zero in experiment B.
    - **C.** negative in experiment A and positive in experiment B.
    - **D.** zero in experiment A and negative in experiment B.

15. Which of the following processes is LEAST likely to be accompanied by a change in temperature?
    - **A.** The kinetic energy of a gas is increased through a chemical reaction.
    - **B.** Energy is transferred to a solid via electromagnetic waves.
    - **C.** A boiling liquid is heated on a hot plate.
    - **D.** A warm gas is mixed with a cold gas.

Answer Key

1. **C**
2. **A**
3. **C**
4. **C**
5. **D**
6. **C**
7. **B**
8. **B**
9. **A**
10. **A**
11. **B**
12. **C**
13. **D**
14. **B**
15. **C**

Detailed explanations can be found at the end of the chapter.

CHAPTER 3

THERMODYNAMICS

In This Chapter

CHAPTER PROFILE

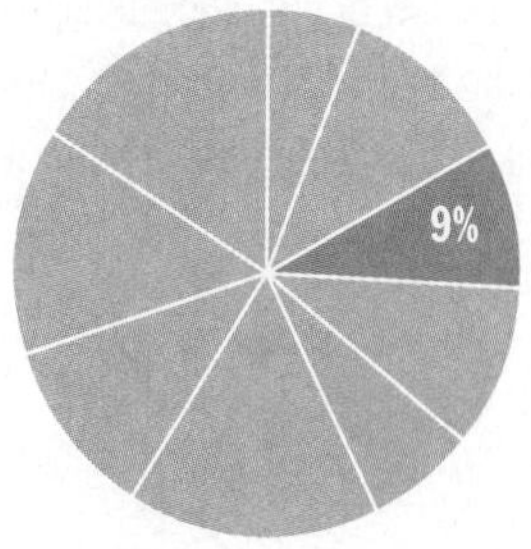

The content in this chapter should be relevant to about 9% of all questions about physics on the MCAT.

This chapter covers material from the following AAMC content categories:

4B: Importance of fluids for the circulation of blood, gas movement, and gas exchange

5E: Principles of chemical thermodynamics and kinetics

Introduction

Thermodynamics is the study of the flow of energy in the universe, as that flow relates to work, heat, entropy, and the different forms of energy. Classical thermodynamics concerns itself only with observations that can be made at the macroscopic level, such as measurements of temperature, pressure, volume, and work. Although the MCAT will test entropy from a thermodynamic rather than probabilistic understanding, we will briefly discuss the statistical model of entropy because it clarifies much of the confusion that arises from a characterization of entropy as a measure of "disorder."

This chapter reviews the laws of thermodynamics with a specific focus on the zeroth, first, and second laws. We will examine how the zeroth law leads to the formulation of temperature scales. Thermal expansion will be discussed as an example of the relationship between thermal energy and physical properties like length, volume, and conductivity. We will then take a moment to examine thermodynamic terminology and functions that are also intimately related to the concepts discussed in Chapter 7 of *MCAT General Chemistry Review*. In the context of the first law—the conservation of energy—we will discuss the relationship between internal energy, heat, and work, and characterize specific heat and heat of transformation. We will also review the various processes by which a system goes from one equilibrium state to another and connect work, discussed in Chapter 2 of *MCAT Physics and Math Review*, with heat. Finally, we will investigate the second law of thermodynamics through the concepts of entropy and its measurement. The third law of thermodynamics is not directly tested on the MCAT, so we will only briefly mention it.

3.1 Zeroth Law of Thermodynamics

LEARNING OBJECTIVES

After Chapter 3.1, you will be able to:

- Explain the zeroth law of thermodynamics
- Predict the relative expansion of an object undergoing a temperature change
- Describe the basis and the significance of the Kelvin scale

KEY CONCEPT

The zeroth law of thermodynamics states the transitive property in thermal systems: If $a = b$ and $b = c$, then $a = c$.

The **zeroth law of thermodynamics** is based on a simple observation: when one object is in thermal equilibrium with another object, say a cup of warm tea and a metal stirring stick, and the second object is in thermal equilibrium with a third object, such as your hand, then the first and third object are also in thermal equilibrium. As such, when brought into thermal contact, no net heat will flow between these objects. Note that thermal contact does not necessarily imply physical contact, as objects can be in thermal contact across space.

Temperature

KEY CONCEPT

Temperature is a physical property of matter related to the average kinetic energy of the particles. Differences in temperature determine the direction of heat transfer.

The formulation of the zeroth law—that no net heat flows between objects in thermal equilibrium, and the corollary that heat flows between two objects *not* in thermal equilibrium—actually arose from studies of temperature. At any given time, all substances have a particular **temperature**. In everyday language, we use the term temperature to describe qualitatively how hot or cold something is, but in thermodynamics, it has a more precise meaning. At the molecular level, temperature is proportional to the average kinetic energy of the particles that make up the substance. At the macroscopic level, it is the difference in temperature between two objects that determines the direction of heat flow. When possible, heat moves spontaneously from materials that have higher temperatures to materials that have lower temperatures. **Heat** itself refers to the transfer of thermal energy from a hotter object with higher temperature (energy) to a colder object with lower temperature (energy). If no net heat flows between two objects in thermal contact, then we can say that their temperatures are equal and they are in **thermal equilibrium**.

Since the 18th century, scales have been developed to quantify the temperature of matter with thermometers. Some of these systems are still in common use, including the **Fahrenheit (°F)**, **Celsius (°C)**, and **Kelvin (K)** scales. Fahrenheit and Celsius are the oldest scales still in common use and are relatively convenient because they are based on the phase changes for water, as shown in Table 3.1. In the Celsius scale, 0° and 100° define the freezing and boiling temperatures of water. In the Fahrenheit scale, these phase change temperatures are defined as 32° and 212°.

	°F	°C	K
Absolute Zero	−460	−273	0
Freezing Point of Water	32	0	273
Boiling Point of Water	212	100	373

Table 3.1 Relevant Points in the Three Major Temperature Scales

The Kelvin scale is most commonly used for scientific measurements and is one of the seven SI base units. It defines as the zero reference point **absolute zero**, the theoretical temperature at which there is no thermal energy, and sets the freezing point of water as 273.15 K. The **third law of thermodynamics** states that the entropy of a perfectly organized crystal at absolute zero is zero. Note that there are no negative temperatures on the Kelvin scale because it starts from absolute zero. Although the Kelvin and Celsius scales have different zero reference points, the size of their units is the same. That is to say, a change of one degree Celsius equals a change of one unit kelvin. Because there are 180 degrees between water's phase changes on the Fahrenheit scale, rather than 100 degrees as on both the Celsius and the Kelvin scales, the size of the Fahrenheit unit is smaller. The following formulas can be used to convert from one scale to another:

$$F = \frac{9}{5}C + 32$$
$$K = C + 273$$

Equation 3.1

where *F*, *C*, and *K* are the temperatures in Fahrenheit, Celsius, and Kelvin, respectively.

MCAT EXPERTISE

The only time Fahrenheit is used routinely on the MCAT is for body temperature, which is 98.6°F or 37°C. In the rare occasion that it is used for a quantitative analysis question, conversions will be given.

Example: If a meteorologist says that the temperature will reach a high of 86°F today, what will be the high temperature in °C and in K?

Solution: To convert from Fahrenheit to Celsius, use:

$$F = \frac{9}{5}C + 32 \rightarrow C = \frac{5}{9}(F - 32)$$
$$C = \frac{5}{9}(86 - 32) = \frac{5}{9}(54) = 30°\text{C}$$

Now convert from Celsius to Kelvin:

$$K = C + 273 = 30 + 273 = 303\text{ K}$$

Thermal Expansion

It has long been noted that some physical properties of matter change when the matter gets hotter or colder. Length, volume, solubility, and even the conductivity of matter change as a function of temperature. The relationship between temperature and a physical property of some matter was used to develop the temperature scales with which we are familiar today. For example, Daniel Fahrenheit developed the temperature scale that bears his name by placing a thermometer filled with mercury into a bath of ice, water, and ammonium chloride. The cold temperature caused the mercury to contract, and when the level in the glass tube stabilized at a lower level, he marked this as the zero reference on the scale. He then placed the same mercury thermometer in a mixture of ice and water (that is, at the freezing point for water). The slightly warmer temperature of this mixture caused the mercury to rise in the glass column, and when it stabilized at this higher level, Fahrenheit assigned it a value of 32°. When he stuck the thermometer under his (or someone else's) tongue, he marked the even higher mercury level as 100° (not 98.6°). The details of how and why Fahrenheit came to choose these numbers (and the history of their adjustment since Fahrenheit first developed the scale) are beyond the scope of this discussion; rather, what is important to note is that a change in some physical property of one kind of matter—in this case, the height of a column of mercury—can be correlated to certain temperature markers, such as the phase changes for water. Once the scale has been set in reference to the decided-upon temperature markers, then the thermometer can be used to take the temperature of any other matter, in accordance with the zeroth law.

REAL WORLD

It is because of thermal expansion that bridges and sidewalks have gaps between their segments; they allow for thermal expansion without damaging integrity.

MNEMONIC

When the temperature of an object changes, its length changes **a lot** ($\alpha L \Delta T$).

Because the property of **thermal expansion** was integral to the development of thermometers, let's look a little more closely at this phenomenon. A change in the temperature of most solids results in a change in their length. Rising temperatures cause an increase in length, and falling temperatures cause a decrease in length. The amount of length change is proportional to the original length of the solid and the increase in temperature according to the equation

$$\Delta L = \alpha L \Delta T$$

Equation 3.2

where ΔL is the change in length, α is the coefficient of linear expansion, L is the original length, and ΔT is the change in temperature. The **coefficient of linear expansion** is a constant that characterizes how a specific material's length changes as the temperature changes. This usually has units of K^{-1}, although it may sometimes be quoted as $°C^{-1}$. This difference is inconsequential because the unit size for the Kelvin and Celsius scales is the same.

Example: A metal rod of length 2 m has a coefficient of linear expansion of 10^{-6} K^{-1}. It is cooled from 1080°C to 80°C. What is the final length of the rod?

Solution: By using the information given in the problem, we can substitute directly into the thermal expansion formula:

$$\Delta L = \alpha L \Delta T = (10^{-6}\ \text{K})(2\ \text{m})(80\ \text{K} - 1080\ \text{K}) = -2 \times 10^{-3}\ \text{m}$$

The negative sign represents a decrease in length. The original length was 2 m; therefore, the final length is $2 - (2 \times 10^{-3}) = 1.998$ m.

Liquids also experience thermal expansion, but the only meaningful parameter of expansion is volume expansion. The formula for volumetric thermal expansion is applicable to both liquids and solids:

$$\Delta V = \beta V \Delta T$$

Equation 3.3

where ΔV is the change in volume, β is the coefficient of volumetric expansion, V is the original volume, and ΔT is the change in temperature. The **coefficient of volumetric expansion** is a constant that characterizes how a specific material's volume changes as the temperature changes. Its value is equal to three times the coefficient of linear expansion for the same material ($\beta = 3\alpha$).

Example: Suppose that a thermometer with 1 mL of mercury is taken from a freezer with a temperature of −25°C and placed near an oven at 275°C. If the coefficient of volume expansion of mercury is 1.8×10^{-4} K^{-1}, by how much will the liquid expand?

Solution: Use the information given to plug into the volumetric expansion formula:

$$\begin{aligned}\Delta V &= \beta V \Delta T = (1.8 \times 10^{-4}\ \text{K}^{-1})(1\ \text{mL})(275°\text{C} - (-25°\text{C})) \\ &= (1.8 \times 10^{-4})(300) = 540 \times 10^{-4}\ \text{mL} = 0.054\ \text{mL}\end{aligned}$$

MCAT CONCEPT CHECK 3.1

Before you move on, assess your understanding of the material with these questions.

1. What is the zeroth law of thermodynamics?

2. What is the maximum distance that two objects can be from one another and still adhere to the zeroth law of thermodynamics?

3. How do the initial length of an object and the amount it expands for a given temperature change relate to one another?

4. True or False: The Kelvin scale is the most accurate measurement method for temperature because it is based on absolute zero.

3.2 Systems

LEARNING OBJECTIVES

After Chapter 3.2, you will be able to:

- Distinguish between closed, isolated, and open thermodynamic systems
- Compare and contrast state and process functions
- List common state functions

Physicists and chemists tend to classify the world on the basis of observable phenomena and interactions between objects. Before moving on, we need to become familiar with some of the jargon that these fields have in common—specifically, thermodynamic systems and state functions. Note that the same jargon is discussed in Chapter 7 of *MCAT General Chemistry Review*.

System Types

A **system** is the portion of the universe that we are interested in observing or manipulating. The rest of the universe is considered the **surroundings**.

Isolated Systems

Isolated systems are not capable of exchanging energy or matter with their surroundings. As a result, the total change in internal energy must be zero. Isolated systems are very rare, although they can be approximated. A bomb calorimeter attempts to insulate a reaction from the surroundings to prevent energy transfer, and the entire universe can be considered an isolated system because there are no surroundings.

Closed Systems

Closed systems are capable of exchanging energy, but not matter, with the surroundings. The classic experiments involving gases in vessels with movable pistons are examples of closed systems. For thermodynamic purposes, most of what will be encountered on Test Day will be a closed system or will approximate a closed system.

Open Systems

Open systems can exchange both matter and energy with the environment. In an open system, not only does the matter carry energy, but more energy may be transferred in the form of heat or work. A boiling pot of water, human beings, and uncontained combustion reactions are all examples of open systems.

State Functions

State functions are thermodynamic properties that are a function of only the current equilibrium state of a system. In other words, state functions are defined by the fact that they are independent of the path taken to get to a particular equilibrium state. The state functions include pressure (P), density (ρ), temperature (T), volume (V), enthalpy (H), internal energy (U), Gibbs free energy (G), and entropy (S). On the other hand, **process functions**, such as work and heat, describe the path taken to get to from one state to another.

MCAT CONCEPT CHECK 3.2

Before you move on, assess your understanding of the material with these questions.

1. Which of the following thermodynamic systems transfer matter? Transfer energy?

System Type	Transfers Matter	Transfers Energy
Closed		
Isolated		
Open		

2. What is the difference between a state function and a process function?
    - State function:

    ____

    - Process function:

    ____

3. List at least five common state functions:
   -
   -
   -
   -
   -

3.3 First Law of Thermodynamics

High-Yield

LEARNING OBJECTIVES

After Chapter 3.3, you will be able to:

- Recall the mathematical relationships between internal energy, work, and heat
- Describe conduction, convection, and radiation
- Draw a graph of the temperature of a solid as it is heated to a gas
- Calculate work for a P–V diagram:

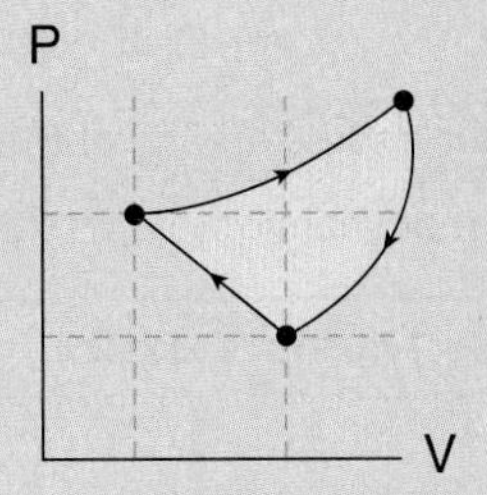

We have already encountered the first law of thermodynamics in our discussion of the conservation of mechanical energy in Chapter 2 of *MCAT Physics and Math Review*. Remember that in the absence of nonconservative forces, the sum of kinetic and potential energies is constant in a system. Now, in our present discussion of thermodynamics, we will look more closely at the relationship between internal energy, heat, and work. Essentially, the **first law of thermodynamics** states that the change in the total internal energy of a system is equal to the amount of energy transferred in the form of **heat** to the system, minus the amount of energy transferred from the system in the form of **work**. The internal energy of a system can be increased by adding heat, doing work on the system, or some combination of both processes. The change in internal energy is calculated from the equation

$$\Delta U = Q - W$$

Equation 3.4

where ΔU is the change in the system's internal energy, Q is the energy transferred into the system as heat, and W is the work done by the system. To use this equation properly, one must carefully apply the following sign convention shown in Table 3.2.

VARIABLE	POSITIVE VALUE	NEGATIVE VALUE
Change in Internal Energy (ΔU)	Increasing temperature	Decreasing temperature
Heat (Q)	Heat flows into system	Heat flows out of system
Work (W)	Work is done by the system (expansion)	Work is done on the system (compression)

Table 3.2 Sign Convention for the First Law of Thermodynamics

The first law is really just a particular iteration of the more universal physical law of energy conservation: energy can be neither created nor destroyed; it can only be changed from one form to another. Because the first law accounts for all work and all heat processes impacting the system, the presence of nonconservative forces poses no problem because the energy transfer associated with friction, air resistance, or viscous drag will be accounted for in the first law equation. For example, when a car "burns rubber," all the smoke and noise coming from the back tires is a clear indication that mechanical energy is not being conserved. However, if we include the energy transfers associated with the frictional forces in our consideration of the change in internal energy of the system, then we can confidently say that no energy has been lost at all: there may be a "loss" of energy from the car as a result of the friction, but that precise amount of energy can be "found" elsewhere—as thermal energy in the atoms and molecules of the surrounding road and air.

KEY CONCEPT

The first law of thermodynamics tells us that an increase in the total internal energy of a system is caused by transferring heat into the system or performing work on the system. The total internal energy of a system will decrease when heat is lost from the system or work is performed by the system.

Heat

In Chapter 2 of *MCAT Physics and Math Review*, we defined work as the process by which energy is transferred as the result of force being applied through some distance. We noted that work and heat are the only two processes by which energy can be transferred from one object to another. As discussed earlier in this chapter, the zeroth law of thermodynamics says that objects in thermal contact are in thermal equilibrium when their temperatures are the same. The corollary of this is the **second law of thermodynamics**: objects in thermal contact and not in thermal equilibrium will exchange heat energy such that the object with a higher temperature will give off heat energy to the object with a lower temperature until both objects have the same temperature at thermal equilibrium. **Heat**, then, is defined as the process by which a quantity of energy is transferred between two objects as a result of a difference

KEY CONCEPT

Heat is the process of energy transfer between two objects at different temperatures and will continue until the two objects come into thermal equilibrium at the same temperature.

in temperature. As we will discuss further in our examination of the second law, heat can never spontaneously transfer energy from a cooler object to a warmer one without work being done on the system.

KEY CONCEPT

One calorie (little c) is the amount of heat required to raise 1 g of water one degree Celsius. One Calorie (big C) is the amount of heat required to raise 1 kg of water 1 degree Celsius, equal to 1000 calories.

The SI unit for heat is the joule (J), which should not be surprising because it is based on energy. Heat can also be measured in the units of calorie (cal), nutritional Calorie (Cal), or the British thermal unit (BTU). The nutritional Calorie ("big C") is not the same thing as the calorie ("little c"); one Calorie is equal to 1000 calories or 1 kcal.

The conversion factors between the units of heat are as follows:

$$1 \text{ Cal} \equiv 10^3 \text{ cal} = 4184 \text{ J} = 3.97 \text{ BTU}$$

Heat Transfer

For energy to be transferred between objects, they must be in thermal contact with each other. This does not necessarily mean that the objects are touching. Like force, energy can travel tremendous distances and does not require a medium to pass through. There are three means by which heat can transfer energy: conduction, convection, and radiation.

Conduction is the direct transfer of energy from molecule to molecule through molecular collisions. As this definition would suggest, there must be direct physical contact between the objects. At the atomic level, the particles of the hotter matter transfer some of their kinetic energy to the particles of the cooler matter through collisions between the particles of the two materials. Metals are described as the best heat conductors because metallic bonds contain a density of atoms embedded in a sea of electrons, which facilitate rapid energy transfer. Gases tend to be the poorest heat conductors because there is so much space between individual molecules that energy-transferring collisions occur relatively infrequently. An example of heat transfer through conduction is the heat that is rapidly, and painfully, conducted to your fingers when you touch a hot stove.

Convection is the transfer of heat by the physical motion of a fluid over a material. Because convection involves flow, only liquids and gases can transfer heat by this means. In convection, if the fluid has a higher temperature, it will transfer energy to the material. Most restaurants and some home kitchens have convection ovens, which use fans to circulate hot air inside the oven. Because the heat is being transferred to the food by both convection and radiation rather than only by radiation, convection ovens cook more rapidly than radiation-only ovens. Convection may also be used to wick heat energy away from a hot object. In laboratory experiments, for example, a running cold-water bath may be used to rapidly cool a reaction.

Radiation is the transfer of energy by electromagnetic waves. Unlike conduction and convection, radiation can transfer energy through a vacuum. Radiation is the method by which the Sun is able to warm the Earth. Many home kitchens have radiant ovens, which use either electrical coils or gas flames to heat the insulated metal box that forms the body of the oven. The hot metal box then radiates the energy through the open space of the oven, where it is absorbed by whatever food is placed inside.

Specific Heat

When heat energy is added to or removed from a system, the temperature of that system will change in proportion to the amount of heat transfer, unless the system is undergoing a phase change during which the temperature is constant. This relationship between heat and temperature for a substance is called the specific heat. The **specific heat (*c*)** of a substance is defined as the amount of heat energy required to raise one gram of a substance by one degree Celsius or one unit kelvin. For example, the specific heat of liquid water is one calorie per gram per unit kelvin $\left(1\ \frac{\text{cal}}{\text{g}\cdot\text{K}}\right)$. Equivalently, this can be expressed as $4.184\ \frac{\text{J}}{\text{g}\cdot\text{K}}$. The specific heat for a substance changes according to its phase. The MCAT will generally provide specific heat values as necessary, although you are expected to know the specific heat of water in calories. The equation that relates the heat gained or lost by an object and the change in temperature of that object is

$$q = mc\Delta T$$

Equation 3.5

where m is the mass, c is the specific heat of the substance, and ΔT is the change in temperature (in Celsius or kelvins). Because the unit size for the Celsius and Kelvin scales is the same, the change in temperature will be the same for temperatures measured in Celsius or kelvins.

MCAT EXPERTISE

The specific heat of water (in calories) is a constant you are expected to know for Test Day. Its value is $1\ \frac{\text{cal}}{\text{g}\cdot\text{K}}$.

MNEMONIC

The equation for heat transfer, given a specific heat, is the same as the test you're studying for! $q = mc\Delta T$ looks a lot like "q equals MCAT."

Heat of Transformation

When a substance is undergoing a phase change, such as from solid to liquid or liquid to gas, the heat that is added or removed from the system does not result in a change in temperature. In other words, phase changes occur at a constant temperature, and the temperature will not begin to change until all of the substance has been converted from one phase into the other. For example, water melts at 0°C. No matter how much heat is added to a mass of ice at 0°C, the temperature of the equilibrated system will not rise until all the ice has been melted into liquid water.

We've determined that adding heat raises the temperature of a system because the particles in that system now have a greater average kinetic energy, and it's true that molecules have greater degrees of freedom of movement in the liquid state than in the solid state (and even more so in the gas state). However, phase changes are related to changes in potential energy, not kinetic energy. The molecules of water in ice, for example, aren't truly frozen in place and unable to move. The molecules rotate, vibrate, and wiggle around. The bonds within each molecule are also free to bend and stretch. Of course, the molecules are held in relatively stable positions by the hydrogen bonds that form between them, but they still have a fairly significant amount of kinetic energy. The potential energy, however, is quite low because of the stability provided by the relative closeness of one molecule to another and by the hydrogen bonds.

Now, think about what happens when one adds heat to ice that is at 0°C. The heat energy causes the water molecules to begin to move away from each other by breaking free of the hydrogen bonds between them. Because the water molecules are being held less rigidly in place, they now have greater degrees of freedom of movement and their average potential energy increases. In statistical mechanics, one would say that this increased freedom of movement permits a greater number of **microstates** for the water molecules. For example, instead of only being able to move up and down or sway side-to-side, a water molecule may now have more freedom of movement and be able to rock forward and back. In gaining additional directions and forms of motion, however, the amount of up-and-down or side-to-side motion must decrease, thus keeping the average kinetic energy of liquid water at 0°C the same as solid water at 0°C. In summary, while liquid water may have a greater number of microstates due to increased freedom of movement, its average kinetic energy is the same as solid water at the same temperature.

BRIDGE

It is important to know the common terms used for phase changes:

- Solid to liquid: fusion or melting
- Liquid to solid: freezing or solidification
- Liquid to gas: boiling, evaporation, or vaporization
- Gas to liquid: condensation
- Solid to gas: sublimation
- Gas to solid: deposition

These phase changes are discussed in Chapter 7 of *MCAT General Chemistry Review*.

When heat energy is added to or removed from a system that is experiencing a phase change, the amount of heat that is added or removed cannot be calculated with the equation $q = mc\Delta T$ because there is no temperature change during a phase change. Instead, the following equation is used:

$$q = mL$$

Equation 3.6

where q is the amount of heat gained or lost from the material, m is the mass of the substance, and L is the **heat of transformation** or **latent heat** of the substance.

REAL WORLD

It is because of the heat of transformation that sweating is such an efficient cooling mechanism. When sweat evaporates, the heat of vaporization is absorbed from the surface of the body. This is also why a hot day seems so much more intense when it is very humid out. The sweat is less likely to evaporate due to the dampness of the environment, so less heat can be lost from the surface of the skin through sweating.

The phase change from liquid to solid (**freezing** or **solidification**) or solid to liquid (**melting** or **fusion**) occurs at the **melting point**. The corresponding heat of transformation is called the **heat of fusion**. The phase change from liquid to gas (**boiling**, **evaporation**, or **vaporization**) or gas to liquid (**condensation**) occurs at the **boiling point**. The corresponding heat of transformation is called the **heat of vaporization**. The relevant heats of fusion and vaporization will be provided on Test Day.

Example: Silver has a melting point of 962°C and a heat of fusion of approximately $1.05 \times 10^5 \frac{\text{J}}{\text{kg}}$. The specific heat of silver is $233 \frac{\text{J}}{\text{kg} \cdot \text{K}}$. Approximately how much heat is required to completely melt a 1 kg silver chain with an initial temperature of 20°C?

Solution: Before melting the chain, we must first heat the chain to the melting point. To figure out how much heat is required, we use this formula:

$$\begin{aligned} q &= mc\Delta T \\ &= (1\text{ kg})\left(233 \frac{\text{J}}{\text{kg} \cdot \text{K}}\right)(942\text{ K}) \approx 200 \times 975 \\ &= 1.95 \times 10^5\text{ J (actual} = 2.19 \times 10^5\text{ J)} \end{aligned}$$

This tells us we have to add 219 kJ of heat to the chain just to get its temperature to the melting point. The chain is still in the solid phase. To melt it, we must continue to add heat in accordance with this formula:

$$q = mL$$
$$= (1\text{ kg})\left(1.05 \times 10^5 \frac{\text{J}}{\text{kg}}\right) = 1.05 \times 10^5\text{ J}$$

The total heat needed to melt the solid silver chain is 219 kJ + 105 kJ = 324 kJ.

Thermodynamic Processes

In the last chapter, we gave significant consideration to work as a change of energy in a system, both as a function of force and displacement and as a function of volume and pressure. We will briefly review the latter and its relationship to heat transfer within a system. Keep in mind that work accomplished by a change in displacement is not likely to be motivated by heat transfer, and any heat transfer that does occur is most likely a result of friction dissipating mechanical energy from the system.

During any thermodynamic process, a system goes from some initial equilibrium state with an initial pressure, temperature, and volume to some other equilibrium state, which may be at a different final pressure, temperature, or volume. These thermodynamic processes can be represented in graphical form with volume on the *x*-axis and pressure (or temperature) on the *y*-axis.

PROCESS	FIRST LAW OF THERMODYNAMICS REDUCES TO:
Isothermal ($\Delta U = 0$)	$Q = W$
Adiabatic ($Q = 0$)	$\Delta U = -W$
Isobaric (constant pressure)	(Multiple possible forms)
Isovolumetric (isochoric) ($W = 0$)	$\Delta U = Q$

Table 3.3 Special Types of Thermodynamic Processes

The MCAT focuses on three particular thermodynamic processes as special cases of the first law (excluding isobaric processes), as shown in Table 3.3. In each of these cases, some physical property is held constant during the process. These processes are **isothermal** (constant temperature, and therefore no change in internal energy), **adiabatic** (no heat exchange), and **isovolumetric** (no change in volume, and therefore no work accomplished; also called **isochoric**). **Isobaric** processes are those that occur at a constant pressure, and are of less focus on the MCAT. Figure 3.1 shows the different types of thermodynamic behaviors for a gas.

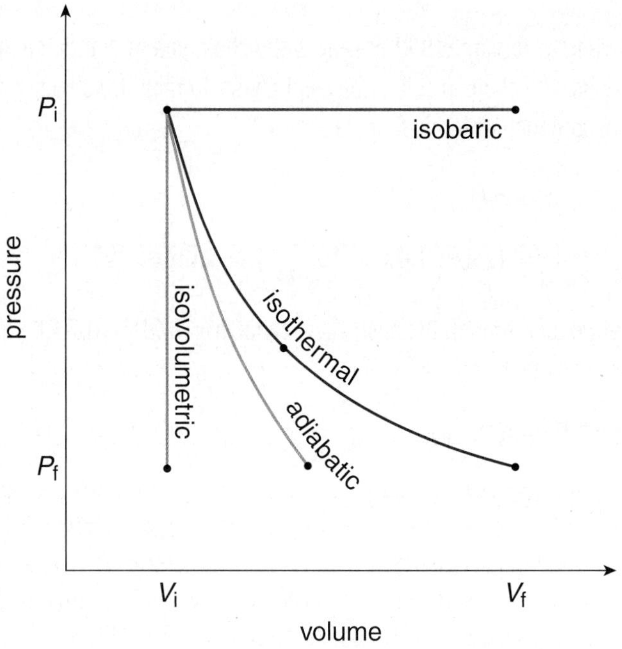

Figure 3.1 Thermodynamic Behaviors of Gases

Figure 3.2 shows a closed-loop thermodynamic process. Because the work on a P–V graph is simply the area under the curve, the work done in this closed-loop process is the area inside the loop.

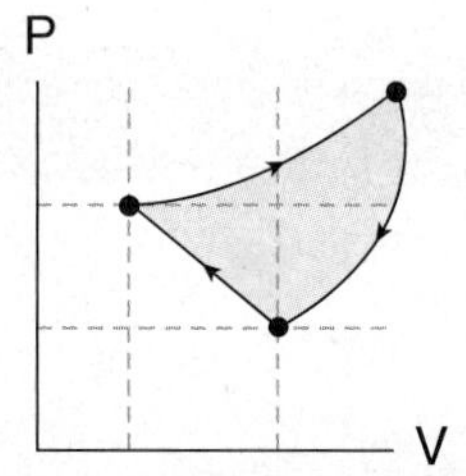

Figure 3.2 A Closed-Loop Process
The work is the area inside the loop.

Example: A gas in a cylinder is kept at a constant pressure of 3.6×10^5 Pa while 300 kJ of heat are added to it, causing the gas to expand from $1.0\ m^3$ to $1.5\ m^3$. Find the work done by the gas and the change in internal energy of the gas.

Solution: The pressure is held constant through the entire process so the work can be found using the equation:

$$W = P\Delta V$$
$$= (3.6 \times 10^5\ \text{Pa})(1.5\ \text{m}^3 - 1.0\ \text{m}^3) = 1.8 \times 10^5\ \text{J}$$

The change in internal energy can be found from the first law of thermodynamics:

$$\Delta U = Q - W = (3 \times 10^5) - (1.8 \times 10^5\ \text{J}) = 1.2 \times 10^5\ \text{J} = 120\ \text{kJ}$$

MCAT CONCEPT CHECK 3.3

Before you move on, assess your understanding of the material with these questions.

1. Describe the relationship between internal energy, work, and heat in words.

---

2. Define the following forms of heat transfer:
   - Conduction:

   - Convection:

   - Radiation:

   ---

3. Draw a representative graph of the temperature of a solid object as it is heated and goes through two phase changes to become a gas.

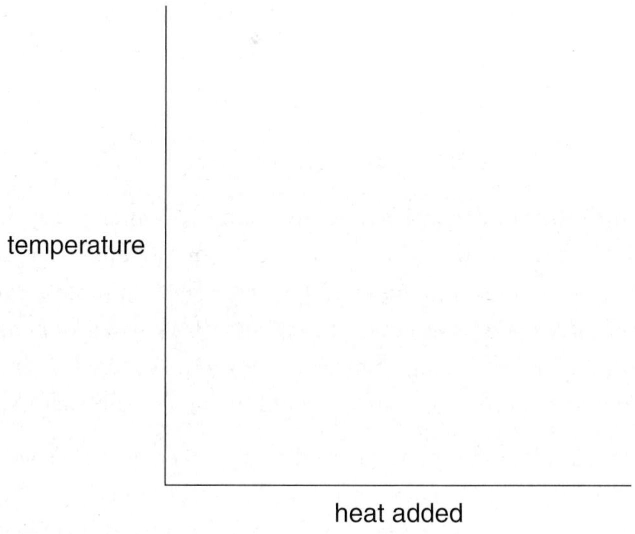

4. How is work calculated in P–V diagrams?

3.4 Second Law of Thermodynamics and Entropy

LEARNING OBJECTIVES

After Chapter 3.4, you will be able to:

- Describe entropy, on both a macroscopic level and in statistical terms
- Explain the relationship between entropy of a system and entropy of the surroundings for any thermodynamic process

The **second law of thermodynamics** states that objects in thermal contact and not in thermal equilibrium will exchange heat energy such that the object with a higher temperature will give off heat energy to the object with a lower temperature until both objects have the same temperature at thermal equilibrium. As such, energy is constantly being dispersed.

Energy Dispersion

Consider each of the following scenarios: hot tea cooling down, a frozen drink melting, iron rusting, buildings crumbling, balloons deflating, and living things dying and decaying. These scenarios share a common denominator. In each of them, energy of some form is going from being localized or concentrated to being spread out or dispersed. The thermal energy in the hot tea is spreading out to the cooler air that surrounds it. The thermal energy in the warmer air is spreading out to the cooler frozen drink. The chemical energy in the bonds of elemental iron and oxygen is released and dispersed as a result of the formation of the more stable, lower-energy bonds of iron oxide (rust). The potential energy of the building is released and dispersed in the form of light, sound, and heat as the building crumbles and falls. The energy of the pressurized air is released to the surrounding atmosphere as the balloon deflates. The chemical energy of all the molecules and atoms in living flesh is released into the environment during the process of death and decay.

Entropy

The **second law of thermodynamics** states that energy spontaneously disperses from being localized to becoming spread out if it is not hindered from doing so. Pay attention to this: *the usual way of thinking about entropy as "disorder" must not be taken too literally, a trap that many students fall into. Be very careful in thinking about entropy as disorder.* The old analogy between a messy (disordered) room and entropy is deficient and may not only hinder understanding but actually increase confusion.

Entropy is the measure of the spontaneous dispersal of energy at a specific temperature: *how much* energy is spread out, or *how widely* spread out energy becomes in a process. In the discussion of microstates earlier, we considered that when ice melts, the freedom of movement of the water molecules increases. If the water remains at the melting point, it will have the same average kinetic energy as molecules of ice; the difference between the two is the number of available microstates. That is, while both water and ice at 0°C have the same kinetic energy, the energy is dispersed over a larger number of microstates in liquid water. Liquid water therefore has higher entropy and, by extension, it is indeed less organized than ice. The equation for calculating the change in entropy is:

$$\Delta S = \frac{Q_{\text{rev}}}{T}$$

Equation 3.7

where ΔS is the change in entropy, Q_{rev} is the heat that is gained or lost in a reversible process, and T is the temperature in kelvin. The units of entropy are usually $\frac{\text{J}}{\text{mol} \cdot \text{K}}$. When energy is distributed into a system at a given temperature, its entropy increases. When energy is distributed out of a system at a given temperature, its entropy decreases.

Example: If, in a reversible process, 5.46×10^4 J of heat is used to change a 200 g block of ice to water at a temperature of 273 K, what is the change in the entropy of the system? (Note: The heat of fusion of ice $= 333 \frac{\text{J}}{\text{g}}$.)

Solution: We know that during a phase change, the temperature is constant; in this case, 273 K. From the information given:

$$\Delta S = \frac{Q_{\text{rev}}}{T} = \frac{5.46 \times 10^4 \text{ J}}{273 \text{ K}} = 200 \frac{\text{J}}{\text{K}}$$

The amount of heat added did not exceed the amount needed to completely melt the block of ice, as calculated by:

$$q = mL = (200 \text{ g})\left(333 \frac{\text{J}}{\text{g}}\right) = 6.66 \times 10^4 \text{ J}$$

Therefore, no heat was applied to change the temperature of the resulting liquid and T remained constant.

Notice that the second law states that energy will spontaneously disperse; it does not say that energy can never be localized or concentrated. However, the concentration of energy will not happen spontaneously in a closed system. Work usually must be done to concentrate energy. For example, refrigerators work against the direction of spontaneous heat flow (that is, they counteract the flow of heat from the "warm" exterior of the refrigerator to the "cool" interior), thereby "concentrating" energy outside of the system in the surroundings. As a result, refrigerators consume a lot of energy to accomplish this movement of energy against the temperature gradient.

The second law has been described as *time's arrow* because there is a unidirectional limitation on the movement of energy by which we recognize *before and after* or *new and old*. For example, you would instantly recognize whether a video recording of an explosion was running forward or backward. Another way of understanding this is

KEY CONCEPT

The universe is a closed, expanding system, so you know that the entropy of the universe is always increasing. The more space that appears with the expansion of the universe, the more space there is for the entire universe's energy to be distributed and the total entropy of the universe to increase irreversibly.

to say that energy in a closed system will spontaneously spread out and entropy will increase if it is not hindered from doing so. Remember that a system can be variably defined to include the entire universe; in fact, the second law ultimately claims that the entropy of the universe is increasing.

$$\Delta S_{\text{universe}} = \Delta S_{\text{system}} + \Delta S_{\text{surroundings}} > 0$$

Equation 3.8

When describing processes, physicists often use terms such as natural, unnatural, reversible, or irreversible. These terms may sometimes be confusing but they are descriptive of observable phenomena. For example, we expect that when a hot object is brought into thermal contact with a cold object, the hot object will transfer heat energy to the cold object until both are in thermal equilibrium (that is, at the same temperature). This is a **natural process** and also one that we would describe as **irreversible**: we are not surprised that the two objects eventually reach a common temperature, but we would be shocked if all of a sudden the hot object became hotter and the cold object became colder. This would be an **unnatural process**.

To define a **reversible reaction**, let's consider a system of ice and liquid water in equilibrium at 0°C. If we place this mixture of ice and liquid water into a thermostat (device for regulating temperature) that is also at 0°C and allow infinitesimal amounts of heat to be absorbed by the ice from the thermostat so that the ice melts to liquid water at 0°C and the thermostat remains at 0°C, then the increase in the entropy of the system (the water) will be exactly equal to the entropy decrease of the surroundings (the thermostat). The net change in the entropy of the system and its surroundings is zero. Under these conditions, the process is reversible. The key to a reversible reaction is making sure that the process goes so slowly—requiring an infinite amount of time—that the system is always in equilibrium and no energy is lost or dissipated. To be frank, no real processes are reversible; we can only approximate a reversible process. Note how physicists define reversible processes: These are processes that can spontaneously reverse course. For example, while water can be put through cycles of freezing and melting innumerable times, ice melting on the warm countertop would not be expected to suddenly freeze if it remains in the warm environment. The liquid water will need to be placed in an environment that is cold enough to cause the water to freeze, and once frozen in the cold environment, the ice would not be expected to begin melting spontaneously. The freezing and melting of water in real life are therefore irreversible processes in *physics* while still being *chemically* reversible.

MCAT CONCEPT CHECK 3.4

Before you move on, assess your understanding of the material with these questions.

1. Describe entropy on a macroscopic level and in statistical terms.
   - Macroscopic:

   ____

   ____

   - Statistical:

   ____

   ____

2. What is the relationship between the entropy of a system and its surroundings for any thermodynamic process?

   ____

   ____

Conclusion

This chapter reviewed the zeroth law of thermodynamics, which reflects the observation that objects at the same temperature are in thermal equilibrium and the net heat exchanged between them is zero. We may consider the zeroth law to be *ex post facto* (after the fact) because it provides the thermodynamic explanation for the function of thermometers and temperature scales, which had been developed many years prior to the law's formulation. We then took some time to define basic thermodynamic terms for systems and state functions. Examination of the first law of thermodynamics revealed that the energy of a closed system (up to and including the universe) is constant, such that the total internal energy of a system (the sum of all its potential and motional energies) equals the heat gained by the system minus the work done by the system. Finally, we carefully investigated the second law of thermodynamics and the concept of entropy. We understand entropy as a measure not only of "disorder" but of the degree to which energy is spread out through a system, up to and including the universe. We now understand that the constant energy of the universe is progressively and irreversibly spreading out and will continue to spread out until there is an even distribution of energy throughout the universe. Many of these concepts will make a reappearance throughout our discussions of general chemistry, and will certainly be seen on the MCAT. In the next chapter, we'll investigate fluids, the final mechanical concept for Test Day.

GO ONLINE

You've reviewed the content, now test your knowledge and critical thinking skills by completing a test-like passage set in your online resources!

CONCEPT SUMMARY

Zeroth Law of Thermodynamics

- The **zeroth law of thermodynamics** states that objects are in thermal equilibrium when they are at the same temperature.
- Objects in thermal equilibrium experience no net exchange of heat energy.
- **Temperature** is a qualitative measure of how hot or cold an object is; quantitatively, it is related to the average kinetic energy of the particles that make up a substance.
- **Thermal expansion** describes how a substance changes in length or volume as a function of the change in temperature.

Systems

- A thermodynamic **system** is the portion of the universe that we are interested in observing, whereas the **surroundings** include everything that is not part of the system.
    - **Isolated systems** do not exchange matter or energy with the surroundings.
    - **Closed systems** exchange energy but not matter with their surroundings.
    - **Open systems** exchange both energy and matter with their surroundings.
- **State functions** are pathway independent and are not themselves defined by a process. Pressure, density, temperature, volume, enthalpy, internal energy, Gibbs free energy, and entropy are all state functions.
- **Process functions** describe the pathway from one equilibrium state to another. Work and heat are process functions.

First Law of Thermodynamics

- The **first law of thermodynamics** is a statement of conservation of energy: the total energy in the universe can never decrease or increase.
- For a closed system, the total internal energy is equal to the heat flow into the system minus the work done by the system.
- **Heat** is the process of energy transfer between two objects at different temperatures that occurs until the two objects come into thermal equilibrium (reach the same temperature).
    - **Specific heat** is the amount of energy necessary to raise one gram of a substance by one degree Celsius or one kelvin.
    - The specific heat of water is $1\ \frac{\text{cal}}{\text{g}\cdot\text{K}}$.
    - During a phase change, heat energy causes changes in the particles' potential energy and energy distribution (entropy), but not kinetic energy. Therefore, there is no change in temperature. This is the **heat of transformation**.

- There are four special types of thermodynamic systems in which a given variable is held constant:
  - For **isothermal processes**, the temperature is constant, and the change in internal energy is therefore 0.
  - For **adiabatic processes**, no heat is exchanged.
  - For **isobaric processes**, the pressure is held constant.
  - For **isovolumetric (isochoric) processes**, the volume is held constant and the work done by or on the system is 0.

Second Law of Thermodynamics and Entropy

- The **second law of thermodynamics** states that in a closed system (up to and including the entire universe), energy will spontaneously and irreversibly go from being localized to being spread out (dispersed).
- **Entropy** is a measure of how much energy has spread out or how spread out energy has become.
- On a statistical level, as the number of available **microstates** increases, the potential energy of a molecule is distributed over that larger number of microstates, increasing entropy.
- Every **natural process** is ultimately **irreversible**; under highly controlled conditions, certain equilibrium processes such as phase changes can be treated as essentially **reversible**.

ANSWERS TO CONCEPT CHECKS

3.1

1. The zeroth law of thermodynamics states that when two objects are both in thermal equilibrium with a third object, they are in thermal equilibrium with each other. By extension, no heat flows between two objects in thermal equilibrium.
2. While there may be a distance at which thermal equilibrium is impractical, there is no theoretical maximum distance. As long as two objects are in thermal contact and at the same temperature, they are in thermal equilibrium.
3. Expansion is a result of an increase in dimension at all points along an object. If an object is initially longer, it will experience a greater expansion. This is also represented in the formula for thermal expansion because there is a direct relationship between length change and the initial length of an object.
4. False. As we will discuss in Chapter 11 of *MCAT Physics and Math Review*, accuracy is related to an instrument, rather than the scale. In addition, Kelvin uses the same scale as Celsius, so there are no practical differences in terms of accuracy.

3.2

1.

System Type	Transfers Matter	Transfers Energy
Closed	No	Yes
Isolated	No	No
Open	Yes	Yes

2. State functions are variables independent from the path taken to achieve a particular equilibrium and are properties of a given system at equilibrium; they may be dependent on one another. Process functions define the path (or how the system got to its state) through variables such as Q (heat) or W (work).
3. State functions include pressure (P), density (ρ), temperature (T), volume (V), enthalpy (H), internal energy (U), Gibbs free energy (G), and entropy (S).

3.3

1. The change in the internal energy of a system is equal to heat put into a system minus the work done by the system. This is the first law of thermodynamics.
2. Conduction is heat exchange by direct molecular interactions. Convection is heat exchange by fluid movement. Radiation is heat exchange by electromagnetic waves, and does not depend on matter.
3.

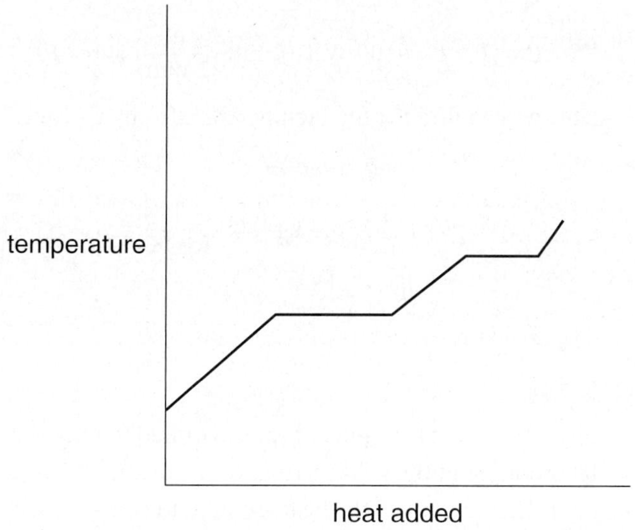

4. In a P–V graph, work is the area under the curve (or within a closed loop).

3.4

1. On a macroscopic level, entropy can be thought of as the tendency toward disorder. Statistically, entropy is the measure of the spontaneous dispersal of energy at a specific temperature, increasing the number of available microstates for a given molecule.
2. The entropy of a system and its surroundings will never decrease; entropy will always either remain constant or increase.

SCIENCE MASTERY ASSESSMENT EXPLANATIONS

1. **C**

The kelvin unit and Celsius degree are the same size; that is, a change of 10 K is equal to a change of 10°C. One degree Celsius is equal to 1.8 degrees Fahrenheit; therefore, 10°C = 18°F.

2. **A**

Because there is essentially only empty space between the Sun and the Earth, the only means of heat transfer is by radiation—electromagnetic waves that propagate across space. When a metal spoon is placed in a pot of hot soup, the molecules in the soup collide with those on the surface of the spoon, thereby transferring heat by conduction. Finally, fire warms the air above it, and the warmed air is less dense than the surrounding air, so it rises. A rising column of warm air means that heat is being transported in the air mass, which is simply the process of convection. The smoke particles ride along with the upward moving air current and create a plume of smoke.

3. **C**

The magnitude of one degree Celsius equals the magnitude of one unit kelvin. Therefore, a change of 100°C is equal to a change of 100 K. We can then find the change in length due to thermal expansion:

$$\Delta L = \alpha L \Delta T = \left(1.1\times10^{-5}\ \text{K}^{-1}\right)(20\ \text{m})(100\ \text{K})$$
$$= 0.022\ \text{m} = 2.2\ \text{cm}$$

Because the rod is originally 2.5 cm above the ground and its length increases by 2.2 cm, we can conclude that it will not touch the ground after the thermal expansion process is completed.

4. **C**

To answer this question, first remember that watts are equal to joules per second; in other words, power is energy transfer over time. In 10 minutes, the tool absorbs the following amount of energy:

$$E = P\times t = (100\ \text{W})(10\ \text{min})\left(\frac{60\ \text{s}}{1\ \text{min}}\right) = 6\times10^4\ \text{J}$$

Now we can find the final temperature from this equation:

$$q = mc\Delta T$$
$$6\times10^4\ \text{J} = (3\ \text{kg})\left(500\ \frac{\text{J}}{\text{kg}\cdot\text{K}}\right)\Delta T$$
$$40^\circ\text{C} = \Delta T$$

The final temperature is thus 20 + 40 = 60°C.

5. **D**

First determine how much heat is required to raise the temperature of the gold earrings to the melting point of gold. Then, calculate the heat required to actually melt the earrings (the latent heat). The total heat required to melt the earrings completely will be the sum of the two heats. The heat required to raise the temperature of the earrings from 25°C to 1064°C is

$$q = mc\Delta T = (0.5\ \text{kg})\left(126\ \frac{\text{J}}{\text{kg}\cdot\text{K}}\right)(1039\ \text{K})$$
$$\approx 60\times1000 = 60\ \text{kJ}$$

Thus, it takes about 60 kJ of heat to bring the earrings to their melting point. The next step is to calculate how much heat is needed to melt the earrings. For this, use the heat of fusion (the latent heat) of gold:

$$q = mL = (0.5\ \text{kg})\left(6.37\times10^4\ \frac{\text{J}}{\text{kg}}\right) = 32\ \text{kJ}$$

So overall, it requires approximately 60 + 32 = 92 kJ of heat to melt the gold earrings. Notice that we can heavily approximate the numbers used in our calculations because the answer choices are so spread out. The closest answer is **(D)**.

6. **C**

The total work done by the cycle is the sum of the work of paths A, B, and C, or the area within the cycle. Because the area bounded by A, B, and C is a triangle with a base of 5 m^3 and a height of 3 Pa, we can calculate the area as $\frac{1}{2}\left(5\ \text{m}^3\right)(3\ \text{Pa}) = 7.5$ J. Clockwise loops tend to do positive work on the environment, while counterclockwise loops do negative work.

7. **B**

To answer the question, make sure you understand all the terms. An adiabatic process means that there is no exchange of heat; in other words, $Q = 0$. When a gas is compressed, positive work is being done *on* the gas (rather than *by* the gas), so the value for work done *by* the gas will be negative ($W < 0$). Based on this, we can determine how the internal energy of the gas changes by using the first law of thermodynamics ($\Delta U = Q - W$). If $Q = 0$ and W is negative, then ΔU is positive.

8. **B**

The entropy of a system can decrease as long as the entropy of its surroundings increases by at least as much. On the other hand, the entropy of an isolated system increases for all real (irreversible) processes. This adheres to the second law of thermodynamics, which says that energy will be dispersed and entropy of the universe will remain constant or increase during all processes.

9. **A**

Calorimeters are our best approximations of isolated systems, where neither energy nor matter is exchanged with the environment. By failing to use an insulating layer and failing to fully contain the system, heat can be exchanged with the environment and matter may be dispersed, creating an open system.

10. **A**

To find the amount of heat needed to bring the substance to its melting point, you can use the specific heat. To heat one mole of the substance one unit kelvin, it would take 1 J of heat. After the substance reaches its melting point, additional heat is needed to actually induce the phase change. Therefore, the total amount of heat required is greater than 1 J.

11. **B**

State functions are any that are independent of the path taken to achieve a given state and which are not themselves defined as a process, such as pressure, density, temperature, volume, enthalpy, internal energy, Gibbs free energy, and entropy. Heat and work are process functions that are pathway dependent.

12. **C**

In this situation, heat will transfer from the warm gas to the metal and then to the cold gas. Convection requires flow of a fluid to cause heat transfer, invalidating **(B)** as an answer. In this case, the gas is not flowing, but rather is in contact with the metal. **(A)** is an invalid answer because heat transfer through radiation is also implausible not only because gases are unlikely to emit heat in the form of waves but also because the radiation would be unlikely to penetrate the thick metal container. Enthalpy, **(D)**, is not a form of heat transfer. Conduction, **(C)**, is the most likely option; it happens when two substances make direct contact with one another. Here, gas A makes contact with the metal container, which makes contact with gas B.

13. **D**

Saying that substance B has a higher internal energy cannot explain the phenomenon because the internal energy is irrelevant; the heat involved in the process is related only to the specific heat, the heat of fusion, and the heat of vaporization. All of the other choices could explain the phenomenon. The heat required to melt the solid is determined by the heat of fusion, **(C)**. The heat required to bring the liquid to its boiling point is determined by the specific heat, **(A)**. The heat required to boil the liquid is determined by the heat of vaporization, **(B)**.

14. **B**

When the ink randomly intersperses throughout the water, the final state is more disordered than the initial state, so the entropy change of the system is positive. When the oil separates from the water, the final state is just as ordered as the initial state (because the oil and the water are still completely separate), so the entropy change is zero. You can also answer this question by noticing the reversibility of the two experiments. Experiment A has a positive entropy change because it is irreversible, while experiment B has no entropy change because the reaction is reversible. According to the second law of thermodynamics, the overall entropy change of a system and its surroundings can never be negative in a thermodynamic process that moves from one equilibrium state to another.

15. **C**

If a substance is undergoing a phase change, any added heat will be used toward overcoming the heat of transformation of the phase change. During the phase change, the temperature will remain constant. Temperature is a measure of the kinetic energy of the molecules in a sample, so a change in kinetic energy, **(A)**, is essentially the same thing as a change in temperature. The heat transfer by radiation described in **(B)** will definitely change the temperature of the solid as long as it is not in the process of melting. **(D)** Describes heat transfer by convection, in which the warm gas will transfer heat to the cold gas until they both reach an intermediate temperature.

Consult your online resources for additional practice. **GO ONLINE**

EQUATIONS TO REMEMBER

(3.1) **Temperature conversions:** $F = \frac{9}{5}C + 32$

$K = C + 273$

(3.2) **Thermal expansion equation:** $\Delta L = \alpha L \Delta T$

(3.3) **Volume expansion equation:** $\Delta V = \beta V \Delta T$

(3.4) **First law of thermodynamics:** $\Delta U = Q - W$

(3.5) **Heat gained or lost (with temperature change):** $q = mc\Delta T$

(3.6) **Heat gained or lost (phase change):** $q = mL$

(3.7) **Entropy and heat:** $\Delta S = \frac{Q_{\text{rev}}}{T}$

(3.8) **Second law of thermodynamics:** $\Delta S_{\text{universe}} = \Delta S_{\text{system}} + \Delta S_{\text{surroundings}} > 0$

SHARED CONCEPTS

Biochemistry Chapter 12
Bioenergetics and Regulation of Metabolism

General Chemistry Chapter 6
Equilibrium

General Chemistry Chapter 7
Thermochemistry

General Chemistry Chapter 8
The Gas Phase

General Chemistry Chapter 12
Electrochemistry

Physics and Math Chapter 2
Work and Energy

CHAPTER 4

FLUIDS

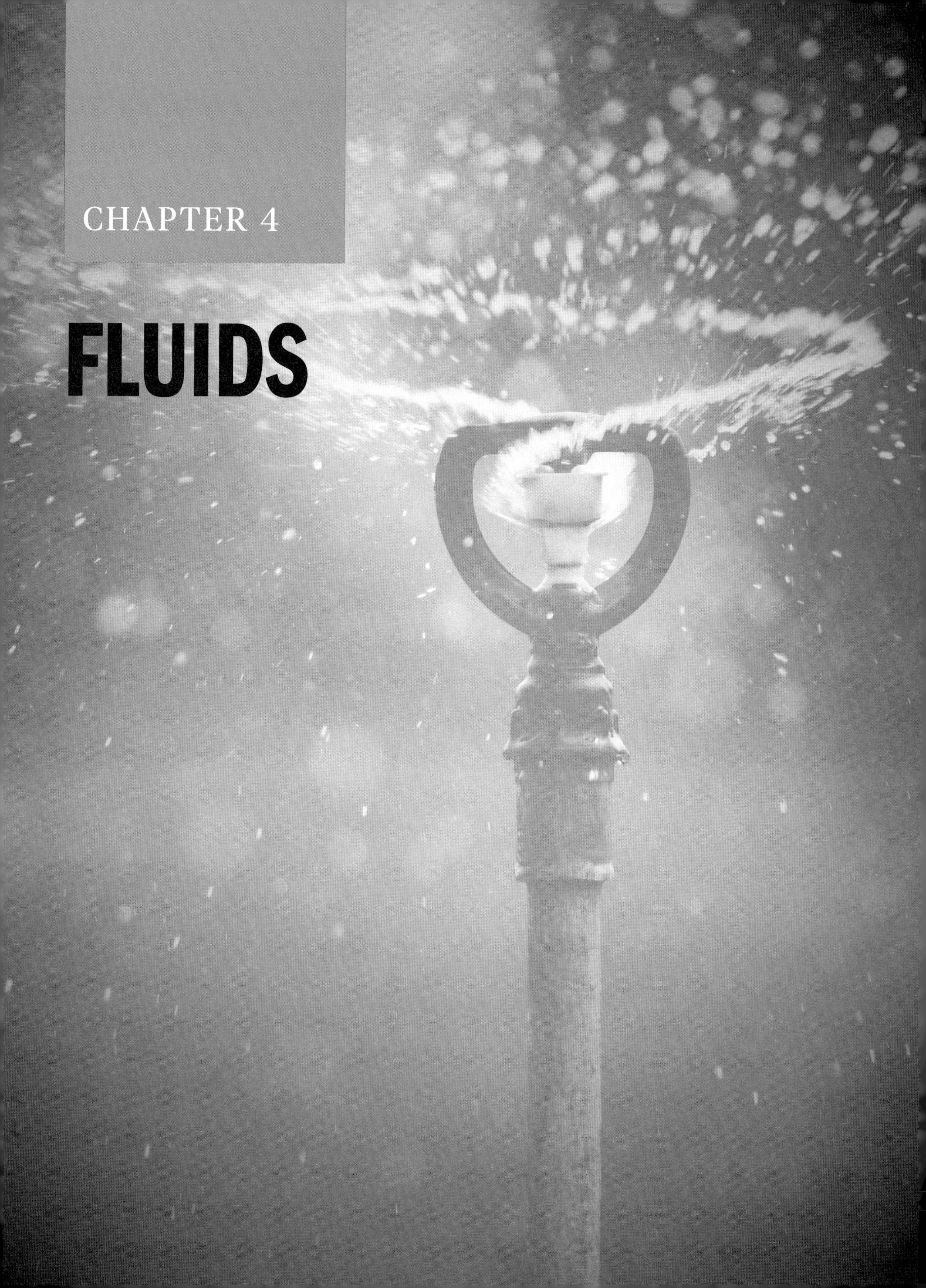

SCIENCE MASTERY ASSESSMENT

Every pre-med knows this feeling: there is so much content I have to know for the MCAT! How do I know what to do first or what's important?

While the high-yield badges throughout this book will help you identify the most important topics, this Science Mastery Assessment is another tool in your MCAT prep arsenal. This quiz (which can also be taken in your online resources) and the guidance below will help ensure that you are spending the appropriate amount of time on this chapter based on your personal strengths and weaknesses. Don't worry though—skipping something now does not mean you'll never study it. Later on in your prep, as you complete full-length tests, you'll uncover specific pieces of content that you need to review and can come back to these chapters as appropriate.

How to Use This Assessment

If you answer 0–7 questions correctly:

Spend about 1 hour to read this chapter in full and take limited notes throughout. Follow up by reviewing **all** quiz questions to ensure that you now understand how to solve each one.

If you answer 8–11 questions correctly:

Spend 20–40 minutes reviewing the quiz questions. Beginning with the questions you missed, read and take notes on the corresponding subchapters. For questions you answered correctly, ensure your thinking matches that of the explanation and you understand why each choice was correct or incorrect.

If you answer 12–15 questions correctly:

Spend less than 20 minutes reviewing all questions from the quiz. If you missed any, then include a quick read-through of the corresponding subchapters, or even just the relevant content within a subchapter, as part of your question review. For questions you got correct, ensure your thinking matches that of the explanation and review the Concept Summary at the end of the chapter.

1. Objects A and B are submerged at a depth of 1 m in a liquid with a specific gravity of 0.877. Given that the density of object B is one-third that of object A and that the gauge pressure of object A is 3 atm, what is the gauge pressure of object B? (Note: Assume atmospheric pressure is 1 atm and $g = 9.8\ \frac{m}{s^2}$.)
   - **A.** 1 atm
   - **B.** 2 atm
   - **C.** 3 atm
   - **D.** 9 atm

2. An anchor made of iron weighs 833 N on the deck of a ship. If the anchor is now suspended in seawater by a massless chain, what is the tension in the chain? (Note: The density of iron is $7800\ \frac{kg}{m^3}$ and the density of seawater is $1025\ \frac{kg}{m^3}$.)
   - **A.** 100 N
   - **B.** 724 N
   - **C.** 833 N
   - **D.** 957 N

3. Two wooden balls of equal volume but different density are held beneath the surface of a container of water. Ball A has a density of $0.5\ \frac{g}{m^3}$, and ball B has a density of $0.7\ \frac{g}{cm^3}$. When the balls are released, they will accelerate upward to the surface. What is the relationship between the acceleration of ball A and that of ball B?
   - **A.** Ball A has the greater acceleration.
   - **B.** Ball B has the greater acceleration.
   - **C.** Balls A and B have the same acceleration.
   - **D.** It cannot be determined from information given.

4. Water flows from a pipe of diameter 0.15 m into one of diameter 0.2 m. If the speed in the 0.15 m pipe is $8\ \frac{m}{s}$, what is the speed in the 0.2 m pipe?
   - **A.** $3\ \frac{m}{s}$
   - **B.** $3.7\ \frac{m}{s}$
   - **C.** $4.5\ \frac{m}{s}$
   - **D.** $6\ \frac{m}{s}$

5. A hydraulic lever is used to lift a heavy hospital bed, requiring an amount of work *W*. When the same bed with a patient is lifted, the work required is doubled. How can the cross-sectional area of the platform on which the bed is lifted be changed so that the pressure on the hydraulic lever remains constant?
   - **A.** The cross-sectional area must be doubled.
   - **B.** The cross-sectional area must be halved.
   - **C.** The cross-sectional area must be divided by four.
   - **D.** The cross-sectional area must remain constant.

6. The figure shown represents a section through a horizontal pipe of varying diameters into which four open vertical pipes connect. If water is allowed to flow through the pipe in the direction indicated, in which of the vertical pipes will the water level be lowest?

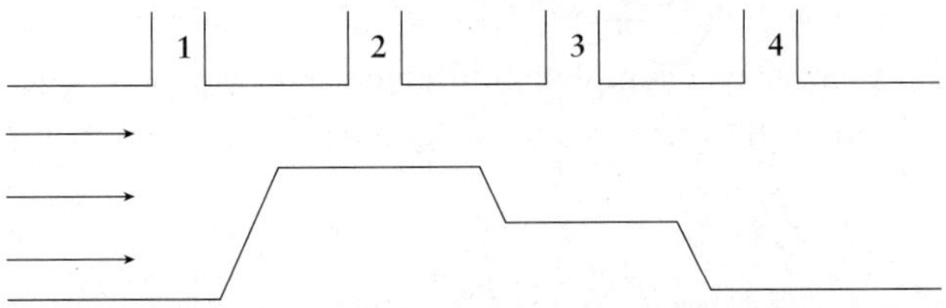

   - **A.** Pipe 1
   - **B.** Pipe 2
   - **C.** Pipe 3
   - **D.** Pipe 4

7. The speed of blood in the aorta is much higher than the speed of blood through a capillary bed. How can this fact be explained using the continuity equation, assuming that we are interested in average flow and that there is no net fluid loss?
   - **A.** The aorta is located higher than the capillary bed.
   - **B.** The pressure in the aorta is the same as the pressure in the capillary bed.
   - **C.** The cross-sectional area of all the capillaries added together is much greater than the cross-sectional area of the aorta.
   - **D.** The cross-sectional area of a capillary is much smaller than the cross-sectional area of the aorta.

8. Which of the following data sets is sufficient to determine the linear speed through an area of a rigid pipe?
   - **A.** The cross-sectional area in another segment of pipe and the cross-sectional area in the region of interest
   - **B.** The Reynolds number, viscosity of the fluid, density, and diameter of the pipe
   - **C.** The radius of the pipe, pressure gradient, viscosity, and length of the pipe
   - **D.** The absolute pressure and density

9. An object with a density of 2 g/cm^3 is submerged to a depth of 25 cm in a container of dichloromethane. If the specific gravity of dichloromethane is 1.33, what is the total pressure exerted on the submerged object?
   - **A.** 3.3 kPa
   - **B.** 104 kPa
   - **C.** 332 kPa
   - **D.** 433 kPa

10. A hydraulic system is designed to allow water levels to change depending on a force applied at the top of the tank as shown. If a force, F_1, of 4 N is applied to a square, flexible cover where $A_1 = 16$, and the area $A_2 = 64$, what force must be applied to A_2 to keep the water levels from changing?

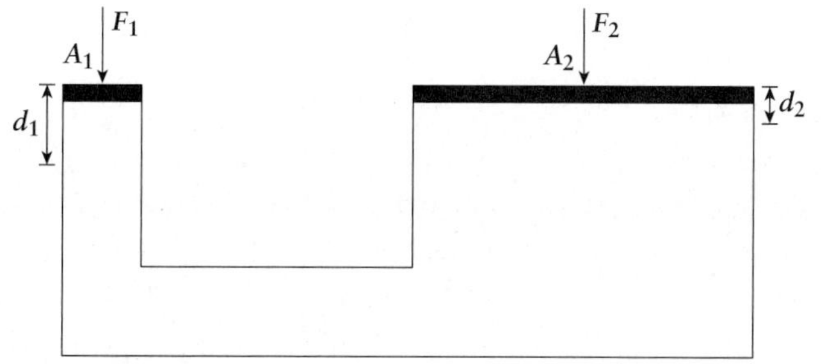

   - **A.** 4 N
   - **B.** 16 N
   - **C.** 32 N
   - **D.** No force needs to be applied.

11. Balls A and B of equal mass (shown below) are fully submerged in a swimming pool. Which ball will produce the greater buoyant force?

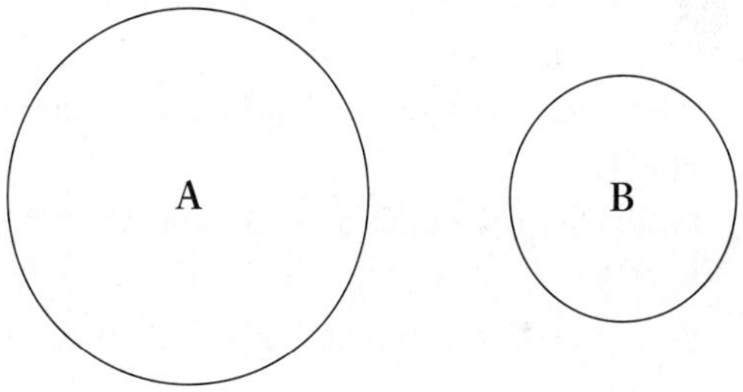

   - **A.** Ball A
   - **B.** Ball B
   - **C.** The forces will be equal.
   - **D.** It is impossible to know without knowing the exact volume of each ball.

12. Which of the following correctly describes blood flow through the circulatory system?
   - **A.** The flow rate is constant.
   - **B.** Pressure created by the heart moves blood through venous circulation.
   - **C.** The volume of blood entering and exiting the heart in a single cycle is equal.
   - **D.** The resistance of an artery is greater than the resistance of an arteriole.

13. A low-pressure weather system can decrease the atmospheric pressure from 1 atm to 0.99 atm. By what percent will this decrease the force on a rectangular window from the outside? (Note: Assume the window is 6 m by 3 m and the glass is 3 cm thick.)
   - **A.** 1%
   - **B.** 10%
   - **C.** $\left(\frac{1}{3}\right)$%
   - **D.** 30%

14. Two fluids, A and B, have densities of x and $2x$, respectively. They are tested independently to assess absolute pressure at varying depths. At what depths will the pressure below the surface of these two fluids be equal?
   - **A.** Whenever the depth of fluid A is one-half that of fluid B
   - **B.** Whenever the depth of fluid A equals that of fluid B
   - **C.** Whenever the depth of fluid A is 2 times that of fluid B
   - **D.** Whenever the depth of fluid A is 4 times that of fluid B

15. A water tower operator is interested in increasing the pressure of a column of water that is applied to a piston. The operator hopes that increasing the pressure will increase the force being applied to the piston. The only way to increase the pressure is to alter the speed of the water as it flows through the pipe to the piston. How should the speed of the water be changed to increase the pressure and force?
   - **A.** Increase the speed
   - **B.** Decrease the speed
   - **C.** Release water intermittently against the pipe
   - **D.** The speed of water will not change pressure at the piston.

Answer Key follows on next page.

Answer Key

1. **C**
2. **B**
3. **A**
4. **C**
5. **A**
6. **B**
7. **C**
8. **C**
9. **B**
10. **B**
11. **A**
12. **C**
13. **A**
14. **C**
15. **B**

Detailed explanations can be found at the end of the chapter.

CHAPTER 4

FLUIDS

In This Chapter

Introduction

Hidden beneath the waves of the Mediterranean Sea, at depths of more than 4,000 meters, lie three lakes. The water in these "seas under the sea" is so salty—five to ten times saltier than the seawater that sits above it—that its extreme density prevents it from mixing with the ocean water above, forming a layer of separation not unlike that between the oil and vinegar in a bottle of salad dressing. These underwater lakes behave eerily like their more common cousins found at sea level. They have tides, shore lines, beach ridges, and swash zones. When deep sea exploratory vessels set down on their surfaces, the vessels bob up and down, causing ripples to emanate outward like a stone dropped in a pond.

Suboceanic lakes and rivers present a particularly fascinating opportunity to illustrate the physics of fluids and solids. This chapter covers the important concepts and principles of fluid mechanics as they are tested on the MCAT. We will begin with a review of some important terms and measurements, including density and pressure. Our next topic will be hydrostatics, the branch of fluid mechanics that characterizes the behavior of fluids at rest. We'll then turn our attention to fluid dynamics, including Bernoulli's equation and the aerodynamics of flight. Finally, the chapter concludes with a discussion of fluid dynamics in physiology, examining the properties that motivate the movement of blood and air within the body.

CHAPTER PROFILE

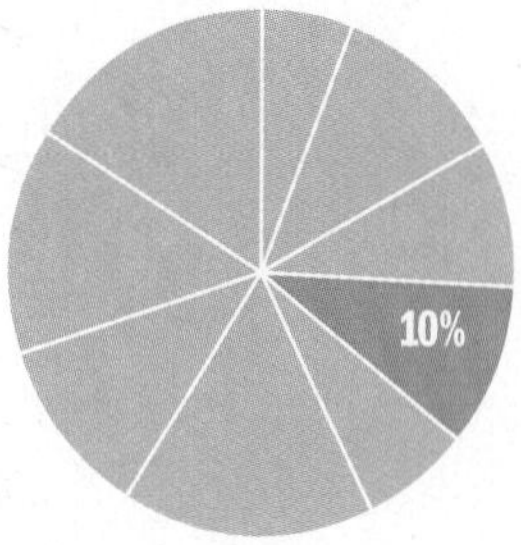

The content in this chapter should be relevant to about 10% of all questions about physics on the MCAT.

This chapter covers material from the following AAMC content categories:

4B: Importance of fluids for the circulation of blood, gas movement, and gas exchange

4E: Atoms, nuclear decay, electronic structure, and atomic chemical behavior

4.1 Characteristics of Fluids and Solids

LEARNING OBJECTIVES

After Chapter 4.1, you will be able to:

- Predict when gauge pressure will be equal to fluid pressure for a column of fluid
- Relate weight and density for an object
- Recall the common units for pressure, as well as the equations for gauge pressure and absolute pressure

Fluids are characterized by their ability to flow and conform to the shapes of their containers. **Solids**, on the other hand, do not flow and are rigid enough to retain a shape independent of their containers. Both liquids and gases are fluids. The natural gas (methane) that many of us use to cook flows through pipes to the burners of our stove and ovens, and the air that we breathe flows in and out of our lungs, filling the spaces of our respiratory tract and the alveoli.

Fluids and solids share certain characteristics. Both can exert forces perpendicular to their surface, although only solids can withstand **shear (tangential) forces**. Fluids can impose large perpendicular forces; falling into water from a significant height can be just as painful as falling onto a solid surface.

Density

All fluids and solids are characterized by the ratio of their mass to their volume. This is known as **density**, which is a scalar quantity and therefore has no direction. The equation for density is

$$\rho = \frac{m}{V}$$

Equation 4.1

where ρ (rho) represents density, m is mass, and V is volume. The SI units for density are $\frac{\text{kg}}{\text{m}^3}$, but you may find it convenient to use $\frac{\text{g}}{\text{mL}}$ or $\frac{\text{g}}{\text{cm}^3}$, both of which may be seen on the MCAT. Remember that a milliliter and a cubic centimeter are the same volume. A word of caution: students sometimes assume that if the mL and the cm^3 are equivalent, then so must be the liter and the m^3. This is absolutely not the case; in fact, there are 1000 liters in a cubic meter. For the MCAT, it is important to know the density of water, which is $1\ \frac{\text{g}}{\text{cm}^3} = 1000\ \frac{\text{kg}}{\text{m}^3}$.

The weight of any volume of a given substance with a known density can be calculated by multiplying the substance's density by its volume and the acceleration due to gravity. This is a calculation that appears frequently when working through buoyancy problems on Test Day:

$$\mathbf{F}_g = \rho V g$$

Equation 4.2

The density of a fluid is often compared to that of pure water at 1 atm and 4°C, a variable called **specific gravity**. It is at this combination of pressure and temperature that water has a density of exactly 1 $\frac{g}{cm^3}$. The specific gravity is given by

$$SG = \frac{\rho}{1\ \frac{g}{cm^3}}$$

Equation 4.3

This is a unitless number that is usually expressed as a decimal. The specific gravity can be used as a tool for determining if an object will sink or float in water, as described later in this chapter.

MCAT EXPERTISE

If an object's density is given in $\frac{g}{cm^3}$, its specific gravity is simply its density as a dimensionless number. This is because the density of water in $\frac{g}{cm^3}$ is 1.

Example: Find the specific gravity of benzene, given that its density is 877 $\frac{kg}{m^3}$.

Solution: The ratio of the density of benzene to the density of water is the specific gravity. Either the numerator must be converted to $\frac{g}{cm^3}$ or the denominator (the density of water) must be given in $\frac{kg}{m^3}$:

$$SG = \frac{\rho}{1000\ \frac{kg}{m^3}} = \frac{877}{1000} = 0.877$$

Pressure

Pressure is a ratio of the force per unit area. The equation for pressure is

$$P = \frac{F}{A}$$

Equation 4.4

where P is pressure, F is the magnitude of the normal force vector, and A is the area. The SI unit of pressure is the **pascal (Pa)**, which is equivalent to the newton per square meter $\left(1\ \text{Pa} = 1\ \frac{N}{m^2}\right)$. Other commonly used units of pressure are millimeters of mercury (mmHg), torr, and the atmosphere (atm). Millimeters of mercury and torr are identical units. The unit of atmosphere is based on the average atmospheric pressure at sea level. The conversions between Pa, mmHg, torr, and atm are as follows:

$$1.013 \times 10^5\ \text{Pa} = 760\ \text{mmHg} \equiv 760\ \text{torr} = 1\ \text{atm}$$

Pressure is a scalar quantity, and therefore has a magnitude but no direction. It is easy to assume that pressure has a direction because it is related to a force, which is a vector. However, note that it is the magnitude of the normal force that is used. No matter where one positions a given surface, the pressure exerted on that surface within a closed container will be the same, neglecting gravity. For example, if we

MCAT EXPERTISE

If you ever forget the units of a variable, you can derive them from equations. You know that pressure equals force over area. Because you know the units of force (N) and area (m^2), you can solve for the base units of pascal by plugging these units into the equation: $\frac{N}{m^2}$.

placed a surface inside a closed container filled with gas, the individual molecules, which are moving randomly within the space, will exert pressure that is the same at all points within the container. Because the pressure is the same at all points along the walls of the container and within the space of the container itself, pressure applies in all directions at any point and, therefore, is a scalar rather than a vector. Of course, because pressure is a ratio of force to area, when unequal pressures are exerted against objects, the forces acting on the object will add in vectors, possibly resulting in acceleration. It's this difference in pressure that causes air to rush into and out of the lungs during respiration, windows to burst outward during a tornado, and the plastic covering a broken car window to bubble outward when the car is moving. Note that when gravity is present, this also results in a pressure differential, which we will explore with hydrostatics later in this chapter.

Example: The window of a skyscraper measures 2.0 m by 3.5 m. If a storm passes by and lowers the pressure outside the window to 0.997 atm while the pressure inside the building remains at 1 atm, what is the net force pushing on the window?

Solution: Because the pressures are different on the two sides of this window, there will be a net force pushing on it in the direction of the lower pressure (outside the window). The difference in pressure itself can be used to determine the net force:

$$\begin{aligned} F_{net} &= P_{net}A \\ &= (P_{inside} - P_{outside})A \\ &= (1 - 0.997 \text{ atm})\left(\frac{1.013 \times 10^5 \text{ Pa}}{1 \text{ atm}}\right)(2.0 \text{ m} \times 3.5 \text{ m}) \\ &\approx (0.003)(10^5)(7.0) = (3 \times 10^{-3})(10^5)(7.0) = 21 \times 10^2 \\ &= 2100 \text{ N (actual} = 2128 \text{ N)} \end{aligned}$$

Absolute Pressure

At this very moment, countless trillions of air molecules are exerting tremendous pressure on our bodies, with a total force of about 2×10^5 N! Of course, we don't actually feel all this pressure because our internal organs exert a pressure that perfectly balances it.

Atmospheric pressure changes with altitude. Residents of Denver (5280 feet above sea level) experience atmospheric pressure equal to 632 mmHg (0.83 atm), whereas travelers making their way through Death Valley (282 feet below sea level) experience atmospheric pressure equal to 767 mm Hg (1.01 atm). Atmospheric pressure impacts a number of processes, including hemoglobin's affinity for oxygen and the boiling of liquids.

Absolute (hydrostatic) pressure is the total pressure that is exerted on an object that is submerged in a fluid. Remember that fluids include both liquids and gases. The equation for absolute pressure is

$$P = P_0 + \rho g z$$

Equation 4.5

where P is the absolute pressure, P_0 is the **incident** or **ambient pressure** (the pressure at the surface), ρ is the density of the fluid, g is acceleration due to gravity, and z is the depth of the object. Do not make the mistake of assuming that P_0 always stands for atmospheric pressure. In open air and most day-to-day situations P_0 is equal to 1 atm, but in other fluid systems, the surface pressure may be higher or lower than atmospheric pressure. In a closed container, such as a pressure cooker, the pressure at the surface may be much higher than atmospheric pressure. This is, in fact, exactly the point of a pressure cooker, which allows food to cook at higher temperatures. This is because the increased pressure raises the boiling point of water in the food, thus reducing the cooking time and preventing loss of moisture.

REAL WORLD

A useful way to remember the two parts of the absolute pressure equation is to think of diving into a swimming pool. At the surface of the water, the absolute pressure is usually equal to the atmospheric pressure (P_0). But if you dive into the pool, the water exerts an extra pressure on you ($\rho g z$), in addition to the surface pressure. You feel this extra pressure on your eardrums.

Gauge Pressure

When you check the pressure in car or bike tires using a device known as a gauge, you are measuring the **gauge pressure**, which is the difference between the absolute pressure inside the tire and the atmospheric pressure outside the tire. In other words, gauge pressure is the amount of pressure in a closed space above and beyond atmospheric pressure. This is a more common pressure measurement than absolute pressure, and the equation is:

$$P_{gauge} = P - P_{atm} = (P_0 + \rho g z) - P_{atm}$$

Equation 4.6

Note that when $P_0 = P_{atm}$, then $P_{gauge} = P - P_0 = \rho g z$ at a depth z.

Example: A diver in the ocean is 20 m below the surface. What is the gauge pressure at that depth? What is the absolute pressure the diver experiences? (Note: The density of sea water is $1025\ \frac{\text{kg}}{\text{m}^3}$.)

Solution: Since the pressure at the surface (P_0) is equal to atmospheric pressure (P_{atm}), we can first solve for gauge pressure using the equation:

$$P_{gauge} = \rho g z = \left(1025\ \frac{\text{kg}}{\text{m}^3}\right)\left(9.8\ \frac{\text{m}}{\text{s}^2}\right)(20\ \text{m})$$
$$\approx (1000)(10)(20)$$
$$= 2 \times 10^5\ \text{Pa}\ (\text{actual} = 2.01 \times 10^5\ \text{Pa})$$

Then, we can solve for absolute pressure using the absolute pressure equation:

$$P = P_{atm} + P_{gauge} = 1.013 \times 10^5\ \text{Pa} + 2.01 \times 10^5\ \text{Pa} = 3.02 \times 10^5\ \text{Pa}$$

MCAT CONCEPT CHECK 4.1

Before you move on, assess your understanding of the material with these questions.

1. How does gauge pressure relate to the pressure exerted by a column of fluid?

2. What is the relationship between weight and density?

3. What is the SI unit for pressure? What are other common units of pressure?
   - SI unit:
   - Other units:

4. True or False: Density is a scalar quantity.

4.2 Hydrostatics

LEARNING OBJECTIVES

After Chapter 4.2, you will be able to:

- Distinguish between cohesion and adhesion
- Predict the appearance of the meniscus of a fluid given knowledge of its cohesive and adhesive properties
- Calculate the buoyant force acting on an object
- Apply the concept of specific gravity
- Solve hydraulic lift problems using Pascal's principle:

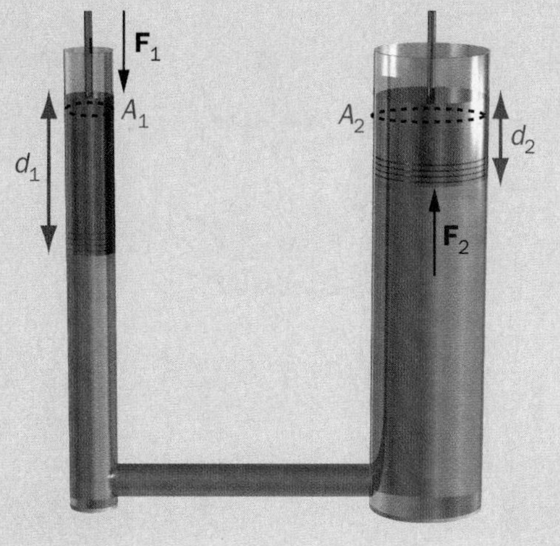

Hydrostatics is the study of fluids at rest and the forces and pressures associated with standing fluids. A proper understanding of hydrostatics is important for the MCAT because the testmakers frequently include passages and questions on hydraulics and buoyancy.

Pascal's Principle

For fluids that are incompressible—that is, fluids with volumes that cannot be reduced by any significant degree through application of pressure—a change in pressure will be transmitted undiminished to every portion of the fluid and to the walls of the containing vessel. This is **Pascal's principle**. For example, an unopened carton of milk could be considered an incompressible fluid in a closed container. If one were to squeeze the container, exerting an increased pressure on the sides of the milk carton, the applied pressure would be transmitted through the entire volume of milk. If the cap were to suddenly pop off, the resulting geyser of milk would be evidence of this increased pressure.

One application of Pascal's principle can be seen in **hydraulic systems**. These systems take advantage of the near-incompressibility of liquids to generate mechanical advantage, which, as we've seen in our discussion of inclined planes and pulleys in Chapter 2 of *MCAT Physics and Math Review*, allows us to accomplish a certain amount of work more easily by applying reduced forces. Many heavy machines use hydraulics, including car brakes, bulldozers, cranes, and lifts.

REAL WORLD

When the air pressure changes above a large body of water, the water level rises or falls to re-establish pressure equilibrium between the air and the water. The surface of a water body directly below a high-pressure air pocket forms a very small but measurable valley of water. A low-pressure air system has the opposite effect, creating a hill of water.

Figure 4.1 shows a simple diagram of a hydraulic lift. Let's determine how such a lift could allow an auto mechanic to raise a heavy car with far less force than the weight of the car. We have a closed container that is filled with an incompressible liquid. On the left side of the lift, there is a piston of cross-sectional area A_1. When this piston is pushed down the column, it exerts a force with a magnitude equal to F_1 and generates a pressure equal to P_1. The piston displaces a volume of liquid equal to A_1d_1 (the cross-sectional area times the distance gives a volume). Because the liquid inside is incompressible, the same volume of fluid must be displaced on the right side of the hydraulic lift, where we find a second piston with a much larger surface area, A_2. The pressure generated by piston 1 is transmitted undiminished to all points within the system, including to A_2. As A_2 is larger than A_1 by some factor, the magnitude of the force, F_2, exerted against A_2 must be greater than F_1 by the same factor so that $P_1 = P_2$, according to Pascal's principle.

$$P = \frac{F_1}{A_1} = \frac{F_2}{A_2}$$

$$F_2 = F_1\left(\frac{A_2}{A_1}\right)$$

Equation 4.7

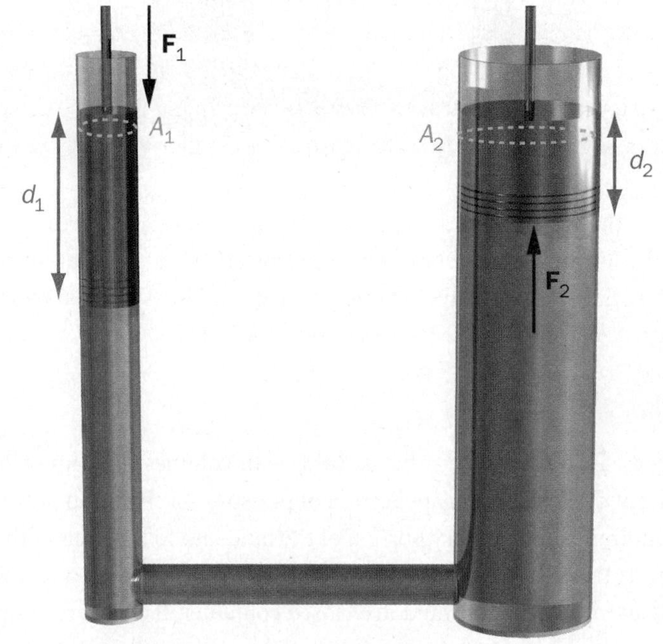

Figure 4.1 Hydraulic Lift

What this series of equations shows us is that hydraulic machines generate output force by magnifying an input force by a factor equal to the ratio of the cross-sectional area of the larger piston to that of the smaller piston. This does not violate the law of energy conservation; an analysis of the input and output work in a frictionless system reveals that there is indeed conservation of energy. As mentioned above, the volume of fluid displaced by piston 1 is equal to the volume of fluid displaced at piston 2.

$$V = A_1 d_1 = A_2 d_2$$
$$d_2 = d_1\left(\frac{A_1}{A_2}\right)$$

Combining the equations for pressure and volume, we can generate an equation for work as the product of constant pressure and volume change, as this is an isobaric process.

$$W = P\Delta V = \frac{F_1}{A_1}(A_1 d_1) = \frac{F_2}{A_2}(A_2 d_2)$$
$$= F_1 d_1 = F_2 d_2$$

This shows us the familiar form of work as the product of the magnitude of force and displacement (times the cosine of the angle between them, which is 0° in this case). Because the factor by which d_1 is larger than d_2 is equal to the factor by which F_2 is larger than F_1, we see that no additional work has been done or unaccounted for; the greater force F_2 is moving through a smaller distance d_2. Therefore, an auto mechanic needs only to exert a small force over a small area through a large distance to generate a much larger force over a larger area through a smaller distance.

KEY CONCEPT

Remember when applying Pascal's principle that the larger the area, the larger the force, although this force will be exerted through a smaller distance.

Example: A hydraulic press has a piston of radius 5 cm, which pushes down on an enclosed fluid. A 50 kg weight rests on this piston. Another piston in contact with this system has a radius of 20 cm. Taking $g = 10\ \frac{\text{m}}{\text{s}^2}$, what force is needed on the larger piston to keep the press in equilibrium?

Solution: Use Pascal's principle:

$$P = \frac{F_1}{A_1} = \frac{F_2}{A_2}$$
$$F_2 = F_1\left(\frac{A_2}{A_1}\right) = m_1 g\left(\frac{\pi r_2^2}{\pi r_1^2}\right) = m_1 g\left(\frac{r_2}{r_1}\right)^2$$
$$F_2 = (50\text{ kg})\left(10\ \frac{\text{m}}{\text{s}^2}\right)\left(\frac{20\text{ cm}}{5\text{ cm}}\right)^2 = (500)(4)^2 = (500)(16) = 8000\text{ N}$$

Archimedes' Principle

You may have heard some version of this story before: Archimedes, a physicist in ancient Greece, was tasked by his king to determine the metallic composition of a certain crown given to the king as a gift. Archimedes knew that he could do this by finding the crown's volume and mass, which would allow him to find its density and compare that density to those of known metals. Weighing the crown would be easy enough, but he was having trouble finding a way to measure its volume without melting it down and ruining its workmanship. Then one day, while getting into his bath, the water that overflowed from the tub gave him the idea to submerge the crown in water and measure the volume of the displaced liquid—*Eureka!*

The principle that derives from the story is one of Archimedes' lasting contributions to the field of physics. **Archimedes' principle** deals with the **buoyancy** of objects when placed in a fluid. It helps us understand how ships stay afloat and why we feel lighter when we're swimming. The principle states that a body wholly or partially immersed in a fluid will be buoyed upwards by a force equal to the weight of the fluid that it displaces.

Just as Archimedes' body and his crown caused the water level to rise in the tub, any object placed in a fluid will cause a volume of fluid to be displaced equal to the volume of the object that is submerged. Because all fluids have density, the volume of fluid displaced will correspond to a certain mass of that fluid. The mass of the fluid displaced exerts a force equal to its weight against the submerged object. This force, which is always directed upward, is called the buoyant force, and its magnitude is given by:

$$F_{\text{buoy}} = \rho_{\text{fluid}} V_{\text{fluid displaced}} g = \rho_{\text{fluid}} V_{\text{submerged}} g$$

Equation 4.8

MCAT EXPERTISE

The most common mistake students make using the buoyancy equation is to use the density of the object rather than the density of the fluid. Remember always to use the density of the fluid itself.

When an object is placed in a fluid, it will sink into the fluid only to the point at which the volume of displaced fluid exerts a force that is equal to the weight of the object. If the object becomes completely submerged and the volume of displaced fluid still does not exert a buoyant force equal to the weight of the object, the object will accelerate downward and sink to the bottom. This will be the case if an object is more dense than the fluid it's in—a gold crown will sink to the bottom of the bathtub because it is denser than water. On the other hand, an object that is less dense than water, such as a block of wood or an ice cube, will stop sinking (and start floating) because it is less dense than water. These objects will submerge enough of their volume to displace a volume of water equal to the object's weight.

KEY CONCEPT

An object will float if its average density is less than the average density of the fluid it is immersed in. It will sink if its average density is greater than that of the fluid.

One way to conceptualize the buoyant force is that it is the force of the liquid trying to return to the space from which it was displaced, thus trying to push the object up and out of the water. This is an important concept because the buoyant force is due to the liquid itself, not the object. If two objects placed in a fluid displace the same volume of fluid, they will experience the same magnitude of buoyant force even if the objects themselves have different masses.

How can one determine how much of a floating object lies below the surface? To do this, one can make comparisons of density or specific gravity. Remember that an object will float, no matter what it is made of and no matter how much mass it has, if its average density is less than or equal to the density of the fluid into which it is placed. If we express the object's specific gravity as a percent, this directly indicates the percent of the object's volume that is submerged (when the fluid is pure water). For instance, the density of ice is 0.92 $\frac{\text{g}}{\text{cm}^3}$, so its specific gravity is 0.92. An ice cube floating in a glass of water has 92 percent of its volume submerged in the water—only 8 percent is sitting above the surface. Therefore, any object with a specific gravity less than or equal to 1 will float in water and any object with a specific gravity greater than 1 will sink in water. A specific gravity of exactly 1 indicates that 100 percent of the object will be submerged but it will not sink.

Example: A wooden block floats in the ocean with half its volume submerged. Find the density of the wood ρ_b. (Note: The density of sea water is 1025 $\frac{\text{kg}}{\text{m}^3}$.)

Solution: The magnitude of the weight of the block of total volume V_b is

$$F_{g,b} = m_b g = \rho_b V_b g$$

The weight of the displaced seawater is the buoyant force and is given by

$$F_{buoy} = m_{water} g = \rho_{water} V_{water} g$$

V_{water} is the volume of displaced water, which is also the volume of the part of the block that is submerged $\left(\frac{V_b}{2}\right)$. Because the block is floating, the buoyant force equals the block's weight:

$$F_{g,b} = F_{buoy}$$

$$\rho_b V_b g = \rho_{water}\left(\frac{V_b}{2}\right) g$$

$$\rho_b = \frac{\rho_{water}}{2} = \frac{1025\ \frac{\text{kg}}{\text{m}^3}}{2} = 512.5\ \frac{\text{kg}}{\text{m}^3}$$

REAL WORLD

At first it may seem strange that cruise ships, constructed of dense metals and weighing thousands of kilograms, can float on water. But remember that any object will float if its average density is less than that of water. The steel hull of the ship would sink by itself, but all the air submerged beneath the water level, between the ship's lower decks, lowers the ship's average density to be less than that of water.

REAL WORLD

The Dead Sea is the deepest hypersaline lake in the world. Having a salt content of about 35 percent, it is almost nine times saltier than the ocean. All of this dissolved salt makes for some of the densest water on the surface of the Earth, with a specific gravity of 1.24. Humans have a specific gravity around 1.1; thus, in most bodies of water, we have a tendency to sink–but in the Dead Sea, one is unable to do anything but float.

Molecular Forces in Liquids

Water striders are insects that have the ability to walk on water. Water striders are able to glide across the water's surface without sinking, even though they are denser than water, because of a special physical property of liquids at the interface between a liquid and a gas. **Surface tension** causes the liquid to form a thin but strong layer like a "skin" at the liquid's surface. Surface tension results from **cohesion**, which is

REAL WORLD

Remember that cohesion occurs between molecules with the same properties. In a container of both water and oil, the water molecules will be cohesive with other water molecules, and the oil will be cohesive with other oil molecules.

the attractive force that a molecule of liquid feels toward other molecules of the same liquid. Consider the intermolecular forces between the separate molecules of liquid water. For those molecules below the surface, there are attractive intermolecular forces coming from all sides; these forces balance out. However, on the surface, the molecules only have these strong attractive forces from the molecules below them, which pulls the surface of the liquid toward the center. This establishes tension in the plane of the surface of the water; when there is an indentation on the surface (say, caused by a water strider's foot), then the cohesion can lead to a net upward force.

Another force that liquid molecules experience is **adhesion**, which is the attractive force that a molecule of the liquid feels toward the molecules of some other substance. For example, adhesive forces cause water molecules to form droplets on the windshield of a car even though gravity is pulling them downward. When liquids are placed in containers, a **meniscus**, or curved surface in which the liquid "crawls" up the side of the container a small amount, will form when the adhesive forces are greater than the cohesive forces. A **backwards (convex) meniscus** (with the liquid level higher in the middle than at the edges) occurs when the cohesive forces are greater than the adhesive forces. Mercury, the only metal that is liquid at room temperature, forms a backward meniscus when placed in a container. Both types of menisci are shown in Figure 4.2.

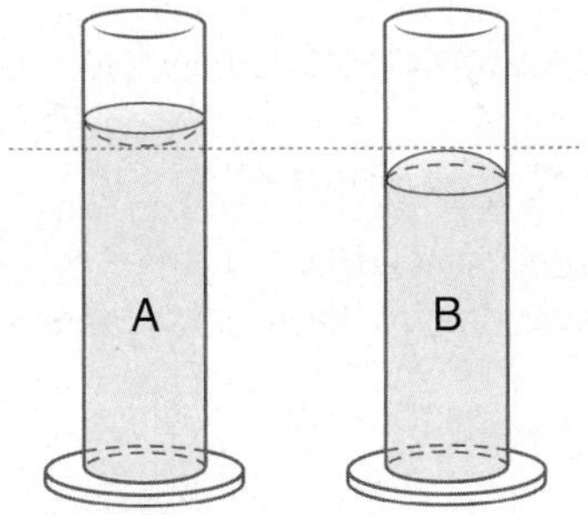

Figure 4.2 Types of Menisci

(A) A concave meniscus (more common); (B) A convex (backwards) meniscus. The dotted line indicates where measurements of depth or volume should be taken with each type of meniscus.

MCAT CONCEPT CHECK 4.2

Before you move on, assess your understanding of the material with these questions.

1. Contrast cohesion and adhesion.
   - Cohesion:

   - Adhesion:

   ---

2. What would the meniscus of a liquid that experiences equal cohesive and adhesive forces look like?

   ---

3. A block is fully submerged three inches below the surface of a fluid, but is not experiencing any acceleration. What can be said about the displaced volume of fluid and the buoyant force?

   ---

4. True or False: To determine the volume of an object by fluid displacement it must have a specific gravity greater than 1.
5. To which side of a hydraulic lift would the operator usually apply a force—the side with the larger cross-sectional area, or the side with the smaller cross-sectional area? Why?

4.3 Fluid Dynamics

High-Yield

LEARNING OBJECTIVES

After Chapter 4.3, you will be able to:

- Describe laminar flow, turbulent flow, dynamic and static pressure, pitot tubes, and viscosity
- Predict the behavior of fluids using the continuity equation, Bernoulli's equation, and the Venturi effect
- Recall the variables involved in flow rate

As the term suggests, **fluid dynamics** is the study of fluids in motion. This is perhaps one of the most fascinating areas of physics because its applications to real life are everywhere. Many aspects of our world, from water delivery to our homes to blood flow through our arteries and veins, can be analyzed and explained (at least in part) by the principles of fluid dynamics. The MCAT presents a relatively simplified version of the topic, making important assumptions such as rigid-walled containers and uniform density of fluids.

Viscosity

KEY CONCEPT

Low-viscosity fluids have low internal resistance to flow and behave like ideal fluids. Assume conservation of energy in low-viscosity fluids with laminar flow.

Some fluids flow very easily, while others barely flow at all. The resistance of a fluid to flow is called **viscosity** (η). Increased viscosity of a fluid increases its **viscous drag**, which is a nonconservative force that is analogous to air resistance. Thin fluids, like gases, water, and dilute aqueous solutions, have low viscosity and so they flow easily. Objects can move through these fluids with low viscous drag. Whole blood, vegetable oil, honey, cream, and molasses are thick fluids and flow more slowly. Objects can move through these fluids, but with significantly more viscous drag.

All fluids (except superfluids, which are not tested on the MCAT) are viscous to one degree or another; those with lower viscosities are said to behave more like ideal fluids, which have no viscosity and are described as **inviscid**. Because viscosity is a measure of a fluid's internal resistance to flow, more viscous fluids will "lose" more energy while flowing. Unless otherwise indicated, viscosity should be assumed to be negligible on Test Day, thus allowing Bernoulli's equation (explained later in this chapter) to be an expression of energy conservation for flowing fluids.

The SI unit of viscosity is the pascal–second $\left(\text{Pa}\cdot\text{s} = \frac{\text{N}\cdot\text{s}}{\text{m}^2}\right)$.

Laminar and Turbulent Flow

When a fluid is moving, its flow can be laminar or turbulent. **Laminar flow** is smooth and orderly, and is often modeled as layers of fluid that flow parallel to each other, as shown in Figure 4.3.

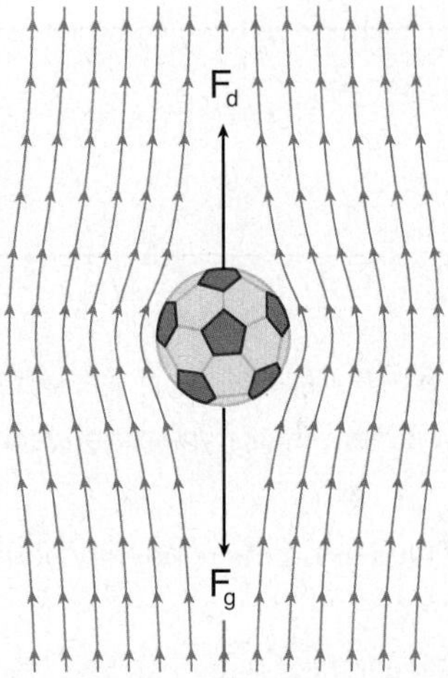

Figure 4.3 Laminar Flow around an Object in a Fluid
When the gravitational force is larger than the buoyant force, an object will sink. Laminar flow is characterized by smooth flow lines around the object.

The layers will not necessarily have the same linear speed. For example, the layer closest to the wall of a pipe flows more slowly than the more interior layers of fluid.

Poiseuille's Law

With laminar flow through a pipe or confined space, it is possible to calculate the rate of flow using **Poiseuille's law**:

$$Q = \frac{\pi r^4 \Delta P}{8\eta L}$$

Equation 4.9

where Q is the flow rate (volume flowing per time), r is the radius of the tube, ΔP is the pressure gradient, η (eta) is the viscosity of the fluid, and L is the length of the pipe. This equation is rarely tested in full; most often, MCAT passages and questions focus on the relationship between the radius and pressure gradient. Note that the relationship between the radius and pressure gradient is inverse exponential to the fourth power—even a very slight change in the radius of the tube has a significant effect on the pressure gradient, assuming a constant flow rate.

Turbulence and Speed

Turbulent flow is rough and disorderly. Turbulence causes the formation of **eddies**, which are swirls of fluid of varying sizes occurring typically on the downstream side of an obstacle, as shown in Figure 4.4.

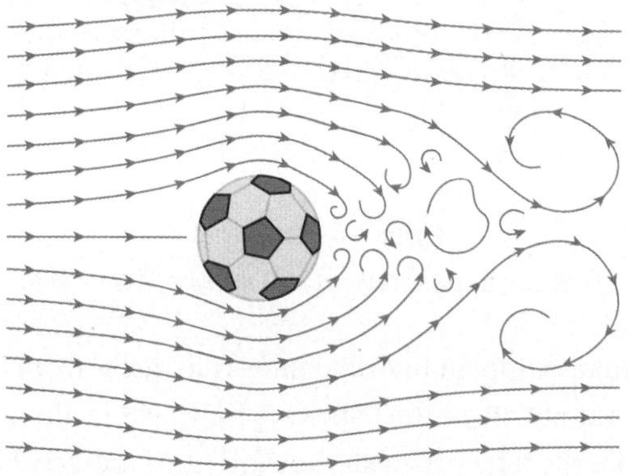

Figure 4.4 Turbulent Flow around an Object in a Fluid
Eddy formation downstream of an object obstructing laminar flow.

In unobstructed fluid flow, turbulence can arise when the speed of the fluid exceeds a certain **critical speed**. This critical speed depends on the physical properties of the fluid, such as its viscosity and the diameter of the tube. When the critical speed for a fluid is exceeded, the fluid demonstrates complex flow patterns, and laminar flow occurs only in the thin layer of fluid adjacent to the wall, called the **boundary layer**. The flow speed immediately at the wall is zero and increases uniformly throughout the layer. Beyond the boundary layer, however, the motion is highly irregular and turbulent. A significant amount of energy is dissipated from the system as a result of the increased frictional forces. Calculations of energy conservation, such as Bernoulli's equation, cannot be applied to turbulent flow systems. Luckily, the MCAT always assumes laminar (nonturbulent) flow for such questions.

For a fluid flowing through a tube of diameter D, the critical speed, v_c, can be calculated as

$$v_c = \frac{N_R \eta}{\rho D}$$

Equation 4.10

where v_c is the critical speed, N_R is a dimensionless constant called the Reynolds number, η is the viscosity of the fluid, and ρ is the density of the fluid. The **Reynolds number** depends on factors such as the size, shape, and surface roughness of any objects within the fluid.

Streamlines

Because the movement of individual molecules of a fluid is impossible to track with the unaided eye, it is often helpful to use representations of the molecular movement called **streamlines**. Streamlines indicate the pathways followed by tiny fluid elements (sometimes called fluid particles) as they move. The velocity vector of a fluid particle will always be tangential to the streamline at any point. Streamlines never cross each other.

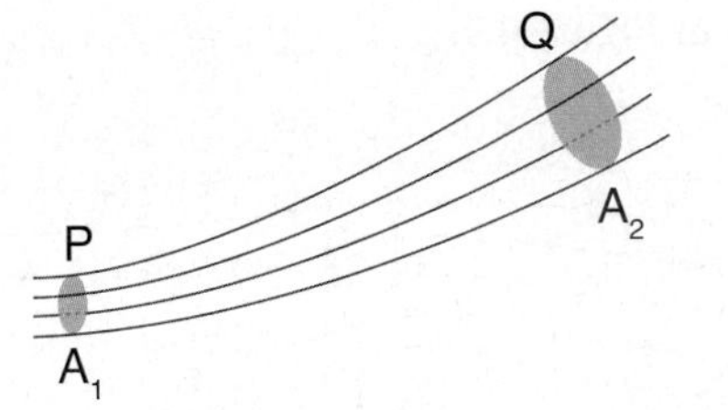

Figure 4.5 Streamlines
The stream's cross-sectional area increases from P to Q.

Figure 4.5 shows a fluid within an invisible tube as it passes from P to Q. The streamlines indicate some, but not all, of the pathways for the fluid along the walls of the tube. You'll notice that the tube gets wider toward Q, as indicated by the streamlines that are spreading out over the increased cross-sectional area. This leads us to consider the relationship between flow rate and the cross-sectional area of the container through which the fluid is moving. Once again, we can assume that the fluid is incompressible (which means that we are not considering a flowing gas). Because the fluid is incompressible, the rate at which a given volume (or mass) of fluid passes by one point must be the same for all other points in the closed system. This is essentially an expression of conservation of matter: if x liters of fluid pass a point in a given amount of time, then x liters of fluid must pass all other points in the system in the same amount of time. Thus, we can very clearly state, without any exceptions, the **flow rate** (that is, the volume per unit time) is constant for a closed system and is independent of changes in cross-sectional area.

While the flow rate is constant, the linear speed of the fluid does change relative to cross-sectional area. **Linear speed** is a measure of the linear displacement of fluid particles in a given amount of time. Notably, the product of linear speed and cross-sectional area is equal to the flow rate. We've already said that the volumetric rate of flow for a fluid must be constant throughout a closed system. Therefore:

$$Q = v_1 A_1 = v_2 A_2$$

Equation 4.11

where Q is the flow rate, v_1 and v_2 are the linear speeds of the fluid at points 1 and 2, respectively, and A_1 and A_2 are the cross-sectional areas at these points. This equation is known as the **continuity equation**, and it tells us that fluids will flow more quickly through narrow passages and more slowly through wider ones. Therefore, in Figure 4.5 earlier, while the flow rate at points P and Q are the same, the linear speed is faster at point P than point Q.

KEY CONCEPT

While flow rate is constant in a tube regardless of cross-sectional area, linear speed of a fluid will increase with decreasing cross-sectional area.

Bernoulli's Equation

Before we cover Bernoulli's equation itself, let's approach a flowing fluid from two perspectives that we've already discussed. First, the continuity equation arises from the conservation of mass of fluids. Liquids are essentially incompressible, so the flow rate within a closed space must be constant at all points. The continuity equation shows us that for a constant flow rate, there is an inverse relationship between the linear speed of the fluid and the cross-sectional area of the tube: fluids have higher speeds through narrower tubes.

Second, fluids that have low viscosity and demonstrate laminar flow can also be approximated to be conservative systems. The total mechanical energy of the system is constant if we discount the small viscous drag forces that occur in all real liquids.

Combining these principles of conservation, we arrive at **Bernoulli's equation**:

$$P_1 + \frac{1}{2}\rho v_1^2 + \rho g h_1 = P_2 + \frac{1}{2}\rho v_2^2 + \rho g h_2$$

Equation 4.12

where P is the absolute pressure of the fluid, ρ is the density of the fluid, v is the linear speed, g is acceleration due to gravity, and h is the height of the fluid above some datum. Some of the terms of Bernoulli's equation should look vaguely familiar. The term $\frac{1}{2}\rho v^2$ is sometimes called the **dynamic pressure**, and is the pressure associated with the movement of a fluid. This term is essentially the kinetic energy of the fluid divided by volume $\left(\rho = \frac{m}{V}\right)$. The term $\rho g h$ looks like the expression for gravitational potential energy, and is essentially the pressure associated with the mass of fluid sitting above some position. Finally, let's consider how the absolute pressure fits into this conservation equation. If one multiplies the unit of pressure $\left(\frac{\text{N}}{\text{m}^2}\right)$ by meters over meters, we obtain $\frac{\text{N}\cdot\text{m}}{\text{m}^3} = \frac{\text{J}}{\text{m}^3}$. Pressure can therefore be thought of as a ratio of energy per cubic meter, or **energy density**. Systems at higher pressure have a higher energy density than systems at lower pressure. Finally, the combination of $P + \rho gh$ gives us the **static pressure**, and is the same equation as that for absolute pressure (although h is used here to imply height above a certain point, whereas z was used earlier to imply depth below a certain point). Bernoulli's equation states, then, that the sum of the static pressure and dynamic pressure will be constant within a closed container for an incompressible fluid not experiencing viscous drag. In the end, Bernoulli's equation is nothing other than a statement of energy conservation: more energy dedicated toward fluid movement means less energy dedicated toward static fluid pressure. The inverse of this is also true—less movement means more static pressure. One example of this principle that you may have previously encountered is how the shape of an airplane's wing helps generate lift, as shown in Figure 4.6.

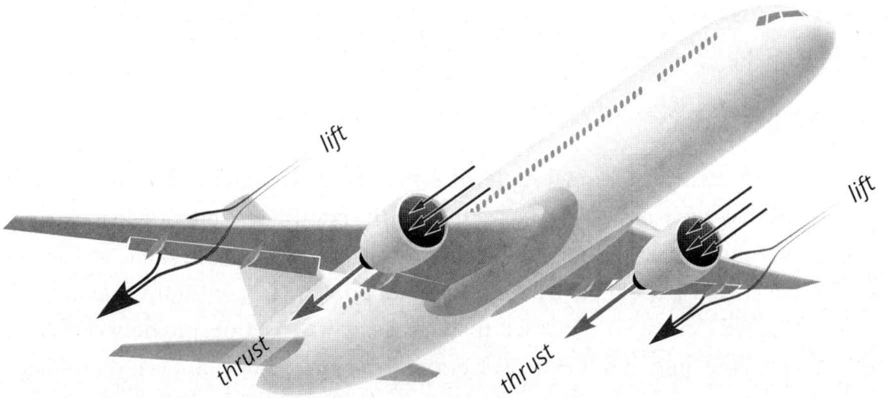

Figure 4.6 Aerodynamics of an Airplane

Propeller and jet engines generate thrust by pushing air backward. In both cases, because the wing top is curved, air streaming over it must travel farther and thus faster than air passing underneath the flat bottom. According to Bernoulli's equation, the slower air below exerts more force on the wing than the faster air above, thereby lifting the plane. Another example of Bernoulli's equation in action is the use of **pitot tubes**. These are specialized measurement devices that determine the speed of fluid flow by determining the difference between the static and dynamic pressure of the fluid at given points along a tube.

A common application of Bernoulli's equation on the MCAT is the **Venturi flow meter**, as shown in Figure 4.7.

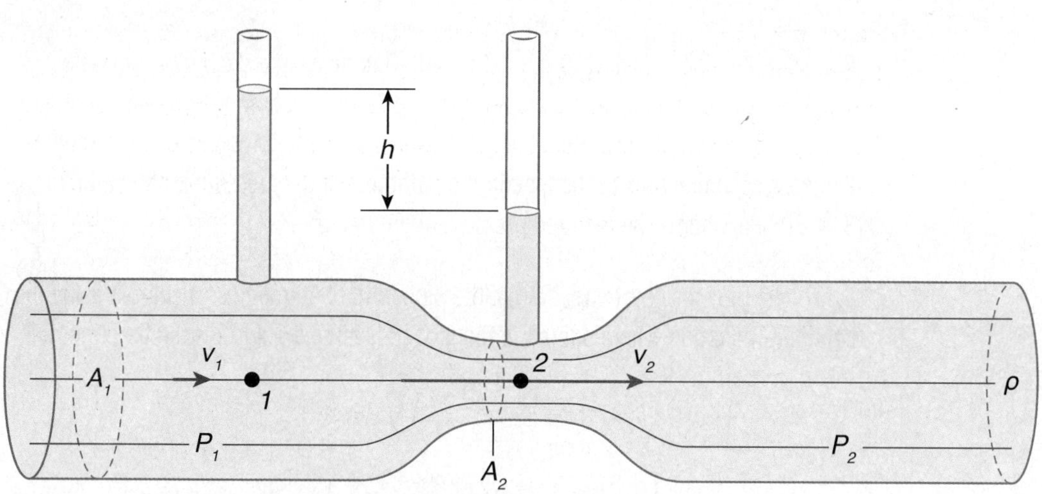

Figure 4.7 Venturi Flow Meter

As the tube narrows, the linear speed increases at point 2. Thus, the pressure exerted on the walls decreases, causing the column above the tube to have a lower height at point 2.

When considering Bernoulli's equation in this example, start by noting that the average height of the tube itself remains constant. Therefore, the ρgh term remains constant at points 1 and 2. Note that the h shown in Figure 4.7 is the difference in height between the two columns at points 1 and 2, not h from Bernoulli's equation, which corresponds to the average height of the tube above a datum. As the cross-sectional area decreases from point 1 to point 2, the linear speed must increase according to the continuity equation. Then, as the dynamic pressure increases, the absolute pressure must decrease at point 2. With a lower absolute pressure, the column of fluid sticking up from the Venturi tube will be lower at point 2. This phenomenon is often called the **Venturi effect**.

Example: An office building with a bathroom 40 m above the ground has its water supply enter the building at ground level through a pipe with an inner diameter of 4 cm. If the linear speed at the ground floor is 2 $\frac{m}{s}$ and at the bathroom is 8 $\frac{m}{s}$, determine the cross-sectional area of the pipe in the bathroom. If the pressure in the bathroom is 3×10^5 Pa, what is the required pressure at ground level?

Solution: The cross-sectional area of the pipe in the bathroom is calculated using the continuity equation, where point 1 is the ground level and point 2 is the bathroom:

$$A_1 v_1 = A_2 v_2 \rightarrow A_2 = \frac{A_1 v_1}{v_2}$$

$$A_2 = \frac{(\pi r_1^2) v_1}{v_2} = \frac{(\pi)(2 \times 10^{-2}\text{ m})^2 \left(2 \frac{\text{m}}{\text{s}}\right)}{\left(8 \frac{\text{m}}{\text{s}}\right)} = \frac{(\pi)(4 \times 10^{-4})(2)}{8}$$
$$= 3.14 \times 10^{-4}\text{ m}^2$$

The pressure can be found from Bernoulli's equation:

$$P_1 + \frac{1}{2}\rho v_1^2 + \rho g h_1 = P_2 + \frac{1}{2}\rho v_2^2 + \rho g h_2$$

$$P_1 = P_2 + \rho\left[\frac{v_2^2 - v_1^2}{2} + g(h_2 - h_1)\right]$$

$$= 3 \times 10^5\text{ Pa} + \left(1000 \frac{\text{kg}}{\text{m}^3}\right)\left[\frac{\left(8 \frac{\text{m}}{\text{s}}\right)^2 - \left(2 \frac{\text{m}}{\text{s}}\right)^2}{2} + \left(9.8 \frac{\text{m}}{\text{s}^2}\right)(40\text{ m})\right]$$

$$\approx 3 \times 10^5 + (1000)\left[\frac{64 - 4}{2} + 400\right] = 3 \times 10^5 + (1000)(430)$$

$$= 3 \times 10^5 + 4.3 \times 10^5 = 7.3 \times 10^5\text{ Pa (actual} = 7.22 \times 10^5\text{ Pa)}$$

MCAT CONCEPT CHECK 4.3

Before you move on, assess your understanding of the material with these questions.

1. Define the following terms:
   - Dynamic pressure:

   ____

   - Static pressure:

   ____

   - Pitot tube:

   ____

   - Viscosity:

   ____

   - Laminar flow:

   ____

   - Turbulence:

   ____

2. How do the following concepts relate to one another: Venturi effect, Bernoulli's equation, and continuity equation? What relationship does each describe?

   ____

3. What effect would increasing each of the following have on flow rate: the radius of the tube, pressure gradient, viscosity, and length of the tube?

   ____

4.4 Fluids in Physiology

LEARNING OBJECTIVES

After Chapter 4.4, you will be able to:

- Recall the conditions in which the continuity equation applies to human circulation
- Describe how total resistance of the airways changes during exhalation
- Compare flow volume and flow rate in different areas of the circulatory system

As a future student of medicine, you may feel that the abstract application of physics and math can often seem unimportant or tedious. However, these disciplines are exceptionally important in physiology. The movement of blood, lymph, and air throughout the body and lungs follow basic principles of fluid dynamics and pressure, with some minor alterations. We will focus primarily on the circulatory system, but also briefly discuss pressure and flow as they relate to gas exchange.

Circulatory System

The circulatory system is a **closed loop** that has a nonconstant flow rate. This nonconstant flow is a result of valves, gravity, the physical properties of our vessels (elasticity, in particular), and the mechanics of the heart. In particular, the nonconstant flow can be felt and measured as a **pulse**. In addition to these features, there is a loss of volume from the circulation as a result of a difference between osmotic (oncotic) and hydrostatic pressures. This fluid is eventually returned to the circulation as a result of lymphatic flow, but it is problematic for applications of the continuity equation. An important point to note is that despite these differences, blood volume entering the heart is always equal to blood volume leaving the heart during a single cycle.

As blood flows away from the heart, each vessel has a progressively higher resistance until the capillaries; however, the total resistance of the system decreases because the increased number of vessels are in parallel with each other. Like parallel resistors in circuits, the equivalent resistance is therefore lower for the capillaries in parallel than in the aorta. Return flow to the heart is facilitated by mechanical squeezing of the skeletal muscles, which increases pressure in the limbs and pushes blood to the heart, and the expansion of the heart, which decreases pressure in the heart and pulls blood in. Finally, the pressure gradients created in the thorax by inhalation and exhalation also motivate blood flow. Venous circulation holds approximately three times as much blood as arterial circulation. Heart murmurs, which result from structural defects of the heart, are heard because of turbulent blood flow.

Respiratory System

The respiratory system is also mediated by changes in pressure, and follows the same resistance relationship as the circulatory system. During inspiration, there is a negative pressure gradient that moves air into the lungs. During expiration, this gradient reverses. An additional point to note is that when air reaches the alveoli, it has essentially no speed.

MCAT CONCEPT CHECK 4.4

Before you move on, assess your understanding of the material with these questions.

1. Under what conditions could the continuity equation be applied to human circulation?

____

____

2. During exhalation, how does the total resistance of the encountered airways change as air leaves the alveoli to escape the nose and mouth?

____

____

____

3. How does flow in the venae cavae relate to flow in the main pulmonary artery?

____

____

Conclusion

The behavior of fluids impacts every moment of our lives. Even if we are nowhere near an ocean or a lake, we are quite literally submerged in a vast expanse of fluid, a mix of gases known as the atmosphere, which exerts forces on all of the surfaces of our bodies. Whenever we take a bath or submerge an object in water, we experience the effect of buoyant forces exerted by the displaced fluid. When we water our gardens, take a shower, or ride in a car with open windows, we experience the speeds, forces, and pressures of a fluid on the move. In the world of medicine, one must consider fluids, flowing and at rest, when evaluating the function of the respiratory and circulatory systems: conditions as varied as asthma and heart murmurs are related to the way in which the body causes fluids to flow. The balance of hydrostatic and oncotic pressures is important for maintaining the proper balance of fluid in the peripheral tissues of the body.

Now that you have the basic concepts of hydrostatics and fluid dynamics, learn to apply them to MCAT passages and questions through your Kaplan practice materials. Don't be intimidated by the seeming complexity of buoyant force problems and applications of Bernoulli's equation. Remember that all fluids, whether liquid or gas, exert buoyant forces against objects that are placed in them as a function of the weight of the fluid displaced. Remember that incompressible fluids demonstrate an inverse relationship between their dynamic pressure (as a function of speed) and their static pressure. This chapter concludes the section of this book focusing on mechanics; in the next two chapters, we'll turn our attention to electrostatics and electricity.

You've reviewed the content, now test your knowledge and critical thinking skills by completing a test-like passage set in your online resources!

GO ONLINE

CONCEPT SUMMARY

Characteristics of Fluids and Solids

- **Fluids** are substances that have the ability to flow and conform to the shape of their containers.
  - Fluids can exert perpendicular forces, but cannot exert shear forces.
  - Liquids and gases are the two phases of matter that are fluids.
- **Solids** do not flow and they retain their shape regardless of their containers.
- **Density** is the mass per unit volume of a substance (fluid or solid).
- **Pressure** is defined as a measure of force per unit area; it is exerted by a fluid on the walls of its container and on objects placed in the fluid.
  - It is a scalar quantity; its value has magnitude only, and no direction.
  - The pressure exerted by a gas against the walls of its container will always be perpendicular (normal) to the container walls.
- **Absolute pressure** is the sum of all pressures at a certain point within a fluid; it is equal to the pressure at the surface of the fluid (usually atmospheric pressure) plus the pressure due to the fluid itself.
- **Gauge pressure** is the name for the difference between absolute pressure and atmospheric pressure. In liquids, gauge pressure is caused by the weight of the liquid above the point of measurement.

Hydrostatics

- **Pascal's principle** states that a pressure applied to an incompressible fluid will be distributed undiminished throughout the entire volume of the fluid.
- **Hydraulic machines** operate based on the application of Pascal's principle to generate mechanical advantage.
- **Archimedes' principle** governs the buoyant force. When an object is placed in a fluid, the fluid generates a **buoyant force** against the object that is equal to the weight of the fluid displaced by the object.
  - The direction of the buoyant force is always opposite to the direction of gravity.
  - If the maximum buoyant force is larger than the force of gravity on the object, the object will float. This will be true if the object is less dense than the fluid it is in.
  - If the maximum buoyant force is smaller than the force of gravity on the object, the object will sink. This will be true if the object is more dense than the fluid it is in.
- Fluids experience **cohesive** forces with other molecules of the same fluid and **adhesive** forces with other materials; cohesive forces give rise to **surface tension**.

Fluid Dynamics

- Fluid dynamics is a set of principles regarding actively flowing fluids.
- **Viscosity** is a measurement of a fluid's internal friction. **Viscous drag** is a nonconservative force generated by viscosity.
- Fluids can move with either **laminar flow** or **turbulent flow**.
  - The rate of laminar flow is determined by the relationships in **Poiseuille's law**.
  - On the MCAT, incompressible fluids are assumed to have laminar flow and very low viscosity while flowing, allowing us to assume conservation of energy.
- The **continuity equation** is a statement of the conservation of mass as applied to fluid dynamics.
- **Bernoulli's equation** is an expression of conservation of energy for a flowing fluid. This equation states that the sum of the **static pressure** and the **dynamic pressure** will be constant between any two points in a closed system.
- For a horizontal flow, there is an inverse relationship between pressure and speed, and in a closed system, there is a direct relationship between cross-sectional area and pressure exerted on the walls of the tube known as the **Venturi effect**.

Fluids in Physiology

- The circulatory system behaves as a closed system with nonconstant flow.
- Resistance decreases as the total cross-sectional area increases.
  - Arterial circulation is primarily motivated by the heart.
  - Venous circulation has three times the volume of arterial circulation and is motivated by the skeletal musculature and expansion of the heart.
- Inspiration and expiration create a pressure gradient not only for the respiratory system, but for the circulatory system as well.
- Air at the alveoli has essentially zero speed.

ANSWERS TO CONCEPT CHECKS

4.1

1. Gauge pressure is equal to the pressure exerted by a column of fluid plus the ambient pressure above the fluid, minus atmospheric pressure. When atmospheric pressure is the only pressure above the fluid column, then gauge pressure equals the fluid pressure.
2. Weight is density times volume and acceleration due to gravity.
3. The SI unit of pressure is the pascal. Other common units include mmHg, torr, and atm.
4. True. Density is directionless, and is thus a scalar quantity.

4.2

1. Cohesion is the attractive force experienced by molecules of a fluid for one another. Adhesion is the attractive force experienced by molecules of a fluid for a different material (usually a solid).
2. If adhesive and cohesive forces are equal, then no meniscus would form and the liquid surface would be flat.
3. The displaced volume is equal to the volume of the block. The buoyant force is equal to the weight of the block, and is equal to the weight of the displaced fluid. By extension, the block and the fluid in which it is immersed must have the same density.
4. False. A fluid with a low specific gravity can be used instead of water to determine volumes of objects that would otherwise float in water.
5. The operator usually applies a force to the side with the smaller cross-sectional area. Because pressure is the same on both sides of the lift, a smaller force can be applied on the smaller surface area to generate the desired pressure.

4.3

1. Dynamic pressure is the pressure associated with flow, and is represented by $\frac{1}{2}\rho v^2$. Static pressure is the pressure associated with position; static pressure is sacrificed for dynamic pressure during flow. A pitot tube is a device that measures static pressure during flow to calculate speed. Viscosity is a measure of the resistance of a liquid to flow. Laminar flow is flow in which there are no eddies and in which streamlines roughly parallel each other. Turbulence is the presence of backflow or current eddies.
2. The continuity equation describes the relationship of flow and cross-sectional area in a tube, while Bernoulli's equation describes the relationship between height, pressure, and flow. The Venturi effect is the direct relationship between cross-sectional area and pressure, and results from the combined relationships of the Bernoulli and continuity equations.

3. Flow rate would increase when increasing either the radius of the tube or the pressure gradient, but would decrease with increasing viscosity or length of the tube.

4.4

1. The continuity equation cannot be applied to human circulation. The presence of pulses, the elasticity of the vessels, and the nature of the pressure gradient preclude this type of analysis. Poiseuille's law should instead be used for isolated segments.
2. Total resistance increases as the air exits the body despite the increase in the diameter of the airways. This is because there are fewer airways in parallel with each other.
3. In theory, there should be equal flow in the venae cavae and the main pulmonary trunk. In reality, the flow in the venae cavae is actually slightly less than in the pulmonary trunk because some of the blood entering the right side of the heart is actually from cardiac (coronary) circulation, not systemic circulation.

SCIENCE MASTERY ASSESSMENT EXPLANATIONS

1. **C**

The absolute and gauge pressures depend only on the density of the fluid, not on that of the object. When the pressure at the surface is equal to atmospheric pressure, the gauge pressure is given by $P_{\text{gauge}} = \rho g z$, where ρ represents the density of the fluid, not the object. These objects are also at the same depth, so they must have the same gauge pressure.

2. **B**

The tension in the chain is the difference between the anchor's weight and the buoyant force because the object is in translational equilibrium: $\mathbf{T} = \mathbf{F}_g - \mathbf{F}_{\text{buoy}}$. The object's weight is 833 N, and the buoyant force can be found using Archimedes' principle. The magnitude of the buoyant force is equal to the weight of the seawater that the anchor displaces:

$$F_{\text{buoy}} = \rho_w V_w g$$

Because the anchor is submerged entirely, the volume of the water displaced is equal to the volume of the anchor, which is equal to its mass divided by its density $\left(V_A = \frac{m_A}{\rho_A}\right)$. We are not given the anchor's mass, but its value must be the magnitude of the weight of the anchor divided by g. Putting all of this together, we can obtain the buoyant force:

$$F_{\text{buoy}} = \rho_{\text{w}} V_{\text{w}} g = \rho_{\text{w}} V_A g = \rho_{\text{w}} \left(\frac{m_{\text{A}}}{\rho_{\text{A}}}\right) g = \rho_{\text{w}} \left(\frac{F_g}{\rho_{\text{A}} g}\right) g = F_g \left(\frac{\rho_{\text{w}}}{\rho_{\text{A}}}\right)$$

$$= 833\ \text{N} \left(\frac{1025\ \frac{\text{kg}}{\text{m}^3}}{7800\ \frac{\text{kg}}{\text{m}^3}}\right) \approx 100\ \text{N}\ (\text{actual} = 109\ \text{N})$$

Lastly, we can obtain the tension from the initial equation $\mathbf{T} = \mathbf{F}_g - \mathbf{F}_{\text{buoy}}$:

$$\mathbf{T} = 833\ \text{N} - 109\ \text{N} = 724\ \text{N}$$

The key to quickly solving this problem on Test Day is recognizing that the answer choices contain an outlier **(A)**, a value slightly less than the weight of the anchor **(B)**, the weight of the anchor **(C)**, and a value slightly higher than the weight of the anchor **(D)**. Since buoyant force is in the same direction as tension and their sum must equal the weight of the anchor, **(B)** is the most likely answer.

3. **A**

Using Newton's second law, $F_{\text{net}} = ma$, we obtain the following equation:

$$F_{\text{buoy}} - mg = ma$$

Thus,

$$a = \frac{F_{\text{buoy}} - mg}{m} = \frac{F_{\text{buoy}}}{m} - g$$

Both balls experience the same buoyant force because they are in the same liquid and have the same volume ($F_{\text{buoy}} = \rho V g$). Thus, the ball with the smaller mass experiences the greater acceleration. Because both balls have the same volume, the ball with the smaller density has the smaller mass ($m = \rho V$), which is ball A.

4. **C**

It is known that water flows faster through a narrower pipe. The speed is inversely proportional to the cross-sectional area of the pipe because the same volume of water must pass by each point at each time interval. Let A be the 0.15 m pipe and B the 0.20 m pipe, and use the continuity equation:

$$v_A A_A = v_B A_B$$

where v is the speed and A is the cross-sectional area of the pipe. Because v is inversely proportional to the cross-sectional area, and the area is proportional to the square of the diameter $A = \pi r^2 = \frac{\pi d^2}{4}$, we obtain the following:

$$v_B = \frac{v_A\left(\frac{\pi d_A^2}{4}\right)}{\left(\frac{\pi d_B^2}{4}\right)} = v_A\left(\frac{d_A}{d_B}\right)^2$$

$$v_B = (8)\left(\frac{0.15}{0.20}\right)^2 = (8)\left(\frac{3}{4}\right)^2$$

$$v_B = (8)\left(\frac{9}{16}\right) = \frac{9}{2} = 4.5\ \frac{\text{m}}{\text{s}}$$

5. **A**

This question tests our understanding of Pascal's principle, which states that a change in pressure applied to an enclosed fluid is transmitted undiminished to every portion of the fluid and to the walls of the containing vessel. We are told that the work required to lift the bed with the patient is double the work needed to lift just the bed. In other words, the force required doubles when both the bed and the patient have to be lifted. To maintain the same pressure, we must double the cross-sectional area of the platform of the hydraulic lever on which the patient and the bed are lifted.

6. **B**

It is not necessary to do any calculations to answer this question. The open vertical pipes are exposed to the same atmospheric pressure; therefore, differences in the heights of the columns of water in the vertical pipes are dependent only on the differences in hydrostatic pressures in the horizontal pipe. Because the horizontal pipe has variable cross-sectional area, water will flow the fastest and the hydrostatic pressure will have its lowest value where the horizontal pipe is narrowest; this is called the Venturi effect. As a result, pipe 2 will have the lowest water level.

7. **C**

The continuity equation states that the flow rate of a fluid must remain constant from one cross-section to another. In other words, when an ideal fluid flows from a pipe with a large cross-sectional area to one that is narrower, its speed increases. This can be illustrated through the equation $A_1 v_1 = A_2 v_2$. If blood flows much more slowly through the capillaries, we can infer that the cross-sectional area is larger. This might seem surprising at first glance, but given that each blood vessel divides into thousands of little capillaries, it is not hard to imagine that adding the cross-sectional areas of each capillary from an entire capillary bed results in an area that is larger than the cross-sectional area of the aorta.

8. **C**

The data given in **(C)** are sufficient to determine the flow rate through Poiseuille's law, which can then be used to determine the linear speed by dividing by the cross-sectional area (which could be determined from the radius, as well). **(A)** would be sufficient if we also knew the flow rate in the other segment of pipe; one could use the continuity equation to determine the linear speed. The data in **(B)** could be used to determine the critical speed at which turbulent flow begins, but there is no indication that there is turbulent flow. The data in **(D)** could be used to determine the depth of an object in a fluid.

9. **B**

To calculate the total pressure, use the hydrostatic pressure formula: $P_{tot} = P_{atm} + \rho gz$. The unit of depth in this equation is meters, so first convert 25 cm to 0.25 m. The specific gravity is equal to the density of a medium divided by the density of water, so, with a specific gravity of 1.33, the density of dichloromethane is 1,330 kg/m^3. Finally, plug in these values and solve for total pressure: $P_{tot} = 101\text{ kPa} + (1{,}330\text{ kg/m}^3)(0.25\text{ m})(10\text{ m/s}^2) = 104\text{ kPa}$, matching **(B)**.

10. **B**

This is a basic restatement of Pascal's principle that a force applied to an area will be transmitted through a fluid. This will result in changing fluid levels through the system. The relationship is stated as $F_2 = \frac{F_1 A_2}{A_1}$. Plugging in the numbers gives an answer of 16 N.

11. **A**

The buoyant force (F_{buoy}) is equal to the weight of water displaced, which is quantitatively expressed as

$$F_{buoy} = m_{\text{fluid displaced}}g = \rho_{\text{fluid}}V_{\text{fluid displaced}}g$$

The volume of displaced fluid is equal to the volume of the ball. The density of the fluid remains constant. Therefore, because ball A has a larger volume, it will displace more water and experience a larger buoyant force.

12. **C**

The volume of blood entering and exiting the heart is always equal in a single cardiac cycle, supporting **(C)** as the correct answer. By contrast, the flow rate of blood through the circulatory system is not constant, as some fluids exit the circulation in tissue and is later returned via the lymphatic system, eliminating **(A)**. Furthermore, the contraction of the heart pushing blood through arterial circulation creates an uneven flow rate which can be observed as the pulse, eliminating **(B)**. Finally, as the diameter of the vessels decreases, resistance increases, and therefore arteries have significantly less resistance to blood flow compared to arterioles, eliminating **(D)**.

13. **A**

This question is a simple application of the definition of pressure, which is force per area. If pressure decreases 1 percent and area does not change, the force will be decreased by 1 percent. Note that the other measurements given do not play a role in our calculations.

14. **C**

The equation for absolute (hydrostatic) pressure is $P = P_0 + \rho gz$, where P_0 is the pressure at the surface, ρ is the density of the fluid, g is acceleration due to gravity, and z is the depth in the fluid. If the density of fluid B is twice that of fluid A, then the depth in fluid A will have to be twice that in fluid B to obtain the same absolute pressure:

$$P_0 + \rho_A g z_A = P_0 + \rho_B g z_B$$
$$(x) g z_A = (2x) g z_B$$
$$z_A = 2 z_B$$

15. **B**

This is a basic interpretation of Bernoulli's equation that states, at equal heights, speed and pressure of a fluid are inversely related (the Venturi effect). Decreasing the speed of the water will therefore increase its pressure. An increase in pressure over a given area will result in increased force being transmitted to the piston.

Consult your online resources for additional practice. GO ONLINE

EQUATIONS TO REMEMBER

(4.1) **Density:** $\rho = \frac{m}{V}$

(4.2) **Weight of a volume of fluid:** $F_g = \rho V g$

(4.3) **Specific gravity:** $SG = \frac{\rho}{1\ \frac{g}{cm^3}}$

(4.4) **Pressure:** $P = \frac{F}{A}$

(4.5) **Absolute pressure:** $P = P_0 + \rho g z$

(4.6) **Gauge pressure:** $P_{gauge} = P - P_{atm} = (P_0 + \rho g z) - P_{atm}$

(4.7) **Pascal's principle:**
$$P = \frac{F_1}{A_1} = \frac{F_2}{A_2}$$
$$F_2 = F_1\left(\frac{A_2}{A_1}\right)$$

(4.8) **Buoyant force:** $F_{buoy} = \rho_{fluid} V_{fluid\ displaced} g = \rho_{fluid} V_{submerged} g$

(4.9) **Poiseuille's law:** $Q = \frac{\pi r^4 \Delta P}{8 \eta L}$

(4.10) **Critical speed:** $v_c = \frac{N_R \eta}{\rho D}$

(4.11) **Continuity equation:** $Q = v_1 A_1 = v_2 A_2$

(4.12) **Bernoulli's equation:** $P_1 + \frac{1}{2}\rho v_1^2 + \rho g h_1 = P_2 + \frac{1}{2}\rho v_2^2 + \rho g h_2$

SHARED CONCEPTS

Biology Chapter 6
The Respiratory System

Biology Chapter 7
The Cardiovascular System

Biology Chapter 8
The Immune System

General Chemistry Chapter 8
The Gas Phase

Physics and Math Chapter 2
Work and Energy

Physics and Math Chapter 3
Thermodynamics

CHAPTER 5

ELECTROSTATICS AND MAGNETISM

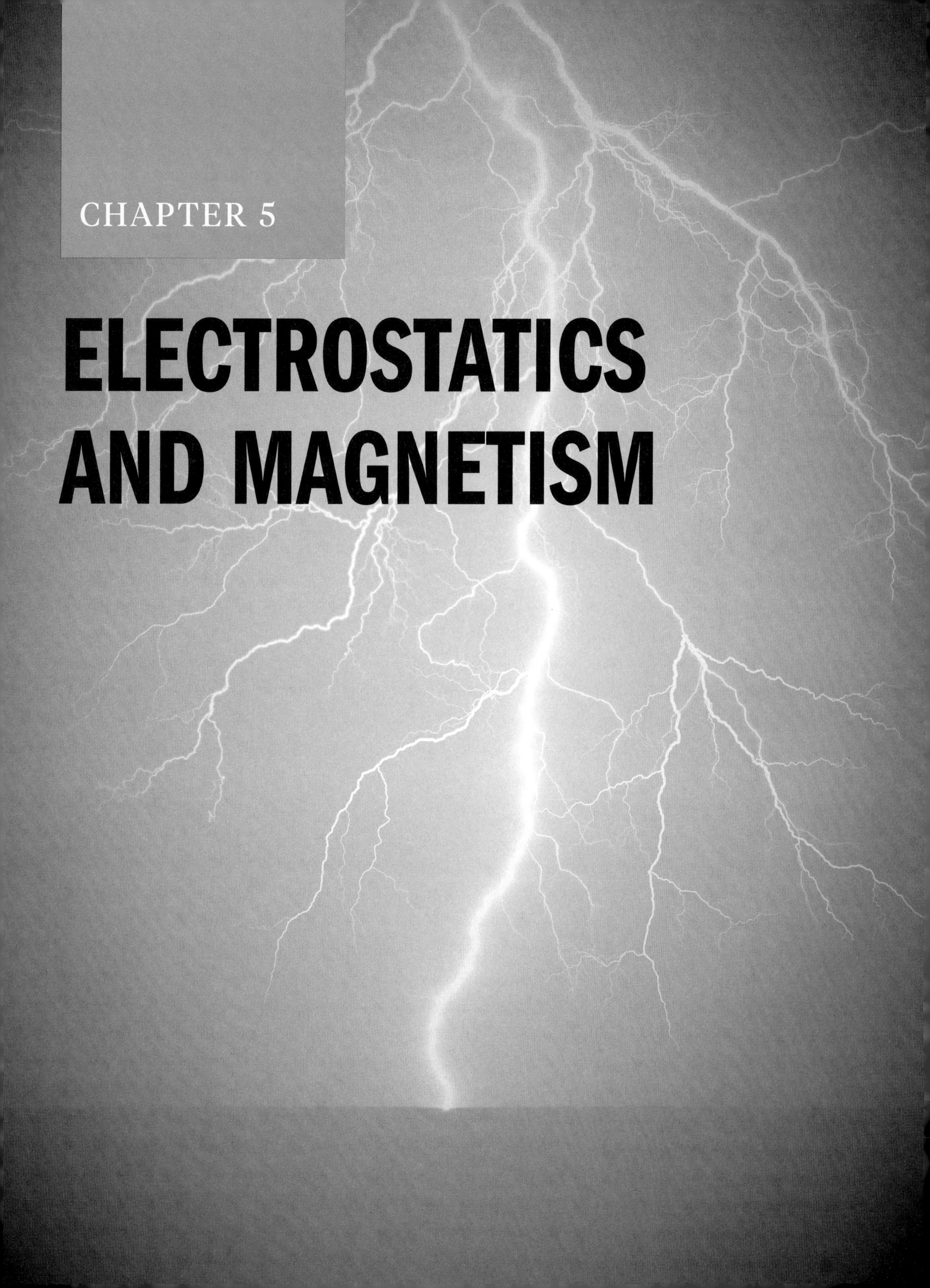

SCIENCE MASTERY ASSESSMENT

Every pre-med knows this feeling: there is so much content I have to know for the MCAT! How do I know what to do first or what's important?

While the high-yield badges throughout this book will help you identify the most important topics, this Science Mastery Assessment is another tool in your MCAT prep arsenal. This quiz (which can also be taken in your online resources) and the guidance below will help ensure that you are spending the appropriate amount of time on this chapter based on your personal strengths and weaknesses. Don't worry though—skipping something now does not mean you'll never study it. Later on in your prep, as you complete full-length tests, you'll uncover specific pieces of content that you need to review and can come back to these chapters as appropriate.

How to Use This Assessment

If you answer 0–7 questions correctly:

Spend about 1 hour to read this chapter in full and take limited notes throughout. Follow up by reviewing **all** quiz questions to ensure that you now understand how to solve each one.

If you answer 8–11 questions correctly:

Spend 20–40 minutes reviewing the quiz questions. Beginning with the questions you missed, read and take notes on the corresponding subchapters. For questions you answered correctly, ensure your thinking matches that of the explanation and you understand why each choice was correct or incorrect.

If you answer 12–15 questions correctly:

Spend less than 20 minutes reviewing all questions from the quiz. If you missed any, then include a quick read-through of the corresponding subchapters, or even just the relevant content within a subchapter, as part of your question review. For questions you got correct, ensure your thinking matches that of the explanation and review the Concept Summary at the end of the chapter.

Questions 1–3 refer to the figure below, in which F represents the electrostatic force exerted on charged particle S by charged particle R.

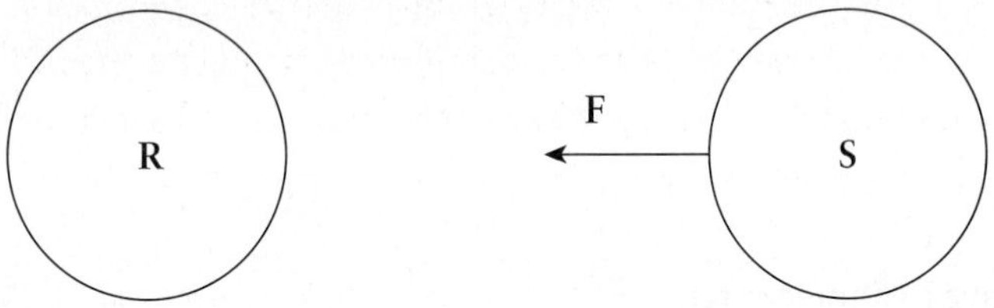

1. In the figure, the magnitude of the electric force on **R** due to **S** is:
   - **A.** $\frac{F}{2}$.
   - **B.** F.
   - **C.** 2F.
   - **D.** 4F.

2. If the distance between the centers of the spheres is halved, the magnitude of the force on **S** due to **R** will be:
   - **A.** $\frac{F}{2}$.
   - **B.** $\frac{F}{4}$.
   - **C.** 2F.
   - **D.** 4F.

3. Assume the direction of **F** is the same direction as the electric field between **R** and **S**. If an electron were placed midway between **R** and **S**, the resultant electric force on the electron would be:
   - **A.** toward **R**.
   - **B.** toward **S**.
   - **C.** upward in the plane of the page.
   - **D.** downward in the plane of the page.

4. If the electric field at a distance r away from charge Q is 36 $\frac{N}{C}$, what is the ratio of the electric fields at r, $2r$, and $3r$?
   - **A.** 9:3:1
   - **B.** 36:9:4
   - **C.** 36:18:9
   - **D.** 36:18:12

5. A positive charge of $+Q$ is fixed at point R a distance d away from another positive charge of $+2Q$ fixed at point S. Point A is located midway between the charges, and point B is a distance $\frac{d}{2}$ from $+2Q$, as shown below. In which direction will a positive charge move if placed at point A and point B, respectively?

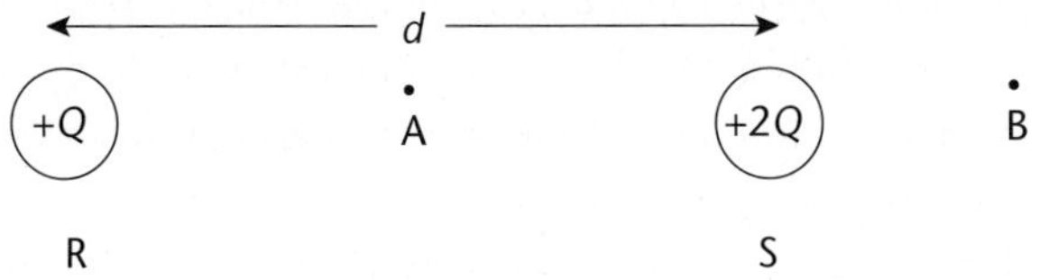

   - **A.** Toward the $+Q$ charge for both
   - **B.** Toward the $+2Q$ charge for both
   - **C.** Toward the $+Q$ charge at point A, and toward the right at point B
   - **D.** Toward the $+2Q$ charge at point A, and toward the right at point B

6. Two parallel conducting plates are separated by a distance d. One plate carries a charge $+Q$ and the other carries a charge $-Q$. The voltage between the plates is 12 V. If a $+2\ \mu C$ charge is released from rest at the positive plate, how much kinetic energy does it have when it reaches the negative plate?
   - **A.** 2.4×10^{-6} J
   - **B.** 4.8×10^{-6} J
   - **C.** 2.4×10^{-5} J
   - **D.** 4.8×10^{-5} J

7. The negative charge in the figure below ($-1\ \mu C$) moves from $y = -5$ to $y = +5$ and is made to follow the dashed line. What is the work required to move the negative charge along this dashed line?

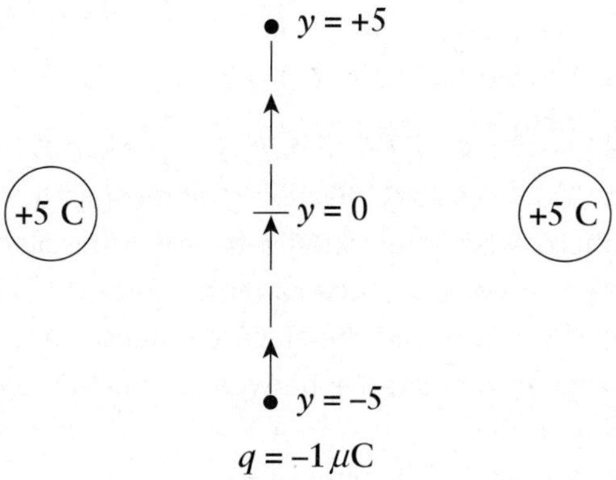

A. -10 J
B. -5 J
C. 0 J
D. 10 J

8. If the magnetic field a distance r away from a current-carrying wire is 10 T, what will be the net magnetic field at r if another wire is placed a distance $2r$ from the original wire (with r in the middle) and has a current twice as strong flowing in the opposite direction?

A. 0 T
B. 15 T
C. 20 T
D. 30 T

9. Given an electric dipole, the electric potential is zero:

A. only at the midpoint of the dipole axis.
B. anywhere on the perpendicular bisector of the dipole axis and at infinity.
C. anywhere on the dipole axis.
D. only for points at infinity.

10. An electron is accelerated over a distance d by an electric potential V. The electric potential applied to this electron is then increased by a factor of 4 and the electron is accelerated over the same distance d. The speed of the electron at the end of the second trial will be larger than at the end of the first trial by a factor of:

A. 16.
B. 8.
C. 4.
D. 2.

11. Which of the following accurately depicts the field lines created by a proton that is moving toward the right on this page?

A.

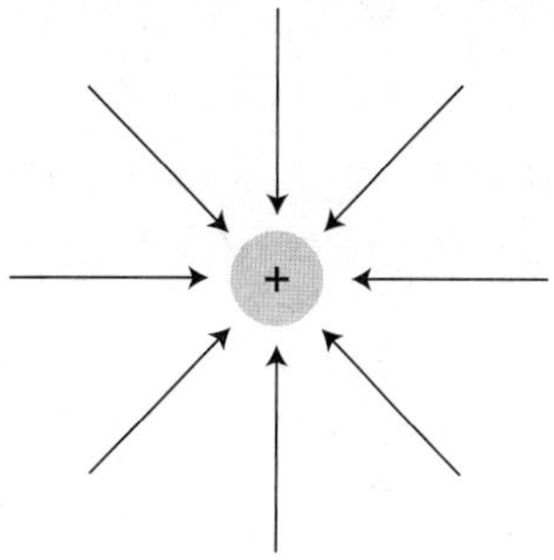

B.

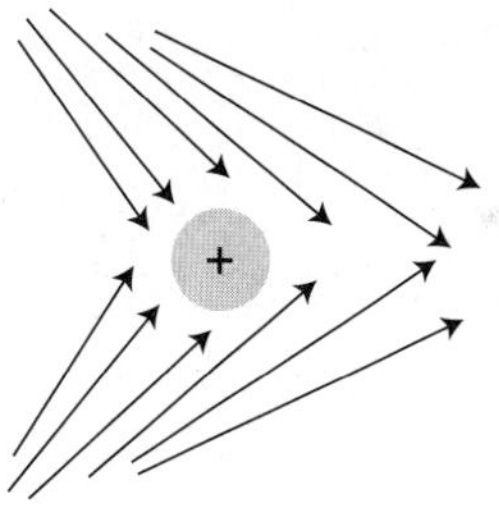

C.

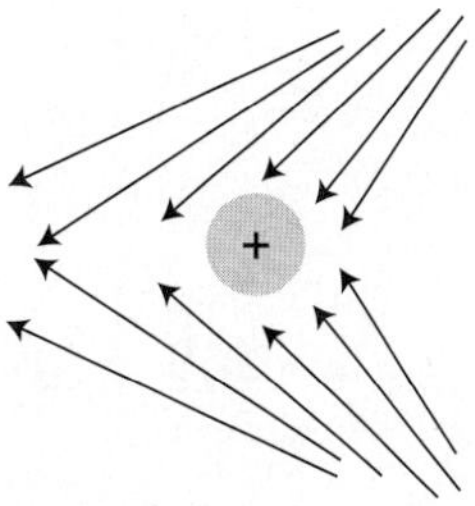

D.

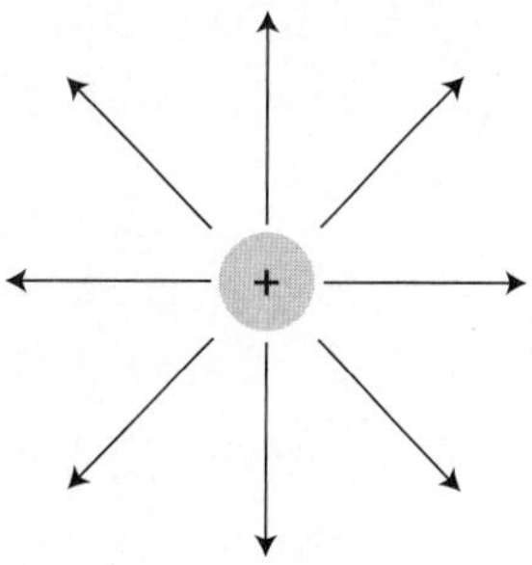

12. A certain 9 V battery is used as a power source to move a 2 C charge. How much work is done by the battery?
   - A. 4.5 J
   - B. 9 J
   - C. 18 J
   - D. 36 J

13. To increase the capacitance of a given capacitor, a dielectric is inserted between the two plates. Dielectrics are materials that block the flow of charge. Which of the following materials would be the best dielectric?
   - A. Salt water
   - B. Steel, an alloy primarily composed of iron
   - C. Glass, an oxide of silica
   - D. Copper

14. A moving negative charge placed in an external magnetic field circulates counterclockwise in the plane of the paper. In which direction is the magnetic field pointing?
   - A. Into the page
   - B. Out of the page
   - C. Toward the center of the circle
   - D. Tangent to the circle

15. Many kinases have divalent cation cofactors to stabilize their interaction with ATP. If the electric potential energy of the cation and ATP is -3.3×10^{-19} J, how would the electric potential energy change if the distance between the cation and ATP were doubled?
   - A. Increase by a factor of 2
   - B. Increase by a factor of 4
   - C. Decrease by a factor of 2
   - D. Decrease by a factor of 4

Answer Key follows on next page.

Answer Key

1. **B**
2. **D**
3. **B**
4. **B**
5. **C**
6. **C**
7. **C**
8. **D**
9. **B**
10. **D**
11. **D**
12. **C**
13. **C**
14. **B**
15. **A**

Detailed explanations can be found at the end of the chapter.

CHAPTER 5

ELECTROSTATICS AND MAGNETISM

In This Chapter

CHAPTER PROFILE

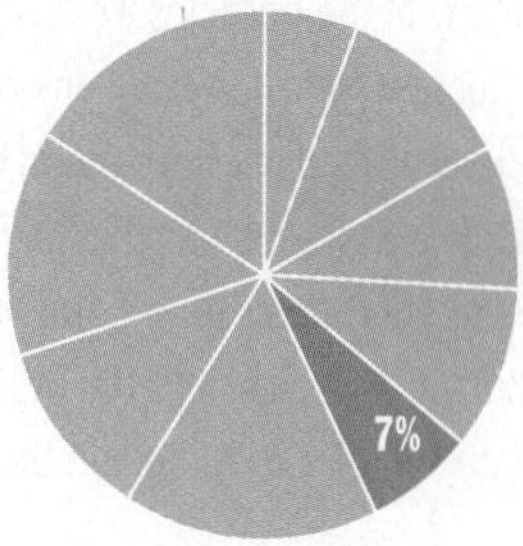

The content in this chapter should be relevant to about 7% of all questions about physics on the MCAT.

This chapter covers material from the following AAMC content category:

4C: Electrochemistry and electrical circuits and their elements

Introduction

Electrostatics is the study of stationary charges and the forces that are created by and which act upon these charges. Without electrical charge, we would not be able to do many of the activities that we enjoy or consider essential to basic living. But living with electrical charge can also be dangerous and even deadly: magnify the small shock you receive from a doorknob after walking across a carpet, and you have the equivalent of a lightning bolt strong enough to stop a heart. This same concept can be used in life-saving therapy as well: cardioversion and defibrillation create a strong electrical current through the heart's conduction system that attempts to resynchronize a pulse.

In this chapter, we will review the basic concepts essential to understanding charges and electrostatic forces including conductors and insulators. We will review Coulomb's law, which describes the attractions and repulsions between charged objects. Next, we will describe the electric fields that all charges create, which allow them to exert forces on other charges. After we've discussed how charges set up these fields, we'll observe the behavior of charges that are placed into these fields. In particular, we will note the motional behavior of these test charges inside a field in relation to the electrical potential difference, or voltage, between two points in space. We can then determine the change in electric potential energy as the charge moves from a position of some electric potential to another. Next, we will describe the electric dipole and solve a problem involving one of the molecular dipoles most important to life on this planet: the water molecule. Finally, we will explore the topic of magnetic fields and forces.

5.1 Charges

LEARNING OBJECTIVES

After Chapter 5.1, you will be able to:

- Contrast the behavior of protons and electrons in charged environments
- Categorize materials, including glass and copper, as conductors or insulators
- Recognize the charge of an electron in coulombs

MCAT EXPERTISE

While many of the particles we discuss in electrostatics are very, very tiny, do not forget that they still do have mass. We can use equations such as the kinetic energy equation when solving problems with charged particles, and the MCAT will sometimes require us to do just that.

Charged subatomic particles come in two varieties. One, the **proton**, has a positive charge; the other, the **electron**, has a negative charge. While opposite charges exert **attractive** forces, like charges—those that have the same sign—exert **repulsive** forces. Unlike the force of gravity, which is always an attractive force, the electrostatic force may be repulsive or attractive depending on the signs of the charges that are interacting.

Most matter is electrically neutral, as a balance of positive and negative charges ensures a relative degree of stability. When charges are out of balance, the system can become electrically unstable. Even materials that are normally electrically neutral can acquire a net charge as result of friction. When you shuffle your feet across the carpet, negatively charged particles are transferred from the carpet to your feet, and these charges spread out over the total surface of your body. The shock that occurs when your hand gets close enough to a metal doorknob allows that excess charge to jump from your fingers to the knob, which acts as a **ground**—a means of returning charge to the earth. **Static charge buildup** or **static electricity** is more significant in drier air because lower humidity makes it easier for charge to become and remain separated.

KEY CONCEPT

The fundamental unit of charge is $e = 1.60 \times 10^{-19}$ C. A proton and an electron each have this amount of charge; the proton is positively charged ($q = +e$), while the electron is negatively charged ($q = -e$).

The SI unit of charge is the **coulomb**, and the fundamental unit of charge is

$$e = 1.60 \times 10^{-19} \text{ C}$$

A proton and an electron each have this amount of charge, although the proton is positively charged ($q = +e$), while the electron is negatively charged ($q = -e$). Even though the proton and the electron share the same magnitude of charge, they do not share the same mass; the proton has a much greater mass than the electron.

Like mass and energy, electric charge is governed by a law of conservation of charge. This law states that charge can neither be created nor destroyed.

Insulators and Conductors

Insulators and conductors vary in their ability to both hold and transfer charges. An **insulator** will not easily distribute a charge over its surface and will not transfer that charge to another neutral object very well—especially not to another insulator. On a molecular level, the electrons of insulators tend to be closely linked with their respective nuclei. By extension, most nonmetals are insulators. Experimentally, insulators serve as dielectric materials in capacitors, as well as in isolating electrostatic experiments from the environment to prevent grounding.

In contrast, when a **conductor** is given a charge, the charges will distribute approximately evenly upon the surface of the conductor. Conductors are able to transfer and transport charges and are often used in circuits or electrochemical cells. Conductors are often conceptualized as nuclei surrounded by a sea of free electrons that are able to move rapidly throughout the material and are only loosely associated with the positive charges. Conductors are generally metals, although ionic (electrolyte) solutions are also effective conductors. Figure 5.1 demonstrates the behaviors of an insulator and a conductor when a negative charge is placed on them.

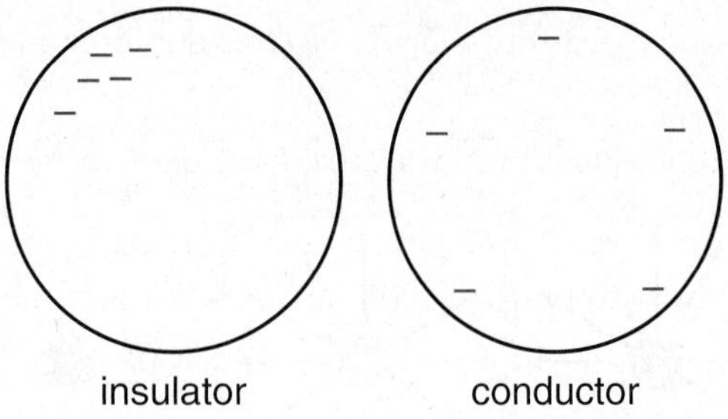

Figure 5.1 A Negatively Charged Insulator and Conductor
Insulators will not distribute charge over their surface; conductors will.

MCAT CONCEPT CHECK 5.1

Before you move on, assess your understanding of the material with these questions.

1. When placed one meter apart from each other, which will experience a greater acceleration: one coulomb of electrons or one coulomb of protons?

____

2. Categorize the following materials as either conductors or insulators: blood, hair, copper, glass, iron, sulfuric acid, and distilled water
   - Conductors:

   ____

   - Insulators:

   ____

3. What is the net charge of an object with one coulomb of electrons and 3 moles of neutrons?

____

5.2 Coulomb's Law

LEARNING OBJECTIVES

After Chapter 5.2, you will be able to:

- Calculate the electric field that a charge generates and the electric force between it and another charge
- Recall the direction in which a negative or a positive electrostatic force will move two charges relative to one another
- Relate distance and charge quantities to electrostatic force and electrostatic field magnitudes
- Apply direction conventions to draw electric fields generated by a charged object:

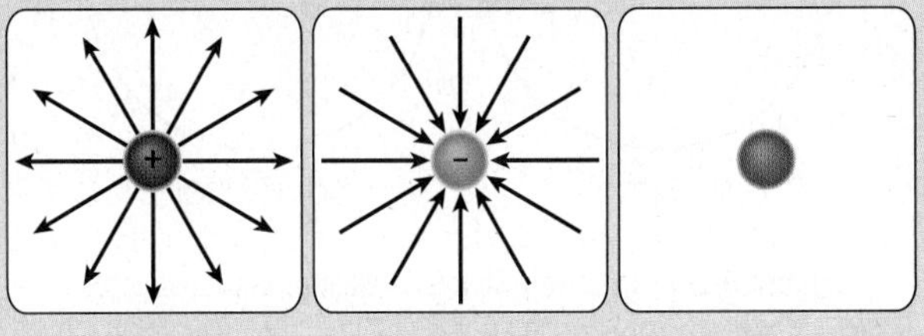

Coulomb's law quantifies the magnitude of the electrostatic force F_e between two charges:

$$F_e = \frac{kq_1q_2}{r^2}$$

Equation 5.1

where F_e is the magnitude of the electrostatic force, k is Coulomb's constant, q_1 and q_2 are the magnitudes of the two charges, and r is the distance between the charges. **Coulomb's constant** (also called the **electrostatic constant**) is a number that depends on the units used in the equation. In SI units, $k = \frac{1}{4\pi\varepsilon_0} = 8.99 \times 10^9 \ \frac{\text{N}\cdot\text{m}^2}{\text{C}^2}$, where ε_0 represents the **permittivity of free space**, $8.85 \times 10^{-12} \ \frac{\text{C}^2}{\text{N}\cdot\text{m}^2}$. The direction of the force may be obtained by remembering that unlike charges attract and like charges repel. The force always points along the line connecting the centers of the two charges.

Example: A positive charge is attracted to a negative charge a certain distance away. The charges are then moved so that they are separated by twice the distance. How has the force of attraction changed between them?

Solution: Coulomb's law states that the force between two charges varies as the inverse of the square of the distance between them. Therefore, if the distance is doubled, the square of the distance is quadrupled, and the force is reduced to one-fourth of what it was originally. Note that it was not necessary to know the distance or the units being used.

A close examination of Coulomb's law reveals that it is remarkably similar in form to the equation for gravitational force. In the electrostatic force equation, the force magnitude is proportional to the charge magnitudes, and this is similar to the proportional relationship between gravitational force and mass. In both equations, the force magnitude is inversely proportional to the square of the distance of separation. These similarities ought to help you remember both equations on Test Day.

BRIDGE

Notice how Coulomb's law looks very similar to the gravitational force equation, but with a different constant and using charge rather than mass. It is this fact that should remind us that this equation is dealing with electrostatic force between two charges, just as the gravitation equation is dealing with the gravitational force between two bodies of mass. The gravitation equation is discussed in Chapter 1 of *MCAT Physics and Math Review*.

Example: Negatively charged electrons are electrostatically attracted to positively charged protons. Because electrons and protons have mass, they will be gravitationally attracted to each other as well. What is the ratio of the electrostatic force to the gravitational force between an electron and proton? (Note: $m_p = 1.67 \times 10^{-27}$ kg, $m_e = 9.11 \times 10^{-31}$ kg, $e = 1.60 \times 10^{-19}$ C, $k = 8.99 \times 10^9 \frac{\text{N} \cdot \text{m}^2}{\text{C}^2}$, and $G = 6.67 \times 10^{-11} \frac{\text{N} \cdot \text{m}^2}{\text{kg}^2}$)

Solution: Both Coulomb's law and the universal law of gravitation state that the attractive forces between the electron and proton vary as the inverse of the square of the distance between them. The ratio between these forces can be calculated by dividing their magnitudes:

$$\frac{F_e}{F_g} = \frac{\left[\frac{kq_1q_2}{r^2}\right]}{\left[\frac{Gm_1m_2}{r^2}\right]} = \frac{kq_1q_2}{Gm_1m_2}$$

Now the values can be plugged in:

$$\frac{F_e}{F_g} = \frac{\left(8.99 \times 10^9 \frac{\text{N} \cdot \text{m}^2}{\text{C}^2}\right)(1.60 \times 10^{-19}\ \text{C})(1.60 \times 10^{-19}\ \text{C})}{\left(6.67 \times 10^{-11} \frac{\text{N} \cdot \text{m}^2}{\text{kg}^2}\right)(1.67 \times 10^{-27}\ \text{kg})(9.11 \times 10^{-31}\ \text{kg})}$$

$$\approx \frac{(9)(1.6)(1.6)(10^{-29})}{(6.67)(1.6)(9)(10^{-69})}$$

$$= \frac{1.6}{6.67} \times 10^{40} \approx \frac{1.6}{6.4} \times 10^{40} = 0.25 \times 10^{40}$$

$$= 2.5 \times 10^{39}\ (\text{actual} = 2.27 \times 10^{39})$$

Note that the electrostatic attraction between the electron and proton is stronger than the gravitational attraction by a factor of almost 10^{40}. Also, note that setting up all of the variables before working out the math simplifies the process because a number of the variables cancel out during the division.

KEY CONCEPT

Electric fields are produced by source charges (Q). When a test charge (q) is placed in an electric field (**E**), it will experience an electrostatic force ($\mathbf{F}_e$) equal to $q\mathbf{E}$.

Electric Field

Every electric charge sets up a surrounding electric field, just like every mass creates a gravitational field. **Electric fields** make their presence known by exerting forces on other charges that move into the space of the field. Whether the force exerted through the electric field is attractive or repulsive depends on whether the stationary **test charge** q (the charge placed in the electric field) and the stationary **source charge** Q (which actually creates the electric field) are opposite charges (attractive) or like charges (repulsive).

The magnitude of an electric field can be calculated in one of two ways, both of which can be seen in the definitional equation for the electric field:

$$E = \frac{F_e}{q} = \frac{kQ}{r^2}$$

Equation 5.2

where E is the electric field magnitude in newtons per coulomb, F_e is the magnitude of the force felt by the test charge q, k is the electrostatic constant, Q is the source charge magnitude, and r is the distance between the charges. The electric field is a vector quantity, and we will discuss the process of determining the direction of the electric field vector in a moment. Look closely: you can see that this equation for the electric field magnitude is derived simply by dividing both sides of Coulomb's law by the test charge q. In doing so, we arrive at two different methods for calculating the magnitude of the electric field at a particular point in space. The first method is to place a test charge q at some point within the electric field, measure the force exerted on that test charge, and define the electric field at that point in space as the ratio of the force magnitude to test charge magnitude $\left(\frac{F_e}{q}\right)$. One of the disadvantages of this method of calculation is that a test charge must actually be present in order for a force to be generated and measured. Sometimes, however, no test charge is actually within the electric field, so we need another way to measure the magnitude of that field.

KEY CONCEPT

By dividing Coulomb's law by the magnitude of the test charge, we arrive at two ways of determining the magnitude of the electric field at a point in space around the source charge.

The second method of calculating the electric field magnitude at a point in space does not require the presence of a test charge. We only need to know the magnitude of the source charge and the distance between the source charge and point in space at which we want to measure the electric field $\left(\frac{kQ}{r^2}\right)$. In this method, we need to know the value of the source charge to be able to calculate the electric field.

By convention, the direction of the electric field vector is given as the direction that a positive test charge would move in the presence of the source charge. If the source charge is positive, then the test charge would experience a repulsive force and would accelerate away from the positive source charge. On the other hand, if the source charge is negative, then the test charge would experience an attractive force and would accelerate toward the negative source charge. Therefore, positive charges have electric field vectors that radiate outward (that is, point away) from the charge, whereas negative charges have electric field vectors that radiate inward (point toward) the charge. These electric field vectors may be represented using field lines, as shown in Figure 5.2.

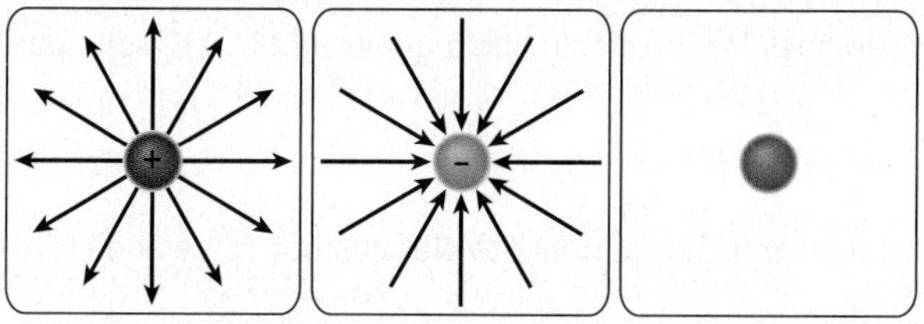

Figure 5.2 Field Lines around a Positive, a Negative, and a Neutral Source Charge

Field lines are imaginary lines that represent how a positive test charge would move in the presence of the source charge. The field lines are drawn in the direction of the actual electric field vectors and also indicate the relative strength of the electric field at a given point in the space of the field. When drawn on a sheet of paper, field lines look like the metal spokes of a bicycle wheel: the lines are closer together near the source charge and spread out at distances farther from the charge. Where the field lines are closer together, the field is stronger; where the lines are farther apart, the field is weaker. Because every charge exerts its own electric field, a collection of charges will exert a net electric field at a point in space that is equal to the vector sum of all the electric fields.

Because electric field and electrostatic force are both vector quantities, it is important to remember the conventions for their direction. If the test charge within a field is positive, then the force will be in the same direction as the electric field vector of the source charge; if the test charge is negative, then the force will be in the direction opposite to the field vector of the source charge.

KEY CONCEPT

Field lines are used to represent the electric field vectors for a charge. They point away from a positive charge and point toward a negative charge. The denser the field lines, the stronger the electric field. Note that field lines of a single charge never cross each other.

MCAT CONCEPT CHECK 5.2

Before you move on, assess your understanding of the material with these questions.

1. What is the electric field midway between two negative charges in isolation?

____

2. What direction does a negative electrostatic force point? What direction does a positive electrostatic force point?

   - Negative electrostatic force:

____

   - Positive electrostatic force:

____

3. Draw the field lines for the electric field generated by an alpha particle $\left({}^{4}_{2}He^{2+}\right)$.

---

4. How do distance and charge relate to electrostatic force and electric field?
   - Electrostatic force:

   - Electric field:

5.3 Electric Potential Energy

LEARNING OBJECTIVES

After Chapter 5.3, you will be able to:

- Describe how a change in electric potential energy will affect the stability of a system
- Calculate electric potential energy
- Compare and contrast electric potential energy with electrostatic force, conceptually and mathematically
- Predict change in electric potential energy given a change in distance

We have already defined potential energy as stored energy that can be used to do something or make something happen. There are different types of potential energy; gravitational, elastic, and chemical are three forms that you will need to know for Test Day. A fourth form is **electric potential energy**. Similar to gravitational potential energy, this is a form of potential energy that is dependent on the relative position of one charge with respect to another charge or to a collection of charges. Electric potential energy is given by the equation

$$U = \frac{kQq}{r}$$

Equation 5.3

If the charges are like charges (both positive or both negative), then the potential energy will be positive. If the charges are unlike (one positive and the other negative), then the potential energy will be negative. Remember that work and energy have the same unit (the joule), so we can define electric potential energy for a charge at a point in space in an electric field as the amount of work necessary to bring the charge from infinitely far away to that point. Because $F_e = \frac{kQq}{r^2}$ and $W = Fd\cos\theta$, if we define d as the distance r that separates two charges and assume the force and displacement vectors to be parallel, then:

$$\Delta U = W = Fd\cos\theta = Fr \times 1 = \left(\frac{kQq}{r^2}\right)r = \frac{kQq}{r}$$

KEY CONCEPT

Electric potential energy is the work necessary to move a test charge from infinity to a point in space in an electric field surrounding a source charge.

Consider two charges: a stationary negative source charge and a positive test charge that can be moved. Because these two charges are unlike, they will exert attractive forces between them. Therefore, the closer they are to each other, the more stable they will be. Opposite charges will have negative potential energy, and this energy will become increasingly negative as the charges are brought closer and closer together. Increasingly negative numbers are actually decreasing values because they are moving farther to the left of 0 on the number line. This decrease in energy represents an increase in stability.

Now let's consider two positive charges. As like charges, these will exert repulsive forces, and the potential energy of the system will be positive. Because like charges repel each other, the closer they are to each other, the less stable they will be. Remember that unlike gravitational systems, the forces of electrostatics can be either attractive or repulsive. In this case, the like charges will become more stable the farther apart they move because the magnitude of the electric potential energy becomes a smaller and smaller positive number.

KEY CONCEPT

The electric potential energy of a system will increase when two like charges move toward each other or when two opposite charges move apart. Conversely, the electric potential energy of a system will decrease when two like charges move apart or when two opposite charges move toward each other.

Example: If a charge of $+2e$ and a charge of $-3e$ are separated by a distance of 3 nm, what is the potential energy of the system? (Note: e is the fundamental unit of charge equal to 1.6×10^{-19} C, and k is the electrostatic constant equal to $8.99 \times 10^9 \frac{\text{N}\cdot\text{m}^2}{\text{C}^2}$.)

Solution: The equation for potential energy is $U = \frac{kQq}{r}$. From the question stem, we know that the charges are $+2e$ and $-3e$, and $r = 3\text{ nm} = 3 \times 10^{-9}$ m. Plugging into the equation, we get:

$$U = \frac{\left(8.99 \times 10^9 \frac{\text{N}\cdot\text{m}^2}{\text{C}^2}\right)(2 \times 1.6 \times 10^{-19}\text{ C})(-3 \times 1.6 \times 10^{-19}\text{ C})}{3 \times 10^{-9}\text{ m}}$$

$$\approx -45 \times 10^{-20}\text{ J} = -4.5 \times 10^{-19}\text{ J (actual} = -4.6 \times 10^{-19}\text{ J)}$$

MCAT CONCEPT CHECK 5.3

Before you move on, assess your understanding of the material with these questions.

1. How does a change in electric potential energy from −4 J to −7 J reflect on the stability of a system?

2. Compare the relationship between electric potential energy and Coulomb's law to the relationship between gravitational potential energy and the universal law of gravitation.

3. How does electric potential energy change between two particles as the distance between them increases?

4. By what factor would electric potential energy change if the magnitude of both charges were doubled and the distance between them was halved?

5.4 Electric Potential

LEARNING OBJECTIVES

After Chapter 5.4, you will be able to:

- Calculate electric potential
- Distinguish between electric potential and voltage
- Predict the movement of a charge relative to a source charge, given the electric potential of the test charge's location
- Relate electric potential to electric potential energy, electric field, and Coulomb's law

Electric potential, discussed here, and electric potential energy, discussed previously, sound like the same (or nearly the same) thing. They are not, although they are very closely related. In fact, **electric potential** is defined as the ratio of the magnitude of a charge's electric potential energy to the magnitude of the charge itself. This can be expressed as:

$$V = \frac{U}{q}$$

Equation 5.4

where V is the electric potential measured in **volts (V)** and $1\text{ V} = 1\frac{\text{J}}{\text{C}}$. Even if there is no test charge q, we can still calculate the electric potential of a point in space in an electric field as long as we know the magnitude of the source charge and the distance from the source charge to the point in space in the field. By dividing $U = \frac{kQq}{r}$ by q, we get:

$$V = \frac{kQ}{r}$$

Equation 5.5

Electric potential is a scalar quantity, and its sign is determined by the sign of the source charge Q. For a positive source charge, V is positive, but for a negative source charge, V is negative. For a collection of charges, the total electric potential at a point in space is the scalar sum of the electric potential due to each charge.

Because electric potential is inversely proportional to the distance from the source charge, a potential difference will exist between two points that are at different distances from the source charge. If V_a and V_b are the electric potentials at points a and b, respectively, then the **potential difference** between them, known as **voltage**, is $V_b - V_a$. From the equation for electric potential above, we can further define potential difference as:

$$\Delta V = V_b - V_a = \frac{W_{ab}}{q}$$

Equation 5.6

where W_{ab} is the work needed to move a test charge q through an electric field from point a to point b. The work depends only on the potentials at the two points a and b and is independent of the actual pathway taken between a and b. Like gravitational force, the electrostatic force is a conservative force.

We've already seen that charges, if allowed, will move spontaneously in whatever direction results in a decrease in electric potential energy. For a positive test charge, this means moving from a position of higher electric potential to a position of lower electric potential. The voltage, $\Delta V = V_b - V_a$, is negative in this case; because q is positive (for a positive test charge), thus, W_{ab} must be negative, which represents a decrease in electric potential energy.

Now let's consider a negative test charge. A negative test charge will spontaneously move from a position of lower electric potential to a position of higher electric potential. The voltage, $\Delta V = V_b - V_a$, is positive in this case; because q is negative (for a negative test charge), W_{ab} must also be negative, which again represents a decrease in electric potential energy. The takeaway: positive charges will spontaneously move in the direction that *decreases* their electric potential (negative voltage), whereas negative charges will spontaneously move in the direction that *increases* their electric potential (positive voltage)—yet, in both cases, the electric potential *energy* is decreasing.

MCAT EXPERTISE

$F_e = \frac{kQq}{r^2}$	$U = \frac{kQq}{r}$
$E = \frac{kQ}{r^2}$	$V = \frac{kQ}{r}$

These are essential equations for Test Day. Know how they relate to each other and when to use them. By memorizing Coulomb's law, you should be able to recreate the table through mathematical manipulation. From left to right, multiply by r; from top to bottom, divide by q.

MNEMONIC

The "plus" end of a battery is the high-potential end, and the "minus" end of a battery is the low-potential end. Positive charge moves from + to − (the definition of current) while negative charge moves from − to +.

KEY CONCEPT

Electric potential is the ratio of the work done to move a test charge from infinity to a point in an electric field surrounding a source charge divided by the magnitude of the test charge.

BRIDGE

Create analogies between mechanics and electrostatics to familiarize yourself with these concepts. Electric field is like a gravitational field, and it exerts forces on charges much like a gravitational field exerts forces on masses. A test charge has a particular electric potential energy at a given electric potential, depending on the magnitude of its charge, much like a mass has a particular gravitational potential energy, depending on the magnitude of its mass. These mechanics concepts are discussed in Chapters 1 and 2 of *MCAT Physics and Math Review*.

MCAT CONCEPT CHECK 5.4

Before you move on, assess your understanding of the material with these questions.

1. What is the difference between electric potential and voltage?

2. How will a charge that is placed at a point of zero electric potential move relative to a source charge?

3. True or False: The units of electric potential energy and electric potential are different.

5.5 Special Cases in Electrostatics

LEARNING OBJECTIVES

After Chapter 5.5, you will be able to:

- Describe equipotential lines and electric dipoles
- Recall the electrical potential at points along the bisector of dipole
- Predict the voltage at two distinct points on an equipotential line
- Predict the behavior of a dipole when exposed to an external field:

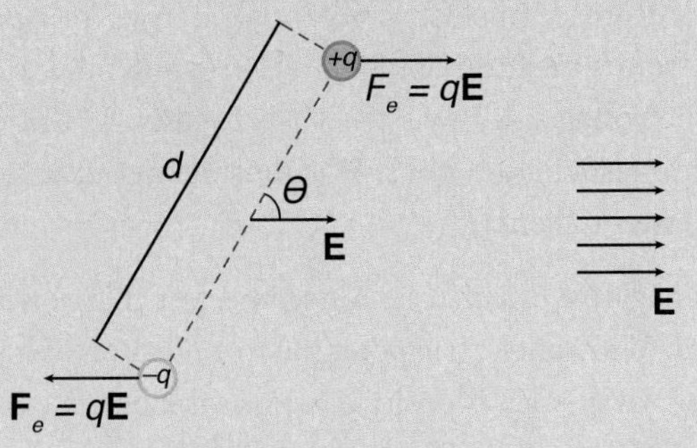

In this section, we will explore some of the unique setups in electrostatics that are common on the MCAT.

Equipotential Lines

An **equipotential line** is a line on which the potential at every point is the same. That is, the potential difference between any two points on an equipotential line is zero. Drawn on paper, equipotential lines may look like concentric circles surrounding a source charge. In three-dimensional space, these equipotential lines would actually be spheres surrounding the source charge. From the equation for electrical potential, we can see that no work is done when moving a test charge q from one point on an equipotential line to another. Work will be done in moving a test charge q from one line to another, but the work depends only on the potential difference of the two lines and not on the pathway taken between them. This is entirely analogous to the displacement of an object horizontally on a level surface. Because the object's height above the ground has not changed, its gravitational potential energy is unchanged. Furthermore, a change in the object's gravitational potential energy will not depend on the pathway taken from one height to another but only on the actual vertical displacement.

BRIDGE

Because the work to move a charge from one equipotential line to another does not depend on the path between them, we know that we are dealing only with conservative forces when moving the charge. Conservative and nonconservative forces are discussed in Chapter 2 of *MCAT Physics and Math Review.*

Example: In the diagram below, an electron goes from point a to point b in the vicinity of a very large positive charge. The electron could be made to follow any of the paths shown. Which path requires the least work to get the electron charge from a to b?

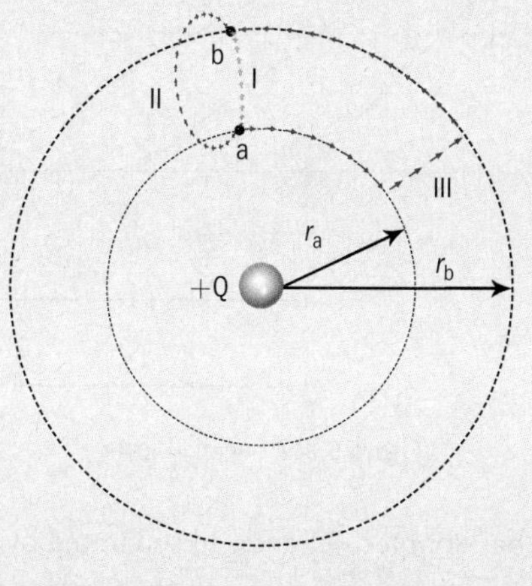

Solution: As stated, the work depends only on the potential difference and not on the path, so any of the paths shown would require the same amount of work in moving the electron from a to b. Note that because the source charge is positive, point b is at a *lower* electrical potential than point a. However, because the test charge is negative, the electrical potential energy is *higher* at point b than point a. This should make sense: the electron will have to gain energy to be moved farther away from positive source charge.

Electric Dipoles

Much of the reactivity of organic compounds is based on separation of charge. The **electric dipole**, which results from two equal and opposite charges being separated a small distance d from each other, can be transient (as in the case of the moment-to-moment changes in electron distribution that create London dispersion forces) or permanent (as in the case of the molecular dipole of water or the carbonyl functional group).

The electric dipole can be visualized as a barbell: the equal weights on either end of the bar represent the equal and opposite charges separated by a small distance, represented by the length of the bar. We'll analyze the generic dipole in Figure 5.3 and then work through the specific example of one of the most important electric dipoles, the water molecule.

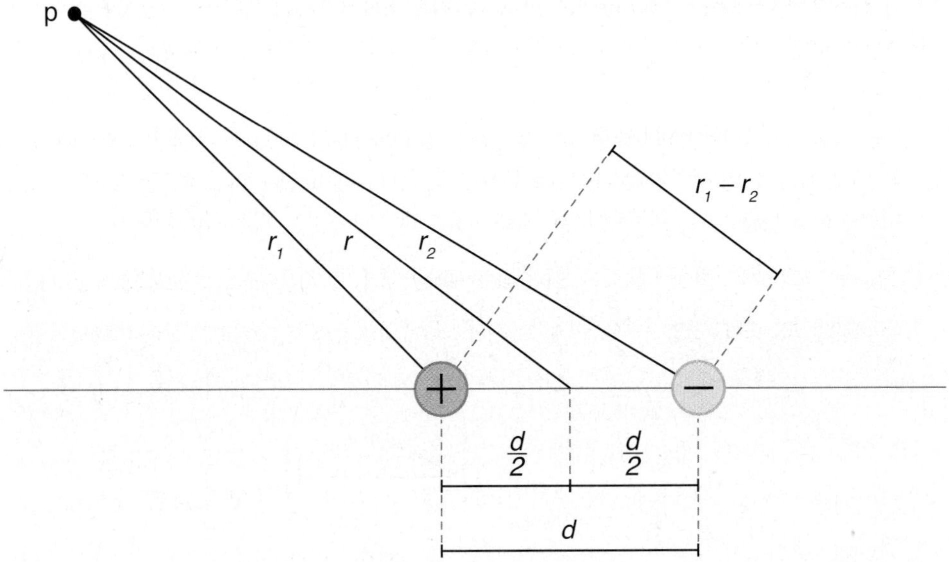

Figure 5.3 A Generic Dipole

The dipole in Figure 5.3 has charges $+q$ and $-q$ separated by a distance d. Notice that $+q$ and $-q$ are source charges, even though they are written in lowercase. Given the dipole, we may want to calculate the electrical potential at some point P near the dipole. The distance between the point in space and $+q$ is r_1; the distance between the point in space and $-q$ is r_2; the distance between the point in space and the midpoint of the dipole is r. We know that for a collection of charges, the electrical potential P is the scalar sum of the potentials due to each charge at that point. In other words:

$$V = \frac{kq}{r_1} - \frac{kq}{r_2}$$
$$= \frac{kq(r_2 - r_1)}{r_1 r_2}$$

For points in space relatively distant from the dipole (compared to d), the product of r_1 and r_2 is approximately equal to the square of r, and $r_1 - r_2$ is approximately equal to $d \cos \theta$. When we plug these approximations into the equation above, we get

$$V = \frac{kqd}{r^2} \cos \theta$$

Equation 5.7

The product of charge and separation distance is defined as the **dipole moment** (**p**) with SI units of C · m:

$$\mathbf{p} = qd$$

Equation 5.8

The dipole moment is a vector, but its direction is defined differently by physicists and chemists. Physicists define the vector along the line connecting the charges (the dipole axis), with the vector pointing from the negative charge toward the positive charge. Chemists usually reverse this convention, having **p** point from the positive charge toward the negative charge. Sometimes, chemists draw a crosshatch at the tail end of the dipole vector to indicate that the tail end is the positive charge.

Example: The H_2O molecule has a dipole moment of 1.85 D. Calculate the electrical potential due to a water molecule at a point 89 nm away along the axis of the dipole. (Note: $k = 8.99 \times 10^9 \frac{\text{N} \cdot \text{m}^2}{\text{C}^2}$ and 1 D (debye) $= 3.34 \times 10^{-30}$ C · m)

Solution: Because the question asks for the potential along the axis of the dipole, the angle θ is 0°. Substitute the values into the equation for the dipole potential and multiply 1.85 D by 3.34×10^{-30} to convert it to C · m:

$$V = \frac{kqd}{r^2} \cos \theta = \frac{kp}{r^2} \cos \theta$$

$$= \frac{\left(8.99 \times 10^9 \frac{\text{N} \cdot \text{m}^2}{\text{C}^2}\right)(1.85 \text{ D})\left(\frac{3.34 \times 10^{-30} \text{ C} \cdot \text{m}}{1 \text{ D}}\right)}{(89 \times 10^{-9} \text{ m})^2}$$

$$\approx \frac{(9)(2)(3)(10^{-21})}{(9 \times 10^{-8})^2} = \frac{(9)(2)(3)(10^{-21})}{(9)(9)(10^{-16})}$$

$$= \frac{(2 \times 10^{-21})}{(3 \times 10^{-16})} = 0.67 \times 10^{-5} \text{ V} = 6.7 \times 10^{-6} \text{ V (actual} = 7.01 \times 10^{-6} \text{ V)}$$

One very important equipotential line to be aware of is the plane that lies halfway between $+q$ and $-q$, called the **perpendicular bisector of the dipole**. Because the angle between this plane and the dipole axis is 90° (and $\cos 90° = 0$), the electrical potential at any point along this plane is 0. The magnitude of the electric field on the perpendicular bisector of the dipole can be approximated as

$$E = \frac{1}{4\pi\varepsilon_0} \times \frac{p}{r^3}$$

Equation 5.9

The electric field vectors at the points along the perpendicular bisector will point in the direction opposite to **p** (as defined directionally by physicists).

The dipole is a classic example of a setup upon which torques can act. In the absence of an electric field, the dipole axis can assume any random orientation. However, when the electric dipole is placed in a uniform external electric field, each of the equal and opposite charges of the dipole will experience a force exerted on it by the field. Because the charges are equal and opposite, the forces acting on the charges will also be equal in magnitude and opposite in direction, resulting in a situation of translational equilibrium. There will be, however, a net torque about the center of the dipole axis:

$$\begin{aligned}\tau &= \left(\frac{d}{2}\right)F_e \sin\theta + \left(\frac{d}{2}\right)F_e \sin\theta \\ &= dF_e \sin\theta \\ &= d(qE) \sin\theta \\ &= pE \sin\theta\end{aligned}$$

Thus, the net torque on a dipole can be calculated from the equation

$$\tau = pE \sin\theta$$

Equation 5.10

where p is the magnitude of the dipole moment ($p = qd$), E is the magnitude of the uniform external electric field, and θ is the angle the dipole moment makes with the electric field. This torque will cause the dipole to reorient itself so that its dipole moment, **p**, aligns with the electric field **E**, as shown in Figure 5.4.

MCAT EXPERTISE

The dipole is a great example of how the MCAT can test kinematics and dynamics in an electrostatics setting. For a dipole at some angle in an external electric field, there will be translational equilibrium, but not rotational equilibrium. This is because the forces are in opposite directions (left and right in Figure 5.4), but the torques are in the same direction (clockwise for both).

MCAT EXPERTISE

The electric dipole is most likely to be tested qualitatively or in the context of a passage or reaction on Test Day. It is unlikely that these mathematical relations will be presented or tested without background.

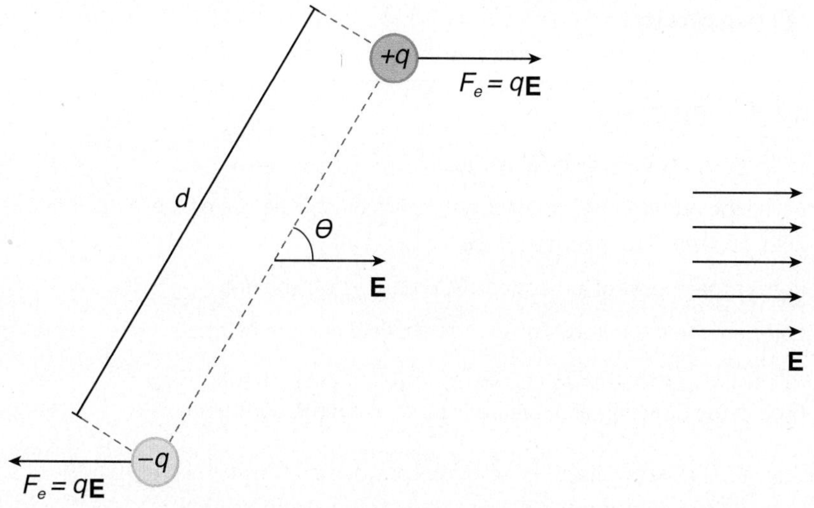

Figure 5.4 Torque on a Dipole from an External Electric Field

MCAT CONCEPT CHECK 5.5

Before you move on, assess your understanding of the material with these questions.

1. Define the following terms:
   - Equipotential lines:

   ___

   - Electric dipole:

   ___

2. What is the voltage between two points on an equipotential line? Will this voltage cause a charge to move along the line?

___

3. Why is the electrical potential at points along the perpendicular bisector of a dipole zero?

___

4. What is the behavior of an electric dipole when exposed to an external electric field?

___

5.6 Magnetism

LEARNING OBJECTIVES

After Chapter 5.6, you will be able to:

- Recall the requirements to have a nonzero electric field, a nonzero magnetic field, or a nonzero magnetic force
- Predict the impact of a magnetic field on a nearby object
- Calculate the magnitudes of a magnetic field and the magnetic force exerted by the field
- Predict the direction of a magnetic force using the right-hand rule:

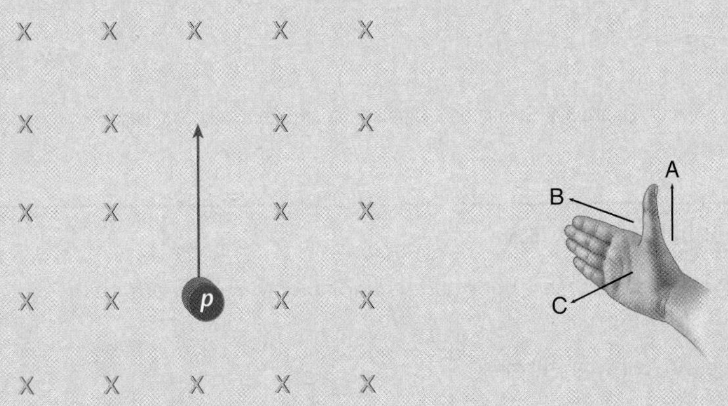

KEY CONCEPT

Any moving charge, whether a single electron traveling through space or a current through a conductive material, creates a **magnetic field.** The SI unit for magnetic field strength is the tesla (T).

Any moving charge creates a **magnetic field**. Magnetic fields may be set up by the movement of individual charges, such as an electron moving through space; by the mass movement of charge in the form of a current though a conductive material, such as a copper wire; or by permanent magnets. The SI unit for magnetic field strength is the **tesla** (**T**), where $1\ \text{T} = 1\ \frac{\text{N} \cdot \text{s}}{\text{m} \cdot \text{C}}$. The size of the tesla unit is quite large, so small magnetic fields are sometimes measured in **gauss**, where $1\ \text{T} = 10^4$ gauss.

All materials can be classified as diamagnetic, paramagnetic, or ferromagnetic. **Diamagnetic materials** are made of atoms with no unpaired electrons and that have no net magnetic field. These materials are slightly repelled by a magnet and so can be called weakly antimagnetic. Diamagnetic materials include common materials that you wouldn't expect to get stuck to a magnet: wood, plastics, water, glass, and skin, just to name a few.

The atoms of both paramagnetic and ferromagnetic materials have unpaired electrons, so these atoms do have a net magnetic dipole moment, but the atoms in these materials are usually randomly oriented so that the material itself creates no net magnetic field. **Paramagnetic materials** will become weakly magnetized in the presence of an external magnetic field, aligning the magnetic dipoles of the material with the external field. Upon removal of the external field, the thermal energy of the individual atoms will cause the individual magnetic dipoles to reorient randomly. Some paramagnetic materials include aluminum, copper, and gold.

Ferromagnetic materials, like paramagnetic materials, have unpaired electrons and permanent atomic magnetic dipoles that are normally oriented randomly so that the material has no net magnetic dipole. However, unlike paramagnetic materials, ferromagnetic materials will become strongly magnetized when exposed to a magnetic field or under certain temperatures. Common ferromagnetic materials include iron, nickel, and cobalt. Bar magnets are ferromagnetic materials with a north and south pole. Field lines exit the north pole and enter the south pole. Because magnetic field lines are circular, it is impossible to have a monopole magnet. If two bar magnets are allowed to interact, opposite poles will attract each other, while like poles will repel each other.

Magnetic Fields

Because any moving charge creates a magnetic field, we would certainly expect that a collection of moving charges, in the form of a current through a conductive wire, would produce a magnetic field in its vicinity. The configuration of the magnetic field lines surrounding a current-carrying wire will depend on the shape of the wire. Two special cases that are commonly tested on the MCAT include a long, straight wire and a circular loop of wire (with particular attention paid to the magnetic field at the center of that loop).

For an infinitely long and straight current-carrying wire, we can calculate the magnitude of the magnetic field produced by the current I in the wire at a perpendicular distance, r, from the wire as:

$$B = \frac{\mu_0 I}{2\pi r}$$

Equation 5.11

where B is the magnetic field at a distance r from the wire, μ_0 is the **permeability of free space** $\left(4\pi \times 10^{-7}\ \frac{\mathrm{T \cdot m}}{\mathrm{A}}\right)$, and I is the current. The equation demonstrates an inverse relationship between the magnitude of the magnetic field and the distance from the current. Straight wires create magnetic fields in the shape of concentric rings. To determine the direction of the field vectors, use a **right-hand rule**. (This is one of two right-hand rules used in magnetism.) Point your thumb in the direction of the current and wrap your fingers around the current-carrying wire. Your fingers then mimic the circular field lines, curling around the wire.

For a circular loop of current-carrying wire of radius r, the magnitude of the magnetic field at the center of the circular loop is given as:

$$B = \frac{\mu_0 I}{2r}$$

Equation 5.12

You'll notice that the two equations are quite similar—the obvious difference being that the equation for the magnetic field at the center of the circular loop of wire does not include the constant π. The less obvious difference is that the first expression gives the magnitude of the magnetic field at any perpendicular distance, r, from the current-carrying wire, while the second expression gives the magnitude of the magnetic field only at the center of the circular loop of current-carrying wire with radius r.

Example: Suppose a wire is formed into a loop that carries a current of 0.25 A in a clockwise direction, as shown here:

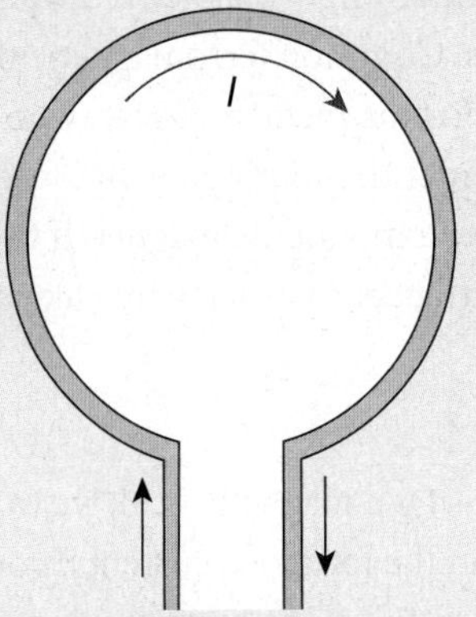

Determine the direction of the magnetic field produced by this loop within the loop and outside the loop. If the loop has a diameter of 1 m, what is the magnitude of the magnetic field at the center of the loop?

Solution: Use the right-hand rule to determine the direction of the magnetic field within and outside the loop, as shown here:

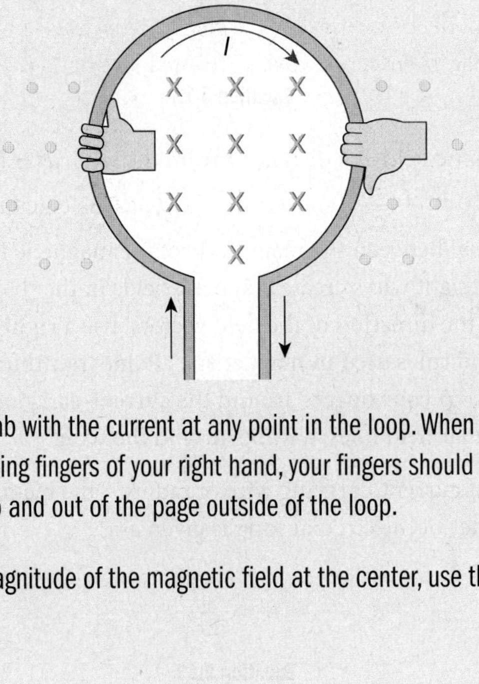

Align your right thumb with the current at any point in the loop. When you encircle the wire with the remaining fingers of your right hand, your fingers should point into the page within the loop and out of the page outside of the loop.

To determine the magnitude of the magnetic field at the center, use the equation for a loop of wire:

$$B = \frac{\mu_0 I}{2r}$$

$$= \frac{\left(4\pi \times 10^{-7} \frac{\text{T} \cdot \text{m}}{\text{A}}\right)(0.25\ \text{A})}{2 \times 0.5\ \text{m}} \approx 3.14 \times 10^{-7}\ \text{T} = 3.14 \times 10^{-3}\ \text{gauss}$$

Magnetic Forces

Now that we've reviewed the ways in which magnetic fields can be created, let's examine the forces that are exerted by magnetic fields on moving charges. Magnetic fields exert forces only on other moving charges. That is, charges do not "sense" their own fields; they only sense the field established by some external charge or collection of charges. Therefore, in our discussion of the magnetic force on moving charges and on current-carrying wires, we will assume the presence of a fixed and uniform external magnetic field. Note that charges often have both electrostatic and magnetic forces acting on them at the same time; the sum of these electrostatic and magnetic forces is known as the **Lorentz force**.

Force on a Moving Charge

When a charge moves in a magnetic field, a **magnetic force** may be exerted on it, the magnitude of which can be calculated as follows:

$$F_B = qvB \sin \theta$$

Equation 5.13

where q is the charge, v is the magnitude of its velocity, B is the magnitude of the magnetic field, and θ is the smallest angle between the velocity vector **v** and the magnetic field vector **B**. Notice that the magnetic force is a function of the sine of the angle, which means that the charge must have a perpendicular component of velocity in order to experience a magnetic force. If the charge is moving parallel or antiparallel to the magnetic field vector, it will experience no magnetic force.

Here we will introduce the second **right-hand rule** that you should practice in anticipation of Test Day. To determine the direction of the magnetic force on a moving charge, first position your right thumb in the direction of the velocity vector. Then, put your fingers in the direction of the magnetic field lines. Your palm will point in the direction of the force vector for a positive charge, whereas the back of your hand will point in the direction of the force vector for a negative charge.

KEY CONCEPT

Remember that sin 0° and sin 180° equal zero. This means that any charge moving parallel or antiparallel to the direction of the magnetic field will experience no force from the magnetic field.

MNEMONIC

Parts of the right-hand rule for magnetic force:

- Thumb—velocity (indicates direction of movement, like a hitchhiker's thumb)
- Fingers—field lines (fingers are parallel like the uniform magnetic field lines)
- Palm—force on a positive charge (you might give a "high five" to a positive person)
- Back of hand—force on a negative charge (you might give a backhand to a negative person)

Example: Suppose a proton is moving with a velocity of 15 $\frac{\text{m}}{\text{s}}$ toward the top of the page through a uniform magnetic field of 3.0 T directed into the page, as shown here:

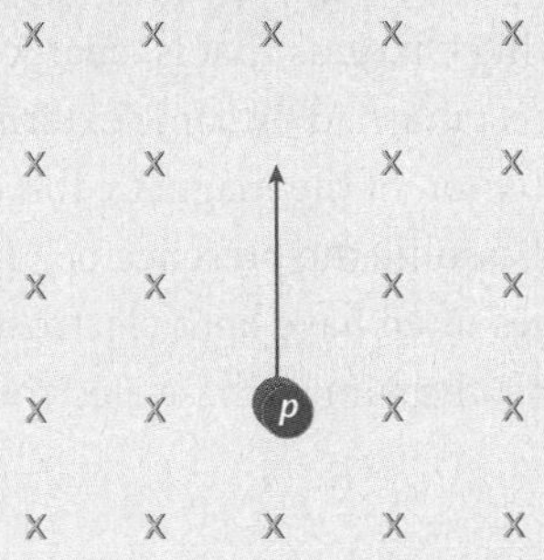

What is the magnitude and direction of the magnetic force on the proton? Describe the motion that will result from this setup. (Note: The charge of a proton is 1.60×10^{-19} C, and its mass is 1.67×10^{-27} kg.)

Solution: Start by determining the magnitude of the force:

$$\begin{aligned} F_B &= qvB \sin\theta \\ &= (1.60 \times 10^{-19}\ \text{C})\left(15\ \tfrac{\text{m}}{\text{s}}\right)(3.0\ \text{T})\sin 90^\circ \\ &= 7.2 \times 10^{-18}\ \text{N} \end{aligned}$$

To determine the direction, use the right-hand rule. Your thumb should point up the page in the direction of **v**. Your fingers should point into the page in the direction of **B**. Protons are positively charged; thus the force, $\mathbf{F}_B$, is in the direction of your palm, which is to the left. Note that $\mathbf{v}$ and $\mathbf{F}_B$ will always be perpendicular to each other; this implies that uniform circular motion will occur in this field, with $\mathbf{F}_B$ pointing radially inward toward the center of the circle.

If the centripetal force is the magnetic force, then we can set these two equations equal to each other:

$$F_c = F_B$$

$$\frac{mv^2}{r} = qvB \sin\theta$$

$$mv = qBr \sin 90^\circ$$

$$r = \frac{mv}{qB} = \frac{(1.67 \times 10^{-27}\ \text{kg})\left(15\ \frac{\text{m}}{\text{s}}\right)}{(1.60 \times 10^{-19}\ \text{C})(3.0\ \text{T})} \approx 5 \times 10^{-8}\ \text{m}\ \left(\text{actual} = 5.2 \times 10^{-8}\ \text{m}\right)$$

Thus, the proton will move in a circle with a radius of 52 nm.

Force on a Current-Carrying Wire

We've just examined the force that can be created by a magnetic field when a point charge moves through the field, so it should not come as a surprise that a current-carrying wire placed in a magnetic field may also experience a magnetic force. For a straight wire, the magnitude of the force created by an external magnetic field, F_B, is:

$$F_B = ILB \sin \theta$$

Equation 5.14

where I is the current, L is the length of the wire in the field, B is the magnitude of the magnetic field, and θ is the angle between **L** and **B**. The same right-hand rule can be used for a current-carrying wire in a field as for a moving point charge; just remember that current is considered the flow of positive charge.

Example: Suppose a wire of length 2.0 m is conducting a current of 5.0 A toward the top of the page and through a 30 gauss uniform magnetic field directed into the page. What is the magnitude and direction of the magnetic force on the wire?

Solution: Because 1 T $= 10^4$ gauss, 1 gauss $= 10^{-4}$ T, and 30 gauss $= 30 \times 10^{-4}$ T $= 3 \times 10^{-3}$ T. The wire is conducting current toward the top of the page, and the magnetic field points into the page; therefore, the current is perpendicular to the magnetic field. The angle between them is $\theta = 90°$. Now, plug into the equation:

$$F_B = ILB \sin \theta$$

$$= (5.0\ \text{A})(2.0\ \text{m})(3 \times 10^{-3}\ \text{T})(\sin 90°)$$

$$= 30 \times 10^{-3} = 3 \times 10^{-2}\ \text{N}$$

To determine the direction, use the right-hand rule. Your thumb should point up the page in the direction of **L**. Your fingers should point into the page in the direction of **B**. Current is a flow of positive charge; thus, the force, $\mathbf{F_B}$, is in the direction of your palm, which is to the left.

MCAT CONCEPT CHECK 5.6

Before you move on, assess your understanding of the material with these questions.

1. What are the requirements to have a nonzero electric field? A nonzero magnetic field? A nonzero magnetic force?

    - Nonzero electric field:

    ___

    - Nonzero magnetic field:

    ___

    - Nonzero magnetic force:

    ___

2. Which would experience a larger magnetic field: an object placed five meters to the left of a current carrying wire, or an object placed at the center of a circle with a radius of five meters? (Note: Assume the current is constant; $\mu_0 = 4\pi \times 10^{-7}\ \frac{\text{T}\cdot\text{m}}{\text{A}}$)

    ___

3. For each of the following combinations of velocity and magnetic field directions, determine the direction of the magnetic force on the given particle:

v	B	Particle	F
Up the page	Left	Electron	
Into the page	Out of the page	Proton	
Right	Into the page	Proton	
Out of the page	Left	Electron	
Down the page	Right	Neutron	

Conclusion

In this chapter, we reviewed the very notion of charge, reminding ourselves that charge comes in two varieties: positive and negative. We also explored the fact that charges travel differently within insulators and conductors. We learned that charges establish electric fields through which they can exert forces on other charges. We relied on similarities between electrical and gravitational systems to better understand Coulomb's law and the nature of the forces that exist between charged particles. Don't forget that electrical forces can be repulsive as well as attractive, which is one of the differences between electrical and gravitational systems. Charges contain electrical potential energy, which we defined as their energy of position with respect to other charges. Charges move within an electric field from one position of electrical potential to another; they will move spontaneously through an electrical potential difference, or voltage, in whichever direction results in a decrease in the charge's electrical potential energy. Then, we considered the geometry of the electric dipole and derived the equation for calculating the electrical potential at any point in space around the dipole. Finally, we considered magnetic fields and forces. In the next chapter, we'll examine moving charges as they interact with circuit elements and complete our understanding of electricity.

GO ONLINE

You've reviewed the content, now test your knowledge and critical thinking skills by completing a test-like passage set in your online resources!

CONCEPT SUMMARY

Charges

- The SI unit of charge is the **coulomb**.
- **Protons** have a positive charge and **electrons** have a negative charge.
  - Both protons and electrons possess the fundamental unit of charge ($e = 1.60 \times 10^{-19}$ C).
  - Protons and electrons have different masses.
- Opposite charges exert **attractive** forces, and like charges exert **repulsive** forces.
- **Conductors** allow the free and uniform passage of electrons when charged.
- **Insulators** resist the movement of charge and will have localized areas of charge that do not distribute over the surface of the material.

Coulomb's Law

- **Coulomb's law** gives the magnitude of the electrostatic force vector between two charges. The force vector always points along the line connecting the centers of the two charges.
- Every charge generates an **electric field**, which can exert forces on other charges.
- The electric field is the ratio of the force that is exerted on a test charge to the magnitude of that charge.
  - Electric field vectors can be represented as **field lines** that radiate outward from positive source charges and radiate inward to negative source charges.
  - Positive test charges will move in the direction of the field lines; negative test charges will move in the direction opposite of the field lines.

Electric Potential Energy

- **Electric potential energy** is the amount of work required to bring the test charge from infinitely far away to a given position in the vicinity of a source charge.
- The electric potential energy of a system will increase when two like charges move toward each other or when two opposite charges move farther apart.
- The electric potential energy of a system will decrease when two opposite charges move toward each other or when two like charges move farther apart.

Electric Potential

- **Electric potential** is the electric potential energy per unit charge.
- Different points in the space of an electric field surrounding a source charge will have different electric potential values.
- Potential difference (**voltage**) is the change in electric potential that accompanies the movement of a test charge from one position to another.
  - Potential difference is path independent and depends only on the initial and final positions of the test charge.
  - The units for both electric potential and voltage are volts.
- Test charges will move spontaneously in whichever direction results in a decrease in their electric potential energy.
  - Positive test charges will move spontaneously from high potential to low potential.
  - Negative test charges will move spontaneously from low potential to high potential.

Special Cases in Electrostatics

- **Equipotential lines** designate the set of points around a source charge or multiple source charges that have the same electric potential.
  - Equipotential lines are always perpendicular to electric field lines.
  - Work will be done when a charge is moved from one equipotential line to another; the work is independent of the pathway taken between the lines.
  - No work is done when a charge moves from a point on an equipotential line to another point on the same equipotential line.
- Two charges of opposite sign separated by a fixed distance, *d*, generate an **electric dipole**.
  - In an external electric field, an electric dipole will experience a net torque until it is aligned with the electric field vector.
  - An electric field will not induce any translational motion in the dipole regardless of its orientation with respect to the electric field vector.

Magnetism

- **Magnetic fields** are created by magnets and moving charges.
- The SI unit for the magnetic field is the **tesla** (**T**; 1 T = 10,000 gauss).
- **Diamagnetic materials** possess no unpaired electrons and are slightly repelled by a magnet.
- **Paramagnetic materials** possess some unpaired electrons and become weakly magnetic in an external magnetic field.
- **Ferromagnetic materials** possess some unpaired electrons and become strongly magnetic in an external magnetic field.
- Magnets have a north and a south pole; field lines point from the north to the south pole.
- Current-carrying wires create magnetic fields that are concentric circles surrounding the wire.
- External magnetic fields exert forces on charges moving in any direction except parallel or antiparallel to the field.
- Point charges may undergo uniform circular motion in a uniform magnetic field wherein the centripetal force is the magnetic force acting on the point charge.
- The direction of the magnetic force on a moving charge or current-carrying wire is determined using the right-hand rule.
- The **Lorentz force** is the sum of the electrostatic and magnetic forces acting on a body.

ANSWERS TO CONCEPT CHECKS

5.1

1. The electrons will experience the greater acceleration because they are subject to the same force as the protons but have a significantly smaller mass.
2. Conductors: blood, copper, iron, sulfuric acid; insulators: hair, glass, distilled water
3. The net charge will be -1 C; neutrons do not contribute charge.

5.2

1. The electric field would be 0 because the two charges are the same. In this case, the fields exerted by each charge at the midpoint will cancel out and there will be no electric field.
2. For a pair of charges, a negative electrostatic force points from one charge to the other (attractive), while a positive electrostatic force points from one charge away from the other (repulsive).
3. 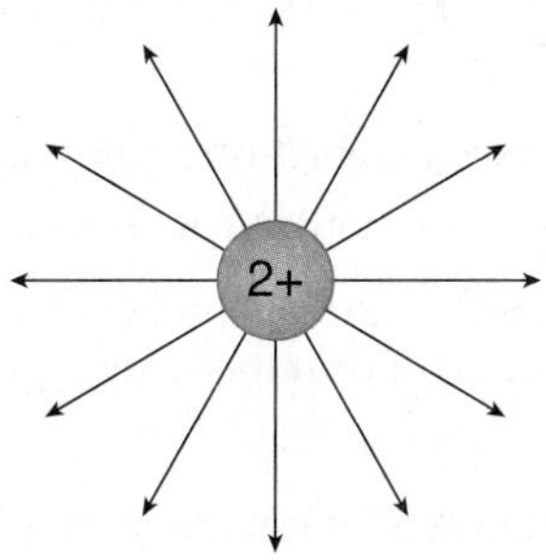

4. Electrostatic force is directly related to each charge and related to the distance by an inverse square relationship. Electric field is unrelated to test charge but is still related to distance by an inverse square relationship. Note that it is the source charge that creates the electric field—not the test charge—so we cannot use the equation $E = \frac{F_e}{q}$ to determine a relationship.

5.3

1. A decrease in potential energy indicates that the system has become more stable. Keep in mind that negative numbers with larger absolute values are more negative, and represent a decrease in value from negative numbers with smaller absolute values (that is, $-4 > -7$ even though $|-4| < |-7|$).
2. Electrical potential energy is Coulomb's law multiplied by distance, whereas gravitational potential energy is the universal law of gravitation multiplied by distance.
3. If both particles have the same charge, the electrical potential energy decreases as distance increases. If the two particles have opposite charges, then the electrical potential energy increases as distance increases.

4. As given by the equation $U = \frac{kQq}{r}$, the electric potential energy would increase by a factor of eight if both charges are doubled and the radius is halved.

5.4

1. Electrical potential is the ratio of a charge's electrical potential energy to the magnitude of the charge itself. Voltage, or potential difference, is a measure of the change in electrical potential between two points, which provides an indication of the tendency toward movement in one direction or the other.
2. A charge will move in such a way to minimize its potential energy. Placing a charge at a point of zero electrical potential does not indicate that there is zero potential difference, so the charge may or may not move—and if it moves, it may move toward or away from the source charge depending on the sign of the source charge and test charge.
3. True. Electrical potential energy is measured in joules (J), while electrical potential and potential difference (voltage) are measured in volts (V).

5.5

1. Equipotential lines are the sets of points within space at which the potential difference between any two points is zero. This is best visualized as concentric spheres surrounding a source charge. An electric dipole is the separation of charge within a molecule such that there is a permanent or temporary region of equal and opposite charges at a particular distance.
2. There is no voltage between two points on an equipotential line, so there will be no acceleration along the line. However, there is a potential difference between different sets of equipotential lines, which can cause particles to move and accelerate.
3. The perpendicular bisector of an electric dipole is an equipotential plane that is perpendicular to the axis of the dipole. As such, the equation $V = \frac{kqd}{r^2} \cos \theta$ is necessarily equal to 0 because $\cos 90° = 0$.
4. A dipole will rotate within an external electric field such that its dipole moment aligns with the field.

5.6

1. To create an electric field, one needs a charge. To create a magnetic field, one needs a charge that must also be moving. To create a magnetic force, one needs an external electric field acting on a charge moving any direction except parallel or antiparallel to the external field.
2. We need not determine the actual values of the magnetic fields in these two cases and can compare the two equations instead. The magnetic field created by the current-carrying wire is given by $B = \frac{\mu_0 I}{2\pi r}$; the magnetic field created by the loop of wire is given by $B = \frac{\mu_0 I}{2r}$ and μ_0, I, and r are the same in both equations. Therefore, the magnetic field at the center of the loop must be larger because the denominator in that equation does *not* include π.
3.

v	B	Particle	F
Up the page	Left	Electron	Into the page
Into the page	Out of the page	Proton	None $(\sin 180° = 0)$
Right	Into the page	Proton	Up the page
Out of the page	Left	Electron	Up the page
Down the page	Right	Neutron	None $(q = 0)$

SCIENCE MASTERY ASSESSMENT EXPLANATIONS

1. **B**

According to Newton's third law, if R exerts a force on S, then S exerts a force with equal magnitude but opposite direction back on R. Therefore, the magnitude of the force on R due to S is F.

2. **D**

The force is inversely proportional to r^2. Cutting the distance in half will therefore multiply the force by 2^2, making it four times its original value:

$$F_{\text{old}} \propto \frac{1}{r^2}$$

$$F_{\text{new}} \propto \frac{1}{\left(\frac{r}{2}\right)^2} = \frac{4}{r^2} = 4 \times F_{\text{old}}$$

3. **B**

An electric field's direction at a given point is defined as the direction of the force that would be exerted on a positive test charge in that position. Because electrons are negatively charged particles, they will therefore feel a force in the opposite direction of the electric field's vector. In this case, because the force points to the left (toward R), an electron will feel a force pointing to the right (toward S) if **E** is in the same direction as **F**.

4. **B**

The first step in answering this question is to remember that the magnitude of the electric field is inversely proportional to the square of the distance:

$$E = \frac{kQ}{r^2} \rightarrow E \propto \frac{1}{r^2}$$

Therefore, if the electric field at radius r, E_r, is 36 $\frac{\text{N}}{\text{C}}$, then the electric field at radius $2r$ will be

$$E_{2r} \propto \frac{1}{(2r)^2} = \frac{1}{4r^2} = \frac{E_r}{4}$$

$$= \frac{\left(36\ \frac{\text{N}}{\text{C}}\right)}{4} = 9\ \frac{\text{N}}{\text{C}}$$

Similarly, the electric field at radius $3r$ is equal to

$$E_{3r} \propto \frac{1}{(3r)^2} = \frac{1}{9r^2} = \frac{E_r}{9}$$

$$= \frac{\left(36\ \frac{\text{N}}{\text{C}}\right)}{9} = 4\ \frac{\text{N}}{\text{C}}$$

Therefore, the ratio of E_r:E_{2r}:E_{3r} is 36:9:4.

5. **C**

A positive charge placed at A will experience two forces: a force to the left due to $+2Q$ and a force to the right due to $+Q$. Because point A is the same distance from $+Q$ and $+2Q$, the force due to $+2Q$ will be larger than that due to $+Q$, and there will be a net force to the left (toward $+Q$). At point B, the forces from both $+Q$ and $+2Q$ will point to the right, so there will be a net force to the right.

6. **C**

Recall that the change in potential energy, ΔU, and the change in potential, ΔV, are related by $W = \Delta U = q\Delta V$. Therefore, $\Delta U = (2 \times 10^{-6}\ \text{C}) \times (-12\ \text{V}) = -2.4 \times 10^{-5}\ \text{J}$. The positive charge is moving from the positive to the negative plate, and is therefore decreasing in potential energy; this is reflected by the fact that the voltage is -12 V rather than $+12$ V. The potential energy that is lost is converted into kinetic energy, so the charge must gain 2.4×10^{-5} J of kinetic energy.

7. **C**

There will be work done in moving the negative charge from its initial position to $y = 0$. However, in moving the negative charge from $y = 0$ to the final position, the same amount of work is done but with the opposite sign. This is because the force changes direction as the electron crosses $y = 0$. Therefore, the two quantities of work cancel each other out. This argument depends crucially on the symmetry of the initial and final positions.

8. **D**

The safest way to answer this question is to quickly draw a diagram:

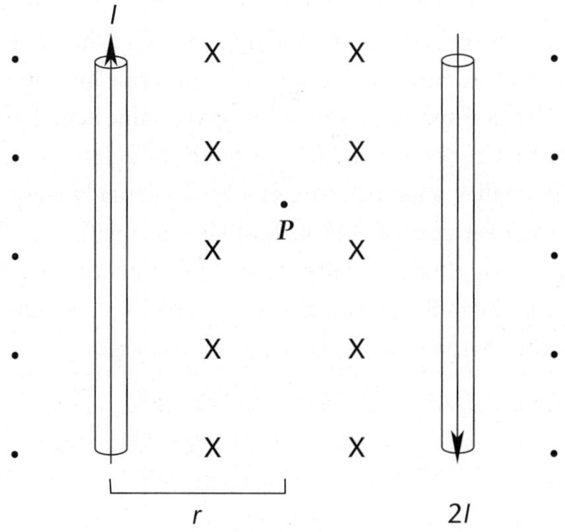

Notice right away that between the two wires, the direction of the magnetic field is the same: into the page. Therefore, because the vector direction is the same, we can just focus on the magnitudes of the two magnetic fields. We know that $B_1 =$ 10 T at a distance r. Consider the relationships in the equation $B = \frac{\mu_0 I}{2\pi r}$. Magnetic field and current are directly proportional, whereas magnetic field and distance are inversely proportional. Therefore, doubling the current will result in double the magnetic field of the first wire, or 20 T. The overall magnitude of the magnetic field is $10\text{ T} + 20\text{ T} = 30\text{ T}$ into the page.

9. **B**

Potential is a scalar quantity. The total potential is the sum of the potentials of the positive and negative charges:

$$V_T = V_+ + V_- = \frac{+kq}{r_+} + \left(\frac{-kq}{r_-}\right)$$

where r_+ and r_- represent the distances from the positive and negative charge, respectively. The sum of these terms will be zero at any point where $r_+ = r_-$. This will be at any point along the perpendicular bisector of the dipole axis, as well as at infinity.

10. **D**

The electric potential (V) is equal to the amount of work done (W) divided by the test charge (q). This means that the potential is directly proportional to the amount of work done, which is equal to the amount of energy gained by the particle; therefore, the overall amount of energy increases by a factor of 4. Because energy is directly proportional to the square of the speed (according to $\frac{1}{2}mv^2$), the speed must increase by a factor of 2.

11. **D**

You should know that the field lines for a positively charged particle will always point away from the particle in a radial pattern, regardless of the direction in which the particle is moving. This is because field lines point in the direction a positive test charge would move in that field (that is, the direction that a force would be exerted on a positive test charge in that field).

12. **C**

Voltage (ΔV) is equal to the quotient of the amount of work done (W) divided by the charge of the particle on which the work is done (q), according to the equation $V = \frac{\Delta U}{q} = \frac{W}{q}$. Because the voltage equals 9 V and the charge equals 2 C, the work done must equal $9\text{ V} \times 2\text{ C} = 18\text{ J}$.

13. **C**

To prevent the flow of charge between the two plates, the dielectric should be an insulative material. Insulative materials contain atoms that tightly bind to their electrons, often nonmetals. Glass is composed of two nonmetals, silicon and oxygen, and would be the best insulator, supporting choice **(C)**. On the other hand, while pure water itself can be an insulator, the presence of ions greatly increases the conductivity of salt water, eliminating **(A)**.

14. **B**

This problem is an application of the right-hand rule. The velocity vector **v** is always tangent to the circle. The magnetic force must always point radially toward the center of the circle. Consider when the negative charge is at the "12 o'clock" position in its circle and apply the right-hand rule. Your thumb points to the left, tangent to the circle at this point. The back of your hand, which represents the force on a negative charge, points down the page, radially toward the center of the circle. Your fingers must point out of the page to get your hand into this position. Therefore, the direction of the magnetic field must be out of the page.

15. **A**

Often, with potential energy, it can be easier to think in terms of common sense, rather than in terms of rigorous mathematical formulas: opposite charges attract. When oppositely charged species like ATP and a cation are moved apart, their potential energy will increase, reflecting the fact that these oppositely charged species would like to move back to a closer distance. Furthermore, the formula for electric potential energy is $U = kQq/r$. From this formula, observe that the relationship between U and r is given by $U \propto 1/r$, meaning that if r is changed by a factor of 2, then U will also change by a factor of 2, and not by a factor of 4. These observations together are enough to justify **(A)** as the correct answer.

For a more mathematically rigorous explanation, consider that the opposite charges of ATP and the cation will cause the output of the formula $U = kQq/r$ to be negative. Then, when the distance between these two charges is doubled, this expression becomes $U = kQq/2r$, which is half as large in magnitude. However, because U is negative for oppositely charged species, a smaller *negative* value actually means that U has *increased*! (Consider: though the magnitude is smaller, a temperature of $-5°C$ is actually *warmer* than a temperature of $-25°C$. Similarly, a U with a smaller negative magnitude actually means higher energy.) In short, doubling the radius means that the energy is also doubled when the charged species have opposite charges.

Consult your online resources for additional practice. GO ONLINE

EQUATIONS TO REMEMBER

(5.1) **Coulomb's law:** $F_e = \frac{kq_1q_2}{r^2}$

(5.2) **Electric field:** $E = \frac{F_e}{q} = \frac{kQ}{r^2}$

(5.3) **Electric potential energy:** $U = \frac{kQq}{r}$

(5.4) **Electric potential (from electric potential energy):** $V = \frac{U}{q}$

(5.5) **Electric potential (from source charge):** $V = \frac{kQ}{r}$

(5.6) **Voltage:** $\Delta V = V_b - V_a = \frac{W_{ab}}{q}$

(5.7) **Electric potential near a dipole:** $V = \frac{kqd}{r^2}\cos\theta$

(5.8) **Dipole moment:** $\mathbf{p} = q\mathbf{d}$

(5.9) **Electric field on the perpendicular bisector of a dipole:** $E = \frac{1}{4\pi\varepsilon_0} \times \frac{p}{r^3}$

(5.10) **Torque on a dipole in an electric field:** $\tau = pE \sin\theta$

(5.11) **Magnetic field from a straight wire:** $B = \frac{\mu_0 I}{2\pi r}$

(5.12) **Magnetic field from a loop of wire:** $B = \frac{\mu_0 I}{2r}$

(5.13) **Magnetic force on a moving point charge:** $F_B = qvB \sin\theta$

(5.14) **Magnetic force on a current-carrying wire:** $F_B = ILB \sin\theta$

SHARED CONCEPTS

General Chemistry Chapter 1
Atomic Structure

General Chemistry Chapter 3
Bonding and Chemical Interactions

General Chemistry Chapter 12
Electrochemistry

Physics and Math Chapter 1
Kinematics and Dynamics

Physics and Math Chapter 2
Work and Energy

Physics and Math Chapter 6
Circuits

CHAPTER 6

CIRCUITS

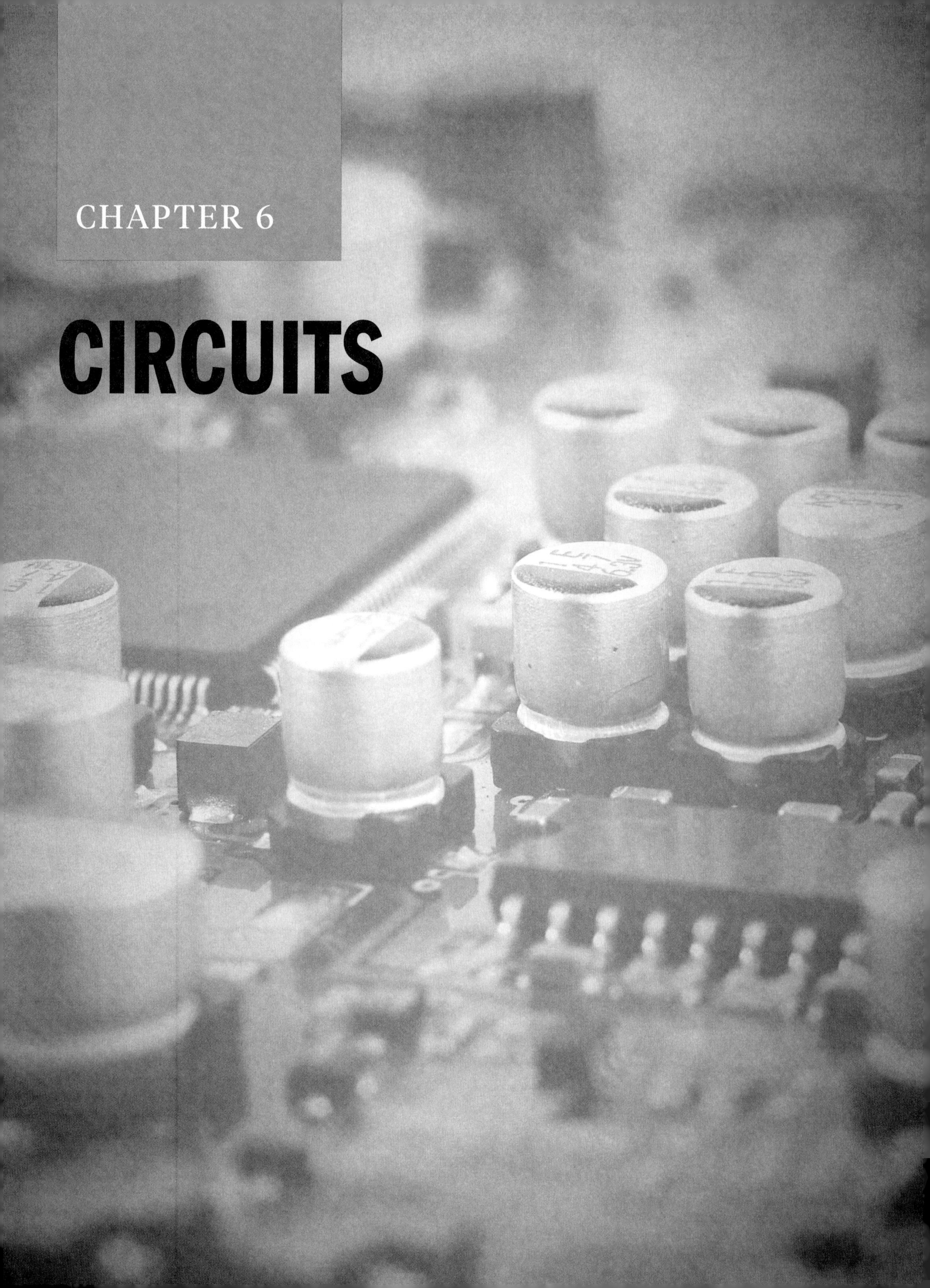

SCIENCE MASTERY ASSESSMENT

Every pre-med knows this feeling: there is so much content I have to know for the MCAT! How do I know what to do first or what's important?

While the high-yield badges throughout this book will help you identify the most important topics, this Science Mastery Assessment is another tool in your MCAT prep arsenal. This quiz (which can also be taken in your online resources) and the guidance below will help ensure that you are spending the appropriate amount of time on this chapter based on your personal strengths and weaknesses. Don't worry though—skipping something now does not mean you'll never study it. Later on in your prep, as you complete full-length tests, you'll uncover specific pieces of content that you need to review and can come back to these chapters as appropriate.

How to Use This Assessment

If you answer 0–7 questions correctly:

Spend about 1 hour to read this chapter in full and take limited notes throughout. Follow up by reviewing **all** quiz questions to ensure that you now understand how to solve each one.

If you answer 8–11 questions correctly:

Spend 20–40 minutes reviewing the quiz questions. Beginning with the questions you missed, read and take notes on the corresponding subchapters. For questions you answered correctly, ensure your thinking matches that of the explanation and you understand why each choice was correct or incorrect.

If you answer 12–15 questions correctly:

Spend less than 20 minutes reviewing all questions from the quiz. If you missed any, then include a quick read-through of the corresponding subchapters, or even just the relevant content within a subchapter, as part of your question review. For questions you got correct, ensure your thinking matches that of the explanation and review the Concept Summary at the end of the chapter.

1. If a defibrillator passes 15 A of current through a patient's body for 0.1 seconds, how much charge goes through the patient's skin?
   - A. 0.15 C
   - B. 1.5 C
   - C. 15 C
   - D. 150 C

2. A student places an ammeter with negligible resistance in parallel with a resistor to determine the amount of current that passes through the resistor. Does the student obtain an accurate reading?
   - A. Yes, because the student used an ammeter with negligible resistance.
   - B. Yes, because the current going through parallel paths is equal.
   - C. No, because the ammeter should have infinite resistance.
   - D. No, because an ammeter in parallel changes the current through the resistor.

3. The resistance of two conductors of equal cross-sectional area and equal lengths are compared, and are found to be in the ratio 1:2. The resistivities of the materials from which they are constructed must therefore be in what ratio?
   - A. 1:1
   - B. 1:2
   - C. 2:1
   - D. 4:1

4. A voltaic cell provides a current of 0.5 A when in a circuit with a 3 Ω resistor. If the internal resistance of the cell is 0.1 Ω, what is the voltage across the terminals of the battery when there is no current flowing?
   - A. 0.05 V
   - B. 1.5 V
   - C. 1.505 V
   - D. 1.55 V

5. A transformer is a device that takes an input voltage and produces an output voltage that can be either larger or smaller than the input voltage, depending on the transformer design. Although the voltage is changed by the transformer, energy is not, so the input power equals the output power. A particular transformer produces an output voltage that is 300 percent of the input voltage. What is the ratio of the output current to the input current?
   - A. 1:3
   - B. 3:1
   - C. 1:300
   - D. 300:1

6. Given that $R_1 = 20\ \Omega$, $R_2 = 4\ \Omega$, $R_3 = R_4 = 32\ \Omega$, $R_5 = 15\ \Omega$, and $R_6 = 5\ \Omega$, what is the total resistance in the setup shown below?

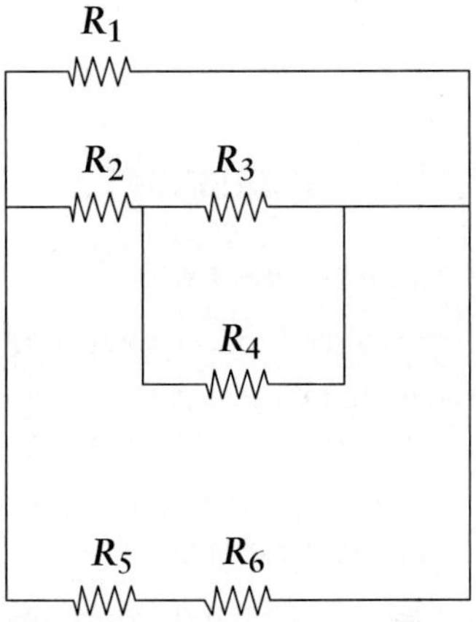

   - A. 0.15 Ω
   - B. 6.67 Ω
   - C. 16.7 Ω
   - D. 60 Ω

7. How many moles of electrons pass through a circuit containing a 100 V battery and a 2 Ω resistor over a period of 10 seconds? (Note: $F = 9.65 \times 10^4 \frac{C}{mol\ e^-}$.)
   - A. 5.18×10^{-3} moles
   - B. 500 moles
   - C. 5.18×10^{3} moles
   - D. 5.2×10^{6} moles

8. In the circuit below, what is the voltage drop across the $\frac{2}{3}$ Ω resistor?

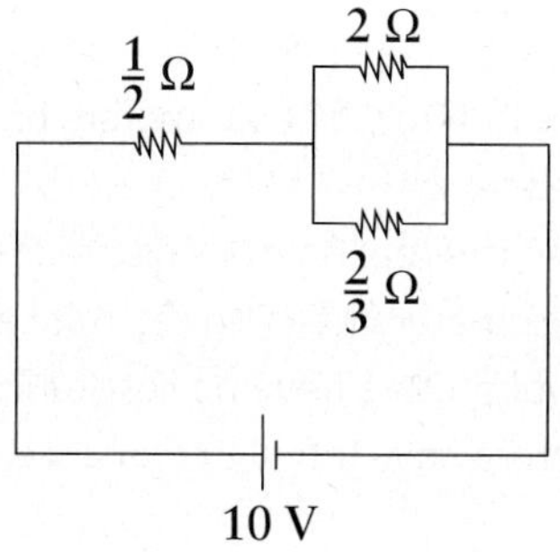

A. $\frac{1}{2}$ V
B. $\frac{2}{3}$ V
C. 5 V
D. 7.5 V

9. If the area of a capacitor's plates is doubled while the distance between them is halved, how will the final capacitance (C_f) compare to the original capacitance (C_i)?
A. $C_f = C_i$
B. $C_f = \frac{1}{2}C_i$
C. $C_f = 2C_i$
D. $C_f = 4C_i$

10. The energy stored in a fully charged capacitor is given by $U = \frac{1}{2}CV^2$. In a typical cardiac defibrillator, a capacitor charged to 7500 V has a stored energy of 400 J. Based on this information, what is the charge on the capacitor in the cardiac defibrillator?
A. 1.1×10^{-5} C
B. 5×10^{-2} C
C. 1.1×10^{-1} C
D. 3.1×10^{6} C

11. A 10 Ω resistor carries a current that varies as a function of time as shown. How much energy has been dissipated by the resistor after 5 s?

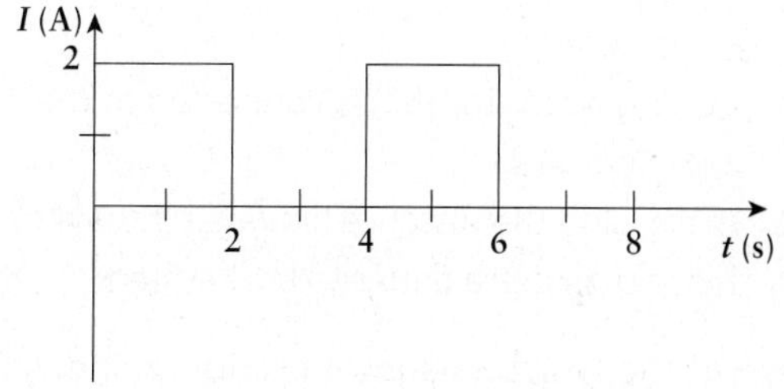

A. 40 J
B. 50 J
C. 120 J
D. 160 J

12. In the figure below, six currents meet at point *P*. What is the magnitude and direction of the current between points *P* and *x*?

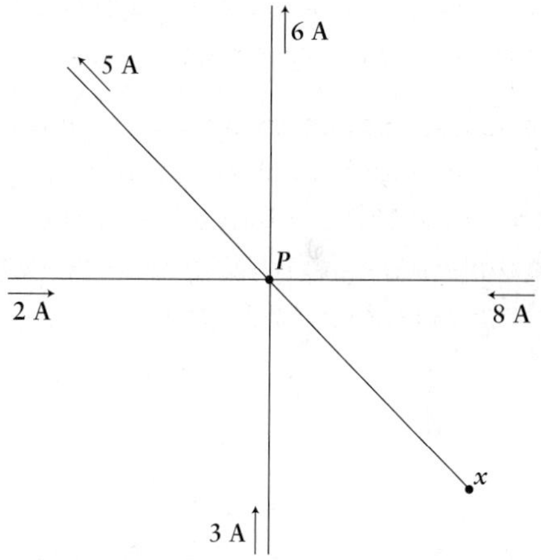

A. 2 A, toward *x*
B. 2 A, toward *P*
C. 10 A, toward *x*
D. 10 A, toward *P*

13. Which of the following will most likely increase the electric field between the plates of a parallel plate capacitor?

A. Adding a resistor that is connected to the capacitor in series

B. Adding a resistor that is connected to the capacitor in parallel

C. Increasing the distance between the plates

D. Adding an extra battery to the system

14. Each of the resistors shown carries an individual resistance of 4 Ω. Assuming negligible resistance in the wire, what is the overall resistance of the circuit?

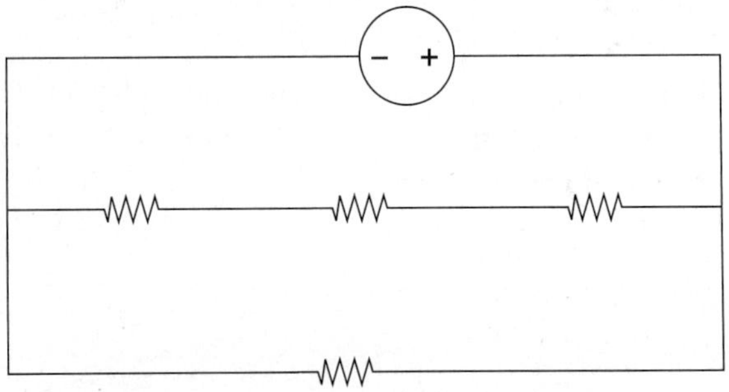

A. 16 Ω

B. 8 Ω

C. 4 Ω

D. 3 Ω

15. Which of the following best characterizes ideal voltmeters and ammeters?

A. Ideal voltmeters and ammeters have infinite resistance.

B. Ideal voltmeters and ammeters have no resistance.

C. Ideal voltmeters have infinite resistance, and ideal ammeters have no resistance.

D. Ideal voltmeters have no resistance, and ideal ammeters have infinite resistance.

Answer Key follows on next page.

Answer Key

1. **B**
2. **D**
3. **B**
4. **D**
5. **A**
6. **B**
7. **A**
8. **C**
9. **D**
10. **C**
11. **C**
12. **A**
13. **D**
14. **D**
15. **C**

Detailed explanations can be found at the end of the chapter.

CHAPTER 6

CIRCUITS

In This Chapter

CHAPTER PROFILE

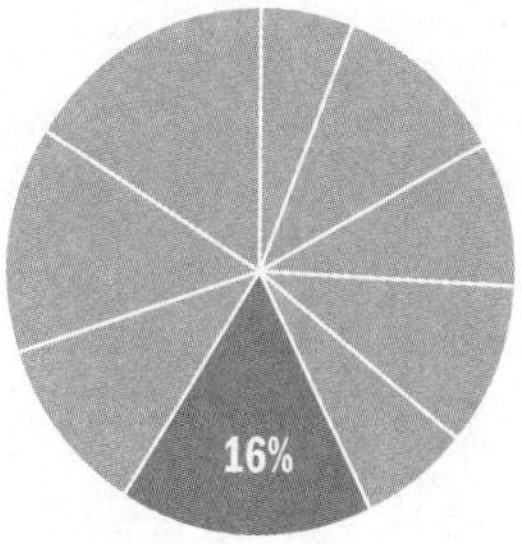

The content in this chapter should be relevant to about 16% of all questions about physics on the MCAT.

This chapter covers material from the following AAMC content category:

4C: Electrochemistry and electrical circuits and their elements

Introduction

Batteries, electric circuits, and electrical equipment pervade our everyday world. Think of any piece of equipment, tool, or toy that has a battery or a power cord, and you've identified an object that depends on the movement of electrons and the delivery of electric potential energy to carry out its function. Turn on a light, watch TV, or toast bread, and you can literally watch electrons at work as they emit light. Electricity is not restricted to the inorganic, material world—even in our bodies, we find electricity serving a key role in a number of physiological functions. Not only do the neurons in our brain and conduction system in our heart rely on electricity, but so does every cell that utilizes mitochondria to carry out oxidative phosphorylation.

This chapter reviews the essentials of circuits. From this broad knowledge base, we will draw on specific topics within circuit theory: conductivity, electromotive force (emf), resistance, power, Kirchhoff's laws, resistors, capacitors, meters, and series and parallel arrangements of circuit components. As you encounter the concepts of this chapter and the equations associated with them, remember this: the MCAT approaches the topic of circuits with a greater emphasis on the concepts than on the math. You will be expected to calculate, say, the equivalent resistance for resistors in series or parallel, but the circuits you encounter on Test Day will, on the whole, be simpler than what you may have seen in your college physics class.

6.1 Current

LEARNING OBJECTIVES

After Chapter 6.1, you will be able to:

- Recall the definitions of current, voltage, electromotive force (emf), and conductivity, and the SI units for each
- Compare the conductivity of two solutions, given their component ions
- Describe the relationship between voltage sources and voltage drop
- Use Kirchhoff's laws to describe the flow of electrons through a circuit

In the last chapter we examined the behaviors of still charges, but in most cases we are interested in the movement of charge, or current. Because of historical conventions, **current** is considered the flow of positive charge—even though only negative charges are actually moving. Any conductive substance may act as a medium through which current can pass.

Conductivity

Conductivity can be divided into two categories: **metallic conductivity**, as seen in solid metals and the molten forms of some salts, or **electrolytic conductivity**, as seen in solutions. **Conductance** is the reciprocal of resistance, a property we will examine in detail later. The SI unit for conductance is the **siemens (S)**, sometimes given as siemens per meter $\left(\frac{\text{S}}{\text{m}}\right)$ for conductivity.

Metallic Conductivity

Some materials allow free flow of electric charge within them; these materials are called electrical conductors. Metal atoms can easily lose one or more of their outer electrons, which are then free to move around in the larger collection of metal atoms. This makes most metals good electrical and thermal conductors. The **metallic bond** has often been visualized as a sea of electrons flowing over and past a rigid lattice of metal cations. While this model is generally appropriate for the MCAT, metallic bonding is more accurately described as an equal distribution of the charge density of free electrons across all of the neutral atoms within the metallic mass.

BRIDGE

Remember that the metals are found on the left side of the periodic table. These are the atoms with the lowest ionization energies; thus, it is easiest for these atoms to lose electrons. Due to this weak hold, electrons are free to move around in the metal, conducting electrical charges. Periodic trends are discussed in Chapter 2 of *MCAT General Chemistry Review*.

Electrolytic Conductivity

While not substantially different from metallic conductivity, it is important to note that electrolytic conductivity depends on the strength of a solution. Distilled deionized water has such a low ion concentration that it may be considered an insulator, while sea water and orange juice are excellent conductors. Conductivity in an electrolyte solution is measured by placing the solution as a resistor in a circuit and measuring changes in voltage across the solution. Because concentration and conductivity are directly related, this method is often used to determine ionic concentrations in solutions, such as blood. One caveat is that conductivity in nonionic solutions is always lower than in ionic solutions. While the concentration of total dissolved solids does relate to conductivity, the contribution of nonionic solids is much, much less important than ion concentration.

Current

Chapter 5 of *MCAT Physics and Math Review* introduced the concept of electrical current: the flow of charge between two points at different electrical potentials connected by a conductor, such as a copper wire. The magnitude of the **current** I is the amount of charge Q passing through the conductor per unit time Δt, and it can be calculated as:

$$I = \frac{Q}{\Delta t}$$

Equation 6.1

The SI unit of current is the **ampère** $\left(1 \text{ A} = 1 \frac{\text{C}}{\text{s}}\right)$. Charge is transmitted by a flow of electrons in a conductor, and because electrons are negatively charged, they move from a point of lower electrical potential to a point of higher electrical potential (and, in doing so, reduce their electrical potential energy). By convention, however, the direction of current is the direction in which positive charge would flow (from higher potential to lower potential). Thus, the direction of current is opposite to the direction of actual electron flow. The two patterns of current flow are **direct current** (**DC**), in which the charge flows in one direction only, and **alternating current** (**AC**), in which the flow changes direction periodically. Direct current is produced by household batteries, while the current supplied over long distances to homes and other buildings is alternating current. Our discussion of circuits will assume direct current, which is tested on the MCAT to the exclusion of alternating current.

A **potential difference** (**voltage**) can be produced by an electrical generator, a galvanic (voltaic) cell, a group of cells wired into a battery, or—as seen in classic science fair projects—even a potato. When no charge is moving between the two terminals of a cell that are at different potential values, the voltage is called the **electromotive force** (**emf** or ε). Do not be misled by this term, as emf is not actually a force; it is a potential difference (voltage) and, as such, has units of joules per coulomb $\left(1 \text{ V} = 1 \frac{\text{J}}{\text{C}}\right)$—not newtons. It may be helpful to think of emf as a "pressure to move" that results in current, in much the same way that a pressure difference between two points in a fluid-filled tube causes the fluid to flow.

BRIDGE

The standard batteries in flashlights and remote controls are examples of galvanic (voltaic) cells. These house spontaneous oxidation-reduction reactions that generate emf as a result of differences in the reduction potentials of two electrodes. Electrochemistry is discussed in Chapter 12 of *MCAT General Chemistry Review*.

Circuit Laws

Currents (and circuits in general) are governed by the laws of conservation. Charge and energy must be fully accounted for at all times and can be neither created nor destroyed. An electric circuit is a conducting path that usually has one or more voltage sources (such as a battery) connected to one or more passive circuit elements (such as resistors). **Kirchhoff's laws** are two rules that deal with the conservation of charge and energy within a circuit.

KEY CONCEPT

Kirchhoff's junction rule is just like a fork in a river. There are a certain number of water molecules in a river, and at any junction, that number has to go in one of the diverging directions; no water molecules spontaneously appear or disappear. The same holds true for the amount of current at any junction.

Kirchhoff's Junction Rule

At any point or junction in a circuit, the sum of currents directed into that point equals the sum of currents directed away from that point. This is an expression of conservation of electrical charge and can be expressed as

$$I_{\text{into junction}} = I_{\text{leaving junction}}$$

Equation 6.2

Example: Three wires (a, b, and c) meet at a junction point P, as shown below. A current of 5 A flows into P along wire a, and a current of 3 A flows away from P along wire b. What is the magnitude and direction of the current along wire c?

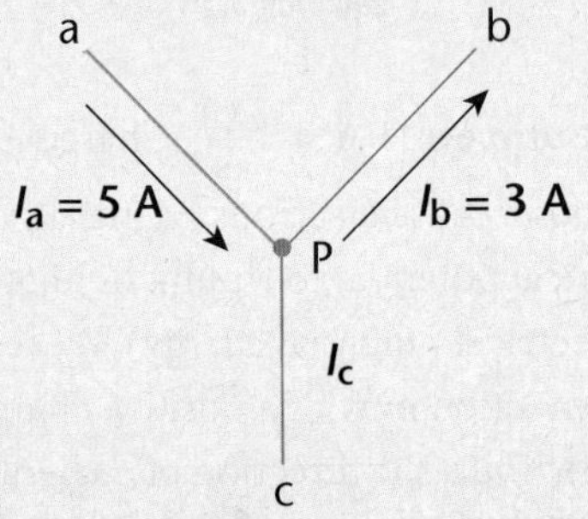

Solution: The sum of currents entering P must equal the sum of the currents leaving P. Assume for now that I_c flows out of P. If we find that it is negative, then we know the current must be going the other direction (into P).

$$I_a = I_b + I_c$$
$$5\text{ A} = 3\text{ A} + I_c$$
$$I_c = 2\text{ A}$$

Thus, a current of 2 A flows out of P along wire c.

Kirchhoff's Loop Rule

KEY CONCEPT

If all of the voltage wasn't "used up" in each loop of the circuit, then the voltage would build after each trip around the circuit, which is impossible.

Around any closed-circuit loop, the sum of voltage sources will always be equal to the sum of voltage (potential) drops. This is a consequence of the conservation of energy. All the electrical energy supplied by a source gets fully used up by the other elements within that loop. No excess energy appears, and no energy disappears that cannot be accounted for. Of course, energy can be changed from one form to another, so the kinetic energy of the electrons can be converted to thermal energy, light, or sound by the particular apparatus that is connected to the circuit. Remember that although

Kirchhoff's loop rule is a consequence of the law of conservation of energy, this law is in terms of voltage (joules per coulomb), not just energy (joules). This can be expressed mathematically as

$$V_{\text{source}} = V_{\text{drop}}$$

Equation 6.3

MCAT CONCEPT CHECK 6.1

Before you move on, assess your understanding of the material with these questions.

1. Define the following terms and provide their SI units.
   - Current:

   - Voltage:

   - Electromotive force (emf):

   - Conductivity:

   ---

2. Which likely has a higher conductivity: 1 *M* glucose or 0.25 *M* NaCl? Why?

   ---

3. True or False: In a circuit, the number of electrons entering a point and leaving that point are the same.

4. True or False: The sum of the voltage sources in a circuit is equal to the sum of the voltage drops in that circuit.

6.2 Resistance

High-Yield

LEARNING OBJECTIVES

After Chapter 6.2, you will be able to:

- Recall how the physical properties of a resistor determine its resistance
- Apply the formulas that connect power to current, voltage, and resistance
- Describe how internal resistance of a battery impacts the circuit system
- Contrast the effects of a resistor on a circuit in series as compared to one in parallel
- Calculate the total resistance of a given circuit:

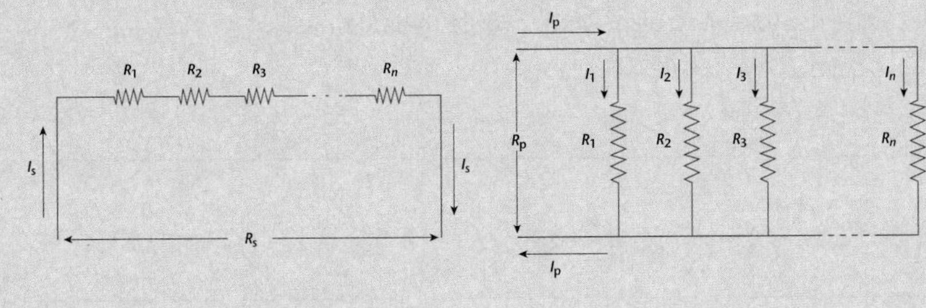

Resistance is the opposition within any material to the movement and flow of charge. Electrical resistance can be thought of like friction, air resistance, or viscous drag: in all of these cases, motion is being opposed. Materials that offer almost no resistance are called conductors, and those materials that offer very high resistance are called insulators. Conductive materials that offer amounts of resistance between these two extremes are called **resistors**.

MCAT EXPERTISE

On the MCAT, the most common resistors you will see outside of generic, unlabeled resistors are light bulbs, although all appliances function as resistors. You may also see resistance applied atypically, as in resistance to air flow in the lungs or to blood moving in the circulatory system. The same mathematical relationships will be useful in both circumstances.

Properties of Resistors

The resistance of a resistor is dependent upon certain characteristics of the resistor, including resistivity, length, cross-sectional area, and temperature. Three of these are summarized by the equation for resistance:

$$R = \frac{\rho L}{A}$$

Equation 6.4

where ρ is the resistivity, L is the length of the resistor, and A is its cross-sectional area. We will explore the effects of each of these variables and temperature in this section.

MCAT EXPERTISE

It is always good practice to be able to derive the units of a variable from equations you know. If you were to solve for resistivity (ρ) in the resistance equation, you'd end up with $\frac{AR}{L}$. Because A is in square meters, R is in ohms, and L is in meters, it simplifies to meters times ohms, which are the units for resistivity.

Resistivity

Some materials are intrinsically better conductors of electricity than others. For example, copper conducts electricity better than plastic, which is why electrical wires have a copper core surrounded by a layer of plastic rather than the other way around. The number that characterizes the intrinsic resistance to current flow in a material is called the **resistivity** (ρ), for which the SI unit is the **ohm–meter** ($\Omega \cdot m$).

Length

According to the resistance equation, the resistance of a resistor is directly proportional to its length. A longer resistor means that electrons will have to travel a greater distance through a resistant material. This factor scales linearly: if a resistor doubles its length, it will also double its resistance.

Cross-Sectional Area

The equation for resistance also demonstrates an inverse proportionality between resistance and the cross-sectional area of the resistor: if a resistor's cross-sectional area is doubled, its resistance will be cut in half. This is because the increase in cross-sectional area increases the number of pathways through the resistor, called **conduction pathways**. The wider the resistor, the more current that can flow. This is analogous to a river, where the wider the river, the less resistance there is to water flow. Note, however, that electrical current does not follow the continuity equation that applies to incompressible fluids ($A_1v_1 = A_2v_2$); it instead obeys Kirchhoff's laws.

Temperature

Although not evident from the resistance equation, most conductors have greater resistance at higher temperatures. This is due to increased thermal oscillation of the atoms in the conductive material, which produces a greater resistance to electron flow. Because temperature is an intrinsic quality of all matter, we can think of the resistivity as a function of temperature. A few materials do not follow this general rule, including glass, pure silicon, and most semiconductors.

Ohm's Law and Power

Now that we've covered voltage, current, and resistance, we can begin to bring these variables together to solve circuits.

Ohm's Law

Electrical resistance results in an energy loss, which reflects a drop in electrical potential. The voltage drop between any two points in a circuit can be calculated according to Ohm's law:

$$V = IR$$

Equation 6.5

where V is the voltage drop, I is the current, and R is the magnitude of the resistance, measured in **ohms (Ω)**. **Ohm's law** is the basic law of electricity because it states that for a given magnitude of resistance, the voltage drop across the resistor will be proportional to the magnitude of the current. Likewise, for a given resistance, the magnitude of the current will be proportional to the magnitude of the emf (voltage) impressed upon the circuit. The equation applies to a single resistor within a circuit, to any part of a circuit, or to an entire circuit (provided one can calculate the equivalent resistance from all of the resistors in the circuit). As current moves through a set of resistors in a circuit, the voltage drops some amount in each resistor; the current (or sum of currents for a divided circuit) is constant. No charge is gained or lost through a resistor; thus, if resistors are connected in series, all of the current must pass through each resistor.

MCAT EXPERTISE

Most batteries on the MCAT will be considered "perfect batteries," and you will not have to account for their internal resistances.

Conductive materials, such as copper wires, act as weak resistors themselves, offering some magnitude of resistance to current and causing a drop in electrical potential (voltage). Even the very sources of emf, such as batteries, have some small but measurable amount of **internal resistance**, r_{int}. As a result of this internal resistance, the voltage supplied to a circuit is reduced from its theoretical emf value by some small amount. The actual voltage supplied by a cell to a circuit can be calculated from

$$V = E_{cell} - ir_{int}$$

Equation 6.6

REAL WORLD

Superconductors, a special class of materials, are the one major exception to the rules of internal resistance. When these elements and compounds are cooled to very low temperatures (usually well below 100 K, but the exact threshold varies by material), the resistivity of the material (ρ) completely dissipates, dropping to zero. Because these materials break a generally applicable law of physics, superconductors have many interesting and unusual applications.

where V is the voltage provided by the cell, E_{cell} is the emf of the cell, i is the current through the cell, and r_{int} is its internal resistance.

If the cell is not actually driving any current (such as when a switch is in the open position), then the internal resistance is zero, and the voltage of the cell is equal to its emf. For cases when the current is not zero and the internal resistance is not negligible, then voltage will be less than emf.

When a cell is discharging, it supplies current, and the current flows from the positive, higher potential end of the cell around the circuit to the negative, lower potential end. Certain types of cells (called **secondary batteries**) can be recharged. When these batteries are being recharged, an external voltage is applied in such a way to drive current toward the positive end of the secondary battery. In electrochemical terms, the cell acts as a galvanic (voltaic) cell when it discharges and as an electrolytic cell when it recharges.

Measuring Power

In Chapter 2 of *MCAT Physics and Math Review*, we briefly mentioned that power is the rate at which energy is transferred or transformed. Power is measured as the ratio of work (energy expenditure) to time and can be expressed as follows:

$$P = \frac{W}{t} = \frac{\Delta E}{t}$$

Equation 6.7

In electric circuits, energy is supplied by the cell that houses a spontaneous oxidation–reduction reaction, which when allowed to proceed (by the closing of a switch, for example), generates a flow of electrons. These electrons, which have electrical potential energy, convert that energy into kinetic energy as they move around the circuit, driven by the emf of the cell. As mentioned above, emf is not a force, but is better thought of as a pressure to move, exerted by the cell on the electrons. Current delivers energy to the various resistors, which convert this energy to some other form, depending on the particular configuration of the resistor.

One recognizable example of resistors at work is the coils inside a toaster. The coils turn red-hot when the toaster is powered on and dissipate thermal energy, which is a direct consequence of the resistance that the coils pose to the current running through them.

The rate at which energy is dissipated by a resistor is the power of the resistor and can be calculated from

$$P = IV = I^2R = \frac{V^2}{R}$$

Equation 6.8

where I is the current through the resistor, V is the voltage drop across the resistor, and R is the resistance of the resistor. Note that these different versions of the power equation can be interconverted by substitution using Ohm's law ($V = IR$).

Resistors in Series and Parallel

Resistors can be connected into a circuit in one of two ways: either in **series**, in which all current must pass sequentially through each resistor connected in a linear arrangement, or in **parallel**, in which the current will divide to pass through resistors separately.

Resistors in Series

For resistors connected in series, the current has no choice but to travel through each resistor in order to return to the cell, as shown in Figure 6.1.

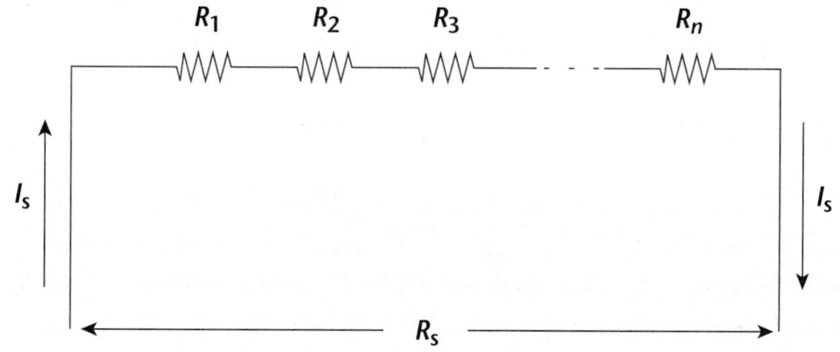

Figure 6.1 Resistors in Series
R_s increases as more resistors are added.

As the electrons flow through each resistor, energy is dissipated, and there is a voltage drop associated with each resistor. The voltage drops are additive; that is, for a series of resistors, $R_1, R_2, R_3, \cdots R_n$, the total voltage drop will be

$$V_s = V_1 + V_2 + V_3 + \cdots + V_n$$

Equation 6.9

MCAT EXPERTISE

These equations for calculating the power of a resistor or collection of resistors are extremely helpful for the MCAT. Commit them to memory—and, more importantly, understand them—and your efforts will be rewarded as points on Test Day.

REAL WORLD

Because power equals voltage times current, power companies can manipulate these two values while keeping power constant. One option is to increase current, which results in a decrease in voltage. The other option would be to increase voltage, thus decreasing the current. Power lines are high-voltage lines, which allows them to carry a smaller current—thus decreasing the amount of energy lost from the system.

KEY CONCEPT

When there is only one path for the current to take, the current will be the same at every point in the line, including through every resistor. Once you know the current of the whole circuit, you can use $V = IR$ to solve for the voltage drop across each resistor (assuming you know the resistances of the resistors).

Because $V = IR$, we can also see that the resistances of resistors in series are also additive, such that

$$R_s = R_1 + R_2 + R_3 + \cdots + R_n$$

Equation 6.10

The set of resistors wired in series can be treated as a single resistor with a resistance equal to the sum of the individual resistances, termed the **equivalent** or **resultant resistance**. Note that R_s will always increase as more resistors are added.

Example: A circuit is wired with one cell supplying 5 V in series with three resistors of 3 Ω, 5 Ω, and 7 Ω, also wired in series as shown below. What is the resulting voltage across and current through each resistor of this circuit, as well as the entire circuit?

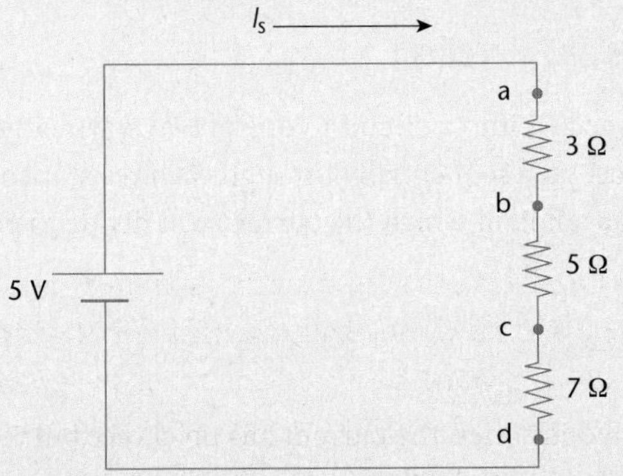

Solution: The total resistance of the resistors is

$$R_s = R_1 + R_2 + R_3 = 3\ \Omega + 5\ \Omega + 7\ \Omega = 15\ \Omega$$

Now use Ohm's law to get the current through the entire circuit:

$$I_s = \frac{V_s}{R_s} = \frac{5\text{ V}}{15\ \Omega} = 0.33\text{ A}$$

Because everything is in series, this is also the current through each circuit element. Now, use Ohm's law for each of the resistors in turn. From a to b, the voltage drop across R_1 is

$$IR_1 = (0.33\text{ A})(3\ \Omega) = 1.0\text{ V}$$

From b to c, the voltage drop across R_2 is

$$IR_2 = (0.33\text{ A})(5\ \Omega) = 1.67\text{ V}$$

From c to d, the voltage drop across R_3 is

$$IR_3 = (0.33\text{ A})(7\ \Omega) = 2.33\text{ V}$$

Resistors in Parallel

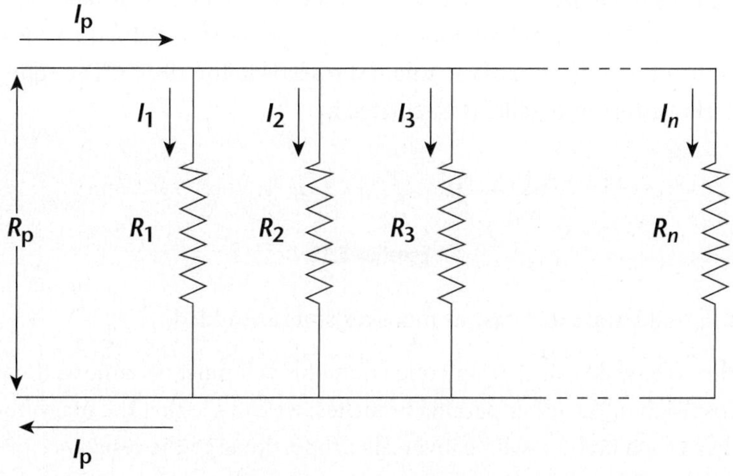

Figure 6.2 Resistors in Parallel
R_p decreases as more resistors are added.

When resistors are connected in parallel, they are wired with a common high-potential terminal and a common low-potential terminal, as shown in Figure 6.2. This configuration allows charge to follow different parallel paths between the high-potential terminal and the low-potential terminal. In this arrangement, electrons have a "choice" regarding which path they will take: some will choose one pathway, while others will choose a different pathway. No matter which path is taken, however, the voltage drop experienced by each division of current is the same because all pathways originate from a common point and end at a common point within the circuit. This is analogous to a river that splits into multiple streams before plunging over different waterfalls, which then come back together to re-form the river at a lower height. If all the water starts at some common height and ends at a lower common height, then it doesn't matter how many "steps" the water fell over to get to the bottom of the falls: the change in height is the same for each stream. In circuits with parallel arrangements of resistors, this is expressed mathematically as:

$$V_p = V_1 = V_2 = V_3 = \cdots = V_n$$

Equation 6.11

While the voltage is the same for all parallel pathways, the resistance of each pathway may differ. In this case, electrons prefer the path of least resistance; in other words, the current will be largest through the pathways with the lowest resistance. In fact, there is an inverse relationship between the portion of the current that travels through a particular pathway and the resistance offered by that pathway.

The resistance equation previously discussed shows us that there is an inverse relationship between the cross-sectional area of a resistor and the resistance of that resistor. Like opening up rush-hour lanes to reduce traffic congestion or performing cardiac bypass to perfuse hypoxic heart tissue, the configuration of resistors

KEY CONCEPT

Remember Kirchhoff's loop rule: if every resistor is in parallel, then the voltage drop across each pathway alone must be equal to the voltage of the source.

in parallel allows for a greater total number of conduction paths, and the effect of connecting resistors in parallel is a reduction in the equivalent resistance. In effect, we could replace all resistors in parallel with a single resistor that has a resistance that is less than the resistance of the smallest resistor in the circuit. The equivalent resistance of resistors in parallel is calculated by

$$\frac{1}{R_p} = \frac{1}{R_1} + \frac{1}{R_2} + \frac{1}{R_3} + \cdots + \frac{1}{R_n}$$

Equation 6.12

Note that R_p will always decrease as more resistors are added.

Because the voltage drop across any one circuit branch must be same as the voltage drops across each of the other parallel branches, we can see that the magnitude of the current in each branch will be inversely proportional to the resistance offered by each branch. This comes directly from Ohm's law. Thus, if a circuit divides into two branches and one branch has twice the resistance of the other, the one with twice the resistance will have half the magnitude of current compared to the other. Remember that the sum of the currents going into each division, according to Kirchhoff's junction rule, must equal the total current going into the point at which the current divides.

Example: Consider two equal resistors wired in parallel. What is the equivalent resistance of the setup?

Solution: The equation for summing resistors in parallel is

$$\frac{1}{R_p} = \frac{1}{R_1} + \frac{1}{R_2}$$

Next, find the common denominator of the right side:

$$\frac{1}{R_p} = \frac{R_2}{R_1 R_2} + \frac{R_1}{R_1 R_2} = \frac{R_1 + R_2}{R_1 R_2}$$

Then, take the inverse:

$$R_p = \frac{R_1 R_2}{R_1 + R_2}$$

This is a special case where $R_1 = R_2$. Substituting in, we get:

$$R_p = \frac{R^2}{2R} = \frac{R}{2}$$

In the example above, we can see that the total resistance is halved by wiring two identical resistors in parallel. More generally, when n identical resistors are wired in parallel, the total resistance is given by $\frac{R}{n}$. Note that the voltage across each of the parallel resistors is equal and that, for equal resistances, the current flowing through each of the resistors is also equal (that is, a current of $\frac{I_{\text{total}}}{n}$ runs through each).

Example: Consider two resistors wired in parallel with $R_1 = 5\ \Omega$ and $R_2 = 10\ \Omega$. If the voltage across them is 10 V, what is the current through each of the two resistors?

Solution: First, the current flowing through the whole circuit must be found. To do this, the equivalent resistance must be calculated:

$$\frac{1}{R_p} = \frac{1}{R_1} + \frac{1}{R_2} = \frac{1}{5\ \Omega} + \frac{1}{10\ \Omega} = \frac{3}{10\ \Omega}$$

$$R_p = \frac{10}{3}\ \Omega$$

Using Ohm's law to calculate the current flowing through the circuit gives

$$I_p = \frac{V_p}{R_p} = \frac{10\ \text{V}}{\left(\frac{10}{3}\ \Omega\right)} = 3\ \text{A}$$

Three amps flow through the combination of R_1 and R_2. Because the resistors are in parallel, $V_p = V_1 = V_2 = 10$ V. Apply Ohm's law to each resistor individually:

$$I_1 = \frac{V_p}{R_1} = \frac{10\ \text{V}}{5\ \Omega} = 2\ \text{A}$$

$$I_2 = \frac{V_p}{R_2} = \frac{10\ \text{V}}{10\ \Omega} = 1\ \text{A}$$

As a check, note that $I_p = 3\ \text{A} = I_1 + I_2$. More current flows through the smaller resistor. In particular, note that R_1, with half the resistance of R_2, has twice the current. Once I_p was found to be 3 A, the problem could have been solved by noting the ratio of the resistances of the two branches.

MCAT EXPERTISE

When approaching circuit problems, the first things you need to find are the total (circuit) values: the total voltage (almost always given as the voltage of the battery), the total (equivalent) resistance, and the total current. To find the total current, first find the total resistance of the circuit.

MCAT CONCEPT CHECK 6.2

Before you move on, assess your understanding of the material with these questions.

1. How does adding or removing a resistor change the total resistance of a circuit with resistors in series? In parallel?

   - Series:

   - Parallel:

   ---

2. What four physical quantities determine the resistance of a resistor?

   -

   -

   -

   -

   ---

3. How does power relate to current, voltage, and resistance?

   ---

4. True or False: The internal resistance of a battery will lower the amount of current it can provide.

5. A circuit is set up with three resistors. The circuit has one branch through R_1, then splits with R_2 and R_3 set up parallel to each other. If $R_1 = 3\ \Omega$, $R_2 = 2\ \Omega$, and $R_3 = 6\ \Omega$, then what proportion of the total current will travel through each resistor? What will be the total resistance of the circuit?

6.3 Capacitance and Capacitors

LEARNING OBJECTIVES

After Chapter 6.3, you will be able to:

- Predict the behavior of a capacitor when charging and discharging
- Describe the impact of a dielectric on capacitance, voltage, and charge
- Recognize the physical properties that impact capacitance of a capacitor
- Contrast the effects of a capacitor on a circuit in series as compared to a circuit in parallel:

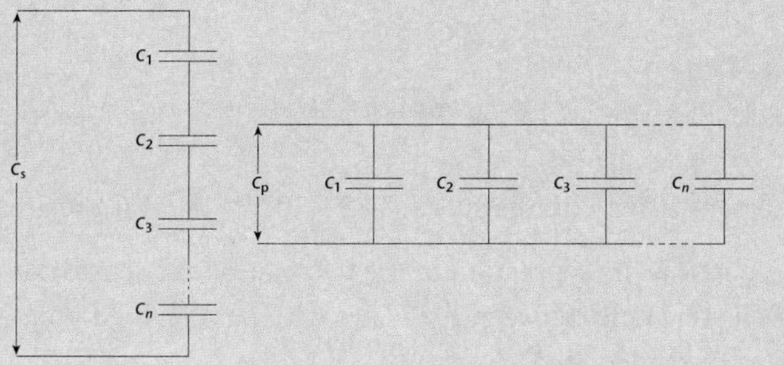

Aside from batteries and resistors, the other major circuit element tested on the MCAT is the capacitor. **Capacitors** are characterized by their ability to hold charge at a particular voltage. There are excellent real-world examples of capacitors. Perhaps the most important capacitor you'll encounter in the clinics is the defibrillator. While a defibrillator is charging, a high-pitched electronic tone sounds as electrons build up on the capacitor. When the defibrillator is fully charged, that charge can be released in one surge of power (after the operator yells *Clear!*). The clouds and the ground during a lightning storm also act as a capacitor, with the charge building up between them eventually **discharging** as a bolt of lightning. The MCAT focuses on a particular type of capacitor called a parallel plate capacitor, and all of our discussion will center on capacitors of this type.

Properties of Capacitors

When two electrically neutral metal plates are connected to a voltage source, positive charge builds up on the plate connected to the positive (higher potential) terminal, and negative charge builds up on the plate connected to the negative (lower potential) terminal. The two-plate system is a capacitor because it can store a particular amount of charge at a particular voltage. The **capacitance** of a capacitor is defined as the ratio of the magnitude of the charge stored on one plate to the potential difference (voltage) across the capacitor. Therefore, if a voltage V is applied across the plates of a capacitor and a charge Q collects on it (with $+Q$ on the positive plate and $-Q$ on the negative plate), then the capacitance is given by

$$C = \frac{Q}{V}$$

Equation 6.13

The SI unit for capacitance is the **farad** $\left(1\text{ F} = 1\dfrac{\text{C}}{\text{V}}\right)$. Because one coulomb is such a large quantity of charge, one farad is a very large capacitance. Capacitances are usually given in microfarads ($1\ \mu\text{F} = 1 \times 10^{-6}\text{ F}$) or picofarads ($1\text{ pF} = 1 \times 10^{-12}\text{ F}$). Be careful not to confuse the farad with the Faraday constant from electrochemistry, F, which is the amount of charge in one mole of electrons $\left(96{,}485\ \dfrac{\text{C}}{\text{mol } e^-}\right)$.

The capacitance of a parallel plate capacitor is dependent upon the geometry of the two conduction surfaces. For the simple case of the parallel plate capacitor, the capacitance is given by

$$C = \varepsilon_0\left(\frac{A}{d}\right)$$

Equation 6.14

where ε_0 is the permittivity of free space $\left(8.85\times10^{-12}\ \dfrac{\text{F}}{\text{m}}\right)$. A is the area of overlap of the two plates, and d is the separation of the two plates. The separation of charges sets up a **uniform electric field** between the plates with parallel field vectors, the magnitude of which can be calculated as

$$E = \frac{V}{d}$$

Equation 6.15

KEY CONCEPT

If you look back to the equations discussed in Chapter 5 of *MCAT Physics and Math Review*, you can see that the equation for E here can be derived from the other fundamental electrostatics equations. If $V = \frac{kQ}{r}$ and $E = \frac{kQ}{r^2}$, then $V = E \times r$. In this setup, r is the distance between the plates, d, so we can rewrite this as $V = Ed$.

The direction of the electric field at any point between the plates is from the positive plate toward the negative plate. If we imagine placing a positively charged particle between the oppositely charged plates, we would expect the particle to accelerate in that same direction. This should not be surprising, as electric field lines always point in the direction that indicates the direction of a force exerted on a positive charge.

Regardless of the particular geometry of a capacitor (parallel plate or otherwise), the function of a capacitor is to store an amount of energy in the form of charge separation at a particular voltage. This is akin to the function of a dam, the purpose of which is to store gravitational potential energy by holding back a mass of water at a given height. The potential energy stored in a capacitor is

$$U = \frac{1}{2}CV^2$$

Equation 6.16

Dielectric Materials

The term **dielectric material** is just another way of saying insulation. When a dielectric material, such as air, glass, plastic, ceramic, or certain metal oxides, is introduced between the plates of a capacitor, it increases the capacitance by a factor called the **dielectric constant** (κ). The dielectric constant of a material is a measure of its insulating ability, and a vacuum has a dielectric constant of 1, by definition. For reference, the dielectric constant of air is just slightly above 1, glass is 4.7, and rubber is 7. These numbers need not be memorized; any relevant dielectric constants will be given on Test Day.

The capacitance due to a dielectric material is

$$C' = \kappa C$$

Equation 6.17

where C' is the new capacitance with the dielectric present and C is the original capacitance.

MNEMONIC

Incorporating the dielectric constant into Equation 6.14 reveals that capacitors are **CA**$\kappa\varepsilon$**d** with charge ($C = A\kappa\varepsilon_0/d$).

KEY CONCEPT

A dielectric material can never decrease the capacitance; thus, κ can never be less than 1.

Dielectrics in Isolated Capacitors

When a dielectric material is placed in an isolated, charged capacitor—that is, a charged capacitor disconnected from any circuit—the voltage across the capacitor decreases. This is the result of the dielectric material shielding the opposite charges from each other. By lowering the voltage across a charged capacitor, the dielectric has increased the capacitance of the capacitor by a factor of the dielectric constant. Thus, when a dielectric material is introduced into an isolated capacitor, the increase in capacitance arises from a decrease in voltage.

Dielectrics in Circuit Capacitors

When a dielectric material is placed in a charged capacitor within a circuit—that is, still connected to a voltage source—the charge on the capacitor increases. The voltage must remain constant because it must be equal to that of the voltage source. By increasing the amount of charge stored on the capacitor, the dielectric has increased the capacitance of the capacitor by a factor of the dielectric constant. Thus, when a dielectric material is introduced into a circuit capacitor, the increase in capacitance arises from an increase in stored charge.

The stored energy in a capacitor is only useful if it is allowed to discharge. The charge can be released from the plates either by discharging across the plates or through some conductive material with which the plates are in contact. For example, capacitors can discharge into wires, causing a current to pass through the wires in much the same way that batteries cause current to move through a circuit. The paddles of the defibrillator machine, once charged, are placed on either side of a patient's heart that has gone into a life-threatening arrhythmia (such as *ventricular fibrillation*). The reason the doctor yells *Clear!* before discharging the paddles is because the current needs to travel through the patient's heart—not through any other people who might be touching the patient and creating a parallel pathway. On a much larger scale, lightning occurs when a very, very large amount of charge exceeds the capacitance of the Earth's surface and the underside of the cloud (the two serving, approximately, as a parallel plate capacitor). The large rapid discharge across the plates of a capacitor is termed a failure of the capacitor, while creating a current through the attached wires is the normal function of a capacitor.

Example: The voltage across the terminals of an isolated 3 μF capacitor is 4 V. If a piece of ceramic having dielectric constant $\kappa = 2$ is placed between the plates, find the new charge, capacitance, and voltage of the capacitor.

Solution: The introduction of a dielectric by itself has no effect on the charge stored on the isolated capacitor. There is no new charge, so the charge is the same as before. The charge stored is therefore given by

$$Q' = Q = CV = (3\ \mu\text{F})(4\ \text{V}) = 12\ \mu\text{C}$$

By introducing a dielectric with a dielectric constant of 2, the capacitance of the capacitor is multiplied by 2 $(C' = \kappa C)$. Hence, the new capacitance is 6 μF.

Now, the new voltage across the capacitor can be determined:

$$V' = \frac{Q'}{C'} = \frac{12\ \mu\text{C}}{6\ \mu\text{F}} = 2\ \text{V}$$

Example: A 3 μF capacitor is connected to a 4 V battery. If a piece of ceramic having dielectric constant $\kappa = 2$ is placed between the plates, find the new charge, capacitance, and voltage of the capacitor.

Solution: This question is very similar to the previous one, but the voltage is held constant here by a battery. Thus, the new voltage is still 4 V.

By introducing a dielectric with a dielectric constant of 2, the capacitance of the capacitor is multiplied by 2 $(C' = \kappa C)$. Hence, the new capacitance is 6 μF.

Now, the new charge on the capacitor can be determined:

$$Q' = C'V' = (6\ \mu\text{F})(4\ \text{V}) = 24\ \mu C$$

Capacitors in Series and Parallel

Just like resistors, capacitors can be arranged within a circuit either in parallel or in series. They can also be arranged with resistors, although this is beyond the scope of the MCAT in most cases.

Capacitors in Series

When capacitors are connected in series, the total capacitance decreases in similar fashion to the decreases in resistance seen in parallel resistors, as shown in Figure 6.3.

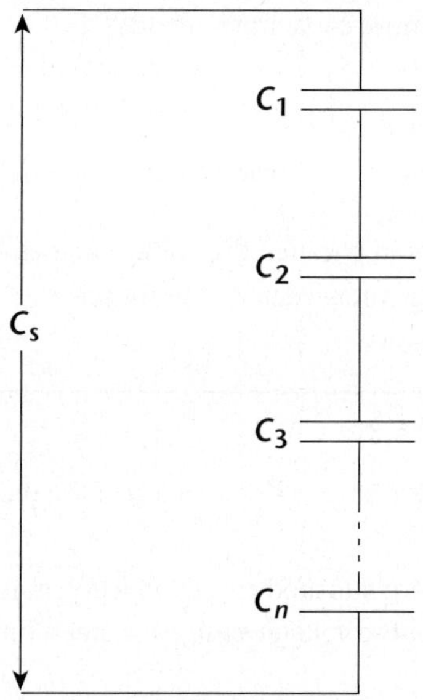

Figure 6.3 Capacitors in Series
C_s decreases as more capacitors are added.

This is because the capacitors must share the voltage drop in the loop and therefore cannot store as much charge. Functionally, a group of capacitors in series acts like one equivalent capacitor with a much larger distance between its plates (in fact, with a distance equal to those of each of the series capacitors added together). This increase in distance, as seen earlier, means a smaller capacitance.

Rather than memorizing the following equations independently, understand the conceptual basis for the mathematics of resistors in series and in parallel, and then simply reverse that mathematical approach for capacitors. The equation for calculating the equivalent capacitance for capacitors in series is

$$\frac{1}{C_s} = \frac{1}{C_1} + \frac{1}{C_2} + \frac{1}{C_3} + \cdots + \frac{1}{C_n}$$

Equation 6.18

which shows that C_s decreases as more capacitors are added. Note that for capacitors in series, the total voltage is the sum of the individual voltages, just like resistors in series.

Capacitors in Parallel

Capacitors wired in parallel, shown in Figure 6.4, produce a resultant capacitance that is equal to the sum of the individual capacitances.

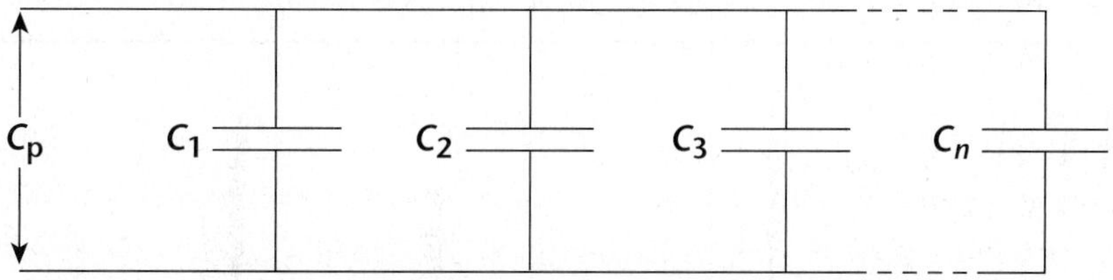

Figure 6.4 Capacitors in Parallel
C_p increases as more capacitors are added.

Therefore, C_p increases as more capacitors are added:

$$C_p = C_1 + C_2 + C_3 + \cdots + C_n$$

Equation 6.19

Just as we saw with resistors in parallel, the voltage across each parallel capacitor is the same and is equal to the voltage across the source.

MCAT CONCEPT CHECK 6.3

Before you move on, assess your understanding of the material with these questions.

1. Assuming the plates are attached by a conducting material, how does a capacitor behave after the voltage source has been removed from a circuit?

____

2. How does a dielectric material impact capacitance? Voltage? Charge?
   - Capacitance:

____

   - Voltage:

____

   - Charge:

____

3. How does adding or removing a capacitor change the total capacitance of a circuit with capacitors in series? In parallel?
   - Series:

____

   - Parallel:

____

4. What physical qualities contribute to the capacitance of a capacitor?

____

6.4 Meters

LEARNING OBJECTIVES

After Chapter 6.4, you will be able to:

- Recall key details about ammeters, voltmeters, and ohmmeters, including what they measure, where they should be placed in a circuit, and their ideal resistances
- Determine whether multiple meters should be placed together in a circuit

Although we've been focused on calculations of hypothetical circuits so far, it's important for us to spend some time considering real ones. While we will not analyze any complex circuits here, it is important to be familiar with **meters**, the devices that are used to measure circuit quantities in the real world.

Ammeters

Ammeters are used to measure the current at some point within a circuit. Using an ammeter requires the circuit to be on, or the current will be 0 A. Ammeters are inserted in series where the current is being measured and use the magnetic properties of a current-carrying wire to cause a visible needle movement or a calibrated display of the current. If there is a particularly high current, this will overwhelm the ammeter, and a special low resistance shunt is used in parallel with the ammeter to allow a reading. Ideally, an ammeter will not change circuit mathematics when it is inserted into the circuit. To do so, it must have an extremely low resistance. Ideal ammeters have zero resistance and no voltage drop across themselves.

Voltmeters

A **voltmeter**, like an ammeter, requires a circuit to be active. Voltmeters also use magnetic properties of current-carrying wires. However, voltmeters are used to measure the voltage drop across two points in a circuit. They are wired in parallel to these two points. Because the goal with any meter is to minimize its impact on the rest of the circuit, and voltmeters are wired in parallel, an ideal voltmeter has infinite resistance.

Ohmmeters

Unlike voltmeters and ammeters, an **ohmmeter** does not require a circuit to be active (in fact, some ohmmeters will give false readings or can be damaged by an active circuit). Ohmmeters will often have their own battery of known voltage and then function as ammeters through another point in the circuit. Because only one circuit element is being analyzed, Ohm's law can be used to calculate resistance by knowing the ohmmeter's voltage and the current created through another point in the circuit.

MCAT CONCEPT CHECK 6.4

Before you move on, assess your understanding of the material with these questions.

1. What do each of the following types of meters measure? Where are they placed in circuits? What are their ideal resistances?

Meter Type	Measures...	Placement	Ideal Resistance
Ammeter			
Voltmeter			
Ohmmeter			

2. True or False: A voltmeter and an ammeter should not be placed in the same circuit.

Conclusion

This chapter covered a lot of material. We began with a review of current, taking special note of the conventional definition of current as the movement of positive charge (when, in fact, negatively charged electrons are actually moving). We considered the basic laws of electricity and circuits: Kirchhoff's laws, which are expressions of conservation of charge and energy, and Ohm's law, which relates voltage, current, and resistance. We defined resistance and analyzed the relationships between resistance and resistivity (directly proportional), resistance and length (directly proportional), and resistance and cross-sectional area (inversely proportional). We also defined capacitance as the ability to store charge at some voltage, thereby storing energy. Throughout, we stressed the importance of the both the conceptual and mathematical treatment of resistors and capacitors in series and in parallel as a major testing topic on the MCAT. Finally, we covered the different meters that can be used to measure circuit quantities.

Electricity is often a challenging concept for MCAT students. Unlike kinematics, thermodynamics, and fluids, which are often more tangible, electricity is often best understood through schematics and models. Take time to review these last two chapters, as they will assuredly pay off as points on Test Day. In the next chapter, we turn our attention to a completely different topic that is no more tangible—but is far more audible: sound.

You've reviewed the content, now test your knowledge and critical thinking skills by completing a test-like passage set in your online resources!

GO ONLINE

CONCEPT SUMMARY

Current

- **Current** is the movement of charge that occurs between two points that have different electrical potentials.
  - By convention, current is defined as the movement of positive charge from the high-potential end of a voltage source to the low-potential end.
  - In reality, it is negatively charged particles (electrons) that move in a circuit, from low potential to high potential.
- Current flows only in **conductive materials**.
  - **Metallic conduction** relies on uniform movement of free electrons in metallic bonds.
  - **Electrolytic conduction** relies on the ion concentration of a solution.
  - **Insulators** are materials that do not conduct a current.
- **Kirchhoff's laws** express conservation of charge and energy.
  - **Kirchhoff's junction rule** states that the sum of currents directed into a point within a circuit equals the sum of the currents directed away from that point.
  - **Kirchhoff's loop rule** states that in a closed loop, the sum of voltage sources is always equal to the sum of voltage drops.

Resistance

- **Resistance** is opposition to the movement of electrons through a material.
- **Resistors** are conductive materials with a moderate amount of resistance that slow down electrons without stopping them.
- Resistance is calculated using the resistivity, length, and cross-sectional area of the material in question.
- **Ohm's law** states that for a given resistance, the magnitude of the current through a resistor is proportional to the voltage drop across the resistor.
- Resistors in circuits can be combined to calculate the equivalent resistance of a full or partial circuit.
  - Resistors in **series** are additive and sum together to create the total resistance of a circuit.
  - Resistors in **parallel** cause a decrease in equivalent resistance of a circuit.
- Across each resistor in a circuit, a certain amount of power is dissipated, which is dependent on the current through the resistor and the voltage drop across the resistor.

Capacitance and Capacitors

- **Capacitors** have the ability to store and discharge electrical potential energy.
- **Capacitance** in parallel plate capacitors is determined by the area of the plates and the distance between the plates.
- Capacitors in series cause a decrease in the equivalent capacitance of a circuit.
- Capacitors in parallel sum together to create a larger equivalent capacitance.
- **Dielectric materials** are insulators placed between the plates of a capacitor that increase capacitance by a factor equal to the material's **dielectric constant**, κ.

Meters

- **Ammeters** are inserted in series in a circuit to measure current; they have negligible resistance.
- **Voltmeters** are inserted in parallel in a circuit to measure a voltage drop; they have very large resistances.
- **Ohmmeters** are inserted around a resistive element to measure resistance; they are self-powered and have negligible resistance.

ANSWERS TO CONCEPT CHECKS

6.1

1. Current is the movement of positive charge through a conductive material over time and is given in ampères $\left(\frac{\text{C}}{\text{s}}\right)$. Voltage is a potential difference between two points and is given in volts $\left(\frac{\text{J}}{\text{C}}\right)$. Electromotive force (emf) refers to the potential difference of the voltage source for a circuit, usually a battery, and is given in volts. Conductivity is the reciprocal of resistance and is a measure of permissiveness to current flow; it is measured in siemens (S).
2. The sodium chloride solution likely has a higher conductivity because it is a salt and will increase the ion content of water. Glucose does not dissociate, and therefore it has a near-zero impact on conductivity.
3. True. This is a restatement of Kirchhoff's junction rule.
4. False. While the voltage sources and voltage drops are equal in any closed loop, this is not necessarily true for the entire circuit. For example, a 9 V battery that powers 10 light bulbs in parallel has a 9 V voltage source and a 9 V drop across each light bulb—a total of 90 V of drop across all of the light bulbs combined.

6.2

1. Adding a resistor in series increases the total resistance of a circuit; removing one in series decreases the total resistance in the circuit. These relationships are reversed in parallel: adding a resistor decreases resistance while removing one increases it.
2. Resistivity, length, cross-sectional area, and temperature all contribute to the resistance of a resistor.
3. Power is related to current, voltage, and resistance through the equations $P = IV = I^2R = \frac{V^2}{R}$.
4. True. The internal resistance will lower the available voltage for the circuit. Lowering the available voltage will also lower current for any given resistance.
5. All current must travel through the first resistor, regardless of its resistance. Since the ratio of resistance for R_2:R_3 is 1:3, the ratio of current passing through them will be 3:1. In other words, $\frac{3}{4}$ of the current will pass through R_2 while $\frac{1}{4}$ of the current will pass through R_3. To calculate the total resistance, first calculate the resistance of the resistors in parallel: $\frac{1}{R_{2+3}} = \frac{1}{2} + \frac{1}{6} = \frac{2}{3} \rightarrow R_{2+3} = 1.5\ \Omega$. Add this to the resistance of R_1 to get the total resistance: 4.5 Ω.

6.3

1. The capacitor discharges, providing a current in the opposite direction of the initial current.
2. A dielectric material will always increase capacitance. If the capacitor is isolated, its voltage will decrease when a dielectric material is introduced; if it is in a circuit, its voltage is constant because it is dictated by the voltage source. If a capacitor is isolated, the stored charge will remain constant because there is no additional source of charge; if it is in a circuit, the stored charge will increase.
3. Adding a capacitor in series decreases the total capacitance of a circuit; removing one in series increases the total capacitance in the circuit. These relationships are reversed in parallel: adding a capacitor increases capacitance while removing one decreases it.
4. Surface area, distance, and dielectric constant all contribute to the capacitance of a capacitor.

6.4

1.

Meter Type	Measures...	Placement	Ideal Resistance
Ammeter	Current	In series with point of interest	0
Voltmeter	Potential difference (voltage)	Parallel with circuit element of interest	∞
Ohmmeter	Resistance	Two points in series with circuit element of interest	0

2. False. Voltmeters and ammeters are designed to have minimum impact on a circuit; thus, they can be used together.

SCIENCE MASTERY ASSESSMENT EXPLANATIONS

1. **B**

Electrical current is defined as charge flow, or in mathematical terms, charge transferred per time: $I = \frac{Q}{\Delta t}$. A 15 A current that acts for 0.1 s will transfer 15 A × 0.1 s = 1.5 C of charge.

2. **D**

To measure the current at any point in a circuit, an ammeter should be placed in series. If placed in parallel, a new path for current would be created, so the measured value would not be reflective of actual current in the circuit. This observation matches **(D)**. Note that an ideal ammeter should have zero resistance so that it has no effect on the current of the circuit.

3. **B**

The resistance of a resistor is given by the formula $R = \frac{\rho L}{A}$. Thus, there is a direct proportionality between resistance and resistivity. Because the other variables are equal between the two resistors, we can determine that if $R_1{:}R_2$ is a 1:2 ratio, then $\rho_1{:}\rho_2$ is also a 1:2 ratio.

4. **D**

This question tests our understanding of batteries in a circuit. The voltage across the terminals of the battery when there is no current flowing is referred to as the electromotive force (emf or ε of the battery). However, when a current is flowing through the circuit, the voltage across the terminals of the battery is decreased by an amount equal to the current multiplied by the internal resistance of the battery. Mathematically, this is given by the equation

$$V = \varepsilon - ir_{\text{int}}$$

To determine the emf of the battery, first calculate the voltage across the battery when the current is flowing. For this, we can use Ohm's law:

$$\begin{aligned} V &= IR \\ &= (0.5\ \text{A})(3\ \Omega) = 1.5\ \text{V} \end{aligned}$$

Because we know the internal resistance of the battery, the current, and the voltage, we can calculate the emf:

$$\begin{aligned} \varepsilon &= V + ir_{\text{int}} \\ &= 1.5\ \text{V} + (0.5\ \text{A})(0.1\ \Omega) \\ &= 1.5 + 0.05 = 1.55\ \text{V} \end{aligned}$$

The answer makes sense in the context of a real battery because its internal resistance is supposed to be very small so that the voltage provided to the circuit is as close as possible to the emf of the cell when there is no current running.

5. **A**

We are told that transformers conserve energy so that the output power equals the input power. Thus, $P_{\text{out}} = P_{\text{in}}$, or $I_{\text{out}}V_{\text{out}} = I_{\text{in}}V_{\text{in}}$. There is therefore an inverse proportionality between current and voltage. If the output voltage is 300% of the input voltage (3 times its amount), then the output current must be $\frac{1}{3}$ of the input voltage. This can be represented as a 1:3 ratio.

6. **B**

The fastest way to tackle these kinds of questions is to simplify the circuit bit by bit. For example, notice that R_3 and R_4 are in parallel with each other and are in series with R_2; similarly, R_5 and R_6 are in series. If we determine the total resistance in each branch, we will be left with three branches in parallel. To start, find the total resistance in the middle branch:

$$\frac{1}{R_{3+4}} = \frac{1}{R_3} + \frac{1}{R_4} = \frac{1}{32\ \Omega} + \frac{1}{32\ \Omega} \rightarrow R_{3+4} = 16\ \Omega$$

$$R_{2+3+4} = R_2 + R_{3+4} = 4\ \Omega + 16\ \Omega = 20\ \Omega$$

Next, take a look at the total resistance in the bottom branch:

$$R_{5+6} = R_5 + R_6 = 15\ \Omega + 5\ \Omega = 20\ \Omega$$

The circuit can now be viewed as three resistors in parallel, each providing a resistance of 20 Ω. The total resistance in the circuit is thus

$$\frac{1}{R_{tot}} = \frac{1}{R_1} + \frac{1}{R_{2+3+4}} + \frac{1}{R_{5+6}} =$$

$$\frac{1}{20\ \Omega} + \frac{1}{20\ \Omega} + \frac{1}{20\ \Omega} \rightarrow \frac{20}{3}\ \Omega = 6.67\ \Omega$$

7. **A**

To determine the moles of charge that pass through the circuit over a period of 10 s, we will have to calculate the amount of charge running through the circuit. Charge is simply current multiplied by time, and the current can be calculated using Ohm's law:

$$V = IR \text{ and } I = \frac{Q}{\Delta t} \rightarrow Q = \frac{V\Delta t}{R}$$

$$Q = \frac{(100\ \text{V})(10\ \text{s})}{2\ \Omega} = 500\ \text{C}$$

Then, calculate the number of moles of charge that this represents by using the Faraday constant and approximating F as $10^5\ \frac{\text{C}}{\text{mol}\, e^-}$:

$$(500\ \text{C})\left[\frac{\text{mol}\ e^-}{10^5\ \text{C}}\right] = 5 \times 10^{-3}\ \text{mol}\ e^-$$

This is closest to **(A)**.

8. **C**

To determine the voltage drop across the $\frac{2}{3}$ Ω resistor, start by calculating the total resistance in the circuit. For the resistors in parallel, the equivalent resistance is

$$\frac{1}{R_p} = \frac{1}{2\ \Omega} + \frac{3}{2\ \Omega} \rightarrow R_p = \frac{1}{2}\ \Omega$$

The total resistance in the circuit is the sum of the remaining resistor and the equivalent resistance of the other two:

$$R_s = \frac{1}{2}\ \Omega + \frac{1}{2}\ \Omega = 1\ \Omega$$

Now that we know the equivalent resistance, we can calculate the total current using Ohm's law:

$$I = \frac{V}{R} = \frac{10\ \text{V}}{1\ \Omega} = 10\ \text{A}$$

Finally, we can determine the voltage drop across the parallel resistors. The voltage drop across the $\frac{1}{2}$ Ω resistor must be $(10\ \text{A})\left(\frac{1}{2}\ \Omega\right) = 5$ V. Therefore, there must be a 5 V drop across both the $\frac{2}{3}$ Ω resistor and 2 Ω resistor, according to Kirchhoff's loop rule. Each of these resistors forms a complete loop in combination with the $\frac{1}{2}$ Ω resistor and 10 V voltage source, and the net potential difference around any closed loop must be 0 V.

9. **D**

This question should bring to mind the equation $C = \varepsilon_0\left(\frac{A}{d}\right)$, where ε_0 is the permittivity of free space, A is the area of the plates, and d is the distance between the plates. From this equation, we can infer that doubling the area will double the capacitance, and halving the distance will also double the capacitance. Therefore, the new capacitance is four times larger than the initial capacitance.

10. **C**

Because the question is asking us to calculate the charge on the capacitor, use the formula $Q = CV$. We are given $V = 7500$ V and can calculate C from the formula for energy, $U = \frac{1}{2}CV^2$:

$$U = \frac{1}{2}CV^2 = \frac{1}{2}\left(\frac{Q}{V}\right)V^2 = \frac{QV}{2}$$

$$Q = \frac{2U}{V} = \frac{2(400\ \text{J})}{7500\ \text{V}} \approx \frac{800}{8000} = 0.1\ \text{C}$$

Thus, the charge is close to 0.1 C, which is closest to **(C)**.

11. **C**

Power is energy dissipated per unit time; therefore, the energy dissipated is $E = P\Delta t$. In the five-second interval during which the resistor is active, it has a 2 A current for three of those seconds. The power dissipated by a resistor R carrying a current I is $P = I^2R$. Therefore, the energy dissipated is

$$E = I^2R\Delta t = (2\ \text{A})^2(10\ \Omega)(3\ \text{s}) = 4 \times 10 \times 3 = 120\ \text{J}$$

12. **A**

Kirchhoff's junction rule states that the sum of all currents directed into a point is always equal to the sum of all currents directed out of the point. The currents directed into point *P* are 8 A, 2 A, and 3 A, so the sum is 13 A. The currents directed out of point *P* are 5 A and 6 A, so the total is 11 A. Because the two numbers must always be equal, an additional current of 2 A must be directed away from point *P* toward point *x*.

13. **D**

The electric field between two plates of a parallel plate capacitor is related to the potential difference between the plates of the capacitor and the distance between the plates, as shown in the formula $E = \frac{V}{d}$. The addition of another battery will increase the total voltage applied to the circuit, which, consequently, will increase the electric field. The addition of a resistor in series will increase the resistance and decrease the voltage applied to the capacitor, eliminating **(A)**. Adding a resistor in parallel will not change the voltage drop across the capacitor and should not change the electric field, eliminating **(B)**. Increasing the distance between the plates, **(C)**, would decrease the electric field, not increase it.

14. **D**

The resistance of the three resistors wired in series is equal to the sum of the individual resistances (12 Ω). This means that the circuit functionally contains a 12 Ω resistor and a 4 Ω resistor in parallel. To determine the overall resistance of this system, use the formula

$$\frac{1}{R_\text{p}} = \frac{1}{R_1} + \frac{1}{R_2} = \frac{1}{12\ \Omega} + \frac{1}{4\ \Omega} = \frac{1+3}{12\ \Omega} \rightarrow R_\text{p} = 3\ \Omega$$

15. **C**

While this is primarily a recall question, it should also be intuitive. Voltmeters are attempting to determine a change in potential from one point to another. To do this, they should not provide an alternate route for charge flow and should therefore have infinite resistance. Ammeters attempt to determine the flow of charge at a single point and should not contribute to the resistance of a series circuit; therefore, they should have no resistance.

Consult your online resources for additional practice. GO ONLINE

EQUATIONS TO REMEMBER

(6.1) **Current:** $I = \frac{Q}{\Delta t}$

(6.2) **Kirchhoff's junction rule:** $I_{\text{into junction}} = I_{\text{leaving junction}}$

(6.3) **Kirchhoff's loop rule:** $V_{\text{source}} = V_{\text{drop}}$

(6.4) **Definition of resistance:** $R = \frac{\rho L}{A}$

(6.5) **Ohm's law:** $V = IR$

(6.6) **Voltage and cell emf:** $V = E_{\text{cell}} - ir_{\text{int}}$

(6.7) **Definition of power:** $P = \frac{W}{t} = \frac{\Delta E}{t}$

(6.8) **Electric power:** $P = IV = I^2R = \frac{V^2}{R}$

(6.9) **Voltage drop across circuit elements (series):** $V_s = V_1 + V_2 + V_3 + \cdots + V_n$

(6.10) **Equivalent resistance (series):** $R_s = R_1 + R_2 + R_3 + \cdots + R_n$

(6.11) **Voltage drop across circuit elements (parallel):** $V_p = V_1 = V_2 = V_3 = \cdots = V_n$

(6.12) **Equivalent resistance (parallel):** $\frac{1}{R_p} = \frac{1}{R_1} + \frac{1}{R_2} + \frac{1}{R_3} + \cdots + \frac{1}{R_n}$

(6.13) **Definition of capacitance:** $C = \frac{Q}{V}$

(6.14) **Capacitance based on parallel plate geometry:** $C = \varepsilon_0\left(\frac{A}{d}\right)$

(6.15) **Electric field in a capacitor:** $E = \frac{V}{d}$

(6.16) **Potential energy of a capacitor:** $U = \frac{1}{2}CV^2$

(6.17) **Capacitance with a dielectric material:** $C' = \kappa C$

(6.18) **Equivalent capacitance (series):** $\frac{1}{C_s} = \frac{1}{C_1} + \frac{1}{C_2} + \frac{1}{C_3} + \cdots + \frac{1}{C_n}$

(6.19) **Equivalent capacitance (parallel):** $C_p = C_1 + C_2 + C_3 + \cdots + C_n$

SHARED CONCEPTS

Biology Chapter 6
The Respiratory System

Biology Chapter 7
The Cardiovascular System

General Chemistry Chapter 12
Electrochemistry

Physics and Math Chapter 2
Work and Energy

Physics and Math Chapter 4
Fluids

Physics and Math Chapter 5
Electrostatics and Magnetism

CHAPTER 7

WAVES AND SOUND

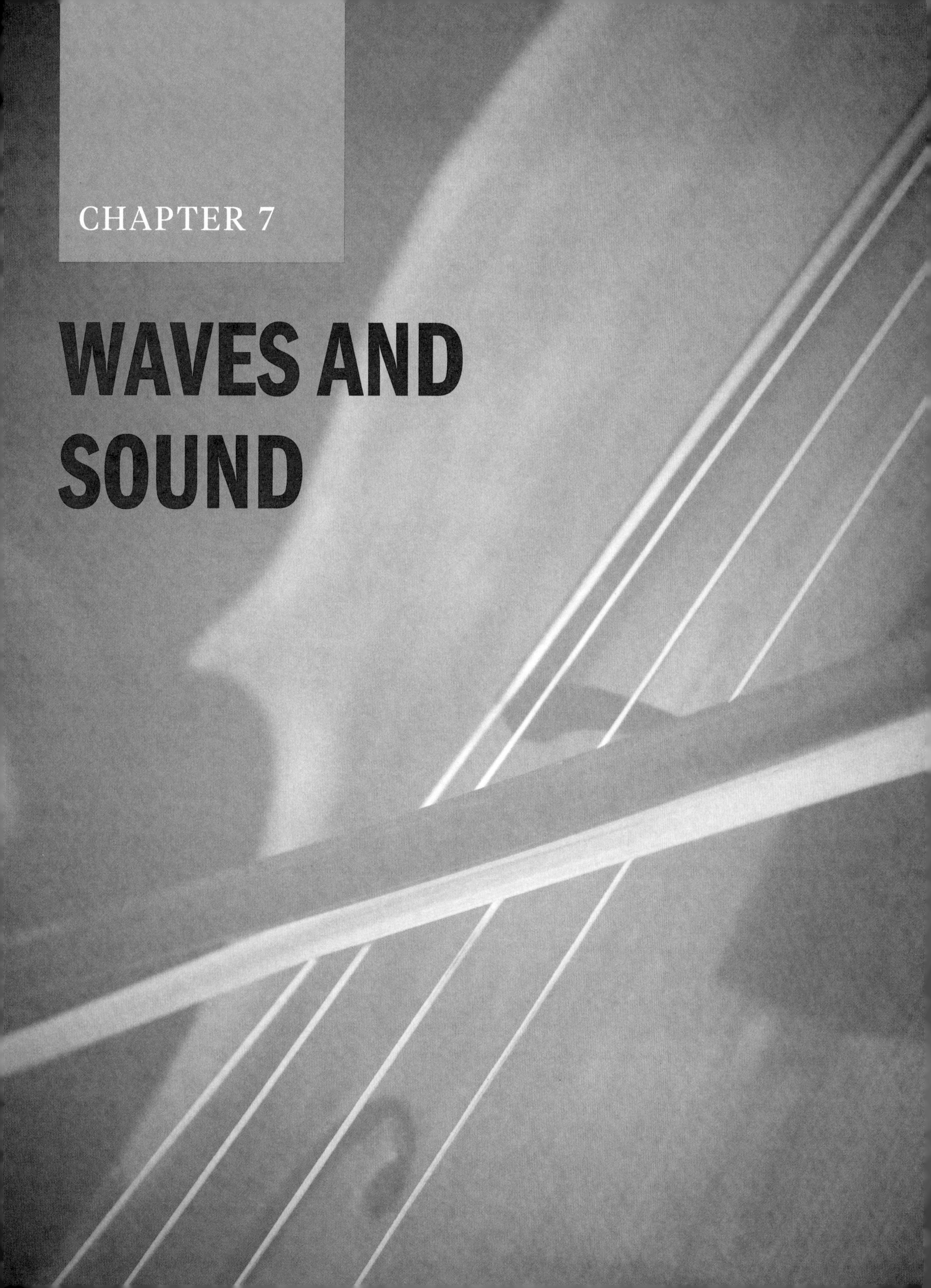

SCIENCE MASTERY ASSESSMENT

Every pre-med knows this feeling: there is so much content I have to know for the MCAT! How do I know what to do first or what's important?

While the high-yield badges throughout this book will help you identify the most important topics, this Science Mastery Assessment is another tool in your MCAT prep arsenal. This quiz (which can also be taken in your online resources) and the guidance below will help ensure that you are spending the appropriate amount of time on this chapter based on your personal strengths and weaknesses. Don't worry though—skipping something now does not mean you'll never study it. Later on in your prep, as you complete full-length tests, you'll uncover specific pieces of content that you need to review and can come back to these chapters as appropriate.

How to Use This Assessment

If you answer 0–7 questions correctly:

Spend about 1 hour to read this chapter in full and take limited notes throughout. Follow up by reviewing **all** quiz questions to ensure that you now understand how to solve each one.

If you answer 8–11 questions correctly:

Spend 20–40 minutes reviewing the quiz questions. Beginning with the questions you missed, read and take notes on the corresponding subchapters. For questions you answered correctly, ensure your thinking matches that of the explanation and you understand why each choice was correct or incorrect.

If you answer 12–15 questions correctly:

Spend less than 20 minutes reviewing all questions from the quiz. If you missed any, then include a quick read-through of the corresponding subchapters, or even just the relevant content within a subchapter, as part of your question review. For questions you got correct, ensure your thinking matches that of the explanation and review the Concept Summary at the end of the chapter.

1. An opera singer has two precisely identical glasses. The singer produces as pure a tone as possible and shatters the first glass at a frequency of 808 Hz. The singer then sings a frequency of 838 Hz in the presence of the second glass. The second glass will likely:
   - **A.** shatter after a longer amount of time because the applied frequency is higher.
   - **B.** shatter after a shorter amount of time because the applied frequency is higher.
   - **C.** not shatter because the applied frequency is not equal to the natural frequency of the glass.
   - **D.** not shatter because higher-frequency sounds are associated with more attenuation.

2. A child is practicing the first overtone on a flute. If the child's sibling covers one end of the flute for a brief second, how will the sound change, assuming that the new pitch represents the first overtone in the new setup?
   - **A.** The pitch of the sound will go up.
   - **B.** The pitch of the sound will go down.
   - **C.** The pitch of the sound will not change.
   - **D.** The change in the pitch depends on the starting pitch.

3. Which of the following is necessarily true regarding frequency, angular frequency, and period of a given wave?
   - **A.** The magnitude of the angular frequency is larger than the magnitude of the period.
   - **B.** The product of the frequency and period is equal to the angular frequency.
   - **C.** The magnitude of the angular frequency is larger than the magnitude of the frequency.
   - **D.** The product of the angular frequency and period is 1.

4. Ultrasound machines calculate distance based upon:
   - **A.** intensity of the reflected sound.
   - **B.** travel time of the reflected sound.
   - **C.** angle of incidence of the sound.
   - **D.** the detected frequency of the sound.

5. The period for a certain wave is 34 ms. If there is a Doppler shift that doubles the perceived frequency, which of the following must be true?
   - **I.** The detector is moving toward the source at a velocity equal to the speed of sound.
   - **II.** The source is moving toward the detector at a velocity equal to half the speed of sound.
   - **III.** The perceived period is 17 ms.
   - **IV.** The perceived period is 68 ms.

   - **A.** III only
   - **B.** I and IV only
   - **C.** II and III only
   - **D.** I, II, and IV only

6. If the speed of a wave is 3 $\frac{m}{s}$ and its wavelength is 10 cm, what is its period?
   - **A.** 0.01 s
   - **B.** 0.03 s
   - **C.** 0.1 s
   - **D.** 0.3 s

7. What is the angular frequency of the third harmonic in a pipe of length 1.5 m with one closed end? (Note: The speed of the sound is approximately 340 $\frac{m}{s}$.)
   - **A.** 170 radians per second
   - **B.** 170π radians per second
   - **C.** 340 radians per second
   - **D.** 340π radians per second

8. A certain sound level is increased by 20 dB. By what factor does its intensity increase?
   A. 2
   B. 20
   C. 100
   D. log 2

9. In some forms of otosclerosis, the stapedial foot plate, which transmits vibrations from the bones of the middle ear to the fluid within the cochlea, can become fixed in position. This limits the displacement of the stapedial foot plate during vibration. Based on this mechanism, which of the following symptoms would most likely be seen in an individual with otosclerosis?
   A. An increase in the perceived volume of sounds
   B. A decrease in the perceived volume of sounds
   C. An increase in the perceived pitch of sounds
   D. A decrease in the perceived pitch of sounds

10. If two waves with the same frequency are 180° out of phase, what is the amplitude of the resultant wave if the amplitudes of the original waves are 5 cm and 3 cm?
   A. 2 cm
   B. 3 cm
   C. 5 cm
   D. 8 cm

11. A student is measuring sound frequencies from the side of a road while walking east. For which of the following situations could the student determine that the difference between the perceived frequency and the actual emitted frequency is zero?
   A. A plane flying directly above the student from east to west
   B. A police car passing the student with its siren on
   C. A person playing piano in a house on the street
   D. A dog barking in a car that moves east

12. In which of the following media does sound travel the fastest?
   A. Vacuum
   B. Air
   C. Water
   D. Glass

13. Shock waves have the greatest impact when the source is traveling:
   A. just below the speed of sound.
   B. exactly at the speed of sound.
   C. just above the speed of sound.
   D. well above the speed of sound.

14. As a teacher approaches a student who is studying with the radio playing loudly nearby, the teacher experiences the Doppler effect. Which of the following statements remains true while the teacher moves closer to the student?
   I. The apparent frequency of the music is increased.
   II. The same apparent frequency would be produced if the teacher were stationary and the student approached at the same speed.
   III. The apparent velocity of the wave is decreased.

   A. I only
   B. II only
   C. I and III only
   D. I, II, and III

15. Ignoring attenuation, how does the intensity of a sound change as the distance from the source doubles?
   A. It is four times as intense.
   B. It is twice as intense.
   C. It is half as intense.
   D. It is one-quarter as intense.

Answer Key

1. **C**
2. **B**
3. **C**
4. **B**
5. **A**
6. **B**
7. **D**
8. **C**
9. **B**
10. **A**
11. **D**
12. **D**
13. **B**
14. **A**
15. **D**

Detailed explanations can be found at the end of the chapter.

CHAPTER 7

WAVES AND SOUND

In This Chapter

CHAPTER PROFILE

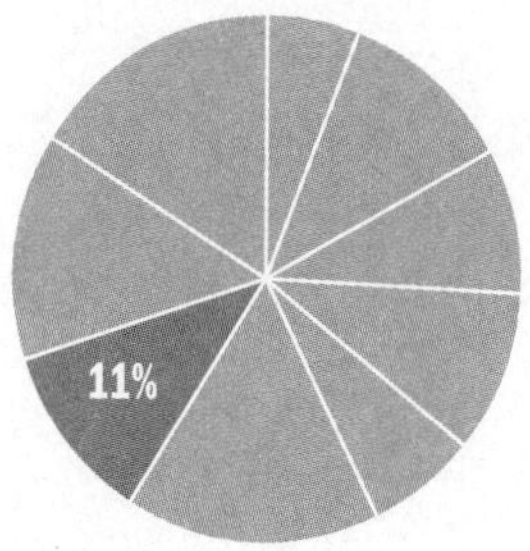

The content in this chapter should be relevant to about 11% of all questions about physics on the MCAT.

This chapter covers material from the following AAMC content categories:

4A: Translational motion, forces, work, energy, and equilibrium in living systems

4D: How light and sound interact with matter

Introduction

As a species, our interactions with sound are amazingly complex. The human ear developed as a means of detecting longitudinal waves carried in the air—this likely served an evolutionary purpose. A rustle in the leaves could indicate not only a potential meal, but also a potential predator. Our brains are highly attuned to analyze the sounds around us, as discussed in Chapter 2 of *MCAT Behavioral Sciences Review*. This includes not only the normal auditory pathway from the pinna through the tympanic membrane, ossicles, cochlea, and vestibulocochlear nerve to the temporal lobe, but also secondary structures such as the superior olive, which helps localize sound, and the inferior colliculus, which is involved in the startle reflex.

Language is also inextricably linked to sound. Through changes in pitch and timbre, we can imply or evoke dozens of complex feelings. Through music, our relationship with sound becomes even more profound. As E.T.A. Hoffman, a musicologist and pedagogue, wrote in his vivid description of Beethoven's opening motif for *Symphony No. 5 in C minor*, op. 67:

Radiant beams shoot through this region's deep night, and we become aware of gigantic shadows which, rocking back and forth, close in on us and destroy everything within us except the pain of endless longing—a longing in which every pleasure that rose up in jubilant tones sinks and succumbs, and only through this pain, which, while consuming but not destroying love, hope, and joy, tries to burst our breasts with full-voiced harmonies of all the passions, we live on and are captivated beholders of the spirits.

Indeed, sound can create entire worlds that we can explore. This chapter, however, aims only to lay the foundation for understanding wave phenomena. The general properties of waves will be introduced, including a discussion of wavelength, frequency, wave speed, amplitude, and resonance. We will also review the interactions of waves meeting at a point in space through constructive and destructive interference and examine the mathematics of standing waves—the means by which musical instruments produce their characteristic sounds. The subject of sound is reviewed as a specific example of the longitudinal waveform with a focus on wave phenomena such as the Doppler effect. Finally, we provide a brief discussion of the use of ultrasound and shock waves in medicine.

7.1 General Wave Characteristics

LEARNING OBJECTIVES

After Chapter 7.1, you will be able to:

- Define key terms applying to waves and sound, such as frequency, pitch, and amplitude
- Distinguish between common examples of transverse and longitudinal waves
- Predict the impact of applying a force at the natural frequency of a given system
- Predict the relative amplitude of a resultant wave created by two interfering waves:

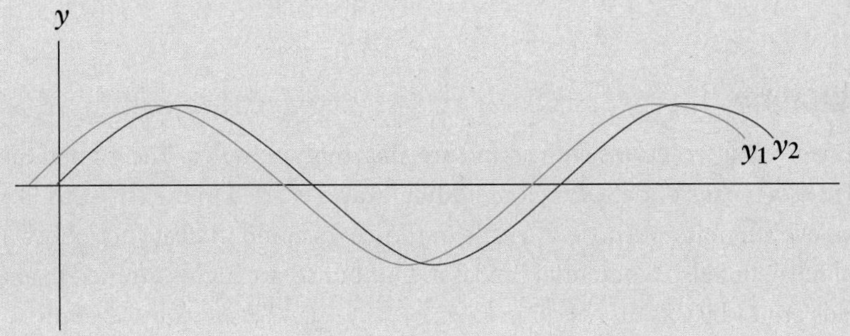

It is important to use a common language when describing waves. We'll establish the terminology associated with wave phenomena, and then spend the rest of this chapter looking at the application of wave principles to sound. In the next chapter, we'll shift our focus to electromagnetic waves.

Transverse and Longitudinal Waves

The MCAT is primarily concerned with **sinusoidal waves.** In these waves, which may be transverse or longitudinal, the individual particles oscillate back and forth with a displacement that follows a sinusoidal pattern. **Transverse waves** are those in which the direction of particle oscillation is perpendicular to the **propagation** (movement) of the wave. To visualize this, consider "The Wave" in a stadium. While "The Wave" moves around the stadium, individuals in the stands do not run around the stadium themselves. Rather, they move perpendicular to the direction of "The Wave"—by standing up and sitting down. More common examples on the MCAT include electromagnetic waves, such as visible light, microwaves, and X-rays. You could also form a transverse wave by attaching a string to a fixed point, and then moving your hand up and down, as is demonstrated in Figure 7.1a. In any waveform, energy is delivered in the direction of wave travel, so we can say that for a transverse wave, the particles are oscillating perpendicular to the direction of energy transfer.

Longitudinal waves are ones in which the particles of the wave oscillate parallel to the direction of propagation; that is, the wave particles are oscillating in the direction of energy transfer. Sound waves are the classic example of longitudinal waves, but because we can't see sound, this waveform is a little more difficult to picture. Figure 7.1b helps us visualize what a longitudinal waveform traveling through air would look like. In this case, the longitudinal wave created by the person moving the piston back and forth causes air molecules to oscillate through cycles of **compression** and **rarefaction** (**decompression**) along the direction of motion of the wave. You could also form a longitudinal wave by laying a Slinky flat on a table top and tapping it on the end.

KEY CONCEPT

Transverse waves have particle oscillation perpendicular to the direction of propagation and energy transfer. Longitudinal waves have particle oscillation parallel to the direction of propagation and energy transfer.

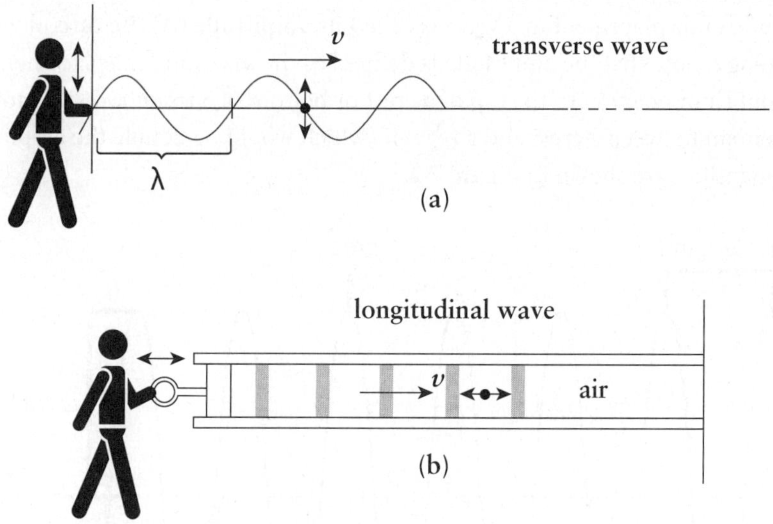

Figure 7.1 Wave Types
(a) Transverse: particles oscillate perpendicular to the direction of propagation; (b) Longitudinal: particles oscillate parallel to the direction of propagation.

Describing Waves

Waves can be described mathematically or graphically. To do so, we must first assign meaning to the physical quantities that waves represent. The distance from one maximum (**crest**) of the wave to the next is called the **wavelength** (λ). The **frequency** (f) is the number of wavelengths passing a fixed point per second, and is measured in **hertz (Hz)** or cycles per second (cps). From these two values, one can calculate the **propagation speed** (v) of a wave:

$$v = f\lambda$$

Equation 7.1

If frequency defines the number of cycles per second, then its inverse—**period** (T)—is the number of seconds per cycle:

$$T = \frac{1}{f}$$

Equation 7.2

Frequency is also related to **angular frequency** (ω), which is measured in radians per second, and is often used in consideration of simple harmonic motion in springs and pendula:

$$\omega = 2\pi f = \frac{2\pi}{T}$$

Equation 7.3

MCAT EXPERTISE

Even if simple harmonic motion in springs and strings (pendula) are not on the formal content lists for the MCAT, it is still important to be familiar with the jargon of wave motion because sound and light (electromagnetic radiation) *are* on those content lists!

Waves oscillate about a central point called the **equilibrium position.** The **displacement** (**x**) in a wave describes how far a particular point on the wave is from the equilibrium position, expressed as a vector quantity. The maximum magnitude of displacement in a wave is called its **amplitude** (***A***). Be careful with the terminology: note that the amplitude is defined as the maximum displacement from the equilibrium position to the top of a crest or bottom of a trough, not the total displacement between a crest and a trough (which would be double the amplitude). These quantities are shown in Figure 7.2.

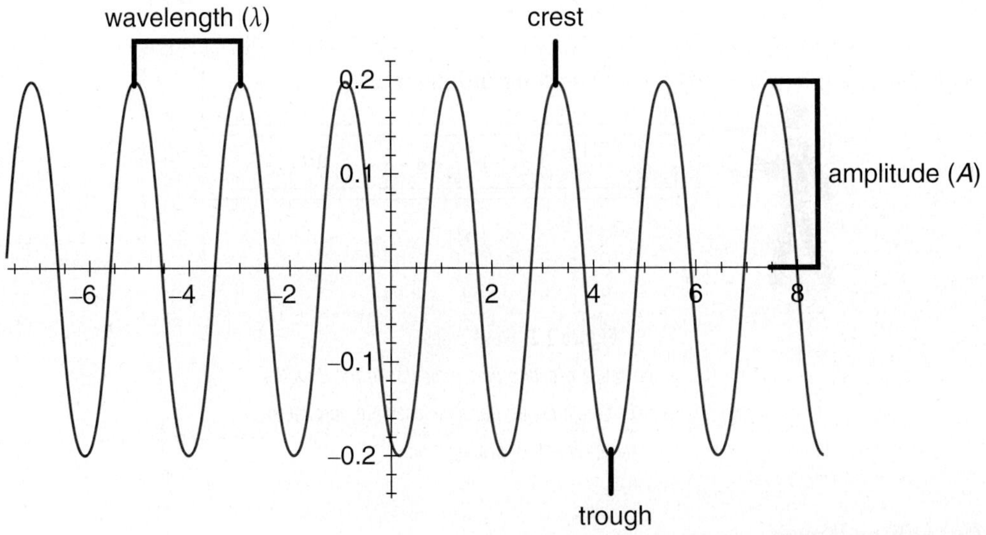

Figure 7.2 Anatomy of a Wave

Phase

When analyzing waves that are passing through the same space, we can describe how "in step" or "out of step" the waves are by calculating the **phase difference.** If we consider two waves that have the same frequency, wavelength, and amplitude and that pass through the same space at the same time, we can say that they are *in phase* if their respective crests and troughs coincide (line up with each other). When waves are perfectly in phase, we say that the phase difference is zero. However, if the two waves travel through the same space in such a way that the crests of one wave coincide with the troughs of the other, then we would say that they are *out of phase*, and the phase difference would be one-half of a wave. This could be expressed as $\frac{\lambda}{2}$ or, if given as an angle, 180° (one cycle = one wavelength = 360°). Of course, waves can be out of phase with each other by any other fraction of a cycle, as well.

Principle of Superposition

The **principle of superposition** states that when waves interact with each other, the displacement of the resultant wave at any point is the sum of the displacements of the two interacting waves. When the waves are perfectly in phase, the displacements always add together and the amplitude of the resultant is equal to the sum of the amplitudes of the two waves. This is called **constructive interference**. When waves are perfectly out of phase, the displacements always counteract each other and the amplitude of the resultant wave is the difference between the amplitudes of the interacting waves. This is called **destructive interference.**

KEY CONCEPT

If two waves are perfectly in phase, the resultant wave has an amplitude equal to the sum of the amplitudes of the two waves. If two equal waves are exactly 180 degrees out of phase, then the resultant wave has zero amplitude.

If waves are not perfectly in phase or out of phase with each other, **partially constructive** or **partially destructive** interference can occur. As shown in Figure 7.3a, two waves that are nearly in phase will mostly add together. While the displacement of the resultant is simply the sum of the displacements of the two waves, the waves do not perfectly add together because they are not quite in phase. Therefore, the amplitude of the resultant wave is not quite the sum of the two waves' amplitudes. In contrast, Figure 7.3b shows two waves that are almost perfectly out of phase. The two waves do not quite cancel, but the resultant wave's amplitude is clearly much smaller than that of either of the other waves.

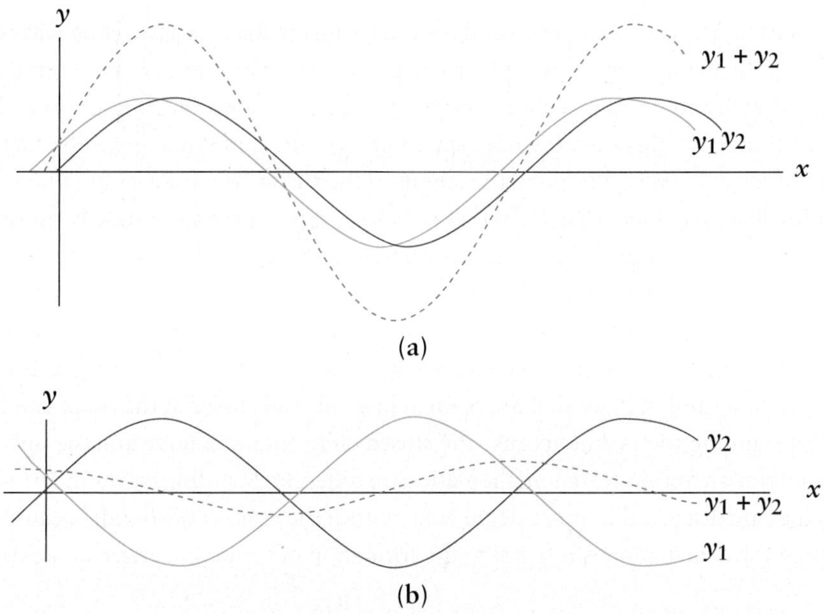

Figure 7.3 Phase Difference

(a) In phase with a difference of almost zero; (b) Out of phase with a difference of almost 180 degrees $\left(\frac{\lambda}{2}\right)$

REAL WORLD

In noise-canceling headphones, pressure waves from noise are canceled by destructive interference. The speaker creates a wave that is 180 degrees out of phase and of similar amplitude. Many frequencies are usually present in the noise, so it is difficult to get perfect noise cancellation.

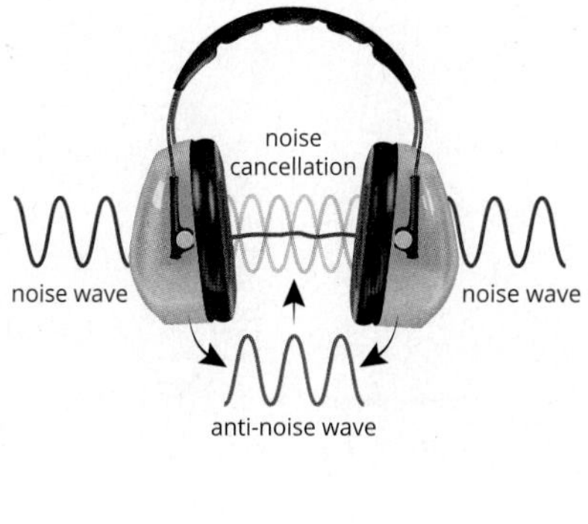

Noise-canceling headphones operate on the principle of superposition. They do not simply muffle sound, but actually capture the environmental noise and, using computer technology, produce a sound wave that is approximately 180 degrees out of phase. The combination of the two waves inside the headset results in destructive interference, thereby canceling—or nearly canceling—the ambient noise.

Traveling and Standing Waves

If a string fixed at one end is moved up and down, a wave will form and travel, or propagate, toward the fixed end. Because this wave is moving, it is called a **traveling wave**. When the wave reaches the fixed boundary, it is reflected and inverted, as shown in Figure 7.4. If the free end of the string is continuously moved up and down, there will then be two waves: the original wave moving down the string toward the fixed end and the reflected wave moving away from the fixed end. These waves will then interfere with each other.

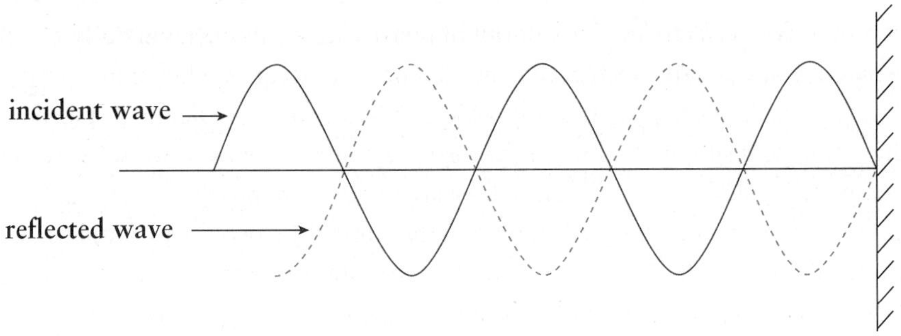

Figure 7.4 Traveling Wave

Now consider the case when both ends of the string are fixed and traveling waves are excited in the string. Certain wave frequencies will cause interference between the traveling wave and its reflected wave such that they form a waveform that appears to be stationary. In this case, the only apparent movement of the string is fluctuation of amplitude at fixed points along the length of the string. These waves are known as **standing waves**. Points in the wave that remain at rest (where amplitude is constantly zero) are known as **nodes**. Points midway between the nodes fluctuate with maximum amplitude and are known as **antinodes**. In addition to strings fixed at both ends, pipes that are open at both ends can support standing waves, and the mathematics relating the standing wave wavelength and the length of the string or the open pipe are similar. Pipes that are open at one end and closed at the other can also support standing waves, but because the closed end contains a node and the open end contains an antinode, the mathematics are different. Standing waves in strings and pipes are discussed in more detail later, within the context of sound, because standing wave formation is integral to the formation of sound in certain contexts.

Resonance

Why are clarinets, pianos, and even half-filled wine glasses considered musical instruments, but not pencils, chairs, or paper? This discrepancy has much to do with the **natural (resonant) frequencies** of these objects. Any solid object, when hit, struck, rubbed, or disturbed in any way will begin to vibrate. Tapping a pencil on a surface will cause it to vibrate, as will hitting a chair or crumpling a piece of paper. Blowing air pressure between a clarinet reed and a mouthpiece, striking a taut piano string, and creating friction on a wine glass's surface will also cause vibration. If the natural frequency is within the frequency detection range of the human ear, the sound will be audible. The quality of the sound, called **timbre**, is determined by the natural frequency or frequencies of the object. Some objects vibrate at a single frequency, producing a pure tone. Other objects vibrate at multiple frequencies that have no relation to one another. These objects produce sounds that we do not find particularly musical, such as tapping a pencil, hitting a chair, or crumpling paper. These sounds are called **noise**, scientifically. Still other objects vibrate at multiple natural frequencies (a **fundamental pitch** and multiple **overtones**) that are related to each other by whole number ratios, producing a richer, more full tone. The human brain perceives these sounds as being more musical, and all nonpercussion instruments produce such overtones. Of note for the MCAT, the frequencies between 20 Hz and 20,000 Hz are commonly audible to young adults, and high-frequency hearing generally declines with age.

The natural frequency of most objects can be changed by changing some aspect of the object itself. For example, a set of eight identical glasses can be filled with different levels of water so that each vibrates at a different natural frequency, producing the eight notes of a diatonic musical scale. Strings have an infinite number of natural frequencies that depend on the length, linear density, and tension of the string.

If a periodically varying force is applied to a system, the system will then be driven at a frequency equal to the frequency of the force. This is known as **forced oscillation**. If the frequency of the applied force is close to that of the natural frequency of the system, then the amplitude of oscillation becomes much larger. This can easily be demonstrated by a child on a swing being pushed by a parent. If the parent pushes the child at a frequency nearly equal to the frequency at which the child swings back toward the parent, the arc of the swinging child will become larger and larger: the amplitude is increasing because the **force frequency** is nearly identical to the swing's natural frequency.

If the frequency of the periodic force is equal to a natural (resonant) frequency of the system, then the system is said to be **resonating**, and the amplitude of the oscillation is at a maximum. If the oscillating system were frictionless, the periodically varying force would continually add energy to the system, and the amplitude would increase indefinitely. However, because no system is completely frictionless, there is always some damping, which results in a finite amplitude of oscillation. In general, **damping** or **attenuation** is a decrease in amplitude of a wave caused by an applied or nonconservative force. Furthermore, many objects cannot withstand the large amplitude of oscillation and will break or crumble. A dramatic demonstration of resonance is the shattering of a wine glass by loudly singing the natural frequency of the glass. This is actually possible with a steady, loud tone—the glass will resonate (oscillate with maximum amplitude) and eventually shatter.

MCAT CONCEPT CHECK 7.1

Before you move on, assess your understanding of the material with these questions.

1. Define the following terms:
   - Wave speed:

   - Frequency:

   - Angular frequency:

   - Period:

   - Equilibrium position:

   - Amplitude:

   - Traveling wave:

   - Standing wave:

   ---
2. If two waves are out of phase at any interval besides 180 degrees, how does the amplitude of the resultant wave compare to the amplitudes of the two interfering waves?

   ---
3. True or False: Sound waves are a prime example of transverse waves.
4. How does applying a force at the natural frequency of a system change the system?

7.2 Sound

High-Yield

LEARNING OBJECTIVES

After Chapter 7.2, you will be able to:

- Explain how sound is produced and transmitted
- Connect amplitude and frequency to their corresponding properties in a sound wave
- Predict changes in apparent frequency based on the movement of two objects in relation to one another
- Calculate key values for sound, including intensity, frequency, apparent frequency, and wavelength in Doppler and pipe systems

Sound is a longitudinal wave transmitted by the oscillation of particles in a deformable medium. As such, sound can travel through solids, liquids, and gases, but cannot travel through a vacuum. The speed of sound is given by the equation

$$v = \sqrt{\frac{B}{\rho}}$$

Equation 7.4

where B is the bulk modulus, a measure of the medium's resistance to compression (B increases from gas to liquid to solid), and ρ is the density of the medium. Because the bulk modulus increases disproportionately more than density as one goes from gas to liquid to solid, sound travels fastest through a solid and slowest through a gas. The speed of sound in air at 20°C is approximately 343 $\frac{\text{m}}{\text{s}}$.

KEY CONCEPT

The speed of sound is fastest in a solid with low density, and slowest in a very dense gas.

Production of Sound

Sound is produced by the mechanical disturbance of particles in a material along the sound wave's direction of propagation. Although the particles themselves do not travel along with the wave, they do vibrate or oscillate about an equilibrium position, which causes small regions of compression to alternate with small regions of rarefaction (decompression). These alternating regions of increased and decreased particle density travel through the material, allowing the sound wave to propagate.

Because sound involves vibration of material particles, the source of any sound is ultimately a mechanical vibration of some frequency. Sound waves can be produced by the vibration of solid objects or the vibration of fluids, including gases. Solid objects that can vibrate to produce musical sound include strings (on a piano, violin, guitar, and so on), metal (bells), or wood bars (xylophone or marimba). Vibration of air within certain objects, including all woodwinds and brass instruments, pipe organs, and even a soda bottle, can also create musical sound. The pitch (frequency) at which the air column within the instrument vibrates is determined by the length of the air column, which can be changed either by covering holes in the instrument or directly changing its length.

The human voice is no less a musical instrument than any of those listed above. Sound is created by passing air between the vocal cords, which are a pair of thin membranes stretched across the larynx. As the air moves past the cords, they vibrate like the double reed of an oboe or bassoon, causing the air to vibrate at the same frequency. The pitch of the sound is controlled by varying the tension of the cords. Adult male vocal cords are often larger and thicker than those of adult females; thus, male voices are commonly lower in pitch.

Frequency and Pitch

We've discussed frequency as the rate at which a particle or wave completes a cycle. Our perception of the frequency of sound is called the **pitch**. Lower-frequency sounds have lower pitch, and higher-frequency sounds have higher pitch. On the MCAT, sound frequencies are usually within the normal range of human hearing, from 20 Hz to 20,000 Hz. Sound waves with frequencies below 20 Hz are called **infrasonic** waves, and those with frequencies above 20,000 Hz are called **ultrasonic** waves. Both dog whistles, which emit frequencies between 20 and 22 kHz, and medical ultrasound machines, which emit frequencies in excess of 2 GHz, are examples of ultrasonic waves.

Doppler Effect

BRIDGE

The Doppler effect applies to all waves, including light. This means that if a source of light is moving toward the detector, the observed frequency will increase. This is called blue shift because blue is at the high-frequency end of the visible spectrum. If the source is moving away from the detector, the observed frequency will decrease, causing red shift. Light and electromagnetic waves are discussed in Chapter 8 of *MCAT Physics and Math Review.*

We've all witnessed the Doppler effect: an ambulance or fire truck with its sirens blaring is quickly approaching from the other lane, and as it passes, one can hear a distinct drop in the pitch of the siren. This phenomenon affecting frequency is called the **Doppler effect**, which describes the difference between the actual frequency of a sound and its perceived frequency when the source of the sound and the sound's detector are moving relative to one another. If the source and detector are moving toward each other, the perceived frequency, f', is greater than the actual frequency, f. If the source and detector are moving away from each other, the perceived frequency is less than the actual frequency. This can be seen from the Doppler effect equation:

$$f' = f\frac{(v \pm v_D)}{(v \mp v_S)}$$

Equation 7.5

where f' is the perceived frequency, f is the actual emitted frequency, v is the speed of sound in the medium, v_D is the speed of the detector, and v_S is the speed of the source. Note the unusual signs in the equation. If memorized in this form, the upper sign should be used when the detector or source is moving *toward* the other object. The lower sign should be used when the detector or source is moving *away* from the other object.

MNEMONIC

Sign convention in the Doppler equation:

- **T**op sign for "**t**oward"
- Bottom sign for "away"

This sign convention is usually the most confusing part of the Doppler effect equation, so let's take a closer look. Imagine the situation presented earlier: you're driving down the street when you hear an ambulance approaching from behind. In this scenario, you are the detector and the ambulance is the sound source. At this time, you would say that you are driving away from the ambulance; even though the ambulance is moving faster and getting closer to you, the direction in which you are driving is still *away* from the ambulance. By this logic, the lower sign (−) should be used in the numerator, which relates to the detector. The driver of the ambulance, on the other hand, would say that the ambulance is driving *toward* you. By this logic, the top sign (−) should be used in the denominator, which relates to the source. In this case, the Doppler effect equation would look like this:

$$f' = f\frac{(v - v_D)}{(v - v_S)}$$

Because $v_S > v_D$, we know that $f' > f$.

Now imagine that the ambulance has passed you and continues to speed down the road. At this point, you would say that you are driving *toward* the ambulance (top sign in the numerator, +), even if you are not going as fast as it is. The ambulance driver would say that the ambulance is driving away from you (bottom sign in the denominator, +) and the corresponding Doppler effect equation would be:

$$f' = f\frac{(v + v_D)}{(v + v_S)}$$

Here, because $v_S > v_D$, $f' < f$. This change in f' from being greater than f to being less than f is perceived as a drop in pitch.

The Doppler effect can be visualized by considering the sound waves in front of a moving object as being compressed, while the sound waves behind the object are stretched out, as shown in Figure 7.5.

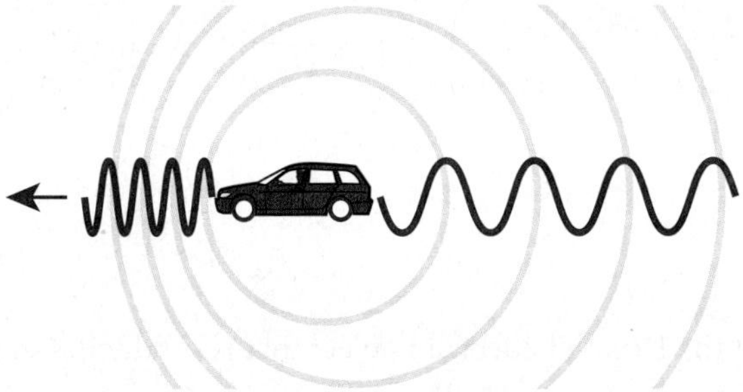

Figure 7.5 The Doppler Effect

The black arrow indicates the direction of motion for the car. In front of the car, crests of the sound wave are compressed together, increasing the frequency (pitch). Behind the car, crests of the sound wave are stretched apart, decreasing the frequency.

The Doppler effect can be used by animals through the process of **echolocation**. In echolocation, the animal emitting the sound (usually a dolphin or bat) serves as both the source and the detector of the sound. The sound bounces off of a surface and is reflected back to the animal. How long it takes for the sound to return, and the change in frequency of the sound, can be used to determine the position of objects in the environment and the speed at which they are moving.

Example: A train traveling south at 216 $\frac{\text{km}}{\text{hr}}$ is sounding its whistle while passing by a stationary observer. The whistle emits sound at a frequency of 1400 Hz. What is the frequency heard by the stationary observer when the train is moving toward the observer, and when the train has passed the observer? (Note: The speed of sound in air is approximately 340 $\frac{\text{m}}{\text{s}}$.)

Solution: To solve this problem, the speed of the train (v_S) must first be converted to $\frac{\text{m}}{\text{s}}$:

$$v_S = 216\ \frac{\text{km}}{\text{hr}}\left[\frac{1\ \text{hr}}{3600\ \text{s}}\right]\left[\frac{1000\ \text{m}}{1\ \text{km}}\right] = 60\ \frac{\text{m}}{\text{s}}$$

When the train is moving toward the stationary observer, the top sign should be used in the denominator. The numerator is simply v because $v_D = 0$. This gives

$$f' = f\,\frac{v}{v - v_S}$$

$$= (1400\ \text{Hz})\left(\frac{340\ \frac{\text{m}}{\text{s}}}{340\ \frac{\text{m}}{\text{s}} - 60\ \frac{\text{m}}{\text{s}}}\right) = 1400\left(\frac{340}{280}\right) = 1400\left(\frac{17}{14}\right) = 1700\ \text{Hz}$$

When the train is moving away from the observer, the sign in the denominator changes. The numerator remains unchanged because the observer is still stationary:

$$f' = f\,\frac{v}{v + v_S}$$

$$= (1400\ \text{Hz})\left(\frac{340\ \frac{\text{m}}{\text{s}}}{340\ \frac{\text{m}}{\text{s}} + 60\ \frac{\text{m}}{\text{s}}}\right) = 1400\left(\frac{340}{400}\right) = 1400\left(\frac{17}{20}\right) = 1190\ \text{Hz}$$

Shock Waves

In a special case of the Doppler effect, an object that is producing sound while traveling at or above the speed of sound allows wave fronts to build upon one another at the front of the object. This creates a much larger amplitude at that point. Because amplitude for sound waves is related to the degree of compression of the medium, this creates a large pressure differential or pressure gradient. This highly condensed wave front is called a **shock wave**, and it can cause physical disturbances as it passes through other objects. The passing of a shock wave creates very high pressure, followed by very low pressure, which is responsible for the phenomenon known as a **sonic boom**. Unlike its depiction in movies and television, a sonic boom can be heard any time that an object traveling at or faster than the speed of sound passes a detector, not just at the point that the speed of sound is exceeded (**Mach 1**). Once an object moves faster than the speed of sound, some of the effects of the shock wave are mitigated because all of the wave fronts will trail behind the object, destructively interfering with each other.

Intensity and Loudness of Sound

The **loudness** or **volume** of a sound is the way in which we perceive its intensity. Perception of loudness is subjective, and depends not only on brain function, but also physical factors such as obstruction of the ear canal, stiffening of the ossicles, or damage to cochlear hair cells by exposure to loud noises or with age. Sound intensity, on the other hand, is objectively measurable. **Intensity** is the average rate of energy transfer per area across a surface that is perpendicular to the wave. In other words, intensity is the power transported per unit area. The SI units of intensity are therefore watts per square meter $\left(\frac{\text{W}}{\text{m}^2}\right)$. Intensity is calculated using the equation

$$I = \frac{P}{A}$$

Equation 7.6

where P is the power and A is the area. Rearranging this equation, we could consider that the power delivered across a surface, such as the tympanic membrane (eardrum), is equal to the product of the intensity I and the surface area A, assuming the intensity is uniformly distributed.

The amplitude of a sound wave and its intensity are also related to each other: intensity is proportional to the square of the amplitude. Therefore, doubling the amplitude produces a sound wave that has four times the intensity.

Intensity is also related to the distance from the source of the sound wave. As sound waves emanate outward from their source, it is as though the waves are pushing against the interior wall of an ever-expanding spherical balloon. Because the surface area of a sphere increases as a function of the square of the radius ($A = 4\pi r^2$), sound waves transmit their power over larger and larger areas the farther from the source they travel. Intensity, therefore, is inversely proportional to the square of the distance from the source. For example, sound waves that have traveled 2 meters from their source have spread their energy out over a surface area that is four times larger than that for identical sound waves that have traveled 1 meter from their source.

The softest sound that a typical human ear can hear has an intensity equal to about $1 \times 10^{-12} \frac{\text{W}}{\text{m}^2}$. The mechanical disturbance associated with the threshold of hearing is remarkably small—the displacement of air particles is on the order of one billionth of a centimeter. At the other end of the spectrum, the intensity of sound at the threshold of pain is $10 \frac{\text{W}}{\text{m}^2}$ and the intensity that causes instant perforation of the eardrum is approximately $1 \times 10^4 \frac{\text{W}}{\text{m}^2}$. This is a huge range, which would be unmanageable to express on a linear scale. To make this range easier to work with, we use a logarithmic scale, called the **sound level** (β), measured in **decibels (dB)**:

$$\beta = 10 \log \frac{I}{I_0}$$

Equation 7.7

BRIDGE

We use logarithms with scales that have an extremely large range. The MCAT will mostly deal with base-ten logarithms (common logarithms). As an example, log 1000 = 3 because $10^3 = 1000$. As another example, log 1 = 0 because $10^0 = 1$. Logarithms are discussed in Chapter 10 of *MCAT Physics and Math Review.*

where I is the intensity of the sound wave and I_0 is the threshold of hearing $\left(1 \times 10^{-12}\ \frac{\text{W}}{\text{m}^2}\right)$, which is used as a reference intensity. When the intensity of a sound is changed by some factor, one can calculate the new sound level by using the equation

$$\beta_f = \beta_i + 10 \log \frac{I_f}{I_i}$$

Equation 7.8

where $\frac{I_f}{I_i}$ is the ratio of the final intensity to the initial intensity.

The sound levels and relative intensities of several sound sources and thresholds are shown in Table 7.1.

SOUND SOURCE	SOUND LEVEL (DB)	INTENSITY $\left(\frac{\text{W}}{\text{M}^2}\right)$
(Threshold of Hearing)	0	1×10^{-12}
Rustling Leaves	10	1×10^{-11}
Whisper	20	1×10^{-10}
Quiet Room at Night	30	1×10^{-9}
Quiet Library	40	1×10^{-8}
Moderate Rainfall	50	1×10^{-7}
Conversational Speech at 1 m	60	1×10^{-6}
Vacuum Cleaner at 1 m	70	1×10^{-5}
Door Slamming	80	1×10^{-4}
Lawn Mower at 1 m	90	1×10^{-3}
Jackhammer at 1 m	100	1×10^{-2}
Loud Rock Concert	110	1×10^{-1}
Thunder	120	1×10^{0}
(Threshold of Pain)	130	1×10^{1}
Rifle at 1 m	140	1×10^{2}
Jet Engine at 30 m	150	1×10^{3}
(Eardrum Perforation)	160	1×10^{4}

Table 7.1 Sound Level and Intensity of Sound Sources and Important Thresholds

Example: A detector with a surface area of 1 square meter is placed 1 meter from a blender. It measures the average power of the blender's sound as being 10^{-3} W. Find the intensity and sound level of the blender, and the ratio of the intensities of the blender and a jet engine. (Note: Assume $\beta_{\text{jet}} = 150$ dB.)

Solution: Intensity is defined as the power per area:

$$I = \frac{P}{A} = \frac{10^{-3}\ \text{W}}{1\ \text{m}^2} = 10^{-3}\ \frac{\text{W}}{\text{m}^2}$$

The sound level can then be calculated from the intensity:

$$\beta = 10 \log \frac{I}{I_0} = 10 \log \left(\frac{10^{-3}\ \frac{\text{W}}{\text{m}^2}}{10^{-12}\ \frac{\text{W}}{\text{m}^2}} \right) = 10 \log 10^9 = 90\ \text{dB}$$

Finally, the ratio of two sound intensities can be found from the difference of their sound levels:

$$\beta_{\text{jet}} = \beta_{\text{blender}} + 10 \log \frac{I_{\text{jet}}}{I_{\text{blender}}}$$

$$150\ \text{dB} = 90\ \text{dB} + 10 \log \frac{I_{\text{jet}}}{I_{\text{blender}}}$$

$$6 = \log \frac{I_{\text{jet}}}{I_{\text{blender}}}$$

$$10^6 = \frac{I_{\text{jet}}}{I_{\text{blender}}}$$

Thus, the jet engine's sound is 1,000,000 times more intense than the blender's sound.

Attenuation

Sound is not transmitted undiminished. Even after the decrease in intensity associated with distance, real world measurements of sound will be lower than those expected from calculations. This is a result of **damping**, or **attenuation**. Oscillations are a form of repeated linear motion, so sound is subject to the same nonconservative forces as any other system, including friction, air resistance, and viscous drag.

The presence of a nonconservative force causes the system to decrease in amplitude during each oscillation. Because amplitude, intensity, and sound level (loudness) are related, there is a corresponding gradual loss of sound. Note that damping does not have an effect on the frequency of the wave, so the pitch will not change. This phenomenon, along with reflection, explains why it is more difficult to hear in a confined or cluttered space than in an empty room: friction from the surfaces of the objects in the room actually decreases the sound waves' amplitudes. Over small distances, attenuation is usually negligible.

MCAT EXPERTISE

Like nonconservative forces, attenuation is generally negligible on Test Day. If it is important for answering a question, the MCAT will make it clear that you should consider the effects of damping (attenuation) on an oscillating system.

Beat Frequency

Sound volume can also vary periodically due to interference effects. When two sounds of slightly different frequencies are produced in proximity, as when tuning a pair of instruments next to one another, volume will vary at a rate based on the difference between the two pitches being produced. The frequency of this periodic increase in volume can be calculated by the equation:

$$f_{beat} = |f_1 - f_2|$$

Equation 7.9

where f_1 and f_2 represent the two frequencies that are close in pitch, and f_{beat} represents the resulting beat frequency.

Standing Waves

Remember that standing waves are produced by the constructive and destructive interference of a traveling wave and its reflected wave. More broadly, we can say that a standing wave will form whenever two waves of the same frequency traveling in opposite directions interfere with one another as they travel through the same medium. Standing waves appear to be standing still—that is, not propagating—because the interference of the wave and its reflected wave produce a resultant that fluctuates only in amplitude. As the waves move in opposite directions, they interfere to produce a new wave pattern characterized by alternating points of maximum displacement (amplitude) and points of no displacement. The points in a standing wave with no fluctuation in displacement are called **nodes**. The points with maximum fluctuation are called **antinodes**.

MNEMONIC

Nodes are places of **No D**isplacement

Not every frequency of traveling wave will result in standing wave formation. The length of the medium dictates the wavelengths (and, by extension, the frequencies) of traveling waves that can establish standing waves. Objects that support standing waves have boundaries at both ends. **Closed boundaries** are those that do not allow oscillation and that correspond to nodes. The closed end of a pipe and the secured ends of a string are both considered closed boundaries. **Open boundaries** are those that allow maximal oscillation and correspond to antinodes. The open end of a pipe and the free end of a flag are both open boundaries.

Strings

Consider a string, such as a guitar or violin string, or a piano wire, fixed rigidly at both ends. Because the string is secured at both ends and is therefore immobile at these points, they are considered nodes. If a standing wave is set up such that there is only one antinode between the two nodes at the ends, the length of the string corresponds to one-half the wavelength of this standing wave, as shown in Figure 7.6a. This is because on a sine wave, the distance from one node to the next node is one-half of a wavelength. If a standing wave is set up such that there are two antinodes between the ends, there must be a third node located between the antinodes, as shown in Figure 7.6b. In this case, the length of the string corresponds to the wavelength of this standing wave. Again, the distance on a sine wave from a node to the second consecutive node is exactly one wavelength. This pattern suggests that the length L of a string must be equal to some multiple of half-wavelengths ($L = \frac{\lambda}{2}, \frac{2\lambda}{2}, \frac{3\lambda}{2}$, and so on).

The equation that relates the wavelength λ of a standing wave and the length L of a string that supports it is:

$$\lambda = \frac{2L}{n}$$

Equation 7.10

where n is a positive nonzero integer ($n = 1, 2, 3$, and so on) called the **harmonic**. The harmonic corresponds to the number of half-wavelengths supported by the string. From the relationship that $f = \frac{v}{\lambda}$ where v is the wave speed, the possible frequencies are:

$$f = \frac{nv}{2L}$$

Equation 7.11

The lowest frequency (longest wavelength) of a standing wave that can be supported in a given length of string is known as the **fundamental frequency** (first harmonic). The frequency of the standing wave given by $n = 2$ is known as the first overtone or second harmonic. This standing wave has one-half the wavelength and twice the frequency of the first harmonic. The frequency of the standing wave given by $n = 3$ is known as the second overtone or third harmonic, as shown in Figure 7.6c. All the possible frequencies that the string can support form its **harmonic series**.

MCAT EXPERTISE

As a shortcut, for strings attached at both ends, the number of antinodes present will tell you which harmonic it is.

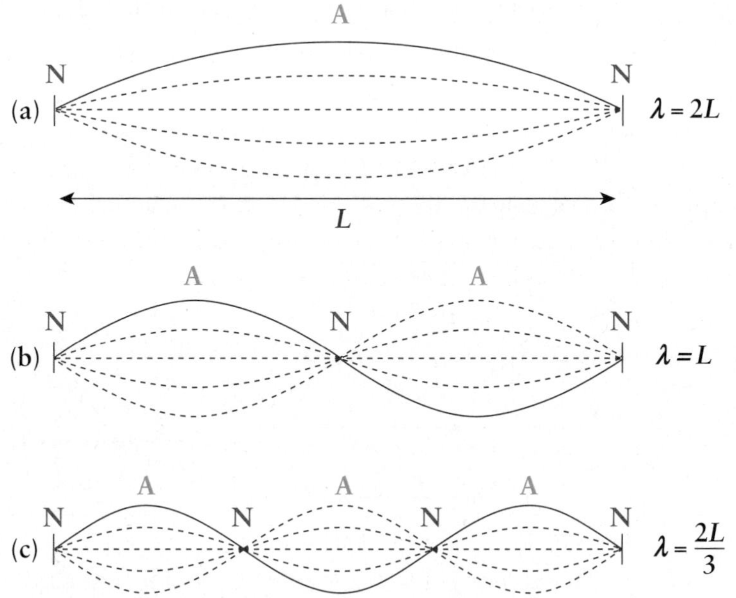

Figure 7.6 First, Second, and Third Harmonics of a String
The harmonic is given by the number of half-wavelengths supported by the string. N = node; A = antinode.

Open Pipes

Pipes can support standing waves and produce sound as well. Many musical instruments are straight or curved tubes within which air will oscillate at particular frequencies to set up standing waves. The end of a pipe can be open or closed. If the end of the pipe is open, it will support an antinode. If it is closed, it will support a node. One end of the pipe must be open at least slightly to allow for the entry of air, but sometimes these openings are small and covered by the musician's mouth—in these cases, they function as a closed end. Pipes that are open at both ends are called **open pipes**, while those that are closed at one end (and open at the other) are called **closed pipes**. The flute functions as an open pipe instrument, while the clarinet and brass instruments are closed pipe instruments. If you are a musician, this may be counterintuitive. The distal end of a flute is open, but the proximal end is closed; however, the mouthpiece of a flute is close enough to this closed end for it to function as an open end. Similarly, while air must pass through the mouthpiece of a reed or brass instrument, the opening is sufficiently small to function as a closed end.

An open pipe, being open at both ends, has antinodes at both ends. If a standing wave is set up such that there is only one node between the two antinodes at the ends, the length of the pipe corresponds to one-half the wavelength of this standing wave, as shown in Figure 7.7a. This is analogous to a string except that the ends are both antinodes instead of nodes. The analogy continues throughout: the second harmonic (first overtone) has a wavelength equal to the length of the pipe, as shown in Figure 7.7b. The third harmonic (second overtone) has a wavelength equal to two-thirds the length of the pipe, as shown in Figure 7.7c. Again, an open pipe can contain any multiple of half-wavelengths; the number of half-wavelengths corresponds to the harmonic of the wave. The relationship between the wavelength λ of a standing wave and the length L of an open pipe that supports it is $\lambda = \frac{2L}{n}$, and the possible frequencies of the harmonic series are $f = \frac{nv}{2L}$, just like a string.

MCAT EXPERTISE

As a shortcut, for open pipes, the number of nodes present will tell you which harmonic it is.

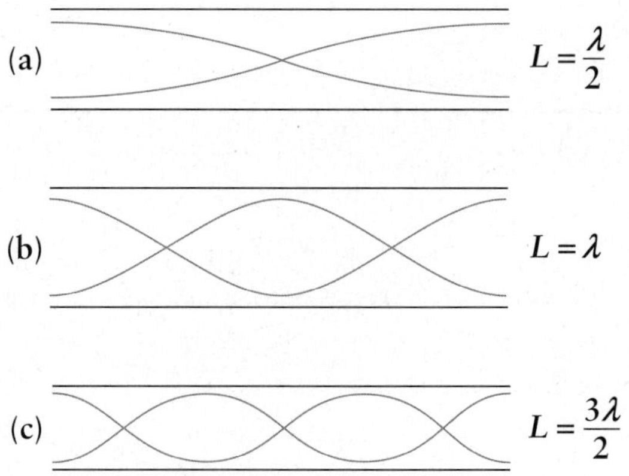

Figure 7.7 First, Second, and Third Harmonics of an Open Pipe
The harmonic is given by the number of half-wavelengths supported by the pipe.

It is worthwhile to note that Figure 7.7 is really a symbolic representation of the first three harmonics in an open pipe. We use the term symbolic because the conventional way of diagramming standing waves is to represent sound waves as transverse, rather than longitudinal, waves (which are much harder to draw).

Closed Pipes

In the case of a closed pipe, the closed end will correspond to a node, and the open end will correspond to an antinode. The first harmonic in a closed pipe consists of only the node at the closed end and the antinode at the open end, as shown in Figure 7.8a. In a sinusoidal wave, the distance from a node to the following antinode is one-quarter of a wavelength. Indeed, unlike strings or open pipes, the harmonic in a closed pipe is equal to the number of quarter-wavelengths supported by the pipe. Because the closed end must always have a node and the open end must always have an antinode, there can only be odd harmonics. This is because an even number of quarter-wavelengths would be an integer number of half-wavelengths—which would necessarily have either two nodes or two antinodes at the ends. The first harmonic has a wavelength that is four times the length of the closed pipe. The third harmonic (first overtone) has a wavelength that is four-thirds the length of the closed pipe, as shown in Figure 7.8b. The fifth harmonic (second overtone) has a wavelength that is four-fifths the length of the closed pipe, as shown in Figure 7.8c. The equation that relates the wavelength λ of a standing wave and the length L of a closed pipe that supports it is:

$$\lambda = \frac{4L}{n}$$

Equation 7.12

where n can only be an odd integers ($n = 1, 3, 5$, and so on). The frequency of the standing wave in a closed pipe is:

$$f = \frac{nv}{4L}$$

Equation 7.13

where v is the wave speed.

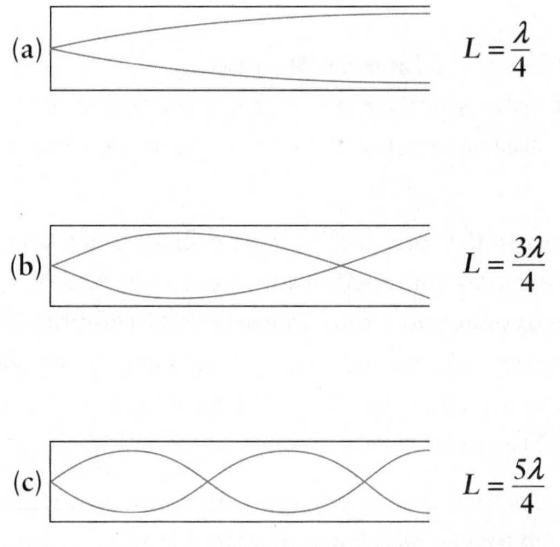

Figure 7.8 First, Third, and Fifth Harmonics of a Closed Pipe
The harmonic is given by the number of quarter-wavelengths supported by the pipe.

MCAT EXPERTISE

Unlike strings and open pipes, one cannot simply count the number of nodes or antinodes to determine the harmonic of the wave in closed pipes. Therefore, when presented with a closed pipe, make sure to actually count the number of quarter-wavelengths contained in the pipe to determine the harmonic.

Ultrasound

Until this point we've focused on sound in the audible range; however, in medicine we can also use sound waves to visualize organs, anatomy, and pathology. This imaging modality can be used for prenatal screening, or to diagnose gallstones and breast or thyroid masses, or for needle guidance in a biopsy. **Ultrasound** uses high frequency sound waves outside the range of human hearing to compare the relative densities of tissues in the body. An ultrasound machine consists of a transmitter that generates a pressure gradient, which also functions as a receiver that processes the reflected sound, as seen in Figure 7.9. Because the speed of the wave and travel time is known, the machine can generate a graphical representation of borders and edges within the body by calculating the traversed distance. Note that ultrasound ultimately relies on reflection; thus, an interface between two objects is necessary to visualize anything. Reflection will be discussed further in the next chapter.

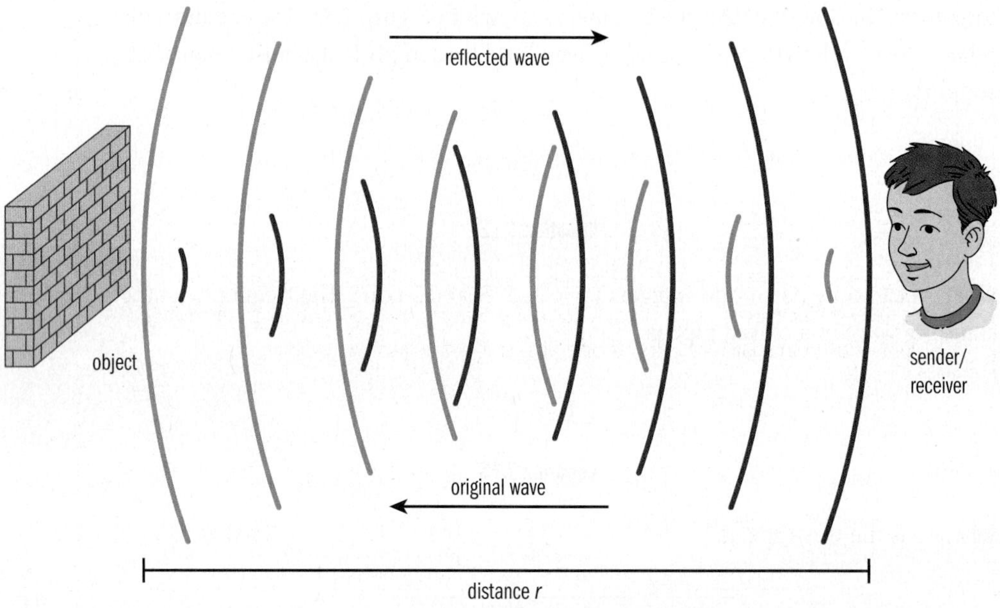

Figure 7.9 Ultrasound
The transmitter (sender) generates a wave, which reflects off of an object and returns to the transmitter (which also functions as a receiver).

Most ultrasound transmitters and receivers are packaged in a single unit. The transmitter and receiver do not function simultaneously, however, because one of the objectives of the system is to reduce interference. In addition to the standard ultrasound, most modern ultrasound machines also have a Doppler mode. **Doppler ultrasound** is used to determine the flow of blood within the body by detecting the frequency shift that is associated with movement toward or away from the receiver.

Ultrasound can also be used therapeutically. Ultrasound waves create friction and heat when they act on tissues, which can increase blood flow to a site of injury in deep tissues and promote faster healing. Focused ultrasound also has a range of applications. Focusing a sound wave using a parabolic mirror causes constructive interference at the focal point of the mirror. This creates a very high-energy wave exactly at that point, which can be used to noninvasively break up a kidney stone (*lithotripsy*) or ablate (destroy) small tumors. Ultrasound can also be used for dental cleaning and destruction of cataracts (*phacoemulsification*). In each case, the ultrasound waves are applied for a sufficient time period to achieve the desired effect.

MCAT CONCEPT CHECK 7.2

Before you move on, assess your understanding of the material with these questions.

1. How is sound produced and transmitted?

____

2. To which properties of a sound wave do amplitude and frequency correspond?
   - Amplitude:

   ____

   - Frequency:

   ____

3. If two objects are traveling toward each other, how does the apparent frequency differ from the original frequency? What if two objects are traveling away from each other? What if one object is following the other?
   - Toward each other:

   ____

   - Away from each other:

   ____

   - One object follows the other:

   ____

4. What phenomena can be detected or treated using ultrasound?

____

5. For each of the following diagrams, label the type of pipe or string it represents, a node and antinode, and the relevant equation relating λ and L:

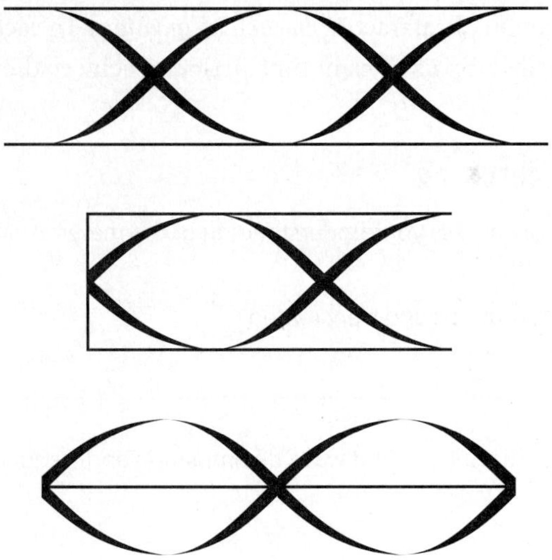

Conclusion

In this chapter, we reviewed the general characteristics of waves, including the phenomena of interference and resonance, and analyzed the characteristics and behaviors of sound as an example of a longitudinal waveform. Sound is the mechanical disturbance of particles creating oscillating regions of compression and rarefaction parallel to the direction of wave movement. The intensity of a sound wave is perceived as the sound level (loudness) of the sound and is measured in decibels. The decibel scale is a logarithmic scale used to describe the ratio of a sound's intensity to a reference intensity (the threshold of human hearing). We also reviewed the Doppler effect and a special case with shock waves. We then reviewed the mathematics governing the formation of standing waves, which are important in the formation of musical sounds in strings, open pipes, and closed pipes. Finally, we discussed a medical application of sound that incorporates many of these topics: ultrasound.

Continue to review these MCAT topics—it's easy to think about sound if you listen to music when you study! Whether you turn on Top 40, smooth jazz, or rococo fugues, the principles of sound production and propagation are key to your enjoyment of these harmonious sounds. Sound, of course, is not the only waveform tested on the MCAT. Light waves (and electromagnetic radiation in general) are heavily tested topics on Test Day—we'll review them in the next chapter.

You've reviewed the content, now test your knowledge and critical thinking skills by completing a test-like passage set in your online resources!

GO ONLINE

CONCEPT SUMMARY

General Wave Characteristics

- **Transverse waves** have oscillations of wave particles perpendicular to the direction of wave **propagation** (e.g., "The Wave," electromagnetic waves).
- **Longitudinal waves** have oscillations of wave particles parallel to the direction of wave propagation (e.g., sound waves).
- **Displacement** (**x**) in a wave refers to how far a point is from the **equilibrium position**, expressed as a vector quantity.
- The **amplitude** (A) of a wave is the magnitude of its maximal displacement.
- The maximum point of a wave (point of most positive displacement) is called a **crest**.
- The minimum point of a wave (point of most negative displacement) is called a **trough**.
- The **wavelength** (λ) of a wave is the distance between two crests or two troughs.
- The **frequency** (f) of a wave is the number of cycles it makes per second. It is expressed in **hertz** (**Hz**).
- The **angular frequency** (ω) is another way of expressing frequency and is expressed in radians per second.
- The **period** (T) of a wave is the number of seconds it takes to complete a cycle. It is the inverse of frequency.
- **Interference** describes the ways in which waves interact in space to form a **resultant wave**.
  - **Constructive interference** occurs when waves are exactly **in phase** with each other. The amplitude of the resultant wave is equal to the sum of the amplitudes of the two interfering waves.
  - **Destructive interference** occurs when waves are exactly **out of phase** with each other. The amplitude of the resultant wave is equal to the difference in amplitude between the two interfering waves.
  - **Partially constructive** and **partially destructive interference** occur when two waves are not quite perfectly in or out of phase with each other. The displacement of the resultant wave is equal to the sum of the displacements of the two interfering waves.
- **Traveling waves** have continuously shifting points of maximum and minimum displacement.
- **Standing waves** are produced by the constructive and destructive interference of two waves of the same frequency traveling in opposite directions in the same space.
  - **Antinodes** are points of maximum oscillation.
  - **Nodes** are points where there is no oscillation.

- **Resonance** is the increase in amplitude that occurs when a periodic force is applied at the **natural** (**resonant**) **frequency** of an object.
- **Damping** is a decrease in amplitude caused by an applied or nonconservative force.

Sound

- **Sound** is produced by mechanical disturbance of a material that creates an oscillation of the molecules in the material.
- Sound propagates through all forms of matter (but not a vacuum).
  - Sound propagates fastest through solids, followed by liquids, and slowest through gases.
  - Within a medium, as density increases, the speed of sound decreases.
- The **pitch** of a sound is related to its frequency.
- The **Doppler effect** is a shift in the perceived frequency of a sound compared to the actual frequency of the emitted sound when the source of the sound and its detector are moving relative to one another.
  - The apparent frequency will be higher than the emitted frequency when the source and detector are moving toward each other.
  - The apparent frequency will be lower than the emitted frequency when the source and detector are moving away from each other.
  - The apparent frequency can be higher, lower, or equal to the emitted frequency when the two objects are moving in the same direction, depending on their relative speeds.
  - When the source is moving at or above the speed of sound, **shock waves** (**sonic booms**) can form.
- Loudness or volume of sound (**sound level**) is related to its **intensity**.
  - Intensity is related to a wave's amplitude.
  - Intensity decreases over distance and some energy is lost to **attenuation** (damping) from frictional forces.
- Strings and **open pipes** (open at both ends) support standing waves, and the length of the string or pipe is equal to some multiple of half-wavelengths.
- **Closed pipes** (closed at one end) also support standing waves, and the length of the pipe is equal to some odd multiple of quarter-wavelengths.
- Sound is used medically in **ultrasound** machines for both imaging (diagnostic) and treatment (therapeutic) purposes.

ANSWERS TO CONCEPT CHECKS

7.1

1. Wave speed is the rate at which a wave transmits the energy or matter it is carrying. Wave speed is the product of frequency and wavelength. Frequency is a measure of how often a waveform passes a given point in space. It is measured in Hz. Angular frequency is the same as frequency, but is measured in radians per second. Period is the time necessary to complete a wave cycle. The equilibrium position is the point with zero displacement in an oscillating system. Amplitude is the maximal displacement of a wave from the equilibrium position. Traveling waves have nodes and antinodes that move with wave propagation. Standing waves have defined nodes and antinodes that do not move with wave propagation.
2. If two waves are perfectly in phase, the amplitude of the resulting wave is equal to the sum of the amplitudes of the interfering waves. If two waves are perfectly out of phase, the amplitude of the resulting wave is the difference of the amplitudes of the interfering waves. Therefore, if the two waves are anywhere between these two extremes, the amplitude of the resulting wave will be somewhere between the sum and difference of the amplitudes of the interfering waves.
3. False. Sound waves are the most common example of longitudinal waves on the MCAT.
4. The object will resonate because the force frequency equals the natural (resonant) frequency. The amplitude of the oscillation will increase.

7.2

1. Sound is produced by mechanical vibrations. These are usually generated by solid objects like bells or vocal cords, but occasionally can be generated by fluids. Sound is propagated as longitudinal waves in matter, so it cannot propagate in a vacuum.
2. The amplitude of a wave is related to its sound level (volume). The frequency of a wave is related to its pitch.
3. When two objects are traveling toward each other, the apparent frequency is higher than the original frequency $\left(f' = f\frac{(v + v_D)}{(v - v_S)}\right)$. When two objects are traveling away from each other, the apparent frequency is lower than the original frequency $\left(f' = f\frac{(v - v_D)}{(v + v_S)}\right)$. When one object follows the other, the apparent frequency could be higher, lower, or equal to the original frequency depending on the relative speeds of the detector and the source $\left(f' = f\frac{(v + v_D)}{(v + v_S)} \text{ or } f' = f\frac{(v - v_D)}{(v - v_S)}\right)$.

4. Ultrasound can be used for prenatal screening or to diagnose gallstones, breast and thyroid masses, and blood clots. It can be used for needle guidance in a biopsy, for dental cleaning, and for treating deep tissue injury, kidney stones, certain small tumors, and cataracts, among many other applications.

5.

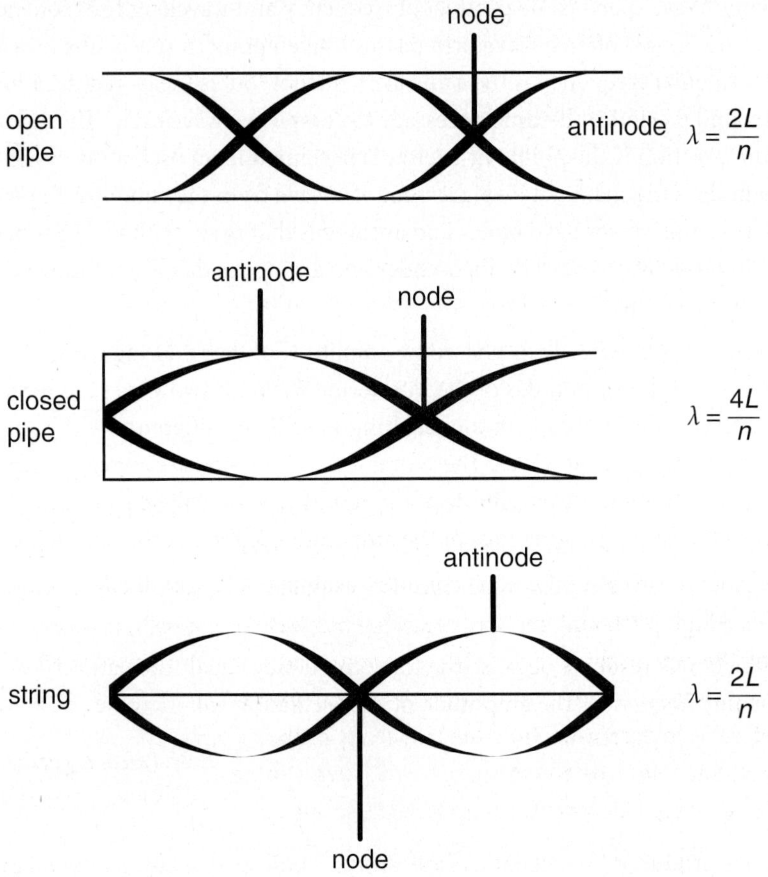

SCIENCE MASTERY ASSESSMENT EXPLANATIONS

1. **C**

If these two glasses are perfectly identical, then the fact that the first glass shattered at 808 Hz tells us that this is very close (if not identical) to the natural (resonant) frequency of the glass. If the singer produces a frequency that is not equal (or very close) to the natural frequency, then the applied frequency will not cause the glass to resonate, and there will not be the increase in wave amplitude associated with resonating objects. Attenuation will increase with increased frequency because there is more motion over which nonconservative forces can damp the sound wave; however, even if sound level was matched to that which shattered the first glass when accounting for attenuation, the glass would still not shatter for the reasons described above, eliminating **(D)**.

2. **B**

This question is testing our understanding of pipes open at one or both ends. To begin, remember that high-frequency sounds have a high pitch and low-frequency sounds have a low pitch. The pipe in this example begins as one that is open on both ends, and then one end is closed off. Our task, therefore, is to determine how the frequency of the second harmonic differs between a pipe that is open at both ends from one of equal length that is open at only one end. For a pipe of length L open at both ends, the wavelength for the second harmonic (first overtone) is equal to L:

$$\lambda = \frac{2L}{n} = \frac{2L}{2} = L$$

In contrast, for a pipe open at one end and closed at the other, the wavelength is equal to $\frac{4L}{3}$:

$$\lambda = \frac{4L}{n} = \frac{4L}{3}$$

Keep in mind that the first overtone for a closed pipe corresponds to the third harmonic, not the second. Thus, when the sibling covers one end of the flute, the wavelength increases. Given that the wavelength and the frequency of a sound are inversely proportional, an increase in wavelength corresponds to a decrease in frequency. Therefore, when the sibling covers one end of the flute, the sound produced by the instrument will be slightly lower in pitch than the original sound.

3. **C**

The angular frequency is related to the frequency through the equation $\omega = 2\pi f$. Therefore, the magnitude of the angular frequency will always be larger than the magnitude of the frequency. The magnitude of the angular frequency may or may not be larger than the magnitude of period; these variables are inversely proportional, eliminating **(A)**. The product of the frequency and the period is always 1 because these two are inverses of each other, eliminating **(B)**. Finally, the product of the angular frequency and period will always be 2π because $\omega = 2\pi f = \frac{2\pi}{T}$, eliminating **(D)**.

4. **B**

Although intensity, **(A)**, could be used to measure distance, time of travel is an easier indication and most commonly used by ultrasound machines. Apparent frequency, **(D)**, is only used in Doppler ultrasound, but is not used to calculate distance. Angle of incidence, **(C)**, can be used to position various structures on the screen of an ultrasound, but is not used to calculate distance.

5. **A**

Period is inversely related to frequency. Because the perceived frequency is doubled, the perceived period must be halved, from 34 ms to 17 ms. While either condition I or II would cause a doubling of the perceived frequency, neither condition must necessarily be true because the opposite could be true instead.

6. **B**

This question is testing our understanding of traveling waves. We know that frequency and wavelength are related through the equation $v = f\lambda$. Frequency and period are inverses of each other, so this equation could be rearranged to solve for period:

$$v = \left(\frac{1}{T}\right)\lambda \rightarrow T = \frac{\lambda}{v} = \frac{(0.1 \text{ m})}{\left(3 \ \frac{\text{m}}{\text{s}}\right)} = 0.03 \text{ s}$$

7. **D**

The angular frequency is related to the frequency of a wave through the formula $\omega = 2\pi f$. Thus, our initial task is to calculate the frequency of the wave. Knowing its speed, we determine the frequency of the wave by first calculating wavelength ($v = f\lambda$). For the third harmonic of a standing wave in a pipe with one closed end, the wavelength is

$$\lambda = \frac{4L}{n} = \frac{4(1.5\text{ m})}{3} = 2\text{ m}$$

The frequency of the wave is therefore

$$f = \frac{v}{\lambda} = \frac{340\ \frac{\text{m}}{\text{s}}}{2\text{ m}} = 170\text{ Hz}$$

Finally, obtain the angular frequency by multiplying the frequency of the wave by 2π:

$$\omega = 2\pi f = 340\pi \text{ radians per second}$$

8. **C**

Let I_i be the intensity before the increase and I_f be the intensity after the increase. Using the equation that relates sound level to intensity, obtain the ratio of I_i to I_f:

$$\beta_f = \beta_i + 10\log\frac{I_f}{I_i} \rightarrow \beta_f - \beta_i = 10\log\frac{I_f}{I_i}$$

$$20\text{ dB} = 10\log\frac{I_f}{I_i}$$

$$2 = \log\frac{I_f}{I_i}$$

$$100 = \frac{I_f}{I_i}$$

9. **B**

Saying that the stapedial footplate has limited displacement during vibration is another way of stating that the amplitude of the vibration has been decreased. Because amplitude is related to intensity, and intensity is related to sound level, the perceived sound level (volume) will be decreased as well. Pitch, described in **(C)** and **(D)**, is related to the frequency of a sound, not its amplitude.

10. **A**

When two waves are out of phase by 180°, the resultant amplitude is the difference between the two waves' amplitudes. In this case, the resulting wave will have an amplitude of 5 cm − 3 cm = 2 cm.

11. **D**

This question is testing you on your understanding of the Doppler effect. A difference of zero between the perceived and the emitted frequencies implies that the source of the sound is not moving relative to the student. If the car in **(D)** is moving at the same speed as the student, then the relative motion between them could be 0. In all of the other cases, the student and the sound source are necessarily moving relative to each other.

12. **D**

Sound is a mechanical disturbance propagated through a deformable medium; it is transmitted by the oscillation of particles parallel to the direction of the sound wave's propagation. As such, sound needs matter to travel through, eliminating **(A)**. The speed of propagation is fastest in solid materials, followed by liquids, and slowest in gases.

13. **B**

Shock waves are the buildup of wave fronts as the distance between those wave fronts decreases. This occurs maximally when an object is traveling at exactly the same speed as the wave is traveling (the speed of sound). Once an object moves faster than the speed of sound, some of the effects of the shock wave are mitigated because all of the wave fronts will trail behind the object, destructively interfering with each other.

14. **A**

Here, an observer is moving closer to a stationary source. The applicable version of the Doppler effect equation is $f' = f\frac{(v + v_D)}{v}$ where v is the speed of the sound. Because the numerator is greater than the denominator, f' will be greater than f; therefore, statement I is true. The scenario described in statement II will produce a similar, but not identical, frequency for the teacher: the frequency formula would be $f' = f\frac{v}{(v - v_S)}$. The apparent frequency will increase, but the increase will not be exactly the same as if the teacher had been moving. Statement III is false because we already know the frequency increases for the teacher—a decrease in velocity would be associated with a decrease in frequency.

15. **D**

Intensity is equal to power divided by area. In this case, area refers to the surface area of concentric spheres emanating out from the source of the sound. This surface area is given by $4\pi r^2$, so as distance (r) doubles, the intensity will decrease by a factor of four.

Consult your online resources for additional practice. GO ONLINE

EQUATIONS TO REMEMBER

(7.1) **Wave speed:** $v = f\lambda$

(7.2) **Period:** $T = \frac{1}{f}$

(7.3) **Angular frequency:** $\omega = 2\pi f = \frac{2\pi}{T}$

(7.4) **Speed of sound:** $v = \sqrt{\frac{B}{\rho}}$

(7.5) **Doppler effect:** $f' = f\,\frac{(v \pm v_D)}{(v \mp v_S)}$

(7.6) **Intensity:** $I = \frac{P}{A}$

(7.7) **Sound level:** $\beta = 10 \log \frac{I}{I_0}$

(7.8) **Change in sound level:** $\beta_f = \beta_i + 10 \log \frac{I_f}{I_i}$

(7.9) **Beat frequency:** $f_{beat} = |f_1 - f_2|$

(7.10) **Wavelength of a standing wave (strings and open pipes):** $\lambda = \frac{2L}{n}$

(7.11) **Frequency of a standing wave (strings and open pipes):** $f = \frac{nv}{2L}$

(7.12) **Wavelength of a standing wave (closed pipes):** $\lambda = \frac{4L}{n}$

(7.13) **Frequency of a standing wave (closed pipes):** $f = \frac{nv}{4L}$

SHARED CONCEPTS

Behavioral Sciences Chapter 2
Sensation and Perception

General Chemistry Chapter 8
The Gas Phase

Physics and Math Chapter 1
Kinematics and Dynamics

Physics and Math Chapter 2
Work and Energy

Physics and Math Chapter 8
Light and Optics

Physics and Math Chapter 10
Mathematics

CHAPTER 8

LIGHT AND OPTICS

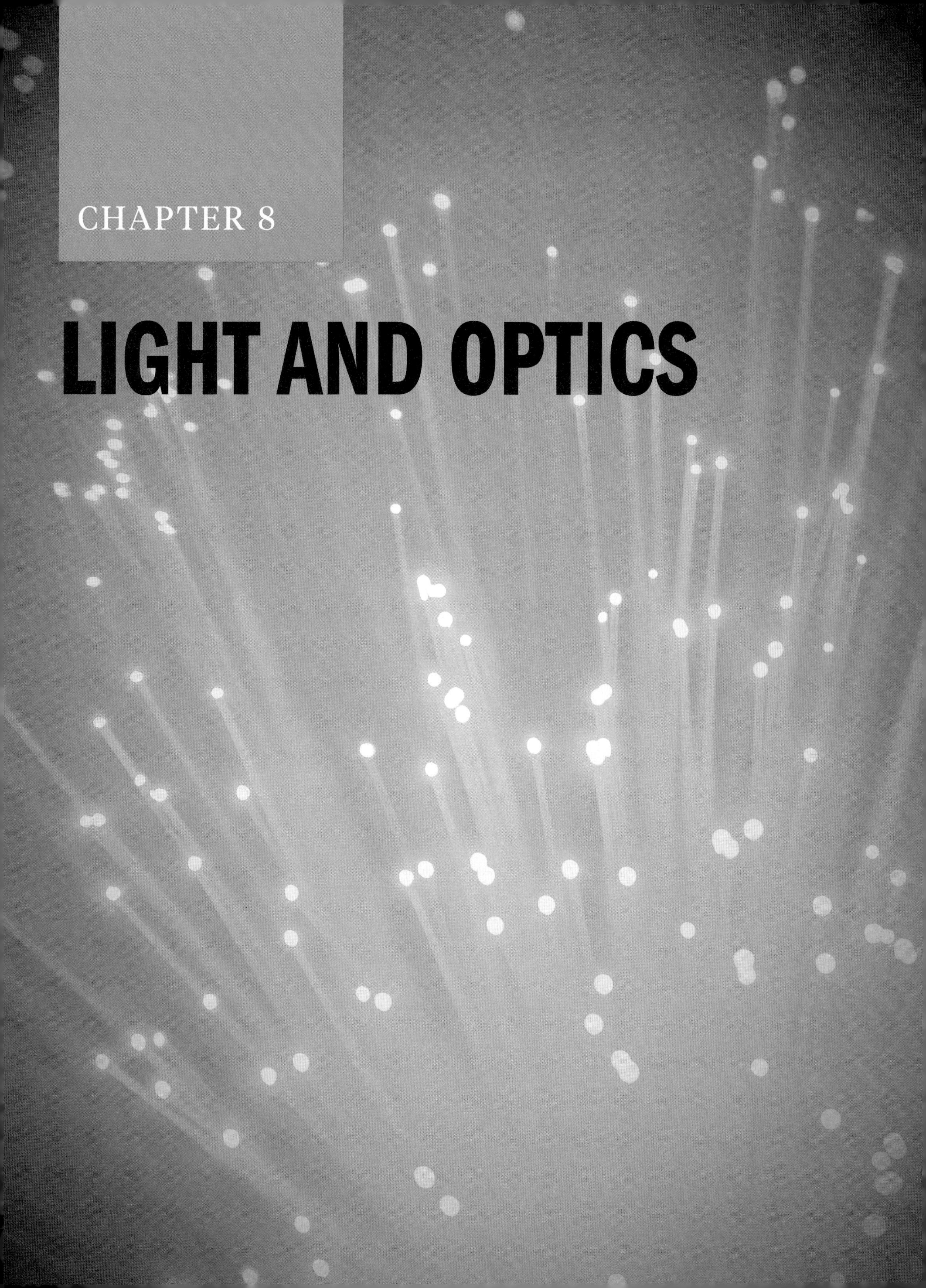

SCIENCE MASTERY ASSESSMENT

Every pre-med knows this feeling: there is so much content I have to know for the MCAT! How do I know what to do first or what's important?

While the high-yield badges throughout this book will help you identify the most important topics, this Science Mastery Assessment is another tool in your MCAT prep arsenal. This quiz (which can also be taken in your online resources) and the guidance below will help ensure that you are spending the appropriate amount of time on this chapter based on your personal strengths and weaknesses. Don't worry though—skipping something now does not mean you'll never study it. Later on in your prep, as you complete full-length tests, you'll uncover specific pieces of content that you need to review and can come back to these chapters as appropriate.

How to Use This Assessment

If you answer 0–7 questions correctly:

Spend about 1 hour to read this chapter in full and take limited notes throughout. Follow up by reviewing **all** quiz questions to ensure that you now understand how to solve each one.

If you answer 8–11 questions correctly:

Spend 20–40 minutes reviewing the quiz questions. Beginning with the questions you missed, read and take notes on the corresponding subchapters. For questions you answered correctly, ensure your thinking matches that of the explanation and you understand why each choice was correct or incorrect.

If you answer 12–15 questions correctly:

Spend less than 20 minutes reviewing all questions from the quiz. If you missed any, then include a quick read-through of the corresponding subchapters, or even just the relevant content within a subchapter, as part of your question review. For questions you got correct, ensure your thinking matches that of the explanation and review the Concept Summary at the end of the chapter.

1. If a light ray has a frequency of 5.0×10^{14} Hz, in which region of the electromagnetic spectrum is it located?
   A. X-ray
   B. UV
   C. Visible
   D. Infrared

2. During the fall, the leaves of some trees change in color from green to red because chlorophyll breaks down, leaving the secondary anthocyanin pigments. Which of the following best describes the light reflected by anthocyanin?
   A. Has a wavelength of 700 m
   B. Has a wavelength of 580 nm
   C. Has a frequency of 4.2×10^{6} Hz
   D. Has a frequency of 4.2×10^{14} Hz

3. An object is placed at the center of curvature of a concave mirror. Which of the following is true about the image?
   A. It is real and inverted.
   B. It is virtual and inverted.
   C. It is real and upright.
   D. It is virtual and upright.

4. In a double slit experiment, what wavelength of light must be used for the second dark fringe to be at an angle of 30° given that the distance between the two slits is 0.3 mm?
   A. 1×10^{-5} m
   B. 6×10^{-5} m
   C. 3.6×10^{-2} m
   D. 6×10^{-2} m

5. A ray of light ($f = 5 \times 10^{14}$ Hz) travels from air into crystal into chromium. If the indices of refraction of air, crystal, and chromium are 1, 2, and 3, respectively, and the incident angle is 30°, then which of the following describes the frequency and the angle of refraction in the chromium?
   A. 5×10^{14} Hz; 9.6°
   B. 5×10^{14} Hz; 57°
   C. 1.0×10^{10} Hz; 9.6°
   D. 1.0×10^{10} Hz; 57°

6. A source of light ($f = 6.0 \times 10^{14}$ Hz) passes through three plane polarizers. The first two polarizers are in the same direction, while the third is rotated 90° with respect to the second polarizer. What is the frequency of the light that comes out of the third polarizer?
   A. 3.0×10^{14} Hz
   B. 6.0×10^{14} Hz
   C. 9.0×10^{14} Hz
   D. Light will not pass through the third polarizer

7. As part of an organic chemistry lab, a student must determine the specific rotation of a chiral product. The student uses a plane polarizer, but accidentally inserts a second polarizer at a 90° angle to the first. What is true of the resulting light if it passes through both polarizers?
   A. It is circularly polarized.
   B. It is twice as plane polarized.
   C. There is no light.
   D. It is the same as when passed through a single polarizer.

8. Which of the following describes the image formed by an object placed in front of a convex lens at a distance smaller than the focal length?
   - **A.** Virtual and inverted
   - **B.** Virtual and upright
   - **C.** Real and upright
   - **D.** Real and inverted

9. A submarine is inspecting the surface of the water with a laser that points from the submarine to the surface of the water and through the air. At what angle will the laser not penetrate the surface of the water but rather reflect entirely back into the water? (Assume $n_{water} = 1.33$ and $n_{air} = 1$.)
   - **A.** 19°
   - **B.** 29°
   - **C.** 39°
   - **D.** 49°

10. A student is analyzing the behavior of a light ray that is passed through a small opening and a lens and allowed to project on a screen a distance away. What happens to the central maximum (the brightest spot on the screen) when the slit becomes narrower?
    - **A.** The central maximum remains the same.
    - **B.** The central maximum becomes narrower.
    - **C.** The central maximum becomes wider.
    - **D.** The central maximum divides into smaller light fringes.

11. Which of the following are able to produce a virtual image?
    - **I.** Convex lens
    - **II.** Concave lens
    - **III.** Plane mirror

    - **A.** I only
    - **B.** III only
    - **C.** II and III only
    - **D.** I, II, and III

12. Monochromatic red light is allowed to pass between two different media. If the incident angle in medium 1 is 30° and the incident angle in medium 2 is 45°, what is the relationship between the speed of the light in medium 2 compared to that in medium 1?
    - **A.** $v_2 = v_1\sqrt{2}$
    - **B.** $v_2\sqrt{2} = v_1$
    - **C.** $v_2 = v_1\sqrt{3}$
    - **D.** $v_2\sqrt{3} = v_1$

13. A scientist looks through a microscope with two thin lenses with $m_1 = 10$ and $m_2 = 40$. What is the overall magnification of this microscope?
    - **A.** 0.25
    - **B.** 30
    - **C.** 50
    - **D.** 400

14. Imagine that a beam of monochromatic light originates in air and is allowed to shine upon the flat surface of a piece of glass at an angle of 60° with the normal. The reflected and refracted beams are perpendicular to each other. What is the index of refraction of the glass?
    - **A.** $\frac{\sqrt{3}}{3}$
    - **B.** 1
    - **C.** 2
    - **D.** $\sqrt{3}$

15. Which of the following will not result in the splitting of white light into its component colors?
    - **A.** Dispersion through a prism
    - **B.** Diffraction through a grating
    - **C.** Refraction within a thin film
    - **D.** Reflection from an ideal convex mirror

Answer Key

1. **C**
2. **D**
3. **A**
4. **B**
5. **A**
6. **D**
7. **C**
8. **B**
9. **D**
10. **C**
11. **D**
12. **A**
13. **D**
14. **D**
15. **D**

Detailed explanations can be found at the end of the chapter.

CHAPTER 8

LIGHT AND OPTICS

In This Chapter

CHAPTER PROFILE

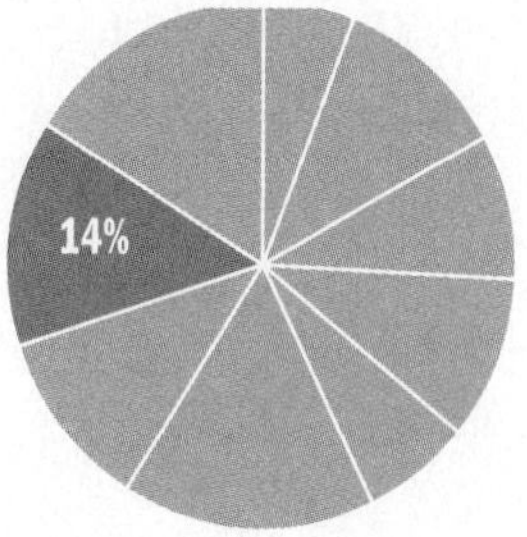

The content in this chapter should be relevant to about 14% of all questions about physics on the MCAT.

This chapter covers material from the following AAMC content category:

4D: How light and sound interact with matter

Introduction

The next time you're browsing your local convenience store, take a look at the security mirrors—the ones that bulge out from the wall, usually above eye level. Looking into one of these mirrors, notice not just that the image you see of the world is distorted but *how* it is distorted: the image is still right-side up, but everything is much smaller than you'd expect, and the curve of the mirror introduces some slopes that are not present in reality. Additionally, you see a much wider field of vision than you would if the mirror were a simple plane mirror. This is why security mirrors are useful: they are a convenient, low-tech solution that allows the cashier to survey the entire store in one glance. All these features result from the fact that the security mirror is a convex, diverging optical system. Parallel light rays that hit the mirror are reflected in multiple directions, which allows observers to see a large field of vision, even if the image is somewhat distorted and the objects in the image are closer than they appear. Indeed, the passenger-side mirror of a car that bears that same message is also a convex mirror, allowing the driver to see a wider view of the other vehicles behind the car.

This chapter will first complete a topic from Chapter 7 of *MCAT Physics and Math Review* by analyzing the transverse waveform of visible light and other electromagnetic (EM) waves. We will then consider in detail the rules of optics, which describe the behavior of electromagnetic waves as they bounce off of and travel through various shapes and compositions of matter. The optical systems covered are those tested on the MCAT: concave and convex mirrors, which produce images by reflection, and concave and convex lenses, which produce images by refraction. To finish, we will discuss the phenomena of thin-slit experiments (diffraction) and light polarization.

8.1 Electromagnetic Spectrum

High-Yield

LEARNING OBJECTIVES

After Chapter 8.1, you will be able to:

- Order the types of electromagnetic radiation, such as X-rays, microwaves, and visible light, from lowest to highest energy
- Describe the properties of electromagnetic waves
- Compare the visible spectrum to the full electromagnetic spectrum

The full **electromagnetic spectrum** includes **radio waves** on one end (long wavelength, low frequency, low energy) and **gamma rays** on the other (short wavelength, high frequency, high energy). Between the two extremes, we find, in order from lowest energy to highest energy, **microwaves**, **infrared**, visible light, **ultraviolet**, and **X-rays**. This chapter will focus primarily on the range of wavelengths corresponding to the visible spectrum of light (400 nm to 700 nm).

Electromagnetic Waves

A changing magnetic field can cause a change in an electric field, and a changing electric field can cause a change in a magnetic field. Because of the reciprocating nature of these two fields, we can see how electromagnetic waves occur in nature. Each oscillating field causes oscillations in the other field completely independent of matter, so electromagnetic waves can even travel through a vacuum.

Electromagnetic waves are transverse waves because the oscillating electric and magnetic field vectors are perpendicular to the direction of propagation. The electric field and the magnetic field are also perpendicular to each other. This is illustrated in Figure 8.1.

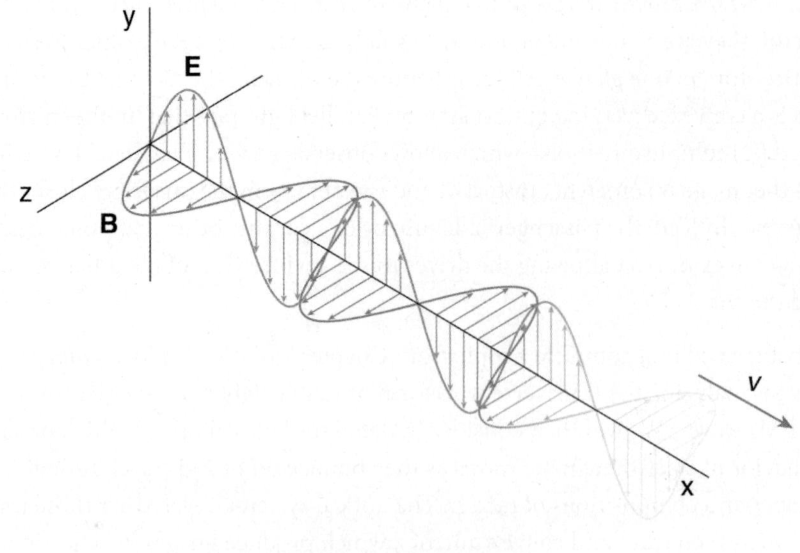

Figure 8.1 Electromagnetic Wave
*The electric field (**E**) oscillates up and down the page; the magnetic field (**B**) oscillates into and out of the page.*

The **electromagnetic spectrum** describes the full range of frequencies and wavelengths of electromagnetic waves. Wavelengths are often given in the following units: mm (10^{-3} m), μm (10^{-6} m), nm (10^{-9} m), and Å (ångström, 10^{-10} m). The full spectrum is broken up into many regions, which in descending order of wavelength are radio (10^9–1 m), microwave (1 m–1 mm), infrared (1 mm–700 nm), visible light (700–400 nm), ultraviolet (400–50 nm), X-rays (50–10^{-2} nm), and γ-rays (less than 10^{-2} nm). The electromagnetic spectrum is depicted in Figure 8.2.

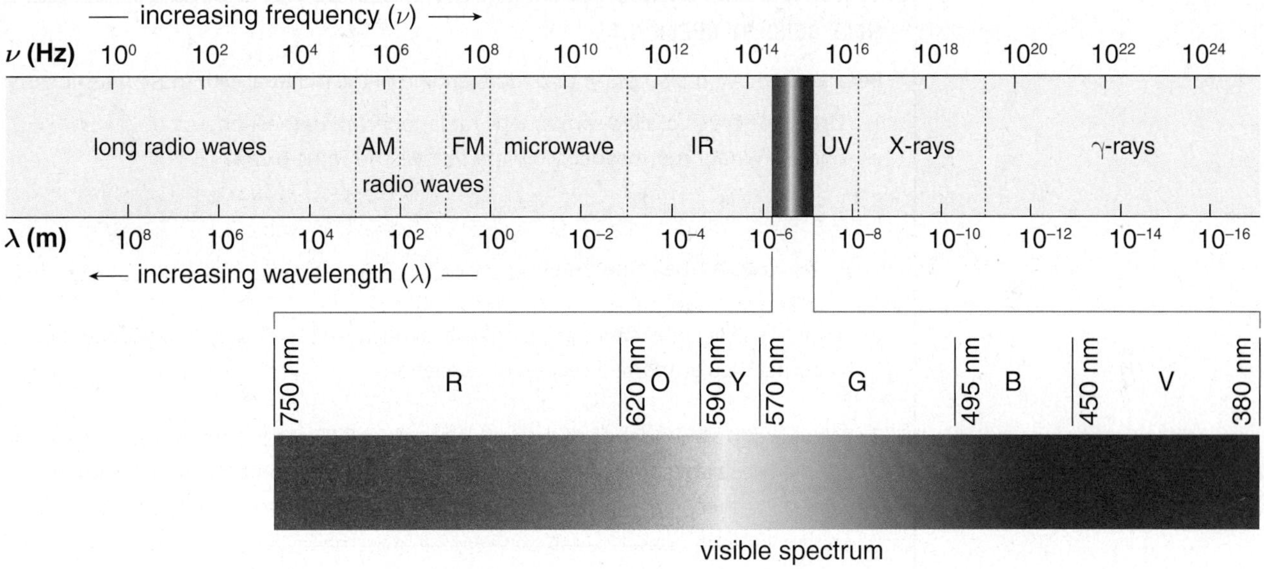

Figure 8.2 The Electromagnetic Spectrum

Electromagnetic waves vary in frequency and wavelength, but in a vacuum, all electromagnetic waves travel at the same speed, called the **speed of light**. This constant is represented by c and is approximately $3.00 \times 10^8 \frac{\text{m}}{\text{s}}$. To a first approximation—and for the purposes of all MCAT-related equations—electromagnetic waves also travel in air with this speed. In reference to electromagnetic waves, the familiar equation $v = f\lambda$ becomes

$$c = f\lambda$$

Equation 8.1

where c is the speed of light in a vacuum and, to a first approximation, also in air, f is the frequency, and λ is the wavelength.

Color and the Visible Spectrum

The only part of the spectrum that is perceived as light by the human eye is the **visible region**. Within this region, different wavelengths are perceived as different colors, with violet at one end of the visible spectrum (400 nm) and red at the other (700 nm).

MNEMONIC

To recall the order of the colors in the visible spectrum, remember the grade-school "rainbow" of **ROY G. BV** (**r**ed, **o**range, **y**ellow, **g**reen, **b**lue, **v**iolet).

MCAT EXPERTISE

Wavelengths in the visible range are common on the MCAT. Remembering the boundaries of the visible spectrum (about 400–700 nm) will save you time and energy on Test Day.

Light that contains all the colors in equal intensity is perceived as white. The color of an object that does not emit its own light is dependent on the color of light that it reflects. Thus, an object that appears red is one that absorbs all colors of light except red. This implies that a red object under green illumination will appear black because it absorbs the green light and has no light to reflect. The term **blackbody** refers to an ideal absorber of all wavelengths of light, which would appear completely black if it were at a lower temperature than its surroundings.

MCAT CONCEPT CHECK 8.1

Before you move on, assess your understanding of the material with these questions.

1. Order the types of electromagnetic radiation from highest energy to lowest energy. What other property of light follows the same trend?

_______ > _______ > _______ > _______ > _______ > _______ > _______

- Also follows the same trend: ______________________

2. True or False: Light waves are longitudinal because the direction of propagation is perpendicular to the direction of oscillation.

3. What are the boundaries of the visible spectrum? How does the range of the visible spectrum compare to the range of the full electromagnetic spectrum?

____

8.2 Geometrical Optics

High-Yield

LEARNING OBJECTIVES

After Chapter 8.2, you will be able to:

- Apply the sign conventions for mirrors and lenses to optics systems
- Describe the bending of light as it moves between media with different refractive indices
- Explain the impact of dispersion effects and aberrations on the behavior of light
- Recall Snell's law and other key optics equations
- Solve optics and Snell's law problems

When light travels through a homogeneous medium, it travels in a straight line. This is known as **rectilinear propagation**. The behavior of light at the boundary of a medium or interface between two media is described by the theory of geometrical optics. Geometrical optics explains reflection and refraction, as well as the applications of mirrors and lenses.

Reflection

Reflection is the rebounding of incident light waves at the boundary of a medium. Light waves that are reflected are not absorbed into the second medium; rather, they bounce off of the boundary and travel back through the first medium. Figure 8.3 illustrates reflection on a plane mirror.

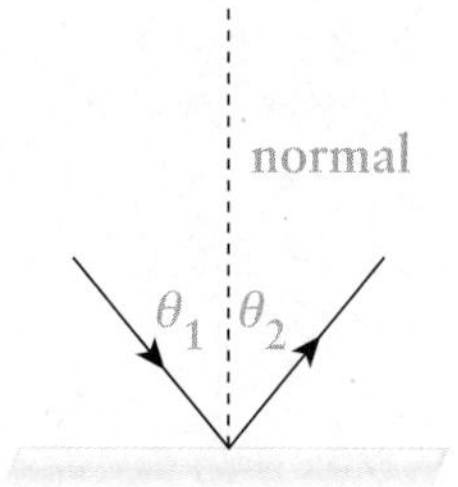

Figure 8.3 Reflection
According to the law of reflection, $\theta_1 = \theta_2$.

The law of reflection is

$$\theta_1 = \theta_2$$

Equation 8.2

where θ_1 is the incident angle and θ_2 is the reflected angle, both measured from the normal. The **normal** is a line drawn perpendicular to the boundary of a medium; all angles in optics are measured from the normal, not the surface of the medium.

Plane Mirrors

In general, images created by a mirror can be either **real** or **virtual**. An image is said to be real if the light actually converges at the position of the image. An image is virtual if the light only *appears* to be coming from the position of the image but does not actually converge there. One of the distinguishing features of real images is the ability of the image to be projected onto a screen.

Parallel incident light rays remain parallel after reflection from a plane mirror; that is, **plane mirrors**—being flat reflective surfaces—cause neither convergence nor divergence of reflected light rays. Because the light does not converge at all, plane mirrors always create virtual images. In a plane mirror, the image appears to be the same distance behind the mirror as the object is in front of it, as shown in Figure 8.4. In other words, plane mirrors create the appearance of light rays originating behind the mirrored surface. Because the reflected light remains in front of the mirror but the image appears behind the mirror, the image is virtual. Plane mirrors include most of the common mirrors found in our homes. To assist in our discussion of spherical mirrors, plane mirrors can be conceptualized as spherical mirrors with an infinite radius of curvature.

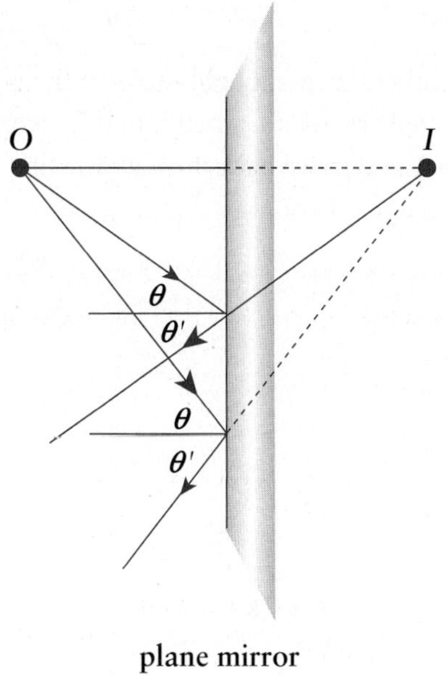

Figure 8.4 Reflection in a Plane Mirror
O is the object and I is the (virtual) image; all incident angles (θ) are equal to their respective reflected angles (θ′).

REAL WORLD

The passenger-side mirrors in cars are an example of convex mirrors (everything appears smaller and farther away); the small circular mirrors used for applying makeup are an example of concave mirrors (everything appears bigger and closer).

MNEMONIC

Con**cave** is like looking into a **cave**.

KEY CONCEPT

Concave mirrors are converging mirrors. Convex mirrors are diverging mirrors. The reverse is true for lenses.

Spherical Mirrors

Spherical mirrors come in two varieties: concave and convex. The word spherical implies that the mirror can be considered a spherical cap or dome taken from a much larger spherically shaped mirror. Spherical mirrors have an associated center of curvature (C) and a radius of curvature (r). The **center of curvature** is a point on the optical axis located at a distance equal to the **radius of curvature** from the vertex of the mirror; in other words, the center of curvature would be the center of the spherically shaped mirror if it were a complete sphere.

If we were to look from the inside of a sphere to its surface, we would see a **concave** surface. On the other hand, if we were to look from outside the sphere, we would see a **convex** surface. For a concave surface, the center of curvature and the radius of curvature are located in front of the mirror. For a convex surface, the center of curvature and the radius of curvature are behind the mirror. Concave mirrors are called **converging mirrors** and convex mirrors are called **diverging mirrors** because they cause parallel incident light rays to converge and diverge after they reflect, respectively.

There are several important lengths associated with mirrors, as shown in Figure 8.5. The **focal length** (***f***) is the distance between the **focal point** (***F***) and the mirror. Note that for all spherical mirrors, $f = \frac{r}{2}$ where the radius of curvature (r) is the distance between C and the mirror. The distance between the object and the mirror is o; the distance between the image and the mirror is i.

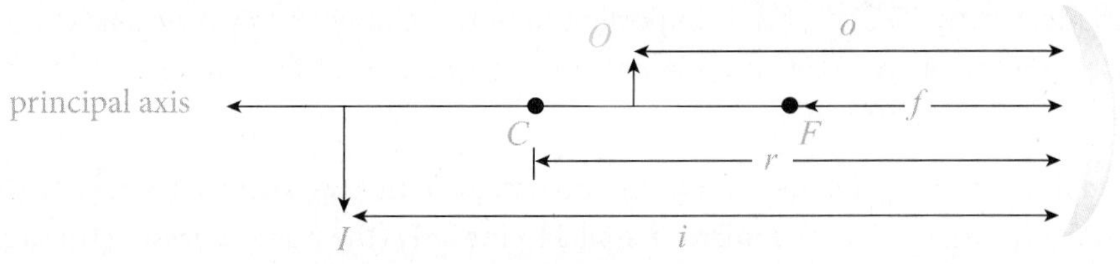

Figure 8.5 Key Variables in Geometrical Optics
The mirror pictured is a concave mirror; light rays are not shown.

There is a simple relationship between these four distances:

$$\frac{1}{f} = \frac{1}{o} + \frac{1}{i} = \frac{2}{r}$$

Equation 8.3

While it is not important which units of distance are used in this equation, it is important that all values used have the *same* units as each other.

On the MCAT, you will most often use this equation to calculate the **image distance** for all types of mirrors and lenses. If the image has a positive distance ($i > 0$), it is a real image, which implies that the image is in front of the mirror. If the image has a negative distance ($i < 0$), it is virtual and thus located behind the mirror. Plane mirrors can be thought of as spherical mirrors with infinitely large focal distances. As such, for a plane mirror, $r = f = \infty$, and the equation becomes $\frac{1}{o} + \frac{1}{i} = 0$ or $i = -o$. This can be interpreted as saying the virtual image is at a distance behind the mirror equal to the distance the object is in front of the mirror.

The **magnification** (***m***) is a dimensionless value that is the ratio of the image distance to the object distance:

$$m = -\frac{i}{o}$$

Equation 8.4

By extension, the magnification also gives the ratio of the size of the image to the size of the object. Following the sign convention given later in Table 8.1, the orientation of the image (upright or inverted) can be determined: a negative magnification signifies an **inverted** image, while a positive value signifies an **upright** image. If $|m| < 1$, the image is smaller than the object (reduced); if $|m| > 1$, the image is larger than the object (enlarged); and if $|m| = 1$, the image is the same size as the object.

Figure 8.6 shows ray diagrams for a concave spherical mirror with the object at three different points. A **ray diagram** is useful for getting an approximation of where an image is. On Test Day, ray diagrams can be helpful for a quick determination of the type of image that will be produced by an object some distance from the mirror (real *vs.* virtual, inverted *vs.* upright, and magnified *vs.* reduced). Ray diagrams should be used with caution, however: under the pressure of Test Day, it can be easy to draw them incorrectly. Therefore, it is important to practice drawing ray diagrams to avoid careless errors on Test Day, and it is also important to be familiar with how to solve optics questions mathematically.

When drawing a ray diagram, there are three important rays to draw. For a concave mirror, a ray that strikes the mirror parallel to the **axis** (the normal passing through the center of the mirror) is reflected back through the focal point (green lines in Figure 8.6 and 8.7). A ray that passes through the focal point before reaching the mirror is reflected back parallel to the axis (red lines). A ray that strikes the mirror at the point of intersection with the axis is reflected back with the same angle measured from the normal (blue lines). In Figure 8.6a, the object is placed beyond *F*, and the image produced is real, inverted and magnified. In Figure 8.6b, the object is placed at *F*, and no image is formed because the reflected light rays are parallel to each other. In terms of the mirror equation, we say that the image distance $i = \infty$ here. For the scenario in Figure 8.6c, the object is placed between *F* and the mirror, and the image produced is virtual, upright, and magnified.

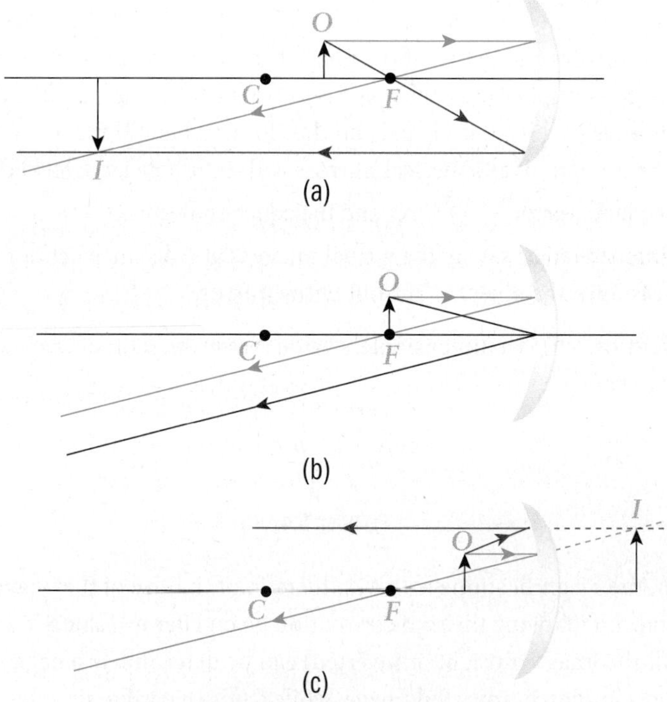

Figure 8.6 Ray Diagrams for Concave (Converging) Mirrors
(a) Object is placed beyond F; (b) Object is placed at F; (c) Object is placed between F and the mirror.

KEY CONCEPT

Any time an object is at the focal point of a converging mirror, the reflected rays will be parallel, and thus, the image will be at infinity.

A single diverging mirror forms only a virtual, upright, and reduced image, regardless of the position of the object. The farther away the object, the smaller the image will be. To quickly remember these rules, recall the convenience store security mirrors mentioned at the beginning of the chapter. The ray diagram of a diverging mirror is shown in Figure 8.7.

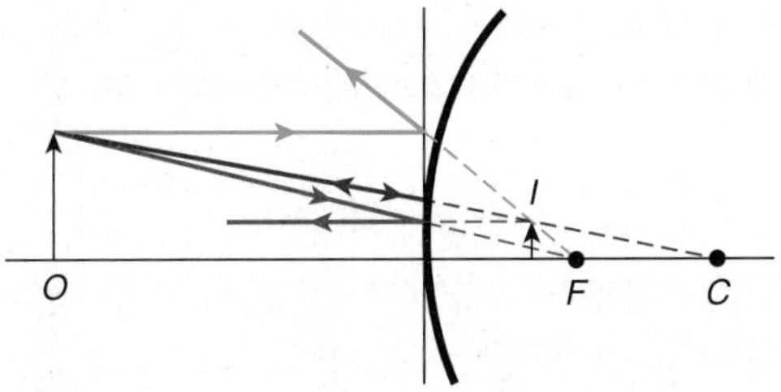

Figure 8.7 Ray Diagrams for Convex (Diverging) Mirrors

Sign Conventions for Mirrors

Table 8.1 provides the sign convention for single mirrors. Note that on the MCAT, for almost all problems involving mirrors, the object will be placed in front of the mirror. Thus, the object distance o is almost always positive.

SYMBOL	POSITIVE	NEGATIVE
o	Object is in front of mirror	Object is behind mirror (extremely rare)
i	Image is in front of mirror (real)	Image is behind mirror (virtual)
r	Mirror is concave (converging)	Mirror is convex (diverging)
f	Mirror is concave (converging)	Mirror is convex (diverging)
m	Image is upright (erect)	Image is inverted

Table 8.1 Sign Convention for a Single Mirror

Example: An object is placed 6 cm in front of a concave mirror that has a 10 cm radius of curvature. Determine the image distance, the magnification, whether the image is real or virtual, and whether it is inverted or upright.

Solution: Use the optics equation:

$$\frac{1}{f} = \frac{1}{o} + \frac{1}{i} = \frac{2}{r}$$

$$\frac{1}{i} = \frac{2}{r} - \frac{1}{o}$$

$$\frac{1}{i} = \frac{2}{10\text{ cm}} - \frac{1}{6\text{ cm}} = \frac{12 - 10}{60} = \frac{2}{60}$$

$$i = \frac{60}{2} = +30\text{ cm}$$

A positive value for i signifies that the image is in front of the mirror and is therefore real. For a single lens or mirror with $o > 0$, a real image will always be inverted.

KEY CONCEPT

To find where the image is (for a mirror), draw the following rays and find a point where any two intersect. This point of intersection marks the tip of the image. If the rays you draw do not appear to intersect, extend them to the other side of the mirror, creating a virtual image.

- Ray parallel to axis ⟶ reflects back through focal point
- Ray through focal point ⟶ reflects back parallel to axis
- Ray to center of mirror ⟶ reflects back at same angle relative to normal

KEY CONCEPT

The focal length of converging mirrors (and converging lenses) will always be positive. The focal length of diverging mirrors (and diverging lenses) will always be negative.

MNEMONIC

Image types with a single lens or mirror (assuming o is positive): **UV NO IR**

- **U**pright images are always **v**irtual
- **No** image is formed when the object is a focal length away
- **I**nverted images are always **r**eal

After determining i, the magnification m can be calculated as:

$$m = -\frac{i}{o} = -\frac{30\text{ cm}}{6\text{ cm}} = -5$$

The negative sign on the magnification confirms that the image is inverted, and the fact that $|m| > 1$ indicates that the image is enlarged.

REAL WORLD

When a pencil (or any straight object) is dipped into a glass of water at an angle, it looks impossibly bent where it intersects the surface of the water because the light reflecting off of the portion of the pencil under water is refracted.

Refraction

Refraction is the bending of light as it passes from one medium to another and changes speed. The speed of light through any medium is always less than its speed through a vacuum. Remember that the speed of light in a vacuum, c, is equal to $3.00 \times 10^8\ \frac{\text{m}}{\text{s}}$. The speed of light in air is just slightly lower that this value; on the MCAT, it is appropriate to use $3.00 \times 10^8\ \frac{\text{m}}{\text{s}}$ for the speed of light in air.

Snell's Law

When light is in any medium besides a vacuum, its speed is less than c. For a given medium

$$n = \frac{c}{v}$$

Equation 8.5

where c is the speed of light in a vacuum, v is the speed of light in the medium, and n is a dimensionless quantity called the **index of refraction** of the medium. The index of refraction of a vacuum is 1, by definition; for all other materials, the index of refraction will be greater than 1. For air, n is essentially equal to 1 because the speed of light in air is extremely close to c. The indices of refraction for a number of common media are shown in Table 8.2. These values are provided only for reference; they need not be memorized.

MEDIUM	INDEX OF REFRACTION (n)
Vacuum	1 (by definition)
Air	1.0003
Ice	1.31
Water	1.33
Acetone	1.36
Ethanol	1.36
Cornea (human)	1.37-1.40
Lens (human)	1.39-1.41
Glass (various types)	1.48-1.93
Diamond	2.42

Table 8.2 Indices of Refraction of Common Media

Refracted rays of light obey **Snell's law** as they pass from one medium to another:

$$n_1 \sin \theta_1 = n_2 \sin \theta_2$$

Equation 8.6

where n_1 and θ_1 refer to the medium from which the light is coming and n_2 and θ_2 refer to the medium into which the light is entering. Note that θ is once again measured with respect to the normal, as shown in Figure 8.8.

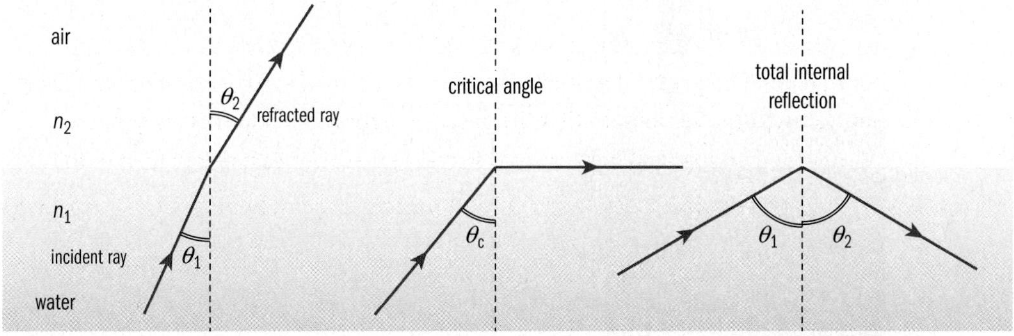

Figure 8.8 Snell's Law

From Snell's law, we can see that when light enters a medium with a higher index of refraction ($n_2 > n_1$), it bends toward the normal ($\sin \theta_2 < \sin \theta_1$; therefore, $\theta_2 < \theta_1$), as shown in Figure 8.9. Conversely, if the light travels into a medium where the index of refraction is smaller ($n_2 < n_1$), the light will bend away from the normal ($\sin \theta_2 > \sin \theta_1$; therefore, $\theta_2 > \theta_1$).

KEY CONCEPT

Remember that when light enters a medium with a higher index of refraction, it bends toward the normal. When light enters a medium with a lower index of refraction, it bends away from the normal.

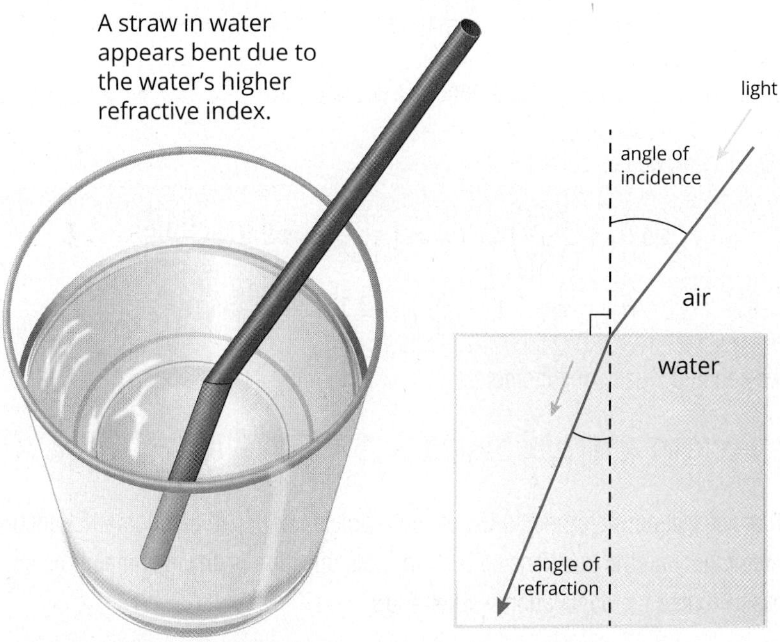

Figure 8.9 Refraction of Light from Air into Water

Example: A penny sits at the bottom of a pool of water ($n = 1.33$) at a depth of 3.0 m. If an observer 1.8 m tall stands 30 cm away from the edge, how close to the side can the penny be and still be visible?

Solution: First, draw a picture of the situation:

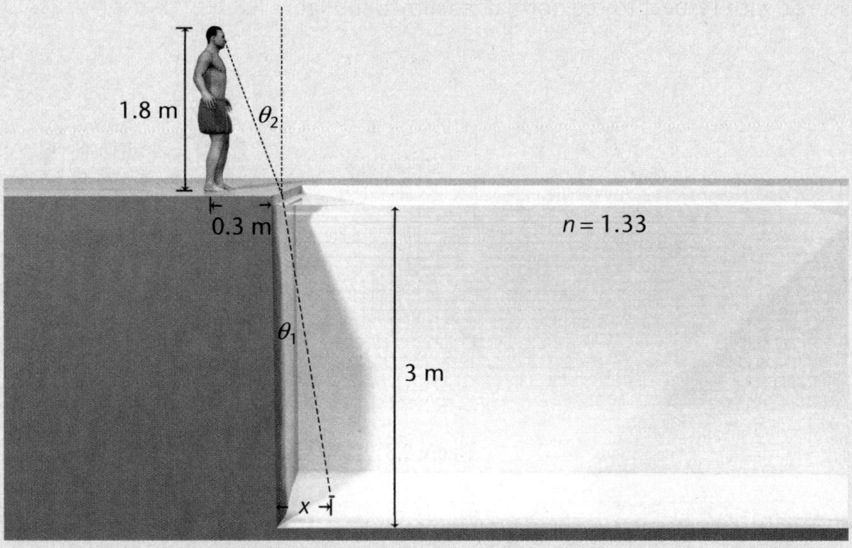

Note that the light is coming from the water ($n_1 = 1.33$) and going into the air ($n_2 \approx 1$), so the light is bent away from the normal ($\theta_2 > \theta_1$). We need to find the angle that the light rays make with the normal to the water's surface:

$$\tan \theta_2 = \frac{0.3\text{ m}}{1.8\text{ m}} = 0.167$$

$$\theta_2 = \tan^{-1} 0.167 = 9.5^\circ$$

Using Snell's law, we can solve for θ_1:

$$\sin \theta_1 = \left(\frac{n_2}{n_1}\right) \sin \theta_2 = \left(\frac{1}{1.33}\right) \sin 9.5^\circ = \frac{0.165}{1.33}$$

$$\theta_1 = \sin^{-1}\left(\frac{0.165}{1.33}\right) = 7.1^\circ$$

Now, we can find x using trigonometry:

$$x = (3\text{ m}) \times \tan \theta_1 = 3 \tan 7.1^\circ = 3 \times 0.124 = 0.37\text{ m} = 37\text{ cm}$$

Note that you will not be expected to calculate precise values of trigonometric functions or inverse trigonometric functions on Test Day. This question is provided mainly as an opportunity to see the application of Snell's law.

Total Internal Reflection

When light travels from a medium with a higher index of refraction (such as water) to a medium with a lower index of refraction (such as air), the refracted angle is larger than the incident angle ($\theta_2 > \theta_1$); that is, the refracted light ray bends away from the normal. As the incident angle is increased, the refracted angle also increases, and eventually, a special incident angle called the **critical angle (θ_c)** is reached, for which the refracted angle θ_2 equals 90 degrees. At the critical angle, the refracted light ray passes along the interface between the two media. The critical angle can be derived from Snell's law if $\theta_2 = 90°$, such that

$$\theta_c = \sin^{-1}\left(\frac{n_2}{n_1}\right)$$

Equation 8.7

Total internal reflection, a phenomenon in which all the light incident on a boundary is reflected back into the original material, results with any angle of incidence greater than the critical angle, θ_c, as shown in Figure 8.10.

KEY CONCEPT

Total internal reflection occurs as the light moves from a medium with a higher refractive index to a medium with a lower one.

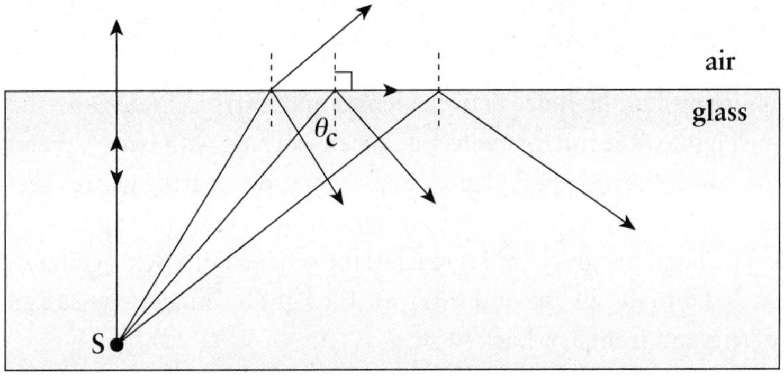

Figure 8.10 Total Internal Reflection
At the incident angle of θ_c, the refracted angle is equal to 90°; at incident angles above 90°, total internal reflection occurs.

Example: From the previous example, suppose another penny is 3 m away from the edge. Will a light ray going from this penny to the edge of the pool emerge from the water?

Solution: The angle made by the second penny's light ray is

$$\theta_1 = \tan^{-1}\left(\frac{\text{opposite}}{\text{adjacent}}\right) = \tan^{-1}\left(\frac{3\text{ m}}{3\text{ m}}\right) = \tan^{-1}(1) = 45°$$

Find the critical angle:

$$\theta_c = \sin^{-1}\left(\frac{n_2}{n_1}\right) = \sin^{-1}\left(\frac{1}{1.33}\right) = \sin^{-1}(0.75) = 48.8°$$

It is not expected on the MCAT that we know the inverse sin of 0.75. However, we do know that $\sin(45°) = \frac{\sqrt{2}}{2} \approx 0.71$. Since $\sin(\theta_c)$ is greater than 0.71, the critical angle must be greater than 45°. Therefore, $\theta_c > \theta_1$ and the light ray will emerge from the pool.

Lenses

There is an important difference between **lenses** and mirrors, aside from the fact that lenses refract light while mirrors reflect it. When working with lenses, there are two surfaces that affect the light path. For example, a person wearing glasses sees light that travels from an object through the air into the glass lens (first surface). Then the light travels through the glass until it reaches the other side, where again it travels out of the glass and into the air (second surface). The light is refracted twice as it passes from air to lens and from lens back to air.

Thin Spherical Lenses

On the MCAT, lenses generally have negligible thickness. Because light can travel from either side of a lens, a lens has two focal points, with one on each side. The focal length can be measured in either direction from the center. For thin spherical lenses, the focal lengths are equal, so we speak of just one focal length for the lens as a whole.

REAL WORLD

Converging lenses (reading glasses) are needed by people who are "farsighted." Diverging lenses (standard glasses) are needed by people who are "nearsighted."

Figure 8.11a illustrates that a converging lens is always thicker at the center, while Figure 8.11b illustrates that a diverging lens is always thinner at the center. The basic formulas for finding image distance and magnification for spherical mirrors also apply to lenses. The object distance o, image distance i, focal length f, and magnification m, are related by the equations $\frac{1}{f} = \frac{1}{o} + \frac{1}{i}$ and $m = -\frac{i}{o}$.

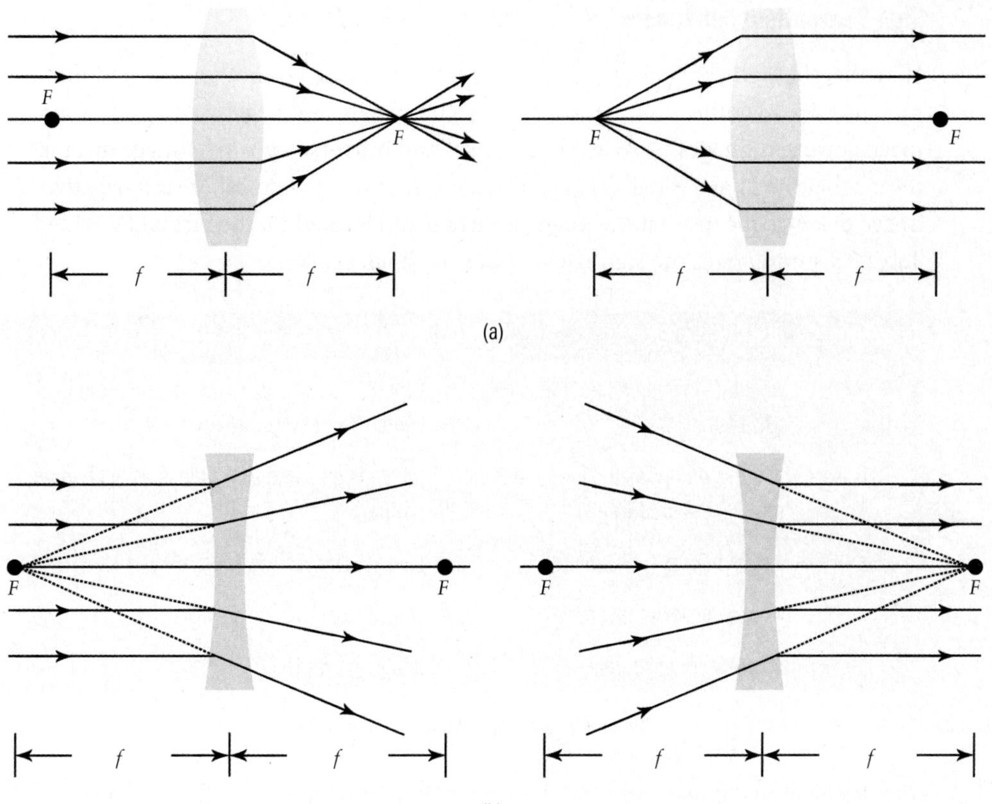

Figure 8.11 Ray Diagrams for Single Lenses
(a) Convex (converging) lenses; (b) Concave (diverging) lenses.

Real Lenses

For lenses where the thickness cannot be neglected, the focal length is related to the curvature of the lens surfaces and the index of refraction of the lens by the **lensmaker's equation**:

$$\frac{1}{f} = (n-1)\left(\frac{1}{r_1} - \frac{1}{r_2}\right)$$

Equation 8.8

where n is the index of refraction of the lens material, r_1 is the radius of curvature of the first lens surface, and r_2 is the radius of curvature of the second lens surface.

The eye is a complex refractive instrument that uses real lenses. The cornea acts as the primary source of refractive power because the change in refractive index from air is so significant. Then, light is passed through an adaptive lens that can change its focal length before reaching the vitreous humor. It is further diffused through layers of retinal tissue to reach the rods and cones. At this point, the image has been focused and minimized significantly, but is still relatively blurry. Our nervous system processes the remaining errors to provide a crisp view of the world.

KEY CONCEPT

To find where the image is (for a lens), draw the following rays and find a point where any two intersect. This point of intersection marks the tip of the image. If the rays you draw do not appear to intersect, extend them to the same side of the lens from which the light came, creating a virtual image.

- Ray parallel to axis → refracts through focal point of front face of the lens
- Ray through or toward focal point before reaching lens → refracts parallel to axis
- Ray to center of lens → continues straight through with no refraction

Sign Conventions for Lenses

Note that the sign conventions change slightly for lenses. For both lenses and mirrors, positive magnification represents upright images, and negative magnification means inverted images. Also, for both lenses and mirrors, a positive image distance means that the image is real and is located on the real (R) side, whereas a negative image distance means that the image is virtual and located on the virtual (V) side. Table 8.3 summarizes the sign conventions for single lenses.

SYMBOL	POSITIVE	NEGATIVE
o	Object is on same side of lens as light source	Object is on opposite side of lens from light source (extremely rare)
i	Image is on opposite side of lens from light source (real)	Image is on same side of lens as light source (virtual)
r	Lens is convex (converging)	Lens is concave (diverging)
f	Lens is convex (converging)	Lens is concave (diverging)
m	Image is upright (erect)	Image is inverted

Table 8.3 Sign Convention for a Single Lens

KEY CONCEPT

It is important to realize that concave mirrors and convex lenses are both converging and thus have similar properties. Convex mirrors and concave lenses are both diverging and also have similar properties.

The designations of real and virtual are often a point of confusion for students because they are on opposite sides when comparing mirrors and lenses. To identify the real side (R), remember that the real side is where light actually goes after interacting with the lens or mirror. For mirrors, light is reflected and, therefore, stays in front of the mirror. Hence, for a mirror, the real side is in front of the mirror, and the virtual side is behind the mirror. For lenses, the convention is different: because light travels through the lens and comes out on the other side, the real side is on the opposite side of the lens from the original light source, and the virtual side is on the same side of the lens as the original light source. Although the object of a single lens is on the virtual side, this does not make the object virtual. Objects are real, with a positive object distance, unless they are placed in certain multiple lens systems in which the image of one lens becomes the object for another (a scenario which is very rarely encountered on the MCAT).

Focal lengths and radii of curvature have a simpler sign convention. For both mirrors and lenses, converging species have positive focal lengths and radii of curvature, and diverging species have negative focal lengths and radii of curvature. Remember that lenses have two focal lengths and two radii of curvature because they have two surfaces. For a thin lens where thickness is negligible, the sign of the focal length and radius of curvature are given based on the first surface the light passes through.

Power

Optometrists often describe a lens in terms of its **power (*P*)**. This is measured in **diopters**, where *f* (the focal length) is in meters and is given by the equation

$$P = \frac{1}{f}$$

Equation 8.9

P has the same sign as *f* and is, therefore, positive for a converging lens and negative for a diverging lens. People who are nearsighted (can see near objects clearly) need diverging lenses, while people who are farsighted (can see distant objects clearly) need converging lenses. Bifocal lenses are corrective lenses that have two distinct regions—one that causes convergence of light to correct for farsightedness (**hyperopia**) and a second that causes divergence of light to correct for nearsightedness (**myopia**) in the same lens.

MCAT EXPERTISE

The MCAT does expect students to understand what myopia and hyperopia are, as well as their corresponding ray diagrams and correction strategies.

Multiple Lens Systems

Lenses in contact are a series of lenses with negligible distances between them. These systems behave as a single lens with equivalent focal length given by

$$\frac{1}{f} = \frac{1}{f_1} + \frac{1}{f_2} + \frac{1}{f_3} + \cdots + \frac{1}{f_n}$$

Equation 8.10

Because power is the reciprocal of focal length, the equivalent power is

$$P = P_1 + P_2 + P_3 + \cdots + P_n$$

Equation 8.11

A good example of lenses in contact is a corrective contact lens worn directly on the eye. In this case, the cornea of the eye (a converging lens) is in contact with a contact lens (either converging or diverging, depending on the necessary correction), and their powers would be added.

For lenses not in contact, the image of one lens becomes the object of another lens. The image from the last lens is considered the image of the system. Microscopes and telescopes are good examples of these systems. The magnification for the system is

$$m = m_1 \times m_2 \times m_3 \times \cdots \times m_n$$

Equation 8.12

REAL WORLD

The human eye typically has an optical power of around 60 diopters. Most contact lens wearers have prescriptions between 0.25 and 8 diopters (both positive and negative). An eye that requires a +8 or −8 prescription still has an optical power that is about 87% of the typical value.

MCAT EXPERTISE

Because the MCAT is a timed test, you will not be given a massive multiple lens system and be expected to make calculations, although the testmaker might test a multiple-lens system conceptually.

Example: An object is 15 cm to the left of a thin diverging lens with a 45 cm focal length as shown below. Find where the image is formed, if it is upright or inverted, and if it is real or virtual. What is the radius of curvature, assuming the lens is symmetrical and is made of glass with a non negligible thickness and an index of refraction of 1.50?

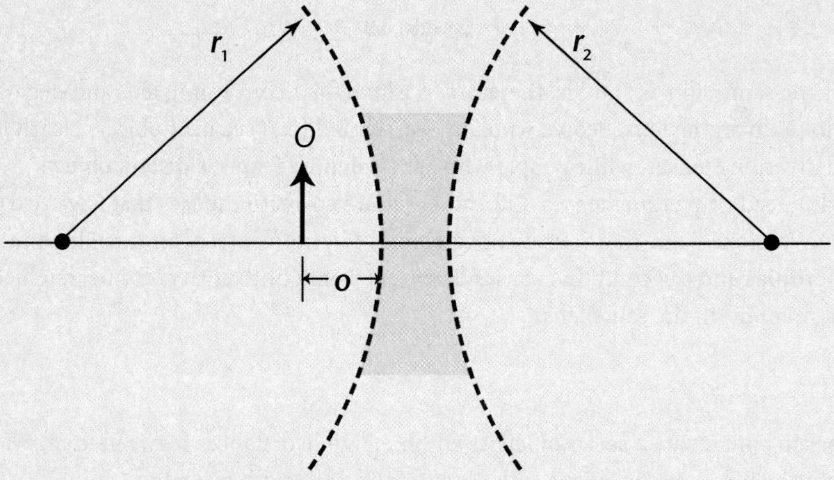

Solution: The image distance (i) is found using the equation

$$\frac{1}{f} = \frac{1}{o} + \frac{1}{i} \rightarrow \frac{1}{i} = \frac{1}{f} - \frac{1}{o}$$

Because the lens is diverging, the focal length has a negative sign ($f = -45$ cm). The object, like any object in a single-lens system, has a positive sign ($o = +15$ cm). Now we can solve for i:

$$\frac{1}{i} = \frac{1}{f} - \frac{1}{o} = \frac{1}{-45\text{ cm}} - \frac{1}{15\text{ cm}} = \frac{-1-3}{45} = \frac{-4}{45}$$

$$i = -\frac{45}{4} = -11.25\text{ cm}$$

The negative sign indicates that the image is on the same side of the light source and is virtual. Remember that for a single lens or mirror, virtual images are always upright.

The thickness of a lens is usually negligible, but we are told otherwise in this question. To determine the radii of curvature, we use the lensmaker's equation. Because the lens is symmetrical, the radii are equal but opposite in sign. As the light progresses from left to right, the first surface of the lens is concave ($r_1 < 0$), and the second surface of the lens is convex ($r_2 > 0$).

$$\frac{1}{f} = (n-1)\left(\frac{1}{r_1} - \frac{1}{r_2}\right) = (n-1)\left(-\frac{1}{r} - \frac{1}{r}\right) = (n-1)\left(\frac{-2}{r}\right)$$

$$r = -2f(n-1)$$

$$= -2(-45\text{ cm})(1.5-1) = 2(45)(0.5) = 45\text{ cm}$$

Spherical Aberration

Spherical mirrors and lenses are imperfect. They are therefore subject to specific types of errors or **aberrations**. **Spherical aberration** is a blurring of the periphery of an image as a result of inadequate reflection of parallel beams at the edge of a mirror or inadequate refraction of parallel beams at the edge of a lens. This creates an area of multiple images with very slightly different image distances at the edge of the image, which appears blurry. This phenomenon can be seen in Figure 8.12.

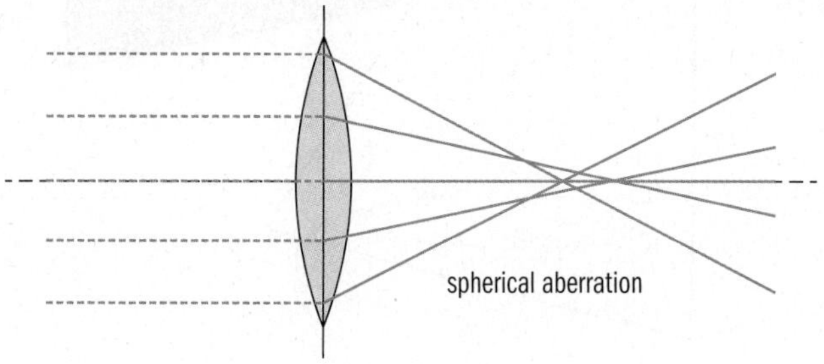

Figure 8.12 Spherical Aberration
Parallel rays are not perfectly reflected or refracted through the focal point, leading to blurriness at the periphery of the image.

Chromatic aberration, discussed below, is predominantly seen in spherical lenses.

Dispersion

As discussed earlier, the speed of light in a vacuum is the same for all wavelengths. However, when light travels through a medium, different wavelengths travel at different speeds. This fact implies that the index of refraction of a medium affects the wavelength of light passing through the medium because the index of refraction is related to the speed of the wave by $n = \frac{c}{v}$. It also implies that the index of refraction itself actually varies with wavelength. When various wavelengths of light separate from each other, this is called **dispersion**. The most common example of dispersion is the splitting of white light into its component colors using a prism.

If a source of white light is incident on one of the faces of a prism, the light emerging from the prism is spread out into a fan-shaped beam, as shown in Figure 8.13. This occurs because violet light has a smaller wavelength than red light and so is bent to a greater extent. Because red experiences the least amount of refraction, it is always on top of the spectrum; violet, having experienced the greatest amount of refraction, is always on the bottom of the spectrum. Note that as light enters a medium with a different index of refraction, the wavelength changes but the frequency of the light does not.

REAL WORLD

If you remember back to conic sections from your precalculus class, it should be no surprise that spherical mirrors and lenses do not focus light perfectly. Parabolas are perfect reflectors, meaning that parallel light rays are reflected perfectly through the focal point. This is used in extracorporeal shock wave lithotripsy, in which a parabolic mirror is positioned with a kidney stone at the focal point. Sound waves are reflected off of the mirror and create enough vibration in the kidney stone to shatter it.

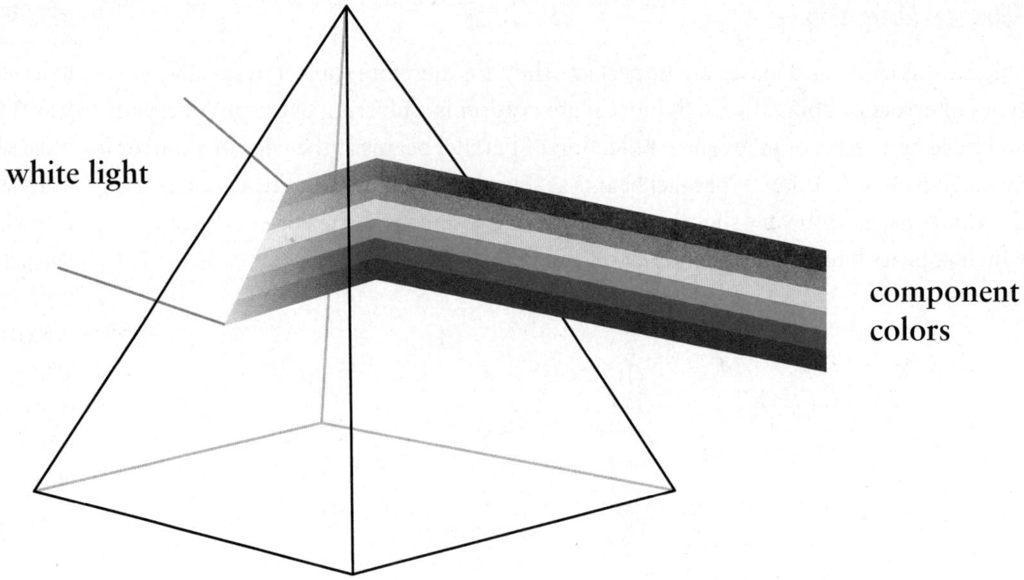

Figure 8.13 Dispersion in a Prism
Due to their different speeds while inside the prism, the various wavelengths of light are refracted to different degrees.

Chromatic Aberration

Chromatic aberration, shown in Figure 8.14, is a dispersive effect within a spherical lens. Depending on the thickness and curvature of the lens, there may be significant splitting of white light, which results in a rainbow halo around images. This phenomenon is corrected for in visual lenses like eyeglasses and car windows with special coatings that have different dispersive qualities from the lens itself.

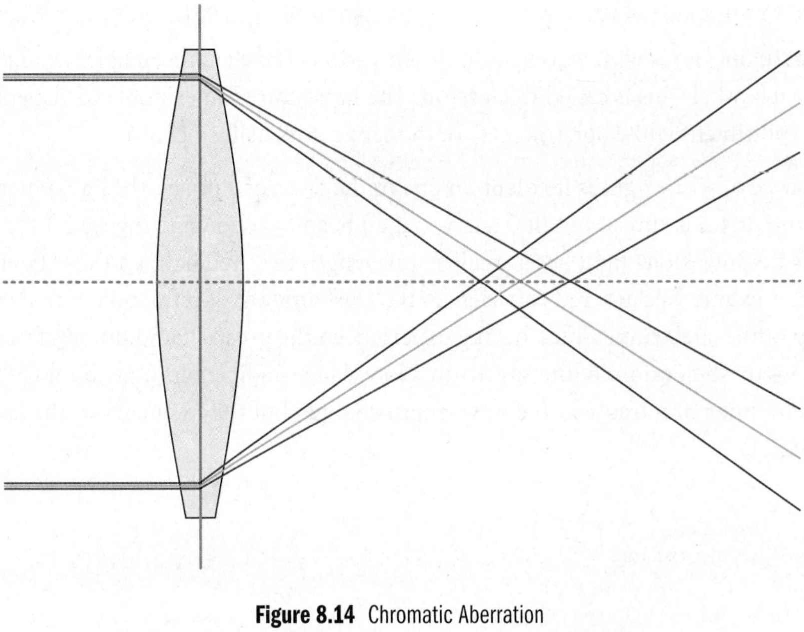

Figure 8.14 Chromatic Aberration
Light dispersion within the glass lens leads to the formation of a rainbow halo at the edge of the image.

MCAT CONCEPT CHECK 8.2

Before you move on, assess your understanding of the material with these questions.

1. Populate the following tables according to the sign conventions for mirrors and lenses:

Mirrors		
Symbol	**Positive**	**Negative**
o		
i		
r		
f		
m		

Lenses		
Symbol	**Positive**	**Negative**
o		
i		
r		
f		
m		

2. True or False: Incident angle is always measured with respect to the normal.

3. Describe the bending of light when moving from a medium with low refractive index to high refractive index, and from a medium with high refractive index to low refractive index:
   - Low *n* to high *n*:

   ____

   - High *n* to low *n*:

   ____

4. Define the following terms:
   - Dispersion:

   ____

   - Aberration:

   ____

5. What are the two mathematical relationships between image distance and object distance?

   ____

8.3 Diffraction

LEARNING OBJECTIVES

After Chapter 8.3, you will be able to:

- Distinguish between the diffraction patterns in single-slit, double-slit, and slit–lens systems
- Recall the wave phenomena that lead to diffraction fringes
- Describe Young's double-slit experiment:

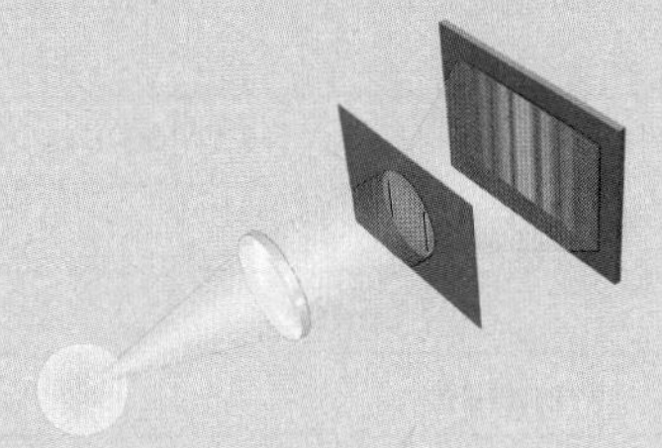

Diffraction refers to the spreading out of light as it passes through a narrow opening or around an obstacle. Interference between diffracted light rays lead to characteristic fringes in slit–lens and double-slit systems. Diffraction and interference are significant evidence for the wave theory of light.

Single Slit

Although it is usually safe to assume that nonrefracted light travels in a straight line, there are situations where light will not actually travel in a straight-line path. When light passes through a narrow opening (an opening with a size that is on the order of light wavelengths), the light waves seem to spread out (diffract), as is shown in Figure 8.15. As the slit is narrowed, the light spreads out more.

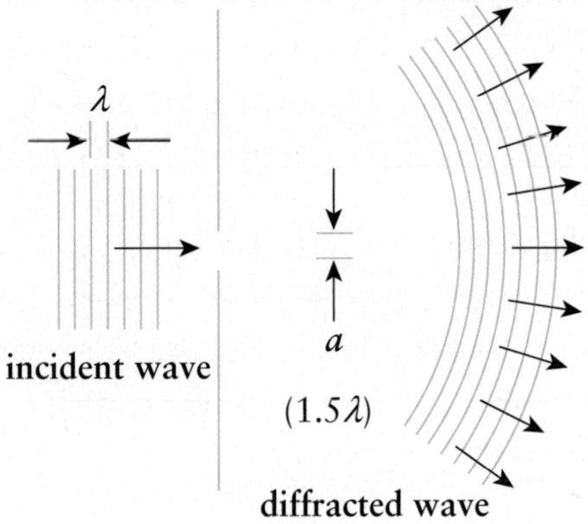

Figure 8.15 Diffraction

Light emerges from a narrow slit in a wide arc, not a narrow beam.

Slit–Lens System

If a lens is placed between a narrow slit and a screen, a pattern is observed consisting of a bright central fringe with alternating dark and bright fringes on each side, as shown in Figure 8.16. The central bright fringe (maximum) is twice as wide as the bright fringes on the sides, and as the slit becomes narrower, the central maximum becomes wider. The location of the dark fringes (minima) is given by the formula

$$a \sin \theta = n\lambda$$

Equation 8.13

where a is the width of the slit, θ is the angle between the line drawn from the center of the lens to the dark fringe and the axis of the lens, n is an integer indicating the number of the fringe, and λ is the wavelength of the incident wave. Note that bright fringes are halfway between dark fringes.

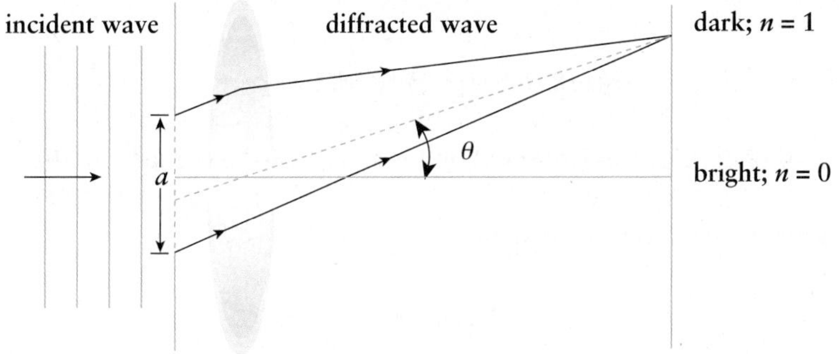

Figure 8.16 Single-Slit Diffraction with Lens

Multiple Slits

When waves interact with each other, the displacements of the waves add together in a process called **interference**, as described in Chapter 7 of *MCAT Physics and Math Review*. In his famous double-slit experiment, Thomas Young showed that the diffracted rays of light emerging from two parallel slits can interfere with one another. This was a landmark finding that contributed to the understanding of light as a wave. Figure 8.17 shows the typical setup for Young's double-slit experiment. When monochromatic light (light of only one wavelength) passes through the slits, an interference pattern is observed on a screen placed behind the slits. Regions of constructive interference between the two light waves appear as bright fringes (maxima) on the screen. Conversely, in regions where the light waves interfere destructively, dark fringes (minima) appear.

BRIDGE

Light is similar to other waveforms; it is affected by constructive and destructive interference when light passes through a slit and a lens, and when light passes through multiple slits. Interference also occurs with sound waves, as discussed in Chapter 7 of *MCAT Physics and Math Review*.

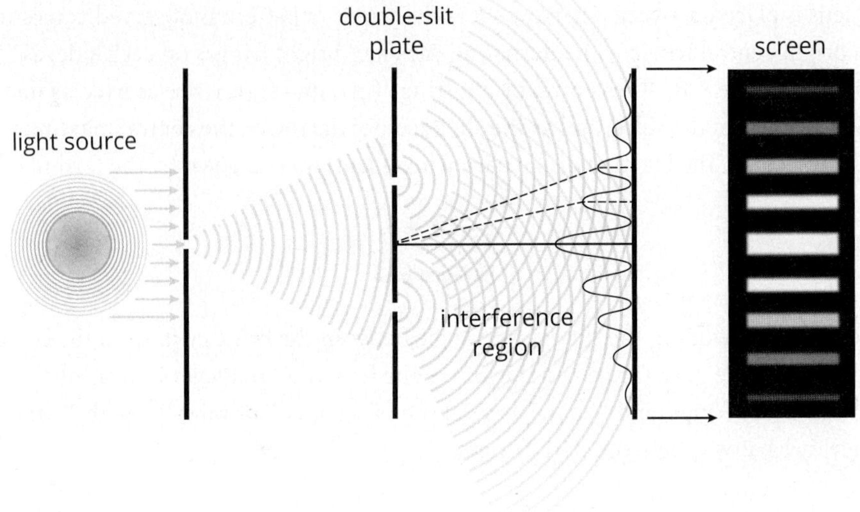

Figure 8.17 Young's Double-Slit Experiment

The positions of dark fringes (minima) on the screen can be found from the equation

$$d \sin \theta = \left(n + \frac{1}{2}\right) \lambda$$

Equation 8.14

where d is the distance between the two slits, θ is the angle between the line drawn from the midpoint between the two slits to the dark fringe and the normal, n is an integer indicating the number of the fringe, and λ is the wavelength of the incident wave. Note that bright fringes are halfway between dark fringes.

Example: In a double-slit experiment, what is the linear distance y between the sixth and eighth minima on the screen? (Note: The wavelength λ is 550 nm, the slits are separated by a distance of 0.14 mm, and the screen is 70 cm from the slits.)

Solution: The position of a dark fringe (minimum) is given by

$$d \sin\theta = \left(n + \frac{1}{2}\right)\lambda$$

We do not know the value of $\sin\theta \left(\frac{\text{opposite}}{\text{hypotenuse}}\right)$. However, for small angles, $\sin\theta \approx \tan\theta$. This is because the length of the hypotenuse is very close to the length of the adjacent side. We do know the value of $\tan\theta \left(\frac{\text{opposite}}{\text{adjacent}}\right)$, so we can substitute it into the equation and still get very close to the correct answer:

$$d \sin\theta = \left(n + \frac{1}{2}\right)\lambda$$

$$d \tan\theta \approx \left(n + \frac{1}{2}\right)\lambda$$

$$d\left(\frac{y}{D}\right) \approx \left(n + \frac{1}{2}\right)\lambda$$

$$y \approx \frac{\left(n + \frac{1}{2}\right)\lambda D}{d}$$

$$y_8 - y_6 \approx \frac{\left(n_8 + \frac{1}{2}\right)\lambda D}{d} - \frac{\left(n_6 + \frac{1}{2}\right)\lambda D}{d}$$

$$\Delta y \approx \frac{(\Delta n)\,\lambda D}{d} = \frac{(2)(550 \times 10^{-9}\text{ m})(0.7\text{ m})}{0.14 \times 10^{-3}\text{ m}} = 550 \times 10^{-5}\text{ m} = 5.5\text{ mm}$$

Diffraction gratings consist of multiple slits arranged in patterns. Diffraction gratings can create colorful patterns similar to a prism as the different wavelengths interfere in characteristic patterns. For example, the organization of the grooves on a CD or DVD act like a diffraction grating, creating an iridescent rainbow pattern on the surface of the disc. Thin films may also cause interference patterns because light waves reflecting off the external surface of the film interfere with light waves reflecting off the internal surface of the film, as shown in Figure 8.18. Common examples of thin films are soap bubbles or oil puddles in wet parking lots. Note that the interference here is not between diffracted rays, but between reflected rays.

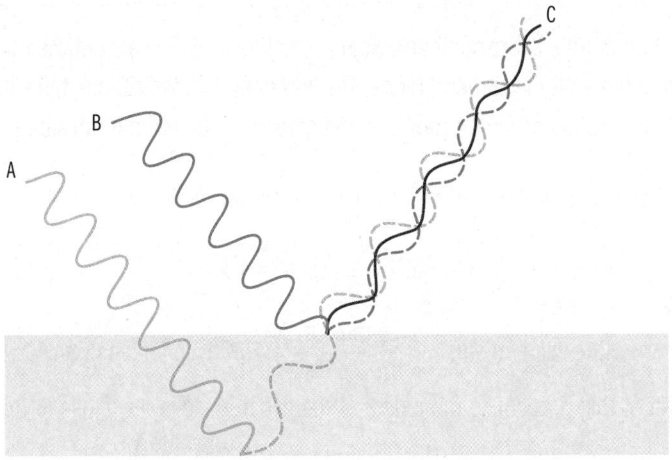

Figure 8.18 Thin Film Interference

Interference patterns, C, occur as light waves reflecting off the external surface of the film, B, interfere with light waves reflecting off the internal surface of the film, A. Note that there would be a small degree of refraction as well, although this is not shown in the image.

BRIDGE

X-ray diffraction and protein crystallography are commonly used to analyze the structure of proteins. These techniques, as well as a number of other protein assays, are discussed in Chapter 3 of *MCAT Biochemistry Review*.

X-Ray Diffraction

X-ray diffraction uses the bending of light rays to create a model of molecules. X-ray diffraction is often combined with protein crystallography during protein analysis. Dark and light fringes do not take on a linear appearance, but rather a complex two-dimensional image. An example of an X-ray diffraction pattern is shown in Figure 8.19.

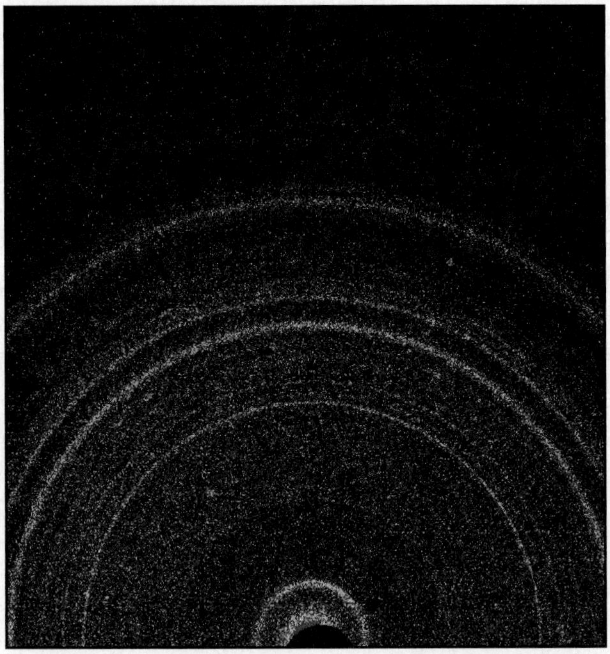

Figure 8.19 X-Ray Diffraction Pattern

MCAT CONCEPT CHECK 8.3

Before you move on, assess your understanding of the material with these questions.

1. How does the diffraction pattern for a single slit differ from a slit with a thin lens?
   - Single slit:

   ___

   - Slit–lens system:

   ___

2. What wave phenomenon do diffraction fringes result from?

   ___

3. How does double-slit diffraction and interference differ from single-slit diffraction?
   - Double-slit:

   ___

   - Single-slit:

   ___

4. True or False: Maxima in diffraction patterns are always equidistant between two minima.

8.4 Polarization

LEARNING OBJECTIVES

After Chapter 8.4, you will be able to:

- Compare and contrast plane-polarized and circularly polarized light
- Describe how a polarized filter impacts the wavelength and/or frequency of light passing through the filter

Plane-Polarized Light

Plane-polarized (or **linearly polarized**) **light** is light in which the electric fields of all the waves are oriented in the same direction (that is, their electric field vectors are parallel). It follows that their magnetic field vectors are also parallel, but convention dictates that the plane of the electric field identifies the plane of polarization. Unpolarized light has a random orientation of its electric field vectors; sunlight and light emitted from a light bulb are prime examples. One of the most common applications of plane-polarized light on the MCAT is in the classification of stereoisomers, as discussed in Chapter 2 of *MCAT Organic Chemistry Review*. The optical

REAL WORLD

Plane-polarized light is used to diagnose a number of diseases. Amyloidosis, caused by the buildup of various forms of misfolded proteins, is diagnosed by biopsy and staining the tissue with Congo red stain; a bright "apple green" color is seen under plane-polarized light. Gout (the precipitation of monosodium urate crystals) and pseudogout (the precipitation of calcium pyrophosphate crystals) are differentiated by their precipitate colors under polarized light: monosodium urate appears yellow and calcium pyrophosphate appears blue when the axis of the crystal is aligned with a polarizer.

activity of a compound, due to the presence of chiral centers, causes plane-polarized light to rotate clockwise or counterclockwise by a given number of degrees relative to its concentration (its **specific rotation**). Remember that enantiomers, as nonsuperimposable mirror images, will have opposite specific rotations.

KEY CONCEPT

The electric fields of unpolarized light waves exist in all three dimensions: the direction of the wave's propagation is surrounded by electric fields in every plane perpendicular to that direction. Polarizing light limits the electric field's oscillation to only two dimensions.

There are filters called polarizers, often used in cameras and sunglasses, which allow only light with an electric field pointing in a particular direction to pass through. If one passes a beam of light through a polarizer, it will only let through that portion of the light parallel to the axis of the polarizer. If a second polarizer is then held up to the first, the angle between the polarizers' axes will determine how much light passes through. When the polarizers are aligned, all the light that passes through the first polarizer also passes through the second. When the second polarizer is turned so that its axis is perpendicular, no light gets through at all.

Circular Polarization

Circular polarization is a rarely seen natural phenomenon that results from the interaction of light with certain pigments or highly specialized filters. Circularly polarized light has a uniform amplitude but a continuously changing direction, which causes a helical orientation in the propagating wave, as shown in Figure 8.20. The helix has average electrical field vectors and magnetic field vectors that lie perpendicular to one another, like other waves, with maxima that fall on the outer border of the helix.

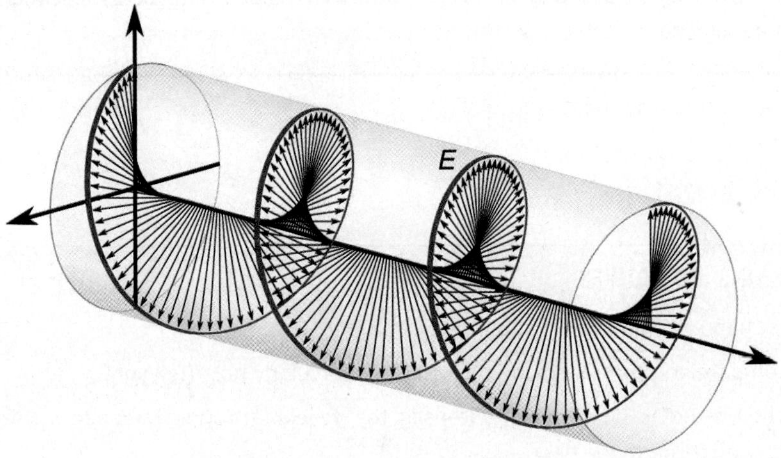

Figure 8.20 Circularly Polarized Light

MCAT CONCEPT CHECK 8.4

Before you move on, assess your understanding of the material with these questions.

1. Contrast plane-polarized and circularly polarized light:
   - Plane-polarized:

   ____

   - Circularly polarized:

   ____

2. How does the application of a polarized filter impact the wavelength of light passing through the filter?

   ____

Conclusion

This chapter illuminated the key behaviors and characteristics of light and optical systems. First, we described the nature of the electromagnetic (EM) wave, noting that we can only perceive light in the visible range (400 nm–700 nm). We then focused on geometrical optics to consider the reflective and refractive behaviors of light, noting the ways in which mirrors reflect light to produce images and lenses refract light to produce images. We acknowledged the fact that light doesn't always travel in straight-line pathways but can bend and spread out through diffraction. We examined the pattern of interference that occurs when light passes through a double slit, as demonstrated in Young's double-slit experiment. Finally, we wrapped up with a discussion on plane-polarized and circularly polarized light. In this chapter, we considered the properties that support the wave theory of light. In the next chapter, we'll explore the photon and properties that support the particle theory of light, as well as other atomic and nuclear phenomena.

GO ONLINE

You've reviewed the content, now test your knowledge and critical thinking skills by completing a test-like passage set in your online resources!

CONCEPT SUMMARY

Electromagnetic Spectrum

- **Electromagnetic waves** are transverse waves that consist of an oscillating electric field and an oscillating magnetic field.
- The two fields are perpendicular to each other and to the direction of propagation of the wave.
- The **electromagnetic spectrum** is the range of frequencies and wavelengths found in EM waves.
- The EM spectrum includes, from lowest to highest energy, **radio waves**, **microwaves**, **infrared**, visible light, **ultraviolet**, **X-rays**, and **γ-rays**.
- The **visible spectrum** runs from approximately 400 nm (violet) to 700 nm (red).

Geometrical Optics

- **Reflection** is the rebounding of incident light waves at the boundary of a medium.
- The **law of reflection** states that the incident angle will equal the angle of reflection, as measured from the normal.
- **Spherical mirrors** have **centers** and **radii of curvature**, as well as **focal points**.
  - **Concave** mirrors are **converging** systems and can produce **real**, **inverted** images or **virtual**, **upright** images, depending on the placement of the object relative to the focal point.
  - **Convex** mirrors are **diverging** systems and will only produce virtual, upright images.
  - **Plane mirrors** also produce virtual, upright images; these images are always the same size as the object. They may be thought of as spherical mirrors with infinite radii of curvature.
- **Refraction** is the bending of light as it passes from one medium to another.
- The speed of light changes depending on the index of refraction of the medium. This speed change causes refraction.
- The amount of refraction depends on the wavelength of the light involved; this behavior causes **dispersion** of light through a prism.
- **Snell's law** (the law of refraction) states that there is an inverse relationship between the index of refraction and the sine of the angle of refraction (measured from the normal).
- **Total internal reflection** occurs when light cannot be refracted out of a medium and is instead reflected back inside the medium.
  - This happens when light moves from a medium with a higher index of refraction to a medium with a lower index of refraction with a high incident angle.
  - The minimum incident angle at which total internal reflection occurs is called the **critical angle**.

- **Lenses** refract light to form images of objects.
    - Thin symmetrical lenses have focal points on each side.
    - Convex lenses are converging systems and can produce real, inverted images or virtual, upright images.
    - Concave lenses are diverging systems and will only produce virtual, upright images.
    - Lenses with non negligible thickness require use of the **lensmaker's equation**.
- The following table summarizes image creation in converging and diverging systems for both mirrors and lenses:

	Converging Systems					Diverging Systems
o* relative to *f	$o > 2f$	$o = 2f$	$2f > o > f$	$o = f$	$o < f$	all object distances
image	real, inverted, reduced	real, inverted, same	real, inverted, magnified	no image	virtual, upright, magnified	virtual, upright, reduced

Diffraction

- **Diffraction** is the bending and spreading out of light waves as they pass through a narrow slit.
- Diffraction may produce a large central light fringe surrounded by alternating light and dark fringes with the addition of a lens.
- Interference supports the wave theory of light.
- **Young's double-slit experiment** shows the constructive and destructive interference of waves that occur as light passes through parallel slits, resulting in minima (dark fringes) and maxima (bright fringes) of intensity.

Polarization

- In **plane-polarized light**, all of the light rays have electric fields with parallel orientation.
- Plane-polarized light is created by passing unpolarized light through a **polarizer**.
- In **circularly polarized light**, all of the light rays have electric fields with equal intensity but constantly rotating direction.
- Circularly polarized light is created by exposing unpolarized light to special pigments or filters.

ANSWERS TO CONCEPT CHECKS

8.1

1. γ-rays > X-rays > ultraviolet > visible light > infrared > microwaves > radio. Frequency follows the same trend as energy, whereas wavelength follows the opposite trend.
2. False. Light waves are transverse because the direction of propagation is perpendicular to the direction of oscillation.
3. Visible light ranges from wavelengths of about 400 nm to 700 nm. This is in comparison to the entire EM spectrum which ranges from wavelengths of nearly 0 to 10^9 m.

8.2

1.

Mirrors		
Symbol	**Positive**	**Negative**
o	Object is in front of mirror	Object is behind mirror (extremely rare)
i	Image is in front of mirror (real)	Image is behind mirror (virtual)
r	Mirror is concave (converging)	Mirror is convex (diverging)
f	Mirror is concave (converging)	Mirror is convex (diverging)
m	Image is upright (erect)	Image is inverted
Lenses		
Symbol	**Positive**	**Negative**
o	Object is on same side of lens as light source	Object is on opposite side of lens from light source (extremely rare)
i	Image is on opposite side of lens from light source (real)	Image is on same side of lens as light source (virtual)
r	Lens is convex (converging)	Lens is concave (diverging)
f	Lens is convex (converging)	Lens is concave (diverging)
m	Image is upright (erect)	Image is inverted

2. True. In optics, incident angles are always measured relative to the normal.
3. Light will bend toward the normal when going from a medium with low n to high n. Light will bend away from the normal when going from a medium with high n to low n; if the incident angle is larger than the critical angle (θ_c), total internal reflection will occur.

4. Dispersion is the tendency for different wavelengths of light to experience different degrees of refraction in a medium, leading to separation of light into the visible spectrum (a rainbow). Aberration (spherical or chromatic) is the alteration or distortion of an image as a result of an imperfection in the optical system.

5. $\frac{1}{f} = \frac{1}{o} + \frac{1}{i}$ and $m = -\frac{i}{o}$

8.3

1. Diffraction through a single slit does not create characteristic fringes when projected on a screen, although the light does spread out. When a lens is introduced into the system, the additional refraction of light causes constructive and destructive interference, creating fringes.
2. Fringes result from constructive and destructive interference between light rays.
3. The image formed during double-slit diffraction contains fringes because light rays constructively and destructively interfere. A single slit forms an image of a wide band of light, spread out from its original beam.
4. True. Maxima and minima alternate in a diffraction pattern. A maximum is equidistant between two minima, and a minimum is equidistant between two maxima.

8.4

1. Plane-polarized light contains light waves with parallel electric field vectors. Circularly polarized light selects for a given amplitude and has a continuously rotating electric field direction.
2. Plane polarization has no effect on the wavelength (or frequency or speed) of light. Polarization *does* affect the amount of light passing through a medium and light intensity.

SCIENCE MASTERY ASSESSMENT EXPLANATIONS

1. **C**

It is unnecessary to memorize the entire electromagnetic spectrum for Test Day; however, it is important to know that the visible spectrum runs from 400–700 nm. We can calculate the wavelength of this light ray:

$$c = f\lambda$$

$$\lambda = \frac{c}{f} = \frac{3 \times 10^8\ \frac{\text{m}}{\text{s}}}{5 \times 10^{14}\ \text{Hz}} = 6 \times 10^{-7}\ \text{m} = 600\ \text{nm}$$

This wavelength falls within the visible spectrum and has a yellow-orange color.

2. **D**

The color of an object is determined by the wavelength of light reflected by that object. Since anthocyanin pigment appears red, it must reflect red light. The frequency of light can be calculated using the equation $c = f\lambda$. Red light has a wavelength of 700 nm, which can be converted to 700×10^{-9} m. Plugging in values yields: $f = (3 \times 10^8) / (700 \times 10^{-9}) = 4.2 \times 10^{14}$ Hz, matching **(D)**. Note that a close eye for units would enable the immediate elimination of **(A)**.

3. **A**

One could solve this question with a ray diagram, but be wary about using ray diagrams on Test Day. It is easy to make small mistakes that cause the light rays not to intersect. Therefore, solve the question using the sign convention. If the object is at the center of curvature, its distance is 2*f*. We can plug into the optics equation:

$$\frac{1}{f} = \frac{1}{o} + \frac{1}{i} \rightarrow \frac{1}{i} = \frac{1}{f} - \frac{1}{o} = \frac{1}{f} - \frac{1}{2f} = \frac{1}{2f}$$

$$i = 2f = r$$

Because *i* is positive, the image is real. For single mirrors or lenses, all real images are inverted.

4. **B**

To calculate the wavelength, use the formula: $d \sin(\theta) = (n + 1/2)\lambda$. Rearrange the formula to solve for wavelength: $\lambda = d \sin(\theta)/(n + 1/2)$. Since the distance is given in millimeters, first convert to meters; $d = 3 \times 10^{-4}$ m. Since the question asks for the second dark fringe, we have $n = 2$. Plugging in the given values yields: $\lambda = (3 \times 10^{-4})\sin(30°)/(2 + 1/2) = 6 \times 10^{-5}$ m, matching choice **(B)**.

5. **A**

This question contains two parts—we have to determine the frequency and the angle of refraction of the light ray. The first part, however, is straightforward because the frequency of a light ray traveling from one medium to another does not change. Because the frequency must be 5×10^{14} Hz, we can eliminate **(C)** and **(D)**. For the angle of refraction, we can either calculate it or determine it using logic. First, the light ray goes from air into crystal; that is, from a low index of refraction to a higher one. According to Snell's law, the angle of refraction will be smaller than the incident angle (closer to the normal). When the light ray moves from crystal to chromium, it again goes from a lower index of refraction into a higher one, thus making the angle of refraction even smaller, eliminating **(B)**. This question could also be answered by calculation using Snell's law, but the calculations are time consuming and unnecessary.

6. **D**

Plane-polarized light is light in which the electric fields of all the waves are oriented in the same direction. Light passing through the first two polarizers will only contain rays with their electric field vectors in the same direction. When it reaches the third polarizer, however, the light will not be able to pass through because all the light rays will be oriented in the direction dictated by the first and second polarizers.

7. **C**

Plane polarizers only allow one specific orientation of the electric field of light to pass through. When plane polarizers are perpendicular to each other, no light can pass through the second polarizer, which supports **(C)** as the correct answer. Note that if two polarizers are aligned, all of the light that passes through the first will also pass through the second; there is no "twice as plane polarized," eliminating **(B)**.

8. **B**

The image produced by a convex lens can be either real or virtual. It is real if the object is placed at a distance greater than the focal point, and virtual if the object is placed at a distance less than the focal point (between the focal point and the lens). Remember that for a single mirror or lens, an image that is real must be inverted and one that is virtual must be upright. In this question, the object is placed in front of the focal point, so the image must be virtual and, therefore, upright. We could also determine this from the optics equation. If $f > o$, then $\frac{1}{f} - \frac{1}{o}$ is negative, and i is therefore negative (virtual).

9. **D**

This question is testing our understanding of total internal reflection. As the laser beam travels from water to air—that is, from a higher to a lower index of refraction—the angle of refraction increases. At the critical angle (θ_c), the angle of refraction becomes 90°; at this point, the refracted ray is parallel to the surface of the water. When the incident angle is greater than the critical angle, all the light is reflected back into the water. The question is asking for the critical angle:

$$\theta_c = \sin^{-1}\frac{n_2}{n_1} = \sin^{-1}\frac{1}{1.33} = \sin^{-1}0.75$$

The inverse sine of 0.75 must be slightly higher than 45° ($\sin 45° = \frac{\sqrt{2}}{2} = 0.707$). 48.59° is the exact answer.

10. **C**

This question is testing our understanding of diffraction. When light passes through a narrow opening, the light waves spread out; as the slit narrows, the light waves spread out even more. When a lens is placed between the narrow slit and the screen, a pattern consisting of alternating bright and dark fringes can be observed on the screen. As the slit becomes narrower, the central maximum (the brightest and most central fringe) becomes wider. This can also be seen in the equation for the position of dark fringes in a slit–lens setup ($a \sin\theta = n\lambda$). As a, the width of the slit, decreases, $\sin\theta$ must increase because $n\lambda$ is constant for a given fringe. If $\sin\theta$ increases, θ necessarily increases, implying that the fringes are spreading farther apart.

11. **D**

All images produced by plane mirrors will be virtual, so statement III is true. The same goes for diverging species (convex mirrors and concave lenses), so statement II is true. Converging species (concave mirrors and convex lenses) can produce real or virtual images, depending on how far the object is from the species, so statement I is also true.

12. **A**

First, the color of the light is irrelevant here; the ratio would be the same even if the specific color were not mentioned. Second, recall Snell's Law: $n_1 \sin\theta_1 = n_2 \sin\theta_2$. Although we don't know the value of n for either medium, you do know the simple relationship $n = \frac{c}{v}$. Replacing n in Snell's law, and canceling out c from both sides, we get:

$$\frac{c}{v_1}\sin\theta_1 = \frac{c}{v_2}\sin\theta_2$$

$$\frac{\sin 30°}{v_1} = \frac{\sin 45°}{v_2}$$

$$\frac{1}{2v_1} = \frac{\sqrt{2}}{2v_2}$$

$$v_2 = v_1\sqrt{2}$$

13. **D**

The overall magnification of a system of multiple lenses is simply the product of each lens's magnification. In this case, that is $10 \times 40 = 400$.

14. **D**

Drawing a diagram is best here. Because the angle given is with respect to the normal, you know that the incident angle must equal 60°. You know that the reflected beam will have an angle of 60° relative to the normal. Therefore, the reflected beam will make an angle of 30° with the plane of the glass. If the reflected and refracted beams are perpendicular to each other, the refracted beam will make a 60° angle with the plane of the glass. $\theta_{\text{refracted}}$ is therefore 30° relative to the normal.

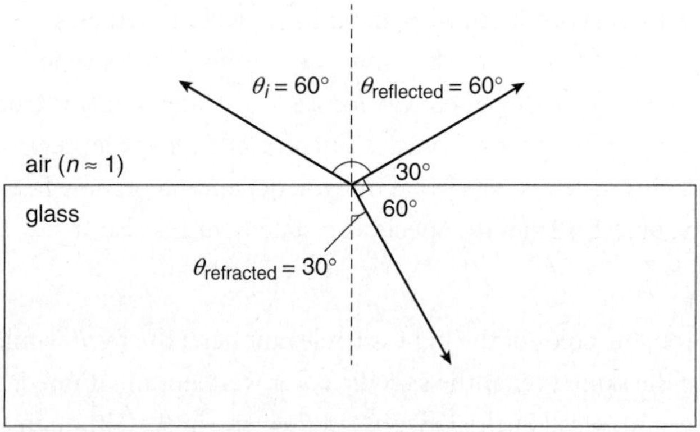

Using $n_1 \sin \theta_1 = n_2 \sin \theta_2$, we have

$$1 \sin 60° = n_2 \sin 30°$$

$$\frac{\sqrt{3}}{2} = n_2 \left(\frac{1}{2}\right)$$

$$\sqrt{3} = n_2$$

15. **D**

Light can be split into its component colors by dispersion, such as that through a prism, eliminating **(A)**. Diffraction by a diffraction grating will also separate colors by their wavelengths, eliminating **(B)**. The refraction of light within a thin film also leads to light dispersion as the different colors are refracted at slightly different angles in the film, eliminating **(C)**. A mirror with significant aberration could lead to a separation of light into its component colors, but we are told that this is an ideal mirror. Thus, **(D)** is the correct answer.

Consult your online resources for additional practice. **GO ONLINE**

EQUATIONS TO REMEMBER

(8.1) **Speed of light from frequency and wavelength:** $c = f\lambda$

(8.2) **Law of reflection:** $\theta_1 = \theta_2$

(8.3) **Optics equation:** $\frac{1}{f} = \frac{1}{o} + \frac{1}{i} = \frac{2}{r}$

(8.4) **Magnification:** $m = -\frac{i}{o}$

(8.5) **Index of refraction:** $n = \frac{c}{v}$

(8.6) **Snell's law:** $n_1 \sin \theta_1 = n_2 \sin \theta_2$

(8.7) **Critical angle:** $\theta_c = \sin^{-1}\left(\frac{n_2}{n_1}\right)$

(8.8) **Lensmaker's equation:** $\frac{1}{f} = (n-1)\left(\frac{1}{r_1} - \frac{1}{r_2}\right)$

(8.9) **Power:** $P = \frac{1}{f}$

(8.10) **Focal length of multiple lens system:** $\frac{1}{f} = \frac{1}{f_1} + \frac{1}{f_2} + \frac{1}{f_3} + \cdots + \frac{1}{f_n}$

(8.11) **Power of multiple lens system:** $P = P_1 + P_2 + P_3 + \cdots + P_n$

(8.12) **Magnification of multiple lens system:** $m = m_1 \times m_2 \times m_3 \times \cdots \times m_n$

(8.13) **Positions of dark fringes in slit–lens setup:** $a \sin \theta = n\lambda$

(8.14) **Positions of dark fringes in double-slit setup:** $d \sin \theta = \left(n + \frac{1}{2}\right) \lambda$

SHARED CONCEPTS

Behavioral Sciences Chapter 2
Sensation and Perception

Biochemistry Chapter 3
Nonenzymatic Protein Function and Protein Analysis

Organic Chemistry Chapter 2
Isomers

Organic Chemistry Chapter 11
Spectroscopy

Physics and Math Chapter 7
Waves and Sound

Physics and Math Chapter 9
Atomic and Nuclear Phenomena

CHAPTER 9

ATOMIC AND NUCLEAR PHENOMENA

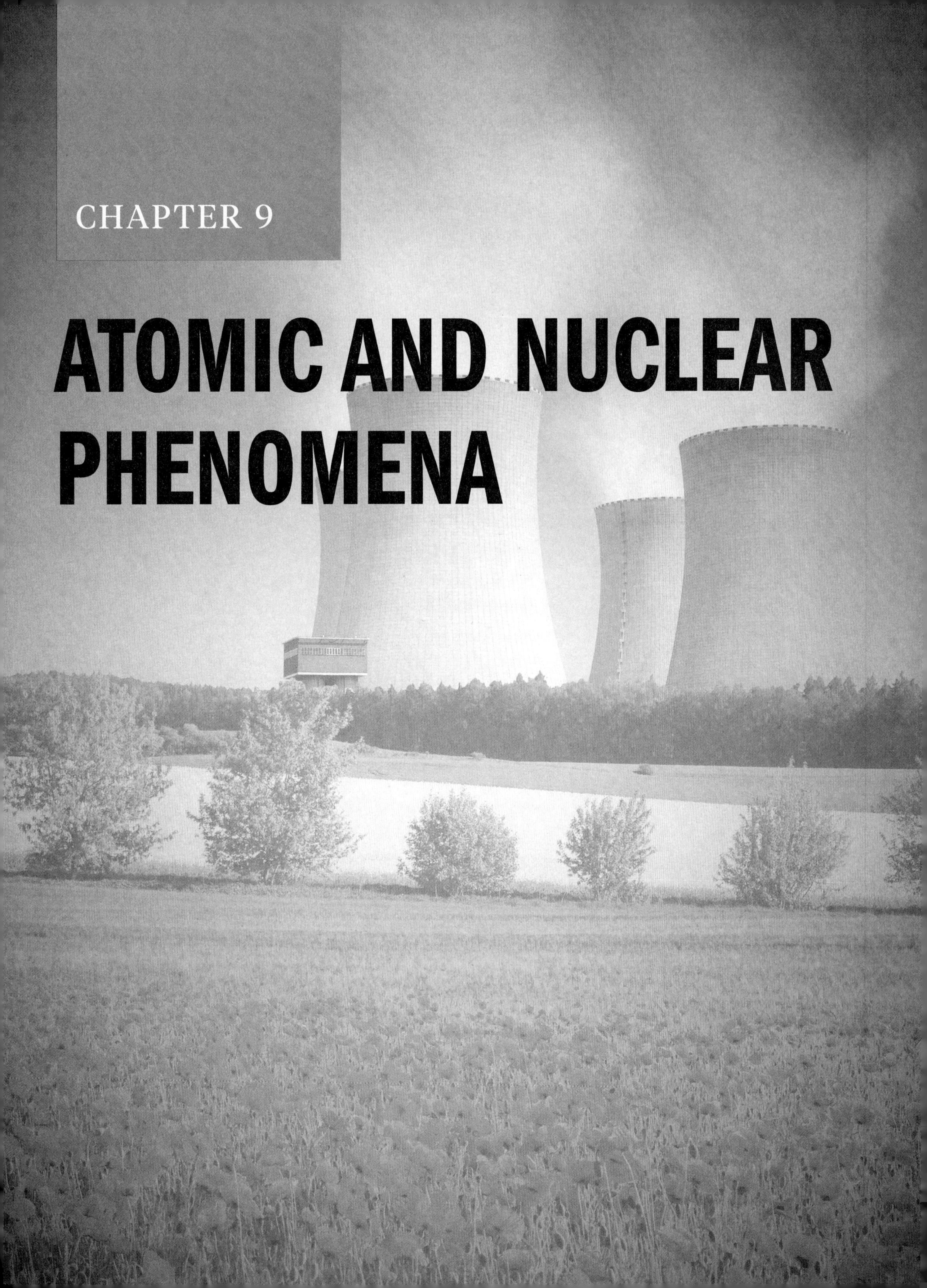

SCIENCE MASTERY ASSESSMENT

Every pre-med knows this feeling: there is so much content I have to know for the MCAT! How do I know what to do first or what's important?

While the high-yield badges throughout this book will help you identify the most important topics, this Science Mastery Assessment is another tool in your MCAT prep arsenal. This quiz (which can also be taken in your online resources) and the guidance below will help ensure that you are spending the appropriate amount of time on this chapter based on your personal strengths and weaknesses. Don't worry though—skipping something now does not mean you'll never study it. Later on in your prep, as you complete full-length tests, you'll uncover specific pieces of content that you need to review and can come back to these chapters as appropriate.

How to Use This Assessment

If you answer 0–7 questions correctly:

Spend about 1 hour to read this chapter in full and take limited notes throughout. Follow up by reviewing **all** quiz questions to ensure that you now understand how to solve each one.

If you answer 8–11 questions correctly:

Spend 20–40 minutes reviewing the quiz questions. Beginning with the questions you missed, read and take notes on the corresponding subchapters. For questions you answered correctly, ensure your thinking matches that of the explanation and you understand why each choice was correct or incorrect.

If you answer 12–15 questions correctly:

Spend less than 20 minutes reviewing all questions from the quiz. If you missed any, then include a quick read-through of the corresponding subchapters, or even just the relevant content within a subchapter, as part of your question review. For questions you got correct, ensure your thinking matches that of the explanation and review the Concept Summary at the end of the chapter.

1. If the work function of a metal is 6.622×10^{-20} J and a ray of electromagnetic radiation with a frequency of 1.0×10^{14} Hz is incident on the metal, what will be the speed of the electrons ejected from the metal? (Note: $h = 6.626 \times 10^{-34}$ J·s and $m_{e^-} = 9.1 \times 10^{-31}$ kg)
   - **A.** $2.62 \times 10^{-6} \frac{m}{s}$
   - **B.** $1.07 \times 10^{-4} \frac{m}{s}$
   - **C.** $9.38 \times 10^{3} \frac{m}{s}$
   - **D.** $3.81 \times 10^{5} \frac{m}{s}$

2. What is the wavelength of a photon that causes an electron to be emitted from a metal with a kinetic energy of 50 J? (Note: The work function of the metal is 16 J, and $h = 6.626 \times 10^{-34}$ J·s)
   - **A.** 1.0×10^{-34} m
   - **B.** 3.0×10^{-27} m
   - **C.** 3.0×10^{-26} m
   - **D.** 1.0×10^{35} m

3. Which of the following statements is inconsistent with the Bohr model of the atom?
   - **A.** Energy levels of the electron are stable and discrete.
   - **B.** An electron emits or absorbs radiation only when making a transition from one energy level to another.
   - **C.** To jump from a lower energy to a higher energy orbit, an electron must absorb a photon of precisely the right frequency such that the photon's energy equals the energy difference between the two orbits.
   - **D.** To jump from a higher energy to a lower energy orbit, an electron absorbs a photon of a frequency such that the photon's energy is exactly the energy difference between the two orbits.

4. When a hydrogen atom electron falls to the ground state from the $n = 2$ state, 10.2 eV of energy is emitted. What is the wavelength of this radiation? (Note: 1 eV = 1.60×10^{-19} J, and $h = 6.626 \times 10^{-34}$ J·s)
   - **A.** 5.76×10^{-9} m
   - **B.** 1.22×10^{-7} m
   - **C.** 3.45×10^{-7} m
   - **D.** 2.5×10^{15} m

5. The figure below illustrates an electron with initial energy of −10 eV moving from point A to point B. What change accompanies the movement of the electron?

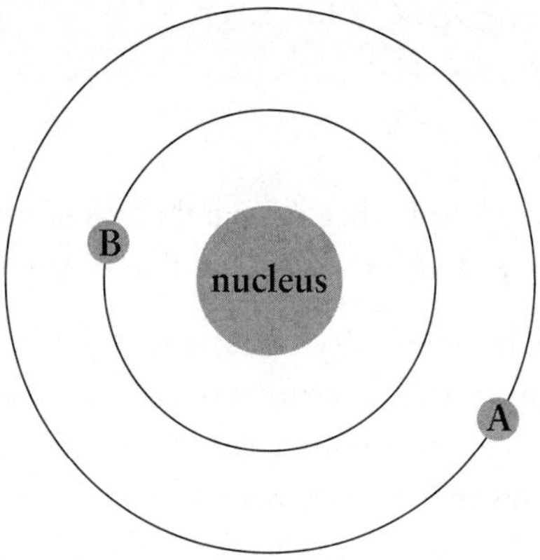

   - **A.** Absorption of a photon
   - **B.** Emission of a photon
   - **C.** Decrease in the atom's work function
   - **D.** Increase in the atom's total energy

6. Which of the following four fundamental forces is primarily responsible for holding the nucleons together?
   - **A.** Binding energy
   - **B.** Strong nuclear force
   - **C.** Electrostatic force
   - **D.** Gravitational force

7. All of the following statements about the photoelectric effect are true EXCEPT:
   - **A.** the intensity of the light beam does not affect the photocurrent.
   - **B.** the kinetic energies of the emitted electrons do not depend on the light intensity.
   - **C.** a weak beam of light of frequency greater than the threshold frequency yields more current than an intense beam of light of frequency lower than the threshold frequency.
   - **D.** for light of a given frequency, the kinetic energy of emitted electrons increases as the value of the work function decreases.

8. What is the binding energy of the argon-40 isotope in MeV? (Note: $m_{proton} = 1.0073$ amu, $m_{neutron} = 1.0087$ amu, $m_{Ar\text{-}40\ nucleus} = 39.9132$ amu, $c^2 = 932\ \frac{MeV}{amu}$)
   A. 0.4096 MeV
   B. 40.3228 MeV
   C. 381.7 MeV
   D. 643.8 MeV

9. Which of the following correctly identifies the following process?

$$^{67}_{31}Ga + e^- \rightarrow {}^{67}_{30}Zn$$

   A. β^- decay
   B. β^+ decay
   C. e^- capture
   D. γ decay

10. Consider the following fission reaction.

$$\underset{1.0087}{^{1}_{0}n} + \underset{10.0129}{^{10}_{5}B} \rightarrow \underset{7.0160}{^{7}_{3}Li} + \underset{4.0026}{^{4}_{2}He}$$

The masses of the species involved are given in atomic mass units below each species, and 1 amu can create 932 MeV of energy. What is the energy liberated due to the transformation of mass into energy during this reaction?
   A. 0.003 MeV
   B. 1.4 MeV
   C. 2.8 MeV
   D. 5.6 MeV

11. Element X is radioactive and decays via α decay with a half-life of four days. If 12.5 percent of an original sample of element X remains after n days, what is the value of n?
   A. 4
   B. 8
   C. 12
   D. 16

12. A graph of an exponential decay process is created. The y-axis is the natural logarithm of the ratio of the number of intact nuclei at a given time to the number of intact nuclei at time $t = 0$. The x-axis is time. What does the slope of such a graph represent?
   A. λ
   B. $-\lambda$
   C. $e^{-\lambda t}$
   D. $\frac{n}{n_0}$

13. A certain carbon nucleus dissociates completely into α-particles. How many particles are formed?
   A. 1
   B. 2
   C. 3
   D. 4

14. The half-life of carbon-14 is approximately 5,730 years, while the half-life of carbon-12 is essentially infinite. If the ratio of carbon-14 to carbon-12 in a certain sample is 25% less than the normal ratio in nature, how old is the sample?
   A. Less than 5,730 years
   B. Approximately 5,730 years
   C. Significantly greater than 5,730 years, but less than 11,460 years
   D. Approximately 11,460 years

15. A nuclide undergoes two alpha decays, two positron decays, and two gamma decays. What is the difference between the atomic number of the parent nuclide and the atomic number of the daughter nuclide?
   A. 0
   B. 2
   C. 4
   D. 6

Answer Key

1. **C**
2. **B**
3. **D**
4. **B**
5. **B**
6. **B**
7. **A**
8. **C**
9. **C**
10. **C**
11. **C**
12. **B**
13. **C**
14. **A**
15. **D**

Detailed explanations can be found at the end of the chapter.

CHAPTER 9

ATOMIC AND NUCLEAR PHENOMENA

In This Chapter

CHAPTER PROFILE

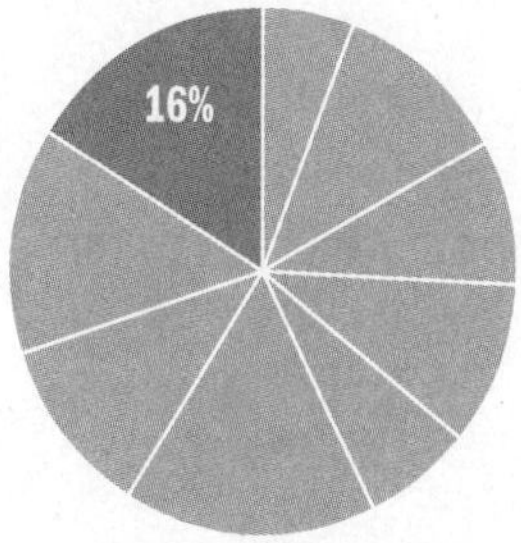

The content in this chapter should be relevant to about 16% of all questions about physics on the MCAT.

This chapter covers material from the following AAMC content categories:

4D: How light and sound interact with matter

4E: Atoms, nuclear decay, electronic structure, and atomic chemical behavior

Introduction

All of life depends on the photoelectric effect. As a photon of light enters the chloroplast in a plant cell, it reacts with chlorophyll, causing the ejection of an electron from certain magnesium-containing dyes. This electron feeds into synthetic pathways that ultimately result in glucose production. While the MCAT does not include photosynthesis in its content lists, its principles are a primary example of the photoelectric effect. It was Albert Einstein who described this effect, and it was this that won him the Nobel Prize—not the theory of relativity. We now use the photoelectric effect in many industrial applications, such as solar panels.

After discussing the photoelectric effect, we will examine nuclear radiation. Nuclear radiation is curiously full of opposites: it can cause life-threatening diseases such as cancer, but it can also be used in the treatment of cancer. It can be used safely for mass power generation, but it can cause untold devastation in meltdowns or weapons of mass destruction. In addition to nuclear radiation, we will examine the strong nuclear force and the equation of mass defect, perhaps the most quoted equation in all of science. At the end of this chapter, we'll have covered all of the physics content tested on the MCAT, and will be ready to move on to mathematics and some skills-based practice.

9.1 The Photoelectric Effect

LEARNING OBJECTIVES

After Chapter 9.1, you will be able to:

- Relate the work function to the energy needed to emit an electron from a metal
- Recall the factor(s) that threshold frequency depends on
- Recognize the phenomena that result from the application of the photoelectric effect:

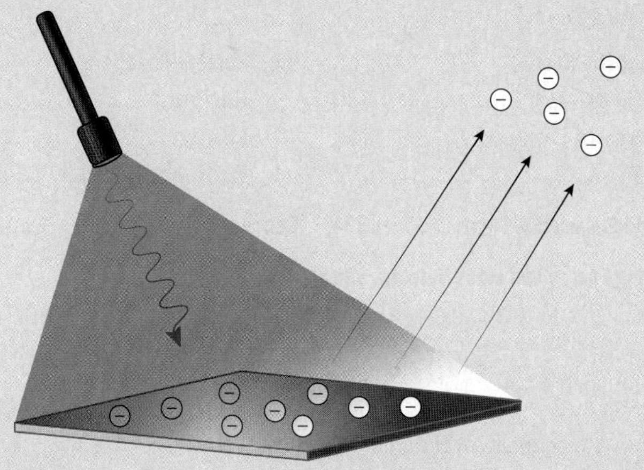

When light of a sufficiently high frequency (typically, blue to ultraviolet light) is incident on a metal in a vacuum, the metal atoms emit electrons. This phenomenon, discovered by Heinrich Hertz in 1887, is called the **photoelectric effect**. As mentioned earlier, Albert Einstein's 1905 explanation of the photoelectric effect won him the Nobel Prize.

Electrons liberated from the metal by the photoelectric effect will produce a net charge flow per unit time, or **current**. Provided that the light beam's frequency is above the threshold frequency of the metal, light beams of greater intensity produce larger current in this way. The higher the intensity of the light beam, the greater the number of photons per unit time that fall on an electrode, producing a greater number of electrons per unit time liberated from the metal. When the light's frequency is above the threshold frequency, the magnitude of the resulting current is directly proportional to the intensity (and amplitude) of the light beam.

Threshold Frequency

The minimum frequency of light that causes ejection of electrons is known as the **threshold frequency,** f_T. The threshold frequency depends on the type of metal being exposed to the radiation. The photoelectric effect is, for all intents and purposes, an "all-or-nothing" response: if the frequency of the incident photon is less than the threshold frequency ($f < f_T$), then no electron will be ejected because the photons do not have sufficient energy to dislodge the electron from its atom. But if the frequency of the incident photon is greater than the threshold frequency

($f > f_T$), then an electron will be ejected, and the maximum kinetic energy of the ejected electron will be equal to the difference between hf and hf_T (also called the work function). Einstein's explanation of these results was that the light beam consists of an integral number of light quanta called **photons.** The energy of each photon is proportional to the frequency of the light:

$$E = hf$$

Equation 9.1

where E is the energy of the photon of light, h is Planck's constant ($6.626 \times 10^{-34}\ \text{J}\cdot\text{s}$), and f is the frequency of the light. Once we know the frequency, we can easily find the wavelength λ according to the equation $c = f\lambda$, as described in Chapter 8 of *MCAT Physics and Math Review.* According to these equations, waves with higher frequency have shorter wavelengths and higher energy (toward the blue and ultraviolet end of the spectrum); waves with lower frequency have longer wavelengths and lower energy (toward the red and infrared end of the spectrum). In nuclear physics, wavelength is commonly measured in nanometers ($1\ \text{nm} = 10^{-9}\ \text{m}$) and ångströms ($1\ \text{Å} = 10^{-10}\ \text{m}$).

KEY CONCEPT

The energy of a photon increases with increasing frequency. The reason that we only discuss electrons being ejected from metals (and not protons or neutrons) is because of the weak hold that metals have on their valence electrons due to their low ionization energies.

Kinetic Energy of Ejected Electrons

If the frequency of a photon of light incident on a metal is at the threshold frequency for the metal, the electron barely escapes from the metal. However, if the frequency of an incident photon is above the threshold frequency of the metal, the photon will have more than enough energy to eject a single electron, and the excess energy will be converted to kinetic energy in the ejected electron. We can calculate the maximum kinetic energy of the ejected electron with the formula:

$$K_{max} = hf - W$$

Equation 9.2

where W is the work function of the metal in question. The **work function** is the minimum energy required to eject an electron and is related to the threshold frequency of that metal by:

$$W = hf_T$$

Equation 9.3

These formulas solve for the maximum kinetic energy of the electron rather than exact kinetic energy because the actual energy can be anywhere between 0 and K_{max}, depending on the specific subatomic interactions between the photon and the metal atom. K_{max} is only achieved when all possible energy from the photon is transferred to the ejected electron.

MCAT EXPERTISE

The photoelectric effect is not frequently tested on the MCAT, but the underlying principles are simple. This is simply another example of energy transfer in which light energy causes an increase in electrical potential energy in the atom—enough to allow the electron to escape. If any energy is "left over," it cannot be destroyed. Rather, it is transferred into kinetic energy in the ejected electron.

BRIDGE

Think of the work function like activation energy, in the sense that it must be matched or exceeded to cause the reaction (escape of an electron) to occur. Activation energy is discussed in Chapter 5 of *MCAT General Chemistry Review.*

Example: If blue light of frequency 6.00×10^{14} Hz is incident on rubidium ($W = 2.26$ eV), will there be photoejection of electrons? If so, what is the maximum kinetic energy that an ejected electron will carry away?
(Note: $h = 6.626 \times 10^{-34}\ \text{J·s} = 4.14 \times 10^{-15}\ \text{eV·s}$)

Solution: If the photons have a frequency of 6.00×10^{14} Hz, each photon has an energy of:

$$E = hf = (4.14 \times 10^{-15}\ \text{eV·s})(6.00 \times 10^{14}\ \text{Hz}) = 2.48\ \text{eV}$$

Clearly then, any given photon has more than enough energy to allow an electron in the metal to overcome the 2.26 eV barrier. In fact, the maximum excess kinetic energy carried away by the electron turns out to be:

$$K = hf - W = 2.48 - 2.26 = 0.22\ \text{eV}$$

In general, the photoelectric effect is strong support for the particle theory of light, which states that light is not a continuous wave but acts as discrete bundles of energy called photons, as shown in Figure 9.1.

MCAT CONCEPT CHECK 9.1

Before you move on, assess your understanding of the material with these questions.

1. How does the work function relate to the energy necessary to emit an electron from a metal?

___

2. What does the threshold frequency depend upon?

___

3. What electrical phenomenon results from the application of the photoelectric effect?

___

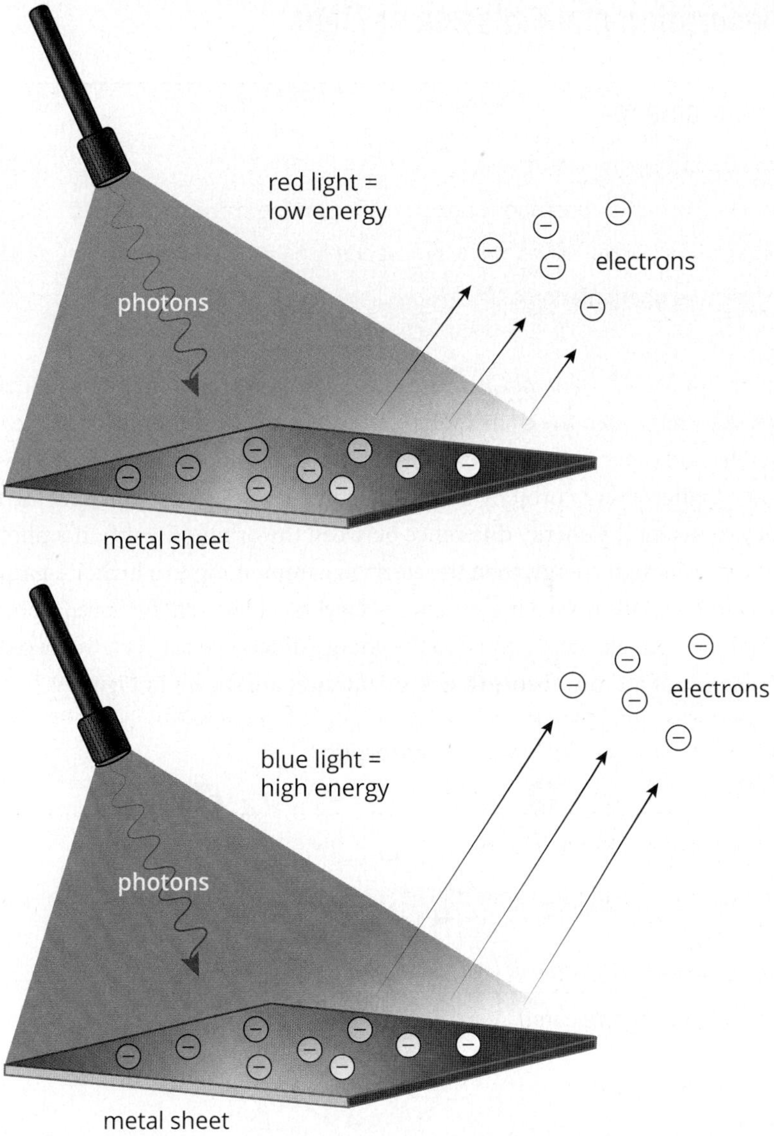

Figure 9.1 The Photoelectric Effect

9.2 Absorption and Emission of Light

LEARNING OBJECTIVES

After Chapter 9.2, you will be able to:

- Describe how the absorption spectrum of a single atom is determined
- Recall when photon emissions are most common during electronic transitions
- Explain the phenomenon of fluorescence

In Chapter 1 of *MCAT General Chemistry Review*, we explored the Bohr model of the atom. As a reminder, the Bohr model states that electron energy levels are stable and discrete, corresponding to specific orbits. An electron can jump from a lower-energy to a higher-energy orbit by absorbing a photon of light of precisely the right frequency to match the energy difference between the orbits ($E = hf$). If a photon does not carry enough energy, then the electron cannot jump to a higher energy level. When an electron falls from a higher-energy level to a lower-energy level, a photon of light is emitted with an energy equal to the energy difference between the two orbits. These processes of **atomic absorption** and **emission** are shown in Figure 9.2.

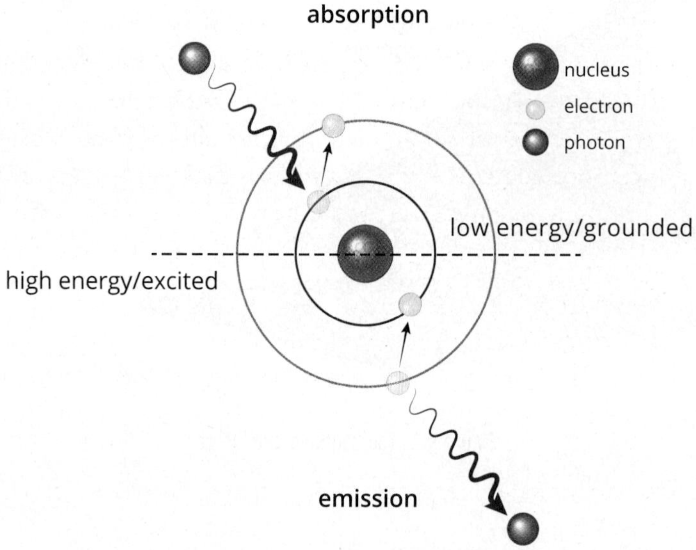

Figure 9.2 Bohr Model: Light Absorption and Emission

BRIDGE

Spectroscopy is discussed in greater detail in Chapter 11 of *MCAT Organic Chemistry Review*.

While information about a single electron is a great foundation for Test Day, in the real world we'll often be handling more complex structures. In organic chemistry, we use **infrared (IR) spectroscopy** to determine chemical structure because different bonds will absorb different wavelengths of light. **UV–Vis spectroscopy** takes this one step further, looking at the absorption of light in the visible and ultraviolet range. Absorption spectra may be represented as a color bar with peak areas of absorption represented by black lines. It can also be shown as a graph with the absolute absorption as a function of wavelength. This is shown in Figure 9.3, which shows the absorption spectrum for the atmosphere across the entire electromagnetic spectrum.

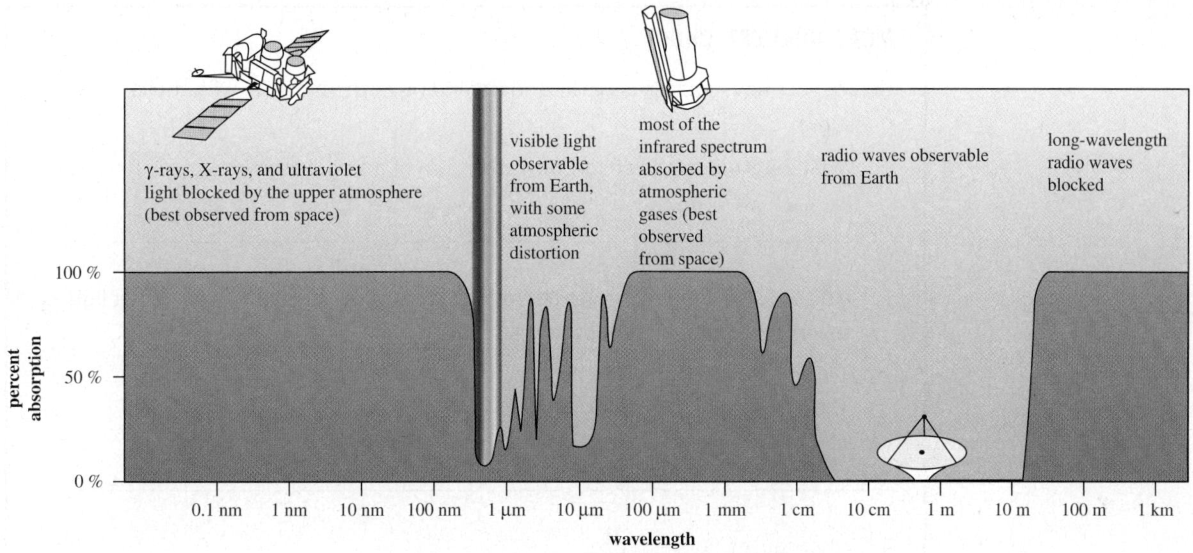

Figure 9.3 Absorption Spectrum of the Atmosphere
The sky is blue because blue light is the least absorbed by atmospheric gases.

Changes in molecular structure can cause dramatic shifts in the absorption patterns of a substance. Consider indicators like phenolphthalein. This indicator has a clear appearance in its acidic state, and thus does not absorb any visible light. In its basic state, it is a bright pink, and thus is absorbing all but the longer wavelengths of visible light—remember that we see the colors that are *not* absorbed. Most indicators contain large organic compounds that have strikingly different absorption patterns based solely on the protonation state of the compound. These compounds often have conjugated double bonds or aromatic ring systems, as this permits the absorption of light from photons in the visible range.

Another phenomenon related to absorption and emission of visible light is **fluorescence**. If one excites a fluorescent substance (such as a ruby, an emerald, or the phosphors found in fluorescent lights) with ultraviolet radiation, it will begin to glow with visible light. Photons of ultraviolet light have relatively high frequencies (short wavelengths). After being excited to a higher energy state by ultraviolet radiation, the electron in the fluorescent substance returns to its original state in two or more steps. By returning in two or more steps, each step involves less energy, so at each step, a photon is emitted with a lower frequency (longer wavelength) than the absorbed ultraviolet photon. If the wavelength of this emitted photon is within the visible range of the electromagnetic spectrum, it will be seen as light of the particular color corresponding to that wavelength. The wide range of colors in fluorescent lights, from the whitish-green of office lighting to the glaring colors of neon signs, is the result of the distinct multi-step emission spectra of different fluorescent materials.

MCAT CONCEPT CHECK 9.2

Before you move on, assess your understanding of the material with these questions.

1. What determines the absorption spectrum of a single atom?

___

2. True or False: Small changes in chemical structure only minimally impact light absorption and emission patterns.

3. During which electronic transitions is photon emission most common?

___

4. What causes fluorescence?

___

9.3 Nuclear Binding Energy and Mass Defect

LEARNING OBJECTIVES

After Chapter 9.3, you will be able to:

- Describe key concepts in nuclear binding energy, including strong nuclear force, mass defect, and binding energy
- Recall the four fundamental forces of nature
- Apply the equation $E = mc^2$

Until this point, we've examined the relationships between electromagnetic radiation and matter—particularly electrons. Now, we'll shift to the energy that is stored in the nucleus, which can be emitted under specific circumstances. While one would assume that the mass of the nucleus is simply the sum of the masses of all of the protons and neutrons within it, the actual mass of every nucleus (other than hydrogen) is slightly smaller than that. This difference is called the **mass defect**. Scientists had difficulty explaining why this mass defect occurred until Einstein characterized the equivalence of matter and energy, embodied by the equation

$$E = mc^2$$

Equation 9.4

where E is energy, m is mass, and c is the speed of light. The mass defect is a result of matter that has been converted to energy. Because of the large exponent on the speed of light—which is squared in the equation—a very small amount of mass will yield a huge amount of energy. For example, the conversion of one gram of mass to energy will produce 89.9 terajoules (1 TJ $= 10^{12}$ joules) or 21.5 billion kilocalories.

When protons and neutrons (**nucleons**) come together to form the nucleus, they are attracted to each other by the **strong nuclear force**, which is strong enough to more than compensate for the repulsive electromagnetic force between the protons. Although the strong nuclear force is the strongest of the four fundamental forces, it only acts over extremely short distances, less than a few times the diameter of a proton or neutron. The nucleons have to get very close together in order for the strong nuclear force to hold them together. The bonded system is at a lower energy level than the unbonded constituents, and this difference in energy must be radiated away in the form of heat, light, or other electromagnetic radiation before the mass defect becomes apparent. This energy, called **binding energy**, allows the nucleons to bind together in the nucleus. Given the strength of the strong nuclear force, the amount of mass that is transformed into the dissipated energy will be a measurable fraction of the initial total mass. The binding energy per nucleon peaks at the element iron, which implies that iron contains the most stable nucleus. In general, intermediate-sized nuclei are more stable than very large or small nuclei.

The **weak nuclear force** also contributes to the stability of the nucleus, but is about one-millionth as strong as the strong nuclear force. The strong and weak nuclear forces constitute two of the four fundamental forces of nature. The other two are electrostatic forces and gravitation.

Example: Measurements of the atomic mass of a neutron and a proton yield these results:

$$\text{proton} = 1.00728 \text{ amu}$$
$$\text{neutron} = 1.00867 \text{ amu}$$

${}^{4}_{2}He$ contains two protons and two neutrons, which should theoretically give a helium nucleus a mass of $2 \times 1.00728 + 2 \times 1.00867 = 4.03190$ amu. However, the true mass of the helium nucleus is 4.00260 amu. What is the mass defect and binding energy of this nucleus? (Note: $c^2 = 932 \frac{\text{MeV}}{\text{amu}}$)

Solution: The difference $4.03190 - 4.00260 = 0.02930$ amu is the mass defect for the helium nucleus. This is the mass that contributed to the binding energy of the nucleus:

$$\begin{aligned} E &= mc^2 \\ &= (0.02930 \text{ amu})\left(932 \frac{\text{MeV}}{\text{amu}}\right) \\ &\approx 0.03 \times 900 = 27 \text{ MeV (actual} = 27.3 \text{ MeV)} \end{aligned}$$

MCAT CONCEPT CHECK 9.3

Before you move on, assess your understanding of the material with these questions.

1. Define the following terms:
    - Strong nuclear force:
    - Mass defect:
    - Binding energy:
2. What are the four fundamental forces of nature?
    -
    -
    -
    -
3. How does the mass defect relate to the binding energy?

9.4 Nuclear Reactions

High-Yield

LEARNING OBJECTIVES

After Chapter 9.4, you will be able to:

- Compare and contrast nuclear fission and nuclear fusion reactions
- Recall the emissions, ΔZ, and ΔA of different radioactive processes
- Recall the type of decay that could be detected in an atomic absorption spectrum
- Predict the number of half-lives necessary for decay of some portion of a radioactive sample:

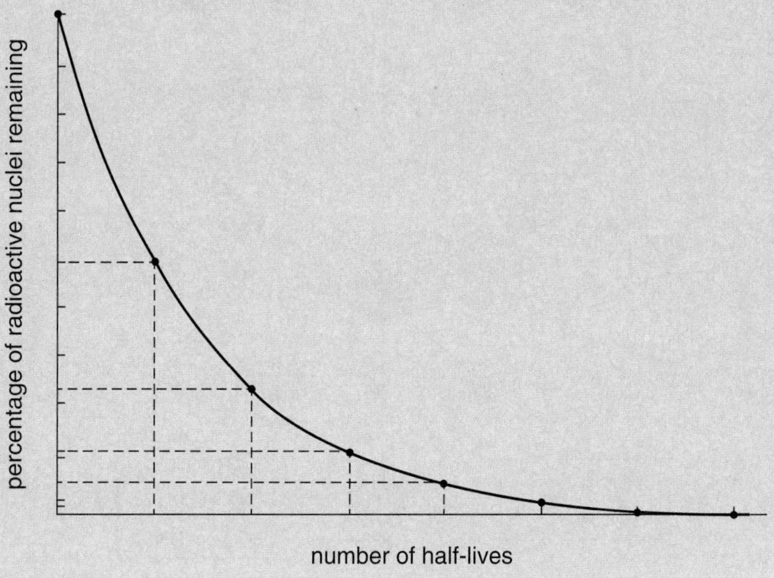

Nuclear reactions, such as fusion, fission, and radioactive decay, involve either combining or splitting the nuclei of atoms. Because the binding energy per nucleon is greatest for intermediate-sized atoms (that is, intermediate-sized atoms are most stable), when small atoms combine or large atoms split, a great amount of energy is released.

When written in **isotopic notation**, elements are preceded by their atomic number as a subscript and mass number as a superscript $\left({}^{A}_{Z}\text{X}\right)$. The **atomic number** (*Z*) corresponds to the number of protons in the nucleus; the **mass number** (*A*) corresponds to the number of protons plus neutrons. When balancing nuclear equations, it is important to balance the number of nucleons on both sides by balancing the atomic numbers and mass numbers.

Fusion

Fusion occurs when small nuclei combine to form a larger nucleus. As an example, many stars (including the Sun) power themselves by fusing four hydrogen nuclei to make one helium nucleus as shown in Figure 9.4. By this method, the Sun produces 3.85×10^{26} joules per second (385 yottawatts), which accounts for the mass defect that arises from the formation of helium nuclei from hydrogen nuclei. Here on Earth, fusion power plants—which are only in developmental stages—generate energy from deuterium $\left(^2_1\text{H}\right)$ and lithium nuclei.

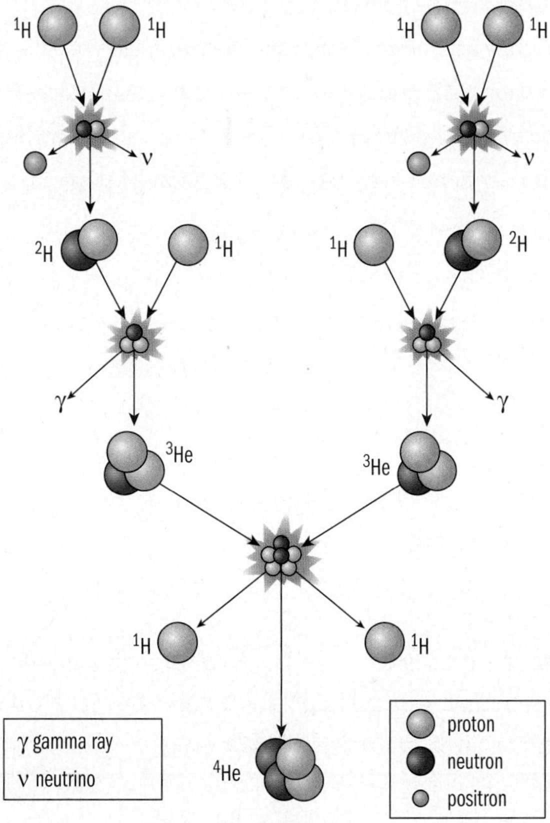

Figure 9.4 Hydrogen Fusion in the Sun, Creating Helium Nuclei

Fission

Fission is a process by which a large nucleus splits into smaller nuclei. Spontaneous fission rarely occurs. However, through the absorption of a low-energy neutron, fission can be induced in certain nuclei. Of special interest are those fission reactions that release more neutrons because these other neutrons will cause a chain reaction in which other nearby atoms can undergo fission. This in turn releases more neutrons, continuing the chain reaction. Such induced fission reactions power most commercial nuclear power plants.

Example: A fission reaction occurs when uranium-235 (U-235) absorbs a low-energy neutron, briefly forming an excited state of U-236, which then splits into xenon-140, strontium-94, and more neutrons. In isotopic notation form, the unbalanced reaction is:

$$^{235}_{92}\text{U} + ^{1}_{0}n \rightarrow ^{236}_{92}\text{U}^{*} \rightarrow ^{140}_{54}\text{Xe} + ^{94}_{38}\text{Sr} + ^{1}_{0}n$$

When balanced, how many neutrons are produced in the last reaction?

Solution: By treating each arrow as an equals sign, the problem is simply asking us to balance the last equation. The mass numbers (A) on either side of each arrow must be equal. This is an application of nucleon number conservation, which says that the total number of neutrons plus protons remains the same, even if neutrons are converted to protons and vice-versa, as they are in some decays. Because $235 + 1 = 236$, the first arrow is indeed balanced. Looking at the atomic numbers, the number of protons are balanced throughout $(92 + 0 = 92 = 54 + 38 + 0)$. To find the number of neutrons, determine how many nucleons remain after accounting for xenon-140 and strontium-94:

$$236 - (140 + 94) = 236 - 234 = 2 \text{ nucleons}$$

Because the protons are balanced, these remaining nucleons are both neutrons. Therefore, two neutrons are produced in this reaction. These neutrons are free to go on and be absorbed by more U-235 and cause more fission reactions. Note that it was not actually necessary to know that the intermediate high-energy state $^{236}_{92}\text{U}^{*}$ was formed.

Radioactive Decay

Radioactive decay is a naturally occurring spontaneous decay of certain nuclei accompanied by the emission of specific particles. On the MCAT, you should be prepared to answer three general types of radioactive decay problems:

1. The integer arithmetic of particle and isotope species
2. Radioactive half-life problems
3. The use of exponential decay curves and decay constants

Isotope Decay Arithmetic and Nucleon Conservation

Let the letters X and Y represent nuclear isotopes. When the **parent nucleus** X undergoes nuclear decay to form **daughter nucleus** Y, the balanced reaction is:

$$^{A}_{Z}\text{X} \rightarrow ^{A'}_{Z'}\text{Y} + \text{emitted decay particle}$$

Equation 9.5

MCAT EXPERTISE

Whenever you approach radioactive decay problems on the MCAT, start by balancing the number of protons (the atomic numbers). Often, wrong answer choices will simply have an error in the number of protons and can be eliminated before even checking the mass numbers.

KEY CONCEPT

Alpha particles do not have any electrons, so they carry a charge of $+2$.

When balancing nuclear reactions, the sum of the atomic numbers must be the same on both sides of the equation, and the sum of the mass numbers must be the same on both sides as well.

Alpha Decay

Alpha decay is the emission of an **α-particle**, which is a ${}^{4}_{2}He$ nucleus that consists of two protons, two neutrons, and zero electrons. The alpha particle is very massive compared to a beta particle and carries double the charge. Alpha particles interact with matter very easily; hence, they do not penetrate shielding (such as lead sheets) very extensively.

The emission of an α-particle means that the atomic number of the daughter nucleus will be two less than that of the parent nucleus, and the mass number will be four less. This can be expressed in the balanced equation:

$${}^{A}_{Z}X \rightarrow {}^{A-4}_{Z-2}Y + {}^{4}_{2}\alpha$$

Equation 9.6

Example: Suppose a parent nucleus X alpha decays as follows:

$${}^{238}_{92}X \rightarrow {}^{A'}_{Z'}Y + \alpha$$

What are the mass number and atomic number of the daughter isotope Y?

Solution: To solve this question, we simply need to balance the atomic numbers and mass numbers:

$${}^{A}_{Z}X \rightarrow {}^{A-4}_{Z-2}Y + {}^{4}_{2}\alpha$$
$${}^{238}_{92}U \rightarrow {}^{234}_{90}Y + {}^{4}_{2}\alpha$$

While it is not necessary to identify the elements to answer the question, answers on the MCAT are usually given with the element's symbol. Y must be thorium (Th) because its atomic number is 90. Therefore, the daughter nucleus is ${}^{234}_{90}Th$.

Beta Decay

Beta decay is the emission of a **β-particle**, which is an electron and is given the symbol e^- or β^-. Electrons do not reside in the nucleus, but they are emitted by the nucleus when a neutron decays into a proton, a β-particle, and an antineutrino ($\overline{\nu}$). Because an electron is singly charged and 1836 times lighter than a proton, the beta radiation from radioactive decay is more penetrating than alpha radiation. In some cases of induced decay (**positron emission**), a **positron** is released, which has the mass of an electron but carries a positive charge. The positron is given the symbol e^+ or β^+. A neutrino (ν) is emitted in positron decay, as well. Note that neutrinos and antineutrinos are not tested on the MCAT, and are therefore omitted in subsequent discussion.

During β^- decay, a neutron is converted into a proton and a β^--particle ($Z = -1$, $A = 0$) is emitted. Hence, the atomic number of the daughter nucleus will be one higher than that of the parent nucleus, and the mass number will not change. This can be expressed in the balanced equation:

$$^{A}_{Z}\mathrm{X} \rightarrow {}^{A}_{Z+1}\mathrm{Y} + \beta^-$$

Equation 9.7

During β^+ decay, a proton is converted into a neutron and a β^+-particle ($Z = +1$, $A = 0$) is emitted. Hence, the atomic number of the daughter nucleus will be one lower than that of the parent nucleus, and the mass number will not change. This can be expressed in the balanced equation:

$$^{A}_{Z}\mathrm{X} \rightarrow {}^{A}_{Z-1}\mathrm{Y} + \beta^+$$

Equation 9.8

KEY CONCEPT

In both types of beta decay, there needs to be conservation of charge. If a negative charge (β^-) is produced, a neutron is converted into a proton to maintain charge. Conversely, if a positive charge (β^+) is produced, a proton is converted into a neutron to maintain charge. Remember that negative beta decay produces a negative β-particle and positive beta decay produces a positive β-particle.

Example: Suppose a promethium-146 nucleus beta-decays as follows:

$$^{146}_{61}\mathrm{Pm} \longrightarrow {}^{A'}_{Z'}\mathrm{Y} + \beta^-$$

What are the mass number and atomic number of the daughter isotope Y?

Solution: Again, balance the atomic numbers and mass numbers:

$$^{146}_{61}\mathrm{Pm} \longrightarrow {}^{A}_{Z+1}\mathrm{Y} + {}^{0}_{-1}\beta^-$$
$$^{146}_{61}\mathrm{Pm} \longrightarrow {}^{146}_{62}\mathrm{Y} + {}^{0}_{-1}\beta^-$$

Y must be samarium (Sm) because its atomic number is 62. Therefore, the daughter nucleus is $^{146}_{62}\mathrm{Sm}$.

Gamma Decay

Gamma decay is the emission of **γ-rays**, which are high-energy (high-frequency) photons. They carry no charge and simply lower the energy of the parent nucleus without changing the mass number or the atomic number. The high-energy state of the parent nucleus may be represented by an asterisk.

This can be expressed in the balanced equation:

$$^{A}_{Z}\mathrm{X}^* \rightarrow {}^{A}_{Z}\mathrm{X} + \gamma$$

Equation 9.9

KEY CONCEPT

Gamma decay questions are the easiest on the MCAT. No changes occur in the mass number or atomic number; only a γ-ray is emitted.

Example: Suppose an excited parent isotope ${}^{A}_{Z}X^*$ gamma decays to ${}^{A'}_{Z'}X$, which then undergoes positron emission to form ${}^{A''}_{Z''}Y$, which in turn alpha decays to ${}^{A'''}_{Z'''}Z$. If Z is americium-241, what is ${}^{A}_{Z}X^*$?

Solution: Because the final daughter nucleus is given, it will be necessary to work backwards through the reactions. The last reaction is the following alpha decay:

$${}^{A''}_{Z''}Y \rightarrow {}^{241}_{95}Am + {}^{4}_{2}\alpha$$

The atomic number of the parent nucleus must be 97, and the mass number is 245. This is berkelium-245. The preceding reaction is the following positron emission:

$${}^{A'}_{Z'}X \rightarrow {}^{245}_{97}Bk + {}^{0}_{+1}\beta^{+}$$

The atomic number of the parent nucleus must be 98, and the mass number is 245. This is californium-245. Finally, the preceding reaction is the following gamma decay:

$${}^{A}_{Z}X^* \rightarrow {}^{245}_{98}Cf + \gamma$$

The atomic number of the parent nucleus must be 98, and the mass number is 245. This is a higher-energy form of californium-245: ${}^{A}_{Z}X^* = {}^{245}_{98}Cf^*$

Electron Capture

Certain unstable radionuclides are capable of capturing an inner electron that combines with a proton to form a neutron, while releasing a neutrino. The atomic number is now one less than the original but the mass number remains the same. **Electron capture** is a rare process that is perhaps best thought of as the reverse of β^- decay:

$${}^{A}_{Z}X + e^- \rightarrow {}^{A}_{Z-1}Y$$

Equation 9.10

Half-Life

In a sample of radioactive particles, the **half-life** $\left(T_{\frac{1}{2}}\right)$ of the sample is the time it takes for half of the sample to decay. In each subsequent half-life, one-half of the remaining sample decays so that the remaining amount asymptotically approaches zero.

MCAT EXPERTISE

Half-life problems are common on the MCAT. Make sure you write them out; it's easy to lose your place when doing them in your head.

Example: If the half-life of a certain isotope is 4 years, what fraction of a sample of that isotope will remain after 12 years?

Solution: If 4 years is one half-life, then 12 years is 3 half-lives. During the first half-life—the first 4 years—half of the sample will decay. During the second half-life (years 4 to 8), half of the remaining half will decay, leaving one-fourth of the original. During the third and final half-life (years 8 to 12), half of the remaining fourth will decay, leaving one-eighth of the original sample. Thus, the fraction remaining after 3 half-lives is $\left(\frac{1}{2}\right)^3 = \frac{1}{8}$.

Exponential Decay

Let n be the number of radioactive nuclei that have not yet decayed in a sample. It turns out that the rate at which the nuclei decay, $\frac{\Delta n}{\Delta t}$, is proportional to the number that remain (n). This suggests the equation

$$\frac{\Delta n}{\Delta t} = -\lambda n$$

Equation 9.11

where λ is known as the decay constant. The solution of this equation tells us how the number of radioactive nuclei changes with time. This is known as an **exponential decay**:

$$n = n_0 e^{-\lambda t}$$

Equation 9.12

where n_0 is the number of undecayed nuclei at time $t = 0$. The decay constant is related to the half-life by

$$\lambda = \frac{\ln 2}{T_{\frac{1}{2}}} = \frac{0.693}{T_{\frac{1}{2}}}$$

Equation 9.13

A typical exponential decay curve is shown in Figure 9.5.

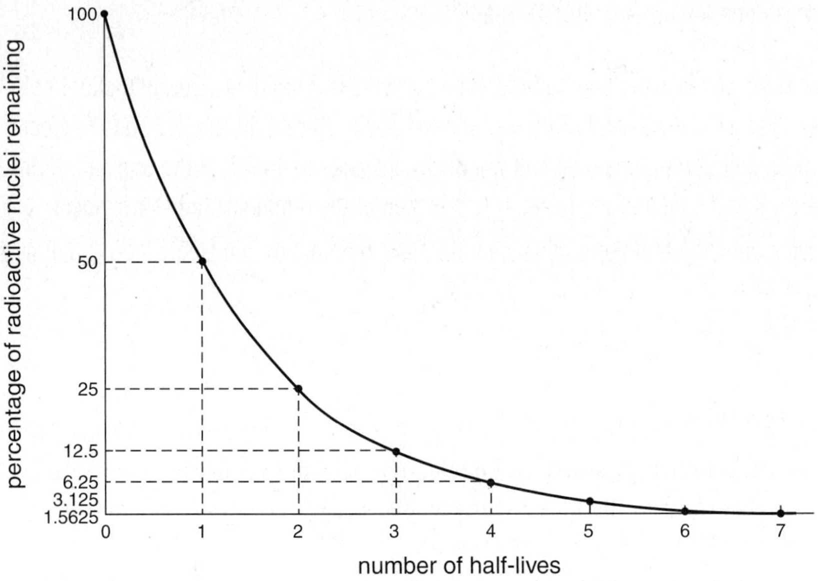

Figure 9.5 Exponential Decay

Example: If at time $t = 0$, there is a 2 mole sample of radioactive isotopes, how many nuclei remain after 45 minutes, assuming a decay constant of 2 hr^{-1}? (Hint: $e^{-\frac{3}{2}} = 0.22$).

Solution: This question is asking for an application of the exponential decay equation:

$$n = n_0 e^{-\lambda t} = n_0 e^{-(2\ \text{hr}^{-1})\left(\frac{3}{4}\ \text{hr}\right)} = n_0 e^{-\frac{3}{2}}$$

Raising Euler's number (e) to an exponent—especially a fractional exponent—is beyond the scope of the math on the MCAT, but the value of $e^{-\frac{3}{2}}$ is 0.22. Thus, 22% of the original 2 mole sample remains. This constitutes 0.44 mol, which, if multiplied by Avogadro's number, gives us the number of nuclei remaining:

$$0.44\ \text{mol} \times 6.02 \times 10^{23}\ \frac{\text{nuclei}}{\text{mol}} = 2.64 \times 10^{23}\ \text{nuclei}$$

MCAT CONCEPT CHECK 9.4

Before you move on, assess your understanding of the material with these questions.

1. True or False: Nuclear fission and nuclear fusion both release energy.
2. Compare and contrast nuclear fission and nuclear fusion reactions:

Nuclear Reaction	Size of Reactant Particles	Change in Nuclear Mass during Reaction (Increase or Decrease)
Fission		
Fusion		

3. Complete the following chart:

Nuclear Reaction	Emits . . .	ΔZ	ΔA
Alpha decay			
Beta-negative decay			
Beta-positive decay			
Gamma decay			
Electron capture			

4. How many half-lives are necessary for the complete decay of a radioactive sample?

5. Which type of nuclear decay could be detected in an atomic absorption spectrum?

Conclusion

Congratulations! You've finished the physics material that will be needed for Test Day. Our last topic was the interaction of energy and matter on the atomic level. We began by examining the photoelectric effect. Further, we took a look at Bohr's model of the hydrogen ion, and made some generalizations about electronic structure and the permissible states in regards to absorption and emission of light energy. We also noted that on a molecular level, small changes in structure can lead to significant shifts in absorption. We studied the interactions of the nucleus with energy, including the prototypical nuclear reactions of fusion and fission. We finished our discussion of nuclear reactions by examining the most common forms of nuclear decay and some of the mathematics for determining half-life or sample remaining. In the next few chapters, we'll focus on building Test Day skills, including MCAT math shortcuts that will make many of these concepts more rewarding.

You've reviewed the content, now test your knowledge and critical thinking skills by completing a test-like passage set in your online resources!

GO ONLINE

CONCEPT SUMMARY

The Photoelectric Effect

- The **photoelectric effect** is the ejection of an electron from the surface of a metal in response to light.
- The **threshold frequency** is the minimum light frequency necessary to eject an electron from a given metal.
    - The **work function** is the minimum energy necessary to eject an electron from a given metal. Its value depends on the metal used and can be calculated by multiplying the threshold frequency by **Planck's constant**.
    - The greater the energy of the incident photon above the work function, the more kinetic energy the ejected electron can possess.
- The ejected electrons create a current; the magnitude of this current is proportional to the intensity of the incident beam of light.

Absorption and Emission of Light

- The **Bohr model of the atom** states that electron energy levels are stable and discrete, corresponding to specific orbits.
    - An electron can jump from a lower-energy to a higher-energy orbit by **absorbing** a photon of light of the same frequency as the energy difference between the orbits.
    - When an electron falls from a higher-energy to a lower-energy orbit, it **emits** a photon of light of the same frequency as the energy difference between the orbits.
- **Absorption spectra** may be impacted by small changes in molecular structure.
- **Fluorescence** occurs when a species absorbs high-frequency light and then returns to its **ground state** in multiple steps. Each step has less energy than the absorbed light and is within the visible range of the electromagnetic spectrum.

Nuclear Binding Energy and Mass Defect

- **Nuclear binding energy** is the amount of energy that is released when **nucleons** (protons and neutrons) bind together.
    - The more binding energy per nucleon released, the more stable the nucleus.
    - The four fundamental forces of nature are the **strong** and **weak nuclear force**, which contribute to the stability of the nucleus, electrostatic forces, and gravitation.
- The **mass defect** is the difference between the mass of the unbonded nucleons and the mass of the bonded nucleons within the nucleus.
    - The unbonded constituents have more energy and, therefore, more mass than the bonded constituents.
    - The mass defect is the amount of mass converted to energy during nuclear fusion.

Nuclear Reactions

- **Fusion** occurs when small nuclei combine into larger nuclei.
- **Fission** occurs when a large nucleus splits into smaller nuclei.
- Energy is released in both fusion and fission because the nuclei formed in both processes are more stable than the starting nuclei.
- **Radioactive** decay is the loss of small particles from the nucleus.
  - **Alpha (α) decay** is the emission of an alpha particle $\left(\alpha, {}_{2}^{4}\alpha, {}_{2}^{4}\text{He}\right)$, which is a helium nucleus.
  - **Beta-negative (β^-) decay** is the decay of a neutron into a proton, with emission of an electron (e^-, β^-) and an antineutrino ($\overline{\nu}$).
  - **Beta-positive (β^+) decay**, also called **positron emission**, is the decay of a proton into a neutron, with emission of a **positron** (e^+, β^+) and a neutrino (ν).
  - **Gamma (γ) decay** is the emission of a gamma ray, which converts a high-energy nucleus into a more stable nucleus.
  - **Electron capture** is the absorption of an electron from the inner shell that combines with a proton in the nucleus to form a neutron.
- **Half-life** is the amount of time required for half of a sample of radioactive nuclei to decay.
- In **exponential decay**, the rate at which radioactive nuclei decay is proportional to the number of nuclei that remain.

ANSWERS TO CONCEPT CHECKS

9.1

1. The work function describes the minimum amount of energy necessary to emit an electron. Any additional energy from a photon will be converted to excess kinetic energy during the photoelectric effect.
2. The threshold frequency depends on the chemical composition of a material (that is, the identity of the metal).
3. The accumulation of moving electrons creates a current during the photoelectric effect.

9.2

1. The energy differences between ground-state electrons and higher-level electron orbits determine the frequencies of light a particular material absorbs (its absorption spectrum).
2. False. Small changes, such as protonation and deprotonation, change in oxidation state or bond order, and others may cause dramatic changes in light absorption in a material.
3. When electrons transition from a higher-energy state to a lower-energy state, they will experience photon emission.
4. Fluorescence is a special stepwise photon emission in which an excited electron returns to the ground state through one or more intermediate excited states. Each energy transition releases a photon of light. With smaller energy transitions than the initial energy absorbed, these materials can release photons of light in the visible range.

9.3

1. The strong nuclear force is one of the four primary forces and provides the adhesive force between the nucleons (protons and neutrons) within the nucleus. Mass defect is the apparent loss of mass when nucleons come together, as some of the mass is converted into energy. That energy is called the binding energy.
2. The four fundamental forces of nature are the strong and weak nuclear forces, electrostatic forces, and gravitation.
3. Mass defect is related to the binding energy such that there is a transformation of nuclear matter to energy with a resultant loss of matter. They are related by the equation $E = mc^2$.

9.4

1. True. While they may seem like inverses of each other, both nuclear fusion and nuclear fission reactions release energy.

2.

Nuclear Reaction	Size of Reactant Particles	Change in Nuclear Mass during Reaction (Increase or Decrease)
Fission	Large (actinides, lanthanides)	Decrease
Fusion	Small (hydrogen, helium)	Increase

3.

Nuclear Reaction	Emits...	ΔZ	ΔA
Alpha decay	Alpha particle $\left(\alpha, {}_{2}^{4}\alpha, {}_{2}^{4}\mathrm{He}\right)$	−2	−4
Beta-negative decay	Electron (e^-, β^-) and antineutrino ($\bar{\nu}$)	+1	0
Beta-positive decay	Positron (e^+, β^+) and neutrino (ν).	−1	0
Gamma decay	Gamma ray (γ)	0	0
Electron capture	Nothing (absorbs an electron from inner shell)	−1	0

4. Because the amount remaining is cut in half after each half-life, the portion remaining will never quite reach zero. This is mostly a theoretical consideration; "all" of a sample is considered to have decayed after 7 to 8 half-lives.

5. Because gamma radiation produces electromagnetic radiation (rather than nuclear fragments), it can be detected on an atomic absorption spectrum.

SCIENCE MASTERY ASSESSMENT EXPLANATIONS

1. **C**

To determine the speed of the electrons ejected, we must first calculate their kinetic energy:

$$\begin{aligned} K &= hf - W \\ &= \left(6.626 \times 10^{-34}\ \text{J·s}\right)\left(1.0 \times 10^{14}\ \text{Hz}\right) - 6.622 \times 10^{-20}\ \text{J} \\ &= (6.626 - 6.622) \times 10^{-20} = 0.004 \times 10^{-20} = 4 \times 10^{-23}\ \text{J} \end{aligned}$$

Now with a value for kinetic energy, we can calculate the speed of the ejected electrons:

$$\begin{aligned} K &= \frac{1}{2}mv^2 \rightarrow v = \sqrt{\frac{2K}{m}} \\ &= \sqrt{\frac{2\left(4 \times 10^{-23}\ \text{J}\right)}{9.1 \times 10^{-31}\ \text{kg}}} \approx \sqrt{\frac{8 \times 10^{-23}}{9 \times 10^{-31}}} \approx \sqrt{10^8} = 10^4\ \frac{\text{m}}{\text{s}} \end{aligned}$$

Notice the wide range in the exponents for the answer choices. While the math in this question may seem complex, this allows us to round significantly.

2. **B**

To determine the wavelength of the light ray, first calculate its frequency from the photoelectric effect equation:

$$\begin{aligned} K &= hf - W \rightarrow f = \frac{K + W}{h} \\ &= \frac{50\ \text{J} + 16\ \text{J}}{6.626 \times 10^{-34}\ \text{J}\cdot\text{s}} \approx \frac{6.6 \times 10^{1}}{6.6 \times 10^{-34}} = 10^{35}\ \text{Hz} \end{aligned}$$

In this case, estimation of Planck's constant makes our calculation much simpler without leading us to a nonviable answer. It is worth attempting an estimation first to avoid doing more work than necessary. Now we can determine the wavelength of the incident ray of light by relating the frequency to the speed of light:

$$c = f\lambda \rightarrow \lambda = \frac{c}{f}$$

$$= \frac{3.00 \times 10^{8}\ \frac{\text{m}}{\text{s}}}{10^{35}\ \text{Hz}} = 3 \times 10^{-27}\ \text{m}$$

3. **D**

The Bohr model is based on a set of postulates originally put forward to discuss the behavior of electrons in hydrogen. In summary, these postulates state that the energy levels of the electron are stable and discrete, and they correspond to specific orbits, eliminating **(A)**. They also state that an electron emits or absorbs radiation only when making a transition from one energy level to another, eliminating **(B)**. Specifically, when an electron jumps from a lower-energy orbit to a higher-energy one, it must absorb a photon of light of precisely the right frequency such that the photon's energy equals the energy difference between the two orbits, eliminating **(C)**. When falling from a higher-energy orbit to a lower-energy one, an electron emits a photon of light with a frequency that corresponds to the energy difference between the two orbits, This is the opposite of **(D)**, which makes it the right answer.

4. **B**

To solve this question correctly, one must be careful with the units. First, convert 10.2 eV to joules:

$$10.2\ \text{eV}\left(1.60 \times 10^{-19}\ \frac{\text{J}}{\text{eV}}\right) \approx 1.6 \times 10^{-18}\ \text{J}$$

Next, to determine the wavelength of the radiation, we can combine the formulas $E = hf$ and $c = f\lambda$:

$$\begin{aligned} E &= hf = \frac{hc}{\lambda} \rightarrow \lambda = \frac{hc}{E} \\ &= \frac{\left(6.626 \times 10^{-34}\ \text{J}\cdot\text{s}\right)\left(3.00 \times 10^{8}\ \frac{\text{m}}{\text{s}}\right)}{\left(1.6 \times 10^{-18}\ \text{J}\right)} \\ &\approx \frac{(4)(3)\left(10^{-26}\right)}{10^{-18}} = 12 \times 10^{-8} = 1.2 \times 10^{-7}\ \text{m} \end{aligned}$$

5. **B**

The electron moves from a higher energy level to a lower energy level; this can only occur if the extra energy is dissipated through the emission of a photon. If the electron moved from B to A, it would absorb a photon and increase the atom's total energy; however, the opposite is occurring, so **(A)** and **(D)** can be eliminated. The work function is the amount of energy required to eject an electron from a material; when moving from A to B, the electrical potential energy of the atom decreases, meaning that more energy will be required to free the electron from the atom, eliminating **(C)**.

6. **B**

The strong nuclear force is the attractive force that holds protons and neutrons together in the nucleus, supporting choice **(B)**. This force is greater than the electrostatic repulsion between protons. Note that binding energy, **(A)**, is not one of the four fundamental forces.

7. **A**

The greater the intensity, the greater the number of incident photons and, therefore, the greater the number of electrons that will be ejected from the metal surface (provided that the frequency of the light remains above the threshold). This means a larger current. Remember that the frequency of the light (assuming it is above the threshold frequency) will determine the kinetic energy of the ejected electrons; the intensity of the light determines the number of electrons ejected per time (the current).

8. **C**

To determine the binding energy, we must first determine the mass defect. The mass defect is simply the masses of each of the protons and neutrons in the unbound state added together minus the mass of the formed argon-40 nucleus (which contains 18 protons and $40 - 18 = 22$ neutrons):

$$\begin{aligned}\text{mass defect} &= (18 \times 1.0073\text{ amu}) + (22 \times 1.0087\text{ amu}) \\ &\quad - 39.9132\text{ amu} \\ &\approx (18 \times 1.007) + (22 \times 1.009) - 39.9132 \\ &= 18.126 + 22.198 - 39.9132 \\ &= 40.324 - 39.9132 \\ &\approx 0.4\ (\text{actual} = 0.4096\text{ amu})\end{aligned}$$

This math was difficult without a calculator, but by rounding one value down (proton) and one value up (neutron) by similar amounts we ended up very near the actual value. Calculating $18 \times 7 = 126$ and $22 \times 9 = 198$ for the decimal values is more manageable than the exact numbers and the spacing of the answer choices allows for our estimation. The binding energy can then be determined from this mass defect:

$$E = mc^2 = 0.4096\text{ amu} \times 932\ \frac{\text{MeV}}{\text{amu}} \approx 0.4 \times 900 = 360\text{ MeV}$$

The closest answer is **(C)**.

9. **C**

This process can be described as electron capture. Certain unstable radionuclides are capable of capturing an inner electron that combines with a proton to form a neutron. The atomic number becomes one less than the original, but the mass number remains the same. Electron capture is a relatively rare process and can be thought of as the reverse of β^- decay. Notice that the equation is similar to that of β^+ decay but not identical because a particle is absorbed, not emitted.

10. **C**

This problem presents a reaction and asks for the energy liberated due to the transformation of mass into energy. To convert mass into energy, we are told that 1 amu can be converted into 932 MeV of energy. All we need to do now is calculate how much mass, in amu, is converted in the reaction. Because we are given the atomic mass for each of the elements in the reaction, this is simply a matter of balancing the equation:

$$\begin{aligned}\text{mass defect} &= (1.0087\text{ amu} + 10.0129\text{ amu}) \\ &\quad - (7.0160\text{ amu} + 4.0026\text{ amu}) \\ &= 11.0216 - 11.0186 \\ &= 0.0030\text{ amu}\end{aligned}$$

Given both the small magnitude of this value and the small difference of the answer choices, it is best to not round at this point of the calculation. This is the amount of mass that has been converted into energy. To obtain energy from mass, we have to multiply by the conversion factor ($1\text{ amu} = 932\text{ MeV}$):

$$E = 0.003 \times 932 \approx 0.003 \times 900 = 2.7\text{ MeV}$$

At this point we were able to round for an easier calculation that keeps us very near the correct answer choice.

11. **C**

Because the half-life of element X is four days, 50% of an original sample remains after four days, 25% remains after eight days, and 12.5% remains after 12 days. Therefore, $n = 12$ days. Another approach is to set $\left(\frac{1}{2}\right)^x = 0.125$, where x is the number of half-lives that have elapsed. Solving for x gives $x = 3$. Thus, 3 half-lives have elapsed, and because each half-life is four days, we know that $n = 12$ days.

12. **B**

The expression $n = n_0 e^{-\lambda t}$ is equivalent to $\frac{n}{n_0} = e^{-\lambda t}$. Taking the natural logarithm of both sides, we get:

$$\ln\left(\frac{n}{n_0}\right) = -\lambda t$$

From this expression, it is clear that plotting $\ln\left(\frac{n}{n_0}\right)$ *vs.* t will give a straight line with a slope of $-\lambda$.

13. **C**

A typical carbon nucleus contains 6 protons and 6 neutrons. An α-particle contains 2 protons and 2 neutrons. Therefore, one carbon nucleus can dissociate into $\frac{6}{2} = 3$ α-particles.

14. **A**

Because the half-life of carbon-12 is essentially infinite, a 25% decrease in the ratio of carbon-14 to carbon-12 means the same as a 25% decrease in the amount of carbon-14. If less than half of the carbon-14 has deteriorated, then less than one half-life has elapsed. Therefore, the sample is less than 5,730 years old. Be careful with the wording here—the question states that the ratio is 25% *less* than the ratio in nature, not 25% *of* the ratio in nature, which would correspond to **(D)**.

15. **D**

In alpha decay, an element loses two protons. In positron decay, a proton is converted into a neutron. Gamma decay has no impact on the atomic number of the nuclide. Therefore, two alpha decays and two positron decays will yield a daughter nuclide with six fewer protons than the parent nuclide.

Consult your online resources for additional practice. GO ONLINE

EQUATIONS TO REMEMBER

(9.1) **Energy of a photon of light:** $E = hf$

(9.2) **Maximum kinetic energy of an electron in the photoelectric effect:** $K_{\text{max}} = hf - W$

(9.3) **Work function:** $W = hf_{\text{T}}$

(9.4) **Mass defect and energy:** $E = mc^2$

(9.5) **Nuclear decay (general form):** ${}_{Z}^{A}\text{X} \rightarrow {}_{Z'}^{A'}\text{Y} + \text{emitted decay particle}$

(9.6) **Alpha decay:** ${}_{Z}^{A}\text{X} \rightarrow {}_{Z-2}^{A-4}\text{Y} + {}_{2}^{4}\alpha$

(9.7) **Beta-negative decay:** ${}_{Z}^{A}\text{X} \rightarrow {}_{Z+1}^{A}\text{Y} + \beta^-$

(9.8) **Beta-positive decay (positron emission):** ${}_{Z}^{A}\text{X} \rightarrow {}_{Z-1}^{A}\text{Y} + \beta^+$

(9.9) **Gamma decay:** ${}_{Z}^{A}\text{X}^* \rightarrow {}_{Z}^{A}\text{X} + \gamma$

(9.10) **Electron capture:** ${}_{Z}^{A}\text{X} \rightarrow e^- \rightarrow {}_{Z-1}^{A}\text{Y}$

(9.11) **Rate of nuclear decay:** $\frac{\Delta n}{\Delta t} = -\lambda n$

(9.12) **Exponential decay:** $n = n_0 e^{-\lambda t}$

(9.13) **Decay constant:** $\lambda = \frac{\ln 2}{T_{\frac{1}{2}}} = \frac{0.693}{T_{\frac{1}{2}}}$

SHARED CONCEPTS

General Chemistry Chapter 1
Atomic Structure

General Chemistry Chapter 2
The Periodic Table

Organic Chemistry Chapter 11
Spectroscopy

Physics and Math Chapter 1
Kinematics and Dynamics

Physics and Math Chapter 2
Work and Energy

Physics and Math Chapter 8
Light and Optics

CHAPTER 10

MATHEMATICS

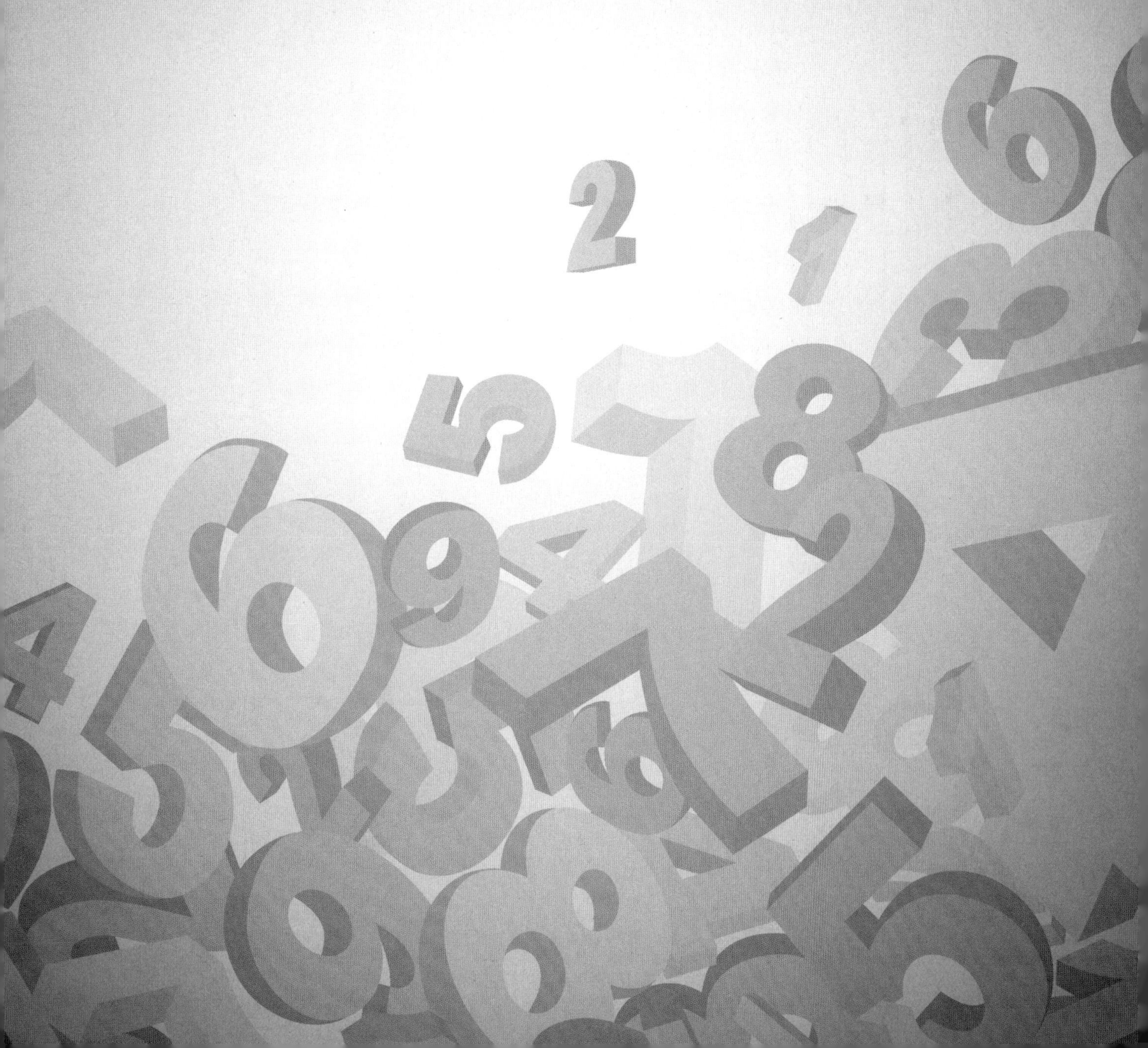

SCIENCE MASTERY ASSESSMENT

Every pre-med knows this feeling: there is so much content I have to know for the MCAT! How do I know what to do first or what's important?

While the high-yield badges throughout this book will help you identify the most important topics, this Science Mastery Assessment is another tool in your MCAT prep arsenal. This quiz (which can also be taken in your online resources) and the guidance below will help ensure that you are spending the appropriate amount of time on this chapter based on your personal strengths and weaknesses. Don't worry though—skipping something now does not mean you'll never study it. Later on in your prep, as you complete full-length tests, you'll uncover specific pieces of content that you need to review and can come back to these chapters as appropriate.

How to Use This Assessment

If you answer 0–7 questions correctly:

Spend about 1 hour to read this chapter in full and take limited notes throughout. Follow up by reviewing **all** quiz questions to ensure that you now understand how to solve each one.

If you answer 8–11 questions correctly:

Spend 20–40 minutes reviewing the quiz questions. Beginning with the questions you missed, read and take notes on the corresponding subchapters. For questions you answered correctly, ensure your thinking matches that of the explanation and you understand why each choice was correct or incorrect.

If you answer 12–15 questions correctly:

Spend less than 20 minutes reviewing all questions from the quiz. If you missed any, then include a quick read-through of the corresponding subchapters, or even just the relevant content within a subchapter, as part of your question review. For questions you got correct, ensure your thinking matches that of the explanation and review the Concept Summary at the end of the chapter.

1. How would the number 17,060 be written in scientific notation?
   A. 1706×10^1
   B. 1.706×10^4
   C. 1.7060×10^4
   D. 0.17060×10^5

2. How does the number of significant digits differ between 14,320,010 and 3.618000?
   A. 14,320,010 has more significant digits than 3.618000
   B. 14,320,010 has fewer significant digits than 3.618000
   C. 14,320,010 has the same number of significant digits as 3.618000
   D. A comparison cannot be made because the numbers are not both in scientific notation.

3. Using the appropriate number of significant digits, what is the answer to the following math problem? (Note: Assume all numbers are the results of measurements.)

$$3.060 \times 4.10 + 200 =$$

   A. 210
   B. 213
   C. 212.5
   D. 212.55

4. Which of the following would be the most appropriate setup for estimating the value 3.6×4.85 for questions in which answer choices differ by a small margin?
   A. 3.5×5
   B. 3.5×4.5
   C. 4×4
   D. 4×5

5. The value of $200^{0.25}$ is closest to:
   A. 4
   B. 14
   C. 50
   D. 800

6. If A and B are real numbers, which of the following equations is INCORRECT?
   A. $A^3 \times B^3 = (AB)^3$
   B. $A^5 \div A^7 = A^{-2}$
   C. $(A^{0.5})^4 + A^2 = 2A^2$
   D. $(A^3)^2 = A^9$

7. How can the value of a natural logarithm be converted to the value of a common logarithm?
   A. The natural logarithm is divided by a constant.
   B. A constant is added to or subtracted from the natural logarithm.
   C. The natural logarithm is raised to an exponent.
   D. The inverse of the natural logarithm is taken.

8. What is the minimum value of $2 \cos \theta - 1$?
   A. -3
   B. -2
   C. -1
   D. 0

9. Which of the following relationships is INCORRECT?
   A. $|\sin \theta \times \cos \theta| < |\sin \theta| + |\cos \theta|$
   B. $\sin \theta \div \cos \theta = \tan \theta$
   C. $\tan 90°$ is undefined
   D. $\sin \theta = \sin (90° - \theta)$

10. What is the approximate pH of a solution with a pK_a of 3.6, [HA] = 100 m*M*, and $[A^-]$ = 0.1 *M*?

(Note: $pH = pK_a + \log \frac{[A^-]}{[HA]}$)

A. 1.6
B. 3.6
C. 5.6
D. 7.6

11. At what temperature do the Fahrenheit and Celsius scales give equal values?

A. 0 K
B. 233 K
C. 313 K
D. 273 K

12. In a certain rigid container, pressure and temperature are directly proportional. If the pressure is changed from 540 torr to 180 torr via a temperature change, by what factor has the temperature changed?

A. 360
B. 3
C. 1
D. $\frac{1}{3}$

13. A 150-pound adult must be given a drug that is dosed at $1.5 \frac{\text{mg drug}}{\text{kg body mass}}$. Approximately how many milligrams of the drug should be administered per dose? (Note: 1 lb = 4.45 N)

A. 33 mg
B. 67 mg
C. 100 mg
D. 225 mg

14. The rate of a reaction is calculated as a change in concentration per time. What are the units of the rate constant, *k*, in a reaction that is second order overall with respect to one species? (Note: A second-order reaction of this type has a rate law with the form rate = $k[A]^2$, where [A] is the concentration of the species.)

A. $\frac{1}{s}$
B. $\frac{M}{s}$
C. $\frac{L}{mol \cdot s}$
D. $\frac{L^2}{mol^2 \cdot s}$

15. One group of people requires a base level of 900 Calories per day plus an additional 12 Calories per kilogram of body mass per day. A second group requires a base level of 500 Calories per day, plus 15 Calories per kilogram of body mass per day. At what mass does the first group and the second group have the same caloric needs?

A. 26 kg
B. 67 kg
C. 133 kg
D. 266 kg

Answer Key

1. **B**
2. **C**
3. **B**
4. **A**
5. **A**
6. **D**
7. **A**
8. **A**
9. **D**
10. **B**
11. **B**
12. **D**
13. **C**
14. **C**
15. **C**

Detailed explanations can be found at the end of the chapter.

CHAPTER 10

MATHEMATICS

In This Chapter

Introduction

Going to the grocery store is not so different from solving an MCAT multiple choice question. You begin the process by determining how much of each item you need in the near future. Once you know what you need, you check what you already have in order to determine the quantity you need to buy to reach your goal. When you get to the store, you compare that amount to the containers on the shelves. Often they won't match exactly. Say, for example, that you need a total of 16 ounces of peas for a recipe. You already have 5 at home, so you only need 11 more. Packages of peas, however, may only come in 10- or 16-ounce packages. At that point, you choose the best one for your needs—the 16-ounce package; better to have a little extra than to run short!

If you've ever shopped in an international grocery store, this process can become even more elaborate because the packaging sizes and currency may not match the units with which you are familiar. You may have never taken the time to consider how intensive one's critical thinking must be to efficiently navigate the grocery store, but recognize that it's the same process you need to use on Test Day. First, figure out what you want (what is the question looking for), what you have (information in a passage, question stem, or outside knowledge), and what's needed (calculations and critical thinking), and then make a decision (by matching your answer, eliminating wrong answer choices, or guessing strategically). In this chapter, we'll be focusing on the calculations and critical thinking of mathematics. The math required for the MCAT is on the level of precalculus. You won't need any derivatives or integrals on Test Day, but rapid application of arithmetic, exponent and logarithm rules, trigonometry, statistics, and graphical analysis may be necessary to navigate the MCAT efficiently. In this chapter, you won't see very much new content, but consider this an opportunity to hone your mathematics skills.

MCAT EXPERTISE

You may note that this chapter and the chapters following do not contain the typical chapter profile, as they aren't directly related to Physics or AAMC content categories. However, this chapter covers fundamental math content required for calculations across all three science test sections. As such, Chapter 10 should be considered a must-review chapter!

10.1 Arithmetic and Significant Figures

LEARNING OBJECTIVES

After Chapter 10.1, you will be able to:

- Convert values to and from scientific notation
- Determine the significant digits within a number, such as: 1,547,200
- Apply rounding techniques in multiplication and division problems

KEY CONCEPT

It is essential to use judicious rounding and math strategies on Test Day to get through the MCAT efficiently. This is particularly true in the *Chemical and Physical Foundations of Biological Systems* section. Do not try to solve for an exact answer–do only as much as you need to be able to choose the right answer choice!

The MCAT often uses numbers that aren't particularly "nice" looking, especially considering that calculators cannot be used on the test. However, the testmakers *also* know that calculators aren't allowed, so even the most complex math still has to be solvable in a reasonable amount of time. We reconcile these two opposing concepts by using a few Test Day tricks: scientific notation, which can help us narrow down the exponent of our answer choice and often gives the answer directly; and judicious estimation, which will differentiate between otherwise similar answers. While significant figures won't lead us to an answer in the way that the other MCAT skills will, it is a testable topic on the MCAT.

Scientific Notation

Scientific notation is a method of writing numbers that takes advantage of **powers of ten**. In scientific notation, a number is written with a **significand** and an **exponent**. This is much easier to conceptualize with an example. Consider the number 217. The math using this number can be somewhat cumbersome. By transforming it into scientific notation (2.17×10^2), the number becomes easier to manipulate because the power of 10 has been pulled out. In this case, 2.17 is the significand (also called the **coefficient** or **mantissa**), and the 2 in 10^2 is the exponent.

The significand must be a number with an absolute value in the range [1,10). This means that it is any real number between -10 and -1 (not including -10) or between 1 and 10 (not including 10). By extension, the significand cannot begin with a 0, nor can it begin with two digits before the decimal point. The exponent, on the other hand, can be any whole number—positive, negative, or 0.

If at any time your calculations are not in scientific notation, consider adjusting them. While there is a small time investment converting to scientific notation, the time saved on subsequent calculations usually makes up for—and often exceeds—this time investment. This is especially true for questions in which the answers differ by powers of ten. The only exception to maintaining scientific notation is in the calculation of square roots, which are discussed later in this chapter.

Significant Figures

Significant figures provide an indication of our certainty of a measurement, and help us to avoid exceeding that certainty when performing calculations. Significant figures are determined by the precision of the instrument being used for measurement. For example, imagine that you are measuring the width of a block of wood with a ruler. The ruler has markings for centimeters and millimeters; you could state with confidence the width of the block in millimeters—say, 55 millimeters.

However, on this ruler, there are no markings smaller than millimeters; you'd be forced to estimate where within the interval between two millimeter markings the block reaches—say 55.2 millimeters. You cannot be 100 percent confident about this decimal, but some information is better than none, and writing it down lets you know that you *were* confident about the first two digits.

In the situation we just described, only the first two digits would be considered significant because we know that they were measured accurately. We can hold on to the third digit during calculations, but by the time we reach a final answer, we need to reduce the answer to an appropriate number of significant figures. To determine the number of significant figures in a number:

- Count all numbers between the first nonzero digit on the left and the last nonzero digit on the right. Any digit between these two markers (including 0) is significant.
- Any zeroes to the left of the first nonzero digit are considered **leading zeroes** and are not significant.
- If there are zeroes to the right of the last nonzero digit *and* there is a decimal point in the number, then those zeroes are significant figures. If there is no decimal point, they are not significant. For example, 3,490 has three significant figures, while 3,490.0 has five.
- For measurements, the last digit is usually an estimation and is not considered significant (as in the example above).

Scientific notation can clarify significant figures when it contains a decimal point. When converting between standard numbers and scientific notation, be sure to maintain the number of significant figures. 100.0 is written in scientific notation as 1.000×10^2, while 100 is written as 1×10^2 because the **trailing zeroes** in the first example are significant while in the second example they are not.

BRIDGE

Significant figures are important because they give an indication of the accuracy of a measurement. Inaccurate measurements can bias research or lead to faulty conclusions. When presented with data, look for accuracy of the measurements in two ways: identifying the number of significant digits in a number, and looking for error margins or statistical significance in graphs. These latter topics are discussed in Chapter 12 of *MCAT Physics and Math Review*.

Math with Significant Figures

Significant figure estimations are most important in the laboratory sciences, particularly analytical chemistry. For multiplication and division, maintain as many digits as possible throughout the calculations so that there is very little rounding error, then round to the number of significant digits that is the same as the *least number of significant digits* in any of the factors, divisors, or dividends. With addition and subtraction, *decimal points are maintained* rather than maintaining significant figures. The convention for decimal points is the same as for significant figures: the answer may have only as many decimal digits as the initial number with the fewest decimal digits.

MCAT EXPERTISE

Most Test Day math (and, by extension, this *Kaplan MCAT Review* series) neglects significant figures in the answer choices. These calculations are only necessary when specified by the question stem or passage.

Example: Determine the volume of a cylinder with a radius that is measured as 7.45 m and a height of 8.323 m. (Note: Use 3.14159 as π, and round the answer to the correct number of significant digits.)

Solution:

$$\begin{aligned} V &= A_{\text{base}} \times h \\ &= (\pi r^2) \times h \\ &= (3.14159)(7.45\text{ m})^2(8.323\text{ m}) \\ &= 1{,}451.249 \end{aligned}$$

Because all of the factors are multiplied, the answer should have the same number of significant digits as the factor with the fewest number of significant digits. In this case, that is the radius, which has only two significant digits (remember that, in the case of measurements, the last digit is an estimate and is not considered significant). Therefore, the correct answer is 1,500 or 1.5×10^3.

Estimation

On Test Day, much of your math will be determined by the answer choices provided. If the answer choices are very close together, there will be minimal opportunity for rounding; when they are far apart, rough estimations are all that are necessary. While estimation of addition and subtraction are relatively simple rounding choices, we'll review a few tricks for multiplication and division.

Multiplication

Consider the following multiplication problem: $(3.17 \times 10^4) \times (4.53 \times 10^5)$. To three significant digits, the answer to this multiplication problem is 1.44×10^{10}, but this precise calculation is beyond the scope of mental math. However, even if the answer choices are close, it is generally acceptable to round to one decimal place, or $(3.2 \times 10^4) \times (4.5 \times 10^5)$. When rounding numbers in multiplication, keep in mind whether the rounded number is larger or smaller than the original number. If one number is rounded up, it is best to round the other number down slightly to compensate. Even with this rounding, the answer still comes out as 1.44×10^{10}.

If the answer choices are *very* far apart—differing by, say, powers of ten—we can adjust the numbers so that one contains only one significant digit, further simplifying the math. In this example, the calculations could be adjusted to $(3 \times 10^4) \times (4.5 \times 10^5)$, or 1.35×10^{10}. This represents an error of 6.25%, which is still close enough to choose the correct answer for most questions on Test Day.

Division

Let's also consider division as an avenue for estimation. While in our multiplication example we adjusted each number in an opposite direction, with division we are attempting to make proportional adjustments in the same direction. Consider the following example:

Example: Estimate the value of $15.4 \div 3.80$.

Solution: Estimations in division should be made by shifting both numbers in the same direction. It is often easier to adjust the divisor first to simplify calculations. If we round the divisor up to 4, we should round the dividend up accordingly. In this case, it makes sense to round the dividend up to 16—which is not only a whole number, but also a multiple of 4. Our estimate is $16 \div 4 = 4$. Note that, despite this very rough adjustment, we are still very close to the true value of 4.05.

KEY CONCEPT

When rounding numbers to be multiplied, round one number up and one number down to compensate. When rounding numbers to be divided, round both numbers in the same direction to compensate.

MCAT CONCEPT CHECK 10.1

1. Describe the process for converting a number into scientific notation. What values are possible for the significand?

___

___

___

2. Highlight or circle the significant digits in the following numbers:

 - 34,600.
 - 0.0003201
 - 1.10
 - 525,600

3. When rounding two numbers containing decimals, in which direction(s) should each number go for multiplication? For division?

 - Multiplication

___

 - Division

___

10.2 Exponents and Logarithms

LEARNING OBJECTIVES

After Chapter 10.2, you will be able to:

- Estimate the square root of a given value, like $\sqrt{1942}$
- Estimate the log value of a given number
- Simplify expressions such as: $(a + 2b)^3$

For many students, exponents and logarithms are topics filed away in the depths of memory. While exponential and logarithmic functions are uncommon for many people in everyday life, a number of science topics and equations regularly tested on the MCAT require use of these concepts, as shown in Table 10.1.

TOPIC	EQUATION	LOCATION IN *KAPLAN MCAT REVIEW* SERIES
Sound level	$\beta = 10 \log \frac{I}{I_0}$	Chapter 7 of *MCAT Physics and Math Review*
Exponential decay	$n = n_0 e^{-\lambda t}$	Chapter 9 of *MCAT Physics and Math Review*
Arrhenius equation for activation energy	$k = Ae^{\frac{-E_a}{RT}}$	Chapter 5 of *MCAT General Chemistry Review*
Gibbs free energy	$\Delta G^\circ_{rxn} = -RT \ln K_{eq}$	Chapter 7 of *MCAT General Chemistry Review*
p scales (pH, pOH, pK_a, pK_b)	$pH = -\log [H^+]$	Chapter 10 of *MCAT General Chemistry Review*
Henderson-Hasselbalch equation	$pH = pK_a + \log \frac{[A^-]}{[HA]}$	Chapter 10 of *MCAT General Chemistry Review*

Table 10.1 Common Exponential and Logarithmic Equations on the MCAT

Exponents

In addition to exponential equations, exponents appear frequently on the MCAT in the context of scientific notation, discussed earlier. Here, we look at the rules of arithmetic with exponents.

Exponent Identities

Only a basic understanding of exponents is necessary for the MCAT, although it can be helpful to know a few values and basic rules. First, any number to the zeroth power is equal to 1:

$$X^0 = 1$$

Equation 10.1

When adding or subtracting numbers with exponents, the true value must be calculated before the addition or subtraction can be performed. For example, $3^2 + 3^2 \neq 6^2$; rather, $3^2 + 3^2 = 9 + 9 = 18$. However, if the base and exponent are the same, we can add the coefficients: $3^2 + 3^2 = (1 + 1) \times 3^2 = 2 \times 3^2 = 18$.

In cases of multiplication and division, the exponents can be manipulated directly, as long as the base number is the same. When multiplying two numbers with the same base, the exponents are added to determine the new number:

$$X^A \times X^B = X^{(A + B)}$$

Equation 10.2

In division, we subtract the exponent of the denominator from the exponent in the numerator to find the exponent in the quotient, as long as all bases are the same:

$$\frac{X^A}{X^B} = X^{(A-B)}$$

Equation 10.3

For a number that is raised to an exponent and then raised again to another exponent, the two exponents are multiplied:

$$(X^A)^B = X^{(A \times B)}$$

Equation 10.4

When a fraction is raised to an exponent, the exponent is distributed to the numerator and denominator:

$$\left(\frac{X}{Y}\right)^A = \frac{X^A}{Y^A}$$

Equation 10.5

Negative exponents represent inverse functions:

$$X^{-A} = \frac{1}{X^A}$$

Equation 10.6

KEY CONCEPT

When adding, subtracting, multiplying, or dividing numbers with exponents, the base must be the same.

For fractional exponents, the numerator can be treated as the exponent, and the denominator represents the root of the number:

$$X^{\frac{A}{B}} = \sqrt[B]{X^A}$$

Equation 10.7

Estimating Square Roots

On Test Day, you may be expected to calculate approximate square roots. To do so, it is useful to be familiar with the values in Table 10.2.

X	X²	X	X²	X	X²	X	X²
1	1	**6**	36	**11**	121	**16**	256
2	4	**7**	49	**12**	144	**17**	289
3	9	**8**	64	**13**	169	**18**	324
4	16	**9**	81	**14**	196	**19**	361
5	25	**10**	100	**15**	225	**20**	400

Table 10.2 Square Values of Integers from 1 to 20

If you are asked to calculate the square root of any number less than 400, you can approximate its value by determining which two perfect squares it falls between. As an alternative method, you can divide the number given to you by known squares to attempt to reduce it:

$$\sqrt{180} = \sqrt{4} \times \sqrt{9} \times \sqrt{5} = 2 \times 3 \times \sqrt{5} = 6\sqrt{5}$$

One can estimate this value by considering that the square root of five is somewhere between 2 and 3 ($2^2 = 4$ and $3^2 = 9$), and is closer to 2 than 3. If we estimate $\sqrt{5}$ to be about 2.2, then $6\sqrt{5} \approx 13.2$, which is congruent with our knowledge that the square root of 180 will be between 13 and 14. The true value of $\sqrt{180}$ is approximately 13.4.

MCAT EXPERTISE

Estimation of square roots and logarithms is generally sufficient to the first decimal place; don't struggle to become more precise because it won't be necessary on Test Day.

If you are using a number in scientific notation, adjust the decimal by one place if necessary so that the exponent is easily divisible by two:

$$\sqrt{4.9 \times 10^{-7}} = \sqrt{49 \times 10^{-8}} = 7 \times 10^{-4}$$

Finally, it is useful to know the values of $\sqrt{2}$ and $\sqrt{3}$:

$$\sqrt{2} \approx 1.414 \text{ (use 1.4)}$$
$$\sqrt{3} \approx 1.732 \text{ (use 1.7)}$$

Equation 10.8

Rules of Logarithms

Logarithms follow many of the same rules as exponents because they are inverse functions. The logarithmic rules are described below:

$$\log_A 1 = 0$$
$$\log_A A = 1$$
$$\log A \times B = \log A + \log B$$
$$\log \frac{A}{B} = \log A - \log B$$
$$\log A^B = B \log A$$
$$\log \frac{1}{A} = -\log A$$

Equations 10.9 to 10.14

It is also useful to know that "p" can be shorthand for −log; thus, $\text{pH} = -\log [\text{H}^+]$, $\text{p}K_\text{a} = -\log K_\text{a}$, and so on.

Example: Derive the Henderson-Hasselbalch equation from the expression for K_a.

Solution:

$$K_\text{a} = \frac{[\text{H}^+][\text{A}^-]}{[\text{HA}]}$$
$$\log K_\text{a} = \log \frac{[\text{H}^+][\text{A}^-]}{[\text{HA}]}$$
$$\log K_\text{a} = \log [\text{H}^+] + \log [\text{A}^-] - \log [\text{HA}]$$
$$-\log [\text{H}^+] = -\log K_\text{a} + \log [\text{A}^-] - \log [\text{HA}]$$
$$\text{pH} = \text{p}K_\text{a} + \log \frac{[\text{A}^-]}{[\text{HA}]}$$

Common vs. Natural Logarithms

Logarithms can use any base, but the most common are base ten, as in our decimal system, and base ***e*** (**Euler's number**, about 2.718). Base-ten logarithms ($\log_{10}$) are called **common logarithms**, whereas those based on Euler's number ($\log_e$ or ln) are called **natural logarithms**. Both common and natural logarithms obey the rules discussed above, but it can be easier to estimate common logarithms because of our familiarity with the decimal number system. Therefore, it is useful to be able to convert between natural logarithms and common logarithms:

$$\log x \approx \frac{\ln x}{2.303}$$

Equation 10.15

KEY CONCEPT

e is Euler's number, which is 2.718281828459045. . . . It is also the base for the natural logarithm.

Estimating Logarithms

When estimating the logarithm of a number, use scientific notation. An exact logarithmic calculation of a number that is not an integer power of 10 is unnecessary on the MCAT. The testmakers are interested, however, in testing your ability to apply mathematical concepts appropriately in solving certain problems. Fortunately, there is a simple method of approximation that can be used on Test Day. If a value is written in proper scientific notation, it will be in the form $n \times 10^m$, where n is a number between 1 and 10. From this fact, we can use logarithm rules to approximate the value:

$$\begin{aligned}\log\left(n \times 10^m\right) &= \log(n) + \log\left(10^m\right)\\ &= m + \log(n)\end{aligned}$$

BRIDGE

A similar concept for estimating logarithms is used in calculations of pH, as described in Chapter 10 of *MCAT General Chemistry Review*. The shortcut is slightly different because we are working with negative logarithms and a negative exponent in the case of pH:

$-\log(n \times 10^{-m}) \approx m - 0.n.$

Because n is a number between 1 and 10, its logarithm will be a decimal between 0 and 1 ($\log 1 = 0$ and $\log 10 = 1$). The closer n is to 1, the closer $\log n$ will be to 0; the closer n is to 10, the closer $\log n$ will be to 1. As a reasonable approximation, one can say that

$$\log(n \times 10^m) \approx m + 0.n$$

Equation 10.16

where $0.n$ represents sliding the decimal point of n one position to the left (dividing n by ten). For example, $\log(9.2 \times 10^8) \approx 8 + 0.92 = 8.92$ (actual $= 8.96$).

MCAT CONCEPT CHECK 10.2

Before you move on, assess your understanding of the material with these questions.

1. Simplify the following expressions:
   - $(a + b)^2 =$ ____________________
   - $\frac{a^2+2a^2}{5a^3} =$ ____________________
   - $\log_a(a) =$ ____________________
   - $\log(a^3) - \log(a) =$ ____________________

2. Estimate $\sqrt{392}$:

____

____

____

3. Estimate log 7,426,135,420:

____

10.3 Trigonometry

LEARNING OBJECTIVES

After Chapter 10.3, you will be able to:

- Explain the appropriate way to orient vectors in vector addition
- Calculate the value of sine, cosine, or tangent for a given right triangle
- Recall the sine, cosine, and tangent values of key angles

Very little trigonometry is required for the MCAT, but a basic understanding of definitions and a strong knowledge of two special right triangles is essential for strong performance, especially on physics material.

Definitions and Relationships

For any given right triangle and angle, there are characteristic values of sine, cosine, and tangent that depend on the lengths of the legs of the triangle and of the hypotenuse, as shown in Figure 10.1.

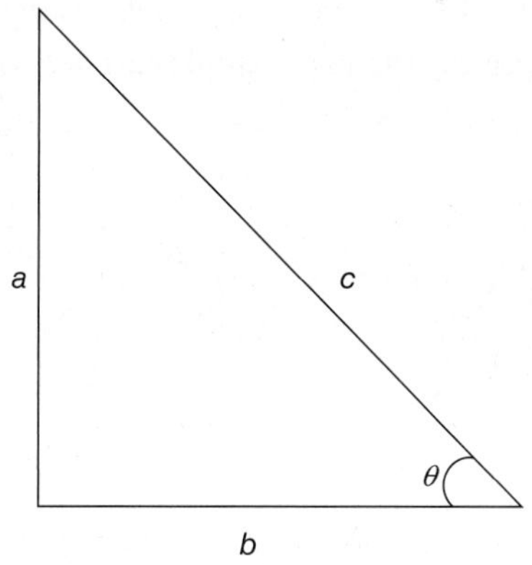

Figure 10.1 Right Triangle and Sides

Sine is calculated as the ratio between the side opposite the angle of interest and the hypotenuse:

$$\sin\theta = \frac{\text{opposite}}{\text{hypotenuse}} = \frac{a}{c}$$

Equation 10.17

Cosine is calculated as the ratio between the side adjacent to the angle of interest and the hypotenuse:

$$\cos\theta = \frac{\text{adjacent}}{\text{hypotenuse}} = \frac{b}{c}$$

Equation 10.18

MNEMONIC

Trigonometric ratios: **SOH CAH TOA:**

- **S**ine = **O**pposite ÷ **H**ypotenuse
- **C**osine = **A**djacent ÷ **H**ypotenuse
- **T**angent = **O**pposite ÷ **A**djacent

KEY CONCEPT

Trigonometric functions are useful for splitting a vector into its components; inverse trigonometric functions are useful for determining the direction of a resultant from its components.

Tangent is calculated as the ratio between the side opposite the angle of interest and the side adjacent to the angle of interest:

$$\tan\theta = \frac{\text{opposite}}{\text{adjacent}} = \frac{a}{b}$$

Equation 10.19

The values of both sine and cosine range from -1 to 1. The values of tangent, however, range from $-\infty$ to ∞.

Each trigonometric function also has an inverse function: **inverse sine** (**sin^{-1}** or **arcsin**), **inverse cosine** (**cos^{-1}** or **arccos**), and **inverse tangent** (**tan^{-1}** or **arctan**). These functions use the calculated value of sine, cosine, or tangent, and yield a numerical value for the angle of interest. For the triangle in Figure 10.1, $\sin^{-1}\left(\frac{a}{c}\right) = \theta$. Inverse trigonometric functions are most likely to appear in questions asking for the direction of a resultant in vector addition or subtraction.

Common Values

On Test Day, you must know the values of sine, cosine, and tangent for all of the angles in the 30–60–90 and 45–45–90 special right triangles, either by memorization or by drawing the triangles. The two triangles are shown in Figure 10.2.

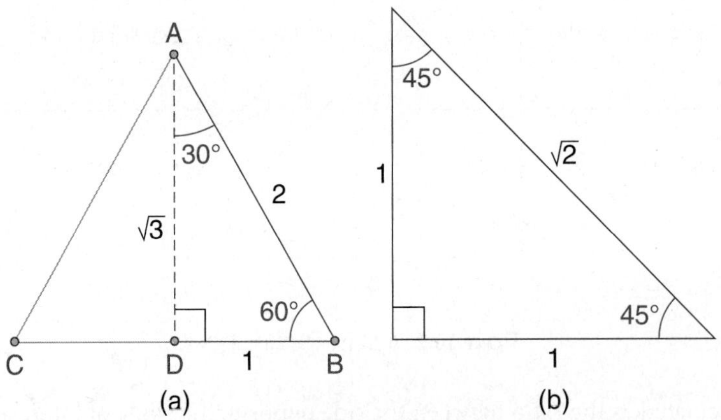

Figure 10.2 Special Right Triangles
(a) 30-60-90; (b) 45-45-90.

Important values of the trigonometric ratios at these angles are shown in Table 10.3.

θ	SIN θ	COS θ	TAN θ
0°	0	1	0
30°	$\frac{1}{2}$	$\frac{\sqrt{3}}{2}$	$\frac{\sqrt{3}}{3}$
45°	$\frac{\sqrt{2}}{2}$	$\frac{\sqrt{2}}{2}$	1
60°	$\frac{\sqrt{3}}{2}$	$\frac{1}{2}$	$\sqrt{3}$
90°	1	0	*undefined*
180°	0	-1	0

Table 10.3 Common Trigonometric Ratios on the MCAT

MCAT CONCEPT CHECK 10.3

Before you move on, assess your understanding of the material with these questions.

1. During vector addition, how is the angle of the resultant calculated?

___

2. How are sine, cosine, and tangent calculated when given the dimensions of a right triangle?
   - Sine:

   ___

   - Cosine:

   ___

   - Tangent:

   ___

3. True or False: Only angles in right triangles have characteristic values of the trigonometric functions.

4. At what angle between 0° and 180° does each trigonometric function have a value of 1?

___

10.4 Problem-Solving

LEARNING OBJECTIVES

After Chapter 10.4, you will be able to:

- Distinguish between direct and inverse relationships
- Convert between metric prefixes
- Solve a system of equations using substitution, setting equations equal, or elimination, such as: $3x + 4y = 17$ and $5x - 2y = 11$

Now that we've examined some individual mathematical skills, let's explore some common problem-solving strategies to approach MCAT questions. The use of relationships and proportionality is especially important in passage-based questions, while unit analysis can help determine which formulas are appropriate for a given question. The use of conversion factors is ubiquitous on the MCAT, as answer choices are often given in different units than the information presented. Algebraic systems are less often required, but may underlie passage interpretation and the approach to some questions.

Use of Relationships

BRIDGE

According to Boyle's law, pressure and volume have an inverse relationship: as one is doubled, the other is cut in half (keeping all else constant). On the other hand, according to Gay-Lussac's law, pressure and temperature have a direct relationship: as one is doubled, so is the other (keeping all else constant).

Relationships are generally indicated in MCAT passages by formulas or the use of proportionality constants. In other cases they may be implied and require a bit more work on our part to calculate ratios. Calculations of this type are based on multiplication and division, but explaining the relationship in words—rather than math—may make it challenging to decode the connections between the variables. In **direct relationships**, increasing one variable proportionately increases the other; as one decreases, the other decreases by the same proportion. In **inverse relationships**, an increase in one variable is associated with a proportional decrease in the other.

Conversions

The MCAT routinely increases the difficulty of a question by requiring the use of conversion factors. Equations may require that variables be in certain formats, or answer choices may differ in units from those given in the question stem. In both cases, it is necessary to convert units. The simplest conversions to perform maintain the same base unit. For example, conversion between grams, kilograms, and milligrams only requires multiplication by an appropriate power of ten. Metric prefixes and their associated powers of ten are found in Table 10.4.

FACTOR	PREFIX	PREFIX ABBREVIATION
10^{12}	*tera-*	T
10^{9}	*giga-*	G
10^{6}	*mega-*	M
10^{3}	*kilo-*	k
10^{2}	*hecto-*	h
10^{1}	*deka-*	da
10^{-1}	*deci-*	d
10^{-2}	*centi-*	c
10^{-3}	*milli-*	m
10^{-6}	*micro-*	μ
10^{-9}	*nano-*	n
10^{-12}	*pico-*	p

Table 10.4 Metric Prefixes

In addition to the conversions that are necessary for changes in prefixes, we must often convert between units, particularly between the British system and SI units. Table 10.5 shows several important conversion factors to recognize on Test Day. Conversion factors (except those for time) should not be memorized; the MCAT will provide them as necessary.

BASE UNIT	EQUIVALENT UNITS
1 mile	5280 feet (ft)
1 ft	12 inches (in)
1 inch (in)	2.54 cm
1 Calorie (Cal)	1000 cal
1 calorie (cal)	4.184 J
1 electron-volt (eV)	1.602×10^{-19} J
1 L	33.8 ounces (oz)
1 pound (lb)	4.45 N
1 atomic mass unit (amu)	1.661×10^{-27} kg

Table 10.5 Common Conversion Factors on the MCAT

Example: A car's speedometer registers a speed of 33 miles per hour. What was its speed in meters per second?

Solution: First convert distance measurements, being careful to cancel them out by arranging numerators and denominators.

$$33\frac{\text{miles}}{\text{hour}}\left(\frac{5280\text{ feet}}{1\text{ mile}}\right)\left(\frac{12\text{ inches}}{1\text{ foot}}\right)\left(\frac{2.54\text{ cm}}{1\text{ inch}}\right)\left(\frac{1\text{ m}}{100\text{ cm}}\right)$$

$$\approx\frac{(33)(5280)(30)}{100}\approx\frac{(1000)(5280)}{100}=52{,}800\frac{\text{m}}{\text{hour}}\left(\text{actual}=53{,}108\frac{\text{m}}{\text{hour}}\right)$$

Then, repeat the procedure with the time measurements.

$$53{,}108\frac{\text{m}}{\text{hour}}\left(\frac{1\text{ hour}}{3600\text{ s}}\right)\approx\frac{540}{36}=\frac{90}{6}=15\ \frac{\text{m}}{\text{s}}\ \left(\text{actual}=14.8\ \frac{\text{m}}{\text{s}}\right)$$

REAL WORLD

It is important to be able to convert between Fahrenheit and Celsius scales in medicine as different hospitals (and different medical records) may use different units. Body temperature is 98.6°F or 37°C. A fever is usually defined as a temperature above 100.4°F or 38°C. Hypothermia is usually defined as a temperature below 95.0°F or 35°C.

One special case of conversions occurs with temperature. Rather than simply multiplying by a conversion factor, there is also a component of addition or subtraction. The following formulas relate the Fahrenheit, Celsius, and Kelvin systems:

$$F=\frac{9}{5}C+32$$

$$K=C+273$$

Equation 10.20

where *F*, *C*, and *K* are the temperatures in degrees Fahrenheit, degrees Celsius, and kelvins, respectively.

Unit Analysis

Unit analysis, also called **dimensional analysis**, may help determine the correct answer even if you forget a relevant formula on Test Day. It can also serve as a double check on one's calculations because the units of the calculated answer must match the units of the answer choices. For example, consider a question in which we are given two quantities: one in $\frac{\text{N}}{\text{C}}$, and the other in volts. The answer choices for the question are all in meters. Even without remembering the equation $V=Ed$, we can infer that we must divide the voltage $\left(1\text{ V}=1\ \frac{\text{J}}{\text{C}}=1\ \frac{\text{N}\cdot\text{m}}{\text{C}}\right)$ by the electric field to get a distance in meters:

$$\frac{\text{N}\cdot\text{m}}{\text{C}}\div\frac{\text{N}}{\text{C}}=\text{m}$$

Dimensional analysis is not a foolproof strategy; it is always better to know the true relationships between variables than to infer them based on units. Still, this strategy can be effective for narrowing down (or even choosing) answer choices on Test Day.

Example: The ejection fraction is the proportion of the blood volume in the left ventricle expelled with each contraction of the heart. A patient is known to have an ejection fraction of 0.6, a cardiac output of 5 $\frac{\text{L}}{\text{min}}$, and a heart rate of 80 $\frac{\text{beats}}{\text{min}}$. What is the volume of blood in this person's left ventricle just prior to contraction?

Solution: A formula was not provided in this question, but we can recognize that the desired answer is a volume. We can start with the cardiac output and heart rate terms to determine the volume ejected per beat.

$$\frac{5\,\frac{\text{L}}{\text{min}}}{80\,\frac{\text{beats}}{\text{min}}} = \frac{1}{16} = 0.0625\,\frac{\text{L}}{\text{beat}}$$

The question also explains that only 60 percent of the blood volume is expelled from the left ventricle per heartbeat. From this, we can determine the volume of blood prior to contraction.

$$0.0625\,\frac{\text{L}}{\text{beat}} = \frac{0.6 \times \text{ventricular volume}}{\text{beat}}$$

$$\frac{0.0625}{0.6}\,\text{L} = \text{ventricular volume} \approx 0.1\text{ L (actual} = 0.104\text{ L)}$$

Algebraic Systems

The last key mathematical skill for Test Day is the ability to solve systems of linear equations. In order to solve a system of equations, there must be at least as many equations as there are variables. Where there is only one variable (which does not truly constitute a system), only one equation is necessary; for example, $6 - x = 1$ reduces to $x = 5$. In contrast, with an equation like $3x + 4y = 17$, there is insufficient data to solve for either variable with only the one equation. If a second equation is introduced, such as $5x - 2y = 11$, then we can solve for both variables using one of three methods: substituting one variable in terms of the other, setting equations equal to each other, or manipulating the equations to eliminate one of the variables.

Substitution

In substitution, we solve for one variable in one of the equations, and then insert this term into the other equation. The steps of this method are listed below.

- Solve for one of the variables in one of the equations:

$$5x - 2y = 11$$

$$y = \frac{5x - 11}{2}$$

- Insert the expression into the other equation:

$$3x + 4\left(\frac{5x - 11}{2}\right) = 17$$

- Isolate the variable and solve the resulting equation:

$$\begin{aligned} 3x + 10x - 22 &= 17 \\ 13x &= 39 \\ x &= 3 \end{aligned}$$

- Solve for the other variable using this value:

$$\begin{aligned} 3(3) + 4y &= 17 \\ 4y &= 8 \\ y &= 2 \end{aligned}$$

Setting Equations Equal

Setting equations equal to one another is a specialized case of substitution. In this method, we solve for the same variable in both equations and then set the two equations equal to each other. The steps of this method are listed below.

- Solve for the same variable in both equations:

$$y = \frac{17 - 3x}{4}$$

$$y = \frac{5x - 11}{2}$$

- Set the equations equal to each other, isolate the variable, and solve for the variable:

$$\begin{aligned} \frac{17 - 3x}{4} &= \frac{5x - 11}{2} \\ 17 - 3x &= 10x - 22 \\ 39 &= 13x \\ 3 &= x \end{aligned}$$

- Solve for the other variable using this value:

$$\begin{aligned} 3(3) + 4y &= 17 \\ 4y &= 8 \\ y &= 2 \end{aligned}$$

Elimination

In elimination, multiply or divide one (or both) of the equations to get the same coefficient in front of one of the variables in both equations. Then, add or subtract the equations as necessary to eliminate one of the variables. The steps of this method are listed below.

- Multiply or divide one (or both) of the equations by a constant so that the coefficient in front of one of the variables in both equations is the same:

$$3x + 4y = 17$$

$$2 \times [5x - 2y = 11]$$

- If the sign of both coefficients is the same, subtract one equation from the other. If the sign is opposite, add the two equations together:

$$\begin{array}{r} 4y + \ \ 3x = 17 \\ -\ 4y + 10x = 22 \\ \hline 13x = 39 \\ x = 3 \end{array}$$

- Solve for the other variable using this value:

$$\begin{aligned} 3(3) + 4y &= 17 \\ 4y &= 8 \\ y &= 2 \end{aligned}$$

Note that each method results in the same answer despite slight differences in the steps taken. As a matter of convention, the answers for systems of equations with the variables x and y are reported as coordinates on the Cartesian plane (x,y); thus, our answer for this system would be (3,2). Systems of equations can have many variables, but it is unlikely that you will encounter a system with more than three variables (x,y,z) on the MCAT.

MCAT CONCEPT CHECK 10.4

Before you move on, assess your understanding of the material with these questions.

1. How are conversions between metric prefixes accomplished? How would a distance be converted from millimeters to kilometers?

____

____

2. What does it mean for two variables to have a direct relationship? An inverse relationship?

   - Direct:

   ____

   - Inverse:

   ____

3. Each of the three methods for solving systems of equations discussed in this chapter solve for one variable, and then use this value to solve for the other. How does each method solve for the first variable?

   - Substitution:

   ____

   - Setting equations equal:

   ____

   - Elimination:

   ____

Conclusion

In this chapter, we reviewed many of the skills that are necessary for successful performance on the MCAT science sections. We began by examining relevant arithmetic calculations for Test Day, including scientific notation and significant figures. We continued our review by examining logarithms and exponents before discussing the most common trigonometric functions and their values. We finished our math review by working on problem-solving skills that will be valuable in your studying and during the MCAT itself. In the next two chapters, we'll review Test Day skills in experimental design and data analysis so that you'll be ready to answer all of the Test Day questions.

You've reviewed the content, now test your knowledge and critical thinking skills by completing a test-like passage set in your online resources!

GO ONLINE

CONCEPT SUMMARY

Arithmetic and Significant Figures

- **Scientific notation** is a method of writing numbers in a way that improves the ease of calculations and the comparability of significant digits.
  - Scientific notation takes the format [significand] $\times$ $10^{[\text{exponent}]}$.
  - The **significand** must be greater than or equal to 1 and less than 10.
  - The **exponent** must be an integer.
- **Significant figures** include all nonzero digits and any trailing zeroes in a number with a decimal point.
  - Measurements are an exception, in that the last digit provided is not significant.
  - In addition and subtraction, reduce the answer to have the same number of decimal places as the number with the fewest number of decimal places.
  - In multiplication and division, reduce the answer to have the same number of significant digits as the number with the fewest number of significant digits.
  - The entire number should be maintained throughout calculations to minimize rounding error.
- Estimation of multiplication and division should be done logically.
  - In multiplication, if one number is rounded up, the other should be rounded down in proportion.
  - In division, if one number is rounded up, the other should also be rounded up in proportion.

Exponents and Logarithms

- **Exponents** are a notation for repeated multiplication. They may be manipulated mathematically, especially when the bases are the same.
- **Logarithms** are the inverse of exponents and are subject to similar mathematical manipulations.
- **Natural logarithms**, which use base ***e*** (**Euler's number**) can be converted into **common logarithms**, which use base 10.

Trigonometry

- Trigonometric relationships can be calculated based on the lengths of the sides of right triangles.
- **Sine** is the ratio of the length of the side opposite an angle to the length of the hypotenuse.
- **Cosine** is the ratio of the length of the side adjacent to an angle to the length of the hypotenuse.
- **Tangent** is the ratio of the side opposite an angle to the side adjacent to it.
- **Inverse trigonometric functions** use the calculated value from a ratio of side lengths to calculate the angle of interest.

Problem-Solving

- In **direct relationships**, as one variable increases, the other increases in proportion.
- In **inverse relationships**, as one variable increases, the other decreases in proportion.
- Conversions between metric prefixes require multiplication or division by corresponding powers of ten.
- Conversions between units of different scales require multiplication or division, and may require addition or subtraction.
- Unit analysis (**dimensional analysis**) can determine the appropriate computation based on given information.
- Algebraic systems may be solved by substitution, setting equations equal, or elimination. The general ideas are the same in each—solve for one variable, and then substitute the variable into an equation to solve for the other—although the specific methods are different.

ANSWERS TO CONCEPT CHECKS

10.1

1. First, determine which digits are significant, as these will be preserved in scientific notation. Then, move the decimal point until the significand is greater than or equal to 1 and less than 10. Finally, determine what power of 10 is necessary for multiplication to restore the original number.
2. 34,600.; 0.0003201; 1.10; 525,600
3. In multiplication, adjust the two decimals in opposite directions. In division, adjust the two decimals in the same direction.

10.2

1.
   - $(a + b)^2 = a^2 + 2ab + b^2$
   - $\frac{a^2 + 2a^2}{5a^3} = \frac{3a^2}{5a^3} = \frac{3}{5a}$
   - $\log_a (a) = 1$
   - $\log\left(a^3\right) - \log(a) = \log \frac{a^3}{a} = \log a^2 = 2 \log a$
2. $\sqrt{392}$ is between $\sqrt{361}$ and $\sqrt{400}$, so the value is between 19 and 20. We can also simplify this radical:

   $$\sqrt{392} = \sqrt{4} \times \sqrt{49} \times \sqrt{2} \approx 14 \times 1.4 = 19.6 \text{ (actual} = 19.8)$$

3. $\log 7{,}426{,}135{,}420 \approx \log(7.4 \times 10^9) \approx 9 + 0.74 = 9.74$ (actual = 9.87). Note that—even with an absurdly large number—we can still get relatively accurate estimations by following basic logarithm rules.

10.3

1. The value of a trigonometric function calculated from the dimensions of the resultant vector is used in the inverse tangent function to calculate the resultant vector angle. Inverse trigonometric ratios, in general, can be used to calculate angles.
2. The sine of an angle is equal to the ratio of the side opposite the angle to the hypotenuse. Cosine is the ratio of the side adjacent to the angle to the hypotenuse. Tangent is the ratio of the side opposite the angle to the side adjacent to the angle.
3. False. Even though calculating the values of sine, cosine, and tangent is more complicated in a triangle that does not contain a right angle, all possible angles do still have characteristic trigonometric values.
4. Sin is equal to 1 at 90°, cos at 0°, and tan at 45°. Many MCAT questions utilize the trend that sin increases going from 0° to 90°, whereas cos decreases over this range.

10.4

1. Conversion between metric prefixes is accomplished by multiplication or division by the appropriate power of ten. To convert from millimeters (10^{-3}) to kilometers (10^{3}), it is necessary to multiply by 10^{-6}. It's wise to double-check your work when converting: a kilometer is a larger unit of distance than a millimeter, so the number of kilometers should be smaller than the number of millimeters.
2. In direct relationships, as one quantity increases, the other also increases in proportion. In inverse relationships, as one quantity increases, the other decreases in proportion.
3. In substitution, solve one equation for one variable in terms of the other; then, substitute this expression into the other equation. In setting equations equal (a modified version of substitution), solve both equations for the same variable and set them equal to each other. In elimination, multiply or divide one (or both) equations so that the coefficient in front of one of the variables is the same in both equations; then, add or subtract the equations to eliminate one of the variables.

SCIENCE MASTERY ASSESSMENT EXPLANATIONS

1. **B**

This question, while overtly testing the ability to use scientific notation, is also checking on the appropriate use of significant digits. Because there is no decimal point, the last zero is not significant and should not be used in scientific notation. The significand in scientific notation should always be between one and ten.

2. **C**

Significant digits include all nonzero digits, all zeroes that are between nonzero digits, and trailing zeroes in any number with a decimal point. In 14,320,010 there is no decimal point; thus, the last zero is insignificant and there are seven significant digits. In 3.618000, all of the digits are significant; thus there are also seven significant digits.

3. **B**

While all digits are preserved during calculations, the final determination of the number of digits is made by both significant figures and decimal places. During multiplication, the answer is maintained to the smallest number of significant digits. During addition, it is maintained to the smallest number of decimal places. By following the order of operations, addition is the last operation; thus we cannot have a decimal in our answer choice. Because multiplication occurred earlier, the result of that multiplication may be shortened according to the two significant figures in 4.10, but not the entire answer.

4. **A**

When estimating the product of two numbers, it is best to round one up while rounding the other down, as in **(A)**. **(B)** and **(D)** each round both numbers in the same direction, which would increase the amount of error in the answer. **(C)** rounds the numbers in opposite directions, but the degree of rounding is significantly larger than in **(A)** and too extreme for answer choices that differ by small amounts.

5. **A**

The fourth root of a number, or a number raised to the one-quarter power, is the square root of the square root of that number:

$$200^{0.25} = 200^{\frac{1}{2} \times \frac{1}{2}} = \sqrt{\sqrt{200}} = \sqrt[4]{200}$$

The square root of 200 should be a bit larger than 14 ($14^2 = 196$); therefore, the fourth root of 200 should be a bit less than 4.

6. **D**

Raising an exponent to another exponent requires multiplying the exponents. Thus, $(A^3)^2 = A^6$.

7. **A**

The relationship between the natural logarithm of a number and the common logarithm of a number is $\log x = \frac{\ln x}{2.303}$. Therefore, the natural logarithm of a number must be divided by the constant 2.303 to obtain the common logarithm of the same number.

8. **A**

The minimum value of the cosine function is -1 ($\cos 180° = -1$). Therefore, the minimum value of $2 \cos \theta - 1$ is $2 \times (-1) - 1 = -3$.

9. **D**

$\sin \theta \neq \sin (90° - \theta)$, although $\sin \theta = \cos (90° - \theta)$. The other statements must all be true. Because sine and cosine values are always between -1 and 1, the product of sine and cosine will always have a magnitude less than 1. The sum of the absolute value of sine and the absolute value of cosine, on the other hand, will always be greater than 1. Therefore, **(A)** can be eliminated. Because sine is the ratio of opposite to hypotenuse and cosine is the ratio of adjacent to hypotenuse, the quotient between the two is the ratio of opposite to adjacent, or the tangent of the angle. Therefore, **(B)** can be eliminated. By the same logic, because $\sin 90° = 1$ and $\cos 90° = 0$, $\tan 90°$ is undefined, eliminating **(C)**.

10. **B**

This question involves both a unit conversion between millimolar values and molar values, and calculation of a logarithm. The relationship between pH and pK_a is described by the Henderson–Hasselbalch equation given in the question stem. 100 mM = 0.1 M, so

$$\text{pH} = pK_a + \log\frac{[\text{A}^-]}{[\text{HA}]} = 3.6 + \log(1) = 3.6$$

11. **B**

This question requires not only unit conversions, but algebra as well. Given that $F = \frac{9}{5}C + 32$, the temperature T can be calculated as:

$$T = \frac{9}{5}T + 32 \rightarrow -\frac{4}{5}T = 32 \rightarrow T = -\frac{5}{4}(32) = -40$$

However, the answers are given in kelvin. $-40°\text{C} + 273 =$ 233 K.

12. **D**

In a direct relationship, a change in one of the variables will be associated with a proportional change in the other. Because the pressure was multiplied by $\frac{1}{3}$, the temperature must also be multiplied by $\frac{1}{3}$. Note that the fractional relationships can only be used with temperatures in kelvin.

13. **C**

Because grams are a unit of mass and pounds are a unit of force, we must first convert pounds to newtons, and then divide by the acceleration due to gravity to find kilograms. The weight of the person in newtons is

$$150 \text{ lb} \times 4.45 \frac{\text{N}}{\text{lb}} \approx 150 \times 4.4 = 600 + 60$$
$$= 660 \text{ (actual} = 667.5 \text{ N)}.$$

This corresponds to a mass of

$$\frac{667.5 \text{ N}}{9.8 \frac{\text{m}}{\text{s}^2}} = \frac{667.5 \frac{\text{kg}\cdot\text{m}}{\text{s}^2}}{9.8 \frac{\text{m}}{\text{s}^2}} \approx 67 \text{ kg}.$$

Now, we can determine the dose:

$$67 \text{ kg}\left(\frac{1.5 \text{ mg drug}}{\text{kg body mass}}\right) \approx 100 \text{ mg}.$$

14. **C**

According to the question stem, the rate of a reaction is measured as a change in concentration over time, and thus has the units $\frac{M}{\text{s}}$, where M (molarity) is measured in moles per liter. However, the rate of the reaction is equal to a rate constant times the concentrations of certain reactants squared. In this case, we know the units of everything except the rate constant and must solve for its units:

$$\text{rate} = k[\text{A}]^2$$
$$\frac{M}{\text{s}} = k[M]^2 \rightarrow k = \frac{1}{M\cdot\text{s}} = \frac{\text{L}}{\text{mol}\cdot\text{s}}$$

15. **C**

This is a system of equations couched in data. From this information, we can construct two equations:

$$C = 900 + 12m$$
$$C = 500 + 15m$$

These equations can be solved by setting them equal:

$$900 + 12m = 500 + 15m$$
$$400 = 3m$$
$$133 \text{ kg} = m$$

Consult your online resources for additional practice. GO ONLINE

EQUATIONS TO REMEMBER

(10.1) **Zero exponent identity:** $X^0 = 1$

(10.2) **Multiplying like bases with exponents:** $X^A \times X^B = X^{(A+B)}$

(10.3) **Dividing like bases with exponents:** $\frac{X^A}{X^B} = X^{(A-B)}$

(10.4) **Raising an exponent to another exponent:** $(X^A)^B = X^{(A \times B)}$

(10.5) **Raising fractions to exponents:** $\left(\frac{X}{Y}\right)^A = \frac{X^A}{Y^A}$

(10.6) **Raising bases to negative exponents:** $X^{-A} = \frac{1}{X^A}$

(10.7) **Raising bases to fractional exponents:** $X^{\frac{A}{B}} = \sqrt[B]{X^A}$

(10.8) **Square root approximations:** $\sqrt{2} \approx 1.414$ (use 1.4)
$\sqrt{3} \approx 1.732$ (use 1.7)

(10.9) **Logarithm of 1 identity:** $\log_A 1 = 0$

(10.10) **Logarithm of base identity:** $\log_A A = 1$

(10.11) **Logarithm of product:** $\log A \times B = \log A + \log B$

(10.12) **Logarithm of quotient:** $\log \frac{A}{B} = \log A - \log B$

(10.13) **Logarithm of exponent-containing expression:** $\log A^B = B \log A$

(10.14) **Logarithm of inverse:** $\log \frac{1}{A} = -\log A$

(10.15) **Conversion of natural to common logarithm:** $\log x \approx \frac{\ln x}{2.303}$

(10.16) **Scientific notation logarithm approximation:** $\log (n \times 10^m) \approx m + 0.n$

(10.17) **Definition of sine:** $\sin \theta = \frac{\text{opposite}}{\text{hypotenuse}} = \frac{a}{c}$

(10.18) **Definition of cosine:** $\cos \theta = \frac{\text{adjacent}}{\text{hypotenuse}} = \frac{b}{c}$

(10.19) **Definition of tangent:** $\tan \theta = \frac{\text{opposite}}{\text{adjacent}} = \frac{a}{b}$

(10.20) **Temperature conversions:** $F = \frac{9}{5}C + 32$
$K = C + 273$

SHARED CONCEPTS

General Chemistry Chapter 5
Chemical Kinetics

General Chemistry Chapter 7
Thermochemistry

General Chemistry Chapter 10
Acids and Bases

Physics and Math Chapter 7
Waves and Sound

Physics and Math Chapter 9
Atomic and Nuclear Phenomena

Physics and Math Chapter 12
Data-Based and Statistical Reasoning

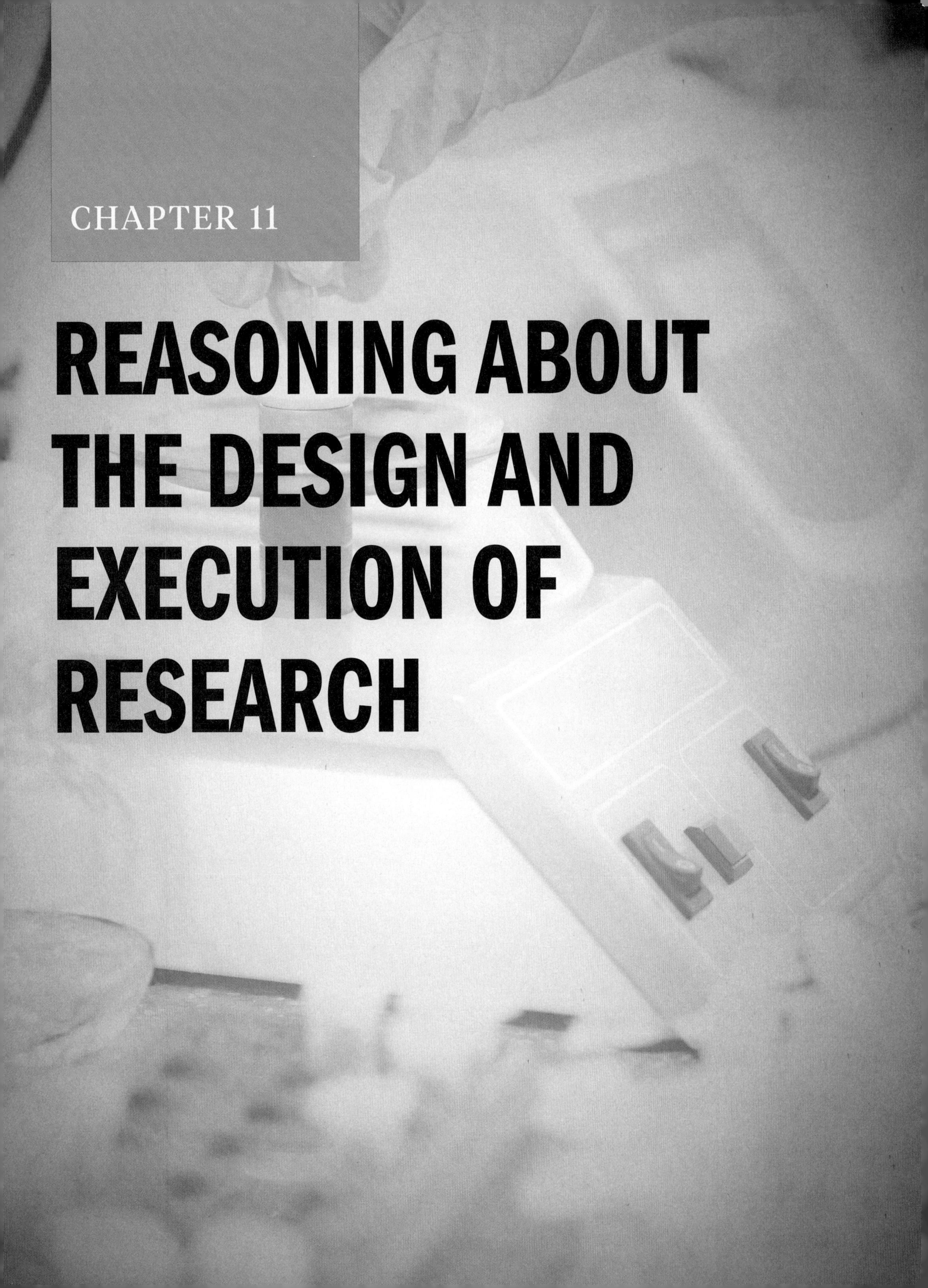

CHAPTER 11

REASONING ABOUT THE DESIGN AND EXECUTION OF RESEARCH

SCIENCE MASTERY ASSESSMENT

Every pre-med knows this feeling: there is so much content I have to know for the MCAT! How do I know what to do first or what's important?

While the high-yield badges throughout this book will help you identify the most important topics, this Science Mastery Assessment is another tool in your MCAT prep arsenal. This quiz (which can also be taken in your online resources) and the guidance below will help ensure that you are spending the appropriate amount of time on this chapter based on your personal strengths and weaknesses. Don't worry though—skipping something now does not mean you'll never study it. Later on in your prep, as you complete full-length tests, you'll uncover specific pieces of content that you need to review and can come back to these chapters as appropriate.

How to Use This Assessment

If you answer 0–7 questions correctly:

Spend about 1 hour to read this chapter in full and take limited notes throughout. Follow up by reviewing **all** quiz questions to ensure that you now understand how to solve each one.

If you answer 8–11 questions correctly:

Spend 20–40 minutes reviewing the quiz questions. Beginning with the questions you missed, read and take notes on the corresponding subchapters. For questions you answered correctly, ensure your thinking matches that of the explanation and you understand why each choice was correct or incorrect.

If you answer 12–15 questions correctly:

Spend less than 20 minutes reviewing all questions from the quiz. If you missed any, then include a quick read-through of the corresponding subchapters, or even just the relevant content within a subchapter, as part of your question review. For questions you got correct, ensure your thinking matches that of the explanation and review the Concept Summary at the end of the chapter.

1. An experimenter is attempting to investigate the effect of a new antibiotic on *E. coli*. The experimenter plates cells and administers one milliliter of the antibiotic. Which of the following is an appropriate negative control in this experiment?
   - **A.** A plate with no cells that was coated with one milliliter of antibiotic
   - **B.** A plate with *E. coli* and no additional treatment
   - **C.** A plate with *E. coli* and one milliliter of isotonic saline
   - **D.** A plate of epithelial cells treated with one milliliter of antibiotic

2. Which of the following would best establish a causal link?
   - **A.** A cross-sectional study using survey data for hand-washing and colds
   - **B.** A case–control study of an exposure during childhood and development of a certain disease later in life
   - **C.** A randomized clinical controlled trial of a new antipyretic drug
   - **D.** An IQ test where the results are later separated by gender

3. An experimenter is attempting to determine the internal energy of a well-known compound. The experimenter cleans the glassware, completes the synthesis, calibrates a bomb calorimeter, and then uses it to measure the appropriate thermodynamic values. One error here is that the experimenter:
   - **A.** did not determine if the compound was novel or if the information has already been determined.
   - **B.** did not have a specific goal at the beginning of the research.
   - **C.** should not be involved in both the synthesis of the compound and later testing.
   - **D.** should have calibrated the calorimeter before the synthesis of the compound.

4. A researcher wishes to generate a parameter for the mean weight of residents of the United States. Which of the following is the most significant concern?
   - **A.** Measuring a person's weight may have psychological consequences and is unethical.
   - **B.** Gathering all of the necessary study participants would be prohibitive.
   - **C.** Knowing the average weight of US residents does not provide any useful information.
   - **D.** Enough studies have already been conducted on this topic to render it unnecessary.

5. A cross-sectional study in which current smoking status and cancer history are assessed simultaneously cannot satisfy which of Hill's criteria?
   - **A.** Strength
   - **B.** Coherence
   - **C.** Plausibility
   - **D.** Temporality

6. After randomization, it is discovered that one group in a study has almost twice as many women as the other. Which of the following is an appropriate response?
   - **A.** Move men and women between groups manually so that they have the same gender profile.
   - **B.** Check the randomization algorithm; if it is fair, continue with the research.
   - **C.** Eliminate all of these subjects because of potential bias and randomize a new cohort.
   - **D.** Keep the current cohort and continue randomizing subjects until the gender profiles are equal.

7. An experimenter is attempting to determine the effects of smoking on very low birth weight (VLBW) and of VLBW on IQ. Which of the following statements is correct?
   - **I.** Smoking is an independent variable.
   - **II.** Smoking is a dependent variable.
   - **III.** VLBW is an independent variable.
   - **IV.** VLBW is a dependent variable.

   - **A.** I only
   - **B.** II and IV only
   - **C.** I, III, and IV only
   - **D.** II, III, and IV only

8. A study is performed on a new medication. Subjects in the experimental group are told about the potential side effects of the medication, while subjects in the placebo group are not. The subjects have no contact with each other and do not know in which group they are placed. The side effects end up being significantly more severe in the treatment group, when seen by the same assessor physician. This is most likely caused by which of the following?

- **A.** Physician unblinding only
- **B.** Patient unblinding only
- **C.** Both physician and patient unblinding
- **D.** Both physician and patient blinding

9. As part of a graduate program entrance exam, a student must submit a grant proposal for a scientific investigation. While the student's hypothesis is well formulated and the student has some preliminary data, the student's proposal is rejected, with the committee reviewing the proposal citing several articles that support the hypothesis. What mistake did the student make in drafting the proposal?

- **A.** The student did not formulate a testable hypothesis.
- **B.** The student did not spend sufficient time reviewing existing studies.
- **C.** The proposed study did not adequately test the hypothesis.
- **D.** The student did not have enough preliminary data.

10. A new study of a weight loss drug uses a radio advertisement to generate study participation. What type of error is most likely to result?

- **A.** Hawthorne effect
- **B.** Selection bias
- **C.** Confounding
- **D.** Detection bias

11. A researcher designing a study has paid for it to be professionally translated into several languages. The researcher discusses the potential risks and benefits with each participant and allows them to bring documentation home for review before committing to the study. This researcher has put special focus on:

- **A.** justice by explaining potential risks.
- **B.** beneficence by describing the potential benefits of the study.
- **C.** respect for persons by acknowledging the subject's perspective and rights.
- **D.** selection bias, by making the recruitment documents inclusive.

12. Which of the following methods would be most appropriate for an initial assessment of hemoglobin saturation during an experiment about breath holding?

- **A.** A pulse oximeter, which uses a small light on an adhesive bandage
- **B.** An arterial cannula, which permits repeated blood draws with a single puncture
- **C.** Repeated venipuncture, because a single puncture would cause data overlap
- **D.** A Swan–Ganz catheter inserted through the femoral artery, which can measure saturation nearest the heart

13. A medical student attempting to impress an attending physician refers to a recent article that says that there is a statistically significant difference in pregnancy length with a new therapy. Which of the following is most likely to be a valid criticism of the article?

- **A.** Medical students usually reference articles in the newest journals, which may be unreliable.
- **B.** The effect didn't change patient outcomes, only a secondary measure.
- **C.** There is a lack of internal validity in the results, despite significance.
- **D.** Selection bias is inherent in the scientific process.

14. Which sample would be the most appropriate participants for a study on hormone replacement therapy for postmenopausal symptoms?

- **A.** Prepubescent girls
- **B.** Premenopausal adult women
- **C.** Pregnant women
- **D.** Postmenopausal women

15. Use of a colorimetric assay to determine protein concentration may be subject to all of the following EXCEPT:

- **A.** the use of standards.
- **B.** measurement error.
- **C.** the Hawthorne effect.
- **D.** systematic error.

Answer Key follows on next page.

Answer Key

1. **C**
2. **C**
3. **A**
4. **B**
5. **D**
6. **B**
7. **C**
8. **A**
9. **B**
10. **B**
11. **C**
12. **A**
13. **B**
14. **D**
15. **C**

Detailed explanations can be found at the end of the chapter.

CHAPTER 11

REASONING ABOUT THE DESIGN AND EXECUTION OF RESEARCH

In This Chapter

Introduction

In the modern world, there are standard places to search for the answers to questions we have: encyclopedias, academic journals, online databases, and other publications. By perusing current research on a topic, we can figure out whether someone else has already asked and answered our question. This is just as true for scientists and other professionals. In many cases, our searches may take us in different directions. This may be as simple as finding additional resources that confirm the answers to our questions; however, research is often more complicated than that. We may find conflicting answers and have to perform critical analysis to determine which data set (and conclusion) was obtained in the most legitimate, unbiased way. Other times, we'll have to find the answers on our own through experiment or observation and data analysis.

In order to generate a consistent body of knowledge, the ways in which scientists generate and search for information must be orderly and uniform. In this chapter, we will discuss the premise of basic science, biomedical, and social sciences research. Our examination will include the necessary criteria for causality, different types of error, and the ethical implications of human subjects research. These research methods are core skills that the MCAT tests—in fact, they constitute one of the four *Scientific Inquiry and Reasoning Skills* on the exam. In addition, their importance will last for the rest of your medical career. As a physician, you will constantly be seeking answers in research to determine prognoses, assess the appropriateness of a

MCAT EXPERTISE

As with the previous chapter, this chapter does not contain any content that falls directly within an AAMC content category. That said, the AAMC has confirmed that a full 10% of the science questions on every MCAT will touch on material in this chapter—and many of those questions will require only information from this chapter, without any other supportive science content. That makes it, point for point, one of the most important chapters in the entire *MCAT Review* series!

treatment modality for a given patient, and answer patients' questions. You may be a researcher yourself in a basic science, clinical, or translational setting. Regardless of your path, evaluating research is critical to the progress of all fields of medicine and will be a key component of your life as a physician.

11.1 The Scientific Method

LEARNING OBJECTIVES

After Chapter 11.1, you will be able to:

- Determine the relative value of a research question by applying the FINER method
- Identify the stages of the scientific method, and evaluate whether they have been appropriately completed
- Evaluate the quality and testability of a hypothesis

The basic paradigm for all scientific inquiry is the scientific method. The **scientific method** is a set of steps that defines the appropriate order of events to structure and carry out an experiment. As such, the scientific method is the established protocol for transitioning from a question to a new body of knowledge. The steps in the scientific method are:

1. **Generate a testable question:** This usually occurs after observing something anomalous in another scientific inquiry or in daily life.
2. **Gather data and resources:** Think back to our introduction; this is the phase of journal and database searches and compiling information. At this step, we as scientists must be careful to look for all information, not just that consistent with our expectations.
3. **Form a hypothesis:** A **hypothesis** is the proposed explanation or proposed answer to our testable question. It is often in the form of an **if–then statement**, which will be tested in subsequent steps.
4. **Collect new data:** This step results from either **experimentation**, which involves manipulating and controlling variables of interest; or **observation**, which often involves no changes in the subject's environment.
5. **Analyze the data:** Look for trends and perform mathematical manipulations to solidify the connections between variables.
6. **Interpret the data and existing hypothesis:** Consider whether the data analysis is consistent with the original hypothesis. If the data is inconsistent, consider alternative hypotheses.
7. **Publish:** Publication provides an opportunity for **peer review**; a summary of what was done during all six prior steps should be included in the publication.
8. **Verify results:** Most experiments are repeated to verify the results under new conditions.

BRIDGE

It is easy to focus on research that agrees with our expectations or opinions, and to ignore research that goes against them. This is an example of confirmation bias at work. Specific types of biases are discussed in Chapter 4 of *MCAT Behavioral Sciences Review* and later in this chapter.

MCAT EXPERTISE

The MCAT will most often test experimental or logical errors during research. Pay particular attention to the scientific method now in order to recognize each area in which an error may occur.

Formulating a testable question often presents students with a challenge because we tend to overreach, creating all-encompassing broad questions; however, in order to form a good testable question, it must be restricted to a relatively narrow area. The same is true of our hypotheses. One might wonder, *Why do hot objects cause injury?* This is not a testable question. In fact, most questions that begin with *Why* are too broad to be testable through a single experiment. In this case, a better, more testable question could be *How do epithelial cells respond to heat* in vivo? Even this question is likely too broad for a single experiment, but it is testable, and we can form related hypotheses. One possible hypothesis would be: *if heat is applied to* in vivo *epithelial cells, then those cells will lyse.* Pay attention to the format of the hypothesis, as the if–then format ensures that it is testable. We will examine other components of the scientific method as they pertain to basic science research, biochemical and biomedical research, and social science research in the relevant sections.

The FINER Method

The **FINER method** for evaluating a research question is a method to determine whether the answer to one's question will add to the body of scientific knowledge in a practical way and within a reasonable time period. The FINER method asks five questions to make this determination.

- Is the necessary research study going to be **feasible**? A question about the response of chemosynthetic bacteria to a particular antibiotic requires access to chemosynthetic bacteria (which are often associated with harsh and difficult environments to access). If the scientist cannot obtain the necessary supplies, then the research is not feasible. Financial or time constraints, or the inability to gather enough subjects are also feasibility concerns.
- Do other scientists find this question **interesting**? This is somewhat subjective, but if there is little interest in the outcome of a particular research question, then the research will have little utility.
- Is this particular question **novel**? If someone has asked this question before, and answered it to the satisfaction of a peer-reviewed journal, then it's now in the confirmatory stages of the scientific method. Barring any anomalies, asking this question again isn't likely to gain new knowledge.
- Would the study obey **ethical** principles? Just because we are capable of carrying out a research study does not mean it is ethically or morally acceptable. If there's an ethical or moral reason not to perform a study, this should dissuade researchers from carrying out the study just as much as an inability to secure funding.
- Is the question **relevant** outside the scientific community? The more people that the research will impact in everyday life, the more important it usually is. There are exceptions, of course—many people might agree that curing a rare fatal illness is more important than improving the odor of a popular perfume, although a much larger group may be impacted by the latter study.

MCAT CONCEPT CHECK 11.1

Before you move on, assess your understanding of the material with these questions.

1. Rank the following research questions from 1 (best) to 3 (worst) using the FINER method and explain your rationale:
   - How long does it take for the Earth to complete one revolution around the Sun?
   - How do medical errors relate to sleep deprivation of medical residents?
   - What is the average lifespan of bacteria in Martian rocks?

   1. ______________________________

      ____

   2. ______________________________

      ____

   3. ______________________________

      ____

2. Errors or biases during publication of results are most likely to affect which stages of the scientific method?

   ____

   ____

   ____

3. True or False: *Most people with hepatitis C acquired it through IV drug use* is an example of a well-formatted hypothesis.

11.2 Basic Science Research

High-Yield

LEARNING OBJECTIVES

After Chapter 11.2, you will be able to:

- Identify common types and sources of error
- Recognize independent and dependent variables and how they are typically displayed graphically
- Explain the importance of the different types of control, including positive and negative controls
- Distinguish between accuracy and precision:

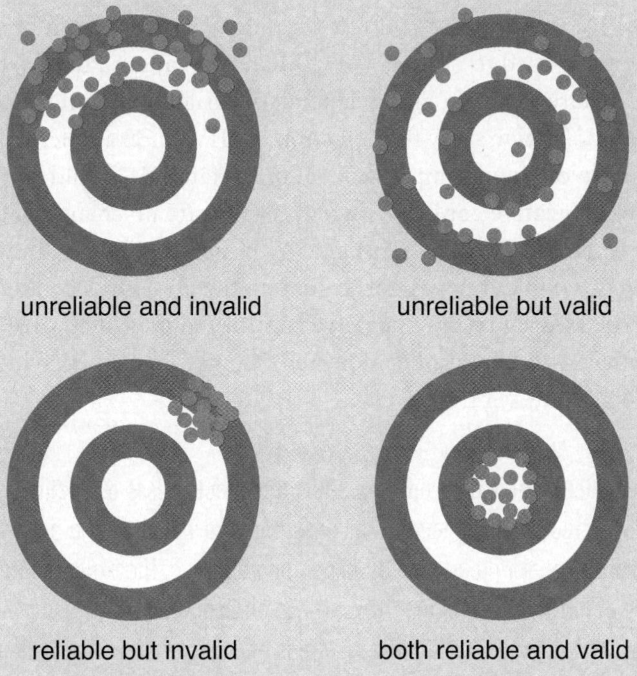

Basic science research—the kind conducted in a laboratory, and not on people—is generally the easiest to design because the experimenter has the most control. Often a causal relationship is being examined because the hypothesis generally states a condition and an outcome. In order to make generalizations about our experiments, we must make sure that the outcome of interest would not have occurred without our intervention, and therefore, we use controls. We must also demonstrate causality, which is relatively simple in basic science research, but less so in other research areas.

Controls

In basic science research, conditions can be applied to multiple trials of the same experiment that are as near to identical as possible. In this way, a **control** or **standard** acts as a method of verifying results. Consider the following experiment: a scientist has an unknown concentration of a basic ammonia solution and wishes to determine the concentration experimentally. The scientist takes a

REAL WORLD

The use of controls also allows investigators to check for contamination of reagents.

standardized solution of hydrochloric acid (made by comparison to a potassium hydrogen phthalate [KHP] standard) and titrates the basic solution in the presence of the same calibrated pH meter used for the hydrochloric acid standardization. The scientist then determines the ammonia concentration from the results of the titration. Because the concentration of the acid used to determine the ammonia concentration was verified against a standard, the scientist can be confident that the calculated ammonia concentration is accurate.

Controls can also be separate experimental conditions altogether. For example, when testing the reaction of a tissue culture to an antibiotic, a separate culture is generally grown and administered an equal quantity of a compound known to be inert, like water or saline. The control corrects for any impact that the simple addition of volume might have had on the experiment. Some experiments have both positive and negative controls for points of comparison or a group of controls that can be used to create a curve of known values. **Positive controls** are those that ensure a change in the dependent variable when it is expected. In the development of a new assay for detection of HIV, for example, administering the test to a group of blood samples known to contain HIV could constitute a positive control. **Negative controls**, in contrast, ensure no change in the dependent variable when no change is expected. With the same assay, administering the test to a group of samples known not to contain the HIV virus could constitute a negative control. In drug trials, a negative control group is often used to assess for the **placebo effect**—an observed or reported change when an individual is given a sugar pill or sham intervention.

Example: A clinical trial is devised to quantify the effectiveness of a retinal scanning system for the detection of Alzheimer's disease. The trial will include a positive control group, a negative control group, and an experimental group. The experimental group is a large sample of individuals who are 70 years old and showing symptoms of Alzheimer's disease. Assuming the retinal scanning system is effective at detecting Alzheimer's disease, rank the groups in decreasing order of percentage of expected disease detection.

Solution: Members of the positive control group should consist of patients who have previously been diagnosed with Alzheimer's disease, whereas members of the negative control group should consist of patients who have previously tested negative for Alzheimer's disease. Therefore, the positive control group and negative control groups should establish the upper and lower bounds of percent detection, respectively. The experimental group is likely to fall between those two extremes. The predicted order is: positive, experimental, and negative.

Causality

The other big advantage to being able to manipulate all of the relevant experimental conditions is that basic science researchers can often establish causality. Causality is an if–then relationship, and is often the hypothesis being tested. In basic science research, we manipulate an **independent variable**, and measure or observe a **dependent variable**. When there is a theoretical or known mechanism that links the independent and dependent variables, a causal relationship can be investigated. If the change in the independent variable always precedes the change in the dependent variable, and the change in the dependent variable does not occur in the absence of the experimental intervention, the relationship is said to be causal.

Example: A test was conducted to determine if water consumption impacts systolic blood pressure in mice. The water consumption and systolic blood pressure of eight mice was tracked for three weeks. The average daily water consumption and the average systolic blood pressure of each mouse is listed in the following table.

Mouse	Average Daily Water Consumption (mL)	Average Systolic Blood Pressure (mmHg)
1	3.9	122
2	3.3	128
3	1.5	146
4	4.7	117
5	6.1	108
6	0.8	153
7	10.3	103
8	8.6	105

The researchers plotted pressure and consumption and obtained the following graph. Identify the independent and dependent variables, and determine if a causal relationship exists between the two.

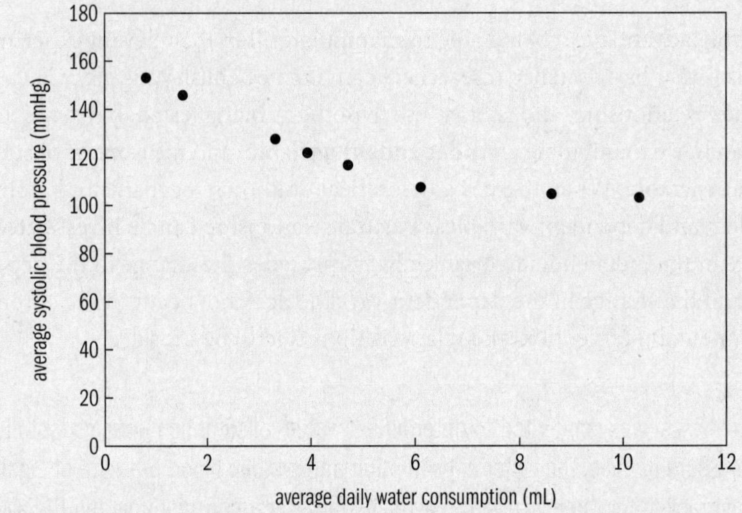

Solution: The independent variable is the "average daily water consumption (mL)" and the dependent variable is the "average systolic blood pressure (mmHg)."

Not enough data is given to determine if a causal relationship exists. More information is needed to determine if the differences in systolic blood pressure occur due to differences in water consumption. It's possible that the mice could have the given systolic blood pressure values even when consuming equal amounts of water.

KEY CONCEPT

The independent variable is the one that the experimenter is manipulating, and the dependent or outcome variable is the one that is being observed. On a graph the independent variable belongs on the *x*-axis and the dependent variable belongs on the *y*-axis.

Error Sources

In basic science research, experimental bias is usually minimal. The most likely way for an experimenter's personal opinions to be incorporated is through the generation of a faulty hypothesis from incomplete early data and resource collection. However, there can be manipulation of the results by eliminating trials without appropriate background, or by failing to publish works that contradict the experimenter's own hypothesis.

The low levels of bias introduced by the experimenter do not eliminate all error from basic science research. Measurements are especially important in the laboratory sciences, and the instruments may give faulty readings. Instrument error may affect accuracy, precision, or both. **Accuracy**, also called **validity**, is the ability of an instrument to measure a true value. For example, an accurate scale should register a 170-pound person's weight as 170 pounds. **Precision**, also called **reliability**, is the ability of the instrument to read consistently, or within a narrow range. The same person standing on a scale that is accurate but imprecise may get readings between 150 and 190 pounds. The same person standing on a scale that is inaccurate but precise may get readings between 129 and 131 pounds, a relatively narrow range. Accuracy and precision are represented in Figure 11.1. Because bias is a **systematic error** in data, only an inaccurate tool will introduce bias, but an imprecise tool will still introduce error. Random chance can also introduce error into an experiment; while **random error** is difficult to avoid, it is usually overcome by using a large sample size.

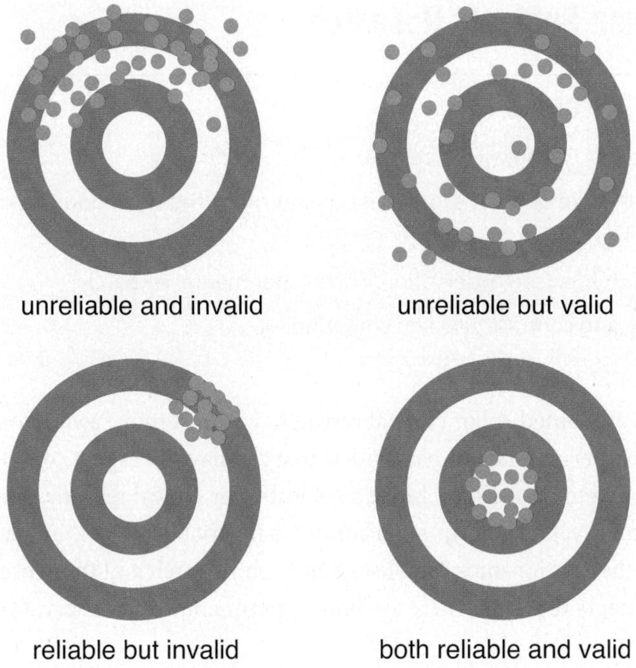

Figure 11.1 Accuracy (Validity) and Precision (Reliability) of Measurements

MCAT CONCEPT CHECK 11.2

Before you move on, assess your understanding of the material with these questions.

1. An experiment with an improperly tared (zeroed) mass balance would suffer from what type of error?

   ____

2. Label the axes and provide representative data for the following situation: An experimenter adds sodium hydroxide to an experimental solution and records the pH. The experimenter finds that the relationship is sigmoidal and that the pH is rising.

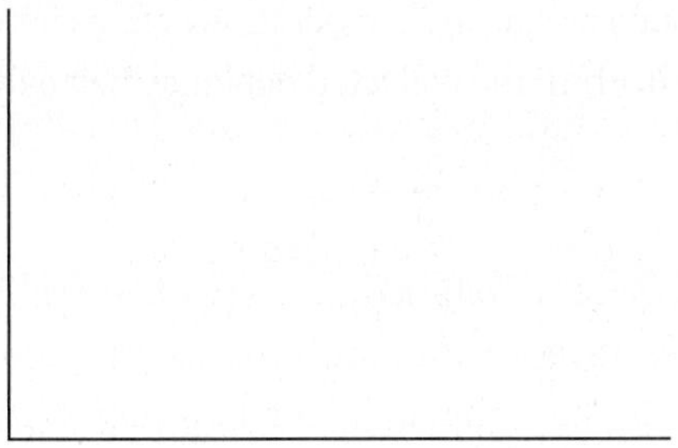

3. What is the purpose of a control during experiments? What characteristic of experimental research would be reduced in the absence of a control?

   ____

11.3 Human Subjects Research

High-Yield

LEARNING OBJECTIVES

After Chapter 11.3, you will be able to:

- Apply Hill's criteria to an experiment to determine the likelihood of a causal relationship
- Distinguish between observational and experimental research
- Compare and contrast bias and confounding

In some cases of biomedical or clinical research, we must move away from petri dishes full of cells or experimental animal models that can have all aspects of their living conditions controlled to research on human subjects. For ethical reasons, which we will discuss later, the level of experimental control is invariably lower than basic science research, and the relationships established by such research will therefore be weaker. In **human subjects research**, there are both experimental and observational studies.

Experimental Approach

In biomedical research, it is possible to perform experiments in which an independent variable is manipulated and an outcome is observed. In these experiments, we are still attempting to elicit a causal relationship. Because subjects are in less-controlled conditions, the data analysis phase is more complicated than in laboratory studies. In clinical and social sciences research, it is often still possible to conduct experiments by manipulating the environment or circumstances of the subject.

Randomization

Randomization is the method used to control for differences between subject groups in biomedical research. Randomization uses an algorithm to determine the placement of each subject into either a control group that receives no treatment or a sham treatment, or one or more treatment groups. A proper randomization algorithm will be equivalent to a coin toss or die roll. Once each individual is assigned to a group, the intervention is performed and the results are measured. Ideally, each group is perfectly matched on conditions such as age and gender; however, as long as there is an appropriate randomization algorithm, the collected data may be analyzed without concern.

Blinding

Because many of the measures in biomedical research are subjective, the perception of the subject and the investigator may be biased by knowing which group the subject is in. To remove this bias, the subjects and/or investigators may be **blinded**, which means they do not have information about which group the subject is in. In **single-blind experiments**, only the patient or the **assessor** (the person who makes measurements on the patient or performs subjective evaluations) is blinded. In **double-blind experiments,** the investigator, subject, and assessor all do not know the subject's group. Without blinding, the **placebo effect** would be greatly reduced in the control group, but still be present in the treatment group.

REAL WORLD

Blinding isn't only useful in drug trials; even sham treatments of acupuncture have been used to blind subjects in randomized controlled trials focusing on the use of acupuncture for musculoskeletal pain.

Data Analysis

In biomedical research, data analysis must account for variables outside of the independent and dependent variables considered. Most often, these include gender and age; lifestyle variables, such as smoking status and body mass index (BMI), and other factors that may affect the measured outcomes. Some of these other factors can be inferred from the initial literature review, although other unexpected **confounding variables** may exist. Software programs can use **binary** (yes *vs.* no, better *vs.* worse), as well as **continuous** (amount of weight lost, percent improvement in cardiac output) or **categorical variables** (state of residence, socioeconomic status) to create a regression model. **Regression analysis** may demonstrate linear, parabolic, exponential, logarithmic, or other relationships, as we will discuss in Chapter 12 of *MCAT Physics and Math Review.*

KEY CONCEPT

Research methods that generate numerical data are quantitative, while those that generate non-numerical data are qualitative; mixed-method research utilizes both.

Observational Approach

We may wish to study certain causal associations for which an experiment cannot be performed for ethical or practical reasons. In such a case, we must draw on the available data and analyze it. **Observational studies** in medicine fit into one of three categories: cohort studies, cross-sectional studies, and case–control studies. These studies often look for the connections between exposures and outcomes. Observational studies do not demonstrate causality, although the tendency toward causality may be demonstrated by Hill's criteria, which we will examine later.

REAL WORLD

Ethnographic studies are observational studies utilized by sociologists. These studies attempt to understand cultures by looking at the complete social environment.

Cohort studies are those in which subjects are sorted into groups based on differences in risk factors (**exposures**), and then assessed at various intervals to determine how many subjects in each group had a certain **outcome**. For example, a study in which 100 smokers and 100 nonsmokers are followed for 20 years while counting the number of subjects who develop lung cancer in each group would be an example of a cohort study.

KEY CONCEPT

A longitudinal study is an observational research method that follows the same subjects over time. Therefore, a cohort study is a form of longitudinal study.

Cross-sectional studies attempt to categorize patients into different groups at a single point in time. For example, a study to determine the prevalence of lung cancer in smokers and nonsmokers at a given point in time would be an example of a cross-sectional study.

Case-control studies start by identifying the number of subjects with or without a particular outcome, and then look backwards to assess how many subjects in each group had exposure to a particular risk factor. For example, a study in which 100 patients with lung cancer and 100 patients without lung cancer are assessed for their smoking history would be an example of a case–control study.

Hill's Criteria

Hill's criteria describe the components of an observed relationship that increase the likelihood of causality in the relationship. While only the first criterion is necessary for the relationship to be causal, it is not sufficient. The more criteria that are satisfied by a relationship, the likelier it is that the relationship is causal. Hill's criteria do not provide an absolute guideline on whether a relationship is causal; thus, for any observational study, the relationship should be described as a **correlation**.

- **Temporality:** The exposure (independent variable) *must* occur before the outcome (dependent variable).
- **Strength:** As more variability in the outcome variable is explained by variability in the study variable, the relationship is more likely to be causal.
- **Dose–response relationship:** As the study or independent variable increases, there is a proportional increase in the response. The more consistent this relationship, the more likely it is to be causal.
- **Consistency:** The relationship is found to be similar in multiple settings.
- **Plausibility:** There is a reasonable mechanism for the independent variable to impact the dependent variable supported by existing literature.
- **Consideration of alternative explanations:** If all other plausible explanations have been eliminated, the remaining explanation is more likely.
- **Experiment:** If an experiment can be performed, a causal relationship can be determined conclusively.
- **Specificity:** The change in the outcome variable is only produced by an associated change in the independent variable.
- **Coherence:** The new data and hypothesis are consistent with the current state of scientific knowledge.

Error Sources

In addition to the measurement error found in basic science research, we must be aware of bias and error introduced by using human subjects as part of an experimental or observational model. As mentioned earlier, bias is a systematic error. As such, it generally does not impact the precision of the data, but rather skews the data in one direction or another. **Bias** is a result of flaws in the data collection phase of an experimental or observational study. **Confounding** is an error during analysis.

Selection Bias

The most prevalent type of bias is **selection bias**, in which the subjects used for the study are not representative of the target population. People who volunteer for a study in a particular area may be significantly different from people who do not volunteer. For example, someone volunteering for a drug trial that requires clinical visits may be healthier or more likely to benefit from the study than someone who does not volunteer because they cannot make it to the hospital.

Selection bias may also apply in cases where one gender is more prevalent in a study than another, or where there are differences in the age profile of the experiment group and the population. Measurement and assessment of selection bias occurs before any intervention.

Detection Bias

Detection bias results from educated professionals using their knowledge in an inconsistent way. Because prior studies have indicated that there is a correlation between two variables, finding one of them increases the likelihood that the researcher will search for the second. For example, high blood pressure (hypertension) and diabetes mellitus are more common among individuals who are obese; thus, a physician may screen patients who are obese for hypertension and diabetes at a higher rate than other patients, inflating the true value of the secondary measurement (although, as described in Chapter 12 of *MCAT Behavioral Sciences Review*, other biases against individuals who are obese actually tend to lead to lower rates of screening and preventative care).

Observation Bias

The **Hawthorne effect**, or **observation bias**, posits that the behavior of study participants is altered simply because they recognize that they are being studied. Often these lifestyle alterations improve the health of the sample population. For example, patients in a study for a given weight loss drug may begin exercising more frequently or may make healthier diet choices, thus artificially increasing the perceived effect of the drug. Because the change in data is systematic and occurs before data analysis, this is an example of bias.

Confounding

Confounding, sometimes inaccurately called confounding bias or omitted variable bias, is a data analysis error. The data may or may not be flawed, but an incorrect relationship is characterized. For example, consider the statement *Having natural red hair leads to a decreased pain tolerance and higher opiate tolerance*. There are two flaws with this statement. First, the statement implies a causal relationship as a result of what would almost certainly be an observational study. Second, consider whether or not this is realistic. How could red hair cause the findings described? According to current research, there is no likely causality between these two. However, a third variable, such as a gene mutation, could potentially cause both parts of this statement. If one measured the degree of red hair pigment and the degree of pain intolerance, there might be a very strong statistical relationship, but there is no causal relationship between the two. These "third-party" variables are called **confounding variables** or **confounders**, as illustrated schematically in Figure 11.2.

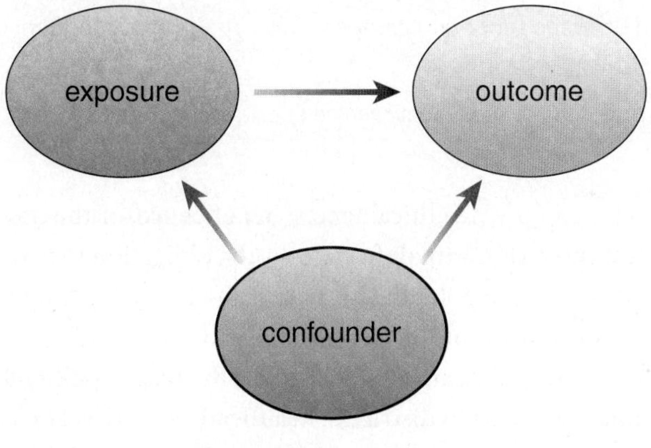

Figure 11.2 Confounding

MCAT CONCEPT CHECK 11.3

Before you move on, assess your understanding of the material with these questions.

1. True or False: A researcher who fails to demonstrate temporality can still provide evidence for a causal relationship by satisfying the rest of Hill's criteria.

2. How does observational research differ from experimental research?
   - Observational research:

   ____

   - Experimental research:

   ____

3. What is the difference between bias and confounding?
   - Bias:

   ____

   - Confounding:

   ____

11.4 Ethics

LEARNING OBJECTIVES

After Chapter 11.4, you will be able to:

- Distinguish between autonomy (medical ethics) and respect for persons (research ethics)
- Predict the ethical issues regarding respect for persons, justice, beneficence, and nonmaleficence within a study
- Distinguish between monetary compensation and coercive influence for a research study
- Recall the populations that must receive special consideration for coercion

In medicine, there are four core ethical tenets: **beneficence**, or the obligation to act in the patient's best interest; **nonmaleficence**, or the obligation to avoid treatments or interventions in which the potential for harm outweighs the potential for benefit; respect for patient **autonomy**, or the responsibility to respect patients' decisions and choices about their own healthcare; and **justice**, or the responsibility to treat similar patients with similar care, and to distribute healthcare resources fairly.

BRIDGE

The key ethical tenets of medicine are also discussed in Chapter 11 of *MCAT Behavioral Sciences Review* in conjunction with an analysis of major institutions in the United States.

In research, these four principles are replaced by a slightly modified set. The *Belmont Report*, a landmark document published by the National Commission for the Protection of Human Subjects of Biomedical and Behavioral Research in 1979, delineates the three necessary pillars of research ethics: respect for persons, justice, and a slightly more inclusive version of beneficence.

Respect for Persons

Respect for persons includes the need for honesty between the subject and the researcher, and generally—but not always—prohibits deception. Respect for persons also includes the process of **informed consent**, in which a patient must be adequately counseled on the procedures, risks and benefits, and goals of a study to make a knowledgeable decision about whether or not to participate in the study. Further, the investigator cannot exert a coercive influence over the subjects, or they will not be acting autonomously. This coercive influence may be the result of a natural power imbalance, such as that between a teacher and a student, or may be the result of an extreme financial incentive or the inability to otherwise receive treatment for a condition. Respect for persons also includes the need to respect the subjects' wishes to continue with or cease participation in a study. The subject may withdraw consent that was previously granted at any time.

Many older studies did not abide by respect for persons. For example, sentinel studies on the severity of untreated syphilis were conducted without the participants' knowledge or consent. Many early psychological and sociological studies involved significant deception, which was not always disclosed after the fact. In current practice, hospital or university **institutional review boards** have put into place systematic protections against unethical studies. **Vulnerable persons**, which include children, pregnant individuals, and prisoners, require special protections above and beyond those taken with the general population. **Confidentiality** is also generally considered as part of respect for persons during research.

REAL WORLD

The Tuskegee syphilis experiment was a notorious forty-year study (1932–1972) by the United States Public Health Service that was fraught with extreme violations of the ethical principle of respect for persons. In this study, African American men living in conditions of poverty were enrolled into a study on the natural progression of syphilis. These men were given sham treatments, barred from accessing appropriate healthcare, and repeatedly deceived by investigators—including the fact that they were never told they had syphilis! This study was so significant in bioethical history that it is actually considered the primary impetus for the writing of the Belmont Report.

Justice

Justice in research applies to both the selection of a research topic and the execution of the research. If we lived in a world where all individuals and all questions were ethically the same, the only just way to determine the selection of a research question would be through random chance. However, we live in a world with morally relevant differences as established by our cultures. **Morally relevant differences** are defined as those differences between individuals that are considered an appropriate reason to treat them differently. For example, age is a significant moral difference in ethical deliberations: all else being equal, a transplant that is as likely to benefit a young child or an older adult might be given to the child because of a longer life expectancy. Population size is often morally relevant in study design because a study that impacts a large population will generally have more potential to do good than one that impacts a small population. In contrast, race, ethnicity, sexual orientation, gender identity, disability status, and financial status are generally not considered morally relevant differences. It should be noted that religion may or may not be a valid moral criterion, depending on the context; for example, certain interventions that are prohibited by a given religion are grounds to avoid that treatment in an individual of that religion—this is in keeping with patient autonomy.

Justice is also important in the selection of subjects and the execution of research. When there is risk associated with a study, it must be fairly distributed so as not to unduly harm any group. This generally corresponds to seeking a diverse group for a study. Note that this also has a side benefit of increasing external validity, which will be discussed later in the chapter. However, the population that is most likely to benefit from the study may be required to bear a greater proportion of the risk. This apparent discrepancy—that all individuals should equally share the burden of risk, and that the target population may assume a higher proportion of risk—is reflective of the fact that likelihood of benefit is a morally relevant difference between individuals. Therefore, in studies in which there is no perceived difference in the likelihood of benefit between individuals, all individuals should assume equal risk; in those for which a particular population is most likely to benefit, that population should assume a higher proportion of risk. Finally, be aware that in some cases, such as drug trials, it may necessary to test the intervention in individuals unaffected by the illness for which the drug has been designed. In this case, the burden of risk falls on a secondary population. This is permissible as long as the potential risks and benefits for the subjects have been addressed through informed consent and respect for persons has been maintained.

Beneficence

Beneficence is the easiest concept to understand in the context of research ethics. It must be our intent to cause a net positive change for both the study population and general population, and we must do our best to minimize any potential harms. This benefit may be as intangible as a feeling of personal satisfaction, and it may be unrelated to the original purpose of the study, such as small financial incentives. It may also be a future benefit if the participant is a member of the target population.

Research should be conducted in the least invasive, painful, or traumatic way possible. For example, a measurement that could be taken with either a finger stick or an indwelling catheter should be taken with a finger stick because it is far less painful and invasive. In addition, in studies comparing two potential treatment options, one cannot approach the research with the knowledge that one treatment is superior to the other. This is termed **equipoise**. If it becomes evident that one treatment option is clearly superior before a study is scheduled to finish, the trial must be stopped because providing an inferior treatment is a net harm.

MCAT CONCEPT CHECK 11.4

Before you move on, assess your understanding of the material with these questions.

1. What is the difference between autonomy in medical ethics and respect for persons in research ethics?

2. During study design, a company wishing to market a drug to individuals with severe diabetes proposes to enroll only individuals with mild diabetes. Which principle of research ethics is the company violating? Are there any research concerns in this proposed study besides ethics?

3. What is the difference between a coercive influence and monetary compensation for a research study?

4. What are some populations that must receive special consideration for coercion?

11.5 Research in the Real World

LEARNING OBJECTIVES

After Chapter 11.5, you will be able to:

- Compare and contrast internal and external validity
- Explain the impact of sample size on generalizability
- Recall the qualities a study must have to justify an intervention

Until this point, we've been discussing research in a vacuum but our goals with any research are application-based. In order to apply the data generated, there are practical concerns that we must consider. For example, we must take into account the statistical strengths and weaknesses of a study, especially those that are related to the differences between the target population and the study sample. We also consider ways in which bias impacts the ability to use study conclusions in the real world, and whether there is any true justification for an intervention.

Populations *vs.* Samples

In statistics and research, we generally work with a sample rather than an entire population. A **population** is the complete group of every individual that satisfies the attributes of interest. Populations may be very large; for example, the population of humans is over seven billion people. In contrast, a population with a large number of qualifiers—for example, the population of females who live in the United States, are between 18 and 30 years old, and who have Darier's disease, a rare skin condition—will be much smaller (in this case, about 100 people). Information that is calculated using every person in a population is called a **parameter**.

Working with a population is generally not feasible, even for smaller groups. Therefore, we make generalizations about populations based on sample data. A **sample** is any group taken from a population that does not include all individuals from the population. Ideally, samples will be representative of the population, and there are several methods of ensuring this. Random samples are generally considered the gold standard, although selecting for certain small subgroups may also be used. Information about a sample is called a **statistic**. With comparatively large or repeated samples, statistics can be used to estimate population parameters. If only a single small sample is taken, then very little information can be gleaned about the population.

REAL WORLD

Drugs undergo continuous evaluation in part because of poor preclinical generalizability. Some marketing changes or additional warnings may become necessary, or a drug may even be taken off the market. These are unforeseen risks or outcomes that only become apparent when the drug becomes available to the entire population.

Generalizability

When analyzing a study, we also look for markers of **internal validity** (or support for causality as discussed earlier) and **external validity**, or **generalizability**. Studies with low generalizability have very narrow conditions for sample selection that do not reflect the target population, whereas studies with high generalizability have samples that are representative of the target population. For example, a psoriasis study with low generalizability might have only participants who were diagnosed within the last year, while a study with high generalizability would have participants with a distribution of time since diagnosis that is similar to the population of all patients who have psoriasis.

Support for Interventions

As future doctors, we are interested in applying research to our patients. To do so, we'll need to consider whether the data is sufficient for the recommendation or exclusion of any therapy or treatment plan.

Statistical *vs.* Clinical Effect

In research, the primary marker of success is being able to generate results that are **statistically significant**—that is, not the result of random chance. However, even the smallest difference between two treatments may be significant mathematically. For example, a decrease in systolic blood pressure of one millimeter of mercury could be statistically significant; however, it is not likely to change patient outcomes. In this way, we must assess whether there is **clinical significance**—a notable or worthwhile change in health status as a result of our intervention.

MCAT CONCEPT CHECK 11.5

Before you move on, assess your understanding of the material with these questions.

1. What is the difference between internal validity and external validity?
   - Internal validity:

   ____

   - External validity:

   ____

2. Why might small samples provide insufficient information about a population?

   ____

   ____

3. What qualities must a study have to provide justification for an intervention?

   ____

   ____

Conclusion

In this chapter, we focused on one of the four *Scientific Inquiry and Reasoning Skills* that will be tested on the MCAT: reasoning about the design and execution of research. We began by reviewing the scientific method and the value of historical data in the formulation of a research question. We then compared the methodology for both basic sciences research and human subjects research, especially with regard to error. We finished our investigation by examining the ethical and practical concerns in research design. The questions for this chapter are designed to allow you to practice this new skill, rather than to test your memorization of this content. In the next chapter, we'll specifically work with data and graphical analysis, another of the *Scientific Inquiry and Reasoning Skills* that will be essential on Test Day.

You've reviewed the content, now test your knowledge and critical thinking skills by completing a test-like passage set in your online resources!

GO ONLINE

CONCEPT SUMMARY

The Scientific Method

- The **scientific method** is a series of eight steps for the generation of new knowledge.
  - The initial steps (generate a testable question, gather data and resources, form a hypothesis) focus on generating a **hypothesis**.
  - The intermediate steps (collect new data, analyze the data, interpret the data and existing hypothesis) focus on testing that hypothesis.
  - The final steps (publish and verify results) relate to providing the results for further testing of the hypothesis.
- The **FINER method** assesses the value of a research question on the basis of whether or not it is feasible, interesting, novel, ethical, and relevant.

Basic Science Research

- Basic science research uses chemicals, cell cultures, or animal subjects and is experiment-based.
- During research, we manipulate **independent variables** and observe changes in the **dependent variable**.
- **Controls** are used to correct for any influences of an intervention that are not part of the model. Controls may be positive or negative.
  - **Positive controls** ensure that a change in the dependent variable occurs when expected.
  - **Negative controls** ensure that no change in the dependent variable occurs when none is expected.
- Basic science research is often the best type for demonstrating causality because the experimenter has the highest degree of control over the experimental conditions.
- Error in basic science research most often results from errors in measurement.
  - **Accuracy** (**validity**) is the quality of approximating the true value.
  - **Precision** (**reliability**) is the quality of being consistent in approximations.

Human Subjects Research

- Human subjects research is subject to ethical constraints that are generally absent in basic science research.
- Experiments may still be performed, but causal conclusions are harder to determine because circumstances are harder to control.

- Much of human subjects research is **observational**.
  - **Cohort studies** record exposures throughout time and then assess the rate of a certain outcome.
  - **Cross-sectional studies** assess both exposure and outcome at the same point in time.
  - **Case–control studies** assess outcome status and then assess for exposure history.
  - Causality in observational studies is supported by **Hill's criteria**, which include temporality, strength, dose–response relationships, consistency, plausibility, consideration of alternative explanations, experiments, specificity, and coherence.
- Error may be in the form of bias, confounding, or random error.
- **Bias** is systematic and results from a problem during data collection.
  - **Selection bias**, in which the sample differs from the population, is most common in human subjects research.
  - **Detection bias** arises from educated professionals using their knowledge in an inconsistent way by searching for an outcome disproportionately in certain populations.
  - The **Hawthorne effect** results from changes in behavior—by the subject, experimenter, or both—that occur as a result of the knowledge that the subject is being observed.
- **Confounding** is an error in data analysis that results from a common connection of both the dependent and independent variables to a third variable.

Ethics

- Medical ethics generally refers to the four principles of **beneficence**, **nonmaleficence**, respect for patient **autonomy**, and **justice**.
- Research ethics were established by the **Belmont Report**.
  - **Respect for persons** includes autonomy, informed consent, and confidentiality.
  - **Justice** dictates which study questions are worth pursuing and which subjects to use.
  - **Beneficence** requires us to do the most good with the least harm. We cannot perform an intervention without **equipoise**—a lack of knowledge about which arm of the research study is better for the subject.

Research in the Real World

- **Populations** are all of the individuals who share a set of characteristics. Population data are called **parameters**.
- **Samples** are a subset of a population that are used to estimate population data. Sample data are called **statistics**.
- **Internal validity** refers to the identification of causality in a study between the independent and dependent variables. **External validity** refers to the ability of a study to be **generalized** to the population that it describes.
- In order to be supported, an intervention must display both statistical and clinical significance.
  - **Statistical significance** refers to the low likelihood of the experimental findings being due to chance.
  - **Clinical significance** refers to the usefulness or importance of experimental findings to patient care or patient outcomes.

ANSWERS TO CONCEPT CHECKS

11.1

1. 1. *How do medical errors relate to sleep deprivation of medical residents?* This is a current topic of investigation and a consensus in the scientific community is still being reached. Medical residents are available for interview, and the research has very relevant outcomes.
   2. *What is the average lifespan of bacteria in Martian rocks?* While it is not very feasible to acquire the Martian rocks, the results would be both novel and interesting.
   3. *How long does it take the Earth to complete one revolution around the Sun?* This question has been asked and answered to the satisfaction of the scientific community. It is neither novel nor interesting (in terms of further research).
2. Errors during publication of current studies adversely affect the quality of future experimentation by providing an incomplete or flawed research base. Without accurate resources, subsequent hypotheses are likely to be flawed.
3. False. While the statement may or may not be true, this is not an easily testable hypothesis. While not required, if–then formatting of a hypothesis necessarily implies a testable relationship between ideas.

11.2

1. This experiment would likely have inaccuracy error but not imprecision error. In other words, the scale would reliably read the same mass or weight, but the mass or weight it reads is not correct. This would lead to bias in the results.
2. 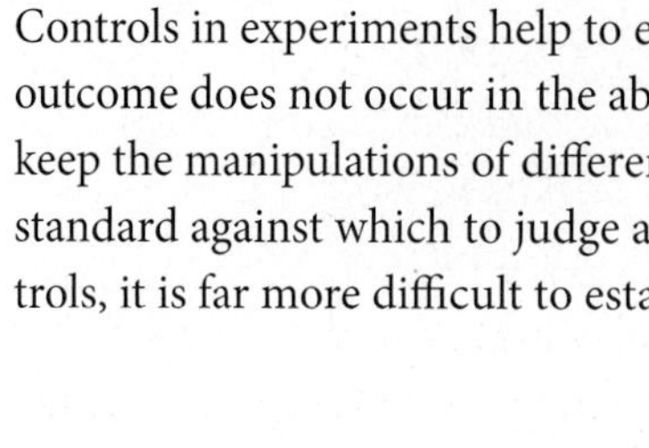

3. Controls in experiments help to establish causality by demonstrating that the outcome does not occur in the absence of an intervention. Controls are used to keep the manipulations of different systems as similar as possible, or as a known standard against which to judge an experimental manipulation. Without controls, it is far more difficult to establish causality.

11.3

1. False. Temporality is the only necessary criterion from Hill's criteria. If temporality is not satisfied, the relationship cannot be said to be causal. The addition of other criteria increases the probability of a causal relationship, assuming that temporality has not been invalidated.
2. Observational research does not involve manipulation of the subjects' environment. It is generally less conclusive and more subjective than experimental research, which does involve manipulation of the subject or environment.
3. Bias is a systematic (unidirectional) error that occurs during the selection of subjects or the measurement and collection of data. Confounding is an error that occurs during data analysis, in which an association is erroneously drawn between two variables because of a shared connection to a third variable.

11.4

1. Autonomy is simply the right of individuals to make decisions on their own behalf and to have those decisions be respected. Respect for persons also requires honesty, confidentiality, informed consent, and freedom from coercion.
2. The company is violating the principle of justice by choosing participants that are not part of the target population. The company is also introducing selection bias.
3. The line between a coercive influence and a compensatory influence is often debated. In general, a compensatory influence is one that does not impact the decision to participate, while a coercive influence is one in which the subject loses autonomy to make the decision to participate.
4. Children, pregnant individuals, and prisoners are considered especially at risk for coercion and thus are granted special protections.

11.5

1. Internal validity is the tendency of the same experiment to produce the same results when repeated, and provides support for causality. External validity is the ability to take the information generated during research and apply it to a larger group. External validity is also called generalizability.
2. Small samples are subject to more random variation than large samples. If only one person is selected, that person may be an outlier, but if a much larger sample is selected, an outlier will have less of an effect on the results.
3. A study must have both statistical significance and clinical significance to provide justification for an intervention. A study without statistical significance may be the result of random chance, whereas one without clinical significance will not impact patients.

SCIENCE MASTERY ASSESSMENT EXPLANATIONS

1. **C**

The purpose of a control is to keep the conditions of two experiments as close as possible to establish causality. In this case, the one milliliter volume addition might have impacted the growth of *E. coli*; thus, we must control for this by administering an equal volume of a theoretically inert compound to a plate of *E. coli*.

2. **C**

An experiment will always establish a clearer causal link than an observational study. **(A)**, **(B)**, and **(D)** are all examples of observational data.

3. **A**

The experimenter has not completed the initial phases of research. There was no data acquisition or refinement, and there was no indication that the question required an experiment to be answered. Were the experimenter doubtful of the validity of the reported value, an experiment could be appropriate—but there is no information to indicate that this is so. Based on the question stem, it is clear that the experimenter had a clear goal, eliminating **(B)**. In human subjects research, tasks may be divided to facilitate blinding, but this is generally unnecessary in basic sciences research, eliminating **(C)**. As long as the calorimeter was calibrated prior to its use, it does not matter when this calibration occurred relative to the synthesis of the compound, eliminating **(D)**.

4. **B**

A parameter is a population measure, so to calculate it, every single member must be measured. Identifying, measuring, and recording data for a population that large—over 300 million—is essentially impossible. Common biometric measures, if not misused, generally neither cause significant psychological harm nor are unethical, eliminating **(A)**. Knowing a mean weight could have major ramifications, including public health measures, medical recommendations, and shifting of body image, eliminating **(C)**. While a number of studies on weight have been performed, there is not yet a parameter describing the entire population, eliminating **(D)**.

5. **D**

Because both the exposure and outcome are measured at the same time, we cannot make any conclusions about temporality. The cancer patient may have only begun smoking after diagnosis, and this type of study doesn't examine that possibility.

6. **B**

Randomization is based on the idea that the results will only vary as a result of random chance as long as the assignment is proper. The appropriate response to a fair algorithm that assigns groups in an unexpected way is to proceed with the research. Participants should never be assigned by the researcher, nor should one continue randomizing samples to achieve a desired outcome—these are likely to introduce more error than leaving unequal groups, eliminating **(A)** and **(D)**. It is unnecessary to drop this entire cohort, assuming the randomization algorithm was fair, eliminating **(C)**.

7. **C**

Two relationships are being assessed. In the relationship between smoking and very low birth weight (VLBW), smoking is the independent variable and VLBW is the dependent variable. In the second relationship, VLBW is being compared to IQ. VLBW is the independent variable here, while IQ is the dependent variable.

8. **A**

Because the same physician sees both the control groups and the experimental groups, there is the potential for the physician to realize which of the groups is receiving which treatment—especially if the subject mentions expected side effects. In this study, patients were not told which group they were in, but if they were assigned to the medication group, they were told about its side effects. If the patients talked to each other they could experience patient unblinding, but we are told they have no communication with each other.

9. **B**

As part of the scientific method, after formulating a testable question, one must search through journals and databases to review the available information. This student likely did not spend sufficient time reviewing existing studies because the review committee was able to cite several studies that had already tested and affirmed the student's hypothesis, meaning that the hypothesis is not scientifically interesting. This observation is consistent with **(B)**. On the other hand, the question stem indicates that the hypothesis was well formulated and that the student had some preliminary data, which eliminates **(A)** and **(D)**. There is no stated criticism of the student's research methods, which eliminates **(C)**.

10. **B**

Requiring subjects to volunteer for a study and to seek the study out will introduce selection bias. The people who end up volunteering listen to the radio, which the general population may not, and are interested in the topic and willing to volunteer. Most studies suffer from selection bias and it is the most common impediment to generalizability.

11. **C**

The behaviors described in the question stem (informing the patient, providing time to make a decision) are consistent with informed consent and autonomy, which are both part of respect for persons.

12. **A**

While it may appear that this question is asking to determine which method is the most accurate or reliable, this is an ethics question. All of these methods (with the exception of venipuncture, **(C)**) measure oxygen saturation. According to the principle of beneficence, we must minimize potential harms associated with our investigations; thus, the noninvasive pulse oximeter should be greatly favored over other measurements for an initial assessment.

13. **B**

Statistical significance is not the same as clinical significance. There are medications that increase the length of pregnancy in preterm labor, but some only do so for a few hours. Because this may not impact patient outcomes, it should not inform treatment decisions.

14. **D**

Samples should always be taken from the target population or population of interest. Given that the target population is postmenopausal women, this group should be used for the sample. Both prepubescent girls and pregnant women are populations with special precautions against coercion, and are not appropriate for this study, eliminating **(A)** and **(C)**. Premenopausal women are unlikely to require hormone replacement therapy unless they have a condition that specifically necessitates it, eliminating **(B)**.

15. **C**

The Hawthorne effect—a change in behavior as a result of the knowledge that one is being observed—is only present with human subjects. Basic science research generally does not suffer from the Hawthorne effect.

Consult your online resources for additional practice. GO ONLINE

SHARED CONCEPTS

Behavioral Sciences Chapter 4
Cognition, Consciousness, and Language

Behavioral Sciences Chapter 8
Social Processes, Attitudes, and Behavior

Behavioral Sciences Chapter 11
Social Structure and Demographics

Behavioral Sciences Chapter 12
Social Stratification

Physics and Math Chapter 12
Data-Based and Statistical Reasoning

CHAPTER 12

DATA-BASED AND STATISTICAL REASONING

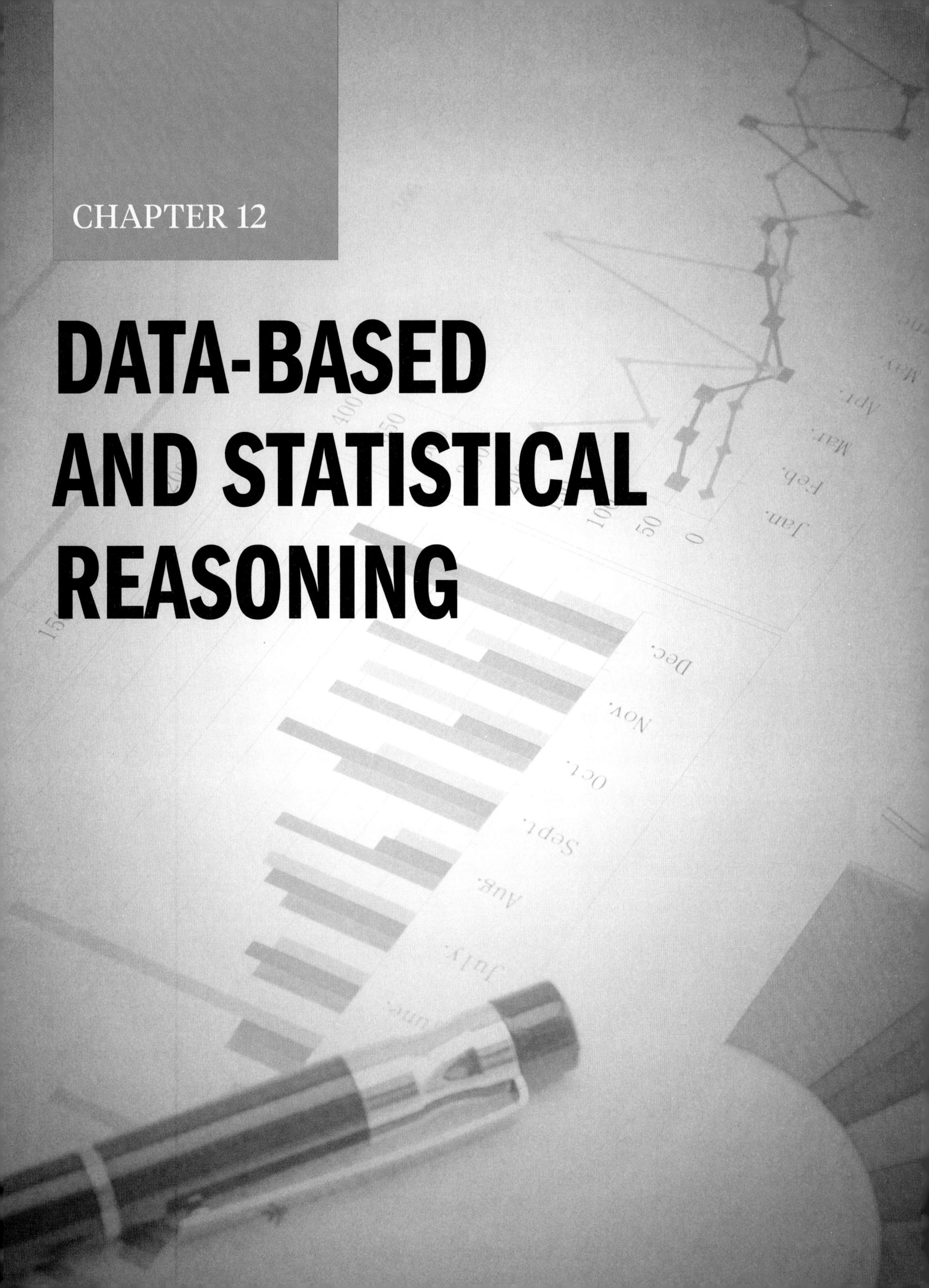

SCIENCE MASTERY ASSESSMENT

Every pre-med knows this feeling: there is so much content I have to know for the MCAT! How do I know what to do first or what's important?

While the high-yield badges throughout this book will help you identify the most important topics, this Science Mastery Assessment is another tool in your MCAT prep arsenal. This quiz (which can also be taken in your online resources) and the guidance below will help ensure that you are spending the appropriate amount of time on this chapter based on your personal strengths and weaknesses. Don't worry though—skipping something now does not mean you'll never study it. Later on in your prep, as you complete full-length tests, you'll uncover specific pieces of content that you need to review and can come back to these chapters as appropriate.

How to Use This Assessment

If you answer 0–7 questions correctly:

Spend about 1 hour to read this chapter in full and take limited notes throughout. Follow up by reviewing **all** quiz questions to ensure that you now understand how to solve each one.

If you answer 8–11 questions correctly:

Spend 20–40 minutes reviewing the quiz questions. Beginning with the questions you missed, read and take notes on the corresponding subchapters. For questions you answered correctly, ensure your thinking matches that of the explanation and you understand why each choice was correct or incorrect.

If you answer 12–15 questions correctly:

Spend less than 20 minutes reviewing all questions from the quiz. If you missed any, then include a quick read-through of the corresponding subchapters, or even just the relevant content within a subchapter, as part of your question review. For questions you got correct, ensure your thinking matches that of the explanation and review the Concept Summary at the end of the chapter.

1. The inclusion of an outlier in statistical analysis will most greatly affect which of the following measurements?
   - **A.** Median
   - **B.** Mode
   - **C.** Mean
   - **D.** All three are equally affected

2. In a sample of hospital patients, the mean age is found to be significantly lower than the median. Which of the following best describes this distribution?
   - **A.** Skewed right
   - **B.** Skewed left
   - **C.** Normal
   - **D.** Bimodal

3. What is the median of the following data set?

   7, 17, 53, 23, 4, 2, 4

   - **A.** 4
   - **B.** 7
   - **C.** 15.7
   - **D.** 23

4. On Santa Cruz island, the available food sources led to disruptive selection in the beak sizes of finches, in which large and small beak sizes were favored over intermediate sized beaks. As a result, few finches have an intermediate sized beak. If a sample of finches were analyzed, what distribution would best describe the distribution of beak size?
   - **A.** Normal
   - **B.** Bimodal
   - **C.** Skewed left
   - **D.** Skewed right

5. A 95% confidence interval will fall within what distance from the mean?
   - **A.** $\pm\sigma$
   - **B.** $\pm 2\sigma$
   - **C.** $\pm 3\sigma$
   - **D.** $\pm 4\sigma$

6. Approximately 20% of people who live in the United States eat fast food at least once per week. A new study conducted by the National Heart Association showed that 48% of US residents have some form of cardiovascular disease. Which of the following hypothetical findings could be used to show that cardiovascular disease is independent of weekly fast food consumption?
   - **A.** Individuals who do not consume fast food do not have cardiovascular disease.
   - **B.** Of the 48% of those who had cardiovascular disease, only half of them ate fast food on a weekly basis.
   - **C.** 9.6% of US residents have cardiovascular disease and consume fast food on a weekly basis.
   - **D.** None of the individuals who consume fast food on a weekly basis develop cardiovascular disease.

7. Which of the following outliers would most likely be the easiest to correct?
   - **A.** A typographical error in data transfer
   - **B.** A measurement error in instrument calibration
   - **C.** A heavily skewed distribution
   - **D.** A correctly measured anomalous result

8. Assume that blonde hair and blue eyes are independent recessive traits. If one parent is a carrier for each gene while the other parent is homozygous recessive for both genes, what is the probability that the first two offspring will both have blonde hair and blue eyes?
   - **A.** 6.25%
   - **B.** 25%
   - **C.** 43.75%
   - **D.** 50%

9. Based on the county-level map below, which of the following statements best represents the data about individuals older than 65 in the continental United States? (Note: The darker the shade of green, the higher the percentage of persons over 65 in the county.)

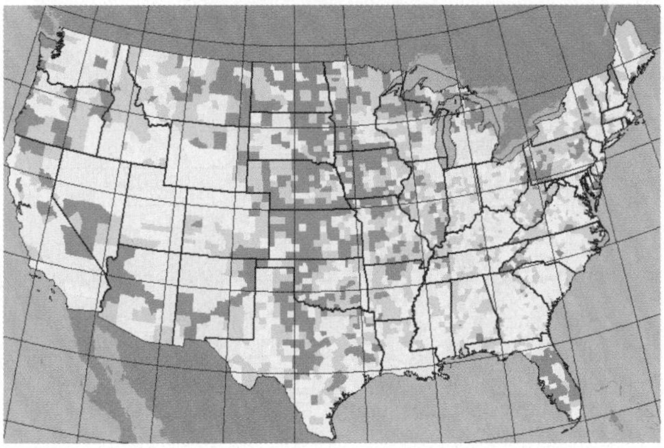

A. Most of the people over 65 in the United States live in the center of the country.
B. Most of the people living in the center of the United States are over 65.
C. The center of the United States tends to have a larger proportion of people over 65.
D. There are more people over 65 moving to the center of the country than elsewhere.

10. As the confidence level increases, a confidence interval:
A. becomes wider.
B. becomes thinner.
C. shifts to higher values.
D. shifts to lower values.

11. Which of the following measures of distribution is most useful for determining probabilities?
A. Range
B. Average distance from mean
C. Interquartile range
D. Standard deviation

12. Are there any outliers on the following box plot?

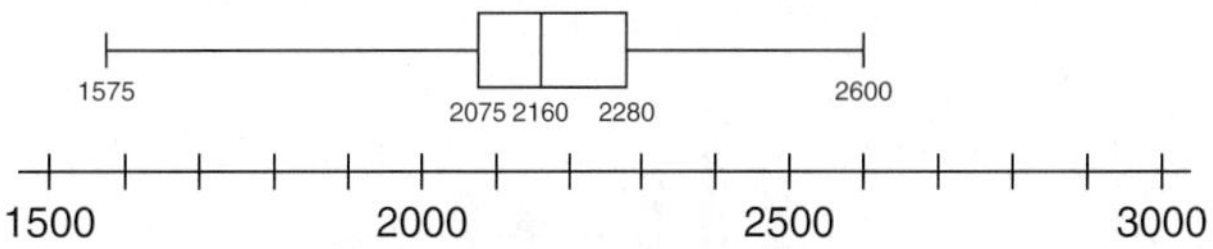

A. Yes; 1575 is an outlier.
B. Yes; 2600 is an outlier.
C. Yes; both 1575 and 2600 are outliers.
D. No; there are no outliers.

13. A gas station attendant notices that there are more lottery tickets sold on the days that a lot of ice cream is sold and hypothesizes that the ingestion of excess glucose leads to an increase in risk-taking behavior. The attendant begins to tally how much ice cream and how many lottery tickets are sold on a daily basis to generate the graph below.

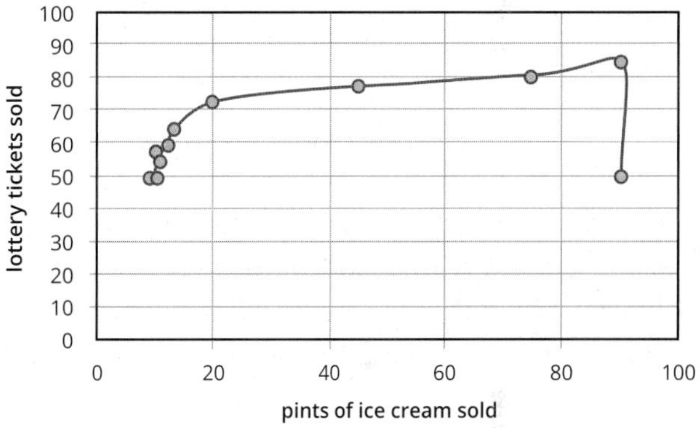

The attendant analyzes the data and concludes that the hypothesis is true. Are there any flaws in this conclusion?
A. No, the number of tickets sold increases as the pints of ice cream sold increase.
B. No, the study is appropriately controlled.
C. Yes, the study is missing a positive control.
D. Yes, the attendant has proved correlation, but not a causal link.

14. The following histogram:

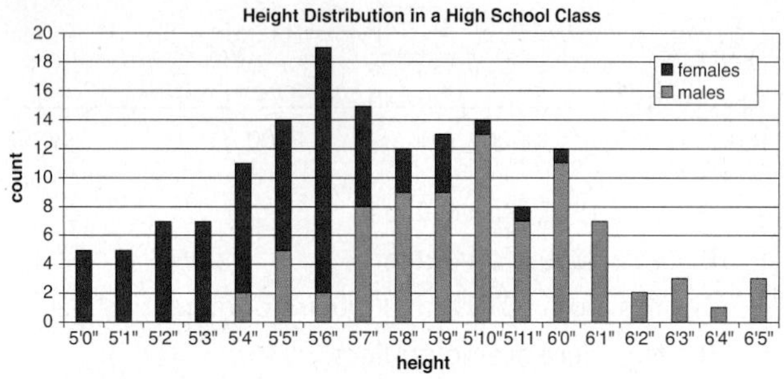

I. contains a bimodal distribution.
II. should be analyzed as two separate distributions.
III. contains one mode.

A. II only
B. I and II only
C. I and III only
D. I, II, and III

15. A cardiologist is investigating a new drug therapy for the treatment of hypertension. The cardiologist measures the baseline blood pressure of several patients, then treats them with the drug for ten weeks, measuring their blood pressure again after this time.

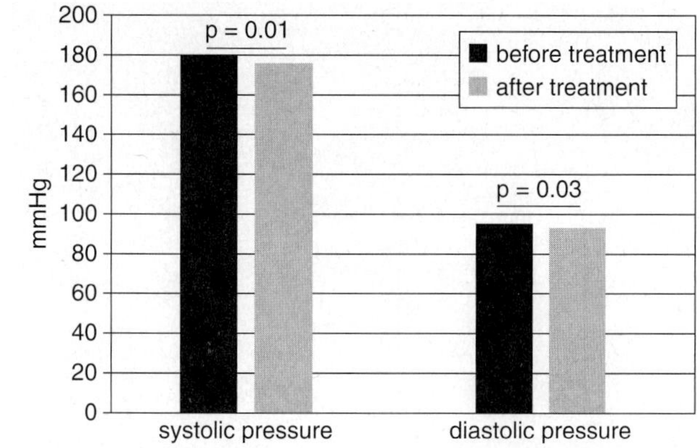

Based on these data, should the doctor advocate for making this drug the standard treatment for hypertension?

A. Yes, there is a statistically significant decrease in blood pressure.
B. Yes, the drug is effective at decreasing blood pressure.
C. No, while statistically significant, the results are not clinically significant.
D. No, the data is not statistically significant.

Answer Key follows on next page.

Answer Key

1. **C**
2. **B**
3. **B**
4. **B**
5. **B**
6. **C**
7. **A**
8. **A**
9. **C**
10. **A**
11. **D**
12. **C**
13. **D**
14. **D**
15. **C**

Detailed explanations can be found at the end of the chapter.

CHAPTER 12

DATA-BASED AND STATISTICAL REASONING

In This Chapter

Introduction

Academic papers are extremely predictable. They generally begin with an abstract that reflects the major points of the rest of the paper. The authors then provide an expanded introduction, materials and methods, data, and discussion. The key to a high-quality research paper is making this discussion unnecessary—any scientists, when given the prior sections, should be led to the same conclusions as those given by the author. The testmakers are keenly aware of this fact. On Test Day, you may be presented with research in the form of an experiment-based passage and part of your task will be inferring the important conclusions that can be supported by the findings of the study.

This chapter covers the last of the *Scientific Inquiry and Reasoning Skills* tested on the MCAT: the statistical analysis of raw data, interpretation of visual representations of this data, and application of data to answer research questions. We'll begin by examining basic statistical principles like distribution types, measures of central tendency, and measures of distribution. We'll also discuss probability, and the semantics of

MCAT EXPERTISE

Chapter 12 does not contain a chapter profile as it does not directly cover any AAMC content categories. That said, just like with Chapter 11 of this book, the AAMC has confirmed that 10% of the science questions on every MCAT will require material in this chapter—and many of those questions will require only information from this chapter, without any other supportive science content. With 10% from Chapter 11 and 10% from Chapter 12, there will be more than 30 questions(!) on your exam that will test one of these two skills.

this branch of mathematics. We'll conclude our discussion of probability and statistics with an exploration of statistical significance in basic hypothesis testing and confidence intervals. Then, we'll move on to the interpretation of charts and graphs. Finally, we'll link all of this information with the skills we gained in the last chapter and assess the future use and validity of studies.

12.1 Measures of Central Tendency

LEARNING OBJECTIVES

After Chapter 12.1, you will be able to:

- Calculate mean, median, and mode for a data set
- Predict the best measure of central tendency for a given data set

Measures of central tendency are those that describe the middle of a sample. How we define *middle* can vary. Is it the mathematical average of the numbers in the data set? Is it the result in a data set that divides the set into two—with half the sample values above this result and half the sample values below? Both of these data can be important, and the difference between them can also provide useful information on the shape of a distribution.

Mean

The **mean** or **average** of a set of data (more accurately, the **arithmetic mean**) is calculated by adding up all of the individual values within the data set and dividing the result by the number of values:

$$\overline{x} = \frac{\sum_{i=1}^{n} x_i}{n}$$

Equation 12.1

where x_i to x_n are the values of all of the data points in the set and n is the number of data points in the set. As we discussed in the last chapter, the mean may be a parameter or a statistic (as is true of all of the measures of central tendency) depending on whether we are discussing a population or a sample. Mean values are a good indicator of central tendency when all of the values tend to be fairly close to one another. Having an **outlier**—an extremely large or extremely small value compared to the other data values—can shift the mean toward one end of the range. For example, the average income in the United States is about $70,000, but half of the population makes less than $50,000. In this case, the small number of extremely high-income individuals in the distribution shifts the mean to the high end of the range.

Example: The following data were collected on the ages of attendees at Ray's birthday party:

23, 22, 25, 22, 22, 24, 36, 20

What is the mean age of the attendees? Is this an appropriate measure for this data?

Solution: The mean is the sum of the data points divided by the number of data points:

$$\overline{x} = \frac{23 + 22 + 25 + 22 + 22 + 24 + 36 + 20}{8} = \frac{194}{8} = 24.25$$

Because the mean is relatively near most of the values collected for this data set, it may be appropriate. Keep in mind, though, that the presence of an outlier and the fact that the mean is greater than all but two of the values collected indicates that the mean has been shifted toward the high end of the range. The presence of a single outlier does not invalidate the mean, but it does make interpretation in context necessary.

Median

The **median** value for a set of data is its midpoint, where half of data points are greater than the value and half are smaller. In data sets with an odd number of values, the median will actually be one of the data points. In data sets with an even number of values, the median will be the mean of the two central data points. To calculate the median, a data set must first be listed in increasing fashion. The position of the median can be calculated as follows:

$$\text{median position} = \frac{(n+1)}{2}$$

Equation 12.2

where n is the number of data values. In a data set with an even number of data points, this equation will solve for a noninteger number; for example, in a data set with 18 points, it will be $\frac{18+1}{2} = 9.5$. The median in this case will be the arithmetic mean of the ninth and tenth items in the data set when sorted in ascending order. The median tends to be the least susceptible to outliers, but may not be useful for data sets with very large ranges (the distance between the largest and smallest data point, as discussed later in this chapter) or multiple modes.

Example: Using the same data from the last question, find the median age of the attendees. Comparing this value to the mean, is the median a better or worse indicator of central tendency in this sample?

Solution: The first step in finding the median is to order the data from smallest to largest. Our original data was:

$$23, 22, 25, 22, 22, 24, 36, 20$$

Reordered, this becomes:

$$20, 22, 22, 22, 23, 24, 25, 36$$

n, the number of data points, is 8, so the median will be the average of the fourth and fifth data points. The median is therefore $\frac{22 + 23}{2} = 22.5$. The median is a better indicator of central tendency for this data than the mean of 24.25. The median is unaffected by the outlier and lies close to most of the values in the data set. One could improve the representativeness of the mean by excluding 36 from the data set, in which case the mean would be 22.6 while the median would be 22.

KEY CONCEPT

The median divides the data set into two groups with 50% of values higher than the median and 50% of values lower than it.

If the mean and the median are far from each other, this implies the presence of outliers or a skewed distribution, as discussed later in this chapter. If the mean and median are very close, this implies a symmetrical distribution.

Mode

The **mode**, quite simply, is the number that appears the most often in a set of data. There may be multiple modes in a data set, or—if all numbers appear equally—there can even be no mode for a data set. When we examine distributions, the peaks represent modes. The mode is not typically used as a measure of central tendency for a set of data, but the number of modes, and their distance from one another, is often informative. If a data set has two modes with a small number of values between them, it may be useful to analyze these portions separately or to look for other variables that may be responsible for dividing the distribution into two parts.

MCAT CONCEPT CHECK 12.1

Before you move on, assess your understanding of the material with these questions.

1. What types of data sets are best analyzed using the mean as a measure of central tendency?

____

____

2. Calculate the mean, median, and mode of the following data set:

25, 23, 23, 6, 9, 21, 4, 4, 2

- Mean: ______________________
- Median: ______________________
- Mode: ______________________

12.2 Distributions

LEARNING OBJECTIVES

After Chapter 12.2, you will be able to:

- Assess whether data without a normal distribution can be analyzed with measures of central tendency and distribution
- Distinguish between normal, skewed, and bimodal distributions
- Describe the relationship between mean, median, and mode in different types of distributions:

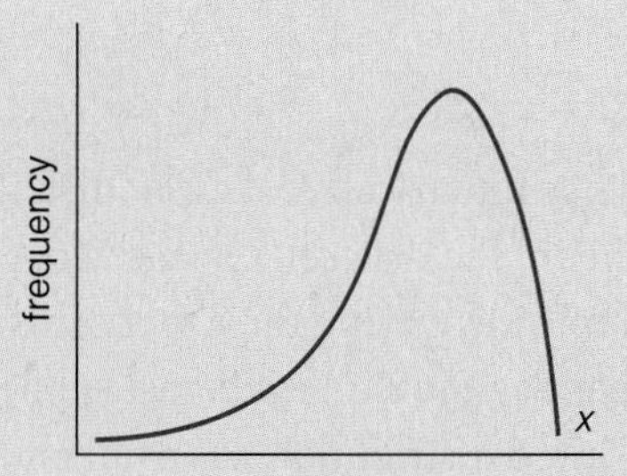

Often a single statistic for a data set is insufficient for a detailed or relevant analysis. In this case, it is useful to look at the overall shape of the distribution as well as specifics about how that shape impacts our interpretation of the data. The shape of a distribution will impact all of the measures of central tendency that we have already discussed, as well as some measures of distribution, which we will examine later.

KEY CONCEPT

The normal distribution and its counterpart, the standard distribution, are the basis of most statistical testing on the MCAT. In the normal distribution, all of the measures of central tendency are the same.

Normal Distributions

In statistics, we most often work with a **normal distribution**, shown in Figure 12.1. Even when we know that this is not quite the case, we can use special techniques so that our data will approximate a normal distribution. This is very important because the normal distribution has been "solved" in the sense that we can transform any normal distribution to a **standard distribution** with a mean of zero and a standard deviation of one, and then use the newly generated curve to get information about probability or percentages of populations. The normal distribution is also the basis for the **bell curve** seen in many scenarios, including exam scores on the MCAT.

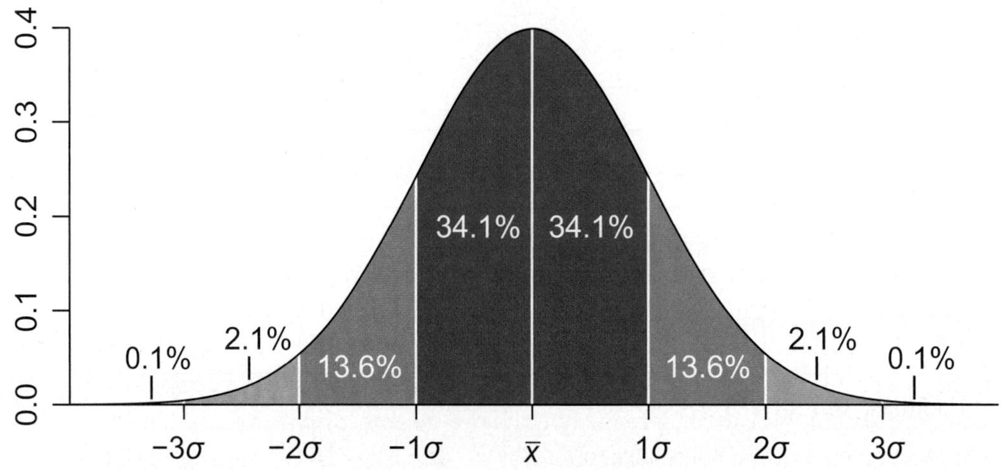

Figure 12.1 The Normal Distribution
The mean, median, and mode are at the center of the distribution. Approximately 68% of the distribution is within one standard deviation of the mean, 95% within two, and 99% within three.

Skewed Distributions

Distributions are not always symmetrical. A **skewed distribution** is one that contains a **tail** on one side or the other of the data set. On the MCAT, skewed distributions are most often tested by simply identifying their type. This is often an area of confusion for students because the *visual* shift in the data appear *opposite* the direction of the skew. A negatively skewed distribution has a tail on the left (or negative) side, whereas a positively skewed distribution has a tail on the right (or positive) side. Because the mean is more susceptible to outliers than the median, the mean of a negatively skewed distribution will be lower than the median, while the mean of a positively skewed distribution will be higher than the median. These distributions, and their measures of central tendency, are shown in Figure 12.2.

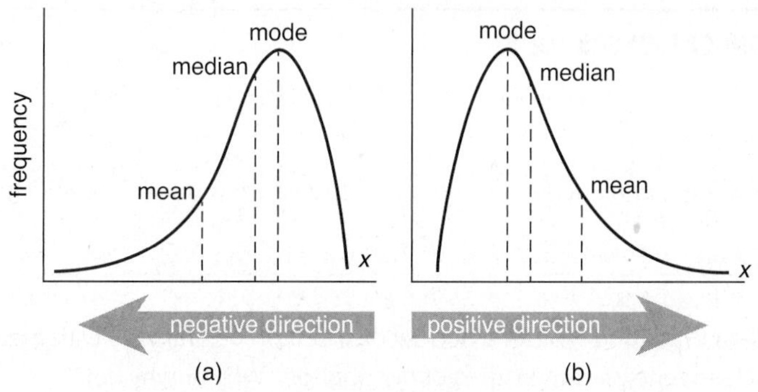

Figure 12.2 Skewed Distributions
(a) Negatively skewed distribution, with mean lower than median;
(b) Positively skewed distribution, with mean higher than median.

KEY CONCEPT

The direction of skew in a sample is determined by its tail, *not* the bulk of the distribution.

Bimodal Distributions

Some distributions have two or more peaks. A distribution containing two peaks with a valley in between is called **bimodal**, as shown in Figure 12.3. It is important to note that a bimodal distribution, strictly speaking, might have only one mode if one peak is slightly higher than the other. However, even when the peaks are of two different sizes, we still call the distribution bimodal. If there is sufficient separation of the two peaks, or a sufficiently small amount of data within the valley region, bimodal distributions can often be analyzed as two separate distributions. On the other hand, bimodal distributions do not *have* to be analyzed as two separate distributions either; the same measures of central tendency and measures of distribution can be applied to them as well.

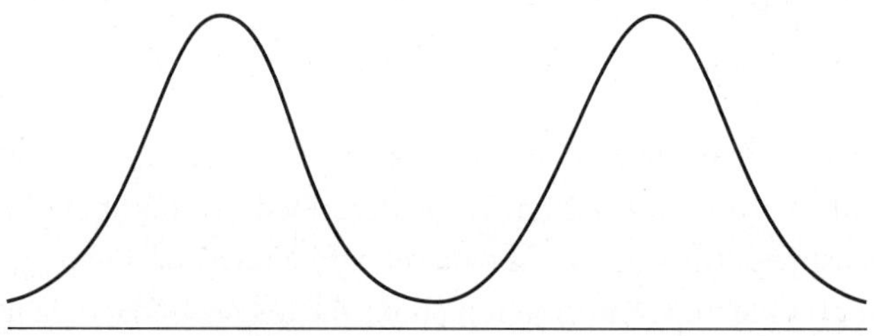

Figure 12.3 Bimodal Distribution

MCAT CONCEPT CHECK 12.2

Before you move on, assess your understanding of the material with these questions.

1. How do the mean, median, and mode compare for a right-skewed distribution?

____

2. Can data that do not follow a normal distribution be analyzed with measures of central tendency and measures of distribution? Why or why not?

____

3. What is the difference between normal or skewed distributions, and bimodal distributions?

____

12.3 Measures of Distribution

LEARNING OBJECTIVES

After Chapter 12.3, you will be able to:

- Identify outliers using interquartile range or standard deviation
- Describe the relationship between range and standard deviation
- Justify whether certain measures of distribution are or are not appropriate for a given situation

Distributions can be characterized not only by their "center" points, but also by the spread of their data. This information can be described in a number of ways. Range is an absolute measure of the spread of a data set, while interquartile range and standard deviation provide more information about the distance that data falls from one of our measures of central tendency. We can use these quantities to determine if a data point is truly an outlier in our data set.

Range

The **range** of a data set is the difference between its largest and smallest values:

$$\text{range} = x_{\text{max}} - x_{\text{min}}$$

Equation 12.3

Range does not consider the number of items of the data set, nor does it consider the placement of any measures of central tendency. Range is therefore heavily affected by the presence of data outliers. In cases where it is not possible to calculate the standard deviation for a normal distribution because the entire data set is not provided, it is possible to approximate the standard deviation as one-fourth of the range.

Interquartile Range

Interquartile range is related to the median, first, and third quartiles. **Quartiles,** including the median (Q_2), divide data (when placed in ascending order) into groups that comprise one-fourth of the entire set. There is some debate over the most appropriate way to calculate quartiles; for the purposes of the MCAT, we will use the most common (and simplest) method:

1. To calculate the position of the first quartile (Q_1) in a set of data sorted in ascending order, multiply n by $\frac{1}{4}$.
2. If this is a whole number, the quartile is the mean of the value at this position and the next highest position.
3. If this is a decimal, round *up* to the next whole number, and take that as the quartile position.
4. To calculate the position of the third quartile (Q_3), multiply the value of n by $\frac{3}{4}$. Again, if this is a whole number, take the mean of this position and the next. If it is a decimal, round up to the next whole number, and take that as the quartile position.

The interquartile range is then calculated by subtracting the value of the first quartile from the value of the third quartile:

$$\text{IQR} = Q_3 - Q_1$$

Equation 12.4

The interquartile range can be used to determine outliers. Any value that falls more than 1.5 interquartile ranges below the first quartile or above the third quartile is considered an **outlier**.

KEY CONCEPT

One definition of an outlier is any value lower than $1.5 \times \text{IQR}$ below Q_1 or any value higher than $1.5 \times \text{IQR}$ above Q_3.

Example: Using the interquartile range, determine whether the 36-year-old from Ray's party is an outlier. The ages are provided in numerical order below for convenience:

20, 22, 22, 22, 23, 24, 25, 36

Solution: In order to determine whether this point is an outlier, we must first determine the interquartile range. To do so, we must determine the first and third quartiles. This data set contains eight values. Multiplying 8 by $\frac{1}{4}$ gives us 2, so the first quartile is the mean of the second and third values in the ordered data set:

$$Q_1 = \frac{22 + 22}{2} = 22$$

Multiplying 8 by $\frac{3}{4}$ gives us 6, so the third quartile is the mean of the sixth and seventh values in the ordered data set:

$$Q_3 = \frac{24 + 25}{2} = 24.5$$

The interquartile range is the difference between these:

$$\text{IQR} = Q_3 - Q_1 = 24.5 - 22 = 2.5$$

Outliers are data values more than 1.5 interquartile ranges below Q_1 or above Q_3. Thus, any value above $24.5 + 1.5 \times 2.5 = 24.5 + 3.75 = 28.25$ or below $22 - 1.5 \times 2.5 = 22 - 3.75 = 18.25$ will be an outlier. 36 is well above 28.25, so it is an outlier in this data set.

Standard Deviation

Standard deviation is the most informative measure of distribution, but it is also the most mathematically laborious. It is calculated relative to the mean of the data. **Standard deviation** is calculated by taking the difference between each data point and the mean, squaring this value, dividing the sum of all of these squared values by the number of points in the data set minus one, and then taking the square root of the result. Expressed mathematically

$$\sigma = \sqrt{\frac{\sum_{i=1}^{n}(x_i - \bar{x})^2}{n-1}}$$

Equation 12.5

where σ is the standard deviation, x_i to x_n are the values of all of the data points in the set, $\bar{x}$ is the mean, and n is the number of data points in the set. The use of $n - 1$ instead of n is mathematically—but not practically—important and the reason for doing so is beyond the scope of the MCAT.

Example: Calculate the standard deviation for the following data set:

1, 2, 3, 9, 10

Solution: First, determine the value of the mean:

$$\overline{x} = \frac{\sum_{i=1}^{n} x_i}{n} = \frac{1+2+3+9+10}{5} = \frac{25}{5} = 5$$

Then, find the difference between each data point and the mean, and square this value. This is a rather tedious project, but is best solved with the use of a table as seen below:

x_i	$x_i - \overline{x}$	$(x_i - \overline{x})^2$
1	-4	16
2	-3	9
3	-2	4
9	4	16
10	5	25

Now we can determine the standard deviation:

$$\sigma = \sqrt{\frac{\sum_{i=1}^{n} (x_i - \overline{x})^2}{n-1}} = \sqrt{\frac{16+9+4+16+25}{4}} = \sqrt{\frac{70}{4}}$$
$$= \sqrt{17.5} \approx 4 \text{ (actual} = 4.18)$$

Keep in mind that when calculating the mean, we use *n* as the denominator, but when calculating standard deviation, we use $n - 1$.

The standard deviation can also be used to determine whether a data point is an outlier. If the data point falls more than three standard deviations from the mean, it is considered an outlier. The standard deviation relates to the normal distribution as well. On a normal distribution, approximately 68% of data points fall within one standard deviation of the mean, 95% fall within two standard deviations, and 99% fall within three standard deviations, as shown in Figure 12.1 earlier. Integration or specialized software can be used to determine percentages falling within other intervals.

KEY CONCEPT

Another definition of *outlier* is any value that lies more than three standard deviations from the mean.

Outliers

While we have already discussed methods for determining if a data point is an outlier, it is useful to know how to approach data with outliers. Outliers typically result from one of three causes:

1. A true statistical anomaly (e.g., a person who is over seven feet tall).
2. A measurement error (for example, reading the centimeter side of a tape measure instead of inches).
3. A distribution that is not approximated by the normal distribution (e.g., a skewed distribution with a long tail).

When an outlier is found, it should trigger an investigation to determine which of these three causes applies. If there is a measurement error, the data point should be excluded from analysis. However, the other two situations are less clear.

If an outlier is the result of a true measurement, but is not representative of the population, it may be weighted to reflect its rarity, included normally, or excluded from the analysis depending on the purpose of the study and preselected protocols. The decision should be made before a study begins—not once an outlier has been found. When outliers are an indication that a data set may not approximate the normal distribution, repeated samples or larger samples will generally demonstrate if this is true.

MCAT EXPERTISE

The existence of outliers is key for determining whether or not the mean is an appropriate measure of central tendency. It may also indicate a measurement error on the part of the investigators.

MCAT CONCEPT CHECK 12.3

Before you move on, assess your understanding of the material with these questions.

1. Compare the method of determining outliers from the interquartile range and from the standard deviation:

   - From interquartile range:

   ____

   - From standard deviation:

   ____

2. How do range and standard deviation generally relate to one another mathematically? Is this relationship accurate for the data set used earlier in this section (1, 2, 3, 9, 10; $\sigma = 4.18$)?

   ____

   ____

3. Why would the average difference from the mean be an inappropriate measure of distribution?

   ____

   ____

12.4 Probability

LEARNING OBJECTIVES

After Chapter 12.4, you will be able to:

- Define independence, mutual exclusivity, and exhaustiveness
- Calculate the probability of an event, or of co-occurrence of multiple independent events

Probability is usually tested on the MCAT in the context of a science question, rather than being tested on its own. In particular, genetics questions involving the Hardy-Weinberg equilibrium and Punnett squares are common applications of probability. Probability also underlies statistical testing, which we will investigate in the next section.

Independence, Mutual Exclusivity, and Exhaustiveness

In probability problems, we must first determine the relationship between events and outcomes. For events, we are most interested in **independence** or **dependence**. Conceptually, **independent events** have no effect on one another. If you roll a die and get a 3, then pick it up and roll it again, the probability of getting a 3 on the second roll is no different than it was before the first roll. Independent events can occur in any order without impacting one another.

KEY CONCEPT

Independent events do not impact each other, so their probabilities are never expected to change.

Dependent events do have an impact on one another, such that the order changes the probability. Consider a container with five red balls and five blue balls. The probability that one will choose a red ball is $\frac{5}{10}$. If a red ball is indeed chosen, then the probability of drawing another red ball is $\frac{4}{9}$. If, however, a blue ball is chosen, then the probability of drawing a red ball is $\frac{5}{9}$. In this way, the probability of the second event (getting a red ball on the second draw) is indeed dependent on the result of the first event.

We are also concerned with whether events are mutually exclusive or not. This term applies to outcomes, rather than events. **Mutually exclusive outcomes** cannot occur at the same time. One cannot flip both heads and tails in one throw, or be both ten and twenty years old. The probability of two mutually exclusive outcomes occurring together is 0%.

Finally, we must consider if a set of outcomes is exhaustive or not. A group of outcomes is said to be **exhaustive** if there are no other possible outcomes. For example, flipping heads or tails are said to be exhaustive outcomes of a coin flip; these are the only two possibilities.

Calculations

For independent events, the probability of two or more events occurring at the same time is the product of their probabilities alone

$$P(\mathrm{A} \cap \mathrm{B}) = P(\mathrm{A\ and\ B}) = P(\mathrm{A}) \times P(\mathrm{B})$$

Equation 12.6

For example, the probability of getting heads on a coin flip twice in a row is the same as the probability of getting heads the first time times the probability of getting heads the second time, or $0.5 \times 0.5 = 0.25$. The probability of two independent events co-occurring is shown diagrammatically in Figure 12.4.

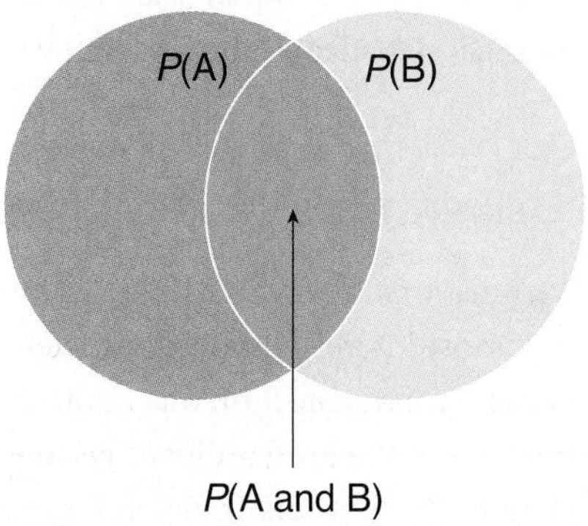

Figure 12.4 Probability of Two Independent Events Co-Occurring
$P(\text{A and B}) = P(\text{A}) \times P(\text{B})$

KEY CONCEPT

In probability, when using the word:

- *and*–multiply the probabilities
- *or*–add the probabilities (and subtract the probability of both happening together)

The probability of at least one of two events occurring is equal to the sum of their initial probabilities, minus the probability that they will both occur.

$$P(\mathrm{A} \cup \mathrm{B}) = P(\mathrm{A\ or\ B}) = P(\mathrm{A}) + P(\mathrm{B}) - P(\mathrm{A\ and\ B})$$

Equation 12.7

Example: In a certain population, 10% of the population has diabetes and 30% is obese. If 7% of the population has both diabetes and obesity, are these events independent? If one chose an individual at random from this population, what would be the probability of that patient having at least one of the two conditions?

Solution: With the numbers given, these events cannot be independent. For independent events, $P(\text{A and B}) = P(\text{A}) \times P(\text{B}) = P(\text{having diabetes}) \times P(\text{being obese}) = 0.1 \times 0.3 = 0.03$. In this population, the probability of having diabetes and being obese is 0.07.

To determine the probability of the individual having at least one of the conditions, we use the “or” equation:

$$P(\text{A or B}) = P(\text{A}) + P(\text{B}) - P(\text{A and B}) = 0.1 + 0.3 - 0.07 = 0.33 \text{ or } 33\%$$

MCAT CONCEPT CHECK 12.4

Before you move on, assess your understanding of the material with these questions.

1. Assume the likelihood of having a male child is equal to the likelihood of having a female child. In a series of ten live births, the probability of having at least one male child is equal to:

____

2. Define the following terms:

- Independence:

____

- Mutual exclusivity:

____

- Exhaustiveness:

____

12.5 Statistical Testing

LEARNING OBJECTIVES

After Chapter 12.5, you will be able to:

- Distinguish between hypothesis tests and confidence intervals
- Recall how p-values are calculated during a hypothesis test
- Predict the outcome of a test given its p- and α-values
- Explain the importance of power in statistical testing

Hypothesis testing and confidence intervals allow us to draw conclusions about populations based on our sample data. Both are interpreted in the context of probabilities, and what we deem to be an acceptable risk of error.

Hypothesis Testing

Hypothesis testing begins with an idea about what may be different between two populations. We have a **null hypothesis,** which is always a hypothesis of equivalence. In other words, the null hypothesis says that two populations are equal, or that a single population can be described by a parameter equal to a given value. The **alternative hypothesis** may be **nondirectional** (that the populations are not equal) or **directional** (for example, that the mean of population A is greater than the mean of population B).

The most common hypothesis tests are *z*- or ***t*-tests**, which rely on the standard distribution or the closely related *t*-distribution. From the data collected, a **test statistic** is calculated and compared to a table to determine the likelihood that that statistic was obtained by random chance (under the assumption that our null hypothesis is true). This is our ***p*-value**. We then compare our *p*-value to a **significance level** (α); 0.05 is commonly used. If the *p*-value is greater than α, then we fail to reject the null hypothesis, which means that there is not a statistically significant difference between the two populations. If the *p*-value is less than α, then we reject the null hypothesis and state that there is a statistically significant difference between the two groups. Again, when the null hypothesis is rejected, we state that our results are statistically significant.

The value of α is the level of risk that we are willing to accept for incorrectly rejecting the null hypothesis. This is also called a **type I error**. In other words, a type I error is the likelihood that we report a difference between two populations when one does not actually exist. A **type II error** occurs when we incorrectly fail to reject the null hypothesis. In other words, a type II error is the likelihood that we report no difference between two populations when one actually exists. The probability of a type II error is sometimes symbolized by β. The probability of correctly rejecting a false null hypothesis (reporting a difference between two populations when one actually exists) is referred to as **power**, and is equal to $1 - \beta$. Finally, the probability of correctly failing to reject a true null hypothesis (reporting no difference between two populations when one does not exist) is referred to as **confidence**. These conditions are summarized in Table 12.1.

		TRUTH ABOUT THE POPULATION	
		H_0 true (no difference)	H_a true (difference exists)
CONCLUSION BASED ON SAMPLE	Reject H_0	Type I error (α)	Power ($1 - \beta$)
	Fail to reject H_0	Confidence	Type II error (β)

Table 12.1 Results of Hypothesis Testing

Confidence Intervals

Confidence intervals are essentially the reverse of hypothesis testing. With a confidence interval, we determine a range of values from the sample mean and standard deviation. Rather than finding a *p*-value, we begin with a desired confidence level (95% is standard) and use a table to find its corresponding *z*- or *t*-score. When we multiply the *z*- or *t*-score by the standard deviation, and then add and subtract this number from the mean, we create a range of values. For example, consider a population for which we wish to know the mean age. We draw a sample from that population and find that the mean of the sample is 30, with a standard deviation of 3. If we wish to have 95% confidence, the corresponding *z*-score (which would be provided on Test Day) is 1.96. Thus, the range is $30 - (3)(1.96)$ to $30 + (3)(1.96) = 24.12$ to

35.88. We can then report that we are 95% confident that the true mean age of the population from which this sample is drawn is between 24.12 and 35.88.

MCAT CONCEPT CHECK 12.5

Before you move on, assess your understanding of the material with these questions.

1. How do hypothesis tests and confidence intervals differ?
   - Hypothesis tests:

   ____

   - Confidence intervals:

   ____

2. If the *p*-value is greater than α in a given statistical test, what is the outcome of the test?

   ____

3. How is the *p*-value calculated during a hypothesis test?

   ____

   ____

4. True or False: Power is the probability of correctly rejecting the null hypothesis.

12.6 Charts, Graphs, and Tables

High-Yield

LEARNING OBJECTIVES

After Chapter 12.6, you will be able to:

- Recognize when data relationships call for transformation into semilog or log-log plots
- Recall the pros and cons of different types of visual data representation, including pie charts, bar graphs, box plots, maps, graphs, and tables
- Distinguish between exponential and parabolic curves

Because your career will be filled with evidence-based medicine, it is important to be able to recognize and interpret data in multiple forms. We have already considered the mathematical side of statistics; now, let's take a look at the visual side. On the MCAT, anticipate that most passages in the sciences will be accompanied by a visual aid in some way—frequently, this will be a chart, graph, or data table.

Types of Charts

Charts present information in a visual format and are frequently used for categorical data.

Pie or Circle Charts

Pie or **circle charts** are used to represent relative amounts of entities and are especially popular in demographics. They may be labeled with raw numerical values or with percent values. The primary downside to pie charts is that as the number of represented categories increases, the visual representation loses impact and becomes confusing. For example, in Figure 12.5, the population of each of the 50 United States and the District of Columbia is presented on a pie chart, but the large number of entities makes the graph incoherent.

MCAT EXPERTISE

Questions about pie charts are likely to be qualitative, asking for the smallest or largest group, or the percentage occupied by one or more groups combined. These questions are unlikely to require additional analysis because pie charts are not dense with information.

BRIDGE

Pie charts are frequently used to present demographic information. Demographics is the statistical arm of sociology and is discussed in Chapter 11 of *MCAT Behavioral Sciences Review*.

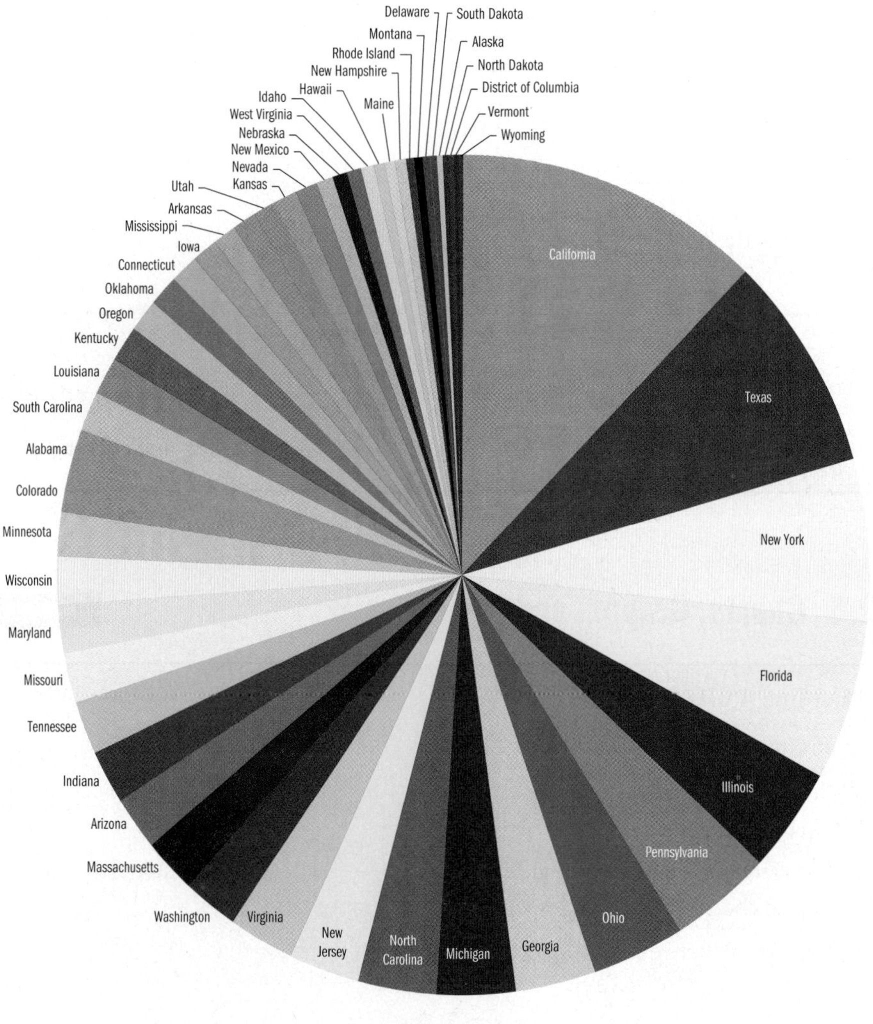

Figure 12.5 Pie Chart of United States Population by State, 2010 Census
Pie charts become difficult to interpret when too many categories are included.

Bar Charts and Histograms

Bar charts and histograms are likely to contain significantly more information than a pie chart for the same amount of page space. **Bar charts** are used for categorical data, which sort data points based on predetermined categories. The bars may then be sorted by increasing or decreasing bar length. The length of a bar is generally proportional to the value it represents. Wherever possible, breaks should be avoided in the chart because of the potential to distort scale. To that end, be wary of graphs that contain breaks; they may be enlarging the difference between bars. Figure 12.6 shows a representative bar graph for causes of cancer death in the United States in 2010.

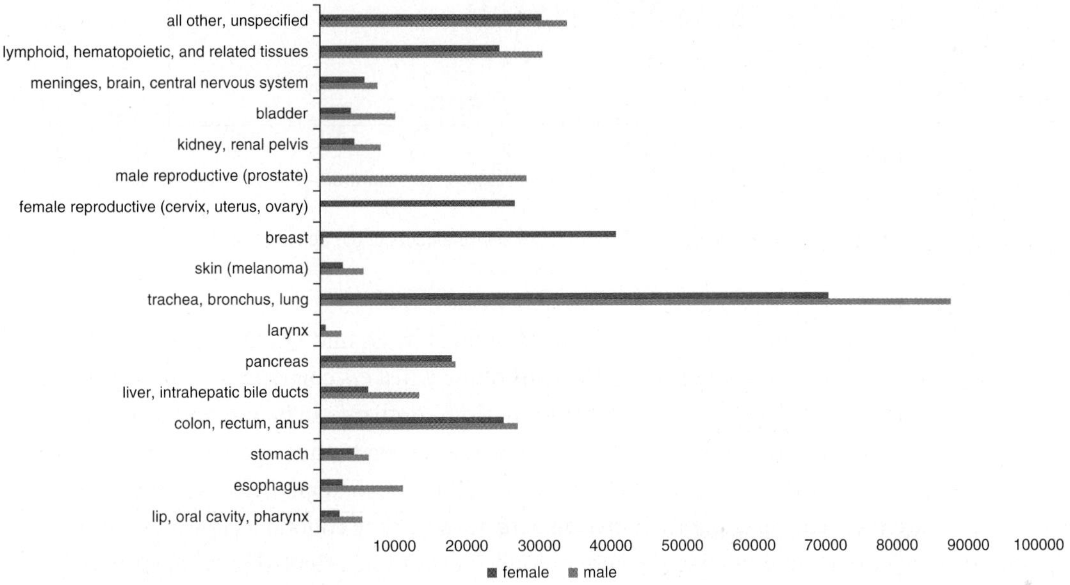

Figure 12.6 Causes of Cancer Death by Type, 2010
Source: *Centers for Disease Control and Prevention National Vital Statistics Reports*

Histograms present numerical data rather than discrete categories. Histograms are particularly useful for determining the mode of a data set because they are used to display the distribution of a data set.

Box Plot

Box plots are used to show the range, median, quartiles and outliers for a set of data. A labeled box plot, also called a **box-and-whisker**, is shown in Figure 12.7.

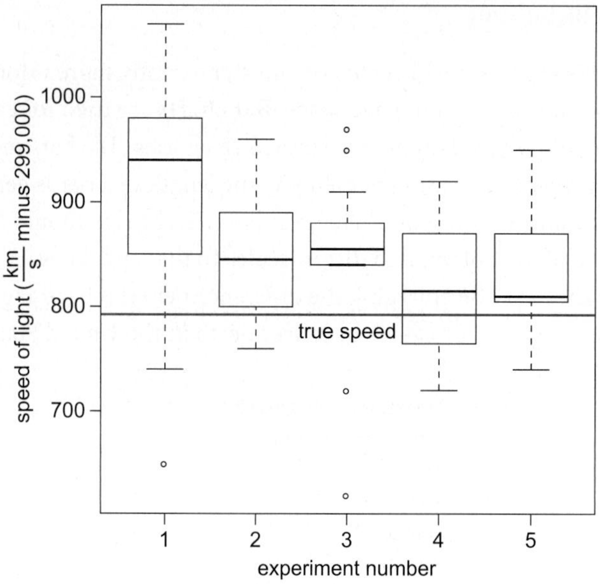

Figure 12.7 Box Plot of Measurements of the Speed of Light

The box of a box-and-whisker plot is bounded by Q_1 and Q_3; Q_2 (the median) is the line in the middle of the box. The ends of the whiskers correspond to maximum and minimum values of the data set. Alternatively, outliers can be presented as individual points, with the ends of the whiskers corresponding to the largest and smallest values in the data set that are still within 1.5 × IQR of the median. Box-and-whisker plots are especially useful for comparing data because they contain a large amount of data in a small amount of space, and multiple plots can be oriented on a single axis.

Maps

In addition to the other forms of charts, data can be illustrated geographically. Maps of health conditions, population density, political districts, and ethnicity are relatively easy to comprehend and may show geographic clustering for some data. The best map data will examine one or at most two pieces of information simultaneously. Any further data may inhibit clarity. A map of population density in each country of the world is shown in Figure 12.8.

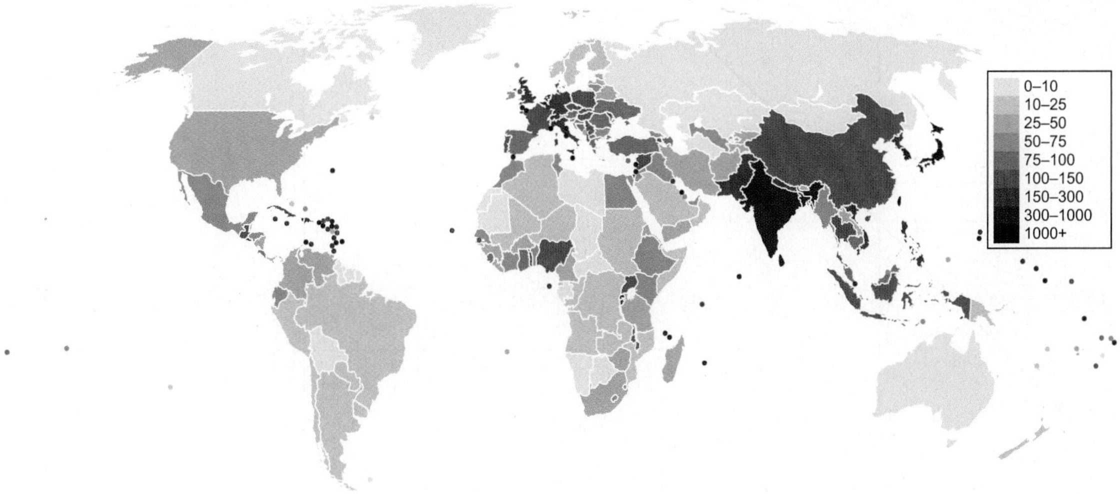

Figure 12.8 Population Density by Country, 2006

Graphs and Axes

While we're all familiar with constructing graphs—especially scatter plots and line graphs—it is important to know some important features and potential stumbling blocks of graphs as we move toward Test Day. When presented with a graph, you should attempt to draw rough conclusions immediately but should not spend time analyzing all of the details of the graph unless asked to do so by a question. The first thing to do when you encounter a graph on Test Day is to look at the axes.

Linear Graphs

Linear graphs show the relationships between two variables. They generally involve two direct measurements and, strictly speaking, do not have to be a straight line. The shape of the curve on this type of graph may be **linear**, **parabolic**, **exponential**, or **logarithmic**. These are shown in Figure 12.9. On Test Day, you should be able to recognize at least these four shapes of graphs.

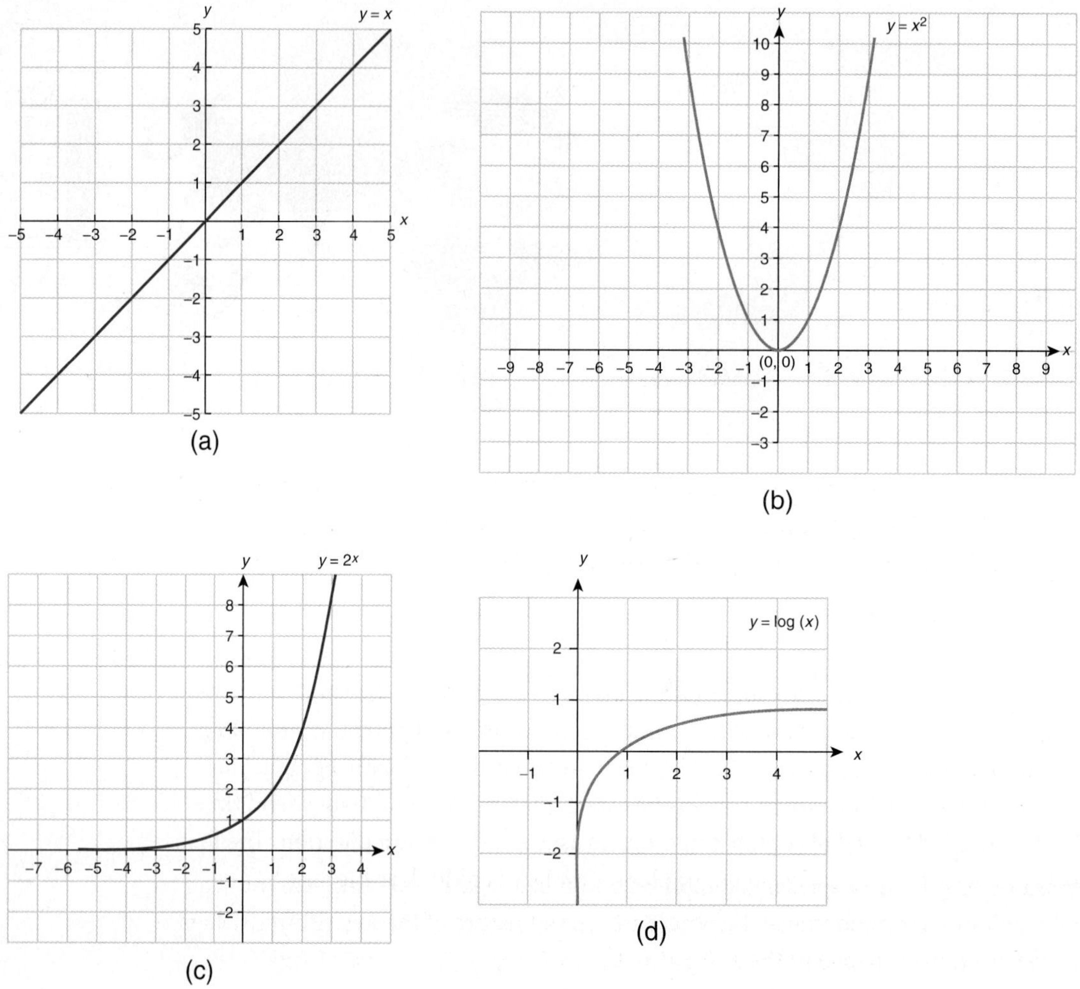

Figure 12.9 Shapes of Common Relationships on a Linear Graph
(a) Linear; (b) Parabolic; (c) Exponential; (d) Logarithmic

MNEMONIC

Slope is like waking up in the morning: Slope is always rise (vertical) over run (horizontal) because you have to get up from bed (rise) before you get moving (run).

The axes of a linear graph will be consistent in the sense that each unit will occupy the same amount of space (the distance from 1 to 2 to 3 to 4 on each axis remains the same size). As with bar graphs, be wary of scale and breaks in axes. Where both the shape of the graph and the graph type are linear, we should be able to calculate the slope of the line. **Slope (*m*)** is the change in the *y*-direction divided by the change in the *x*-direction for any two points:

$$m = \frac{\text{rise}}{\text{run}} = \frac{\Delta y}{\Delta x}$$

Equation 12.8

Example: Calculate the slope of the line in the graph shown below.

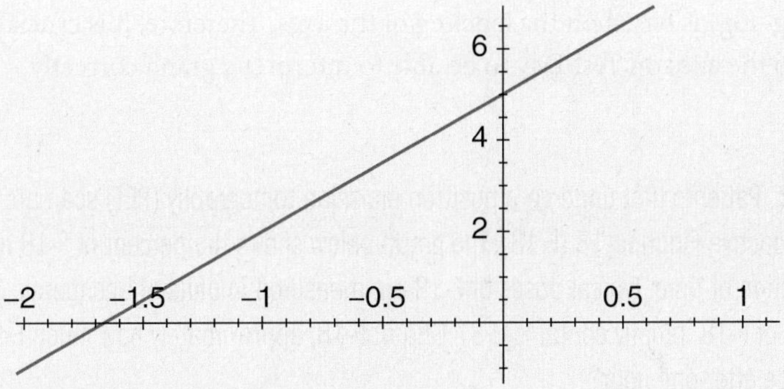

Solution: The slope of a line is equal to the difference in the values of two points in the *y*-direction divided by the difference in the values of the same two points in the *x*-direction. The *x*- and *y*-intercepts are generally good choices because one of the values will be zero for each point:

$$m = \frac{y_2 - y_1}{x_2 - x_1} = \frac{0 - 5}{-1.66 - 0} = \frac{-5}{-1.66} = \frac{5}{\frac{5}{3}} = 3$$

Semilog and Log-Log Graphs

Semilog graphs are a specialized representation of a logarithmic data set. They can be easier to interpret because the otherwise curved nature of the logarithmic data is made linear by a change in the **axis ratio**. In semilog graphs, one axis (usually the *x*-axis) maintains the traditional unit spacing. The other axis assigns spacing based on a ratio, usually 10, 100, 1000, and so on. The multiples may be of any number as long as there is consistency in the ratio from one point on the axis to the next. Figure 12.10 shows an example of a semilog plot.

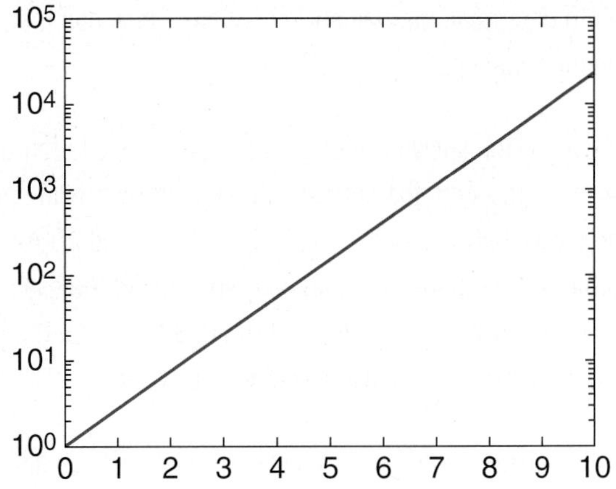

Figure 12.10 A Semilog Plot

KEY CONCEPT

The axes on a graph will determine which type of plot is being used, and provide key information about the underlying relationship between the relevant variables.

In some cases, both axes can be given a different axis ratio to create a linear plot. When both axes use a constant ratio from point to point on the axis, this is termed a **log–log graph**. Note that the difference between these three plot types (linear, semilog, and log–log) is based on the labeling of the axes. Therefore, it is crucial to pay attention to the axes on Test Day to be able to interpret a graph correctly.

Example: Patients that undergo a positron emission tomography (PET) scan are injected with radioactive Flouride-18 (F-18). The graph below shows the percent of F-18 remaining as a function of time. Typical doses of F-18 are measured in units of becquerels (Bq). If a syringe of F-18 initially contains 0.37 GBq of F-18, approximately how much F-18 is in the syringe after one hour?

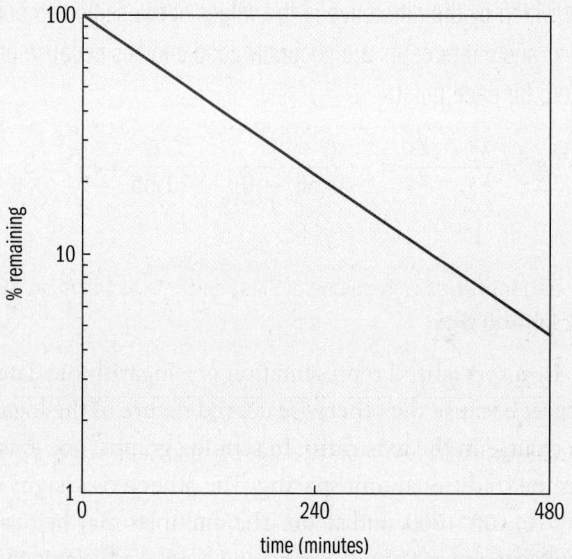

Solution: Notice that the values on the *y*-axis are equally spaced and multiples of ten. That means the *y*-axis is logarithmic. The *x*-axis is linear so the graph is a semilog plot. Use the graph to determine the percent remaining, which can then be used to determine the amount remaining.

Start by finding one hour (the known value) on the *x*-axis. It is one-fourth of the distance between 0 and 240 minutes. Find the corresponding point on the line and then note the location on the *y*-axis. Between each *y*-axis label (1, 10, and 100) the axis is divided equally *in value*, although the marks are unequally spaced. So the eight axis markers between 10 and 100 represent 20, 30, 40, 50, 60, 70, 80, and 90. The point at one hour corresponds to about the third mark below 100, or 70%.

To find the amount of F-18 remaining, the original amount must be multiplied by 0.70. Therefore the correct answer is approximately 0.26 GBq.

Interpreting Tables

Unlike with graphs, you should only take a brief moment to glance at the title of a table before approaching Test Day questions. Tables are more likely to contain disjointed information than either charts or graphs because they often contain categorical data or experimental results. Tables that do not have unusual data values (zeroes, outliers, changes in a trend, and so on) should be approached especially briefly.

When a table does contain significant organization (for example, listing results progressively), this structure is likely to be relevant while answering questions. For example, a trend that suddenly appears or disappears will often require an explanation.

Additionally, when provided with data in the form of a table, you should be able to convert it to a rough graph or to a linear equation. The MCAT may test on the interpretation of slope without actually providing a graph.

MCAT CONCEPT CHECK 12.6

Before you move on, assess your understanding of the material with these questions.

1. What type of data relationship is least likely to require transformation into a semilog or log–log plot?

___

2. Fill in the following table with the pros and cons of each type of visual data representation:

Type of Visual Aid	Pros	Cons
Pie Chart		
Bar Graph		
Box Plot		
Map		
Graph		
Table		

3. How do exponential and parabolic curves differ in shape?
   - Exponential:

___

   - Parabolic:

___

12.7 Applying Data

LEARNING OBJECTIVES

After Chapter 12.7, you will be able to:

- Distinguish between correlation and causation
- Relate the statistical results of a study to the impact of those findings on scientific knowledge and policy change

Finally, we have reached the discussion section of an academic paper, in which the data that we have gathered and interpreted is applied to the original problem. We can then begin drawing conclusions and creating new questions based on our results. Because much of this was covered in the discussion on experimental methods in Chapter 11 of *MCAT Physics and Math Review*, we will be terse in our review here.

Correlation and Causation

As discussed previously, we must be careful with our wording when discussing variable relationships. **Correlation** refers to a connection—direct relationship, inverse relationship, or otherwise—between data. If two variables trend together, that is as one increases so does the other, there is a positive correlation. If two variables trend in opposite directions (one increases as the other decreases) there is a negative correlation. These relationships can be quantified with a **correlation coefficient**, a number between -1 and $+1$ that represents the strength of the relationship. A correlation coefficient of $+1$ indicates a strong positive relationship, a value of -1 indicates a strong negative relationship, and a value of zero indicates no apparent relationship.

Correlation does not necessarily imply **causation**; we must avoid this assumption when there is insufficient evidence to draw such a conclusion. If an experiment cannot be performed, we must rely on Hill's criteria, discussed in Chapter 11 of *MCAT Physics and Math Review*. Remember that the only one of Hill's criteria that is uniformly necessary for causation is temporality.

In the Context of Scientific Knowledge

When interpreting data, it is important that we not only state the apparent relationships between data, but also begin to draw connections to other concepts in science and to our background knowledge. At a minimum, the impact of the new data on the existing hypothesis must be considered, although ideally the new data would be integrated into all future investigations on the topic. Additionally, we must develop a plausible rationale for the results. Finally, we must make decisions about our data's impact on the real world, and determine whether or not our evidence is substantial and impactful enough to necessitate changes in understanding or policy.

Example: A textbook publisher wanted to study the effectiveness of a new Advanced Placement (AP) study aid. From 2006 to 2015 the researchers recruited high schools across the country to participate, and randomly assigned each school to a group—those who received the study aid (Group A) and those who did not (Group B). Grades were tracked in AP Statistics over a 10 year time period. On which three years was there a statistically significant difference between the two groups, and a high likelihood of passing for those who used the study aid?

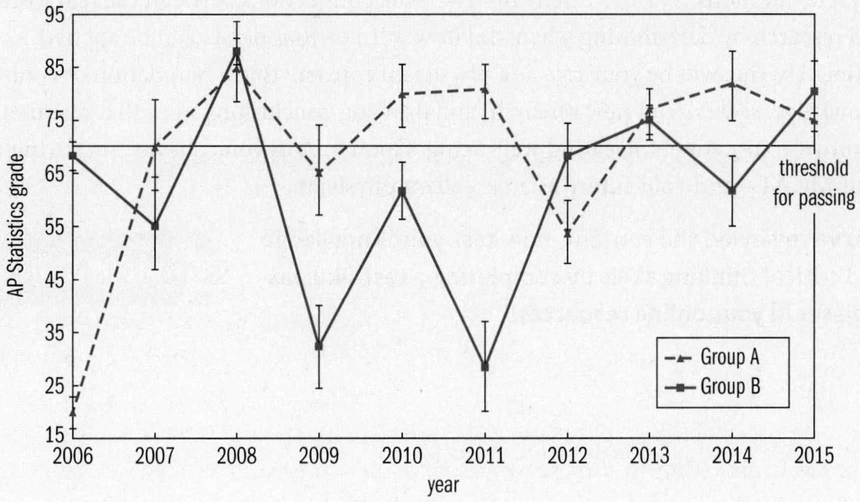

Average AP Grades by Group
Error bars show the 95% CI

Solution: In order to support the claim that the study aid helps students pass the AP exam, the evidence should show a statistically significant difference between those who received the aid and those who did not. Further, the true score (which should be within the confidence interval 95% of the time) of those who received the aid should be above passing and the true score of those who did not should be below passing. The data from 2010, 2011, and 2014 fit the description and provide the best support.

MCAT CONCEPT CHECK 12.7

Before you move on, assess your understanding of the material with these questions.

1. True or False: Statistical significance is sufficient criteria to enact policy change.

2. True or False: Two variables that are causally related will also be correlated with each other.

Conclusion

Congratulations on completing *MCAT Physics and Math Review*! While it has been a challenging journey, you are now equipped with all of the physics content knowledge and *Scientific Inquiry and Reasoning Skills* (SIRS) you need to perform well on Test Day. We completed our discussion of the MCAT SIRS by covering the transformation of raw data to actionable information. When taking the MCAT, these concepts may present themselves as the opportunity to use statistical methods and interpretation to draw conclusions, as well as the analysis of figures used as adjuncts to passages and discrete questions. We also briefly reviewed the connections between the real world and research by determining when and how our newfound data can be applied. Ultimately, this will be your role as a physician: constructing a foundation of content knowledge, seeking out new research, and drawing conclusions from that research to improve your patients' lives and well-being. Good luck as you continue preparing for your MCAT—and your future as an excellent physician.

You've reviewed the content, now test your knowledge and critical thinking skills by completing a test-like passage set in your online resources!

GO ONLINE

CONCEPT SUMMARY

Measures of Central Tendency

- **Measures of central tendency** provide a single value representation for the middle of a group of data.
- The **arithmetic mean** or **average** is a measure of central tendency that equally weighs all values; it is most affected by outliers.
- The **median** is the value that lies in the middle of the data set. Fifty percent of data points are above and below the median.
- The **mode** is the data point that appears most often; there may be multiple (or zero) modes in a data set.

Distributions

- Distributions have characteristic features that are exemplified by their shape. Distributions can be classified by measures of central tendency and measures of distribution.
- The **normal distribution** is symmetrical. The mean, median, and mode are all the same in the normal distribution.
    - The **standard distribution** is a normal distribution with a mean of zero and a standard deviation of one; it is used for most calculations.
    - 68% of data points occur within one standard deviation of the mean, 95% within two, and 99% within three.
- **Skewed distributions** have differences in their mean, median, and mode; the skew direction is the direction of the **tail** of the distribution.
- **Bimodal distributions** have multiple peaks, although not necessarily multiple modes, strictly speaking. It may be useful to perform data analysis on the two groups separately.

Measures of Distribution

- **Range** is the difference between the largest and smallest values in a data set.
- **Interquartile range** is the difference between the value of the **third quartile** and **first quartile**; interquartile range can be used to determine outliers.
- **Standard deviation** is a measurement of variability about the mean; standard deviation can also be used to determine outliers.
- **Outliers** may be a result of true population variability, measurement error, or a non normal distribution.
- Procedures for handling outliers should be formulated before the beginning of a study.

Probability

- The probability of **independent events** does not change based on the outcomes of other events.
- The probability of a **dependent event** changes depending on the outcomes of other events.
- **Mutually exclusive outcomes** cannot occur simultaneously.
- When a set of outcomes is **exhaustive**, there are no other possible outcomes.

Statistical Testing

- **Hypothesis tests** use a known distribution to determine whether a hypothesis of no difference (the **null hypothesis**) can be rejected.
- Whether or not a finding is statistically significant is determined by the comparison of a ***p*-value** to the selected **significance level (α)**. A significance level of 0.05 is commonly used.
- **Confidence intervals** are a range of values about a sample mean that are used to estimate the population mean. A wider interval is associated with a higher **confidence level** (95% is common).

Charts, Graphs, and Tables

- **Pie charts** (**circle charts**) and **bar charts** are both used to compare categorical data.
- **Histograms** and **box plots** (**box-and-whisker plots**) are both used to compare numerical data.
- Maps are used to compare up to two demographic indicators.
- **Linear**, **semilog**, and **log–log** plots can be distinguished by their axes.
- **Slope** can be calculated most easily from linear plots.
- Tables may contain related or unrelated categorical data.

Applying Data

- **Correlation** and **causation** are separate concepts that are linked by Hill's criteria.
- Data must be interpreted in the context of the current hypothesis and existing scientific knowledge.
- Statistical and practical significance are distinct.

ANSWERS TO CONCEPT CHECKS

12.1

1. The mean is the best measure of central tendency for a data set with a relatively normal distribution. The mean performs poorly in data sets with outliers.
2. Mean: $\frac{25+23+23+6+9+21+4+4+2}{9}=\frac{117}{9}=13$

   Median: The fifth position of 2, 4, 4, 6, 9, 21, 23, 23, 25 is 9

   Mode: There are two numbers that each appear twice: 4 and 23. These are both modes of this data set.

12.2

1. The mean of a right (positively) skewed distribution is to the right of the median, which is to the right of the mode.
2. Any distribution can be mathematically or procedurally transformed to follow a normal distribution by virtue of the central limit theorem, which is beyond the scope of the MCAT. Regardless, a distribution that is not normal may still be analyzed with these measures.
3. Bimodal distributions have two peaks, whereas normal or skewed distributions have only one.

12.3

1. Outliers can be defined as data points more than $1.5 \times$ IQR below Q_1 or above Q_3. They can also be defined as data points more than 3σ above or below the mean. The cutoff values calculated through the two methods are likely to be different, and the selection of one method over the other is one of preference and study design. In general, the use of the standard deviation method is superior.
2. Where the data are not available, the range can be approximated as four times the standard deviation. For this data set, the relationship fails. The range is 9, which is only a little more than twice the standard deviation. This is because the data set does not fall in a normal distribution.
3. The average distance from the mean will always be zero. This is why, in calculations of standard deviation, we always square the distance from the mean and then take the square root at the end—it forces all of the values to be positive numbers, which will not cancel out to zero.

12.4

1. Simplify this question by rewording it as the probability of *not* having all female children. Having at least one male child and having all female children are mutually exclusive events, and no other possibilities can occur. Thus, the probability of having all female children is $(0.5)^{10}$ and the probability of having at least one male child is $1 - (0.5)^{10}$, or 99.90%.
2. Independence is a condition of events wherein the outcome of one event has no effect on the outcome of the other. Mutual exclusivity is a condition wherein two outcomes cannot occur simultaneously. When a set of outcomes is exhaustive, there are no other possible outcomes.

12.5

1. Hypothesis tests are used to validate or invalidate a claim that two populations are different, or that one population differs from a given parameter. In a hypothesis test, we calculate a p-value and compare it to a chosen significance level (α) to conclude if an observed difference between two populations (or between a population and the parameter) is significant or not. Confidence intervals are used to determine a potential range of values for the true mean of a population.
2. If the p-value is greater than α, then we fail to reject the null hypothesis.
3. After the test statistic is calculated, a computer program or table is consulted to determine the p-value of the statistic.
4. True. Power is the probability that the individual rejects the null hypothesis when the alternative hypothesis is true for the population.

12.6

1. Linear relationships can be analyzed without any data or axis transformation into semilog or log–log plots.
2.

Type of Visual Aid	Pros	Cons
Pie Chart	Easily constructed; useful for categorical data with a small number of categories.	Easily overwhelmed with multiple categories. Difficult to estimate values with circles.
Bar Graph	Multiple organization strategies. Good for large categorical data sets.	Axes are often misleading because of sizeable breaks.
Box Plot	Information-dense; can be useful for comparison.	May not highlight outliers or mean value of a data set. Only useful for numerical data.
Map	Provide relevant and integrated geographic and demographic information.	May only be used to represent at most two variables coherently.
Graph	Provide information about relationships. Useful for estimation.	Axis labels and logarithmic scales require careful interpretation.
Table	Categorical data can be presented without comparison. Does not require estimation for calculations.	Disorganized or unrelated data may be presented together.

3. Exponential and parabolic curves both have a steep component; however, exponential curves have horizontal asymptotes and become flat on one side while parabolic curves are symmetrical and have steep components on both sides of a center point.

12.7

1. False. As discussed in the last chapter, there must be practical (clinical) as well as statistical significance for a conclusion to be useful.
2. True. While two variables that are correlated are not necessarily causally related, all variables that are causally related must be correlated in some way (direct relationship, inverse relationship, or otherwise).

SCIENCE MASTERY ASSESSMENT EXPLANATIONS

1. **C**

The mean is computed by taking the sum of all of the data points and dividing by the total number of data points. If a very large data point was included, the sum would be significantly larger, inflating the mean. This observation justifies **(C)**. On the other hand, since the median is the middle number and the mode is the most common value, the inclusion of outliers would have minimal effect on these measures.

2. **B**

The mean is to the left of the median, which implies that the tail of the distribution is on the left side; therefore, this distribution is skewed left. It would be expected that there would be a low plateau on the left side of the distribution, which accounts for the shift in the mean.

3. **B**

The median is the central data point in an ordered list. Because this data set has seven numbers, the central point will be in the fourth position. Reordered, the list reads: 2, 4, 4, 7, 17, 23, 53. Thus, the median is 7. **(A)**, 4, is the mode while **(C)**, 15.7, is the mean.

4. **B**

Based on the population description in the question stem, we would expect to see a large number of finches with small beaks, a very small number of finches with intermediate beaks, and a large number of finches with large beaks. This pattern is consistent with a bimodal distribution, choice **(B)**.

5. **B**

Approximately 95% of values fall within two standard deviations ($\pm 2\sigma$) of the mean for a normal distribution. A confidence interval is constructed using the same values. Approximately 68% of the values are within one standard deviation, and 99% are within three standard deviations, eliminating the other answer choices.

6. **C**

When two events are independent of each other, the probability of them occurring simultaneously is equal to the product of the probability of each occurring separately. Thus, for weekly fast food consumption and prevalence of cardiovascular disease to be independent, the probability of both occurring must be (20%)(48%) = 9.6%, supporting **(C)**. While **(D)** is a tempting answer choice, a lack of cardiovascular disease among people who eat fast food would not imply independence of these factors, rather it would imply that fast food consumption actually decreases or eliminates the likelihood of cardiovascular disease.

7. **A**

Because the error is in data transfer, the original source of data can be consulted to allow for the inclusion of the correct data point. An error in instrument calibration may introduce bias; while this should not affect the standard deviation of a sample, it would certainly affect the mean. The instrument would have to be recalibrated, and the relevant data points would have to be measured again to correct for this type of outlier, eliminating choice **(B)**. A skewed distribution is one that has a long tail. In this case, it may be more challenging to determine if a particular value is an outlier or simply a value in the long tail of the distribution. Repeated sampling or a large sample size is usually required to determine if a sample is truly skewed, eliminating choice **(C)**. An anomalous result is challenging to interpret, and how to correct for the result may be unclear. In some cases, the result should be inflated or weighted more heavily to reflect its significance; in other cases, it should be interpreted as a regular value. In still other cases, it is appropriate to drop the anomalous result. This decision should ideally be made before the study even begins, but this still certainly requires more consideration than simply checking a result from one's original data set, eliminating choice **(D)** and making choice **(A)** correct.

8. **A**

Because one parent is homozygous for both traits, we are only concerned with the other parent. This parent has a 50% chance of transmitting each independent trait, and thus a 25% chance of transmitting both $\left(\frac{1}{2} \times \frac{1}{2} = \frac{1}{4}\right)$. This probability is the same for both pregnancies because they are independent events; thus, the probability that both children exhibit both traits is: $\frac{1}{4} \times \frac{1}{4} = \frac{1}{16} = 0.0625 = 6.25\%$.

9. **C**

With data about percentages, we can only draw conclusions about percentages. Thus any information about number of people, as in **(A)**, is incorrect. This map shows us that a higher percentage of the residents in the middle of the country are over 65 in comparison to other parts of the country. There are, of course, exceptions to this rule, including Florida, the Pacific Coast, and parts of Appalachia, which are all in the top category. Even so, there appears to be a clustering of counties with a high percentage of individuals over 65 in the middle of the country. We also cannot say that most of the population is over 65 in any place on this map because we are not given actual values for the percentages. There may be a plurality, but there is insufficient information to posit a majority, eliminating **(B)**. The map gives no indication of migration patterns, so we can also eliminate **(D)**.

10. **A**

To increase the confidence level, one must increase the size of the confidence interval to make it more likely that the true value of the mean is within the range. Therefore, the confidence interval must become wider.

11. **D**

Standard deviation is the most common measure of distribution. It is the most closely linked to the mean of a distribution and can be used to calculate p-values, which are probabilities (specifically, p-values are the probability that an observed difference between two populations is due to chance).

12. **C**

Outliers can be determined with respect to the interquartile range, Q3–Q1. The interquartile range for this box plot is 2280 – 2075, or 205. Values that are 1.5 times IQR below Q1 or above Q3 are considered outliers. 2075 – 1.5 times 205 is approximately 2075 – 300, or 1775 (actual = 1767.5). Therefore, 1575 is an outlier. 2280 + 1.5 times 205 is approximately 2580 (actual = 2587.5). Therefore, 2600 is also an outlier.

13. **D**

The attendant hypothesized that glucose in ice cream was the cause of the increase in risk-taking behavior and designed an observational study. While there was an increase in lottery ticket sales with an increase in ice cream sales, this relationship is a correlation. Correlation does not prove causation. Thus, the conclusion that glucose was the cause is a significant flaw, making **(D)** the correct answer.

14. **D**

Because the histogram contains two peaks with a valley in between, it is a bimodal distribution. The color separation of two distinct populations provides evidence that there is a qualitative difference in the data between the two peaks, thus the data should be analyzed according to gender. There is indeed only one mode, at 5′6″. This is the measurement with the largest number of corresponding data points.

15. **C**

When considering whether the findings of a study merit policy change, both the statistical and clinical significance must be evaluated. In comparing the difference in both the systolic and diastolic blood pressure before and after treatment, the effect of the drug is minimal. While the results are statistically significant, it is very unlikely that this small reduction would lead to a significant clinical improvement. Thus, the doctor should not advocate, making **(C)** the correct answer.

Consult your online resources for additional practice. GO ONLINE

EQUATIONS TO REMEMBER

(12.1) **Arithmetic mean:** $\bar{x} = \frac{\sum_{i=1}^{n} x_i}{n}$

(12.2) **Median position:** median position $= \frac{(n+1)}{2}$

(12.3) **Range:** range $= x_{max} - x_{min}$

(12.4) **Interquartile range:** IQR $= Q_3 - Q_1$

(12.5) **Standard deviation:** $\sigma = \sqrt{\frac{\sum_{i=1}^{n}(x_i - \bar{x})^2}{n-1}}$

(12.6) **Probability of two independent events co-occurring:**
$P(\text{A} \cap \text{B}) = P(\text{A and B}) = P(\text{A}) \times P(\text{B})$

(12.7) **Probability of at least one event occurring:**
$P(\text{A} \cup \text{B}) = P(\text{A or B}) = P(\text{A}) + P(\text{B}) - P(\text{A and B})$

(12.8) **Slope:** $m = \frac{\text{rise}}{\text{run}} = \frac{\Delta y}{\Delta x}$

SHARED CONCEPTS

Behavioral Sciences Chapter 11
Social Structure and Demographics

Biology Chapter 12
Genetics and Evolution

General Chemistry Chapter 5
Chemical Kinetics

Physics and Math Chapter 1
Kinematics and Dynamics

Physics and Math Chapter 10
Mathematics

Physics and Math Chapter 11
Reasoning About the Design and Execution of Research

GLOSSARY

Aberration–Visual alterations as the result of an imperfect optical device; may be chromatic or spherical.

Absolute pressure–The actual pressure at a given depth in a fluid, including both ambient pressure at the surface and the pressure associated with increased depth in the fluid; also called hydrostatic pressure.

Absolute zero–The theoretically coldest temperature at which all atomic movements would halt (0 K).

Acceleration–The rate of change in the velocity of an object; related to force through mass and measured in $\frac{m}{s^2}$.

Accuracy–The tendency for data to represent the true answer; also known as validity.

Adhesion–The intermolecular force between molecules of a liquid and molecules of another substance.

Adiabatic–A thermodynamic process that occurs with no heat exchange.

Air resistance–The resistance that opposes the motion of a falling object.

Algebraic system–A method for determining the values of variables that are the same in two or more equations by relating them to each other.

α-particle–A helium nucleus $\left({}^4_2\text{He}\right)$ emitted during alpha decay.

Alternating current (AC)–In circuits, a pattern of current flow that changes direction periodically.

Ammeter–A device used to measure current within a circuit.

Amplitude–The maximum displacement from the equilibrium point during wave or oscillatory motion.

Antinode–A point of maximum displacement in a standing wave.

Archimedes' principle–States that a body immersed in a volume of fluid experiences a buoyant force equal to the weight of the displaced fluid.

Atomic absorption–Process in which an electron jumps from a lower to a higher energy orbit by absorbing a photon of light.

Atomic emission–Process by which an electron falls from a higher to a lower energy level and emits a photon of light.

Atomic number–The number of protons in the nucleus of a given element.

Attenuation–The loss of energy of a propagating wave as a result of nonconservative forces; also known as damping.

Autonomy–The ethical principle that states that individuals have the right to make decisions about their own healthcare.

Beat frequency–The difference between the frequencies of two interacting sound waves.

Beneficence–The ethical principle that states that practitioners should always act in their patients' best interests; in research ethics, also states that a research project should create a net positive change for both the study population and general population.

β-particle–An electron emitted during β^- decay, or a positron emitted during β^+ decay.

Bernoulli's equation–An equation that relates static and dynamic pressure for a fluid to the pressure exerted on the walls of a tube and the speed of the fluid.

Bias–A result of flaws in the data collection phase of an experimental or observational study that typically skews data within a study.

Bimodal distribution–A distribution of data with two peaks and a valley in between them.

Blackbody–An ideal absorber of all wavelengths of light.

Blinding–Withholding information about a research subject's group assignment from the subject or evaluator to remove some potential bias from the results.

Boiling point–The temperature at which the vapor pressure of a liquid equals the ambient (incident) pressure, usually atmospheric pressure; the temperature at which the liquid boils.

Boundary layer–A region of laminar flow in an otherwise turbulent system that occurs at the very edges of the vessel.

Box-and-whisker plot–A visual representation of the range of data, quartiles, and the interquartile range; may contain outliers as separate points.

Buoyancy–The upward force that results from immersion in a fluid; described by Archimedes' principle.

Capacitance–A measure of the ability of a capacitor to store charge; the magnitude of the charge on one plate divided by the potential difference between the plates; measured in farads (F).

Capacitor–Two conducting surfaces that store charges of equal magnitude but opposite sign when connected to a voltage source.

Case-Control Study–An observational study that starts by identifying subjects with a given outcome, then looks for correlations to specific exposures within the group.

Causation–A relationship between two variables in which one (at least partially) depends on the other in order to occur.

Center of gravity–A point such that the entire force of gravity acting on an object can be thought of as acting at that point.

Center of mass–The point that acts as if the entire mass of an object was concentrated at that point.

Centripetal acceleration–The acceleration of an object that travels in a circle; it is always directed toward the center of the circle if the object is in uniform circular motion.

Centripetal force–The force responsible for centripetal acceleration; usually a result of gravity, tension, or a normal force.

Charges–Entities that can influence the environment through electrostatic forces or be influenced by electrostatic forces, measured in coulombs (C).

Chromatic aberration–A dispersive effect within a spherical lens.

Circular motion–A form of motion that occurs when forces cause an object to move in a circular pathway.

Cohesion–The intermolecular forces experienced between the molecules of a liquid.

Cohort study–An observational study in which subjects are sorted into groups based on different exposures, and then assessed at various intervals to determine outcome.

Concave–A surface that has a similar curvature to the interior of a sphere.

Condensation–The phase transition from a gas to a liquid.

Conductance–In the transfer of charge, the degree to which an object conducts electricity. Conductance can be metallic or electrolytic.

Conduction–In thermodynamics, the transfer of heat by physical motion of a fluid over a material.

Conduction pathway–a route for current to take through a resistor.

Conductor–A material that allows the free movement of electrical charge; one with very low or zero resistance.

Confidence–A statistical indicator of the likelihood that acquired results did not occur by random chance; equal to $1 - \alpha$.

Confounding–An error that results when a causal variable is associated with two other variables in a study but is not accounted for; may falsely indicate that the two variables are associated.

Conservative force–A force that does not cause energy to be dissipated from a system, such as gravity, electrostatic forces, and springs (approximately conservative); pathway independent and associated with a potential energy function.

Control–A set of experimental conditions meant to ensure that the results of the experimental group are a result of the intervention.

Convection–Heat transfer as a result of bulk flow of a fluid over an object.

Converging–The tendency to move parallel light rays toward one another; concave mirrors and convex lenses converge parallel light to a focal point.

Convex–A surface that has a similar curvature to the exterior of a sphere.

Correlation–The degree to which two variables have a relationship with one another.

Correlation coefficient–A numerical value between -1 and $+1$ that indicates how strong a relationship is between two variables.

Coulomb's law–Relates the electrostatic force between two charged particles to their charges and the distance between them.

Critical angle–The angle above which any incident light will undergo total internal reflection; occurs when light is moving from a material with a higher refractive index to one with a lower refractive index.

Critical speed–The speed above which flow of a fluid will be turbulent.

Cross-sectional study–An observational study in which patients are categorized into different groups at the same point in time.

Current–The orderly movement of charge, often in a circuit; measured by convention as the direction that positive charge would flow within the circuit, and measured in ampères (A).

Decay constant–The proportionality constant between the rate at which radioactive nuclei decay and the number of radioactive nuclei remaining.

Density–A measure of mass per unit volume; useful for buoyancy calculations and usually measured in $\frac{g}{cm^3}$, $\frac{kg}{m^3}$, or $\frac{g}{mL}$.

Dependent variable–The measured or observed variable in an experiment that is affected by manipulations of the independent variable.

Detection bias–An error in data collection that results from the tendency to look more carefully for certain outcomes because a known association with that outcome exists.

Diamagnetic material–A material made of atoms with no unpaired electrons that have no net magnetic field.

Dielectric material–An insulating material used to increase capacitance.

Diffraction–The spreading or bending of light rays.

Dipole moment–In electrostatics calculations, the product of charge and separation distance.

Direct current (DC)–In circuits, a pattern of current in which charge flows in only one direction.

Direct relationships–A relationship in which increasing one variable proportionately increases the other.

Dispersion–The separation of light into its component wavelengths when passing through a medium, such as a prism.

Displacement–The vector representing the straight-line distance and direction from an initial point; not necessarily equal to total distance traveled, and measured in meters.

Diverging–The tendency to move parallel light rays away from one another; convex mirrors and concave lenses diverge parallel light rays from a focal point.

Doppler effect–Quantifies the perceived change in frequency of sound due to relative movement between the source and detector (observer).

Double-blind experiment–Experiment in which both the assessor and the subject do not know the subject's group.

Dynamics–In kinematics and dynamics, the study of forces and torques.

Efficiency–In machines, the ratio of useful work output compared to work input.

Electric dipole–A separation of equal and opposite charge by a small distance; can be seen in polar molecules.

Electric field–A region generated by an electric charge or multiple charges that can exert a force on another charge brought into the field; measured in $\frac{N}{C}$.

Electric meters–Devices used to measure circuit quantities like current, potential difference, or resistance.

Electric potential–A measure of electric potential energy per unit charge, given in volts (V); differences in electric potential (voltage) also drive current as the electromotive force in a circuit.

Electric potential energy–A form of potential energy that is dependent on the relative position of one charge with respect to another charge or to a collection of charges.

Electromagnetic radiation–A form of energy composed of oscillating electric and magnetic fields perpendicular to each other and perpendicular to the direction of propagation; includes visible light and other types of transverse waves, and can travel through a vacuum.

Electromagnetic spectrum–The full range of frequencies and wavelengths of electromagnetic waves.

Electromotive force–The difference in electric potential (voltage) that drives current in a circuit or battery.

Electron–A subatomic particle that remains outside the nucleus and carries a single negative charge.

Electron capture–A process in which an unstable atom absorbs an inner electron that combines with a proton to form a neutron, while releasing a neutrino.

Electrostatics–The study of stationary charges and the forces that are created by (and act upon) these charges.

Energy–The capacity to do work or transfer heat, measured in joules (J).

Entropy–A statistical measure of the distribution of unusable energy or heat; randomness introduced to a system, measured in $\frac{J}{g \cdot K}$.

Equilibrium–The state at which the net torque or net force is equal to zero, such that there is no acceleration.

Equipoise–The state of not knowing whether there is a difference between two interventions; ethically necessary for comparative study of the interventions.

Equipotential lines–Regions within an electric field with equal electric potential; movement from one point on these lines to another causes no change in the energy of the system.

Excited state–Describes an atom in which an electron occupies an energy state above the minimum energy (ground) state.

Exhaustive–Describes a set of outcomes that leave no room for other possible outcomes.

External validity–The ability to apply findings of a research study to other populations; also called generalizability.

Ferromagnetic material–A material made of atoms with unpaired electrons that become strongly magnetized when exposed to an external magnetic field.

Field line–A visual representation of the electric field; points to the direction a force would be exerted on a positive test charge in the electric field.

FINER method–A way to determine the usefulness of a research question on the basis of feasibility, interest, novelty, ethics, and relevance.

Fission–The splitting of a large nucleus into smaller nuclei with the release of energy.

Flow rate–The volume per unit time of a fluid in motion.

Fluid–A material that conforms to the shape of its container and that can flow.

Fluid dynamics–The study of fluids in motion.

Fluorescence–A process in which the electrons of certain substances are excited to higher energy levels by high-frequency photons, and then emit visible light as the energy is released in two or more steps back to the ground state.

Focal length–The distance from a mirror or lens to the focal point.

Focal point–The point at which rays of light parallel to the axis of a mirror or lens converge, or from which they appear to diverge when reflected by a mirror or refracted by a lens.

Force–A push or a pull, measured in newtons (N).

Free fall–A system in which the only force is gravity.

Freezing–The phase transition from liquid to solid; also called solidification.

Frequency–The rate at which a recurring event occurs; usually measured in hertz (Hz).

Friction–A nonconservative force that arises from the interactions between two surfaces in contact.

Fundamental frequency–The first harmonic of a pipe, string, or other standing wave.

Fusion–The merging of small nuclei into a larger nucleus with the release of energy.

γ-rays–High-energy photons released during gamma decay; part of the electromagnetic spectrum.

Gauge pressure–Pressure above and beyond atmospheric pressure.

Gravitational potential energy–A form of potential energy dependent on the relative position of an object within a gravitational field.

Gravity–An attractive force between two objects that depends on their masses and the distance between them.

Ground–A means of returning charge to the earth.

Ground state–The lowest energy state of an atom.

Half-life–The amount of time it takes for one-half of a sample of radioactive nuclei to decay.

Harmonic series–The set of frequencies that can create standing waves in a given pipe or string.

Hawthorne effect–The tendency for research participants to change their behavior because they know they are being observed.

Heat–The transfer of thermal energy; measured in joules (J), calories (cal), or kilocalories (kcal or Cal).

Heat of transformation–The amount of heat necessary to cause a phase transition of a unit mass of a substance at the characteristic temperature and pressure of that phase transition; also called latent heat.

Hill's criteria–A systematized way of evaluating evidence for causality; only temporality is absolutely necessary to demonstrate causality.

Histogram–A visual representation for numerical data; related to a bar chart.

Hydraulic system–A simple machine that exerts mechanical advantage using an incompressible fluid; based on Pascal's principle and conservation of energy.

Hydrostatics–The study of fluid systems at rest.

Hyperopia–Farsightedness, or the ability to see distant objects while nearby objects are unfocused or blurry.

Hypothesis testing–A statistical method used to compare results between groups or to a theoretical value with a given level of confidence.

Image–The region where light rays converge or appear to converge after being reflected from a mirror or passing through a lens.

Independent variable–The manipulated variable in an experiment that affects measurements or observations of the dependent variable.

Index of refraction–A ratio of the speed of light in a vacuum to the speed of light in a given medium.

Inertia–An object's resistance to a change in its motion when a force is applied.

Informed consent–An ethical requirement for treatments or research, which requires that the patient or participant is able to understand the procedure and its consequences and alternatives; related to autonomy.

Infrared–A region of the electromagnetic spectrum that is not visible; may be perceived as heat.

Infrasonic–Sound that has a frequency that is lower than the range of human hearing.

Insulator–A material that resists the movement of charge because the electrons are tightly associated with their nuclei.

Intensity–The average rate of energy expenditure (power) per unit area, measured in $\frac{\text{W}}{\text{m}^2}$; in waves, intensity is related to the amplitude of the wave.

Interference–Interactions between waves traveling in the same space; may be constructive (waves adding together), destructive (waves cancelling each other), partially constructive, or partially destructive.

Internal validity–The ability to infer causality from a study or to replicate its results under the same conditions.

Interquartile range–A measure of distribution of a sample; outliers lie at least 1.5 interquartile ranges below Q_1 or above Q_3.

Inverse relationship–A relationship in which an increase in one variable is associated with a proportional decrease in the other.

Inverted–Describes an image that is upside down relative to the object; in single-mirror or single-lens systems, inverted images are always real.

Irreversible–A thermodynamic process that is extraordinarily unfavorable in reverse, usually as a result of changes in entropy.

Isobaric–A thermodynamic process that occurs under constant pressure.

Isothermal–A thermodynamic process that occurs under constant temperature.

Isotopes–Atoms of a given element with different numbers of neutrons and therefore different mass numbers.

Isovolumetric–A thermodynamic process that occurs under constant volume; also called isochoric.

Justice–The ethical principle that states that practitioners should fairly distribute healthcare resources, and which requires that differences in treatment choices between individuals are only due to morally relevant differences.

Kinetic energy–The energy of movement, which depends on both mass and speed; measured in joules (J).

Kinetic friction–The friction that exists between a sliding object and the surface over which the object slides.

Kirchhoff's laws–Rules that describe the conservation of charge and conservation of energy within an electric circuit; includes the junction rule and loop rule.

Laminar flow–Smooth flow within a fluid; characterized by streamlines that do not cross each other and an absence of backwards movement.

Lenses–Devices that act to create an image by refracting light; usually have spherical surfaces.

Logarithm–The inverse function of exponentiation; logarithmic scales are often used to mask large absolute differences between quantities by presenting them as small scale differences.

Longitudinal wave–A wave in which the oscillation of the material is parallel to the direction of propagation; sound is a classic example.

Lorentz force–The sum of the electrostatic and magnetic forces acting on a charge.

Loudness–Perceived intensity of a sound, which correlates with sound level; measured in decibels (dB).

Magnetic field–Field created by a moving charge.

Magnetic force–A force that is exerted when a charge moves in a magnetic field, provided the charge has a perpendicular component of velocity in comparison to the magnetic field vector.

Magnification–Apparent increase or decrease in size of an image as a result of forming the image with a converging or diverging system.

Mass–A measure of inertia or of the amount of "stuff" in an object; measured in kilograms.

Mass defect–The difference between the sum of the masses of unbound nucleons forming a nucleus and the mass of that nucleus in the bound state.

Mass number–The sum of the number of protons and neutrons in an atom; also called the atomic mass.

Mean–The average of a group of data; specifically, the arithmetic mean.

Measures of central tendency–Measures that describe the middle of a sample.

Mechanical advantage–The reduction in input force required to accomplish a desired amount of output work using a simple machine.

Median–The central value of a data set.

Melting–The phase transition from solid to liquid; also known as fusion.

Metric system–A system of measurements based on the powers of ten; most commonly used in scientific disciplines.

Microwaves–Long-wavelength electromagnetic radiation capable of inducing vibration in bonds.

Mode–The most common data point in a data set.

Monochromatic–Electromagnetic radiation wherein the wavelength is the same for all incident photons.

Mutually exclusive–Describes outcomes that cannot occur simultaneously.

Myopia–Nearsightedness, or the ability to see nearby objects while distant objects are unfocused or blurry.

Natural frequency–The frequency at which a system resonates; also called the resonant frequency.

Natural process–In thermodynamics, a process which would occur as expected in nature.

Newton's first law–The first law, also called the law of inertia, states that an object will remain at rest or move with a constant velocity if there is no net force on the object. This law thus accounts for the conservation of mechanical energy.

Newton's second law–This law states that any acceleration is the result of the sum of the forces acting on the object and its mass.

Newton's third law–This law states that any two objects interacting with one another experience equal and opposite forces as a result of their interaction.

Node–A point of zero displacement of a standing wave.

Nonconservative force–A force that causes energy to be dissipated from a system, such as friction, air resistance, and viscous drag; pathway dependent.

Nonmaleficence–The ethical principle that states that practitioners have an obligation to avoid treatments or interventions in which the potential for harm is greater than the potential for good.

Normal–A line perpendicular to the surface of interest.

Normal force–The force that two surfaces in contact exert on each other that is perpendicular to the plane of contact.

Nucleon–A proton or neutron.

Null hypothesis–The hypothesis of no difference; given enough statistical evidence, the null hypothesis may be rejected.

Observational study–A study that looks for the connection between exposures and outcomes without demonstrating causality.

Ohmmeter–A device used to measure resistance.

Ohm's law–Relates voltage, current, and resistance for a given circuit element.

Outlier–A data point that deviates significantly from the perceived pattern of distribution; depending on the context, an outlier may be disregarded, analyzed normally, or given disproportionate weight when calculating statistics.

Parallel–An arrangement of circuit elements in which the current can go through one element or the other, but not through both.

Paramagnetic material–A material made of atoms with unpaired electrons that will become weakly magnetized in the presence of an external magnetic field.

Parameter–A measure of population data.

Pascal's principle–States that pressure applied to a noncompressible fluid is distributed equally to all points within that fluid and the walls of the container.

Period–The amount of time it takes for a wave or oscillation to complete one cycle, measured in seconds; the inverse of frequency.

Phase difference–The difference in phase between waves with the same frequency, referenced at the same point.

Photoelectric effect–A phenomenon in which light of sufficiently high frequency incident on a metal in a vacuum causes the metal to emit electrons.

Pitch–A perception of sound that results from its frequency; as frequency increases, pitch gets higher.

Pitot tubes–Measurement devices for pressure or flow rate of a dynamic fluid system.

Plane mirrors–Reflecting surfaces with an infinite radius of curvature, which results in equal image and object distances.

Plane-polarized light–Electromagnetic radiation in which all of the electric field vectors are oriented parallel to one another.

Poiseuille's law–Relates viscosity, tube dimensions, and pressure differentials to the rate of flow between two points in a system.

Population–The group of all individuals who have certain specified characteristics.

Positron–Antiparticle of an electron; it has the same mass as an electron and the opposite charge (e^+ or β^+).

Potential difference–The difference of electric potential between two distinct points, measured in volts (V); also called voltage.

Potential energy–Energy associated with position, measured in joules (J); includes gravitational, elastic, chemical, and electrical forms.

Power–Rate at which work is accomplished, or energy expenditure per unit time; measured in watts (W). In statistics, the probability of correctly rejecting a false null hypothesis.

Precision–The tendency of measurements to agree with one another; also called reliability.

Pressure–The ratio of force to the area over which it is applied; measured in pascals (Pa), millimeters of mercury (mmHg) or torr, or atmospheres (atm).

Principle of superposition–When waves interact with each other, the displacement of the resultant wave at any point is the sum of the displacements of the two interacting waves.

Process functions–Physical quantities that depend on the path taken to get from one state to another; include work and heat.

Propagation–In waves and sound, the movement of a wave.

Proton–A subatomic particle that carries a single positive charge and has a mass slightly less than 1 amu.

Pythagorean theorem–Relationship between the three sides of a right triangle: the square of the hypotenuse is equal to the sum of the squares of the other two sides.

Quantum–A discrete bundle of energy such as the photon.

Quartiles–Values that separate data in ascending order into four evenly sized groups.

Radiation–A method of heat transfer that relies on electromagnetic waves; can occur in a vacuum.

Radioactive decay–A naturally occurring spontaneous decay of certain nuclei accompanied by the emission of specific particles.

Radio waves–Very long wavelength electromagnetic radiation.

Random error–In an experiment, error caused by natural variation in subjects and data points that can be reduced in impact by increasing sample size.

Randomization–A method of reducing bias and confounding during research in which participants are assigned to a group by a random number generator or similar method; participants or researchers cannot choose the groups.

Range–The difference between the smallest number in a data set and the largest.

Ray diagram–Visual representation of a geometrical optics system.

Real–Describes an image on the same side of a lens or mirror as the refracted or reflected light that can be projected on a screen; in single-mirror or single-lens systems, real images are always inverted.

Rectilinear propagation–A phenomenon in which light travels in a straight line when passing through a homogeneous medium.

Reflection–The return of light rays from a medium at an angle equal to the incident angle.

Refraction–The bending of light rays as a result of a change in the index of refraction between media.

Resistance–A measure of the opposition to current flow through a material, measured in ohms (Ω); the inverse of conductance.

Resistivity–A measure of the intrinsic resistance of a material independent of its shape or size; resistivity generally increases with temperature.

Resonance–Oscillation at maximum amplitude as the result of a periodically applied force at the natural (resonant) frequency of an object.

Respect for persons–A principle of research ethics that encompasses autonomy and informed consent.

Resultant–The sum, difference, or product of vector mathematics; also refers to the sum or difference of two waves.

Right-hand rule–A method for determining the direction of a vector that is the product of two vectors.

Rotation–The turning of an extended body about an axis or center.

Sample–A subset of a population that is used to make generalizations about the population as a whole.

Scalar–A mathematical quantity that lacks directionality.

Scientific method–A systematized way of evaluating data and investigating new hypotheses.

Scientific notation–A mathematical representation of quantities as multiples of powers of ten.

Selection bias–Occurs when research participants differ from the general population in a meaningful way.

Series–An arrangement of circuit elements in which the current must go through all of the elements.

Shear forces–Also called tangential forces, forces exerted on the surface of an object that are parallel to the surface of the object.

Shock wave–The buildup of wave fronts that occurs when the source is travelling at or above the speed of sound.

Significant figures–A tool for maintaining appropriate levels of precision when performing mathematical calculations.

Simple machine–A basic mechanical device for applying a force. The six simple machines include inclined planes, wedges, wheel and axle systems, levers, pulleys, and screws.

Single-blind experiment–An experiment in which only the subject or the assessor is blinded, but the other party is aware of the treatment the subject is receiving.

Snell's law–Relates the incident angle, refracted angle, and indices of refraction for two media.

Solid–A material with distinct boundaries and strong intermolecular forces capable of resisting shear forces.

Sound–The perception of longitudinal waves of pressure changes in air and other media.

Source charge (*Q*)–In electrostatics, the charge that creates the electric field.

Specific gravity–The ratio of an object's density to the density of water; unitless.

Specific heat–The relationship between thermal energy and temperature change per unit mass of a substance, measured in $\frac{\text{J}}{\text{g}\cdot\text{K}}$.

Speed–The ratio of distance traveled to time; at any given point, instantaneous speed is the magnitude of instantaneous velocity; measured in $\frac{\text{m}}{\text{s}}$.

Spherical aberration–A blurring of the periphery of an image as a result of inadequate reflection of parallel beams at the edge of a mirror or lens.

Spherical mirror–A mirror that causes convergence or divergence of light rays incident upon its surface.

Standard deviation–A measure of distribution of data from the mean of a sample; outliers lie at least three standard deviations above or below the mean.

Standing waves–Waveforms with steady nodes and antinodes formed from the interference of incident and reflected waves at a boundary.

State functions–Physical quantities that can be determined based on the state of an object, such as pressure, density, temperature, volume, enthalpy, internal energy, Gibbs free energy, and entropy; pathway independent.

Static friction–The friction that exists between a stationary object and the surface upon which it rests.

Statistic–A measure of sample data.

Streamlines–Visual representations of the movement of fluid during laminar flow.

Strong nuclear force–One of the four fundamental interactions; it is responsible for the binding of protons and neutrons together in the nucleus.

Surface tension–The result of the cohesive forces in a liquid creating a barrier at the interface between a liquid and the environment.

Surroundings–Everything that is not being measured as part of a given system.

System–The observed and quantified region of the universe of interest to the experimenter. Systems can be isolated (unable to exchange energy or matter with their surroundings), closed (able to exchange energy with their surroundings), or open (able to exchange matter and energy with their surroundings).

Systematic error–An error in an experiment that is typically caused by measuring instruments and creates a flaw in data that cannot be offset by increasing the data pool.

Temperature–A measure of the average kinetic energy of particles in a substance; measured in degrees Fahrenheit (°F), degrees Celsius (°C), or kelvins (K).

Temporality–A necessary criterion for causality; the independent variable must occur before the dependent variable.

Terminal velocity–The velocity at which air resistance is equal to gravitational force and no acceleration occurs for an object in free fall.

Test charge (*q*)–In electrostatics, the charge placed in an electric field.

Thermal equilibrium–Equilibrium of thermal energy that exists when no heat flows between two objects in thermal contact.

Thermal expansion–An increase in length or volume of a substance as a result of an increase in temperature.

Threshold frequency–The minimum frequency of light that causes ejection of electrons.

Timbre–The quality of sound produced by an instrument.

Torque–The primary motivator for rotational movement that combines force, lever arm, and the angle between them; measured in N·m.

Total internal reflection–A phenomenon in which all the light incident on a boundary is reflected back into the original material.

Total mechanical energy–The sum of an object's potential and kinetic energies.

Translation–Motion through space without rotation.

Transverse wave–A wave that propagates in a direction perpendicular to the direction of oscillation.

Traveling wave–A wave that propagates through a medium with changes in the locations of crests and troughs.

Turbulent flow–Fluid movement that does not follow parallel streamlines; has backflow, eddies, and swirls.

Type I error–An error in conclusion in which the null hypothesis is incorrectly rejected.

Type II error–An error in conclusion in which the experimenter fails to correctly reject the null hypothesis.

Ultrasonic–Above the frequencies that a human ear can hear.

Ultrasound–A treatment and diagnostic modality using ultrasonic waves for medical purposes.

Ultraviolet–A region of the electromagnetic spectrum that is not visible; primarily responsible for the damaging effects of sunlight on skin.

Unnatural process–In thermodynamics, a process that does not undergo naturally predicted changes in heat/energy over time.

Upright–Describes an image that is the same orientation as the object; in single-mirror or single-lens systems, upright images are always virtual.

Vaporization–The phase transition from liquid to gas; also called boiling or evaporation.

Vector–A mathematical quantity that has both magnitude and direction.

Velocity–The rate of change in the displacement of an object; measured in $\frac{m}{s}$.

Venturi effect–Describes the relationship between the continuity equation and Bernoulli's equation; as the cross-sectional area of a tube decreases, the speed of the fluid increases, and the pressure exerted on the walls of the tube decreases.

Virtual–Describes an image on the opposite side of a lens or mirror as the refracted or reflected light; in single-mirror or single-lens systems, virtual images are always upright.

Viscosity–A measure of the resistance to flow in a fluid.

Viscous drag–A nonconservative force exerted by fluids in a manner proportional to the viscosity of the fluid.

Visible region–The part of the electromagnetic spectrum visible to the human eye.

Voltmeter–A device used to measure voltage.

Wavelength–The distance between two corresponding points of successive cycles in a waveform, measured in meters.

Weak nuclear force–One of the four fundamental interactions; it is responsible for radioactive decay and contributes to nuclear stability.

Weight–The force of gravity acting on an object.

Work–A function of the applied force and the distance through which it is applied or the pressure and volume changes in a gas system; work is the use of energy to accomplish something and is measured in joules (J).

Work–energy theorem–States that net work is equal to the change in energy (usually kinetic energy) of an object.

X-rays–A type of electromagnetic radiation; primarily used for medical imaging.

Zeroth law of thermodynamics–If two thermodynamic systems are in thermal equilibrium with a third system, they are in thermal equilibrium with each other.

INDEX

Note: Material in figures or tables is indicated by italic *f* or *t* after the page number.

C

G

H

I

J

K

L

M

T

U

V

W

X

Y

Z

ART CREDITS

Chapter 4 Cover—Image credited to sakhorn. From Shutterstock.

Figure 4.6—Image credited to lvcandy. From Getty Images. Modified from source.

Chapter 5 Cover—Image credited to Piotr Krzeslak. From Shutterstock.

Chapter 6 Cover—Image credited to Jelena Aloskina. From Shutterstock.

Chapter 7 Cover—Image credited to Andreea Dragomir. From Shutterstock.

Chapter 8 Cover—Image credited to Juan J. Jimenez. From Shutterstock.

Chapter 9 Cover—Image credited to Vaclav Volrab. From Shutterstock.

Chapter 10 Cover—Image credited to zphoto. From Shutterstock.

Chapter 11 Cover—Image credited to Serg Zastavkin. From Shutterstock.

Chapter 12 Cover—Image credited to Zorabc. From Shutterstock.

Figure 12.1—Image credited to User: Mwtoews. From Wikimedia Commons. Copyright © 2007. Used under license: CC-BY-2.5.

Notes

Notes

Notes

Notes

Notes

Notes

Notes